Cancer Nursing
A COMPREHENSIVE TEXTBOOK

Second Edition

Ruth McCorkle, Ph.D., F.A.A.N.
Professor
School of Nursing
University of Pennsylvania
Philadelphia, Pennsylvania

Marcia Grant, D.N.Sc., F.A.A.N.
Research Scientist and Director
Nursing Research and Education
City of Hope National Medical Center
Duarte, California

Marilyn Frank–Stromborg, Ed.D., J.D., A.N.P., F.A.A.N.
Professor and Nurse Practitioner
Northern Illinois University
School of Nursing
DeKalb, Illinois

Susan B. Baird, M.P.H., M.A., R.N.
Director of Nursing and Patient Services
Fox Chase Cancer Center
Philadelphia, Pennsylvania

W.B. SAUNDERS COMPANY
A Division of Harcourt Brace & Company
Philadelphia London Toronto Montreal Sydney Tokyo

W.B. SAUNDERS COMPANY

A Division of Harcourt Brace & Company

The Curtis Center
Independence Square West
Philadelphia, Pennsylvania 19106

NOTICE

Cancer nursing is an ever-changing field. Standard safety precautions must be followed, but as new research and clinical experience broaden our knowledge, changes in treatment and drug therapy become necessary or appropriate. The editors of this work have carefully checked the generic and trade drug names and verified drug dosages to ensure that the dosage information in this work is accurate and in accord with the standards accepted at the time of publication. Readers are advised, however, to check the product information currently provided by the manufacturer of each drug to be administered to be certain that changes have not been made in the recommended dose or in the contraindications for administration. This is of particular importance in regard to new or infrequently used drugs. It is the responsibility of the treating physician and health care providers, relying on experience and knowledge of the patient, to determine dosages and the best treatment for the patient. The editors cannot be responsible for misuse or misapplication of the material in this work.

THE PUBLISHER

Library of Congress Cataloging–in–Publication Data

Cancer nursing: a comprehensive textbook/[edited by] Ruth McCorkle
    . . . [et al.]. — 2nd ed.
        p.   cm.
    Rev. ed. of: Cancer nursing/Susan B. Baird, Ruth McCorkle,
Marcia Grant. 1991.
    Includes bibliographical references and index.
    ISBN 0–7216–5668–4
    1. Cancer—Nursing. I. McCorkle, Ruth, 1941-
    [DNLM: 1. Neoplasms—nursing. 2. Oncologic Nursing. WY 156
C2192 1996]
RC266.B334 1996
610.73'698—dc20
DNLM/DLC
                                                                95-42807

CANCER NURSING A COMPREHENSIVE TEXTBOOK   ISBN 0–7216–5668–4

Copyright © 1996 by W.B. Saunders Company

Printed in the United States of America

Last digit is the print number: 9   8   7   6   5   4   3   2   1

To my children—Amanda, David, Nicholas, John, and Jesse.
For the joy and energy they give me every day.
Ruth McCorkle

To the memory of my mother, Henrietta Moeller, and to the support
of my husband, Stuart and daughter, Susan.
Marcia Grant

To Brian Kenneth Wilk, born 10/12/73, and died 4/28/94.
Born with a smile on his lips and a laugh to dispel all cares.
Marilyn Frank-Stromborg

To my daughter Leslie and my grandsons Alex and Anthony,
for the love and joy they add to my life.
Susan Baird

Ruth McCorkle, Ph.D., F.A.A.N., is a Professor of Nursing at the University of Pennsylvania School of Nursing. In addition, she is Associate Director of Cancer Control at the University of Pennsylvania Comprehensive Cancer Center and Director of the Center for Advancing Care in Serious Illness. Her career began as a Clinical Nurse Specialist in Oncology in Iowa. Subsequently, she has established a nationally recognized graduate program in cancer nursing. She is also internationally known for her research with patients living with cancer and the measurement of patient and family outcomes to improve the quality of their lives.

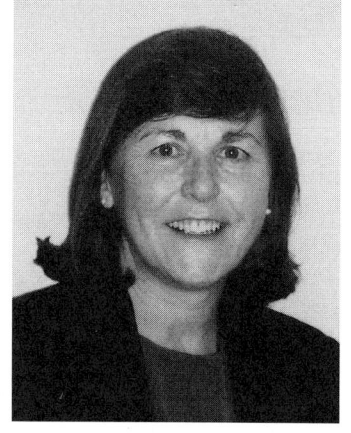

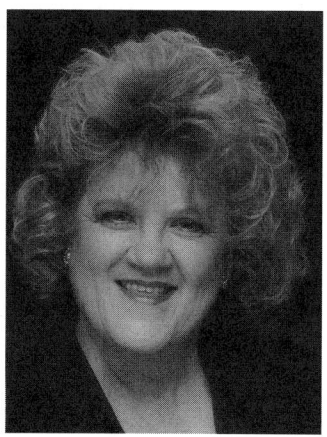

Marcia Grant, D.N.Sc., F.A.A.N., is Research Scientist and Director, Nursing Research and Education at the City of Hope National Medical Center in Duarte, California. She received her doctoral degree from the Department of Physiological Nursing, University of California San Francisco, and has written and lectured extensively on quality of life and symptom management in the care of patients with cancer. She was the recipient of the 1990 Oncology Nursing Society/Roche Distinguished Service Award. She is on the editorial board for *Seminars in Oncology Nursing*. Dr. Grant is also the recipient of the 1996 Oncology Nursing Society Chiron Excellence in Writing Award.

Marilyn Frank-Stromborg, Ed.D., J.D., A.N.P., F.A.A.N., is Professor and Nurse Practitioner at Northern Illinois University School of Nursing, DeKalb, Illinois. Her clinical background includes three years in the U.S. Air Force nurse corps and continuous part-time employment as a nurse practitioner for the last 12 years. Her academic credentials include numerous publications, as well as multiple large-scale–funded research projects in the areas of identifying the psychosocial needs and the health promoting activities of ambulatory cancer patients, instrument development, and minority health issues. She has been active in the Oncology Nursing Society and has served on the board of directors and as secretary. One of the highest honors that the Oncology Nursing Society can bestow on a member is the Mara Mogenson Flaherty Lectureship, and Dr. Stromborg received this honor as well as the 1991 ONS/Ross Laboratories Award for Excellence in Cancer Nursing Education.

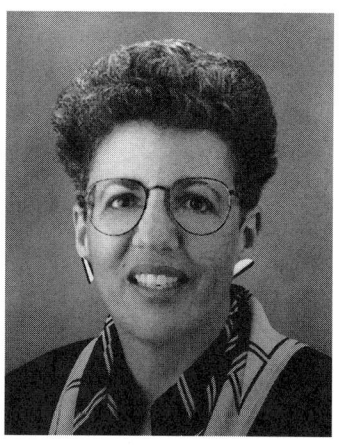

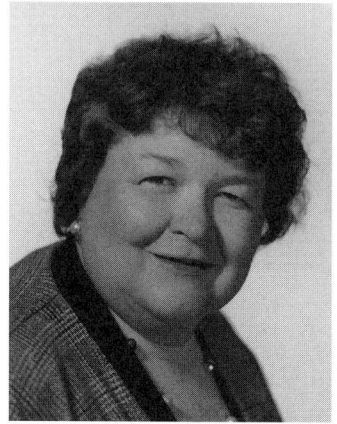

Susan B. Baird, M.P.H., M.A., R.N., is Director of Nursing and Patient Services at the Fox Chase Cancer Center, Philadelphia, Pennsylvania. She has served as Chief of the Cancer Nursing Service at the Clinical Center, National Institutes of Health and as Associate Director for Cancer Control at the Norris Cotton Cancer Center, Dartmouth-Hitchcock Medical Center, Hanover, New Hampshire. She has received the Distinguished Service Award from both the American Cancer Society and the Oncology Nursing Society. She has also received the Linda Arenth Outstanding Administrator Award from the Oncology Nursing Society. She served as editor of the *Oncology Nursing Forum*, the official publication of the Oncology Nursing Society, from 1979 to 1991.

Contributors

Elizabeth J. Abernathy, M.S.N., R.N.
Consulting Clinical Associate, Duke University, Durham, North Carolina
Biologic Response Modifiers

Terri B. Ades, B.S.N., R.N., O.C.N.
Director, Detection and Treatment/Nursing, American Cancer Society, Atlanta, Georgia
Developing Strategies for Public Education in Cancer; Cancer Organizations

Madalon Amenta, Dr.P.H., M.P.H., M.N., B.A.
Executive Director, Hospice Nurses Association, Pittsburgh, Pennsylvania
Hospice Services: The Place of Hospice Care in Cancer Treatment

Susan B. Baird, M.P.H., M.A., R.N.
Director of Nursing and Patient Services, Fox Chase Cancer Center, Philadelphia, Pennsylvania
Cancer Nursing as a Specialty; When a Colleague Has Cancer

Barbara A. Barhamand, M.S., R.N., A.O.C.N.
Oncology Clinical Nurse Specialist and Practice Manager, Hematology Oncology Consultants, Ltd., Naperville, Illinois
Documentation Issues in Cancer Nursing

Bill Barrick, M.S.N., R.N.
Head Nurse, HIV Research Outpatient Program, Warren Grant Magnuson Clinical Center, National Institutes of Health, Bethesda, Maryland
AIDS and the Spectrum of HIV Disease

Sandra Mitchell Beddar, M.Sc.N., C.N.P., A.O.C.N.
Nurse Practitioner, Hematology-Oncology and Bone Marrow Transplantation, Roswell Park Cancer Institute, Buffalo, New York
Abnormalities in Hemostasis and Hemorrhage

Katrina Bertin-Matson, M.S.N., R.N., O.C.N.
Guest Lecturer, Graduate Division Oncology Tract, University of Pennsylvania School of Nursing; Interim Associate Clinical Director, Surgical Nursing and Nurse Manager, Gynecology-Oncology, University of Pennsylvania Medical Center, Philadelphia, Pennsylvania
Gynecologic Cancers

Linda K. Birenbaum, Ph.D., R.N.
Senior Scientist, Chiles Research Institute; Administrative Coordinator, Columbia River Oncology Program, Portland, Oregon
Immobility

Jean K. Brown, Ph.D., R.N.
Assistant Professor, State University of New York Buffalo School of Nursing, Buffalo, New York
Role Clarification: Rights and Responsibilities of Oncology Nurses

Jennifer Dunn Bucholtz, M.S., R.N., O.C.N.
Adjunct Faculty, University of Delaware, Department of Advanced Nursing Science, Newark, Delaware; Faculty Associate, Johns Hopkins School of Nursing; Clinical Specialist, Johns Hopkins Oncology Center, Baltimore, Maryland
Central Nervous System Tumors

Nancy Burns, Ph.D., R.N., F.A.A.N.
Professor and Director, Center for Nursing Research, University of Texas Arlington School of Nursing, Arlington, Texas
Body Image Changes

Mary E. Callaghan, M.N., R.N., O.C.N.
Clinical Nurse Specialist, Hematology/Oncology/Bone Marrow Transplantation, Green Hospital of Scripps Clinic, La Jolla, California
Leukemia

Colette Carson, M.N., B.S., B.S.N.
Oncology Clinical Nurse Specialist, Gene Therapy, Sidney Kimmel Cancer Center, La Jolla, California
Hodgkin's Disease and Non-Hodgkin's Lymphomas

Kathryn Ann Caudell, Ph.D., R.N.
Assistant Professor, University of New Mexico College of Nursing, Albuquerque, New Mexico
Cancer Biology: Molecular and Cellular Aspects

Terry Chamorro, M.N., R.N.
Assistant Clinical Professor, University of California Los Angeles; Project Manager, Clinical Information Systems, Nursing Research and Development, Cedars-Sinai Medical Center, Los Angeles, California
Legal Responsibilities of the Nurse

Stephanie Chang, M.N., R.N., O.C.N.
Assistant Professor of Nursing, Graduate Program, University of California Los Angeles; Oncology Clinical Nurse Specialist and Bone Marrow Transplant Coordinator, University of California Los Angeles Medical Center, Los Angeles, California
Soft Tissue Sarcomas and Bone Cancers

Cynthia C. Chernecky, Ph.D., R.N.
Associate Professor of Nursing, University of Wisconsin Osh Kosh, Osh Kosh, Wisconsin
Complications of Advanced Disease

Bernadine Cimprich, Ph.D., R.N.
Assistant Professor, University of Michigan School of Nursing, Ann Arbor, Michigan
Symptom Management: Loss of Concentration

Ann M. Collins-Hattery, M.S., R.N., A.O.C.N.
Oncology Clinical Nurse Specialist, Hahnemann University Hospital, Philadelphia, Pennsylvania
Multiple Myeloma

Paul H. Coluzzi, M.D., M.P.H.
Director, Physician Services, Vitas Healthcare Corporation, Anaheim Hills, California
Supportive Care Services

Mary E. Cooley, M.S.N., C.R.N.P.
Doctoral Student and Oncology Clinical Nurse Specialist, University of Pennsylvania School of Nursing, Philadelphia, Pennsylvania
Role Implementation in Cancer Nursing; Unknown Primary Malignancies

Nessa Coyle, M.S., R.N.
Associate in Nursing, Columbia University School of Nursing; Director, Supportive Care Program, Department of Neurology and Pain Services, Memorial Sloan-Kettering Cancer Center, New York, New York
Pharmacologic Management of Cancer Pain

Linda J. Cuaron, M.N., R.N., O.C.N.
Research Nurse Coordinator, Puget Sound Blood Center, Seattle, Washington
Cancer Biology: Molecular and Cellular Aspects

Gregory A. Curt, M.D.
Clinical Director, National Cancer Institute, Bethesda, Maryland
Implementation of Clinical Trials

B. Joyce Davison Ph.D.(C.), M.N., B.N., R.N.
Steve Fonyo Doctoral Research Student, National Cancer Institute of Canada, Toronto, Ontario, Canada
Decision Making

Marie Steenberg De Stefano, M.S.N., R.N., O.C.N.
Administrative Director of Oncology, Delaware County Memorial Hospital, Drexel Hill, Pennsylvania; Board Member, American Cancer Society, Media, Pennsylvania
Gynecologic Cancers

Grace E. Dean, M.S.N., R.N.
Research Specialist, Department of Nursing Research and Education, City of Hope National Medical Center, Duarte, California
Infection; Nondrug Pain Interventions

Lesley F. Degner, Ph.D., M.A., B.N., R.N.
Professor, University of Manitoba Faculty of Nursing; Nurse Scientist-in-Residence, St. Boniface General Hospital Research Centre, Winnipeg, Manitoba, Canada
Decision Making

Marylin Dodd, Ph.D., M.N., B.S.N.
Professor, University of California San Francisco, San Francisco, California
Self-Care

Karen Hassey Dow, Ph.D., R.N., F.A.A.N.
Associate Professor, University of Central Florida School of Nursing, Orlando, Florida; Clinical Nurse Specialist and Researcher, Holmes Regional Medical Center, Melbourne, Florida
Radiation Oncology

Karin Dufault, S.P., Ph.D., M.S.N.
Advisory Board, Seattle University School of Nursing; Chair of Board of Directors, Sisters of Providence Health System, Seattle, Washington
Immobility

Jacqueline Fawcett, Ph.D., F.A.A.N.
Professor, University of Pennsylvania School of Nursing, Philadelphia, Pennsylvania
Assessment of Function

Jayne I. Fernsler, D.S.N., R.N., O.C.N.
Associate Professor, Medical-Surgical Nursing, University of Delaware College of Nursing, Newark, Delaware
Developing Strategies for Public Education in Cancer

Betty Rolling Ferrell, Ph.D., F.A.A.N.
Associate Research Scientist, City of Hope National Medical Center, Duarte, California
Nondrug Pain Interventions

Rosemary Ford, B.S., B.A., R.N.
Outpatient Nurse Manager, Fred Hutchinson Cancer Research Center, Seattle, Washington
Marrow Transplant and Peripheral Blood Stem Cell Transplantation

Marilyn Frank-Stromborg, Ed.D., J.D., A.N.P., F.A.A.N.
Acting Chair and Professor, Northern Illinois University School of Nursing, DeKalb, Illinois
Cancer Nursing as a Specialty; Evaluating Cancer Risks and Preventive Oncology; Cancer Screening and Early Detection; Recovering from the Experience of a Family Member's Illness and Death; Legal Responsibilities of the Nurse

Brandi Funk, B.S.N., R.N.
Research Specialist, City of Hope National Medical Center, Duarte, California
Nondrug Pain Interventions

Betty Bierut Gallucci, Ph.D.
Professor, Department of Biobehavioral Nursing and Health Systems, University of Washington School of Nursing, Seattle, Washington
Cancer Biology: Molecular and Cellular Aspects

Barbara B. Germino, Ph.D.
Associate Professor and Chair, Department of Adult and Geriatric Health, University of North Carolina Chapel Hill, Chapel Hill, North Carolina
Cancer and the Family

Barbara Given, Ph.D., R.N., F.A.A.N.
Professor and Director, Research Center, Michigan State University College of Nursing; Associate Director, Cancer Prevention and Control, Cancer Center, Michigan State University College of Human Medicine, East Lansing, Michigan
Family Caregiver Burden From Cancer Care

C. William Given, Ph.D.
Professor and Assistant Chairperson for Research, Department of Family Practice, Michigan State University College of Human Medicine, East Lansing, Michigan
Family Caregiver Burden From Cancer Care

John Godwin, M.D., M.S.
Assistant Professor of Medicine and Pathology, Loyola University Chicago; Full-time Faculty Physician and Associate Director, Clinical Hematology Laboratories, Foster G. McGaw Hospital, Maywood, Illinois
Blood Component Therapy

Sara C. Gold, M.S.N., R.N., O.C.N.
Education Coordinator, Cedars-Sinai Comprehensive Cancer Center, Los Angeles, California
Colorectal Cancer

Michelle Goodman, M.S., R.N.
Assistant Professor, Rush University College of Nursing; Oncology Clinical Nurse Specialist, Rush Cancer Institute, Rush-Presbyterian–St. Luke's Medical Center, Chicago, Illinois
Delivery of Cancer Chemotherapy

Christine Grady, Ph.D., R.N.
Assistant Director for Clinical Science, National Institute of Nursing Research, National Institutes of Health, Bethesda, Maryland
AIDS and the Spectrum of HIV Disease

Marcia Grant, D.N.Sc., F.A.A.N.
Director and Research Scientist, Department of Nursing Research and Education, City of Hope National Medical Center, Duarte, California
Cancer Nursing as a Specialty; Alterations in Nutrition; Survivorship and Quality of Life Issues

Patricia E. Greene, M.S.N., R.N., F.A.A.N.
National Vice President, Patient Services, American Cancer Society, Atlanta, Georgia
My Mother's Struggle with Endometrial Cancer: Coping from a Distance

Eva R. Greimel, Ph.D.
Clinical Psychologist, Department of Obstetrics and Gynecology, University Hospital, Auenbruggerplatz, Austria
Survivorship and Quality of Life Issues

Jennifer L. Guy, B.S., R.N.
Administrator for Oncology, Regional Oncology Center, Park Medical Center, Columbus, Ohio
Medical Oncology—The Agents

Mel R. Haberman, Ph.D., R.N., F.A.A.N.
Director of Research, Oncology Nursing Society, Pittsburgh, Pennsylvania; Assistant Staff Scientist, Fred Hutchinson Cancer Research Center, Seattle, Washington
Cancer Nursing Research Today

Douglas Haeuber, M.S.N., M.A., R.N.
Staff Nurse, Medical Oncology, Stanford University Medical Center, Stanford, California
Infection

Gloria A. Hagopian, Ed.D., R.N.
Associate Professor, University of North Carolina Charlotte College of Nursing, Charlotte, North Carolina
Patient and Family Education

Marilyn D. Harris, M.S.N., B.S.N.
Executive Director, Visiting Nurse Association of Eastern Montgomery County, Department of Abington Memorial Hospital, Willow Grove, Pennsylvania
Home Care Services

Margaret McLean Heitkemper, Ph.D., M.N., B.S.N.
Professor, Department of Physiological Nursing, University of Washington, Seattle, Washington
Living with the Consequences of a Spouse's Cancer

Karen Billars Heusinkveld, Dr.P.H., R.N.
Associate Professor, University of Texas Arlington School of Nursing, Arlington, Texas
Evaluating Cancer Risks and Preventive Oncology

Laura J. Hilderley, M.S., R.N.
Clinical Nurse Specialist, Radiation Oncology Services of Rhode Island, Warwick, Rhode Island
Radiation Oncology

Barbara Carlile Holmes, M.S.N., R.N., O.C.N.
Doctoral Candidate, University of Texas Austin, Austin, Texas; Oncology Nursing Consultant, San Antonio, Texas
Body Image Changes

Linda Edwards Hood, M.S.N., B.S.N., R.N., O.C.N.
Clinical Associate Faculty, Duke University Medical Center; Head Nurse, Oncology Treatment Center, Duke Comprehensive Cancer Center, Duke University Medical Center, Durham, North Carolina
Biologic Response Modifiers

Susan Molloy Hubbard, B.S., M.P.A., R.N.
Director, International Cancer Information Center, Associate Director, National Cancer Institute, National Institutes of Health, Bethesda, Maryland
The Biology of Invasion and Metastases

Barbara A. Ingram, R.Ph.
Oncology Pharmacist, Regional Oncology Center Park Medical Center, Columbus, Ohio
Medical Oncology—The Agents

Ryan R. Iwamoto, M.N., R.N., C.S.
Clinical Instructor, Department of Physiological Nursing, University of Washington, Seattle, Washington; Clinical Instructor, Seattle University School of Nursing, Seattle, Washington; Instructor, Educational Development and Health Sciences Division, Bellevue Community College, Bellevue, Washington; Clinical Nurse Specialist, Section of Radiation Oncology, Virginia Mason Medical Center, Seattle, Washington
Alterations in Oral Status

Linda A. Jacobs, M.S.N., B.S.N., R.N.
Clinical Faculty, Oncology Graduate Program, University of Pennsylvania School of Nursing, Philadelphia, Pennsylvania
The Phenomenon of Fatigue and the Cancer Patient

Barbara A. Jagels, B.S.N., R.N.
Assistant Nurse Manager, Outpatient Department, Fred Hutchinson Cancer Research Center, Seattle, Washington
Marrow Transplant and Peripheral Blood Stem Cell Transplantation

Patricia F. Jassak, M.S., R.N., O.C.N.
Joint Practice Research Coordinator and Manager, Rush Cancer Institute, Rush-Presbyterian–St. Luke's Medical Center, Chicago, Illinois
Blood Component Therapy

Jean Jenkins, M.S.N., R.N.
Clinical Nurse Specialist Consultant, Medical Genetics Branch, National Center for Human Genome Research, National Institutes of Health, Bethesda, Maryland
Implementation of Clinical Trials

Bonnie Mowinski Jennings, COL, D.N.Sc., F.A.A.N.
Assistant Chief, Department of Nursing and Director, Inpatient Quality Management Group, Madigan Army Medical Center, Tacoma, Washington
The Generation of Stress in the Provision of Care

Bonny Libbey Johnson, M.S.N., R.N., O.C.N.
Clinical Trials Coordinator, University of Connecticut Health Center, Farmington, Connecticut
Endocrine Cancers

Marjorie Kagawa-Singer, Ph.D., M.N., R.N.
Assistant Professor, Community Health Sciences and Asian American Studies Center, University of California Los Angeles School of Public Health, Los Angeles, California
Cultural Systems

Mark H. Kawachi, M.D., B.S., F.A.C.S.
Assistant Professor, Department of Urology, University of Southern California School of Medicine, Los Angeles, California; Urologic Oncologic Surgery, City of Hope National Medical Center, Duarte, California
Genitourinary Cancers

Catherine A. Kefer, M.J., R.N., O.C.N.
Research, Rush Cancer Institute, Rush-Presbyterian–St. Luke's Medical Center, Chicago, Illinois; Oncology Research Coordinator and Educator, Westlake Community Hospital, Oak Park Hospital, Melrose Park, Illinois
Blood Component Therapy

Cynthia R. King, M.S.N., R.N., C.N.A.
Senior Associate and Doctoral Candidate, University of Rochester School of Nursing; Owner and Nurse Consultant, Special Care Consultants, Rochester, New York
Alternative Cancer Therapies

M. Tish Knobf, M.S.N., R.N., F.A.A.N.
Associate Professor, Yale University School of Nursing, New Haven, Connecticut; Doctoral Student, University of Pennsylvania, Philadelphia, Pennsylvania; Oncology Clinical Nurse Specialist, Ambulatory Service, Yale New Haven Hospital, New Haven, Connecticut
Breast Cancers

Elise C. Kohn, M.D.
Chief, Signal Transduction and Prevention Unit, Laboratory of Pathology, National Cancer Institute, Bethesda, Maryland
The Biology of Invasion and Metastases

Ruth Krech-Fritskey, M.S.N.
Oncology Clinical Nurse Specialist, Cleveland Clinic Foundation, Cleveland, Ohio
Complications of Advanced Disease

Margaret A. Lamb, Ph.D., R.N.
Associate Professor, Department of Nursing, University of New Hampshire, Durham, New Hampshire
Sexuality and Sexual Functioning

Patricia J. Larson, D.N.Sc., R.N.
Associate Professor and Director of Oncology Graduate Program in Nursing, University of California San Francisco, San Francisco, California
The Generation of Stress in the Provision of Care

Connie J. Leek, M.S.N., R.N.C., O.C.N.
Clinical Assistant Professor of Nursing, Department of Nursing, University of Southern California, Los Angeles, California; Clinical Educator, City of Hope National Medical Center, Duarte, California
Genitourinary Cancers

Elise L. Lev, Ed.D., R.N., C.S.
Assistant Professor, Rutgers, The State University of New Jersey College of Nursing, Newark, New Jersey
Loss and Bereavement

Esther Muscari Lin, M.S.N., B.S.N., R.N., A.O.C.N.
Advanced Practice Oncology Nurse, Clinician Five, University of Virginia Cancer Center, Charlottesville, Virginia
Abnormalities in Hemostasis and Hemorrhage

Ada M. Lindsey, Ph.D.
Dean and Professor, University of Nebraska Medical Center College of Nursing, Omaha, Nebraska
Lung Cancer

Alice J. Longman, Ed.D., R.N., F.A.A.N.
Professor Emerita, University of Arizona College of Nursing, Tucson, Arizona
Skin Cancers

Virginia R. Martin, M.S.N., R.N., A.O.C.N.
Clinical Director, Ambulatory Care, Fox Chase Cancer Center, Philadelphia, Pennsylvania
Delivery of Cancer Chemotherapy

Mary S. McCabe, B.S., B.A., R.N.
Special Assistant to Associate Director, Cancer Therapy Evaluation Program, National Cancer Institute, Bethesda, Maryland
Cancer Legislation

Margo McCaffery, M.S., R.N., F.A.A.N.
Consultant in the Nursing Care of Patients with Pain, Los Angeles, California
Pain Assessment

Ruth McCorkle, Ph.D., F.A.A.N.
American Cancer Society Professor and Director, Center for Advancing Care in Serious Illness, University of Pennsylvania School of Nursing, Associate Director, Cancer Control, Philadelphia, Pennsylvania
Cancer Nursing as a Specialty; Loss and Bereavement; Surviving Breast Cancer; Psychosocial Aspects of Cancer; Cancer Nursing Education Today

Joanne McDonald, M.A., B.S.N.
Director of Clinical and Patient Education, Fred Hutchinson Cancer Research Center, Seattle, Washington
Marrow Transplant and Peripheral Blood Stem Cell Transplantation

Marianne McLaughlin-Hagan, M.S.N., R.N., O.C.N.
Formerly Clinical Nurse Specialist, Fox Chase Cancer Center, Philadelphia, Pennsylvania
Gastric and Related Cancers

Curtis Mettlin, Ph.D.
Chief of Epidemiologic Research, Roswell Park Cancer Institute, Buffalo, New York
The Causes of Cancer

Christine Miaskowski, Ph.D., R.N., F.A.A.N.
Associate Professor and Chair, Department of Physiological Nursing, University of California San Francisco, San Francisco, California
Oncologic Emergencies

Arthur M. Michalek, Ph.D.
Assistant Director for Educational Affairs and Associate Dean, Roswell Park Graduate Division, University of Buffalo Roswell Park Cancer Institute, Buffalo, New York
The Causes of Cancer

Karin J. Mitchell-Supplee, B.S.N., R.N., C.C.R.N.
Critical Care Education Specialist, Fred Hutchinson Cancer Research Center, Seattle, Washington
Marrow Transplant and Peripheral Blood Stem Cell Transplantation

Darlene W. Mood, Ph.D., M.A., B.Med.
Professor and Associate Dean for Research and Director, Center for Health Research, Wayne State University College of Nursing; Adjunct Medical Staff, Department of Otolaryngology, Harper Hospital, Detroit, Michigan
The Diagnosis of Cancer: A Life Transition

Kathi H. Mooney, Ph.D., R.N., A.O.C.N., F.A.A.N.
Professor, University of Utah College of Nursing, Salt Lake City, Utah
Cancer Nursing Research Today

Lee E. Mortenson, M.S., M.P.A., D.P.A.
Executive Director, Association of Community Cancer Centers; President and Chief Executive Officer, ELM Services, Inc., Rockville, Maryland
Understanding Cancer Reimbursement

Judith K. Much, M.S.N., R.N., A.O.C.N.
Oncology Clinical Nurse Specialist and Psychosocial Resource Nurse, Fox Chase Cancer Center, Philadelphia, Pennsylvania
When a Colleague Has Cancer

Donna Edwards Neumark, M.S.N., B.A., R.N.
Instructor, Michigan State University College of Nursing; Research Associate, Michigan State University, East Lansing, Michigan
Surgical Oncology

Brenda M. Nevidjon, M.S.N., R.N.
Associate Chief Operating Officer for Patient Care Services, Duke University Medical Center, Durham, North Carolina
Ambulatory Care Services

Laurel L. Northouse, Ph.D., R.N., F.A.A.N.
Associate Professor, Wayne State University College of Nursing, Detroit, Michigan
Interpersonal Communication Systems

Peter G. Northouse, Ph.D.
Professor, Department of Communication, Western Michigan University, Kalamazoo, Michigan
Interpersonal Communication Systems

Denise M. Oleske, Ph.D., R.N.
Associate Professor, Department of Health Systems Management, Rush University, Chicago, Illinois
Epidemiologic Principles for Cancer Nursing Practice

Sharon J. Olsen, M.S., R.N.
Lecturer, Johns Hopkins University School of Nursing; Joint Appointment, Cancer Prevention and Screening, Johns Hopkins Oncology Center, Baltimore, Maryland
Cancer Screening and Early Detection

Maureen E. O'Rourke, M.S., O.C.N.
Doctoral Student, University of North Carolina Chapel Hill, Chapel Hill, North Carolina
Cancer and the Family

Faith D. Ottery, M.D., Ph.D.
President, Society for Nutritional Oncology Adjuvant Therapy; Program Director, Nutritional Oncology–Cancer Recovery Center, Philadelphia, Pennsylvania
Gastric and Related Cancers

Geraldine V. Padilla, Ph.D.
Professor and Associate Dean for Research, University of California Los Angeles School of Nursing; Associate Director for Community Research, Jonsson Comprehensive Cancer Center, University of California Los Angeles, Los Angeles, California
Survivorship and Quality of Life Issues

Gayle Giboney Page, D.N.Sc., M.N., B.S.N.
Assistant Professor, Ohio State University College of Nursing, Columbus, Ohio
Pain: Physiologic Aspects

Carol Ann Parente, M.S.N., R.N., C.R.N.P.
Adult Nurse Practitioner, Visiting Nurse Association of Eastern Montgomery County, Department of Abington Memorial Hospital, Willow Grove, Pennsylvania
Home Care Services

Jeannie Pasacreta, Ph.D., R.N.
Lecturer, University of Pennsylvania School of Nursing; Psychiatric Consultation Liaison Nurse, University of Pennsylvania Medical Center, Philadelphia, Pennsylvania
Psychosocial Aspects of Cancer

Mary Pickett, Ph.D., R.N.
Research Assistant Professor, University of Pennsylvania School of Nursing; Associate Director, Center for Advancing Care in Serious Illness, Research Dissemination Unit, University of Pennsylvania, Philadelphia, Pennsylvania
Symptoms of the Dying

Joan A. Piemme, M.N.Ed., R.N., F.A.A.N.
HIV Coordinator, Veterans Administration Medical Center, Martinsburg, West Virginia
Cancer Legislation

Barbara F. Piper, D.N.Sc., R.N., O.C.N., F.A.A.N.
Associate Clinical Professor, Department of Physiological Nursing, University of California San Francisco School of Nursing; Oncology Clinical Nurse III and Evening Charge Nurse, University of California San Francisco Mount Zion Medical Center, San Francisco, California
The Phenomenon of Fatigue and the Cancer Patient

Russell K. Portenoy, M.D.
Associate Professor of Neurology, Cornell University Medical College; Director, Analgesic Studies, Pain Service, Memorial Sloan-Kettering Cancer Center, New York, New York
Pharmacologic Management of Cancer Pain

Janice Post-White, Ph.D., R.N.
Assistant Professor and American Cancer Society Professor of Oncology Nursing, University of Minnesota School of Nursing, Minneapolis, Minnesota
Principles of Immunology

Fredrica Preston, R.N.C., N.P., A.O.C.N.
Oncology Nurse Practitioner, North Shore Cancer Center, Peabody, Massachusetts
Cancer Nursing Education Today

Jean L. Reese, Ph.D., R.N.
Associate Professor, University of Iowa College of Nursing, Iowa City, Iowa
Head and Neck Cancers

Michelle Rhiner, M.S.N., R.N., N.P., O.C.N.
Nurse Practitioner, Supportive Care Services, City of Hope National Medical Center, Duarte, California
Supportive Care Services

Lynne M. Rivera, M.S.N., R.N.
Research Specialist, Department of Nursing Research and Education, City of Hope National Medical Center, Duarte, California
Infection; Pain Assessment

Linda Robinson, M.S.N., R.N., C.S.
Doctoral Candidate, University of Pennsylvania School of Nursing, Philadelphia, Pennsylvania
Loss and Bereavement

Kim Rohan, M.S., R.N.
Patient Services Coordinator, Edward Hospital, Naperville, Illinois
Evaluating Cancer Risks and Preventive Oncology

Mary E. Ropka, Ph.D., R.N.
Associate Professor, Virginia Commonwealth University School of Nursing, Richmond, Virginia
Alterations in Nutrition

Charlene Sakurai, B.A., R.N., O.C.N.
Clinical Support Specialist, AMGEN, Thousand Oaks, California
Colorectal Cancer

Linda Sarna, D.N.Sc., R.N., F.A.A.N.
Assistant Professor and American Cancer Society Professor of Oncology Nursing, University of California Los Angeles School of Nursing, Los Angeles, California
Lung Cancer

Judith M. Saunders, D.N.Sc., F.A.A.N.
Assistant Professor, Department of Nursing, University of Southern California, Los Angeles, California
My Story: Responding to Severe Cervical Dysplasia

Wanda Sebastian, B.S.N., R.N., O.C.N.
Clinical Educator, City of Hope National Medical Center, Duarte, California
Genitourinary Cancers

Vivian R. Sheidler, M.S., R.N.
Research Associate in Oncology, Johns Hopkins University School of Medicine; Clinical Associate, Johns Hopkins University School of Nursing; Clinical Nurse Specialist, Neuro Oncology, Johns Hopkins Oncology Center, Baltimore, Maryland
Central Nervous System Tumors

Gayle H. Shiba, M.S.N., B.S.N., R.N.
Doctoral Candidate, Department of Physiological Nursing, University of California San Francisco, San Francisco, California
Self-Care

Mathew Jay Soltis, B.S.
Research Fellow, Signal Transduction and Prevention Unit, Laboratory of Pathology, National Cancer Institute, Bethesda, Maryland
The Biology of Invasion and Metastases

Diane L. Spatz, Ph.D., M.S.N., B.S.N., R.N.C.
Clinical Nurse Specialist-Research, University of Pennsylvania School of Nursing, Philadelphia, Pennsylvania
Role Implementation in Cancer Nursing

Liz Sullivan, M.N., R.N., O.C.N., A.N.P.
Assistant Clinical Professor, University of California Los Angeles School of Nursing, Los Angeles, California; Clinical Educator and Nurse Practitioner, City of Hope National Medical Center, Duarte, California
Genitourinary Cancers

Lorraine Tulman, D.N.Sc., F.A.A.N.
Associate Professor, University of Pennsylvania School of Nursing, Philadelphia, Pennsylvania
Assessment of Function

Deborah Lowe Volker, M.A., R.N., O.C.N.
Director of Nursing Staff Development, University of Texas, M.D. Anderson Cancer Center, Houston, Texas
Cancer Nursing Education Today

Frances E. Walker, M.S.N., R.N., A.O.C.N.
Nursing Care Coordinator, Thomas Jefferson University Hospital, Philadelphia, Pennsylvania
Delivery of Cancer Chemotherapy

Pamela G. Watson, Sc.D., R.N.
Professor and Chairman, Department of Nursing, Thomas Jefferson University College of Allied Health Sciences; Professor, Rehabilitation Medicine, Thomas Jefferson University Jefferson Medical College, Philadelphia, Pennsylvania
Rehabilitation Services

Faith Norcross Weintraub, M.S.N., R.N., C.R.N.P.
Adjunct Clinical Faculty, University of Pennsylvania; Adult Nurse Practitioner, Division of Gastrointestinal Surgery, University of Pennsylvania Medical Center, Philadelphia, Pennsylvania
Surgical Oncology

M. Linda Workman, Ph.D., R.N., O.C.N., F.A.A.N.
Associate Professor of Nursing, Case Western Reserve University Frances Payne Bolton School of Nursing, Cleveland, Ohio; American Cancer Society Professor of Oncology Nursing, American Cancer Society, Ohio Division, Dublin, Ohio
Gene Therapy

Donna Yancey, D.N.S., R.N.
Assistant Professor, Purdue University School of Nursing, West Lafayette, Indiana
Symptoms of the Dying

Connie Henke Yarbro, B.S.N., R.N.
Clinical Associate Professor, University of Missouri Columbia School of Medicine, Columbia, Missouri; Editor, *Seminars in Oncology Nursing*
The History of Cancer Nursing

Joyce M. Yasko, Ph.D., R.N.
Professor, Oncology Nursing, University of Pittsburgh; Associate Director, University of Pittsburgh Cancer Institute; Clinical Administrator, University of Pittsburgh Medical Center, Pittsburgh, Pennsylvania
Role Implementation in Cancer Nursing

Foreword

The second edition of *Cancer Nursing: A Comprehensive Textbook* provides a broad scope and a wealth of information for the neophyte in cancer nursing as well as the experienced practitioner. The second edition contains 85 chapters organized in 11 units. The chapters are grouped within specific units in a methodical manner, providing ready reference and a complete treatise on cancer nursing. Each chapter concludes with a pertinent bibliography. Illustrations, graphs, and charts are also included.

The textbook begins with chapters on cancer nursing as a specialty, nursing roles, and historical development of cancer nursing to provide a frame of reference. Nursing care related to the major areas of the cancer continuum—early detection, prevention, diagnosis, treatment, rehabilitation, and continuity of care—are then covered. Special chapters on ambulatory care, self-care, and hospice reflect current changes in the delivery of nursing care. As more people survive cancer, the need to help the survivors and their families has become evident. Access to resources is extremely important.

The use of case studies by nurse leaders reflects the contributors' experiences with cancer and their recommendations for enhancing patient and family outcomes. These kinds of personal accounts are important because they make us realize that nurses play a critical role in helping others cope with the experiences at many levels of care. The case studies point out that regardless of how expert we might be in the field of cancer nursing, whenever cancer touches us, the same individual and family reactions and emotions occur as they do in lay individuals. At times like these, we may need to be made aware of the need for help and accept it. These case studies also point out the necessity for allowing adequate time for loss and bereavement.

The second edition of the textbook has been greatly expanded by additional chapters covering new, expanding areas. These include new areas related to gene therapy, immunology, and major nursing problems including confusion and hemorrhage associated with cancer and cancer therapies. There are several very important chapters on pain focusing on the current clinical efforts related to the national pain initiative. These new chapters include the physiologic aspects of pain, assessment, and pharmacologic and non-pharmacologic pain management. Every nurse who cares for patients with cancer needs to know this information.

One unit includes adult cancers organized by cancer sites plus the hemopoietic aspects of cancer and HIV/AIDS. This unit will be of great value to the clinician who is responsible for planning nursing care based on pathophysiology, diagnosis, and treatment. Current cancer nursing research is also integrated throughout the textbook and should be of value not only to the researcher, but to the practitioner who must use research findings to enhance patient care outcomes.

Contributors to the textbook are national leaders in the field of cancer nursing and cancer. The reader will recognize these individuals as experts and specialists in their fields of practice, education, and research in various work settings. Many will be recognized for their research efforts in cancer nursing and as contributors to the current body of literature. The growth of cancer nursing education programs is described. Educational opportunities are identified and scholarships available through the American Cancer Society and the Oncology Nursing Society are described. Masters and doctorally prepared nurses are needed to plan, deliver, and conduct clinical research and aspects of care as well as to work in multidisciplinary teams.

This comprehensive textbook is a must for every student, practicing nurse, and others in the cancer nursing field. This textbook is essential reading and will help to prepare nurses for the many changes resulting from healthcare reform. Health educators, managed care staff, and health coordinators will find the text very useful. This text should be in every health science nursing library for reference of authentic current material in the field. National legislation, scientific and clinical research, and medical advances have had a definite impact on cancer nursing. Modern cancer nursing is far removed from when I began my career in cancer nursing in 1950.

The tremendous growth and explosion of knowledge in cancer nursing has been captured in this text under one cover. It represents a tremendous contribution to cancer nursing. Sincere congratulations and gratitude are in order for the authors and editors. This is a textbook to be proud of. It supports the concept that for anyone practicing today in the field of cancer nursing current education and information are a necessity not an option.

RENILDA HILKEMEYER

Preface

Since release of the first edition in 1991, *Cancer Nursing: A Comprehensive Textbook* has been the book that educators and students select, the resource text that oncology clinical nurse specialists value, and the ready reference source for the skilled clinician. Our team of editors for the second edition has changed and expanded. Our backgrounds and areas of expertise are varied yet complementary, and serve to address the ever changing and expanding scope of cancer nursing practice. A challenging position as nursing administrator at Fox Chase Cancer Center in Philadelphia demanded Susan Baird's full attention. She has continued, however, to contribute her wealth of cancer nursing experience to the book, particularly her perspective as an administrator in rapidly changing times.

Ruth McCorkle and Marcia Grant continue to lend their years of experience as clinicians, educators, and researchers. We were especially fortunate to recruit Marilyn Frank-Stromborg as an editor for this edition. Because of her eclectic background as an educator, researcher, nurse practitioner, and lawyer, Marilyn lends multifaceted and unique knowledge and perspective to the text. The depth of respect and admiration that we have for each other as individuals and as nursing professionals continues to be strong and in large part accounts for the success and value accorded *Cancer Nursing* as a comprehensive text that synthesizes the diverse and fluid nature of nursing knowledge in the field.

As editors, our intent continues to be to encompass the broad spectrum of responsibilities and practice arenas within cancer nursing while incorporating current theory, the latest research, and the most up-to-date issues to affect clinical practice. Several challenges to meeting our high standards for this second edition include incorporating into the text the profound changes in our health care delivery system and how they have affected nursing roles, practice settings, and quality patient care. Concurrent with changes in the delivery of health care, a virtual explosion of information and knowledge regarding cancer etiology and treatment has occurred. A prime example of this phenomenon is in the area of genetic vulnerability to specific cancers and gene therapy. While new knowledge is exciting and promising, it has produced new and challenging legal and ethical issues. Clear expectations and guidelines regarding professional behaviors and practices have not kept pace with the rapid expansion of knowledge. This text provides beginning guidelines, direction, and discussion of these important aspects of practice. We believe that inclusion of these issues places the second edition of *Cancer Nursing* on the "cutting edge" of some of the most pressing problems facing health care delivery today.

The second edition of *Cancer Nursing* acknowledges and addresses the currents of social and economic change serving as the basis for health care reform. The period spanning the middle of the twentieth century during which patients routinely have been cared for in acute care hospitals may turn out to be a brief aberration in social and medical history. Before this time, patients were cared for primarily at home by their families. Today, rapid reform of the health care system is removing patients from the hospital and returning them home once again. Although at face value this change seems positive, simultaneous changes in the needs of our nation's health care consumers have highlighted large gaps and deficiencies in the system. Dramatic advances in science and technology allow us to keep patients alive longer despite complex and chronic health problems, yet these problems have created new problems and challenges.

The burden of care increasingly falls on patients and families who are usually unprepared to manage the physical and emotional demands inherent in chronic health problems. Additional issues that stem from reform of our health care system include: reduced usage of inpatient beds with resultant changes in nursing roles and practice settings; a shift in the burden of care from hospital to home often with inadequate or unaffordable follow-up services resulting in emotional and financial strain on patients and families; and increasingly aggressive treatments used in cases where there is questionable benefit and within the context of diminishing resources leading to new legal and ethical questions that are unparalleled in medical history. The preceding issues are but some of the current aspects of cancer care addressed in the text. The effect of these problems on patients, families, providers, and society is great, yet effective strategies for managing results of health care reform are quite small.

There are many people to recognize for their contributions to the second edition of this book. The authors accomplished their chapters with enthusiasm despite busy schedules and many professional demands. They were selected as contributors because they are the leading experts in the field and they remain our trusted colleagues. We greatly appreciate the assistance of Barbara Nelson Cullen, Senior Editor for Nursing Books at W.B. Saunders Company, who has provided tremendous encouragement and support. As was true with the first edition, we continued to receive competent, enthusiastic help from the people at W.B. Saunders Company—Francine Rosenthal and Marie Pelcin. We would also like to thank Chris Cook from Cracom Corporation for her editorial assistance.

The release of the second edition of *Cancer Nursing* could not have come at a better time. With all of the change and upheaval occurring in health care, the presence amid an atmosphere of uncertainty, nurses have more opportunities than ever to influence the lives and care of those affected by cancer. As always our hope is that this book will aid nurses in their efforts.

RUTH MCCORKLE
MARCIA GRANT
MARILYN FRANK-STROMBORG
SUSAN B. BAIRD

Contents

CHAPTER 17

Cancer Screening and Early Detection   265

CHAPTER 18

The Diagnosis of Cancer: A Life Transition . . 298

UNIT V
Cancer Treatment: Therapies and Physical Support Approaches

CHAPTER 19

Surgical Oncology   315

CHAPTER 20

Radiation Oncology   331

CHAPTER 21

Medical Oncology—The Agents   359

CHAPTER 22

Delivery of Cancer Chemotherapy   395

CHAPTER 23

Biologic Response Modifiers   434

CHAPTER 24

Gene Therapy   458

UNIT VI
Effects of Common Adult Cancers

CHAPTER 44

AIDS and the Spectrum of HIV Disease   . . . 870

CHRISTINE GRADY
BILL BARRICK

UNIT VII
CANCER AS AN ILLNESS

CHAPTER 45

My Story: Responding to Severe Cervical Dysplasia   887

JUDITH M. SAUNDERS

CHAPTER 46

Surviving Breast Cancer   893

RUTH McCORKLE

CHAPTER 47

Living with the Consequences of a Spouse's Cancer 899

MARGARET McLEAN HEITKEMPER

CHAPTER 48

Recovering from the Experience of a Family Member's Illness and Death 902

MARILYN FRANK-STROMBORG

CHAPTER 49

When a Colleague Has Cancer 907

JUDITH K. MUCH
SUSAN B. BAIRD

CHAPTER 50

My Mother's Struggle with Endometrial Cancer: Coping from a Distance   914

PATRICIA E. GREENE

UNIT VIII
MANAGEMENT OF MAJOR CLINICAL NURSING PROBLEMS

CHAPTER 51

Alterations in Nutrition 919

MARCIA GRANT
MARY E. ROPKA

UNIT IX
COMMUNICATION, EDUCATION, AND RESEARCH

UNIT X
THE DELIVERY OF CANCER CARE SERVICES: RESOURCES AND REFERRAL SYSTEMS

UNIT I
NATURE AND SCOPE OF CANCER NURSING

CHAPTER
1

Cancer Nursing as a Specialty

Ruth McCorkle • Marcia Grant • Marilyn Frank-Stromborg • Susan B. Baird

SPECIALIZATION IN NURSING

Cancer nursing is a unique nursing specialty. It draws on a knowledge base rich in physiologic, psychologic, social, and cultural concepts. It encompasses disease that occurs in people of all ages and both sexes. It is concerned with managing the symptoms caused more frequently by the medical treatment than by the disease itself. It spans care settings ranging from health promotion centers to acute care settings, ambulatory care clinics and primary care offices, home care agencies, and hospice arrangements. Care approaches are complicated by the negative stigma that continues to surround cancer and that causes people to dread the diagnosis and to be uncomfortable talking with others about the disease.

It takes a special kind of nurse to pursue as a career the care of people at risk for developing cancer or patients living with cancer. Cancer nurses are dedicated, intelligent, and caring nurses. It is not uncommon for patients to feel as the following patient felt as she wrote her thanks to the cancer nursing inpatient unit staff:

This is the first time that I have ever been in a hospital in my life. It was very hard to come and deal with my leukemia. I had been a picture of good health up to about six weeks ago. I want to acknowledge particularly my nurses for the way they have cared for me and the way they have supported me through the toughest six days of my life. You nurses have made the difference for me during this time. Your commitment to me and this institution has often times inspired me right above the pain I was enduring at the time. You nurses arrived many times like angels to minister to me and take away my pain. Your warm words and kind hearts motivate me to get better so that I can share my life and kind words with others. You are a blessing from God and I know He will reward you for your efforts.

The idea of specialization in nursing is not new, but the recognition of specialization and the definition of its continuation have been evolving (American Nurses' Association, 1980; Hamric, 1989). Specialty groups arise from a focus on a specific disease, such as cancer; a specific kind of treatment, such as surgical treatment; or a specific phase of treatment, such as intensive care. Specialization within nursing has evolved because of the extensive and specific body of knowledge necessary to give safe and thorough care to a specific group of patients, such as patients with cancer (Lynaugh & Fairman, 1989).

Content on cancer nursing care has been taught in nursing programs since the early 1900s, but recognition of cancer nursing as a specialty emerged with the education for cancer nursing care sponsored by the Clinical Education Grants Program of the National Cancer Institute (Craytor, 1982). The preparation of nurses through this program led to an increasing number of nurses who considered themselves cancer nursing specialists.

The effort of these specialists was critical in the formation in 1975 of a national organization for cancer nurses, the Oncology Nursing Society (ONS). This organization established the specialization and provided support at the national level with national congresses that included sessions on clinical practice, education, and research. (See Chapter 2 for an in-depth development of the history of cancer nursing.)

One of the major activities of the Oncology Nursing Society that has further cemented the specialization of cancer nursing has been the development in 1984 of the Oncology Nursing Certification Corporation. The sole purpose of this corporation is to develop, administer, and evaluate a program for the certification of oncology nurses. The certification examination tests the oncology nursing knowledge base of the professional nurse. The first generalist examination was offered in 1985 and resulted in 1384 oncology-certified nurses. As of Spring 1995 there were more than 15,000 oncology nurses certified at the generalist level. In addition, at the 1995 annual congress, the advanced oncology nursing certification examination was offered for the first time.

The specialization of cancer nursing is recognized by both the nursing profession and a variety of health care professionals in related fields. In academic settings, recognition of the specialty is evident through the establishment of cancer nursing specialty programs at the master's, doctoral and post-doctoral levels.

Current activity within the specialty of cancer nursing includes the identification and formation of many subspecialty groups. The special interest groups, a recent development within the Oncology Nursing Society, include such diverse subspecialties and interests as bone marrow transplantation, vascular access devices, and advanced research. Thus the specialty continues to grow. Subspecialty areas are being revised continually, depending on influential factors from the clinical arena and education and research settings.

The specialty can be further described in relation to the philosophy of practice and other factors that continue to influence the shape and nature of cancer nursing.

PHILOSOPHY OF PRACTICE

In helping people through periods of their lives that are so stressful and full of consequence, nurses become involved in the planning and implementing of care as a collective group of professionals and as individuals. Giving and receiving support among nurses and other professionals is essential as patient, family, and professional goals are identified and met. It is very useful for nurses to explicitly identify a philosophy of practice for themselves as individuals and as a collective group and review it periodically to strengthen their practice. A philosophy represents the "ideals" of the nursing staff within a given care environment. Box 1–1 presents an example of a nursing philosophy developed by nurses on an oncology nursing inpatient unit at the University of Washington Health Care Center in Seattle.

COMPONENTS OF THE PHILOSOPHY OF CANCER NURSING

The philosophy of cancer nursing incorporates the importance of collaboration with all members of the health care team, the primacy of the person at risk for cancer or person who has developed cancer and the family member as decision makers, and the education and research responsibility of staff within individual health care institutions. It is recommended that the philosophy developed as a collective effort be adopted as a multidisciplinary philosophy by all health care professionals within a specific unit or facility. In this way they can continue to strive for the highest quality of care and for the recognition of patients as human beings with unique needs.

Because patients and families in our society may, generally speaking, have problems coping with the crisis of the threat of cancer, a cancer diagnosis, or the recurrence of cancer, the development of person-cen-

---

Box 1–1. *Nursing Philosophy of 8-South*

In accordance with the philosophy of University Hospital and the Department of Nursing services, we, the nursing staff of 8-South, believe that our primary responsibility lies with the patient and with the patient's family. We subscribe to the philosophy of primary nursing in providing for and concerning ourselves with the physical, psychosocial, and spiritual needs of the patient. We acknowledge the special needs of the patient with cancer and are dedicated to the relief of symptoms of cancer and to its treatment, as well as to the promotion of comfort. We uphold the right of patients as individuals to have the opportunity to obtain information about their disease, prognosis, treatment, and available alternatives. We believe that the patient should be the primary participant in the decision-making process. In conjunction with this belief, we believe that all patients have a right to accept or refuse treatment and to receive support for the decisions they make.

We believe that families and individual patients have the need of continual support when their self-images, their social roles, and their functions undergo change. In this way, the patient can live to capacity and die with dignity. Patients and their families must have continual support during periods of adjustment and during times of grief.

We acknowledge the importance of collaboration with other members of the health team within the hospital, clinics, and community. In an effort to provide excellence of care, we have the responsibility to share knowledge, to participate continually in continued education, and to assist and support our colleagues in their research efforts. To this end, it is our intention to be flexible in our approaches and to be receptive to the creative ideas of others. Through an atmosphere of collaboration, we wish to promote an environment of mutual trust, respect, and support for health providers.

From McCorkle, R. (1979). A new beginning: The opening of a multidisciplinary cancer unit. Part I. *Cancer Nursing, 2,* 201–209. Reproduced by permission.

tered services is needed to provide assistance with the immediate and long-term consequences of these singular events (Benoliel & McCorkle, 1978; Krouse & Krouse, 1984; Weisman & Worden, 1976–1977). Persons with cancer have a right to know what is happening to them and to participate in the decisions that affect their lives. Further, by virtue of their positions in the health care system, professional nurses can readily assume leadership in developing and implementing services designed explicitly to achieve the goal of personalized patient care. By no means do nurses provide all care needed by patients and families, but nurses are ideally suited by educational background and position to provide coordination of care and problem-focused support services to patients and families undergoing changes in their lives (Benoliel & McCorkle, 1978).

To provide such services, nurses must be able to cope with their own feelings and reactions to cancer and with patients' potential decline, be knowledgeable about the psychosocial impact of these events on family systems and family relationships, be skilled in the use of communication strategies that promote collaboration among the many health care providers likely to be involved, and be clinically competent in the delivery of health services to all members of the family (Tornberg, Burns McGrath, & Quint Benoliel, 1984). To implement such services, nurses must be knowledgeable about the community resources available to assist with different types of family problems. To make these services available on an ongoing basis, nurses must be able to collaborate with one another and have continuing access to a socially supportive system of human relationships. Caplan (1974) believes that persons whose experience of living brings them into frequent contact with emotional crisis and strain are able to function more effectively when they have regular contact with a social network that provides consistent communication, appropriate rewards, and feedback about their performance. In view of this belief, mutual support and consultation among nurses are essential elements in the provision of cancer care to patients and families.

A CARE VERSUS CURE COMMITMENT

Nurses have a long history of concern for the rights of individuals to have access to basic health care resources that promote their health and well-being (Benoliel & McCorkle, 1977; McCorkle, 1980). Current evidence suggests that a major issue for the human community in the twenty-first century continues to center on the unbalanced distribution of health care resources between cure- and care-oriented services. The current United States health care system is a reflection of the interplay among several factors. Although there are strong efforts to decrease specialization in medicine, it is a system of multiple providers from various professions and occupations. At present, it continues to be a system organized around the primacy of life-saving activity. Differences and priorities in care and in the meaning of caregiving characterize the various professional groups. Among the same professional groups,

differences exist in manifest power to influence decisions. Finally, the health care system is not responsive to the rights and responsibilities of professions other than those of medicine (Benoliel, 1972).

In a profound sense, the health care system shows an imbalance in the priorities given to the goals of cure and care. The differences in these goals were formulated by Benoliel (1976) and continue to be relevant today. They include the following:

> Cure centers on the diagnosis and treatment of disease; in contrast, care is concerned with the welfare and well-being of the person. Cure deals with the objective aspects of the case whereas care is concerned with the subject and meaning of the disease experience and the effects of treatment on the person. Cure has many origins and signs and instrumentation "doing to" people. Care has its root in human compassion, respect for the need of the vulnerable and "doing with" people. Although care as a spouse is important, cure is the goal around which the health care system is organized.

Historically, influences on nursing and the social context of practice have affected nurses' perceptions of themselves and the value of their contribution to health care. Nurses have been socialized to believe that cure activities are more important than care activities and take precedence over them on a day-to-day basis. Nurses have also been socialized to believe that they have less to offer the public than medicine in terms of service. In addition, nurses may have low self-esteem and lack self-confidence in many areas of their work, and these attitudes perpetuate a subservient working relationship with physicians. The many different phases of cancer care offer nurses opportunities to initiate and take responsibility for patient care activities, more so than with other diseases. The majority of patients seen by nurses is shifting from the hospital to the community and patients in these new practice arenas will require ongoing monitoring and management strategies. It is at these times that nurses can make deliberate shifts in their approaches to patients to respond to their care needs as a priority. Concurrently, nurses will become more comfortable with patients, and subsequently their confidence will increase. In addition, their explicit actions will increase the visibility of their role responsibilities for themselves, patients, and other professional caregivers.

Major issues for nurses in the twenty-first century include action to reverse nurses' invisibility as major contributors to effective health care outcomes, to secure identified reimbursement for services rendered by nurses, and to promote the growth of professionalism in nurses through encouragement of effective relationships among all groups of professionals. Nurses must be willing to assume positions of power in the health care system and to use their power as a means of bringing about change in the system. Nurses must assume true leadership for the accountability for quality and cost outcomes of nursing practice and nursing services. Nurses must now move into developing an approach to peer review that focuses on actual practices of nurses and not on what is recorded on the patient care records. Nurses need to assume responsibility for defining practice and behaviors that are important to produce effective patient and family outcomes in the care arena.

INFLUENCING FACTORS

The development of a specialty practice within the health care professions is moved and guided by a variety of influencing factors. Some specialties can trace their emergence to events such as the development of a specific technology. The initial availability of renal dialysis, for example, prompted a need for knowledgeable caregivers—nurses who could both manage chronic yet life-threatening illness and carry out the dialysis procedure. The availability of a specific technology then separated the patient population with renal failure from the general medical-surgical population.

Other specialties emerged more gradually and were based on a growing body of knowledge and care approaches that limited care delivery to a specific population or care setting, such as public or occupational health. A few specialties have formally recognized new or expanded roles for nurses, such as nurse midwives or nurse anesthetists. Yet other specialties have a narrow range of functions, often procedural rather than disease focused, such as operating room nursing or intravenous therapy nursing. Change for these groups focuses on improvement of procedures and techniques. To a certain extent, the growth of oncology nursing is due to a major social investment in a serious health care problem (Lynaugh & Fairman, 1989).

Medical and nursing specialties carve out specific territories or boundaries of disease or care. Once identified, further development occurs with various factors affecting ongoing refinement. Factors likely to influence cancer nursing as a specialty in the twenty-first century include health care reform, the changing role of the nurse, the emergence of scientific and technologic advances, ethical issues impacting the specialty, and the structuring of groups and processes for networking and developing leadership.

HEALTH CARE REFORM

The 1990s have been marked by debates related to changes in health care reform. There have been numerous proposals discussed at various levels, including the White House, government agencies, insurance companies, and health care delivery systems. Common themes that run through many of the proposals include: universal coverage, consumer choice, managed care, single payer, insurance reform, tax increase vs. tax relief, employer mandates, health care bureaucracy, and elimination of preexisting disease clauses. During this same time period, government- and business-driven trends in health care have occurred that have resulted in hospitals admitting fewer patients and significantly shortening lengths of stay. As a result, care delivery models in hospitals have shifted toward more ambulatory, community-based, and home-care services. In addition, health care reform may dramatically alter the profile of the health care system. Included in the health care reform agenda is the need to dramatically decrease the number of medical specialists, including oncologists. Consequently, the role of the oncologist may change, thereby impacting the role of the oncology nurse. These trends mean that nurses must acquire new perspectives, sensitivity, and team-building skills. These skills have not been previously required in providing health care. The growth of managed care has increased the emphasis on cost, health promotion, and disease prevention. Oncology nurses must learn that everything they do in relation to health care is being translated into four factors: access, quality, cost, and outcomes.

It is not clear what the final changes in health care reform will look like in the twenty-first century, but it is recognized that these changes are intended to improve access and health care services for all. Special attention will be directed toward health promotion and the prevention of illness, to decreasing health care costs, and to the care of underserved groups (Oermann, 1994). It is clear that no matter what kind of health care system is put in place, there will continue to be fewer dollars coming into health care institutions to provide quality care. Oncology nurses must be among the voices informing the public and legislators that just decreasing health care costs without regard for quality and outcomes will not solve many of these problems.

The national goal at the federal level is to dramatically decrease the number of specialists and increase the number of physicians involved in primary care. There are several reasons given for this goal and they are: (1) it is believed that having fewer specialists available to treat patients will decrease health care costs, (2) primary care physicians will be viewed as "gate keepers" and given the task of making it more difficult to access specialty care, and (3) having more specialists requires more equipment to support their practices; fewer specialists will result in less equipment and support personnel. Fewer oncologists will impact nursing practice and alter the traditional nursing role. It has been postulated that the oncologist will assume a director role with nurses in expanded roles carrying case loads, monitoring patients' side-effects and deciding when to contact the physician as well as medically managing these patients.

It is argued that decreasing the number of specialists available for patients to access will help decrease the money spent for health care. It is further argued that much of the treatment sought from specialists could be delivered by the primary care physician. The decrease in the number of oncologists will alter the traditional role of the oncology nurse, particularly those nurses with advanced educational preparation. Advanced practice nurses may be required to carry their own patient load of oncology patients, follow written practice guidelines, and act as "gate keepers" in terms of deciding when the oncology patient needs to see the oncologist.

Health care over the last decade has moved out of the hospital and into the community. More and more oncology treatments are being done on an outpatient basis. Those oncology patients who are hospitalized spend significantly less time in the hospital than similar conditions merited several years ago. It has become routine for oncology patients to spend the majority of their diagnosis, treatment, and terminal care in an outpatient or home setting. Today, home care includes very sophisticated treatments that once were done only in the acute care setting. Specialized home care agencies can bring into the home complicated, high-technology oncology procedures. The oncology nurse will need to become comfortable delivering care in the non-acute care setting. The fastest growing segment of the health care system is home care and this may prove to be the major employer of oncology nurses in the coming years. Consequently, much of the care of patients is assumed by family members as caregivers who are often ill equipped to assume this role. This demand on family members is not a new occurrence, but the role of care-giving has dramatically shifted from one of promoting convalescence to actively providing high-technology care in the home (McCorkle et al., 1993). A nursing outcome of increasing importance is the rate of unscheduled readmissions for symptoms such as uncontrolled pain (Grant, Ferrell, & Rivera, in press).

Health care reform emphasizes cost containment at all levels. Unfortunately, quality of care is often missing from discussions of cost containment. The actual impact of cost cutting measures on the patient and family are frequently missing from any discussion. Oncology nurses need to articulate and keep focusing discussions of health care reform on the issue of quality of care. The most appropriate time to discuss quality of care for the patient and family is before cost containment measures have been instituted. It is essential that oncology nurses maintain and articulate their patient advocate role in any discussion of health care changes.

Across the country hospitals and health care institutions in both urban and rural settings are downsizing and restructuring. The driving force behind these changes is the increasing emphasis on the economics of health care. Downsizing has resulted in nurses being laid off or retiring early. The assumption that "a nurse will always have a job" has been seriously challenged in some areas of the country. In some parts of the country, nurses are being cross trained to perform the functions of other health care workers. For instance, the hospital may eliminate the IV Team, Respiratory Therapist Team, or the EKG Team and have nurses on each unit pick up these skills.

Overall economics will drive the delivery of health care. Changes that occur in the health care system will most likely be done for economic reasons. This may or may not result in positive changes for nursing. The restructuring and downsizing of health care institutions has tended to result in less employment opportunities for nurses; what further economic changes bring to the nursing profession remains to be seen.

CHANGING ROLE OF THE NURSE

Nursing's Agenda for Health Care Reform (National League for Nursing [NLN], 1991) emphasizes the movement of health care toward the community and the important role of nurses in providing primary health care within community-based systems. Oncology nurses will function increasingly as members of integrated teams of health professionals in the provision of this care. Leading nursing organizations, such as the American Association of Colleges of Nursing (AACN, 1993) advocate an expanded role for nurses in the future, particularly in community-based primary care.

While health care reform emphasizes primary care provided within community-based systems, this shift toward the community as a setting for practice is already evident in cancer care. Oncology nurses are caring for increasing numbers of cancer patients, many with acute illnesses and complex needs, in ambulatory clinics, physicians' offices, and patients' homes. Advanced practice specialists increasingly are becoming frontline health care providers by combining their roles of clinical nurse specialists and nurse practitioners. In the future, oncology nurses will have a greater role in caring for the community's health needs and participating in primary care within community settings.

The care available for patients with cancer is immensely complex. One way to illustrate that complexity and its implications for nurses is to look at the treatment for cancer. Few patients receive only surgery, radiation, or chemotherapy; multimodal treatment is the norm. Even within one treatment modality approaches are often complex. Chemotherapy regimens, for example, use combinations of agents. The increased effectiveness of combined agents was first demonstrated in the treatment of advanced Hodgkin's disease (DeVita, Serpick, & Carbone, 1970) and now the use of combinations of agents is commonplace. Although combined modalities have obvious beneficial outcomes, their complexity was an early focus of attention within the specialty and continues to pose challenges for nurses.

First, nurses must understand how each modality affects the others in combined treatments and what modifications are necessary because treatments are being combined; this knowledge is important because of complications that may arise with the disease process or because of the presence of another chronic or acute disease that has its own treatment. To provide care, the nurse must understand each treatment modality. Nurses specializing in one treatment modality must have close communication with nurses working in other modalities to assist in care planning that will promote continuity and ensure safety in care.

Second, because of the specialized body of knowledge within each modality, subspecialties have emerged. Although the separation of medical, surgical, and radiation oncology has been recognized for several years, recent advances in treatment have prompted the emergence of other treatment subspecialties such as bone marrow transplantation and biotherapy. Intensive care support for patients experiencing multisystem failure has influenced both the creation of intensive care units for these patients and the development of oncology critical care as a newer subspecialty. As the emphasis on decreasing medical specialization occurs, it is unclear whether nurses will be adequately prepared to care for the multiple needs of these patients. Oncology nurses must assume complete accountability for remaining current with the evolving body of knowledge regarding the latest advances in cancer care. This point is especially relevant in light of changes in patient profiles, merged positions, and subsequent increased nursing demands.

Finally, nurses interact with a broad variety of providers who are involved in the delivery of complex care. In a multidisciplinary approach to care, nurses learn from and are influenced by the role and contributions other providers make in complex cancer care.

Each practice setting offers the nurse a slightly different variation in the provision of care. For example, the nurse new to oncology may find the structure of the inpatient setting supportive. Resources are usually abundant, and the new nurse is assisted by and can learn from the experience of others. A more experienced nurse may prefer the flexibility and autonomy in practice that is usually available through home care and ambulatory clinics. Assessment skills and problem solving abilities are routinely tested, and the veteran nurse can draw on previous experience to develop care approaches for the patient and family.

As experience with different cancer care delivery systems builds, nurses are able to share these experiences and begin to compare care across settings. Policy adjustments, procedure modifications, cost studies, and cross-setting collaboration can result. The cancer chemotherapy and venous access guidelines developed and published by the Oncology Nursing Society (1988, 1990) are examples of the kinds of work that can be accomplished across settings and that result in specific direction for the oncology nurse providing direct care.

As health care moves out of the hospital and into the community, nurses are being forced to seek employment in outpatient and community settings. The nursing curricula of undergraduate nursing education is being changed to reflect the increasing emphasis on outpatient/home care settings. The acute care setting is increasingly being limited to intensive care patients. Thus nurses in the acute care setting are expected to have intensive care skills that can be delivered to very sick patients. At the same time federal and managed care guidelines require that patients be discharged from the hospital as soon as possible. Homes are also becoming acute care settings and nurses must carry over these sophisticated skills into the home. Nurses must also assume responsibility for teaching family members to care for the complex and ongoing needs of patients in the home.

Nurses in the acute care settings are also being expected to supervise nonprofessional workers who are delivering health care at the bedside. In some settings these nonprofessional workers, called Registered Care Technicians (RCT), have been hired to replace nurses.

There is tremendous controversy surrounding the use, supervision, and replacement of nurses with RCTs. Oncology nurses are not immune from this controversy.

Nursing education at the graduate level has undergone dramatic change in the last few years. There has been a national move to prepare more nurse practitioners and advanced practice nurses. This movement has been fueled by several changes occurring in the practice arena. These changes include the restructuring of clinical nurse specialist (CNS) jobs into case management positions or the elimination of the role, the opening of nurse practitioner positions in settings that historically were hostile to nurses in expanded roles, and the proposed health care agenda that predicts that nurses in advanced practice roles would be employed to deliver primary care and serve as "gate keepers" along with physician assistants and physicians. See Chapter 3 for a comprehensive discussion of the evolving nurses' roles in oncology.

SCIENTIFIC AND TECHNOLOGIC ADVANCES

Through practice, education, and research a large body of knowledge related to cancer nursing and cancer nursing care has been developed. Because all aspects of cancer care are in a continual state of redefinition and refinement, the body of scientific knowledge that supports cancer nursing practice is also changing and expanding. Nurses entering or practicing in cancer care today need a variety of resources to build their knowledge base initially and then to remain current. In recent years, the cancer nursing literature has proliferated. Numerous texts and journals are readily available. Many nurses have access to computerized databases, such as the National Cancer Institute's Physician Data Query (PDQ) (Deininger, Collins, & Hubbard, 1989). Orientation and staff development programming (Stuckey, 1983), continuing education offerings (Bushy & Kost, 1990; Donaldson et al., 1988), expansion of cancer content in basic education programs (Mooney & Dudas, 1987; Sarna & McCorkle, in press), and increased availability of graduate preparation in oncology (Hinds, 1989; Mooney, 1994) all reflect a strong educational base for this specialty (see Chapter 71). The number of opportunities for doctoral studies and post-doctoral fellowships increased in the late 1980s and 1990s, especially with increased funding provided by professional organizations (ONS), federal agencies (National Institute for Nursing Research, NINR; National Cancer Institute, NCI), and lay organizations (American Cancer Society, ACS).

Concurrently, there have been a number of major breakthroughs in medical science that continue to have a direct relationship to the knowledge base of oncology nurses. One important example has been the recent discovery of the BRCA1 gene for breast cancer (Miki et al., 1994). Before the twenty-first century, "predictive" presymptomatic genetic testing of diseases that might manifest themselves later in life may be commonplace. If advances in gene mapping continue, the public will generate new expectations of medicine and nursing.

Knowledge of the susceptibility gene BRCA1 (Miki et al., 1994) and the simultaneous condition that no definitive course of preventive action is known, raises concerns that life altering information has the potential to cause psychologic and social harm, not only to the present generation, but also to future generations (Kolata, 1994a). With the discovery of the BRCA1 and the proximate inevitability of genetic screening of breast cancer susceptibility, the demand for testing may become very high. As a result there will be concerns about the social and psychologic risk/benefit to the "worried well", the "asymptomatic ill", and it can be certain that high risk women and others will seek genetic testing (Feldman, 1994) or join clinical prevention trials even though they may not have a full understanding of the outcomes of such screening/testing or trial participation. Another complex issue is the potential ability of screening to alert people at increasingly earlier stages of their susceptibility to a specific disease, without the concomitant ability to provide a prevention or a definitive cure for the disease, and this issue has already been raised in the lay print media (Kolata, 1994b).

There is no question that scientific advances such as genetic testing and their potential consequences will enhance the professional opportunities for oncology nurses. The critical question is whether oncology nurses will seize these opportunities and lead the way for the clinical care that will be needed, especially the psychosocial and economic issues that will occur. These issues remain as challenges for nurses and other professionals in the future.

The delivery of health care has been influenced tremendously by the explosion in health care technology. The application of this technology in cancer care is obvious throughout the disease continuum. Newer detection and monitoring methods such as scans, imaging devices, and tumor markers have influenced the role of nurses who prepare patients for testing, oversee various aspects of detection, monitor outcomes, and assist patients and families in understanding the results and implications of such testing.

The development and testing of new antineoplastic agents and new combinations of existing agents have tremendous impact on the roles of the oncology nurse. Nurses are involved in every aspect of these trials and have gradually assumed increased responsibility. For example, the technologic explosion in delivery and monitoring devices for chemotherapy has allowed care settings to shift. The nurse who once had to master a particular line or pump for chemotherapy infusions on the inpatient unit may now be teaching patients and families to deal with this equipment at home. This is a tremendous responsibility that includes both assessing the abilities of family members to solve problems and to cope with complications that may arise, and determining when the patient and family are adequately prepared to assume this role. In addition, experimental or investigational protocols have been extended into a variety of community settings, creating new pressures for nurses who heretofore may not have been involved in any type of clinical research study.

This involvement necessitates a redefinition of practice roles.

Merely keeping up with scientific and technologic advances is a challenge. For example, scientific inquiry into immunotherapy and biotherapy has forced cancer nurses to keep their knowledge base about the immune system and related pathophysiologic processes up to date. Because change in these content areas is continual, nurses specializing in cancer care must identify avenues for continued learning.

Many technologic advances result in equipment options. Changing technologies may offer opportunities to influence purchasing decisions. Nurses may be asked, for example, to compare the efficiency of two pumps in terms of the frequency of problems each presents and the nursing time required to correct the problem. Nurses may be asked to consider whether the pump that seems best in the hospital is also best for home use. Nurses may need to assist patients and families in making decisions about product and care alternatives. Manufacturers of equipment and pharmacologic agents also seek information from nurses about their needs and about their experiences with specific products. Many manufacturers of cancer drugs and equipment have oncology nurses as employees for these purposes, and several have product advisory boards through which this information is sought.

ETHICAL AND LEGAL ISSUES IMPACTING THE SPECIALTY

There are changes occurring in the greater American society that may impact the practicing oncology nurse and create difficult ethical situations. For instance, the anti-immigration movement in some parts of the country has resulted in legislation designed to deny education and health care to illegal immigrants and to mandate the reporting of illegal immigrants who attempt to secure these services. Oncology nurses may be confronted with the ethical dilemma of whether or not to report the immigration status of their patient.

The 1990s have been marked by a series of controversies concerning informed consent, medical misconduct and falsification of medical research data. Attention has been focused on the Breast Cancer Prevention Trial (BCPT) which was approved for implementation by the National Surgical Adjuvant Breast and Bowel Project (NSABP) in February, 1991. NSABP is one of the National Cancer Institute's (NCI) 13 cooperative groups and is the sponsor of the BCPT that started accrual of participants April 29, 1992 (Broder, 1992; Fisher & Redmond, 1991; NCI, 1992). During the congressional hearing for the BCPT (Broder, 1994), the lay public learned that Dr. Poisson, a Canadian investigator with the NSABP, was involved in scientific misconduct (Crewdson, 1994). Subsequently, a cascade of problems was brought to light: the audit of additional NSABP sites revealed poor record keeping, missing data, and the falsification of data. The Office of Research Integrity (ORI) became involved; the head of the NSABP was fired and several senate and congressional hearings took place and the media offered almost daily accounts of the events as they unfolded. One of the consequences of these events has been that the original contract that was made by subjects when they volunteered to participate in the BCPT has been altered by the necessity for a revised consent form, detailing a description of the risks and benefits.

The continuation of the BCPT raises larger scientific and societal concerns—concerns related to the ethics of having healthy subjects in clinical trials, concerns related to the role of the lay media, and questions about the meaning of prevention, early detection, high risk, and side effects. There is also clear evidence that ethical issues are a major concern of the diagnostic and treatment aspects of cancer. Oncology nurses in advanced practice roles need to be aware that one of the emerging litigation issues is "failure to diagnose" (Osuch & Bonham, 1994; Wynstra, 1994). Advanced practice nurses (APN) who are in primary prevention or primary care settings are vulnerable to these types of suits. The oncology APN will need to adhere to the recommended screening guidelines of national organizations and to stay abreast of any recommended changes in these guidelines. The most familiar type of "failure to diagnose" suit involves breast lesion(s) and the practitioner's failure to diagnose breast cancer. Protocols and written practice guidelines that specifically address the process the APN should follow when evaluating suspicious lesions or symptoms need to be developed.

Another issue that is being litigated is referral delay. This issue frequently arises with patients who are in health maintenance organizations (HMOs) who have symptoms consistent with a diagnosis of cancer and are denied the opportunity to see a specialist in a timely manner. HMOs face intense pressure to contain costs; therefore, according to some critics, they may be unable to maintain quality. HMOs and other managed care plans must be monitored to see whether they restrict only unnecessary care or cross the crucial boundary between services that may be omitted or not prescribed and those that the patient genuinely needs. This question is especially critical for cancer. The patient has the best chance of survival if diagnosis is timely and accurate, and treatment appropriate. If a health care provider restricts the resources necessary to accomplish these goals, needless mortality may result (Greenwald, 1992).

As health care reform is implemented, patients are receiving complex and highly technical treatments in outpatient and home settings, resulting in additional ethical issues. For example, in 1994, massive overdoses of anti-cancer drugs given to two women with breast cancer who were undergoing experimental treatment at Dana-Farber Cancer Institute in Boston resulted in one patient dying and the other having irreversible heart damage. The Federal Health Care Financing Administration, an agency in the Department of Health and Human Services, found serious deficiencies in patient care and poor supervision of its doctors and nurses at the cancer institute. Specifically, in the review of 40 patient medical records, they found that in 27 cases "supervision and evaluation of nursing care was not consistently comprehensive." Interviews with nurses found that they were often poorly informed about treatment plans for individual patients, in part because such plans were not included in patient records. Eight of 14 medication administration reports reviewed by the reviewers found "errors in nursing transcription of orders and lack of written evidence that medications were administered in accordance with physician orders and/or established protocols" (Altman, 1995).

The ONS has taken the initiative to prevent and handle many of these issues in a proactive way. For example, guidelines for monitoring scientific integrity and procedures for responding to allegations of scientific misconduct have been approved and are designed to help nurses identify potential threats to the scientific integrity of specific projects and clinical practice. Statements of vision and core values for ONS are being developed from documents prepared by the Ethics Advisory Council, the Leadership Task Force and the Work Analysis Working Group. These statements will articulate the oncology nursing perspective consistent with the American Nurses Association Code of Ethics. The ONS Ethics Advisory Council will use these statements as they prepare ONS documents related to emerging ethical and legal issues. The first issues to be addressed are assisted suicide and euthanasia and are under review by the ONS membership.

STRUCTURING OF GROUPS AND PROCESSES

The development of cancer nursing as a specialty has been aided by the overall specialty movement within nursing (Lynaugh & Fairman, 1989) and by specific efforts within cancer care. The American Cancer Society and the Oncology Nursing Society have been vital and continued forces in these efforts. In the past decade, the American Cancer Society has strengthened its emphasis on nursing and provided valuable programming and scholarship assistance. As the professional nursing organization for cancer nurses, the Oncology Nursing Society sees its mission as promoting excellence in oncology nursing by promoting professional standards, exchanging information, encouraging specialization, fostering professional development, and maintaining a responsive organizational structure and function (Oncology Nursing Society, 1990). Major efforts affect practice, education, research, and administration activities across the United States and abroad. For example, the development of the Oncology Nursing Certification Corporation and the offering of certification in oncology nursing give nurses a tangible credential in their chosen specialty. The Oncology Nursing Certification Corporation has continued to set the standard for practice by developing certification that recognizes advanced preparation in the specialty. There is now ongoing dialogue to debate the need for certification in subspecialties of oncology nursing.

Both organizations, ONS and ACS, have national and local programs. Perhaps the most valuable yet least easily defined activity made possible through these organizations is the opportunity to build both formal and informal networks for information sharing and program building. Efforts include fostering advanced preparation, developing new care initiatives, and influencing public policy. Networking efforts in nursing have also been developed and formalized in some of the cancer cooperative study groups. These groups provide for collaboration among nurses working on specific medical research initiatives and have the potential to generate important questions for research.

Significant progress in multidisciplinary efforts has been made through state cancer pain initiative movements. The national effort began in 1984 when a group of professionals in Wisconsin met to discuss the idea of formulating a state cancer pain initiative; two years later, the Wisconsin Cancer Pain Initiative was formally organized (Dahl & Joranson, 1990). There are formalized pain initiatives in 45 states. Most states hold an annual statewide meeting to mobilize health professionals and to share information about pain management strategies. A major goal of the state cancer pain initiatives (SCPIs) in 1994 was to implement a strategic plan to obtain optimal dissemination and media coverage of the Clinical Practice Guideline developed by the Agency for Health Care Policy and Research (AHCPR) (Dahl, 1995).

The completion of the clinical practice guidelines for acute cancer pain is an excellent example of successful collaboration among disciplines. The guidelines were developed by a multidisciplinary panel of clinicians, patients, researchers, and experts in health policy. The cancer pain guideline provides a synthesis of scientific research and expert judgment to make recommendations on pain assessment and management. Approximately 470 health care professionals and 70 patients were involved in the process of developing the guideline for cancer pain (AHCPR, 1994).

FUTURE DIRECTIONS

Health care and social trends, both in general and in nursing specifically, exert a tremendous influence on the practice arena. Nurses at all levels and in all settings should be aware of and understand the ramifications of these agents of change. Some issues that seem especially important are recruiting and retaining nurses within the specialty, monitoring the quality of care delivered to patients, and defining and promoting nursing roles in underserved areas.

RECRUITMENT AND RETENTION OF NURSES

Over time, oncology nursing has overcome its stigma among specialty choices—early studies of career preferences of senior students always placed cancer at the bottom (Barckley, 1985). Students exposed to cancer care in their clinical experiences will have witnessed skilled clinicians making vital contributions to patient care. Students should be exposed to the tremendous variety of nursing roles available along the disease continuum. Given the decreased number of young adults choosing nursing as a career, efforts to increase the visibility and satisfaction of cancer nursing must be undertaken. Realistic expectations for orientation must be developed and opportunities to supplement beginning skills must be ensured.

The recruitment of experienced nurses into cancer care provides a tremendous challenge with stiff competition. Gullatte and Levine (1990) note that retention of skilled nurses should receive as much emphasis as recruitment to avoid high staff turnover and the resultant need for more recruitment. The complexity of care of patients with cancer can benefit from the presence of nurses with a wide variety of backgrounds. The increasing number of older patients with cancer, for example, offers a good opportunity for the geriatric clinician to apply previous skills to a new subpopulation.

QUALITY OF CARE

Access to quality care regardless of geographic setting is a commonly cited goal in cancer care and a focus of many funded programs. Nurses frequently express concern about the quality of care that is available and delivered to patients with cancer. Indeed, many of the efforts within the specialty have been undertaken as efforts to improve or ensure the quality of care. Increased complexities of care, variety in the preparation of care providers, the need for continuity across care settings, and cost-containment measures have stimulated efforts to ensure that quality of care remains an important consideration in decision making.

Although many definitions of quality of care exist, the initiatives of private and regulatory bodies seem to be defining quality of care by both cost containment and efficient utilization of services. It is likely that national initiatives and those within individual facilities will stress quality of care in setting standards. Cancer nurses can make use of opportunities that may arise to participate in setting the definitions, criteria, and measuring approaches used to evaluate quality of care (Baird & Mortenson, 1990).

The beginnings of the specialty of cancer nursing were marked by the demonstration of how much nurses could do for their patients and how many ways they could address patient concerns. Primarily because of economic considerations, nurses must now find ways to demonstrate how little they can do for patients and still achieve satisfactory ends (Baird & Mortenson, 1990). Comparing care approaches, evaluating delivery systems, and demonstrating cost effectiveness are important areas for practice and research efforts, but these areas must include quality outcomes. Efforts in these areas have the potential to substantially influence cancer nursing as a specialty.

DEFINING AND PROMOTING NURSING ROLES

Developments within the specialty of cancer nursing have stimulated the creation of a number of roles for nurses. Although the majority of cancer nurses are now employed by hospitals and function in fairly traditional roles, many alternative opportunities offer varied patient populations, work settings, or role functions. More and more cancer care is delivered outside of traditional hospital settings (Sandrik,

1990), and as a result more cancer nurses will be forced to work in ambulatory care, office practice, and home care.

The modification of position descriptions and procedures for alternative care sites, and the development and implementation of standards of care within these settings are major nursing challenges. Because fewer nurses may be engaged in these roles or settings in any specific geographic location, mechanisms for effective communication across settings and with other providers are essential to give nurses in new roles the assistance they need. One of the most important channels nurses may use for communication in the future may be the Internet and other computer systems. These systems are already being used for information exchange about the latest research findings. As sufficient numbers of nurses function in newer roles or with specific populations, communication networks must evolve. The variety of special interest groups being developed within the ONS attest to the need for collaboration and communication. These groups can identify areas of need and can move to meet these through educational programming, publishing, and research.

There is no question that cancer nursing research will become a major factor in enhancing cancer nursing practice and in clarifying nurses' roles and their relationships to patient and family outcomes in the future. This process is strengthened by ONS and its strong commitment to research. In March 1995, ONS released a grant announcement to fund multi-institutional research development grants in Cancer Related Fatigue called the Fatigue Initiative Through Research and Education (FIRE). The grant initiative evolved from a State-of-the-Knowledge Conference on Fatigue sponsored by ONS. The outcomes of the conference were published as an article entitled "Fatigue and the cancer experience: The state of the knowledge" (Winningham et al., 1994). The initiative is funded by the Oncology Nursing Foundation and Ortho Biotech, Inc. The initiative supports three developmental grants of $50,000 each to be funded in 1995-1996 and one grant of $500,000 to run from 1997 to 2000.

Another recommendation that evolved from the State-of-the-Knowledge Conference was a call for Clinical Research Scholars sponsored by the Oncology Nursing Foundation. The program is designed to foster the development of Centers of Excellence in Oncology Nursing Research. The ultimate goal of the scholars program is to improve care given to persons with cancer and their families by fostering the development of a scientific base for practice and the utilization of research by oncology nurses. Applications are peer-reviewed by nationally recognized researchers and awarded for 2 consecutive years. These research activities will enhance the collaborative efforts among oncology nurses and with other disciplines.

SUMMARY

Cancer nursing offers many varied professional opportunities. Skilled nurses practice in every aspect of care. Although the specialty is fairly young, it is extremely well established in terms of educational opportunities, practice role delineations, delivery of specialized care, research initiatives, and publications. Cancer nursing is an interactive practice well received and respected by other disciplines. As an integral part of the health care system, cancer nursing will be influenced by a variety of factors with further refinement of the specialty and numerous challenges and rewards.

REFERENCES

Altman, L. (1995, May 31). Federal officials cite deficiencies at Harvard hospital. *New York Times*, p. A16.

American Association of Colleges of Nursing. (1993). *Addressing nursing education's agenda for the 21st century*. (Position statement). Washington, DC: Author.

American Nurses' Association. (1980). *Nursing: A social policy statement*. Kansas City, MO: Author.

Baird, S. B., & Mortenson, L. E. (1990). Economic concerns in the changing health care delivery system. *Cancer, 65*(3, Suppl.), 766–769.

Barckley, V. (1985). The best of times and the worst of times: Historical reflections from an American Cancer Society national nursing consultant. *Oncology, 12*(1, Suppl.), 16–18.

Benoliel, J. Q. (1972). Institutionalized practices of information control. In E. Freidson & J. Lorber (Eds.), *Medical men and their work* (pp. 220–238). Chicago: Aldine-Atherton.

Benoliel, J. Q. (1976). Overview: Care, cure, and the challenge of choice. In A. M. Earle (Ed.), *The nurse as caregiver for the terminal patient and his family* (pp. 9–30). New York: Columbia University Press.

Benoliel, J., & McCorkle, R. (1977, May 10). Ethical consideration in treatment. In *Proceedings of the Second National Conference on Cancer Nursing*. New York: American Cancer Society.

Benoliel J. Q., & McCorkle, R. (1978). A holistic approach to terminal illness. *Cancer Nursing, 1*, 143–149.

Broder, S. (1992, May 6). Breast Cancer Prevention Trial takes off. In Smigel, K. *Journal of the National Institutes of Health, 84*, 669–670.

Broder, S. (1994, April 13). National Cancer Institute on Scientific Fraud at NSABP. Subcommittee on Oversight and Investigations Committee on Energy and Commerce. Statement. Washington, D.C.

Bushy, A., & Kost, S. (1990). A model of continuing education for rural oncology nurses. *Oncology Nursing Forum, 17*, 207–211.

Cancer Pain Management Guideline Panel. (1994). *Clinical practice guideline, number 9—Management of cancer pain*. U.S. Department of Health and Human Services, Agency for Health Care Policy and Research. Washington, DC: U.S. Department of Health and Human Services.

Caplan, G. (1974). *Support systems and community mental health*. New York: Behavioral Publications.

Craytor, J. (1982). Highlights in education for cancer nursing. *Oncology Nursing Forum, 9*(4), 51–59.

Crewdson, J. (1994, March 13). Fraud: Some research into breast cancer faked. *Chicago Tribune*, pp. 1A, 7A.

Dahl, J. (1995). State cancer pain initiatives: A progress report. *APS Bulletin, 3*, 20–22.

Dahl, J., & Joranson, D. (1990). The Wisconsin cancer pain initiative. *Advances in Pain Research and Therapy, 16*, 499–503.

Deininger, H., Collins, J. L., & Hubbard, S. M. (1989). Nurses and PDQ: What's in it for you? *Oncology Nursing Forum, 16,* 547–552.

DeVita, V. T., Serpick, A. A., & Carbone, P. P. (1970). Combination chemotherapy in the treatment of advanced Hodgkin's disease. *Annals of Internal Medicine, 73,* 881–895.

Donaldson, W. S., Glass, E. C., Helmick, F., Ezzone, S., Kellerstraus, B., & Stevenson, B. (1988). Determining continuing education priorities in cancer management for nurses. *Oncology Nursing Forum, 15,* 625–630.

Feldman, G. (1994, October 12). When women know too much. *New York Times,* p. A23.

Fisher, B., & Redmond, C. K. (1991, December 20). *NSABP Protocol P-1: A clinical trial to determine the worth of tamoxifen for preventing breast cancer.* University of Pittsburgh, PA.

Grant, M., Ferrell, B., & Rivera, L. (in press). Unscheduled readmissions for uncontrolled symptoms: A health care challenge for nurses. *Nursing Clinics of North America.*

Greenwald, H. (1992). *Who survives cancer?* Berkeley: University of California Press.

Gullatte, M. M., & Levine, N. M. (1990). Recruitment and retention of oncology nurses. *Oncology Nursing Forum, 17,* 419–423.

Hamric, A. B. (1989). History and overview of the CNS role. In A. B. Hamric & J. A. Spross (Eds.), *The clinical nurse specialist in theory and practice* (2nd ed., pp. 3–18). Philadelphia: W. B. Saunders Co.

Hinds, P. (1989). Survey of graduate programs in cancer nursing. *Oncology Nursing Forum, 16*(6), 881–887.

Kolata, G. (1994a, September 26). Should children be told if genes predict illness? *New York Times,* pp. A1, A14.

Kolata, G. (1994b, November 8). New ability to find cancers: A mixed blessing? *New York Times,* pp. C1, C12.

Krouse, T. K., & Krouse, J. E. (1984). Careplan for retaining the new nurse. *Nursing Management, 15*(2), 30–33.

Lynaugh, J., & Fairman, J. (1989). Caring for the chronically ill: Historical perspectives. *American Nephrology Nurses' Association Journal, 16,* 192–196.

McCorkle, R. (1980). An ethical dilemma: Information control in cancer care. *Bioethics Quarterly, 2,* 148–158.

McCorkle, R., Yost, L., Jepson, C., Malone, D., Baird, S., & Lusk, E. (1993). A cancer experience: Relationship of patient psychosocial responses to caregiver burden over time. *Psycho-Oncology, 2,* 21–32.

Miki, Y., Swenson, J., Shattuck-Eidens, D., Futreal, P. A., Harshman, K., Tavtigian, S., et al. (1994, October 7). A strong candidate for the breast and ovarian cancer susceptibility gene BRCA1. *Science, 266,* 66–71.

Mooney, K. (1994). *The master's degree, curriculum guide.* (3rd ed.). Pittsburgh: American Cancer Society and Oncology Nursing Society.

Mooney, M., & Dudas, S. (1987). Undergraduate independent study in cancer nursing. *Oncology Nursing Forum, 14*(1), 51–53.

National Cancer Institute. (1992, April 29). *Cancer facts* (pp. 1–15). Bethesda, MD: Office of Cancer Communications.

National League for Nursing. (1991). *Nursing's agenda for health care reform.* New York: Author.

Oermann, M. (1994). Reforming nursing education for future practice. *Journal of Nursing Education, 33*(5), 215–218.

Oncology Nursing Society. (1988). *Cancer chemotherapy guidelines (Modules I–V).* Pittsburgh: Author.

Oncology Nursing Society. (1990). *Access device guidelines (Modules I–III).* Pittsburgh: Author.

Osuch, J. R., & Bonham, V. L. (1994). The timely diagnosis of breast cancer. *Cancer Supplement, 74*(1), 271–278.

Sandrik, K. (1990, February 5). Oncology: Who's managing outpatient programs? *Hospitals,* pp. 32–37.

Sarna, L., & McCorkle, R. (in press). A cancer nursing curriculum guide for baccalaureate nursing education. *Cancer Nursing.*

Stuckey, P. A. (1983). Orientation to an oncology unit. *Oncology Nursing Forum, 10*(4), 226–229.

Tornberg, M. J., Burns McGrath, B., & Quint Benoliel, J. (1984). Oncology transition services: Partnerships of nurses and families. *Cancer Nursing, 7*(2), 131–137.

Weisman, A. D., & Worden, J. W. (1976–1977). The existential plight in cancer: Significance of the first 100 days. *International Journal of Psychiatry in Medicine, 7,* 1–15.

Winningham, M., Nail, L., Burke, M., Brophy, L., Cimprich, B., Jones, L., Pickard-Holley, S., Rhodes, V., St. Pierre, B., Beck, S., Glass, E., Mock, V., Mooney, K., & Piper, B. (1994). Fatigue and the cancer experience: The state of the knowledge. *Oncology Nursing Forum, 21*(1), 23–36.

Wynstra, N. A. (1994). Breast cancer: Selected legal issues. *Cancer Supplement, 74*(1), 491–511.

The History of Cancer Nursing

Connie Henke Yarbro

Understanding the emergence of oncology nursing as a specialty allows an appreciation of the tremendous progress made to date and may provide directions on how to achieve still more in the future. Humans knew about and feared cancer for at least 1000 years before Hippocrates, when the Edwin Smith papyrus described what must have been a malignant tumor and advised, "There is no treatment" (Shimkin, 1977). All anyone could offer was supportive care; rational cancer nursing had to await the emergence of rational science.

MILESTONES IN THE HISTORY OF CANCER RESEARCH AND CARE

EIGHTEENTH CENTURY

The eighteenth century has been identified as the Age of Reason in the development of medicine and the biomedical sciences (Shimkin, 1977). Before the eighteenth century, no distinction was made between scientific thought and metaphysical concepts; medicine rested on philosophic thinking (Kardinal & Yarbro, 1979). However, patterns of incidence were emerging. In 1713 Ramazzini noted more cases of breast cancer in nuns when compared with other women. Snuff was associated with cancer, and in 1775 Percivall Pott described scrotal cancer in chimney sweeps. The black bile theory as a cause of cancer was dispelled after more than 1000 years. A rationale for cancer surgery began to develop. The first facility for cancer patients opened in 1740 in Rheims, France, but was moved in 1779 to the outskirts of Rheims because residents were concerned about the contagiousness of cancer (Shimkin, 1977). In 1792 the Middlesex Hospital in London (considered by many to be the first cancer institute) established a cancer ward to study the natural history of cancer and to investigate new methods of treatment.

NINETEENTH CENTURY

The nineteenth century marked the modern beginnings of discovery in the biomedical sciences and the development of cancer care facilities.

FACILITIES

In 1851 the Royal Marsden Hospital was established in London to treat cancer patients exclusively. The New York Cancer Hospital, founded by James M. Sims in 1884, became Memorial Hospital for Treatment of Cancer and Allied Disease in 1899 and is known today as Memorial Sloan-Kettering Cancer Center. In 1898 the New York state legislature appropriated $10,000 for the study of causes, mortality, and treatment of cancer with the establishment of the New York State Pathological Laboratory at the University of Buffalo. In 1911 it became the New York State Institute for the Study of Malignant Diseases and was renamed Roswell Park Memorial Institute in 1946, after its first director. In 1890, what may be considered the first hospice for cancer patients in America was established in New York with the opening of St. Rose's Free Home for Incurable Cancer.

CANCER AND ITS TREATMENT

Discoveries of this period provided the foundation for the future refinement of cancer therapy. The introduction of anesthesia in 1846 and antisepsis in 1867 allowed advances in surgery. New surgical approaches for cancer began in the late 1880s and of significance was William S. Halsted's radical mastectomy for breast cancer in 1894. Wilhelm Conrad Roentgen's discovery of x-rays in 1895 was followed by Marie Curie's discovery of radium in 1898. In that same year, Paul Erhlich, considered the founder of modern chemotherapy, was searching for useful agents against cancer (Shimkin, 1977). The only chemical agent that had been used successfully against cancer was arsenic (Zubrod, 1979).

Nursing Practice

The period of 1890 to 1900 was a time of considerable growth in American nursing. The need for trained nurses became apparent during the Civil War, and the first school of nursing, New England Hospital School of Nursing, opened in Boston in 1872. The number of nursing schools increased rapidly to approximately 400 by 1900. The head nurse was the only graduate nurse on the unit and taught the students who provided the care (Kramer, 1987). Graduate nurses practiced in the hospital, the district, or the home, but home care predominated.

Twentieth Century

The first half of the twentieth century is noted for the use of ionizing radiation in the diagnosis and treatment of cancer and the extension of surgical procedures. The second half of the century is noted for significant progress in systemic chemotherapy, increased understanding of cell biology, and advanced technology that allowed research proliferation.

Early 1900s

At the turn of the century, cancer was considered incurable, and many people thought it was contagious. In one of the first articles in the nursing literature on cancer, Rice (1902) stated, "While cancer has not yet been classed with the transmissible diseases, there are authentic cases where a wife has been infected with cancer by her husband and vice versa." She also noted cancer's prevalence in certain geographic locations, and she designated Buffalo, New York, as "a veritable tropic of cancer." Indeed, the belief that cancer was an infectious disease was so common that some nurses refused to care for patients with the disease (Transmission, 1907). In 1906 C. P. Childe, a British physician, wrote the first book to inform the public about cancer: *The Control of a Scourge* (Ross, 1987). Note that the word *cancer* was not used in the title.

The death rate from cancer was 90 per cent. Although prevention of cancer was not the focus during this period of time, one physician asserted that the development of cancer was due to excessive and faulty nutrition (Scovil, 1915). He recommended exercise, avoidance of coffee and alcohol, and a vegetarian diet with the exception of butter.

The organizational fight against cancer began when the American Association for Cancer Research was established in 1907. In 1913 the American Society for the Control of Cancer, known today as the American Cancer Society (ACS), was established to educate the lay public about cancer. In that same year, the first cancer article aimed at the general public appeared in the *Ladies' Home Journal.* Author Samuel Hopkins Adams encouraged women to be watchful of themselves and to report any suspicious symptoms (Ross, 1987; Shimkin, 1977). The word *cancer* was rarely printed in newspapers or magazines or discussed openly in society. Women were often too frightened and inhibited to discuss symptoms with their physicians. Despite a high mortality rate from gynecologic and breast cancer (King, 1988), the average time between the discovery by the patient and the seeking of medical advice was 1 year, with longer delays noted for men (Control of Cancer, 1919). In addition, many doctors did not recognize early symptoms. For example, vaginal discharges were not investigated; cancers of the rectum were treated as hemorrhoids; and cancers of the oral cavity were misdiagnosed as syphilis (American Society, 1924). To increase physician awareness, the American Society for the Control of Cancer and the American Medical Association published *Essential Facts about Cancer for the Medical Profession* in 1919 (American Society, 1924).

Cancer nursing in the early 1900s was primarily concerned with bedside care and comfort measures for surgical patients, because surgery was the major treatment method. Most patients presented with advanced cancer and encountered numerous difficulties, yet nurses used ingenuity to address individual problems. One nurse modified a Kelly pad to manage the patient's excessive discharge from the bowels and bladder (New Use, 1916) (Box 2–1). A physician shared with nurses a formula for removing the offensive odor from their hands after changing dressings of patients with inoperable cancers (Cumston, 1900) (Box 2–2). Nurses providing home care also had to improvise and economize. Tucker (1915) reported caring for a patient with pelvic cancer that caused bladder and rectal fistulas. Pads were not thick enough to prevent the bedsheets from getting wet. She improvised by using an air cushion

---

Box 2–1. *New Use for a Kelly Pad*

Dear Editor: While nursing a case of cancer, where there was excessive discharge from both bladder and bowels, the patient using cloths and sanitary pads which caused discomfort and chafing, as well as much washing of cloths and bed linen, I thought of trying a Kelly pad. I procured a surgeon's size, which is smaller than the obstetric size, and was more comfortable, relieving the patient's back from pressure. I made pads of cotton batting and cheesecloth, large squares, which I placed inside the pad. When they were wet, they were removed and burned, thus eliminating all washing and keeping the patient dry and comfortable. The results far exceeded my expectations, the patient's suffering and distress being much lessened. The pad could be used in many cases where there is continuous discharge or drainage.
District of Columbia.   **C.E.**

with newspapers underneath and muslin wrapped around the cushion and newspapers. When soiled, only the muslin needed cleaning, which meant a great saving on laundry expenses. As a home nurse, she was provided a budget to carry out her work but was expected to save as much as possible. She recommended that nurses in private work keep an account of everything ordered in case questions were raised about the bills.

1920s

General hospitals often refused to care for patients with chronic diseases, placing a priority on patients with acute conditions. The average hospital stay for all cases was 2 weeks, but cancer patients required terminal care for periods of 4 to 5 months (Eaves & Associates, 1928). The state of Massachusetts, concerned about facilities to care for patients with inoperable cancers, established Pondville Hospital for cancer patients in 1927. For 2 to 3 months after the opening of Pondville, there was no x-ray equipment, the operating room was not ready, and radium had not arrived, but "we showed what good nursing could do" by cleaning up sloughing lesions and reducing infection (Daland, 1969).

Affluent families could afford trained nurses to provide care at home for family members with advanced disease. This demand for nurses often created competition between private duty nursing and hospital nursing for graduates of the nearly 2000 training schools (Lynaugh & Fagin, 1988). Home care for patients with cancer was an important issue, and emphasis began to be placed on the care of patients by public health nurses.

The Boston Community Health Association evaluated the care of 181 cancer patients by nurses of their association, and 628 histories were obtained from surviving relatives (Eaves & Associates, 1928). Approximately 78 per cent of the cancer patients had a hopeless outlook; superstition and misunderstanding by patients and family members prevailed. These attitudes were reinforced by physicians and nurses who practiced deception and concealment that subsequently promoted fear and disgrace. The nursing care required for these patients was demanding and stressful. Nausea and incontinence were major problems, and care focused on surgical dressing changes, enemas, douches, catheter care, nourishment by means of tubes, and pain relief. A home care visit cost $0.85 (Eaves & Associates, 1928); hospital care was $1.50 per day if paid by the patient or $2.50 per day if paid by the city or town (Daland, 1969); and the average salary of the public health nurse was $135.00 per month (Tatterhall, 1928).

In 1927 the American Society for the Control of Cancer adopted the slogan, "Fight Cancer with Knowledge," emphasizing the development of cancer committees within state medical societies to educate physicians (Nursing Advisory Committee, 1948a; Ross, 1987). The attitudes of the medical profession warranted criticism because delays in detection and treatment by approximately 10 per cent of the medical profession were considerable (American Society, 1924–1925). Examples of medical misinformation sound shocking today: a woman with breast cancer was told by her physician to "wait until it begins to bleed and then come back, and I will tell you what to do." Bleeding from a cancerous uterus was ascribed to "a return of menstruation," "rheumatism," or "a cold in the pelvis." Other familiar sayings were, "It is your menopause"; "Don't bother it till it bothers you"; and "Go home and forget it" (American Society, 1924–1925).

In 1928, 158 nurses attended a symposium on cancer at Harvard Cancer Research Hospital (Ross, 1928). Ross (1928) reported that many of the nurses were dissatisfied because speakers gave them no reassurance of positive cures, leaving them with little hope for progress. The literature had little information about nursing care for the cancer patient, but Ross provides some insight regarding patient attitudes and nursing care. Ignorance and superstition contributed to suffering, and many patients spent their earnings on quacks. She reported that excessive use of morphia (morphine) in homebound cancer patients was an unnecessary evil and argued that morphia should be used only to help patients through a special crisis because coal tar products and sedatives could keep patients comfortable (Ross, 1928).

1930s

The convention of considering 5-year end results in cancer as an indication of cure became the basis of clinical statistical consideration (Shimkin, 1977). In the 1930s fewer than one in five patients were alive 5 years after diagnosis.

In 1931 a physician and a nurse from the Massachusetts State Department of Public Health studied the habits of 387 patients with cancer and 387 patients in a control group (Lombard & McDonald, 1931). Alcohol use and heavy smoking were identified in the cancer group, but no significant difference in food groups eaten by the patients was noted between the two groups. There was also an average 6-month delay in the notification of symptoms to medical authorities in the cancer group. The role of the public health nurse as an important member of the anticancer network was emphasized with regard to patient advocacy, assessment, and follow-up care (Fischel, 1931).

Cancer organizations made considerable progress in the 1930s. The American College of Surgeons established standards for the evaluation of cancer patients. In 1935 the International Union Against Cancer (UICC) was established, and the American Society for the Control of Cancer established the Women's Field Army to educate women about cancer symptoms. Later the Field Army educated both men and women and used lay public volunteers to augment the professional health educators (Nursing Advisory Committee, 1948a; Ross, 1987) (Fig. 2–1). The National Cancer Institute (NCI) was established through an act of Congress on August 5, 1937. In addition, the first course for nurses in radiotherapy began at the Christie Hospital in Manchester, England, in 1938.

Nursing education in the 1930s was in a state of unrest, with movement from an apprentice-type training program to a more formal educational base for practice (Craytor, 1982). Nursing education, which was controlled by hospitals, was not on an equal level with other forms of specialized education. Salaries were low, and nurses worked 12-hour shifts. A proposed scheme of 8-hour shifts was opposed by hospital administrators, who were worried that money would be lost and that other personnel would want an 8-hour schedule (Editorial, 1934).

Cowan (1934), Education Director of Women's Hospital in New York City, published a paper, "Modern Cancer Nursing," that provided some indication of cancer nursing practice in those days. She stressed the importance of nurses' attention to the mental attitude of patients with cancer, including teaching control of pain using mental hygiene measures, personal hygiene measures, and drugs. Nursing care of hemorrhage and strangulation in head and neck cancers was also discussed. Care of the bowels in patients with colon cancer aimed to increase elimination through colonic irrigations with salt solution 1 to 2 times per day.

1940s

One in four patients with cancer was alive 5 years after diagnosis. Chemotherapeutic agents gained recognition. The discovery of the antitumor activity of nitrogen mustard, an agent of the chemical warfare program, was made at Yale by Goodman et al. (1946). The

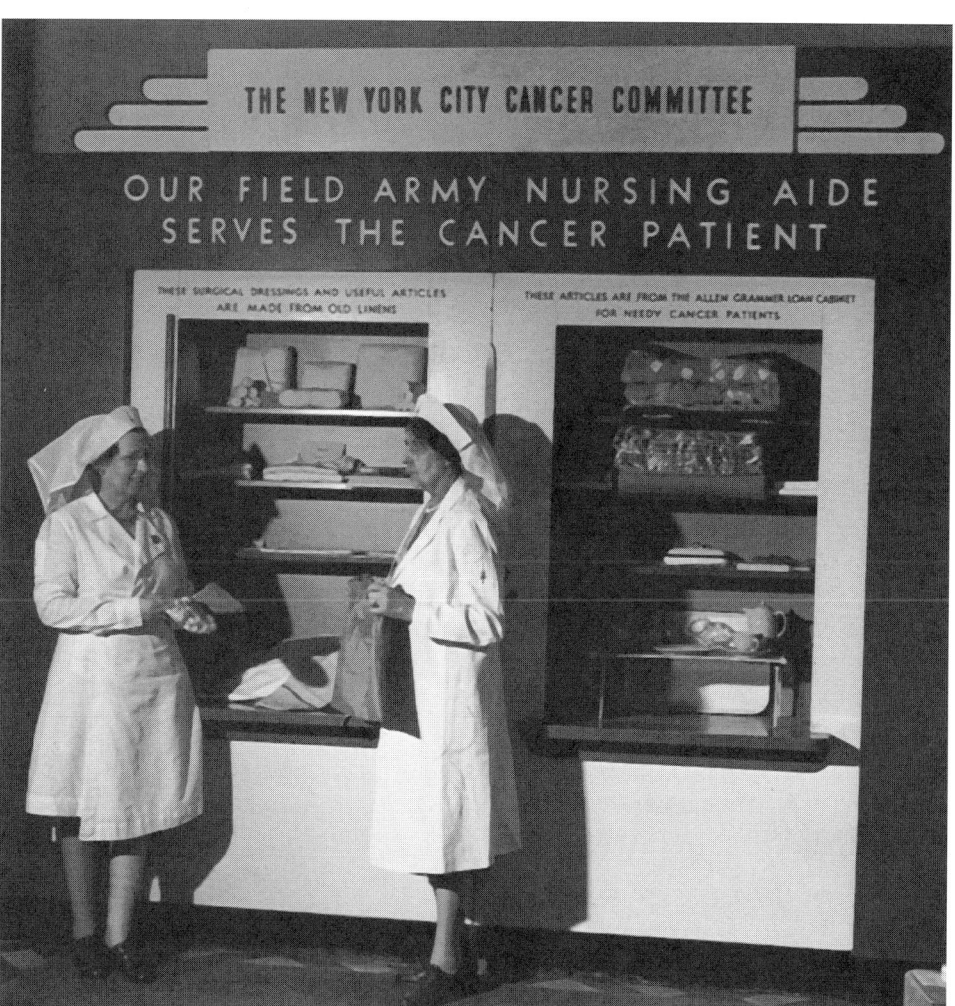

FIGURE 2–1. As the American Cancer Society expanded its Field Army program, volunteers augmented nurses' efforts. (Courtesy of the American Cancer Society.)

first patient treated with it had far advanced lymphosarcoma. In 1947, Sidney Farber of the Children's Hospital in Boston achieved the first remission in a 10-year-old boy, using the antineoplastic agent aminopterin—an important milestone in the development of chemotherapy. Prevention and early detection were promoted through breast self-examination and development of the Papanicolaou test. In 1944 the American Society for the Control of Cancer became the American Cancer Society and began to emphasize cancer research as well as cancer education.

During the 1940s the demand increased for nurses to implement new therapies and procedures and to develop resources for World War II. The hospital became the center for health care delivery, but a shortage of nurses existed. Aides and auxiliary workers filled the gap, and practical nursing came into being.

It is probably fair to state that the development of cancer nursing as a specialty had its real beginnings in the decade of the forties, with a primary emphasis on cancer nursing education. This decade was also significant because the first leaders in cancer nursing could be identified.

The Nursing Section of the Cancer Control Branch of the National Cancer Institute was established in 1948. Rosalie Peterson, named Senior Nurse Officer and Chief Public Health Nursing Consultant of the Cancer Control Division, had a significant impact on cancer nursing education. Because of investigations in 1947 that revealed nurses' limited knowledge of cancer, home care, and rehabilitation and their beliefs that cancer was always fatal, Peterson became actively involved in courses on cancer treatment and diagnosis for nursing instructors. She taught cancer care to public health nurses and awarded grants in 1949 to the School of Public Health at the University of Minnesota and the Columbia University Teachers College to enrich the graduate education curriculum (Peterson, 1948, 1956; Peterson & Walker, 1949).

The first university course in cancer nursing specialization was taught by Katherine Nelson in 1947 at Teachers College, Columbia University in New York (Craytor, 1982). The year-long course provided 16 academic credit hours toward a master of arts degree. Anne Ferris, Director of Nursing at Memorial Hospital, initiated the idea for this course and secured a grant of $30,000 from the New York City Committee of the ACS (Craytor, 1982). Elizabeth Walker and Nelliana Best assisted in the teaching, and the clinical practicum was held at Memorial Hospital.

On April 30, 1948, the Nursing Advisory Committee of the American Cancer Society had its first meeting (Table 2–1). Margorie Schlotterbeck was the first nursing consultant for the ACS, followed by Claire Richmond in 1955, Virginia Barckley in 1962, and Patricia Greene in 1981. The nursing committee made recommendations and advised on projects that were under way and on those that needed to be developed. Responding to an increased emphasis by the ACS on professional education, the nursing committee began work on films, an exhibit, and criteria and standards for

TABLE 2–1. *Members of the First American Cancer Society Nursing Advisory Committee, 1948*

Katherine Nelson, Chair	Columbia University Teachers College, New York
Hedwig Cohen	National Organization of Public Health Nursing
Montrose Williams*	
Fraziska Glienke*	
Irene Carn	League of Nursing Education
Anne Ferris	Memorial Hospital, New York
Ruth Smith*	
Rosalie Peterson	National Cancer Institute
Ethel Chandler*	
Caroline Keller	Memorial Hospital, New York
Marjorie Schlotterbeck	American Cancer Society

*Affiliations unknown.

scholarships for nurses (Nursing Advisory Committee, 1948a, 1948b). The ACS-sponsored workshops were launched. A course in cancer control was held at the University of Washington School of Nursing for 25 nurses (Patterson, 1948). Caroline Keller, Director of Nursing, and Margaret Coleman, Director of Nursing Education, both at Memorial Hospital, and Dr. Vera Fry, Dean at New York University, established 4- to 6-week oncologic nursing workshops twice a year for registered nurses, who were recruited through ACS state divisions (Co-operating, 1949–1950; E. Wolf, personal communication, 1982).

Documentation of cancer nursing practice and care was still minimal in the 1940s, but some insights into care and concerns during that time are available. Hopp (1941) discussed the role of the roentgenologic nurse in cancer treatment and diagnosis, stating that there was "no special routine to follow in caring for these patients and efforts to combat side effects of nausea and vomiting had not been entirely successful." Lemon juice, sour wine sipped slowly, and ginger ale were used for nausea, vomiting, and anorexia. Glienka and Kress (1944b) reported that most cancer deaths occur in the home and that cobra venom was used to control pain. Urea was used to eliminate or decrease odors in malodorous lesions of the breast (Glienke & Kress, 1944a). Cockerill (1948) cited the importance of understanding the fears, reactions, and problems of the individual with cancer.

Home care of patients with cancer was also a concern (Biehusen, 1956; Ferguson, 1948). The Connecticut Division of the ACS developed a cancer nursing reimbursement plan for visiting nurse and public health agencies, allocating $20,000 in 1947 to support nursing services in tumor clinics at $1.50 per hour and nursing visits to the home at $1.00 per visit (Biehusen, 1956). Connecticut was the first state to formally establish a nursing committee in any division of ACS.

1950s

The cobalt 60 unit was developed in the early 1950s, and Best (1950) described the role of the nurse with this new treatment method. In 1955 the NCI developed a national chemotherapy program devoted to testing chemicals that might be effective against cancer. Multimodality treatment approaches replaced single-modality treatment for cancer.

Cancer nursing education continued to improve, and cancer nursing activities increased tremendously. Hilkemeyer (1982), who was a consultant in nursing education to the Bureau of Cancer Control, Missouri Division of Health, from 1950 to 1955 and became Director of Nursing for M.D. Anderson Hospital and Tumor Institute, stated, "the 1950's was an era when the nursing profession was concerned about who we were and what we should be doing."

In 1950 Peterson and two other NCI instructors conducted a 3-week institute at the University of Minnesota for 30 nursing instructors from across the country. In 1951 Peterson published a series of articles outlining in-service education for cancer nursing care (Peterson, 1951a, 1951b, 1951c). The following year the NIH funded five pilot studies for education in cancer nursing (Farrell, 1953; Peterson, 1956). The first grant awarded went to Skidmore College for the integration of cancer nursing throughout the basic curriculum. Doris Diller wrote the proposal while taking a research course at Columbia. She and Francis Brady, a fellow faculty member at Skidmore, constructed a test to measure knowledge about cancer among nursing students over 3 successive years (Craytor, 1982). Diller received a grant from the NCI to conduct the cancer knowledge investigation in 100 schools (Diller, 1957). Her efforts stimulated interest and emphasized the need for cancer nursing in the basic nursing curriculum.

Cancer nursing education activities flourished during this era. Dr. Rosemary Bouchard, Norma Owens, and Inga Thornblad of the Department of Education at New York University implemented workshops on oncologic nursing (Craytor, 1982) and collaborated with Memorial Hospital for the Treatment of Cancer and Allied Diseases by offering a year-long cancer nursing internship program for foreign nurses. Hilkemeyer established 5-day institutes on cancer nursing for public health nurses and an in-service education program at Ellis Fischel Cancer Hospital in Columbia, Missouri (Hilkemeyer & Kinney, 1956).

Outside of major centers, a small number of nurses were volunteering for the ACS, reporting on what had been learned about cancer care and cancer nursing. The dedication to volunteer work by these nurses helped spread the word. As Edith Wolf (personal communication, 1982), Associate Director of Nursing Education at Memorial Hospital from 1950 to 1969, stated, "Today, one would receive honoraria for all the hard work but my only thought was to get the information to where it would help those who cared for the patients so their lives would be better."

The ACS nursing committee remained active during the 1950s, with an increased focus on nursing practice and collaboration with the ACS divisions. The ACS published *A Cancer Source Book for Nurses,* and the minutes from the committee's meeting on March 13, 1957, reported that 63 graduate and 263 undergraduate scholarships or fellowships were awarded to nurses by the ACS divisions (Nursing Advisory Committee, 1957). Chairpersons of the ACS Nursing Advisory Committee during the 1950s were Elizabeth Stobo, Vera Fry, and Julia Hereford. In 1958 the committee surveyed 30 graduate programs; only New York University and Columbia University Teachers College offered advanced programs in cancer nursing and an undergraduate level course. Boston University, University of California at Los Angeles, Teachers College, and New York University were the only schools that identified a faculty member as a cancer nursing specialist (Nursing Advisory Committee, 1958).

While cancer nursing education was moving ahead, the practice arena was encountering unique problems. A nursing shortage existed, and Caroline Keller, Director of Nursing at Memorial Hospital for the Treatment of Cancer and Allied Diseases, decided to go to Argentina to recruit nurses. Through an indirect connection with the Perons and the social reform activity of Evita Peron, women were recruited from the streets to be trained as nurses. Subsequently, Edith Wolf spent 2 years on the monumental task of educating 13 young women in American culture and cancer nursing (Wolf, personal communication, 1982). At that time, she reported "my mail was heavy, no one outside of Memorial had ever heard of a colostomy irrigation [developed by their chief of gastric surgery] and nurses were clamoring for this information." Wolf provides insights into nursing practice at that time: "Patients were not told they had cancer, we always said tumor or growth" (Wolf, personal communication, 1982). Meanwhile, Mary Patterson at Memorial Hospital recruited a volunteer pianist and initiated arm exercise classes for mastectomy patients (Higgenbotham, 1957) (Figs. 2–2 and 2–3).

Considerable progress was made in the 1950s in defining cancer nursing. Craytor, in her master's thesis in 1959, defined the well-prepared nurse as a co-worker of the health care team. This work subsequently led to a demonstration project that illustrated the value of a team (physician, nurse, and social worker) to deal with the problems of cancer care (Craytor, 1982). Nelson continued her crusade for cancer nursing. In a letter to Claire Richmond, nursing consultant for ACS, at the renewal of her cancer nursing education grant, Nelson (1959) stated "If we believe that there should be a small number of highly prepared nurse consultants and teachers in cancer nursing, these nurses should be sought out, encouraged to get this preparation and return to their agencies better able to help in the preparation of nurse practitioners in the nursing care of patients with late stage cancer. Cancer nursing is at a crossroads, it either has to be given up as an undesirable thing or it must be looked at critically and really supported."

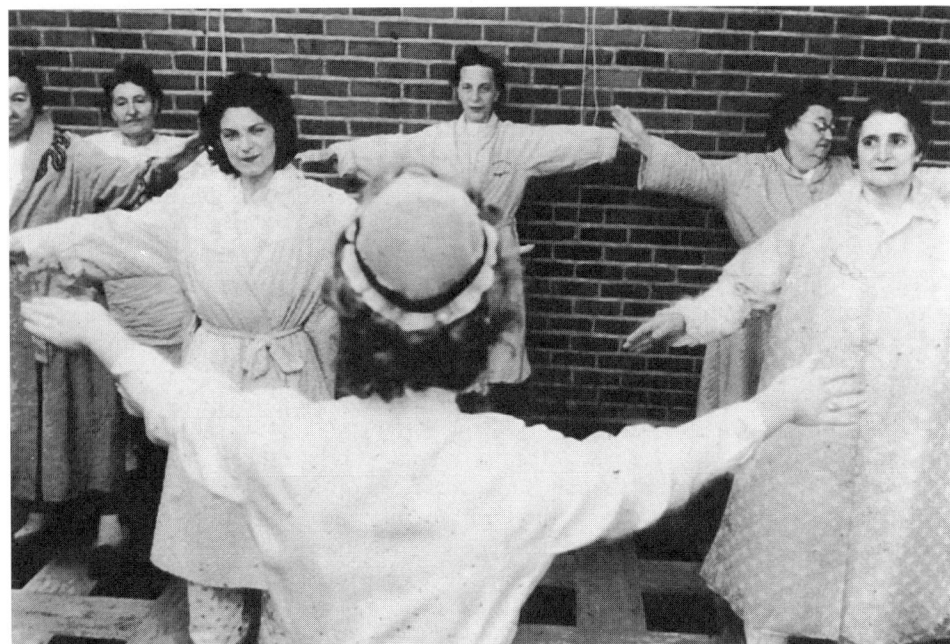

FIGURE **2–2.** An exercise class for mastectomy patients. (Courtesy of the Oncology Nursing Society, historical files.)

1960s

Oncology Comes of Age. Cancer statistics improved: one of three individuals was now alive 5 years after diagnosis. The clinical trials program established by the NCI led to the development and discovery of other active agents in the 1960s. Skipper, Schabel, and Wilcox (1964) established guiding principles in chemotherapy that were related to cellular kinetics. Frei, Freireich, Gehan and colleagues (1961) pioneered the first effective combination chemotherapy for treatment of leukemia. Adjuvant chemotherapy, begun in the 1950s, first proved useful in 1965 (Zubrod, 1979). In 1964, the American Society of Clinical Oncology was established to create a forum for the new specialty of medical oncology.

Specialization of Nursing. A distinct growth in nursing specialization paved the road for oncology nursing as a specialty. Coronary care units, surgical intensive care units, dialysis units, burn units, and medical intensive care units necessitated a change in nursing roles to clinical nurse specialists or nurse clinicians (Donahue, 1985) and the need for such specialists (Leone, 1965).

This specialty role was not clear to many. Physician members of the ACS Professional Education Committee wanted to know what defined cancer nursing and

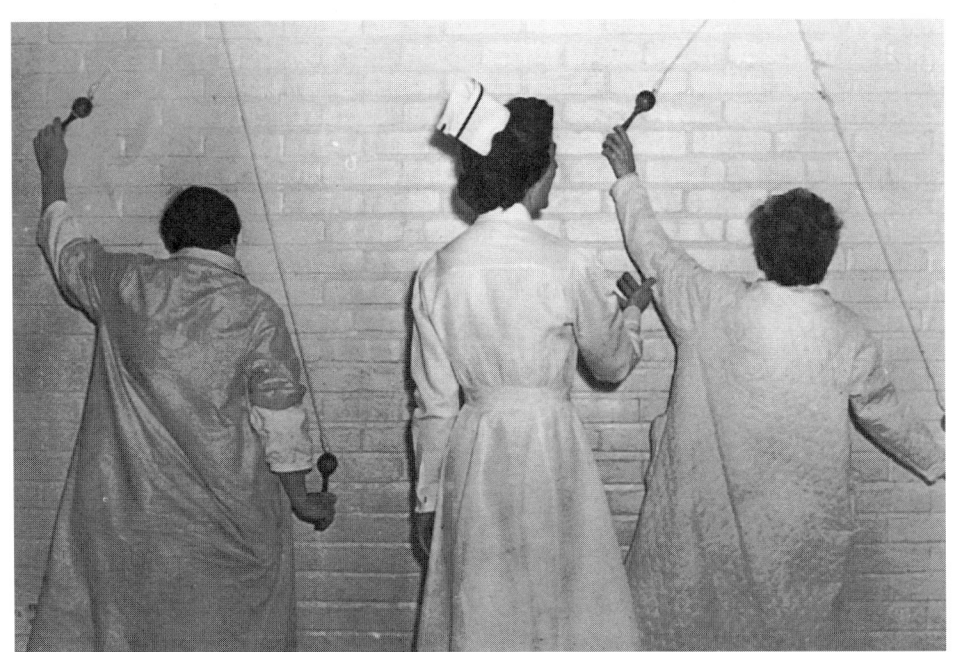

FIGURE **2–3.** Mastectomy patients performing arm exercises. (Courtesy of the Oncology Nursing Society, historical files.)

how it differed from other nursing. In response, the ACS nursing committee dropped the term *cancer nursing* in favor of *nursing care of cancer patients* (Nursing Advisory Committee, 1960). However, with a beginning emphasis placed on oncology nursing practice in the later 1960s, it was becoming clear what constituted cancer nursing.

The first expanded nursing roles in oncology were those associated with sophisticated clinical trials of new chemotherapeutic agents (Hubbard & Donehower, 1980). Initially, the nurse in a clinical trial team primarily collected patient data for the clinical trial. But gradually the nurse's role changed as patients found the nurse a better source of counsel than an unfamiliar member of the medical house staff or the busy clinical investigator. The clinical investigator found that the research nurse was often a better source of information regarding the subtleties of patient status. Thus before there was an oncology nurse or a medical oncology specialty, a symbiotic relationship grew between two professionals whose special training was acquired on the job (Henke, 1980).

As this symbiosis and interdependence grew, the nursing role was expanded far beyond technical or task-oriented functions. The nurse often became the liaison between the clinical investigator and other services gradually added to the cancer care team (e.g., social work, pastoral care, rehabilitation).

What began as a clinical research team was gradually recognized as a better approach to providing cancer care. Cancer patients as a group began to benefit from this improved system of care, and the oncology nurse became a central figure in the new team approach to cancer care. There were two consequences. As oncologists entered practice in community hospitals, they took with them the team approach and the expanded role for the oncology nurse. Also, as the identity of oncology nursing was formalized, hospital nursing services began to seek out and establish positions for nurses in this emerging specialty (Henke, 1980). One of the first institutions to formally recognize the role of oncology nursing was St. Jude Children's Research Hospital in Memphis by establishing the position of pediatric oncology nurse practitioner in 1969. Andi Wood, Ellen Shanks, Clara Mason, and Shirley Stagner were the first nurses to function in this role (Greene, 1983). They subsequently developed a 3-month fellowship in childhood cancer nursing to share their experiences with other nurses.

The nursing literature expanded concerning nursing care of the patient with cancer. Wolf (1964, 1968) stressed the importance of the role of the nurse in education for patients with cancer, emphasizing the need to teach patients self-care. The ACS published *Care of Your Colostomy: A Source Book of Information* in 1964. There was considerable focus on care of the dying patient (Barckley, 1964, 1967; Kübler-Ross, 1969). The first textbook, edited by Bouchard, *Nursing Care of the Cancer Patient,* was published in 1967. The landmark clinical nursing research study by Quint (1963) identified the psychological needs of women who had breast cancer and were treated with radical

mastectomy (Box 2–3). The nurse's role in home care (Hammond, 1964) and the early detection of breast and cervical cancer were also discussed (Lewison, 1965; Leyshon, 1966).

1970s

In 1971 Congress passed the National Cancer Act, the first law by any nation to make the conquest of cancer a national priority. National funding for cancer rose from $233 million in 1971 to $379 million in 1972 and to more the $1 billion over the next 12 years (Ross, 1987). Comprehensive cancer centers expanded from

---

Box 2–3. *Exploratory Investigation of the Process of Adjustment Following Mastectomy*

Principal Investigator: Lulu W. Hassenplug, Dean, School of Nursing, University of California, Los Angeles Project Director: Jeanne C. Quint, Junior Research Nurse

This 2-year study investigated the process by which a woman adjusts to the loss of a breast because of cancer. Attention was directed toward understanding how women came to terms with two changes precipitated by the surgery: the defeminizing change in body appearance and the decision concerning camouflage and concealment; and the knowledge of having cancer and the impact of an uncertain future. All women admitted to the hospital for breast biopsy were potential subjects. Initial contacts with subjects were made the evening before surgery, and data were collected by participant observation during the hospital stay. Interviews occurred at 2 weeks, 6 weeks, 3 months, 6 months, and between the tenth and eleventh month. Interview guides for the home interviews were based on a combination of previously identified areas of importance and salient events or experiences observed by the nurse fieldworkers during their contacts with the women and their families. Data were obtained from 21 women over an 18-month period. Categories and category relationships were established using the constant comparative method of data analysis. The women ranged in age from 38 to 79 years, with a median of 57. Ten were married; ten were widows, and one was divorced. Six received medical supervision from private physicians, and the others from nonprivate medical services. Death and dying became integral parts of the lives of these women; for all of them, life expectancy was foreshortened. Three patterns of adjustment were found: (1) those who faced an uncertain future with satisfactory wound healing and physical recovery; (2) those who faced an ambiguous future associated with a nonhealing incision or persistent physical discomfort; and (3) those who underwent physical regression and death. Interactional difficulties for the women were associated with complex organizational structure and unspoken death concerns of all participants.

This study was supported by NIH Grant MH 05495 and was conducted under sponsorship of the School of Nursing, University of California, Los Angeles, between September 1, 1961, and August 31, 1963.

three to 20 centers during the 1970s, and clinical trials began to enter community hospitals by the late 1970s.

Combination drug regimens were used with drugs reconstituted and administered by nurses. The use of scalp vein needles and bolus injections were common practice, and little consideration was given to safety factors for reconstitution and administration.

The management of chemotherapy side effects was a trial and error process. For nausea and vomiting, if one antiemetic did not work, another was tried. Combination antiemetic regimens were unheard of. The development of guidelines for care was just beginning.

Patient education materials were almost nonexistent, which meant that nurses had to spend considerable time on verbal instruction and on developing appropriate patient resources. In addition, considerable time was spent with patients and families in overcoming the myths associated with cancer. Some still thought cancer was contagious and a death sentence with few options available.

Oncology nurses rose to the opportunities at hand, which built on the groundwork that had already been laid. Barckley (1982) summed it up best when she wrote, "The nineteen seventies, when the seeds sown by so many came to a full bloom, were a kind of richness."

Cancer Nursing Education. Nurses were being encouraged to enter the field of cancer nursing, and the future challenges and opportunities for this specialty were emphasized (Hilkemeyer, 1974; Koons, 1976; Leininger, 1977; Marino, 1976; Miller, 1976; Nelson, 1974). The American Cancer Society sponsored a 6-week summer experience for senior nursing students to encourage them to enter cancer nursing (Barckley, 1971). In 1971 the NCI supported a 10-week work-study program in cancer nursing at the NIH Clinical Center in collaboration with the ACS. In 1973 the Division of Cancer Control and Rehabilitation at the NCI funded 18 oncology nursing education programs for a 5-year period. These programs developed curricula and materials covering general and specialized aspects of cancer care for continuing education programs and for undergraduate- and graduate-level courses. More than 16,000 nurses were reached through these programs (L. Lunceford, personal communication, April 2, 1982). Graduate education in cancer nursing was also being developed at the University of California at Los Angeles by Anayis Derdiarin and at the University of Washington by Jeanne Quint Benoliel and Ruth McCorkle (Craytor, 1982). In 1979 the NCI funded two postmaster's fellowship programs in oncology nursing education at San Jose State University and the University of Alabama.

Cancer Nursing Organizations. In 1973 the ACS sponsored the First National Cancer Nursing Conference in Chicago, the first major cancer conference *for* cancer nurses organized by cancer nurses. Lisa Marino, at the University of Chicago and Shirlee Koons, Director of Nursing at the Mountain States Tumor Institute in Boise, coordinated a small meeting after the conference to discuss the idea of a national organization for oncology nurses. The 20 nurses present agreed that an organization was needed. During 1974 Connie Henke

(Yarbro), University of Alabama Comprehensive Cancer Center, worked with Marino to establish a communications network of oncology nurses. Koons published and distributed the first newsletter in 1974. By January 1975, 400 cancer nurses had been identified. At the same time, Patricia Greene was spearheading a move to identify pediatric oncology nurses. On November 3, 1974, the Association of Pediatric Oncology Nurses came into being, with Greene serving as the first president (Greene, 1983). In May 1975, a nursing session was held at the meetings of the American Society of Clinical Oncology and the American Association for Cancer Research in San Diego, and the decision was made to establish a formal national organization. The initial four officers were Lisa Begg Marino, president; Cindy Mantz (Cantril), vice president; Daryl Maass (Mathers), secretary; and Connie Henke (Yarbro), treasurer. In July 1975, the Oncology Nursing Society was officially incorporated in the state of Illinois; by the end of the year there were more than 400 members (Yarbro, 1984).

Progress was also being made internationally with cancer nursing. England established its Oncology Nursing Society under the auspices of the Royal College of Nursing, and Switzerland established an oncology nurses interest group within their nursing association in 1978 (Ash, 1983). In the fall of 1978, the first International Cancer Nursing Conference was sponsored by the Royal Marsden Hospital and Nursing Mirror in London. South Africa held its first national cancer nursing conference in 1979.

Cancer Nursing Research. In 1973 Marilyn Oberst from Memorial Sloan-Kettering surveyed a panel of 575 nurses to determine the priorities for clinical research in cancer nursing. The highest priorities were for research on problems related to the side effects of cancer treatment and relief of the physical discomfort experienced by the patient (Oberst, 1978) (Box 2–4). MacVicar (1975) studied the problems experienced by families after the onset of metastatic disease in the male spouse. Lewis, Firsich, and Parsell (1979) developed a tool to assess the outcomes of cancer patients who received chemotherapy, and McCorkle and Young (1978) developed and tested a symptom distress scale to assess ways in which patients cope or fail to cope with their cancer therapy. The NCI also funded the work of several cancer nurse researchers: Ida Martinson, "Home Care for the Child with Cancer"; Jane Dixon, "Nursing Interventions in Nutrition of Cancer Patients"; Gail Hongladorum, "Community-Based Cancer Nursing Education Program"; and Denise Oleske, "Demonstration Project: Home Nursing for Cancer Patients" (L. Lunceford, personal communication, April 2, 1982).

Cancer Nursing as a Specialty. The rapid growth of oncology nursing was influenced by increased funding for cancer research; medical, scientific, and technologic advances; public interest in cancer; and changes in the nursing profession. Cancer nursing literature increased with the development of two professional journals devoted to cancer nursing: *Oncology Nursing Forum*, official journal of the Oncology Nursing Society, and *Cancer Nursing*. The Oncology Nursing Society grew

Box 2–4. *Priorities for Cancer Nursing Research*

1. Determine effective methods of relieving chemotherapy or radiation induced nausea and vomiting.
2. Study nursing interventions for the relief of pain in individuals with cancer.
3. Establish discharge planning and follow-up programs that effectively mobilize patient, family, and community resources.
4. Identify nursing interventions that assist patients and families in coping with grief and impending death during the preterminal and terminal stages of disease.
5. Find effective ways to prevent or treat stomatitis resulting from chemotherapy.
6. Determine the most effective techniques for venipuncture, maintenance of intravenous lines, and preservation of veins for patients receiving long-term antibiotic or chemotherapy.
7. Delineate modifications in the physical plant, nursing care program, and policy that will promote comfort and dignity for the hospitalized terminally ill individual.
8. Establish effective analgesia protocols for patients with cancer.
9. Develop more effective methods of psychological support for patients and families at various stages of disease and cancer treatment.
10. Clarify the dying patient's rights to make decisions about a health care program and establish more effective mechanisms for the exercise of those rights.

Adapted from Oberst, M. (1978). Priorities in cancer nursing research. *Cancer Nursing, 1,* 281–290.

rapidly to more than 2000 members by 1979, gave national stature to the collective force of nurses involved in cancer care, and provided a forum for the development of cancer nursing activities. One of the major activities was the development of *Outcome Standards for Cancer Nursing Practice* (Oncology Nursing Society and American Nurses' Association, 1979).

1980s

The 1980s witnessed significant growth in all aspects of oncology and oncology nursing. Half of all cancer patients were cured. There were dramatic changes in the delivery of cancer care. There was a dramatic shift in cancer care from the academic setting to the community setting with approximately 80 per cent of cancer patients treated by community-based oncologists (Cheson, 1991). The NCI-funded grant program to develop cancer centers in community hospitals, which had begun in 1976, evolved into the Community Clinical Oncology Program (CCOP) in 1983. Because community hospitals were managing the majority of patients with cancer, their contributions to clinical trials increased until they were contributing more patients to collaborative group studies than the university centers (Yarbro & Yarbro, 1993).

This decade also witnessed the beginnings of what was to be called health care "reform" in the next decade. In 1984 the federal government formally endorsed the "competitive health care model" as a means of controlling the spiraling cost of health care. Diagnosis-related groups (DRGs) changed reimbursement patterns and resulted in a shift from inpatient to outpatient chemotherapy.

Cancer nursing expanded to meet the unending challenges of providing increased levels of cancer care. Their roles expanded beyond the walls of the hospital as nurses began to subspecialize in such areas of cancer as radiation therapy, bone marrow transplantation, home care, hospice care, outpatient care, pain management, and others. An increase in cancer nursing texts and journals occurred, with the *Journal of the Association of Pediatric Oncology Nursing* and *Seminars in Oncology Nursing* joining the ranks of cancer nursing journals.

Cancer Nursing Education. Given (1980) noted that "if we are to be more than a technical practice field, our profession must be built upon a scientific base and body of knowledge. Our education system must prepare nurses for oncology." In 1980 there were 13 graduate programs in cancer nursing. In 1981 the American Cancer Society established scholarships for masters-level preparation and 5 years later began to provide scholarship support at the doctoral level. By the end of the 1980s there were 44 graduate programs in cancer nursing in the United States (ONS Education Committee, 1988)

The *Outcome Standards for Cancer Nursing Education: Fundamental Level* developed by the ONS in 1982 laid the groundwork for addressing all levels of preparation with the publication of the *Standards of Oncology Nursing Education: Generalist and Advanced Practice Levels* (ONS Education Committee, 1995).

Certification has had an important influence on cancer nursing education. In 1981 the ONS established a task force to explore the feasibility of certification of oncology nurses, which led to the establishment of the Oncology Nursing Certification Corporation in 1984. The first offering of the oncology nursing certifying examination was April 30, 1986, and by the end of the decade there were more than 8000 oncology certified nurses (OCNs).

Cancer Nursing Organizations The Oncology Nursing Society grew to more than 15,000 members and 135 local chapters across the country. The activities of the society were varied and widespread and had a major influence on the expansion of oncology nursing as a specialty area of nursing. In 1981 the ONS reached a significant milestone with the establishment of the Oncology Nursing Foundation. The Foundation was established to educate the public and provide scholarships for education in cancer nursing and grants for cancer nursing research (Yarbro, 1982).

The specialty of cancer nursing was also expanding at the international level. The sponsors of the Second International Cancer Nursing Conference in London in 1980 (*Nursing Mirror* and Royal Marsden Hospital) held a 2 day seminar at Leeds Castle, Kent, to review the past two conferences and discuss plans for future conferences (Ash, 1983). Twenty-one people representing international cancer nursing interests defined the parameters of future international cancer nursing conferences, which began to be held every 2 years beginning in 1984.

During the Third International Conference on Cancer Nursing held in Melbourne, Australia, in 1984, the International Society of Nurses in Cancer Care (ISNCC) was founded under the presidency of the late Robert Tiffany of the Royal Marsden Hospital. The aims of ISNCC are to support and enhance developments in cancer nursing worldwide, develop networks among cancer nurses throughout the world, assist in the establishment of national oncology societies, and communicate with nurses in those countries where no such organization exists. Every 2 years the Society sponsors, in association with the host association, an international conference that attracts approximately 2000 nurses from more than 60 countries.

Oncology nursing has become an integral part of the International Cancer Congresses sponsored by the International Union Against Cancer (UICC) through regular program presentations (Ash, 1983). In addition, the UICC Nursing Committee has developed programs to disseminate basic cancer information to developing countries.

Cancer Nursing Research. Nurses have always played an important role in cancer research, but cancer *nursing* research to codify and test a body of knowledge that guides our practice of nursing care was minimal in the early 1980s. McCorkle and Lewis (1980) noted, "if nursing research is in its infancy, cancer nursing research is in its prenatal period." Cancer nurses rose to the challenge, and significant progress was made in cancer nursing research during this decade.

The research priorities of cancer nursing have been identified and revised over the years. The ONS Research Committee surveyed the membership's research priorities and interests in 1981, 1984, and 1989 (Grant & Stromborg, 1981; McGuire, Frank-Stromborg, & Varricchio, 1984; Funkhouser & Grant, 1989). The major areas of cancer nursing research activity include pain, patient education, coping, stress, home care, self-care, and quality of life (Grant, Paddilla, & Ferrell, 1993).

1990s

What had begun in the 1980s as modest cost-control measures designed to reduce the spiraling costs of health care reached a culmination in the 1990s, when managed care reimbursement policies began to significantly influence the kinds of cancer care delivered. Precertification before hospital admission became routine for much nonemergency cancer care. This decade saw the application in the community of a number of technologic innovations such as high-dose chemotherapy with stem cell rescue, immunotherapy, growth factor stimulation of bone marrow after chemotherapy, and the emergence of genetic engineering. These high-cost procedures often precipitated a battle between third-party payers striving to control costs and physicians striving to maximize the efficacy of cancer management. The oncology nurse was often caught in the middle.

In 1994 the ONS membership reached 24,500 members, there were 179 local chapters, and attendance at annual congresses increased to 5000. Certification of oncology nurses increased to 13,700. Cancer nurses, although educated and organized better than ever before, now faced new challenges. Collective political action was needed to ensure appropriate federal and state policies toward such issues as mammography reimbursement, insurance coverage for patients on clinical trials, smoking in public places, and many other important concerns. The shift from inpatient care to the outpatient setting resulted in a major change in the nursing needs of the patient with cancer. New priorities in patient education resulted from the complex reimbursement regulations mandated by managed care organizations. In some communities where the "marketplace" was "mature," competitive bidding began to lead to patients being forced to change from one oncologist to another even during the course of their intricate multimodality treatment regimens. These and other changes placed new stresses on the oncology nurse.

At the time of this writing, the health care delivery system is in a major state of change and the outcome is far from clear. Where cancer care is to be given is uncertain, how it will be paid for is not yet decided, and the battle between the advocates of a primary care "gate-keeper" and those who support a strong role for the specialist is not yet resolved. One thing, however, seems settled beyond a doubt. Whatever the resolution of health care "reform," the cancer nurse will continue to be the person on the front line between the patient and the delivery system who deals with those intimate human needs that must be dealt with to humanize a complex system.

SUMMARY

The progress made against cancer over the past centuries has been eclipsed by that of the past 25 years. From a cancer nursing perspective, the late 1940s, 1950s, and 1960s were crusades for cancer nursing with major emphasis on education. Very few cancer nurses are aware of what the early cancer nursing leaders contributed; they received very little recognition for their accomplishments. Hilkemeyer (1982) stated, "What many of us did was a real struggle to try to get things accomplished, but if we had never done those initial things we wouldn't be where we are today." In the past few years, information has been collected from some of these leaders about the past; unfortunately, some of them have died, and we are too late to learn what they could share with us. However, we take the legacies they left us and move forward. Cancer nursing history is a record of pioneering, a proud heritage.

REFERENCES

American Society for the Control of Cancer. (1924). *Essential facts about cancer: A handbook for the medical profession.* New York: Author.

American Society for the Control of Cancer. (Ca. 1924–1925). *Its objects and methods and some of the visible results of its work.* New York: Author.

Ash, C. R. (1983). Cancer nursing: An international perspective. *Oncology Nursing Forum, 10*(2), 69–72.

Barckley, V. (1964). Enough time for good nursing. *Nursing Outlook, 12,* 44–48.

Barckley, V. (1967). Crises in cancer. *American Journal of Nursing, 67,* 278–280.

Barckley, V. (1971). Workstudy program in cancer nursing. *Nursing Outlook, 19,* 328–330.

Barckley, V. (1982). The best of times and the worst of times. *Oncology Nursing Forum, 9,* 54–56.

Best, N. (1950). Radiotherapy and the nurse. *American Journal of Nursing, 50,* 140–143.

Biehusen, I. (1956). Cancer nursing is expensive. *Nursing Outlook, 4,* 438–441.

Bouchard, R. (1967). *Nursing care of the cancer patient.* St. Louis: C. V. Mosby Co.

Cheson, B. D. (1991). Clinical trials program. *Seminars in Oncology Nursing, 7,* 235–242.

Cockerill, E. E. (1948). The cancer patient as a person. *Public Health Nursing, 40,* 78–83.

The control of cancer. (1919). *American Journal of Nursing, 19,* 293.

Co-operating in cancer nursing education (1949–1950). Brochure from Memorial Hospital and Department of Nursing Education, New York University.

Cowan, M. (1934). Modern cancer nursing. *Trained Nurse, 92,* 243–255.

Craytor, J. K. (1982). Highlights in education for cancer nursing. *Oncology Nursing Forum, 9,* 51–58.

Cumston, C. G. (1900). A new formulae used in surgical nursing. *American Journal of Nursing, 1,* 13–14.

Daland, E. M. (1969). *Pondville hospital 1927–1969.* Walpole, MA: Massachusetts Department of Public Health.

Diller, D. (1957). *An investigation of learning in ninety-one selected schools of nursing (3rd rep.).* New York: Skidmore College.

Donahue, M. P. (1985). *Nursing, the finest art.* St. Louis: C. V. Mosby Co.

Editorial. (1934). *Trained Nurse, 92,* 278–279.

Eaves, L., & Associates. (1928). Nursing cancer patients in their home. *New England Journal of Medicine, 198,* 240–246.

Farrell, M. (1953). Experimentation in teaching cancer nursing. *Nursing Research, 2,* 41.

Ferguson, M. (1948). The public health nurse and the cancer program. *Public Health Nursing, 40,* 343–346.

Fischel, E. (1931). The public health nurse's responsibility in relation to cancer. *Public Health Nurse, 23,* 334–337.

Frei, E. III, Freireich, E. T., Gehan, E., et al. (1961). Studies of sequential and combination antimetabolite therapy in acute leukemia: 6-mercaptopurine and methotrexate. *Blood, 18,* 431–454.

Funkhouser, S. W., & Grant, M. M. (1989). 1988 ONS survey of research priorities. *Oncology Nursing Forum, 16,* 413–416.

Given, B. (1980). Education of the oncology nurse: The key to excellent patient care. *Seminars in Oncology, 7,* 71–79.

Glienke, F., & Kress, L. C. (1944a). The cancer patient: Giving bedside care in the home. *American Journal of Nursing, 44,* 434–443.

Glienke, F., & Kress, L. C. (1944b). The cancer patient: Planning for and introducing home care. *American Journal of Nursing, 44,* 351–354.

Goodman, L. S., Wintrobe, M. W., Dameshek, W., Goodman, M. J., Gilman, A., & McLennan, M. T. (1946). Nitrogen mustard therapy. Use of methyl-bis (beta-chloroethyl) amine hydrochloride for Hodgkin's disease, lymphosarcoma, leukemia and certain allied and miscellaneous disorders. *Journal American Medical Association, 132,* 126–132.

Grant, M., Padilla, G., & Ferrell, B. (1993). Cancer nursing research. In S. L. Groenwald, M. H. Frogge, M. Goodman, C. H. Yarbro (Eds.), *Cancer Nursing Principles and Practice* (pp. 1599–1613). Boston, MA: Jones and Bartlett Publishers.

Grant, M., & Stromborg, M. (1981). Promoting research collaboration: ONS research committee survey. *Oncology Nursing Forum, 8*(2), 48–53.

Greene, P. E. (1983). The Association of Pediatric Oncology Nurses: The first ten years. *Oncology Nursing Forum, 10,* 59–63.

Hammond, B. (1964). Home care improvisations. *Nursing Outlook, 64,* 49–51.

Henke, C. (1980). Emerging roles of the nurse in oncology. *Seminars in Oncology, 7,* 4–8.

Higgenbotham, S. (1957). Arm exercises after mastectomy. *American Journal of Nursing, 12,* 1573–1574.

Hilkemeyer, R. (1974). Cancer nursing: The state of the art. *Proceedings of the National Conference on Cancer Nursing* (pp. 1–6). New York: American Cancer Society.

Hilkemeyer, R. (1982). A historical perspective in cancer nursing. *Oncology Nursing Forum, 9,* 47–56.

Hilkemeyer, R., & Kinney, H. (1956). Teaching cancer nursing. *Nursing Outlook, 4,* 177–180.

Hopp, M. (1941). Roentgen therapy and the nurse. *American Journal of Nursing, 41,* 431–444.

Hubbard, S. M., & Donehower, M. G. (1980). The nurse in a cancer research setting. *Seminars in Oncology, 7,* 9–17.

Kardinal, C. G., & Yarbro, J. W. (1979). A conceptual history of cancer. *Seminars in Oncology, 6,* 396–408.

King, M. (1988). Volunteerism: Still a tradition in America. *Cancer News,* (Winter), 16–18.

Koons, S. B. (1976). Bicentennial forecast: The future of cancer nursing. *RN, 39,* 23–34.

Kramer, M. (1987). Identity in nursing. *ResMedica* (St. Louis, St. John's Mercy Medical Center) *3,* 3–8.

Kübler-Ross, E. (1969). *On death and dying.* New York: Macmillan Co.

Leininger, M. (1977). Roles and directions in nursing and cancer nursing. *Proceedings of the Second National Conference on Cancer Nursing* (pp. 6–16). New York: American Cancer Society.

Leone, L. (1965). The attack on heart disease, cancer and stroke—Is nursing ready. *American Journal of Nursing, 65,* 68–72.

Lewis, F. M., Firsich, S. C., & Parsell, S. (1979). Clinical tool development for adult chemotherapy patients: Process and content. *Cancer Nursing, 2,* 99–108.

Lewison, E. F. (1965). The nurse's role in early detection of cancer of the breast. *Nursing Forum, 4,* 82–86.

Leyshon, V. N. (1966). Taking cervical smears in the home. *Nursing Times, 62,* 361–362.

Lombard, H., & McDonald, E. (1931). Complete records and control of cancer. *Public Health Nursing, 23,* 532–533.

Lynaugh, J. E., & Fagin, C. M. (1988). Nursing comes of age. *Image, 20,* 184–190.

MacVicar, M. (1975). *The effect of cancer in the male spouses on the family.* Unpublished doctoral dissertation. Ohio State University, Columbus.

Marino, L. B. (1976). Cancer patients: Your special role. *Nursing, 76, 6,* 25–29.

McCorkle, R., & Lewis, F. M. (1980). Research in cancer nursing. *Seminars in Oncology, 7,* 80–87.

McCorkle, R., & Young, K. (1978). Development of a symptom distress scale. *Cancer Nursing 1,* 373–378.

McGuire, D., Frank-Stromborg, M., & Varricchio, C. (1985). 1984 ONS research committee survey of membership's research priorities. *Oncology Nursing Forum, 12*(2), 99–103.

Miller, S. A. (1976). Is oncology nursing the challenge you are looking for? *Nursing 76, 6,* 70–72.

Nelson, K. R. (1959, March 20). Letter to Claire Richmond, Nursing Committee of American Cancer Society.

Nelson, K. R. (1974). The future in cancer nursing. *Proceedings of the National Conference on Cancer Nursing* (pp. 141–145). New York: American Cancer Society.

New use for a kelly pad [Letter to the Editor]. (1916). *American Journal of Nursing, 16,* 536.

Nursing Advisory Committee minutes. (1948a, April 30). New York: American Cancer Society.

Nursing Advisory Committee minutes. (1948b, October 18). New York: American Cancer Society.

Nursing Advisory Committee minutes. (1957, March 13). New York: American Cancer Society.

Nursing Advisory Committee minutes. (1958, October 20). New York: American Cancer Society.

Nursing Advisory Committee minutes. (1960, October 24). New York: American Cancer Society.

Oberst, M. (1978). Priorities in cancer nursing research. *Cancer Nursing, 1,* 281–290.

Oncology Nursing Society and American Nurses' Association. (1979). *Outcome Standards for Cancer Nursing Practice.* Kansas City, MO: American Nurses' Association.

Oncology Nursing Society Education Committee. (1988). Survey of graduate programs in cancer nursing. *Oncology Nursing Forum, 15,* 825–831.

Oncology Nursing Society Education Committee. (1995). *Standards of Oncology Nursing Education: Generalist and Advanced Practice Levels.* Pittsburgh, PA: Oncology Nursing Society.

Oncology Nursing Society. (1982). *The Outcome Standards for Cancer Nursing Education at the Fundamental Level.* Pittsburgh, PA: Oncology Nursing Society.

Patterson, L. (1948). Cancer institute. *Public Health Nursing, 40,* 83.

Peterson, R. (1948). Public health nursing in the cancer control program of the U.S. Public Health Service. *Public Health Nursing, 40,* 74–77.

Peterson, R. (1951a). Inservice education in cancer nursing. *Public Health Nursing, 43,* 255–258.

Peterson, R. (1951b). Inservice education in cancer nursing. *Public Health Nursing, 43,* 331–333.

Peterson, R. (1951c). Inservice education in cancer nursing. *Public Health Nursing, 43,* 386–389.

Peterson, R. (1956). Federal grants for education in cancer nursing. *Nursing Outlook, 4,* 103–105.

Peterson, R., & Walker, E. (1949). Integrating nursing service. *Hospitals, 23,* 61.

Quint, J. (1963). Impact of mastectomy. *American Journal of Nursing, 53,* 88–92.

Rice, F. (1902). Tumors. *Trained Nurse, 29,* 89–90.

Ross, E. (1928). How can we help in the control of cancer? *Public Health Nursing, 20,* 13–16.

Ross, W. (1987). *Crusade: The official history of the American Cancer Society.* New York: Arbor House.

Scovil, E. R., (1915). The medical aspects of cancer. *American Journal of Nursing, 15,* 855.

Shimkin, M. B. (1977). *Contrary to nature.* (DHEW Publication No. [NIH] 76–720). Washington DC: U.S. Government Printing Office.

Skipper, H. E., Schabel, F. M., & Wilcox, W. S. (1964). Experimental evaluation of potential anticancer agents. XIII. On the criteria and kinetics associated with the "curability" of experimental leukemia. *Cancer Chemotherapy Reports, 35,* 3–11.

Tatterhall, L. M. (1928). Salaries of public health nurses. *Public Health Nurse, 20,* 244–251.

The transmission and cure of cancer. (1907). *American Journal of Nursing, 7,* 200.

Tucker, L. E. (1915). Needed economies for a long case. *American Journal of Nursing, 15,* 293.

Wolf, E. S. (1964). Where hope comes first. *Nursing Outlook, 12,* 52–54.

Wolf, E. S. (1968). Nurse clinician in a specialty hospital. *Nursing Outlook, 16,* 41.

Yarbro, C. H. (1982). President's message. *Oncology Nursing Forum, 9*(4), 8.

Yarbro, C. H. (1984). The early days: Four smiles and a post office box. *Oncology Nursing Forum, 11,* 79–85.

Yarbro, C. H., & Yarbro, J. W. (1993). Historial development of cancer programs. *Seminars in Oncology Nursing, 9,* 3–7.

Zubrod, C. G. (1979). Milestones in curative chemotherapy. *Seminars in Oncology, 6,* 490–505.

CHAPTER

3

Role Implementation in Cancer Nursing

Mary E. Cooley • Diane L. Spatz • Joyce M. Yasko

Oncology nursing is one of the most dynamic specialties available for nurses. New developments in science and technology have created exciting options for the prevention, early detection, treatment, and palliation of cancer. To provide the complex care that patients with a potential or actual diagnosis of cancer and their families require, an in-depth knowledge base is necessary. Oncology nurses have responded to the challenge of high technologic care by developing a sophisticated level of expertise that incorporates a caring and holistic approach to care. This chapter discusses the development and implementation of the oncology nursing role, presents current trends in the advanced practice nursing role, and highlights future issues in implementation of the oncology nurses' role.

PROFESSIONAL NURSING PRACTICE IN ONCOLOGY

Because cancer is such a prevalent disease, three levels of nursing practice have evolved to provide cancer services. These levels include the generalist nurse, the oncology nurse, and the advanced practice oncology nurse (Tiffany, 1987).

The generalist nurse has undergone basic preparation as a registered professional nurse. Additional training in oncology is usually acquired through work experience and attending continuing education activities. Although individuals with cancer are part of the generalist's practice, they form only one part of the caseload of patients. This nurse practices in a variety of settings such as home care, nutrition support, infusion therapy, and community hospitals, and provides care to the majority of individuals with cancer.

The oncology nurse provides specialized care to individuals with a potential or actual diagnosis of cancer and their families. Therefore, a cancer-specific knowledge base and clinical competence in cancer care must be acquired in addition to completion of a basic nursing program (McNally, Somerville, Miakowski, & Rostad, 1991). Certification in basic oncology nursing is strongly recommended. Traditionally, oncology nurses have practiced in acute care settings and have provided care to patients who were receiving active treatment. Today, however, oncology nursing extends to all care settings (Stalsbroten & Baird, 1991).

The advanced practice oncology nurse requires in-depth knowledge in oncology and provides expert care to individuals with a potential or actual diagnosis of cancer and their family members. A master's degree is the minimum educational requirement for advanced practice nursing (ONS, 1990). The traditional role of the advanced practice nurse in oncology was the oncology clinical nurse specialist. Recent trends, however, have introduced the role of the oncology nurse practitioner. The differences and similarities as well as the controversies surrounding these roles are discussed later in this chapter.

THE DEVELOPMENT OF EXPERT ONCOLOGY NURSING PRACTICE

Oncology nursing is a practice discipline. Therefore, it is essential to identify strategies to assist nurses in making a transition from the student role to clinician.

Creative programs that combine practice and education are necessary to facilitate the development of oncology nurses who have expertise in the many facets of cancer care.

Benner's (1984) work, *From Novice To Expert: Excellence and Power in Clinical Nursing Practice,* provides a framework to discuss the development of the oncology nursing role. Benner (1984) identified the differences in the clinical performance and situation appraisal of beginning and expert nurses using the Dreyfus (1980) model of skill acquisition. This model proposes that one moves through five levels of proficiency when developing a new skill: novice, advanced beginner, competent, proficient, and expert.

Novice. The novice is at the beginning level of clinical practice. This nurse has learned principals and theory but has no practical experience to guide decision making. As a result, reliance on strict rules and objective measurable phenomena such as temperature, heart rate, and blood pressure are necessary to guide actions.

Advanced Beginner. The advanced beginner is able to demonstrate marginally acceptable performance. Although these nurses have begun to accumulate practical experience, they still need assistance in setting priorities and in making accurate assessments.

Competent. Competent nurses begin to base their interventions on conscious, deliberate planning and long-range goals. They are able to differentiate attributes of a situation that are important from those that can be ignored. A feeling of mastery over clinical problems begins to emerge after working in similar clinical situations for 2 to 3 years.

Proficient. The proficient nurse has developed a solid foundation in clinical practice and begins to see the situation as a whole rather than discrete aspects. As a result of rich clinical experiences, the proficient nurse is able to detect nuances of a situation and identify the most important aspects of the clinical situation. This stage of development usually takes 3 to 5 years of working in similar clinical situations.

Expert. The expert practitioner, with many years of clinical experience, perceives the situation as a whole and is able to immediately and accurately identify the problem. This nurse is recognized for quick action and keen clinical judgment. The term "Critical incidents" has been coined by Benner (1984) to capture those situations where the expert nurses' intervention made a crucial difference in the patient's outcome. Benner (1984) believes that systematic evaluation of the critical incidents of expert practitioners is an important step in clinical knowledge development.

Benner's framework was used to evaluate the role and the clinical competency of advanced practice nurses. Fenton (1985) examined the performance of clinical nurse specialists in a hospital setting. This study verified the high level of skill acquisition in these practitioners and further expanded Benner's domains. Additional areas of skilled performances were identified; these included the presence of teaching and providing emotional support to staff nurses, acting as change agents within the organization, and providing expert advice to other members of the health care team. In a similar study, Brykcznski (1989) evaluated the role and clinical competency of nurse practitioners in an ambulatory care setting using Benner's framework. Findings from the study supported a high level of skill acquisition of these practitioners and expanded Benner's domains for skills specific for nurse practitioners. The new domains that were specific for the nurse practitioner included management of patient health/illness status and providing expert advice to other health care providers.

Benner's (1984) model also identifies the teaching and learning needs of the nurse at each level of proficiency. The novice and advanced beginner need close supervision and guidance to develop strong clinical skills. Basic physical and psychosocial assessment, clinical decision making, psychomotor skill acquisition (i.e., venipuncture), and effective interpersonal communication have been identified as the most important learning needs during this time (Johnson, Cohen, & Hull, 1994). Preceptor programs have been effective in helping novice nurses make a successful transition to the competent stage of proficiency (Cooper, 1990).

Although competent nurses begin to have a sense of mastery over clinical problems, they lack the speed and flexibility of the proficient nurse. Both the competent and proficient nurse need to develop complex competencies. Interactive methods of learning such as the use of decision making games, case studies, and nursing rounds have been suggested as methods to help competent and proficient nurses increase their clinical skills (Benner 1984; Cobb & Cooley, 1986; Lin et al., 1993). For these nurses to progress to the expert level of practice, however, mentoring is essential (Cooper, 1990). Johnson et al. (1994) identified that mentoring was an important aspect of developing expertise in oncology nursing. Role modeling and providing information and interpersonal support were the most helpful mentoring behaviors. Faculty members or clinical nurse specialists were the individuals most likely to provide mentoring in the clinical setting.

THE DEVELOPMENT OF A KNOWLEDGE BASE IN ONCOLOGY NURSING

Oncology nursing is a complex, multifaceted discipline that deals with the physical, psychosocial, and economic impact of the potential or actual diagnosis of cancer. To provide optimal patient care, the development and cultivation of a knowledge base for practice is essential. Formal academic educational programs, continuing education activities, mentor-protege relationships, government and community resources, and certification in oncology nursing are various methods to promote learning.

ACADEMIC PREPARATION

UNDERGRADUATE ACADEMIC EDUCATIONAL PROGRAMS

Participating in formal academic educational programs is generally the first step in acquiring a knowledge base in nursing. However, content in oncology nursing is not presented in the majority of undergraduate programs in the United States (Brown, 1983). This absence may be the result of the integrated or medical model approach to nursing education or the inadequate numbers of undergraduate faculty prepared in oncology nursing. Ways that oncology nursing can be taught at the undergraduate level are formalized courses, integrated content, and electives in oncology nursing—all with planned clinical experiences. An elective in oncology may be taken along with the basic curriculum or after graduation. Courses of this nature are a comprehensive foundation for specialization in oncology nursing.

A survey completed in 1983 by Brown found that only 19 per cent of undergraduate nursing programs included formalized courses, clinical experiences, or both in cancer nursing and that if cancer nursing was included in the curriculum, little time was devoted to this content (Brown, 1983). In a survey conducted by Mayer and Yasko (1990), a survey of masters-prepared oncology nurses revealed that the number of masters programs in oncology nursing has expanded from 13 in 1981 to 45 in 1988. However, the masters-prepared nurses who were functioning in faculty roles had fewer formalized educational courses and less clinical experience than those in clinical nurse specialist and nursing administrator roles. The results of this study further illustrate the fact that students are being taught by teachers who have not had academic preparation in oncology nursing. It is unlikely that the trend of inadequate preparation in oncology nursing will be reversed in the near future. A concentrated effect to remedy the present situation must be made. Providing continuing education courses for nursing educators, developing the undergraduate electives in oncology nursing, and influencing undergraduate faculty to include oncology nursing content are but a few of the possible actions that can be taken to remedy the situation. Pierce (1992) suggests that since undergraduate students are prepared to practice as generalist nurses and provide the majority of care to patients with cancer, there must be a minimal level of competency regarding cancer care that includes knowledge of the most common cancers, their associated risk factors, prevention, early detection, diagnostic interventions, and basic treatment options. Further development into expert oncology nurses must be undertaken by the individual nurse and the nursing service administrators that employ the nurse. See Chapter 71 for discussion of other strategies to gain knowledge in oncology nursing.

ADVANCED PRACTICE ACADEMIC EDUCATIONAL PROGRAMS

Progression to the advanced practice of oncology nursing usually occurs as a result of increased knowledge, a sound practice base, and advanced (masters or doctoral level) educational preparation. In addition to providing an advanced knowledge base, a graduate-level education program also provides preparation in the theoretic basis of nursing practice, the trends and issues that have an actual or potential impact on nursing, the process of nursing research, and the theories that influence advanced nursing practice such as conflict, role, change, stress, learning, organizational management, and system theories. Deciding to enter a graduate-level nursing program requires a large amount of time, energy, and money. Although choosing a program that is best suited to the nurses' needs may not be easy, there are several resources that may be helpful. The Oncology Nursing Society's Education Committee compiles a list of graduate programs in cancer nursing on a regular basis (Brown & Hinds, 1994). In addition, Hagopian and McCorkle (1993), experienced educators in oncology nursing, published an article that provides practical advice on choosing a graduate program in the United States.

CONTINUING EDUCATION

Seminars, courses, and programs of variable length and content are available in most geographic areas. Continuing education programs that meet content and evaluation criteria are reviewed and awarded approval for a specified number of content hours by a provider of continuing education in nursing accredited by the regional accrediting committee of the American Nurses' Association. Continuing education courses should be reviewed to determine whether accreditation has been obtained. This is an essential step to ensure quality.

While attending continuing education programs, participants should identify areas of inadequate knowledge and focus their efforts on obtaining the necessary knowledge and incorporating it in their practice of oncology nursing. A Gaps and Contracts method can be utilized to ensure that this occurs. During a continuing education program, the nurse identifies gaps between current practices and what is being presented during the program. At the completion of the program, nurses list the gaps identified in order of importance and develop a contract—written or mental—that includes the methods, resources, and time required to incorporate the newly acquired knowledge into their individual practices or the practices of the oncology nurses working in a specific agency (Barg, McCorkle, Robinson, Yasko, Jepson, & McKeehan, 1992; Donovan, Wolpert, & Yasko, 1981).

Continuing education courses or seminars offer an excellent opportunity to learn from those who have advanced competence in oncology nursing. Continuing education programs in oncology nursing served as the formalized introduction to oncology nursing for the majority of those who call themselves oncology nurses today. History reveals that the first formalized oncology nursing educational courses were continuing education programs. In the mid 1970s, when oncology nursing was beginning to organize, the National Cancer Institute (NCI) released a request for a proposal to develop oncology nursing educational programs. The proposal was designed to include continuing education programs that provided a foundation in oncology nursing, master's programs that provided advanced preparation in oncology nursing, and a continuing education program that focused on the prevention and early detection of cancer and taught nurses to utilize early detection skills in their practice of oncology nursing. Academic sites throughout the nation were funded to carry out these efforts. The programs that developed as a result of this NCI effort provided a network of educational resources and prepared nurses to care for persons with cancer.

Participating in independent study is an essential ingredient in obtaining a knowledge base in oncology nursing. A number of written and audiovisual educational resources exist in oncology nursing. Written resources include oncology nursing textbooks, curriculum resources, self-learning modules, educational resources developed by pharmaceutical or medical supply companies, articles in refered journals, journals devoted entirely to oncology nursing, newsletters sponsored by professional organizations and pharmaceutical companies, and educational resources from the Oncology Nursing Society, the NCI, and the American Cancer Society (ACS).

Developing a resource library is an essential component of independent study. Each person has a limited amount of financial resources to allocate to developing a library; therefore, time should be spent reviewing the available resources before purchases are made. Access to a health center or hospital library is also essential for obtaining journals, textbooks, and other educational resources.

Independent study is essential to achieve and maintain competence in oncology nursing. A knowledge explosion is occurring in cancer research and cancer nursing. Only through consistent, disciplined, independent study will a comprehensive knowledge base be achieved and maintained.

ACCESS TO A MENTOR

A mentor is needed throughout a professional career. A mentor is a professional nurse who has expertise in oncology nursing and who is willing to share that expertise with others—someone who is interested in helping other nurses become the best that they can be. A mentor does not compete but rather takes pleasure in seeing others be and become. Every professional needs a mentor who will give positive and negative feedback, pave the way for opportunities to occur, and offer unconditional support, advice, and counsel. The goal of a mentor-protégé relationship is to help the protégé reach the level of the mentor faster than the mentor and with less difficulty. One outgrows specific mentors but never the need for a mentor.

Mentor-protégé relationships rarely just happen; they must be initiated, developed, and cultivated. Nurses must identify potential mentors who exemplify the kind of oncology nurse that they would like to emulate. They then communicate their perceptions to the would-be mentors, ask if they would be willing to support, teach, and counsel, and then foster the relationship by giving the mentors feedback on how the information provided has been utilized and what outcomes have been achieved. It is important for nurses to ac-

knowledge their mentors as they achieve their goals and to multiply the benefits received by becoming mentors to other nurses who have less knowledge, experience, or both. Becoming mentors to oncology nurses is one of the most effective ways to advance the practice of oncology nursing. This process is both a professional right and a responsibility.

GOVERNMENT AND COMMUNITY AGENCIES

Government and community agencies are a major source of educational resources and opportunities for the development of a knowledge base. Examples of agencies that produce a variety of written resources, support groups, educational services, and opportunities are the following:

- American Cancer Society: National, state, and local units. The ACS provides continuing education programs and written resources for health professionals, patients and families, and the public. Scholarships for graduate education (master's and doctoral programs) are also available, as are professorships in oncology nursing. A local unit can be contacted for information.
- National Cancer Institute: Cancer centers and cancer information services funded by the NCI are valuable resources. The nearest cancer information center can be reached by calling 1-800-4-CANCER. This service provides information on cancer pathology, prevention, early detection, treatment and rehabilitation, and community resources, as well as information on how to effectively utilize the health care system.
- Cancer centers, university health systems, and community hospitals also provide educational seminars and on-site clinical experiences. Each community also has local resources such as Make Today Count, the Ostomy Association, and others. These resources are usually listed in the telephone directory or are available through the social services department of local hospitals.

The key factors in developing and maintaining a comprehensive knowledge base in oncology nursing are to utilize as many educational resources as possible, capture every teachable moment, learn from those who have gone before, be consistent and thorough, and never stop learning. There is no substitute for a comprehensive knowledge base. Without it one cannot achieve competence as an oncology nurse or enter advanced practice roles. The time, effort, and money expended to develop and maintain a comprehensive knowledge base are sound investments in one's career.

CERTIFICATION AS AN ONCOLOGY NURSE

Certification is a credential used by the health professions to communicate that a person has the knowledge and experience to care for a specific patient population. The requirement for certification in oncology nursing communicates to the public, patient and family consumers, and other health professionals that specialized knowledge and clinical experience are needed to care safely and effectively for persons with cancer. There are two types of certification, basic and advanced practice, available through the oncology nursing certification corporation. When a nurse obtains certification via the Oncology Nursing Certification Corporate Examination, it communicates that the nurse has the knowledge and experience to care for persons with cancer and has the privilege of using the OCN (oncology certified nurse) or the AOCN (advanced oncology certified nurse) credential. Certification examinations are offered several times each year by the Educational Testing Service of Princeton, New Jersey. Information regarding eligibility criteria and location of testing sites can be obtained by contacting the Oncology Nursing Certification Corporation.

IMPLEMENTATION OF THE ROLE OF THE ONCOLOGY NURSE

Since its inception, oncology nursing has developed a wide array of innovative and creative roles. The four main components of the oncology nursing role are: clinical practice, education, administration, and research. The role components for the advanced practice oncology nurse are direct caregiver, coordinator, consultant, educator, researcher, and administrator. An additional role that is important for both the oncology nurse as well as the advanced practice nurse is that of collaborator and partner in a multidisciplinary team. Implementation of the nursing role varies depending on the educational preparation of the individual nurse, the patient population, and the practice setting. McMillian, Heusinkveld, and Spray (1995) recently demonstrated the differences and similarities between oncology nurses and advanced practice oncology nurses. A role delineation study was undertaken to define advanced clinical practice in oncology nursing. Six hundred thirty-seven masters-prepared oncology nurse clinicians and 619 baccalaureate nurses who were in the first 4 years of certification as oncology nurses responded to a survey. The survey consisted of 190 items that ascertained the frequency with which they performed direct caregiver, consultant, administrator/coordinator, researcher, and educator behaviors. Results of the survey demonstrated that direct clinical care and the educator role were performed most often by both groups, and these behaviors were believed to be the most important to their practice. The consultant and research behaviors illustrated the differences between the groups as they were reported more frequently in the advanced practice nurses.

Although clinical practice and educational activities are reported as the most frequent behaviors for both the oncology nurse and the advanced practice nurse, there is evidence that implementation of these roles differ. The American Nurses' Association and Oncology Nursing Society (1987) has developed outcome standards and guidelines for practice that provide the nurse with a framework for assessment. There are 11 common problems that occur in individuals with a potential or actual diagnosis of cancer. Using this framework,

the oncology nurse performs a comprehensive assessment that includes physical, psychosocial, and financial aspects of care. The advanced practice nurse shares these skills with the oncology nurse but often focuses on providing effective symptom management (McGee, Powell, Broadwell, & Clark, 1987). In addition to these skills, however, the advanced practice nurse may need to conduct a comprehensive history and physical examination, order laboratory tests, write prescriptions, and/or initiate referrals to other health care providers (Maxwell, 1979; Sawyers, 1993). Similarly, psychomotor skills required by the oncology nurse and the advanced practice nurse may differ. Several surveys were conducted in ambulatory care and revealed the psychomotor skills that oncology nurses performed most frequently were care of catheters, ports and pumps, dressing changes, venipuncture, administration of intravenous medications, chemotherapy, and blood products (Barhamand, 1991; ONS, 1991). Although there are no published reports of the psychomotor skills that advanced practice nurses perform, anecdotal evidence in the literature suggest that these nurses prescribe chemotherapy medications according to protocols and perform bone marrow biopsies and lumbar punctures (Lin, 1994; Maxwell, 1979; Sawyers, 1993).

Educational activities are central to the role of the oncology nurse. Educating patients and families about self-care behaviors related to treatment modalities, developing structured educational programs, and implementing support groups have been identified as the most frequent activities (Barhamand, 1991; Garvey & Kramer, 1983). The oncology nurse is often described as the "anchor" of the health care team and has the most consistent contact with patients and their family members (Pluth, 1993). Developing mutually agreeable goals between the nurse and the patient is an important aspect of care. Promoting patient autonomy in making health care decisions and supporting their desired goals for care is the essence of oncology nursing practice (Steeves, Cohen, & Wise, 1994). Advanced practice nurses may share similar educational activities but often provide support to the staff nurse for complex patient teaching and teach other nurses and precept graduate students in oncology nursing (Hagopian, Ferszt, Jacobs, & McCorkle, 1992).

Oncology nurses have primary responsibility for coordinating the care of patients and communicate their patient assessment to other health care providers (McCorkle, 1979). Administrative duties are common in many areas of practice and include participating in continuous quality improvement and committees. Advanced practice nurses are often involved in helping to develop policies and procedures in the clinical area. They may also coordinate the care for complex patient populations (Lin, 1993).

Collaboration is inherent to the role of oncology nurses. Building interdisciplinary relationships is essential if the health disciplines are to work as a team. Teamwork does not just happen; it is based on trust in, respect for, and dependence on team members and the realization that the whole is more efficient and effective than any one of its parts. Each discipline has a unique role to play, and it is the responsibility of members of that discipline to communicate to other team members a description of that role so that expectations will be grounded in reality. Often there are grey areas in which no one has official responsibility but that several team members want to claim as their responsibility; sometimes just the opposite occurs, and no one on the team wants to take responsibility for these grey areas. When this situation occurs, open negotiation with team members should occur so that expectations will be consistent and all responsibilities will be accounted for. Building relationships with members of other disciplines also provides a source of knowledge, support, and acceptance. The greater the amount of interdisciplinary communication and intervention, the greater will become the awareness, understanding, and acceptance of the role and responsibilities of oncology nursing.

Developing relationships with individuals holding administrative positions, such as chief executive officers, fiscal officers, and others within the employing agency, is essential if oncology nurses are to be involved, understood, and allowed to grow and develop. Oncology nurses must take every opportunity to communicate with individuals in administrative roles about the needs of persons with cancer and their families, the resources that are needed to provide an optimal level of care, and the methods to recruit and retain qualified oncology nurses. Oncology nurses can assist the administrative staff in meeting the goals that they have set for the employing agency. They should not wait to be invited to participate. Nurses can join together and submit written proposals to develop programs, to decrease the cost of care, to improve the efficiency and effectiveness of care, and to recruit and retain qualified nurses.

It is beneficial to develop an attitude of working with administrative personnel to accomplish agency goals and to teach them and demonstrate for them how oncology nurses can assist in the process. This strategy not only will facilitate the acceleration of the power and status of oncology nursing within the agency but also will assist in the process of promoting this attitude in administrators nationally.

Research activities of nurses vary depending on the setting. Oncology nurses often provide care to patients undergoing intensive research protocols or may be part of the research team. Since the beginning of oncology nursing, nurses have been an integral part of the research team. Recently, oncology nurses have assumed roles as data managers for clinical trials (White-Hershey & Nevidjon, 1990). As early as 1980, McCorkle and Lewis (1980) advocated a role for nurses as primary investigators. Although advanced practice nurses are involved with disseminating research findings, evidence from a recent survey identified that nurses would like to increase their activity in research (McMillian, Heusinkveld, & Spray, 1995). Competing demands from the clinical area provide barriers to effective implementation of the research role. This is an area of the oncology nurse's role that needs further development to advance the profession.

There is evidence to suggest that oncology nurses' and advanced practice nurses' work closely together in the clinical area and that their skills often complement each other. Both roles are essential for further development of the profession. An excellent example of collegial role development is provided by Watson (1993) (Box 3–1). In an innovative program, a rural cancer outreach program was developed that utilized the

---

Box 3–1. *Role Development in a Rural Cancer Outreach Program*

Watson, A. C. (1993). The role of the psychosocial oncology CNS in a rural cancer outreach program. *Clinical Nursing Specialist, 7,* 259–265.

Purpose: (1) Describe the implementation of an urban-rural nurse oncology program. (2) Describe the role of the psychosocial oncology clinical nurse specialist in implementing the program.

Data Sources: Published reports, journal articles, anecdotal report.

Setting: A rural cancer outreach program was initiated by Massey Cancer Center, Medical College of Virginia, Virginia Commonwealth University, Richmond, Virginia, to bring state-of-the-art cancer treatment to rural Virginians in their own communities.

Data Synthesis: The goals of the program were to: (1) Provide cancer care to all patients in the rural community. (2) Keep patients functional in their own communities. (3) Educate rural physicians and nurses to provide the care. (4) Develop economically viable cancer care services for rural hospitals. (5) Develop community-based initiatives to address prevention, detection, and treatment of cancer.

Rural oncology nurses provide day-to-day physiologic and psychologic support to cancer patients in their own communities by giving chemotherapy, monitoring lab values, managing central and peripheral venous access devices, and assessing psychologic and rehabilitative needs of families with cancer. The clinical nurse specialists provide periodic on-site clinical and educational support and are available for consultation on a daily basis by telephone and fax support.

The psychosocial oncology clinical nurse specialist described the implementation of the clinician, consultant, networker, coach, educator, change agent, supervisor, and research subroles.

Conclusions: Implementation of the program was successful. Collaboration among rural nurses, clinical nurse specialists, and a multidisciplinary team provided quality, competent health care through a rural outreach program.

Implications: Recommendations for research in rural nursing cancer care emerged from the implementation of this program and included development and implementation of nurse-managed clinics, study of reimbursement issues for advanced practice nurses in rural areas, and further exploration into urban nurse-rural nurse collaboration.

skills of both oncology nurses and advanced practice nurses to provide care to individuals in a rural setting.

McDonnell and Ferrell (1992) reported the results of the Oncology Life Cycle Task Force. This task force was convened by the Oncology Nursing Society to help understand the oncology nurse's role and patterns of recruitment and retention. Ten key concepts were identified that influenced the implementation of the nurse's role (Figure 3–1). Concepts such as the essence of oncology nursing, nurses' involvement with patients and families, the importance of influential people to provide mentoring, and the role diversity within oncology nursing have been highlighted in previous discussion. Several other areas noted in the model warrant discussion. The need for a supportive environment, the nature of the work, and the opportunity for specialization are important considerations.

Effective implementation of the role of the oncology nurse requires a supportive environment that will promote the personal and professional development of the nurse and allow one to provide nursing care that results in effective patient and family outcomes. Developing a personal philosophy of cancer care is a necessary first step in identifying a supportive environment. It is recommended that each nurse develop a personal philosophy of oncology nursing and a positive concept of the unique and essential role of oncology nurses. A philosophy of nursing is a person's prescribed beliefs about what oncology nursing is and what it is not. It is necessary for an oncology nurse to be in touch with personal beliefs, because these beliefs form the foundation of practice. If a nurse believes that oncology nursing is holistic in nature and includes physiologic as well as psychologic care but agency policy states that psychologic care is to be referred to other disci-

plines, or if providing psychological care is not rewarded or viewed as important by the nurse's peers or agency, then a conflict will occur between personal beliefs about the practice on a daily basis. These conflicts can cause discomfort, dissatisfaction, and burnout in the work environment. Many researchers have described burnout as unfulfilled job expectations—when what the individual thought a job would be differs from what it actually is (Dolan, 1987; McElroy, 1982); in other words, a person's philosophy of care cannot be fulfilled in the work environment. An exercise that will help to clarify personal beliefs and values is to write a philosophy of nursing by completing the sentence, "I believe oncology is . . .." Once written, the philosophy of oncology nursing can be a method of keeping in touch with one's beliefs. A philosophy can be altered or expanded as one's scope of knowledge and experience grows (see Chapter 1).

Working in an environment that supports the nurses' beliefs about oncology nursing is important because of the nature of the work. Cohen and Sarter (1992) conducted a study as part of the Oncology Life Cycle Task Force goals to understand the nurses' role (Box 3–2). Nurses in this study described working with patients with cancer "as being on the front lines of a war against death, disfigurement, and intense human suffering" (Carter & Sarter, 1992, p. 1485). A typical day was full of surprises. Handling physiologic emergencies, recognizing potential life-threatening errors, and "being there" for patients in emotional distress were the most important elements of their practice. Given the nature of these stressors, a supportive work environment and the need for balancing personal and professional roles are necessary.

There is an enormous variety of roles and opportunities for specialization within oncology nursing. Nurses work in all types of positions: staff nurse, office nurse, school nurse, advanced practice nurse, and research nurse, and in all types of settings: ambulatory care, physician offices, schools, hospitals, and home care/hospice. Specialization in oncology has evolved in response to the diverse practice settings, complex patient populations, and multiple treatment modalities. The Oncology Nursing Society is an organization that promotes specialization in oncology nursing and offers numerous opportunities for professional development. Membership in the oncology nursing society provides nurses with a journal subscription, educational opportunities, local networking through chapter activities, and national networking through special interest groups. The special interest groups were developed to support the members' interest for specialization within oncology nursing (Table 3–1).

ADVANCED PRACTICE IN ONCOLOGY NURSING

The advanced practice role in oncology nursing has undergone tremendous change within the last several years. The traditional advanced practice nurse in oncology was the clinical nurse specialist. Recent trends,

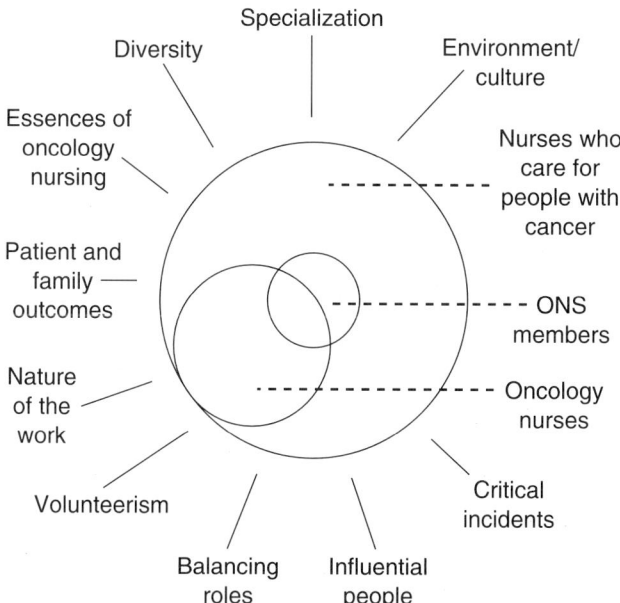

FIGURE 3–1. Essential concepts of the life cycle of the oncology nurse. (From McDonnell, K., & Ferrell, B. [1992]. ONS life cycle task force report: The life cycle of the oncology nurse. *Oncology Nursing Forum, 19,* 1545–1550.)

Box 3–2. *Oncology Nurses' View of Their Work*

Cohen, M. Z., & Sarter, B. (1992). Love and work: Oncology nurses' view of the meaning of their work. *Oncology Nursing Forum, 19,* 1481–1486.

Purpose: Obtain a better understanding of how nurses caring for cancer view their work.

Sample: Twenty-three nurses working in a hospital who provided care to patients with cancer.

Methods: Phenomenologic interviews and participant observation of 23 nurses in one hospital were conducted by the investigators.

Each area's nursing director identified nurses who might be willing to discuss their work and who, in the director's opinion, could provide insights into oncology nursing. Additional nurses were identified by the researchers during participant interviews.

Cohen conducted more than 200 hours of participant observation on each unit and shift of one cancer hospital. In addition, interviews were conducted using phenomenologic techniques with 23 nurses working in this hospital. Interviews were tape-recorded, transcribed verbatim, and independently analyzed by the authors using phenomenologic techniques.

Results: The typical day for staff nurses comprised handling the unexpected, organizing and coordinating multiple tasks, setting priorities, and monitoring and assessing patients.

The typical day for charge nurses comprised trying to maintain staff morale, coordinating the flow of patients and caregivers, making equitable assignments, coping with short staffing, handling unexpected problems, and "keeping track" of everything.

The essence of cancer nursing, identified through critical incidents, was successfully handling physiologic emergencies, recognizing potential for patients in emotional distress, and having empathy for patients' experiences.

The difficulties that nurses encountered with their work included poor staffing, unexpected crisis, patient deaths, balancing work and personal life, and difficult medical staff.

The rewards that nurses experienced in their work included patients becoming well and patients' gratitude for emotional support.

Conclusions: Oncology nursing requires the performance, prioritization, and coordination of multiple, complex tasks. Nurses must handle frequent physiologic and psychologic crises. Therefore, monitoring the patient for sudden problems and life-threatening errors is essential. Although stressful, oncology nursing carries many rewards.

---

however, have introduced the role of the oncology nurse practitioner. There has been controversy in the oncology nursing community and the nursing profession over whether these roles should become blended into a singular advanced practice nursing role. Both of these roles evolved approximately 25 years ago. The historic development, differences, and similarities between roles and the move toward a blended role are discussed. The resulting professional and legal implications for advanced practice follow.

TABLE 3–1. *Oncology Nursing Society Special Interest Groups*

Advanced Nursing Research	Hospice
Ambulatory/Office Nursing	Lymphedema Management
Biotherapy	Management
Bone Marrow Transplant	Nurse Practitioner
Cancer Program Development and Management	Pain Management
	Patient Education
	Pediatrics
Cancer Rehabilitation	Prevention/Early Detection
Chemotherapy	Psychoneuroimmunology
Clinical Nurse Specialist	Psychosocial
Clinical Trial Nurses	Radiation
Critical Care	Spiritual Care
Ethics	Staff Education
HIV/AIDS	Surgical Oncology
Home Care	Survivorship
	Transcultural Nursing Issues

CLINICAL NURSE SPECIALIST

The clinical nurse specialist movement grew out of the need to improve patient care. The role was envisioned as a way to keep expert clinicians at the bedside. Programs were based in university settings and offered clinical specialization at the master degree level. The scope of practice included providing direct care and psychosocial support to patients about how to manage health care problems, serving as a role model to staff, providing consultation to staff about patient care issues, and conducting research on nursing practice outcomes (Steele & Fenton, 1988). Although implementation of this role was slow to start, clinical nurse specialists have begun to document the quality and cost-effectiveness of their care. Naylor and Brooten (1993) provide an excellent review of research conducted on the role of clinical nurse specialists. Multiple studies demonstrate that clinical nurse specialists improve patient outcomes and provide cost savings in a variety of vulnerable, high-cost populations.

In a landmark study by Brooten et al. (1986) the efficacy of clinical nurse specialists in caring for low birth weight infants after early discharge was demonstrated. In a randomized clinical trial, one group of very low birth weight infants was discharged earlier than hospital routine; the control group had no special interventions. For families in the early discharge group, instruction, counseling, home visits, and daily on-call availability of a perinatal clinical nurse specialist were provided. Families in the control group received routine care provided by the institution. The families followed in this study were primarily economically disadvantaged, poorly educated, and received public health insurance.

In the clinical nurse specialist, early discharge group, infants were able to be discharged at a mean of 11 days earlier, 200g less in weight and 2 weeks younger than the control group. No significant differences in rehospitalizations, acute care visits, or growth and development outcomes were found between the early discharge and the control group. Hospital charges were 27 per cent less and physician charges 22 per cent less for the early discharge nurse followed group.

Brooten et al. predicted that if just *half* of all very low birth weight infants born in the United States would receive this clinical nurse specialist service, the possible savings using conservative estimates would be $167 million dollars.

Naylor adapted Brooten's "Quality Cost Model of Transitional Care" for the elderly, including cancer patients. The clinical nurse specialist provided comprehensive discharge planning for the elderly patient and their primary caregiver and a minimum of two phone contacts in the 2 weeks after discharge. In the clinical nurse specialist followed group, there was a decrease in the total number of hospital readmissions, and the time between rehospitalizations was increased. Due to the success of this study, Naylor has now expanded the services of the clinical nurse specialist to include home visiting of these patients (Naylor, 1990).

In the oncology specialty, clinical nurse specialist care has also been demonstrated to be effective. McCorkle et al. (1989) conducted a randomized clinical trial to assess the effects of home nursing care for patients with progressive lung cancer. There were three groups: 1) home care by clinical nurse specialists, 2) home care by professional nurses, and 3) no home care.

The groups receiving nursing care had less symptom distress and more functional independence 6 weeks longer than the control group. The group followed by the clinical nurse specialist had significantly fewer hospitalizations for symptoms and complications of malignancy (McCorkle et al., 1989). In America, large amounts of money are spent on the aging population, especially during the last 2 weeks of life. By using a clinical nurse specialist, patients were able to be kept at home with family members at much lower health care costs (McCorkle, 1987). Programs such as this demonstrate improved quality of life for the terminally ill patient and a reduction in the cost of health care.

NURSE PRACTITIONER

The nurse practitioner movement grew out of a perceived shortage of primary care physicians. Although the first program was developed at the University of Colorado, most of the early programs were certificate programs. Many of the early nursing educators were not supportive of this role, because they believed that the role was too closely aligned with medical practice. Over time, however, the education of nurse practitioners has slowly moved back into a university setting. At

the present time, most of the nurse practitioner programs are offered at the master's degree level of education. Within the nurse practitioner's scope of practice, the nurse practitioner provides direct care, performs history and physical examinations, orders diagnostic tests, diagnoses common problems, initiates treatment, prescribes medications, and educates patients and families about how to manage health care.

The U.S. Congress Office of Technology Assessment (1986) found the quality of nurse practitioner care to be as good as or better than care provided by physicians. Additionally, nurse practitioners were found to have better communication, counseling, and interviewing skills than physicians have. Safriet (1992) also supports the high-quality cost effectiveness of nurse practitioners and advocates their use to increase access to primary care.

The Office of Technology Assessment report (1986) and Safriet's analysis (1992) of advanced practice nursing both are landmark publications that cite the effectiveness of nurse practitioners. Additionally, multiple examples of nurse practitioners' effects on outcomes are published in the health care literature; therefore only two articles are cited that highlight different areas of expertise of nurse practitioners.

Over the past decade, the findings of several demonstration projects confirm that the use of geriatric nurse practitioners in nursing homes substantially improves patient outcomes and ensures a more rational system of care without increasing cost. The Mountain States Health Corporation, based in Idaho, conducted a project to recruit, train, and place geriatric nurse practitioners in 13 western states between 1976 and 1986. After training and placement, two groups of nursing homes were compared for quality of care and services utilization. Thirty nursing homes that employed geriatric nurse practitioners and 30 control nursing homes were matched. Favorable changes in the nurse practitioner group were seen in two out of eight activity of daily living measures, five out of 18 nursing therapies, and two of six drug therapies. Additionally there was some reduction in hospital admissions and the total number of days for admissions in the nursing homes with geriatric nurse practitioners (Kane et al., 1988, 1989). These findings suggest the usefulness of nurse practitioners in this capacity.

Ramsay, McKenzie, and Fish (1982) examined two groups of patients with hypertension. One group (*n* = 40) underwent follow-up by physicians at a clinic, and the other group (*n* = 40) received nurse practitioner care at a clinic. Demographic and clinical characteristics of the two groups were not significantly different. The study findings indicated that patients cared for by nurse practitioners had better quality outcomes (Ramsay et al., 1982). A significant difference in weight reduction was documented with patients cared for by nurse practitioners as compared with those cared for by physicians. The patients in the nurse practitioner clinic had significantly lower blood pressures after 12 months of care. Attrition rates were similar for both groups but were particularly high in patients not receiving medication in the physician clinic (Ramsay et al., 1982).

The cumulative evidence demonstrates that nurse practitioners provide cost-effective care that substitutes for physician services for many different patient populations. More important, nurse practitioners can provide primary, acute, and long-term care services to people of all ages. As more roles for nurse practitioners evolve in oncology nursing, it will be important to document outcomes affected by the role.

BLENDED ROLE BETWEEN CLINICAL NURSE SPECIALIST AND NURSE PRACTITIONER

Historically, the clinical nurse specialist worked in the hospital setting, and the nurse practitioner worked in the outpatient setting. With a move toward outpatient care and an emphasis on cost-effectiveness, these roles have begun to converge, and this distinction is no longer true (Hockenberry-Eaton & Powell, 1992). The newsletters of the ANA council of the clinical nurse specialist and the council for primary care featured an editorial examining the similarities and differences between the advanced practice roles in 1986 (Sparacino & Durand, 1986). As a result of this initial exploration into the advanced practice roles, the ANA executive committee convened a joint meeting to discuss a merger of the two councils. Subsequently, the councils were combined in 1991 and formed a singular advanced practice council.

There has been much controversy over the future role of the advanced practice nurse. Although the ANA made a decision to merge the clinical nurse specialist and nurse practitioner councils, not all specialty organizations within nursing have followed this initiative. The Oncology Nursing Society continues to maintain separate special interest groups for advanced practice nurses (Table 3–1). The similarities and the differences between these roles are discussed, and controversies surrounding blending of the roles are presented. Several studies have demonstrated that the roles are more similar than they are dissimilar and that the core content between graduate programs differs primarily by increased emphasis on history taking, physical assessment skills, and pharmacology in the nurse practitioner programs (Elder & Bullough, 1990; Forbes, Rafson, Spross, & Kozlowski, 1990). Many agree that these

skills should be a comprehensive part of any clinical program for advanced practice nurses and that a blending of the roles is a natural evolution of the role.

Fenton and Brykcznski (1993) compared results of qualitative studies that evaluated the role and competencies of clinical nurse specialists and nurse practitioners. The results of this study demonstrated that although there were similarities of the roles, there were also distinct differences (Table 3–2). Page and Arena (1994) express concern over the move toward a combined role, fearing that nursing will lose its focus as a caring profession and shift laterally into medical roles. Similarly, McCaffrey-Boyle (1994a) emphasized that there is little discussion of maintaining the clinical nurse specialist subrole proficiencies in blending the advanced practice nursing roles.

There are no easy answers to the current controversies surrounding the evolution of the advanced practice roles. Oncology nursing is seated by a window of opportunity. There is a need to demonstrate that we can provide quality, cost-effective care. Oncology nursing must examine its priorities in providing care to patients with a potential or actual diagnosis of cancer and their families and evaluate how we can best position ourselves in the current health care environment. McCorkle (1977) suggested that oncology nursing is a challenge not to be taken lightly. There is evidence to suggest that advanced practice nurses in oncology are in need of nurse practitioner skills. It is essential, however, to maintain a focus on specialty care that provides a caring, holistic approach. Educational programs that provide this focus are needed to help us meet the challenges that lie ahead.

LEGAL AND PROFESSIONAL ISSUES IN ADVANCED PRACTICE

Proponents of blending the role of the clinical nurse specialist and nurse practitioner suggest that unity would increase our political power, thereby enhancing opportunities for reimbursement, prescribing ability, and increasing public acceptance by decreasing confusion over the many types of advanced practice nurses. A brief review of these issues is summarized.

TABLE 3–2. *Distinctions and Similarities in the Practice of Nurse Practitioners and Clinical Nurse Specialists*

DISTINCTIVE PRACTICE OF NURSE PRACTITIONER	SIMILARITIES OF PRACTICE BETWEEN NURSE PRACTITIONER AND CLINICAL NURSE SPECIALIST	DISTINCTIVE PRACTICE OF CLINICAL NURSE SPECIALIST
Primary care	Patient advocate	Specialty care
73% of time spent in direct care	Physician collaboration	52% of time spent in direct care
Perform history and physical exam	Interprofessional collaboration	Conduct support groups
Prescribe medications	Provide emotional and informational	Teach and role model for staff nurses
Initiate treatment	support to patient and family	Participate in policy and procedure
Provider of care	Advanced health assessment	development
Health promotion, illness prevention, long term management of chronic, stable conditions	Clinical decision making	Facilitator of care (Case Manager) Acute and intense period of illness

(Data from Fenton, M. V., & Brykczynski, K. A. [1993]. Qualitative distinctions and similarities in the practice of clinical nurse specialists and nurse practitioners. *Journal of Professional Nursing, 9,* 313–326.)

Third-Party Reimbursement

Reimbursement reform is necessary to enable nurses to be directly reimbursed for their services by the insurance provider (Safriet, 1992). Because states regulate the insurance industry, reimbursement of the advanced practice nurse varies based on state statutes. Federal reimbursement and reimbursement in some states currently occurs for certified nurse midwives and nurse practitioners. However, there are many limitations and restrictions on which services are reimbursable. Also, the current level of reimbursement for advanced practice nursing services is lower than physician reimbursement in most states and from the federal government (Safriet, 1992).

States that have not done so already should enact nondiscrimination requirements for health insurance and contracts. This step would ensure that any service covered by the policy would be covered if provided by the APN as long as it is within the scope of practice (Safriet, 1992). These nondiscrimination requirements would extend to payment also, so that if direct reimbursement is available to one type of provider, it is available to all. Finally, all states should extend their Medicare regulations to reimburse APNs services. This would include services provided by nurse practitioners, midwives, clinical specialists, and nurse anesthetists (Safriet, 1992).

Prescriptive Authority

The ability to prescribe medications and the stipulations surrounding prescribing practices are marked with great differences dependent on the state in which one practices. The two primary areas of difference from state to state are the degree of professional autonomy and the range of drugs that the advanced practice nurse is authorized to prescribe (Pearson, 1992). Unfortunately, much of the current regulation in each state has been molded by organized medicine. Physicians are controlling nursing's prescriptive practices. The American Medical Association's position is that physicians should directly supervise prescriptive abilities and limit the types of drugs that advanced practice nurses may prescribe (Pearson, 1992).

Nurses, however, do possess adequate pharmacologic knowledge. Advanced practice nurses are educated regarding pharmacology pertinent to their specialty area. Additionally, all nurses receive a broad pharmacologic basic education in their baccalaureate programs. In the health care literature, there are few reports of APN's misusing their prescriptive authority. In fact, nurse practitioners are more likely to opt for alternative treatment before prescribing medication (Safriet, 1992).

Role Definition and Regulation

The first step in decreasing confusion is to come to an agreement in using one term, that being the "advanced practice nurse," to cover the range of individuals providing such nursing care. The term "advanced practice nurse" encompasses nurse practitioners and clinical nurse specialists in any specialty area, certified registered nurse anesthetists, and certified nurse midwives. Safriet (1992) recommends the following definition of the advanced practice nurse that was adapted from the Alaska Nurse Practice Act (Alaska Statute Sec. 08.68.410).

> "A registered nurse licensed to practice in this state who, because of specialized education and experience is authorized (certified) to perform acts of prevention, (medical) diagnosis, and the prescription of (medical) therapeutic or corrective measures under regulations adopted by the Board of Nursing" (p. 479).

This definition is broad enough to encompass the various types of advanced practice nursing, and the direct regulation of advanced practice nurses could be carried out by the Board of Nursing alone. The definition would legally recognize the role of the advanced practice nurse, and it empowers the Board of Nursing to develop and implement regulations specifically applicable to the advanced practice nurse (Safriet, 1992).

Currently, the regulations and control over advanced practice nurses vary widely from state to state (Board of Medicine, Joint Committees, Board of Nursing, or a combination). Implementation of a standard definition and sole regulating body can greatly decrease disparities in scope of practice and role responsibilities. Nursing can best determine the role, scope of practice, and necessary regulatory mechanisms for the advanced practice nurse, not physicians or other professions. It is essential that the profession come to agreement on this issue and actively pursue becoming the sole regulating body for advanced practice nurses.

FUTURE ISSUES FOR IMPLEMENTATION OF THE ROLE OF THE ONCOLOGY NURSE

The delivery of health care is changing rapidly in this country. There has been an emphasis on providing quality health care in a cost-effective manner. Although oncology nurses have made major strides in developing and implementing roles that are integral to providing health care to patients with a potential or actual diagnosis of cancer and their families, anticipation of future trends in health care is essential for a secure future. According to McCaffrey-Boyle, Engelking, and Harvey (1994), two major trends in health care, the pervasiveness of cancer and increased cost of technology-driven health care, will affect the future roles of oncology nurses.

Coile (1992) predicts that cancer will become the leading cause of death by the year 2000. The pervasiveness of cancer in our society will be affected by trends towards increasing age. The number of elderly in our population is expected to increase from 12 per cent currently to 21 per cent by the year 2030 (Spencer, 1989). The incidence of cancer increases markedly with age. Unfortunately, older individuals often present with more advanced stages of disease (Holmes & Hearne, 1981). Therefore, an emphasis on the prevention and early detection of cancer is essential. Nurses will need to broaden their knowledge about the elderly and health promotion to provide effective services and meet the special psychoeducational needs of this population.

The increased cost of technology-driven health care has caused a shift in the patterns of health care delivery. Aggressive cancer treatments, once reserved for the hospital, are now being delivered in the outpatient and home care setting. Oncology nurses will find a changing job market. There will be fewer opportunities in the acute care setting and an emphasis on ambulatory care. As a result, oncology nurses and advanced practice nurses must define new roles. McCaffrey-Boyle (1994b) predicts that new hybrids of nurses, such as gero-oncology intensivist and community cancer care consultant, will emerge from these trends. The need for advanced practice nurses will continue to increase dramatically. Promoting continuity of care for patients will be a major emphasis for nurses. Documenting advanced practice oncology nurses effectiveness in providing quality, cost-effective care must assume a priority in future clinical and research efforts.

REFERENCES

American Nurses' Association and Oncology Nursing Society. (1987). *Standards of oncology nursing practice.* Kansas City: American Nurses' Association.

Barg, F. K., McCorkle, R., Robinson, K., Yasko, Y. M., Jepson, C., & McKeehan, K. M. (1992). Gaps and contract: Evaluating the diffusion of new information. Part 1. A description of the strategy. *Cancer Nursing, 15,* 401–405.

Barhamand, B. (1991). A survey of the role, benefits, and realities of the office based oncology nurse. *Oncology Nursing Forum, 18,* 31–37.

Benner, P. (1984). *From novice to expert: Excellence and power in clinical nursing practice.* Menlo Park: Addison-Wesley Publishing Co.

Brooten, D., Kumar, S., Butts, P., Finkler, S., Bakewell-Sach, S., Gibbons, A., & Delivoria-Papadopoulos, M. (1986). A randomized clinical trial of early hospital discharge and home follow-up of very low birthweight infants. *New England Journal of Medicine, 315,* 934–939.

Brown, J. K. (1983). Survey of cancer nursing education in U.S. schools of nursing. *Oncology Nursing Forum, 10,* 82–83.

Brown, J. K., & Hinds, P. (1994). Assessing master's programs in oncology nursing. *Oncology Nursing Forum, 21,* 1239–1248.

Brykczynski, K. A. (1989). An interpretive study describing the clinical judgement of nurse practitioners. *Scholarly Inquiry for Nursing Practice, 3,* 75–104.

Cobb, S. C., & Cooley, M. E. (1988). Nursing rounds: Idea to reality. *Oncology Nursing Forum, 15,* 23–27.

Cohen, M. Z., & Sarter, B. (1992). Love and work: Oncology nurses' view of the meaning of their work. *Oncology Nursing Forum, 19,* 1481–1490.

Coile, R. (1992). *Health trends 1992. Special report.* Santa Clara, CA: The Health Forecaster Group.

Cooper, M. D. (1990). Mentorship: The key to the future of professionalism in nursing. *Journal of Perinatal and Neonatal Nursing, 4,* 71–77.

Dolan, N. (1987). The relationship between burnout and job satisfaction in nurses. *Journal of Advanced Nursing, 12,* 3–12.

Donovan, M. L., Wolpert, P., & Yasko, J. (1981). Gaps and contracts: An evaluation strategy. *Nursing Outlook, 29,* 467–471.

Dreyfus, S. E., & Dreyfus, H. L. (1980). *A five-stage model of the mental activities involved in directed skill acquisition.* Unpublished report supported by the Air Force Office of Scientific Research, USAF (Contract F49620-79-C-0063), University of California at Berkeley.

Elder, R., & Bullough, B. (1990). Nurse practitioners and clinical nurse specialists: Are the roles merging? *Clinical Nurse Specialist, 4,* 78–84.

Fenton, M. V. (1985). Identifying competencies of clinical nurse specialists. *Journal of Nursing Administration, 15,* 31–37.

Fenton, M. V., & Brykczynski, K. A. (1993). Qualitative distinctions and similarities in the practice of clinical nurse specialists and nurse practitioners. *Journal of Professional Nursing, 9,* 313–326.

Forbes, K., Rafson, J., Spross, J. A., & Kozlowski, D. (1990). Clinical nurse specialist and nurse practitioner core curriculum survey results. *Nurse Practitioner, 15,* 45–48.

Garvey, E., & Kramer, R. (1983). Improving cancer patients' adjustment to infusion chemotherapy: Evaluation of a patient education program. *Cancer Nursing, 6,* 373–378.

Hagopian, G. A., Ferszt, G., Jacobs, L., & McCorkle, R. (1992). Preparing clinical preceptors to teach master level students in oncology nursing. *Journal of Professional Nursing, 8,* 295–300.

Hagopian, G. A., & McCorkle, R. (1993). Choosing a master's program in cancer nursing in the United States. *Cancer Nursing, 16,* 473–478.

Hockenberry-Eaton, M., & Powell, M. (1992). Merging advanced practice roles: The NP and CNS. *Journal Pediatric Health Care, 2,* 158–159.

Holmes, F., & Hearne, E. (1981). Cancer stage to age relationship: Implications for cancer screening in the elderly. *Journal of American Geriatrics Society, 29,* 55–57.

Johnson, C. R., Cohen, M. Z., & Hull, M. M. (1994). Cultivating expertise in oncology nursing: Methods, mentors, and memories. *Oncology Nursing Forum, 21*(Suppl.), 27–34.

Kane, R. A., Kane, R. L., Arnold, S., Garrad, J., McDermott, S., & Kepferle, L. (1988). Geriatric nurse practitioners as nursing home employees: Implementing the role. *The Gerontologist, 28* 469–477.

Kane, R. L., Garrad, J., Skay, C. L., Radosevich, D. M., Buchanan, J. L., McDermott, S. M., Arnold, S. B., & Kepferle, L. (1989). Effects of a geriatric nurse practitioner on process and outcome of nursing home care. *American Journal of Public Health, 17,* 1271–1277.

Lin, E. M. (1994). A combined role of clinical nurse specialist and coordinator: Optimizing continuity of care in an autologous bone marrow transplant program. *Clinical Nurse Specialist, 8,* 48–55.

Lin, E. M., Aikin, J. L., Bailey, W., Fitzgerald, B., Mings, D., Mitchell, S., & Rigby, B. J. (1993). Improving ambulatory oncology nursing practice: An innovative educational approach. *Cancer Nursing, 16,* 53–62.

Maxwell, M. B. (1979). Nurse practitioner chemotherapy clinic. *Cancer Nursing, 1,* 211–218.

Mayer, D., & Yasko, J. (1990). Burnout in oncology administration educators and clinical nurse specialists. Unpublished manuscript.

McCaffrey-Boyle, D. (1994a). Where is the missing piece of the jigsaw puzzle? *Clinical Nurse Specialist, 8,* 117–121.

McCaffrey-Boyle, D. (1994b). New identities: The changing profile of patients with cancer, their families and their professional caregivers. *Oncology Nursing Forum, 21,* 55–61.

McCaffrey-Boyle, D., Engelking, C., & Harvey, C. (1994). Making a difference in the 21st century: Are oncology nurses ready? *Oncology Nursing Forum, 21,* 53–55.

McCorkle, R. (1977). Oncology nursing—a challenge not to be taken lightly. *Oncology Nursing Forum, 4,* 1–4.

McCorkle, R. (1979). A new beginning: The opening of a multidisciplinary cancer unit, Part 1. *Cancer Nursing, 1,* 201–209.

McCorkle, R. (1987). Complications of early discharge from hospitals. In American Cancer Society. *Proceedings of the Fifth National Conference—Human Values and Cancer.* New York: American Cancer Society.

McCorkle, R., Benoliel, J., Donaldson, G., Georgiadon, F., Moinpour, C., & Goodel, B. (1989). A randomized clinical trial of home nursing care for lung cancer patients. *Cancer, 64,* 1375–1382.

McCorkle, R., & Lewis, F. M. (1980). Research in cancer nursing. *Seminars in Oncology, 7,* 80–87.

McDonnell, K. K., & Ferrell, B. R. (1992). ONS life cycle task force report: The life cycle of the oncology nurse. *Oncology Nursing Forum, 19,* 1545–1550.

McElroy, A. (1982). Burnout—A review of the literature with application to cancer nursing. *Cancer Nursing, 5,* 211–217.

McGee, R. F., Powell, M. L., Broadwell, D. C., & Clark, J. C. (1987). A delphi survey of oncology clinical nurse specialist competencies. *Oncology Nursing Forum, 14,* 29–34.

McMillian, S. C., Heusinkveld, K. B., & Spray, J. (1995). Advanced practice in oncology nursing: A role delineation study. *Oncology Nursing Forum, 22,* 41–56.

McNally, J. C., Somerville, E. T., Miakowski, C., & Rostad, M. (1991). *Guidelines for oncology nursing practice.* Philadelphia: W.B. Saunders Co.

Naylor, M. (1990). Special feature: An example of a research grant application—comprehensive discharge planning for the elderly. *Research in Nursing and Health, 13,* 327–347.

Naylor, M., & Brooten, D. (1993). The roles and functions of clinical nurse specialists. *Image, 25,* 73–78.

Oncology Nursing Society. (1990). *Standards of advanced practice in oncology nursing.* Pittsburgh: Oncology Nursing Press.

Oncology Nursing Society. (1991). *National survey of salary, staffing, and professional practice patterns in ambulatory oncology.* Pittsburgh: Oncology Nursing Press.

Page, N. E., & Arena, D. M. (1994). Rethinking the merger of the clinical nurse specialist and the nurse practitioner roles. *Image, 26,* 315–318.

Pearson, C. J. (1992). 1991–92 update: How each state stands on legislative issues affecting advanced nursing practice. *Nurse Practitioner, 17,* 14–23.

Pierce, M. (1992). Undergraduate preparation of the oncology nurse. *Oncology Nursing Forum, 19,* 1234–1237.

Pluth, N. (1993). Continuity of care for patients and families through health care systems. In P. C. Buchsel & C. H. Yarbo, (Eds.), *Oncology nursing in the ambulatory setting: Issues in models of care.* Boston: Jones & Bartlett.

Ramsay, V. A., McKenzie, J. K., & Fish, D. G. (1982). Physicians and nurse practitioners, do they provide equivalent health care? *American Journal of Public Health, 73,* 55–56.

Safriet, B. (1992). Health care dollars and regulatory sense: The role of advanced practice nursing. *Yale Journal on Regulation, 9,* 417–488.

Sawyers, J. E. (1993). Defining your role in ambulatory care: Clinical nurse specialist or nurse practitioner? *Clinical Nurse Specialist, 7,* 4–7.

Sparacino, P. S. A., & Durand, B. (1986). Editorial on specialization in advanced practice. *Momentum, 4,* 1–4.

Spencer, G. (1989). *Projections of the population of the United States, by age, sex, and race: 1988–2330.* Washington, D.C.: U.S. Government Printing Office, Current Population Reports, series p-25, No. 1018.

Stalsbroten, V. L., & Baird, S. B. (1991). Introduction to cancer nursing care. In S. Baird, M. G. Donehower, V. L. Stalsbroten, & T. B. Ades (Eds.), *A cancer source book for nurses.* Atlanta: American Cancer Society.

Steele, S., & Fenton, M. (1988). Expert practice of clinical nurse specialists. *Clinical Nurse Specialist, 2,* 45–52.

Steeves, R., Cohen, M. Z., & Wise, C. T. (1994). An analysis of critical incidents describing the essence of oncology nursing. *Oncology Nursing Forum, 21*(Suppl.), 19–26.

Tiffany R. (1987). The development of cancer nursing as a specialty. *International Nursing Review, 34,* 35–42.

U.S. Congress Office of Technology Assessment. (1986). *Nurse practitioners, physician assistants, and certified nurse midwives: A policy analysis.* (Health technology case study 37) GTA-HCS-37 Washington, D.C. : U.S. Government Printing Office.

Watson, A. C. (1993). The role of the psychosocial oncology clinical nuse specialist in a rural cancer outreach program. *Clinical Nurse Specialist, 7,* 259–265.

White-Hershey, D., & Nevidjon, B. (1990). Fundamentals for oncology nurse/data managers—Preparing for a new role. *Oncology Nursing Forum, 17,* 317–327.

CHAPTER 4

Cultural Systems

Marjorie Kagawa-Singer

Oncology nurses are increasingly faced with the frustrations and rewards of working with patients, families, and fellow staff members from cultures different than their own. Cultural differences have always affected interactions between patients and nurses, but culture heretofore has not been used as an integrating, fundamental dimension of cancer care. Culture is not a singular characteristic to be added on to a laundry list of items such as language, religion, culture and so forth. Rather it is the core element with which the cancer experience is constructed.

This chapter provides a broader, culturally based framework within which to view the human response to cancer. Definitions of the constituent elements of this framework are provided, and each of the major domains in cancer care that are affected by cultural variances are briefly described. The intent of the discussion of cultural differences in each domain is to demonstrate that "normal" and "adaptive" behavior is defined only within its appropriate cultural context: an *ethnorelative* as opposed to an *ethnocentric* perspective.

The cancer experience cannot be understood as an objective event separated from its cultural context. Culture is the milieu in which all human life occurs and it affects every aspect of the cancer experience for patient, family, and nurse.

The domains of the cancer experience that appear to be universal and influenced by cultural differences are listed in Table 4–1. Seeking the cause and meaning for one's cancer appears to be a universal drive. Individuals, their families, and community seek an order to the chaos imposed by a cancer diagnosis and direction on how potential suffering should be borne. Each cultural group also has different styles of communication, and both age and gender establish specific parameters

TABLE 4–1. *Cultural Domains of Influences in the Response to Cancer*

Meaning of cancer
  Etiology
Suffering
Communication
  Verbal
  Nonverbal
  Truth-telling
  Ethics
  Decision making
Age
Gender
Life roles/quality of life/spirituality
Side effects
  Drug metabolism
Body image and sexuality
  Significance of body parts
Pain
Disability/impairment
Dependency/social support
Tragedy of death
  End-of-life decision making
Family and family dynamics

for what are considered appropriate topics of discussion, and with whom, when, and how such interactions can occur. The life stage and role responsibilities of the person with the disease also modulates the impact of the disease on the patient and family. Culture also prescribes who is appropriate to provide social support and what form this support should take to be considered appropriate and acceptable.

Attitudes toward the side effects of treatment, concepts of body image, sexuality, and the response to pain also vary according to cultural norms and expectations regarding suffering, private behavior, and interactions with authority figures. Racial differences in the pharmacodynamics and pharmacokinetics of drug metabolism indicate additional areas of assessment that must be incorporated into oncology nursing practice to better assist patients and families to control the side effects of treatment.

Perceptions of disability and dependency are also integrated into individual and family identity according to cultural precepts. Moreover, even the concept of who constitutes family and the dynamics that occur within the family unit in response to cancer differ cross-culturally. Death, a universal phenomenon, is conceptualized and commemorated in distinct fashion from group to group, and finally, quality of life and spirituality may also be defined by different parameters.

Each of these domains will be discussed in more detail later, but the framework in which these elements are presently assessed is currently monocultural. Culture appears to be erroneously perceived either as being synonymous with race or as being a discreet, disconnected factor such as diet or religion. An organizing theoretic framework is needed to correct this misperception and encompass the multiple domains listed above into an integrated cultural context.

THEORETIC FRAMEWORK

Figure 4–1 depicts an ecologic framework of the factors that form the cancer experience for patients, families, and nurses. This model has four nested dimensions that each contain several continuums denoting the presence or absence or abundance or scarcity of its domain. Beginning at the outermost layer, the environment contains elements such as the region of residence, environmental resources such as transportation, and availability and accessibility of health care services (Johnson & Sargent, 1990; McElroy & Townsend, 1989). The second layer consists of social, political, and class constraints, and the third layer contains interpersonal structures of family, group, and social network. The innermost dimensions contain the individual cancer variables such as the site and stage of the disease, age of the patient, and degree of acculturation and assimilation of the individual into the host culture. The variables in all four layers interact simultaneously to define the individual's experience of cancer.

Each of the 16 domains listed in Table 4–1 are part of basic nursing assessments, but a culturally informed assessment requires that the entire complex of elements be considered within its specific cultural context. As an example, a kaleidoscope contains a given set of pieces like the domains. Each time the kaleidoscope is turned, the patterns change as the colored pieces assume different positions of dominance and are reflected as varying angles off the mirrors. Such is the case with cultural groups. All human groups face the same set of issues in life, but each group has established a different angle of refraction depending upon its environmental constraints, resources, and world view, that emphasizes different elements or priorities within the set of issues. One particular pattern may not be inherently better than another. Each has its own validity and integrity.

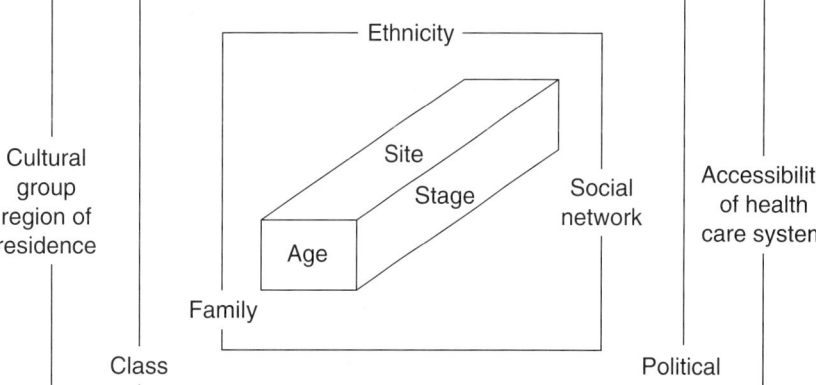

FIGURE **4–1.** Ecologic model for a cultural context in oncology nursing.

The test of each pattern or response to cancer is its usefulness in adapting to the situation. The author proposes that adaptation is a process that is designed to meet three basic, universal needs: security, self-integrity, and a sense of belonging (Erickson, 1963; Kagawa-Singer, 1994a; Maslow, 1973). Security is a sense of physical and emotional safety. Self-integrity is a sense of self-worth as a contributing, productive member of one's social network, and a sense of belonging is a genetically coded aspect of humans as social animals (Drotar, 1991). Humans are designed to belong to a group and be cared for and cared about. When these three needs are met, an individual has a sense of quality in his or her life. Each culture, however, uniquely provides for these needs for its members. It is the task of the nurse to conduct a cultural assessment to determine, *with* the patient and family, how best to incorporate their beliefs and practices into a plan of care that would be culturally appropriate and acceptable.

DEFINING CULTURE

Culture is a tool that operationalizes a group's world view into symbols of beliefs, values, and practices that its members learn to use to ensure their well-being. It identifies a group of people as a unique population with a common identity. A group's world view organizes the universe into a cohesive comprehensible vision of reality. Their religion, life philosophy, or both transform their world view into symbols of beliefs and values that can be used to derive meaning in life and a purpose for being.

The two functions of culture are (1) the *integrative,* which provides the beliefs and values that give an individual a sense of purpose in life and identity, and (2) the *functional,* the rules for behavior that support an individual's sense of self-worth and maintain group function and welfare (Jones, 1976). These common beliefs and rules for behavior provide consistency and predictability for its members in everyday social interactions as well as for those inevitable stressful life events such as sickness and death (Hallowell, 1955).

The integrative and functional functions of culture are like the warp and woof of a tapestry. Weaving is a universal technique, but the patterns that emerge from each group of people are culturally identifiable. For example, Persian, French, and Chinese rugs all have distinct characteristics. Concepts of beauty such as color, balance, symmetry, and the subjects chosen to display in the tapestries are culturally defined and symbolically express the ethos of the culture. The significance of this analogy is that the two functions of culture and the beliefs, values, and proscriptions for behavior are woven like individual threads into a whole, rich, cultural fabric. A thread can be taken out and compared across cultural groups for its inherent structure, but its specific function and integrity are incomprehensible unless seen within the pattern of the entire cultural fabric from which it came.

Taken out of context, a belief or behavior may be misinterpreted or even disregarded as unnecessary or maladaptive, especially if evaluated against a different standard. In clinical practice, nurse/patient miscommunication occurs when the nurse disassembles the patient's cultural tapestry and analyzes it according to the template of the nurse's culture. The essence and rationality of the original pattern is lost. If interventions are instituted with such a one-sided, ethnocentric perspective, the patient or family would likely feel misunderstood, and the prescribed intervention would probably fail. For example, the Muslim cultural edict against telling a Muslim patient that he or she has a terminal diagnosis or providing anticipatory grief counseling is antithetical to the U.S. concept of patient autonomy. Yet, within the context of the religious beliefs of Muslims, to do so would be unethical. Thus, even though grief, bereavement, and mourning are universal reactions to dying and to the loss of loved ones, the manner and meaning in which this occurs and the proper moral protocol for its observance are culturally distinct (Kagawa-Singer, 1994).

Nurses are beginning to recognize how the differences in beliefs and values held by other cultural or ethnic groups affect practice. Difficulties arise, however, when the U.S. system, as one system and one way of treating disease and illness, is considered the right way. Experience in compliance clearly indicates that knowledge and behavior are not directly related (Haynes, Taylor, & Sackett, 1979). Just because patients and families know the rationale for a medical regimen, it is no guarantee that they will follow it. Patients will incorporate medical treatment recommendations if these changes fit into their belief system, are relevant to their lives at this point in time, the lifestyle changes required are seen as worth the effort, and they have the resources to do so (Steffensen & Colker, 1982).

Learning to respect cultural differences requires viewing the health care beliefs and practices of other cultural and ethnic groups as *equally valid* within their own context: an *ethnorelative* perspective (Dana, 1993). A "gold standard" for the evaluation of appropriate behavior does not exist. Empirically, the practices may not be equally efficacious, but we must respect the integrity of the patient's belief system. The nurse's task is to provide the patient and family with as much information as possible for them to understand what is recommended and then to negotiate with them to achieve the most useful and acceptable course of action. If we subscribe to the value of patient autonomy, then we must be supportive of the right of the patient and family to disagree with us and modify our recommendations in accordance with their needs.

U.S. MEDICINE: A CULTURAL SYSTEM

An important first step in the process of developing cross-cultural expertise in oncology is to recognize that the health care system in the United States is itself a cultural system that reflects the values of one cultural group and thus may be too restrictive for a multicultural society. For example, the use of space is culturally determined (Hall & Whyte, 1963). Private rooms are valued in most hospitals, for privacy is important in standard U.S. society. In many other cultures a private room is seen as punitive for its isolation.

The Judeo-Christian values of the standard ethos in the United States are also expressed in the three basic values of the American health care system: (1) life is sacred and should be preserved at all cost, (2) autonomous decision-making ability should be promoted, supported, and preserved, and (3) no one should suffer (Silberfarb, 1982). The sanctity of life is part of the Jewish faith and the Old Testament of the Christian Bible (Mark & Roberts, 1994). Our intensive care units and organ transplant services speak to this belief.

The values of autonomy in decision making, individuality, and self-reliance are reflected in our support of patient's rights through the legal establishment of advanced directives, legal power of attorney, the Patient Self Determination Act, and informed consents. Orem's model of self-care clearly articulates this ethos in which nursing efforts are directed towards the maintenance, restoration, or development of the patient's independence through self-care (Feathers, 1989).

The recent enhanced efforts for pain control exemplify the dedication by U.S. health practitioners to relieve patient suffering (AHCPR, 1992, 1994), and much of oncology nursing research focuses on symptom management as in this volume in the section on major clinical nursing problems.

In contrast, the basic values of interdependency, collectivism, and community have been described as the cultural ethos of Canada (Clark, 1991) and, in fact, are held by most peoples in the world other than those who believe in the standard U.S ethos. For example, the health care values held by Japanese Americans are that (1) individual life is not sacred—the welfare of the group must be considered, (2) decisions are made by consensus—one would be considered rude to make decisions alone without consideration of the effect such decisions would have on those who are closest in one's life, and (3) suffering in life is inevitable. The basic tenet of Buddhism, which structures Japanese culture, is that all life is suffering. One strives to overcome this suffering through diligence and selflessness. Values that differ among cultures are not mutually exclusive. Rather the emphasis, prioritization, and patterns of use are culturally distinct.

Two additional examples of misunderstandings of cultural behaviors demonstrate how important it is to ascertain the patient's and family's perspective within their cultural context before intervening. One very ill, elderly, nonEnglish-speaking Muslim patient was thought to be confused because he fell out of bed several times a day. To his apparent dismay, he was put into restraints. His family explained to the staff that he was trying to face Mecca to pray five times a day as his religion required. The nurses then turned his bed to face

the desired direction, and the "noncompliant" and "confused" behavior ceased.

The last example concerned an elderly Russian immigrant who was admitted for severe abdominal pain and jaundice. The doctors informed the family that he had terminal pancreatic cancer and would live only a few more months. The doctors wanted to debulk the tumor to relieve the man's pain; but the family did not want their father to know his diagnosis, for they felt the news would be too depressing and it would hasten his death. To be respectful of the family's wishes, the surgical informed consent form that the man signed read, "removal of gallbladder stones." Sometimes, as in the last example, even correct understanding does not resolve the issue. The ethical and legal ramifications of cross-cultural issues can become even more complicated.

These examples highlight the implicit cultural bases of our hospital policies and clinical approaches. Until we recognize the culturally based infrastructure of our health care system, we will not be able to fully respond to the needs of patients and their families with cultural backgrounds different from that of the standard U.S. ethos.

CROSS-CULTURAL CONCEPTS AND TERMINOLOGY

A few additional concepts are useful as a basis when beginning to navigate in this expanded dimension of cross-cultural practice.

GENERALIZE/STEREOTYPE

Stereotypes may not only be misleading, but they may also be harmful, for they blind us to the uniqueness of each individual. On the other hand, *generalizations* are entrees into each person's life. Generalizations can be used as hypotheses about a group that can then be tested with specific individuals for its applicability (Geissler, 1994). Each person uses the general guides provided by his or her ethnic tapestry and then weaves his or her own unique pattern using borrowed and created ideas as well. Additional intragroup variables must also be considered in the assessment, such as immigrant, refugee, or American-born status, level of acculturation, socioeconomic status, degree of assimilation, language fluency, age, and gender.

ACCULTURATION/ASSIMILATION

Acculturation is the ability to function comfortably in another culture. Individuals learn the rules of behavior of the other culture to a degree that enables them to function with ease (Berry, 1980). The end of the acculturation process is often mistaken to be assimilation. *Assimilation* means that individuals give up the beliefs, values, material culture, and practices of their native group and adopt those of the host culture. In fact,

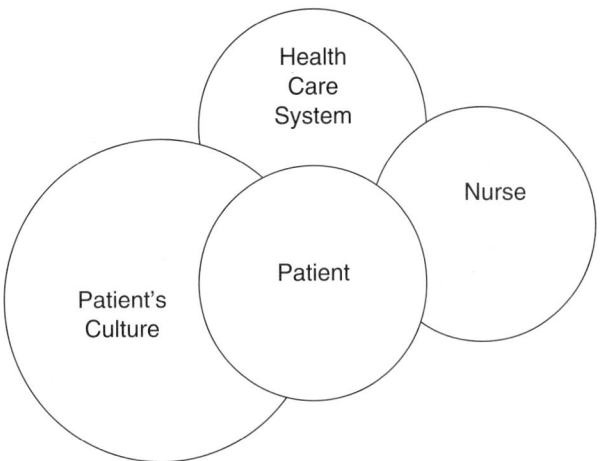

FIGURE 4–2. Intersection of cultural belief systems for the patient, the patient's culture, the nurse, and the American health care system.

most individuals become at least bicultural. That is, they hold two or more sets of cultural beliefs and practices and often become quite adept at functioning comfortably in multiple cultures. Indeed, some degree of blending occurs as well. The degree of blending of cultures is partly personal choice but to a larger extent is constrained by historic and social forces beyond an individual's control, such as racism or class discrimination (Berreman, 1982).

In illness, the different sets of cultural values both within the patient as well as between patients and health care practitioners sometimes conflict, and confusion, frustration, and miscommunication are common. Figure 4–2 depicts the patient/health care system intersections: the patient's system of beliefs will intersect to varying degrees with his or her own larger ethnic group and may intersect to varying degrees with that of the U.S. health care system, just as the belief system of nurses may intersect to varying degrees with that of the patient and the health care system. The degree of congruence between belief systems determines the facility with which communication will occur. The smaller the degree of intersection, obviously, the less likely it is that there will be mutual areas of understanding, and successful communication will require a much more conscious effort on the part of practitioners, patient, and family.

ETIC/EMIC

Etic refers to the outsider's perspective and interpretation of observable behavior. *Emic* refers to the insider's interpretation and meaning behind the actions. The task in providing effective care to patients and families from different cultures is to elicit their emic interpretation of the cancer experience. Nurses then compare their etic interpretation with the patient's emic perspective to verify the nursing assessment.

DISEASE/ILLNESS

Differentiating between disease and illness is helpful when determining the patient's and family's interpretation of the recommended regimen for cancer prevention, screening, early detection, treatment, rehabilitation, or end-of-life decisions (Chrisman, 1991; Eisenberg, 1977; Fabrega, 1972). *Disease* is the observable, measurable aspects of cancer using the nosology of the health care system used by the patient and family. *Illness* is the meaning of the experience created by the disease. Oncology nurses develop expertise in assessing both aspects, but the disease dimension is less variable among patients and families than the illness dimension. A major portion of nursing time is spent on meeting the needs of patients and families created by cultural differences in the illness response to the disease because of their different beliefs, values, and proscriptions for behavior.

ETHNICITY

An *ethnic group* is a self-identified cultural group that resides within another society and has beliefs, values, and rules that permit appropriate interactive behavior among its members (DeVos & Romanucci-Ross, 1982). *Ethnicity* is an individual's self-identification with a group as well as identification by others in and outside the group. Ethnic identity is recognized as the nonbiologic characteristics inherited through socialization. The relevance of ethnic identity to oncology practice is that one's ethnic group provides the individual with a sense of social belonging, self-worth, and ultimate loyalty (Berreman, 1982). Thus to overlook or discount ethnicity would be to deny an individual's sense of self and sources of support (Kagawa-Singer & Chung, 1994).

As nurses, we belong to at least four cultures. We are, first of all, members of the ethnic group(s) into which we were born. Second, each of us has been socialized into the culture of the biomedical health care system, which has values, beliefs, and precepts for behavior that may be quite variant from our native ethnic groups. Third, we have been further socialized into the subculture of nursing in the United States. As Leininger's (1993) work has shown, appropriate caring behavior by nurses varies significantly among countries. When nurses trained elsewhere come to the United States to practice, or nurses from the United States go abroad or even into different ethnic enclaves within the United States, differences in beliefs, values, and interpersonal styles can be a source of frustration. Moreover, interdisciplinary conflicts often arise because of differences in professional world views. Fourth, each of us is male or female and obtains validation of self and a sense of self-worth by different criteria (Tavris, 1982). Because of these gender differences, men and women bring different aspects of caring to a clinical interaction (Leininger, 1970). Unfortunately, in the United States we tend to minimize these differences when they could be used as complementary strengths (Tannen, 1990).

RACE

The term *race* has been associated with phenotypically identifiable groups but technically refers to biologic variations among groups. Moreover, within phenotypically identified groups, biologic variations are often greater than group variations (Montagu, 1945, 1962). The usefulness of race as a group identifier is limited to approximately 10 per cent of variation in cancer incidence, such as familial traits (Fraumeni, Hoover, Devesa, & Kinlen, 1989).

The remaining 85 to 90 per cent of cancers are attributed to lifestyle factors such as diet, environmental exposures, and work-related toxins (Fraumeni et al., 1989). Lifestyle is most frequently determined by one's ethnicity, social class status, or both. Therefore unless specific biologic differences are discussed, this chapter will refer to only ethnic or cultural differences.

DEVELOPING A CULTURAL CONTEXT IN NURSING PRACTICE

Thus far this chapter has outlined the basic concepts of a cultural framework for oncology nursing. This next section describes how culture affects specific dimensions of the cancer experience.

The pathophysiology of cancer is probably universal, and the treatments in first world countries result in similar physical side effects. Table 4–1 listed the major dimensions of the cancer experience that are probably modified by cultural differences. Oncology nurses must develop skills in understanding these dimensions within the integrity of the cultural groups most represented in their practice to effectively reduce the burden of cancer on the patient and the family.

MEANING OF THE DISEASE

Humans seek a rationale for seemingly irrational suffering that has befallen them and try to extract meaning from their misfortune (Mishel, Padilla, Grant, & Sorenson, 1991). The meaning ascribed to the cancer experience is dependent upon the patient's and family's world view or cultural organization of reality. Cancer connotes unpredictability and chaos. Individuals draw upon their cultural background for guidance on how to bear the emotional and physical suffering caused by the disease. How each cultural group views the cause of cancer provides direction for the proper emotional and behavioral response. For example, if the cause is by capricious supernatural forces, fear and guilt may be overriding responses and propitiation for the offense would be the logical reaction, whereas if the cancer is sent from a Supreme Being as punishment, one might be remorseful and resigned in order to regain grace in this life or the next.

COMMUNICATION

Transcultural experiences create additional complexity for accurate communication and greater potential for miscommunication because of differences in language, rules of communication, syntax, gender, and age issues.

The first challenge to the nurse is to establish rapport with the patient and family (Northouse & Northouse, 1992). Establishing rapport requires a fundamental ability to show respect for the individual and listen for his or her verbal and nonverbal concerns. If trust and confidence are not established, it is unlikely subsequent interventions for physical, emotional, or social assistance will be of any benefit.

The same guides for appropriate communication as described elsewhere in this volume apply to transcultural communication, but the different nuances of culturally proscribed rules of nonverbal as well as verbal communication must be considered. For example, even when the patient speaks English, the level of fluency must be established. Patients/families may understand and speak everyday conversational English, but their knowledge of biomedical terminology and concepts of Western anatomy and physiology may be quite limited. The level of education will also modify the type of vocabulary used. Moreover, talking with a patient or family member about a diagnosis as emotionally laden as cancer may further reduce their ability to comprehend what is being discussed. The individual and family may prefer to discuss their disease and treatment options in their native language for both emotional comfort as well as to ensure understanding.

Rules of appropriate communication are quite stringently prescribed in most cultures. It has been said that greater than 80 per cent of communication is nonverbal. In U.S. ethos, however, more emphasis and value are placed on the rational, verbal aspects of communication than on the emotional and nonverbal aspects. Although we do interpret and feel nonverbal behavior in Euro-American culture, nonverbal communication does not have the veracity and importance it does in most other cultures (Gudykunst & Ting-Toomey, 1988). Concepts of proper use of space, time, privacy, and touch (by whom, under what circumstances, and what the character of the touch means) also differ significantly among groups (Hall & Whyte, 1976).

The specific language itself can be a barrier if the patient and nurse speak different languages. Significant within-language variations exist that also affect the effectiveness of communication: the level of usage, that is, degree of sophistication of the user; the medium, that is, visual, written, verbal, and nonverbal; rules of communication, for example, gender differences in terminology used and acceptability of subject matter to be discussed and superior-subordinate rules of behavior and language; correctness and appropriateness of translation and translator; and finally, with written material, the level of reading and the size of the print must be considered.

Many languages have a male and female syntax. Translations and translators must be fluent enough in the language to know how to use the correct vocabulary. Accordingly, with some cultures, sexually related topics are not to be discussed in mixed company even when they concern discussion of the cancer diagnosis and treatment. Usually, however, these rules are waived between physician and patient, but awareness of this is essential for nurses (the majority of whom are female) and especially when a translator is being used. The translator should be of the same sex as the patient (especially if they are not also a physician and of the same social class as the patient and family), and preferably, not a family member because family members may interpret rather than translate, depending upon their desire to protect the patient and upon their own understanding of medical terminology.

Social class differences can be significant barriers to communication when the translator is of a lower class than the patient/family. In many cultures this situation places the translator in a position of authority. Such a social transposition can be viewed as rude and insulting by the patient and family and can be awkward for the translator as well.

Communication etiquette is often unconscious, but its effect is powerful. For example, eye contact is another aspect of communication that often causes ill feelings and frustrations for the participants using different rules of conduct for "respectful" behavior. In the standard U.S. culture, direct eye contact is valued. A person's character is judged by their ability to make and keep eye contact during a discussion. Moreover, such eye contact communicates interest and attention. In contrast, many hierarchically structured societies consider direct eye contact by a subordinate to a superior to be aggressive and extremely rude. In these cultures subordinates show their respect and sensitivity to the individual in authority by dropping their eyes.

Touch is a different language of communication with its rules and boundaries. For example, a single Asian Indian woman is not permitted to touch a man, as in shaking hands. Instead, the palms of the hands are placed together with fingers extended as in prayer close to the chest, and a greeting is given with a slight bow. A male physician or nurse who greets a traditional Asian Indian woman by shaking her hand may unknowingly create discomfort and a barrier to further communication. In Iran, women seek care for gynecologic problems from female physicians. Seeking care in the United States from female gynecologists may be more problematic because of limited availability. It is possible that Iranian women may delay seeking attention for symptoms because of the strong religious and social edicts of interactions between men and women in that culture, but clinically, Persian women seem to be making the transition to male gynecologists fairly smoothly.

Suffering

Suffering is subjective, but its meaning, that is, the perceived reason for its presence, and the acceptable mode for its expression are culturally formed. To accurately assess the existence, nature, and severity of both emotional and physical distress, potential variations in cultural interpretations must be known (Angel &

Thoits, 1987; Mechanic, 1972). For example, in the U.S. ethos, a cancer diagnosis is often seen as a personal affront (Erwin, 1984; Peters-Golden, 1982) rather than a fate that must be silently endured, as in Hispanic cultures (Perez-Stable, Sabogal, Ortera-Sabogal, Hiatt, & McPhee, 1992). Concepts of proper demeanor will indicate how suffering should be expressed, such as vocally and demonstrative as in some Middle Eastern cultures (Reizan & Meleis, 1986) or silently and stoically as in Old Yankee cultures (Zborowski, 1952; Zola, 1966).

Side Effects

Cancer therapy often results in toxic side effects. Oncology nurses focus a major portion of their practice and research on the amelioration of side effects (see Unit VIII in this volume). To increase the effectiveness of nursing interventions, more effort must be devoted to elicit the emic interpretation of the side effects of treatment for different ethnic groups. If the assessment is more accurate, patients and families will probably feel that they are able to communicate with the nurse, and the chances are greater that effective and culturally acceptable interventions will be provided.

Much of the public believes that cancer therapy is worse than the disease itself, and this belief dissuades them from receiving optimum care. They may delay in seeking care for fear something will be found or, once they have received a diagnosis, these individuals might decline adjuvant or more aggressive therapy because of the anticipated side effects of therapy. Although this mystique is not confined to ethnic minority populations, this belief, which may have some relationship to physiologic differences, is compounded by cultural concepts about the cause of cancer and often places ethnic groups at higher risk of being underserved[1] (Underwood, Hoskins, Tarshemicka, Morris, & Williams, 1994; Burstin, Lipsitz, & Brennan, 1992).

Drug Metabolism

Recent research indicates that racial differences exist in both the pharmacodynamics and pharmacokinetics of certain classes of drugs that may be used in cancer care such as anesthetics, analgesics, and psychotropics (Lin, Poland, & Hakasaki, 1993). Enzymatic variations, for example, in acetylation (Murray

---

[1]The American Cancer Society, California Division adopted the following definition for the Underserved (February, 1993):

The underserved is broadly defined as those who encounter barriers to optimal cancer care (education, prevention, detection, treatment, and rehabilitation). The underserved includes, but is not limited to, individuals and their children who are indigent; working poor without adequate medical insurance; elderly; homeless; undocumented residents; those who have limited literacy and language ability; persons with disabilites and those whose cultureal beliefs and practices may pose barriers to using Western biomedical techniques.

& Reidy, 1990; Weber, 1987), and differences in protein binding (Otten, Schadel, Cheung, Kaplan, Busto, & Sellers, 1993), and microsomal variations (Zhou, Koshakji, & Silberstein, 1989) exist among racial groups. These variations, however, can also be influenced by dietary components (Anderson, Conney, & Kappas, 1992), and a growing literature in cancer care points to both protective and risk factors according to dietary intake. Ethnicity and diet are intertwined. Thus some of the variation in metabolism may be due to dietary influences and not to racial variations alone (Hunter et al., 1993; King & McCay, 1983; Willett, Stampfer, Colditz, Rosner, & Speizer, 1990).

Clinically, patients of different ethnic groups have reported responses to medications that may be biologically linked (Houghton, Aun, Gin, & Lau, 1992; Katz, Norman, Seed, & Conrad, 1969). For example, Asian patients have long reported excess sedation from anesthesia, pain, and antiemetic medications. Such patients have sometimes reported that they discontinued taking the medications prescribed to alleviate the side effects of chemotherapy, because the side effects of the agents employed were worse than the chemotherapeutic side effects themselves (Zhou, Sheller, Nu, Wood, & Wood, 1993).

It is possible that there are variations in the metabolism of medications used to treat the side effects of chemotherapy. This has not yet been studied, but it is an area that should be addressed. If the variations in the response to the medications used to treat the side effects of therapy occur, such knowledge would enable practitioners to better tailor the treatments (Levy, 1993).

PAIN

The recent publication of the AHCPR Pain Guidelines (AHCPR, 1992, 1994) stresses the point that pain is whatever the individual says it is and occurs whenever the individual says it does. The practitioner's responsibility is to accurately assess and effectively treat the pain. Practitioners are encouraged to note cultural differences, yet no explanation is provided regarding what these differences might be and how to effectively intervene.

A paucity of literature exists on cultural differences in pain perception, expression, and intervention, and expansion of this knowledge has not been sought for oncology practice (Cleeland, Ladinsky, & Serlin, 1988; Garro, 1990; Lipton & Marbach, 1984). For instance, in the mid-1950s and early 1960s, the seminal work by Zborowski (1952) and Zola (1966) indicated significant differences in symptom presentation and the meaning of pain by three white ethnic groups in the New England area: Old Yankee, Italian, and Jewish. Davitz, Sameshima, and Davitz (1976) also demonstrated differences in six cultures in attitudes towards pain and symptom presentation: Vietnamese, Japanese, Taiwanese, Thai, Puerto Rican, and U.S. American.

Less literature exists on the practitioner's response to cultural differences in pain assessment and treatment (Mayer & McWhorter, 1989; Samelson, Speers, Ferguson, & Bennett, 1994). Todd, Samaroo, and Hoffman (1993) conducted a study of the administration of pain medications for patients who had had long bone fractures and noted that Hispanic patients received significantly less medication for the same fractures as did a matched group of white patients. Language communication did not seem to be an issue, because a Spanish translator was always available in the emergency room. The authors speculated on the possibility of variances in symptom presentation by the patients as well as interpretation of symptoms by the staff.

Individual expressions of pain range from stoicism to very vocal and demonstrative expressions. These differences, however, are characteristic of cultural groups as well. Nurses need to be knowledgeable of both cultural and idiosyncratic variations in pain expression to accurately assess levels of distress from pain and provide adequate pain control. As yet, however, little information exists on the differences in the meaning of cancer pain by different cultural groups, the cross-cultural validity of the behavioral cues used to indicate the levels of pain, and issues of the cross-cultural validity of the assessment tools themselves (Adams, 1993).

GENDER

Research on illness behavior has noted significant gender differences in health care system utilization, disease incidence (e.g., lung cancer), and treatment response. Women utilize the health care system more frequently than men and seek care at earlier stages for symptoms, but in some instances the woman's symptoms or style of presentation is discounted (Healy, 1991). Cross-culturally, women (mothers) are the major health care decision-makers in the family as well as the caretakers (Finerman, 1983; Sargent, 1982).

Men and women also seem to use different modes of coping (Kagawa-Singer, 1988; Murphy, 1986). Research in psychosocial oncology is just beginning to study this area in relationship to ethnicity. Gender role expectations and restrictions vary between cultures, and nursing interventions based in the Euro-western culture may not be appropriate in other cultural groups. Additionally, some ethnic differences may not be apparent unless gender and ethnicity are studied simultaneously (Kagawa-Singer, 1988).

Gender differences in response to analgesias indicate that premenopausal women require larger doses of morphine for pain control than men because of competition of binding sites with estrogen (Da Silva & Hall, 1992; Islam, Cooper, & Bodnar, 1993). This fact may be complicated by racial enzymatic variations in drug response as noted earlier (Kalow, 1992).

AGE AND LIFE ROLES

Studies have indicated that patients older than 60 years of age experience less dysphoria from the cancer experience than younger adults (Ganz, Schag, & Heinrich, 1985). The association with age and degree of distress appears to be related to the differences in the impact of cancer according to life roles and one's normal lifestyle. The degree of disruption to one's normal lifestyle seems to determine how difficult the experience will be. Northouse (1994) and Schain (1992) have used a developmental approach to study stress associated with cancer and have documented that young adults experience the greatest stress compared with middle-aged or older adults because of competing demands of career and young children. The response to the cancer and its sequelae by the rest of the family and community is also influenced by the age of the patient and the cultural value of each developmental stage. In one study of the relative tragedy of the death of a family member, Anglo families listed the death of a young child (aged 1 to 7 years) as most tragic compared with Mexican, African-American, or Asian families, who listed the death of a young adult as most tragic and ranked the death of a child (aged 1 to 7 years) third or fourth (Kalish & Reynolds, 1976).

Although developmental theory appears to provide a better context to identify the potential stresses posed by cancer for the individual and his or her family, a larger cultural context would provide greater accuracy. Health was defined by a group of older Anglo- and Japanese-American patients receiving chemotherapy as the ability to be a productive, integral part of their social network (Kagawa-Singer, 1993). Their ability to cope with the cancer experience was ameliorated by their ability to continue functioning according to their life roles (mother, father, nurturer, worker) and was less tied to their physical status. Most subjects were coping well, but the style of coping of each ethnic group would have been inappropriate for the other.

A major mode of meeting the three basic needs of every individual, namely security, self-worth, and belonging, was fulfillment of life responsibilities. Western biomedicine has focused on physical functioning as an outcome for health care, but the quality of the life preserved by biomedical technology seems to be of greater concern for patients (Litwin, 1994). Such evidence indicates that studies of age differences combined with ethnic variations should be conducted (Goldstein & Teng, 1991; Koukouras et al., 1991).

BODY IMAGE AND SEXUALITY

The physical body is a metaphor that expresses the ethos of each culture (Scheper-Hughs & Lock, 1987). In the United States a mechanistic view of the body enables us to define life and death according to measurable parameters such as brain death. Other cultures, which view the body as a microcosm of the universe, such as with Native American and traditional Chinese medicine (Lock, 1980), imbue life and body parts with much greater spiritual significance than standard U.S. society explicitly acknowledges. Native Americans and Chinese may be very resistant to removal of body parts, for it would interfere with their spiritual wholeness.

Additionally, for example, the significance of different body parts differs among cultures. In Japan, traditionally the most beautiful part of a woman was the nape of the neck. Life energy or the "soul" resides in the "belly" or the hypogastric area, whereas in Western society the soul resides in the area of the heart. Thus the significance of stomach or colon cancer may have very different connotations in Japan than it does in the United States. In France, the liver has greater symbolic significance for concepts of health and emotional well-being than in the United States. Such concepts of the body are alien to the Western mechanistic, functional view of the body with its interchangeable parts (heart, lung, knees, hips). Little research has sought to delve into the effect of these variations, but the symbolic meaning of the organ or body part may have deep significance and thereby influence the magnitude of the impact of the cancer experience.

A diagnosis of cancer, probably for all patients, requires a redefinition and transformation of one's self-image (Kagawa-Singer, 1988), and sexuality, in all its components of self-identity (physical, emotional, social, and spiritual), will also be affected (Bos, 1986; Darty & Potter, 1984). Sexuality is an area that has long been overlooked in oncology nursing research, and no studies have been found that address the impact of cancer on the sexuality of women in other than Euro-western cultures. For example, the symbolic and functional meaning of the uterus or cervix for a young, unmarried woman in many traditional cultures such as Japanese or Native American holds social as well as biologic significance, for her marriageability is severely reduced.

Notably, however, the rules of communication on the subject of sexuality regarding gender and age of discussants are even more stringently applied than the other domains presented thus far. In some cultures the mother or husband may not be the appropriate individual to translate for a nonEnglish-speaking young woman, whereas in others, such as the Hispanic/Latino cultures, it may be more appropriate. In others, an elder of the same sex from the community may be the designated counsel for a young woman or man.

DISABILITY/IMPAIRMENT

Views toward the disabled vary cross-culturally, and depending upon the disability, reactions can range from disdain to deification (Kagawa-Singer, 1994b). In general, cancer appears to carry a stigma and is surrounded in fatalism both in the United States and internationally (Sontag, 1977).

Even if the disease is successfully treated and the sequelae of treatment are not visible, a history of cancer can affect the social status of the family in some communities. For example, a history of breast cancer in the family can reduce the marriageability of its single members. A young, single, Asian-Indian women in India with a history of breast cancer may be unmarriageable.

Social forces that shape the attitudes and behaviors toward the sick and disabled are often far removed from the biologic reality. What cannot be changed physically is invested with meaning for the members of that society—meaning derived from the moral structure of their cultural world view. Public education efforts in ethnic communities must identify the cultural view of cancer in each of the communities. Otherwise, both the mode and the message may be irrelevant, and the educational efforts will have little or no effect on the intended audience.

CONCEPTS OF HEALTH, WELL-BEING, AND QUALITY OF LIFE

The Western biomedical model focuses upon physiologic integrity as a construct for health. Recent quality of life measurements, however, indicate that individual health status, well-being, or both are much more subjectively defined and tend to emphasize role fulfillment over physical integrity (Gill & Feinstein, 1994; Kagawa-Singer, 1993). To understand health behavior regarding screening, early detection, and emotional responses to the cancer experience, oncology nurses must elicit the patient and family's definition of health and how the cancer would affect this concept.

DEATH AND DYING

The classic function of the dying process is to foster the acceptance of death as a natural event and ensure the continuity of the community. In hospitals the human experience of dying typically is decontextualized from tradition, lineage, and accepted dogma (Irish, 1994), because death signifies that our medical system has failed.

Every culture has rituals to guide its members, both the dying and the bereaved, through this final life transition (Pagli & Abramovitch, 1984). Rituals reaffirm the symbolic fit of members into society and provide predictability, stability, and security during this transition. These rituals also provide instructions on how to appropriately channel grief and provide social support to the patient and to the family members.

In the United States grief and bereavement counseling in oncology for the patient and the family is structured within the beliefs and values of the standard white Judeo-Christian North American culture (Parry, 1990). The grief practices of other cultures sometimes conflict with hospital policies, which are designed to guide family members and patients to achieve an "acceptable death": controlled, quiet, and detached (Kellahear, 1990). Their pain is respected by providing them the valued commodity in the Euro-western culture of privacy. This attitude is observed when the terminal patient is moved to a private room—this practice is also designed to protect the feelings of the other patients and families by removing the physical reminder that cancer too often leads to death. In practice, however, privacy often isolates the family from care and support. The private room for the dying is often farthest from the nurse's station on the unit and farthest from the waiting area of the unit where families often obtain informal support from family members of other patients. Also, hospital policy and rules often restrict the number of visitors who can be in the room at any one time. Despite the words spoken by staff, this practice is often interpreted by patients and families as abandonment and loss of hope.

The philosophy of hospice counters this practice of isolating the dying and the bereaved and supports the patient and the family through this transition. Yet the structure of hospice in the United States has a Euro-Christian base. As would be expected, this is the population best supported by its services, for the predominant hospice population is Caucasian (>90%) (Mor & Masterson-Allen, 1988; Pawling-Kaplan & O'Connor, 1989). Because of the philosophic basis and structure of support for the dying, the fears of other ethnic individuals and families of dying alone or suffering intensely cannot be easily allayed in our system, for actions speak louder than words.

The cultural assumptions that underlie practices and laws surrounding end-of-life decisions in the standard U.S. ethos are not shared by other cultures. For example, in the Islamic culture it is felt to be unethical to discuss the possibility of death before its occurrence because to do so means that humans are interfering with the Will of Allah. In some cultures major life decisions are no longer made by the elderly, for these individuals have absolved themselves of the responsibility and expect and want someone else to make such decisions on their behalf. Cultural groups differ, however, on who this individual is. It usually is not the spouse but rather the eldest son or daughter, brother, or tribal elder. This information is essential to obtain and is ethically challenging considering the legal edicts in this country on advanced directives and informed consent (Klessig, 1992).

FAMILY/DEPENDENCY AND SOCIAL SUPPORT

Social support in illness has been found to be of major importance in supporting an individual's coping ability (DiMatteo & Hays, 1981; Dunkel-Schetter, 1984), but the magnitude of this effect is equivocal. One confounding factor may be that subjects in psychosocial oncology studies tend to be treated as a homogeneous group, with an underlying assumption that family and social support are universally defined (Kagawa-Singer, 1988). Some studies, however, such as Zola's and Zborowski's on pain, indicate that the "white" population is not homogenous. Ignoring intragroup and intergroup variations may result in inconclusive findings in statistical analyses.

In ethnic cultures other than the standard U.S. culture, family is defined much more broadly than the nuclear or immediate family (Ell, Mantell, & Hamovitch, 1988). Ritual kin such as godparents and the clergy of one's religious group, and fictive kin, those whom one chooses to be part of one's family, are integral to one's life and self-identity, and a patient-designated representative from this extended group must be included in health care decision making. Nurses must be more aware of this broader concept of family and include them as the major support system, for they will often be of great assistance in guiding the patient through the cancer experience.

The construct of social support itself also appears to differ. Who provides social support, what is considered appropriate and desired, and when it is provided are culturally determined. For example, in oncology practice emotional support in the form of expression of feelings is often assumed to be paramount in helping the patient cope with the experience (Lazarus & Folkman, 1984). In many cultures, however, material support and "doing for" the individual is more appropriate and expresses emotional support without words (Uba, 1994). In such cultures talking about dysphoric emotions creates greater distress, because it will not change the situation and is often felt to be more harmful to the individual (Reynolds, 1989). Efforts by nurses to encourage expression of dysphoric emotions and sharing of intimate feelings can often be counterproductive. More culturally appropriate and acceptable modes of providing social support must be identified and supported if they are more effective (Wellisch, Kagawa-Singer, & Reid, 1995).

SPIRITUALITY

Spirituality provides individuals an ability to see beyond themselves and appreciate a pattern, a continuity in life that includes all those they care about and provides them a reason for being. Important for nursing care, spirituality is often cited by patients as their greatest source of strength. Overall, however, this has been an area long overlooked in cancer care (Ferrell, Schmidt, Rhiner, & Fonbuena, 1992; Ferrell, Schmidt, Rhiner, Whitehead, Fonbuena, & Forman 1992). Weisman (1984) and Doi (1985) both noted that mortality can be accepted when individuals realize that their lives may be transient but that they remain irreplaceable in their social networks. Again, support of the spiritual sustenance provided by a culture's world view, such as that of the American Indians, or its symbolic form of organized religions, such as Catholicism, should be better integrated into practice (Brown-Saltzman, 1994).

PREVENTION AND TREATMENT CHOICES

One of the major purposes of culture is to ensure the survival of its members. To this end, each cultural group defines health and well-being, identifies the causes of disease and misfortune, and prescribes appropriate and effective treatment. Because these practices are so fundamental to the existence of the group and have proven to be effective in ensuring the group's survival through generations, we can understand the tenacity with which individuals hold to these indigenous beliefs and practices.

Of more immediate concern to oncology practice is that patients are often simultaneously using the three systems of care present in most cultures: (1) popular, which consists of family, social network, and community, (2) folk, which consists of indigenous healers or complementary therapies, and (3) professional, which consists of the formal health care system as well as Western biomedicine (Kleinman, 1980). Most patients will be using at least two of the systems simultaneously, and sometimes all three. The patient and family's cultural background and material as well as emotional re-

sources affect the behaviors used to prevent disease, identify symptoms that warrant help-seeking behavior, designate the appropriate system from which to seek assistance, and affect willingness and ability to comply or adhere to the prescribed medical regimen. A good overview of these cultural beliefs and practices is provided in *Cancer Prevention in Minority Populations* by Frank-Stromborg and Olsen (1993).

The rationale behind the popular and folk systems of care are based within each group's cultural world view. As such, these are integrated, logical systems that by and large have worked to keep its members well, but conventional practice in biomedicine has discounted much of traditional health practices as unscientific. More damaging responses to patients have occurred when these indigenous practices were perceived as mere superstitions. Patients report having been negatively judged for discussing these practices, so they usually avoid any mention of the practices they are using or treatments they are receiving.

Indigenous practices are designed to counteract what the group believes to be the cause of the cancer. The etiology may be natural, as in accidents or infectious diseases, supernatural, as in spirits or gods, or metaphysical, such as winds or energy forces. Western biomedicine addresses the natural causes well but offers very little for the treatment of supernatural or metaphysical causes. Patients may well utilize Western biomedicine for the symptoms of the disease, but often they will use biomedical doctors to treat the symptoms of the disease and indigenous practitioners to heal them from the source of the imbalance that made them vulnerable to the disease in the first place (Fabrega, 1972).

Professional practitioners of traditional health systems such as Chinese Medicine and Ayurvedic Medicine have a long history of empiric success in treating disease. Cancer patients who utilize these modalities, such as acupressure, spiritual balancing through movement or meditation, and herbs, often report benefit. Difficulties can arise, however, when some of these herbal remedies negatively interact with Western biomedical medications. The active ingredients in many of the natural herbs are unknown. Even when the chemical structure is known, the interaction with chemotherapeutic agents or medications used to treat the side effects of therapy is not known. It is important, therefore, to ask in a nonjudgmental fashion about use of complementary health practices so that potential problems can be avoided.

Health practitioners must assess whether the practice is helpful, neutral, or harmful (Tripp-Reimer & Afifi, 1989). Nurses should support those practices that are helpful or neutral, for even biologically neutral practices serve psychologically and socially supportive functions. Changes in maladaptive or harmful practices need to be negotiated with the patient and family for their welfare. When working with patients and families from any culture different than the nurses' own, knowledge of these three systems helps to develop culturally respectful interventions at all stages of the cancer care continuum.

1. Knowledge of group
2. Observation and openness
3. Patience
4. Facilitation

ACHIEVING CULTURALLY BASED CARE

A variety of cross-cultural assessment tools or guides have been devised (Tripp-Reimer, Brink, & Saunders, 1984). Some focus on the individual and others on the community level, and they should be incorporated into the general nursing assessment. None, however, focuses specifically on patients with cancer.

Table 4–2 lists the four basic steps needed to use any of the established cross-cultural assessment tools. The elements and process of a culturally based assessment are the same as in any basic nursing assessment. The fundamental difference is that all of the elements are consciously placed within the group's own whole cultural fabric and are not gathered as separate concepts to be evaluated within the Euro-western framework (Kagawa-Singer & Chung, 1994). Briefly, the first step requires gaining substantial *knowledge* about the ethnic groups most represented in a particular practice. A basic knowledge can be gained from reading, but much of the subcultural knowledge will be obtained from informed community leaders.

The general knowledge gained in step 1 must be tested in the second step, *observation and openness.* Patients and families provide the specific, personal information required to develop a plan of care.

Nurses can use the types of questions listed in Table 4–3 to elicit the patient's and family's understanding of the disease and expectations about treatment and outcomes (Kleinman, 1980; Kleinman, Eisenberg, & Good, 1978; Weiss et al., 1992). This list of questions is not meant to be exhaustive, but it indicates the exploration that is required to get a sense of the client's emic perspective. The questions should be woven into the interview and framed in such a way that they are not threatening to the patient or family (Kagawa-Singer & Chung, 1994; for a more extensive and validated tool to document the explanatory model, see Weiss et al., 1992).

The third step is *patience.* This step is perhaps one of the most difficult to achieve because of the structural constraints on nursing time. Nonetheless, with patients from other cultures, it is essential. It takes time to build trust and confidence between the nurse and patients from cultures different than the nurses, especially when the social and historic context of ethnic minorities and class differences in the United States is considered. Often patients and families will divulge little personal information at the first few meetings, because they are

1. What do you think has caused your problem?
2. Why do you think it started when it did?
3. What do you think your sickness does to you? How does it work in your body?
4. How severe is your sickness? Will it have a long or a short course?
5. What kind of treatment do you think you should receive?
6. What are the most important results you hope to receive from this treatment?
7. What are the chief problems your sickness has caused for you?
8. What do you fear most about your sickness?

assessing the nurse's competence, trustworthiness, credibility, and respect for them. The nurse's actions must match the words used.

The last step is *facilitation.* The nurse must work with the cancer care team to draw upon the richness of the patient's cultural background to negotiate mutually acceptable goals and the means to achieve them. To do so the nurse must recognize and respect the cultural construct of the patient and family as having equal validity as that of the biomedical model. Negotiation will succeed if the patient and family feel that the cancer team is working on their behalf *with* them.

SUMMARY

The cancer experience for patients, families, and nurses occurs within a cultural context. Most of the time we are unaware of the cultural milieu in which we live, for it is our world. Transcultural interactions bring to the fore the arbitrariness of this cultural context. This chapter has provided an overview of culture as a fundamental, integrating dimension of cancer care, has described how culture modifies the major domains of the cancer experience, and has suggested how nurses can use the overarching theory of culture to incorporate the variations discussed.

Use of a culturally based framework that encompasses the biologic, psychologic, and social forces that affect the cancer experience for individuals would enable nurses to refine their critical thinking ability. Assessments would be based within the reality of the patient and family, the interventions negotiated would be more relevant and acceptable, and the criteria used to evaluate the effectiveness of practice would also have a greater likelihood of accuracy.

Cross-cultural knowledge also widens the horizon of possibilities to solve the problems created by the cancer experience. Different cultures provide alternative approaches, and such experience increases the number of options for "right" ways to solve the multitude of problems and reduce the stresses created by the cancer experience.

Expertise in cross-cultural nursing progresses from *cultural sensitivity,* where awareness of differences exists and syntax and/or behavior changes as necessary, to *cultural relativism*, where concepts or interventions must hold relevance to the group targeted, and finally to *cultural competence* in which the nurse, in partnership with the patient and family, systematically integrates and translates cultural understanding into acceptable, appropriate actions. Development of cultural competence in oncology nursing practice would then enable nurses to administer culturally and socially appropriate and acceptable care for all patients.

REFERENCES

Adams, J. (1993). Pain assessment has many cultural aspects. *Oncology Nursing Society Special Interest Group Newsletter, Pain Management: Sharing Our Expertise*, December, p. 7.

Agency for Health Care Policy and Research, Public Health Service, U.S. Department of Health and Human Services. (1992). *Acute pain management: Operative or medical procedures and trauma. Clinical practice guideline*. AHCPR Pub. No. 92-0032. Rockville, MD: Author.

Agency for Health Care Policy and Research, Public Health Service, U.S. Department of Health and Human Services. (1994). *Management of cancer pain. Clinical practice guideline No. 9*. AHCPR Publication No. 94-0592. Rockville, MD: Author.

Anderson, K., Conney, A., & Kappas, A. (1992). Nutritional influences on chemical biotransformations in humans. *Nutrition Reviews, 40*, 161–169.

Angel, R., & Thoits, P. (1987). The impact of culture on the cognitive structure of illness. *Culture, Medicine & Psychiatry, 11*, 465–494.

Berreman, G. (1982). Bazar behavior: Social identity and social interaction in urban India. In G. Devos & L. Romanucci-Ross (Eds.), *Ethnic identity: Cultural continuities and change* (pp. 71–150). Chicago: The University of Chicago Press.

Berry, J. W. (1980). Acculturation and varieties of adaptation. In A. M. Padilla, (Ed.), *Acculturation: Theories and models and some new findings*. Boulder, CO: Westview Press.

Bos, G. (1986). Sexuality of gynecological cancer patients: Quantity and quality. *Journal of Psychosomatic Obstetrics and Gynecology, 5*, 217–224.

Brown–Saltzman, K. A. (1994). Tending the spirit. *Oncology Nursing Forum, 21*(6), 1001–1006.

Burstin, H. R., Lipsitz, S. R., & Brennan, T. A. (1992). Socioeconomic status and risk for substandard medical care. *Journal of the American Medical Association, 268*, 2383–2387.

Chrisman, N. (1991). Cultural system. In S. B. Baird, R. McCorkle, & M. Grant (Eds.), *Cancer nursing: A comprehensive textbook* (pp. 45–54). Philadelphia: W. B. Saunders.

Clark, P. G. (1991). Ethical dimensions of quality of life in aging: Autonomy vs collectivism in the United States and Canada. *The Gerontologist, 31*, 631–639.

Cleeland, C. S., Ladinsky, J. L., & Serlin, R. C. (1988). Multidimensional measurement of cancer pain: Comparisons of US and Vietnamese patients. *Journal of Pain and Symptom Management, 3*, 23–27.

Da Silva, J. A., & Hall, G. M. (1992). The effects of gender and sex hormones on outcome in rheumatoid arthritis. *Baillieres Clinical Rheumatology, 6*, 196–219.

Dana, R. H. (1993). *Multicultural assessment perspectives for professional psychology*. Boston: Allyn & Bacon.

Darty, T. E., & Potter, S. J. (1984). Social work with challenged women: Sexism, sexuality and the female cancer experience. *Journal of Social Work & Human Sexuality, 2*, 83–100.

Davitz, L. J., Sameshima, Y., & Davitz, J. (1976). Suffering as viewed in six different cultures. *American Journal of Nursing, 76*, 1296–1297.

DeVos, G., & Romanucci-Ross, L. (Eds.). (1982). *Ethnic identity: Cultural continuities and change*. Chicago: The Univeristy of Chicago Press.

DiMatteo, M. R., & Hays, S. (1981). Social support and serious illness. In B. H. Gottlieb (Ed.), *Social networks and social support* (pp. 117–148). Beverly Hills, CA: Sage Publications.

Doi, T. (1985). *The anatomy of self: The individual versus society*. Tokyo: Kodansha Internaltional, Ltd.

Drotar, D. (1991). The family context of nonorganic failure to thrive. *American Journal of Orthopsychiatry, 61*, 23–34.

Dunkel-Schetter, C. (1984). Social support and cancer: Findings based on patient interviews and their implications. *Journal of Social Issues, 40*, 77–98.

Eisenberg, L. (1977). Psychiatry and society: A sociobiological synthesis. *New England Journal of Medicine, 296*, 903–910.

Ell, K. O., Mantell, J. E., & Hamovitch, M. B. (1988). Socioculturally sensitive intervention for patients with cancer. *Journal of Psychosocial Oncology, 6*, 141–155.

Erickson, E. H. (1963). *Childhood and society*. New York: Norton.

Erwin, D. O. (1984). *Fighting cancer, dying to win: The American strategy for creating a chronic sick role*. Unpublished doctoral dissertation, Southern Methodist University.

Fabrega, H. (1972). Medical anthropology. In B. J. Siegel (Ed.), *Biennial review of anthropology*. Stanford, CA: Stanford University Press.

Frank–Stromborg, M., & Olsen, S. J. (Eds.). (1993). *Cancer prevention in minority populations: Cultural implications for health care professionals*. St Louis, MO: Mosby–Year Book, Inc.

Feathers, R. L. (1989). Orem's Self-Care Nursing Theory. In J. Riehl-Sisca (Ed.), *Conceptual models for nursing practice* (3rd ed., pp. 369–376). Norwalk, CT: Appleton & Lange.

Ferrell, B., Schmidt, G. M., Rhiner, M., & Fonbuena, P. (1992). The meaning of quality of life for bone marrow transplant survivors. Part 2. *Cancer Nursing, 15*(4), 247–253.

Ferrell, B., Schmidt, G. M., Rhiner, M., Whitehead, C., Fonbuena, P., & Forman, S. J. (1992). The meaning of quality of life for bone marrow transplant survivors. Part 1. *Cancer Nursing, 15*(3), 153–160.

Finerman, R. D. (1983). Experience and expectation: Conflict and change in traditional family health care among the Quichua of Saraguro. *Social Science and Medicine, 17*, 1291–1298.

Fraumeni, J. F., Jr., Hoover, R. N., Devesa, S. S., & Kinlen, L. J. (1989). Epidemiology of cancer. In V. T. Devita Jr., S. Hellman, & S. A. Rosenberg (Eds.), *Cancer: Principles and practice of oncology* (3rd ed., pp. 196–235). Philadelphia: J. B. Lippincott.

Ganz, P., Schag, C., & Heinrich, R. (1985). The psychosocial impact of cancer on the elderly: A comparison with younger patients. *American Geriatric Society, 33*, 429–435.

Geissler, E. M. (1994). *Pocket guide to cultural assessment*. St. Louis: Mosby–Year Book, Inc.

Garro, L. C. (1990). Culture, pain and cancer. *Journal of Palliative Care, 6*, 34–44.

Gill, T. M., & Feinstein, A. R. (1994). A critical appraisal of the quality of quality-of-life measurements. *Journal of the American Medical Association, 272*, 619–626.

Goldstein, M. K., & Teng, N. N. H. (1991). Gynecologic factors in sexual dysfunction of the older woman. *Clinics in Geriatric Medicine, 7*, 41–61.

Gudykunst, W. B., & Ting-Toomey, S. (1988). *Culture and interpersonal communication*. Newbury Park, CA: Sage Publications.

Hall, E. T., & Whyte, W. F. (1976). Intercultural communication: A guide to men of action. In P. Brink (Ed.), *Transcultural nursing: A book of readings* (pp. 44–62). Englewood Cliffs, NJ: Prentice-Hall, Inc.

Hallowell, A. I. (1955). *Culture and experience.* Philadelphia: University of Pennsylvania Press.

Haynes, R. H., Taylor, D. W., & Sackett, D. L. (Eds.). (1979). *Compliance in health care.* Baltimore: Johns Hopkins University Press.

Healy, B. (1991). The Yentl syndrome. [Editorial]. *New England Journal of Medicine, 325,* 274–275.

Houghton, I. T., Aun, C. S. T., Gin, T., & Lau, J. T. F. (1992). Inter-ethnic differences in postoperative Pethidine requirements. *Anaesthesia Intensive Care, 20,* 52–55.

Hunter, D. J., Manson, J. E., Colditz, G. A., Stampfer, M. J., Rosner, B., Hennekens, C. H., Speizer, F. E., & Willett, W. C. (1993). A prospective study of the intake of vitamins C, E, and A and the risk of breast cancer. *The New England Journal of Medicine, 329,* 234–240.

Irish, P. B. (1994). *Ethnic variation on dying.* Bristol, PA: Taylor & Francis Publishing.

Islam, A. K., Cooper, M. L., & Bodnar, R. J. (1993). Interactions among aging, gender, and gonadectomy effects upon morphine antinociception in rats. *Physiology and Behavior, 54,* 45–53.

Johnson, T. M., & Sargent, C. F. (Eds.). (1990). *Medical anthropology: Contemporary theory and method.* New York: Praeger Press.

Jones, W. T. (1976). World-views and Asian medical systems: Some suggestions for further study. In C. Leslie (Ed.), *Asian medical systems* (pp. 253–379). Berkeley: University of California Press.

Kagawa-Singer, M. (1988). Bamboo and oak: The influences of culture on adaptation to cancer between Japanese-American and Anglo-American patients. Unpublished dissertation, University of California Los Angeles.

Kagawa-Singer, M. (1993). Redefining health: Living with cancer. *Social Science and Medicine, 37,* 295–304.

Kagawa-Singer, M. (1994a). Quality of life: Cross-cultural differences. Unpublished manuscript.

Kagawa-Singer, M. (1994b). Cross–cultural views of disability. *Rehabilitation Nursing, 19,* 362–365.

Kagawa-Singer, M. (1994). Diverse cultural beliefs and practices about death and dying in the elderly. *Gerontology & Geriatrics Education, 15,* 101–116.

Kagawa-Singer, M., & Chung, R. C-Y. (1994). A paradigm for culturally based care in ethnic minority populations. *Journal of Community Psychology, 22,* 192–208.

Kalish, R. A., & Reynolds, D. K. (1976). *Death and ethnicity: A psychocultural study.* Los Angeles, CA: Ethel Percy Andrus Gerontology Center.

Kalow, W. (Ed.). (1992). *Pharmacogenetics of drug metabolism.* New York: Pergamon Press.

Katz, R. L., Norman, J., Seed, R. F., & Conrad, L. (1969). A comparison of the effects of suxamethonium and tubocurarine in patients in London and New York. *British Journal of Anaesthesia, 41,* 1041–1047.

Kellahear, A. (1990). *Dying of cancer: The final year of life.* Chur & London: Harwood Academic Publishers.

King, M. M., & McCay, P. B. (1983). Modulation of tumor incidence and possible mechanisms of mammary carcinogenesis by dietary oxidants. *Cancer Research, 43*(Suppl), 2485S–2490S.

Kleinman, A. (1980). *Patients and healers in the context of culture: An exploration of the borderland between anthropology, medicine, and psychiatry.* Berkely, CA: University of California Press.

Kleinman, A., Eisenberg, L., & Good, B. (1978). Culture, illness and care: Clinical lessons from anthropological and cross-cultural research. *Annals of Internal Medicine, 88,* 251–258.

Klessig, J. (1992). The effect of values and culture on life-support. *Western Journal of Medicine Special Edition, 157,* 316–322.

Koukouras, D., Spiliotis, J., Schopa, C. D., Dragotis, K., Kalfarentzos F, Tzoracoleftherakis, E., & Androulakis, J. (1991). Radical consequence in the sexuality of male patients operated for colorectal carcinoma. *European Journal of Surgical Oncology, 17,* 285–288.

Lazarus, R. S., & Folkman, S. (1984). *Stress appraisal and coping.* New York: Springer.

Leininger, M. (1970). *Nursing and anthropology: Two worlds to blend.* New York: John Wiley & Sons, Inc.

Leininger, M. (1993). Towards conceptualization of transcultural health care systems: Concepts and a model. *Journal of Transcultural Nursing, 4,* 32–40.

Levy, R. (1993). *Ethnic & racial differences in response to medicines: Preserving individualize therapy in managed pharmaceutical programs.* Reston, VA: National Pharmaceutical Council.

Lin, K-M, Poland, G., & Nakasaki, G. (Eds.). (1993). *Psychopharmacology and psychobiology of ethnicity.* Washington, DC: American Psychiatric Press.

Lipton, J. A., & Marbach, J. J. (1984). Ethnicity and the pain experience. *Social Science and Medicine, 19,* 1279–1298.

Litwin, M. (1994). Quality time: Prostate cancer. *Advances: Jonsson Comprehensive Cancer Center, UCLA, 3,* 14–15.

Lock, M. (1980). *East Asian medicine in urban Japan.* Berkeley, CA: University of California Press.

Mark, N., & Roberts, L. (1994). Ethnosensitve techniques in the treatment of the Hasidic patient with cancer. *Cancer Practice, 2,* 202–208.

Maslow, A. H. (1973). A theory of human motivation. In R. J. Lowry (Ed.), *Dominance, self-esteem, self-actualization: Germinal papers of A. H. Maslow* (pp. 153–174). Montery, CA: Brooks/Cole Publishing Company.

Mayer, W. J., & McWhorter, W. P. (1989). Black/white differences in non-treatment of bladder cancer patients and implications for survival. *American Journal of Public Health, 79,* l772–774.

McElroy, A., & Townsend, P. K. (1989). *Medical anthropology in ecological perspective* (2nd ed.). Boulder, CO: Westview Press.

Mechanic, D. (1972). Social psychologic factors affecting the presentation of bodily complaints. *New England Journal of Medicine, 286,* 1132–1139.

Mishel, M. H., Padilla, G., Grant, M., & Sorenson, D. S. (1991). Uncertainty in illness theory: A replication of the medicating effects of mastery and coping. *Nursing Research, 40,* 236–240.

Montagu, A. (1945). *Man's most dangerous myth: The fallacy of race.* New York: Columbia University Press.

Montagu, A. (1962). The concept of race. *American Anthropologist, 64,* 919–928.

Mor, V., & Masterson-Allen, S. (1988). The hospice model of care for the terminally ill. *Advances in Psychosomatic Medicine, 13,* 119–134.

Murphy, J. M. (1986). Trends in depression and anxiety: Men and women. *Acta Psychiatrica Scandinavica, 73,* 113–127.

Murray, M., & Reidy, G. (1990). Selectivity in the inhibition of mammalian cytochromes P-450 by chemical agents. *Pharmacology Review, 42,* 2–101.

Northouse, L. (1994). The family impact of cancer in women. In *American Cancer Society, Third national conference on cancer nursing research, abstracts* (pp. 6–A). Newport Beach, CA: American Cancer Society.

Northouse, L. L., & Northouse, P. G. (1992). *Health communication: Strategies for health professionals* (2nd ed.). Norwalk, CT: Appleton & Lange.

Otten, S. V., Schadel, M., Cheung, S. W., Kaplan, H. L., Busto, U. E., & Sellers, E. M. (1993). CYP26D6 phenotype determines the metabolic conversion of dydrocodone to hydromorphone. *Clinical Pharmacology & Therapeutics, 54,* 463–472.

Pagli, P., & Abramovitch, H. (1984). Death: A cross cultural perspective. *Annual Review of Anthropology, 13,* 385–417.

Parry, J. K. (Ed.). (1990). *Social work practice with the terminally ill.* Springfield, IL: Charles C. Thomas.

Pawling-Kaplan, M., & O'Connor, P. (1989). Hospice care for minorities: An analysis of a hospital based inner city palliative care service. *American Journal of Hospice Care, 6,* 13–21.

Perez-Stable, E. J., Sabogal, F., Otero-Sabogal, R., Hiatt, R. A., & McPhee, S. J. (1992). Misconceptions about cancer among Latinos and Anglos. *Journal of American Medical Association, 268,* 3219–3223

Peters-Golden, H. (1982). Breast cancer: Varied perceptions of social support in the illness experience. *Social Science and Medicine, 16,* 438–491.

Reizan, A., & Meleis, A. I. (1986). Arab-Americans' perceptions of and responses to pain. *Critical Care Nurse, 6,* 30–37.

Reynolds, D. K. (1989). Meaningful life therapy. *Culture, Medicine and Psychiatry, 13,* 457–463.

Samelson, E. J., Speers, M. A., Ferguson. R., & Bennett, C. (1994). Racial differences in cervical cancer mortality in Chicago. *American Journal of Public Health, 84,* 1007–1009.

Sargent, C. F. (1982). *The cultural context of therapeutic choice.* Dordrecht, Netherlands: Reidel Publishing Company.

Schain, W. (1992). *The impact of cancer and cancer treatment on sexuality and reproductive function.* Paper presented at the Psychosocial Oncology: Enhancing Patient and Family Care Conference, Beverly Hills, CA: Cedars-Sinai Comprehensive Cancer Center.

Scheper–Hughes, N., & Lock, M. (1987). The mindful body: A prolegomenon to future work in medical anthropology. *Medical Anthropology Quarterly, 1,* 6–41.

Silberfarb, P. M. (1982). Research in adaptation to illness and psychosocial intervention. *Cancer, 1*(Suppl.), 1921–1925.

Sontag, S. (1977). *Illness as metaphor.* New York: Vintage Books.

Steffensen, M. S., & Colker, L. (1982). Intercultural misunderstanding about health care. *Social Science and Medicine, 16,* 1949–1954.

Tannen, D. (1990). *You just don't understand: Women and men in conversation.* New York: Ballantine Books.

Tavris, C. (1982). *Anger: The misunderstood emotion.* New York: Simon & Schuster, Inc.

Todd, K. H., Samaroo, N., & Hoffman, J. R. (1993). Ethnicity as a risk factor for inadequate emergency department analgesia. *Journal of American Medical Association, 269,* 1537–1539.

Tripp-Reimer, T., & Afifi, L. A. (1989). Cross-cultural perspectives on patient teaching. *Nursing Clinics of North America, 24,* 613–619.

Tripp-Reimer, T., Brink, P., & Saunders, J. M. (1984). Cultural assessment: Content and process. *Nursing Outlook, 32,* 78–82.

Uba, L. (Ed.). (1994). *Asian Americans: Personality, patterns, identity, and mental health.* New York: Guilford Press.

Underwood, S. M., Hoskins, D., Tarshemicka, C., Morris, K., & Williams, A. (1994). Obstacles to cancer care: Focus on the economically disadvantaged. *Oncology Nursing Forum, 21,* 47–52.

Weber, W. W. (1987). *The acetylator genes and drug responses.* New York: Oxford University Press.

Wellisch, D. K., Kagawa-Singer, M., & Reid, S. L. (1995). Variations in social support between Asian- and Anglo-American women with breast cancer. (In preparation).

Weisman, A. D. (1984). *The coping capacity.* New York: Human Sciences Press.

Weiss, M. G., Doongaji, D. R., Siddharha, S., Wypij, D., Pathare, S., Bhatawdekar, M., Bhave, A., Sheth, A., & Fernandes, R. (1992). The Explatory Model Interview Catalogue (EMIC): Contributions to cross-cultural research methods from a study of leprosy and mental health. *British Journal of Psychiatry, 1600,* 819–830.

Willett, W. C., Stampfer, M. J., Colditz, G. A., Rosner, B. A., & Speizer, F. E. (1990). Relation of meat, fat and fiber intake to the risk of colon cancer in a prospective study among women. *New England Journal of Medicine, 323,* 1664–1672.

Zhou, H. H., Koshakji, R. P., & Silberstein, D. J. (1989). Racial differences in drug response. *New England Journal of Medicine, 320,* 565–570.

Zhou, H. H., Sheller, J. R., Nu, H., Wood, M., & Wood, A. J. J. (1993). Ethnic differences in response to morphine. *Clinical Pharmocology & Therapeutics, 54,* 507–513.

Zborowski, M. (1952). Cultural components in response to pain. *Journal of Social Issues, 3,* 16–30.

Zola, I. K. (1966). Culture and symptoms: An analysis of patients presenting complaints. *American Sociological Review, 31,* 615–630.

UNIT II
CONCEPTUAL THEMES BASIC TO CANCER NURSING

CHAPTER
5

Self-Care

Marylin Dodd • Gayle H. Shiba

Although self-care always has been the predominate form of health and illness care delivery, health care professionals only recently have begun to view individuals as active participants in their care. Partnerships between individuals, patients, and their families and health professionals may be not only desirable but may be essential to improve access and quality of care and to ensure greater accountability and lower cost (Levin, Katz, & Holst, 1976). Realizing these advantages, an increasing number of health professionals and lay person groups vigorously support the belief that self-care is the key to health and illness care.

Self-care has been investigated by several disciplines: social medicine, medical sociology, economics, and nursing. In nursing, the predominant theory of Orem's Self-Care Deficit Theory of Nursing (S-CDTN) has been used to provide the theoretic basis for self-care studies. The purpose of this chapter is to present Orem's S-CDTN and the published empiric work that has described and tested different components of the theory in the oncology population.

OREM'S SELF-CARE DEFICIT THEORY OF NURSING

Central to the philosophy of S-CDTN is the belief that there is always a need for self-care, and one has both the ability and responsibility to meet those needs. Orem's S-CDTN includes three related smaller theories:

(1) self-care, (2) self-care deficits, and (3) nursing systems (Orem, 1991). To understand the overall theory of S-CDTN, a review of each of these smaller theories is necessary, because the relationships among these theories is pivotal for understanding any one of the theories.

Factors have been identified that affect both an individual's ability to do self-care and the amount and type of self-care needed. These factors are defined as *basic conditioning factors* and include but are not limited to age, gender, developmental stage, health state, sociocultural orientation, family systems factors, patterns of living, environmental factors, resource availability, and adequacy (Orem, 1991). Basic conditioning factors can affect all three theories.

SELF-CARE

The first theory of self-care includes the concepts of self-care, therapeutic self-care demand, and self-care agency.

SELF-CARE

Self-care "is the practice of activities that individuals initiate and perform on their own behalf in maintaining life, health, and well-being" (Orem, 1991, p. 117). Self-care is purposeful and conducted to meet self-care requisites (needs) of individuals themselves or others in need of care (dependent care).

THERAPEUTIC SELF-CARE DEMAND

Therapeutic self-care demands are the self-care actions necessary to meet known self-care requisites (needs). Orem states that the therapeutic self-care demands are the "summation of measures of self-care required at moments in time or for some duration" (Orem, 1991, p. 65). These actions are initiated to fulfill an individual's self-care requisites (needs) or are the reasons a person initiates self-care.

Orem has identified three categories of self-care requisites: universal, developmental, and health deviation requisites. Universal self-care requisites are common to all humans and include both physiologic and psychosocial needs. Eight universal requisites are the maintenance of air, water, food, elimination, rest, and activity; prevention of hazards; and promotion of functioning. These requisites represent self-care activities to support human structure, functioning, and development (Orem, 1991).

Developmental self-care requisites are based on age and stage of life. At times, developmental requisites are viewed as specialized universal self-care requisites that relate to developmental processes or new requisites resulting from a situation or condition (e.g., pregnancy) (Orem, 1991).

Health deviation self-care requisites are uniquely individual and result from a health problem or condition. These requisites can be associated with medical diagnostic and treatment measures. Orem (1991) states "the characteristics of health deviations as conditions extending over time determine the kinds of care demands that individuals experience as they live with the effects of pathologic conditions . . ." (p. 133).

SELF-CARE AGENCY

Self-care agency is the acquired ability or power of the individual to engage in self-care and includes a composite of capabilities and limitations of the individual for meeting his or her therapeutic self-care demands. Central to self-care agency is the individual's experience, understanding, critical reflection, and clinical judgment. Three components have been identified for self-care agency: (1) foundational capabilities, (2) power components, and (3) capabilities for specific self-care (Orem, 1991). These three types of abilities are hierarchically arranged.

Foundational capabilities and dispositions are those abilities that come into play when an individual performs *any* deliberate action, not just those limited to self-care. The power components are the set of enabling capabilities that relate specifically to the engagement of self-care. Finally, the capabilities for specific self-care (estimative, transitional, and productive) are the most focused component of self-care agency. Both the power components and the capabilities for specific self-care are directly related to self-care.

SELF-CARE DEFICIT

The theory of self-care deficit is central to the S-CDTN, because this is where the need for nursing is identified. Patients experience self-care deficits when they are unable to fully care for themselves. Self-care deficit is the "relationship between self-care agency and therapeutic self-care demands of individuals in which capabilities for self-care, because of existent limitations, are not equal to meeting some or all of the categories of their therapeutic self-care demands" (Orem, 1991, p. 173). Actual or potential self-care deficits need to exist for nursing care to be required.

NURSING SYSTEMS

The third theory, nursing systems, is the relationship between the patient and the nurse within the overall theory of S-CDTN. Nursing systems theory is based on the capabilities and needs of the patient to perform self-care. Nursing systems are classified as (1) wholly compensatory, (2) partly compensatory, and (3) supportive-educative. The wholly compensatory nursing system is needed when the patient is completely unable to engage in self-care activities. For example, a critically ill oncology patient in the intensive care unit (ICU) may require a wholly compensatory nursing system. The partly compensatory nursing system occurs when both the patient and the nurse mutually engage in self-care activities. Finally, the supportive-educative nursing system is when the patient is able to learn to perform therapeutic self-care activities but needs assistance and support in learning to do so.

A REVIEW OF THE STUDIES THAT HAVE USED OREM'S S-CDTN

Selected studies in this section will be described, along with how they are placed within Orem's theory and how the findings elucidate the theory. There were 12 published self-care studies found that used primarily the theory of self-care, only one study that used the theory of self-care deficit, and nine studies that used primarily the theory of nursing systems.

SELF-CARE: TWELVE STUDIES
SELF-CARE (BEHAVIORS)

1. Dodd (1984a, 1988) conducted a descriptive study whose purpose was to determine the patterns of self-care behaviors in breast cancer patients who were experiencing side effects of chemotherapy. Thirty patients who were initiating their first course of a selected adjuvant chemotherapy protocol were obtained from six oncologists in private practice. The descriptive design was longitudinal with repeated measures. Three instruments were used in the study: State-Trait Anxiety Inventory, Multidimensional Locus of Control Scale, and the Self-Care Behavior Log. At the initiation of chemotherapy the patients completed the questionnaires and were taught how to record in the log the side effects of treatment and their self-care behaviors. These recordings had two components: first, the

self-care behaviors the patients performed to prevent the side effects from occurring; and second, the behaviors they performed to manage a side effect once it occurred. At the next cycle of chemotherapy (approximately 3 weeks later) patients were contacted to inquire how they were doing and whether recording in the log was presenting any difficulties. Three weeks later (approximately 6 weeks after initiating treatment) the patients were again contacted to complete the questionnaires and to return their completed logs.

The theoretic basis of the study was provided by Orem's S-CDTN. The focus on self-care behaviors was directly derived from self-care theory. The Therapeutic Self-Care Demand's Health-Deviation Requisites (TS-CD, H-DReq) were the side effects of chemotherapy. The study variables that were possible correlates of self-care behaviors (i.e., demographic characteristics, anxiety, and locus of control) are viewed as Orem's Basic Conditioning Factors (bcfs).

The findings of this study corroborated an earlier study by Dodd (1982, 1984a). Patients did not know what self-care behaviors were helpful to either prevent the side effects or to manage them once they occurred (Dodd, 1984a, 1988). They often waited until the side effects were severe and persistent before initiating self-care. Some patients believed the side effects were to be endured and were reluctant to complain about the treatment. Finally, patients cited themselves most frequently as the source of information for their self-care behaviors; the nurse was cited infrequently. State anxiety decreased significantly during the study period and was significantly related to the number of self-care behaviors. There were no other significant relationships between the other bcfs and number of self-care behaviors.

2. A parallel study was conducted by the same investigator with 30 patients receiving radiation therapy for a variety of types of cancer (Dodd, 1984b). The findings of this study corroborate the overall pattern of self-care behaviors in the earlier investigations (Dodd, 1982, 1984a, 1988). Because of space limitations, this and other studies are summarized in Table 5–1.

3. Robinson and Posner (1992) conducted a study to determine the needs and the self-care interventions of patients who had received at least one previous treatment of Biologic Response Modifier therapy. Their second purpose was to determine the extent to which the needs and self-care interventions identified by patients compared with those perceived by their family members and nurses. Sixteen patients with various types of cancer participated in the study and experienced fatigue. The descriptive, cross-sectional design consisted of open-ended questions to obtain data on patients' self-care needs and interventions. The investigators developed a demographic data form and an Analysis of High-Intensity Self-Care Needs and Intervention survey that was specific for fatigue. The questionnaires were completed by the patients and designated family members within 1 week of the patient's first unsolicited report of fatigue as a side effect of biotherapy. The nurse's questionnaire was completed within 48 hours of the patient's reporting the onset of the symptom.

The investigators described components of Orem's S-CDTN theory that related to the study. The symptom of fatigue could be placed within the theory as a TS-CD, H-DReq. The demographic and disease data are viewed as bcfs, with the self-care interventions being derived from Self-Care theory.

Patients rated the symptom of fatigue as moderate to severe, with notable changes in their employment status caused by the fatigue. Neither the type of Biologic Response Modifier therapy received nor the dosage (bcfs) correlated significantly with the degree or the duration of fatigue (TS-CD, H-DReq). There was considerable disparity between the patients' and nurses' ratings of fatigue, with less disparity between the patients' and family members' ratings. Patients identified self-care interventions that are common knowledge and have been reported by others. A new finding was the identification by the patient of interventions others could do (Dependent Care) to reduce the fatigue. No analyses were provided for the relationships between the bcfs and self-care interventions. The investigators concluded that there appears to be some difficulty for the patient in identifying potentially useful interventions for fatigue (reflecting a self-care deficit). Unfortunately, the nurses and family members reported that they had no idea which interventions may prove beneficial. With this finding the adequacy of the Nursing System and Dependent Care seems in doubt.

4. Musci and Dodd (1990) conducted a study whose purposes were to describe the self-care behaviors initiated by patients and family members and to determine the relationship between patients' and family members' affective states, family functioning, and self-care behaviors. The sample included 42 patients and their family members. The inclusion of family members occurred for the first time in self-care studies in the oncology population. The patients were beginning their first course of chemotherapy at a large tertiary hospital's outpatient clinic. The correlational design was longitudinal, extending over three Cycles of chemotherapy (approximately 12-16 weeks) with repeated measures. The instruments used were: Profile of Mood States (affective states), F-COPES (family functioning), and the Self-Care Behavior Log (self-care behaviors). Consenting patients identified a family member who was most involved in their care. The POMS was completed by the patients and family members at each Cycle, the F-COPES was completed by patients and family members at Cycle 2 only, and the Self-Care Behavior Log was completed on an ongoing basis by the patients.

The conceptual framework for the study was provided by Coping and Stress theory for both the

TABLE 5–1. ***Studies that Tested Orem's Theory of Self-Care***

REFERENCE	PURPOSE/SAMPLE	METHODS/DESIGN	SELECTED FINDINGS

1. Dodd, M. J. (1984a, 1988)	• To determine the patterns of self-care behaviors
	• 30 women with breast cancer who were initiating CTX
		• Descriptive, longitudinal
		• Variables measured:
		  a) anxiety
		  b) control
		  c) self-care behaviors
			• Low self-care behaviors
			• Delay initiating behaviors
			• Anxiety significantly related to number of self-care behaviors

2. Dodd, M. J. (1984b)	• To determine the patterns of self-care behaviors
	• 30 patients with selected types of cancer who were initiating RT
		• Descriptive, longitudinal
		• Variables measured:
		  a) anxiety
		  b) control
		  c) self-care behaviors
			• Low self-care behaviors
			• Significant positive relationship between patients' knowledge and self-care behaviors
			• Significant positive relationship between distress and self-care activity
			• Significant correlations between control and effectiveness of self-care

3. Robinson & Posner (1992)	• To determine the needs and self-care interventions of patients receiving biologic response modifiers • To compare these needs and interventions among patient, family members, and nurses • 16 patients with various types of cancer	• Descriptive, cross-sectional • Variables measured: a) fatigue	• Patients reported moderate to severe fatigue, that was not related to dosage or duration of therapy • There was disparity between the patients' and nurses' ratings of fatigue • Self-care interventions were common knowledge

4. Musci & Dodd (1990)	• To describe the self-care behaviors initiated by patients and family members
	• To determine the relationship between patients' and family members' affective state, family functioning, and self-care behaviors
	• 42 patients and their family members
		• Correlational, longitudinal, with repeated measures
		• Variables measured:
		  a) affective states
		  b) family functioning
		  c) self-care behaviors
		  d) side effects
			• Female patients performed a greater diversity of self-care behaviors and relied on medications to control their side effects less often than male patients
			• Length of illness was significantly associated with greater self-care
			• Only at Time 1 did two affective states significantly predict the number of self-care behaviors, severity of the side effects consistently predicted self-care behaviors

5. Dodd et al. (1992)	• To describe the side effects experienced and self-care behaviors performed
	• To determine relationships of selected bcfs and side effects and self-care
	• 69 patients with selected types of cancer who were initiating CTX
		• Correlational, longitudinal with repeated measures
		• Variables measured:
		  a) demographic, disease, and treatment
		  b) side effects
		  c) self-care behaviors
			• Older patients perceived their self-care as less effective than younger patients
			• Performance status scores correlated positively with overall self-care behaviors
			• Number of CTX agents received and health status were significant predictors of the number of side effects

6. Rhodes et al. (1988)	• To examine the relationship between self-reported symptoms and Self-Care Agency
	• 20 patients who had experienced six cycles of CTX
		• Descriptive, retrospective data
		• Variables measured:
		  a) symptomatology
		  b) self-care
			• Tiredness and weakness most interfered with self-care activities
			• Specific self-care activities were obtained for tiredness and weakness

7. Hanucharurnkul (1989)	• To determine whether self-care can be predicted jointly by social support and selected bcfs
	• 112 patients with selected types of cancer who were receiving RT
		• Correlational, cross-sectional
		• Variables measured:
		  a) demographic, disease, and treatment
		  b) social support
			• Occupational prestige and social support were significant predictors of self-care
			• Stage and site of cancer predicted self-care indirectly through social support

TABLE 5–1. *Studies that Tested Orem's Theory of Self-Care* Continued

REFERENCE	PURPOSE/SAMPLE	METHODS/DESIGN	SELECTED FINDINGS

8. Dodd & Dibble (1993)	• To determine predictors (bcfs and power components) of self-care behaviors over time
	• 127 patients with cancer who were initiating high morbidity CTX agents
		• Correlational, longitudinal
		• Variables measured:
		  a) performance status
		  b) CTX knowledge
		  c) self-care abilities
		  d) perceived self-efficacy
		  e) health promoting behaviors
		  f) affective state
		  g) self-care behaviors
			• Patients with lower performance status, less social support, and higher anxiety performed significantly more self-care behaviors

9. Kubricht (1984)	• To identify the Therapeutic Self-Care Demands of outpatients
	• 30 patients receiving RT
		• Descriptive, cross-sectional
		• Variables measured:
		  a) changes in lives since RT began
		  b) demographic, disease, and treatment
			• Patients identified an average of over 18 Therapeutic Self-Care Demands

10. Oberst et al. (1991)	• To describe the Self-Care Burden (TS-CD, H-DReqs)
	• To identify antecedent factors that contribute to the Self-Care Burden
	• To test a model
	• 72 patients with cancer who were receiving RT
		• Descriptive, correlational, cross-sectional
		• Variables measured:
		  a) self-care burden
		  b) symptom distress
		  c) bcfs
			• Patients were receiving help with self-care, most often spouse
			• Dependency and symptom distress were the primary predictors of health-deviation self-care burden
			• Symptom distress and dependency were the best predictors of universal self-care burden
			• Greater symptom distress and health-deviation self-care burden in patients with recurrent disease

11. Munkres et al. (1992)	• To determine how much the personal meaning of the situation mediates the effects of personal characteristics, illness characteristics, and self-care burden (TS-CD, H-DReqs) on emotional outcomes
	• 60 patients (28 with initial cancer and 32 with recurrent cancer) receiving CTX
		• Descriptive, correlational, cross-sectional
		• Variables measured:
		  a) symptom distress
		  b) self-care burden
		  c) family hardiness
		  d) appraisal of illness
		  e) affective states
		  f) personal illness characteristics
			• Symptom distress accounted for 26% of variance in universal self-care burden, with economic status and dependency contributing an additional 12% and 7% respectively

12. Rhodes et al. (1987)	• To describe patterns of nausea and vomiting and distress (TS-CD, H-DReqs)
	• 309 patients with cancer who were initiating CTX
		• Descriptive, time series
		• Variables measured:
		  a) nausea and vomiting
		  b) demographic, disease, and treatment
			• 71% experienced little or no nausea, with 84% having their vomiting well controlled by 48 hours
			• Three distinct antiemetic patterns emerged

individual and families, and Orem's S-CDTN. The primary focus of the study was self-care behaviors, so Self-Care theory was central to the investigation. Because the patients kept the Self-Care Behavior Log, the families Dependent Care was infrequently reported. Orem's bcfs (demographic and disease characteristics, family functioning, and affective states of both patients and families) played an important role as potential predictors of self-care behaviors. TS-CD, H-DReqs were the side effects experienced by the patients, with the severity rating of the side effects being a dimension of this requisite.

Some patients experienced a remarkable TS-CD, H-DReq, in the severity of side effects (averaged from 3.7 to more than 3.8 on a five-point Likert scale). There were modest numbers of self-care behaviors performed, but the patients' ratings of effectiveness were moderately high. A gender (bcf) difference was observed, with women performing a greater diversity of self-care behaviors and relying on medications for side effect control less often than men. The length of illness (bcf of experience) was significantly associated with greater self-care behaviors. These last two findings are noteworthy in that gender and length of illness have not been found to relate to self-care behaviors in other investigations. The affective states subscales (bcfs) of depression (negative) and vigor (positive) predicted the number of self-care behaviors at Cycle 1 only. However, the severity of the side effects (TS-HD, H-DReq), consistently predicted fewer self-care behaviors.

5. The purposes of a study conducted by Dodd, Dibble, and Thomas (1992) were twofold: to describe the side effects experienced by patients who were beginning chemotherapy and the self-care behaviors they performed, and to determine the relationships of selected bcfs with the side effects and self-care behaviors. This study was a part of a larger study of Coping and Self-Care of Patients and Their Families (RO1 NR01441) and is summarized in Table 5–1.

6. Rhodes, Watson, and Hanson (1988) conducted a study whose purpose was to examine the relationship between self-reported symptoms and Self-Care Agency perceived by patients receiving antineoplastic chemotherapy (as stated in abstract). Later in the text the stated purpose was, "to examine the relationship between patients' symptoms and their self-care activities . . ." (p. 187). Still later, another purpose statement was given . . . "what symptoms they were able to identify as interfering with Self-Care Activities (note *not* Self-Care Agency), and what modification of self-care activities was taken to alleviate . . ." (p. 188). Some insight into this confusion in terms is provided in their Figure 2, where the investigators combine Self-Care Agency and Self-Care Abilities into one concept.

   The sample for the study included 20 patients who had completed six cycles of chemotherapy and were part of a larger study ($N = 329$). The design was descriptive with retrospective data being obtained in patient telephone interviews. The interview schedules were developed by the investigators and used open-ended questions regarding symptoms and self-care. The patients were interviewed by phone twice by a research assistant. Schedule A interviews asked about symptoms, self-care, and effectiveness of the self-care activities. Schedule B ($n = 11$) contained more in-depth questions and was audiotaped and transcribed. Sample items included: "tell me about tiredness, fatigue, and weakness after receiving your chemotherapy"; "how it affected your life and daily care"; and self-care activities.

   Rhodes and her colleagues view the symptoms experienced by patients as a component of health state, whereas Dodd and her colleagues and others view these as TS-CD, H-DReqs. Whether bcfs (health state) is what a person brings to the situation, or what happens during the event that is being studied is not clear in Orem's theory.

   Under the heading of "Symptoms that most interfere with Self-Care Abilities," it is noted that tiredness and weakness were identified as the symptoms that most interfered with self-care activities (note Self-Care, not Self-Care Agency). There is a detailed description of the specific self-care activities for tiredness and weakness. One category of activities for decreasing expenditure of energy was given as increasing dependence on others. This strategy would directly relate to Orem's Dependent Care provided by others.

7. The study by Hanucharurnkul (1989) stands out from the others presented in this chapter in that it was the first to plan apriori to test some of Orem's propositions as they relate not only to bcfs but also to Dependent Care. The purpose of this study was to determine whether self-care can be predicted jointly by social support and selected bcfs of age, marital and socioeconomic status, living arrangements during treatment, and stage and site of cancer. The sample included 112 adult patients with cervical or head and neck cancer who were receiving radiation therapy in outpatient clinics in Bangkok, Thailand. These patients had received at least 15 treatments before being entered into the study. The design was correlational, cross-sectional. Selected instruments were the Self-Care Behavior Questionnaire, which listed 41 self-care behaviors, the Social Support Questionnaire, the Norbeck Social Support Questionnaire, and socioeconomic questions. Patients completed the questionnaires in the clinic.

   Orem's S-CDTN provided the theoretic framework for the study. With the occurrence of cancer and its treatment, the investigator sees the patients as having to meet modified Universal, Developmental, and Health-Deviation Self-Care Requisites to maintain life, health, and well-being. This is consistent with Orem's concept of Therapeutic Self-Care Demands, as is the investigator's viewing Dependent Care as including social support. Dependent Care may be needed especially from family members and health care providers to meet complex self-care requisites. Dependent Care as defined by Orem and Taylor (1986) is action performed by an adult to meet the components of the dependent's self-care requisites. Dependent Care in this study was conceptualized as being in the form of social support that includes informational, emotional, and tangible support (Wortman, 1984). Orem postulates that the presence of a social support system as an environmental resource may facilitate self-care. The components of Orem's theory that fit with this study are Self-Care theory (self-care behaviors), bcfs (socio-economic questions), Dependent Care (social support), and TS-CD, H-DReq (side effects of radiotherapy).

   The investigator concluded that socioeconomic ("occupational prestige") a bcf, and social support (Dependent Care) were significant predictors of self-care (behaviors). The stage and site of cancer predicted self-care indirectly through social support. The investigator proposed a buffering effect of social support. These findings support Orem's theory in part in that the socioeconomic and social support as available resources affect the initiation and continuation of self-care behaviors.

8. Dodd and Dibble (1993) replicated and extended the work of Hanucharurnkul (1989). The purpose of this study was to determine the predictors of self-care over time in patients receiving chemotherapy. The primary questions were: what are the significant bcfs of self-care (behaviors), and what are the significant

power components of self-care (behaviors)? This study was part of a larger randomized control trial (Dodd et al., 1986–1990). The sample consisted of 127 adults with cancer who were receiving their first dose of specific types of chemotherapy agents (chosen because of reported high morbidity) from 18 health care settings in California. The design was longitudinal-correlational. Instruments used in the study included Karnofsky Performance Status, Chemotherapy Knowledge Questionnaire, Exercise of Self-Care Agency, Perceived Self-Efficacy Scale, Health Promoting Lifestyle Profile, Profile of Mood States, and the Self-Care Behavior Checklist. An instrument packet was given to patients by the office/clinic nurse at the time of the first chemotherapy cycle. A research nurse collected the completed packet at the patients' homes during nadir of the chemotherapy. At Cycles 2, 3, and 4 data again were collected in this same manner.

Orem's S-CDTN provided the theoretic framework for the study. The TS-CD, H-DReqs from the experienced side effects provided the stimulus for self-care. Selected bcfs included age, gender, years of schooling, health state (performance status, type of cancer, and stage), health care system factors (chemotherapy treatment, and side effects), family system factors (social support), and patterns of living (health promoting lifestyles). The Power Components of the concept of Self-Care Agency included:

- ability to maintain attention and exercise requisite vigilance with respect to self-care and internal conditions (self-care abilities, perceived self-efficacy, and affective states)
- controlled use of available physical energy for self-care operations (self-care abilities)
- ability to reason within a self-care frame of reference (self-care abilities)
- motivation towards self-care (self-care abilities, perceived self-efficacy)
- ability to acquire technical knowledge about self-care (self-care abilities).

The components of Orem's theory that are evident in this study are primarily Self-Care theory (self-care behaviors), the selected predictors of the bcfs and Power Components (PCs) of the concept of Self-Care Agency, and to a lesser extent the TS-CD, H-DReqs resulting from the experienced side effects of treatment.

Patients with lower performance status (bcf), less social support (bcf), more schooling (bcf), and high anxiety (PC) performed significantly more self-care (behaviors). The performance status is viewed by Orem as part of the health state; with a better health state it would be expected that the individual would be more capable of greater self-care. In this study a significant negative correlation existed between the performance scores and the number of side effects experienced. The side effects were viewed by the investigators to be a stimulus for self-care activity.

Orem conceptualized social support to be a resource that facilitates self-care. However, in this study those patients with less social support performed more self-care. The investigators propose that those patients with less social support may mobilize more self-care on their own behalf as a result of having fewer options to meet their requisites for care. The finding that patients with more years of schooling performed more self-care is consistent with Orem's view of education being a personal resource or asset for self-care. Finally, the finding of higher anxiety was a significant predictor of self-care. Perhaps the more vigilant state (as reflected in higher anxiety) may be conducive to greater activity by some patients.

THERAPEUTIC SELF-CARE DEMAND (THREE CATEGORIES OF REQUISITES)

- **Universal Self-Care Requisites**
- **Developmental Self-Care Requisites**
- **Health Deviation Self-Care Requisites**

9. Kubricht's (1984) study identified the Therapeutic Self-Care Demands expressed by outpatients receiving radiation therapy. The sample consisted of 30 patients who had completed half of their treatments. A descriptive survey was utilized in the cross-sectional study. An open-ended interview technique asked the patients for changes that occurred in their lives since the radiation therapy began. These interviews were conducted by the investigator and were audiotaped and transcribed.

Radiation therapy, physiology, Orem's concept of Therapeutic Self-Care Demand, and Magoon's constructivist methodology were synthesized as a foundation for the study. It was postulated that Orem's Therapeutic Self-Care Demand was experienced with both the physiologic and psychologic changes that occurred during treatment and that these changes would result in activation of the patients' Self-Care Agency. The investigators used Orem's Universal Self-Care Requisites to categorize the qualitative data. Also included were selected bcfs of age, gender, race, education, number of weeks of treatment, location of the treatment, and others. These factors were not used for comparative analyses of the Therapeutic Self-Care Demands of this sample.

Patients were very able to identify their Therapeutic Self-Care Demands; on average they identified more than 18. The majority of responses (20 per cent) related to the Universal Self-Care Requisites category called protection from hazards. All of the categories of the Universal Self-Care requisites were represented in the patients' responses. A question that remains to be answered is, since the patients reported changes that had occurred after beginning their treatment, are these changes Universal Self-Care Requisites or Health-Deviation Self-Care Requisites? If it is the latter, then using the categories of Universal Self-Care Requisites for the data analyses is inconsistent.

10. Oberst, Hughes, Chang, and McCubbin (1991) conducted a study of 72 patients with cancer who were receiving radiation therapy. Their purposes included to describe the self-care burden (SCB) of these patients and the difficulty or distress associated with them, to identify antecedent illness and personal and resource factors that contribute to the SCBs, and to test a model of the effects of SCBs, symptom distress, and appraisal of the meaning of illness on mood. The study used a descriptive correlational design that was cross-sectional. Instruments included the Self-Care Burden Scale and the modified Symptom Distress Scale. Other characteristics of the illness situation were assessed on the basis of patients' self-report. Patients took the questionnaires home to complete and returned them, usually within the week, to the radiation therapy department.

Although conceptually this study was guided by a cognitive appraisal model of stress and coping, the investigators presented a review of self-care studies where Orem's theory provided the theoretic framework. Self-Care Burden was a major variable in this study and was defined as a product of self-care demands. Orem's concept of Therapeutic Self-Care Demands does not have a similar notion of burden. The Self-Care Burden Scale was developed by the investigators to assess the extent of the self-care demands and the difficulty of meeting those demands. The personal characteristics selected were derived from cognitive appraisal theory but could have been labeled as bcfs of Orem's theory.

More than half of the sample were receiving help with self-care, most often from a spouse. Among the health-deviation self-care tasks, "coming to treatment" was the most demanding, and self-treatment such as skin care was the most difficult. Universal self-care activities that were the most disrupted by treatment were social and recreational activities. Path analysis revealed that dependency and to a lesser extent, symptom distress, were the primary predictors of health-deviation self-care burden. This finding is in contrast to a later study where dependency predicted universal self-care burden (Munkres et al., 1992). Symptom distress (and to a lesser extent, dependency) was the best predictor of universal self-care burden. This finding was corroborated in the later study (Munkres et al., 1992) and is puzzling in that symptom distress more directly relates to the sequela of cancer and its treatment. Should disruptions in, for example, air, food, and social activities caused by cancer and its treatment and the burden of managing these disruptions be classified as Universal Self-Care or Health-Deviation Self-Care Requisites? Finally, Health-Deviation along with three other variables explained 55 per cent of the variance of affective mood dysfunction. This mood state could be broadly interpreted as a health outcome as a result of self-care in Orem's theory. Un-

fortunately, self-care activities were not measured in this study but no doubt were being performed by these patients.

11. Munkres, Oberst, and Hughes (1992) undertook a later study to examine response differences in people receiving chemotherapy for initial versus recurrent cancer and to determine how much the personal meaning/appraisal of the situation mediates the effects of personal characteristics, illness characteristics, and self-care burden on emotional outcomes. Because of space limitations, this study is summarized in Table 5–1.

12. Rhodes, Watson, Johnson, Madson, and Beck (1987) conducted a study whose purpose was to describe patterns of nausea and vomiting occurrence and distress that emerged during six consecutive cycles of selected initial antineoplastic chemotherapy drug regimens. The study is summarized in Table 5–1.

SELF-CARE AGENCY (THREE COMPONENTS)

- **Foundational capabilities**
- **Power components (10)**
- **Capabilities for specific self-care (three levels)**
  - **(a)   Estimative capabilities**
  - **(b)   Transitional capabilities**
  - **(c)   Productive capabilities**

No studies were found.

SELF-CARE DEFICIT: ONE STUDY

1. Fernsler (1986) conducted a study where the purpose was to compare patient and nurse perceptions of the patients' self-care deficits associated with cancer chemotherapy in an outpatient setting. Thirty patients and their assigned five nurses provided the convenience sample. The descriptive design was used in this cross-sectional study. Two semistructured interview schedules were developed by the investigator for the patient and the nurse. Patients were interviewed before their chemotherapy treatment, and the nurses were interviewed as soon as possible after the patients' treatment. Interviews were audiotaped and transcribed verbatim.

Self-care concepts (Orem), perceptual theory of behavior, and constructivist methodology were used as the framework for the study. Specifically, the interview schedules were developed from Orem's theory. The investigator used for her qualitative data analyses Orem's categories of Universal Self-Care Requisites instead of the Health Deviation Self-Care Requisites. Because her sample included persons with cancer who were receiving treatment, the use of Universal rather than Health-Deviation Requisites was not discussed. Selected bcfs (race, gender, number of chemotherapy agents) were used for subgroup analyses of the data. The primary focus of this study is Orem's theory of Self-Care Deficits, with a secondary focus of Self-Care, specifically Therapeutic Self-Care Demand of the experienced side effects of treatment, and selected bcfs.

Fernsler found that patients generally perceived more self-care deficits than did nurses in the categories of problems with the physical side effects of treatment. The greatest number of responses were for the category of activity and rest. Nurses perceived slightly more patient deficits than did patients in the categories of psychosocial problems. The study summary is found in Table 5–2.

NURSING SYSTEMS (ACTIONS): NINE STUDIES

1. Dodd (1982, 1982a, 1983, 1984) conducted a study whose purposes were to test different types of information (drug, side effect management techniques [SEMT], or a combination of the two) on patients' knowledge of chemotherapy, self-care behaviors, and affective states. The sample included patients with cancer who had at a minimum received 2 weeks of their initial chemotherapy. In this experimental study the investigator randomly assigned the patients to one of four groups (the experimental conditions mentioned previously, and the control group). Instruments selected for the dependent variables included the Chemotherapy Knowledge Questionnaire (chemotherapy knowledge), the Self-Care Behavior Questionnaire (self-care behaviors), and the Profile of Mood States (affective states). The investigator conducted all the preintervention interviews; she administered the questionnaires, then presented the information to the three patients in the experimental group and spent equal time with the patients in the control group but did not impart drug or SEMT information. The information was given in written form to the patients. Four to 9 weeks later, data collectors (nurses working in the referral sites) who were blind to the patients' assigned group conducted the second interview, in which the patients again completed the questionnaires.

   The theoretic framework for the study was provided by theories of Coping and Stress, Control, and Orem's S-CDTN. The informational interventions (Nursing Systems theory, Supportive-Educative) provided the prerequisite elements suggested by Orem to be necessary for self-care such as side effect drug information and suggestions for self-

care activities for Health-Deviation Requisites. Bcfs of demographic and disease characteristics were assessed for their influence on the dependent variables, and if significant, for their equal distribution across the four groups at Time 1. The primary emphasis of the study was to enhance self-care activities, treatment-related knowledge, and the general health outcome of affective states.

The hypotheses were supported in part. Patients who received drug information (either alone or in combination with SEMT) knew significantly more about their treatment. Patients who received SEMT information (either alone or in combination with drug information) performed significantly more self-care behaviors. Patients who received combined information knew significantly more about their treatment and performed significantly more self-care behaviors but did not have better affective states than patients in the other three groups. That the types of information provided to these patients made a significant difference in their knowledge and self-care would be expected by Orem's theory, but this expectation would extend to the affective state as well.

2. Dodd (1988a) conducted another experimental study whose purposes were twofold. One purpose was to test three hypotheses about the effects of two different schedules of presenting Side Effect Management Techniques (SEMT) information (before and after the occurrence of experienced side effects) on patients' self-care behavior. The second purpose was to determine the influence of selected potential moderator variables on patients' self-care behavior. Sixty patients who were beginning their initial course of chemotherapy for selected types of cancer constituted the sample. Instruments selected for this study were STAI (State-Trait Anxiety Inventory), Multidimensional Health Locus of Control, and the Self-Care Behavior Log. Patients were randomly assigned to two experimental conditions: Schedule A intervention consisted of presenting SEMT information on the potential side effects the patient was susceptible to develop, *before* the development of any of these side effects. Schedule B intervention consisted of presenting SEMT information on the patient's experienced side effects *after* the development of any of these side effects. Measurement of the potential moderating variables of Anxiety and Control occurred once at the initiation of treatment and 6 weeks later at the comple-

TABLE 5–2. *Study that Tested Orem's Theory of Self-Care Deficit*

REFERENCE	PURPOSE/SAMPLE	METHODS/DESIGN	SELECTED FINDINGS
1. Fernsler (1986)	• To compare patient and nurse perceptions of the patient's self-care deficits • 30 outpatients receiving CTX and 5 nurses	• Descriptive, cross-sectional • Variables measured: 　a) demographic, disease, treatment 　b) self-care deficits	• Patients reported more self-care deficits related to physical side effects of CTX • Nurses reported more patient deficits related to psychosocial problems

tion of Cycle 2. Measurement of the dependent variable of self-care behaviors that were the patients' self-report occurred throughout the study period.

The theoretic framework for the study was provided by Stress and Coping, and Orem's S-CDTN. The primary focus of the study was Nursing Systems theory, Supportive-Educative, to enhance self-care behaviors (Self-Care theory). The potential moderating variables of anxiety and control are bcfs that were tested for their influence on self-care. The experienced side effects are the stimulus for self-care and as such are Therapeutic Self-Care Demands, specifically Health-Deviation Self-Care Requisites.

The hypotheses were supported in part. The Schedule A SEMT information resulted in greater self-care behaviors, both for preventing the side effects and for managing the side effects once they occurred. This effect is consistent with Orem's theory. Schedule A did not result in a significant decrease in the delay of initiating the self-care behaviors nor in the severity and distress of the side effects. The bcfs of anxiety and control were not significantly related to self-care behaviors, but patients in the Schedule A group were significantly more anxious at Cycle 1 and had a significant reduction in their anxiety scores by the completion of Cycle 2.

3. The next investigation was a parallel study to the experimental study just described with the following exceptions: the sample included 60 patients with cancer who were receiving initial radiation therapy; in place of a Schedule B SEMT information there was a control group who received standard care; and the control instrument selected was a cancer-specific version of the Multidimensional Health Locus of Control scale (Dodd, 1987). The study is summarized in Table 5–3.

4. In a study by Hagopian (1991) the purpose was to investigate the effects that structured patient educational information (weekly newsletter) had on the knowledge, side effects, and self-care behaviors of patients with cancer who were receiving radiation therapy. Fifty-two patients constituted the control group, and they were randomly selected from a list of patients who had completed treatment for cure. How the 51 patients in the experimental group were selected was not described. The study used the post-test-only control group design. The instruments selected were the Radiation Side Effect Profile (RSEP), a knowledge test, and a demographic data form. The experimental group also completed the newsletter survey form. After completion of their treatment, patients in the control group were sent a letter and questionnaires to complete and return by mail. Once all the data were collected from the control group, the weekly newsletter was introduced into the clinic. After the newsletter had been distributed for 6 weeks and a group of patients had completed treatment, data were collected from the experimental group in the

same manner as used with the control group. It was hypothesized that the intervention would increase knowledge and increase self-care behaviors that would lead to a decrease in the severity of side effects.

The content of the newletter used Orem's overall principles of Supportive-Educative Nursing System and was specific to radiation therapy. The work of other theorists were used also by the investigator in developing the newsletter content. Patient knowledge about the health situation is one of the power components of the concept of Self-Care Agency. The data collected on self-care behaviors lean heavily on the theory of Self-Care. Because the severity of side effects is an outcome variable in this study, it is difficult to place it as a bcf of health state or a Therapeutic Self-Care Demand that would possibly provoke greater mobilization of the patients' self-care agency. The bcfs are usually thought to be the resources and characteristics that individuals bring to the situation, not the outcome of intervention as is seen in an individual's health state. However, Denyes (1988) contends that because Orem describes health both in terms of general state of wholeness and integrity *and* of health-deviations, data from measures of these are considered as possible health outcomes. The primary focus of this study is Nursing Systems theory (Supportive-Educative), with secondary emphasis on Self-Care Agency, the power component of knowledge, Self-Care (behaviors), and selected bcfs (e.g., age, gender, years of school) that were used in the analyses to test the similarities between the two groups. The question of where in this study the severity of side effects belongs in Orem's theory persists.

Patients who read the newsletter (experimental group) demonstrated significantly increased treatment knowledge, but they did not perform more self-care behaviors or have decreased severity of their side effects. This is not the result expected based on Orem's theory. The patients found the newsletter helpful but still cited the radiation oncologist as the most frequent source of their information. The investigator did not comment on the design, which has considerable threats to the internal validity of the study. The major assumption of the post-test-only control group is that the patients in both groups are the same on salient study variables. Hagopian compared the two groups of patients on some study variables but perhaps was limited in determining significant differences by the small sample size.

5. Hagopian and her colleagues conducted two other intervention studies (Hagopian & Rubenstein, 1990; Weintraub & Hagopian, 1990) that used an experimental design and tested the effectiveness of weekly phone calls and nurse consultation sessions. Both interventions resulted in nonsignificant outcomes and are summarized in Table 5–3.

6. Hiromoto and Dungan (1991) conducted an evaluation study designed to measure the effectiveness of

TABLE 5–3. *Studies that Tested Orem's Theory of Nursing Systems*

REFERENCE	PURPOSE/SAMPLE	METHODS/DESIGN	SELECTED FINDINGS
1. Dodd (1982, 1982a, 1983, 1984)	• To test different types of information on patients' knowledge, self-care behaviors, and affective states • 48 patients with cancer receiving CTX	• Experimental, blind • Variables measured: a) CTX knowledge b) self-care behaviors c) affective states d) demographic, disease, treatment	• Patients knew significantly more CTX information and performed significantly more self-care behaviors • The interventions did not significantly improve affective states
2. Dodd (1988a)	• To test different schedules of information on patients' self-care behaviors • To determine the influence of selected variables on self-care behavior • 60 patients with selected types of cancer initiating CTX	• Experimental, blind • Variables measured: a) anxiety b) control c) self-care behaviors d) demographic, disease, treatment	• Patients performed significantly more self-care behaviors if given the information prior to developing side effects • Anxiety and control were nonsignificantly related to self-care behaviors
3. Dodd (1987)	• To test different schedules of information on patients' self-care behaviors • To determine the influence of selected variables on self-care behavior • 60 patients with cancer initiating RT	• Experimental, blind • Variables measured: a) anxiety b) control c) self-care behaviors d) demographic, disease, treatment	• Patients performed significantly more selected self-care behaviors • Anxiety and control were nonsignificantly related to self-care behaviors • Significant decreases in anxiety
4. Hagopian (1991)	• To test the effects of a weekly newsletter on knowledge, side effects, and self-care behaviors • 103 patients with cancer who were receiving RT	• Post-test only, control group design • Variables measured: a) side effects b) self-care behaviors c) knowledge d) demographics	• Patients knew significantly more about their treatment but did not perform more self-care behaviors or have decreased severity of their side effects
5. Hagopian & Rubenstein (1990)	• To test the effects of weekly telephone calls on patients' well-being • 55 patients with cancer receiving RT for cure	• Experimental design with repeated measures • Variables measured: a) anxiety b) side effects c) coping strategies	• The intervention failed to demonstrate an effect on patients' well-being
6. Weintraub & Hagopian (1990)	• To test the effects of nursing consultation sessions on anxiety, experienced side effects, and helpfulness of self-care strategies • 56 patients with cancer receiving RT for cure	• Experimental design with repeated measures • Variables measured: a) side effects b) anxiety c) self-care behaviors	• The intervention failed to demonstrate a significant effect
7. Hiromoto & Dungan (1991)	• To test the effectiveness of contract learning on active participation in health care • Case study sample of 5 persons with cancer receiving CTX	• Evaluation study • Variables measured: a) learning needs b) self-care activities	• 4 of 5 patients benefited from the contract learning
8. Weinrich (1990)	• To determine variables that predict whether older persons will participate in fecal occult blood screening • 171 participants of a congregate meal program	• Quasi-experimental • Variables measured: a) demographic b) functioning	• 47% of the participants submitted specimens for occult blood testing • Predictors were women, abilities in functioning, and previous occult blood testing
9. Maddox (1991)	• To explore the validity of teaching older women the practice of breast self-examination (BSE) using the method of return demonstration • 75 women attending a senior citizen's center	• Quasi-experimental • Variables measured: a) confidence in participants' perceptions b) frequency of BSE c) accuracy of BSE d) knowledge	• Women felt significantly more confident in performing BSE • There were subgroup differences in confidence, frequency, and accuracy

contract learning in a "casestudy" sample of five persons with cancer who were receiving chemotherapy in a private oncology/hematology clinic. The study is summarized in Table 5–3.

7. The study by Weinrich (1990) is exceptional in that it is only one of two studies that has used Orem's theory to investigate cancer screening practices. The purpose of this study was stated as "to determine variables that predict whether older persons will participate in fecal occult blood screening" (p. 716). The investigation did however, have an intervention component to it and an outcome variable (specimen for occult blood). The sample include 171 participants of a congregate meal program from 11 different sites. The design was described as "descriptive one-group," but participants did receive the ACS's colorectal cancer education slide tape presentation. A 33-item instrument was developed by the author from the literature and from existing instruments. The instrument included data about the potential predicting variables (e.g., demographic, sensory loss, instrumental activities of daily living). A group of interviewers (four elderly, with two being white and two being black; a premedical student, and the author) collected data, then the colorectal health education program was presented. Instructions were provided on how to provide a stool specimen, and a Hemocult Kit was distributed. Six days later the author collected the specimen, and sent a mail reminder to participants who had not provided a specimen.

As already mentioned, Orem's theory provided the conceptual framework for the study. The potential predictor variables for the colorectal screen specimen can be considered bcfs, with the self-care practice of screening part of Self-Care theory. The author identifies the Nursing System's Supportive-Educative component as reflected in the educational program and teaching. She also identifies the higher risk of older persons for colorectal cancer as an increased Therapeutic Self-Care Demand.

Forty-seven per cent of the participants submitted specimens for occult blood testing. Analyses of the data revealed several significant predictors: women were more likely to return a specimen; some abilities in activities of daily living (e.g., use of telephone, shopping, and cleaning house); and previous participation in occult blood testing. The author views the results of this study as supportive of Orem's theory in that the 47 per cent of the participants who provided a specimen is well above this practice in the general older population. She concludes that there is an obvious need for more supportive-educative interventions in this at-risk group.

8. This is the second study that used Orem's theory to test an intervention to affect health screening practices (Maddox, 1991). The overall purpose was to explore the validity of teaching older women the practice of breast self-examination (BSE), using the method of return demonstration. The investigator examined how the nursing intervention affected confidence level, frequency, and accuracy of performing breast self-examination. The study is summarized in Table 5–3.

CLINICAL IMPLICATIONS

Cancer and its treatment produce therapeutic self-care demands such as symptoms and side effects. These demands for many patients result in a self-care deficit, because without supplemental interventions patients are not very knowledgeable or active with their self-care.

A beginning profile of patients most in need of self-care intervention is suggested in research findings. Patients who experience more severe side effects and disruptive affective (mood) states are at risk for having a greater self-care deficit. In addition, patients who are more recently diagnosed and receiving treatment appear to need more focused assistance with their self-care.

The patients' abilities to perform self-care (self-care agency) is an area that has been understudied. Many of the elements of the power components (i.e., readiness to learn, attention, motivation, and functional abilities) are assessed by nurses in their practice. There are many diverse instruments that measure individual elements of the power components, but to rely solely on instruments to measure all of the power components is impractical for both patients and nurses. Instead, the clinician is advised to continue to interview (ask questions) to ascertain the adequacy of patients' abilities to perform self-care.

The usefulness of providing self-care interventions (knowledge, self-care skills, and support) has clearly been demonstrated in earlier studies. Patients who received self-care interventions did perform greater self-care activities. However, it is not the goal of self-care to have individuals merely active in their self-care; they should be practicing effective self-care. The evidence for self-care resulting in decreased morbidity (symptoms and side effects status) has been more clearly observed in clinical practice than documented in empiric studies. Nonetheless the benefits of providing relevant information, self-care skills, and support in a timely manner are self-evident, and these nursing actions should continue.

REFERENCES

Denyes, M. J. (1988). Orem's model used for health promotion: Directions for research. *Advances in Nursing Science, 11,* 13–21.

Dodd, M. J. (1982). Assessing patient self-care for side effects of cancer chemotherapy. *Cancer Nursing, 5,* 447–451.

Dodd, M. J. (1982a). Chemotherapy knowledge in patients with cancer: Assessment and informational interventions. *Oncology Nursing Forum, 9,* 39–44.

Dodd, M. J. (1983). Self-care for side effects of cancer chemotherapy: An assessment of nursing interventions. *Cancer Nursing, 6,* 63–67.

Dodd, M. J. (1984). Measuring informational intervention for chemotherapy and self-care behavior. *Research in Nursing and Health, 7,* 43–50.

Dodd, M. J. (1984a). Self-care for patients with breast cancer to prevent side effects of chemotherapy: A concern for public health nursing. *Public Health Nursing, 1*, 202–209.

Dodd, M. J. (1984b). Patterns of self-care in cancer patients receiving radiation therapy. *Oncology Nursing Forum, 10*, 23–27.

Dodd, M. J., Lindsey, A. M., Larson, P., Musci, E., Thomas, M., Dibble, S., Hudes, M., Hauck, W., & Kato, F. (1986–1990). Coping and self-care of cancer families: Nurse prospectus. *Final Report*, RO1 NR01441.

Dodd, M. J. (1987). Efficacy of proactive information on self-care in radiation therapy patients. *Heart and Lung, 16*, 538–544.

Dodd, M. J. (1988). Patterns of self-care in patients with breast cancer. *Western Journal of Nursing Research, 10*, 7-14.

Dodd, M. J. (1988a) Efficacy of proactive information on self-care in chemotherapy patients. *Patient Education and Counseling, 11*, 215–225.

Dodd, M. J., Dibble, S. L., & Thomas, M. L. (1992). Self-care for patients experiencing cancer chemotherapy side effects: A concern for home care nurses. *Home Healthcare Nurse, 9*, 21–26.

Dodd, M. J., & Dibble, S. L. (1993). Predictors of self-care: A test of Orem's model. *Oncology Nursing Forum, 20*, 895–901.

Fernsler, J. (1986). A comparison of patient and nurse perceptions of patients' self-care deficits associated with cancer chemotherapy. *Cancer Nursing, 9*, 50–57.

Hagopian, G. A. (1990). The measurement of self-care strategies of patients in radiation therapy. In O. L. Strickland, & C. F. Waltz (Eds.), *Measurement of Nursing Outcomes: Vol. 4. Measuring client self-care and coping skills* (pp. 45–57). New York: Springer Publishing Co.

Hagopian, G. A. (1991). The effects of a weekly radiation therapy newsletter on patients. *Oncology Nursing Forum, 18*, 1199–1203.

Hagopian, G. A., & Rubenstein, J. H. (1990). Effects of telephone call interventions in patients' well-being in a radiation therapy department. *Cancer Nursing, 13*, 339–344.

Hanucharurnkul, S. (1989). Predictors of self-care in cancer patients receiving radiotherapy. *Cancer Nursing, 12*, 21–27.

Hiromoto, B. M., & Dungan, J. (1991). Contract learning for self-care activities. *Cancer Nursing, 14*, 148–154.

Kubricht, D. W. (1984). Therapeutic self-care demands expressed by outpatients receiving external radiation therapy. *Cancer Nursing, 7*, 43–52.

Levin, L., Katz, A., & Hoist, E. (1976). *Self-Care*, New York: Prodist.

Maddox, M. A. (1991). The practice of breast self-examination among older women. *Oncology Nursing Forum, 18*, 1367–1371.

Munkres, A., Oberst, M. T., & Hughes, S. H. (1992). Appraisal of illness, symptom distress, self-care burden, and mood states in patients receiving chemotherapy for initial and recurrent cancer. *Oncology Nursing Forum, 19*, 1201–1209.

Musci, E., & Dodd, M. J. (1990). Predicting self-care with patients and family members' affective states and family functioning. *Oncology Nursing Forum, 17*, 394–400.

Oberst, M., Hughes, S. H., Chang, A. S., & McCubbin, M. A. (1991). Self-care burden, stress appraisal, and mood among persons receiving radiotherapy. *Cancer Nursing, 14*, 71–78.

Orem, D. E., & Taylor, S. (1986). Orem's general theory of nursing. In P. Winstead-Fry (Ed.), *Casestudies in Nursing Theory* (pp. 37–71). New York, NY: National League for Nursing.

Orem, D. E. (1991). Nursing. *Concepts of Practice.* St. Louis, MO: Mosby Year Book.

Rhodes, V. A., Watson, P. M., Johnson, M. H., Madsen, R. W., & Beck, N. C. (1987). Patterns of nausea, vomiting, and distress in patients receiving antineoplastic drug protocols. *Oncology Nursing Forum, 14*, 35–44.

Rhodes, V. A., Watson, P. M., & Hanson, B. M. (1988). Patients' descriptions of the influence of tiredness and weakness on self-care abilities. *Cancer Nursing, 11*, 186–194.

Robinson, K. D., & Posner, J. D. (1992). Patterns of self-care needs and interventions related to biological response modifier therapy: Fatigue as a model. *Seminars in Oncology Nursing, 8*(Suppl), 17–22.

Weinrich, S. P. (1990). Predictors of older adults' participation in fecal occult blood screening. *Oncology Nursing Forum, 17*, 715–720.

Weintraub, F. N., & Hagopian, G. A. (1990). The effect of nursing consultation on anxiety, side effects, and self-care of patients' receiving radiation therapy. *Oncology Nursing Forum, 17*(Suppl), 31–38.

Wortman, C. (1984). Social support and the cancer patient. *Cancer, 53*(Suppl), 2339–2363.

6

Assessment of Function

Jacqueline Fawcett • Lorraine Tulman

Cancer is a serious illness that can have a substantial impact on the patient's functioning for a prolonged period of time. Indeed, cancer treatments such as surgery, chemotherapy, radiation therapy, hormonal therapy, and immunotherapy may alter functioning in usual activities for many months or even years. Remissions and recurrences of cancer also alter functioning. Consequently a major focus of the nursing assessment of cancer patients is to determine and compare their past and current levels of functioning. Furthermore Dudas (1991) pointed out that rehabilitation for cancer focuses on improving the bodily functions and physical abilities that are so frequently altered by cancer and its treatment.

The purposes of this chapter are to identify the effects of cancer and its treatment on functioning, examine the ways in which assessment of functioning has been defined and measured in the cancer nursing literature, and propose a schema for the comprehensive nursing assessment of functioning in cancer patients.

EFFECTS OF CANCER ON FUNCTIONING

Functioning is frequently modified for many cancer patients before, during, and even after the diagnostic and treatment phases of the illness. For example, investigators have reported that almost 50 per cent of patients with soft-tissue sarcoma stated that chemotherapy interfered with their lives and that approximately one quarter of the women who survive breast cancer and one third of cancer patients with advanced disease experience a decline in functioning (Allen, Mor, Raveis, & Houts, 1993; Arzouman, Dudas, Ferrans, & Holm, 1991; Irvine, Brown, Crooks, Roberts, & Browne, 1991).

Performance of basic activities of daily living, such as eating, bathing, dressing, walking, and exercising,

frequently are impeded during the postoperative period or during chemotherapy or radiation therapy (Brink, 1988; Jacobs, Ross, Walker, & Stockdale, 1983; Oberst, Hughes, Chang, & McCubbin, 1991; O'Hare, Malone, Lusk, & McCorkle, 1993; Sarna, 1993). Many cancer patients also experience difficulty performing the usual activities associated with their domestic, social, and vocational roles (Brink, 1988; Loescher, Clark, Atwood, Leigh, & Lamb, 1990; Northouse, 1989; Northouse & Swain, 1987; Sarna, 1993; Welch-McCaffrey, Hoffman, Leigh, Loescher, & Meyskens, 1989).

For example, both male and female cancer patients who are receiving radiation therapy experience a decline in household activities, out-of-home activities such as errands, shopping, and banking, social activities, and recreational activities (Oberst et al., 1991). Similarly, many cancer patients receiving outpatient chemotherapy experience a decline in their performance of basic activities of daily living as well as decreased activity in the areas of heavy housekeeping, shopping, and household business (Allen et al., 1993; Guadagnoli & Mor, 1991). Allen et al. (1993) reported that 37 per cent of their sample of men and women beginning chemotherapy or radiation therapy had needs related to meal preparation, 38 per cent of the men and 41 per cent of the women had needs related to light housework, 44 per cent of the men and 61 per cent of the women had needs related to heavy housework, 39 per cent of the men and 52 per cent of the women had needs related to shopping, 20 per cent of the men and 30 per cent of the women had needs related to transportation, and 25 per cent of the men and 26 per cent of the women had needs related to filling out forms.

Moreover, cancer patients experiencing chemotherapy-induced emesis experience a substantial decline in the performance of household tasks, enjoyment of meals, and socializing with family and friends, as well as maintaining other daily and recreational activities

(Lindley et al., 1992). In addition, many patients with cancer-related pain experience substantial reductions in such areas of functioning as cooking, dressing/undressing, bathing, reading, and interacting with family members (Strang, 1992). Also, survivors of bone marrow transplants for malignant disease typically experience some decline in activities associated with virtually all life roles, ranging from hobbyist to worker or student. The smallest reported percentages of decline are in activities associated with the roles of family member (3 per cent), friend (5 per cent), and home maintainer (8 per cent), whereas the largest percentages are in the activities associated with the roles of student (27 per cent) or worker (24 per cent) (Baker, Curbow, & Wingard, 1991).

Noteworthy are recent research findings suggesting that systematic nursing assessment and appropriate nursing interventions during adjuvant therapy may prevent or limit a decline in functioning. Larson, Lindsey, Dodd, Brecht, and Packer (1993), for example, reported that lung cancer patients remained ambulatory and were able to maintain most of their usual activities of daily living while they were undergoing radiation therapy. Sarna (1993) found that lung cancer patients who were receiving chemotherapy had less of a decline in functioning over a 1-month period than did the patients who were not. Sarna speculated that the untreated patients might not receive the same "vigilant nursing assessment" (p. 722) and subsequent nursing intervention as patients in active treatment.

EMPLOYMENT ISSUES

Cella (1987) pointed out that "at least half of all [cancer] survivors are interested or engaged in gainful employment" (p. 65). Yet one study revealed that only one half of the women previously employed were able to return to work within 4 months of diagnosis (Silberfarb, Maurer, & Crouthamel, 1980). Although many men and women who survive cancer return to work in a caring atmosphere (Childre, 1992), many others encounter major forms of employment discrimination including dismissal, failure to hire, demotion, denial of promotion, undesirable transfer, denial of benefits, and hostility (Dow, 1991; Hoffman, 1991). In fact, return to usual occupational activities may be prevented or impeded by employer bias and discrimination, hostility, fear of contagion, and shunning from co-workers (Berry & Catanzaro, 1992; Brown & Tai-Seale, 1992; Gerlach, Gambosi, & Bowen, 1990; Hoffman, 1991; Leigh, 1992; Loescher et al., 1990; Smith & Lesko, 1988). Clearly, Clark and Landis's (1989) characterization of the cancer survivor's reentry into the work role as a crisis is appropriate. An important effect of cancer-related work discrimination is insurance coverage, which frequently is tied to employment. When the cancer survivor is unable to return to work or find a new position because of discrimination, major difficulties usually are encountered in securing new health insurance coverage (Clark & Landis, 1989; Ganz, 1990). In addition, life insurance coverage may be difficult or impossible to secure, waiting periods for coverage may be excessively extended, or premiums may be prohibitive (Quigley, 1989; Silberner, 1989).

GENDER ISSUES

Although family norms have been changing in recent years, women continue to assume not only the major responsibility for household management but also for organizing social activities involving friends, relatives, and community organizations (Benin & Agostinelli, 1988). Consequently, despite the fact that husbands frequently have to adjust their own activities when their wives are diagnosed with cancer, the wives typically have more adjustment problems in the areas of domestic, social, and vocational activities (Northouse, 1989; Northouse & Swain, 1987). For example, women breast cancer patients who carry a disproportionate share of household responsibilities before the diagnosis still have the most responsibility after diagnosis, even though family members assume more responsibility during the treatment and recovery period. In fact, the distribution of responsibilities typically reverts to the prediagnosis pattern within a year (Green, 1986).

DEFINITIONS OF FUNCTIONING

An analysis of the literature dealing with the effects of cancer on functioning revealed that the term has a vast range of meaning, from the ability to independently walk a short distance to the independent performance of the array of activities associated with one's life roles. Table 6–1 presents several definitions of functioning that were found in the cancer nursing literature as well as tools used to assess functioning.

A systematic review of the purpose and content of tools used to assess functioning revealed that some measure the person's *ability to perform* activities, whereas others measure the *actual performance* of those activities (Richmond, McCorkle, Tulman, & Fawcett, 1995). Furthermore at least one tool—the Physical Functioning Scale (Stewart & Ware, 1992)—includes an item measuring the individual's satisfaction or dissatisfaction with his or her current level of activity. Moreover, the type and range of activities assessed vary from tool to tool.

In addition, although functioning typically refers to physical function (Fucile, 1992), some definitions of functioning extend far beyond the physical performance of activities associated with various life roles to domains such as communication, mental health, cognition, emotional status, pain, general health perceptions, and socioeconomic resources (Brink, 1988; Fucile, 1992; Hughes, 1993; Larson et al., 1993; McGill & Paul, 1993; Sarna, 1993; Thomas & Dodd, 1992). Finally, some tools are regarded as objective measures, and others are regarded as subjective measures of functioning (Sarna, 1993). Objective measures employ observer ratings of the cancer patient, whereas subjective

TABLE 6–1. *Examples of Definitions and Measures of Functioning Found in the Cancer Nursing Literature*

DEFINITION	ASSESSMENT TOOL	USED BY
Needing help or assistance from other people to perform activities or roles that under ordinary circumstances adults can do by themselves	Enforced Social Dependency Scale (Benoliel, McCorkle, & Young, 1980)	O'Hare et al., 1993
The person's need for help and assistance in personal and social activities	Enforced Social Dependency Scale	Sarna et al., 1993
Physical, social, and role (worker, student, and/or homemaker) functioning, mental health, health perceptions, and pain	Medical Outcomes Study General Health Survey-Short Form (Stewart & Ware, 1992)	Hughes, 1993
The person's view of his or her limitations in physical activities (self-care, mobility, ambulation, physical activity) owing to health problems, and the degree of satisfaction or dissatisfaction with the current activity level	Medical Outcomes Study General Health Survey-Short Form—Physical Functioning Scale (Stewart & Ware, 1992)	Sarna, 1993
Impact of cancer and its treatment on independent function (normal activity, self-care, need for assistance, need for special care)	Karnofsky Performance Status Scale (Karnofsky & Burchenal, 1949)	Larson et al., 1993; Sarna, 1993; Schumacher et al., 1993; Thomas & Dodd, 1992
Impact of cancer on ambulation, daily activities, recreation, working, pain, weight loss, and problems with fit of clothing	Cancer Inventory of Problem Situations—Physical Functioning Superscale (Schag et al., 1983)	Sarna, 1993
Social resources, economic resources, mental health, physical health, and activities of daily living	Functional Assessment Inventory (Pfeiffer et al., 1981)	Thomas & Dodd, 1992
Ability to eat, dress and undress, care for appearance, walk, get in and out of bed, and perform basic hygiene	Functional Assessment Inventory—Physical Activities of Daily Living Subscale (Pfeiffer et al., 1981)	Larson et al., 1993
Ability to use the telephone, get to places beyond walking distance, go shopping for groceries, prepare own meals, perform housework, take own medications, and manage own money	Functional Assessment Inventory—Instrumental Activities of Daily Living Subscale (Pfeiffer et al., 1981)	Larson et al., 1993
Degree of impairment of mental health, physical health, and activities of daily living	Functional Assessment Inventory—Overall Health Rating Subscale (Pfeiffer et al., 1981)	Larson et al., 1993
Current level of functioning	Eastern Cooperative Oncology Group/Zubrod Performance Status Score (Stanley, 1980)	Longman et al., 1992

measures are self-reports that typically are completed by the patient.

The lack of distinction between the ability to perform and the actual performance of activities has created considerable confusion with regard to what aspect of functioning actually is assessed and what functional outcomes of interventions are actually evaluated. In addition, the lack of consistency in the range and type of activities, as well as in the domains of function, assessed by various tools has created confusion with regard to the comprehensiveness of the assessment. Moreover, the lack of consistency in the way in which some tools have been administered has created confusion with regard to the interpretation of data obtained. For example, the Karnofsky Performance Status Scale (Karnofsky & Burchenal, 1949) typically is scored by

an observer and is therefore regarded as an objective measure of functioning. Schumacher, Dodd, and Paul (1993) and Thomas and Dodd (1992), however, asked patients to rate themselves on the Karnofsky Scale, thereby yielding a subjective self-report of functioning.

COMPREHENSIVE ASSESSMENT OF FUNCTIONING

A comprehensive schema for assessment of functioning in cancer patients would take into account both ability and performance across a wide array of activities. The development of such a schema in our program of research has been guided by the Roy Adaptation Model of Nursing (Roy & Andrews, 1991).

TABLE 6–1. *Examples of Definitions and Measures of Functioning Found in the Cancer Nursing Literature* Continued

DEFINITION	ASSESSMENT TOOL	USED BY
Present functioning in the areas of toileting, feeding, dressing, grooming, physical ambulation, and bathing	Physical Self-Maintenance Scale (Lawton & Brody, 1969)	Longman et al., 1992
Present functioning in the areas of ability to use the telephone, do housekeeping, and do laundry; mode of transportation; responsibility for own medications; and ability to handle finances	Instrumental Activities of Daily Living Scale (Lawton & Brody, 1968)	Longman et al., 1992
Degree of alteration in lifestyle with regard to changes in daily activities	Investigator developed survey questionnaire—Item II	Post-White, 1986
Activities of daily living and work limitations	Quality of Life Questionnaire—Subscales 1A and 1B (Aaronson et al., 1986)	Ostchega et al., 1988
Global measure of the functional status of cancer patients	Functional Living Index-Cancer (Schipper et al., 1984)	Arzouman et al., 1991
Global measure of the quality of life	Functional Living Index-Cancer	Monahan, 1988
Self-care, mobility, ambulation, bowel and bladder dysfunction, communication, cognition, social interaction, and emotion	Functional Independence Measure (UDS Data Management Service, 1990)	Fucile, 1992
The individual's perception of health, support, and independence in six domains: activities of daily living, cognitive, personal adjustment, physical health, social, and time use	Philadelphia Geriatric Center Multilevel Assessment Instrument (Lawton & Moss, 1983)	McGill & Paul, 1993
Performance of usual personal care, household and family, occupational, and social and community activities	Inventory of Functional Status-Cancer (Tulman et al., 1991)	Tulman et al., 1991
The level at which a person is functioning in any of a variety of areas such as physical health, activities of daily living, self maintenance, role activity, social activity, and emotional status	Investigator developed semistructured interview schedule: items include perceived health status, symptoms (pain, nausea, appetite, sleep problems, mobility problems, diarrhea, constipation, tiredness, loss of concentration, depression, irritability, appearance), and activities (eating, dressing, walking and movement, traveling, bathing, toileting, home activities, work activities, recreational activities, communication)	Brink, 1988

THE ROY ADAPTATION MODEL OF NURSING

The Roy Adaptation Model depicts the individual as an adaptive system who interacts with constantly changing environmental stimuli (Fig. 6–1). Those stimuli are categorized as focal, which refers to the stimuli most immediately confronting the person; contextual, which refers to contributing factors in the situation; and residual, which refers to other unknown factors that may influence the situation. When the factors making up residual stimuli become known, they are considered focal or contextual stimuli.

Individuals respond to stimuli through regulator and cognator coping mechanisms. The regulator mechanism encompasses basic neural, chemical, and endocrine channels that process stimuli in an automatic, unconscious manner. The cognator mechanism encompasses four cognitive-emotive channels for stimulus processing: perceptual/information processing, learning, judgment, and emotion.

The outcomes of coping are observed in one biologic and three psychosocial response modes. The biologic mode of adaptation, called the physiologic mode, is concerned with basic needs requisite to maintaining the physical and physiologic integrity of the human system. The psychosocial modes of adaptation include role function, self-concept, and interdependence. The role function mode is concerned with people's performance of roles on the basis of their positions within society. The self-concept mode deals with people's conceptions of their physical and personal selves. The interdepen-

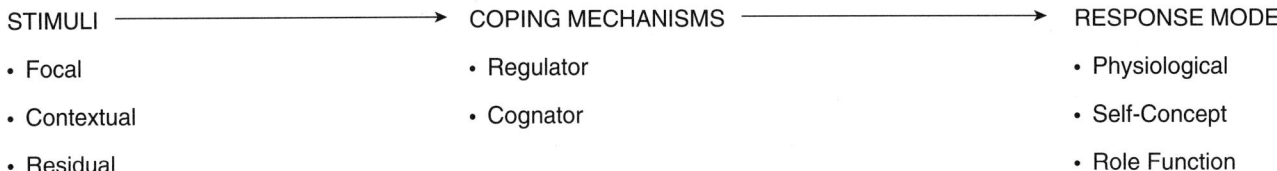

FIGURE 6–1. The Roy Adaptation Model of nursing.

dence mode deals with development and maintenance of satisfying affectional relationships with significant others as well as the provision and receipt of social support. The four modes are interrelated, such that responses in any one mode may act as a stimulus in one or all of the other modes. Responses to environmental stimuli are judged as adaptive or ineffective. Adaptive responses meet the goals of survival, growth, reproduction, and mastery. Ineffective responses do not meet those goals.

THE ROLE FUNCTION RESPONSE MODE

Functioning, within the context of the Roy Adaptation Model, may be viewed as role function mode responses. The role function mode directs attention to activities associated with a person's primary, secondary, and tertiary roles (Banton, 1965) (Fig. 6–2).

A person's primary or basic role determines most of the activities engaged in at a particular developmental stage, taking gender and age into account. Examples of a primary role are a young adult woman who is 25 years old and a middle-aged man who is 50 years old. Activities associated with the primary role encompass basic activities of daily living (Katz, Ford, & Moskowitz, 1963) such as bathing, grooming, dressing, elimination, and eating.

A person's secondary or general roles are taken on to fulfill the developmental tasks of each stage of life. Examples of secondary roles are sister, student, husband, father, and accountant. Activities associated with secondary roles include intermediate activities of daily living (Lawton & Brody, 1969) such as housekeeping, food preparation, use of transportation, shopping, and advanced activities of daily living (Reuben & Solomon, 1989) such as working and going to school.

A person's tertiary or independent roles are chosen freely, although they frequently are extensions of secondary roles. Examples include charity fund raiser, member of a professional organization, swimmer, and golfer. Activities associated with tertiary roles include advanced activities of daily living (Reuben & Solomon, 1989) such as engaging in hobbies and participating in social and religious groups.

Responses in the role function mode encompass both the ability to perform activities and tasks that are important for independent living, and the actual performance of activities and tasks crucial to the fulfillment of roles within one's current life circumstances. Accordingly, assessment of functioning encompasses two dimensions—functional ability and functional status (Fig. 6–3).

Functional Ability. The dimension of functional ability refers to the actual or potential capacity to perform activities normally expected of a person at a certain age (Nagi, 1991). Individuals have limitations in functional ability if they are unable to independently perform an action or activity in the manner or in the range considered normal. The inability to perform activities within the range considered normal may be temporary or permanent, static or dynamic.

Functional Status. The dimension of functional status refers to a person's actual performance of activities associated with his or her current life roles. Functional status has to be assessed in relation to societal expectations regarding performance of activities typically ascribed to various roles at various stages of life. Limitations in functional status are said to occur when there is "a discrepancy between individual performance and average [expected] role performance" (Moriarty, 1975, p. 15).

INSTRUMENTAL AND EXPRESSIVE COMPONENTS OF FUNCTIONING

In keeping with the Roy Adaptation Model, each activity associated with each role should be evaluated with regard to its instrumental and expressive components (Parsons & Shils, 1951). The instrumental components are the physical capacity to perform the activity and the actual extent to which it is performed, that is, functional ability and functional status. The expressive components are the person's feelings, attitudes,

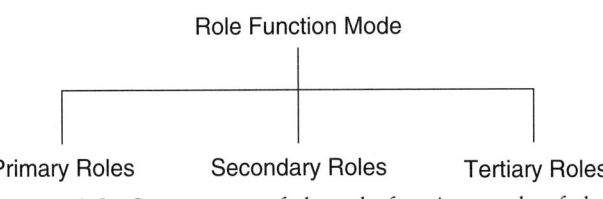

FIGURE 6–2. Components of the role function mode of the Roy Adaptation Model.

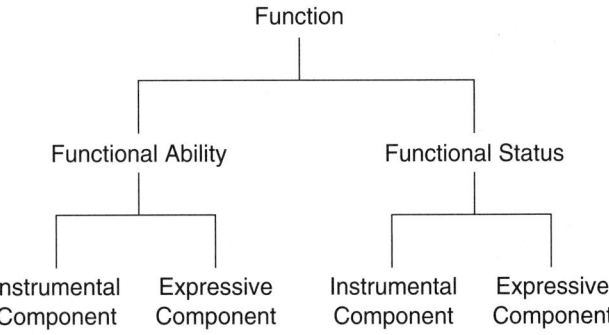

FIGURE 6–3. The two dimensions of function and their components.

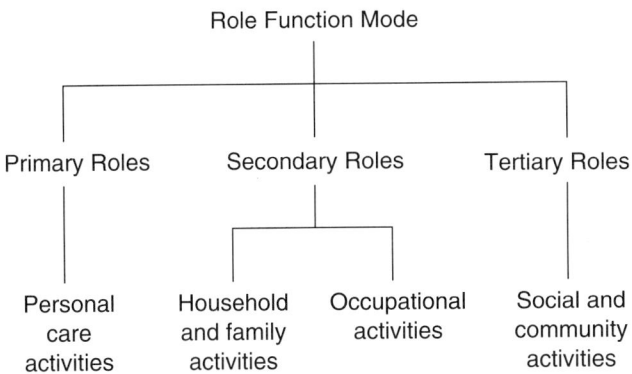

FIGURE 6–4. Types of activities associated with primary, secondary, and tertiary roles.

likes, or dislikes about his or her level of functional ability and functional status (see Fig. 6–3).

A COMPREHENSIVE ASSESSMENT TOOL

The Comprehensive Inventory of Functioning-Cancer (CIF-CA) is currently being developed (Tulman & Fawcett, 1994–1995). This assessment tool is an extension of the Inventory of Functional Status-Cancer (IFS-CA) (Tulman, Fawcett, & McEvoy, 1991), which was designed to measure the cancer patient's current performance of usual personal care, household and family, occupational, and social and community activities. Both tools include subscales that reflect the primary, secondary, and tertiary roles of the Roy Adaptation Model role function response mode (Fig. 6–4).

When completed, the CIF-CA will include four sections: Functional Ability-Instrumental Component, Functional Ability-Expressive Component, Functional Status-Instrumental Component, and Functional Status-Expressive Component. Each section will include the following subscales: Personal Care Activities, Household and Family Activities, Occupational Activities, and Social and Community Activities. Examples of the items for the subscales in each section are listed in Table 6–2.

McGill and Paul (1993) also used the Roy Adaptation Model of Nursing to guide assessment of what they called functional status. They viewed functional status in a global manner rather than solely within the context of the role function mode. They asserted that the approach to functional status reflected in the Philadelphia Geriatric Center's Multilevel Assessment Instrument (MAI) (Lawton & Moss, 1983) is congruent with the Roy Adaptation Model, because that approach "focuses on the individual's perception of health, support, and independence rather than on medical cure and treatment" (p. 1208). They maintained that six of the seven domains of the MAI are congruent with the four response modes of the Roy Adaptation Model. The six domains they identified are activities of daily living, cognitive, personal adjustment, physical health, social, and time use. McGill and Paul did not, however, explain which domain of the MAI was linked with which Roy Adaptation Model response mode.

Although McGill and Paul's (1993) work is conceptually interesting, the approach we have taken in the development of the CIF-CA is to provide an in-depth assessment of functioning within the context of the role function response mode of the Roy Adaptation Model. A complete assessment of the cancer patient using the Roy Adaptation Model would go beyond assessment of functioning by incorporating other tools specifically designed to provide in-depth assessments of relevant focal and contextual stimuli, the regulator and cognator coping mechanisms, and all aspects of the physiologic, self-concept, and interdependence modes. For example, an in-depth assessment of the interdependence response mode would require consideration of the types of and changes in the patient's relationships with significant others, the degree of his or her satisfaction with those relationships, the extent of and satisfaction with the patient's social support network, and the patient's ability to provide support for others.

TABLE. 6–2. *The Comprehensive Inventory of Functioning-Cancer: Directions and Sample Items*

DIRECTIONS	SAMPLE ITEMS

Section I: Functional Ability-Instrumental Component
Please indicate the extent to which you are *currently able* to do each of the activities listed below, using the scale of 1 = not at all, 2 = some of the time, 3 = most of the time, 4 = all of the time
Section II: Functional Ability-Expressive Component
Please indicate the extent to which you *want to be able* to do each of the activities listed below, using the scale of 1 = less, 2 = the same amount, 3 = more
Section III: Functional Status-Instrumental Component
Please indicate the extent to which you are *currently doing* each of the activities listed below, using the scale of 1 = not at all, 2 = some of the time, 3 = most of the time, 4 = all of the time
Section IV: Functional Status-Expressive Component
Please indicate the extent to which you *want to do* each of the activities listed below, using the scale of 1 = less, 2 = the same amount, 3 = more
	Personal care activities
	  Take walks
	  Spend time relaxing
	Household and family activities
	  Tend to the needs of my children
	  Clean the house
	Occupational activities
	  Work all of the hours my job requires
	  Carry out my job responsibilities
	Social and community activities
	  Participate in volunteer or service organizations
	  Go out with friends

IMPLICATIONS FOR PRACTICE

Cancer and its treatment may have profound effects on the patient's functioning in activities associated with his or her life roles. The Roy Adaptation Model of Nursing provides a comprehensive guide for the assessment of cancer patients' functioning by incorporating instrumental and expressive components of functional ability and functional status.

The CIF-CA can easily be used in clinical practice as a paper and pencil tool that is completed by the cancer patient during office or clinic visits. It also may be used as the basis for a structured interview of the patient during face-to-face encounters with the nurse or during telephone conversations. It is recommended that the CIF-CA be administered periodically to track changes in functioning during the course of treatment and recovery.

The importance of comprehensive nursing assessment directed toward functioning in usual activities is underscored by the strong association between functioning and survival in cancer patients (Schonwetter, Teasdale, Storey, & Luchi, 1990) as well as the association between functioning and the quality of the cancer patient's life (Foreman & Kleinpell, 1990; Gotay, Korn, McCabe, Moore, & Cheson, 1992; Holmes & Dickerson, 1987; Sarna, Lindsey, Dean, Brecht, & McCorkle, 1993). Furthermore nursing assessment of cancer patients' functioning provides the basis for planning and implementing appropriate nursing interventions directed toward assisting cancer patients to adjust to changes in the performance of their usual activities, to facilitate their performance of new cancer-related activities, and to promote their optimal functioning in all of those activities before, during, and after cancer treatment. In addition, nursing assessment of cancer patients' functioning provides a baseline for evaluation of the outcomes of nursing and medical interventions.

ACKNOWLEDGMENTS. The contributions of Nelda Samarel, Diana Newman, Geraldine Paier, April Hazard Vallerand, Therese Richmond, Lenore Kurlowitz, and Bonnie Graff to our understanding of the concept of function are gratefully acknowledged.

REFERENCES

Aaronson, N. K., Van Dan, F. S. A. M., Bakker, W., VanZandwijk, N., Stewart, A. L., & Yarnold, J. J. (1986). Multi-dimensional approach to the measurement of quality of life in lung cancer clinical trials. In N. K. Aaronson, J. Beckmann, S. Bernheing, & R. Zittoun (Eds.), *Quality of life in cancer EORTC monograph series.* New York: Raven Press.

Allen, S. M., Mor, V., Raveis, V., & Houts, P. (1993). Measurement of need for assistance with daily activities: Quantifying the influence of gender roles. *Journal of Gerontology, 48,* S204–S211.

Arzouman, J. M. R., Dudas, S., Ferrans, C. E., & Holm, K. (1991). Quality of life of patients with sarcoma postchemotherapy. *Oncology Nursing Forum, 18,* 889–894.

Baker, F., Curbow, B., & Wingard, J. R. (1991). Role retention and quality of life of bone marrow transplant survivors. *Social Science and Medicine, 32,* 697–704.

Banton, M. (1965). *Roles: An introduction to the study of social relations.* New York: Basic Books.

Benin, M. H., & Agostinelli, J. (1988). Husbands' and wives' satisfaction with the division of labor. *Journal of Marriage and the Family, 50,* 349–361.

Benoliel, J. Q., McCorkle, R., & Young, K. (1980). The development of a social dependency scale. *Research in Nursing and Health, 3,* 3–10.

Berry, D. L., & Catanzaro, M. (1992). Persons with cancer and their return to the workplace. *Cancer Nursing, 15,* 40–46.

Brink, H. L. (1988). The impact of advanced cancer on the functional status of patients attending oncology clinics in selected urban areas. *Curationis, 11*(3), 11–16.

Brown, H. G., & Tai–Seale, M. (1992). Vocational rehabilitation of cancer patients. *Seminars in Oncology Nursing, 8,* 202–211.

Cella, D. F. (1987). Cancer survival: Psychosocial and public issues. *Cancer Investigation, 5,* 59–67.

Childre, F. (1992). From your patient to our employees: Nurses working together. In *Surviving cancer. Survivorship: Getting patients back to the business of living* (pp. 47–52). Atlanta, GA: American Cancer Society.

Clark, J. C., & Landis, L. L. (1989). Reintegration and maintenance of employees with breast cancer in the workplace. *AAOHN Journal, 37,* 186–193.

Dow, K. H. (1991). The growing phenomenon of cancer survivorship. *Journal of Professional Nursing, 7,* 54–61.

Dudas, S. (1991). Rehabilitation of the patient with cancer. *Journal of Enterostomal Therapy, 18,* 61–67.

Foreman, M. D., & Kleinpell, R. (1990). Assessing the quality of life of elderly persons. *Seminars in Oncology Nursing, 6,* 292–297.

Fucile, J. (1992). Functional rehabilitation in cancer care. *Seminars in Oncology Nursing, 8,* 186–189.

Ganz, P. A. (1990). Current issues in cancer rehabilitation. *Cancer, 65,* 742–751.

Gerlach, R. W., Gambosi, J. R., & Bowen, R. H. (1990). Cancer survivors' needs reported by survivors and their families. *Journal of Cancer Education, 5,* 63–70.

Gotay, C. C., Korn, E. L., McCabe, M. S., Moore, T. D., & Cheson, B. D. (1992). Quality-of-life assessment in cancer treatment protocols: Research issues in protocol development. *Journal of the National Cancer Institute, 84,* 575–579.

Green, C. P. (1986). Changes in responsibility in women's families after the diagnosis of cancer. *Health Care of Women International, 7,* 221–239.

Guadagnoli, E., & Mor, V. (1991). Daily living needs of cancer outpatients. *Journal of Community Health, 16,* 37–47.

Hoffman, B. (1991). Employment discrimination: Another hurdle for cancer survivors. *Cancer Investigation, 9,* 589–595.

Holmes, S., & Dickerson, J. (1987). The quality of life: Design and evaluation of a self-assessment instrument for use with cancer patients. *International Journal of Nursing Studies, 24,* 15–24.

Hughes, K. K. (1993). Psychosocial and functional status of breast cancer patients: The influence of diagnosis and treatment choice. *Cancer Nursing, 16,* 222–229.

Irvine, D., Brown, B., Crooks, D., Roberts, J., & Browne, G. (1991). Psychosocial adjustment in women with breast cancer. *Cancer, 67,* 1097–1117.

Jacobs, C., Ross, R. D., Walker, I. M., & Stockdale, F. E. (1983). Behavior of cancer patients: A randomized study of the effects of education and peer support groups. *American Journal of Clinical Oncology, 6,* 347–350.

Karnofsky, D. A., & Burchenal, H. H. (1949). The clinical evaluation of chemotherapeutic agents in cancer. In C. M. MacLeod (Ed.), *Evaluation of chemotherapeutic agents* (pp. 191–205). New York: Columbia University Press.

Katz, S., Ford, A. S., & Moskowitz, R. W. (1963). The index of ADL: A standardized measure of biological and psychosocial function. *Journal of the American Medical Association, 185,* 914–919.

Larson, P. J., Lindsey, A. M., Dodd, M. J., Brecht, M., & Packer, A. (1993). Influence of age on problems experienced by patients with lung cancer undergoing radiation therapy. *Oncology Nursing Forum, 20,* 473–480.

Lawton, M. P., & Brody E. M. (1969). Assessment of older people: Self-maintaining and instrumental activities of daily living. *Gerontologist, 9,* 179–186.

Lawton, M. P., & Moss, M. S. (1983). *Philadelphia Geriatric Center Multilevel Assessment Instrument manual.* Philadelphia: Philadelphia Geriatric Center.

Leigh, S. (1992). Myths, monsters, and magic: Personal perspectives and professional challenges of survival. *Oncology Nursing Forum, 19,* 1475–1480.

Lindley, C. M., Hirsch, J. D., O'Neill, C. V., Transau, M. C., Gilbert, C. S., & Osterhaus, J. T. (1992). Quality of life consequences of chemotherapy-induced emesis. *Quality of Life Research, 1,* 331–340.

Loescher, L. J., Clark, L., Atwood, J. R., Leigh, S., & Lamb G. (1990). The impact of the cancer experience on long-term survivors. *Oncology Nursing Forum, 17,* 223–229.

Longman, A. J., Atwood, J. R., Sherman, J. B., Benedict, J., & Shang, T. (1992). Care needs of home-based cancer patients and their caregivers: Quantitative findings. *Cancer Nursing, 15,* 182–190.

McGill, J. S., & Paul, P. B. (1993). Functional status and hope in elderly people with and without cancer. *Oncology Nursing Forum, 20,* 1207–1213.

Monahan, M. L. (1988). Quality of life of adults receiving chemotherapy: A comparison of instruments. *Oncology Nursing Forum, 15,* 795–798.

Moriarty, J. B. (1975). Disability concepts: Implications for research. In E. B. Whitten (Ed.), *Pathology, impairment, functional limitations, and disability - Implications for practice, research, program and policy development and service delivery* (pp. 15–20). Washington, DC: National Rehabilitation Association.

Nagi, S. (1991). Disability concepts revisited: Implications for prevention. In A. M. Pope & A. R. Tarlov (Eds.), *Disability in America: Toward a national agenda for prevention* (pp. 309–327). Washington, DC: National Academy Press.

Northouse, L. L. (1989). A longitudinal study of the adjustment of patients and husbands to breast cancer. *Oncology Nursing Forum, 16,* 511–516.

Northouse, L. L., & Swain, M. A. (1987). Adjustment of patients and husbands to the initial impact of breast cancer. *Nursing Research, 36,* 221–225.

Oberst, M. T., Hughes, S. H., Chang, A. S., & McCubbin, M. A. (1991). Self-care burden, stress appraisal, and mood among persons receiving radiotherapy. *Cancer Nursing, 14,* 71–78.

O'Hare, P. A., Malone, D., Lusk, E., & McCorkle, R. (1993). Unmet needs of black patients with cancer posthospitalization: A descriptive study. *Oncology Nursing Forum, 20,* 659–664.

Ostchega, Y., Donohue, M., & Fox, N. (1988). High-dose cisplatin–related peripheral neuropathy. *Cancer Nursing, 11,* 23–32.

Parsons, T., & Shils, E. (Eds.). (1951). *Toward a general theory of action.* Cambridge, MA: Harvard University Press.

Pfeiffer, E., Johnson, T. M., & Chiofolo, R. C. (1981). Functional assessment of elderly subjects in four service settings. *Journal of the American Geriatrics Society, 29,* 433–437.

Post-White, J. (1986). Glucocorticosteroid–induced depression in the patient with leukemia or lymphoma. *Cancer Nursing, 9,* 15–22.

Quigley, K. M. (1989). The adult cancer survivor: Psychosocial consequences of cure. *Seminars in Oncology Nursing, 5,* 63–69.

Reuben, D. R., & Solomon, D. H. (1989). Assessment in geriatrics: Of caveats and names. *Journal of the American Geriatrics Society, 37,* 570–572.

Richmond, T., McCorkle, R., Tulman, L., & Fawcett, J. (1995). Measuring function. In M. Frank-Stromborg & S. Olsen (Eds.), *Instruments for clinical nursing research* (2nd ed). Boston: Jones & Bartlett.

Roy, C., & Andrews H. A. (1991). *The Roy Adaptation Model: The definitive statement.* Norwalk, CT: Appleton and Lange.

Sarna, L. (1993). Fluctuations in physical function: Adults with non-small cell lung cancer. *Journal of Advanced Nursing, 18,* 714–724.

Sarna, L., Lindsey, A. M., Dean, H., Brecht, M., & McCorkle, R. (1993). Nutritional intake, weight change, symptom distress, and functional status over time in adults with lung cancer. *Oncology Nursing Forum, 20,* 481–489.

Schag, C. A., Heinrich, R. L., & Ganz, P. O. (1983). Cancer inventory of problems situations: An instrument for assessing cancer patients' rehabilitation needs. *Journal of Psychosocial Oncology, 1,* 11–25.

Schipper, H., Clinch, J., McMurray, A., & Levitt, M. (1984). Measuring the quality of life of cancer patients: The Functional Living Index-Cancer: Development and validation. *Journal of Clinical Oncology, 2,* 472–483.

Schonwetter, R. S., Teasdale, T. A., Storey, P., & Luchi, R. J. (1990). Estimation of survival time in terminal cancer patients: An impedance to hospice admissions? *Hospice Journal, 6*(4), 65–79.

Schumacher, K. L., Dodd, M. J., & Paul, S. M. (1993). The stress process in family caregivers of persons receiving chemotherapy. *Research in Nursing and Health, 16,* 395–404.

Silberfarb, P. M., Maurer, L. H., & Crouthamel, C. S. (1980). Psychosocial aspects of neoplastic disease: I. Functional status of breast cancer patients during different treatment regimens. *American Journal of Psychiatry, 137,* 450–455.

Silberner, J. (1989). First, you beat the cancer. Next, you get employers and insurers to believe it. *U. S. News World Report,* November 6, 97–99.

Smith, K., & Lesko, L. M. (1988). Psychosocial problems in cancer survivors. *Oncology, 2,* 33–44.

Stanley, K. L. (1980). Prognostic factors for survival in patients with lung cancer. *Journal of the National Cancer Institute, 65,* 24–32.

Stewart, A. L., & Ware, J. E. (1992). *Measuring functioning and well-being: The Medical Outcomes Study approach.* Durham, NC: Duke University Press.

Strang, P. (1992). Emotional and social aspects of cancer pain. *Acta Oncologica, 31,* 323–326.

Thomas, M. L. & Dodd, M. J. (1992). The development and testing of a nursing model of morbidity in patients with cancer. *Oncology Nursing Forum, 19,* 1385–1396.

Tulman, L., & Fawcett, J. (1994–1995). *Functional status outcomes in female cancer patients.* Research in progress. University of Pennsylvania Research Foundation.

Tulman, L., Fawcett, J., & McEvoy, M. D. (1991). Development of the Inventory of Functional Status–Cancer. *Cancer Nursing, 14,* 254–260.

UDS Data Management Service. (1990). *Uniform data system for medical rehabilitation: Rehabilitation follow-up coding sheet.* Buffalo, NY: SUNY South Campus.

Welch-McCaffrey, D., Hoffman, B., Leigh, S. A., Loescher, L. J., & Meyskens, F. L. (1989). Surviving adult cancers. Part 2: Psychosocial implications. *Annals of Internal Medicine, 111,* 517–524.

Decision Making

B. Joyce Davison • Lesley F. Degner

PARTICIPATION IN DECISION MAKING
INFORMATION AND DECISION MAKING
INFORMATION INTERVENTIONS

CLINICAL GUIDELINES
SUMMARY

Medical consumerism emphasizes the importance of people assuming more bargaining power in their relationships with health care professionals. This process involves consumers actively listening to what the professional has to say, actively questioning the professional and seeking additional information if required, and subsequently taking responsibility for making their own health-related decisions. Current support for this ideal of medical consumerism is based on the assumption that most people desire some degree of control over treatment decisions and that exercising such control will have a positive influence on their survival and quality of life (Degner & Aquino-Russell, 1988). However, there is no empiric evidence to support the assumption that such activism is effective for all people. Indeed, several investigators have suggested that an individualized approach may be both more appropriate and more effective (Degner & Beaton, 1987; Degner & Sloan, 1992; Forrow, Wartman, & Brock, 1988). Forcing people to take more responsibility in decision making than they feel comfortable in assuming may actually be another approach to prescribing roles in health care.

The current emphasis on increased patient involvement in health care decision making can be attributed largely to current ethical, legal, and social concerns of a consumer conscious society. Ethically, the provision of information is necessary in a society that supports patient autonomy and self-determination. Legally, informed consent places respect for a patient's self-determination at the center of the physician-patient relationship and recognizes that an active role in treatment decision making is often the best guarantee that these decisions will promote well-being (Forrow, Wartman, & Brock, 1988). Socially, patients as health consumers are advocating a more equal relationship with health care professionals. Although the patient's desire for information and the use of such information for the purpose of decision making has been studied by many researchers, it is still not understood whether the provision of information necessarily leads to more patient involvement in the decision making process or even

whether such involvement is appropriate for all individuals (Northouse & Wortman, 1990).

PARTICIPATION IN DECISION MAKING

Investigators have produced conflicting findings regarding the type and degree of participation that patients prefer to have in medical decision making. Although advocacy of shared decision making by patients and clinicians is supported in theory, many clinicians doubt whether patients actually want to participate in medical decision making. Clinicians frequently maintain that patients should not participate in decision making because they do not have the knowledge required to participate in making critical choices, and that even if patients did, they might suffer psychologic harm if the outcomes of the decision they made were negative (Degner & Beaton, 1987). There is little empiric evidence to support these beliefs.

Some early studies suggested that the general public as well as patients with cancer may prefer a collaborative role in medical treatment decision making. For example, a random sample of 200 Canadians surveyed by Vertinsky, Thompson, and Uyeno (1974) concluded that although the majority of respondents did not wish to take the entire responsibility for medical decision making, they also did not wish to be entirely passive in the patient/physician relationship. A similar study by Haug and Lavin (1981), which surveyed 466 members of the general public and 86 physicians, found that a substantial proportion of the public wished to assume a consumerist position and take some responsibility for medical decision making. In 1980 Cassileth, Zupkis, Sutton-Smith, and March conducted a survey of 300 patients with metastatic cancer to determine information and decision making preferences. Two thirds of the patients indicated a preference for participating in medical decisions. Hack, Degner, and Dyck (1994) examined the relationships between preferences for involvement in decision making and preferences for information in a group of 35 women with early stage breast cancer. The investigators found that 80 per cent of the women in this study preferred either an active or collaborative role in choosing their treatment.

Further evidence that patients may prefer a pattern of shared decision making was provided by several investigators. Strull, Lo, and Charles (1984) studied a group of hypertensive patients and concluded that better assessment of individual preferences for information, discussion, and decision making authority may result in enhanced patient participation in decision making. These conclusions were supported by Greenfield, Kaplan, and Ware (1985), who found that providing a group of ulcer disease patients with detailed information and encouraging them to participate in decision making resulted in them being more involved in the patient-physician interaction and assuming a more active role in decision making. Robinson and Whitfield (1985) also reported that a group of surgery patients gained a more accurate understanding of the suggested treatment when they were encouraged to ask the physician questions about the treatment recommendations. Recent studies of women with breast cancer have found that both women and their husbands who were offered choice of treatment (lumpectomy vs. mastectomy) had lower anxiety levels irrespective of the choice they made when compared with patients whose surgeon made the treatment choice (Fallowfield, Hall, Macguire, & Baum, 1990; Morris & Royle, 1988).

INFORMATION AND DECISION MAKING

In most oncology settings, health professionals believe they should provide the information needed by cancer patients to actively participate in treatment decision making (Northouse & Wortman, 1990). However, research findings have consistently demonstrated that the majority of patients cared for in such settings were dissatisfied with the kind of information, amount of information, or both that they received from physicians and nurses (Degner, Jerry, & Till, 1991). These patients also have been found to experience difficulties in obtaining information they needed to achieve meaningful participation in decision making (Messerli, Garamendi, & Romano, 1980; Strull et al., 1984).

Several investigators have identified the information needs of cancer patients, but few have conducted studies to determine the best methods of delivering this information for the purpose of increasing participation in treatment decision making. Previous investigators (Feldman, 1976; Greenleigh Associates, 1979; Jones, 1981; Weisman & Wordon, 1976) reported that information desired by cancer patients falls into four major categories (in hierarchic order): disease, personal, family, and social. After they received a diagnosis, the informational needs cancer patients perceived as necessary for effective coping with each of these categories

were identified as follows: disease-related—diagnosis, tests, treatments, and prognosis; personal-related—impact of the disease and/or the treatments on their physical well-being and ability to function, their psychologic well-being, and emotional stability, their job/career, and their plans/goals for the future; family-related—impact on spouse/significant other, children, parents, and siblings; and social-related—contractual, leisure, and intimate relationships.

Derdiarian conducted several studies (1986, 1987) to identify the informational needs of recently diagnosed cancer patients. The information requirements of the patients studied were reported to be related to the four categories of disease, personal, family, and social. Although in the 1986 study Derdiarian indicated few differences in the informational needs among the patients related to age, gender, and stage of cancer, in her 1987 study she reported that men in general attached more importance to information about tests, physical well-being, and spouse. The older adults tended to need less information on relationships with spouse, parents, and career than the younger subjects. Patients with local and regional disease also were found to need more information than those with disseminated disease. Because no other differences were found when the patients were stratified according to gender, stage of life, marital status, education, time lag since first symptoms, and having read about cancer, she concluded that the results of the study would be useful to provide a baseline to predict the informational needs of these patients in the future course of their treatment. In the 1986 study Derdiarian concluded that although more research is needed, the information needs of recently diagnosed cancer patients may be universal.

An extensive review of the literature carried out in Canada identified items of information that were important to people with cancer generally and, more particularly, with breast cancer (Degner, Farber, & Hack, 1989). The literature revealed the nine major areas of importance for women with breast cancer included physical, psychologic and social aspects of care and treatment and included information on the spread of disease, likelihood of cure, impact on social life, effect on family and friends, self-care, sexual attractiveness, treatment options, risk to family of getting the same disease, and treatment side effects. Likelihood of cure, spread of disease, and treatment options have been found to be the three most important information needs of both breast cancer patients (Bilodeau & Degner, in press; Luker, Beaver, Leinster, Owens, Degner, & Sloan, in press) and men with prostate cancer (Davison, Degner, & Morgan, in press). Information concerning sexual attractiveness (females) and sexual function (males) was ranked last in these studies. Although these findings support Derdiarian's conclusion that information needs may be universal among various cancer populations, they also demonstrate that cancer patients, if given a choice, prefer to receive information pertaining to these three items.

Several investigators have shown there are significant benefits to providing cancer patients with information. Some of these benefits include increasing participation in treatment decision making and satisfaction with treatment choice (Cassileth et al., 1989); increasing satisfaction with the medical consultation (Damian & Tattersall, 1991); gaining control and coping with the stress of diagnosis (Fisher & Britten, 1993); decreasing levels of anxiety, mood disturbance, and affective distress (Rainy, 1985); increasing ability to cope during and after treatment (Johnson, Nail, Lauver, King, & Keys, 1988); and assisting in communication of illness-related information to family (Hogbin & Fallowfield, 1989; Johnson & Adelstein, 1991; Reynolds, Sanson-Fisher, Poole, Harker, & Byrne, 1981).

Cancer patients have been found to vary with respect to the extent to which they want to be involved in the decision making process (Cassileth et al., 1980; Sutherland, Llewellyn-Thomas, Lockwood, Tritchler, & Till, 1989). Several investigators (Cassileth et al., 1980; Hack et al., 1994; Sutherland et al., 1989) found a positive relationship between decision making and identified information needs in cancer patients, with those preferring more active roles in decision making desiring more information. It also has been suggested that patients who prefer a more active role in treatment decision making may require different types and amounts of information than may patients who are concerned primarily with coping with the effects of the treatment(s) and disease (Degner & Sloan, 1992). However, patients who assume a more active role in treatment decision making do experience significant benefits over their more passive counterparts. Some of these benefits include increased satisfaction with treatment decisions; increased satisfaction with care received, less anxiety and depression both pre-operatively and post-operatively; and a higher degree of hope (Cassileth et al., 1989; Cassileth et al., 1980; Morris & Royle, 1988).

Certain sociodemographic characteristics have been reported to have an impact on the preferred role in treatment decision making. Blanchard, LaBrecque, Ruckdeschel, and Blanchard (1988) reported older men and married cancer patients preferred a less active role in decision making. Cassileth et al. (1980) reported older, less educated cancer patients preferred the physician to make treatment decisions. These findings also were supported by Degner and Sloan (1992), who reported older, less educated patients were found to prefer less control in decision making, and being an older man with a cancer of the reproductive system was a significant predictor of preferring a passive role in decision making.

Researchers have produced conflicting findings regarding the impact of stage of disease on the preference for information and preferred role in treatment decision making. Cassileth et al. (1980) reported that cancer patients whose prognosis was positive preferred an active role in treatment decision making and detailed information. However, Blanchard et al. (1988) reported that cancer patients who preferred an active role in decision making had a poor prognosis. Ende, Kazis, Ash, and Moskowitz (1989) reported the desire of medical patients to make treatment decisions decreased as the severity of the illness increased. The clinical hypothesis that sicker cancer patients prefer less control in treatment decision making was not supported in the study conducted by Degner and Sloan (1992).

INFORMATION INTERVENTIONS

A review of the literature revealed that six main methods had been used to provide information to patients. The first method of providing written information to cancer patients through various methods (pamphlets, supplementary information, letters, and access to charts) has been shown to increase their satisfaction with the treatment choice made and ability to make treatment decisions (Cassileth et al., 1989), increase their satisfaction with the medical consultation (Damian & Tattersall, 1991), and assist them in gaining control and coping with the stress of having cancer (Fisher & Britten, 1993). Providing newly diagnosed male cancer patients and their spouses with an individualized information package was reported to significantly increase their satisfaction with the information they received (Derdiarian, 1989). Ellis, Hopkin, Leitch, and Crofton (1979) also reported that the provision of supplementary, written information to a group of medical patients increased their understanding and recall of information.

The provision of taped information (audio or audiovisual) to cancer patients before the treatment consultation has been reported to result in a decreased level of anxiety, less mood disturbance, less affective distress (Rainy, 1985), and an increased ability in coping during and after treatment (Johnson et al., 1988). However, Rainy (1985) reported there was no difference in the level of knowledge as a result of this intervention.

Studies involving the benefits of providing cancer patients with an audiotape of their medical consultation have produced conflicting results. Several investigators have reported that providing cancer patients with an audiotape of the initial treatment consultation with their physician assisted in communication of illness-related information to family (Hogbin & Fallowfield, 1989; Johnson & Adelstein, 1991; Reynolds et al., 1981). Still others reported that cancer patients found the tapes to be a source of new information, assisted them in recalling information (Hogbin & Fallowfield, 1989; Johnson & Adelstein, 1991), decreased their anxiety about the future treatment (Hogbin & Fallowfield, 1989), and was recognized as a way to cope with their illness (Johnson & Adelstein, 1991). Reynolds and associates (1981) found that providing a tape recording of the consultation had no effect on recall of information or patient satisfaction. Dunn et al. (1993) reported that although audiotapes of the initial consultation increased satisfaction with the medical consultation, they had limited potential to increase recall of information and had no effect on psychologic adjustment to cancer. However, North, Cornbleet, Knowles, and Leonard (1992) found this approach increased the retention of information and decreased levels of anxiety in a group of patients with advanced carcinoma. Physicians have also been reported to plan their treatment discussion more carefully when they knew they were being audiotaped (Hogbin & Fallowfield, 1989; Johnson & Adelstein, 1991).

The fourth method of assisting patients to formulate questions to ask the physician has been shown to increase older medical patients' satisfaction with medical care (Merkel, Rudisill, & Nierenberg, 1983), increase the number of questions asked (Robinson & Whitfield, 1985; Roter, 1984) and increase the understanding and recall of information (Robinson & Whitfield, 1985). Greenfield et al. (1985) reported question-asking did not have an effect on medical patients' satisfaction. However, when a group of cancer patients received this intervention, Gotcher and Edwards (1990) reported their satisfaction with the information and the quality of their communication was increased and as a result of the improved communication, they were able to manage their fears better. Neufeld, Degner, and Dick (1993) also reported that a nursing intervention which included assisting female cancer patients to identify questions to ask the physician was effective in assisting them to participate in treatment decision making to the extent they desired.

The literature has also shown that spouses or significant others play an important role in providing support to the cancer patient (Jassak, 1992; Kesselring, Lindsay, Dodd, & Lovejoy, 1986; Rose, 1990; Ward, Leventhal, Easterling, & Love, 1991), and assistance in treatment decision making (Dermatis & Lesko, 1991). Although the presence of a family member in a patient-physician interaction has also been reported to result in the physician spending more time with the patient and providing more information, it was not found to have an impact on patient satisfaction or quality of life (LaBrecque, Blanchard, Ruckdeschel, & Blanchard, 1991). Referral to community information resources such as patient support groups was identified as a way to empower cancer survivors to be advocates for themselves and for other cancer patients experiencing similar experiences (Gray & Doan, 1990). Research to examine the role of community cancer support groups in information-sharing and decision making was identified as lacking. Information telephone networks were identified as a way to supplement the information provided by health care professionals to cancer patients and their families, but it was suggested that alternative approaches were required to reach older men especially if they lived in rural areas. Empirically based studies related to the effect of including significant others in information sharing and referral of patients to community information resources (such as cancer support groups) were identified as lacking. A summary of the four most investigated interventions and the outcomes of these interventions as related to cancer populations can be found in Table 7–1.

CLINICAL GUIDELINES

Certain sociodemographic and treatment/disease factors have been identified as indicators of whether cancer patients prefer their physician to make all treatment decisions. For example, cancer patients who more recently received a diagnosis (Davison et al., 1995; Degner & Sloan, 1992), were older (Blanchard et al., 1988; Cassileth et al., 1980; Degner & Sloan, 1992; Sutherland et al., 1989), married (Blanchard et al., 1988), and less educated (Cassileth et al., 1980; Degner & Sloan, 1992) have been found to prefer to delegate decisional responsibility to their physician. Controversy exists over the relationship between prognosis and extent to which cancer patients wish to participate in decision making. For example; Cassileth and colleagues

---

TABLE 7–1. *Information Interventions and Outcomes*

1. **Provision of Written Information**
   - Increased satisfaction with treatment choice and ability to make treatment decisions (Cassileth et al., 1989)
   - Increased satisfaction with medical consultation (Damian & Tattersall, 1991)
   - Assistance in gaining control and coping with stress of having cancer (Fisher & Britten, 1993)
   - Increased satisfaction with information received (Derdiarian, 1989)

2. **Provision of Taped Information (Audio or Audiovisual)**
   - Decreased levels of anxiety, less mood disturbance, less affective distress (Rainy, 1985)
   - Increased ability to cope during and after treatment (Johnson et al., 1988)

3. **Patients Provided With Audio Tape of Medical Consultation**
   - Assistance in communication of illness-related information to family (Hogbin & Fallowfield, 1989; Johnson & Adelstein, 1991; Reynolds et al., 1981)
   - Source of new information and assistance in recalling information (Hogbin & Fallowfield, 1989; Johnson & Adelstein, 1991)
   - Decreased anxiety about future treatment (Hogbin & Fallowfield, 1989)
   - Assisted in coping with illness (Johnson & Adelstein, 1991)
   - Increased satisfaction with medical consultation (Dunn et al., 1993)
   - Physicians planned treatment discussion more carefully (Hogbin & Fallowfield, 1989; Johnson & Adelstein, 1991)
   - Increased retention of information and reduced levels of anxiety (North et al., 1992)

4. **Assisting Patients Formulate Questions to Ask Physician**
   - Increased satisfaction with information and quality of communication, and better management of fears (Gotcher & Edwards, 1990)
   - Assistance in treatment decision making (Neufeld et al., 1993)

TABLE 7–2. *Potential Roles in Treatment Decision Making*

A. I prefer to make the final selection about which treatment I will receive.
B. I prefer to make the final selection of my treatment after seriously considering my doctor's opinion.
C. I prefer that my doctor and I share responsibility for deciding which treatment is best for me.
D. I prefer that my doctor makes the final decision about which treatment will be used, but seriously considers my opinion.
E. I prefer to leave all decisions regarding my treatment to my doctor.

reported patients with a favorable prognosis preferred a more active role in decision making, and Blanchard and colleagues reported those patients with a poorer prognosis were more active. The clinical hypothesis that sicker patients with cancer prefer less control in treatment decision making was not supported by Degner and Sloan. Although these predictors were found to be significant, individual assessment of preferences to participate in decision making remains the best clinical approach.

Neufeld, Degner, and Dick (1993) described a nursing intervention designed to provide decisional support for cancer patients who wanted to participate in medical decision making. The intervention consisted of assessing the extent to which patients preferred to participate in decision making, helping them to identify questions to ask the physician, and supporting them in getting the information they wanted. This intervention was tested and found to be effective in an oncology clinic setting with women who had a confirmed diagnosis of breast or gynecologic cancer. Although further research is required to determine the effectiveness of this intervention, it is suggested that having patients select their preferred role in treatment decision making

(see Table 7–2) would be helpful in assisting clinicians assess the extent to which each patient prefers to participate. An abstract of Degner and Sloan's (1992) study demonstrates how these statements have been used to measure role preferences of cancer patients who have recently received a diagnosis (see Box 7–1).

The types of information found to be important to cancer patients were identified in this chapter. The question is how can we assist these patients to get the information they want? Three types of clinical interventions to assess the kind and amount of information that cancer patients want to have or avoid to satisfy their degree of involvement in decision making have been identified. The first method includes providing each patient with a list of the different information needs, as previously identified by cancer patients, and asking them to identify the type and amount of information they want about each category. A card sort procedure of information categories, similar to the decision making card sort used by Degner and Sloan (1992), have also been shown to be an effective way of determining information preferences (Hack et al., 1994). The clinician could then provide them with written information on each of the identified categories.

Assisting patients in formulating questions to ask the physician also has been shown to be an effective approach. Table 7–3 lists some of the questions cancer patients could use to get the information they require. It is suggested that providing such a list of questions to patients would assist them to obtain the type and amount of information they wanted when they met with their physician to discuss treatment options. These questions were adapted from a booklet published by the National Coalition for Cancer Survivorship (1991).

The third method includes providing each patient with the opportunity to have his or her treatment consultation with the physician audio- or videotaped. Such an intervention would allow patients to review the information they received, share information about their disease and treatment with their family, and assist them

---

Box 7–1. *Abstract of Degner and Sloan's Study*

Degner, L. F., & Sloan, J. A. (1992). Decision making during serious illness: What role do patients really want to play? *Journal of Clinical Epidemiology, 45,* 941–950.

Purpose/Objectives: To determine what roles people actually want to assume in selecting cancer treatments.
Setting: Two tertiary referral cancer clinics in Winnipeg, Manitoba, Canada.
Design: Survey.
Sample: 436 newly diagnosed cancer patients and 482 members of the general public.
Methods: Preferences were elicited using two card sort procedures, each of which described five potential roles in decision making.
Findings: The majority (59 per cent) of patients wanted physicians to make treatment decisions on their behalf, but 64 per cent of the public thought they would want to select their own treatment if cancer developed. Most patients (51 per cent) and members of the public (46 per cent) wanted their physician and family to share responsibility for decision making if they were too ill to participate. Sociodemographic variables accounted for only 15 per cent of variance in preferences.
Conclusions: The findings suggested that the impact of being diagnosed with a life-threatening illness may influence preferences to participate.
Implications for Nursing Practice: Given the small proportion of variance in preferences accounted for by sociodemographic variables, individual assessment of preferences to participate in treatment decision making remains the best clinical approach.

TABLE 7–3. *List of Questions to Ask to Obtain Information About Treatment Options*

1. Considering the type and extent of cancer I have, as well as my age, lifestyle, and other factors, what treatment options are available?
2. Are there any treatment options that can be performed on a home therapy basis?
3. Which treatment option(s) do you recommend?
4. What is the goal of treatment (example: cure, shrink tumor so it can be treated by other means, extend life, reduce pain)?
5. How many patients have you treated with this type of cancer in the last 12 months?
6. What types of doctors do you think will need to be involved in treating me?
7. Would it be helpful for me to talk with someone who has been treated for this kind of cancer?

For Each Treatment Option:
1. Please explain what the treatment is.
2. What are the short-term and long-term risks?
3. What are the side effects (example: temporary, long-term, delayed—those which may not occur until perhaps later)?
4. What can I do to prevent or lessen the side effects?
5. How will the treatment option affect my other medical problems?
6. What side effects should I report to you during or after treatment?
7. How will the treatment affect my ability to work or perform other activities that are necessary or important to me?
8. Will the treatment hurt or be uncomfortable?
9. What can be done to prevent or lessen the discomfort?
10. How long will this treatment take?
11. How and when will you be able to determine whether this treatment accomplishes its intended goal?
12. Will the treatment affect me emotionally or sexually?
13. What will my quality of life be like during and after treatment?
14. After the treatment ends, what medical care will I receive to determine whether the cancer recurs or spreads in the future?
15. Should I get a second opinion from another doctor?
16. How can I make plans to get help at home during my recovery, or help with care for my spouse?

in decision making. It is believed that a combination of these three clinical interventions would assist cancer patients obtain the type and amount of information they require and enable them to assume a more active role in the decision making process.

SUMMARY

Cancer patients are faced with a complexity of diagnostic and treatment choices from the earliest point of entry into the health care system. For those at risk of getting cancer, there may be choices about preventative changes in lifestyle or undergoing anxiety-producing diagnostic procedures. These life events suggest an opportunity for patients to exercise their autonomy and individual preferences in making treatment decisions. Few investigators have studied the effect of implementing one or more of these information interventions in the clinical area for the purpose of assisting cancer patients in the treatment decision making process. Cassileth and colleagues (1989) were the only investigators who studied the effect of provision of written information (to a group of cancer patients who had recently received a diagnosis) on participation in treatment decision making. There is an overwhelming need for randomized clinical research studies to be conducted in this area. The results of such studies will contribute a great deal to our understanding of how nurses can assist cancer patients to make the difficult decisions they face.

REFERENCES

Bilodeau, B., & Degner, L. F. (in press). *Information needs, sources of information, and decisional roles in women with breast cancer. Oncology Nursing Forum.*

Blanchard, C. G., LaBrecque, M. S., Ruckdeschel J. C., & Blanchard, E. B. (1988). Information and decision-making preferences of hospitalized adult cancer patients. *Social Science Medicine, 27,* 1139–1145.

Cassileth, B. R., Soloway, M. S., Vogelzang, N. J., Schellhammer, P. S., Seidmon, W. J., Hait, H. I., & Kennealey, G. T. (1989). Patients' choice of treatment in stage D prostate cancer. *Urology, 33* (Suppl 5), 57–62.

Cassileth, B. R., Zupkis, R. V., Sutton-Smith, K., & March, V. (1980). Information and participation preferences among cancer patients. *Annals of Internal Medicine, 92,* 832–836.

Damian, D., & Tattersall, M. H. N. (1991). Letters to patients: Improving communication in cancer care. *The Lancet, 338,* 923–925.

Davison, B. J., Degner, L. F., & Morgan, T. R. (in press). *Information and decision making preferences of men with prostate cancer. Oncology Nursing Forum.*

Degner, L. F., & Beaton, J. I. (1987). *Life-death decisions in health care.* New York: Hemisphere Publishing.

Degner, L. F., Farber, J. M., & Hack, T. F. (1989). *Communication between cancer patients and health care professionals; an annotated bibliography.* Winnipeg, Manitoba; National Cancer Institute of Canada.

Degner, L. F., Jerry, M., & Till, J. (1991). Terry Fox workshop on patient-health professional communication in cancer. *Canadian Medical Association Journal, 144,* 1417–1418.

Degner, L. F., & Sloan, J. A. (1992). Decision making during serious illness: What role do patients really want to play? *Journal of Clinical Epidemiology, 45,* 941–950.

Derdiarian, A. K. (1986). Informational needs of recently diagnosed cancer patients. *Nursing Research, 35,* 276–281.

Derdiarian, A. K. (1987). Information needs of recently diagnosed cancer patients: Part 2: Method and description. *Cancer Nursing, 10,* 156–163.

Derdiarian, A. K. (1989). Effects of information on recently diagnosed cancer patients' and spouses' satisfaction with care. *Cancer Nursing, 12,* 285–292.

Dermatis, H., & Lesko, L. M. (1991). Psychosocial correlates of physician-patient communication at time of informed consent for bone marrow transplantation. *Cancer Investigation, 9,* 621–628.

Dunn, S. M., Butow, P. N., Tattersall, M. H. N., Jones, Q. J., Sheldon, J. S., Taylor, J. J., & Sumich, M. D. (1993). General information tapes inhibit recall of the cancer consultation. *Journal of Clinical Oncology, 11,* 2279–2285.

Ellis, D. A., Hopkin, J. M., Leitch, A. G., & Crofton, Sir J. (1979). "Doctors' orders": Controlled trial of supplementary, written information for patients. *British Medical Journal,* 456.

Ende, J., Kazis, L., Ash, A., & Moskowitz, M. A. (1989). Measuring patients' desire for autonomy: Decision making and information-seeking preferences among medical patients. *Journal of General Internal Medicine, 4,* 23–30.

Fallowfield, L. J., Hall, A., Macquire, G. P., & Baum, M. (1990). Psychological outcomes of different treatment policies in women with early breast cancer outside of a clinical trial. *British Medical Journal, 310,* 575–580.

Feldman, S. (1976). *Work and cancer health histories—a study of the experiences of recovered patients* (Report). San Francisco, CA: California Division, American Cancer Society, 36–52.

Fisher, B., & Britten, N. (1993). Patient access to records: Expectations of hospital doctors and experiences of cancer patients. *British Journal of General Practice, 43,* 52–56.

Forrow, L., Wortman, S. A., & Brock, D. W. (1988). Science, ethics, and the making of clinical decisions. *Journal of the American Medical Association, 259,* 3161–3167.

Gotcher, J. M., & Edwards, R. (1990). Coping strategies of cancer patients: Actual communication and imagined interactions. *Health Communication, 2,* 255–266.

Gray, R. E., & Doan, B. D. (1990). Empowerment and persons with cancer: Politics in cancer medicine. *Journal of Palliative Care, 6,* 33–45.

Greenfield, S., Kaplan, S., & Ware, J. E. (1985). Expanding patient involvement in care: Effect on patient outcomes. *Annals of Internal Medicine, 102,* 520–528.

Greenleigh Associates. (1979). *Report on the social, economic, and psychological needs of cancer patients in California: Major findings and implications* (Report). San Francisco, CA: California Division, American Cancer Society, 40–116.

Hack, T. F., Degner, L. F., & Dyck, D. G. (1994). Relationship between preferences for decisional control and illness information among women with breast cancer: A quantitative and qualitative analysis. *Social Science Medicine, 39,* 279–289.

Haug, M. R., & Lavin, B. (1981). Practitioner or patient: Who's in charge? *Journal of Health and Social Behavior, 22,* 212–229.

Hogbin, B., & Fallowfield, L. (1989). Getting it taped: The "bad news" consultation with cancer patients. *British Journal of Hospital Medicine, 41,* 330–333.

Jassak, P. F. (1992). Families: An essential element in the care of the patient with cancer. *Oncology Nursing Forum, 19,* 871–876.

Johnson, I. A., & Adelstein, D. J. (1991). The use of recorded interviews to enhance physician-patient communication. *Journal of Cancer Education, 6,* 99–102.

Johnson, J. E., Nail, L. M., Lauver, D., King, K. B., & Keys, H. (1988). Reducing the negative impact of radiation therapy on functional status. *Cancer, 61,* 46–51.

Jones, J. S. (1981). Telling the right patient. *British Medical Journal, 283,* 291–292.

Kesselring, A., Lindsey, A. M., Dodd, M. J., & Lovejoy, N. C. (1986). Social network and support perceived by Swiss cancer patients. *Cancer Nursing, 9,* 156–163.

LaBrecque, M. S., Blanchard, C. G., Ruckdeschel, J. C., & Blanchard, E. B. (1991). The impact of family presence on the physician-cancer patient interaction. *Social Science Medicine, 33,* 1253–1261.

Luker, K. A., Beaver, K., Leinster, S. J., Owens, R. G., Degner, L. F., & Sloan, J. A. (in press). The information needs of women newly diagnosed with breast cancer. *Journal of Advanced Nursing.*

Merkel, W. T., Rudisill, J. R., & Nierenberg, B. P. (1983). Preparing patients to see the doctor: Effects on patients and physicians in a family practice center. *Family Practice Research Journal, 2,* 147–163.

Messerli, M. L., Garamendi, C., & Romano, J. (1980). Breast cancer: Information as a technique of crisis intervention. *American Journal of Orthopsychiatry, 50,* 728–731.

Morris, J., & Royle, G. T. (1988). Offering patients a choice of surgery for early breast cancer: A reduction in anxiety and depression in patients and their husbands. *Social Science Medicine, 26,* 583–585.

National Coalition for Cancer Survivorship (1991). *Teamwork: The cancer patients guide to talking with your doctor.* Silver Spring, MD: Author.

Neufeld, K. R., Degner, L. F., & Dick, J. A. M. (1993). A nursing intervention to foster patient involvement in treatment decisions. *Oncology Nursing Forum, 20,* 631–635.

North, N., Cornbleet, M. A., Knowles, G., & Leonard, R. C. (1992). Information giving in oncology: A preliminary study of tape-recorder use. *British Journal of Clinical Psychology, 31,* 357–359.

Northouse, L. L., & Wortman, C. B. (1990). Models of helping and coping in cancer care. *Patient Education and Counseling, 15,* 49–64.

Rainy, L. C. (1985). Effects of preparatory patient education for radiation oncology patients. *Cancer, 56,* 1056–1061.

Reynolds, P. M., Sanson-Fisher, R. W., Poole, A. D., Harker, J., & Byrne, M. J. (1981). Cancer and communication: Information-giving in an oncology clinic. *British Medical Journal, 282,* 1449–1451.

Robinson, E. J., & Whitfield, M. J. (1985). Improving the efficiency of patients' comprehension monitoring: A way of increasing patients' participation in general practice consultations. *Social Science Medicine, 21,* 915–919.

Rose, J. H. (1990). Social support and cancer: Adult patients' desire for support from family, friends, and health professionals. *American Journal of Community Psychology, 18,* 439–465.

Roter, D. L. (1984). Patient question asking in physician-patient interaction. *Health Psychology, 3,* 395–409.

Strull, W. M., Lo, B., & Charles, G. (1984). Do patients want to participate in medical decision making? *Journal of the American Medical Association, 252,* 2990–2994.

Sutherland, H. J., Llewellyn-Thomas, H. A., Lockwood, G. A., Tritchler, D. L., & Till, J. E. (1989). Cancer patients: Their desire for information and participation in treatment decisions. *Journal of the Royal Society of Medicine, 82,* 260–263.

Vertinsky, I. B., Thompson, W. A., & Uyeno, D. (1974). Measuring consumer desire for participation in clinical decision making. *Health Services Research, 9,* 121–134.

Ward, S., Leventhal, H., Easterling, D., & Love, R. (1991). Social support, self-esteem, and communication in patients receiving chemotherapy. *Journal of Psychosocial Oncology, 9,* 95–116.

Weisman, A. L., & Worden, W. J. (1976). *Coping and vulnerability in cancer patients.* (Report of Project Omega, Department of Psychiatry, Harvard Medical School.) Boston, MA: Massachusetts General Hospital.

Cancer and the Family

Barbara B. Germino • Maureen E. O'Rourke

In this era of cost containment and health care reform, cancer care is increasingly being delivered in outpatient and community settings while those hospitalized for treatment are being discharged much earlier. Persons with cancer often depend on their families and others at home for various kinds of help and support. The experiences of cancer and cancer treatment have significant impact not only on the patient but also on the patient's family. Knowledge of how cancer affects family systems has never been more crucial to nursing practice, because families are much more involved with providing support and care throughout the illness, often during remissions and recurrences, and frequently for long periods of time. Nurses are central in helping families live with the changes and disruptions cancer and treatment for cancer may cause in their lives.

WHO IS THE PATIENT'S FAMILY?

The patient's family traditionally has been defined in the health care literature as those persons related by blood, marriage, or adoption. In many studies of families with children, the mother has been the informant for the entire family, providing a "window" into the family system, but the window provided by the mother's perspective excluded the perspectives of other family members, including adult children (Feetham, 1984).

For purposes of clinical practice it is most useful to allow patients to define and describe their own families. Those who function as family members may or may not be related to the patient in the traditional sense, even though they live in the patient's household. For some people, friends, neighbors, partners, and lovers may be as likely to be considered family as are spouses, children, parents, grandparents, siblings, and other relatives.

THE FAMILY AS A SYSTEM

STRUCTURE AND FUNCTION OF FAMILY SYSTEMS

Those who function as family for the patient are part of a social system in which members have ties to one another, have ongoing interactions with one another, are interdependent, have some common history or frame of reference that ties them together, and share some goals. Family systems, like other systems, are more than simply the sum of their parts. They are composed of subsystems (e.g., spouses, mother-daughter pairs) of members who have unique ties and relationships. A variety of factors help to shape the rules by which the family system deals with other systems and with events that affect it. The structure of the family (i.e., the members of the system and their roles), the relationships among family members, the family's history and past experiences, and the family's culture, religion, and social environment all combine to influence family functioning. Family rules guide the behavior of individual system members as well as the operations of the family unit. The rules may be implicit or explicit; they often relate to issues of communication, for example, who talks to whom about what or what kinds of family issues may be discussed with nonfamily members. Family rules reflect the family's values. Loyalty, privacy, relationships among family members, honesty, and child rearing are all examples of issues around which families often develop rules. In the situation of cancer, family rules about privacy may, for instance, affect who is told about the cancer, how much they are told, and when. Such rules may have been helpful to the family system in the past, but when extra support is needed, they may prove less helpful.

FAMILY SYSTEM BOUNDARIES

The extent to which family systems are open to outsiders is a reflection of family system boundaries. The nature and extent of a family's relationship with other systems in its environment are governed by its boundaries.

Families define boundaries to keep what they perceive as disruptive influences out of the family, protecting themselves. At the same time families maintain some contact with the external world to obtain support and assistance. Because families are information-processing systems, they must find ways to manage and evaluate information from outside their boundaries. So boundaries can help them to filter information as well as regulate the distance between them and other systems (Quinn & Herndon, 1986). The context or environment in which the family lives, then, is not only the physical environment or geographic location but also the other social systems with which the family interacts: extended family, neighborhood, community, and local health care systems are all examples of such systems. Information about family boundaries is crucial to nurses attempting to assist families in dealing with cancer. Validating or making explicit family rules about boundaries can help families clarify feelings and behaviors and to solve problems about getting the needs of individuals met while maintaining and enhancing family functioning. For example, the clinician can ask about families' rules such as those about expressing anger, sharing guilt, and keeping secrets. By doing so, not only will there be a better understanding of the family by the clinician, but a clearer view of problem areas may be identified for families, and a starting place for intervention may be achieved.

FRAMEWORK FOR CONSIDERING CANCER AND FAMILIES

In discussing cancer and families, it is helpful to look at a few of the factors that may influence the impact of such a potentially life-threatening illness. The specific kind of cancer diagnosis and treatment, the timing and trajectory of the illness, the personal meaning of experiences for those involved, the nature of human responses during the cancer experience, and the caregiving demands and costs are all important factors in considering families with cancer (Fig. 8–1) (Oberst & Scott, 1988).

IMPACT OF SPECIFIC CANCER DIAGNOSIS

BODY IMAGE CHANGES

The experience of cancer is shaped to some extent by the particular kind of cancer and its implications for change. The alteration of one's body or the loss of a body part are significant changes about which much has been written. How persons view their bodies, themselves as persons, and their sexuality are all important issues in the impact of cancer-related physical changes. Studies of self-image and body image in people with cancer have focused primarily on women with mastectomies and hysterectomies and on men and women who have had ostomy surgery (Donahue & Knapp, 1977; Frank-Stromborg & Wright, 1984; Gallagher, 1972). The kinds of surgery that cause visible or symbolic changes in the body have been shown to be related, at least for a time, to negative changes in the patient's self-image and body image, to grief reactions, and to changes in relationships (Woods & Earp, 1978). However, it has become clear that initially devastating physical changes may be integrated into a changed view of oneself, that such changes take time—sometimes years—and that relationships with significant people, especially spouses and partners, can be extremely important and positive as mediators of that impact. The

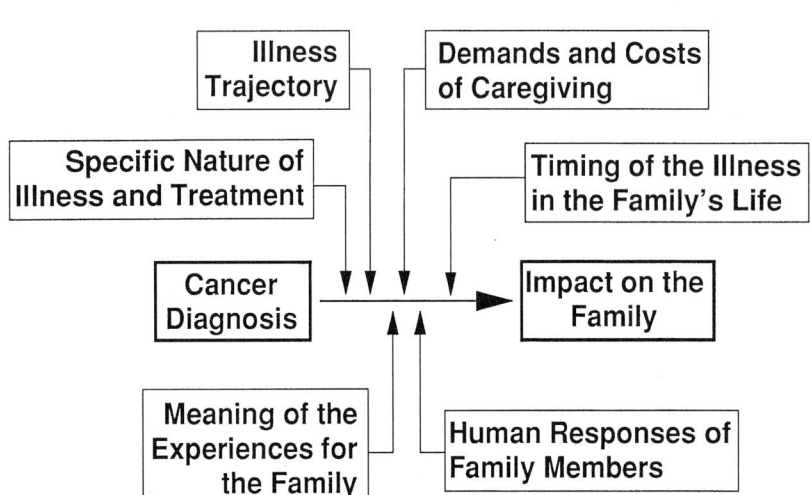

FIGURE 8–1. The impact of cancer on the family. (Design by Larue Coats, Ph.D., The Design Center, University of North Carolina—Chapel Hill School of Nursing.)

visibility of physical changes may accentuate or minimize the social impact of cancer and the extent to which it affects relationships with others.

SOCIAL IMPACT OF PHYSICAL CHANGES

The extent to which physical changes affect important areas of functioning may make a crucial difference in their social impact, both on the person experiencing them and on the family. If the patient has experienced major physical changes such as loss of a breast or creation of an ostomy but is still able to carry on functions that are personally important, the impact of the physical changes on relationships may not be as extensive as it is when function is lost. At least one study of women with breast cancer indicated that the women who carried a disproportionate share of household and family responsibilities shifted some of that responsibility to their families and friends during recovery from surgery and during chemotherapy and radiation treatments; within 6 or 12 months after diagnosis, however, the women had returned to their prediagnosis levels of responsibility (Green, 1986). The physical changes of cancer and cancer treatment can be significant ones in the cancer experience, but professional caregivers may tend to focus on them sometimes to the exclusion of broader issues that cross diagnostic boundaries. For instance, some evidence suggests that the quality of life for patients with physically devastating kinds of cancer may at times be low but overall may be perceived by the patient as being quite good despite symptom distress and an uncertain future (Frank-Stromborg & Wright, 1984; Germino & Dalton, 1986).

SPECIFIC TYPE OF CANCER AND FAMILIES

Much of the family research has been done with mixed samples of families representing many, often unspecified cancer diagnoses. The emphasis has clearly been less on the specific kind of cancer and treatment than on the impact of the potentially life-threatening group of illnesses that cancer represents. There are some notable exceptions in studies of women with breast cancer and their families.

The family has been described as providing a crucially important context or environment for the woman with breast cancer, the quality of that environment (in this case indicated by tension and conflict) being directly related to the woman's adjustment to her illness over time (Spiegel, Bloom, & Gottheil, 1983). The family's adaptation to breast cancer after the initial diagnostic and early treatment period is characterized by complex feelings. Northouse (1989) studied husbands of women who had had mastectomies for breast cancer and found that during an 18 month period, despite improvement in their mood and role functioning, these spouses maintained elevated levels of distress equal to those at 3 and 30 days after the mastectomy. Zahlis and Shands (1993) confirmed the finding that approximately one fourth of partners of women with breast cancer, 18 months after diagnosis, continued to describe negative feelings and effects of the illness on their daily lives. The subjects in their study, unlike those in Northouse's earlier work, had generally had lumpectomies rather than mastectomies. Specific fears identified across these studies include, most commonly, the fear of recurrence. Going to follow-up appointments, finding a new lump, or experiencing a symptom like back pain can precipitate increases in anxiety and even "flashbacks" to the earlier experiences. Partners are anxious not only about the possibility of recurrence but also about dealing with the emotional responses they anticipate in their wives (Zahlis & Shands, 1993). In addition to the cancer, families in their daily lives were generally dealing with unrelated but concurrent stressors that were already present at the time of diagnosis (Zahlis & Shands, 1991). Marital problems, which may have preexisted at some level before the woman's diagnosis, may increase in intensity and have been described as difficulty communicating and change in the quality of the couple's intimate relationship (Andersen, 1990; Schain, 1988; Zahlis & Shands, 1993).

The extent to which coping behaviors of women with breast cancer and their husbands affect one another in the process of adjusting to breast cancer and treatment is a question that has not been well studied and one which has potential importance for nursing intervention designed to help partners enhance their coping strategies and behaviors. The results of a small study of couples within the first year of dealing with breast cancer indicated that the husband's coping behaviors and his rating of the relationship were the best predictors of the wife's psychologic distress. The husband's distress depended on a combination of his own and his wife's coping behaviors (Hannum, Giese-Davis, Harding, & Hatfield, 1991). It is important then, that caregivers dealing with these families over time pay attention to the quality of relationships within the family as well as to individual family members' responses. Such findings reinforce the importance of learning to assess and intervene with the family as a system rather than only as individuals.

Other issues in the family's adaptation to breast cancer over time may include a sense of powerlessness in the face of the disease, a powerlessness that may be accentuated in situations in which family members do not feel a part of the decision making process. Ambivalence toward the patient and toward aspects of the treatment experience has been described as a normal response to disruption in family routines and threatened expectations (Lewis, Ellison, & Woods, 1985). Lewis and colleagues describe families experiencing breast cancer as living two lives: the life related to the illness and its contingencies and the life of being a family that must deal with the needs of all its members. Some of the latter needs may conflict with the special care and attention needed by the patient (Lewis et al., 1985).

Many studies have contained mixed or unspecified samples of patients and their families, and the body of work on psychosocial issues in breast cancer has grown much more quickly than research on other specific kinds of cancer. In this chapter we have used breast cancer as an example of how a specific type of cancer diagnosis is important as part of a framework for considering the impact of cancer on families. More information about how other specific cancers may affect the family is emerging and will need to be considered by clinicians asking how cancer affects the family.

TIMING AND TRAJECTORY OF CANCER IN THE FAMILY'S LIFE

TIMING OF CANCER IN THE FAMILY'S LIFE

The timing of a cancer diagnosis in the context of both the individual's life and the life of the family are additional factors to be considered in attempts to understand the potential impact of cancer. The family life cycle, for instance, has been used as an organizing framework for examining the effects of chronic illness on the family (Eisenberg, Sutkin, & Jansen, 1984). Families coping with cancer experience a variety of different concerns, threats, and challenges, some of which are related to where they are developmentally. Developmental phases identified for families include the youngest family, young families, families with adolescents and young adults, and aging families. In today's families these phases are often blurred, and the developmental needs of families and the interface of these needs with those imposed by cancer have not been well studied. In the same way that newly married young couples striving to create an enduring new system must cope with issues of separation from their family of origin, a cancer diagnosis may propel patients and spouses back to intimacy with their siblings and parents rather than with each other (Rait & Lederberg, 1990). Family decision making may be affected by parental influence, which may conflict with the spouse's legal prerogative. The family life cycle framework has not been well tested, and research on many contemporary family groups has not been conducted. However, developmental factors may be important in the impact of cancer on a family and should be included in clinical assessment.

The largest proportion of family-focused oncology literature focuses on families coping with a child's cancer. Such families must continue to meet the specific developmental needs of healthy siblings while trying to incorporate the cancer experience into family life. Illness-related demands such as transportation, child care, financial, and caregiving burdens have been identified in numerous studies. There are conflicting data regarding the impact of cancer on the quality of the partners' marital relationships (Barbarin, Hughes, & Chester, 1985; Rose, 1987). A growing body of literature exists examining the effects of a cancer diagnosis on the health of siblings (Martinson, Gilliss, Colaizzo, Freeman, & Bossert, 1990). Additionally recent literature has focused on the impact of a parental diagnosis of cancer on children. Issel, Ersek, and Lewis (1990) interviewed 81 children (aged 6 to 20 years) whose mothers had received a cancer diagnosis within the preceding 2.5 years. Their interviews revealed age and developmental differences in the coping strategies utilized by children, with younger children attempting to help more at home and older children being more likely to express their feelings and concerns. Common to all

of the children were attempts to maintain normalcy and avoid the illness. Adolescents who had lost a parent from cancer have reported experiencing increased isolation and reliance on peers, family, and friends for support (Berman, Cragg, & Kuenzig, 1988). The impact of the initial diagnosis and coping throughout the disease trajectory related to the developmental needs of family members have not been systematically described.

For adult children coping with a parental diagnosis of cancer, role and relationship concerns have been identified as a major issue (Germino & Funk, 1993). More specifically, role changes like taking on the new role of support person to the ill parent were a struggle as was balancing the demands of a parent's illness and the demands of their own lives, including meeting their own developmental needs. Unresolved relationship issues with parents generated ambivalence, confusion, and concern for many. With the growing emphasis on gerontologic oncology and the realization that approximately 60 per cent of cancers occur in the over-65 age group, there is clearly a need for additional research with older families.

The timing of cancer for families may be important not only in terms of their developmental phase of the family and of individual members but also in terms of other stresses in the family's lives. Cancer may be more difficult for families to accept and deal with during critical transitions such as marriage, the birth of a child, or the beginning of retirement. For many families losses of friends and family members, children leaving home, financial difficulties, moving, and other illnesses occur along with cancer. Both normative changes and strains can and do often occur simultaneously. Family stress theory suggests that an accumulation of stressors can disrupt even the strongest family's ability to continue functioning well (McCubbin & Patterson, 1983).

CANCER ILLNESS TRAJECTORY

The trajectory of an illness refers not only to the course of the illness, its "unfolding over time," but also to the handling or management of the work of the illness and the impact on those involved (Strauss et al., 1984). The family's experiences with cancer change over time, and patients and families experience a sequence of problems as they cope with new demands imposed by their illness. Using available research literature, Sales (1991) revised Northouse's earlier model of a cancer trajectory to reflect six phases. The initial phase includes diagnosis and hospitalization; the adaptation phase has been separated into posthospital, adjuvant treatment, and recurrence; and the terminal phase remains as originally described. In today's health care system, for many people with cancer there is never a hospitalization, so these phases need to be interpreted as only a guide for possibilities; many other trajectory patterns may characterize the current clinical realities. Research on the family response to a cancer diagnosis is limited, but concerns of families focus heavily on the diagnostic process, treatment, emotional, and existential issues and the future (Cooper, 1984; Germino, Funk, Burman, & May, 1994; Gotay, 1984; Mah & Johnston, 1993). Some studies have indicated that male spouses have difficulty dealing with their wives' emotional distress (Gotay, 1984; Zahlis & Shands, 1993) and that acute stress reactions including shock, denial, fear, and depression are more pronounced among spouses than patients (Cooper, 1984).

Numerous researchers have documented the reactions and needs of families during the adaptation or treatment phase of the cancer illness trajectory. The demands of cancer and cancer treatment as well as the burdens imposed on family caregivers contribute to shaping the trajectory of illness that families must manage. Demands range from managing physical care needs and role changes required to deal with the illness to coping with new emotional demands of family members upon each other (Lewis, 1986; Lewis et al., 1985; Stetz, 1987). At least one study has indicated that families who are able to adapt to such demands with shifting and expanding roles and effective communication experience less disruption and conflict over time (Vess, Moreland, & Schwebel, 1985).

Consistent with family systems theory, Northouse and Swain (1987) noted that both breast cancer patients and their spouses reported comparable levels of emotional distress immediately after surgery and that distress levels remained high 30 days postoperatively. In an extension of this longitudinal study, Northouse (1990) reported persistent psychologic distress in patients and spouses 18 months after surgery. Oberst and James (1985) found the spouses of gastrointestinal and genitourinary cancer patients were more anxious than the patients during hospitalization and attributed this to fatigue and greater role responsibilities. In following a cohort of patients with cancer and their family caregivers from hospital discharge through 6 months after hospitalization, McCorkle et al. (1993) noted that although by 3 and 6 months after hospitalization, patients' conditions stabilized or improved, caregivers continued to report similar levels of burden. In addition, patient psychosocial responses had strong positive correlations with the financial impact on caregivers, the impact on caregiver schedules, and their physical caregiving responsibilities. These findings are also congruent with family stress theory and the concept of "pileup" as described by McCubbin & Patterson (1983).

We have only begun to study the impact of the recurrence of cancer after long periods without any signs of disease and find that recurrence may be, from the patient's and family member's perspective, more difficult than the initial diagnosis. Chekryn (1984) reported that some patients and spouses avoided discussing the possible outcomes of the recurrence with each other, particularly when the outcome may be death. Although some subjects reported that recurrence had fostered increased marital cohesion, many reported a lack of shared meaning about the cancer recurrence and experienced uncertainty, grief, feelings of injustice, fear, and anger. More recently, Given and Given (1992) followed patients and family caregivers for a 6-month period to determine the psychologic impact of breast cancer recurrence in comparison with the reactions of patients recently given a breast cancer diagnosis and their family caregivers. They concluded

that family caregivers experienced more psychologic distress than patients and that new vs. recurrent disease status did not have a differential effect on this outcome. The paucity of prospective longitudinal research hinders our understanding of the family experience of recurrent disease and hampers our planning of appropriate family-centered interventions. This lack of research regarding cancer recurrence is surprising, because fear of recurrence is recognized as an almost universal issue.

Because of advances in both diagnostic procedures and treatment, more patients are living longer, and the issue for many cancer survivors becomes one of rehabilitation—of learning to cope with a chronic illness rather than an illness that has been "cured" and no longer exists among patients and their family members (Sales, 1991). Few studies describe the experience of rehabilitation and adaptation to cancer as a chronic illness. Available findings suggest that a family's adjustment to a child-rearing mother's breast cancer changes positively over time in two areas—a decrease in illness-related demands on the family and improvement in the marriage. However, the patient's depressive mood, family functioning, and coping seem not to improve during the rehabilitative period after treatment is over. This lack of improvement has implications for caregivers following families over time, because these women and their families may need more intensive support services during a period when traditional services have generally been less available (Lewis & Hammond, 1992).

As large clinical trials have become available to many patients outside of major cancer centers, there is a need to better understand what Stetz (1993) has called "survival work," or the experiences of patients and their families involved in experimental treatment for cancer. Quality of life issues become important, including informed consent, engagement in the protocol, monitoring of symptoms, and carrying on or living with the cancer (Stetz, 1993).

Descriptions of family experiences during the terminal phases of cancer predominate in the oncology nursing research literature. The central preoccupation of families during this phase is meeting the patient's physical needs (Hinds, 1985; Stetz, 1987). Studies have revealed frustration regarding the lack of information, skills, and tangible resources needed, coupled with feelings of exhaustion and isolation (Sales, 1991). Stetz (1987) reported that spouses averaged spending 23 hours daily at home, with 75 per cent of spouses never leaving the house at all. Hull (1989) reviewed 13 studies addressing family needs and supportive nursing behaviors during terminal care. Across care settings and studies she found that families regarded information about their relatives' conditions and interventions to enhance patient comfort as most supportive to them. Interestingly, families viewed interventions that encouraged them to ventilate their own feelings as least supportive.

A number of variables have been examined in an attempt to predict family grief responses including the location of death, type and reason for death, and degree of preparation for death. Additional variables that may affect the grief experience include family presence at the time of death and the speed with which the cancer illness trajectory progressed. In a recent study of spousal bereavement, high- and low-risk groups (for poor bereavement outcomes) were identified with validity both before and after the spouse's death (Robinson, McCorkle, Lev, & Nuamah, 1994). The investigators found support for variables identified by Parkes (1975) as differentiating those at high and low risk for psychologic distress after the death of a spouse. Systematic knowledge about family grief reactions is beginning to grow, then, and is foundational to the planning of effective intervention strategies. Findings do suggest that bereavement intervention can be started as soon as possible, even before the anticipated death (Robinson et al., 1994).

In summary, published evidence suggests that the family's cancer experience changes over time. Although Northouse's (1984) and Sales' (1991) conceptualizations of the needs of families over the cancer illness trajectory provide a useful organizational framework, inclusion of a preventive phase in this trajectory has become necessary. Nurses are now challenged to assist families in coping with the implications of genetic risk analysis and chemopreventive clinical trials. Research is currently lacking in this area. Little is known about families' experiences with recurrent disease and with issues of survivorship and rehabilitation. Last, many studies have focused on family as the traditional marital dyad and have not included the responses and needs of young or adult children or even

a broader conceptualization of family as defined by the patients themselves.

COSTS OF CANCER TO THE FAMILY

Part of the impact of cancer on the family involves the costs of cancer care. Regardless of socioeconomic status, almost all families experiencing cancer and cancer treatment have financial problems. Even those who are well insured can be financially devastated by substantial gaps in coverage (Berkman & Sampson, 1993). With few exceptions, studies that focus on costs of cancer care to families take into account only outlays of cash for hired labor or costs attributable to loss of employment (Given, Given, & Stommel, 1994) (Box 8–1). Family involvement in care activities has not been well described. As many people with cancer are treated as outpatients, with home care often supplementing family caregiving for periods of time, costs would seem to be less than those of hospitalization. This idea has recently been challenged by a study of the costs of cancer home care to families. When family labor is included in calculations of costs, average cancer home care costs for a 3-month period were only slightly lower than the average costs of nursing home care. There is substantial variation in home care costs as well, which appears to be unrelated to the specific cancer diagnosis, type of treatment, or time since diagnosis. It is instead a function of the patient's functional status and the family living arrangements (Stommel, Given, & Given, 1993). In another study the same investigators followed a sample of 62 women with new or recurrent

---

Box 8–1. *Family and Out of Pocket Costs for Women with Breast Cancer*

Given, B. A., Given, C. W., & Stommel, M. (1994). *Cancer Practice, 2(3),* 187–193.

Purposes/Objectives: To review the literature indicating the types of costs borne by patients and families; to classify and measure these costs; and to compare patients who survive at least 3 months after their observation and their families with patients who die during the succeeding 3-month period and their families.

Design: Longitudinal descriptive panel study.

Setting: Community cancer treatment centers.

Sample: 62 women with new or recurrent breast cancer and their caregivers. Forty-nine were breast cancer survivors (mean age 56) and their 49 caregivers (mean age 55); 13 were breast cancer nonsurvivors (mean age 55) and their 13 caregivers (mean age 51).

Methods: Telephone interviews and mailed questionnaires were completed by patients and their caregivers at intake and at 3 and 6 months.

Measures: Costs of care to families of women with breast cancer were operationalized as out-of-pocket expenditures, labor costs of the primary caregiver, and labor costs of "other" family members (nonprimary caregivers). Family primary caregivers included spouses, adult children, relatives, and others who provided tangible assistance to the woman with breast cancer. They did not have to reside in the same household.

Findings: Data are presented for the out-of-pocket costs, primary family caregiver and "other" family labor costs, and total costs. Considering all costs, the 3-month average was $2720 (SD, $3314) for the survivors and $7905 (SD $5448) for the decedents. Regressions of costs on predictors were performed; survivors' status and patient dependencies in activities of daily living were the only significant predictors.

Conclusions: Family care costs need to be considered along with the formal and direct reimbursable medical costs as an essential component of breast cancer care cost.

Implications for Nursing Practice: Other than loss of income to family members, little attention has been given to costs incurred by women with breast cancer and their families. Informal costs such as the family labor for patient care and non-reimbursed out-of-pocket expenditures to care for the patient with breast cancer need to be considered. Practitioners need to consider patient and family time, variation based on stage of disease, and where the patient is in treatment. Before assuming that a family can deal with home care, the question of how much care and cost the family would assume should be addressed.

breast cancer, collecting data at baseline and at 3-month intervals on informal costs, including family labor for patient care and nonreimbursed out-of-pocket expenditures for the patient. Terminally ill patients incurred the greatest costs in addition to loss of family members' income. These costs to patients averaged, for 3 months, $7905, while family survivors incurred average 3-month costs of more than $2700. The predictors of family and out-of-pocket costs were the patient's dependency in activities of daily living, along with their survival status (Given et al., 1994).

Still to be studied are what have been called "quality-of-life" costs, such as promotions denied, reduced work effort, and decline in productivity in the home not related to patient care. Some of these costs, like loss of promotion opportunities, could result in further long-term losses to family income as well as to family well-being (Given et al., 1994). Home care may seem to be less expensive than care in an institution, because the work of the family usually is neither acknowledged nor counted as it is in calculating acute care costs. For breast cancer as well as other types of cancers with long and sometimes uncertain trajectories as well as aggressive,

longer term treatment, nonmedical direct costs, costs in morbidity, and psychosocial and family costs should be considered as a potentially significant segment of total cancer costs (Given et al., 1994). Oncology teams guiding the care of cancer patients and their families need to consider the amount of care the family assumes and its informal costs in money, time, and energy to appreciate the full economic impact of cancer on families.

MEANING OF THE EXPERIENCE

PERSONAL MEANING OF THE CANCER EXPERIENCE

The personal meaning of the cancer experience for those involved is a third major factor in how it affects family members and the family as a unit. Meaning is the individual's perception of the potential significance of an event, such as the occurrence of cancer, for the self and for one's plan of action. Meaning may be anywhere on a continuum from negative to positive, is derived over time, and may change over time (Germino, Fife, & Funk, 1995) (Box 8–2). The individual percep-

---

BOX 8–2. *Cancer and the Partner Relationship: What is its Meaning?*

Germino, B., Fife, B., & Funk, S.G. (1995). *Seminars in Oncology Nursing, 11,* 43–50.

Purposes/Objectives: To review relevant work on the meaning of illness for spouses or partners as well as for the dyad and to describe and explain the importance of the meaning of cancer within the partner relationship. The results of the two studies presented here support the following premises: meaning within the dyad is both shared and divergent, partners' perceptions may affect one another, and meaning may influence both individual and dyadic adjustment.

Design: Two studies are presented. Both are secondary analyses from larger studies. One is an exploratory qualitative study that used a cross-sectional design to study adult families within the first 6 months after diagnosis. The other was a quantitative cross-sectional study of patients and partners who were at four specific points on the illness trajectory: diagnosis, first remission, first recurrence, and metastatic disease.

Sample: The first study includes 50 patients newly diagnosed with breast, lung, or colorectal cancer and their spouses; the second includes 412 patients with a variety of specific cancer diagnoses and 175 partners; the data were not paired.

Methods: In the first study interviews included open-ended and semi-structured questions. Patients and spouses were interviewed separately and simultaneously in their home. In the second study structured interviews composed of a set of pencil and paper measures were the method of data collection.

Measures: In the first (qualitative) study, there were no structured measures. Interviews were designed to test the content validity of a previously constructed and tested instrument, the Family Concerns Inventory. In the second (quantitative) study, meaning was measured by the constructed meaning scale, emotional response by the Bi-Polar Profile of Mood States; adjustment variables by the Psychological Adjustment to Illness Scale; personal control by the Mastery Scale; and the partner relationship variables such as communication and marital satisfaction by the Dyadic Adjustment Scale.

Findings: Findings pointed to the importance of meaning in the adjustment of individuals as well as the dyad. Interview data indicated that patients and their partners searched for meaning in the illness that would decrease its threat. There were both similarities and differences in the specific meaning the illness held for patients and partners. Statistical analyses indicated that patients do not view the illness from a more negative perspective than partners, or vice versa. Furthermore, based on the scores obtained using the constructed meaning scale, both groups held a fairly positive perspective. Statistical analyses also demonstrated the significance of meaning to specific aspects of adjustment.

Conclusions: The importance of considering meaning in care that is directed toward the prevention of problems within the dyad that can occur as a result of coping with the stress of cancer is clear. Prevention through ongoing monitoring of individual meaning and early psychosocial intervention is worth considering.

Implications for Nursing Practice: Nurses are often in a position to be able to assess the meaning the illness has for individuals, and this kind of information can provide some indication of their ability to adjust to the stress with which they are forced to live. When individuals view their illness from a highly negative perspective with great anxiety and without hope, it is important to monitor this attitude and to make referrals for psychosocial intervention if and when this seems warranted. It is crucially important to care for the partners of patients as well as the patients themselves—a challenge since they may be less accessible and their needs less apparent. Finally, the need for communication between patients and their partners during this difficult time seems important to adjustment. Even if they see the illness differently, partners need to respect and support one another.

tions of the patient and family members involved, their view of the events related to the cancer, the implications of those events, their past experiences with illness and with loss as well as their encounters with the health care system, the changes that occur for them during the cancer experience, and the fears and concerns that emerge along the way all contribute to the derivation of meaning from the cancer experience.

Part of the meaning of cancer in Western society, despite public education and advances in effective treatment, continues to be its life-threatening nature and the threat of loss of well-being, of a future, and of one's life. The search for meaning in cancer has been described as an internal and external dialogue involving "questions about the personal experience of a life circumstance, such as cancer, in order to give the experience purpose and to place it in the context of a total life pattern" (O'Connor, Wicker, & Germino, 1990, p. 168). The process of finding meaning involves the reworking and redefining of past meaning while simultaneously looking for meaning in the current situation. In a study of 50 adults with newly diagnosed breast, lung, or colorectal cancer (O'Connor et al., 1990), six issues involved in seeking the personal meaning of cancer experiences were identified. *Seeking an understanding of the significance of the cancer for their lives* was an important part of the process and included asking such questions as, "Why me?" A second issue was the *consequences of the cancer* including lifestyle changes, the possibility of suffering and death, being unable to carry out important roles, and how the cancer would affect their families and those close to them. Also common to the subjects in this study was a taking stock or reflecting on their lives and relationships, including a judgment of what their life had meant. In this study the process of redefining meaning was exemplified by subjects' descriptions of *changes in attitudes towards themselves, towards others and towards life.* The other two issues in the personal search for meaning were identified as *learning to live with the cancer* (usually in multiple ways) and *finding sources of hope.*

Because the meaning of cancer is personal and unique to each patient and family member dealing with it, the issues that are of importance to any one member of a family may not be the primary focus for others. For example, some people may focus primarily on reviewing their past life, others may focus on current relationships, and others on the future. Family members may or may not share the same meaning of cancer (Chekryn, 1984). In addition, individuals find meaning through a variety of processes. For some the questions are asked of the self, an internal dialogue. For others it is helpful and important to raise the questions and discuss alternative answers or lack of answers with another. Frankl (1959), who wrote about the personal search for meaning from his experiences in a concentration camp and later used his ideas in counseling others, described three ways in which humans find meaning in their lives: by creative work, by experiencing something or someone that leads to goodness and love, and by transforming personal tragedy into a triumph.

COMPLEXITY OF MEANING FOR FAMILIES

It is in trying to understand the meaning of the cancer experience for families that we see just how complex the impact of cancer can be. Family members, even while living in the same household, may indeed have different perceptions of the situation, difference priorities of fear and concern, and different needs (Germino, 1984; Germino & Dalton, 1986; Gotay, 1984; Lewis et al., 1985; Mah & Johnston, 1993). For instance, although the initial period after a cancer diagnosis is made has been considered to be one of the most stressful for patients and their families (Northouse, 1984), the nature and timing of that stress may differ for those involved. Women who had mastectomies have reported that the preoperative period was the most stressful (Stolar, 1982), whereas their families saw the immediate postoperative period as most stressful for them (Stolar, 1982; Wellisch, 1981).

In studies of patients' and adult family members' concerns after cancer diagnosis, all family members shared common concerns about the patient, but each family member also had unique concerns. The patients tended to worry most about physical symptoms (especially fatigue), spouses were most concerned about their own anxiety, and adult children were expending the most energy dealing with existential concerns generated by the threatened loss of a parent (Germino, 1984; Germino & Funk, 1987–1989, 1993). Similarly, Gotay (1984) found that both in the early diagnostic and advanced illness periods, patients and spouses shared a fear of cancer and a concern for the patient's emotional upheaval, but their other concerns differed.

Family members' concerns are complex in that they not only reflect particular topics or issues but also have a focus or referent person. In other words, they may focus on themselves in one area and on other family members in other areas. Patients have been reported to be most concerned about their own symptoms, their care and treatment, and their futures. However, they also worry about the futures of their spouses and adult children, their spouses' physical health, and the need to depend on others (Germino, 1984; Germino & Funk, 1987–1989).

Differing perceptions are reflected in studies of families in which a member had breast cancer. In one study of the perception of demands the cancer imposed, clear differences were evident among family members. The women in this study, for instance, saw the illness as imposing many more demands than the men did (Lewis et al., 1985).

Although we are beginning, through studying family members, to unravel the complexity that is the meaning of cancer to families, we do not yet know very much about how the meaning of cancer relates to a family's responses and functioning, particularly in the ability of the family unit to provide continuing support to patients while continuing to meet other family members' needs and managing family maintenance tasks. The experiences of family members who are caregivers for persons with cancer are important to assess, because heavy illness demands over a prolonged period of time may affect their health and well-being. Caregiving may also have positive effects. One study of caregivers whose spouses had advanced cancer indicated that those who saw caring for their ill partners as giving them a sense of purpose in life had a more positive view of their own health (Stetz, 1987).

Everyone who is a part of the family system must struggle with how to integrate the cancer experience and its meanings into their lives. The meaning of cancer to the family is the context in which this adjustment process occurs (Germino et al., 1995; Lewis, Woods, Hough et al., 1989; Lewis & Hammond, 1992; Lewis, 1993; Lewis, Hammond, & Woods, 1993). "The family's adjustment to cancer involves, among other things, dealing with a myriad of changes including changes in their basic views of their lives and their world. Family members must somehow integrate the changes brought on by the illness, and in so doing, comprehend the meaning for themselves as individuals and for the family as a whole. This may involve challenging long held assumptions, changing the way they view themselves, their life and their relationships, reexamining values, and addressing fears and concerns" (Germino et al., 1995 p. 43; Lewis, 1993; Feldman, 1974; Stetz, Lewis, & Primomo, 1986).

UNCERTAINTY

Uncertainty in illness, the inability to determine the meaning of illness-related events (Mishel, 1988), is present when patients and their families lack information about what is happening to them, when they do not understand information they are given, when they are not sure how to manage their symptoms, and when treatment-related events are strange, unfamiliar, or unexpected (Mishel, 1988). Uncertainty characterizes the experience of cancer for many patients and families. For the patient uncertainty may interfere with self-care (Mishel, 1988). The patient's prognosis, the outcomes of the cancer and cancer treatment, the possibility of recurrence, and the unpredictability of future illness contribute to threaten the family's psychological control over the cancer (Lewis, 1986). Uncertainty about the impact of the cancer experience on the family and on each family member's future is present in the early period after diagnosis, in the years of living with cancer, in the advanced stages of illness, and at recurrence (Chekryn, 1984; Germino & Funk, 1987–1989; Gotay, 1984; Lewis, 1986). In patients with breast cancer, uncertainty appears to be present from the time of diagnosis to at least 5 years after treatment (Mishel, Hostetter, King, & Graham, 1984). In the cancer literature uncertainty is often mentioned and has been described as an important influence on the patient's experience with illness (Hilton, 1989). Among patients being treated for various cancers, uncertainty has been associated with negative mood states such as anxiety and depression (Mishel et al., 1984; Mishel & Braden, 1987; Richardson et al., 1987). Among people with cancer and other chronic illnesses, poorer quality family relationships, leisure activities, sexual relationships,

self-help, and sense of control have all been reported as outcomes of uncertainty (Braden, 1990; Christman, 1990; Mishel & Sorenson, 1991; Mishel, Padilla, Grant, & Sorenson, 1991).

Patients' support systems can assist them in reducing uncertainty if support persons are not immobilized by dealing with their own uncertainties resulting from a family member's illness. Family members' own uncertainties must be addressed before they are able to deal with the patient's concerns. Uncertainty about the patient's functional status, symptoms, outcomes of treatment, possible recurrence, financial resources and future goals have been identified by families as inherent in experiencing a cancer diagnosis and treatment (Black, 1989; Chekryn, 1984; Lewis, 1986; Northouse, 1984).

FAMILY RESPONSES TO CANCER

ACTIVE FAMILY RESPONSES TO CANCER

Finally, the impact of cancer involves human responses to the experience. The impact of cancer on patients and families can range from mildly disruptive to totally overwhelming. What is impressive, however, is the resilience of many families, their ability to find within themselves the emotional resources to deal with what must be dealt with. Clearly there are exceptions, but both clinical observation and research are encouraging. Families often respond actively and positively to events that affect them. Many will actively seek information and make cognitive or role changes that allow them to adapt to the demands of the cancer and treatment. Families are often primary sources of support and assistance at the time of the cancer diagnosis (Germino & Funk, 1987–1989; Lewis, 1986; Mishel & Braden, 1987). There is some research indicating that nursing intervention designed to assist patients in this process can be very effective in facilitating adaptation. For instance, the work of McHenry, Allen, Mishel, and Braden (1993) in designing and testing an uncertainty management intervention that has demonstrated effectiveness with women with breast cancer indicates that patient adaptation can be enhanced by assistance in managing the many uncertainties of breast cancer and treatment. Such interventions with families are currently being tested in research in progress.

The human abilities to be hopeful and optimistic, to endure discomfort, to work at keeping life normal in the midst of major disruption, to live with uncertainty, to maintain a sense of humor, and to grieve for what has been lost and then go on with life are all positive examples of the scope of active human responses to cancer. Many families appear to have significant success in dealing with the disruptions of cancer, maintaining important family functions by shifting roles and responsibilities, and by striving to keep as much of family life as normal as possible.

DIFFICULTIES DEALING WITH CANCER

Families who have difficulty dealing with cancer may be those whose perceptions of the illness, ongoing problems, and limited or ineffective resources prevent the system from adapting to the changes and uncertainties the cancer experience may precipitate. Major problems of family functioning and family communication when combined with the potential stressors of a cancer diagnosis may be more disruption than the system can bear. Patients and family members have been reported to have difficulty communicating with one another during the time after the diagnosis (Wortman & Dunkel-Schetter, 1979), as indicated by little or no discussion of emotional concerns (Jamison, Wellisch, & Pasnau, 1978). Family members also have reported difficulties obtaining information from health care providers and difficulties with the manner in which the information is given (Bond, 1982a, 1982b). In other situations an accumulation of stressors has been found to be associated with less family adaptability (Gilliss & Gortner, 1987). The family's resources for all kinds of support and the extent to which family system boundaries are open to outside help may be important in determining how well that family continues to function through stressful cancer-related experiences. Other family response issues that may have an impact on the outcome of cancer experiences for the family include (1) emotional strain, (2) the physical demands of caring for the patient, (3) adverse effects of cancer on family lifestyle, including financial pressures, (4) lack of availability of health and support services for families, and (5) problems with sexuality and intimacy (Lewis, 1986).

EFFECTS OF HUMAN RESPONSES ON THE IMPACT OF THE CANCER

It is important to view human responses in cancer both as part of the impact of the illness on the family and as affecting what that impact will be. The responses of family members to the demands of illness on emotional, physical, social, spiritual, and financial resources may vary. Roles and relationships within the system may be altered as well. The balance of meeting ongoing family system needs as well as dealing with the demands of cancer, cancer treatment, and the changes they precipitate is a precarious one. Enough energy must be coming into the family system to replenish the tremendous amount of energy that may be expended on dealing with all of these issues. Such energy may be replenished by the support and caring of others, from the family's religious faith and spirituality, from the family's strengths and past success in dealing with difficult times, and from finding meaning in the cancer experiences that can be incorporated into the family's life.

Although much work remains to be done in studying family responses to cancer, it is reasonable to hypothesize that families, like individuals, can respond effectively to cancer experiences if the nature and quality of major stresses and strains in their functioning allow them the energy and resources to deal with the additional burdens of cancer-related experiences. Research on life events has taught us that individuals can tolerate multiple stressful events and not become ill if support from others is available and is sufficient to buffer that stress (Stetz, 1987). With these issues in mind, the as-

sessment of families and the planning of care that complements and supports the family's ability to respond to the demands of cancer is a challenge for current and future cancer nursing (Northouse, 1988).

SUMMARY

As cost containment puts people with cancer more and more often in the care of their families, knowledge of family systems under stressful conditions will become increasingly important. Family social systems are more than the sum of their parts. They are complex and changing units that are influenced by their structure, their history, their culture, their social environment, and the relationships within the system. Family rules guide the behavior of family members and determine the way the family system operates both internally and in its relationships with outsiders. Rules reflect family values and often relate to family communication within the system and with those outside its boundaries. To understand the impact of cancer on families, it is helpful to utilize a framework that assists in identifying some key factors that may influence the impact of the illness and treatment on the family. The specific kind of cancer diagnosis and treatment, the timing and trajectory of the illness in the context of the family's life, the meanings of cancer experiences for individual family members and the family system, the nature of human responses during the cancer experiences, and the caregiving demands and costs are important factors to consider in working with families throughout the trajectory of cancer.

REFERENCES

Andersen, B. (1990). How cancer affects sexual functioning. *Oncology 4*, 81–88.

Barbarin, O. A., Hughes, D., & Chesler, M. A. (1985). Stress, coping and marital functioning among parents of children with cancer. *Journal of Marriage and the Family, 47*, 473–480.

Berkman, B. J. & Sampson, S. E. (1993). Psychosocial effects of cancer economics on patients and their families. *Cancer, 72*, (Suppl.) 2846–2849.

Berman, H., Cragg, C. E., & Kuenzig, L. (1988). Having a parent die of cancer: Adolescents' reactions. *Oncology Nursing Forum, 17*, 5–10.

Black, R. B. (1989). Challenges for social work as a core profession in cancer services. *Social Work in Health Care, 12*, 1–14.

Bond, D. (1982a). Communicating with families of cancer patients 1: The relatives and doctors. *Nursing Times, 78*, 962–965.

Bond, D. (1982b). Communicating with families of cancer patients 2: The nurses. *Nursing Times, 78*, 1027–1029.

Braden, C. J. (1990). Learned self–help response to chronic illness experience: A test of three alternative learning theories. *Scholarly Inquiry for Nursing Practice: An International Journal, 4*, 23–40.

Chekryn, J. (1984). Cancer recurrence: Personal meaning, communication and marital adjustment. *Cancer Nursing, 7*, 491–498.

Christman, N. (1990). Uncertainty and adjustment during radiotherapy. *Nursing Research, 39*, 17–20.

Cooper, E. T. (1984). A pilot study on the effects of the diagnosis of lung cancer on family relationships. *Cancer Nursing, 7*, 491–498.

Donahue, V., & Knapp, R. C. (1977). Sexual rehabilitation of gynecologic cancer patients. *Obstetrics and Gynecology, 49,* 118–121.

Eisenberg, M. G., Sutkin, L. C., & Jansen, M. A. (Eds.). (1984). *Chronic illness and disability through the lifespan: Effects on self and family (Vol. 4).* In T. E. Backer (Ed.), *Springer series on rehabilitation.* New York: Springer.

Feetham, S. (1984). Family research: Issues and directions for nursing. In H. H. Werley & J. Fitzpatrick (Eds.), *Annual Review of Nursing Research: Vol. 2.* New York: Springer.

Feldman, D. J. (1974). Chronic disabling illness: A holistic view. *Journal of Chronic Disease, 27,* 287–291.

Frank-Stromborg, M., & Wright, P. (1984). Ambulatory cancer patients' perceptions of the physical and psychosocial changes in their lives since the diagnosis of cancer. *Cancer Nursing 7,* 117–129.

Frankl, V. E. (1959). *Man's search for meaning; An introduction to logotherapy.* Boston: Beacon, 1959.

Gallagher, A. (1972). Body image changes in the patient with a colostomy. *Nursing Clinics of North America, 6,* 669.

Germino, B. (1984). Family members' concerns after cancer diagnosis. *Dissertation Abstracts International, 44,* 3358B. (University of Washington).

Germino, B., & Dalton, J. (1986). Quality of life in patients with lung cancer. *Oncology Nursing Forum, 13* (Suppl.), 97.

Germino, B., Fife, B., & Funk, S. G. (1995). Cancer and the partner relationship: What is its meaning? *Seminars in Oncology Nursing, 11,* 43–50.

Germino, B. & Funk, S. G. (1987–1989). *Development of the family concerns inventory.* Grant funded by the National Center for Nursing Research, National Institutes of Health, #1RO1BR01331–01A1.

Germino, B. B., & Funk, S. G. (1993). Impact of a parent's cancer on adult children: Role and relationship issues. *Seminars in Oncology Nursing, 9,* 101–106.

Germino, B., Funk, S. G., Burman, S., & May, A. (Under review, 1995). Cancer as a family experience: Concerns of family members in the first six months.

Gilliss, C., & Gortner, S. (1987). *Family functioning after cardiac surgery.* Paper presented at the National Conference on Family Relations, Atlanta, GA.

Given, B., Given, C., & Stommel, M. (1994). Family and out of pocket costs for women with breast cancer. *Cancer Practice 2,* 187–193.

Given, G., & Given, C. W. (1992). Patient and family caregiver reaction to new and recurrent breast cancer. *Journal of the American Medical Women's Association, 47,* 201–206.

Gotay, C. (1984). The experience of cancer during early and advanced stages: The view of patients and their mates. *Social Science and Medicine, 18,* 605–613.

Green, C. P. (1986). Changes in responsibility in women's families after the diagnosis of cancer. *Health Care for Women International 7,* 221–239.

Hannum, J. W., Giese-Davis, J., Harding, K., & Hatfield, A. K. (1991). Effects of individual and marital variables on coping with cancer. *Journal of Psychosocial Oncology 9,* 1–21.

Hilton, B. A. (1989). The relationship of uncertainty, control, commitment, and threat of recurrence to coping strategies used by women diagnosed with breast cancer. *Journal of Behavioral Medicine 12,* 39–54.

Hinds, C. (1985). The needs of families who care for patients with cancer at home: Are we meeting them? *Journal of Advanced Nursing, 10,* 575–581.

Hull, M. M. (1989). Family needs and supportive nursing behaviors during terminal cancer: A review. *Oncology Nursing Forum 16,* 787–792.

Issel, L. M., Ersek, M., & Lewis, F. M. (1990). How children cope with mother's breast cancer. *Oncology Nursing Forum, 17,* 5–10.

Jamison, K. R., Wellisch, D. K., & Pasnau, R. (1978). Psychosocial aspects of mastectomy: The woman's perspective. *American Journal of Psychiatry 135,* 432–436.

Lewis, F. M. (1986). The impact of cancer on the family: A critical analysis of the research literature. *Patient Education and Counseling 8,* 269–289.

Lewis, F. M. (1993). Psychosocial transitions and the family's work in adjusting to cancer. *Seminars in Oncology Nursing 9,* 127–129.

Lewis, F. M., Ellison, E., & Woods, N. F. (1985). The impact of breast cancer on the family. *Seminars in Oncology Nursing 1,* 206–213.

Lewis, F. M., & Hammond, M. A. (1992). Psychosocial rehabilitation of the family to breast cancer: A longitudinal analysis. *Journal of the American Medical Women's Association, 47,* 194–200.

Lewis, F. M., Hammond, M. A., & Woods, N. F. (1993). The family's functioning with newly diagnosed breast cancer in the mother: Development of an explanatory model. *Journal of Behavioral Medicine, 16,* 351–359.

Lewis, F. M., Woods, N. F., Hough, E. E., & Bensley, L. S. (1989). Family functioning with chronic illness in the mother: The spouse's perspective. *Social Science and Medicine, 29,* 1261–1269.

Mah, M. A., & Johnston, C. (1993). Concerns of families in which one member has head and neck cancer. *Cancer Nursing 16,* 382–387.

Martinson, I. M., Gilliss, C., Colaizzo, D. C., Freeman, M., & Bossert, E. (1990). Impact of childhood cancer on healthy school-age siblings. *Cancer Nursing, 13,* 183–190.

McCorkle, R., Yost, L. S., Jepsdon, C., Malone, D., Baird, S., & Lusk, E. (1993). A cancer experience: Relationship of patient psychosocial responses to care-giver burden over time. *Psycho-Oncology 2,* 21–32.

McCubbin, H., & Patterson, J. (1983). The family stress process: The double ABCX model of family adjustment and adaptation. In H. McCubbin, M. Sussman, & J. Patterson (Eds.), *Advances and developments in family stress theory and research.* New York: Haworth.

McHenry, J., Allen, C., Mishel, M. H., & Braden, C. J. (1993). Uncertainty management for women receiving treatment for breast cancer. In S. G. Funk, E. Tornquist, M. Champagne, & R. Wiese. (Eds.). *Key aspects of caring for the chronically ill: Hospital and home.* New York: Springer.

Mishel, M. H. (1988). Uncertainty in illness. *Image, 200,* 225–232.

Mishel, M. H., & Braden, C. (1987). Uncertainty: A mediator between support and adjustment. *Western Journal of Nursing Research, 9,* 43–47.

Mishel, M. H., Hostetter, T., King, B., & Graham, V. (1984). Predictors of psychosocial adjustment in patients newly diagnosed with gynecological cancer. *Cancer Nursing, 7,* 291–299.

Mishel, M. H., Padilla, G., Grant, M., & Sorenson, D. S. (1991). Uncertainty in illness theory: A replication of the mediating effects of mastery and coping. *Nursing Research, 40,* 236–240.

Mishel, M. H., & Sorenson, D. S. (1991). Uncertainty in gynecological cancer: A test of the mediating functions of mastery and coping. *Nursing Research, 40,* 167–171.

Northouse, L. (1984). The impact of cancer on the family: An overview. *International Journal of Psychiatry in Medicine, 14,* 215–242.

Northouse, L. (1988). A longitudinal study of the adjustment of patients and husbands to breast cancer. *Oncology Nursing Forum, 16,* 511–516.

Northouse, L. (1989). A longitudinal study of the adjustment of patients and husbands to breast cancer. *Oncology Nursing Forum, 16,* 511–516.

Northouse, L. (1990). A longitudinal study of the adjustment of patients and husbands to breast cancer. *Oncology Nursing Forum, 17* (Suppl), 39–45.

Northouse, L., & Swain, M. (1987). Adjustment of patients and husbands to the initial impact of breast cancer. *Nursing Research, 36,* 221–225.

Oberst, M., & James, R. (1985). Going home: Patient and spouse adjustment following cancer surgery. *Topics in Clinical Nursing, 7,* 46–57.

Oberst, M. T., & Scott, D. T. (1988). Postdischarge distress in surgically treated cancer patients and their spouses. *Research in Nursing and Health, 11,* 223–233.

O'Connor, A., Wicker, C., & Germino, B. B. (1990). Understanding the cancer patient's search for meaning. *Cancer Nursing, 13,* 167–175.

Parkes, C. M. (1975). Determinants of outcome following bereavement. *Omega, 6,* 303–323.

Quinn, W. H., & Herndon, A. (1986). The family ecology of cancer. *Journal of Psychosocial Oncology, 4,* 45–59.

Rait, D., & Lederberg, M. (1990). The family of the cancer patient. In J. C. Holland & J. H. Rowland (Eds.), *Handbook of Psychooncology: The psychological care of the patient with cancer* (pp. 585–597). New York: Oxford University Press.

Richardson, J. L., Marks, G., Johnson, C. A., Graham, J. W., Chan, K. K., Selser, J. N., Kisbaugh, C., Barranday, Y., & Levine, A. M. (1987). Path model of multidimensional compliance with cancer therapy. *Health Psychology, 6,* 183–207.

Robinson, L. A., McCorkle, R., Lev, E., & Nuamah, I. (1994, in press). A prospective longitudinal investigation of spousal bereavement examining Parkes' predictive variables of negative bereavement outcomes. *Journal of Palliative Care.*

Rose, D. B. (1987). Assessing families of school aged children with cancer. In M. Leahey & L. M. Wright (Eds.), *Families and life-threatening illness.* Springhouse, PA: Springhouse.

Sales, E. (1991). Psychosocial impact of the phase of cancer on the family: An updated review. *Journal of Psychosocial Oncology, 9,* 1–17.

Schain, W. (1988). The sexual and intimate consequences of breast cancer treatment. *CA, 38,* 154–161.

Spiegel, D., Bloom, J. R., & Gottheil, E. (1983). Family environment as a predictor of adjustment to metastatic breast cancer. *Journal of Psychosocial Oncology, 1,* 30–33.

Stetz, K. M. (1987). Caregiver demands during advanced cancer. *Cancer Nursing, 10,* 260–268.

Stetz, K. M. (1993). Survival work: The experience of the patient and the spouse involved in experimental treatment for cancer. *Seminars in Oncology Nursing, 9,* 121–126.

Stetz, K. M., Lewis, F. M., & Primomo, J. (1986). Family coping strategies and chronic illness in the mother. *Family Relations, 35,* 515–522.

Stolar, E. (1982). Coping with mastectomy: Issues for social work. *Health and Social Work, 7,* 26–34.

Stommel, M., Given, C., & Given, B. (1993). The cost of cancer home care to families. *Cancer, 71,* 1867–1874.

Strauss. A. L., Corbin, J., Fagerhaugh, S., Glaser, B., Maines, D., Suczek, B., & Wiener, C. (1984). *Chronic illness and the quality of life* (2nd ed.). St. Louis: C. V. Mosby Co.

Vess, J., Moreland, J., & Schwebel, A. (1985). A follow-up study of role functioning and the psychological environment of two families of cancer patients. *Journal of Psychosocial Oncology, 2,* 1–14.

Wellisch, D. K. (1981). Family relationships of the mastectomy patient: Interactions with the spouse and children. *Israel Journal of Medical Science, 17,* 993–996.

Woods, N. F., & Earp, J. (1978). Women with cured breast cancer: A study of mastectomy patients in North Carolina. *Nursing Research, 27,* 279–285.

Wortman, C., & Dunkel-Schetter, G. (1979). Interpersonal relationships and cancer: A theoretical analysis. *Journal of Social Issues, 35,* 120–156.

Zahlis, E., & Shands, M. (1991). Breast cancer: Demands of the illness on the patient's partner. *Journal of Psychosocial Oncology, 9,* 75–93.

Zahlis, E., & Shands, M. (1993). The impact of breast cancer on the partner 18 months after diagnosis. *Seminars in Oncology Nursing, 9,* 83–87.

Family Caregiver Burden From Cancer Care

Barbara Given • C. William Given

The reduction in length of stays in acute care settings and the treatment in outpatient ambulatory care settings has shifted ongoing and supportive cancer care responsibilities to patients and their families (Bender, Weinert, Faulkner, & Quimby 1989; Given, Given, & Stommel, 1994; Hileman & Lackey, 1992; Kornblith, Herr, Ofman, Scher, & Holland, 1994; Mor, Masterson-Allen, Houts, & Siegel, 1992; Northouse, 1988; Northouse & Swain, 1987; Oberst & James, 1984; Oberst & Scott, 1988). These factors cause a need for assistance as patients experience sequelae and symptom distress caused by chemotherapy and radiation. Because of this need for assistance, families are now providing the majority of supportive and continuing cancer care. Clearly the availability of this informal support system, that is, the family, a system that is willing and able to assist and provide care to the patients, has to be considered as a part of the cancer health care system. Care to individuals with cancer by family members may be accomplished at lower health system costs, but this care is not without personal and family costs and burden to family members involved. Emotional, social, physical, and financial costs may affect the overall family member well-being. The reactions of family members to the care requirements need to be understood as they undertake personal and intimate care tasks, make decisions and judgments, and supervise and monitor the effects of treatment and overall health status.

Models of caregiver burden and distress outcomes have been proposed by numerous researchers as a way to provide a framework for integrating disparate and fragmented research knowledge (Biegel, Sales, & Schultz, 1991; Given & Given, 1991, 1994; Pallett, 1990; Pearlin, Mullan, Semple, & Skaff, 1990). These models, however, have been applied to patients who are

frail and chronically ill, elderly, or have dementia. Although most of these models are not cancer-related, they provide a perspective for review as they are related to cancer care.

In this chapter the model that will be used for discussion of factors contributing to caregiver responses to care of family members with cancer is found in Figure 9–1. These factors relate to how family members deal with the distress associated with ongoing and continuous care for individuals with cancer. There are background and social context variables for the patient and caregiver that include age, gender, marital status, occupation, education, socioeconomic and living arrangements, and previous caregiver-patient relationships. Stressors of the care situation relate to disease and treatment and include site, type, and stage of cancer as well as the functional disability, symptom distress, treatment, and resultant patient needs and care requirements. Other care-related stresses and strains include the impact of disease and treatment on patient and family member—family, work, social, and personal roles. Care roles and demands may permeate the whole life of the family members as well as that of the patient (Stetz, 1987).

The formal and informal systems of care that support the dyad influence the demands of the patient and the caregiver. This care role in conjunction with other demands may result in multidimensional responses in physical, economic, and mental burdens and role adaptations to the family member directly involved in care (Young & Kahana, 1989; Zarit, Todd, & Zarit, 1986). Researchers continue to search for the mediating factors such as coping, social support, and other strategies that mediate the stressor of providing care to family members (Pearlin et al., 1990; Schumacher, Dodd, &

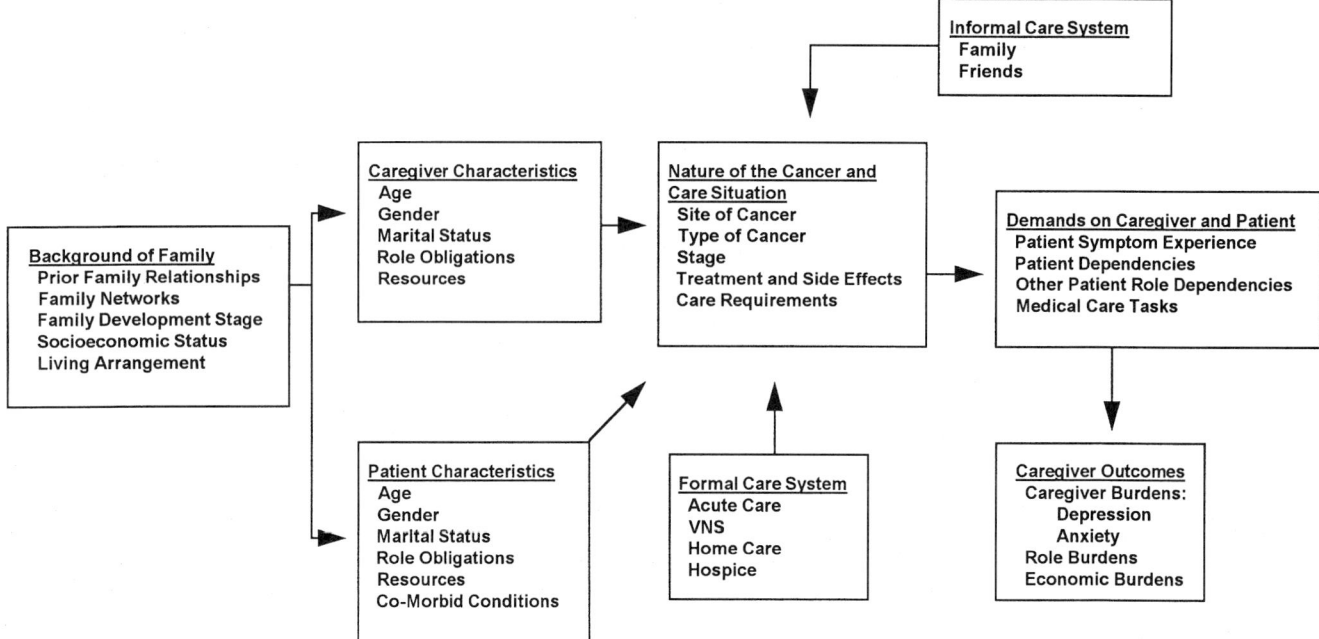

FIGURE 9–1. Continuing cancer care demands and family caregiver burden.

Paul, 1993; Wright, Clipp, & George, 1993). The following description focuses on the factors related to family members' caregiver burden, that is, reactions and distress of those providing care to cancer patients during the ongoing and supportive phase. The description is based on the model described. We start with the definition of caregiver burden and responses and then focus on factors that lead to or affect such factors or burdens.

DEFINITION OF CAREGIVER BURDEN AND RESPONSES— THE OUTCOME

Considerable effort has been expended toward conceptualizing, identifying, and measuring the reaction and distress that families experience related to their caregiving roles. The provision of care to a family member is generally described as a burden, strain, or stressor and produces negative psychologic and emotional responses or alters physical health status in the person providing care (Hooyman, Gonyea, & Montgomery, 1985; Poulshock & Deimling, 1984). *Caregiver burden*, or *caregiver strain* have been the terms most often used to describe the persistent hardships or the physical, psychologic, social, financial, and emotional responses and stress that can be experienced by family members providing continuing and supportive cancer care (Oberst & Scott, 1988; Oberst, Thomas, Gass, & Ward, 1989; Stetz, 1989; Stommel, Wang, Given, & Given, 1992).

Caregiver burden and distress include strain brought about by direct care tasks, administration of complex medical treatments, medication, and procedures, assisting with daily activities, discrepancies in care role expectations, disruption of personal routines, and the sense of overload in role obligations (Montgomery, Stull & Borgatta, 1985; Northouse, 1989; Oberst & Scott, 1988; Schultz, Fello, & Love, 1989; Schultz, Tompkins, & Rau, 1988). The ability of the patient to perform self-care activities and the amount of supervision or assistance required of the caregiver have been related to the burdens of care. In addition to responsibilities for administration of complex treatments, family members monitor changes in health status and potential complications (McCorkle, Benoliel, Donaldson, Georgiadou, Moinpour, & Goodell, 1989; Siegel, Raveis, Houts, & Mor, 1991; Stommel, Given, & Given, 1990; Yost, McCorkle, Buhler-Wilkerson, Schultz, & Lusk, 1993). Burdens may be related to the amount of time or hours of care per day that must be devoted to caring, the inability to control timing of tasks, the intimacy of the tasks of care, or to the anxiety surrounding monitoring and observing for new signs and symptoms. Caregivers of individuals with cancer are concerned about their ability to provide physical care, keep the patient comfortable, and meet the patient's emotional needs. Family members continue to express a need for information. Information needs include current patient status, patient progress, and prognosis. The emotional strain and lack of resources to meet patient needs may serve as the etiology of caregiver distress (Carey, Oberst, McCubbin, & Hughes, 1991; Given, Stommel, Collins, King, & Given, 1990; Oberst et al., 1989).

Oberst and James (1984), Oberst et al. (1989), and Stetz (1987, 1989) reported that the pervasive sense of uncertainty regarding what is happening to the patient, as well as the open-ended nature of the caring process resulting from periods of treatment, disease remission, maintenance, and recurrence, leads to increased strain and distress among family members of cancer patients.

The diagnosis and treatment of cancer may affect numerous dimensions of the family life as well, especially for the primary family caregiver as alterations in organization of roles, domestic routines, patterns of communication, self-esteem, disruption, independence, and family cohesion occur (Lewis, Ellison, & Woods, 1985; Lewis, Woods, Hough, & Bensley, 1989; Northouse & Swain, 1987; Oberst & James, 1984; Pederson & Valanis, 1989; Thorne, 1984; Woods, Lewis, & Ellison, 1989). The provision of direct care imposes restrictions on other family role responsibilities and social activities and influences the manner in which the family member views care tasks. In addition, changes and restrictions in work roles and career opportunities coupled with economic costs such as loss of patient and family income and out-of-pocket expenses reflect additional burdens of family caregivers that must be considered (Given, Stommel, Given, Osuch, Kurtz, & Kurtz, 1993; Siegel, Raveis, Mor, & Houts, 1991). Time spent by the family members providing care is time not spent in other family-, social-, or work- related activities and must be considered as a social cost of care. These role stresses and conflicts caused by tensions created in relationships may add to the distress of the caregiver (Stommel et al., 1990). These stresses and conflicts may be particularly problematic at certain stages of family or individuals' development as well as at certain career stages. Social and leisure restrictions, confinement, and perceived abandonment by others contribute to family member responses to care.

Emotional reactions such as frustration, anxiety, anger, depression, lack of privacy, lack of personal time and energy, and decreased satisfaction in relationships with family members may result from the involvement in care (Montgomery et al., 1985; Siegel, Raveis, Houts, & Mor, 1991). Northouse and Peters-Golden (1993) and Oberst and James (1984) documented anger, guilt, physical problems, and fatigue described by family members of cancer patients. Physical and mental exhaustion and sleep disorders occur. Goldberg (1978) reported that spouses of patients with lung cancer were susceptible to depression if their own interest and involvement in the social environment was limited. These negative reactions and distress influence the caregivers' view, the way in which they forego normal activities, and the way in which they view their own current emotional and physical well-being and overall quality of life (Given et al., 1993; Northouse, 1989, 1990; Oberst & Scott, 1988; Oberst et al., 1989).

Montgomery, Stull, and Borgatta (1985) classified the burdens experienced by family caregivers as subjective and objective. Objective burden relates to disruptions of family life caused by the patient's illness and to the time and effort required for the care. Objective burden includes activity restrictions, time spent on types of assistance and tasks, and financial resources expended. Subjective burden pertains to the amount of "felt strain" experienced by the family member in areas such as emotional status, physical status, finan-

cial, and work domains (Montgomery, Gonyea, & Hooyman, 1985).

Negative emotional reactions among families providing care are generally assessed by self-report using standardized depression scales or symptom check lists: Beck depression index (Beck & Beck, 1972), Center for Epidemiological Studies-Depression (CES-D) (Radloff, 1977), Zung depression scale (Zung, 1965), Brief Symptom Inventory (BSI) (Derogatis & Spencer, 1982), or Symptom Checklist (SCL) (Derogatis, Lipman, & Covi, 1973). Negative caregiving reactions also include depression, burden, and caregiver stress that occur with the ongoing commitment to the provision of care.

In summary, caregiver burden and distress can be defined as a multidimensional biopsychosocial reaction resulting from an imbalance of care demands and requirements relative to physical, social, emotional, and financial resources available to the individual providing care and support to a family member with cancer that have a direct effect on caregiver well-being. Negative emotional reactions include caregivers' views of the future, their beliefs about the quality of their present lives, the role conflicts that occur, and how caring is causing them to forego normal activities for persons their age. Family caregiving may be burdensome, but it is part of a set of normative responsibilities of family members, and in many cases caregiving is carried out with love, personal commitment, and obligation on the part of the family member for long periods, often years.

Family members' reactions to the patient, tasks of care, and the impositions of the disease and treatment on their daily and family lives need to be determined to adequately plan and assist families with continued cancer care (McCorkle et al., 1989; Northouse, 1989; Oberst & Scott, 1988; Robinson, 1990; Stetz, 1989; Stommel et al., 1990). As we examine the needs that families must address when caring for patients at home, it is essential to consider the impact that care has upon each member of the family, how those impacts vary depending upon who provides the care, the other demands that caregivers face upon their time, the information they have, the amount of assistance from others available to caregivers, and the family developmental stage.

POSITIVE CAREGIVER REACTIONS

Reactions to providing care to individuals with cancer may be both positive and negative, and it is important to mention positive caregiver reactions (George & Gwyther, 1986; Lawton, Moss, Kleban, Glicksman, & Rovine, 1991). In contrast with negative responses, the positive aspects of providing cancer care, although not well documented and seldom mentioned, need to be considered. Families describe a sense of competency, a feeling of satisfaction, and a sense of meaning associated with providing care resulting from the accomplishment of care tasks. Positive responses by the family member result from a sense of well-being and the knowledge that one is successfully fulfilling a valued responsibility and personal challenge while meeting care needs of a family member. Special meaning and experiences can result. This positive response that has been labeled "competency" comes from the mutuality and reciprocities in the relationship with the care recipient (Archbold, Stewart, Greenlick, & Harvath, 1990). Mutuality and preparedness for the tasks of caring have been suggested by Archbold et al. to explain variation in caregiver strain. Mutuality is the gratification in the relationships and meaning in the care situation and the caregiver's ability to perceive the patient as reciprocating by virtue of existence. High levels of mutuality enable the caregivers to continue caregiving despite difficult situations and to moderate their responses (Hirshfeld, 1983).

Lawton et al. (1991) described mastery of caregiving as important to a positive view of ability to provide care. Mastery helps to reduce feelings of uncertainty to help individuals gain a sense of control and a more clearly defined situation (Younger, 1991). Uncertainty reduces one's sense of personal resources to manage a situation (Mishel & Sorenson, 1991). Archbold et al. (1990) showed that mutuality, a positive relationship with the care receiver, and preparedness were predictive of less caregiver role strain. Those providing care found providing care meaningful. Preparedness to care relates to confidence in ability to manage care activities and may lead to feelings of competence in the care tasks. Those with high levels of confidence in their ability may report lower strain (Haley, Levine, Brown, & Bartolucci, 1987). Certain strains were not reduced by mutuality and preparedness in such areas as lack of resources, economic burden, and worry. Strain from direct care, increased tension, and global strain, however, were reduced with mutuality and preparedness.

Relationships during care represent important rewards of caregiving and enable the family member to find meaning in the care situation (Cartwright, Archbold, Stewart, & Limandri, 1994; Montgomery, Gonyea, & Hooyman, 1985). Positive response and sense of well-being about the care situation may buffer further stress (Miller, 1989; Stommel et al., 1990). The positive reactions to care must be considered further. Work by Given, Given, and Stommel (1994) indicates that caregivers can exhibit positive and negative strains at the same time. Family members may find their caregiving activities fulfilling and rewarding but still acknowledge the impact of caring upon their overall lives. Future work needs to be directed toward better understanding the relationship between the rewards of caring and how those rewards modify strains in the caregiving roles.

BACKGROUND CHARACTERISTICS OF THE FAMILY

ROLE RELATIONSHIPS

In addition to the examination of the characteristics of patient and caregiver, the overall role relationships and previous relationships between the dyad need to be considered. Family caregiving is a stressful normative expectation feeling of obligation and attachment, and families assume these caregiving responsibilities as a part of family expectations that support the commitment to family (Brody, 1985; Cicirelli, 1992; Vess, Moreland, & Schwebel, 1985). Family caregiving tasks must be placed within a historic context, because bonds of affection and reciprocity that sustain caregiving take root in past relationships. Although multiple members may be involved in providing care for individuals with cancer, there is usually one person primarily responsible for the direct care and coordination of care. If the care is for a parent, this individual is usually female (see Living Arrangements). Both recipient and giver of care bring a history of interactions that may enhance or complicate the caregiving process. Therefore it is important to consider not only the influence of relationship type but also the quality of the relationship in terms of its impact and the intensity of feeling generated by dyadic interactions. The impositions of the cancer care on family lives need to be determined to plan meaningful assistance that will enable them to continue providing home care during the treatment and illness trajectory (Blank, Clark, Longman, & Atwood, 1989). The art of caregiving poses stresses and challenges to those providing care. The quality of the patient/family caregiver relationship may influence the burden that results from the care. Family cohesion or conflict may reflect the way families usually function and are now compounded in response to the challenges of cancer care. Social integration of care into their usual role may influence the effectiveness of care and the resultant strain (Zarit & Pearlin, 1993).

DEVELOPMENTAL STAGE

Family developmental stage may influence family response and availability because roles often conflict with, compete with, and are disrupted by care demands (Gray-Price & Szczesny, 1985; Kristjanson, 1986, 1989; Kristjanson & Ashcroft, 1994). Families experience different concerns and problems based on where they are in the developmental stage (Brody, 1981; Hileman & Lackey, 1992; Nugent, 1988). If caregiving is required "off time" in younger families, care challenges are even more burdensome, because not only are they unexpected but also the support needed or usual approach may not be available. It is a nonnormative time. In a recent review of more than 200 articles by Kristjanson and Ashcroft (1994), research, and theoretic writings between 1970 and 1991, family developmental stage was one of the four dimensions of the family cancer experience. Kristjanson (1986, 1989) described how distress to the family may be greater during a transition from one developmental stage to another, and this stage is when most family dysfunction is likely to occur. Galloway (1990) reported that adult children (20 to 39 years) who experienced death of a parent suffered grief and turmoil. Kirshling (1987) and Kristjanson and Ashcroft (1994) suggest that financial demands of the illness itself, the loss of a wage earner, and social implications of widowhood are the major problems facing family caregivers during middle age.

The role of primary caregiver may exacerbate existing family tensions or inflame new ones. Some members may be alienated. Such tensions may eliminate potential sources of help and add to family division and rivalry. Deterioration in sibling relationships among children because of resentment over levels of involvement in parent care may be a significant source of stress (Horowitz, 1985). Differences in subjective value that caregiving spouses attach to the tangible support that they receive from their sons and daughters also create discord, which adds to stress and sometimes alters continued family support. Research shows that perceived *patient* status, not caregiver need, dictates whether continued other family support is provided over time to the caregiver and the patient. Caregiver burden or distress may exist, but secondary levels of caregivers may abrogate their responsibilities if they perceive that patient status has improved or has not deteriorated (Given, Given, Stommel, & Linn, 1994).

Adult children who provide parent care, for example, may be caught between their work life, professional careers, and their own family roles as well as the care demands. Responsibilities to parents with cancer may at times take precedence over responsibility to spouse, children, or others because the care of a parent with cancer is seen as the more pressing and immediate need. If a spouse caregiver is not available, an adult daughter generally assists with the care of the parent or parent-in-law with cancer. These women as caregivers then become sandwiched between their spouse, children, and their own career roles, which may add to increased stress and conflict as they strive to deal with the competing role demands. The demand of middle-aged families who themselves have a family member such as a spouse with cancer find cancer care difficult as jobs, careers, family roles, stage of life, and implications of widowhood face them. Families, especially during the mid-life stage, take on vacated roles of the individual with cancer (Buehler & Lee, 1992). Family caregiver's sense of role obligation, role relief, and role conflict to the care role need to be assessed.

Needs arise from domains in lifestyle functioning *and* developmental stage, such that patients who are more socially active and involved may require more assistance with their care activities to compensate for the additional roles they must try to balance. If this is correct, then family caregivers of middle-aged cancer patients may have more needs for assistance with care than older individuals.

Barnes, Given, and Given (1992) found that working daughters did not provide less total care to the patient than those who did not work. Working daughters providing parent care, however, did spend less time assisting with personal and self-care needs of the parent and had assistance with that care either from family members or purchased it from formal systems or agencies. These caregiver daughters reported less personal time for themselves, less social activities, and less privacy.

Family members with other role obligations and responsibilities and those who are employed are reported to experience withdrawal from work, have work absences, or reduction in work productivity or other role involvement as a means of controlling their caregiver burden and distress. For some caregivers, however, employment provides respite from ongoing cancer care activities and serves as a buffer to distress. Social interaction outside the home such as in work settings may provide emotional support as well as respite (Barusch & Spaid, 1989; Brody, 1985). To provide care for the middle-aged cancer patient, family caregivers often make changes in their own employment situation and add parent care to their other family responsibilities. Women more than men appear likely to give up work roles. Among middle-aged caregivers in a study by Given and Given (1991), 16 per cent quit jobs, 17 per cent took leaves, 36 per cent decreased hours worked, 39 per cent missed days worked, and 7 per cent took early retirement. More than 40 per cent of the working caregivers had an alteration in work schedule necessitated by the provision of cancer care. Although employment is less of an issue for many elderly spouse caregivers who are retired, it remains an important issue for adult children who are caring for elderly parents.

AGE

Intergenerational caregivers (adult children) are more likely to suffer role conflicts because of multiple competing role demands, whereas intragenerational caregivers suffer from caregiver role entrenchment. Elderly spouse caregivers may have fewer defined current roles to perform than adult children caregivers and may respond to demands of cancer care by isolating themselves from social and family roles to become completely focused on the care of their spouses. This isolation allows little change from daily routine and focuses all of the caregiver energy on the cancer care experience. Isolation reduces the opportunity for diversion and renewal and may affect the caregiver responses to the long-term provision of care and ultimately their physical and mental health.

Older and aging families living with cancer, however, may have other problems related to care tasks because of decreased physical abilities that may be due to comorbid conditions such as cardiovascular disease, isolation of those assisting with care, diminished family resources, and family caregiver health problems of their own. Older family members who provide care may need help with physical care and administration needs. This may lead not only to an increase in caregiver distress but to patient dependency as well. Decreased personal physical abilities, isolation, and decreased financial resources of the older caregiver contribute to overall strain and stress.

LIVING ARRANGEMENTS

When adult children provide care, living arrangements may be altered either temporarily or permanently so they can manage the care of the patient. The patient may move into the home to facilitate care, or family members may move into the home of the patient to provide care. Secondary caregivers are also much more involved in parent care than spousal care situations. When a patient is widowed, single, or divorced, more caregivers are involved. In a study of 315 patients with cancer, Olson (1989) and Wellisch et al. (1988) found that home care was provided by one caregiver in 66 per cent of cases when the patient was married, that among widowed patients one caregiver was involved in only 24 per cent of the situations, and that among single or divorced patients one caregiver was involved in only 29 per cent and 30 per cent, respectively, of these situations. Clearly, 60 per cent to 70 per cent of patients with no spouse caregivers have more than one individual involved in their care. Thus others, generally female, assist with care when a spouse is not available.

SOCIOECONOMIC STATUS

Cancer care is most burdensome to those with low incomes if there are substantial out-of-pocket costs, because they have limited financial resources. Unemployed individuals may experience more distress because they may have fewer resources and capacity to respond to the distress (Mor, Guadagnoli, & Wool, 1988). Davis-Ali, Chesler, and Chesney (1993) indicated in their research that perhaps families with cancer who have higher incomes do not concern themselves with financial hardships of cancer.

CHARACTERISTICS OF THE CAREGIVER

For caregivers as well as patients, age, gender, employment, financial status, marital status, living arrangements, and usual roles also have to be considered. For the caregiver, however, these age and gender characteristics directly influence availability, capability, and willingness to assist with cancer care. The disposition of the family caregiver such as optimism or hardiness may affect the caregiver burden and reaction to care (Kurtz, Kurtz, Given, & Given, 1993). Those who have the most positive dispositions, that is, optimism, perceive less caregiver burden and depression about the care provided.

The common family caregiving situation for cancer patients involves women older than 55 years of age with support primarily from other family members and to a lesser extent friends or neighbors and from one family member who also usually shares the household with the care recipient. As a consequence of the longevity of women, elderly women with cancer are generally cared for by adult children, whereas older men are generally cared for by their spouse. In the absence of both spouses and children, patients with cancer are cared for by nieces and nephews or grandchildren. These patients with more distant relatives for caregivers are at greater risk for institutionalization when they become dependent. If adult children provide care, there is generally one child who assumes the major care role, generally an adult daughter.

Caregivers of younger patients may report more distress from care than those caring for older patients (Given et al., 1993; Schumacher et al., 1993). Schu-

macher et al. found that caregivers of young male patients with lower functional status and lower levels of efficacy experienced more strain than caregivers with older patients.

Gender has been shown to cause burdens differentially. Female caregivers may be more adversely affected by their caregiving role functions than are male caregivers, a pattern that holds among caregivers of physically impaired, stroke, heart disease, and cancer patients (Haley et al., 1987, Robinson, 1990; Siegel, Raveis, Mor, & Houts, 1991; Mor, Guadagnoli, & Wool, 1988). Spousal caregivers appear to be at particular risk for caregiver burden, because they typically provide the most extensive and comprehensive care, maintain their role longer, tolerate greater levels of disability among family members than adult children and other nonspousal caregivers, and experience more lifestyle adjustment and exhibit lower levels of well-being (George & Gwyther, 1986; Siegel, Raveis, Houts, & Mor, 1991). When the caregiver is not the spouse, the obligations and expectations may be lower, and they may not accept willingly the personal cost of providing care. The more distant the relative, the less obligated they are to provide care (Barusch & Spaid, 1989; Given et al., 1993; Pruchno & Potashnik, 1989; Schumacher et al., 1993). The level of depression among caregivers is highest for wives, followed by daughters, then other female caregivers, then sons, and then husband caregivers (Stommel et al., 1990).

Caregivers who live with the person with cancer may be more depressed than those who live in separate households (Stommel & Kingry, 1991). Income and overall financial concerns cause problems to caregivers during long periods of caregiving (Clipp & George, 1990) as meager resources are used. The educational level and financial resources of the family members may enable them to access resources and serve as a basis when entering the care situation. Individuals with low incomes and who were unemployed have been shown to have a greater risk for emotional distress, as overall the resources available to them are most tenuous.

Family members' finances and economic resources are affected by cancer care. Stommel, Given, and Given (1993) have summarized how shortened lengths of hospital stays and shifts toward outpatient care coupled with increases in women in the labor force intensify the economic consequences of caring for cancer patients in the home. Stommel et al. (1993) have shown how physical dependencies, most likely to be associated with shorter lengths of hospital stay, can influence the costs of family labor associated with home care. Given, Given, and Stommel (1994) describe the informal costs of continuing cancer care. Substantial out-of-pocket costs, loss of income, and family labor costs may occur and contribute to the cost burden. Out-of-pocket expenses for transportation, clothing, and phone as well as wages for both patient and caregiver lost because of cancer care may cause substantial burdens to families. Houts et al. (1984) described costs for treatment weeks and nontreatment weeks. Patients living at a distance reported more transportation costs and younger patients more wages lost. Patients with lower incomes often spent more than 50 per cent of their weekly incomes on nonreimbursable care expenses.

Perry and Roades de Meneses (1989) found that fully half of their caregivers were having difficulty maintaining their work roles while assisting with a family member who had cancer. Given and Given (1991) estimated the lost work hours resulting from caregiving for patients with cancer. Employment confirms both economic as well as personal benefits to the caregiver and his or her family. As family members take leaves of absence, miss work, or leave early to provide care, they may be sacrificing economic rewards and benefits as well as diversion from caring and the loss of self-esteem and personal rewards.

Given, Given, and Stommel (1994) calculated the average hours of family labor during a 3-month period devoted to caring for 191 middle-aged cancer patients with solid tumors. The average daily involvement for cancer care was approximately 5 hours, or 35 hours per week—nearly equivalent to a full-time job. Patient dependency and not duration of disease or site of cancer influenced the amount of family hours of care required.

Caregivers adapt employment to manage and meet caregiving obligations (Anastas, Gibeau, & Larson, 1990; Franklin, Ames, & King, 1994; Neal, Chapman, Ingersol-Dayton, & Emlen, 1993; Scharlach & Boyd, 1989). Employment adaptation among family caregivers may take place early in the course of caring. Changes may include short-term adjustments such as arriving late, leaving early, missing work without pay, taking sick or personal days, or altering work hours. Some take a leave of absence, whereas others quit work to provide care (Given, Given, & Stommel, 1994). Siegel, Raveis, Mor, and Houts (1991) suggest that financial burdens appear less stressful and easier to adjust to than those in emotional, social, and physical realm.

CHARACTERISTICS OF THE PATIENT

The age, gender, employment, marital status, role obligations, and resources of the patient need to be considered in examination of the caregiver burden. Developmental stage of the individual and gender of the patient influence the response that one brings to the diagnostic and treatment situation. How this relates to care has been discussed previously. Age not only affects how one responds to an "on time" diagnosis but may influence availability of support from the family and the assistance available. Because women live longer than men they often have more difficulty getting assistance. Gender may influence the usual tasks of care in the household that have to be realigned when cancer is diagnosed in a patient. Role obligations and resources (social, family, personal, work, and financial) of the patient need to be considered. Usual roles of the patient to be taken over or given up because of the effects of the disease and treatment need to be assessed. Living arrangements influence usual daily activities and roles within the home and who is available to assist the pa-

tient with needed care. The previous functional or mental status of the patient has been considered important to the patterns and consequences of family role in cancer care. (The cancer-related status and influence will be discussed in the disease-related section.) Comorbid conditions of the patient, however, do need to be determined, because they may confound the impact of disease and treatment on the functional status, capacity, and subsequent care requirements of the patient. Thus patient age, gender, employment, and living arrangements, as well as comorbid and cancer disease state conditions need to be determined because they may directly influence care requirements and demands as well as relationships with the caregiver.

CAREGIVING AND CARE CONTEXT—THE EFFECT ON CAREGIVER BURDEN

NATURE OF DISEASE AND TREATMENT— ILLNESS TRAJECTORY

Other than the work of Bender et al. (1989), Given et al. (1990), and Yost et al. (1993), who have focused on the continuing care needs of the patient and the family (Woods et al., 1989), most of the knowledge about stage of illness and family issues relates to diagnosis, acute care, late stages of illness, or death. The illness and treatment that makes care necessary is integral to determining the potential or risks for caregiver reactions and distress. The stage of cancer, the length of illness, phase in treatment trajectory, symptom experience, impacts of cancer and treatment on functional and mobility status, and role changes of the patient will influence cancer care demands on families (Given et al., 1993). The care demands take place in the context of the other roles of the family caregiver, adding complexity to the care situation; hence the potential for strain and stress exists. The care demands and direct and indirect requirements change over time in response to the stage of the disease and treatment plan. Changes in disease control, treatment, or care requirements may reinforce the uncertainty of the illness and serve as a source of the caregivers distress (Mishel & Sorenson, 1991; Oberst & James, 1984; Oberst et al., 1989). A long terminal phase among cancer patients, particularly patients with brain tumors (Biegel et al., 1991), was associated with symptoms of depression and emotional distress in family caregivers.

Several small-scale studies have shown that recurrent disease causes caregivers distress (Wright et al., 1993). Little work has been done with family reaction in the recurrent phase of illness (Chekryn, 1984; Given & Given, 1992; Weisman & Worden, 1986). Chekryn studied the meaning of cancer to patients and spouses and found that recurrence posed uncertainty, grief, fear, and anger, but no evidence of increased marital dysfunction. More recent reports, however, by Schumacher et al. (1993) and Given and Given (1992) indicate that recurrent disease as compared with new disease was related to lower levels of strain or distress in family members. Given and Given (1992) and Schumacher et al. (1993) could find no evidence that new versus recurrent disease influenced family health status or level of depression. This might suggest that caregivers may adapt to stress of caregiving during the course of a chronic illness or that other factors relate to distress (Townsend, Noelker, Deimling, & Bass, 1989). Instead of the presence of recurrence, patient's level of immobility was most stressful for the caregivers.

However, Schumacher et al. (1993) found that depression among caregivers for patients with recurrent disease was significantly related to gender, perceived adequacy of social support, and coping efficacy. Caregivers of patients who were more independent perceived higher levels of social support. This social support seemed to mediate the relationship between functional status and depression. Caregivers of male patients with less social support and coping were more depressed. Caregivers are more likely to experience transient moods and negative reactions, but only a modest percentage actually experience clinical depression. Moreover, the level of impairment or disease status may not contribute to depression directly but rather through the caregiver-perceived stress and burden (Schumacher et al., 1993).

Reactions of families in the early phase of diagnosis, treatment, and threat of illness have been documented by Oberst and James (1984) and Oberst and Scott (1988) and in the work of Northouse (1988). Constancy in adjustment, that is, change in patient status—either improvement or deterioration—may influence the family response over time. If the conditions change because of remission and exacerbation, necessitating change in the family reaction or care responsibilities, the negative reaction and stress and strain may occur (Lloyd & Coggles, 1990; Loomis & Wood, 1983). Change adds stress, and constant adaptations require more work, negotiation, and adjustment of the family members within the patient care system.

CARE TASKS AND DEMANDS ON THE CAREGIVER

Care requirements depend on the functional and psychologic level of the patient. In addition, the treatment activities and stages of the disease influence how the patient responds to the cancer. These care requirements beyond the capacity of the patient are then translated to caregiver demands for care. Involvement in care tasks is described in relationship to patient functional disability, activities such as bathing, dressing, and eating, and instrumental activities of daily living such as cleaning, laundry, and transportation.

Family members provide a wide range of care and provide care during the day, at night, on weekends, as well as on demand. With the chronicity of cancer this family care demand may occur for a number of years. In addition, the intensity and frequency of involvement varies with treatment type and phase and stage of disease. Changes in care tasks occur with progression of disease and disability and range from providing transportation to assuming responsibility for personal care

such as dressing and bathing. Involvement in care includes a number of dimensions: the frequency of tasks performed, the nature of the tasks, the hours of care provided each day, and the predictability of timing tasks and support received from other family members (McCorkle & Wilkerson, 1991).

Tasks of care seem to cover those related to physical care (Grobe, Ahmann, & Ilstrup, 1982; Grobe, Ilstrup, & Ahmann, 1981; Houts et al., 1988; McCorkle & Wilkerson, 1991; Mor et al., 1988; Wright & Dyck, 1984), nutrition (Houts, Yasko, Kahn, Schelzel, & Marconi, 1986; Houts et al., 1988), emotional support, spiritual support (Houts et al., 1988), social support (Houts et al., 1986), housekeeping sources (Grobe et al., 1981, 1982; Mor et al., 1988; Oberst et al., 1989), transportation (Blank et al., 1989; Grobe et al., 1981, 1982; Houts et al., 1986, 1988; Oberst et al., 1989) and financial assistance (Blank et al., 1989; Houts et al., 1986, 1988; Mor et al., 1988; Mor, Masterson-Allen, Houts, & Siegel, 1992; Mor, Masterson-Allen, Siegel, & Houts, 1992). The involvement in each of these categories often depends on patient disease status and the level of physical functioning.

Family involvement in cancer care includes direct assistance for self-care and activities such as shopping, transportation, money management, and arranging for treatments and services. However, symptom management and control become a major focus for both the patient and the family as they struggle to manage the symptoms of disease and side effects from ongoing treatment (Dodd, 1984a, 1984b; Given & Given, 1991; Given, Given, Stommel, & Linn, 1994; McCorkle, Yost, & Jepson, 1983; McCorkle & Wilkerson, 1991; Nail, Greene, Jones, & Flannery, 1989). Symptom distress influences social and physical function of the family member, curtails caregiver-patient interaction, and affects role interactions with others. Patients' symptom distress also may lead to such emotional responses as anger, frustration, or depression, which then affect the demands on the family caregiver.

Blank et al. (1989), Ferrell, Wenzl, and Wisdom (1988), Ferrell, Wisdom, and Schneider (1989), Ferrell, Rhiner, Cohen, Grant, and Rozek (1991), and Hull (1989) have all studied pain management by families and believe that it presents one of the most intractable problems for family caregivers and accounts for substantial anxiety and frustration.

Family caregivers assist in both nonpharmacologic and pharmacologic pain management. With regard to pharmacologic management for pain, for example, caregivers are involved in deciding *what* medication to use for pain relief and *when* to give medications, day and night; reminding and encouraging the patient to take the medication; and *keeping* records about decisions, dosages, and pain assessment for themselves and to report to health-care professionals.

With respect to nonpharmacologic pain management, family caregivers assist patients to position themselves by using pillows, with ambulation, or apply lotions and ointments or heat and cold to painful areas of the body. Family caregivers report that simply being present, touching, distracting, or talking to patients may help to manage pain. Nonpharmacologic pain interventions are often acquired through trial-and-error approaches and may not be the result of instruction from the health care professionals (Ferrell et al., 1991).

Families' involvement (assistance) in patients care management ranges from direct care to complex monitoring and decision making to emotional comforting. Each form of involvement demands different skills, organizational capacities, role demands, and psychologic strengths from family members.

Families must interact and negotiate with the health-care system to obtain information, services, and equipment and with family and friends to mobilize support for assistance with care. In addition, families make financial decisions regarding the purchasing of supplies, medications, and equipment (Mor et al., 1988; Tringali, 1986; Wellisch, Landsverk, Guidera, Pasnau, & Fawzy, 1983; Wright & Dyck, 1984). Cancer involves family members in such responsibilities as making judgments and decisions regarding when and how to obtain care: coordinating care, medication administration, symptom management, supervision of care, and counseling and comforting patients. Most of these activities require a more sophisticated and complex level of decision making than that with which family members are familiar. Thus they need assistance from the professionals to be prepared to care.

Tasks of care often depend on location in the illness or treatment trajectory. Mor (1987) found that patient need was related to the duration of the disease and pain experience. Buehler and Lee (1992) found that the longer the dying trajectory and the greater the patient deterioration, the greater the caregiver burden.

Oberst et al. (1989) found that the most demanding activities included providing transportation, giving emotional support, and doing extra household activities. McCorkle and Wilkerson (1991) found that during a 6-month period, even though patient symptoms and functional abilities improved, caregivers continued to report that they were providing assistance to patients. Caregivers still had to modify schedules to assist patients to deal with cancer and cancer treatments, provide care during the night, and be available for care 24 hours a day. Carey et al. (1991) reported on levels of burden in a population of cancer patients receiving chemotherapy. Care demands contribute differentially to burden among caregivers. Providing emotional support to the patient was the most demanding and the most difficult for the family members and produced the most burden. Providing transportation was time-consuming but not difficult and therefore was less of a burden. Lowest burden scores were present for personal and direct care activities. Indirect care such as managing illness-related finances, extra housework, and errands were moderately time-consuming and difficult and thus produced moderate burden (Carey et al., 1991). Older caregivers (Carey et al., 1991) were less likely to have mood disturbance and viewed caregivers as benign or beneficial, perhaps because of expectations of care roles in their lives.

Given and Given (1991, 1994) report that symptom management, providing support and encouragement, and dealing with the patient's emotional status and psychologic distress required the most caregiver assistance. These activities, along with managing symptoms and structuring care activities, consumed more caregiver time than assistance with self-care and direct care. The number and severity of such symptoms as fatigue, decreased appetite, nausea, and vomiting influenced patients' mobility, which in turn was related to caregivers' burden.

Stommel et al. (1990) explain depression as the distress related to symptoms of the disease or treatment and, to a *lesser extent,* by the loss of physical function experienced by the patient. Patients' dependencies in tasks of daily living, symptom severity, and immobility had a direct effect on the impact of caring on family members' daily schedule and subsequently on caregiver depression.

Oberst and Scott (1988) found that psychosocial response to the surgical experience was not a self-limiting event that resolved within a short period in a group of cancer patients. Family dyads had ongoing associated distress up to 18 months after initial treatment. Distress may continue even after the patient's status improves (Given et al., 1993; McCorkle & Wilkerson, 1991). The greater the demands of the patient's illness (objective) are on the family caregiver, the stronger the burden is. Severity and duration of patient illness, symptoms, and physical decline are thought to account for negative responses in the caregiver. In the terminal stages, families may be overwhelmed with the demands of illness plus the poor prognosis (Cassileth, Lusk, Strouse, Miller, Brown, & Cross, 1985) and threat of approaching death. The patient's own reaction to illness appear to influence the family member burden, and at times family member distress equals or exceeds that of the patient (Carey et al., 1991; Given et al., 1990; Wellisch et al., 1988). This may be mediated by care demands and patient symptoms and disability.

Research findings on the effect of patient functional status on caregiver strain and distress have been mixed. Severity of functional impairment (e.g., activities of daily living, cognitive and social functioning) and severity of symptoms may be significantly related to depression or caregiver well-being (Clipp & George, 1990; George & Gwyther, 1986; Given et al., 1993; Mor, 1987; Oberst et al., 1989). Most researchers have found that impaired cognitive function produces higher negative caregiver outcomes than impaired physical functioning among patients (Carey et al., 1991). Thus the literature suggests that family caregivers may adapt to the demands in physical functioning placed upon them, but the caring for patients with cognitive deficits produces high and sustained levels of caregiver burden.

Corbin and Strauss (1988) describe how cancer superimposes "illness-related work" upon "everyday life work" of the family members. Cancer patients can be time-consuming, labor-intensive, and stressful (Given et al., 1994; Kiecolt-Glaser, Glaser, Shuttleworth, Dyer, Ogrocki, & Speicher, 1987; Kiecolt-Glaser, Dura, Speicher, Trask, & Glaser, 1991; Lewis et al., 1989; McCorkle et al., 1989; Northouse, 1989; Northouse &

Swain, 1987; Oberst & Scott, 1988; Pederson & Valanis, 1989; Stetz, 1989; Woods et al., 1989; Yost et al., 1993). The extent and industry of "work" may not be the burdensome concerns; it may be the pervasive nature and wear and tear and unpredictability that cause the distress. The continued uncertainty associated with adjustment in role as well as disease and treatment trajectories appears to be distressing to family members. Illness-related work contains within it the emotional burdens of caring and the reorganizing of established role relationships such as parenting and work. This distress may be more problematic for the family member who tries to maintain all his or her normatively defined roles than for the elderly caregiver, who may have fewer pressing daily role demands (Given & Given, 1991, 1994).

The *level* of distress reported by individuals with cancer may not differ substantially from that of family members, but the *timing* of distress may vary among caregivers. Patient distress may occur earlier because of diagnosis and initial treatment, whereas the distress of the family caregiver may occur later in the course of the illness and ongoing treatment (Grobe et al., 1981, 1982; McCorkle & Wilkerson, 1991; Northouse, 1988; Stommel et al., 1990) and may continue to be present during stable periods (Lewis et al., 1989) of disease and treatment as well as during periods of recurrence or active treatment.

The dynamic of patient need and resolution of problems may require continued family involvement beyond the formal treatment (Carey et al., 1991; Mor, Masterson-Allen, Houts, & Siegel, 1992; Mor, Masterson-Allen, Siegel, & Houts, 1992). Family caregivers' psychologic responses are related, at least in part, to the level of mood disturbance, behavior change, overall distress, and depression among the cancer patients (Billings, 1985; Cassileth et al., 1985; Hinds, 1985; McCorkle et al., 1989; Northouse, 1990; Stommel et al., 1990). That is, caregivers strain is related to patient distress.

As the family caregiver deals with the care situation it is the formal and informal care system that provides support to them and may moderate the distress as they provide continuing and supportive care during the long cancer care trajectory.

FORMAL CARE SYSTEM

Factors that influence and are supportive to families and reduce caregiver burden include formal and informal care. These are described. Formal sources of supportive care for cancer patients and their families fall into three categories: acute care, skilled home care after discharge from the hospital; general outpatient and clinic services, usually related to the source of adjuvant therapy such as chemotherapy and radiation; and care provided through community-based agencies and general physician office practice. Community-based agencies provide such services as home health aides and transportation or nutrition assistance. When some aspect of home care is beyond the capacity of

families, health care professionals must turn to skilled home care agencies or other formal sources of home care. Skilled home care services must be ordered by a physician, and to be eligible for these services, patients must be homebound or require procedures that can be done only by a skilled home care nurse. This means that except for brief periods of time, home care services are not available to assist families with care. Formal agencies do not substitute for the care that family members provide.

Many patients and families are unaware of the existence of these agencies or are uncertain about how to find them or to gain access; other families may be reluctant to acknowledge that they need help (see Chapter 74 for a complete description on Home Care). These factors seem to account for the relatively infrequent use of community agencies by cancer patients and their families until late-stage disease. Socially adept caregivers will be able to identify and secure agency services more easily than those who have few social skills. Nurses need to identify formal sources of care and to evaluate the capacity and type of services provided to ensure that they can meet the needs of cancer patients. These types of services often need to be legitimized to the family by the health care professional (Guadagnoli, Rice, & Mor, 1991).

Oncology outpatient clinic services are often targeted toward the delivery of adjuvant therapy. The extent to which comprehensive services and concern for the total plan of care occurs in these settings varies. Beyond the oncology clinic where therapy is received, cancer patients and their families often do not have readily available services to address symptom management, treatment information, equipment operation, monitoring, emotional or informational needs, and skill development. It is essential that nurses in ambulatory care settings realize the importance of their role to the ongoing supportive care needs of family caregivers.

Formal assistance and support programs have not been shown to reduce depression or increase caregiver morale (Knight, Lutzky, & Macofsky-Urban, 1993; Lawton et al., 1991; Toseland & Rossiter, 1989). These programs have not, however, been focused or targeted and most often are not directed to family members but are directed instead to direct patient care activities. Therefore it is necessary to match referral to appropriate support groups for caregivers to those special support groups designed to deal with caregivers' emotional needs.

Health care professionals must be sensitive to the changes in family needs, eligibility criteria for services, as well as the costs of such care to the family. Reimbursement often determines which community health care services can be provided; thus the service that is offered does not always match the patient's actual need. The need to coordinate among different agencies to obtain needed services may become tedious and necessitate considerable effort by the family. Few case management services exist for cancer patients but may be necessary given the rapid move to ambulatory and managed care.

Family support to caregivers varies based on family developmental stage and stage of illness. In the literature "other" support beyond the primary caregiver, other family and friends, may provide assistance, but this often wanes over time independent of patient and family needs for assistance. The amount of social support provided by secondary caregivers to support family members may be influenced by severity and length of illness, and literature suggests that over time secondary caregivers leave the care situation (Given, Given, Stommel, Collins, King, & Franklin, 1992).

Informal support may lead to respite or assistance in care tasks, but there is little evidence that instrumental (Clipp & George, 1990; Lawton et al., 1991) support is related to decreased caregiver burden. Managing others to provide care may actually add to the distress of the caregiver. Most studies have documented that perceived quality and perceived adequacy of family and friend support is more important than actual quality of support received (Clipp & George, 1990; Robinson, 1989). Thus, even though studies of informal and formal support are confusing and unclear, it is important that presence or absence and perceived need be addressed in the care of cancer patients. These are probably mediators in the process of care and caregiver stress. Dimensions of family support have been described in previous sections.

The final section of this chapter will be devoted to strategies and interventions that should be assistive to family caregivers to reduce their burden and distress.

STRATEGIES TO ASSIST FAMILY CAREGIVERS TO REDUCE CAREGIVER BURDEN AND DISTRESS

The model outlined in Figure 9–1 provides a guide for selecting the strategies to assist family caregivers to provide care for a family member with cancer. Nurses need to assess, plan, implement, and evaluate the needs of the family caregiver based on the following considerations: (1) the type and stage therapy, (2) the patient characteristics and status, (3) caregivers' characteristics and needs for information and skill acquisition to implement rehabilitation, manage symptoms, monitor status, operate equipment, provide physical care, coordinate services, and address patients' emotional needs, (4) the manner in which families have chosen to organize informal home care, and (5) extent and level of family caregiver distress and burden. A careful consideration of each of these factors is important to the planning and implementation of care. The family caregiver as well as the patient must be considered an integral collaborative member of the cancer care team (Given & Given, 1989). The family caregiver should be involved in all components of care management and decisions and understand how they and their patient are to work and communicate with the health care professionals. Transition care between hospital and home should be carefully considered after diagnosis because the type

and scope of family involvement is often set at that time. The needs of the caregiver to provide care must be determined.

A detailed, individualized assessment should be conducted to plan for each phase of care with families. Modifications in the plan need to be made as changes in care demands arise, in each new phase of illness and treatment as new informational and skill needs emerge, and as services are provided in outpatient settings and community agencies. Outpatient care and medical plans of care and therapy should be integrated with the informal home care provided by the family member who is the responsible coordinator for ongoing and supportive patient care.

Assessments should always include family caregivers' perceptions of patients' needs and how best to meet them. Because family members identify information as a top priority need, the provision of information by the nurse is important to family members. Family caregivers want accurate and dependable information about diagnosis, prognosis, treatment, and expected stage and trajectory. (Hull, 1989; Kristjanson, 1986; Stiles, 1990). Family caregivers desire information to help them gain predictability of the disease and treatment situation (Dyck & Wright, 1985; Northouse & Swain, 1987).

Caregivers' progress reports on the patient should be considered and evaluated carefully. This will enable the nurse to discuss with family members alternative methods for meeting care goals within the resources and skill levels of the family. There is a need to determine for the family care provider the impact of caregiving responses over time and to determine how reactions occur, accumulate, wax, and wane. How altered responses to changes in extent and intensity of involvement or deterioration in patient status caused by disease and treatment need to be determined. Repeat assessments allow all participants—that is, the patient, family, and nurses—to revise strategies and care approaches as new problems emerge or old ones are resolved.

Nurses should consider family caregiver and patient background characteristics when developing a plan of care. The age and frailty of the primary caregiver as well as the family stage may affect how self-care activities and household chores along with the cancer care tasks are allocated. Anticipating the demands of each family member's other social and work roles and how these can be accomplished while meeting the added care demands will make care tasks more reasonable. Families need assistance to examine all the family and household roles, to identify where conflicts are likely to arise, the sources of these conflicts, who can help to alleviate them, and what can be done to deal with role overload or role conflict. Family conferences may be a useful strategy to help families examine and deal with family role conflicts.

The gender and relationship of the caregiver may also be a concern. Adult children may be reluctant to assist parents with intimate and personal care activities such as bathing and toileting. When thrust into caregiving roles, older men may be less able to carry out such tasks as cooking, laundry, and household chores. Working caregivers may need special assistance from home care agencies or from other family members if they are to maintain their employment and ensure that the patient care needs are met. Consideration of these factors is important to assessment and planning.

A plan for the care of cancer patients should link the clinical course of the disease and treatment with a set of outcome goals and special care requirements. Family members need to clearly understand their role in the care. This partnership between the formal and informal system acknowledges the resources and contributions of the family caregiver, accepts their methods of organizing care, and allows for negotiations regarding how care is to be delivered. Key elements of the plan can then be implemented, and requisite information can be provided, and skills can be taught to those family members who will be responsible for implementation of these activities.

The emotional needs of the family should be monitored and plans made to assist them to cope with frustration, anxiety, and depression. Caregiver efforts and contributions should be acknowledged at every contact and their reactions and feelings determined. What are the difficulties, stresses, strains, and burdens experienced? Current relationships and difficulties with the patient should be discussed. Caregivers should be encouraged to talk about feelings, especially guilt, anger, and resentment, so that they realize that expression is acceptable and that these feelings are normal. Interventions can include teaching the patient and caregiver to identify their feelings, perceptions, and interpretations that contribute to distress, to recognize usual emotional responses and to determine which responses are helpful, and to learn behaviors that manage responses in a constructive way. It is critical to determine whether the caregivers feel supported by both the formal and informal systems or what additional support they think is necessary. Encouragement of the caregivers to attend to their own self care and personal needs is essential.

Family caregiver personal resources may be valuable. Caregivers who remain optimistic may interpret the care experience less negatively. Scheier and Carver (1987) indicate that this resource may be related more to problem-focused coping than emotional focus; thus it may be useful to modify family reactions and stresses to caring. Given et al. (1993) found that optimism played an important role in caregiving and was an influential predictor of variation in caregiver depression and care burden. Optimism and other enduring traits may help to specify which family members may be successful in handling caregiver burden and which ones may need assistance from the health care system.

It is critical to watch for signs and symptoms of excessive burden and stress that require intervention. Assessment at regular intervals is important, and special attention should be paid to transition times such as after hospitalization, the beginning of treatment, recurrence, and moving to advanced disease with emphasis on palliative and terminal care. At each stage caregivers must learn to relax, talk, and identify targeted support groups, counseling, and respite that can help them through the specific stage at the time in the trajectory. Participation in their own social and leisure activities should be encouraged despite their report of extreme fatigue, because this may provide the respite that enables them to continue care.

During all phases of care, providing family caregivers with information on the disease, treatment, symptoms, and side effects, as well as how to manage symptoms is of paramount concern. Written information and guides assist family members to understand and recall useful strategies. Written information should, however, never take the place of open, ongoing verbal communication. Information alone may be insufficient. Caregivers may need reassurance and support when new or difficult problems arise. Family members may not be ready to hear or comprehend new information until the need for it actually exists; thus reiteration of new plans for care need to be made as the patient moves to a new level in the trajectory.

Education and information should be provided in a timely fashion relative to the stage of the disease and the phase of treatment symptom management and resources. Information obtained directly from nurses and physicians will reduce the possibility that families have to search outside the "system" for information that may be difficult for them to interpret or run counter to the treatment care plan. Confusion about care may actually disrupt the channels of communication between professional and family caregivers and result in negative caregiver reactions and burden. Increasing the knowledge will create in the family caregiver a sense of control, competence, confidence, and security over the care situation and reduce anxiety and distress, which will enable them to manage care problems.

In addition to information about the disease and treatment, family members need to know more about the emotional aspects of cancer and recovery. Family caregivers frequently observe signs of patients' suffering and are uncertain how to help. Family members need to be prepared to address the patient's anxiety, anger, or depression as well as physiologic signs and symptoms and side effects from treatment that occur. It is not uncommon for family members to express as the biggest concern patient comfort and concern for symptom control. Therefore one of the important strategies that caregivers need assistance with is to ensure that patients are kept comfortable. Caregivers need to understand strategies for symptom management. The acquisition of caregiving skills, the changes in demands of care across time, and the impact of preparedness for care tasks on the caregivers' reactions need to be determined. Change in the reactions of caregivers as they become more prepared or master the tasks and demands of caregiving need to be assessed and documented. A sense of mastery will help reduce ambiguity or lack of predictability and facilitate use of personal and other resources.

As the care demands continue for long periods of time, family caregivers need to be given permission to discontinue some aspects of care, involve others (including formal sources of care), or quit their caregiving roles entirely. They also need to understand through communication and interaction with the nurses that it is acceptable to ask for help from the formal or informal care system and that they are not a failure when they do so.

Effective discharge planning and referral to home health care and community health services or case management strategies may assist family (McCorkle et al., 1989) members to deal with caregiver burdens. Current work suggests that use of these services, however, is associated with increased age (Yost et al., 1993) and not patient or caregiver need. Need for services may exist beyond aggressive treatment or radical surgery. Examination of how and when discharge planning can be used based on family needs is a necessary part of continuing cancer care.

Nurses can help to anticipate problems and prevent caregiver distress by helping the caregivers to identify and mobilize support and resources and to explore barriers to using this support. Mobility and availability of support to provide care and fluctuations in patients and caregiver need suggest necessity of ongoing appraisal of family situation based on family, age, employment, and gender factors as well as patient disease and treatment status. Social support to family caregivers can be supplied from other family members or friends in the form of tangible or intangible assistance or formally from professional services. Assessing needed social support and teaching effective coping strategies in the actual caregiving environment may be more successful than formalized group intervention (Quayhagen & Quayhagen, 1989). Home health aides, homemakers, volunteers, as well as family members should be considered as resources to help the caregiver.

Respite for the caregiver is an important component of home care and should be included as part of the overall plan. Respite can be done through family friends and support groups as well as community agencies. Respite may include relief from direct care, the provision of instrumental activities, or transportation. Arranging for respite is important. A few hours of respite from care each week that enables the caregiver some personal time may enable them to *continue* providing care for long periods of time often necessitated by cancer care trajectory. Caregivers with high social skills are able to mobilize social support in the environment more effectively and need to be encouraged to seek out assistance. Those caregivers without strong social skills should be identified and receive assistance. Ideally, a case manager needs to be responsible to assist the family to obtain care resources across the cancer care trajectory. Only with continuity can the family continue to be prepared, develop problem-solving skills, enhance their own family communication, and explore alternative strategies as the care situation changes.

To reduce family burden and to ensure that treatment compliance is not compromised, providers need to be sensitive to *"care problems"* of families. Family caregivers need to be assessed for family capacity and ability to provide and continue cancer care. Family caregivers need to be continuously assessed for caregiver burden. Those caregivers most at risk for needing assistance from the formal care system are those who are emotionally challenged and those with limited social, family, and financial resources. If there is evidence of lack of mutuality between the patient and the caregiver, we should help the family member explore alternatives to direct care.

Interventions need to be dynamic and responsive as the family moves through multiple transitions that are characterized by periods of uncertainty, role change, emotional change, and varying care demands resulting from the nature of the disease and treatment. Different family types require different forms of assistance at different phases of the illness. To meet the family caregiver's needs, the nurse must determine whether the demand experienced is a consequence of an uncontrollable phenomenon. When there is little caregivers can do in the care situation, caregivers need to be taught coping strategies rather than skills or procedures to provide the care. Nurses need to attend to the "burden" the care imposes. Recognizing problems and helping families to set limits on their care responsibilities assumes an important role for families during the supportive cancer care period so they can reevaluate their commitment and capacity to care.

SUMMARY

Cancer in a family member creates demands not *previously* experienced by most family members. The pattern of care demands vary in magnitude and type and change numerous times depending on the stage of illness and phase of treatment. Interventions directed toward the family need to be dynamic and responsive as the family moves through multiple transitions that are characterized by periods of uncertainty, role change, emotional change, and varying care demands resulting from the nature of the disease and treatment. Nursing interventions to assist families to anticipate illness demands and to gain a sense of self-competence and self-esteem may facilitate their ability to continue care and may influence the level of caregiver burden. Families need assistance to reframe their perception of the caregiving experience so that they focus on the strengths they bring to the care situation.

The focus on caregiver burden has been such that the caregiver is viewed as the subject of concern. This is certainly appropriate; however, in this time of cost containment and dramatic shifts in care from the formal to the informal system, we believe that burdens exhibited by the caregivers may also have profound impact upon patient care outcomes. Caregivers who are highly stressed, anxious, or depressed are less able to provide high-quality home care for patients. With the shifts in care from the formal to the home, the responsibilities of family members have changed as well. Today and in the foreseeable future, family members will be engaged in more than just custodial care. Caregivers are the managers of pain and observers of subtle changes or deteriorations in healing, the early signs of infection, dehydration, potassium imbalance, and a host of other problems that, if not identified early on, will lead to expensive care and to extended periods of caring in the home. Therefore it is critical that family caregivers be supported and their levels of burden monitored. Just as "burnout" in the formal caregiving settings has taken on meaning, burden in the family system can lead to poor patient outcomes as well. As more care moves under capitated programs, it is less likely that managed systems will want or can afford poor patient and caregiver outcomes such as repeat hospitalization for patients and extended periods of work loss, which will count against the managed care ability to keep persons in the work force.

Interventions for family caregivers will be successful if they are tailored to patient and caregiver characteristics, family background, informal and formal care, support, care situations and demands, knowledge, and beliefs about expected outcome and their ability to carry out needed care. Meeting the needs of the family caregiver may prevent or minimize caregiver burden and distresses. Nurses need to gain an understanding of the role and demands of the multiple factors that influence the family cancer care system. The goal of care is to restore or promote meeting the needs of the patient with cancer and the family caregiver, thereby enhancing the quality of life for families living with cancer and limiting the caregiver burden experienced.

REFERENCES

Anastas, J. W., Gibeau, J. L., & Larson, P. J. (1990). Working families and eldercare: A national perspective in an aging America. *Soc-Work, 35,* 405–411.

Archbold, P. G., Stewart, B. J., Greenlick, M. R., & Harvath, T. (1990). Mutuality and preparedness as predictors of caregiver role strain. *Research Nursing Health, 13,* 375–384.

Barnes, C. L., Given, B. A., & Given, C. W. (1992). Caregivers of elderly relatives: Spouses and adult children. *Health and Social Work, 17,* 282–289.

Barusch, A. S., & Spaid, W. M. (1989). Gender differences in caregiving: Why do wives report greater burden? *Gerontologist, 29,* 667–676.

Beck, A. T., & Beck, R. W. (1972). Screening depressed patients in family practice: A rapid technique. *Postgraduate Medicine, 52,* 1–85.

Bender, L., Weinert, C., Faulkner, L., & Quimby, R. (1989). *Montana families living with cancer.* Bozeman, MT: College of Nursing, Montana State University.

Biegel, D. E., Sales, E., & Schultz, R. (1991). *Family caregiving in chronic illness* (pp. 62–163). Newbury Park, CA: Sage.

Billings, J. A. (1985). Symptom control, support, and hospice-in-the-home. *Outpatient management of advanced cancer* (pp. 115–172). Philadelphia: JB Lippincott.

Blank, J. J., Clark, L., Longman, A. J., & Atwood, J. R. (1989). Perceived home care needs of cancer patients and their caregivers. *Cancer Nursing, 12,* 78–84.

Brody, E. M. (1981). Women in the middle and family help to older people. *The Gerontologist, 25,* 19–29.

Brody, E. M. (1985). The Donald P. Kent Memorial Lecture. Parent care as a normative family stress. *The Gerontologist, 25,* 19–29.

Buehler, J., & Lee, H. (1992). Exploration of home care resources for rural families. *Cancer Nursing, 15,* 299–308.

Carey, P. J., Oberst, M. T., McCubbin, M. A., & Hughes, S. (1991). Appraisal and caregiving burden in family members caring for patients receiving chemotherapy. *Oncology Nursing Forum, 18,* 1341–1348.

Cartwright, J. C., Archbold, P. G., Stewart, B. J., & Limandri, B. (1994). Enrichment processes in family caregiving to frail elders. *Esthetics and the Art of Nursing, 17,* 31–43.

Cassileth, B. R., Lusk, E. J., Strouse, T. B., Miller, D. S., Brown, L. L., & Cross, P. A. (1985). A psychological analysis of cancer patients and their next-of-kin. *Cancer, 55,* 72–76.

Chekryn, J. (1984). Cancer recurrence: Personal meaning, communication, and marital adjustment. *Cancer Nursing, 1,* 491–498.

Cicirelli, V. (1992). *Family caregiving autonomous and paternalistic decision making* (Vol. 186). Thousand Oaks, CA: Sage.

Clipp, E. C., & George, L. K. (1990). Caregiver needs and patterns of social support. *Journal of Gerontology, 45,* S102–S111.

Corbin, J., & Strauss, A. (1988). *Unending work: Managing chronic illness at home.* San Francisco, CA: Josey Bass Publishers.

Davis-Ali, S., Chesler, M., & Chesney, B. (1993). Recognizing cancer as a family disease: Worries and support reported by patients and spouses. *Social Work in Health Care, 19,* 45–65.

Derogatis, L. R., Lipman, R. S., & Covi, L. (1973). SCL-90: An outpatient psychiatric rating scale: Preliminary report. *Psychopharmacology Bulletin, 9,* 13–28.

Derogatis, L. R., & Spencer, P. M. (1982). *The Brief Symptom Inventory (BSI). Administration, Scoring and Procedures Manual I.* Baltimore: Clinical Psychometrics Research.

Dodd, M. (1984a). Self-care for patients with breast cancer to prevent side effects of chemotherapy: A concern for public health nursing. *Public Health Nursing, 1,* 202–209.

Dodd, M. (1984b). Patterns of self care in cancer patients receiving radiation therapy. *Oncology Nursing Forum, 11,* 23–27.

Dyck, S., & Wright, K. (1985). Family perceptions: The role of the nurse throughout an adult's cancer experience. *Oncology Nursing Forum, 12,* 53–56.

Ferrell, B., Rhiner, M., Cohen, M., Grant, M., & Rozek, A. (1991). Pain as a metaphor for illness. *Oncology Nursing Forum, 18,* 1315–1321.

Ferrell, B., Wenzl, C., & Wisdom, C. (1988). The pain management team: Five years' experience. *Oncology Nursing Forum, 15,* 285–289.

Ferrell, B., Wisdom, C., & Schneider, C. (1989). Quality of life as an outcome variable in the management of cancer pain. *Cancer, 63,* 2321–2327.

Franklin, S., Ames, B. D., & King, S. (1994). Acquiring the family eldercare role: Influence on female employment adaptation. *Research on Aging, 16,* 27–42.

Galloway, S. C. (1990). Young adults' reactions of the death of a parent. *Oncology Nursing Forum, 17,* 899–904.

George, L. K., & Gwyther, L. P. (1986). Caregiver well being: A multidimensional examination of family caregivers of demented adults. *The Gerontologist, 26,* 253–259.

Given, B., & Given, C. W. (1989). Compliance among patients with cancer. *Oncology Nursing Forum, 12,* 71–77.

Given, B., & Given, C. W. (1991). Family caregivers of cancer patients. In S. Hubbard, P. Greene, & M. Knobf (Eds.), *Current issues in cancer nursing practice* (pp. 1–9). Philadelphia: W.B. Saunders Co.

Given, B., & Given, C. W. (1992). Patient and family caregiver reaction to new and recurrent breast cancer. *Journal of the American Medical Women's Association, 47,* 201–212.

Given, B. A., Given, C. W., Stommel, M. (1994). Family and out-of-pocket costs for women with breast cancer. *Cancer Practice, 2,* 187–193.

Given, B., Given, C. W., Stommel, M., & Linn, C. S. (1994). Predictors of use of secondary carers used by the elderly following hospital discharge. *Journal of Aging & Health 6,* 353–376.

Given, B., Stommel, M., Collins, C., King, S., & Given, C. W. (1990). Responses of elderly spouse caregivers. *Research in Nursing and Health, 13,* 77–85.

Given, C. W., Given, B., Stommel, M., Collins, C., King, S., & Franklin, S. (1992). The caregiver reaction assessment (CRA) for persons with chronic physical and mental impairments. *Research in Nursing & Health, 15,* 271–283.

Given, C. W., & Given, B. A. (1994). The home care of a patient with cancer. In E. Kahana, D. E. Biegel, & M. L. Wykle (Eds.), *Family caregiving across the lifespan* (pp. 240–261). Thousand Oaks, CA: Sage.

Given, C. W., Stommel, M., Given, B., Osuch, J., Kurtz, M., & Kurtz, J. C. (1993). The influence of cancer patients' symptoms and functional states on patients' depression and family caregivers' reaction and depression. *Health Psychology, 12,* 277–285.

Goldberg, P. (1978). *Manual of the general health questionnaire.* Windsor: NFER-Nelson Publishing Co.

Gray-Price, H., Szczesny, S. (1985). Crisis intervention with families of cancer patients: A developmental approach. *Topics in Clinical Nursing, 7,* 58–70.

Grobe, M. E., Ahmann, D. L., & Ilstrup, D. M. (1982). Needs assessment for advanced cancer patients and their families. *Oncology Nursing Forum, 9,* 26–30.

Grobe, M. E., Ilstrup, D., & Ahmann, D. (1981). Skills needed by family members to maintain the care of an advanced cancer patient. *Cancer Nursing, 4,* 371–375.

Guadagnoli, E., Rice, C., Mor, V. (1991). Cancer patients' knowledge of and willingness to use agency-based services: Toward application of a model of behavioral change. *Journal of Psychosocial Oncology, 9,* 1–21.

Haley, W. E., Levine, E. G., Brown, S. L., & Bartolucci, A. A. (1987). Stress, appraisal, coping, and social support as predictors of adaptational outcome among dementia caregivers. *Psychology & Aging, 2,* 323–330.

Hileman, J. W., & Lackey, N. R. (1992). Identifying the needs of home caregivers of patients with cancer. *Oncology Nursing Forum, 19,* 771–777.

Hinds, C. (1985). The needs of families who care for patients with cancer at home: Are we meeting them? *Journal of Advanced Nursing, 10,* 575–581.

Hirshfeld, M. (1983). Homecare vs. institutionalization: Family caregiving and senile brain disease. *International Journal of Nursing Studies, 20,* 23–32.

Hooyman, N., Gonyea, J., & Montgomery, R. (1985). The impact of in-home services termination of family caregivers. *The Gerontologist, 25,* 141–145.

Horowitz, A. (1985). Sons and daughters as caregivers to older parents: Differences in role performance and consequences. *Gerontologist, 25,* 612–617.

Houts, P., Lipton, A., Harvey, H., Martin, B., Simmonds, M., Dixon. R., Longo, S., Andrews, T., Gordon, R., Meloy, J., & Hoffman, S. (1984). Nonmedical costs to patients and their families associated with outpatient chemotherapy. *Cancer, 53,* 2388–2392.

Houts, P. S., Yasko, J. M., Kahn, S. B., Schelzel, G. W., & Marconi, K. M. (1986). Unmet psychological, social, and economic needs of persons with cancer in Pennsylvania. *Cancer, 58,* 2355–2361.

Houts, P. S., Yasko, J. M., Simmonds, M. A., Kahn, S. B., Schelzel, G. W., Marconi, K. M., & Bartholomew, M. J. (1988). A comparison of problems reported by persons with cancer and their same sex siblings. *Journal of Clinical Epidemiology, 41,* 875–881.

Hull, M. M. (1989). Family needs and supportive nursing behaviors during terminal care: A review. *Oncology Nursing Forum, 16,* 787–792.

Kiecolt-Glaser, J. K., Dura, J. R., Speicher, C. E., Trask, O. J., & Glaser, R. (1991). Spousal caregivers of dementia victims: longitudinal changes in immunity and health. *Psychosomatic Medicine, 53,* 345–362.

Kiecolt-Glaser, J. K., Glaser, R., Shuttleworth, E. E., Dyer, C. S., Ogrocki, P., & Speicher, C. E. (1987). Chronic stress and immunity in family caregivers of Alzheimer's disease victims. *Psychosomatic Medicine, 49,* 523–535.

Kirshling, J. M. (1987). Intervening with middle-aged families and terminal cancer. In M. Leahey, & L.M. Wright (Eds.), *Families and life threatening illness* (pp. 287–309). Springhouse, PA: Springhouse.

Knight, B., Lutzky, S., & Macofsky-Urban, F. (1993). A meta-analytic review of interventions for caregiver distress: Recommendations for future research. *The Gerontologist, 33,* 240–248.

Kornblith, A., Herr, H., Ofman, U., Scher, H., & Holland, J. (1994). Quality of life of patients with prostate cancer and their spouses. *Cancer, 73,* 2791–2802.

Kristjanson, L. J. (1986). Indicators of quality of palliative care from a family perspective. *Journal of Palliative Care, 1*(2), 8–17.

Kristjanson, L. J. (1989). Quality of terminal care: Salient indicators identified by families. *Journal of Palliative Care, 5*(1), 21–30.

Kristjanson, L. J., & Ashcroft, T. (1994). The family's cancer journey: A literature review. *Cancer Nursing, 17,* 1–17.

Kurtz, M. E., Kurtz, J. C., Given, C. W., & Given, B. (1993). Loss of physical functioning among cancer patients: A longitudinal view. *Cancer Practice, 1,* 275–281.

Lawton, M. P., Moss, M., Kleban, M. H., Glicksman, A., & Rovine, M. (1991). A two-year factor model of caregiving appraisal and psychological well-being. *Journal of Gerontology, 46,* P181–189.

Lewis, F. M., Ellison, E. S., & Woods, N. F. (1985). The impact of breast cancer on the family. *Seminars in Oncology Nursing, 1,* 206–213.

Lewis, F. M., Woods, N. F., Hough, E. E., & Bensley, L. S. (1989). The family's functioning with chronic illness in the mother: The spouse's perspective. *Social, Science & Medicine, 29,* 1261–1269.

Lloyd, C., & Coggles, L. (1990). Psychological issues for people with cancer and their families. *Cancer Journal of Occupational Therapy, 57,* 211–215.

Loomis, M. E., & Wood, D. J. (1983). Cure: The potential outcome of nursing care. *IMAGE: Journal of Nursing Scholarship, 15,* 4–7.

McCorkle, R. (1988). A prospective and concurrent study of spouse bereavement. (Final Report No. NR01626, NCNR, NIH). Philadelphia: University of Pennsylvania.

McCorkle, R., Benoliel, J. Q., Donaldson, G., Georgiadou, F., Moinpour, C., & Goodell, B. (1989). A randomized clinical trial of home nursing care for lung cancer patients. *Cancer, 64,* 1375–1382.

McCorkle, R., & Wilkerson, K. (1991). Home care needs of cancer patients and their caregivers. (Final Report No. NR01914). Philadelphia: University of Pennsylvania School of Nursing.

McCorkle, R., Yost, L. S., Jepson, C., et al. (1983). A cancer experience: Relationship of patient psychosocial responses to caregiver burden over time. *Journal of Psychosocial Oncology, 2,* 21–32.

Miller, B. (1989). Adult children's perceptions of caregiver stress and satisfaction. *Journal of Applied Gerontology, 8,* 275–293.

Mishel, M. H., & Sorenson, D. S. (1991). Uncertainty in gynecological cancer: A test of the mediating functions of mastery and coping. *Nursing Research, 40,* 167–171.

Montgomery, R., Stull, D. E., & Borgatta, E. F. (1985). Measurement and the analysis of burden. *Research on Aging, 7,* 137–152.

Montgomery, R. V., Gonyea, J. G., & Hooyman, N. R. (1985). Caregiving and the experience of subjective and objective burden. *Family Relations, 34,* 19–26.

Mor, V. (1987). Cancer patients' quality of life over the disease course: Lessons from the real world. *Journal of Chronic Disease, 40,* 535–544.

Mor, V., Guadagnoli, E., & Wool, M. (1988). The role of concrete services in cancer care. *Advances in Psychosomatic Medicine, 18,* 102–118.

Mor, V., Masterson-Allen, S., Houts, P., & Siegel, K. (1992). The changing needs of patients with cancer at home. *Cancer, 69,* 829–838.

Mor, V., Masterson-Allen, S., Siegel, K., & Houts, P. (1992) Determinants of need and unmet need among cancer patients residing at home. *Health Services Research, 27,* 337–360.

Nail, L. M., Greene, D., Jones, L. S., & Flannery, M. (1989). Nursing care by telephone: Describing practice in an ambulatory oncology center. *Oncology Nursing Forum, 16,* 387–395.

Neal, M., Chapman, N., Ingersol-Dayton, B., & Emlen, A. (1993). *Balancing work and caregiving for children, adults and elders.* Newburg, CA: Sage.

Northouse, L. L. (1988). Social support in patients' and husbands' adjustment to breast cancer. *Nursing Research, 37,* 91–95.

Northouse, L. L. (1989). A longitudinal study of the adjustment of patients and husbands to breast cancer. *Oncology Nursing Forum, 16,* 511–516.

Northouse, L. L. (1990). A longitudinal study of the adjustment of patients and husbands to breast cancer. *Oncology Nursing Forum, 17,* 39–43.

Northouse, L. L., & Peters-Golden, H. (1993). Cancer and the family: Strategies to assist spouses. *Seminars in Oncology Nursing, 9,* 74–82.

Northouse, L. L., & Swain, M. A. (1987). Adjustment of patients and husbands to the initial impact of breast cancer. *Nursing Research, 36,* 221–225.

Nugent, L. S. (1988). The social support requirements of family caregivers of terminal cancer patients. *Cancer Journal of Nursing Research, 20,* 45–58.

Oberst, M. T., & James, R. H. (1984). Going home: Patient and spouse adjustment following cancer surgery. *Top Clinical Nurse, 7,* 46–57.

Oberst, M. T., & Scott, D. W. (1988). Post discharge distress in surgically treated cancer patients and their spouses. *Research In Nursing & Health, 11,* 223–233.

Oberst, M. T., Thomas, S. E., Gass, K. A., & Ward, S. E. (1989) Caregiving demands and appraisal of stress. *Cancer Nursing, 12,* 209–215.

Olson, M. (1989). Family participation in post hospital care: Women's work. *Journal of Psychosocial Oncology, 7,* 77–93.

Pallett, P. (1990). A conceptual framework for studying family caregiver burden in Alzheimer's type dementia. *IMAGE: Journal of Nursing Scholarship, 22,* 52–58.

Pearlin, L. I., Mullan, J. T., Semple, S. J., & Skaff, M. M. (1990). Caregiving and the stress process: An overview of concepts and their measures. *Gerontologist, 30,* 583–594.

Pederson, L. M., & Valanis, B. G. (1989). The effects of breast cancer on the family: A review of the literature. *Psychosocial Oncology, 6,* 95–117.

Perry, G. R., & Roades de Meneses, M. (1989). Cancer patients at home: Needs and coping styles of primary caregivers. *Home Healthcare Nurse, 7,* 27–30.

Poulshock, S. W., & Deimling, G. T. (1984). Families caring for elders in residence: Issues in the measurement of burden. *Journal of Gerontology, 39,* 230–239.

Pruchno, R. A., & Potashnik, S. L. (1989). Caregiving spouses: Physical and mental health in perspective. *Journal of the American Gerontological Society, 37,* 697–705.

Quayhagen, M. P., & Quayhagen, M. (1989). Differential effects of family-based strategies on Alzheimer's disease. *Gerontologist, 29,* 150–155.

Radloff, L. S. (1977). The CES-D scale: A self-report depression scale for research in the general population. *Applied Psychology Measurement, 1,* 385–401.

Robinson, K. (1990). The relationship between social skills, social support, self-esteem and burden in adult caregivers. *Journal of Advanced Nursing, 15,* 788–795.

Robinson, K. M. (1989). Predictors of depression among wife caregivers. *Nursing Research, 38,* 359–363.

Robinson, L., McCorkle, R., Lev, E., & Nuamah, I. (In press). A Prospective Longitudinal Investigation of Spousal Bereavement Examining Parkes' Predictive Variables of Negative Bereavement Outcomes. *Journal of Palliative Care.*

Scharlach, A. E., & Boyd, S. L. (1989). Caregiving and employment: Results of an employment survey. *The Gerontologist, 29,* 383–387.

Scheier, M. F., & Carver, C. S. (1987). Dispositional optimism and physical well-being: The influence of generalized outcome expectancies on health. *Journal of Personality, 55,* 169–210.

Schultz, R., Fello, M., & Love, J. (1989). Grant entitled "Living with homecare cancer patients and caregivers." National Institutes of Health (NCI).

Schultz, R., Tompkins, C. A., & Rau, M. T. (1988). A longitudinal study of the psychosocial impact of stroke on primary support persons. *Psychological Aging, 3,* 131–141.

Schumacher, K. L., Dodd, M. J., & Paul, S. M. (1993). The stress process in family caregivers of persons receiving chemotherapy. *Research in Nursing & Health, 16,* 395–404.

Siegel, K., Raveis, V., Houts, P., & Mor, V. (1991). Caregiver burden and unmet patient needs. *Cancer, 68,* 1131–1140.

Siegel, K., Raveis, V. H., Mor, V., & Houts, P. (1991). The relationship of spousal caregiver burden to patient disease and treatment-related conditions. *Annals of Oncology, 2,* 511–516.

Stetz, K. M. (1987). Caregiving demands during advanced cancer: The spouse's needs. *Cancer Nursing, 10,* 260–268.

Stetz, K. M. (1989). The relationship among background, characteristics, purpose of life, and caregiving demands on perceived health of spouse caregivers. *Scholarly Inquiry for Nursing Practice: An International Journal, 3,* 133–153.

Stiles, M. K. (1990). The shining stranger: Nurse-family spiritual relationship. *Cancer Nursing, 13,* 235–245.

Stommel, M., Given, C. W., & Given, B. (1990). Depression as an overriding variable explaining caregiver burden. *Journal of Aging Health, 2,* 81–102.

Stommel, M., Given, C. W., & Given, B. (1993). The cost of cancer home care to families. *Cancer, 71,* 1867–1874.

Stommel, M., & Kingry, M. (1991). Support patterns for spouse-caregivers of cancer patients: The effect of the presence of minor children. *Cancer Nursing, 14,* 200–205.

Stommel, M., Wang, S., Given, C. W., & Given, B. (1992). Confirmatory factor analysis (CFA) as a method to assess measurement equivalence. *Research in Nursing & Health, 15,* 399–405.

Thorne, S. (1984). The family cancer experience. *Cancer Nursing, 8,* 285–291.

Toseland, R. W., & Rossiter, C. M. (1989). Group interventions to support family caregivers: A review and analysis. *Gerontologist, 29,* 438–448.

Townsend, A., Noelker, L., Deimling, G., & Bass, D. (1989). Longitudinal impact of interhousehold caregiving on adult childrens' mental health. *Psychology and Aging, 4,* 393–401.

Tringali, C.A. (1986). The needs of family members of cancer patients. *Oncology Nursing Forum, 13,* 65–70.

Vess, J., Moreland, J., & Schwebel, A. I. (1985). Understanding family role reallocation following a death: A theoretical framework. *Omega, 16,* 115–128.

Weisman, A. D., & Worden, J. W. (1986). The emotional impact of recurrent cancer. *Journal of Psychosocial Oncology, 3,* 5–16.

Wellisch, D., Wolcott, D. L., Pasnau, R. O., Fawzy, F. I., & Landsverk, J. (1988). An evaluation of the psychosocial problems of the homebound cancer patient: Relationship of patient adjustment to family problems. *Journal of Psychosocial Oncology, 7,* 55–76.

Wellisch, D., Landsverk, J., Guidera, K., Pasnau, R. O., & Fawzy, F. (1983). Evaluation of psychosocial problems of the homebound cancer patient: Methodology and problem frequencies. *Psychosomatic Medicine, 45,* 11–21.

Woods, N. F., Lewis, F. M., & Ellison, E. S. (1989). Living with cancer: Family experiences. *Cancer Nursing, 12,* 28–33.

Wright, K., & Dyck, S. (1984). Expressed concerns of adult cancer patients' family members. *Cancer, 7,* 371–374.

Wright, L., Clipp, E., & George, L. (1993). Health consequences of caregiver stress. *Medicine, Exercise, Nutrition and Health, 2,* 181–195.

Yost, L. S., McCorkle, R., Buhler-Wilkerson, K., Schultz, D., & Lusk, E. (1993). Determinants of subsequent home health care nursing service use by hospitalized patients with cancer. *Cancer, 72,* 3304–3312.

Young, R. F., & Kahana, E. (1989). Specifying caregiver outcomes: Gender and relationship aspects of caregiving strain. *Gerontologist, 29,* 660–666.

Younger, J. B. (1991). A theory of mastery. *Advanced Nursing Science, 14,* 76–89.

Zarit, S. H., & Pearlin, L. I. (1993). Family caregiving: Integrating informal and formal care systems for care. In S. H. Zarit, L. I. Pearlin, & K. Schaie (Eds.), *Caregiving systems: Formal and informal helpers* (pp. 303–316). New Jersey: Eilbaum & Associates.

Zarit, S. H., Todd, P. A., & Zarit, J. M. (1986). Subjective burden of husbands and wives as caregivers: A longitudinal study. *Gerontologist, 26,* 260–266.

Zung, W. (1965). A self-rating depression scale. *Archives of General Psychiatry, 12,* 63–70.

Loss and Bereavement

Elise L. Lev • Linda Robinson • Ruth McCorkle

The study of bereavement has expanded since Lindemann's classic study of survivor's recovery after disaster (Lindemann, 1944). Research indicates that grief follows loss, symptoms of grief vary among individuals, and the outcome may be adaptive or maladaptive. Although the terms "grief" and "bereavement" have been used interchangeably, grief refers to the response following many types of loss. Bereavement is the period after death in which patterns of grieving occur.

Osterweis, Solomon, and Green (1984), in an Institute of Medicine report, noted that nurses can provide useful information to families of the bereaved, help them to understand grief reactions that are normal, and identify abnormal reactions. Continued contact with the recently bereaved was recommended in the same report to demonstrate concern, provide emotional support, assist families in organizing to provide support, and assess survivor's health adjustment.

THEORETIC PERSPECTIVES

The predominance of the bereavement research conducted during the past 5 decades has examined the experience after conjugal loss. The published works of Colin Murray Parkes evolved from his experience with cancer patients and combine to form a descriptive theory of spousal bereavement pertinent in its scope to clinicians across many disciplines. Parkes, a clinical and research psychiatrist, defines grief as a "process of realization, of making psychologically real an external event which is not desired and for which coping plans do not exist" (1970, p. 465). Parkes considers bereavement to be a psychosocial transition. This broad philosophic frame of reference has been shared by nurse researchers in the field of bereavement. Benoliel (1985) stated that for the majority of people, reaction to loss is an adaptive process characterized by emotional and behavioral upset.

Many theories of bereavement have been reported in the literature reflecting diverse philosophic perspectives. Parkes' theory of bereavement was selected to frame this chapter based on its broad philosophic scope and pertinence to bereavement after cancer deaths. Findings reported by other bereavement investigators will be integrated into the discussion of Parkes' body of work.

HEALTH EFFECTS OF BEREAVEMENT

One of Parkes' earliest studies examined, through a retrospective review of medical records, the number of physician visits sought by London widows after their husband's death compared with the number of visits sought before the death. It was shown that there was a 63 per cent rise in physician consultation visits among three quarters of the sample during the first 6 months of bereavement (Parkes, 1964).

A subsequent study compared bereaved widows and widowers to nonbereaved control subjects on indexes of health and emotional disturbance. In this study bereaved subjects differed significantly from control subjects in sleep disturbances, appetite and weight changes, and consumption of alcohol, tobacco, and tranquilizers (Parkes, 1972).

The relationship between health effects and bereavement has been further examined by other bereavement researchers. Clayton (1990) asserted that the essence of the morbidity of bereavement occurs because of the increased use of alcohol, tranquilizers, hypnotics, cigarettes, and other substances. Increased mortality occurs in the first year of bereavement in men younger than 75 years of age, but mortality did not increase in women or parents during the first year. Pathologic grief, defined as a continued depressive symptom, occurred in approximately 15 per cent of bereaved persons when they were initially widowed.

Bartrop, Lockhurst, Lazarus, Kiloh, and Penny (1977) were the first investigators to report a relationship between bereavement and decreased lymphocyte stimulation 8 weeks after bereavement. Schleifer, Keller, Camerino, Thomton, and Stein (1983) also found depressed lymphocyte stimulation in widowers within 2 months after the death of their spouse as compared with prebereavement lymphocyte stimulation. Linn, Linn, and Jensen (1984) found significant lymphocyte reduction in bereaved men. Spratt and Denney (1991) reported that bereaved parents showed significantly decreased T-suppresser cells when compared with control subjects during the first 8 months of bereavement. Consistently, bereaved family members demonstrate depressed immune status within days to months after the death. These results underscore Parkes' early suspicions that bereavement may leave survivors vulnerable to increased symptoms and an illness episode.

PHASES OF GRIEVING

From the earliest studies it has been apparent that bereavement is not an event, but rather a process. To determine what constitutes the "normal" process of bereavement, it has been necessary to study and describe the experience of bereaved individuals over time. Parkes' (1970) longitudinal investigation following London widows for 13 months provided description of the psychologic reaction to and process of grieving.

This process is characterized by four general phases: (1) numbness, (2) yearning and protest, (3) disorganization, and (4) recovery. Numbness characterizes the initial reaction to death most frequently experienced. During this initial phase episodes of panic or distress alternate with periods of numbness. For the widows in Parkes' (1970) study, this phase persisted for 5 to 7 days.

In the second phase, yearning and protest, the bereaved widows experienced two opposing drives. The first drive was that of intense pining for their deceased husbands. Parkes (1970) believed pining to be the singular feature of grief that distinguishes it from other affective states. Pining is a form of separation anxiety whereby the bereaved individual attempts to recover the lost person despite the futility in doing so. The theoretic explanation for this phenomenon is based on Bowlby's Attachment Theory (1973). Crying is common in this phase and may reflect an unconscious attempt to be reunited with the lost person just as an infant uses crying to signal needs to a parent who is temporarily out of sight (Parkes, 1970).

In Parkes' study the widows described being drawn to places and things they associated with their husbands. They also reported being preoccupied with thoughts of their husband particularly in the early months of bereavement and near the anniversary of the death. The "protest" drive experienced during this phase is characterized by feelings of anger and guilt as well as a sense of restless energy. It was not uncommon for the widows to direct their anger at health care providers in an effort to somehow assign blame for their loss. The time frame for the "phase of yearning and protest" was less uniform than that of numbness. However, behaviors characteristic of yearning and protest were most common between the second to fourth weeks of bereavement.

The phase after yearning and protest is that of disorganization. This phase is characterized by apathy and aimlessness. Subjects could not yet view the future with a positive outlook. In his study Parkes found that after 13 months of bereavement, two thirds of his sample were still in this phase. This finding was unexpected given that earlier investigators suggested the process of bereavement occurred in a shorter time frame.

Parkes did not refer to recovery in the 1970 investigation describing the phases of bereavement. He believed the 13 month duration of the study did not allow enough time to observe recovery in most of the widows in the sample. Later he designed investigations to follow subjects for 2 to 4 years (1972). Parkes refers to recovery in general as the time when the intensity, frequency, and duration of the "pangs" of grief diminish. Recovery occurs in varying lengths of time depending upon unique aspects of the relationship that are lost (Parkes, 1985). Parkes points out, however, that although recovery can be expected for the bereaved, grief never clearly ends.

The phases of bereavement described by Parkes provide a clinically useful model as shown in Table 10–1.

While time frames for and specific characteristics of bereavement phases are highly individualized, this model provides direction in the planning and development of nursing interventions to assist the bereaved. With Parkes' model as a guide, nursing care can be specific to the symptoms and behaviors characteristic of the varying phases of bereavement rather than provide standard bereavement interventions regardless of the phase. The clinical outcomes of phase-specific bereavement interventions could then be tested, further expanding upon Parkes' model.

VARIABLES AFFECTING BEREAVEMENT

To gain increased understanding as to why some people recover from bereavement without intervention and others suffer long-term effects, it has been necessary to investigate variables believed to influence bereavement outcomes. Multiple variables related to both the deceased and the bereaved have been found to affect patterns of grieving. Although it is impossible to present all of the variables shown to influence bereavement in the scope of a chapter, three broad categories of variables will be considered with respect to bereavement outcomes: time, type of relationship, and social support.

TIME

Time has been shown to be a very important variable when bereavement outcomes are considered. Time has been studied in terms of time elapsed since the death, the time available to anticipate and prepare for a death, and the timeliness of death in the life cycle.

TABLE 10–1. *Phases of Bereavement and Nursing Implications*

	NUMBNESS ⟶	YEARNING AND PROTEST ⟶	DISORGANIZATION ⟶	RECOVERY
Characteristic symptoms	Panic attacks alternating with periods of numbness	*Yearning* • Crying • Preoccupied with thoughts of deceased • Desire to be near objects or places associated with deceased *Protest* • Restlessness • Angry outbursts • Feelings of guilt	• Apathy • Hopelessness • Helpfulness • Depressed mood • Social withdrawal	• Pangs of grief diminish • Appetite returns • Sexual interests return
Nursing care	Encourage support system to be available to bereaved without hovering. Reassure family that "numbness" does not reflect indifference or mental illness	Allow/encourage ventilation Encourage use of community support groups Reassure family that searching behaviors are normal Discourage family from disposing of articles of the deceased's in attempts to be helpful Avoid defensiveness when anger is directed toward health care	Assist bereaved to problem solve Offer positive reinforcement on decision making Monitor physical status: • Nutritional intake • Weight loss • Sleep disturbances • Substance abuse	Acknowledge new strengths and skills gained having survived a significant loss Reassure bereaved that grief never fully ends and that anniversary reactions can be expected Memorial rituals may be helpful and should be explored

There is a great deal of debate over how long "normal" bereavement lasts. A number of investigations of spousal bereavement have examined the relationship between time elapsed since the loss of the deceased and bereavement outcomes (Bowling, 1988–1989; Demi, 1984a; Jacobs, Kasl, Ostfeld, Berkman, & Charpentier, 1986; Jacobs, Kasl, Ostfeld, Berkman, Kosten, & Charpentier, 1986; Klerman & Izen, 1977; Thompson, Breckenridge, Gallagher, & Peterson, 1984; Vezina, Bourque, & Belanger, 1988; Windholz, Marmar, & Horowitz, 1985; Zisook & Shuchter, 1985). In general, these investigations support Parkes' (1970) early findings of a general decrease in symptoms and psychologic distress 4 to 5 months after the loss of a spouse.

Vachon, Rogers, Lyall, Lancee, Sheldon, & Freeman (1982) reported that a high proportion of those widows who are symptomatic at 4 months after their loss continue to have difficulty at 1 year or longer. Parkes and Brown (1972), in an investigation using a nonbereaved control group, found that subjects who were bereaved for 1 year remained distinguishable from the nonbereaved by depression and autonomic symptoms. A steady decline in depression and autonomic symptoms continued until 3 years after the death.

Parkes (1975) also investigated the relationship between the length of time spousal survivors had to prepare for the death and bereavement outcomes. Widows who had had a shorter time to prepare for the death of their spouse experienced negative bereavement outcomes characterized by a "depressive symptom complex" still present 13 months after the death. Parkes (1975) noted that the widow or widower who was prepared for the death made a better adjustment during the period of bereavement than the widow or widower who was not prepared for the death of the spouse.

With respect to the variable of time, an appropriate death was defined as one that was anticipated, occurring in the natural order of life, in an older person. An inappropriate death was defined as one that occurred outside of the expected life cycle, in a young person, and was not anticipated.

RELATIONSHIP

Another important variable influencing bereavement is the relationship that was lost. Different relationships meet varying needs across the life span. It follows that the particularities of the relationship of the deceased to the mourner can influence the grief experience. Although it is impossible to rank relationship losses in order of their bereavement severity, it may be possible to better understand particular bereavement responses by considering the relationship that was lost. Bugen posits that two dimensions of a relationship are predictive of bereavement outcome: the degree of closeness and the mourner's perception of preventability of the death (1977).

Bereavement following the loss of specific kinship and conjugal relationships have been the most often studied. As previously mentioned, most of what is known about bereavement is based on conjugal loss. Fulton (1987) noted in a large descriptive study of bereavement responses, that surviving spouses and parents reported symptoms of grief, whereas adult children, after the death of a parent, reported no disturbance in life pattern. Sanders (1979–1980) found significantly higher intensities of grief in parents surviving the death of their child when compared with bereavement responses after the death of a spouse or parent.

These investigations, while supporting the fact that bereavement differs after the loss of different relationships, are few in number and scope. Bereavement after the loss of other important relationships such as siblings, grandparents, and friends deserve further study. Bereavement care can then be modified to meet individual needs when more is learned about the grief process after the loss of key relationships.

SOCIAL SUPPORT

Social support, a concept with multiple components, is another important variable in bereavement research. The presence of support network factors were shown to differentiate those "at risk" from those who were bereaved after both a cancer death and a death from another cause (Vachon et al., 1982). Vachon further asserted that there must be a balance between the amount of support offered and the threat engendered by a particular situation. Support that is offered but does not correspond with the needs of the individual may not be perceived by the individual as helpful (Vachon & Stylianos, 1988). Despite the fact that hundreds of studies investigated social support, many areas such as the analysis of helpful and unhelpful behaviors between bereaved persons and supportive others are in need of research (Davidowitz & Myrick, 1984). The timing of support as well as costs and benefits of being a support person (Kessler, McLeod, & Wethington, 1983; Parkes & Weiss, 1983) are also in need of further research.

Social support may be lacking for the bereaved after deaths from stigmatized causes such as suicide, alcoholism, and acquired immunodeficiency syndrome (AIDS), or after deaths of stigmatized relationships. Fears of being judged by others may lead bereaved individuals to become withdrawn and isolated. When a person experiences loss of a meaningful and significant attachment and is restricted from openly acknowledging the loss, grief is disenfranchised; preventing the mourner from receiving social support.

The AIDS crisis has given increased recognition of the need to explore grief reactions that had previously been disenfranchised such as the loss of an ex-spouse, the loss of a lover in an extramarital affair, the loss of a person with whom the bereaved has co-habitated, and the loss of a lover of the same gender (Doka, 1989).

VARIABLES PREDICTIVE OF NEGATIVE OUTCOMES

With retrospective analyses, numerous variables such as those just described and others beyond the scope of this chapter have been found to correlate with negative bereavement outcomes. This knowledge has been useful toward understanding the phenomenon of bereavement in hindsight. However, this knowledge is not sufficient to assist the clinician in making a judgment prospectively as to which individuals who are to become bereaved are more likely to need help than others.

To that end Parkes conducted an investigation to identify the variables most predictive of negative bereavement outcomes. Parkes examined correlations between assessments of psychologic state after bereavement and subsequent appraisals of recovery (Parkes & Weiss, 1983). With discriminant function analysis on data obtained in a descriptive longitudinal study of spousal bereavement, Parkes identified variables that were highly predictive of negative bereavement outcomes. This analysis led to the development of an eight item instrument shown in Box 10–1. The variables most predictive of negative bereavement outcomes include young age, low socioeconomic status, lack of preparation for the death, clinging or pining, anger, self-reproach, lack of family support, and clinician's prediction of negative outcome. Subjects are rated on each of the items, and a total score is calculated. Higher scores indicate higher risk for negative bereavement outcomes. A total score of 18 or greater indicates the subject is at high risk for negative bereavement outcomes. Additionally, any subject receiving a 4 or 5 on the clinician's prediction for outcome is considered high risk regardless of total score (Parkes & Weiss, 1983). The validity of Parkes' instrument was supported with an independent sample as described in Box 10–2.

Knowledge of key variables placing individuals at risk for negative bereavement outcomes allows clinicians working with the bereaved to identify those at greatest risk for negative bereavement outcomes and to prioritize the distribution of resources available to assist the bereaved toward recovery. The instrument developed by Parkes is intended for clinical application, because it can be quickly completed and scored.

GRIEF IN SURVIVORS OF CANCER PATIENTS

The unique aspects of a death from cancer may complicate the process of the survivor's bereavement. Shubin (1978) reported that cancer widows reported more anger and helplessness than widows whose hus-

---

Box 10–1. *Bereavement Risk Index*

A. Age of key person (applies only if key person is spouse)
1. 75+
2. 66-75
3. 56-65
4. 46-55
5. 15-45

B. Occupation of principle wage-earner of key person's family
1. Professional and executive
2. Semiprofessional
3. Office and clerk
4. Skilled manual
5. Semiskilled manual
6. Unskilled manual

C. Length of key person's preparation for patient's death
1. Fully prepared for long period
2. Fully prepared for less than 2 weeks
3. Partly prepared
4. Totally unprepared

D. Clinging or Pining
1. Never
2. Seldom
3. Moderate
4. Frequent
5. Constant
6. Constant and intense

E. Anger
1. None (or normal)
2. Mild irritation
3. Moderate—occasional outbursts
4. Severe—spoiling relationships
5. Extreme—always bitter

F. Self-Reproach
1. None
2. Mild—vague
3. Moderate—some clear self reproach
4. Severe—preoccupied with self blame
5. Extreme—major problem

G. Family
1. Warm—will give full support
2. Doubtful
3. Family supportive but lives at distance
4. Family not supportive
5. No family

H. How will key person cope?
1. Well—normal grief and recovery without special help
2. Fair—probably get by without special help
3. Doubtful—may need special help
4. Badly—requires special help
5. Very Badly—requires urgent help

From *Recovery From Bereavement* by Colin Murray Parkes & Robert S. Weiss. Copyright (c) 1983 by Colin Murray Parkes and Robert S. Weiss. Reprinted by permission of BasicBooks, a division of HarperCollins Publishers, Inc.

bands died of cardiovascular disease. Parkes' model provides some guidance as to why this would occur given that circumstances surrounding death can greatly influence bereavement outcomes. For example, cancer treatment perceived by a family to have been ineffective or mismanaged could place families at high risk for negative bereavement outcomes.

The burden of caring for the cancer patient may also influence bereavement. Bass and Bowman (1990) examined two competing hypotheses about the relationship between care-related strain and the difficulty adjusting to an ill relative's death. One hypothesis suggested that family members who perceive caregiving as stressful will experience some relief when their relative dies, because care responsibilities end. An alternative hypothesis posits the opposite relationship, suggesting that greater strain on family members during the pa-

tient's illness results in greater strain during bereavement. Panel data from spouse and adult-child caregivers collected before and after the death supported the second hypothesis. Respondents who appraised caregiving as more difficult with negative caregiving consequences for the family, assessed bereavement as more difficult with greater bereavement strain for the family.

Biegel, Sales, and Schulz (1991) suggested that the demands of providing care to relatives for prolonged periods of time may affect the roles of caregivers in a number of ways. The most frequently studied symptoms among caregivers are those indicating depression, burden, and physical morbidity (Given, Stommet, Given, Osuch, Kurtz, & Kurtz, 1993). A scale to measure caregiver burden was described by Given, Given, Stommet, Collins, King, and Franklin (1992).

Box 10–2. *An Investigation of Spousal Bereavement*

Robinson, L. A., Nuamah, I. F., Lev, E., & McCorkle, R. (in press). A prospective longitudinal investigation of spousal bereavement examining Parkes and Weiss' Bereavement Risk Index. *Journal of Palliative Care.*

The purpose of this study was (1) to describe spousal bereavement both prospectively and longitudinally and (2) to examine the validity of the Bereavement Risk Index (BRI) published by Parkes and Weiss. Using the Brief Symptom Inventory (BSI), psychological distress was measured in 46 subjects across five time intervals starting before a spousal death and ending 25 months after the death. The criterion related validity of Parkes' instrument to discriminate between those at high and low risk for psychologic distress was supported during measurements taken within 2 months of the patient's diagnosis (prior to death), at 6 weeks after the death, and 6 and 13 months thereafter. These findings support the need for early identification of individuals at high risk for negative bereavement outcomes even before the death.

There appears to be a relationship between cancer patients' psychologic states, diagnoses, and losses in functioning and the well-being or depression of their caregivers including immediate family (Baider & De-Nour, 1988; Ryan, 1987). Researchers focusing on the impact of cancer on the patient and the family identified lung cancer, which has a rapid course and poor prognosis, as being different from cancer of a much longer duration and a greater chance for cure or remission (Ryan, 1987). In addition, because at least 80 per cent of all lung cancer is caused by smoking and is thus preventable, survivors' feelings of guilt and blame may complicate bereavement. Results of a pilot study indicated that problematic alternations in marital and family relationships occurred in patients with lung cancer and that the needs of the spouse often were unmet (Cooper, 1984). Communication problems between spouses were reported. Twice as many spouses as patients reported the presence of signs of stress such as nervousness, sleeplessness, loss of appetite, inability to concentrate, and irritability. Spouses reported they felt helpless as they saw their mates' deterioration.

BEREAVEMENT INTERVENTION

It is important to now move beyond description of the phenomenon of bereavement and begin to plan interventions that will alleviate suffering among survivors. It is clear from the review of the literature that not all bereaved persons require formal intervention to facilitate recovery. It has been suggested that intervention is only warranted for subjects with high-risk factors who may not return to prebereaved status as time elapses (Windholz et al., 1985).

Parkes has described three broad models of bereavement care available in the United States: professional care, mutual support groups and hospice care (1987). Professional care is private care usually provided by a mental health professional. This type of care is expensive and therefore not accessible to many. Mutual support is characterized by a nonprofessional group format. This model of bereavement care is inexpensive but may not be suitable to individuals who resist joining groups or are intimidated by them. Hospice care is limited to the relatives of patients who have died under the care of a hospice.

Bereaved persons may enter the health care system by self-referral or when a nurse or other health professional identifies the need for bereavement intervention in family members of dying patients. Crisis intervention, one type of intervention for bereaved persons, focuses on the characteristic course of a particular crisis such as the death of a loved one. Specific interventions aimed at adaptive resolution of the crisis may be given in individual or group therapy before or after the death of the patient. Emphasis is placed on the decreased adjustment of the person in crisis and the processes needed to regain a precrisis or higher level of functioning (Aguilera & Messick, 1978).

Parkes and Parkes (1984) investigated the effects of bereavement care provided to spouses of cancer patients during the period of time that the patient was dying. Subjects receiving bereavement care at St. Christopher's Hospice suffered significantly less anxiety after the death of their spouse when compared with subjects at other local hospitals who had received no bereavement care.

To evaluate the effects of a comprehensive program of care for cancer patients (Cameron & Parkes, 1983) on bereaved family members, 20 close relatives of patients who had died in a palliative care unit (PCU) were compared with a matched group of 20 relatives of patients who had died of cancer in other units of the same teaching hospital. Interviewed by telephone 2 weeks and 1 year after the death of the patient, relatives of patients in the PCU reported fewer psychologic symptoms and less lasting grief and anger than relatives of patients who had died elsewhere. Factors during the patients' dying that were thought to have contributed to more positive outcomes for the bereaved included successful relief of pain, awareness by relatives of the coming death of the patient, and support given to relatives during bereavement.

The efficacy of bereavement counseling for widows thought to have a poor outcome was supported when, after 13 months, significantly more were found to have progressed favorably than those in a control group who received no counseling. Counseling included encouraging the bereaved to recall and recount in detail the events that led up to the loss, the circumstances surrounding the loss, and experiences since the loss. The history of the relationship including satisfactions and deficiencies were also reviewed. It was found that until the bereaved had progressed in the review of the past and reorientation towards the future, giving advice did far more harm than good (Bowlby, 1977). Raphael (1982) reported that support from health professionals both before and after the death of the patient resulted in increased well-being for the bereaved.

Sociocultural influences may affect grief and should be considered when planning bereavement interventions. Cultural influences on bereavement may interact with economic variables, social support variables, or both in ways that enhance or decrease bereavement. Pickett (1993) described a method of achieving more culturally appropriate intervention strategies with patients and families experiencing loss and grief. There is a paucity of research investigating cultural and ethnic variables of bereavement, despite the fact that differences in traditions of various groups have been described (Osterweis et al., 1984).

Regardless of the method of intervention selected, it is important to monitor the response of the bereaved to the care provided. Demi (1984b) has suggested the following goals when evaluating the success of programs targeted to bereaved persons: (1) decreased emotional pain, (2) recognition, expression, and acceptance of feelings, (3) increased understanding of the grief process, (4) recognition of the normal manifestations of grief, (5) development of healthy coping behaviors, (6) acceptance of the reality and irreversibility of death, (7) development of a support system, (8) development of a realistic memory of the deceased, (9) promotion of personal growth, (10) reinvestment of oneself in life, (11) recognition of one's own strengths and weaknesses, and (12) reestablishment of a spiritual belief system.

Much still needs to be learned to plan and implement bereavement interventions that best fit with the individual needs of the person who has suffered a loss. Regardless of the model or particular implementation strategy employed, there is encouraging evidence of the value in offering such care to those who are most distressed.

IMPLICATIONS FOR NURSING PRACTICE

Throughout the cancer illness trajectory there are critical points where health professionals have opportunities to intervene with those who will survive. Based on the review of the literature it is possible for practicing nurses to identify persons at high risk of suffering prolonged and negative bereavement outcomes (see Box 10–3). Although the responsibility for health professionals' involvement with family members may seem obvious, recent literature has cited problems in this area (Osterweis et al., 1984). Nurses interact with both the dying and survivors of the dying more than other health professionals (Kalish, 1985), and therefore they seem likely to be the health care professional to provide counseling and assistance. However, nurses' own fears of death may be nonverbally expressed through depersonalized modes of care fragmenting the care of the dying patient and soon-to-be bereaved family (Lev, 1986). Providing opportunities to deal with existential questions assists family members to communicate concerns, seek meaning, and provide an opportunity to bring closure to life with the patient (Benoliel, 1993).

Although facilitating separation from the dying patient may be accomplished by providing opportunities for the patient and family members to communicate (Osterweis et al., 1984), it is critical for the nurse to assess the patient's and family's individual needs. Some families desire open communication with the dying member, whereas other families do not (Hinton, 1980). In families that normally avoid discussion of emotionally laden issues, this pattern most likely will be repeated when one member is dying. Family members may try to protect one another from the painful awareness of death. Not all families need to communicate about death. Those who have comfortable, agreed-upon patterns of avoiding discussion of feelings within the family may cope effectively with silence. Fifty-nine per cent of widows who reported not having discussed death with their partner said that it made no difference in terms of their later adjustment during the period of bereavement (Vachon et al., 1977). This suggests that nondiscussion of death may be an effective coping mechanism for some people. Clayton (1990) asserted further that no data currently exist supporting the idea that painful feelings are best dealt with by being expressed.

IMPLICATIONS FOR NURSING RESEARCH AND THEORY DEVELOPMENT

Parkes' published works provide a descriptive theory of spousal bereavement, the content of which has been well supported by other investigators. Parkes' philosophic view of bereavement as both a social and emotional event is consistent with nursing's general frame of reference, contending that the person can not be viewed outside the context of his or her environment. Descriptive theory is, however, the most basic type of theory in that it only states what is (Fawcett & Downs, 1992).

The current challenge to nurses working with the bereaved is to build on descriptive theory to examine the why's of bereavement. By studying the relationships between concepts identified by Parkes and others, explanatory and predictive theories of bereavement may be generated.

Whether bereavement research is designed to describe or test variables, methods of measurement must be given serious consideration. The need to measure various components of bereavement to facilitate further study of the phenomenon has been acknowledged (Lev, Munro, & McCorkle, 1993; Parkes, 1975, 1985; Sanders, 1989). A short version of an instrument measuring bereavement was reported to be a concise, valid, and reliable measure sensitive to the grief experience that may be useful for assessing bereavement in clinical settings (Box 10–4).

SUMMARY

Despite striking improvements in the care of dying people and their families in recent years, care for the bereaved is provided as an episodic luxury (Osterweis et al., 1984; Potocky, 1993). While additional research is needed to demonstrate outcomes of specific bereavement interventions, care must be initiated now for the newly bereaved. Evidence has been presented indicating that when bereavement care is provided to persons at special risk, there is a reduction in pathologic consequences. Clinicians caring for dying patients have an

---

Box 10–3. *Variables Placing Individuals at High Risk for Negative Bereavement Outcomes*

Survivor characteristics

- Young age
- Closely related to deceased (spouse, parent, child, sibling)
- History of depressive illness or otherwise compromised health status
- Lack of social support
- Low socioeconomic status

Circumstances surrounding death

- Short length of illness
- Untimeliness of death in the expected lifecycle

Box 10–4. *An Instrument Measuring Bereavement*

Lev, E., Munro, B. H., & McCorkle, R. (1993). A shortened version of an instrument measuring bereavement. *International Journal of Nursing Studies, 30,* 213–226.

The purpose of this study was to develop a tool to measure the grief experience. The Grief Experience Inventory (GEI) (Sanders et al., A Manual for the Grief Experience Inventory. C. M. Sanders, Charlotte, NC [1979]) was revised according to Parkes' (Bereavement: Studies of Grief in Adult Life. International Universities Press, New York [1972]) framework. Four hundred eighteen subjects who had been primary caregivers for significant others before the loss of the person through death completed Revised Grief Experience (RGEI) questionnaires. The internal consistency reliability (coefficient alpha) for the RGEI was 0.93. A principal components factor rotation was performed yielding a four-factor solution consistent with the theoretic structure (Parkes, 1972). Results demonstrated that the RGEI is a concise, valid, and reliable measure sensitive to the grief experience.

---

opportunity to assess family members for the variables placing them at high risk for negative bereavement outcomes and to make referrals for bereavement care for those who need it during the patient's recovery and thereafter.

It has been the intent in this chapter to present an overview of the bereavement literature in the context of Parkes' model to help nurses better understand the impact of bereavement on family members after a death. Too often nursing care ceases with the death of the patient, leaving bereaved family members alone in their suffering. Cancer nurses, by virtue of their close involvement with dying patients and professional preparation, are in an ideal position to recognize those family members at greatest risk for negative bereavement outcomes and to initiate bereavement care.

REFERENCES

Aguilera, D. C., & Messick, J. M. (1978) *Crisis intervention: Theory and intervention.* St. Louis: C.V. Mosby.

Baider, L., & De-Nour, A. T. (1988). Adjustment to cancer: Who is the patient—the husband or the wife? *Israel Journal of Medical Sciences, 24,* 631–636.

Bartrop, R. W., Lockhurst, E., Lazarus, L., Kiloh, L. G., & Penny, R. (1977). Depressed lymphocyte function after bereavement. *Lancet, 1,* 834–836.

Bass, D. M., & Bowman, K. (1990). The transition from caregiving to bereavement: The relationship of care-related strain and adjustment to death. *Gerontologist, 30,* 35–42.

Benoliel, J. Q. (1985). Loss and adaptation: Circumstances, contingencies, and consequences. *Death Studies, 9,* 217–235.

Benoliel, J. Q. (1993). Personal care in an impersonal world. In J. D. Morgan (Ed.) *Personal care in an impersonal world: A multidimensional look at bereavement.* Amityville, NY: Baywood Publishing Co.

Biegel, D. E., Sales, E., & Schulz, R. (1991). *Family caregiving in chronic illness.* Newbury Park, CA: Sage Publications.

Bowlby, J. (1973). *Attachment and loss, Vol. 2.* Anger. New York: Basic Books.

Bowlby, J. (1977). The making and breaking of affectional bonds: Some principles of psychotherapy. *British Journal of Psychiatry, 130,* 421–431.

Bowling, A. (1988–1989). Who dies after widow(er)hood? A discriminant analysis. *Omega Journal of Death and Dying, 19,* 135–153.

Bugen, L. A. (1977). Human grief: A model for prediction and intervention. *American Journal of Orthopsychiatry, 47,* 196–206.

Cameron, J., & Parkes, C. M. (1983). Terminal care: Evaluation of effects on surviving family of care before and after bereavement. *Postgraduate Medicine Journal, 59,* 73–78.

Clayton, P. J. (1990). Bereavement and depression. *Journal of Clinical Psychiatry, 51,* 34–38.

Cooper, E. T. (1984). A pilot study on the effects of the diagnosis of lung cancer on family relationships. *Cancer Nursing, 7,* 301–308.

Davidowitz, M., & Myrick, R. D. (1984). Responding to the bereaved: An analysis of "helping" statements. *Research Record, 1,* 35–42.

Demi, A. S. (1984a). Social adjustment of widows after a sudden death: Suicide and non-suicide survivors compared. *Death Education, 8(suppl),* 9–11.

Demi, A. S. (1984b). Hospice bereavement program: Trends and issues. In S. H. Schraff (Ed.), *Hospice: The nursing perspective* (pp. 131–151). New York: The National League for Nursing.

Doka, K. J. (1989). *Disenfranchised grief.* Lexington, MA: Lexington Books.

Fawcett, J., & Downs, F. S. (1992). *The relationship of theory and research* (2nd ed.). Philadelphia: F.A. Davis.

Fulton, R. (1987). The many faces of grief. *Death Studies, 11,* 243–256.

Given, C. W., Given, B., Stommet, M., Collins, C., King, S., & Franklin, S. (1992). The caregiver reaction assessment (CRA) for caregivers to persons with chronic physical and mental impairments. *Research in Nursing and Health, 15,* 271–283.

Given, C. W., Stommet, M., Given, B., Osuch, J., Kurtz, M. E., & Kurtz, J. C. (1993). The influence of cancer patients' symptoms and functional states on patients' depression and family caregivers' reaction and depression. *Health Psychology, 12,* 277–285.

Hinton, J. (1980). The cancer ward. *Advances in Psychosomatic Medicine, 10,* 78–98.

Jacobs, S., Kasl, S., Ostfeld, A., Berkman, & Charpentier, P. (1986). The measurement of grief: Age and sex variation. *British Journal of Medical Psychology, 59,* 305–310.

Jacobs, S. C., Kasl, S. V., Ostfeld, A. M., Berkman, L., Kosten, T. R., & Charpentier, P. (1986). The measurement of grief: Bereaved versus non-bereaved. *The Hospice Journal, 2,* 21–36.

Kalish, R. A. (1985). *Death, grief, and caring relationships.* Monterey, CA: Brooks/Cole Publishing Co.

Kessler, R. C., McLeod, J. D., & Wethington, E. (1983). The costs of caring: A perspective on the relationship between sex and psychological distress. In I. G. Sarason & B. R. Sarason (Eds.), *Social support: Theory, research and applications.* The Hague: Martinus.

Klerman, G. L., & Izen, J. E. (1977). The effects of bereavement and grief on physical health and general well-being. *Advances in Psychosomatic Medicine, 9,* 63–104.

Lev, E. L. (1986). Effects of course in hospice nursing: Attitudes and behaviors of baccalaureate school of nursing undergraduates and graduates, *Psychological Reports, 59,* 847–858.

Lev, E. L., Munro, B. H., & McCorkle, R. (1993). A shortened version of an instrument measuring bereavement. *International Journal of Nursing Studies, 30,* 213–226.

Lindemann, E. (1944). Symptomatology and management of acute grief. *American Journal of Psychiatry, 101,* 141–148.

Linn, M. W., Linn, B. S., Jensen, J. (1984). Stressful events, dysphoric mood, and immune responsiveness. *Psychological Reports, 54,* 219–222.

Osterweis, M., Solomon, F., & Green, M. (1984). *Bereavement: Reactions, consequences and care.* Report of the Institute of Medicine, National Academy Press.

Parkes, C. M. (1964). Recent bereavement as a cause of mental illness. *British Journal of Psychiatry, 110,* 198–204.

Parkes, C. M. (1970). The first year of bereavement: A longitudinal study of the reaction of London widows to the death of their husbands. *Psychiatry, 33,* 449–461.

Parkes, C. M. (1972). *Bereavement: Studies of grief in adult life.* New York: International Universities Press.

Parkes, C. M. (1975). Unexpected and untimely bereavement: A statistical study of young Boston widows and widowers. In B. Schoenberg, I. Gerber, A. Wiener, A. H. Kutscher, D. Peretz, & A. C. Carr (Eds.), *Bereavement: Its psychosocial aspects.* New York: Columbia University Press.

Parkes, C. M. (1985). Bereavement. *British Journal of Psychiatry, 146,* 11–17.

Parkes, C. M. (1987). Models of bereavement care. *Death Studies, 11,* 257–261.

Parkes, C. M., & Brown, R. J. (1972). Health after bereavement: A controlled study of young Boston widows and widowers. *Psychosomatic Medicine, 3,* 449–461.

Parkes, C. M., & Parkes, J. (1984). 'Hospice' versus 'hospital' care—Re-evaluation after 10 years as seen by surviving spouses. *Postgraduate Medicine Journal, 60,* 120–124.

Parkes, C. M., & Weiss, R. S. (1983). *Recovery from Bereavement.* New York: Basic Books.

Pickett, M. (1993). Cultural awareness in the context of terminal illness. *Cancer Nursing, 16,* 102–106.

Potocky, M. (1993). Effective services for bereaved spouses: A content analysis of the empirical literature. *Health and Social Work, 18,* 288–301.

Raphael, B. (1982). *The Anatomy of Bereavement.* New York: Basic Books.

Robinson, L., Nuamah, I., Lev, E., & McCorkle, R. (in press). A prospective longitudinal investigation of spousal bereavement examining Parkes and Weiss' Bereavement Risk Index. *Journal of Palliative Care.*

Ryan, L. S. (1987). Lung cancer: Psychosocial implications. *Seminars in Oncology Nursing, 3,* 222–227.

Sanders, C. M. (1979–1980). A comparison of adult bereavement in the death of a spouse, child and parent. *Omega, 10,* 303–322.

Sanders, C. M. (1989). *Grief: The mourning after.* New York: John Wiley & Sons.

Schleifer, S. L., Keller, S. E., Camerino, M., Thomton, J. C., & Stein, M. (1983). Suppression of lymphocyte stimulation following bereavement. *Journal of the American Medical Association, 250,* 374–377.

Shubin, S. (1978). Cancer widows—a special challenge. *Nursing, 8,* 56–60.

Spratt, M. L., & Denney, D. R. (1991). Immune variables, depression, and plasma cortisol over time in suddenly bereaved parents. *Journal Neuropsychiatry Clinical Neuroscience, 3,* 299–306.

Thompson, L. W., Breckenridge, J. N., Gallagher, D. G., & Peterson, J. (1984). Effects of bereavement on self-perceptions of physical health in elderly widows and widowers. *Journal of Gerontology, 39,* 309–314.

Vachon, M. L., Freedman, A. F., Rogers, J., Lyall, W., & Freeman, S. (1977). The final illness in cancer: The widow's perspective. *Canadian Medical Association Journal, 117,* 1151–1157.

Vachon, M., Rogers, J., Lyall, W. A., Lancee, W. J., Sheldon, A., & Freeman, S. J. (1982). Predictors and correlates of adaptation to conjugal bereavement. *American Journal of Psychiatry, 139,* 998–1002.

Vachon, M. L. S., & Stylianos, S. (1988). The role of social support in bereavement. *Journal of Social Issues, 44,* 175–190.

Vezina, J., Bourque, P., Belanger, Y. (1988). Spousal loss: Depression, anxiety and well being after grief periods of varying lengths. *Canadian Journal on Aging, 7,* 391–396.

Windholz, M. J., Marmar, C. R., & Horowitz, M. J. (1985). A review of the research on conjugal bereavement: Impact on health and efficacy of intervention. *Comprehensive Psychiatry, 26,* 433–447.

Zisook, S., & Shuchter, S. (1985). Time course of spousal bereavement. *General Hospital Psychiatry, 7,* 95–100.

UNIT III
CANCER AS A DISEASE

Epidemiologic Principles for Cancer Nursing Practice

Denise M. Oleske

The increased life expectancy of the United States population is one indicator of the health of the nation. However, this phenomenon raises new challenges—namely, the increased likelihood of health problems associated with an aging society and problems stemming from technology and associated lifestyles that in themselves may promote chronic diseases such as cancer. Epidemiology is the study of the distribution and determinants of disease in a population. In addition, its methods assist in the identification of factors associated with the development of cancer. This chapter discusses the application of epidemiologic principles relevant to nursing practice that aid in understanding the cancer problem and guide in the formulation of approaches to control it.

CLASSIFICATION SYSTEMS

Because *cancer* is a term that represents a process common to a very heterogeneous group of diseases, it is particularly important to be able to distinguish cases and classify them according to their type. Epidemiology has been in the forefront in stimulating efforts to improve the definition and classification of cancer. Currently, cancers are typically classified at diagnosis by anatomic site, cell type, and stage. The most widely used scheme for classifying cancers according to anatomic site is contained in the publication *The Inter-*

national Classification of Diseases, 9th revision (ICD-9). Each anatomic site is assigned a four-digit code, the first three digits indicating the general anatomic site and the fourth digit designating a subsite. Table 11–1 contains a list of the ICDs associated with neoplasia. Internationally accepted nomenclature for the histologic categorization of tumors is documented in the International Histological Classification of Tumors (World Health Organization, 1988–1992). The procedures generally followed for staging of a solid tumor are those described by the American Joint Committee on Cancer (Beahrs, Henson, Hutter, & Kennedy, 1992). Cancer stage may be based on clinical findings alone or include the observations made during a surgical procedure with the results of histopathologic studies. For some cancers additional laboratory information may be important in classification—for example, karyotyping in leukemia. The more exactly a neoplasm may be defined, the more precisely cancer epidemiologists may be able to identify its associated risk and prognostic factors.

DATA SOURCES FOR EPIDEMIOLOGIC RESEARCH

Data for epidemiologic research in cancer may be obtained either through existing systems or through the collection of primary data in surveys or other types of

TABLE 11–1. *Tabular List of Major Headings for Neoplasia in ICD-9*

CATEGORY OF MALIGNANT NEOPLASM	ICD-9 CODES
Lip, oral cavity, and pharynx	140–149
Digestive organs and peritoneum	150–159
Respiratory and intrathoracic organs	160–165
Connective tissue, skin, and breast	170–175
Genitourinary organs	179–189
Other, unspecified sites	190–199
Lymphatic and hematopoietic tissue	200–208
In situ	230–234

ICD-9, *International Classification of Diseases,* 9th Rev. (U.S. Department of Health and Human Services, 1989.)

studies. A number of resources useful to persons conducting epidemiologic studies are available. Those commonly utilized in cancer epidemiology studies are described in the following sections.

DECENNIAL CENSUS

Each decade the Bureau of the Census seeks to count each person in the United States according to "usual place of residence." In attempting to derive specific information about the population, a core set of questions is asked about each person within the housing unit contacted, and from a subset of these units a more detailed questionnaire is administered. The items covered on the core set are the following: name, household relationship, sex, race, age, marital status, Hispanic origin, and some characteristics of housing. Information on ancestry, previous residence, occupation, poverty status, and education are obtained from a sample. Data from the census are useful for constructing a demographic profile of the community of interest as well as serving as the denominator in calculating demiologic rate measures for geopolitically defined populations.

THE NATIONAL DEATH INDEX

Mortality information is useful for a variety of reasons in epidemiologic studies, including monitoring of vital status and outcomes of participants in prospective studies and in clinical trials. A central source of death record information called the National Death Index (NDI) is maintained by the National Center for Health Statistics (NCHS), and this index can assist investigators in these efforts (Calle & Terrell, 1993). To use this service, the investigator needs to complete an application form ensuring that the data are for health research and that provisions are made for maintaining confidentiality. Data files containing subjects' names and pertinent identification criteria are forwarded to the NDI, where the names are sought in the NDI's file. Computer reports returned may contain some false matches, thus requiring that death certificates be obtained from a state Vital Records Division to confirm the information received. The cost of the computerized service is nominal, and turn-around time for handling requests is short.

THE SEER PROGRAM

The principal source of national estimates of cancer incidence for the United States is the SEER (Surveillance, Epidemiology, and End Results) Program. Nine regional areas participate in this program and collect detailed information on the incidence and mortality of malignant neoplasms. The areas involved in the SEER program are Metropolitan Atlanta, Metropolitan Detroit, San Francisco-Oakland SMSA, the Seattle-Puget Sound area, and the entire states of Connecticut, Hawaii, Iowa, New Mexico, and Utah. The information collected for each cancer case includes demographic characteristics of the patient, anatomic site, histologic cell type, extent of disease at the time of diagnosis, treatment data, and vital status over time (Miller et al., 1993). From an epidemiologic perspective, the national cancer incidence data from the SEER program help identify demographic groups with exceptionally high or low risk of getting cancer. Population-based site-specific mortality and survival data also are accumulated in this program. From these data etiologic hypotheses and prognostic indicators can be generated, and effects of progress in treatment and programs geared to those target groups for cancer prevention and early detection can be developed. And, because SEER serves as a population-based surveillance system, the effects of cancer control measures may be evaluated.

CANCER REGISTRY

A cancer registry is one means of gathering data about the disease process and treatment efforts. It comprises the listing of cancer patients and the administrative system by which this listing is maintained and updated. The registry maintains only those data that are not likely to change: demographic characteristics (age at diagnosis of cancer, race, and sex), tumor characteristics at diagnosis (site, histology, stage), and general type of treatment. Most registries in the United States are hospital-based and have a service-oriented focus. Registries began with the intent of being a type of medical audit system to ensure quality care for cancer patients by recording information on the treatment process. Registries can also be a source of population-based control samples for experimental studies (Klawansky et al., 1991). Hospitals participating in the American College of Surgeons (ACS) cancer registry program are required to collect information on the histologic diagnosis obtained before treatment. In addition, registries are required to query physicians each year regarding the vital status of each treated patient, thereby promoting the continued follow-up of patients after the initiation of treatment. For epidemiologic purposes the hospital tumor registry is a useful source for the identification of incident cases in a case-control study. It is necessary, however, to be cautious in the use of cancer registries in instances in which more than one hospital serves a geographic area. In these circumstances patients may be listed in more than one registry because of second opinions, transfers for therapy resources, changes of physician, and so forth.

POPULATION SURVEYS

The National Health Survey was enacted through congressional legislation in 1956 to obtain periodic information about the health status and health needs of the United States population. This activity is carried out through the NCHS. Random samples of households are selected for the Health Interview Survey, in which questions are asked on acute and chronic conditions, activity limitations, and visits to a hospital, doctor, or dentist. Through the Health Examination Survey, random samples for the population are selected for a complete physical examination, which includes laboratory testing as well as electrocardiograms and pulmonary function testing. The National Health and Nutrition Examination Survey (NHANES), conducted from 1971 to 1975, represents the first time that interview and physical examination data were linked. In a random sample of the population, a detailed medical history was obtained and a dietary questionnaire was administered; in addition, the patient underwent a standardized medical examination in which blood and urine specimens were taken to obtain nutrient levels. These survey results provide prevalence information on the rates of illness and health problems of the United States population by geographic region. Excluding nonmelanoma skin cancer, the prevalence rate of all types of cancer was 3230 per 100,000 population. This means that approximately 3.2 per cent of adults in the U.S. are survivors of cancer, the largest proportion of which are women with breast cancer (Table 11–2).

In addition to periodic surveys of the health of the United States population, the NCHS also periodically surveys hospitals, skilled care facilities, and home care agencies to obtain information on utilization rates and personnel. Among persons diagnosed as having cancer, hospitalization rates and length of stay are declining in all age groups and for most cancer types (Graves, 1990, 1994). Changes in the financing of health care and the shift to the delivery of services in nonhospital settings have stimulated these trends. In 1992, the average length of hospital stay for cancer patients was 8.5 days. The length of stay for cancer patients increases after age 14 years with persons aged 65 years and over experiencing an average length of hospital stay of 9.0 days. The rate of inpatient hospital utilization for malignant neoplasms also declined from 68.4 per 100,000 population in 1988 to 62.2 per 100,000 in 1992. Data on the rates of health care utilization may be used to represent levels of realized access to health care in an area. They may also assist in the planning of facilities and personnel for delivering health care.

THE BEHAVIORAL RISK FACTOR SURVEILLANCE SYSTEM

The Behavioral Risk Factor Surveillance System (BRFSS) was started by the Centers for Disease Control and Prevention in 1984 for the purpose of rapidly obtaining continuous information on the prevalence rates of personal behaviors associated

TABLE 11–2. *Prevalence of Cancer Per 100,000 Population, Individuals 18 Years of Age and Older, By Gender, United States, 1987*

CANCER SITE/TYPE	GENDER		TOTAL
	MALE	FEMALE	
Digestive	655	489	568
Colon/rectum	378	312	343
Other digestive	283	177	227
Lung/larynx	199	90	142
Melanoma	136	83	108
Breast, female	—	1332	1332
Genital, total female	—	1914	1914
Cervix	—	775	775
Corpus	—	926	926
Ovary	—	125	125
Other	—	102	102
Genital, total male	388	—	388
Prostate	324	—	324
Testis	61	—	61
Bladder	169	70	117
Kidney	103	44	72
Hodgkin's disease	44	53	49
Leukemia/other lymphoma	99	120	110
All other sites	275	382	331
Total*	1930	4402	3230

*Total excludes nonmelanoma skin cancers.

(Data from Byrne, J., Kessler, J. G., & Devesa, S. S. (1992). The prevalence of cancer among adults in the United States: 1987. *Cancer, 96,* 2154–2159.)

TABLE 11–3. *Prevalence of Behavioral Risk Factors Among Adults ≥ 18 Years of Age in the Total Population vs. Selected High Risk Population Subgroups, 1991*

Overweight
   Total 23.4%
   African-American 39.0%
No Leisure Activity
   Total 28.0%
   Low Income 37.3%
Smoking
   Total 23.0%
   High School or Less 28.1%
No Breast Examination or Mammography*
   Total 42.2%
   Low Income 58.6%
Never Had a Pap Smear[†]
   Total 20.3%
   Less Than High School 30.6%

*Women ages ≥ 50 years having clinical breast examination and mammography during the previous 2 years.
[†]Women with an intact uterine cervix.
(Data from Siegel, P. Z., Frazier, E. K., Mariolis, P., Brackbill, R. M., & Smith, C. (1993). Behavioral risk factor surveillance, 1991: Monitoring progress toward the nation's year 2000 health objectives. *Morbidity and Mortality Weekly Review, 42(SS-4),* 1–20.)

with the leading causes of death in the United States (Centers for Disease Control [CDC], 1985). The personal behaviors monitored include current smoking status, alcohol consumption, hypertension, compliance with treatment, seat belt use, physical activity, being overweight, obtaining Papanicolaou smears, routine mammograms, and stool testing for blood. Within the 47 states participating in the system, approximately 100 adults per month are selected for interview by random digit dialing. In contrast to the Health Interview Survey, this system is designed to yield valid estimates at the state level of selected behavioral risk factors over time so that trends in selected behaviors can be monitored. For example, this system has identified that people from both Kentucky and Tennessee are lagging behind those from the other states in cessation of smoking, with 30.2 and 28.1 per cent, respectively, of their adult populations being current smokers, compared with the average prevalence of 23.0 per cent among other reporting states (Siegel, Frazier, Mariolis, Brackbill, & Smith, 1993). The prevalence of smoking and other behavioral risk factors are displayed for the total population and for select high risk population subgroups in Table 11–3. This database is also useful for states in estimating the impact of intervention programs for changing behavior patterns associated with the development of cancer.

CANCER OCCURRENCE

Today cancer is the second leading cause of death in the United States, accounting for 23.7 per cent of all deaths (Table 11–4). Using data sources such as those previously mentioned, nurses may compile descriptive statistics to assess the nature and magnitude of the cancer problem in their own communities. The most common descriptive measures used in cancer epidemiology are rates. A rate measures the frequency of events on a population and can be used to characterize the incidence (new cases), prevalence (total number of cases), or mortality (deaths) in a population. A rate is computed as follows:

$$\text{rate per } 10^k = E(t)/P(t) \times 10^k$$

where E = number of events occuring in the population during a specified period of time (t)

   P = population in the same area at the same time (t) in which the events were expected to occur

TABLE 11–4. *Death Rates and Per Cent of Total Deaths for the 10 Leading Causes, United States, 1991*

RANK ORDER	CAUSE OF DEATH (NINTH REVISION INTERNATIONAL CLASSIFICATION OF DISEASES, 1975)	RATE PER 100,000 POPULATION	PER CENT OF TOTAL DEATHS
. . .	All causes	860.3	100.0
1	Diseases of heart	285.9	33.2
2	Malignant neoplasms, including neoplasms of lymphatic and hematopoietic tissue	204.1	23.7
3	Cerebrovascular diseases	56.9	6.6
4	Chronic obstructive pulmonary diseases and allied conditions	35.9	4.2
5	Accidents and adverse effects	35.4	4.1
. . .	Motor vehicle accidents	17.3	2.0
. . .	All other accidents and adverse effects	18.2	2.1
6	Pneumonia and influenza	30.9	3.6
7	Diabetes mellitus	19.4	2.3
8	Suicide	12.2	1.4
9	Human immunodeficiency virus infection	11.7	1.4
10	Homicide and legal intervention	10.5	1.2

(From National Center for Health Statistics [1994]. *Health United States, 1993.* Hyattsville, MD.)

10^k = a unit of population to which the rate applies expressed as a power of 10.

Thus, if there were 340 new cases of lung cancer in a community with 300,000 persons, the incidence rate per 100,000 population would be:

$$340/300,000 \times 100,000 = 113.3 \text{ per } 100,000$$

A rate may be crude, referring to the total number of events in a population, specific, referring to a population subgroup, or adjusted. Adjustment involves weighting specific rates of the populations to be compared by the numbers of persons in the corresponding subgroup of a standard population for the variables whose effect is to be removed, typically age. These measures may be used simultaneously to assess the cancer problem in a population by addressing the questions: In whom does it occur (person)? Where does it occur? (place)? When does it occur (time)? Examples of the use of rates as descriptive measures in assessing the cancer problem follow.

PERSON

AGE

For most types of cancer, incidence and mortality rates increase dramatically with increasing age (Table 11–5). This means that both the risk of developing cancer and the risk of dying of it increase as people get older. In addition, each cancer type has a unique age pattern with respect to the onset and mortality associated with it. Figure 11–1A–C displays the age-specific mortality patterns associated with cancers of the breast, Hodgkin's disease, and cancer of the testis to illustrate these concepts.

TABLE 11–5. *Age-Specific and Age-Adjusted* Cancer Mortality Rates Per 100,000 Population, United States, Selected Years, 1950 Through 1990*

AGE	1950	1975	1990
All ages, age-adjusted	158.1	162.3	174.0
<5	11.1	5.2	3.2
5–14	6.6	4.7	3.1
15–24	8.5	6.6	4.8
25–34	19.8	14.6	12.1
35–44	64.2	53.9	44.7
45–54	175.2	179.2	161.5
55–64	394.0	423.2	441.9
65–74	700.0	769.8	871.2
75–84	1160.9	1156.0	1344.5
≥85	1450.7	1437.9	1752.9

*Rates are age-adjusted to the 1970 U.S. standard population.
(Data from Miller, B. A., Gloeckler Ries, L. A., Hankey, B. F., Kosary, C. L., Harras, A., Devesa, S. S., & Edwards, B. K. (1993). *Cancer Statistics Review: 1973–1990* (NIH Pub. No. 93-2789). Bethesda, MD: National Cancer Institute.)

GENDER AND RACE/ETHNICITY

Historically, there have been marked differences in cancer incidence and mortality between males and females and among the races and ethnic groups. The overall age-adjusted incidence and mortality from cancer are generally higher among men than among women for all races (Table 11–6). Variations by race/ethnicity are apparent when examining specific cancer mortality rates. Of concern is the fact that death rates among African-Americans, both male and female, are higher than among any other racial/ethnic group in the United States (Figure 11–2). These rates suggest the need for additional studies with respect to cultural factors and aspects of the health care system. The profoundly higher cancer mortality rates in African-Americans also suggest the need to increase efforts in the delivery of health care for cancer prevention, detection, and access to treatment.

LIFESTYLE

Over the years, a long list of individual lifestyle factors have been found to be associated with various types of cancers. Table 11–7 summarizes these. It is estimated that 80 per cent of the total cancer mortality may be due to lifestyle factors (Doll, 1990). Therefore, most, if not all, of the cancer mortality may be preventable. Epidemiologic rate measures of exposure prevalence may be used to monitor a community's progress toward the reduction of cancer mortality presumed to be linked with certain lifestyles.

GENETIC PREDISPOSITION

Genetic factors by themselves are thought to be responsible for only a small percentage of types of cancer. An understanding of the mechanisms for heritable cancers is gained from examining the patterns of cancer occurrence in certain high-risk populations such as those with familial polyposis (colon cancer), dysplastic nevus syndrome (malignant melanoma), and albinos (basal cell carcinoma). In addition, the identification of a single case of any of these conditions should signal the nurse to have the parents, siblings, and possibly children of the patient's family also be examined and counseled regarding their high risk. Cancers with onset earlier than expected, such as premenopausal breast cancer, are also thought to have a heritible component (Kelsey, 1993).

PLACE

Definitions of place considered in cancer epidemiology are those areas defined by latitude and longitude. Analyses commonly focus on comparison of geopolitical units (urban-rural; intercountry, and so forth) and physical units (areas of different soil types, elevations, water sources). Examination of disease rates by some unit of place is useful in developing hypotheses concerning the cause of the disease under investigation. Research on the role of diet in cancer had been stimulated by studies of intercountry comparisons of mortality rates from colon cancer. From

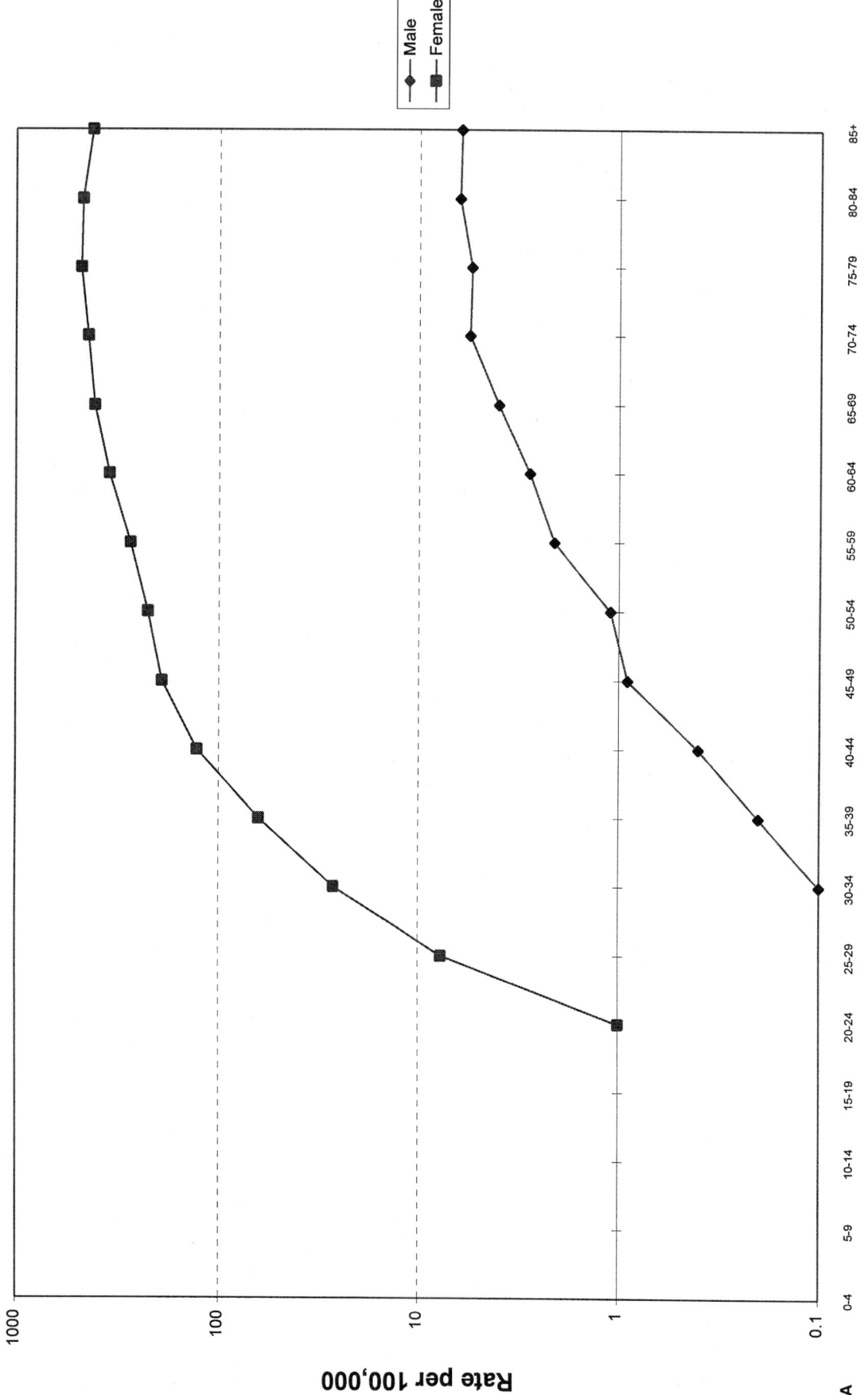

FIGURE 11-1. Age-specific cancer incidence rates, SEER, 1986–90. A, Breast. B, Hodgkin's disease. C, Testis. (Data from Miller, B. A., Gloecker Ries, L. A., Hankey, B. F., Kosary, C. L., Harras, A., Devesa, S. S., & Edwards, B. K. (1993). *Cancer Statistics Review: 1973–1990* [NIH Pub. No. 93-2789]. Bethesda, MD: National Cancer Intitute. *Continued*

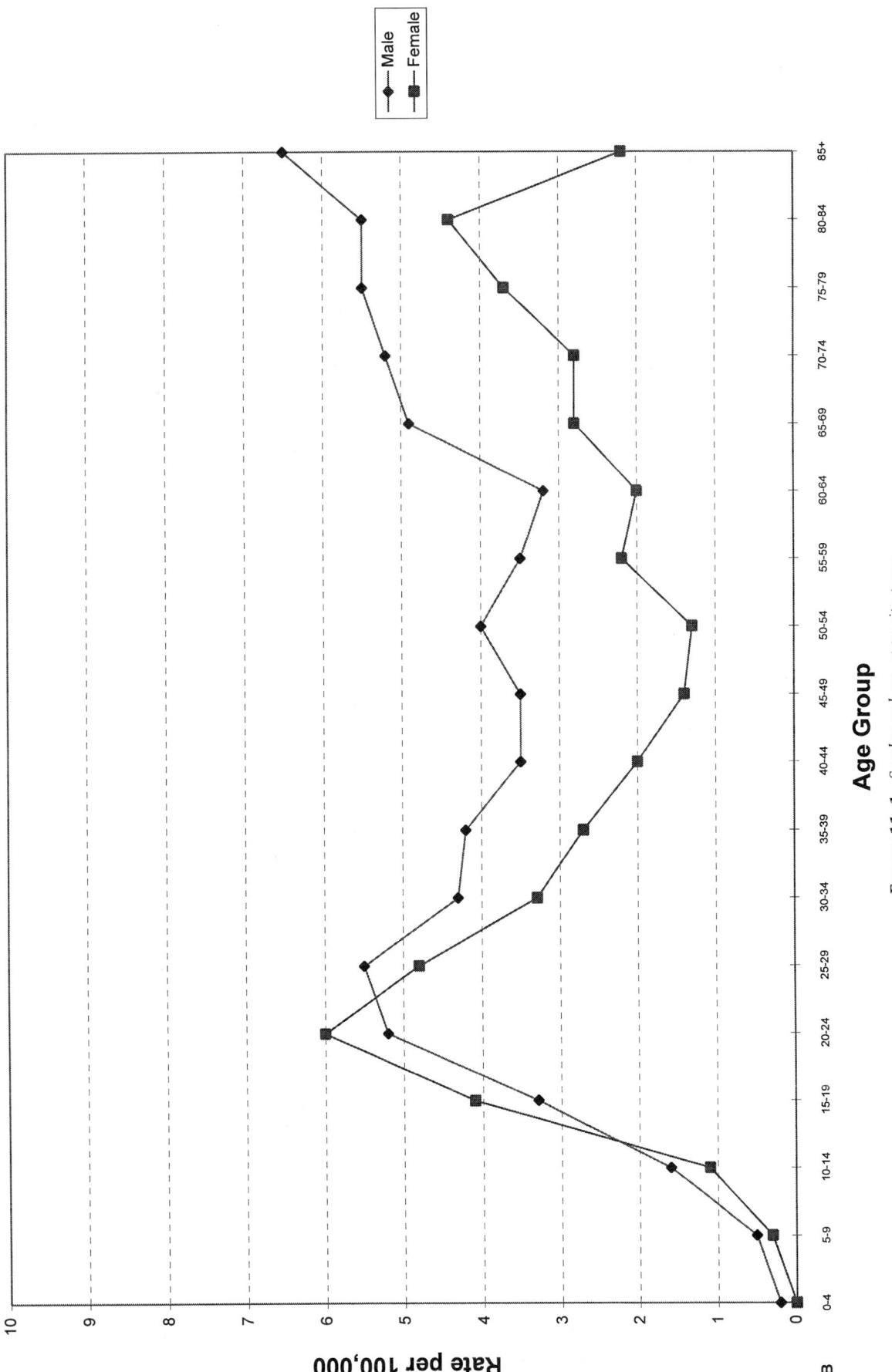

FIGURE 11–1. *See legend on opposite page*

125

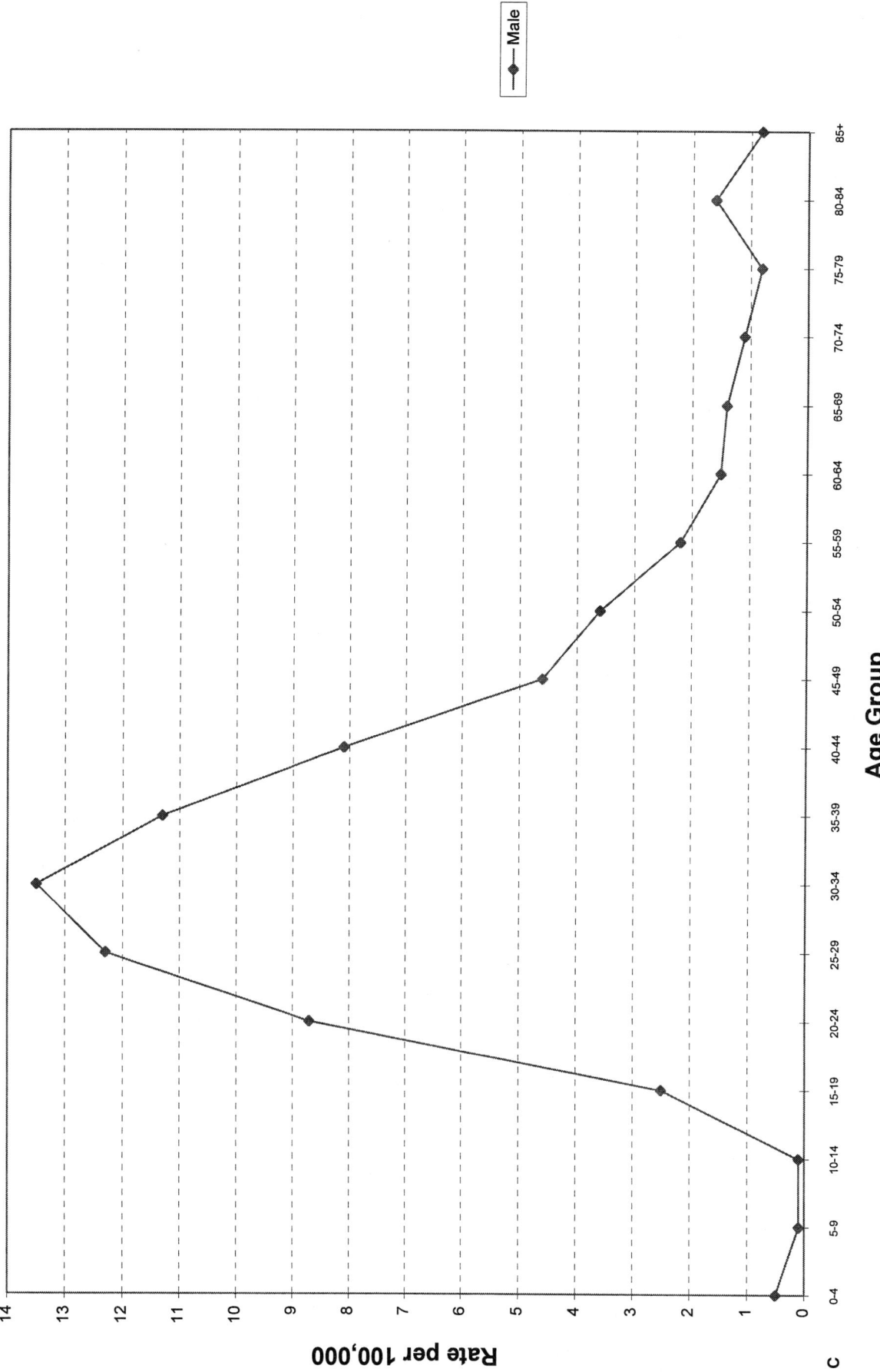

FIGURE 11–1. *See legend on page 124.*

TABLE 11–6. *Age-Adjusted* Incidence and Mortality Rates Per 100,000 Population for Major Cancer Sites/Types by Gender, 1986-1990, United States*

SITE OR TYPE	INCIDENCE			MORTALITY		
	TOTAL	MALE	FEMALE	TOTAL	MALE	FEMALE
Oral cavity and pharynx	10.9	16.5	6.2	3.0	4.7	1.7
Digestive system, total	78.0	98.4	62.8	40.9	53.1	32.0
Colon/rectum	49.0	59.7	41.2	19.4	23.9	16.3
Larynx	4.6	8.1	1.7	1.4	2.5	0.5
Lung and bronchus	57.8	82.6	39.3	48.7	74.9	29.5
Melanoma	10.9	12.8	9.5	2.2	3.0	1.5
Breast	59.5	0.9	108.4	15.4	0.2	27.4
Female, total genital	25.7	—	47.2	8.5	—	15.0
Cervix uteri	4.6	—	8.7	1.7	—	3.0
Corpus uteri	11.4	—	20.9	1.1	—	1.8
Male, total genital	47.0	113.1	—	9.7	25.5	—
Prostate	44.4	10.7	—	9.5	25.0	—
Testis	2.2	4.4	—	0.1	0.3	—
Urinary system, total	26.2	43.0	13.8	6.8	10.8	4.1
Urinary bladder	18.0	32.1	7.8	3.4	6.1	1.6
Kidney	8.5	11.8	5.9	3.4	4.9	2.3
Brain and nervous system	6.2	7.3	5.3	4.1	5.1	3.4
Thyroid	4.8	2.5	6.0	0.4	0.3	0.4
Hodgkin's disease	2.8	3.3	2.4	0.6	0.8	0.5
Non-Hodgkin's lymphoma	13.9	17.1	11.2	6.0	7.5	4.9
Multiple myeloma	4.3	5.2	3.6	2.9	3.6	2.4
Leukemias	9.9	13.1	7.6	6.3	8.4	4.9
All sites	382.2	450.4	340.0	172.4	220.0	140.6

*Incidence and mortality rates are per 100,000 and are age-adjusted to the 1970 U.S. standard population.
(From Miller, B. A., Gloeckler Ries, L. A., Hankey, B. F., Kosary, C. L., Harras, A., Devesa, S. S., & Edwards, B. K. [1993]. *Cancer Statistics Review: 1973–1990*. Bethesda, MD: National Cancer Institute.)

these comparisons, it was observed that developing nations had substantially lower colon cancer mortality than industrialized nations. Associations between environment and disease can be further explored descriptively using an ecologic approach whereby disease rates are correlated with exposure levels of groups rather than individuals. Figure 11–3 illustrates this methodology, showing the strong positive relationship between breast cancer mortality and the percentage of dietary calories from fat. The states that exhibit the highest colon/rectum mortality rates for females (Figure 11–4) are similar to those that have high female

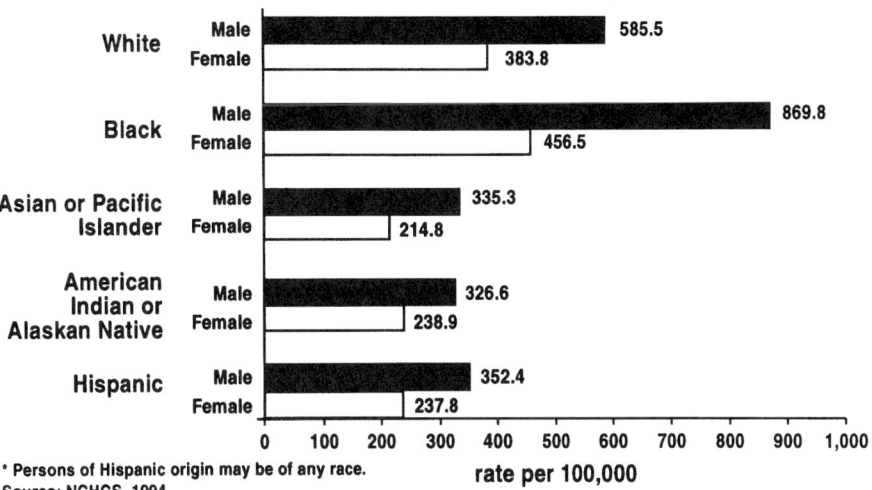

FIGURE 11–2. Age-adjusted death rates for malignant neoplasms according to race, Hispanic origin, persons 45 years and older, United States, 1989–91. (Data from National Center for Health Statistics. [1994]. *Health, United States, 1993*. Hyattsville, MD: Public Health Service.)

TABLE 11-7. *Lifestyle Factors Associated with Various Types of Cancer*

LIFESTYLE FACTOR	CAUSAL RELATION ACCEPTED BY IARC*	STRONGLY SUGGESTED OR POSSIBLE CAUSAL RELATION
Smoking	Bronchi Oral cavity Oropharynx and hypopharynx Esophagus Larynx Pancreas Renal pelvis Bladder	Renal body Stomach Cervix uteri Marrow Liver Nose
Alcohol	Oral cavity Pharynx, other than nasopharynx Larynx Esophagus Liver	Breast Rectum
Excess calories leading to obesity	Corpus uteri, gallbladder	Breast
Aflatoxin	Liver	
High fat content		Breast, colon, rectum, prostate
High meat content		Rectum
Nitrates/nitrites		Stomach

Exposure to sunlight
  Regular
  Untanned skin
	
	Exposed skin squamous and basal cell
	Melanoma	

Sexual intercourse with multiple partners	Cervix uteri, vagina, vulva, penis, anus	

*IARC, International Agency for Research on Cancer.
(Adapted from Doll, R. [1990]. Lifestyle: An overview. *Cancer Detection and Prevention, 14,* 589–594.)

breast cancer mortality rates (Figure 11–5). Observations generated from such studies further support the statement that certain dietary components, such as fats, are related to cancer in humans.

Place is useful not only in identifying etiologic factors associated with personal lifestyle or cultural practices but also in exploring associations whereby some natural features of the environment or contamination of the environment by human action represent a carcinogenic threat to human populations.

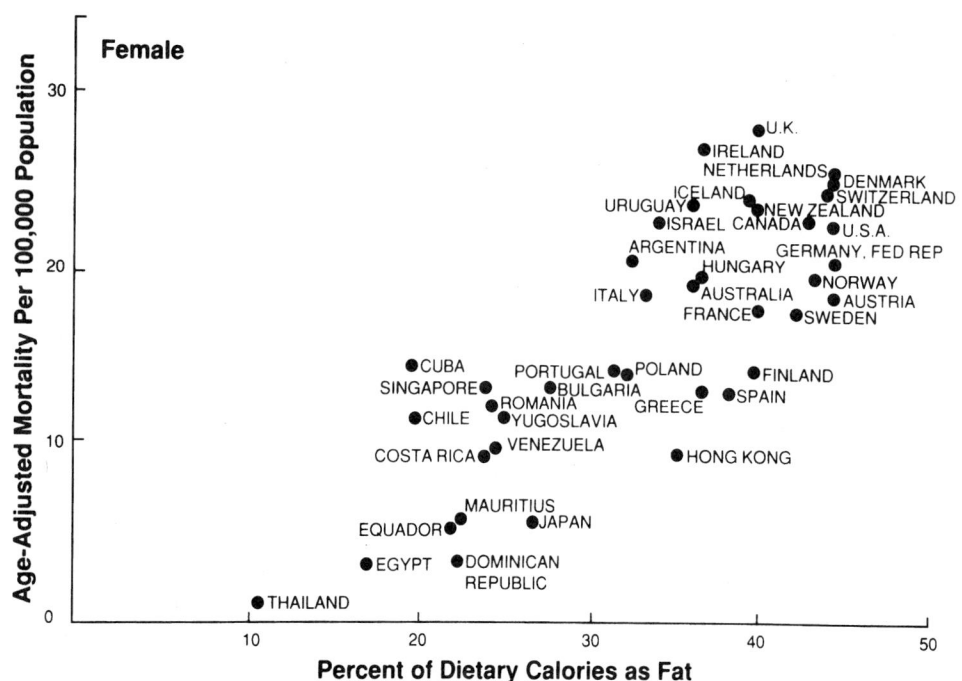

FIGURE 11–3. International correlation between the percentage of dietary calories from fat and the age-adjusted mortality from breast cancer. (Data from Greenwald, P. [1994]. Experience from clinical trials in cancer prevention. *Annals of Medicine, 26,* 73–80. Reproduced by permission.)

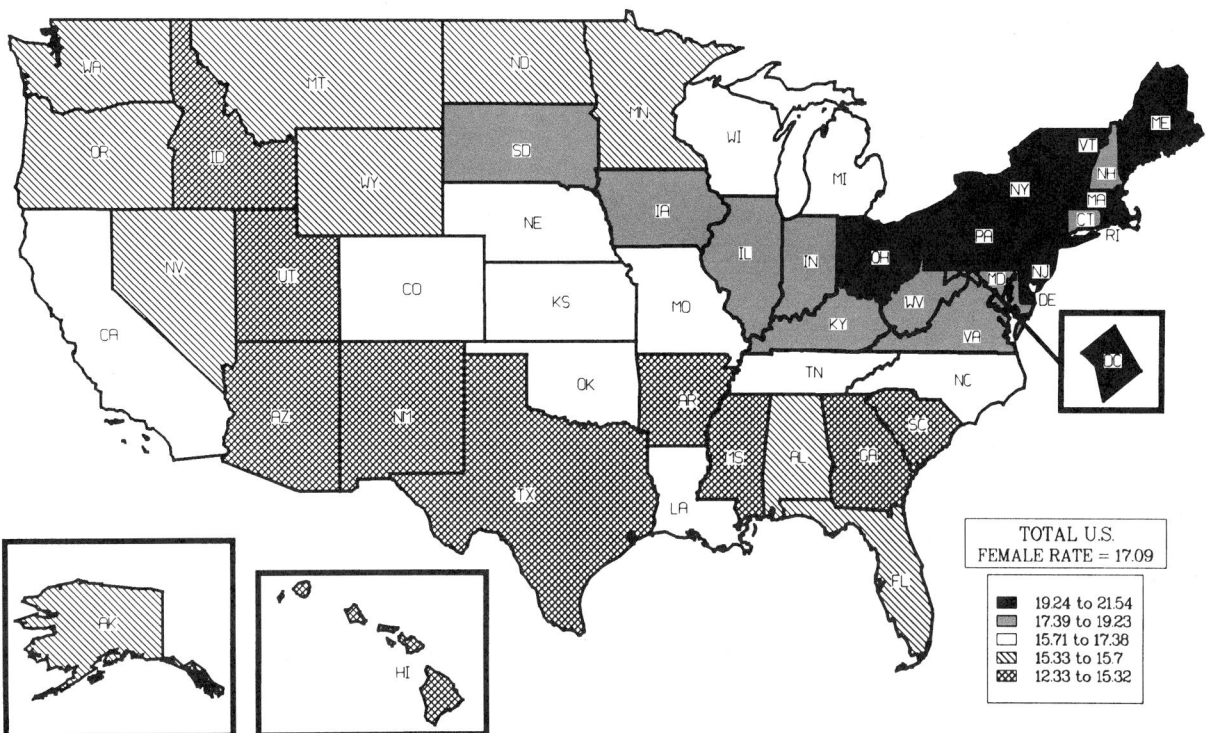

FIGURE 11–4. Average annual age-adjusted cancer mortality rates per 100,000 population, United States, 1984–88, colon and rectum, all races, females. (Data from Gloeckler Ries, L. A., Hankey, B. F., Miller, B. A., Hartman, A. M., & Edwards, B. K. [1991]. *Cancer statistics review 1973–1988* [DHHS Pub. No. NIH 91-2789]. Bethesda, MD: National Cancer Institute.)

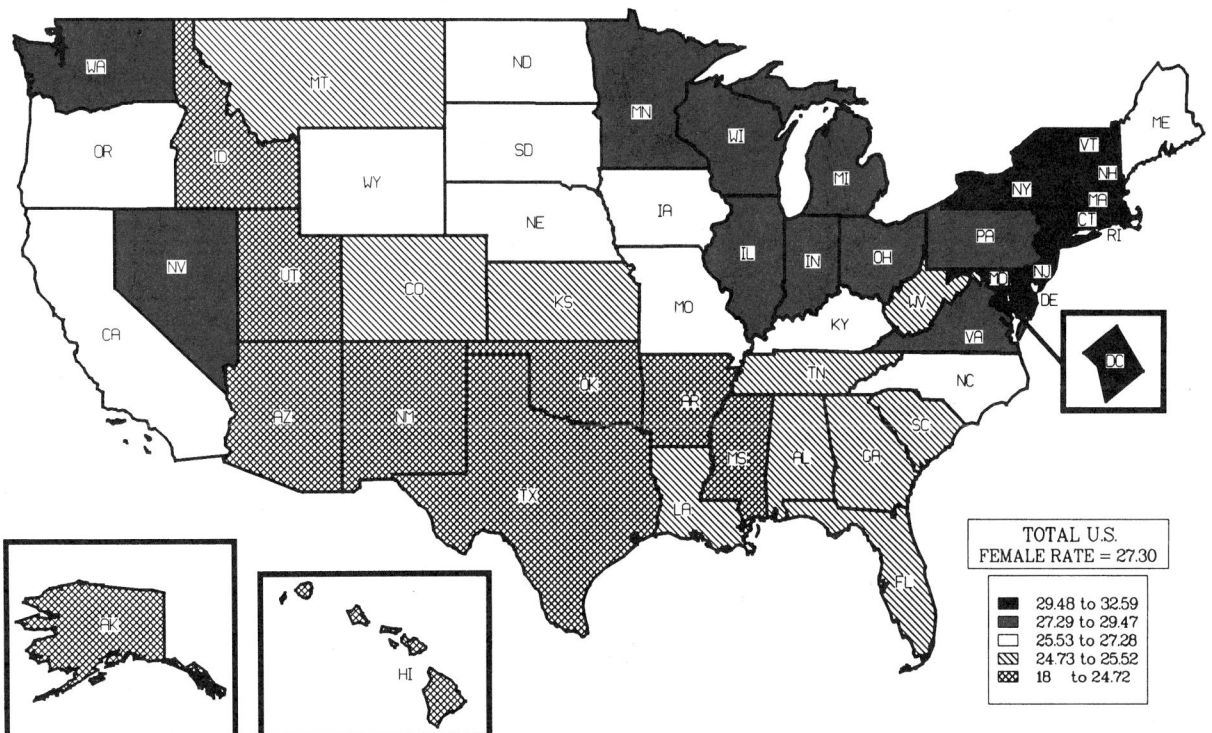

FIGURE 11–5. Average annual age-adjusted cancer mortality rates per 100,000 population, United States, 1984–88, breast, all races, females. (Data from Gloeckler Ries, L. A., Hankey, B. F., Miller, B. A., Hartman, A. M., & Edwards, B. K. [1991]. *Cancer statistics review 1973–1988* [DHHS Pub. No. NIH 91-2789]. Bethesda, MD: National Cancer Institute.)

TIME

Variations in cancer incidence rates over time indicate changes in the prevalence of known or suspected etiologic factors that give rise to the observed rates or progress in controlling or treating the disease. Between 1973 and 1986–1990, the total age-adjusted cancer incidence rate increased from 317.5 to 382.2 per 100,000 population. Of all the cancer types, the largest increase in incidence has been observed for melanomas of the skin (Figure 11–6). Increases in voluntary sun exposure, the use of artificial tanning devices, and the depletion of the protective ozone layer may contribute to this increase.

Differential mortality rates between males and females over time for the various cancer types have also been apparent. The largest increase is found to occur in lung cancer in women who experienced a 545.4 per cent rise in mortality between 1950 and 1990. Among men, the increase was 222.2 per cent. The trends offset gains in survival achieved for cancer of other sites, such as the decrease of 75.1 per cent in mortality from cancer of the uterine cervix and of 3.8 per cent in mortality from endometrial cancer in women, and the declines of 74.6 per cent in stomach cancer and lip cancer for both sexes during the same time period. White and nonwhite differentials in mortality from cancer over time are also noted. The percentage increase in mortality between 1973 and 1990 from cancer has been greater among African-Americans than whites for a number of cancer sites including: non-Hodgkin's lymphoma, multiple myeloma, prostate, lung (male), kidney and renal pelvis, breast, pancreas, larynx, colon/rectum, and oral cavity/pharynx (Figure 11–7). The steep increase in mortality among African-Americans is attributable to the higher cancer incidence rates and lower survival, particularly among African-American males.

In summary, mortality rates, prevalence rates, and incidence rates, when available, can be used to rank order the specific cancer types occurring in a community, and identify population subgroups at high risk for a particular cancer type, and they therefore serve as a guide for targeting cancer control interventions and evaluating the effects of these over time.

ANALYTIC EPIDEMIOLOGIC STUDIES

Etiologic hypotheses are generated with epidemiologic rate measures. These hypotheses are then tested with analytic epidemiologic studies. In addition, analytic studies are utilized for refining knowledge of risk factors. Most cancer epidemiologic studies use an observational design as the analytic approach. The primary purpose of observational studies is to identify which exposures are associated with the cancer type under investigation. Design types that are classified as observational include cross-sectional studies, prospective studies (concurrent or historical), and case-control studies. The major distinguishing feature among these design types is the time element—that is, when the exposure occurred relative to the disease outcome at the time the study is being conducted. Experimental studies nay also be utilized to test etiologic hypotheses. Generally, the purpose of experimental epidemiologic studies is to determine whether intervention, aimed at eliminating or modifying a risk factor, prevents disease.

CROSS-SECTIONAL STUDY

In a *cross-sectional study*, the relationship between diseases and the variables of interest are examined as they exist in the group at one specific time. Data pertaining to the presence or absence of disease and the

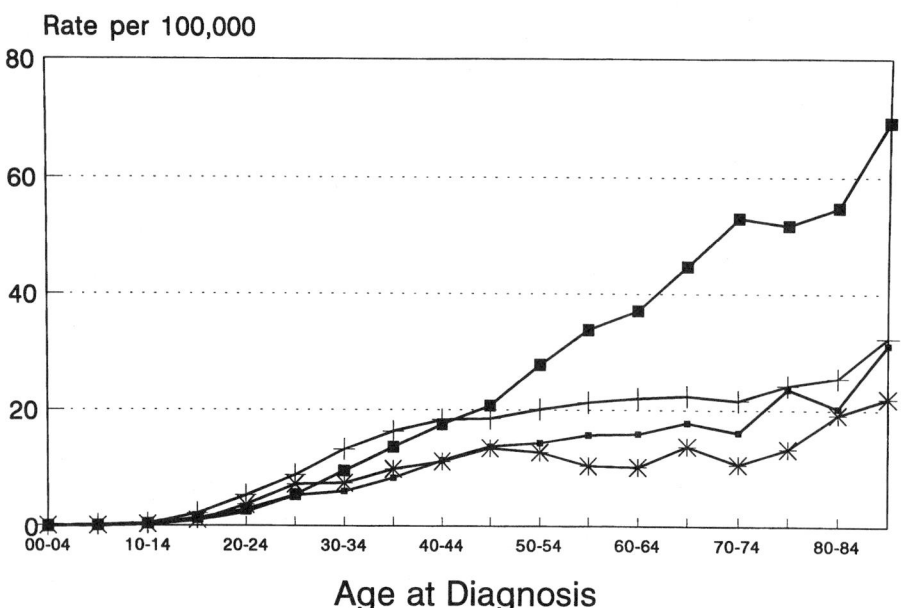

Rate per 100,000

FIGURE 11–6. Melanoma of the skin. SEER incidence by age and gender, whites, 1973–1975 vs. 1988–1990. (Data from Miller, B. A., Gloeckler Ries, L. A., Kosary, C. L., Harras, A., Devesa, S. S., & Edwards, B. K. [1993]. *SEER cancer statistics review 1973–1990* [NIH Publication No. 93-2789]. Bethesda, MD: National Cancer Institute.)

Age at Diagnosis

➤ Male 1973-75 ■ Male 1988-90 ✳ Female 1973-75 ✛ Female 1988-90

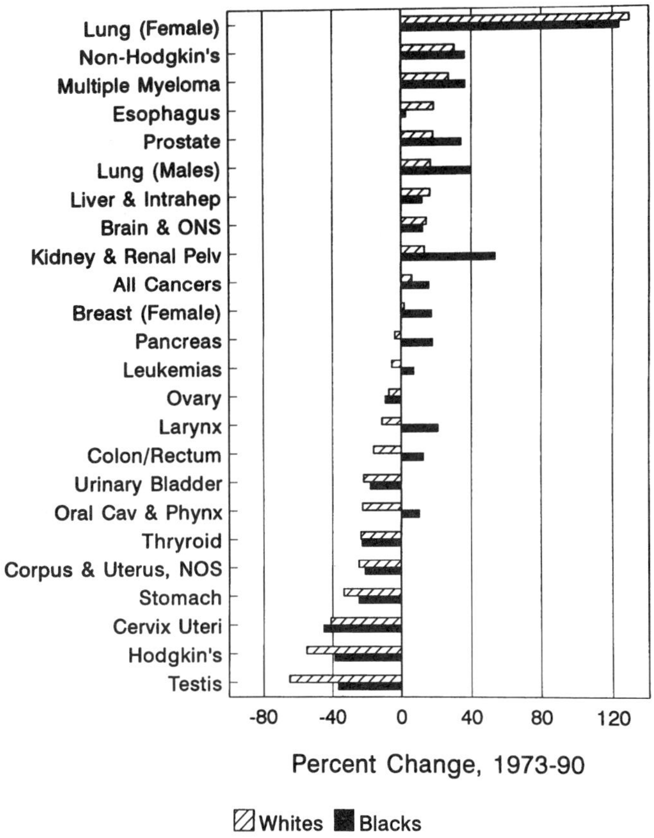

FIGURE 11–7. Trends in U.S. mortality rates, 1973–1900, by primary cancer site, whites and blacks, all ages. (Data from Miller, B. A., Gloeckler Ries, L. A., Kosary, C. L., Harras, A., Devesa, S. S., & Edwards, B. K. [1993]. *SEER cancer statistics review 1973–1990* [NIH Publication No. 93-2789]. Bethesda, MD: National Cancer Institute.)

presence or absence of exposure factors are obtained from each member of the study population or from a representative sample. Descriptive epidemiologic measures obtained in a cross-sectional study are prevalence rates of disease and/or exposure and odds ratios (computed in the same manner as for a prospective study). The surveys conducted by the NCHS are examples of cross-sectional designs.

PROSPECTIVE STUDY

A *prospective study* (concurrent study) consists of observing over time a group of volunteers (cohort) who are initially free of the disease under investigation. This group is heterogeneous with respect to the exposure factor or factors that are of interest. The incidence of the disease subsequently identified in the cohort can be directly related to various exposure levels. Cohorts may also be assembled to represent a group that existed at some point in the past whose membership may be reconstructed. This type of prospective study is termed *historical prospective*. This design is acceptable exposure if the factors and disease outcomes of interest were adequately documented or are accessible through other sources during the time period of interest. This is possible in large, "stable" populations such as clients in a Health Maintenance Organization (HMO), employees of an industry, or students from a certain school. Although a prospective study can determine whether the risk factor under investigation precedes the disease, it requires a long period of time to conduct and a large num-

ber of participants to obtain a sufficient number of people with the outcome variables of interest for analysis.

A number of important prospective studies in cancer epidemiology have been conducted. Examples of cohorts used and the exposure factors studied are: (1) concurrent: American Cancer Society Cancer Prevention Studies: volunteers (family history, air pollution, pesticides, smoking, alcohol consumption, diet, drug usage, and occupations and occupational exposures) (Anonymous, 1992); (2) historical prospective: steelworkers' cohort (coke oven emissions and lung cancer) (Rockette & Redmond, 1985); medical specialists (occupational radiation exposure and leukemia) (Seltser & Sartwell, 1965).

In a prospective study, the degree of the relationship between exposure to a factor and a disease is measured by either the relative risk (RR) or the odds ratio (OR) (Table 11–8A). Mathematically, the RR is defined as follows:

$$RR = \frac{\text{Incidence rate in exposed}}{\text{Incidence rate in nonexposed}}$$

Substituting in data from Table 11–8B, the RR of lung cancer associated with a high vitamin A index (≥5) for the 45- to 54-year-old age group is

$$RR = 4/1809 \div 4/690 = 0.38$$

With a baseline value of 1, indicating no difference in the disease incidence rates of the exposed and nonexposed, the RR of 0.38 obtained may be interpreted to mean that those with a high vitamin A index are at

TABLE 11–8A. *Computation of Odds Ratios (OR) and Relative Risk (RR)*

	DISEASE STATUS	
EXPOSURE STATUS	DISEASE	NO DISEASE
Exposed	a	b
Not Exposed	c	d

Exposure OR (case-control study) = (a/c) / (b/d)
Disease OR (cross-sectional, prospective study) = (a/b) / (c/d)
RR (prospective study) = (a/a+b) / (c/c+d)

lower risk of having disease. In this situation, the exposure of interest is said to be "protective."

The OR for a prospective study is defined as the ratio of the odds of the disease among the exposed to the odds of disease among those without the exposure. Using the data from Table 11–8B, the computation of the OR is mathematically represented as $4/1805 \div 4/686 = 0.38$. Thus it can be seen that the OR is a close approximation of the RR and yields a similar conclusion when the frequency of the outcome is low, that is, that lung cancer is less likely to occur among those with a high vitamin A index.

The major disadvantages of a prospective study are the cost and effort associated with a study that is long-term and large scale. Loss of participants in follow-up and death occurring from causes other than the disease being investigated are other limitations. Thus, this study design is not employed unless an association that is consistently detected in cross-sectional or case-control studies needs to be confirmed.

CASE-CONTROL STUDY

A case-control study compares the prevalence of a risk (exposure) factor among persons with the disease under investigation to that observed in a control group without the disease. An important design consideration is that both cases and controls must be representative of some defined population base. This may be achieved by either selecting all known incident cases of a disease within a certain time period or selecting a random sample of them. Controls may be selected either through a random sample from the same population group from

which the cases arose or through some matching strategy (e.g., pairwise or frequency matching).

The case-control approach is commonly used in cancer epidemiology because it can be implemented quickly to test etiologic hypotheses, even with a small number of cases. Some examples of case-control studies investigating the role between cancer and previous exposure to carcinogenic substances are exemplified in the work of Herbst, Ulfelder, and Poskanzer, (1963) (diethylstilbestrol and vaginal adenocarcinoma); Lowengart et al. (1987) (fathers with occupational exposure to chlorinated solvents after birth of child and risk of leukemia in their children); and Doll and Hill (1952) (cigarette smoking and lung cancer). Box 11–1 contains an abstract illustrating the study design features and conclusions drawn from a case-control study.

The primary measure of the degree of the relationship between exposure and disease in a case-control study is the OR because incidence rates cannot be derived from a case-control study. As demonstrated earlier, the OR is an approximation of the relative risk when the outcome is rare, and hence it is sometimes referred to as the estimated relative risk in case-control studies. The OR derived from a case-control study represents the likelihood of exposure among the cases relative to the likelihood of exposure among the controls. An OR = 1 is the reference level, with values of the OR >1 indicating that cases were more likely to have the exposure (risk factor) than the controls. An OR <1 indicates that the factor under investigation exerts a protective effect among the case groups. The OR is a descriptive measure of the strength of the association between a risk factor and a disease, which may be statistically evaluated to determine whether the OR derived represents a significant effect. It is a measure that can be used to compare the risk factor-disease relationships, regardless of whether the study was cross-sectional, prospective, or case-control. Table 11–8 illustrates how the crude OR is derived from a case-control study for two variables (a 2 × 2 table) and may be compared with the computation of an OR for a cross-sectional study and prospective study. The OR may be "adjusted"—that is, weighted—to control for the effect of confounding variables. A confounding variable is one that is associated with both the exposure and the disease. When it is present, it is unequally distributed among the exposed and the unexposed such that it distorts the apparent magnitude of risk. In Table 11–9 crude and adjusted ORs are displayed to represent the likelihood of in situ cancer of the uterine cervix developing from cigarette smoking among three age groups. Adjustment for confounding decreased the values of the ORs. In addition, the confidence interval (CI) can be computed for an OR to evaluate the reliability and statistical significance of this measure. This interval relates the range in which the true OR is thought to be within a specified level of confidence (usually 95 per cent). The wider the range is, the more imprecise the OR is. A CI whose limits contain 1 indicates that the OR is not statistically significantly different from the reference level (e.g., OR = 1.6; 90 per cent CI of 0.7 and 3.7). When the lower limit of the CI is higher than 1, the OR is el-

TABLE 11–8B. *Incidence of Lung Cancer First Diagnosed in 1968–1972 by Vitamin A Index, Men Aged 45–54 Years*

	VITAMIN A INDEX	
LUNG CANCER	≥5	<5
Yes	4	4
No	1805	686
Total	1809	690

(Data from Bjelke, E. (1975). Dietary vitamin A and human lung cancer. *International Journal of Cancer, 15,* 561–565.)

Box 11–1. *Smoking and Carcinoma In Situ of the Uterine Cervix*

Lyon, J. L., Gardner, M. D., West, D. W., Stanish, W. M., & Herbertson, R. M. (1983). Smoking and carcinoma in situ of the uterine cervix. *American Journal of Public Health, 73,* 558–562.

A case-control study was conducted by Lyon et al. (1983) to investigate the relationship between cigarette smoking and carcinoma in situ of the uterine cervix. Cases were residents of the metropolitan area of Utah identified through the Utah Cancer Registry (a population-based registry) and were all histologically diagnosed between 1975 and 1977 as having squamous cell carcinoma in situ of the cervix. Controls were selected from the same geographic area using random digit dialing and were frequency matched to obtain an approximately equal number of cases and controls in each county and age category. Through personal interviews of the cases and controls, information was obtained concerning pregnancy, sexual behavior, types of birth control, use of alcohol and tobacco, previous illness, and demographics. The relationship between exposure to selected risk factors and in situ carcinoma of the uterine cervix was evaluated using crude and adjusted odds ratios. Even after adjusting for the confounding effects of age, lifetime number of sex partners, and other well-established risk factors, cases were 3.5 times more likely to have been smokers than controls.

---

evated statistically significantly (e.g., OR = 17; 90 per cent CI of 6.5 and 44). When the upper limit of the CI is lower than 1, the OR is significantly less than the reference level.

Although case-control studies have more advantages, several sources of bias may be encountered that may lead to either an artificial increase or a decrease in the OR obtained. Because information on previous exposure is typically obtained by self-report, recall bias is a major limitation of this design. Bias may also arise in the selection of cases or controls. For example, a hospital control series might yield an overestimate of exposure if the exposure under investigation is associated with hospitalization. This was identified as a limitation of early case-control studies of smoking and lung cancer, with the result that the effect of cigarette smoking was initially underestimated because cigarette smoking

is associated with many diseases whose courses are likely to lead to hospitalization, such as chronic obstructive pulmonary disease. To eliminate this problem, the selection of hospital controls from patients with a wide variety of diagnoses or from the population at large should be considered.

RANDOMIZED CLINICAL TRIAL

A randomized clinical trial is an experiment involving human volunteers that determines which intervention is superior among various alternatives. The features of this design type are randomization, control, and manipulation. This design is also prospective in nature as the entire study group is followed over time and monitored for the occurrence of the outcomes of interest. In cancer epidemiology, the intervention usually

---

TABLE 11–9. *Computation of the Odds Ratio (OR) in a Case-Control Study of Smoking and Carcinoma in Situ of the Uterine Cervix*

AGE GROUP	SMOKING STATUS	CASES	CONTROLS	CRUDE OR[a]	ADJUSTED OR* (90 PER CENT CI)[b]
20–29	Yes	41	6	28.0	17 (6.5, 44)
	No	13	53		
30–39	Yes	66	25	5.9	3.1 (1.87, 5.5)
	No	37	83		
40+	Yes	23	14	2.8	1.6 (0.7, 3.7)
	No	37	62		
Total	Yes	130	45 ⎫	6.6	3.5 (2.3, 5.2)
	No	87	198 ⎭		

$$\text{OR (20–29)} = \frac{41 \times 53}{13 \times 6} = 28.0$$

$$\text{OR (30–39)} = \frac{66 \times 83}{37 \times 25} = 5.9$$

$$\text{OR (40+)} = \frac{23 \times 62}{37 \times 14} = 2.8$$

[a]OR = Odds ratio.
[b]CI = Confidence interval.
*Adjusted for lifetime number of sex partners and religion.
(From Lyon, J. L., Gardner, M. D., West, D. W., Stanish, W. M., & Herbertson, R. M. [1983]. Smoking and carcinoma *in situ* of the uterine cervix. *American Journal of Public Health, 73,* 558–562. Reproduced by permission.)

Box 11–2. *Reduction in Mortality from Breast Cancer After Mass Screening with Mammography*

Tabar, L., Gad, A., Holmberg, L. H., Ljungquist, U., Fagerberg, C. J. G., Baldetorp, O., Lundstrom, B., & Manson, J. C. (1985). Reduction in mortality from breast cancer after mass screening with mammography. *Lancet, 1*, 829–832.

A randomized controlled clinical trial was conducted in two counties in Sweden to investigate the efficacy of mass screening by mammography in reducing breast cancer mortality (Tabar et al., 1985). Within the counties, 19 blocks were selected that represented socioeconomic homogeneity. The populations of the blocks were divided into units of roughly equal size and randomly assigned either to receive screening every 2 or 3 years depending on their age or to a control group in which screening was not offered. Women older than the age of 40 in each block entered the study at the same time, having been sent individual letters inviting them to participate before the start of each screening round. A total of 162,981 women entered the study and were followed for an average of 6 years. At the end of the study, the relative risk (RR) of dying of breast cancer was significantly reduced in the group screened with mammography (RR = 0.69, 95% CI: 0.51, 0.92). The relative risk of developing a stage II or more advanced breast cancer in the screened group was also significantly reduced (RR = 0.75, 95% CI: 0.65, 0.87). This study demonstrates that early detection utilizing mammography is effective in reducing mortality from breast cancer.

---

consists of the modification of host characteristics (e.g., chemoprevention), lifestyle changes (e.g., diet modification), or screening (e.g., mammography) to prevent the disease. The intervention efficacy can be evaluated through a variety of approaches, including conventional statistical methods, measures of effect used in prospective studies, and survival analysis. If the hypothesized effect is demonstrated, additional evidence is garnered for the causal relationship between a risk factor and the disease under investigation. Sources of bias in this study design include that generated when withdrawal from participation or loss to follow-up occurs. Bias emerging from the documentation of the study outcomes may be minimized by "blinding" the participant and the observer as to the participant's study group assignment. Box 11–2 contains an abstract describing a clinical trial to evaluate the efficacy of screening by mammography in the reduction of breast cancer mortality. Illustrated in Table 11–10 are selected clinical trials that were conducted or are in progress to evaluate the efficacy of chemoprevention for human cancers. Often the objective of chemoprevention trials is to achieve regression of the precursor lesions associated with the occurrence of a cancer type in the risk group. However, chemoprevention is also being evaluated to prevent tumor recurrence.

In a clinical trial, *survival analysis* is often employed to help judge the efficacy of an intervention. Survival analysis is a technique for estimating and comparing the probability that a particular outcome will occur (e.g., development of a cancer, disease recurrence, or death) in various treatment groups, and hence, for evaluating their efficacy. Survival analyses may also be used to identify which disease and host characteristics influence the probability that the outcome being monitored will occur. These characteristics are called *prognostic factors*. Johnston-Early et al. (1980) utilized this technique to examine the relationship of smoking cessation on survival in a group of persons with small-cell lung cancer, all treated with the same protocol. These investigators found that those who quit smoking either before or at the time of diagnosis had a significantly greater median survival time than those who continued

to smoke (Figure 11–8). The implication of this survival analysis is that cigarette smoking is a prognostic factor—that is, it is associated with a lower probability of survival among those with lung cancer. Thus, even at the time of diagnosis of a cancer, it is not too late to advise the patient to stop smoking. Knowledge of expected probability of survival can serve as a guide for health professionals in making realistic short-term and long-term plans for cancer patients. Clues concerning disease causation may also be generated from knowledge of prognostic factors. For example, the marked differences in survival between premenopausal and postmenopausal women treated with chemotherapy observed in several countries led to epidemiologic studies, which subsequently identified different risk factor relationships for the two types of breast cancer (Helmrich et al., 1983; Lubin, Ruder, Wax, & Modan, 1985). The SEER program publishes results of survival analyses for various cancer types by cancer stage, treatment modality, race, and gender (see Figure 11–9). Nurses should refer to the results of such data to aid in the formulation of realistic long- and short-term goals for cancer patients.

CAUSALITY

Generally, hypotheses concerning a risk factor are generated from clinical or field observations, descriptive statistics, or both. An association between a risk factor and a disease is not declared by the scientific community without rigorous and extensive evaluation of the relationship. For this purpose, cross-sectional, case-controlled, and prospective studies, laboratory investigations, and clinical trials are conducted. The results from these studies are then examined to determine whether evidence for causality exists. The criteria used to evidence causality are (1) strength of association—the larger the value of a measure of the association (relative risk, odds ratio, attributable risk, correlation, or regression coefficient), the higher the likelihood of a causal relationship; (2) dose-response relationship—increasing levels of an exposure factor result in a corresponding rise in disease occurrence (Fig. 11–10); (3) de-

TABLE 11–10 *Selected Chemoprevention Branch Clinical Trials, National Cancer Institute, Division of Cancer Prevention and Control*

TARGET SITE	STUDY POPULATION	STUDY AGENT(S)
All	Male physicians	β-Carotene: 50 mg QOD Aspirin: 325 QOD
Bladder	Resected superficial tumours	4-HPR* (Fenretinide): 200 mg/day
Breast	S/P Stage I breast cancer	4-HPR* (Fenretinide): 200 mg/day
Breast	Proliferative breast disease	Tamoxifen: 20 mg/day
Cervix	CIN† I, II, III	β-trans Retinoic Acid: 0.372%
Cervix	CIN† I, II	β-Carotene: 30 mg/day
Cervix	CIN† I, II, III	β-Carotene: 30 mg/day
Cervix	CIN† III	4-HPR*: 200 mg/day
Cervix	CIN† III	DFMO‡
Colon	Previous colon adenoma	β-Carotene: 30 mg/day Ascorbic Acid: 1 g/day α-Tocopherol: 400 mg/day
Colon	Previous colon adenoma	Calcium carbonate: 3 g/day
Colon	Previous colon adenoma	Wheat bran: 13, 5 or 2 g/day Calcium carbonate: 0.25 or 1.50 g/day
Colon	Previous colon adenoma	Piroxicam: 7.5 mg/day vs. placebo
Colon	Previous colon adenoma	DFMO‡: Phase I varying doses
Colon	Previous colon adenoma	Calcium carbonate: 3 or 5 g/day
Colon	Familial adenomatous polyposis	Sulindac: 150 mg BID
Colon	Previous colon cancer	β-Carotene: 30–180 mg/day
Colon	Previous colon polyp	Calcium: 1200 mg/day
Colon	Patients s/p Duckes' A & B1 colon cancer	Omega-3 Fatty Acids: 10 g/day
Colon		DFMO‡: Phase I varying doses
Colon	Previous colon adenoma	Sulindac: 150 mg BID
Colon	Normal volunteers	Acarbose: 200 mg TID
Colon	Previous neoplastic adenoma of the colon	Aspirin: 80 or 325 mg/day
Colon	Previous adenoma of the colon or colon cancer	Aspirin: 81 or 325 mg/day
Colon	Previous colon adenoma	DFMO‡: 0.065 g/m, 0.125 g/m, 0.25 g/m day
Colon & prostate	Previous colon adenoma, stage A/B prostate cancer, serum PSA 3–10	DFMO‡: 0.5 g/day
Head & neck	Previous head & neck cancer	13-cis Retinoic Acid: 30 mg/day year 1; 15 mg/day years 2 & 3
Lung	Men, exposed to asbestosis	Retinol: 25,000 IU every other day β-Carotene: 50 mg/day
Lung	Chronic smokers	13-cis Retinoic Acid: 1.0 mg/kg/day
Lung	Cigarette smokers	β-Carotene: 30 mg/day Retinol: 25,000 IU/day
Lung	Men, asbestosis	β-Carotene: 50 mg/day Retinol: 25,000 IU every other day
Lung	Women, smokers	β-Carotene: 50 mg QOD Vitamin E: 600 mg QOD
Oral cavity		β-Carotene α-Tocopherol Retinol
Oral cavity	Oral leukoplakia	13-cis Retinoic Acid: 0.5 mg/kg/day year 1; 0.25 mg/kg/day years 2 & 3 vs. β-Carotene: 30 mg/day + Retinol: 25,000 IU/day
Prostate	PSA >4, negative prostate biopsy	4-HPR*: 100 or 200 mg/day
Skin	Albinos in Tanzania	β-Carotene: 100 mg/day
Skin	Previous BCC§ or squamous cell cancer of the skin	β-Carotene: 30 mg/day
Skin	Previous BCC§ of skin	Retinol: 25,000 IU/day 13-cis Retinoic Acid: 0.15 mg/kg
Skin	Actinic keratosis	Retinol: 25,000 IU/day
Skin	Actinic keratosis	4-HPR*

*4-HPR, All-*trans*-N-4(hydroxyphenyl)retinamide.
†Cervical intraepithelial neoplasia.
‡DFMO, 2-difluoromethylornithine.
§BCC, basal cell carcinoma.
(From Greenwald, P. [1994]. Experience clinical trials in cancer prevention. *Annals of Medicine, 26,* 73–80. Reproduced by permission.)

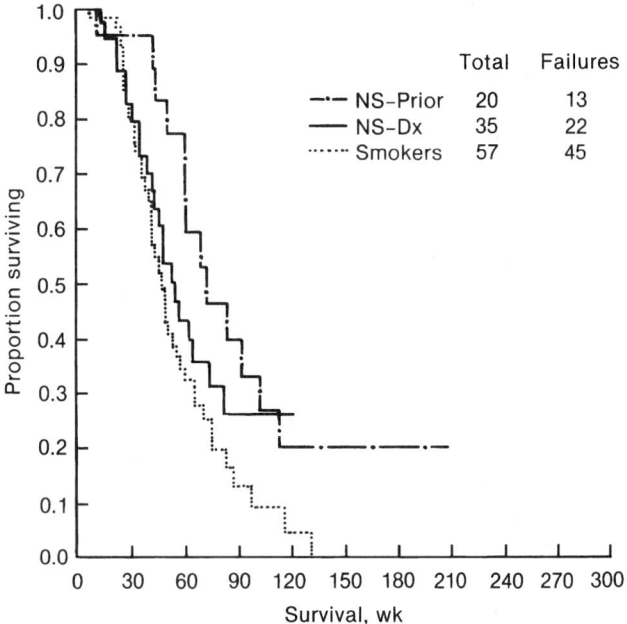

FIGURE 11-8. Survival analysis of 112 individuals meeting the National Cancer Institute-Vetrans Administration Medical Oncology Branch small-cell lung cancer treatment protocol. *NS-Prior*, Non-smokers prior to diagnosis; *NS-Dx*, stopped smoking prior to diagnosis. (From Johnston-Early, A. et al. [1980]. Smoking abstinence and small cell lung cancer survival. *Journal of the American Medical Association, 224*, 2175–2179. Copyright 1980, American Medical Association.)

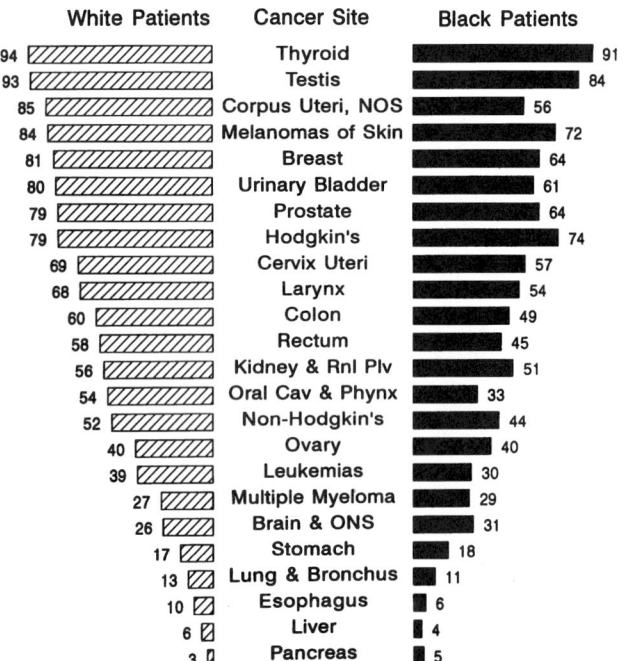

FIGURE 11-9. Five-year relative survival rates (per cent) SEER Program, 1983–98, whites and blacks. (Data from Miller, B. A., Gloeckler Ries, L. A., Hankey, B. F., Kosary, C. L., Harras, A., Devesa, S. S., & Edwards, B. K. [1993]. *Cancer statistics review: 1973–1990.* [NIH Pub. No. 93-2789]. Bethesda, MD: National Cancer Institute.)

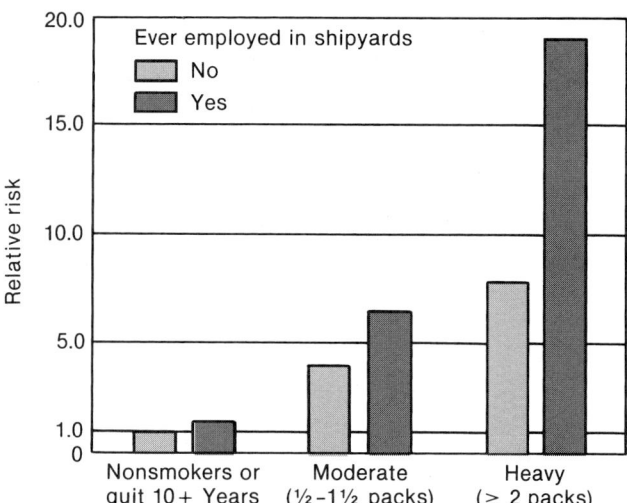

FIGURE 11-10. Case-control study of lung cancer among shipyard workers, by smoking status. (From Blot, W. J., Harrington, M., Toledo, A., Hoover, R., Heath, C. W., & Fraumeni, J. F., Jr. [1978]. Lung cancer after employment in shipyards during World War II. *New England Journal of Medicine, 299*, 620–624. Reproduced by permission of the *New England Journal of Medicine.*)

tection of the association in other populations and using different study methods and designs; (4) temporality—the factor must precede the disease, allowing for any period of induction and latency; (5) specificity—the degree to which a specific causal factor is related to or produces a single disease; and (6) coherence—biologic support exists for the relationship between a risk factor and disease (e.g., pathology studies, laboratory experiments), including how disease progression differs in those with continued exposure versus those whose exposure is discontinued. In addition, the relationship between a risk factor and a disease must be found to be statistically significant, but only after ruling out the effects of bias and confounding variables. The relationship between cigarette smoking and lung cancer is said to be causal, having met all the foregoing criteria (U.S. Department of Health and Human Services, 1982). However, the relationship between dietary factors and human cancer is still being investigated. Increasingly, meta-analysis is being used to evaluate a body of literature to evaluate the nature of the relationship between a risk factor and a cancer type. Meta-analysis summarizes and evaluates the statistical significance of the measure of the relationship (an OR or RR) from a comprehensive search of the pool of the available published studies that meet predetermined criteria for inclusion in the analysis. Because meta-analysis is a retrospective look at data, its results should be carefully reviewed before the results are accepted as fact.

To provide accurate information on cancer prevention to patients and families or to the lay community, the oncology nurse should be able to interpret the scientific literature in terms of the evidence it contains to support a causal relationship between the disease of concern and the risk factors thought to be associated with it.

SUMMARY

Cancer epidemiology goes beyond identification of risk factors and studies of causes. For nurses, it provides (1) a framework for assessing the needs of a community, (2) data to guide in the formulation of short-term and long-term goals for cancer patients, and (3) a means for the evaluation of interventions aimed at the control of cancer.

REFERENCES

Anonymous. (1992). Cancer prevention study II. The American Cancer Society prospective study. *Statistical Bulletin, 73,* 21–29.

Beahrs, O. H., Henson, D. E., Hutter, R. V. P., & Kennedy, B. J. (Eds.) (1992). *Manual for staging of cancer* (4th ed.). Philadelphia: J.B. Lippincott.

Blot, W. J., Harrington, M., Toledo, A., Hoover, R., Heath, C. W., & Fraumeni, J. F., Jr. (1978). Lung cancer after employment in shipyards during World War II. *New England Journal of Medicine, 299,* 620-624.

Bjelke, E. (1975). Dietary Vitamin A and human lung cancer. *International Journal of Cancer, 15,* 561-565.

Byrne, J., Kessler, J. G., & Devesa, S. S. (1992). The prevalence of cancer among adults in the United States: 1987. *Cancer, 96,* 2154–2159.

Calle, E. E., & Terrell, D. D. (1993). Utility of the National Death Index for ascertainment of mortality among cancer prevention study II participants. *American Journal of Epidemiology, 137,* 235–241.

Centers for Disease Control. (1985). Behavioral risk factor surveillance in selected states. *Journal of the American Medical Association, 256,* 697–698.

Doll, R. (1990). Lifestyle: An overview. *Cancer Detection and Prevention, 14,* 589–594.

Doll, R., & Hill, A. B. (1952). A study of the aetiology of carcinoma of the lung. *British Medical Journal, 1,* 1451–1455.

Graves, E. J. (1990). 1988 Summary: National Hospital Discharge Survey. *Advance data from vital and health statistics.* No. 185. Hyattsville, MD: National Center for Health Statistics.

Graves, E. J. (1994). 1992 Summary: National Hospital Discharge Survey. *Advance data from vital and health statistics.* no. 249. Hyattsville, MD: National Center for Health Statistics.

Greenwald, P. (1994). Experience from clinical trials in cancer prevention. *Annals of Medicine, 26,* 73–80.

Helmrich, S. P., Shapiro, S., Rosenberg, L., Kaufman, D. W., Slone, D., Bain, C., Miettinen, O. S., Stolley, P. D., Rosenshein, N. B., Knapp, R. C., Leavitt, T., Schottenfeld, D., Engle, R. L., & Levy, M. (1983). Risk factors for breast cancer. *American Journal of Epidemiology, 117,* 35–45.

Herbst, A. L., Ulfelder, H., & Poskanzer, D. C. (1963). Adenocarcinoma of the vagina: Association of maternal stilbestrol therapy with tumor appearance in young women. *New England Journal of Medicine, 284,* 878–881.

Johnston-Early, A., Cohen, M. H., Minna, J. D., Paxton, L. M., Fossieck, B. E., Ihde, D. C., Bunn, P. A., Matthews, M. J., & Makuch, R. (1980). Smoking abstinence and small cell lung cancer survival. *Journal of the American Medical Association, 244,* 2175–2179.

Kelsey, J. (1993). Breast cancer epidemiology: Summary and future directions. *Epidemiologic Reviews, 15,* 256–263.

Klawansky, S., Burdick, E., Adams, M., Bollini, P., Orza, M., Falotico-Taylor, J. (1991). Use of the SEER cancer registry for technology assessment. *International Journal of Technology Assessment in Health Care, 7,* 134–142.

Lowengart, R. A., Peters, J. M., Cicioni, C., Buckely, J., Bernstein, L., Preston-Martin, S., & Rappaport, E. (1987). Childhood leukemia and parents' occupational and home exposures. *Journal of the National Cancer Institute, 79,* 39–46.

Lubin, F., Ruder, A. M., Wax, Y., & Modan, B. (1985). Overweight and changes in weight throughout adult life in breast cancer etiology. *American Journal of Epidemiology, 122,* 579–588.

Lyon, J. L., Gardner, M. D., West, D. W., Stanish, W. M., & Herbertson, R. M. (1983). Smoking and carcinoma *in situ* of the uterine cervix. *American Journal of Public Health, 73* 558–562.

Miller, B. A., Gloeckler Ries, L. A., Hankey, B. F., Kosary, C. L., Harras, A., Devesa, S. S., & Edwards, B. K. (1993). *Cancer Statistics Review: 1973–1990.* National Cancer Institute. NIH Pub. No. 93-2789. Bethesda, MD.

National Center for Health Statistics. (1994). *Health, United States, 1993.* Hyattsville, MD: Public Health Service.

Reis, L. A. G., Hankey, B. F., Miller, B. A., Hartman, A. M., & Edwards, B. K. (1991). *Cancer statistics review 1973–1988* (DHHS Pub. No. NIH 91-2789). Bethesda, MD: National Cancer Institute.

Rockette, H. E., & Redmond, C. K. (1985). Selection, follow-up and analysis in the Coke Oven Study. *National Cancer Institute Monograph, 67,* 89–94.

Seltser, R., & Sartwell, P. E. (1965). The influence of occupational exposure to radiation on the mortality of American radiologists and other medical specialists. *American Journal of Epidemiology, 81,* 2–22.

Siegel, P. Z., Frazier, E. L., Mariolis, P., Brackbill, R. M., & Smith, C. (1993). Behavioral risk factor surveillance, 1991: Monitoring progress toward the nation's year 2000 health objectives. *Morbidity and Mortality Weekly Review, 42(SS–4),* 1–20.

Tabar, L., Gad, A., Holmberg, L. H., Ljungquist, U., Fagerberg, C. J. G., Baldetorp, O., Lundstrom, B., & Manson, J. C. (1985). Reduction in mortality from breast cancer after mass screening with mammography. *Lancet, 1,* 829–832.

U.S. Department of Health and Human Services, Public Health Service. (1982). *The health consequences of smoking-cancer.* (NIH Pub. No. DHHS [PHS] 82-50179). Washington, DC, U.S. Government Printing Office.

U.S. Department of Health and Human Services, Public Health Service. (1989). *International Classification of Diseases, 9th Rev., Clinical Modification.* DHHS Pub. No. (PMS) 89-1260. Washington, DC, U.S. Government Printing Office.

World Health Organization. (1988–1992). *WHO International Histological Classification of Tumors,* (2nd ed.). Berlin-New York: Springer-Verlag.

CHAPTER
12

The Causes of Cancer

Curtis Mettlin • *Arthur M. Michalek*

Cancer in some forms occurs in virtually every higher organism. It has been recorded as a human malady since early history, and archaeologic evidence suggests it afflicted humans throughout prehistory. In modern times cancer is observed in every geographic region and culture and occurs in varying form and intensity in every subgroup of age, sex, and race. Although some view cancer as an antagonist or aberration of nature, its nearly universal occurrence as a biologic phenomenon suggests that cancer is among the most common processes of nature. As such, scientists believe that we can understand cancer using the same kinds of tools we use to understand other natural phenomena—that by observation and reason, we can identify the cause of cancer and, as a result, possibly learn to prevent or modify its occurrence of natural course.

This ultimate goal, however, has proved elusive. Understanding fully the processes by which the cell is stimulated to seemingly unregulated growth, loses its inhibition to grow in the presence of other cells and tissues, and ceases its harmonious contribution to the functioning of the organism remains only partly understood. The term for this fundamental process is *carcinogenesis. Etiology* refers to the study of the causes that initiate the process of carcinogenesis. Carcinogenesis and etiologic research each are sciences in their own right with a unique body of theory and specialized terminology. A glossary of related terminology is presented in Table 12–1.

Understanding the natural history of cancer has important implications for health care professionals. It can help their role as a public health agent in educating the public on risk reduction and disease prevention. Knowledge of the principles of cause and prevention also permit the specialist in cancer to contribute to public policy in matters relating to cancer risk such as environmental protection, workplace safety, and safe use of medicines and medical procedures. Finally, understanding the processes of cancer cause and prevention enable the health care provider to advise patients and their families on how to reduce their risk of cancer.

HISTORIC PERSPECTIVE

The study of carcinogenesis has many historic landmarks. These have been reviewed by Shimkin (1977) and Holleb and Randers-Pehrson (1987). Herein, we note a few of the events that these authors and others have seen in retrospect as significant in the history of cancer research.

The first phase of the history of carcinogenesis has numerous examples of astute clinical observations linking some form of cancer with a suspected causative factor. Ramazzini of Padua, Italy, reported in 1713 that breast cancer occurred more frequently among nuns, and we now recognize nulliparity as a risk factor for this disease. In 1775 the English surgeon Percivall Pott described the common occurrence of scrotal cancer among chimneysweeps related to their chronic exposure to soot. Harting and Hesse (1879) investigated the high frequency of respiratory diseases among miners in

TABLE 12–1. *Glossary of Carcinogenesis Research Terms*

Analytic epidemiology:	Hypothesis testing investigative method used to study the association among the dependent variable, disease, and possible causative variables in a defined human population
Carcinogenesis:	Process resulting in abnormal cell expression characteristic of malignant transformation, including loss of contact inhibition and mitotic inhibition
DNA repair:	Process of preventing carcinogenesis by restoring alternations in DNA caused by environmental insult and the natural loss of structure
Descriptive epidemiology:	Hypothesis generating research method used to characterize a study population with respect to demographics, general exposures, behaviors, and health status
Etiology:	Study of all factors preceding development of disease
Genome:	Diploid set of chromosomes that contribute a complete group of hereditary factors
Genotoxin:	Clinical, physical, or biologic factor capable of damaging the genome
Initiation:	The early stage process of cellular transformation induced by an agent that causes irreversible molecular alteration of the genetic component of the cell
Latency:	Quiescent interval between initiation and cellular proliferation characteristic of cancer
Mutagen:	Chemical, physical, or biologic factor that induces genetic mutations
Oncogene:	Gene that is capable of causing malignant transformation of cells
Promotion:	Later stage process of carcinogenesis involving the enhancement of the expression of previously initiated genetic alteration
Synergy:	Enhancement of the effects of multiple carcinogens or promoters resulting from their combined occurrence
Tumor suppressor genes:	Genes having the ability to regulate growth and inhibit carcinogenesis
Vectors:	Factors or situations that lead to exposure to potential disease causes

the Black Forest regions. Their careful investigation and classification of causes of death clearly linked the occurrence of lung cancer with the mining environment. Ludwig Rehn observed an epidemic of bladder cancer among workers in the aniline dye industry, and his 1895 observations are considered an important event in the development of modern industrial hygiene.

Although the importance of clinical observation in identifying potential sources of risk continues in present day medicine, other important lines of inquiry have developed in parallel. The movement of cancer research into the laboratory was accelerated by the development of methodologies that enabled the transplantation of tumors from one animal or species to another and by Yamagiwa and Ichikawa's observation (1918) that cancer could be induced in the ear of the rabbit by repeated application of coal tar. The ability to observe important living malignant processes in a setting other than the whole animal was made possible by the development of systems for observing malignant transformation of cells in culture and for studying mutagenesis in the bacteria assay developed by Ames, Durston, Yamasaki, and Lee (1973).

The systematic inquiries of epidemiologists and statisticians have also been important. Early classics in this field include Rigoni-Stern's (1842) analyses of late eighteenth-century deaths in Verona showing breast cancer to be five times more common in nuns than among other women. Modern classics include Wynder and Graham's case-controlled study (1950) strongly linking lung cancer to cigarette smoking and the several studies conducted by Selikoff and associates linking mesothelioma and lung cancer to occupational asbestos exposure (Selikoff, Hammond, & Churg, 1964, 1968; Selikoff, Churg, & Hammond, 1965; Selikoff, Hammond, & Seidman, 1973).

In addition to the efforts of individual investigators, credit for progress in this field must be given to the public health officials who have developed the modern systems of cancer reporting and registration, which permit monitoring of disease trends by characteristics of time, person, and place. The first large-scale cancer registry in the United States was established in Connecticut in 1935, and national surveys of the occurrence of cancer were undertaken by the National Cancer Institute in 1937 and 1947.

MODERN CARCINOGENESIS RESEARCH

Although the early carcinogenesis research involved investigative tools that were few and relatively simple, the modern era involves a large number of disciplines and investigative approaches. Most research on cancer cause and prevention, however, can be classified according to whether it is conducted on cells or molecular constituents, whole animals, or human populations (the level of observation). Cellular and animal research are typically experimental, whereas research with humans is usually observational. Each has advantages and disadvantages, and each has made unique contributions to our current understanding of carcinogenesis.

LEVELS OF OBSERVATION

CELLULAR-MOLECULAR

The most fundamental level of understanding carcinogenesis is at the cellular or, even more accurately, the molecular level. Although the typical clinical presentation of cancer is as a mass or as disseminated disease, we know that it is possible for such extensive growths to originate from a single malignant cell. For example, it is possible to induce leukemia in a mouse experimentally by the injection of a single leukemic cell (Furth & Kahn, 1937). In naturally occurring cancers, the cancer cell is not acquired exogenously but arises intrinsically from the transformation of a normal cell to a cancer cell. Something affects the normal cell to cause it eventually to express two traits that are basic to cancer: unregulated growth and loss of function.

In the normal cell, both the pattern of growth and the nature of cell function are genetically regulated, and a significant aspect of carcinogenesis is the alteration of specific genes regulating growth and function. The genes themselves are the unique sequences occurring within the DNA making up the genome. Modern techniques of molecular biology have made it possible to describe, locate, and reproduce the specific biochemical sequences that constitute individual genes. Approximately 50 genes have been found capable of cell transformation; however, only 20 of these genes have been found in human tumors (Weinberg, 1994). These transformed genes are known collectively as *oncogenes*. Genes that have not yet been transformed to their oncogenic state are called *proto-oncogenes*. The change in the gene that leads to malignant transformation may be the result of one of many different processes including environmental insult by chemicals, viruses, or radiation. It also is possible to inherit an oncogene that is incomplete or altered. Proto-oncogenes are necessary and are involved in normal cell growth. Once transformed to oncogenes, they ignore signals resulting in uncontrolled growth.

Just as some genes are capable of initiating cancer, others appear to have the ability to regulate and stop growth. These regulatory genes are called *tumor suppressor genes*. These genes are capable of turning off cell growth. If defective, the cell is allowed to proliferate wildly. Thus, cancer may result from an oncogene turning on or the failure of a tumor suppressor to turn off. One particular tumor suppressor gene that has received a great deal of attention is the p53 gene. This gene is present in many human tumors including lung, colon, breast, oral, and bladder cancers. It is possible that many other types of cancer are related to this particular tumor suppressor gene. There is no doubt that a plethora of other oncogenes and tumor suppressor genes remain to be discovered.

The discovery of oncogenes and tumor suppressor genes represent major advances in carcinogenesis research. This knowledge combined with many other pieces of information about the nature and function of the cell and its components provides an understanding of basic events of cancer. However, understanding an event does not necessarily lead to the ability to predict its occurrence or modify the ultimate course of events.

Vogelstein and Kinzler (1993) have reviewed the complex interplay between oncogenes and tumor suppressor genes. The number of genes that may be involved in human cancer are several, and there may be multiple ways by which they may be activated or inactivated. This apparently occurs in colon cancer, a cancer that proceeds through defined morphologic stages from normal to neoplastic. A number of mutation/losses in both oncogenes and tumor suppressors are involved in this pathway (Fearon & Vogelstein, 1990). Preventive measures for specific cancers cannot yet be precisely targeted to specific genes or pathways of genetic transformation. The potential of using knowledge of these genes to diagnose cancer or to identify persons who harbor exceptional susceptibility to cancer by virtue of their genetic makeup may be the most immediate application of these technologies. Moreover, their identification and role in light of the epidemiologic approach may shed further light on the carcinogenic pathway.

ANIMAL MODELS

The fundamental processes of cancer may occur within the cell, but the actual pathologic condition always involves the entire living organism. The progressive development of cancer after the required alteration has occurred in the genome can be highly variable. The tumor cell may be recognized and destroyed by surrounding cells, the proliferation of the tumor cell may be accelerated or retarded, and the growing tumor may have a greater or lesser malignant character. In addition, the impact of potential sources of damage to the genome may be greatly influenced by the natural defenses of the organism. Host immunity to viruses and the ability to metabolize chemical carcinogens are both examples of the body's interfering with processes that theoretically would result in cancer. Because of these and many other similarly complex processes, it always has been important that carcinogenesis be studied in vivo.

For obvious ethical reasons, however, the opportunities to conduct carcinogenesis experiments on humans are not possible. To carry out experimental carcinogenesis in whole living organisms, researchers have developed a number of models of human cancer in lower mammals. The rat and mouse are often used because most common human cancers can be induced in similar form in rodents. In addition to being able to produce analogous cancers in test animals, use of small species with a brief natural life span allows the researcher to study large populations economically in relatively short periods of time. Also, it is possible to control in the experimental animal factors which would be uncontrollable in human populations. For example, animals can be selected by their pedigrees to be particularly susceptible to induction of a given tumor type.

In spite of the important things that can be learned about human cancer from animal models, some caution must be used in extrapolating findings from one species to another. There are few, if any, biologic universals. That which is true for one type of organism may not be true for another. For example, certain dyes that are carcinogenic to humans do not cause cancer in rodents. Saccharin, an artificial sweetener, shown to be highly carcinogenic in an animal model, has not been shown to be carcinogenic in human populations (Hoover & Strasser, 1980). Conversely, alcohol and asbestos both cause cancer in humans but not in test animals. The dosage levels used in animal experimentation typically are far greater than those humans experience, and extrapolation from levels of risk observed in the laboratory to those actually encountered in the environment often is difficult. Finally, the controlled experimental situation does not duplicate the complex environment in which human populations exist. All of the interactions or antagonisms among multiple sources of risk that occur in real life are impossible to simulate in the laboratory.

HUMAN POPULATION RESEARCH

Although the risks of experimental carcinogenesis research are too great to justify exposure of human populations, it is possible to identify "natural experiments," which can tell us much about the processes of cancer causation in populations. These natural experiments occur when some segment of a population is exposed to risk while another is not. For example, the influence of an industrial hazard may be evaluated by studying the disease experience of persons who worked directly with the hazard compared with those who did not. Similarly, the effects of a habit of living, such as a dietary practice or cigarette smoking, may be studied by comparing groups that have the habit compared with those who do not. Another approach is to study populations whose exposures change over time. Changes in the disease experience of migrating populations as they move from one region and culture to another or changes in the risk of disease within a region as the environment or habits of the population change are both common research topics. The roles of nonexperimental epidemiologic research designs in cancer research were discussed in Chapter 11, and the strengths and weaknesses of these methods have been examined in detail elsewhere (Mettlin, 1988).

The traditional view of epidemiology as a nonexperimental approach to cancer has changed, as it is now being applied to the evaluation of protective factors. The discovery of possible mechanisms of cancer inhibitors in the diet or of synthetic origin has given rise to the concept of *chemoprevention* and the possibility that clinical trials of potential preventive agents may be conducted. Such trials truly are experimental in nature and are closely modeled on the principles of the clinical trial (see Chapter 25). They also are similar to the large-scale intervention trials that have been conducted in the field of cardiovascular disease prevention and control. Such trials are difficult because they can require that large populations be studied over a long period of time. Their high cost will likely ensure that prevention trials will be undertaken only selectively, after other research methods have suggested a high likelihood of effectiveness for the intervention to be studied.

The distinction between research at the cellular-molecular level and human population research also has been revised. A new level of inquiry is emerging that links the expertise of the laboratory investigator with that of the epidemiologist. These hybrid approaches, known as molecular epidemiology, use modern molecular techniques to study the distribution of changes in the human genome across populations. For example, Perera et al. (1993) report on the ameliorating affects of specific vitamins in a case-control study of lung cancer while also assessing specific exposures. They noted an inhibitory effect of certain vitamins on DNA adduct formation. This finding further supports the use of molecular epidemiology in the study of intermediary end points rather than waiting longer periods of time for cancers to develop.

MULTISTEP CARCINOGENESIS

INITIATION, PROMOTION, AND LATENCY

Although the starting point of cancer development may be the mutation or damage of the genome, the progression from that origin is not simple. It is not usually the actual cell in which the malignant transformation has occurred that expresses the disorganized pattern of growth characteristic of cancer. Cancer growth may not occur until many generations of descendants from the affected cell have passed. For example, the atomic bomb explosions in Japan represented an exposure to carcinogenic radiation that occurred at a single point in time and which was not repeated. The excesses of leukemia and other cancers, however, did not occur until several years after the radiation exposure, long after the exposed cells and tissues had been replaced by new growth. The time from first insult to cancer expression is termed *latency*. What occurs during this period is unclear. Does the affected gene become immortalized and held in check for years and then become phenotypically expressed? Or is it during this time that the cellular genome is receiving a series of insults resulting in chromosomal loss or damage? This would characterize latency not as a period of quiescence, but one in which the "multihit" stage of carcinogenesis occurs.

It follows from the ability of cancer to remain latent for long periods that events other than the initial damage to the genetic makeup of the cell may be necessary for the full development of cancer. It has been shown repeatedly in laboratory experiments that carcinogenesis may involve multiple steps. Berenblum (1941) theorized that carcinogenesis is a two-step process. The first step, in which the cell is transformed so that it or its progeny are capable of behaving as cancer, is termed *initiation*. The second event, that which causes initiated cells to begin the unregulated proliferation leading to tumor formation, is termed *promotion*. Advances in molecular biology have given us a more complete understanding of the multiple steps involved in initiation and promotion.

Many carcinogens are known to be complete carcinogens, capable of both initiating and promoting the development of cancer. Some agents appear, however, only to be capable of promotion. Croton oil, for example, does not cause skin tumors when applied to mouse skin, but when it is applied to the skin after application of the initiator benz(a)pyrene, tumors occur more rapidly than are observed with benz(a)pyrene alone. Initiators may be of chemical, physical, or biologic origin. They act by causing irreversible damage to the molecular structure of the genetic component of the cell. In contrast, promoters influence the expression of the genetic code buy may not alter the genetic code itself. Thus promoters may not have the irreversible effects of initiators, tending to influence the expression of cancer only at the time of their presence.

The multistep model of carcinogenesis has many implications for human cancer. It may explain why persons can be exposed to a number of different known carcinogens in the environment without any of them immediately, or ever, resulting in cancer. The exposure to an initiator(s) may not set into motion the events required for cancer to develop. Multistage carcinogenesis also has important implications for cancer prevention. It suggests that many people, if not all, by the time they reach a certain age, bear cells for which the first stage of carcinogenesis already has occurred. It is likely that many of the factors regarded as sources of human cancer risk are promoters rather than complete carcinogens. Alcohol, hormones, and dietary fat all are agents that do not act as carcinogens in the experimental setting but do appear to promote the occurrence of cancer in human populations.

FAMILIAL CANCERS

The first reported association of a human cancer with a genetic aberration was chronic myeloid leukemia and the Philadelphia chromosome (Nowell & Hungerford, 1960). Since then a number of other translocations resulting in the activation of oncogenes have been described (Evans, 1993). As newer, more sensitive molecular biologic techniques are developed, understanding of the genetic link to disease will increase. Sometimes cancers cluster within a family because of common environmental exposures, and sometimes it is because of genetic inheritance.

One of the best known models involving genetic inheritance is Knudson's two-hit model of carcinogenesis. Some other well studied conditions and their associated cancers include polyposis of the colon and colon cancer, dysplastic nevi and melanoma, and von Recklinghausen disease and neurofibromatosis. Breast cancer, a common cancer in developed countries, also has been found to cluster in families. For those families in which there is a genetic link, the disease appears earlier in life in succeeding generations. Earlier age at cancer diagnosis is a common feature of genetically linked cancers. The most significant syndrome reported to date is the Li-Fraumeni Syndrome. This syndrome is an autosomal dominant disorder involving chromosome 17p and the p53 tumor suppressor gene. It involves multiple cancer sites including soft tissue sarcoma, breast cancer, osteosarcoma, leukemia, and adrenocortical carcinoma. Again, this syndrome involves earlier age at cancer diagnosis. The study of genetic disorders not only aids us in our understanding of cancer but ultimately will aid us in the prevention and treatment of cancers in affected individuals.

THE IMPORTANCE OF DOSE

The evidence on the differences between initiators and promoters suggests clearly that not all sources of cancer risk exert their effects in the same way. It also is known from experimental data that there is a wide range of potency for different agents in initiating or promoting cancer. The weakest known carcinogen requires a dose a million times greater than the most powerful carcinogen to achieve the same biologic effect (Ames, 1983a). An example of a very potent carcinogen is *aflatoxin*, a toxin produced by a mold found on stored agricultural products. A weak carcinogen may be saccharin, its potency being so low that there is uncertainty about whether it truly is carcinogenic in humans.

This broad range of carcinogenic potency is another means by which we may explain how the human species is able to survive in an environment in which some exposure to carcinogens is certain. Some levels of risk to which humans are exposed are so low that they probably never lead to cancer in the normal life span. This knowledge of the importance of dose can have important implications for efforts to control environmental exposure to carcinogens, with strong carcinogens potentially deserving greater attention than weak ones.

ANTICARCINOGENS AND INHIBITORS

Until relatively recently, the focus of prevention and carcinogenesis research has been on discovery and control of carcinogens and promoters, those substances and exposures that increase cancer risk. Within the last decade, however, there has been strong interest in the discovery and evaluation of substances, natural and synthetic, that have protective effects. Researchers have identified a small number of these substances called anticarcinogens or inhibitors, but the number that eventually may be discovered may equal or exceed the number of carcinogens and promoters in the environment. These discoveries would provide yet another explanation for the natural defenses against cancer, and if some agents are proved safe and effective in clinical use, provide additional tools to practice prevention in populations at risk for cancer.

An anticarcinogen exerts its effect by preventing cancer initiation and suppressing the expression of pathology. The search for these protective factors has focused mainly on natural substances occurring in the human diet. Of these, the anticarcinogenic antioxidants and the inhibiting vitamin A compounds have been most studied. Ames (1983b) theorizes that antioxidants in the diet act as defense mechanisms against the oxygen radicals, which are major contributors to DNA damage. Examples of antioxidants in the diet include vitamin E, beta-carotene, selenium, glutathione, and ascorbic acid (vitamin C). Epidemiologic studies have demonstrated that antioxidants may inhibit carcinogenesis. Vitamin A is seen as protective for a number of epithelial tissues. Interview studies have shown that lung cancer patients report less frequent consumption of food sources of vitamin A in comparison with healthy control subjects (Mettlin, Graham, & Swanson, 1979). Similar effects have been reported for bladder and breast cancers.

Studies such as these have led to the conduct of large prospective studies aimed at measuring the chemopreventive effects of a number of agents. There are currently seven different organ systems targeted for chemopreventive trials. The sites and agents under review include colon and antiinflammatories such as aspirin, prostate and testosterone inhibitors such as finasteride, lung and retinoids/carotinoids, breast and antiestrogens, bladder and antiinflammatories and antiproliferatives, oral and retinoids/carotenoids, and cervix with retinoids/antiproliferatives (Kelloff, 1994). Colon cancer is particularly well suited for such investigation given its well-documented histopathology and progression from adenoma (benign) to carcinoma sequence. Colon cancer is associated with hyperproliferation of colonic cells; thus antiproliferative agents would seem a logical choice in preventing this disease, Suh, Mettlin, and Petrelli (1993) noted in a case control study that individuals reporting regular aspirin use had reduced risk compared with nonusers of developing colorectal polyps.

TYPES OF CARCINOGENS

The agents and materials in the human environment that are capable of acting as carcinogens can be categorized as physical, chemical, or biologic. Physical factors known to play a role in carcinogenesis include ultraviolet radiation from sunlight, ionizing radiation, and inhaled or embedded particles and fibers. Other physical forces under investigation for which the data are less convincing include microwave radiation and electromagnetic fields. Chemical carcinogens include compounds found in nature as well as those developed synthetically for commercial and medical uses. The biologic factors that generated the greatest interest are the several viruses now linked to different cancers.

ULTRAVIOLET RADIATION

Skin cancer is the most common of all cancers, and its high incidence in regions of high sunlight exposure and among workers in outdoor occupations provides epidemiologic evidence of a cause and effect association. It is estimated that no less than 65 per cent of melanomas are due to sun exposure (Armstrong & Kricker, 1993). The association has been defined more clearly as involving ultraviolet radiation (UVR) on the basis of animal experimentation. The association is dose dependent; therefore, protective measures that reduce exposure to sunlight reduce risk. Individuals who burn easily are at greater risk for skin cancer than individuals who tan (White, Kirkpatrics, & Lee, 1994). In fact, tanning during childhood has been found to be protective. Skin pigmentation is a natural defense to UVR damage, and the human cell appears to have mechanisms to repair UVR-induced damage to the DNA. This repair capability is not present among persons with the inherited disease xeroderma pigmentosum, who have hypersensitivity to sunlight and high risk of developing skin cancers, including melanoma.

MICROWAVE RADIATION AND ELECTROMAGNETIC FIELDS (EMF)

Microwave radiation is employed as a means of electronic communication and rapid food preparation. The energy of microwave radiation is too low to affect chemical bonds or cause DNA damage, and this form of radiation is not likely to be carcinogenic (Shore, 1988).

The link between EMFs and cancer was first reported by Wertheimer and Leeper (1979) who observed an association of childhood leukemia in areas of high tension wiring. Since then a myriad of studies have been undertaken yielding equivocal results. Large numbers of persons are exposed to EMFs from household electrical wiring, appliances, electrical transmission lines, and electrical production. Although there are known biologic effects of EMFs, the effects are not clearly carcinogenic. Feychting and Ahlbom (1993), in a large Swedish study, reported that children residing in close proximity to high-tension wires were two and a half times more likely to develop leukemia. Persons in occupations involving high exposure to EMFs, such as power linemen and electronic engineers, have been surveyed with respect to cancer risk, and the data do suggest some greater leukemia risk. In another Swedish study conducted by Floderus et al. (1993), 104 cases of chronic lymphocytic leukemia were analyzed among men in reference to estimated occupational EMF exposure. They observed increasing risk with increasing EMF exposure. Although these data support an EMF cancer connection, other comprehensive studies refute the association. A prospective cohort study by Verkasalo et al. (1993) of more than 100,000 boys and girls in Finland failed to observe any excess cases of cancer in general or from leukemia or lymphoma. Many EMF studies have been criticized as being methodologically weak because of their inability to measure accurately long-term exposure to EMFs. Whether there is significant risk to human populations remains an unresolved research tissue.

IONIZING RADIATION

The cancer risks of ionizing radiation are well documented. Even in the early days of experimentation with radiography and radium, the risks of skin cancer and leukemia were suspected. Early radiologists experienced higher rates of death from leukemia, and the workers who painted radium on watch dials to give them luminescence suffered high rates of osteosarcoma of the jaw. Much of our knowledge about the effects of ionizing radiation on humans comes from careful investigations of the populations of Hiroshima and Nagasaki, who survived the blast effects of the only two nuclear weapons ever used in warfare.

In studies just mentioned, it was possible to study the effects of dose according to distance from the blast epicenter and to examine the interactions of age and sex with exposure. Follow-up studies have shown that survivors are at greater risk of leukemia as well as a dose-related increase for cancers of the esophagus, stomach, and colon. A significantly increased risk also was observed for cancers of the lung, breast, ovary, and urinary tract, as well as multiple myeloma (Shimizu, Schull, & Kato, 1990).

It has also been observed that individuals exposed in utero experienced heightened risk of cancers, whereas individuals conceived after the blast did not (Yoshimito, 1990). However, these studies report on the long term sequelae to a single, massive exposure. Most common exposures tend to be of lower levels for longer periods of time.

Persons exposed occupationally before the dangers were recognized and the large atomic bomb-exposed populations all represent examples of high exposure to radiation. Some segments of the United States population continue to have high levels of exposure to radiation. Uranium miners are an example, as are persons receiving radiation therapy. There also has been a recognition that many homes can harbor high levels of radon gas, the result of seepage of the gases from the rock formations on which the homes are built (Council on Scientific Affairs, 1987). Pershagen et al. (1994) reported significantly elevated risk of lung cancer with cumulative and time-weighted residential radon exposure. These findings are in close agreement to what would be expected based on data from uranium miners. Most populations, however, are exposed to much lower doses of radiation, principally from medical radiographs, naturally occurring radiation, nuclear power production, past atmospheric weapons tests, and other minor sources.

Shore (1988) has estimated the distribution by source of the ionizing radiation to which the United States population is exposed annually. Table 12–2 shows that, for the average person in the population, the largest single source of radiation is medical diagnostic procedures followed closely in rank by natural sources. Other sources are one twentieth to one thousandth as significant as contributors to risk. All sources considered, Shore estimates that between 0.5 and 3.5 per cent of all cancer deaths in the United States are the result of radiation exposure. The risk associated with radiation from diagnostic medical procedures should be weighed relative to the health benefits derived from these procedures. This assessment has been done in the case of mammography, for example, with the analyses suggesting that the risks of not detecting breast cancer far exceed the risks of the screening procedure (American Cancer Society, 1980).

PARTICLES AND FIBERS

A form of physical carcinogen different from radiation is that of solid bodies embedded in tissue. Asbestos is the most well known such carcinogen, with higher rates of lung cancer and mesothelioma found among workers involved with the mining, manufacturing, or installation of asbestos products (Wagner, Sleggs, & Marchand, 1960). The mechanisms of particulate carcinogenesis are not well understood. Animal studies have shown that fibers such as chyrsotile injected intrapleuraly produce mesothelioma (Van de Meeren et al., 1992). This form of asbestos also is known to cause chromosomal aberrations (Jourand, 1991). The mechanism appears to be complex, involving both physical and chemical parameters. It is possible that asbestos particles act in the same manner, with the surface of the fiber interfering with normal patterns of cellular growth and proliferation. The fibers, to the extent that they perforate the cell's protective membrane, might also act as conduits for other carcinogens to enter the cell.

CHEMICALS

Chemical carcinogens may act as initiators, promoters, or both. The potential of certain chemicals to initiate carcinogenesis is believed to arise from their ability to affect the chemical bonding within the cellular DNA, causing the deletion of segments or the inclusion of disruptive genetic information. It is known that the host organism can influence significantly the course of chemical carcinogenesis by metabolizing substances to more or less carcinogenic forms and by repairing or failing to repair the DNA damage (Miller, 1978).

Chemical carcinogens can be identified by a variety of laboratory test procedures, including short-term assays such as the Ames test, which detects mutagenicity, and whole animal assays. With new chemicals continually being discovered, these laboratory testing procedures can help protect the public against exposure to new carcinogenic substances. In spite of the importance of these test systems, most of our knowledge about chemicals carcinogenic to humans comes from studies of chemicals in the workplace. Table 12–3 lists some chemicals known to be carcinogenic or potentially carcinogenic to humans. Other chemicals are suspected of being human carcinogens from laboratory and other studies, and the International Agency for Research on Cancer (IARC) has identified chemicals requiring spe-

TABLE 12–2. *Annual Exposures to Ionizing Radiation for the United States Population*

SOURCE	DOSE (MREM/YR), TOTAL POPULATION
Medical diagnostic procedures	90
Natural background (cosmic, terrestrial, and internal)	80
Atmospheric weapons tests	5
Nuclear power plants (nearby residents)	<0.1
Television sets	0.5
Airline travel	0.5

(Adapted from Shore, R. E. [1988]. Electromagnetic radiations and cancer: Cause and prevention. *Cancer, 62*, 1747–1754. Reproduced by permission of J. B. Lippincott Co.)

TABLE 12–3. *Chemicals Known to be Carcinogenic or Potentially Carcinogenic*

Associated Neoplasms	Chemicals
Lung	Beryllium
	bis(chlormethyl)ether
	Chromium
	Coal tar and pitch
	Iron and steel founding
	Mustard gas
Lung and skin	Arsenic
	Benzo(a)purene
	Soots
Lung and bladder	Aluminum production
Lung and pleura	Asbestos
Lung and prostate	Cadmium
Lung, skin, kidney	Coke production
Lung, nasal cavity	Nickel compounds
Lung, liver, brain	Vinyl chloride
Bladder	4-Aminobiphenyl
	Auramine manufacture
	Benzidine
	2-Napthalymine
	Rubber manufacture
Bone marrow	Benzene
Bone marrow, nasal sinus	Boot and shoe manufacture
Skin	Mineral oils
	Shale oils

(Data from Shields, P. G., & Harris, C. C. [1993] Principles of carcinogenesis: Chemical. In V. T. DeVita Jr., S. Hellman, & S. Rosenberg [Eds.], *Cancer: Principles and practice of oncology* [4th ed., p. 205.] Philadelphia: J. B. Lippincott Co.)

cial attention because of their potential carcinogenicity in humans (International Agency of Research on Cancer (IARC), 1982; Tomatis et al., 1978).

VIRUSES

The role of bacterial and viral infections in cancer etiology has engendered a great deal of speculation over the years. The first viral cause of cancer to be identified was Rous's discovery of a virus associated with sarcomas in chickens. Although discoveries of feline and mouse leukemia viruses followed, the identification of human cancer viruses was slower in coming. Burkitt's lymphoma, a tumor found mainly in subtropical Africa, eventually was found to be associated with the Epstein-Barr virus. Liver cancer, common in underdeveloped regions, as well as nasal lymphomas have been linked to the hepatitis B virus. Viruses are believed to be capable of inducing cancer by their ability to integrate segments of genetic information into the human chromosome.

Modern techniques of molecular biology, most notably PCR (Polymerase Chain Reaction), have made the detection of new classes of viruses possible. Best known of the viruses associated with human cancer is human immunodeficiency virus (HIV). HIV-positive individu-

als are known to be at risk for certain malignancies such as Kaposi's sarcoma (Safai, Diaz, & Schwartz, 1992). Human papilloma virus (HPV) is of greater concern because of its prevalence in the population. Laboratory and epidemiologic evidence show that HPV causes most cases of cervical intraepithelial neoplasia (Schiffman et al., 1993). Eluf-Neto et al. (1994) demonstrated an odds ratio of 69.7 for HPV and cervical cancer. HPV has also been associated with cancers of the penis, vulva, and oral cavity.

VECTORS OF EXPOSURE

Laboratory investigations have identified a wide range of potential carcinogens and possible mechanisms of carcinogenesis, but that information does not necessarily reflect the true nature of cancer as a public health phenomenon. Many laboratory carcinogens are not usually encountered in the environment, and the infinitely variable mix of harmful materials to which a population may be exposed cannot be recreated in the laboratory setting. To better describe the causes of cancer in human populations, it is necessary to shift focus from the underlying biologic mechanisms to the circumstances and situations that expose persons to carcinogens or promoters. These situations or circumstances are known to epidemiologists as *vectors of exposure.*

It is possible to prevent or control disease without knowing the fundamental processes involved by controlling vectors of exposure. A classic example is Snow's discovery of the transmission of cholera via the nineteenth-century London water system many years before the organism causing the disease was identified. A more recent example is the knowledge that cigarette smoking is the vector for lung cancer, even though the specific carcinogens in tobacco smoke that lead to the disease have not been completely delineated.

The vectors of human cancer risk can be classified broadly into those of inherited, lifestyle, or environmental natural. Of these, the lifestyle and environmental vectors of risk are believed to offer the greatest opportunities for prevention, because an inherited susceptibility to cancer currently cannot be modified. Lifestyle is the constellation of habits and behaviors customary to a person or population. Diet, tobacco and alcohol use, sexual conduct, and childbearing patterns are all culturally influenced aspects of lifestyle. Environmental vectors include exposures to natural and artificial radiation as well as chemicals and biologic agents in the air, water, or workplace. Generally speaking, lifestyle risks are those to which persons subject themselves by their own acts, whereas environmental risks are experienced involuntarily.

The relative significance of these different vectors of exposure is an important question, because it helps define how people may best reduce their risks of cancer and it also indicates what kinds of governmental, industrial, or other public actions might be beneficial. Doll and Peto (1981) have calculated estimates of the proportions of cancer that are attributable to different vectors of exposure. The public's opinion may be that

TABLE 12–4. *Proportions of Cancer Deaths Attributed to Various Factors*

FACTORS OR CLASS OF FACTORS	PERCENTAGE OF ALL CANCER DEATHS	
	BEST ESTIMATE	RANGE OF REASONABLE ESTIMATES
Tobacco	30	25–40
Diet	35	10–70
Reproductive and sexual behavior	7	1–13
Occupation	4	2–8
Pollution	2	<1–5
Medicines and medical procedures	1	0.5–3

(Data from Doll, R., & Peto, R. [1981]. The causes of cancer. *Journal of the National Cancer Institute, 66,* 1191–1308.)

air and water pollution, toxic dump sites, and carcinogens in the workplace are the greatest hazards, but the figures in Table 12–4 suggest that the most important sources of cancer risk in the United States are of lifestyle origin, namely, smoking and diet. Some of the evidence for each of these vectors of exposure will be reviewed. The roles of tobacco, diet, and sexual reproductive practices, although they are among the most important vectors, are discussed only briefly here because they are examined in detail in Chapter 16.

TOBACCO

The role of tobacco in cancer causation is perhaps the best understood aspect of the cancer problem. Lung cancer is the leading cause of cancer deaths in men and women in the United States, and an estimated 85 per cent of all lung cancer is attributable to cigarette smoking (United States Public Health Service [USPHS], 1982). Cigarette use also contributes to the occurrence of cancers of the mouth, larynx, esophagus, bladder, kidney, uterine, cervix, and pancreas.

DIET

Although our knowledge of the role of diet in cancer causation and prevention is less certain than that for tobacco, the overall importance of diet may ultimately prove to be greater. This importance, in part, is because the effects of smoking are mainly on the respiratory organs, but the effects of diet can potentially cause cancer in every organ system. Moreover, although everyone eats, not everyone smokes.

The evidence for dietary factors comes from multiple sources. Many differences in cancer rates among groups or regions are correlated with differences in dietary practices. Similarly, trends in diets across time have been linked to trends in the risk for certain cancers. Persons with cancer report histories of dietary practices that differ from those of comparable persons who did not develop the disease. In addition, labora-

tory experiments have shown that tumor growth in animals may be affected by many different kinds of dietary manipulation. The current list of dietary cancer preventers include carotenoids, antioxidants such as vitamins C and E, fiber, and flavinoids. Whether these agents are best consumed naturally or via supplements is under study.

REPRODUCTIVE AND SEXUAL BEHAVIOR

Nulliparity, age at menarche, and later age at first birth increase a woman's risk of breast cancer (Kelsey, Gannon, & John, 1993). Pregnancy is related to risk of developing cancers with estrogen sensitivity, suggesting that the effect is the result of the influence of pregnancy on the production and distribution of endogenous hormones. Risk of cervical cancer has repeatedly been demonstrated to be associated with multiple sex partners, early age of first intercourse, history of sexually transmitted diseases, and presence of HPV (Brinton et al., 1993). Ovarian cancer risk has been found to be reduced in women taking oral contraceptives (Gross & Schlesselman, 1994).

OCCUPATION

In addition to the chemical risks listed in Table 12–3, work environments can involve exposure to ionizing and UVR as well as to a variety of fibers and dusts. Asbestos is the most common occupational carcinogen, because asbestos products were at one time used so commonly in different construction and industrial applications. Lung cancer is the most common tumor linked to occupational exposures, but cancers of virtually every type have been linked to different carcinogens found in the workplace. The problem is not necessarily an industrial problem. Farmers are exposed to pesticides, herbicides, and animal populations that may harbor viruses. Despite extensive data on occupational risks, Doll and Peto (1981) estimate the proportion of cancers attributable to occupational exposures is small relative to some of the other factors they considered. However, their importance lies not only in the risks workers are exposed to but in the fact that these exposures eventually are transmitted to the general population.

POLLUTION

The natural environment is a vector of exposure to a number of different chemical contaminants (Swanson, 1988). Air pollution originates from motor vehicles, manufacturing, and power generation, among other sources. "Indoor air pollution" results from home heating, tobacco use, radon, and sometimes seepage of natural gases. Water supplies are contaminated by known carcinogens from manufacturing, by leakage from hazardous dump sites, and by the byproducts of mining, agriculture, and forestry work.

Although it is possible to detect the presence of carcinogens throughout our natural environment, there is little evidence that any significant portion of the cancer burden in the United States results from ambient pollutants. This is perhaps because the dose of carcinogens to which the population is exposed is so low. Ames (1983b) has estimated, for example, that it is necessary to breathe severely polluted air for 2 weeks to inhale the amount of particulate matter inhaled by smoking just a single cigarette. He further suggests that the levels of carcinogens humans ingest from pesticides and water pollution pales in comparison to carcinogenic exposure from natural foods and their preparation. On the other hand, it is possible that part of the risk of environmental pollution is overlooked because the entire population is exposed to some level of risk and, lacking a point of reference for the nonexposed, the true effect cannot be gauged.

MEDICINES AND MEDICAL PROCEDURES

As noted earlier, medical radiographs are a major vector of exposure to ionizing radiation, and several drugs and chemicals used in medicine have carcinogenic potential. Table 12–5 lists a number of carcinogens found in pharmaceuticals. The estrogens are perhaps the most significant of this list because of the numbers of women who have been exposed through use of oral contraceptives or replacement estrogens taken at menopause. Estrogens are carcinogenic in animal models and thought to be carcinogenic to humans, especially after long-term use (Lupuleseu, 1993). Unopposed estrogens increase risks of breast cancer. Oral contraceptive use, however, has not shown to significantly increase the risk for breast cancer and may, in fact, reduce risk for endometrial ovarian cancer. (Jordan, Jeng, Catherino, & Parker, 1993). Replacement estrogens, in contrast, have been linked to endometrial

TABLE 12–5. *Selected Pharmaceutical Agents with Known or Potential Human Carcinogenicity*

AGENT	HUMAN ORGAN AFFECTED
Phenacetin	Kidney
Chloramphenicol	Bone marrow
Cloronaphazine	Bladder
Bischloroethylnitrosourea	Bone marrow
Busulphan	Bone marrow
Chlorambucil	Bone marrow
Chlorzotocin	Bone marrow
Melphalan	Bladder, bone marrow
Nitrogen mustard	Bone marrow
8-Methoxypsoralen & UVA	Skin
Testosterone	Skin
Nonsteroid estrogen	Liver, vagina, cervix
Estrogen replacement	Endometrium
Azothioprine	Lymphatic
Cyclosporine	Lymphatic

(Adapted from Shields, P. G., & Harris, C. C. [1993]. Principles of carcinogenesis: Chemical. In V. T. DeVita Jr., S. Hellman, & S. Rosenberg [Eds.], *Cancer: Principles and practice of oncology* [4th ed., p. 209.] Philadelphia: J. B. Lippincott Co. Reproduced by permission.)

cancer (Herrinton & Weiss, 1993). At one time diethylstilbestrol (DES) was prescribed to prevent miscarriage. Women exposed in utero were later shown to be at high risk for vaginal cancers. Women given DES during pregnancy may also be at increased risk of breast and endometrial carcinoma (Marselos & Tomatis, 1992). Some antineoplastic drugs have proved to have carcinogenic potential, and medical practice often involves balancing a small future risk against greater, immediate benefit. Personnel involved in mixing and handling antineoplastic agents sometimes demonstrate acute reactions (Valanis, Vollmer, Labuhn, & Glass, 1993), and if these procedures are done improperly, the patients present with chromosome aberrations (Oestreicher, Stephana, & Giatzel, 1990).

TYPES OF PREVENTION

PRIMARY, SECONDARY, AND TERTIARY PREVENTION

Given the complexity of cancer causes, no single intervention aimed at preventing cancer can be expected to address the problem completely. Cancer prevention requires multidisciplinary approaches carried out at different levels. Cancer prevention has been divided into three stages according to the stage of the natural history of the disease. *Primary* prevention refers to efforts to block the cancer during carcinogenesis, before initiation, or no later than the promotion stage. Regulation of carcinogens, cessation of smoking, and dietary change all are primary prevention measures. *Secondary* prevention efforts are undertaken after the onset of pathology but before signs and symptoms are present. Screening of asymptomatic persons to detect unsuspected cancers at a time when their treatment may be most effective is the goal of secondary prevention. *Tertiary* prevention is not aimed at prevention of disease but at interventions to prevent serious consequences of the disease. Prompt appropriate treatment and rehabilitation are both examples of tertiary interventions. Tertiary prevention aims at prolongation and enhancement of quality of life.

FUTURE DIRECTIONS

Research on the causes of cancer has progressed greatly. Much of this progress is attributable to the melding of clinical, laboratory, and public health perspectives. The future course of research and development in cancer prevention may further reflect this trend toward multidisciplinary efforts. These efforts will no doubt be enhanced by the exponential growth of our knowledge in molecular biology and the human genome. In addition, based on present understanding of fundamental processes, future efforts may tend more toward development of practical interventions. This may be particularly true with respect to the development of chemopreventive interventions. Until such clinical interventions are proved safe and effective, traditional reliance on early detection and avoidance of exposure to carcinogens will remain the most effective tools of prevention at our disposal.

REFERENCES

American Cancer Society. (1980). Guidelines for the cancer related checkup: Recommendations and rationale. *CA-Cancer Journal for Clinicians, 30,* 4–50.

Ames, B. N. (1983a). The detection of environmental mutagens and potential carcinogens. *Cancer, 53,* 2034–2039.

Ames, B. N. (1983b). Dietary carcinogens and anticarcinogens. Oxygen radicals and degenerative diseases. *Science, 221,* 1256–1264.

Ames, B. N., Durston, W. E., Yamasaki, E., & Lee, F. D. (1973). Carcinogens as mutagens: A simple test system combining liver homogenates for activation and bacteria for detection. *Proceedings of the National Academy of Sciences. U.S.A., 70,* 2281–2285.

Armstrong, B. K., & Kricker, A. (1993). How much melanoma is caused by sun exposure? *Melanoma Research, 3,* 395–401.

Berenblum, I. (1941). The mechanism of carcinogenesis: A study of the significance of cocarcinogenic action and related phenomena. *Cancer Research, 1,* 807–814.

Brinton, L. A., Herrero, R., Reeves, W. C., deBritton, R. C., Gaitan, E., & Tenorro, R. (1993). Risk factors for cervical cancer by histology. *Gynecologic Oncology, 51,* 299–300.

Council on Scientific Affairs. (1987). Radon in homes. *Journal of the American Medical Association, 258,* 668–672.

Doll, R., & Peto, R. (1981). The causes of cancer. *Journal of the National Cancer Institute, 66,* 1191–1308.

Eluf-Neto, J., Booth, M., Munoz, N., Bosch, F. S., Meijer, C. J., & Walboomers, J. M. (1994). Human papillomavirus and invasive cervical cancer in Brazil. *British Journal of Cancer, 69,* 114–119.

Evans, H. J. (1993). Molecular genetic aspects of human cancers: The Frank Rose lecture. *British Journal of Cancer, 68,* 1051–1060.

Fearon, E. R., & Vogelstein, B. (1990). A genetic model for colorectal tumorigenesis. *Cell, 61*(5), 759–767.

Feychting, M., & Ahlbom, A. (1993). Magnetic fields and cancer in children residing near Swedish high-voltage power lines. *American Journal of Epidemiology, 138,* 467–481.

Floderus, B., Persson, T., Steuland, C., Wennberg, A., Ost, A., & Knave, B. (1993). Occupational exposure to electromagnetic fields in relation to leukemia and brain tumors: A case-control study in Sweden. *Cancer Causes and Control, 4,* 465–476.

Furth, J., & Kahn, M. C. (1937). The transmission of leukemia of mice with a single cell. *American Journal of Cancer, 31,* 276–282.

Gross, T. P., & Schlesselman, J. J. (1994). The estimated effect of oral contraceptive use on the cumulative risk of epithelial ovarian cancer. *Obstetrics Gynecology, 83,* 419–424.

Harting, F. H., & Hesse W. (1879). Der Lungenkrebs, die Bergkrankheit in den Schneeberger Gruben. *Vrtljschr Gerlichtl Med, 30,* 296–309.

Herrinton, L. J., & Weiss, N. S. (1993). Postmenopausal unopposed estrogens: Characteristics of use in relation to the risk of endometrial carcinomas. *Annals of Epidemiology, 3,* 308–318.

Holleb, A. I., & Randers-Pehrson, M. B. (Eds.). (1987). *Classics in oncology.* New York: American Cancer Society.

Hoover, R. N., & Strasser, P. H. (1980). Artificial sweeteners and human bladder cancer. *Lancet, 1,* 837.

International Agency of Research on Cancer (1982). *Chemicals, industrial processes and industries associated with cancer in humans.* (IARC Monographs, Supplement 4). Lyon: Author.

Jordan, V. C., Jeng, M. H., Catherino, W. H., & Parker, C. J. (1993). The estrogenic activity of synthetase progesterins used in oral contraceptives. *Cancer, 71* (Suppl. 4), 1501–1505.

Jourand, M. C. (1991). Observations on the carcinogenicity of asbestos fibers. *Annals of the New York Academy of Sciences, 643,* 258–270.

Kelloff, G. J., Boone, C. W., Steele, V., Crowell, J. A., Lubet, R., & Sigman, C. C. (1994). Progress in cancer chemoprevention: Perspectives on agent selection and short-term clinical intervention trials. *Cancer Research, 54* (Suppl. 7), 2015S–2024S.

Kelsey, J. L., Gannon, M. D., & John, E. M. (1993). Reproductive factors and breast cancer. *Epidemiology Reviews, 15,* 36–47.

Lupuleseu, A. (1993). Estrogen use and cancer risk: A review. *Experimental & Clinical Endocrinology, 101,* 204–214.

Marselos, M., & Tomatis, L. (1992). Diethylstilseotrol: I, pharmacology, toxicology and carcinogenicity in humans. *European Journal of Cancer, 28A,* 1182–1189.

Mettlin, C. (1988). Descriptive and analytical epidemiology: Bridges to cancer control. *Cancer, 62,* 1680–1687.

Mettlin, C., Graham, S., & Swanson, M. (1979). Vitamin A and lung cancer. *Journal of the National Cancer Institute, 62,* 1435–1438.

Miller, E. C. (1978). Some current perspectives on chemical carcinogenesis in humans and experimental animals: Presidential address. *Cancer Research, 38,* 1479–1496.

Nowell, P. C., & Hungerford, D. A. (1960). A minute chromosome in human chronic granulocytic leukemia. *Science, 132,* 1497.

Oestreicher, V., Stephana, G., & Giatzel, M. (1990). Chromosome and SCE analysis in peripheral lymphocytes of persons occupationally exposed to cytostatic drugs handled with and without use of safety covers. *Mutation Research, 242,* 271–277.

Perera, F. P., Tang, D., Grinberg-Funes, R. A., Blackwood, M. A., Dickey, C., Blaner, W., & Sanfella, R. M. (1993). Molecular epidemiology of lung cancer and the modulation of markers of chronic carcinogen exposure by chemopreventive agents. *Journal of Cellular Biochemistry, 17F,* 119–128.

Pershagen, G., Akerblaou, G., Axelson, O., Claveniza, B., Damber, L., Desai, G., Enflo, A., Lagarde, F., Mellander, H., & Svartengren, M. (1994). Residential radon exposure and lung cancer in Sweden. *New England Journal of Medicine, 330,* 159–164.

Pott, P. (1775). *Chirurgical observations relative to the cataract, the polypus of the nose, the cancer of the scrotum, the different kinds of ruptures, and the mortification of the toes and feet.* London: Hawes, Clarke, & Collins.

Ramazzini, B. (1713). *De Morbis Artificum, Diatriba* [Diseases of Workers] (p. 191). (W. C. Wright, Trans., 1964). New York: Hafner.

Rehn, L. (1895). Blasengeschwultse bei Fuchin-Arbeiten. *Arch Klin Chir, 50,* 588–600.

Rigoni-Stern, D. A. (1842). Fatti statistici relativi alli malattie cancerose. *Gior Servire Prop Path Terap, 2,* 507–512.

Safai, B., Diaz, B., & Schwartz, J. (1992). Malignant neoplasms associated with human immunodeficiency virus infection. *CA- Cancer Journal for Clinicians, 42,* 74–95.

Schiffman, M. H., Bauer, H. M., Hoover, R. N., Glass, A. G., Cadell, D. M., Rush, B. B., Scott, D. R., Sherman, M. E., Kurman, R. J., & Wacholder, S. (1993). Epidemiologic evidence showing that human papillomavirus infection causes most cervical intraepithelial neoplasia. *Journal of the National Cancer Institute, 85,* 958–964.

Selikoff, I. J., Churg, J., & Hammond, E. C. (1965). Relationship between exposure to asbestos and mesothelioma. *New England Journal of Medicine, 272,* 560–565.

Selikoff, I. J., Hammond, E. C., & Churg, J. (1964). Asbestos exposure and neoplasia. *Journal of the American Medical Association, 143,* 329–336.

Selikoff, I. J., Hammond, E. C., & Churg, J. (1968). Asbestos exposure, smoking, and neoplasia. *Journal of the American Medical Association, 204,* 106–112.

Selikoff, I. J., Hammond, E. C., & Seidman, H. (1973). Cancer risk of insulation workers in the United States. In: International Agency for Research on Cancer. *Biological effects of asbestos* (pp. 209–216). Lyon: Author.

Shields, P. G., & Harris, C. C. (1993). Principles of carcinogenesis: Chemical. In V. T. DeVita Jr., S. Hellman, & S. Rosenberg (Eds.), *Cancer: Principles and practice of oncology.* (4th ed., pp. 200–221). Philadelphia: J.B. Lippincott Co.

Shimizu, Y., Schull, W. J., & Kato, H. (1990). Cancer risk among atomic bomb survivors: The RERF Life Span Study. *Journal of the American Medical Association, 264,* 601–604.

Shimkin, M. B. (1977). Some historical landmarks in cancer epidemiology. *Contrary to nature.* (DHEW Publication No. [NIH] 76-720, pp. 60–74). Washington, DC, U.S. Department of Health, Education and Welfare, Public Health Service. National Institute of Health.

Shore, R. E. (1988). Electromagnetic radiations and cancer: Cause and prevention. *Cancer, 62,* 1747–1754.

Suh, O., Mettlin C., & Petrelli N. (1993). Aspirin use, cancer, and polyps of the large bowel. *Cancer, 72,* 1171–1177.

Swanson, G. M. (1988). Cancer prevention in the workplace, and natural environment: A review of etiology, research design, and methods of risk detection. *Cancer, 62,* 1725–1746.

Tomatis, L., Agthe, C., Bartsch, H., Huff, J., Montesano, R., Saracci, R., Walker, E., & Wilbourn, J. (1978). Evaluation of the carcinogenicity of chemicals: A review of the monograph program of the International Agency for Research on Cancer. *Cancer Research, 38,* 877–885.

United States Public Health Service, (1982). *The health consequences of smoking. A report of the Surgeon General of the Public Health Service, U.S. Department of Health and Human Services, Office on Smoking and Health.* Washington, DC: U.S. Government Printing Office.

Valanis, B. G., Vollmer, V. M., Labuhn, K. T., & Glass, A. G. (1993). Association of antineoplastic drug handling with acute adverse effects in pharmacy personnel. *American Journal of Hospital Pharmacy, 50,* 455–462.

Van de Meeren, A., Fleury, J., Nebut, M., Monchaux, G., Janson, X., & Jaurand, M. C. (1992). Mesothelioma in rats following intrapleural injection of chrysotile and phosphorylated chyrsotile. *International Journal of Cancer, 50,* 937–942.

Verkasalo, P. K., Pukkala, E., Hongisto, M. Y., Valjus, J. E., Jarvinen, P. K., Heikkila, K. V., & Koskenuvuo, M. (1993). Risk of cancer in Finnish children living close to power lines. *British Medical Journal, 307,* 895–899.

Vogelstein, B., & Kinzler, K. W. (1993). The multistep nature of cancer. *Trends in Genetics, 9*(4), 138–141.

Wagner, J. C., Sleggs, C. A., & Marchand, P. (1960). Diffuse pleural mesothelioma and asbestos exposure in North Western Cape Province. *British Journal of Industrial Medicine, 17,* 260–271.

Weinberg, R. A. (1994). Oncogenes and tumor suppressor genes. *CA-Cancer Journal for Clinicians, 44,* 160–170.

Wertheimer, N., & Leeper, E. (1979). Electrical wiring configurations and childhood cancer. *American Journal of Epidemiology, 109,* 273–284.

White, E., Kirkpatrics, C. S., & Lee, J. A. (1994). Case-control study of malignant melanoma in Washington State. I. Constitutional factors and sun exposure. *American Journal of Epidemiology, 139,* 857–868.

Wynder, E. L., & Graham, E. A. (1950). Tobacco smoking as possible etiologic factor in bronchogenic carcinoma: Study of six-hundred and eight-four proved cases. *Journal of the American Medical Association, 143,* 329–336.

Yamagiwa, K., & Ichikawa, K. (1918). Experimental study of the pathogenesis of carcinoma. *Journal of Cancer Research, 3,* 1–29.

Yoshimito, Y. (1990). Cancer risk among children of atomic bomb survivors: A review of RERF epidemiologic studies. *Journal of the American Medical Association, 264,* 596–600.

Cancer Biology: Molecular and Cellular Aspects

Kathryn Ann Caudell • Linda J. Cuaron • Betty Bierut Gallucci

Cancer is a disease of genetic and molecular changes leading to altered states of cellular differentiation, proliferation and death. Although there are a number of variations in the macro- and microscopic characteristics of different cancers, they do have similar features that determine the way in which they grow and behave. This chapter provides a historical overview of molecular biology, discusses the process of cell division, the genetic and molecular factors that initiate the development of tumor cells and the potential for gene therapy. Recent developments are discussed within the context of previous accomplishments. Clinical examples are often given after the basic biologic discussion as a bridge from the laboratory to the clinical arenas.

AN OVERVIEW

DEFINITIONS

Pitot (1986) distinguishes between *cancer* and *neoplasms,* referring to the clinical entity as a cancer and the basic biologic processes underlying the disease as a neoplasia. The word tumor is defined as "any swelling" (Stedman, 1982) and was originally referred to as "a

swelling caused by inflammation" (Cotran, Kumar, & Robbins, 1994b, p. 241). Neoplasms also can cause swelling or tumors, but in recent times, however, tumor is referred to as a neoplasm.

Pitot's specific definition of a neoplasm is as follows: "A neoplasm is a heritably altered, relatively autonomous growth of tissue" (Pitot, 1986). This physiologic definition proposed by Pitot emphasizes the concept of tissue, autonomy, and growth. Autonomy implies that some normal regulatory controls over cell growth and division are lacking. The term *relatively* is included because cancer cells are not completely independent of all regulatory processes. If they were, such tumors as breast and prostate cancers would not respond to hormonal therapies.

Sir Rupert Willis, a noted British oncologist, defines neoplasm as "an abnormal mass of tissue, the growth of which exceeds and is uncoordinated with that of the normal tissues and persists in the same excessive manner after cessation of the stimuli which evoked the change" (Cotran et al., 1994b, pp. 241–242). This definition is similar to that of Pitot's in that the mass is described as uncoordinated or autonomous. It is important to note, however, that this autonomy is "virtual" because neoplasms, like all cells, require nutritional support from the host.

Other definitions emphasize, or imply, that cellular abnormalities are crucial to the definition of neoplasia. This is not surprising because the basic building block of all tissue is the cell. Bonfiglio and Terry (1983) defined cancer as "a disease of the cell in which the normal mechanisms of control of growth and proliferation are disturbed. This results in distinctive morphologic alterations of the cell and aberrations of tissue patterns." These morphologic differences and aberrations (in which the cells in the malignant tissue appear immature or less differentiated) are clues for the pathologist, who helps determine the presence or absence of a malignancy.

Although there are several definitions of cancer and neoplasia, selecting the most appropriate definition will depend ultimately on the individual's framework. One useful perspective is to define cancer or neoplasia as a process. In this way the conceptualization is broad enough to include all the aspects of this disease as studied both in the clinical and in the laboratory setting.

THE NATURAL HISTORY OF CANCER

Some well-known phenomena can help us understand that cancer is a process—not one event or one alteration, but a series of events. The discoveries of the histologic features of malignant growth led to the development of a classification system around 1900 (Rather, 1978). However, even with these established features, tissue alterations were discovered that could not be placed into either normal or neoplastic categories. Instead these intermediate lesions were considered to represent the sequential changes leading from the normal cell and tissue structure to the neoplastic ones. These forms included metaplasia, dysplasia, and carcinoma in situ (Fig. 13–1). This purported sequence helped to emphasize that the development of cancer has a natural history and that the clinical manifestations are often the final stages in a series of events (Correa, 1982; Goldfarb, 1983).

In metaplasia a normal differentiated cell type is replaced by another normal differentiated cell type. Typically metaplasia is induced by an irritant, and once the irritant is removed, the tissue reverts back to its normal state. Dysplasia, on the other hand, is "a loss in the uniformity of the individual cells as well as a loss in their architectural orientation" (Cotran et al., 1994b, p. 247). Characteristics of dysplastic cells include (1) the cells generally are found in the epithelia, (2) they exhibit pleomorphism, (3) they contain abnormally large nuclei for the cell, (4) mitoses may occur at all levels of the epithelium. Normally, higher proliferative rates occur in the basal level. (Cotran et al., 1994). Carcinoma in situ occurs when the dysplastic changes become more pronounced and involve all layers of the stratified epithelium (Fig. 13–1).

Studies of metastases provide a second example of cancer as a process. Metastasis is possible because cancer cells invade the blood vessels, withstand the natural immune mechanisms while traveling in the vessels, attach to capillary walls, enter tissue, and grow in the new milieu of the metastatic site. Each of the steps listed and perhaps a dozen others may involve genetic changes in the cell. Indicators of genetic changes include the formation of new clones of malignant cells, the activation of new enzymes, and the expression of new molecules on the cell surface and the loss of others (see Chapter 15, Fig. 15–1). Because most primary cancers can now be controlled by current therapies, understanding of the steps involved in metastasis should lead to better or more effective life-saving therapies (Fidler & Hart, 1982; Hart, 1986; Sukumar, Carney, & Barbacid, 1988; Wolberg, 1983).

Current knowledge of cancer as a clinical phenomenon is based on results of investigations ranging from the biochemical to the cellular and continues to the level of multiple physiologic interactions in the whole individual. This very brief outline of the molecular biology of cancer illustrates the complexity of the processes involved. Currently our understanding is evolving at so rapid a rate that it is difficult for any one individual to keep pace with all the new developments.

CANCER: A DISEASE OF ALTERED CELL DIFFERENTIATION

In normal growth and development, a cell becomes more specialized or committed to a particular line of development, and it acquires new characteristics. Differentiation is the process that results in readily observable changes in cellular characteristics. These changes are irreversible, self-perpetuating, and passed on to the daughter cells. Because most cells contain the entire genome, differentiation is the result of expression of certain genes and the repression of others (Alberts et al., 1989b; Ruddon, 1981; Watson, Hopkins, Roberts, Steitz, & Weiner, 1987).

Differentiated cells are mature cells that perform the functions of the particular tissues that they comprise. In the adult, undifferentiated cells (not totally committed) are known as pluripotent cells, precursor cells, or stem cells. Cells with the least amount of differentiation are found in the embryo. The fertilized egg is a totipotent cell and undergoes primary differentiation. As a cell becomes more differentiated, its potential becomes more restricted (Fig. 13–2). Totally differentiated cells often lose their ability to replicate, implying that the fate of the mature cell is death. Examples of fully differentiated cells are red blood cells, neurons, muscle cells, and helper T lymphocytes (Alberts et al., 1989b; Ruddon, 1981; Watson et al., 1987).

The most obvious reason why cancer is considered an altered differentiation state is that many neoplasms resemble undifferentiated tissue. For instance, both neoplastic and embryonic cells often are rapidly dividing, are motile, and have similar markers on their cell surfaces, such as carcinoembryonic antigen. Conversely, the most differentiated cells generally have lost their ability to divide.

One way of visualizing the differentiation process is to consider the development of a red blood cell in the

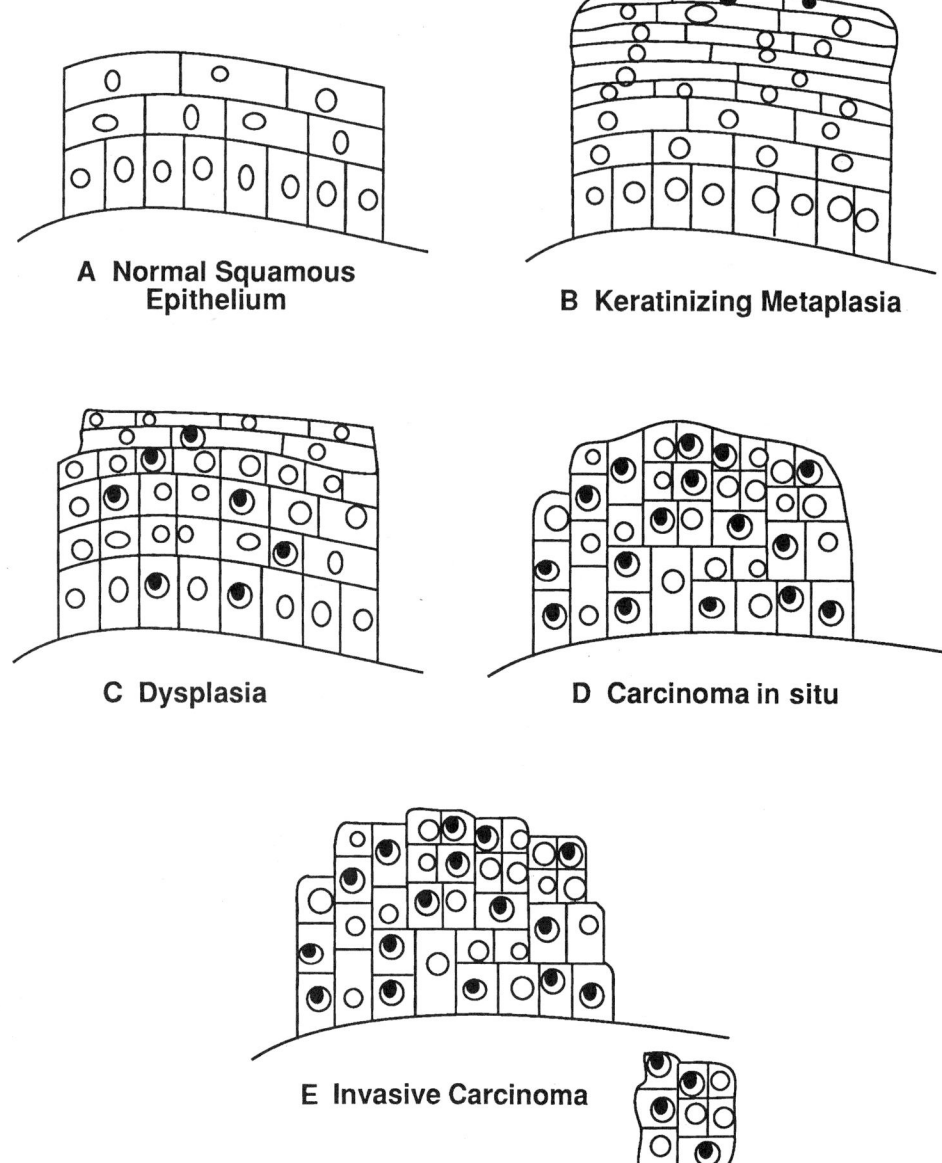

A Normal Squamous Epithelium

B Keratinizing Metaplasia

C Dysplasia

D Carcinoma in situ

E Invasive Carcinoma

FIGURE 13–1. The lesions that are presumably antecedent to invasive carcinoma: metaplasia, dysplasia, carinoma in situ. **A,** Normal endocervical epithelial differentiation, from a columnar basal cell to a flat, mature surface cell. **B,** Metaplasia: normal epithelium replaced by a keratinizing epithelium that is typical of skin and areas of irritation. **C,** Dysplasia: some atypical cells, but the surface is flattened and contains mature cells. **D,** Carcinoma in situ: total loss of differentiation with many atypical and dividing cells. **E,** Invasive carcinoma: malignant cells can be found beneath the basal lamina in the connective tissue.

adult (see Fig. 13–3). The stem cell resides in the bone marrow. This stem cell (pluripotent stem cell) has the capability to generate cell lines that will form any one of the blood cells (i.e., red blood cells as well as many of the white blood cells). As differentiation proceeds, some of the daughter cells of this stem cell acquire the cytologic characteristics of the mature cell, and they become committed (terminal differentiation) to a particular cell line. These cytologic features may be identified by a variety of cytologic and biochemical characteristics. The mature red blood cell will be anucleated, will be packed with hemoglobin, and will circulate in the blood (Alberts et al., 1989b; Greaves, 1986; Ruddon, 1981; Sachs, 1987; Watson et al., 1987).

Neoplasia can develop at any point in the process of differentiation. A cancer of the cell line leading directly to the red blood cell (at the point of terminal differentiation) is a erythroleukemia, a rare leukemia (Fig. 13–3). An example of a leukemia occurring in the cells

at an earlier stage of differentiation is acute myelogenous leukemia. In this disease the cells possess staining characteristics and markers of immature cells. During the natural history of many cancers, as the malignant cells grow and divide, they often lose more and more of their mature characteristics. In the natural history of erythroleukemia, this shift to a less differentiated cell type appears as the myeloblastic leukemia phase of the disease (Greaves, 1986; Oishi, 1983; Ruddon, 1981; Sachs, 1987).

Knowledge of differentiation prompts the obvious question: does induction of differentiation reduce the ability of malignant cells to divide? In the mouse erythroleukemia model, the addition of dimethylsulfoxide (DMSO) (as well as other chemicals such as retinoic acid) is capable of inducing some differentiation. While the leukemic cells are exposed to DMSO, the cells take on characteristics of a more mature cell (Pitot, 1986). Some of these differentiation agents have been tested in

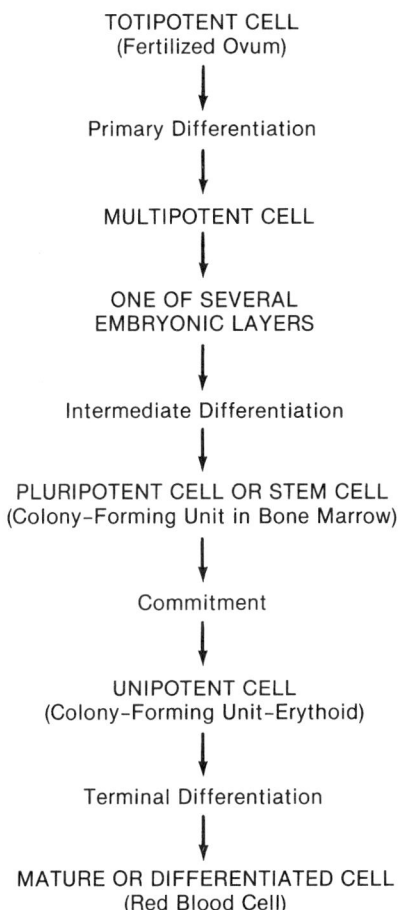

FIGURE 13–2. An example of how differentiation results in the production of red blood cells. Differentiation occurs many times in the life history of a cell. Each step in differentiation further limits the potential of the cell. The most differentiated cell is one that cannot divide and is destined to die.

human clinical trials (Hawkins, 1993; Pitot, 1986; Ruddon, 1981). Retinoids have not been successful in treating advanced malignancies. However, there have been some successes such as in the treatment of acute promyelocytic leukemia. Clinical treatment with trans-retinoic acid has resulted in a few complete remissions, and the promyelocytic cells express more mature differentiation antigens, and their proliferative ability is decreased (Hawkins, 1993).

Differentiation also refers to the degree to which the cells of neoplasms appear comparable, both morphologically and functionally, to normal cells. For example, tumors that are classified as well differentiated contain cells that resemble normal cells of the original tissue, whereas undifferentiated tumors have unspecialized, primitive-appearing cells. In the case of benign tumors, it is frequently difficult to distinguish benign tumor cells from normal cells. In this case, the clinical feature that distinguishes the two is the accumulation of benign cells into a mass surrounded by a fibrous capsule separating the tumor from the normal tissue (Cotran et al., 1994b).

One of the hallmarks of neoplasia is the lack of differentiation or anaplasia. Anaplastic cells and their nuclei are pleomorphic, that is, they vary in size and shape. The nuclei also contain large amounts of DNA and are disproportionate in size for the cell. These cells also exhibit a high rate of mitoses, which is not always indicative that the cells are neoplastic (Cotran et al., 1994b). However the mitotic figures in neoplastic cells are often bizarre with tripolar, quadripolar or multipolar spindles.

CLASSIFICATION OF TUMORS

The definitive diagnosis of cancer is made by the pathologist after he or she examines cells and tissues obtained at biopsy or from cytologic procedures. Classification of the tumor type is based on tissue and cellular staining. Differences in cytoplasmic and nuclear

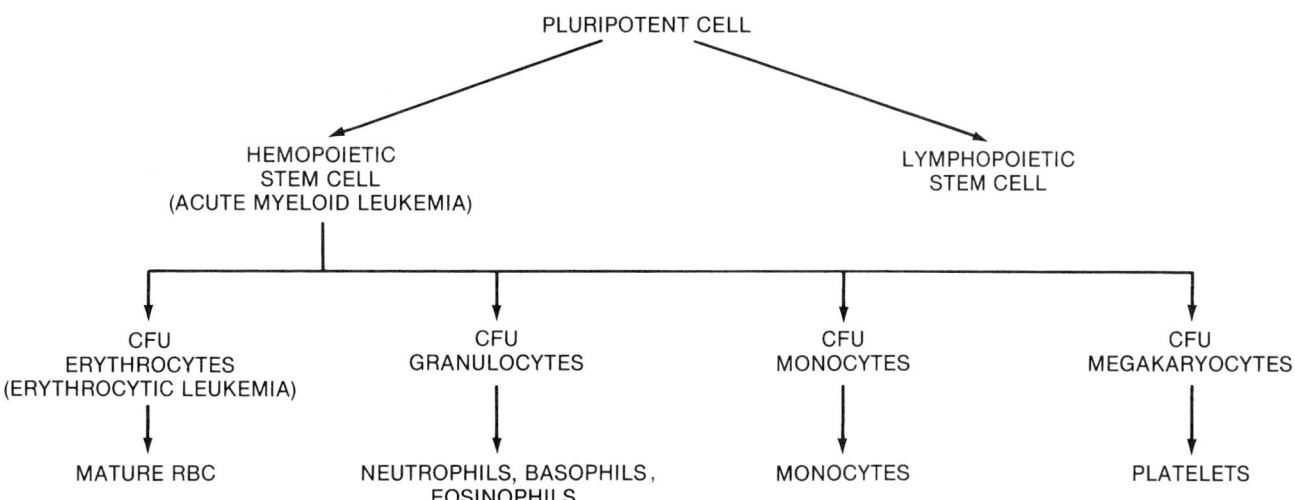

FIGURE 13–3. An expansion of Figure 13–2. An outline of differentiation in a hemopoietic cell line. The differentiation stages are noted in which erythrocytic leukemia and acute myeloid leukemia occur. *CFU,* colony-forming units; *RBC,* red blood cells.

TABLE 13–1. *Some Examples of the Differences Between Benign and Malignant Tumors*

PROPERTY	BENIGN TUMORS	MALIGNANT TUMORS
Growth	Slow expansile	Invasive
Differentiation	Fully differentiated	Immature, not differentiated
Metastasis	Absent	Present
Cytoplasm	Normal, uniform	Irregular in size and shape, pleomorphic
	Regular is size and shape	Basophilic
Nucleus	DNA content euploid	DNA content euploid to aneuploid
	Infrequent mitosis	Frequent mitosis
		Many nucleoli
Paraneoplastic syndromes	Absent	Present in many cases; for example anorexia, cachexia

staining distinguish one cell type from another and identify their stages of *differentiation*. A malignant neoplasm of epithelial tissue is classified as a *carcinoma*, as an *adenocarcinoma* if the tissue of origin has both epithelial and glandular components, and as a *sarcoma* if the tissue of origin is connective tissue. Likewise, benign tumors also follow a similar schema for classification. In most cases, benign tumors are classified by adding the suffix "oma" to the cell of origin. For example, a benign tumor of glandular origin is an adenoma; that of fibrous connective tissue is a fibroma. (For a list of selected characteristics of benign and malignant tumor types and a simple classification system, see Table 13–1 and Table 13–2.) Classification of the tumor type is imperative before decisions can be made about the most appropriate type of treatment (Bonfiglio & Terry, 1983; Cotran et al., 1994b).

In addition to assigning a classification to a tumor, a grade will frequently be given. The grade of a tumor is based on the degree of differentiation of the cells. A grade of 1 is given to a neoplasm that is well differentiated (i.e., one that appears similar to the specialized tissue from which it arose). The highest grade of 4 is given to a neoplasm that appears so undifferentiated (anaplastic) that it is difficult to identify the tissue of origin. It is thought that the degree of differentiation of a tumor is correlated with its growth rate. For example,

undifferentiated tumors grow more rapidly than a more differentiated tumor. Again, while this is generally true, there are incidences where malignant tumors apparently dormant for a number of years suddenly begin to proliferate rapidly, causing death in a short time (Cotran et al., 1994b). For many tumors, the higher the grade or the less differentiated the tumor is, the poorer the prognosis is (Bonfiglio & Terry, 1983).

Determination of grades between the two extremes of well differentiated and poorly differentiated tumor is difficult. Subjectivity and experience of the decision maker plays a role. Currently pathologic reports tend to emphasize the description of the tumor and not the assignment of a numeric grade. New advances in laboratory medicine, such as the development of flow cytometry, which can automatically characterize the DNA content of thousands of cells at one time and estimate the number of dividing cells, may lead to better prognostic indicators than the grade of the tumors.

TRANSFORMATION—A METHOD FOR UNDERSTANDING NEOPLASIA

Through histologic techniques, pathologists were able to distinguish malignant cells from normal cells. But it would seem profitable to study cell differentia-

TABLE 13–2. *Selected Examples of Benign and Malignant Tumors*

TISSUE OF ORIGIN	BENIGN TUMORS	MALIGNANT TUMORS
Epithelial	Adenoma	Adenocarcinoma
Glandular	Polyp, papilloma	Carcinoma
Epithelial		
Connective		
Bone	Osteoma	Osteosarcoma
Fibrous	Fibroma	Fibrosarcoma
Fat	Lipoma	Liposarcoma
Smooth muscle	Leiomyoma	Leiomyosarcoma
Striated muscle	Rhabdomyoma	Rhabdomyosarcoma
Hematopoietic		
Erythrocytes		Erytholeukemia
Lymphocytes		Lymphocytic leukemia
Lymphatic tissue		Malignant lymphoma, Hodgkin's disease
Plasma cell		Multiple myeloma
Pigmented cells	Nevus	Melanoma
Neural	Neuroma	Glioblastoma

Box 13–1. *Types of Cells*

Normal cells transferred from the animal into tissue culture undergo only a fixed number of divisions. For instance, skin cells will undergo approximately 50 to 100 divisions before the culture dies out.

From a *culture* of normal cells, some cells arise that can undergo repeated divisions. Once this process becomes established the culture is called a *cell line*. Even though this cell line is *immortal*, it does not have other biologic characteristics of a true malignancy. One of the easiest cell lines to establish in culture is the fibroblast. Much of the original transformation work was done on fibroblasts even though tumors of this cell type are very rare in humans (Alberts et al., 1983; Pardee, 1982; Pitot, 1986; Ruddon, 1981; Watson et al., 1987).

Transformed cells are cells derived from established cell lines and are essentially immortal (i.e., they can undergo repeated cell divisions). These lines can be kept in culture for years without dying if the proper culture conditions are maintained. They also have cytoplasmic and nuclear characteristics of malignant cells (Alberts et al., 1983; Pardee, 1982; Pitot, 1986; Ruddon, 1981; Watson et al., 1987).

---

tion and carcinogenesis in isolation from the influence of all the other supporting structures and physiologic processes of the host, as in cell cultures. However, malignant tissue from actual patients is not always available, nor is it the best experimental system.

As early as the 1920s, when modern biochemistry was emerging, neoplastic cells were removed from the animal or the patient and brought to the laboratory, where attempts were made to cultivate them (in vitro cell culture studies). These neoplastic cells then were examined with respect to their properties. Attempts were also made to sequence the changes characteristic of the neoplastic process. But these cells already had a long "malignant history" (Alberts et al., 1989b; Pardee, 1982; Pitot, 1986; Ruddon, 1981; Watson et al., 1987). The initiating events occurred at an early stage, and it was difficult to unravel the chain of events.

To overcome these problems and in an attempt to study the earliest stages of oncogenesis, normal cells were established in culture (cell lines) and were then exposed to carcinogens (chemicals, viruses, or radiation). These cultured cells subsequently developed characteristics of malignant cells; this process was termed *transformation*. Because these cells are not derived from a tumor in a human or an animal, they are termed transformed rather than malignant cells (see Box 13–1) (Alberts et al., 1989b; Pardee, 1982; Pitot, 1986; Ruddon, 1981; Watson et al., 1987).

Methodologic problems also exist when studying carcinogenesis and the neoplastic phenotype via transformation. Criteria were established to help ensure that what was happening in culture (in vitro) was similar to the neoplastic process in vivo. One of the main criteria is the ability of transformed cells to establish a tumor in an appropriate animal model. The putatively transformed cells are injected into an animal, and if a tumor results, then transformation is said to have occurred. This definitive experiment is not always done because of the expense and time commitment. Some of the reported examples of cellular changes may not be exclusively associated with the neoplastic phenotype but rather are correlated with normal cell division (Alberts et al., 1989b; Pardee, 1982; Pitot, 1986; Ruddon, 1981; Watson et al., 1987). However, studies of transformation have led to insights into neoplasia and the ability to distinguish critical events in oncogenesis.

Many of the characteristics of the transformed and malignant cell can now be attributed to changes in the genome (Pardee, 1982).

CHARACTERISTICS OF TRANSFORMED CELLS

The physically obvious features of size, shape, and orientation and the growth characteristics of transformed cells distinguish them from normal cell lines (see Fig. 13–4 and Chapter 15, Fig. 15–1). Transformed cells in culture have basophilic cytoplasm, irregular cellular outlines, and large nuclei that contain multiple nucleoli. Mitotic figures are more numerous in transformed cell lines than in a normal cell line. In addition, transformed cells differ from normal cells in such im-

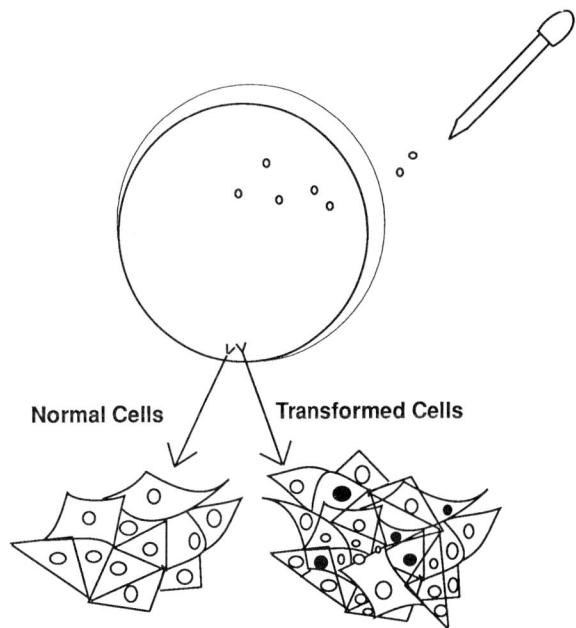

FIGURE 13–4. A schematic representation of normal cells in culture and transformed cells in culture. Cells are deposited onto a Petri dish containing suitable growth media. Normal cells exhibit contact inhibition. Transformed cells are more diverse with respect to their cytoplasmic and nuclear characteristics; they can form mulitlayers, and they lack contact inhibition.

portant characteristics as mobility and growth requirements (Alberts et al., 1989b; Pardee, 1982; Pitot, 1986; Ruddon, 1981; Watson et al., 1987).

THE CELL SURFACE

The study of the cytoplasmic membrane adds an important dimension in the study of transformation because (1) loss of contact inhibition is linked to changes in the cell surface, (2) establishment of metastatic deposits depends on the ability of the tumor cells to invade and move, (3) hormones and growth factors often act at the surface, and tumor cells often lose the ability to be regulated by these factors, and (4) it is at the surface that the immune system will or will not recognize the cell as altered (Nicolson & Poste, 1974; Pitot, 1986; Ruddon, 1981).

The cytoplasmic membrane is also the interface between the cell and the extracellular medium. The cell membrane consists of lipids (phospholipids), proteins, and carbohydrates bound to either the lipid or the protein components. Molecules in the membrane can move or rearrange themselves. Tumor cells have a greater fluidity, perhaps owing to changes in the lipid composition. This property of malignant cells may in the future be exploited by the packaging of chemotherapeutic agents into liposomes. These liposomes (spheres with an outer lipid layer and an internal core of drugs) are more readily taken up by the malignant cell membrane than by the normal cell membrane. Thus the malignant cells would receive a greater dosage of the chemotherapeutic agent than normal cells (Nicolson & Poste, 1974; Pardee, 1982; Ruddon, 1981).

The cell surfaces of transformed cells express new antigens (molecules) not present in the normal cell type. These antigens are called tumor-associated antigens in animal models; in human cells they are oncofetal antigens, viral antigens, or tumor-associated molecules. Two examples of oncofetal antigens used in monitoring patients are carcinoembryonic antigen and α-fetoprotein. Other antigens, or surface molecules, are absent in transformed cells. It has been proposed that the loss or shedding of tumor antigens or antigen-antibody complexes might form blocking factors and prevent the immune cells or molecules from attaching to malignant cells (Nicolson & Poste, 1974; Pitot, 1986; Ruddon, 1981; Watson et al., 1987).

CYTOPLASMIC STRUCTURES

Much has been written about the differences in the cytoplasmic structures and metabolic processes of transformed cells and their normal counterparts. As in the case of the cytoplasmic membrane, it is not clear at this point which changes are a result of transformation and which initiate transformation. To ask the question in another way, at which stage of oncogenesis do these events occur? With our increased understanding of oncogenes, the sequence of cytoplasmic and nuclear events is being unraveled.

Warburg's hypothesis is given here as an example of cytoplasmic changes in transformation. But for every cytoplasmic structure and metabolic pathway, a similar story holds:

1. When the phenomenon is first investigated, it seems to hold for all the cases investigated. As more experiments are done, exceptions are found owing to the extreme heterogeneity of neoplasms.
2. It is difficult to determine which alterations in the cytoplasm and cell membrane are primary and which are secondary events in transformation.

The mitochondrial changes and the intermediary metabolism of glucose were among the first cellular systems investigated, starting with Warburg's work in the 1920s and 1930s. Warburg developed an elaborate hypothesis of carcinogenesis based on the observation that malignant cells utilized anaerobic glycolysis to a greater extent than normal cells (i.e., malignant cells consumed less oxygen and produced more lactic acid than normal cells). Warburg proposed that carcinogens poisoned the mitochondria, allowing the more primitive cells (those with fewer mitochondria) to survive. Mitochondria generate adenosine triphosphate (ATP) via oxidative phosphorylation. Because the more primitive cells could survive in oxygen-poor environments, Warburg contended that it was from this population the malignant cells arose (Pardee, 1982; Pitot, 1986; Watson et al., 1987). His observations still stand today. However, the present theoretic framework is very different. Currently the interpretation would be that tumor cells survive in oxygen-poor environments because of oncogenesis rather than the lack of oxygen being the initiator. It must be remembered that during Warburg's time it was not known which molecules in the cell were the repository of genetic information, and therefore his reasoning was logical. With the rapid increase in knowledge of oncogenesis today, how many current ideas will be rejected even 5 years from now?

CONTACT INHIBITION: ONE PROPERTY OF TRANSFORMED CELLS

Normal cell lines in culture exhibit a property known as contact inhibition, that is, when a cell line is plated onto a Petri dish, the cells will keep growing and dividing until the bottom of the dish is covered with cells, and then division stops. This monolayer of cells will orient themselves with respect to one another. Transformed cells, on the other hand, do not stop dividing. Instead, they move over and pile on top of one another until a multilayered culture is formed (see Fig. 13-4). This lack of contact inhibition is thought to be the result of two independent properties of the cell, mobility and replication (Pardee, 1982; Pitot, 1986; Ruddon, 1981; Watson et al., 1987).

First, transformed cells are more mobile and do not adhere to other cells as well as do normal cells. This property is linked to changes in the plasma membrane of the transformed cell as well as to alteration in the cytoplasmic skeletal elements. Normal cells, however, will form tight junctions and other areas of close contact with cells of their own type. Second, as already noted, transformed cells do not stop dividing and therefore grow to a high density in culture. This ability to grow in conditions unfavorable to normal cell lines often signals when transformation has occurred.

THE CELL CYCLE AND APOPTOSIS: A PRELUDE TO UNDERSTANDING THE MOLECULAR EVENTS IN TRANSFORMATION AND CARCINOGENESIS

To adequately understand the molecular biology of transformation and the theories underlying the treatment and diagnosis of cancer, one needs to examine the different types of cells according to their proliferative ability and the processes that occur during the cell cycle. According to one of the classification schemas, there are three types of cells: (1) the continuously dividing or labile cells, (2) the quiescent cells, and (3) the nondividing or permanent cells. The labile cells continually replace cells that are being destroyed either via natural cell death or injury. These cells are found in surface epithelia, hematopoietic tissues, and mucosa such as the columnar epithelia of the gastrointestinal tract, and the transitional epithelium of the urinary tract (Cotran et al., 1994a).

Quiescent cells are characterized by a low level of cellular division but can rapidly divide when exposed to stimuli such as injury or inflammation. Cells of this type are found in the glandular organs of the body, the mesenchymal cells, which includes fibroblasts, and the vascular endothelium. Nondividing cells have permanently left the cell cycle and are incapable of mitosis.

Nerve, skeletal, and cardiac muscle cells constitute this type of cell (Cotran et al., 1994a) (see Box 13–2 for a glossary of terminology).

THE CELL CYCLE

The cell cycle consists of four major phases whose processes sequentially result in cell division or mitosis (see Fig. 13–5). Between mitotic phases, an interphase period or elapse time occurs. During this phase, elaborate preparations for mitosis are taking place. Three phases make up the interphase: G_1, S, and G_2. Interphase begins with the G_1, during which time many of the enzymes necessary for DNA synthesis are made. In the S phase, the cellular DNA component doubles in preparation for division. During the G_2 phase, RNA is synthesized, and specialized proteins as well as the mitotic spindle are manufactured. The M phase, which is the shortest phase of the cell cycle lasting approximately one half hour to 1 hour, is made up of four stages: prophase, metaphase, anaphase, and telophase. During the prophase, the chromosomes increase in thickness and begin to clump together. The chromosomes then line up in the center of the cell during the metaphase. This is followed by anaphase, during which time segregation of the chromosomes to the centrioles occurs. Finally, during telophase, the cell divides, producing two daughter cells (Alberts et al., 1989b; Dorr & Von Hoff, 1994).

Autoradiography is the technique by which the time of DNA synthesis in the cell cycle is determined. The method utilizes ^{3}H-thymidine, a radioactive precursor needed by all cells in the synthesis of DNA, either in-

---

Box 13–2. *Glossary of Terms*

General terminology

Neoplasm: An abnormal mass of tissue, the growth of which exceeds and is uncoordinated with that of the normal tissues and persists in the same excessive manner after cesssation of the stimuli, which evoked the change.

Tumor: Any swelling.

Cancer: A disease of the cell in which the normal mechanisms of control of growth and proliferation are disturbed and results in distinctive morphologic alterations of the cell and aberrations of tissue patterns.

Differentiation: The process that results in readily observable changes in cellular characteristics that are irreversible, self-perpetuating, and passed on to daughter cells. The cells are mature and perform the functions of the particular tissues that they comprise.

Undifferentiation: Not differentiated. The cells are primitive, immature, enbryonic cells that have no special structure or function.

Anaplasia: Lack of differentiation. The cells are pleomorphic, and their nucei contain large amounts of DNA and are disproportionate in size to the cell.

Dysplasia: A loss in the uniformity of the individual cells and in their architectural orientation. The cells are found in the epitheilia, exhibit pleomorphism, contain large nuclei for the cell, and higher mitoses rates occur throughout epithelium.

Metaplasia: The abnormal transformation of an adult, fully differentiated tissue of one kind into a differentiated tissue of another kind.

Proliferative cell types

Labile cells: Continuously dividing cells that replace cells that are constantly being destroyed either by apoptosis or injury.

Quiescent cells: Characterized by a small amount of cellular division. Can rapidly divide when exposed to stimuli such as injury or inflammation.

Permanent cells: Nondividing cells that have left the cell cycle and are incapable of mitosis.

Stem cell: A pluripotent cell from which all blood cells originate.

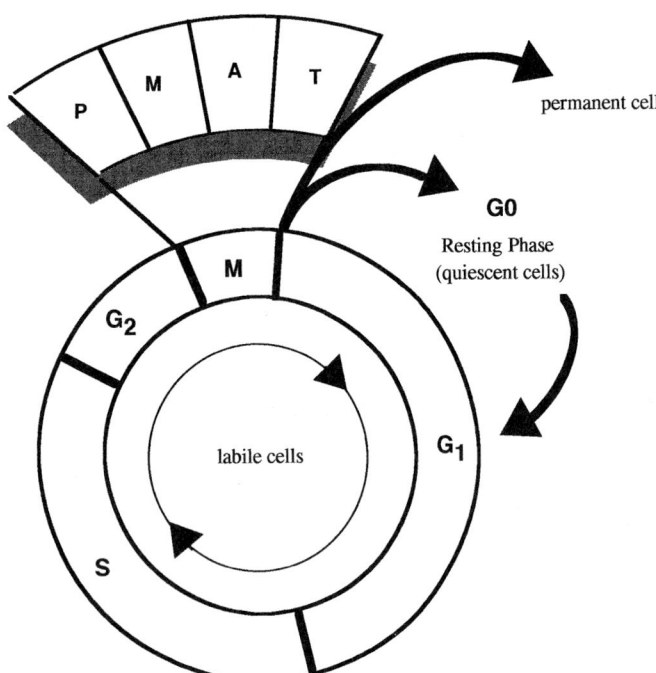

Figure 13–5. A visual representation of the cell cycle consisting of four major phases: G_1, S, G_2, and M. Four subphases are contained within the mitosis phase: prophase (P), metaphase (M), anaphase (A), and telophase (T).

jected into the animal (in vivo) or added to the culture medium of cells (in vitro). If an injection of ^{3}H-thymidine is administered to the culture medium and autoradiographs are prepared at various time points after the injection, it is possible to determine the four phases of the cell cycle and the duration of each phase. Cells that are in the S phase at the time of injection are the first to be radiolabeled because DNA is being synthesized. The duration of G_2 is determined by measuring the time it takes the cells to reach the M phase from the S phase. Then, the duration of the entire cell cycle can be determined by measuring the time it takes the radiolabeled cells to reappear in the M phase. Finally, by subtracting the durations of the S, G_2, and M phases from the total cell cycle time, the duration of the G_1 is determined. The cell cycle can vary considerably in time among cells, ranging from as little as 8 hours to more than 1 year in adults. In addition, a resting phase, G_0, also occurs, during which time the cell is not committed to actual cell division (Alberts et al., 1989b; Dorr & Von Hoff, 1994).

GROWTH FACTORS, CHECKPOINTS, CYCLINS, AND THE CELL CYCLE

What regulates the cell cycle? It is only with the discovery of growth factors, oncogenes, and tumor suppressor genes that a coherent picture is evolving. To induce a cell into division, growth factors must be present in the serum or be produced by the cells. *Growth factors* are polypeptides that either set the stage for proliferation, that is, make cells in the G_0 or G_1 phase competent for division, or stimulate DNA synthesis in the competent cells. Growth factors also influence many other cellular properties such as differentiation and cell motility.

Many growth factors bind to receptors on the cell membrane. The binding of these growth factors results in conformational changes of the molecule in the membrane and change in enzymatic activity inside the cell. Other growth factors such as steroids are transported across the cell and bind to cytoplasmic receptors and are then transported to the nucleus. In either case the growth factor acts as a signal and sets off a chain of reactions inside the cell that ultimately leads to cell division (Cotran et al., 1994a).

This chain of reactions is called *signal transduction* and acts via a second messenger (the first messenger being the growth factor). Three mechanisms have been proposed to explain the transduction of the signal from the surface membrane to the cytoplasm and nucleus. The first is the activation of protein kinases, which generate cyclic nucleotides such as cyclic adenosine monophosphate (cAMP) and cyclic guanosine monophosphate (cGMP). The second involves endocytosis (engulfing and incorporation) of the complexed hormone and receptor. The third mechanism involves the influx into the cytoplasm of small ions such as calcium and magnesium. Phospholipase C, GTP-binding proteins, and serine threonine kinase are some of the molecules involved. The end result of signal transduction is regulation of gene transcription, mRNA processing and degradation, protein synthesis, and DNA synthesis—all of which ultimately leads to cell division (Alberts et al., 1989b; Cotran et al., 1994a; Watson et al., 1987). In turn, signal transduction is regulated by another series of proteins or *growth inhibitors*, which are often the cellular phosphatases.

There are several control points during the cell cycle that, given environmental conditions, influence the continuation of growth. For instance, in the G_1 phase there is a restriction or *checkpoint* where the growth of the cells may be temporarily stopped if the environmental conditions are not favorable. If the cells pass this point, they are committed to complete the cell cycle (Alberts et al., 1989; Hartwell, Leland, & Kastan, 1994; Hartwell & Weinert, 1989; Marx, 1991). Before the checkpoint the cell needs growth factors to grow; after the checkpoint the cell continues with the cell cycle and eventually divides even if growth factors are absent. The checkpoints are then important processes to examine in cellular transformation, since tumor cells can often proceed in the cell cycle independent of the availability of growth factors.

The *cyclins* are a class of proteins that regulate the activity of the kinases, which trigger the events in the cell cycle. (Kinases are enzymes that phosphorylate proteins, that is, add a phosphate group to the protein.) There are four sets of cyclins, and there may be others. The cyclins complex with cellular kinases and drive the cell from one phase of the cell cycle to the next. The D cyclins and its kinase are probably activated by growth factors. Cyclin E or A in late G_1 activates a kinase, which results in DNA replication. Other cyclins activate a kinase that signals the initiation of S phase. If cyclins at the checkpoints do not bind to the kinases then the cell cannot proceed to the S phase of the cycle. During the cell cycle, for mitosis to occur, DNA is replicated, protein synthesis is induced, the nuclear membrane dissolves, condensation and packaging of chromosomes occur, and the cytoskeleton reorganizes. This orderly sequence of events and the accurate replication of DNA during the cell cycle is dependent on these tightly regulated systems of both positive and negative feedback loops (Hartwell & Kastan, 1994).

The activity of the genes that control the checkpoints are integrated with DNA repair mechanisms and surveillance of the spindle structures of mitosis. For instance, the checkpoint of the G_1 to S phase detects DNA damage. If defective DNA is present, then the cell stops replicating the DNA, and G_1 is arrested. This is accompanied by a rise in the p53 protein levels. One function of p53 is to turn on other genes, some of which control cell death. If the checkpoints were impaired, this could lead to chromosomal rearrangements, deletions, amplification, and translocations. Spindle defects could lead to loss or gain of whole chromosomes or a change in ploidy. All these defects are commonly seen in tumor progression (Hartwell & Kastan, 1994).

APOPTOSIS

To maintain a stable number of cells in a tissue, not only must cell growth, division, and differentiation occur, but also must cell death (Fig. 13–6). Apoptosis is normal programmed cell death and is distinguishable from necrosis (cell death due to an injury). In apoptosis the chromatin material of the nucleus condenses, and the nucleus fragments. The cell fragments and separates into discrete membrane bound apoptotic bodies, which are then phagocytosed. External stimuli can also induce apoptosis. Irradiation, deprivation of growth factors, lymphotoxin, tumor necrosis factor, and glucocorticoids all stimulate the cell to undergo apoptosis.

STEM CELL

⇓

PROLIFERATION

⇓

DIFFERENTIATION

⇓

CELL POPULATION

⇓

SENESCENCE

⇓

APOPTOSIS

⇓

DEATH

FIGURE 13–6. The number of cells in a population is a balance of two different rates: proliferation and apoptosis or programmed cell death. Neoplasia can be the result of genetic changes that control either of these two processes. The increase number of cells seen in neoplasms are then the result of increase of cell proliferation or a decrease in cell death.

Apoptosis does not induce an inflammatory response and therefore is not accompanied by pain. In necrosis, swelling of the organelles occurs rather than condensation. There is membrane damage, rupture of the cytoplasmic membrane, and inflammation. The genes that control apoptosis are of interest not only to the oncologists but also the gerontologists. Perhaps some of the aging processes are under control of the apoptotic genes (Cotran et al., 1994b).

As in the regulation of the cell cycle, there are positive and negative modulators of apoptosis. The positive genetic modulators of apoptosis inhibit growth, are called growth arrest genes, and are closely related to the genes activated by DNA damage. They may also be activated in the process of differentiation and called primary response genes. The negative modulators of apoptosis promote cell survival and inhibit apoptosis. In a cell the balance of the positive and negative modulators determines whether a cell will survive and proliferate or differentiate and die (Hoffman & Liebermann, 1994).

GENE REPLICATION AND TRANSCRIPTION

The cell cycle and apoptosis are controlled by numerous genes, and defects in these genes can lead to transformation or the development of a malignant cell. Before the discussion of oncogenes and cancer suppressor genes, it may be helpful to review gene replication and transcription.

The human genome is composed of 23 pairs of different chromosomes, for a total of 46 chromosomes. One set of chromosomes is inherited from the mother,

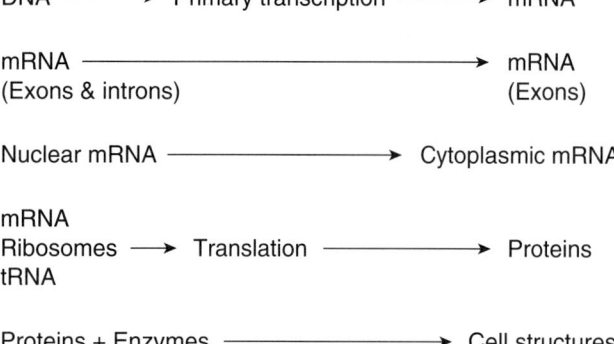

DNA ⟶ Primary transcription ⟶ mRNA

mRNA ⟶ mRNA
(Exons & introns)   (Exons)

Nuclear mRNA ⟶ Cytoplasmic mRNA

mRNA
Ribosomes ⟶ Translation ⟶ Proteins
tRNA

Proteins + Enzymes ⟶ Cell structures
& function

FIGURE 13–7. Major sequence of reactions in gene expression. The genetic code is translated into cellular structure, which determines cellular function. *DNA,* deoxyribonucleic acid; *mRNA,* messenger RNA, a polymer of nucleotides (A,U,G,C) and is decoded to form proteins; *tRNA,* transfer RNA; enzymes: proteins or RNA chains capable of facilitating a specific chemical reaction.

the other set from the father. Each chromosome consists of two highly coiled strands of deoxyribonucleic acid (DNA) that are held together by chemical bonds. DNA chains can be very large, totaling 1 million to 1 billion atoms. Genetic information is conveyed by the arrangement of the nucleotide sequence in each DNA chain. The construction of genetic information can be compared to a description of written language. Symbols or letters (nucleotides) guided by rules (chemical bonds) and punctuation (enzymes, promotor and suppressor genes) can be combined in numerous ways (codons and exons) to create innumerable words (genes). These words can be arranged in countless sentences (DNA, RNA, proteins) to create paragraphs and poems (cellular structure), chapters and books (complex organisms).

The process of interpreting a gene's information is called gene expression (Fig. 13–7). The first step in gene

expression is transcription or the transferring of the genetic code from DNA to ribonucleic acid (RNA). Transcription is mediated by an enzyme called RNA polymerase, which causes the DNA to start unwinding at the beginning of a gene. The enzyme then begins to assemble RNA chains using nucleotides that match the DNA sequence. The newly formed RNA maintains its sequence as it "peels off" the DNA chain. The unwound segment of DNA then resumes its original location reforming the double helix.

Before leaving the nucleus for the cytoplasm, the RNA is processed, leaving only coding regions of the RNA strand (exons). The product, messenger RNA, enters the cytoplasm, where it is used to generate polypeptides (polymers of amino acids). Proteins are often composed of more than one polypeptide chain. The process of generating polypeptide chains from RNA is called translation (Alberts et al., 1989a; Berg & Singer, 1992; Mathews & van Holde, 1990) (see Fig. 13–8).

Gene expression is far from simple. Approximately 100 enzymes are involved in synthesizing the bases adenine, guanine, tyrosine, and cytosine, and connecting them to the sugars and phosphates prior to their insertion in the newly formed DNA strand. Other enzymes repair gaps and breaks in the DNA strand, unwind the strands so that replication can occur, and twist the strands so that the complementary base pairs can be correctly connected (Edlin, 1984). During DNA replication approximately 109 nucleotides are copied and their bases correctly aligned within a half an hour to 1 hour. Mistakes in this replication process can lead to mutations that are subsequently copied in all future generations of the cell line. In some cases, the mutation might result in the inactivation of a crucial protein, therefore causing cell death and loss of the mutation. In other incidences, the mutation may take place in a nonessential region on the gene and be considered a silent gene (Alberts et al., 1989a) (see Fig. 13–8). Other mutations may result in the production of abnormal proteins or abnormal gene expression and lead to transformation.

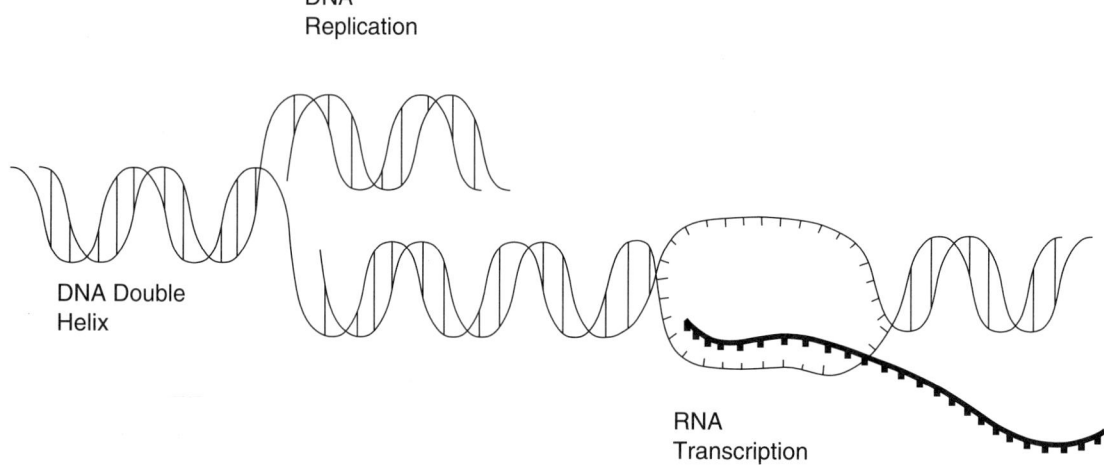

FIGURE 13–8. DNA double helix undergoing replication and transcription. The individual DNA strands are connected by base pairs. During replication, complementary strands of DNA are produced. During transcription, the two DNA strands separate while an RNA strand is synthesized. After transcription, the DNA strands reanneal and the RNA strand separates from the helix.

ONCOGENIC STUDIES: STUDIES AT THE SINGLE GENE LEVEL

In general, three main types of genes are involved in the development of malignant characteristics (Klein & Klein, 1985). The first type is the oncogene, which actively induces the development of a tumor or transformation in cell culture. The second type is the tumor suppressor gene or antioncogene. The loss or the inactivity of the tumor suppressor gene permits the development of a tumor. The p53 gene, a positive modulator of apoptosis, and the breast cancer susceptibility gene BRCA1 are considered tumor suppressor genes. A great deal of the evidence for oncogenes and antioncogenes derives from the study of heritable forms of cancer, such as retinoblastoma and breast and colon cancers (Marx, 1994). The third type is the modulating genes that are involved in the modification of tumor-host interactions and are therefore involved in tumor progression. An example of these genes are the ones for angiogenesis and antiangiogenesis factors involved in the metastatic process.

To some extent the classification of the genes involved in transformation is a bit arbitrary. To date, oncogenes consist of genes that code for growth factors or hormone receptors at the cell surface, the transduction of growth signals from the cell membrane to the nucleus, transcription factors, which enhance the synthesis of messenger RNA and regulate gene activity, DNA repair enzymes, which are also involved in transcription and apoptosis, and for tissue differentiation. To date, approximately 70 oncogenes and 12 tumor suppressor genes have been described (Marx, 1994).

The growth in this field is so rapid and these molecules are so central to the cell cycle, differentiation, and cell death that it is impossible to discuss all of them and their activities here. Just as discovering the differences between normal and tumor cells in terms of biochemistry and cytology led to new discoveries and theories, so too this new area of molecular biology has led to remarkable insights into normal cell cell biology, developmental biology, neurobiology, and immunology. As in early eras, some of these newly described differences between normal cells and malignant cells will most likely be the result of transformation, but others will be necessary and sufficient for the development of a malignancy.

Because single genes cannot be visualized even by the most sensitive chromosomal banding techniques, transformation studies are used to detect the presence of a gene or altered forms of the gene (Heim & Mitelman, 1987; Kahn & Graf, 1986; Klein & Klein, 1985; Nowell, 1988; Pitot, 1986; Teich, 1986; Watson et al., 1987). Other methods and discoveries that were key to the unraveling of the mysteries of oncogenes were the identification of restriction enzymes (that cleave DNA strands at specific sequences), polymerase chain reaction (permits detection of extremely small quantities of DNA or RNA and amplifies a copy of DNA 2^{30} times), sequencing of the human genome, and using recombinant DNA to develop transgenic animals.

DETECTION OF ONCOGENES

Oncogenes are studied by introducing a gene into cells growing in culture and noting whether the cells then undergo transformation. The genes causing the transformation can be obtained from two sources, tumor viruses or malignant cells (Table 13–3). These studies have provided a great deal of evidence that the critical event in carcinogenesis is a genetic change.

Oncogenes were first studied in retroviruses approximately 20 years ago. These viruses can induce the formation of multiple tumors in infected animals and transform cells in culture. The genetic material of retroviruses is RNA, and once inside a cell the viral RNA is used as a template to form viral DNA. The viral DNA can then induce the formation of more viral particles or become incorporated into the host's genetic material and remain latent. While studying the genes of these viruses, it became possible to separate the gene that caused transformation from the viral genes. The oncogene could by itself induce transformation. (Klein & Klein, 1985; Nowell, 1988; Pitot, 1986; Teich, 1986).

In 1976 Stehelin, Varmus, Bishop, and Vogt discovered that viral oncogenes were very similar, if not identical, to normal cellular genes. These cellular genes were termed *cellular oncogenes (c-onc)*, or proto-oncogenes. It appears that at some point in its evolutionary history, the retrovirus captured the cellular oncogene and incorporated it into viral genome. This was an exciting discovery since, "it told us that the cell contains genes that have an oncogenic potential" (Marx, 1994, p. 1942). The oncogene, it was thought, conferred an advantage to the virus, and therefore the oncogene was conserved in the viral genome.

Cellular oncogenes were found in every species that has been studied. Indeed, the structure of cellular oncogenes has been found to be similar no matter where found, from mammalian to yeast to fruit fly cells. This evolutionary conservation means that these genes are very important and serve essential functions in the cell. In this sense, the term oncogene does not adequately

TABLE 13–3. *Examples of Oncogenes, Their Origins, and the Chromosome(s) on Which They Are Located*

ONCOGENE	ORIGIN*	CHROMOSOME(S)
abl	Abelson murine leukemia	9
erbB	Avian erythroblastosis	7
fms	Feline sarcoma	5
met	Human osteosarcoma	3
myc	Avian myelocytomatosis	8
L-myc	Human lung carcinoma	1
N-myc	Human neuroblastoma	2
ras	Murine sarcoma (several types)	6, 11, 12
N-ras	Human neuroblastoma	1
sis	Simian sarcoma	22

*Virally induced tumor or the tumor in which the oncogene was discovered.

describe the function of these genes but rather describes how they were first investigated (Heim & Mitelman, 1987; Kahn & Graf, 1986; Nowell, 1988; Teich, 1986; Watson et al., 1987).

Another method used to study or "see" oncogenes is termed *transfection*. In this technique, DNA from malignant cells, either human or experimentally induced tumors, is introduced into normal cultured cells. Some of the recipient cells will then undergo transformation and acquire a malignant phenotype (Bar-Sagi & Feramisco, 1986; Gebhardt & Foulkes, 1986; Hanafusa, 1986; Watson, Tooze, & Kurtz, 1983). The gene that caused the transformation is then cloned and analyzed. These types of experiments proved that oncogenes were not a manifestation of a rare viral infection but were also present in spontaneously arising tumors (Cotran et al., 1994b).

Murray et al. (1981) and Krontiris and Cooper (1981) reported that DNA from bladder cancer induced transformation in a transfection assay. Later this gene turned out to be the homologue of the viral oncogene *ras* (murine sarcoma virus). In this case the difference between the oncogene and the proto-oncogene (normal cellular gene) was a point mutation. A change in a single nucleotide base was enough to substitute one amino acid for another in the protein and convert a normal gene to an oncogene. The ras oncogene is frequently activated in common cancers such as in 90 per cent of pancreatic adenocarcinomas, 50 per cent of colon and thyroid cancers, and 30 per cent of lung adenocarcinomas (Cotran et al., 1994b; Marx, 1994). Other mechanisms for producing oncogenes have since been discovered.

FORMATION OF ONCOGENES AND TUMOR SUPPRESSOR GENES

How do oncogenes and tumor suppressor genes differ from their normal cellular counterparts—that is, if they do? Theoretically, two major mechanisms can be responsible for the activation of oncogenes. The first involves the *regulation* of the gene and the second the *alteration of the structure* of the gene itself. Oncogenes, like all other genes, are regulated, and the decoupling of the regulation of the oncogene could result in overexpression of the gene. This probably occurs in the *c-myc* gene in Burkitt's lymphoma, in which there appears to be a physical uncoupling of the gene from its regulator.

In Burkitt's lymphoma a reciprocal *chromosomal translocation* may lead to the proto-oncogene, c-myc, to be placed together in proximity to the immunoglobulin promoter or enhancer elements. This new location presumably leads to relentless stimulation of the gene and production of increased levels of the c-myc protein product in the cell. In chronic myelogenous leukemia the c-abl proto-oncogene is translocated and inserted into another gene in a different chromosome. This chromosomal translocation results in structural change. The c-able gene is fused to another gene, and a new gene that codes for a novel protein is formed (Phillips & Nuwayhid 1993). This protein might be the ideal

target for developing chemotherapeutic or immunologic agents, since normal cells do not possess this novel protein.

Another process, called *gene amplification,* occurs when multiple copies of the gene are made; this could also lead to overexpression of the oncogene. For some oncogenes, it appears that a *mutation* (structural change) has occurred. Therefore, the oncogene differs from its normal counterpart by one or more DNA bases. This seems to be the case with the *ras* oncogene. In addition, major structural changes are seen in other oncogenes such as the abl gene in chronic myeloid leukemia (Heim & Mitelman, 1987; Kahn & Graf, 1986; Klein & Klein, 1985; Nowell, 1988; Phillips & Nuwayhid, 1993; Pitot, 1986; Teich, 1986; Watson et al., 1987).

Insertional mutagenesis occurs when strong gene promoters are inserted next to an oncogene. This leads to activation and dysregulation of the gene (Cotran et al., 1994b). *Deletion* of tumor suppressor genes can occur by the loss of a whole chromosome or a loss of part of a chromosome or a mutation that inactivates the gene. The loss of both retinoblastoma genes (Rb), one on each of the pair of chromosome 13, leads to a loss of function and tumorgenesis. The loss of Rb genes is seen in retinoblastoma and Wilm's tumor.

However, it is unlikely that activation of only one oncogene in a cell is *sufficient* to trigger the development of a malignant phenotype. One of the requirements needed to induce transformation or a malignancy is the activation of the oncogene in a particular cell type. In addition, the cell probably must be in a particular state of differentiation; otherwise activation will be of no consequence. Because carcinogenesis involves multiple steps, a particular oncogene probably is responsible for only one of several necessary genetic changes (Heim & Mitelman, 1987; Kahn & Graf, 1986; Klein & Klein, 1985; Nowell, 1988; Pitot, 1986; Teich, 1986; Watson et al., 1987).

ONCOGENES AND THEIR PRODUCTS

How do oncogenes contribute to the initiation and development of a tumor? The answer to this question is under intense investigation at this time. What is known is that (1) families of oncogenes exist, and the actions of one family will be different from those of the others; (2) growth factors, receptors for growth factors, the transduction of the growth factor signal, inhibition of the growth factor signals, and apoptotic genes are all major candidates for initiating transformation; (3) tumor development involves the sequential activation of oncogenes—that is, the activation of more than one oncogene is necessary for tumor progression; and (4) many oncogenes are located at chromosomal breakpoints (Cotran et al., 1994b; Kahn & Graf, 1986; Schlessinger, 1986; Schwab, 1986).

GROWTH FACTORS

The *sis* oncogene of simian sarcoma virus codes for the β chain of platelet-derived growth factor (PDGF), which also is a potent mitogen of fibroblasts and smooth muscle cells (Cotran et al., 1994b; Heldin & Westermark, 1986). PDGF is produced by several tumor types including astrocytomas and osteosarcomas. In this case, the *sis* oncogene may allow the cells to produce their own growth factor. In addition, these tumors also express receptors for PDGF, and this can result in autocrine stimulation. Thus the tumor cell can escape regulation. In cell cultures PDGF cannot stimulate growth on its own. It confers "competence" on the cell to progress through the cell cycle and perhaps to work at the checkpoints early in G_1 (Mendelsohn & Lippman, 1993).

GROWTH FACTOR RECEPTORS

The next step in the sequence of events that lead to growth and proliferation of the cell is activation of the growth factor receptor. The viral oncogene *erbB* is a mutation of the gene coding for the epidermal growth factor (EGF) receptor (Heldin & Westermark, 1986). An increased expression of EGF receptors is seen in breast, lung, head and neck, and bladder cancers. In breast cancer the presence of EGF receptor is correlated with a poor prognosis. The disease-free survival and total survival are shorter in women who are EGF receptor-positive than in those who are EGF receptor-negative (Mendelsohn & Lippman, 1993). Perhaps the amplification of the receptor genes and the overexpression of the protein receptor in the breast cancer cell makes the cell very sensitive to the presence of small amounts of growth factors and therefore more aggressive (Cotran et al., 1994b). The HER2/NEU oncogene codes for a growth factor receptor that is homologous but distinct from EGF receptor. Gene amplification and overexpression of this oncogene are also harbingers of a poor prognosis in breast cancer. In addition to breast cancer, HER2/NEU oncogene is overexpressed in tumors of the lung, ovary, and stomach (Mendelsohn & Lippman, 1993; van de Vijver, 1993).

SIGNAL TRANSDUCTION

After a growth factor binds to a growth factor receptor, then the complex of factor and receptor changes its shape and a sequence of reactions take place at the membrane, in the cytoplasm, and then in the nucleus. This signal transduction is carried out by different types of proteins, two of which are the tyrosine kinases and the guanosine triphosphate binding proteins.

Many of the known retroviral oncogenes had kinase activity, including *v-src* (Rous sarcoma virus), mos, *raf, src, fes,* and *fms.* Tyrosine kinases are found at the epidermal growth factor receptors. This type of evidence suggests that an altered cellular oncogene results in a disturbed pathway for growth signals, which then results in uncontrolled cellular division (Kahn & Graf, 1986; Schlessinger, 1986; Schwab, 1986). The *abl* oncogene found in chronic myeloid leukemia and some acute lymphoblastic leukemias has tyrosine kinase activity (Cotran et al., 1994b; Marx, 1994).

The oncogenes of the *ras* family were found to be efficient in inducing the metastatic phenotype (Egan et al., 1987; Marshall, 1986). After introducing them into a fibroblast cell line, the cells were transformed and when subsequently injected into nude mice created metastatic lesions in the lungs (Egan et al., 1987). In humans mutation of the ras gene is the ". . . single most common abnormality of dominant oncogenes" (Cotran et al., 1994b, p. 261). Normally ras proteins cycle between their quiescent or inactive state to an active state. The protein binds to guanosine diphosphate while it is inactive and then exchanges GDP for GTP when activated by the binding of a growth factor to its receptor. Mutated ras proteins appear to be stuck in the active state and excite the regulators of cell proliferation such as protein kinase C (Cotran et al., 1994b). The ras oncogenes have been associated with bladder, breast, and lung cancer (Phillips & Nuwayhid, 1993).

NUCLEAR REGULATION

Eventually the signal for growth and proliferation induces changes in the nucleus. Proteins of the *myc, myb,* and *fos* oncogenes are located in the nucleus and control transcription of growth genes. The *myc* oncogene is associated with the cell moving from the G_0 to the G_1 state and proliferation. The normal protein is transiently expressed; when the cell receives a signal to divide, it binds to DNA and rapidly returns to baseline levels. The *myc* oncogene is amplified in Burkitt's lymphoma and neuroblastoma. Overexpression of the myc protein is associated with a poor prognosis in neuroblastoma.

TUMOR SUPPRESSOR GENES AND THEIR PRODUCTS

Antioncogenes have also been termed *recessive cancer genes* or *tumor suppressor genes.* They were first discovered in hereditary cancers, notably in hereditary retinoblastoma. Less is known about the gene products of the tumor suppressor genes than about those of the oncogenes. Antioncogenes involve gene deletion or inactivation as compared with oncogenes, which are involved in gene activation (Friend, Dryja, & Weinberg, 1988; Knudson, 1985; Phillips & Nuwayhid, 1993; Wyke & Green, 1986).

In hereditary retinoblastoma, both copies of the normal tumor suppressor gene (both alleles) are absent; therefore, the development of this malignant tumor in genetic terminology is named recessive. The existence of only one of the tumor suppressor genes, Rb gene, would prevent the development of the tumor. (That is, the antitumor state of the cell is the dominant state.) Knudson first hypothesized this in 1971 with his two-step model of carcinogenesis (Knudson, 1983, 1985, 1987).

In the Knudson model, the first step in carcinogenesis in persons with hereditary cancer occurs in the germ line of cells. Therefore, this defect is present in all the cells of the body at birth. The second step (the second mutation, or second deletion) then occurs in the somatic cell, and only when this second genetic change occurs does the malignant phenotype develop in the cell and in each of the daughter cells. Because the first genetic change is present in all cells of the body, there is a greater likelihood for multiple primaries. In nonhereditary cancers, both genetic changes must occur in the somatic cells, so these cancers appear later in life in comparison with the hereditary forms, and there is less chance for multiple primaries to occur (Knudson, 1977, 1983, 1985, 1987).

The normal Rb gene is involved in preventing cells from moving to the S phase. It appears that the Rb gene product binds to transcription factors. When the cell is stimulated by growth factors or cyclins, the Rb gene product releases the transcription factors, synthesis of DNA can occur, and then mitosis occurs. If this gene is mutated, uncontrolled cycling occurs since the transcription factors are not regulated. (Cotran et al., 1994b) Loss of the Rb gene or loss of its activity occurs in retinoblastoma, osteosarcoma, and cancers of the breast, prostate, and lung (Cotran et al., 1994b; Harbour et al., 1988).

Loss of tumor suppressor activity of the p53 gene has been detected in 50 per cent of lung cancers, 30 to 50 per cent of breast cancers, and 70 per cent of colon cancers. These three cancers are the most commonly occurring human cancers. The p53 gene has been called a "molecular policeman" and "guardian of the genome" (Cotran et al., 1994b, p. 269). The p53 gene appears to arrest the cells in the G_1 phase, that is, it stops them from completing the cell cycle until damaged DNA is repaired. If the DNA repair mechanism fails, then the p53 seems to trigger apoptosis or cell death. This would prevent mutations from becoming fixed in a cell. In tumors the p53 gene appears mutated and codes for abnormal p53 protein which can be detected by special staining methods. It may be that this loss of functional ability allows additional mutations and eventually transformation to occur (Cotran et al., 1994b).

The pathways of inhibition of cell proliferation are less understood than those for promotion. But there is evidence that tumor suppressor genes will be involved with contact inhibition, downregulation of signal transduction, and regulation of gene activity. Perhaps once the regulation of these pathways can be identified, then a more coherent picture of the contribution of both oncogenes and tumor suppressor genes to the development of cancer will be possible. This will then change the current view of cancer as consisting of hundreds of different diseases to one of groups of cancers with similar genetic and molecular pathogenesis.

TRANSGENIC MICE OR GENE STUDIES AT THE WHOLE ORGANISM LEVEL

As discussed earlier, studies of transformation have certain advantages over the study of carcinogenesis in animals. Yet the question always arises: are studies of cells in culture relevant to carcinogenesis in animals or humans? The development of transgenic mice is a bridge between these two types of experimental orientations.

Transgenic mice are defined as, "mice in which the genome of each cell contains specific DNA sequences that were introduced experimentally during early em-

bryogenesis" (Hanahan, 1986, p. 348). Genes, such as oncogenes, are injected into the pronuclei of fertilized eggs of mice. The injected gene integrates into the egg genome. The eggs then are implanted into a pseudopregnant mouse, and approximately 20 per cent of the mice born will express the injected oncogene (Fig. 13–9). The second and third generations of these mice may also inherit the injected gene, if the oncogene was incorporated into the germ line cells (eggs and sperm). Therefore, clones of animals can be developed that express the oncogene(s) of interest (Hanahan, 1986).

The oncogenes that are transferred can be either the "natural" oncogene with its normal regulatory component attached or a hybrid or recombinant oncogene. In the hybrid form, the oncogene is fused to a regulatory component of an unrelated gene (enhancer component). The fusion increases the potential of the oncogene to be expressed in a specific tissue (Hanahan, 1986).

In one experiment, Ornitz, Hammer, Messing, Palimiter, and Brinster (1987) linked the early genes of the SV-40 virus with the rat elastase gene (enhancer component). The early genes of the simian virus 40 contain the T-antigen genes, which transform cultured cells, reduce contact inhibition, and reduce the serum growth factor requirements (Ornitz et al., 1987). The regulatory component of the rat elastase gene ensures that the acinar (exocrine) cells of the pancreas express the T-antigen genes or oncogenes. Elastase is one of the proteins that is normally produced and released by the acinar cells of the pancreas (Ornitz et al., 1987).

In the resulting strains of mice that expressed the T antigen gene, the animals who reached 3 months of age developed pancreatic cancer. The natural stages of development of this tumor were followed. The newborn mice had hyperplastic pancreatic acini by the time they were 2 weeks old. At 10 weeks the mice had pancreatic tumor masses. Death from pancreatic cancer occurred between 10 and 23 weeks of age. Metastatic lesions rarely occurred, but seeding of tumor cells into the peritoneal cavity was fairly common (Ornitz et al., 1987).

These investigators demonstrated that early in life, the acinar cells expressed the T-antigen gene and that the architecture of the tissue was reasonably normal. This was interpreted as the preneoplastic state. When the tumor nodules start to develop, the acinar cells no longer manufacture those proteins that signify a mature or differentiated state and the amount of T-antigen RNA production increased. At this same time, the chromosome numbers in the tumor cells become aneuploid. (Aneuploidy occurs when the cell has an abnormal number of chromosomes. The number is not a multiple of the haploid or diploid number. An example of aneuploidy occurs when a human cell contains 31 or 61 chromosomes.) These investigators suggested that the chromosomal loss results in an alteration of the regulation of growth (Ornitz et al., 1987). The loss may be similar to the loss of antioncogenes in retinoblastoma. The deregulation of growth confers a growth advantage, and numerous tumor nodules are formed in the pancreas.

This experiment exemplifies the current state of the art in understanding the molecular events in the development of tumors. The investigators started with a known gene, then induced its expression in an animal. What resulted in the offspring is a tumor that develops through all the pathologic stages found in human tumors, from hyperplasia to frank carcinoma, from euploid to aneuploid cells. This elegant animal model may help to shed some light on the development of pancreatic tumors, which for humans has a very poor prognosis.

The knowledge of oncogenes, however, has not been translated as quickly into clinical applications. Probably the first benefits from oncogene research will result in new and better diagnostic tests. For instance, the protein coded by the Philadelphia chromosome is unique and is not manufactured by normal cells. If techniques are developed to identify this as truly a cancer marker (that is, this protein is not made by any normal tissue or in other diseases), the diagnosis of chronic myeloid leukemia will be made easier. Identification of the other unique proteins produced in the different stages of neoplastic progression eventually might lead to new therapeutic approaches for the treatment of cancer. If these therapies are directed at true differences between cancer cells and normal cells, toxicities of cancer therapy might be reduced, and the patient would receive the ultimate benefit, a better quality of life.

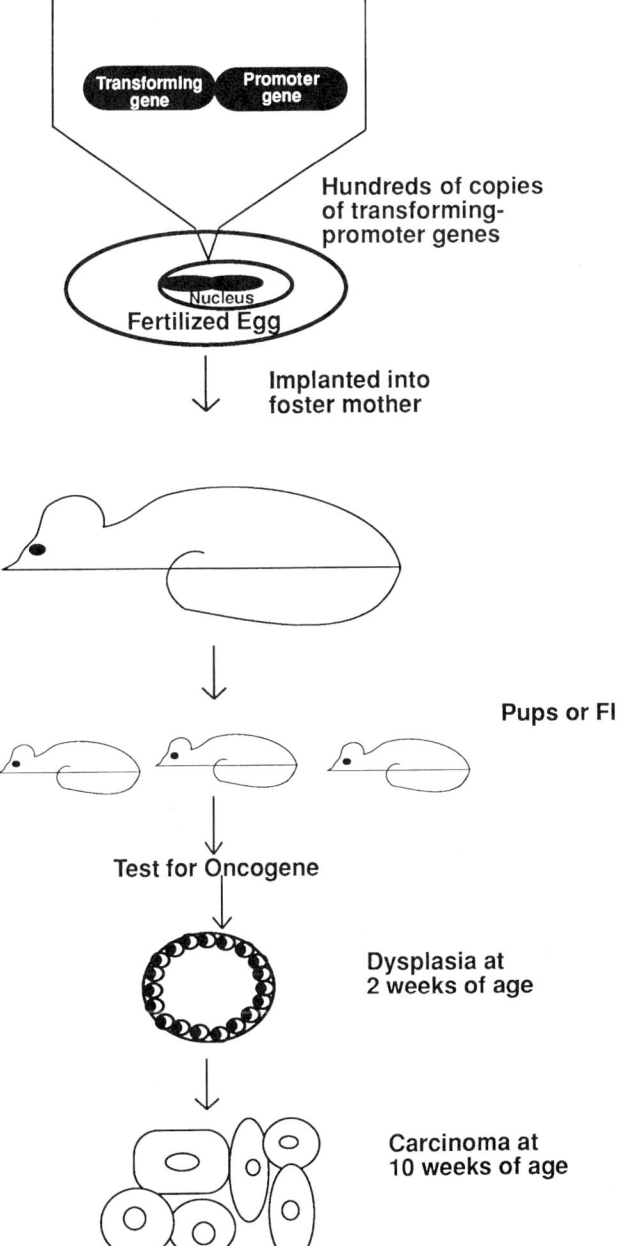

GENE THERAPY AND ITS POTENTIAL

If cancer is a result of genetic aberrations and inadequate immune functioning, is gene therapy for cancer a futuristic expectation? Ongoing clinical trials are being conducted for melanoma, prostate cancer, and renal cell cancer using gene transfer techniques. If these clinical trials are successful, then cancer therapies in the future will be highly specific and targeted to the patient's own tumor.

GENE THERAPY

Gene therapy was described as treating disease "... by transfer of genetic material into specific cells of a patient..." (Mulligan, 1993, p. 926). Gene therapy was first proposed for the treatment of inborn errors of metabolism, where the function of a single gene is disrupted (Table 13–4). Examples of these types of diseases are severe combined immunodeficiency disease or sickle cell anemia. Today gene therapy is being used to add genes to cells to enhance their function or to improve a specific characteristic (Anderson, 1992). For instance, the Il-2 gene is added to natural killer cells to enhance their ability to kill malignant cells, and the gene for granulocyte-macrophage colony stimulating factor is added to prostate cancer cells to make a patient-specific tumor vaccine.

FIGURE 13–9. In transgenic mice, hundreds of copies of the transforming gene fused to the promoter gene are introduced into the nucleus of the fertilized egg. The fertilized egg is implanted into a pseudopregnant female. A few of the first generation of progeny will contain the oncogene, which then leads to the development of a malignancy.

TABLE 13–4. *Requirements for a Disease to be Treated by Gene Therapy*

1. The cause of the disease is at the genetic level
2. Clones of the relevant gene are available
3. Target tissue or cells are easily obtained
4. A significant number of target cells accept the gene
5. The relevant gene is integrated, expressed, and functions normally
6. The probability of stimulation of an oncogene is low

In theory there are two general approaches to genetic modification in humans. The first approach is to change a gene in the somatic (body) cells. Alteration of somatic cells does not cause a change in heritable traits. Altering genes to produce heritable changes involves manipulation of germ cells (ova and sperm). These germ cells are sequestered early in development and are thus protected. There are no studies underway to alter germ cells in humans. Today there are multiple gene therapy clinical trials on three continents with many more awaiting approval, all involving somatic cell lines (Anderson, 1992).

Gene therapy involves several steps. Cells are removed, cultured in a suitable medium, and altered using a vector containing the desired gene. The modified cells are then reintroduced into the patient. Some of the technical issues in gene therapy research include development of methods for gene delivery with and without having to remove the cells from the body and understanding the specific gene actions once the cells are reintroduced into the recipient (Rosenberg, Anderson, & Blaese et al., 1992).

BIOLOGIC DELIVERY

Biologic delivery of genes is done with the help of viral vectors (Fig. 13–10). Retroviral and adeno-associated viral vectors are most frequently used in ex vivo gene therapy. Ex vivo therapy involves the removal of the target cells from the patient and altering the cells in a laboratory culture. The alteration by which the desired gene along with the viral genes (recombinant DNA) are incorporated into the target cell DNA is call *transduction*. Then the cells with the recombinant DNA are reintroduced into the patient (Mulligan, 1993). There are advantages and disadvantages in using viral vectors in humans. Viruses that have been studied include retroviruses, adenoviruses and herpes viruses.

Retroviral vectors are advantageous because of their ability to stably transduce close to 100 per cent of the target cells. To obtain this high percentage, the target cells must have appropriate receptors for the virus on their plasma membranes, a cell population that can be induced to divide, and a vector capable of proliferating within the target cell. For human therapy, recombinant "replication-defective" viruses are being developed to inhibit their ability to perpetuate an infection or to spread to other cells once the cells are reintroduced into the patient (Anderson, 1992; Ogasawara & Rosenberg, 1993).

Adenoviruses (cold viruses) can efficiently infect nondividing cells. They are relatively stable and withstand purification and concentration. However, in cells that are easily infected, adenoviral infection often leads to lysis of the cells. In nonpermissive cells (where lysis is inhibited) the virus or the recombinant DNA is not efficiently integrated. In cell culture adenoviral infection can lead to "malignant" transformation of the cell line. Herpes viruses vectors hold promise for delivery of recombinant DNA into the central nervous system. However, it appears that even replication-incompetent

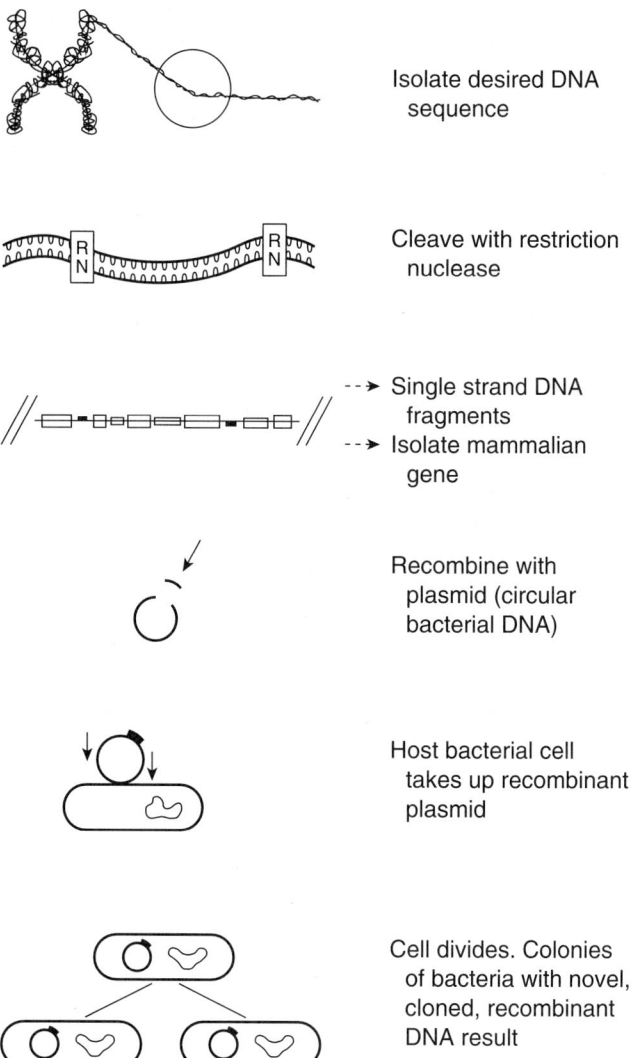

Isolate desired DNA sequence

Cleave with restriction nuclease

- -→ Single strand DNA fragments
- -→ Isolate mammalian gene

Recombine with plasmid (circular bacterial DNA)

Host bacterial cell takes up recombinant plasmid

Cell divides. Colonies of bacteria with novel, cloned, recombinant DNA result

FIGURE 13–10. Recombinant DNA technique, also called gene splicing, involves isolating the DNA sequence of interest and incorporating the isolated sequence into another genome. In this example the recombinant DNA is incorporated into a bacterial cell and cloned.

herpes viruses can still express gene products that are toxic to the cell. Work to prevent the expression of these genes is an important area of research (Mulligan, 1993).

PHYSICAL DELIVERY

There are physical techniques for inserting the relevant gene into the recipient's cells (Fig. 13–11). Electroporolation is a process that involves the use of electric shock to improve the efficiency of DNA uptake by cells (Berg & Singer, 1992). DNA-encapsulating liposomes are being used in at least one clinical trial to introduce DNA in cells of individuals with cystic fibrosis. A mechanical device called a "gene gun" uses high-pressure helium to inject micromolecular plasmid-coated genes into large areas of solid tissue (Tang & Carbone, 1993). The advantage of the physical tech-

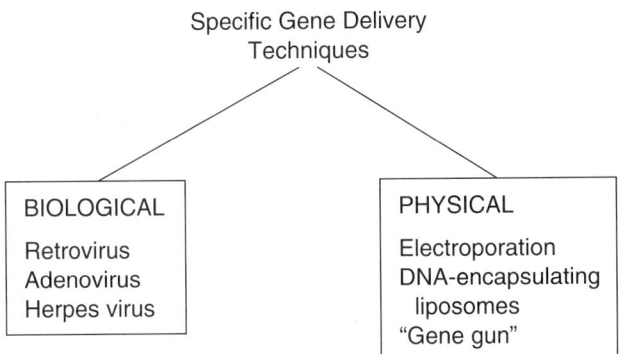

FIGURE 13–11. Gene delivery techniques include biologic and physical methods.

niques for delivery of genes is that they are potentially safer than viral vectors.

POTENTIAL USES OF GENE THERAPY FOR THE TREATMENT OF CANCER

In the treatment of cancer, gene therapy could be used to alter the tumor cells themselves or the immune system or bone marrow stem cells (Rosenberg, Anderson, Blaese et al., 1993; Varmus & Weinberg, 1993). In animal models, it is possible to manipulate the immune system to eliminate tumors. However, in humans, once the diagnosis of cancer has been made, the immune system has already failed to destroy the tumor (Stites & Terr, 1991). Researchers are currently modifying lymphocytes by gene therapy to enhance their ability to kill tumor cells (Schendel & Gansbacher, 1993). Genetic modification of tumor cells is being directed at (1) increasing their susceptibility to drugs, (2) increasing their ability to stimulate an immune response, (3) increasing their sensitivity to lymphocyte killing, and (4) blocking the expression of oncogenes. One aim of modification of normal bone marrow cells is to make them more resistant to chemotherapeutic agents (DeVita, Hellman, & Rosenberg, 1993).

MODIFICATION OF LYMPHOCYTES

TILs AND IL-2: INCREASING IMMUNE RESPONSES

Tumor-infiltrating lymphocytes (TILs) are cytotoxic T cells that recognize certain tumor epitopes (specific areas of the antigen) and thus "home" to the tumor. TILs have been used in clinical trials, in conjunction with interleukin-2 (IL-2) in the treatment of solid tumors. The genetic modification of this effector cell involves transducing the TIL cell with tumoricidal cytokine genes such as tumor necrosis factor (TNF). The homing ability of TIL cells and addition of TNF genes would presumably result in increased secretion of TNF at the site of the tumor thereby killing the tumor without damage to normal tissue (DeVita et al., 1993; Rosenberg, Anderson, Asher et al., 1992).

MODIFICATION OF TUMOR CELLS

SUICIDE GENES: INCREASING SUSCEPTIBILITY TO DRUGS

The function of a suicide gene is to make the cell expressing that gene more sensitive to a cytocidal drug (Johnston & Hoth, 1993). An example of a suicide gene is herpes simplex virus thymidine kinase (HSV-tk) gene. The gene is introduced into the tumor cell. When the gene is expressed, the tk enzyme is found in the cytoplasm of the cell. Theoretically, if the drug gancyclovir is introduced into the patient, the HSV-tk enzyme converts the drug to a more toxic metabolite. Cells that would not have this gene would be more resistant to the effects of gancyclovir. This technique may be valuable in reducing primary tumors that are localized or require sophisticated surgery such as glioblastoma multiforme (Caruso et al., 1993; Tang & Carbone, 1993).

CYTOKINE GENES: INCREASING IMMUNOGENICITY

Cytokines mediate complex interactions among lymphoid, inflammatory, hematopoietic, and other cells. They assist in cell-to-cell communication, regulate immune function, and act in both an autocrine and paracrine fashion (Kuby, 1992). Numerous cytokines including IL-2, IL-4, IL-6, IL-7, TNF, IFN, and GM-CSF have been shown to arrest tumor growth after the particular cytokine gene was transferred into tumor cells. The advantage of introducing cytokine genes into tumor cells is that there is continual release of lethal factors into the tumor with little systemic effect. Additionally, the cytokines locally activate the appropriate effector cell to mount a greater immune response to the tumor (DeVita et al., 1993; Tang & Carbone, 1993).

CLASS I MHC GENES: INCREASING IMMUNOGENICITY

The products of the MHC genes are associated with immune responses and the discrimination between self and foreign molecules. Class I MHC molecules are on practically all nucleated cells, and they present antigen to cytotoxic (killer) T lymphocytes (Abbas, Lichtman, & Pober, 1991). Introducing MHC class I genes in tumor cells may enhance the signaling process and tumor antigen recognition by T cells. This would then stimulate a chain of reactions leading to the release of cytokines and the destruction of nearby tumor cells (Borden & Schlom, 1993).

ANTISENSE OLIGONUCLEOTIDES: BLOCKING ONCOGENES

Oncogenes induce and maintain the malignant phenotype of a cell. When an oncogene is overexpressed, hundreds of copies of the gene are present in the cell. Not only are hundreds of copies of the gene present but the messenger RNA level is increased just as is the level of the protein product of that gene. The aim of antisense therapy would be to prevent the expression of the oncogene.

Antisense molecules are complementary copies of DNA or RNA to a particular gene. Theoretically, antisense DNA could bind to the coding DNA strand to prevent the manufacture of RNA (transcription). Or antisense DNA could become incorporated into the genome and manufacture antisense m-RNA that would bind to the normal messenger RNA and prevent either primary transcription or protein synthesis. Other antisense strategies include manufacturing antisense RNA and directly delivering it to the target cells, where it would interfere with translation; designing antisense oligonucleotides that would form triple helices with DNA; or combining antisense molecules with chemotherapeutic agents (Israel, 1993).

PHASE I: THERAPEUTIC TRIALS FOR CANCER

Phase I safety trials are underway to determine (1) if a TIL cell can be transduced with either the tumor necrosis factor gene or the IL-2 gene, (2) if the transduced cell homes to its tumor origin, and (3) if the transduced cells provide high doses of cytokines locally while avoiding systemic side effects. Because most TIL cells are trapped in liver, spleen, and lungs before they reach tumor sites, the potential for large concentrations of the cytokines producing undesired and unacceptable levels of side effects is an issue.

The first phase I trials used TIL cells transduced with the TNF gene. The cells were infused twice weekly, and the dose was escalated. After the first three patients were treated, then in another trial the transduced cells with both the TNF and NeoR gene were infused. The presence of the NeoR allowed the transduced cells to be selectively grown in culture. The lymphocytes were removed from the patient, grown in culture, and exposed to a vector containing both the TNF and NeoR genes. These cultures contain some lymphocytes that were successfully transduced and others that were not. Then a neomycin analog was added to the culture. The analog kills normal mammalian cells but not the cells with the NeoR gene. Thus, the culture resulted in a higher percentage of transduced cells, and the overall production of TNF was greater. Other modifications of the therapy included the exogenous administration of IL-2 to the patient and the addition of another gene to the vector, which increased the secretion of TNF. Then patients received the transduced TIL cells. Of these patients, six had failed previous TIL therapy. One patient had an objective response that at the last report had continued for 2 years (Rosenberg, Anderson, Blaese et al., 1993).

Another ongoing set of clinical trials involves transducing the patient's tumor cell with either TNF or IL-2. In this protocol the transduced tumor cells are (1) injected into the thigh of a patient; (2) 3 weeks later they are surgically removed to check for any growth of the tumor cells; (3) the draining lymph nodes are resected to recover lymphocytes that are grown in IL-2; and (4) the cultured lymphocytes are reinfused into the patient (adoptive immunity). The tumor cells serve to immunize the patient against the tumor. The recovered lymphocytes are more likely to be reactive against the tumor and serve as a form of adoptive immunotherapy. From the prior animal studies it was learned that tumor cells with cytokine genes first grew at the injected site and then regressed. At last report in none of the patients did the transduced tumor cells grow, and one patient had a partial regression. This ongoing trial has shown that transduced tumor cells can be rejected and has helped to prove the safety of administration of gene-modified tumor cells (Rosenberg, Anderson, Blaese et al., 1993).

A new trial with prostate cancer has been announced. The patient's tumor cells would be excised, grown in culture, and transduced with GM-CSF. Then the transduced cells would be radiated so that they could not divide but would remain functional. The autologous cells then would be given back to the patient as a vaccine. It is hoped that the GM-CSF would stimulate the patient's own immune system to recognize and destroy any remaining tumor cells. Similar trials are ongoing in melanoma and renal cell cancer with established tumor cells in culture. The patient receives cultured transduced tumor cells that are a histocompatible match. Tumor antigens, mutated oncogene products, and novel fusion proteins resulting from chromosomal translocations are all potential immunogenic sequences that could be used in the future in specific vaccination protocols (Foa et al., 1994).

SUMMARY

The molecular biology methods that are currently being used to study cancer are relatively new, and large gaps still exist in our knowledge. Currently it is impossible to distinguish all the events between the initiation of carcinogenesis and the development of the metastatic lesion. However, the pace of our understanding of the events of carcinogenesis has quickened at an unprecedented rate. These findings should result in new therapeutic agents. Gene therapy and these scientific developments are receiving considerable media attention. The public is becoming increasingly knowledgeable about the progress of science and technology. Oncology nurses in all settings may expect that cancer patients will want to know what these new developments mean and what future treatments may be available to them.

REFERENCES

Abbas, W., Lichtman, A., & Pober, J. (1991). *Cellular and molecular immunology* (pp. 115–137). Philadelphia: W. B. Saunders Co.

Alberts, B., Bray, D., Lewis, J., Raff, M., Roberts, K., & Watson, J. D. (1989a). *Molecular biology of the cell* (2nd ed., pp. 95–134). New York: Garland Publishing, Inc.

Alberts, B., Bray, D., Lewis, J., Raff, M., Roberts, K., & Watson, J. D. (1989b). *Molecular biology of the cell* (2nd ed., pp. 727–790). New York: Garland Publishing, Inc.

Alberts, B., Bray, D., Lewis, J., Raff, M., Roberts, K., & Watson, J. D. (1989c). *Molecular biology of the cell* (2nd ed., pp. 879–950). New York: Garland Publishing, Inc.

Anderson, W. (1992). Human gene therapy. *Science, 256,* 808–813.

Anderson, W. F. (1992). (Editorial) Uses and abuses of human gene transfer. *Human Gene Therapy, 3,* 1–2.

Bar-Sagi, D., & Feramisco, J. R. (1986). Induction of membrane ruffling and fluid-phase pinocytosis in quiescent fibroblast by *ras* protein. *Science, 233,* 1061–1068.

Berg, P., & Singer, M. (1992). *Dealing with genes: The language of heredity* (p. 269). Mill Valley, CA: University Science Books.

Bonfiglio, T. A., & Terry, R. (1983). The pathology of cancer. In P. Rubin (Ed.), *Clinical oncology: A multidisciplinary approach* (6th ed., pp. 20–29). New York: American Cancer Society.

Borden, E., & Schlom, J. (1993). Williamsburg conference on biological and immunological treatments for cancer, 1992. *Journal of the National Cancer Institute, 85*(16), 1288–1293.

Caruso, M., Panis, Y., Gagandeep, S., Houssin, D., Salzmann, J., & Klatzmann, D. (1993). Regression of established macroscopic liver metastases after in situ transduction of a suicide gene. *Proceedings of the National Academy of Science, 90,* 7024–7028.

Correa, P. (1982). Morphology and natural history of precursor lesions. In D. Schottenfeld & J. F. Fraumeni (Eds.), *Cancer epidemiology and prevention* (pp. 90–118). Philadelphia: W. B. Saunders Co.

Cotran, R. S., Kumar, V., & Robbins, S. L. (1994a). *Robbin's pathologic basis of disease* (5th ed., pp. 35–50). Philadelphia: W. B. Saunders Co.

Cotran, R. S. Kumar, V., & Robbins, S. L. (1994b). *Robbin's pathologic basis of disease* (5th ed., pp. 241–303). Philadelphia: W. B. Saunders Co.

DeVita, V. T., Hellman, S., & Rosenberg, S. A. (1993). Gene therapy of cancer. In V. T. DeVita, S. Hellman, & S. A. Rosenberg (Eds.), *Cancer: Principles and practice of oncology* (4th ed., pp. 2598–2613). Philadelphia: J. B. Lippincott Co.

Dorr, R. T., & Von Hoff, D. D. (Eds.). (1994). *Cancer chemotherapy handbook* (2nd ed., pp. 3–9). Norwalk: Appleton & Lange.

Edlin, G. (1984). *Genetic principles. Human and social consequences* (pp. 97–115). Boston: Jones and Bartlett Publishers, Inc.

Egan, S. E., Wright, J. A., Jarolim, L., Yanagihara, K., Bassin, R. H., & Greenberg, A. H. (1987). Transformation by oncogenes encoding protein kinases induces the metastatic phenotype. *Science, 238,* 202–205.

Fidler, I. J., & Hart, I. R. (1982). Principles of cancer biology: Biology of cancer metastasis. In V. T. DeVita, S. Hellman, & S. A. Rosenberg (Eds.), *Cancer: Principles and practice of oncology* (pp. 80–92). Philadelphia: J. B. Lippincott Co.

Foa, R., Guarini, A., Cignetti, A., Cronin, K., Rosenthal, F., & Gansbacher, B. (1994). Cytokine gene therapy: A new strategy for the management of cancer patients. *Natural Immunity, 13,* 65–75.

Friend, S. H., Dryja, T. P., & Weinberg, R. A. (1988). Oncogenes and tumor-suppressing genes. *New England Journal of Medicine, 318,* 618–622.

Gebhardt, A., & Foulkes, J. G. (1986). Transformation by the v-abl oncogene. In P. Kahn & T. Graf (Eds.), *Oncogenes and growth control* (pp. 114–119). New York: Springer-Verlag, Inc.

Goldfarb, S. (1983). Pathology of neoplasia. In S. B. Kahn, R. R. Love, C. Sherman, & R. Chakrovorty (Eds.), *Concepts in cancer medicine* (pp. 127–142). New York: Grune & Stratton, Inc.

Greaves, M. F. (1986). Biology of human leukaemia. In L. M. Franks & N. M. Teich (Eds.), *Introduction to the cellular and molecular biology of cancer* (pp. 40–62). Oxford: Oxford University Press.

Hanafusa, H. (1986). Activation of the *c-src* gene. In P. Kahn & T. Graf (Eds.), *Oncogenes and growth control* (pp. 100–105). New York: Springer-Verlag, Inc.

Hanahan, D. (1986). Oncogenesis in transgenic mice. In P. Kahn & T. Graf (Eds.), *Oncogenes and growth control* (pp. 349–363). New York: Springer-Verlag, Inc.

Harbour, J. W., Lai, S.-L., Whang-Peng, J., Gazdar, A. F., Minna, J. D., & Kaye, F. J. (1988). Abnormalities in structure and expression of the human retinoblastoma gene in SCLC. *Science, 241,* 353–356.

Hart, I. R. (1986). The spread of tumors. In L. M. Franks & N. M. Teich (Eds.), *Introduction to the cellular and molecular biology of cancer* (pp. 27–39). Oxford: Oxford University Press.

Hartwell, L. H., & Kastan, M. B. (1994). Cell cycle control and cancer. *Science, 266,* 1821–1828.

Hartwell, L. H., & Weinert, T. A. (1989). Checkpoints: Controls that ensure the order of cell cycle events. *Science, 246,* 629–634.

Hawkins, M. J. (1993) Investigational Agents. In V. T. DeVita, S. Hellman, & S. A. Rosenberg (Eds.), *Cancer principles and practice of oncology* (4th ed., pp. 349–374). Philadelphia: J. B. Lippincott Co.

Heim, S., & Mitelman, F. (1987). *Cancer cytogenetics* (p. 309). New York: Alan R. Liss, Inc.

Heldin, C. H., & Westermark, B. (1986). Role of PDGF-like growth factors in autocrine stimulation of growth of normal and transformed cells. In P. Kahn & T. Graf (Eds.), *Oncogenes and growth control* (pp. 43–50). New York: Springer-Verlag, Inc.

Hoffman, B. & Liebermann, D. A. (1994). Molecular controls of apoptosis: Differentiation/growth arrest primary response genes, proto-oncogenes, and tumor suppressor genes as positive and negative modulator. *Oncogene 9,*1807–1812.

Israel, M. A. (1993). Molecular approaches to cancer therapy. In G. F. Vande Woude & G. Klein (Eds.), *Advances in cancer research* (Vol. 61, pp. 57–84). San Diego: Academic Press.

Johnston, M., & Hoth, D. (1993). Present status and future prospects for HIV therapies. *Science, 260,* 1286–1291.

Kahn, P., & Graf, T. (Eds.). (1986). Malignant transformation as a multistep process. In P. Kahn & T. Graf (Eds.), *Oncogenes and growth control* (pp. 292–293). New York: Springer-Verlag, Inc.

Klein, G., & Klein, E. (1985). Evolution of tumours and the impact of molecular oncology. *Nature, 315,* 190–195.

Knudson, A. G. (1977). Genetic predisposition to cancer. In H. H. Hiatt, J. D. Watson, & J. A. Wisten (Eds.), *Origins of human cancer. Book A. Incidence of cancer in humans* (pp. 45–54). Cold Spring Harbor, NY: Cold Spring Harbor Laboratory.

Knudson, A. G. (1983). Hereditary cancers of man. *Cancer Investigation, 1,* 187–193.

Knudson, A. G., Jr. (1985). Hereditary cancer, oncogenes and antioncogenes. *Cancer Research, 45,* 1437–1442.

Knudson, A. G., Jr. (1987). A two-mutation model for human cancer. In G. Klein (Ed.), *Advances in viral oncology* (Vol. 7, pp. 1–17). New York: Raven Press.

Krontiris, T. G., & Cooper, G. M. (1981). Transforming activity of human tumor DNA's. *Proceedings of the National Academy of Sciences USA, 78,* 1181–1184.

Kuby, J. (1992). *Immunology* (pp. 245–270). New York: W. H. Freeman.

Marshall, C. J. (1986). The ras gene family. In P. Kahn & T. Graf (Eds.), *Oncogenes and growth control* (pp. 192–199). New York: Springer-Verlag, Inc.

Marx, J. (1991). The cell cycle: Spinning farther afield. *Science, 252,* 1490–1492.

Marx, J. (1994). Oncogenes reach a milestone. *Science, 266,* 1942–1944.

Mathews, C. K., & van Holde, K. E. (1990). *Biochemistry* (pp. 91–121). Redwood City, CA: The Benjamin/Cummins Publishing Co.

Mendelsohn, J., & Lippman, M. E. (1993). Principles of molecular cell biology of cancer: Growth factors. In V. T. DeVita, S. Hellman, & S. A. Rosenberg (Eds.), *Cancer principles and practice of oncology* (4th ed., pp. 114–133). Philadelphia: J. B. Lippincott Co.

Mulligan, R. (1993). The basic science of gene therapy. *Science, 260,* 926–931.

Murray, M. J., Shilo, B. Z., Shih, C., Cowing, D., Hsu, H. W., & Weinberg, R. A. (1981). Three different human tumor cell lines contain different oncogenes. *Cell, 25,* 355–361.

Nicolson, G. L., & Poste, G. (1974). The cancer cell: Dynamic aspects and modifications in cell-surface organization parts 1 and 2. *New England Journal of Medicine, 295,* 197–203, 253–258.

Nowell, P. C. (1988). Molecular events in tumor development. *New England Journal of Medicine, 319,* 575–577.

Ogasawara, M., & Rosenberg, S. (1993). Enhanced expression of HLA molecules and stimulation of autologous human tumor infiltrating lymphocytes following transduction of melanoma cells with γ-interferon genes. *Cancer Research, 53,* 3561–3568.

Oishi, N. (1983). The leukemias. In S. G. Kahn, R. R. Love, C. Sherman, & R. Chakrovorty (Eds.), *Concepts in cancer medicine* (pp. 597–617). New York: Grune & Stratton, Inc.

Ornitz, D. M., Hammer, R. E., Messing, A., Palimiter, R. D., & Brinster, R. L. (1987). Pancreatic neoplasia induced by SV40 T antigen expression in acinar cells of transgenic mice. *Science, 238,* 188–193.

Pardee, A. B. (1982). Principles of cancer biology: Cell biology and biochemistry of cancer. In V. T. DeVita, S. Hellman, & S. A. Rosenberg (Eds.), *Cancer: Principles and practice of oncology* (pp. 59–72). Philadelphia: J. B. Lippincott Co.

Phillips, C. A. & Nuwayhid, N. F. (1993) The malignant state: The molecular, cytogenetic and immunologic basis of cancer. In G. Weiss, *Clinical oncology* (pp. 3–10). Norwalk, CT: Appleton & Lange.

Pitot, H. C. (1986). *Fundamentals of oncology* (3rd ed., p. 532). New York: Marcel Dekker, Inc.

Rather, L. J. (1978). *The genesis of cancer: A study in the history of ideas* (p. 262). Baltimore: Johns Hopkins University Press.

Rosenberg, S., Anderson, W., Blaese, M, Ettinghausen, S. E., Hwu, P., Karp, S. E., Kasid, A., Mule, J. J., Parkinson, D. R., Salo, J. C., Schwartzentruber, D. J., Topalian, S. L., Weber, J. S., Yannelli, J. R., Yang, J. C., & Linehan, W. M. (1992). Immunization of cancer patients using autologous cancer cells modified by insertion of the gene for interleukin-2. *Human Gene Therapy, 3,* 75–90.

Rosenberg, S., Anderson, W., Asher, A., Blaese, M., Ettinghausen, S. E., Hwu, P., Kasid, A., Mule, J. J., Parkinson, D. R., Schwartzentruber, D. J., Topalian, S. L., Weber, J. S., Yannelli, J. R., Yang, J. C., & Linehan, W. M. (1992). Immunization of cancer patients using autologous cancer cells modified by insertion of the gene for tumor necrosis factor. *Human Gene Therapy, 3,* 57–73.

Rosenberg, S., Anderson, W. F., Blaese, M., Hwu, P., Yannelli, J. R., Yang, J. C., Topalian, S. L., Schwartzentruber, D. J., Weber, J. S., Ettinghausen, S. E., Parkinson, D. N., & White, D. E. (1993). The development of gene therapy for the treatment of cancer. *Annals of Surgery, 218*(4), 455–464.

Ruddon, R. W. (1981). *Cancer biology* (p. 344). New York: Oxford University Press.

Sachs, L. (1987). The molecular control of blood cell development. *Science, 238,* 1374–1379.

Schendel, D., & Gansbacher, B. (1993). Tumor-specific lysis of human renal cell carcinomas by tumor-infiltrating lymphocytes: Modulation of recognition through retroviral transduction of tumor cells with interleukin-2 complementary DNA and exogenous α interferon treatment. *Cancer Research, 53,* 4020–4025.

Schlessinger, J. (1986). Regulation of cell growth by the EGF receptor. In P. Kahn & T. Graf (Eds.), *Oncogenes and growth control* (pp. 77–84). New York: Springer-Verlag, Inc.

Schwab, M. (1986). Amplification of proto-oncogenes and tumor progression. In P. Kahn & T. Graf (Eds.), *Oncogenes and growth control* (pp. 332–339). New York: Springer-Verlag, Inc.

Stedman, T. L. (1982). *Stedman's medical dictionary* (4th ed., p. 1501). Baltimore: Williams & Wilkins.

Stehelin, D., Varmus, H. E., Bishop, J. M., & Vogt, P. K. (1976). DNA related to the transforming genes(s) of avian sarcoma viruses is present in normal avian DNA. *Nature, 260,* 170–173.

Stites, D., & Terr, A. (1991). *Basic and clinical immunology* (pp. 580–587). Norwalk, CT: Appleton & Lange.

Sukumar, S., Carney, W. P., & Barbacid, M. (1988). Independent molecular pathways in initiation and loss of hormone responsiveness of breast carcinoma. *Science, 240,* 524–526.

Tang, D., & Carbone, D. (1993). Potential application of gene therapy to lung cancer. *Seminars in Oncology, 20*(4), 368–373.

Teich, N. M. (1986). Oncogenes and cancer. In L. M. Franks & N. M. Teich (Eds.), *Introduction to the cellular and molecular biology of cancer* (pp. 200–228). Oxford: Oxford University Press.

van de Vijver, M. J. (1993). Molecular genetic changes in human breast cancer. *Advances in Cancer Research, 61,* 25–56.

Varmus, H., & Weinberg, R. (1993). *Genes and the biology of cancer.* New York: Scientific American Library.

Watson, J. D., Hopkins, N. H., Roberts, J. W., Steitz, J. A., & Weiner, A. M. (1987). *Molecular biology of the gene: Vol. II. Specialized aspects* (4th ed., pp. 747–1163). Menlo Park, CA: The Benjamin/Cummings Publishing Company, Inc.

Watson, J. D., Tooze, J., & Kurtz, D. T. (1983). *Recombinant DNA: A short course* (p. 260). New York: Scientific American Books, W. H. Freeman & Co.

Wolberg, W. H. (1983). Metastasis. In S. B. Kahn, R. R. Love, C. Sherman, & R. R. Chakrovorty (Eds.), *Concepts in cancer medicine* (pp. 149–156). New York: Grune & Stratton, Inc.

Wyke, J. A., & Green, A. R. (1986). Suppression of the neoplastic phenotype. In P. Kahn & T. Graf (Eds.), *Oncogenes and growth control* (pp. 341–345). New York: Springer-Verlag, Inc.

CHAPTER
14

Principles of Immunology

Janice Post-White

This chapter provides an overview of the immune system and immune interactions involved in cancer outcome. The content addresses a small fraction of knowledge available on the role the immune system plays in controlling cancer. The purpose is to provide basic principles of immunology to help understand the role the immune system plays in the onset and progression of cancer and the role immunologic therapies have in cancer control.

ORGANIZATION AND FUNCTION OF THE IMMUNE SYSTEM

STIMULUS RESPONSE SYSTEM

The primary function of the immune system is to recognize and eliminate foreign substances from the body. These foreign substances may be infectious microbes such as viruses, bacteria, fungi, protozoa, and parasites, a tissue allograft, or innocuous environmental substances such as pollens or foods. Foreign substances that are recognized as being nonself act as a stimulus to trigger the immune response. Foreign substances that bind antibody are referred to as antigens. Two critical steps in ridding the body of foreign substances include recognizing the pathogen as foreign and then mounting a response to eliminate it.

A variety of immune responses are required to deal with different types of foreign substances, depending on the pathogen and the site of invasion. If the antigen remains localized in the skin, a local inflammatory response triggers regional lymph nodes to mount an immune response. If the antigen traverses the mucosal barriers of the respiratory or gastrointestinal tract, lymphoid tissue of the tonsils or Peyer's patches in the gut produce antibodies that recognize and fight the invading pathogen. The antigen also may enter the bloodstream directly, initiating an immune response from the spleen. Because lymphocytes travel throughout the bloodstream and lymphatic system, all pathogens generally cause some degree of systemic response. As a result, the symptoms observed in response to a foreign substance are a response to both the pathogen itself and the immune system activation by the pathogen.

The immune response is a complex network of cell to cell recognition, signaling, interaction, and lysis. The immune system can fail in its performance of recognizing foreign cells as self and nonself and of balancing the signals for immune activation or suppression, which may result in immunopathologic reactions such as cancer, autoimmune disease, immunodeficiency, and hypersensitivity. Different cells have different roles in this stimulus-response system. Intercellular communication is the key to maintaining the balance between immune activation and feedback regulation.

NONSPECIFIC AND SPECIFIC IMMUNITY

There are two primary types of immune response to foreign substances: nonspecific (innate) immunity and specific (acquired or adaptive) immunity. These two responses involve different immune cells and signaling mediators (Table 14–1).

Nonspecific immunity, also called innate or natural immunity, is present from birth and is available on short notice to protect the individual from foreign substances. Components of nonspecific immunity include physical barriers such as the skin and mucous membranes, which prevent penetration; chemical influences such as pH and lysozyme enzyme secretion, which damage bacterial cell walls; internal elements such as complement and acute-phase proteins that target bacterial infection; and interferons and natural killer cells that bind to and kill viruses and cancer cells. Macrophages, polymorphonuclear lymphocytes (PMNs), and natural killer (NK) cells are the primary immune cells involved in nonspecific immunity. These cells prevent invasion of pathogens and respond immediately to destroy and eliminate any foreign substances.

Specificity and immunologic memory are unique to specific immunity. Also referred to as acquired or adaptive immunity, specific immunity requires recognition of a pathogen from a previous encounter. Macrophages and lymphocytes are the primary immune cells involved in specific immunity. T lymphocytes recognize the pathogen, which is processed and presented by the macrophages in the form of an antigen, and then signal

B lymphocytes to produce antibodies with specificity against the foreign substance. These antibodies remain "on call" and respond when the individual is reexposed to the identical foreign substance. This response, called memory, improves with each successive encounter and is the mechanism for lifelong immunity and vaccinations.

CELL DEVELOPMENT AND MATURATION

The principal cells of the immune system are lymphocytes and mononuclear phagocytes. Lymphocytes are the only immunocompetent cells capable of specific recognition of antigens. Mononuclear phagocytes are critical for host defense in nonspecific immunity and are involved in recognition and activation of specific immunity.

Lymphocytes differentiate and mature in the thymus and bone marrow (the primary lymphoid organs). The thymus provides the microenvironment necessary for the maturation of T cells, and the bone marrow is the primary site for pluripotent stem cell and B lymphocyte development and maturation. In the thymus, T lymphocytes differentiate, acquire new functions and surface antigens, and then emigrate to peripheral tissues. The thymus grows until puberty and then gradually involutes. It decreases from 0.27 per cent to 0.02 per cent of total body weight between the ages of 5 and 15 years (Kamani & Douglas, 1991).

In the bone marrow, stem cells differentiate into mature lymphocytes and progenitors of hematologic cells. In response to growth factors (cytokines), the progenitors then divide and differentiate into phagocytic cells (neutrophils and monocytes), erythrocytes, platelets, and eosinophils. The bone marrow produces one billion lymphocytes daily (Kamani & Douglas, 1991). After maturation, these lymphocytes are released into circulation to the secondary lymphoid organs: the spleen, lymph nodes, and Peyer's patches of the ileum. Lymphocytes continuously circulate through the vascular and lymphatic channels from one lymphoid organ to another.

SURFACE MARKERS AND RECEPTORS

Markers and receptors appear on the immune cell surface during maturation. Receptors differ from surface markers in that receptors are a functional macromolecule with a known binding affinity for a specific antigen (Kamani & Douglas, 1991). Lymphocytes have multiple surface markers that differentiate lymphocyte subsets and their functions. Various monoclonal antibodies recognize these surface markers and are labeled as cluster of differentiation (CD) according to the International Workshop on Human Leukocyte Differentiation Antigens.

For example, the surface markers CD4 and CD8 generally define the helper (CD4) and suppressor/cytotoxic (CD8) functions of T cells. All T lymphocytes form rosettes with sheep erythrocytes (CD2); this marker is used to identify human T cells. Similarly, when B lymphocytes are activated by a signal from T lymphocytes, they differentiate into antibody secreting

TABLE 14–1. *Comparison of Nonspecific and Specific Immunity*

CHARACTERISTIC	NONSPECIFIC IMMUNITY	SPECIFIC IMMUNITY
Primary role	Prevent invasion of pathogen Eliminate foreign substance	Specificity for pathogen Immunologic memory
Response-generated	Immediate First encounter for pathogen Present from birth Phagocytosis Inflammation	Response to a specific antigen Second encounter stronger response Humoral and cellular immunity
Immune cells	Macrophage Polymorphonuclear Neutrophils (PMN) Natural killer (NK) cells	Macrophages Lymphocytes (T and B)
Soluble factors	Interferons Complement Acute phase proteins (CRP) Lysozyme enzymes	Antibodies Cytokines

cells that produce one of five classes of immunoglobulins (Ig): IgM, IgG, IgD, IgE, and IgA. In addition to one or more of these surface markers, B lymphocytes also may carry receptors for antigen-antibody complexes, complement, and Epstein Barr virus as well as other surface antigens that define the cell's specific activity. Cells use these surface markers and receptors to signal one another and to carry out their functions of recognition, binding, and killing.

Tumor-associated antigens are antigens that usually are also found on normal cells of the same or other lineages (Herlyn, Menrad, & Koprowski, 1990). Initiating an immune response against a tumor depends on the ability of surface markers to initiate an antigenic response. Antigens on tumor cells take various forms. In comparison with their normal counterparts, tumor cells may express antigens that are absent on normal cells, are "unmasked" on tumor cells but masked on normal cells, or are present only in earlier cell development, such as oncofetal or embryonic cells (Benjamini & Leskowitz, 1988).

COMPONENTS OF IMMUNE RESPONSE

The immune response has three primary components: phagocytosis, in which the invading substance is ingested and destroyed by individual immune cells; inflammation, in which cells and proteins defend the body against infection and repair tissue damage; and cellular or humoral immunity, in which antigen specific responses are mediated by either serum antibodies (humoral) or T lymphocytes (cellular) (Table 14-2). Each response protects the body against foreign pathogens. Phagocytosis and inflammation are predominantly nonspecific immune responses, and humoral and cellular immunity are characteristic of specific immunity.

PHAGOCYTOSIS

Phagocytosis is the ingestion and destruction of invading foreign substances by individual cells. Monocytes, macrophages, and polymorphonuclear leukocytes (also called neutrophils or PMNs), assume the primary role of phagocytosis. When mononuclear phagocytes circulate in the blood, they are referred to as monocytes; when they reside in tissues, they are called macrophages. Macrophages are found in connective tissues, lungs, liver, nervous system, serous cavities, bones and joint, and lymphoid organs. The major function of macrophages is engulfment and ingestion of particles by phagocytosis. They actively kill bacteria, fungi, and tumor cells.

Macrophages respond to their environment through receptors for immunoglobulin (IgG, IgE) and complement (C3b, C5a), growth factors (M-CSF, GM-CSF), lipoproteins, peptides, and polysaccharides (Broide, 1991). Binding of these receptors to their antigens initiates macrophage proliferation, chemotaxis to the site of invasion, phagocytosis, and secretion of products that stimulate other cells (interleukin 1 and tumor necrosis factor), and assist with cell killing (enzymes and oxidative metabolites). Because macrophages bear class II MHC antigens, they also play an important role

TABLE 14–2. *Components of Immune Response*

	PHAGOCYTOSIS	INFLAMMATION	HUMORAL IMMUNITY	CELLULAR IMMUNITY
Purpose of response	Injest and destroy pathogen	Defend against infection Repair tissue damage	Protective against bacterial invasion (extracellular)	Protective against viruses, tumors, parasites, nonself antigens (intracellular)
Mechanism of response	Attach to particle Release destructive enzymes Generate toxic oxygen products	Neutrophils migrate to site (chemotaxis), Phagocytize Recruit inflammatory cells Activate complement	IgG, IgM neutralize bacterial toxins, (opsonization) Activate complement	Macrophage presents antigen to T cell, T cell binds to target, releases enzymes, releases cytokines to signal macrophages and B cells
Type of response	Nonspecific	Nonspecific	Specific	Specific
Immune cells involved	Monocytes Macrophages Neutrophils (PMNs)	Neutrophils Eosinophils Basophils Macrophages Mast cells Platelets	B lymphocytes Macrophages	T lymphocytes Macrophages NK cells
Mediators of response	IgG, IgE Complement GM-CSF, M-CSF Lipoproteins Peptides Polysaccharides TNF Lysozyme enzymes	Histamine Complement Coagulation proteins	Antibodies (IgG, IgM, IgA, IgD, IgE) Complement Bradykinins	Cytokines (Interleukins, Interferons, TNF)

in cellular immunity by processing and presenting antigen to T lymphocytes (referred to as antigen presenting cells, APC).

Macrophages and neutrophils carry out their phagocytic function by attaching to and surrounding the particle, releasing destructive enzymes from the cytoplasmic granules, and generating toxic oxygen products. Macrophages produce tumor necrosis factors that enhance phagocytosis and killing properties of macrophages and neutrophils. Neutrophil phagocytosis also is enhanced by the presence of complement and IgG antibody, but they are not required. Macrophages have longer life spans than neutrophils; the cytokines they produce signal neutrophils to the site.

INFLAMMATION

The inflammatory immune response is the mechanism by which the body defends against infection and repairs tissue damage. The process of inflammation involves increased capillary permeability via histamine release, which results in edema and increased circulating leukocytes in the blood or lymph. Several types of immune cells can induce inflammation, including neutrophils, eosinophils, basophils, macrophages, mast cells, and platelets. Other proteins also participate in the inflammatory response and include complement, coagulation, fibrinolysis, and kinin pathways.

Neutrophils predominantly appear during the early stage of inflammation; macrophages generally arrive 8 to 12 hours after onset to phagocytize the debris. Neutrophils move by chemotaxis (migrating to particles to be ingested), phagocytize by recognizing, attaching to, and engulfing particles, and kill by releasing cytoplasmic granules and generating oxidative metabolism. Similar to macrophages, most peripheral blood neutrophils have cell surface receptors for IgG and the complement fragment C3b, which help the neutrophil respond to early infection and amplify the inflammatory response. In addition to phagocytosis, monocytes and macrophages have the unique ability to produce endogenous pyrogens (including IL-1 and prosta-glandins) responsible for fever. And in the presence of helper T cells, macrophages form granulomas around dead tissue and invaders, a hallmark of delayed type hypersensitivity reactions.

Mast cells (in tissue) and basophils (circulating) are granulocytes that act as primary inflammatory mediators by increasing vascular permeability and recruiting other inflammatory cells. Mast cells are prevalent in the skin, lungs, gastrointestinal tract, and mucus membranes, and have a primary role in IgE-mediated (allergic) inflammation. Both mast cells and basophils have histamine-containing cytoplasmic granules and cell surface IgE receptors. Eosinophils also carry IgE and complement receptors and respond during inflammation but are specific for allergy and parasite infection. Platelets remain intravascular and participate in inflammation by producing mediators and clotting and growth factors. They may also aggregate and trap leukocytes.

HUMORAL AND CELLULAR IMMUNITY

Humoral immunity is the principal protective specific immune response against bacteria (Abbas, Licht-

man, & Pober, 1991). Humoral immunity is mediated by serum antibodies, which are immunoglobulins that bind individually to specific antigens. Both IgG and IgM antibodies neutralize bacterial toxins, which prevents their binding and promotes clearance, and both activate complement, which enhances phagocytosis and mediates acute inflammation.

Humoral immunity plays a major role against infection with most gram-positive and some gram-negative organisms. The critical step in inhibiting bacterial growth is quick opsonization by antibody and activation of complement (Unanue & Benacerraf, 1984). Antibodies also play a role in neutralizing toxins and some viruses such as diptheria and tetanus toxin and polio viruses. There is an age-related decrease in antibody response, which is thought to be related to a defect in antibody function more so than a decrease in numbers of antibody available (Dubey & Yunis, 1991). The levels of antibody remain similar, except for a relative increase of IgA and IgG with age.

Cellular immunity (also called cell-mediated immunity) also is antigen-specific but relies on T lymphocytes instead of B cells to mediate the immune response. T lymphocytes have the unique capability to mount an immune response to organisms that invade *within* the cells, whereas B lymphocytes primarily target extracellular organisms. Some examples of intracellular organisms that initiate T cell response are parasites, such as tuberculosis, leprosy, and toxoplasma, and retroviruses, such as human immunodeficiency virus (HIV) and cytomegalovirus (CMV). T lymphocytes also mount an immune response to foreign antigens presented in grafts or transplants. Graft rejection is specific and requires memory; it takes approximately 14 days for a mouse to reject a first graft of allogeneic skin (Kimball, 1990). This ability to differentiate self from nonself emanates from the T cell recognition of their targets in association with the major histocompatibility complex (MHC), which are genes that encode cell surface antigens.

Like humoral immunity, cell-mediated immunity also relies on other nonspecific immune components such as macrophages. When a macrophage presents an antigen to a T cell, the T cell becomes activated and releases lymphokines (cytokines released by lymphocytes), which signal other T cells and B cells and attract and activate more macrophages. T cells do not produce antibody, but they do signal B lymphocytes to proliferate and produce antibody to assist with cell-mediated immunity. Figure 14–1 depicts the cellular interactions involved in humoral and cellular immunity. The macrophage initiates responses by presenting the antigen in context of MHC to T cells.

SUMMARY

Specific (acquired) immune responses usually involve both humoral and cellular immunity. The B and T lymphocytes also interact with components of nonspecific immunity, such as macrophages and natural killer cells, to destroy invaders. Usually the invader is a bacteria or a virus, but immunity also may be directed

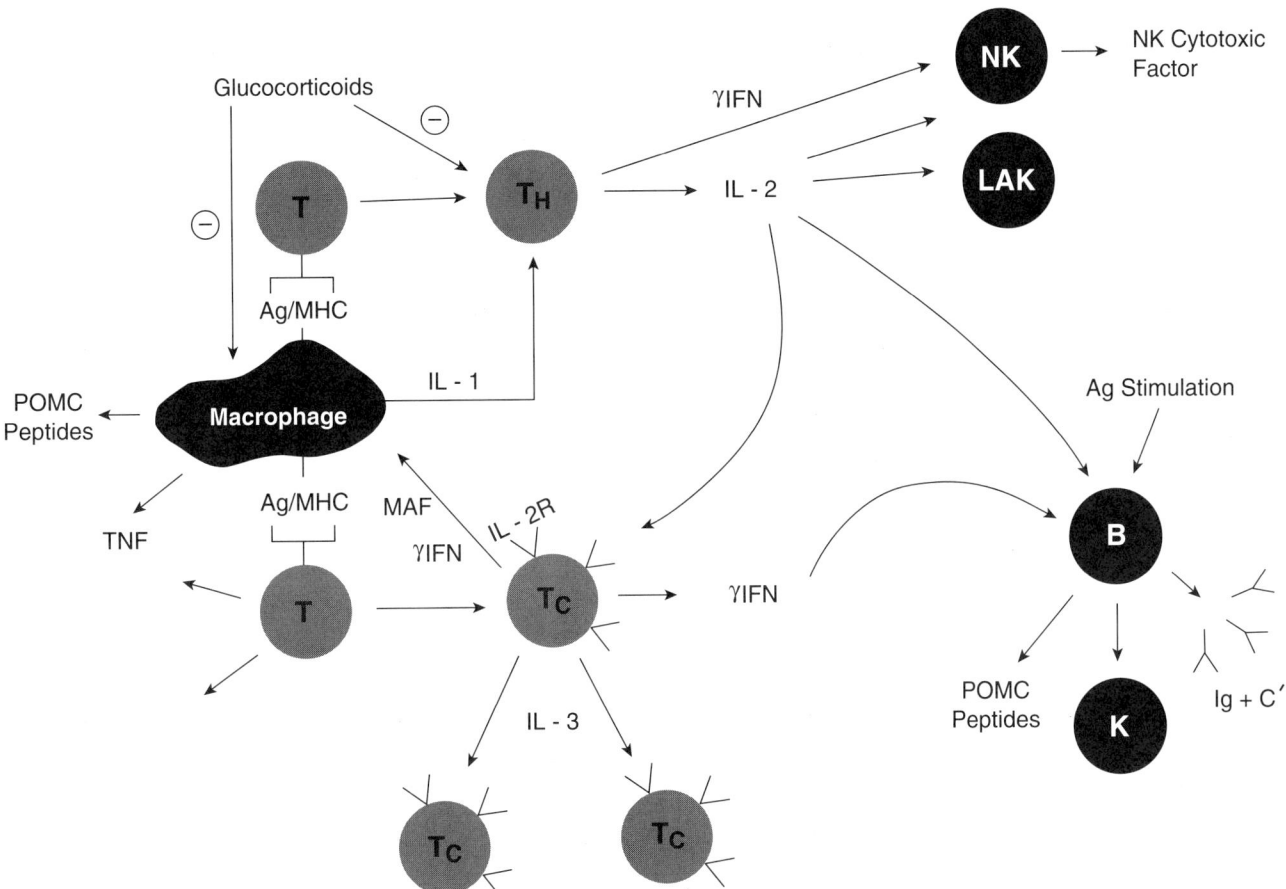

FIGURE 14–1. Cellular interactions involved in humoral and cell-mediated immunity. T_C = cytotoxic T cell; T_H = helper T cell; NK = natural killer cell; LAK = lymphokine-activated killer cell; K = killer cell; Ig = immunoglobulin; C' = complement; Ag = antigen; IL = interleukin; IFN = interferon; POMC = proopiomelanocortin.

against tumor cells, which have surface antigens that are recognized as foreign and can induce an immune response against themselves. The following two sections will address in detail how humoral and cellular immunity fight invaders and tumor cells.

ANTIGEN-ANTIBODY INTERACTIONS

The primary function of antibody is to bind antigen. Specificity of this interaction is an important component of the immune response. The immune system has the ability to discriminate among different antigenic sites (called epitopes) and respond to only those that necessitate a response rather than to mount a random response to all antigens (Benjamini & Leskowitz, 1988). Binding of antibody to antigen initiates secondary effector functions (complement fixation, phagocytosis) that result in killing of foreign cells. Two types of molecules are involved in the recognition of foreign antigen: B cell antigen receptors (immunoglobulins) and T cell antigen receptors (TCR). B cell response (humoral immunity) requires antigen-antibody interactions. T cell response (cell-mediated immunity) does not require antibody but can result in activation of B

cells to produce antibody. Immunoglobulins are produced in large quantities after stimulation of B cells (through contact with antigen) into plasma cells.

ANTIBODY STRUCTURE AND FUNCTION

Immunoglobulins consist of two identical heavy and two identical light chains linked by disulfide bonds (Fig. 14–2). The heavy chains determine the immunoglobulin class, and the light chains determine binding site for antigens. Both chains consist of constant (C) regions and variable (V) regions. The constant region (also referred to as the Fc fragment) allows antibody to perform biologic functions, and the variable region (referred to as the Fab fragment) provides diversity in the foreign bodies that are recognized and responded to. Because an antibody molecule is symmetric, with two identical Fab antigen-binding sites, two antigenic determinants can bind one antibody molecule. The advantage of a single antibody molecule crossreacting with more than one antigenic determinant is that fewer number of different antibodies are needed to mount an immune response.

The diversity of antibody recognition and function can be attributed to three regions of variation: isotypic,

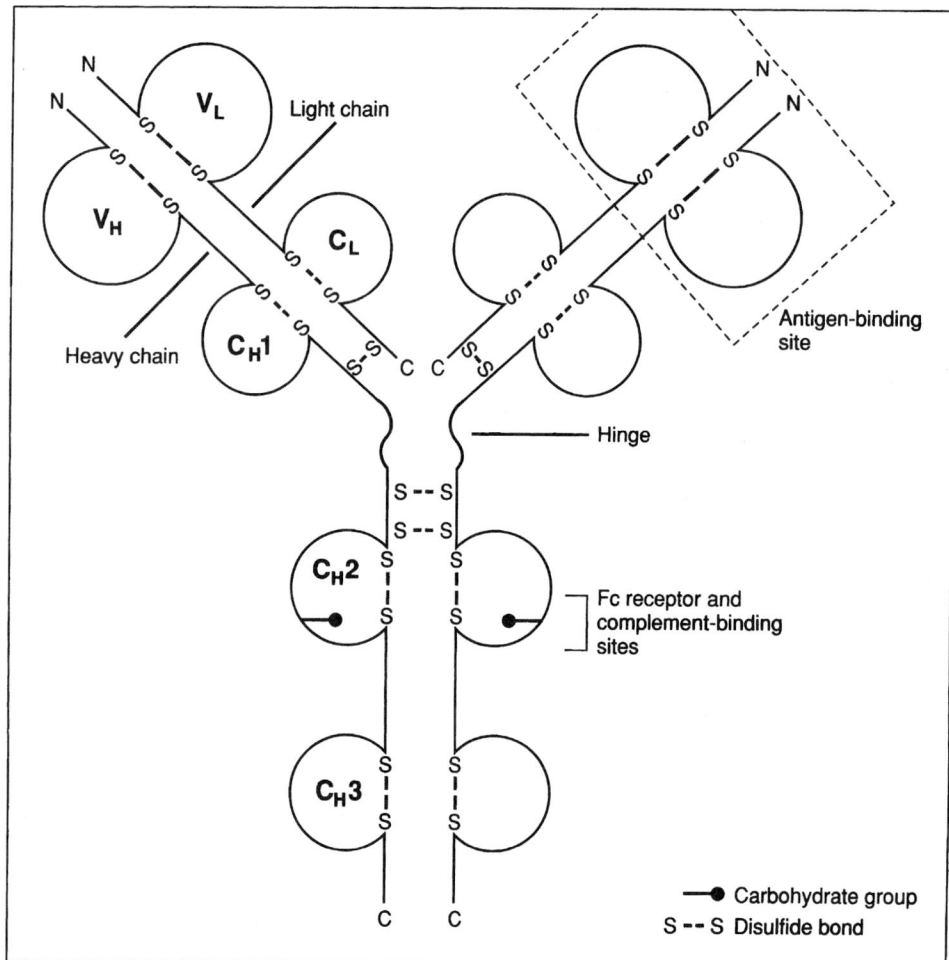

FIGURE 14–2. Schematic diagram of an immunoglobulin molecule. In this drawing of an IgG molecule, the antigen-binding sites are formed by the juxtaposition of V_L and V_H domains. The locations of complement and Fc receptor-binding sites within the heavy chain constant regions are approximations. S — S refers to intrachain and interchain disulfide bonds; N and C refer to amino and carboxy termini of the polypeptide chains, respectively. (Reproduced with permission from Abbas, A. K., Lichtman, A. H., & Pober, J. S. [1994]. *Cellular and molecular immunology* [2nd ed., p. 39]. Philadelphia: W. B. Saunders Co.)

allotypic and idiotypic. Isotypic variation varies among species and refers to the different heavy and light chain classes; allotypic variants occur within the same species and are markers for Mendelian inheritance; and idiotypic sites vary within the individual and confer specificity to each antibody molecule. It is this idiotypic region that determines which antigen the antibody will bind to. Within these variable regions are short polypeptide segments that make up hypervariable regions, the site where antibody binds antigen. These hypervariable regions determine specificity and are exposed to antigen when the immunoglobulin changes its configuration in response to antigen presentation.

Diversity in antibody specificity is achieved through extensive gene rearrangements that code for the variable regions (V) of the heavy and light chains, and the constant (C), joining (J), and diversity (D) regions of the heavy chain. Multiple gene combinations coding the C,V,D, and J regions, along with somatic mutations and gene splicing, produce numerable variations in antigen specificity. Through these active DNA rearrangements, the immune system generates unlimited antibody diversity from a small amount of chromosomal DNA.

In contrast to this potential diversity, all of the antibody produced from a single B lymphocyte has identical antigen specificity. These monoclonal antibodies have the same precise specificity for a given antigen determination site (epitope) and are useful in laboratory procedures, diagnostic tests, and cancer immunotherapy. For example, injecting radiolabeled, tumor-specific, monoclonal antibodies into individuals with cancer allows visualization of tumor metastases by CAT scan as the circulating specific antibody seeks out and attaches to the tumor antigens.

ANTIGEN-ANTIBODY BINDING

Antigen-antibody binding involves weak, noncovalent forces of molecular interactions (ionic, hydrogen-bonding, hydrophobic) (Benjamini & Leskowitz, 1988). Because the binding is weak, there has to be a close fit between the antigen and antibody combining site (similar to a lock and key). The low energy involved in the binding contributes to the ability to dissociate the antigen from the antibody by a low or high pH, high salt concentrations, or cyanates (Benjamini & Leskowitz, 1988). Therefore, the cellular environment is important to antibody effector functions.

Other factors involved in antigen-antibody binding include affinity and avidity. Affinity is determined by the attraction, or intrinsic association constant, of the antibody for the antigen at one site. For example, the amino acid sequence of the binding site (hypervariable region) may vary among antibodies with the same specificity. The antigen will still bind, but the affinity, or strength of binding, will be stronger in those sites with the closest match of amino acids. Whereas affinity is determined by the individual binding site, avidity refers to the total binding strength at multiple sites. When the antigen has many sites for binding (epitopes), the avidity is determined by the sum of the binding strengths of all epitopes.

Many laboratory assays can test the ability of antibody to recognize antigen and the strength of the binding and can measure the amount of antibody or antigen present. Assays that measure minute amounts of antibody or antigen-antibody complexes include immunoelectrophoresis, radioimmunoassay (RIA), enzyme-linked immunosorbent assay (ELISA), radioimmuno-absorbent assay (RAST), and immunofluorescence. Tumor antigens can be detected in several ways, depending on the type of antigen and location of the tumor. One example of a detectable tumor antigen is high concentrations in serum of monoclonal immunoglobulins of a certain isotype or the presence of light chains of these immunoglobulins (Bence-Jones proteins) in the urine. The concentration of these myeloma proteins in the blood or urine is reflective of the tumor mass. Table 14–3 displays a description of these assays and examples of their clinical use.

ANTIBODY-MEDIATED IMMUNE RESPONSE

Foreign antigens that enter the body activate B lymphocytes by binding to the membrane immunoglobulin (Ig) on B cells, which are located mostly in the spleen, lymph nodes, and mucus membranes, and at the site of entry. In the primary immune response, there is a latent period in which B cells make contact with the antigen, proliferate, differentiate, and secrete antibody. Because resting B cells express only IgM and IgD (which is rarely secreted), IgM is the dominant antibody class secreted in the primary immune response. Other immunoglobulin isotypes (IgG, IgA, IgE) appear with second exposure to the same antigen as a result of isotype switching. The secondary antibody response exhibits memory; therefore antibodies appear more rapidly than in the primary response. There also is a greater level of IgG than IgM and a higher affinity of antibody to its antigenic epitope with the secondary immune response (Fig. 14–3).

TABLE 14–3. *Laboratory Tests of Antigen-Antibody Binding*

TEST	WHAT IS MEASURED	CLINICAL EXAMPLE	INTERPRETATION
Agglutination reactions	Aggregation of particulate Ag by cross-linking with Ab	Coombs test (direct and indirect) detects Ab to red blood cells	Positive in transfusions that produce Ab, hemolytic anemia
Precipitation reactions	Ab and soluble Ag are mixed; they crosslink, lose solubility, and precipitate; measures equivalence of Ag to Ab	High-density lipoprotein (HDL) cholesterol; Staphylococcus A	Quantifies levels
Immunoelectrophoresis	Moves, separates and quantifies proteins in an electrical field	Serum immunoglobulin and other protein levels	Peak IgM levels may indicate early infection; myeloma produces Bence Jones protein
Radioimmunoassays (RIA)	Radioactively labeled Ag reacts with Ab to determine the ratio of bound to unbound Ab or Ag	Quantitate tumor markers	Carcinoembryonic antigen (CEA) elevated in colorectal, breast, pancreatic CA. Alpha fetoprotein (AFP) elevated in germ cell, testicular, liver CA
Enzyme-linked immunosorbent assay (ELISA)	Enzyme is linked to an Ab; colored substrate measures activity of bound enzyme, which is reflective of bound Ab	Quantitate HIV and hepatitis A antibodies; cytokine levels	Screening for HIV; measures levels of circulating interleukins, interferon-α
Radioimmunoabsorbent assay (RAST)	Solid phase radioimmunoassay to detect IgE Ab bound to Ag in an allergic individual	Test for IgE antibody to individual foods suspected of causing allergy	Higher levels indicate allergy to substance
Immunofluorescence	Fluorescently labeled specific Ab added to target Ag and amount of fluorescence measured	Quantification of serum T, B and NK cells	Low CD4 (helper T) count, diagnosis of AIDS (CD4 functions as receptor for HIV)

Ab = antibody
Ag = antigen

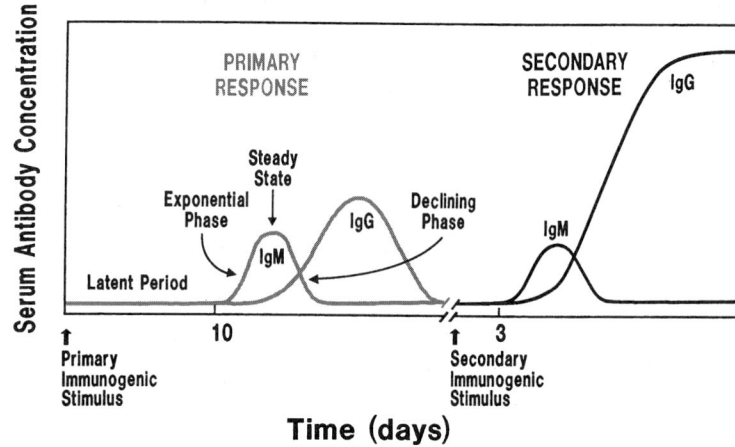

FIGURE 14–3. Antibody response to antigen on first and subsequent exposures. (From Benjamini, E., & Leskowitz, S. [1988]. *Immunology: A short course* [p. 155]. New York: Alan R. Liss, Inc. Copyright© 1988 by Alan R. Liss, Inc. Reprinted by permission of John Wiley & Sons, Inc.)

Contact with an antigen does not automatically elicit an immune response. Factors such as the amount of antigen, the timing of the antigen exposure, the route of invasion, and the "foreignness" to the host determine the body's response to the antigen. When a bivalent antiimmunoglobulin antibody or an antigen with two or more identical epitopes does cross-link to a B cell, a series of effector responses are triggered. After a progression of biochemical and cellular responses (Abbas et al., 1991), messenger RNA is increased and B cells enlarge and move from a resting (G_0) phase to a proliferating (G_1) phase of the cell cycle. Within 12 to 24 hours after stimulation, B cells express increased levels of membrane receptors for helper T cell-derived cytokines (Abbas et al., 1991). If the antigen is a protein, the B cell processes and presents the protein on its surface in combination with class II MHC molecules, which can be recognized by helper T lymphocytes. Nonprotein antigens like polysaccharides and lipids can induce antibody responses without antigen-specific helper T cells. Once the antigen and antibody bind in a complex, effector functions induce destruction of the foreign body through complement activation.

COMPLEMENT AND KININ ACTIVATION

The complement and kinin cascades are involved in the effector response of immune activation. Complement designates a group of more than 25 plasma and cell membrane proteins that cause lysis, mediate opsonization of cells, and help regulate inflammatory responses. In general (and briefly), antigen-antibody complexes (particularly IgG and IgM) activate the classic complement pathway, whereas no antibody is needed for activation of the alternative pathway. The proteins in each pathway interact in a precise sequence. Once C3 is formed, the pathways merge to ultimately form C5–9 proteins, which result in cell membrane lysis, chemotaxis, opsonization, and antigen adherence.

The kinin system (also called kallikrein system) is another humoral amplification system. It is activated by

factor XII and results in the formation of bradykinins that cause vasodilation and smooth muscle contraction. The kinin system is activated in inflammation and is thought to be partially responsible for asthma, angioedema, and pain of pancreatitis (Frank, 1991).

SUMMARY

Cellular cooperation is important in the antibody response. In actuality, both B and T cells participate in humoral immunity. B cells produce the antibody and T cells respond to B cell antigen presentation. Macrophages also play an important role in humoral and cellular immune responses through their surface receptors for antibody and complement and by functioning as an antigen presenting cell (APC) and secreting membrane proteins that promote T cell activation.

CELL-MEDIATED IMMUNITY

Cell-mediated immunity (CMI) involves immune responses carried out primarily by T lymphocytes, although macrophages and antibody also play a role. An important role of T lymphocytes is the ability to discriminate between self and nonself by recognition of the MHC (major histocompatibility complex) molecule on the antigen presenting cell. Presentation of an antigen in the context of MHC activates the T cell to release lymphokines, which attract and activate monocytes, macrophages, and other lymphocytes. The antigen may be foreign tissue, viruses or mycobacteria, a soluble protein, or a chemical capable of penetrating the skin. In contrast to the immediate B cell response, the first contact with an antigen requires 1 to 2 weeks to mount a cell-mediated response (Benjamini & Leskowitz, 1988).

T CELL RECEPTOR STRUCTURE AND FUNCTION

Processing of antigen by macrophages or B cells is a critical step in activating T lymphocytes to proliferate

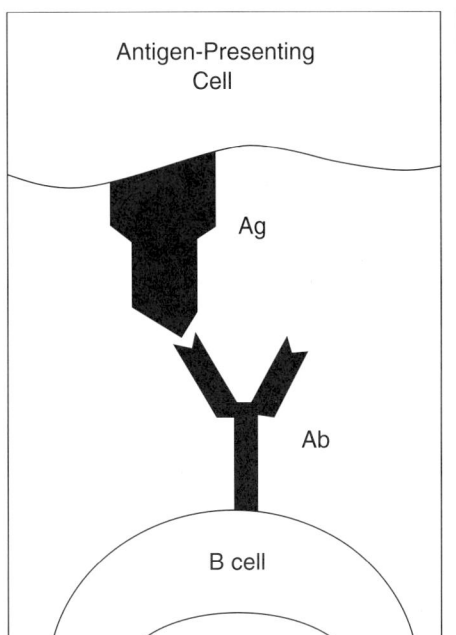

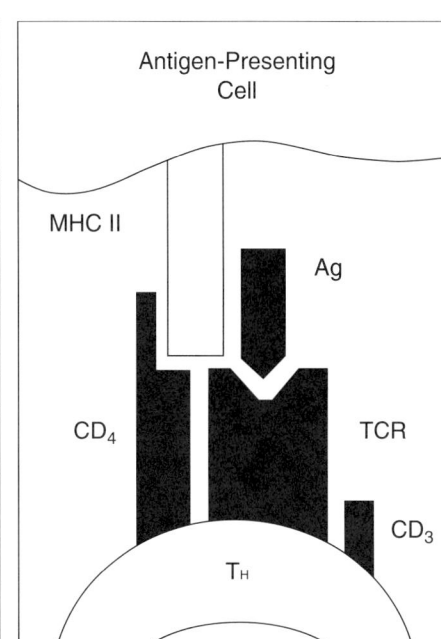

FIGURE 14–4. Antigen presentation to B cells and helper T cells.

and produce lymphokines. The macrophage or B cell ingests the antigen by phagocytosis or pinocytosis, cleaves the antigen into peptide fragments that contain the antigenic site (epitope), and presents the epitope on its cell surface, where it forms a noncovalent bond with the class II MHC molecule. T cells recognize only antigens presented in conjunction with the MHC molecule. Therefore, a prerequisite for all antigen presenting cells (APC) is the presence of class II MHC molecules on the cell surface. Cells that meet this criteria include macrophages, B cells, and dendritic cells (Benjamini & Leskowitz, 1988).

Once presented, a receptor on the helper T cell recognizes the epitope in conjunction with the MHC receptor on the APC. Presentation of the antigen by the APC to the B or T cell is shown in Figure 14–4. The T cell receptor (TCR) is composed of two chains (α and β) that define its variable region. A third component of the TCR, CD3, is required for the expression of the TCR on the T cell surface. The genes that encode the TCR are formed from rearrangements of the VDJ regions, as in the immunoglobulin genes. A second receptor on the T cell surface recognizes the MHC glycoprotein associated with the epitope of the foreign substance. This complex T cell receptor mechanism prevents binding of free antigen, which would activate the immune response indiscriminantly; this role is reserved for the immediate response of antibody and B cells.

MHC RESTRICTION

There are three classes of antigens involved in the MHC: class I antigens, the histocompatibility molecules that provoke an antibody response and include HLA-A, B, and C regions; class II antigens, which encode in the D region and stimulate lymphocytes; and class III antigens, which emanate from the C region and consist of complement components. For successful trig-

gering of T cells, the APC must be identical at the HLA region to the T cell that responds to the antigen (Benjamini & Leskowitz, 1988).

Helper T cells (CD4) recognize antigens in conjunction with class II MHC molecules, and cytotoxic T cells (CD8) recognize antigens presented with class I MHC molecules. Class I molecules are present on all nucleated cells and are recognized by the host CD8 T lymphocytes during graft rejection. If a genetic difference exists at the MHC loci, a rejection reaction ensues in which lymphocytes and monocytes invade the area and trigger an inflammatory reaction, which leads to destruction of vessels, necrosis, and breakdown of the grafted tissue (because deprived of nutrients). Figure 14–5 demonstrates how T cells mediate graft rejection. The activation of helper/inducer (CD4) T cells by alloantigen is pivotal to allograft rejection (Stites, Terr, & Parslow, 1994). Class II molecules are similarly responsible for graft versus host (GVH) reaction in bone marrow transplantation. GVH occurs when mature immunocompetent T cells are transfused into an allogeneic recipient that is unable to reject them. The donor T cells proliferate and attack host organ and tissue cells that carry class II MHC products.

The MHC association of antigens determine which subset of T cells is selectively activated. Extracellular antigens activate class II restricted CD4 cells, which stimulate proliferation and phagocytosis, whereas endogenous antigens (viruses) activate class I restricted CD8 T cells, which lyse cells producing these intracellular antigens. Thus, different forms of antigens selectively stimulate the T cell population that is most effective at eliminating that type of antigen (Abbas et al., 1991).

Specific immunity to tumor-associated antigens provides the basis for the theory of immune surveillance. Hypothetically, the immune system is thought to be able to recognize transformed cells as nonself and stim-

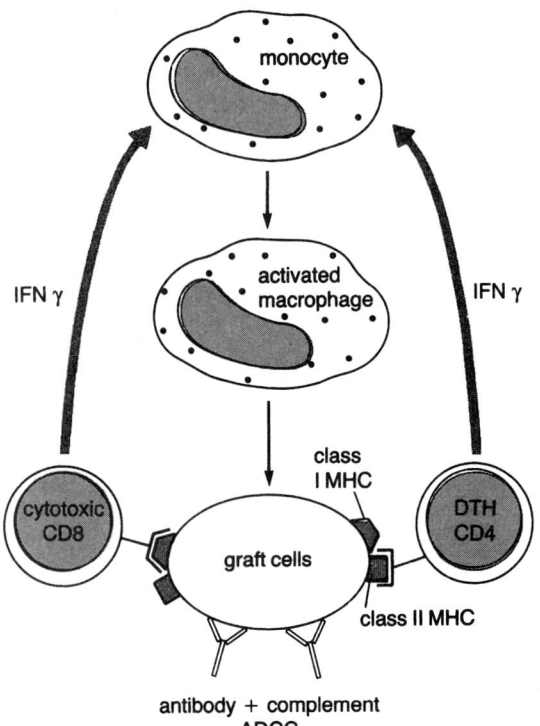

FIGURE 14–5. Effector mechanisms of allograft rejection. (From Stites, D. P., Terr, A. I., & Parslow, T. G. (1994). *Basic and clinical immunology* (8th ed., p. 748). Norwalk, CT: Appleton & Lange. Printed by permission.)

TABLE 14–4. *Humoral and Cell-mediated Immune Response to Tumors*

Humoral Responses	Immune Components Involved
Complement activated lysis Phagocytosis	IgM, IgG, B cells, Macrophages, complement, antitumor Ab
Antibody-mediated loss of adhesion	Antibodies specific to tumor antigens
Cell-mediated Responses	**Immune Components Involved**
Tumor-specific cytotoxicity	Cytotoxic T lymphocytes with specificity for tumor antigen
	Helper T lymphocytes assist
Antibody-dependent cell-mediated Cytotoxicity (ADCC)	Tumor-specific antibodies, B cells, K cells (non T, non B lymphocytes) with Fc receptors
Macrophage killing	IFN-γ secreted by helper T lymphocyte (antigen specific)
Natural killer cell cytotoxicity	Interferon activated

ulate killing by immune effector cells. Whether the immune system maintains surveillance over malignant transformed cells is debated. It is likely that several immune components play a role in preventing development of some malignancies (Unanue & Benacerraf, 1984) and that natural killer cells participate in immune surveillance by direct lysis of malignant cells. Table 14–4 outlines the different types of humoral and CMI responses and the immune components involved. Cell-mediated immune responses generally are more specific and directed toward tumor targets than are humoral immune responses.

CELL-MEDIATED IMMUNE RESPONSE

The effector function of the cell-mediated immune response involves an array of immune molecules and cytokine mediators. Macrophages play an important role in CMI by functioning as APCs and secreting membrane proteins that promote T cell activation. T cell receptor recognition of antigen results in activation of T cell helper and suppressor activity, cytotoxicity, and possibly, natural killer (NK) cell activity (Roitt, Brostoff, & Male, 1993). Helper T cells direct specificity and effector mechanisms, whereas the cells involved in direct killing include macrophages, cytotoxic

T cells, natural killer (NK), and lymphoid killer (K) cells. Cytotoxic T cells kill target cells either because they are infected or because they are recognized as nonself (Roitt et al., 1993). T cell-mediated lysis is independent of antibody and complement but dependent on cell-to-cell contact, TCR binding, presence of magnesium, calcium, and glucose, and shared MHC gene products with the target cell (Henney & Gillis, 1984). The three phases of killing include binding to the target, release of enzymes that modify the target, and cell death.

HELPER T CELL RESPONSE

Binding of the MHC and antigen complex is the first signal to the helper T cell. A second signal, interleukin 1 (IL-1), is required to activate the helper T cell. This cytokine is produced by macrophages and induces the helper T cell to produce IL-2 receptors on its surface. Once activated, the helper T cell secretes IL-2 and other soluble lymphokines that activate B cells and cytotoxic T cells. While proliferating, T cells release several lymphokines, including macrophage chemotactic factor, which attracts monocytes and macrophages to the T cell response site; migration inhibiting factor (MIF), which makes monocytes adherent to cell walls; macrophage activating factor (MAF), which enhances killing ability of macrophages; and lymphotoxin, which has been shown to kill some tumor cells.

Helper T cells consist of at least two subtypes that have different surface markers and carry out different functions. Helper T "inducer" cells (CD4+, Leu 8+) induce mature helper and suppressor cells and helper T "helper" cells (CD4+, Leu 8–) activate antibody production. Similarly, suppressor T cells (CD8) can be subdivided into "true suppressor cells" (CD8+, CD11+), which activate antibody production, or cytotoxic T cells (CD8+, CD11–), which directly lyse target cells. These subtype functions of the helper T and suppressor T cell overlap, providing dual coverage for some immune responses and a feedback mechanism to control immune responsiveness.

OTHER CMI EFFECTOR CELLS

Several cell lines have nonspecific, MHC-unrestricted killing, including natural killer (NK) and lymphokine activated killer (LAK) cells. Natural killer cells are large granular lymphocytes that act as effector cells to spontaneously lyse target (including tumor) cells. NK cells function independently of antibody or specific recognition and are not MHC-restricted. They have no TCR or immunoglobulin as surface antigen receptors. They have membrane-bound granules that contain acid hydrolases, which lyse cells to which they directly bind. This nonspecific lysis is important in eliminating viral and cancer cells from the body. The ability of NK cells to kill tumor cells is enhanced by interferons, tumor necrosis factor (TNF), and IL-2. NK cells also release interferon-γ (IFN-γ), IL-1, and GM-CSF, which are important in regulating other immune responses and stimulating hematopoiesis. Some NK cells also recognize and lyse target cells coated with IgG antibodies. This mechanism is referred to as antibody-dependent cellular cytotoxicity (ADCC) or killer (K) cell activity.

Resting NK cells also express the α-chain of the IL-2 receptor, which when activated by IL-2 transforms the NK cell to a lymphokine-activated killer (LAK) cell. LAK cells kill a broader spectrum of tumor targets than NK cells and play a role in control of tumor metastases.

ASSAYS OF CELL-MEDIATED IMMUNE RESPONSE

Counting or quantifying T or NK cells or subsets provides clinical information that can help in diagnosing and understanding immunodeficiency diseases or T cell leukemias and lymphomas, in evaluating immunocompetence in autoimmune diseases, or in detecting cellular changes in HIV infection and organ or bone marrow transplantation. Functional assays (such as NK and LAK cytotoxicity) that measure the ability of lymphocytes to proliferate or kill targets in response to a stimulus have little clinical application at this time. They do, however, provide information on cellular interactions and the integrity of immune cells to respond to specific antigens. Examples of lymphocyte assays and their applications are shown in Table 14–5.

SUMMARY

One of the major functions of cell-mediated immunity is to defend against viruses and bacteria that can live within cells. Antibodies cannot reach intracellular pathogens. Therefore, the elaborate mechanism of recognizing the antigen as foreign and mounting a cellular response is the responsibility of T lymphocytes. Cell-mediated immune responses are more localized than antibody responses and require direct contact of the T lymphocyte with its target. Lymphokines assist in signaling accessory cells and other immune cells to aid in the killing of targets. Because T cell recognition is MHC-restricted, T lymphocytes can usually differentiate host cells from foreign antigen. Allograft rejection is a clear example of self and nonself recognition of T cells.

TABLE 14–5. *Cellular Immune Lymphocyte Assays*

TEST	WHAT IS MEASURED	CLINICAL AND RESEARCH APPLICATION
Fluorescence	DNA cell kinetic analysis/ploidy assays (cell cycle phase)	Breast cancer, phase of division of cells (clinical indicator) In all stages of colorectal cancer, no change measured in NK or T cell number from presurgery to 6 months postsurgery; only B cell number increased[a]
Lymphocyte activation (cytotoxicity assays)	Quantification of ability to kill radiolabeled tumor cells in vitro (NK, LAK, T cells)	Not used clinically Increases in LAK and monocyte cytotoxicity measured in response to imagery group intervention over 4 months[b] PHA stimulated T cell response was greater at 2 weeks post breast biopsy than pre biopsy or 1 week post[c]
Mixed leukocyte reaction (MLR)	Measures the reaction of T cells of one individual to MHC antigens from another individual	Determines ability of a host to react to a donor's tissue (clinical indicator of histocompatibility for transplant)
Delayed type hypersensitivity (DTH) skin tests	T cell recognition and response 24 and 48 hours after antigen is injected intradermally (not subcutaneously)	Determines immunocompetence (anergy may be clinically determined in immunosuppression, some cancers, and some immunodeficiency diseases)

[a] Tax et al., 1994
[b] Post-White, 1991
[c] Owen, 1992

REGULATION OF THE IMMUNE RESPONSE

The immune system has feedback control mechanisms that are critical to regulating the immune response. Mediators and cellular interactions suppress as well as augment the immune response. Self-tolerance, a form of immune suppression, prevents the body from mounting an immune response to itself and explains why a mother does not reject her fetus and why autoimmune diseases are an exception instead of a rule (Benjamini & Leskowitz, 1988). Disturbances in these regulatory mechanisms can create immunodeficiencies or hypersensitivities and can be caused by genetic defects, hormonal imbalances, or infection. Acquired immune deficiency syndrome (AIDS) is an example of a defect in the ability of the immune system to respond to foreign antigen secondary to viral (HIV) infection.

CELLULAR REGULATION
DYSREGULATION OF IMMUNE ENHANCEMENT

T and B lymphocytes and accessory cells activate the immune response when they respond to antigens. Examples of the importance of this immune enhancement are natural immunity to infectious organisms or foreign substances and protection against diseases through immunizations. Humoral and cellular immunity, however, can be detrimental when activated without normal feedback controls. For example, antigen-antibody complexes can augment the immune response by activating complement, resulting in cell injury, inflammation, and antibody deposition in arteries and tissues. Acute serum sickness and systemic lupus erythematosus (SLE) are prototypes for immune complex-mediated disorders. Several autoimmune disorders occur when autoantibodies develop to self-tissues, such as in autoimmune hemolytic anemia and myasthenia gravis, or to foreign antigens that cross-react with self proteins, such as in rheumatic fever and rheumatoid arthritis. T lymphocytes normally maintain self-tolerance but may become autoreactive and cause tissue injury, such as in insulin-dependent diabetes mellitus or autoimmune thyroiditis. These inflammatory reactions and autoimmune diseases are examples of dysregulation, or a lack of inhibition, of the immune response. Recognition of self and immunologic tolerance are two immune mechanisms that help to regulate the immune response.

IMMUNOLOGIC TOLERANCE

During an immune response, two pathways are activated—one to eliminate the foreign substance and one to suppress or regulate the immune response (Hood, Weissman, Wood, & Wilson, 1984). Immunologic tolerance is an immune control mechanism in which there is a diminished or absent ability to mount a specific cell-mediated or humoral immune response. Tolerance is more likely to occur with either large or small doses of antigen, a weakly immunogenic antigen, inability of macrophages to phagocytize antigen, a lack of lymphocytes (such as an induced immunosuppression), or inhibition of cell-to-cell interactions by cytokine mediators (Roitt et al., 1993; Benjamini & Leskowitz, 1988).

Tolerance can be favorable when preventing rejection of foreign tissue grafts or reducing hypersensitivity to self. Tolerance can be undesirable, however, when tumor cells remain unrecognized. Tumor cells can evade immune response by modulating their antigens and evading recognition, by secreting soluble antigens that block antibodies, or by secreting prostaglandins that directly suppress immune responses. Antigen-specific suppressor T lymphocytes also have been found in tumors (Benjamini & Leskowitz, 1988), producing a form of tolerance to tumor in distant sites (North, 1985). Immunity to tumors is T cell-mediated and not antibody-mediated. However, antibody-tumor antigen complexes can block the cytotoxic effect of T cells on large tumors, which creates a general depression in immunity (Sjogren, 1985).

Antigen-processing cells are central to development of tolerance. If the processing cell is bypassed, some form of tolerance is induced (Benjamini & Leskowitz, 1988). Tolerance is easily induced in newborns because they have small or absent populations of these accessory cells.

T and B lymphocytes also are involved in tolerance. Examples of downregulation of antibody include endogenous production of IgG to suppress IgM and exogenously administered anti-D antibody to Rh-negative mothers in cases of Rhesus (Rh) incompatibility. Several mechanisms are thought to be responsible for antibody downregulation. Competition for antigen and a higher affinity of IgG for antigen can suppress IgM production. In antibody blocking, high doses of antibody block the interaction of the antigen epitope from the B cell receptor specific to that antigen. In receptor cross-linking, low doses of antibody cross-link with the B cell's Fc receptors and prevent antibody synthesis. Tolerance only occurs to the Fc portion of antibody, which exists in large numbers. Antigen-antibody complexes also can inhibit immune responses. It has been postulated that in patients with cancer, circulating immune complexes composed of antibody and tumor cell antigens can suppress immune responses by cross-linking the B cell's Fc receptor with the antigen receptor (Roitt et al., 1993).

T cell tolerance occurs earlier and lasts longer than B cell tolerance. Tolerance in T cells is mediated either by clonal deletion, in which T cells lack one specific reactivity, or by the presence of suppressor T cells with specificity for the antigen. Helper T cells appear to play an important role in immune regulation through their cytokine production. The production of cytokines (IL-4, IL-10, IFN-γ) signals upregulation or downregulation of other cells and may explain the suppression observed when high doses of autoantigen are administered. An example of this is in allergy desensitization, where increasing increments of antigen, known to induce an IgE response in the individual, is injected, producing a T cell response and IFN-γ-induced IgE suppression.

CYTOKINE MEDIATORS

Cytokines are hormone-like peptides or glycopeptides that are required for the generation of an effective immune response. They provide a communication network among immune cells, are mediators of natural immunity, provide protection against viral infection, and initiate the inflammatory response to bacterial antigens. There are several categories of cytokines, including interferons, interleukins, colony-stimulating factors (CSFs), and tumor necrosis factor (TNF), which function as regulators of immune and inflammatory responses (Table 14–6). They control growth, mobility, and differentiation of leukocytes and other cells. T and B cells must be activated to produce and secrete cytokines, which are highly specific and potent. Cytokines are rapidly secreted but circulate briefly. They exert their effects primarily by binding to specific receptors on target cells.

Cytokines provide both enhancing and suppressing immune regulating feedback. For example, IL-10 and IL-4 upregulate humoral immune responses and downregulate cell-mediated immune response, particularly suppressing the two subsets of helper T cells. Cytokines also can "switch off" the response to another cytokine by acting through a different receptor (Roitt et al., 1993). For example, IL-1 and IFN-γ may have an upregulating synergistic effect with TNF, contributing to cachexia and septic shock (Cerami, 1992). IL-13 is thought to downregulate IL-1 by acting through the IL-4 receptor to stimulate neutrophils to produce IL-1 receptor antagonist, resulting in an antiinflammatory function (Aversa et al., 1993). IL-1 also has a direct inhibitor, which competes with IL-1 for IL-1 receptors (Whicher & Evans, 1990).

Cytokines have demonstrated effectiveness against tumors and have been cloned and used to enhance immune activation against tumors. Paciotti and Tamarkin (1988a, 1988b) measured direct inhibitory effects of IL-1 and IL-2 on hormone-dependent breast cancer cell lines. The most encouraging results are with interferon-α in hairy-cell leukemia and IL-2 in renal cell carcinoma and melanoma. Preliminary studies with LAK or tumor-infiltrating lymphocytes (TIL) plus IL-2 indi-

TABLE 14–6. *Cytokines and Their Role in Immune Response*

CYTOKINE	IMMUNE CELL SOURCE	PRIMARY ACTIVITY	IMMUNE EFFECTS
IL-1	Macrophages, monocytes	Augments T and B lymphocytes	Inflammatory Stimulate hematopoiesis
IL-2	Helper T lymphocytes NK cells	T and B cell growth factor	Stimulates T, NK cells and LAK activity
IL-3	T lymphocytes	Hematopoietic growth factor	Stimulate hematopoiesis
IL-4	Helper T lymphocytes	T and B cell growth factor Promotes mast cell growth	Stimulates IgE reactions
IL-5	Helper T lymphocytes	B cell growth factor IgA enhancing factor	Stimulates B cells and eosinophils
IL-6	Fibroblasts Macrophages, monocytes	B cell growth factor	Augments inflammation
IL-7	Stromal cells	Pre B and pre T cell growth factor	Stimulates B and T cell proliferation
IL-8	Macrophages	Neutrophil-activating and chemotactic factor	Attracts neutrophils and T lymphocytes
IL-9	Activated T lymphocytes	T cell growth factor Mast cell growth factor	Stimulate erythropoietin
IL-10	Helper T_2 lymphocytes	Cytokine inhibitory factor	Inhibits cytokine synthesis Modulates B cell and macrophage activity
IL-11	Bone marrow stromal cells	Blast cell growth factor	Stimulate hematopoiesis, acute phase response, neuron generation
IL-12	Monocytes, macrophages, B lymphocytes, mast cells	NK stimulatory factor	Stimulates NK, LAK, T cell activity Activates macrophages through IFN-γ
IL-13	Activated T lymphocytes	Antiinflammatory factor	Stimulate macrophage expression and B cells, inhibit ADCC, nitric oxide production
G-CSF	Monocytes	Myeloid growth factor	Generates neutrophils
M-CSF	Monocytes	Macrophage growth factor	Generates macrophages
GM-CSF	T lymphocytes	Monomyelocytic growth factor	Myelopoiesis
IFN (αβγ)	Leukocytes, fibroblasts, T lymphocytes, NK cells	Antiviral, antiproliferative, immunomodulating	Stimulates macrophages, NK cells
TNF α	Macrophages T lymphocytes	Inflammatory Tumoricidal	Necrosis of tumor cells
TGF β	Platelets, bone	Immunosuppression	Wound healing, bone repair

cated a greater response of tumors than with IL-2 alone (Rosenberg et al., 1988). These results have not been as promising as initially anticipated, however. Activating immune responsiveness is not necessarily curative, and biologic therapies are associated with acute (and sometimes life-threatening) side effects. The use of biologic therapies for supportive measures has shown more promise. Colony-stimulating factors (GM-CSF, G-CSF), which stimulate hematopoiesis, have been effective in shortening the period of aplasia after bone marrow transplantation and high-dose chemotherapy regimens (Roitt et al., 1993).

HORMONAL REGULATION

Many endocrine organs appear to be involved in some aspect of the immune regulatory process. Lymphocytes have estrogen receptors. Estrogens can be both immunostimulating by enhancing synthesis of antibodies and immunoinhibiting by suppressing cell-mediated immune responses. Estrogen treatment inhibits NK cell function and T cell-mediated cutaneous de-

layed hypersensitivity reactions, cancer immune surveillance, and graft rejection (Grossman, 1991). Women taking estrogen (with or without progesterone) and men taking diethylstilbestrol (DES) for prostatic cancer have similar depressions in cellular immune responses (Grossman, 1991). Although the clinical implications are unclear, tamoxifen has been shown to reduce NK function and helper T cell numbers in women with breast cancer who were on tamoxifen for 1 to 3 years. (Robinson, Rubin, Mekori, Segal, & Pollack, 1993). Estrogen also may play a role in autoimmune diseases, which are more prevalent in women than in men, possibly because of the inhibition of suppressor T cell response, which normally shuts off immune enhancement. Both androgens and progesterone also suppress CMI and are thought to be dependent on estrogens to produce this immunosuppression (see Box 14–1).

Glucocorticosteroids (i.e., cortisol) suppress both cellular and humoral immunity. They appear to inhibit cytokine production, particularly IL-1, IL-2, IL-4, and IFN-γ, which contributes to suppression of T cell and NK cytotoxicity, reduced B cell production of antibody

---

Box 14–1. *The Role of Tamoxifen in Activating LAK Cells to Lyse Adenocarcinoma of the Breast*

Albertini, M. R., Gibson, D. F. C., Robinson, S. P., Howard, S. P., Tans, K. J., Lindstrom, M. J., Robinson, R. R., Tormey, D. C., Jordan, V. C., & Sondel, P. M. (1992). Influence of estradiol and tamoxifen on susceptibility of human breast cancer cell lines to lysis by lymphokine-activated killer cells. *Journal of Immunology, 11*:30–39.

Rationale and Purpose: With the somewhat seemingly universal prescribing of tamoxifen for breast cancer, it seems appropriate that this group of researchers set out to determine the actual effects of tamoxifen on both estrogen receptor-positive and -negative breast cancer tumors. Because tamoxifen is a cytostatic compound, continuous therapy is required and is only effective if the tumor cells remain hormone-dependent. Because some patients with estrogen receptor-negative tumors can also have antitumor responses with tamoxifen therapy, the investigators thought that mechanisms other than hormone-inhibiting effects may be contributing to tamoxifen's effectiveness. Therefore, the purpose of their study was to evaluate combination hormonal and immunotherapeutic treatments for breast cancer. They hypothesized that IL-2 therapy, in combination with tamoxifen, could induce LAK cells to kill tumor cells.

Sample and Methods: Normal donors and six patients with melanoma, renal cancer, and lymphoma enrolled in an IL-2 clinical trial donated blood samples. The blood was incubated with breast cancer tumor cell lines (estrogen receptor-positive and -negative) and a control medium (estrogen free), a medium containing tamoxifen, or medium with both estradiol and tamoxifen. The ability of the patients' lymphocytes to kill the tumor cells and the phase of cell cycle were determined.

Results: As expected, cells from the estrogen-positive tumor cell line stimulated with estradiol alone increased their proliferation; the percentage of cells in S phase also was higher. When tamoxifen was added with estradiol, the estradiol-induced growth was inhibited. In addition, the estradiol-stimulated tumor cells were more susceptible to lysis by activated LAK cells. When tamoxifen was added, the percentage of lysis was reduced, but it was still higher than in the control group. In estrogen receptor-negative tumor cell lines, however, the addition of either estradiol, tamoxifen, or control had no effect. If estradiol was given with tamoxifen, there was a slightly higher (significantly) ability to lyse tumor cells. Comparison of in vivo administration of IL-2 and in vitro activation of LAK cells with IL-2 indicated that in vitro activation was more effective in inducing tumor lysis. The addition of a monoclonal antibody, with known activity against breast adenocarcinoma, significantly boosted in vivo IL-2 stimulated LAK activity in estrogen-positive and -negative tumor cells incubated with estradiol, tamoxifen, estradiol plus tamoxifen, and even the control group. A more inconsistent and smaller effect was seen when the monoclonal antibody was added to in vitro stimulated IL-2 LAK cells.

Conclusions and Implications: These results suggest that tamoxifen may decrease the sensitivity of breast cancer cells to lysis by LAK cells. However, because tamoxifen also inhibits the growth of estrogen-dependent cancer cells, the advantage of using tamoxifen to prevent growth may outweigh the risk of reducing lysis once the tumor grows. And because tamoxifen was more effective than control alone, in patients with low estrogen levels, tamoxifen may actually enhance IL/LAK cell therapy. The estrogen receptor-negative tumor cells were less susceptible to lysis by LAK. They did, however, respond significantly when incubated with both estradiol and tamoxifen, possibly reflecting the greater amount of immune activation with in vitro activation by IL-2. The boosting of lysis by the monoclonal antibody occurred independent of hormonal therapy, suggesting that lysis is due to intrinsic differences in recognition or activation. The authors conclude that long-term therapy with tamoxifen could be improved by adding IL-2 and possibly monoclonal antibody to facilitate antibody-dependent cellular cytotoxicity (ADCC).

and suppressed inflammatory role of macrophages. When given in high doses for treatment of lymphomas, glucocorticoids cause lysis of circulating lymphocytes (Barrett, 1988). Other hormones, such as thyroid hormones (T_3 and T_4) and pituitary hormones (somatotropin and prolactin), exert opposite effects to augment both cellular and humoral immune response.

An example of the effects of hormonal regulation on immune response is seen in pregnancy. Pregnancy (with its concommitent increase of estrogen and progesterone) significantly depresses the cellular immune response but does not greatly affect the humoral immune response (Grossman, 1991). During pregnancy there is a decrease in T cell number and function, which prevents maternal rejection of fetal antigens. There also is a decrease in NK number (function is thought to remain the same), which contributes to the increase in viral infections observed during gestation. Conversely, serum immunoglobulin concentrations increase. Three to 6 months postpartum, the reduction in sex steroid levels stimulates immune reactivity (Grossman, 1991).

ENVIRONMENTAL REGULATION

In addition to internal regulation by feedback inhibition, tolerance, and the regulatory effects of hormones and cytokines, the nervous system also influences immune response. The immune system shares with the central nervous system its ability to signal other cells via the hypothalamus-pituitary-adrenal (HPA) axis. The interaction between the nervous and immune system is bidirectional and thought to be influenced by behavioral and emotional conditions. Stress is the classic example of environmental effects on immune function. Although stress itself probably does not directly alter immune function, the individual's reaction to the stress (stressors) can create physical, immunologic, and emotional responses. Stress stimulates adrenal and inhibits gonadal function, producing different immunologic effects in males and females (Grossman, 1991).

STRESS AND EMOTIONAL RESPONSES

Stress has been associated with alterations in humoral and cellular immunity, including decreased response to antigens, reduced lymphocyte-mediated cytotoxicity and delayed hypersensitivity, and suppressed antibody responses and graft-versus-host disease (Yirmiya et al., 1991). The key to the complex regulation of the immune response by adrenal and hormonal influences involves the effects of corticotropin-releasing hormone (CRH) on adrenocorticotropic hormone (ACTH). The amygdala is an area in the limbic system that responds to emotional states, is rich in neuropeptides, and innervates specific brainstem catecholaminergic cells that control response to stressors through communication with the hypothalamus (Gray, 1991). The hypothalamus secretes corticotropin-releasing hormone (CRH), which signals the release of adrenocorticotropin-releasing hormone (ACTH) from the pituitary and immunosuppressive cortisol from the adrenal gland

(Fig. 14–6). ACTH and CRH respond to stress-ors and act indirectly and directly on immune function. CRH suppresses NK cytotoxicity directly (Irwin, Vale, & Britton, 1987), and ACTH directly inhibits antibody production, interferes with macrophage-mediated tumoricidal activity, modulates B cell function, and suppresses IFN-γ (Heijnan, Kavelaars, & Ballieux, 1991). NK and LAK cells defend against cancer and are reduced in individuals undergoing long-term stressors (Esterling, Kiecolt-Glaser, Bodnar, & Glaser, 1993). NK and LAK cytotoxicity have been shown to increase in response to psychologic interventions such as relaxation (Fawzy et al., 1990) and imagery (Post-White, 1991). The exact response to stressors is variable, however, and depends (in animals) on the timing of the stressor (Justice, 1985), the chronicity and intensity of the stressor, and the controllability of the animal to respond (Monjan, 1981; Yirmaya et al., 1991). Measuring immune effects to stressors in humans is even more complex.

Cytokines produced by the immune system and central nervous system also provide feedback to the hypothalamus (Blalock, Harbour-McMenamin, & Smith, 1985). Because immune cells do not directly reach the central nervous system, these mediators assist in neurohormone regulation of immune responses to physical and emotional states. IFN-α attenuates the effect of stressors by decreasing plasma corticosterone concentrations (Saphier & Roerig, 1993) and altering hypothalamic and hippocampal electrical activity (Dyck & Greenberg, 1991). Several cytokines, such as IL-6, IL-1, and TNF, also have direct feedback effects on the hypothalamus or pituitary, which can alter activity of brain neurons and endocrine tissues (Coleman, Lombard, & Sicard, 1992). The cognitive dysfunction associated with biologic response modifiers (particularly interferon-α and IL-2) can be partly explained by the competition with neurotransmitters for receptor binding in the central nervous system, endorphin opioid-like effects, and increased neuroendocrine hormone levels, such as β-endorphin and ACTH (Bender, 1994).

Immune control of cancer has been tentatively linked with coping style, stress, and emotional well-being (Jemmott & Locke, 1984; Ader, Felten, & Cohen, 1991). Psychologic processes thought to influence cancer progression through immunosuppression include hopelessness (Schmale & Iker, 1966), helplessness (Levy & Wise, 1988), repressive coping style (Antoni & Goodkin, 1988) and depression (Levy & Wise, 1988; Persky, Kempthorne-Rawson, & Shekelle, 1987). Negative emotional states may be the common denominator through which psychosocial events contribute to increased fatigue (Belza, Henke, Yelin, Epstein, & Gilliss, 1993) immunosuppression, infections, and cancer (Kiecolt-Glaser & Glaser, 1991). Very little research exists, however, to validate or explain the role of psychologic states on immune function and cancer. There are anecdotal reports and research studies to both support and negate the role of psychologic state in cancer. Because psychoneuroimmune interactions are complex and coping responses are individualized, validating these relationships requires scientific rigor, large sample sizes, and replication of results (see Box 14-2).

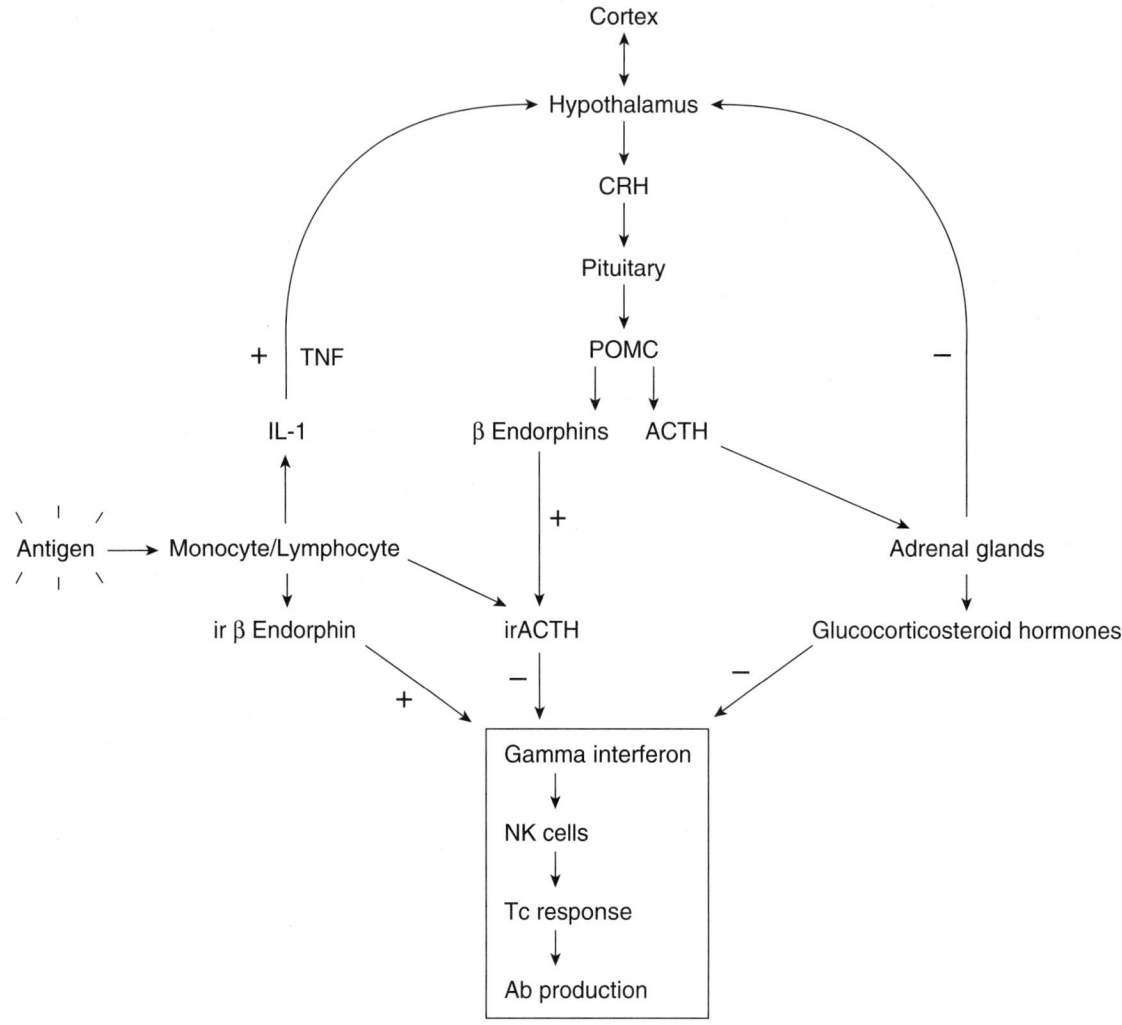

FIGURE 14–6. Immunoregulatory pathway of endorphins and ACTH. CRH = corticotropin releasing hormone; POMC = prooplomelanocortin; ACTH = adreno-corticotropic hormone; IL-1 = interleukin 1; Ir = immune reactive; TNF = tumor necrosis factor. (Adapted from Post-White, J., & Johnson, M. [1991]. Complementary nursing therapies in clinical oncology: Relaxation and imagery. *Dimensions in Oncology Nursing, 5*(2), 15–20.)

OTHER FACTORS

Circadian rhythm, nutritional state, and age are other factors that contribute to regulation of the immune response. Circadian rhythm has been known to alter gonadal steroid, thymic hormone, and glucocorticoid levels. Both sex steroids and glucocorticoids are lowered during the dark phase. Melatonin, which is synthesized in the dark, inhibits the release of CRH, thereby reducing levels of immunosuppressive ACTH. Maximal cellular and humoral response occurs during the dark phase when most people sleep (glucocorticoid levels are lowered and thymic hormone levels are raised). Interestingly, acute sleep loss of 64 hours was associated with leukocytosis and increased NK activity in a study of 20 male and female healthy volunteers (Dinges et al., 1994). This unexpected increase was thought to be secondary to nonspecific activation of macrophages and IL-1 release, resulting in activation of T cells and IL-2 release.

Increasing age contributes to changes in immune function. There is a decline in T and NK cell response, lower IL-2 and IFN-γ production, reduced responses of antibodies to particular antigens, and reduced suppressor T cell populations to regulate immune responses. Consequently, older adults tend to have greater bacterial and some viral infections and an increase in autoimmune diseases. Reduced T cell and NK functions can partially explain the increased incidence of some cancers with age.

Nutritional state can have a significant influence on immune response also. Protein-calorie malnutrition is a common cause of immune deficiency and results in reduced CMI, phagocytosis, and complement. The age of the individual influences the immune defects observed; thymic atrophy occurs in malnourished children, resulting in long-lasting immunosuppression. Vitamin and mineral deficiencies also contribute to immune dysfunction. Iron deficiency may impair lymphocyte func-

---

Box 14–2. *NK Cell Activity and Mood Predicts Recurrence*

Levy, S. M., Herberman, R. B., Lippman, M., D'Angelo, T., & Lee, J. (1991). Immunological and psychosocial predictors of disease recurrence in patients with early-stage breast cancer. *Behavioral Medicine, 17*(2), 67–75.

Study Purpose and Methods: Characteristics most commonly used to predict breast cancer outcome include age, number of positive lymph nodes, size of primary tumor, estrogen and progesterone receptor concentration, cell nuclear grade, and degree of cell differentiation. In this study, the authors hypothesize that cellular immune function and psychosocial factors can also determine survival from breast cancer. They tested the relationship between NK cell activity, perceived social support, and mood states in 90 women with stage I and II breast cancer. The women were assessed 5 days, 3 months, and 15 months after surgery and were followed for five or more years later. A baseline structured interview assessed for perceived social support. Women also completed the Profile of Mood States (POMS) and had blood drawn for NK cell activity and estrogen receptor protein measurement at baseline, 3 months, and 15 months. All women had completed therapy by 15 months.

Results: Of the 29 women with recurrent disease, nine of them had local recurrences. The women with local recurrence were eliminated from the analysis. The mean time to recurrence was 35 months. NK activity was a strong predictor of recurrence, while psychosocial factors predicted how soon the women would recur. Women with higher NK cell activity at baseline (after surgery) were more likely to have recurrence, whereas women with higher NK cell activity at 15 months were the least likely to have recurrent disease. The lower the baseline NK cell activity and the larger the tumor size were, the lower the follow-up NK was, which related to increased recurrence. Psychologic distress at baseline was predictive of earlier recurrence (along with more positive nodes). Older age and better support also predicted longer time to recurrence.

Conclusions and Implications: In this study, NK cell activity after adjuvant therapy was particularly important in preventing recurrence. Once recurrence occurs, however, mood state and psychologic support may predict progression of disease. Although the sample size was relatively large at baseline, approximately 50% of the patients were lost to follow-up, which is a particular problem with this type of longitudinal research. Because of potential bias in the subjects not followed, this study needs to be replicated to validate the results. It provides preliminary evidence, however, for the role of the mind in influencing immune function and cancer outcome.

---

tion and reduce cytokine release, zinc is an important enzyme cofactor in DNA synthesis and cell repair, and selenium and vitamin E inhibit tumorigenesis and retard tumor growth in animals (Dubey & Yunis, 1991). Other vitamins, including A, B_6, B_{12}, folic acid, and C, also contribute to either cellular or humoral immunity or both.

SUMMARY

Multiple factors influence immune regulation. Immune enhancement is critical to survival and resistance to disease. Immune suppression and tolerance provide the feedback necessary to maintain regulation of immune activation. Much of the immune cellular cooperation is mediated by cytokines and an intricate balance of immune activation and suppression. Several other factors are also important in maintaining immune regulation, including response to stress, circadian rhythm, age, nutritional state, and gender.

FUTURE DIRECTIONS

Future directions in immunology include continued investigation into cellular interactions and discovery of new mediators and relationships. The desire for new methods of vaccinations (i.e., for AIDS), alternative transplant opportunities, and regulatory control of autoimmune diseases will drive the search for innovative advances. One exploration proposed for the next 5 years is determining how tumor cells can be genetically

engineered in vitro and introduced into the body to create an effective immune response against specific cancer cells (Schwartz, 1994).

The first step in developing immunoenhancing effects against tumor cells was nonspecific, such as activating macrophages with bacillus Calmette-Guerin (BCG). In the second stage, cytokines were added to boost the effects of biologic agents (LAK/IL-2). New approaches currently under investigation include active immunization with tumor vaccines and genetically modified tumor cells and immunization with monoclonal antiidiotype antibodies (Ritz, 1994). The p53 gene can inhibit tumor growth by preventing DNA damage and can encourage abnormal cell development in its mutant state. Much work is being done to determine the role of p53 and how it triggers or controls tumor growth in colorectal, lung, and breast cancer. Immunotherapy trials also are being done with conjugating antitumor antibodies to radioisotopes or toxic molecules. Toxins such as ricin or diphtheria toxin are highly potent inhibitors of protein synthesis and are clinically useful if bound in low doses to tumor-specific antibodies. In this therapy it is critical that the antibody be highly specific to avoid killing nontumor cells and that the antibody reaches the target cell before clearance by phagocytosis (Abbas et al., 1991).

Creative ways in using cytokines to stimulate immune response include administering IL-2 after bone marrow transplant (autologous and T cell-depleted allogeneic) to reduce the risk of relapse (Soiffer et al., 1992) and transfecting tumor cells with cytokine genes and transplanting the conjugate back into the individual to produce immunostimulatory cytokines at the tumor site (Abbas et al., 1991).

Other implications for cancer treatment include advances in immunotherapy and immunodiagnostics. The emergence (and availability) of highly specific, antitumor, monoclonal antibodies greatly improves the ability to target immune responses to specific antigens. Tailor-making cancer treatments to the individual tumor is a way of taking advantage of the body's complex immune interactions to target a specific immune response.

REFERENCES

Abbas, A. K., Lichtman, A. H., & Pober, J. S. (1991). *Cellular and molecular immunology.* Philadelphia: W.B. Saunders Co.

Ader, R., Felten, D. L., & Cohen, N. (1991). *Psychoneuroimmunology* (2nd ed.). San Diego: Academic Press.

Albertini, M. R., Gibson, D. F. C., Robinson, S. P. Howard, S. P., Tans, K. J., Lindstrom, M. J., Robinson, R. R., Tormey, D. C., Jordan, V. C., & Sondel, P. M. (1992). Influence of estradiol and tamoxifen on susceptibility of human breast cancer cell lines to lysis by lymphokine-activated killer cells. *Journal of Immunology, 11,* 30–39.

Antoni, M. H., & Goodkin, K. (1988). Life stress and moderator variables in the promotion of cervical neoplasia: I: Personality facets. *Journal of Psychosocial Research, 32,* 327–338.

Aversa, G., Punnonen, J., Cocks, B. G., de Waal Malefyt, R., Vega, F., Zurawski, S. M., Zurawski, G., & de Vries, J. E. (1993). An interleukin 4 (IL-4) mutant protein inhibits both IL-4 or IL-13-induced human immunoglobulin G4 (IgG4) and IgE synthesis and B cell proliferation: Support for a common component shared by IL-4 and IL-13 receptors. *Journal of Experimental Medicine, 178,* 2213–2218.

Barrett, J. T. (1988). *Textbook of immunology* (5th ed.). St. Louis: C. V. Mosby.

Belza, B. L., Henke, C. J., Yelin, E. H., Epstein, W. V., & Gilliss, C. L. (1993). Correlates of fatigue in older adults with rheumatoid arthritis. *Nursing Research, 42,* 93–99.

Bender, C. M. (1994). Cognitive dysfunction associated with biological response modifier therapy. *Oncology Nursing Forum, 21,* 515–523.

Benjamini, E., & Leskowitz, S. (1988). *Immunology: A short course.* New York: Alan R. Liss, Inc.

Blalock, J. E., Harbour-McMenamin, P., & Smith, E. M. (1985). Peptide hormones shared by the neuroendocrine and immunologic systems. *Journal of Immunology, 135,* 858–861.

Broide, D. H. (1991). Inflammatory cells: Structure and function. In D. P. Stites & A. I. Terr (Eds.), *Basic and Clinical immunology* (pp. 141–153). Norwalk, CT: Appleton & Lange.

Cerami, A. (1992). Inflammatory cytokines. *Clinical Immunology and Immunopathy, 62*(1), S3–S10.

Coleman, R. M., Lombard, M. F., Sicard, R. E. (1992). *Fundamental immunology* (2nd ed.). Dubuque, IA: Wm C Brown Publ.

Dinges, D. F., Douglas, S. D., Zaugg, L., Campbell, D. E., McMann, J. M., Whitehouse, W. G., Orne, E. C., Kapoor, S. C., Icaza, E., & Orne, M. T. (1994). Leukocytosis and natural killer cell function parallel neurobehavioral fatigue induced by 64 hours of sleep deprivation. *Journal of Clinical Investigation, 93,* 1930–1939.

Dubey, D. P., & Yunis, E. J. (1991). Aging and nutritional effects on immune functions in humans. In D. P. Stites & A. I. Terr (Eds.), *Basic and clinical immunology* (pp. 190–196). Norwalk, CT: Appleton & Lange.

Dyck, D. G., & Greenberg, A. H. (1991). Immunopharmacological tolerance as a conditioned response: Dissecting the brain immune pathways. In R. Ader, D. Felten, & N. Cohen (Eds.), *Psychoneuroimmunology* (pp. 663–684). San Diego: Academic Press.

Esterling, B. A., Kiecolt-Glaser, J. K. I., Bodner, J. C., & Glaser, R. (1993). Stress-associated modulation of natural killer cell cytotoxicity *in vitro* by interferon-gamma and interleukin-2 in elderly care givers of Alzheimer's disease patients. *Research Perspectives in Psychoneuroimmunology IV.* Abstract. Boulder, CO. April.

Fawzy, F. L., Kemeny, M. E., Fawzy, N. W., Elasnoff, R., Morton, D., Cousins, N., & Fahey, J. L. (1990). A structured psychiatric intervention for cancer patients: Part II; Changes over time in immunologic measures. *Archives of General Psychiatry, 47,* 729–735.

Frank, M. M. (1991). Complement & kinin. In D. P. Stites & A. I. Terr (Eds.), *Basic and clinical immunology* (pp. 161–174). Norwalk, CT: Appleton & Lange.

Gray, T. S. (1991). Amygdala: Role in autonomic and neuroendocrine responses to stress. In J. A. McCubbin, P. G. Kaufmann, & C. B. Nemeroff, (Eds.), *Stress, neuropeptides and systemic disease* (pp. 37–55). San Diego: Academic Press.

Grossman, C. J. (1991). Immunoendocrinology. In F. S. Greenspan (Ed.), *Basic and clinical endocrinology* (pp. 40–52). Norwalk, CT: Appleton & Lange.

Heijnen, C. J., Kavelaars, A., & Ballieux, R. E. (1991). Proopiomelanocortin-derived peptides in the modulation of immune function. In R. Ader, D. Felten, & N. Cohen (Eds.), *Psychoneuroimmunology* (pp. 429–446). San Diego: Academic Press.

Henney, C. S., & Gillis, S. (1984). Cell-mediated cytotoxicity. In W. E. Paul (Ed.), *Fundamental immunology* (pp. 669–684). New York: Raven Press.

Herlyn, M., Menrad, A., Koprowski, H. (1990). Structure, function, and clinical significance of human tumor antigens. *Journal of the National Cancer Institute, 82,* 1883–1889.

Hood, L. E., Weissman, I. L., Wood, W. B., & Wilson, J. H. (1984). *Immunology* (2nd ed.). Menlo Park, CA: Benjamin/Cummings Publ. Co.

Irwin, M., Vale, W., & Britton, K. (1987). Central corticotropin releasing factor suppresses natural killer cytotoxicity. *Brain, Behavior, and Immunity, 1,* 81–87.

Jemmott, J. B., & Locke, S. E. (1984). Psychosocial factors, immunologic mediation, and human susceptibility to infectious diseases: How much do we know? *Psychological Bulletin, 95,* 78–108.

Justice, A. (1985). Review of the effects of stress on cancer in laboratory animals: Importance of time of stress application and type of tumor. *Psychological Bulletin, 1,* 108–138.

Kamani, N. R., & Douglas, S. D. (1991). Structure and development of the immune system. In D. P. Stites & A. I. Terr (Eds.), *Basic and clinical immunology* (pp. 9–33). Norwalk, CT: Appleton & Lange.

Kiecolt-Glaser, J. K., & Glaser, R. (1991). Psychosocial factors, stress, disease, and immunity. In R. Ader, D. L. Felton, & N. Cohen (Eds.), *Psychoneuroimmunology* (2nd ed.), (pp. 847–868). San Diego: Academic Press.

Kimball, J. W. (1990). *Introduction to immunology* (3rd ed.). New York: Macmillan

Levy, S. M., & Wise, B. D. (1988). Psychosocial risk factors and cancer progression. In C. L. Cooper (Ed.), *Stress and breast cancer,* (pp. 348–353). Chinchester: Wiley & Sons.

Monjan, A. A. (1981). Stress and immunologic competence: Studies in animals. In R. Ader, (Ed.), *Psychoneuroimmunology* (pp. 185–228). New York: Academic Press.

North, R. J. (1985). Down-regulation of the antitumor immune response. *Advances in Cancer Research, 45,* 1–43.

Owen, D. (1992). *Emotional distress, coping behavior, and immunity in women undergoing breast biopsy.* Dissertation. Case Western Reserve University, Cleveland, OH.

Paciotti, G. F., & Tamarkin, L. (1988a). Interleukin-1 directly regulates hormone dependent breast cancer cell proliferation *in vitro. Molecular Endocrinology, 2,* 459–464.

Paciotti, G. F., & Tamarkin, L. (1988b). Interleukin-2 differentially affects the proliferation of a hormone-dependent and a hormone-independent human breast cancer cell line *in vitro* and *in vivo. Anticancer Research, 8,* 1233–1240.

Persky, V. W., Kempthorne-Rawson, J., & Shekelle, R. B. (1987). Personality and risk of cancer: 20 year follow-up of the Western Electric Study. *Psychosomatic Medicine, 49,* 435–449.

Post-White, J. (1991). *The effects of mental imagery on emotions, immune function, and cancer outcome.* University of Minnesota (University Microfilms No. 9205462).

Ritz, J. (1994). Tumor immunity: Will new keys unlock the door? *Journal of Clinical Oncology, 12,* 237–238.

Robinson, E., Rubin, D., Mekori, T., Segal, R., Pollack, S. (1993). In vivo modulation of natural killer cell activity by tamoxifen in patients with bilateral primary breast cancer. *Cancer Immunology Immunotherapy, 37,* 209–212.

Roitt, I., Brostoff, J., & Male, D. (1993). *Immunology* (3rd ed.). St. Louis, MO: Mosby

Rosenberg, S. A., Packard. B. S., Aebersold, P. M., Solomon, D., Topalian, S. L., Tay, S. T., Simon, P., Lotze, M. T., Yang, J. C., Seipp, C. A., Simpson, C., Carter, C., Bock, S., Schwartzentruber, D., Wei, J. P., & White, D. E. (1988). Use of tumor-infiltrating lymphocytes and interleukin-2 in the immunotherapy of patients with metastatic melanoma. *The New England Journal of Medicine, 319,* 1676–1680.

Saphier, D., & Roerig, S. C. (1993). Central nervous system effects of alpha-interferon. *Research Perspectives of Psychoneuroimmunology IV.* Abstract. Boulder, CO, April.

Schmale, A. H., & Iker, H. P. (1966). The effect of hopelessness and the development of cancer. *Journal of Psychosomatic Medicine, 28,* 714–721.

Schwartz, R. H. (1994). Immunology. *Journal of NIH Research, 6,* 68–69.

Sjogren, H. O. (1985). Tumour immunology. In L. A. Hanson & H. Wigzell (Eds.), *Immunology* (pp. 120–126). London: Butterworths.

Soiffer, R. J., Murray, C., Cochran, K., Cameron, C., Wang, E., Schow, P. W., Daley, J. F., & Ritz, J. (1992). Clinical and immunologic effects of prolonged infusion of low-dose recombinant interleukin-2 after autologous and T-cell-depleted allogeneic bone marrow transplantation. *Blood, 79,* 517–526.

Stites, D. P., Terr, A. I., & Parslow, T. G. (1994). *Basic and clinical immunology* (8th ed.). Norwalk, CT: Appleton & Lange.

Tax, A. W., Orsi, A. J., Lafferty, M. A., Barsevick, A., Luborsky, L., Prystowsky, M., Nahass, D. M., Lowery, B., & McCorkle, R. (1994). A descriptive study of immune status in patients undergoing colorectal surgery. *Oncology Nursing Forum, 21,* 1539–1544.

Unanue, E. R., & Benacerraf, B. (1984). *Textbook of immunology* (2nd ed.). Baltimore, MD: Williams & Wilkins.

Webster, E. L., Tracey, D. E., & De Souza, E. B. (1991). Upregulation of interleukin-1 receptors in mouse AtT-20 pituitary tumor cells following treatment with corticotropin-releasing factor. *Endocrinology, 129,* 2796–2798.

Whicher, J. T., & Evans, S. W. (1990). Cytokines in disease. *Clinical Chemistry, 36,* 1269–1281.

Yirmiya, R., Shavit, Y., Ben-Eliyahu, S., Gale, R. P., Liebeskine, J. E., Taylor, A. N., & Weiner, H. (1991). Modulation of immunity and neoplasia by neuropeptides released by stressors. In J. A. McCubbin, P. G. Kaufman, & C. B. Nemeroff (Eds.), *Stress, neuropeptides, and systemic disease* (pp. 262–280). San Diego: Acedemic Press.

15

The Biology of Invasion and Metastases

Mathew Jay Soltis • *Susan Molloy Hubbard* • *Elise C. Kohn*

How tumor cells form metastases is one of the most important questions in cancer biology. Despite numerous advances in the existing therapeutic approaches of surgery, radiation, and chemotherapy, alone or in combination, approximately 550,000 Americans will die of cancer in 1995, and there will be an estimated 1,252,000 newly diagnosed cases in 1995, making cancer the second leading cause of death in the United States (American Cancer Society, 1995). The vast majority of cancer patients are not cured by modern therapy and will die from the direct effects of their cancers or, less commonly, from complications associated with treatment (Fidler, 1990). A metastasis is a focus of malignant tumor at a site other than the primary tumor. Greater than 30 per cent of patients bearing common epithelial and mesenchymal malignancies harbor overt metastatic dissemination at the time of diagnosis. An additional 30 per cent to 40 per cent have occult metastases that are apparent only later in the course of disease. Although it is generally appreciated that certain tumors have unique patterns of dissemination, it is not yet possible to predict the metastatic potential of an individual tumor (Plesnicar, 1989; Sugarbaker, 1981). Even tumors of identical size and histologic type can have markedly different metastatic properties. Autopsy studies have demonstrated that disseminated metastatic disease is prevalent in most patients at the time of cancer-related death. To a large extent, an inability to alter the cancer-related mortality rates may be attributed to the fact that only a small percentage of newly diagnosed patients can potentially be cured by local therapeutic modalities (Sugarbaker, 1981). This fact argues for more attention to prevention and early cancer detection and also for the development of therapeutic strategies to combat the formation and progression of tumor invasion and metastasis. Thus, a familiarity with the biologic processes and pathways of cancer metastasis is crucial in defining prognosis and uncovering new therapeutic possibilities for cancer patients.

All neoplasms are characterized by some independence of the host tissue requirements for space and nutrients. The cells of most benign tumors remain encased within a defined area. Thus, tissues are generally damaged only when the mass grows large enough to encroach on vital organ function. Malignant tumors are characterized by the ability to invade; this may be manifest even when the primary tumor is only microscopic. Metastases have the potential themselves to metastasize. Detectable metastatic disease is often accompanied by a large number of micrometastases disseminated from the primary and metastatic sites. It is this ability to invade and metastasize that forms the principal functional characteristic that distinguishes malignant neoplasms from benign tumors.

Recent advances in molecular and cell biology have led to the identification of cellular properties and genetic factors that influence tumor cell invasion, dissemination, and metastasis formation in experimental systems. Experimental data on how these mechanisms operate are providing much needed information on the fundamental properties that enable cancer cells to invade and metastasize. Elucidation of both the cellular and molecular biology of the invasive and metastatic phenotype continues to be a principal and crucial focus of current cancer research. Future therapeutic strategies are now being targeted to key steps in the processes of invasion and metastasis, with the express purposes of accurate early detection, prediction of metastatic spread, and eradication of occult and overt metastatic disease.

CELLULAR PROPERTIES THAT INFLUENCE INVASION AND METASTASIS

The development of metastases is a dynamic process that occurs as a complex cascade of events involving gene expression, anatomic factors, host-microenvironment interactions, and intrinsic tumor cell properties, all working in concert (Bishop, 1987; Fidler & Balch, 1987; Frost & Fidler, 1986; Lapis, Liotta, & Rabson, 1986; Liotta, 1989; Liotta, Steeg, & Stetler-Stevenson, 1991; Schirrmacher, 1985). Although large numbers of cancer cells may be found circulating in the bloodstream of cancer patients, as many as 10^7 to 10^9 cells per day, the frequency of successful metastasis is very low (Galves, 1983; Galves, Huben, & Weiss, 1988). Experimental evidence indicates that less than 0.01 per cent of tumor cells in the bloodstream successfully become established as metastases (Fidler & Balch, 1987; Fidler, Gersten, & Riggs, 1977; Weiss & Ward, 1983). Disseminated tumor cells that cannot complete all of the steps in the metastatic cascade are eliminated by host defenses. The process of metastasis is not random; rather, it is a cascade of linked steps that must be negotiated by tumor cells if a metastasis is to develop. Selected genes appear to be important in enabling this small population of metastatic cells to perform the function of metastasis. These genes are not always linked to the proliferation rate of the primary tumor, as studies have indicated that tumor growth and metastatic behavior may be under individual control mechanisms (Minniti et al., 1992; Muschel, Williams, Lowy, & Liotta, 1985; Waterfield, 1989). The cells that successfully metastasize and establish secondary sites represent a small and select subpopulation of cells with unique genetic and biologic properties that are not shared by all cells within the primary tumor mass. Some of these important metastasis pathways, genes, and properties will be highlighted below.

INTERACTIONS WITH THE EXTRACELLULAR MATRIX

The mammalian organism is composed of a series of tissue compartments separated from each other by the two components of the extracellular matrix (ECM): interstitial stroma and basement membrane (Hay, 1982; Stracke, Murata, Aznavoorian, & Liotta, 1994). These boundaries are actively traversed by metastasizing cells in the progression of invasive tumors. The interstitial stroma is an acellular network that provides the support for blood vessels, lymphatic tissue, and nerves in a background of collagenous and fibrillar proteins. Organ parenchymal cells are attached to a basement membrane, which in turn is anchored to the interstitial stroma. The basement membrane forms a formidable barrier to all types of cell movement.

The extracellular matrix is a dense latticework composed of collagens and elastin that is embedded in a ground substance composed of glycoproteins and proteoglycan. This meshwork forms a three-dimensional supporting scaffold that isolates tissue compartments, mediates cell attachment, determines tissue architecture, and serves as a mechanical barrier to invasion. The spacing, orientation, and charge of matrix components influence the filtration of soluble macromolecules through the matrix. Regulatory signals are transmitted from matrix components through specific cell surface receptors. These receptors enable matrix components to exert chemical and mechanical influences on the shape and biochemistry of the cell and play an important role in cell morphology, mitogenesis, and cytodifferentiation (Hay, 1982; Liotta, 1987, 1989; Wicha, Liotta, Garbisa, & Kidwell, 1980).

The molecular composition of the ECM has been shown to be tissue specific. Each unique set of matrix components identifies the tissue of origin and helps create the organization and physical properties of that tissue (Stetler-Stevenson, Aznavoorian, & Liotta, 1993). Collagens are the major structural elements in the ECM. Multiple collagens have been identified, cloned, and sequenced, and each differs chemically, genetically, and immunologically. Collagens may be broken down into functional categories. The interstitial collagens (types I, II, and III) are present in fibrous and stromal structures (types I and III) and cartilage (type II) and form tightly ordered fibrils. Other types of collagen (types IV and V) are arranged in nonfibrous structures. Types IV and V collagen make the scaffolding for the basement membranes (Kuhn et al., 1985).

Basement membranes contain three major components: types IV and V collagen, laminin, and specific proteoglycans (Hay, 1982; Stracke et al., 1994; Wicha et al., 1980). These molecules bind together to form homogeneous sheets that resist simple penetration of cells. Sheets of basement membrane form the interface between the organ parenchymal cells and the interstitial connective tissue. Normal epithelial cells require a basement membrane for anchorage and growth (Hay, 1982; Kleinman, Klebe, & Martin, 1981; Stracke et al., 1994; Wicha et al., 1980). In benign neoplasms and carcinoma in situ, the tumor cells do not penetrate the epithelial basement membrane; the primary difference between these noninvasive cells and the advanced invasive state of malignant cells is in cellular regulation. A transition occurs from in situ carcinoma to invasive cancer when tumor cells penetrate the basement membrane and invade into the interstitial stroma. This action of invasion is the hallmark of tumor metastasis.

Tumor cell interaction with the extracellular matrix occurs at multiple stages in the metastatic cascade (Barsky, Siegal, Jannotta, & Liotta, 1983; Forster, Talbot, & Critshley, 1984; Liotta, 1986, 1987, 1989; Liotta, Mandler et al., 1986; Liotta, Rao, & Barsky, 1983; Liotta, Thorgeirsson, & Garbisa, 1982). During the transition from in situ to invasive carcinoma, changes in the organization and distribution of the epithelial basement membrane occur as tumor cells locally invade and penetrate the basement membrane and enter the underlying interstitial stroma. During intravasation and extravasation, tumor cells must also penetrate the vascular subendothelial basement membrane. After extravasation from the circulation, tumor cells must traverse the perivascular interstitial stroma to establish a metastatic focus in the target organ.

For example, the proliferative disorders of the breast, are characterized by disorganization of the normal epithelial stromal architecture. Benign disorders are characterized by a continuous basement membrane separating the breast epithelium from the tissue stroma (Kleinman et al., 1981). In contrast, invasive breast carcinomas consistently exhibit defective extracellular basement membranes with zones of matrix loss in the regions of the invading tumor cells (Barsky et al., 1983; Liotta, Rao, & Wewer, 1986; Siegel, Barsky, Terranova, & Liotta, 1981). This phenomenon occurs in all types of carcinomas. The extent of basement membrane loss has been correlated with an increased incidence of metastases and poor 5-year survival rates for breast cancer patients and has been used as an indicator of occult dissemination (Forster et al., 1984).

CELL SURFACE MEMBRANE DETERMINANTS

Certain intrinsic physico-chemical properties appear to be cellular determinants of metastatic potential (Fig. 15–1). Comparisons of normal cells, embryonic cells, and metastatic tumor cells in experimental models have implicated a number of cell surface factors as partial determinants of metastatic potential. Cell membrane proteins, in particular glycoproteins, may have functions as enzymes, transporters, antigens, and cell surface receptors (Hynes, 1981; Hynes & Lander, 1992; Nicolson, 1987; Stracke, Kruzsch, Unsworth, Arestad, & Cioce, 1992). The regulated distribution of cell surface proteins is an important feature of normal differentiated cells. The cytoskeleton, comprising membrane-associated microtubules and microfilaments, regulates the distribution of cell surface receptors and effector proteins within the membrane. Disruption and changes in number or type of cell surface receptors and effector proteins, as in cancer cells, may result in marked changes in cell behavior. Alterations in the cell surface, depicted in Figure 15–1, have been shown to develop during neoplastic transformation. These alterations are thought to contribute to loss of growth control, increased cell motility, altered patterns of cell recognition, modified cell adhesion, and the development of cellular and biochemical properties that enable tumor cells to overcome mechanical barriers to invasion.

Cell-cell communication is a crucial factor in growth control. When normal mammalian cells are grown in culture, they migrate away from the center of the colony in an orderly radial pattern until continuous cell contact is made; then motility and further proliferation ceases abruptly (Abercrombie, 1975). This phenomenon, known as density-dependent growth feedback, serves to regulate normal cell growth and to suppress tissue invasion. Other mechanisms that are involved in environmental regulated growth control include parameters such as adhesion molecule specificity, anchorage-dependent growth, and cell orientation, which enable normal cells to organize and remain as functional units (Fig. 15–1). Defects in these feedback mechanisms and alterations in the tumor cell-host interactions are thought to contribute to the relentless

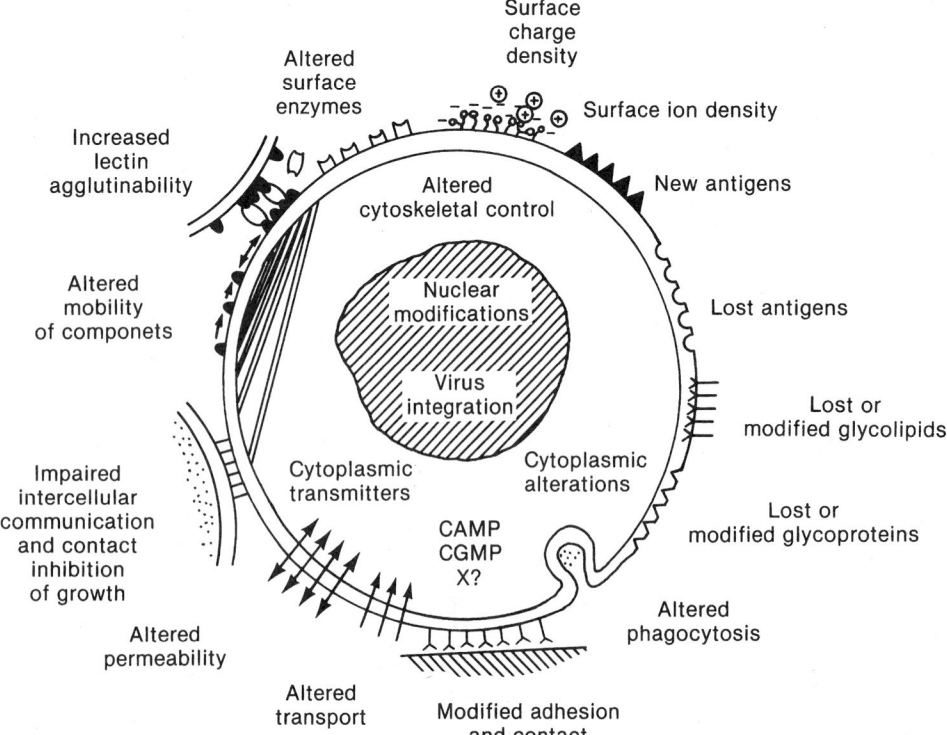

FIGURE 15–1. Alterations in cell surface properties that contribute to tumor cell invasion and metastasis. The interaction of tumor cells with their environment is mediated by cell surface constituents. A wide variety of celluar feedback mechanisms and recognition systems are medated by molecules on the cell surface. Alterations in the cell surface contribute to loss of growth control, increased cell motility, altered patterns of cell recognition, diminished cell cohesion, and development of cellular and biochemical properties that enable tumor cells to overcome mechanical barriers to invasion and metastasis.

growth and invasive behavior demonstrated by metastatic cancer cells (Table 15–1) (Plesnicar, 1989).

Although tumor growth may be promoted by alterations of the cell cycle, tumor growth may also be enhanced by autocrine stimulation. Autocrine, or self-stimulatory, growth involves the secretion of and response to endogenously produced proteins and chemical factors (Anzano, Roberts, Smith, Sporn, & De-Larco, 1983; Bishop, 1987; Todaro, Fryling, & De-Larco, 1980). The action of autocrine growth factors depends on the presence of functional receptors on the surface of the cells that can respond to the self-produced growth factors, therefore creating an autocrine loop. Autocrine growth factor expression has been directly and indirectly linked to changes in cellular genes, proto-oncogenes, that cause neoplastic growth when damaged or activated (Bishop, 1987). The autocrine growth loop has led to the postulation and more recently to proof of autocrine motility loops (Liotta, 1986; Minniti et al., 1992; Stracke et al., 1992). Autocrine stimulation may propagate and instigate the development of primary tumors, but it may also stimulate a cascade of events that result in metastatic dissemination.

THE FIVE-STEP MODEL OF INVASION AND METASTASIS

Tumor cells must overcome multiple barriers to complete the metastatic cascade (Table 15–1). Currently, focused investigation is underway to study the specific steps of the metastatic cascade. While these steps are complex in vivo, the processes of invasion can be broken down and studied in five distinct events: adhesion to endothelial cell basement membrane components, local proteolytic destruction of the basement membrane, migration through this barrier into secondary sites, proliferation, and angiogenesis or neovascularization (Fig. 15–2) (Liotta Rao, et al., 1986; Liotta et al., 1991). Each step of this cascade can be analyzed independently in the laboratory. This discussion will focus on the steps of the invasion cascade, the genes that drive the process, and novel therapeutic and diagnostic strategies targeted at tumor invasion, metastasis, and angiogenesis.

INVASION OF THE EXTRACELLULAR MATRIX

Local stromal invasion by tumor cells is a prerequisite for successful metastasis and represents the crucial step in the metastatic cascade. In its earliest stages, local invasion may appear as direct tumor extension. At some point, however, cells or clumps of cells become detached from the primary tumor and infiltrate the surrounding interstitial spaces. Among the mechanisms believed to play a role in local invasion by neoplastic cells are decreased cell-to-cell adhesion, increased cell motility, and the release of chemotactic substances and matrix-degrading enzymes by neoplastic cells and host inflammatory cells (Day, Myers, Stansly, Garattini, & Lewis, 1977; Fidler, Gersten, & Hart, 1978; Hart, 1981; Liotta, 1986; Liotta et al., 1991; Muller, Wolf, Abecassis, Millon, & Engelmann, 1993). Physical and biochemical properties that facilitate the invasion of normal stroma also enable tumor cells to penetrate lymphatic channels and blood vessels, promoting their dissemination to distant sites (Table 15–1). Once the cells are arrested in the capillary bed of a target organ, these invasive properties enable tumor cells to extravasate from the vasculature and infiltrate the perivascular stroma and the parenchyma of the target organ.

Normal cells exhibit a variety of behavioral characteristics during embryogenesis that closely resemble

TABLE 15–1. *Tumor Cell-Host Interactions During the Metastatic Cascade*

A. Tumor Event	Potential Mechanisms
Tumor initiation and promotion	Gene activation, amplification or mutation, loss of suppressor gene function, loss of chromosomes, genetic and epigenetic instability
Angiogenesis	Autocrine and paracrine angiogenic factors
Uncontrolled proliferation	Autocrine and paracrine growth factors
Evasion of host defenses	Evasion of immunologic surveillance, altered antigen profile
Resistance to drug therapies	Amplification of drug resistance genes, altered metabolism profiles

B. Metastasis Event	Potential Mechanisms
Invasion	Expression and activation of metastasis-associated genes and signaling pathways
Adhesion	Tumor cell binding to platelets, clotting factors, ECM components, and CAMs
Proteolysis	Increase in MMPs, plasminogen activators, heparinases, and cathepsins, altered balance of endogenous inhibitors: TIMP and PAI-1
Motility	Autocrine motility factors, growth factor and ECM attractants, autotaxin
Colony formation at secondary site	Growth and angiogenic factors

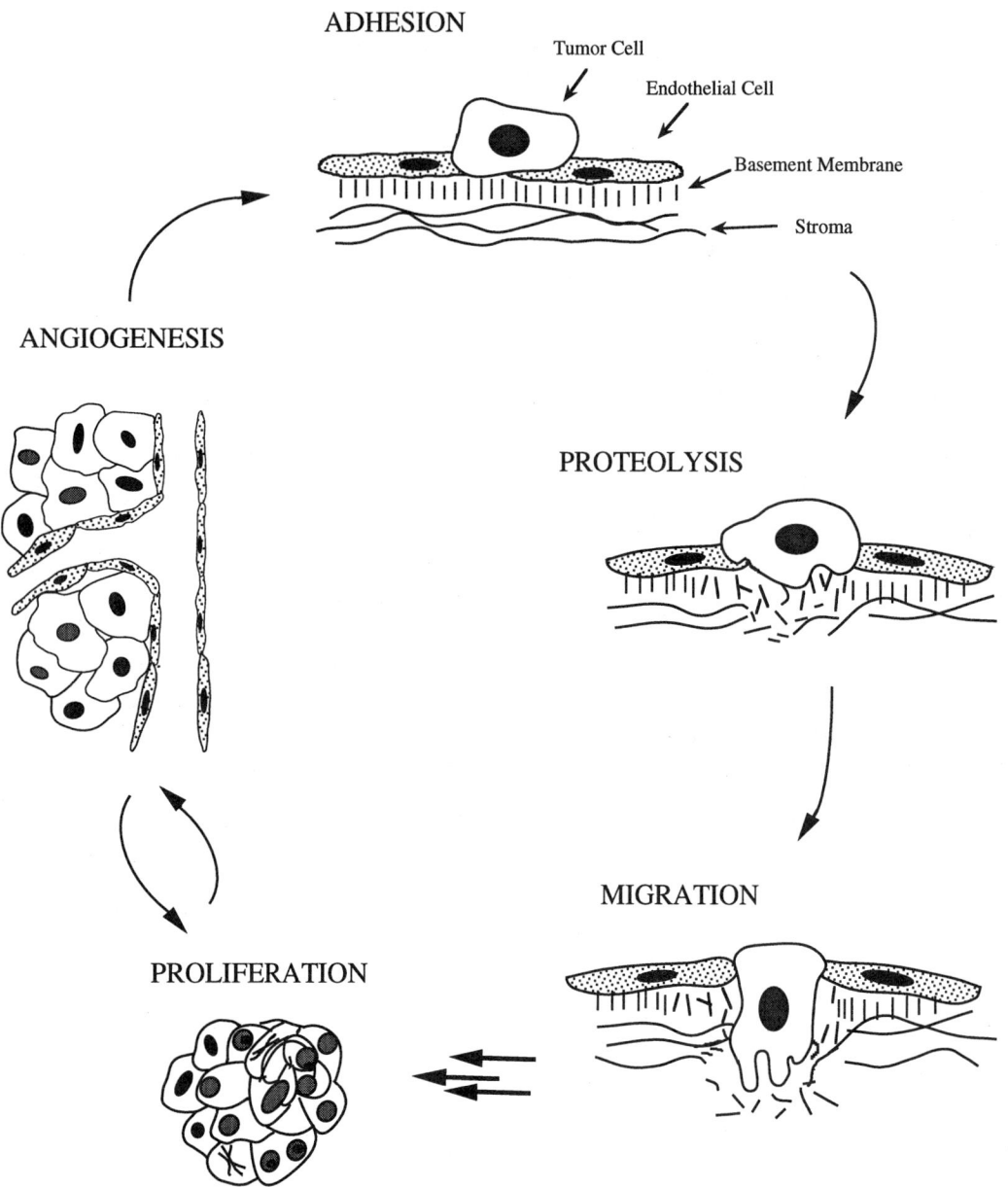

ADHESION

Tumor Cell

Endothelial Cell

Basement Membrane

Stroma

ANGIOGENESIS

PROTEOLYSIS

MIGRATION

PROLIFERATION

FIGURE 15–2. The metastatic cascade. The metastatic cascade involves the primary tumor growth, migration from primary site, adhesion to endothelial cells and the basement membrane, the retraction of endothelial cells, local proteolysis of the basement membrane and interstitial stroma, tumor cell migration into secondary sites, and proliferation at the metastatic site. It both begins and ends with the stimulation of angiogenesis.

invasion and metastasis. However, embryonic cells are regulated by genetic signals that limit these behaviors to those required for the development of organ systems and for normal functional relationships with other tissues. In the mature adult, only special cells such as leukocytes, endothelial cells, and fibroblasts remain endowed with the ability to infiltrate tissues that are normally not freely permeable to cell migration. Aberrant control of the physiologic process of regulated invasion accounts for the ability of malignant tumor cells to actively invade the stroma. These facts suggest that the capacity for invasive behavior is encoded in the genome but is not generally expressed in the mature organisms

except under special conditions. Neoplastic transformation may represent such a circumstance.

A sequence of biochemical events occurs during tumor cell invasion of the extracellular matrix (Barsky et al., 1983; Kalebic, Garbisa, Glaser, & Liotta, 1983; Liotta, 1986, 1987, 1989; Liotta et al., 1982; Terranova, Liotta, Russo, & Martin, 1982; Liotta et al., 1983; Liotta, Abe, Gehron, & Martin, 1979; Liotta, Kleinerman, Catanzara, & Rynbrandt, 1977; Liotta, Kleinerman, & Saidel, 1974; Liotta, Mandler, et al., 1986). This process occurs in several phases, depicted in Figure 15–2. The first step is tumor cell attachment via cell surface receptors that bind to specific matrix glycoproteins, laminin, fibronectin, type IV collagen, and other adhesion molecules. The anchored tumor cell then either secretes proteolytic enzymes or induces host cells to secrete enzymes that degrade the matrix in a highly localized region close to the tumor cell surface. The amount of active enzyme in the local area outbalances natural protease inhibitors present in the serum and the matrix and secreted by the tumor cell itself. In blood vessels the local release of these enzymes induces the active retraction of endothelial cells along the endothelial basement membrane and exposes basement membrane to which the tumor cell attaches itself and directs proteolytic dissolution (Fig. 15–2). Next, the tumor cell migrates through the degraded matrix into or out of the stromal vasculature. Continued invasion of the matrix occurs by cyclic repetition of these steps. Directional migration of tumor cells invading the extracellular matrix is influenced by chemotactic factors derived from the serum, and the organ parenchyma. Thus, tumor cells that disseminate hematogenously are a select subpopulation of cells that have the biochemical capability to adhere to, degrade vascular basement membranes, and pass through the degraded membrane.

ADHESION AND ATTACHMENT FACTORS

There are two types of cellular adhesion: cell-matrix adhesion and cell-cell adhesion. Cell-matrix adhesion may involve cell binding to the matrix component glycoproteins such as laminin, type IV collagen, and fibronectin. In vitro, when cells bind to tissue culture plastic, they create their own matrix by secreting these components into the media. Cell-cell adhesion involves cell binding to other cells through cell surface components. A major mechanism by which cells attach to the extracellular matrix is through receptors for matrix glycoproteins (Fig. 15–1) (Liotta, 1986, 1987, 1989; Yamada et al., 1985). These attachment factors form a bridge between the tumor cell surface and other structural components of the extracellular matrix. Many models indicate the first step in invasion is the tumor cell interaction with basement membrane (Fidler & Radinsky, 1990; Liotta et al., 1991). Multiple matrix proteins can also serve as attachment factors demonstrating cooperativity in the metastatic phenotype to enhance the metastatic potential of individual cells. Attachment factors may be synthesized by the cell that is attaching to the extracellular matrix, or the cell may have receptors for and bind to attachment factors already present in the matrix.

In vitro assays developed for evaluating biochemical events that occur during attachment have revealed that type IV collagen, fibronectin, and laminin are the matrix components that are actively involved in tumor cell adhesion. Laminin is a large, complex glycoprotein that is a major constituent of all basement membranes. It has a distinctive cruciform shape that enables it to bind to multiple matrix components and to play a key role in cell attachment to basement membrane (Barsky, Rao, Hyams, & Liotta, 1984; Charpin et al., 1986; Forster et al., 1984; Liotta, 1986, 1987, 1989; Liotta, Rao, & Wewer, 1986). Highly metastatic cells show a distinct preference for attachment to laminin (Barsky, Rao, Hyams, & Liotta, 1984; Kalebic et al., 1983; Yamada et al., 1985). Laminin has also been shown to be a chemoattractant for tumor cells and may promote cell growth (Castronovo, Taraboletti, & Sobel, 1991; Vlodavsky, Fuks, Bar-Ner, Ariav, & Schirrmacher, 1983).

The laminin receptor family is involved in cell-matrix adhesion. Laminin receptors appear to be present in higher numbers but with fewer occupied receptors in human carcinomas (Barsky, Rao, Hyams, & Liotta, 1984; Barsky et al., 1983; Charpin et al., 1986; Forster et al., 1984; Terranova, Rao, & Kalebic, 1983; Terranova, Hujanen, & Martin, 1986; Yamada et al., 1985). In animal models tumor cells selected for the ability to attach to basement membrane via laminin demonstrate a tenfold increase in hematogenous metastases (Liotta et al., 1983). Preincubation of tumor cells with laminin can increase hematogenous metastases, whereas treating the cells with the receptor-binding fragment of the 67kD laminin receptor markedly inhibits or abolishes metastases from hematogenously introduced tumor cells (Gehlsen, Sillner, & Evgvall, 1988; Liotta et al., 1983; Terranova, Williams, & Liotta, 1984).

Integrins are a diverse family of membrane glycoprotein cell surface receptors that also mediate normal and tumor cell adhesion (Hynes, 1992; Schwartz, 1993). Integrins are formed of dimers of one α and one β subunit; various noncovalent combinations of these dimers give rise to a family of receptor combinations conferring specificity and function depending on the type α and β subunits linked together (Albelda, 1993; Hynes, 1992). The cytoplasmic domain of integrins has been implicated in binding to and mediating interactions with the cytoskeleton, whereas the extracellular domains bind to collagens, laminin, fibronectin, vitronectin, and other matrix components. The binding of integrins to extracellular substrates is in many instances mediated by recognition of the target amino acid sequence RGD (arginine, glycine, aspartic acid), present in glycoproteins that integrins bind (Hynes, 1992). The integrin-mediated binding of RGD peptides in pancreatic acinar cells stimulates multiple intracellular signals, including an increase in intracellular calcium and the activation of the enzyme phospholipase C (Somogyi, Lasic, Vukicevic, & Banfic 1994). Altered expression of several integrins has been correlated with enhanced invasive ability (Albelda et al., 1990; Gehlsen, Davis, & Sriramaro, 1992; Seftor et al., 1992). Several investigators have shown increased expression of the α_V-β_3 vitronectin receptor in malignant melanoma and chemically transformed cells correlates with invasiveness (Dedhart & Saulnier, 1990; Natali, Nicotra, Cavaliere, & Bigotti, 1993; Seftor et al., 1992). This integrin has also been suggested to be involved in the process of angiogenesis (Brooks, Clark, & Cheresh, 1994). A recent study has shown that in vivo the α_5-β_1 integrin, which binds to fibronectin, functions as a metastasis suppressor gene (Giancotti & Ruoshlati, 1990). When α_5-β_1 was overexpressed in hamster ovary cells, this integrin increased the production of fibronectin, inhibited migration, and prevented tumor formation when injected subcutaneously into mice, further suggesting a functional role as a metastasis suppressor (Giancotti, & Ruoshlati, 1990).

CD44 is an example of another factor that mediates cell-matrix interaction and is involved in metastasis (East & Hart, 1993). CD44 is a transmembrane extracellular proteoglycan receptor specific for hyaluronic acid. Current data suggests that CD44 binds to collagen type IV. Studies have correlated elevated expression of CD44 with high metastatic potential and have found that increasing expression of this factor correlates with increased metastatic potential in human melanoma and in rat carcinoma cells (Birch, Mitchell, & Hart, 1991; Gunther et al., 1991). Monoclonal antibodies have been used in vivo to inhibit metastasis in several different CD44 expressing cells (Merzak, Koochekpour, & Pilkington, 1994; Seitser et al., 1993). Experimental evidence has suggested a significant reduction in expression of CD44 in cells that are metastatic. Thus, the level of CD44 expression in tumors and the measurable CD44 serum concentrations may be a functional indicator of tumor burden and metastatic disease (Guo et al., 1994; Tarin & Matsumura, 1993).

Cellular adhesion molecules, or CAMs, are also involved in tumor cell-cell adhesion, adhesion to the endothelial cells, and to the basement membrane (Takeichi, 1990, 1993). The detachment of the tumor cells from the primary, and reattachment to endothelial cells are crucial initial steps in the metastatic cascade. There are several mediators of this balance, but the cadherin class of CAMs appears to be very important in metastasis. The cadherin family contain transmembrane proteins with extracellular domains that mediate adhesion to other cells. Intracellular small molecular weight proteins, such as the α and β catenins, interact with the intracellular domains of the cadherins and transmit adhesion signals from the ECM (Rubinfield et al., 1993; Peifer, 1993). There are three subtypes of cadherins in mammals (P-placental, N-neural, and E-epithelial cadherins). All mediate cell-cell binding in an extracellular calcium ion-dependent fashion (Takeichi, 1990, 1993). Endothelial cells as well as individual metastasizing cells are known to express different levels and subtypes of CAMs (Pauli et al., 1990). When E-cadherin was overexpressed in highly metastatic epithelial tumor cells, the recipient cells had increased cadherin mediated cell-cell interactions, were less invasive, and produced fewer metastases in animal models (Uleminckx, Vackat, Mareel, Fiers, & Van Roy, 1991). These data indicate that E-cadherin functions as a metastasis-suppressor gene (Mareel, Van Roy, & DeBaetselier, 1990). Studies have shown that decreased levels of expression of E-cadherin levels correlate with invasiveness and poor survival rates for bladder and breast cancers. (Bringuier et al., 1993; Oka et al., 1993).

Cell-cell and cell-matrix interactions are a key aspect of the process of invasion and metastasis. In addition to the specificity of the molecules themselves, the loss or location of adhesion molecules and matrix fragments plays a crucial role in adhesion and also migration steps of metastasizing cells. Thus, adhesion is not only regulated by cell surface determinants on the metastasizing cell but also by the basement membrane and the surrounding cell interactions within the tumor.

PROTEOLYTIC ENZYMES

For tumor cells to successfully metastasize, they must traverse the extracellular matrix. This active process is facilitated by enzymes that can degrade the major components of the ECM, called proteinases. Cellular proteinases, when unregulated, may exert destructive effects on the extracellular matrix. These enzymes have long been known to play a key role in tumor invasion and metastasis (Roblin, 1981; Strauli, 1980; Liotta et al., 1991). Proteolytic enzymes secreted by tumor cells play an important role in the degradation of collagens type I, II, III, IV, and V, fibronectin, elastin, and matrix glycoproteins, which abound in the perivascular basement membrane and the adjacent interstitial stroma. One important class of proteolytic enzymes are the collagenases, enzymes that preferentially digest collagen. Tumor cells can either produce and secrete collagenases, secrete latent forms of these enzymes to be converted to active collagenase by lysosomal proteases such as plasmin and cell surface activators, or stimulate secretion by other cells (Sato et al., 1994). The collagenases that are most commonly associated with metastatic potential are called matrix metalloproteinases (MMPs) (Stetler-Stevenson et al., 1993).

There are several classes of collagenases, but all function similarly, as metal ion-dependent, neutral pH hydrolases (Stetler-Stevenson et al., 1993). There are several classes of matrix metalloproteinases that are catagorized based upon their preferential collagen substrates. The type IV collagenases, a 72kD form, MMP-2, or gelatinase A, and the 92kD form MMP-9, or gelatinase B, cleave the amino acid terminal portion of basement membrane collagen (Stetler-Stevenson et al., 1993). MMP-2 can also degrade types V, VII, IX, X collagens. The expression of MMP-2 has been shown to be increased in multiple tumorgenic cell lines and in human colonic adenocarcinoma, further implicating the breakdown of the ECM as a crucial step in the progression of metastasis (Brown, Levy, Margulies, Liotta, & Stetler-Stevenson, 1990; Levy et al., 1991). Interstitial collagenase (MMP-1) and the stromelysins (MMP-3 and 11) can proteolyze interstitial and stromal collagens and cleave the carboxy terminus of the collagen molecule. Type IV collagen, the structural element of the basement membrane, is resistant to the interstitial collagenases. The expression of type IV collagenase has been correlated with the metastatic phenotype in a wide variety of human cancers including colon cancer, breast cancer, lung cancer, and thyroid cancer (Levy & Cioce, 1991; Garbisa et al., 1987; Tryggvason, Hoyhtya, & Pyke, 1993; Ura et al., 1989). Expression of the MMP-9 collagenase can be induced in primary culture rat embryo fibroblast cells by transfecting them with the *H-ras* oncogene (Muschel, Williams, Lowy, & Liotta, 1985; Pozzatti et al., 1986). The stromelysin family of MMPs, composed of stromelysin 1, 2, and 3, and matrilysin, have been found to be elevated in many metastatic tumors (Basset, Bellocq, Wolf, Stoll, & Hutin, 1990; Muller et al., 1993; Pajouh et al., 1991). Stromelysins are similar to the gelatinases in enzyme structure but have different substrate preferences.

As with many steps in the metastatic cascade, regulation of MMP activity is not limited to only gene expression and proteinase production. Recent investigation has characterized two different inhibitors of metalloproteinases that act as negative regulators to balance the action of MMPs. Tissue inhibitors of metalloproteinases (TIMPs) have been cloned, sequenced, and characterized as small molecular weight proteins that bind to the MMPs and inhibit their proteolytic activity (Goldberg et al., 1989; Kleiner, Tuuttila, Tryggvasson, & Stetler-Stevenson, 1993; Stetler-Stevenson, Krutzsch, & Liotta, 1989). Although related in structure and function, TIMP-1 and TIMP-2 are encoded by separate genes and are regulated independently of one another. Both of these inhibitors have been shown to be functionally active in vitro and in vivo in multiple systems by binding to select MMPs in a one-to-one ratio and inhibiting their proteolytic function (Fig. 15–3) (Alvarez, Carmichael, & DeClerck, 1990; DeClerck et al., 1992; Testa, 1992). TIMP-2 can selectively bind and prevent activation of latent MMP-2 and can inhibit the active form of all MMPs. TIMP-1 cannot inhibit the activity of the latent MMPs and is less selective in its inhibitory function (Stetler-Stevenson et al., 1993). The biochemical properties and the strong correlation of overexpression of MMPs and underexpression of TIMPs in many metastatic tumors suggests that this balance should be investigated further as a diagnostic marker to tumor type and metastatic ability. Analysis of function and regulation of both TIMPs and MMPs will give a better understanding of the role they play in cancer and possibilities for intervention.

A number of other proteinases that are bound to or released from the cell surface appear to facilitate tumor invasion through local proteolysis. Another hydrolytic enzyme that is augmented in tumor cells and plays a role in invasive behavior is tissue plasminogen activator (Roblin, 1981; Strauli, 1980; Thorgeirsson, Turpeenniemi-Hujanen, & Liotta, 1985). Plasminogen activator converts the serum proenzyme plasminogen into the proteinase plasmin. Plasmins can hydrolyze and activate a variety of serum and cellular proteins including MMP-2. Malignant cells have been found to have increased amount of plasminogen activator (Dano, Andreason, & Grondahl-Hansen, 1985). The binding of urokinase plasminogen activator to its receptor has been shown to localize the activity of this enzyme and increase the amount of active enzyme (Pollanen, Stephens, & Vaheri, 1991). The amount and binding of urokinase to its receptor has been correlated to metastatic ability in vitro (Hollas, Blasi, & Boyd, 1991; Mohanam et al., 1993). Levels of urokinase plasminogen activator mRNA in human primary lung and breast carcinomas have been demonstrated to be elevated at least six times over those seen in controls of normal tissue (Sappino, Busso, Belin, & Vassali, 1987).

As with the TIMPs, inhibitors of plasminogen have also been described. Plasminogen activator inhibitor-1 (PAI-1) is a glycoprotein that inhibits the plasminogen activator family through covalently binding to the plasmin enzyme at the active site blocking the entrance of the substrates of plasminogen (Sumiyoshi et al., 1992). High levels of tissue PAI-1 have been found to correlate positively with increasing metastatic potential and relapse rate in primary breast cancer patients (Grondahl-Hansen et al., 1993; Foekens et al., 1994). A multivariate analysis of a large cohort of breast cancer patients has shown that PAI-1 was the strongest prognostic factor for early relapse for both node-negative and node-positive patients. The usage of PAI-1 as an indicator for prognostic purposes in breast cancer was thus proposed (Foekens et al., 1994).

FIGURE 15–3. Matrix metalloproteinase, MMP-2, is inhibited by tissue inhibitor of metalloproteinases-2, TIMP-2. The tumor cell secretes MMP-2 to facilitate proteolytic degradation of the basement membrane and interstitial stroma. MMP-2 function is inhibited by the tumor cell-secreted TIMP-2, which binds in a equimolar ratio.

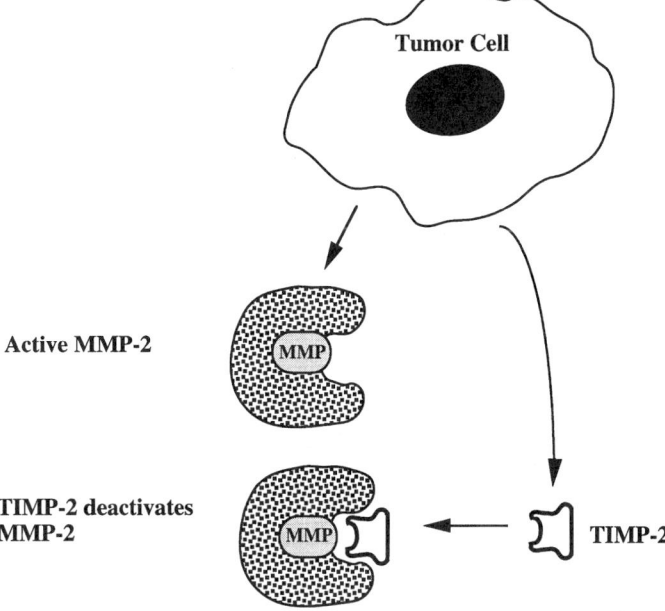

The cysteine proteases, cathepsins B, D, and L, also play a role in cancer progression and metastasis (Sloane, Rozhin, & Jonson, 1986). Cathepsins may degrade proteoglycan, another important component of the subendothelial basement membrane, and the perivascular connective tissue. The family of cathepsins are lysosomal acidic proteases that are expressed in the membranes of malignant cells and are secreted by human tumors grown in culture. High levels of cathepsin B and D in the stroma have been linked to poor survival rates and increased metastatic dissemination in breast cancer patients (Johnson, Torri, Lippman, & Dickson, 1993; Tandon, Clark, Chamness, Chirgwin, & McGuire, 1990; Weiss, Liu, Ahlering, Dubeau, & Droller, 1990). Hence, expression and activity of the different families of proteolytic enzymes may provide a useful marker for prognosis and identification of invasive cells (Table 15–2).

LOCOMOTION

Active migration of normal cells occurs during embryogenesis, wound-healing, and vascular development, but most cells differentiating under normal conditions generally lose this capacity. Pseudopodia, cytoplasmic processes formed by extention of microfilament bundles are the leading edge of cell migration. Proteins on the surface of these cytoplasmic processes have been shown to contain receptors for specific substrates such as ECM proteins. Cell motility occurs as attachments to these substrates are made and broken (Guirguis, Margulies, Taraboletti, Schiffmann, & Liotta, 1987; Raz & Geiger, 1982). Local factors in the host microenvironment may influence migratory behaviors by stimulating directional locomotion, or chemotaxis. In chemotaxis, tumor cells move preferentially along a positive attractant gradient in the direction of growth factors, such as the insulin family and the granulocyte-macrophage colony-stimulating factor (Kohn, Francis, Liotta, & Schiffmann, 1990; Stracke & Kohn, 1988), tumor-derived motility factors (Liotta, 1986; Evans, Walsh, & Kohn, 1991; Stracke et al., 1992) and ECM components, such as type IV collagen, laminin, and flbronectin (Aznaroovian & Stracke, 1990). Malignant mesothelioma cells, for example, have been shown to both migrate in the direction of a solid motility factor gradient, haptotaxis, and to chemotax to growth factors (Klominek, Robert, & Sundquist, 1993; McCarthy, Basera, Palm, Sas, & Furcht, 1985).

Although host-derived chemoattractants undoubtedly contribute to the directional tumor cell migration and perhaps organ homing, their actions do not sufficiently explain the initiation of tumor cell locomotion or the sustained migration of highly invasive tumor cells. A search for active mechanisms of tumor migration has led to the identification of a new class of proteins that are produced endogenously and profoundly

TABLE 15–2. *Clinically Important Markers of Invasion and Metastasis*

MARKER	POSSIBLE DIAGNOSTIC USE	THERAPEUTIC POTENTIAL
Matrix metalloproteinases	Activity and gene expression increased in many tumors compared with normal tissue	Drug target of synthetic inhibitor BB-94. Administration of recombinant TIMP protein. CAI inhibits MMP expression and activity
Plasminogen activator	Increased expression in invasive breast cancer	
Plasminogen activator-Inhibitor-1	Prognostic factor for early relapse in node-negative and node-positive breast cancer	
Cathepsins	Increased cathepsin B1 production with increased grade and stage of breast cancer. Cathepsin D correlated with disease-free survival, overall survival, and stage of breast cancer	
CD44	Elevated levels of CD44 correlate with high metastatic potential	
Integrins	Increased expression of multiple integrins correlates with invasiveness of breast cancers	Inhibitory peptides in preclinical development
Cadherins	Loss of E-cadherin expression correlates with high risk of metastasis	
Motility factors	AMF correlated with stage and grade in bladder cancer	Inhibition of ectokinases to alter motility
Angiogenesis	Microvessel counts and density correlate with prognosis in breast, prostate, and ovary cancer	Use of AGM-1470, CAI, and thalidomide as angiogenesis inhibitors
Growth factor receptor	Increased levels correlate with prognosis and tumor stage	Use of tyrphostins as therapeutic modulator of growth factor receptor kinases
NM-23	Levels inversely correlated with metastatic potential and survival, in node-negative breast carcinoma	

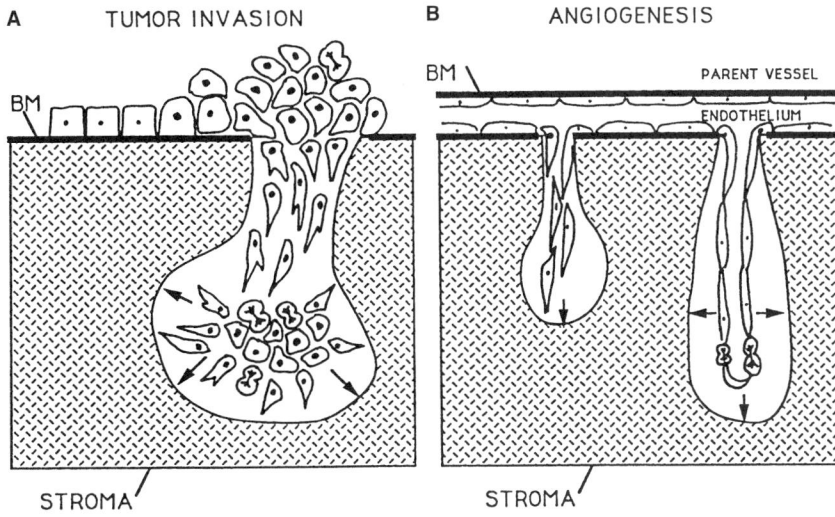

FIGURE 15–4. The functional similarity of tumor invasion and angiogenesis. **A,** Transition from in situ to invasive carcinoma is tumor invasion into the basement membrane (BM) and migration into the interstitial stroma. Proliferation of tumor expands the secondary colony. **B,** Angiogenesis involves dissolution of the parent vessel basement membrane and endothelial migration into the stroma towards the angiogenic stimulus. Proteolysis of the stroma permits expansion of the sprout diameter and lumen formation. Proliferation of endothelial cells is required for elongation of the vascular tree.

stimulate the intrinsic motility of tumor cells (Liotta, Mandler, et al., 1986; Stracke et al., 1992; Evans, Walsh, & Kohn, 1991). These autocrine motility factors stimulate both random and directional tumor cell motility. They may also exert a paracrine recruiting effect on adjacent tumor cells (Nicolson, 1993) (Table 15–1). Autocrine motility factor (AMF) was the first tumor cell-derived factor to be discovered. Breast cancer cells were shown to extend pseudopodia towards a gradient of AMF and migrate in response to AMF attraction (Guirguis et al., 1987; Liotta & Schiffmann, 1988). Besides setting the cell in motion, pseudopodia contain receptors that act as the cell's eyes, guiding it to its destination. One of these receptors recognizes and binds to laminin in the basement membrane. AMF-induced pseudopodia in human breast cancer cells were shown to have a twenty-fold increase in laminin receptor numbers on their plasma membrane, suggesting receptor recruitment (Guirguis et al., 1987). This increase in laminin receptors facilitates attachment of tumor cells to the basement membrane. Autotaxin, a human melanoma cell-derived AMF, was recently purified, cloned, and sequenced (Stracke et al., 1992). Autotaxin is a novel protein that functions as an ectokinase/pyrophosphatase, representing a new category of metastasis-associated enzymes. Further investigation into autotaxin and other motility factors will aide the understanding of tumor locomotion and motility.

ANGIOGENESIS

Tumor growth is limited by the ability of nutrients and waste products to diffuse into and out of the tumor mass efficiently. Metastasis may also be limited by the availability of conduits for dissemination. Experiments have demonstrated that tumor implants cannot grow more than a few millimeters in overall diameter without the development of new blood vessels for the delivery of gases and nutrients (Fig. 15–4) (Folkman, 1994; Folkman & Shing, 1992, Folkman, Watson, Ingber, & Hanahan, 1989). Before neovascularization, tumors have no vascular access to shed cells. Avascular tumors

have a much lower probability of metastasizing than tumors in which neovascularization has occurred. In experimental systems, malignant cells are found in the effluent of implanted tumors only after tumor vascularization has taken place (Liotta et al., 1974). As the tumor becomes vascularized, the number of cells released into the circulation increases. In fact, in experimental systems, the rate of tumor cell release into the vasculature can be related mathematically to the number of pulmonary metastases that develop (Liotta, Saidel, & Kleinerman, 1976).

The rate of hematogenous spread has also been correlated with tumor vascularity in clinical situations. Small cell carcinoma of the lung and undifferentiated carcinoma of the thyroid gland, which all arise in highly vascular beds, frequently develop early metastatic dissemination and lead to widespread blood-borne metastases to highly vascular organs such as the bone marrow, lung, and brain (Table 15–3). However, it may be possible for small populations of tumor to remain in an avascular phase for prolonged periods as dormant

TABLE 15–3. *Clinically Observed Patterns of Metastasis*

PRIMARY TUMOR TYPE	FREQUENT SECONDARY SITES
Breast	Lymph nodes, lung, liver, bone, brain, contralateral breast
Lung cancer	Liver, bone, brain, lung, bone marrow, lymph nodes
Gastrointestinal carcinomas	Lymph nodes, liver, lung
Ovary cancer	Lymph nodes, serosal surfaces, liver, lung
Prostate cancer	Bone, lymph nodes, lung, liver
Melanoma	Brain, liver, bone, lymph nodes, lung
Soft-tissue sarcoma	Lung, liver, lymph nodes
Head and neck	Lymph nodes, lung

metastases (Folkman & Shing, 1992). Immunologic defenses that keep tumor growth in check, dependence on exogenous hormones or autocrine growth factors may also play important roles in tumor dormancy (Schirrmacher, 1985).

Tumor cells have been found to secrete multiple angiogenic substances that cause the host to make new blood vessels (Folkman, 1981, 1994; Furcht, 1986). Several angiogenic factors have been recently characterized and studied extensively with endothelial cell models in vivo and in vitro. A valuable in vivo model of angiogenesis is stimulation of vessel formation into the normally avascular rabbit cornea. Tumor implants or angiogenesis factors placed on the cornea induce the ingrowth of blood vessels from the cornea towards the implant (Folkman & Tyler, 1992). Newly formed tumor-associated blood vessels are often defective with pores and interrupted basement membranes, which may facilitate tumor cell dissemination. Insulin-like growth factor-1 and basic-fibroblast growth factors (bFGF) have been shown to be the most potent stimulators of angiogenesis (Grant et al., 1993; Moscatelli, 1986). These cytokines can be produced either by the endothelial cells themselves or by surrounding tumor cells, stimulating endothelial cells to respond to angiogenic factors in a paracrine signaling fashion (Folkman & Shing, 1992; Hori et al., 1991). A recent study has demonstrated that angiogenesis can be inhibited in vitro by TIMP-1, further demonstrating the relationship between angiogenesis and metastasis (Johnson et al., 1994). Because of the importance of angiogenesis in the metastatic process, therapeutic intervention at this point may prevent further metastatic growth and slow disease progression.

Until recently, physiologic blood concentrations of the cytokine bFGF could not be assayed. An ELISA detection scheme has been developed to assay the amount of bFGF in urine, which enables the accurate prediction of tumor angiogenic state (Nguyen et al., 1994; Soutter, Nguyen, Watanabe, & Folkman, 1993). Increased levels of bFGF were found in the urine of patients with breast, lung, prostrate, and other tumors (Nanus et al., 1993; Nguyen et al., 1994). The receptor for this important cytokine also has been found to be overexpressed in human pancreatic cancers (Yamanaka et al., 1993). Another newly developed diagnostic tool is microvessel density count as an indicator of tumor angiogenesis. In this procedure biopsy slides are studied by staining for endothelial cells with antibodies to target vessel factors, for example, factor VIII, or von Willebrand's factor, and then the microvessels are quantitated (Vartanian & Weidner, 1994). A positive correlation has been found with increasing microvessel density and p53 expression, tumor size, lymphatic vessel invasion, and intratumoral endothelial cell proliferation in node-negative breast cancer (Gasparini et al., 1994; Weidner et al., 1992). In addition, increased microvessel numbers have been shown to correlate with poor prognosis in prostate cancers and ovarian cancers (Gasparini et al., 1994; Weidner et al., 1992; Weidner, Carroll, Blumenfeld, & Folkman, 1993). This correlation may enable the usage of microvessel counts as an indicator of patients at high risk for cancer. These diagnos-

tic techniques, focused on the angiogenesis step in the metastatic cascade, will aide in detection and prognosis of cancer.

PATTERNS AND ASSOCIATED RISK FACTORS FOR DISSEMINATION

Three basic patterns of metastatic spread exist: direct extension, lymphatic dissemination, and hematogenous spread. However, these mechanisms are not mutually exclusive within a single tumor or metastasis. The body contains numerous microscopic anatomic connections that permit free passage of tumor cells, facilitating metastatic spread by more than one route. In fact, tumor cell dissemination via one mechanism often facilitates metastasis through others.

Anatomic routes of direct tumor extension involve infiltration of interstitial spaces, coelomic and epithelial cavities, and cerebrospinal spaces. Until the 1970s, tumor invasion and metastasis was thought to be a passive outcome, produced by enlarging tumors that compressed and destroyed host tissues and created pressure gradients that favored tumor cell invasion. However, simple growth pressure does not account for the differences in invasive behavior between rapidly growing benign and malignant tumors. Breast fibroadenomas and uterine leiomyomas often generate significant growth pressure but never invade or metastasize. Mechanical pressure alone cannot explain how the tumor cells traverse organ parenchyma and connective tissue as well as other mechanical barriers, nor the discontinuous invasion of tumor cells frequently identified on serial histologic sectioning. Furthermore, experimental data from in vitro invasion assays have clearly demonstrated that pressure alone is not sufficient for invasion (Gabbert, 1985; Mareel, 1983). Mechanical forces appear to assist invasion rather than serve as the primary mechanism. In addition, response to cytokines, growth and motility factors, and the local environment signal the tumor cells to voluntarily proceed forward, either directly or through vascular conduits (Table 15–1).

Involvement of the regional lymph nodes draining a cancer may be one of the first clinical signs of metastasis other than disruption of the basement membrane. Most sites of nodal metastases are easily explained by anatomic and mechanical considerations. However, the mechanisms that enhance and control lymphatic spread are still poorly understood. Tumors generally lack a well-formed lymphatic network. Communication between tumor cells and lymphatic channels generally occurs only at the tumor periphery and not within the tumor mass. Tumor cells entering the lymphatic drainage are carried to regional lymph nodes, where they lodge in the large lymphatics of the subcapsular sinus. Initially, regional lymph nodes may exert a barrier effect, impeding the dissemination of tumor cells into the lymphatic system. Experimental data reveal that within 10 to 60 minutes after tumor cells arrest in a lymph node, a significant fraction of the tumor cells detach and enter the efferent lymphatics (Fisher & Fisher, 1966). These tumor cells eventually end up in the regional or systemic venous drainage owing to the existence of numerous lymphatic-hematogenous communications. As a result, regional lymph nodes do not function as true mechanical barriers to tumor dissemination, and it is likely that lymphatic and hematogenous dissemination ultimately occurs in parallel. Nonspecific host defenses, such as macrophages and natural killer cells, may then play a role in the elimination of circulating tumor cells and in the destruction of micrometastases. At some point in the metastatic cascade, lymph nodes lose their ability to filter and destroy tumor cells. Numerous physiologic and immunologic factors have been implicated, but the basic mechanisms responsible for this loss have still not been elucidated. Factors such as the intensity and duration of challenge by tumor cells also appear to play a role in the development of nodal involvement. Although tumor-specific antigens have been identified in animal models and more recently in melanoma patients on immunotherapy protocols at the National Cancer Institute, it remains unclear what antigens actually play roles in human tumor development and metastasis (Frost & Kerbel, 1983; Hanna & Key, 1982; Rosenberg, 1994).

There is considerable evidence that the immune system has both inhibitory and stimulatory effects on tumor growth, and these effects can be manifest simultaneously (Fidler, 1974; Fidler et al, 1977). The increased incidence and virulence of cancer in immunosuppressed patients has suggested that some tumors develop and metastasize more readily when the immune system is suppressed (Krueger, Tallent, Richie, & Johnson, 1985). Data from animal studies suggest that an activated immune system can significantly enhance the development of metastases by selecting out weakly antigenic cell lines, leading to the proliferation of tumor cells that the host's immune system does not recognize as foreign. The relative lack of antigenicity may enable tumor cells to evade macrophages and other elements of the cell-mediated immune system in the circulation. Factors that determine whether a stimulatory or an inhibitory immune response will predominate are not known for certain but may involve the properties that are specific to a particular tumor antigen, the mode of presentation, and the initial site of interaction with host immune cells.

Hematogenous dissemination is a complex process that requires tumor cells to penetrate into and then leave blood vessels disseminating to distant organs. Data from experimental systems indicate that vascularized tumors shed malignant cells constantly as they grow, often releasing millions of cells without producing metastases (Fidler, 1970; Fidler et al., 1978; Weiss, 1983). Thus, the mere presence of tumor cells in the bloodstream does not predict metastasis. To establish a metastasis, circulating tumor cells must be able to evade host defenses, survive mechanical trauma in the bloodstream, and lodge in the venous or capillary bed of the target organ (Cady et al., 1976; Lindberg, 1972; Shah, Cendron, & Farr, 1976). Circulating tumor cells utilize a variety of means to lodge in the vessels of the target organ, where they may initiate metastatic colonies. Approximately 80 per cent of tumor cells circulate as single cells and attach directly to intact endothelial cell surfaces or to preexisting regions of exposed subendothelial basement membrane (Liotta,

1987). Emboli of circulating tumor cells or tumor cells aggregated with leukocytes, fibrin, or platelets can directly embolize in precapillary venules by mechanical impaction. The formation of a fibrin-platelet complex is thought to protect tumor cells within the emboli from host defenses and to facilitate successful attachment to the vascular epithelium. Having become arrested in a blood vessel, a tumor cell must then actively invade the vascular wall and interstitial stroma to reach the parenchyma of the target organ and must possess the ability to grow in that foreign soil (Fig. 15–5). Cancer

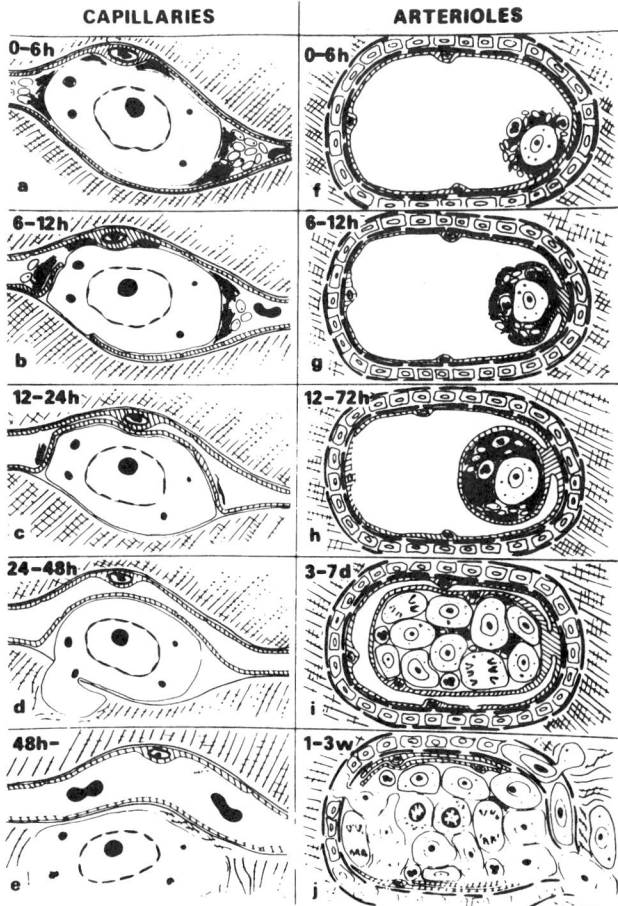

FIGURE 15–5. Extravasation of tumor cells. Steps during hematogenous extravasation of tumor cells differ, depending on whether the tumor cells arrest in capillaries or venules *(left panels)* versus arterioles *(right panels)*. In the capillaries, tumor cells, coated with platelets and fibrin, adhere loosely to the endothelial *(EN)* surface **A**, causing the endothelial cells to retract **B** and exposing the underlying basement membrane *(BM)* *(small arrow)*. Tumor cells attached to the exposed basement membrane are covered by endothelial cells **C** and separated from the blood stream. After a period of time, local dissolution of the basement membrane occurs and is followed by protusion of tumor cell pseudopodia **D–E** and ultimately by extravasation of the whole tumor cell. Arteriole arrest of tumor cells is also associated with fibrin and platelets **F**, but it does not induce endothelial retraction. Instead, the surrounding endothelium covers the tumor cell emboli and expands as the colony grows **G–I**. After 2 to 3 weeks, the tumor colony disrupts the endothelium and exposes the basement membrane **J**. Invasion of the arteriole wall follows.

cells that simply become attached to blood vessel surfaces never establish metastases in distant parenchyma, although they may shed additional tumor emboli into the circulation if they survive and grow on the endothelial surface. Growth in the target organ parenchyma requires the development of a vascular network and continued evasion of host immune and nonimmune defenses.

SIZE AND METASTATIC POTENTIAL

Dogma says that the metastatic potential of many common solid epithelial tumors is statistically related to the size of the primary tumor (Sugarbaker, 1981). Notable exceptions exist including microscopic ocular melanomas and varied carcinomas that disseminate with no detectable primary tumor. Metastases generally do not develop until a primary tumor reaches approximately 1 cm^3 in size (10^9 cells) (Weiss, 1983). Although the reasons for this are not completely clear, it is possible that more aggressive tumor cells evolve in larger tumors by accumulated genetic changes during multiple cell divisions. Larger tumors may also provide a greater antigenic burden that favors the survival of disseminated cells. In breast cancer, if the tumor is less than 1 cm in diameter, less than 25 per cent of the patients will have axillary nodal metastases; however, if the tumor is greater than 3 cm in diameter, more than 50 per cent of the patients will have axilliary lymph node metastases. Once the tumor reaches 5 cm, more than 80 per cent of the patients have auxilliary metastases. Still, up to 20 per cent to 25 per cent of patients with small node-negative primary breast tumors may die of disseminated disease (Sugarbaker, 1981). Mesenteric metastases from colorectal carcinomas also are related to tumor size. Tumors less than 3 cm in diameter have a 22 per cent incidence of regional nodal metastases. If the tumor is 5 to 7 cm in diameter, the incidence of nodal metastases rises to 53 per cent (Sugarbaker, 1981). Tumor size is also a predictive factor in melanoma as those that are less than 1.5 mm in thickness have a risk of regional lymph node metastases of approximately 7 per cent. If the primary tumor is greater than or equal to 1.5 mm, the risk for regional lymph node metastases rises to 23 per cent (Balch, Soong, & Murad, 1979). Although this size relationship appears to be a sustained and valid rule in most cases, it is important to note that there are many other critical determinants of tumor cell aggressiveness. It is the complex genetic and environmental balance, along with size, that determines outcome. Size may merely be a marker of accumulated genetic alterations and mutations.

ANATOMIC LOCATION

The distribution of metastases also varies with the anatomic location of the primary tumor (Liotta, 1989; Sugarbaker, 1981). The most frequent location of distant metastasis in many cancer cell types appears to be the first capillary bed encountered by the circulating tumor cells (Schirrmacher, 1985; Sugarbaker, 1981). Although the complete circulation eventually passes through the heart and lungs, the shunting of tumor cells through different vascular pathways predisposes certain organs to develop hematogenous metastasis in given patterns (Fig. 15–5). For example, tumor cells in the systemic venous system spread to the lungs as the first capillary bed encountered, whereas cancers disseminating via the portal venous system frequently cause liver metastases, and those arising in the lung find the first capillary bed in the systemic circulation, frequently causing brain, liver, and bone metastases. In addition, the vertebral venous system, Batson's plexus, drains venous blood from the pelvis to the base of the skull with communicaion at many different levels. This plexus plays an important role in determining metastases from the genitourinary, breast, and head and neck primary sites. A series of illustrative examples is given in Table 15–3 (Liotta, 1989; Schirrmacher, 1985; Sugarbaker, 1981).

ORGAN TROPISM FOR METASTASES

The location of metastases does not always correlate with patterns of blood flow or the locations of capillary beds. An explanation why some tumors preferentially metastasize to specific organs was first set forth by Paget in 1873. He hypothesized that metastases to a particular organ were the result of properties of the tumor cell—the seed, or the organ—the soil. Autopsy statistics and modern research models have shown that both the seed and the soil are important. Although 50 to 60 per cent of metastatic sites can be explained by the circulatory anatomy, many cannot be predicted on the basis of anatomic considerations alone. Examples of tumor organ tropism include ocular melanoma, which frequently metastasizes to the liver, and clear cell kidney carcinomas, which preferentially spread to bone and thyroid. A number of theoretic mechanisms have been developed to explain organ tropism (Liotta, 1987; Shah et al., 1976; Sugarbaker, 1981). These mechanisms include preferential growth in specific organs due to local growth and environmental factors that are present in the target organ, selective adherence to the endothelium of certain target organs, and the presence of chemotactic factors that diffuse from the target organ and cause circulating tumor cells to extravasate from the vasculature and aggregate in the target organ. Evidence exists that tumor cells contain organ-specific receptors that can discriminate between various vascular beds and cause preferential homing to certain organs. These data suggest that organ tropism may be genetically determined. Experimental evidence indicates that the metastatic potential of individual tumor cells in a primary tumor is quite variable and that different patterns of preferential metastasis exist among the cells in an individual tumor (Fidler & Balch, 1987; Fidler et al., 1978; Fidler & Hart, 1982; Nicolson, 1978; Poste, 1986).

BIOLOGIC HETEROGENEITY

Biologic heterogeneity is an important concept in tumor biology and is basic to the pathogenesis of metastasis as well as the inherent problems associated with the treatment of metastatic disease. Even tumors that arise from a single transformed cell have been shown to contain a heterogeneous population of abnormal cells by the time that they are detectable clinically (Fig. 15–6). The generation of biologic heterogeneity in tumors and tumor metastases is attributable to genetic instability that is either inherent in malignant cells or acquired during tumor growth (Fialkow, 1979; Fidler & Balch, 1987; Fidler & Hart, 1982; Fidler & Nicolson, 1976; Foulds, 1975; Frost & Fidler, 1986; Nicolson, 1987; Nowell, 1986; Poste, 1986). Genetic instability may be a result of accumulated spontaneous somatic mutations at random intervals, which produce permanent and irreversible changes in cellular DNA that are inherited by cell progeny. Phenotypic changes also contribute to biologic heterogeneity. Genotypic and phenotypic variations are clinically manifested by heterogeneity with regard to growth rates, karyotypic abnormalities, cell surface receptors, marker enzymes, a variety of cellular and biochemical properties, and responsiveness to radiotherapy and chemotherapy. Highly malignant subpopulations are thought to arise spontaneously as a result of accumulated changes. The heterogeneity of a tumor with regard to metastatic potential has been demonstrated and widely confirmed in experimental systems (Fig. 15–6).

METASTATIC SUPPRESSION AND THERAPEUTIC INTERVENTION

GENES AND METASTASIS

Cancer is a disease that results from accumulated genetic and biochemical alterations that cause normal cells to transform into tumors that in turn abandon normal constraints and become hyperproliferative, invasive, and metastatic. Gene expression and protein function are controlled by a balanced regulation in normal cells. This important balance is often upset by aberrant signaling in tumor cells, which may be due to gene overexpression, mutational loss, or other biochemical changes in the malignant phenotype. Studies have identified several key genes involved in the metastatic phenotype (Mareel, Van Roy, & DeBaetselier, 1990; Nicolson, 1984). These genes may be either metastasis suppressor genes whose loss results in increased metastatic potential, or genes that are increased in expression, altering the balance of regulatory events that control normal cells. Alterations in the production and function of metastasis-associated genes, TIMPs, MMPs, integrins, ECM components, cadherins, and others may have significant effect on downstream pathways (Table 15–2) (Sobel, 1990).

The first defined metastasis tumor suppressor gene was NM-23, located on chromosome 17q (Steeg et al., 1988). NM-23 has been correlated in vivo and in vitro with metastasis suppressor activity, but no effects on tumorgenicity have been demonstrated (Leone, Flatow et al., 1991; Leone, Mcbride et al. 1991). NM-23 expression has been shown to be significantly lower in metastatic cells compared with malignant but nonmetastatic controls (Steeg et al., 1988). Decreased expression of NM-23 was shown to correspond with decreased survival and increased metastatic potential in lymph node-negative breast cancers, suggesting that it may be useful as a molecular marker of metastasis. The NM-23 gene codes for a nucleotide diphosphate kinase. NDP-kinases are phosphate shuttles for nucleotide phosphorylation. The abnormal wing disk gene, *awd*, of *Drosophila* has almost complete sequence homology to NM23, suggesting the phylogenetic importance of this gene (Liotta & Steeg 1990; Rosengard et al., 1989). NM23 has also been shown to transcriptionally activate the expression of the *c-myc* oncogene, which itself is a DNA binding protein that acts as a promoter for transcription (Postel, Berderich, Flint, & Ferrone, 1993).

One of the well-characterized tumor-associated genes is the *Ha-ras*-oncogene, a member of the small

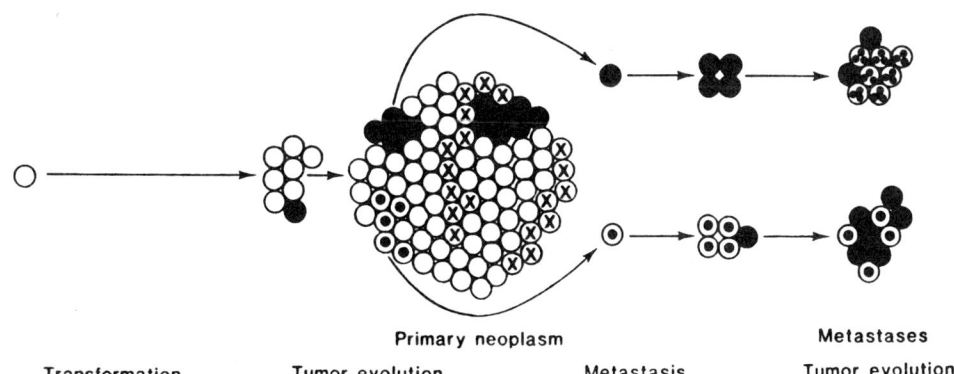

FIGURE 15–6. The origin of biologic heterogeneity in a tumor and its metastases. Many tumors are unicellular in origin but are composed of a biologically heterogeneous population of cells by the time they are detectable. The generation of cellular diversity within a tumor is attributable to genetic instability that either is inherent in malignant cells or is acquired during tumor growth. Highly malignant cell clones that are capable of metastasis are thought to arise during this process. Metastases may arise from different progenitor cells within a heterogeneous parent tumor, which leads to tumor cell heterogeneity within and among metastases.

guanine nucleotide family. The *Ha-ras* oncogene transfected NIH-3T3 cells have been shown to cause increased expression and activity of type IV collagenase, cathepsins B and L, and decreased expression and activity of TIMP-1 and TIMP-2 (as reviewed by Chambers & Tuck, 1993). The altered expression of *Ha-ras* may account for the ECM proteolytic activity in metastasizing cells. In addition to *Ha-ras,* other oncogenes have been shown to induce the metastatic phenotype, including *mos, raf,* and *src* (Egan et al., 1987; Seiki, Sato, Liotta, & Shiffman, 1991). In contrast, studies with the nuclear oncogenes *c-myc* and mutated p53 have demonstrated tumorgenicity and aberrant growth but have not shown direct effects on the classical metastasis phenotype (Egan et al., 1987). Differences among the classes of oncogenes further stresses the independence of the growth and the metastasis pathways.

The DCC (deleted in colon carcinoma) gene has been proposed as a tumor suppressor gene (Vogelstein, 1988). DCC has been shown to function as an adhesion molecule; it has an immunoglobulin domain in its structure, as found in the classical CAM molecules (Narayanan et al., 1992). DCC may play a role in the maintenance of cell adhesion, with control of cell proliferation and anchorage-independent growth (Iino et al, 1994; Narayanan et al., 1992). Clinical studies have shown that the expression of DCC is lost frequently in hepatic and lymphatic metastases, but expression patterns of DCC were not found to be changed in noninvasive carcinomas (Iino et al., 1994). Understanding the regulation and control of the genes primary in creating and maintaining the metastatic phenotype will lead to an improved knowledge and clinical targets.

METASTASIS AS A TARGET FOR THERAPEUTIC INTERVENTION

The complex cellular processes such as metabolism, protein expression, proliferation, and apoptosis are regulated by a dynamic balance between positive and negative signals. Advances in understanding transmembrane, cytoplasmic, and nuclear signaling have led to the identification of novel genes and proteins and have suggested new approaches to intervention (Tables 15–2 and 15–4). Transmembrane signal transduction is the process by which external signals are passed into the cell and processed through a series of membrane and intracellular events, resulting in a nuclear signal that drives the cellular response. Studies of the complex cascades of cell signaling have revealed that cancer is a disease where genetic alterations lead to aberrant signaling systems. Many of the genes involved in invasion and metastasis are controlled by these altered signaling systems. Several novel therapeutic strategies for prevention and treatment are currently focused on signaling pathway targets of cytokines, ECM receptors and components, transcription factors, ion fluxes, phosphorylation and dephosphorylation, and lipid metabolism, with the hopes to control tumor growth, angiogenesis, invasion, and metastasis (Cole & Kohn, 1993; Powis, 1991; Chabner, 1993).

Three classes of transmembrane signaling exist through which cells respond to cellular and environmental signals. These are phosphorylation/dephosphorylation, ion shifts through the membrane channels or transporters, and activation of guanine nucleotide-binding (G) protein signaling catalysts (Berridge, 1987; Cole & Kohn, 1993; Whitfield, 1992; Yarden & Ulrich, 1988). Both regulation of gene expression, and protein production and activity in normal cells may be mediated through the molecular switches of phosphorylation and dephosphorylation. Three amino acids are targets for phosphorylation: serine, threonine, and tyrosine. Several new drugs have been designed to focus at selected phosphorylation events. Enhanced tyrosine phosphorylation activity has been associated with proliferative state of cancer (Bishop, 1987). Tyrphostins are a series of synthetic compounds that inhibit select kinases which phosphorylate tyrosine residues (Levitzki & Gilon, 1991; Lyall et al., 1989). Substitutions in the primary structure of these compounds can confer markedly different kinase specificity. One tyrphostin

TABLE 15–4. *Invasion and Metastasis Therapeutics Under Development*

DRUG	THERAPEUTIC EFFECT	MECHANISM OF ACTION	CLINICAL STATUS
CAI	Inhibits adhesion, proteolysis, migration, and growth, antiangiogenic	Inhibits select nonvoltage-gated calcium influx and calcium mediated pathways	In clinical trial
AGM-1470	Antiangiogenic	Unknown, possible cell cycle blocker	In clinical trial
Thalidomide	Antiangiogenic	Unknown	In clinical trial
Tamoxifen	Antiproliferative, antiangiogenic	Mixed function estrogen agonist Inhibits protein kinase C	Wide use for cancer treatment In clinical cancer prevention trial
Staurosporine	Inhibits growth, invasion, and adhesion	Inhibits protein kinases C and A	PKC inhibitors in clinical trial
Bryostatin	Inhibits growth and metastasis	Modulates PKC activity	In clinical trial
Tyrphostins	Inhibits growth and metastatic phenotype	Inhibits growth factor stimulated-tyrosine phosphorylation	Preclinical development
BB-94	Inhibits proteolysis and invasion, anti-angiogenic	Inhibits MMP-2 activity	In clinical trial

has been demonstrated to slow tumor cell proliferation through the inhibition of the epidermal growth factor (EGF) receptor kinase (Yaish, Gazit, Gilon, & Levitzki, 1988). EGF cytokine signaling is important in autocrine growth stimulation and the anchorage-independent phenotype of multiple cancer cell types.

A second phosphorylation event is mediated by the protein kinase C family (PKC), enzymes that phosphorylate serine or threonine amino acid residues. The signal transduction pathways of many ligands, including growth factors, neurotransmitters, and ECM components include activation of PKC family members (Nishizuka, 1988). Several factors have implicated this family of kinases in the regulation of cancer metastasis. Diacylglycerol, a lipid second messenger produced by transmembrane signal transduction pathways, is the physiologic activator of PKC; it has been found to be elevated in many oncogene-transformed cells (O'Brian & Ward, 1989). The lipid-binding site of PKC also binds the potent tumor promoter phorbol 12-myristate 13-acetate (PMA), a phorbol ester (Kikkawa, Kishimoto, & Nishizuka, 1989; Nishizuka, 1988). Phorbol esters stimulate PKC by causing the translocation from the cytosol to the plasma membrane, where active PKC can function (Hata, Akita, Suzuki, & Ohno, 1993). Increasing activity and expression levels of PKC have been demonstrated to correlate with invasion and metastasis (Gopalakrishna & Barsky, 1988). Inhibition of PKC function by drug modulators has linked PKC activity to the metastasis properties of adhesion, surface receptor phosphorylation, and tumor growth (Dumount, Jones, & Bitonti, 1992; Isakov, Gopas, Priel, Segal, & Altman, 1991; Liu et al., 1992; Stanwell, Gescher, Bradshaw, & Pettit, 1994). PKC is thus a good target for therapeutic intervention. Several inhibitors and modulators of PKC function have been isolated and studied.

Originally isolated from *Streptomyces* spp. staurosporine is a potent PKC inhibitor that acts at the ATP-binding site of PKC. Staurosporine has been shown to inhibit the invasion and metastasis of human bladder carcinoma in vivo (Schwartz et al., 1990). Staurosporine inhibits key metastasis-related activity of adhesion and may modulate MMP-9 production (Liu et al., 1992; Ries, Kolb, & Petrides, 1994). The PKC inhibitor, bryostatin, is a macrocyclic polylactone isolated from sea mosses. This compound functions in a somewhat opposite fashion to that of staurosporine by binding to the phorbol ester-binding site of PKC and initally activating PKC before downregulating the enzyme (Berkow & Kraft, 1985). Although bryostatin binds with high affinity to the same PKC site as phorbol esters, bryostatin does not have the tumor-promoting effects of phorbol esters; rather it inhibits proliferation and prevents PKC function both in vivo and in vitro (Schuchter et al., 1993). Phase one clinical trials of bryostatin-1 are currently underway in the United Kingdom and are to begin in the United States. The nonsteroidal antiestrogen compound tamoxifen has been shown to inhibit PKC at high doses (Couldwell et al., 1993; Edashige, Sato, Akimaru, Yoshioka, & Utsumi, 1991). However, the striking efficacy of this drug

in breast cancer studies is at low doses where the activity of tamoxifen is linked to a mixed agonist and antagonist estrogenic activity. Tamoxifen has also been shown to be an inhibitor of angiogenesis and thus may also have antimetastatic activity (Davisdon & Abeloff, 1994; Parazzini, Colli, Scatigna, & Tozzi, 1993).

Synthetic inhibitors of matrix metalloproteinases have been developed to target the crucial metastasis and angiogenesis steps of matrix degradation. BB-94, a low molecular weight peptide compound that binds to MMP-9 with high affinity and to other MMPs at a lower affinity. BB-94 functions to inactivate the proteolytic site of MMP enzyme by altering the coordination of the zinc atom cofactor (Davies, Brown, East, Crimmin, & Balkwill, 1993). This binding mimics the function of the physiologic protein inhibitor TIMP. BB-94 has been effective in controlling in vitro tumor metastasis and prolonging survival of nude mice (Davies et al., 1993). Clinical trials of this compound are now underway in Europe and the United States.

Angiogenesis in the setting of malignancy is a key step in metastatic progression (Weidner, Semple, Welch, & Folkman, 1991). The process of angiogenesis may be a selective target for cancer therapy. Early work with angiostatic steroids and heparin proved unsuccessful, due to both toxicity and poor clinical efficacy. Further research identified several agents with antiangiogenic activity in vitro (Fotsis et al., 1993). One of the members of the new angiogenesis inhibitor class AGM-1470, a synthetic analog of the fungal product, fumagillin, potently inhibits the proliferation and migration of endothelial cells in vitro and in vivo (Yamaoka et al., 1993). It has also been shown to inhibit tumor cell proliferation in vivo and in vitro. Clinical trials for toxicity are currently in progress for patients with solid tumors and with HIV-related Kaposi's sarcoma. Thalidomide, a newly defined inhibitor of angiogenesis, was initially developed as a sedative for pregnant women in the 1950s. Thalidomide was removed from the market after it was found to cause the serious congenital deformity, phokomyelia. The suggested mechanism of action for the teratogenic activity of thalidomide is the inhibition of angiogenesis as limb development occurs in the first trimester, the same time during which thalidomide was taken (D'Amato, Loughnan, Flynn, & Folkman, 1994). The isoflavonoid, genistein, is a member of a dietary-derived class of antiangiogenic compounds. This compound has been isolated from the urine of people taking high soy diets and was demonstrated to be antiangiogenic (Fotsis et al., 1993). Genistein is an inhibitor of tyrosine phosphorylation (Fotsis et al., 1993), however, its inhibiton of tyrosine phosphorylation has not yet been functionally linked to its antiangiogeneic effects.

Calcium and other ions may function as signaling messengers (Cole & Kohn, 1994; Whitfield, 1992). Small changes in the balance of these ions can significantly alter the biochemical events of signaling and thus cell function. The identification and characterization of a novel inhibitor of both nonvoltage-gated calcium influx and metastasis, CAI, created a tool with which to study the role of calcium-mediated signaling events in invasion, metastasis and angiogenesis. Calcium-mediated events have been shown to be important in all components of invasion and metastasis: angiogenesis (Somogyi et al., 1994), adhesion (Kohn, Sandeen, & Liotta, 1992; Lehel, Lasic, Vukicevic, & Banfic, 1994), proteolysis (Kohn, Jacobs et al., 1994), migration (Savarese, Russell, Fatatis, & Liotta, 1992; Stossel, 1993), and proliferation (Kohn et al. 1992; Nordstrom, Nevanlinna, & Anderson, 1994). CAI is now in clinical trials and is the first signal transduction therapy agent targeted to cancer (Cole & Kohn, 1994; Spoonster & Kohn, 1994; Kohn & Liotta, 1990).

CAI, a small molecular weight hydrophobic drug, was shown to selectively alter the signal transduction pathways of calcium influx and the calcum-dependent activity of phospholipase A2 and phospholipase C-γ enzymes (Felder, Ma, Liotta, & Kohn, 1991; Felder, MacArthur, Ma, Gusovsky, & Kohn, 1993; Gusovsky, Lueders, Kohn, & Felder, 1993; Kohn et al., 1992). No inhibition of calcium-independent events such as activation of phospholipase C-β or adenylyl cyclase were observed (Felder et al., 1991; Gusovsky et al., 1993). The cellular effects of CAI include cytostatic inhibition of proliferation of a broad array of human cancer cell types in vitro in monolayer culture and in soft agar colony-forming assays (Kohn & Liotta, 1990; Kohn et al., 1992; Kohn, Felder et al., 1994). A structural-activity relationship analysis using a family of CAI analogs linked the antisignaling effects of CAI to its antiproliferative effects in a similar concentration range (Felder et al., 1991; Kohn, Felder et al., 1994). Use of these effective antisignaling concentrations of CAI resulted in inhibition of tumor cell adhesion and migration in response to extracellular matrix components, and expression and function of MMP-2 (Kohn, Jacobs et al., 1994). The dose-dependent inhibition of MMP-2 activity suggested a novel role for intracellular calcium homeostasis in the regulation of MMP-2 activity (Kohn, Jacobs et al., 1994) . CAI has been shown to be antiangiogenic in vitro and in vivo. It has been shown to inhibit the adhesion, motility, collagenolytic activity, and proliferation of human endothelial cells (Kohn, Alessandro, Spoonster, Wersto, & Liotta, 1995). The proposed mechanisms of signal transduction inhibition and the modulation of each of the distinct steps in the metastatic cascade led to animal efficacy experiments to test both antimetastatic and antiproliferative effects of CAI in human xenografts models.

The 5R *Ha-ras*-transfected rat embryo fibroblast cell line has been shown to form pulmonary metastases when injected into the tail vein of nude mice (Pozzatti et al., 1986). CAI pretreatment of 5R cells and the human colon cancer cell line HT29 resulted in marked reduction in the number and the size of pulmonary metastases when compared with vehicle treated cells (Kohn et al., 1992). Oral administration of CAI to mice was found to yield plasma concentrations of 2 to 20 uM. A2058 human melanoma cells were inoculated into the subcutaneous tissue of mice and oral CAI was administered daily beginning 3 to 7 days after inocula-

tion. Approximately 40 per cent of inoculated sites did not develop tumors in the treated group, whereas all animals in the vehicle-treated group had readily measurable tumors with exponential growth. Progression and metastatic potential of human ovarian cancer, OVCAR3, xenografts were inhibited by oral administration of CAI (Kohn et al., 1992). Animal weight, tumor masses, microscopic parenchymal metastases, and extent of ascites were decreased in the treated group of OVCAR3-bearing animals. Histologic analysis of the tumors revealed pulmonary micrometastases only in the vehicle-treated group; no pulmonary micrometastases were seen in the CAI treatment group. No evidence of normal tissue damage was seen grossly or at histologic review in the animal experiments. Preclinical studies demonstrated minimal toxicity with oral administration of CAI in multiple animal species. Presently, CAI is in phase I clinical trial, and further clinical investigation is planned. CAI is the first example where both a biochemical target, calcum-mediated signaling, and a cellular target, metastasis, were used as a screen for novel therapeutics for cancer treatment.

SUMMARY

The mechanisms thought to play a role in tumor invasion and metastases have progressed from the simple passive mechanical hypothesis of force driving invasion to the characterization of a highly complex cascade of active biochemical and genetic events mediated by a multiplicity of signal transduction pathways and molecular systems. In parallel with our widened understanding of invasion and metastasis, we have expanded our understanding of the roles of tumor heterogeneity and the molecular events that modulate metastases. Oncogenic activation of gene expression and protein production can confer unique cellular and biochemical properties on tumor cells to enable them to metastasize. Research will continue to identify cellular and biochemical properties that are uniquely augmented or lost in metastatic cells, such as matrix-degrading enzymes, cell surface receptors, metastasis-suppressor genes, and altered signal transduction pathways. This knowledge coupled with the resolution of the genes and signaling control mechanisms underlying the metastatic phenotype will identify new targets for the development of more effective diagnostic, therapeutic, and prevention tools to combat cancer.

REFERENCES

Abercrombie, M. (1975). The contact behavior of invading cells. In *Cellular membranes and tumor cell behavior*. 28th Annual Symposium on Fundamental Cancer Research (pp. 21–37). Baltimore: Williams & Wilkins.

Albelda, S. M. (1993). Role of integrins and other cell adhesion molecules in tumor progression and metastasis. *Laboratory Investigation, 68,* 4–17.

Albelda, S. M., Mette, S. A., Elder, D. E., Stewart, R. M., Damjanovich, L. et al. (1990). Integrin distribution in malignant melanoma: Association of the B-3 subunit with tumor progression. *Cancer Research, 50,* 6757–6764

Alvarez, O. A., Carmichael, D. F., & DeClerck, Y. A. (1990). Inhibition of collagenolytic activity and metastasis of tumor cells by a recombinant human tissue inhibitor of metalloproteinases. *Journal of the National Cancer Institute, 7,* 589–595.

American Cancer Society (1995). Cancer statistics, 1995. *CA: A Cancer Journal for Clinicians, 45,* 8–30.

Anzano, M. A., Roberts, A. B., Smith, J. M., Sporn, M. B., & DeLarco, J. E. (1983). Sarcoma growth factor from conditioned medium of virally transformed cells is composed of both types of transforming growth factors. *Proceedings of the National Academy of Sciences, USA, 80,* 6264–6268.

Aznavoorian, S., & Stracke, M. L. (1990). Signal transduction for chemotaxis and hapotaxis by matrix macromolecules in tumor cells. *Journal Cell Biology, 110,* 1427–1438.

Balch, C. M., Soong, S., & Murad, T. (1979). A multifactorial analysis of melanoma. II. Prognostic factors of clinical stage I disease. *Surgery, 86;* 343–347.

Barsky, S. H., Rao, C. N., Hyams, D., & Liotta, L. A. (1984). Characterization of a laminin receptor from human breast tissue. *Breast Cancer Research and Treatment, 4,* 181–188.

Barsky, S. H., Siegal, G. P., Jannotta, F., & Liotta, L. A. (1983). Loss of basement membrane components by invasive tumors but not their benign counterparts. *Laboratory Investigation, 49,* 140–148.

Basset, P., Bellocq, J. P., Wolf, C., Stoll, I., Hutin, P. (1990). A novel metalloproteinase gene specifically expressed in stromal cell of breast carcinoma. *Nature, 348,* 699–704.

Berkow, R. L., & Kraft, A. S. (1985). Bryostatin, a non-phorbol macrocylic lactone, activates intact human polymorphonuclear leukocytes and binds to the phorbol ester receptor. *Biochemistry and Biophysics ACTA, 131,* 1109–1116.

Berridge, M. (1987). Inositol trisphosphate and diacylglycerol: Two interacting second messangers. *Annual Review of Biochemistry, 56,* 159–193.

Bishop, J. M. (1987). The molecular genetics of cancer. *Science, 235,* 305–311.

Bringuier, P., Umbas, R., Schaafsma, H., Karthaus, H., Debruyne, F., & Schalken, J. (1993). Decreased E-cadherin immunoreactivity correlates with poor survival in patients with bladder tumors. *Cancer Research, 53,* 3241–3245.

Brooks, P. C., Clark, R. A. F., & Cheresh, D. A. (1994). Requirement of vascular integrin a_V-b_3 for angiogenesis. *Science, 264,* 569–571.

Brown, P., Levy, A., Margulies, I., Liotta, L., & Stetler-Stevenson, W. (1990). Independent expression and cellular processing of M_r 72,000 type IV collagenase and interstitial collagenase in human tumorigenic cell lines. *Cancer Research, 50,* 6184–6191.

Birch, M., Mitchell, S., & Hart, I. R. (1991). Isolation and characterization of human melanoma cell variants expressing high and low levels of CD44. *Cancer Research, 51,* 6660–6667.

Cady, B., Sedgwick, C., Meissner, W. A., Bookwalter, J. R., Romagosa, V., & Werber, J. (1976). Changing clinical, pathologic, therapeutic, and survival patterns in differentiated thyroid carcinoma. *Annals of Surgery, 184,* 541–546.

Castronovo, V., Taraboletti, G., & Sobel, M. E. (1991). Functional domains of the 67-kDa laminin receptor precursor. *Journal of Biological Chemistry, 266,* 20440–20446

Chabner, B. A. (1993). Biological basis for cancer treatment. *Annals of Internal Medicine, 118,* 633–637.

Chambers, A. F., & Tuck, A. B. (1993). Ras-responsive genes and tumor metastasis. *Critical Reviews in Oncogenisis, 4,* 95–114.

Charpin, C., Lissitzky, J. C., Jacquemier, J., Lavaut, M. N., Kopp, F., Pourreau-Schneider, N., Martin, P. M., & Toga, M. (1986). Immunohistochemical detection of laminin in 98 human breast carcinomas: A light and electron microscopic study. *Human Pathology, 17,* 355–365.

Cole, K., & Kohn, E. C. (1994). Calcium-mediated signal transduction: Biology, biochemistry, and therapy. *Cancer and Metastasis Reviews, 13,* 31–44.

Couldwell, W. T., Weiss, M. H., DeGiorgio, C. M., Weiner, L. P., Hinton, D. R., Ehresmann, G. R., Conti, P. S., & Apuzzo, M. L. (1993). Clinical and radiographic response in a minority of patients with recurrent malignant gliomas treated with high-dose tamoxifen. *Neurosurgery, 32,* 485–489.

D'Amato, R. J., Loughnan, M. S., Flynn E., & Folkman, J. (1994). Thalidomide is an inhibitor of angiogenesis. *Proceedings of the National Academy of Sciences, USA, 91,* 4082–4085.

Dano, K., Andreasen, P. A., & Grondahl-Hansen, J. (1985). Plasminogen activators, tissue degradation and cancer. *Advances in Cancer Research, 44,* 139–142 .

Davidson, N. E., & Abeloff, M. D. (1994). Adjuvant therapy of breast cancer. *World Journal of Surgery, 18,* 112–116.

Davies, B., Brown, P. D., East, N., Crimmin, M. J., & Balkwill, F. R. (1993). A synthetic matrix metalloproteinase inhibitor decreases tumor burden and prolongs survival of mice bearing human ovarian carcinoma xenografts. *Cancer Research, 53,* 2087–2991.

Day, S. B., Myers, W. P., Stansly, P., Garattini, S., & Lewis, M. G. (Eds.). (1977). *Cancer invasion and metastasis: Biologic mechanism and therapy.* New York: Raven Press.

DeClerk, Y. A., Perez, N., Shimada, H., Boone, T. C., Langley, K. E., & Taylor, S. M. (1992). Inhibition of invasion and metastasis in cells transfected with an inhibitor of metlloproteinases. *Cancer Research, 52,* 701–708.

Dedhart, S., & Saulnier, R. (1990). Alterations in integrin receptor expression on chemically transformed human cells: Specific enhancement of laminin and collagen receptor complexes. *Journal of Cell Biology, 110,* 481–489.

Division of Cancer Prevention and Control. (1986). In P. Greenwald, & E. Sondik (Eds.), *Cancer control objectives for the nation: 1985–2000. NCI Monographs 2,* 1–105.

Dumont, J., Jones, W., Bitonti, A. (1992). Inhibition of experimental metastasis and cell adhesion of B16F1 melanoma cells by inhibitors of protein kinase C. *Cancer Research, 52,* 1195–1200.

East, J. A., & Hart, I. R. (1993). CD44 and its role in tumor progression and metastasis. *European Journal of Cancer, 29A,* 1921–1992.

Edashige, K., Sato, E. F., Akimaru, K., Yoshioka, T., & Utsumi, K. (1991). Nonsteroidal antiestrogen suppresses protein kinase C—its inhibitory effect on interaction of substrate protein with membrane. *Cell Structure and Function, 16,* 273–281.

Egan, S. E., Wright, J. A., Jarolim, L., Yanagihara, K., Bassin, R. H., & Greenberg A. H. (1987). Transformation by oncogenes encoding protein kinases induces metastatic phenotype. *Science, 238,* 202–205.

Evans, C., Walsh, D., & Kohn, E. (1991). An autocrine motility factor secreted by the dunning R-3327 rat prostatic adenocarcinoma cell subtype AT2.1. *International Journal of Cancer, 49,* 109–113.

Felder, C. C., Ma, A. L., Liotta, L. A., & Kohn, E. C. (1991). The antiproliferative and antimetastatic compound L651582 inhibits muscarinic acetylcholine receptor-stimulated calcium influx and arachidonic acid release. *Journal of Pharmacology and Experimental Therapeutics, 257,* 967–971.

Felder, C. C., MacArthur, L., Ma, A. L., Gusovsky, F., & Kohn, E. C. (1993). Tumor-suppressor function of muscarinic acetylcholine receptors is associated with activation of receptor-operated calcium influx. *Proceedings of the National Academy of Sciences, USA, 90,* 1706–1710.

Fialkow, P. J. (1979). Clonal origin of human tumors. *Annual Review of Medicine, 30,* 135–176.

Fidler, I. J. (1970). Metastasis: Quantitative analysis of distribution and fate of tumor emboli labeled with ^{125}I-5-iodo-2'-deoxyuridine. *Journal of the National Cancer Institute, 45,* 773–782.

Fidler, I. J. (1974). Immune stimulation-inhibition of experimental cancer metastasis. *Cancer Research, 34,* 491–498.

Fidler, I. J. (1990). Critical factors in the biology of human cancer metastasis: Twenty-eight G. H. A. Clowes memorial award lecture. *Cancer Research, 50,* 6130–6138.

Fidler, I. J., & Balch, C. M. (1987). The biology of cancer metastasis and implications for therapy. *Current Problems in Surgery, 24,* 129–209.

Fidler, I. J., Gersten, D. M., & Hart, I. R. (1978). The biology of cancer invasion and metastasis. *Advances in Cancer Research, 28,* 149–160.

Fidler, I. J., Gersten, D. M., & Riggs, C. W. (1977). Quantitative analysis of tumor-host interaction and the outcome of experimental metastasis. In S. B. Day, W. P. Myers, P. Stansly, S. Garattini, & M. G. Lewis (Eds.), *Cancer invasion and metastasis: Biological mechanisms and therapy* (pp. 277–304). New York: Raven Press.

Fidler, I. J., & Hart, I. R. (1982). Biologic diversity in metastatic neoplasms: Origins and implications. *Science, 217,* 998–1003.

Fidler, I. J., & Nicolson, G. L. (1976). Organ selectivity for implantation, survival and growth of B-16 melanoma variant tumor lines. *Journal of the National Cancer Institute, 57,* 1199–1202.

Fidler, I. J., & Radinsky, R. (1990). Genetic control of cancer metastasis. *Journal of the National Cancer Institute, 82,* 166–168.

Fisher, B., & Fisher, E. R. (1966). The relationship of hematogenous and lymphatic tumor cell dissemination. *Surgery, Gynecology, & Obstetrics, 122,* 791–798.

Foekens, J. A., Schmitt, M., VanPutten, W. L. J., Peters, H., Kramer, M. D., Janicke, F., & Klijn, J. G. M. (1994). Plasminogen activator inhibitor-1 and prognosis in primary breast cancer. *Journal of Clinical Oncology, 12,* 1648–1658.

Folkman, J. (1981). Tumor angiogenesis. *Cancer Biology Reviews, 2,* 175–199.

Folkman, J. (1994). Angiogenesis and breast cancer. *Journal of Clinical Oncology, 12,* 441–443.

Folkman, J., & Shing, Y., (1992). Angiogenesis. *Journal of Biological Chemistry, 267,* 10931–10934.

Folkman, J., Watson, K., Ingber, D., & Hanahan, D. (1989). Introduction of angiogenesis during the transition from hyperplasia to neoplasia. *Nature, 399,* 58–61.

Forster, S. J., Talbot, I. C., & Critshley, D. R. (1984). Laminin and fibronectin in rectal adenocarcinoma: Relationship to tumor grade, stage and metastasis. *British Journal of Cancer, 50,* 51–61.

Fotsis, T., Pepper, M., Adlercreutz, H., Fleischmann, G., Hase, T., Montesano, R., & Schweigerer, L. (1993). Genistein, a dietary-derived inhibitor of in vitro angiogenesis. *Proceedings of the National Academy of Sciences, USA, 90,* 2690–2694.

Foulds, L. (1975). *Neoplastic development.* New York: Academic Press.

Frost, P., & Fidler, I. J. (1986). Biology of metastasis. *Cancer, 58,* 550–553.

Frost, P., & Kerbel, R. S. (1983). Immunology of metastasis. Can the immune response cope with tumor dissemination? *Cancer and Metastasis Reviews, 2,* 375–378.

Furcht, L. T. (1986). Critical factors controlling angiogenesis: Cell products, cell matrix, growth factors. *Laboratory Investigation, 55,* 505–509.

Gabbert, H. (1985). Mechanisms of tumor invasion: Evidence from in vivo observations. *Cancer and Metastasis Reviews, 4,* 283–310.

Galves, D. (1983). Correlation between circulating cancer cells and incidence of metastases. *British Journal of Cancer, 48,* 665–673.

Galves, D., Huben, R. P., & Weiss, L. (1988). Haematogenous dissemination of cells from renal adenocarcinomas. *British Journal of Cancer, 57,* 32–35.

Garbisa, S., Pozzatti, R., Muschel, R. J., Saffiotti, U., Ballin, M., Goldfarb, R. H., Khoury, G., & Liotta, L. A. (1987). Secretion of type IV collagenolytic protease and metastatic phenotype: Induction by transfection with *c-Ha-ras* but not *c-Ha-ras* plus *AD2-E1A1. Cancer Research, 47,* 1523–1528.

Gasparini, G., Weidner, N., Bevilacqua, P., Maluta, S., Dalla-Palma, P., Caffo, O., Bardareschi M., Boracchi, P., Marubini, E., & Pozza, F. (1994). Tumor microvessel density, p53 expression, tumor size, and peritumoral lymphatic microvessel invasion and relevant prognostic markers in node-negative breast carcinoma. *Journal of Clinical Oncology, 12,* 454–466.

Gehlsen, K. R., Davis, G. E., & Sriramaro, P. (1992). Integrin expression in human melanoma cells with differing invasive and metastatic properties. *Clinical and Experimental Metastasis, 10,* 110–120.

Gehlsen, K. R., Sillner, L., & Evgvall, E. (1988). The human laminin receptor is a member of the integrin family of cell adhesion receptors. *Science, 241,* 1228–1229.

Giancotti, F., & Ruoshlati, E. (1990). Elevated levels of the A_5B_1 fibronectin receptor suppress the transformed phenotype of chinese hanster ovary cells. *Cell, 60,* 849–859.

Goldberg, G. I., Marmer, B. L., Grant, G. A., Eisen, A. Z., Wilhelm, A., & He, C. (1989). Human 72-kilodalton type IV collagenase forms a complex with a tissue inhibitor of metalloproteinases designated TIMP-2. *Proceedings of the National Academy of Sciences, USA, 86,* 8207–8211.

Gopalakrishna, R., & Barsky, S. H. (1988). Tumor promoter-induced membrane-bound protein kinase C regulates hematogenous metastasis. *Proceedings of the National Academy of Sciences, USA, 85,* 612–616.

Grant, M. B., Mames, R. N., Fitzgerald, C., Ellis E. A., Aboufriekha, M., & Guy, J. (1993). Insulin-like growth factor-1 acts as an angiogenic agent in rabbicorena and reina: Comparative studies with basic fibroblasts growth factor. *Diabetologica, 36,* 282–291.

Griffiths, J. D., McKinna, J. A., Rowbotham, H. D., Tsolakidis, P., & Salsbury, A. J. (1973). Carcinoma of the colon and rectum: Circulating malignant cells and five-year survival. *Cancer, 31,* 226–230.

Grondahl-Hansen, J., Christensen, I. B., Rosenquist, C. et al. (1993). High levels of urokinase-type plasminogen activator (uPA) and its inhibitor PAI-1 in cytosolic extraces of breast carcinomas are associated with poor prognosis. *Cancer Research, 53,* 2513–2521.

Guirguis, R., Margulies, I., Taraboletti, G., Schiffmann, E., & Liotta, L. (1987). Cytokine-induced pseudopodial protrusion is coupled to tumour cell migration. *Nature, 329,* 261–263.

Gunther, U., Hofman, M., Rudy, W., Reber, S., Zoller, M., Haubmann, I., Matzu, S., & Zoller, M. (1991). A new variant of glycoprotein cd44 congers metastatic potential to rat carcinoma cells. *Cell, 65,* 13–24.

Guo, Y., Liu, G., Wang, X., Jin, D., Wu, M., Ma, J., & Sy, M. (1994). Potential use of soluble CD44 in serum as indicator of tumor burden and metastasis in patients with gastric or colon cancer. *Cancer Research, 54,* 422–426.

Gusovsky, F., Lueders, J. E., Kohn, E. C., & Felder, C. C. (1993). Muscarinic receptor-mediated tyrosine phosphorylation of phospholipase C-√. *Journal of Biological Chemistry, 268,* 7768–7772.

Hanna, M. G., & Key, M. E. (1982). Immunotherapy of metastases enhances subsequent chemotherapy. *Science, 217,* 367–369.

Hart, I. R. (1981). Mechanisms of tumor cell invasion. *Cancer Biology Review, 2,* 29–58.

Hata, A., Akita, Y., Suzuki, K., & Ohno, S. (1993). Functional divergence of protein kinase C (PKC) family members. PKC gama differs from PKC alpha and -beta II and nPKC epsilon in its competence to mediate-12-O-tetradecanoyl phorbol 13-acetate (TPA)-responsive transcriptional activation through a TPA-response element. *Journal of Biological Chemistry, 268,* 9122–9129.

Hay, E. D. (1982). *Cell biology of extracellular matrix.* New York: Plenum Press.

Hollas, W., Blasi, F., & Boyd, D. (1991). Role of the urokinase receptor in facilitating extracellular matrix invasion by cultured colon cancer. *Cancer Research, 51,* 3690–3695.

Hori, A., Sasada, R., Matsutani, E., Naito, K., Sakura, Y., Fujita, T., & Kozai, Y. (1991). Suppression of solid tumor growth by immunoneutralizing monoclonal antibody against basic fibroblast growth factor. *Cancer Research, 51,* 6180–6184.

Hynes, R. (1992). Integrins: Versatility, modulation, and signaling in cell adhesion. *Cell, 69,* 11–25.

Hynes, R. O. (1981). Relationships between fibronectin and the cytoskeleton. In G. Poste, & G. L. Nicolson (Eds.), *Cytoskeleton elements and plasma membrane organization: Cell surface reviews* (Vol. 7, pp. 97–139). Amsterdam: Elsevier-Biomedical Press.

Hynes, R., & Lander, A. (1992). Contact and adhesive specificities in the associations, migrations, and targeting of cells and axons. *Cell, 63,* 303–322.

Iino, H., Fukayama, M., Maeda, Y., Koike, M., Mori, T., Takahashi, T., Kikuchi-Yanoshita, R., Miyaki, M., Mizuno, S., & Watanabe, S. (1994). Molecular genetics for clinical management of colorectal carcinoma. 17p, 18q, and 22q loss of heterozygosity and decreased DCC expression are correlated with the metastatic potential. *Cancer, 73,* 1324–1331.

Isakov, N., Gopas, J., Priel, E., Segal, S., & Altman, A. (1991). Effect of protein kinase C activating tumor promoters on metastases formation by fibrosarcoma cells. *Invasion Metastasis, 11,* 14–24.

Johnson, M., Kim, H., Chesler, L., Tsao-Wu, G., Bouck, N., & Polverini, P. (1994). Inhibition of angiogenesis by tissue inhibitor of metalloproteinase. *Journal of Cell Physiology, 160,* 194–202.

Johnson, M., Torri, J., Lippman, M., & Dickson, R. (1993). The role of cathepsin D in the invasiveness of human breast cancer cells. *Cancer Research, 53,* 873–877.

Kalebic, T., Garbisa, S., Glaser, B., & Liotta, L. A. (1983). Basement membrane collagen: Degradation by migrating endothelial cells. *Science, 221,* 281–283.

Kikkawa, U., Kishimoto, A., & Nishizuka, Y. (1989). The protein kinase family: Heterogeneity and its implications. *Annual Review of Biochemistry, 58,* 31–44.

Kleiner, D. E., Tuuttila, A., Tryggvasson, K., & Stetler-Stevenson, W. G. (1993). Stability anaylsis of latent and active 72-kDa type IV collagenase: The role of tissue inhibitor of metalloproteinases-2 (TIMP-2). *Biochemistry, 32,* 1583–1592.

Kleinman, H. K., Klebe, R. J., & Martin, G. R. (1981). Role of collagenous matrices in the adhesion and growth of cells. *Journal of Cell Biology, 88,* 473–482.

Klominek, J., Robert, K. H., & Sundqvist, K. G. (1993). Chemotaxis and haptotaxis of human malignant mesothelioma cells: Effects of fibronectin, laminin, type IV collagen, and an autocrine motility factor-like substance. *Cancer Research, 53,* 4376–4382.

Kohn, E. C., Alessandro, R. A., Spoonster, J., Wersto, R., & Liotta, L. A. (1995). Angiogenesis: Role of calcium mediated signal transduction. *Proceedings of the National Academy of Sciences, USA, 92,* 1307–1311.

Kohn, E. C., Felder, C. C., Jacobs, W., Holmes, K. A., Day, A., Freer, R., & Liotta, L. A. (1994). Structure-function analysis of signal and growth inhibition by carboxyamino-triazole, CAI. *Cancer Research, 54,* 935–942.

Kohn, E. C., Francis, E., Liotta, L., & Schiffmann, E. (1990). Heterogeneity of the motility responses in malignant tumor cells: A biological basis for the diversity and homing of metastatic cells. *International Journal of Cancer, 46,* 287–292.

Kohn, E. C., Jacobs, W., Kim, Y., Alessandro, R., Stetler-Stevenson, W., & Liotta, L. (1994). Calcium influx modulates expression of matrix metalloproteinase-2 (72-kDa type IV collagenase, gelatinase A). *The Journal of Biological Chemistry, 269,* 21505–21511.

Kohn, E. C., & Liotta, L. A. L651582 (1990). A novel antiproliferative and antimetastatsis agent. *Journal of the National Cancer Institute, 82,* 54–60

Kohn, E. C., Sandeen, M. A., & Liotta, L. A. (1992). In vivo efficacy of a novel inhibitor of selected signal transduction pathways including calcium, arachidonate and inositol phosphates. *Cancer Research, 52,* 3208–3212.

Krueger, T. C., Tallent, M. B., Richie, R. E., & Johnson, H. K. (1985). Neoplasia in immunosuppressed renal transplant patients: A 20-year experience. *Southern Medical Journal, 78,* 501–506.

Kuhn, K., Glanville, R., Babel, W., Qian, R., Dieringer, H., Voss, T., Siebold, B., Oberbaumer, I., Schwarz, U., & Yamada, Y. (1985). The structure of type IV collagen. *Annals New York Academy of Sciences,* 14–24.

Lapis, K., Liotta, L. A., & Rabson, A. S. (Eds.). (1986). *Biochemistry and molecular genetics of cancer metastasis.* The Hague: Martinus Nijhoff.

Lehel, S., Lasic, Z., Vukicevic, S., & Banfic, H. (1994). Collagen type IV stimulates an increase in intracellular Ca^{2+} in pancreatic acinar cells via activation of phospholipase C. *Biochemistry Journal, 299,* 603–611.

Leone, A., Flatow, U., King, C. R., Sandeen, M. A., Margulies, I. M. K., Liotta L. A., & Steeg, P. S. (1991). Reduced tumor incidence, metastatic potential and cytokine responsiveness of nm23 transfected melanoma cells. *Cell, 65,* 25–35.

Leone, A., McBride, O. W., Weston, A., Wang, M. G., Anglard, P., Cropp, C. S., Goepel, J. R., Lidereau, R., Callahan. R., Linehan, W. M., Ress, R. C., Harris, C. C., Liotta L. A., & Steeg, P. S. (1991). Somatic allelic deletion of nm23 in human cancer. *Cancer Research, 51,* 2490–2493.

Levitzki, A., & Gilon, C. (1991). Tyrphostins as molecular tools and potential antiproliferative drugs. *Trends in Pharmacological Sciences, 12,* 171–174.

Levy, A., & Cioce, V. (1991). Increased expression of the Mr 72,000 type IV collagenase in human colonic adenocarcinoma. *Cancer Research, 51,* 439–444.

Levy, A., Cioce, V., Sobel, M., Garbisa, S., Grigioni, W., Liotta, L., & Stetler-Stevenson, W. (1991). Increased expression of the Mr 72,000 type IV collagenase in human colonic adenocarcinoma. *Cancer Research, 51,* 439–444.

Lindberg, R. (1972). Distribution of cervical lymph node metastases from squamous cell carcinoma of the upper respiratory and digestive tracts. *Cancer, 29,* 1446–1449.

Liotta, L. A. (1986). Tumor invasion and metastases—role of the extracellular matrix: Rhoads Memorial Award Lecture. *Cancer Research, 46,* 1–7.

Liotta, L. A. (1987). Overview of the biology of cancer invasion and metastases. In S. A. Rosenberg (Ed.), *Surgical treatment of metastatic cancer* (pp. 1–36). Philadelphia: J. B. Lippincott Co.

Liotta, L. A. (1989). Biology of metastasis. In W. N. Kelley (Ed.), *Textbook of internal medicine* (pp. 1148–1152). Philadelphia: J. B. Lippincott Co.

Liotta, L. A., Abe, S., Gehron, P., & Martin, G. R. (1979). Preferential digestion of basement membrane collagen by an enzyme derived from a metastatic murine tumor. *Proceedings of the National Academy of Sciences, USA, 76,* 2268–2276.

Liotta, L. A., Kleinerman, J., Catanzara, P., & Rynbrandt, D. (1977). Degradation of basement membrane by murine tumor cells. *Journal of the National Cancer Institute, 58,* 1427–1439.

Liotta, L. A., Kleinerman, J., & Saidel, G. M. (1974). Quantitative relationships of intravascular tumor cells, tumor vessels, and pulmonary metastases following tumor implantation. *Cancer Research, 34,* 997–1002.

Liotta, L. A., Mandler, R., Murano, G., Katz, D. A., Gordon, R. K., Chiang, P. K., & Schiffmann, E. (1986). Tumor cell autocrine motility factor. *Proceedings of the National Academy of Sciences, USA, 83,* 3302–3306.

Liotta, L. A., Rao, C. N., & Barsky, S. H. (1983). Tumor invasion and the extracellular matrix. *Laboratory Investigation, 49,* 636–649.

Liotta, L. A., Rao, C. N., & Wewer, U. M. (1986). Biochemical interactions of tumor cells with the basement membrane. *Annual Review of Biochemistry, 55,* 1037–1057.

Liotta, L. A., Saidel, G., & Kleinerman, J. (1976). Stochastic model of metastases formation. *Biometrics, 32,* 535–550.

Liotta, L. A., & Schiffmann, E. (1988). Autocrine motility factors. In V. T. DeVita, S. A. Hellman, & S. A. Rosenberg (Eds.), *Important advances in oncology* (pp. 17–30). Philadelphia: J. B. Lippincott Co.

Liotta, L. A., & Steeg, P. S. (1990). Slews to the function of nm23 and Awd proteins in development, signal transduction, and tumor metastasis provided by studies of Dictostelium discoideum. *Journal of the National Cancer Institute, 82,* 1170–1172.

Liotta, L. A., Steeg, P. S., & Stetler-Stevenson, W. G. (1991). Cancer metastasis and angiogenesis: An imbalance of positive and negative regulation. *Cell, 64,* 327–336.

Liotta, L. A., Thorgeirsson, U. P., & Garbisa, S. (1982). Role of collagenases in tumor cell invasion. *Cancer and Metastasis Reviews, 1,* 277–288.

Liu, B., Renaud, C., Nelson, K., Chen, Y., Bazaz, R., Kowynia, J., Timar, J., Diglio, C., & Honn, K. (1992). Protein-kinase-C inhibitor calphostin C reduces B16 amelanotic melanoma cell adhesion to endothelium and lung colonization. *International Journal of Cancer, 52,* 147–152.

Lyall, R., Zilberstein, A., Gazit, A., Gilon, C., Levitzki, A., & Schlessinger, J. (1989). *Journal of Biological Chemistry, 264,* 14503–14509.

Mareel, M. M. (1983). Invasion in vitro: Methods of analysis. *Cancer and Metastasis Reviews, 2,* 201–219.

Mareel, M. M., Van Roy, F. M., & DeBaetselier, P. (1990). The invasive phenotypes. *Cancer Metastasis Reviews, 9,* 45–62

McCarthy, J. B., Basera, M. L., Palm, S. L., Sas, D. F., & Furcht, L. T. (1985). Stimulation of haptotaxis and migration of tumor cells by serum spreading factors. *Cancer Metastasis Reviews, 4,* 125–152.

Merzak, A., Koocheckpour, S., & Pilkington, G. (1994). CD44 mediates human glioma cell adhesion and invasion in vitro. *Cancer Research, 54,* 3988–3992.

Minniti, C. P., Kohn, E. C., Grubb, J. H., Sly, W. S., Oh, Y., Muller, H. L., Rosenfeld, R. G., & Helman, J. L. (1992). The insulin-like growth factor II (IGF-II)/mannose 6-phosphate receptor mediates IGF-II-induced motility in human rhabdomyosarcoma cells. *The Journal of Biological Chemistry, 267,* 9000–9004.

Mohanam, S., Sawaya, R., McCutcheon, I., Ali-Osman, F., Boyd, D., & Rao, J. (1993). Modulation of *in vitro* invasion of human glioblastoma cells by urokinase-type plasminogen activator receptor antibody. *Cancer Research, 53,* 4143–4147.

Muller, D., Wolf, C., Abecassis, J., Millon, R., & Engelmann A. (1993). Increased stromelysin 3 gene expression is associated with increased local invasiveness in head and neck squamous cell carcinomas. *Cancer Research, 53,* 165–169.

Muschel, R. J., Williams, J. E., Lowy, D. R., & Liotta, L. A. (1985). Harvey *ras* induction of metastatic potential depends upon oncogene activation and type of recipient cell. *American Journal of Pathology, 121,* 1–8.

Nanus, D., Schmitz-Drager, B., Motzer, R., Lee, A., Vlamis, V., Cordon-Cardo, C., Albino, A., & Reuter, V. (1993). Expression of basic fibroblast growth factor in primary human renal tumors: Correlation with poor survival. *Journal of the National Cancer Institute, 85,* 1597–1599.

Narayanan, R., Lawlor, K. G., Schaapveld, Q. J., Cho, K. R., Vogelstein, B., Tran, P. B. V., Osborne, M. P., & Telang, N. T. (1992). Antisense RNA to the putative tumor suppressor gene DCC transforms Ratt 1a fibroblasts. *Oncogene, 7,* 553–561.

Natali, P. G., Nicotra N. A., Cavaliere, R., & Bigotti, A. (1993). Integrin expression in cutaneous malignant melanoma: Association of the alpha3/beta1 Heterodimer with tumor progression. *International Journal of Cancer, 54,* 68–72.

Nguyen, M., Watanabe, H., Budsen, A., Richie, J., Hayes, D., & Folkman, J. (1994). Elevated levels of an angiogenic peptide, basic fibroblast growth factor, in the urine of patients with a wide spectrum of cancers. *Journal of the National Cancer Institute, 86,* 356–361.

Nicolson, G. (1993). Paracrine and autocrine growth mechanisms in tumor metastasis to specific sites with particular emphasis on brain and lung metastasis. *Cancer and Metastasis Reviews, 12,* 325–343.

Nicolson, G. L. (1978). Experimental tumor metastasis: Characteristics and organ specificity. *Bioscience, 28,* 441–447.

Nicolson, G. L. (1984). Generation of phenotypic diversity and progression in metastatic tumors. *Cancer Metastasis Reviews, 3,* 25–42.

Nicolson, G. L. (1987). Tumor cell instability, diversification, and progression to the metastatic phenotype: From oncogene to oncofetal expression. *Cancer Research, 47,* 1473–1487.

Nishizuka, Y. (1986). Studies and perspectives of protein kinase C. *Science, 233,* 305–311.

Nishizuka, Y. (1988). The molecular heterogeneity of protein kinase C and its implications for cellular regulation. *Nature, 334,* 661–665

Nordstrom, T., Nevanlinna, H., & Anderson, L. C. (1994). Mitosis-arresting effect of calcium cancer inhibitor SK&F 96365 on human leukemia cells. *Experimental Cell Research, 202,* 487–494.

Nowell, P. C. (1986). Mechanisms of tumor progression. *Cancer Research, 46,* 2203–2207.

O'Brian, C. A., & Wark, N. E. (1989). Biology of the protein kinase C family. *Cancer Metastasis Reviews, 8,* 199–214.

Oka, H., Shiozaki, H., Kobayashi, K., Inoue, M., Tahara, H., Kobayashi, T., Takatsuka, Y., Matsuyoshi, N., Hirano, S., Takeichi, M., & Mori, T. (1993). Expression of E-cadherin cell adhesion molecules in human breast cancer tissues and its relationship to metastasis. *Cancer Research, 53,* 1696–1701.

Paget, J. (1863). *Lectures on surgical pathology.* London: Longman, Brown, Green, & Longmans.

Pajouh, M. S., Nagle, R. B., Breathnach, R., Finch, J. S., Brawer, M. K., & Bowden, G. T. (1991). Expression of metalloproteinase genes in human prostrate cancer. *Journal of Cancer Research and Clinical Oncology, 117,* 144–150.

Parazzini, F., Colli, E., Scatigna, M., & Tozzi, L. (1993). Treatment with tamoxifin and progestins for metastatic breast cancer in postmenopausal women: A quantitative review of published randomized clinical trials. *Oncology, 50,* 483–489.

Pauli, B. U., Augestin-Voss, H. G., El-Saddam, M. E., et al. (1990). Organ preferances of metastasis. The role of endothelial cell adhesion molicules. *Cancer Metastisis Review, 9,* 175–189.

Peifer, M. (1993). Cancer, catenins, and cuticle pattern: A complex connection. *Science, 262,* 1667–1668.

Plesnicar S. (1989). Mechanisms of development of metastases. *Critical Reviews Oncogenesis, 1,* 175–194.

Pollanen, J., Stephens, R. W., & Vaheri, A. (1991). Directed plasminogen activation at the surface of normal malignant cells. *Advanced Cancer Research, 57,* 273–328.

Postel, E. H., Berderich, S. J., Flint, S. J., & Ferrone, C. A. (1993). Human c-myc transcription factor PuF identified as nm23-H2 nucleoside diphosphate kinase, a candidate suppressor of tumor metastasis. *Science, 261,* 487–480

Poste, G. (1986). Pathogenesis of metastatic disease: Implications for current therapy and for the development of new therapeutic strategies. *Cancer Treatment Reports, 70,* 183–198.

Powis, G. (1991). Signaling targets for anticancer drug development. *Trends in Pharmacological Sciences, 12,* 188–194

Pozzati, R., Williams, J. E., Lowry, D. R., Padmanbhan, R., Howard, B., Liotta L. A., & Khoury, G. (1986). Primary rat embryo cells transformed by one or two oncogenes show different metastatic potentials. *Science, 232,* 223–227.

Raz, A., & Geiger, B. (1982). Altered organization of cell-substrate contacts and membrane-associated cytoskeleton in tumor cell variants exhibiting different metastatic capabilities. *Cancer Research, 42,* 5183–5190.

Ries, C., Kolb, H., Petrides, P. (1994). Regulation of 92-kd gelatinase release in HL-60 leukemia cells: Tumor necrosis factor-alpha as an autocrine stimulus for basal- and phorbol ester-induced secretion. *Blood, 83,* 3638–3646.

Roblin, R. (1981). Contributions of secreted tumor cell products to metastasis. *Cancer Biology Reviews, 2,* 59–92.

Rosenberg, S. A. (1994). Modern combined modality management of Hodgkin's disease. *Current Opinion in Oncology, 6,* 470–472.

Rosengard, A. M., Krutzsch, H. C., Shearn, A., Briggs, J. R., Barker, E., Margulies, I. M. K., King, C. R., Liotta, L. A., & Steeg, P. S. (1989) Reduced Nm23 Awd protein in tumor metastasis and aberrant *Drosophila* development. *Nature, 342,* 177–180.

Rubinfeld, B., Souza, B., Albert, I., Muller, O, Chamberlain, S., Masiarz, F., Munemitsu, S., & Polakis, P. (1993). Association of the APC gene product with B-catenin. *Science, 262,* 1731–1734.

Sappino, A. P., Busso, B., Belin, D., & Vassali, J. D. (1987). Increase of urokinse type plasminogen activator gene expression in human lung and breast carcinomas. *Cancer Research, 47,* 4043–4046.

Sato, H., Takino, T., Okada, Y., Cao, J., Sinagawa, A., Yamamoto, E., & Seiki, M. (1994). A matrix metalloproteinase expressed on the surface of invasive tumor cells. *Nature, 370,* 61–65.

Savarese, D. M. F., Russel, J. T., Fatatis, A., & Liotta, L. A. (1992). Type IV collagen stimulates an increase in intracellular calcium: Potential role in tumor cell motility. *Journal of Biological Chemistry, 267,* 21928–21935.

Schirrmacher, V. (1985). Cancer metastasis: Experimental approaches, theoretical concepts, and impacts for treatment strategies. *Advances in Cancer Research, 43,* 1–73.

Schuchter, L. M., Esa, A. H., Stratford, M. W., Laulis, M. K., Pettit, G. R., & Hess, A. D. (1993). Successful treatment of murine melanoma with Bryostatin 1. *Cancer Research, 51,* 682–687.

Schwartz, G., Redwood, S., Ohnuma, T., Holland, J., Droller, M., & Liu, B. (1990). Inhibition of invasion of invasive human bladder carcinoma cells by protein kinase C inhibitor staurosporine. *Journal of the National Cancer Institute, 82,* 1753–1756.

Schwartz, M. (1993). Signaling by integrins: implications for tumorigenesis. *Cancer Research, 53,* 1503–1506.

Seftor, R. E., Seftor, E. A., Gehlsen, K. R., Stetler-Stevenson, W. G., Brown, P. D. et al. (1992). Role of the alpha-v-beta-3 integrin in human melanoma cell invasion. *Proceedings of the National Academy of Sciences, USA, 89,* 1557–1561.

Seiki, M., Sato, H., Liotta, L. A., & Schiffman, E. (1991). Comparison of autocrine mechanisms promoting motility in two metastatic cell lines: Human melanoma and ras-transfected NIH3T3 cells. *International Journal of Cancer, 49,* 717–720.

Seitser, S., Arch, R., Reber, S., Komitowski, D., Hofman, M., Ponta, H., Herrlich, P., Matzku, S., & Zoller, M. (1993). Prevention of tumor metastases formation by antivariant CD44. *Journal of Experimental Medicine, 177,* 443–455.

Shah, J. T., Cendon, R. A., & Farr, H. W. (1976). Carcinoma of the oral cavity. Factors affecting treatment failure at the primary site and neck. *American Journal of Surgery, 132,* 504–509.

Siegel, G. P., Barsky, S. H., Terranova, V. P., & Liotta, L. A. (1981). Stages of neoplastic transformation of human breast tissue as monitored by dissolution of basement membrane components. *Invasion and Metastases, 1,* 54–70.

Sloane, B. F., Rozhin, J., & Jonson, K. (1986). Cathepsin B: Association with plasma membrane in metastatic tumors. *Proceedings of the National Academy of Sciences, USA, 83,* 2483–2487.

Sobel, M. E. (1990). Metastasis suppressor genes. *Journal of the National Cancer Institute, 82,* 267–276.

Somogyi, L., Lasic, Z., Vukicevic, S., & Banfic, H. (1994). Collagen type IV stimulates an increase in intracellular Ca++ in pancreatic acinar cells via activation of phospholipase C. *Biochemistry Journal, 299,* 603–611.

Soutter, A., Nguyen, M., Watanabe, H., & Folkman, J. (1993). Basic fibroblast growth factor secreted by an animal tumor is detectable in urine. *Cancer Research, 53,* 5297–5299.

Spoonster, J., & Kohn, E. (1994). Carboxyamido-triazole: A novel approach to chemotherapy. *Contemporary Oncology, 6,* 38–46.

Stanwell, C., Gescher, A., Bradshaw, T., & Pettit, G. (1994). The role of protein kinase C isoenzymes in the growth inhibition caused by bryostatin 1 in human A549 lung and MCF-7 breast carcinoma. *International Journal of Cancer, 56,* 585–592.

Steeg, P. S., Bevilaqua, G., Kopper, I., Thorgeirsson, U. P., Talmadge, J. E., Liotta, L. A., & Sobel, M. E. (1988). Evidence for a novel gene associated with low tumor metastatic potential. *Journal of the National Cancer Institute, 80,* 200–204.

Stetler-Stevenson, W., Aznavoorian, S., & Liotta, L. (1993). Tumor cell interactions with the extracellular matrix during invasion and metastasis. *Annual Review of Cell Biol., 9,* 541–573.

Stetler-Stevenson, W. G., Krutzsch, H. C., & Liotta, L. A. (1989). Tissue inhibitor of metalloproteinase (TIMP-2). *Journal of Biological Chemistry, 264,* 17374–17378.

Stossel, T. P. (1993). On the crawling of cells. *Science, 260,* 1086–1093.

Stracke, M. L., & Kohn, E. C. (1988). Insulin-like growth factors stimulate chemotaxis in human melanoma cells. *Biochemical and Biophysical Research Communications, 153,* 1076–1083.

Stracke, M. L., Kruzsch, H. C., Unsworth, E. J., Arestad, A., & Cioc, C. (1992). Identification, purification, and partial sequence analysis of autotaxin, a novel motility-stimulating protein. *Journal of Biological Chemistry, 267,* 2524–2529.

Stracke, M. L., Murata, J., Aznavoorian, S., & Liotta, L. A. (1994). The role of the extracellular matrix in tumor cell metastasis. *In Vivo, 1,* 49–58.

Strauli, P. (1980). Proteinases and tumor invasion. In P. Strauli, A. J. Barrett, & A. Bauci (Eds.), *Proteinases and tumor invasion* (pp. 215–222). New York: Raven Press.

Sugarbaker, E. V. (1981). Patterns of metastasis in human malignancies. *Cancer Biology Reviews, 2,* 235–278.

Sumiyoshi, K., Serizawa, K., Urano, T., Takada, Y., Takada, A., & Baba, S. (1992). Plasminogen activator system in human breast cancer. *International Journal of Cancer, 3,* 345–348.

Takeichi, M. (1990). Cadherins: A molecular family important in selective cell-cell adhesion. *Annual Review of Biochemistry, 59,* 237–253.

Takeichi, M. (1993). Cadherins in cancer: Implications for invasion and metastasis. *Current Opinion in Cell Biology, 5,* 806–811.

Tandon, A., Clark, G., Chamness, C., Chirgwin, J., & McGuire, W. (1990). Cathepsin D and prognosis in breast cancer. *New England Journal of Medicine, 322,* 297–302.

Tarin, D., & Matsumura, Y. (1993). Deranged activity of the CD44 gene and other loci as biomarkers for progression to metastatic malignancy. *Jounral of Cellular Biochemisitry Supplement, 17G,* 173–185.

Terranova, V. P., Hujanen, E. S., & Martin, G. R. (1986). Basement membrane and the invasive activity of metastic tumor cells. *Journal of the National Cancer Institute, 77,* 311–316.

Terranova, V. P., Liotta, L. A., Russo, R. G., & Martin, G. R. (1982). Role of laminin in the attachment and metastasis of murine tumor cells. *Cancer Research, 42,* 2265–2273.

Terranova, V. P., Rao, C. N., & Kalebic, T. (1983). Laminin receptor on human breast carcinoma cells. *Proceedings of the National Academy of Sciences, USA, 80,* 444–451.

Terranova, V. P., Williams, J. E., & Liotta, L. A. (1984). Modulation of the metastatic activity of melanoma cells by laminin and fibronectin. *Science, 226,* 982–984.

Testa, J. E. (1992). Loss of the metastatic phenotype by human epidermoid carcinoma cell line, HEp-3, is accompanied by increased expression of tissue inhibitor of metalloproteinases 2. *Cancer Research, 52,* 5597–5603.

Thorgeirsson, U. P., Turpenniemi-Hujanen, T., & Liotta, L. A. (1985). Cancer cells, components of basement membranes, and proteolytic enzymes. *International Review of Experimental Pathology, 27,* 203–234.

Todaro, G. J., Fryling, C., & De Larco, J. E. (1980). Transforming growth factors produced by certain human tumor cells: Polypeptides that interact with epidermal growth factor receptors. *Proceedings of the National Academy of Sciences, USA, 77,* 5258–5263.

Tryggvason, K., Hoyhtya, M., & Pyke, C. (1993). Type IV collagenases in invasive tumors. *Breast Cancer Research and Treatment, 24,* 209–218.

Uleminckx, K., Vackat, L., Mareel, M., Fiers, W., & Van Roy, F. V. (1991) Genetic manipulation of E-cadherin expression by epithelial tumor cells reveals an invasion suppressor role. *Cell, 66,* 107–119.

Ura, H., Bonfil, R. D., Reich, R., Reddel, R., Pfeifer, A., Harris, C. C., & Klein, A. J. P. (1989). Expression of type IV collagenase and procollagen genes and its correlation with the tumorgenic, invasive, and metastatic abilities of oncogene-

transfomed human bronchial epithelial cells. *Cancer Research, 49,* 4615–4621.

Vartanian, R., & Weidner, N. (1994). Correlation of intratumoral endothelial cell proliferation with microvessel density (tumor angiogenesis) and tumor cell proliferation in breast carcinoma. *American Journal of Pathology, 144,* 1188–1194.

Vlodavsky, I., Fuks, Z., Bar-Ner, M., Ariav, Y., & Schirrmacher, V. (1983). Lymphoma cell-mediated degradation of sulfated proteoglycans in the subendothelial extracellular matrix: Relationship to tumor cell metastasis. *Cancer Research, 43,* 2704–2711.

Vogelstein, B. (1988). Genetic alterations during colorectal-tumor development. *New England Journal of Medicine, 319,* 525–532.

Waterfield, M. D. (1989). Altered growth regulation in cancer. *British Medical Bulletin, 45,* 570–581.

Weidner, N., Carroll, P., Blumenfeld, W., & Folkman, J. (1993). Tumor angiogenesis correlates with metastasis in invasive prostate carcinoma. *American Journal of Pathology, 143,* 401–409.

Weidner, N., Folkman, J., Pozza, F., Bevilacqua, P., Allred, E., Moore, D., Meli, S., & Gasparini, G. (1992). Tumor angiogenesis: A new significant and independent prognostic indicator in early-stage breast carcinoma. *Journal of the National Cancer Institute, 84,* 1875–1887.

Weidner, N., Semple, J. P., Welch, W. R., & Folkman, J. (1991). Tumor angiogenisis and metastasis-correlation in invasive breast carcinoma. *New England Journal of Medicine, 324,* 1–8.

Weiss, L. (1983). Random and non-random processes in metastasis and metastatic inefficiency. *Invasion and Metastases, 3,* 193–207.

Weiss, L., & Ward, P. M. (1983). Cell detachment and metastasis. *Cancer Metastasis Reviews, 2,* 111–123.

Weiss, R., Liu, B., Ahlering, T., Dubeau, L., & Droller, M. (1990). Mechanisms of human bladder tumor invasion: Role of protease cathepsin B. *The Journal of Urology, 144,* 798–804.

Whitfield, J. (1992). Calcium signals and cancer. *Critical Reviews in Oncogenesis, 3,* 55–90.

Wicha, M. S., Liotta, L. A., Garbisa, S., & Kidwell, W. R. (1980). Basement membrane collagen requirements for attachment and growth of mammary epithelium. *Experimental Cell Research, 124,* 181–190.

Yaish, P, Gazit, A., Gilon, C., & Levitzki, A. (1988). Blocking of EGF-dependent cell proliferation by EGF receptor kinase inhibitors. *Science, 4880,* 933–935.

Yamada, K. M., Akiyam, S. K., Hasegawa, T., Humphries, M. J., Kennedy, D. W., Nagata, K., Urushihara, H., Olden, K., & Chen, W. T. (1985). Recent advances in research on fibronectin and other cell attachment factors. *Journal of Cell Biochemistry, 28,* 79–97.

Yamanaka, Y., Friess, H., Buchner, M., Beger, H., Uchida, E., Onda, M., Kobrin, M., & Korc, M. (1993). Overexpression of acidic and basic fibroblast growth factors in human pancreatic cancer correlates with advanced tumor stage. *Cancer Research, 53,* 5289–5296.

Yamaoka, M., Yamamoto, T., Masaki, T., Ikeyama, S., Sudo, K., & Fujita, T. (1993). Inhibition of tumor growth and metastasis of rodent tumors by the angiogenesis inhibitor O-(Chloroacetyl-Carbamoyl)fumagillol (TNP-470; AGM-1470). *Cancer Research, 53,* 4262–4267.

Yarden, Y., & Urlich, A. (1988). Growth factor receptor kinases. *Annual Review of Biochemistry, 57,* 443–478.

CHAPTER

16

Evaluating Cancer Risks and Preventive Oncology

Marilyn Frank-Stromborg • Karen Billars Heusinkveld • Kim Rohan

In 1995, approximately 1,252,000 Americans will be diagnosed with cancer. Nonmelanoma skin cancer and carcinoma in situ have not been included in these statistics. The incidence of nonmelanoma skin cancer adds an additional 800,000 cases. In 1995, approximately 547,000 individuals will die of these cancers (American Cancer Society, 1995). Cancer will surpass heart disease as the number one cause of death by the year 2000 (Greenwald & Sondek, 1986). Certainty is growing about which agents start the abnormal process leading to cancer. Recent evidence leads to the inescapable conclusions that cancer is not entirely inevitable and that individual lifestyles may influence its occurrence. Lifestyle habits of tobacco use, diet and nutrition, and sexual practices have been found to influence the frequency of cancer.

CANCER CONTROL

A national commitment to cancer prevention and early detection is reflected in the National Cancer Institute's goal of reducing cancer mortality by 50 per cent by the year 2000 (Greenwald & Sondek, 1986). A substantial part of the solution to the cancer problem at the present time lies within the grasp and responsibility of each individual. The current trend and growing sensitivity of the public to cancer prevention and early de-

tection has awakened in oncology nursing a new commitment to educate the public concerning risk factors and guidelines. Cancer nurses must help individuals redefine their life goals and expectations and learn to manage new health and self-care practices, thereby helping them to become more active participants in their own health care. Nurses represent an extraordinary potential for expanding health education in cancer prevention in all realms of health care. Nurses work with clients and families in all stages of health and illness and in a variety of health care settings, including hospitals, clinics, industry, and schools within rural, urban, and inner-city communities. Nurses can make a difference.

Cancer prevention uses three major approaches: education, regulation, and host modification. Education is intended to reduce the cancer-causing behaviors of individuals and practices of society through the translation of scientific findings into sound, practical advice. Education programs should "include provision for antismoking messages to reduce lung cancer, the promotion of sun avoidance and the use of sun blockers to reduce skin cancer, the modification of diet to prevent colon cancer and possibly breast and prostate cancers, the adoption of practices in the workplace to reduce exposure to chemical carcinogens, and the modification of sexual practices to prevent cervical cancer and cancers related to acquired immunodeficiency syndrome" (Cole & Amoateng-Adjepong, 1994, p. 8).

Some environmental carcinogens cannot be avoided by individual behavior modification and education programs. Hence, the regulation approach is needed. The United States Environmental Protection Agency and other agencies provide regulations and guidelines intended to minimize carcinogens in the environment. The regulatory approach is being used to prohibit the sale of tobacco to minors, to prohibit smoking in many public places, and to impose taxes on tobacco products. In the future, the regulatory efforts will also focus on technology that will permit alteration of the genomes of plants and animals, thereby reducing some of these carcinogens. The third and latest approach of cancer prevention is host modification. This requires immunization and chemoprevention methods (Cole & Armoateng-Adjepong, 1994). Much of the research in these areas will have important implications for nurses in prevention and early detection efforts.

Statistics on cancer help us understand how much we have accomplished in cancer control. For three major sites of cancer—lung, breast, prostate—the statistics are encouraging. The educational efforts to reduce smoking have reflected a decrease in incidence of lung cancer and the start of a decrease in mortality trends. The efforts to improve early detection of breast and prostate cancer have resulted in an increase in the incidence of early-detected cases, which should ultimately reduce mortality for these two sites.

CHALLENGES FOR NURSING RESEARCH

There are many challenges for nursing research to continue our progress toward cancer control. To focus on preventative care, additional nursing research is needed with a preventative emphasis, focusing on individual health beliefs and behavior changes, the effects of the nurse/patient interaction, and the individuals being active partners in their health plans. We need to identify the needs of different populations and target interventions that are specific to that population. As all nurses know, not all groups are alike, and not all interventions should look alike. Research is also needed to determine accessibility of cancer control information and services to specific populations, to know the range of prevention and early detection services that are needed, and to know how to best work with specific populations.

Oncology nurses must continue research on how best to help individuals to consistently, rationally, and freely take action to prevent cancer. A full understanding of these factors is a prerequisite for the planning or revision of any cancer prevention/early detection educational programs. Nursing research is also needed to provide data on which to determine public policy and on how nurses can best influence public policy in cancer control.

Because of the increased cost of health care in the United States, more emphasis will be placed on managing the utilization of health care services. The reform in the health care system—both private and public—is resulting in greater attention being paid to early detection and prevention of illness. The emphasis of managed care on controlling cost and cost reduction requires the modification of the behaviors of providers and consumers. This is being accomplished by using financial penalties and rewards. With a priority of managed care systems on cancer control through prevention and early detection, nurses will have a greater responsibility in the health care system. The consumer will be required to take more responsibility for his own personal health and for making informed health decisions. Nurses must focus on helping people become informed and to help themselves. An informed consumer can exert a strong influence on quality and cost-effectiveness of the health care system.

The economics of the health care system in the past focused on illness care, to the exclusion of emphasis on prevention and early detection. Nurses must now shift from the predominant focus on illness and cure to an orientation on wellness and care. With increasing interest and value on health and wellness by individual employers and business consortiums, providers of care are putting more emphasis on preventative care indicators such as numbers of mammograms, prostate screenings, and pap smears as well as emphasis on tobacco control. This gives added importance to the efforts in cancer prevention and early detection that nurses have been doing. Nurses must be more aware of guidelines for preventative care and early detection in the managed care arena. Nurses, with knowledge and skills in assessment, establishing priorities, intervention, and evaluation are major players in the new health care environment. It is nurses who assess groups to determine prevention and detection needs; it is nurses who plan prevention and early detection programs to meet these needs; it is nurses who evaluate outcomes of these programs. A nursing research focus toward prevention, detection, and health care policy will be essential for career control.

FRAMEWORKS FOR PREVENTION

The relatively low levels of public participation in preventive health behaviors and screening for cancer have been extensively documented. The belief that the problem of prevention is mainly a failure of the health professional to communicate pertinent factual information to the public about the condition has been discounted for some time. Over 30 years ago, Hochbaum noted that ample evidence "points to the conclusion that while information is often one of several necessary conditions for rational behavior, it is rarely sufficient to produce it" (1960, p. 13).

Many frameworks for health education for a variety of health problems and situations have been developed and evaluated. By careful consideration of behavioral and attitudinal factors, nurses can have an impact by promoting compliance with prevention guidelines. The Health Belief Model and the PRECEDE model, a discussion of which follows, may be helpful in health education efforts.

HEALTH BELIEF MODEL

The health belief model may have considerable value in explaining and predicting an individual's cancer prevention behavior. The model holds that individuals who exhibit the appropriate combination of beliefs will take action to prevent and detect illness in the absence of symptoms. It hypothesizes that for an individual to take any action or engage in any health behavior, minimal levels of relevant health motivation and knowledge must be present.

The individual's readiness to be concerned about the particular health issue and to comply with recommended behavior is determined by a perceived susceptibility to the possible illness and a perception of the probable severity of the illness. If the individual believes in both the likelihood of personal susceptibility to the disease and the likelihood that the consequences of the disease will be serious, he or she must then evaluate the benefits or barriers to the health action.

Benefits as defined in the health belief model are beliefs in the efficacy of the health behavior or effectiveness of the health action in relation to the illness; *barriers* are the physical, financial, and psychologic costs of engaging in that behavior. To take the health action, the individual must perceive that the benefits outweigh the barriers (Fig. 16–1).

Specifically, the health belief model (Becker & Rosenstock, 1975) contains the following elements:

1. *Individual Perceptions:* The individual's subjective state of readiness to take action, which is determined by both perceived likelihood of *susceptibility* to the particular illness and perceptions of the probable *severity* of the consequences (organic and social) of contracting the disease.
2. *Modifying Factors:* A cue to action, which must occur to trigger the appropriate health behavior; this stimulus can be either internal (e.g., symptoms) or external (e.g., interpersonal interactions, mass media communications).
3. *Likelihood of Action:* The individual's evaluation of the advocated health behavior in terms of its feasibility and efficaciousness (i.e., an estimate of the action's potential *benefits* in reducing susceptibility or severity) weighs against perceptions of physical, psychological, financial, and other costs or *barriers* involved in the proposed action (p. 25).

This approach to health behavior relates the perceived susceptibility and severity of the particular illness to the health action the individual will take. Perceived susceptibility or perceived likelihood of occurrence are known to vary widely among individu-

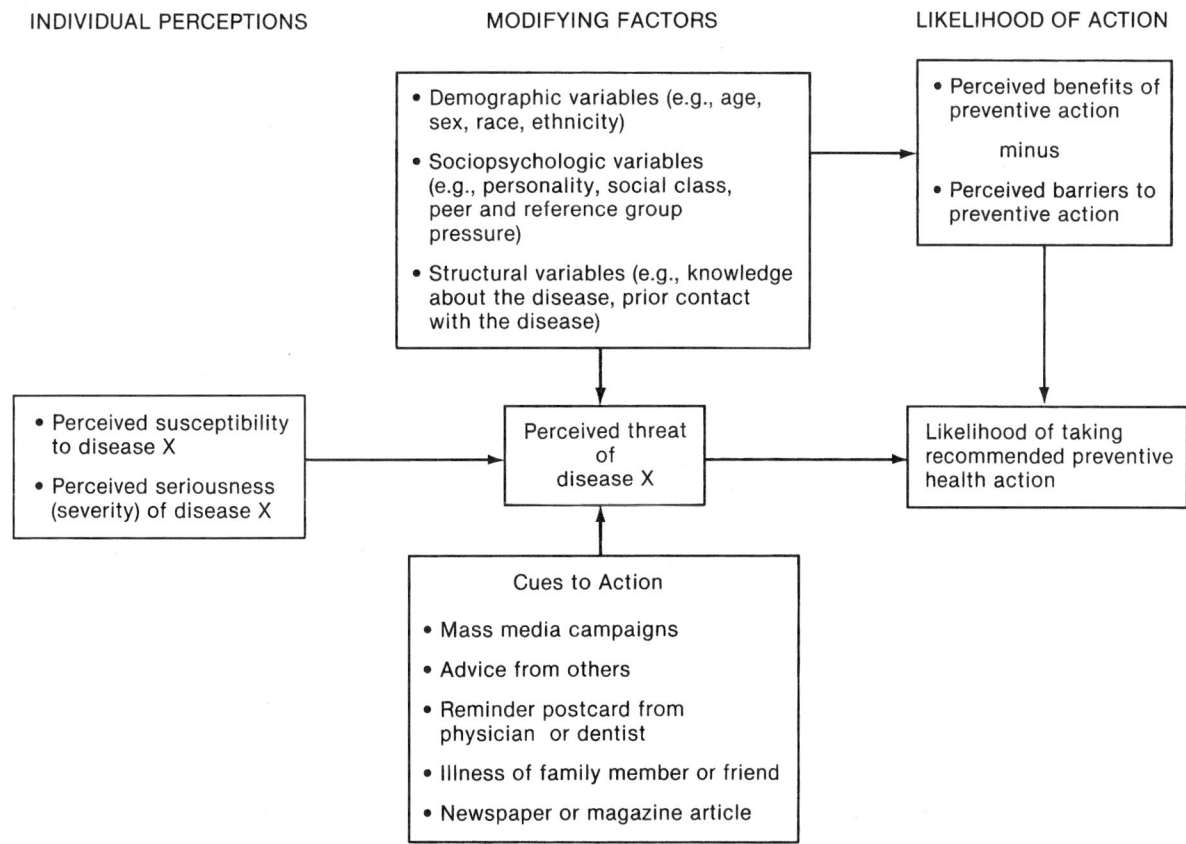

FIGURE 16–1. The health belief model as predictor of preventive health behavior. (From Becker, M. H., Drachman, R. H., & Kirscht, J. P. [1975]. A field experiement to evaluate various outcomes to continuity of physician care. *American Journal of Public Health, 64,* 1062–1070. Reproduced by permission.)

als. At one extreme are individuals who deny any possibility of contracting a particular illness, and at the other extreme are individuals who feel a real danger of contracting a particular illness. Perceived seriousness of a given illness varies among individuals; it may be seen in terms of a reduction in physical or mental functioning for long periods of time, a permanent disability, or a cause of death. Perceived seriousness of a condition may have even broader or more complex implications, such as effects on career, family life, and social relationships. A smoker's perception of the risk of getting cancer from smoking may influence a decision to quit.

A health action directed toward cancer prevention and early detection can lower the individual's perceived susceptibility to cancer and reduce the perceived severity of the illness. According to the model, the expectation of success of the health action for an individual in a particular situation is a function of the perceived benefits of taking the action minus the effects of the barriers that inhibit taking the action. Barriers for an individual may be expressed in terms of physical, psychological, sociologic, and economic costs. The health benefits of quitting smoking must outweigh the relaxation and stress reduction associated with smoking.

The cue to action makes the individual become conscious of feelings and to begin thinking about how to deal with the threat of cancer. Thus the likelihood of taking action is predicted to be predicated on the individual's belief that the comparable benefits of the protective action outweigh the inconvenience, discomfort, or undesired consequences of taking that action. Motivation as a necessary condition for action is assumed in the health belief model and is operationalized as the psychological state of readiness to take specific action and as the extent to which a particular health action is believed to be beneficial in reducing the threat (Rosenstock, 1966).

Taking a specific action is a function of the individual's evaluation of several sets of factors, including the individual's assessment of susceptibility to a given disease and the individual's evaluation of the severity of the condition. Perceived threat in the model is the individual's estimation of the chances of the condition worsening if health advice is not followed. Modifying factors, including sociodemographic and structural characteristics and cues to action such as media and advice from others are included in the model. The specific combination of these factors for an individual results in an increased or decreased probability that the recommended health action will be undertaken.

PRECEDE MODEL

The PRECEDE model, designated by Green, Kreuter, Deeds, and Partridge (1980), is a framework that nurses may find useful in cancer prevention education programs in community settings. The basic tenet of the model is that health behavior is a voluntary behavior and that the reason for a behavior change must be understood by those whose behavior is in question.

The framework PRECEDE (which stands for *predisposing, reinforcing,* and *enabling causes* in *educational diagnosis* and *evaluation*) asks what behavior precedes each health benefit and what causes precede each health behavior. PRECEDE utilizes a deductive approach that starts with the final consequences and works back to the original causes. The PRECEDE model directs the initial attention to outcomes rather than to inputs and encourages the asking of "why" questions before the asking of "how" questions. By beginning with the final outcome, one determines what must precede that outcome by determining what causes that outcome. The factors important to an outcome must be diagnosed before interventions are designed. If this is not done, the interventions may be based on guesswork and run a greater risk of being misdirected and ineffective.

The PRECEDE model identifies seven phases (Fig. 16–2). Phase 1—epidemiologic diagnosis—delineates the extent, distribution, and causes of a health problem in a population. Quality of life is assessed by looking at some of the social problems and concerns of the people in the population. The demands of social problems in a given community are good barometers of the community's quality of life. Phase 2—social diagnosis—identifies the specific high-priority health problems that appear to be contributing to the social problems. Available data and data generated by appropriate investigations for vital indicators and dimensions of the health problem are used. Phase 3—behavioral diagnosis—delineates the specific health behaviors that appear to be linked to the health problem. Preventive actions, utilization, consumption patterns, compliance, self-care, economics, genetics, and environment are assessed in this phase. These behaviors and dimensions are identified specifically and are carefully ranked.

Phase 4—educational diagnosis—requires the sorting and categorizing of predisposing, enabling, and reinforcing factors that have a direct impact on the health problem. Predisposing factors are attitudes, beliefs, and perceptions that facilitate or hinder health behaviors. Enabling factors are barriers such as limited facilities, lack of income or health insurance, and inadequate personnel or community resources. The skills and knowledge required for a desired behavior to occur are also enabling factors. Reinforcing factors are those related to feedback from others concerning health behaviors. The feedback may either encourage or discourage the behavioral change. In Phase 5—prioritizing—the relative importance of each of the factors and available resources is determined. These factors are the focus of the intervention.

Phase 6—administrative diagnosis—is the actual development and implementation of a program. Based on knowledge of limitations of resources, time constraints, and abilities, the appropriate educational interventions are determined. Administrative problems and resources are assessed. Phase 7—evaluation—is not a phase unto itself but is considered an integral and continuous part of the entire framework. It begins with clearly stated program and behavioral objectives in the diagnostic phases and ends with evaluation of

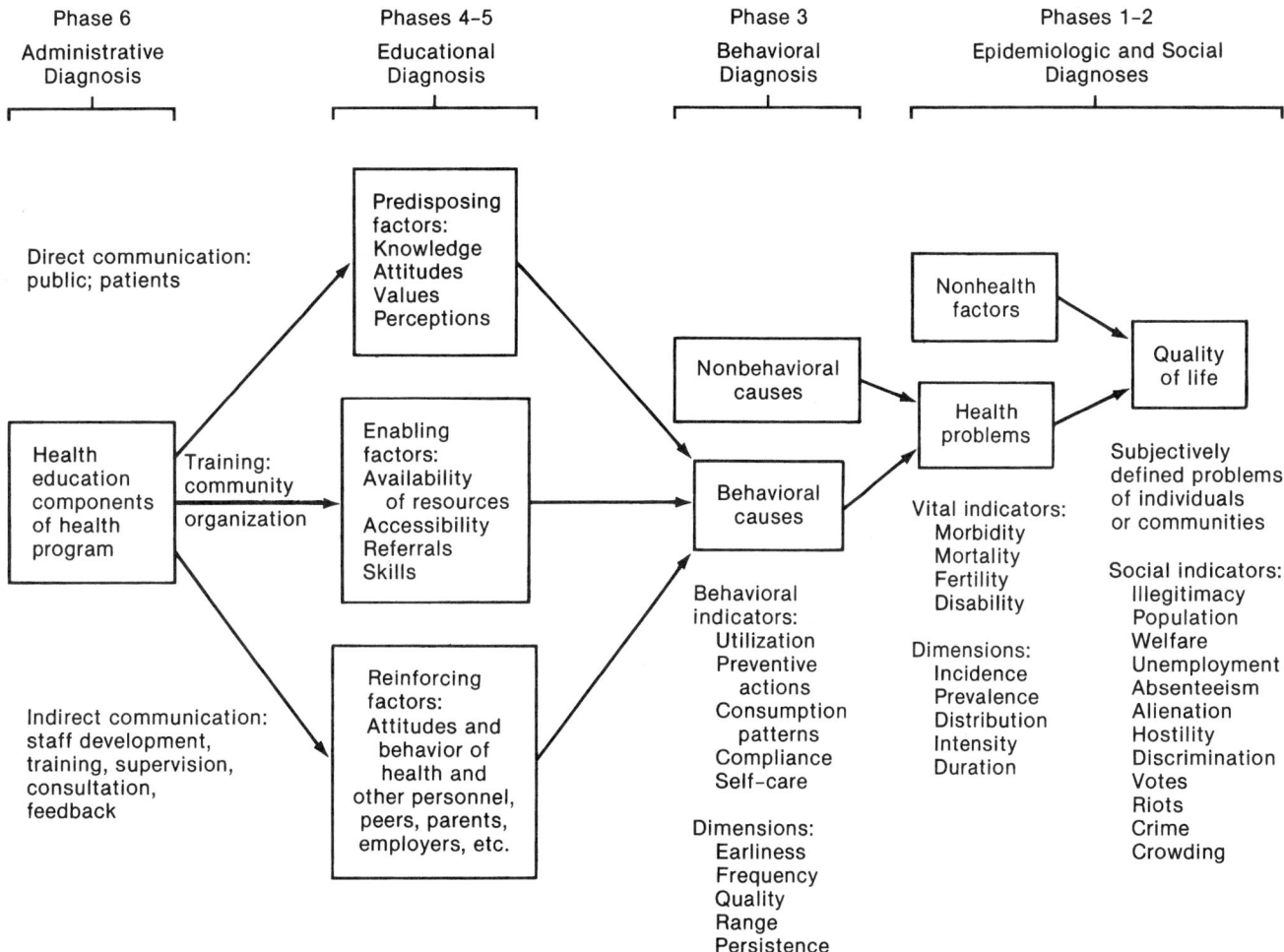

Phase 6	Phases 4–5	Phase 3	Phases 1–2
Administrative Diagnosis	Educational Diagnosis	Behavioral Diagnosis	Epidemiologic and Social Diagnoses

FIGURE 16–2. PRECEDE framework. (From Green, L. W., Kreuter, M. W., Deeds, M. W., & Partridge, K. B. [1980]. *Health education planning. A diagnostic approach.* Palo Alto, CA: Mayfield Publishing Co. Reproduced by permission.)

long-range goals of improved quality of life and social benefits.

PRECEDE requires epidemiologic, social-survey, and demographic data for the identification of major social and health problems in a group. Those problems that are important enough to the group to be targets of the cancer prevention education program are the focus of health education.

DEFINITION OF TERMS

To help individuals take an active role in their health, an understanding of risk factors for cancer is important.

Many terms are used in discussing the risks for developing cancer. *Risk* is the potential realization of unwanted consequences of an event; it is the probability of injury or death. Both the probability of occurrence of an event and the magnitude of its consequence are involve (Rowe, 1986, p. 4). *Risk factor* is an element of personal behavior or genetic makeup or an exposure to a known cancer-causing agent that increases a person's chances of developing a particular form of cancer (White, 1986, p. 184). Hazard is another term that is frequently used in discussions of cancer risk. *Hazard* implies the existence of some threat, whereas risk implies both the existence of a threat and the potential for its occurrence. An example of a hazard is vinyl chloride; its toxicity in terms of amount of exposure and incidence of cancer is documented. However, until vinyl chloride has a pathway to humans or to the environment, it poses no risk.

Because living itself involves risks, there is no such thing as a zero-risk situation, only ones that involve involuntary and voluntary risks. For instance, although risks are involved in crossing streets, eating calorie-rich desserts, and adding extra automobile driving time to a daily routine, most people routinely undertake one or more of these activities, because the benefits outweigh the risks or because the risks (an accident or obesity) are so minimal. Smoking is a classic example of a *voluntary risk*, in which 30 per cent of the American population participate, whereas air pollution is an example of an *involuntary risk* (Ernster, 1987; Stokes, 1987).

Risk factors play a significant part in any discussion of cancer causation and prevention. Alcohol consumption, smoking, and typical American diet practices are all personal risk factors (voluntary risks) that have been linked to cancer mortality. Elimination of smoking would reduce lung cancer deaths by an estimated 83 per cent, modification of the Western diet could reduce cancer mortality by 30 per cent, and elimination of alcohol consumption could cut approximately 5 per cent of cancer deaths in the United States (Costanza, Frederick, Green, & Patterson, 1986; Newell & Vogel, 1987). Air pollution (involuntary risk) that disturbs the stratospheric ozone layer may significantly increase the solar ultraviolet radiation that reaches the earth, thereby causing an increase in skin cancer of 60 per cent or more in the twenty-first century (Sternburg, 1983).

There are many *classifications of risk factors*, including those by Senie (1986), who classifies them into exogenous factors (environmental and lifestyle) and endogenous factors (host factors); Burack and Drelichman (1982), who classify risk factors into three categories: (1) genetic and familial, (2) personal, or (3) group; and Ash et al. (1982), who divide risk factors into behavioral-environmental factors (controlled or minimized by the individual or society) and host factors (individuals' physical attributes and inherited characteristics). Although occupational exposures have been studied intensively, the proportion of cancers attributable to exposures in the workplace has been estimated to be only 6 per cent, whereas the proportion attributable to lifestyle factors may be more than 80 per cent (Senie, 1986). Risk factors may be individual or group attributes. A *high-risk group* is one that shares risk factors due to its members' common genetic makeup, socioeconomic status, habits, occupation, geographic location, medical treatments, culture, or race or ethnic background (Table 16–1 lists examples of high-risk groups in each of these categories). Because African-Americans have the highest incidence and mortality rates for all cancers combined among the major racial and ethnic groups in the United States, they are an example of a high-risk group (National Cancer Institute, 1986). In contrast, Mormons are an example of a low-risk group, with cancer mortality and incidence rates significantly below the average rate experienced by the U.S. white population in the United States (Enstrom & Kanim, 1983).

IDENTIFICATION AND QUANTIFICATION OF RISK FACTORS

For some activities, risk is not difficult to determine. It is possible to estimate accurately the risks of accidental death due to driving a car or riding a bicycle because historic statistical data are available and because demonstrating the causal connection between injury and these types of activities is not very difficult. Determination of the causes of cancer is much more complex. Cancer appears to be characterized by a latency of onset, making it difficult to determine reliably a direct cause-and-effect relationship between exposure and incidence (Baeck & Eisenberg, 1985). The fact that the development of cancer is thought to be a multistage process further complicates attempts to identify the causes of cancer. Other barriers to the determination of risk factors are that (1) it is difficult to determine many individual risk factors for cancer because they tend to be multiple and interactive, (2) an individual risk factor may have multiple consequences, and (3) if little evidence exists on the connection between risk behavior and a specific pathologic process, the causal relationship may be unclear (Hirschman & Leventhal, 1983).

When a substance is suspected of directly or indirectly causing cancer, human epidemiologic studies or animal studies are utilized to determine whether the substance is a carcinogen and whether it poses a risk to humans. The study by Rinsky et al. (1987) is an example of an epidemiologic study to determine quantitatively the association between a suspected carcinogen and the development of cancer. This study examined the association between benzene exposure and leukemia by looking at the mortality rate of a cohort of rubber workers who were exposed to benzene. A typical animal study to determine risk is the long-term inhalation assays in rodents to determine the carcinogenic potential of formaldehyde (Squier & Cameron, 1984). The National Research Council details four steps in carcinogenic risk assessment.

Hazard Identification. Evidence of potential carcinogenic risk from environmental chemicals derives from four sources: epidemiologic studies of human populations, bioassay of animals, short-term tests for genotoxicity or cell transformation, and chemical structure relationships to known carcinogens. They are designed to answer questions such as the following. Is this substance a carcinogen? What type of carcinogen is it? What is the nature and strength of the evidence supporting this evaluation? (Robbins, 1978).

Dose Response Assessment. This relationship is the estimation of the potency of a chemical substance that is measured by evaluating the relationship between ad-

TABLE 16–1. *Example of Categorizations of High-Risk Groups*

Category	Example	Resultant Cancer
Genetic	Xeroderma pigmentosum	Skin
	Familial polyposis	Colon
Geographic	Transkei, Africa	Esophageal
	Japan	Gastric
	Sections of India	Oral
Socioeconomic	High socioeconomic status in U.S.	Breast
	Low socioeconomic status in U.S.	Cervical
Habits	Smoking	Lung cancer
	Chewing betel	Oral
Iatrogenic	Diethylstilbestrol	Vaginal
Occupational	Individuals who work with vinyl chloride	Angiosarcoma of the liver

(From Clemmesen, J. [1987]. Parameters for identification of high-risk groups. In H. Nieburgs [Ed.], *Prevention and detection of cancer, Part I, Prevention. Vol. 2. Etiology* [pp. 1513–1516]. New York: Marcel Dekker, Inc.)

ministered or received dose and incidence of cancer. This step almost always involves high-to-low dose extrapolation and frequently involves extrapolation from experimental animals to humans.

The dose-response relationship *quantitatively* defines the role of the dose of a chemical in evoking a biologic response. In the absence of the chemical, no response is seen. As the chemical is introduced into the system, the response is initiated at the threshold dose and increases in intensity as the dose is raised. Ultimately a dose is reached beyond which no further increase in response is observed (Snyder, 1984).

Exposure Assessment. For each potential route of exposure, an effort must be made to evaluate the frequency, magnitude, and duration of an exposure event and the number and susceptibility of people affected.

Risk Assessment. This measurement involves combining the information on dose-response with that on exposure to derive estimates of the probability that the hazards associated with a substance or activity will be realized under the conditions of exposure experienced by the population group of interest (Baeck & Eisenberg, 1985, pp. 672–673; Rodricks & Tardiff, 1984, pp. 9–10).

INDIVIDUAL RISK FACTORS

Once a substance (or a habit, occupation, or geographic location) is identified as a risk factor, the task for the health professional is to determine the *individual's* risk factors and assist that individual in reducing the risks. Existing evidence suggests that (1) individuals at risk for cancer are often unaware of their risk, (2) health professionals may not be familiar with those factors associated with the highest cancer risk, and (3) methods to reduce cancer risk have been underapplied because of lack of knowledge, funds, or motivation among patients and health professionals. The traditional health history and physical examination is one method of obtaining the individual's cancer-risk profile. Specialized cancer-risk assessment forms have been developed that concentrate on the known risk factors for specific cancer sites. Examples of risk factors from a typical cancer-risk assessment form follow (Faulkenberry, 1983):

Breast:

_____ Family history of breast cancer

_____ No children or first birth after age 30

_____ Obesity

_____ High dietary fat intake

_____ Personal history of ovarian or endometrial cancer

_____ Early menarche or late menopause

Another approach that has been advocated for *identifying* and *quantifying* an individual's risk factors is the

Health Hazard Appraisal (HHA) or Health Risk Appraisal (HRA). Dr. Lewis C. Robbins is generally credited with developing HRA. His work on cervical cancer and heart disease prevention during the late 1940s led him to the idea of keeping a record of a patient's health hazards to use as a guide to encouraging preventive efforts and then to the creation of a simple health hazard chart that could give the medical examination a more prospective orientation (Schoenbach, 1987; Stokes, 1987). The HHA is a simple approach to estimating personal risk (i.e., an individual's chance for developing cancer) and providing the basis for practical advice to persons wishing to reduce that risk. By explaining risk factors to people in terms of their chances of dying in the next 10 years, the health professional is describing the risk in terms the individual can understand easily. The actual risk factor value is derived by comparing the mortality rate for an individual associated with a specific behavior or characteristic (e.g., a cigarette smoker) with the mortality rate for an individual who does not have this behavior or characteristic (a nonsmoker of the same age, sex, and race) (Ross, 1981). An HHA can be achieved by a simple hand computation or a computerized appraisal. At present, more than 52 different instruments are available (Healthfinder, 1985). Sample questions from the HHA are the following:

How often do you examine your breasts for lumps? (women only)

_____ Monthly

_____ Once every few months

_____ Rarely or never

Did your mother, sister, or daughter have breast cancer? (women only)

_____ Yes

_____ No

_____ Not sure

_____ Not applicable

It must be noted that HRAs have been criticized in the literature in terms of the reliability of the approach (Sacks, Krushat, & Newman, 1980) and the validity of HRA risk scores (Schoenbach, 1987). However, Schoenbach acknowledges that "HHA, as a vehicle for what might be termed 'prospective health assessment,' potentially has a number of very desirable qualities for health professionals: preventive orientation, systemic approach, ability to emphasize modifiable factors, and grounding in current scientific knowledge" (1987, p. 410). Preliminary studies document that changes in behavior do occur as a result of HHA programs.

In summary, the nurse has several options for obtaining a history that will delineate persons at high risk for cancer from lifestyle habits, occupational exposure, or family history ("at-risk" asymptomatic individuals).

Identifying risk factors is important because preventive teaching cannot occur unless the risks are known by both the at-risk individual and the health professional. Those individuals who are at risk for cancer can be targeted for screening, more intensive follow-up, and behavior modification. The approaches that can be used are as follows:

1. A standard health questionnaire: the clinician can probe for more information when indicated.
2. A health screening flow sheet that indicates risk factors and behaviors most important to consider in preventing disease and maintaining good health.
3. A customized history questionnaire (self-administered or used as an interview tool) that is designed to elicit risk factors for cancer and is usually site-specific.
4. Computerized questionnaires that ensure standardization of medical records, provide a comprehensive history, are time-effective, and yield a concise and legible printout (Burack & Drelichman, 1982).

Regardless of the approach taken, no one method should be seen as an end in itself. The most important element in risk identification is the rapport established between the nurse and the individual so that questions are understood and complete information is obtained. Above all, the results of risk identification must be translated into sound practical advice that the individual can follow. The effort that the nurse expends to identify the major risk factors for cancer is the first step in managing those risks successfully.

ASSESSING INDIVIDUAL RISK THROUGH IDENTIFYING PREDISPOSING FACTORS OR SUSCEPTIBILITIES

Individuals can be described according to an infinite number of variables. The variables that have been evaluated in studies to determine cancer risks range from increasing age to past occupations. Recognition that the identification of high-risk individuals or groups provides a key to the ultimate reduction of cancer incidence and mortality through opportunities for surveillance, early detection and treatment, etiologic research, and preventive measures is increasing. The delineation of high-risk individuals or groups may come from clinical studies, animal and laboratory studies, or epidemiologic studies. It is clear that advances will be needed in risk identification before a major impact can be made on clinical and public health practices (Fraumeni, 1975).

The incidence, prevention, and early detection in major cancer sites with an emphasis on the related role for each will be discussed.

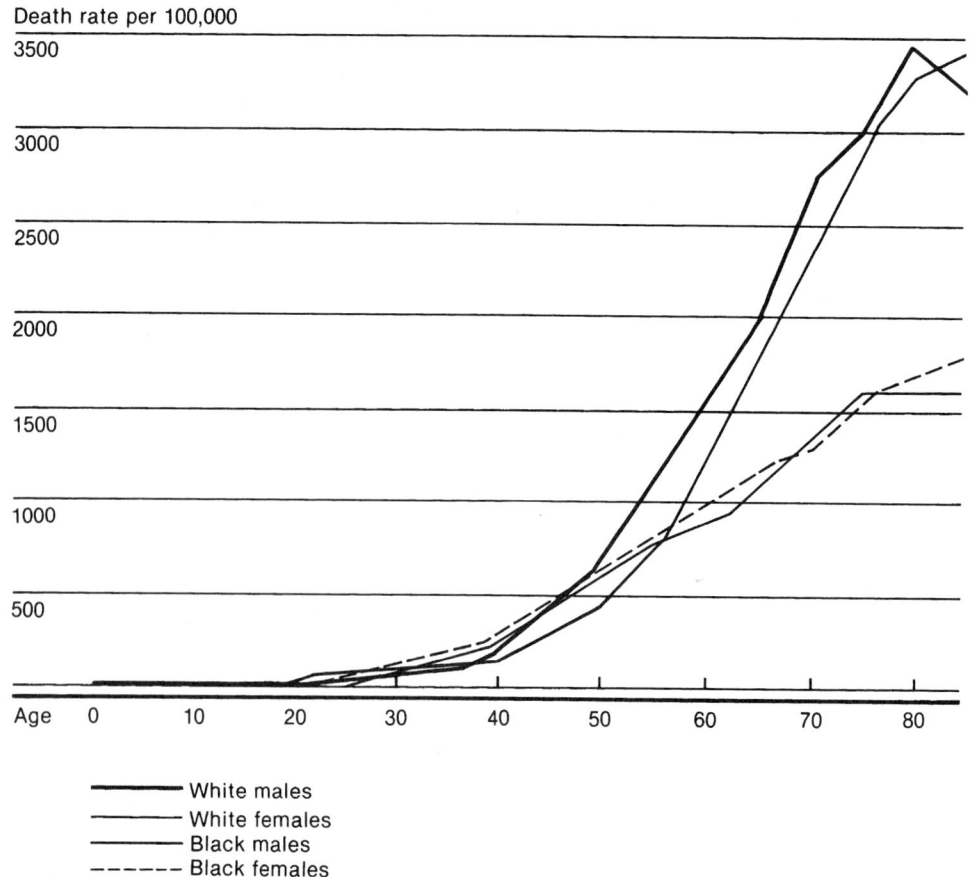

FIGURE 16–3. Average annual age-specific cancer incidence per 100,000 U.S. population by race and sex, all sites combined, 1973–1977. (From Surveillance of Epidemiology and End Results Program.)

AGE

Cancer is predominantly a disease of middle and old age; this finding is graphically depicted in Figure 16–3. Cancer occurs most frequently between the ages of 60 and 65 years (Page & Asire, 1995). However, the incidence rate for the majority of cancers increases continually after the first decade of life; the older a person becomes, the more likely he or she is to develop cancer. After 85 to 90 years of age, both incidence and mortality from all forms of cancer decline for both white males and females. The probability that a 65-year-old man will develop cancer in the next 5 years is 1 in 14, compared with 1 in 700 for a 25-year-old. The incidence rate for all sites of cancer combined rises steadily throughout life until it peaks at 2308 per 100,000 in persons aged 85 years and older (Birdsell, 1986).

The types of cancers seen in aging men and women differ considerably from those found in younger individuals. The classification of *elderly* is defined as individuals older than 65 years of age. Cancer of the breast, colon, and lung are *less aggressive* in the elderly than in the young, whereas cancer of the prostate and thyroid, leukemia, and melanoma are *more aggressive* in the elderly than in the young. Cancer of the vulva and chronic lymphocytic leukemia characteristically occur in the elderly. When the median age for the occurrence of the most common kinds of cancer is examined, the effect of age becomes readily apparent: the median age for breast cancer is 60 years; the median age for lung cancer is 65 years; and the median age for colon and prostate cancer is 70 years. The three leading cancer sites for aging men are lung, prostate, and colon-rectum; for aging women they are breast, lung, and colon-rectum (Silverberg & Lubera, 1987). Cancers of the stomach, colon, rectum, prostate, and breast account for more than 50 per cent of the invasive carcinomas in patients older than aged 60 years. Table 16–2 details the mortality figures for the most common cancers among different age groups.

The importance of these facts is underscored by the demographic changes that are occurring in the United States. Nearly 23 million Americans are older than aged 65 years, and they represent 11 per cent of the population (Ouslander & Beck, 1982). The elderly population will double to nearly 50 million by the year 2030, but those older than 75 years of age will increase more rapidly, with the number older than 85 years of age expected to triple (Somers, 1978). As we progress into the twenty-first century, a greater proportion of our society will be older than 65 years of age. This development has important implications for nurses. It is essential that nurses use any contact with the elderly to educate them about early cancer detection and to determine individual risk factors and perform physical assessments, if appropriate. Furthermore, the elderly

TABLE 16–2. *Reported Deaths for the Five Leading Cancer Sites for Males and Females by Age, United States, 1991*

ALL AGES	UNDER 15	15–34	35–54	55–74	75+
Males					
All cancer	All cancer	All cancer	All cancer	All cancer	All cancer
272,380	982	3,699	27,529	142,089	98,067
Lung	Leukemia	Leukemia	Lung	Lung	Lung
91,690	350	661	8,741	55,890	26,896
Prostate	Brain & CNS	Non-Hodgkin's	Colon & rectum	Colon & rectum	Prostate
33,564	252	lymphomas	2,393	13,888	20,909
Colon & rectum	Endocrine	501	Non-Hodgkin's	Prostate	Colon & rectum
28,178	111	Brain & CNS	lymphomas	12,306	11,686
Pancreas	Non-Hodgkin's	414	1,726	Pancreas	Pancreas
12,375	lymphomas	Skin	Brain & CNS	6,730	4,299
	64	298	1,577	Esophagus	Bladder
Leukemia	Connective tissue	Hodgin's disease	Pancreas	4,600	3,698
10,194	46	233	1,298		
Females					
All cancer	All cancer	All cancer	All cancer	All cancer	All cancer
242,277	727	3,434	29,302	111,419	97,388
Lung	Leukemia	Breast	Breast	Lung	Lung
52,068	260	660	9,188	30,154	16,400
Breast	Brain & CNS	Leukemia	Lung	Breast	Colon & rectum
43,583	220	432	5,372	19,900	15,727
Colon & rectum	Endocrine	Uterus	Colon & rectum	Colon & rectum	Breast
29,017	69	343	1,999	11,117	13,834
Ovary	Connective tissue	Brain & CNS	Uterus	Ovary	Pancreas
13,247	33	328	1,978	6,720	6,637
Pancreas	Bone	Non-Hodgkin's	Ovary	Pancreas	Ovary
13,161	28	lymphomas	1,779	5,669	4,601
		209			

(From Wingo, P. A., Tong, T., & Bolden, S. [1995]. Cancer statistics, 1995. *CA: A Cancer Journal for Clinicians, 45*(1), 8–30.)

should be educated about the need for regular physical examinations to detect cancer in the early stages rather than after symptoms have occurred. Also, they should be educated in techniques that can help in the early detection of cancer, for example, performing breast self-examinations, inspecting the skin under dentures, and reporting changes in skin lesions.

GENDER

Sex differences in risk for cancer are commonly observed for most cancers. Some of the observed sex differences are explainable because they are related to different occupations and lifestyles. The causes of other sex differences in rates for such cancers as thyroid and kidney cancer and Hodgkin's disease are unknown. Sexual factors, pregnancy, or both are thought to contribute substantially to the pathogenesis of a large group of cancers (e.g., breast, uterus, ovary, cervix, penis) (Henderson, Gerkins, & Pike, 1975). The causes of cancer of the prostate and testis are at present unknown. Comparing the worldwide incidence of cancer among men and women indicates that cancer is generally less common among women. The risk factors for cancer of the breast, uterus, ovary, cervix, and penis are discussed in the following sections.

SKIN CANCER

Incidence. Skin cancer, primarily caused by exposure to sunlight, is the most common type of cancer among whites in the United States (Kopf, 1988). The incidence of skin cancer has risen 1500 per cent over the past 50 years (Lawler, 1990). In 1995, an anticipated 800,000 people will be diagnosed with basal and squamous cell skin cancer and 34,100 with melanoma, 90 per cent of which are thought to be related to sun exposure (Wingo, Tong, & Bolden, 1995). In the United States, one in six individuals will develop skin cancer during the course of their lifetime (Moulds, 1992). Australia has the highest incidence of melanoma in the world. In 1982 the incidence was 18 per 100,000 in males and 17.6 in females. The lifetime risk of contracting melanoma in Australia is 1 in 52 for men and 1 in 58 for women (Girgis, Campbell, Redman, & Sanson-Fisher, 1991).

There are three basic types of skin cancer: basal cell carcinoma, squamous cell carcinoma, and melanoma. The nonmelanoma types (basal and squamous) are highly curable, having a survival rate of 96 to 99 per cent with early detection and proper treatment (White & Faulkenberry, 1985). Basal cell carcinoma is the most common type of skin cancer followed by squamous cell and melanoma. When melanoma is detected early (Breslow measure of ≤1 mm), it is curable by surgery alone (NIH Consensus Development Panel on Early Melanoma, 1992). However, advanced melanoma has a high mortality rate. For white men and women, the incidence of melanoma has been rising sharply worldwide, doubling each decade during the past 30 years (Kelly, 1991; Kopf, Rigel, & Friedman, 1982). Melanoma is increasing faster than any other

cancer except for lung cancer. It comprises 3 per cent of cancers diagnosed in the United States and will result in an estimated 7200 deaths in 1995 (American Cancer Society, 1995).

Risk Factors. Sunlight (ultraviolet radiation) is regarded as the probable factor in the pathogenesis of skin cancer and of primary melanoma of the skin of white persons. The National Academy of Sciences has stated that for a Caucasian population living at 40 degrees latitude (Philadelphia) no less than 40 per cent of the melanomas and 80 per cent of the squamous and basal cell carcinomas are caused by ultraviolet radiation. Cosmic irradiation varies by roughly a factor of two based on the altitude at which one lives; people living at higher altitudes receive more exposure. Likewise, exposure varies with latitude; people living closer to the equator receive more exposure (*The dark side*, 1986).

There are multiple precancerous skin lesions. A precancerous lesion may be defined as a morphologically altered tissue in which cancer is more likely to occur than in its apparently normal counterpart. If left alone, precancerous lesions will progress to invasive cancer.

These precancerous lesions of the skin are (1) actinic (solar) keratosis, which consists of dysplasias of the upper layers of the epidermis that are squamous cell, white, scaly, keratotic lesions (Amonette & Buker, 1992); (2) Bowen's disease (squamous cell), which is a dysplasia of the basal layers of the dermis that is considered a carcinoma in situ; the lesions are flat, reddish, scaly patches with superficial erosions (Sherman, 1983); (3) arsenical keratosis; (4) Queyrat's erythroplasia, which occurs on the penis and is identical to carcinoma in situ of the skin; lesions are raised, red, and velvet in appearance (Haynes, Mead, & Goldwyn, 1985); and (5) extramammary Paget's disease, which can affect any part of the skin in which epidermis and sweat glands coexist.

Melanoma of the skin is relatively rare in populations with dark skin color, but it is also rare in the populations of Latin America and eastern Asia, which are not particularly pigmented (Boffetta & Parkin, 1994). The exception is melanomas of the sole of the foot, which seem to occur at the same rate in different ethnic groups.

Skin cancer is among the most age-dependent of all cancers. Americans over the age of 65 years account for more than half of all the new cases of skin cancer diagnosed each year (Pollack, 1992). Table 16–3 lists the specific risk factors for melanoma and nonmelanoma.

Prevention. Skin cancer is highly preventable by avoiding, limiting, or protecting against sun exposure. Clinical examination, self-examination, and biopsy of suspicious lesions are the major methods of early detection.

Prevention is the key to reduction in the incidence of skin cancer and requires that nurses educate, assess, screen, detect, and act as role models. Prevention begins with educating the public about the warning signs, risk factors, measures to decrease sun exposure, and skin self-examination. The reduction of ultraviolet (UV) exposure has been a difficult practice for individuals to understand because of past societal pressure for

TABLE 16–3. *Risk Factors for Skin Cancer*

TYPES OF SKIN CANCER	RISK FACTORS
Melanoma (MacKie, Freudenberger, & Aitchison, 1989; Rhodes, Weinstock, Fitzpatrick, Mihm, & Sober, 1987)	Persistently changed or changing mole (strong risk factor): change in color, increase in diameter, increase in height, change in borders, sensation, consistency, surrounding skin, shape. Adulthood (risk increases with age). One or more large or irregular pigmented lesions (dysplastic moles and lentigo maligna). Congenital moles (benign pigmented nevi > 2mm diameter). Caucasian race. Previous cutaneous melanoma. Cutaneous melanoma in parents, children, or siblings. Immunosuppression. Sun sensitivity. Excess sun exposure, especially during childhood episodes of severe sunburn. Presence of freckles or tendency to freckle. Use of artificial ultraviolet sources.
Nonmelanoma (Gray, 1985; Haynes, Mead, & Goldwyn, 1985; Sherman, 1983)	Caucasians who are fair skinned, red-headed with freckles, and live in sunny climates. Long-term exposure to the sun or indoor tanning. Arsenical drugs applied to the skin. Premalignant lesions (actinic keratosis, arsenical keratosis, Bowen's disease, leukoplakia). Psoriasis patients treated with psoralens and untraviolet radiation (PUVA). Occupations involving chemical, arsenicals, pesticides, polycyclic aromatic hydrocarbons, coal tar and pitch, soot, liquid tar and paraffin, oils and petroleum. Ionizing radiation used in medical and dental procedures. Genetic conditions (xeroderma pigmentosum, albinism, multiple basal cell carcinoma).

(From Frank-Stromborg, M. & Rohan, K. [1992]. Nursings' involvement in the primary and secondary prevention of cancer. *Cancer Nursing*, 15[2], 79–108.)

"bronzed" skin. Caucasians with red or blond hair, blue or green eyes, fair skin that burns easily, and a positive familial history of skin cancer are at increased risk for the development of skin cancer (Lawler, 1990). Cumulative exposure is related to nonmelanoma skin cancer development, whereas intermittent sun exposure (weekend tanning) is associated with a higher risk of melanoma (Lawler & Schreiber, 1989).

The American Cancer Society, the Skin Cancer Foundation, and the American Academy of Dermatology recommend the following general precautions to decrease the risks of skin cancer:

1. Avoid sun exposure between 10 AM and 2 PM (11 AM to 3 PM during daylight savings time) in the summer months, when ultraviolet rays are most intense.
2. Wear a hat, tightly woven protective clothing, and sunglasses when exposed to the sun.
3. Before sun exposure, apply a sunscreen with a sun protection factor of 15 or more. Specifically it is recommended that individuals use liberal amounts of sunscreen (at least an ounce), reapply sunscreens every 2 to 4 hours, and use physical sunscreens on high-risk areas of the body such as the nose, shoulders, and tops of ears (Wells, 1989).

In addition to general precautions, the following additional information should be shared:

1. Exposure to the sun should not exceed 15 to 30 min/day; as one becomes tan, time out of doors may gradually increase.
2. Ultraviolet rays penetrate clouds on cloudy days, so sunscreen should always be used.

3. When swimming, waterproof sunscreens that are effective for 80 minutes through swimming or perspiration should be used.
4. The risk for burning is increased when one is exposed to snow, because snow reflects ultraviolet rays.
5. Ultraviolet radiation increases with proximity to the equator.
6. Certain drugs increase photosensitivity, for example, tetracycline, and birth control pills. Thus, high-risk persons should inquire about the drugs they are taking.
7. Men should be sure to apply sunscreens to the tops of their ears and bald scalp areas.
8. Sun damage is cumulative over a lifetime. Children should be taught to use sunscreens at an early age (Sturm & Hanke, 1992).

Early Detection. The key to long-term survival with skin cancer is early detection before metastasis occurs. Skin cancer is readily visible and easy to detect. Nurses have multiple opportunities to examine clients' skin and report suspicious lesions. A clinical examination should include inspection and palpation of the entire body. Any suspicious areas should be documented and the patient referred for further evaluation. Patients should be instructed on self-examination with emphasis placed on the ABCD system. Clinical features of de novo pigmented lesions suggestive of melanoma include *Asymmetry, Border* irregularity, *Color* variegation, and *Diameter* greater than 6 mm in diameter, the size of a pencil eraser. Figure 16–4 illustrates the earliest warning signs of malignant melanoma using the ABCD system. Other changes that should alert the clin-

A
Asymmetry

B
Border

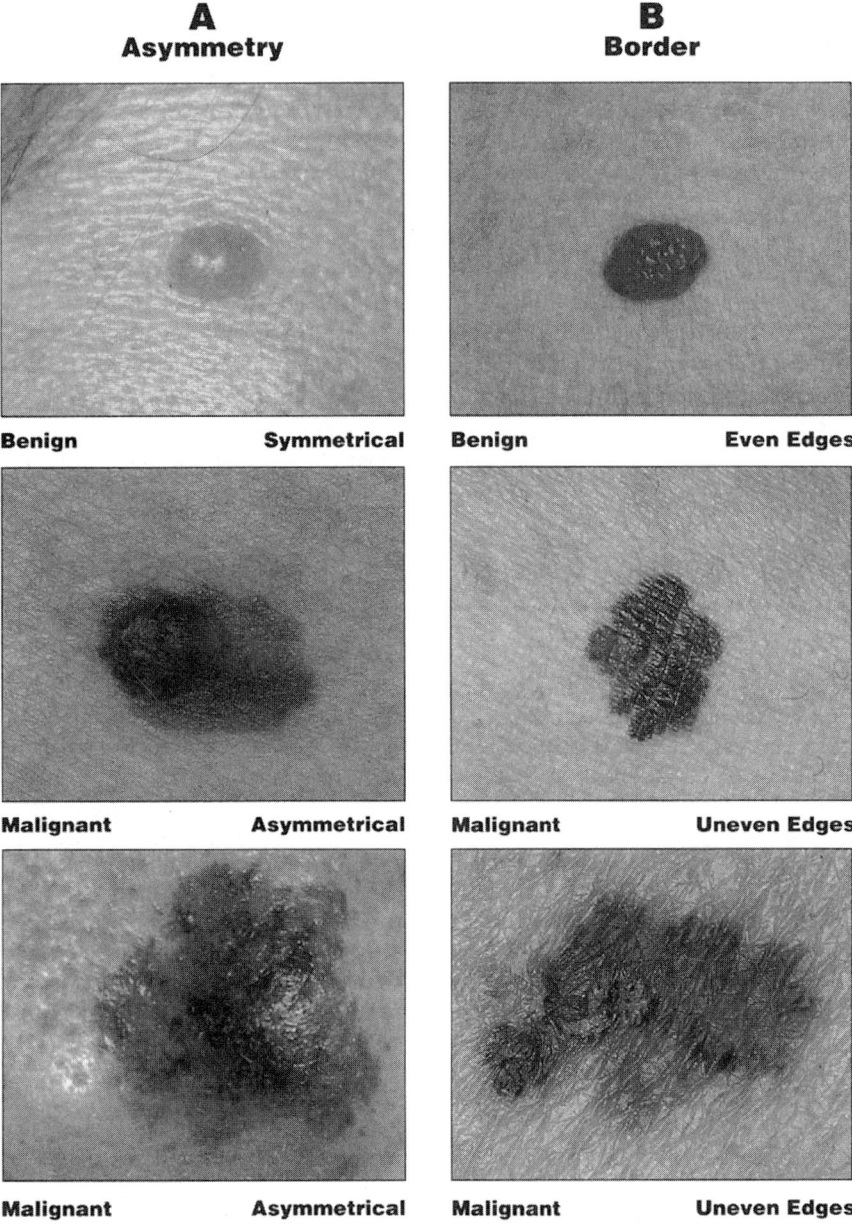

Benign   Symmetrical

Benign   Even Edges

Malignant   Asymmetrical

Malignant   Uneven Edges

Malignant   Asymmetrical

Malignant   Uneven Edges

FIGURE 16–4. **A,** Some forms of early malignant melanoma are asymmetrical, meaning a line drawn through the middle will not create matching halves. Moles are round and symmetric. **B,** The borders of early melanomas are frequently uneven, often containing scalloped or notched edges. Common moles have smooth even boarders.

ician to possible melanoma are itchiness, tenderness, redness, swelling, softening, or hardening of moles (Friedman, Rigel, & Kopf, 1992).

Nursing Roles. A review of the literature indicated that nurses are actively involved in educating the public about skin cancer and the risks of ultraviolet exposure. Nurses have (1) planned, implemented, participated in, and evaluated skin cancer screening programs in the employment and community setting; (2) coordinated clinics for pigmented lesions and individuals who are at high risk for skin cancer; (3) published articles on the prevention of skin cancer for the public; and (4) conducted research designed to determine approaches to effective primary prevention (Koh, Lew & Prout, 1989; Lawler, 1990; Lawler & Schreiber, 1989; Olsen, Fieser, Conte, & Schroeter, 1987; Poniatowski, 1990).

The role of the nurse in screening for melanoma was detailed by Larson (1986), Madsen (1988), and Buck-

ley and Cody (1990). This role was described as educational in terms of teaching patients to recognize their own skin changes, modify sun exposure, and participate in surveillance and early detection programs. Nurses were also urged to include in their assessment questions about first-degree relatives having either melanoma or large, unusual-looking moles (Larson, 1986). Coody (1987), at M.D. Anderson Hospital and Tumor Institute, also discussed the role of the Special Risk Nurse in a Special Risk Clinic. The Special Risk Nurse is responsible for "obtaining risk assessment information, providing genetic and behavioral modification and surveillance counseling, instructing patients in cancer screening techniques and coordinating clinical and basic science cancer control research" (Coody, 1987). The high-risk clinic at M.D. Anderson Hospital was designed for families with familial cancer syndromes (polyposis coli, dysplastic nevi, cancer of the

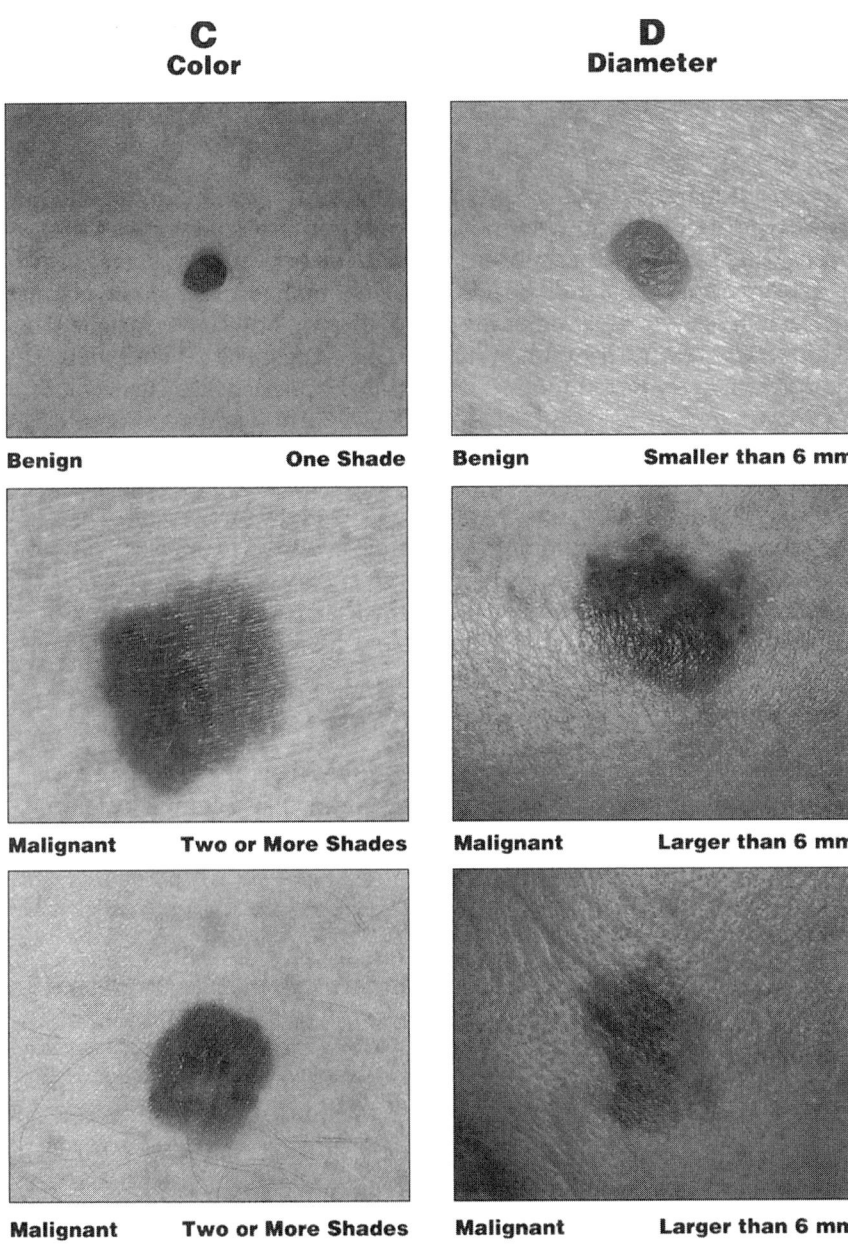

FIGURE 16–4 *Continued* **C,** Different shades of brown or black are often the first sign of a malignant melanoma. Common moles usually have a single shade of brown. **D,** Common moles are usually less than 6 mm in diameter (1/4"), the size of a pencil eraser. Early melanomas tend to be larger than 6mm. (From Friedman, R. J., Rigel, D. S., & Kopf, A. W. [1992]. The ABCDs of moles and melanomas. *Primary Care and Cancer, 12*(7), 16–17.)

colon). Fraser, at the Cancer Nursing Service, National Institutes of Health, also detailed the role of a nurse working with high-risk individuals for malignant melanoma. The educational role of the nurse was stressed by Fraser (1981, 1982) and includes providing high-risk individuals "with the knowledge, skills, support, and motivation needed to prevent and control melanoma" (Fraser, 1981, p. 92). McGuire (1979, 1985), in her discussion of the educational and psychosocial needs of families with hereditary cutaneous malignant melanoma, supports the educational roles of the nurse that Fraser advocated when working with this group of high-risk clients. She stated that nurses must continue to act as role models, practice "sun sensibility," and continue to educate patients, colleagues, friends, families, and the community at large.

The public has many misconceptions about the safety of indoor tanning because tanning booths have been incorrectly advertised as safe and capable of providing protection to the skin from further ultraviolet B (UVB) damage. Stewart (1990) therefore advocates that nurses take an active role in educating the public about the implications of indoor tanning and preventing skin damage. Such education should include the information that tanning represents the body's response to injury, causes premature aging, and may cause increased damage to areas of the body not normally exposed to the sun.

An innovative approach to educating the general public and screening for early skin cancer was discussed by Anderson and Munson (1990). The oncology nursing staff at North Memorial Medical Center in Minnesota designed and implemented a day-long skin cancer fair. This fair, titled "Be Smart in the Sun: Slip, Slop, Slap," was designed to provide an on-site, educational program to present information on the incidence, risk factors, early detection, and prevention of skin cancer. The fair included displays, music, refreshments, give-aways of sun protection materials, colorful posters, handouts, mini lectures, and consultation sessions with on-staff dermatologists. Organizers used a quiz to measure participants' knowledge of sun protection to evaluate the effectiveness of the fair.

The "Slip! Slop! Slap!" message was originally developed in 1981 in Australia by the Anti-Cancer Council of Victoria. It stands for slip on a shirt, slop on some sunscreen, and slap on a hat (Education about skin cancer, 1988). A Slip! Slop! Slap! kit was made available to Australian primary schools, t-shirts with this message were worn by life guards, and television messages were designed for the Australian population.

Nurses have been involved in conducting research to determine the most effective methods of educating individuals at risk for skin cancer. Kersey and Kroll (1985) conducted a sunscreen counseling project with 31 people with malignant melanoma, dysplastic nevus syndrome, or both. In this project, the physician or nurse counseled these high-risk patients in measures to prevent a second primary skin cancer. A pretest-posttest research design demonstrated that this multidisciplinary approach to cancer prevention increased the awareness of the danger of ultraviolet rays and use of sunscreens.

Owen (1989) also studied the psychosocial aspects of having a history of melanoma. Her research findings point out that intervention strategies to promote melanoma-preventive health practices must stress the benefits of performing skin self-examination and to minimize the perceived barriers to observing this primary preventive practice.

The nursing role for helping to lower the incidence of skin cancer would be to modify sun-seeking behavior (indoor and outdoor tanning). The nursing assessment should identify individuals who use tanning booths, document their history of sun exposure and family history of skin diseases (especially genetically related diseases such as dysplastic nevus syndrome), and assess the skin for suspicious lesions/moles that warrant a physician referral. Routine skin self-examination should be taught to all individuals who are frequent users of indoor tanning booths.

LUNG CANCER

Incidence. Lung cancer is estimated to be the leading cause of cancer death in both males and females in the United States. It is estimated that 169,900 persons will be diagnosed with this cancer in 1995 and that an estimated 157,400 will die from it (Wingo et al., 1995). Laryngeal cancer will account for an estimated 4090 cancer deaths and the diagnosis of 11,600 cases in 1995, with the prevalence higher in men than women (Wingo et al., 1995). It is estimated that 82 per cent of laryngeal cancers are due to cigarette smoking (Bartecchi, MacKenzie, & Schrier, 1994). The same type of statistics are true for oral cancers. The incidence of oral cancer among smokers ranges from 2 to 18 times that

among people who have never smoked. About 93 per cent of oral-cavity tumors in men and 61 per cent of such cancers in women are related to tobacco use, the greatest risk being in tobacco users who regularly use alcohol (Bartecchi et al., 1994). Epidemiologic evidence clearly supports that lung and laryngeal cancers are preventable cancers. Worldwide it is estimated that 1 million to 1.5 million cancer cases per year are attributable to tobacco use. Specifically, 80 to 90 per cent of lung cancers would be prevented and 85 per cent of laryngeal cancers would be prevented (Sasco, 1991). More than 80 per cent of lung cancer cases occur in smokers.

Risk Factors. In 1990, an estimated 89.9 million (50.1 per cent) U.S. adults were ever smokers, and 45.8 million (22.8 per cent) were current smokers. Approximately 44.1 million (49.1 per cent of all smokers ever) were former smokers in 1990 (Cigarette smoking among adults—United States, 1990). The prevalence of smoking was highest among persons aged 25 to 44 years, American Indians/Alaskan Natives, non-Hispanics, and persons with fewer than 12 years of education. Even more disturbing is the fact that projections suggest that 100,000 youths 12 years of age are habitual smokers, and the age at which first experimentation with smoking occurs is decreasing.

Occupational exposures to carcinogens in conjunction with smoking multiply the risk of cancer. It is recommended that a thorough occupational history be obtained during the health history when the patient is a smoker or has a history of smoking. People who smoke in a contaminated work atmosphere may inhale more of an ambient toxin than they would if they were breathing normally. Another underappreciated aspect of smoking in the workplace is how the heat generated by cigarettes can turn harmless substances into harmful ones (Uncovering occupational illness, 1990).

Asbestos workers who smoke have four to five times the risk for lung cancer as other smokers and more than 50 times the risk of those who neither smoke nor are exposed to asbestos (Greenwald & Sondek, 1986). The following additional facts are known about tobacco use:

1. Individuals who smoke filtered, low-tar cigarettes have a lower lung cancer risk than individuals who smoke nonfiltered, high-tar cigarettes.
2. Smoking prevalence rates for African-Americans are higher than for all other racial groups.
3. Smoking prevalence is high among blue-collar workers and the unemployed; prevalence of smoking decreases among men as income increases.
4. Rates for lung cancer are rising more sharply in women than in men.
5. Smokers who have quit for 15 or more years have a lung cancer mortality rate between one and two times that of nonsmokers.

While it is acknowledged that tobacco use is a major cause of cancers of the larynx, oral cavity, lung, and esophagus, it is also linked with increased incidence of cancers of the bladder, pancreas, and kidney.

There has been debate over the years about the risk of lung cancer when an individual is exposed to environmental tobacco smoke (ETS) (Harvey & Beattie, 1993). However, recent studies have found an elevated risk of lung cancer among individuals who have never smoked but are living with someone who smokes cigarettes (Fontham et al., 1994; Stockwell, Goldman, Lyman, Noss, & Armstrong, 1992). It is estimated that in the United States between 2500 and 8400 of the approximately 12,200 annual deaths from lung cancer that are not due to smoking may be attributable to environmental tobacco smoke. The majority of smoke given off from a lit cigarette is sidestream smoke rather than smoke that is inhaled. "Sidestream and mainstream smoke contain many of the same air contaminants. Sidestream smoke has more particles with smaller diameters, and these particles are therefore more likely to be deposited in the most distant regions of the lungs" (Bartecchi et al., 1994 p. 907). Recently it has been documented that infants of passive smokers are at risk of measurable exposure to cigarette smoke. Hair accumulation of cigarette smoke constituents have been found in the hair of newborn infants of passive smoking mothers (see Box 16–1) (Eliopoulos et al., 1994). It is important to note that environmental tobacco smoke has recently been classified as a known human lung carcinogen, or a "group A" carcinogen, under the EPA's system of carcinogen classification.

There is controversy about the relationship of indoor radon and the development of lung cancer. "Indoor exposure to radon seems to present a real risk and is probably the second most important cause of lung cancer. Radon exposure may be responsible for about 10,000 lung cancer deaths per year . . . While the risk from smoking is considerably larger, radon exposure may be the most significant risk factor for the nonsmoker that can be readily reduced" (Harley & Harley, 1990, p. 274).

Early Detection. Prevention is the best method of controlling lung and laryngeal cancers, because these cancers are asymptomatic in the early stages and are not presently amenable to early detection. Mass screening using chest radiography and sputum cytology remains controversial; large-scale studies are being conducted to determine the efficacy of such measures. The scope of the controversy is evident in two recent articles that assert the value of screening. Bechel, Kelley, Petty, Patz, and Saccomanno (1994) argue that sputum cytologic testing should be used as a case-finding tool, particularly in heavy smokers and those with occupational risks. While Bechel et al. reported improved survival, they did not document decreased mortality (Bechel et al., 1994). Furthermore, the recent reevaluation of data from the Early Lung Cancer trial and case mortality analyses by Chu and Smart suggest that "screening radiography alone may reduce lung cancer mortality by 10 per cent, or about 15,000 persons, in the United States annually" (Karsell & McDougall, 1993). Past screening trials using routine sputum cytology and chest radiography have not reduced lung cancer-related mortality.

To date, the American Cancer Society (ACS) and the U.S. Preventive Services Task Force recommend primary prevention in terms of smoking cessation rather than screening programs for lung cancer. Furthermore, the American College of Physicians, Canadian Task Force, and the U.S. Preventive Services Task Force do not recommend routine chest radiography for lung cancer nor selective x-rays for cigarette smokers during the periodic health examination (Sox, 1994).

New techniques of analyzing sputum cytology may result in the ACS and other groups' changing their recommendations about early detection of lung cancer. A group of researchers have developed an immunostaining technique for sputum cytologies. Their premise is that immunostaining with a panel of monoclonal antibodies may result in a more sensitive technique for identifying malignant cells than conventional morphologic criteria (Mittman & Roby, 1991). Support for this premise is documented in their study showing staining of atypical but not malignant sputum specimens with monoclonal antibodies that recognize lung cancer-associated antigens. Specimens obtained with the monoclonal antibodies stained an average of 24 months before the development of clinical lung cancer (Mulshine, Treston, & Scott, 1991).

Box 16–1. *Accumulation of Cigarette Smoke Constituents in the Hair of Newborn Infants of Passive Smoking Mothers*

Eliopoulos C., Klein J., Phan M. K., Knie B., Greenwald M., Chitayat D., Koren G. (1994). Hair concentrations of nicotine and cotinine in women and their newborn infants. *JAMA*, 271(8), 621–623.

Purpose/Objectives: To measure maternal and neonatal hair concentrations of nicotine and cotinine in 94 mother-infant pairs. Mothers in the study included mothers who were nonsmokers, passive smokers, and active smokers.

Data Source: Mothers who were active smokers, passive smokers, and nonsmokers and their infants 1 to 3 days after delivery in Toronto, Canada. Hair samples were taken from the infants and their mothers.

Data Synthesis: Passive smoking mothers and their infants had significantly higher hair concentrations of both nicotine and cotinine than nonsmoking mothers and their infants. Active smoking mothers had significantly higher hair concentrations of nicotine and cotinine than nonsmoking mothers. Infants of smoking mothers had significantly higher hair concentrations of nicotine and cotinine than infants of nonsmoking mothers.

Conclusions: Provides biochemical evidence that infants of passive smokers are at risk of detectable exposure to cigarette smoke. This reflects long-term systemic exposure to these toxins and perinatal risks.

Nursing Implications: This study points out the need for nurses to be actively involved in educating young women about the known hazards of smoking both when pregnant and after pregnancy. The results of this study need to be communicated to mothers as yet more scientific proof about the effect of the parent's smoking on the vulnerable infant.

The hope is that once cellular changes of the lung are identified, active therapy, as with β-carotene and other vitamin A compounds, may achieve a complete reversal of atypical cells for those patients at risk for the development of lung cancer. However, a recent, large-scale, randomized, double-blind, placebo-controlled, primary-prevention trial to determine whether daily supplementation with α-tocopherol, β-carotene, or both reduced lung cancer incidence showed that there was no reduction of this cancer. The dietary supplementation was taken by male smokers for 5 to 8 years (The Alpha-Tocopherol, Beta Carotene Cancer Prevention Study Group, 1994). Further chemoprevention studies are being proposed in an attempt to determine whether dietary supplementation will lower the incidence of lung cancer.

Nursing Role. Nurses have been instrumental in the implementation of (1) smoke-free legislation and the creation of smoke-free employment settings, (2) smoking cessation counseling, antismoking education, and structured smoking-cessation programs, (3) antismoking educational programs designed for employees in the employment setting and for children in school settings, and (4) research to determine nurses' smoking behaviors and attitudes toward smoking. The literature review documented that nurses were actively and assertively disseminating information on the disease potential of smoking in employment, educational, health-care, and community settings. Furthermore, nurses are increasingly acting as positive role models by refraining from smoking and by actively working at creating nonsmoking environments in both their employment and home settings (Janerich, Thompson, Varela et al., 1990).

Because research has clearly documented that attitudes of health professionals may influence patients to start or stop smoking, there has been extensive writing and research about the smoking habits of nurses and their smoking-related attitudes. Studies of the percentage of nurses who smoke have shown that the prevalence was lower than the prevalence reported in a national sample of adult females yet higher than that for some male health professionals (Burns, Stotts & Henderson, 1988; Gritz & Kanim, 1986; Johnston-Early, 1983). The National Clearinghouse for Smoking and Health surveyed nurses in 1976 and found that 39 per cent of the nurses smoked. These data contrast with the 1986 research conducted by several nurse researchers that reported smoking rates of 24.3 per cent among Minnesota registered nurses, 28 per cent among nurses in western New York (Wagner, 1985), and 19.5 per cent among oncology nurses in southern California.

The decline in smoking among health professionals is further verified in a 1991 study comparing the cigarette smoking among physicians, registered nurses, and licensed practical nurses. They reported that cigarette smoking had declined from 18.8 per cent to 3.3 per cent among physicians, from 31.7 per cent to 18.3 per cent among registered nurses, and from 37.1 per cent to 27.2 per cent among licensed practical nurses (Nelson et al., 1994).

It is encouraging that many researchers have found that the smoking cessation rate among registered nurses

is increasing (Burns et al., 1988; Casey, Haughey, Dittmar, O'Shea, & Brasure, 1989). In a comparison study of critical care nurses and medical-surgical nurses, DeMello, Hoffman, Wesmiller, & Zullo (1989) found that oncology clinical specialists had the lowest prevalence of cigarette smoking among the nursing groups. The importance of having more nurses stop smoking is based on research that has consistently shown that nurses who smoke are less likely to teach or positively influence patients who smoke (DeMello et al., 1989; Feldman & Richard, 1986; Gritz & Kanim, 1986).

A key step toward cancer control is to decrease tobacco use and prevent the initiation of tobacco use among youth. But preventing death and disease from tobacco use is not as simple as it sounds. The greatest threat to cancer death is tobacco use among youth. Approximately 28 per cent of high school students in the U.S. currently smoke, and 21 per cent of high school males use smokeless tobacco. The use of tobacco by youth has reached epidemic proportions and promises to exact a high price in disease, death, and dollars.

Smoking is not a passing phase for adolescents. Research indicates that most adolescents who regularly smoke are addicted to nicotine, and the majority continue to smoke as adults. Health problems caused by smoking are a function of the intensity and frequency of tobacco use, making early onset of smoking particularly tragic. The younger one begins to smoke, the more likely they are to smoke heavily as an adult and suffer serious health consequences.

How can nurses combat tobacco use among youth? Acting as advocates and role models, nurses can participate in education, clinical interventions, community programs, and implementation of public policies. *Healthy People 2000: National Health Promotion and Disease Prevention Objectives* offers these objectives related to tobacco and youth.

1. Decrease the initiation of cigarette smoking by youth.
2. Decrease the proportion of children who are regularly exposed to tobacco smoke at home.
3. Decrease smokeless tobacco use.
4. Establish tobacco-free environments and include tobacco use prevention in the curricula of all schools.
5. Enact comprehensive state laws that prohibit or restrict smoking in the workplace and enclosed public places.
6. Enforce state laws prohibiting the sale and distribution of tobacco products to youth.
7. Increase the number of states with plans to reduce tobacco use, especially among youth.
8. Eliminate or severely limit all forms of tobacco product advertising and promotion to which youth are likely to be exposed.
9. Increase the proportion of health care providers who routinely advise on tobacco cessation and provide assistance and follow-up for all of their tobacco-using patients.

Nurses must become ever more proactive in tobacco control among youth. Education, clinical interventions, community service, and public policy are ways nurses can contribute to Objectives 2000.

Teaching youth about tobacco is a special challenge for nurses. Research has shown that providing information about the health consequences of tobacco has little effect on youth. However, educational efforts emphasizing social influences, norms, and skills training such as assertiveness training are found to be effective. This approach focuses on the skills needed to interpret advertising and its impact on the thought processes of the young. Nurses can assist school teachers in developing and teaching a program that is appropriate for the ethnic culture of children and the ages of the children. Other activities are working with churches and synagogues to focus on youth tobacco counseling and education.

Nurses can initiate a tobacco intervention program for youth in the workplace setting and assist in tobacco counseling and education programs. Nurses must assess tobacco use in a youth health history and discuss the importance of avoiding tobacco by emphasizing cosmetic effects (stained teeth and fingernails, foul-smelling breath and clothes) and decreased physical endurance due to tobacco use. For youth who already use tobacco, nurses must provide tobacco cessation counseling, which includes setting a quit date and positive support when quitting. Time is the critical barrier to implementing prevention activities; seize the moment.

Nurses can work with community agencies and groups to determine tobacco control needs and concerns and to determine the level of services currently available to decrease tobacco use among youth and adults. Nurses must develop community relationships to work toward elimination of tobacco sponsorship of sporting events or tobacco billboards near schools or neighborhoods, especially in minority neighborhoods.

The purpose of public policy is to promote a smokeless environment. Most tobacco-free advocacy efforts have been state and federal level legislation. However, state and federal laws regarding tobacco control have met a tough barrier with the tobacco lobby and have been difficult to pass. Nurses must continue to be involved in state and national tobacco control issues and must make every effort to continually contact nationally and state-elected representatives. Nationwide, tremendous activity in tobacco-control public policy has been generated at the local level rather than at the state and federal levels, particularly in the area of public smoking. Local communities are in a position of making decisions regarding what policies to pursue and how to pursue them. Nurses need to be involved in these local decisions and take a leadership role in providing direction for public policy in their communities. Working with the school board, city counselpersons, and county officials will be necessary and will take all the communication and negotiation skills that the nurse has. Individually, nurses can make a difference and collectively, through collaboration, nurses can make an even larger impact!

Nurses have planned and implemented multiple educational approaches and used diverse settings to deliver antismoking messages. Troxler (1989) advocates having oncology nurses present smoking prevention programs in the junior high school setting, because they are perceived by the students as "experts." Knudsen, Schulman, Fowler, and Van Den Hoek (1984) described a smoking cessation program with patients who had non-small cell tumors surgically resected. They noted the physical and psychosocial benefits these patients experienced when they stopped smoking. "Stop-smoking education for the lung cancer patient may be used to reach another important group, his family and friends" (Knudsen et al., 1984, p. 33). Nurses are also increasingly focusing their research on the difficulties encountered by individuals attempting to stop smoking (Steuer & Wewers, 1989).

The advent of the transdermal nicotine patch system has been successful in helping some smokers quit. A study by Hurt et al. (1994) documented that nurses play an important role in assisting people who are using a nictone patch quit-smoking system. It was found that smoking cessation can be achieved using nicotine patch therapy *combined* with physician intervention, nurse counseling, follow-up, and relapse prevention. The nurse counseling occurred weekly either in person or via the phone.

Nurses in other countries have also been involved in designing antismoking educational campaigns, conducting individual smoking cessation counseling, and assisting government efforts to create nonsmoking environments. Bultz, Scott, & Taenzer (1988) described a successful smoking cessation clinic instituted at the Tom Baker Cancer Centre in Calgary, Canada. This smoking cessation clinic has had 700 participants since it was started 6 years ago. Eighty per cent of their graduates were not smoking at the 6-month follow-up visit, and 77 per cent were not smoking at the 1-year follow-up visit. They point out that "nurses and other health professionals who take up the challenge of leading similar programs can learn from their model" (Bultz et al., 1988). Their smoking cessation program includes teaching quitting behaviors as well as helping smokers adjust to and enjoy a nonsmoking lifestyle.

Shugg (1984) conducted a study of smoking habits and attitudes toward smoking in over 900 nurses in Tasmania, Australia. She reported many of the same findings in Australian nurses that have been documented in U.S. nurses: (1) nurses who smoked were less likely to encourage smokers to quit; (2) nurses who smoked were more likely to underestimate the effect of smoking as a cause in smoking-related ailments; and (3) nurses in the area of Australia had a smoking rate close to double that of Australian doctors.

Cahill (1980) of the Canadian Cancer Society described the role of five Industrial Cancer Education nurses in the province of Ontario. The Industrial Cancer Education nurses visit employment settings and present a short talk, film, and a smoking demonstration by "Smoking Sam" designed to demonstrate the amount of tar and nicotine accumulated from one cigarette. After the presentation, the nurse is available for private counseling with employees who have cancer-related concerns. This model has been successfully adopted in the United States and was reported by Mettlin, McCoy, Nuchereno, and Murphy (1980).

Grobbelaar (1990) advocates that nurses must "play a leading role in anti-smoking campaigns, and in the developing countries in the negotiation for legislation to regulate advertising." It is evident from the literature review that nurses both in the United States and in other countries have responded to the statement by the Surgeon General of the United States: "Cigarette smoking is the chief, single, avoidable cause of death in our society and the most important public health issue of our time." Nurses are involved in all aspects of helping the public to stop smoking and are actively working to create smoke-free environments at the local, regional, state, and national level (Mettlin et al., 1980).

COLORECTAL CANCER

Incidence. Cancers of the colon and rectum (colorectal) are diseases associated with economically developed countries. For example, the highest death rates occur in western Europe, New Zealand, and North America; the lowest death rates are in Africa, Asia, and most Latin American countries (Page & Asire, 1985). The countries with the lowest rates for gastric and esophageal cancers carry the highest rates for colorectal cancer and vice versa. It is estimated that 156,700 U.S. citizens will develop colorectal cancer in 1995, and 55,300 will die of the disease (Wingo et al., 1995).

When colorectal cancer is detected and treated in an early, localized stage, the 5-year survival rate is 84 per cent as compared with 56 per cent and 6 per cent with regional and distant metastasis, respectively (Hirayama, 1979). Therefore, early detection substantially alters the mortality rates in colorectal cancer. Colorectal cancers can develop in the intestinal tract from the cecum to the anus; most tumors occur in the descending colon, rectosigmoid area, and rectum (Leffall, 1981).

Risk Factors. Risk assessment is a crucial component of any screening modality (White, 1986b). There are two high-risk groups in the United States for the development of colorectal cancer: the elderly and the African-American population. The incidence of colorectal cancer rises sharply after 50 years of age, and incidence rates are equal for both sexes. The incidence of colorectal cancer begins to increase at 40 years of age and doubles at age 50 and each following decade until age 80, when the incidence stabilizes (Page & Asire, 1985). Survival rates and age at diagnosis of colorectal cancer have a definite relationship. Although 98 per cent of all colorectal cancers occur in individuals ≥40 years of age, the mortality rates are much higher in individuals ≤40, especially children (Messner, Gardner, & Webb, 1986). Tumors in the young tend to be more poorly differentiated and make possible a decreased number of potentially curative resections (Messner & Gardner, 1985).

Individual risk factors for the development of colorectal cancer include a family history of polyposis syndromes (familiar polyposis, Gardner's syndrome, Peutz-Jegher's syndrome, and juvenile polyposis), a history of chronic ulcerative colitis, cured colorectal cancer, genital cancer (for women), and adenomatous polyps, and individuals whose diets are high in total fat and low in dietary fiber (Messner & Gardner, 1985; Messner et al., 1986; Weinrich, Blesch, Dickson, Nussbaum, & Watson, 1989).

Individual risk factors also include having first-degree relatives with common colorectal cancer. This risk is greater if diagnosis was at an early age and is greater when other first-degree relatives are affected (St. John et al., 1993). Fuchs et al. (1994) did a prospective study of over 32,000 men and 87,000 women investigating the relationship of family history of colorectal and risk of developing cancer and reported the same type of association.

> ... the majority of people with a family history of colorectal cancer, particularly those who are 60 years or older, the excess risk of colorectal cancer is not large. Nevertheless, the increased risk among younger people with a family history supports the recommendation of the American Cancer Society that people with a family history of colorectal cancer undergo earlier screening (Fuchs et al., 1994, p. 1673).

Colorectal cancers begin as polyps that are benign for years and eventually degenerate to malignancy. This process is believed to take 25 years (Messner et al., 1986). Adenomatous polyps are present in 5 to 10 per cent of all individuals >45 years of age (Messner et al., 1986). Malignant degeneration of these polyps increases as the size of the polyp surpasses 0.5 cm. Sugarbaker, MacDonald, and Querllson (1982) list several arguments for an adenomatous polyp-to-cancer transition, including the following:

1. Patients who are kept polyp-free remain cancer free.
2. Incidence of cancer increases as number of polyps increases.
3. The peak age at which polyps are diagnosed precedes that for cancer by about approximately 5 years.
4. A similar distribution of polyps and cancer occurs within the large bowel. Not all colon polyps undergo malignant transformation, but the more polyps are allowed to grow for a longer time to larger size, the greater is the chance that cancer will develop from them.

Winawer et al. (1993) report that removing polyps via colonoscopy resulted in a lower-than-expected incidence of colorectal cancer. This study involved a large group of patients who had one or more adenomas of the colon or rectum removed and then were followed by periodic colonoscopy for an average of 5.9 years. During this period of time, the incidence of colorectal cancer was ascertained. Winawer et al. (1993) write that these results support the view that colorectal adenomas progress to adenocarcinomas. Table 16–4 shows recommended screening for colorectal cancer for low- and high-risk individuals.

Villous adenomas have a 40 to 50 per cent chance of undergoing malignant transformation (Simon,

TABLE 16–4. *Recommended Screening for Colorectal Cancer for Both Low-Risk and High-Risk Individuals*

RISK FACTOR	RISK OF DEVELOPING COLORECTAL CANCER	RECOMMENDED SCREENING
Asymptomatic persons not at high risk		Annual digital rectal examination from age 40; annual fecal occult blood test from age 50; and sigmoidoscopy beginning at age 50 to be repeated every 3 to 5 years after two consecutive annual normal examinations (see Box 16–1 for research study related to screening)
Family history of familial polyposis coli or Gardner's syndrome	Approaches 110% by 40 years of age	Biannual screening with fecal occult blood tests beginning at age 10 years, with annual flexible sigmoidoscopy beginning by age 15 years; at age 45 years, screening frequency may be relaxed if patient is asymptomatic
Cancer family syndrome	Risk in first-degree relative approaches 50%	Periodic colonoscopy beginning in the third decade of life, recommended every 3 years, and annual fecal occult blood testing
History of one or two first-degree relatives with colorectal cancer	Twofold to threefold increase in risk for colorectal cancer	Yearly fecal occult blood testing and periodic flexible sigmoidoscopy beginning at age 40 years
History of ulcerative colitis	After 30 years' duration, overall culmulative risk is 50%	Biannual screening colonoscopy beginning after 8 years of disease with frequency increased to annually after 15 years of disease
History of colorectal cancer or adenomatous polyps	Additional carcinomas found in 4 to 5% of patients with colorectal cancer	Periodic colonoscopic examination along with annual fecal occult blood testing for follow-up of all patients who have had either a cancer or a polyp detected
History of endometrial, ovarian, or breast cancer	Twofold increase in risk for colorectal cancer	Perodic screening sigmoidoscopy and annual fecal occult blood testing

(Data from DeCosse, 1988; Selby & Friedman, 1989; Vessey, 1985.)

1985). Villous polyps may produce mucus in the stool, but there are often no warning signs until malignant transformation occurs. This points to the need for detection of the presence of these polyps and the removal before transformation occurs (Messner et al., 1986).

Prevention. Primary prevention involves the modification of diet. The ACS has recommended (1) eating a diet low in fat (<30 per cent of total caloric intake) that includes a variety of fruits and vegetables on a daily basis; (2) increasing the intake of high-fiber foods; (3) limiting alcoholic beverages and salt-cured nitrite-cured foods; and (4) avoiding obesity (The Work Study Group on Diet, Nutrition, and Cancer, 1991). Having a polypectomy also decreases the risk of malignant transformation and the development of colorectal cancer (Update of ACS guidelines, 1989).

Research into the etiology and prevention of cancer has been an important branch of research for several decades. In the course of this research, epidemiologists have reported large differences in cancer incidence and mortality among countries and have suggested that these differences are largely due to environmental factors. Some leading scientists and national advisory bodies have proposed that dietary patterns are among the important environmental determinants of human cancer (Birdsell, 1986). Cancer patterns in migrating populations provided further compelling data. Japanese in Japan have a tenfold higher mortality rate from stomach cancer than do Americans in the United States, but Japanese who have migrated to Hawaii or the United States mainland and their succeeding generations have progressively lowered mortality rates from stomach cancer.

Dietary factors are associated with cancers of the gastrointestinal tract (esophagus, stomach, colon, rectum, pancreas, and liver) and some sex- and hormone-specific sites (breast, prostate, ovaries, and endometrium). The dietary components that have been implicated in the development of cancer are summarized in Table 16–5. Table 16–6 lists the National Institutes of Health's suggestions on how to increase fiber and reduce fat in the daily diet.

Poor dietary practices including inadequate intake of fiber and important micronutrients are thought by some scientists to be as significant as tobacco smoking in causing cancer. About 27 per cent of all cancer deaths are caused by lung cancer; the vast majority caused by smoking. Another 30 per cent of all cancer deaths are due to cancer of the colon-rectum, breast, and prostate. For these three cancers, dietary practices are implicated as risk factors. The consensus of investigators is that as much as 25 to 35 per cent of cancer mortality is related to dietary factors (Greenwald & Sondek, 1986). Estimates of risk from diet range from 10 to 70 per cent. These estimates are based on a large number of studies, although the exact magnitude of the association and the biologic mechanisms involved are uncertain. As Weinhouse (1986) points out, much of the information on the relationship between diet and development of cancer is inferential. Although convincing associations have been found between cancer and

TABLE 16–5. *Dietary Components and Their Known or Suspected Relationship to Cancer*

DIETARY COMPONENT	ANATOMIC SITE AFFECTED	MECHANISM	DISCUSSION	YEAR 2000 DIETARY OBJECTIVES
Fat	Breast, colon, endometrium, and prostate cancers associated with diets high in fat.	May act as promoter: exact mechanism unknown.	Dietary polyunsaturated vegetable oils promote tumorigenesis in animals, saturated fats and polyunsaturated fish oils either have little effect or are inhibitory. Total fat intake accounts for 40% of total calories in U.S. diet compared with only 20% in Japanese diet.	Per capita daily consumption of fat will decrease from 40 to 25% or less of total calories.
Fiber	Colon cancer associated with diets low in fiber.	Production of short-chain fatty acids (products of fiber fermentation), regulation of energy intake, dilution of colonic contents, and absorption of bile acids decreases production of mutagens in stool.	No consistent thread of evidence through either human or experimental data that confers an unequivocally protective role on fiber in general or some specific fiber or fiber component in particular (Kritchevsky, 1986). Inverse association between eating vegetables and occurance of colon cancer. U.S. diet includes only 15 to 20 g of fiber a day: 25 to 30 g a day is recommended.	Per capita consumption of fiber from grains, fruits, and vegetables will increase from 8 to 12 g per day to 20 to 30 g per day.
Vitamin C (ascorbic acid)	Inverse association between fresh fruit/vegetable consumption and stomach and esophagus cancer.	Animal studies show vitamin C can inhibit formation of carcinogenic *N*-nitroso compounds from ingested nitrates. Ascorbic acid plays key role in maintenance of immune system.		
Vitamin E		Blocks formation of carcinogenic nitroso compounds. Laboratory studies show may inhibit tumorigenesis.	No evidence that megadoses protect individuals against cancer. Vitamin E, a fat-soluble vitamin, is potentially toxic in high doses.	
Vitamin A*	Inverse association between dietary vitamin A or carotenoids and cancers of the oral cavity, urinary bladder, pharynx, larynx, and lung.	Carotenoids have a potent antioxidant effect and reduce cancer risk by preventing tissue damage due to oxidation. Retinoids have potent hormone-like effects on cell growth and differentiation: in vitro studies show they can reverse keratinization and other premalignant changes.	Fat-soluble, stored in liver, and toxic in high doses.	
Selenium	Inverse correlation between selenium intake and cancer, specifically of the head and neck.	May be mediated through an increase in the activity of the selenium-dependent enzyme glutathione peroxidase.	Selenium in high doses is toxic.	
Cured, pickled, and smoked foods	Inverse relationship between pickled, cured, and smoked foods and stomach cancer.	Formation of nitrosamines occurs in vitro during curing processes and has been demonstrated to occur in animals in vivo. Evidence of carcinogenicity of nitrosamines is not conclusive.	Nitrates and nitrites are used as preservatives in many foods as curing agents. Smoking and pickling foods produce higher levels of polycyclic aromatic hydrocarbons and *N*-nitroso compounds. Cyclic aromatic hydrocarbons are mutagenic, carcinogenic, or both. Fish and beef cooked at high temperatures produced mutagenic activity from the breakdown products of proteins and amino acids. Formed only with temperatures of 250° C or greater.	Minimize consumption of foods preserved by salt curing (including salt pickling or smoking). Avoid frying and high-temperature cooking.
Protein	Dietary protein associated with breast, endometrium, prostate, colon, rectum, pancreas, and kidney cancers.	Laboratory studies with animals have demonstrated carcinogenesis can be suppressed by a dietary level of protein at or below the minimum required for optimal growth. Chemically induced carcinogenesis seems to be enhanced as protein intake is increased up to 2 or 3 times the normal requirement.	Because there is a strong correlation between intake of fat and protein in the Western diet, it is difficult to separate protein from fat as an independent cancer risk factor.	

Carotenoids are provitamins or natural precursors of vitamin A. *Retinoids,* or preformed vitamin A, occur only in foods of animal origin.
(Data from Carroll, Braden, Bell, & Kalamegham, 1986; DeVita, 1985; Greenwald, 1985; Greenwald, Sondik, & Lynch, 1986; Hennekens, Mayrent, & Willett, 1986; Kritchevsky, 1986; Newell, 1985; Page & Asire, 1985; Palmer, 1986).

TABLE 16–6. *Suggestions to Increase Fiber and Reduce Fat in the Daily Diet*

To *increase* dietary fiber, select the following:	Select the following *less often:*
1. Bakery products such as bran muffins, whole-wheat crackers, rye, bagels, and pumpernickel 2. Breakfast cereals such as shredded wheat, whole-grain or whole-wheat flake cereals 3. Foods made with whole-grain flours such as waffles and pancakes 4. All fruits and vegetables with the skins on 5. All dried peas and beans	1. Refined bakery and snack foods such as croissants, chips, and pastries
To *decrease* fat, select the following: 1. Lower fat, poultry, fish, and meat (water-packed canned fish, chicken, and turkey) 2. Beef, veal, lamb, and pork cuts trimmed of all fat and no visible fat in meat 3. Low-fat or skim milk dairy products (mozzarella, ricotta, sherbet, low-fat yogurt) 4. Peas and beans 5. "Diet" and low-fat salad dressings and low-fat margarine 6. Prepare food by baking, oven broiling, boiling, stewing, poaching, stir frying, simmering, and steaming	Select the following *less often:* 1. Tuna packed in oil, poultry with skin, duck, and goose 2. Luncheon meats 3. Beef, veal, lamb, and pork with fat and marbling 4. Nuts and seeds 5. Full-fat dairy products (butter, sweet cream, sour cream) 6. Hard cheeses, full-fat soft cheeses such as cream cheese, and ice cream 7. Mayonnaise, gravies, butter sauces over vegetables, and salad oils 8. Preparing food by deep-fat frying: adding cream or butter to vegetables 9. Snack and bakery foods such as doughnuts, pies, cakes, cookies, brownies, chips, granola, and croissants

(From U.S. Department of Health and Human Services. [1985]. *Diet, nutrition and cancer prevention: A guide to food choices* [NIH Publication No. 85–2711]. Washington, DC: U.S. Government Printing Office. This is an excellent publication for lay people that offers practical advice on following a cancer-prevention diet.

dietary practices throughout the world, association is not necessarily equatable with causation.

The delineation of dietary risk factors is not simple. Creasey (1985, p. 6) details some of the reasons, including the following:

1. Carcinogenesis is a multistage process that takes a long time to complete; initiating events may have occurred decades before the cancer appears
2. Conclusions from dietary surveys involving individuals who have cancer are misleading, because the disease changes dietary habits.
3. Prospective studies are rare, and blind-double-blind experiments used in typical clinical trials are impossible to perform.

4. The elevated incidence of a cancer may be the result of two or more factors in combination rather than one alone.
5. The type of role played by dietary factors may affect the ease with which an association can be demonstrated.

Chemoprevention, another approach to primary prevention, involves the use of specific pharmacologic agents to inhibit carcinogenesis. Giovannucci, Rimm, Stampfer, Colditz, and Ascherio (1994) report data suggesting that regular aspirin use may decrease the incidence of disease and death from colorectal cancer. They found that regular use (≥2 times per week) was associated with a decreased risk for colorectal cancer and that consistent aspirin use further reduced the risk.

Early Detection. The ACS guidelines for the detection of colorectal cancer for the average-risk asymptomatic individuals includes annual digital rectal examination beginning at age 40 years, annual stool blood tests beginning at age 50, and sigmoidoscopy every 3 to 5 years beginning at age 50 (American Cancer Society, 1989). The digital rectal examination can detect 12 to 15 per cent of colorectal cancers (Leffall, 1981). Serial guaiac testing provides a safe, convenient, cost-effective means of detecting colonic lesions in the asymptomatic individual. Three separate specimens are recommended while the individual adheres to a meat-free, high-residue diet for 24 hours before the first stool specimen is obtained and during the next 3 days of specimen collection (Simon, 1985).

Sigmoidoscopy is recommended for high-risk individuals at more frequent intervals and must be initiated at an earlier age than for individuals with average risk. In high-risk individuals, sigmoidoscopy should begin 5 years before the youngest family member was diagnosed with colorectal cancer (Lindberg, 1987).

Mandel et al. (1994) reported a 33 per cent reduction in mortality from colorectal cancer in people who were offered annual occult-blood testing with *rehydrated slides* and colonoscopic follow-up in individuals with positive test results. This result was accompanied by a shift to the detection of earlier stage cancers and improved survival in those in whom cancer developed as compared with the control group (Mandel et al., 1994). However, controversy surrounds the results of this prospective, randomized trial. Lang and Ransohoff (1994) argue that one third to one half of the mortality reduction observed from Fecal Occult Blood testing (FOBT) screening in the Minnesota study conducted by Mandel et al. may be attributable to chance selection for colonoscopy.

There is ongoing debate about recommendations involving periodic colonoscopic surveillance. Specifically Ransohoff, Lang, and Kuo (1991) question the recommendation that patients who have had an adenomatous colon polyp removed have periodic colonscopic surveillance at fixed and regular intervals. They argue that routinely surveying persons who had a single small adenoma removed may be excessively costly and not indicated.

It is anticipated that in the future, genetic testing of stools may be used to detect neoplasia by identifying mutated genes, and genomic DNA may be studied in blood to identify inherited susceptiblity (Winawer, 1993). It is known that colorectal tumors shed large numbers of neoplastic cells into the colonic lumen.

> About 40 per cent of colorectal carcinomas and adenomas over 1 cm in diameter carry K-ras mutations, and the data suggest that such mutations arise early in colorectal carcinogenesis. Consequently, the technique* might be applicable to screening for colorectal tumors in symptom-free individuals, especially since both right and left colonic lesions were detectable (Screening for colorectal cancer by stool DNA analysis, 1992, p. 1141).

Nursing Role. Colorectal screening has been found to be beneficial in identifying lesions in a localized stage of the disease process. Occupational health nurses or cancer education nurses (CENs) have been successful in providing occupationally based programs of cancer health education. For example, Messner and Gardner (1985) realized an 80 per cent compliance rate in serial guaiac stool screening in the work setting. The authors attribute this high compliance to the close, therapeutic relationship established by these nurses with the clients and their families.

Several authors have addressed the issues of detection in the elderly and the special educational and physiologic considerations in this population (Frank-Stromborg, 1986; Messner & Gardner, 1985; Stromborg, 1982). It has been demonstrated that the elderly require teaching about screening and dietary modifications and require assistance with screening. The elderly have traditionally used health-care professionals only in times of illness and have not been taught the benefits of preventative care. Therefore, an important role for nurses is to be involved in planning and implementing educational programs for elderly groups that present the benefits of cancer prevention and early detection.

Incidence and mortality rates are higher and survival rates lower for African-Americans than for whites. Frank-Stromborg, Johnson, and McCorkle (1987) developed workshops for African-American nurses that included information about cancer epidemiology in African-American U.S. citizens, cultural attitudes toward cancer, and early detection techniques for this population. Continuation of these workshops designed specifically for African-American nurses throughout the United States and related research by Olsen and Frank-Stromborg (1991b) documented the positive impact of the educational intervention on the African-American community. Many of the nurses who attended the workshops have planned, implemented, and evaluated community-based cancer prevention and early detection programs, they have disseminated information from the workshops back to the communities in which they live. The hope is that ultimately the activities of these nurses will lower the incidence rates and increase the survival rates among African-American U.S. citizens.

Mitchell-Beren, Dodds, Choi, and Waskerwitz (1989) attempted to influence the incidence of colorectal cancer in the African-American population by implementing a prevention, screening, and evaluation program in community churches. Volunteer nurses from the Michigan Black Nurses' Association presented the educational component of the program in 20 community churches. These authors found positive dietary changes after the program. In addition, participants increased their fiber intake, decreased their consumption of fat and alcohol, and decreased smoking. However, there was a low response to the serial stool testing required for screening. The authors attributed the low response rate to the dietary restrictions necessary for the testing. These authors contend that church-based educational programs are both beneficial and effective in an African-American population.

Dietary habits develop early in life, during adolescence, and possibly earlier. Krohner, McBurney, and Wadelin (1988) found few studies or programs that focused on the prevention of colon cancer by educating children about diet during their formative years. Results of their survey of the health beliefs about colon cancer and dietary practices of parents and their sixth, seventh, and eigth grade children lead them to suggest that oncology nurses need to be involved in the development of cancer prevention curriculum for adolescents. This is obviously an area that deserves much more research and educational pursuits if colorectal cancer is to be eradicated.

Several nurses have been involved in programs designed specifically for high-risk colorectal patients (Beck, Breckenridge-Potterf et al, 1988; Fitzsimmons, Conway, Madsen, Lappe, & Coody, 1989; Fitzsimmons, Kriegler, Shea, & Lynch, 1987; Harbora & Kamitoma, 1985; Lappe & Fitzsimmons, 1988; Tyner & Loney, 1989). Lappe and Fitzsimmons (1988) conducted a research study of compliance with prescribed cancer surveillance measures with individuals who were members of cancer-prone families. They used their findings to develop more effective interventions to increase compliance with prescribed cancer surveillance measures. Fitzsimmons et al. (1989) noted that the nurse working with high-risk families is in a "pivotal role by teaching surveillance and early detection measures, assisting in role-playing situations, explaining hereditary cancer risk factors, supporting families through the ambivalence of a diagnosis of a hereditary disease, and by fostering positive coping behaviors in general" (Fitzsimmons et al., 1989).

Harbora and Kamitoma (1985), two nurses working with a medical oncologist and an endoscopist, investigated a colonoscopy program designed to detect second primaries in colorectal patients after curative surgery. Nurses were responsible for "the initial presentation of the study and the coordination between various nursing departments, medical personnel and participants to ensure the smooth and efficient running of the program" (Harbora & Kamitoma, 1985).

Several institutions in the United States provide educational programs that train nurses to perform sigmoidoscopy (Rosevelt & Frankl, 1984; Schroy, Wig-

---

*Polymerase chain reaction techniques were used to detect Kirsten ras oncogene mutations in DNA purified from stool.

gins, Winawer, Diaz, & Lightdale, 1988; Spencer & Ready, 1977). Rosevelt and Frankl (1984) discussed the program at the Southern California Permanent Health Plan for nurse practitioners. This program consisted of 3 half-days per week for a period of 1 month. The nurse practitioners were taught the use of a 60-cm fiberoptic sigmoidoscope. A research study by Schroy et al. (1988) compared the diagnosis of nurse practitioners performing 40-cm videosigmoidoscopy with the videotape review by physician endoscopists. The nurse practitioners performed the sigmoidoscopy at Memorial Sloan-Kettering Cancer Center, New York. "Near excellent concordance (k = 0.72) was observed between the nurse practitioner's findings and those of the physician. Using the physician's review as the standard, overall sensitivity and specificity of the nurse practitioner's examinations were 75 per cent and 94 per cent, respectively" (Schroy et al., 1988).

Beck et al. (1988) participated in a multidisciplinary program of targeted prevention in Utah. In this program using the public school system, a family risk profile questionnaire was developed for Utah high school students taking health science classes. A program was developed where the students and their families complete the questionnaire and return it to the school. The questionnaire data are analyzed, and the results regarding risk for disease are mailed to consenting families. High-risk families (high risk for heart disease, cancer, stroke, diabetes) are referred to their local health departments for follow-up by a professional nurse. The authors note that targeting families at risk is a cost-effective approach to cancer prevention and that their Family High-Risk Program provides an example of an innovative way for nurses to participate in targeted cancer prevention (Beck et al., 1988).

Nurses have been involved in planning, implementing, and evaluating multiple, creative, and nontraditional community-wide educational and screening programs for colorectal cancer (Post-White, Herzan, & Drew, 1988; Wilkes & Bersani, 1983). For instance, the Metro Minnesota ONS chapter participated in public education health fairs held at seven sites that attracted 700 people (Post-White et al., 1988). Their role was to educate the public about how to adopt a cancer prevention diet. Their evaluation of the project indicated that the majority of individuals who responded to their survey (38 per cent response rate) had made dietary changes in the 2 weeks after the health fair. The nurses at the Department of Cancer Control and Epidemiology of Roswell Park Memorial Institute working with the Erie County Unit of the ACS distributed Guaiac or Hemoccult II R Test kits at five shopping malls over a 3-day period and had 3822 kits returned (a 48 per cent return rate) (Wilkes & Bersani, 1983). One hundred seven of the returned slides were positive (2.8 per cent). Follow-up information was available on 91 persons, and 72 had some evidence of pathology, five of which were colorectal cancers.

This review has shown that nurses are actively involved in multiple areas of primary and secondary prevention of colorectal cancer. They are educating individuals in the dietary modifications necessary to decrease the incidence of this cancer. Nurses are also encouraging individuals to follow the guidelines established by the ACS through community-based, creative, nontraditional educational offerings. Furthermore, they are educating individuals about serial guaiac testing, sigmoidoscopy, and the rationale for digital rectal examinations. In selected institutions in the United States, nurses and nurse practitioners are performing fiberoptic sigmoidoscopy. Research documents that specially trained nurses performing fiberoptic sigmoidoscopy has significantly expanded the number of elderly people who could be screened (Spencer & Ready, 1977). The literature documents that nurses are involved with individuals from families at increased risk for development of colorectal cancer through specialized clinics and programs. Research conducted by nurses with high-risk populations have found that the needs of these individuals are diverse and the psychosocial implications are far-reaching (Coody, 1987).

TESTICULAR CANCER

Incidence. Testicular cancer is a rare form of cancer, accounting for only 1 per cent of all cancers in males (Frank, Keys, & McCune, 1983); however, it is the most common neoplasm found in white males between the ages of 15 and 24 years (Einhorn et al., 1982). Recently, there has been a dramatic increase in the incidence of testicular cancer but a downward trend in death rates, which is probably due to the advances in testicular cancer management (Einhorn et al., 1982). In 1995, 7100 males are estimated to have been diagnosed with this cancer, while only 370 deaths are projected (Wingo et al., 1995).

There are four major types of testicular neoplasms, the most common being seminomas, which account for 40 per cent of testicular cancer (Richie, 1993). Seminomas are derived from the epithelial cells that line the seminiferous tubules. Seminomas are generally the least aggressive and most treatable of testicular tumors. Seminomas are rarely diagnosed before age 16 years and have a peak incidence early in the fourth decade (Culp, Boatman, & Wilson, 1973). Fifteen to 20 per cent of testicular tumors are embryonal carcinomas (Rubin & Bakemeier, 1978). These tumors tend to be more aggressive and metastasize early in the disease process (Rubin & Bakemeier, 1978). They occur most frequently in males 20 to 26 years of age (Pierce & Abell, 1970). Teratocarcinomas account for 20 to 25 per cent of testicular neoplasms and are equally as aggressive as embryonal carcinomas (Rubin & Bakemeier, 1978). Teratocarcinomas are composed of several embryonic cell types believed to persist throughout childhood and young adulthood. The frequency of this tumor is equal during the first 6 decades of male life. The most aggressive and lethal testicular tumor is the choriocarcinoma, which fortunately represents only 1 per cent of testicular neoplasms (Rubin & Bakemeier, 1978). This cell type mimics cells found in the uterus during pregnancy and is most frequently observed in the 30- to 40-year old group (Rubin & Bakemeier, 1978). Fortunately 5-year survival rates for all testicular cancers is 88 per cent, and if localized the rate rises to 96 per cent. These statistics demonstrate the benefits of early detection of testicular tumors.

Risk Factors. There is a fourfold increase in the incidence of testicular cancer in white males as compared with African-American or Asian males 15 to 40 years of age (Einhorn et al., 1982). The most significant predisposing factor for testicular cancer is cryptorchidism (Einhorn et al., 1982; Frank et al., 1983). The estimates for this increased risk range from five to 48 times that of normally descended testicles. If the testes fail to descend or descend after the age of 6 years, either surgically or of their own accord, the chance of developing testicular cancer is 11 to 45 per cent (Rubin & Bakemeier, 1978). Other risk factors are thought to include hereditary predisposition, inguinal hernias, congenital anomalies of the genitourinary tract, atrophy of testes related to viral infections (e.g., mumps), extra hormones, estrogen or progesterone, maternal ingestion of diethylstilbestrol during pregnancy, high social economic status, and trauma (Einhorn et al., 1982; Frank et al., 1983; Rubin & Bakemeier, 1978). In mothers exposed to diethylstilbestrol (DES), there is a two-and-one half- to fivefold increase in the risk of testicular cancer in the son (Gerchufsky, 1995). There has been uncertainty as to whether trauma draws attention to the tumor or precedes the tumor (Marty & McDermott, 1983); however, urologists presently believe that trauma does not contribute to testicular cancer (Gerchufsky, 1995).

Prevention. Surgical correction of cryptorchidism is the only preventative practice known to reduce the risk of testicular cancer. Encouraging vaccination in the prevention of mumps would also reduce risk; otherwise, the risk factors for testicular cancer are beyond human control; therefore, early detection is the key.

Early Detection. A thorough assessment should include questions to elicit any subjective symptomatology and risk factors for testicular cancer. Testicular cancer signs and symptoms include (1) firm, nontender mass on the front or side of the testicle, (2) dragging sensation in the groin, (3) heavy feeling in the testicle, (4) accumulation of fluid or blood in the scrotal sac, and (5) pain in an advanced stage of the disease (Carlin, 1986; Frank et al., 1983; Williams, 1981). It is advocated that all men 15 to 50 years of age be taught to perform monthly testicular self-examination (TSE). All physical examinations should include an assessment of the testes. Transillumination is advisable for any testicular swelling and is helpful in distinguishing cystic from solid masses. Testicular cancer rarely transilluminates light (Williams, 1981).

Nursing Role. The best defense against testicular cancer is a well-educated male population that practices TSE and understands the importance of seeking medical attention when a lump is discovered. Authorities advocate that education about testicular cancer and TSE begin in physical education classes in grammar schools or in activities involved with sports (Conklin, Klint, Morway, Sawyer, & Shephard, 1978; Marty & McDermott, 1983). Nurses have conducted research on the effectiveness and feasibility of incorporating TSE

into high school and college curriculums (Conklin et al., 1978; Marty & McDermott, 1983; Rudolf & Quinn, 1988; Stack, 1979). For instance, Stack (1979) developed a plan and teaching tool that would involve educators and could be used to teach high school students about testicular cancer. Rudolf and Quinn (1988) conducted a quasiexperimental study of knowledge of testicular cancer before and after a nursing educational program. They found that the college men in the study were lacking in knowledge about testicular cancer and TSE and that there was a significant increase in knowledge and practice of performing TSE after the nursing program. Rudolf and Quinn (1988) also demonstrated the effectiveness of a testicular educational program in terms of increasing the practice of TSE; 63 per cent of the college men started this self-examination technique after attending the program.

Several nurse researchers have investigated the knowledge level and testicular self-examination practices of men at risk for this cancer (Fraser, 1983; Reno, 1988; Rudolf & Quinn, 1988). Fraser (1983) found that the men from five families at high risk for testicular cancer knew little about their increased risk or how or why to do TSE. Because of the frequent findings that men generally know little about testicular cancer and how to do TSE, many feel TSE has not received the exposure that breast self-examination has received. This is perceived by some as an injustice to men (Goldering, 1986; Trevelyan, 1989). In Blesch's study of 233 professional men, 61 per cent showed moderate knowledge of testicular cancer, and 31 per cent knew about TSE. Only 9.5 per cent practiced TSE (Blesch, 1986).

Lack of knowledge about TSE is not limited to lay individuals. Stanford (1987) conducted a research study in England and found that 64.5 per cent of the nurses surveyed did not remember being taught TSE at their schools of nursing. The sample was composed of 60 nurses at a Sussex hospital. In addition, few of the nurses knew the risk factors associated with testicular cancer. Although two thirds of the nurses saw teaching TSE as part of their role, very few had ever taught it. Stanford (1987) wrote that female nurses who are concerned about embarrassing the patient (or being embarrassed themselves) should offer the patient the choice of discussing TSE with a nurse of either sex. Warren and Pohl (1990), in a study of nurse practitioners in Michigan, found that nurses were not using the opportunities that they had with male patients to teach TSE. Conroy (1986) surveyed unit nurses in a large Chicago research hospital and found that few of the nurses knew about testicular cancer or taught TSE to patients. Inservices and assigned readings were given on TSE and follow-up showed that the educational intervention for the nurses increased both the number of patients they assessed in terms of teaching them TSE and the number of men taught this self-examination practice.

This review has shown that there is a need for nurses to educate themselves, their colleagues, and their patients about testicular cancer and TSE. The major deterrent to early detection and treatment is young men's lack of knowledge of the great danger of testicular cancer and the lack of awareness of the need for regular self-examination. Nurses who work in the military, in occupational health settings, in physicians' offices, and in educational settings are in ideal clinical settings for teaching TSE and providing education that will dispel the myths that contribute to delay once a testicular lump is found (White, 1986). There is a need to include TSE techniques in health education classes, just as breast self-examination is now routinely included in these classes. Nurse researchers have shown that educational interventions are successful in increasing both knowledge about this cancer and practice of TSE.

ORAL CANCER

Incidence. In 1995, there will be an estimated 28,150 new cases of oral cancer (Wingo et al., 1995). Cancers of the oral cavity include cancers of the mouth, pharynx, tongue, and lip. Oral cancer is prevalent in men between the ages of 50 and 70 years (Mashberg & Samit, 1989).

Internationally, India has one of the highest rates for oral cancer. In Bombay, 55 per cent of the cancers in men and 25 per cent in women are in the oral cavity and pharynx (Sankaranarayanan, Duffy, Day, Nair, & Padmakumary, 1989). A comparison with the incidence of oral cancer in India and England illustrates the high rate of this cancer in India. The rate for men in India is 10.5 per 100,000 compared with 4.9 per 100,000 for men in England and 7.9 per 100,000 for women in India and 3.0 per 100,000 for women in Oxford, England (Jayant & Ycole, 1987, Sanghvi, 1981).

Risk Factors. Risk increases with age and is associated primarily with the use of tobacco and alcohol. The high rate of oral cancers in India are primarily attributed to the use of tobacco. Specifically in India, high-risk individuals tend to engage in either Bidi smoking (Bidi is a local cigarette manufactured by wrapping coarse tobacco dust in a dried temburni leaf), Hookah smoking (a smoking practice started in India at the end of sixteenth century; tobacco is seasoned by mixing it with molasses and the smoke is passed through water), or pan-tobacco-chewing (a mixture of fresh betel leaf smeared with aqueous lime and sliced dry or fresh arecanut) (Gray, 1985; Jayant & Ycole, 1987). Although not as prevalent as cigarette smoking and drinking, the habitual use of cigars, pipes, and chewing tobacco or snuff does contribute to the frequency of the disease (Winn, 1988).

Other risk factors attributed to the development of oral cancer are chronic irritation from broken or decayed teeth, long-term occupational exposure to the sun (such as experienced by ranchers, fishermen, and farmers), and general dietary deficiencies (Frank-Stromborg, 1991).

The majority of oral cancers cause no symptoms in their early stages; however, the initial signs are an oral lesion and local discomfort. Oral lesions that merit a physician's attention because they may be premalignant are leukoplakia (white patch) and erythroplasia (granular, red lesion). Any findings of lesions, swelling, ulceration, areas of tenderness or bleeding, abnormal textures, and limited motion of the tongue should cause suspicion of oral cancer. Marked cervical adenopathy may also suggest oral cancer.

Early Detection. Detection of these cancers at an early stage (<1 cm in diameter) provides a high cure rate. Unfortunately, 60 per cent of these cancers are at an advanced stage when they are discovered (Mashberg & Samit, 1989). Systematic examination of the oral cavity and biopsy are the primary method for early detection.

Prevention. The prevention of oral cancer is best accomplished by the avoidance of smoking, intake of alcohol, avoidance of chewing tobacco, and health maintenance of the teeth or dental appliances (e.g., dentures, bridges).

Nursing Roles. A review of 13 years of the abstracts submitted to the Oncology Nursing Society (ONS) for presentation at the Annual ONS Congress showed only two abstracts related to the prevention and early detection of oral cancer. Both abstracts dealt with research conducted by nurses in the area of oral cancer prevention and early detection.

Klatt-Ellis (1988) surveyed high school students, grades 9 to 12, to determine their usage and knowledge of the health implications of smokeless tobacco. Her findings showed a heavy usage of smokeless tobacco among boys (37 per cent) and the need for more surveys of this type in high schools in different geographic areas. "Information gleaned from an assessment study such as this can guide educational programming in the high-school setting" (Klatt-Ellis, 1988).

A similar type of research approach was taken by Schulmeister (1986). In collaboration with a dentist, 200 adults from the dental practice were surveyed about the symptoms of oral cancer and related risk factors. Data showed widespread misconceptions about the early symptoms of oral cancer and total lack of knowledge about conducting oral self-assessments. When given a pamphlet explaining how to conduct oral self-assessment, the majority of these adults stated they would probably not do it because "sores are so common." These findings led Schulmeister to advocate that "teaching, screening and detecting oral cancer by oncology nurses is critically needed" (1986).

White (1983, 1986), White, Cornelius, Judkins, and Patterson (1978), Frank-Stromborg (1986, 1991), and Frank-Stromborg and Cohen (1990) have published extensively in the area of the nurse's role in primary and secondary prevention of cancer and propose a multiplicity of roles related to oral cancer for nurses. Nurses should (1) routinely obtain information from patients regarding their risk factors for oral cancer, (2) when appropriate, conduct an oral assessment using the physical assessment techniques of inspection and palpation, (3) teach all high-risk individuals oral self-assessment and emphasize the importance of this self-examination technique, (4) stress the relationship of tobacco and alcohol to the development of oral cancer, and (5) make community referrals to assist high-risk individuals who are interested in stopping use of tobacco, decreasing alcohol intake, or both.

The literature review documented that nurses who were involved in the prevention and early detection of oral cancer tended to be functioning in ambulatory settings exclusively devoted to screening for cancer (Nelson-Manen & Krebs, 1991; O'Rourke, Gypson, & Weitberg, 1986; Warren & Pohl, 1990). Nurses in traditional settings (e.g., staff nursing, public health nursing, occupational nursing) do not appear to be using available opportunities to conduct risk assessments and oral examinations or to be providing instruction in oral self-assessment and the relationship between risk factors and the development of oral cancer.

GASTRIC CANCER

Incidence. Gastric carcinoma has been declining in incidence in developing countries over the past several decades. During the 1930s it was the leading cause of cancer-related deaths among men in the United States and was the third leading cause of cancer-related deaths in women. Over the last 50 years, the incidence and mortality in the United States has decreased by 70 per cent for men and 80 per cent for women. Although gastric cancer has decreased dramatically, it still remains one of the leading causes of death (ranking fifth) in older men (55 to 74 years of age) (Bongiorno, 1988; Charnley, Tannenbaum & Correa, 1982). The American Cancer Society (ACS) estimated that for 1995 there will be a total of 22,800 new cases and 14,700 deaths a year (Wingo et al., 1995). Of the total estimated new cases, 14,000 are projected to occur in men and 8800 in women; of the total 14,700 estimated deaths, 8800 are projected to occur in men and 5900 in women.

In stark contrast to the decreasing incidence of stomach cancer in westernized countries, gastric cancer in Japan, Singapore, China, the former Soviet Republics, Israel, Finland, Colombia, and Chile ranks foremost among all cancers (Charnley et al., 1982). Although migrants from high-risk areas generally retain a higher incidence of gastric cancer than the indigent population when living in a low-risk area, their children experience the lower incidence of the adopted country. It is hypothesized that the risk of developing gastric cancer may be determined by the environment in the first two decades of life (Mayer, 1988). See Table 16–7 for the international range of incidence for common cancers.

Risk Factors. The risk factors for gastric cancer include socioeconomic status, physical changes in the mucosa of the stomach, and genetic and environmental factors. Men are twice as likely as women to develop stomach cancer, with 60 per cent of cases occurring in persons over 65 years of age (Nomura, 1982). The incidence is highest in nonwhites and those in the lower socioeconomic strata. Persons with type A blood have a 10 per cent increased risk. Environmental factors include phenol exposure, high sodium intake, cigarette smoking, and high alcohol intake. Several stomach conditions such as pernicious anemia, atrophic gastritis, gastric ulcer, surgery for benign gastric disease, and intestinal metaplasia are also known risk factors (Mikulin & Hardcastle, 1987).

Although gastric cancer tends to be asymptomatic in its early stage, there are some symptoms that are

TABLE 16–7 *International Range of Incidence for Common Cancers*

SITE OF ORIGIN OF CANCER	HIGH-INCIDENCE AREA	LOW-INCIDENCE AREA
Skin (chiefly nonmelanoma)	Australia, Queensland	India, Bombay
Esophagus	Iran, northeast section	Nigeria
Lungs and bronchus	England	Nigeria
Stomach	Japan	Uganda
Cervix uteri	Colombia	Israel
Prostate	United States	Japan
Liver	Mozambique	England
Breast	Canada, British Colombia	Israel
Colon	United States, Connecticut	Nigeria
Corpus uteri	United States, California	Japan
Buccal cavity	India, Bombay	Denmark
Rectum	Denmark	Nigeria
Bladder	United States, Connecticut	Japan
Ovary	Denmark	Japan
Nasopharynx	Singapore	England
Pancreas	New Zealand	India, Bombay
Larynx	Brazil, São Paulo	Japan
Pharynx	India, Bombay	Denmark
Penis	Parts of Uganda	Israel

(Modified from Doll, R., & Peto, R. [1981]. The causes of cancer: Quantitative estimates of avoidable risks of cancer in the United States today. *Journal of the National Cancer Institute, 66,* 1191–1308.)

known to herald the occurrence of this cancer. The initial symptom is indigestion, with the most common presenting symptoms being increasing frequency and intensity of epigastric pain, vomiting, and dysphagia (Mikulin & Hardcastle, 1987).

Prevention. At present, it would appear that the most effective prevention of stomach cancer is through dietary interventions. It is estimated that 15 to 20 per cent of all stomach cancers could be prevented by specific dietary changes (Wahrendorf, 1987). In general, researchers recommend that individuals living in high-risk areas reduce their intake of foods that are salty, smoked, and high in starch and nitrites, and increase the number of fruits and vegetables that are high in vitamin C.

Early Detection. There are no randomized, controlled studies that document the benefits of regular periodic patient screening for gastric cancer. However, mass screening of the population for malignant gastric lesions has been undertaken for a number of years in Japan, because in that country more deaths are due to gastric cancer than all other cancers combined. Screening in Japan involves radiographic studies to identify suspicious lesions followed by gastroscopy (Charnley et al., 1982). In China, a new method, the occult blood bead detector, is being piloted. The occult blood bead detector is a small plastic container on a string that is swallowed by the patient, lies in the stomach for a few minutes, and then is brought back up. Inside the small plastic container is an indicator that changes color in the presence of blood. This method is inexpensive and practical and promises to be an effective method of screening high-risk populations (Zin et al., 1988).

Nursing Role. There are several specific actions nurses can take in terms of the primary prevention of gastric cancer. These actions include being knowledgeable about the risk factors for this cancer, the research-based recommended dietary changes, and screening procedures to decrease the risk. Because it is believed that the risk of developing gastric cancer is determined by exposures in the first 2 decades of life, educational programs should be aggressively targeted to parents of young children (Frank-Stromborg, 1989). These educational programs should detail the specific dietary changes that will lower an individual's risk and should be incorporated into the family's dietary lifestyle. When dietary changes are recommended, it is best to keep any suggestions simple, practical, and cost-effective.

A review of 13 years of abstracts submitted to the ONS for presentation at the Annual ONS Congress, as well as the abstract books and proceedings of the second through the sixth International Conference on Cancer Nursing, showed no abstracts related to the primary and secondary prevention of gastric cancer. Although gastric cancer is one of the leading causes of cancer-related deaths in many countries of the world, it would appear that this is not an area in which nurses outside of the United States are involved in primary and secondary prevention. Although the incidence of gastric cancer has dramatically decreased in the United States, this picture may change with the aging of the American population, because increasing age is a significant risk factor for this cancer (Charnley et al, 1982).

ESOPHAGEAL CANCER

Incidence. The same pattern reported for gastric cancer is found with esophageal cancer in terms of incidence in the United States versus other countries. Although cancer of the esophagus is rare in whites in the United States, the incidence for African-American men in Detroit, San Francisco, and Alameda, California, are exceedingly high (Day & Munoz, 1982).

The epidemiology of esophageal cancer is unusual because of the wide variation in incidence, even within close geographic confines. For instance, there is a region referred to as the esophageal cancer belt located in Central Asia that includes the provinces of Henan, Hebei, and Shanzi of Northern China; Northern Iran; and Soviet Central Asia. In areas only a few hundred miles from the esophageal cancer belt, the disease is extremely rare (Tollefson, 1985). Economic factors do not seem to be responsible for the uneven distribution, because although such cancer is endemic among rural people with the limited diets and impoverished agriculture of Southern Africa, Central Asia, and Northern China, esophageal cancer is almost absent in other, similarly economically deprived areas of the world (Kibblewhite, Van Rensburg, Laker, & Rose, 1984).

Another unusual feature of this cancer is that although it has been known in some countries for hundreds of years, it is newly documented in others. Esophageal cancer in Northern Iran has been recognized for more than 800 years (Shadirian, 1987). In contrast, within the last 12 years, this cancer has become the most common cancer in black men in parts of South Africa.

Risk Factors. The risk factors for esophageal cancer are generally divided into exogenous causative factors and those relating to host susceptibility.

The most prominent exogenous causative factors in Northern America and Western Europe are smoking and drinking. In both regions, these two factors account for 90 per cent or more of the risk for esophageal cancer (Day & Munoz, 1982). Studies have shown that alcohol and tobacco are synergistic factors, increasing the risk of esophageal cancer (Tollefson, 1985).

Although excessive use of alcohol plays an important role in the causation of esophageal cancer in westernized individuals, alcohol seems to play little or no role in the major endemic areas of the world (Gayal, 1983). However, the practice of smoking opium pipes followed by the scraping out of the pipes and eating the remains is a common practice in the esophageal cancer belt for both men and women (Ghadinan et al., 1986). It is hypothesized that the ingestion of opium pyrolysates may be a risk factor because of the geographic parallel between opium use and esophageal cancer incidence (Ghadinan et al., 1986).

Another exogenous risk factor implicated for esophageal cancer is drinking excessively hot beverages (Hirayama, 1979). For example, *mate,* a hot drink taken through a metal tube that brings the hot infusion into the posterior part of the tongue where it is immediately swallowed, has been implicated in the development of esophageal cancer in parts of South America (Munoz et al., 1987). Nutritional deficiencies also have been linked to the development of esophageal cancers (Day & Munoz, 1982; Tollefson, 1985; Van Rensberg, Bradshaw, Bradshaw, & Rose, 1985).

Dysphagia is an initial symptom of esophageal cancer, but this symptom does not occur until at least 60 per cent of the esophageal circumference is infiltrated with cancer (Mayer, 1988). Dysphagia and weight loss are the initial symptoms of esophageal cancer in 90 per cent of patients.

Prevention. The exogenous factors that must be reduced in high-risk populations are smoking cigarettes, excessive intake of alcohol, use of opium, ingestion of excessively hot food and drinks, and smoking a pipe and swallowing the remaining tobacco juice. To date, both early detection and secondary prevention do not appear to be effective in decreasing mortality from esophageal cancer; thus, primary prevention assumes an even more important role in any discussion of this cancer.

Early Detection. At present there are no early detection methods available, and the early detection of esophageal cancer is rare. The esophogram with esophagoscopy is the mainstay of diagnosis (Mayer, 1988). It is recommended that esophagoscopy be performed in all patients complaining of weight loss and dysphagia and that a biopsy be taken with brushings of any suspicious lesions (Mayer, 1988).

Nursing Role. Mackel and Greski (1990) discuss the nurse's role related to the early detection of esophageal cancer. The Tucson Veteran's Medical Center set up a nursing clinic to follow patients with Barrett's esophagus. Barrett's esophagus, a complication of chronic gastroesophageal reflux, is an acquired premalignant condition of the esophagus. Many of the patients in this clinic are smokers, or heavy alcohol drinkers. The nursing role in this clinic includes early cancer detection, patient education, lifestyle and risk-factor modification, symptom control, and assistance with chemoprevention trials being conducted with this high-risk population.

Pervan (1988), a nurse in the Republic of South Africa, writes about the high incidence of esophageal cancer in this region as well as the enormous difficulties of instituting early detection measures with rural Africans. Rural Africans are at high risk for this cancer due to their diet of maize, which is low in vitamin B content and tends to be infected with aflatoxin, and their high incidence of smoking. She cites the need for involvement of oncology nurses in community education at the grass roots level, which incorporates the tribal healer as well as the health beliefs of the African culture.

In general, the role of the nurse in the primary prevention of esophageal cancer involves taking an active part in the prevention and cessation of all forms of smoking and alcohol abuse and the education of high-risk individuals about the dangers of routinely eating and drinking excessively hot foods or beverages. Although it is recommended that the nurse provide prevention-oriented education at the individual level, it is recognized that the prevention of cancer of the esophagus necessitates a broader, more comprehensive approach (Frank-Stromborg, 1989). Nurses can assume an active role in working with the government in establishing primary prevention programs at the local and national levels.

PROSTATE CANCER

Incidence. Prostate cancer is now the number one cancer in males in the United States and has the third highest death rate. It is estimated that there were 244,000 new cases of prostate cancer in 1995, with 40,400 cancer deaths anticipated (Wingo et al., 1995). Current estimates indicate that a 50-year-old American man has an approximately 40 per cent chance of developing microscopic prostate cancer during his lifetime, a 10 per cent chance of being diagnosed with the disease, and a 2 per cent to 3 per cent chance of dying of prostate cancer (Garnick, 1993).

African-American males in the United States have the highest incidence of prostate cancer in the world. The etiology remains unclear. Japanese-American men have the lowest incidence (Haenvel & Kurihara, 1968). Less than 1 per cent of prostate cancer patients are <50 years of age, and the incidence and mortality rise with age thereafter (Murphy et al., 1982). However, younger men have a more aggressive disease at time of diagnosis as compared with the older prostate cancer patient (Petersen, 1986). See Table 16–8 for the cancer incidence in different ethnic or racial groups.

Risk Factors. Other risk factors include increasing age, race, familial history, alcohol intake, high-fat diet, diet low in green and yellow vegetables, exposure to cadmium or fertilizer, and occupations in the tire and rubber industry (Hayes, Bogdanovicz, & Schroeder, 1988; Murphy, 1988; White, 1986). A recent study reported an association between vasectomy and subsequent risk of prostate cancer (Giovannucci et al.,

TABLE 16–8. *Cancer Incidence in Different Ethnic or Racial Groups*

RACIAL OR ETHNIC GROUP	CANCERS UNIQUE TO GROUP
African-Americans	*Highest incidence* rates for esophagus, colon, larynx, lung (male), multiple myeloma, pancreas, prostate, female breast (woman under age 40). Highest incidence rate for all cancers combined. Overall cancer rate: Male = 487.9 per 100,000, 1978–1981 Female = 290.3 per 100,000, 1978–1981
Native Americans	*Highest incidence* rate for cancers of the cervix uteri. Native Americans have stomach cancer rate twice as high as that for whites. Male native American men have highest rate for gallbladder cancer in the world and lowest rate of lung cancer in the world. *Lowest incidence* rates for cancers of the bladder, colon, rectum, larynx, male and female lung, female breast, corpus uteri, pancreas, ovary. Overall cancer rate: Male = 172.3 per 100,000, 1978–1981 Female = 155.5 per 100,000, 1978–1981
Native Hawaiians	*Highest incidence* rates for cancer of the female breast, ovary, corpus uteri, stomach, and lung (female). *Highest incidence rate* of breast cancer in the world. Overall cancer rate: Male = 390.9 per 100,000 Female = 336.5 per 100,000
Japanese-Americans	*Highest incidence* rates for rectal cancer, colon and rectum combined. *Lowest incidence* for cervix uteri and multiple myeloma. Stomach cancer rate is twice as high as that for whites. Overall cancer rates: Male = 300.4 per 100,000, Hawaii Female = 225.5 per 100,000, San Francisco
Hispanics	*Lowest rate* for cancer of esophagus. Overall cancer rate: Male = 279.8 per 100,000, New Mexico Male = 245.2 per 100,000, Puerto Rico Female = 218.4 per 100,000, New Mexico Female = 181.3 per 100,000, Puerto Rico

(Data from *Cancer Facts and Figures for Minority Americans,* 1986; Clemmesen, 1987; Cook-Mozaffari, 1985; Enstrom & Kanim, 1983; National Cancer Institute, 1986; Page & Asire, 1985.)

1993). The biological mechanism underlying the increased risk "may be related to a diminished secretory rate of prostatic fluid following vasectomy, or, alternatively, to the postvasectomy immune response to sperm antigens, which may cross-react with tumor-associated antigens and suppress tumor immunosurveillance mechanisms" (Giovannucci et al., 1993).

A sexually transmitted infectious agent has been hypothesized in the development of prostate cancer, because several studies have shown a higher incidence of prostate cancer in sexually hyperactive or promiscuous men as compared with controls and among men whose sexual partners had cervical cancer (Badalament & Drago, 1991). However, it should be pointed out that epidemiologic evidence for the sexually transmitted agent hypothesis is sparse.

Prostate cancer appears to result from an interplay between endogenous hormones and environmental influences that include, most prominently, dietary fat (Pienta & Esper, 1993). There is a high correlation between the incidence of breast and prostate cancer, and both types of cancer are higher in more developed countries. This has suggested that environmental factors, such as a diet high in animal fat, may be important in the promotion of these two types of cancers.

Prevention. Prevention includes a diet low in fat and avoidance of alcohol consumption. Because of their high incidence, educational efforts must be directed toward elderly African-American males (Murphy, 1988). Work is being done to reach this group of individuals by educating African-American nurses to disseminate the information in their communities (Frank-Stromborg, Johnson, & McCorkle, 1987).

The Prostate Cancer Prevention Trial (PCPT) is being sponsored by the National Cancer Institute and is the first large-scale prostate cancer prevention study for men aged 55 and older. The PCPT will enroll 18,000 men to determine whether the drug finasteride will prevent prostate cancer. Finasteride is currently being used to treat benign prostatic hyperplasia. All men enrolled in this study will take one pill per day for up to 7 years, either a 5-mg dose of finasteride or a placebo (American Cancer Society Cancer Response System, 1994).

Early Detection. Prostate cancer is insidious, and frequently few symptoms are noted until dissemination occurs. Early symptoms may include difficulty in starting the urinary stream, frequent, interrupted, and painful urination, dribbling, bladder retention, and hematuria. These symptoms are also found with prostatic enlargement, which is common in older men. Most symptoms are related to advanced disease and include ureteral obstruction with anuria, urinary retention, uremia, anemia, azotemia, anorexia, or bone pain from metastatic disease. New onset of impotence or less firm penile erections should alert the health professional to the possibility that prostate cancer may be present and is involving periprostatic tissue involved in erectile function (Garnick, 1993). Loss of penile erection may not be elicited in the health history because the man assumes it is a normal part of aging.

The ACS recommends annual digital rectal examinations after the age of 40 years. It has been well established that screening asymptomatic men over the age of 50 by digital rectal examination increases the detection rate for prostate cancer. The use of prostate-specific antigen (PSA) and transrectal ultrasound are being investigated for their role in early diagnosis of prostate cancer (Catalona et al., 1991; Drago, 1989; Lee, Torp-Pedersen, & Siders, 1989; Virji, Mercer, & Herberman, 1988). The early findings support PSA in conjunction with other screening techniques, because PSA may be elevated in a large percentage of patients with benign prostatic hypertrophy (Catalona et al., 1991; Drago, 1989; Murphy, 1988). Transrectal ultrasound has shown some promising results detecting twice as many cancers as digital rectal examination alone (Lee et al., 1989). The role that PSA and transrectal ultrasound will play in the early detection of prostate cancer remains to be seen (Bostwick, 1989).

There is national debate about the value of screening asymptomatic men for prostatic cancer. Gerber, Thompson, Thisted, and Chodak (1993) argue that routine screening for prostate cancer by annual digital rectal examination alone is insufficient to prevent significant mortality from this disease. Lange (1993) and the ACS National Prostate Cancer Detection Project (1993) contend that for now the periodic prostate examination should be encouraged and include both a DRE and PSA serum level determination. However, Lange does acknowledge that there is no proof that detecting more "early" prostate cancer can improve the quality and quantity of life. Krahn et al. (1994) calculated life expectancy, quality-adjusted life expectancy, and cost-utility ratios for unselected and high-prevalence populations. Their findings resulted in the following:

> Our analysis does not support using PSA, TRUS, or DRE to screen asymptomatic men for prostatic cancer. Screening may result in poorer health outcomes and will increase costs dramatically. Assessment of comorbidity, risk attitude, and valuation of sexual function may identify individuals who will benefit from screening, but selecting high-prevalence populations will not improve the benefit of screening (p. 773).

The National Cancer Institute is presently conducting a randomized prospective study of the effect of screening on prostate cancer mortality to resolve some of the above issues (Kramer, Brown, Prorok, Potosky, & Gohagan, 1993).

Nursing Role. It was not possible to locate any reports devoted solely to the nursing role in preventing or detecting prostate cancer. Rather, there are several reports about nurse-run screening/prevention clinics that included screening for prostate cancer. Stoltzfus and Ashby (1990) reported a mobile screening program that was a joint venture between the City of Hope National Medical Center and the ACS. This mobile screening program is designed to educate and screen individuals within the workplace, senior citizen centers, and community ethnic groups. A nurse practitioner conducted the examination, which included screening for testicular, prostate, and rectal cancer. In 34 months of operation, 10,500 persons have been educated and nearly 7700 individuals screened, with a 25.9 per cent referral rate for suspicious findings. Nelson-Manen and Krebs (1991) reopened a nurse-run cancer prevention/screening clinic that evaluates the cancer risk and concerns of healthy, asymptomatic adults. The nursing role in this clinic includes performing a cancer risk assessment and physical examination and teaching risk reduction. In 8 months of operation, 100 healthy adults have been seen and about one third referred to a specific physician or to another clinic for follow-up.

Because prostate cancer is the primary cancer in men, the role of the nurse in prevention and early detection of this cancer is essential (Martin, 1990). The literature review clearly demonstrated the limited involvement of nurses in the education, counseling, and screening of men for this cancer. It is important that nurses find ways to disseminate information on prostate cancer to the African-American male population and encourage their participation in early detection programs. The best way to reduce the mortality from prostate cancer is by diagnosing men when they are asymptomatic and by continuing nursing research into the best means of attaining this goal.

BREAST CANCER

Incidence. Cancer of the breast is the most common malignancy among women and is rare among men. It occurs most frequently in white females. Breast cancer is the second leading cause of cancer-related deaths among women, with an estimated 184,400 new cases in 1995 and 46,240 lives being lost in 1995 (Wingo et al., 1995). The rates of breast cancer have been steadily increasing in the U.S., since formal tracking of cases through registries started in the 1930s. Breast cancer can occur anytime after menarche but occurs rarely before 20 years of age and primarily after age 40. Postmenopausal women are at greatest risk (Schatzkin et al., 1989a). There has been an upsurge in the incidence of breast cancer that began in the early 1980s. While much of this surge is attributed to the increased use of mammography screening, the large increase that has occurred over the past half century appears to be real. "Breast cancer is clearly continuing to increase, especially among postmenopausal women, and will require even greater attention on the part of researchers and clinicians" (Harris, Lippman, Veronesi, & Willett, 1992).

Risk Factors. Breast cancer appears to be related to a constellation of risk factors rather than to any single factor. However, established risk factors include older age, birth in North America or Northern Europe, a family history of breast cancer (especially if both the mother and a sister of the woman have had breast cancer at early ages), the presence of hyperplastic epithelial cells in fluid aspirated from the nipple, nodular densities on a mammogram, biopsy-confirmed benign proliferative breast disease, a history of cancer in one breast, radiation to the chest in moderate-to-high doses, obesity (for breast cancer diagnosed in postmenopausal women), and the demographic characteristics of high social class, never having been married, urban residence, white race (for breast cancer diagnosed after the

age of 50), and African-American race (for breast cancer diagnosed before the age of 40) (DuPont et al., 1994; Kelsey & John, 1994). See Table 16–9 for established and probable risk factors for breast cancer.

There are conflicting data on the relationship between the consumption of alcohol and the risk of breast cancer, as well as the use of birth control pills, estrogen replacement, and increased risk of breast cancer (Gambrell, 1990; Schatzkin et al., 1989; Willett et al., 1987). There are studies that have shown that moderate alcohol consumption is associated with an elevation in the risk of breast cancer (Schatzkin et al., 1987), and there are also studies that have found no association between alcohol and breast cancer (Bultz et al., 1988; Harris & Wynder, 1988; Good news for women who booze . . ., 1988). The same type of debate has revolved around the use of birth control pills and increased risk of breast cancer (The Cancer and Steroid Hormone Study . . ., 1986; Longman & Buehring, 1987). Although it has been demonstrated that unopposed estrogens increase a woman's risk of endometrial adenocarcinoma and that cyclic addition of progestogen reduces it, the impact of the sex hormones on the pathogenesis of breast cancer remains highly controversial. Gambrell (1990) writes that 30 reports investigating the relationship between postmenopausal estrogen replacement and carcinoma of the breast failed to demonstrate a clear relationship in any direction.

It has been widely believed that lactation has no effect on the incidence of breast cancer. However, recent research has found a relationship between lactation and the development of breast cancer, but the reduction in risk of breast cancer occurred only among premenopausal women, not postmenopausal women with a history of lactation (Newcomb et al., 1994).

The relationship between dietary fat and the risk of breast cancer continues to be studied (Holmberg et al., 1994; Schatzkin et al., 1989; Willett et al., 1987). There are marked international differences in rates of breast cancer that highly correlate with national per capita fat consumption. The lower the national per capita consumption of fat is, the lower the rate of breast cancer is in that country. Kelsey and Gammon (1991), in an excellent review article on the epidemiology of breast cancer, stated that "with the exception of obesity, none of the established risk factors readily leads to opportunities for primary prevention" (p. 158).

Another risk factor for breast cancer is lobular carcinoma in situ. Lobular carcinoma in situ (lobular CIS) has been cited as a precancerous lesion and is diagnosed by microscopic examination of the specimen. Some clinicians prefer the term *atypical lobular hyperplasia*. It arises within the end parts of the lobule. Lobular CIS is characterized by clusters of anaplastic small cells of high nuclear grade that lie within lobules. For a woman with lobular CIS, the risk of developing homolateral breast cancer is approximately 70 per cent in 24 years, and the chance of developing carcinoma of the opposite breast is approximately 40 per cent. This precancerous lesion has a tendency to involve both breasts, either synchronously or asynchronously. Lobular carcinoma of the breast seems to require years before progressing

TABLE 16–9. *Established and Probable Risk Factors for Breast Cancer*

RISK FACTOR	COMPARISON CATEGORY	RISK CATEGORY	TYPICAL RELATIVE RISK	STUDY
Family history of breast cancer	No 1st degree relatives affected	Mother affected before the age of 60	2.0	Nurses' Health Study*
		Mother affected after the age of 60	1.4	Nurses' Health Study*
		Two 1st-degree relatives affected	4–6	Gail et al. (1989)
Age at menarche	16 yr	11 yr	1.3	Kampert et al. (1988)
		12 yr	1.3	
		13 yr	1.3	
		14 yr	1.3	
		15 yr	1.1	
Age at birth of 1st child	Before 20 yr	20–24 yr	1.3	White (1987)
		25–29 yr	1.6	
		≥30 yr	1.9	
		Nulliparous	1.9	
Age at menopause	45–54 yr	After 55 yr	1.5	Trichopoulos et al. (1972)
		Before 45 yr	0.7	
		Oophorectomy before 35 yr	0.4	
Benign breast disease	No biopsy or aspiration	Any benign disease	1.5	Willett et al. (1987)
		Proliferation only	2.0	Dupont & Page (1985)
		Atypical hyperplasia	4.0	Dupont & Page (1985)
Radiation	No special exposure	Atomic bomb (100 rad)	3.0	Boice & Monson (1977)
		Repeated fluoroscopy	1.5–2.0	McGregor et al. (1977)
Obesity	10th percentile	90th percentile:		Tretli (1989)
		Age, 30–49 yr	0.8	
		Age, ≥50 yr	1.2	
Height	10th percentile	90th percentile:		Tretli (1989)
		Age, 30–49 yr	1.3	
		Age, ≥50 yr	1.4	
Oral contraceptive use	Never used	Current use†	1.5	Romieu et al. (1989)
		Past use†	1.0	
Postmenopausal estrogen-replacement therapy	Never used	Current use all ages	1.4	Colditz et al. (1990)
		Age, <55 yr	1.2	
		Age, 50–59 yr	1.5	
		Age, ≥60yr	2.1	
Alcohol use	Nondrinker	Past use	1.0	Longnecker et al. (1988)
		1 drink/day	1.4	
		2 drinks/day	1.7	
		3 drinks/day	2.0	

*Unpublished prospective data were obtained from Graham Colditz (personal communication).
†Relative risks may be higher for women given a diagnosis of breast cancer before the age of 40.
(From Harris, J. R., Lippman, M. E., Veronesi, U., & Willett, W. [1992]. Breast cancer. *New England Journal of Medicine, 327*[5], 319–328. Reprinted by permission of *The New England Journal of Medicine.* Copyright 1992, Massachusetts Medical Society.)

to invasive carcinoma, and some lesions never progress to cancer.

The average woman in America is estimated to have a one in nine chance of developing breast cancer during her lifetime (Fennelly, 1994). The cumulative probability of breast cancer over the fifth or sixth decades of life (approximately 1.5 per cent and 1.8 per cent, respectively, or 3.3 per cent for the entire 20-year span) is a one in 30 risk. Certain factors may increase or decrease this "average" risk of breast cancer. However, 70 to 80 per cent of all women with breast cancer have *no known risk factors*. The longitudinal study by Seidman, Stellman, and Mushinski (1982) of 570,000 white American women found that when they considered

known risk factors alone or in combination, the risk factors explained only 21 per cent of the breast cancer risk among women aged 30 to 54 years and 29 per cent of the risk among women aged 55 to 84 years: "We have not appreciably increased our ability to identify substantial numbers of truly 'high-risk' women. From the point of view of the clinician, *all women should be treated as being at appreciable risk for breast cancer*" (Seidman et al., 1982, p. 311).

Berg (1984) supports the Seidman study's statement by saying ". . . for health maintenance, every woman with breast tissue must be considered at high risk for breast cancer, whatever that implies at her particular age" (p. 590). Bulbrook et al. (1986) conducted a prospective study of 15,000 women and found that there was a *small subset* of women who were at high risk for the development of breast cancer. Women who are nulliparous or have a first child at or after 28 years of age have a high proportion of their blood E_2 (estradiol) not bound to protein or a low concentration of sex hormone-binding globulin, and have high-risk Wolfe grades on mammograms appear to be at considerable risk for breast cancer. However, a combination of classic, endocrinologic, and radiologic risk factors *failed to identify 70 per cent* of the potential breast cancer cases.

To date, no one factor or combination of factors has been found that can predict the occurrence of breast cancer in any one individual, although major risk factors have been identified. When asking about major risk factors, the nurse should remember that, regardless of the responses, all women should be considered at risk for this cancer.

The physical signs that most strongly suggest cancer of the breast are dimpling; flattening of the nipple; abnormal contours of the breast; peau d'orange; a palpable, hard, poorly circumscribed nodule fixed to the skin or underlying tissue; and palpable hard, fixed nodes in the axillae or supraclavicular region.

Prevention. Presently the state of the art in reference to the prevention of breast cancer limits any definitive recommendations. Many known risk factors are beyond our ability to modify or manipulate (e.g., hereditary). However, there is presently a randomized clinical trial, NCI/National Surgical Adjuvant Breast and Bowel Project (NSABP) Breast Cancer Prevention Trial (BCPT), that is investigating the prevention of breast cancer in high-risk women with the use of Nolvadex (tamoxifen citrate). There will be 16,000 women enrolled in this study; half the women will receive the drug during the 5 years of the study, and half the women will receive a placebo. The results of the BCPT with tamoxifen will be closely studied to see whether the drug prevents cancer in high-risk women (Loescher & Hazelkorn, 1993).

There are other preventative trials being conducted across the county and world to determine whether breast cancer can be prevented. These trials are:

1. National Cancer Institute Women's Health Trial Feasiblity Study in Minority Populations. Study being done to determine whether low-fat diet in minority women decreases the risk of breast and colon cancer in women ages 45 to 69 years of age.
2. National Institutes of Health Women's Health Initiative. This is a broad study looking at the prevention of cancer, heart disease, and osteoporosis in 150,000 women age 50 to 79 years of age. Interventions involve hormone replacement therapy, diet, and supplementation of calcium plus vitamin D.
3. Prevention of Contralateral Breast Cancer with Fenretinide (4-HPR). Study looking at the effectiveness of 4-HPR in preventing contralateral breast cancer in disease-free women ages 35 to 65 years who have been treated for early-stage breast cancer.
4. The Royal Marsden Pilot Trial. Double-blinded, placebo-controlled trial to evaluate tamoxifen

solely as a chemopreventive agent for breast cancer (Loescher & Hazelkorn, 1993).

Early Detection. Breast self-examination (BSE), physical examination, and mammography are three major methods for the screening and early detection of breast cancer. Approximately 80 to 90 per cent of all breast lesions are discovered by women themselves; thus, BSE is an important method of early detection of breast cancer.

There are multiple issues with breast screening of asymptomatic females that limit the ability to say with certainty that detecting cancers at a very early stage will decrease mortality from the disease. These issues are:

1. lead-time bias
2. length-time bias
3. overdiagnosis bias
4. selection bias

Lead-time bias means that lethal cancers are detected sooner, but the end result, mortality, does not change. *Length-time bias* is present when slow-growing cancers are detected that are less likely to be lethal. *Overdiagnosis bias* is present when tumors of questionable malignant potential are detected. *Selection bias* is present in any screening program by virtue of the fact that those who come for screening may have different risk factors than those who do not come for screening. Randomized clinical trials are successful in removing these bias and have resulted in significant change in recommendations about the age to start baseline mammography (Harris, Lippman, Veronesi, & Willett, 1992).

For the early detection of breast cancer, the ACS recommends monthly BSE, a baseline mammogram between 40 and 49 years of age, mammogram every 1 to 2 years from ages 40 to 49 years, and yearly mammograms for women >50 years of age (Mettlin & Smart, 1994) and a yearly clinical breast examination by a health-care provider. The ACS recommendations differ from those of the National Cancer Institute (NCI). The NCI omits any recommendation for mammography and clinical breast examination for women aged 40 to 49 years because of the lack of agreement among experts on the role of routine screening mammography for this age group. The United Kingdom recommends single-view mammography performed every 3 years in all women between 50 and 64 years of age. Canada recommends that mammography be performed every 2 years in women between 50 and 69 years of age (Harris et al., 1992).

The debate regarding when a woman should have baseline mammography and yearly mammography stems from research conducted in Canada and Sweden (Baines, 1994; Nyström, Rutquist, & Wall, 1993). Five randomized trials of breast cancer screening with mammography were done in Sweden and involved 282,777 women who were followed for 5 to 13 years. Among women aged 40 to 74 years who participated in the breast cancer screening with mammography, the relative reduction in breast cancer mortality was 24 per cent. The greatest benefit was among women aged 50 to 69 years, who showed a relative reduction of 29 per cent in breast cancer mortality (Nyström et al., 1993).

The Canadian National Breast Screening Study showed no reduction in breast cancer mortality after 7 years in women screened with mammography who were 40 to 49 years of age (Baines, 1994). "Further, mammography did not achieve an incremental mortality benefit over and above clinical examination in women 50 to 59 years old, although it did achieve higher rates of cancer detection" (Baines, 1994, p. 326). Further adding to the controversy is a meta-analysis conducted by Kerlikowske, Grady, Rubin, Sandrock, and Emster (1995). Kerlikowske analyzed 13 studies (nine randomized controlled trials and four case-control studies) that had appeared in the literature from 1966 to 1993. They reported similar findings about the long-term benefits of screening mammography as the Swedish researchers did.

> Screening mammography significantly reduces breast cancer mortality in women aged 50 to 74 years after 7 to 9 years of follow-up, regardless of screening interval . . . There is no reduction in breast cancer mortality in women aged 40 to 49 years after 7 to 9 years of follow-up. Screening mammography may be effective in reducing breast cancer mortality in women aged 40 to 49 years after 10 to 12 years of follow-up, but the same benefit could probably be achieved by beginning screening at menopause or 50 years of age (Kerlikowske et al., 1995, p. 149).

Recently there has been increasing debate about the merit of BSE. A recurring criticism is the lack of prospective randomized controlled trials to establish the effectiveness of BSE in reducing breast cancer mortality (Diem & Rose, 1985; Frank & Mai, 1985). Studies measuring the effectiveness of treatment after screening by BSE have been retrospective or descriptive in design. Most retrospective BSE data have been from women who have developed breast cancer, raising questions of recall bias.

The most recent and widely quoted study to support the argument that regular BSE does improve survival was conducted by Foster et al. (1978), in which they investigated the relationship of BSE to survival in 1004 newly diagnosed breast cancer patients. Survival at 5 years was 75 per cent for women who had practiced BSE versus 57 per cent for those who had not. Furthermore, they found that 90 per cent of the women who performed BSE detected their own breast cancers, and 50 per cent of the lesions were <2 cm in diameter when diagnosed. In contrast, 54 per cent of the women who never examined themselves discovered their cancers accidentally.

Nursing Role. A review of the literature documented the involvement of nurses in every conceivable aspect of the early detection of breast cancer. More literature was found in this area than for any other cancer site. The literature reflects the following:

1. Nurses have conducted an extensive amount of research into the factors that facilitate and impede BSE (Champion, 1988; Crooks & Jones, 1989; Glenn & Moore, 1990; Hallal, 1982; Hirshfeld-Bartek, 1982; Massey, 1986; Nichols, 1983; Olson & Mitchell, 1989; Schmitt & Krebs, 1987). The majority of these research studies have investigated the practice of BSE as it relates to the Health Belief Model (Champion, 1985, 1987; Hallal, 1982; Hirshfield-Bartek, 1982; Redeker, 1989; Rutledge & Davis, 1988; Wyper, 1990).

2. Nurses have investigated BSE in selected groups of women, including women in rural settings (Gray, 1990), elderly women (Coleman, 1990; Williams, 1988), black women (Nemcek, 1989; Willis, Davis, Cairns, & Janiszewski, 1989), Chinese-American women (Lovejoy, Jenkins, Wu, Shankland, & Wilson, 1989), Mexican-American women (Gonzalez, 1990; Longman, Modiano-Revah, & Saint-Germain, 1990), women who have had breast cancer (Facciponti & Cartwright, 1988; Muller, 1988), the daughters of women who have had breast cancer (Doyle & Simonich, 1991; Schulmeister, 1985), and adolescents (Kitson, 1989; Sheehan, Michalek, & Cassidy, 1981).

3. Nurses have investigated the BSE practices of nurses, their ability to detect breast lesions, and their attitudes toward this practice (Cole & Gorman, 1984; Haughey et al., 1984; Kumar, 1990).

4. Nurses have investigated performance issues related to the practice of BSE (Edgar, 1985; Esparza & Kean, 1980; Kitson, Brenner, & Brooks, 1983; Lierman, 1990) as well as different methods of teaching BSE (Marty, McDermott, & Gold, 1983; Smith, 1991).

5. Nurses have organized, conducted, and described breast cancer early-detection programs in multiple settings, including programs in home-care settings (Williams, 1989), employment settings (Grindal, 1983; Marley, 1982; Simon & Worthen, 1989; Styrd, 1982), hospital settings (Case, 1984; Kalinowki, Goodman, & Lawler, 1986; Kelley, Hoffman, & Newton, 1988), primary educational settings (Tyson, 1980), and specialty clinics for high-risk women or women with breast lesions (Ammirata, Bordeaux, & Ferguson, 1989; Calzone, Saran, & Sommerfield, 1986; Carpenter, 1989; Ellerhorst-Ryan, 1985; Larpenteur, 1989; Nielsen, 1989; Tranin & Fabian, 1991; Wilcox, 1979; Wilcox, Ziegeld, Hoopes, & Ashley, 1990).

The literature review documented that nurses can and are promoting change in the performance of BSE (Shamian & Edgar, 1987). Unfortunately, it has been found that nurses were not consistently assessing their clients' BSE performance or technique (Clarke & Sandler, 1989; Sawyer, 1986). Cretain (1989) suggested that before nurses can motivate women to practice consistent BSE, they must become more motivated toward this practice themselves. Sawyer (1986) reported that nurses who practiced BSE regularly were more likely to ask their clients about BSE than were nurses who did not self-examine regularly. The employment setting has been shown to provide an environment conducive to learning and promoting BSE (Brailey, 1986; Styrd, 1982). Both high attendance and long-term compliance rates have been reported in BSE educational programs offered in the workplace. In the BSE program reported by Styrd (1982), >60 per cent of the eligible female employees indicated that they had performed BSE on a monthly basis since attending the program, and the difference between their BSE practice before the program and after the program was statistically significant. Long-term follow-through established relationships and peer support are felt to promote BSE when programs are offered in the workplace. (The reader is referred to an in-depth discussion of BSE in Olsen & Frank-Stromborg, 1991a.)

Other nurses have investigated the approaches to teaching BSE (Marty, McDermott, & Gold, 1983) and have found modeling and guided practice to be the most effective method of teaching BSE. Multiple expanded roles for nurses in the early detection of breast cancer have been advocated, including the following.

1. Having a nurse coordinate all activities connected with a mobile mammography van to a population with limited access to preventive health care (Nielsen, 1989).
2. Having a clinical nurse specialist in a clinic devoted exclusively to diseases of the breast take a risk assessment history, conduct a breast examination, and provide one-on-one BSE instruction (Kelley et al., 1988).
3. Having a nurse practitioner evaluate clients in a clinic for women with breast masses, provide breast education, and refer suspicious lesions (Wilcox, 1979).
4. Training staff nurses to provide individualized BSE instruction to hospitalized patients (Kalinowki et al., 1986).
5. Having nurses expand their role in a breast care center to include involvement in marketing strategies, data collection, statistical analysis, and the management of operational areas (Calzone et al., 1986).

Many continuing education programs are being offered that are designed to certify the nurse in teaching BSE, conducting breast examinations, or both. Typical of these are the Breast Cancer Education Program sponsored by Roswell-Park Memorial Institute, New York. They have a 3-hour breast self-examination certification program for nurses and health educators. This program includes pretests and posttests, lectures, films, slides, and simulated practice with breast models. Participants who are qualified according to a score on a test and demonstrated ability on the breast models are given a certificate indicating that they are certified to teach a BSE (Breast Cancer Education Program). Similar educational approaches have been instituted in other areas of the country, including Ohio (Gill, 1989), Maryland (Riese, 1983), California (Coleman, McCarthy, & Mullins, 1986), and Texas (Toth & Heusinkveld, 1979).

The role of nurses in mammography has become important in the last several years. Nurses have tried to find ways of providing low-cost mammograms for high-risk females. Many women, as well as insurance companies, have not accepted mammography as a useful tool in early detection of breast cancer. Nurses are

educating and must continue to educate women through the media, as in the television-promoted mammography screening project in Chicago (Winchester, Lasky, Sylvester, & Maher, 1988).

Nurses must also act politically with insurance companies and the government in developing low-cost mammograms for women. Cost and lack of understanding are seen as the two major deterrents to mammography (Breast Cancer Education Program).

GYNECOLOGIC CANCER

CERVICAL CANCER

Incidence. There has been a decline in the incidence of invasive cancer of the cervix over the past 30 years, undoubtedly due to the extensive use of the Papanicolaou test (Pap smear) for early diagnosis. The 1995 estimated new cases of invasive cervix uteri cancer are estimated to be 15,800, with 4800 estimated deaths (Wingo et al., 1995). The incidence of cervical cancer in the United States is almost two and one half times higher in African-American women than in white women, and the mortality is almost three times higher in African-Americans. However, Native American women have a higher incidence of cervix uteri cancer than do African-American women (National Cancer Institute, 1986).

With the use of Pap smears, more cases of preinvasive lesions of the cervix are being detected, and the incidence of stage II and III invasive carcinoma of the cervix is significantly reduced (Cashavelly, 1987). The increased use of Pap smears has also led to more cervical lesions being detected in the early stages, particularly in young sexually active women (Sadeghi, Hseih, & Gunn, 1984).

Risk Factors. Studies have shown that women with certain behavioral and physical characteristics are at increased risk for the development of cervical cancer. The frequency and length of exposure to these risk factors increase the risk of developing a lesion (Lovejoy, 1987). Factors considered to increase one's risk of cervical cancer include certain genital infections (human papillomaviruses [HPV] and herpes-simplex-2), chemical carcinogens (nicotine, oral contraceptives, diethylstilbestrol [DES], immunosuppressive drugs, chemotherapy, and alcohol), lifestyle habits (multiple sexual partners, intercourse before age 20, poor hygiene), and male sexual partners (smokers, multiple partners, visits to prostitutes, penile warts) (Cashavelly, 1987; Herrero et al, 1990; Lovejoy, 1987).

There are two types of lesions identified as precancerous that involve the cervix. These are dysplasia and carcinoma in situ. Dysplasia refers to lesions involving less than the full thickness of the epithelium; carcinoma in situ refers to lesions involving the full thickness. Dysplasias are subdivided into very mild, mild, moderate, and severe, depending on the extent of involvement of the epithelium. In a different classification system (cervical intraepithelial neoplasia nomenclature), three types of lesions are described: atypical cells involving (1) less than one third of the epithelium (CIN 1), (2) one third to two thirds of the epithelium (CIN 2), and (3) the full thickness of the epithelium (CIN 3) (Lovejoy, 1987, p. 2). See Table 16–10 for known or suspected risk factors for cervical cancer.

Prevention. Several factors have been suggested in lowering the risk of precancerous lesions. Barrier-type contraceptives, that is, condoms and diaphragms, have been shown to lower the risk of precancerous lesions and may facilitate regression of lesions (Richardson & Lyon, 1981). Vasectomy for males and taking daily allowances of vitamin A, β-carotene, and vitamin C by women have also been supported in the literature (Romney et al, 1981; Swan & Brown, 1979).

Early Detection. Regular pelvic examinations and Pap smears are the best methods for early detection of cervical cancer, and women of all ages should be instructed on the importance of these measures. A discrepancy arises as to the recommended frequency of Pap smears and pelvic examinations. The ACS recommends that "all women who are or who have been sexually active or have reached age 18, should have an annual Pap smear and pelvic examination. After a woman has had 3 or more consecutive satisfactory normal annual examinations, the Pap test may be performed less frequently at the discretion of her physician" (Ameri-

can Cancer Society, 1989, p. 79). The American College of Obstetrics and Gynecology recommends annual cytologic screenings for most women, and the screening interval should be an informed choice determined by both the patient and her physician (Romney et al., 1981). An ACS survey has shown that only 30 per cent of U.S. females have annual Pap smears (American Cancer Society, 1978).

Fahs, Mendelblatt, Schechter, & Muller (1992) analyzed the costs and benefits of screening for cervical cancer. Their results agree with the recommendations of the United States Preventive Services Task Force that after a woman who is 65 years of age or older has a documented history of negative Papanicolaou smears, screening is inefficient and can cease.

High-risk women, that is, those who have had syphilis, gonorrhea, genital herpes, or HPV infection, must be alert to the necessity of having at least yearly Pap smears. Women with vulvar condyloma acuminatum should be referred for a thorough examination of the vagina, cervix, and perirectal epithelium and the possibility of colposcopic examination. It also is recommended that these women and their infected male partners have frequent follow-up examinations to detect precancerous conditions caused by a latent virus in

TABLE 16–10. *Known or Suspected Risk Factors for Uterine Cervical Cancer*

RISK FACTOR	EXPLANATION	MAY REDUCE RISK
Genital Infections		
Human papillomaviruses	Strong relationship between genital warts and precancerous lesions.	Treatment of infections and frequent survillance. Barrier methods of birth control (condoms).
Herpes simplex virus II (HSV II)	Women with genital HSV II infections are at greater risk of developing precancerous lesions.	Barrier methods of birth control (condoms).
Multiple Sexual Partners	May relate to high protein content of sperm in some men. Risk may be due to immunosuppressive effects or chronic immune stimulation of sperm of different partners.	Limit number of sexual partners.
Immunosuppression	Persons with multiple medical conditions (e.g., cancer, scleroderma) that cause suppression of the immune system and transplant surgery patients are at increased risk.	
Type of Contraception Used	Use of barrier methods of contraceptives (condom or diaphragm) associated with low risk; oral contraceptives increase risk.	Barrier methods, especially if multiple sexual partners.
Smoking by the Female (?)	One study found female smokers who were monogamous had a risk 7 times that of nonsmoking women of developing precancerous lesions.	Stop smoking.
Characteristics of Male Sexual Partner	Penile warts and cancer; multiple sexual partners; sexual intercourse with prostitutes; previous wives with precancerous or invasive cervical cancer.	
Racial and Religious Group Membership	Religious differences noted—Jews, Mormons, and Seventh-Day Adventists have low risk. Related to low prevalence of divorce, use of barrier methods, and intercourse confined to marriage. High incidence in Latin America.	
Coital Factors(?)		
Douching frequently; poor hygiene; intercourse during menses	Douching may relate to use of coal tar derivatives in douching solution. Orthodox Jews who abstain during menses rarely develop invasive cervical cancer.	

(Data from Hendershot, 1983; Henderson, Gerkins, & Pike, 1975; Lovejoy, 1987; Page & Asire, 1985; Shanmugaratnam, 1985.) The reader is referred to Lovejoy (1987) for an excellent in-depth discussion of the risk factors for cervical cancer.

clinically and histologically normal tissue (Bender, 1988). Women whose Pap smears indicate the presence of warty infections such as koilocytotic cells or those who show cells consistent with squamous papilloma or warty atypia also should be referred to a physician for further evaluation (Jones & Saigo, 1986). Unfortunately, there has been a dramatic increase in the incidence of HPV nationally and internationally, and these women constitute a high-risk group for cervical cancer.

ENDOMETRIAL CANCER

Incidence. In 1995, it is estimated that 32,800 women were diagnosed with endometrial cancer, and 5900 women will die from the disease (Wingo et al, 1995). There was a large increase in the incidence in the 1970s due to the widespread sale of estrogens as replacement therapy for menopausal symptoms. The use of estrogens increased until around 1975, when it began to decrease after reports appeared of estrogen use associated with endometrial cancer.

Risk Factors. The risk factors associated with endometrial cancer include obesity, age >40 years, few or no children, infertility, early menarche, late menopause, estrogen therapy, and high socioeconomic status (Page & Asire, 1985; Sherman, 1983). The risk of this cancer is clearly age-related; the disease usually affects women 55 to 69 years of age with the median age for diagnosis in white women being 61 and in African-American women 64 (Dunn, 1981; Vecchia, Franceschi, Decarli, Galius, & Tognoni, 1984). Some authorities believe women who use "sequential" birth control pills have double the risk of endometrial cancer as women who use other forms of birth control (Persky et al., 1990; Schlaff & Rosenshein, 1985; Shapiro et al., 1985). Sequential birth control pills have been removed from the U.S. market. Use of oral contraceptives that contain both estrogen and progesterone in each pill for at least 1 year have a protective effect against endometrial cancer. Early symptoms of endometrial cancer include postmenopausal vaginal bleeding, spotting, and a watery discharge.

Estrogen therapy was introduced in the United States in the 1930s, and estrogens were suspected of contributing to the development of endometrial carcinoma early on (Schlaff & Rosenshein, 1985). The hormone estrogen was popular with menopausal women because it helped to control menopausal symptoms such as hot flashes or thinning of the vaginal lining, which caused painful sexual intercourse. From 1963 to 1973 the sale of estrogens as replacement therapy (e.g., Premarin) rose fourfold, and a rise in the incidence of endometrial cancer was noted by researchers beginning in 1969. The use of estrogens for the treatment of menopausal symptoms increased until around 1975, when it began to decrease after reports appeared that associated estrogen use with endometrial cancer.

It is now believed that estrogens are not carcinogenic but are promoters in the process of malignancy. Because the risk of endometrial cancer was found to rise with increasing dose, it is suggested that the therapy be of as short a duration and at as low a dose as possible (Vessey, 1985). There is clinical evidence periodic administration of a progestin (cyclic progestogen therapy) will protect postmenopausal women who are receiving estrogen replacement therapy from developing endometrial cancer. Table 16–11 lists the known or suspected risk factors for endometrial cancer.

Early Detection. Endometrial cancer can be detected early; however, the Pap smear is not an effective method for detection of this cancer (Gusberg, 1988). The ACS recommends that women with risk factors for endometrial cancer should have an endometrial tissue sample examined at menopause. For this reason an annual suction curettage is recommended for menopausal women and women who have taken estrogen without progesterone modification for a prolonged period after menopause. Suction curettage can provide an excellent sample and in most cases can be performed in the office without need for anesthesia (Gusberg, 1988; White, Cornelius, Judkins, & Patterson, 1978).

OVARIAN CANCER

Incidence. Ovarian cancer is the most lethal of the gynecologic tumors, accounting for an estimated 26,600 women who developed ovarian cancer and 14,500 women who died of the disease in 1995 (Wingo et al., 1995). There has been a decline in the incidence of ovarian cancer in younger women, whereas the incidence of this disease has increased in women over the age of 50 years. Ovarian cancer occurs more frequently in white females of European and North American origin than in African-American or Oriental women (Page & Asire, 1985; Barber, 1986).

Risk Factors. High-risk women are those who have delayed onset of child-bearing; low parity, particularly with a history of infertility; nulliparity; a history of breast cancer; two or more first-degree relatives with a history of ovarian cancer; high socioeconomic status; and several spontaneous abortions (Rubin & Peterson, 1985; Barber, 1986; Cancer and Steroid Hormone Study, 1986; Runowicz, 1992; Rossing, Daling, Weiss, & Moore, 1994). The use of oral contraceptives, which create a hormonal balance similar to that of pregnancy (suppression of ovulation), has been found to decrease the risk of epithelial ovarian cancer (Henahan, 1900; Ozols, 1991). Rossing et al. (1994) reported that prolonged use of clomiphene, an ovulation-inducing medication, may increase the risk of a borderline or invasive ovarian tumor.

Family history is reported to affect only a small proportion of women with the disease (one to three per cent) (Runowicz, 1992). However, Carlson and colleagues write that age and family history are the most important risk factors for ovarian cancer. They estimate that women with a family history of a hereditary ovarian cancer syndrome represent a small subgroup that is at highest risk, with a lifetime probability of ovarian cancer of up to 50 per cent (Carlson, Skates, & Kinger, 1994). See Table 16–12 for known or suspected risk factors for ovarian cancer and Table 16–13 for other genetic conditions associated with increased cancer risk.

TABLE 16–11. *Major Risk Factors for Corpus Uteri Cancer*

RISK FACTOR	EXPLANATION	MAY REDUCE RISK
Estrogen replacement therapy	Prolonged, continuous exposure of the endometrium to estrogen stimulation increases risk to 6 to 7 times for post-menopausal women. Risk increases with duration of use and dosage of replacement estrogens. Women who have taken conjugated estrogen for 1 or more years remain at increased risk for at least 10 years after they discontinue use.	Cyclic progestogen therapy with estrogen therapy reduces risk.
Obesity	Obese women (30% more than normal weight for height) are twice as likely to develop endometrial cancer. Risk increases with increasing weight. Obese women, particularly after menopause, have higher levels of estrogens in blood. Tallness, coupled with obesity, also increases risk.	Maintain ideal body weight.
Fertility	Women who have four or more children are 1.3 times as likely to develop endometrial cancer.	
Conditions associated with continuous estrogenic status	Polycystic ovary syndrome (Stein-Leventhal), thecagranulosa cell tumors, infertility secondary to failure of the ovulatory mechanism.	Treatment of medical condition.
High socioeconomic status	More affluent women use replacement estrogens more frequently than less affluent women.	
Birth control pills	Women who use "sequential" birth control pills have double the risk of endometrial cancer as women who use other forms of birth control. Sequential pills have been removed from the American market. Women who use combination pills (estrogen and progesterone in each pill) for at least 1 year have one half the risk of endometrial cancer as women who do not use this form of birth control. Decreased risk persisted for at least 10 years after discontinuing use and was most notable in nulliparous women.	Avoidance of sequential birth control pills.
Late natural menopause Turner's syndrome(?) Family history of endometrial cancer		

(Data from Dunn, 1981; Henderson, Gerkins, & Pike, 1975; Lynch & Lynch, 1978; Page & Asire, 1985; Rubin & Peterson, 1985; Schlaff & Rosenshein, 1985; Shapiro, Kelly, Rosenberg, Kaufman, Helmrich, Rosenshein, Lewis, Knapp, Stolley, & Schottenfeld, 1985; Vessey, 1985)

Early Detection. The rectovaginal examination is an effective method of detecting early asymptomatic ovarian tumors. Women considered at high risk should have an annual rectovaginal examination. At initial diagnosis, approximately 60 to 70 per cent of ovarian cancers have already reached stage III or IV (Barber, 1986). Barber (1986) reported that an early sign of ovarian cancer is the postmenopausal palpable ovary syndrome. "Palpation of what is interpreted as a normal-sized ovary in the premenopausal woman represents an ovarian tumor in the postmenopausal woman."

It was announced at the seventh international meeting on advances in the applications of monoclonal antibodies in clinical oncology that "a single determination of elevated serum CA-125 levels using monoclonal antibodies in conjunction with abnormal pelvic ultrasound is a highly specific method of detecting epithelial ovarian carcinoma in postmenopausal women" (Ozols, 1991). Currently, in patients who have a significantly increased risk for ovarian cancer a combination approach is being investigated. The combination approach involves taking serial serum CA-125 levels, doing transvaginal ultrasound examinations, and performing routine rectovaginal examinations.

The NIH Consensus Development Panel on Ovarian Cancer (1995) reported that there is no evidence to support routine screening in women with no family history or other high risk factors. Furthermore, screening with ultrasonography or CA 125 radioimmunoassay is not recommended for women with two or more first-degree relatives (Carlson et al., 1994; NIH Consensus Development Panel on Ovarian Cancer, 1995).

Prevention. The role of prophylactic oophorectomies is controversial at this time and it may not entirely eliminate the risk of ovarian cancer. Some authors recommend prophylactic oophorectomy in women with family histories of two or more first-degree relatives with ovarian cancer (Runowicz, 1992). In women with a hereditary ovarian cancer syndrome, the lifetime risk of ovarian cancer is approximately 40 per cent. For this group of women, it is recommended that after childbearing is completed (or by 35 years of age), prophylactic bilateral oophorectomy be done to reduce their significant risk (NIH Consensus Development Panel on Ovarian Cancer, 1995).

Nursing Role. In the United States, nurses have served multiple roles, from role modeling, to education, to performing gynecologic examinations (Goodman,

TABLE 16–12. *Known or Suspected Risk Factors for Ovarian Cancer*

RISK FACTOR	EXPLANATION	MAY REDUCE RISK
Lack of childbearing	Several pregnancies confer more protection than one pregnancy. Women who have had a child are half as likely to get ovarian cancer as nulliparous women. Pregnancy suppresses ovulation. "Incessant" ovulation increases risk. Delayed childbearing may also increase risk of ovarian cancer.	Having children at a young age.
History of breast cancer	Twice the expected risk of developing ovarian cancer. Women who have had ovarian cancer are three to four times more likely to develop breast cancer.	
Type of birth control utilized	*Decreased risk* with use of oral contraceptives; protective effect evident for women who used oral contraceptives for as little as 3 to 6 months; protective effect continued for 15 years after use ended.	Use of oral contraceptives.
Exposure to asbestos and talc	Conflicting data on risk of ovarian cancer and talc. Stronger evidence on risk of asbestos and ovarian cancer.	
High socioeconomic status and living in a western country	May relate to high-fat diet or small number or absence of children.	
Irradiation of pelvic organs (also mentioned in the literature)		

(Data form Barber, 1986; Cancer and Steroid Hormone Study, 1987; Earhart, 1983; Page & Asire, 1985; Rawson, 1978; Rubin & Peterson, 1985; Schlaff & Rosenshein, 1985.)

1982; Stalker, 1985; White et al., 1978). Multiple continuing education programs to prepare nurses for a role in cancer screening and detection have been offered throughout the United States. One of the earliest continuing education programs, starting in 1976, was offered at M.D. Anderson Hospital and Tumor Institute in Texas. Originally the course was 3 weeks long, and continues with the addition of week-long modules, for example, a module instructing nurses in screening for pelvic cancer (White et al., 1978). Similar programs to prepare nurses in conducting gynecologic examinations but no longer being offered, were "Cancer Prevention: A Course for Nurse Practitioners" offered by Memorial Sloan-Kettering Cancer Center, New York City, and a course titled "Focus on Cancer: Prevention and Early Detection" developed by the University of Washington for nurse practitioners and physicians assistants (*Focus on cancer*, 1984; Gianella, 1985; Stalker, 1985).

Role modeling involves practicing the preventive measures recommended by the ACS for Pap and pelvic examinations. McMillan (1990) surveyed RNs in southwest Florida and found that the majority of nurses (57 per cent) who responded to her survey reported having had a Pap test within the past 3 years; an additional 22 per cent had had a hysterectomy and thus were not eligible for cervical smear.

Nurses have been involved in educating women who are at increased risk for cervical cancer (D'Onofrio, 1979; Lovejoy, 1987; Mitchell, Sandella, & White, 1992; St. Pierre, 1988) as well as conducting research studies with these high-risk women (Graham & Leigh, 1984; Walczak, 1983). St. Pierre (1988) writes that women diagnosed with condyloma acuminatum lesions have special educational needs that

nurses should address. She makes the point that the nurse's involvement in meeting the special educational needs of these high-risk women will facilitate the woman's sense of well-being throughout the experience. Graham and Leigh (1984) discussed the role of the research nurse in a chemoprevention study designed to abrogate or suppress cervical preneoplastic changes. They pointed out that the role of the nurse includes all aspects of the research process, including developing a toxicity scale for assessing vulvar, vaginal, and cervical toxicity; providing informational and emotional support to the patient; and assessing the objective responses to the chemoprevention agents. In the early 1980s, Walczak (1983) investigated the date of the most recent Pap smear for a group of women with invasive cervical cancer. Walczak's study was conducted in response to the revised ACS recommendations for the frequency of Pap smears. Her study indicated that the overwhelming majority of women had not had a Pap smear 10 or more years before the diagnosis of cervical cancer. She wrote that these findings support the importance of nurses being involved in patient education that emphasizes participation in gynecologic screening programs.

Elderly women are another group with whom nurses have targeted their educational efforts, research, and clinical practice (Blesch, 1990; Denny, Koren, & Wisby, 1989; Melillo, 1985; Nussbaum, 1990; Weinrich & Nussbaum, 1984; Weinrich & Weinrich, 1990). The study of Denny et al. (1989) found that there are unmet gynecologic health needs in older women. "Nurses can respond to the need of older women for gynecological health care by providing: screening for common gynecological health problems; education on

TABLE 16–13. *Genetic Conditions Associated with Increased Cancer Risk*

GENETIC CONDITION	ASSOCIATED CANCER
Familial polyposis coli (dominant inheritance)	Colon carcinoma
Gardner's syndrome (dominant inheritance)	Colon carcinoma, osteomas
Peutz-Jeghers syndrome (dominant inheritance)	Gastrointestinal carcinoma
Familial Wilms's tumor (dominant inheritance)	Wilms's tumor
Cancer family syndrome (dominant inheritance)	Mostly adenocarcinoma of colon, endometrium
Familial retinoblastoma (dominant inheritance)	Retinoblastoma
Ataxia telangiectasia (dominant inheritance)	Lymphoid neoplasm
Fanconi's anemia (recessive inheritance)	Acute myelomonocytic leukemia, hepatoma
Xeroderma pigmentosum (recessive inheritance)	Basal and squamous cell cancer of skin
Retinoblastoma, bilateral	Sarcoma
Multiple lipomatosis	Skin cancer
Hereditary pancreatitis	Carcinoma of pancreas
Familial, juvenile, and neonatal cirrhosis	Hepatocellular carcinoma
Familial hydronephrosis	Congenital sarcoma of kidney
Fibrocystic pulmonary dysplasia	Bronchial adenocarcinoma
Albinism (recessive inheritance)	Skin cancer
Polycythemia vera	Acute myelocytic leukemia
Dyskeratosis congenita	Leukoplakia with squamous cell carcinoma
Torre's syndrome	Diverse gastrointestinal and urogenital cancers
Klinefelter's syndrome	Breast cancer risk approaches the risk in normal women and is approximately 66 times the risk in normal men
Gonadal dysgenesis	Gonadal malignancy—risk is 25 per cent
Turner's syndrome	Tumors of neural crest origin and brain and pituitary tumors. Endometrial cancer but only with prolonged estrogen therapy
Cryptorchidism	Testicular cancer
Glutathione reductase deficiency	Leukemia
Kostmann's syndrome (infantile genetic agranulocytosis)	Acute monocytic leukemia
Bloom's syndrome (recessive inheritance)	Acute nonlymphocytic leukemia, gastrointestinal tumors
Neurofibromatosis or von Recklinghausen's disease (dominant inheritance)	Neurologic sarcomas, gliomas, Wilms' tumor, rhabdomyosarcoma, myeloid leukemia
Nevoid basal cell carcinoma syndrome (dominant inheritance)	Medulloblastoma, basal cell carcinomas, ovarian fibrosarcoma
Down's syndrome	Acute leukemia—risk increased 11 times in children with Down's syndrome
XY gonadal dysgenesis (sex-linked recessive, a male-limited dominant)	Gonadoblastoma, dysgerminoma
Mixed gonadal dysgenesis	Gonadoblastoma
Testicular feminization (sex-linked recessive)	Gonadoblastoma

(Data from Anderson, 1975; Meadows & Li, 1983, pp. 17–24; Meisner, 1983, pp. 167, 168, 169; Mulvihill, 1975, p. 21; Rawson, 1978.)

self-care practices related to gynecological health; and referral for interventions outside nursing's scope of practice" (p. 35). Melillo (1985) set up a mobile health van designed to educate and screen elderly women for breast, uterine, and cervical cancer. Nurse practitioners and nurses in the mobile health van provided risk assessment, preventive education, and physical examinations for all women and referred abnormal findings. When discussing the mobile health van designed specifically for elderly women, Melillo wrote that this " . . . cost-effective and relevant cancer screening clinic for elderly women focused on a nursing model and is one form of a nurse-managed and client-centered health care that may positively influence future health behaviors" (1985).

Weinrich and Weinrich (1990) demonstrated knowledge deficits related to cancer's early warning signals, the relationship between aging and cancer, and the similarities between some aging changes and cancer symptoms in a group of elderly men and women, They wrote that their results emphasize that nurses must be involved in cancer programs for less educated, low-income, older African-American persons. Nussbaum (1990) reported similar findings in terms of the lack of knowledge about facts about cancer and the use of cancer screening tests in a sample of poor, elderly African-American females who were surveyed as they attended congregate meal sites.

The involvement of nurses in the early detection of cervical cancer is most urgently needed in developing countries. For instance, invasive cervical carcinoma is the most common genital malignancy in South Africa (du Toit, 1985; Searle, 1980). Cervical cancer is also a frequently occurring cancer in eastern and western Africa (Benjamin & Pritchard, 1987; Mitchley, 1984) and is recognized as a leading cause of death in women throughout Latin America and the Caribbean (de Llueca, 1987). In South Africa the Department of Gynecology of the Faculty of Medicine of the University of Stellenbosch and the Tygerberg Hospital conducted a special course in cervical cytology for nurses (du Toit, 1985). The nurses were required to take a written, oral, and practical examination at the end of the course before being awarded a certificate of competency. In 12 years these specially trained nurses have taken 48,426 smears and detected 370 genital malignancies. "In approximately 60 per cent of these patients, the lesions were still in the in situ or very early invasive stage and therefore easily amenable to treatment" (du Toit, 1985).

Nurses are actively involved in obtaining Pap smears in other countries as well. Gillatt (1984) wrote in 1984 that there were 32 health centers in Ireland and each of these centers has a Cervical Smear Test Clinic staffed by public health nurses who were trained to take cervical smears as well as to teach breast self-examination. In Finland, each municipality has at least one maternal and child welfare clinic where Pap smears are taken by specially trained public health nurses (Massingberd, 1988). In 1987, 149,505 women were screened by these Finnish nurses, and 55 cases of invasive cancer were detected. Tuladhar (1990) wrote that nurses could serve an important role in lowering the high uterine cancer rate in Nepal by educating and screening women. However, nurses are prevented from doing so because of a number of barriers including the low visibility of nurses in Nepal.

In summary, in terms of cervical cancer, nurses are involved in identifying high-risk women, counseling on early detection and risk reduction measures, performing examinations, and providing women with information. There was far less information on the role nurses were assuming in terms of the prevention and early detection of uterine and ovarian cancer. If the incidence of gynecologic cancer is to be decreased, more nurses will need to be educated for an active role in the primary and secondary prevention of this cancer. More nursing research is needed in terms of investigating the most effective educational methods of reaching "hard-to-reach" women: high-risk women, poor women, elderly women, and minority women. Table 16–14 provides an overview of cancer prevention, screening, and detection activities.

COMMUNITY-BASED PROGRAMS

Nurses who have cancer prevention and early detection information and health education framework knowledge can promote effective strategies for cancer control in their communities and specifically for those who are at high risk for cancer. All nurses need to be cancer-prevention and detection nurses. Nurses who are not always thought of as cancer nurses are critical to the overall community cancer control efforts. School nurses, occupational health nurses, nurses in private physicians' offices, nurses in ambulatory care, and health department nurses are of prime importance to community cancer control programs.

At this time, a comprehensive program for cancer prevention and detection education among nurses does not exist. Nurses receive information on cancer prevention and detection during their formal academic preparation, at conferences and workshops, and through the literature. Health education in cancer prevention and detection for nurses is in its infancy and must be addressed. A conscious effort must be made to reach all nurses in all practice settings.

To ensure that nurses have and use cancer prevention and detection information in their practices, a nurse work group can be established in each community. The work group would include nurse leaders from a variety of practice areas (hospitals, schools, health departments, physician offices, industry, ambulatory clinics, and private practice) in the community. A group of nurses whose special clinical practice is in oncology should be the initiators of the work group. They would invite nurse leaders in various practice settings in the community to meet and discuss issues and possible strategies. The work group would plan for dissemination of cancer prevention and detection information to all nurses. This dissemination could be done formally, through established nursing groups, or informally, through the workplace. Nurses in the local work group would know the nurses in practice settings similar to their own and would know the strengths, needs, and concerns of these nurses.

Because the work group nurses will represent a variety of health care settings in the community, they will know not only the needs for nurse education but also the health needs of the community for cancer prevention and detection. The work group would plan for dissemination of cancer control information to all nurses and help nurses with health education strategies and evaluation. By using the community-based nurse work group process, the commitment to cancer control would be strengthened.

SUMMARY

Early detection and prevention cancer efforts by nurses have not been promoted in the health care system. However, with reform in health care emphasizing wellness, nurses have an opportunity to take a leading role in reducing cancer mortality. If the year 2000 goals for cancer control are to be obtained, nurses will have to be a major part of these efforts. A concerted effort must be made to encourage clinicians and nurse researchers to focus on cancer prevention and early detection. Appropriate lifestyle changes and limiting exposure to known carcinogens will be essential. Cancer prevention is the best defense against cancer. Every nurse must address limiting tobacco use, helping people change questionable dietary habits, and educating people concerning early detection. Nurses have an exceedingly important role in helping ourselves, individuals, groups, and communities change behaviors. If we are willing to use the knowledge we now have about cancer prevention and early detection, we will be well on the road to the elimination of cancer.

TABLE 16–14. **Cancers: Prevention, Screening and Detection**

| TYPE OF CANCER | PREVENTION PRACTICES | 1995 ACS SCREENING RECOMMENDATIONS | HIGH-RISK FACTORS | DETECTION | | | |
				HISTORY	EARLY SIGNS AND SYMPTOMS	DIAGNOSTIC TECHNIQUES
Skin	Reduce ultraviolet exposure, use sunscreens and protective clothing	Monthly self-examinations, professional examination (>20 yr of age every 3 yrs, >40 yr of age every year)	Caucasian w/red or blond hair, blue or green eyes, fair skin, positive familial history of skin cancer	Changes in moles, unhealed sores	Change in symmetry, border, color, or diameter of a mole; skin lesions; unhealed sores	Biopsy of lesions
Oral	Avoid smoking and smokeless tobacco, limit alcohol intake, practice good oral and dental hygiene	Monthly oral self-examination for high risk individuals, annual dental checkups	Poor dental hygiene, tobacco use	Tobacco and/or alcohol use, oral lesions or sore, dental problems	Oral lesions or pain, leukoplakia, erythroplasia, limited motion of tongue, marked cervical adenopathy	Biopsy, exfoliative cytology
Gastric	Avoid salty, smoked, starchy, and high-nitrate foods, and eat fruits, vegetables, and foods high in vitamin C	None	Nonwhite, lower socioeconomic strata, blood type A, male	Stomach conditions, pernicious anemia, atrophic gastritis, gastric ulcer, surgery for benign gastric disease, intestinal metaplasia	Indigestion, epigastric pain, vomiting, dysphagia	Endoscopy, biopsy
Esophageal	Avoid tobacco, alcohol, opium, excessively hot foods and beverages	None	Smoking, drinking, smoking opium pipes, ingestion of *mate*	Smoking, alcohol use, diet	Dysphagia	Esophogram esophagoscopy
Colorectal	Avoid animal fat intake; consume fiber	Digital rectal exam (≥40 yr annually) stool guaiac slide test (≥50 yr annually), sigmoidoscopy (≥50 yr every 3–5 yr), more frequently for high-risk individuals, beginning 5 yr before youngest diagnosed family member	Family history, polyposis syndrome, chronic ulcerative colitis, cured colorectal, female genital cancer, history adenomatous polyps	Family history, diet	Changes in bowel habits, anemia, rectal bleeding, vague abdominal pain, rectal pain, anorexia, weight loss, change in diameter of stool	Rectal exam, proctosigmoidoscopy, colonoscopy, barium enema with contrast
Testicular	Surgically correct crytochidism, get mumps vaccine	Monthly testicular self-examination	Uncorrected crythochidism, white male	Swollen painful testicle, history of undescended testicle, history of mumps, mother with DES	Enlarged testicle, nodule or mass, scrotal "heaviness," pain	Physical exam, transillumination, biopsy

DES, diethylstilbestrol.
(From Frank-Stromborg, M. & Rohan, K. [1992]. Nursings' involvement in the primary and secondary prevention of cancer. *Cancer Nursing*, 15[2], 79–108.)

Continued on following page.

TABLE 16–14. Cancers: Prevention, Screening and Detection Continued

TYPE OF CANCER	PREVENTION PRACTICES	1995 ACS SCREENING RECOMMENDATIONS	HIGH-RISK FACTORS	DETECTION			
				HISTORY	EARLY SIGNS AND SYMPTOMS	DIAGNOSTIC TECHNIQUES
Prostate	Avoid alcohol and fat intake; eat green and yellow vegetables	Annual rectal exam over age 40 yr	African-American elderly North American	Exposure to cadmium or fertilizer, occupation in tire/rubber industry	Difficulty initiating stream, frequent, interrupted or painful urination, dribbling, urinary retention, hematuria	Transrectal ultrasonography, PSA levels, biopsy
Cervical	Limit number of sexual partners	Annual pap test and pelvic exam for women who are sexually active or ≥18 yr of age; after three or more consecutive normal annual exams, the pap test can be done less frequently at discretion of physician	Multiple sexual partners, intercourse before age 20 yr, poor hygiene, genital infection (HPV and herpes simplex-2)	Sexual history, vaginal bleeding or discharge	Abnormal bleeding	Pap smear, colposcopy w/biopsy
Endometrial	Avoid obesity	Yearly pelvic exam	Obesity, >40 yr of age, few or no children, infertility, early menarche, late menopause, estrogen therapy	Vaginal bleeding or discharge, menstrual history	Abnormal bleeding or discharge, abdominal pain or mass	Endometrial tissue sampling
Ovarian		Bimanual vaginal exam annually	Delayed onset of childbearing, low parity, history of breast cancer, familial history of ovarian cancer, several spontaneous abortions	Child-bearing history, familial history of ovarian, oral contraceptive use	Abdominal pain or mass	Bimanual pelvic exam, pap smear, laparotomy
Lung and laryngeal	Avoid smoking and second-hand smoke	None	Smoking, asbestos worker	Smoking history, work exposure	Cough, pleuritic chest pain	Chest radiography or computed tomography, bronchoscopy w/ washings and biopsy, sputum cytology
Breast	Avoid fat intake and obesity	Monthly self-examination, annual professional exam, mammogram every 1–2 yr ages 40–49, and annually after 50 yr of age; screening mammography should begin by age 40	Genetic predisposition, fibrocystic disease, obesity, nulliparity, adverse normal milieu	Mother, grandmother, aunt, sister with breast cancer, child-bearing history, fibrocystic disease	Dimpling, flattening of nipple, abnormal contours of the breast, peau d'orange, palapable mass	Mammography, biopsy

REFERENCES

American Cancer Society. (1978). *Facts and figures.* New York: Author.

American Cancer Society. (1989a). Survey of physician's attitudes and practices in early cancer detection. *CA: A Cancer Journal for Clinicians, 40,* 79.

American Cancer Society. (1989b). *Summary of current guidelines for the cancer-related checkup: Recommendations.* New York: Author.

American Cancer Society Cancer Response System. (1994). Prostate cancer prevention trial. 02/11/94.

American Cancer Society. (1995). *Cancer facts and figures.* Atlanta: Author.

Ammirata S., Bordeaux-Ferguson, I. (1989). Development of a breast cancer screening clinic in a research setting (Abstract 130). *Oncology Nursing Forum, 16*(Suppl.), 161.

Amonette, R. A., & Buker, J. L. (1992). Actinic keratosis: The most common precancer. *Primary Care & Cancer, 12*(7), 18–26.

Anderson, D. (1975). Familial susceptibility. In J. Fraumeni (Ed.), *Persons at high risk of cancer. An approach to cancer etiology and control* (pp. 39–54). New York: Academic Press.

Anderson S., & Munson, N. (1990). Skin cancer fair in the hospital setting (Abstract 268). *Oncology Nursing Forum, 17,* 204.

Ash, C., Oberst, M., Stalker, M., Park, D. Avellanet, C., & Glasel, M. (1982). *Cancer prevention: A course for nurse practitioners.* New York: Memorial Sloan-Kettering Cancer Center, Division of Nursing.

Badalament, R. A., & Drago, J. R. (1991). Prostate cancer. *DM, 37,* 203–268.

Baeck, M. L., & Eisenberg, M. (1985). Carcinogenic risk assessment: Concepts and issues. *Maryland Medical Journal, 34,* 672–674.

Baines, C. J. (1994). The Canadian national breast screening study: A perspective on criticisms. *Annals of Internal Medicine, 120,* 326–334.

Barber, H. (1986). Ovarian cancer. *CA: A Cancer Journal for Clinicians, 36,* 149–183.

Bargoil, S. (1991). Skin cancer prevention: "Do you know which sunscreen to use?" (Abstract 1351). *Oncology Nursing Forum, 18,* 383.

Bartecchi, C. E., MacKenzie, T. D., & Schrier, R. (1994). The human costs of tobacco use (First of two parts). *New England Journal of Medicine, 330*(13), 907–912.

Bechel, J., Kelley, W., Petty, T., Patz, D., & Saccomanno, G. (1994). Outcome of 51 patients with roentgenographically occult lung cancer detected by sputum cytologic testing: A community hospital program. *Archives of Internal Medicine, 154,* 975–980.

Beck, S, Breckenridge-Potterf, S., Wallace, S., Ware, J., Asay, E., & Giles, R. (1988). The family high-risk program: Targeted cancer prevention. *Oncology Nursing Forum, 15,* 301-306.

Becker, M. H., Drachman, R. H. & Kirscht, J. P. (1975). A field experiment to evaluate various outcomes to continuity of physician care. *American Journal of Public Health, 64,* 1062–1070.

Becker, M. H., & Rosenstock, I. M. (1975). Socio-psychological research on determinants of prevention health behavior. In *The Fogarty International Center Series on the Teaching of Preventative Medicine. The behavioral sciences and prevention medicine: Opportunities and dilemmas* (p. 4). Bethesda, MD: National Cancer Institute.

Bender, M. (1988). A clinician's guide to genital papillomavirus infection. *Current Concepts in Skin Disorders,* Fall, 1–6.

Benjamin, E. V., & Pritchard, A. P. (1987). Professional education in Africa and the Middle East. *Cancer Nursing, 10,* 207–211.

Berg, J. (1984). Clinical implications of risk factors for breast cancer. *Cancer, 53,* 589–591.

Birdsell, J. (1986). Cancer in the aged. In D. Welch-McCaffrey (Ed.), *Nursing considerations in geriatric oncology.* Columbus, OH: Adria Laboratories.

Blesch, K. S. (1990). Cervical cancer screening in older women: Issues and interventions (Abstract 120). *Oncology Nursing Forum, 17,* 167.

Blesch, K. S. (1986). Health beliefs about testicular cancer and self-examination among professional men. *Oncology Nursing Forum, 13,* 29–33.

Boffetta, P., & Parkin, D. M. (1994). Cancer in developing countries. *CA: A Cancer Journal for Clinicians, 44*(2), 81–89.

Boice, J. D., Jr, & Monson, R. R. (1977). Breast cancer in women after repeated fluoroscopic examinations of the chest. *Journal of the National Cancer Institute, 59,* 823–832.

Bongiorno, C. (1988). Appropriate prevention and detection of gastrointestinal neoplasms in the elderly. *Clinics in Geriatric Medicine, 4,* 223–233.

Bostwick, D. G. (1989). The pathology of early prostate cancer. *CA: A Cancer Journal for Clinicians, 39,* 376–393.

Brailey, L. J. (1986). Effects of health teaching in the workplace on women's knowledge, beliefs, and practices regarding breast self-examination. *Research in Nursing and Health, 9,* 223–231.

Breast Cancer Education Program. Buffalo, New York: Roswell-Park Memorial Institute.

Buckley, M., & Cody, B. (1990). Prevention and early detection of skin cancer: A comprehensive overview (Abstract 225). *Oncology Nursing Forum, 17,* 194.

Bulbrook, R. D., Hayward, J. L., Wang, D. Y., Thomas, B. S., Clark, G., Allen, D., & Moore, J. W. (1986). Identification of women at high risk of breast cancer. *Breast Cancer Research and Treatment, 7*(Suppl.), 7–10.

Bultz, B., Scott, J., & Taenzer, P. (1988). Successful smoking cessation. *Cancer Nursing, 11,* 18–20.

Burack, R. C., & Drelichman, A. (1982). *Risk assessment through the patient interview: A model emphasizing cancer prevention (Module IX),* Detroit: Wayne State University School of Nursing.

Burns, N., Stotts, C., & Henderson, A. (1988). Smoking among nurses in Texas (Abstract 39). *Proceedings of the thirteenth annual congress of the Oncology Nursing Society* (p. 111). Pittsburgh, PA, May 4–7.

Cahill, L. M. (1980). Industrial cancer education service. In: R. Tiffany, (Ed.), *Cancer nursing update. Proceedings of the 2nd international cancer nursing conference,* (pp. 42–44). London: Bailliere Tindall.

Calzone, K., Saran, P., & Sommerfield, D. (1986). Establishing a multi-disciplinary breast care center. Meeting the challenge (Abstract 128P). *Oncology Nursing Forum, 13,* 87.

Cancer facts and figures for minority Americans, 1986. (1986). New York: American Cancer Society.

Cancer and Steroid Hormone Study of the Centers for Disease Control and the National Institute of Child Health and Human Development. (1986). Oral-contraceptives and the risk of breast cancer. *New England Journal of Medicine, 315,* 405–411.

Cancer and Steroid Hormone Study of the Centers for Disease Control and the National Institute of Child Health and Human Development. (1987). The reduction in risk of ovarian cancer associated with oral-contraceptive use. *New England Journal of Medicine, 316,* 650–655.

Carlin, P. J. (1986). Testicular self-examination: A public awareness program. *Public Health Reports, 101,* 98–102.

Carlson, C. T. (1991a). Prevention, screening and detection. In S. E. Otto (Ed.), *Oncology nursing* (pp. 28–37). St. Louis: C. V. Mosby.

Carlson, C. T. (1991b). Diagnosis and staging. In S. E. Otto (Ed.), *Oncology nursing* (pp. 38–48). St. Louis: C. V. Mosby.

Carlson, K. J., Skates, S. J., & Singer, D. (1994). Screening for ovarian cancer. *Annals of Internal Medicine, 121*(2), 124–132.

Carpenter, L. C. (1989). Breast health awareness: A collaborative county-wide project (Abstract 59). *Oncology Nursing Forum, 16*(Suppl.), 143.

Carroll, K., Braden, L., Bell, J., & Kalamegham, R. (1986). Fat and cancer. *Cancer, 58,* 1818–1825.

Case, C. (1984). Teaching breast self-examination in hospitals (Abstract 103). *Oncology Nursing Forum, 11*(Suppl.), 75.

Casey, F., Haughey, B., Dittmar, S., O'Shea, R., & Brasure, J. (1989). Smoking practices among nursing students: A comparison of two studies. *Journal of Nursing Education, 28,* 397–401.

Cashavelly, B. J. (1987). Cervical dysplasia. An overview of current concepts in epidemiology, diagnosis, and treatments. *Cancer Nursing, 10,* 199–206.

Catalona, W., Smith, D., Ratliff, T., Dodds, K. M., Coplen, D. E., Yuan, J. J., Petros, J. A., & Andriole, G. L. (1991). Measurement of prostate-specific antigen in serum as a screening test for prostate cancer. *New England Journal of Medicine, 324,* 1156–1161.

Champion, V. (1985). Use of the health belief model in determining frequency of breast self-examination. *Advances in Nursing Science, 8,* 373–379.

Champion, V. (1987). The relationship of breast self-examination to health belief model variables. *Advances in Nursing Science, 10,* 37S–82S.

Champion, V. (1988). Attitudinal variables related to intention, frequency, and proficiency of breast self-examination in women 35 and over. *Advances in Nursing Science, 11,* 283–291.

Charnley, S., Tannenbaum, S., & Correa, P. (1982). Gastric cancer: An etiologic model. In P. MaGee (Ed.), *Nitrosamines and human cancer* (pp. 503–522). Cold Spring Harbor, NY: Cold Spring Harbor Laboratory.

Cigarette smoking among adults—United States, 1990. (1992). *Journal of the American Medical Association, 267*(23), 3133.

Clarke, D. E., & Sandler, L. S. (1989). Factors involved in nurses' teaching breast self-examination. *Cancer Nursing, 12,* 41–46.

Clemmesen, J. (1987). Parameters for identification of high-risk groups. In H. Nieburgs (Ed.), *Prevention and detection of cancer. Part I. Prevention. Vol 2. Etiology* (pp. 1513–1516). New York: Marcel Dekker, Inc.

Colditz, G. A., Stampfer, M. J., Willett, W. C., Hennekens, C. H., Rosner, B., & Speizer, F. E. (1990). Prospective study of estrogen replacement therapy and risk of breast cancer in postmenopausal women. *Journal of the American Medical Association, 264,* 2648–2653.

Cole, C. F., & Gorman, L. M. (1984). Breast self-examination: Practices and attitudes of registered nurses. *Oncology Nursing Forum, 11,* 37–41.

Cole, P., & Amoateng-Adjepong, Y. (1994). Cancer prevention: Accomplishments and prospects. *American Journal of Public Health, 84,* 8–9.

Coleman, C., McCarthy, P., & Mullins, A. (1986). Toward standardization in clinical breast examination (Abstract 235). *Oncology Nursing Forum, 13,* 113.

Coleman, E. A. (1990). Efficacy of breast self examination teaching methods among the aging (Abstract 13A). *Oncology Nursing Forum, 17,* 141.

Conklin, M., Klint, K., Morway, A., Sawyer, J. R., & Shephard, R. (1978). Should health teaching include self-exam of the testes? *American Journal of Nursing, 12,* 2073–2074.

Conroy, C. (1986). A pilot project implementing breast self-exam (BSE) and testicular self-exam (TSE) teaching on one hospital unit (Abstract 52). *Oncology Nursing Forum, 13,* 68.

Coody, D. (1987). Special risk clinic (Abstract 35A). *Oncology Nursing Forum, 14,* 90.

Cook-Mozaffari, P. (1985). The geography of cancer. In M. P. Vessey & M. Gray (Eds.), *Cancer risks and prevention* (pp. 15–43). Oxford: Oxford University Press.

Costanza, M., Frederick, L., Green, H., & Patterson, W. B. (1986). Cancer prevention and detection: Strategies for practice. In *Cancer manual* (7th ed., pp. 14–35). Boston: American Cancer Society, Massachusetts Division, Inc.

Creasey, W. A. (1985). *Diet and Cancer.* Philadelphia: Lea & Febiger

Cretain, G. K. (1989). Motivational factors in breast self-examination. Implications for nurses. *Cancer Nursing, 12,* 250–256.

Crooks, C. E., & Jones, S. D. (1989). Educating women about the importance of breast screenings: The nurse's role. *Cancer Nursing, 12,* 161-164.

Culp, D. A., Boatman, D. L., & Wilson, V. B. (1973). Testicular tumors: 40 years of experience. *Journal of Urology, 110,* 548–553.

The dark side of the sun. (1986, June 9). *Newsweek,* 60–64.

Day, N., & Munoz, N. (1982). Esophagus. In D. Schottenfeld & J Fraumeni (Eds.), *Cancer epidemiology and prevention* (pp. 596–623). Philadelphia: W. B. Saunders Co.

DeCosse, J. (1988). Early cancer detection. Colorectal cancer. *Cancer, 62,* 1787–1790.

de Llueca, L. A. (1987). Teaching of cancer nursing in Latin America. A pilot study. *Cancer Nursing, 10,* 200–206.

DeMello, D. J., Hoffman, L. A., Wesmiller, S. W., & Zullo, T. G. (1989). Smoking and attitudes toward smoking among clinical nurse specialists, critical care nurses, and medical-surgical nurses. *Oncology Nursing Society, 16,* 795–799.

Denny, M. S., Koren, M. E., & Wisby, M. (1989). Gynecological health needs of elderly women. *Journal of Gerontology Nursing, 15,* 33–37.

DeVita, V. (1985). Cancer as a preventable disease. *Maryland Medical Journal, 34,* 41–43.

Diem, G., & Rose, D. (1985). Has breast self-examination had a fair trial? *New York State Journal of Medicine, 85,* 479–480.

Doll, R., & Peto, R. (1981). The causes of cancer: Quantitative estimates of avoidable risks of cancer in the United States today. *Journal of the National Cancer Institute, 66,* 1191–1308.

D'Onofrio, M. (1979). Prevention and early detection of cervical cancer by evaluation of the abnormal Pap smear (Abstract 133). *Proceedings of the fourth annual congress of the Oncology Nursing Society* (p. 45). Pittsburgh, PA. May 17–19.

Doyle, M. A., & Simonich, W. (1991). Comparison of breast self examination (BSE) practices in women with breast cancer versus women with a non-breast primary (Abstract 193). *Oncology Nursing Forum, 18,* 392.

Drago, J. (1989). The role of new modalities in the early detection and diagnosis of prostate cancer. *CA: A Cancer Journal for Clinicians, 39,* 326–336.

Dunn, L. (1981). Endometrial cancer increasing but highly curable. *Diagnosis, 3,* 39–50.

Dupont, W. D., Page, D. L., Parl, R., Vnencar-Jones, C., Plummer, W. D., Rados, M. S., & Schuyler, P. A. (1985). Risk factors for breast cancer in women with proliferative breast disease. *New England Journal of Medicine, 312,* 146–151.

du Toit, J. P. (1985). The role of the nurse in the early detection of cervical carcinoma in a developing country. *Cancer Nursing, 8,* 121–127.

Earhart, R. (1983). Cancer of the ovary. In S. B. Kahn, R. Love, C. Sherman, & R. Chakravorty (Eds.), *Concepts in cancer medicine* (pp. 483–491). New York: Grune & Stratton, Inc.

Edgar, L. (1985). A systematic means of evaluating the quality of BSE (Abstract 125). *Oncology Nursing Forum, 12,* 70.

Education about skin cancer. Australia. (1988). *International Cancer News, 11,* 9–12.

Einhorn, L. H., Paulson, D. F., & Pickham, M. T., et al. (1982). Testicular carcinoma. In V. DeVita, S. Helman, & S. Rosenberg (Eds.), *Cancer principles and the practice of oncology* (pp. 786–822). Philadelphia: J. B. Lippincott.

Eliopoulos, C., Klein, J., Phan, M., Knie, B., Greenwald, M., Chitayat, D., & Koren, G. (1994). Hair concentrations of nicotine and cotinine in women and their newborn infants. *Journal of the American Medical Association, 271*(8), 621–623.

Ellerhorst-Ryan, J. (1985). Breast consultation center multidisciplinary model for care of women with breast disease (Abstract 160). *Oncology Nursing Forum, 12*(Suppl.), 79.

Enstrom, J., & Kanim, L. (1983). Populations at low risk. In G. Newell (Ed.), *Cancer prevention in clinical medicine* (pp. 49–78). New York: Raven Press.

Ernster, V. (1987). Trends in tobacco use and cancer risk. In *Proceedings of the second national conference on cancer prevention and detection.* New York: American Cancer Society.

Esparza, D. M., & Kean, T. J. (1980). Performance issues in breast self-examination (Abstract 60). *Proceedings of the Fifth Annual Congress of the Oncology Nursing Society.* (p. 48). San Diego, CA, May 28–30.

Facciponti, C. A., & Cartwright, F. (1988). Identifying barriers to breast self examination practice in post mastectomy patients (Abstract 235). *Proceedings of the thirteenth annual congress of the Oncology Nursing Society* (p. 160). Pittsburgh, PA, May 4–7.

Fahs, M., Mandelblatt, J., Schechter, C., & Muller, C. (1992). Cost effectiveness of cervical cancer screening for the elderly. *Annals of Internal Medicine, 117,* 520–527.

Faulkenberry, J. (1983). Cancer prevention and detection: Risk assessment. The medical history. *Cancer Nursing, 7,* 388–401.

Feldman, B., & Richard, E. (1986). Prevalence of nurse smokers and variables identified with successful and unsuccessful smoking cessation. *Research in Nursing and Health, 9,* 131–138.

Fennelly, D. W. (1994). Current approaches to the diagnosis and treatment of breast cancer. *Directions in Psychiatry, 14,* 1–8.

Fitzsimmons, M. Conway, T., Madsen, N., Lappe, J., & Coody, D. (1989). Hereditary cancer syndromes: Nursing's role in identification and education. *Oncology Nursing Forum, 16,* 87–94.

Fitzsimmons, M., Kriegler, M., Shea, P., & Lynch, H. (1987). Hereditary cancers: Implications for nursing practice (Abstract 223A). *Oncology Nursing Forum, 14,* 137.

Focus on cancer: Prevention and early detection longitudinal evaluation. Final report. (NCI Contract NO1-CN-95483). (1984). Seattle, WA: University of Washington.

Fontham, E., Correa, P., Reynolds, P., & Wu-Williams, A., et al. (1994). Environmental tobacco smoke and lung cancer in nonsmoking women. A multicenter study. *Journal of the American Medical Association, 271*(22), 1752–1759.

Foster, R. S., Lang, S. P., Costanza, M. C., Worden, J. K., Haines, C. R., & Yates, J. W. (1978). Breast self-examination and breast cancer stage. *New England Journal of Medicine, 299,* 265–270.

Frank, I. N., Keys, H. M., & McCune, C. S. (1983). Urologic and male genital cancers. In P. Ruben (Ed.), *Clinical oncology* (pp. 198–220). New York: American Cancer Society.

Frank, J, & Mai, V. (1985). Breast self-examination in young women: More harm than good? *Lancet, 2,* 654–657.

Frank-Stromborg, M. (1986). The role of the nurse in early detection of cancer: Population sixty-six years of age and older. *Oncology Nursing Forum, 13,* 66–74.

Frank-Stromborg, M. (1989). The epidemiology and primary prevention of gastric and esophageal cancer. A worldwide perspective. *Cancer Nursing, 12,* 53–64.

Frank-Stromborg, M. (1991). Evaluating cancer risk. In S. Baird, R. McCorkle, & M. Grant, (Eds.), *Cancer nursing: A comprehensive textbook* (pp. 155–189). Philadelphia: W. B. Saunders Co.

Frank-Stromborg, M., & Cohen, R. (1990). Assessment and intervention for cancer prevention and detection. In: S. Groenwald, M. Frogge, M. Goodman, & C. Yarbro (Eds.), *Cancer nursing principles and practice,* (2nd ed., pp. 119–160) Boston: Jones & Bartlett.

Frank-Stromborg, M., Johnson, J., & McCorkle, R. (1987). A program model for nurses involved with cancer education of black Americans. *Journal of Cancer Education, 2,* 145–151.

Fraser, M. (1981). Self-care: A plan for melanoma-prone families (Abstract 193). *Proceedings of the sixth annual congress of the Oncology Nursing Society.* (p. 92). Baltimore, May 4–6.

Fraser, M. (1982). The role of the nurse in the prevention and early detection of malignant melanoma. *Cancer Nursing, 5,* 351–360.

Fraser, M. (1983). Familial testicular cancer: Nursing management (Abstract 115). *Proceedings of the eighth annual congress of the Oncology Nursing Society.* (p. 75). San Diego, May 18–21.

Fraumeni, J. (1975). Preface. In J. Fraumeni (Ed.), *Persons at high risk of cancer. An approach to cancer etiology* (p. xvi). New York: Academic Press.

Friedman, R. J., Rigel, D. S., & Kopf, A. W. (1992). The ABCDs of moles and melanomas. *Primary Care & Cancer, 12*(7), 16–17.

Fuchs, C. S., Giovannucci, E. L., Colditz, G. A., Hunter, D. J., Speizer, F. E., & Willett, W. C. (1994). A prospective study of family history and the risk of colorectal cancer. *New England Journal of Medicine, 331,* 1669–1674.

Gail, M. H., Brinton, L. A., & Byar, D. P., et al. (1989). Projecting individualized probabilities of developing breast cancer for white females who are being examined annually. *Journal of the National Cancer Institute, 81,* 1879–1886.

Gambrell, R. D. (1990). Estrogen-progestogen replacement and cancer risk. *Hospital Practice, March,* 81–100.

Garnick, M. B. (1993). Prostate cancer: Screening, diagnosis, and management. *Annals of Internal Medicine, 118,* 804–818.

Gayal, R. (1983). Disease of the esophagus. In R. Petersdorf, R. Adams, E. Braunwald, K. Isselbacher, T. Martin, & T. Wilson (Eds.), *Harrison's principles of internal medicine* (10th ed. pp. 1687–1697). New York: McGraw-Hill.

Gerber, G. S., Thompson, I. M., Thisted, R., & Chodak, G. W. (1993). Disease-specific survival following routine prostate cancer screening by digital rectal examination. *Journal of the American Medical Association, 269,* 61–64.

Gerchufsky, M. (1995). Testicular cancer. An underemphasized disease. *ADVANCE for Nurse Practitioners, 3*(1), 21–24.

Ghadinan, P., Stein, G., Gorodetzky, C., Roberfroid, M., Mahon, G., & Bartsch, H. (1986). Oesophageal cancer studies in the Caspian littoral of Iran: Some residual results, including opium use as a risk factor. *International Journal of Cancer, 35,* 593–597.

Gianella, A. (1985). Teaching cancer prevention and detection. *Cancer Nursing, 8*(Suppl 1), 9–12.

Gill, M. J. (1989). Breast self-exam, instructor training program: A unique strategy for instructor education (Abstract 82). *Oncology Nursing Forum, 16*(Suppl.), 149.

Gillatt, A. (1984). Aspects of oncology nursing in the community of Ireland. In *Cancer nursing in the '80s. Proceedings of 3rd international conference on cancer nursing* (pp. 173–177). Melbourne, Australia: The Cancer Institute/Peter MacCallum Hospital and the Royal Melbourne Hospital.

Giovannucci, E., Tosteson, T. D., Speizer, F. E., Ascherio, A., Vessey, M., & Colditz, G. (1993). A retrospective cohort study of vasectomy and prostate cancer in US men. *Journal of the American Medical Association, 269,* 878–882.

Giovannucci, E., Rimm, E. B., Stampfer, M. F., Colditz, G. A., Ascherio, A., & Willett, W. C. (1994). Aspirin use and the risk for colorectal cancer and adenoma in male health professionals. *Annals of Internal Medicine, 121,* 241–246.

Girgis, A., Campbell, E., Redman, S., & Sanson-Fisher, R. (1991). Screening for melanoma: A community survey of prevalence and predictors. *Medical Journal of Australia, 154,* 338–343.

Glenn, B., & Moore, L. (1990). Relationship of self-concept, health locus of control and perceived cancer treatment options to the practice of BSE. *Cancer Nursing, 13,* 361–365.

Goldering, J. M. (1986). Equal time for men: Teaching testicular self-examination (Editorial). *Journal of Adolescent Health Care, 7,* 273–274.

Gonzalez, J. (1990). Factors related to frequency of breast self-examination among low income Mexican American women. *Cancer Nursing, 13,* 134–142.

Good news for women who booze—CDC finds no breast cancer increase. (1988). *Cancer Letter, 14,* 6–7.

Goodman, M. (1982). A cancer screening and detection program in Texas. *Nursing Times, November 3,* 1855–1858.

Graham, V., & Leigh, S. (1984). Chemoprevention of cervical dysplasia: A research nurse's unique role (Abstract 128). *Oncology Nursing Forum, 11*(Suppl.), 81.

Gray, M. (1990). Factors related to practice of breast self-examination in rural women. *Cancer Nursing, 13,* 100–107.

Gray, N. (1985). Cancer risks and cancer prevention in the third world In M. P. Vessey, & M. Gray, (Eds.), *Cancer risks and prevention.* Oxford, England: Oxford University Press.

Green, L. W., Kreuter, M. W., Deeds, M. W., & Partridge, K. B. (1980). *Health education planning: A diagnostic approach.* Palo Alto, CA: Mayfield Publishing Co.

Greenwald, P. (1985). Diet and cancer prevention. *Maryland Medical Journal, 34,* 44–49.

Greenwald, P., & Sondek, E. (Eds.). (1986). *Cancer control objectives for the nation: 1985–2000.* (NIH Publication No. 86-2880). Washington, DC: U. S. Government Printing Office.

Greenwald, P., Sondek, E., & Lynch, B. (1986). Diet and chemoprevention in NCI's research strategy to achieve national cancer control objectives. *Annual Review of Public Health, 7,* 267–291.

Grindal, A. (1983). BSE: A model in health education. *Occupational Health Nursing, 31,* 20–22.

Gritz, E., & Kanim, L. (1986). Do fewer oncology nurses smoke? *Oncology Nursing Forum, 13,* 61–64.

Grobbelaar, W. (1990). Tobacco abuse as an issue in cancer prevention in Africa (Abstract 28). Sixth international conference on cancer nursing (p. 6). Amsterdam, August.

Gusberg, S. B. (1988). Detection and prevention of uterine cancer. *Cancer, 62,* 1784–1786.

Haenvel, W., & Kurihara, M. (1968). Studies of Japanese migrants. 1. Mortality from cancer and other diseases among Japanese in the United States. *Journal of the National Cancer Institute, 40,* 43–68.

Hallal, J. C. (1982). The relationship of health beliefs, health locus of control, and self concept to the practice of breast self-examination in adult women. *Nursing Research, 31,* 137–142.

Harbora, D., & Kamitoma, V. (1985). Development of a colonoscopy program for high risk colorectal patients following curative surgery (Abstract 13). *Oncology Nursing Forum, 12,* 43.

Harley, N. H., & Harley, J. H. (1990). Potential lung cancer risk from indoor radon exposure. *CA: A Cancer Journal for Clinicians, 40,* 265–276.

Harris, J. R., Lippman, M. E., Veronesi, U., & Willett, W. (1992). Breast cancer. *New England Journal of Medicine, 327*(5), 319–328.

Harris, R. E., & Wynder, E. L. (1988). Breast cancer and alcohol consumption. *MMA, 259,* 2867–2871.

Harvey, J., & Beattie, E. (1993). Lung cancer. *Clinical Symposia, 45*(3), 2–32.

Haughey, B. P., Marshall, J. R., Mettlin, C., Nemoto, T., Kroldart, K., & Swanson, M. (1984). Nurses' ability to detect nodules in silicone breast models. *Oncology Nursing Forum, 11,* 37–42.

Hayes, R., Bogdanovicz, J., & Schroeder, F., DeBruijn, A., Raatgever, J., Van der Maas, P., Oishi, K., & Yoshida, O. (1988). Serum retinol and prostate cancer. *Cancer, 62,* 2021–2026.

Haynes, H., Mead, K., & Goldwyn, R. (1985). Cancers of the skin. In V. DeVita, S. Hellman, & S. A. Rosenberg (Eds.), *Cancer. Principles and practice of oncology* (2nd ed. pp. 1343–1370). Philadelphia: J. B. Lippincott.

Healthfinder. (1985). National Health Information Clearinghouse, Office of Disease Prevention and Health Promotion. Washington, DC: U. S. Department of Health and Human Services.

Henahan, J. (1990). Screening detects ovarian cancer. *Oncology Biotechnology News, 4,* 1.

Hendershot, G. (1983). Coitus-related cervical cancer risk factors: Trends and differentials in racial and religious groups. *American Journal of Public Health, 73,* 299–301.

Henderson, B., Gerkins, V., & Pike, M. (1975). Sexual factors and pregnancy. In J. Fraumeni (Ed.), *Persons at high risk of cancer. An approach to cancer etiology and control* (p. xx). New York: Academic Press.

Hennekens, C., Mayrent, S., & Willett, W. (1986). Vitamin A, carotenoids, and retinoids. *Cancer, 58,* 1837–1841.

Herrero, R., Brinton, L. A., Reeves, W., Brenes, M., Tenorio, F., Britton, R., Gaitan, E., Garcia, M., & Rawls, W. (1990). Sexual behavior, venereal diseases, hygiene practices, and invasive cervical cancer in a high-risk population. *Cancer, 65,* 380–386.

Hirayama, T. (1979). Diet and cancer. *Nutrition and Cancer, 1,* 67–81.

Hirshfield-Bartek, J. (1982). Health beliefs and their influence on breast self-examination practices in women with breast cancer. *Oncology Nursing Forum, 9,* 77–81.

Hirshfield-Bartek, J. (1988). Health beliefs and their influence on breast self-examination practices in women with breast cancer (p. 161). Oncology Nursing Society. Pittsburgh, PA, May 4–7.

Hirschman, R., & Leventhal, H. (1983). The behavioral science of cancer prevention. In S. B. Kahn, R. Love, C. Sherman, & R. Chakravorty (Eds.), *Concepts in cancer medicine* (pp. 229–240). New York: Grune & Stratton, Inc.

Hochbaum, G. M. (1960). Modern theories of communication. *Children, 7,* 13–18.

Holmberg, L., Ghlander, E., Byers, T., Zack, M., Walk, A., Bergstrom, R., Bergkrist, L., Thurfjell, E., Bruce, A., & Adami, H. (1994). Diet and breast cancer risk. *Archives of Internal Medicine, 154,* 1805–1811.

Hurt, R. D., Dale, L. C., Fredrickson, P. A., Caldwell, C. C., Lee, G. A., Offord, K. P., Lauger. G. G., Marusic, Z., Neese, L. W., & Lundberg, T. G. (1994). Nicotine patch therapy for smoking cessation combined with physician advice and nurse follow-up. *Journal of the American Medical Association, 271,* 595–600.

Janerich, D., Thompson, W. D., Varela, L., Greenwald, P., Chorost, S., Tucci, C., Zaman, M., Melamed, M., Kiely, M., & McKneally, M. (1990). Lung cancer and exposure to tobacco smoke in the household. *New England Journal of Medicine, 323,* 632–636.

Jayant, K., & Ycole, B. (1987). Cancers of the upper alimentary and respiratory tracts in Bombay, India: A study of incidence over two decades. *British Journal of Cancer, 56,* 847–852.

Johnston-Early, A. (1983). Nurses and smoking: We've got to call it "quits" (p. 99) (Abstract 213). *Proceedings of the eighth annual congress of the Oncology Nursing Society.* San Diego, CA, May 18–21.

Jones, W., & Saigo, P. (1986). The "atypical" Papanicolaou smear. *CA: A Cancer Journal for Clinicians, 36,* 237–242.

Kalinowki, B., Goodman, M., & Lawler, P. (1986). An individualized approach to teaching BSE to hospitalized women (Abstract 111). *Oncology Nursing Forum, 13,* 83.

Kampert, J. B., Whittemore, A. S., & Paffenbarger, R. S., Jr. (1988). Combined effect of childbearing, menstrual events, and body size on age-specific breast cancer risk. *American Journal of Epidemiology, 128,* 962–979.

Karsell, P. & McDougall, J. (1993). Diagnostic tests for lung cancer. *Mayo Clinic Proceedings, 68,* 288–296.

Kelley, C., Hoffman, S., & Newton, M. (1988). Breast cancer screening: A collaborative nursing practice model between oncology and women's health (p. 116) (Abstract 58A). *Proceedings of the thirteenth annual congress of the Oncology Nursing Society.* Pittsburgh, PA, May 4–7.

Kelly, P. (1991). Melanoma/skin cancer awareness campaign (Abstract 36A). *Oncology Nursing Forum, 18,* 332.

Kelsey, J. L., & Gammon, M. D. (1991). The epidemiology of breast cancer. *CA: A Cancer Journal for Clinicians, 41,* 146–165.

Kelsey, J. L, & John, E. M. (1994). Lactation and the risk of breast cancer. *New England Journal of Medicine, 330*(2), 136–137.

Kerlikowske, K., Grady, D., Rubin, S. H., Sandrock, C., & Ernster, V. L. (1995). Efficacy of screening mammography: A meta-analysis. *Journal of the American Medical Association, 273,* 149–154.

Kersey, P., & Kroll, B. (1985). Be sunsible! (Abstract 17P). *Oncology Nursing Forum, 12*(Suppl.), 44.

Kibblewhite, M., Van Rensburg, S., Laker, M., & Rose, E. (1984). Evidence for an intimate geochemical factor in the etiology of esophageal cancer. *Environmental Research, 33,* 370–378.

Kitson, J. K. (1989). Breast self exam and the high risk adolescents (Abstract 280). *Oncology Nursing Forum, 16*(Suppl.), 198.

Kitson, J. K., Brenner, R., & Brooks, S. (1983). Everyone's doing it, but are they doing it right: Breast self exam (p. 69) (Abstract 91). *Proceedings of the eighth annual congress of the Oncology Nursing Society.* May 18–21.

Klatt-Ellis, T. (1988). Adolescent use and knowledge of smokeless tobacco: Implications for school programming (p. 126) (Abstract 100). *Proceedings of the thirteenth annual congress of the Oncology Nursing Society.* Pittsburgh, PA, May 4–7.

Knudsen, N., Schulman, S., Fowler, R., & Van Den Hoek, J. (1984). Why bother with stop-smoking education for lung cancer patients? *Oncology Nursing Forum, 11,* 30–33.

Koh, H. K., Lew, R. A., & Prout, M. N. (1989). Screening for melanoma/skin cancer: Theoretic and practical considerations. *Journal of the American Academy of Dermatology, 20,* 159–172.

Kopf, A. W. (1988). Prevention and early detection of skin cancer/melanoma. *Cancer, 62,* 1791–1795.

Kopf, A., Rigel, D., & Friedman, R. (1982). The rising incidence and mortality rates of malignant melanoma. *Journal of Dermatologic Surgery and Oncology, 8,* 760–761.

Krahn, M. D., Mahoney, J. E., Eckman, M. H., Trachtenber, J., Pauker, S. G., & Detsky, A. S. (1994). Screening for prostate cancer. A decision analytic view. *Journal of the American Medical Association, 272*(10), 773–780.

Kramer, B. S., Brown, M. L., Prorok, P. C., Potosky, A. L., & Gohagan, J. K. (1993). *Annals of Internal Medicine, 119*(9), 914–923.

Kritchevsky, D. (1986). Diet, nutrition, and cancer. *Cancer, 58,* 1830–1836.

Krohner, K. M., McBurney, B. H., & Wadelin, J. W. (1988). Assessing cancer prevention learning needs of parents and their 6th, 7th and 8th grade children. *Oncology Nursing Forum, 15,* 59–64.

Kumar, T. (1990). The nurse's role in breast cancer screening—Yugoslavia (p. 49) (Abstract S5). *Sixth international conference on cancer nursing.* Amsterdam, August.

Lang, C. A., & Ransohoff, D. F. (1994). Fecal occult blood screening for colorectal cancer. Is mortality reduced by chance selection for screening colonoscopy? *Journal of the American Medical Association, 271*(13), 1011–1013.

Lange, P. H. (1993). The next era for prostate cancer. Controlled clinical trials. *Journal of the American Medical Association, 269*(1), 95–96.

Lappe, J., & Fitzsimmons, M. (1988). Compliance variables in hereditary colon cancer families (p. 133) (Abstract 128). *Proceedings of the thirteenth annual congress of the Oncology Nursing Society.* Pittsburgh, PA, May 4–7.

Larpenteur, M. (1989). Mobile mammography: An on-site educational and diagnostic opportunity for breast cancer detection (Abstract 44). *Oncology Nursing Forum, 16*(Suppl.), 139.

Larson, R. (1986). The role of the nurse in the melanoma screening process (Abstract 91). *Oncology Nursing Forum, 13,* 78.

Lawler, P. E. (1990). The prevention of skin cancer, a nursing challenge. *Cancer Nursing News, 8,* 1–2.

Lawler, P. E., & Schreiber, S. (1989). Cutaneous malignant melanoma: Nursing's role in prevention and early detection. *Oncology Nursing Forum, 16,* 345–352.

Lee, F., Torp-Pedersen, S., & Siders, D. (1989). The role of transrectal ultrasound in the early detection of prostate cancer. *CA: A Cancer Journal for Clinicians, 39,* 337–360.

Leffall, L. D. (1981). Colorectal cancer-prevention and detection. *Cancer, 47,* 1170–1172.

Lierman, L. (1990). Efficacy of breast self-examination: Methodological issues related to measurement (Abstract 128). *Oncology Nursing Forum, 17,* 169.

Lindberg, S. C. (1987). Adult preventive health screening: 1987 update. *Nurse Practitioner, 12,* 19–41.

Littrup, P. J., Goodman, A. C., & Mettlin, C. J. (1993). The investigators of the American Cancer Society-National Prostate Cancer Detection Project. The benefit and cost of prostate cancer early detection. *CA: A Cancer Journal for Clinicians, 43*(3), 134–149.

Loescher, L., & Hazelkorn, K. (1983). Development of a skin cancer early detection and prevention program (p. 65) (Abstract 75J). *Proceedings of the eighth annual congress of the Oncology Nursing Society.* San Diego, CA, May 18–21.

Longman, A. J., Modiano-Revah, M., & Saint-Germain, M. (1990). Breast cancer prevention for older hispanic women (Abstract 80). *Oncology Nursing Forum, 17,* 157.

Longman, S. M., & Buehring, G. C. (1987). Oral contraceptives and breast cancer. In vitro effect of contraceptive steroids on human mammary cell growth. *Cancer, 59,* 281–287.

Longnecker, M. P., Berlin, J. A., Orza, M. J., & Chalmers, T. C. (1988). A meta-analysis of alcohol consumption in relation to risk of breast cancer. *Journal of the American Medical Association, 260,* 652–656.

Lovejoy, N. C. (1987). Precancerous lesions of the cervix: Personal risk factors. *Cancer Nursing, 10,* 2–14.

Lovejoy, N. C., Jenkins, C., Wu, T., Shankland, S., & Wilson, C. (1989). Developing a breast cancer screening program for Chinese-American women. *Oncology Nursing Forum, 16,* 181–192.

Lynch, H., & Lynch, P. (1978). Constitutional factors and endometrial carcinoma. In H. Nieburgs (Ed.), *Prevention and detection of cancer. Part I. Prevention. Vol 2. Etiology* (pp. 2105–2117). New York: Marcel Dekker, Inc.

Mackel, C., & Greski, P. (1990). Barrett's esophagus: A model for monitoring and intervening in preneoplasia (Abstract 105). *Oncology Nursing Forum, 17,* 164.

MacKie, R., Freudenberger, T., & Aitchison, T. C. (1989). Personal risk-factor chart for cutaneous melanoma. *Lancet, 2,* 487–490.

Madsen. (1988). Cutaneous malignant melanoma, dysplastic nevi, and heredity (p. 129) (Abstract 1111). *Proceedings of the thirteenth annual congress of the Oncology Nursing Society.* Pittsburgh, PA, May 4–7.

Mandel, J. S., Bond, J. H., Church, T. R., Snover, D. C., & Bradley, G. M. (1994). Reducing mortality from colorectal cancer by screening for fecal occult blood. *New England Journal of Medicine, 328,* 1365–1371.

Marley, L. (1982). Knowledge of cancer facts among workers following an educational program. *Occupational Health Nursing, 30,* 16–17, 42.

Martin, J. P. (1990). Male cancer awareness: Impact of an employee education program. *Oncology Nursing Forum, 17,* 59–64.

Marty, P. J., & McDermott, R. J. (1983). Teaching about testicular cancer and testicular self-examination. *Journal of School Health, 53,* 351–356.

Marty, P. J., McDermott, R. J., & Gold, R. S. (1983). An assessment of three alternative formats for promoting breast self-examination. *Cancer Nursing, 6,* 207–211.

Mashberg, M., & Samit, A. (1989). Early detection, diagnosis, and management of oral and oropharyngeal cancer. *CA: A Cancer Journal for Clinicians, 39,* 67–87.

Massey, V. (1986). Perceived susceptibility to breast cancer and practice of breast self-examination. *Nursing Research, 35,* 183–185.

Massingberd, K. (1988). The role of nurses in a comprehensive cancer screening program for women in Finland (pp. 135–137). In A. P. Pritchard (Ed.), *Cancer nursing: A revolution in care.* Proceedings of the fifth international conference on cancer nursing. London, September.

Mayer, R. (1988). Gastrointestinal cancer. In E. Rubenstein & D. Federman (Eds.), *Scientific American Medicine* (pp. 1–17). New York: Scientific American.

McGregor, H., Land, C. E., & Choi, K., et al. (1977). Breast cancer incidence among atomic bomb survivors, Hiroshima and Nagasaki, 1950–69. *Journal of the National Cancer Institute, 59,* 799–811.

McGuire, D. B. (1979). Familial cancer and the role of the nurse. *Cancer Nursing, 2,* 443–452.

McGuire, D. B. (1985). Preventive health practices and educational needs in families with hereditary melanoma. *Cancer Nursing, 8,* 29–36.

McMillan, S. (1990). Nurses' compliance with American Cancer Society guidelines for cancer prevention and detection. *Oncology Nursing Forum, 17,* 721–727.

Meadows, A., & Li, F. (1983). The practicing etiologist. In G. Newell (Ed.), *Cancer prevention in clinical medicine* (pp. 17–24). New York: Raven Press.

Meisner, L. (1983). Genetic factors in human cancer. In S. B. Kahn, R. Love, C. Sherman, & R. Chakravorty (Eds.), *Concepts in cancer medicine* (pp. 165–176). New York: Grune & Stratton, Inc.

Melillo, K. D. (1985). Who needs health maintenance. *Journal of Gerotology Nursing, 11,* 18–21.

Messner, R. L., & Gardner, S. S. (1985). Colorectal cancer screening in the workplace. *Occupational Health Nursing, 33,* 561–565.

Messner, R. L., & Gardner, S. S. (1985). Stop a killer with early detection. *Journal of Gerontology Nursing, 11,* 8–10, 13–14.

Messner, R. L., Gardner, S. S., & Webb, D. D. (1986). Early detection—the priority in colorectal cancer. *Cancer Nursing, 9,* 8–14.

Mettlin, C., McCoy, V., Nuchereno, F., & Murphy, G. (1980). The role and impact of the cancer education nurses in industrial health programs. *Oncology Nursing Forum, 28,* 18–22.

Mettlin, C., & Smart, C. R. (1994). Breast cancer detection guidelines for women aged 40 to 49 years: Rationale for the American Cancer Society reaffirmation of recommendations. *CA: A Cancer Journal for Clinicians, 44*(4), 248–255.

Mikulin, T., & Hardcastle, J. (1987). Gastric cancer—delay in diagnosis and its causes. *European Journal of Cancer and Clinical Oncology, 23,* 1683–1690.

Mitchell-Beren, M. E., Dodds, M. E., Choi, K. L., & Waskerwitz, M. (1989). A colorectal cancer prevention, screening and evaluation program in community black churches. *CA: A Cancer Journal for Clinicians, 39,* 115–118.

Mitchell, M. F., Sandella, J. A., & White, L. (1992). Cervical cancer: The role of the human papillomavirus. *Current Issues in Cancer Nursing Practice Updates, 1*(1), 1–9.

Mitchley, J. (1984). Western Cape: Cultural aspects of cancer nursing. In: *Cancer nursing in the 80's* (pp. 154–155). Proceedings of 3rd international conference on cancer nursing. Melbourne, Australia: The Cancer Institute/Peter MacCallum Hospital and the Royal Melbourne Hospital.

Mittman, C., & Roby, T. J. (1991). Current status of sputum cytology in the detection of lung cancer. *Primary Care & Cancer, January,* 15–22.

Moulds, M. (1992). Sun alert America: The Foundation's national skin cancer prevention initiative. *Primary Care & Cancer, 12*(7), 13–15.

Muller, D. (1988). Breast self-exam as a tool in the early detection of breast cancer recurrence at the primary site (p. 147) (Abstract 185). *Proceedings of the thirteenth annual congress of the Oncology Nursing Society.* Pittsburgh, PA, May 4–7.

Mulshine, J., Treston, A., Scott, F., Avis, M., Boland, C., Phelps, R., Kasprzyk, P., Nakanishi, Y., & Cuttitta, F. (1991). Lung cancer: Rational strategies for early detection and intervention. *Oncology, 5,* 25–37.

Mulvihill, J. (1975). Congenital and genetic diseases. In J. Fraumeni (Ed.), *Persons at high risk of cancer. An approach to cancer etiology and control* (pp. 3–37). New York: Academic Press.

Munoz, N., Victona, C., Crespi, M., Saul, C., Braga, N., & Conrea, P. (1987). Hot mate drinking and precancerous lesions of the esophagus: An endoscopic survey in Southern Brazil. *International Journal of Cancer, 39,* 708–709.

Murphy, G. (1988). Urologic cancer. *Cancer, 62,* 1800–1807.

Murphy, G. P., Natarajan, N., Pontes, J. E., Schmitz, R. L., Smart, C. R., & Mettlin, C. (1982). The national survey of prostate cancer in the United States by the American College of Surgeons. *Journal of Urology, 127,* 928–934.

National Cancer Institute. (1986). *Cancer among blacks and other minorities: Statistical profile* (NIH Publication No. 86-2785). Washington, DC: U. S. Government Printing Office.

Nelson, D., Giovino, G., Emont, S., Brackbill, R., Cameron, L., Peddicord, J., & Mowery, P. (1994). Trends in cigarette smoking among US physicians and nurses. *Journal of the American Medical Association, 271,* 1273–1275.

Nelson-Manen, P., & Krebs, L. (1991). Designing and implementing a nurse-run cancer screening/prevention clinic (Abstract 270A). *Oncology Nursing Forum, 18,* 357.

Nemcek, N. (1989). Factors influencing black women's breast self-examination practice. *Cancer Nursing, 12,* 339–343.

Nemcek, N. (1990). Health beliefs and breast self-examination among black women. *Health Values, 14,* 41–53.

Newcomb, P. A., Storer, B. E., Longnecker, M., Mittendorf, R., Greenberg, E. R., Clapp, R. W., Burke, K., Willett, W., & MacMahon, B. (1994). Lactation and a reduced risk of premenopausal breast cancer. *New England Journal of Medicine, 330*(2), 81–87.

Newell, G. (1985). Epidemiology of cancer. In V. DeVita, S. Hellman, & S. Rosenberg (Eds.), *Cancer. Principles and practice of oncology* (2nd ed, pp. 151–182). Philadelphia, PA: J. B. Lippincott Co.

Newell, G., & Vogel, V. (1987). Personal risk factors: What do they mean? *Proceedings of the Second National Conference on Cancer Prevention and Detection.* New York: American Cancer Society.

Nichols, S. (1983). 1. The South Hampton breast study—implications for nurses. *Nursing Times,* December 14, 24–27.

Nielsen, B. B. (1989). The nurse's role in mammography screening. *Cancer Nursing, 12,* 271–275.

NIH Consensus Development Panel on Early Melanoma. (1992). Diagnosis and treatment of early melanoma. *Journal of the American Medical Association, 268*(10), 1314–1319.

NIH Consensus Development Panel on Ovarian Cancer. (1995). Screening, treatment, and follow-up. *Journal of the American Medical Association, 273*(6), 491–497.

Nomura, A. (1982). Stomach cancer. In: D. Schottenfeld & J. Fraumeni (Eds.), *Cancer epidemiology and prevention* (pp. 624–637). Philadelphia, PA: W. B. Saunders.

Nussbaum, J. (1990). Cancer knowledge, screening behaviors and data sources among elderly blacks (Abstract 254). *Oncology Nursing Forum, 17,* 201.

Nyström, L., Rutquist, L. E., & Wall, S. (1993). Breast cancer screening with mammography: Overview of Swedish randomised trials. *Lancet, 341,* 973–978.

Olsen, T. G., Fieser, T. A., Conte, E. T., & Schroeter, A. L. (1987). Skin cancer screening—a local experience. *Journal of the American Academy of Dermatology, 16,* 637–641.

Olsen, S, & Frank-Stromborg, M. (1991a). Cancer screening and early detection. In S. Baird, R. McCorkle & M. Grant (Eds.), *Cancer nursing. A comprehensive textbook* (pp. 190–218). Philadelphia, PA: W. B. Saunders.

Olsen, S, & Frank-Stromborg, M. (1991b). Practical applications for improving the quality of life of African-Americans (Abstract 137A). *Oncology Nursing Forum, 18,* 343.

Olson, R. L., & Mitchell, E. S. (1989). Self-confidence as a critical factor in breast self-examination. *Journal of Obstetrics and Gynecology Neonatal Nursing, Nov/Dec,* 476–81.

O'Rourke, A., Gypson, B., & Weitberg, A. (1986). Developing a cancer screening center (Abstract 163). *Oncology Nursing Forum, 14,* 13.

Ouslander, J., & Beck, J. (1982). Defining the health problems of the elderly. In L. Breslow, J. Fielding, & L. Lave (Eds.), *Annual Review of Public Health, 3,* 55–84.

Owen, P. (1989). Health beliefs and preventive practices among adults with a history of melanoma (Abstract 68A). *Oncology Nursing Forum, 16*(Suppl.), 145.

Ozols, R. (1991). The current status of the treatment of ovarian cancer. *Mediguide Oncology, 11,* 1–5.

Page, H., & Asire, A. L. (1985). *Cancer rates and risks.* (3rd ed.). Washington, D. C.: U. S. Government Printing Office, NIH Publication No. 85-691.

Palmer, S. (1986). Dietary considerations for risk reduction. *Cancer, 58,* 1949–1953.

Persky, V., Davis, F., Barrett, R., Ruby, E., Sailer, C., & Levy, P. (1990). Recent time trends in uterine cancer. *American Journal of Public Health, 80,* 935–939.

Pervan, V. (1988). Cultural aspects of oesophageal cancer (pp. 125–126). *Proceedings of the fifth international conference on cancer nursing.* London, September 4–9.

Petersen, R. O. (1986). Prostate neoplastic disorders. (pp. 613–667). In R. Peterson & B. Stein (Eds.), *Urologic pathology.* Philadelphia, PA: J. B. Lippincott,.

Pienta, K. J., & Esper, P. S. (1993). Risk factors for prostate cancer. *Annals of Internal Medicine, 118,* 793–803.

Pierce, A. B., & Abell, M. R. (1970). Embryonal carcinoma of the testis. *Pathology Annual, 1,* 27–60.

Pollack, S. V. (1992). Skin cancer and aging. *Primary Care & Cancer, 12*(7), 25–26.

Poniatowski, L. (1990). Guarding against skin cancer. *Health Journal-Magazine of RUSH-Anchor,* Summer 22–23.

Post-White, J. Herzan, D., & Drew, D. (1988). Prevention of dietary associated cancer (p. 107) (Abstract 21). *Proceedings of the thirteenth annual congress of the Oncology Nursing Society.* Pittsburgh, PA, May 4–7.

Ransohoff, D. F., Lang, C., & Kuo, S. (1991). Colonoscopic surveillance after polypectomy: Considerations of cost effectiveness. *Annals of Internal Medicine, 114*(3), 177–182.

Rawson, R. (1978). Identification of tumor susceptibility of individuals at high risk for the development of cancer. In H. Nieburgs (Ed.), *Prevention and detection of cancer. Part I. Prevention. Vol. 2. Etiology* (pp. 1493–1512). New York: Marcel Dekker, Inc.

Redeker, N. (1989). Health beliefs, health locus of control and the frequency of practice of breast self-examination in women. *Journal of Obstetrics and Gynecology Neonatal Nursing, 18,* 45–51.

Reno, D. R. (1988). Men's knowledge and health beliefs about testicular cancer and testicular self-exam. *Oncology Nursing Forum, 11,* 112–117.

Rhodes, A., Weinstock, M., Fitzpatrick, T., Mihm, M., & Sober, A. (1987). Risk factors for cutaneous melanoma: A practical method of recognizing predisposed individuals. *MMA, 258,* 3146–3154.

Richardson, A. C., & Lyon, J. B. (1981). The effect of condom use on squamous cell cervical intraepithelial neoplasia. *American Journal of Obstetrics and Gynecology, 140,* 909–913.

Richie, J. P. (1993). Detection and treatment of testicular cancer. *CA: A Cancer Journal for Clinicians, 43*(3), 151–175.

Riese, N. E. (1983). Design and implementation of a statewide breast self examination program (BSE) (p. 75) (Abstract 114). *Proceedings of the eighth annual congress of the Oncology Nursing Society.* San Diego, CA, May 18–21.

Rinsky, R., Smith, A., Hornung, R., Filloon, T., Young, R., Okun, A., & Landrigan, P. (1987). Benzene and leukemia: An epidemiologic risk assessment. *New England Journal of Medicine, 316,* 1044–1050.

Robbins, L. (1978). Evaluation of risk factors in cancer prevention. In H. Nieburgs (Ed.), *Prevention and detection of cancer: Part I. Prevention, Vol 2, Etiology,* (pp. 2099–2143). New York: Marcel Dekker, Inc.

Rodricks, J., & Tardiff, R. (1984). Conceptual basis for risk assessment. In J. Rodricks & R. Tardiff (Eds.), *Assessment and management of chemical risks,* (pp. 1–12). ACS Symposium Series. Washington, DC: American Chemical Society.

Romieu, I., Willett, W. C., & Colditz, G. A., et al. (1989). Prospective study of oral contraceptive use and the risk of breast cancer in women. *Journal of the National Cancer Institute, 81,* 1313–1321.

Romney, S. L., Palan, P. R., & Duttagupta, C., et al. (1981). Retinoids and the prevention of cervix dysplasia. *American Journal of Obstetrics and Gynecology, 141,* 890–894.

Rosenstock, I. M. (1966). Why people use health services. *Milbank Memorial Fund Quarterly, 44,* 94–127.

Rosevelt, J., & Frankl, H. (1984). Colorectal cancer screening by nurse practitioner using 60-cm flexible fiberoptic sigmoidoscope. *Digestive Diseases and Sciences, 29,* 161–163.

Ross, C. (1981). Health hazard appraisal. In L. Schneiderman (Ed.), *The practice of preventive health care* (pp. 26–36). Menlo Park, CA: Addison-Wesley Publishing Co., Inc.

Rossing, M. A., Daling, J. R., Weiss, N. S., Moore, D. E. & Self, S. G. (1994). Ovarian tumors in a cohort of infertile women. *New England Journal of Medicine, 331,* 771–776.

Rowe, W. (1986). Identification of risk. In A. Brigger (Ed.), *Risk and reason: Risk assessment in relations to environmental mutagens and carcinogens* (pp. 3–22). New York: Alan R. Liss.

Rubin, G., & Peterson, H. (1985). Researchers can now investigate long-term effects of OCs on cancer. *Contraceptive Technology Update, 6,* 7–12.

Rubin, P., & Bakemeier, R. F. (1978). *Clinical oncology for medical students and physicians.* New York: American Cancer Society.

Rudolf, V. M., & Quinn, K. M. (1988). The practice of TSE among college men: Effectiveness of an educational program. *Oncology Nursing Forum, 15,* 45–48.

Runowicz, C. (1992). Advances in the screening and treatment of ovarian cancer. *CA: A Cancer Journal for Clinicians, 42*(6), 327–349.

Rutledge, D., & Davis, G. (1988). Breast self examination compliance and the Health Belief Model. *Oncology Nursing Forum, 15,* 175–179.

Sacks, J., Krushat, M., & Newman, J. (1980). Reliability of the health hazard appraisal. *American Journal of Public Health, 70,* 730–732.

Sadeghi, S. B., Hseih, E. W., & Gunn, S. W. (1984). Prevalence of cervical intraepithelial neoplasia in sexually active teenagers and young adults. *American Journal of Obstetrics and Gynecology, 148,* 726–729.

Sanghvi, L. (1981). Cancer epidemiology: The Indian scene. *Journal of Cancer Research and Clinical Oncology, 99,* 1–14.

Sankaranarayanan, R., Duffy, S., Day, N., Nair, M., & Padmakumary, G. (1989). A case-control investigation of cancer of the oral, tongue and the floor of the mouth in southern India. *International Journal of Cancer, 44,* 617–621.

Sasco, A. J. (1991). World burden of tobacco-related cancer. *The Lancet, 338,* 123–124.

Sawyer, P. F. (1986). Breast self-examination: Hospital-based nurses aren't assessing their clients. *Oncology Nursing Forum, 13,* 44–48.

Schatzkin, A., Carter, C. L., & Green, S. B., et al. (1989a). Is alcohol consumption related to breast cancer? Results from the Framingham heart study. *Journal of the National Cancer Institute, 81,* 31–35.

Schatzkin, A., Greenwald, P., Byar, D., & Clifford, C. K. (1989b). The dietary fat-breast cancer hypothesis is alive. *Journal of the American Medical Association, 261,* 3284–3287.

Schatzkin, A., Jones, Y. D., Hoover, R. N., Taylor, P., Brinton, L. A., Ziegler, R., Harvey, E. B., Carter, C. L., Licitra, L., DuFour, M., & Larson, D. B. (1987). Alcohol consumption and breast cancer in the epidemiologic follow-up study of the first national health and nutrition examination survey. *New England Journal of Medicine, 316,* 1169–1173.

Schlaff, W. B., & Rosenshein, N. B. (1985). Estrogens and endometrial cancer. *Maryland Medical Journal, 34,* 57–62.

Schmitt, R. M., & Krebs, L. U. (1987). Motivational factors affecting oncology nurses' practice of breast self-examination (Abstract 211A). *Oncology Nursing Forum, 14,* 134.

Schoenbach, V. (1987). Appraising health risk appraisal. *American Journal of Public Health, 77,* 409–411.

Schroy, P., Wiggins, T., Winawer, S., Diaz, B., & Lightdale, C. (1988). Video endoscopy by nurse practitioners: A model for colorectal screening. *Gastrointestinal Endoscopy, 34,* 390–394.

Schulmeister, L. (1985). Performance of BSE by daughters of women with breast cancer (Abstract 8A). *Oncology Nursing Forum, 12*(Suppl.), 41.

Schulmeister, L. (1986). Screening for oral cancer: Collaborating with dentistry (Abstract 32A). *Oncology Nursing Forum, 13,* 63.

Screening for colorectal cancer by stool DNA analysis. *The Lancet, 339*(May 9, 1992), 1141–1142.

Searle, C. (1980). Aspects of oncology nursing in remote countries with traditional cultures and unsophisticated health communities (pp. 28–33). In R. Tiffany (Ed.), *Cancer nursing update. Proceedings of the second international cancer nursing conference.* London: Bailliere Tindall.

Sehroy, P., Wiggins, T., Winawer, S., Diaz, B., & Lightdale, C. (1988). Videoendoscopy by nurse practitioners: A model for colorectal screening. *Gastrointestinal Endoscopy, 34,* 390–394.

Seidman, H., Stellman, S., & Mushinski, M. (1982). A different perspective on breast cancer risk factors: Some implications of nonattributable risk. *CA: A Cancer Journal for Clinicians, 32,* 301–311.

Selby, J., & Friedman, G. (1989). Sigmoidoscopy in the periodic health examination of asymptomatic adults. *Journal of the American Medical Association, 26,* 595–601.

Senie, R. (1986). Assessment of carcinogenesis through epidemiologic and environmental investigations. *Seminars in Oncology Nursing, 2,* 154–160.

Shadirian, P. (1987). Food habits of the people of the caspian littoral of Iran in relation to esophageal cancer. *Nutrition and Cancer, 9,* 147–157.

Shamian, J., & Edgar, L. (1987). Nurses as agents for change in teaching breast self-examination. *Public Health Nursing, 4,* 29–34.

Shanmugaratnam, K. (1985). Prevention and early detection of cancer. *Cancer Detection and Prevention, 8,* 431–445.

Shapiro, S., Kelly, I., Rosenberg, L., Kaufman, D. W., Helmrich, Schottenfeld, D. S. P., Rosenshein, N., Lewis, J., Knapp, R., & Stolley, P. D. (1985). Risk of localized and widespread endometrial cancer in relation to recent and discontinued use of conjugated estrogens. *New England Journal of Medicine, 313,* 969–972.

Sheehan, A. P., Michalek, A. M., & Cassidy, M. H. (1981). Outcomes of a BSE program for adolescents (p. 92) (Abstract 191). *Proceedings of the sixth annual congress of the Oncology Nursing Society.* Baltimore, MD, May 4–6.

Sherman, C. (1983). Skin cancer. In S. B. Kahn, R. Love, C. Sherman, & R. Chakravorty, (Eds.), *Concepts in cancer medicine* (pp. 557–563). New York: Grune & Stratton.

Shugg, D. (1984). Smoking and cancer the size of the problem—what can a nurse do? In: *Cancer nursing in the 80's. Proceedings of the third international conference on cancer nursing* (pp. 86–89). Melbourne, Australia: The Cancer Institute/Peter MacCallum Hospital and the Royal Melbourne Hospital.

Silverberg, E., & Lubera, J. (1987). Cancer statistics, 1987. *CA: A Cancer Journal for Clinicians, 37,* 2–19, 20–25.

Simon, J. (1985). Occult blood screening for colorectal carcinoma. A critical review. *Gastroenterology, 88,* 820–837.

Simon, R. C., & Worthen, N. (1989). Breast health: A strategy for increasing employee awareness and participation in self care (Abstract 380A). *Oncology Nursing Forum, 16*(Suppl.), 223.

Smith, P. E. (1991). A comparison of two educational methods for teaching women about breast cancer and early detection and their effects on knowledge, attitudes, and behavior (Abstract 205). *Oncology Nursing Forum, 18,* 394.

Snyder, R. (1984). Basic concepts of the dose-response relationship. In J. Rodricks & R. Tardiff (Eds.), *Assessment and management of chemical risks* (pp. 37–55). ACS Symposium Series. Washington, DC: American Chemical Society.

Somers, A. R. (1978). The high cost of care for the elderly: Diagnosis, prognosis, and some suggestions for therapy. *Journal of Health Politics Law, 3,* 163–180.

Sox, H. C. (1994). Preventive health services in adults. *New England Journal of Medicine, 330*(22), 1589–1595.

Spencer, R., & Ready, R. (1977). Looking ahead: Utilization of nurse endoscopists for sigmoidoscopic examination. *Diseases of the Colon and Rectum, 20,* 94–96.

Squier, R. & Cameron, L. (1984). An analysis of potential carcinogenic risk from formaldehyde. *Regulatory Toxicology and Pharmacology, 4,* 107–129.

St. John, D. J., McDermott, F. T., Hopper, J. L., Debney, E. A., Johnson, W., & Hughes, E. (1993). Cancer risk in relatives of patients with common colorectal cancer. *Annals of Internal Medicine, 118*(10), 785–790.

St. Pierre, B. (1988). Special needs of women with a potentially malignant cervical lesion (p. 109) (Abstract 32). *Proceedings of the thirteenth annual congress of the Oncology Nursing Society.* Pittsburgh, PA, May 4–7.

Stack, T. D. (1979). Testicular cancer—the need for education and early detection (p. 45) (Abstract 84). *Fourth annual congress proceedings of the Oncology Nursing Society.* New Orleans, May 17–19.

Stalker, M. (1985). Evaluation of a cancer prevention project. *Cancer Nursing, 8*(Suppl 1), 13–16.

Stanford, J. (1987). Testicular self-examination: Teaching, learning and practice by nurses. *Journal of Advanced Nursing, 12,* 13–19.

Sternburg, J. K. (1983). Identification and management of risk factors for cancer. In S. B. Kahn, R. Love, C. Sherman, & R. Chakravorty (Eds.), *Concepts in cancer medicine* (pp. 241–253). New York: Grune & Stratton, Inc.

Steuer, J. D., & Wewers, M. E. (1989). Cigarette craving and subsequent coping responses among smoking cessation clinic participants. *Oncology Nursing Forum, 16,* 193–198.

Stewart, D. S. (1990). Indoor tanning: The nurses role in preventing skin damage (pp. 79–94). In C. Reed-Ash & L. Jenkins (Eds.), *Enhancing the role of cancer nursing.* New York: Raven.

Stockwell, H., Goldman, A., Lyman, G., Noss, C., Armstrong, A., Pinkman, P. A., Candelora, E., & Brusa, M. (1992). Environmental tobacco smoke and lung cancer risk in nonsmoking women. *Journal of the National Cancer Institute, 84,* 1417–1422.

Stokes, J. (1987). The methods of clinical prevention. In H. Vanderschmidt, D. Koch-Weser, & P. Woodbury (Eds.), *Handbook of clinical prevention* (pp. 29–58). Baltimore, MD: Williams & Wilkins.

Stoltzfus, S., & Ashby, A. (1990). Bringing cancer prevention and detection to the workplace utilizing a mobile screening unit (Abstract 199P). *Oncology Nursing Forum, 17,* 187.

Stromborg, M. (1982). Early detection of cancer in the elderly: Problems and solutions. *International Journal of Nursing Studies, 9*(3), 139–156.

Sturm, B. R., & Hanke, C. W. (1992). 13 ways to protect yourself from the sun. *Primary Care & Cancer, 12*(7), 45–46.

Styrd, A. M. (1982). A breast self-examination program in an occupational health setting. *Occupational Health Nursing, 30,* 33–35.

Sugarbaker, P. H., MacDonald, J. S., & Querllson, L. L. (1982). Colorectal cancer. In V. T. Devita, Jr., S. Hellman, & S. A. Rosenberg (Eds.), *Cancer: Principles and practice of oncology* (pp. 640–723). New York: J. B. Lippincott.

1989 Survey of physicians' attitudes and practice in early cancer detection. (1990). *CA: A Cancer Journal for Clinicians, 40,* 77–101.

Swan, S. H., & Brown, W. (1979). Vasectomy and cancer of the cervix (Letter). *New England Journal of Medicine, 301,* 46.

The Alpha-Tocopherol, Beta Carotene Cancer Prevention Study Group (1994). The effect of vitamin E and beta carotene on the incidence of lung cancer and other cancers in male smokers. *New England Journal of Medicine, 330,* 1029–1035.

The Cancer and Steroid Hormone Study of the Centers for Disease Control and the National Institute of Child Health and Human Development. (1986). Oral-contraceptive use and the risk of breast cancer. *New England Journal of Medicine, 315,* 405–411.

The Work Study Group on Diet, Nutrition, and Cancer (1991). American Cancer Society Guidelines on Diet, Nutrition, and Cancer. *CA: A Cancer Journal for Clinicians, 41*(8), 334–338.

Tollefson, L. (1985). The use of epidemiology, scientific data, and regulatory authority to determine risk factors in cancer of some organs of the digestive system. 2. Esophageal cancer. *Regulatory Toxicology and Pharmacology, 5,* 255–275.

Toth, M., & Heusinkveld, K. (1979). "BSE and feel free": A certification program for RN's (p. 52) (Abstract 112). *Proceedings of the Oncology Nursing Society.* New Orleans, May 17–19.

Tranin, A. S., & Fabian, C. (1991). The development and implementation of a nurse managed high risk breast cancer screening program (Abstract 248). *Oncology Nursing Forum, 18,* 399.

Treti, S. (1989). Height and weight in relation to breast cancer morbidity and mortality: A prospective study of 570,000 women in Norway. *International Journal of Cancer, 44,* 23–30.

Trevelyan, J. (1989). Well men. *Nursing Times, 85,* 46–47.

Trichopoulos, D., MacMahon, B., & Cole, P. (1972). Menopause and breast cancer risk. *Journal of the National Cancer Institute, 48,* 605–613.

Troxler, I. J. (1989). A model for an adolescent smoking prevention program (Abstract 245). *Oncology Nursing Forum, 16*(Suppl.), 190.

Tuladhar, S. (1990). Role of nurses in early detection of uterine cancer (p. 2) (Abstract 9). *Sixth international conference on cancer nursing.* Amsterdam, August.

Tyner, R., & Loney, M. (1989). Colorectal screening project: An educational program for a population at risk in a metropolitan area (Abstract 154P). *Oncology Nursing Forum, 16*(Suppl.), 167.

Tyson, S. (1980). Cancer nurses' role in public education in Queensland (pp. 44–46). In R. Tiffany (Ed.), *Cancer nursing update. Proceedings of the second international cancer nursing conference.* London, England: Bailliere Tindall.

Uncovering occupational illness. (1990). *Emergency Medicine, February, 15,* 22–44.

U. S. Department of Health and Human Services (1985). *Diet, nutrition and cancer prevention: A guide to food choices* (NIH Publication No. 85-2711). Washington, DC: U. S. Government Printing Office.

Update of ACS guidelines for detection of colorectal cancers-sigmoidoscopy. (1989). *CA: A Cancer Journal for Clinicians, 39,* 317.

Van Rensburg, S., Bradshaw, E., Bradshaw, D., & Rose, E. (1985). Oesophageal cancer in Zulu men, South Africa: A case-control study. *British Journal of Cancer, 51,* 399–405.

Vecchia, C., Franceschi, S., Decarli, A., Galius, G., & Tognoni, G. (1984). Risk factors for endometrial cancer at different ages. *Journal of the National Cancer Institute, 73,* 667–671.

Vessey, M. (1985). Exogenous hormones. In M. P. Vessey, & M. Gray (Eds.)., *Cancer risks and prevention* (pp. 166–194). Oxford: Oxford University Press.

Virji, M., Mercer, D., & Herberman, R. (1988). Tumor markers in cancer diagnosis and prognosis. *CA: A Cancer Journal for Clinicians, 38,* 104–126.

Wagner, T. (1985). Smoking behavior of nurses in western New York. *Nursing Research, 34,* 58–60.

Wahrendorf, W. (1987). An estimate of the proportion of colorectal and stomach cancer which might be prevented by certain changes in dietary habits. *International Journal of Cancer, 40,* 625–628

Walczak, J. R. (1983). The frequency of Pap smear screening and its relevance to nursing practice (p. 103) (Abstract 229). *Proceedings of the eighth annual congress of the Oncology Nursing Society.* San Diego, May 18–21.

Warren, B., & Pohl, J. (1990). Cancer screening practices of nurse practitioners. *Cancer Nursing, 13,* 143–151.

Weinhouse, S. (1986). The role of diet and nutrition in cancer. *Cancer, 58,* 1791–1794.

Weinrich, S. P., & Weinrich, M. C. (1990). Cancer knowledge among elderly individuals. In C. Reed-Ash & J. Jenkins (Eds.), *Enhancing the role of cancer nursing.* New York: Raven, 217–233.

Weinrich, S. P., & Nussbaum, J. (1984). Cancer in the elderly: Early detection. *Cancer Nursing, 7,* 475–482.

Weinrich, S. P., Blesch, K. S., Dickson, G. W., Nussbaum, J. S., & Watson, E. J. (1989). Timely detection of colorectal cancer in the elderly. Implications of the aging process. *Cancer Nursing, 12,* 170–176.

Wells, P. (1989). Sunscreens supplement body's natural defenses. *Oncology Nursing News,* (Missouri Division Nursing Education Committee), *Summer,* 4–5.

White, E. (1987). Projected changes in breast cancer incidence due to the trend toward delayed childbearing. *American Journal of Public Health, 77,* 495–497.

White, L. N. (1986a) Cancer prevention and detection: From twenty to sixty-five years of age. *Oncology Nursing Forum, 13,* 59–64.

White, L. N. (1986b). Cancer risk assessment. *Seminars in Oncology Nursing, 2,* 184–190.

White, L. N. (1983). The nurse's role in cancer prevention. In G. R. Newell, (Ed.), *Cancer prevention in clinical medicine* (pp. 91–111). New York: Raven.

White, L. N., Cornelius, I., Judkins, A., & Patterson, J. (1978). Screening of cancer by nurses. *Cancer Nursing, 1,* 15–20.

White, L. N., & Faulkenberry, I. (1985). Screening by nurse clinicians in cancer prevention and detection. *Current Problems in Cancer, 9,* 1–42.

Wilcox, P. (1979). A new clinic for women with breast masses (p. 65) (Abstract 167). *Proceedings of the Oncology Nursing Society.* New Orleans, May 17–19.

Wilcox, P., Ziegeld, C., Hoopes, N., & Ashley, B. (1990). Beyond breast cancer screening: The nursing role in breast lesion evaluation program (BLEP) (Abstract 226A). *Oncology Nursing Forum, 17,* 194.

Wilkes, B., & Bersani, G. (1983). Development of a community colorectal cancer program (p. 66) (Abstract 79). *Proceedings of the eighth annual congress of the Oncology Nursing Society.* San Diego, May 18–21.

Willett, W. C., Stampfer, M. J., Colditz, G. A., Rosner, B. A., Hennekens, C. H., & Speizer, F. E. (1987). Dietary fat and the risk of breast cancer. *New England Journal of Medicine, 316,* 22–28.

Williams, H. A. (1981). Screening for testicular cancer. *Pediatric Nursing, 7,* 38–40.

Williams, D. (1988). Factors affecting the practice of breast self-examination in older women. *Oncology Nursing Forum, 15,* 611–615.

Williams, R. D. (1989). Breast cancer detection in home health care of the older woman. *Home Healthcare Nurse, 8,* 25–29.

Willis, M. A., Davis, M., Cairns, N. U., & Janiszewski, R. (1989). Interagency collaboration: Teaching breast self-examination to black women. *Oncology Nursing Forum, 16,* 171–180.

Winawer, S. J. (1993). Colorectal cancer screening comes of age. *New England Journal of Medicine, 328(19),* 1416–1417.

Winchester, D. P., Lasky, H. J., Sylvester, J., & Maher, M. L. (1988). A television-promoted mammography screening pilot project in the Chicago metropolitan area. *CA: A Cancer Journal for Clinicians, 38,* 291–309.

Wingo, P., Tong, T., & Bolden, S. (1995). Cancer statistics, 1995. *CA: A Cancer Journal for Clinicians, 45,* 8–30.

Winn, D. (1988). Smokeless tobacco and cancer: The epidemiologic evidence. *CA: A Cancer Journal for Clinicians, 38,* 236–243.

Wyper, M. (1990). Breast self-examination and the Health Belief Model: Variations of a theme. *Research in Nursing and Health, 13,* 421–428.

Zin, D., Wang, S., Yuan, F., Tang, M., Li, M., & Zhang, Z. (1988). Screening for upper digestive tract cancer with an occult bead detection. *Cancer, 62,* 1030–1034.

Cancer Screening and Early Detection

Sharon J. Olsen • Marilyn Frank-Stromborg

Controlling cancer requires cancer prevention, risk assessment, screening for preclinical disease, followed by early detection of disease or surveillance. *Primary cancer prevention* efforts thwart the biologic onset of cancer by altering personal susceptibility or by preventing exposure to cancer-causing agents (see Chapter 16). *Secondary prevention* employs the use of selective screening strategies to detect preclinical cancer in the asymptomatic individual at a time when cancer is presumed to be localized for the purpose of decreasing morbidity and mortality. *Risk assessment* is a critical component of primary and secondary prevention. It involves thorough documentation of the client's medical history, lifestyle characteristics, work and exposure history, and analysis of any familial/genetic predisposition to cancer. Risk assessment should guide recommendations for primary and secondary prevention. *Early detection* employs the use of various diagnostic tests to rule out or confirm the presence of cancer in asymptomatic persons. *Surveillance* is the regular, ongoing monitoring of individuals who have already been identified as high risk. This chapter focuses on current basic and clinical research in the secondary prevention of cancer, specifically, cancer screening and early detection. Its aim is to provide a foundation for understanding and adapting cancer screening and early detection in clinical practice among asymptomatic individuals.

NURSING MANDATES AND INVOLVEMENT

The National Cancer Institute (NCI), Division of Cancer Prevention and Control, in its *Cancer Control Objectives for the Nation: 1985–2000*, directs health care providers to "inform patients of the value of cancer screening and recommend utilization of efficacious screening procedures" (1986, p. 31). The Oncology Nursing Society (ONS) publishes standards of oncology nursing practice for the generalist and the advanced practice nurse to guide nurses in providing population-specific cancer screening and early detection (ANA-ONC, 1987; ONS, 1989a, 1989b).

Nursing efforts in secondary prevention are broad and varied. Nurses aid in case finding and inform clients of guidelines and frequencies for selective screening tests and examinations. They counsel and educate clients about how to recognize the warning signs and symptoms of cancer, perform self-examination techniques, and modify unhealthy lifestyles. They develop, implement, and evaluate school-based, work site, and community cancer-control activities and reinforce screening recommendations previously received from other health care providers. More recently, nurses have provided anticipatory guidance regarding molecular screening and lifestyle predispositions for cancer. Nurses are actively involved in exploring the impact of biopsychosocial variables on screening behaviors through research.

Regarding actual participation in cancer screening, Entrekin and McMillan (1993) found that in a sample of more than 2500 nurses in Florida, only 55.7 per cent of advanced practice nurses, 65.7 per cent of oncology nurses, and 66 per cent of staff nurses agreed they should be responsible for cancer prevention and detection. In general, nurses were not teaching screening to the majority of their patients, nor were they personally involved in many screening activities. Barriers to screening included limited time, knowledge, and opportunity to do screening. Results of this study suggested the need for more cancer prevention and screening content in graduate, undergraduate, and continuing education courses for nurses.

DEFINITIONS

SCREENING AND EARLY DETECTION

The term *screening* is frequently used synonymously with "early detection" or "secondary prevention." For *screening* and *early detection,* finding cancer while it is still localized and curable is the common goal; however, there is an important distinction between them. *Early detection* refers to an attempt to diagnose cancer in a curable stage, whereas cancer *screening* is just one of the strategies used to achieve this goal (Miller, 1986b). According to the American Cancer Society ". . . early detection ideally should be a continuous day-by-day process of self-observation and heightened awareness. It implies a degree of individual responsibility for self-care together with ready access to medical facilities for diagnosis and treatment. It means paying attention to symptoms and seeking prompt help should anything unusual be detected. Cancer *screening,* on the other hand, must be done intermittently or periodically by a health care professional" (Miller, 1986b, p. 16). Screening for cancer involves the use of examinations and tests to search for and identify disease in asymptomatic persons (Eddy, 1985, 1986; Hakama, 1986). A person is considered asymptomatic if he or she is not aware of any signs or symptoms of cancer (Eddy, 1985). In some cases, cancer can be detected in a premalignant state (e.g., leukoplakia of the mouth, dysplasia of the cervix, and adenomas of the colon). More commonly, a lesion has already developed into a cancer by the time it is discovered (e.g., breast cancer). There are three implicit assumptions underlying screening for most cancers: that the tests are capable of detecting cancers before the appearance of signs or symptoms; that these tests will find a greater proportion of cancers in early stages; and that persons with cancers detected through screening will have higher survival rates and tend to live longer after diagnosis and treatment (Eddy, 1986).

MASS SCREENING

Mass screening involves the general population. The main purpose of mass screening is to reduce cancer mortality. Very large populations and large numbers of health care practitioners must be mobilized, and issues such as long-term compliance, cost of test vs. benefit offered, and untoward morbidity (perhaps even mortality) from tests with low sensitivity and specificity make such testing prohibitive. Four ongoing European trials are currently attempting to evaluate a possible reduction in mortality from colorectal cancer by screening for fecal occult blood using Hemoccult-II (Kronborg et al., 1992). Taken together, the trials include more than 300,000 asymptomatic persons. The studies began in 1985 and will be completed in 1996.

SELECTIVE SCREENING

Selective screening is targeted at persons with risk factors that predict for high disease prevalence—that is, high-risk groups. Selective screening involves surveillance and is the attentive follow-up of persons at risk for cancer with the intent to detect any premalignant or malignant condition early (Patterson, 1986). Underlying selective screening is the presumption that no matter how carefully designed a screening program may be, it will have finite resources and, therefore, the yield and subsequently the cost-benefit ratio of such efforts will be greater when targeted to high-risk persons.

Risk factors may be divided into the following categories: age, symptoms, signs, historic risk factors, and environmental and occupational risk factors. It is possible and desirable to target select populations at risk. For instance, it is known that the incidence of cancer of the prostate rises eight times between the ages of 45 and 54 years, whereas for the testis, the incidence remains the same. Lung cancer almost triples, and colon cancer more than doubles for the same age group. Historic risk factors, such as family history of breast cancer, polyposis coli, or maternal use of diethylstilbestrol (DES) during gestation; personal risk factors, such as ulcerative colitis, undescended testes, and leukoplakia; and exposure to environmental and occupational carcinogens all influence the risk factor pattern for any particular person.

Carriers of certain cancer genes (e.g., ataxia-telangiectasia) and certain members of cancer families can have an unusually high risk of developing specific cancers, often at unusually early ages. In some of these individuals, precursor states, such as dysplastic nevus syndrome; can identify genetic predisposition to cancer and can lead to appropriate measures for disease prevention and early detection (Li, 1986). Frank-Stromborg and Heusinkveld have detailed for the reader risk factors associated with specific cancers in Chapter 16. The NCI lists the following as high-risk persons: those with a strong family history of cancer of the breast, ovaries, and colon, or melanoma; adolescent boys and young men (testicular cancer); and those exposed to known environmental or occupational carcinogens.

CASE FINDING

Case finding is "the detection of disease by means of tests or procedures that are undertaken by health workers on clients who are consulting for unrelated symptoms. (This means that the 'case finder' is responsible for the investigation and follow-up of high-risk persons identified in this way)" (Canadian Task Force on the Periodic Health Examination, 1979, p. 1203). Case finding provides opportunities for identifying symptoms and changes in risk factors. The screening guidelines developed by major medical organizations are not for population screening outside the framework of medical care but are really for case finding within that framework (Winawer, 1995).

CANCER CONTROL

According to NCI's Division of Cancer Prevention and Control (1986), cancer control consists of two components: screening and communication. This group suggests that screening be aimed at cancer detection in large populations, including symptomatic and asymptomatic individuals. Communication involves educating the public and, in particular, those persons at risk, about cancer and cancer prevention, and motivating them to indulge in behaviors that are associated with lowered risk for cancer.

IMPORTANT SCREENING TEST FEATURES

Widespread application of a cancer screening test requires a clear understanding of any possible early detection benefit. Generally agreed upon criteria provide guidelines for determining whether specific tests are suitable for screening. These guidelines take into consideration the magnitude of the impact of the disease on society, clinical acceptance of the test in practice, and text accuracy (Table 17–1). At this time, no perfect test exists, and potential risks associated with cancer screening tests can include cost, unnecessary morbidity for those with false-positive results, potential overtreatment of borderline lesions, and false reassurance secondary to false negative test results.

GUIDELINES FOR SCREENING

Decisions regarding who to screen, when to begin screening, and at what intervals continue to be controversial. Guidelines may be evidence-based (Canadian Task Force on Periodic Health Examination, World Health Organization Collaborating Centre for the Prevention of Colorectal Cancer, Agency for Health Care Policy and Research, U. S. Preventive Services Task Force) or a combination of evidence-based and expert opinion (American Cancer Society, various medical specialty organizations, i.e., The American College of Radiology, American College of Physicians, American College of Gastroenterology). Guidelines may or may not address average and high-risk population screening needs. Though many organizations agree on certain guidelines, some disagreement continues. This lack of expert and organizational consensus is compounded by differences in opinion among practitioners. As a result, national cancer screening recommendations tend to vary both within and between clinical practice settings, including cancer control programs in cancer centers.

Findings from a recent study (Czaja, McFall, Warnecke, Ford, & Kaluzny, 1994) of more than 3400 community physicians regarding their cancer screening practices concluded that (1) community physicians accept the idea of screening even when screening is not recommended; (2) physicians tend to accept the most heavily publicized guidelines even when they differ from recommendations by their own professional societies (in this case the American Cancer Society and NCI guidelines were preferred); and (3) economic considerations, perceived test reliability, patient acceptance, and demands or limitations in the practice setting all affected recommendations. Surgeons tended to favor more aggressive screening than family physicians and internists; gynecologists most consistently favored aggressive screening for cancer in women; and older physicians and those in solo practice tended to favor outmoded procedures such as routine chest x-ray examinations and to be more conservative about screening intervals.

AMERICAN CANCER SOCIETY

In general, the most well-known cancer screening guidelines are offered by the American Cancer Society (Levin & Murphy, 1992) (Table 17–2). The Society clearly states that its guidelines are "not rules" and apply only to individuals without symptoms. Surveillance of high-risk patients is left to physician-patient collaboration and determined on an individual basis.

NATIONAL CANCER INSTITUTE

Screening statements (Table 17–3) and the Working Guidelines for Early Cancer Detection (Table 17–4) from the National Cancer Institute are based on various levels of published scientific evidence and collective clinical experience (NCI, 1994). Data upon which the NCI screening guidelines were developed are available at no charge from the Physician's Data Query service of the National Cancer Information Service (1-800-4-CANCER). This information is regularly updated.

CANADIAN NATIONAL TASK FORCE

The Canadian Task Force on the Periodic Health Examination recommends an age- and gender-specific plan for lifetime health assessments for all Canadians (Table 17–5). This national health protection package recommends detection tests (i.e., blood pressure measurement and fecal occult blood testing) for various diseases, including cancer. It also specifies related interventions (i.e., immunization and counseling). This task force regards their recommendations as minimal standards, clearly recognizing that high-risk individuals require more than the recommended interventions.

BENEFITS AND RISKS OF SCREENING

Screening asymptomatic adults for cancer is a valuable activity, but it has associated risk and costs. The *benefits* include improved prognosis for some cases, but

TABLE 17–1. *Critical Features and Bias of Cancer Screening Tests That Guide Clinical Use*

CRITICAL FEATURES AND BIAS	RATIONALE
I. Clinical Impact of the Disease The cancer must be highly prevalent and a source of significant morbidity and mortality. Treatment for cancer must be available such that, when applied, it is more effective for preclinical disease than disease that is symptomatic.	To warrant risks and costs associated with any screening program. Effective treatment for early-stage disease should ultimately translate into decreased mortality from the disease.
II. Clinical Acceptance The test must be safe, convenient (preferably readily available during health care visits), acceptable to the public and relatively low cost.	To enhance compliance and utilization, and minimize short/long-term side effects.
III. Accuracy Sensitivity: the percentage of persons with cancer who have positive screening tests; ideal screening tests are 100% sensitive. Specificity: the percentage of persons without cancer who have negative screening tests; ideal screening tests are 100% specific. Predictive value: *Positive predictive value:* the percentage of persons with a positive screening test who actually have cancer. *Negative predictive value:* the percentage of persons with a negative screening test who clearly do not have cancer.	Tests with low sensitivity run the risk of falsely reassuring patients who may in fact have false-negative test results. Tests with low specificity can overwhelm diagnostic services, result in prohibitive follow-up costs, and expose individuals to the risk of unnecessary diagnostic workups, potentially resulting in substantial physical and psychologic morbidity and possible mortality.
IV. Bias	These three biases invalidate comparisons of stage distribution or survival between series of asymptomatic screen-detected cancers and series of detected cancers that were symptomatic. Well-designed, randomized, controlled trials generally control for these biases.
Lead-time bias: occurs when cancer is detected earlier but the detection does not affect mortality. In this case, the survival time appears to be longer but actually is not. The appearance of improved survival in screen-detected cases that results from moving the diagnosis forward by screening merely lengthens the interval from diagnosis to death rather than lengthening life.	This bias is most notable when short follow-up periods, such as 5-year survival rates are used. Lead-time bias is determined by the sensitivity of the test, the testing interval, and the duration of the preclinical stage.
Length bias: at any point in time, a population will consist of persons with aggressive and symptomatic disease and asymptomatic, less aggressive cancers. Screening will identify both but, because a greater proportion have less aggressive disease, it appears that survival is lengthened because the average life span observed increases.	The improved survival in the screened population derives at least in part from the growth properties of the tumor rather from the benefits of the screening program.
Prognostic selection bias: can occur if patients undergoing screening have better health habits than the general population or have lower mortality or longer survival because they are more resistant to the tumor or more compliant with therapy.	

(Data from Eddy, 1986; Frame, 1986; Hakama, 1986; Love et al., 1984; Patterson, 1986; Selby & Friedman, 1989.)

TABLE 17-2. *Summary of American Cancer Society Recommendations for the Early Detection of Cancer in Asymptomatic People*

	POPULATION		
TEST OR PROCEDURE	SEX	AGE	FREQUENCY
Sigmoidoscopy, preferably flexible	M & F	50 and over	Every 3 to 5 yrs
Fecal occult blood test	M & F	50 and over	Every yr
Digital rectal examination	M & F	40 and over	Every yr
Prostate specific antigen	M	50 and over	Every yr
Pap test	F	All women who are or who have been sexually active, or have reached age 18, should have an annual Pap test and pelvic examination. After a woman has had three or more consecutive satisfactory normal annual examinations, the Pap test may be performed less frequently at the discretion of her physician	
Pelvic examination	F	18–40	Every 1–3 yrs with Pap test
		Over 40	Every year
Endometrial tissue sample	F	At menopause, women at high risk*	At menopause
Breast self-examination	F	20 and over	Every month
Clinical breast examination	F	20–40	Every 3 yrs
		Over 40	Every yr
Mammography**	F	40–49	Every 1–2 yrs
		50 and over	Every yr
Health counseling and cancer checkup***	M & F	Over 20	Every 3 yrs
	M & F	Over 40	Every yr

*History of infertility, obesity, failure to ovulate, abnormal uterine bleeding, or estrogen therapy.
**Screening mammography should begin by age 40.
***To include examination for cancers of the thyroid, testicles, prostate, ovaries, lymph nodes, oral region, and skin.
(From Levin, B. & Murphy, G. P. [1992]. Revision of American Cancer Society recommendations for the early detection of cancer. *CA-A Cancer Journal for Clinicians*, 42(5), p. 298; and American Cancer Society [1994]. *Cancer facts and figures*. Atlanta: ACS.)

TABLE 17-3. *National Cancer Institute Screening Statements*

Breast cancer	
Ages 40–49 yrs:	There is insufficient evidence to make an informed decision regarding the efficacy of screening in women.
Ages 50–69 yrs:	There is strong evidence that screening on a regular basis is efficacious.
Ages 70+ yrs:	Clinical trials offer no information on efficacy of screening in women, though risk of disease increases with age and there is no known upper age limit at which screening ceases to be effective.
Cervical cancer	Evidence strongly suggests a decrease in mortality from regular screening with Pap tests in women who are sexually active or who have reached 18 years of age. The upper age limit at which to cease screening is unknown.
Colorectal cancer	Annual guaiac-based fecal occult blood testing using hydrated stool specimens in people over the age of 50 yrs decreases mortality from colorectal cancer.
	Evidence suggests that a decrease in mortality occurs with regular screening by sigmoidoscopy in people over the age of 50. There is insufficient evidence to determine the optimal interval for such screening.
Ovarian cancer	There is insufficient evidence to establish that screening with serum markers such as CA-125 levels, transvaginal ultrasound, or pelvic examinations results in decreased mortality.
Prostate cancer	There is insufficient evidence to establish that a decrease in mortality occurs with screening by digital rectal examination, transrectal ultrasound, or serum markers including prostate-specific antigen.
Skin cancer	There is evidence from ecologic studies to establish that a decrease in mortality occurs with routine examination of the skin.
Testicular cancer	There is insufficient evidence to suggest that screening results in a decrease in mortality.

TABLE 17–4. *Working Guidelines for Early Cancer Detection, National Cancer Institute*

GUIDELINES	BASES FOR GUIDELINES
Breast Cancer	
Physicians should encourage their female patients to do monthly breast self-examination.	Breast cancer is the most frequent cancer in women and is second only to lung cancer as the leading cause of death from cancer.
Physicians are encouraged to do clinical breast examinations on all female patients in whom they are doing a periodic examination.	Early stage breast cancer has an excellent survival rate (90%).
Beginning at the age of 40 yrs, a mammogram should be encouraged for the patient every 1 to 2 yrs until the age of 50 yrs, after which it should become annual.	Mammography and physical examination are proven methods of detecting early breast cancer.
In women with a personal history of cancer, mammography should be encouraged on an annual basis.	Mortality has been reduced in randomized screening trials using mammography and physical examination.
Cervical Cancer	
All women who are or have been sexually active, or who have reached age 18 yrs, should have an annual Papanicolaou test and pelvic examination. After a woman has had three or more consecutive satisfactory normal annual examinations, the Papanicolaou test may be performed less frequently at the discretion of her physician.	The Papanicolaou test has been proven to decrease mortality.
	The general recommendation has been changed back to yearly because of the change in sexual practices and recent observations on papillomavirus.
Colorectal Cancer	
A rectal examination should be included as a part of the periodic health examination.	Colorectal cancer is the second leading cause of death from cancer. The majority of patients have advanced disease at diagnosis.
At the age of 50 yrs, annual fecal occult blood testing and a sigmoidoscopy every 3 to 5 yrs should be done.	Removal of premalignant lesions whose natural history leads to cancer will decrease incidence and eventual mortality.
The physician should identify, for special surveillance, high-risk patients, including those with a strong family history of colon cancer, or with a personal history of polyps, colon cancer, or inflammatory bowel disease.	Early testing of asymptomatic patients results in the detection of adenomatous polyps, increased numbers of early stage cancers, and decreased numbers of advanced stage cancers.
Oral Cancer	
Oral examination, including palpation of the tongue, floor of the mouth, salivary glands, and lymph nodes of the neck should be performed as part of the periodic health examination.	Cancers of the oral cavity and pharynx are a major cause of death from cancer in the United States.
Special attention should be given to those at high risk owing to tobacco and alcohol use.	This is a region of the body that is generally accessible to examination by the patient, the dentist, and the physician.
	Oral cancer occurs predominantly in patients who smoke cigarettes or chew tobacco or consume considerable amounts of alcohol.
	An oral examination looking for leukoplakia and early cancer should be a part of every periodic health examination in a dentist's or physician's office without additional cost.
	The routine examination of symptomatic and asymptomatic patients results in the detection of earlier stage cancers.
	Treatment outcome is better in patients with early stage disease.

Note: As of April 1990, no changes have been made in these guidelines, per telephone conversations with Charles R. Smart, M.D., Chief of the Early Detection Branch, Division of Cancer Prevention and Control, National Cancer Institute, Bethesda, MD.

(Modified from Early Detection Branch, Division of Cancer Prevention and Control [1987, December 17]. *Working guidelines for early cancer detection: Rationale and supporting evidence to decrease mortality.* Bethesda, MD: National Cancer Institute.)

not all; the possibility of less pain, disfigurement, and disability; less radical treatment to cure some cancers; reassurance for those with negative test results; fiscal savings if less radical treatment/intervention is needed; and lower follow-up costs for surveillance compared with long-term treatment for disease (Chamberlain, 1983; Eddy, 1986; Miller, 1986a). Regarding costs, a recent report by the Office of Technology Assessment (1995) concluded that colorectal cancer screening employing any of the following strategies, annual fecal occult blood testing, regular flexible sigmoidoscopy or colonoscopy, or double-contrast barium enema, was clearly cost-effective for screening average-risk adults beginning at age 50. Alternatively, Optenberg and Thompson (1990) have concluded that mass screening for prostate cancer is prohibitively expensive.

Risks may be direct, such as radiation or perforation, or indirect, such as false-positive test results. Selby (1995) concluded from his review that the perforation rate for flexible sigmoidoscopy was less than 1 in 5000. A danger following false-negative screening is that symptoms may be ignored, resulting in delayed diagnosis and a poorer prognosis. In addition, a more complex and costly workup may be required. A longer and perhaps more emotionally and financially costly period of observation may be inevitable if the screening test is

TABLE 17–4. *Working Guidelines for Early Cancer Detection, National Cancer Institute* Continued

GUIDELINES	BASES FOR GUIDELINES
Prostate Cancer Annual digital rectal examination of the prostate should be performed on all men over 40 yrs of age. More specific education and training should be given to physicians in the detection of prostate cancer.	Prostate cancer is a significant health problem for men in terms of both morbidity and mortality. With the advancing age of the United States population, the overall impact of prostate cancer on the national health will increase. Despite improved understanding of the biologic potential of prostate cancer as it relates to histologic grade and tumor volume, the need to treat or diagnose a given case of prostate cancer cannot be proved at this time. It follows, then, that rigorous statistical validation or cost-effectiveness of any current screening test as a matter of national rather than personal health policy cannot be accomplished at this time. It is clear that disease-free survival is increased in patients treated for localized versus advanced prostate cancer (length and lead times biases notwithstanding). Until we can predict the biologic potential of a given tumor, attempts to decrease morbidity and mortality from prostate cancer require a uniform screening method for earlier detection of disease. Given the imperfections of every available method, routine annual digital rectal examination for men over 40 years of age appears to be the most reasonable screening test for prostate cancer with regard to overall efficiency, noninvasiveness, morbidity, availability, and cost. A continued search for more precise methods for the early detection of curable *and* biologically active prostate cancer is warranted.
Skin Cancer (Melanoma) Based on the recommendation of the American Academy of Dermatology, all persons should be encouraged to examine their skin thoroughly on a regular basis. Primary care physicians should be encouraged to examine the skin as part of the periodic health examination. Further public and professional education should be promoted on the early detection of skin cancers and in particular malignant melanoma.	Melanoma in the United States makes up 2% of all malignancies and 1% of cancer deaths (slightly more than for cancer of the cervix). The incidence has increased more rapidly than that for any other cancer in recent years. Education of the public and physicians has resulted in earlier detection, improved survival, and stabilization of mortality in other countries. The examinations are a part of usual medical practice and have no cost implications.
Testes Cancer Periodic (monthly) testicular self-examination should be encouraged. Routine palpation of the testicles by a physician during physical examination should be carried out as part of the health examination.	This is a rare disease in an organ that is readily accessible to examination by the individual person. Although germ cell testicular tumor is relatively uncommon, it is a significant cause of cancer-related morbidity and mortality in young men. Testis cancer has uniformly high virulence. Testis cancer is very responsive to therapy. The morbidity and cost to achieve cure is lower for low stage and low volume of disease compared to advanced disease. Treatment failures are more often associated with bulky late-stage disease. Diagnosis by simple palpation, which is noninvasive, inexpensive, and nonmorbid, should be easily taught to health professionals and to the male population with a high positive predictive value.

capable of detecting presymptomatic cases. Finally, longer periods of morbidity for patients in whom prognosis is unaltered and the risk of overtreatment of borderline abnormalities cannot be minimized.

Substantial psychologic and monetary costs can be associated with the risks of screening. Direct costs include the physician or clinic charge for the visit; direct costs of the test or examination, including pro-

cessing and interpretation; morbidity and mortality from the test itself; and the dollar cost of diagnostic evaluation of persons with false-positive screening test results. Indirect costs include those incurred while going for the screening test (e.g., time lost from work, babysitting, automobile gasoline, parking fees) and the nonfinancial costs of inconvenience, anxiety, discomfort, and psychologic stress if early screening incurs no

TABLE 17–5. *Guidelines for Screening for Cancer, Canadian National Task Force*

CONDITION, AGE	MANEUVER	RECOMMENDATION*
Breast Cancer		
40–49	Annual physical breast examination	C
50–59	Annual mammography and physical breast examination	A
≥ 60	Annual mammography and physical breast examination	B
≤ 40	Teach breast self-examination	C
Cervical Cancer		
18–35; sexually active	Annual Papanicolaou smear	B (based on 1976 recommendations)
> 35–60; sexually active	Papanicolaou smear every 5 yrs	
35 +; high risk	Women whose contact with the health care system is through venereal disease clinics or penal institutions should not be discouraged from having smears more frequently than every 5 yrs if they request them	
> 60	If a woman has had repeated satisfactory smears without significant atypia, she may stop having Papanicolaou smears	
Colorectal Cancer		
< 40; with NO known risk factors	No routine recommendations	C
> 40; with NO known risk factors	No routine recommendations; however, evidence does not warrant stopping the use of fecal occult blood testing or sigmoidoscopy where it already exists	C
People with two or more first-degree relatives with colorectal cancer	Periodic colonoscopy (beginning at age 40 yrs)	C
People with one first-degree relative with colorectal cancer detected after age 40 yrs	Fecal occult blood testing and sigmoidoscopy (beginning at age 40 yrs)	C
Women with a history of endometrial, ovarian, or breast cancer	Periodic sigmoidoscopy	C
People with a history of colorectal cancer, adenomatous polyps, or ulcerative colitis of 10-years' duration	Periodic colonoscopy	
Family members of patients with familial polyposis	Periodic sigmoidoscopy at an early age, followed by periodic colonoscopy after age 30 yrs	
Prostate Cancer	Digital palpation per rectum	C
	Prostate specific antigen	C
Testis Cancer	Clinical examination of testes	C
Bladder Cancer	Cytologic urine analysis for high-risk groups: workers occupationally exposed to bladder carcinogens, smokers. Frequency based on clinical judgment	D for general population; B for high-risk groups
Hodgkin's Disease	Physical examination and x-ray studies	C
Oral Cancer	Visual examination of males and all smokers annually beginning at age 65 yrs	C
Skin Cancer Including Melanoma	Counseling to reduce exposure and foster use of sunscreens and periodic skin examination at appropriate intervals on the basis of clinical judgment	D for general population; B for high-risk groups

*A There is good evidence to support the recommendation that the condition be specifically considered in a periodic health examination.

B There is fair evidence to support the recommendation that the condition be specifically considered in a periodic health examination.

C There is poor evidence regarding the inclusion of the condition in a periodic health examination, and recommendations may be made on other grounds.

D There is fair evidence to support the recommendation that the condition be excluded from consideration in a periodic health examination.

(Modified from Canadian Task Force. [1979, November 3]. The periodic health examination. *Canadian Medical Association Journal, 121,* 1195, 1206–1246; Canadian Task Force on Cervical Cancer Screening Programs. [1982, October 1]. Cervical cancer screening programs: Summary of the 1982 Canadian task force report. *Canadian Medical Association Journal, 127,* 581–589; Canadian Task Force. [1986, April 1]. The periodic health examination: 2. 1985 update. *Canadian Medical Association Journal, 134,* 724; Canadian Task Force on the Periodic Health Examination. [1989, August 1]. The periodic health examination: 2. 1989 update. *Canadian Medical Association Journal, 141,* 209–216. Reprinted with permission of the Health Services Directorate, Health Services and Promotion Branch, Department of National Health and Welfare and the *Canadian Medical Association Journal;* Canadian Task Force on The Periodic Health Examination. [1991]. Periodic health examination, 1991 update: 3. Secondary prevention of prostate cancer. *Canadian Medical Association Journal, 145,* 413–428.)

prolonged survival benefit (Eddy, 1985; Love, Leventhal, Hughes, & Fryback, 1984). Pain cannot be underestimated as a substantial direct cost of, for example, endometrial tissue biopsy. Eddy (1985) suggests that the pain associated with this procedure will be mild for 70 per cent of women but moderate to severe for the majority of nulliparous women.

THE POTENTIAL FOR SCREENING TO REDUCE CANCER MORTALITY

The goal of screening is to reduce mortality. It is generally agreed that the strongest evidence is provided by randomized, controlled, clinical trials using mortality as an end point. Evidence from studies that are controlled but not randomized, such as case-control studies and those with historic controls, is generally weaker but still useful.

The best results currently available from screening trials indicate that screening can potentially reduce mortality from breast cancer by about 30 per cent, colon and rectal cancers by about 30 to 40 per cent, cervical cancer by about 90 per cent, melanoma (through public awareness of early detection) by 20 per cent, and oral cancer in high-risk persons by 20 per cent (NCI, 1994). Few data are available to estimate the effect of screening on mortality from cancers of the stomach, esophagus, bladder, or liver; however, Eddy (1986) predicts that if only a 10 per cent reduction were possible, the potential value of early detection would be that a screening program in 1977 could have saved about 750 million person-years of life throughout the world, and by the year 2000 almost 1000 million person-years of productive life could be saved for each year of screening.

DEVELOPING SCREENING PROGRAMS

A rapid increase in the number of screening programs initiated in primary, secondary, and tertiary care settings is occurring today. Increasingly, nurses are becoming more actively involved in the development, implementation, and ongoing operation of these programs. It is clear that the use of a screening test as part of an office visit does not constitute a screening program (Prorok & Connor, 1986). Several authors (Eddy, 1986; Love & Olsen, 1985; Prorok & Connor, 1986) have provided suggestions and guidelines for the development of comprehensive and well-designed screening programs. According to Prorok and Connor (1986), a screening program depends on the organizational entity, the specialized facility dedicated to carrying out a screening protocol, and the personnel to ensure that it is followed. It includes an outreach or recruitment program for a target population or populations; the necessary equipment and personnel to perform, evaluate, and monitor the quality control of the screening tests; and sufficient resources to follow up positive and suspicious results with appropriate action.

Eddy (1986) emphasizes that the following conditions should be considered when developing a screening program:

1. A formal analysis should be performed to estimate the effectiveness, risks, and costs of screening the selected populations.
2. The screening program should be planned as part of an integrated and holistic health care program.
3. Screening should be limited to circumstances in which the principles of screening are adhered to.
4. Screening should be applied selectively to those persons most likely to benefit.
5. The risks as well as the expected benefits of screening should be explained to the prospective subjects. The risks include any possible complications of the examination procedures and the possibility of false-positive and false-negative test results.
6. The program should be organized to ensure high-quality examinations and to minimize costs.
7. Facilities should be available to follow, diagnose, and treat people who have positive results on examination.
8. Records should be kept to monitor the program's quality and success.

Love and Olsen (1985) specify a prescriptive framework for organizing and integrating cancer prevention strategies into clinical practice. Four goals for a comprehensive screening and early detection program that relies on interdependent and complementary clinical practice between nursing and medicine are described. The first goal is to designate specific staff responsibilities. Initially, this requires staff agreement on a philosophy of client care and designation of the policies of the practice. A philosophy that is receptive to and promotes self-care encourages clients to take control of their own health and provides them with open access to health care information and education in specialized skills. Designated staff responsibilities may vary from program to program but should be limited only by practitioner competence and creativity or organizational necessity.

Development of a medical records system to facilitate staff work is the second goal. A detailed database for each client permits in-depth and accurate analysis of risk factors, planning of personalized and comprehensive screening and health education, and facilitates regular follow-up. The third goal entails the definition of specific screening and detection behaviors and attitudes for both clients and staff. Consensus must be reached regarding which screening tests and frequency guidelines will be regularly monitored and promoted by the practice. Health education protocols and educational media must be agreed on. The goals of ancillary, nursing, and medical staff must all be directed toward these common goals to present a holistic and unified clinical practice milieu committed to the importance of primary prevention, cancer screening, and early detection. Finally, the fourth goal emphasizes staff education. Love and Olsen (1985) suggest that commitment to a practice-wide continuing education system that legitimizes and promotes personal as well as profes-

TABLE 17–6. *Guidelines for Culturally Sensitive Screening*

Learn to recognize signs that indicate patient's use of traditional healers (i.e., presence of amulets, particular marks on the skin, medicine bundles, religious articles around wrists or necks). Never remove these articles without permission.

Proceed slowly and respectfully. Tell patient what you are/will be doing and how it relates to the problem of concern. Educate patient about own body, normal physiology, and self-examinations during exam.

Attend to modesty and dignity. Use similarly gendered practitioners for intimate examinations. Drape adequately. Expose only one body part at a time. This minimizes embarrassment, retains dignity, and prevents chilling, which some believe can cause illness and disease. Be aware of cultural beliefs concerning sexuality and how the practitioner's touch might be perceived as inappropriate.

Give permission to ask questions. Some cultures out of deference to authority and concern for maintaining harmony will not disagree, ask questions, or seek clarification.

Give permission to express pain or discomfort so patient may retain dignity in presence of strangers.

Learn to recognize normal variations in skin tones and mucous membranes in African-Americans.

Advise patients of disposition of body fluids or samples. Some traditional cultures believe these can be maliciously used to allow evil spirits, illness, or disease to enter the body; others believe cutting the flesh can disrupt harmony. Determine whether beliefs require that samples be returned.

Advocate for special needs of culturally diverse individuals. Seek out *appropriate* translators/interpreters. Arrange, negotiate for, and/or facilitate access to necessary follow-up.

(Data from Frank-Stromborg, M., & Olsen, S. J. [1993]. *Cancer prevention and screening in minorities: Cultural implications for health care providers.* St. Louis: Mosby.)

sional education is mandatory for personal growth, continued job satisfaction, and the delivery of up-to-date and high-quality client care.

SCREENING MEDICALLY UNDERSERVED, LOW-INCOME, AND ETHNICALLY DIVERSE POPULATIONS

During the last decade, increasing emphasis has been placed on screening underserved, low-income, and ethnically diverse populations (USDHHS, 1985; ACS, 1989). Poverty has been identified as the most compelling risk factor for higher cancer incidence, lower survival, and higher cancer mortality among medically underserved U. S. citizens (Adams & Kerner, 1982; Baquet, Horm, Gibbs, & Greenwald, 1991; Baquet & Ringen, 1985; Bassett & Krieger, 1986; Butler, King, & White, 1983; Freeman, 1981; Gregorio, Cummings & Michalek, 1983; Satariano, Belle, & Swanson, 1986; Subcommittee on Cancer in the Economically Disadvantaged, ACS, 1986). Poverty leads to illiteracy, unemployment, poor or substandard housing, inadequate health care, and inadequate or substandard nutritional status. Illiteracy limits exposure to health messages that recommend screening and early detection. Inadequate or substandard housing and diet modify immunologic status and increase exposures and risk factors. Finally, access to quality and consistent screening, early detection, and follow-up care is significantly compromised in this population.

National surveys have found that African-Americans tend to underestimate the prevalence of cancer, tend to be more pessimistic than whites about their chances for survival should they get cancer, and are less likely to believe that early detection makes a difference or that existing treatments are effective. A comprehensive national survey conducted by the ACS in 1985

found that, in comparison with the general population, Hispanics (1) believe to a lesser degree that early detection increases the chances of cure, (2) were less aware of the warning signals and specific cancer tests, and (3) were somewhat more fearful of developing cancer. Other important barriers included that Spanish was the language spoken by 63 per cent of the people at home, the majority had a clear preference for information in Spanish, one third had no medical insurance, and the majority were most comfortable with Spanish-speaking male physicians (A study of Hispanics' attitudes, 1985). Belonging to a minority group would appear to be a significant barrier to early cancer detection owing to knowledge deficits and pessimism about the disease as well as language barriers to obtaining cancer information.

Guidelines for culturally sensitive and specific screening with the medically underserved, poor, and ethnically diverse populations have been described in depth elsewhere (Frank-Stromborg & Olsen, 1993; Freeman, Muth, & Kerner, 1995; Olsen & Frank-Stromborg, 1993; Palos, 1994). The nurse can facilitate cooperation, willingness to return for future examinations, and trust and openness by following a few generic guidelines (Table 17–6).

CRITICAL FACTORS IN SCREENING

The following section will review nursing, patient, and system factors (beliefs, practices, knowledge, barriers, and facilitators) currently associated with screening for selective cancers.

SCREENING FOR BREAST CANCER

Lillington, Padilla, Sayre, and Chelbowski (1993) examined the role of the nurse in breast cancer (BC) screening. Nurses (sample = 2800) reported BC knowledge deficits (36 per cent) for risk factors (36 per cent) and signs and symptoms (35 per cent); 85 per cent believed that nursing had a role in breast cancer screening and early detection. Only 27 per cent performed clinical breast examination; 61 per cent assessed for risk factors. Common barriers to screening included work setting obstacles (64 per cent), knowledge and skill deficits (57 per cent), lack of patient education materials (51 per cent), uncertainty about RN vs. MD role in cancer control, and time constraints (42 per cent).

Champion (1995) recently reviewed the data correlating barriers and benefits with compliance with mammography guidelines and found ample evidence for positive correlation. Barriers included fear of radiation, fear of results, knowledge deficits, time, and expense. Elderly, minority, and women of lower socioeconomic class have reported fewer motivations and greater barriers to mammographic screening (Roetzheim et al., 1993). Kornguth et al. (1993) concluded that giving women control over the amount of compression applied during mammography resulted in good to excellent compression and an image at least as good as that produced with technologist-applied compression. Lerman and Schwartz (1993) concluded from their review of the literature that women at high risk for breast cancer have high levels of psychologic distress and persistent and intrusive worries about developing breast cancer and that a substantial proportion do not adhere to breast cancer screening guidelines.

Factors that appear to promote adherence to mammography screening include presentation with persuasive messages that emphasize personal responsibility for screening (Rothman, Salovey, Turvey, & Fishkin, 1993); reminding physicians to send computer reminders to patients (Burack et al., 1994); providing women with tailored messages to alter their beliefs and information regarding screening (Champion, 1994); mailing women an individually tailored mammography screening recommendation letter (Kendall & Hailey, 1993; Skinner, Strecher, & Hospers, 1994). For older, low-income, inner-city women, the provision of vouchers for obtaining mammograms increased examination participation, but fear, lack of transportation, and finances remained significant barriers to screening.

Social support has been identified as a positive predictor of breast self-examination (BSE) practice by six authors (Edwards, 1980; Kang & Bloom, 1993; Laughter et al., 1981; Lierman, Kasprzyk, & Benoliel, 1991; Lierman, Powell-Cope, Benoliel, Georgiadou, & Young, 1994; Rutledge & Davis, 1988). Important aspects of social support included physician encouragement, peer and family support, social network, and social pressure.

SCREENING FOR CERVICAL CANCER

Cervical cancer (CC) screening rates in the United States vary by race, socioeconomic status, and age. In a 1988 National Survey of Family Growth ($n = 8450$ women), 67 per cent of those 15 to 44 years of age had had a Pap test or pelvic examination (Wilcox & Mosher, 1993). Predictors of low CC screening included women who were not sexually active, women with little education or low income, women of Native American, Hispanic, and Asian/Pacific Islander descent, older African-American women, women with no usual source of health care, and women with a lack of physician recommendation (Austin, Baron, & Gates, 1993; Calle, Flanders, Thun, & Martin, 1993; Mayer et al., 1992; Wilcox & Mosher, 1993).

Factors that have been demonstrated to facilitate CC screening include (1) screening elderly, poor, African-American women during routine primary care visits in hospital clinics (Mandelblatt, Traxler, Lakin, Kanetsky, & Kao, 1993), and (2) using nurses and public health workers to increase CC knowledge and access to free screening and follow-up, when needed, among low-income African-American women (Ansell, Lacy, Whitman, Chen, & Phillips, 1994). Yancey and Walden (1994) suggest that video modalities can be effective in increasing knowledge and promoting screening in low-income African-Americans.

A 3-year study in Maryland that mandated offering CC screening to hospitalized women found that despite legislation, inpatient CC screening rates mirrored outpatient patterns and that elderly and low-income women continued to go unscreened (Klassen, Celentano, & Weisman, 1993).

The use of nurse practitioners in CC screening has resulted in improved adherence to screening follow-up in women with abnormal Paps (Gifford & Stone, 1993; Hartz, 1995; Marcus et al., 1992). Most nurse practitioner colposcopy clinics have served to extend care to patients falling in the 185 to 200 per cent poverty rate.

SCREENING FOR COLORECTAL CANCER

The most recent population-based study of fecal occult blood testing (FOBT) and sigmoidoscopy screening was conducted from 1987 to 1989 in 4915 citizens of Minnesota (Bostick, Sprafka, Virnig, & Potter, 1993). Among men and women 50 to 65 years of age, 77 per cent had had a digital rectal examination; 52.5 per cent an FOBT; and 48.3 per cent a sigmoidoscopy.

Rates for colorectal cancer (CRC) screening with FOBT or flexible sigmoidoscopy (FS) are not consistent, and we have only scanty data on factors that facilitate or impede participation. Macrea et al. (1984) found the following in their study of 581 persons offered FOBT: (1) real and perceived susceptibility to CRC was positively related to acceptance of the FOBT kit and (2) perceived barriers to taking the FOBT kit ("Embarrassing to test bowel action with the Hemoccult test" and "It would cause worry to test bowel action") contributed significantly to explaining differences between compliers and noncompliers.

Lack of perceived individual need to participate in screening programs for CRC has been reported by others (Silman & Mitchell, 1984; Spector, Applegate, Olmstead, DiVasto, & Skipper, 1981). Spector et al. found in their study of 202 clinic patients that nonvolunteers were more likely to deny that they could have cancer and objected to specific aspects of the early detection programs, such as sampling stool.

In 1983, a survey of the American public found a general lack of confidence in the early detection of CRC ("Cancer of the colon"). CRC was seen as a male problem, believed to be a crippling disease, and believed to be well advanced with poor survival chances when it was discovered. Alternatively, Farrands, Hardcastle, Chamberlain, and Moss (1984) found that participants in a CRC screening program were more likely to have positive attitudes toward preventive health practices, were better informed about serious illnesses, and were more optimistic and less frightened about cancer.

Farrands et al. (1984) found that more women than men accepted the FOBT and that the participation rate in people over age 65 years was lower than for younger people. The observation that women and individuals in younger age groups are more likely to participate in colorectal screening was also found in a study by Box, Nichols, Lailemand, Pearson, and Vakil (1984). In 1978, the best compliance rate achievable for FOBT by Elwood, Erickson, and Lieberman was 28.7 per cent (total sample size = 11,115). This was during a group meeting of volunteers attending a regular AARP meeting where the purpose of the test was discussed and kits were distributed to requestors. A mass screening program for FOBT with more than 156,000 persons resulted in a 35 per cent response rate (Morris et al., 1991). Interventions included 121 minutes of televised ads and regional notification of more than 5000 physicians. Myers et al. (1991) found that it took an advance letter, a FOBT screening kit, a reminder letter, a self-held booklet, an instruction call, and a reminder call to achieve a 48 per cent compliance rate with FOBT in more than 2200 members of an IPA/HMO. In a study of FOBT use among 617 African-Americans, social support favorably predicted screening with FOBT (Kang & Bloom, 1993). In a recent pilot study Weinrich, Weinrich, Boyd, Atwood, and Cervenka (1994) examined the impact of adapting a CRC screening program (FOBT) to the aging needs of older, poor, and African-American adults (*n* = 135). Adaptations included demonstration and practice with the procedure. Participation in screening was significantly higher than the 5 to 34 per cent rates reported in the literature for socioeconomically disadvantaged populations.

McCarthy and Moskowitz (1993) found that 84 per cent of men and 65 per cent of women who were scheduled and confirmed for FS actually had the examination. Preprocedural and postprocedural surveys revealed that patients (*n* = 105) found the procedure significantly less embarrassing and painful than expected. They also found that 91 per cent of those who had previous FS repeated the examination. A postcard reminder to more than 760 patients over age 50 years resulted in only 1.3 per cent of patients receiving FS (Petravage & Swedberg, 1988). Kelly and Shank (1992) did not find the combined use of educational materials and a phone reminder to increase compliance with their recommendation to have FS (*n* = 333). Holt (1991) concluded that the only factor that correlated with his patients (*n* = 20) having FS was physician recommendation.

Several studies have examined the use of nurses to screen for CRC using FS. They conclude that with sufficient training and education, registered nurses can perform FS safely, efficiently, accurately, and competently (DiSario & Sanowski, 1993; Maule, 1994). Others suggest that the use of nurses to perform FS (1) is a viable economic alternative to the use of physicians to perform screening FS (Spencer & Ready, 1977; Maule, 1994) and (2) maximizes access to the test for at risk populations (Schroy, Wiggins, Winawer, Diaz, & Lightdale, 1988). Patient satisfaction with nurse administered examinations has been favorable (Roosevelt & Franki, 1984; Gertler, Murray, Akashi, & Jonas, 1991; DiSario & Sanowski, 1993), and female patients often expressed relief at being examined by another women.

SCREENING FOR PROSTATE CANCER

Clinical use of the prostate-specific antigen (PSA) blood test to screen for prostate cancer (PC) has garnered significant national attention and controversy. Recent research suggests that the use of the PSA for mass screening can lead to possible overdiagnosis, resulting in the treatment of clinically nonsignificant PC, significant patient morbidity, and significant financial health care burden. Nurse practitioners in Michigan (*n* = 97) believed that screening and counseling men about prostate, testicular, and colorectal cancer was not consistent with their role (Warren & Pohl, 1990).

Data from the 1993 Kentucky Health Survey (*n* = 661) concluded that 92 per cent of that sample had heard of prostate cancer but that 67 per cent had never heard of the PSA test despite significant national media attention (Mainous & Hagen, 1994). Ninety-four per cent of the men who had the test recommended by their physician had undergone the test, suggesting the significant acceptability of this inexpensive and easy-to-obtain blood test.

Data from five sites during the 1991 Prostate Cancer Awareness Week screening events demonstrated that screening offerings in major medical centers primarily attracted white males who already practiced adequate screening (Demark-Wahnefried, Catoe, Pasket, Robertson, & Rimer, 1993).

Currently an important role for nursing surrounding PC screening is informing men about the current controversy regarding PSA use and the potential outcomes of treatment and assisting them to make a truly informed decision.

SELF-EXAMINATION TECHNIQUES

The self-examination techniques that are utilized in early detection of cancer are BSE, testicular self-examination (TSE), self-administered Hemoccult testing, and oral self-examination. Hemoccult testing is designed to detect occult blood in the stool, and oral self-examination has been recommended for persons at risk for oral lesions (e.g., heavy smokers, those with a history of leukoplakia or erythroplakia). Breast self-examination and self-administered Hemoccult testing have received the most intensive investigation and questioning, whereas there is a dearth of information or research on TSE and oral self-examination. Because breast and colorectal cancer are two of the leading causes of cancer deaths in the United States, subsequent discussion of self-examination techniques will focus primarily on BSE and self-administered Hemoccult testing.

BREAST SELF-EXAMINATION

THE BREAST SELF-EXAMINATION DEBATE

For many years BSE has been advocated for all women as a screening technique for detecting breast cancers in the early clinical stage and thereby reducing mortality. It has been argued that BSE should be taught in connection with yearly physical examinations or other health-related encounters. There are two major arguments for encouraging BSE.

1. Research has documented that between 85 and 90 per cent of all breast cancers are discovered by women themselves (Chie & Chang, 1994).
2. The National Institutes of Health-American Cancer Society Breast Cancer Detection Demonstration Projects reported that 17 per cent of the breast cancers were detected during intervals between visits (termed interval cancers) (Foster, Costanza, & Worden, 1985). Higher percentages of interval cancers have been reported by Tabar, Fagerberg, Gad, Holmberg, and Thomas, (1985), who found that 20 to 25 per cent of breast cancers were detected in the interval between annual mammograms, clinical breast examinations, or both.

Breast self-examination was believed to be a cost-effective early-detection method because it required no special equipment, needed no appointment with a health professional, and could be done in the privacy of a woman's home at her convenience. A series of Gallup surveys conducted for the ACS over the last decade have indicated a steady increase in women's awareness of BSE; it is now nearly universal at 95 per cent (Van Parijs & Eckhardt, 1984). However, even though most women have heard of BSE, only 15 to 40 per cent are reported to perform it monthly (O'Malley & Fletcher, 1987).

More recently, there has been increasing debate about the merit of BSE. A recurring criticism is the lack of prospective randomized controlled trials to establish the effectiveness of BSE in reducing breast cancer mortality (Diem & Rose, 1985; Frank & Mai, 1985). Studies measuring the effectiveness of treatment after screening by BSE have been retrospective or descriptive in design (Table 17–7). Most retrospective BSE data have been from women who have developed breast cancer, raising questions of recall bias. However, this criticism is being addressed by a prospective, randomized, controlled trial being conducted by the World Health Organization in Russia. A population of more than 193,000 women aged 40 to 64 years has been defined in Moscow and St. Petersburg and randomized to study and control groups. This study is expected to last for 15 years. A key issue of the study is compliance of the population with BSE and reduction of mortality from breast cancer.

The most recent and widely quoted study to support the argument that regular BSE does improve survival was done by Kurebayashi, Shimozuma, and Sonoo (1994), in which they investigated the relationship of BSE to survival in Japanese breast cancer patients. They found a positive relationship between more frequent BSE and an earlier clinical stage. For women who performed BSE monthly the mean maximum tumor diameter was 1.7 cm compared with 2.5 cm for women who occasionally practiced BSE and 3.0 cm for women who did not do BSE. At 34 months, 0 per cent of the women who practiced regular BSE had died compared with 3.8 per cent of women who occasionally did BSE and 7.6 per cent of women who did not do BSE.

RISKS OF BREAST SELF-EXAMINATION

Although it is rare to see any discussion of the risks of performing BSE, Frank and Mai (1985) argue that this self-examination technique does pose some potential risks to women.

1. Some women experience considerable anxiety when they examine their bodies for cancer.
2. There are potential risks of false reassurance (false-negative results) from BSE when a woman finds nothing. The sensitivity of BSE (the ability to detect a cancerous lump present in breast tissue) has been estimated to be 26 per cent, compared with an estimated sensitivity of 75 per cent for the combination of mammography and clinical breast examination (these estimates are from the Breast Cancer Detection Demonstration Project data) (O'Malley & Fletcher, 1987).
3. False-positive results are expensive, are time-consuming, and result in unnecessary medical tests. A Finnish study found that in 56,177 women aged 20 to 80 years who were taught BSE, 750 women came to medical attention with breast symptoms in the first year and 300 in the second year of the study. Gastrin (1980) found a 99 per cent likelihood that a breast abnormality found by BSE was benign (predictive value for cancer of BSE in this study was 12 per cent). The results of another large-scale study in England indicated that only 43 cancers were identified from a total of 717 self-referrals (of 14,827 women), giving a predictive value for a positive BSE finding of 6 per cent (Holliday, Roebuck, & Doyle, 1983).

Because the evidence that BSE's accuracy (sensitivity and specificity) "appears to be considerably inferior to that of the combination of clinical breast examination and mammography," the United States Preventive Services Task Force makes no recommendation about the inclusion or exclusion of teaching BSE during the periodic health examination (1987, p. 2196). This task force (1987) also states that it endorses the following World Health Organization statement about BSE.

> There is insufficient evidence that BSE as applied to date is effective in reducing mortality from breast cancer. Therefore BSE screening programmes are not at present recommended as public health policy, although there is equally insufficient evidence to change them where they already exist (p. 2196).

TABLE 17-7. Descriptive Studies of the Effectiveness of Treatment Following Screening by Breast Self-Examination (BSE)

Source, Year	Data	No.	Tumor Size and Nodal Involvement by BSE Practice — BSE Performance Frequency	%	Tumor Size, Mean or % < 2 cm	No Nodal Involvement, %	Tumor Stage by Detection Method — Stage or Tumor Size by Detection Method	%	BSE Detection/ ACC* Ratio	Significance Stage by Detection Method
Foster et al., 1978	Vermont Breast Cancer Network, 1975–1977	335	1/mo	25	1.97 cm	60	NA*		NA	NA
			<1/mo	28	2.47 cm	57				
			NE	47	3.59 cm	43				
Greenwald et al., 1978	Regional Breast Cancer Program, Northeastern New York & Western Massachusetts, 1975–1977	293	Yes	28	NA	NA	Pathologic stage 0, 1		1.29	NS*
			No	72			BSE	22		
							ACC	17		
Smith et al., 1980	Cancer Surveillance System, Seattle, 1977	230	> 2/yr	61	23%	NA	Pathologic stage 0, 1		NA	NA
			≤ 2/yr	39	22%		BSE > 2/yr	59		
							BSE ≤ 2/yr	58		
Senie et al., 1981	Memorial Sloan-Kettering Cancer Center, 1976–1978	1216	1/mo	29	47%	64	NA		NA	NS†
			<1/mo or NE*	71	43%	58				
Huguley & Brown, 1981	Georgia Cancer Management Network, 1975–1979	2092	1/mo	34	47%‡	57‡	Pathologic stage 0, 1		1.23	NA
			<1/mo	33	37%‡	41	BSE	27		
			NE	33			ACC	22		
Feldman et al., 1981	Brooklyn Breast Cancer Demonstration Network, 1975–1979	996	1/mo	19	56%‡	53	NA		NA	NA
			<1/mo	22	39%§	54				
			Rarely	26		42				
			NE	33		38				
Tamburini et al., 1981	Instituto Nationale Tumori, Milan, Italy, 1978–1979	500	1/mo	11	37%‡	59‡	NA		NA	NA
			<1/mo	24	21%‡	49				
			NE	65						
Gould-Martin et al., 1982	Los Angeles County Cancer Surveillance Program, 1976–1977	274	≥ 6/yr	43	NA	59‡	In situ or localized		0.89	NA
			< 6/yr	22		64	BSE	52		
			NE	35			ACC	59		
Hislop et al., 1984	British Columbia Cancer Registry, 1980–1982	416	1/mo	54	21%*	85‡	NA		NA	NA
			<1/mo	18	14%					
			NE	28						
Owen et al., 1985	Oklahoma Hospitals Breast Cancer Control Network, 1975–1977	2063	NA		NA	78	In situ or localized		1.12	NA
							BSE	58		
							ACC	52		
Smith & Burns, 1985	Iowa SEER, 1980–1982	365	≥ 2/yr	56	NA	NA	In situ or localized		1.18	NS
			< 2/yr	44			BSE	59		
							ACC	50		

*ACC indicates accidental patient detection; NA = not available; NS = not significant; NE = never.
†Nonsignificance noted but data not presented.
‡Monthly and less than monthly BSE categories combined.
§Rarely and never BSE categories combined.
(From O'Malley, M., & Fletcher, S. [1987]. Screening for breast cancer with breast self-examination. *Journal of the American Medical Association, 257,* 2197–2203. Copyright 1987, American Medical Association.)

Until there is definitive evidence on the long-term benefits or lack of long-term benefits of BSE, nurses should continue teaching this self-examination practice. Many researchers suggest that BSE will contribute to earlier detection of breast cancer and thereby will save lives. Although no proof exists that periodic BSE reduces mortality due to breast cancer, there is evidence to support this theory. Foster et al. (1985) caution that the degree of certainty that may be possible with randomized controlled trials would likely not be worth the cost of such studies with this approach. They make the point that prospective randomized studies do not provide 100 per cent certainty and are costly and time-consuming, as well as being difficult to control for all extraneous variables. For instance, it would be impossible to control for information sharing that could occur through television, radio, and the printed media.

RESEARCH IN BREAST SELF-EXAMINATION

The literature is replete with studies investigating the characteristics of women who practice and do not practice BSE. In general, women more likely to engage in BSE practice are younger, are better educated, are oriented toward prevention, have higher perceived vulnerability to breast cancer, and have been shown how to perform BSE by a health professional (Adams & Kerner, 1982; Hirshfield-Bartek, 1982; Bennett, Lawrence, Fleischman, Gifford, & Slack, 1983; Cole & Goman, 1984; Hallal, 1982; Kegeles, 1985; Massey, 1986; McCusker & Morrow, 1980; Perez, Fair, Ihde, & Labrie, 1985; Salazar, 1994). Nurses need to be cognizant of these characteristics when instructing women in this technique. A woman who does not believe in the value of early detection of cancer or who thinks that her chances of developing cancer are remote may not practice BSE. Thus teaching BSE should include a discussion of these attitudes as well as efforts to (1) promote the benefits of the early detection of breast cancer and (2) point out the research documenting that all women over the age of 35 in the United States should consider themselves at risk for breast cancer (Seidman, Stellman, & Mushinski, 1982).

Figure 17–1 is the United States National Institutes of Health (NIH)-recommended technique for BSE. All BSE instruction should include an opportunity for the woman to repeat the demonstration under the supervision of the nurse or health care professional doing the teaching. This gives the health professional the opportunity to increase the woman's confidence in her ability to do BSE as well as correct any mistakes in technique. Several different educational approaches have been used to improve BSE practice.

Group Approaches. Kegeles and Grady (1982) suggested that group procedures could improve knowledge, specific skills, and perhaps the quality of BSE but that it was uncertain whether they increased BSE frequency. Other evaluations of group approaches included 6-month follow-ups. However, whether performance would be sustained after 6 months was unclear. Marty, McDermott, and Gold (1983) and Boyle, Michalek, Bersani, Nemoto, and Mettlin (1981)

exemplify the BSE research on the group approach. Marty and associates (1983) randomly assigned 219 female college students to one of three groups. One group was given ACS pamphlets on BSE, one group was exposed to discussions by a facilitator who covered breast disease and models of BSE, and one group was assigned to a program containing the features of modeling with the addition of guided practice. The group exposed to modeling and guided practice had more positive attitudes about the benefits of BSE than the other two groups ($p < 0.01$) and a higher practice frequency on follow-up ($p < 0.05$).

Wilkes's approach (1983) was two-tiered. The first part was presented to nurses and included didactic (lecture) and psychomotor practice. At the end of the experience, nurses could become certified instructors in BSE. The intent was to have the nurses become active teachers in BSE programs to lay women and their partners. The second portion was a model for programs presented in the community to lay audiences. This program included lectures, pamphlets, and breast models for practicing on. At the 3-month follow-up they found the following:

1. In a sample of 110 nurses, 97 per cent reported practicing BSE 3 months after instruction, with 85 per cent doing so at least monthly.
2. In a sample of 305 lay people, 82 per cent reported regular practice, with 87 per cent reporting at least monthly practice. However, at the 6-month follow-up, fewer than 25 per cent of the certified nurses had taught BSE. The reasons for lack of participation were not enough time, lack of confidence, never being asked, and not feeling comfortable in front of groups.

Wilkes writes that nurses who take the course in the future should be told that it is expected that they will promote and teach BSE to others.

Individual Approaches. Kegeles and Grady (1982) reviewed the literature related to individual approaches to teaching BSE. They report that this method appeared successful in attracting both low users of health services and women at high risk for cancer. As with the group approach, the individual approach has attempted to increase the frequency of BSE with some success up to 6 months' duration (Kegeles, 1985). Three studies typify the individual approach. Shamian and Edgar (1987) designed a quasi-experimental, one-group pretest-posttest study to determine the role of nurses as agents for change in teaching BSE. Data were collected from 223 women who had been exposed to a predetermined educational program (posters, charts, group session) and one-to-one teaching by nurse-clinicians. Their findings, based on a pretest, posttest, and 6-month follow-up, concluded that nurses influenced positively the factual and proficiency knowledge base of clients as well as the frequency of BSE practice. At the pretest, 13 per cent of the women were regular practitioners and at the 6-month follow-up after the educational intervention, 52 per cent of the women were regular practitioners. Although nurses have the potential to positively influence women to practice

Breast Self-Examination

Breast self-examination (BSE) should be done once a month so that you become familiar with the usual appearance and feel of your breasts. Familiarity makes it easier to notice any changes in the breast from one month to another. Early discovery of a change from what is "normal" is the main idea behind BSE. The outlook is much better if you detect cancer in an early stage.

If you menstruate, the best time to do BSE is 2 or 3 days after your period ends, when your breasts are least likely to be tender or swollen. If you no longer menstruate, pick a particular day, such as the first day of the month, to remind yourself it is time to do BSE.

Some women do the next part of the exam in the shower because fingers glide over soapy skin, making it easy to concentrate on the texture underneath.

Here is one way to do BSE:

1. Stand before a mirror. Inspect both breasts for anything unusual such as any discharge from the nipples or puckering, dimpling, or scaling of the skin.

The next two steps are designed to emphasize any change in the shape or contour of your breasts. As you do them, you should be able to feel your chest muscles tighten.

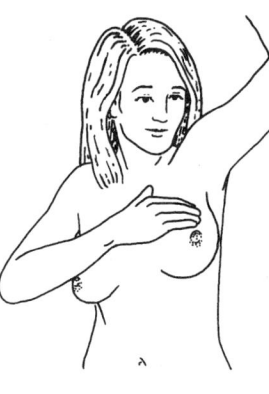

4. Raise your left arm. Use three or four fingers of your right hand to explore your left breast firmly, carefully, and thoroughly. Beginning at the outer edge, press the flat part of your fingers in small circles, moving the circles slowly around the breast. Gradually work toward the nipple. Be sure to cover the entire breast. Pay special attention to the area between the breast and the underarm, including the underarm itself. Feel for any unusual lump or mass under the skin.

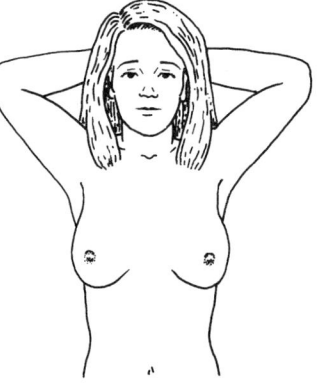

2. Watching closely in the mirror, clasp your hands behind your head and press your hands forward.

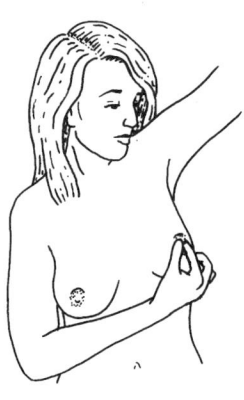

5. Gently squeeze the nipple and look for a discharge. (If you have any discharge during the month—whether or not it is during BSE—see your doctor.) Repeat steps 4 and 5 on your right breast.

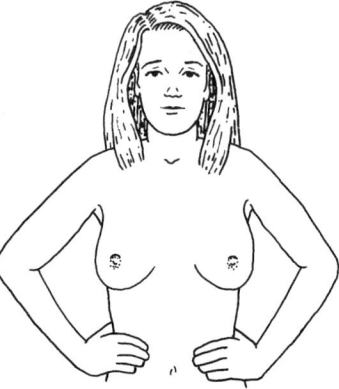

3. Next, press your hands firmly on your hips and bow slightly toward your mirror as you pull your shoulders and elbows forward.

6. Steps 4 and 5 should be repeated lying down. Lie flat on your back with your left arm over your head and a pillow or folded towel under your left shoulder. This position flattens the breast and makes it easier to examine. Use the same circular motion described earlier. Repeat the exam on your right breast.

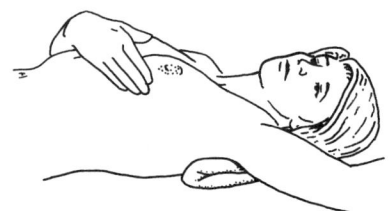

FIGURE 17–1. Recommendations for conducting breast self-examination. (From National Institutes of Health. [1983]. *Breast cancer: We're making progress every day* [USDHHS Publication No. NIH 83–2409]. Bethesda, MD; National Cancer Institute.)

BSE, Entrekin and McMillan (1993) found that nurses were *not* teaching BSE. They assessed 2348 nurses in terms of their knowledge and involvement in the prevention and early detection of cancer (i.e., breast, prostate, skin). Most nurses reported using early detection of cancer practices (teaching BSE, performing skin examinations) 0 to 20 per cent of the time with their patients. It is encouraging to note that the majority of nurses (66 per cent) believe that cancer prevention is part of the role of the staff nurse. Lillington et al. (1993) also surveyed a large group of nurses ($n = 1117$ responses) about their knowledge and involvement in cancer prevention and early detection of breast cancer. In their study, approximately 50 per cent of the nurses taught women about BSE and health promotion activities. Both of these studies document that nurses are missing opportunities to provide this valuable health promotion information to their clients.

Studies evaluating BSE practice commonly focus on frequency (Morrison, 1992). Studies of proficiency suffer from a lack of valid proficiency measurement techniques. Four studies have evaluated the concordance among various BSE assessment modalities. Newcomb, Olsen, Roberts, Storer, and Love (1995), Stephanek and Wilcox (1990) and Howe (1980) found no relationship between procedural assessment (an expanded verbal evaluation) and lump detection in a silicone model. Mamon and Zapka (1985) observed a significant correlation between self-report and observed performance (0.62, p <0.01) but self-report as measured by written self-report underestimated a woman's demonstrated BSE practice. Because BSE practice tends to vary not only within but also between subjects, a truly valid assessment of BSE proficiency may be impossible to obtain (Newcomb, et al, 1995). In light of this concern, data concerning BSE efficacy and utilization may warrant reconsideration.

The research by Coleman, Riley, Fields, and Prior (1991) is representative of studies that have compared the individual vs. the group approach. The goal of the research was to determine whether there is a difference in BSE performance between women taught BSE individually using self-modeling in addition to a breast model (experimental group) and women taught BSE in a group using only a breast model (control group). The researchers administered a pretest, posttest, and a posttest 3 months later. Analysis showed that women in the experimental group performed BSE significantly more proficiently than women in the control group.

Whereas the definitive research on the impact of BSE on survival still needs to be done, nurses are urged to use every opportunity both during work and in the community to encourage and educate women in BSE. Even though, as this review has shown, there are risks and significant questions to be answered about BSE, it would appear that it is better to err on the side of overcaution than to abandon the practice entirely.

SELF-ADMINISTERED HEMOCCULT TESTING

Colorectal cancer incidence and mortality among men and women in the United States are second only to those of lung cancer. However, the same concerns that are raised about BSE are raised about Hemoccult (blood in stool) testing. Does early detection of colorectal cancer through Hemoccult testing result in a decrease in mortality from that disease? A large-scale randomized prospective study was conducted in Minnesota to answer this question. More than 45,000 volunteers were assigned to one of the following three groups:

1. Screened for occult blood every other year.
2. Screened annually for occult blood.
3. Not screened at all (control group).

The study represents the only true prospective randomized controlled study on this topic in the United States. It is important to note that the use of a parallel control group should eventually permit assessment of cancer outcome relatively free of lead time, length, and selection biases. The Minnesota study showed a benefit of 33 per cent reduction in mortality with annual testing but essentially no difference in mortality for people screened every 2 years vs. no screening (Mandel et al., 1993).

The original guaiac test depended on the reaction between a colorless dye (gum guaiac) and hemoglobin in the presence of hydrogen peroxide to yield a blue color. This test resulted in a high number of both false-positive and false-negative results (Alquist, McGill, & Schwartz, 1984). The test has a false-positive rate of 2 to 3 per cent, a false-negative rate of 20 to 31 per cent, and predictive values for adenomas and cancer of 22 to 58 per cent (De Cosse, Tsioulias, & Jacobson, 1994). At present, most of the tests are done with guaiac-impregnated cards that have the advantage of permitting some storage before they are tested. In the Hemoccult test gum guaiac is impregnated in a test paper, and hydrogen peroxide is provided in a developer solution. The resultant phenolic oxidation of guaiac in the presence of blood yields a blue color (Simon, 1985). However, there are still problems with false-positive and false-negative results, including the following:

1. False-negative results can be due to the ingestion of an oxidizing agent such as ascorbic acid or to a delay of more than 5 days in developing the test.
2. The test appears to be more sensitive for cancer than for adenoma because the false-negative rate is higher for adenoma (Winawer, 1983). Studies of laboratory FOBT suggest a sensitivity of 25 to 40 per cent for cancers and approximately 10 per cent for detecting adenomatous polyps greater than 1 cm (Montgomery, 1994).
3. The reaction is not specific for human hemoglobin, and contamination can occur with dietary vegetable peroxidases and meat, causing false-positive results.
4. Aspirin, iron, and cimetidine can give false-positive reaction.
5. Research indicates that these tests do not detect the portion of hemoglobin that is converted to porphyrins in the gut (Alquist et al., 1984).
6. Rehydration of slides increases the possibility of false-positive results (Simon, 1985). (See Chapter 16

for an in-depth research study on the value of rehydration of fecal occult blood slides.)

Numerous causes for false-negative test results exist, including the fact that not all tumors cause bleeding, occult blood may not be uniformly distributed in the feces, and the test simply does not detect fecal blood losses of less than 20 ml/day. Simon (1985) writes that at least 33 per cent and perhaps 50 per cent of colorectal cancers in a screened population can be missed. Thus the sensitivity of occult blood testing (the proportion of diseased subjects who have a positive result) is low, probably only in the 50 to 65 per cent range.

Compliance is another significant problem in any discussion of early detection of colorectal cancer. Reported compliance rates based on literature reviews vary tremendously. Morrow, Way, Hoagland, and Cooper (1982) report compliance rates between 30 and 80 per cent, Box, Nichols, Lailemand, Pearson, and Vakil (1984) between 27 and 42 per cent in asymptomatic people and 92.5 per cent in symptomatic patients, and Simon (1985) a low of 15 per cent to a high of 98 per cent, with most in the 50 to 70 per cent range. Three studies that most carefully document compliance with Hemoccult testing reported compliance rates ranging from 22 per cent to less than 30 per cent (Elwood et al., 1978; Morrow et al., 1982; Winchester et al., 1980).

The Third International Symposium on Colorectal Cancer held in 1983 issued recommendations for obtaining fecal occult blood tests; these are provided in Box 17–1. Other recommendations designed to decrease false-negative and false-positive results include (1) women should not be tested during or immediately following a menstrual period (Rakel, 1983), and some clinicians recommend that people should eat plenty of fruits and vegetables and moderate amounts of fiber-containing foods to stimulate colorectal lesions to bleed (Leffall, 1981). To date the value of a high-residue diet

during the 3 days of testing has never been validated (Simon, 1985). Several new tests designed to remedy problems encountered with the widely used Hemoccult tests are available commercially.

1. *HemoQuant.* HemoQuant is a quantitative test that measures human blood loss with a high degree of sensitivity and specificity and is designed to enhance clinical validity. The advantages of this test are that (1) it is unaffected by stool hydration and storage, dietary peroxidases (which reduce false-positive results), iron, and ascorbic acid; (2) it detects both upper and lower gastrointestinal bleeding with equal sensitivity (Simon, 1985); (3) it does not require dietary prescription and thus it may result in higher compliance rates (Winawer, Schottenfeld, & Sherlock, 1985). A disadvantage is that it requires greater stool sampling than present tests do. Comparisons of HemoQuant with Hemoccult by several researchers have resulted in conflicting data. St. John et al. (1992) compared Hemoccult II and HemoQuant tests regarding their specificity and sensitivity in screening for colorectal cancer. They report that the HemoQuant test's performance characteristics in the detection of colorectal cancer were less satisfactory than those of Hemoccult II. In contrast, a prospective study conducted by Ahlquist et al. (1993) reports low sensitivities for both tests:

> Fecal blood screening failed to detect more than 70 per cent of colorectal cancers and more than 90 per cent of polyps. . . . HemoQuant and Hemoccult proved to be similarly insensitive for colorectal neoplasia (Ahlquist et al., 1993, p. 1265).

2. *Immunochemical Detection.* A test developed by Songster, Barrows, and Jarrett (1980) is reported to detect human hemoglobin and not be affected by animal heme, drugs, or foodstuffs. This test eliminates dietary and chemical restrictions placed on people who participate. The researchers report that

---

Box 17–1. *Recommendations on Performing a Fecal Occult Blood Test from the Third International Symposium on Colorectal Cancer, 1983*

1. The patient should avoid rare red meat and high peroxidase foods for 3 days *before* and during testing. High peroxidase foods include broccoli, turnip, rare red meat, cauliflower, parsnip, cabbage, potato, and cantalope. These foods can give a false-positive reaction.
2. Vitamin C, iron tablets, and nonsteroidal anti-inflammatory drugs should be avoided. Vitamin C will give a false-negative reaction.
3. The delay between preparation and laboratory testing should not exceed 6 days.
4. Slides should *not* be rehydrated. Rehydrating the stool samples by adding a drop of water to them induces false-positive reactions.
5. Two samples of each of three consecutive stools should be tested *(six smears).* Increasing the number of samples tested from each stool will make up for the nonuniform distribution of blood in stools, especially from left-sided lesions. The sample size must be sufficient to produce a detectable blue color; patients must be instructed to cover the whole test slide with fecal material.
6. *Important:* A single positive smear should be considered a positive test and lead to the recommended work-up, even in the absence of dietary restrictions. Having the patient repeat the slide testing is not recommended.

Data from Gnauck, R., MacRae, F., & Fleisher, M. [1984]. How to perform a fecal occult blood test. *CA: A Cancer Journal for Clinicians, 34,* 130–133.

the smear is stable for up to 30 days; however, there is a 24- to 48-hour delay between receiving and interpreting the test. It is technically very simple and may enhance specificity (Winawer et al., 1985).

3. *Immunochemical Test* (using blood serum). Louvard from the Pasteur Institute in Paris has developed a simple, inexpensive, immunochemical blood test that relies on the determination of the blood level of villin. Villin is a protein found mainly in the absorptive cells of the small and large intestines, as well as in the duct cells of the pancreas and biliary system and the cells of kidney proximal tubules. Cells of other organs contain little to no villin. Preliminary data show that false-positive results do not exceed 10 per cent and false-negative results are as high as 50 per cent. If the ratio of false-negative results is reduced, this test could become a major tool for the diagnosis of colorectal cancer (Dorozynski, 1987).

While the Minnesota study (Mandel et al., 1993) has documented that annual screening using FOBT is effective, Sox (1994) argues that FOBT is inefficient. The present method of obtaining fecal occult blood (Hemoccult slides) has low sensitivity and requires dietary and drug restrictions to avoid false-positive and false-negative results. For screening and early detection, it is most important to avoid false-negative findings; thus tests with high sensitivity are desired. Low compliance rates have been reported in a majority of large-scale screening programs, and compliance has been shown to decrease with age. Many of the issues raised about BSE are also raised with self-administered occult blood testing. Until definitive answers are known, nurses are urged to use every professional encounter to educate and motivate people over the age of 40 years (or earlier if they have known risk factors) to participate in colorectal screening for cancer.

Because compliance decreases with advancing age, special education and motivation efforts need to be directed toward elderly persons who live alone.

TESTICULAR SELF-EXAMINATION

Although cancer of the testes accounts for only about 1 per cent of all male cancers, it is the most common type of cancer in men between 20 and 36 years of age. Two groups of men have a greater risk of developing testicular cancer: those whose testes have not descended into the scrotum and those whose testes descended after the age of 6. Testicular cancer is 10 to 40 times more likely to develop in these men (National Cancer Institute, 1985).

Ten years ago, testicular cancer was often fatal because it spread rapidly to vital organs, particularly the lungs. Recent advances in treatment have made cancer of the testes one of the most curable cancers, especially if detected and treated promptly.

The most common symptom of testicular cancer is a painless scrotal mass. Mild testicular pain, a dull ache, and dragging sensation in the lower abdomen, groin, or scrotum are other symptoms of testicular cancer (Ganong & Markovitz, 1987). Benign conditions that can be confused with testicular tumors include hydrocele, varicocele, spermatocele, torsion, and hematoma (Reno, 1988). Although never evaluated systematically as a screening or early-detection method, it is generally thought that regular TSE will provide the opportunity for early diagnosis of testicular cancer.

Studva (1983) suggests professional clinical testicular examination be performed in the following manner. The client should be examined in both the supine and the standing positions. In the supine position, suspected varicocele can be ruled out because this entity will collapse when the client is lying down with the scrotum elevated. The firmness and weight of a testicular tumor can be evaluated best in the upright position. Orderly examination of the intrascrotal contents is recommended. If the client has symptoms, the uninvolved testis should be examined first to serve as a baseline. The testes should be carefully palpated between the thumb and first two fingers. Generally, the glands are fairly uniform in size and consistency and move freely. Any area of induration, nodularity, or irregularity should be considered a tumor until proved otherwise. The epididymis and the spermatic cord should be palpated along their entire course.

Nine studies have investigated knowledge about testicular cancer and practice of TSE. The findings of these studies are summarized in Table 17–8. In general, it continues to be true that most men are not knowledgeable about testicular cancer or TSE, nor do they regularly practice this skill (Walker, 1993). Ganong and Markovitz (1987) suggest that lack of knowledge may be the consequence of (1) a general denial among young men that they are "at risk" for any health problem, (2) failure to actively seek out information about personal health care or to have regular checkups in this age group, or (3) lack of awareness about testicular cancer by health care providers or their hesitation to discuss this potentially embarrassing subject with their male clients. Reasons cited by subjects for not practicing TSE included forgetfulness, not remembering the proper technique, not feeling it was necessary to do it at their age, not concerned about getting cancer at this time, and too busy (Reno, 1988; Rovinski, 1980).

Nurses can help to decrease the current testicular cancer and TSE information gap that exists among young men. First and foremost, nurses' personal knowledge deficits must be filled. Then creative approaches to educating these men need to be investigated. Integrating men's health issues into school health curricula needs further exploration, as does reaching the young men through health fairs. The effectiveness of educating late grade school and junior high school boys (boys who are most likely to have required health examinations for school) about TSE also needs to be examined. Finally, the influence of regular TSE on testicular cancer mortality has not been investigated and clearly needs further study if monthly self-examination technique for all men is to be recommended, given that only about 1 per cent of the population will develop this disease.

TABLE 17–8. *Studies of Men's Knowledge of Testicular Cancer and TSE*

REFERENCE	SAMPLE	METHODOLOGY	FINDINGS
Conklin et al. (1978)	90 randomly chosen college men (ages 18–23 yrs).	Interview developed by the researchers.	75% had never heard of TC; none knew how to do TSE; 75% said they would probably do TSE.
Cummings, Lampone, Mettlin, & Potes, (1983)	266 male students (ages 17–41 yrs); convenience sample drawn from health courses.	Questionnaire; investigated knowledge.	42% knew age at greatest risk; 52% did not know any symptoms; 16% had heard of TSE but only 33% of these had done TSE; 88% interested in learning TSE.
Goldenring & Purtell (1984)	147 male college athletes (ages 18–23 yrs).	Interviews during physical examination; investigated knowledge and practice.	12.9% knew TC was most common in their age group; 9.5% had been taught TSE; 6.1% had done TSE.
Ostwald & Rothenberger (1985)	577 male high school and college students.	Questionnaire developed by researchers was given to men who viewed a slide tape on TSE; investigated knowledge and practice.	61% had heard of TC; 54% had no information about TSE; 14% did TSE regularly; 75% of a follow-up group did TSE after instruction.
Thornhill et al. (1986)	395 Irish men (ages 21–65 yrs), selected because they had more education and were from higher SES groups.	Mailed questionnaire to 500 men (395 responded).	32% unaware of TSE; 87% did not know high-risk ages; 72% did not know any symptoms; 8% knew of TSE; 5% did TSE regularly; 90% wanted more information.
Blesch (1986)	Random sample of 129 men drawn from a group of 3300 professional men employed in a telecommunications firm.	Mailed questionnaire developed by the researcher sent to 233 men; investigated practice, knowledge, and relationship of health beliefs to TSE and TC.	61% had heard of TC; 31% knew of TSE; 9.5% practiced TSE; 96% said lack of knowledge was a barrier to doing TSE.
Ganong & Markovitz (1987)	A convenience sample of 64 male college students (ages 18–36 yrs).	Survey-questionnaire investigated knowledge and intention to do TSE.	18% had heard of TSE; 5% had done TSE; 49 of 50 who never heard of TSE wanted to learn about it; exposure to brief printed information increased intentions to perform TSE this week and this month ($p < 0.001$).
Reno (1988)	Convenience sample of 126 male college students.	Questionnaire measured knowledge and beliefs about TSE and TC.	12 reported TSE practice, and of these 41% practiced monthly; 87% of the 114 who did not practice TSE had not heard of TSE; 88.9% reported that if given TSE information, they would practice TSE.
Rudolph & MacEwen-Quinn (1988)	Convenience sample of 64 male college students (ages 17–24 yrs).	Modified Blesch's questionnaire; assessed TSE practice before and after video tape and didactic program.	Before education, 22% claimed TSE practice; 8 weeks after intervention there was no significant increase in TC knowledge, but 39 of the initial 61 who never practiced TSE did so after the education session.

TC = Testicular cancer; TSE = testicular self-examination; SES = socioeconomic status.
(Modified with permission from Ganong, L. H., & Markovitz, J. [1987]. Young men's knowledge of testicular cancer and behavioral intentions toward testicular self-exam. *Patient Education & Counseling, 9,* 253.)

DIAGNOSTIC TECHNIQUES

The early detection of cancer is the attempt to diagnose cancer in its earliest, most treatable stage. Clearly screening is an important strategy for achieving this goal. However, certain diagnostic techniques must also be employed to rule out or confirm the actual presence of a cancer. The following section details the nurse's role in diagnosis.

OBTAINING THE HISTORY

Frequently the first contact a person has with the health care system is with a nurse. The nurse establishes the tone of future interactions and obtains the initial health history. When obtaining the health history, it is important to inquire into risk factors for cancer that are related to the chief complaint. It is not uncommon for people to supply vague, nondescriptive complaints in the hope that the physician will find nothing wrong. They may in fact have very specific signs and symptoms that they consciously withhold from the health professional, particularly if they are frightened. Therefore, when taking a health history, the nurse needs to carefully question the person about any early signs, symptoms, and risk factors for cancer specifically related to the chief complaint as well as other cancer-related risk factors.

Elements of the history that are important aids to the clinician include the family, social, occupational, and medical histories (Kahn, 1983). A complete sexual history also provides important information. For instance, women at risk for cancer of the reproductive organs can be identified when a thorough and complete gynecologic and sexual history has been obtained. Because early age of first intercourse, multiple sexual partners, and a history of human papillomavirus (HPV) infection are key risk factors for cervical cancer, it is important that the nurse include questions about these areas. Chapter 16 details the known risk factors and early signs and symptoms for individual cancers.

ELEMENTS OF A COMPLETE HISTORY

The history should contain questions that will enable the nurse to identify known risk factors for cancer. Identification of risk factors is essential for effective client education as well as for alerting the other health professionals about potential problem areas. "Risk factors also form the basis for a hypothesis about what might be wrong with the patient even before details of the history of the present illness completely unfold" (Kahn, 1983, p. 270).

Family History. A family history should include information about acute and chronic illnesses of blood relatives and exact causes of deaths. Cancer should be specifically inquired about, including asking about the presence of "tumors" and "growths."

Social History. Significant risk factors for cancer include tobacco, alcohol, and drug use. If the client has any of these habits, the length of use, amounts, complications from use of the substance, side effects, and

attempts to quit should be detailed. Sexual history should include the number of partners, type of sexual protection commonly used (such as barrier methods), history of venereal disease, specifically condyloma and herpes simplex, abnormal Papanicolaou smears, and follow-up. A residential history should be obtained and exposure to environmental pollutants in these residences determined. Military experience and known military exposures (e.g., to Agent Orange) should also be inquired about of both men and women. An occupational history is frequently included in the social history and includes asking about the person's lifetime area of employment, work locations, work materials used in the occupational setting, illness of other workers, carcinogenic exposures if known, and required safety procedures or equipment to avoid exposures. A history of hobbies or leisure-time activities and toxic materials to which the client may have been exposed while working on hobbies should be also obtained.

Health History. Ideally, the following information should be obtained: all prior acute and chronic illnesses and their treatments; past x-ray treatments, including treatments for acne, swollen tonsils, and enlarged thymus (a practice abandoned in the 1950s); maternal use of diethylstilbestrol (DES); blood transfusions; past surgeries; all prior medications (including birth control pills); vitamins, over-the-counter drugs; relevant dietary practices and, if appropriate, a history of obesity; reproductive history, including mensus and menopause history.

When obtaining the history, questions should be phrased in a manner that will ensure the client will understand. Shortridge and McLain (1979) suggest that, when asking about the review of systems for the urinary system,

> . . . rather than asking "Do you have any hesitance?" ask instead a more specific symptoms-oriented question such as "Do you have to wait for your stream to begin?" or "Does your stream stop while you still have the urge to void/urinate?" Such phrasing is more apt to uncover subtle symptoms of obstruction otherwise overlooked.

It is important to remember that cultural beliefs influence not only health practices but also perceptions of what merits medical attention. For instance, a man who believes or has been told by friends that a growing feeling of heaviness in his scrotum is a sign of increasing virility will not perceive this symptom to merit medical attention. Nurses must make a conscious effort to acquaint themselves with the folk beliefs and health practices of different cultural groups, particularly those with whom they come into contact. Open-ended questions during the health assessment encourage the client to express his or her health beliefs; in addition, the nurse may be able to identify myths and misconceptions relating to the chief complaint and present illness. One method of encouraging sharing of culturally determined health beliefs is to open a discussion with the statement, "Many people believe that . . ." Frequently people are reticent to share their health beliefs with health professionals because they are afraid they will be laughed at, so the nurse should avoid value judgments. By openly identifying and acknowledging that a health belief is held by many people, the nurse makes it easier for the client to admit he or she also believes these statements to be true. Once misconceptions are identified, the nurse has a professional and moral obligation to alter false opinions that will prevent early detection of cancer and facilitate corrective education. However, as with any effective teaching, it should take place when the learner is receptive.

PHYSICAL EXAMINATION AND DIAGNOSTIC TESTING

The process of history taking and physical examination leads to formulation of a differential diagnosis by the physician. It is at this point that laboratory and radiologic tests designed to aid in the determination of a correct diagnosis are ordered. Table 17–9 lists the sensitivity and specificity of commonly used approaches to the diagnosis of cancer. Some diagnostic testing can be done during the physical examination (e.g., the Papanicolaou smear). However, most testing necessary to confirm the diagnosis of cancer requires the person to return to the health care setting for additional testing. Table 17–10 lists the physical assessment and diagnostic tests for each anatomic site used to confirm cancer. Although this table includes many recommended physical assessment techniques, the reader is referred to any standard physical assessment textbook for a more comprehensive discussion and to Tables 17–2, 17–4 and 17–5 for the recommended screening frequencies. The anatomic system(s) to which the chief complaint and present illness refer should be examined meticulously, as should common sites of metastasis.

The physical examination should be thorough and include all four of the cardinal techniques of physical assessment: inspection, palpation, percussion, and auscultation. Cancer is diagnosed using appropriate combinations of the following: cytologic methods, biochemical tests, radiographic techniques, clinical examination, and endoscopy.

NURSING RESPONSIBILITIES

Early detection of cancer is a complex issue that involves many separate decisions on the part of both the consumer and the health professional. On the one hand, health care professionals must actively strive to integrate cancer screening and detection into their day-to-day clinical practices. On the other hand, it is incumbent on the individual to make a conscious decision to seek the services of a health professional for a cancer detection examination or test or to report a suspicious symptom. The suspicious sign or symptom may have been discovered through the decision to engage in a cancer detection self-examination technique (e.g., BSE, TSE), or it may have been discovered accidentally. Once the person has contacted a health professional, the health professional in turn must judge how extensive the history, physical examination, and laboratory tests will be. If a suspicious symptom or finding is present, a tentative hypothesis about its cause is formulated.

The previous discussion has clearly shown that there is tremendous variation in who decides to practice cancer detection self-examination techniques, who decides to seek the services of health care professionals for early detection of cancer, and what diagnostic tests can be used in the detection of cancer. The task of the

TABLE 17–9. *Tests in the Diagnosis of Cancer*

TEST	DIAGNOSIS	STAGING	SENSITIVITY	SPECIFICITY	PV
I Routine blood or urine studies (complete blood count, urine, multiphasic biochemical screen)	+	–	Fair-good	Fair-poor	Low
II Routine x-ray studies (chest, intravenous pyelogram, upper and lower gastrointestinal series, mammogram) (only chest radiograph is used in staging)	+	– to +	Good-excellent	Good	Medium
III Special x-ray or imaging and endoscopic studies (ultrasonography, computed tomography, lymphangiography, angiography)	+	+	Good-excellent	Good	High
IV Radionuclide scanning (liver, bone, gallium)	–	+	Good	Poor	Low
V Biochemical markers (acid phosphatase, beta chorionic gonadotropin, alpha± = fetoprotein, carcinoembryonic antigen)	+ to –	+	Good-excellent	Good-excellent	High

PV = Predictive value in diagnosis of symptomatic patients.
+ = Useful; – = not useful; ± = may be useful selectively.
(From Kahn, S. B. [1983]. Cancer diagnosis. In S. Kahn, R. Love, C. Sherman, & R. Chakravorty [Eds.], *Concepts in cancer medicine* [pp. 267–287]. New York: Grune & Stratton, Inc. Reproduced by permission.)

TABLE 17–10. *Cancer Detection: Physical Examination and Diagnostic Testing*

SITE	PHYSICAL EXAMINATION	DIAGNOSTIC TESTING
Cervical cancer ("ACS modified guideline," 1987; Perez, Knapp, Disaia, & Young, 1985; Smith, Clarke-Pearson, & Creasman, 1985).	**Vagina:** Evaluate consistency of cervix, check for presence of papilloma, Bartholin's cysts, unusual vaginal discharge and tissue friability; evaluate depth of vaginal fornices; check size, position, and mobility of uterus; evaluate color, discharge, and presence of any lesions. **Rectum:** Evaluate elasticity and softness of parametrium; evaluate Douglas' pouch (retro-uterine pouch)—normally not palpable; evaluate consistency and shape of cervix; evaluate size, position, and mobility of uterus.	**Papanicolaou smear:** Cytologic examination of exfoliated cervical cells; sample taken from transition zone, ectocervix, and endocervix. **Colposcopy:** The vagina and cervix are washed with acetic acid to highlight abnormal tissue and then examined with magnifying instrument; colposcopy is done following an abnormal Papanicolaou smear or the presence of cervical lesions; a directed biopsy may be done if abnormal tissue is found. **Conization:** A cone-shaped excision is made of the abnormal areas of the cervix. **Biopsy:** In the presence of gross lesions, multiple punch biopsies are taken.
Endometrial cancer	**Vagina:** Palpate vagina, sub-uretheral areas, and meatus to detect metastases. **Rectum:** Palpate cul-de-sac of Douglas, noting consistency and thickening; palpate rectum for extension of neoplasm.	**Endometrial biopsy:** Use a Novack curette or less widely used Gravlee jet washer to obtain specimens. **Suction curettage:** Tissue is obtained from endometrial cavity. **Fractional dilatation and curettage (D & C):** This is done if endometrial pathology is suspected.
Vaginal cancer	**Inspect** vulva and palpate vagina, noting areas of induration; note vaginal bands and cervical structural changes; rotate speculum to visualize entire vagina (vividly red focal areas should arouse suspicion).	**Colposcopy:** Colposcopy is used for directed biopsies of abnormal sites in the vagina.
Ovarian cancer (Khan, Slack, & Cosgrove, 1985; Sargris, 1983; Young, Knapp, Fules, & Disaia, 1985)	**Inspect** for skin signs of abdominal distention, contour for distention, masses (generalized or symmetrical or asymmetrical), bulging flanks. **Palpate** for masses and tenderness. **Percussion:** Solid tumor is dull to percussion and fluid wave will be dull to percussion. **Bimanual pelvic examination:** Palpate adnexa for masses; any enlargement in a premenarchal or postmenopausal woman should be evaluated; solid, bilateral, or fixed masses greater than 10 cm should raise suspicion of malignancy; palpate cul-de-sac via rectovaginal examination (nodularity in cul-de-sac is suspect).	**Ultrasound:** Used in prestaging assessment of suspected ovarian cancer and preoperatively to assess degree of tumor extension in pelvic, abdominal, and retroperitoneal regions; high level of accuracy in detecting tumors. **Lymphangiography:** For prestaging evaluation of women known or suspected to have ovarian cancer. **Computed tomography:** Computed tomography (CT) provides additional diagnostic and staging information.
Breast cancer (Carlile & Hadaway, 1985; Paulus, 1987)	**Inspection:** Sitting with arms at the side, sitting with arms elevated, sitting with pectoral muscle contraction, sitting bending forward. **Palpation:** Inspect breasts with patient in sitting and supine positions with superficial palpation for thickening and temperature changes, and with deeper palpation for lesions; palpate with patient in sitting position for women with pendulous breasts and women with present or past complaints of breast masses; supine: have women lie in left and right lateral decubitus positions to check for lesions between ribs. **Examine** nipples for discharge and fix discharge for cytologic examination.	**Film-screen mammography or xeromammography:** These methods detect noninvasive or invasive cancers smaller than 0.5 cm. **Galactography:** Used in evaluation of nipple discharge; detects papillomas; water-soluble contrast medium is injected into duct. **Pneumocystography:** Mammography is performed after removal of fluid and introduction of air into a breast cyst; this is definitive in the detection of intracystic tumors.

Continued on following page.

TABLE 17–10. *Cancer Detection: Physical Examination and Diagnostic Testing* Continued

SITE	PHYSICAL EXAMINATION	DIAGNOSTIC TESTING
Stomach cancer (Macdonald, Cohn, & Gunderson, 1985; Thompson, 1985)	**Abdominal examination:** Inspect contour for ascites, peristaltic waves (which move from left to right), pallor of mucous membranes indicating anemia, jaundice. **Palpate abdomen:** Check painless mass in epigastrium (cancer of stomach is palpable to left of midline). Nodular liver may indicate metastasis to liver; ovarian mass (Krukenberg tumors) may indicate metastasis to ovaries; check for umbilical metastasis. **Percussion of abdomen:** Check for dullness, ascites, fluid wave, shifting dullness, puddle test done for small amounts of fluid in the abdomen; palpate nodes in supraclavicular region (Virchow's node is usually on the left) and axillary region. **Rectal examination:** Palpate cul-de-sac for metastasis. **Skin:** Inspect skin for acanthosis nigricans (suggests cancer of the stomach). Acanthosis nigricans is brown to black pigmentation of the skin.	**Double-contrast barium studies:** Reported to miss 8 to 10% of gastric cancers; combination of air and barium enables radiologist to better visualize colonic mucosa. **Fiberoptic endoscopy:** Supplemented by biopsy and cytology techniques, this is judged to be superior to barium examination; sensitivity reported to be 100% and specificity is 99%. **Gastric biopsy:** Take specimens from suspected lesions or ulcers; diagnostic accuracy as high as 96%. **Cytology:** Obtain specimens of gastric walls using brushing technique, gastric washings, or endoscopic jet wash technique. Accuracy rates are reported to be over 90%.
Liver cancer (Cody, Macdonald, & Gunderson, 1985)	**Abdomen:** Inspect for masses, signs of portal hypertension, jaundice; palpate liver—note tenderness and surface consistency (hard, nodular, irregular masses or masses adjacent to the liver are suspicious for cancer); percuss liver borders, fist percussion of liver for tenderness, percuss for fluid; palpate extremities for edema. **Respiratory tract:** Impairment of air entry in right basal segments may be heard in cancer of the liver; check for restriction of diaphragmatic movement on the right side with a friction rub in cancer of the liver. **Skin:** Inspect for signs suggesting cirrhosis—e.g., spider angiomas, palmar erythemia, gynecomastia in males, sparse axillary, pubic, and pectoral hair in men.	**Serum alkaline phosphatase:** This enzyme is elevated in 70 to 80% of patients with hepatic metastases. **Alpha-fetoprotein (AFP) assay:** This is useful in diagnosis and follow-up of people with hepatocellular carcinoma; AFP strongly associated with hepatocellular carcinoma; reports suggest that 75 to 90% of people with primary hepatic cancer have levels above the normal values of 20 to 40 ng/ml. **Posterior-anterior and lateral chest x-ray films:** These depict the shape of diaphragm. **Radionuclide liver scanning:** This demonstrates whether the liver has an abnormality consistent with hepatoma. **Biopsy:** Biopsy may be considered to establish a tissue diagnosis.
Lung cancer (Grant, 1985; Menna, Higgins, & Glatstein, 1985)	**Palpation:** Palpate supraclavicular region for lymphadenopathy; palpate liver for nodularity, indicating metastatic spread. **Wheeze:** Any unilateral wheeze merits further evaluation.	**PA (posterior-anterior) chest x-ray film:** PA and lateral films should be obtained if a lesion is seen on PA film; conventional and computed tomography also are done in presence of peripheral opacity. **Cytology:** Examination of 3-day pooled sputum has identified cancer in persons with normal chest radiographs. **Flexible fiberoptic bronchoscopy:** This technique provides a visual examination of the interior of the bronchi and, when used with bronchial washings, the combined technique gives an overall accuracy of 79% with a false-positive rate of 0.8%. **Transthoracic fine needle aspiration biopsy:** This new procedure is done under fluoroscopic guidance and can diagnose intrapulmonary and solitary pulmonary nodules; research shows low false-positive and false-negative results.

TABLE 17–10. *Cancer Detection: Physical Examination and Diagnostic Testing* Continued

SITE	PHYSICAL EXAMINATION	DIAGNOSTIC TESTING
Colorectal cancer (Boyle, Michatek, Bersani, Nemoto, & Mettlin, 1981; Sugarbaker, Gunderson, & Wittes, 1985; Thompson, 1987)	**Rectum:** Palpate entire circumference of anorectal segment for masses and ask patient to strain while examining, palpate Blumer's rectal shelf, check for occult blood in stool. **Abdomen:** Inspect contour for distention or masses, use light palpation for subcutaneous nodules or signs of metastatic cancer (enlarged nodular liver, bilateral ovarian tumors, umbilical metastases); percuss for ascites, distention, or areas of dullness indicating masses.	**Fecal occult blood testing:** The patient collects stool samples for 3 days using Hemoccult slides; these slides are designed to detect blood in the stool when a chemical is applied. **Barium enema x-ray studies:** Barium plus air contrast is recommended over single-contrast technique because the latter can miss up to 40% of polypoid lesions and 20% of carcinomas; reports suggest that barium and air contrast technique can detect 92% of cancers. **Proctosigmoidoscopy:** This technique finds lesions low in rectum; approximately 55% of colon cancers occur within 25 cm of anal verge. **Flexible sigmoidoscopy:** Physician can see 50 to 60 cm of colon, and biopsy and polyp removal can be performed. Nearly two thirds of cancers seen with this instrument. **Colonoscopy:** If barium enema shows lesions, additional lesions are often found at colonoscopy; can provide specimens for cytologic examination (biopsy, brushing, or washing); polypectomy can also be done; entire colon can be visualized.
Skin cancer (Finley, 1986)	**Inspection:** Entire skin. Note size, shape, color, surface, location, sensations, and surrounding skin of any lesions: note development of any itchiness or irritation. **Malignant melanoma:** Inspect back above the waist; head, scalp, and neck; finger and toe webs and soles of feet in deeply pigmented people; the skin between the border of mucous membranes and body orifices; fingernails. Any pigmented nevus that grows rapidly, ulcerates, bleeds or becomes infected should be considered a possible melanoma. Persons with dysplastic nevus syndrome and high-risk characteristics should be examined routinely (see Chapter 16 for specific recommendations).	**Biopsy:** Definitive diagnosis can be made.
Thyroid cancer (Brennan & Macdonald, 1985)	**Inspect:** Inspect neck, especially on swallowing, for mass or asymmetry; palpate cervical lymph nodes, salivary glands, and thyroid gland, (noting size, contour, symmetry, consistency); masses should be evaluated for firmness, fixation irregularity, or pain; indirect laryngoscopy should be done.	**Biopsy:** Biopsy of the thyroid nodule is the only unequivocal diagnostic tool; percutaneous needle biopsy can provide tissue for histologic analysis; fine-needle aspiration is used to obtain tissue for cytologic examination. **Ultrasonography:** Ultrasonography is used to distinguish benign from malignant thyroid lesions. **Thyroid scintigram:** This is useful in demonstrating size, shape, and position of lesions detected clinically; with both ultrasound and radionuclide methods, tumors of 0.5 cm can be detected.

Continued on following page.

TABLE 17–10. *Cancer Detection: Physical Examination and Diagnostic Testing* Continued

SITE	PHYSICAL EXAMINATION	DIAGNOSTIC TESTING
Testicular cancer (Einhorn, Donohue, Peckham, Williams, & Loehrer, 1985; Hogan, 1983)	**Palpation:** Palpate the scrotum and testicles with both hands while patient stands; note size, shape, consistency, tenderness, and weight of testicles; weight differential between testicles is a clue to malignancy—tumor will feel weighty. Testicle feels neither hard nor soft—it has a somewhat rubbery consistency; surface should be smooth and free of lumps except for the ductus deferens; common sites for tumors are on the testicular anterior and lateral surfaces; check for hydrocele. **Transillumination:** When scrotum is transilluminated, tumors do not permit passage of light, but cysts do; palpate abdomen to check for retroperitoneal lymph node involvement; metastatic nodes usually lie at the level of, or slightly caudal to, the umbilicus; palpate supraclavicular node area for evidence of metastasis.	**Ultrasonography:** This technique is reported to distinguish a solid mass from a cystic mass and to be able to show whether the mass involves testis or epididymis or both. **Serum markers (AFP and beta-human chorionic gonadotropin):** When measured together one or the other will be positive 85% of the time in men with testicular cancer; not sufficiently sensitive to be relied on alone and not used in early detection. Definitive diagnosis is by removal of testes and pathologic analysis.
Prostate cancer (Gann, Hennekens, & Stampfer, 1995; Staff, 1987; Perez, Fair, Ihde, & Labrie, 1985)	**Rectal examination:** With patient in knee-chest position, evaluate anal sphincter (which is relaxed in prostate cancer); when palpating prostate, note size, median furrow, surface, shape, consistency, mobility, and sensitivity; cancer is usually a nontender, palpable hard nodule on posterior surface; palpable lymph nodes in groin and supraclavicular region suggest metastasis.	**Digital rectal examination:** Earliest stage detectable by rectal examination is Stage B disease; however, digital rectal examination is judged to be the best method of early detection. **Prostate-specific antigen:** PSA has the highest validity of any circulating cancer screening marker. Blood levels are increased when normal glandular structure is disrupted by benign or malignant tumor or inflammation. **Needle biopsy:** Needle biopsy is the standard method to diagnose tumor in United States; aspiration biopsy is the preferred method in Europe. **Transrectal ultrasonography:** This method currently is in testing state to assess its value in early detection; it is useful in detecting tumor invasion through the prostatic capsule (anteriorly).
Bladder cancer (Cetrin, 1983; Richie, Shipley, & Yagoda, 1985)	Tumor may be palpated suprapubically; bladder can be best felt by rectal or vaginal palpation under anesthesia.	**Urinary cytology:** This test may lead to presumptive diagnosis of bladder cancer. **Cytoscopy:** Cytoscopic examination and transurethral biopsy confirm the diagnosis. **Ultrasonography:** This technique is used in staging to assess invasion of the bladder wall by cancer.
Detection of cancer in general (Van Der Werf, 1987)		**Water-suppressed nuclear magnetic resonance (NMR) spectroscopy:** Blood test should be done when lipoprotein widths are measured. Differences will be noted between persons with benign and malignant tumors, and in persons with tumors and without tumors. This method is in the investigative stage.

nursing profession is to continue to identify the barriers to early detection that occur in persons and groups and to design, implement, and evaluate interventions that will assist in removing or decreasing these barriers. For example, research has shown that the elderly have significant delay in reporting the signs and symptoms of cancer owing to transportation difficulties, lack of financial resources, assumptions that the signs and symptoms are part of the normal aging process, and reluctance to undergo cancer treatments. Designing inexpensive early detection programs for the elderly in which the screeners go out into the community is one method to decrease barriers created by transportation needs and lack of financial resources. These programs could be offered in Golden Age Clubs, nursing homes, residential centers for the elderly, food gathering centers, and day care centers for the elderly.

The nurse needs to recognize that the barriers to early detection differ in geographic location and with different racial, ethnic, religious, and socioeconomic groups. What works with one group of people in one part of the country may not work equally well somewhere else. Thus it is essential that the nurse be familiar with the research on the barriers to early detection found in the groups he or she works with the most.

Nurses need to consider using creative as well as cost-effective, nontraditional approaches when designing cancer early detection programs. For instance, the church is the focal point of the political and social activities in the typical African-American community, and most African-American churches have a health-oriented guild within the church structure. Early detection programs could be held in these churches using nurses and other health care professionals who are church members. This community-based approach has been used in the past with other diseases commonly found in African-Americans (e.g., sickle cell anemia, hypertension) and has proved to be effective in involving the "hard to reach" person.

From 1985 to 1987, the ONS conducted a series of 2-day regional cancer prevention–early detection workshops for African-American nurses. These workshops were funded by the NCI for the following purposes:

1. Increasing the knowledge and skill level of African-American nurses in primary and secondary prevention of cancer.
2. Increasing their level of community-based participation in activities related to primary and secondary prevention of cancer.
3. Fostering positive attitudes toward cancer prevention and early detection.

The results from the workshops clearly indicate that nurses brought about significant changes in attitudes toward the early detection and prevention of cancer, increased the level of participation of the workshop participants in community-based activities, and resulted in increased cancer-related knowledge and skills (Frank-Stromberg, Johnson, & McCorkle, 1987). A partial list of the nontraditional settings and cancer-related activities implemented by workshop participants is given in Box 17–2.

Compliance, a significant issue in any discussion of cancer self-examination practices, is another area that merits further attention and research. Nurses can increase compliance by addressing the issue in a forthright manner. When teaching self-examination techniques, the nurse needs to spend time understanding how people feel about the technique, what barriers prevent them from practicing it, what is needed to help them practice it, and what benefits they feel are inherent in the procedure. These areas need to be discussed

---

Box 17–2. *Examples of Nontraditional Settings and Cancer-Related Activities of Nurses Participating in NCI-Sponsored Black Nurses Regional Cancer Prevention–Early Detection Workshops from 1985 to 1987*

1. Implemented screening programs in food pantries and feeding centers.
2. Organized church-sponsored educational and screening programs through the nursing guild.
3. Organized a multistate church program that designated 1 month "Cancer in Black Americans." The month was filled with educational programs as well as screening programs.
4. Organized cancer-related programs in local schools, Parent-Teacher Organizations, family planning, and Parents-Too-Soon programs.
5. Designed health fairs that included cancer-related activities in collaboration with local African-American sororities.
6. Contacted African-American political organizations in the community and designed and implemented community education programs that focused on educating the community about cancer and the importance of early detection. The progam was designed to use block volunteers who would go door-to-door.
7. Offered cancer-oriented educational and screening programs in work settings with the cooperation of the local unions and site management.
8. Contacted local veterans groups and offered cancer-related programs to the membership.
9. Designed and implemented both educational and screening programs in low-income housing. Programs focused on the elderly in these settings and offered transportation to the program.
10. Offered special cancer screening programs during the evening and on weekends at local store-front free health clinic.
11. Designed and implemented a hospital-based multimedia educational approach (posters, slide-tape programs, announcements over loudspeakers, newspaper articles, TV spots) focusing on early detection of cancer in African-Americans. These programs were targeted to hospital employees, hospital patients, and their families.

with the person learning the technique, and consumer (rather than health professional)-generated solutions should be encouraged.

Nurses need to keep abreast of new research findings documenting whether cancer self-examination techniques (e.g., BSE, Hemoccult testing, TSE) make a difference in decreasing cancer mortality. Currently, there are no definitive answers to this question; however, it is recommended that self-examination techniques be taught to high-risk persons (Chapter 16 details high-risk persons or groups).

The health history can be used as a vehicle for identifying high-risk individuals. When appropriate, nurses with physical assessment skills can use these skills to conduct an examination designed for early cancer detection. All nurses with physical assessment skills can be involved in community-based programs designed to detect cancer in the early stages as well as provide education on cancer self-examination techniques. As has been demonstrated from the NCI-funded African-American nurses' regional workshops, nurses can carry out cost-effective early detection programs in both traditional and nontraditional settings and attract people typically difficult to reach. The importance of offering programs in nontraditional settings is shown by the research on participation in early detection programs; nonparticipants are less educated, have lower incomes, and are older than participants (Van Parijs & Eckhardt, 1984). Because these demographic variables are associated with higher risk for various cancers, lack of participation presents a serious challenge to cancer education.

A final example of using nursing to offer early cancer detection programs is found in a report on cancer nurses in action ("Nurse helps promote screening services," 1987). Screening clinics in a small rural hospital were set up on a monthly basis and included mammary and cervical, skin, male genitourinary, oral, head and neck, and colorectal cancers. These clinics were coordinated by a nurse with special training in early cancer detection physical assessment techniques. This nurse formulated risk assessments, taught cancer self-examination techniques, and conducted site-specific physical examinations.

REFERENCES

Adams, M., & Kerner, J. (1982). Evaluation of promotional strategies to solve the problem of underutilization of a breast examination/education center in a New York City Black community. *Issues in Cancer Screening and Communications, 83,* 151–161.

Alquist, D., McGill, D., & Schwartz, S. (1984). HemoQuant: A new quantitative assay for fecal hemoglobin. *Annals of Internal Medicine, 101,* 297–309.

Ahlquist, D., Wierand, H., Moertel, C., McGill, D., Loprinzi, C. I., O'Connell, M. J., Mailliard, J. A., Gerstner, J. B., Pandya, K., & Ellefson, D. B. (1993). Accuracy of fecal occult blood screening for colorectal neoplasia. *Journal of the American Medical Association, 269*(10), 1262–1267.

American Cancer Society. (1989). *Cancer in the poor: A report to the nation. Findings of regional hearings conducted by the ACS.* (Report No. 89-3M-No. 0216). Atlanta: Author.

American Cancer Society. (1994). *Cancer facts and figures.* Atlanta: ACS.

American Nurses Association and Oncology Nursing Society. (1987). *Standards of oncology nursing practice.* Kansas City, MO: American Nurses' Association.

Ansell, D., Lacy, L., Whitman, S., Chen, E., & Phillips, C. (1994). A nurse-delivered intervention to reduce barriers to breast and cervical cancer screening in Chicago inner-city clinics. *Public Health Reports, 109*(1), 104–11.

A study of Hispanics' attitudes concerning cancer and cancer prevention (1985). Unpublished manuscript prepared for the American Cancer Society, Atlanta, GA, by Clark, Martire, and Bartolomeo, Inc.

Austin, R. M., Baron, P. L., & Gates, C. E. (1993). Opportunities for enhanced cervical and breast screening referral in Charleston County. *Journal–South Carolina Medical Association, 89*(7), 323–8.

Baquet, C. R., Horm, J. W., Gibbs, T., & Greenwald, P. (1991). Socioeconomic factors and cancer incidence among blacks and whites. *Journal of the National Cancer Institute, 83*(8), 551–557.

Baquet, C., & Ringen, K. (1985). Cancer control in blacks: Epidemiology and NCI program plans. In L. Mortenson, P. Engstrom, & P. Anderson (Eds.), *Advances in cancer control: Health care financing and research.* New York: Alan Liss, Inc.

Bassett, M., & Krieger, N. (1986). Social class and black-white differences in breast cancer survival. *American Journal of Public Health, 76,* 1400–1403.

Bennett, S., Lawrence, R., Fleischmann, S., Gifford, C., & Slack, W. (1983). *Journal of the American Medical Association, 249,* 488–491.

Blesch, K. (1986). Health beliefs about testicular cancer and self-examination among professional men. *Oncology Nursing Forum, 13,* 29–33.

Bostick, R. M., Sprafka, J. M., Virnig, B. A., & Potter, J. D. (1993). Knowledge, attitudes, and personal practices regarding prevention and early detection of cancer. *Preventive Medicine, 22*(1), 65–85.

Box, V., Nichols, S., Lailemand, R., Pearson, P., & Vakil, P. (1984). Haemoccult compliance rates and reasons for non-compliance. *Public Health, London, 98,* 16–25.

Boyle, M., Michalek, A., Bersani, G., Nemoto, T., & Mettlin, C. (1981). Effectiveness of a community program to promote early breast cancer detection. *Journal of Surgical Oncology, 18,* 183–188.

Brennan, M., & Macdonald, J. (1985). Cancer of the endocrine system. In V. DeVita, S. Hellman, & S. Rosenberg (Eds.), *Cancer: Principles and practice of oncology* (2nd ed., pp. 1179–1241). Philadelphia: J. B. Lippincott Co.

Burack, R. C., Gimotty, P. A., George, J., Stengle, W., Warbasse, L., & Moncrease, A. (1994). Promoting screening mammography in inner-city settings: A randomized controlled trial of computerized reminders as a component of a program to facilitate mammography. *Medical Care, 32*(6), 609–24.

Butler, L., King, G., & White, J. (1983). Communications strategies, cancer information and black populations: An analysis of longitudinal data. In *Progress in cancer control IV: Research in the cancer control* (pp. 171–182). New York: Alan Liss, Inc.

Calle, E. E., Flanders, W. D., Thun, M. J., & Martin, L. M. (1993). Demographic predictors of mammography and Pap smear screening in US women. *American Journal of Public Health, 83*(1), 53–60.

Canadian Task Force. (1982). Cervical cancer screening programs summary of the 1982 Canadian task force report. *Canadian Medical Association Journal, 127,* 581–588.

Canadian Task Force on the Periodic Health Examination. (1979). The periodic health examination. *Canadian Medical Association Journal, 121,* 1193–1248.

Carlile, T., & Hadaway, E. (1985). Screening for breast cancer. In B. A. Stoll (Ed.), *Screening and monitoring of cancer* (pp. 135–152). New York: John Wiley & Sons, Inc.

Chamberlain, J. (1983). Screening for cancer. *Journal of Applied Medicine, 9,* 11–15.

Champion, V. L. (1994). Strategies to increase mammography utilization. *Medical Care, 32*(2), 118–29.

Champion, V. (1995). Development of a benefits and barriers scale for mammography utilization. *Cancer Nursing, 18*(1), 53–9.

Chie, W., & Chang, K. (1994). Factors related to tumor size of breast cancer at treatment in Taiwan. *Preventive Medicine, 23*(1), 91–97.

Citrin, D. (1983). Bladder cancer. In S. Kahn, R. Love, C. Sherman, & R. Chakravorty (Eds.), *Concepts in cancer medicine* (pp. 493–502). New York: Grune & Stratton, Inc.

Cody, B., Macdonald, J., & Gunderson, L. (1985). Cancer of the hepatobiliary system. In V. DeVita, S. Hellman, & S. Rosenberg (Eds.), *Cancer: Principles and practice of oncology* (2nd ed., pp. 741–770). Philadelphia: J. B. Lippincott Co.

Cole, C., & Goman, L. (1984). Breast self-examination: Practices and attitudes of registered nurses. *Oncology Nursing Forum, 11*(5), 37–41.

Coleman, E., Riley, M., Fields, F., & Prior, B. (1991). Efficacy of breast self-examination teaching methods among older women. *Oncology Nursing Forum, 18*(3), 561–566.

Conklin, M., Klint, K., Morway, A., Sawyer, J. R., & Shepard, R. (1978). Should health teaching include self-examination of the testes? *American Journal of Nursing, 78,* 2073–2074.

Cummings, K. M., Lampone, D., Mettlin, C., & Potes, J. (1983). What young men know about testicular cancer. *Preventive Medicine, 12,* 326–330.

Czaja, R., McFall, S. L., Warnecke, R. B., Ford, L., & Kaluzny, A. D. (1994). Preferences of community physicians for cancer screening guidelines. *Annuals of Internal Medicine, 120*(7), 602–608.

DeCosse, J., Tsioulias, G., & Jacobson, J. (1994). Colorectal cancer: Detection, treatment, and rehabilitation. *CA-A Cancer Journal for Clinicians, 44*(1), 27–42.

Demark-Wahnefried, W., Catoe, K. E., Pasket, E., Robertson, C. N., & Rimer, B. K. (1993). Characteristics of men reporting for prostate cancer screening. *Urology, 42*(3), 269–74.

Diem, G., & Rose, D. (1985). Has breast self-examination had a fair trial? *The New York State Journal of Medicine, 85,* 479–480.

DiSario, J. A., & Sanowski, R. A. (1993). Sigmoidoscopy training for nurses and resident physicians. *Gastrointestinal Endoscopy, 39*(1), 29–32.

Division of Cancer Prevention and Control (1986). Screening. In P. Greenwald & E. Sondik (Eds.), *Cancer control objectives for the nation: 1985–2000.* NCI Monograph, NIH Publication 86–2880. Bethesda, MD: National Institutes of Health.

Dorozynski, A. (1987). Test for early detection of colorectal cancer under development. *Oncology & Biotechnology News, 1*(2), 3.

Early Detection Branch Division of Cancer Prevention and Control (1987, December 27). *Working guidelines for early cancer detection rationale and supporting evidence to decrease mortality.* Bethesda, MD: National Cancer Institute.

Eddy, D. A. (1985). Screening for cancer in adults. *CIBA Foundation Symposium 110,* 88–109.

Eddy, D. M. (1986). Secondary prevention of cancer: An overview. *Bulletin of the World Health Organization, 64,* 421–429.

Edwards, V. (1980). Changing breast self-examination behavior. *Nursing Research, 29,* 301–306.

Einhorn, L., Donohue, J., Peckham, M., Williams, S., & Loehrer, P. (1985). Cancer of the testes. In V. DeVita, S. Hellman, & S. Rosenberg (Eds.). *Cancer: Principles and practice of oncology* (2nd ed., pp. 979–1011). Philadelphia: J. B. Lippincott Co.

Elwood, T., Erickson, A., & Lieberman, S. (1978). Comparative educational approaches to screening for colorectal cancer. *American Journal of Public Health, 68,* 135–138.

Entrekin, N., & McMillan, S. (1993). Nurses' knowledge, beliefs, and practice related to cancer prevention and detection. *Cancer Nursing, 16*(6), 431–9.

Farrands, P. A., Hardcastle, J., Chamberlain, J., & Moss, S. (1984). Factors affecting compliance with screening for colorectal cancer. *Community Medicine, 6,* 12–19.

Feldman, J. G., Carter, A. C., Nicastri, A. D., & Hostat, S. T. (1981). Breast self-examination, relationship to stage of breast cancer at diagnosis. *Cancer, 47,* 2740–2745.

Finley, C. (1986). Malignant melanoma: A primary care perspective. *Nurse Practitioner, 11,* 18–38.

Foster, R., Costanza, M., and Worden, J. (1985). The current status of research in breast self-examination. *The New York State Journal of Medicine, 85,* 480–482.

Foster, R. S., Lang, S. P., Costanza, M. C., Worden, J. K., Haines, C. R., & Yates, J. W. (1978). Breast self-examination and breast cancer stage. *New England Journal of Medicine, 299,* 265–270.

Frank, J., & Mai, V. (1985). Breast self-examination in young women: More harm than good? *Lancet, 2,* 654–657.

Frank-Stromborg, M., Johnson, J., & McCorkle, R. (1987). A program model for nurses involved with cancer education of black Americans. *Journal of Cancer Education, 2,* 145–151.

Frank-Stromborg, M., & Olsen, S. J. (1993). *Cancer prevention and screening in minorities: Cultural implications for health care providers.* St. Louis, MO: Mosby.

Freeman, H. (1981). *Cancer mortality: A socio-economic phenomenon.* American Cancer Society's Twenty-Third Science Writers' Seminar. New York: American Cancer Society.

Freeman, H. P., Muth, B. J., & Kerner, J. F. (1995). Expanding access to cancer screening and clinical follow-up among the medically underserved. *Cancer Practice, 3*(1), 19–30.

Gann, P., Hennekens, C., & Stampfer, M. (1995). A prospective evaluation of plasma prostate-specific antigen for detection of prostate cancer. *Journal of the American Medical Association, 273*(4), 289–94.

Ganong, L. H., & Markovitz, J. (1987). Young men's knowledge of testicular cancer and behavioral intentions toward testicular self-exam. *Patient Education and Counseling, 9,* 251–261.

Gastrin, G. (1980). Program to encourage self-examination for breast cancer. *British Medical Journal, 2,* 193.

Gifford, M. S., & Stone, I. K. (1993). Quality, access, and clinical issues in a nurse practitioner colposcopy outreach program. *Nurse Practitioner, 18*(10), 25–34.

Goldenring, J. M., & Purtell, E. (1984). Knowledge of testicular cancer risk and need for self-examination in college students: A call for equal time for men in teaching of early cancer detection techniques. *Pediatrics, 74,* 1093–1096.

Gould-Martin, K., Paganini-Hill, A., Casagrande, C., Mack, T., & Ross, R. K. (1982). Behavioral and biological determinants of surgical stage of breast cancer. *Preventive Medicine, 11,* 429–440.

Grant, I. (1985). Screening for lung cancer. In B. A. Stoll (Ed.), *Screening and monitoring cancer* (pp. 119–133). New York, John Wiley & Sons, Inc.

Greenwald, P., Nasca, P. C., Lawrence, C. E., Horton, J., McGarrah, M. S., Gabrielle, T., & Carlton, K. Estimated effect of breast self-examination and routine physician examinations on breast cancer mortality. (1978). *New England Journal of Medicine, 299,* 271–273.

Gregorio, D., Cummings, M., & Michalek, A. (1983). Delay, stage of disease, and survival among white and black women with breast cancer. *American Journal of Public Health, 73,* 590–593.

Guinan, P., Sharifi, R., & Bush, I. (1984, January). Prostate cancer: Tips toward earlier detection. *Your Patient & Cancer,* 37–42.

Hakama, M. (1986). Scientific basis of screening in early detection. *Cancer Detection and Prevention, 9,* 139–143.

Hallal, J. (1982). The relationship of health beliefs, health locus of control, and self-concept to the practice of breast self-examination in adult women. *Nursing Research, 31,* 137–142.

Hartz, L. E. (1995). What's happening, quality of care by nurse practitioners delivering colposcopy services. *Journal of the American Academy of Nurse Practitioners, 7*(1), 23–27.

Hirschfield-Bartek, J. (1982). Health beliefs and their influence on breast self-examination practices in women with breast cancer. *Oncology Nursing Forum, 9,* 77–81.

Hislop, T. G., Coldman, A. J., & Skippen, D. H. (1984). Breast self-examination: Importance of technique in early diagnosis. *Canadian Medical Association Journal, 131,* 1349–1352.

Holt, W. S. Jr. (1991). Factors affecting compliance with screening sigmoidoscopy. *Journal of Family Practice, 32*(6), 585–9.

Hogan, T. (1983). Testicular germ cell cancers. In S. Kahn, R. Love, C. Sherman, & R. Chakravorty (Eds.), *Concepts in cancer medicine* (pp. 513–525). New York: Grune & Stratton, Inc.

Holliday, H., Roebuck, E. J., & Doyle, P. J. (1983). Initial results from a programme of BSE. *Clinical Oncology, 9,* 11–16.

Howe, H. L. (1980). Proficiency in performing breast self-examination. *Patient Counseling in Health Education, 2,* 151.

Huguley, C. N., & Brown, R. L. (1981). The value of breast self-examination. *Cancer, 47,* 989–995.

Kang, S. H., & Bloom, J. R. (1993). Social support and cancer screening among older black Americans. *Journal of the National Cancer Institute, 85*(9), 737–42.

Khan, O., & McCready, V. R. (1985). Isotope imaging in staging and monitoring. In B. A. Stoll (Ed.), *Screening and monitoring cancer* (pp. 31–46). New York: John Wiley & Sons, Inc.

Khan, O., Slack, N., & Cosgrove, D. (1985). Ultrasound imaging in staging and monitoring. In B. A. Stoll (Ed.), *Screening and monitoring cancer* (pp. 79–94). New York: John Wiley & Sons, Inc.

Kahn, S. B. (1983). Cancer diagnosis. In S. B. Kahn, R. Love, C. Sherman, & R. Chakravorty (Eds.), *Concepts in cancer medicine* (pp. 267–283). New York: Grune & Stratton, Inc.

Kegeles, S. S. (1985). Education for breast self-examination: Why, who, what and how? *Preventive Medicine, 14,* 702–720.

Kegeles, S. S., & Grady, K. E. (1982). Behavioral dimensions in cancer control. In D. Schottenfeld & J. G. Fraumeni (Eds.), *Cancer epidemiology and prevention* (pp. 1049–1063). Philadelphia: W. B. Saunders Co.

Kelly, R. B., & Shank, J. C. (1992). Adherence to screening flexible sigmoidoscopy in asymptomatic patients. *Medical Care, 30*(11), 1029–42.

Kendall, C., & Hailey, B. J. (1993). The relative effectiveness of three reminder letters on making and keeping mammogram appointments. *Behavioral Medicine, 19*(1), 29–34.

Kiefe, C. I., McKay, S. V., Halevy, A., Brody, B. A. (1994). Is cost a barrier to screening mammography for low-income women receiving Medicare benefits? A randomized trial. *Archives of Internal Medicine, 154*(11), 1217–24.

Klassen, A. C., Celentano, D. D., & Weisman, C. S. (1993). Cervical cancer screening in hospitals: The efficacy of legislation in Maryland. *American Journal of Public Health, 83*(9), 1316–20.

Kornguth, P. J., Rimer, B. K., Conaway, M. R., Sullivan, D. C., Catoe, K. E., Stout, A. L., Bracket, J. S. (1993). Impact of patient-controlled compression on the mammography experience. *Radiology, 186*(1), 99–102.

Kronborg, O., Fenger, C., Pedersen, S. A., Hem, J., Bertlesen, K., & Olsen, J. (1992). Causes of death during the first 5 years of a randomized trial of mass screening for colorectal cancer with fecal occult blood test. *Scandinavian Journal of Gastroenterology, 27,* 47–52.

Kurebayashi, J., Shimozuma, K., & Sonoo, H. (1994). The practice of breast self-examination results in the earlier detection and better clinical course of Japanese women with breast cancer. *Surgery Today, 24*(4), 337–41.

Lailemand, R., Vakil, P., Pearson, P., & Box, V. (1984). Screening for asymptomatic bowel cancer in general practice. *British Medical Journal, 288,* 31–33.

Laughter, D. C., Kean, T. J., Drean, K. D., Esparza, D., Hortobaqyi, G., Judkins, A., Levitt, D. Z., Marcus, C., & Selberberg, Y. (1981). The breast self-examination practices of high risk women: Implications for patient education. *Patient Counseling and Health Education, 3,* 103–107.

Leffall, L. (1981). *Early diagnosis of colorectal cancer.* New York: American Cancer Society Publication, No. 3311-PE.

Lerman, C., & Schwartz, M. (1993). Adherence and psychological adjustment among women at high risk for breast cancer. *Breast Cancer Research & Treatment, 28*(2), 145–55.

Levin, B., & Murphy, G. P. (1992). Revision of American Cancer Society recommendations for the early detection of cancer. *CA-A Cancer Journal for Clinicians, 42*(5), 298.

Li, F. P. (1986). Genetic and familial cancer: Opportunities for prevention and early detection. *Cancer Detection and Prevention, 9,* 41–45.

Lierman, L. M., Kasprzyk, D., & Benoliel, J. Q. (1991). Understanding adherence to breast self-examination in older women. *Western Journal of Nursing Research, 13,* 46–66.

Lierman, L. M., Powell-Cope, G., Benoliel, J. Q., Georgiadou, F., & Young, H. M. (1994). Using social support to promote breast self-examination performance. *Oncology Nursing Forum, 21*(6), 1051–7.

Lillington, L., Padilla, G., Sayre, J., & Chlebowski, R. (1993). Factors influencing nurses' breast cancer control activity. *Cancer Practice, 1*(4), 307–314.

Love, R. R., Leventhal, H., Hughes, B. S., & Fryback, D. G. (1984). *Cancer prevention for clinicians, course text.* Madison, WI: Board of Regents of the University of Wisconsin System.

Love, R. R., & Olsen, S. J. (1985). An agenda for cancer prevention in nursing practice. *Cancer Nursing, 8,* 329–338.

Macdonald, J., Cohn, I., & Gunderson, L. (1985). Cancer of the stomach. In V. DeVita, S. Hellman, & S. Rosenberg (Eds.), *Cancer principles and practice of oncology* (2nd ed., pp. 659–690). Philadelphia: J. B. Lippincott Co.

Macrea, F., Hill, D., St. John, J., Ambikatathy, A., Garner, J., & Ballarat General Practitioner Research Group. (1984). Predicting colon cancer screening behavior from health beliefs. *Preventive Medicine, 13,* 115–126.

Mamon, J., & Zapka, J. (1985). Determining validity of measuring the quality of breast self-examination. *Evaluation in the Health Professions, 8,* 55–68.

Mainous, A. G., & Hagen, M. D. (1994). Public awareness of prostate cancer and the prostate-specific antigen test. *Cancer Practice, 2*(3), 217–21.

Mandel, J. S., Bond, J. H., Church, T. R., Snover, D. C., Bradley, G. M., Schuman, L. M., & Ederer, F. (1993). Reducing mortality from colorectal cancer by screening for fecal occult blood. *New England Journal of Medicine, 328,* (19) 1365–71.

Mandelblatt, J., Traxler, M., Lakin, P., Kanetsky, P., & Kao, R. (1993). Targeting breast and cervical cancer screening to elderly poor black women: Who will participate? The Harlem Study Team. *Preventive Medicine, 22*(1), 20–33.

Marcus, A. C., Crane, L. A., Kaplan, C. P., Reading, A. E., Savage, E., Gunning, J., Bernstein, G., & Berek J. S. (1992). Improving adherence to screening follow-up among women with abnormal Pap smears: Results from a large clinic-based trial of three intervention strategies. *Medical Care, 30*(3), 216–30.

Marty, P., McDermott, R., & Gold, R. (1983). An assessment of three alternative formats for promoting breast self-examination. *Cancer Nursing, 6,* 207–211.

Massey, E. (1986). Perceived susceptibility to breast cancer and practice of breast self-examination. *Nursing Research, 35,* 183–185.

Maule, W. F. (1994). Screening for colorectal cancer by nurse endoscopists. *New England Journal of Medicine, 330*(3), 183–7.

Mayer, J. A., Slymen, D. J., Drew, J. A., Wright, B. L., Elder, J. P., Williams, S. J. (1992). Breast and cervical cancer screening in older women: The San Diego Medicare Preventive Health Project. *Preventive Medicine, 21*(4), 395–404.

McCarthy, B. D., & Moskowitz, M. A. (1993). Screening flexible sigmoidoscopy: Patient attitudes and compliance. *Journal of General Internal Medicine, 8*(3), 120–5.

McCusker, J., & Morrow, G. (1980). Factors related to the use of cancer early detection techniques. *Preventive Medicine, 9,* 388–397.

Menna, J., Higgins, G., & Glatstein, E. (1985). Cancer of the lung. In V. DeVita, S. Hellman, & S. Rosenberg (Eds.), *Cancer: Principles and practice of oncology* (2nd ed., pp. 507–598). Philadelphia: J. B. Lippincott Co.

Miller, A. B. (1986a). Screening for cancer: Issues and future directions. *Journal of Chronic Diseases, 39,* 1067–1077.

Miller, D. G. (1986b). Cancer prevention: Steps you can take. In A. I. Holleb (Ed.), *The American Cancer Society Cancer Book* (pp. 15–40). Garden City, NY: Doubleday & Co.

Montgomery, K. (1994). Recommendations for screening for cancer in women. *IM,* April, 78–88.

Morris, J. B., Stellato, T. A., Guy, B. B., Gordon, N. H., & Berger, N. A. (1991). A critical analysis of the largest reported mass fecal occult blood screening program in the United States. *American Journal of Surgery, 161*(1), 101–105.

Morrison, A. S. (1992). *Screening in chronic diseases.* Oxford: Oxford University Press.

Morrow, G., Way, J., Hoagland, A., & Cooper, R. (1982). Patient compliance with self-directed hemoccult testing. *Preventive Medicine, 11,* 512–520.

Myers, R. E., Ross, E. A., Wolf, T. A., Bolshem, A., Jepson, C., Millner, L. (1991). Behavioral interventions to increase adherence in colorectal cancer screening. *Medical Care, 29*(10), 1039–1050.

National Cancer Institute (1985). *Testicular self-examination.* Bethesda, MD: U.S. Department of Health and Human Services, Public Health Service, National Institutes of Health, NIH Publication No. 86–2636.

National Cancer Institute. (1994). *PDQ Cancer Screening/ Prevention Summary,* Bethesda, MD: NIH.

Newcomb, P. A., Olsen, S. J., Roberts, F. D., Storer, B. E., & Love, R. R. (1995). Assessing breast self-examination. *Preventive Medicine, 24,* 255–258.

Office of Technology Assessment. (1995). *Cost-effectiveness of colorectal cancer screening in average-risk adults.* Washington, DC: Congress of the U.S. Publication No. BP-H-146.

Olsen, S. J., & Frank-Stromborg, M. (1993). Cancer prevention and early detection in ethnically diverse populations. *Seminars in Oncology Nursing, 9*(3), 198–209.

O'Malley, M., & Fletcher, S. (1987). Screening for breast cancer with breast self-examination. A critical review. *Journal of the American Medical Association, 257,* 2196–2203.

Oncology Nursing Society. (1989a). *Standards of oncology education, patient/family and public.* Pittsburgh: Author.

Oncology Nursing Society. (1989b). *Standards of oncology nursing education, generalist and advanced practice levels.* Pittsburgh: Author.

Optenberg, S. A., & Thompson, I. M. (1990). Economics of screening for carcinoma of the prostate. *Urologic Clinics of North America, 17*(4), 719–37.

Ostwald, S. K., & Rothenberger, J. (1985). Development of a testicular self-examination program for college men. *Journal of the Association of Community Hospitals, 33,* 234–239.

Owen, W. L., Hoge, A. F., Asal, N. R., Anderson, P. S., Owne, A. S., & Cucchiara, A. J. (1985). Self-examination of the breast: Use and effectiveness. *Southern Medical Journal, 78,* 1170–1173.

Palos, G. (1994). Cultural heritage: Cancer screening and early detection. *Seminars in Oncology Nursing, 10*(2), 104–113.

Patterson, W. B. (1986). Screening for colorectal cancer in asymptomatic patients. In G. Steele & R. R. Osteen (Eds.), *Colorectal cancer: Current concepts in diagnosis and treatment* (pp. 138–152). New York: Marcel Dekker, Inc.

Paulus, D. (1987). Imaging in breast cancer. *Cancer, 37,* 133–150.

Perez, C., Fair, W., Ihde, D., & Labrie, F. (1985). Cancer of the prostate. In V. DeVita, S. Hellman, & S. Rosenberg (Eds.). *Cancer: Principles and practice of oncology* (2nd ed., pp. 929– 964). Philadelphia: J. B. Lippincott Co.

Perez, C., Knapp, R., DiSaia, P., & Young, R. (1985). Gynecologic tumors. In V. DeVita, S. Hellman, & S. Rosenberg (Eds.), *Cancer: Principles and practice of oncology* (2nd ed., pp. 1013–1081). Philadelphia: J. B. Lippincott Co.

Petravage, J., & Swedberg, J. (1988). Patient response to sigmoidoscopy recommendations via mailed reminders. *Journal of Family Practice, 27*(4), 387–389.

Prorok, P. C., & Connor, R. J. (1986). Screening for the early detection of cancer. *Cancer Investigation, 4,* 225–238.

Rakel, R. (1983, December). A clinician's guide: Tips on fecal occult blood testing. *Your Patient and Cancer, 3*(12), p. 23.

Reno, D. R. (1988). Men's knowledge and health beliefs about testicular cancer and testicular self-examination. *Cancer Nursing, 11,* 112–117.

Richie, J., Shipley, W., & Yagoda, A. (1985). Cancer of the bladder. In V. DeVita, S. Hellman, & S. Rosenberg (Eds.), *Cancer: Principles and practice of oncology* (2nd ed., pp. 915–928). Philadelphia: J. B. Lippincott Co.

Roetzheim, R. G., VanDurme, D. J., Brownlee, J. J., Herold, A. H., Woodard, L. J., & Blair, C. (1993). Barriers to screening among participants of a media-promoted breast cancer screening project. *Cancer Detection & Prevention, 17*(3), 367–77.

Roosevelt, J., & Frankl, H. (1984). Colorectal cancer screening by nurse practitioner using 60cm flexible fiberoptic sigmoidoscope. *Digestive Diseases & Sciences, 29*(2), 161–3.

Rothman, A. J., Salovey, P., Turvey, C., & Fishkin, S. A. (1993). Attributions of responsibility and persuasion: Increasing mammography utilization among women over 40 with an internally oriented message. *Health Psychology, 12*(1), 39–47.

Rovinski, C. (1980). Nurses and cancer's seven warning signals. *Cancer Nursing, 3,* 53–55.

Rudolph, V. N., & MacEwen-Quinn, K. L. (1988). The practice of TSE among college men: Effectiveness of an educational program. *Oncology Nursing Forum, 15*(1), 49–58.

Rutledge, D. N., & Davis, G. T., (1988). Breast self-examination compliance and the health belief model. *Oncology Nursing Forum, 15,* 175–179.

Salazar, M. (1994). Breast self-examination beliefs: A descriptive study. *Public Health Nursing, 11*(1), 49–56.

Sargis, N. (1983). Detecting ovarian cancer: A challenge for nursing assessment. *Oncology Nursing Forum, 10*(2), 48–52.

Satariano, W., Belle, S., & Swanson, M. (1986). The severity of breast cancer at diagnosis: A comparison of age and extent of disease in black and white women. *American Journal of Public Health, 76,* 779–782.

Schroy, P. C., Wiggins, T., Winawer, S. J., Diaz, B., Lightdale, C. J. (1988). Video-endoscopy by nurse practitioners: A model for colorectal cancer screening. *Gastrointestinal Endoscopy, 34*(5), 390–4.

Seidman, H., Stellman, S. D., & Mushinski, M. H. (1982). A different perspective on breast cancer risk factors: Some implications of the nonattributable risk. *Cancer, 32,* 301–313.

Selby, J. V. (1995). Clinical trials of screening sigmoidoscopy. In A. M. Cohen & S. J. Winawer (Eds.), *Cancer of the colon, rectum & anus.* New York: McGraw Hill.

Semiglazov, V., Sagaidak, V., Moiseyenko, V., & Mikhailov, E. (1993). Study of the role of breast self-examination in the reduction of mortality from breast cancer. The Russian Federation/World Health Organization Study. *European Journal of Cancer, 29a*(14), 2039–46.

Senie, R. T., Rosen, P. P., Lesser, M. L., & Kinne, D. W. (1981). Breast self-examination and medical examination related to breast cancer stage. *American Journal of Public Health, 71,* 583–590.

Shamian, J., & Edgar, L. (1987). Nurses as agents for change in teaching breast self-examination. *Public Health Nursing, 4*(1), 29–34.

Shanmugaratnam, K. (1985). Prevention and early detection of cancer. *Cancer Detection and Prevention, 8,* 431–445.

Shortridge, L., & McLain, B. (1979). Primary care and prostate cancer. *The Nurse Practitioner, 4,* 25.

Silman, A., & Mitchell, P. (1984). Attitudes of non-participants in an occupational based programme of screening for colorectal cancer. *Community Medicine, 6,* 8–11.

Simon, J. (1985). Occult blood screening for colorectal carcinoma: A critical review. *Gastroenterology, 88,* 820–837.

Skinner, C. S., Strecher, V. J. & Hospers, H. (1994). Physicians' recommendations for mammography: Do tailored messages make a difference? *American Journal of Public Health, 84*(1), 43–9.

Smith, E. B., Clarke-Pearson, D., & Creasman, W. (1985). Screening for cervical cancer. In B. A. Stoll (Ed.), *Screening and monitoring cancer* (pp. 153–165). New York: John Wiley & Sons, Inc.

Smith, E. M., Francis, A. M., & Polissar, L. (1980). The effect of breast self-exam practices and physician examinations on extent of disease at diagnosis. *Preventive Medicine, 9,* 409–417.

Songster, C. L., Barrows, G. H., & Jarrett, D. D. (1980). Immunochemical detection of human fecal occult blood. In S. J. Winawer, D. Schottenfeld, & P. Sherlock (Eds.), *Colorectal cancer: Prevention, epidemiology, and screening* (pp. 193–204). New York: Raven Press.

Sox, H. (1994). Preventive health services in adults. *New England Journal of Medicine, 330*(22), 1589–95.

Spector, M., Applegate, W., Olmstead, S., DiVasto, P., & Skipper, B. (1981). Assessment of attitudes toward mass screening for colorectal cancer in a Veterans Administration hospital. *American Journal of Surgery, 145,* 89–93.

Spencer, R. J., & Ready, R. L. (1977). Utilization of nurse endoscopiest for sigmoidoscopic examinations. *Diseases of the Colon and Rectum, 20*(2), 94–100.

Spitzer, W. O. (1984). The periodic health examination. *Canadian Medical Association Journal, 130,* 1276–1292.

St. John, D., Young, G., McHutchinson, J., Deacon, M., et al. (1992). Comparison of the specificity and sensitivity of Hemoccult and HemoQuant in screening for colorectal neoplasia. *Annals of Internal Medicine, 117*(5), 376–382.

Staff. (1987, November 27). ACS modifies guidelines for Pap test frequency: Physician discretion. *Cancer Letter,* p. 6.

Staff. (1987, March 6). New prostate cancer detection group to study potential of ultrasound. *Cancer Letter,* p. 4.

Staff. (1987, March). Nurse helps promote screening services at community hospital. *Cancer Nursing Letter,* p. 5.

Stephanek, M. E., & Wilcox, P. (1990). Breast self-examination among women at increased risk: Assessment of proficiency. *Cancer, 1,* 591–596.

Studva, K. V. (1983, December). Cancer prevention and detection: Testicular cancer. *Cancer Nursing, 6,* 468–485.

Subcommittee on Cancer in the Economically Disadvantaged. (1986). *Cancer in the economically disadvantaged. A special report.* New York: American Cancer Society.

Sugarbaker, P., Gunderson, L., & Wittes, R. (1985). Colorectal cancer. In V. DeVita, S. Hellman, & S. Rosenberg (Eds.), *Cancer: Principles and practice of oncology* (2nd ed., pp. 795–884). Philadelphia: J. B. Lippincott Co.

Swanson, D. (1987). Why you should conscientiously promote testicular self-examination. *Consultant, 27,* 142–147.

Tabar, L., Fagerberg, C. J. G., Gad, A., Holmberg, H. L., & Thomas, B. A. (1985). Reduction in mortality from breast cancer after screening with mammography. *Lancet, 1,* 829–832.

Tamburini, M., Massara, G., Bertario, L., Re, A., & Dipietro, S. (1981). Usefulness of breast self-examination for an early detection of breast cancer. Results of a study on 500 breast cancer patients and 652 controls. *Tumori, 67,* 219–224.

Thompson, H. (1985). Screening for stomach cancer. In B. A. Stoll (Ed.), *Screening and monitoring cancer* (pp. 167–193). New York: John Wiley & Sons, Inc.

Thompson, W. (1987). Imaging strategies for tumors of the gastrointestinal system. *Cancer, 37,* 165–185.

Thornhill, J. A., Conroy, R. M., Kelly, D. B., Walsh, A., Fennelly, J. J., & Fitzpatrick, J. M. (1986). Public awareness of testicular cancer and the value of self-examination. *British Journal of Medicine, 293,* 480–481.

U. S. Department of Health and Human Services. (1985). *Report of the Secretary's Task Force on Black & Minority Health. Vol 1. Executive Summary.* Bethesda, MD: National Institutes of Health.

U. S. Preventive Services Task Force. (1987). Recommendations for breast cancer screening. *Journal of the American Medical Association, 257,* 2196.

Van Der Werf, M. (1987). New diagnostic technique for cancer to enter clinical trials. *Oncology and Biotechnology News, 1*(3), 18.

Van Parijs, L. G., & Eckhardt, S. (1984). Public education in primary and secondary cancer prevention. *Hygie, 3,* 16–28.

Walker, R. (1993). Modeling and guided practice as components within a comprehensive testicular self-examination educational program for high school males. *Journal of Health Education, 24*(3), 12–8.

Warren, B., & Pohl, J. M. (1990). Cancer screening practices of nurse practitioners. *Cancer Nursing, 13*(3), 143–51.

Weinrich, S. P., Weinrich, M. C., Boyd, M. D., Atwood, J., & Cervenka, B. (1994). Teaching older adults by adapting for aging changes. *Cancer Nursing, 17*(6), 494–500.

Wilcox, L. S., & Mosher, W. D. (1993). Factors associated with obtaining health screening among women of reproductive age. *Public Health Reports, 108*(1), 76–86.

Wilkes, B. (1983). The development of a two-tier BSE educational program. In *Progress in cancer control III: A regional approach* (pp. 127–131). New York: Alan Liss, Inc.

Wilkinson, G., & Wilson, J. (1983). An evaluation of demographic differences in the utilization of a cancer information service. *Social Science Medicine, 17,* 169–175.

Winawer, S. (1995). Surveillance overview. In A. M. Cohen & S. J. Winawer (Eds.), *Cancer of the colon, rectum & anus.* New York: McGraw Hill.

Winawer, S. J. (1983). Detection and diagnosis of colorectal cancer. *Cancer, 51,* 2519–2524.

Winawer, S. J., Schottenfeld, D., & Sherlock, P. (1985). Screening for colorectal cancer: The issues. *Gastroenterology, 88,* 841–844.

Winchester, D. P., Schull, J. H., Scanlon, E. F., et al. (1980). A mass screening program for colorectal cancer using chemical testing for occult blood in the stool. *Cancer, 45,* 2955–2958.

Yancey, A. K. & Walden, L. (1994). Stimulating cancer screening among Latinas and African-American women. A community case study. *Journal of Cancer Education, 9*(1), 46–52.

Young, R., Knapp, R., Fuks, Z., & DiSaia, P. (1985). Cancer of the ovary. In V. DeVita, S. Hellman, & S. Rosenberg (Eds.), *Cancer: Principles and practice of oncology* (2nd ed., pp. 1083–1117). Philadelphia: J. B. Lippincott Co.

The Diagnosis of Cancer: A Life Transition

Darlene W. Mood

A MODEL OF THE CANCER EXPERIENCE

In most cultures, the word *cancer* carries with it a threatening and frightening connotation (Holland, 1982; Krant, 1976; Lierman, 1988; Weisman, 1979a). Although each individual may have a personal meaning for cancer, the cross-culturally shared meaning with its many negative features affects the way people react when confronted with a cancer experience. This includes not only the persons who are patients or their families but also the many health professionals with whom they interact and the larger network of persons who constitute the world in which they live. Basic human relationships are significantly altered: communication barriers may arise between spouses, parents and children may become dishonest with one another, health providers may avoid discussing certain topics with the client, employers may become fearful and lose confidence in their formerly valued employee. The personal discovery that one has cancer often involves major and dramatic shifts in peoples' lives. This chapter examines the transition that occurs when a person experiences the first signs and symptoms and then reaches the stage of formal diagnosis of cancer. This chapter also addresses the psychosocial effects of that transition as well as some factors that facilitate or serve as barriers to making the transition. Finally, the nursing implications of the transition and associated factors are discussed.

Several models have been proposed in the psychosocial oncology literature to describe the cancer experience (Giacquinta, 1977; Weisman, 1979b). One

very practical model, shown in Figure 18–1, was first proposed by Holland (1982) and later elaborated on by Saunders and McCorkle (1985). In this model, the patient experiencing some symptoms seeks medical consultation and then goes through a series of tests and evaluations, which result in a cancer diagnosis. This is the first transition. At this point, depending on the site and stage of the disease, a curative treatment attempt is made. In the most satisfactory of outcomes, the cancer is completely responsive to the treatment, and the patient never experiences a recurrence and is cured (course A). However, there are two other possible outcomes after the curative attempt. In the first (course B), the cancer is initially or partially responsive to the treatment but later recurs or spreads to other parts of the body, or both. The duration of the response could be very brief and limited (e.g., days or weeks) or it could last for many years. The other outcome after the curative attempts is no response (course C). Both clinical courses B and C generally follow a trajectory of progressive disease and then death. These final steps also constitute course D. In this clinical course, no curative attempt is ever made, and the disease progresses to death.

Each of the arrows in Figure 18–1 could be considered a transition stage in the cancer experience. This chapter focuses on the first of these transitions, namely, the transition that takes the individual from being a person without cancer through a personal discovery that "I do have cancer" (a formal cancer diagnosis). This transition has three phases: becoming aware of the first signs and symptoms, obtaining a formal diagnosis, and planning for treatment. The entire transition may

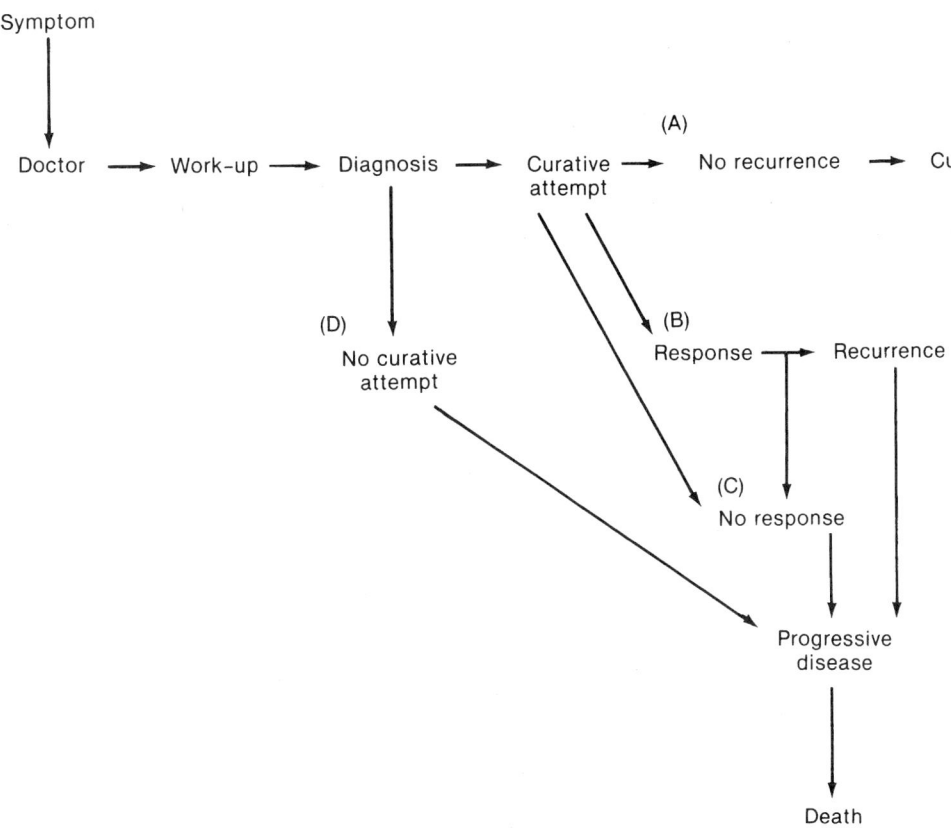

FIGURE **18-1.** Possible clinical courses of cancer. (From Holland, J. [1982]. Psychologic aspects of cancer. In J. Holland & E. Frei III [Eds.], *Cancer medicine.* Philadelphia: Lea & Febiger. Reproduced by permission.)

be accomplished in several weeks, or it may take months or years to complete, depending on a great number of personal and situational factors.

THE FIRST SIGNS

Biologically, the change from being cancer free to having a cancerous condition is a very slow process occurring silently within the individual person's physical structure. It is not known with certainty what causes the abnormal cells to develop and multiply. Diet, environmental contamination, lifestyle choices, stress, and heredity have all been implicated in carcinogenesis. It has been proposed, in fact, that abnormal cells capable of producing a cancer are produced regularly in the body but that the body's alert immune system monitors for these abnormal cells and destroys them before they become a cancer (LeShan, 1966; Simonton, Matthews-Simonton, & Creighton, 1978). Within this theoretic framework, then, the occurrence of cancer represents a failure of the body's immune system to function effectively. Psychologic as well as physical triggers of this process have been proposed (Borysenko, 1982; LeShan, 1966; Thomas & Greenstreet, 1973). The avoidance of cancer, in turn, is achieved in part through the physical and perhaps psychologic maintenance of the effectively functioning immune system (Simonton et al., 1978).

Whatever the causes of cancer are, the biologic shift that occurs is believed to differ significantly from the psychosocial transition. Although the cancer cells usu-

ally divide and grow undetected over a long period of time, the person is unaware of those processes until some event brings them to sudden awareness.

What are some of the events that people experience that catapult them from the belief that they are cancer-free to the suspicion and discovery that they have cancer? The most sudden shift is the self-detection of an obvious sign or symptom. For example, a woman is showering and she finds a lump in her breast that she does not recall having felt before; a man faces the mirror shaving and notices an unevenness between the two sides of his neck; a person notes blood in the urine or feces. These common first signs trigger an awareness that something may be wrong and generally place the person in a state of hyperalertness that eventually will lead to some action. The rapidity of each individual's response will depend on many factors.

Other signs and symptoms commonly are first detected by the person but are not so obvious in their association with cancer, for example, a persistent cough or sore throat, or shortness of breath. Sometimes a cut or bruise that just will not heal, as it would have in the past, is noticed first. The appearance of, or changes in the appearance of, skin moles may be an initially unrecognized sign. Changes in bladder or bowel habits may be attributed to many different causes. Although pain frequently is difficult to ignore, rarely would cancer be considered as the first explanation. Extreme fatigue likewise may be the initial sign noticed. These less obvious manifestations are often overlooked as the individual waits for them to disappear. However, when these events are signals of cancer, they persist; eventually, the person becomes aware of the potential threat and enters the already mentioned state of hyperalertness likely to lead at some point to action.

A final possible situation occurs when a person with no known signs and symptoms of cancer, often in apparent good health, enters the health care system for a routine examination or acute care of an unrelated health problem. In the course of examination, something occurs that makes the health provider suspicious. This may be the unusual results of a blood test or an x-ray study, or it may be the discovery of a sign that had not been detected by the patient or client. Such discoveries may lead to further testing that, even before the physician has shared the findings with the person, may raise anxieties because the testing is recognized as extraordinary.

Therefore, it is clear that although people may detect the first signs of cancer themselves or discover the suspicious signs of cancer during a totally unrelated interaction with the health care system, the discovery is virtually always an unexpected event. It catches the person off guard and generally unprepared to cope with its meaning and threat.

RESPONDING TO THE THREAT

Conventional wisdom would dictate that, given a sign or symptom that suggests the possibility of cancer or a persistent symptom that will not go away, the person involved would seek medical advice and diagnosis. In fact, how the person responds to these first signs will depend on many factors. During this early phase of cancer detection, people struggle to make sense of the symptoms they are experiencing. Often these initial symptoms are ambiguous, and symptom meaning can consist of highly speculative attributions about the underlying cause. Mechanic (1972) suggested that symptom attributions generally are loosely constructed hypotheses or hunches until clinical confirmation is made. It is not uncommon for people to attribute their initial symptoms to minor illnesses (Comaroff & Maguire, 1981). People tend to normalize their symptoms within the context of everyday life experience (Chrisman & Kleinman, 1980).

Eventually symptoms come to interfere with daily activities of living or otherwise cause the person to seek care from a primary health provider. Zola's research (1973) documented that symptoms that persisted beyond an expected time frame and that interfered with vocational or daily activities often guided the decision to seek health care.

Other factors affect the person's responses to first signs: *personal characteristics*, such as age and gender; *financial issues*, such as income and insurance; *psychologic makeup*, including coping resources and typical coping patterns; *social considerations*, such as family structure, social network and support, and work status; and the person's configuration of *knowledge, experience, and attitudes*, including awareness of the implications of the symptoms, valuing the importance of early

diagnosis, previous experience with the health care system, spiritual orientation including religious beliefs and practices, personal existential philosophy, and beliefs about or experiences with cancer. Any of the factors can either facilitate or impede the person's response to the initial alerting event signaling the possibility of cancer. The speed or delay in seeking diagnosis and treatment has been referred to as *lag time* (Weisman, 1979a; Worden & Weisman, 1975) and is further divided into (1) the period of time between the alerting event and the first health provider contact, referred to as *patient delay*; and (2) the time between the first health provider contact and the initiation of treatment, or *diagnostic delay* (Marshall & Funch, 1986).

PERSONAL CHARACTERISTICS

Characteristics such as age, gender, ethnic background, and level of education are associated with people's response to a threatening health or illness signal. For example, younger and middle-aged persons are more likely to use prevention and detection services in the absence of symptoms (National Center for Health Statistics [NCHS], 1986). This may be a function of the fact that screening programs generally are directed toward women in their reproductive years (Given & Given, 1989). Young adults have longer periods of patient delay than older persons. This response may be attributable to less awareness of the significance of the symptoms, disbelief or denial of susceptibility or that something serious could be wrong, less adequate insurance, and less time. As a group, middle-aged persons have the shortest lag times. Lierman (1988) reported that the women in her sample who sought medical attention for their symptoms of breast cancer quickly (less than 4 weeks) were significantly younger (59.8 years) than those who delayed a year or more (71.8 years). The data on patient delay among the elderly are less clear. Older persons spend more time interacting with the health care system in response to a greater number of somatic complaints. This can result in shorter lag times, especially if there is a personal history of cancer (Mettlin, Reese, & Murphy, 1980). As all subjects in Lierman's study were at least 50 years old and would be considered "older" in the general population, her finding that 60 per cent of the women had short or intermediate delay times is consistent with the description that older persons have shorter lag times. It has been noted, however, that older persons tend to practice fewer cancer detection behaviors (Holmes & Hearne, 1981) and fail to seek specific cancer examinations on the assumption that their interactions with providers for other health problems are sufficient to identify signs of cancer (Given & Given, 1989). Also, cancer symptoms in the elderly can easily be confused with signs of normal aging (Frank-Stromborg, 1986). These observations may explain why elderly persons are found to have more advanced disease at the time of diagnosis (Holmes & Hearne, 1981). Delay may be extended also if the elderly person has less education and limited financial resources and insurance benefits (Funch, 1985). Thus age does appear to be a significant factor in lag time, but the relationship is complex and nonlinear.

Gender is another significant factor in determining a person's response to signs of illness. Verbrugge (1979a, 1982) points out that, in general, women are more likely than men to seek medical attention, but their health problems are likely to be of a less serious or life-threatening nature. Women use more prevention and detection services (NCHS, 1986), perhaps because cancer screening programs are more likely to be directed toward them (Given & Given, 1989). Men have more serious chronic health conditions, a higher incidence of injuries, more long-term disability, and ultimately a shorter life span. Because women are more likely to utilize the health care system, they might be expected to seek treatment more promptly than men. However, in one examination of women's health care practices and cancer, McCorkle (1989) reported that women showed significant delays in seeking treatment for a variety of cancer symptoms. For example, between 20 and 35 per cent of women who discovered a lump in their breasts waited months or even more than a year to seek treatment. These findings are consistent with those reported by Funch (1985), Funch and Francis (1982), and Lierman (1988). Among colorectal cancer patients of both genders, the sexes differed in both patient delay and diagnostic delay (Marshall & Funch, 1986). In both components of lag time, delay was longer for women. A variety of explanations for these differences have been proposed, and Lierman (1988) expressed particular concern over the fact that many of the causes of delay were a function of health providers' differential response to women's symptoms rather than to delays caused by the women themselves. Even women who sought prompt medical attention did not necessarily receive prompt diagnosis and treatment.

McCorkle (1989) also summarized the controversial findings in studies of women's practice of breast self-examination (BSE). She concluded that there is some tendency for women who practice BSE to delay seeking treatment on discovery of a symptom. This might suggest that the practice of BSE, at least for these women, is motivated more by fear than by a positive attitude of self-care. In addition, McCorkle noted that further delays may be related to age, education, physical stature, and past experience with breast cancer.

Education also is a factor in the promptness with which people respond to their initial symptoms. Persons with less education are more likely to delay seeking treatment (Funch, 1985; Germino & McCorkle, 1985). Ethnicity also has been associated with differences in response to warning signs. Degree of trust in the health care system often is a key factor in determining whether persons will seek out standard medical care or choose to try folk cures (Long, 1993). Nonwhite persons are more likely to delay than are whites (Lauver, 1994; Long, 1993; Vernon, Telley, Neale, & Steinfeldt, 1985). African-Americans have been described as more fatalistic than Caucasians, although Matthews, Lannin, and Mitchell (1994) argue that such labeling is highly counterproductive and leads to ineffective intervention attempts. Research has shown,

nonetheless, that African-Americans are more likely to believe cancer myths, to have less knowledge regarding cancer prevalence or early cancer warning signs, and to question if cancer is even an African-American health problem; they are less likely to believe that early detection makes a difference (EVAXX, 1981; Long, 1993; National Cancer Institute, 1986; Olsen & Frank-Stromborg, 1994; U.S. Department of Health and Human Services [USDHHS], 1986). Other findings, however, attribute these apparent racial or ethnic differences to poverty (American Cancer Society [ACS], 1989; Boring, Squires, & Heath, 1992; Freeman & Wasfie, 1989).

FINANCIAL CONSIDERATIONS

Financial resources are clearly a significant factor affecting persons' response to their cancer symptoms (Houts et al., 1985). Persons from lower socioeconomic classes tend to have significantly longer delays in seeking diagnosis (Hackett, Cassem, & Raker, 1973; Lewis & Bloom, 1978–1979). An American Cancer Society (ACS) report on cancer in the poor (1989) concluded that economically disadvantaged Americans have severely limited access to health care and health insurance, and they obtain care only at great personal sacrifice. Furthermore, the care they receive is often inadequate, insensitive, and at times irrelevant to their needs (Long, 1993). Thus the poor face many barriers to responding to their cancer symptoms, and they sometimes appear to believe that the outcomes are not worth the effort required.

People need not be poverty stricken, however, to feel constraints in their cancer health care. For example, the relatively high cost of a mammogram has been reported to be one reason for not using this valuable detection procedure (Crooks & Jones, 1989). Whether the person has health insurance is another important consideration. Uninsured and underinsured persons are likely to delay seeking diagnosis and treatment. Even with health insurance, out-of-pocket expenses for transportation, meals away from home, hotel costs during outpatient care in a distant city, and other costs not covered by insurance are a serious burden to families on limited incomes, especially for single-parent families and the elderly on fixed incomes. Loss of time from work poses an additional financial problem. These threats of financial burden are likely to lead to delay in seeking medical attention, especially if the symptoms are not painful or visible. Financial resources clearly become a direct factor in the decision to take advantage of some of the latest but most expensive diagnostic procedures or to obtain more complex cancer treatment, such as bone marrow transplants.

PSYCHOLOGIC MAKEUP

When people suddenly recognize that a symptom may be a possible indicator of cancer, their response will be influenced by their complex psychologic makeup. Although the literature on the role of psychosocial factors in predicting the onset of cancer is growing (Cunningham, 1985; Fox, 1983; Greer & Morris, 1975; Morris & Greer, 1980; Stams & Steggles, 1987), few investigators have discussed these factors in association with delay in seeking diagnosis or treatment (Levy, 1985). People tend to respond to the threat of cancer in much the same way they have responded to other crises in their lives (Holland, 1976; Worden & Weisman, 1975). Generally, persons who have used denial as a major coping mechanism can be expected to delay longer in seeking treatment (Greer, 1974; Magarey, Todd, & Blizard, 1977), although these findings are not undisputed. Delay may also be a function of the unwillingness of individuals to become dependent on their health providers or family (Hammerschlag, Fisher, De Cosser, & Kaplan, 1964). Weisman points out that delay may be consistent with a "trait of independent self-reliance" just as well as "fearful procrastination" (1979a, p. 15). This mixture of coping strategies may explain why some investigators have found no differences between deniers and acceptors in their length of delay in seeking treatment (Watson, Greer, Blake, & Sharpnell, 1984). Intellectualization, isolation, guilt, anxiety, and depression also have been associated with delay in seeking diagnosis and treatment (Gold, 1964; Krant, 1981; Magarey et al., 1977). Fear of the diagnosis of cancer, of the treatment modalities, and of pain or disfigurement have all been implicated in delay (Crooks & Jones, 1989; Gold, 1964). Fear also may explain why some women engage in self-detection behaviors but delay seeking diagnosis when they find a possible symptom (McCorkle, 1989). Assessing psychologic factors associated with delay is very difficult because the subjects needed for a prospective study of this topic are unknown until they enter the health care system. By this time, they will have gone through a number of steps in their decision making that may alter their psychologic state and interfere with their ability to accurately reproduce their feelings at the time of the discovery of symptoms.

SOCIAL CONSIDERATIONS

Family dynamics, marital status, social support, and work status are among the social factors believed to be associated with response to warning signs of cancer. Married women who discover a breast lump become concerned about their spouses' reaction to the lump or to the loss of the breast; mothers worry about how their children will react (Lambert & Lambert, 1979; Verbrugge, 1979b). Family members, reluctant to see their elderly family member subjected to aggressive therapies for cancer, may delay seeking diagnosis (Given & Given, 1989).

Members of a person's social network can play a major role in reducing delay. Wool (1986), in her study that compared women with breast lumps who delayed longer than 3 months (extreme deniers) with women who sought medical attention more promptly, observed that the deniers were significantly more likely to see the doctor only if encouraged to do so by a relative or friend. Yet family members may inadvertently support delaying behavior because they are more likely to share

common values and characteristics. Salloway and Dillon (1973) found that persons with more *friends* in their social networks were less likely to delay seeking health care than persons with large *family* networks. Giacquinta (1977) has described in detail the family's stresses and concerns when a member has cancer. Some of these problems may contribute to patient delay in seeking health care.

KNOWLEDGE, EXPERIENCE, AND ATTITUDES

A person experiencing a signaling event must have the knowledge that a lump in the breast or a wound that does not heal has meaning that should not be overlooked. To this end, agencies such as the National Cancer Institute (NCI) and the ACS invest large sums of money and effort into public education. Research has shown that increasing people's understanding of the importance of screening and detection can also increase their likelihood of their partaking in them (Crooks & Jones, 1989; Kegeles, 1969). Nonetheless, many persons remain unaware of many of the publicized danger signs, with elderly persons who are at greater risk being even less knowledgeable than the population as a whole (Weinrich & Weinrich, 1986). Many women, for example, remain uneducated regarding BSE despite having at least occasional Papanicolaou smears. Only about 15 per cent of women aged 50 years old and older obtain recommended annual mammograms (Crooks & Jones, 1989). The vast majority of women of all ages, races, and socioeconomic status fail to follow breast screening guidelines (Long, 1993). Thus lack of knowledge continues to be a serious source of delay in seeking medical attention for a signaling event.

Knowledge, however, is never enough in and of itself. Knowing is not always accompanied by the desirable health behavior. Among women who have been taught BSE, few carry out this easy practice regularly, although it has repeatedly been shown to be associated with the discovery of tumors at an earlier stage. There is also some question of whether women who report performing BSE are actually following the recommended procedures accurately. Nurses may be even less likely than women in general to practice BSE on a regular basis. This may be an act of denial related to nurses' expressed fears of cancer therapies (Mood, Brenner, & Richardson, 1985) but it can be reversed through focused educational experiences (Post-White, Carter, & Anglism, 1993). Women who do practice BSE know the possible meaning of a breast lump, but those who have more knowledge regarding breast cancer are sometimes *more* likely to delay seeking medical treatment (Owens, Duffy, & Ashcroft, 1985). Similarly, it was found that when women detected lumps in their breast by BSE, they were more likely to delay (Gould-Martin, Paganini-Hill, Casagrande, Mack, & Ross, 1982). Thus it would seem that some knowledge can interact with other factors to become another source of delay.

Beliefs and attitudes can affect a person's responses to many aspects of life. These include individual spiritual beliefs, which may be religious but may also derive from a personal existential philosophy. Some evidence exists that religiosity—measured by the extent to which a person affiliates with a religious group, engages in religious activities, and reports that religious experiences influence beliefs about life and death—is associated with significantly less fear of death (Mood & Van Fossen, 1983; Wendt, 1989). Reducing fear and inspiring hope (Miller, 1985) may be one important way of reducing delay in seeking health care when confronted by threatening symptoms. Although beliefs held by some religious groups deter their followers from seeking professional health care, most mainstream religions in the United States support prompt and active intervention.

Beliefs specifically related to health may also affect people's health behaviors. In particular, their belief in their susceptibility to illness or its potential seriousness are among the factors that influence the decision to seek medical advice (Cox, 1982; Kegeles, 1969; Rosenstock, 1974).

One important factor that influences beliefs and attitudes is past experience with the health care system (Holland, 1982). Persons who have had limited experience may have an idealized image of the system—a "Dr. Marcus Welby syndrome"—which may lead them to seek medical assistance more readily but perhaps more naively. If men and women with prior experience judge that they have received good health care in the past and they feel a sense of trust in their care providers, they may be inclined to contact them more rapidly. If, on the other hand, their experience has been one of poor communication, fear, painful interventions without adequate preparation or explanation, or a sense of anonymity within a large uncaring system, they are less likely to seek help promptly. This is especially evident in the research that has examined the beliefs and behaviors of persons of color and/or poverty (Lauver, 1994; Long, 1993).

Even more influential in persons' decisions to seek care than their general experience with health care systems is their experience with, and resulting attitudes and beliefs about, cancer. Many persons still believe that a cancer diagnosis is a death sentence (Holland, 1982; Krant, 1976). To the extent they recognize that their signaling event is a cancer risk sign, they may be afraid of confirming their worst fears. Fear of cancer treatment, when thought of as mutilating surgery or cancer-producing radiation, or even as treatments causing nausea and hair loss, can be as intense as the fear of cancer itself (Holland, 1976; Leis & Pilnik, 1974; Vettese, 1976). Furthermore, persons who have experienced the death of a family member or close friend from cancer are more likely to delay seeking diagnosis of a possible cancer symptom even if they regularly engage in cancer detection behavior (Funch, 1985; Hackett et al., 1973). However, experience may interact with age to reverse this trend because older persons with a personal history of cancer seek medical care more promptly (Mettlin et al., 1980).

Thus it is clear that knowledge is important, but it is not always enough to ensure prompt action in the face of symptoms. Experience also is important and interacts with knowledge to form beliefs and attitudes that may help or hinder the person's motivation to take action. When knowledge or experience or both lead to a fearful reaction, the result may be patient delay.

OTHER FACTORS

A variety of other factors have been shown to be related to the person's decision to take prompt action or to delay seeking treatment. One factor that generally hastens a decision to act is the severity of any symptoms. Pain is a major motivator to seeking treatment. Symptom distress heightens the person's awareness of the possible seriousness of the condition and tends to interfere with the use of denial (Germino & McCorkle, 1985). It should be noted, however, that even extreme symptoms can be seen in some deniers. For example, a woman with a draining lesion in the breast delayed seeking medical attention for 7 years and finally did so only when another, more serious condition made it necessary (Lierman, 1988). Her beliefs and attitudes were such that although she knew the potential seriousness of her symptoms from the start, and although her mother had died of breast cancer, she chose to close her eyes to the situation and delay professional care.

Stage of disease also has been associated with the speed with which treatment is sought, although the relationship is not a clear one. Advanced disease is generally associated with greater symptom distress, which is more likely to lead to prompt seeking of treatment. On the other hand, as shown earlier, women who practice BSE and seek prompt treatment are significantly more likely to have early-stage breast cancer (Crooks & Jones, 1989; Funch, 1985; McCorkle, 1989).

Some physical characteristics may also be important. For example, Funch (1985) found that women with large breasts delayed seeking care longer than women with small breasts. Funch offered no explanation of this finding, so that it is unclear whether women with large breasts were more embarrassed or self-conscious about their breast size, or whether it was perhaps a more general issue of weight. Whatever the specific dynamics are, Funch's findings suggest that body image may affect health care decisions.

In summary, then, it is clear that people can become aware of the first signs of cancer in a variety of ways. They may discover an obvious symptom; they may experience a sign or symptom that is not immediately obvious but which, over time, is clearly different from their past experience; or the first signs may be found by a health care provider in the course of providing unrelated health care or routine checkups. In whatever manner the first signs become known to the person, there is an experience of sudden awareness that opens a door to the personal discovery of a new life role; that is, the transition from being a person without cancer to being a person with cancer, or at least suspected cancer. The transition is not really complete until a formal diagnosis and treatment plan are obtained. Individual responses to this first step in the transition vary widely, with some persons moving quickly to seek diagnosis and treatment and others delaying in taking health care action. Many factors, both internal and external to the person, have been shown to be related to that critical decision. What is not known at this time is the relative importance of these factors and whether these findings, many of which are based on studies of women, are similar for men. It is also unclear which factors would have the greatest impact on altering attitudes, behaviors, and outcomes if systematic nursing interventions were planned to facilitate such changes.

THE DIAGNOSIS

The many factors that propel or impede individual responses to the first signs of cancer have been reviewed. If those signs are obvious, the degree of certainty regarding the diagnosis may be high even before the person obtains a formal diagnosis. More often, however, the signs are equivocal. For example, most breast lumps are benign. Similarly, virtually any sign or symptom of cancer could also be a sign or symptom of something else. Therefore, the real impact of this first transition comes with a formal diagnosis. The conditions under which the diagnosis is made and then shared with the patient can have a significant effect on patients' reactions, the meanings they ascribe to their diagnosis, their ability to cope with this new dimension in their lives, and their later behavior. Therefore, the diagnosis of cancer will be considered from the perspectives of both the professionals who make and give the diagnosis and the persons (i.e., patients and family) who receive the diagnosis.

GIVING THE DIAGNOSIS: PROFESSIONAL ATTITUDES AND ACTIONS

In the United States, the prevailing practice among health professionals in the field of oncology is to provide patients with an accurate description of their diagnosis and treatment plans. However, this is a relatively new phenomenon that began in the late 1960s. A survey of physicians conducted in 1961 reported that 90 per cent said they did not disclose a cancer diagnosis to the patient (Novack et al., 1979; Oken, 1961). By 1977, physicians' attitudes and behavior regarding disclosure had changed dramatically, with 97 per cent reporting that it was better to inform patients of their cancer diagnoses, treatment options, and realistic expectations for outcomes (Israel, 1978; Novack et al., 1979). However, as Holland (1976) points out, physicians must deal with their own feelings about cancer when faced with the decision of what to tell their patients. Many times, these practitioners have not resolved their own fears and anxieties, resulting in behavior that is sometimes overly protective and paternalistic or sometimes overly blunt and cold. Therefore, although a very high proportion of physicians now favor disclosing accurate diagnostic and treatment information to their patients, their actual behavior in practice may reflect a much more limited change in approach from earlier years.

Nurses also show some discrepancy between their attitudes and practices with respect to sharing information with patients. Nurses who were asked about their attitudes and experiences with dying patients consistently expressed a belief in openness and honesty with all patients as long as the patients were mentally competent (Castles & Murray, 1979). When asked about their behavior, however, many nurses described practices that were not consistent with their stated belief. They offered many different reasons—for example, "there's a policy here against it," "the patients don't want to hear about that stuff," "I don't really have enough time for that." In a secondary linguistic analysis of these nurses' responses, it was found that in every one of the 40 interviews evaluated, the nurses were more likely to substitute the pronoun *it* for terms such as *cancer, tumor,* and *death* than for less negative terms such as *nursing care* or *temperature* (Mood, 1980). This highly consistent finding was interpreted as an unconscious linguistic mechanism that allowed the nurses to avoid the use of unpleasant words while continuing to discuss the topic. These findings have since been replicated in a study of staff nurses, half of whom worked in oncology units (Mood et al., 1985). The oncology nurses were just as likely to manifest linguistic signs of avoidance and denial as were the general medical or surgical nurses.

The high disclosure rates reported by American physicians are not typical of the disclosure practices in other parts of the world. In Great Britain and Europe, as well as the eastern world, many physicians continue to adhere to the practice of withholding the cancer diagnosis from patients (Israel, 1978), sometimes causing bitter disputes among international colleagues. This nondisclosure practice continues even though as long ago as 1959, Aitken-Swan and Easson reported that 66 per cent of a sample of 231 British patients with various early-stage curable cancers approved of having been given an accurate diagnosis. Remembering that this study was conducted at a time and place in which disclosure was virtually unheard of, the fact that only 12 per cent of the patients said they would have preferred not to have been told was quite amazing. The remaining 22 per cent were neutral in their opinions. Patients who were contacted a second time more than a year later tended to adhere to their original reaction, with a high proportion of the patients continuing to approve of the disclosure practice.

An interesting observation reported by Aitken-Swan and Easson (1959) is that one of the negative consequences of nondisclosure, especially to early-stage cancer patients, is that the general public never learns that cancer is a curable disease. If the experience of the general public is that all persons with cancer die (because persons with curable cancers never had their diseases labeled as such), the belief that people always die of cancer is reinforced. Patients in the Aitken-Swan and Easson study reported that friends and relatives would not believe them when they shared their diagnoses and favorable prognoses.

Thus the giving of a cancer diagnosis is an important step. It involves physicians, nurses, and other health care providers coming to grips with their own beliefs regarding cancer and death and how these beliefs may be affecting their disclosure practices. The speed, clarity, and care with which the diagnosis is made, the attitudes and behaviors of the health care providers during the diagnostic workup period, and the manner in which the diagnosis is finally given have a major impact on the patient, the family and friends, and even the public at large.

RECEIVING THE DIAGNOSIS: PATIENTS' AND FAMILIES' RESPONSES

Despite the more open disclosure practices of American physicians and broad programs of public education to increase the awareness of cancer as curable or avoidable by lifestyle changes such as stopping smoking and watching the diet, cancer is still more dreaded than any of the other major life-threatening illnesses (Matthews et al., 1994). Krant (1976) suggests that this fear is due to the fact that people associate cancer not only with likely death but also with protracted pain and disability. Cancer "is equated with a withering away of life's essential elements, and is associated with foul smells, feelings of dirtiness, hopeless irrevocability, severe and relentless pain, and eventual death after weeks and months of this suffering" (p. 270).

Although very little research has addressed the question of people's reactions to a diagnosis of cancer, the many anecdotal reports and articles based on clinical experience paint a grim picture of shock, disbelief, fear, depression, sadness, and hopelessness (Hagopian, 1993; Krant, 1981). Fear and panic are the most common initial reactions at this time (Novotny, Hyland, Coyne, Travis, & Pruyner, 1984). The response to the cancer diagnosis has been described as similar to grief reactions often seen in the face of disaster or great threatened losses (Holland, 1976, 1986). This seems to be especially true when surgery is the recommended treatment, perhaps because of the threat of mutilation (Vettese, 1976). Loss of self-determination or of a sense of control can also accompany the intense emotional reactions (Fountain, 1985; Vettese, 1976), which in turn can lead to withdrawal, anxiety, and agitation (Giacquinta, 1977).

In one descriptive study of patients' reactions to their cancer diagnoses, Weisman and Worden (1976–1977) summarized the experience of 120 patients in the first 100 days after their diagnosis. They describe this time frame as the period of "existential plight in can-

cer." *Existential plight* consists of two substages: *impact distress* (the initial immediate response to the diagnosis) and *existential plight proper* (the first 3 to 4 months after diagnosis, which often includes patients' completion of primary treatment). During these 100 days, patients in Weisman and Worden's study completed a series of questionnaires and interviews, including standardized and investigator-developed instruments. Patients' responses indicated that this is a period of great emotional impact. However, the intensity and duration of the initial distress varied widely—from brief and transient discomfort to extreme and continuing anxiety, depression, anger, and desperation. These investigators noted that it was sometimes difficult to detect the level of distress from overt signs, an observation substantiated by other reports (Jamison, Wellisch, & Pasnau, 1978; Maguire, 1975, 1985).

During the initial period after diagnosis, Weisman and Worden found that patients' concerns focused more on existential issues of life and death than on any other of the areas assessed, including patients' health, work and finances, religion, self, and relationships with family and friends. Earlier, Benoliel (Quint, 1963) had made a similar observation of the primacy of existential concerns among women following mastectomy. In later studies, she and her colleagues (McCorkle & Benoliel, 1983) again reported findings consistent with Weisman and Worden's description.

Although it is not unusual, then, to observe extreme emotional reactions as the first response to a cancer diagnosis, it is nonetheless important to assess the nature of the patient's response carefully. Holland (1982) recommends that an assessment of psychologic and social resources be included as part of the medical history because the initial reactions are often predictive of later adjustment (Graydon, 1988; Morris, Greer, & White, 1977; Northouse, 1984; Weisman & Worden, 1976–1977) and can identify those persons at risk and in greatest need of psychosocial intervention (Weisman, Worden, & Sobel, 1980; Worden, 1983). Hagopian (1993) provides a basis for such an assessment in her review of some of the major issues patients consider in appraising the threat the cancer diagnosis represents (Box 18–1). Such assessments must be done with caution, however. Although a large proportion of patients retrospectively describe the diagnostic period as the most stressful of their entire cancer experience, many

---

Box 18–1. *Cognitive Strategies Used in Adapting to a Cancer Diagnosis*

Hagopian, G. A. (1993). Cognitive strategies used in adapting to a cancer diagnosis. *Oncology Nursing Forum, 20,* 759–763.

Adapting to a cancer diagnosis requires much time, energy, and effort. Patients, who often feel stressed and vulnerable, use several cognitive processes to help protect themselves and adapt to the illness. Denial, attributions, downward comparison, reappraisal of life, and developing a sense of mastery are some of the common emotion-focused strategies or cognitive processes used to allow patients to adapt to the disease and to a changed life. Before intervening, nurses must assess the presence of these processes and the intensity with which they are being used. Nursing interventions include cognitive restructuring, assisting with problem solving, giving information in small amounts, listening, and expressing care and concern.

did not or could not share their feelings with either family members or health professionals at the time (Jamison et al., 1978; Maguire, 1975, 1985). This may be an example of what Lazarus (1979) refers to as "positive denial," a coping strategy persons use to delay dealing consciously with the threat of a situation to be able to get through the situation. When newly diagnosed cancer patients appraise the diagnosis as demanding more coping abilities than they feel they can muster, positive denial allows them some time to gather their resources and reappraise the situation as more manageable. During the time they are using positive denial effectively, patients are not likely to be able to report the distress because they cannot allow themselves to think about it, in much the same way as persons who perform heroic deeds block out thoughts of danger so that they can carry out their acts of bravery. Later, upon reflection, cancer patients, like heroes, are able to provide a retrospective report of their intense distress, as seen in the studies noted earlier by Jamison and colleagues (1978) and Maguire (1975, 1985). This may explain why some investigators observe low levels of distress in the responses to questionnaires from newly diagnosed patients, contrary to expectations (Edlund & Sneed, 1989; Mood & Bickes, 1989). It suggests that the timing of assessments may be an important factor in the findings obtained. Age appears to be another important factor affecting this assessment as well, with younger persons (under 50 years old) showing more psychologic distress than older persons (over 70 years) (Edlund & Sneed, 1989).

Another common reaction at the time of diagnosis is the fear of abandonment (Fountain, 1985); patients often fear that they will lose the love and support of their family and friends. In turn, these "significant others" are frequently at a loss as to how to communicate effectively. Fears of discussing sensitive issues are common and can sometimes lead to a "conspiracy of silence" (Weisman & Hackett, 1961). Emotional reactions, physical symptoms, and treatment demands can disrupt the intimacy of the family and a couple's sexual relationship. Because of the significant impact of the cancer diagnosis on the persons closest to the patient, cancer is often described as a disease of the family system (Giacquinta, 1977; Lewandowski & Jones, 1988; Marino, 1981; Northouse, 1984, 1989; Weisman, 1979a; Woods, Lewis, & Ellison, 1989). Oncology nursing in particular often defines the family unit rather than the individual patient as the client. This is a critical distinction because the responses of the patient's significant others are critical to the patient's own response (Litman, 1974). As family system theory would suggest, when one family member makes a significant life transition, each of the other members must make his or her own parallel transition. Studies of the reactions of family members to the patient's cancer diagnosis are limited (Gotay, 1984; Northouse, 1984, 1989; Northouse, Jeffs, Cracchiolo-Caraway, Lampman, & Dorris, 1995). It has been reported that the family's concerns during this initial phase focus on providing support for the patient, on being assured that the patient is receiving the best possible care, and on gathering information to better understand what is happening (Dyck & Wright, 1985; Lewandowski & Jones, 1988). Often it is the family who is the first to be informed of the cancer diagnosis, and not uncommonly their initial reaction is to want to withhold the information from the patient. Holland (1976) suggests that this is a response to the family's own inability to accept the diagnosis. However, by the time the diagnosis is shared with the patient, the family has had some time to adjust to the initial shock.

Family members share the existential concerns of the patients as well as their own concerns about how their lives will change with the illness and possible death of the patient (Giacquinta, 1977; Northouse, 1989; Northouse et al., 1995). This experience can precipitate many dysfunctional family dynamics. Family members have some painful issues of their own to resolve. They need to find the time to support the ill member, take on added role responsibilities that the ill member is unable to fulfill, and still maintain their own life roles. They may experience emotions they find unacceptable. For example, they may feel relieved that they are not the one with the illness. They may resent some aspects of the patient's past behavior that they perceive to be a cause of the cancer (e.g., smoking). They also may experience anger toward the ill person for becoming ill and altering their lives. These are feelings that they will have difficulty acknowledging or sharing and will often need assistance to resolve. If the patient is a child, siblings will feel abandoned as parents spend long hours away from home and are not physically or emotionally able to meet their needs. Thus the impact of the cancer diagnosis is more far-reaching than the reactions of the patient alone.

Although reports in the literature clearly communicate the devastating emotional impact of a cancer diagnosis on the patient and family, some evidence suggests that, at times, there are positive reactions as well. First, as described earlier, Weisman and Worden's study (1976–1977) of patients' reactions during the first 100 days after diagnosis indicated that a significant proportion (50 to 60 per cent) of patients adjust well to their diagnosis and cope effectively without intervention. Investigators who have examined patients' reactions to cancer have found that many persons report positive coping strategies, such as taking firm action and finding something favorable about the situation (Gotay, 1984), maintaining optimism about the future and meaning in their lives (Mages et al., 1981), and having an active determination to recover (Hughes, 1982). It has been proposed that nursing interventions be designed to assist patients to redefine the threat of cancer diagnosis into one or more of these more positive appraisals (Hagopian, 1993). It has also been proposed that denial may have a beneficial effect, at least for a period of time, in assisting persons to cope effectively with a threatening situation (Forester, Kornfeld, & Fleiss, 1978; Lazarus, 1979; Watson et al., 1984). Frank-Stromborg and her associates (Stromborg, Wright, Segella, & Diekmann, 1984) reported that 27 per cent of the responses provided by 340 ambulatory cancer patients who were asked to recall their feelings after receiving their cancer diagnosis were classified as reflecting positive attitudes (e.g, "I decided to make the best of it" and "I decided to conquer the cancer"). In a later instrument development study, a sample of 441 ambulatory cancer patients in active treatment responded to a 36-item questionnaire assessing their reactions to their cancer diagnosis (Frank-Stromborg, 1989). The questionnaire contained both negative and positive items. Respondents readily endorsed the positive as well as negative items.

Thus it appears that responses to a diagnosis of cancer can be positive as well as negative. This raises some interesting questions that will need to be addressed in future research:

1. Are reports of devastating emotional reactions exaggerated, perhaps by observers' bias; that is, do professionals who expect patients to be devastated by a cancer diagnosis merely see what they expect to see? Alternatively, are the apparent positive reactions now being reported actually a form of denial that can be reported only retrospectively as emotionally traumatic?
2. Are attitudes toward cancer changing with greater openness and more public education and media attention? Will patients no longer receive reactions of disbelief when they share their cancer diagnosis and favorable prognosis with family and friends?
3. Do health care providers continue to give "mixed messages" to patients and family about the appropriateness of sharing feelings?

Oncology nursing research may be able to provide answers to these questions by accurately assessing patients' reactions over time, and by identifying some of the factors that predict or explain those reactions, and by testing the effectiveness of interventions designed to alleviate or effectively cope with the reactions to a cancer diagnosis.

The Meaning of the Diagnosis

There is increasing evidence that the human experience of receiving a diagnosis of cancer elicits a wide array of personal and social meanings. The process of seeking clinical confirmation for symptoms of a cancer diagnosis is characterized by a series of ambiguous situations. People are often unprepared for several aspects of the experience, including the urgency that surrounds the diagnostic workup, the new experience of being hospitalized and subjected to a series of diagnostic tests, and the eventual disclosure of the life-threatening diagnosis. Northouse et al. (1995) reported that women undergoing breast biopsy, the majority of which result in the diagnosis of benign disease, reported nearly three times more anxiety and two times more depression than the general population norms.

During the clinical diagnostic period, people may have limited access to information about their health condition. Many clinicians are guarded about the information they disclose until a substantive diagnosis is established. An alternative approach is to keep patients informed of the ongoing nature of the diagnostic experience. This approach would allow health professionals to minimize the uncertainty that is generated by a deficiency in information.

Building explanatory models of cancer during the early-phase centers on the process of transforming clinical knowledge into personal terms. People may search for the cause of their cancer. They may struggle with the question, "Why me?" It is an effort in which both the patient and the family members engage as each tries to understand what he or she is experiencing. Answers are sought to the questions of why this is happening to this person at this time. This search for meaning may represent a basic spiritual need (Highfield & Cason, 1983; Sodestrom & Martinson, 1987). Thus seeking the meaning of a cancer diagnosis represents a normal human response. It is an effort to find hope and purpose, sometimes through prayer (Miller, 1985; Sodestrom & Martinson, 1987). Within a nursing conceptual framework, patients and their families are exercising their self-care abilities (Hanucharurnkul, 1989; Orem, 1995).

The search for meaning has also been described as an attempt to use cognitive resources to gain intellectual mastery over the emotional reactions to the cancer process (Berckmann & Austin, 1993; Giacquinta, 1977; Lewandowski & Jones, 1988). People may formulate beliefs about how the illness works as a disease process, and they may gather information to estimate the severity of the illness condition. For family members, this search for meaning may also include an effort to reassure themselves that they are not subject to the same sources of vulnerability and therefore at great risk for developing cancer themselves. The meaning people ascribe to their diagnoses may even affect their bodies' response to their disease and treatment (Simonton et al., 1978).

Personal Meaning

Cognitive reappraisals are a key component of peoples' personal construction of the illness experience. Reappraisals lead to an interpretive change in personal meaning. When a person is confronted with illness, he or she must evolve and develop new "meaning" to understand and give order or coherence to life. This is often a period of profound reorganization of personal goals and priorities. Cognitive reappraisals also demonstrate the person's resilience to adapt to the adverse situation and the ability to construe some personal benefit from a tragic situation (Hagopian, 1993). Specifically, these reappraisals allow the person to assign positive meanings to the situation. Reappraisals such as "take things day by day," "appreciate each day to its fullest," and "there must be some purpose to this" are generated to redefine the situation so that some of its threatening aspects can be diminished. Another reappraisal strategy is for people to make social comparisons of their own situation with that of others who are living through similar experiences (Hagopian, 1993; Taylor, 1983). When a person takes notice that another patient with a similar diagnosis is not doing so well, *downward comparison* is used to enhance the first person's self-esteem. In contrast, an *upward compari-*

son allows the individual to emulate as a positive role model someone who is perceived as coping effectively.

SOCIAL MEANING

A number of social implications occur with the confirmation of the cancer diagnosis. As the person integrates a set of personal meanings about the experience, a self-identity evolves within a social environment. Additional meanings are derived from social transactions with others. One of the most difficult social interactions that occurs is the disclosure of the diagnosis to family and friends. It is not uncommon for the person to want to protect significant others from the devastating news. Giacquinta (1977) points out that this information may be shared prematurely, before the patient and the immediate family have had adequate opportunity to process the information and their initial reactions themselves. It is difficult, under these circumstances, to derive the support and sense of courage that can come when the social sharing is timed more appropriately.

CAUSAL ATTRIBUTIONS

Causal attributions are defined as naive perceptions or common-sense explanations for events or experiences (Berckman & Austin, 1993; Frieze & Bar-Tal, 1978). A growing body of research argues that people search for reasons why important and unexpected events happen. Such searching is carried out by persons attempting to understand their own life situations or by larger groups within society. The latter is sometimes called *research* and has resulted in causal attributions for cancer such as "smoking causes cancer" and "breast cancer is hereditary." The reasons we identify, both individually and collectively, are interpreted by each person, influencing the way the event is perceived. Causal search may be a necessary prerequisite for the full interpretation of the emotions linked to important events such as a diagnosis of cancer (Weiner, 1979). Additionally, expectations for the future are determined by the causal attributions of past events.

When people ask "Why me?" they are attempting to ascribe a cause to an event or an experience. Events that are considered stressful, those that are not expected, or situations in which the goal is not attained tend to prompt causal thinking. Taylor (1983) has proposed that one part of the coping process involves finding meaning in an event, such as a cancer diagnosis, and this search can involve a search for a cause.

Causal search, however, was not found to be related to adjustment in a sample of 78 women with breast cancer who were interviewed about 2 years after their operations (Taylor, Lichtman, & Wood, 1984). The responses about causal thinking were prompted by a question asking subjects to share their hunches or theories about how they got their cancer. Patients' recollections about when causal thinking occurred in relation to time of diagnosis, and patients' beliefs about the controllability of their cancer were assessed, as were the patients' psychologic and overall adjustments. Patients also were asked to rate their agreement with 22 potential causes listed on a questionnaire.

Although 95 per cent of subjects eventually ascribed a cause, few patients (28 per cent) reported making attributions at the time of diagnosis, with 71 per cent indicating that causal thinking was not important at that time. During recovery and at the time of the study, 41 per cent believed causal thinking was important. Adjustment was generally unrelated to the specific causes either from the interview or from the attributional questionnaire. No attempt was made to relate these findings to variables such as patient delay (Taylor et al., 1984).

Gotay (1984) also found that neither the process of causal search nor the specific attribution was related to adjustment. She interviewed 42 early-stage gynecologic patients within 2 weeks of their cancer diagnosis and 31 advanced-stage gynecologic or breast patients who had been diagnosed from several months to 10 years before the interview. Subjects were asked if they had ever asked "Why me?" with respect to cancer and, if so, what answer they reached. A structured attributional measure also was used, which asked subjects to assign a percentage of blame to four factors: "yourself; the kind of person you are," "things you have done," "the environment and other people," and "chance."

In response to the open-ended question, 26 (62 per cent) early-stage and 16 (52 per cent) advanced-stage patients indicated they had asked "Why me?". "Chance" was the most common response of early-stage subjects, and "God's will" was identified most commonly by advanced-stage patients. Chance was also the most common attribution in the structured survey, with 64 per cent of early-stage patients and 56 per cent of advanced-stage subjects choosing that response. It is interesting to note that all patients, including the 42 per cent who either had not asked "Why me?" or had asked it and failed to answer it, chose an attribution on the structured questionnaire. Gotay (1984) reached a somewhat different conclusion than Taylor and colleagues (1984). She interpreted her findings to mean that patients may avoid making connections between cancer and its perceived causes because of the frightening nature of the disease. This interpretation is supported in a study of patients with cancers of the head and neck. Patients were significantly less willing to endorse items reflecting personal responsibility for their cancer than similarly worded items that addressed their health in general, despite the fact that for most of them, smoking and excessive use of alcohol are major causative factors. The cancer-specific items may have been more threatening (Mood & Parzuchowski, 1986).

Berckman and Austin (1993) introduced the concept of perceived control into their study of causal attribution and adjustment in patients with lung cancer. They found that perceived control, which they defined as the belief that a cognitive strategy could change an aversive event, was positively correlated with both internal and external causal attributions, but not with adjustment. Contrary to Taylor et al. (1984) and Gotay (1984), Berckman and Austin did find significant, but negative, correlations between both internal and external causal attribution and various aspects of adjustment. However, the magnitude of these relationships was small.

Thus whereas the search for meaning has been described as a universal response to a cancer diagnosis, the specific focus on causal attributions is not, especially at the time of diagnosis. Only 28 per cent of patients in the study by Taylor and associates (1984) and 62 per cent of the early-stage patients in the Gotay study (1984) reported making such inferences early in their cancer experience. Furthermore, whether or not they attempted such attribution and regardless of the causes they identified, little relationship was found between these factors and various measures of coping and adjustment.

In summary, then, the diagnostic stage of the transition to becoming a person with cancer is a difficult and emotional one for all persons involved. Physicians, nurses, and other health professionals struggle with issues of how best to carry out the complicated diagnostic workup, balancing the desire to avoid unnecessary anxiety for patients with the patient's right to a fair and accurate description of what is being done. Patients and their families, during the diagnostic workup period, struggle with the uncertainties and ambiguities of what is readily recognized as an unusual process. If they are aware that a cancer diagnosis is the probable or even likely outcome of this process, they have already begun the period of existential plight, with its intense concern for life and death matters.

With the completion of the diagnostic workup, the professionals confront the challenge of disclosing the cancer diagnosis to the patient and family. This can raise many anxieties in the professional, who has often learned to cope with these feelings by suppressing them. In the process, many professionals develop styles of talking to patients that involve little feeling or empathy. Patients and their families, in turn, often are unable to show or communicate their intense emotional reactions, which are the signs of the initial impact of the diagnosis.

Although most patients experience an initial reaction of shock, fear, and anxiety, many find the actual diagnosis to be a relief from the previous uncertainty. Knowing what they face, they are now able to draw on their personal and social resources as they reappraise their situation. In their search for meaning, they find strengths in themselves and those around them as well as challenges in the experience. At this point, they are ready to complete the transition by entering the last stage and making plans for their treatment.

PLANNING FOR TREATMENT

With the firm establishment of the cancer diagnosis, the planning for treatment begins. If patients have been given a clear understanding of their condition while being encouraged to maintain hope, the initial reaction of shock, fear, and desperation can give way to a sense of optimism at this time (Holland, 1982). Most patients understand that the first course of treatment offers the best chance for cure or durable remission. Any sense of "fighting spirit" or determination to "beat the cancer" can be seen most prominently at this time.

The three major treatment options are surgery, chemotherapy, and radiation therapy. These methods may be used alone, concurrently or sequentially, or in combination with other forms of therapy such as immunotherapy. Some evidence suggests that both individual and group psychotherapy or counseling and various types of other nonmedical interventions may also be beneficial when used in combination with the traditional medical interventions (Bellert, 1989; Cousins, 1979; Mast, Meyers, & Urbanski, 1987; Siegel, 1986; Simonton et al., 1978). Whatever therapeutic regimen is planned, however, the most critical factors in patient care at this time are keeping them informed and actively participating in their own care and helping them to cope with the demands of the disease and its treatment (Mood & Bickes, 1989; Mood, Templin, & Marcil, 1995). Helping patients to understand that they have treatment alternatives and to evaluate the risk-benefit ratios of those alternatives is important. Personal, nonmedical factors will need to be weighed against survival statistics and physical side effects in determining the relative risks and benefits (Valanis & Rumpler, 1985). For example, body image may be the critical variable in a woman's decision to elect lumpectomy with radiation therapy over mastectomy for the treatment of her early-stage breast cancer.

Treatment planning is also a time when patients' readiness to cooperate and endure even pain and discomfort are at their highest point (Holland, 1982). It is an especially suitable time for patient teaching and preparation for self-care, before the side effects of treatment, the adjustment demands of the disease, and the recurring anxieties about living and dying return. At this point, persons who just days or weeks ago had no awareness of the silent biologic changes taking place in their bodies have now made the critical life transition through the personal discovery of themselves as a *person with cancer*.

NURSING IMPLICATIONS

Nursing's role in facilitating this first critical transition in the cancer experience is carried out at three levels: *direct care* to persons involved in making this transition; *indirect care* to other clients through patient education and cancer risk assessment; and *self-care* in the recognition, assessment, and resolution of the nurse's own unhealthy or negative attitudes in working and living with cancer.

DIRECT CLIENT CARE

The first opportunity to provide direct patient care occurs when the person with symptoms comes to the health care system. The initial stage of the diagnostic process often involves a series of clinical assessments and laboratory procedures. This battery of tests can be quite complex and frightening to the patient and the family. Ambiguity and uncertainty are high. One of the important interventions the nurse can provide at this time is to review the diagnostic test battery with the patient and family, describing each of the procedures to be followed, the time demands each procedure will require, the order in which the procedures will be done, any special preparation the patient needs to make in advance of the procedures, the discomforts that might accompany any of the tests, and any self-care measures or suggestions that might facilitate the patient's adjustment to the experience. Unless it is contraindicated, the purpose of each test and what information will be gained by the test should also be given. Providing an opportunity for patients to preview the laboratories where large unfamiliar equipment is to be used is very helpful. This can be accomplished either by a visit to the laboratory or through visual aids. Also, it has repeatedly been demonstrated that information on sensation (i.e., descriptions of what patients can expect to experience through the senses of sight, hearing, smell, taste, and touch) is an important and beneficial element in preparatory information (Johnson & Leventhal, 1974; Johnson, Rice, Fuller, & Endress, 1978). Preparatory information can help familiarize the patient with what to expect and reduce the *fear of the unknown* (Mood, Cook, & Chadwell, 1988). It can also assist patients and family members to recognize that fear is a normal reaction to the threatening experiences they are having.

Encouraging a family member or friend to participate in preparatory information sessions can have many benefits. First of all, it sets a model for collaboration between patient and significant others that encourages communication and coping with the demands of the experience. It also allows the nurse to meet other important persons in the patient's life and gain greater insight into the patient's level of coping and available resources. Finally, because the increased anxiety typically experienced at this time is likely to reduce the patient's ability to assimilate the information, it is helpful to have someone close to the patient also hear what is said. This associate can then assist the patient in reviewing, recalling, and applying the content as needed through the complex set of procedures. Preparatory information provided by the nurse is helpful even if it is a review of information already given by other members of the professional team. Again, most likely because of disruptions in the patient's cognitive functioning, a good deal of information is lost on first hearing. A review by the nurse can significantly increase the amount of information the patient recalls (Dodd & Mood, 1981). Recommendations for oncology nurses preparing educational programs for newly diagnosed patients have been provided in the literature (Anderson, 1989; Derdiarian, 1987a, 1987b; Mood et al., 1988). Determining patients' and family members' reasons for wanting information (e.g., preparing for a procedure versus reducing anxiety) may also assist nurses to tailor the message (Hinds, Streater, & Mood, in press).

The period of the diagnostic workup is especially delicate psychologically. The nurse, as well as the other members of the professional team, must strike a balance between honesty on the one hand and premature diagnosis on the other. When a cancer diagnosis is in doubt, it does not serve the client well to emphasize that particular possibility. At the other extreme, when cancer is a virtual certainty and the diagnostic battery is being run to determine the exact nature of the disease

or the extent of spread, then refusing to mention cancer serves no useful purpose for the client. Nurses can assist with clarifying information about treatment alternatives and treatment expectations. Persons with cancer should be allowed to participate in the choices and decisions regarding the treatment of their illness and how it will affect their lives and the lives of their families (McCorkle & Germino, 1984; Northouse, in press; Valanis & Rumpler, 1985). Assisting the client to maintain a sense of optimism and hopefulness is essential under any circumstance. This is sometimes best achieved by responding to the client's spiritual needs (Highfield & Cason, 1983; Miller, 1985; Sodestrom & Martinson, 1987).

Once the patient and family receive the formal diagnosis, the nurse can play a major role in assisting them to respond effectively to this crisis. This often involves listening carefully to the patients' and family members' perceptions of what their needs are. It has been shown repeatedly that these needs are not always what the nurse thinks they are (Dyck & Wright, 1985; Larson, 1987; Young-Brockapp, 1982). Giacquinta (1977) identifies five goals for nursing intervention during this stage: fostering *hope* to meet the hurdle of despair, fostering *cohesion* in response to a sense of isolation, fostering *security* against the feelings of vulnerability, fostering *courage* to deal with the crisis first within the family and then with others outside the immediate circle, and fostering *problem-solving skills* to cope with the sense of helplessness. Treating the family as the client will give the patient the benefit of a supportive environment at home, where most of the patient's day-to-day living will occur (Litman, 1974), in addition to the hospital, clinic, or other treatment facility where the professional team provides care.

INDIRECT PATIENT CARE

In addition to the nursing care provided directly to patients and their families as they begin their cancer experience, nurses in many different settings can indirectly assist with the first transition in a number of ways. First of all, nurses play an active role in public education regarding health promotion and cancer prevention. As patient educators, nurses teach all kinds of persons in all kinds of settings about lifestyle choices and lifestyle changes that can reduce cancer risks and improve health in general. Early diagnosis is a major point to be made in this context. The fact that cancer can be a curable disease is an important message. Nurses also teach the various self-examination techniques for both men and women, such as testicular or breast self-examination (BSE). Introducing more men and women to the use of these easy practices, developing teaching strategies that communicate the simplicity of their use in addition to their importance, and helping persons who do practice the techniques to understand the importance of taking action immediately on finding any suspicious sign or symptom are nursing actions that could have a major impact on what stage some cancers are in at the time of diagnosis. Nurses are in a position to provide cancer education programs in occupational and community settings (Crooks & Jones, 1989; Frank-Stromborg, 1988) as well as to friends, family, professional colleagues, and students (Post-White et al., 1993). School nurses teaching these techniques to high school—or even junior high school—boys and girls could produce future generations of adults for whom these cancer detection practices are as common as brushing teeth.

In addition to general public education, nurses can use their interactions with the clients they see for other purposes as opportunities for cancer risk assessment. The one-to-one interaction in the nurse-client contact is a superior basis for discussing lifestyle changes and planning individualized programs that may be suitable for that particular client. For example, determining a woman's willingness and ability to do BSE cannot easily be achieved across a stage when addressing an audience; it can be approached more readily when providing maternity care or administering a flu shot.

Especially important in the one-to-one contacts that nurses have with clients is the cancer risk assessment and the identification of factors that might predict who is likely to delay seeking diagnosis if symptoms do appear. The woman with a family history of breast cancer needs more careful assessment and education regarding her increased risk. Obese persons need to know that they increase their risk of cancer in addition to their other health risks by not decreasing their fat intake. However, the nurse also needs to be aware that overweight persons may also be at greater risk for delay in seeking health care advice when symptoms occur if they are generally embarrassed or self-conscious about their bodies. Similarly, people with a fierce sense of individualism may be as likely to delay seeking care as the denier or the fearful procrastinator (Weisman, 1979a). Nurses who identify clients who might fit any of these patterns can be alert to signs of concern, or they can take a more aggressive stance in alerting the client to the dangers of delay. Through assessment of cancer risk and assessment of risk for delay, nurses can indirectly promote their clients' initial transitions should they have to confront the cancer experience.

PROFESSIONAL SELF-CARE

The third level at which nurses can help their clients is thorough self-assessment and resolution of their own fears and negative attitudes toward cancer. Nurses are, after all, members of the society at large and as such carry with them many of the culturally shared values and attitudes. Often, negative attitudes can go unrecognized because they are shared by so many people around them. In a study of nurses' attitudes toward death, the nurses often mentioned cancer and projected how they might handle the situation if they themselves had cancer (Mood et al., 1985). It was clear that, like the public at large, many nurses shared the belief that a cancer diagnosis is a death sentence; that it would be one of the worst possible ways to die; and that if they were so unfortunate as to have cancer themselves, they would forego any therapy and let "nature take its course." Nurses employed on oncology units were as likely to express these negative attitudes toward cancer as their nononcology colleagues. It must be asked what effect these attitudes may have on the care these nurses provide to their patients. Can the nurse who is so fearful of cancer discuss cancer openly with a patient? Does the nurse use linguistic devices of avoidance and inadvertently communicate high levels of anxiety to patients (Mood, 1980; Mood et al., 1985)? At present, these questions have not been adequately studied. However, it is likely that the nurse who is fearful of cancer, its treatment, and its sequelae will not be able to provide the best nursing care.

The solution to this problem lies in its recognition. Taking an introspective approach and assessing one's own feelings and attitudes about cancer is the important first step. No one has to maintain a false professional demeanor in the privacy of his or her own thoughts. It is a measure of professionalism to engage in self-assessment. If areas needing attention are recognized, seeking the information, peer support, or counseling necessary to resolve the fears and apprehensions will lead to a transition for the nurse, and the end result will be a person who can provide optimal oncology nursing care for clients at any stage of the cancer experience.

REFERENCES

Aitken-Swan, J., & Easson, E. (1959). Reactions of cancer patients on being told their diagnosis. *British Medical Journal, 1,* 779–783.

American Cancer Society. (1989). A summary of the American Cancer Society report to the nation: Cancer in the poor. *CA: Cancer Journal for Clinicians, 39,* 263–265.

Anderson, J. L. (1989). The nurse's role in cancer rehabilitation: Review of the literature. *Cancer Nursing, 12,* 85–94.

Bellert, J. L. (1989). A therapeutic approach in oncology nursing. *Cancer Nursing, 12,* 65–70.

Berckman, K. L., & Austin, J. K. (1993). Causal attribution, perceived control, and adjustment in patients with lung cancer. *Oncology Nursing Forum, 20,* 23–30.

Boring, C. C., Squires, T. S., & Heath, C. W. (1992). Cancer statistics for African-Americans. *CA -A Cancer Journal for Clinicians, 42,* 7–17.

Borysenko, J. Z. (1982). Behavioral-physiological factors in the development and management of cancer. *General Hospital Psychiatry, 4,* 69–74.

Castles, M. R., & Murray, R. (1979). *Dying in an institution.* New York: Appleton-Century-Crofts.

Chrisman, N. J., & Kleinman, A. (1980). Health beliefs and practices. In S. Thernstrom, A. Orlov, & O. Handlin, (Eds.), *Harvard encyclopedia of American ethnic groups.* Cambridge: Harvard University Press.

Comaroff, J., & Maguire, P. (1981). Ambiguity and the search for meaning: Childhood leukemia in the modern clinical context. *Social Science and Medicine, 15,* 115–123.

Cox, C. (1982). Interaction model of client health behavior: Theoretical prescription for nursing. *Advances in Nursing Science, 5*(1), 41–56.

Crooks, C. E., & Jones, S. D. (1989). Educating women about the importance of breast screenings: The nurse's role. *Cancer Nursing, 12,* 161–164.

Cousins, N. (1979). *Anatomy of an illness as perceived by the patient.* New York: W. W. Norton.

Cunningham, A. J. (1985). The influence of mind on cancer. *Canadian Psychology, 26,* 13–29.

Derdiarian, A. (1987a). Informational needs of recently diagnosed cancer patients: A theoretical framework. Part I. *Cancer Nursing, 10,* 107–115.

Derdiarian, A. (1987b). Informational needs of recently diagnosed cancer patients: Method and description. Part II. *Cancer Nursing, 10,* 156–163.

Dodd, M. J., & Mood, D. W. (1981). Chemotherapy: Helping patients to know the drugs they are receiving and their possible side effects. *Cancer Nursing, 4,* 311–318.

Dyck, S., & Wright, K. (1985). Family perceptions: The role of the nurse throughout an adult's cancer experience. *Oncology Nursing Forum, 12,* 53–56.

Edlund, B., & Sneed, N. V. (1989). Emotional responses to the diagnosis of cancer: Age-related comparisons. *Oncology Nursing Forum, 16,* 691–697.

EVAXX, Inc. (1981). *A study of black Americans' attitudes toward cancer and cancer tests.* New York: American Cancer Society.

Forester, B. M., Kornfeld, D. S., & Fleiss, J. (1978). Psychiatric aspects of radiotherapy. *American Journal of Psychiatry, 135,* 960–963.

Fountain, M. J. (1985). Psychosocial support for the person experiencing cancer. *Orthopedic Nursing, 4,* 33–35.

Fox, B. H. (1983). Current theory of psychogenic effects on cancer incidence and prognosis. *Journal of Psychosocial Oncology, 1,* 17–31.

Frank-Stromborg, M. (1986). The role of the nurse in early detection of cancer: Population 66 years of age and older. *Oncology Nursing Forum, 13,* 107–115.

Frank-Stromborg, M. (1988). Nursing's role in cancer prevention and detection: Vital contributions to attainment of the Year 2000 goals. *Cancer, 62,* 1833–1838.

Frank-Stromborg, M. (1989). Reaction to the diagnosis of cancer questionnaire (RDCQ): Development and psychometric evaluation. *Nursing Research, 38,* 364–369.

Freeman, H. P., & Wasfie, T. J. (1989). Cancer of the breast in poor black women. *Cancer, 63,* 2562–2569.

Frieze, I., & Bar-Tal, D. (1978). Attribution theory: Past and present. In I. H. Frieze, D. Bar-Tal, & J. S. Carroll (Eds.), *New approaches to social problems.* San Francisco: Jossey-Bass Publishers.

Funch, D. P. (1985). The role of patient delay in the evaluation of breast self-examination. *Journal of Psychosocial Oncology, 2(3),* 31–39.

Funch, D. P., & Francis, A. M. (1982). Issues in the early detection and rehabilitation of breast cancer patients. In C. Mettlin & G. P. Murphy (Eds.), *Issues in cancer screening and communications* (pp. 219–229). New York: Alan R. Liss, Inc.

Germino, B., & McCorkle, R. (1985). Acknowledged awareness of life-threatening illness. *International Journal of Nursing Studies, 22,* 33–44.

Giacquinta, B. (1977). Helping families face the crisis of cancer. *American Journal of Nursing, 77,* 1585–1588.

Given, B., & Given, C. W. (1989). Cancer nursing for the elderly: A target for research. *Cancer Nursing, 12,* 71–77.

Gold, M. A. (1964). Causes of patient delay in diseases of the breast. *Cancer, 17,* 564–577.

Gotay, C. C. (1984). The experience of cancer during early and advanced stages: The views of patients and their mates. *Social Science and Medicine, 18,* 605–613.

Gould-Martin, K., Paganini-Hill, A., Casagrande, C., Mack, T., & Ross, R. K. (1982). Behavioral and biological determinants of surgical stage of breast cancer. *Preventive Medicine, 11,* 429–440.

Graydon, J. E. (1988). Factors that predict patients' functioning following treatment for cancer. *International Journal of Nursing Studies, 25,* 117–124.

Greer, S. (1974). Psychological aspects: Delays in the diagnosis of breast cancer. *Proceedings of the Royal Society of Medicine, 67,* 470–479.

Greer, S., & Morris, T. (1975). Psychological attributes of women who develop breast cancer: A controlled study. *Journal of Psychosomatic Research, 19,* 147–153.

Hackett, T. P., Cassem, N. H., & Raker, J. W. (1973). Patient delay in cancer. *New England Journal of Medicine, 289,* 14–20.

Hagopian, G. A. (1993). Cognitive strategies used in adapting to a cancer diagnosis. *Oncology Nursing Forum, 20,* 759–763.

Hammerschlag, C. A., Fisher, S., De Cosser, F., & Kaplan, E. (1964). Breast symptoms and patient delay: Psychological variables involved. *Cancer, 17,* 1480–1485.

Hanucharurnkul, S. (1989). Predictors of self-care in cancer patients receiving radiotherapy. *Cancer Nursing, 12,* 21–27.

Highfield, M. F., & Cason, C. (1983). Spiritual needs of patients: Are they recognized? *Cancer Nursing, 6,* 187–192.

Hinds, C., Streater, A., & Mood, D. (in press). Functions and preferred methods of receiving information related to radiotherapy: Perceptions of cancer patients. *Cancer Nursing.*

Holland, J. C. (1976). Coping with cancer: A challenge to the behavioral sciences. In J. W. Cullen, B. H. Fox, & R. N. Isom (Eds.), *Cancer: The behavioral dimensions.* New York: Raven Press.

Holland, J. C. (1982). Psychologic aspects of cancer. In J. C. Holland & E. Frei III (Eds.), *Cancer medicine* (pp. 1175–1184). Philadelphia: Lea & Febiger.

Holland, J. C. (1986). Doctors should be aware of patients' emotional responses to cancer. *Oncology Times, 8(4),* 1.

Holmes, F., & Hearne, E. (1981). Cancer stage-to-age relationships: Implications for cancer screening in the elderly. *Journal of the American Geriatric Society, 19,* 55–57.

Houts, P. S., Harvey, H. A., Simmonds, M. A., Marshall, M., Gottlieb, R., Lipton, A., Martin, B. A., Dixon, R. H., Gelman, E. S., & Valdevia, D. (1985). Characteristics of patients at risk for financial burden because of cancer and its treatment. *Journal of Psychosocial Oncology, 3(2),* 15–22.

Hughes, J. (1982). Emotional reactions to the diagnosis and treatment of early breast cancer. *Journal of Psychosomatic Research, 26,* 277–281.

Israel, L. (1978). *Conquering cancer.* New York: Random House.

Jamison, J. R., Wellisch, D. K., & Pasnau, R. P. (1978). Psychological aspects of mastectomy. I. The woman's perspective. *American Journal of Psychiatry, 135,* 432–436.

Johnson, J. E., & Leventhal, H. (1974). Effects of accurate expectations and behavioral instructions on reactions during a noxious medical examination. *Journal of Personality and Social Psychology, 29,* 710–718.

Johnson, J. E., Rice, V. H., Fuller, S. S., & Endress, M. P. (1978). Sensory information instruction in a coping strategy and recovery from surgery. *Research in Nursing and Health, 1,* 4–17.

Kegeles, S. S. (1969). A field experimental attempt to change beliefs and behavior of women in an urban ghetto. *Journal of Health and Social Behavior, 10,* 115–124.

Krant, M. J. (1976). Problems of the physician in presenting the patient with the diagnosis. In J. W. Cullen, B. H. Fox, & R. N. Isom (Eds.), *Cancer: The behavioral dimensions* (pp. 269–274). New York: Raven Press.

Krant, M. J. (1981). Psychosocial impact of gynecological cancer. *Cancer, 48,* 608–612.

Lambert, V. A., & Lambert, C. E. (1979). *The impact of physical illness.* Englewood Cliffs, NJ: Prentice-Hall, Inc.

Larson, P. J. (1987). Comparison of cancer patients' and professional nurses' perceptions of important nurse caring behaviors. *Heart and Lung, 16,* 187–192.

Lauver, D. (1994). Care-seeking behavior with breast cancer symptoms in Caucasian and African-American women. *Nursing in Research and Health, 17,* 421–431.

Lazarus, R. S. (1979, November). Positive denial: The case for not facing reality. *Psychology Today,* pp. 44–60.

Leis, H., & Pilnik, S. (1974). Breast cancer: A therapeutic dilemma. *AORN Journal, 19,* 813–820.

LeShan, L. (1966). An emotional life history associated with neoplastic disease. *Annals of the New York Academy of Science, 125,* 780–795.

Levy, S. M. (1985). *Behavior and cancer: Lifestyle and psychosocial factors in the initiation and progression of cancer.* San Francisco: Jossey-Bass.

Lewandowski, W., & Jones, S. L. (1988). The family with cancer. *Cancer Nursing, 11,* 313–321.

Lewis, F. M., & Bloom, J. R. (1978–1979). Psychosocial adjustment to breast cancer: A review of selected literature. *International Journal of Psychiatry in Medicine, 9,* 1–17.

Lierman, L. M. (1988). Discovery of breast changes: Women's responses and nursing implications. *Cancer Nursing, 11,* 352–361.

Litman, T. J. (1974). The family as a basic unit in health and medical care: A social-behavioral overview. *Social Science and Medicine, 8,* 495–519.

Long, E. (1993). Breast cancer in African-American women: Review of the literature. *Cancer Nursing, 16,* 1–24.

Magarey, C. J., Todd, P. B., & Blizard, P. J. (1977). Psychosocial factors influencing delay and breast self-examination in women with symptoms of breast cancer. *Social Science and Medicine, 11,* 229–232.

Mages, N. L., Castro, J. R., Fobair, P., Hall, J., Harrison, I., Mendelsohn, G., & Wolfson, A. (1981). Patterns of psychosocial response to cancer: Can effective adaptation be predicted? *International Journal of Radiation Oncology Biology Physics, 7,* 385–392.

Maguire, P. G. (1975). The psychological and social consequences of breast cancer. *Nursing Mirror, 140,* 54–57.

Maguire, P. (1985). The psychological impact of cancer. *British Journal of Hospital Medicine, 34,* 100–103.

Marino, L. (1981). *Cancer nursing.* St. Louis: C. V. Mosby Co.

Marshall, J. R., & Funch, D. P. (1986). Gender and illness behavior among colorectal cancer patients. *Women and Health, 11,* 67–82.

Mast, D., Meyers, J., & Urbanski, A. (1987). Relaxation techniques: A self-learning module for nurses: Unit I. *Cancer Nursing, 10,* 141–147.

Matthews, H. F., Lannin, D. R., & Mitchell, J. P. (1994). Coming to terms with advanced breast cancer: Black women's narratives from eastern North Carolina. *Social Science Medicine, 38,* 789–800.

McCorkle, R. (1989). Women and cancer. In R. Tiffany (Ed.), *Oncology for nurses and health care professionals* (2nd ed., Vol. 2, pp. 281–292). London: Harper & Row, Publishers.

McCorkle, R., & Benoliel, J. Q. (1983). Symptom distress, current concerns, and mood disturbance after diagnosis of life-threatening disease. *Social Science and Medicine, 17,* 431–438.

McCorkle, R., & Germino, B. (1984). What nurses need to know about home care. *Oncology Nursing Forum, 12,* 63–69.

Mechanic, D. (1972). Social psychological factors affecting the presentation of bodily complaints. *New England Journal of Medicine, 286,* 1132–1139.

Mettlin, C., Reese, P., & Murphy, G. P. (1980). Care-seeking behavior among positive screenees. *Preventive Medicine, 9,* 518–524.

Miller, J. F. (1985). Inspiring hope. *American Journal of Nursing, 85,* 22–25.

Mood, D. W. (1980). Linguistic indicators of attitudes toward death and dying: A measure of denial? In M. A. Simpson (Ed.), *Psycholinguistics in clinical practice* (pp. 260–291). New York: Irvington Press.

Mood, D. W., & Bickes, J. T. (1989). Strategies to enhance self-care in radiation therapy. *Oncology Nursing Forum, 16*(Suppl.), 143.

Mood, D. W., Brenner, P. S., & Richardson, C. (1985). *Linguistic indicators of nurses' attitudes toward aging and dying.* Paper presented at the Eighth Annual Research Symposium, Sigma Theta Tau, Ann Arbor, MI.

Mood, D. W., Cook, C. A., & Chadwell, D. K. (1988). Increasing patients' knowledge of radiation therapy. *International Journal of Radiation Oncology Biology Physics, 15,* 989–993.

Mood, D. W., & Parzuchowski, J. (1986). Health and illness versions of the Multidimensional Health Locus of Control scales. Proceedings of the Great Lakes Oncology Nursing Conference, Lansing, MI.

Mood, D. W., Templin, T., & Marcil, L. (1995, March). *Using contingency contracting to maintain nutritional status in head and neck cancer.* (Poster session.) Presented at the 16th Annual Meeting of the Society of Behavioral Medicine, San Diego, CA.

Mood, D. W., & Van Fossen, M. (1983). *Assessment of children's development of the concept of death.* Annual report, Nursing Research Emphasis Grant, Wayne State University, Detroit, MI.

Morris, T., & Greer, S. (1980). A "Type C" for cancer? Low trait anxiety in the pathogenesis of breast cancer [Abstract 102]. *Cancer Detection and Prevention, 3,* 114.

Morris, T., Greer, S., & White, P. (1977). Psychological and social adjustment to mastectomy. *Cancer, 40,* 2381–2387.

National Cancer Institute. (1986) *Cancer among blacks and other minorities: Statistical profile* (NIH Publication No. 86-2785). Bethesda, MD: National Institutes of Health.

National Center for Health Statistics. (1986). Use of selected preventive care procedures, United States, 1982. *Vital and health statistics.* Series 10, #157 (U.S. Department of Health and Human Services, Publication No. (PHS) 86-1585. Public Health Service). Washington, DC: U.S. Government Printing Office.

Northouse, L. (1984). The impact of cancer on the family: An overview. *International Journal of Psychiatry in Medicine, 14,* 215–242.

Northouse, L. (1989). A longitudinal study of the adjustment of patients and husba6nds to breast cancer. *Oncology Nursing Forum, 16,* 511–516.

Northouse, L. L., Jeffs, M., Cracchiolo-Caraway, A., Lampman, L., & Dorris, G. (1995). Emotional distress reported by women and husbands prior to a breast biopsy. *Nursing Research, 44,* 196–201.

Novack, D. H., Plumer, R., Smith, R. L., Ochitill, H., Morrow, G. R., & Bennett, J. M. (1979). Changes in physicians' attitudes toward telling the cancer patient. *Journal of the American Medical Association, 241,* 897–900.

Novotny, E., Hyland, J., Coyne, L., Travis, J., & Pruyner, H. (1984). Factors affecting adjustment to cancer. *Bulletin of the Menninger Clinic, 48,* 318–328.

Oken, D. (1961). What to tell cancer patients: A study of medical attitudes. *Journal of the American Medical Association, 175,* 1120–1128.

Olsen, S. J., & Frank-Stromborg, M. (1994). Cancer prevention and screening activities reported by African-American nurses. *Oncology Nursing Forum, 21,* 487–494.

Orem, D. E. (Ed.). (1995). *Nursing: Concepts of practice* (5th ed.). St. Louis: C.V. Mosby Co.

Owens, R. G., Duffy, J. E., & Ashcroft, J. J. (1985). Women's response to detection of breast lumps: A British study. *Health Education Journal, 44,* 69–70.

Post-White, J., Carter, M., & Anglism, M. A. (1993). Cancer prevention and early detection: Nursing students' knowledge, attitudes, personal practices, and teaching. *Oncology Nursing Forum, 20,* 743–749.

Quint, J. C. (1963). The impact of mastectomy. *American Journal of Nursing, 63,* 88–92.

Rosenstock, J. M. (1974). Historical origins of the Health Belief Model. *Health Education Monographs, 2,* 328–335.

Salloway, J. C., & Dillon, P. B. (1973). A comparison of family networks and friend networks in health care utilization. *Journal of Community Family Studies, 4,* 131–141.

Saunders, J. M., & McCorkle, R. (1985). Models of care for persons with progressive cancer. *Nursing Clinics of North America, 20,* 365–377.

Siegel, B. S. (1986). *Love, medicine, and miracles.* New York: Harper & Row Publishers, Inc.

Simonton, O. C., Matthews-Simonton, S., & Creighton, J. L. (1978). *Getting well again.* New York: Bantam Books.

Sodestrom, K. E., & Martinson, I. M. (1987). Patients' spiritual coping strategies: A study of nurse and patient perspectives. *Oncology Nursing Forum, 14,* 41–46.

Stams, H. J., & Steggles, S. (1987). Predicting the onset or progression of cancer from psychological characteristics: Psychometric and theoretical issues. *Journal of Psychosocial Oncology, 5*(2), 35–46.

Stromborg, M., Wright, P., Segalla, M., & Diekmann, J. (1984). Psychological impact of the cancer diagnosis. *Oncology Nursing Forum, 11,* 16–22.

Taylor, S. E. (1983, November). Adjustment to threatening events: A theory of cognitive adaptation. *American Psychologist,* pp. 1161–1173.

Taylor, S. E., Lichtman, R. R., & Wood, J. V. (1984). Attributions, beliefs about control, and adjustment to breast cancer. *Journal of Personality and Social Psychology, 46,* 489–502.

Thomas, C. B., & Greenstreet, R. L. (1973). Psychobiological characteristics in youth as predictors of five disease states: Suicide, mental illness, hypertension, coronary heart disease and tumor. *Johns Hopkins Medical Journal, 132,* 16–43.

U.S. Department of Health and Human Services (1986). *Report of the Secretary's task force on black and minority health.* Vol IV. Cancer. Washington, DC: U.S. Government Publications Office.

Valanis, B. G., & Rumpler, C. H. (1985). Helping women to choose breast cancer treatment alternatives. *Cancer Nursing, 8,* 167–175.

Verbrugge, L. M. (1979a). Female illness rates and illness behavior: Testing hypotheses about sex differences in health. *Women and Health, 4,* 61–79.

Verbrugge, L. M. (1979b). Marital status and health. *Marriage and Family, 41,* 267–285.

Verbrugge, L. M. (1982). Sex differentials in health. *Public Health Report, 97,* 417–437.

Vernon, S. W., Telley, B. C., Neale, A. V., & Sternfeldt, L. (1985). Ethnicity, survival, and delay in seeking treatment for symptoms of breast cancer. *Cancer, 55,* 1563–1571.

Vettese, J. M. (1976). Problems of the patient confronting the diagnosis of cancer. In J. W. Cullen, B. H. Fox, & R. N. Isom (Eds.), *Cancer: The behavioral dimensions* (pp. 275–280). New York: Raven Press.

Watson, M., Greer, S., Blake, S., & Sharpnell, K. (1984). Reaction to a diagnosis of breast cancer: Relationship between denial, delay, and rates of psychological morbidity. *Cancer, 53,* 2008–2012.

Weiner, B. (1979). A theory of motivation for some classroom experiences. *Journal of Educational Psychology, 71,* 3–25.

Weinrich, S. P., & Weinrich, M. C. (1986). Cancer knowledge among elderly individuals. *Cancer Nursing, 9,* 301–307.

Weisman, A. D. (1979a). *Coping with cancer.* New York: McGraw-Hill Book Co.

Weisman, A. D. (1979b). A model for psychosocial phasing in cancer. *General Hospital Psychiatry, 1,* 187–195.

Weisman, A. D., & Hackett, T. (1961). Predilection to death. *Psychosomatic Medicine, 23,* 232.

Weisman, A. D., & Worden, J. W. (1976–1977). The existential plight in cancer: Significance of the first 100 days. *International Journal of Psychiatry in Medicine, 7,* 1–15.

Weisman, A. D., Worden, J. W., & Sobel, H. J. (1980). *Psychosocial screening and intervention with cancer patients: Final report of the Omega Project (CA 19797).* Bethesda, MD: National Cancer Institute.

Wendt, P. (1989). *Ethnicity, parental anxiety, and religiosity: Their relationship to children's death concept development and death anxiety.* Unpublished master's thesis, Wayne State University, College of Nursing, Detroit, MI.

Woods, N. F., Lewis, F. M., & Ellison, E. S. (1989). Living with cancer: Family experiences. *Cancer Nursing, 12,* 28–33.

Wool, M. S. (1986). Extreme denial in breast cancer patients and capacity for object relations. *Psychotherapy and Psychosomatics, 46,* 196–204.

Worden, J. W. (1983). Psychosocial screening of cancer patients. *Journal of Psychosocial Oncology, 1*(4), 1–10.

Worden, J. W., & Weisman, A. D. (1975). Psychosocial components of lagtime in cancer diagnosis. *Journal of Psychosomatic Research, 19,* 69–79.

Young-Brockapp, D. (1982). Cancer patients' perceptions of five psychosocial needs. *Oncology Nursing Forum, 9,* 31–35.

Zola, I. K. (1973). Pathways to the doctor— from person to patient. *Social Science and Medicine, 7,* 677–689.

UNIT V
CANCER TREATMENT: THERAPIES AND PHYSICAL SUPPORT APPROACHES

CHAPTER

19

Surgical Oncology

Faith Norcross Weintraub • Donna Edwards Neumark

As many as 90 per cent of all patients with cancer will undergo a surgical procedure during the course of their care (Daly, Wanebo, & DeCosse, 1993). Surgical oncology involves the application of surgical techniques in the diagnosis, staging, palliation, management, and cure of cancer. Historically, surgery was the only method of cancer treatment, and it remains the best option for some malignancies. Specifically, it is a local treatment approach especially effective in the cure and management of solid tumors. Today, the importance of individualizing treatment using a multimodality approach is widely recognized as having the greatest potential for improvements in disease-free survival and positive patient outcomes. Decisions to treat cancer with surgery are based on careful consideration of the natural biology of the disease, stage of disease, physiologic and psychosocial status of the patient, expected rehabilitation potential, and efficacy and availability of adjuvant treatment.

Nurses in a variety of health care settings are responsible for providing care to patients and families experiencing cancer surgery. Development of a comprehensive nursing plan often requires the coordinated efforts of nurses from multiple settings and builds on basic surgical and oncology principles as well as psychosocial and rehabilitation concerns.

HISTORY OF SURGERY IN CANCER

Surgery is the oldest method used to treat cancer. Through the ages, surgical oncology emerged in accordance with current beliefs about the causes of cancer and its mechanisms for spreading. Ancient Egyptian documents describe the excision of tumors as early as 1600 B.C. During the time of Hippocrates (460 to 375 B.C.), cancer was described by the word "carcinos," meaning "crab." Its cause was linked to black bile, consistent with the prevalent belief of characterizing disease by one of the body's four humors: phlegm, yellow bile, blood, and black bile (Kardinal & Yarbro, 1979). Hippocrates classified cancer as either malignant ulcers or occult tumors, and although he advocated against treatment of the hidden disease, superficial tumors were sometimes treated with surgery, cauterization, and purging of the black bile (Hill, 1979; Robinson, 1986). Although distorted through time, these humoral theories remained the primary basis for cancer treatment through the Middle Ages. Medieval times produced few new ideas about the causes of cancer or its treatment. European physicians in the 1200s described radical cutting away of breast cancers, with removal of the entire affected part, including "the veins and the roots" (Hill, 1979).

Eventually, beliefs about the causes of cancer, the way it spread, and subsequent treatments were based on discoveries of human anatomy, circulation, and the lymphatic system. Surgeons of the Renaissance period believed that cancer was a local disease yet understood that it sometimes spread to other parts of the body. Removal of a malignancy in the mid-1600s included excision of local lymph nodes, if possible, and ligation of blood vessels supplying the tumor (Hill, 1979).

Scientific advances and discoveries during the eighteenth and nineteenth centuries led to a more sophisticated understanding about the cellular nature of cancer and methods of metastatic spread by local infiltration. In addition, the links between carcinogenic exposure and host predisposition were recognized. Other predisposing causes of cancer, including age, body parts, and heredity were identified (Hill, 1979; Robinson, 1986). The early 1800s marked the first successful excision of a benign ovarian mass. Although cancer was still widely treated by surgical excision, differentiation between benign and malignant lesions was becoming increasingly clear (Robinson, 1986).

The success of surgery in the treatment of cancer was enhanced by two major scientific developments of the nineteenth century. First was the introduction of general ether anesthesia. Second, perioperative morbidity and mortality were greatly reduced by the understanding of the microbial basis of infection, leading to the widespread use of antiseptic techniques (Moffat & Ketcham, 1994; Rosenberg, 1993). With these developments, as well as refinement of surgical instruments, the pace and scope of surgery greatly expanded its role in treating malignancies. In the late 1800s, Albert Bilroth performed the first gastrectomy, laryngectomy, and esophagectomy. The radical mastectomy was described by Halsted in 1890 and included the first example of the elective removal of clinically uninvolved local lymph nodes (Pilch, 1984). Within the first half of the twentieth century, excision of cancers of the rectum, head and neck, prostate, uterus, lung, pancreas, and colon were reported. In addition, neurosurgical procedures aimed at pain relief, such as a cordotomy, were being performed.

Surgical advances in the mid-1900s resulted from improvements in supportive measures, including blood transfusion, improved anesthesia, antibiotics, and refinement of technical skills, thus allowing procedures

that were more extensive, such as pelvic exenteration and hemipelvectomy (Hill, 1979; Pilch, 1984). These early attempts at cure were superradical, often yielding severe functional and social consequences, yet not always resulting in improved survival (Moffat & Ketcham, 1994).

CURRENT TRENDS

The 1980s and 1990s yielded increased understanding of the genetic and molecular basis of cancer, more knowledge about mechanisms of metastasis, development of new chemotherapeutic and biologic agents, and the use of prognostic indicators, such as tumor-specific antigens, which may help determine cancer treatment selection (Engelking, 1994). In the last decades of the twentieth century, surgery continues to be the treatment of choice for some patients with localized disease. However, the trend in all areas of cancer management, including surgery, appears to be towards reducing invasiveness and minimizing toxicity (Engelking, 1994; Moffat & Ketcham, 1994).

IMPACT OF TECHNOLOGY

Technologic advances have affected the nature of cancer care by providing for the benefits of surgery without many of the postoperative complications. Internal stapling devices used in thoracic, abdominal, and gynecologic surgery for closure and anastomosis have decreased the incidence of postoperative anastomotic leaks (Rothrock, 1991). Electrocautery, or "bovie," blends cutting and coagulating currents, reduces blood loss, and improves operating times (Cox, 1986). The CUSA knife (Cavitron ultrasonic surgical aspirator), used to remove lesions from the liver, brain, and spinal cord, has an ultra-high frequency oscillating tip that shatters tissue with high water content, aspirates debris, and leaves vascular and ductal structures intact (Cox, 1986). Endoscopic equipment, lasers, and videography are state-of-the art surgical approaches of the late twentieth century, and increased applications for laparoscopic procedures, laser surgery, photodynamic therapy, and radioimmunoguided surgery are anticipated in the future (Cohen et al., 1991; Engelking, 1994; Greene, 1993; Pass et al., 1994). At times, radical surgery may still be necessary. Advances in reconstructive and microvascular techniques have helped reduce the degree of disablement and disfigurement. Nonetheless, patients undergoing any surgical procedure for treatment, control, or prevention of a malignancy may still experience both functional and psychosocial difficulties.

FACTORS INFLUENCING THE SELECTION OF SURGERY FOR CANCER TREATMENT

Multiple factors affect the decision to offer surgery as a cancer treatment. Treatment goals, tumor location, tumor growth rate, invasiveness and metastatic potential, surgical risk, quality of life, and available personnel and services are all considered during the collaborative decision-making process prior to surgery.

Nurses are instrumental during the initial planning process. They have major roles in ensuring that patients and families receive and understand the goals of treatment options explored, the advantages and disadvantages of appropriate options, as well as anticipated postoperative and long-term outcomes as they relate to the individual patient.

Combined therapy is recommended when it is the best option for local and distant disease control while preserving cosmesis and function. Multiple clinical trials for solid tumors are ongoing and vary by the treatments used and role of preoperative verses postoperative adjuvant therapy. Nurses as well as physicians have a role in encouraging patients to participate in clinical trials when appropriate (Rosenberg, 1993).

TREATMENT GOALS

The primary goal of cancer surgery is the complete eradication of local and regional tumor (Eilber, 1990). Other goals for surgery may include palliation or intervention for oncologic emergency situations. The first and foremost concern in cancer care today is achieving a "cure." The ability to provide a potential for cure is dependent on early diagnosis and the effectiveness of the initial treatment plan. The initial plan of care should be based on the biology and natural history of the disease, the extent of known disease, and the known treatment options available with the potential to eliminate all viable cancer cells.

TUMOR LOCATION

Defining the exact location of a tumor with diagnostic approaches that may include video endoscopy, magnetic resonance imaging, computed tomography, angiography, and physical examination is paramount to the treatment planning process. Projected functional, cosmetic, and rehabilitative outcomes are based partly on tumor location. Large tumors with poor vascular supplies and central necrosis are less responsive to radiation and chemotherapy, and their location therefore supports an initial surgical approach. The size of the surgical procedure is directly related to tumor location and defined by the neighboring tissues and structures that may need to be removed en bloc to eradicate all viable cancer cells. In some instances tumors will be inoperable because of their proximity to vital structures.

TUMOR CELL KINETICS

GROWTH RATE

The anticipated rate of tumor growth influences the decision to recommend surgery as a single treatment modality over a multimodality approach. The growth rate of a tumor is dependent on the cell cycle activity of the tissue of origin, the number of cells within the cell cycle, and the rate of cell loss (Lind, 1992). Unlike chemotherapy and radiation therapy, which are most effective for tumors with rapidly dividing cells, surgery is most successful for tumors that are slow-growing and consist of cells with long cell cycles because they tend to be locally confined (Kalinowski, 1992).

INVASIVENESS

The preoperative workup is based partly on an understanding of the natural progression of the disease and the degree of suspicion for local invasion that affects the ability of the surgeon to remove the tumor en bloc with a sufficient margin of normal tissue. The surgical oncologist must know where to look intraoperatively for spread of disease. In instances where tumors are less invasive, there is now support for conservative surgical approaches that preserve function and cosmesis (Daly et al., 1993). The extent of invasion determines surgical margins and provides the rationale for an aggressive, radical surgical procedure, which is justified when it is the best chance for local control of invasive disease (Witt & Marshall, 1991). Tumors can invade vascular structures, perineural tissue, bone, or adjacent vital organs, eliminating any possibility for a curative resection.

METASTATIC POTENTIAL

Treatment planning is also influenced by the potential for metastatic spread of disease. An understanding of the major anatomic sites at greatest risk for metastasis and the anticipated disease-free interval influence the choice and sequencing of treatment modalities. Carcinoma in situ has a very low incidence of subsequent metastasis, and some cancers are expected to metastasize within 6 months to 2 years. The increased knowledge of how cancer spreads explains why outcomes were less favorable with radical surgical approaches alone and supports the use of combining local, regional, and systemic treatment. It is suggested that the incidence of micrometastasis is 70 per cent by the time a tumor has grown large enough to be clinically or radiologically identified (Rosenberg, 1993). More patients die of complications directly related to distant metastasis than local or regional failure.

SURGICAL RISK

GENERAL STATE OF HEALTH

One's general state of health is considered when determining the role for cancer surgery. Today age alone is less likely to be a limiting factor in this decision process and is replaced by consideration of current quality-of-life issues. Other areas of concern include general health habits, host resistance, nutritional status, and the extent of preexisting medical conditions such as cardiac, pulmonary, kidney, or endocrine disease. In oncology, special consideration is also given to the use of prior treatment modalities. For example, a history of prior radiation therapy may increase problems with wound closure and healing.

ANESTHESIA

Modern anesthetic techniques have advanced options in surgical oncology and have contributed to a decrease in length of stay. Regional anesthesia is a reversible blockade of pain and includes local field blocks, peripheral nerve blocks, and topical, epidural, and spinal anesthetic approaches. General anesthesia is a reversible state of loss of consciousness achieved by chemical agents that act directly on the brain and can be induced by using intravenous and inhalation anesthetic agents. Frequently, neuromuscular blocking agents are used to relax muscles. The potential effects of general anesthesia on bone marrow depression and immunosuppression are considered prior to surgery (Rosenberg, 1993). Specifically, it may be necessary to delay surgery after chemotherapy administration until laboratory monitoring demonstrates bone marrow recovery.

QUALITY OF LIFE

In today's health care environment the quality of care delivered must be defined by clinical outcomes that address quality-of-life concerns. Standard and experimental treatment options are scrutinized based on morbidity and mortality rates, length of stay, comparisons of anticipated disease-free and long-term survival rates, cosmetic and functional outcomes, as well as the patient's ability to return to work and to have a satisfying, productive lifestyle.

ACCESS TO CARE

Access and availability of potential treatment options have an impact on the surgical procedure proposed. While the general surgeon plays a major role in cancer surgery, access to a surgical oncologist and a tertiary medical center may be necessary for radical operations or those requiring microvascular reconstruction. In some instances radiation therapy may be the initial treatment of choice but may not be available for the patient. Many practitioners today express concerns regarding the ever increasing impact of health care reform and managed care plans on limiting access to specific institutions and treatment options.

BASIC SURGICAL PRINCIPLES APPLIED TO SURGICAL ONCOLOGY

It is important for nurses to have a basic knowledge of the principles of surgery most applicable in surgical oncology today. Eilber (1985) described these cardinal principles as they apply to the surgery of cancer. They have evolved over time with advances in cancer cell biology, surgical instrumentation and technique, as well as philosophic changes in the importance of clinical outcomes. Incorporation of these practices in routine cancer surgery has had an impact on improved disease-free and long-term survival as well as quality-of-life outcomes (see Table 19–1).

THE SCOPE OF CANCER SURGERY

Developments in complementary fields of medicine and patient care have increased the scope of surgery. Advances in critical care, nutritional support, anesthesia, pain management, and antibiotic coverage have all

TABLE 19–1. *Principles to Enhance Surgical Outcomes*

Surgery should not be done if the outcome is unsuitable for the individual.

The surgeon should do as much surgery as possible to eradicate the tumor, tempered with the belief to always do as small a procedure as therapeutically possible.

Reconstruction and rehabilitation are essential components of quality clinical outcomes.

Maximum exposure of the tumor intraoperatively facilitates adequate accessibility necessary to achieve normal tissue margins and evaluation of spread of disease.

A bloodless surgical field is important for gross observation at all times. This can be achieved with careful hemostasis and suction.

Human tissue is friable, requires special attention to blood supply at all times, and should be handled delicately especially if previously irradiated.

Attention to the "no-touch technique" minimizes tumor seeding and potential for local recurrence. This includes early ligation of tumor blood supply and minimal palpation of the tumor.

Free tumor cells in the operative field can be source for local recurrence and metastasis. Careful surgical techniques that include glove changes, instrument and extensive wound irrigation with cytotoxic agents (5 per cent formaldehyde, hypotonic saline) will reduce risk of seeding.

Skill and patience are required prior to beginning the tumor resection to define all tumor margins and draining lymphatics. All vessels are to be ligated early to prevent potential escape of tumor cells in the general circulation.

Curative resection or en bloc resection encompasses the primary tumor, regional lymph nodes, and intervening lymphatic channels.

Sutures and anastomosis should be placed in nonirradiated, disease free tissue.

The anastomosis should be made in an area with minimal tension to the incision.

If a second area of the body requires surgical intervention at the time of tumor excision, all gloves and instruments must be changed.

(Data from Cox, C. E. [1986]. Principles of operative surgery: Antisepsis, technique, sutures, and drains. In D. C. Sabiston [Ed.], *Textbook of surgery* [13th ed., pp. 244–258]. Philadelphia: W.B. Saunders; Daly, J. M., Wanebo, H., & DeCosse, J. J. [1993]. Principles of surgical oncology. In P. Calabresi & P. S. Schein [Eds.], *Medical oncology basic principles and clinical management of cancer* [2nd ed., pp. 237–251]. New York: McGraw-Hill; Eilber, F. R. [1985]. Principles of cancer surgery. In C. M. Haskell [Ed.], *Cancer treatment* [2nd ed.]. Philadelphia: W.B. Saunders; Eilber, F. R. [1990]. Principles of cancer surgery. In C. M. Haskell [Ed.], *Cancer treatment* [3rd ed., pp. 9–15]. Philadelphia: W.B Saunders.)

helped improve the potential outcomes from surgery. Technical developments in endoscopic and laser surgery have minimized the extent of some surgical procedures. Conversely, improved surgical instrumentation now allows for major surgical resections for isolated metastatic disease. Multimodality therapy has become the mainstay in cancer care. All of these advances have contributed to improvements in surgical morbidity, mortality, and quality of life. Today nurses in almost every area of health care are being introduced to oncology through these advances in surgery.

The shift in emphasis away from single-modality treatment has not detracted from the significant and expanding role of surgery in the management of the patient with malignant disease. Table 19–2 gives examples of the variety of surgical procedures currently used in cancer care.

DIAGNOSIS

While a cancer diagnosis may be suspected from physical examination or radiologic examination, confirmation needs to be established from a tissue sample. In many instances it is necessary to obtain the histologic diagnosis and grade of disease to optimize the initial plan of care (Turner, 1994). The differential diagnosis helps to determine which biopsy procedure to perform. Biopsy techniques include needle aspiration, percutaneous needle aspiration/biopsy, needle biopsy, exfoliative cytology, shave biopsy, punch biopsy, incisional biopsy, excisional biopsy, and endoscopic biopsy (Szopa, 1992). The biopsy should be located so any fur-

ther surgical interventions will encompass the site. Minimal dissection, careful hemostasis at the biopsy site, and attention to avoid contaminating new tissue planes during the procedure will minimize the risk for spread of disease. A representative sample should be obtained from the periphery of the suspicious mass in an effort to encompass cells at the interface of malignant and normal tissue (Elias, 1989). Proper handling and orientation of the tissue is imperative for accurate diagnosis. Sufficient tissue must be obtained for flow cytometry, histochemical stains, and electron microscopy when indicated. Orientation of the specimen with inked or sutured margins is also helpful. Table 19–3 describes the advantages and disadvantages of the various biopsy procedures.

STAGING

Surgical staging may be used to establish the extent of disease in an effort to maximize treatment options. The classic examples include staging laparotomy for Hodgkins disease and ovarian cancer (Szopa, 1992). A knowledge of the biologic nature of the specific cancer aids the surgeon in evaluation of all tissue and organs that could potentially harbor disease. Multiple tissue and fluid samples are taken for cytologic and pathologic review. Second-look surgery for ovarian cancer is also indicated to stage disease and determine treatment response after completion of the initial treatment plan. It may also be considered for patients with colorectal cancer who on sequential follow-up are found to have a rising cancer embryonic antigen (CEA) and a negative metastatic workup (Daly et al., 1993; Moffat & Ketcham, 1994).

TREATMENT OF THE PRIMARY TUMOR

Surgery is the primary treatment of choice for tumors that are localized or regionally contained, do not invade major organ or vascular structures, and are not associated with distant metastatic disease. The extent of the primary resection for disease that has the potential for local invasion includes an en bloc resection of the primary tumor, regional lymph nodes, and intervening lymphatic channels (Daly et al., 1993). The extent of the deep, medial, and lateral margins is dictated by the specific disease and can range from 2 to 5 cm (Eilber, 1990). The optimal treatment approach is one that eradicates all viable tumor cells, maintains tissue and organ function, and minimizes alteration in appearance.

PALLIATION

The goal of palliative surgery is to minimize symptoms of disease and relieve suffering. Consideration to undergo surgery is based on the pace of the disease, life expectancy, and expected outcomes. Preoperative education and support for both patients and family members needs to be consistent with information given by the surgical team and should reinforce the palliative na-

TABLE 19–2. *Surgical Approaches to Cancer Care*

INTERVENTION	EXAMPLE
Diagnosis	Breast biopsy
Staging	Staging laparotomy
	Second-look laparotomy
Primary tumor resection	Curative resection (colon resection)
Reconstruction, rehabilitation	Breast reconstruction
	Ileal conduit formation
	Microvascular flaps
Palliative	Gastrojejunostomy
	Choledochojejunostomy
Adjuvant	Venous access device
	Intraarterial pumps
Complications of other methods	Lysis of adhesions due to radiation
	Bowel resection for proctitis
Resection of metastases	Hepatic resection
	Pulmonary resection
Cytoreductive	Ovarian carcinoma
	Abdominal soft-tissue sarcomas
Emergencies	Obstruction
	Surgical decompression
Cancer prevention	Colectomy (familial polyposis)
	Orchidopexy (testicular)

TABLE 19–3. *Surgical Biopsy Techniques*

TECHNIQUE	USES IN CANCER CARE	ADVANTAGES	DISADVANTAGES
Fine-needle aspiration 20–22 gauge	Retrieves cells vs tissue Used when high suspicion for malignancy Used for solid, palpable lesions Examples: breast, thyroid, cervical adenopathy	Quick Avoid surgical scar Local anesthesia Outpatient	Need trained cytologist False-negative results Cannot be used to diagnose lymphoma, sarcoma
Percutaneous needle aspiration 20–23 gauge	Retrieves cells vs tissue Used for solid, nonpalpable lesions Radiologic localization, CT, MRI, U/S, Mammogram Examples: lung, breast	May avoid need and cost of surgery Local anesthesia Outpatient	False-negative results Cannot be used to diagnose lymphoma, sarcoma Special stains procedures cannot be done
Core needle biopsy 14–20 gauge Trucut automated biopsy gun	Retrieves tissue Used for both palpable and nonpalpable lesions through radiographic approach Examples: pancreas, liver, stereotactic breast biopsy, retroperitoneum	Avoids surgical scar Local anesthesia Outpatient	Need technically trained and skilled personnel Risk injury to adjacent structures Risk tumor cell seeding along biopsy tract
Incisional biopsy	Obtain wedge of tissue for solid, large mass Example: head and neck tumors, liver	Obtain tissue diagnosis when mass too large to easily remove surgically Local and/or IV sedation	Necessitates scar Requires OR time Bleeding at site Risk of infection
Excisional biopsy	Solid, palpable mass Removal of complete lump with little or no planned margin	Day surgery Remove all gross disease	Risk of infection Requires scar
Endoscopic biopsy	Used for solid mass in lumen Used to obtain cytologic brushings and/or tissue	Avoids surgical procedure Can place scar cosmetically Day surgery	Pain and trauma associated with scope
Laparoscopic biopsy	Used to sample tissue— abdomen, pelvis, lymphadenopathy, pancreas, liver	May avoid need for more major surgery Decreased length of stay	Decreased ability to assess complete abdomen

ture of the procedure. Some indications for palliative surgery include relief of pain, ablative surgery, relief of gastrointestinal, urinary, or respiratory obstruction, and the management of fungating wounds.

SURGERY FOR METASTATIC DISEASE

In selected cases there is a place for resection of isolated metastases. This is usually performed when cure will be affected and when the cancer is controlled at the primary site. The psychologic as well as physical status of the patient before surgery is an important consideration. Other factors that influence the decision to intervene surgically are the nature of the tumor, the disease-free interval, and the tumor doubling time. Isolated metastases in the bone, liver, lung, and brain have been resected with an approximate 25 per cent cure rate (Eilber, 1990; Moffat & Ketcham, 1994).

CYTOREDUCTION

This role for surgery is controversial and should be considered only when other effective treatment modal-

ities are available to control the remaining residual disease. Cytoreduction is the surgical resection of bulky disease reducing tumor cell mass to a level that will render chemotherapy, immunotherapy, radiation therapy, and host defenses more effective. Its surgical role has been most effective in the management of Burkitts lymphoma and ovarian cancer (Rosenberg, 1993; Szopa, 1992).

ONCOLOGY EMERGENCIES

The decision to intervene surgically in oncologic emergencies is often highly controversial and an ethical dilemma. Whatever the procedure, the optimal result should be to relieve symptoms and improve the quality of the patient's remaining life. Emergency surgery is used in instances of gastrointestinal hemorrhage, spinal cord compression, and exsanguinating hemorrhage from arterial blowout. Astute nursing assessment in identifying oncology patients at risk and a review of advanced directives with patients and families can lead to a more supportive plan of care if emergencies requiring surgical intervention develop.

ADJUVANT THERAPY/SUPPORTIVE

A number of malignant conditions and cancer treatments require surgical intervention. Examples include placement of therapeutic devices, radioactive implants, or supportive devices such as implantable access catheters and feeding tubes.

Surgery may also be indicated for the management of complications due to adjuvant therapy such as fistulas, abscesses, obstructive symptoms, or tissue impairment.

RECONSTRUCTIVE OR REHABILITATIVE SURGERY

Radical surgical resections can result in defects that cannot be repaired satisfactorily by simple wound closure. Complicating these technical difficulties is the effect radical surgery can have on the quality of life of the cancer patient. Traditionally, reconstructive surgery was often delayed to allow the patient to be monitored for recurrence of the disease. Early reconstruction is now often performed and preferred. Advances in microvascular surgery and the ability to transfer free skin, muscle, and tissue for wound closure and prosthetic reconstruction have improved the rehabilitation outcome from radical, curative surgical resections (Rosenberg, 1993).

PROPHYLACTIC SURGERY

In the area of cancer prevention there are certain clinical settings in which the use of surgery can be effective such as in the management of cervical cancer. This condition can be readily detected through simple cytologic screening, and limited surgical excision or laser techniques can effectively reduce spread of the disease.

Surgery is also used in the management of certain familial diseases. In the case of familial polyposis coli, colectomy may be advocated to prevent colon cancer. Breast cancer is another malignant disease with a strong familial link. Approximately 9 per cent of women with breast cancer demonstrate hereditary causation. Certain women with a very high risk may become candidates for prophylactic mastectomy as a treatment alternative to surveillance (Fitzsimmons, Conway, Madsen, Lappe, & Coody, 1989).

IMPLICATIONS FOR NURSING MANAGEMENT

Many factors contribute to the challenge of caring for the person with cancer who is having surgery. Nurses have to be knowledgeable in general surgical nursing and must possess a sound background in oncologic principles, effects of radiation and chemotherapy treatment, and knowledge of the disease process with its potential physical and psychosocial sequelae. As in any interaction with a patient or family, it is vital to remember that everyone has different needs, values, and beliefs surrounding cancer and cancer treatment. Whether intended to prevent, diagnose, control, or eliminate cancer, any surgical procedure causes the patient and family to confront a new array of concerns related to survival, pain, disability, and the impact of surgery on future lifestyle and relationships. The nurse must integrate physiologic, psychosocial, financial, and rehabilitative needs to maximize the effects of surgical interventions for cancer.

ISSUES IN PREOPERATIVE CARE

Dimensions of care that can be the focus of preoperative nursing interventions include clarifying information, discussing potential sources of support, teaching about preoperative, surgical, and postoperative routines, and identifying issues related to follow-up care. The patient should be instructed about the use of any equipment, pulmonary exercises, coughing techniques, and pain management options. Involving the family or other caregivers is essential for promoting acceptance of the disease and in recovery from surgery (Bagg, 1988). In a retrospective study, women who underwent major gynecologic surgery for cancer reported that it would have been beneficial for a partner to participate fully in all the preoperative information sessions (Corney, Everett, Howells, & Crowther, 1992) (see Box 19–1).

Physiologic factors that may increase complications related to surgery must be assessed. A comprehensive physical examination, critical laboratory tests, and di-

---

BOX 19–1. *Care Needs of Patients Undergoing Surgery For Gynecologic Cancer*

Corney, R., Everett, H., Howells, A., & Crowther, M. (1992). The care of patients undergoing surgery for gynaecological cancer: The need for information, emotional support and counselling. *Journal of Advanced Nursing, 17,* 667–671.

Sample: One hundred and five women who had undergone a radical vulvectomy (N=28), a Wertheim's hysterectomy (n=69), or a pelvic exenteration (n=8) in the last 5 years. Forty partners were also interviewed.

Measures: Semistructured interviews were conducted by one of the authors; Hospital Anxiety and Depression Scale.

Findings: The interviews revealed a large proportion of the women remained depressed and anxious following surgery, and many reported ongoing sexual problems. Many of the women and some of the partners would have liked to receive more information prior to the surgery, especially about the physical and psychologic effects that may occur postoperatively.

Limitations: Patients were all under the care of one consultant and hospital team, so results may not be generalized to other situations. Specific demographic information about the patients and time since surgery were not reported.

agnostic data unique to surgery are obtained, and arrangements for autologous blood donations should be made if necessary. Also, the patient's age must be considered. Older people have normal physiologic changes related to aging that may contribute to potential postoperative complications (Szopa, 1992). Nonetheless, the impact of general health status on operative mortality is probably a better predictor of postoperative complication potential (Rosenberg, 1993). Preexisting conditions such as cardiovascular, pulmonary, renal, neurologic, gastrointestinal, or liver disease can contribute to perioperative morbidity. For the patient who has a suspicion of cancer or is undergoing treatment, altered laboratory values, cardiovascular compromise, immunosuppression, or anemia increase the likelihood of complications.

Lifestyle activities such as smoking, alcohol, or drug use can also influence the patient's postoperative course (Szopa, 1992). Patients should be encouraged to refrain from smoking, and for some, preoperative pulmonary therapy may be indicated to decrease postoperative pulmonary complications (Sideranko, 1993). A current medication history should be obtained, and instructions regarding taking usual medications prior to surgery should be clarified. Nonsteroidal antiinflammatory medications taken within 7 days of surgery increase the risk for bleeding complications and should be discontinued until further evaluations in the postoperative period.

CONSIDERATION OF PRIOR CANCER THERAPIES

Knowledge of the patient's treatment plan and previous chemotherapy or radiation must be known. Newer clinical trials support the preoperative use of adjuvant therapy for curative treatment. While preoperative chemotherapy and radiotherapy are designed to reduce tumor size and improve resectability, these therapies may increase the likelihood of postoperative complications (Sideranko, 1993). Bleomycin, methotrexate, and busulfan can contribute to prolonged pulmonary toxicity and prolong efforts to wean from mechanical ventilation postoperatively. When high concentrations of oxygen are given to surgical patients previously treated with bleomycin, the risk of respiratory failure increases (Polomano, Weintraub, & Wurster, 1994). Previous treatment with cardiotoxic drugs increases the perioperative and postoperative risk of congestive heart failure and pulmonary edema (Kalinowski, 1992). Bleomycin, doxorubicin, alkylating agents, and corticosteroids all delay wound healing. Elective surgery should be scheduled no sooner than 1 to 2 weeks after chemotherapy administration (Daly et al., 1993).

The timing interval between surgery and radiation therapy is generally longer than for chemotherapy and is 5 to 6 weeks. Prior radiation therapy will affect healing if the surgical wound is in the treatment field and can contribute to fistula development, rejection of tissue grafts, anastomotic leaks, obstruction, and hemorrhage. Reinforcement of the anastomotic site and additional coverage of major blood vessels at risk for rupture are surgical precautions that can reduce postoperative complications (Eilber, 1990).

Another area that should be assessed is the patient's previous surgical experience, including type of surgery, response to anesthesia, and postoperative complications (Szopa, 1992).

ISSUES IN POSTOPERATIVE CARE

The postoperative plan of care is influenced by the surgical setting, the specific surgical procedure performed, intraoperative events, and the patient's preexisting health (Daly & Cady, 1993). Exposure to prior cancer therapies and the physiologic changes directly related to the cancer process place all surgical patients at an increased risk for the development of problems. A description of the major surgical procedures performed for cancer and site-specific nursing implications are listed in Table 19–4. Guidelines for the assessment and management of the more serious problems that can potentially develop as a result of radical cancer surgery are identified in Table 19–5.

Surgical specialists have made significant contributions to advances in nutrition support, perioperative pain management, and wound care. More detailed information specific to these problems as they relate to surgical oncology follow.

NUTRITION SUPPORT FOR THE SURGICAL ONCOLOGY PATIENT

Nutritional disorders have a significant impact on postoperative recovery. Surgical oncology patients often present with protein-calorie malnutrition. Contributing factors include the disease process, anorexia, dysphagia, prior chemotherapy and radiation therapy, and increased catabolic requirements. Preoperative malnutrition is associated with poor surgical outcomes including an increased incidence of sepsis, wound dehiscence, ileus, and increased length of stay (Chen, Souba, & Copeland, 1991). The increased incidence of postoperative complications is believed to be related to impaired immune competence, which is reduced with malnutrition (Smith & Mullen, 1991).

Perioperative support for surgical oncology patients presenting with protein-calorie malnutrition has significantly reduced postoperative morbidity and mortality. Earlier fears that nutrition support would stimulate tumor growth have not been substantiated. Patients who have lost more than 15 per cent of their body weight during a 3- to 4-month period or who weigh less than 85 per cent of ideal body weight and who are well hydrated but have a serum albumin of less than 3 gm/100 ml should be considered for perioperative nutrition support (Fischer, 1992). The route of administration is based on treatment goals as well as the functional status of the gastrointestinal tract. Methods of nutrition support include oral diets, enteral tube feedings, peripheral vein infusion, and total parenteral nutrition (TPN). Newer tubes that are easier to pass orally or from the nares, as well as advances in percutaneous endoscopic gastrostomy have expanded the use of en-

TABLE 19–4. *Major Surgical Procedures with Associated Nursing Needs*

Surgical Procedure	Tissue Excised	Postoperative Complications and Functional Changes	Associated Perioperative Teaching/Care
Modified/radical head and neck procedures (may be laryngectomy, radical neck dissections, glossectomy, maxillectomy, mandibulectomy)	Dependent upon location of tumor (often includes myocutaneous free flap reconstruction using muscles such as gracilis, rectus abdominis, latissimus dorsi, pectoralis; may require node resection)	Airway management, secretion management, hemorrhage, wound seromas, cellulitis or abscess, neurologic dysfunction; paresthesia and anesthesia in certain areas, mobility changes (tongue, lips, shoulder), communication changes, tracheostomy, altered ingestion, swallowing difficulty	Cosmesis, nutritional support, tracheostomy and laryngectomy care, control of secretions, communication, intimacy issues, odor control
Lobectomy	Lung lobe	Pain, pneumothorax, atelectasis, pleural effusion, bronchospasm, bronchopleural fistula, pulmonary embolus, infection, cardiac arrhythmias, empyema, impaired mobility	Respiratory care, nutritional support, pain management
Mastectomy (modified radical)	Breast parenchyma, nipple-areolar complex, ipsilateral axillary lymph nodes, pectoralis minor muscle	Lymphedema, decreased ROM of affected arm, phantom breast sensation, arm paresthesia, loss of ability for breast stimulation, body image	Intimacy issues, arm care, arm exercises
Esophagectomy (thoracic or abdominal approach)	Esophagus with mobilization of stomach for reanastamosis; more radical approach includes thoracic duct; zygos vein and intercostal veins or arteries	Hemorrhage, postoperative fistula, anastomotic leak, reflux, esophagitis, infection/sepsis, prolonged swallowing dysfunction, gastroesophageal reflux, esophagitis, pneumothorax, atelectasis and pneumonia, pulmonary emboli, dumping syndrome, early satiety	Speech therapy, swallowing therapy, jejunostomy feedings
Total gastrectomy	Stomach, mesentery, associated lymph nodes	Pneumonia, anastomotic leak, hemorrhage, reflux, small-bowel obstruction, vitamin B12 deficiency	Nutritional issues
Gastroduodenostomy (Bilroth I)	Portion of duodenum, distal stomach, pylorus, lymphatic vessels; stomach anastomosed to jejunum	As with gastrectomy, dumping syndrome	Nutritional issues
Bilroth II	Antrum, pylorus, portion of jejunum, circulating structures, lymph nodes, remaining stomach anastomosed to jejunum	As with gastrectomy, dumping syndrome, diarrhea, vitamin deficiency	Nutritional issues
Whipple (Pancreatoduodenectomy)	Head of pancreas, duodenum, antrum, gall bladder and bile duct; remaining biliary tract and pancreas anastomosed to jejunum, gastrojejunostomy performed, vagotomy	Fistula, hemorrhage, anastomotic leakage, cardiopulmonary problems, wound infection, sepsis, renal failure, maldigestion, diarrhea, hyperglycemia	Nutritional issues, tube feedings, diabetic teaching

Continued on following page.

TABLE 19–4. *Major Surgical Procedures with Associated Nursing Needs* Continued

SURGICAL PROCEDURE	TISSUE EXCISED	POSTOPERATIVE COMPLICATIONS AND FUNCTIONAL CHANGES	ASSOCIATED PERIOPERATIVE TEACHING/CARE
Esophagogastrectomy	Lower esophagus, omentum, stomach (partial to total), supporting lymph and circulatory structures	Respiratory complications, pulmonary edema, atelectasis, pneumonia, pulmonary embolus, anastomotic leak, infection, reflux, cardiac arrhythmias, fluid shifts, reflux, dysphagia	Pain management, nutritional issues, jejunostomy feedings
Abdominal hysterectomy	Uterus	Loss of orgasmic uterine contractions, loss of reproductive capacity	Reproductive and intimacy issues
Radical hysterectomy	Uterus, upper ⅓ vagina, ovaries, fallopian tubes, broad ligaments, parametrial tissue	Potential voiding dysfunction, vaginal dryness, decreased depth of vagina, loss of uterine capacity with deep penetration, loss of reproductive capacity, hormonal changes	Reproductive and intimacy issues
Radical vulvectomy	Clitoris, mons fat pad, vulva and inguinal nodes	Immobility, skin integrity, lymphedema, decreased ROM lower extremities, areas of perineal anesthesia, introital stenosis, decreased lubrication, large postoperative wound, eliminative changes	Intimacy issues, wound care, altered urinary flow, body image
Total pelvic exenteration	All female reproductive organs, lymph nodes, bladder and distal ureters, rectum, distal sigmoid colon, perineum, pelvic floor, peritoneal and levator muscles; (often necessitates formation of an artificial bladder and/or colostomy)	Hemodynamic instability, hemorrhage, deep vein thrombosis, large postoperative wound, ureteral leak or fistula, pelvic seroma and abscess formation, neurologic complications, pulmonary edema or emboli, infection/sepsis, small bowel obstruction, no vaginal intercourse (without reconstruction), two ostomies, loss of reproductive capacity, changes in sexual function, elimination, body image	Reproductive and intimacy issues, ostomy and vaginal care, cosmesis, body image
Right and transverse colectomy	Anatomic resection of the ascending colon with its attendant mesentery, vascular and lymphatic supply	Diarrhea, anastomotic leak, intraabdominal abscess, staphyloccal enteritis, large-bowel obstruction, rectal oozing, potential sexual dysfunction	Ostomy teaching, nutritional issues, body image
Left colectomy and sigmoid resection	Distal, transverse, descending colon, sigmoid colon, and mesocolon	As with right and transverse colectomy	Ostomy teaching, nutritional issues, body image
Radical prostatectomy	Prostate from bladder neck to apex, seminal vesicles and vas deferens, lymph nodes	Bladder spasms, infections, thromboembolism, impotence, incontinence, rectal injury, blood loss	Intimacy issues, elimination issues, catheter care, perineal exercises
Radical cystectomy with construction of urinary diversion	Anterior pelvic organs with reanastomosis of ureters to a segment of resected bowel; prostate, seminal vesicles, bladder, visceral peritoneum and perivesicle fat in men; urethra, bladder, cervix, anterior vaginal wall, vaginal cuff, uterus, ovaries, fallopian tubes and anterior pelvic peritoneum in women	Bowel obstruction, fistula formation, pyelonephritis, urine leakage from anastomotic sites, vascular infarction, necrosis of conduit or stoma, wound infection, stomal strictures, ureterointestinal stenosis, frequent urinary tract infections, urinary calculi formation	Elimination issues, ostomy care, body image issues, intimacy issues

TABLE 19–5. *General Acute Care Issues for the Surgical Oncology Patient*

NURSING DIAGNOSIS	GOALS	INTERVENTIONS
Alteration in fluid volume secondary to intraoperative fluid losses and bleeding	Restore hemodynamic stability; promote tissue repair	Monitor vital signs and hemodynamic pressures for hypovolemia Report decreases in BP, CVP, PAP, CO, MAP, and increase in HR Monitor urine output hourly and report output <30 ml/hr Monitor and record quantity and and consistency of fluid from drains and NG tube Monitor IV solutions and rates Observe S/S electrolyte imbalance Assess for signs of central and/or peripheral edema Assess for cold clammy skin, poor skin turgor, and dry mucous membranes Replace fluid losses with isotonic solutions as ordered Administer blood products as ordered Document responses to fluid therapy
Alteration in respiratory status secondary to mechanical ventilation, decreased vital capacity, infection, aspiration, pulmonary fibrosis, excessive sedation and mechanical obstruction	Promote optimal respiratory function	Assess character of respiratory rate, depth, rhythm, and use of accessory muscles Auscultate lung fields and note type/location of adventitious sounds Assess cardiac rate and rhythm for signs of hypoxia (sinus tachycardia and ventricular ectopy) Obtain, evaluate, and report to physician results of ABGs Monitor CXR results Assess and treat hypothermia Monitor response to pain medication (for pain relief, respiratory status and BP) Provide information, emotional support and a quiet environment to reduce anxiety Turn patient every 2 hours to maintain optimal ventilation and prevent atelectasis Position patient in semihigh Fowlers to promote adequate gas exchange Coordinate chest physical therapy per institutional protocol Teach coughing and deep breathing Demonstrate use of incentive spirometry Administer mucolytic agents for thick tenacious secretions Provide humefied air as needed Tracheal suctioning per institutional policy Be aware of early signs/symptoms of ARDS: tachypnea, dyspnea, restlessness, hypoxia and respiratory alkalosis
Alteration in cardiovascular status secondary to intraoperative fluid losses, bleeding, fluid/electrolyte losses, and prior treatment antracyclines	Ensure optimal cardiac function and restoration of circulatory volume and components	Monitor vital signs frequently and report HR, BP and respiratory changes Monitor direct hemodynamic parameters, MAP, PAP, CO and report abnormality to physician Replace electrolytes per institution protocal Evaluate for potential changes in rate/rhythm Administer vasopressors and antiarrhythmic agents if required and prescribed Check capillary filling in finger and toes for adequate tissue perfussion
Impaired blood coagulation secondary to perioperative transfusions, cancer process, and prior treatments	Restore hematologic function	Monitor laboratory values: Hgb Hct, platelets, PT, PTT, fibrinogen level, factor assays II, V, VII Administer vitamin K as ordered Administer FFP, platelets, whole blood and PRBCs as ordered Assess for early signs of DIC: oozing, petchiae, CNS changes, venous distention, tachycardia, skin color changes, decreased BP, acral cyanosis hematuria, decreased urine output and abdominal pain
Potential for infection secondary to surgery, disruption in mechanical barrier, malnutrition, prior radiation and/or chemotherapy, malignancy-induced immunosuppression	Prevent development of sepsis	Monitor vital signs per institution policy; report increases in temperature, HR, and RR to physician Monitor WBC and report abnormalities Assess fluid from closed drainage systems every shift and report changes in quantity, color, consistency, or order When suspicious send drainage for C/S Maintain aseptic technique when caring for drains, invasive lines, and incision Assess nutritional parameters and institute nutritional support as indicated to decrease risk of infection Inspect skin integrity and treat pressure sores to maintain barrier protection Inspect skin at operative site for warmth and blanching Administer postoperative IV antibiotics as ordered Teach family clean techniques when caring for wounds, drains, and lines Monitor for early signs of sepsis: warm flushed skin, tachycardia, pounding pulse, tachypnea, decreased BP, irritability, and restlessness

ARDS = adult respiratory distress syndrome; BP = blood pressure; CO = cardiac output; RR = respiratory rate; FFP = fresh frozed plasma; Hct = hematocrit; PT = prothrombin time; PTT = partial prothrombin time; WBC = white blood count; CVP = central venous pressure; MAP = mean arterial pressure; PRBC = packed red blood cells; DIC = disseminated intravascular coagulation; PAP = pulmonary arterial pressure; HR = heart rate, ABG = arterial blood gas; Hgb = hemoglobin; CNS = central nervous system; C/S = culture and sensitivity; S/S = signs and symptoms.
(Adapted from Polomano, R., Weintraub, F. N., & Wurster, A. [1994]. Surgical critical care for cancer patients. *Seminars in Oncology Nursing, 10,* 165–176.)

teral nutrition in surgery. The diversity of elemental products available demonstrates advances in the application of clinical biochemistry to the field (Dudrick, 1991). Support is continued throughout postoperative recovery and can be reduced as patients progress from clears to a regular diet. Research is ongoing to identify those patients who will best benefit from continued postoperative support once discharged home.

PAIN MANAGEMENT

One major concern and fear patients and families associate with surgery is the experience of pain. This is true regardless of the complexity of the procedure. Some basic considerations specific to the nurse's role in pain management during cancer surgery are discussed here. For more detailed information refer to both the chapter on pain and individual chapters by disease site.

Preoperative and preprocedure teaching can decrease anxiety and level of pain. Descriptions of sensations likely experienced during and after procedures are useful. Written and verbal information about all available postoperative pain management options should be reviewed preoperatively and a plan of care documented in the chart. Identification and attention to psychosocial needs may also minimize perception of pain. Nonpharmacologic strategies including relaxation, visualization, and massage should also be addressed (Acute Pain Mangement Guideline Panel, 1992).

One potential mistake nurses can make is misinterpreting the origin of the patient's pain. Variables important to include in the pain assessment are intensity, onset, location, duration, actions that aggravate or relieve the pain, as well as the effect of current treatments. The nurse needs to question whether the pain fits with the patient's disease and treatments received. If not, consideration of emergent medical problems should be ruled out.

Today traditional perioperative pain management is being redefined. Intermittent dosing is now known to

be less effective than continuous patient-controlled analgesia (PCA) (Gilbert, 1990). It is suggested that improvements in adequate perioperative pain management will increase patient satisfaction and decrease length of stay (Lubenow & Ivankovich, 1991). For these reasons pain management is of major concern for surgeons, anesthesiologists, and surgical nurses. Many institutions are creating multidisciplinary perioperative pain services (Gilbert, 1990). Early research is also beginning to demonstrate the safe and effective use of continuous epidural analgesia outside intensive monitored settings (Fulk & Hadley, 1990; Polomano, Blumenthal, Schiavone-Gatto, & O'Brien, 1993). Research is ongoing to define the role for interpleural and perineural local anesthetics as well as transmucosal and nasal aerosol narcotic delivery systems (Gilbert, 1990).

WOUND MANAGEMENT

A considerable amount of attention during the postoperative period is directed to the care of surgically created and preexisting wounds. Wound healing occurs in overlapping stages and is dependent on a variety of host and operative factors (see Tables 19–6 and 19–7). Decreases in the postoperative length of stay have necessitated that nurses in ambulatory and home care settings develop expertise in wound management.

There are four classifications of surgical wounds. A clean wound occurs when aseptic technique has not been violated, there is no sign of infection, and the wound is closed to heal by primary intention. A clean-contaminated wound occurs when the respiratory, gastrointestinal, or genitourinary tract is entered but no break in aseptic technique occurred and there is no intraoperative sign of infection. Primary closure is also possible, and closed-system drainage may be employed. Wounds are contaminated when a break in aseptic technique occurs. Infection or gross spillage from the gastrointestinal tract as in a perforated bowel occurs. Such wounds are left open to heal by secondary intention.

TABLE 19–6. *Stages of Wound Healing*

STAGE	TIME	EVENT	CELLS
Inflammation			
Protection	0–2 hrs	Hemostasis	Platelets Erythrocytes Leukocytes
Debridement	0–4 days	Phagocytosis	Neutrophils Macrophages
Proliferative	1–4 days	Epitheliazation	Keratinocytes
Collagen synthesis from fibroblasts; increased tensile strength	2–7 days	Neovascularization	Endothelial
of wound	2–22 days	Collagen synthesis	Fibroblasts
	2–20 days	Contraction	Myofibroblasts
Maturation			
Scar remodeling and strengthening	21 days–2 yr	Collagen Lysis and re-synthesis	Fibroblasts

(Adapted from Wysocki, A. B. [1989]. Surgical wound healing. A review for perioperative nurses. *AORN Journal, 49,* 506.)

TABLE 19–7. *Factors Affecting Wound Healing*

OPERATION	PATIENT
Length of operation	Age
Length of preoperative admission	Obesity
	Malnutrition
Surgical technique	Immunosuppression
Preparation of operative site	Prior radiation
Intraoperative antibiotics	Prior chemotherapy
Suture material	Connective tissue disorder
Mechanical stress	Liver disease
Wound tension	Peripheral vascular disease
Vascular supply tissue	Diabetes
Tissue oxygenation	Hypovolemia
Presence of devitalized tissue	Vitamin deficiency (C, A, B, K)
Foreign bodies	Steroid use
	Vasopressors
	Vasoconstrictors
	Hypoxia

(Adapted from Barbul, A. [1992]. Postoperative wound infection. In J. L. Cameron [Ed.], *Current surgical therapy* [4th ed., pp. 960–967]. St. Louis: Mosby-Year Book; Wysocki, A. B. [1989]. Surgical wound healing. A review for perioperative nurses. *AORN Journal, 49,* 508.)

Healing by granulation and scar formation occurs slowly in a process known as wound contraction. If after 4 to 5 days there is no sign of wound infection, edges may be approximated and healing occurs by delayed primary closure or third intention. Dirty or infected wounds are the result of a previous trauma or involve an existing clinical infection. These wounds may be surgically debrided and left to heal by secondary intention (Henry, 1991; Weigel, 1992).

Assessment of surgical wounds is critical to determine the appropriate treatment. Wound assessment and documentation should address the location and direction of the wound, the length, width, and depth of the wound including the presence of sinus tracts in open wounds, the stage of tissue involvement, and a description of the wound's base, edges, and exudate. The overall incidence of postoperative wound infection is 5 to 10 per cent, but for contaminated or dirty wounds it can be as high as 40 per cent (Barbul, 1992; Daly et al., 1993). Wound complications can increase the patient's length of stay, necessitate reoperation, delay adjuvant treatment, and lead to sepsis if not treated appropriately. Potential complications such as wound dehiscence, necrotizing fasciitis, and gas gangrene should be considered.

Dressings are used to protect, immobilize, enhance comfort, and maintain a moist environment. Debridement of dead tissue and prevention of fluid collections are part of good wound management. It is now known that irrigation with solutions such as full-strength povidone-iodine and wet-to-dry dressings disrupt normal wound healing and base granulation tissue and should be used only when debridement is necessary. New treatment options that include alginate dressings should be considered. Alginate is known to absorb exudate without disrupting wound healing (Barbul, 1992). Dressings

may also incorporate drains. Penrose drains are passive, can be advanced, and are placed to drain by gravity. Most often a closed low-suction drainage system is used. Such drains exit the body from a separate stab wound made at the time of surgery. Percutaneous, closed, low-suction drainage systems are popular today and can be used to drain the chest, abdomen, and pelvis (Cox, 1986; Henry, 1991). Guidelines for nursing care based on wound classification and current market products are included in Table 19–8.

PSYCHOSOCIAL CONCERNS AND REHABILITATION AFTER SURGERY

People undergoing surgery for cancer report a great deal of distress, especially in the times between the first medical indication that something is wrong and obtaining the cancer diagnosis and between the discovery of cancer and the operation (Corney et al., 1992; Wainstock, 1991). Comprehensive and ongoing assessment, beginning during the person's first contact with the health care delivery system, can facilitate the provision of individualized care and result in positive physical and psychosocial outcomes.

Psychosocial examination, including exploration of concerns and assessment of the current level of coping, is vital prior to and throughout the surgical experience (Szopa, 1992). Important nursing interventions include encouraging use of usual coping strategies and support systems and assisting in identification of other potential resources. Knowledge of the patient's home environment, financial status, self-care capabilities, support personnel, support services, and employment status can yield valuable information (Szopa, 1992). Offering emotional support while administering care, and providing explanations that may allay anxiety are imperative.

Before surgery is performed, it is important to be aware of any physical or psychosocial limitations that may interfere with an individual's ability to actively participate in postoperative care (Hossan & Striegel, 1993). Familiarity with the intended surgical procedure, possible complications, and associated perioperative care is vital to provide accurate information for the patient and the family and to anticipate postoperative needs (see Table 19–4). Key areas that need to be addressed in the preoperative period include length of hospital stay, physical and psychosocial needs at hospital discharge, and an approximate time frame for returning to normal activities of daily living. Often, the benefits and outcome of surgery may not be known until the final pathology report is available, which may take up to 5 to 7 days. Waiting increases the anxiety experienced during this period (McQuarrie, 1992).

A perioperative plan of care should reflect problems commonly seen in surgical patients with cancer, as well as one that is individualized to meet specific patient needs (Langston, 1992). There are special considerations for the person undergoing a radical procedure, especially if loss of a body part or loss of function is expected. For example, women undergoing gynecologic surgery or men having a prostatectomy may be con-

TABLE 19–8. *Wound Classifications and Nursing Management Guidelines*

DESCRIPTION	GOAL	DRESSING CHOICES	SUGGESTED FREQUENCY FOR DRESSING CHANGES

Red:
Pink to red with shiny granulation tissue
Edges pearly white
	Protection	Superficial:
		  Hydrocolloid
		  Transparent film
		  Hydrogel
		Deep:
		  Moist gauze or kling; saline
		    preferred solution*
		  Calcium alginate
			
			3–5 days, 1–2 if thin
			12–48 hrs
			12–24 hrs
			
			4–8 hrs
			
			every 24 hrs

Yellow: Yellow to gray necrotic tissue or thick exudate Edges erythematous and edematous	Cleansing	Wet to damp gauze; saline preferred solution†	4–8 hrs

Black:
Black, gray, or brown necrotic tissue that
  adheres to wound
Pus may be evident
Edges erythematous, edematous
	Debridement	Surgical debridement with
		  instruments
		Wet to moist gauze dressing
		  with saline solution or
		  transparent film
			Assessment as indicated
			
			4–8 hrs

*Betadine and Dakin's solutions are toxic to healthy cells in red wound; antiseptic solution not necessary.
†Systemic antibiotics anti-microbial treatment of choice.
(Copyright 1988 The American Journal of Nursing Company. Reprinted from *American Journal of Nursing*, October, 1988, vol. 88. Used with permission. All rights reserved.)

cerned about sexual dysfunction, incontinence, and loss of sexual desire. Discussions about these issues and referrals for sexual counseling may benefit both the patient and partner (Corney et al., 1992; Maxwell, 1993). Undergoing surgery for head and neck cancer may result in some degree of cosmetic deformity, loss of some mouth dexterity, and diminished clarity of speech. It is important to reassure the patient that convalescence and rehabilitation will be longer than with other surgical experiences and will be ongoing even after hospital discharge (McQuarrie, 1992). Discharge plans that include collaboration among multiple rehabilitation services will continue to maximize outcomes after hospitalization.

Rehabilitation and positive clinical outcomes are no longer afterthoughts of cancer surgery but driving forces in the treatment decision process. Surgical nurses are challenged to create environments that minimize preoperative complications and length of stay. Barrere (1992) identified the benefits for both patients and ambulatory surgery nurses when an oncology clinical nurse specialist was consulted to provide information and support to patients and families after they were told of the cancer diagnosis. Critical pathways, clinical practice guidelines, and care maps need to reflect timely teaching to patients and families about wound management and care of external drains and lines that will remain after hospital discharge. The initiation of early community referrals for specialized home health care is imperative.

Nurses can contribute to advances in rehabilitative care though research that addresses the ongoing needs of patients experiencing cancer surgery. Oberst & Scott (1988) were some of the first nurse researchers to document that distress after cancer surgery continues long after hospital discharge (see Box 19–2). Yost, Mc-

Corkle, Wilkerson, Schultz, and Lusk (1993), explored the use of home health care services after hospitalization for cancer and concluded that home health care nurses need to be skilled in the management of cancer symptoms and complex problems commonly experienced by patients during their postoperative recovery.

Health care delivery systems that utilize nurses by services or that allow for the continued delivery of care across settings have the potential to further improve postoperative clinical outcomes. More research is needed to clarify patient and family needs in the immediate discharge period prior to the initiation of adjuvant therapies. Utilization of patient/family education materials, postdischarge telephone follow-up protocols, and nurse-scheduled consultations should be based on identified needs with the main goal of supporting rehabilitation potential.

FACING THE FUTURE OF SURGICAL ONCOLOGY NURSING

Specialization in oncology has occurred within the multidisciplinary framework that is most beneficial to the person with cancer. Surgical oncology, with its distinctive body of knowledge, evolved as a subspecialty within general surgery (Balch, 1992). Within oncology nursing, surgical oncology also emerged as a recognized area of specialization. The Surgical Oncology Special Interest Group was established as part of the Oncology Nursing Society (ONS) in 1991 to facilitate networking of members in this subspecialty area. Its mission is to develop a knowledge base and educational products to promote excellence in surgical oncology nursing (Oncology Nursing Society, 1993). Specifically, nurses in surgical oncology must incorporate knowledge of the chronic disease process and its impact on physiologic,

---

Box 19–2. *Postdischarge Distress in Surgical Cancer Patients*

Oberst, M. T., & Scott, D. W. (1988). Postdischarge distress in surgically treated cancer patients and their spouses. *Research in Nursing and Health, 11,* 223–233.

Sample: Forty patient-spouse dyads (N=80); 31 men and nine women in the patient group. All were recently diagnosed as having bowel or urinary system cancer. Mean age of patient group 59.9 years, spouse group 54.4 years. Half the patient group had a permanent ostomy (N=20).

Measures: Brief Symptom Inventory (BSI); State Trait Anxiety Inventory; Vulnerability Scale; and semistructured interviews following a COPE format at 10, 30, 60, 90, and 180 days after discharge.

Findings: Minimal variation between patients and spouses in intensity of distress. Results suggest that the crisis of initial cancer treatment is not resolved, even when the prognosis is favorable, until 3 to 6 months after discharge. The majority of spouses displayed a degree of anger, frustration, or fatigue at 2 months after discharge, and at 90 and 180 days had raised BSI scores.

Limitations: Small study of patient-spouse pairs with similar diagnosis who received care at the same urban cancer center; therefore, it is difficult to draw parallels with patients with cancer at other sites. The patient group was predominantly male, and therefore gender differences could have affected results. The majority of respondents were middle or upper class with annual incomes above the national average.

---

biologic, and psychosocial processes into all aspects of perioperative care.

The restructuring of cancer care delivery and health care economics have widespread implications for surgical oncology nurses and contribute to the challenge of providing optimal perioperative care to the person with cancer (Harvey, 1994). With complex multimodality treatments, shortened hospital stays, and invasive procedures occurring more often in outpatient settings, continuity of care is difficult to maintain. Ensuring that the patient and family receive all the pertinent information, undergo necessary physical and diagnostic testing, as well as receive optimal psychosocial care requires creativity, flexibility, and coordination of care.

The ultimate goal, to provide optimal care to people with cancer having surgery, remains unchanged. Nurses working in surgical oncology need to remain abreast of scientific and technologic advances that affect cancer care delivery to provide expert consultation about clinical problems that are unique to this population. In addition, oncology nurses need to be involved in collaborative research to document the physical and psychosocial outcomes of surgery on people with cancer and their caregivers, and the effects of nursing interventions on these outcomes.

Early intervention, anticipation of needs, and efficient utilization of resources are essential to providing high-quality, cost-effective care (Harvey, 1994). Oncology nurses must take the initiative in establishing environments in which the patient and family can ask questions and receive information while living with cancer. Basic principles of patient teaching and patient advocacy can contribute to positive short- and long-term outcomes for the person with cancer undergoing surgery.

REFERENCES

Acute Pain Management Guideline Panel. (1992). *Acute pain management: Operative or medical procedures and trauma. Clinical practice guidelines.* (AHCPR Pub. NO. 92–0032). Rockville, MD: Agency for Health Care Policy and Research, Public Health Service, U.S. Department of Health and Human Services.

Bagg, A. M. (1988). Whipple's procedure: Nursing guidelines. *Critical Care Nurse, 8*(5), 34–45.

Balch, C. M. (1992). Surgical oncology in the 21st century. *Archives of Surgery, 127,* 1272–1277.

Barbul, A. (1992). Postoperative wound infection. In J. L. Cameron (Ed.), *Current surgical therapy* (4th ed., pp. 960–967). St. Louis, MO: Mosby-Year Book.

Barrere, C. C. (1992). Breast biopsy support program: Collaboration between the oncology clinical nurse specialist and the ambulatory surgery nurse. *Oncology Nursing Forum, 19,* 1375–1379.

Chen, M. K., Souba, W. W., & Copeland, E. M. (1991). Nutritional support of the surgical oncology patient. *Hematology/Oncology Clinics of North America, 5,* 125–145.

Cohen, A. M., Martin, E. W., Lavery, I., Daly, J., Sardi, A., Aitken, D., Bland, K., Mojzisik, C., & Hinkle, G. (1991). Radioimmunoguided surgery using Iodine 125 B72. 3 in patients with colorectal cancer. *Archives of Surgery, 126,* 349–352.

Corney, R., Everett, H., Howells, A., & Crowther, M. (1992). The care of patients undergoing surgery for gynaecological cancer: The need for information, emotional support and counselling. *Journal of Advanced Nursing, 17,* 667–671.

Cox, C. E. (1986). Principles of operative surgery: Antisepsis, technique, sutures, and drains. In D. C. Sabiston (Ed.), *Textbook of surgery* (13th ed., pp. 244–258), Philadelphia: W.B. Saunders Co.

Cuzzell, J. (1988). The new RYB color code. *American Journal of Nursing, 88,* 1342–1346.

Daly, J. M. & Cady, B. (1993). Introduction. In J. M. Daly & B. Cady (Eds.), *Atlas of surgical oncology.* St. Louis, MO: Mosby-Year Book.

Daly, J. M., Wanebo, H. & DeCosse, J. J. (1993). Principles of surgical oncology. In P. Calabresi & P. S. Schein (Eds.), *Medical oncology basic principles and clinical management of cancer* (2nd ed., pp. 237–251). New York: McGraw-Hill.

Dudrick, S. J. (1991). Preface—current strategies in surgical nutrition. *The Surgical Clinics of North America, 71,* xi–xii.

Eilber, F. R. (1985). Principles of cancer surgery. In C. M. Haskell (Ed.), *Cancer treatment* (2nd ed.). Philadelphia: W.B. Saunders Co.

Eilber, F. R. (1990). Principles of cancer surgery. In C. M. Haskell (Ed.), *Cancer treatment* (3rd ed.), (pp. 9–15). Philadelphia: W.B. Saunders Co.

Elias, E. G. (1989). *Handbook of surgical oncology* (pp. 1–15). Boca Raton, FL: CRC Press.

Engelking, C. (1994). New approaches: Innovations in cancer prevention, diagnosis, treatment, and support. *Oncology Nursing Forum, 21,* 62–71.

Fischer, J. E. (1992). Metabolism in surgical patients: Protein, carbohydrate, and fat utilization by oral and parenteral routes. In D. C. Sabiston & H. K. Lyerly (Eds.), *Textbook of surgery pocket companion* (pp. 56–62). Philadelphia: W.B. Saunders Co.

Fitzsimmons, M. L., Conway, T. A., Madsen, N., Lappe, J. M., & Coody, D. (1989). Hereditary cancer syndromes: Nursing's role in identification and education. *Oncology Nursing Forum, 16,* 87–94.

Fulk, C., & Hadley, J. C. (1990). Something for pain: New trends in epidural analgesia. *Journal of Post Anesthesia Nursing, 5,* 247–253.

Gilbert, H. C. (1990). Pain relief methods in the postanesthesia care unit. *Journal of Post Anesthesia Nursing, 5,* 6–15.

Greene, F. L. (1993). Laparoscopic surgery in cancer treatment. In V. T. DeVita, S. Hellman, & S. A. Rosenberg (Eds.), *Important advances in oncology* (pp. 157–166). Philadelphia: Lippincott.

Harvey, C. (1994). New systems: The restructuring of cancer care delivery and economics. *Oncology Nursing Forum, 21,* 72–77.

Henry, J. (1991). Wound healing, dressings and drains. In M. H. Meeker, & J. C. Rothrock (Eds.), *Alexander's care of the patient in surgery* (9th ed.), (pp. 141–145). St. Louis: Mosby Year Book.

Hill, G. J. (1979). Historic milestones in cancer surgery. *Seminars in Oncology, 6,* 409–427.

Hossan, E., & Striegel, A. (1993). Carcinoma of the bladder. *Seminars in Oncology Nursing, 9,* 252–266.

Kalinowski, B. H. (1992). Surgical therapy. In S. L. Groenwald, M. H. Frogge, M. Goodman, & C. H. Yarbro (Eds.), *Cancer nursing principles and practice* (3rd ed.), (pp. 222–234). Boston: Jones & Bartlett.

Kardinal, C. G. & Yarbro, J. W. (1979). A conceptual history of cancer. *Seminars in Oncology, 6,* 396–408.

Langston, W. G. (1992). Surgical resection of lung cancer. *Nursing Clinics of North America, 27,* 665–678.

Lind, J. (1992). Tumor cell growth and cell kinetics. *Seminars in Oncology Nursing, 8,* 3–9.

Lubenow, T. R. & Ivankovich, A. D. (1991). Postoperative epidural analgesia. *Critical Care Nursing Clinics of North America, 3,* 25–31.

Maxwell, M. B. (1993). Cancer of the prostate. *Seminars in Oncology Nursing, 9,* 237–251.

McQuarrie, D. G. (1992). Head and neck cancer. *AORN Journal, 56,* 79–97.

Moffat, F. L., & Ketcham. A. S. (1994). Surgery for malignant neoplasia: The evolution of oncologic surgery and its role in the management of cancer patients. In R. J. McKenna & G. P. Murphy (Eds.), *Cancer surgery* (pp. 1–20). Philadelphia: Lippincott.

Oberst, M. T., & Scott, D. W. (1988). Postdischarge distress in surgically treated cancer patients and their spouses. *Research in Nursing and Health, 11,* 223–233.

Oncology Nursing Society. (1993). *Surgical oncology SIG strategic plan.* Pittsburgh: Oncology Nursing Society.

Pass, H. I., DeLaney, T. F., Tochner, Z., Smith, P., Temeck, B., Pogrebniak, H., Kranda, K., Russo, A., Friaus, W., Cole, J., Mitchell, J., & Thomas, G. (1994). Intrapleural photodynamic therapy: Results of a phase I trial. *Annals of Surgical Oncology, 1,* 28–37.

Pilch, Y. H. (1984). *Surgical oncology.* New York: McGraw-Hill.

Polomano, R., Blumenthal, N., Schiavone-Gatto, P., & O'Brien, J. (1993). Recommendations and guidelines for developing policies and procedures for care of patients receiving continuous epidural/narcotics/local anesthetics for postoperative pain with or without patient-controlled analgesia. *Med-Surg Nursing, 2,* 195–196.

Polomano, R., Weintraub, F. N., & Wurster, A. (1994). Surgical critical care for cancer patients. *Seminars in Oncology Nursing, 10,* 165–176.

Robinson, J. O. (1986). History of surgical oncology. In R. J. McKenna & G. P. Murphy (Eds.), *Fundamentals of surgical oncology* (pp. 14–27). New York: Macmillan.

Rosenberg, S. A. (1993). Principles of surgical oncology. In V. T. DeVita, S. Hellman, & S. A. Rosenberg (Eds.), *Cancer principles and practice of oncology* (4th ed., pp. 238–247). Philadelphia: Lippincott.

Rothrock, J. C. (1991). Sutures, needles, and instruments. In M. H. Meeker, & J. C. Rothrock (Eds.), *Alexander's care of the patient in surgery* (9th ed., pp. 114–140.), St. Louis, MO: Mosby Year Book.

Sideranko, S. (1993). Esophagogastrectomy. *Critical Care Nursing of North America, 5,* 177–184.

Smith, L. C., & Mullen, J. L. (1991). Nutritional assessment and indications for nutritional support. *The Surgical Clinics of North America, 71,* 449–457.

Szopa, T. J. (1992). Implications of surgical treatment for nursing. In J. C. Clark & R. F. McGee (Eds.), *Core curriculum for oncology nursing* (2nd ed., pp. 309–318). Philadelphia: W.B. Saunders Co.

Turner, A. F. (1994). Radiographically guided techniques of biopsy. In R. J. McKenna & G. P Murphy (Eds.), *Cancer surgery* (pp. 21–33). Philadelphia: Lippincott.

Wainstock, J. M. (1991). Breast cancer: Psychosocial consequences for the patient. *Seminars in Oncology Nursing, 7,* 207–215.

Weigel, R. J. (1992). Wound healing: Biologic and clinical features. In D. C. Sabiston, & H. K. Lyerly (Eds.), *Textbook of surgery pocket companion* (pp. 80–85). Philadelphia: W.B. Saunders Co.

Witt, T. R., & Marshall, J. S. (1991). The "mega" operation. In S. P. Economou, T. R. Witt, D. J. Deziel, T. J. Saclarides, E. D. Staren, & S. D. Bines (Eds.), *Adjuncts to cancer surgery* (pp. 233–235). Philadelphia: Lea & Febiger.

Wysocki, A. B. (1989). Surgical wound healing : A review for perioperative nurses. *AORN Journal, 49,* 502–505.

Yost, L. S., McCorkle, R., Wilkerson, K. B., Schultz, D. & Lusk, E. (1993). Determinants of subsequent home health care nursing service use by hospitalized patients with cancer. *Cancer, 72,* 3304–3312.

CHAPTER
20

Radiation Oncology

Laura J. Hilderley • Karen Hassey Dow

Radiation therapy is the use of high-energy, ionizing radiation, or x-rays, to treat cancer. The specialty of radiation oncology is a highly sophisticated subspecialty firmly grounded in basic science that has developed into a clinical science over the past 100 years. To achieve treatment goals, patient, family, and members of the radiation oncology team must fully discuss the risks vs. the benefits of therapy. In addition, treatment options should be presented and discussed.

The day to day practice of radiation oncology requires interdisciplinary collaboration among the radiation oncologists, physicists, therapists, and oncology nurses. Nursing practice is firmly established in radiation oncology and has made great strides over the past 10 years. One of the earliest documented studies on the role of nursing in radiation included a survey of 179 radiation facilities that employed at least one oncology nurse (Grant, Dodd, Hilderley, & Patterson, 1984). A study of that summary appears in Box 20–1. In 1990 the Radiation Oncology Special Interest Group (SIG) was chartered with 153 members. In 1994 the number grew to more than 500 members. As the number of nurses has increased, so too has the scope of their contribution to patient care. The Radiation SIG, through its various Work Groups has generated a number of useful documents. The first of these was the *Manual for Radiation Oncology Nursing Practice and Education* (Bruner, Iwamoto, Keane, & Stroll, 1992). The Documentation Work Group published a nursing assessment and documentation form in 1994 available in both hard copy and computer software format (ONS, 1994).

BOX 20–1. *Radiation Oncology Nursing Role*

Grant M., Dodd, M., Hilderley, L., & Patterson, P. (1984). Radiation oncology nurses' role: A national survey. *Oncology Nursing Forum Supplement: Proceedings of the Tenth Annual Congress, 11*(2), 107.

Sample: 414 institutions with radiation oncology departments from throughout the United States (respondents from a total of 1088 institutions on the mailing list).

Methodology: A 133-item questionnaire in four parts: (1) description of the facility, (2) description of department personnel, (3) demographic information about the nurse, and (4) specific functions of the nurse. 110 functions were listed in part 4, and these were further defined as to (a) person primarily responsible for that function, (b) whether nurse assumes this function if others are not available, (c) nurse's priority for the function, and (d) nurse's willingness to perform function.

Findings:

Number of institutions with no nurse: 235
Number of institutions with one nurse: 146
Number of institutions with more than one nurse: 33
Number of nurses increased with size of institution
Lines of authority in general were tied to radiation oncology department; however, as number of nurses increases, ties with nursing department increase
Average age of nurse: 35 yr

Educational preparation:	nonbaccalaureate	55%
	baccalaureate	23%
	graduate	9%
	vocational (LPN)	13%
Job satisfaction:	not at all	0%
	a little satisfied	2%
	somewhat satisfied	20%
	very satisfied	75%
Functions with highest priority ratings:	side-effect management	
	patient counseling	
	teaching patient before treatment	
	dietary counseling	
	nursing assessment	

Functions for which the nurse was responsible, but rated as low priority and was unwilling to perform:
assisting physician with examination
teaching radiation therapy technology students
conducting collaborative research

Guidelines for Radiation Safety developed by the SIG Radiation Safety Work Group (Bucholtz, 1995) has provided a valuable resource to nurses and other health care providers.

Currently within the Radiation SIG, a Research Work Group is testing a radiation therapy skin assessment tool and promoting collaborative research among its members. Another Work Group is developing the framework for a nursing quality assessment and improvement program in radiation oncology. Clearly, nurses and nursing practice have a vital role in radiation oncology.

This chapter provides an overview of radiation therapy, with a discussion of the scientific concepts of radiation physics and tumor biology that underlie treatment. The chapter also includes a review of the critical role of oncology nursing in education, support, management of side effects, and improving quality of life for patients and their families who are undergoing this cancer treatment modality.

PRINCIPLES OF RADIATION PHYSICS

The therapeutic goal of radiation oncology is to deliver a precise dose of ionizing radiation to a specific tumor volume while sparing the surrounding healthy tissue (Kijewski, 1994). Ideally radiation will result in eradication of tumor, repair of healthy tissue, and maintenance or improvement of quality of life for the patient.

Radiation treatment is based on several physical and biologic principles. When subjected to ionizing radiation, the living organism responds in a generally predictable manner. Irradiated cells are either destroyed or rendered incapable of reproduction.

All living matter is composed of molecules, the basis of which is the atom. An atom consists of two parts: a nucleus containing protons with a positive charge and neutrons with no charge, and the shell or shells composed of electrons (with negative charge) that circle in orbit around the nucleus. Figure 20–1 illustrates the structure of stable and radioactive atoms. In a stable atom, the number of negative electrons equals the number of positive protons in the nucleus; this balance between protons and electrons maintains the stability of the atom. Ionizing radiation disrupts the atom's stability by displacing electrons (ejecting them from their orbital position) and triggering a process of physical and chemical change that leads ultimately to cell injury or death.

Ionizing radiation is part of the electromagnetic spectrum, whose scale ranges from radio and

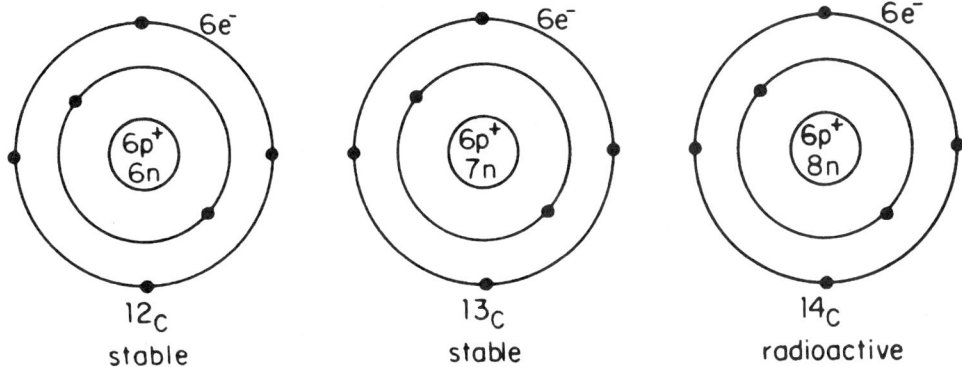

FIGURE 20–1. Composition of atoms of matter: in the stable atom, electrons are equal to the number of protons. Nuclides with the same number of protons but different number of neutrons are called isotopes. (Reprinted by permission of the publisher from Shapiro, J. [1981]. *Radiation protection: A guide for scientists and physicians* [2nd ed.]. Cambridge, MA: Harvard University Press, Copyright © 1972, 1981, 1990 by the President and Fellows of Harvard College.)

microwaves of very long length at one end of the spectrum to ionizing radiation of relatively short wavelength at the opposite end of the spectrum. The penetrating power of ionizing radiation depends on the energy of that radiation and the composition of the tissue being traversed. Thus radiotherapy equipment of varying energies is needed to meet particular needs (Tables 20–1 and 20–2).

Tissue density is a major factor in the effectiveness of ionizing radiation. As the radiation penetrates body tissue, interactions occur and energy is released. Linear energy transfer (LET) is the rate at which energy is deposited per unit distance. The significance of LET is seen in the degree of cell damage that occurs when ionizing events are closely spaced as opposed to the degree of damage in those that are more widely separated.

TABLE 20–1. *Teletherapy Equipment and Its Use*

EQUIPMENT	EMISSION	BEAM CHARACTERISTICS AND RADIOBIOLOGIC EFFECTS	CLINICAL APPLICATION, ADVANTAGES, DISADVANTAGES
Kilovoltage 40–150 kV	X-rays	Superficial, limited range, poor skin tolerance	Skin cancers or other very superficial lesions, if electrons are not available
Orthovoltage 150–1000 kV	X-rays	Deep penetration, high skin dose, high bone absorption	Limited, owing to poor skin tolerance and potential for bone necrosis
Cesium-137 radioisotope (600 kV)	Gamma rays	Large source size with large penumbra	Long half-life; low energy and output; used in head and neck treatment
Megavoltage or Supervoltage Cobalt-60 1.25–2 MeV	Gamma rays	Deeply penetrating; skin-sparing due to maximum dose build-up beneath the skin; produces penumbra area at edge of beam that receives less dose	Deep-seated tumors; ease of mechanical operation Slower dose-rate (longer treatment time) as source decays
Linear Accelerators 4–20 MeV	Photons	Deeply penetrating; skin-sparing; increased versatility and precision of dose distribution	Deep-seated tumors; large field capability; complex electronics with tendency for "down-time"
6–30 MeV	Electrons (optional)	Electrons give maximum dose on skin and a few centimeters beneath, falling off rapidly thereafter	Skin lesions, chest wall recurrence, superficial nodes
Betatron 10–30 MeV	Electrons	High-velocity electrons with deep penetration	High dose rate with shorter treatment time; limited field size; bulky equipment; low dose rate photons
18-40 MeV	X-rays	High-energy photons	

(From Hilderley, L. [1992]. Radiation oncology: Historical background and principles of teletherapy. In K. Hassey Dow & L. Hilderley [Eds.], *Nursing care in radiation oncology* [pp. 3–15]. Philadelphia: W. B. Saunders Co.)

TABLE 20–2. *High Linear Energy Transfer (LET) and Heavy Charged Particle Beams*

ENERGY SOURCE	BEAM CHARACTERISTICS AND RADIOBIOLOGIC EFFECTS	USE IN CLINICAL TRIALS
Fast Neutrons 16–50 MeV deuterons	Fixed field size and beam position; wide penumbra; absorbed dose decreases exponentially with depth; low OER; RBE is higher with small dose increments	Advanced cancers of the head and neck, pelvis, gliomas, and melanoma; esophageal cancer and osteosarcomas
Protons and Helium Ions 600 MeV	Precise dose distribution with ability to deliver very high tumor dose with sparing of adjacent normal tissues; RBE and OER similar to those obtained with gamma and photon sources	Pituitary tumors, chondrosarcoma, cordoma; abdominal and pelvic tumors; soft-tissue sarcomas; head and neck tumors
Negative Pi-Mesons 40–70 MeV	Absorbed dose increases slowly with depth, then rises sharply; lower OER; enhanced RBE	Head and neck tumors, brain, prostate, pancreas; skin metastases

OER = Oxygen enhancement ratio; RBE = relative biologic effectiveness.
(From Hilderley, L. [1992]. Radiation oncology: Historical background and principles of teletherapy. In K. Hassey Dow & L. Hilderley [Eds.], *Nursing care in radiation oncology* [pp. 3–15]. Philadelphia: W. B. Saunders Co.)

This difference in cell damage as influenced by LET is known as the relative biologic effectiveness or RBE (Griffin, 1987).

PRINCIPLES OF RADIOBIOLOGY

TARGET THEORY

The exact mechanism of cell killing or cell damage by ionizing radiation has been the subject of research for many years. The actual mechanism by which radiation energy causes biologic damage is a highly complex sequence of events. *Target theory* proposes that radiation damage is the result of both direct and indirect hits (Coleman, Beard, Hlatky, Kwok, & Bump, 1994; Travis, 1975). A *direct hit* refers to damage to DNA, the critical target. Results of a direct hit are (1) change or loss of a base (thymine, adenine, guanine, or cytosine), (2) breakage of the hydrogen bond between the two chains of the DNA molecule, (3) breaks in one or both chains of the DNA molecule, and (4) cross-linking of the chains after breakage.

An *indirect hit* refers to the ionization of water, the medium surrounding the molecular structures within the cell. Ionizing radiation absorbed by water molecules initiates a series of chemical interactions, the most important of which is production of the hydroxyl radical, OH. This free radical is now available to combine with others, forming new and potentially cytotoxic agents. Because water is the predominant substance in any tissue, the likelihood that indirect hits and resulting cell injury will occur is greater than that for direct damage to the DNA structure. Box 20–2 illustrates the sequence of events in the ionization of water by radiation.

THE FOUR Rs OF RADIOBIOLOGY

Radiation effect at the cellular level is a function of the cell's response to the damaging effects of ionization. Although the goal of treatment is to destroy tumor tissue, healthy tissue must be preserved. Fractionation of dose is based upon the following four Rs of radiobiology: repair, repopulation, redistribution, and reoxygenation.

REPAIR

Fractionated radiation doses should allow repair of sublethal damage. Between daily treatment fractions, the normal tissue is able to repair radiation injury, whereas tumor cells are less likely to do so.

REPOPULATION

Repopulation of normal cells through mitosis after repair of radiation injury allows continued proliferation of normal tissue. Tumor cells are less likely to undergo mitosis because of inability to repair sublethal damage.

REDISTRIBUTION

Ionizing radiation is believed to be most effective during the mitotic stage of the cell cycle. With each successive dose of radiation, more cells are likely to be in actual mitosis through cycle delay, therefore increasing the effectiveness of each dose. Normal cells are much less likely to be delayed or redistributed in their cycle than tumor cells.

REOXYGENATION

Well-oxygenated cells are more sensitive to radiation effect than hypoxic cells. Protracted fractionation of dose allows reoxygenation and therefore enhances radiosensitivity of tumor cells, which may have been hypoxic.

BIOLOGIC RESPONSE TO RADIATION

Response to radiation occurs at the cellular level, triggering a sequence of biologic events that result in tissue injury, destruction, or ultimate repair. Some of the earliest work in radiobiology was that of Bergonie and Tribondeau (1959), who theorized that radiosensi-

---

Box 20–2. *Ionization of Water Molecules*

Water, which constitutes 80 per cent of the mammalian cell content, undergoes a series of chemical reactions when exposed to ionizing radiation. In the following, water (HOH) is converted to hydrogen peroxide (H_2O_2).

The final products of the ionization of water molecules (HOH) by radiation are an ion pair (H^+, OH^-) and free radicals (H, OH), which are capable of damaging the cell. The ionization of water is shown in the following steps:

$$HOH \xrightarrow{\text{Radiation}} HOH^+ + e^-$$

The free electron (e^-) is then captured by another available water molecule and, as shown in the next step, forms the second ion:

$$HOH + e^- \rightarrow HOH^-$$

Because the two ions (HOH^+, HOH^-) produced by these reactions are unstable, rapid breakdown occurs (in the presence of other normal water molecules), forming yet another ion and a free radical as follows:

$$HOH^+ \rightarrow H^+ + OH$$

$$HOH^- \rightarrow OH^- + H$$

Although the resulting ion pair (H^+, OH^-) have some potential for cellular damage through chemical reactions, they are more likely to recombine and form water (HOH). The free radicals (H, OH) are extremely reactive, and they too may simply recombine to form water. However, free radicals appear to be more likely to undergo chemical interactions with other free radicals, forming cytotoxic agents, as shown in this reaction:

$$OH + OH \rightarrow H_2O_2 \text{ (hydrogen peroxide)}$$

Free radicals that result from the interaction of radiation with water are capable of triggering a variety of chemical reactions within the cell and are therefore believed to be a major factor in the production of damage in the cell.

From Hilderley, L. (1993). Radiotherapy. In S. L. Groenwald, M. H. Frogge, M. Goodman, & C. H. Yarbro (Eds.), *Cancer nursing: Principles and practice* (3rd ed., pp. 235–269). ©1993 Boston: Jones and Bartlett Publishing. Reprinted with permission.

---

tivity is directly related to the reproductive capacity of a cell. This theory was based on their experiments on rat testes, in which they successfully destroyed the germ cells, leaving the interstitial and supporting cells of the seminiferous tubules intact.

RADIOSENSITIVITY

Radiosensitivity refers to the degree and speed of response to radiation of any given tissue, whether it is tumor tissue or normal healthy tissue. Within the cell cycle, radiosensitivity also varies. According to Hall (1994), cells are most sensitive at or close to mitosis, resistance is usually greatest in the latter part of the S phase, if G_1 has an appreciable length, a resistant period is evident early in G_1 followed by a sensitive period toward the end of G_1, and the G_2 phase is usually sensitive to radiation, perhaps as sensitive as the M phase.

Radiosensitivity varies with the type of tumor as well as with its size and location. Some malignant lesions generally classified as radiosensitive include seminoma, acute lymphocytic leukemia, Hodgkin's disease, and lymphomas. Among the more radioresistant tumors are squamous cell carcinomas, ovarian tumors, soft-tissue sarcomas, and gliomas.

Similarly, normal tissues and organs can be classified according to degree of radiosensitivity, based on parenchymal hypoplasia. Lymphoid organs, bone marrow, gonads, skin, and mucous membranes are highly radiosensitive. Those organs and tissues categorized as having a low degree of radiosensitivity (relatively radioresistant) include mature bone and cartilage, liver, thyroid gland, muscle, brain, and spinal cord.

RADIOCURABILITY

Radiocurability is a term used to describe the ability to eradicate tumor at the local or regional site. Unfortunately, radiosensitivity does not necessarily equate with radiocurability. Some of the most radiosensitive tumors are also among the most anaplastic and undifferentiated (metastasizing early and rapidly) and thus are not radiocurable.

RADIATION TECHNIQUES

Two major methods of delivering radiation therapy are used: teletherapy and brachytherapy. Teletherapy makes use of a machine (such as a linear accelerator) to deliver ionizing radiation from outside the body. Brachytherapy involves placement of a radioactive source within or close to the tissue to be treated, such as the interstitial or intracavitary techniques used in the treatment of oral and gynecologic cancers.

TELETHERAPY

Teletherapy (from *tele*, Greek prefix meaning at a distance) is external radiation treatment given with a machine or source at some distance from the target site. Early machines had a kilovoltage in the range of 40 to 150 kV and produced x-rays with minimal penetration because of their low energy. Between 1920 and 1940, orthovoltage equipment, with a range of 180- to 250-kV energy, was introduced, providing the capability to treat much more deeply seated tumors. Healthy tissues were not spared, however, and poor skin tolerance combined with late bone necrosis limited the therapeutic value of orthovoltage equipment.

Nuclear research in the era of World War II led to technology that helped to develop radioactive sources for therapeutic use. In the early 1940s, radiation therapy entered the supervoltage era. Atomic reactors made Cobalt-60 a more readily available source, and the betatron and linear accelerator were developed. The betatron was the first generator of supervoltage x-rays used therapeutically, and this machine was favored for its ability to produce high energy at a relatively low cost. There were disadvantages, however, including the low intensity of the beam and the physical massiveness of the equipment required to produce the x-rays.

Cobalt-60 was first used in a teletherapy unit in 1951. Cobalt machines became the standard source for deep therapy and were utilized in most radiotherapy treatment centers. Their major advantage is the relative simplicity of the equipment, which requires minimal maintenance (time and cost) and is highly reliable.

The linear accelerator (Linac) evolved out of the electronics era of the 1960s and 1970s and is widely used today. An example of a linear accelerator is shown in Figure 20–2. These highly sophisticated machines operate on the principle of rapid acceleration of electrons in a vacuum. As the electrons strike a metal target such as tungsten, photons are produced. Photons are the equivalent of gamma rays and x-rays, differing only in their means of production. Some linear accelerators are dual-purpose, capable of emitting either electrons or photons. If electrons are used, the metal target is removed from the path of the accelerated electrons, allowing them to emerge from a narrow window in the vacuum tube, targeted directly at the treatment site. Table 20–1 lists low LET standard teletherapy equipment, types of emissions, beam char-

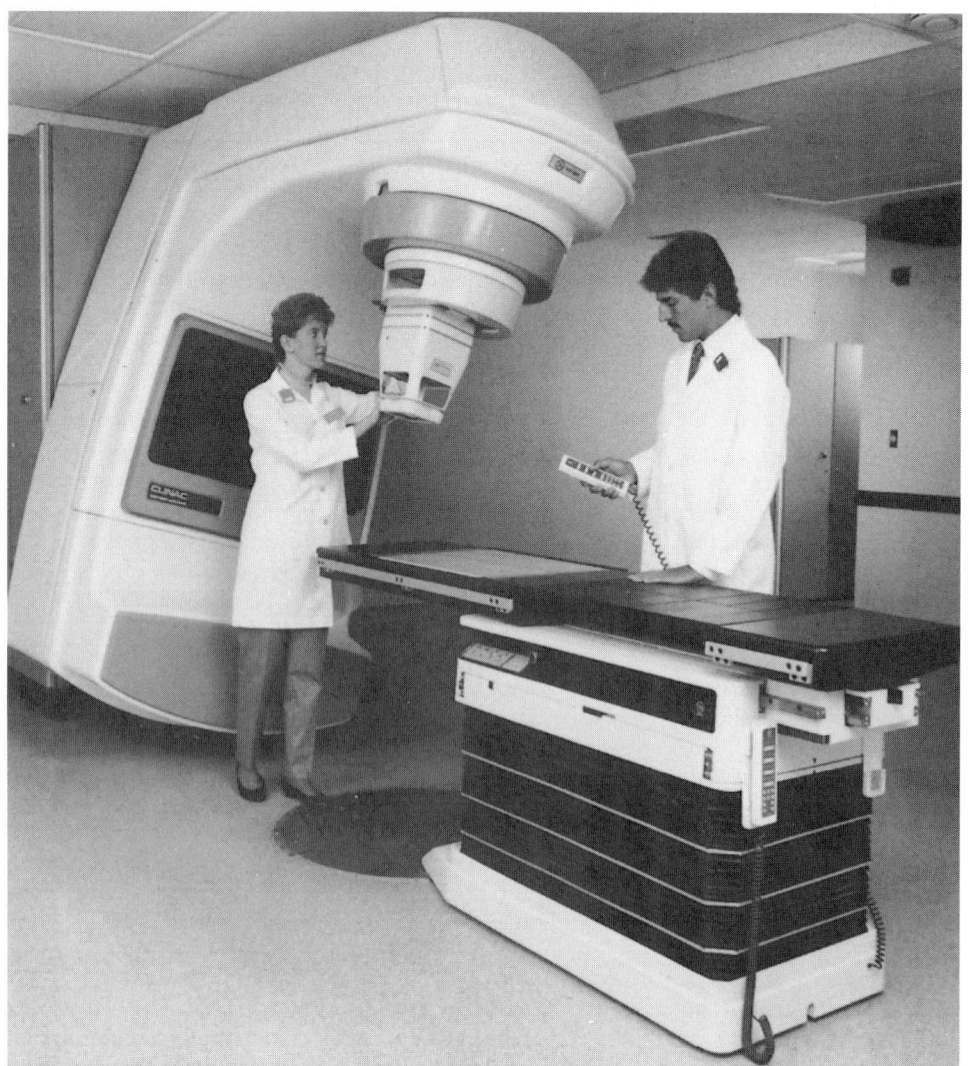

FIGURE 20–2. A Varian Clinac 2100 C linear accelerator with x-ray energies ranging from 6 to 18 Mv and electron beams from 4 to 20 MeV. (Varian Associates, Inc., Palo Alto, CA. Reproduced by permission.)

acteristics, and clinical applications as well as limitations.

HIGH LET AND HEAVY CHARGED PARTICLE BEAMS

Megavoltage teletherapy equipment, as described previously, is the most common means of delivering radiation therapy. In some situations, a distinct therapeutic advantage can be gained through the use of heavy charged particle beams or high linear energy transfer (LET) radiations (Munzenrider & Crowell, 1994). Characteristics of high LET and heavy charged particle beams are described in Table 20–2. The two major advantages to these sources of ionizing radiation are (1) deposition of large doses of radiation in small volumes of tissue with sparing of surrounding normal tissue (by proton beams, heavy ions, and negative pi mesons), and (2) biologic advantages, including more effective killing of hypoxic cells and decreased fluctuation in radiosensitivity throughout the cell cycle (by fast neutrons, heavy ions, and pi mesons) (Griffin, 1987; Munzenrider & Crowell, 1994).

The physical and biologic advantages of high LET and heavy charged particle beams are offset somewhat by the complexity and costs of the equipment and facilities required. However, it is generally agreed (Griffin, 1987; Munzenrider & Crowell, 1994) that despite slow accumulation of data, the sparsity of population groups in any given tumor category, and the complexity and cost of equipment, research into the clinical application of high LET and charged particle beam therapy should continue and expand.

GOALS OF RADIATION THERAPY IN CANCER MANAGEMENT

Radiation therapy has multiple applications in cancer treatment. It may be given (1) with curative intent, (2) to help control local disease, (3) as an adjuvant to surgery, chemotherapy, or biologic therapy, and (4) as palliative treatment. Radiation dosage terminology is listed in Table 20–3.

Curative radiation therapy generally refers to a situation in which this modality is the primary treatment, as in treating skin cancers or early-stage breast, laryngeal, or prostate cancers (Marks & Sessions, 1987; Million, Cassisi, & Wittes, 1985; Perez, 1987). Generally, if radiation is the primary treatment, extensive surgery can be avoided, thus sparing the patient from the significant physical and psychologic side effects of radical surgery. When the intent is curative and radiation is the primary method being used, the treatment course is generally longer and the dose is higher than in a palliative situation. Curative doses of 45 to 70 Gy given over 6 to 8 weeks are usual. For example, when radiation is combined with minimal surgery (breast-conserving surgery) in a woman with early-stage breast cancer, the intent is cure, and doses range between 46 and 50 Gy (Levitt & Perez, 1987; Mendenhall, Ames, Sarrazin, & Veronisi, 1991; Wilson, 1989).

Radiation therapy is also used to *control* local disease and is often combined with chemotherapy and surgery in achieving local and regional control. For example, control of locally advanced breast cancer and head and neck cancer is greatly enhanced by combining radiotherapy with adjuvant chemotherapy (Phillips, 1994). Radiation is unquestionably effective in control of microscopic nodal disease (Richter, Share, & Goodman, 1985).

Adjuvant therapy is given to enhance or assist the primary method of treatment. For example, radiation is used in an adjuvant manner when it is given preoperatively for early colorectal cancers. In this instance, the purpose of the radiation is to sterilize microscopic disease beyond the surgical margins, to reduce tumor bulk, to reduce the likelihood of residual tumor cell implants, and to avoid the need for regional lymphadenopethy. A second example of the use of adjuvant radiotherapy is in treating sanctuary sites (central ner-

---

TABLE 20–3. *Radiation Dosage Terminology*

In 1985 the International Commission on Radiation Units and Measurements (ICRU) designated several new terms related to radiation dose. Medical and nursing literature began to reflect these changes in the late 1980s. Therefore, for clarity, both the old and the new terms are listed here.

Becquerel (Bq): Unit of measure for the amount of activity of a radioactive nuclide in a particular energy state. One becquerel equals one nuclear disintegration per second. The becquerel replaces the former unit designation *curie*. (1 Bq $= 2.7 \times 10^{-11}$ Ci)

Curie (Ci): Unit of measure formerly used to describe the rate of nuclear disintegration of a radioactive source. This unit is now called a becquerel (Bq). (1 Ci $= 3.7 \times 10^{10}$ Bq)

Gray (Gy): Unit of radiation dose (one joule per kilogram). Measure of the energy deposited by radiation in an absorbing medium. The gray has replaced the term *rad*. 1 gray equals 100 cGy equals 100 rad. (1 rad equals 1 cGy)

Rad (r): Acronym for *r*adiation *a*bsorbed *d*ose. One rad equals an energy absorption of 100 ergs per gram of absorber. In 1985, the term gray (Gy) became the official term for radiation absorbed dose, replacing the rad. One gray equals 100 rad, and 1 cGy equals 1 rad.

Rem: Acronym for *r*oentgen *e*quivalent—*m*an, the term used to measure the dose equivalent of ionizing radiation when considering radiation safety and radiation protection rather than therapeutic radiation dose. Dose in rem equals dose in rad × quality factor (QF). The QF has a different value for different radiations. Rem has been replaced by the term *sievert* (Sv). (1 rem = 0.01 Sv)

Roentgen (R): Unit of exposure to ionizing radiation: refers to the ability of x-rays to ionize air.

Sievert (Sv): The unit of dose equivalent of ionizing radiation is equivalent to one joule per kilogram. The Sv has replaced the term *rem* and is used in radiation protection and radiation safety when quantifying occupational exposure. (1 Sv = 100 rem)

vous system) in patients with acute lymphocytic leukemia, whose primary treatment is chemotherapy. Radiation facilitates transfer of the chemotherapeutic agent across the blood-brain barrier, which is composed of the perivascular glial membrane and vascular endothelium.

Approximately one half of all patients treated with radiation therapy are treated for *palliation* of symptoms. Treatment to sites of bone metastases is very effective in relieving pain as well as in restoring mobility in some situations. Pain attributable to pressure or obstruction of a hollow viscus by bulky lesions can also be palliated with radiotherapy. Other situations requiring palliation include bleeding, necrosis, ulceration, superior vena caval (SVC) syndrome, central nervous system metastases, and functional obstruction (respiratory, gastrointestinal, genitourinary). When radiation treatment is needed in an emergency situation (SVC syndrome, spinal cord compression, bronchial obstruction, hemorrhage), it is generally given with palliative intent as well.

Principles of palliative treatment include use of a short, sometimes intensive course of treatment to achieve a rapid result. Treatment is generally completed in 1 or 2 weeks, and it may be discontinued if palliation has been achieved before the prescribed course is completed. This is especially important if quality of life is diminished or disturbed more by the daily travel to the treatment facility than by the symptoms being palliated. The nurse has an important role in observing the patient's response and communicating with the radiotherapist regarding the patient's total situation.

STEPS TO DELIVERY OF RADIATION THERAPY

CONSULTATION

The patient's initial visit to the radiation therapy facility is for consultation, assessment, and discussion of the role of radiation in his or her treatment. A family member or significant other should be encouraged to accompany the patient to help provide information as well as to reinforce information given by the caregivers. During this visit, a complete history is taken, a physical examination is performed, and a plan of radiation is described. Diagnostic studies and pathology reports may be reviewed before the consultation, and they may also be presented for discussion at a multidisciplinary tumor conference.

Ideally, the radiation oncology nurse meets with the patient on the consultation visit (Hilderley, 1980, 1991). In addition to performing a nursing assessment, the nurse may begin the physical orientation to the radiation facility, initiate patient and family education about the proposed treatment and potential side effects, and provide both physical and emotional support as needed. By establishing contact on this first visit, the radiation oncology nurse becomes a resource for both the patient and the staff in providing continuity throughout treatment and follow-up.

TREATMENT PLANNING

Before radiation treatments can be started, a series of steps are taken to define the treatment target, ensure the accuracy of daily setups, and protect healthy tissues from radiation injury. The radiation therapist, physics staff members, and radiation oncologist are involved in a process termed *simulation*.

In simulation the target volume is localized and defined by using x-rays, scans, and physical landmarks. The patient is positioned exactly as he or she will be positioned for the actual treatment, using coordinate points on the body to ensure alignment. This process takes place using a simulator machine, which mimics the physical characteristics of the teletherapy machine but does not deliver ionizing radiation. Figure 20–3 illustrates an example of a treatment simulator.

Immobilization devices such as casts (or other molded materials), head holders, or restraints may be needed to ensure accurate positioning. Need for such devices is determined during simulation, and the appropriate devices are prepared.

Skin markings are needed to define the target or portal. During simulation, ink marks are placed to indicate the area of treatment as well as to mark the coordinate points as a guide to proper positioning. These markings may be left in place for a period of days until accuracy of positioning has been verified. At a later point, permanent tattoos are placed to identify the field and coordinate points, at which time the ink markings may be removed. Tattoos are very tiny, discrete, permanent dots that are barely visible to the casual observer.

Lead blocks are often needed to help shape the radiation beam and block radiation from reaching organs and tissues adjacent to the tumor site. A radiation beam is rectangular, and its size can be changed by adjusting the collimater on the machine. However, because treatment portals are not always rectangular in shape, lead blocks must be prepared for positioning between the beam source and the patient to block areas within the beam that are not to be treated.

Computerized treatment plans based on measurements and radiographs taken during simulation as well as on beam characteristics are now a routine part of treatment planning. These computer-generated plans help to determine the final treatment prescription, which includes description of the treatment field or fields, total dose, daily dose fraction, and elapsed time.

RADIATION TREATMENTS

When simulation and treatment planning are complete, the patient begins a course of therapy that ranges from 2 to 8 weeks, with the average course lasting 5 weeks. Treatments are given on a daily basis, 5 days per week. Altered fractionation regimens (such as two treatments per day, fewer than five treatments per week, or single hemibody treatments of very large doses) may be employed in special situations. Two treatments per day (separated by at least 4 hours) may

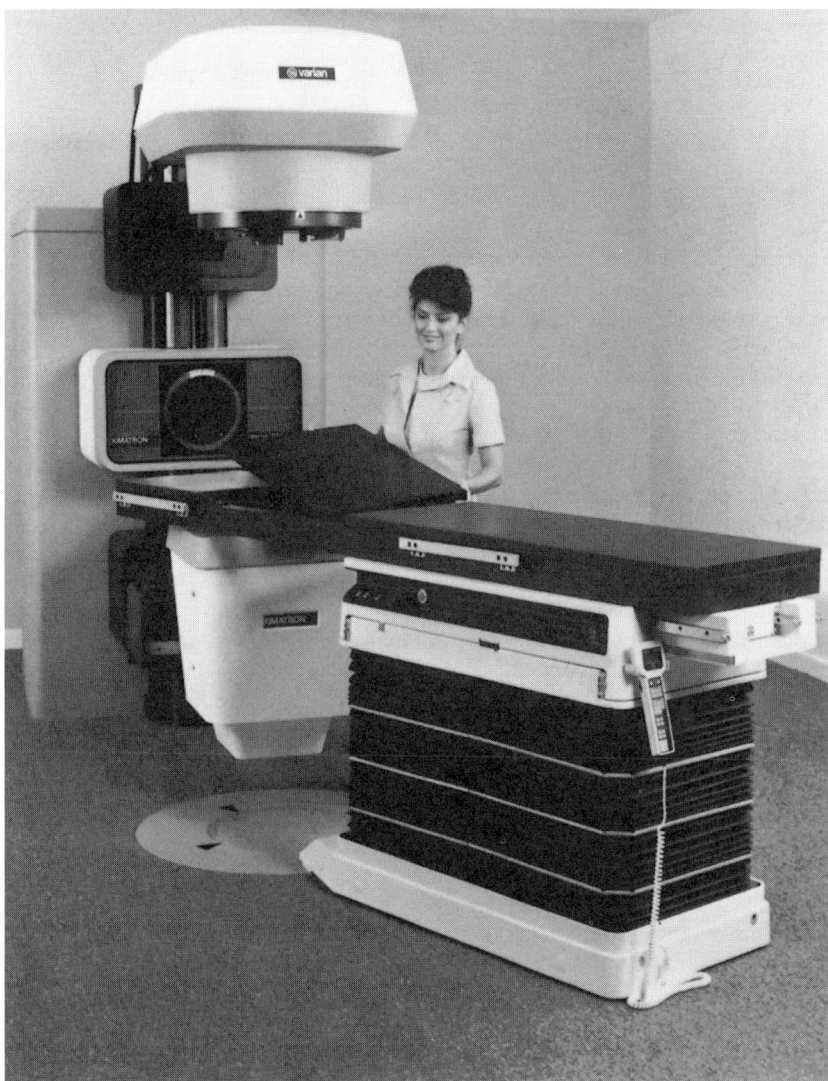

FIGURE 20–3. A Varian Ximatron™ C-Series radiation therapy simulator. (Varian Associates, Inc., Palo Alto, CA. Reproduced by permission.)

be used for a particularly radioresistant tumor. Severely debilitated patients or those with transportation problems may be treated three or four times per week. Widespread bony metastasis can be effectively treated with a single dose of 500 cGy to the upper, middle, or lower hemibody. The reader is referred to Dudjak (1992) for details of treatment with altered fractionation and nursing implications.

TREATMENT PROCESS

Teletherapy treatments take only a few minutes of actual radiation exposure and require approximately 10 minutes in the treatment room altogether. Most of this time is spent in positioning the patient and the machine, then repositioning the beam to a second, third, or fourth angle to treat each prescribed field. For example, treatment of the uterus or prostate is generally done using the four-field box technique, which employs anterior, posterior, and two lateral fields. Some treatments are more complex, requiring multiple angles or changing the patient's position (for example, supine to prone), and therefore take longer to complete. Others are very simple setups in which only a single field is utilized and the treatment is completed in a few minutes.

Periodic beam films (also called check films or portal films) are taken to ensure the accuracy of the setup. A beam film is a radiograph taken through the treatment beam that is then compared with the original simulation films to evaluate positioning and technique. This process takes a few extra minutes on the treatment table, and patients mistakenly think that this film will show changes such as tumor shrinkage. Careful explanation of the process and its purpose is important.

Treatment machines are very large and may be somewhat noisy, but patients can be assured that there is no pain or sensation of any kind during the treatment. People expect to feel heat, tingling, or some other sensation, but this does not happen. Some discomfort may result from positioning or from lying on a very firm table, however. An example of a linear accelerator is shown in Figure 20–2.

Treatments are given by a team of registered radiation therapists who have an important role both in patient care and in the technical delivery of the prescribed treatment. Therapists see the patient daily (the radiation oncology nurse and radiation oncologist may not) and can therefore monitor any alterations in either physical or emotional status. Patients are then referred to the nurse or physician for management of problems.

During a course of treatment, the patient is usually seen and examined by the radiation oncologist or radiation oncology nurse (or both) at least once per week. This status check (on-therapy review) serves to monitor the progress of treatment, to assess reactions, and to offer supportive physical and emotional interventions. It is vital that patients and their families understand the importance of completing the prescribed course of therapy. Nurses are in an excellent position to effectively support patients throughout a lengthy treatment course, thus helping to ensure compliance and completion (Oberst, Hughes, Chang, & McCubbin, 1991).

Patients can expect to be weighed each week during therapy and to have a complete blood count (CBC) and platelet count obtained weekly as well. In some treatment centers, radiation therapy patients are also seen and assessed by other members of the cancer care team on a regular basis. Oncology social workers, nutritionists, physical therapists, dentists, and psycho-oncologists are valuable resources. In addition to working with individual patients, these professionals also are participants in conferences that are held to review patient progress.

THE POSTTREATMENT PERIOD

When a course of treatment is completed, the radiation therapy patient is again examined by the radiation oncologist and radiation oncology nurse. The appropriate physical examination is followed by review of posttreatment instructions and discussion of changes that can be expected in the coming weeks. The radiation oncology nurse has primary responsibility for patient education and side-effects management, often maintaining close telephone contact with the patient after treatment ends. Referrals to the appropriate community agencies are made, and in addition the nurse serves as a consultant on radiation patient care to nurses in these agencies as well as to the inpatient nursing staff (Hilderley, 1980, 1991).

Most radiation oncologists follow the treated patient with periodic checkups for varying periods of time. Particularly if radiation is the primary treatment (early breast, head and neck, and skin cancers), the radiation oncologist may remain as the patient's primary cancer physician.

Posttreatment evaluation varies in scope from a physical examination to multiple radiographic studies. Patients are eager for concrete evidence that their cancer is either gone or greatly reduced in size. Obviously, this cannot always be assessed, because treatment may have been either prophylactic or adjuvant, in which case there was no measurable tumor in the first place. When a definable tumor mass has been treated, an obvious change, shrinkage, and improvement in symptoms may be immediately noticed. Conversely, it may take weeks or months after treatment for tumor shrinkage to be measurable. These are frustrating times for the patient, during which nursing support and patient education continue to be important.

SIDE EFFECTS AND THEIR MANAGEMENT

Radiation therapy is local treatment delivered to those structures located within the target volume. Most treatment fields encompass a limited volume or area of the body, with the exception of total body irradiation (TBI), used before bone marrow transplantation or hemibody treatment for extensive bone metastases. Most physical side effects of radiation therapy are confined to those tissues and organs within the path of the radiation beam. Onset, severity, and duration of reactions can be correlated with the cell renewal characteristics of the target tissue, total dose, fractionation, concomitant therapies, nutritional status, and volume of tissue irradiated.

Side effects, which occur during a course of treatment and up to 6 months afterward, are considered acute reactions. Those that occur or persist after 6 months are categorized as late or chronic effects. Acute radiation reactions develop as a result of radiation effect on cell renewal tissues of the skin and mucous membranes. The mucosa of the oropharynx, small intestine, rectum, bladder, and vagina is often affected and produces some of the more severe reactions seen. Size and number of doses (fractionation) and the length of course (protraction) are the factors that influence the severity of acute side effects (Rubin, Constine, & Nelson, 1992). Acute effects usually resolve fairly quickly when treatment is completed as the rate of new cell proliferation returns to normal and cell destruction ends.

Late or chronic effects of ionizing radiation—which persist or occur 6 months or more after treatment—are frequently unrelated to the occurrence or severity of acute reactions. Late effects appear to be closely related to *total* dose of radiation and *size* of dose fraction. In contrast to acute reactions, the damage seen in late effects is thought to be related to injury to stromal vasculature or to endothelial cells rather than solely to the cell renewal system. In addition to specific organ damage (blindness, transection of the spinal cord), such late effects as necrosis, ulceration, and fibrosis may be seen. Table 20–4 lists major site-specific early and late effects of radiation therapy.

Management of radiation-induced physical side effects is a primary function of the radiation oncology nurse (Strohl, 1988, 1990). The concept of *local treatment—local effect* is very important in planning and providing nursing care. Most side effects can be predicted, and patients can therefore be prepared with

TABLE 20–4. *Major Acute and Chronic Side Effects of Radiation Therapy*

SITE	ACUTE EFFECT	CHRONIC EFFECT
Skin	Erythema (3000–4000 cGy); dry desquamation, moist desquamation (4500–6000 cGy)	Fibrosis, atrophy, telangiectasia, permanent darkening of skin
Oral cavity	Change and loss of taste, dryness, mucositis (3000–4000 cGy)	Permanent xerostomia, permanent taste alterations, dental caries
Esophagus	Pain, esophagitis	Fibrosis
Stomach	Nausea and vomiting (125 cGy)	Obstruction, ulceration, fibrosis
Intestines	Diarrhea (2000 – 3000 cGy)	Malabsorption strictures, necrosis (6000–7000 cGy)
Kidney		Radiation nephritis
Bladder	Cystitis (3000 cGy)	Fibrosis, contracted bladder (6500–7000 cGy)
Bone marrow	↓ White blood cells and platelets	May be chronic anemia especially with combined modality treatment
Respiratory system	Pneumonitis (2500–3000 cGy)	Fibrosis
Cardiovascular system	Rare reports of pericarditis, myocarditis	Fibrosis
Central nervous system	Edema and inflammation	Infarction, occlusion, necrosis
Brain and spinal cord		
Peripheral nerves		
Eyes		Cataracts
Bone and cartilage (child)		Growth disturbances if growth plate of bone is in field (2000–3000 cGy)
Gonads		
Spermatogonia	↓ Sperm count after 90–120 days; temporary sterility (100–300 cGy)	
Ovary	Sterility (500–1000 cGy) depends on age	

(From Strohl, R. [1988]. The nursing role in radiation oncology: Symptom management of acute and chronic reactions. *Oncology Nursing Forum, 15*[4], 431. Reprinted by permission.)

appropriate self-care behaviors. Patient knowledge of what to expect and when to expect it usually helps to reduce anxiety, particularly among patients who have preconceived ideas about radiation therapy. Most patients benefit as much from learning what *will not* happen as what to anticipate.

COMMON ACUTE SIDE EFFECTS OF RADIATION THERAPY: SYMPTOM MANAGEMENT

SKIN REACTIONS

Regardless of body site, radiation must penetrate skin to reach its target within the body. Skin reaction varies from very mild erythema to moist desquamation, and some patients exhibit no skin changes at all. Various systems have been used to categorize skin reactions (Hilderley, 1983), and each treatment facility devises a method of skin care that seems most effective in minimizing both discomfort and any permanent skin changes.

Some of the basic principles of care include the following:

1. Avoid friction, pressure, and thermal extremes.
2. Cleanse treated site gently, using mild soap.
3. Avoid using any skin care products other than those recommended by the radiation oncologist or nurse.

An example of skin care instructions for the patient is shown in Table 20–5. When reactions become very intense, with moist desquamation (owing to high dose, surface treatment, enhancement by concomitant medications), special procedures may be needed. These measures might include daily flushing and cleansing followed by application of topical agents or dressings, or both. Occlusive dressings should not be used because they tend to inhibit healing. Moisture- and vapor-permeable dressings help to promote healing. Care must be taken to avoid placing tape on irradiated skin, because each time it is removed, the skin beneath is further traumatized.

Some of the topical agents currently used for brisk erythema and moist desquamation include vitamin A and D ointment, suspensions or ointments containing petrolatum, aloe, or lanolin, and silver sulfadiazine (Dini et al., 1993).

Most radiation skin reactions heal very well when appropriate care is taken. A severe reaction that includes moist desquamation may result in increased pigmentation of that skin. Sitton (1992a, 1992b) presents a thorough discussion of the biology of radiation skin reaction and summarizes current practices in skin care. The Radiation SIG is currently involved in a multisite study with the goal of standardizing care of radiation skin reactions.

ALOPECIA

When the head is irradiated, alopecia (either partial or complete) will occur. Doses between 30 and 35 Gy cause temporary hair loss, with regrowth starting approximately 1 month after treatment. Rate of re-

TABLE 20–5. *Skin Care During Radiation*

Skin over the area where you are receiving radiation therapy needs to be treated with gentle care. During your course of radiation treatment, please follow these guidelines:

Keep the treated area dry and free from irritation.

Do not wash the treated area until 2 or 3 days after the start of your radiation treatments.

Do not remove the lines or ink marks that have been placed on your skin until the end of radiation treatments.

When permitted, wash the treated skin gently, using a mild soap, and rinse well before patting dry. Always use warm or cool water, *not* hot water.

Do not apply any lotions, creams, alcohol, aftershave, perfume, deodorants, or other skin preparations in the treated area.

Do not apply heating pads and hot-water bottles directly on treated skin.

Avoid friction, that is, avoid clothing that is tight or may rub over the treated skin such as tight shirt collars, ties, undergarments, belts.

Men should use an electric razor if they are receiving treatment to the face or neck area. Do not use aftershave.

If treated skin becomes reddened or tender, you may apply a thin layer of vitamin A and D ointment. Be sure to let us know when redness occurs. If further irritation develops, we will give you special instructions or medications for skin care.

Protect the treatment area from exposure to direct sunlight. While you are receiving a course of therapy, do not sunbathe or spend more than a few minutes in the bright sun if the treated area is exposed. We will give you special instructions about future sun exposure when you finish your course of treatment.

(Reproduced by permission from Philip G. Maddock and Laura Hilderley, Radiation Oncology, Warwick, Rhode Island.)

growth varies, but most patients will have a reasonable regrowth in 6 to 9 months. At higher doses (40 Gy and above) to the scalp, alopecia is usually permanent.

Radiation-induced alopecia is not preventable. However, care of the hair and scalp is important in minimizing skin reaction. Use of a mild shampoo, followed by thorough rinsing and gentle towel drying, is recommended. Patients should avoid hair dryers, curling devices, chemicals (for coloring or curling), and even vigorous brushing of the hair. Any of these will hasten the inevitable hair loss but, more important, will likely enhance skin reaction on the scalp. Areas particularly susceptible to erythema and desquamation include the forehead and periauricular tissues. Care of the scalp follows general guidelines for skin care. In addition, patients may want to purchase a wig or use hats, turbans, or scarves. Protection of the scalp from summer sun, as well as protection from heat loss via the bare scalp in winter, should be part of patient education content.

The Look Good, Feel Better Program cosponsored by the Cosmetic, Toiletry and Fragrance Association Foundation (CTFA) and the National Cosmetology Association (NCA) in conjunction with the American Cancer Society (ACS) provides excellent tips, suggestions, and support for individuals wishing to maintain their appearance during radiation treatment. Inquiries about this program can be made through local units of the ACS.

MUCOSITIS

Mucosa of the respiratory, digestive, and genitourinary tracts is sensitive to radiation. Mucous membranes undergo continuous proliferation, and when cell renewal cannot replace cell loss as a result of radiation exposure, mucositis occurs (Dudjak, 1987; Iwamoto, 1992).

Intraoral and pharyngeal reactions include xerostomia, taste alterations, mucosal erythema, and mucositis. Severity is dose-related, with onset of symptoms occurring at doses of 20 to 25 Gy. Oral care includes use of a soft toothbrush and frequent rinsing with water, saline solution, or nonalcohol-containing oral care preparations. Elixir of benadryl and water in a 1-ounce to 1-quart solution makes a mild, soothing rinse. Inspection of the oral cavity and assessment for candidiasis should be done regularly. Nystatin (Mycostatin) (tablets or suspensions) or ketoconazole tablets can be prescribed for candidiasis.

Dental consultation before treatment is essential for patients who will be receiving treatments to the oral cavity. Salivary changes can lead to late radiation caries, particularly after high doses to the mouth or oral cavity. Dental prophylaxis, fluoride treatments, and coverage with antibiotics before any dental extractions or other oral surgery procedures are recommended after treatment.

ESOPHAGITIS

Esophagitis can occur when the chest is irradiated. Onset of symptoms is usually marked by a sensation of "a lump in the throat" or an object stuck in the esophagus. This can be due to edema or to spasm of the esophageal musculature, triggered by the presence of food attempting to pass the irritated mucosa. Within a few days, true esophagitis with dysphagia develops, and the patient experiences pain, particularly when attempting to eat (Wilson, Herman, & Chubon, 1991).

Antacids and mild anesthetic agents may be helpful in relieving symptoms; however, until treatment is completed and healing takes place, the discomfort remains.

Dietary adjustments are necessary when intraoral or esophageal mucositis occurs. Protein and calorie requirements may be met with the use of liquid food supplements and soft foods. In addition, the diet should be bland to avoid further local irritation (Iwamoto, 1992).

NAUSEA AND VOMITING

Treatment to the abdomen, particularly to large fields, can cause nausea and vomiting. Patients receiving spinal irradiation (especially to the thoracic and lumbar vertebrae) may also have nausea, and occasionally patients will experience nausea after lower abdominal or pelvic field radiation. Nausea and vomiting are not, however, an inevitable side effect of radiation therapy. Even when treatment is expected to produce these distressing symptoms, reaction can be minimized or prevented with the use of antiemetics. The prescribed medication should be taken before treatment and repeated as necessary. In addition, a light diet should be consumed before treatment and for several hours afterward.

Patients experiencing nausea and vomiting related to radiation therapy treatments need support and encouragement (as well as combination antiemetics), emphasizing that these distressing symptoms often will decrease as treatments proceed. The new patient may have an element of anxiety, which enhances the potential for radiation-induced nausea. It is not unusual for nausea to either disappear or decrease in severity as the treatment course progresses. The body adjusts to the treatment, the patient relaxes, and nausea is no longer a significant problem.

DIARRHEA

Patients at risk for radiation-induced diarrhea include those receiving treatment to the abdomen or pelvis (McCarthy, 1992). Changes in the epithelial layer of the small bowel are related to the highly proliferative nature of the cells of the columnar epithelium. Normal cell loss coupled with radiation-induced cell injury results in flattening or loss of the villi. This in turn decreases the absorptive surface area of the intestine, leading to diarrhea. Cramping, increased flatus, and a feeling of distention sometimes accompany diarrhea.

The diarrhea is usually dose-related and occurs after doses of 18 to 30 Gy. Patients with previous abdominal surgery, colitis, ileitis, or other bowel disorders are more likely to develop radiation-related diarrhea, and symptoms will develop at a lower dose. Diarrhea is usually controlled with dietary modification (low-residue diet) and various antidiarrheal medications. When treatments are completed, several weeks to months may elapse before the intestinal lining recovers and returns to normal function. During this recovery period, it is especially important that the patient maintain a low-residue diet, adding other foods back into the diet on a very gradual basis. For some patients, certain foods (such as corn, legumes, or milk products) may no longer be tolerated by the irradiated bowel.

Nursing management of diarrhea requires frequent patient assessment and reinforcement of dietary and medication instructions. As with any dietary adjustments, it is important to include the person responsible for meal preparation in the teaching plan.

FATIGUE

Fatigue is a common occurrence in the person receiving radiation therapy (Aistars, 1987; Greenburg, Sawicka, Eisenthal, & Ross, 1992; Kobashi-Schoot, Hanewald, van Dam, & Bruning, 1985; Piper, Lindsey, & Dodd, 1987). Although many patients are able to perform their normal daily activities in addition to coming for treatment each day, most will report feeling fatigued as the treatment course progresses.

Theories presented to explain the occurrence of fatigue include (1) increased metabolic rate, (2) the presence of toxic breakdown products as a result of cell injury or death, (3) energy expenditure required for tissue repair, and (4) the tiring effects of travel to and from the radiation facility on a daily basis.

Patients should be told they may experience fatigue as treatment progresses; if not forewarned, they may become concerned that their fatigue is an indication of tumor progression. They may also fail to respond to the need for increased rest, thinking that to do so means giving in to the disease itself. Many patients are able to carry out all normal daily activities (including work) throughout a course of treatment; others are unable to perform their usual daily tasks.

Although it is anticipated that volume of tissue irradiated will influence degree of fatigue, other variables can cause fatigue as well, such as recent surgery, low hemoglobin level, travel time or distance, length of treatment course, and total dose of radiation. Haylock and Hart (1979) reported on one of the first studies of fatigue in cancer patients. Thirty patients were surveyed on a daily basis throughout their course of treatment. In addition to noting a significant increase in fatigue level over the course of treatment, a strong correlation was seen between certain physical symptoms and fatigue level, supporting the belief that the cause of radiation fatigue is physiologic rather than psychologic.

Fatigue in oncology patients was the focus of an Oncology Nursing Society State-of-the-Knowledge Conference on Fatigue held in 1992 (Winningham et al., 1994). Participants in this conference reviewed and analyzed existing knowledge on the subject, presented clinical practice guidelines, and proposed potential topics for further research.

Patients receiving radiation treatment constitute a large portion of the cancer patient population. This group is particularly vulnerable to fatigue because of the necessity for daily travel to a treatment center for periods ranging from 2 to 7 weeks.

Nursing interventions for the patient experiencing radiation-related fatigue include monitoring blood counts, nutritional assessment and support, education regarding the need for increased rest and sleep, and emotional support and encouragement throughout this difficult period. Patients need to know that fatigue may last for several months after treatment is completed. Assurance that fatigue is common and will ultimately subside may be the most helpful nursing intervention of all.

ALTERATIONS IN FERTILITY AND SEXUALITY

Menopausal symptoms and changes in fertility are particularly problematic for young women receiving radiation therapy to the pelvis. The ovaries are sensitive to the effects of radiation at a total radiation dose as low as 2000 cGy. Menopausal effects include hot flashes, amenorrhea, dyspareunia, loss of libido, and irritability (Feldman, 1989). Gynecologic patients treated with brachytherapy (radioactive implant to the vagina, uterus, or both) are at risk for vaginal dryness, adhesions, and occlusion. Nursing interventions include careful instruction on use of a vaginal dilator and stressing there must be long-term compliance with this procedure. Although an individual may not be concerned about maintaining vaginal patency for sexual purposes, it is essential that patency is maintained to facilitate pelvic examination in follow-up.

Dow, Harris, and Roy (1994) evaluated treatment outcome and quality of life in women treated with radiation after breast-conserving surgery and radiation. Twenty-three women with subsequent pregnancies were compared with a matched group of 23 women who did not become pregnant. Results of this study were consistent with previous reports that demonstrated no difference in recurrence or distant metastases between patients with or without subsequent pregnancies. In addition, both groups of women perceived that they were able to adjust well after treatment. This study provides support for decision making when women treated for breast cancer with radiation are considering pregnancy. Chapter 62 in this text provides detailed pathophysiology, psychosocial factors influencing sexual functioning, and care plans for alterations in sexuality and sexual functioning.

INFORMATION NEEDS

Radiation therapy has long been characterized as mysterious, frightening, and poorly understood, especially by the lay public. This is understandable when one realizes that public exposure to information about radiation as a treatment modality has been primarily focused on the few accidents or incidents that occur and on personal stories of severe reactions to treatment.

Fortunately, this negative attitude is changing. As public awareness and education lead to a better understanding of radiation therapy and its applications, individuals referred for radiation therapy are better prepared.

Oncology nurses often provide the bulk of patient/family education in radiation therapy. Ideally, the radiation oncology nurse meets with each new patient at the time of initial visit to initiate the teaching process. In addition to providing verbal information, teaching booklets, pamphlets, and video and audio tapes are used to supplement and reinforce discussion.

A sampling of patient education materials developed by nurses for radiation oncology patients is shown in Table 20-6. Sporkin (1987) described a newsletter prepared for radiation oncology patients, and Hagopian (1991) also describes a weekly radiation therapy newsletter that helped to increase patient knowledge and understanding while reducing treatment-related anxiety.

COMFORT MEASURES

Nursing care in radiation oncology addresses the many needs of both patient and family as they experience the process of radiation treatment. In addition to symptom management for the various physical effects of both treatment and disease as previously discussed, provision of comfort is also essential. The Oncology Nursing Society *Standards of Oncology Nursing Practice* (ONS, 1987) lists provision of comfort as one of the 11 standards on which practice is based.

Comfort is sometimes defined narrowly as the absence of pain. Pain management is a major aspect of care for many oncology patients, particularly when palliative treatment is being given. Chapters 55 to 58 in this text address the entire subject of pain and pain management. Beyond pain management, however, the concept of comfort is particularly applicable in radiation oncology.

Provision of comfort addresses aspects such as education, advocacy, compassion, and caring. How we teach, what setting we use, patient and family perceptions of our interest in them—all are measure of the comfort that we provide. Bucholtz (1994) thoroughly examined the concept of comfort in nursing and detailed specific needs and interventions to ensure comfort for both child and family during radiation therapy.

Patients of all ages, each with their own unique needs, wants, and personalities require comfort measures that nurses can provide. From running interfer-

TABLE 20-6. *Sampling of Patient Education Materials for Radiation Oncology Patients*

AUTHOR OF MATERIALS	CONTENTS
Brandt, 1989	Definitions; treatment description; questions/answers; safety precautions; oral care; diet/food lists; skin care; follow-up.
Jordan & Buck, 1991	Drawings (anatomy); photos (treatment equipment and procedures); instructions preprocedure and postprocedure.
Lydon, McDonald-Lynch, Marshall, & Villaneuva, 1989	Definitions; questions/answers; treatment description; preadmission and postdischarge instructions; side effects.
Mast & Mood, 1990	Description of procedure (with emphasis on self-care measures); illustrations.
Myers, Davidson, Hutt, & Chatham, 1987	Sample teaching plans; patient instruction sheets re: precautions for leukopenia and thrombocytopenia.
Richards & Hiratzka, 1986	Questions/answers re: use of vaginal dilator, sexual activity, douching; photo of dilator.
Skalla & Lacasse, 1992	Questions/answers re: defining, identifying, and understanding fatigue; suggestions for controlling fatigue.
Witt, 1987	Questions/answers re: radiation, equipment, diet, side-effects, skin care, blood tests, sterility, late effects.

ence in resolving scheduling problems to escorting the bewildered elderly through the department, providing comfort should be a standard of nursing practice in radiation oncology.

BRACHYTHERAPY

Discussion to this point has dealt primarily with the principles of radiobiology, physics, treatment planning, and treatment with *teletherapy*. Nursing care as presented thus far also is specific to the patient receiving teletherapy.

A second method of treatment uses radioactive sources in the technique known as *brachytherapy*. This method of treatment is based on somewhat different principles of radiation biology and has very different implications for nursing because of the need for radiation safety and protection.

Brachytherapy had its beginnings in 1904 when Pierre Curie loaned a small quantity of radium to a physician who used the radioactive source to prepare surface applicators in the treatment of skin lesions (Glasgow & Perez, 1987). Brachytherapy is the form of internal radiation therapy in which a radioactive isotope or radionuclide is placed directly on or adjacent to tumors. Brachytherapy techniques are used for surface (or plaque), interstitial, or intracavitary application. Brachytherapy delivers a high radiation treatment dose to a specified tumor volume with a rapid fall-off in radiation dose to adjacent normal tissues.

Uses of Brachytherapy

Brachytherapy (BRT) techniques may be used alone or in combination with external radiation, chemotherapy, surgery, hyperthermia (Brandt & Harney, 1989), radiation sensitizers, and laser therapy (Shea, Allen, Tharratt, Chan, & Siefkin, 1993) to improve local tumor control, preserve vital organ function (Masters, Steger, & Bown, 1991), manage symptoms occurring with recurrent or inoperable disease (McDermott, Gutin, Larson, & Sneed, 1990), and/or control of disease in previously irradiated sites (Arai et al., 1992;

Brandt & Harney, 1989; Clark & Martinez, 1990; Glicksman & Leith, 1988; Goffinet, Cox, Clark, Fu, Hilaris, & Ling, 1988; Hall & Brenner, 1991; Marsh, Colvin, Zinreich, Jackson, & Lee, 1993; Schray, Gunderson, Sim, Pritchard, Shives, & Yeakel, 1990). Table 20–7 lists various applications of brachytherapy.

Improving Local Tumor Control

Brachytherapy may be combined with external beam treatment to improve the local control of tumors. One of the oldest uses of brachytherapy combined with external beam radiation is in the treatment of gynecologic malignancies. Brady, Rotman, and Calvo (1993) reported that innovative uses of intracavitary and interstitial brachytherapy have dramatically reduced the incidence of local failure associated with gynecologic cancers.

Breast Cancer. One of the most innovative applications of brachytherapy combined with x-ray therapy to improve local control was in the treatment of breast cancer. Generally, a total dose of 4600 cGy was administered to the breast with an iridium-192 implant to boost the tumor site. However, in recent years, breast implants have been replaced with electron boost therapy, which provides comparable local control of disease (Recht, Triedman, & Harris, 1991). Another advantage is that patients are spared a hospitalization and can receive electron treatments on an outpatient basis (Mast & Mood, 1990; McCarthy, 1987).

Prostate Cancer. Brachytherapy techniques have been used in the treatment of prostate cancer to improve local control (Greenburg, Petersen, Hansep-Peters, & Baylinson, 1990; Lannon, el-Araby, Joseph, Eastwood, & Awad, 1993; Porter & Forman, 1993; Vijverberg et al., 1993). Brachytherapy consists of either temporary interstitial implantation of iridium-192 or permanent brachytherapy using interstitial implantation of iodine-125 or palladium-103 sources (Porter & Forman, 1993). Insertion of the radioactive sources can be accomplished in an open or closed procedure using either a suprapubic or perineal retropubic approach. The use of ultrasound imaging has also improved the afterloading of iridium-192 or iodine-125

TABLE 20–7. *Applications of Brachytherapy*

TYPE OF APPLICATION	DISEASE	RADIOISOTOPES USED
Sealed Sources		
Intracavitary	Cervical cancer	Radium-226, cesium-137
	Uterine cancer	Radium-226, cesium-137
Interstitial	Breast cancer	Iridium-192
	Prostate cancer	Iodine-125, gold-198
	Head and neck cancer	Iridium-192, cesium-137
Surface	Choroid cancer	Iodine-125
	Pterygium	Strontium-90
Unsealed Sources		
Oral	Hyperthyroidism	Iodine-131
Intravenous	Polycythemia vera	Phosphorus-32
Intrapleural	Mesothelioma	Phosphorus-32
	Malignant pleural effusion	Gold-198
Intraperitoneal	Ovarian cancer	Phosphorus-32

catheters into the prostate gland (Prestidge, Butler, Shaw, & McComas, 1994). Ultrasound imaging helps to visualize the entire path of the catheter placement for optimal placement and identifies the prostate, seminal vesicles, bladder neck, urethra, and rectum, thus minimizing morbidity. The newer technique of remote afterloading has significantly reduced radiation exposure and protection problems associated with manually loaded radioactive sources.

Preserving Vital Organ Function

Preserving vital organ and limb function can be accomplished with brachytherapy techniques (Mazeron, Crook, Martin, Peynegre, & Pierquin, 1989). For example, treatment of soft tissue sarcomas generally requires amputation of the involved limb (Schray et al., 1990). Brachytherapy using iridium-192 has been combined with limb-sparing surgical resection and has demonstrated effective local control of disease (Shiu, Hilaris, Harrison, & Brennan, 1991). In addition, the preservation of limbs and vital organs has added considerably to the patient's quality of life. Brachytherapy controlled 70 per cent of tumors that were adjacent to or had invaded a major neurovascular bundle and played a significant role in preventing local recurrence. Serious wound complications were also decreased by postponing the loading of radiation sources until after the fifth postoperative day (Shiu et al., 1991).

Oropharyngeal Cancer. Iridium-192 implants have been used following standard external radiation for cancers of the oropharynx (Mazeron et al., 1989). Excellent local control rates have been achieved for these cancers with preservation of function and minimal xerostomia.

Intraocular Melanoma. Intraocular melanoma by radioactive eye plaque brachytherapy techniques spares the individual from enucleation (Brady et al., 1988).

Meningioma. Due to the many problems with repeated surgical procedures in the treatment of primary and recurrent skull base meningiomas, interstitial radiation using iodine-125 seed implantation has been used (Kumar, Patil, Syh, Chu, & Reeves, 1993). Fifteen patients received a minimum tumor dose between 100 and 500 Gy at a low dose rate (LDR) of 0.05 to 0.25 Gy per hour. With a median follow-up of 29 months, 11 patients achieved a complete response. No early or late complications from radiation were observed. The authors concluded that interstitial radiation with iodine-125 seeds was an effective, safe, and relatively easy method to treat skull base meningiomas.

Malignant Brain Tumors. Since conventional external beam radiation is limited by normal brain tissue tolerance, brachytherapy techniques have been a useful alternative in the treatment of brain tumors. Cranial interstitial radiation using iodine-125 seeds into the tumor bed via a sterotactic technique have decreased the use of repeated surgical procedures and has lessened the complications associated with surgery (Ostertag, 1989; Willis, Rittenmeyer, & Hitchon, 1986). Brachytherapy techniques for malignant brain lesions have not improved survival but have been useful in decreasing symptoms associated with the disease (Musolino, Mer-

ckaert, Munari, Daumas-Duport, & Chodkiewicz, 1989).

Treating Recurrent or Inoperable Cancers

Salvage brachytherapy techniques have been used to treat recurrent or inoperable cancers (Choo et al., 1993; Randall, Evans, Greven, McCunniff, & Doline, 1993). Lung brachytherapy in combination with external beam radiation and surgery can improve local tumor control in advanced-stage disease, with no increase in pulmonary complications but only modest survival advantage (Hilaris & Martini, 1988). Patients with symptomatic airway obstruction have limited therapeutic options. Several brachytherapy techniques have been used to relieve airway obstruction (Goldman et al., 1993). These include intraluminal iridium-192 radiation (Nori, 1993; Paradelo, Waxman, Throne, Beller, & Kopecky, 1992) and permanent radioactive seed implants. Pisch, Berson, Harvey, Mishra, and Beattie (1994) evaluated the use of absorbable mesh for suturing of radioactive seeds for tumors in the chest wall. After thoracotomy and tumor resection, a layer of absorbable mesh was sutured to the tumor bed. Nylon afterloading catheters were sutured into the mesh, and a second layer of mesh was sutured on top of the catheters. This technique provided adequate anchor for catheters in areas of scant tissue or in large surgical areas.

Controlling Disease in Previously Irradiated Sites

Interstitial reirradiation for recurrent gynecologic cancers was reported by Randall et al. (1993). Thirteen patients (median age of 70 years) with recurrent or new primary gynecologic malignancies after previous radiation underwent interstitial reirradiation. This technique was an effective treatment for selected patients, especially elders and those who are not candidates for additional surgery. Another advantage of brachytherapy over radical surgery is the potential to preserve organ structure and function. Iridium-192 was used in 20 patients with recurrent or persistent neck metastasis from primary head and neck cancer (Choo et al., 1993). Fifteen patients had control of tumor with few treatment side effects.

Maulard et al. (1994) reported on 28 patients with prior radiation to the oropharynx for squamous cell carcinoma of the tonsil, soft palate, or both. Salvage brachytherapy consisted of two split course implants delivering 35 and 30 Gy, respectively, approximately 1 month apart. Twenty-three patients achieved complete remission. Brachytherapy provided an effective option for salvage treatment in patients with recurrent and second cancers in the tonsillar region even in those having previous high-dose radiation.

Radioactive Sources and Properties

Radioactive sources and their unique properties make them especially suitable for brachytherapy (Maddock, 1987). Standard radioactive sources most often used include iridium-192, cesium-137, iodine-125, and gold-198. Newer radioactive sources include palladium-103 (Anderson, Moni, & Harrison, 1993) and a neutron-emitting isotope, californium-252. As discussed earlier in this chapter, an atom is unstable when the balance between protons and neutrons is unequal (see Fig. 20–1). Nuclides with the same number of protons but a different number of neutrons are called isotopes. Some isotopes are radioactive and occur naturally, such as radium-226; others are produced artificially in atomic reactors by bombarding stable elements with neutrons. Examples of artificially produced isotopes are iridium-192, cobalt-60, and phosphorus-32.

RADIOACTIVE DECAY

The process in which an unstable isotope transforms to a stable one is known as radioactive decay or disintegration. Radioactive decay products are called α and β particles and γ rays. The rate of radioactive decay is constant, as the number of atoms that disintegrate per unit of time is proportional to the number of radioactive atoms.

α **Particle Decay.** An unstable nucleus may eject an α particle that consists of two protons and two neutrons. α particles are very heavy and have a charge of +12. α particles have high LET, and when they travel through matter, they lose energy at a very fast rate when they collide with electrons in their path. Because of their high LET, α particles cannot penetrate more than 0.04 mm into tissue. Generally, radioisotopes that are α emitters are not used in brachytherapy. However, byproducts of radium decay can be α emitters as in the case of radium-226, which is radon gas. When radon is inhaled, it can cause damage to the lung.

β **Particle Decay.** β particles are moderate- to high-speed electrons with a charge of −1 that are emitted by atoms when they release energy. Kinetic energies of β particles range from a few thousand to several million volts. β particles, like α particles, have high kinetic energy and high LET so that their range of penetration in tissue is limited to the outer layers of skin. Phosphorus-32 and strontium-90 are two examples of pure β emitters used in brachytherapy.

γ **Radiation.** Radioactive sources may also decay by emitting excess energy in the form of γ rays. γ rays are electromagnetic radiation emitted as packets of energy called photons. γ rays and β particles are often ejected together from nuclei of atoms. γ rays travel at the speed of light. Because of their penetrating power, γ emitters (cesium-137, gold-198, iodine-131, radium-226) comprise the largest number of radioisotopes used in brachytherapy.

MECHANISM OF RADIATION INJURY

α and β particles and γ rays produce damage by transferring energy to living matter. They ionize molecules in cells to cause physical and chemical changes that affect the biologic processes responsible for reproduction. Irradiated cells are either destroyed or rendered incapable of reproduction.

The extent of radiation injury depends primarily on the type of energy transfer. Energy transfer may be either directly or indirectly ionizing. α and β particles are directly ionizing radiations. Because they are electrically charged, they produce ionization at small intervals along their paths through collision.

γ rays are indirectly ionizing. Unlike charged particles, they have no electrical charge. Energy loss does not occur until γ rays interact with an atom, an electron, or a nucleus in their path. γ rays then transfer energy to directly ionizing particles such as electrons. Electrons are ionized, liberated from the atom, and proceed to ionize other particles in their path. The net result is that indirectly ionizing γ rays transfer energy to directly ionizing particles deep in tissue, more penetrating than what directly ionizing particles can reach from outside the atom. As noted earlier, because γ emitters possess the greatest capacity to produce damage deep in tissue, they are the most useful in brachytherapy. However, they also present the greatest hazard to care providers. Table 20–8 lists commonly used radioisotopes in brachytherapy and their physical properties.

Half-life. The half-life of a radioactive isotope refers to the time it takes for it to decay to 50 per cent of its activity. Half-lives vary among the elements and range from several days (gold-198) to more than 1600 years (radium-226). A particular radioisotope is selected for either temporary or permanent use on the basis of its half-life. For example, gold-198 has a half-life of less than 3 days and can be inserted permanently. Cesium-137 has a half-life of 30 years and is thus used as a temporary implant (Table 20–8).

NEW AND PROMISING RADIOACTIVE SOURCES

Newer forms of radioactive sources include palladium-103 and the neutron-emitting radioactive substance, californium-252.

PALLADIUM-103

Palladium-103 radioactive seeds are a promising alternative to iodine-125 seeds. This isotope has been used in permanent implants that require a higher initial

TABLE 20–8. *Radioisotopes and Their Properties*

RADIOISOTOPE	SYMBOL	HALF-LIFE	TYPE OF EMISSION
Cesium-137	^{137}Cs	30 yr	Beta, gamma
Gold-198	^{198}Au	2.7 days	Beta, gamma
Iodine-125	^{125}I	60 days	Beta, gamma
Iodine-131	^{131}I	8 days	Beta, gamma
Iridium-192	^{192}Ir	74.4 days	Beta, gamma
Phosphorus-32	^{32}P	14.3 days	Beta
Radium-226	^{226}Ra	1620 yr	Alpha, gamma
Strontium-90	^{90}Sr	28.1 yr	Beta

(From National Council on Radiation Protection and Measurements. [1972]. NCRP Report #40. *Protection against radiation from brachytherapy sources.* Washington, DC: Author. Reproduced by permission.)

treatment dose. The advantage of palladium is that it provides better radiation protection than iodine seeds (Anderson et al., 1993).

CALIFORNIUM-252 NEUTRON BRACHYTHERAPY

Maruyama et al. (1991) and Maruyama, van Nagell, Yoneda, DePriest, and Kryscio (1993) reported on a clinical trial using the neutron-emitting radioactive isotope, californium-252 (Cf-252), in the treatment of 218 patients with cervical cancer. The initial trial began with advanced-stage (III and IV) cervical cancer and was extended to include patients with unfavorable presentations, stage IB bulky tumors, or barrel-shaped tumors. Five-year survival for patients using neutron Cf-252 implant before conventional external beam treatment was 46 per cent vs. 19 per cent for Cf-252 after external beam treatment or conventional brachytherapy using cesium-137. Neutron treatment before external photon treatment demonstrated better outcomes for all stages of disease. Neutron brachytherapy was effective in producing a rapid response and improved local control in bulky, barrel, or advanced cervical cancers.

In a follow-up study, Cf-252 was used in 31 patients with medically inoperable uterine cancer or with advanced disease (Maruyama et al., 1993). Patients were in generally poor medical conditions and had multiple chronic medical illnesses. Cf-252 provided for a short implant treatment time (few hours), was usable in a small number of insertions, and demonstrated its usefulness in treating large-volume tumors.

BRACHYTHERAPY TECHNIQUES

Brachytherapy techniques include conventional or standard low-dose rate (LDR) radiation, high-dose rate (HDR) radiation, permanent implantation, and radionuclide therapy. These techniques may be used in the treatment of different solid tumors to achieve local tumor control (Erickson & Wilson, 1993; Finan, Hoffman, Greenberg, Roberts, Cavanagh, & Fiorica, 1993).

CONVENTIONAL LOW-DOSE RATE TECHNIQUES (LDR)

Conventional low-dose brachytherapy uses the temporary insertion of sealed radioactive sources such as iridium-192 and cesium-137. When LDR techniques are used rather than external beam radiation, the radiobiologic principles of repair, repopulation, redistribution, and reoxygenation have related but different implications (Glicksman, 1987; Glicksman & Leith, 1988). For example, sublethal damage accumulation will decrease with LDR brachytherapy. Thus, the *repair* of tumor cells in the radiated volume is hampered, rendering a smaller proportion of tumor cells to repair radiation damage. LDR blocks a greater percentage of tumor cells in the G_2 phase of the cell cycle, which has a higher susceptibility to radiation damage. During LDR, cellular proliferation can occur. However, when new tumor cells cycle into the G_2 phase, these cells are blocked and damaged by the radiation. With the *redistribution* of a significant proportion of the tumor cell population into G_2, a net sensitization effect to radiation occurs. The *repopulation* of tumor cells during LDR results in a blocked progression through the cell cycle. LDR requires less oxygen to eradicate tumor cells. Thus, brachytherapy techniques may be more effective in treating anoxic tumors than conventional, fractionated, external beam radiation (Glicksman, 1987; Hall, 1994).

LDR Afterloading and Radiation Safety. Sealed, temporary sources such as iridium-192 and cesium-137 do not present a potential radiation contamination problem. Because of their relatively long half-lives, these sources are inserted into body tissue or cavities for a specified time period and are then removed. LDR afterloading techniques involve the insertion of an empty applicator device during an operative procedure and the afterloading of the radioactive source once the patient returns to the hospital room. While standard LDR afterloading techniques reduce radiation exposure, there are still significant costs incurred as a result of patient hospitalization.

Patients with radioactive implants must have a private room with private bath. Some institutions have specially designed radiation precaution rooms with built-in lead shields lining the walls of the room. In institutions that are not equipped with special radiation rooms, the radiation safety officer may designate rooms that are suitable for patients with radioactive implants. These are usually located at the ends of halls or corridors where there is less radiation exposure to occupants of adjacent rooms (National Council on Radiation Protection and Measurements [NCRP], 1989).

Nursing Care Guidelines. Nursing care should be preplanned so that as much direct care as possible is provided during the period before loading the radioactive source (Hassey, 1985; Lowdermilk, 1990; Randall, Drake, & Sewchand, 1987). Brandt (1991) discusses the informational needs of 22 patients receiving brachytherapy. Informational needs most frequently identified were (1) how to manage side effects and maintain comfort, (2) identifying the cause of current symptoms, and (3) how the implant could affect their symptoms. Brandt reported a high correlation between the number of informational needs and stage of disease. Patients with advanced disease had fewer informational needs than those with early-stage disease.

Once the implant is loaded, time spent in the room must be minimized and distance maximized. The many teaching pamphlets and booklets available today stress the need for patient self-care activities during the implant period.

Patients with gynecologic implants will require additional care because they must remain on complete bedrest. The head of the bed may be elevated approximately 30 degrees, and patients can log roll from side to side. Patients will also require Foley catheter care and in addition will not be able to have a bowel movement during the implant period.

Patients do not generally experience significant pain at the implant site; however, they experience discomfort such as pressure at the implant site and may have an urge to void. Pain medication may be given to relieve discomfort. Recently, Miller reported on the use of an innovative undergarment to keep the applicator implant in place without the use of tape or sutures (Miller, personal communication, 1994).

The implant period can be tedious, and patients may wish to have visitors. However, certain visiting restrictions will apply. Federal regulations limit the radiation dose exposure to the general public at 500 millirems (5 mSv) per year (Table 20–9) (NCRP, 1993). Therefore, each visitor must be limited to approximately one-half hour visit per day. A distance of at least 6 feet must be maintained between visitors and the radioactive source. Pregnant women and children under the age of 18 years are prohibited from visiting patients with implants.

While all necessary precautions are taken to improve radiation safety, there are extreme and unusual circumstances in which a radioactive source becomes dislodged. A pair of long-handled forceps and a lead container should always be present in the patient's room. The forceps must be used to retrieve the source, which should then be placed in the lead container. The radioactive source should never be touched with bare hands. The radiation oncologist and radiation safety officer should be notified immediately in the event of a dislodged source or applicator (Bucholtz, 1992a; Hassey, 1985).

TABLE 20–9. *Recommendations on Limits for Exposure to Ionizing Radiation*

	DOSE
Occupational exposure (annual)	
Effective dose equivalent limit	5.0 rem/yr
Dose equivalent limits for tissues and organs:	
Lenses of eyes	15.0 rem/yr
All others (red bone marrow, breasts, lungs, gonads, skin, and extremities)	50.0 rem/yr
Guidance: Cumulative exposure	1 rem × age in yr
Public exposure (annual)	
Effective dose equivalent limit	0.1 rem/yr
Effective dose equivalent limit, infrequent exposure	0.5 rem/yr
Education and training exposures	
Effective dose equivalent limit	0.1 rem/yr
Dose equivalent limit for lens of eye, skin, and extremities	5.0 rem/yr
Embryo-fetus exposures	
Total dose equivalent limit	0.5 rem/yr
Dose equivalent limit in a month	0.05 rem/yr
Negligible individual risk level (annual)	
Effective dose equivalent per source or practice	0.001 rem/yr

(From National Council on Radiation Protection and Measurements. [1993]. NCRP Report #116. *Recommendations on limits for exposure to ionizing radiation.* Bethesda, MD: Author. Reproduced by permission.)

The removal of sealed sources does not present a contamination hazard. However, all linens and dressings should be kept in the patient's room during the course of the implant to ensure safe disposal of the radioisotope used (in case of dislodgment, for example). Linen and dressings can be disposed of in the usual manner once the source is removed and accounted for.

Summary of LDR. While LDR brachytherapy provides additional benefits to eradicate or control tumors, the major disadvantages are the expense of inpatient hospitalization and radiation exposure to health care providers. In recent years, high dose rate brachytherapy techniques using a remote afterloading device have been developed and are gaining in popularity and use over LDR brachytherapy.

HIGH-DOSE RATE REMOTE AFTERLOADING TECHNIQUES (HDR)

High-dose rate brachytherapy is an innovative method of delivering a high dose, short duration of radiation therapy. HDR has several distinct advantages over conventional LDR brachytherapy: (1) HDR improves radiation safety, (2) decreases treatment times, (3) allows for outpatient scheduling, and (4) is cost-effective. A remote afterloading device used with HDR spares health care providers from exposure to ionizing radiation. Radiation treatment times are decreased because a high dose rate of radiation of 0.5 to 5.0 Gy/minute can be delivered in one treatment, which allows for fewer treatments and obviates the need for required hospitalization and bedrest (Edmundson et al., 1993; Jordan & Buck, 1991; Jordan & Mantravadi, 1991; Stitt, 1992).

HDR brachytherapy is a cost-effective treatment for gynecologic cancer (Bastin et al., 1993). Investigators surveyed 150 radiation therapy centers across the United States to analyze treatment costs incurred for anesthesia use and hospitalization and perioperative morbidity and mortality associated with LDR and compared with costs incurred for HDR intracavitary brachytherapy. Ninety-five (63 per cent) centers responded. Results indicated a 244 per cent higher overall charge for LDR treatment compared with HDR. The majority of costs were related to inpatient and operating room expenses. Investigators also found that HDR had the advantage of cost-shifting to the radiation therapy department.

HDR Compared With LDR in Control of Local Disease. HDR was compared with LDR with regard to effectiveness in local control of disease and occurrence of late complications (Brenner, Huang, & Hall, 1991; Khoury, Bulman & Joslin, 1991). Arai et al. (1992) reported on a 20-year experience comparing HDR afterloading with conventional LDR intracavitary radiation in 1022 patients with squamous cell cervical carcinoma. Five-year survival rates across all stages of disease between the two groups were comparable. In addition, severe or late complications to the rectosigmoid colon, bladder, and small intestine were 4.1 per cent, 1.2 per cent and 1.1 per cent, respectively. These late effects occurred less often with HDR than LDR.

Orton, Seyedsadr, and Somnay (1991) analyzed data from a survey of 56 institutions treating a total of more than 17,000 patients with cervical cancer and compared HDR with LDR. Results showed an improved 5-year survival, lower morbidity, and reduction of radiation "hot spots" to the rectum and bladder with HDR. Arterbery (1993) also found that HDR techniques decrease rectal and bladder dose in cervical cancer when compared with standard LDR. Arterbery reported that LDR had less effective local control of advanced cervical cancer than HDR intracavitary brachytherapy. While HDR has not demonstrated an improved survival advantage when compared with LDR brachytherapy, the practical advantages of HDR may account for its increasing use and popularity.

HDR and Vaginal Cancer. Nanavati, Fanning, Hilgers, Hallstrom, & Crawford (1993) reported on the use of HDR in 13 patients with primary stage I and II vaginal cancer; the median age was 65 years. Patients were treated with external beam radiation (4500 cGy) and HDR brachytherapy (2000 to 2800 cGY in 3 to 4 fractions). All 13 patients had a complete response, and local control was achieved in 12 patients with no acute or chronic intestinal or bladder late effects. The authors concluded that HDR produced a high response rate, good local control, and comparable survival with minimal complications.

Palliating Symptoms Using HDR. Twenty-two patients with advanced esophageal cancers were compared using manually afterloaded LDR cesium-137 or remote afterloaded HDR iridium-192 (Harvey, Fleischman, Bellotti, & Kagan, 1993). Investigators found that LDR total dose of 2000 cGy in 3 fractions was comparable to HDR total dose of 1250 cGy in 1 fraction with respect to relief of dysphagia and maintenance of esophageal patency. Investigators also found that HDR improved patient comfort because of the reduced time spent in the hospital. They stressed that HDR has distinct advantages for patients with poor physical conditions and shortened life expectancy.

HDR intraluminal brachytherapy has been effective in the treatment of malignant airway obstruction caused by lung cancer (Chang, Horvath, Peyton, & Ling, 1994; Marsh et al., 1993). Investigators used an average of 7 Gy at a radius of 1 cm from the center of the source that was delivered by iridium-192. Patients received 3 fractions on a biweekly basis. HDR was effective in relieving dyspnea, cough, hemoptysis, and postobstructive pneumonia. The authors concluded that HDR was effective in palliating symptoms related to malignant airway obstruction despite no definitive increase in survival.

Use of HDR in Phase I/II Trials. HDR was also used in combination with interstitial hyperthermia in the treatment of anal cancer in a phase I/II study (Kapp, Kapp, Stuecklschweiger, Berger, & Geyer, 1994). Fourteen patients with primary cancer of the anal canal were treated with split-course external beam radiation, one or two interstitial iridium-192 HDR implants (6 to 8 Gy), and interstitial hyperthermia. HDR and hyperthermia were well tolerated, and complete responses were seen in 11 (78.5 per cent) patients. Sphincter function was maintained in 50 per cent of patients.

HDR Use in Treating Infants and Children. Radiation poses particular problems in the treatment of infants and young children (Bernstein & Laperriere, 1990; Black et al., 1993; Bucholtz, 1992b). External beam radiation is generally avoided in the young due to adverse long-term complications. Conventional LDR brachytherapy techniques are also limited because of the additional radiation exposure incurred by nurses and parents. Limited but successful use of HDR remote brachytherapy was reported by Nag, Grecula, and Ruymann (1993). Seven children with rhabdomyosarcoma were treated with multiagent chemotherapy, organ preservation surgery, and HDR. A minimal dose of 36 Gy HDR was given twice a day for 3 days. Treatments were delivered on an outpatient basis, and each treatment session lasted for 2 to 5 minutes. HDR treatments required shorter sedation and less immobilization compared with standard LDR brachytherapy. With a reported median follow-up of 30 months, all children were alive. Acute side effects were seen in the skin; patients had relatively good organ growth and function during the short follow-up period. While initial reports are encouraging, researchers caution that HDR in young children should be restricted to controlled clinical trials until the effect on long-term morbidity and efficacy can be established.

Summary of HDR. HDR is a promising and highly effective alternative to LDR brachytherapy. It is increasingly being used as a cost-effective alternative to LDR brachytherapy because of its lower cost, decreased hospitalization, low to nonexistent radiation exposure, and use in a wide variety of cancers and patient conditions.

PERMANENT INSERTION OF BRACHYTHERAPY SOURCES

Permanent insertion of radioactive isotopes such as gold-198 and iodine-125 in combination with external beam radiation has been used in the treatment of prostate, lung, and brain cancers. Lannon et al. (1993) reported on 180 patients with stage A2-C prostate cancer followed for 5 years. Actuarial 10-year disease-free survival was 83 per cent and 91.3 per cent for stages A2 and B1, respectively. Vijverberg et al. (1993) reported on transperineal ultrasound-guided iodine-125 implantation for localized prostate cancer with favorable local control results.

Conventional radiation in the treatment of brain tumors is limited because of the narrow margin between tumor sensitivity and healthy brain sensitivity. Iodine-125 seeds for permanent implant have demonstrated effectiveness in local tumor control. Ostertag (1989) reported on 170 patients with differentiated gliomas and other anaplastic gliomas, glioblastomas, ependymomas, and papillomas. Iodine-125 implants were recommended for slowly proliferating, differentiated, nonresectable tumors in functionally critical areas. Interstitial radiation using iodine-125 seeds has also been used in the treatment of pediatric malignant astrocytoma (Black et al., 1993).

Nursing Care Guidelines. Sealed, permanent implants such as gold-198 and iodine-125 seeds have a short half-life, so they may be inserted permanently into tissues such as the prostate. During hospitalization, patients' activities are restricted to their room. They should be encouraged in self-care activities such as bathing and grooming. There are no dietary restrictions. Patients may bring in reading materials and other diversionary materials during the implant period. Since radioactive gold-198 or iodine-125 seeds decay rapidly, patients may be discharged home within a few days after implantation. However, radiation dose levels must be less than 30 mCi (111 × 10^7 Bq) of activity before patients may be discharged from the hospital (NCRP, 1974).

Radionuclide Therapy. While most radioactive sources are sealed or encased within an outer sheath of material such as platinum, some radioactive sources are best used unsealed in a colloidal suspension that will be placed in direct contact with tissues. Radionuclide therapy may be administered orally (iodine-131 for thyroid cancer); intravenously (phosphorus-32 for polycythemia vera); intrapleurally (phosphorus-32 for lung cancer); or intraperitoneally (phosphorus-32 for ovarian cancer). Radionuclide therapy using specific tumor-seeking radiopharmaceuticals are increasingly being used because the procedures are noninvasive and there are relatively few or nonexistent side effects compared with chemotherapy and external beam therapy (Hoefnagel, 1991).

Nursing Care Guidelines. Because radiopharmaceuticals are unsealed sources, they require special radiation precautions. For example, iodine-131 is orally administered in a "radioactive cocktail" drink that is odorless and tasteless. Patients are admitted to the hospital for a short 2- to 3-day stay. During hospitalization, patients' activities are restricted to their room. There are no dietary or self-care restrictions. Iodine-131 is excreted in feces, urine, vomitus, saliva, sweat, and other body fluids. Since many patients experience intense itching during the time the radioactive iodine is excreted, they should be encouraged to increase fluid intake, take showers as often as needed, and void regularly. Nurses should wear rubber gloves while providing direct care. Patients should also be instructed to flush the toilet several times after each bowel movement or urination.

Since linen and patient gowns may be contaminated, they must be stored in a separate isolation bag. Other articles in the room, such as telephone, call light, and floors, must be covered with plastic. Disposable plastic or paper products should be used for dietary trays and utensils (NCRP, 1974). In addition, patients should not be encouraged to bring in any belongings or personal effects from home, since these items will need to be disposed of separately when the patient is discharged from the hospital.

STANDARDS FOR RADIATION SAFETY

With the improvements in brachytherapy techniques, nurses have decreased their radiation exposure significantly. Yet nurses continue to fear radiation exposure because of misconceptions and misunderstandings about radiation (Sedhmo & Yanni, 1985; Sticklin, 1994). It is important to maintain meticulous radiation safety practices. Sticklin (1994) described the innovative development, implementation, and evaluation of an educational program to prepare nurses to care for patients receiving brachytherapy. Particular attention was given to nurses of childbearing age. The teaching session included information about knowledge and a discussion about the nurses' fears and concerns.

Federal regulations mandate that maximum permissible dose for whole-body occupational exposure is 5000 millirem (50 mSv) per year, or 3000 millirem (30 mSv) in a 3-month period (NCRP, 1993). Standards are based on risk-vs.-benefit criteria and account for factors such as age, occupational versus nonoccupational exposure limits, and critical organ exposure. The recommendations on limits of exposure to ionizing radiation are listed in Table 20–9.

Since many nurses caring for implant patients are of childbearing age, the recommendation that allows dose accumulation of up to 3000 millirem (30 mSv) in a 3-month period will not apply. Maximum permissible dose for women of reproductive capacity is 1250 millirem (12.5 mSv) per quarter, equal to 5000 millirem (50 mSv) a year delivered at an even rate. Under these conditions, the dose to an embryo during the critical first 2 months of organogenesis would normally be less than 1 rem (0.01 Sv) (NCRP, 1977). However, it is strongly recommended that any nurse who is pregnant or suspects that she is pregnant should refrain from caring for implant patients.

Regardless of maximum limits, occupational exposure should be "as low as reasonably achievable" or ALARA. In practice, nurses working with patients treated with LDR brachytherapy receive less than 100 millirem (1 mSv) or 2 per cent of the maximum permissible dose limit per year. Dose levels in this range can be achieved through close monitoring by the radiation safety officer and radiation oncologist, and careful adherence to radiation safety principles by nursing staff (Jankowski, 1992).

PRINCIPLES OF TIME, DISTANCE, AND SHIELDING

The way in which nurses can keep radiation exposure limits as low as reasonably achievable is to follow three key principles of time, distance, and shielding.

Time. The longer the time of radiation exposure is, the greater the amount of absorbed radiation is. Minimum exposure time must be stressed because no one can feel the presence of radiation or any physical discomfort to remind them to limit their exposure (i.e., working) times. Generally, nurses are limited to one-half hour per shift of direct time with the patient (Hassey, 1987). Thus, preplanning direct care activities at the bedside will help to decrease time of radiation exposure.

Distance. Radiation exposure and distance are inversely related. That is, the intensity of radiation decreases as the square of the distance from the source increases. The following rule can be used to calculate exposure: amount of radiation exposure at 1 m from the radioactive source times distance squared equals the amount of radiation exposure at any distance from the source times distance squared.

Nurses can maximize their distance from the radioactive sources in several ways. First, they can stand at the doorway of the patients' rooms when talking to patients or providing indirect care. Second, when providing direct care, it is best to stand at the head of the bed rather than at the side or foot of the bed for patients with gynecologic implants. Third, nurses need to preplan their activities and to complete their tasks as efficiently as possible when in the patient's room.

Shielding. The type of shielding device used in brachytherapy depends on the type of particle or γ ray. The maximum thickness that particles can penetrate is called the range. Owing to their short range in tissue, α particles cannot penetrate the outermost layers of skin. A thin sheet of paper is sufficient to stop α particles. α particles, therefore, are not an external hazard.

Most β particles are not external hazards because they cannot penetrate the outermost layer of skin. For example, the range in tissue of phosphorus-32 is 0.8 cm.

γ rays are indirectly ionizing, and a percentage of γ rays can pass through any shield. The percentage of radiation that can penetrate decreases as the thickness of the shield increases. The effectiveness of shielding for γ rays is expressed in terms of half-value layers. A half-value layer is the thickness required for a shield to reduce the intensity of γ rays by a factor of 2 (Noz & Maguire, 1979; Shapiro, 1981).

Lead shields are used to decrease radiation exposure; however, their success can be variable. Many nurses complain that lead shields are cumbersome to work around, necessitating increased time and decreased distance from the radioactive source. Other nurses wish to have lead shields placed in a patient's room because they serve as a reminder that radiation is present and motivates them to work as efficiently as possible.

Personnel Monitoring Devices

Personnel monitoring devices, which are required by law, offer a measure of radiation safety and protection. Devices do not protect the individual from radiation exposure; rather, they provide a record of exposure. Monitoring is done in several ways and depends on the type and level of radiation exposure and the cost and reliability of the monitoring device. Records of exposure are generally kept by the radiation safety officer.

Nurses must always wear a monitoring device when caring for patients with implants. Several types of monitoring devices or detectors are used for personnel and environmental monitoring. These include the nuclear emulsion monitor or film badge, the thermolumines-

cent dosimeter detector (TLD) or ring badge, and the pocket ion-chamber dosimeter. Monitoring devices are intended to provide an accurate record of *occupational* exposure and should not be worn outside the hospital (Khan, 1984; Noz & Maguire, 1979; Shapiro, 1981).

The film badge is the most widely used personnel monitor because it is accurate, reliable, and inexpensive to use. A film badge should not be shared. The film consists of a photographic emulsion mounted in a plastic holder. It provides a measure of whole body exposure. The film darkens in proportion to exposure to radiation. A film badge must be changed every month owing to fading of the film.

The TLDs are used for personnel monitoring in the same way as film badges. Owing to their small size, TLDs are especially useful for monitoring doses of radiation to the hand, hence the term *ring badge*. They contain a thermoluminescent powder such as lithium fluoride. Electrons in the lithium are raised to an excited state when exposed to the radioactive source. The excited energy appears in the form of visible light, and the amount of light is proportional to the energy absorbed by the radiation. The major disadvantage of TLDs is that a permanent record of exposure cannot be kept.

Pocket ion-chamber dosimeters are shaped like pens and are attached to clothing. These ionization chambers must be charged before being used. Exposure of the chamber to radiation results in loss of the charge proportional to the amount of radiation exposure. These self-reading monitors provide immediate information on the amount of exposure. The nurse records the reading on the pocket ion-chamber before entering the patient's room, wears the device while in the room, and then records a reading when leaving the patient's room. As with TLDs, once readings are taken and values recorded, it is not possible to double-check exposure information.

The Geiger-Mueller counter (G-M counter) is used for surveying a patient's room. Survey meters are not used for personnel monitoring because they do not measure exposure or dose rate. The device responds to the presence of ionizing particles by producing electrical pulses that are triggered by the transfer of energy of the radioisotope to electrons in the G-M counter. The G-M counter is the most popular of survey meters owing to its ease of operation, sensitivity, and reliability.

Summary of Brachytherapy

The shift from LDR to HDR brachytherapy has dramatically changed the way in which this modality is delivered. Increasingly, patients will receive HDR that will decrease cost and expense, decrease radiation exposure hazards, and avoid expensive hospitalization.

SPECIALIZED RADIATION THERAPY TECHNIQUES

Radiation techniques that are used in specialized centers include intraoperative radiation (Smith, 1992), hyperthermia (Bahman & Perez, 1985; Seegenschmiedt, Sauer, Miyamoto, Chalal, & Brady, 1993; Valdagni, Fei-Fei, & Kapp, 1988), radiation sensitizers (Coleman, Beard, Hlatky, Kwok, & Bump, 1994; McGinn & Kinsella, 1994; Noll, 1992), and proton beam treatment (Suit & Urie, 1992). These specialized techniques are most often used in a controlled clinical trial setting rather than in standard direct care practice. The techniques are not used alone; rather, they are most often used in combination with standard external beam or brachytherapy treatments.

INTRAOPERATIVE RADIATION THERAPY (IORT)

Intraoperative radiation therapy (IORT) delivers a high dose of radiation directly to the tumor bed without damaging normal structures in the beam pathway. This technique is used in several centers across the United States and in other countries (Close, Morris, & Nguyen, 1993; Hilaris & Martini, 1988; Kinsella & Sindelar, 1985; Nori, 1993; Noyes et al., 1992; Shipley, Kaufman, & Prout, 1987; Smith, 1992).

IORT is accomplished by surgically exposing a tumor-bearing organ, excising the diseased portion, and then delivering a single high dose of radiation directly to the tumor bed. Radiation is delivered via a conventional teletherapy machine through a specially constructed adapter, which is placed in very close proximity to the opened surgical site. This procedure takes place with the fully anesthetized and surgically exposed patient being monitored by the surgical team. Because noninvolved organs such as the intestine can be packed out of the pathway of the radiation beam, little or no radiation effect is seen in adjacent organs. Thus side effects are virtually nonexistent despite the high treatment dose. After the radiation dose has been delivered, the incision is closed, and the patient is transferred to the recovery unit.

IORT can be delivered either in the operative suite, with a dedicated therapy machine, or in the radiation oncology department. Treatment given in any other locale outside the surgical suite requires elaborate planning and preparation, because the fully anesthetized patient must be transported through the hospital corridors.

Most IORT is given prophylactically after surgical removal of bulk disease or as adjuvant therapy in locally advanced carcinomas, such as colorectal, gastric, pancreatic, and soft-tissue sarcomas (Kinsella & Sindelar, 1985). Shipley et al. (1987) reported that IORT using either an iridium-192 implant or a large single dose of electrons was safe and resulted in cure of bladder cancers with preservation of bladder function in more than 75 per cent of patients with solitary tumors that have not invaded the bladder muscle. Once the patient recovers from surgery, an additional course of external beam therapy is usually given.

HYPERTHERMIA

Heat is known to be cytotoxic, and when it is applied at temperatures high enough to produce cell death, this effect is seen in normal as well as tumor tissues (Perez & Emami, 1989). Heat is not selective; therefore, it is not useful as a single agent in cancer treatment. The use of controlled hyperthermia combined with radiation therapy has been shown to achieve tumor cell killing without excess toxicity to normal tissues.

Several factors combine to produce the desired biologic effect of hyperthermia plus radiation therapy:

1. Hyperthermia is known to be most effective during the S phase of the cell cycle, when radiation is least effective.
2. Hypoxic cells that are generally radioresistant are heat-sensitive.
3. Heat inhibits repair of radiation injury (Valdagni et al., 1988).

Thus three of the four Rs of radiobiology—repair, redistribution, and reoxygenation—are enhanced by the addition of hyperthermia to radiation therapy.

Hyperthermia is administered by several techniques, the choice of technique usually depending on the volume of tissue to be heated. Standard techniques include the use of ultrasound, microwaves, immersion in a heated bath, perfusion, and interstitial probe implants (Bahman & Perez, 1985; Guy & Chou, 1983).

Nurses caring for patients receiving hyperthermia therapy may have multiple responsibilities, including surgical assistance with probe implantation, monitoring treatment tolerance, and assessing posttreatment response for research protocols (Brandt, 1989). However, primary nursing interventions are focused on provision of patient and family education, emotional support, and symptom management (Wojtas, 1992).

CHEMICAL MODIFIERS OF RADIATION EFFECT

Radiosensitizers and radioprotectors are chemical compounds used to modify the effect of radiation on cells and tissues. Since the early 1970s, clinical trials using a variety of compounds have been used (Coleman et al., 1994; Fowler, 1985; Hellman, 1985; Noll, 1992; Wasserman & Kligerman, 1987). The rationale for the use of radiosensitizers is based on the knowledge that many tumors have hypoxic portions that are highly radioresistant (oxygen effect). Chemical radiosensitizers are drugs that take the place of oxygen in hypoxic cells to enhance radiation effectiveness. Compounds in current use include SR-2508, RO-03-8799, metronidazole, misonidazole, and desmethylmisonidazole.

Pyrimidine analogs (BUdR, IUdR) are also useful as radiosensitizers. These substances are very readily incorporated into DNA and subsequently inhibit the repair of sublethal damage (Fowler, 1985; Hellman, 1985; McGinn & Kinsella, 1994; Phillips, 1994). Perfluorocarbons are a third group of chemical modifiers that absorb high amounts of oxygen when exposed to hyperbaric conditions, then release oxygen when environmental oxygen is low. These compounds, therefore, serve as an oxygen transport vehicle, bringing oxygen to hypoxic tumors and enhancing the radiation effect.

Thiol depletors such as diethyl maleate (DEM) and butionine sulphoximine (BSO) act to deplete intracellular glutathione (GSH) prior to irradiation. The presence of GSH tends to protect against radiation damage and decreases the radiosensitivity of tumor cells. When used in combination with radiosensitizing agents, thiol depletors have enhanced tumor response in the laboratory setting (Fowler, 1985; Phillips, 1994; Wasserman & Kligerman, 1987).

Protecting normal tissue while enhancing tumor radiosensitivity is a therapeutic challenge. Compounds that serve as radioprotectors must be selective to the healthy tissue to obtain the desired results. Sulfhydryl compounds are the major group of radioprotectors currently under investigation and are described as scavengers in their affinity for the products of irradiated water (Wasserman & Kligerman, 1987). Repair of the critical molecules damaged by ionization is facilitated by donation of a hydrogen atom from the sulfhydryl compound. The radioprotective compound WR 2721 (a cystamine analog) is the subject of numerous investigations (Fowler, 1985).

Whenever therapies are combined to produce greater cytotoxicity, side effects are also increased. In addition, radiosensitizers characteristically have their own specific side effects of neurotoxicity and affect both the central and peripheral nervous systems. Prominent among these effects are peripheral neuropathy, somnolence, confusion, and transient coma. Gastrointestinal effects (nausea and vomiting) are also frequently seen (Noll, 1992).

Patient and family education in preparation for treatment with chemical modifiers is essential. Radiation oncology nurses are the best sources of providing information, assisting the patient and family to cope with the physical and emotional effects of treatment, and managing symptoms (Noll, 1992).

SUMMARY

Radiation therapy, whether used alone as the primary treatment of cancer or combined in a multimodality approach, has a major role in oncology. Patients today may have options for treatment in which they are given a choice between surgery or radiation therapy (early breast and laryngeal cancers) when either option has equal probability of cure or local control. Others may not have the same choice but are referred for radiation treatment because of its known palliative effects in advanced disease. Nurses caring for oncology patients in all settings have a responsibility to assist the patient and family by providing accurate information about radiation therapy. The scientific rationale of radiation oncology has been presented here as background for the science, art, and practice of oncology nursing intervention in care of the person receiving radiation.

REFERENCES

Aistars, J. (1987). Fatigue in the cancer patient: A conceptual approach to a clinical problem. *Oncology Nursing Forum, 14*(6), 25–30.

Anderson, L., Moni, J., & Harrison, L. (1993). A nomograph for permanent implants of palladium-103 seeds. *International Journal of Radiation Oncology, Biology, Physics, 27*(1), 129–135.

Arai, T., Nakano, T., Morita, S., Sakashita, K, Nakamura, Y., & Fukuhisa, K. (1992). High-dose-rate remote afterloading intracavitary radiation therapy for cancer of the uterine cervix: A 20-year experience. *Cancer, 69*(1), 175–180.

Arterbery, V. (1993). High-dose rate brachytherapy for carcinoma of the cervix. *Current Opinion in Oncology, 5*(6), 1005–1009.

Bahman, E., & Perez, C. (1985). Interstitial thermoradiotherapy: An overview. *Endocurietherapy/Hyperthermia Oncology, 1*, 35–40.

Bastin, K., Buchler, D., Stitt, J., Shanahan, T., Pola, Y., Paliwal, B., & Kinsella, T. (1993). Resource utilization. High dose rate versus low dose rate brachytherapy for gynecologic cancer. *American Journal of Clinical Oncology, 16*(3), 256–263.

Bergonie, J., & Tribondeau, L. (1959). Interpretation of some results of radiotherapy and an attempt at determining a logical technique of treatment. *Radiation Research, 2*, 587.

Bernstein, M., & Laperriere, N. J. (1990). A critical appraisal of the role of brachytherapy for pediatric brain tumors. *Pediatric Neurosurgery, 16*(4-5), 213–218.

Black, P., Tarbell, N., Alexander, E., Rockoff, M., Zhan, M., Loeffler, J., & Alexander, E. (1993). Stereotactic techniques in managing pediatric brain tumors. *Childs Nervous System, 9*(6), 343–346.

Brady, L., Markoe, A., Amendola, B., Karlsson, U., Micaily, B., Shields, J., & Augsburger, J. (1988). The treatment of primary intraocular malignancy. *International Journal of Radiation Oncology, Biology, Physics, 15*(6), 1355–1361.

Brady, L., Rotman, M., & Calvo, F. (1993). New advances in radiation oncology for gynecologic cancer. *Cancer, 71*(4), 1652–1659.

Brandt, B. (1989). What you should know about radiation implant therapy to the head and neck. *Oncology Nursing Forum, 16*(4), 579–582.

Brandt, B. (1991). Informational needs and selected variables in patients receiving brachytherapy. *Oncology Nursing Forum, 18*(7), 1221–1227.

Brandt, B., & Harney, J. (1989). An overview of interstitial brachytherapy and hyperthermia. *Oncology Nursing Forum, 16*(6), 833–841.

Brenner, D., Huang, Y., & Hall, E. (1991). Fractionated high dose-rate versus low dose-rate regimens for intracavitary brachytherapy of the cervix: Equivalent regimens for combined brachytherapy and external irradiation. *International Journal of Radiation Oncology, Biology, Physics, 21*(6), 1415–1423.

Bruner, D., Iwamoto, R., Keane, K., & Strohl, R. (Eds.). (1992). *Manual for radiation oncology nursing practice and education.* Pittsburgh: Oncology Nursing Society.

Bucholtz, J. (1992a). Radiation therapy. In J. Clark & R. McGee (Eds.), *Core curriculum for oncology nursing* (pp. 319–328). Philadelphia: W. B. Saunders Co.

Bucholtz, J. (1992b). Issues concerning the sedation of children for radiation therapy. *Oncology Nursing Forum, 19*(4), 649–655.

Bucholtz, J. (1994). Comforting children during radiotherapy. *Oncology Nursing Forum, 21*(6), 987–994.

Bucholtz, J. (Ed.). (1995). *Guidelines for radiation safety.* Pittsburgh: Oncology Nursing Society.

Chang, L., Horvath, J., Peyton, W., & Ling, S. (1994). High dose rate afterloading intraluminal brachytherapy in malignant airway obstruction of the lung. *International*

Journal of Radiation Oncology, Biology, Physics, 28(3), 589–596.

Choo, R., Grimard, L., Esche, B., Crook, J., Genset, P., & Odell, P. (1993). Brachytherapy of neck metastases. *Journal of Otolaryngology, 22*(1), 54–57.

Clark, D., & Martinez A. (1990). An overview of brachytherapy in cancer management. *Oncology, 4*(9), 39–46.

Close L., Morris, T., & Nguyen, P. (1993). Intraoperative versus interstitial radiotherapy: A comparison of morbidity in the head and neck. *Laryngoscope, 103*(3), 231–246.

Coleman, C. N., Beard, C. J., Hlatky, L., Kwok, T. R., & Bump, E. (1994). Biochemical modifiers: Hypoxic cell sensitizers. In P. M. Mauch & J. S. Loeffler (Eds.), *Radiation oncology technology and biology* (pp. 56–89). Philadelphia: W. B. Saunders Co.

Dini, D., Macchia, R., Gozza, A., Bertelli, G., Forno, G., Guenzi, M., Bacigalupo, A., Scolaro, T., & Vitale, V. (1993). Management of acute radiodermatitis. Pharmacological or nonpharmacological remedies. *Cancer Nursing, 16*(5), 366–370.

Dow, K. H., Harris, J. R., & Roy, C. (1994). Pregnancy after breast conserving surgery and radiation therapy for breast cancer. *Journal of the National Cancer Institute Monograph, 16*, 131–138.

Dudjak, L. (1987). Mouth care for mucositis due to radiation therapy. *Cancer Nursing, 10*(3), 131–140.

Dudjak, L. (1992). Alternatives in dose fractionation and treatment volume. In K. Hassey Dow & L. Hilderley (Eds.), *Nursing care in radiation oncology* (pp. 285–294). Philadelphia: W.B. Saunders Co.

Edmundson, G., Rizzo, N., Teahan, M., Brabbins, D., Vicini, F., & Martinez. (1993). Concurrent treatment planning for outpatient high dose rate prostate template implants. *International Journal of Radiation Oncology, Biology, Physics, 27*(5), 1215–1223.

Erickson, B., & Wilson, J. (1993). Nasopharyngeal brachytherapy. *American Journal of Clinical Oncology, 16*(5), 424–443.

Feldman, J. (1989). Ovarian failure and cancer treatment: Incidence and interventions for premenopausal women. *Oncology Nursing Forum, 16*(5), 651–657.

Finan, M., Hoffman, M., Greenberg, H., Roberts, W., Cavanagh, D., & Fiorica, J. (1993). Interstitial radiotherapy for early stage vaginal cancer. A new method of tumor localization. *Journal of Reproductive Medicine, 38*(3), 179–182.

Fowler, J. (1985). Chemical modifiers of radiosensitivity—theory and reality: A review. *International Journal of Radiation Oncology, Biology, Physics, 11*, 665–674.

Glasgow, G., & Perez, C. (1987). Physics of brachytherapy. In C. Perez & L. Brady (Eds.), *Principles and practice of radiation oncology* (pp. 213–251). Philadelphia: J. B. Lippincott Co.

Glicksman, A. (1987). Radiobiologic basis of brachytherapy. *Seminars in Oncology Nursing, 3*, 3–6.

Glicksman, A., & Leith, J. (1988). Radiobiological considerations of brachytherapy. *Oncology, 2*(1), 25–32.

Goffinet, D., Cox, R., Clarke, D., Fu, K., Hilaris, B., & Ling, C. (1988). Brachytherapy. *American Journal of Clinical Oncology, 11*(3), 342–354.

Goldman, J., Bulman, A., Rathmell, A., Carey, B., Muers, M., & Joslin, C. (1993). Physiological effect of endobronchial radiotherapy in patients with major airway occlusion by carcinoma. *Thorax, 48*(2), 110–114.

Grant, M., Dodd, M., Hilderley, L., & Patterson, P. (1984). Radiation oncology nurses' role: A national survey. *Oncology Nursing Forum Supplement: Proceedings of the Ninth Annual Congress, 11*(2), 107.

Greenburg, D., Sawicka, J., Eisenthal, S., & Ross, D. (1992). Fatigue syndrome due to localized radiation. *Journal of Pain & Symptom Management, 7*(1), 38–45.

Greenburg, S., Petersen, J., Hansep-Peters, I., & Baylinson, W. (1990). Interstitially implanted I125 for prostate cancer using transrectal ultrasound. *Oncology Nursing Forum, 17*(6), 849–854.

Griffin, T. (1987). High linear energy transfer and heavy charged particles. In C. A. Perez & L. W. Brady (Eds.), *Principles and practice of radiation oncology* (pp. 298–309). Philadelphia: J. B. Lippincott Co.

Guy, A., & Chou, C. K. (1983). Physical aspects of localized heating by radiowaves and microwaves. In F. Storm (Ed.), *Hyperthermia in cancer therapy* (pp. 279–304). Boston: G. K. Hall.

Hagopian, G. (1991). The effects of a weekly radiation therapy newsletter on patients. *Oncology Nursing Forum, 18*(7), 1199–1203.

Hall, E. (1993). The Janeway Lecture 1992. Nine decades of radiobiology: Is radiation therapy any the better for it? *Cancer, 71*(11), 3753–3766.

Hall, E. (1994). *Radiobiology for the radiologist*. Philadelphia: J. B. Lippincott Co.

Hall, E., & Brenner, D. (1991). George Edelstyn Memorial Lecture: Needles, wires and chips—advances in brachytherapy. *Clinical Oncology, 4*(4), 249–256.

Harvey, J., Fleischman, E., Bellotti, J., & Kagan, A. (1993). Intracavitary radiation in the treatment of advanced esophageal carcinoma: A comparison of high dose rate vs. low dose rate brachytherapy. *Journal of Surgical Oncology, 52*(2), 101–104.

Hassey, K. (1985). Demystifying care of patients with radioactive implants. *American Journal of Nursing, 85*, 788–792.

Hassey, K. (1987a). Principles of radiation safety and protection. *Seminars in Oncology Nursing, 3*(1), 23–29.

Hassey, K. (1987b). Radiation therapy for rectal cancer and the implications for nursing. *Cancer Nursing, 10*(6), 311–318.

Haylock, P., & Hart, L. (1979). Fatigue in patients receiving localized radiation. *Cancer Nursing, 2*, 461–467.

Hilaris, B., & Martini, N. (1988). The current state of intraoperative interstitial brachytherapy in lung cancer. *International Journal of Radiation Oncology, Biology, Physics, 15*(6), 1347–1354.

Hilderley, L. (1980). The role of the nurse in radiation oncology. *Seminars in Oncology, 7*, 39–47.

Hilderley, L. (1983). Skin care in radiation therapy: A review of the literature. *Oncology Nursing Forum, 10*(1), 51–56.

Hilderley, L. (1991). Nurse-physician collaborative practice: The clinical nurse specialist in a radiation oncology private practice. *Oncology Nursing Forum, 18*(3), 585–591.

Hoefnagel, C. (1991). Radionuclide therapy revisited. *European Journal of Nuclear Medicine, 18*(6), 408–431.

Iwamoto, R. (1992). Altered nutrition. In K. Hassey Dow & L. Hilderley (Eds.), *Nursing care in radiation oncology* (pp. 69–95). Philadelphia: W. B. Saunders Co.

Jankowski, C. (1992). Radiation protection for nurses, regulations and guidelines. *Journal of Nursing Administration, 22*(2), 30–35.

Jordan, L., & Buck, S. (1991). A teaching booklet for patients receiving high dose rate brachytherapy. *Oncology Nursing Forum, 18*(7), 1235–1238.

Jordan, L., & Mantravadi, R. (1991). Nursing care of the patient receiving high dose rate brachytherapy. *Oncology Nursing Forum, 18*(7), 1167–1171.

Kapp, K., Kapp, D., Stuecklschweiger, G., Berger, A., & Geyer, E. (1994). Interstitial hyperthermia and high dose rate brachytherapy in the treatment of anal cancer: A phase I/II study. *International Journal of Radiation Oncology, Biology, Physics, 28*(1), 189–199.

Khan, F. M. (1984). *The physics of radiation therapy.* Baltimore: Williams & Wilkins.

Khoury, G., Bulman, A., & Joslin, C. (1991). Long term results of Cathetron high dose rate intracavitary radiotherapy in the treatment of carcinoma of the cervix. *British Journal of Radiology, 64*(767), 1036–1043.

Kijewski, P. (1994). Three-dimensional treatment planning. In P. M. Mauch & J. S. Loeffler (Eds.), *Radiation oncology, technology and biology* (pp. 10–33). Philadelphia: W. B. Saunders, Co.

Kinsella, T. J., & Sindelar, W. F. (1985). Newer methods of cancer treatment: Intraoperative radiotherapy. In V. T. DeVita, S. Hellman, & S. A. Rosenberg (Eds.), *Cancer: Principles and practice of oncology* (2nd ed., pp. 2293–2304). Philadelphia: J. B. Lippincott Co.

Kobashi-Schoot, J., Hanewald, G., van Dam, F., & Bruning, P. (1985). Assessment of malaise in cancer patients treated with radiotherapy. *Cancer Nursing, 8*(6), 306–313.

Kumar, P., Patil, A., Syh, H, Chu, W., & Reeves, M. (1993). Role of brachytherapy in the management of the skull base meningioma. Treatment of skull base meningiomas. *Cancer, 71*(11), 3726–3731.

Kusler, D., & Rambur, B. (1992). Treatment for radiation-induced xerostomia. An innovative remedy. *Cancer Nursing, 15*(3), 191–195.

Lannon, S., el-Araby, A., Joseph, P., Eastwood, B., & Awad, S. (1993). Long-term results of combined interstitial gold seed implantation plus external beam irradiation in localised carcinoma of the prostate. *British Journal of Urology, 72*(5), 782–791.

Levitt, S. H., & Perez, C. A. (1987). Breast cancer. In C. A. Perez & L. W. Brady (Eds.), *Principles and practice of radiation oncology* (pp. 730–792). Philadelphia: J. B. Lippincott Co.

Lowdermilk, D. (1990). Nursing care update: Internal radiation therapy. *NAACOG Clinical Issues in Perinatal Womens Health Nursing, 1*(4), 532–540.

Lydon, J., McDonald-Lynch, A., Marshall, I., & Villanueva, W. (1989). Patient teaching about hyperthermia. *Oncology Nursing Forum, 16*(6), 855–860.

Maddock, P. (1987). Brachytherapy sources and applicators. *Seminars in Oncology Nursing, 3*(1), 15–22.

Marks, J. E., & Sessions D. G. (1987). Carcinoma of the larynx. In C. A. Perez & L. W. Brady (Eds.), *Principles and practice of radiation oncology* (pp. 598–618). Philadelphia: J. B. Lippincott Co.

Marsh, B., Colvin, D., Zinreich, E., Jackson, J., & Lee, D. (1993). Clinical experience with an endobronchial implant. *Radiology, 189*(1), 147–150.

Maruyama, Y., van Nagell, J., Yoneda, J., DePriest, P., & Kryscio, R. (1993). Clinical evaluation of 252cf neutron intracavitary therapy for primary endometrial adenocarcinoma. *Cancer, 71*(12), 3932–3937.

Maruyama, Y., van Nagell, J., Yoneda, J., Donaldson, E., Gallion, H., Powell, D., & Kryscio, R. (1991). A review of californium-252 neutron brachytherapy for cervical cancer. *Cancer, 68*(6), 1189–1197.

Mast, D., & Mood, D. (1990). Preparing patients with breast cancer for brachytherapy. *Oncology Nursing Forum, 17*(2), 267–270.

Masters, A., Steger, A., & Bown, S. (1991). Role of interstitial therapy in the treatment of liver cancer. *British Journal of Surgery, 78*(5), 518–523.

Maulard, C., Housset, M., Delanian, S., Ucla, L., Rozec, C., Chauvenic, L., & Baillet, F. (1994). Salvage split course brachytherapy for tonsil and soft palate carcinoma: Treatment techniques and results. *Laryngoscope, 104,* 359–363.

Mazeron, J., Crook, J., Martin, M., Peynegre, R., & Pierquin, B. (1989). Iridium 192 implantation of squamous cell carcinomas of the oropharynx. *American Journal of Otolaryngology, 10*(5), 317–321.

McCarthy, C. (1987). The role of interstitial implantation in the treatment of primary breast cancer. *Seminars in Oncology Nursing, 3*(1), 47–53.

McCarthy, C. (1992). Altered patterns of elimination. In K. H. Dow & L. Hilderley (Eds.), *Nursing care in radiation oncology* (pp. 126–148). Philadelphia: W. B. Saunders Co.

McDermott, M., Gutin, P., Larson, D., & Sneed, P. (1990). Interstitial brachytherapy. *Neurosurgery Clinics of North America, 1*(4), 801–824.

McGinn, C. J., & Kinsella, T. J. (1994). Biochemical modifiers: Nonhypoxic cell sensitizers. In P. M. Mauch & J. S. Loeffler (Eds.), *Radiation oncology, technology and biology* (pp. 90–112). Philadelphia: W. B. Saunders Co.

Mendenhall, N. P., Ames, F. C., Sarrazin, D., & Veronisi, U. (1991). Postoperative irradiation following breast-conserving surgical procedures. In K. I. Bland & E. M. Copeland (Eds.), *The breast* (pp. 781–816). Philadelphia: W. B. Saunders Co.

Million, R. R., Cassisi, N. J., & Wittes, R. E. (1985). Cancer of the head and neck. In V. T. DeVita, S. Hellman, & S. A. Rosenberg (Eds.), *Cancer: Principles and practice of oncology* (Vol. 1, 2nd ed., pp. 407–506). Philadelphia: J. B. Lippincott Co.

Munzenrider, J. E., & Crowell, C. (1994). Charged particles. In P. M. Mauch & J. S. Loeffler (Eds.), *Radiation oncology, technology and biology* (pp. 34–55). Philadelphia: W. B. Saunders Co.

Musolino, A., Merckaert, P., Munari, C., Daumas-Duport, C., & Chodkiewicz, J. (1989). Stereotactic endocavitary treatment of cysts and pseudocyst of glioma. Preliminary report. *Journal of Neurosurgical Sciences, 33*(1), 107–141.

Myers, J. S., Davidson, J., Hutt, P., & Chatham, S. (1987). Standardized teaching plans for management of chemotherapy and radiation side-effects. *Oncology Nursing Forum, 14*(5), 95–99.

Nag, S., Grecula, J., & Ruymann, F. (1993). Aggressive chemotherapy, organ-preserving surgery, and high-dose-rate remote brachytherapy in the treatment of rhabdomyosarcoma in infants and young children. *Cancer, 72*(9), 2769–2776.

Nanavati, P., Fanning, J., Hilgers, R., Hallstrom, J., & Crawford, D. (1993). High-dose-rate brachytherapy in primary stage I and II vaginal cancer. *Gynecologic Oncology, 51*(1), 67–71.

National Council on Radiation Protection and Measurements. (1972). *NCRP report #40: Protection against radiation from brachytherapy sources.* Washington, DC: Author.

National Council on Radiation Protection and Measurements. (1973). *NCRP report #37: Precautions in the management of patients who have received therapeutic amounts of radionuclides.* Washington, DC: Author.

National Council on Radiation Protection and Measurements. (1974). *NCRP report #39: Basic radiation protection criteria.* Washington, DC: Author.

National Council on Radiation Protection and Measurements. (1989). *NCRP report #105: Radiation protection for medical and allied health personnel.* Bethesda, MD: Author.

National Council on Radiation Protection and Measurements. (1993). *NCRP report #116: Recommendations on limits for exposure to ionizing radiation.* Bethesda, MD: Author.

Noll, L. (1992). Chemical modifiers of radiation therapy. In K. Hassey Dow & L. Hilderley (Eds.), *Nursing care in radiation oncology*, Philadelphia: W. B. Saunders Co.

Nori, D. (1993). Intraoperative brachytherapy in non-small cell lung cancer. *Seminars in Surgical Oncology, 9*(2), 99–107.

Noyes, R., Weiss, S., Krall, J., Sause, W., Owens, J., Wolkov, H., Langiano, R., Hanks, G., & Hoffman, J. (1992). Surgical complications of intraoperative radiation therapy: The radiation therapy oncology group experience. *Journal of Surgical Oncology, 50,* 209–215.

Noz, M., & Maguire, G. (1979). *Radiation protection in the radiologic and health sciences.* Philadelphia: Lea & Febiger.

Oberst, M., Hughes, S., Chang, A., & McCubbin, M. (1991). Self-care burden, stress appraisal, and mood among persons receiving radiotherapy. *Cancer Nursing, 14*(2), 71–78.

Oncology Nursing Society. (1987). *ONS/ANA standards of oncology nursing practice.* Kansas City, MO: American Nurses Association.

Oncology Nursing Society (1994). *Radiation therapy patient care record: A tool for documenting nursing care* (GLRD9401). Pittsburgh: Oncology Nursing Society.

Orton, C., Seyedsadr, M., & Somnay, A. (1991). Comparison of high and low dose rate remote afterloading for cervix cancer and the importance of fractionation. *International Journal of Radiation Oncology, Biology, Physics, 21*(6), 1425–1434.

Ostertag, C. (1989). Stereotactic interstitial radiotherapy for brain tumors. *Journal of Neurosurgical Sciences, 33*(1), 83–89.

Paradelo, J., Waxman, M., Throne, B., Beller, T., & Kopecky, W. (1992). Endobronchial irradiation with 192IR in the treatment of malignant endobronchial obstruction. *Chest, 102*(4), 1072–1074.

Perez, C. A. (1987). Carcinoma of the prostate. In C. A. Perez & L. W. Brady (Eds.), *Principles and practice of radiation oncology* (pp. 867–898). Philadelphia: J. B. Lippincott Co.

Perez, C. A., & Emami, B. (1989). Clinical trials with local (external and interstitial) irradiation and hyperthermia. Current and future perspectives. *Radiologic Clinics of North America, 27*(3), 525–542.

Phillips, T. L. (1994). Biochemical modifiers: Drug-radiation interactions. In P. M. Mauch & J. S. Loeffler (Eds.), *Radiation oncology, technology and biology* (pp. 113–151). Philadelphia: W. B. Saunders, Co.

Piper, B., Lindsey, A., & Dodd, M. (1987). Fatigue mechanisms in cancer patients: Developing nursing theory. *Oncology Nursing Forum, 14*(6), 17–23.

Pisch, J., Berson, A., Harvey, J., Mishra, S., & Beattie, E. (1994). Absorbable mesh in placement of temporary implants. *International Journal of Radiation Oncology, Biology, Physics, 28*(3), 719–722.

Porter, A., & Forman, J. (1993). Prostate brachytherapy. An overview. *Cancer, 71*(3), 953–958.

Prestidge, B., Butler, E., Shaw, D., & McComas, V. (1994). Ultrasound guided placement of transperineal prostatic afterloading catheters. *International Journal of Radiation Oncology, Biology, Physics, 28*(1), 263–266.

Randall, M., Evans, L., Greven, K., McCunniff, A., & Doline, R. (1993). Interstitial reirradiation for recurrent gynecologic malignancies: Results and analysis of prognostic factors. *Gynecologic Oncology, 48*(1), 23–31.

Randall, T., Drake, D., & Sewchand, W. (1987). Neurooncology update: Radiation safety and nursing care during interstitial brachytherapy. *Journal of Neuroscience Nursing, 19*(6), 315–320.

Recht, A., Triedman, S., & Harris, J. (1991). The "boost" in the treatment of early-stage breast cancer: Electrons versus interstitial implants. *Frontiers of Radiation Therapy and Oncology, 25,* 169–179.

Richards, S., & Hiratzka, S. (1986). Vaginal dilatation post-pelvic irradiation: A patient education tool. *Oncology Nursing Forum, 13*(4), 89–91.

Richter, M. P., Share, F. S., & Goodman, R. L. (1985). Principles of radiation therapy. In P. Calabresi, P. S. Schein, & S. A. Rosenberg (Eds.), *Medical oncology: Basic principles and clinical management of cancer* (pp. 280–291). New York: Macmillan Publishing Co.

Rubin, P., Constine, L. S., & Nelson, D. F. (1992). Late effects of cancer treatment. In C. A. Perez & L. W. Brady (Eds.), *Principles and practice of radiation oncology* (2nd ed., pp. 124–172). Philadelphia: J. B. Lippincott Company.

Schray, M., Gunderson, L., Sim, F., Pritchard, D., Shives, T., & Yeakel, P. (1990). Soft tissue sarcoma: Integration of brachytherapy, resection, and external radiation. *Cancer, 66*(3), 451–456.

Sedhmo, L., & Yanni, M. (1985). Radiation therapy and nurses' fears of radiation exposure. *Cancer Nursing, 8*(2), 129–134.

Seegenschmiedt, M., Sauer, R., Miyamoto, C., Chalal, J., & Brady, L. (1993). Clinical experience with interstitial thermoradiotherapy for localized implantable pelvic tumors. *American Journal of Clinical Oncology, 16*(3), 210–222.

Shapiro, J. (1981). *Radiation protection: A guide for scientists and physicians* (2nd ed.). Cambridge, MA: Harvard University Press.

Shea, J., Allen, R., Tharratt, R., Chan, A., & Siefkin, A. (1993). Survival of patients undergoing Nd:YAG laser therapy compared with Nd:YAG laser therapy and brachytherapy for malignant airway disease. *Chest, 103*(4), 1038–1031.

Shipley, W., Kaufman, S., & Prout, G. (1987). Intraoperative radiation therapy in patients with bladder cancer. A review of techniques allowing improved tumor doses and providing high cure rates without loss of bladder function. *Cancer, 60*(7), 1485–1488.

Shiu, M., Hilaris, B., Harrison, L., & Brennan, M. (1991). Brachytherapy and function-saving resection of soft tissue sarcoma arising in the limb. *International Journal of Radiation Oncology, Biology, Physics, 21*(6), 1485–1492.

Sitton, E. (1992a). Early and late radiation-induced skin alterations. Part I: Mechanisms of skin changes. *Oncology Nursing Forum, 19*(5), 801–807.

Sitton, E. (1992b). Early and late radiation-induced skin alterations. Part II: Nursing care of irradiated skin. *Oncology Nursing Forum, 19*(6), 907–912.

Skalla, K. A., & Lacasse, C. (1992). Patient education for fatigue. *Oncology Nursing Forum, 19*(10), 1537–1541.

Smith, R. (1992). Intraoperative radiation therapy. In K. Hassey Dow & L. Hilderley (Eds.), *Nursing care in radiation oncology.* Philadelphia: W. B. Saunders Co.

Sporkin, E. (1987). A newsletter for radiation therapy patients [Abstract]. *Oncology Nursing Forum, 14*(2, Suppl.) 149.

Sticklin, L. A. (1994). Strategies for overcoming nurses' fear of radiation exposure. *Cancer Practice, 2*(4), 275–278.

Stitt, J. (1992). High-dose-rate intracavitary brachytherapy for gynecologic malignancies. *Oncology, 6*(1), 59–70.

Strohl, R. (1988). The nursing role in radiation oncology: Symptom management of acute and chronic reactions. *Oncology Nursing Forum, 15,* 429–434.

Strohl, R. (1990). Radiation therapy. Recent advances and nursing implications. *Nursing Clinics of North America, 25*(2), 309–329.

Suit, H., & Urie, M. (1992). Proton beams in radiation therapy. *Journal of the National Cancer Institute, 84*(3), 155–164.

Travis, E. (1975). *Primer of medical radiobiology*. Chicago: Year Book Medical Publishers.

Valdagni, R., Fei-Fei, L., & Kapp, D. (1988). Important prognostic factors influencing outcome of combined radiation and hyperthermia. *International Journal of Radiation Oncology, Biology, Physics, 15,* 959–972.

Vijverberg, P., Blank, L., Dabhoiwala, N., de Reijke, T., Koedooder, C., Hart, A., Kurth, K., & Gonzalez, D. (1993). Analysis of biopsy findings and implant quality following ultrasonically-guided 125I implantation for localised prostatic carcinoma. *British Journal of Urology, 72*(4), 470–477.

Wasserman, T. H., & Kligerman, M. (1987). Chemical modifiers of radiation effect. In C. A. Perez & L. W. Brady (Eds.), *Principles and practice of radiation oncology* (pp. 360–376). Philadelphia: J. B. Lippincott Co.

Willis, D., Rittenmeyer, H., & Hitchon, P. (1986). Intracranial interstitial radiation. *Journal of Neuroscience Nursing, 18*(3), 153–156.

Wilson, J. F. (1989). The breast. In W. T. Moss & J. D. Cox (Eds.), *Radiation oncology: Rationale, technique, results* (6th ed., pp. 312–350). St. Louis: C. V. Mosby Co.

Wilson, P., Herman, J., & Chubon, S. (1991). Eating strategies used by persons with head and neck cancer during and after radiotherapy. *Cancer Nursing, 14*(2), 98–104.

Winningham, M. L., Nail, L. M., Barton-Burke, M., Brophy, L., Cimprich, B., Jones, L. S., Pickard-Holley, S., Rhodes, V., St. Pierre, B., Beck, S., Glass, E. C., Mock, V. L., Mooney, K. H. & Piper, B. (1994). Fatigue and the cancer experience: The state of the knowledge. *Oncology Nursing Forum, 21*(1), 23–36.

Witt, M. (1987). Questions on colon and rectum radiation therapy. *Oncology Nursing Forum, 14*(3), 79–82.

Wojtas, F. (1992). Hyperthermia and radiation therapy. In K. Hassey Dow & L. Hilderley (Eds.), *Nursing care in radiation oncology*. Philadelphia: W. B. Saunders Co.

CHAPTER
21

Medical Oncology—The Agents

Jennifer L. Guy • Barbara A. Ingram

Medical oncology focuses on the systemic management of malignant disease by the use of antineoplastic medications, commonly referred to as chemotherapy. Chemotherapy is "the treatment of disease by chemical agents; first applied to the use of chemicals that attack the causative organisms unfavorably but do not harm the patient" (*Dorland's illustrated medical dictionary*, 1994). Chemotherapy administered to patients for the management of confined or disseminated malignant disease is the focus of this discussion.

Today many diseases are curable with chemotherapy. Prolonged disease-free intervals and increased survival times have been documented with chemotherapeutic intervention for a number of tumors (Table 21–1). For other tumors, chemotherapy can help to control pain and ease suffering.

The clinical management of medical oncology patients is based on an understanding of the principles of chemotherapeutic intervention and of the host factors that determine the choice of drugs, dose, route, and schedule, as well as knowledge of the agents and their acute and delayed toxicities.

HISTORIC PERSPECTIVES

The concept of using chemicals to treat malignant disease dates to the sixteenth century, when heavy metals were used systemically to treat cancers. They were mostly ineffective and extremely toxic, and thus they were discarded until the resurgence of the use of arsenic in 1865 in the treatment of chronic leukemias (Burchenal, 1977). Today heavy metals such as cisdiamminedichloroplatinum (cisplatin) are a mainstay in the treatment of solid tumors.

Chemotherapy evolved from the unlikely province of chemical warfare. During World War I, soldiers were observed to suffer severe bone marrow suppression,

aplasia, and death after exposure to sulfur mustard gas. World War II fostered the recognition of the therapeutic application of alkylating agents to the treatment of malignancy (Gilman & Phillips, 1946; Zubrod, 1979). Nitrogen mustard was the first antineoplastic drug to undergo clinical trials; it was shown to produce significant therapeutic effect in patients with tumors of the lymphoid organs (Gilman, 1963; Gilman & Phillips, 1946). Folic acid antagonists were shown to be effective in acute leukemia in children by Farber, Diamond, Mercer, Sylvester, and Wolfe (1948) (Box 21–1). Thioguanine and mercaptopurine were synthesized and were found to produce remissions in antifolate-resistant acute leukemia (Burchenal, 1977).

TABLE 21–1. *Impact of Chemotherapy in Malignant Disease*

CURABLE	IMPROVED SURVIVAL
Choriocarcinoma	Small-cell carcinoma of the lung
Acute lymphoblastic leukemia (children)	Ovarian carcinoma
Embroyonal rhabdomyosarcoma	Breast carcinoma
Wilms' tumor	Osteosarcoma
Diffuse histiocytic lymphoma	Multiple myeloma
Germinal testicular carcinoma	Chronic leukemia (lymphocytic and myelogenous)
Burkitt's lymphoma	
Hodgkin's disease	Non-Hodgkin's lymphoma
Ewing's sarcoma	Soft-tissue sarcomas
Acute myelogenous leukemia	Neuroblastoma

(Data from DeVita, V. T., Jr. [1993]. Principles of Chemotherapy. In V. T. DeVita, S. Hellman, & S. A. Rosenberg [Eds.], *Cancer: Principles and practice of oncology* [4th ed., pp. 276–292]. Philadelphia: J. B. Lippincott; and Skeel, R. T. [1991]. *Handbook of Cancer Chemotherapy* [pp. 6–121]. Boston: Little, Brown, & Co.)

Box 21–1. *An Early Chemotherapy Study*

Farber, S., Diamond, L. K., Mercer, R. D., Sylvester, R. F., & Wolfe, J. A. (1948). Temporary remissions in acute leukemia in children produced by folic acid antagonist, 4-aminopteroyl-glutamic acid (aminopterin). *New England Journal of Medicine, 238,* 787–793.

Sample: Sixteen children with acute leukemia, many of whom were moribund at the onset of therapy. Five case reports are detailed, all with bone marrow confirmation of acute leukemia.

Treatment: Aminopterin was administered at a dose of 0.5 to 1.0 mg IM daily for variable periods of time in the cases detailed. Some subjects concomitantly received liver extract and folic acid in an attempt to prevent toxicity.

Results: Ten of the 16 children responded to treatment with aminopterin as evaluated by improvement in peripheral blood counts, bone marrow blast counts, splenomegaly, hepatomegaly, and lymphadenopathy, and improvement in performance status. Six patients failed to respond. Remissions were temporary. Toxicity included stomatitis with early ulceration, which was reversible.

Conclusions: Aminopterin induces temporary remissions in children with acute leukemia, but produces "significant" toxicity, which "may make continued use of the drug impossible." The authors state "these studies justify the search for other antagonists to folic acid which are less toxic and may be even more powerful."

Limitations: Variable amounts of aminopterin were administered for variable periods of time. In an attempt to control toxicity, liver extract and folic acid were administered to some subjects. No distinction is made between acute lymphoblastic and acute myelogenous leukemia. Limitations of the study emanate from technologies extant at the time the investigation was undertaken.

Significance: This study documented the efficacy of antimetabolites in hematologic malignancies. Performance status was carefully assessed; improvement in performance status was a parameter of response. This study employed the concept of "rescue" of normal cells, albeit primitive, from the effects of antimetabolites. Toxicity was evaluated critically and considered prohibitive by the authors. The study lends insight into the evolution of clinical investigations and discoveries in cancer chemotherapy.

In the 1950s, antibiotics were resurrected as cytotoxic agents. Also, 5-fluorouracil was synthesized, setting the stage for the use of purine and pyrimidine analogs, which remain a cornerstone of cancer therapy today. During this decade, asparaginase was isolated from *Escherichia coli,* paving the way for the use of enzymes in cancer treatment.

Rosenberg and coworkers demonstrated the effect of platinum coordinate complexes in the 1960s, initially in bacteria, then in lymphosarcoma and solid tumors (Rosenberg, Krigas, & Van Camp, 1965; Rosenberg, Trosko, Mansour, & Van Camp, 1969). In the late 1960s and early 1970s, multidrug chemotherapy regimens were found to improve remission rates without inducing undue toxicity. The use of chemotherapy in combination with other methods of cancer treatment also came into clinical practice in this decade (see Chapter 22).

The 1970s and 1980s were dedicated to the synthesis and clinical testing of available agents, alone and in combination, and the continued screening and synthesis of new agents. In addition, interest piqued in developing analogs of known efficacious agents such as doxorubicin in hopes of decreasing toxicity, increasing activity, or both. These efforts have been fruitful; a dozen new agents became available in the 1990s and are included in this chapter. The antineoplastic effects of biologic response modifiers were identified in the 1980s and further investigated in the 1990s, better defining their role in oncologic therapeutics. Currently, drug development is emphasizing new agents such as Taxol with novel mechanisms of action, often attempting to exploit recent knowledge about mechanisms of drug resistance. The availability of growth factors has revolutionized the science of cancer chemotherapy, avoiding some toxicities (sepsis, neutropenic fever), minimizing others (anemia), and motivating the development of new interventions such as peripheral stem cell transplants. Concurrently, new toxicities may be identified as dose intensity increases (Armitage & Antman, 1992).

The current armamentarium of antineoplastics consists of more than 60 agents used as treatment for a broad spectrum of diseases collectively known as cancer. Pharmacologic considerations (doses, routes, schedule), disease variables (biologic behavior, primary site, stage, histology), and patient factors (age, organ system function) result in multiple permutations and combinations of therapeutic interventions, many yet to be studied.

DRUG DEVELOPMENT

The identification of compounds with antitumor activity and their subsequent development into clinically useful and available agents began in the 1930s with Shear's efforts at the National Cancer Institute (NCI) (Zubrod, 1984). In 1955, at the direction of the United States Congress, the NCI established the Cancer Chemotherapy National Service Center (CCNSC), and a national drug development program was initiated.

The first step in drug development is the recognition of potential antineoplastic effect and synthesis of the active compound. Agents are then screened using in vitro and in vivo tumor panels. Currently, the NCI alone screens over 10,000 compounds a year (DeVita, 1993). Of those screened, less than 1 per cent ultimately undergo clinical evaluation.

Once an agent has shown antineoplastic activity in the screening process, it must be produced and synthesized in a clinically usable formulation, a challenge sometimes insurmountable despite positive tumor screens. Preclinical toxicology testing of active compounds is accomplished in mouse models to establish the lethal dose; a reproducible lethal dose in 10 per cent of the rodents (LD_{10}) is acceptable for initial human use. Because some clinically significant toxic effects of antineoplastics have not been consistent between rodent and human systems, further evaluation is accomplished in dogs, with which better human correlation has been shown. This phase of preclinical testing includes pathologic examination of the tissue to define the mechanisms of toxicities. The progress of a new agent through preclinical testing is summarized in Figure 21–1.

HOW ANTINEOPLASTICS WORK

Malignant tumors are characterized by cell division, which is no longer controlled as it is in normal tissue. Normal cells cease dividing when they come into contact with like cells, a mechanism known as contact inhibition (Korsmeyer, 1993). Malignant cells lose this ability. However, cancer cells continue to move through the cell cycle, progressing from a resting state (G_0) through mitosis (M). A malignant tumor is composed of millions of cells with various proportions of cells distributed through the five phases of the cell cycle at any one time. The proportion of cells actively dividing at any given time constitutes the growth fraction of the tumor. The time required for a malignant tumor to increase cell number by 100 per cent is referred to as the doubling time. Cell cycle time refers to the time required for a single cell to progress through the cell cycle and reproduce itself (Schackney, 1985).

Cytotoxicity depends on halting cellular biochemical functions that allow cell replication. The higher the proportion of dividing cells or the shorter the time it takes for the cell to divide, the more likely it is that chemotherapy will induce tumor regression. Table 21–2 classifies common tumors according to their cell cycle time and compares them with the division rates of normal tissues (Schackney, 1985; See-Lasley & Ignoffo, 1981). Rapidly dividing normal cells are most often adversely affected by chemotherapy.

Table 21–3 delineates the phases of the cell cycle and their duration, cellular activities, and sensitivity to chemotherapy. The resting phase, G_0, is highly variable in duration. The higher the proportion of cells in this phase is, the longer the doubling time will be. Phases G_1, S, and G_2 are preparatory to the mitotic (M) phase, at which point cell division occurs. Normal cells then differentiate, whereas malignant cells reenter G_0 and continue to divide. Newer approaches to chemotherapy focus on agents that potentiate cellular differentiation (Cheson, Chun, Friedman, & Jasperse, 1986). Retinoic acids have rendered acute progranulocytic leukemia (APL) reversible by differentiating the leukemic cells to normal mature granulocytes.

Antineoplastics may be classified according to the point in the cell cycle at which they exert their effect. Agents that are lethal only if the cell is dividing are considered cell cycle–specific. If a drug's activity is restricted to one specific phase (i.e., G_1, S, G_2, or M) of the cell cycle, it is considered phase-specific as well. If the drug is effective only on resting cells (G_0), it is cycle-nonspecific. Recruitment refers to motivating cells to leave G_0 and enter the growth phases of the cell cycle in which they are susceptible to cell cycle–specific and phase-specific agents (Dorr & Fritz, 1980; Dorr & Von Hoff, 1994; Schackney, 1985). This may be accomplished by rapid reduction in the dividing cell population, which mobilizes nondividing cells into an active growth phase (Schackney, 1985).

For example, aggressive regimens for the treatment of non-Hodgkin's lymphoma (M-BACOD, PRO-MACE-MOPP) involve rapid cytoreduction by day 1 therapy, followed by nonmyelosuppressive agents on day 14, when the nondividing cells have been recruited into the active growth phases, G_1, S, G_2, and M. Alternatively, tumors with a high percentage of cells in G_0 or a long cell cycle time will experience greater lethality from cell cycle–nonspecific agents. Some antineoplastics act on both resting and cycling cells and are classified as cell cycle–specific and phase-nonspecific. Antineoplastic effect may also be demonstrated in more than one phase of the cell cycle. Table 21–4 provides an overview of the cell cycle and phase activity of the five major classes of antineoplastics.

Scheduling and punctual administration are imperative to obtain optimal effects on the cell cycle. The rationale for continuous infusion of chemotherapy is based on exposing tumor cells to the drug as they enter the phase of the cell cycle during which the drug exerts its effect. Agents designed to enhance cell synchronization or recruitment must be administered at times con-

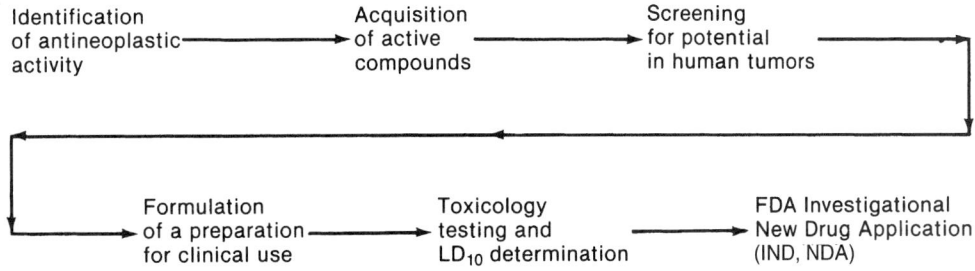

FIGURE 21–1. Preclinical development of antineoplastics. LD_{10}, lethal dose in 10 per cent of mice tested; *FDA*, Food and Drug Administration; IND, Investigational New Drug; NDA, New Drug Application.

TABLE 21–2. *Comparative Cell Cycle Times*

Doubling time	Short	Intermediate	Long
Cell cycle time	Hours to days	Weeks	Months
Normal cell	Gastrointestinal mucosa	Skin	Liver
	Mucous membrane	Hair follicles	Kidney
	Bone marrow		
Malignancies	Burkitt's lymphoma	Small-cell lung cancer	Breast cancer
	Germ-cell tumors	Hodgkin's disease	Colon cancer
	Acute myelogenous leukemia	Non-Hodgkin's lymphoma	Lung cancer (non-small-cell)

(Data from See-Lasley, K., & Ignoffo, R. J. [1981]. *Manual of oncology therapeutics*. St. Louis: C. V. Mosby Co.; and Schackney, S. E. [1985]. Cell kinetics and cancer chemotherapy. In P. Calabresi, P. S. Schein, & S. A. Rosenberg [Eds.], *Medical oncology: Basic principles and practice of oncology* [2nd ed., pp. 2008–2013]. Philadelphia: J. B. Lippincott Co.)

sistent with data on the cell cycle time to effect cell kill (Schackney, 1985). For example, aggressive regimens for the treatment of non-Hodgkin's lymphoma (M-BACOD, PROMACE-MOPP) involve rapid cytoreduction by day 1 therapy, followed by nonmyelosuppressive agents on day 14, when the nondividing cells have been recruited into the active growth phases, G_1, S, G_2, and M.

Tumor burden at the onset of chemotherapy has prognostic implications for its success in eradicating the tumor. Antineoplastics induce cell kill by first-order kinetics (i.e., the same proportion of cells are killed with each subsequent exposure to the lethal agent). The absolute number of cells killed by a second exposure to a lethal drug is smaller than the number killed with the first exposure, assuming a constant fraction of actively dividing cells. However, as tumor burden increases, the rate of growth slows, decreasing the number of cells in active division. Sensitivity to cycle-specific agents then decreases (Dorr & Fritz, 1980; Schackney, 1985).

In 1979, Goldie and Coldman described a model of spontaneous tumor cell mutations, demonstrating that a mass of fewer than 1 million cells may contain clones with variable antineoplastic sensitivity. The Goldie-Coldman hypothesis explains why curability of a small tumor cannot always be ensured despite treatment. The earliest possible institution of chemotherapy may minimize the development of resistant clones and increase curability. Alternation of different, non-cross-resistant agents and regimens is aimed at killing resistant clones.

The Goldie-Coldman hypothesis explains the variation of response that can be observed among identically treated patients with tumors of the same primary site, stage, and histologic features (Schackney, 1985).

Additional mechanisms of tumor cell resistance have been described: amplification of genetic control, development of alternate metabolic pathways allowing cell survival, and antineoplastic alteration of cellular chromosomes that increases genetic instability and mutation rate (Schackney, 1985). For example, gene amplification has been documented to produce resistance to methotrexate. Tumor cells previously exposed to prolonged low doses of methotrexate (2.5 mg weekly for 3 years) have been shown to expand the genetic sequence that controls the production of dihydrofolate reductase (Trent, Buick, Horna, Olson, & Schimke, 1984). Thus increasing amounts of this enzyme are produced that are no longer inhibited by standard doses of methotrexate.

DRUG RESISTANCE

Although not completely understood, the tumor cell has the ability to innately express a cellular membrane protein, p-glycoprotein, which is controlled by the multidrug resistance gene (MDR). P-glycoprotein (Pgp) actively effluxes antineoplastics from the cell, thus preventing them from reaching their intracellular site of action. Pgp may be intrinsic to the tumor cell, thus conferring a primary resistance of at least some of the

TABLE 21–3. *Phases of the Cell Cycle*

ANTINEOPLASTIC SENSITIVITY	PHASE	CELLULAR EVENTS	DURATION
±	→G_0 ↓	Resting (cells not committed to cell division)	Highly variable
+	G_1 ↓	RNA and protein synthesis (enzymes produced that are necessary for DNA synthesis)	18–30 hr
+	S ↓	DNA synthesis	18–20 hr
+	G_2 ↓	RNA, protein synthesis (specialized)	2–10 hr
+	←M ↓	Mitosis (cell division)	0.5–1 hr
±	Differentiation	Permanently nondividing cells that will die, resulting in expected cell loss	

TABLE 21–4. *Effect of Antineoplastics on Cell Cycle Phases**

CELL CYCLE PHASE	ANTINEOPLASTICS ACTIVE IN THIS PHASE
G_0	Nitrosoureas, alkylating agents
G_1	Enzymes, steroids, hormones, antibiotics, alkylating agents
S	Antimetabolites, hydroxyurea
G_2	Antibiotics, antimetabolites
M	Plant alkaloids

*Major effect of each class is in the designated phase of the cell cycle. Alkylating agents, nitrosoureas, and many antitumor antibiotics are also active throughout the cell cycle.

malignant clones; it may be acquired as the result of genetic changes such as chromosomal translocations, deletions, mutations, or amplifications, induced by exposure to prior antineoplastic administration. The overproduction of Pgp results in multidrug resistance (MDR) and usually confers resistance to predominately the natural products (antibiotics, vinca alkaloids, podophyllotoxins) but may also result in resistance to antimetabolites and synthetic compounds (Booser & Hortobagyi, 1994).

The identification of Pgp has led to attempts to overcome MDR by the administration of agents known to prevent binding of the antineoplastic to the Pgp receptor. Agents such as calcium channel blockers, cyclosporines, some hormones, and quinines are currently being investigated for their ability to overcome resistance by administration in conjunction with antineoplastics. To date, the problems incumbent in this approach have been the toxicities of the sensitizing agents. Research is ongoing (Chaudhary & Robinson, 1991; Cimoli, De Sessa, Parodi, Russo, & Valenti, 1994; Cordon-Cardo et al., 1990; Dalton, 1993; Georges, Ling, & Sharom, 1990; Nooter & Sooneveld, 1994).

Another identified mechanism of drug resistance involves the ability of intracellular enzymes known as topoisomerases to change, rendering the cells resistant to antineoplastics that inhibit topoisomerase activity. Topoisomerases are required for the dissociation and subsequent realignment of the DNA strands during cellular replication. Investigational agents such as the camptothecins (topotecan) and available agents (etoposide, doxorubicin) inhibit topoisomerase activity, resulting in cell death; however, changes in the amount of topoisomerase required for DNA strand alignment, development of alternate pathways, or changes in the configuration of the enzyme may render the topoisomerase inhibitors ineffective (Alton & Harris, 1993; Creemers, Lund, & Verweij, 1994).

While some mechanisms of drug resistance are well understood, this knowledge has not affected our ability to overcome them in the clinic. It is hoped that increasing understanding of the molecular and genetic basis of resistance will result in clinically useful approaches to preventing or circumventing resistance (Liu & D'Arpa, 1992; Morrow & Cowan, 1993).

PRINCIPLES OF CHEMOTHERAPY ADMINISTRATION

Chemotherapy may be administered as a single agent palliatively. For example, busulfan is used to lower the white blood cell count in the chronic phase of chronic myelogenous leukemia and in high doses in preparation for bone marrow transplant. Hydroxyurea alone may then be administered to control leukocytosis and splenomegaly in the accelerated phase. It should be noted that single-agent chemotherapy does not cure cancer, with the exception of the use of methotrexate in choriocarcinoma (DeVita, 1993).

Combinations of antineoplastic agents are more effective than single agents in tumors that are responsive (i.e., sensitive) to multiple agents. Agents selected for inclusion in combination chemotherapy regimens must be individually active against the targeted tumor type and ideally be synergistic with the agents used in the regimen. Multiagent regimens should include non-cross-resistant drugs and agents that act at different points in the cell cycle. The classic example of these principles is the MOPP regimen (mechlorethamine [Mustargen], vincristine [Oncovin], procarbazine, and prednisone) for the treatment of Hodgkin's disease (Box 21–2) (DeVita, Carbone, & Serpick, 1970). To circumvent the problem of drug resistance, alternation of regimens may be used, such as the alternation of MOPP with doxorubicin (Adriamycin), bleomycin, vinblastine (Velban), and dacarbazine (ABVD) in Hodgkin's disease (Bonadonna, Santoro, & Valagussa, 1986). Alternating non-cross-resistant agents improves cell death rate by affecting clones resistant to alternate agents. Recent understanding of mechanisms of drug resistance have suggested using known, less effective regimens prior to known regimens with greater efficacy to attempt to obliterate resistant clones that may grow during treatment with the most lethal regimen (DeVita, 1993; Norton & Day, 1991).

Chemotherapy may be administered as the primary curative modality, an example of which is the cisplatin, vinblastine (Velban), and bleomycin (PVB) regimen in the treatment of testicular cancer (Einhorn, 1981) or the MOPP regimen in the treatment of Hodgkin's disease (De Vita et al., 1970). In childhood lymphoblastic leukemia, chemotherapy is the primary curative modality.

Control of malignant disease may be accomplished with chemotherapy when improved survival can be demonstrated. Doxorubicin-containing regimens, hormonal chemotherapy, alkylating agents, and the cyclophosphamide, methotrexate, and 5-fluorouracil (CMF) regimen are effective in prolonging disease-free intervals after potentially curative surgery and in inducing remissions in metastatic breast cancer (Osbourne, 1989). In multiple myeloma, vincristine, melphalan, cyclophosphamide, and prednisone (VMCP), vincristine, carmustine (BCNU), doxorubicin (Adriamycin), and prednisone (VBAP) induce remission, can result in remarkable pain relief, and prolong life.

Palliation may be accomplished with chemotherapy. Hydroxyurea may produce a decrease in splenomegaly and splenic pain in chronic myelogenous leukemia

---

Box 21–2. *An Early Combination Chemotherapy Study*

DeVita, V. T., Carbone, P. P., & Serpick, A. A. (1970). Combination chemotherapy in the treatment of advanced Hodgkin's disease. *Annals of Internal Medicine, 73,* 881–895.

Sample: Forty-four patients with histologically confirmed Hodgkin's disease, Stages III and IV, who had no more than one prior dose of single-agent chemotherapy, or who had relapsed after primary radiation therapy; 20 women; 23 men; mean age 31 years (range, 12 to 69 years); 8 Stage III; 35 Stage IV. One patient was not evaluable.

Treatment: Thirty-two patients were treated with vincristine, 1.4 mg/m^2 IV on days 1 and 8; nitrogen mustard, 6 mg/m^2 IV, days 1 and 8; procarbazine, 100 mg/m^2 PO, days 1 through 14; prednisone, 40 mg/m^2 PO, days 1 through 14 during the first and fourth courses only. Twelve patients had cyclophosphamide substituted for nitrogen mustard at a dose of 650 mg/m^2 IV on days 1 and 8. Cycles were repeated at 28-day intervals. Dose adjustments for subsequent courses were made by sliding scale titrated to blood counts on day 29. Patients were evaluated after six courses of therapy.

Results: Two patients died after their initial course of treatment both as a result of rapid necrosis of tumor. Thirty-five patients (81 per cent) achieved a complete remission; six patients responded to treatment but failed to attain a complete remission. Survival time was markedly increased for patients attaining a complete remission. Toxicity included leukopenia, thrombocytopenia, anemia, neurotoxicity, nausea, vomiting, and alopecia. All of these were tolerable and reversible.

Significance: This study documented that combinations of antineoplastics could be administered without undue toxicity and could induce significant, durable responses. DeVita and co-workers also found that prolonged therapy (6 months) was efficacious in inducing remission, as opposed to the standard approach (at that time) of declaring treatment failures after 4 to 6 weeks of chemotherapy.

(CML). Chemotherapy may produce dramatic pain relief in multiple myeloma and in breast cancer.

As an adjunct to curative surgical resection, chemotherapy has been shown to improve the disease-free interval and survival in breast cancer. The success of adjuvant chemotherapy depends on effective agents used in patients with minimal tumor burden (Box 21–3). Studies in colon cancer document that improvement in the disease-free interval and survival may also be accomplished in this malignancy with the use of

---

Box 21–3. *An Example of Adjuvant Chemotherapy*

Bonadonna, G., Bajetta, E., Brambilla, C., Brugnatelli, L., Brusamolino, E., DeLena, M., Musumeci, R., Rossi, A., Tancini, G., Valagussa, P., & Veronesi, U. (1976). Combination chemotherapy as an adjuvant treatment in operable breast cancer. *New England Journal of Medicine, 294,* 405–410.

Sample: Three hundred ninety-one women with primary breast cancer. All patients had conventional or extended radical mastectomy for potentially curable disease. Only patients with T1a through T2b and one or more histologically positive axillary lymph nodes without distant metastases (M0) were included. Patients with fixed primary tumors (T3B1-T4) and clinically obvious nodal disease (N2-N3) were excluded.

Experimental Design: Patients were stratified by age, number of positive axillary nodes, and type of mastectomy and were randomized to receive 12 cycles of chemotherapy or no further treatment after mastectomy. The cyclophosphamide, methotrexate, and 5-fluorouracil (CMF) regimen was used: cyclophosphamide, 100 mg/m^2 orally on days 1 through 14; methotrexate, 40 mg/m^2 IV on days 1 and 8; 5-fluorouracil, 600 mg/m^2 IV on days 1 and 8. Cycles were repeated at 28-day intervals. Women over 65 years of age were treated at reduced doses. Dose decreases were made for toxicity; no dose escalations were allowed in the absence of toxicity. Both the treatment and the control groups were monitored with serial laboratory and radiographic studies to detect recurrence (local, regional, or distant), the end point of the study. Three hundred eighty-six patients were evaluable, 179 in the control group and 207 in the treatment group.

Results: After 27 months of study, 24 per cent of patients in the control group and 5.3 per cent in the treatment group had relapsed ($p<10^{-4}$). Relapse was more frequent in patients with greater than four positive nodes (40.7 per cent in the control group compared with 8.8 per cent in the treatment group). Recurrence occurred at distant sites in 81.5 per cent of the relapsing patients. Both premenopausal and postmenopausal patients benefited from CMF in terms of relapse-free interval. Toxicity was acceptable and consisted of myelosuppression, variable degrees of alopecia, oral mucositis, conjunctivitis, cystitis, and amenorrhea.

Significance: Bonadonna and colleagues demonstrated a statistically significant reduction in recurrence rate in women treated with prolonged (12 cycles) combination chemotherapy (CMF) following radical mastectomy for primary breast cancer with nodal metastases. Adjuvant combination chemotherapy improved disease-free interval irrespective of menopausal status. Toxicity of chemotherapy resulted in a decrement in performance status in fewer than approximately 10 per cent of the patients.

Limitations: At the time of publication the major limitation of this study was the short follow-up time, 27 months from the initiation of the study. Thus, the impact of improved disease-free interval on the rate of survival could not be determined. However, by 1990, it has become clear that a prolonged disease-free interval affects survival. In addition, the primary surgical procedure was extended or conventional radical mastectomy; thus, extrapolation to lesser surgical procedures must be done cautiously.

chemotherapy as an adjunct to surgery (Friedman & Hamilton, 1988; Moertel et al., 1990). Similar improvements have been accomplished in rectal cancer by the use of both chemotherapy and local radiation therapy interdigitated after curative resection (Cohen, Friedman, & Minsky, 1993).

Chemotherapy may be employed preoperatively in an attempt to convert nonresectable disease to resectable disease. Preoperative chemotherapy, sometimes referred to as neoadjuvant therapy, is currently being studied in bladder and breast cancer (Scher, Herr, & Yagoda, 1988). In localized but nonresectable non-small-cell lung cancer (stages IIIa and IIIb), chemotherapy and concurrent or sequential radiation therapy are rendering some tumors resectable and have been shown to prolong survival. Studies to define the optimal regimen and sequences are in progress (Green, 1993).

CLASSIFICATION OF ANTINEOPLASTICS

Cancer chemotherapy agents are classified into five categories on the basis of their mechanism of action, derivation, and chemical structure. Although agents may be assigned to a given group, individual agents may exhibit properties that overlap with other classes. The following discussion of the five main categories will emphasize the clinically important agents within each class. Table 21–5 presents a more comprehensive alphabetic listing by generic name of commercially available contemporary antineoplastics and also provides data on availability, storage and stability, route of administration, and acute and delayed toxicity. Figure 21–2 summarizes the mechanisms of action and the major sites of activity of each agent within the biochemical pathways leading to cellular proliferation.

ALKYLATING AGENTS

Alkylating agents, the oldest class of antineoplastics, act by substituting an alkyl group ($R-CH_2-CH_2$) for a hydrogen atom in organic compounds. The ultimate effect is an abnormal cross-linking of DNA base pairs that results in cell death or mutation by altering the decoding and replication process. The mutagenic property of alkylating agents is potentially carcinogenic. Six chemical classes of alkylating agents are known (Table 21–6).

Alkylating agents are most active in the G_0 or resting cell; they are non-cell-cycle–specific. The oral aklylators (cyclophosphamide, chlorambucil, melphalan, busulfan) are frequently administered as single agents on a daily schedule, with a break in therapy being titrated to bone marrow suppression. High-dose intermittent use may take place with busulfan in chronic myelogenous leukemia and with chlorambucil, melphalan, and cyclophosphamide in myeloma. Because the absorption of the oral alkylators is variable, they should be taken consistently on an empty stomach (Burton et al., 1986). Recently, an IV preparation of melphalan has been marketed, which should find utility in patients unable to take the oral formulation.

Cyclophosphamide may be administered intravenously at high doses (0.5 to 1.5 g/m^2) in preparation for bone marrow transplantation (see Chapter 27). Intravenous cyclophosphamide, in conventional doses, moderately high doses with growth factor support, and in pretransplant conditioning regimens can produce a syndrome of inappropriate secretion of antidiuretic hormone (SIADH), an oncologic emergency (see Chapter 66). Cyclophosphamide is metabolized to its active form in the liver and excreted via the kidneys. Hemorrhagic cystitis may result from both oral and intravenous administration owing to its excretion in the urine.

Ifosfamide, a recently marketed alkylator, is similar in structure to, but distinct from cyclophosphamide. It has significant bladder toxicity consisting of hemorrhagic cystitis that can be prevented by the concurrent administration of MESNA. Currently it is a mainstay of chemotherapy for soft-tissue sarcomas and is being used in combination with other agents in lung cancer, ovarian cancer, and the non-Hodgkin's lymphomas (Dorr & Von Hoff, 1994).

MESNA may be useful in avoiding radiation therapy-induced cystitis. It is believed to act as a reducing agent, inactivating metabolic byproducts that are toxic to the urothelium (Plowman & Trott, 1987).

The most important clinical role for mechlorethamine (nitrogen mustard) is in the treatment of Hodgkin's disease in the MOPP regimen (De Vita et al., 1970) and its variants. Mechlorethamine may be used for intracavitary instillation to control malignant pleural and pericardial effusions. It may also be applied topically in mycosis fungoides and skin cancers. If extravasation occurs, nitrogen mustard causes severe tissue necrosis. Treatment of extravasation is detailed in Chapter 22. Mechlorethamine is unstable when reconstituted and must be administered promptly (Dunagin, 1982).

Thiotepa is a sulfur-containing compound enjoying a resurgence of use intravenously in breast cancer and intravesicularly in early bladder cancer (see Chapter 22). Thiotepa and hexamethylmelamine are the only clinically important agents in their chemical class. Hexamethylmelamine, structurally similar to the methylenemelamines, is now commercially available and is known to have activity in ovarian cancer resistant to classical alkylators.

Busulfan has its primary effect on cells of the granulocytic series and thus is used in chronic myelogenous leukemia; it has not proved useful in acute myelogenous leukemia. Because busulfan affects the stem cell, it can produce a marked bone marrow hypoplasia, which may progress to aplasia, an effect also seen less frequently with chlorambucil. Very high-dose busulfan (4 mg/kg/day for 4 days) may be used in preparation for bone marrow transplantation; seizures have been reported with this dose (Hartmann et al., 1986).

Dacarbazine must be transformed to its active metabolite in the liver. It may be administered as a high-dose bolus or at lower doses on sequential days; a short continuous infusion may increase the exposure of cells in G_0 phase. Dacarbazine is active in melanoma,

Text continued on page 380.

TABLE 21–5. *Drug Data*

DRUG AND AVAILABILITY*	STORAGE AND STABILITY	ADMINISTRATION	TOXICITY—ACUTE	TOXICITY—DELAYED
ALDESLEUKIN (interleukin-2, IL-2, Proleukin) Injection: 22×10^6 unit vial	Unreconstituted: Refrigeration Diluted: Room temperature or refrigerated, 48 hr Other: preservative-free; do not filter	IV, SC	Pulmonary congestion (54%); Dyspnea (52%); pulmonary edema (10%); hypotension (85%); sinus tachycardia (70%); arrhythmia (22%); bradycardia (7%); nausea vomiting (87%); diarrhea (76%); mental status change (73%); dizziness (17%); sensory dysfunction (10%); seizure (1%); ogliuriasanuria (76%); BUN elevation (63%); creatinine elevation (61%); proteinuria (12%); hematuria (9%); pruritus (48%); erythema (41%); rash (26%); dry skin (15%); urticaria (2%); fever/chills (89%); pain (54%); fatigue/malaise (53%); edema (47%); headache (12%)	Elevated bilirubin (64%); elevated transaminase (56%); elevated alkaline phosphatase (56%); jaundice (11%); ascites (4%); anemia (22%); thrombocytopenia (64%); leukopenia (34%); coagulation disorders (10%); leukocytosis (9%); eosinophilia (6%); alopecia (1%); hypomagnesemia (16%); acidosis (16%); hypocalcemia (15%); hypophosphotemia (11%); hypokalemia (9%); hyperuricemia (9%); hypoalbuminemia (8%); hypoproteinemia (7%); infection (23%); weight gain (>10%) (23%); exfoliative dermatitis (14%); stomatitis (32%); anorexia (27%); GI bleeding (13%); constipation (5%)
ALTRETOMINE (hexamethylmelamine, HXM, HMM, Hexalen) Capsules: 50 mg	Store at controlled room temperature, 15–30° C (59–86°F)	PO	Mild to moderate nausea and vomiting (32%); severe nausea and vomiting (1%); seizures (1%)	Elevated alkaline phosphatase (9%); mild peripheral neuropathy (22%); moderate to severe peripheral neuropathy (9%); anorexia (1%); leukopenia (5%); thrombocytopenia (9%); anemia (33%); elevated serum creatinine (7%); elevated BUN (9%)
AMINOGLUTETHIMIDE (Cytadren) Tablets: 250 mg	Room temperature	PO	Drowsiness (40%); skin rash (17–20%); dizziness (14%); nausea and anorexia (10–13%); ataxia (10%); vomiting (3–10%); pruritus (5%); fever (5%); headache (5%); orthostatic hypotension (3%); myalgia (3%); tachycardia (2.5%)	Hypothyroidism (occasional); virilization (occasional); hepatotoxicity; elevated liver function test results, cholestatic jaundice (rare); myelosuppression (rare)
AMSACRINE (Amsidine, AMSA, n-AMSA) Injection: 50 mg/ml 1.5 ml ampule with 20 ml vial of L-lactic acid diluent INVESTIGATIONAL, NCI Group C	Undiluted: Refrigeration Diluted: Room temperature, 8 hr	Slow IV infusion; PO in some investigational studies	Phlebitis; skin rashes; mild nausea, vomiting, diarrhea; mucositis; anorexia; anaphylaxis; local allergic reactions	Dose-limiting leukopenia; elevated serum alkaline phosphatase; elevated serum bilirubin; cardiac arrythmias; congestive heart failure; rare peripheral neuropathy and CNS effects
ASPARAGINASE (Elspar); Injection: 10,000 IU vial *Erwinia* asparaginase (Porton asparaginase)	Unreconstituted: Refrigeration Elspar: Reconstituted: Refrigeration, 8 hr	Intra-arterial, IVP, IV infusion, IM	Nausea (30%); vomiting (30%); anorexia (30%); hypersensitivity reactions (20–35%); anaphylaxis after one to four doses	Myelosuppression: leukopenia (100%) (nadir day 4 to 7), thrombocytopenia (30%) (nadir day 5 to 10); hepatotoxicity: fatty metamor-

This information is adapted from Grant Medical Center (1987). *Chemotherapy: A data compendium.* It is intended to provide a reference to specific agents, addressing drug names, availability, storage and stability, administration, and toxicity.

PO, oral; IVP, intravenous push; IV, intravenous; IM, intramuscular; D_5W, 5% dextrose in water; SC, subcutaneous; BUN, blood urea nitrogen; SGOT, serum glutamic-oxaloacetic transaminase; SIADH, syndrome of inappropriate secretion of antidiuretic hormone; CHF, congestive heart failure; CNS, central nervous system; ECG, electrocardiogram; LDH, lactic dehydrogenase; FBS, fasting blood sugar; SGPT, serum glutamic-pyruvate transaminase; HPA, hypothalamic-pituitary-adrenal axis; MU, million units; CSF, cerebrospinal fluid; MI, myocardial infarction; CVA, cardiovascular accident; UTI, urinary tract infection.

*Explanation and interpretation of format is as follows, using aminoglutethimide as an example:

Aminoglutethimide is also known as Cytadren (drugs may have more than one generic name), and is available in 250-mg tablets. It may be stored at room temperature. Administration is by mouth. Acute toxicities include drowsiness, occurring in 40% of patients receiving it. Delayed toxicities include hypothyroidism, which occurs occasionally.

The information relative to stability and toxicity has been compiled from a variety of sources; in this changing field of medical oncology, data are subject to constant change. The reader should update them with current sources.

TABLE 21–5. *Drug Data* Continued

DRUG AND AVAILABILITY*	STORAGE AND STABILITY	ADMINISTRATION	TOXICITY—ACUTE	TOXICITY—DELAYED
INVESTIGATIONAL Injection: 10,000 IU vial	Diluted: Refrigeration, 8 hr Erwinia: Reconstituted: Room temperature, 20 days; refrigeration, 20 days Diluted: Diluted to a concentration of 35 IU/ml: room temperature, 4 days; refrigeration 4 days		(3.3%), after five or more doses (32%); hyperglycemia	phosis (42–87%), elevated liver function test results (50%); hypercholesterolemia (85%); neurotoxicity: personality changes (66%), somnolence, lethargy (33%), confusion (10%); clotting disorders (60%); azotemia (30%); proteinuria (15%); pancreatitis (5%)
5-AZACITIDINE (5-AC, Mylosar) Injection: 100 mg vial INVESTIGATIONAL, NCI Group C	Unreconstituted: Refrigeration Diluted: Room temperature, 8 hr Other: Dilute only in Ringer's lactate solution and dilute within 30 min of reconstitution	IVP, SC, IV infusion	Nausea and vomiting (often severe); drug fever; hypotension; rash; stomatitis	Dose-limiting leukopenia; thrombocytopenia; anemia; hepatic toxicity; asthenia; rhabdomyolysis Drug is contraindicated in patients with hepatic metastases, serum albumin <3 gm/100 ml, serum glutamicoxolacetic transaminase >120 IU/ml
BLEMOYCIN (Blenoxane) Injection: 15 units/ampule	Unreconstituted: Refrigeration Reconstituted: Room temperature, 14 days; refrigeration, 28 days Diluted: Room temperature, 24 hours in D_5W, 0.9% NaCl, or D_5W containing heparin, 100 to 1000 units/ml	Intra-arterial, intrapleural, IVP, IV infusion, SC, IM	Fever and chills (30%); hypersensitivity reaction (20–50%); nausea and vomiting (15%); anorexia and weight loss (common); anaphylaxis (rare)	Pulmonary toxicity (10–40%); pneumonitis (8%), fibrosis (1%); dermatologic toxicity (25–50%): hyperpigmentation (25%), skin peeling (10%), nail banding (10%), alopecia (50%); stomatitis (15%); ulceration (10%); radiation recall (occasional)
BUSULFAN (Myleran) Tablets: 2 mg	Room temperature	PO	Hypersensitivity reaction (rare); nausea and vomiting (rare); diarrhea (rare)	Myelosuppression: leukopenia (100%) (nadir day 7), thrombocytopenia (70%) (nadir day 11 to 30, recovery day 24 to 54); hyperpigmentation (5–10%); pulmonary toxicity: interstitial fibrosis (2.5–11.5%); hyperuricemia; cataract formation (rare); gonadal suppression: amenorrhea, azoospermia, gynecomastia (rare); alopecia (rare)
CARBOPLATIN (CBDCA) (Paraplatin) Injection: 150-mg vial 450 mg vial 50 mg vial	Unreconstituted: Refrigeration, 1 year Reconstituted: Refrigeration, 24 hr; room temperature, 24 hr Diluted: Refrigeration, 24 hr; room temperature, 24 hr Other: Light sensitive	Intraperitoneal, intra-arterial, IV infusion	Nausea and vomiting	Myelosuppression: leukopenia, thrombocytopenia, erythrosuppression; ototoxicity; renal failure (reversible); hyperuricemia
CARMUSTINE (BCNU, BiCNU) Injection: 100-mg vial	Unreconstituted: Refrigeration, 2 yr Reconstituted: Room temperature, 6 hr; refrigeration, 24 hr Diluted: Refrigeration, 48 hr when diluted in 500 ml 0.9% NaCl or D_5W Other: Light sensitive	Intraarterial, topical, IV infusion	Nausea and vomiting (80%); facial flushing (frequent); vein irritation (frequent)	Myelosuppression: leukopenia (100%) (nadir 5 to 6 weeks), thrombocytopenia (100%) (nadir 4 to 5 weeks); hepatotoxocity: mild changes in liver function tests (26%), bilirubinemia (5–25%); nephrotoxicity; elevated BUN (10%), renal failure or interstitial nephritis (9%); pulmonary toxicity; interstitial fibrosis

Continued on following page.

TABLE 21–5. *Drug Data* Continued

Drug and Availability*	Storage and Stability	Administration	Toxicity—Acute	Toxicity—Delayed
CARMUSTINE—cont'd				(1.3–30%); pigmentation at injection site (occasional); neurotoxicity with intra-arterial administration (4–31%)
CHLORAMBUCIL (Leukeran) Tablets: 2 mg	Room temperature Light sensitive	PO	Nausea and vomiting (10%); hypersensitivity reactions (rare)	Myelosuppression: leukopenia (100%) (nadir day 14 to 20, recovery day 28 to 42), thrombocytopenia (100%) (nadir day 10 to 14, recovery day 21); hepatotoxicity (rare): elevated SGOT and alkaline phosphatase levels, cholestatic hepatitis; alopecia (occasional); exfoliative dermatitis (rare); interstitial pneumonitis and fibrosis (rare); hyperuricemia
CISPLATIN (Platinol, CACP, DDP) Injection: 10-mg and 50-mg vials	Unreconstituted: Room temperature, 2 yr Reconstituted: Room temperature, 20 hr Diluted: Room temperature, 20 hr Other: Do not refrigerate after reconstitution as the drug may precipitate; light sensitive	Intra-arterial, intraperitoneal, IVP, IV infusion	Nausea and vomiting (100%); seizures (9%); hypersensitivity reactions (1–20%)	Myelosuppression: leukopenia (36%) (nadir day 18 to 23, recovery day 29), thrombocytopenia (5%) (nadir day 14, recovery day 21), anemia (25–30%); hemolytic anemia (rare); nephrotoxicity; elevated creatinine level (40%), elevated BUN (30%), acute tubular necrosis (25%); ototoxicity (30%); tinnitus (9%), deafness (6%); hyperuricemia (30%); neurotoxicity, peripheral neuritis (6%); hyperpigmentation (occasional)
CLADRIBINE (Leustatin, 2-CdA, 2-chlorodeoxyadenosine) Injection: 1 mg/ml, 10 ml vial	Unreconstituted: Refrigerated Diluted: Room temperature, 8 hr	IV	Nausea (28%); rash (22%); headache (22%); injection site reaction (19%); vomiting (13%)	Neutropenia (70%); fever (≥100°F) (69%); infection (28%); anemia (37%); anorexia (17%); fatigue (11%); thrombocytopenia (12%); abnormal breath-sounds (11%); cough (10%); diarrhea (10%); purpura (10%); myalgia (7%)
CYCLOPHOSPHAMIDE (Cytoxan, Neosar, Endoxan) Injection: 100-mg, 200-mg, 500-mg, 1-g, and 2-g vials Tablets: 25 mg and 50 mg	Tablets: Room temperature Unreconstituted: Room temperature Reconstituted: Room temperature, 24 hr; refrigeration, 6 days Diluted: Room temperature, 24 hr	Intraperitoneal, intrapleural, PO, IVP, IV infusion	Nausea and vomiting (50–90%, dose dependent); anorexia; diarrhea; stomatitis	Myelosuppression: leukopenia (100%) (nadir day 8 to 15, recovery day 17 to 28), thrombocytopenia (20%) (nadir day 10 to 14, recovery day 21); reversible alopecia (50%); gonadal suppression (10–33%); SIADH (20%); hemorrhagic cystitis (7–12%); cardiotoxicity; hemolytic anemia; pulmonary toxicity (rare): interstitial fibrosis; hyperuricemia; radiation recall (occasional); nail changes (frequent)
CYTARABINE (Cytosar-U, ARA-C, cytosine arabinoside) Injection: 100-mg and 500-mg vials	Unreconstituted: Controlled room temperature (15° C to 30° C) Reconstituted: Controlled room temperature, 48 hr; do not refrigerate solution after reconstitution	Intrathecal, intraperitoneal, IVP, IV infusion, IM, SC	Nausea and vomiting (15–20%); diarrhea (20–25%); fever and chills (10–20%); skin rash (20%); anaphylaxis (rare)	Myelosuppression: leukopenia (100%) (first nadir day 7 to 9, recovery day 12; second nadir day 15 to 24, recovery day 34), thrombocytopenia (100%) (nadir day 12 to 15, recovery day 25), anemia, megaloblastosis; hepatotoxocity: ele-

TABLE 21–5. *Drug Data* Continued

DRUG AND AVAILABILITY*	STORAGE AND STABILITY	ADMINISTRATION	TOXICITY—ACUTE	TOXICITY—DELAYED
CYTARABINE—cont'd	Diluted: Room temperature, 8 days			vated liver function tests (30–50%); stomatitis (30–50%); hyperuricemia; reversible alopecia (occasional)
DACARBAZINE (DTIC-Dome, DTIC, imidazole carboxamide) Injection: 100-mg and 200-mg vials	Unreconstituted: Refrigeration Reconstituted: Room temperature, 8 hr; refrigeration, 72 hr Diluted: Room temperature, 8 hr; refrigeration, 24 hr Other: Light sensitive	Intra-arterial, IVP, IV infusion	Nausea and vomiting (90%), anorexia (90%); vein irritation; anaphylaxis (rare); facial flushing (occasionally); paresthesias	Myelosuppression: leukopenia (30–50%), thrombocytopenia (30–50%) (nadir day 10 to 14, recovery day 24), anemia; flu-like syndrome of fever, malaise, and myalgia; alopecia; skin rash; hepatotoxicity, elevated liver enzymes (50%); vein thrombosis, necrosis (rare)
DACTINOMYCIN (Actinomycin D, Cosmegen) Injection: 0.5-mg vial	Unreconstituted: Room temperature Reconstituted: Use immediately Other: Light sensitive	Isolated perfusion, IVP, IV infusion	Nausea and vomiting, mild (80%), moderate to severe (20%); drug fever; anaphylaxis (rare)	Myelosuppression: leukopenia (55%), thrombocytopenia (47%), anemia (50%) (nadir day 14 to 21, recovery day 21 to 28); dermatologic reactions: follicular acne (80–90%), erythema, desquamation, hyperpigmentation (occasional), rash, reversible alopecia (47%); inflammation and ulceration of oral and GI mucosa (5–30%); diarrhea (3–5%); radiation recall (common); gonadal suppression; amenorrhea, azoospermia
DAUNORUBICIN (Cerubidine, DNR, daunomycin, rubidomycin) Injection: 20-mg vial	Unreconstituted: Room temperature Reconstituted: Room temperature, 24 hr; refrigeration, 48 hr Diluted: Room temperature, 24 hr Other: Light sensitive	IVP, IV infusion	Nausea and vomiting (50%); fever and chills (33%); local irritation (occasional)	Myelosuppression: leukopenia (90%) (nadir day 8 to 10, recovery day 21), thrombocytopenia (90%) (nadir day 4 to 15, recovery day 15 to 21); alopecia (90%); phlebitis (30%); diarrhea (25%); gonadal suppression: azoospermia (25%), amenorrhea (40%); stomatitis (15%); skin rash (6%); cardiotoxicity: arrhythmias (30%), CHF (2–5%), cardiomyopathy (1%); hyperuricemia; radiation recall reaction; nail changes (occasional)
DIETHYLSTILBESTROL (DES, stilbestrol) Tablets: 0.1 mg, 0.25 mg, 0.5 mg, 1 mg, and 5 mg (regular or enteric-coated) Other: Also available as cream, lotion, powder, or suppositories Diethystilbestrol diphosphate (Stilphostrol, fosfestrol) Tablets: 50 mg Injection: 250 mg/5 ml ampules	Tablets: Room temperature Injection: Room temperature Diluted: Room temperature, 24 hr Other: Light sensitive Protect from freezing	PO, IM, IV infusion, topical, and intravaginal	Diarrhea (12%); nausea (9%); anorexia (3%); vomiting (2%); headache (1%); glucose intolerance	Gynecomastia (80%), breast tenderness (69%); elevated liver function test results (37%); fluid retention (18%); thromboembolic disorders (18%), thrombophlebitis (7%), pulmonary emboli (5%); skin pigment changes (3%); lassitude (3%), mental depression (2%); hypercalcemia (10%)
DOCETAXEL (Taxotere) Injection: 80 mg/2 ml vial INVESTIGATIONAL	Undiluted: Refrigertion Diluted: Room temperature, 8 hr Other: Protect from light; maximum concentration is 0.3 mg/ml in D_5W	IV	Anaphylactoid-like reactions (flushes, pruritus, rigors); phlebitis; rash; mild to moderate nausea, vomiting and diarrhea; hand and foot syndrome.	Dose-limiting neutropenia; thrombocytopenia; alopecia; pleural effusion; peripheral edema; asthenia; peripheral neuropathy

Continued on following page.

TABLE 21–5. *Drug Data* Continued

DRUG AND AVAILABILITY*	STORAGE AND STABILITY	ADMINISTRATION	TOXICITY—ACUTE	TOXICITY—DELAYED
DOXORUBICIN (ADR. Adriamycin, Rubex) Injection: 10-mg and 50-mg vials	Unreconstituted: Room temperature Reconstituted: Room temperature, 24 hr; refrigeration, 48 hr Diluted: Room temperature, 24 hr; refrigeration, 48 hr Other: Light sensitive	Intra-arterial, intraperitoneal, IVP, IV infusion, intravesicular	Nausea and vomiting (45%); cardiotoxicity: ECG changes and arrhythmias (33%); lacrimation (25%); phlebitis (5–10%); fever and chills (5%); anaphylaxis (rare); local skin reactions (3%); pink urine and perspiration	Myelosuppression: leukopenia (100%) (nadir day 10 to 14, recovery day 21), thrombocytopenia (30–40%) (nadir day 14, recovery day 21 to 24), anemia (nadir day 14, recovery day 21); reversible alopecia (85–100%); stomatitis (75%); cardiotoxicity: CHF (1–31%, cumulative dose dependent); radiation recall reaction; hyperuricemia; gonadal suppression: amenorrhea, azoospermia; hyperpigmentation (10%); nail changes
ESTRAMUSTINE (Emcyt) Capsules: 140 mg	Refrigerate Light sensitive	PO	Nausea (16%); diarrhea (13%); gastrointestinal upset (12%); hypertension; glucose intolerance	Gynecomastia (76%), breast tenderness (71%); hepatotoxicity: elevated liver function test results (38%); fluid retention (20%); hypercalcemia
ETOPOSIDE (VePesid, VP-16-213) Injection: 50 mg/2.5-ml vial, 100 mg/5-ml vial Capsules: 50 mg	Capsules: Room temperature Injection: Unreconstituted: Room temperature Diluted: Room temperature for either 96 hr (0.2 mg/ml) or 48 hr (0.4 mg/ml)	IV infusion, PO	Nausea and vomiting (31%); diarrhea (13%); anorexia (13%); anaphylactic-like reactions (2%); hypotension (2%); stomatitis (1%)	Myelosuppression: leukopenia (60%) (nadir day 7 to 14, recovery day 20), thrombocytopenia (28%) (nadir day 9 to 16, recovery day 20); alopecia (20%); hepatotoxicity (3%); CNS toxicity (somnolence and fatigue) (3%); peripheral neuropathy (paresthesias) (0.7%)
FLOXURIDINE (FUDR) Injection: 500-mg vial	Unreconstituted: Room temperature Reconstituted: Refrigerated, 14 days Diluted: Room temperature, 24 hr	Intra-arterial, IV infusion	Gastrointestinal toxicity: gastritis (60%), abdominal pain (30%), diarrhea (15%), nausea and vomiting, anorexia; stomatitis (56%); erythema at injection site; fever; CNS toxicity: lethargy, malaise, weakness	Hepatotoxicity, elevated liver function test results (54%), hepatitis (23%); gastrointestinal ulceration (8%); myelosuppression: leukopenia (57%) (nadir day 21, recovery day 30), thrombocytopenia, anemia; alopecia; skin rash (10%), photosensitivity, hyperpigmentation
FLUDARABINE (Fludara, Fludarabine phosphate) Injection: 50 mg	Undiluted: Refrigerated Diluted: Room temperature, 8 hr	IV	Nausea and vomiting (36%); diarrhea (15%); anorexia (7%); stomatitis (9%); rash (15%); pruritus (1%); myalgia (7%); tumor lysis (1%); headache (3%)	Fever (60%); chills (11%); fatigue (10%); infection (33%); malaise (8%); weakness (9%); paresthesia (4%); visual disturbance (3%); hearing loss (2%); depression (1%); cough (10%); dyspnea (9%); edema (8%); abnormal renal function test (1%); leukopenia (59%); anemia (60%); thrombocytopenia (55%)
FLUOROURACIL (5-FU, 5-fluorouracil, Fluorouracil, Adrucil) Injection: 500 mg/10-ml vial Topicals: 1% cream and 1% solution (Fluoroplex); 2% and 5% solutions, and 5% cream (Efudex)	Undiluted: Room temperature Diluted: Room temperature, 36 hr Other: Do not refrigerate or freeze; light sensitive	PO, IVP, IV infusion, topical	Nausea and vomiting (20% with weekly schedule, 50–90% with high-dose schedule); anorexia (30–50%); cardiotoxicity (ECG changes) (1.7%)	Myelosuppression: leukopenia (100%) (nadir day 9 to 14, recovery day 21 to 25), thrombocytopenia (nadir day 7 to 17, recovery day 30); oral and gastrointestinal ulceration (4–8%, weekly; 60–75%, high-dose); diarrhea (5%, weekly; 30–80%, high-dose); alopecia (5–10%, weekly; 5–50%, high-dose); excessive lacrimation (30%); dermatologic reac-

TABLE 21–5. *Drug Data* Continued

DRUG AND AVAILABILITY*	STORAGE AND STABILITY	ADMINISTRATION	TOXICITY—ACUTE	TOXICITY—DELAYED
FLUOROURACIL—cont'd				tions; scaling (10–20%), rash (5%), hyperpigmentation (frequent); radiation recall (frequent); cerebellar ataxia (5%); gonadal suppression: amenorrhea, azoospermia; nail changes (occasional)
			Toxicities are for systemic adminstration only	
FLUOXYMESTERONE (Halotestin) Tablets: 2 mg, 5 mg, and 10 mg	Room temperature Protect from light	PO	Nausea (30–40%); headache; anaphylaxis (rare)	Virilization (56%); fluid retention and electrolyte imbalance (50%); hypercalcemia (10%); hepatotoxicity (9%); elevated liver function test results, cholestatic jaundice, hepatic neoplasms, peliosis hepatis; menstrual irregularities, gynecomastia
FLUTAMIDE (Eulexin) Capsules: 125 mg	Store at 2–30° C (36–86°F)	PO	Nausea and vomiting (11%); diarrhea (12%); other GI disturbance (6%); drowsiness, depression, anxiety, and nervousness (1%)	Gynecomastia (9%); hot flashes (61%); loss of libido (36%); impotence (33%); elevated liver function tests, rare; elevated serum creatinine, rare; edema (4%); anemia (6%); leukopenia (3%); thrombocytopenia (1%)
			Toxicities for Eulexin are when in combination with a LHRH agonist	
GEMCITABINE HCL (LY18011 HCL) Injection: 200 mg, 100 mg INVESTIGATIONAL	Unreconstituted: Room temperature, 24 hr Other: Reconstituted with unpreserved 0.9% NaCl. Dilute with 0.9% NaCl; due to stability problems, doses of 2500 mg/m² or greater must be diluted in at least 1000 ml 0.4% NaCl and infused over at least 4 hrs.	IV	Reversible skin rash, mild nausea and vomiting, flu-like syndrome, fever. (Febrile episodes seen in 50% patients within 6–12 hours of 1st dose).	Thrombocytopenia, rare anemia, negative effect on erythropoiesis.
GOSERELIN ACETATE (Zoladex) Injection: Device 3.6 mg sustained release/28 days	Room temperature	SC	Pain at injection site	Hot flashes (62%), sexual dysfunction (21%), decreased erections (18%), lower urinary tract symptoms (13%), lethargy (8%), pain flare (8% in first 30 days of treatment), edema (7%), rash (6%), diaphoresis (6%), CHF (5%), anorexia (5%), dizziness (5%), insomnia (5%), nausea (5%), hypertension, acute MI, chest pain, CVA, arrhythmia, peripheral vascular symptoms (1–5%), anxiety, depression, headache (1–5%), constipation, diarrhea, vomiting, ulcer (1–5%), anemia (1–5%), gout, hyperuricemia, weight gain (1–5%), chills, fever (1–5%), urinary obstruction, UTI (1–5%), breast swelling, tenderness (1–5%)

Continued on following page.

TABLE 21–5. *Drug Data* Continued

DRUG AND AVAILABILITY*	STORAGE AND STABILITY	ADMINISTRATION	TOXICITY—ACUTE	TOXICITY—DELAYED
HYDROXYUREA (Hydrea) Capsules: 500 mg Injection: 2-g vial INVESTIGATIONAL	Capsules: Room temperature Unreconstituted: Room temperature Reconstituted: Refrigeration, 72 hr	IVP, IV infusion, PO	Nausea and vomiting (25%); dermatologic reactions (20%); rash, facial erythema (occasional), pruritus; diarrhea (10%); constipation; anorexia	Myelosuppression (nadir day 7, recovery day 14 to 21); leukopenia (70%), thrombocytopenia (20%), anemia (34%), megaloblastosis (90%); reversible alopecia (frequent); neurologic disturbances: headache, dizziness, disorientation, hallucinations, convulsions; stomatitis (occasional); hyperuricemia; nail changes (occasional); radiation recall reaction (frequent); drug fever; gonadal suppression: amenorrhea, azoospermia
IDARUBICIN (Idamycin, IDA) Injection: 5 mg, 10 mg vials)	Unreconstituted: Room temperature Reconstituted: Refrigeration, 7 days room temperature, (15–30° C, 50–86° F) 72 h	IV	Nausea and vomiting (82%); abdominal cramps and diarrhea (73%); headache (20%)	Infection (95%); alopecia (77%); hemorrhage (63%); mucositis (50%); rash, erythema of hands and feet (46%); mental changes (41%); pulmonary (39%); fever (26%); cardiovascular (16%); peripheral neuropathy (7%); seizure (4%); severe myelosuppression in all patients
IFOSFAMIDE (Isophosphamide, Ifet) Injection: 1-g and 3-g vials See Mesna	Unreconstituted: Room temperature Reconstituted: Room temperature, 7 days; refrigeration, 6 weeks Diluted: Diluted to a concentration between 0.6 mg/ml and 16 mg/ml; room temperature, 7 days; refrigeration, 6 weeks Other: Will liquefy at temperatures above 35° C	IVP, IV infusion	Nausea and vomiting (10–15%); hematuria, gross and microscopic (50%)	Myelosuppression: leukopenia (12%) (nadir day 10, recovery day 18), thrombocytopenia (6%); hemorrhagic cystitis (29%), acute tubular necrosis (high doses); reversible alopecia (50%); neurotoxicity at high doses (10%), lethargy, convulsions; hepatic enzyme elevations
INTERFERON-αA-2a (IFN-αA, I Roferon-AFLA) Injection: 3 MU/1-ml and 18 MU/3-ml vials	Refrigeration Do not freeze Room temperature, 24 hr	IV, IM, SC Intraperitoneal, intralesional	Fever (98%); fatigue (89%); myalgias (73%); headache (71%); chills (64%); anorexia (46%); nausea (32%), diarrhea (29%); vomiting (10%); hypotension (6%)	Myelosuppression: leukopenia (69%) (nadir day 22), thrombocytopenia (42%) (nadir day 17), neutropenia (58%); hepatotoxicity: elevations in SGOT (78%), alkaline phosphatase (48%), LDH (47%), bilirubin (31%); nephrotoxicity: proteinuria (25%), elevated uric acid (15%), elevated serum creatinine (10%), elevated BUN (10%); hypocalcemia (51%); elevated FBS (39%); elevated serum phosphorus (17%); dizziness (21%); confusion (10%); paresthesias (6%); numbness (6%); lethargy (3%); edema (3%); hypertension (<3%); chest pain (<3%); arrhythmias (<3%); skin rash (18%); dryness or inflammation of the oropharynx (16%); dry skin or pruritus (13%); partial alopecia (8%); weight loss (14%); change in taste (13%); diaphoresis

TABLE 21–5. *Drug Data* Continued

DRUG AND AVAILABILITY*	STORAGE AND STABILITY	ADMINISTRATION	TOXICITY—ACUTE	TOXICITY—DELAYED
INTERFERON-αA-2a— cont'd				(8%); transient impotence (6%); arthralgia (5%); inflammation at injection site (rare)
INTERFERON-α A-2b (IFN-α2; IFN-2; 2-interferon, Intron A) Injection: 3-MU, 5-MU, 10-MU, and 25-MU vials	Unreconstituted: Refrigeration, 24 months Reconstituted: Refrigeration, 30 days; room temperature, 24 hr	IV, IM, SC Intraperitoneal, intralesional	"Flu-like" symptoms: fever, chills, fatigue, malaise, tachycardia, myalgias, and headache (98%); nausea (46%); vomiting (29%); hypotension (14%); hypertension (3%); diarrhea (27%)	Myelosuppression: leukopenia (18%), thrombocytopenia (18%), granulocytopenia (20%), anemia (4%); hepatotoxicity: elevated SGOT and SGPT (10%), elevated alkaline phosphatase (6%), elevated lactic dehydrogenase (3%); elevated BUN (1%); CNS effects: somnolence (14%), confusion (12%), coma (rare); arrhythmia or tachycardia (3%); skin rash (12%)
LEUCOVORIN (leucovorin calcium, folinic acid, citrovorum factor, Wellcovorin, 5-formyltetrahydrofolate) Tablets: 5 mg and 25 mg Injection: 3-mg/1 ml ampule; 50-mg vial; 5 mg/1 ml, 1-ml and 5-ml ampules	Tablets: Room temperature Unreconstituted: Room temperature Reconstituted: Preserved, 7 days; unpreserved, use immediately (or within 8 hr) Diluted: 24 hr Other: Light sensitive; protect from freezing	IM, PO, IVP, IV infusion	Hypersensitivity reactions (rare)	None reported; delayed toxicities of stomatitis, mucositis, diarrhea occur from use in combination with antimetabolites
LEUPROLIDE (leuprolide acetate, Lupron, Lupron depot) Injection: 5 mg/ml and 14 mg/2.8-ml vials	Refrigerate until dispensed Store unrefrigerated solution below 30° C Protect vial from light—store vial in carton until use	SC, IM (depot only)	Vasomotor hot flashes (40–70%); increased bone pain (10%); myalgia (<3%); renal disturbances: hematuria, dysuria, flank pain, polyuria, increased BUN and serum creatinine (<3%); CNS disturbances: dizziness (6%), pain (5%), headache (5%), paresthesia (3%); blurred vision, lethargy, insomnia, memory disorder, sour taste, numbness (<3%); gastrointestinal: anorexia (2%), constipation (3%), nausea and vomiting (5%); erythema, ecchymosis, and irritation at the injection site (occasional)	Impotence and decreased libido (frequent); gynecomastia or breast tenderness (3%); amenorrhea or vaginal bleeding (occasional); testicular atrophy (<3%); cardiovascular: peripheral edema (8%), congestive heart failure (1%), thrombophlebitis, phlebitis, or pulmonary embolus (1%); respiratory effects: difficulty in breathing, pleural rub, worsening of pulmonary fibrosis (rare); decreased hematocrit and hemoglobin (<3%); asthenia (<3%); fatigue (<3%); fever (<3%); facial swelling (<3%); rash (<3%); hives (<3%); hair loss (<3%); itching (<3%)
LOMUSTINE (CCNU, CeeNU) Capsules: 10 mg, 40 mg, and 100 mg	Room temperature Avoid storage temperature above 40° C	PO	Nausea and vomiting (90%); anorexia	Myelosuppression: leukopenia (65%) (nadir day 42, recovery day 49 to 56), thrombocytopenia (90%) (nadir day 28, recovery day 35 to 42), anemia (nadir 4 to 7 weeks); hepatotoxicity: elevated transaminase levels (35%); stomatitis (frequent); alopecia; pulmonary fibrosis; renal toxicity
MECHLORETHAMINE (nitrogen mustard, HN₂, Mustargen) Injection: 10-mg vial	Unreconstituted: Room temperature Reconstituted: Use immediately (within 1 hr) Other: Less stable in neutral or alkaline solutions	Intracavitary, intralesional, IVP, topical	Nausea and vomiting (95%); fever and chills (30–40%); diarrhea (10%); anorexia; weakness; headache; skin rash (occasional); metallic taste; phlebitis; anaphylaxis (rare); stomatitis (frequent). Toxicities are for	Myelosuppression; leukopenia (100%) (nadir day 10, recovery day 21 to 28), thrombocytopenia (100%) (nadir day 10, recovery day 21 to 28); gonadal suppression: amenorrhea (79%), azoospermia (88%); alope-

Continued on following page.

TABLE 21–5. *Drug Data* Continued

DRUG AND AVAILABILITY*	STORAGE AND STABILITY	ADMINISTRATION	TOXICITY—ACUTE	TOXICITY—DELAYED
			systemic and intracavitary administration	cia (75%); hyperuricemia
MEDROXYPROGRES-TERONE ACETATE (Provera, Amen, Curretab) Injection: 100 mg/ml, 5-ml vials; 400 mg/ml, 2.5-ml and 10-ml vials; 400 mg/1-ml syringes (Depo-Provera) Tablets: 2.5 mg and 10 mg	Injection: Room temperature; protect from freezing Tablets: Room temperature	IM, PO	Sterile abscesses (30%); nausea (10–20%); glucose intolerance (7%); local pain at injection site: anorexia; CNS toxicity: headache, dizziness, fatigue, insomnia, somnolence, nervousness	Fluid retention (30%), cushingoid facies (26%), weight gain (25%); hypercalcemia (10%); rash (7%); thromboembolic disorders; menstrual irregularities; alopecia; photosensitivity; skin pigment changes; hepatotoxicity; jaundice, elevated liver function tests; breast tenderness, galactorrhea; depression
MEGESTROL ACETATE (Megace, Pallace) Tablets: 20 mg and 40 mg	Room temperature	PO	None reported	Weight gain (10–20%); fluid retention (10–20%)
MELPHALAN (PAM, L-PAM, phenylalanine mustard, L-sarcolysin, Alkeran) Tablets: 2 mg Injection: 50 mg vial	Tablets: Room temperature Injection: Unreconstituted: Room temperature below 25° C, or refrigeration Reconstituted: Room temperature, 15 to 30 min Diluted: Room temperature, 15 to 30 min Other: Light sensitive	Regional perfusion, IV, PO	Nausea and vomiting (high dose: 30%; divided doses: 10%); diarrhea (10%); hypersensitivity reactions (2.4%)	Myelosuppression: leukopenia (65%) (nadir day 21 to 25, recovery day 28 to 42), thrombocytopenia (75%) (nadir day 21 to 25, recovery day 28 to 42), anemia (75%) (nadir day 8 to 10, recovery day 42 to 50); alopecia (4%); stomatitis (1%); pulmonary pneumonitis and fibrosis (rare); skin rash; hyperuricemia; gonadal suppression; amenorrhea, azoospermia; nail changes (occasional)
MERCAPTOPURINE (6-mercaptopurine, 6MP, Purinethol) Tablets: 50 mg Injection: 500-mg vial, INVESTIGATIONAL	Tablets: Room temperature Injection: Unreconstituted: Room temperature Reconstituted: Room temperature, 21 days Diluted: Room temperature, 3 days Other: Light sensitive	IVP, IV infusion, PO	Nausea and vomiting (25%); anorexia (25%); drug fever (5%); diarrhea	Myelosuppression: leukopenia (nadir day 14, recovery day 21), thrombocytopenia (nadir day 14, recovery day 21), anemia; hepatotoxicity: cholestatic jaundice (33%), elevated transaminases (15%), hepatic necrosis (rare); skin rash (5–10%); stomatitis (rare); depressed cellular immunity; radiation recall (occasional); pulmonary interstitial fibrosis (rare); gonadal suppression: amenorrhea, azoospermia
MESNA (Mesnex) Injection: 100 mg/ml in 200 mg, 400 mg and 1 gm ampules	Undiluted: Room temperature Diluted: Room temperature, 24 hr Other: Compatible when combined with ifosfamide or cyclophosphamide in the same infusion container; for PO use, may be diluted in cold drinks or juices	IV, PO	Mild GI effects (nausea, diarrhea); bad taste in mouth	None identified to date
METHOTREXATE (MTX, amethopterin, Mexate) Tablets: 2.5 mg Injection: Preserved and preservative-free: 5 mg/2-ml, 50 mg/2-ml, 100 mg/4-ml, and 200 mg/8-ml vials Powder for injection: Preservative-free: 20-mg,	Tablets: Room temperature Injections: Room temperature Unreconstituted: Room temperature Reconstituted: Room temperature, 7 days Diluted: Room temperature, 7 days	Intra-arterial, intrathecal, IVP, IV infusion, PO, IM	Nausea and vomiting (low-dose, 10%; high-dose 65%); hypersensitivity reactions (10%); diarrhea (5–10%)	Myelosuppression: leukopenia (30%) (first nadir day 4 to 7, recovery day 7 to 13; second nadir day 12 to 21, recovery day 15 to 29), thrombocytopenia (30%) (nadir day 5 to 7, recovery day 15 to 27), anemia (nadir day 6 to 13); stomatitis (10–40%); hepatotoxi-

TABLE 21–5. *Drug Data* Continued

DRUG AND AVAILABILITY*	STORAGE AND STABILITY	ADMINISTRATION	TOXICITY—ACUTE	TOXICITY—DELAYED
METHOTREXATE—cont'd 50-mg, 100-mg, and 250-mg vials INVESTIGATIONAL FORMS: Powder for injection (preservative free): 50-mg and 1-g vials Tablet: 50 mg				city: elevated transaminase levels (20%), periportal fibrosis (27%), cirrhosis (19%); conjunctivitis (14%); skin rash (10% with high doses); alopecia (5–10%); gastrointestinal ulceration (5%); renal failure (5% with high doses); pneumonitis (1%); hyperpigmentation (occasional); radiation recall (frequent); depressed cellular immunity; hyperuricemia; gonadal suppression: amenorrhea, azoospermia
MITOMYCIN (mitomycin-C, MTC, MMC, Mutamycin) Injection: 5-mg and 20-mg vials	Unreconstituted: Room temperature Reconstituted: Room temperature, 7 days; refrigeration, 14 days Diluted: In D_5W, 3 hr; in 0.9% NaCl, 12 hr; in sodium lactate, 24 hr (solution concentration, 20–40 µg/ml) Other: Light sensitive	Intra-arterial, intravesicular, IVP, IV infusion	Nausea and vomiting (75%); diarrhea (20%); anorexia (14%); fever (14%)	Myelosuppression: leukopenia (50%) (nadir day 25, recovery day 32 to 39), thrombocytopenia (40%) (nadir day 28, recovery day 42 to 49), anemia (3%); stomatitis (20%); pulmonary toxicity (5–12%); dyspnea with nonproductive cough, pulmonary infiltrates; skin rash (5–10%); nephrotoxicity (1–10%); elevated BUN and serum creatinine (2%), glomerular sclerosis; hemolytic uremic syndrome; general debilitation; cardiotoxicity; CHF; nail banding (rare)
MITOTANE (o.p′-DDD, Lysodren) Tablets: 500 mg	Room temperature Light sensitive	PO	Nausea (80%); vomiting (80%); diarrhea (80%); anorexia (80%); skin rash (15%); visual disturbances (3%)	Hypouricemia (100%); hyperlipoproteinemia (55%); CNS effects (40%); decreased memory (50%), lethargy and somnolence (25%), dizziness or vertigo (15%), mental depression; arthralgia (19%); gynecomastia (17%); leukopenia (7%)
MITOXANTRONE (DHAD, dihydroxyanthracenedione dihydrochloride, Novantrone) Injection: 10 mg/5-ml, 20 mg/10-ml, and 30 mg/15-ml ampules	Undiluted: Room temperature Diluted: Room temperature, 48 hr Other: Storage under refrigeration may cause formation of a precipitate, which will redissolve on warming to room temperature	IV infusion	Nausea (31%); vomiting (19%); drug fever (42%)	Myelosuppression: leukopenia (50%) (nadir day 10 to 12, recovery day 21), anemia (17%), thrombocytopenia (12%) (nadir day 8 to 16, recovery day 21); elevated liver function tests (33%); mucositis (25%); alopecia (20%); diarrhea (10%); cardiotoxicity
PACLITAXEL (Taxol) Injection: 30 mg/5 ml vial	Undiluted: Refrigeration Diluted: Room temperature, 27 hr Other: Final concentration when diluted should be 0.3–1.2 mg/ml; use glass container only with non-PVC administration set containing 0.22 um in-line filter	IV	Nausea and vomiting (59%); diarrhea (43%); mucositis (39%); hypersensitivity reaction (41%); bradycardia (10%); hypotension (23%); abnormal ECG (30%); myalgia (55%)	Neutropenia <2,000 (92%), <500 (67%); leukopenia <4,000 (93%), <1,000 (20%); thrombocytopenia <100,000 (27%), <5,000 (10%); anemia <11 (90%), <8 (24%); infection (35%); bleeding (19%); peripheral neuropathy (62%); alopecia (82%); elevated bilirubin (8%); elevated alkaline phosphatase (23%); elevated AST (16%)
PEGASPARGASE (Oncaspar)	Undiluted: Refrigeration	IV, IM	Hypersensitivity reaction (acute anaphylaxis, bron-	Leukopenia, thrombocytopenia, anemia, severe hemo-

Continued on following page.

TABLE 21–5. *Drug Data* Continued

DRUG AND AVAILABILITY*	STORAGE AND STABILITY	ADMINISTRATION	TOXICITY—ACUTE	TOXICITY—DELAYED
PEGASPARGASE—cont'd Injection: 750 IU/ml, 5 ml vial	Do not use if frozen Use immediately when drawn up or diluted Other: Do not shake, do not freeze		chospasm, dyspnea, urticaria, edema, hives, swelling, chills, fever, rash); nausea and vomiting; malaise	tolytic anemia, clinical hemorrhage, and elevated liver function tests (1–5%); elevated BUN and creatinine (61%); clinical pancreatitis (1%); hyperglycemia (3%); thrombosis (4%); anorexia, mucositis, arthralgia, paresthesias, seizures, mental status changes, and nail changes (1–5%)
PENTOSTATIN (Nipent, DCF, 2-deoxycoformycin) Injection: 10 mg vial	Unreconstituted: Refrigeration Diluted: Room temperature, 8 hr Other: If diluted in a larger volume of 0.9% NaCl or D_5W, keep concentration between 0.18–0.33 mg/ml; patient should be prehydrated with 500–1000 ml $D_5/0.45$ NaCl and post-hydrated with 500 mg D_5W	IV	Nausea and vomiting (22–53%); anorexia (16%); diarrhea (15%); rash (26%); pruritus (3–10%); headache (3%)	Leukopenia (60%); anemia (35%); thrombocytopenia (32%); fever (42%); infection (36%); fatigue (29%); allergic reaction (11%); weight loss (3–10%); elevated LDH (3–10%); elevated hepatic liver enzymes (19%); cough (17%); lung disorder (12%); GU disorder (15%); myalgia (11%); abnormal vision (3–10%); ear pain (3–10%); neuropathy (<3%)
PLICAMYCIN (Mithracin) Injection: 2.5-mg vial	Unreconstituted: Refrigeration Reconstituted: Room temperature, use immediately Diluted: Room temperature, 4 to 6 hr	IV infusion	Nausea and vomiting (90%); fever (15–83%); facial flushing (3%); diarrhea (2%); anorexia	Myelosuppression (nadir day 5 to 10, recovery day 10 to 18); thrombocytopenia, leukopenia (6%); hepatotoxicity: elevated enzyme levels (90%), necrosis; dermatologic reactions (33%); facial blushing, thickening of facial features; nephrotoxicity; proteinuria (20–40%), elevated BUN and serum creatinine (20–40%), tubular necrosis (20%); stomatitis (15%); nervousness, irritability (6–75%); bleeding syndrome (5–12%); hypocalcemia; metallic taste: reversible alopecia
PREDNISONE Tablets: 1 mg, 2.5 mg, 5 mg, 10 mg, 20 mg, 25 mg, and 50 mg Syrup: 5 mg/5 ml	Room temperature	PO	Gastrointestinal distress	HPA axis suppression: Cushing's disease (depression, moon facies, truncal obesity, striae, bruises, muscle weakness); fluid and electrolyte disturbances; increased appetite; impaired wound healing; masked signs of infection; decreased glucose tolerance; mental disturbances ranging from euphoria to psychoses; acne; osteoporosis
PROCARBAZINE (Matulane) Capsules: 50 mg	Room temperature Protect from moisture	PO	Nausea and vomiting (75–95%); anorexia (75%); diarrhea (10%); hypersensitivity reactions; skin rash (5%); urticaria (5%); pneumonitis (rare)	Myelosuppression: leukopenia (100%) (nadir day 25 to 36, recovery day 36 to 50), thrombocytopenia (100%) (nadir day 21, recovery day 28), anemia (5%); alopecia (18%); CNS depression (10%); stomatitis (6–10%); peripheral neuropathy (5%); interstitial pneumonitis and fibrosis (rare); gonadal suppression: amenorrhea, azoospermia

TABLE 21–5. *Drug Data* Continued

DRUG AND AVAILABILITY*	STORAGE AND STABILITY	ADMINISTRATION	TOXICITY—ACUTE	TOXICITY—DELAYED
STREPTOZOCIN (STZ, Zanosar) Injection: 1-g vial	Unreconstituted: Refrigeration Reconstituted: Refrigeration, 96 hr; room temperature, 48 hr Diluted: Refrigeration, 96 hr; room temperature, 48 hr Other: Protect from light	Intra-arterial, IVP, IV infusion	Nausea and vomiting (90%); diarrhea; glucose intolerance (6–60%); local necrosis (occasional)	Nephrotoxicity (65%); proteinuria (50–73%), tubular necrosis (30–40%); hypophosphatemia (25%); azotemia; glycosuria (80%); renal tubular acidosis (25%); hepatotoxicity; elevated liver function tests (67%), hypoalbuminemia, jaundice; myelosuppression; anemia (20%), leukopenia (5%) (nadir day 14, recovery day 21), thrombocytopenia (5%) (nadir day 14, recovery day 21)
TAMOXIFEN (Nolvadex) Tablets: 10 mg	Room temperature Protect from light and heat	PO	Nausea and vomiting (10–20%); hot flashes (25%); headache	Myelosuppression: leukopenia, transient (10%) (nadir day 10), thrombocytopenia, transient (10%) (nadir day 12), anemia (26%); lethargy (26%); bone and tumor pain (20%); sodium and fluid retention (80–90%); skin rash (4%); menstrual irregularities (2%); hypercalcemia (2%); hypercoagulability
TENIPOSIDE (Vumon, VM-26) 50 mg/5 ml ampules	Undiluted: Refrigeration Diluted: Room temperature Other: Dilute only in D₅W or 0.9% NaCl to 0.1, 0.2, or 0.4 mg/ml Stability: 1 mg/ml–4 hrs stability; <1 ml/ml–24 hrs. Incompatible with heparin; use only non-DHEP containers and tubing; observe solution for precipitation; reduce dose for hepatic/renal impairment, and in Down's syndrome; avoid phenothiazines.	IV infusion only	Anaphylaxis; fever (3%); hypersensitivity reactions (chills, flushing, bronchospasm, tachycardia, urticaria, hypertension and hypotension) (5%); seizures (rare); nausea and vomiting (29%); mucositis (76%); diarrhea (33%)	Leukopenia (89%); neutropenia (95%) thrombocytopenia (85%); anemia (88%); alopecia (9%); peripheral neuropathy (1%); hepatotoxicity, and metabolic abnormalities (all <1%)
TESTOLACTONE (Teslac) Injection: 500-mg vial Tablets: 50 mg	Injection: Room temperature, protect from freezing Tablets: Room temperature	PO, IM	Nausea and vomiting (30–40%); diarrhea (8%); anorexia; increased blood pressure	Sodium and fluid retention (50%); hypercalcemia (10%); paresthesias; skin rash; glossitis; alopecia; nail growth disturbance; hepatotoxicity; jaundice
THIOGUANINE (6-TG, 6-thioguanine) Tablets: 40 mg Injection: 75-mg vial, INVESTIGATIONAL	Tablets: Room temperature Injection: Unreconstituted: Refrigeration Reconstituted: Refrigeration, 24 hr Diluted: Room temperature, 24 hr; refrigeration, 24 hr	IV, PO	Nausea and vomiting (16%); anorexia; stomatitis; diarrhea; rash	Myelosuppression; leukopenia (100%) (nadir day 14 to 28), thrombocytopenia (100%) (nadir day 14, recovery day 21), anemia; hepatotoxicity; elevated liver function tests (11%), cholestatic jaundice (6%); veno-occlusive disease; hyperuricemia; decreased vibrational sensitivity; unsteady gait; gonadal suppression: amenorrhea, azoospermia

Continued on following page.

TABLE 21–5. *Drug Data* Continued

DRUG AND AVAILABILITY*	STORAGE AND STABILITY	ADMINISTRATION	TOXICITY—ACUTE	TOXICITY—DELAYED
THIO-TEPA (Triethylenethiophosphoramide, TSPA, TESPA) Injection: 15-mg vial	Unreconstituted: Refrigeration Reconstituted: Refrigeration, 5 days Diluted: Room temperature, 24 hr	Intravesicular, intra-arterial, intratumor, intrathecal, intracavity, ophthalmic; IVP, IV infusion, topical	Local pain (10–20%); nausea and vomiting (10–15%); anorexia; stomatitis; dizziness; tightness of throat; hypersensitivity reactions (rare); hives, skin rash, anaphylaxis	Myelosuppression: thrombocytopenia (80%), anemia (50%) (nadir day 14, recovery day 28), leukopenia (40%); hyperuricemia; alopecia (occasional); gonadal suppression: amenorrhea, azoospermia; hyperpigmentation (occasional)
VINBLASTINE (VLB, Velban) Injection: 10-mg vial Tablets: 5 mg, INVESTIGATIONAL	Tablets: Refrigeration Injection: Unreconstituted: Refrigeration Reconstituted: refrigeration, 30 days Diluted: Room temperature, 24 hr Other: Light sensitive	IVP, IV infusion, PO	Nausea and vomiting (20%); anorexia (20%); headache: paresthesias (10%); jaw pain (10%); diarrhea or constipation (20%); fever; local necrosis (occasional)	Myelosuppression (nadir day 5 to 9, recovery day 14 to 21); leukopenia (100%) (nadir day 5 to 10, recovery day 12 to 24), thrombocytopenia (100%), anemia (50%) (nadir day 10, recovery day 17); neurotoxicity (10–20%); peripheral neuritis, numbness, areflexia (10%); depression; convulsions; dermatologic effects: phototoxicity, dermatitis, reversible alopecia (occasioinal); stomatitis (frequent); hyperuricemia; gonadal suppression: amenorrhea, azoospermia
VINCRISTINE (Oncovin, VCR) Injection: 1 mg/1-ml, 2 mg/2-ml, and 5 mg/5-ml vials	Undiluted: Refrigeration Diluted: Room temperature, 24 hr; refrigeration, 24 hr	IVP, IV infusion	Nausea (6%); jaw pain; fever; local vein irritation (occasional)	Peripheral neuritis (100%); areflexia (50–100%); reversible alopecia (90%); bowel dysfunction (33%); paralytic ileus (5–10%); myelosuppression (nadir day 4 to 5, recovery day 7), leukopenia (5%); stomatitis (frequent); SIADH (rare); hyperuricemia; gonadal suppression: amenorrhea, azoospermia
VINDESINE (Eldisine®, vindesine sulfate, enisone, VDS, DVA) Injection: 5 mg vial with sterile diluent INVESTIGATIONAL	Unreconstituted: Refrigeration 2–8° C for 30 days Diluted: In D₅W or 0.9% NaCl Room temperature, 24 hr Other: Precipitation occurs at pH >6, therefore, do not dilute in multi-electrolyte solutions	IVP, IV infusion	Jaw pain, rare; skin rash; nausea and vomiting; stomatitis, rare	Leukopenia (dose-limiting, nadir in 7 days, recovery in 14 days); thrombocytopenia; less severe than leukopenia; peripheral neuropathy (may be dose-limiting); muscle weakness, rare; loss of deep tendon reflexes, rare constipation; vertigo, rare; alopecia; paralytic ileus, rare
VINORELBINE (Vinorelbine tartrate, Navelbine®) Injection: 10 mg/ml 1 ml vial, 10 mg/ml 5 ml vial	Undiluted: Store at 2–8° C (36–46° F); also stable for 72 hr at room temperature (15–30°C; 59–86°F); protect from light Diluted: 24 hr at room temperature (5–30°C; 41–86°F) Other: Dilute in D₅W or 0.9% NaCl to concentration of 1.5–3 mg/ml for IVP or concentration of 0.5–2 mg/ml for IV infusion	IVP, IV infusion	Nausea (33–50%); vomiting (14–23%); diarrhea (28–38%); constipation (13–20%); injection site reaction (21–38%); phlebitis (5–10%); jaw pain, rare	Granulocytopenia (80–96%); leukopenia (81–99%); thrombocytopenia (4–6%); anemia (77–87%); elevated bilirubin (9–14%); elevated SGOT (54–75%); peripheral neuropathy (21–31%); dyspnea (3–9%); alopecia (12%); interstitial pulmonary changes, rare; loss of deep tendon reflexes, rare

D_5W note: reconstituted in text above refers to D_5W.

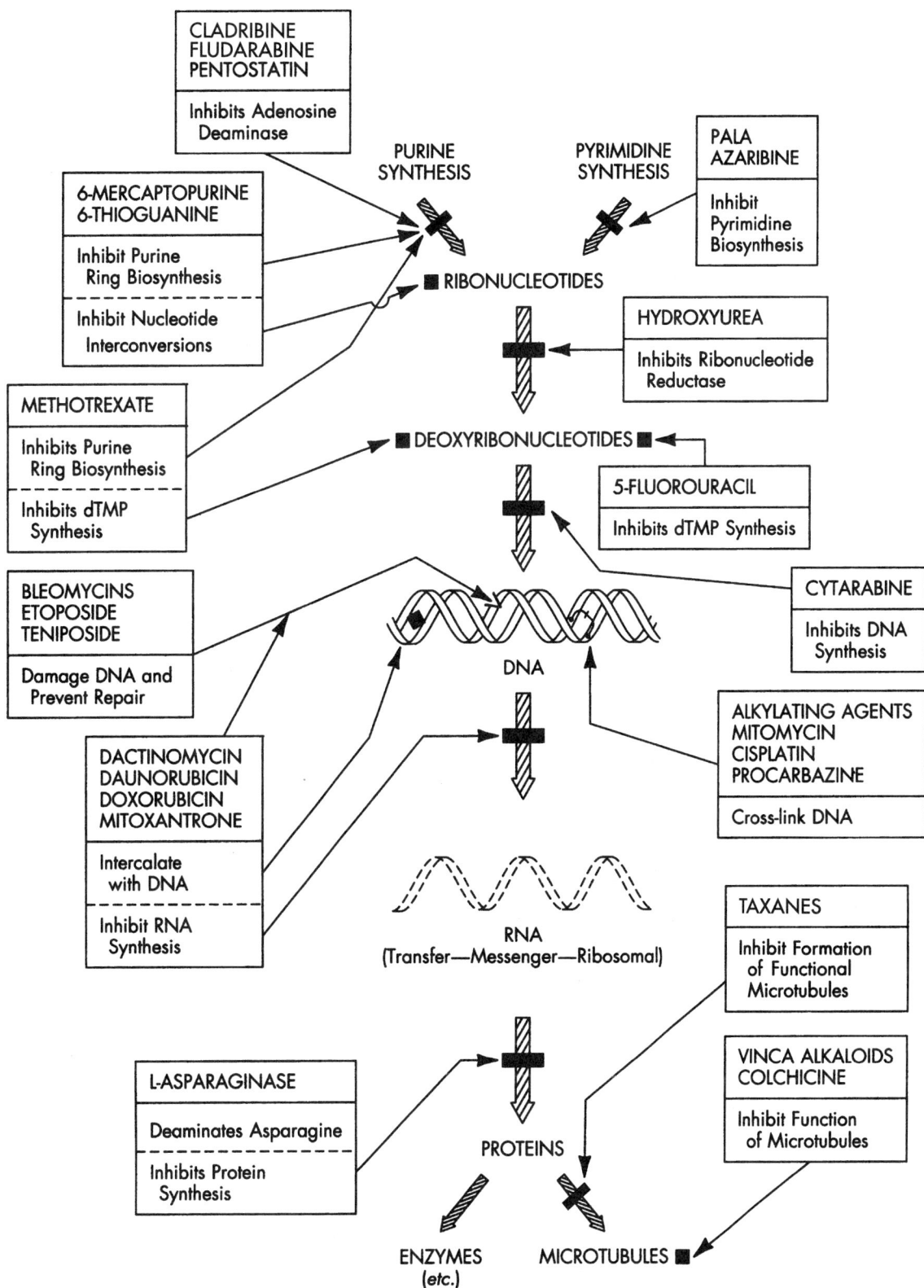

FIGURE 21–2. Summary of the mechanisms and sites of action of chemotherapy agents. (Adapted with permission from Gillman, A. G., Nies, A. S., Rall, T. W., & Taylor, P. [1993]. *Goodman and Gillman's the pharmacological basis of therapeutics.* New York: McGraw-Hill, Inc. Reproduced with permission of The McGraw-Hill Companies.)

TABLE 21–6. *Chemical Classes of Alkylating Agents*

CLASS	AGENTS	CLINICAL USE
Mustard derivatives	Mechlorethamine Cyclophosphamide Chlorambucil Melphalan Ifosfamide	Hodgkin's disease, non-Hodgkin's lymphoma, chronic leukemia, acute lymphocytic leukemia, myeloma, cancers of breast, ovary, skin, lung, prostate
Ethylenimines	Thiotepa Hexamethylmelamine	Breast, bladder cancers (intravesicular) Ovarian cancer
Alkyl sulfonates	Busulfan	Chronic myelogenous leukemia
Triazenes	Dacarbazine derivatives	Melanoma, Hodgkin's disease, sarcoma
Nitrosoureas	BCNU, CCNU Streptozocin	Myeloma, Hodgkin's disease, non-Hodgkin's lymphoma, brain tumors, melanoma, gastric cancer, islet cell cancer, carcinoid, acute leukemia
Metal salts	Carboplatin Cisplatin	Lung, testis, ovary, head and neck, acute leukemias, non-Hodgkin's lymphoma

sarcoma, and Hodgkin's disease. It can be hepatotoxic, the clinical manifestations of which must be differentiated from hepatic metastases (Sutherland & Krementz, 1981).

Unlike the other alkylators, nitrosoureas are lipid-soluble and cross the blood-brain barrier. They are useful in the treatment of primary brain tumors. Nitrosoureas are non-cross-resistant with other alkylators; their effect is on the G_0 (resting) phase of the cell cycle. The nitrosoureas produce delayed bone marrow suppression (5 to 6 weeks after administration) owing to the long half-lives of their active metabolites. The investigational drug methyl-CCNU is active in colorectal cancer; however, it has been associated with the development of acute myelogenous leukemia (Boice et al., 1983).

Streptozocin is a unique natural product with specificity for pancreatic exocrine cells. Its primary use is in the treatment of islet cell carcinoma of the pancreas; it may be effective in other endocrine malignancies. Hypoglycemia is an acute complication of therapy; chronically, glucose intolerances can occur, requiring the use of insulin or oral diabetic agents. Blood and urine sugar levels must be evaluated frequently. Streptozocin is excreted renally and is nephrotoxic. Renal tubular acidosis may occur, identified by electrolyte imbalances preceded by proteinuria.

Use of the platinum complexes, the first inorganic compounds employed in human malignancy, had almost been abandoned when diuresis was found to be effective in preventing their nephrotoxicity. These complexes are classified as aklylators; however, their inhibition of DNA synthesis takes place by a different mechanism than that of classic alkylators. Cisplatin persists in tissues for months due to protein binding; thus the toxicities of cisplatin mimic those of heavy metal poisoning: nephrotoxicity, peripheral neuropathy, seizures, ototoxicity, and anemia. Concomitant administration of fluids and maintenance of adequate urinary output during and immediately after administration is imperative to avoid renal damage. Protein-bound cisplatin is slowly released from these binding sites located in the protein associated with nerve tracts, resulting in cumulative and delayed peripheral neuropathy, which often worsens after the drug is stopped. The combination of taxol and cisplatin increases both the incidence and severity of peripheral neuropathy, which may be dose-limiting (Holden & Felde, 1987). Hypomagnesemia and hypocalcemia may occur from renal tubular damage; oral and intravenous supplementation is utilized (Cooley, Abrahm, & Davis, 1994; Gonzalez & Villasanta, 1982; McCauley, Begent, Newlands, & Phillips, 1982). Concomitant administration of intravenous magnesium may prevent this toxicity. Less frequently, hypophosphatemia, hypokalemia, and other manifestations of renal tubular damage (Fanconi's syndrome-like picture) may occur and require dietary supplements.

The platinum complexes have rendered nonseminomatous testicular cancer curable and have prolonged survival in other tumors. Cisplatin is used in many solid tumors; its use is currently being extended to non-Hodgkin's lymphoma. Clinically active analogues have been synthesized. Carboplatin is the first platinum analog to become commercially available. One of the advantages of carboplatin over cisplatin is its lack of protein binding and thus, lack of the associated toxicities of renal tubular damage, ototoxicity, and peripheral neuropathy. It is less emetogenic than cisplatin and appears to be of equal efficacy in a number of tumors. However, it is more myelosuppressive, inducing markedly more thrombocytopenia than its parent compound. This has led to investigation of new dosing schemas such as that proposed by Calvert which project the concentration of drug over time, known as the area under the curve (AUC). Dosing is calculated based upon desired AUC and the patient's glomerular filtration rate (Calvert et al., 1989). Some authors propose that AUC dosing will minimize the thrombocytopenia associated with carboplatin that has been observed with standard mg/M^2 dosing (Wittes, 1992). Anemia may occur with carboplatin due to impairment of erythropoiesis but is generally less recalcitrant than that induced by cisplatin.

Currently nine platinum analogs are being investigated, many with activity in platinum-resistant cell lines in vitro. Some have side effects differing from cisplatin and carboplatin, such as neutropenia, while others induce dose-limiting neurotoxicity (ormaplatin) or nephrotoxicity (zeniplatin). However, their early activity in head and neck, cervical, and colon cancers motivate further study (Christian, 1992).

The selection of alkylators for clinical use must consider the patient's hepatic function (biotransformation), renal function (excretion), bone marrow reserves (myelosuppression), and inherent alkylator sensitivity of the tumor. Because of the mutagenic, teratogenic, and carcinogenic capabilities of alkylators, patient age and childbearing capability should also be considered (Kyle, 1982).

PLANT ALKALOIDS

The plant alkaloids are so named because they are extracted from foliage. Clinically efficacious agents are listed in Table 21–7.

The vinca alkaloids are extracted from the periwinkle plant *(Catharanthus rosea)*. These cell-cycle-specific, phase-specific compounds arrest mitosis (M); in addition, they also inhibit DNA synthesis (S) and RNA synthesis (G_2). Although they are chemically similar, vincristine and vinblastine are non-cross-resistant and exhibit a difference in spectrum of efficacy and toxicity. Vinorelbine has less neurotoxicity but more hematologic toxicity than vincristine and vinblastine (Besenval, Delgado, Demarez, & Krikorian, 1989; Krikorian, Bore, Bromet, Cano, & Rahmani, 1989).

All vinca alkaloids are administered intravenously and are vesicants (see Chapter 22). Continuous infusions of these agents are being investigated to determine whether increasing exposure to increasing numbers of cells in the M phase will increase tumor cell kill (Guy et al., 1990, Yap et al., 1980). Because they are vesicants, continuous infusion administration via a central line is recommended. Neurotoxicity, manifested acutely as constipation, urinary retention, and jaw pain (the latter uncommon), occurs with all vinca alkaloids, most frequently with vincristine and least with vinorelbine. Peripheral neuritis occurs with cumulative doses; its onset is heralded by paresthesias of the fingers and toes, which can progress to generalized sensorimotor weakness. This neuropathy generally is reversible and

disappears once the drug is discontinued but may take months to abate. Bone marrow suppression and gastrointestinal toxicity (nausea, vomiting, mucositis) are more frequent with vinblastine and vinorelbine. The latter, when combined with cisplatin in the treatment of non-small-cell lung cancer, has resulted in promising response rates but with significant myelosuppression and peripheral neuropathy (Armand & Marty, 1989; Besenval et al., 1989).

Podophyllotoxins, derived from the May apple plant, act in the M phase to inhibit mitosis and in the G_2 phase to inhibit entry into the M phase. These cycle- and phase-specific agents can also act in the late G_2 and S phases by inhibition of topoisomerase II, an enzyme required for DNA replication. Etoposide is effective in testicular cancer and lung cancer (small-cell and non-small-cell); recently its use has expanded to the hematologic malignancies, ovarian cancer, and radiosensitization. Intravenous administration may be associated with significant hypotension, necessitating monitoring of blood pressure. Slowing the infusion rate prevents clinically significant hypotensive events. An oral form of etoposide is now available and has been used in lung cancer (small-cell and non-small cell), ovarian and germ cell tumors, cancers of the head and neck, and AIDS-related lymphomas; hypotension is rare with oral administration. Tenopiside is useful in acute monocytic leukemia and in childhood acute lymphoblastic leukemia. It is available as an intravenous preparation only. Its role in other malignancies is being studied.

The podophyllotoxins are extensively protein-bound. Hemolytic anemia has been reported. Monitoring of serial hemoglobin levels, urine occult blood, and Coomb's test may identify this uncommon reaction (Doll & Weiss, 1985; Habibi et al., 1982).

The plant alkaloids are metabolized by the liver and excreted by both the liver and the kidney. Because they are natural products, allergic reactions are known to occur, including anaphylaxis. Recent reports have included type II hypersensitivity reactions with etoposide, which consist of hypertension and dyspnea, which can be managed with steroids and antihistamines; these reactions do not always recur on rechallenge. Allergic reactions have also been reported with the oral preparation (Kasperek & Black, 1992).

TABLE 21–7. *Plant Alkaloids*

CLASS	AGENTS	CLINICAL USE
Vinca alkaloids	Vincristine Vinblastine	Acute leukemia, Hodgkin's disease, non-Hodgkin's lymphoma, myeloma, Burkitt's lymphoma, breast cancer, Wilm's tumor, testicular cancer
	Vindesine*	Lung, esophageal, colorectal, breast cancers, lymphoma, leukemias
	Vinorelbine	Lung, breast and ovarian cancers
Podophyllotoxins	Etoposide Tenisopide	Non-Hodgkin's lymphoma, acute myelogenous leukemia, acute lymphoblastic leukemia, testicular and lung cancers
Taxanes	Taxol	Ovarian, breast, gastric and lung cancer, malignant melanomas, and cancer of unknown primary
	Taxotere*	Lung, breast, ovarian, and pancreatic cancers

*Investigational

The taxanes are the newest plant products derived from the *Taxus* (yew) species. Like the vinca alkaloids, these compounds act in the M phase to inhibit mitosis. The taxanes exert their primary effect by inducing formation of nonfunctional microtubules, effectively paralyzing the cell from further replication. Taxol, currently the only commercially available taxane, is a natural product made from Pacific yew bark, while the investigational agent taxotere is a semisynthetic preparation, derived in part from the needles of the European yew (Chabner, 1993).

The major clinical use for taxol today is in the treatment of refractory ovarian and breast cancers; research is ongoing in other solid tumors and is encouraging in lung cancers. Both taxol and taxotere require an organic solubilizing agent that result in the potential for severe allergic reactions characterized by hypotension, flushing, and dyspnea. Thus, current practice dictates pretreatment with corticosteroids and histamine blockers (commonly cimetidine and diphenhydramine), which usually avoid acute anaphylaxis. Arrhythmias, predominately asymptomatic bradycardia, are common but usually revert with slowing of the infusion rate and are of little clinical consequence. The physical properties of taxanes require administration in glass containers through nonpolyvinyl chloride containing tubing (nitroglycerin tubing), using a 0.22 μm in-line filter. Vigorous flushing of central lines and implanted ports is necessary to avoid buildup of precipitates. When combined with other agents (cisplatin and adriamycin), the sequence of administration may have important implications for the degree of toxicity induced (Rowinsky et al., 1991).

Like other plant-derived antineoplastics, the taxanes cause neurotoxicity consisting of peripheral neuropathy, which is potentiated when administered in combination with cisplatin. Central neurologic effects have also been observed, including visual changes. Most commonly seen with 3-hour infusions of taxol, "flashing lights" (photopsia) resolve spontaneously without sequelae but may recur on rechallenge (Arbuck, 1994).

The metabolism of the taxanes is probably hepatobiliary but is poorly understood at present. The taxanes represent a promising new class of plant alkaloids with unique mechanisms of action and activity (Rowinsky, Donehower, & McGuire, 1993).

ANTITUMOR ANTIBIOTICS

Species of the soil fungus *Streptomyces* produce natural products with antineoplastic activity called antitumor antibiotics (Table 21–8).

The anthracyclines act in multiple phases of the cell cycle and are considered cell-cycle–specific and phase-nonspecific. Their action on DNA (intercalation) interferes with DNA synthesis and DNA-directed production of RNA and DNA. The anthracyclines are biotransformed to their active metabolites in the liver; they exhibit tissue binding and a prolonged half-life. Excretion is primarily hepatic. Pretherapy liver dysfunction may preclude their use or mandate dose reductions. Anthracyclines are vesicants and are administered on an intermittent bolus schedule; however, weekly low-dose administration of doxorubicin has been shown to have equal efficacy with less toxicity (cardiac, gastrointestinal, alopecia) in some tumors (Legha et al., 1982; Weiss & Manthel, 1977). Continuous infusions of doxorubicin have been especially useful in soft-tissue sarcomas; in this case, administration via a central line is mandatory due to its vesicant properties.

The cardiotoxicity of the anthracyclines is dose-limiting. The mechanism is a direct effect on the myocardium, resulting in left ventricular hypertrophy and a clinical cardiomyopathy, which may be manifested as congestive heart failure (Unverferth et al., 1981). For doxorubicin, the incidence is 10 per cent at doses in excess of 550 mg/m^2. Research is ongoing to find agents that protect the myocardium; Zinecard (dexrazoxane) is one example. Also, continuous infusions may decrease the incidence of anthracycline-induced cardiotoxicity (Galassi, 1992; Legha et al., 1982; Myers et al., 1983). Monitoring is accomplished with baseline and serial electrocardiograms (ECGs) and measurements of left ventricular function (resting and stress-multigated analysis [MUGA], echocardiography); endomyocardial biopsy may be useful in selected patients (Bristow, Billingham, Lopez, Mason, & Winchester, 1982). Acute cardiotoxicities are manifested as transient ECG changes and arrhythmias, which usually occur in patients with preexisting heart disease; rarely, acute pericarditis may occur (Bristow et al., 1982; Kaszyk, 1986).

TABLE 21–8. *Antibiotics*

CLASS	AGENT	CLINICAL USE
Anthracyclines	Doxorubicin Daunomycin Mitoxantrone	Acute leukemia, Hodgkin's disease, non-Hodgkin's lymphoma, chronic lymphocytic leukemia, breast cancer, sarcoma, ovarian and lung cancers, hepatoma
	Idarubicin	Acute myelogenous leukemia, acute lymphoblastic leukemia
Chromomycins	Dactinomycin Plicamycin	Melanoma, sarcoma, testicular cancer, choriocarcinoma, malignant hypercalcemia
Miscellaneous	Mitomycin	Colonic, rectal, gastric cancers, pancreatic adenocarcinomas, testicular, breast, cervical cancers, cloacogenic, vulvar, head and neck, bladder cancers (intravesicular), lung cancer
	Bleomycin	Hodgkin's disease, non-Hodgkin's lymphoma, melanoma, cervical, anal, head and neck, testicular cancers

Because anthracyclines act in all phases of cell growth, they exhibit toxicities in multiple organ systems: gastrointestinal, mucosal, hair follicles, bone marrow, and gonads. Their derivation from microbes predisposes patients to allergic reactions, which range from local cutaneous reactions to anaphylaxis. The local cutaneous reactions must be differentiated from frank extravasation (see Chapter 22).

The anthracyclines, particularly doxorubicin, are a mainstay of chemotherapy for both hematologic malignancies and solid tumors. During the last decade, efforts have been directed at the production of analogues with equivalent efficacy but less toxicity (Crossley, 1984; Weiss, 1992). Mitoxantrone induces significantly less toxicity (nausea, vomiting, alopecia) than doxorubicin, but the incidence of cardiotoxicity is nearly equivalent to that of doxorubicin at equipotent doses. Mitoxantrone turns the urine blue and the serum green (Crossley, 1984). Idarubicin and daunomycin are the newest available anthracyclines, having their primary utility in the treatment of acute myelogenous leukemia, and have a toxicity profile similar to the other agents in this class (Berman et al., 1991).

The chromomycins act by the same mechanisms as the anthracyclines; they are cell-cycle–specific and phase-nonspecific. Their chemical structure is markedly different, and they do not induce cardiotoxicity. Both available chromomycins are administered intravenously and may be associated with local and systemic allergic reactions; skin necrosis occurs with extravasation. Dactinomycin is useful in melanomas, gastrointestinal tumors, germ cell tumors, sarcomas, and lung cancer. Plicamycin is most commonly utilized in a low-dose schedule by intravenous infusion for the control of malignancy-associated hypercalcemia. Chronic administration in this situation results in bone marrow suppression and may exacerbate the myelosuppressive effect of agents given for control of the underlying malignancy. A thickening of facial features and renal and hepatotoxicity occur with chronic use for hypercalcemic control (Dorr & Fritz, 1980; Dorr & Von Hoff, 1994). Plicamycin is rarely used for its direct antitumor effects because of its significant toxicities at tumoricidal doses.

Mitomycin C must be biotransformed intracellularly into an active alkylating agent. Interestingly, alkylator-resistant tumors are often sensitive to mitomycin, whereas mitomycin-resistant cells rarely are sensitive to other alkylating agents. Blue in solution, mitomycin is administered intravenously and is a known vesicant without accepted antidote. Bone marrow suppression is dose-limiting and cumulative. Excretion is via the bile and kidney; a selective effect may occur on the glomerulus, resulting in renal failure. Hemolytic uremic syndrome, manifested by rising creatinine levels, elevation of liver function tests, specifically LDH, hemolytic anemia, and thrombocytopenia, has been described with prolonged repetitive mitomycin C administration. This syndrome is often fatal. Plasmapheresis may be used in its control (Doll & Weiss, 1985; Verway, Boven, Pinedo, & van der Meulen, 1984). Mitomycin C is used in adenocarcinomas of the gastrointestinal tract, breast cancer, non-small-cell lung cancer, and intravesicularly in superficial bladder cancer (Batts, 1992).

Unlike the other antibiotics, bleomycin exerts its best effect on slowly proliferating cells and has phase specificity in G_1 (RNA and protein synthesis) and M (mitosis). It may also induce scission of the DNA strand. Agents that act by intercalation appear to potentiate its cytotoxicity. Experimentally, bleomycin has been used to synchronize cells into the G_2 and S phases for attack by other phase-specific antineoplastics.

Myelosuppression from bleomycin is mild. Allergic reactions, including anaphylaxis, constitute its most clinically significant toxicity and test doses are recommended. Temperatures over 38.5° C (101° F) and chills occur acutely and may be controlled by the administration of antipyretics. Because bleomycin is concentrated in the keratin, palmar and plantar erythema, hyperpigmentation, and nail changes occur. Pulmonary fibrosis, developing from a dose-related pneumonitis, may be heralded by the development of rales and dyspnea. Pulmonary infiltrates appear on chest radiographs (Ginsberg & Comis, 1982; Seipp, 1985). Serial measurements of diffusing lung capacity for carbon monoxide (DLCO) corrected for hemoglobin are helpful in detecting early bleomycin lung toxicity. Bleomycin is not a vesicant. Its primary route of administration is intravenous; topical preparations may be used in cutaneous malignancies. Intracavitary administration may control malignant effusions. The affinity of this agent for squamous epithelium has fostered its use in the treatment of tumors of this origin (cervical, head and neck, vulvular cancers, melanoma, cloacogenic carcinoma) and in Hodgkin's disease, non-Hodgkin's lymphoma, and germ cell tumors of the testis.

ANTIMETABOLITES

This group exerts its effect by interrupting cellular metabolic function. These agents are structurally similar to intracellular substances; the cell incorporates them into essential sites of cellular metabolism and then is unable to continue to divide. Antimetabolites are classified by the compounds with which they interfere (Table 21–9).

Antimetabolites are phase-specific in the S phase. They are most effective in tumors with a high growth fraction. The first documented cure of a malignant tumor (choriocarcinoma) by chemotherapy occurred with methotrexate in 1956 (Li, 1979).

Methotrexate binds the enzyme dihydrofolate reductase (DHR), making it unavailable for the conversion of folic acid to tetrahydrofolic acid, which is required for DNA, RNA, and protein synthesis; cellular growth is stopped. Because only minuscule amounts of DHR are required, sufficient amounts of methotrexate must be administered to bind all the DHR.

The inhibition of production of tetrahydrofolic acid (calcium leucovorin, folinic acid) also occurs in normal cells and thus prohibits their proliferation. Cells of the gastrointestinal mucosa and bone marrow are most commonly affected, producing mucositis of the oral

TABLE 21–9. *Antimetabolites*

CLASS	AGENTS	CLINICAL USE
Folic acid antagonist	Methotrexate	Acute lymphoblastic leukemia, non-Hodgkin's lymphoma, breast cancer, sarcoma, head and neck and colon cancers, choriocarcinoma, testicular and bladder cancers
Pyrimidine antagonist	5-Fluorouracil Floxuridine Cytarabine 5-Azacytidine*	Acute leukemia, chronic leukemia, and colonic, gastric, esophageal, pancreatic, pulmonary, cloacogenic, breast, and skin cancers
Purine antagonist	6-Mercaptopurine 6-Thioguanine	Acute leukemia
Adenosine deaminase inhibitor	Cladribine	Hairy cell leukemia, non-Hodgkin's lymphoma, cutaneous T-cell lymphoma, acute and chronic lymphocytic leukemias, mycosis fungoides
	Fludarabine	Chronic lymphocytic leukemia, non-Hodgkin's lymphoma, macroglobulinemic lymphoma, prolymphocytic leukemia, hairy cell leukemia, Hodgkin's lymphoma, cutaneous T-cell lymphoma, mycosis fungoides
	Pentostatin	Hairy cell leukemia, chronic lymphocytic leukemia, mycosis fungoides, acute lymphoblastic leukemia, lymphoblastic lymphoma, and adult T-cell leukemia

*Investigational

cavity and gastrointestinal tract and bone marrow depression.

To maximize the antimetabolic effect in tumor cells without undue toxicity, variability in cell cycle times between malignant and normal cells and differential mechanisms of transport into the cells between methotrexate and tetrahydrofolate can be used to enhance the tumoricidal effects of methotrexate. Administration of high, potentially lethal doses of methotrexate must be followed by a carefully timed administration of calcium leucovorin. Ideally, methotrexate will block the production of tetrahydrofolic acid in tumor cells more rapidly than in normal cells; the subsequent administration of calcium leucovorin will then allow its differential incorporation into normal cells, allowing them to continue with normal cellular function. The result should be maximal tumor cell kill with minimal toxicity to the patient. Carefully timed administration of methotrexate and leucovorin rescue are imperative. If oral forms of calcium leucovorin rescue are prescribed, the patient must be carefully observed for interference with its absorption (vomiting, malabsorption). If gastrointestinal absorption is compromised, parenteral administration is indicated. Serum methotrexate levels should be monitored to guide the duration and dose of leucovorin rescue. High (greater than 0.5 g/M^2) and intermediate (100 mg/M^2) doses of methotrexate with leucovorin rescue are used in osteogenic sarcoma, non-Hodgkin's lymphoma, head and neck tumors, soft-tissue sarcomas, and breast, colorectal, and gastric cancers.

Methotrexate is also administered orally and intramuscularly. Intrathecal administration is useful in the prevention of leptomeningeal leukemia and in the treatment of leptomeningeal carcinomatosis (see Chapter 22). Unlike the other pyrimidine analogues, methotrexate does not require biotransformation. Its excretion is primarily renal. Renal dysfunction may exacerbate its toxicities or require reduced doses. Methotrexate precipitates in the kidney at pH of less than 5; urine alkalinization (with sodium bicarbonate or Diamox) may be utilized. Methotrexate is highly protein-bound and accumulates in third-space fluids. It is bound to drugs such as salicylates, sulfonamides, tetracycline, and probenecid. Protein-bound methotrexate is released slowly, resulting in delayed toxicities. Methotrexate may be hepatotoxic, as manifested by mild elevations in liver function test results; continued administration may result in cirrhosis (Perry, 1982). Long-term administration of methotrexate may result in pulmonary fibrosis; this is uncommon.

The pyrimidine antagonists act as irreversible enzyme inhibitors. 5-fluorouracil (5-FU) inhibits thymidylate synthetase, which is essential for DNA synthesis. 5-fluorouracil is metabolized intracellularly to its active component after intravenous administration. Bolus and continuous infusion schedules are repeated at weekly or monthly intervals.

In the late 1980s, there was a resurgence of interest in 5-FU. Constant, continuous, low-dose infusions of 5-FU have been used to provide an uninterrupted inhibition of thymidylate synthetase in cells advancing to the S phase (O'Connell, 1987). The active metabolite of 5-FU, FdUMP, requires tetrahydrofolate (leucovorin) to bind thymidylate synthetase, precluding the synthesis of thymidine, which is required for DNA synthesis. The exogenous administration of leucovorin further inhibits the formation of thymidine. This observation has resulted in the widespread use of leucovorin to potentiate the activity of 5-fluorouracil in the treatment of gastrointestinal malignancies. The administration of methotrexate prior to 5-FU increases the formation of the active metabolite of 5-FU. The combination is useful in the treatment of gastric and colorectal cancers with or without the administration of leucovorin rescue (Nordic Gastrointestinal Tumor Adjuvant Therapy Group, 1989; Wils et al., 1986). Other agents, such as the interferons, are also being used for their ability to modulate the effects of 5-FU.

The combination of 5-FU and leucovorin may result in a secretory diarrhea, which may or may not be accompanied by oral mucositis. This 5-FU cholera syndrome can be life-threatening but is reversible by vigorous fluid and electrolyte replacement; subcutaneous octreotide should also be used to control diarrhea. Further treatment with the combination of 5-FU and folinic acid should be adjusted downward after an episode of this syndrome.

The toxicities of 5-FU result from action on rapidly dividing cells with high growth fraction (bone marrow, gastrointestinal mucosa). Skin toxicity, manifested as photosensitivity, palmar and plantar erythema, and hyperpigmentation, may occur. (In fact, 5-fluorouracil may be used topically in the treatment of skin cancers.) Somnolence, ataxia, and pyramidal tract signs also may be seen. These generally revert with discontinuation of the drug; persistence demands evaluation for an alternative cause (brain stem metastases, cerebrovascular accident). Floxuridine also inhibits thymidylate synthetase. It is most often used for the treatment of hepatic metastases from colorectal carcinoma (Bruckner & Motwani, 1991). Prolonged administration may induce a chemical hepatitis in addition to the toxicities commonly seen with 5-FU (Skeel, 1991).

Cytarabine is a pyrimidine antagonist that blocks the action of DNA polymerases. It is phase-specific and is most effective by continuous infusion although commonly administered on an intermittent IV schedule in combination with other agents. Cytarabine is a mainstay in the induction of remission in acute myelogenous leukemia, in which it may be used in standard doses (200 mg/M²/24 hr) or high doses (3 to 6 g/M²/day). Low, subcutaneous doses have been utilized to try to improve blood counts in myelodysplasia. Cytarabine may also be administered intrathecally for the control of leukemic and nonleukemic leptomeningeal carcinomatosis. Intrathecal administration is required to achieve cerebrospinal fluid concentrations that are tumoricidal. Maintenance regimens in acute myelogenous leukemia utilize intermittent subcutaneous administration. Cytarabine crosses the blood-brain barrier; the high-dose regimens are associated with high central nervous system (CNS) concentration and thus increased frequency of CNS toxicity. Pellagra-like symptoms (diarrhea, dementia, dermatitis), conjunctivitis, cerebellar signs, seizures, and hepatic dysfunction may occur at both standard and high doses, but their incidence increases with increasing dose. Prophylactic dexamethasone eye drops should be used to minimize ocular toxicity.

Gemcitabine, structurally similar to cytarabine arabinoside, is currently undergoing phase II and III testing in a number of solid tumors. In 1995, it became available for the treatment of refractory or relapsed adenocarcinoma of the pancreas. Objective responses have been described in head and neck, ovarian, renal, breast, and advanced pancreatic cancers, as well as with small-cell lung cancer. This drug achieves a 20-fold higher intracellular concentration and has a longer duration of action than cytarabine due to its higher membrane penetration and enhanced binding to its tar-get enzyme deoxycitadine kinase (Dorr & Von Hoff, 1994).

Azacytidine, an investigational inhibitor of pyrimidine metabolism, exerts its action and toxicity through mechanisms similar to those of cytarabine; however, its instability in solution limits its clinical utility. It is currently restricted to the treatment of acute myelogenous leukemia and is available through the Group C acquisition program of the NCI. Rhabdomyolysis has been associated with its use (Cline & Haskell, 1980).

6-Mercaptopurine (6-MP) and thioguanine (6-TG) compete with purines in the leukemic cell. Xanthine oxidase is required for the degradation of 6-MP; concomitant administration of allopurinol requires dose reduction. Both purine antagonists require biotransformation to their active components, and both are excreted renally (Langevin, Greenberg, Koren, & Soldin, 1987). The available oral forms are mildly emetogenic; intravenous preparations are available investigationally. Myelosuppression is common with both agents and represents their dose-limiting toxicity. Cholestatic jaundice may occur with progression to hepatic necrosis being reported with 6-MP (Perry, 1982). Cross-resistance occurs between the two drugs. 6-Mercaptopurine is active in the treatment of acute myelogenous leukemia and in combination with methotrexate in maintenance regimens for acute lymphoblastic leukemia. Thioguanine is most valuable in acute myelogenous leukemia (Dorr & Fritz, 1980).

Adenosine analogs are the newest group of antimetabolites to come into clinical utility. Three agents are currently available; fludarabine phosphate (Fludara), 2-chlorodeoxyadenosine (CdA, cladarabine), and deoxycoformycin (DCF, pentostatin). These agents exert their antitumor effects by competing with or inhibiting the enzyme adenosine deaminase, which is prevalent in cells of lymphoid lineage. Fludarabine and pentostatin are most useful in the treatment of B-cell malignancies (chronic lymphocytic leukemia, low-grade non-Hodgkin's lymphoma), while cladarabine is effective in hairy cell leukemia. These agents are also used in the treatment of malignancies of T-cell lineage such as cutaneous T-cell lymphomas (mycosis fungoides) (Olin, Dombek, Gremp, Hebel, & Kastrup, 1994).

Nephrotoxicity is common with pentostatin but may be avoided with vigorous hydration and avoidance of concomitant nephrotoxic agents. Pulmonary toxicity, manifested by dyspnea, and interstitial infiltrates on chest x-ray films may occur with fludarabine but has not been problematic with cladarabine or pentostatin. Cutaneous toxicity consisting of dry skin and keratoconjunctivitis may occur with CdA and DCF. All adenosine analogs induce significant myelosuppression, predominantly anemia, and thrombocytopenia. Hemolytic anemia has been reported with the adenosine deaminase inhibitors (Doll & Weiss, 1985).

MISCELLANEOUS ANTINEOPLASTICS

A few clinically useful agents exist today whose mechanisms of action are poorly defined or unique (Table 21–10). Procarbazine, an oral agent, inhibits

TABLE 21–10. *Miscellaneous Agents*

CLASS	AGENTS	CLINICAL USE
Monoamine oxidase inhibitor	Procarbazine	Hodgkin's disease
		Brain tumors
		Lung cancer
Ribonucleotide reductase inhibitor	Hydroxyurea	Chronic myelogenous leukemia
		Acute myelogenous leukemia
		Acute lymphoblastic leukemia
Adrenocortical steroid inhibitor	Mitotane	Adrenocortical cancer
Enzyme	L-Asparaginase	
	Pegasparaginase	Acute lymphoblastic leukemia

monoamine oxidase and, therefore, exhibits the clinical effects of other monoamine oxidase inhibitors. Procarbazine's primary role is in the treatment of Hodgkin's disease in the well-known MOPP regimen (DeVita et al., 1970).

The toxicities of procarbazine include myelosuppression, allergic skin rashes, pleuropulmonary reaction with occasional pneumonitis and fibrosis, and hemolytic anemias with formation of Heinz bodies in erythrocytes (Cline & Haskell, 1980). Ataxia, orthostatic hypotension, urticaria, and neuropathies may occur. Because procarbazine inhibits monoamine oxidase, concomitant administration of tricyclic antidepressants, sympathomimetics, or foods high in tyramine (aged cheese, chocolate, Chianti wine, dark beer) may result in hypertensive episodes. Similarly, procarbazine may yield a disulfiram-like reaction with the concomitant ingestion of alcohol, including medications containing alcohol (e.g., cough syrup, cold preparations).

Hydroxyurea inhibits ribonucleotide reductase, phase specifically (S). It is used in chronic leukemia and as emergency therapy for rapid lysis of blasts in patients with acute leukemia (both myelogenous and lymphocytic) who have blast levels that interfere with circulatory function. In the latter situation, simultaneous administration of allopurinol is indicated to prevent the development of tumor lysis syndrome (see Chapter 66) (Hughes, 1987). Hydroxyurea is also used to control blood counts in other myeloproliferative disorders, such as essential thrombocytosis. Leukophoresis may be used concomitantly to decrease splenic size in advanced myelofibrosis and chronic myelogenous leukemia. Hydrea is non-cross-resistant with busulfan. Toxicities include bone marrow depression, predominantly of the leukocytes; thrombocytopenia is less common. However, patients with massive splenomegaly may exhibit pronounced thrombocytopenia before and during therapy, owing to splenic sequestration of platelets. Skin reactions (hyperpigmentation, scaly atrophy, nail changes) and erythema and swelling of the hands and face may occur. Alopecia is possible. Neurologic disturbances including headaches, dizziness, disorientation, hallucinations, and seizures have been reported. An investigational parenteral preparation is available.

Mitotane, a derivative of the insecticide DDT, has a single antineoplastic indication: malignant carcinoma of the adrenal gland. Mitotane binds to the mitochondria in the cells of the adrenal cortex, preventing the conversion of cholesterol to steroids. Spironolactone potentiates its activity and should not be administered concomitantly. The onset of action after oral daily administration of mitotane may not be clinically detectable for 2 to 3 months after initiation of therapy.

The toxic manifestations of mitotane include nausea, vomiting, diarrhea, anorexia, orthostatic hypotension, and skin rashes. Visual disturbances, decreased memory, lethargy, somnolence, dizziness, vertigo, and mental depression occur because mitotane's lipid solubility allows it to cross the blood-brain barrier. Adrenal insufficiency should be anticipated. Patients experiencing trauma, infections, or shock must be treated with supplemental corticosteroids; mitotane should be discontinued during this period.

Asparaginase is an enzyme that acts by destruction of extracellular supplies of L-asparaginine, resulting in the death to tumor cells that lack the ability to produce this essential amino acid. Asparaginase may block some cells in G_1 or S, but it is generally considered cell-cycle phase-nonspecific. Asparaginase is extracted from *E. coli*; anaphylaxis is the most dangerous toxicity. Pretreatment skin tests should be administered, and test doses should be given; in the event of hypersensitivity reactions, desensitization regimens must be administered before a therapeutic dose. Skin testing should be repeated when doses are given after long separations in time. Asparaginase has also been isolated from *Erwinia caratovora,* a plant parasite. Allergic intolerance to the *E. coli* preparation may require using the *Erwinia* preparation, which is available investigationally from the NCI. The enzymatic nature of asparaginase results in some unique toxicities; hypercholesterolemia, hyperglycemia, decreased synthesis of clotting factor, and neurotoxicity manifested as personality changes, somnolence, lethargy, and confusion may occur. Azotemia and proteinuria may develop; rarely, pancreatitis has been reported. Asparaginase has its current role in the treatment of acute lymphoblastic leukemia and is incorporated into most induction regimens (Capizzi & Holcenberg, 1993).

A modified L-asparaginase, pegasparaginase, has been developed that has decreased immunogenicity and a longer plasma half-life. It is indicated in patients requiring asparaginase who are intolerant of the natural products.

HORMONALLY ACTIVE AGENTS

Many tumors arise from hormonally active tissues; manipulations of the hormonal milieu are used to inhibit their growth. Hormonal manipulations are based on the observation that tumor cells contain surface receptors for specific hormones required for cellular growth. The hormones are then transported intracellularly, where they exert their effects. Antineoplastic hormonal manipulations include obliterating host production of the required hormone, blocking the hormone receptors with competing agents, and substituting chemically similar agents for the active hormone, which cannot be utilized by the tumor cell. The hypothalamic hormones (LHRH, somatostatin) are now available and are proving useful in the management of many hormonally active tumors (Schally, 1994). Hormonal cancer chemotherapeutics are summarized in Table 21–11.

Adrenocorticosteroids have direct antineoplastic effects in hematologic malignancies. Agents that block the production of adrenocorticosteroids are also used in the treatment of hormonally active cancers. Because aminoglutethimide induces a medical adrenalectomy, cortisone must be administered simultaneously and supplemental corticosteroids must be given during periods of distress or gastrointestinal malfunction. They are also required in patients with an absent or malfunctioning pituitary gland.

Megestrol acetate (Megace) has been helpful in alleviating the anorexia associated with malignancy, its therapy, and the weight loss associated with AIDS. The reader is referred to endocrinology texts for in-depth discussion of the hormones; their toxicities do not differ substantially when used in the treatment of malignant disease.

DIFFERENTIATING AGENTS

The most clinically useful agents in this class are cisretinoic and all-transretinoic acid. The retinoic acids, vitamin A derivatives, induce a differentiation in promyelocytic leukemia (APL) by a noncytotoxic mechanism (Miller & Dmitrovsky, 1993; Parkinson, Cheson, Friedman, Smith, & Stevenson, 1992; Tallman & Wiernik, 1992). These orally administered drugs have a toxicity profile similar to high-dose vitamin A, including dry skin, photosensitivity, and hepatotoxicity. 13-cis-retinoic acid is not quantitated by a standard vitamin A level. Accutane is the commercially available retinoid.

TABLE 21–11. *Hormonally Active Agents*

CLASS	AGENTS	CLINICAL USE
Estrogens	DES Estradiols Estramustine* Chlorotrianisene Premarin	Breast cancer, prostate cancer
Progestins	Megestrol acetate Medroxyprogesterone Hydroxyprogesterone caproate Depo-Provera	Appetite stimulant, breast cancer, endometrial cancer, renal cell cancer
Androgens	Fluoxymesterone Oxymetholone Testolactone Testosterone	Breast cancer, myelodysplasia ("preleukemia")
Antiestrogens	Tamoxifen Toremifen**	Breast cancer, endometrial cancer, melanoma, brain tumors
Antiandrogens	Flutamide	Prostate cancer
LHRH blockers	Leuprolide Goserelin acetate Leuprolide depot	Breast cancer, prostate cancer
Steroids	Prednisone Dexamethasone Methylprednisone Predhisolone Methylprednisolone Cortisone Hydrocortisone	Hodgkin's disease, non-Hodgkin's lymphoma, myeloma, breast cancer, acute leukemia, chronic leukemia, prior to Taxol
Steroid blockers	Aminoglutethimide Mitotane	Breast cancer, prostate cancer Adrenal cortex cancer

LHRH, Lutenizing hormone-releasing hormone; DES, diethylstilbestrol.
*DES conjugated to mechlorethamine.
**Investigational.

Recently, vaginally administered 13-cis-retinoic acid has been shown to reverse premalignant lesions of the cervix (Graham et al., 1986). Research is ongoing using the retinoids in chemoprophylaxis in hairy leukoplakia and in combination with the biologics and antineoplastics in the treatment of a variety of malignancies.

BIOLOGIC ANTINEOPLASTICS

Biologic response modifiers entered cancer chemotherapy clinical trials in the 1980s (Abernathy, 1987). Currently interleukin-2 (IL-2) is the only commercially available interleukin. It is effective in renal cell carcinoma and melanoma and is used both as a single agent and in combination with antineoplastic regimens. The discovery that the interleukins activate lymphocytes in vivo, coupled with improvements in technology allowing in vitro activation and subsequent administration to patients, have opened new areas of investigation into the interactions of biologic products and the classic antineoplastics. Much research is ongoing and is required to better define the role of such therapeutic interventions in the treatment of malignant disease (DeVita, Hellman, & Rosenberg, 1991).

The use of growth factors to minimize the myelosuppression of classic antineoplastics are an example of the impact of the biologics on the science of cancer chemotherapy (Schuchter, Luginbuhl, & Meropol, 1992). Currently, available agents include granulocyte colony-stimulating factor (GCSF), which stimulates production of neutrophils, and granulocyte macrophage colony-stimulating factor (GMCSF), which increases both neutrophils and macrophages. To be utilized effectively (i.e., dosed through the granulocyte nadir), the recovery time of these cells needs to be known. Table 21–12 gives the nadirs and recovery times after administration of specific drugs. Additional agents have been identified with the ability to stimulate the pleuripotent stem cell and thus simultaneously alleviate chemotherapeutic effects on all hematopoietic cells with a single agent; its availability will further affect the delivery of cancer therapies, allowing an increase in dose intensity (Hryniuk, 1988). Dose intensity will, no doubt, uncover additional toxicities such as the suspicion of an increased incidence of acute leukemias, which have recently been identified in dose-intense adjuvant breast cancer trials (Abrams & Smith, 1994).

Simultaneously, improved ability to synthesize and administer more specific monoclonal antibodies have opened new horizons in the evaluation of patients with cancer, in the control of symptoms such as bone pain, and in offering therapeutic potential. Chapter 23 discusses the biologic response modifiers and their role in cancer therapy.

NEW HORIZONS

The 1980s saw the initiation of investigations into alternative delivery mechanism of chemotherapy. High-dose chemotherapy with autologous bone marrow transplantation (see Chapter 27) and regional chemotherapy (arterial infusions for liver metastases and brain tumors and limb perfusions in melanoma), are currently under investigation. Clonogenic assays, or tumor stem cell assays, have been developed that incubate fresh tumor cells with antineoplastic agents in

TABLE 21–12. *Nadir and Recovery Time in Drug-Induced Myelosuppression*

CATEGORY	DRUG	NADIR OF GRANULOCYTES (DAYS)	RECOVERY (DAYS)
Primarily myelosuppressive toxicity	Mechlorethamine	7–15	28
	Melphalan	10–12	—
	Busulfan	11–13	24–54
	Carmustine	26–30	35–49
	Lomustine	40–50	60
	Cytarabine	12–14	22–24
	Vinblastine	5–9	14–21
	Etoposide	10–14	16–21
Myelosuppressive toxicity plus other toxicities	Cyclophosphamide	8–14	18–25
	5-Fluorouracil	7–14	20–30
	Mercaptopurine	7	14–21
	Methotrexate	7–14	14–21
	Actinomycine-D	15	22–25
	Procarbazine	25–36+	25–50+
	Doxorubicin	6–13	21–24
	Dacarbazine	21–28	28–35
	Mitomycin-C	28–42	42–56
Rarely cause granulocytopenia	Vincristine	4–5	7
	Bleomycin	—	—
	Asparaginase	—	—
	Cisplatin	—	—
	Hormones	—	—

(Reprinted with permission from Haskell, C. M. [1990]. *Cancer treatment* [3rd ed., pp. 21–43]. Philadelphia: W. B. Saunders Co.)

vitro to determine effective agents for use in vivo. These have been disappointing to date but may be refined, allowing improved selection of effective chemotherapy for individual patients.

Additional approaches to multidisciplinary therapy, such as hyperthermia and perioperative chemotherapy (preoperatively, during, or immediately postoperatively), will doubtlessly be explored through the end of the century (Berger, 1986; Scher et al., 1988). Hyperthermia, used to increase the core temperature of the tumor before treatment with radiation therapy or chemotherapy in an effort to enhance cell kill, will continue to be studied. Radiosensitization, the use of chemotherapy to improve the efficacy of radiation therapy, will be refined (Beard, Coleman, & Kinsella, 1993).

Other agents, such as hematoporphyrin esters combined with light, may prove directly cytotoxic and are expected to have a role in defining surgical margins, in detecting recurrent disease, and in palliation (Ball, 1987; Imamura et al., 1994; Kitzrow, 1992; McCaughan et al., 1992; Whelan et al., 1993). Photodynamic therapy is based on preferential uptake of the ester by tumor cells, which then can be activated by light to create toxic radicals, resulting in cell death. Lung, bladder, esophageal, and cutaneous tumors have been controlled with photodynamic therapy (Penning & Dubbelman, 1994). Minimizing the toxicities of antineoplastics by general or selective protection of target organs with medication is an evolving area of investigation (Table 21–13) (Chapman, 1982; Myers et al., 1983).

TABLE 21–13. *Common Organ System Toxicities of Antineoplastics**

Organ System	Toxicity	Class of Agent					
		AA	PA	A	AM	M	H
Gastrointestinal (Conrad, 1986; Coons, Larson, Leventhal, Love, & Nerenz, 1987; Dorr & Fritz, 1980; Mitchell & Schein, 1982)	Nausea, vomiting (Duigon, 1986; Needleman, 1987; Sallan & Cronin, 1985; See-Lasley & Ignoffo, 1981)	1–4	1–2	3	2	3–4	1
	Diarrhea	1	1	1	2–3	1	1
	Constipation	1	2	1	1	1	1
	Mucositis	1–2	1	2	3–4	1	1
Hepatotoxicity (Perry, 1992; Seipp, 1985)	Elevated LFT results	1	1	1	2	1	1
	Cholestatic jaundice	1	1	2	2	1	1
	Hepatitis	1	1	1	2	1	1
Bone marrow (Grant Medical Center, 1987; Hoagland, 1982)	Leukopenia	4	4	4	4	1–4	1
	Thrombocytopenia	2–3	1–4	2–3	2	1–4	1
Cutaneous (Doll & Weiss, 1985; Dunagin, 1982; Lovejoy, 1979; Parker, 1987; Weiss, 1982)	Rash	1	1	2–3	2–3	2–3	1
	Nail changes	1	1	1–2	2	1	1
	Hyperpigmentation	1	1	1–2	1–3	1	1
	Radiation recall	1	1	2	2	1	1
	Alopecia (Dean, Griffith, & Salmon, 1979; O'Brien, Pearson, Schwartz, & Zelson, 1970; Parker, 1987; Seipp, 1985)	1–4	1	1–4	1–4	1	1
Pulmonary (Buzdar et al., 1980; Ginsberg & Comis, 1982; Wickham, 1986)	Allergic pneumonitis	1	1	1	2	2	2
	Pulmonary fibrosis	1–2	1	1–2	1	1	1
Genitourinary (Lydon, 1986; Schilsky, 1982; Verway et al., 1984)	Kidney (Schilsky, 1982)	2–4	1	1	2–4	1	1
	Bladder	1	1	1	1	1	1
Cardiac (Kaszyk, 1986; Myers et al., 1983; Unverferth et al., 1981; Von Hoff, Piccart, & Rozencweig, 1982)	Myocardial damage	1	1	2	1	1	1
	Electrocardiographic changes	1	1	2	1	1	1
Neurologic (Conrad, 1986; Holden & Felde, 1987; Kaplan & Wiernik, 1982; Lopez & Agarwal, 1984)	Central nervous system	1	1–3	1	2	2	1
	Peripheral nerves	1	1–3	1	2	1	1
Reproductive (Chapman, 1982; Grant Medical Center, 1987; Seipp, 1985; Wilkes, Burke, & Ingwersen, 1994)	Gondal function	2–3	?	1–3	?	1–2	1–4

*Based on reported incidence and the likelihood of occurrence in general medical oncology practice.

LFT, liver function tests; AA, alkylating agents; PA, plant alkaloids; A, antibiotics; AM, antimetabolites; M, miscellaneous; H, hormones.

1, Rare; incidence range, 0–19%; 2, Occasional; incidence range 20–49%; 3, Common; incidence range, 50–75%; 4, Frequent; incidence range, greater than 75%; ?, Requires further definition. When ranges are given, there is marked variability among drugs, doses, routes, and patients.

Advances in the application of currently available antineoplastics will be based on improved understanding of tumor kinetics and mechanisms of drug resistance, allowing efficacious drug selection, dosing, and scheduling (DeVita, 1993; DeVita, Hellman, & Rosenberg, 1988).

Also, phase II trials are ongoing to study liposomal drug delivery, which is the encapsulation of therapeutic agents within microscopic closed vesicles, consisting of phospholipid bilayers. Liposomes preferentially distribute to areas of inflammation and neoplasm and to organs of the reticuloendothelial system, especially the liver and spleen. Interest in this novel method of drug delivery is currently focused on encapsulated doxorubicin and daunorubicin, which have been shown in preliminary testing to have less cardiotoxicity than their nonencapsulated counterparts and therefore the potential to overcome cardiac limitations on the cumulative dosing of these agents (Balazsovits et al., 1989; Bangham, 1992; Cowens et al., 1993; Ostro, 1992).

New strategies will be developed to enhance the mechanisms of cell death (Berger, 1986). Methods to manipulate oncogene expressions to improve antineoplastic sensitivity will be identified (Vesell, 1985). Improved knowledge about the mechanisms of resistance will allow the development of non-cross-resistant agents and regimens (Berger, 1986; DeVita, 1993). New techniques in molecular genetics have resulted in genetic engineering approaches to the treatment of malignancies and have led to a resurgence of interest in cancer vaccines (Cohen, 1993).

Chemotherapy is a mainstay of cancer treatment. It is a continually and constantly changing modality whose role is well established in some malignancies and is evolutionary in others. As the predominant systemic therapy for malignant disease, chemotherapy will continue to play a major role in oncologic therapeutics.

ACKNOWLEDGMENT. The authors thank Dr. Jerry T. Guy for his advice and support in the preparation of this manuscript, Nancy Cohen and Debra Milks for their assistance with literature review, and Sherri Starrett for assistance in preparation of the manuscript.

REFERENCES

Abernathey, E. (1987). Biotherapy: An introductory overview. *Oncology Nursing Forum Supplement, 14*(6), 13–15.

Abrams, J., & Smith, M. (1994). Letter: Acute myeloid leukemia following doxorubicin and cyclophosphamide: Increased risk for dose-intensive regimens? *Investigator's Letter, NCI, NIH, DHHS, PHS.*

Alton, P. A., & Harris, A. L. (1993). The role of DNA topoisomerases II in drug resistance. *British Journal of Haematology, 85,* 241–245.

Arbuck, S. G. (1994). Memorandum: Paclitaxel and visual abnormalities. *Department of Health and Human Services.*

Armand, J. P., & Marty, M. (1989). Navelbine: A new step in cancer therapy? *Seminars in Oncology, 15*(2) (Suppl. 4), 41–45.

Armitage, J. O., & Antman, K. H. (1992). *High-dose cancer therapy.* Baltimore: Williams & Wilkins.

Balazsovits, J. A. E., Bally, M. B., Cullis, P. R., Falk, R. E., Ginsberg, R. S., McDonell, M., & Mayer, L. D. (1989). Analysis of the effect of liposome encapsulation on the vesicant properties, acute and cardiac toxicities, and antitumor efficacy of doxorubicin. *Cancer Chemotherapy and Pharmacology, 23,* 81–86.

Ball, K. (1987). Photodynamic therapy of malignant tumors. *Today's OR Nurse, 9*(6), 9–15.

Bangham, A. D. (1992). Liposomes: Realizing their promise. *Hospital Practice, 27*(12), 51–62.

Batts, C. N. (1992). Adjuvant intravesical therapy for superficial bladder cancer. *The Annals of Pharmacotherapy. 26,* 1270–1276.

Beard, C. J., Coleman, C. N., & Kinsella, T. J. (1993). Radiation sensitizers. In V. T. DeVita, S. Hellman, & S. A. Rosenberg (Eds.), *Cancer: Principles and practice of oncology* (4th ed., pp. 2701–2713). Philadelphia: J. B. Lippincott Co.

Berger, N. (1986). Cancer chemotherapy: New strategies for success. *Journal of Clinical Investigation, 78,* 1131–1135.

Berman, E., Andreeff, M., Clarkson, B., Gabrilove, J., Gee, T., Gulati, S., Heller, G., Jhanwar, S., Keefe, D., Kempin, S., Kolitz, J., McKenzie, S., Mayer, K., O'Reilly, R., Penenberg, D., Raymond, V., Reich, L., Santorsa, J., Schluger, A., Trainor, K., & Young, C. (1991). Results of a randomized trial comparing idarubicin and cytosine arabinoside with daunorubicin and cytosine arabinoside in adult patients with newly diagnosed acute myelogenous leukemia. *Blood, 77*(8), 1666–1674.

Besenval, M., Delgado, M., Demarez, J. P., & Krikorian, A. (1989). Safety and tolerance of navelbine in phase I-II clinical studies. *Seminars in Oncology, 26*(2) (Suppl. 4), 37–40.

Boice, J. D., Chen, T. T., Ellenberg, S. S., Fraumeni, J. F., Greene, M. H., Keehn, R. J., Killen, J. Y., & McFadden, E. (1983). Leukemia and preleukemia after adjuvant treatment of gastrointestinal cancer with semustine (methyl-CCNU). *The New England Journal of Medicine, 309*(18), 1079–1084.

Bonadonna, G., Bajetta, E., Brambilla, C., Brugnatelli, L., Brusamolino, E., DeLena, M., Musumeci, R., Rossi, A., Tancini, G., Valagussa, P., & Veronesi, U. (1976). Combination chemotherapy as an adjuvant treatment in operable breast cancer. *The New England Journal of Medicine, 294,* 405–410.

Bonadonna, G., Santoro, A., & Valagussa, P. (1986). Alternating non-cross-resistant combination chemotherapy or MOPP in Stage IV Hodgkin's disease. *Annals of Internal Medicine, 104,* 739–746.

Booser, D. J., & Hortobagyi, G. N. (1994). Anthracycline antibiotics in cancer therapy: Focus on drug resistance. *Drugs, 47*(2), 223–258.

Bristow, M. R., Billingham, M. E., Lopez, M. B., Mason, J. W., & Winchester, M. A. (1982). Efficacy and cost of cardiac monitoring in patients receiving doxorubicin. *Cancer, 50,* 32–41.

Bruckner, H. W., & Motwani, B. T. (1991). Chemotherapy of advanced cancer of the colon and rectum. *Seminars in Oncology, 18*(5), 443–461.

Burchenal, J. H. (1977). The historical development of cancer chemotherapy. *Seminars in Oncology, 4*(2), 135–148.

Burton, N. K., Aherne, G. W., Barnett, M. J., Douglas, I., Evans, J., Lister, T. A. (1986). The effect of food on the oral administration of 6-mercaptopurine. *Cancer Chemotherapy and Pharmacology, 18,* 90–91.

Buzdar, A. U., Blumenschein, G. R., Hortobagyi, G. N., Legha, S. S., Luna, M. A., & Tashima, C. K. (1980). Pulmonary toxicity of mitomycin. *Cancer, 45,* 236–244.

Calvert, A. H., Boxall, F. E., Burnell, M., Gore, M. E., Gumbrell, L. A., Judson, I. R., Newell, D. R., O'Reilly, S., Siddik, Z. H., & Wiltshaw, E. (1989). Carboplatin dosage: Prospective evaluation of a simple formula based on renal function. *Journal of Clinical Oncology, 7(11),* 1748–1756.

Capizzi, R. L., & Holcenberg, J. S. (1993). Asparaginase. In J. F. Holland (Ed.), *Cancer medicine* (3rd ed., pp. 796–804). Philadelphia: Lea & Febiger.

Chabner, B. A. (1993). Anticancer drugs. In V. T. DeVita, S. Hellman, & S. A. Rosenberg (Eds.), *Cancer: Principles and practice of oncology* (4th ed., pp. 325–417). Philadelphia: J. B. Lippincott Co.

Chapman, R. M. (1982). Effect of cytotoxic therapy on sexuality and gonadal function. *Seminars in Oncology, 9(1),* 84–94.

Chaudhary, P. M., & Robinson, I. B. (1991). Expression and activity of p-glycoprotein, a multidrug efflux pump, in human hematopoietic stem cells. *Cell, 66,* 85–94.

Cheson, B. D., Chun, H. G., Friedman, M. A., & Jasperse, D. M. (1986). Differentiating agents in the treatment of human malignancies. *Cancer Treatment Reviews, 13,* 129–145.

Christian, M. C. (1992). The current status of new platinum analogs. *Seminars in Oncology, 19(6),* 720–733.

Cimoli, G., DeSessa, F., Parodi, S., Russo, P., & Valenti, M. (1994). Circumvention of atypical multidrug resistance with tumor necrosis factor. *Japanese Journal of Cancer Research, 85,* 135–138.

Cline, M. J., & Haskell, C. M. (1980). *Cancer chemotherapy.* Philadelphia: W. B. Saunders Co.

Cohen, A. M., Friedman, M. A., & Minsky, B. D. (1993). Rectal cancer. In V. T. DeVita, S. Hellman, & S. A. Rosenberg (Eds.), *Cancer: Principles and practice of oncology* (4th ed). Philadelphia: J. B. Lippincott.

Cohen, J. (1993). Cancer vaccines get a shot in the arm. *Science, 262,* 841–843.

Conrad, K. J. (1986). Cerebellar toxicities associated with cytosine arabinoside: A nursing perspective. *Oncology Nursing Forum, 13(5),* 57–59.

Cooley, M. E., Abrahm, J., & Davis, L. (1994). Cisplatin: A clinical review. *Cancer Nursing, 17(4),* 283–293.

Coons, H. L., Larson, S., Leventhal, D. R., Love, R. R., & Nerenz, D. R. (1987). Anticipatory nausea and emotional distress in patients receiving cisplatin-based chemotherapy. *Oncology Nursing Forum, 14(3),* 31–35.

Cordon-Cardo, C., Bertino, J. R., Boccia, J., Casals, D., Melamed, M. R., & O'Brien, J. P. (1990). Expression of the multidrug resistance gene product (p-glycoprotein) in human normal and tumor tissues. *The Journal of Histochemistry and Cytochemistry, 38(9),* 1277–1287.

Cowens, J. W., Brenner, D. E., Creaven, P. J., Ginsberg, R., Greco, W. R., Ostro, M., Petrelli, N., Pilkiewics, F., & Tung, Y., (1993). Initial clinical (phase I) trial of TLC D-99 (doxorubicin encapsulated in liposomes). *Cancer Research, 53,* 2796–2802.

Creemers, G. J., Lund, B., & Verweij, J. (1994). Topoisomerase I inhibitors: topotecan and irenotecan. *Cancer Treatment Reviews, 20,* 73–96.

Crossley, R. J. (1984). Clinical safety and tolerance of mitoxantrone. *Seminars in Oncology, 11(3)* (Suppl. 1), 54–58.

Dalton, W. S. (1993). Overcoming the multidrug-resistant phenotype. In V. T. DeVita, S. Hellman, & S. A. Rosenberg (Eds.), *Cancer: Principles and practice of oncology* (4th ed., pp. 2655–2666). Philadelphia: J. B. Lippincott Co.

Dean, J. C., Griffith, K. S., & Salmon, S. E. (1979). Prevention of doxorubicin-induced hair loss with scalp hypother-mia. *The New England Journal of Medicine, 301(26),* 1427–1429.

Depierre, A., Dabouis, G., Dalphin, J. C., Garnier, G., Jacoulet, P., & Lemarie, E. (1989). Efficacy of navelbine (NVB) in non-small cell lung cancer (NSCLC). *Seminars in Oncology, 16(2, Suppl. 4),* 26–29.

DeSpain, J. D. (1992). Dermatologic toxicity of chemotherapy. *Seminars in Oncology, 19(5),* 501–507.

DeVita, V. T., Jr. (1993). Principles of chemotherapy. In V. T. DeVita, S. Hellman, & S. A. Rosenberg (Eds.), *Cancer: Principles and practice of oncology* (4th ed., pp. 276–292). Philadelphia: J. B. Lippincott Co.

DeVita, V. T., Jr., Carbone, P. P., & Serpick, A. A. (1970). Combination chemotherapy in the treatment of advanced Hodgkin's disease. *Annals of Internal Medicine, 73,* 881–895.

DeVita, V. T., Hellman, S., & Rosenberg, S. A. (1988). *Important advances in oncology 1988.* Philadelphia: J. B. Lippincott Co.

DeVita, V. T., Hellman, S., & Rosenberg, S. A. (1991). *Biologic therapy of cancer.* Philadelphia: J. B. Lippincott Co.

Doll, D. C., & Weiss, R. B. (1985). Hemolytic anemia associated with antineoplastic agents. *Cancer Treatment Reports, 69(7-8),* 777–782.

Dorland's illustrated medical dictionary (28th Ed.) (1994). Philadelphia: W. B. Saunders Co.

Dorr, R. T., & Fritz, W. L. (1980). *Cancer chemotherapy handbook.* New York: Elsevier Science Publishing Co.

Dorr, R. T., & Von Hoff, D. D. (1994). *Cancer chemotherapy handbook* (2nd ed.). Connecticut: Appleton & Lange.

Duigon, A. (1986). Anticipatory nausea and vomiting associated with cancer chemotherapy. *Oncology Nursing Forum, 13(1),* 35–40.

Dunagin, W. G. (1982). Clinical toxicity of chemotherapeutic agents: Dermatologic toxicity. *Seminars in Oncology, 9(1),* 14–22.

Einhorn, L. H. (1981). Testicular cancer as a model for a curable neoplasm: The Richard and Linda Rosenthal Foundation Award lecture. *Cancer Research, 41,* 3275–3280.

Farber, S., Diamond, L. K., Mercer, R. D., Sylvester, R. F., & Wolfe, J. A. (1948). Temporary remissions in acute leukemia in children produced by folic acid antagonist, 4-aminopteroyl-glutamic acid (aminopterin). *The New England Journal of Medicine, 238(23),* 787–792.

Friedman, M., & Hamilton, J. M. (1988). Progress in adjuvant therapy of large bowel cancer. In V. T. DeVita, S. Hellman, & S. A. Rosenberg (Eds.), *Important advances in oncology 1988* (pp. 273–296). Philadelphia: J. B. Lippincott Co.

Galassi, A. (1992). The next generation: new chemotherapy agents for the 1990s. *Seminars in Oncology Nursing, 8(2),* 83–94.

Georges, E., Ling, V., & Sharom, F. J. (1990). Multidrug resistance and chemosensitization: Therapeutic implications for cancer chemotherapy. *Advances in Pharmacology, 21,* 185–220.

Gilman, A. (1963). The initial clinical trial of nitrogen mustard. *American Journal of Surgery, 105,* 574–578.

Gilman, A., & Phillips, F. J. (1946). The biological actions and therapeutic applications of b-chloroethyl amines and sulfides. *Science, 103(2675),* 409–415.

Gilman, A. G., Nies, A. S., Rall, T. W., & Taylor, P. (1993). *Goodman and Gilman's: The pharmacological basis of therapeutics.* New York: McGraw-Hill.

Ginsberg, S. J., & Comis, R. L. (1982). The pulmonary toxicity of antineoplastic agents. *Seminars in Oncology, 9(1),* 34–51.

Goldie, J. H., & Coldman, A. J. (1979). A mathematical model for relating the drug sensitivity of tumors to their spontaneous mutation rate. *Cancer Treatment Reports, 63*(11–12), 1727–1733.

Gonzalez, C., & Villasanta, U. (1982). Life-threatening hypocalcemia and hypomagnesemia associated with cisplatin chemotherapy. *Obstetrics and Gynecology, 59*(6), 732–734.

Graham, V., Surwit, E. S., Weiner, S., et al. (1986). Phase II trial of beta-all-trans-retinoic acid for intraepithelial cervical neoplasia delivered via a collagen sponge and cervical cap. *Western Journal of Medicine, 145,* 192–195.

Grant Medical Center. (1987). *Chemotherapy: A data compendium.* Columbus: Author.

Green, M. R. (1993). Chemotherapy and radiation in the nonoperative management of stage III non-small-cell lung cancer: the right chemotherapy works in the right setting. In V. T. DeVita, S. Hellman, & S. A. Rosenberg (Eds.), *Important advances in oncology 1993* (pp. 125–137). Philadelphia: J. B. Lippincott Co.

Guy, J. T., Boyd, J. F., Fleming, T., Hynes, H. E., Pollock, T. W., Pugh, R. P., Rivkin, S. E., & Saiers, J. H. (1990). 5-Day vinblastine infusion for pancreatic adenocarcinoma, a phase II Southwest Oncology Group study. *Investigational New Drugs, 7,* 199–200.

Habibi, B., Baumelou, A., Lopez, M., Marteau, R., Salmon, C., Serdaru, M., & Vonlanthen, M. D. (1982). Immune hemolytic anemia and renal failure due to teniposide. *The New England Journal of Medicine, 306*(18), 1091–1093.

Hartmann, O., Beaujean, F., Benhamoa, F., Flamant, F., Kalifa, C., Lemerle, J., Patte, C., & Pico, J. L. (1986). High-dose busulfan and cyclophosphamide with autologous bone marrow transplantation support in advanced malignancies in children: A phase II study. *Journal of Clinical Oncology, 4*(12), 1804–1810.

Haskell, C. M. (1990). *Cancer treatment* (3rd ed., pp. 21–43). Philadelphia: W. B. Saunders Co.

Hoagland, H. C. (1982). Hematologic complications of cancer chemotherapy. *Seminars in Oncology, 9*(1), 95–102.

Holden, S., & Felde, G. (1987). Nursing care of patients experiencing cisplatin-related peripheral neuropathy. *Oncology Nursing Forum, 14*(1), 13–19.

Hryniuk, W. M. (1988). The importance of dose intensity in the outcome of chemotherapy. In V. T. DeVita, S. Hellman, & S. A. Rosenberg (Eds.), *Important advances in oncology 1988.* Philadelphia: J. B. Lippincott Co.

Hughes, C. (1987). Tumor lysis syndrome: A serious complication of chemotherapy. Implications for the I.V. nurse. *National Intravenous Therapy Association, 10*(2), 112–114.

Imamura, S., Fukuoka, M., Kudo, S., Kusunoki, Y., Masuda, N., Matsui, K., Negoro, S., Ryu, S., Takada, M., & Takifuju, N. (1994). Photodynamic therapy and/or external beam radiation therapy for roentgenologically occult lung cancer. *Cancer, 73*(6), 1608–1614.

Kaplan, R. S., & Wiernik, P. H. (1982). Neurotoxicity of antineoplastic drugs. *Seminars in Oncology, 9*(1), 103–130.

Kasperek, C., & Black, C. D. (1992). Two cases of suspected immunologic-based hypersensitivity reactions to etoposide therapy. *The Annals of Pharmacotherapy, 26,* 1227–1229.

Kaszyk, L. K. (1986). Cardiac toxicity associated with cancer therapy. *Oncology Nursing Forum, 13*(4) 81–88.

Kitzrow, C. (1992). Photodynamic therapy for bronchial and esophageal tumors. *AORN Journal, 55*(6), 1483–1492.

Korsmeyer, S. J. (1993). Programmed cell death: Bcl-2. In V. T. DeVita, S. Hellman, & S. A. Rosenberg (Eds.), *Important advances in oncology.* Philadelphia: J. B. Lippincott Co.

Krikorian, A., Bore, P., Bromet, M., Cano, J. P., & Rahmani, R. (1989). Pharmacokinetics and metabolism of navelbine. *Seminars in Oncology 1993. 16*(2, Suppl. 4), 21–25.

Kyle, R. A. (1982). Second malignancies associated with chemotherapeutic agents. *Seminars in Oncology, 9*(1), 131–142.

Langevin, A. M., Greenberg, M., Koren, G., & Soldin, S. J. (1987). Pharmacokinetic case for giving 6-mercaptopurine maintenance doses at night. *Lancet, 2,* 505–506.

Legha, S. S., Benjamin, R. S., Blumenschein, G. R., Ewer, M., Freireich, E. J., Mackay, B., Rasmussen, S. L., Valdivieso, M., & Wallace, S. (1982). Reduction of doxorubicin cardiotoxicity by prolonged continuous intravenous infusion. *Annals of Internal Medicine, 96,* 133–139.

Li, M. C. (1979). The historical background of successful chemotherapy for advanced gestational trophoblastic tumors. *American Journal of Obstetrics and Gynecology, 135,* 266–272.

Liu, L. F., & D'Arpa, P. D. (1992). Topoisomerase-targeting antitumor drugs: mechanisms of cytotoxicity and resistance. In V. T. DeVita, S. Hellman, & S. A. Rosenberg (Eds.), *Important advances in oncology 1992.* Philadelphia: J. B. Lippincott Co.

Lopez, J. A., & Agarwal, R. P. (1984). Letter: Acute cerebellar toxicity after high-dose cytarabines associated with CNS accumulation of its metabolite, uracil arabinoside. *Cancer Treatment Reports, 68*(10), 1309–1310.

Lovejoy, N. C. (1979). Preventing hair loss during Adriamycin therapy. *Cancer Nursing, 2,* 117–121.

Lydon, J. (1986). Nephrotoxicity of cancer treatment. *Oncology Nursing Forum, 3*(2), 68–77.

McCaughan, J. S., Brown, D. G., Guy, J. T., Hawley, P. C., Hicks, W. J., Laufman, L. R., & Williams, T. E. (1992). Photodynamic therapy: An eight-year experience. In B. W. Henderson, & T. J. Dougherty (Eds.), *Photodynamic therapy: Basic principles and clinical applications* (pp. 323–331). New York: Marcel Dekker, Inc.

McCauley, V. M., Begent, R. H. J., Newlands, E. S., & Phillips, M. E. (1982). Prophylaxis against hypomagnesemia induced by cisplatinum combination chemotherapy. *Cancer Chemotherapy and Pharmacology, 9,* 179–181.

Miller, W. H., & Dmitrovsky, E. (1993). Retinoic acid and its rearranged receptor in the treatment of acute promyelocytic leukemia. In V. T. DeVita, S. Hellman, & S. A. Rosenberg (Eds.), *Important advances in oncology* (pp. 81–90). Philadelphia: J. B. Lippincott Co.

Mitchell, E. P., & Schein, P. S. (1982). Gastrointestinal toxicity of chemotherapeutic agents. *Seminars in Oncology, 9*(1), 52–64.

Moertel, C. G., Emerson, W. A., Fleming, T. R., Glick, J. H., Goodman, P. J., Haller, D. G., Laurie, J. A., MacDonald, J. S., Mailliard, J. A., Tormey, D. C., Ungerleider, J. S., & Veeder, M. H. (1990). Levamisole and fluorouracil for adjuvant therapy of resected colon carcinoma. *The New England Journal of Medicine, 322*(6), 352–358.

Morrow, C. S., & Cowan, K. H. (1993). Mechanisms of antineoplastic drug resistance. In V. T. DeVita, S. Hellman, & S. A. Rosenberg (Eds.), *Cancer: Principles and practice of oncology* (4th ed., pp. 340–346). Philadelphia: J. B. Lippincott Co.

Myers, C., Bonow, R., Corden, B., Doroshow, J., Epstein, S., Jenkins, J., Locker, G., & Palmeri, S. (1983). A randomized controlled trial assessing the prevention of doxorubicin cardiomyopathy by N-acetylcysteine. *Seminars in Oncology, 10*(1) (Suppl. 1), 53–55.

Needleman, R. (1987). Chemotherapy: An overview of nausea and vomiting in the cancer patient: Etiology and management of serious complications of chemotherapy. *Amer-

ican Association of Occupational Health Nursing Journal, 35(4), 179–182.

Nooter, K., & Sonneveld, P. (1994). Clinical relevance of p-glycoprotein expression in haematological malignancies. *Leukemia Research,* 18(4), 233–243.

Nordic Gastrointestinal Tumor Adjuvant Therapy Group. (1989). Superiority of sequential methotrexate, fluorouracil, and leucovorin to fluorouracil alone in advanced symptomatic colorectal carcinoma: a randomized trial. *Journal of Clinical Oncology,* 7(10), 1437–1446.

Norton, L, & Day, R. (1991). Potential innovations in scheduling in cancer chemotherapy. In V. T. DeVita, S. Hellman, & S. A. Rosenberg (Eds.), *Important advances in oncology* (pp. 57–73). Philadelphia: J. B. Lippincott Co.

O'Brien, R., Pearson, H. A., Schwartz, A. D., & Zelson, J. H. (1970). Scalp tourniquet to lessen alopecia after vincristine. *The New England Journal of Medicine,* 283(26), 1469.

O'Connell, M. J. (1987). Antipyrimidines: 5-Fluorouracil and 5-Fluoro-2'-deoxyuridine. In J. J. Lokich (Ed.), *Cancer chemotherapy by infusion* (pp. 117–122). Chicago: Precept Press, Inc.

Olin, B. R., Dombek, C. E., Gremp, J. L., Hebel, S. K., & Kastrup, E. K. (1994). *Drug facts and comparisons.* St. Louis: Wolters Kluwer Co.

Osbourne, C. K. (1989). Breast cancer. In R. Wittes (Ed.), *Oncologic therapeutics* (pp. 201–211). Philadelphia: J. B. Lippincott Co.

Ostro, M. J. (1992). Drug delivery via liposomes. *Drug Therapy,* April, 61–65.

Parker, R. (1987). The effectiveness of scalp hypothermia in preventing cyclophosphamide-induced alopecia. *Oncology Nursing Forum,* 14(6), 49–53.

Parkinson, D. R., Cheson, B. D., Friedman, M. A., Smith, M. A., & Stevenson, H. C. (1992). Trans-retinoic acid and related differentiation agents. *Seminars in Oncology,* 19(6), 734–741.

Penning, L. C., & Dubbelman, T. (1994). Fundamentals of photodynamic therapy: Cellular and biochemical aspects. *Anti-Cancer Drugs,* 5, 139–146.

Perry, M. C. (1982). Hepatotoxicity of chemotherapeutic agents. *Seminars in Oncology,* 9(1), 65–74.

Perry, M. C. (1992). *The chemotherapy source book.* Baltimore: Williams & Wilkins.

Plowman, P. N., & Trott, K. (1987). Mesna and total body irradiation. *Lancet,* Jan 17, 167.

Rosenberg, B., Krigas, T., & VanCamp, L. (1965). Inhibition of cell division in *Escherichia coli* by electrolysis products from a platinum electrode. *Nature,* 205, 698–699.

Rosenberg, B., Trosko, J. E., Mansour, V. H., & VanCamp, L. (1969). Platinum compounds: A new class of potent antitumor agents. *Nature,* 222, 385–386.

Rowinsky, E. K., Donehower, R. C., & McGuire, W. P. (1993). The current status of taxol. In W. J. Hoskins, C. A. Perez, & R. C. Young (Eds.), *Principles and practice of gynecologic oncology updates.* Philadelphia: J. B. Lippincott Co.

Rowinsky, E. K., Gilbert, M. R., McGuire, W. P., Noe, D. A., Grochow, L. B., Forastiere, A. A., Ettinger, D. S., Lubejko, B. G., Clark, B., Sartorius, S. E., Cornblath, D. R., Hendricks, C. B., & Donehower, R. C. (1991). Sequences of taxol and cisplatin: a phase I and pharmacologic study. *Journal of Clinical Oncology,* 9(9), 1692–1703.

Sallan, S. E., & Cronin, C. M. (1985). Nausea and vomiting. In V. T. DeVita, Jr., S. Hellman, & S. A. Rosenberg (Eds.), *Cancer: Principles and practice of oncology* (2nd ed., pp. 2008–2013). Philadelphia: J. B. Lippincott Co.

Schackney, S. E. (1985). Cell kinetics and cancer chemotherapy. In P. Calabresi, P. S. Schein, & S. A. Rosenberg (Eds.), *Medical oncology: Basic principles and clinical management of cancer* (pp. 41–60). New York: Macmillan.

Schally, A. V. (1994). Hypothalamic hormones: From neuroendocrinology to cancer therapy. *Anti-Cancer Drugs,* 5, 115–130.

Scher, H. I., Herr, H. W., & Yagoda, A. (1988). Neoadjuvant M-VAC (methotrexate, vinblastine, doxorubicin, and cisplatin) effect on the primary bladder lesion. *Journal of Urology,* 139, 470–474.

Schilsky, R. L. (1982). Renal and metabolic toxicities of cancer chemotherapy. *Seminars in Oncology,* 9(1), 75–83.

Schuchter, L. M., Luginbuhl, W. E., & Meropol, N. J. (1992). The current status of toxicity protectants in cancer therapy. *Seminars in Oncology,* 19(6), 742–751.

See-Lasley, K., & Ignoffo, R. J. (1981). *Manual of oncology therapeutics.* St. Louis: C. V. Mosby Co.

Seipp, C. A. (1985). Hair Loss. In V. T. DeVita, Jr., S. Hellman, & S. A. Rosenberg (Eds.), *Cancer: Principles and practice of oncology* (2nd ed., pp. 2007–2008). Philadelphia: J. B. Lippincott Co.

Skeel, R. T. (1991). *Handbook of cancer chemotherapy* (pp. 6–121). Boston: Little, Brown, & Co., Inc.

Sutherland, C. M., & Krementz, E. T. (1981). Hepatic toxicity of DTIC. *Cancer Treatment Reports,* 65(3-4), 321–322.

Tallman, M. S., & Wiernik, P. H. (1992). Retinoids in cancer treatment. *Journal of Clinical Pharmacology,* 32, 868–888.

Trent, J. M., Buick, R. N., Horna, R. C., Jr., Olson, S., & Schimke, R. T. (1984). Cytologic evidence for gene amplification in methotrexate-resistant cells obtained from a patient with ovarian adenocarcinoma. *Journal of Clinical Oncology,* 2(1), 8–15.

Unverferth, D. V., Baba, N., Balcerzak, S. P., Magorien, R. D., Tallay, R. L., & Unverferth, B. P. (1981). Human myocardial morphologic and functional changes in the first 24 hours after doxorubicin administration. *Cancer Treatment Reports,* 65(11-12), 1093–1097.

Verwey, J., Boven, E., Pinedo, H. M., & van der Meulen, J. (1984). Recovery from mitomycin C-induced hemolytic uremic syndrome: A case report. *Cancer,* 54(12), 2878–2881.

Vesell, E. S. (1985). Genetic host factors: Determinants of drug response [Letter to the Editor]. *New England Journal of Medicine,* 313(4), 261–262.

Von Hoff, D. D., Piccart, M., & Rozencweig, M. (1982). The cardiotoxicity of anticancer agents. *Seminars in Oncology,* 9(1), 23–33.

Weiss, R. B. (1982). Hypersensitivity reactions to cancer chemotherapy. *Seminars in Oncology,* 9(1), 5–13.

Weiss, R. B. (1992). The anthracyclines: Will we ever find a better doxorubicin? *Seminars in Oncology,* 19(6), 670–686.

Weiss, A. J., & Manthel, R. W. (1977). Experience with the use of Adriamycin in combination with other anticancer agents using a weekly schedule with particular reference to lack of cardiac toxicity. *Cancer,* 40, 2046–2052.

Whelan, H. T., Schmidt, M. H., Segura, A. D., et al. (1993). The role of photodynamic therapy in posterior fossa brain tumors: A preclinical study in a canine glioma model. *Journal of Neurosurgery,* 79, 562–568.

Wickham, R. (1986). Pulmonary toxicity secondary to cancer treatment. *Oncology Nursing Forum,* 13(5), 69–76.

Wilkes, G. M., Burke, M. A., & Ingwersen, K. (1994). *Oncology nursing drug reference.* Boston: Johnes & Bartlett Publishers.

Wils, J., Bleiberg, Dalesio, Blijham, Mulder, Planting, Splinter, & Duez. (1986). An EORTC gastrointestinal group evaluation of the combination of sequential methotrexate and 5-fluorouracil, combined with adriamycin in advanced measurable gastric cancer. *Journal of Clinical Oncology,* 4(12), 1799–1803.

Wittes, R. E. (1992). *Manual of oncologic therapeutics.* Philadelphia: J. B. Lippincott Co.

Yap, H. Y., Blumenschein, G. R., Hortabagyi, G. N., Kanting, M. J., Loo, T. L., & Tashima, C. K. (1980). Vinblastine given as a continuous 5-day infusion in the treatment of refractory breast cancer. *Cancer Treatment Reports, 64,* 279–283.

Zubrod, C. G. (1979). Historic milestones in curative chemotherapy. *Seminars in Oncology,* 6(4), 490–505.

Zubrod, C. G. (1984). Origins and development of chemotherapy research at the National Cancer Institute. *Cancer Treatment Reports,* 68(1), 9–19.

Delivery of Cancer Chemotherapy

Virginia R. Martin • Frances E. Walker • Michelle Goodman

Today the schedule, method, and route of chemotherapy administration varies as greatly as the health care setting in which it is delivered. Professionals responsible for the administration of chemotherapy must possess a wealth of knowledge and multiple skills that match the variety of routes and methods of chemotherapy administration. Today, more than ever, nurses are challenged to possess all the latest information and proficiency to ensure safe and competent administration of antineoplastic agents.

Administration of chemotherapy is similar to the administration of other medication; the nurse is responsible for checking the order from the physician, preparing the proper dose, using aseptic technique, being knowledgeable about the drug and its side effects, and administering it properly. Chemotherapy is unique in that it is administered using a variety of routes and requires special equipment. Special precautions must be observed during the preparation and administration of chemotherapy. Incorrect administration of chemotherapy could have devastating effects; thus, chemotherapy administration should be done by qualified nurses and physicians.

This chapter discusses issues pertinent to chemotherapy administration. The issues include routes of administration, devices used during administration, the process of chemotherapy administration including vein selection, pretreatment assessment, documentation, and patient education, and the administration issues of safety and handling and extravasation.

ROUTES OF ADMINISTRATION

There are two fundamental routes of chemotherapy administration: systemic and regional. The route of administration chosen is an important variable in optimal drug delivery. The goal of systemic chemotherapy is to attain a drug concentration sufficient to achieve a therapeutic cytotoxic effect in presumed or proven metastatic disease without causing excessive toxicity to normal tissues. Systemic chemotherapy may be given orally, intravenously, subcutaneously, or intramuscularly (Dorr,1994). Systemic chemotherapy fails at times to adequately control disease. A limitation of systemic chemotherapy is the inability to deliver a sufficient concentration of the drug without causing undue toxicity to normal tissues. Theoretically, regional chemotherapy can enhance the dose-response curve by increasing the concentration at the tumor site and lowering the systemic drug exposure (Goodman,1991; Keizer & Pinedo,1985). The most common methods of regional drug delivery are intraventricular, intraperitoneal, intraarterial, intravesicular, and intrapleural. Regardless of the route chosen, however, it is imperative that chemotherapeutic agents are administered safely and that this administration is accompanied by appropriate patient and family education (Dorr,1994).

SYSTEMIC

ORAL

The oral route is used for chemotherapeutic agents that are well absorbed and nonirritating to the gastrointestinal tract (Brown & Hogan, 1990). Before the oral route is chosen, however, the following factors must be considered: (1) availability of the medication in oral form, (2) patency and functioning of the gastrointestinal tract, (3) presence of nausea, vomiting, or diarrhea, (4) patient's state of consciousness, (5) patient's ability and willingness to comply with the schedule (Burke, 1991). To avoid an accidental overdose, only enough medication for a single course of treatment should be prescribed at a time (Holmes, 1994).

Oral chemotherapy has been used in large part because of the convenience of administration and the decrease in the cost and toxicity of the drug(s). However, as with all oral medication, the availability and concentration of oral neoplastic agents can be incomplete and erratic for drugs that are poorly soluble, slowly absorbed, unstable, or extensively metabolized by the liver (Goodman, 1991). Drugs metabolized by the liver are specifically a problem for patients who have questionable liver or renal function (Holmes, 1994). Table 22–1 lists the most commonly administered oral antineoplastic agents, their doses and schedules, side effects, and pharmacokinetics (Pharmacists Subcommittee, 1984; Dorr & Fritz, 1980; Goodman, 1991; Hubbard & Seipp, 1985).

The issue of compliance is a critical area for future studies (Dorr, 1994). Recent research has demonstrated that noncompliance with oral therapy is a serious problem (Barofsky, 1984; Levine et al.,1987). Levine et al. found full compliance with oral medications was remarkedly low among outpatients with treatable cancers. These authors used three implementation packages to increase compliance: combination of education, home psychologic support and restructuring, and training in pill-taking. An initial compliance rate of 16.8 per cent increased to 44 to 48 per cent with intervention. Oral chemotherapy administration requires skillful assessment and education of the patient and family because of the potential for noncompliance. Assessment should include the patient's cognitive and emotional functioning, social support, physical abilities, and willingness to comply with the treatment plan (Holmes, 1994). Strategies for educating patients and their families are discussed in detail in a later section of the chapter.

INTRAVENOUS

Chemotherapy may be given intravenously by several methods: (1) intravenous (IV) push (direct-push method, two-syringe technique), (2) IV sidearm (IV side port, IV Y-site), (3) mini-infusion (IV piggyback), (4) IV infusion, and (5) continuous IV infusion via one of a variety of mechanical devices. The IV push method is the administration of the chemotherapeutic agent(s) directly into a vein through a single syringe (per antineoplastic agent), with the use of an additional syringe for flushing purposes. Administration of the drug(s) from a syringe through a sideport or a Y-site of a freely running IV line is referred to as an IV sidearm. A mini-infusion, long called an IV piggyback, is the administration of the chemotherapeutic agent diluted in a secondary IV bag, usually in 50 to 100 ml diluent. The secondary line is usually attached to a needle and primary line or heparin lock and is removed when not in use. IV infusion is the administration of the chemotherapy diluted in the main IV bag, usually in 250 to 1000 ml of IV solution. Continuous infusions are frequently mixed in solutions from 50 to 250 cc.

The choice of an intravenous method of administration is based on the following facts (Goodman, 1991): (1) vesicant properties of the drug(s) (i.e., the tendency of the drug to cause tissue damage if infiltrated), (2) potential vein irritation of the drug(s), (3) potential for immediate or delayed complications of the drug(s), (for example anaphylaxis, hypertension, or hypotension), and (4) the logistics of the specific treatment protocol. These facts should be reflected in the insitutional/ agency policies and procedures (Goodman, 1991).

Most chemotherapy, including vesicants and nonvesicants, is administered by IV push. The main controversy over which intravenous method to employ usually concerns the administration of vesicants. Both the IV push and the IV sidearm methods are considered safe for the administration of vesicants; however, the IV push (two-syringe) method is preferable because venous pressure (resistance) and blood return are more easily assessed with this method. The IV push method permits more precise and direct control of the fluid into the vein. A very important point is that all drugs, vesicant and nonvesicant, should be injected directly into a peripheral vein only after ample flushing with normal saline is performed to ascertain adequate blood flow and venous integrity (Goodman, 1991).

Short-term infusions, 30 minutes to 6 hours, are indicated when the chemotherapeutic agents produce complications or undesirable side effects when given the IV push method (i.e., drug requires too much diluent to be given IV push). Examples of drugs that should be given by short-term infusions include cyclophosphamide, carboplatin, ifosfamide, Ara-C, etoposide, cisplatin, 5-FU, and taxol.

Long-term infusions, 6 to 8 hours or longer, including continuous infusions, are increasing because of the accumulating knowledge of the advantages of this method. Continuous infusions have demonstrated advantages in (1) overcoming drug resistance and thereby minimizing toxic effects while enhancing tumor response, (2) maximizing the intracellular levels of the drug by prolonging exposure to low extracellular levels of the drug(s), (3) enhancing the transport mechanisms of the cell membrane through saturation process provided by continuous infusion therapy, and (4) avoiding peak plasma levels and thereby minimizing toxic effects (Goodman, 1991).

In the past 10 years, continuous infusional schedules have been used for virtually every class of antineoplastic agent and have demonstrated an improved therapeutic index by reduced or altered toxicity (e.g.,

TABLE 22–1. *Oral Antineoplastic Agents*

DRUG AND DISEASE INDICATIONS	DOSE AND SCHEDULE	SIDE EFFECTS: ACUTE OR DELAYED	PHARMACOKINETICS	COMMENTS
CYCLOPHOS- PHAMIDE (Cytoxan, Endoxan) Breast cancer Multiple myeloma Small-cell lung cancer	Tablets: 50-mg Dose: 1–5 mg/kg/day 60–120 mg/m^2 Adjust dose in presence of renal dysfunction	Nadir: 7–14 days Bone marrow suppression (BMS) Anorexia, nausea, and vomiting Alopecia Hemorrhagic cystitis with gross or microscopic hematuria Amenorrhea Sterility	Activated in the liver Oral absorption in 1 hour 30% of drug excreted unchanged in urine	Vigorous hydration (3 L/day). Encourage frequent voiding to prevent hemorrhagic cystitis (a sterile inflammation of the urinary bladder). If patient complains of burning on urination or bladder incontinence, urinalysis may reveal occult blood. Control by withdrawal of the drug and hydration. May take pills in divided doses early in the day and with meals or all at one time. Better tolerated with cold foods. Barbiturates and other inducers of hepatic microsomal enzymes may enhance toxicity, e.g., cimetidine. Allopurinol may enhance BMS.
CHLORAMBUCIL (Leukeran) Leukemia Hodgkin's disease Breast cancer Ovarian cancer	Tablets: 2-mg white Dose: 4–8 mg/m^2/day × 3–6 weeks 16 mg/m^2/week every 4 weeks	Nadir: 7–10 days Severe BMS Slight nausea and vomiting Occasional dermatitis Abdominal liver function Pulmonary fibrosis with prolonged use Second malignancy Sterility	Hepatic metabolism to active compound Renal excretion of 50% of unchanged drug	Good oral aborption. Concomitant barbiturate administration may enhance toxicity. Marrow suppression may be prolonged.
BUSULFAN (Myleran) Leukemia	Tablets: 2-mg white Dose: 4–12 mg/day; for several weeks	Nadir: 10–30 days delayed marrow recovery Potentially teratogenic Pulmonary fibrosis with long-term use Dermatologic hyperpigmentation Gynecomastia Amenorrhea	Well absorbed Extensive hepatic metabolism to inactive compounds Renal excretion	Bone marrow recovery may be delayed; therefore caution is advised with long-term use. Hydration and allopurinol may be indicated to prevent hyperuricemia. Total cumulative dose: 600 mg. Long-term daily administration is not recommended owing to the risk of second malignancies with chronic alkylating agents.
6-THIOGUANINE Leukemia	Tablets: 40 mg; green/ yellow Dose: 80–100 mg/m^2 Reduce dose if stomatitis occurs	Nadir: 7–28 days Stomatitis Diarrhea Hepatotoxicity	Variable, incomplete absorption Hepatic metabolism Renal excretion	Administer on an empty stomach. Does not require dose reduction when used in conjunction with allopurinol.
6-MERCAPTOPURINE (6 MP) Leukemia	Tablets: 50 mg Dose: 80–100 mg/m^2/day Titrate dose based on blood counts Reduce dose in presence of hepatic or renal dysfunction	Nadir: 10–14 days Nausea, vomiting Mucositis Diarrhea Drug fever Intrahepatic cholestasis Pulmonary toxicity with prolonged use	Incomplete oral absorption Hepatic inactivation Renal excretion 10% unchanged in 24 hours	Protect pills from light. Administer as single dose on an empty stomach. Increased toxicity with allopurinol (reduce dose by one third to one fourth of the original dose). Administer with caution to patients on sodium warfarin (Coumadin). Monitor liver function tests.

Continued on following page.

TABLE 22–1. *Oral Antineoplastic Agents* Continued

DRUG AND DISEASE INDICATIONS	DOSE AND SCHEDULE	SIDE EFFECTS: ACUTE OR DELAYED	PHARMACOKINETICS	COMMENTS
HEXAMETHYLME-LAMINE Lung cancer Ovarian cancer Lymphomas	Capsules: 50–100-mg cream-colored (in 4 divided doses) Dose: 240–320 mg/m^2/day	Nadir: 21–28 days Acute liver toxicity is dose limiting; nausea and vomiting are dose-related Mild BMS Abdominal cramping Diarrhea Peripheral neuropathies Agitation, confusion	Variable absorption Rapid metabolism Urine excretion 90% in 72 hours	Pyridoxine 50 mg/day may decrease neuropathy. Take with food, prophylactic antiemetics. May worsen vincristine-related peripheral neuropathy.
L-PHENYLANINE MUSTARD (Melphalan, Alkeran) Multiple myeloma Ovarian cancer Breast cancer	Tablets: 2-mg white Dose: 0.1–0.15 mg/kg/day × 2–3 weeks Reduce dose with hepatic or renal impairment	Nadir: 10–18 days Nausea and vomiting usually mild Dermatitis Pulmonary fibrosis Long-term therapy can result in acute leukemia	Hepatic metabolism Renal excretion 20–35% (10% unchanged) 20–50% excreted in feces within 6 days	Protect pills from sunlight. Take on an empty stomach. BMS may be cumulative in older patients.
SEMUSTINE (MeCCNU) (not currently available)	Capsules: 100 mg: black/brown 50 mg: brown 10 mg: white Dose: 100–150 mg/m^2/day every 6–8 weeks	Nadir: 28–42 days Severe cumulative BMS Hepatotoxicity Alopecia Severe nausea and vomiting 5–8 hours after dosing Second malignancy	Well-absorbed Rapid hepatic metabolism Crosses into cerebrospinal fluid (CSF)	Refrigerate: take on an empty stomach, just before bedtime. Pretreat with aggressive antiemetic regimen.
LOMUSTINE (CCNU) Brain cancer Lymphomas	Capsules: 100mg: green/green 40 mg: green/purple 10 mg: purple Dose: 100–130 mg/m^2 every 6–8 weeks	Nadir: 28–42 days Severe cumulative BMS Nausea and vomiting 4–6 hours after dosing Anorexia Alopecia Stomatitis Hepatotoxicity	Absorbed rapidly (<60 minutes) Hepatic metabolism Renal excretion of 50% in 24 hours and 75% in 96 hours Crosses into CSF	Dispense one dose at a time to prevent accidental overdose. Take on an empty stomach just before bedtime. Pretreat with aggressive antiemetics. Protect pills from heat and humidty.
HYDROXYUREA (Hydrea) Chronic myelocytic leukemia Melanoma Head and neck cancer	Capsules: 500 mg Dose: 80 mg/kg/day every third day 750–1000 mg/m^2/day × 5 Decrease dose in presence of renal dysfunction Store in tight container in a cool environment	Nadir: 13–17 days Acute nausea and vomiting Chronic and severe anemia Neurologic seizures and hallucinations Dermatitis Dysuria Azotemia	Well-absorbed Hepatic metabolism Renal excretion of 80% of compound in 12 hours Crosses into CSF	Concomitant radiation, and/or 5-FU, or both, may enhance neurotoxicity. Dysuria and renal impairment may occur. Consider pretreatment with allopurinol.

(From Goodman, M. [1991]. Delivery of cancer chemotherapy. In S. B. Baird, R. McCorkle, & M. Grant [Eds.], *Cancer nursing: A comprehensive textbook* [pp. 291–320]. Philadelphia: W. B. Saunders Co.)

doxorubicin, fluorouracil, ifosfamide, platinum analogs) or increased tumor cell killing (e.g., fluorouracil, etoposide, cladribine). Although there are few phase III trials comparing continuous infusion versus push administration, the evidence is clear that toxicity is altered and therapeutic benefit is not diminished by continuous infusion schedules of drug administration (Anderson & Lokich 1994).

REGIONAL

Regional chemotherapy is the direct administration of an anticancer drug into a tumor-bearing region of the body to achieve greater regional drug exposure than achieved by systemic administration (Ensminger, 1993). The direct administration is possible when the region is accessible by an arterial blood supply or an anatomically distinct space (Ensminger,1993). Regional chemotherapy can be divided into two categories: administration into a third-space regional compartment (CSF, pleural space, pericardial space, and peritoneal cavity) or intrarterial infusion into the artery feeding a tumor-bearing organ or body region (Ensminger,1992). The goal of this type of therapy is to attempt to produce a higher cell kill by injecting directly into the tumor site. The concept behind giving drugs regionally is to increase the concentration locally and perhaps reduce the amount reaching the systemic circulation, thus widening the therapeutic index (Sainsbury, 1991). Drugs having a high total body clearance and those

TABLE 22–1. *Oral Antineoplastic Agents* Continued

DRUG AND DISEASE INDICATIONS	DOSE AND SCHEDULE	SIDE EFFECTS: ACUTE OR DELAYED	PHARMACOKINETICS	COMMENTS
VP-16-213 (Etoposide, VePesid) Lung cancer Testicular cancer	Capsules: 50 mg Dose: 2 × the intravenous dose or 100–200 mg/m²/day over 3–5 days every 3–4 weeks	Nadir: 7–14 days (white blood cell count) Nausea and vomiting: 9–16 days (platelets) Alopecia Bone marrow suppression is dose limiting	Renal and hepatic metabolism Incomplete and variable absorption	Nausea is mild though can be more severe with oral route than with intravenous route.
PROCARBAZINE (Matulane) Hodgkin's disease	50-mg capsules Dose: 100 mg/m²/day × 14 days every 4 weeks; reduce dose in presence of hepatic or renal dysfunction	Nadir: 4 weeks Bone marrow suppression, nausea, vomiting, and diarrhea gradually subside; flu-like syndrome, paresthesias, neuropathies, dizziness, and ataxia	Well absorbed from the gastrointestinal tract Metabolized in the liver with a biologic half-life of about 1 hr 70% of the drug is eliminated by 24 hr in the urine, 5% appears as unchanged drug	Drug and food interactions can occur. Central nervous system (CNS) depression can occur with concomitant administration of procarbazine and CNS depressants. Hypertensive crisis can occur when procarbazine is administered with certain antidepressants (tricyclics and monoamine oxidase inhibitors) and tyramine-rich foods. Severe nausea and vomiting can occur if taken with ethanol, mixed drinks, and beer.
METHOTREXATE Squamous-cell carcinoma Lung cancer	Tablets: 2.5 mg Dose: 2.5–10 mg/day PO or 15–30 mg/day PO × 5 days every 1–3 weeks	Nadir: 7–10 days Nausea and anorexia can occur; stomatitis and ulcerations can occur and are dose-limiting	Serum half-life is 2–4 hr Excreted by the kidneys	Dose is reduced with renal impairment; dosing on an empty stomach may enhance bioavailability. Excretion may be impaired in patients with simultaneous administration or weak acids such as salicylates or vitamin C; oral dosing is generally well tolerated. Avoid administration of methotrexate with ketoprotein or probenecid because toxicity of methotrexate may be enhanced.

that are highly bound or inactivated after one pass through the region are suitable for regional chemotherapy. Intraarterial and intraperitoneal are the most widely practiced areas of regional drug delivery. Other methods of regional chemotherapy administration include intraventricular or intrathecal, intravesicular, and intrapleural.

INTRAPERITONEAL

Intraperitoneal chemotherapy is used for anticancer drug delivery directly into the peritoneum. Intraperitoneal chemotherapy (IP) is controversial and has been studied extensively over the past 2 decades, particularly as a treatment for low-volume ovarian cancer (Markman, 1985). Even though it has been demonstrated that a pharmacologic advantage exists when this mode of administration is chosen, a subsequent decrease in cancer has not yet been demonstrated. Historically,

intraperitoneal chemotherapy was used to treat malignant ascites (Doane,1993). Research interest was renewed when models showed the drug concentration was as much as 10 to 1000 times greater than plasma administration (Dedrik et al., 1978; Malloy, 1991). The peritoneal membrane enables a prolonged malignant cell exposure to the drug and the peritoneal cavity acts as a reservoir for the drug. Holding the drug in the peritoneal cavity allows for a sustained assault on the tumor with a much slower clearance of the agent than if it was administered into the plasma (Surbone & Myers, 1988; Zook-Enck, 1990).

Drugs administered IP are absorbed two ways: (1) by the visceral peritoneum, mesentery, and omentum, which results in drainage to the portal venous system, and (2) by the parietal peritoneum and lymphatic system, which leads to drainage to the systemic circulation (Koeller & Fields, 1994). The ideal drug to be used is

TABLE 22–2. *Single and Combination Agents Used in IP Therapy*

Single Chemotherapeutic Agents Used in Intraperitoneal Therapy
5-Fluorauracil
Cisplatin
Doxorubicin
Mitoxantrone
Carboplatin
Melphalan
Bleomycin
Methotrexate
Cytosine Arabinoside
Taxol

Combination Agents Used in Intraperitoneal Therapy
Cisplatin and Doxorubicin
Cisplatin, Cytarabine, and Bleomycin
Cisplatin and Cytarabine
Cisplatin and Etoposide

Biologic Agents Used in Intraperitoneal Therapy
Bacillus Calmette-Guerin
α, β, and γ Interferon
Interleukin-2

one that has a large systemic circulation clearance and a small peritoneal clearance. Most of the fluid and chemotherapy is then absorbed by the portal vein en route to the liver, where it is metabolized. This route decreases the toxic systemic effects and allows any liver metastasis to get exposed. Intraperitoneal route allows peak drug levels that could not be tolerated systemically to be reached; therefore the antitumor effect is increased, and systemic effects are decreased. For IP to be most effective, the disease should be limited to the peritoneal cavity.

Both chemotherapeutic and biologic agents are being investigated using the IP route. A list of the agents used in intraperitoneal therapy is shown in Table 22–2.

Intraperitoneal access devices deliver the agent directly into the cavity. The most widely used intraperitoneal access devices are temporary in-dwelling catheters, intraperitoneal implantable ports, and in-dwelling Tenckhoff catheters.

A temporary single-use catheter can be placed percutaneously and then removed at the end of each infusion of chemotherapy (Hoff 1991; Runowicz, Dottino, & Shafir 1986). Consideration must be given to the length of time the catheter will be in place and the frequency of drug instillation when deciding whether this catheter should be chosen.

The Tenckhoff catheter is a soft, flexible, silicone tube filled with one or two Dacron cuffs. The catheter is inserted at the time of laparotomy or percutaneously. The tip of the catheter is inserted at the tumor site in the peritoneum, and the cuffs are tunneled and placed in the subcutaneous tissue. A stab incision brings the catheter to an external exit site (Fig. 22–1).

The PORT-A-CATH is a totally implantable system. It consists of a stainless-steel port sutured to the fascia over the lower edge of the rib cage at the midclavicular line. The port is attached to a silastic catheter with multiple holes at the distal end. The catheter is tunneled in the same fashion as the Tenckhoff catheter. The port must be accessed with a noncoring Huber needle. The port can be used for draining ascites or obtaining peritoneal fluid specimens, although it can be difficult to withdraw fluid.

The Tenckhoff catheter is usually selected for cyclic intraperitoneal therapy. Complications with the Tenckhoff catheter most commonly seen are microbial peritonitis and occlusion (Hoff, 1987; Jenkins, 1985; Piccart, Speyer, & Markman 1985; Runowicz et al., 1986; Surbone & Myers, 1988; Zook-Enck, 1990). Other less common complications are: exit site infections, leakage of fluid around the catheter and chemical peritonitis (Brenner,1986; DeGraff et al,1988; Hoff,1987; Jenkins,1985; Piccart,Speyer,Markman, et al,1985; Swenson & Erickson,1986; Zook-Enck,1990). The literature supports the idea that the increased frequency of access or disconnection of the catheter increases the infection rate (Jenkins,1985; Kaplan et al., 1985; Markman, 1985; Markman,1986; Ostechega et al.,1985; Zook-Enck,1990). Developing standards and implementation of procedures and standards for the catheter can decrease the risk of infection. Maintaining strict sterile technique should be the goal, and minimizing the frequency of accessing the delivery system is important.

The incidence of infection has also been noted to be reduced if chemotherapy is delivered once a month rather than by dialysis exchange (Kaplan et al., 1985; Nguyen,Averette, & Wyble, 1993) and when a totally implanted system, that is, PORT-A-CATH, is used (Nguyen et al., 1993; Pfeile & Howell,1984; Piccart et al., 1985). A group of authors designed a modified Tenckhoff catheter that was larger, longer, and had more perfusion holes (Nguyen et al., 1993). There were infections, inflow obstructions, bowel perforation, and incidence of leakage with this new catheter. Although the incidence of inflow obstruction was reduced compared with the standard Tenckhoff, it was not statistically significant, and these authors recommend further evaluation of this new catheter design. The authors recommend unused catheters should be electively removed because of the risk of delayed bowel perforation (Nguyen et al., 1993).

A descriptive study by Almadrones and Yerys highlighted their institution's experience with a totally implanted system for intraperitoneal therapy. Problems evaluated were catheter function (ability to inject, drain, or both), incidence and degree of pain during procedure, incidence of infection, and medical and nursing procedures used to manage catheter dysfunction (Almadrones & Yerys,1990). The review supported the literature that supports the use of the implanted port over the Tenckhoff catheter because of patient preference and a lower incidence of infection (Almadrones & Yerys,1990; Brenner, 1986; Hoff,1987; Pfeifle & Howell,1984; Piccart et al.,1985; Swenson & Eriksson,1986).

The administration procedure for intraperitoneal therapy uses a peritoneal dialysis set with Y tubing (Doane,Fischer, & McDonald, 1990). A Y tubing setup supports the theory of allowing the rapid infusion of

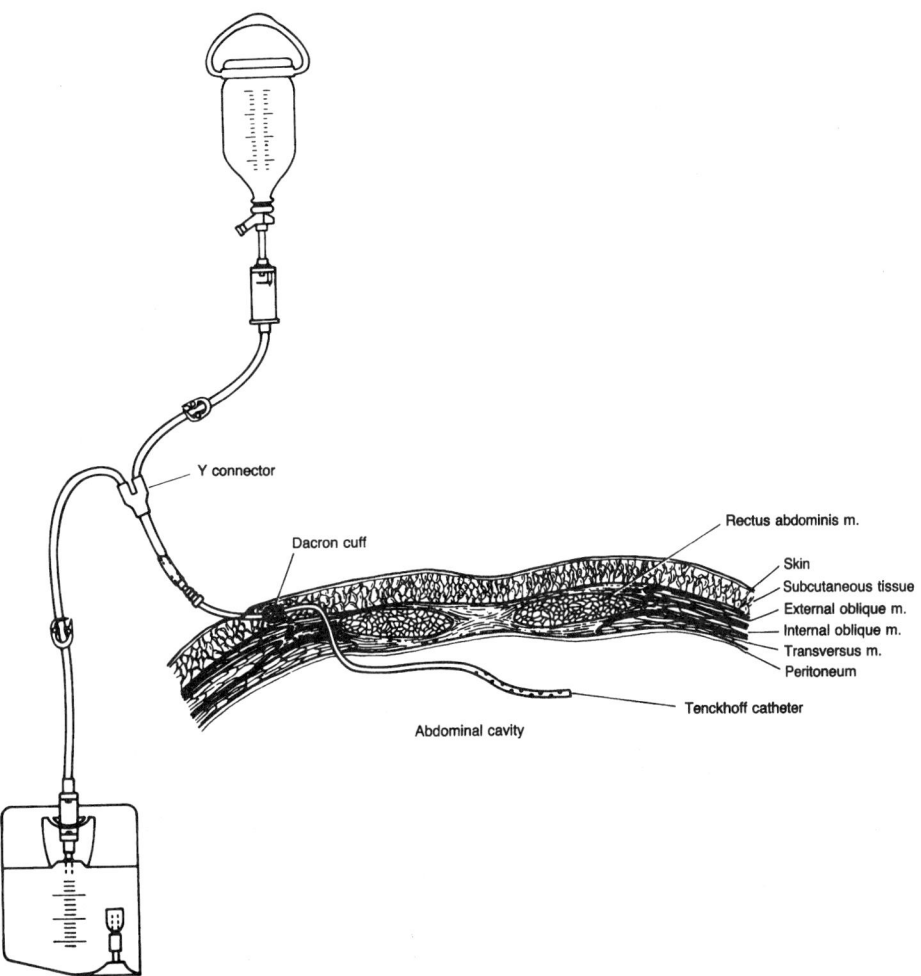

Y connector

Dacron cuff

Rectus abdominis m.
Skin
Subcutaneous tissue
External oblique m.
Internal oblique m.
Transversus m.
Peritoneum

Tenckhoff catheter

Abdominal cavity

FIGURE 22–1. Placement of Tenckhoff catheter for administration of intraperitoneal chemotherapy. (From DeVita, V. T. & Hellman, S. [Eds.]. [1985]. *Cancer: Principles and practice of oncology* [2nd ed., p. 1102]. Philadelphia: J. B. Lippincott Co. Reproduced by permission.)

intraperitoneal chemotherapy. One end of the tubing goes to the patient, and the other two ends are for administration and drainage. Concurrent medications are given to protect specific organs or to prevent general systemic toxicities (e.g., sodium thiosulfate with cisplatin or IV leucovorin with methotrexate). Chemotherapy is infused over a short interval and allowed to dwell up to 23 hours and is then drained. Sometimes treatment allows the chemotherapy to be reabsorbed, so draining is not required. Institutional procedures need to be established for chemotherapy administration as well as care of the external catheter or implanted port.

Nursing management includes decreasing discomfort or pain involved with the installation of the drug or fluid. Other side effects noted are bloating, abdominal pressure, frequent urination, shortness of breath, and diminished appetite, which are noted to be temporary and associated with the large volume of fluid instilled (Almadrones & Yerys, 1990). Patient education plays a large role in intraperitoneal chemotherapy. Alleviating anxiety regarding treatment, reducing complications from the side effects of therapy, and increasing patient compliance are all important outcomes. The

nurse should provide information on the insertion of the catheter, list potential postinsertion complications, and use a demonstration model for reinforcement of catheter teaching. Each patient needs to understand the rationale, the potential side effects during and after the procedure, and the side effects of the chemotherapy agent used for treatment.

INTRAVENTRICULAR/INTRATHECAL

Intraventricular or intrathecal administration of chemotherapy is used when the drugs need to reach the cerebral spinal fluid (CSF). The blood-brain barrier does not allow for the penetration of many systemically administered chemotherapeutic agents. This can cause a problem for patients with tumors that are likely to metastasize to the meninges. Intraventricular therapy, drug therapy into the CSF space, has an established role for prophylaxis in childhood acute lymphocytic leukemia (ALL) and the treatment of established leptomeningeal cancer. With the use of intrathecal administration of chemotherapy, the relapse rate in ALL (a disease with a propensity to relapse in the CNS) has decreased to less than 10 per cent (Koeller & Fields,

1994). Drug administration to the CSF is performed either by lumbar puncture or by intraventricular administration using a subcutaneous implanted reservoir. The Ommaya reservoir is the most common of such devices. This reservoir is a domed device with an attached catheter. It is placed in the subcutaneous tissue of the scalp, and the catheter is threaded into a lateral ventricle (Fig. 22–2). Antimetabolites, including methrotrexate and cytarabine and the alkylating agent thiotepa, have been used most commonly for intrathecal administration. The most common volume administered intrathecally is 5 to 10 ml. Nurses who administer chemotherapy by this device should follow institutional procedures for intrathecal administration. Procedures are necessary to ensure proper sterile technique, since infection can be a serious complication.

INTRAARTERIAL

Intraarterial drugs are administered through a catheter that rests in the arterial blood vessel supplying the tumor. The history of arterial chemotherapy is

noted when Klopp accidently injected nitrogen mustard into the brachial artery in 1950 (Klopp et al., 1950; Sainsbury, 1991). The affected hand was noted to be red and desquamated; the other hand was not affected. Intraarterial chemotherapy has been used for head and neck cancers, limb sarcoma, limb melanoma, liver metastasis, gastric cancer, pancreatic cancer, brain tumors, and recurrent pelvic tumors and breast cancer (Sainsbury,1991). Intraarterial chemotherapy can also be combined with hyperthermia.

Angiography is employed to demonstrate the blood supply to a particular tumor-bearing area. The artery or vein is then cannulated. There are two types of devices used in this treatment. The first is an external catheter placed by a radiologist. These external catheters are small and temporary. If a femoral site is to be used, a patient's mobility should be restricted to prevent catheter kinking. The site must be assessed regularly for bleeding. The catheter is removed after the therapy is completed. The second method is an implanted pump placed surgically in the subcutaneous tis-

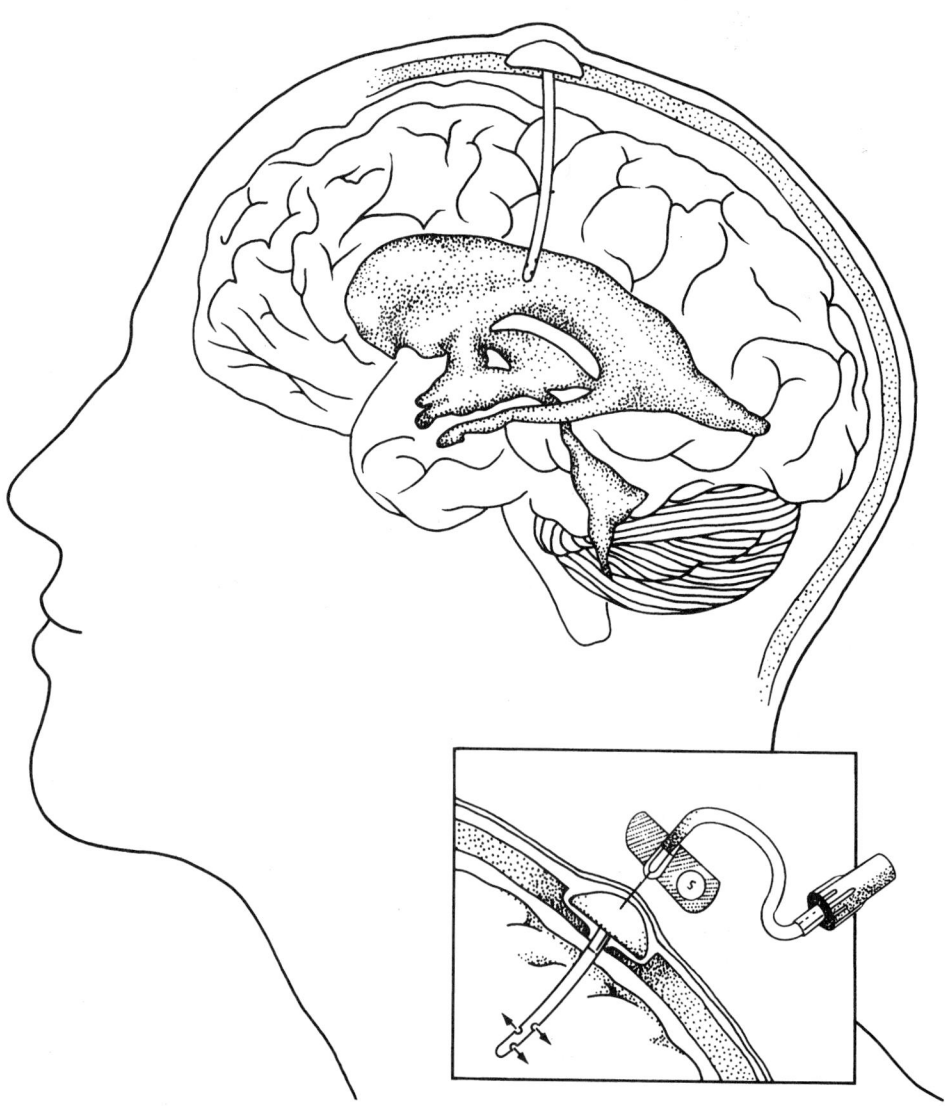

FIGURE 22–2. Ommaya reservoir. (Drawing by Pamela Townsend.)

sue. There are various types of pumps available, and their function and maintenance requirements are model-dependent (see section on infusion pumps). The pump is filled with chemotherapy or saline and infuses the targeted organ. Patency of the catheter lumen is maintained by continuous pump infusion or intermittent heparinization (Goodman, 1991).

The main advantage of intraarterial administration is related to total body clearance of a given drug, its extraction fraction, and blood flow (Sainsbury, 1991). The largest application of intraarterial chemotherapy has been hepatic arterial infusions for colorectal cancer metastatic to the liver (Ensminger, 1993). Requirements for regional infusions for colorectal liver metastasis are a drug with the appropriate pharmacokinetics, the catheter placement to infuse the entire tumor, and a safe and reliable drug delivery system (Dworkin & Allen-Marsh, 1991). The rationale behind hepatic-arterial chemotherapy is based on the vascular pattern of hepatic metastasis. The metastasis is found to be supplied by the hepatic artery rather than the portal vein. Hepatic arterial chemotherapy has been around for 30 years and is currently the most effective therapy for unresectable hepatic colorectal metastasis (Dworkin & Allen-Marsh, 1991). Response rates are higher than for any other therapy, but no clear survival advantages compared with systemic chemotherapy have been demonstrated (Dworkin & Allen-Marsh, 1991).

A patient education pamphlet for intraarterial chemotherapy infusion was developed by Camp-Sorrell. This pamphlet explains the purpose of intraarterial chemotherapy infusions, the procedure for placement of the catheter, and what to expect from the procedure. The author also developed a companion nursing teaching guide and checklist to ensure a consistent level of teaching and documentation of the teaching provided (Camp-Sorrell,1990).

INTRAVESICULAR

Intravesicular administration is the installation of chemotherapy agents directly into the bladder for superficial and invasive bladder cancer. The drugs used include thiotepa, doxorubicin, mitomycin, euthoglucid (epodyl), and bacillus calmette-guarin (BCG). BCG is the most commonly used and the most effective (Lamm, 1992). Long-term benefits of intravesicular administration are elusive, and the superficial bladder cancer recurrence rate averages 88 per cent in individuals who survive 15 years (Kilbridge & Kantoff, 1994; Lamm,1992).

Intravesicular chemotherapy is usually administered by an RN or MD in an office or hospital setting. Pretreatment urine culture and IVP are performed because intravesicular chemotherapy cannot be done if infection or bladder obstruction is present. A urinary catheter is inserted, and then the drug is instilled from a syringe slowly for 30 minutes. The patient remains supine for about 2 hours, turning from side to side for better distribution. Patients are asked to try and retain solution for 2 hours before voiding. If the drug BCG is used, the patient stays until first void so the contaminated urine can be properly disposed. Chemotherapy agents produce side effects, with cystitis being the most

frequently seen side effect. Patients should be instructed to drink as much fluid as possible for the first 48 hours to flush the bladder (Moore et al., 1993).

INTRAPLEURAL

Chemotherapy administration directly into the pleural cavity has been done for many years for the purpose of sclerosing malignant pleural effusions caused by cancers. Malignant effusions can result from cancers of the breast or lung and leukemias and lymphomas. The most frequently used agents for this purpose are doxycycline, mechlorethamine, thiotepa, and talc.

More recently, it has been advocated that tumors confined to the pleural cavity be directly treated with chemotherapy because of the demonstrated pharmacokinetic advantages and antitumor activity demonstrated with intraperitoneal chemotherapy administration. It has been shown that the pharmacokinetics of intrapelural drug administration is similar to intraperitoneal chemotherapy administration (Bogliolo, Lerza, Bottino, et al., 1991; Koeller & Fields, 1994; Rusch, Figlin, Godwin, et al., 1991). Agents used for intrapleural chemotherapy administration include bleomycin, mitoxantrone, doxorubicin, mitomycin-C, cisplatin, etoposide, BCG, and interferon-γ (Koeller & Fields,1994).

ADMINISTRATION DEVICES

VENOUS ACCESS DEVICES

In recent years, the role of the central venous access device in the administration of cancer therapy has increased. Cancer therapy requires frequent venous access, prolonged therapy, use of sclerosing agents, and administration of large volumes of fluid. The multiple venipunctures can cause vein deterioration and increase patient anxiety. Placement of a venous access device early in the course of therapy allows easy administration of vesicants and irritants while decreasing the risk of extravasation. Peripheral access is preserved, and patient anxiety associated with frequent venipunctures is decreased (Berman, Chisolm, DeCarvalho, et al., 1993).

Oncology nurses often act as consultants to nurses in other specialties, because venous access devices are also used with persons with AIDS, sickle cell anemia, burns, Crohn's disease, osteomyelitis, and other illnesses. Nurses must be able to use these devices safely in various care settings and to recognize complications and intervene appropriately if they occur (Wickham,1990).

Three types of venous access devices (VADs) are currently available: tunneled, nontunneled, and venous access ports. Tunneled catheters and totally implanted venous access ports are most often chosen for long-term access, but nontunneled catheters are also used in many settings.

Tunneled central venous catheters include a Dacron cuff around which granulation tissue forms, actually helping to hold the catheter in place. The 4- to 10-inch tunnel through which the catheter is channeled serves to prevent the easy passage of bacteria from the skin into the vein. The cuff is also thought to help stop bacteria from traveling along the subcutaneous portion of the catheter (Reymann, 1993). Central venous catheters are surgically implanted via the subclavian or jugular vein with the tip terminating in the superior vena cava near the right atrium (Tenenbaum & Scelsi, 1994).

Nontunneled or short-term VADs have no cuff and do not pass through a subcutaneous tunnel. This places the patient with this type of device at increased risk for infection, catheter-related sepsis, or both (Tenenbaum & Scelsi, 1994).

A port is a hollow housing containing a compressed latex septum over a portal chamber that is connected via a small tube to a silicone or polyurethane catheter which is inserted into a blood vessel (Reymann, 1993).

Tunneled catheters and venous access port catheters have several features in common, including catheter material and catheter placement. Tunneled catheters are constructed of silicone, or less often, polyurethane. These materials are less thrombogenic than polyethylene and polyvinylchloride (Cervera et al., 1989; Pottecher,Forrler,Picardat, et al., 1984). Polyurethane catheters have thinner walls and small external diameters. All catheters are radiopaque, so fluoroscopy or regular radiographs can be used to determine correct catheter placement after insertion or any time catheter displacement is suspected.

Catheters are usually inserted into one of the major veins of the upper neck or chest. The brachial or cephalic vein may be used in the case of nontunneled catheters or completely implanted peripheral devices (Fig. 22–3). The distal catheter tip is advanced to the superior vena cava at or above the junction of the right atrium. The position of the catheter must be confirmed by fluoroscopy or radiograph. Some conditions preclude cannulation of the superior vena cava. In such instances, a tunneled catheter or venous access port is placed via the saphenous vein and advanced in the inferior vena cava. The port in such a system would be located on the top of the thigh or in the abdomen, whereas a catheter would be tunneled upward to exit higher in the abdomen. The abdominal exit site is preferred because of a possibility of increased risk of infection for catheters exiting in the inguinal area (Reed,Neuman,deJongh, et al., 1983).

VADS are similarly versatile for infusion therapy. Any of them may be used for bolus injections or continuous intravenous infusions of virtually any intravenous solution, including fluids, medications, total

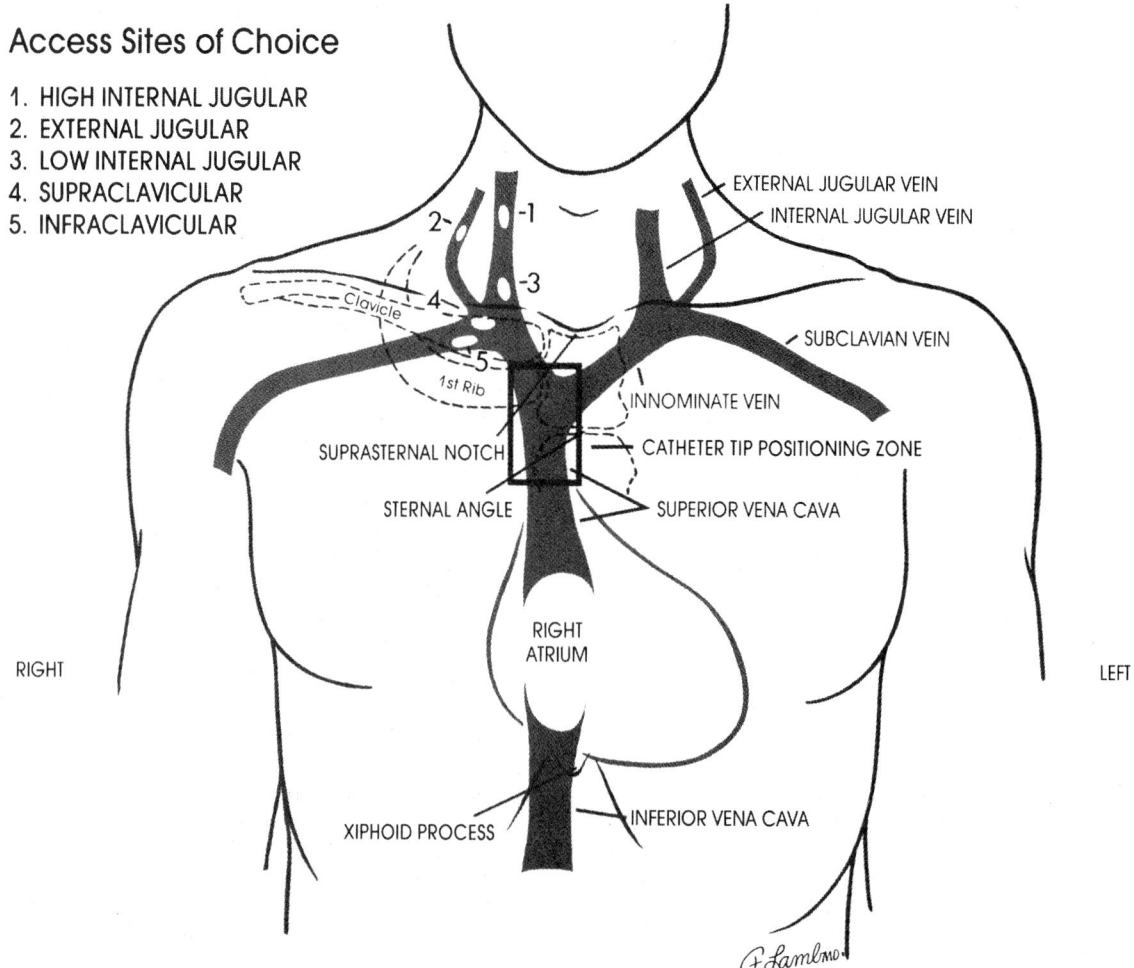

FIGURE 22–3. Anatomic location of vascular access catheters. (Courtesy of Cook, Inc, Bloomington, IN.)

parental nutrition (TPN), blood, and blood components.

Blood sampling is possible with any VAD, although routine blood sampling is not recommended with nontunneled catheters. Blood sampling may be obtained for any test except partial thromboplastin time and activated partial thromboplastin time. These two tests may be seriously prolonged when drawn from heparinized VADs (Almadrones, Godbold, Raaf, et al., 1987; Barton & Poon, 1986). The patient who has a catheter inserted for coagulation profiles will need a catheter that does not require heparin to maintain patency.

TYPES OF DEVICES

Nontunneled Catheters. Nontunneled catheters have the smallest lumen and external diameter. These catheters terminate in the superior vena cava or the right atrium. Most are inserted by a physician at the bedside or in the clinic into the subclavian or jugular vein and are usually 15- to 19-gauge for adults (Holmes, 1994).

Many clinicians consider nontunneled catheters short-term devices, because they enter the vein 1 inch from the exit site. With proper care, however, they can be maintained for extended periods and offer several advantages. Nontunneled catheters can be inserted in outpatient nonsurgical settings. If the catheter becomes damaged or a catheter-related infection is suspected, it can be replaced by an over-the-wire technique. Furthermore, some have suggested that small catheters may be associated with a lower incidence of phlebitis and venous thrombosis (Horattas, Wright, Fenton, et al., 1988; Lokich, Bothe, Benotti, et al., 1985; Rutherford, 1988).

The disadvantages of nontunneled catheters include care requirements as well as the deleterious effects they have on activities and body image. Aseptic technique is required for dressing changes. All persons who have a peripheral catheter require assistance with catheter care. Generally catheters are flushed daily with heparinized saline, dressings are changed every 2 to 7 days, and T connectors and injection caps are changed weekly. Care costs, which may be borne totally by the patient, are high. The presence of an external catheter generally precludes activities such as swimming, and a peripheral catheter exiting at the antecubital fossa may limit arm movement. In addition, some persons may object to a catheter exiting on the arm or high on the chest (Wickman, 1990).

Along with their use for immediate access in emergency situations, nontunneled central venous catheters are also used in oncology patients who have a need for multiinfusional therapy beyond the capabilities of an existing tunneled central venous catheter or implantable port. For instance, a multilumen subclavian catheter might be placed in an acute leukemic patient on chemotherapy, hydration, antibiotics, TPN, blood products, and other medications, or in a patient on a complex investigational drug protocol including bone marrow transplant or peripheral blood stem cell transplantation. The triple-lumen central catheter can augment the long-term device during a hospitalization and be removed prior to discharge (Reymann, 1993).

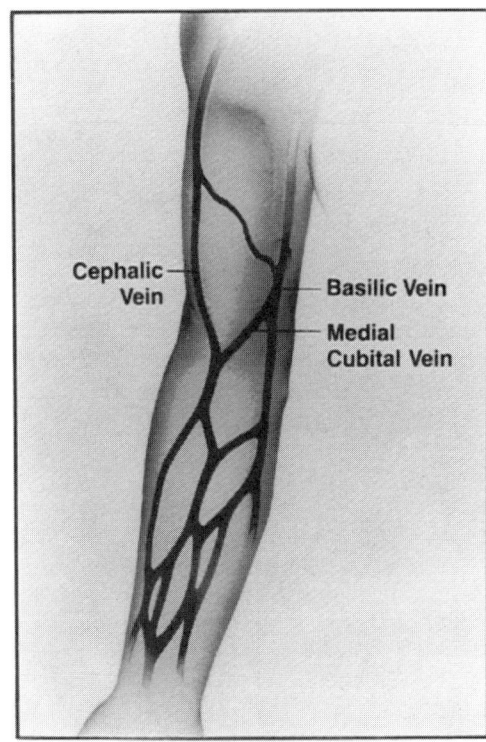

FIGURE 22–4. Vessels commonly accessed for peripherally central placement. (Courtesy of BARD Access Systems; Salt Lake City, UT.)

For long-term use, the gap that existed between the trauma caused by subclavian lines and the investment in a long-term tunneled catheter or port has been closed with the use of peripherally inserted central catheters (PICCs) (Hadaway, 1990). From the patient's viewpoint, the PICC is the least expensive and most easily inserted long-term central venous catheter. The PICC requires self-care capabilities and often even a caregiver, since it is located at the antecubital fossa, and self-care has to be one handed. These small-gauge, thin-walled catheters are inserted at the antecubital fossa into the basilic or cephalic vein (Figs. 22–4 and 22–5). The procedure is usually performed by a physician or a specially trained nurse at the bedside, and the catheter can be advanced into the superior vena cava; x-ray verification of placement is required. In some situations, the PICC line may be advanced only as far as the axillary or subclavian veins. In these cases, x-ray verification of placement is not necessarily required but is preferred, especially for vesicant administration.

PICCs are ideal for short-term access, 1 week to several months; in patients with adequate antecubital veins, self-care capabilities, and the need for a wide variety of intravenous therapies, including antibiotics, chemotherapy, TPN, and analgesics. The thin, flexible nature of the catheter does not lend itself well to blood drawing, but it is not contraindicated and may be successfully achieved with gentle application of pressure via the syringe used for blood drawing. The complication rate is similar to that for other VADs in terms of infection, clotting, and malfunction (Graham et al.,

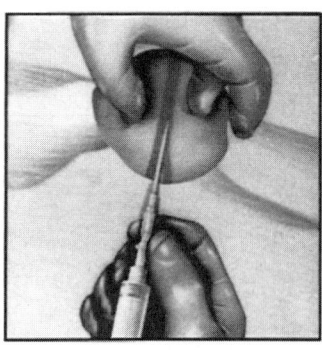
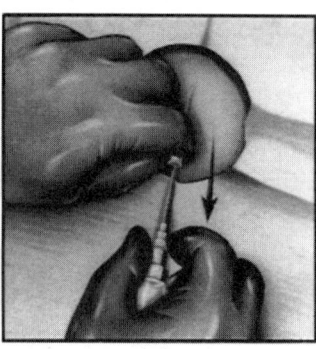
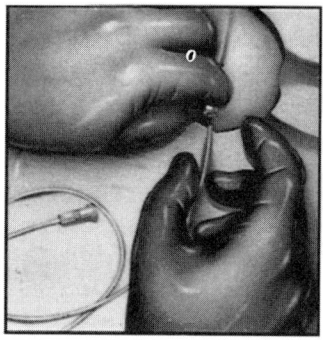
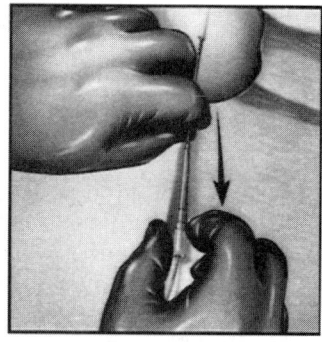

1 Select vein, prep, drape and measure according to hospital procedure, wash gloves prior to touching catheter. Prime catheter through flushing stylet. Insert introducer catheter assembly into selected vessel using standard technique. Observe flashback in flashback chamber.

2 Remove needle from the introducer catheter assembly leaving introducer catheter in place.

3 Have patient turn head toward venipuncture side to help prevent improper cannulation. Insert Groshong®PICC into vessel through the introducer catheter to predetermined depth—use catheter markings as guide. If difficulty is encountered, arm movement or irrigation through priming stylet may assist in catheter advancement.

4 Remove the introducer catheter from the vein, leaving the Groshong PICC in place. Slide introducer catheter to distal end of Groshong PICC.

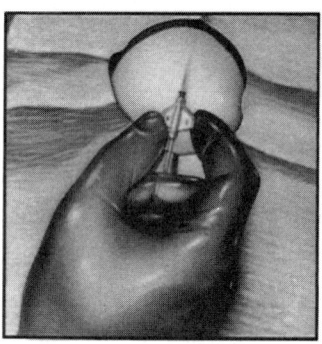
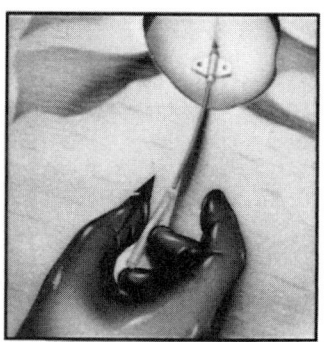
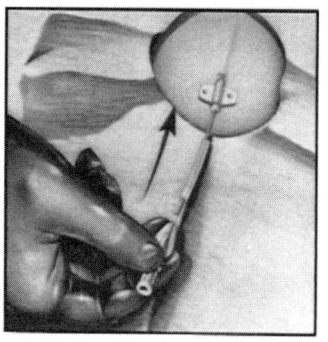
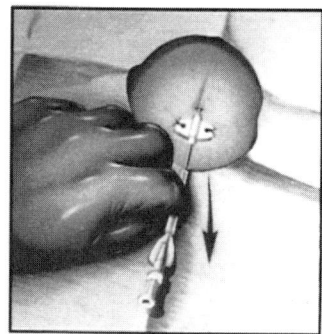

5 Place stabilization wing around PICC Catheter at the venipuncture site. Secure wing using suture or tape. Remove flushing stylet from PICC Catheter, slide introducer catheter off PICC, trim catheter to desired length.

6a Apply catheter hub. **Step 1:** Slide oversleeve onto the PICC Catheter.

6b **Step 2:** INSERT the connector into the catheter using the stylet as a guide. Remove the stylet from connector.

6c **Step 3:** Slide the oversleeve up over the connector to secure the catheter in place. Aspirate blood sample to confirm patency and irrigate with 10cc normal saline. Attach injection cap or connect to an IV line. Confirm placement radiographically.

FIGURE 22–5. Key steps for insertion of the single lumen PICC catheter. (Courtesy of BARD Access Systems, Salt Lake City, UT.)

1991; Gullatte, 1989; May & Davis,1988). Some studies suggest a higher rate of phlebitis. Meticulous attention to sterile technique during insertion and rinsing the powder off the gloves prior to handling the PICC seem to decrease these complications (Masoorli & Angeles, 1990).

Tunneled Catheters. The tunneled central venous catheter provides safe and reliable long-term access, months to years, with a low incidence of infection. It is suitable for almost all hematology/oncology patients and many others as well. It continues to be well accepted and has been modified by the various manufacturers who now market similar devices (Reymann, 1993).

Broviac (Broviac,Cole, & Schribner, 1973) developed the first tunneled catheter for patients who required long-term TPN, and Hickman and colleagues (Hickman et al., 1979) developed a larger, more versatile catheter for patients undergoing bone marrow transplantation. Virtually all tunneled catheters are large-bore and constructed of thick-walled silicone. One exception is the thin-walled silicone Groshong catheter.

Tunneled catheters usually exit the body midway between the nipple and the sternum and are tunneled for several inches to the cannulated vein. All catheters have a Dacron cuff that lies about 2 inches from the exit site. The cuff becomes enmeshed with scar tissue, which secures the catheter in place. The cuff also may decrease the risk of organisms ascending the catheter to induce infection. It is not possible to determine whether the true risk of infection is lower with tunneled catheters versus nontunneled catheters, because no prospective, randomized trials comparing infection rates have been done (Reymann,1993).

Tunneled catheters are versatile and can be used for intermittent bolus or continuous IV therapy. Single-

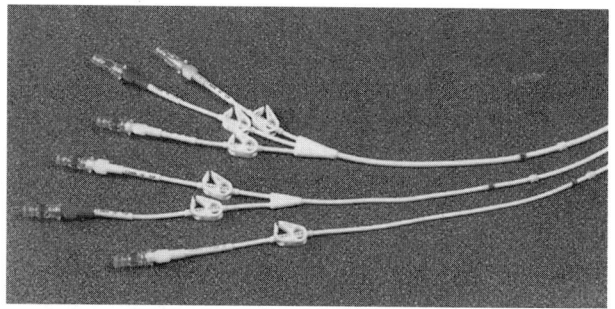

FIGURE 22–6. Single-lumen, double-lumen, and triple-lumen Hickman®catheters (C. R.Bard, Inc.), with VitaCuff (Vitaphore Corp.). (Photographs courtesy of Bard Access Systems.)

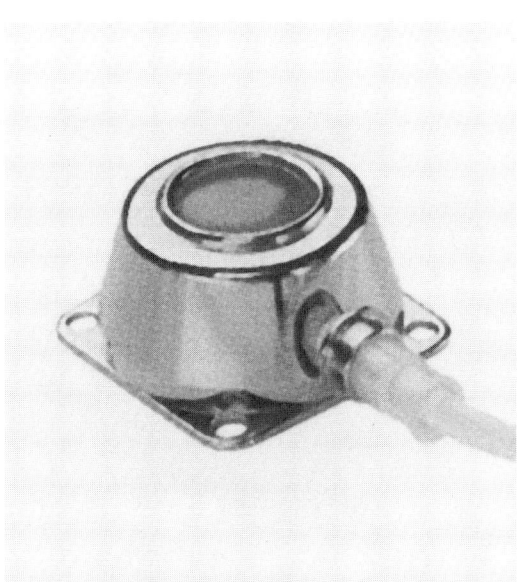
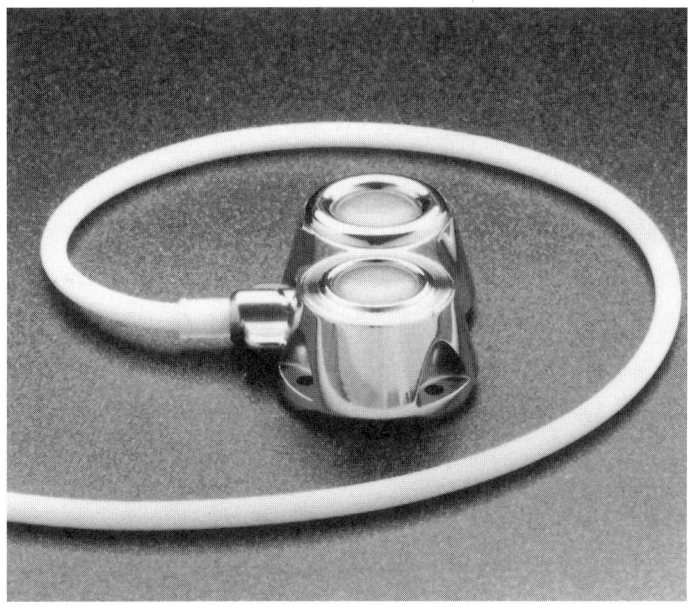

A   B

FIGURE 22–7. **A,** Single-lumen PORT-A-CATH®. **B,** Dual-lumen PORT-A-CATH®. (Courtesy of SIMS Deltec, Inc., St. Paul, MN.)

lumen, double-lumen, and even triple-lumen catheters are available (Fig. 22–6). The average number of lumens necessary for therapy should be determined before placement so that the patient does not have to undergo repeated peripheral intravenous cannulation or care for unneeded catheter lumens.

Tunneled catheters are more expensive to place, but maintenance costs are generally less than those of nontunneled devices. Patients need to keep a gauze or occlusive dressing over the exit site until it has healed (3 to 4 weeks). Once the site has healed, a nonimmunocompromised patient may not need to cover the site. The catheter should always be taped to the chest wall to prevent inadvertent displacement or catheter damage.

Caring for the tunneled catheters can be fairly expensive and includes dressings and dressing supplies, syringes, normal saline, and heparin flush solutions. Heparin flush concentrations as well as the amount and frequency of flushes has generally been selected empirically. Groshong catheters are flushed with normal saline once a week or after use to maintain patency (Wickham, Purl, & Welker, 1992).

Venous Access Ports. Venous access ports consist of a catheter attached to a plastic or metal (stainless steel or titanium) port or ports (Fig. 22–7). Both lie completely beneath the skin. The port consists of a dense silicone septum overlying a small reservoir. Many brands of ports are available, and most have a septum that lies perpendicular to the skin. Most septums feel somewhat similar to the palpating fingers. Three devices differ from the "standard" ports: the Norport SP (Nolfold Medical, Skokie, IL), the S.E.A. Port (Harbor Medical Devices, Boston, MA), and the P.A.S. Port (Pharmacia Deltec, St. Paul, MN).

The P.A.S. Port is a top-access port that is implanted into the forearm, and the catheter is advanced to the central venous system through the basilic or cephalic vein (Fig. 22–8). The Norport SP is a single-lumen skin parallel port that is cannulated with a straight needle straight on, whereas the S.E.A. Port is a double-lumen port that is cannulated from either or both sides (Fig. 22–9). The manufacturers of side-access ports claim this design decreases the risk of needle dislodgement and subsequent extravasation.

The surgical technique used to place ports is similar to the one used for placing tunneled catheters. The catheter is cut to the appropriate length and advanced into the superior vena cava. The attached port is sutured into a subcutaneous pocket. Although adequate subcutaneous tissue over the port is necessary to preclude erosion through the skin, a larger problem is excess adipose tissue over the port, which makes cannulation difficult. Some physicians allow the port to be used immediately after placement, whereas others require the port not to be used until postoperative swelling has resolved. Ports are accessed with noncoring, deflected-tip needles, which allow the septum to reseal when the needle is withdrawn (Fig. 22–10). Side access ports are accessed with straight needles, and top-access ports are accessed with 90-degree needles or tack-type needles, most of which have a short length of preattached tubing.

A port may be preferable to an external catheter because of versatility, low maintenance between use, and a lesser effect on the patients' activities, body image, and cosmesis. On discontinuation of use, or every 4 to 8 weeks when not in use, ports are flushed with 2 to 3 ml heparinized saline (1200 U/ml). Because no part of the system exits the body, there are generally no activity restrictions between use except heavy contact sports. A lower risk of infection is suggested with ports than with external catheters (Decker & Edwards, 1988; May & Davis, 1988), but very few ran-

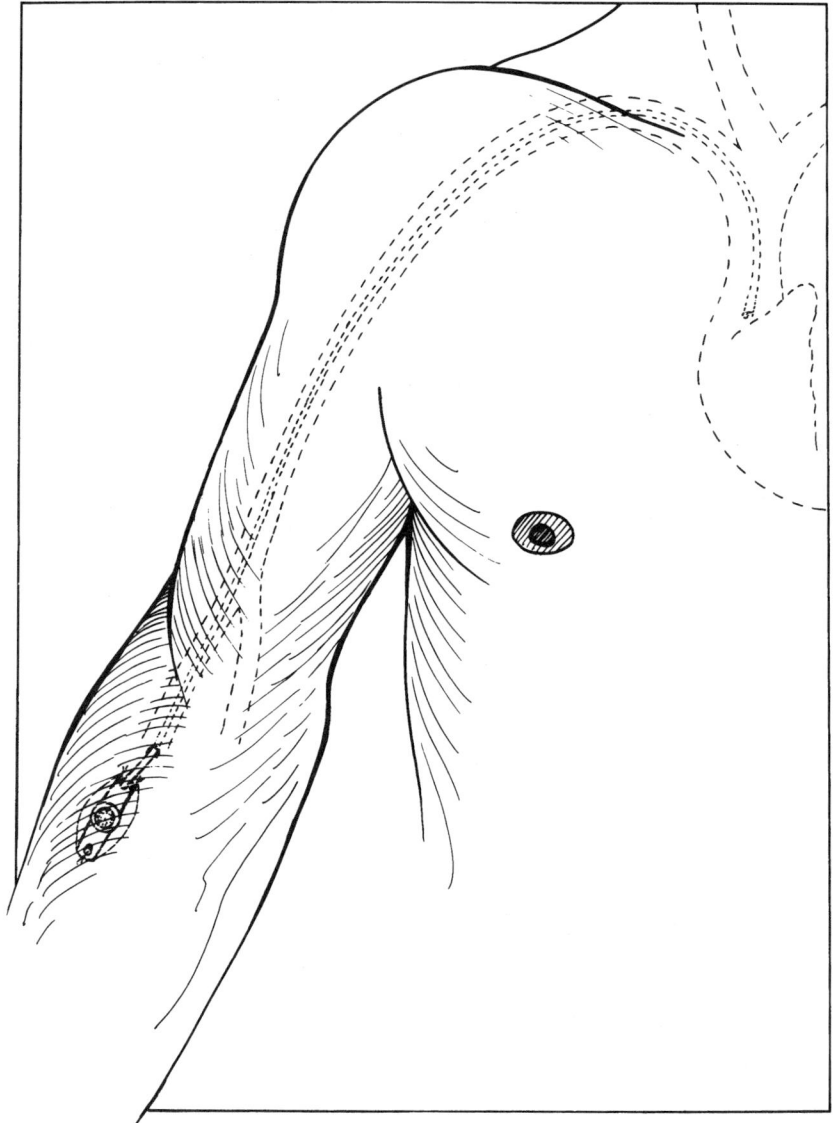

FIGURE 22–8. Placement site of P.A.S. PORT® system. (Courtesy of SIMS Deltec, Inc., St Paul, MN.)

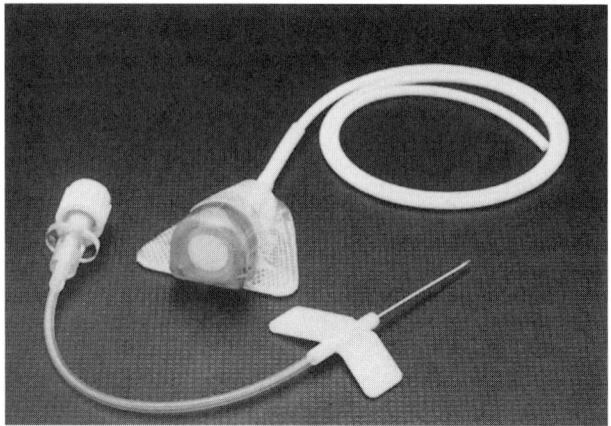

FIGURE 22–9. Norport-SP: a side entrance port. (Courtesy of Norfolk Medical Products, Inc., Skokie,IL.)

Accessing The System

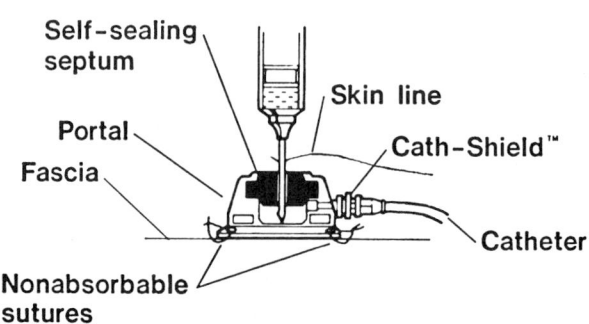

FIGURE 22–10. PORT-A-CATH® cross section with Huber point needle in place. (Courtesy of SIMS Deltec, Inc., St Paul, MN.)

domized studies have confirmed a lower infection rate with ports.

Ports are the most expensive VAD to place. However, maintenance costs are so low that the cost difference between ports and tunneled catheters evens out in about 6 months. Another potential disadvantage is the needle stick necessary for accessing a port, which should be discussed with patients before a decision is made to have a port inserted (Wickham, 1990).

COMPLICATIONS

Complications of VADs can occur during or at any time after placement. Although the relative risk for any complication may be greater or less with a given VAD, the nurse must remember that the potential for a given complication exists for every patient and every catheter. Occlusions, both intraluminal and extraluminal, are common complications with VADs. Other frequently reported complications are infection, catheter thrombosis and extravasation (Wickham, 1990).

Intraluminal Occlusions. The complete inability to withdraw blood or infuse fluid in a VAD is most commonly the result of blood clot within the catheter. It can also be caused by incompatible drugs or lipids that have crystallized, precipitated, or obstructed the catheter. Blood clots can build up over time (i.e., sluggish catheter) but can also appear suddenly, for instance, in a port that is accessed only monthly. Drug precipitates tend to be more directly related to a recent infusion and are seen more often with TPN and lipids (Breaux et al., 1987). The following measures are used to prevent intraluminal occlusions.

1. Maintain positive pressure within the catheter when flushing.
2. Advise patient to avoid excessive manipulation of external catheters.
3. Vigorously flush with at least 20 cc of sterile saline after any blood has gotten into the catheter.
4. Document each patient's VAD experience, and adjust concentration, volume, and frequency of heparinized flush as needed.
5. Question patient and family regarding actual catheter maintenance activities to assess compliance with recommended care and usage.
6. Flush between each drug with at least 10 cc of plain IV fluid to avoid incompatible drug admixture.
7. Vigorously flush catheter every 8 to 12 hours when administering TPN or lipids.
8. Avoid administering IV fluid or TPN containing visible precipitants (Hurtubise,Bottino, & Lawson, et al., 1980).

In the case of ports, the inability to infuse or aspirate usually is due to needles being improperly placed in the septum rather than the portal. Advancing the needle into the portal will usually solve the problem.

Management of an occluded catheter when a blood clot is suspected involves the installation of streptokinase or urokinase, which is almost universally successful (Hurtubise et al., 1980; Lawson, 1982; Wachs, 1990). Urokinase is less antigenic than streptokinase and is preferred by many practitioners. A dose of urokinase (5000 U in 1 to 3 ml) is instilled using a 3 ml or larger syringe and a gentle to and fro motion. The catheter is then clamped for 30 minutes, after which an attempt is made to aspirate the catheter contents. If successful, the catheter is flushed and used; if unsuccessful the procedure is repeated (Bagnall et al., 1989). If a second installation of urokinase is unsuccessful, a variety of options exist: a 24-hour lock of urokinase, continuous infusions of urokinase for 4 to 24 hours (Bagnall et al., 1989; Curnow et al., 1985), and t-PA tissue plasminogen activator, which remains investigational (Atkinson,Bgnall, & Gomperts,1990). If TPN is not involved and a specific drug is known or suspected to be causing the occlusion, a pharmacist should be consulted about possible agents that might dissolve the precipitant and enable it to be aspirated from the catheter.

Extraluminal Occlusions. Catheter sluggishness or partial occlusion can be due to two extraluminal phenomena: fibrin sheath formation and thrombosis. The catheter position can also affect flow, so a partial occlusion in the absence of pain should first be managed by instructing the patient to change positions, raise the arms, deep breathe, and/or cough. Each of these might release the open lumen of the catheter from the vein wall and allow easy flushing and blood withdrawal. If the catheter flushes easily but backflow is very sluggish or nonexistent, fibrin sheath formation or thrombosis should be considered. Fibrin sheaths can form at the lumen of the catheter and extend like a sleeve around the catheter. Fibrin sheaths can be dissolved by instilling urokinase (5000 to 10,000 U) into the catheter with an extended dwell time of 1 to 24 hours (Wickham et al., 1992).

Venous thrombosis can be caused by a variety of factors including endothelial injury, hypercoagulability, multiple catheters, catheter stiffness (i.e., polyvinyl chloride), catheter size (i.e., larger bore), and catheter placement (i.e., left side or in a smaller vein). The incidence of catheter thrombosis with clinical symptoms appears to be as high as 10 per cent (Groeger,Lucas, & Coit,1991; Wickham et al., 1992) (Box 22–1), whereas incidence of extraluminal occlusion in the absence of thrombosis could be as high as 50 per cent (Groeger et al., 1991). The signs and symptoms that are present are related to impaired blood flow and can include edema of the neck, face, shoulder or arm; prominent superficial veins; neck pain; tingling of the neck, shoulder or arm; and skin color or temperature changes. A variety of radiographic studies can be used to diagnose and treat thrombosis accurately.

Management of venous thrombosis usually involves anticoagulants or thrombolytic agents. A central or peripheral infusion of urokinase for 4 to 24 hours has been successful in many cases (Bagnall et al., 1989; Curnow et al., 1985; Fraschini et al., 1987). It is recommended that all lumens of a multilumen catheter be treated. The serum fibrinogen level should be maintained at 80 to 100 mg/dl by titration of the urokinase (Fraschini et al., 1987). Prophylactic administration of low-dose warfarin (1 mg/day) appears to prevent or decrease the incidence of thrombus formation (Bern et al., 1986; Bern et al., 1990).

BOX 22–1. *Causes of Tunneled Catheter Thrombosis*

Brown-Smith, J. K., Stoner, M. H., & Barley, Z. A. (1990). Tunneled catheter thrombosis: Factors related to incidence. *Oncology Nursing Forum, 17*(4), 543–549.

Sample: The sample consisted of two cohorts: (1) 145 tunneled catheters using 5 ml daily of 100U/ml heparin flush, and (2) 51 catheters using 10 cc/daily of 100 U/ml heparin flush. Data were also collected for an additional 98 catheters (transitional) utilizing a combination of regimen #1 and #2 from adjacent time periods. The entire sample therefore consisted of 294, 1.6 mm internal diameter, single-lumen, open-ended tunneled catheters placed in a subclavian vein. No evidence of venous thrombosis was detected at the time of placement. Ninety-five per cent of the catheters were placed at a community acute care hospital. Care of all study catheters was supervised by health care professionals at the community hospital. Seven per cent of the catheters (12/162) from flush #1 regimen, 2% (2/53) from flush #2 regimen and 7% (7/105) from the transitional regimen sample were dropped from the study, either because they were lost to follow-up or did not conform to the eligibility criteria.

All the flush #1 regimen (*n*=145) catheters were clear silastic, while those of flush #2 regimen (*n*=51) were radiopaque silastic. The transitional catheters were both clear (*n*=42) and radiopaque (*n*=56) silastic.

The two cohorts were compared for catheter-related thrombosis (CRT) incidence. All 294 catheters were evaluated for CRT incidence in relation to internal catheter tip location and chemotherapy infusate volume. As in other cohort studies, every eligible catheter from each time period was included in the investigation.

Measures: The study used a quasiexperimental cohort design with medical records providing pretest data for the first cohort. The cohorts varied in concentration of heparin and volume of flush. Flush #1 regimen utilized 5 ml of 10U/ml heparin daily (50 units total), and flush #2 regimen consisted of 10 ml 100U/ml heparin daily (1000 U daily). Descriptive statistics were used to examine the association of two variables with tunneled catheter thrombosis: internal tip location (optimal and suboptimal) and chemotherapy infusate volume (high or low). All catheters were followed for 12 months from catheter insertion date or until removal of the catheter or client death, if less than 12 months.

Findings:
- Within the two cohorts, there are a large number of categories that preclude meaningful analysis (i.e., diagnosis, chemotherapy regimen, placement surgeon).
- Variables that could be examined to compare the two cohorts at baseline include subject age and gender, catheter longevity, and chemotherapy ratio.
- No significant differences were detected between the two groups in any of these baseline characteristics.
- The incidence of CRT in the flush #1 group was 17% compared with a rate of 14% in the flush #2 group. There was no significant difference in these incidence rates.
- The CRT incidence for the transitional sample was 22% (22/98) and 18% for all VADs. Based on the similarities demonstrated among the three catheter groups, the total of 294 catheters were used together in all additional analyses.
- CRT incidence in relation to catheter tip location was examined in the 107 clients in whom radiopague catheters were placed. More thrombosis occurred in suboptimally placed catheters (62%) than in optimally placed catheters (16%). This difference was statistically significant.
- An analysis of CRT incidence related to chemotherapy infusate volume demonstrated that the incidence rates were not statistically significant between the high-volume and the low-volume groups.
- The incidence of thrombosis for side of catheter placement was compared. For the entire sample, 11% of right-sided catheters thrombosed compared with 25% rate of thrombosis in left-sided catheters. This represents a statistically significant difference.

Limitations:
- Potential threats to validity for the study include selection factors and differential catheter loss.
- Comparisons of data collected over a long period of time can involve unknown, confounding variables.
- Flush regimens warrant further study utilizing randomized designs.
- Factors of VAD care in need of investigation include CRT incidence as it relates to specific cancer diagnoses, chemotherapy regimens, infusate volumes, chemotherapy administration technique, and client coagulation history.

Infection. Sepsis is the most common complication associated with long-term central venous catheterization. Patients receiving chemotherapy are particularly susceptible to local as well as systemic infection (Lopez, 1992).

Long-term central venous catheters are designed to minimize the risk of infection compared with short-term venous catheters, but it still occurs in 2.7 to 60 per cent of devices (Groeger et al., 1991; Press, Ramsey, Larson, et al., 1984; Schuman, Winters, & Gross, et al., 1985). Infections can occur locally (on the skin), in the catheter tunnel/port pocket, or systemically. Infec-

tions are more common in patients with neutropenia (500 or less granulocytes), those with multilumen catheters, and those receiving TPN or chemotherapy.

Local infections at the catheter exit site or over the skin around the port needle insertion site usually are due to organisms on the skin such as *Staphylococcus aureus* and *Staphylococcus epidermis*. Symptoms can include redness, warmth, discomfort, and exudate. Management includes culture of the area, increased frequency of dressing changes with meticulous site care, and administration of appropriate oral or IV antibiotics (Groeger et al., 1991; Press et al., 1984; Wickham et al., 1992). The needle should be removed from an implantable port if a skin infection occurs over the port, and it should not be reaccessed until the infection clears.

Infections in the catheter tunnel or port pocket usually involve a variety of different organisms and are manifested by redness, edema, tenderness or discomfort, exudate, skin warmth, and/or fever. Appropriate IV antibiotic therapy is initiated after cultures have been taken, including aspiration of any port pocket exudate (Groeger et al., 1991; Press et al., 1984; Wickham et al., 1992). If the causative organism is identified and appropriate antiinfective therapy fails to resolve the infection, consideration should be given to removal of the device.

Systemic infections can be thrombus-related or caused by intraluminal catheter colonization with a wide variety of infective organisms. Signs and symptoms include fever and chills. Blood cultures are taken through the device as well as peripherally and can be positive either in the device or from both routes. Administration of appropriate antibacterial or antifungal therapy is initiated, and blood cultures are repeated. Failure to resolve the infection is cause to consider removal of the device (Groeger et al., 1991; Press et al., 1984).

Preventing infection is a primary concern when caring for all types of VADs. Attention should be focused on the techniques used in routine maintenance, and care should be taken to employ measures to decrease the risk of infection. A new technologic development is the VitaCuffR (Vitaphore, San Carlos, Calif.), which is impregnated with silver ions and can be attached to any catheter before insertion to provide an antimicro-

bial barrier within the catheter tunnel. It has been reported to decrease the incidence of catheter infections (Flowers, Schwenzer, & Kopel et al., 1989). Another preventive measure is the flushing of a device with a heparinized vancomycin solution instead of a heparinized saline solution. No toxicities have been noted, and no patients have experienced bacteremia due to intraluminal colonization of vancomycin-susceptible organisms, although infection due to other organisms has occurred (Schwartz, Hendrickson, & Roghmann, et al., 1990).

Other Complications. Occlusions and device malfunctions can occur for a variety of other reasons, and careful assessment of the device when occlusion occurs should always include malposition or breakage. Catheters can be kinked, compressed by tumor, compressed between the rib and clavicle, malpositioned due to patient manipulation, malpositioned for other reasons, severed, punctured, split, or separated (Gebarski & Gebarski, 1984; Lafreniere, 1991; Lum & Soski, 1989) (Box 22–2). The port access needle can be embedded in the septum, inaccurately placed into the side of the port or catheter instead of the portal housing, or become dislodged from the port and remain under the skin.

Thrombus formation can result in a retrograde flow of blood or fluid along the catheter tract, with subsequent extravasation into the subcutaneous tissues. Infusion of drugs into a severed, punctured, or separated catheter can also result in extravasation (Groeger et al., 1991). As is discussed elsewhere in this chapter, extravasation of vesicants into the chest wall or thorax can result in severe deformity, loss of function, or

---

Box 22–2. *Relationship Between Catheter Malposition and Superior Vena Cava Thrombosis*

Puel, V., Caudry, M., LeMetayer, P., Baste, J. C., Midy, D., Marsault, C., Demeaux, H., & Maire, J. P. (1993). Superior vena cava thrombosis related to catheter malposition in cancer chemotherapy given through implanted ports. *Cancer,* 72(7), 2248-2252.

Sample: The sample comprised 379 patients. The cases were selected according to the following criteria: chemotherapy actually administered at the oncology department where the study was conducted; patients followed by a senior member of the oncology staff; and exact catheter position assessable on routine postimplantation chest radiographs.

Measure: To assess the role of catheter position, the routine chest radiographs of 379 patients who received chemotherapy through venous access devices and who received follow-up between December 1985 and December 1990 were reviewed. Four groups (upper left, upper right, lower left, lower right) were defined according to the level of the catheter tip (innominate veins or upper half of the vena cava versus lower half of the vena cava or auricula) and to the side of port implantation. No attempt was made to detect occult thrombosis. Only symptomatic thromboses were accounted for in the current study; a;; were confirmed by cavagraphy. In patients complaining of shoulder or retrosternal pain, thrombosis was suspected, because this symptom was triggered or enhanced by injection into implanted device.

Findings:
- Ten patients developed symptomatic venous thrombosis (superior vena cava in 9 patients, left subclavian in 1 patient).
- A strong correlation existed between catheter position and incidence of thrombosis: upper left, 8/28 (28.6%); upper right 1/33 (3%); lower right 1/68 (1.5%); and lower left, 0/250.
- Since 1988, this study group has insisted on replacement of malpositioned catheters and has observed fewer thromboses (2/191 versus 8/188).

Conclusions:
- The current study suggests that patients with left-sided ports and catheter tips lying in the left upper part of the vena cava are at high risk for severe thrombotic complications.
- Implantation of venous access ports cannot be delegated to inexperienced surgeons and correct positioning is essential in preventing vena cava thrombosis.

death. Therefore, no vesicant therapy should ever be initiated into any device whose function is questionable (Reymann, 1993).

INFUSION PUMPS

There is a wide variety of commercially available external pumps. For infusions in the hospital, larger pumps supported on wheeled IV stands are generally utilized. These larger pumps generally have built-in monitoring capabilities and are also able to infuse large volumes of fluid (Ensminger, 1992). These pumps ensure the regulation of infusion rates and help troubleshoot problems with peripheral and central intravenous catheters. They are therefore most useful in the administration of chemotherapy infusions not given by IV push or IV sidearm methods (Fig. 22–11 for an example of an external pump).

Recently infusion pumps for delivering and controlling ambulatory continuous intravenous infusion have become widely available. These infusion pumps include battery-driven syringe and peristaltic pumps, elastomeric balloon pumps, and implantable volatile liquid vapor-powered pumps (Carlson, 1992).

Chemotherapy may be administered via an ambulatory infusion pump as a short-term infusion, over several hours to several days, or as a long-term infusion, over a day, weeks, or months. The pump allows for the safe, effective administration of chemotherapy and gives the client maximum independence and participation in self-care. Many clients may continue to work and participate in day-to-day activities with fewer restrictions while receiving a continuous infusion via the pump.

Most pumps contain a battery as the power source, and many can be adapted to function on AC electrical current as well. Other features common to most include a reservoir, a pump mechanism, a programmer, a prime mover, and a method of connecting the pump to the patient. Elastomeric pumps include a reservoir with pumping pressure and delivery tubing.

The major types of ambulatory infusion devices are external systems including peristaltic and elastomeric balloon pumps and implantable systems.

EXTERNAL AMBULATORY

These devices are used in conjunction with a vascular access device (e.g., central venous catheter, port, peripherally inserted central catheter (PICC) line, or epidural catheter).

Peristaltic Infusion Pumps. These pumps function by use of a peristaltic mechanism, which compresses the administration tubing to force fluid at a predetermined rate through the delivery pathway (Fig. 22–12). The flow is controlled and monitored by a computer microprocessor, and a variety of delivery rates and modes are available. Medication can be delivered from an internal reservoir, or some models allow connection to a standard IV bag. There are types of peristaltic infusion pumps that function by using a linear peristaltic action in which mechanical, fingerlike projections massage the tubing and move fluid along. Power sources and battery types vary. Most peristaltic action pumps

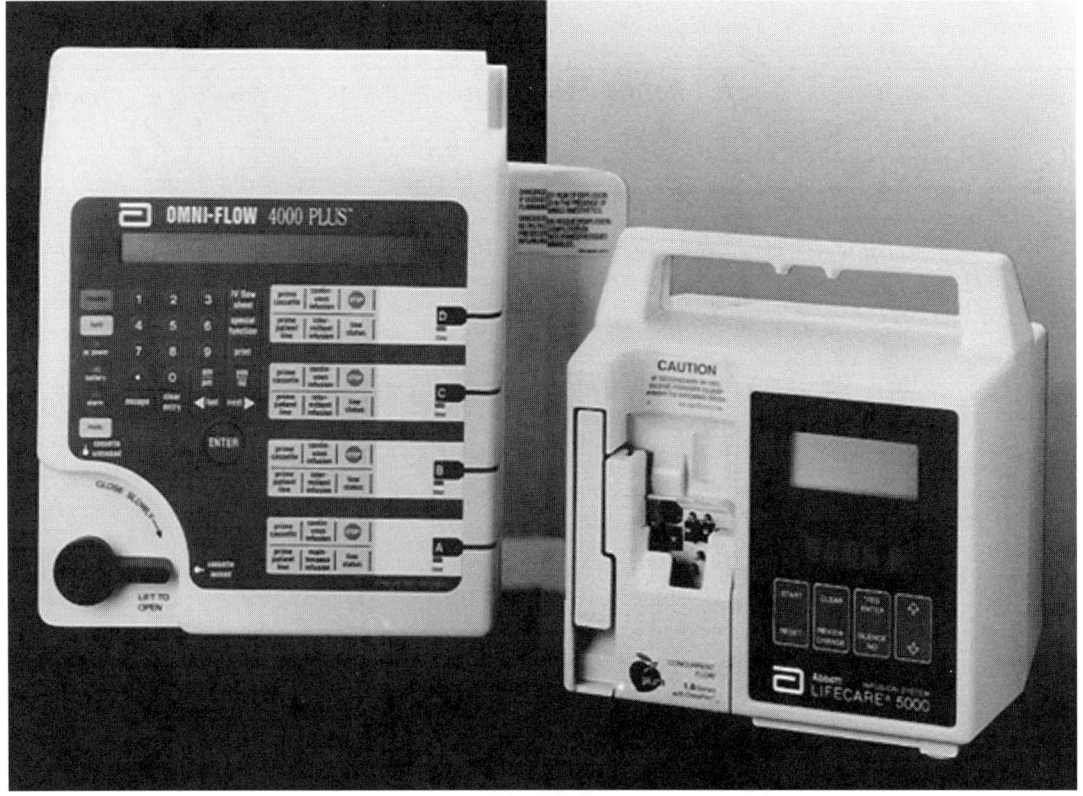

FIGURE 22–11. Omni-Flow and Plum external pumps. (Courtesy of Abbott Laboratories, North Chicago, IL.)

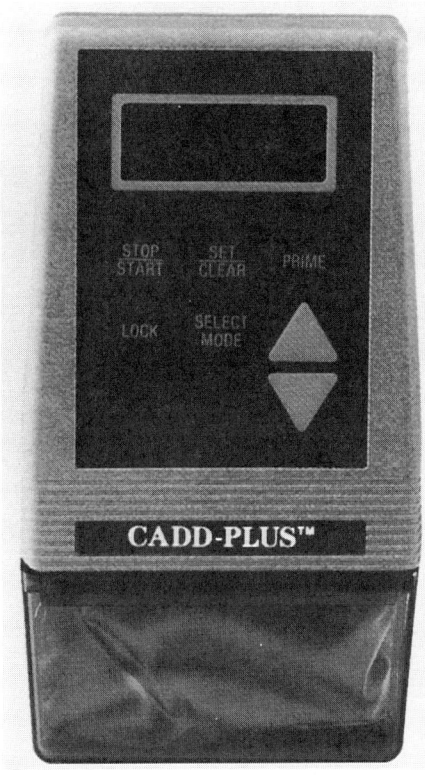
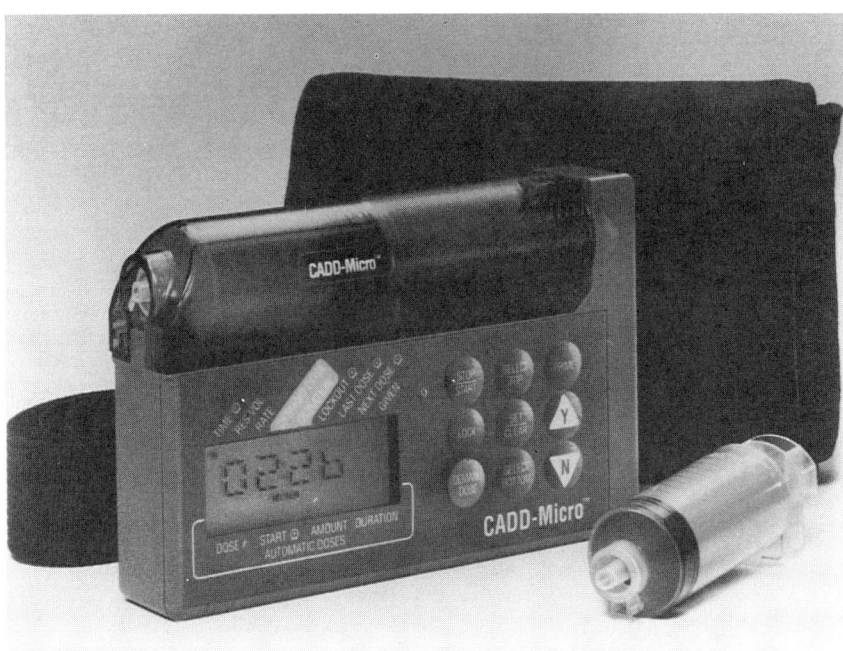

A **B**

FIGURE 22–12. Peristaltic infusion pumps. **A,** CADD-PLUS ® Pump. **B,** CADD-Micro ® pump. (Courtesy of SIMS Deltec, Inc., St Paul, MN.)

weigh between 9.7 and 16 ounces and can be worn in a pouch by the ambulatory patient.

Elastomeric Reservoirs/Pumps. Elastomeric reservoirs are lightweight, nonelectronic, disposable units that come in a variety of shapes. Each unit contains an outer shell and an inner elastomeric "balloon" reservoir. The reservoir stores medication and provides the pumping pressure to force the solution through the delivery tubing. A flow restrictor keeps fluid flowing at a constant rate. It should be noted that flow rate accuracy is calculated for normal saline solution at room temperature. Increased environmental or body temperature or contact between the fluid flow tubing and the patient's skin may increase the flow rate. A more viscous solution (e.g., 5 per cent dextrose in water) may flow at a slightly slower rate. Some models have options such as filter or a patient control module.

IMPLANTABLE INFUSION SYSTEMS

An implantable infusion system consists of a pump and an outlet catheter and has no external components. It is used for continuous regional infusion of chemotherapy or other medications (e.g., analgesics) into a localized space (see section on regional administration of chemotherapy). Two pumps currently in use, the Infusaid model 400 and the SynchroMed Infusion System, each function in a

different manner (Fig. 22–13). A third, the Therex pump, is in clinical trial.

Patient Selection and Education for External Ambulatory Infusion Pumps. Patients with ambulatory continuous infusion pumps must be able to operate the pump, handle related equipment, monitor for side effects, and troubleshoot problems that may occur. The following are criteria for selecting appropriate patients: (1) patient ability and desire to learn, (2) adequate support at home, (3) an organized teaching program, (4) follow-up by nurses with specific expertise to ensure patient compliance, (5) reliable vascular access via catheter, port, or reservoir, (6) drugs that are stable for several days at room temperature, and (7) patient desire for ambulatory or outpatient therapy (Tenenbaum & Scelsi, 1994).

Nursing Care of the Patient with an External Ambulatory Infusion Pump. Nursing care of the patient with an ambulatory infusion pump includes client assessment and education regarding medications and equipment used. The patient/significant other must be provided with information to be able to perform the following: (1) flush the catheter, (2) change IV bags or medication cassettes, and (3) understand the basic operation and maintenance of the pump. Most companies provide external pumps with written patient education information. It includes identification of all the pump parts, instructions on changing the battery, instructions on how to start and stop the

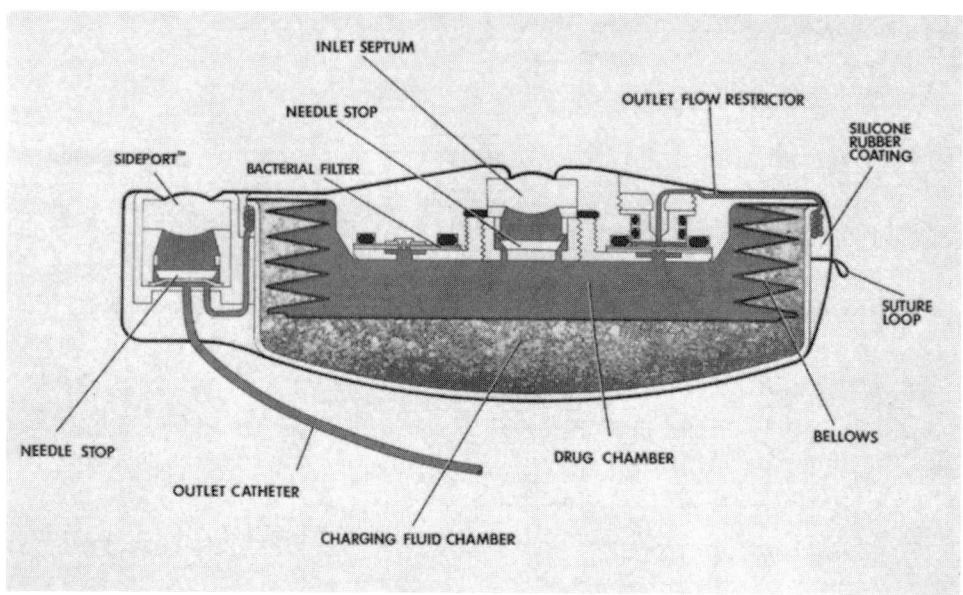

FIGURE 22–13. Infusaid model 400 implantable pump, internal view. (Courtesy of Shiley Infusiad,Inc., Norwood,MA.)

pump, explanation of what pump signals mean and a troubleshooting chart with possible actions to be taken, and information on changing the medication cassette. Nursing education to the patient and family must include chemotherapy safety in the home, cleanup of chemotherapy spills, how to flush the central venous access line in case of emergency, and emergency phone numbers to call.

PROCESS OF CHEMOTHERAPY ADMINISTRATION

INFORMED CONSENT

It is the physician's responsibility to obtain the informed consent necessary for chemotherapy administration. The purpose of consent is fivefold: (1) to explain the possible treatment-related side effects or risks, (2) explain the expected benefits and goals of therapy, (3) identify if the treatment is research-oriented, (4) explain whether alternate forms of therapy are available, and (5) let patients know of their right to refuse or withdraw from therapy (Reymann,1993). The nurse will restate the plan, teach about the side effects, and provide reassurance about the treatment plan. The purpose of a signature demonstrates the patients' understanding of the proposed therapy and their voluntary agreement to participate in the treatment.

PRETREATMENT ASSESSMENT

Before attempting venous access and drug delivery, it is important to consider that the patient has received adequate preparation about the treatment, including education, the treatment schedule, and possible side effects. Nurses must perform a thorough assessment of

the patient's understanding of the scheduled therapy. Goodman has outlined specific steps for nurses to follow before attempting venous access and delivery of the chemotherapy drug (Table 22–3).

VEIN SELECTION AND CANNULATION

Only a person knowledgeable and trained in venipuncture and chemotherapy administration should administer chemotherapy. If the patient has a preexisting peripheral IV line, nonvesicant agents may be administered through this line provided there are no signs or symptoms of phlebitis and the blood return is adequate. If the blood return is absent or sluggish or if the IV line has been in place for longer than 24 hours, a new line should be established. If the patient is receiving a vesicant agent and has a preexisting peripheral IV line in place, it is safe to use the preexisting line, provided blood return is adequate and venous irritation or phlebitis is absent. This practice is especially prudent when the patient has small, fragile veins. If any doubt exists as to the integrity of the vein, a new IV line should be established before injecting the drug. Table 22–4 lists important issues to consider in vein selection and cannulation (Goodman,1991).

DOCUMENTATION

Documentation of the administration of chemotherapy in any setting should be done in accordance with the guidelines of drug administration. Special attention should be made to record the condition of the site of the chemotherapy infusion, as extravasation is a possible occurrence and could not be noted until hours after the procedure. A sample documentation form from an ambulatory chemotherapy infusion unit is shown in Figure 22–14. Documentation forms developed should

TABLE 22–3. *Steps in Pretreatment Assessment*

1. If the patient is receiving chemotherapy for the first time, make sure he or she has received adequate instruction regarding the treatment plan and that the patient feels sufficiently informed.
2. If treatment is of an investigational nature, verify that an informed consent has been signed and that the patient feels sufficiently informed.
3. Check the drug dosage against the physician's order. The order should include the patient's name, name of the drug or drugs, frequency of administration, and, if appropriate, rate of administration. Most drug doses are based on a calculation of milligrams per kilogram or on a body surface area (m^2). Body surface area is based on a calculation of the individual's ideal body weight and height. Obesity, ascites, or other factors such as the loss of a limb are important considerations in dose adjustment. Consider whether the dose and route of administration seem appropriate for the patient.
4. Check the patient's most recent laboratory test results. The complete blood count (CBC) including the platelet count should be within normal limits or within the limits specified in the research protocol. A dose modification or treatment delay may be needed if the CBC is below the normal limits.
5. If the white blood count (WBC) is low, calculate the absolute granulocyte count (AGC) to determine the patient's ability to fight infection. The AGC is computed by multiplying the precentage of neutrophils and bands by the total WBC. When the AGC is less than 1200 cells/mm^3, treatment with myelosuppressive agents is generally not recommended. An AGC of less than 1000 cells/mm^3 is associated with a more severe risk of infection.
6. Consider the way each drug is metabolized or eliminated. If there is any clinical or laboratory evidence of organ dysfunction (e.g. liver or kidney), the pharmacokinetics or pharmacodynamics of the drug may be hindered, leading to excessive toxicity. Dose reductions or treatment delays may be warranted.
7. Consider any pretreatment antiemetics, hydration, or measures to minimize side effects.
8. Check to see if emergency equipment, including materials to manage an allergic reaction or extravasation, is available. If a vesicant is being injected, review the policy and procedure on management of an extravasation. Be prepared to manage an allergic response should one occur.
9. Ensure adequate lighting and patient comfort. A call light or similar method of communication should be available if the patient is left unattended or is receiving an infusion.
10. Review the patient's medication history, including over-the-counter drugs. Be alert to drug incompatibilities, drug interactions, and additive toxicities.

(From Goodman, M. [1991]. Delivery of cancer chemotherapy. In S. B. Baird, R. McCorkle, & M. Grant [Eds.], *Cancer nursing: A comprehensive textbook* [pp. 291–320]. Philadelphia: W.B. Saunders Co.)

include an assessment piece and be outlined in an efficient format to ease the documentation process. Always include the status of the patient at discharge, the education materials given to the patient, and the patient's comprehension of the instructions given.

PATIENT AND FAMILY EDUCATION

Although it is assumed that the cancer patient will accept treatment readily, it is important to present the treatment plan in a manner that ensures attention to his or her specific needs. This includes assessment of the patient's and family's capability to provide self-care measures needed to control chemotherapy's side effects. Likewise, assessment of their ability to recognize expected untoward reactions and report those needing immediate care should be done. Treatment education begins when options are presented to the patient and is a process that is ongoing. Time for patients' questions to be answered is critical, and the individual patient and family teaching must be specific to the treatment plan chosen. Health care personnel should outline the plan and begin to explain the chemotherapy, drug names, how they will receive them, and how often the treatment is to be given. During the initial assessment phase obtain a baseline assessment of all systems and include the patient's fears, anxieties, and coping skills. Social support is key to success, and cognitive abilities are important to assess.

The nursing role is defined by the ONS Outcome Standards of Oncology Education; Patient and Family (ONS,1982). Assessment of the patients must also include their individual responses to the diagnosis, their communication style, their ability to read and comprehend information, the family status, lifestyle, and treatment outcome expectations. Certain environmental concerns should be addressed when teaching is initiated. The area in which the teaching is being done needs to be quiet and relaxed for optimal teaching. Ask the patients about their concerns and observe the body language of the individuals for clues about their coping styles. Make sure that the process of education is documented; most settings use a checklist type of form for ease of documentation. Additional written tools may help reinforce the teaching, such as drug information sheets or cards and chemotherapy packets. Written information also helps family members who were not present when patient education is done.

ADMINISTRATION ISSUES

EDUCATIONAL PREPARATION OF THOSE WHO ADMINISTER CHEMOTHERAPY

It is the recommendation of the Oncology Nursing Society (ONS) that all antineoplastic agents be administered by professional nurses who have received specialized training in chemotherapy administration. This recommendation has been based on ensuring optimal quality of care and patient safety. ONS's Cancer Chemotherapy Guidelines provide a framework for the development of a cancer chemotherapy course. The guidelines are divided into two major parts: (1) the didactic component, which includes the basic science of chemotherapy; principles of chemotherapy administration,including preparation, handling, and administration of the drugs and nursing assessment and management principles; and documentation recommendations;

TABLE 22–4. *Issues to Consider in Vein Selection and Cannulation*

1. Selecting the proper site for venipuncture should begin with a careful, systematic assessment of all available arm veins. Extra time spent selecting the proper vein usually results in successful venous access, whereas a hurried approach can result in inadequate venous distention, vein collapse, and repeated needle insertions. Full visibility of the arms unencumbered by constricting jewelry or clothing aids in determining venous access, as does good lighting and a firm surface on which to place the arm.

2. All equipment required to achieve venipuncture and secure the line should be assembled before attempting venipuncture. Because this step requires the handling of chemotherapy drugs, in particular, the removal of Luer-Lock caps from the syringes containing the drugs, the nurse should put on any personal protective equipment at this time. The Occupational Safety and Health Administration has issued guidelines and recommendations for handling cytoxic drugs (Occupational Safety and Health Administration, 1986). It is recommended to wear a disposable gown made of lint-free, low-permeability fabric with a closed front, long sleeves, and elastic or knit cuffs. In some institutions nurses do not wear gowns to administer chemotherapy, preferring instead to wear a lab coat or uniform. Most experienced clinicians are confident in their ability to handle the drugs during administration and feel gowns are unnecessary. Nurses who are less experienced and handle or administer chemotherapy infrequently are advised to wear gowns (Miller, 1988). Wearing disposable, surgical latex gloves is unquestionably a minimal precaution that should be taken during equipment assembly and venipuncture.

3. During vein selection, the nurse should avoid venipuncture in any arm with possible or proven compromised circulation (e.g., phlebitis, lymphedema due to tumor invasion or axillary dissection, and prior trauma to veins such as drug extravasation). The risk for drug extravasation is increased when drugs are infused into an arm with evidence of superior vena cava syndrome or compromised circulation or into phlebitic veins that are inflamed and irritated.

4. To preserve venous integrity over time, the nurse should begin distally and, if possible, alternate venipuncture sites. In general, veins of the dorsum of the hand are preferred because they are easy to visualize and stabilize. However, the favored site for the administration of vesicant agents is the forearm. The forearm has more underlying muscle and tissue to protect vital nerves and provide tissue coverage, if necessary, in the event of surgical management of an extravasation. If no obvious vein is found in the forearm, the dorsum of the hand is a good second choice, followed by the wrist area. A large vein on the dorsum of the hand is preferred to a small vein in the forearm. The antecubital fossa is generally avoided for vesicant drug administration. If the drug infiltrates into this area, the signs and symptoms are difficult to detect early. Consequently, severe structural and functional problems can occur, with damage to nerves and tendons in and around the antecubital area. With the advent of numerous Vascular Access Devices (VADs), it is no longer reasonable or safe to resort to administering vesicant agents in the area of the antecubital fossa.

5. If an obvious site for venipuncture is not apparent by observation or palpation following the use of traditional methods of venous distention (tourniquet, vein percussion, heat), a colleague should be consulted before attempting venipuncture. Also, seek assistance after two unsuccessful attempts to secure adequate venous access. Consider whether the patient should have a VAD placed before receiving the drug.

6. A cannula should be selected that is appropriate for both the length of the therapy and the patient's available veins. A 25- or 23-gauge scalp vein needle (butterfly) is ideal for direct-push (two-syringe technique) or short-term infusions (30-60 minutes). A plastic thin-walled catheter is appropriate for more lengthy infusions such as for blood components or hydration regimens that last 2 to 3 hours (Knobf & Fischer, 1989). The site is sterilized by a 1-minute alcohol rub or a povidine-iodine and alcohol rub. To avoid contaminating the area, do not repalpate before venipuncture. Once the scalp vein needle enters the vein and blood return is obvious, release the tourniquet and attach a syringe of saline to the tubing. Tape the phalanges of the needle securely without obstructing the entrance of the needle. Aspirate the air from the tubing and flush the catheter with 7 to 10 ml of saline to ensure that the needle has not punctured the vein. Palpate the site gently and observe for swelling or any evidence of infiltration. The chemotherapy is injected slowly to prevent undue pressure on the vein wall. Check for blood return after every 1 to 2 ml of solution is administered. Flush the vein with 3 to 5 ml of saline between agents and with 5 to 7 ml of saline before removing the needle.

7. If the drug is to be given via the side arm of a freely running IV line, any dressing hindering visualization of the site should be removed. The size of the needle attached to the syringe must be smaller than the size of the needle in the patient's vein to permit the IV solution to drip while the drug is being injected. Otherwise fluid backs up in tubing and make this method of drug delivery no different from straight push using the two-syringe technique. Ensure a blood return by lowering the infusion bag or by aspirating blood into the tubing.

8. When injecting a vesicant into the side arm of a peripheral IV line, the line should not be infusing with the aid of an infusion pump because of the increased potential for extravasation and the impossibility of quickly reversing the direction of drug flow in the event of a possible extravasation.

9. If a drug in combination is known to be associated with rapid onset of nausea and vomiting (e.g., high-dose cyclophosphamide or cisplatin), it is generally administered last. If a vesicant is to be given along with an infusion, it should be given first in anticipation of perivenous irritation from movement during the time of the infusion. The order of administration of drugs (vesicant first or last) has associated rationale for either way, but hospital regency policy should be followed either way. Regardless of the order of the drugs, the line should be flushed with saline before changing drugs and at the end of the treatment.

10. The entire course of the vein should be visible during the injection and infusion. Observe for any evidence of vein irritation. The patient is encouraged to report any feelings of pain, itching, or burning during the treatment.

11. A vesicant agent should not be injected distal to a previous puncture site.

12. Vesicant agents should not be infused as a mini-infusion or continuous infusion into a peripheral vein. Regardless of its dilution, the drug has the potential to cause tissue destruction if infiltration occurs. Given the ease of insertion of the numerous short-term and long-term VADs, infusing a vesicant agent into a peripheral vein places the patient at unnecessary risk for drug extravasation and tissue damage. If an infusion of a vesicant is required to achieve the optimum therapeutic result, a central venous access line, as a tunneled, a nontunneled, or an implanted device, should be inserted before initiating therapy.

(From Goodman, M. [1991]. Delivery of cancer chemotherapy. In S. B. Baird, R. McCorkle, & M. Grant [Eds.], *Cancer nursing: A comprehensive textbook* [pp. 291–320]. Philadelphia: W.B. Saunders Co.)

FOX CHASE CANCER CENTER — INFUSION ROOM ORDER FORM/NURSING FLOW SHEET

FOR PHYSICIAN:

DIAGNOSIS _____ PERFORMANCE STATUS _____

ALLERGY: NONE/DRUGS _____

HEIGHT _____ WEIGHT _____ BSA_____

PROTOCOL PATIENT: NO   YES   PROTOCOL # _____ SEQ _____

CHECK COUNTS BEFORE GIVING THERAPY: NO( ) YES( ) N/A( )

WBC _____ GRAM#_____ PLT _____ MG _____

H/H _____ / _____ BUN/CREAT _____ / _____

LYTES: _____ / _____ / _____ / _____

INFORMED CONSENT (DATE) _____ ORDERS: (CYCLE #_____)

CHEMO MEDS: _____

PRE-MEDICATIONS:

DATES OF TREATMENT: _____

DOSE MODIFICATION: _____ PHYSICIAN SIGNATURE: _____

	NURSING ASSESSMENT	NURSING DOCUMENTATION
DATE		
TIME IN		
1. B/P		
2. TEMP		
3. PULSE		
4. WEIGHT		
5. MODE OF ARRIVAL		
6. PERFORM/STATUS		
7. NAUSEA		
8. VOMITING		
9. DIARRHEA		
10. CONSTIPATION		
11. STOMATITIS		
12. PAIN		
13. SKIN		
14. ALOPECIA		
15. GU		
16. NUTRITION		
17. PULMONARY		
18. NEURO-SENSORY		
19. NEUROMOTOR		
20. NEUROCORTICAL		
21. NEUROCEREBELLAR		
22. NEUROMOOD		
23. NEUROHEADACHE		
24. WBC		
25. HGB		
26. PLT		
27. OTHER _____		
28. PERIPH IV SITE		
29. BLOOD RETURN		
30. LOCAL REACTION		
31. VAD		
32. UROKINASE		
33. EDUCATION		
34. D/C STATUS		
35. MODE/DISCHARGE		
36. ACCOMPANIED BY		
37. TIME OUT		
38. RN INITIALS		

FIGURE 22–14. Documentation of chemotherapy administration. (Reproduced with permission from Fox Chase Cancer Center, Philadelphia, PA.)

Continued on next page.

	ASSESSMENT LEVEL	0	1	2	3	4
5	Mode of Arrival	Ambulatory	Wheelchair	Litter		
6	Performance Status	Normal Activity	Symptoms but Ambulatory	In Bed >50% of time	100% Bedridden	
7	Nausea	NONE	Able to eat Reasonable Intake	Intake not Sig., but can eat	No Sig. Intake	----------
8	Vomiting	NONE	1/24 hr.	2-5/24 hr.	6-10/24 hr.	>10/24 hr. or needs IV fluids
9	Diarrhea	NONE	2-3/24 hr.	4-6/24 hr. or mod. cramps	7-9/24 hr. or incontinence or sev. cramping	≤10/24 hr. or Bloody or need IV fluids
10	Constipation	NONE	MILD	MODERATE	SEVERE	ILEUS
11	Stomatitis	NONE	Painless Ulcers Erythema, or Mild Soreness	Painful Erythema Edema, or Ulcers but can eat	Painful Erythema Edema, or Ulcers cannot eat	Needs IV Fluids
12	Pain	O/NONE	1 - 3	4 - 6	7 - 10	----------
13	Skin	No change	Scattered Mucular or papular rash or Erythema-Asymptomatic	Level I with Pruritus or other assoc. symptoms	Generalized symptomatic rash	Exfoliative dermatitis or ulcerating
14	Alopecia	No Loss	Mild Loss	Pronounced or Total	----------	----------
15	GU	No Symptoms	Burning	Frequency	Loss of Control	Bleeding
16	Nutrition	Normal-no change in intake or no. wt. loss	Less intake than prior to treatment wt. within 10 lbs.	Minimal intake >10 lbs. wt. lost	No nutritional intake	----------
17	Pulmonary	NONE or No △	Intermittent Dyspnea	Dyspnea on Signif. Exertion	Dyspnea at Normal Activity	Dyspnea at Rest
18	Neuro-Sensory	NONE or No △	Mild Paresthesias	Mild or Med. Sensory loss Mod. Paresthesia	Severe Sensory loss or paresthesia interfere with function	----------
19	Neuro-Motor	NONE or No △	Subjective weakness	Mild object Weakness no impairment of function	Object Weakness with impaired function	----------
20	Neuro-Cortical	NONE	Mild Somnolence or aggitation	Moderate Somnolence or aggitation	Severe Somnolence aggitation, confusion disorientation or hallucination	Seizures toxic psychosis
21	Neuro-Cerebellar	NONE	Slight incoordination	Intention tremor dysmetria, slurred speech, nystagmus	Locomotor staxis	----------
22	Nero-Mood	No△	Mild Anxiety or Depression	Mod. Anxiety or Depression	Severe anxiety or Depression	Suicidal ideation
23	Neuro-Headache	NONE	MILD	Mod. or Severe but transient	Unrelenting and severe	----------
28	Periph IV Site indicate (R/L/further information)	Not Used	Hand	Wrist	Anticub.	Forearm
29	Blood Return	Yes	No			
30	Local reaction	NONE	PAIN	Pain & Swelling with inflammation or phlebitis	Ulceration	----------
31	VAD	NONE	H/B	Vascular Port	Implant. Pump	Other
32	Urokinase	Not Needed	Cath. Flushes Bld. Return	Cath. Flushes/no Bld. return. MD notified	Flow study Done	----------
33	Education	N/A	Verbal/understanding confirmed	Verbal/Materials understanding confirmed	Demonstration/understanding confirmed	Demonstration/materia is understanding confirmed
34	Discharge Status	Non-Sedated	Sedated	Admitted	----------	----------
35	Mode of Discharge	Ambulatory	Wheelchair	Litter	----------	----------
36	Accompanied by	Self	Other	----------	----------	----------

FIGURE 22–14. *Continued*

and (2) the clinical practicum, which includes the clinical skills the practitioner must demonstrate before being qualified to administer chemotherapy (ONS, 1988). The successful development and evaluation of a course based on these guidelines has been reported by Welch-McCafferty (Brown & Hogan, 1990; Welch-McCafferty, 1985).

Formal chemotherapy certification programs are common today, and they vary in length from several days to several weeks. Most commonly the course involves components of classroom teaching or self-learning modules. Programs should include a posttest to verify learning and some type of supervised clinical demonstration of the skill, such as a skills checklist.

Since antineoplastic agents have potentially life-threatening side effects, this formal education process needs to be instituted, and those attending should receive documentation of participation. Additional information that may help design a program specific to your agency's needs can be found (Belcher,1987; Brown & Hogan, 1990; Fernsler, 1987; Fischer, Knobf, & Durivage, 1993; Itano,1987; McMillan, 1987; Volker, 1987). Chemotherapy can be administered in a variety of settings today, including the hospital, home, or a physician's office. Regardless of the setting, the nurse is considered qualified only after adequate educational preparation has taken place.

SAFETY AND HANDLING

Cancer chemotherapy drugs are toxic to all cells, and the carcinogenic, teratogenic, and mutagenic nature of these agents has been well documented in animal models and patients (Stellman & Zoloth, 1986). In 1979, mutagenic activity was first found in the urine of nurses involved in cancer chemotherapy (Falck et al., 1979). Since then, additional studies have been conducted to measure changes in the complete blood count (Jochimsen et al., 1988); to measure sister chromatid exchanges in lymphocytes (Jordan et al., 1986; Ostereicher, Stephan, & Glatzel, 1990; Sardas, Gok, Karakaya, 1991; Sarto et al., 1990); to measure urinary thioethers (Burgaz, Ozdamar, Karakaya, 1988; Sarto et al., 1990); and to screen for urinary mutagens (Caudell et al., 1988; Venitt et al., 1984). Additionally, case studies report a variety of symptoms related to exposure to cytotoxic drugs. These symptoms include blurred vision, skin discoloration, sloughing or necroses of the skin, allergic responses, mucus membrane irritation, dizziness, liver damage, gastrointestinal tract problems, renal problems, and headaches (Curran, 1989; McDiarmid, 1990; McDiarmid & Egan, 1988; OSHA,1986; Zimmerman et al., 1981). Two studies showed possible reproductive hazards for health care workers handling cytotoxic agents and not using protective equipment (McDonald et al., 1988; Selevan,Lindbohm, & Hornung, 1985). Even though the results have been conflicting and inconclusive and the degree and magnitude of risk are difficult to ascertain, all the literature supports the fact that a risk does exist. These drugs represent an occupational hazard, and guidelines for handling chemotherapy should be followed.

Exposure to chemotherapy may occur during drug preparation, administration, or disposal. Health care employees potentially at risk for exposure include pharmacists, nurses, physicians, and housekeeping and maintenance personnel. It is believed that the extent of health risk to employees who handle chemotherapy drugs is a combination of exposure time, amount and method of exposure, and class of drug (Goodman,1991). Inhalation, absorption, and ingestion are the main routes of exposure. Effects of exposure may be short- or long-term. Short-term effects are usually seen within hours or days afterward, and examples include dermatitis or hyperpigmentation. Long-term effects, although still inconclusive, include chromosomal abnormalities, carcinogenicity, and partial alopecia.

In 1983, guidelines were developed by the Occupational Safety and Health Administration (OSHA), the Oncology Nursing Society (ONS), and the American Society of Hospital Pharmacists (OSHA,1986). The purpose of these guidelines is to protect health care personnel, patients, and the environment from unnecessary exposure to these potentially hazardous substances (Mayer,1992; National Study Commission on Cytotoxic Exposure,1984, ONS,1988). The recommendations are aimed at minimizing the risks of absorption through direct skin contact and inhalation. These recommendations and guidelines are offered as standards to be incorporated into the institution's policies and procedures and are summarized in Table 22–5 (Goodman,1991).

It remains the responsibility of all who handle chemotherapy to remain cognizant of the latest information regarding safety and handling. More research is needed to evaluate the risk as well as the issues involved in implementing these guidelines. Nurses are often the central health care workers involved in developing policies and procedures for chemotherapy drug administration and as a result need to possess all the latest information as it becomes available.

Each institution has certain responsibilities with respect to the administration of chemotherapy agents. It is responsible to define agency policies and procedures consistent with professional and federal recommendations to minimize risks to personnel; to orient all agency personnel who may come in contact with antineoplastic agents about the potential risks and the agency policies and procedures; to review their policies and procedures at periodic intervals; and to include compliance policies and procedures as a component of the agency quality assurance program (Tenenbaum, Ellsworth-Wolk, & Hawthorne, 1994).

In 1991, occupational health personnel of a health maintenance organization in Southern California formed a Regional Occupational Health Committee (ROHC) to examine safety and health issues related to occupational hazards of chemotherapy (Parillo,1994). The group concluded that the OSHA work practice guidelines, although specific for areas that address personal protective equipment, training, and waste disposal, were not specific in the section addressing medical surveillance. The ROHC decided to examine the medical surveillance of health care workers who handle cytotoxic drugs and provide an appropriate, consistent, occupational surveillance program at 10 of their regional facilities. The ROHC identified five areas of concern that needed to be addressed when developing the regional surveillance procedure. These concerns and recommendations are as follows:

1. Which health care workers will be covered by this procedure? Those identified were those who administer or prepare the drugs and anyone who might have an accidental exposure.
2. What baseline data will be obtained? A physical examination, liver function tests, creatinine, CBC,

TABLE 22–5. *Guidelines for Safe Handling and Disposal of Antineoplastic Agents*

A. Drug Preparation
1. All antineoplastic drugs should be prepared by specially trained individuals in a centralized area to minimize interruptions and risk of contamination
2. Drugs are prepared in a class II biologic safety cabinet (vertical laminar air-flow hood) with vents to the outside, if possible. The blower is left on 24 hours a day, 7 days a week. The hood is serviced regularly according to the manufacturer's recommendation.
3. Eating, drinking, smoking, and applying cosmetics in the drug preparation area are prohibited.
4. The work surface is covered with a plastic absorbent pad to minimize contamination. This pad is changed immediately in the event of contamination and at the completion of drug preparation each day or shift.
5. The prescribed drug is prepared using aseptic technique according to the physician's order, other pharmaceutic resources, or both.
6. Disposable surgical latex unpowdered gloves are used when handling the drugs. Gloves should be changed hourly or immediately if torn or punctured.
7. A disposable long-sleeved gown made of lint-free fabric with knitted cuffs and a closed front is worn during drug preparation.
8. A thermoplastic (Plexiglas) face shield or goggles and a powered air-purifying respirator should be used if a biologic safety cabinet is not available.
9. Because exposure can result when connecting and disconnecting intravenous (IV) tubing, when injecting the drug into the IV line, when removing air from the syringe or infusion line, and when leakage occurs at the tubing, syringe, or stopcock connection, priming of all IV tubing is carried out under the protection of the hood.
10. Other measures to guard against drug leakage during drug preparation include venting the vial and using large-bore needles, Luer-Lock fittings, and sterile gauze or sponge around the neck of the vial during needle withdrawal. Aerosolization may also be minimized by attaching an aerosol protection device (CytoGuard, Bristol-Myers) to the vial of drug before adding the diluent.
11. Once reconstituted, the drug is labeled according to institutional policies and procedures; the label should include the drug's vesicant properties and antineoplasstic drug warning.
12. Antineoplastic drugs are transported in an impervious packing material and are marked with a distinctive warning label.
13. Personnel responsible for drug transport are knowledgeable of procedures to be followed in the event of drug spillage.

B. Drug Administration
1. Chemotherapeutic agents are administered by registered professional nurses who have been specially trained and designated as qualified according to specific institutional policies and procedures.
2. Before administering the drugs, the nurse ensures that informed consent has been given and clarifies any misconception the patient might have regarding the drugs and their side effects.
3. Appropriate laboratory results are evaluated and found to be within acceptable levels (e.g., complete blood count, renal and liver function).
4. Measures to minimize side effects of the drugs are carried out before drug administration (e.g., hydration, antiemetics and antianxiety agents, and patient comfort).

(Data from Oncology Nursing Society, 1988; Sotaniemi, Sutinen, Arranto, Sutinen, Sotaniemi, Lehtola, & Pelkonen, 1983, U.S. Department of Labor, 1986.)

and cancer risk factor questionnaire were recommended.
3. What periodic monitoring will be necessary, and at what interval will it be conducted? Three questions related to cytotoxic drug exposure were developed, and if the answer was yes to any question, it required follow-up; the monitors were to be done annually.
4. How will exposure incidence be handled? Was exposure ingested, inhaled, or absorbed? If so, a physical examination and repeat laboratory tests would be obtained.
5. What documentation forms will be necessary and where will the collected information be maintained? A form was developed, and it was determined it would be filed in the health care worker's records and the occupational health department.

Implementation of this program has been met with varied success, as all administrators at these facilities are not convinced of the need. The author's facility has

implemented the form for 1 full year, and it has been found to take less time than the previous ones. The ROHC continues to work for consistency in medical surveillance. Greater use of protection was seen during drug preparation than drug administration, and the larger and high-volume hospitals implemented more of these recommendations and the private offices and home care, the least (Parillo,1994).

Regardless of site, reasonable policies and procedures should be developed and implemented that will cover the relative risk to people and the environment. Research is still needed to evaluate the issues involved in implementing the guidelines, and it is the responsibility of all those who handle chemotherapy to remain cognizant of the latest information (see Box 22–3 for a chapter's results with safe handling practices).

EXTRAVASATION

Extravasation is the infiltration or leakage of an intravenous chemotherapeutic agent into the local tis-

TABLE 22–5. *Guidelines for Safe Handling and Disposal of Antineoplastic Agents* Continued

5. An appropriate route for drug administration is ensured according to the physician's order.
6. Personal protective equipment is worn, including disposable latex surgical gloves and a disposable gown made of a lint-free, low-permeability fabric with a closed front, long sleeves, and elastic or knit closed cuffs (optional).
7. The work surface is protected with a disposable absorbent pad.
8. The drug or drugs are administered according to established institutional policies and procedures.
9. Documentation of drug administration, including any adverse reaction, is made in the patient's medical record.
10. A mechanism for identification of patients receiving antineoplastic agents is established for the 48-hour period following drug dispensing.
11. Disposable surgical unpowdered latex gloves and a disposable gown are worn when handling body secretions such as blood, vomitus, or excreta from patients who received chemotherapy drugs within the previous 48 hours.
12. In the event of accidental exposure, remove contaminated gloves or gown immediately and discard according to official procedures.
13. Wash the contaminated skin with soap and water.
14. Flood an eye that is accidentally exposed to chemotherapy with water or isotonic eye wash for at least 5 minutes.
15. Obtain a medical evaluation as soon as possible after exposure and document the incident according to institutional policies and procedures.

C. Drug Disposal
1. Regardless of the setting (hospital, ambulatory care, or home), all equipment and unused drugs are treated as hazardous and are disposed of according to the insitution's policies and procedures.
2. All contaminated equipment including needles are disposed of intact to prevent aerosolization, leaks, and spills.
3. All contaminated materials used in drug preparation are disposed of in a leak-proof, puncture-proof container with a distinctive warning label and are placed in a sealable 4-mil polyethylene or 2-mil polypropylene bag with appropriate labeling.
4. Linen contaminated with bodily secretions of patients who have received chemotherapy within the previous 48 hours is placed in a specially marked laundry bag, which is then placed in an impervious bag that is marked with a distinctive warning label.
5. In the event of a spill, personnel should don double surgical latex unpowdered gloves; eye protection; and a disposable gown made of a lint-free, low-permeability fabric with a closed front, long sleeves, and elastic or knit closed cuffs.
6. Small amounts of liquids are cleaned up with gauze pads, whereas larger spills (more than 5 ml) are cleaned up with absorbent pads.
7. Small amounts of solids or spills involving powder are cleaned up with damp cloths or absorbent pads.
8. The spill area is cleaned three times with a detergent followed by clean water.
9. Broken glassware and disposable contaminated materials are placed in a leak-proof, puncture-proof container and then placed in a sealable 4-mil polyethylene or 2-mil polypropylene bag and marked with a distinctive warning label.
10. Contaminated reusable items are washed by specially trained personnel wearing double surgical unpowdered latex gloves.
11. The spill should be documented according to established institutional policies and procedures.

sue surrounding the administration site, which may result in local tissue damage. Chemotherapy drugs are one group of drugs that may cause tissue damage or extravasation. Drugs that are associated with severe necrosis when extravasated are known as vesicants, whereas those associated with less severe burning or inflammation are known as irritants. A vesicant is a medication that has the potential to cause cellular damage or tissue destruction if leakage into subcutaneous tissue occurs. Sloughing of tissue, prolonged pain, infection, and/or loss of mobility are potential injuries caused by the extravasation of vesicants (Montrose,1987). In contrast, an irritant is a medication that may produce pain and inflammation at the administration site or along the path of the vein by which it is administered. The reaction caused by an irritant is often classified as a flare reaction. A flare is a raised, red streak along the course of a vein, which may be mistaken for extravasation. Table 22–6 lists the known vesicants and irritants.

Once extravasation occurs, tissue damage of varying degrees ensues. The actual clinical course of tissue destruction is variable depending on the drug itself, the concentration, the amount extravasated, and the specific measures utilized to manage the infiltration. The tissue damage may appear initially to be minimal as a result of the indolent course of most extravasations. Gradually, after 3 to 5 days, the area appears inflamed and is painful to the touch, providing evidence of cellular destruction. After 12 to 14 days, the actual extent of damage is usually evident with frank ulceration, demarcation, and eschar formation (Montrose, 1987). The damage to underlying structures (tendons and nerves) may lead to functional impairment. Infection and cellulitis can result in progressive tissue damage and limb dysfunction.

The reported incidence of inadvertent chemotherapy extravasation ranges from 1 to 6 per cent of all toxic reactions to chemotherapy (Goodman,1991, Ignoffo & Friedman, 1980; Larsen, 1982; Laughlin, Landeen, & Habal,1979; Montrose,1987). Differences in occurrence may be related to inexperience or lack of knowledge of the signs and symptoms of extravasation. Current recommendations are that these drugs be administered according to established policies and procedures by persons who are specially trained in chemotherapy drug administration (ONS,1992). The factors that affect the risk of extravasation are (1) the skill of the practitioner, (2) the condition of the vein, (3) the drug administration technique, (4) the order of

---

Box 22–3. *Safe Handling Practices*

Mahon,S. M., Casperson,D. S., Yackzan,S., et al.(1994). Safe handling practices of cytotoxic drugs: The results of a chapter survey. *Oncology Nursing Forum, 21*(7), 1157–1165.

Purpose: To describe how nurses from a local Oncology Nursing Society (ONS) chapter implement Occupational Safety and Health Administration (OSHA) guidelines for handling cytotoxic drugs in their individual practices and to identify barriers to implementing these guidelines.

Method: Mailed survey consisting of 48 questions with demographic questions as well.

Sample: 103 nurses, 83 of whom handle cytotoxic drugs. Mean years in oncology nursing, 7.5.

Findings:
- Subjects used protective equiment when preparing and administering drugs but type of equipment and frequency of use did not specifically meet OSHA guidlelines.
- Rates of compliance with guidelines were better with management of spills and disposal of equipment.
- Verbal instruction for patients and families were given but very few provided written instructions.
- Barriers identified included lack of time, problems with availability, and concerns about patient reactions.

Conclusions:
- Barriers must be overcome.
- Better, safe practices must be incorporated to ensure nurses' safety.
- More education of family members of patients receiving these drugs.

TABLE 22–6. *List of Known Vesicants and Irritants*

GENERIC NAME (BRAND NAME)	DESCRIPTION
Amsacrine (AMSA-PD)	Vesicant
Carmustine (BiCNU, BCNU)	Irritant
Cisplatin (Platinol)	Irritant
Dacarbazine (DTIC-Dome)	Irritant
Dactinomycin (Actinomycin-D)	Vesicant
Daunomycin (Daunorubicin, Cerubidine)	Vesicant
Doxorubicin (Adriamycin, Rubex)	Vesicant
Epirubicin (Pharmorubicin)	Vesicant
Etoposide (VePesid)	Irritant
Idarubicin (Idamycin)	Vesicant
Mechlorethamine, Nitrogen Mustard (Mustargen)	Vesicant
Mitomycin-C (Mutamycin)	Vesicant
Paclitaxel (Taxol)	Irritant
Plicamycin (Mithracin)	Irritant
Streptozocin (Zanosar)	Irritant
Teniposide (V,-26, Vumon)	Irritant
Vinblastine (Velban, Velbe, Velsar)	Vesicant
Vincristine (Oncovin, Vincasar)	Vesicant
Vindesine (Eldesine)	Vesicant

vesicant administration, (5) the site of venous access, and (6) the use of a preexisting IV line. Table 22–7 summarizes strategies that are effective in the prevention of extravasation.

The signs and symptoms of extravasation can be pain, stinging, and burning, but these symptoms cannot always be present. Nursing observation during vesicant administration is crucial. If swelling or diffuse induration, resistance to intravenous flow, or the absence of a blood return are present, a thorough investigation must be done. Also, the presence of a blood return will not guarantee an infiltration has not occurred, because the needle may extend partially through the posterior wall of the vein and could allow for a subtle leakage of a vesicant. Any slight change in appearance of the area or tissue surrounding the insertion site is sound reason to stop the administration of the agent and restart it in another vein. Additionally, if no change is observed in the area around the insertion site but a patient complains of pain, stinging, or burning, this needs to be investigated further.

Whenever extravasation involving a vesicant agent is suspected, the administration of the agent should be discontinued first. Aspiration of the tubing contents for any remaining drug is done immediately. If a peripheral catheter has been used, it should be removed. If a vascular device was in use, surgical or radiologic evaluation of the catheter or implanted device is recommended.

The use of antidotes in extravasation is controversial. Each health care agency should develop a procedure for antidote usage. It has been recommended that application of warm compresses be used for extravasation by vinca alkaloids to allow for dispensation of the agent. For agents such as doxorubicin, cold compresses are recommended to cause vasoconstriction to localize the drug that leaked into the tissue. If a peripheral site was used, elevation of the affected extremity should be done as soon as possible. Use of the limb should not be restricted, and activity should be resumed with a scheduled follow-up (Dorr, 1994).

TABLE 22–7. *Extravasation of Vesicant Antineoplastic Agents: Preventive Strategies*

RISK FACTOR	PREVENTIVE STRATEGY	RATIONALE
Skill of the Practitioner	Chemotherapy administration only done by registered nurses who are specifically trained and supervised.	Procedures for management of extravasation vary according to the drug infiltrated. Certain drugs (streptozocin or BCNU) may cause a burning sensation during infusion, which is normal. However, it is abnormal and indicative of a problem if burning occurs during infusion of drugs such as doxorubicin and mitomycin.
	No attempts by practitioner to do procedures beyond his or her expertise. Practitioners are skillful in venipuncture. Practitioners are knowledgeable of the signs and symptoms of extravasation and drug therapy. Practice is based on institutional policies and procedures that are routinely updated to meet the changinng standards and methods of practice.	Procedures change rapidly. Techniques need to be learned and mastered before assuming responsibility for administration of chemotherapy. The definition of customary care in the community helps dictate standard of practice.
Condition of the Veins • Small fragile veins • Access limited owing to axillary surgery, vein thrombosis, prior extravasation • Long-term drug therapy • Multiple vein punctures	Use conventional methods for venous distention such as heat and percussion. Assess all available arm veins. Assess veins in a methodical fashion, taking time to select the most appropriate vein. If practitioners do not feel confident in their ability to cannulate a person's veins successfully, they should seek the assistance of a colleague. After attempting one or two injections without success, the practitioner should seek the assistance of a colleague before trying again. A patient who consistently needs two or more attempts to secure venous access should be considered a candidate for a VAD. The time to place a VAD is before an extravasation, not after.	Risk of vesicant drug seepage exists with repeated venipuncture. Multiple vein injections lead to thrombosis and limited availability. Before the advent of vascular access devices (VADs), multiple venous injections to administer a drug might have been accepted as the only method of drug administration. This is no longer the case. Instead, treatment should be delayed until a VAD can be placed. Most VADs can be used immediately or within 24 to 48 hours, so delay in drug therapy is not usually an issue.
Drug Administration Technique	Vesicant agents are never given as continuous infusions into a peripheral vein.	The risk of infiltration of a vesicant from a peripheral vein infusion is great owing to the following: 1. Blood return is not assessed frequently. 2. The longer the infusion, the greater the possibility of needle dislodgment. 3. The patient can move the extremity, which could dislodge the intravenous (IV) cannula. 4. Even a small amount of vesicant can cause tissue damage. 5. Infiltration can be subtle and difficult to detect until a large volume has infiltrated. 6. The patient may be sedated from an antiemetic and be unable to report sensations associated with extravasation. 7. The pump forces drug into the tissues.
	If peripheral line in on a controlled infusion pump, disconnect pump before injection of chemotherapy. When a vesicant is to be given as a continuous infusion, the drug should be infused via an externally based central venous catheter whenever possible.	When an implanted port already exists, the patient is taught to check the needle three times a day to ensure placement during continuous infusion of a vesicant. The incidence of vesicant drug extravasation from ports used for continuous infusion is well documented and presents a risk to be avoided, if possible.
	Vesicant agents are most commonly administered using the two-syringe technique or through the side port of a free-flowing peripheral intravenous line.	The two-syringe technique allows for proper assessment of blood flow and resistance in the vein. A scalp vein needle causes minimal vein irritation.

Continued on following page.

TABLE 22–7. **Extravasation of Vesicant Antineoplastic Agents: Preventive Strategies** Continued

RISK FACTOR	PREVENTIVE STRATEGY	RATIONALE
Drug Administration Technique— cont'd	**Two-Syringe Technique** 1. Select an appropriate vein. 2. Begin a new intravenous line using a scalp vein needle (25 or 23 gauge). 3. Access vein using a single approach. 4. Flush line with 8 to 10 ml of saline. Assess for brisk, full blood return and any evidence of infiltration. Check for swelling at the site, redness or pain, and lack of blood return. 5. Once access is assured, switch to syringe of chemotherapy. 6. Dilute drugs according to the package insert. 7. Inject drugs slowly and with minimal resistance. 8. Assess for blood return every 1 to 2 ml of infusion. 9. Irrigate with 3–5 ml of saline between each drug and 8–10 ml at the completion of the infusion of the drug or drugs.	A subtle leak can be caused by accidentally piercing the vein before accessing it; avoid searching for a vein with repeated approaches. Increasing the dilution increases the time it takes to administer the drug, thus increasing risk of infiltration. The speed of the injection is determined by the resistance in the vein. Resistance will vary depending on the size of the needle used.
	Side-arm Technique 1. Ensure proper venous access site. The IV fluid should be additive free. 2. Cannula used to access the vein should be at least a 20 gauge to ensure an adequate blood return and fluid flow. 3. Secure cannula but do not obstruct entrance site. 4. Pinch off tubing and assess for blood return. 5. Test the vein with 50 to 100 ml to ensure an adequate and swift drip on infusion. 6. With IV fluid continuing to drip, slowly inject vesicant into IV line. 7. Do not allow vesicant to flow backwards. 8. Do not pinch off tubing except to assess for blood return. 9. Assess for blood return every 1 to 2 ml of injection. 10. Flush scalp vein needle with saline at the completion of injection.	The main rationale for the side-arm technique is the added dilution of the drug by the continuous drip of the IV fluid. Common pitfalls: 1. Not using a large enough cannula for a brisk infusion of infusate. 2. Vesicant backs up into IV line. 3. Intravenous line has to be pinched off to inject vesicant, which defeats the purpose. 4. Clinician tends to take eyes off of the site of drug infusion to watch fluid drip more than with two-syringe technique.
Order of Vesicant Drug Administration *Note:* Sequencing is probably unimportant. The most critical issue is adequately testing the vein with saline (8–10 ml) before administering any drug (vesicant or nonvesicant).	Give vesicant first. Give vesicant between two nonvesicants. Give vesicant last.	Vascular integrity decreases over time. Practitioner's assessment skills are most acute initially. Patient may be more sedated from antiemetic and less able to report changes in sensation at infusion site as time goes on. Chemotherapy is irritating to the veins. Nonvesicants are presumed to be less irritating than vesicants. Because venous spasm occurs early during the injection, it is less likely to be confused with pain or extravasation if vesicant is given last. It is assumed that because the vein tolerated the nonvesicants, it will also tolerate the vesicant.
Site of Venous Access Choosing the best vein	VADs, including tunneled catheters, implanted ports, and nontunneled central venous catheters, are indicated when patients have small, frail veins and are in need of long-term indefinite chemotherapy, continuous infusion or vesicant drugs, or both.	VADs are important options for patients with poor venous access. Externally based catheters are ideal for continuous infusion of vesicant chemotherapeutic agents because the risk of extravasation is very minimal.

(From Goodman, M. [1991]. Delivery of cancer chemotherapy. In S. B. Baird, R. McCorkle, & M. Grant [Eds.], *Cancer nursing: A comprehensive textbook* [pp. 291–320]. Philadelphia: W. B. Saunders Co.)

TABLE 22–7. *Extravasation of Vesicant Antineoplastic Agents: Preventive Strategies* Continued

RISK FACTOR	PREVENTIVE STRATEGY	RATIONALE
Site of Venous Access—cont'd	Although a VAD is a good way to prevent extravasation, it is not indicated just because someone is receiving a vesicant drug.	Expert technique and a knowledgeable clinician are the most cost-effective and safe means of administering vesicant drugs.
	Peripheral access is optimal in the large veins of the forearm, especially the posterior basilic vein. After these, the metacarpal veins of the dorsum of the hand are easy to access and stabilize. The veins over the wrist are risky because of potential damage to tendons and nerves should extravasation occur. *Note:* A large straight vein over the dorsum of the hand is preferable to a smaller vein of the forearm.	Veins in the forearm are large and adequately supported by surrounding tissue. Adequate tissue exists around veins to provide coverage and promote healing should a problem occur.
	The antecubital fossa is to be avoided for vesicant drug administration. If the antecubital fossa appears to be the only vein available for access, the patient needs an access device. Hold chemotherapy—insert VAD.	The area is dense with tendons and nerves. Seepage of a vesicant can be subtle and go unnoticed. Damage here can result in loss of structure and function. Risking extravasation and subsequent tissue damage is not worth the temptation to give "just one more treatment" before considering other options. There is no evidence that delaying chemotherapy for 24 hours in selected cases is detrimental to the overall outcome.
	Avoid administering chemotherapy in lower extremities.	Risk for thrombosis is increased when chemotherapy is given in lower extremities.
Using a Preexisting IV Line	Do not use a preexisting peripheral intravenous line if any of the following are true: 1. The IV cannula was placed more than 12 hours earlier. 2. The site is reddened, swollen, or sore, or there is evidence of infiltration. 3. The site is over or around the wrist. 4. Evidence of blood return is sluggish or absent. 5. The IV fluid runs erratically and the IV seems positional. If the IV fluid runs freely; the blood return is brisk and consistent; and the site is without redness, pain, or swelling, then there is no reason to inflict unnecessary pain by injecting the patient again.	It is unreasonable to disregard the potential for a perfectly adequate venous access line because it was not started by the person administering the vesicant drug. Our ability to assess the vein and evidence of blood return should be adequate to ensure the practitioner of an adequate and safe venous access.
	Prior dressings must be carefully removed over the cannula insertion site to fully visualize the vein during injection of the vesicant agent.	Dressings and tape can severely impede both visually and tactilely an assessment for an extravasation.

COMMON VESICANT DRUGS AND ANTIDOTE USE

Anthracyclines. The anthracyclines classified as vesicants are doxorubicin, daunomycin, and dactinomycin. Doxorubicin has a reported extravasation incidence from 0.5 per cent (Laughlin,Landeen, & Habal,1979) to 6.5 per cent (Bailock,Howser, & Hubbard,1979). Doxorubicin can also cause a local venous flare reaction in to up 3 per cent of cases (Etcubanas & William, 1974; Souhami & Feld, 1978; Vogelzang,1979). The flare reaction is a local erythematous streaking and inflammation that can continue up to 30 minutes after the drug infusion

and is accompanied by itching along the course of the vein. The flare reaction does not warrant any local therapy, because it resolves in 20 to 30 minutes.

A severe ulceration can result from the infiltration of doxorubicin or daunomycin in the subcutaneous tissues. Symptoms, which include severe pain and swelling, are usually immediate in onset. Major changes in tissue occur within 3 days and can persist up to 12 weeks or longer (Coleman, Wlaker, & Didolkar,1983).

Doxorubicin skin reactions can also "recall" or synergize with prior radiotherapy-induced skin toxicity, prior doxorubicin therapy, or both (Dorr, 1994). Thus, repeated doxorubicin injections can sometimes cause previously healed extravasation sites to react with pain, swelling, and rarely, tissue necrosis, even though the drug being administered is in a vein distal to the prior site (Dorr, 1994).

A variety of pharmacologic approaches have been evaluated to treat doxorubicin and daunomycin extravasations. A true antidote does exist, DHM3, but it is not available for clinical use (Averbach et al., 1985, 1986; Averbach et al.,1988). A common therapy has been the local injection of corticosteroids such as hydrocortisone. However, corticosteroid therapy does not have a clear pharmacologic rationale for being an anthracycline antidote (Cohen,1979; Luedke,Kennedy, & Rietschel,1979; Petro et al., 1979), and in high concentrations these corticosteroids can do damage locally (Dorr, Alberts, & Chen,1980).

Dimethyl sulfoxide (DMSO) has been evaluated as a topical antidote and has shown complete protection from doxorubicin in the pig and rat model (Desai & Teres 1982; Svingen et al.,1981). Olver et al. (1988) showed an efficacy rate of 98 per cent with 1.5 ml DMSO applied topically every 6 hours for 14 days.

Topical cooling or the immediate application of ice for 20 to 60 minutes four to six times a day is effective for doxorubicin extravasation (Dorr, Alberts, & Stone,1985; VanSloten-Harwood & Bachur, 1987). Additional accumulation of drug concentration to the infiltrated site is limited by vasoconstriction as a result of the cold application. Another study of the treatment of tissue extravasation of antitumor agents reported that ice applied for 20 minutes four times a day for 3 days as well as elevation of the limb resulted in 89 per cent of patients requiring no further therapy (Larsen,1985).

If there is residual pain and swelling at the site 2 weeks after the event, surgical follow-up is recommended (Larsen, 1982). Wide local excision may be needed, because pharmacologic studies have documented prolonged local retention of high concentrations of the drug (Dorr et al.,1989; Garneck et al.,1981; Sonneveld,Wasserman, & Nooter,1984). The development of an open ulcer is a very late stage of extravasation development and should not be used as criterion for surgical or reconstructive therapy.

Mitomycin-C. Mitomycin-C is a severe vesicant that can cause delayed extravasation symptoms in patients. Delay of tissue toxicity for up to 3 months following extravasation of mitomycin-c is noted (Aizawa & Tagami,1987; Wood & Ellerhorst-Ryan, 1984), and there are reports of reactions occurring distally to the site of injection (Johnston-Early & Cohen, 1981). Ulcers from mitomycin extravasation are painful and enlarge slowly over weeks. Sunlight can aggravate the lesions, and surgical debridement is necessary once lesions appear.

Ineffective antidotes tried experimentally include corticosteroids, sodium thiosulfate, hyaluronidase, and vitamin E (Dorr, 1994). Also, neither topical cooling nor topical heating was found to be effective. Topical DMSO provided partial to complete protection in the mouse model (Dorr et al., 1986) and in three clinical cases (Alberts & Dorr, 1991). A 99 per cent solution was applied to the site every 6 hours for at least 14 consecutive days (Alberts & Dorr, 1991).

Vinca Alkaloids. The vinca alkaloids can cause serious soft-tissue ulcers. Pain is usually noted first, followed by cellulitis, phlebitis, and/or local inflammation over 3 to 5 days. In a matter of weeks, the blisters can progress to necrotic ulcers. Sometimes these lesions can heal. Effective antidote measures include immediate warm compresses for 30 to 60 minutes, then alternately off and on every 15 minutes for 1 day. Hyaluronidase has been shown to be highly effective at preventing ulcers in the mouse model (Dorr & Alberts, 1985). Ineffective antidotes include cooling, leucovorin, diphenhydramine, hydrocortisone bicarbonate, and vitamin A (Dorr, 1994).

Etoposide and teniposide, although classified as irritants rather than vesicants, produce local venous reactions similar to the vinca alkaloids. The local reactions can consist of phlebitis, urticaria, or erythema. In small ulcers produced in mice, the enzyme hyaluronidase was found to be completely effective to prevent these lesions from progressing (Dorr & Alberts, 1983).

Cisplatin. Cisplatin rarely produces extravasation necrosis, but it has been noted when large amounts of highly concentrated cisplatin solutions are extravasated. An effective cisplatin antagonist is sodium thiosulfate (Howell & Taetle, 1980). Probably no therapy is needed for cisplatin extravasation unless a large volume (>20 ml) of concentrated solution (>0.5 mg/ml) is extravasated.

Mechlorethamine. Mechlorethamine (nitrogen mustard) is a severe vesicant and if extravasated causes immediate severe pain and protracted necrosis. These lesions require treatment, as they can widen and have delayed healing for months if untreated (Chait & Dinner, 1975). The preferred antidote is one installation of sterile isotonic sodium thiosulfate in a one sixth molar concentration. This antidote binds with and inactivates the nitrogen mustard by forming nontoxic thioethers that can then be excreted in the urine (Chait & Dinner, 1975). Neither heat nor cool applications aid in mechlorethamine ulcer healing.

NURSING ROLE

Extravasations can occur from physiologic reasons as well as poor venipuncture technique. Elderly patients with fragile, small-diameter veins are at high risk as well as those patients with superior vena cava syndrome or those who have obstructed venous drainage due to axillary surgery. A previously irradiated site is also at an increased risk. A nurse must gather information during initial assessment, as all these factors are important to consider prior to chemotherapy administration. It is recommended to avoid the antecubital fossa and the wrist and hand. In the antecubital fossa it is difficult to see extravasation as it occurs. It is also recommended to not puncture the same vein repeatedly. The optimal site is the forearm.

Nurses are often the first to recognize extravasation, and therefore it is important to have a treatment protocol written and approved. A kit or tray for extravasation treatment should be available (Table 22–8). Acute observation and prompt treatment can prevent severe necrosis. Surgical/plastics consultation may be needed for debridement and repair. Recovery from extravasation can be long and painful, so it is most important to recognize extravasation early and treat it aggressively.

SETTINGS

Patient selection for the setting for chemotherapy administration is important to the success of treatment and follow-through. Such selection necessitates knowledgeable assessment of the patients' performance status and their support systems at home. Continual reassessment of the patients and their environment should be maintained throughout the treatment period. Today chemotherapy administration can be safely done in the hospital, the office or outpatient setting, or in the patient's home. Certain criteria must be in place for the transition to either outpatient or home, but certainly many obstacles have been met, and chemotherapy administration is no longer limited to a hospital stay.

OUTPATIENT, OFFICE/AMBULATORY

The outpatient setting, compared with an inpatient facility, is designed to provide the comfort of familiar surroundings and the convenience of fewer administrative procedures. Patients thus encounter the same staff,which allays anxieties while developing relationships with the caregivers. Treatment is such that ambulatory/office settings promote a more normal routine, since the patients' schedules are planned to accommodate work, family obligations, and social events. Prolonged waiting for laboratory results and chemotherapy preparation should be eliminated by the assignment of a staff member to perform both such clinical functions. The costs generally are less than inpatient hospital charges.

Modern outpatient facilities have been developed to accommodate the needs of patients and their families during chemotherapy administration. Many facilities provide reclining chairs or venipuncture chairs with armrest, movable overhead lighting, video libraries, and refreshments (Behrend & Sklaroff, 1993). A call light should be accessible for patient needs. Creating an environment that is conducive to patient care thus has become an important focal point for these facilities.

Treatment rooms can be arranged for single or multiple patients. Patient privacy is preferable; at the least a curtain should be provided in group treatment areas. Diversions such as televisions, audio headsets, movie videos, magazines, as well as educational material that describes the management of side effects common to cancer treatment should be available. The facility must be wheelchair- and stretcher-accessible and have an appropriate number of well-placed lavatories. Appropriate containers should be provided for chemotherapy waste. Outpatient chemotherapy limits hospitalization costs and decreases direct treatment costs to patients. An important aspect to outpatient treatment is quality of life. Hopefully, quality of life is improved by being able to return home after the treatment and resume a more normal routine.

HOME INFUSION PROGRAMS

Home care has evolved to a very sophisticated level due to chronicity of cancer and the transition of care from hospital to home. Technologic advances have made home chemotherapy administration more available. Complex infusion therapy is now commonly self-administered by a family member in the home. Ambulatory infusion pumps and VADs have paved the way for home infusions. High technologic services and agencies have been created for home infusion therapy. Today, almost everything given via simple IV push to complex multidrug infusions is being done at home. Palmer and Myers reported their experiences giving intensive consolidation chemotherapy to adults with

---

TABLE 22–8. *Suggested Contents of an Emergency Extravasation Tray (Kit)*

- Disposable latex gloves (talc-free, 0.007–0.009″ thick)
- Needles—18 gauge; 25 gauge; filter needles (2 each)
- Syringes—tuberculin; 3 cc; 5 cc; 10 cc; 20 cc
- One-inch paper tape; 2 sterile 4x4s; alcohol wipes; 4 Telfa pads; hot pack; cold pack
- Local anesthestic—lidocaine, ethyl chloride
- Diluent—1 each: 30 ml bacteriostatic 0.9% sodium chloride injection; 30 ml bacteriostatic water.
- Hydrocortisone or other steroid cream—1% topical
- Antidotes—10% sodium thiosulfate
  –Hydrocortisone solution (100-ml vial)
  –Sodium bicarbonate (100-ml vial)
  –Dexamethasone 4mg/ml
  –Dimethyl sulfoxide 50–100% topical
  –Hyaluronidase 150 U (store in refrigerator)
- Extravasation record
- Policy and procedure for extravasation management

(Reprinted with permission from Tenenbaum,L., Ellsworth-Wolk,J., & Hawthorne,J. [1994]. Preparation, administration, and safe disposal of chemotherapeutic agents. In L. Tenenbaum, [Ed.], *Cancer chemotherapy and biotherapy: A reference guide*. Philadelphia: W.B. Saunders Co.)

acute lymphoblastic leukemia in an outpatient setting and in the home (Palmer & Myers, 1990). This successfully demonstrated that complex treatments could be given in the home. Some drugs would not be appropriate to administer at home, for example, those with a high anaphylactic potential, those that require intense hydration, or those that cause severe myelosuppression.

Obvious benefits of receiving treatments in the home include a better quality of life; patients may keep their jobs more easily, spend more time with their family in their own environment, maintain a normal lifestyle, be more involved in decision making about their care, and feel less vulnerable (Brown, 1985; Lampert,Schulmeister, & Bodnar,1993). Nurses in home care need skills in performing venipuncture and accessing implanted devices and in the administration of chemotherapy. The agency has to have policies and standards for chemotherapy administration, and many use ONS's standards as the basic criteria. Laboratory and pharmacy support must be available to successfully administer chemotherapy at home. Policies and procedures must follow standards of nursing practice and should include a quality assurance program. Informed consent has to include that the patient agrees to accept therapy in a nonmedical setting. There must be a 24-hour telephone service available for patients who have problems. Table 22–9 illustrates the contents of a home chemotherapy administration kit contents (Parker, 1992). Also, a spill kit needs to be available in the home, and the nurse needs to teach the patient and family how to use it.

Careful assessment criteria must be in place for home infusion patients. Table 22–10 lists criteria for

TABLE 22–9. *Contents of a Home Chemotherapy Administration Kit*

SUPPLIES	MEDICATIONS
Normal Saline	Heparin flush
10 cc vials	Anaphalaxsis:
500 cc bags	Benadyl 50 mg IV
Needles	Benadryl 50 mg po
Regular 20 gauge	Hydrocortisone 50 mg IV
Noncoring for access	Epinenphrine 1 : 1000 IV
devices	Extravasation Antidote
Butterfly 20 gauge	Hyaluronidase (Wydase)
Syringes	for vinca alkaloids
5 cc	
10 cc	
Heparin Lock Caps	
Intravenous Tubing	
Alcohol pads	
Tourniquet	
Latex Gloves	
Mask	
Airway	
Cold Pack	
Puncture proof container	
4 × 4 gauze	
Band aids	

(Reproduced with permission from Parker, G. G. [1992]. Chemotherapy administration in the home. *Home Health Care Nurse, 10* [1], 32.)

TABLE 22–10. *Criteria for Patient Selection for Home Infusion Therapy*

- The patient's diagnosis and therapy is appropriate for home infusion therapy.
- The patient is clinically stable.
- Consistent infusion access is available.
- The patient or family/caregiver demonstrates proficiency and competency in maintaining the access device, drug admixture and storage, infusion techniques, therapy monitoring, and recognizing potential side effects of the therapy prior to unsupervised drug infusion in the home.
- The home has adequate space and facilities for storage of drugs, infusion supplies, and equipment.
- A telephone is available in the home, or one is easily accessible.
- The patient and caregiver are motivated and desire to have therapy in the home setting.
- The patient understands the therapy and rationale (informed consent).

(Reproduced with permission from Lampert,A. I., Schulmeister,L, & Bodnar,K. [1993]. Home infusion therapy. In P.C. Buschel & C.H. Yarbro [Eds.], *Oncology nursing in the ambulatory setting: Issues and models of care* [p. 261]. © 1993 Boston: Jones and Bartlett. Reproduced with permission.)

patient selection for home infusion therapy. A patient's medical history has to be documented by the nurse. Those patients with multiple, chronic, unstable health problems should not be considered. Many agencies require the patient to have received the drug the first time in a hospital or office setting, There needs to be no history of anaphylaxsis, and the patient needs to *not* be historically noncompliant. Supports must be in place, there has to be a qualified caregiver, and family and patients must understand all instructions. Electricity, plumbing, and telephone services are needed in the home as well.

Patient education includes first assessing the patient's disease process, then assessing the patient's ability to understand instructions. Then the nurse must evaluate the family and the environment. Patients need an initial overview of the treatment plan and then written step-by-step instructions. Return demonstrations by the patient may be useful. Be aware of the resources available, and document all activities. Communication and coordination are crucial to successful management of patients outside an acute care setting. The nurse must also provide education about infection control and waste management. Universal precautions need to be implemented. It is recommended that contaminated waste should be labeled and incinerated at a high temperature by a waste management company. Timing of supplies must be well coordinated, and patients should be instructed to keep supplies out of reach of pets and children. Patient education must include the planned treatment regimen, the schedule, the method in which drug will be given, signs and symptoms to report, information on posttreatment care, and information about the 24-hour resource program.

Reimbursement for Home Infusion Therapy. Insurers consider on a case-by-case management approach. If there is a significant cost savings, insurers may change an initial denial to a claim. Medicare currently does reimburse for home infusion on a limited basis, and investigational/clinical trial studies usually are not covered. The cost-effectiveness of home infusion therapy has been documented (Balinsky & Nesbitt,1989; Brown,1985; Lampert et al.,1993; Smith,1986).

A well-coordinated effort is essential between caregivers to make chemotherapy administration successful in any setting. Physicians and nurses must work together collaboratively, and communication must remain open and free-flowing between settings. This type of collaboration will enable achievement of a common goal, making it possible for patients to resume as much of their normal lives as possible while undergoing treatment.

SUMMARY

As cancer therapies have evolved to higher levels of sophistication, the nurses' level of expertise has needed to develop at the same pace. Any examiniation of the numerous ways of administering chemotherapy as well as the various types of chemotherapy administration, the settings in which it is administered, and the types of patients to whom it is administered demonstrates the degree of precision that is demanded of oncology nurses. The education nurses must receive has to keep pace with the demands of this continually growing field. The ever-changing nature of cancer care also lends itself easily to innovation, which provides endless opportunity for nurses to make a significant impact on the lives of patients and each other.

REFERENCES

Aizawa,H., & Tagami,H. (1987). Delayed tissue necrosis due to mitomycin-c. *Acta Dermato-Venereologica (Stockholm)* 67,364–366.

Alberts,D. S., Dorr,R. T. (1991). Case report:Topical DMSO for mitomycin-c induced skin ulceration. *Oncology Nursing Forum, 19,*693–695.

Almadrones, L.,Godbold,J., Raaf,J., et al. (1987). Accuracy of activated partial thromboplastin time drawn through central venous catheters. *Oncology Nursing Forum, 14*(2),15–18.

Almadrones,L., & Yerys,C. (1990). Problems associated with the administration of intraperitoneal therapy using the port-a-cath system. *Oncology Nursing Forum, 17*(1),75–80.

Anderson, N., & Lokich, J. J. (1994). Cancer chemotherapy and infusional scheduling. *Oncology, 8*(5), 99–116.

Atkinson, J. B., Bagnall, H. A., & Gomperts, E. (1990). Investigational use of tissue plasminogen activator (t-PA) for occluded central venous catheters. *Journal of Parenteral & Enteral Nutrition, 14,* 310–311.

Averbach,S. D., Boldt,M., Gaudino,G., et al (1988). Experimental chemotherapy-induced skin necrosis in swine:Mechanistic studies of anthracycline antibiotic toxicity and protection with a radical dimer compound. *Journal of Clinical Investigation, 81,*142–148.

Averbach,S. D., Gaudino,G., Koch,T. H. et al (1985). Radical dimer rescue of toxicity and improved therapeutic index of adriamycin in tumor-bearing mice. *Cancer Research, 45,*6200–6204.

Averbach,S. D., Gaudino,G, Koch,T. H., et al (1986). Doxorubicin-induced skin necrosis in the swine model:Protec-

tion with a novel radical dimer. *Journal of Clinical Oncology, 4*(1),88–94.

Bagnall, H. A.,Gomperts,E., Atkinson,J. B., et. al. (1989). Continuous infusion of low-dose urokinase in the treatment of central venous catheter thrombosis in infants and children. *Pediatrics, 83*(6),963–966.

Bailock,A. L., Howser,D. M., & Hubbard,S. M. (1979). Nursing management of adriamycin extravasation. *American Journal of Nursing, 137,*94–96.

Balinsky, W., & Nesbitt, S. (1989). Cost-effectiveness of outpatient parental antibiotics: A review of the literature. *American Journal of Medicine, 87,*301–305.

Barofsky, I. (1984). Therapeutic compliance and the cancer patient. *Health Education, 10,* 43–56.

Barton, J. C., & Poon, M. C. (1986). Coagulation testing of hickman catheter blood in patients with acute leukemia. *Archives of Internal Medicine, 146,*2165.

Behrend, S. W., & Sklaroff, R. B. (1993). The evolving profile of the office oncology nurse. In P. Buschel, & C. H. Yarbro, (Eds.), *Oncology nursing in the ambulatory setting.* Philadelphia: Jones and Bartlett Publishers.

Belcher, A. E. (1987). Developing continuing education programs in cancer nursing: Defining content and methods. *Oncology Nursing Forum,14,*65–67.

Berman, A.,Chisolm,L., DeCarvalho,M., et al. (1993). Programmed instruction:Cancer chemotherapy intravenous administration. *Cancer Nursing, 16*(2), 145–160.

Bern, M. M.,Bothe,A. Jr, Bistriani,B., et al. (1986). Prophylaxis against central venous thrombosis with low-dose warfarin. *Surgery,99*(2),216–221.

Bern, M. M.,Lokich,J. J., Wallach,S. R., et al.(1990). Very low doses of warfarin can prevent thrombosis in central venous catheters—randomized prospective trial. *Annals of Internal Medicine, 112,* 423–428.

Bogliolo,G. V., Lerza,R., Bottino,G. B., et al (1991). Regional pharmacokinetic selectivity of intrapleural cisplatin. *European Journal of Cancer, 27,*839–842.

Breaux, C. W. Jr.,Duke,D., Georgeson,K. E., et al. (1987). Calcium phosphate crystal occlusion of central venous catheters used for total parental nutrition in infants and children: Prevention and treatment. *Journal of Pediatric Surgery,22*(9),829–832.

Brenner,D. E. (1986). Intraperitoneal chemotherapy: A review. *Journal of Clinical Oncology, 4*(7),1135–1147.

Broviac, J. W., Cole, J. J., & Schribner, B. H. (1973). A silicone rubber atrial catheter for prolonged parenteral alimentation. *Surgical Gynecologic Obstetrics, 136,* 602.

Brown, J. (1985). Ambulatory services: The mainstay of cancer nursing care. *Oncology Nursing Forum, 12,*57–59.

Brown, J. K., & Hogan, C. M. (1990). Chemotherapy. In S. L. Groenwald, M. H. Frogge, M. Goodman, & C. H. Yarbro (Eds.), *Cancer nursing: Principles and practice* (2nd ed.), (pp. 230–283). Boston: Jones and Bartlett.

Brown-Smith,J. K., Stoner,M. H., & Barley,Z. A. (1990). Tunneled catheter thrombosis: Factors related to incidence. *Oncology Nursing Forum 17*(4),543–549.

Burgaz,S., Ozdamar,Y. N., & Karakaya,A. E. (1988). A signal assay for the detection of genotoxic compounds:Applications on the urines of cancer patients on chemotherapy and of nurses handling cytotoxic drugs. *Human Toxicology 7,*557–560.

Burke, M. B. (1991). Principles of chemotherapy administration and drug delivery systems. In M. B. Burke, G. M. Wilkes, D. Berg, C. K. Bean, & K. Ingwersen (Eds.), *Cancer chemotherapy: A nursing process approach* (pp. 375–423). Boston: Jones and Bartlett.

Camp-Sorrell,D. (1990). Intra-arterial chemotherapy infusion. *Oncology Nursing Forum, 17*(1),103–105.

Carlson, R. W. (1992). Continuous intravenous infusion chemotherapy In M. C. Perry (Ed.), *The chemotherapy sourcebook* (pp.232–249). Baltimore: Williams & Wilkins.

Caudell,K. A., Vredevor,D. L., Dietrick,M. F., et al. (1988). Quantification of urinary mutagens in nurses during potential antineoplastic agent exposure: A pilot study with concurrent environmental and dietary control. *Cancer Nursing*, 11,41–50.

Cervera,M., Dolz, M., Herreaz,J. V., et al (1989). Evaluation of the elastic behavior of central venous PVC, polyurethane and silicone catheters. *Physical Medicine Biology*, 34,177.

Chait,L. A., & Dinner,M. I. (1975). Ulceration caused by cytotoxic drugs. *South African Medical Journal*, 49,1935–1936.

Cohen,M. H. (1979). Amelioration of adriamycin skin necrosis: An experimental study. *Cancer Treatment Reviews*, 63(6),1003–1004.

Coleman,J. J., Wlaker,A. P., & Didolkar,M. S. (1983). Treatment of adriamycin skin ulcers: A prospective controlled study. *Journal of Surgical Oncology*, 22,129–135.

Curnow, A.,Idowu,J.,Behrens,E., et al.(1985).Urokinase therapy for Silastic catheter induced intravascular thrombis in infants and children. *Archives of Surgery*,120(11), 1237–1240.

Curran, C. F. (1989). Accidental exposure to fluoruracil (Letter to the editor). *Oncology Nursing Forum*, 16,468.

Decker,M. D., & Edwards, K. M. (1988). Central venous catheter infections. *Pediatric Clinics of North America*, 35,579.

Dedrik,R. L., Myers,C. E., Burgay,P. M., et al. (1978). Pharmacologic rationale for peritoneal drug administration in the treatment of ovarian cancer. *Cancer Treatment Reviews*, 62,1–9.

DeGraff, P. W., Mellema, M. M., tenBokkel Huinink, W. W., et al. (1988). Complications of Tenckhoff catheter implantation in patients with multiple previous intraabdominal procedures for ovarian carcinoma. *Gynecologic Oncology*, 29,43–49.

Desai, M. H., & Teres, D. (1982). Prevention of doxorubicin-induced skin ulcers in the rat and pig with dimethyl sulfoxide (DMSO). *Cancer Treatment Reviews*, 66(6), 1371–1374.

Doane, L. S. (1993). Administering intraperitoneal chemotherapy using a peritoneal port. *Nursing Clinics of North America*, 28(4), 885–897.

Doane, L. S., Fischer, L. M., & McDonald, T. W. (1990). How to give intraperitoneal chemotherapy. *American Journal of Nursing*, 58–64.

Dorr, R. T. (1994). Pharmacologic management of vesicant chemotherapy extravasations. In R. T. Dorr, & D. D. Von Hoff (Eds.), *Cancer chemotherapy handbook* (2nd ed., pp. 109–118) Norwalk, CT: Appleton & Lange.

Dorr, R. T., & Alberts, D. S. (1983). Skin ulceration potential with therapeutic anticancer activity for epipodophyllotoxin commercial diluents. *Investigational New Drugs*, 1,151–159.

Dorr, R. T., & Alberts, D. S. (1985). Vinca alkaloid skin toxicity: Antidote and drug disposition studies in the mouse. *Journal of the National Cancer Institute*, 74,113–120.

Dorr, R. T., Alberts, D. S. & Chen, H. S. G. (1980). The limited role of corticosteroids in ameliorating experimental doxorubicin skin toxicity in the mouse. *Cancer Chemotherapy and Pharmacology*, 5,17–20.

Dorr, R. T., Alberts, D. S., & Stone, A. (1985). Cold protection and heat enhancement of doxorubicin skin toxicity in the mouse. *Cancer Treatment Reviews*, 69(4), 431–437.

Dorr, R. T., Dordal, M. S., Koenig, L. M., et al (1989). High doxorubicin tissue levels in a patient experiencing extravasation during a four day infusion. *Cancer* 64(12), 2462–2464.

Dorr, R. T., & Fritz,W. L. (1980). *Cancer chemotherapy handbook*. New York: Elsevier North-Holland, Inc.

Dorr, R. T., Soble, M., Liddal, J. D., et al (1986). Mitomycin-c skin toxicity studies in the mouse. *Journal of the National Cancer Institute*, 74,113–120.

Dworkin, M. J., & Allen-Marsh, T. G. (1991). Regional infusion chemotherapy for colorectal hepatic metastasis—where is it going? *Cancer Treatment Reviews*, 18,213–224.

Ensminger, W. D. (1992). Intraarterial therapy. In M. C. Perry (Ed.), *The chemotherapy sourcebook* (pp. 256–271). Baltimore: Williams & Wilkins.

Ensminger, W. D. (1993). Regional chemotherapy. *Seminars in Oncology*, 20(1),3–11.

Etcubanas, E., & William, J. R. (1974). Uncommon side effects of adriamycin (NSC-123127). *Cancer Chemotherapy Reports*, 58(6),757–758.

Falck, K., Groh, P., Sorsa, M., et al (1979). Mutogenicity in urine of nurses handling cytostatic drugs (Letter). *Lancet*, 1(8128),1250–1251.

Fernsler, J. (1987). Developing continuing education programs in cancer nursing. An overview. *Oncology Nursing Forum*, 14,59–60.

Fischer, D. S., Knobf, M. T., & Durivage, H. J. (1993). The cancer chemotherapy handbook (4th ed.). St. Louis: Mosby-Yearbook, Inc.

Flowers, R. H. III,Schwenzer,K. J., Kopel,R. F., et al. (1989). Efficacy of an attachable subcutaneous cuff for the prevention of intravascular catheter-related infection. *Journal of the American Medical Association*, 261(6),878–883.

Fraschini, G.,Jadeja,J., Lawson,M., et al. (1987). Local infusion of urokinase for the lysis of thrombosis associated with permanent central venous catheters in cancer patients. *Journal of Clinical Oncology*, 5(4),672–678.

Garneck, M., Israel, M., Knetarpal, I. V. et al (1981). Persistence of anthracycline levels following dermal and subcutaneous adriamycin extravasation (Abstract) *Proceedings of the American Society of Clinical Oncology*, 22,173.

Gebarski, S. S., & Gebarski, K. S. (1984). Chemotherapy port "twiddler's syndrome": A need for preinjection radiography. *Cancer*, 54, 38–39.

Goodman, M. (1991). Delivery of cancer chemotherapy. In S. B. Baird, R. Corkle, M. Grant, (Eds.), *Cancer nursing: A comprehensive textbook* (pp. 291–320). Philadelphia: W. B. Saunders Co.

Graham, D. R.,Keldermans,M. M., Klemm,L. W., et al. (1991). Infectious complications among patients receiving home intravenous therapy with peripheral, central or peripherally placed central venous catheters. *American Journal of Medicine*, 91(3B),9S–100S.

Groeger, J. S.,Lucas, A. B., & Coit, D. (1991). Venous access in the cancer patient. In V. T. DeVita, S. Hellman, & S. A. Rosenberg (Eds.), *Principles and practice of oncology* (pp. 1–14). Philadelphia: Lippincott.

Gullatte, M. M. (1989). Managing an implanted infusion device. *Registered Nurse, January*, 45–49.

Hadaway, L. C. (1990). An overview of vascular access devices inserted via the antecubital area. *Journal of Intravenous Nursing*, 13, 297–306.

Hickman, R. O.,Buckner,C. O., Clift,R. A., et al.(1979). A modified right atrial catheter for access to the venous system in marrow transplant recipients. *Surgical Gynecologic Obstetrics*, 148(6),871–875.

Hoff, S. T. (1987). Concepts in intraperitoneal chemotherapy. *Seminars in Oncology Nursing*, 3(2),112–117.

Hoff, S. T. (1991). Nursing perspectives on intraperitoneal chemotherapy. *Journal of Intravenous Nursing, 14*(5),309–314.

Holmes, B. C. (1994). Administration of cancer chemotherapy agents. In R. T. Dorr & D. D. Von Hoff (Eds.), *Cancer chemotherapy handbook* (2nd ed., pp. 58–94). Norwalk, CT: Appleton & Lange.

Horattas, M. C., Wright, D. J., Fenton, A. H.,et al (1988). Changing concepts of deep venous thrombosis of the upper extremity—report of a series and review of the literature. *Surgery, 104*,561.

Howell, S. B., & Taetle, R. (1980). Effect of sodium thiosulfate on cisdichlorodiammineplatinum (II) toxicity and antitumor activity in Lizio leukemia. *Cancer Treatment Reviews, 64*(4/5),611–616.

Hubbard, S. M., & Seipp, C. A. (1985). Administration of cancer treatments: Practical guide for physicians and oncology nurses. In V. T. DeVita, S. Hellman, & S. A. Rosenberg (Eds), *Cancer principles and practice of oncology* (pp.2189–2222). Philadelphia: Lippincott.

Hurtubise, M. R.,Bottino,J. C., Lawson,M.,et al.(1980). Restoring the patency of occluded central venous catheters. *Archives of Surgery, 115*(2),212–213.

Ignoffo, R. J., & Freidman, M. A. (1980). Therapy of local toxicities caused by extravasation of cancer chemotherapeutic drugs. *Cancer Treatment Reviews 7*,17–27.

Itano, J. (1987). Developing continuing education programs in cancer nursing: Developing educational objectives. *Oncology Nursing Forum, 14*,62–65.

Jenkins, J. (1985). Managing intraperitoneal chemotherapy:A medical, nursing and personal challenge. *Seminars in Oncology, 12*(3),97–100.

Jochimsen, P. R., Corder, M. P., Lachenbruch, P. A., et al (1988). Preparation and administration of chemotherapy:Haematological consequences for hospital based nurses. *Medical Toxicology, 3*,59–63.

Johnston-Early, A., & Cohen, M. (1981). Mitomycin-c induced skin ulceration remote from infusion site. *Cancer Treatment Reviews, 65*,5–6.

Jordan, D. K., Jochimsen, P. R., Lachenbruch, P. A., et al (1986). Sister chromatid exchange analysis in nurses handling antineoplastic drugs. *Cancer Investigations, 4*, 101–107.

Kaplan, R. A., Markman, M., Lucas, W. E., et al (1985). Infectious peritonitis in patients receiving intraperitoneal chemotherapy. *American Journal of Medicine, 78*,49–53.

Keizer,J. H., & Pinedo,H. M. (1985). Cancer chemotherapy: Alternate routes of drug administration—a review. *Cancer Drug Delivery, 2*,147–169.

Kilbridge, K. L., & Kantoff, P. (1994). Intravesicular therapy for superficial bladder cancer: Is it a wash? *Journal of Clinical Oncology, 12*(1),1–4.

Klopp, G. T., Alford, T. C., Bateman, J., et al (1950). Fractionated intra-arterial cancer chemotherapy. *Annals of Surgery, 132*,811–832.

Koeller,J. M., & Fields,S. (1994). Alternate routes of chemotherapy administration. In R. T. Dorr, & D. D. Van Hoff (Eds.), *Cancer chemotherapy handbook* (2nd ed., pp. 95–108). Norwalk, CT: Appleton & Lange.

Lafreniere, R. (1991). Indwelling subclavian catheters and a visit with the "inched-off sign." *Journal of Surgical Oncology, 47*, 261–264.

Lamm, D. L. (1992). Long-term results of intravesical therapy for bladder cancer. *Urologic Clinics of North America, 19*(3), 573–580.

Lampert, A. I., Schulmeister, L., & Bodnar, K. (1993). Home infusion therapy. In P. B. Buschel, & C. H. Yarbro (Eds.), *Oncology nursing in the ambulatory setting* (pp. 248–272). Boston: Jones and Bartlett.

Larsen, D. L. (1982). Treatment of tissue extravasation of antitumor agents. *Cancer, 49*,1796–1799.

Larsen, D. L. (1985). What is the appropriate management of tissue extravasation by antitumor agents? *Plastic and Reconstructive Surgery, 75*,397–402.

Laughlin, R. A., Landeen, J. M., & Habal, M. B. (1979). The management of inadvertent subcutaneous adriamycin infiltration. *American Journal of Surgery, 137*,408–412.

Lawson, M.,(1982). The use of urokinase to restore the patency of occluded central venous catheters. *American Journal of Intravenous Therapeutic Clinical Nutrition, 9*, 29–31.

Levine, A. M.,Richardson,J. L, Marks,G., et al. (1987). Compliance with oral drug therapy in patients with hematologic malignancy. *Journal of Clinical Oncology,5*(9),1469–1476.

Lokich, J. L., Bothe, A., Benotti, P., et al (1985). Complications and management of implanted venous access catheters. *Journal of Clinical Oncology, 3*,710.

Lopez, M. J. (1992). Central venous access for chemotherapy. In M. C. Perry (Ed.), *The chemotherapy sourcebook* (pp. 780–797). Baltimore: Williams & Wilkins.

Luedke, D. W., Kennedy, P. S., & Rietschel, R. L. (1979). Histopathogenesis of skin and subcutaneous injury induced by adriamycin. *Plastic and Reconstructive Surgery, 63*(4),463–465.

Lum, P. S., & Soski, M. (1989). Management of malpositioned central venous catheters. *Journal of Intravenous Nursing, 12*, 356–365.

Mahon, S. M., Casperson, D. S., Yackzan, S., et al (1994). Safe handling practices of cytotoxic drugs:The results of a chapter survey. *Oncology Nursing Forum, 21*(7),1157–1165.

Malloy, J. (1991). Administering intraperitoneal chemotherapy a new approach. *Nursing '91, January*,58–62.

Markman, M. (1985). Melphalan and cytarabine administered intraperitoneally as single agents and combination intraperitoneal chemotherapy with cisplatin and cytarabine. *Seminars in Oncology, 12*(3),33–37.

Markman, M. (1986). Infectious considerations in intracavitary chemotherapy. *Infect Surg, 5*,304–306.

Masoorli, S., & Angeles, T. (1990). PICC lines: The latest home care challenge. *Registered Nurse, January*, 44–51.

May, G. S., & Davis, C. (1988). Percutaneous catheters and totally implantable access systems: A review of reported infection rates. *Journal of Intravenous Nursing, 11*, 97–103.

Mayer, D. (1992). Hazards of chemotherapy. *Cancer Supplement, 70*(4), 988–992.

McDiarmid, M. A. (1990). Medical surveillance for antineoplastic agents handlers. *American Journal of Hospital Pharmacy, 47*, 1061–1065.

McDiarmid, M., & Egan, T. (1988). Acute occupational exposure to antineoplastic agents. *Journal of Occupational Medicine, 30*,984–987.

McDonald, A. D., McDonald, J. C.,Armstrong, B., et al (1988). Congenital defects and work in pregnancy. *British Journal of Industrial Medicine, 45*,581–588.

McMillan, S. C. (1987). Developing continuing education programs in cancer nursing: Program evaluation. *Oncology Nursing Forum, 14*,67–70.

Montrose, P. A. (1987). Extravasation management. *Seminars in Oncology Nursing, 3*(2),128–132.

Moore, S., Newton, M., Grant, E. G., et al (1993). Treating bladder cancer: New methods, new management. *American Journal of Nursing, May*, 32–39.

National Study Commission on Cytotoxic Exposure. (1984). *Recommendations handling cytotoxic agents*. Providence, Rhode Island.

Nguyen, H. A., Averette, H. E., Wyble, L. (1993). Preliminary experience with a modified tenckhoff catheter for intraperitoneal chemotherapy. *Journal of Surgical Oncology, 52,*237–240.

Occupational Safety & Health Administration. (1986). *Work practice guidelines for personnel dealing with cytotoxic drugs.* (Instruction). (OSHA Publication 8-1.1), Washington, D.C.: Department of Labor.

Oliver, I. N., Aisner, J., Hament, A., et al (1988). A prospective study of topical dimethyl sulfoxide for treating anthracyclin extravasation. *Journal of Clinical Oncology, 6*(11),1732–1735.

Oncology Nursing Society. (1982). *Outcome standards for cancer patient education.* Pittsburgh: Oncology Nursing Society.

Oncology Nursing Society. (1988). *Cancer chemotherapy guideline: Module I,II,III, IV.* Pittsburgh: Oncology Nursing Press.

Oncology Nursing Society (1992). *Cancer chemotherapy guidelines: Module V.* Pittsburgh, PA: Oncology Nursing Press.

Ostechega, Y., Gianola, F., Jenkins, J., et al (1985). *Prospective assessment of exit site care for the patient with a tenckhoff catheter.* Presented at the 4th Cancer Nursing Research Conference, Hawaii.

Ostreicher, U., Stephan, G., & Glatzel, M. (1990). Chromosome and SCE analysis in peripheral lymphocytes of persons occupationally exposed to cytotoxic drugs handled with and without safety covers. *Mutation Research, 242,*271–277.

Palmer, P., & Myers, F. J. (1990). An outpatient approach to the delivery of intensive consolidation chemotherapy to adults with acute lymphoblastic leukemia. *Oncology Nursing Forum, 17,*553–558.

Parillo, V. L. (1994). Documentation forms for monitoring occupational surveillance of healthcare workers who handle cytotoxic drugs. *Oncology Nursing Forum, 21*(1),115–118.

Parker, G. G. (1992). Chemotherapy administration in the home. *Home Health Care Nurse, 10*(1),30–36.

Petro, J. A., Graham, W. P. III, Miller, S. H., et al (1979). Experimental and clinical studies of ulcers induced with adriamycin. *Surgical Forum, 30,*535–537.

Pfeile, C. E., & Howell, S. B. (1984). Totally implantable systems for peritoneal access. *Journal of Clinical Oncology, 2*(11),1277–1280.

Pharmacists Subcommittee and Consultants of the American Cancer Society. (1984). *Cancer chemotherapeutic agents.* Oakland, CA: ACS, California Division, Inc.

Piccart, M. F., Speyer, J. L., & Markman, M. (1985). Intraperitoneal chemotherapy: Clinical experience at five institutions. *Seminars in Oncology, 12*(3),90–96.

Pottecher, T., Forrler, M., Picardat, P., et al.(1984). Thrombogenicity of central venous catheters: prospective study of polyethylene, silicone and polyurethane catheters with phlebography or postmortem examination. *European Journal of Anaesthesiology, 1,*361.

Press, O. W., Ramsey, P. G., Larson, E. B., et al. (1984). Hickman catheter infections in patients with malignancies. *Medicine (Baltimore), 63*(4), 189–200.

Puel, V., Caudry, M., LeMetayer, P., Baste, J. C., Midy, D., Marsault, C., Demeaux, H., & Maire, J. P. (1993). Superior vena cava thrombosis related to catheter malposition in cancer chemotherapy given through implanted ports. *Cancer, 72*(7),2248–2252.

Reed, W. P., Neuman, K. A., deJongh, C., et al (1983). Prolonged venous access for chemotherapy by means of the hickman catheter. *Cancer, 52,*185.

Reymann, P. E. (1993). Chemotherapy: Principles of administration. In S. L. Groenwald, M. H. Frogge, M. Goodman, & C. H Yarbro (Eds.), *Cancer nursing: principles and practice,* (3rd ed., pp. 293–330). Boston: Jones and Bartlett.

Runowicz, C. D., Dottino, P. R., & Shafir, M. K. (1986). Catheter complications associated with intraperitoneal chemotherapy. *Gynecologic Oncology, 24,*41–50.

Rusch, V. W., Figlin, R., Godwin, D., et al (1991). Intrapleural cisplatin and cytarabine in the management of malignant pleural effusions: A lung cancer study group trial. *Journal of Clinical Oncology, 9,*313–319.

Rutherford, C. (1988). A study of single lumen peripherally inserted central line catheter dwelling time and complications. *Journal of Intravenous Nursing, 11,*69.

Sainsbury, R. (1991). Intra-arterial chemotherapy for breast cancer. *British Journal of Surgery, 78,*769–770.

Sardas, S., Gok, S., & Karakaya, A. E. (1991). Sister chromatid exchange in lymphocytes of nurses handling antineoplastic agents. *Toxicology Letters, 55,*311–315.

Sarto, F., Trevisan, A., Tomanin, R., et al (1990). Chromosomal aberrations sister chromatid exchanges, and urinary thioethers in nurses handling antineoplastic drugs. *American Journal of Industrial Medicine, 18,*689–694.

Schuman, E. S., Winters, V., Gross, G. F., et al. (1985). Management of hickman catheter sepsis. *American Journal of Surgery, 149*(5),627–628.

Schwartz, C., Hendrickson, K. J., Roghmann, K., et al. (1990). Prevention of bacteremia attributed to luminal colonization of tunnelled central venous catheters with vancomycin-suspectible organisms. *Journal of Clinical Oncology, 8*(9),1591–1597.

Selevan, S. G., Lindbohm, M. L., & Hornung, R. W. (1985). A study of occupational exposure to antineoplastic drugs and fetal loss in nurses. *New England Journal of Medicine, 313,*1173–1178.

Smith, P. (1986). Quality standards in high tech IV home care. *Caring, 591*–594.

Sonneveld, P., Wasserman, H. A., & Nooter, K. (1984). Long persistence of doxorubicin administration. *Cancer Treatment Reviews, 68*(6),895–896.

Sotaniemi, E. A., Sutinen, S., Arranto, A. J., Sutinen, S., Sotaniemi, K. A., Lehtola, J., & Pelkonen R. O. (1983). Liver damage in nurses handling cyotostatic agents. *Acta Medica Scandinavica, 214,* 181–189.

Souhami, L. Jr., & Feld, R. (1978). Urticaria following intravenous doxorubicin administration. *Journal of the American Medical Association, 240*(15),1624–1626.

Stellman, J., & Zoloth, S. (1986). Cancer chemotherapeutic agents as occupational hazards: A literature review. *Cancer Investigations, 4,*127–135.

Surbone, A., & Myers, C. E. (1988). Principles and practice of intraperitoneal therapy. *Antibiotic Chemotherapy, 40,*14–25.

Svingen, B. A., Powis, G., Appel, P. L., et al (1981). Protection against adriamycin-induced skin necrosis in the rat by dimethy sulfoxide and atocopherol. *Cancer Research, 41,*3395–3399.

Swenson, K. K., & Eriksson, J. H. (1986). Nursing management of intraperitoneal chemotherapy. *Oncology Nursing Forum, 12*(5),33–39.

Tenenbaum, L., Ellsworth-Wolk, J., & Hawthorne, J. L. (1994). Preparation, administration, and safe disposal of chemotherapeutic agents. In L. Tenenbaum (Ed.), *Cancer chemotherapy and biotherapy: A reference guide* (2nd ed., pp. 15–43). Philadelphia: W. B. Saunders Co.

Tenenbaum, L., & Scelsi, D. B. (1994). Central venous access devices. In L. Tenenbaum (Ed.), *Cancer chemotherapy and biotherapy* (pp. 411–497). Philadelphia: W. B. Saunders Co.

U.S. Department of Labor, Office of Occupational Medicine, Occupation Safety and Health Administration. (1986). *Work practice guidelines for personnel dealing with cytotoxic (antineoplastic) drugs.* (Publication No. 8.1.1). Washington, DC: Author.

Van Sloten-Harwood, K., & Bachur, N. (1987). Evaluation of dimethyl-sulfoxide and local cooling as antidotes for doxorubicin extravasation in a pig model. *Oncology Nursing Forum, 14*(1),39–44.

Venitt, S., Crofton-Sleigh, C., Hunt, J., et al. (1984). Monitoring exposure of nursing and pharmacy personnel to cytotoxic drugs:Urinary mutation assays and urinary platinum as markers of absorption. *Lancet,8368,*74–77.

Vogelzang, N. J. (1979). "Adriamycin flare":A skin reaction resembling extravasation. *Cancer Treatment Reviews, 63*(11/12),2067–2069.

Volker, D. (1987). Developing continuing education programs in cancer nursing: Learning needs assessment. *Oncology Nursing Forum, 14,*60–62

Wachs, T. (1990). Urokinase administration in pediatric patients with occluded central venous catheters. *Journal of Intravenous Nursing, 13,* 100–102.

Welch-McCafferty, D. (1985). Rationale, development and evaluation of a chemotherapy certification course for nurses. *Cancer Nursing, 8,*255–262.

Wickham, R. S. (1990). Advances in venous access devices and nursing management strategies. *Nursing Clinics of North America, 25*(2), 345–361.

Wickham, R., Purl, S., & Welker, D. (1992). Long-term central venous catheters: Issues for care. *Seminars in Oncology Nursing, 8,* 133–147.

Wood, H. A., & Ellerhorst-Ryan, J. M. (1984). Delayed adverse skin reaction associated with mitomycin-c administration. *Oncology Nursing Forum, 11*(4), 14–18.

Zimmerman, P. F., Larsen, R. K., Barkley, E. W., et al. (1981). Recommendations for the safe handling of injectable antineoplastic drug products. *American Journal of Hospital Pharmacy, 38,*1693–1695.

Zook-Enck,D. L. (1990). Intraperitoneal therapy via the Tenckhoff catheter; prevention and management of complications. *Journal of Intravenous Nursing, 13*(6),375–382.

Biologic Response Modifiers

Linda Edwards Hood • Elizabeth J. Abernathy

The scientific and medical community over the last decade has begun to recognize biotherapy as the fourth treatment modality for patients with cancer, the other three being surgery, chemotherapy, and radiation therapy (Wujcik, 1993). With an excess of 300 active clinical trials of biologics and over 25 agents approved for clinical practice, the impact of biotherapy is seen throughout the oncology practice (*Physicians' Data Query*, 1994). Biotherapy is based largely on the manipulation of the immune system in an effort to control cancer. Other biologic systems, such as the hematopoietic system, may be modulated through the use of biologic response modifiers (BRMs). If through the use of BRMs the body's innate ability to protect and heal itself can produce antitumor activity, then biotherapy will become the prominent treatment for cancer.

Biotechnology is defined by the FDA as a technique that uses living organisms or a part of a living organism to produce or modify a product, to improve a plant or animal, or to develop a microorganism to be used for a specific purpose. Advances in biotechnology are making a tremendous contribution to the understanding and treatment of cancer and a host of other diseases (Wordell, 1991). At the heart of biologic therapy in cancer is the search for the understanding of the human body's contribution to the cancer. What caused the cancer? Was it a breakdown in the immune response that enabled the cancer to become established and replicate? Is it the role of the immune system to recognize malignant growth and release an immune response to destroy and clear it from the body? Is the cancer a result of a deficiency or mutation of the body's genetic composition? Or is the cancer the product of the environment and our body's response to the toxins that pollute our world? The answer is probably a combination of all the above and may be related to still undefined concepts. Certainly, it appears that gaining more knowledge on biotherapy science is the right track to understanding the mystery of cancer (Abernathy, 1994).

MECHANISM OF ACTION

Biologic response modifiers are being researched both clinically and in the laboratory. Even after extensive research, the mechanism of action of many of the agents is not clearly defined. Table 23–1 lists some of the more frequently used agents and their recognized modes of antitumor activity or combinations of activities. Several of the agents have multiple antitumor activities; thus for these agents, it is difficult to determine which antitumor activity capabilities are the most essential. For example, interferon acts both as an immunomodulator and as a cytotoxic agent with direct activity on cancer cells (Trotta, 1986).

Biologic response modifiers can be classified into three major divisions: (1) agents that restore, augment, or modulate the host's immunologic mechanisms, (2) agents that have direct antitumor activity, and (3) agents that have other biologic effects (agents that interfere with tumor cells' ability to metastasize or survive, differentiating agents, or agents that affect cell transformation) (Clark & Longo, 1986).

Included in the classification of BRMs are many cytokines and monoclonal antibodies. Gene therapy may also be considered biotherapy, since it attempts to alter the body's biologic response to obtain a therapeutic effect.

Cytokines are a network of chemical messengers that when released from the body's immune system cells have the ability to regulate immune and other biologic functions. All cytokines are BRMs and pleiotropic in that they have many, often overlapping, functions (Traynor, 1992). Interferons, interleukins, colony-stimulating factors, and tumor necrosis factor are all

TABLE 23–1. *Functions of Biologic Response Modifiers*

AGENT	MODE OF ACTION
Lymphokines (IL 2, interferon-γ)	I
Nonspecific immunomodulating agents (bacille Calmette-Guérin, *Corynebacterium parvum*)	I
Active specific immunizations with tumor cells	I
Interferon or interferon inducers (e.g., alpha, beta, gamma/poly: ICLC, Sendai virus)	I/C
Adoptive immunotherapy (lymphokine-activated killer cells)	C
Tumor necrosis factor	C
Metastasis preventors (laminin fragments and anticoagulation agents)	C
Growth factors (granulocyte colony-stimulating factor, granulocyte-macrophage colony-stimulating factor, erythropoietin)	B

I = immunomodulation; C = direct cytotoxic or cytostatic effect; B = other biologic effects.

cytokines. If a particular cytokine is produced by a lymphocyte, it is referred to as a lymphokine; cytokines produced by monocytes are called monokines (Rumsey & Rieger, 1992).

HISTORIC BACKGROUND

There is considerable overlap between BRM therapy and immunotherapy. William B. Coley, a surgeon who practiced at New York's Memorial Hospital from 1891 until 1936, is responsible for some of the most interesting early work using the principles of immunotherapy, although the scientific foundations of his research were not clearly defined at the time. At the death of a young female patient with a malignancy, the disheartened Dr. Coley began searching hospital records for clues to explain why, after a cancerous tumor was surgically removed, some patients appeared to be cured, whereas others relapsed very quickly. He found a positive correlation between patients who developed severe infections following surgery and those who remained tumor-free for a prolonged time.

To induce an infectious response in cancer patients, Dr. Coley first used live bacteria and later filtered toxins with mixed therapeutic success. Coley's toxins, as they were known, were used clinically until 1975 and provide the background data for tumor necrosis factor (TNF), a BRM that is being clinically researched today. These toxins may have acted as immunotherapy to boost the immune system to recognize, destroy, or clear tumor cells from the body (Goodfield, 1984).

Although the concept of immunotherapy was developed in the 1800s, its application to cancer therapy gained popularity only in the last 2 decades. In the 1960s, many clinical trials were initiated using injections of bacterial agents, such as Bacillus Calmette-Guérin (BCG), methanol-extracted residue (MER), and *Corynebacterium parvum*. It was hypothesized that exposure to these agents would elicit a nonspecific immune response, thus boosting the body's ability to destroy foreign invaders such as tumor cells. These experiments produced positive results in selected laboratory animal tumor models (Oldham, 1983).

In 1969, Mathe and Amiel reported successful results of immunotherapy in a small clinical trial of patients with acute lymphoblastic leukemia. Although this success was never replicated, hundreds of clinical trials of nonspecific bacterial agents were conducted. Viruses were used to stimulate tumor cells to produce products to fight the tumor, which were injected in an attempt to stimulate an immune response to the tumor cell. Tumor cells and their products were used to try to stimulate the specific immunity of the patient and to activate either humoral or cell-mediated immunity to slow tumor growth.

Although some results of these clinical trials were positive, the majority were very discouraging, and by the late 1970s, the majority of clinicians had a negative attitude toward immunotherapy (Terry & Rosenberg, 1982). It has been suggested that a lack of understanding of immunologic responses and related physiologic and pathophysiologic mechanisms contributed to the failure of these earlier trials (Oldham & Smalley, 1983). The 1980s clearly brought about tremendous advancements in biologic therapy. Many new technologies that supported biotherapy were either defined or refined with the assistance of the sophisticated computers that allowed researchers to gain knowledge at such a rapid rate. The development of hybridoma technology and recombinant deoxyribonucleic acid technology allowed researchers to explore biologics. The production of purified BRMs was simplified and the quality standardized. With nine biologic agents approved by the FDA (see Table 23–2) and more than 25 agents active in clinical trials, it is apparent that biologics have made significant impact on cancer therapy.

BRM CLASSIFICATIONS

Major technologic advances in the last decade have expanded the ability to study biologics (Fig. 23–1). Recombinant DNA gene cloning and increased sophistication of computers and other laboratory equipment enabled the determination of interferon's molecular structure, the examination of its biologic activity, and, subsequently, the mass production of it in large quantities. The recombinant method involves the isolation of DNA from the human gene responsible for interferon production (Fig. 23–2). DNA is then implanted into altered bacteria, which produce mass quantities of interferon, unlike cultured "human" interferon obtained by the Cantell method. The Cantell method involved viral inoculation of large vats of human leucocytes obtained by harvesting the buffy coat of leucocytes from donated blood. The leucocytes reacted by secreting a mixture containing many types of interferons and proteins together in the vat, which was then harvested. Recombinant interferons consist of only the one subtype of interferon that was coded on the DNA.

TABLE 23–2. *Approved Biologic Agents*

AGENT	TRADE NAME	GENERIC NAME	APPROVED INDICATIONS	DATE
CSFs				
G-CSF	Neupogen	Filgrastin	Chemotherapy-induced myelosuppression	1991
GM-CSF	Leukine	Sargramostim	Post-ABMT for lymphoid malignancy engraftment failure	1991
EPO	Epogen Procrit	Epoietin alfa	Anemia; chronic renal failure; AZT treated HIV infection; chemotherapy-related	1989
Interferon				
Alpha			Hairy cell leukemia, condyloma, AIDS-related Kaposi's sarcoma, chronic hepatitis	1986
Beta			Multiple sclerosis	1992
Gamma			Chronic granulomatous disease	1992
Interleukin				
IL-2	Proleukin	Aldesleukin	Metastatic renal cell carcinoma	1992
Monoclonal Antibodies				
Oncoscint		Oncoscint	Diagnostic testing for ovarian & colorectal cancer	1993
OKT-3		Orthoclone	Treatment of acute cell-mediated rejection in organ transplants.	1986

This ability to make large quantities of purified human interferon proteins facilitated clinical trials that began in the late 1970s. All cytokines currently in clinical trials are produced by the recombinant method.

Another important advance refined in the 1980s was hybridoma technology (Fig. 23–3), which has made possible the development of clones of cells that produce specific antibodies against one antigen. *Monoclonal antibodies* (MoAbs) are antibodies developed to bind with specific types of cancer cells. They are used directly in cancer therapy and diagnosis and indirectly in the isolation and purification of other BRMs (Foon, Bernhard, & Oldham, 1982).

Clinically, interferons have been more extensively studied than any other BRM. Approved by the FDA in 1986 for therapeutic use in patients with hairy cell leukemia (Clark & Longo, 1987), interferon-α continues to be studied in many phase II and III trials that have examined various indications, dosages, schedules, and routes of administration. Clinical trials of interferon-γ and interferon-β have supported their approval for certain disorders. Research on the use of interferon in combination with radiation therapy, chemotherapy, and other biologics is also under way (see Chapter 21).

In the last 10 years, considerable attention has been focused on another biologic, interleukin-2 (IL-2). This BRM, a lymphokine produced by T lymphocytes, is being examined for direct antitumor activity as well as in an exciting approach to immunotherapy: adoptive immunotherapy. Adoptive immunotherapy has been defined as a "treatment approach in which cells with antitumor reactivity are administered to a tumor-bearing host and mediate either directly or indirectly the regression of established tumor" (Rosenberg et al., 1985, p. 1485). With this approach, IL-2 mixes with human peripheral blood lymphocytes and generates cells termed *lymphokine-activated killer cells* (LAK) cells that are capable of killing tumor cells. A group of

cytokines that stimulate cellular growth in the hematopoietic system, termed colony-stimulating factors (CSFs), have made a tremendous impact in cancer care over the past decade. Three colony-stimulating factors have received FDA approval and are being used frequently to support patients with cancer.

For more than a century and particularly since Coley's work, the antitumor effects of bacterial cell products have been recognized (Oettgen & Old, 1987). In 1975, researchers isolated an agent and named it *tumor necrosis factor* (TNF) for its ability to induce hemorrhagic necrosis in tumor cells without harming normal tissues. Severe toxicity has limited the ability to explore clinical applications in depth.

The approach to testing cytotoxic agents clinically has been to establish the maximum tolerated dose (MTD) in phase I trials (see Chapter 25). With BRMs, the MTD as well as the optimal immunomodulatory dose (OID) must be determined, because lower doses of some biologics may be more effective in altering various aspects of the immune response than higher doses, or the agent may be effective by different mechanisms at different doses.

MONOCLONAL ANTIBODIES

Monoclonal antibody technology holds great promise for the development of treatments that are specific for the various types of cancer. The immune system has the ability to recognize unfamiliar antigens (molecules of protein and glycoproteins located on tumor cells) and to produce antibodies that target these particular antigens. This capability provides the potential for targeting treatment specifically to tumor cells, sparing normal cells.

Monoclonal antibodies (MoAb) are high molecular weight proteins produced by a clone of cells. The clone of cells originate from a single parent cell and produce

KEY EVENTS IN BIOTHERAPY

Late 1800's
Coley's toxins

Early 1900's
Ehrlich's "Magic bullet" Theory

1957
Interferon discovered—Issacs and Lindenmann

1960's
Non-specific immunotherapy with BCG &
C. Parvum

1970's
Negative results for many clinical trials

1975
Hybridoma technology—Kohler & Milstein-MoAbs

1979
NCI established the BRMP (Biological Response
Modifier Program)

1981
Recombinant DNA technology

1980's
Clinical trials with recombinant cytokines

1984
IL-2 + LAK trials

1986
FDA approval for 1st BRM=Alpha Interferon

1980-1990's
Many clinical trials with cytokines, especially growth
factors

1989
Gene therapy for humans

1990's
FDA approval for IL-2, G-CSF, GM-CSF, EPO, Beta
& Gamma Interferon, Oncoscint

1990's
Tumor suppressor genes and oncogenes isolated

FIGURE 23–1. Key events in biotherapy.

only the particular antibody to which the parent cell was sensitive. Monoclonal antibodies therefore will target only one specific antigen and potentially can be used to differentiate cells possessing that antigen from other normal cell antigens.

Historic Background. At the turn of the century, Paul Ehrlich, a pioneer of antibacterial agents, applied the phrase "the magic bullet" to the possible targeting of antibodies to tumors (Ehrlich, 1900). Early studies involved administration of sera from recovered cancer patients to patients with active tumors. Occasional short-lived tumor responses in patients with melanoma and renal cell carcinoma were reported. Failure to fully achieve the anticipated success may have been due to two factors. First, the sera contained minute amounts of specific antibody, and second, the sera contained many other products and impurities that may have blocked beneficial effects (Moldawer, & Murray, 1985). Two events confirmed the technology to identify with precision antigens located on tumor cells and revived interest in monoclonal antibodies. These events are the purification of the carcinoembryonic antigen (CEA) and studies by Goldenberg and colleagues on the localization of radiolabeled antibodies in colorectal carcinomas (Pimm, 1987).

The immune system normally scouts the body for any nonself substances or antigens. Ordinarily when an antigen is recognized and the immune reaction is initiated, various antibody-producing cells are stimulated to secrete several different antibodies that attach to receptors located on the antigen's cell wall. These different antibodies are polyclonal, since they are produced by a variety of cells.

In the late 1970's Kohler and Milstein (1975) developed a method of producing antigen-specific monoclonal antibodies from cloned cells or hybridomas from mice that had been inoculated with tumor cells. This breakthrough allowed scientists to develop large quantities of identical antibodies specific to a desired antigen.

To make a monoclonal antibody by the hybridoma technique (Fig. 23–3), mice are injected with an antigen that causes their immune systems to react and initiate the production of antibodies. Antibody-producing lymphocytes are harvested from the spleen's reservoir and isolated. Each lymphocyte, which is capable of producing only one antibody, is fused to a mouse myeloma cell. Myelomas are tumors of plasma cells (mature antibody-producing B cells) that live for a very long time. The fused spleen and myeloma cells, called hybridomas, can produce a large quantity of antibody. The antibody that is produced by the hybridoma is isolated and tested to determine whether it possesses the desired specificity. If it does, the hybridoma is grown in culture, producing large quantities of one specific purified antibody; this process explains the reason for the name *monoclonal* antibodies (Gallucci, 1985).

With the advances made in the 1975-1985 decade in monoclonal antibody technology and the ability to identify antigens on tumor cells with precision, clinical immunology surpassed the progress of the previous 3 decades. Now monoclonal antibodies can be utilized for a variety of uses (Table 23–3). Approval for a diagnostic murine monoclonal antibody (OncoScint; Cytogen, Princeton, NJ) that is used to detect ovarian and colorectal tumors was granted in 1992, becoming the first monoclonal antibody approved for clinical use.

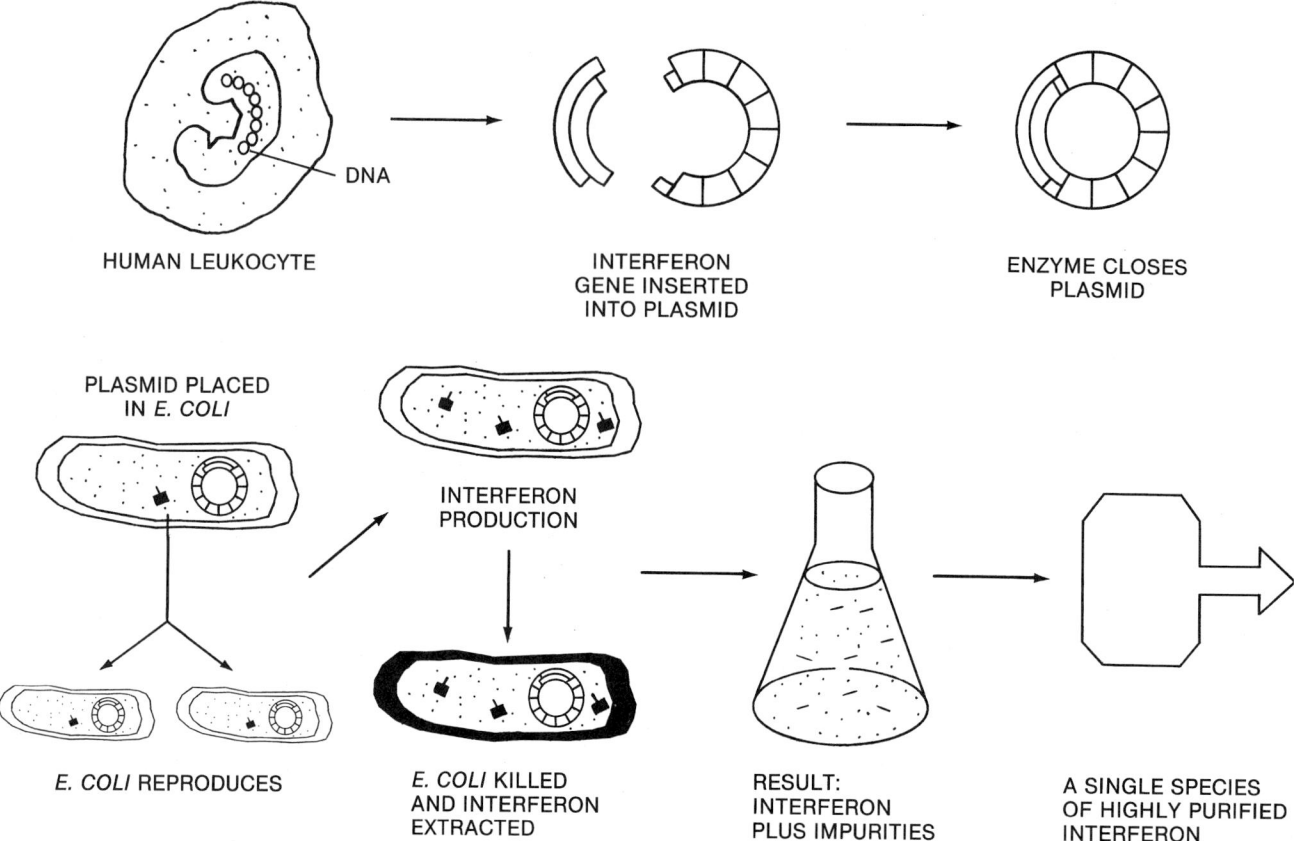

HUMAN LEUKOCYTE

INTERFERON
GENE INSERTED
INTO PLASMID

ENZYME CLOSES
PLASMID

PLASMID PLACED
IN *E. COLI*

INTERFERON
PRODUCTION

E. COLI REPRODUCES

E. COLI KILLED
AND INTERFERON
EXTRACTED

RESULT:
INTERFERON
PLUS IMPURITIES

A SINGLE SPECIES
OF HIGHLY PURIFIED
INTERFERON

FIGURE 23–2. Recombinant DNA production of highly purified human interferon-alpha-2b. (Schering Corporation. Reproduced by permission. Copyright © 1986. Schering Corporation. All rights reserved.)

Monoclonal antibodies are used alone as tumor vaccines or as carriers of agents such as cytotoxic drugs, toxin molecules, and diagnostic or therapeutic radioisotopes (Goldenberg, 1994).

Mechanism of Action. The central issue regarding the potential of monoclonal antibodies is whether tumor-specific antigens exist or whether antigens possessed by tumors are shared with normal tissues. To induce a specific immune response, the tumor cells must express an antigen specific to or associated with the tumor. Monoclonal antibodies attach to antigens on the tumor cell surface and are recognized by circulating immune cells. The tumor cell may then be destroyed directly by normal immune responses of the cytotoxic cell.

Some tumor cells possess antigens on their cell membranes that are capable of eliciting an immune response in the host. However, because tumors are derived from the transformation of normal cells, it cannot be assumed that tumors carry antigens that are unique or foreign. In fact, tumor cells usually share antigens with the cells of the parent organ from which the tumor arose. Some tumor cells possess antigens that are normally displayed only on fetal tissues, for example, carcinoembryonic antigen, which is associated with colon carcinomas and is found on normal fetal gut cells during the first 2 trimesters of pregnancy, or α_1-fetoprotein, which is secreted by hepatocellular carcinomas. Other tumor-associated antigens include differentiation antigens, such as the protein antigens on malignant melanoma cells, carbohydrate antigens expressed by carcinomas of breast and ovary, and glycolipid antigens in colorectal cancer (Baldwin & Byers, 1987).

The immune response against tumor-associated antigens can occur in different ways. These responses include formation of antibody against antigen and the attachment of various immune cells (stimulated killer lymphocytes and macrophages) to the antibody that is bound to the tumor.

Tumors can escape immunologic attack in a number of ways. Tumor cells can shed their surface antigens or alter their appearance within 2 hours of monoclonal antibody exposure, an effect that can last up to 36 hours (Dillman, 1994; Oldham, 1983). Or circulating tumor antigen may bind with the monoclonal antibody, blocking its receptor sites and thus preventing it from reaching the tumor cell. Blocking factors may be released by tumor cells to coat the tumor cell surface antigens, preventing recognition and destruction of tumor (Dillman, 1994; Oldham, 1983). Immune complexes composed of the linked antibody and antigen may be drawn into the cell, where detection of the tumor cell antigen becomes hidden from the immune effector cells. Antigens bound by antibodies create a large complex that is unable to penetrate very deep into the tumor; therefore, only a small proportion of the tumor cells are attacked. Tumors are heterogeneous, with metastases displaying different antigens than the

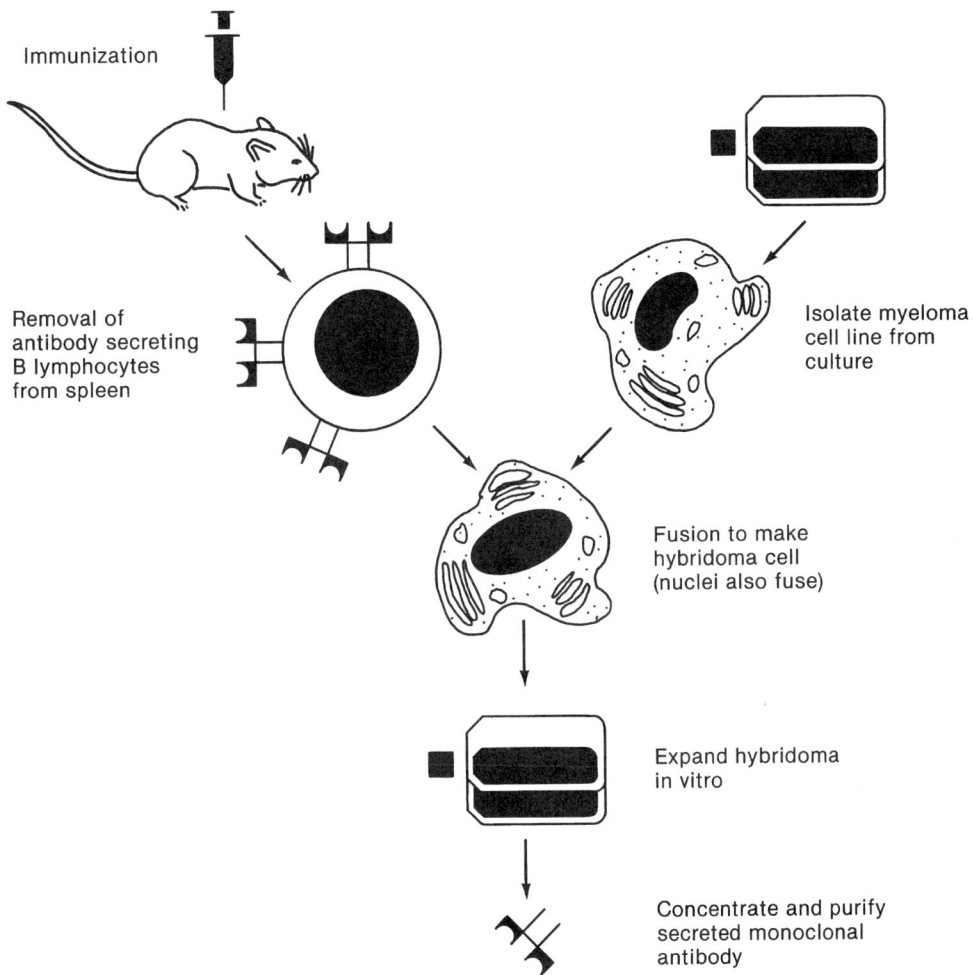

FIGURE 23–3. The hybridoma technology. (From NeoRx Corporation. K. A. Foon, M.D. Application of monoclonal antibodies in the diagnosis and therapy of cancer, 1988. Reproduced by permission.)

TABLE 23–3. *Uses of Monoclonal Antibodies*

Diagnostic
1. Early detection of cancer by identifying surface markers of tumor cells and circulating tumor-associated antigens
2. Identification and disabling of activated lymphocytes involved in organ transplant rejection and graft-versus-host disease
3. Identification of lymphocyte antigens and correlation of their functions in the immune response
4. Identification of dysfunction of components of the immune system in cancer and other immune-related diseases
5. Identification of function, isolation, or blockage of growth factors, tumor factors, and other biologic response modifiers, ultimately allowing for manipulation of the immune response
6. Delivery of radioactive isotopes directly to tumor sites, allowing scans to visualize the tumor

Therapeutic
1. Delivery of immunotoxins—target to tumor
   a. toxic agents, such as ricin
   b. chemotherapy, such as doxorubicin and daunomycin
   c. radioactive isotopes for both diagnostic scans and therapeutic delivery of radiation

primary tumor, such that one specific monoclonal antibody may not recognize all of the areas of tumor in one individual. Also neoplastic cells survive with minimal accessibility to blood supply; thus, it is difficult for monoclonal antibodies to reach many tumor cells.

Clinical Applications. The use of antibodies to mediate specific toxicity for the cancer cell through recruitment of cell-mediated immunity and activation of the complement system is under investigation. Tumor regressions have been reported in lymphoma, melanoma, neuroblastoma, and in severe B-cell lymphoproliferative disorders occurring after transplantation (Dillman, 1994). Antibody fragments and immunoglobulins are also being studied to take advantage of their smaller size to better penetrate the tumor. Greater potential is attributed to the ability to link many types of molecules to monoclonal antibodies. Cancer treatment can be enhanced through the use of monoclonal antibodies as carriers to deliver drugs, toxins, and radioactive substances, specifically to the area of tumor (Moldawer & Murray, 1985).

The use of monoclonal antibodies to detect early or preinvasive tumor by examining serum samples for surface antigens also holds great promise in the fight against cancer. For example, pathologic diagnosis of testicular carcinoma in situ, melanoma cells, and lymphoma cells is facilitated by monoclonal antibodies. Monoclonal antibodies also will be used to confirm the existence of tumor-associated antigens.

Currently monoclonal antibodies are used to purge the bone marrow of neoplastic cells before reinfusion for bone marrow transplantation. Monoclonal antibodies can identify and then disable activated lymphocytes that are responsible for transplant rejection or graft-versus-host disease without causing overall suppression of the immune mechanisms of the host (Baldwin & Byers, 1987). The use of monoclonal antibodies to correlate distinct lymphocyte surface antigens with specific functions would allow an understanding of the pathophysiology of immune dysfunction in cancer and other immune-related diseases. This can be accomplished by using a monoclonal antibody to block a certain receptor for a particular cell or cytokine. Once the receptor has been blocked, the effect on the immune response can be determined, establishing the role of the selected cell or cytokine in the normal immune response.

The ability of monoclonal antibodies to identify, isolate, or block growth factors, tumor factors, or other biologic response modifiers may play an important role in the understanding of their function on the development and maintenance of the cell that has undergone neoplastic transformation and how tumor cells may go undetected by the immune system (Thor, Weeks, & Schlom, 1986). Monoclonal antibodies may be used to manipulate the immune system to specifically interfere with the activity of growth factors induced by the tumor. They may also be used to block other factors secreted by the tumor that induce immunosuppression by increasing numbers of suppressor lymphocytes (Dillman, 1994).

Immunotoxins are created by the linkage of toxins to monoclonal antibodies. Linkages of anthracyclines, vinca alkaloids, folic acid antagonists, and a variety of natural toxins, such as ricin, are underway. The toxin bound to the monoclonal antibody attaches to the antigenic receptor on the tumor cell membrane and then penetrates into the cytoplasm by endocytosis through smooth invaginations or coated pits of the plasma membrane. Once inside the tumor cell's cytoplasm, protein synthesis is inactivated, and cell killing results (Baldwin & Byers, 1987). The therapeutic effect of immunotoxins is limited by the ability of these large toxin-to-antibody complexes to be internalized into the cell membrane. Additionally before utilization of immunotoxins, technology must provide techniques to ensure that the monoclonal antibody will securely hold the toxin until it reaches the tumor cell; otherwise, normal cells will be eliminated by the toxin molecule.

Where monoclonal antibodies are linked to radioactive isotopes, scanning for areas of monoclonal antibody localization on tumor cells can determine if and where tumor recurrence exists. Such use could also guide surgeons regarding the extent of surgery needed to yield a total tumor resection. Studies with many radiolabeled monoclonal antibodies show that only a proportion of the total antibody dose actually localizes into the tumor. A large proportion of intravenously administered monoclonal antibody remains in the circulation or is distributed in the reticuloendothelial system such as the lungs, liver, and spleen where the circulation pools blood (Morgan & Foon, 1986). However, when therapeutic doses of radiation are linked to monoclonal antibodies, radiation can be emitted to local areas of tumor. Regional administration into a body cavity is an effective method for delivery of radioactive monoclonal antibodies in both diagnostic and therapeutic procedures (Goldenberg, 1994).

Targeting of drugs conjugated to monoclonal antibodies may increase therapeutic efficacy by improved localization, retention of drug in tumors, and by reducing normal tissue toxicity (Baldwin & Byers, 1987). Although there exists great promise in the diagnosis and treatment of cancer, a few problems have surfaced. Toxicity to normal cells, although generally mild, has occurred when they are used with patients.

Side Effects. Side effects associated with monoclonal antibodies have not been major (Table 23–4), and usually were associated with the initial one or two administrations or with rapid intravenous infusions exceeding 5 to 10 mg/hr. The development of HAMA (human antimouse antibodies) has been noted where murine monoclonal antibodies are used. Because the murine monoclonal antibodies are foreign, large molecular weight, protein molecules, they can evoke the host's immune allergic response. The reaction related to HAMA usually occurs 2 to 3 weeks after the initial monoclonal antibody dose and is unrelated to dose or rate of administration (Goldenberg, 1994). The host may produce antibodies against the injected monoclonal antibodies that inactivate their therapeutic effect. The use of chimeric or humanized monoclonal antibodies may decrease the occurrence of antibodies (Jakobsen, 1987). With some of the human monoclonal antibodies, mild erythema at the injection site is the only side effect noted.

TABLE 23–4. *Side Effects Associated with Monoclonal Antibodies*

COMMON	RARE (RATE-RELATED)
Fever, chills, rigors	Bronchospasm, wheezing, dyspnea
Urticaria, pruritis, rash	Hypotension
Myalgias/arthralgias	Hypersensitivity (allergic) reactions
Nausea & vomiting, diarrhea	Anaphylaxis
Development of HAMA (human antimouse antibody) with serum sickness	Tumor flare (warmth and tenderness of lymph nodes)

Side effects of immunotoxin (monoclonal antibodies linked with toxins) included a dose-limiting capillary leak syndrome manifested by a drop in serum albumin, weight gain, and fluid shifts resulting in mild edema and hypovolemia (Baldwin & Byers, 1987; Goldenberg, 1994). The linked toxins have shown that they can be administered in large quantities with less toxicity than when they are administered as a single agent. Close observation for severe toxicities may indicate that the toxin has become detached from the MoAb molecule.

Safety Issues. See the discussion of nursing care and management of BRM patients later in this chapter for guidelines for the administration, assessment, education, and support of patients receiving monoclonal antibodies. Additionally, the determination about the development of anti-MoAb antibodies such as HAMA should be made by the clinical laboratory prior to subsequent administrations of the monoclonal antibody to prevent severe hypersensitivity reactions such as bronchospasm and anaphylactic shock.

Where radiolabeled monoclonal antibodies are utilized, the handling and disposal of radioactive substances and of the patient's body fluids are important safety issues. Knowledge of the radioactive element and its half-life should be shared with individuals involved in the clinical care of the patient, although the doses of radioactivity in most cases are not high enough to require isolation. Badges that register the amount of radioactivity to which a health care member is exposed should be worn. Also, radiation safety teams should monitor the emissions of radioactivity from the patient. Body fluids, blood samples drawn, and other procedures expose the health care member to increments of excreted radioactivity. Lead shields and lead-lined specimen containers can be utilized to further minimize individual exposure. The patient's contact with family members and particularly with small children or pregnant women may be limited for a period of time following the administration of the monoclonal antibody.

INTERFERON

Interferon (IFN) is a family of cytokines that are glycoproteins produced as part of the cell-mediated immune response of the T lymphocyte after activation by viruses or tumor cells. Interferon is named for its antiviral ability to interfere with the spread of viral infection by affecting the synthesis of viral RNA and protein; it has been found to possess antitumor and immunomodulatory potential as well. Interferon has potent effects on the immune system as an "immunological hormone" (Gutterman, 1988). It is considered to be the prototype BRM, a natural human protein that can alter the body's immune response to result in detrimental effects to the tumor with little toxicity to normal tissues.

Historic Background. Since the early 1900's, it has been known that viral infection with one agent could prevent simultaneous infection with a second agent. In 1957 Issacs and Lindenmann discovered an agent with antiviral properties and called it "interferon" (Linden-

mann, 1982). The production of this agent initially was an expensive and tedious process that yielded insufficient and impure supplies of interferon. Also, interferon was species-specific, which meant that preclinical laboratory research with animals was not useful in predicting toxicity and biologic effects in humans. When the antitumor properties of interferon were discovered, however, the press heralded interferon as a potential miracle cure, and investment capital quickly was provided for its study and production (Gresser & Tovey, 1978).

Interferon refers to a family of small glycoproteins of three general types based on the type of cell and the substance that stimulates the interferon production. Their names are designated by the Greek letters α, β, and γ. All three are antigenically distinct and possess separate biologic and chemical properties, but all share the ability to prevent viral spread.

Interferon-α is produced by viral, bacterial, or tumor cell stimulation of leukocytes, including T and B lymphocytes, macrophages, natural killer cells, and large granular lymphocytes (Hooks & Detrick, 1985). A single gene exists for the production of interferon-β and interferon-γ; therefore, only one type of each exists. Interferon-β is produced by stimulation of fibroblast or epithelial cells. Interferon-γ is produced by helper and suppressor T lymphocytes as an integral part of the immune response.

Mechanism of Action. Interferon affects the body's immune response, initiated by binding to a specific cell surface receptor, and triggering a cascade of cellular events. The particular biochemical response generated by interferon depends on the type of interferon involved, the responding cell, and the agent against which interferon is reacting—virus, parasite, or tumor.

Antiviral. Interferon was originally identified for its antiviral properties: it is able to induce an antiviral state when a virus attaches to a cell membrane. Interferon stimulates the production of various factors that protect cells from a second simultaneous infection. Interferon also prevents further viral RNA and protein replication, halting the virus' ability to spread to other body cells (Higgins, 1984).

Antitumor. Direct antitumor effects that involve inhibition of tumor growth and cell division have been identified. As interferon contacts a tumor cell receptor site, it triggers a number of reactions that arrest or delay the stages of cell division, primarily G_0-G_1 (Goldstein & Laszlo, 1986; Higgins, 1984). Interferon also influences the production of other cellular products, enzymes, and lymphokines. These other products can result in differentiation of the malignant cell, alterations in malignant cell phenotype and metabolism, or inhibition of important genes, such as oncogenes. Inhibition of oncogene expression can accompany changes in morphology of some cell lines that have undergone neoplastic transformation with loss or decrease in tumorigenicity, inhibition of cell proliferation, and return to normal growth of these cells (Clark & Longo, 1987).

Immunomodulatory. Interferon causes some indirect effects, influencing various immunomodulatory aspects of both cellular and humoral immunity. Some of these effects include the stimulation of cytotoxic T lymphocytes, macrophages, and natural killer cells as well as phagocytic activity. Interferon also increases the expression of tumor-associated antigens on the tumor cell membrane, which causes the tumor cells to be more recognizable (Goldstein & Laszlo, 1986; Higgins, 1984). B lymphocytes are directed by interferon to differentiate into antibody-producing plasma cells. Overall, interferon influences a number of immune activities that enhance the body's ability to recognize and rid itself of tumor growth.

Clinical Applications

Interferon-α. Interferon-α was initially approved by the FDA in June 1986 for use against *hairy cell leukemia* (HCL). Hairy cell leukemia is a rare, chronic form of B-cell leukemia that is highly sensitive to small amounts of interferon. Hairy cell leukemia is named for the many hairlike projections of cytoplasm that extend from the walls of lymphoid cells. The symptoms of HCL are fatigue, anemia, easy bruising, and frequent infections. As with other leukemias these symptoms are caused by crowding of the bone marrow, which prevents production of normal blood cells. Prior to the discovery of interferon's effectiveness, patients would be observed for several years when the HCL remained asymptomatic. In about half of these patients the symptoms would progress, at which point the usual treatment was splenectomy. Forty per cent of those undergoing a splenectomy have relapses within 2 years, at which point few interventions effectively control the disease. Patients then die of infections or bleeding (Balmer, 1990).

Hairy cell leukemia responds to interferon-α in a reported 67 to 90 per cent of patients at low doses of 2 to 3 IU/m^2 after 6 to 10 months of daily or 3 times per week administration (Goldstein & Laszlo, 1986; Oldham, 1985). Responses are evidenced by improvement in hematologic parameters, with increases in platelet counts, production of normal leukocytes, and resolution of anemia. Forty per cent of those responding will have relapses between 4 and 36 months after interferon-α is discontinued, which indicates the need for maintenance therapy or reinduction to maintain remissions (Hansen & Borden, 1992).

Chronic myelogenous leukemia (CML) in the benign or chronic phase has also been found to respond to interferon-α. The benign or chronic phase of this disease is characterized by large numbers of leukocytes in the blood, giving the appearance of "purulent blood." The benign phase lasts an average of 3.5 years despite current chemotherapy. The accelerated phase and blastic crisis follow the chronic phase with their course little affected by chemotherapy (Melin & Ozer, 1992). Chronic myelogenous leukemia is associated with increased cytogenetic abnormalities, such as the presence of the Philadelphia chromosome and activation of various oncogenes and growth factors (Gutterman, 1988).

Complete hematologic responses in CML are achieved at a rate of about 70 per cent in patients treated with interferon-α. Continued interferon use also induces prolonged suppression of the Philadelphia chromosome and reversal of some cytogenetic abnormalities. These response rates with correction of cytogenetic abnormalities have lasted for more than 3 years as the patients in remission continue to be followed (Gutterman, 1988). There is an increased response rate if treatment is started within 6 months of diagnosis.

Interferon-α is also indicated for use against acquired immunodeficiency syndrome (AIDS)-related Kaposi's sarcoma. Classic Kaposi's sarcoma is a relatively rare tumor of older men, usually considered to be benign. It appears as flat, macular lesions, primarily in the lower extremities, that are faint pink to reddish-purple. The incidence of this malignancy in young male homosexuals has increased, an observation that, in fact, led to the awareness of the AIDS epidemic in the early 1980's. Kaposi's sarcoma is a multifocal cancer of the skin and connective tissue that does not metastasize to internal organs; however, its spread along the epithelial linings of the visceral mucosa is a poor prognostic indicator.

In Kaposi's sarcoma the response to interferon includes the flattening or disappearance of the lesions with no evidence of disease on biopsy of prior Kaposi's sarcoma sites. The response is dose-related, with 28 to 40 per cent of the responses occurring with high doses (18 to 36 IU/day three times per week). Interferon-α does not correct the immune deficiencies of AIDS but does suppress human immunodeficiency virus (HIV), and the incidence of opportunistic infections in responders is reported to decrease. However, toxicities are considerable and require dose reductions in one third of the patients who have significant fatigue, malaise, and neutropenia (Balmer, 1990).

Other hematologic disorders that show responsiveness to interferon-α when combined with chemotherapy include nodular non-Hodgkin's lymphoma, chronic lymphocytic leukemia, cutaneous T-cell lymphoma, and multiple myeloma. Solid tumors have shown less responsiveness to interferon, but some significant responses have been seen in renal cell carcinoma, malignant carcinoid tumors, superficial bladder cancer with intravesical instillation, in ovarian carcinoma with intraperitoneal administration, and in colon cancer with interferon enhancing the effect of 5-fluorouracil. For more detailed discussions of clinical indications for the use of interferon-α, comprehensive review articles are available (Balmer, 1990; Goldstein & Laszlo, 1986; Gutterman, 1988; Hansen & Borden, 1992; Kirkwood & Ernstoff, 1984; Moldawer & Figlin, 1995).

Interferon-α has also been studied in a number of nononcologic illnesses. Results have been dramatic in interferon treatment of some conditions induced by viral infections, such as the hepatitis virus and the papovavirus, which causes genital and laryngeal warts. Use of interferon-α successfully reduces growth of laryngeal warts, postponing the need for repeated surgeries to maintain a clear airway. The antiviral effect of interferon inhibits replication of the hepatitis B virus (HBV). Remissions of chronic hepatitis B treated with at least 6 months of interferon-α are reported to be of long duration and with loss of the viral hepatitis B surface antigen (Moldawer & Figlin, 1995).

Interferon-β. Interferon-β is very similar to interferon-α, although modest in both its antiviral activity and its toxicities. Interferon-β (Betaseron; Chiron Corporation) received Food and Drug Administration approval for the nononcologic use to decrease the frequency of relapsing-remitting multiple sclerosis. Small subcutaneous doses of this recombinant form of interferon-β have been shown to decrease visual problems, partial paralysis, tremors, lack of coordination, and memory loss (Anonymous, 1993). Some promising activity in primary brain tumors (gliomas) has been seen with interferon-β (Balmer, 1990). Trials currently focus on the synergistic effects of interferon-β given concomitantly with chemotherapy or other biologic agents (Balmer, 1990; Moldawer & Figlin, 1995).

Interferon-γ. Interferon-γ plays an integral role in the normal immune response, and it has several different biologic effects that differentiate it from either interferon-α or interferon-β. It has more of an activation effect on macrophages and demonstrates a much higher cytotoxic effect in vitro through its role in regulating cytotoxic T cells (Vilcek, Kelker, Jumming, & Yip, 1985). The toxicity profile with interferon-γ is similar to interferon-α. In addition, prolonged systolic hypotension, which in some cases lasts up to 24 hours after interferon-γ administration, will result in dose reductions. Headaches also are more common and may reach dose-limiting severity.

Although early clinical trials of interferon-γ used as a single agent have failed to yield tumor regressions, it has been shown to suppress growth and differentiation and to interact with other interferons, TNF, and interleukins to produce antiproliferative effects (Gutterman, 1988). Continued trials that study interferon-γ as adjuvant therapy or in combination with other biologics and chemotherapy will define its role in the future.

Side Effects. Toxicity frequently occurs at doses of higher than one IU, and severity increases with larger doses (Table 23–5). Tolerance to the acute side effects develop after the first one to three doses of interferon. See the section on "Management of Toxicities" for detailed discussion of side effects. Long-term administration of high doses (greater than 15 IU) may result in cumulative, dose-limiting toxicities. These dose-limiting toxicities include unacceptable fatigue, anorexia with weight loss, confusion, and occasionally liver transaminase elevations (Kirkwood & Ernstoff, 1984). Other less frequent toxic effects that are transient and reversible with cessation of therapy include nausea, hypotension, central nervous system depression, somnolence, electroencephalogram changes, and proteinuria. Acute cardiac failure with arrhythmias and acute ischemic events are evidence of a rare life-threatening toxicity. Caution is required in administering high doses of interferon to those with a strong history of cardiovascular disease.

COLONY-STIMULATING FACTORS

The body's blood cell production is a never ending cycle that is strictly regulated by a complex system of checks and balances innate to the human body. Mature red cells, white cells, and platelets circulating in the blood stream are short-lived and in need of continuous replacement. At the core of this system exists a group of molecules called hematopoietic colony-stimulating factors (CSFs) that mediate the proliferation, maturation, regulation, and activation of mature blood cells (Haeuber & Spross, 1991).

All of the blood cells originate from pluripotent hematopoietic stem cells located primarily within the bone marrow. Stem cells are primitive cells capable of giving birth to cells that will proliferate and further differentiate to become functional mature blood cells, replacing old cells or increasing the cell pool as body conditions render. It is also capable of reproducing itself to replace those stem cells that become committed to differentiation (Applebaum, 1993). The factors that control the behavior of the pluripotent stem cell are not well understood. However, much is known about how the proliferation and differentiation of committed hematopoietic progenitors is controlled. This process of blood production and differentiation is referred to as hematopoiesis (Fig. 23–4).

CSFs direct the proliferation and differentiation of committed hematopoietic progenitors by binding to receptors on their target cells. The cellular response depends on the particular target; the immature cell will typically proliferate and begin to differentiate into mature cells whereas in mature cells, the response is to become functionally activated (Metcalf, 1989).

CSFs, which are classified as cytokines, generally are named after the cell lineage they affect (Crosier & Clark, 1992). GM-CSF is a growth factor that affects both granulocytes and macrophages, whereas G-CSF is a growth factor affecting only granulocytes. However, an overlap of effects from these factors most likely occurs. Interleukins, substances released from white blood cells that assist in the regulation of the activity of other white blood cells, may function either directly as CSFs or indirectly by binding to target cells and activating them to release CSFs (Applebaum, 1993). Interleukin-3 is an example of an interleukin that functions directly as a CSF. Table 23–6 presents the growth factors currently in clinical trials.

Erythropoietin. Red blood cell production (erythropoiesis) is dependent on the hormone-like glycoprotein,

TABLE 23–5. *Interferon Side Effects*

FREQUENT	LESS COMMON
Acute	
Fever (to 40°C)	Nausea and vomiting
Chills (and rigors)	Diarrhea
Headaches	Hypotension
Chronic	
Fatigue	Central nervous system changes:
Malaise	Confusion
Anorexia (taste change)	Depression
Weight loss	Electroencephalogram changes
Mild leukopenia	Mild hepatic dysfunction
Mild thrombocytopenia	Proteinuria
	Cardiac arrhythmias

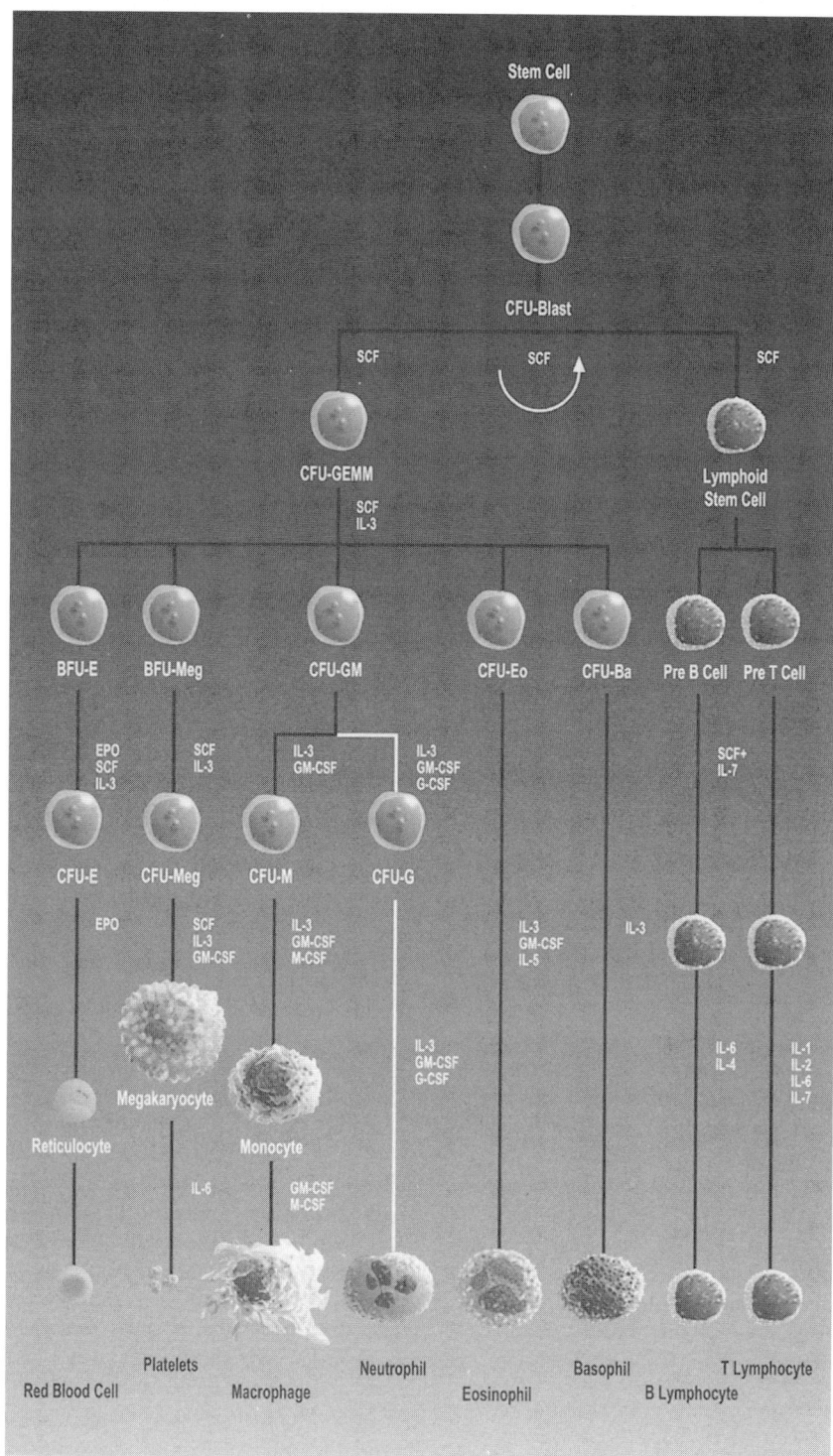

FIGURE **23–4.** Hematopoiesis. (© 1993 Amgen Inc., Amgen Center, Thousand Oaks, CA 91320.)

erythropoietin (EPO). It regulates erythropoiesis by binding to the receptors on the erythroid precursors undergoing differentiation in the bone marrow, thus stimulating the release of reticulocytes and increasing hemoglobin synthesis (Erslev,1991) (Fig. 23–5).

Erythropoiesis is regulated by EPO in response to tissue oxygenation in the kidneys. When the oxygenation levels decline, the kidneys respond by releasing EPO into circulation; the EPO is filtered through the bone marrow and stimulates the erythroid precursors (St. Germain, 1992). Epoetin alfa is a glycoprotein manufactured by recombinant DNA technology and is produced by mammalian cells containing the EPO gene. In 1989 Epoetin alfa became the first CSF to receive FDA approval for clinical use. It currently is approved for patients with chronic renal failure, Aids-

TABLE 23–6. *Approved and Investigational Hematopoietic Growth Factors*

Growth Factor	Generic Name (Trade Name[s])	Side Effects
Approved		
Epo	Epoetin-alfa (Epogen, Procrit)	Flulike symptoms with arthralgias and myalgias. Occasional headache and bloodshot eyes
G-CSF	Filgrastim (Neupogen)	Bone pain in areas of high bone marrow reserve, rare allergic reactions with rash, urticaria, facial edema, dyspnea, hypotension, tachycardia
GM-CSF	Sargamostim (Leukine, Prokine)	Fever, dose-related fluid retention, dyspnea, myalgias, joint pain, bone pain
Investigational		
	Molgrastim (Leucomax)	Fever, fluid retention, dyspnea, myalgias, joint pain, bone pain
M-CSF	M-CSF (Macstim, Macrolim)	Fever, rash, headache, facial flushing, myalgias, photophobia (thrombocytopenia, chest tightness, wheezing may occur with *Escherichia coli* product)
IL-3		Dose-related fever, chills, headache, bone pain, facial flushing, nausea and vomiting
SCF		Local injection site reaction, dermatologic reactions, occasional cough, sore throat, throat tightness and hypotension
PIX 321 (GM-CSF/IL-3 fusion protein)	GM-CSF+ IL-3 (Pixikine)	Local injection site reaction, headache, chest pain, asthenia

Epo = Erythropoietin; G-CSF = Granulocyte colony-stimulating factor; GM-CSF = Granulocyte-macrophage colony stimulating factor; M-CSF = Macrophage colony-stimulating factor; IL-3 = Interleukin-3; SCF = Stem cell factor.
(Adapted with permission from Foon, K. [1993]. The cytokine network. *Oncology, 7*[12], 11–16.)

related anemia, or cancer chemotherapy-related anemia (Haeuber, 1993). Current research in this area includes the use of EPO to increase RBC production in patients before surgery in an attempt to harvest and store their blood for autologous perioperative transfusions, thus avoiding donor transfusions that carry safety and immunologic concerns (Henry, 1992).

Clinical Applications. Research was conducted on the effect of EPO in patients with cancer chemotherapy-induced anemia based on the success of EPO in treating anemia in patients with chronic renal failure and zidovudine-treated HIV-infected patients. Abels reported in 1991 on a double-blind, placebo controlled, multisite study of 131 anemia patients receiving chemotherapy (Abels, 1992). Patients received either 150 U/kg Epoetin alfa or a placebo as a subcutaneous injection three times weekly for 12 weeks. Results were statistically significant in the group that received Epoetin alfa for a rise in hematocrit during months 2 and 3 and for a lower transfusion requirement. Patients in this study tolerated the EPO therapy very well (Abels, 1992).

Nursing Considerations. The recommended starting dose for cancer patients on chemotherapy is 150 U/kg administered subcutaneously three times a week. The patient's hematocrit level should be monitored every week. If after 8 weeks the hematocrit has decreased or remained unchanged, the dose can be increased up to a maximum dose of 300 U/kg three times a week. Patients who do not respond after a month on 300 U/kg usually will not respond. Once the hematocrit reaches 36 to 40 per cent, the dose should be maintained and monitored periodically (Rieger, 1993).

Instruct patients that it usually takes 2 to 4 weeks for their anemia to respond to EPO. Erythropoiesis requires a good supply of iron and protein, and patients should be instructed on a diet high in these elements. Supplemental iron is necessary for some of the patients (Rieger, 1993). Side effects typically are not a problem; however, a small percentage of patients will experience a rise in their blood pressure (Abels,1992).

G-CSF and GM-CSF. The leading cause of death from cancer is infection, and now with the ability to prevent or diminish neutropenia the potential to influence death from infection exists (Pizzo & Meyers, 1989). Chemotherapy-induced neutropenia is the most common type of neutropenia seen in cancer patients. It has been well established that the risk of infection is related to both the severity and duration of neutropenia. With prolonged neutropenia the risk of primary infection increases, and the risk of secondary opportunistic infections, mainly fungus, is accelerated (Applebaum, 1993). Research has documented anywhere from 25 to 56 per cent of patients receiving chemotherapy will have a febrile neutropenic episode; the average number of episodes per patient is three (Bodey, Buckley, Sathe, & Freireich, 1966) . A second problem associated with chemotherapy-related neutropenia is that the chemotherapy regimen must often be reduced, because patients cannot tolerate the bone marrow suppression. Dose intensity has been shown to be closely correlated to tumor response and patient survival. However, patients often receive less intensive regimens because of the fear of neutropenia (Hyrniuk, Figueredo, & Goodyear, 1987).

Clinical Applications. GM-CSF and G-CSF are two growth factors that are widely used to prevent and

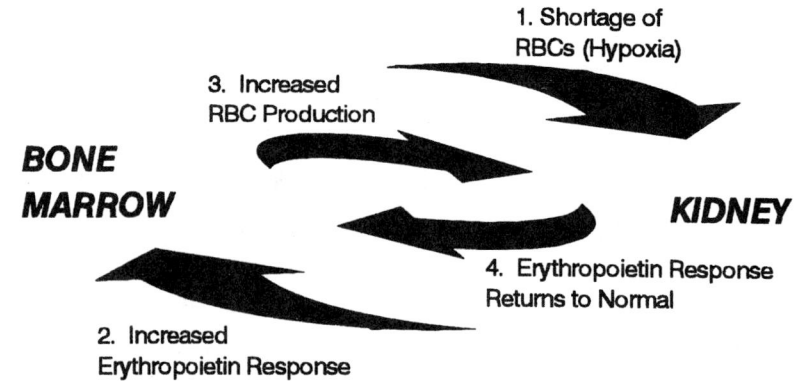

FIGURE 23–5. Red blood cell–oxygen demand feedback loop. (From Ortho Biotech, Inc., Raritan, NJ.)

treat neutropenia. Both G-CSF and GM-CSF have demonstrated the therapeutic ability of increasing the neutrophil count and decreasing the episodes of febrile neutropenia in patients who have received chemotherapy (Crawford, Ozer, & Johnson, 1990; Herrmann et al., 1989). However, each agent appears to have different biologic characteristics. G-CSF appears to influence neutrophil production, whereas GM-CSF stimulates monocytes as well as eosinophils and neutrophils, thus providing wider coverage of pathogens (Applebaum, 1993).

The possibility of stimulation of tumor growth by CSF's has been documented as a theoretic concern. It is reported that CSF's can stimulate myeloid leukemia cells to proliferate in culture and that small-cell carcinoma of the lung may have low levels of receptors for either G-CSF or GM-CSF. Currently, no data exists in published literature to support this risk in the clinical setting (Baldwin et al., 1989; Estey, 1994; Ohno et al., 1990).

The use of CSFs after bone marrow transplants is a rapidly evolving practice, since bone marrow transplantation is usually associated with weeks of severe pancytopenia before the rescue marrow begins to repopulate the marrow and restore the circulating cell population. Despite aggressive supportive care, life-threatening infections occur in approximately one third of the patients (Nienhuis et al., 1987). The use of growth factors to shorten the period of pancytopenia has been widely studied.

There are a number of published studies documenting the use of GM-CSF in patients after autologous marrow transplantation. The results of the studies support that GM-CSF can be beneficial in aiding in the recovery of neutrophil counts, thus reducing infection and allowing the patient to be released sooner from the hospital (Nemunaitis et al., 1991). In one study the use of GM-CSF resulted in a $12,000 savings per patient in related medical costs. There are less data regarding G-CSF in this population; however, studies suggest similar medical and cost-saving effects of G-CSF as with GM-CSF (Peters et al., 1988).

The use of CSF's after allogeneic transplantation is more complicated due to the sensitive immunologic relationship of the host and the donor. Since CSFs may stim-

ulate certain cells of the immune system, the possibility exists of increasing rejection because of this stimulation (Powles et al., 1990). However, allogeneic transplants carry a higher risk of infections than autologus transplants due to the prolonged neutropenic period following transplant, so the potential benefit from CSF's is great. Encouraging results have been documented in using GM-CSF in donor-related transplants as well as unrelated matched transplants. The period of neutropenia was shortened, and the incidence of graft-vs.-host disease was not increased (Nemunaitis et al., 1991).

Other CSF's are currently being studied in the BMT population. Refractory thrombocytopenia remains a deadly complication in some transplants, and the search for an agent, possibly thrombopoietin, to stimulate megakaryocytes is ongoing (Burris, 1993). Several of the interleukins have been used alone and in combination with other CSF's in an effort to better stimulate the bone marrow (see Interleukin section). CSF's, such as G-CSF and GM-CSF, have been given to patients before peripheral stem cell harvest to increase the numbers of stem cells circulating in peripheral blood. This increases the harvest of stem cells that can be frozen and later transfused to the patient (Nemunaitis, 1993).

Nursing Considerations. G-CSF and GM-CSF appear to be well tolerated at doses up to 32 μg/kg. At higher doses GM-CSF produces a wider variety of systemic toxicities than G-CSF (Beveridge & Miller, 1993). Both agents have been administered by subcutaneous and intravenous routes. Typically patients are started on these agents after chemotherapy is completed and continue receiving the factor until their predicted nadir has occurred. Many of the patients at home will need to inject themselves with the growth factor several times a week.

Reimbursement Issues. CSF's are expensive and may be difficult for patients to be reimbursed if they are receiving the agent for off-label use. There are also a number of reimbursement issues that surround patients when they receive the growth factors at home. For example, Medicare patients receive reimbursement for their growth factors only if the injections are administered in a physician's office. Most of the pharmaceutical companies marketing the growth factors have excellent resources on reimbursement issues.

INTERLEUKINS

Interleukins are a group of cytokines (lymphokines and monokines) named for their ability to "interlink" cells in vivo—especially cells of the immune system, such as lymphocytes, natural killer cells, macrophages, and also hematopoietic cells. By interlinking cells of the immune system, interleukins aid in the control of the behavior of these cells. Interleukins can be CSF's, such as interleukin 3, or by interacting with their target cells they can enable their target cells to release CSF's, thus having an indirect effect on hematopoiesis.

At least a dozen interleukins have been identified. In addition to IL-2, which has received the most investigation, IL-1, IL-3, IL-4, IL-6, and IL-11 are also being studied clinically. In this ever-changing area of biotherapy we can expect other interleukins to rapidly be clinically introduced.

Interleukin-1. IL-1 represents a family of polypeptides produced by macrophage fibroblasts, endothelial cells, and smooth-muscle cells that exhibits a wide variety of biologic activities. Two molecular forms of IL-1—IL-1α and IL-1β—were isolated in purification of human IL-1 (Foon, 1993). IL-1 plays an important immunoregulatory role through a spectrum of activities including (1) activation of T cells to produce IL-2 and other cytokines, (2) induction of fibroblast proliferation, (3) induction of fever, (4) enhancement of antibody responsiveness through stimulation of helper T cells and B cells, (5) enhancement of cytotoxicity of lymphocytes, (6) induction of tumor-cell markers, and (7) provision of radioprotective properties (Zsebo et al., 1988). Early clinical data have yielded the potential for pronounced toxicity similar to IL-2 that was reversible when the agent was stopped (Burris, 1993). Both IL-1α and IL-1β are currently in clinical trials.

Interleukin-3. IL-3 is produced principally by activated T lymphocytes, and its activities appear to be that of a growth factor. It is able to stimulate early hematopoietic progenitors, including myeloid, erythroid, and megakaryocytic precursors, as well as augment the activities of mature targets, such as eosinophils and monocytes. Early clinical trials with IL-3 have shown a modest increase in white cells, mostly lymphocytes and eosinophils, and an increase in platelet counts. Preliminary trials using the "steel" factor, which is a fusion molecule of GM-CSF and IL-3, suggest that this combination may prove very beneficial in stimulating platelet recovery (Miller et al., 1993). Side effects from IL-3 appeared dose-dependent and included chills, facial flushing, and mild bone pain (Burris, 1993).

Interleukin 4. IL-4, known as the B cell stimulating factor, appears to be a B cell regulator with some activity on select T lymphocytes and macrophages. It is being tested in certain B cell malignancies such as multiple myeloma and indolent B cell lymphomas. It is synergistic when given with G-CSF, EPO, and IL-1 (Paul, 1987).

Interleukin 6. IL-6 may have positive clinical effects on increasing platelet recovery. Preclinical studies in murine models suggest that IL-6 also may have antitumor effects. Clinical data support that when IL-6 is administered in conjunction with intensive chemotherapy regimens, there is an increased platelet recovery in a shorter period of time (Weber et al., 1993).

Interleukin 11. IL-11 seems to hold promise in its ability to produce platelet-enhancing activity. Studies are currently examining these properties in the transplant population. Researchers are also examining the production of cytokine cocktails that would include several cytokines which exhibit synergistic effects when given together. IL-11 is being tested in one of these cocktails with GM-CSF (Burris, 1993).

Interleukin 2. Interleukin 2 is a lymphokine that is a BRM (peptide hormone); it is secreted by T lymphocytes, which are capable of directing the function of other cells in the area of an immune response. Interleukin-2 directs the T lymphocytes to multiply into clones capable of performing during an immune response (Morgan, Ruscetti, & Gallo, 1976). Clinical studies indicate antitumor response with high doses of IL-2 (Lotze et al.,1986).

Historic Background. IL-2 was initially described by Morgan et al. in 1976 as "T cell growth factor." These investigators noted that IL-2 was a small protein that had the ability to sustain the proliferation in vitro of activated T lymphocytes. Although its biology is not fully understood, the protein has been purified, and its gene has been cloned in the past 10 years. The gene for IL-2 has been expressed in bacteria, and recombinant IL-2 is now commercially available for biologic and pharmacologic studies (Morgan et al., 1976).

Mechanism of Action. IL-2 acts as a growth factor by binding to specific receptors on T lymphocytes and triggering the proliferation of activated T lymphocytes. IL-2 supports the proliferation of activated T lymphoctes. IL-2 supports the proliferation of natural killer cells and augments various other T-cell functions. IL-2 is also capable of activating cytotoxic effector cells that secrete a host of secondary cytokines such as TNF, IL-1, IL-6, and interferon γ. In vitro, the administration of IL-2 has corrected the immune deficit in the athymic nude mouse (Rosenberg et al., 1985). In vitro, some of the immunologic abnormalities have been reversed in patients with AIDS. Studies have demonstrated that human lymphocytes incubated with IL-2 develop the ability to lyse human tumor cells in the laboratory. High doses of IL-2 have also been shown to lyse tumor cells in mice (Rosenberg et al., 1985).

Clinical Applications. After evaluating the positive in vitro responses, researchers at the National Cancer Institute's surgery branch began a series of human clinical trials (Rosenberg et al., 1985). In 1984, Rosenberg began treating a series of patients with a combination of IL-2 cells and cells that had been harvested from the patient and incubated in the laboratory with IL-2, referred to as LAK cells (Box 23–1). IL-2 and LAK cell therapy is known as adoptive immunotherapy. This term implies that there is a transfer of active immunologic cells with the potential to directly or indirectly induce an antitumor response in the patient with a tumor (Rosenberg et al., 1985).

BOX 23–1. *Interleukin-2*

Rosenberg, S. A., Lotze, M. T., Muul, L. M., Leitman, S., Chang, A. E., Ettinghausen, S. E., Matory, Y. L., Skibber, J. M., Shiloni, E., Vetto, J. T., Seipp, C. A., Simpson, C., & Reichert, C. M. (1985). Observations on the systemic administration of autologous lymphokine-activated killer cells and recombinant interleukin-2 to patients with metastatic cancer. *New England Journal of Medicine, 313,* 1485–1492.

This research report was the first to relate the promising effects of administering interleukin-2 (IL-2) and lymphokine-activated killer cells (LAK) to patients with refractory cancer. In this study, 25 patients with metastatic cancer who had failed standard therapy were treated. Patients received both LAK cells, generated from lymphocytes obtained through serial leukapheresis, and up to 90 doses of IL-2.

More than a 50 per cent volume regression was observed in 11 of the 25 patients. One patient with metastatic melanoma obtained a complete remission of 10 months' duration. Partial responses occurred in nine patients with pulmonary or hepatic metastases from melanoma and colon or renal cell cancer and in one patient with a primary unresectable lung adenocarcinoma. Severe toxicities were reported in this study.

More than 50 per cent of all patients gained in excess of 10 per cent of their weight from fluid retention. Pulmonary interstitial edema was seen in 20 patients, and two of these 20 patients required intubation. Fever, chills, and malaise were seen in almost all of the patients. A generalized erythematous rash was seen in 17 of the 25 patients. Adverse effects in all patients disappeared promptly after the IL-2 administration ended.

The process of treating patients with IL-2 and LAK cells was initially very complex (Fig. 23–6). Patients were admitted and placed on high doses of IL-2, which increases the number of lymphocytes in the body (100,000 U/kg intravenously three times per day for days 2 through 6 of the first week). The second week involved 5 days of lymphocytopheresis, the purpose of which was to obtain sufficient quantities of lymphocytes to incubate with IL-2 in the laboratory cultures. These lymphocytes then produced LAK cells that were infused back into the patient (in the same manner as other cell transfusions). On the last day of pheresis, the patient received IL-2 again in the same doses as the first week, as well as the first round of LAK cell infusions. This complex 2-week process was continued for three doses daily of IL-2 plus LAK cells (Jassak & Stricklin, 1986).

The initial results published in December 1985 reported significant tumor responses in patients with malignant melanoma, colon carcinoma, and metastatic renal cell carcinoma (Rosenberg et al., 1985). Researchers became very optimistic that IL-2 given with LAK cells could be a breakthrough in cancer treatment (Bylinsky, 1985). The media picked up on the excitement, and soon most papers and news magazines were carrying the story of the "breakthrough." Because this treatment was associated with significant toxicity, many centers throughout the world began to experiment with different approaches using IL-2 in an attempt to increase tumor kill and decrease toxicity.

The same group of researchers from the National Cancer Institute began looking at a group of T lymphocytes that invade tumors. The researchers excised the tumor and harvested the group of T cells. The tumor-infiltrating lymphocytes (TILs) were then expanded in IL-2 in the laboratory. Studies have shown these cells to be 50 to 100 times more potent than LAK cells in lysing tumor cells (Simpson, Seipp, & Rosen-

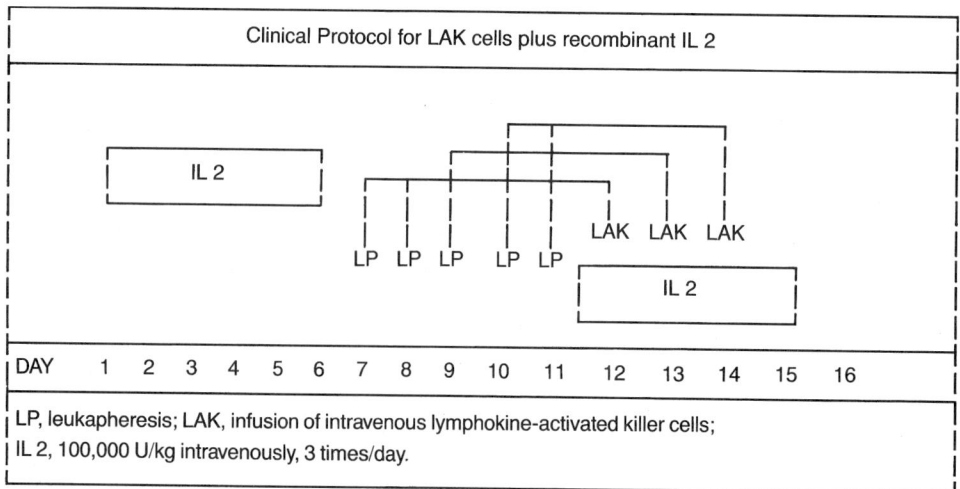

FIGURE 23–6. Schedule for administration of interleukin 2 (IL-2) and lymphokine-activated killer (LAK) cells. (Adapted from Simpson, C., Seipp, L. A., Rosenberg, S. A. [1988]. The current status and future applications of interleukin-2 and adoptive immunotherapy in cancer treatment. *Seminars in Oncology Nursing, 4*[2]:132–141.)

berg, 1988). Tumor-infiltrating lymphocytes are administered in the same manner as LAK cells, through a central catheter. Initial published results indicated a 35 to 40 per cent response rate for patients with metastatic melanoma; however, updated reports indicate a much lower response rate with short response duration (Sznol & Parkinson, 1994).

A subsequent review of all known clinical trials using high-dose rIL-2 to treat patients with metastatic renal cell carcinoma documented objective antitumor responses in 36 (14 per cent) of 255 patients. This included 12 (5 per cent) complete and 24 (9 per cent) partial responses. Actuarial analysis projected that 78 per cent of responding patients would remain free of disease progression for 1 year; 55 per cent would remain progression-free for 18 months. Based on the safety and efficacy data, the FDA approved rIL-2 (aldesleukin, proleukin) in May 1992 for the treatment of good performance metastatic renal cell carcinoma patients (Fisher, 1993).

Several years of clinical trials with IL-2, including dose and schedule modifications and combinations with other biologics and chemotherapy, have shown more limited antitumor activities than researchers had predicted (Sznol & Parkinson, 1994). It is suggested that because of the severe toxicities associated with IL-2, doses clinically cannot be increased to the degree necessary to yield antitumor results (Rosenberg, 1992). Lower doses of IL-2 have been administered on an outpatient basis to renal cell patients who were not eligible for the high-dose therapy. Similar results were obtained with the lower doses as would have been obtained with high-dose treatment (Caligiuri, 1993). Researchers searching for the optimal method of administering IL-2 have combined it with other cytokines such as interferon α. Combining IL-2 with other cytokines has not resulted in a substantial increase in tumor response over that of IL-2 alone (Sznol, Thurn, & Parkinson, 1993). Combination of IL-2 and chemotherapy has yielded higher response rates in patients with metastatic melanoma than IL-2 alone; however, the medium duration of response is short (lasting 5 to 7 months) (Sznol & Longo, 1993). The combination of chemotherapy to IL-2 must be further evaluated to understand the contribution the combination may offer.

Current research is concentrating on reducing the toxicity associated with high doses of IL-2 by adding other agents to mitigate its toxicity without affecting the antitumor activity (Lotze, Agarwala, Kirkwood, 1994). Nitric oxide synthetase inhibitors, amino guanidine (to reduce hypotension), and inhibitors of TNF such as pentoxifylline have been shown to reduce IL-2 toxicity without affecting tumor response (Thompson, Bianco, Benyunes, Neubaur, & Fefer, 1993).

Enhanced cytokine therapy through the use of gene therapy is being examined with IL-2. This involves inserting the gene for IL-2 in TIL cells and reinfusing the cells back to the patient. It is thought that when the TIL cells migrate back to the tumor site they will release the IL-2, delivering a dose directly to the tumor site (Rosenberg, 1992). It is too early to make any clinical predications on this method.

Side Effects. Therapy with high doses of IL-2 can be very difficult for patients to tolerate because of the severe toxicity associated with it. The toxicity is generally dose-dependent and is cummulative in effect, escalating in severity the longer a patient receives the treatment. Performance status declines markedly over time. Careful pretherapy assessment is essential in selecting patients that will have the best tolerance for the therapy. In general the more compromised patients are before therapy, especially if their morbidity involves heart, lung, kidneys or liver, the less likely they will be to tolerate the therapy. Patient and family education should explain the therapy, the potential side effects, and the treatment of side effects before beginning the treatment (Rieger, Weatherly & Rumsey, 1993).

Every body system is affected by IL-2 toxicity. Like all other BRMs individuals react differently with the agent; however, dose and schedule appears to influence the toxicity. The concomitant use of adoptive immunotherapy, other BRMs, or chemotherapy will also influence the effect of IL-2. The mechanism by which IL-2 produces the side effects is not fully understood. It has been shown that IL-2 can produce some of the side effects; however, it may be the release of other cytokines mediated by IL-2 that produces the majority of the ill effects (Rieger et al., 1993). Table 23–7 summarizes the side effects, and the nursing management of these patients is discussed in the final section of this chapter.

TUMOR NECROSIS FACTOR

Tumor necrosis factor (TNF) was named on the basis of its ability to cause necrosis of established tumors in the mouse. Tumor necrosis factor is a monokine produced by activated macrophages and specialized circulating phagocytic monocytes that selectively kills neoplastic cells.

Historic Origin. Tumor necrosis factor evolved from the investigations with Coley's toxins in the early 1900's. Coley noted that a recurrent sarcoma, which had continued to regrow after five resections within 3 years, regressed following two episodes of an unusual bacterial infection. Coley began investigations with toxins derived from heat-killed bacteria. Several patients, primarily sarcoma cases, experienced tumor regressions. Side effects included nausea and vomiting, headache, malaise, and fever, which disappeared in 1 to 2 days (Coley, 1893). One of Coley's toxins was refined by Shear, Turner, Perrault, and Shovelton (1943) and was much more potent in inducing hemorrhage and necrosis in mouse tumor implants. This refined endotoxin was located in the cell wall of gram-negative bacteria.

The name *tumor necrosis factor* was chosen because this toxin appeared to specifically affect the tumor without causing undesirable effects to normal tissues (Oettgen & Old, 1987). Tumor necrosis factor, which is comparable to the interferon system, most likely consists of a whole family of cytotoxic factors. Two genetic sequences have been identified, one for lymphotoxin and one for cachectin. Chronic infections

TABLE 23–7. *Side Effects of Interleukin-2*

SIGNS AND SYMPTOMS	COMMENTS
Flulike Syndrome	
Fever	Peaks at 39°–40°C.
Chills	Onset 2–4 hrs. after administration; rigors possible; may be produced by a hypothalmic-gassed stress response or by release of lymphokines/monokines.
Myalgia/arthralgia	At high doses, may be due to accumulation of IL-2-induced cells or cytokine deposits in joint spaces.
Headache	Enhanced by fever and chills.
Malaise	
Gastrointestinal	
Nausea, vomiting, diarrhea, mucositis, xerostomia, anorexia	Acute or chronic, dose-related, cumulative toxicities; may produce generalized inflammation of mucosal lining; may require prophylaxis for GI bleeding.
Integumentary	
Dryness, erythematous rash, pruritus, desquamation	Pruritus may occur without rash.
Neurologic/Psychologic	
Confusion, irritability, impaired memory, expressive aphasia, sleep disturbances, depression, psychoses, hallucination	Mental status changes may be enhanced by anxiety, sleep deprivation, and/or an intensive care environment.
Cardiovascular	
Capillary leak syndrome	Dose-related (>100,000 U/kg).
Peripheral edema, ascites, weight gain	Decreased systemic vascular resistance results in shift of fluid from intravascular to interstitial spaces, including organs.
Arrhythmias	Mostly atrial; occasional supraventricular tachycardia, myocarditis, chest pain; rare sudden cardiac death.
Hypotension	Causes decreased tissue oxygenation and renal blood flow.
Pulmonary	
Dyspnea, tachypnea	Dose-related.
Pulmonary edema	Acute at onset; results in decreased oxygen diffusion to alveoli; occasional pulmonary infiltrates on chest x-ray; excessive fluid replacement is contraindicated.
Cough	
Nasal congestion	
Renal/Hepatic	
Oliguria, proteinuria, increased serum creatinine and GUM, elevated liver function tests (serum bilirubin, SGOT, SGPT, LDH, alkaline phosphatase)	Direct tubular-cell toxicity and decreased renal blood flow; cumulative dose effect.
Hematologic	
Anemia/thrombocytopenia	Cumulative, dose-related; occasional abnormalities in coagulation studies.

(Adapted from Dudjak, L. A., & Yasko, J. M. [1990]. Biological response modifier therapy. In J. M. Yasko & L. A. Dudjak [Eds.], *Biological response modifier therapy: Symptom management* [pp. 3–24]. Pittsburgh: Park Row.)

and cancer have been noted to cause severe wasting with negative calorie and nitrogen balance leading to death. It is hypothesized that this wasting results from the effects of cachectin (Beutler & Cerami, 1987).

Mechanism of Action. The production of TNF by mononuclear phagocytes is induced by most infectious agents, including virus particles and some of the other biologics. Tumor necrosis factor is the mediator of general inflammation and septic shock. Its induction of necrosis appears to be related to its ability to diminish tissue perfusion. It alters hemostatic properties of vascular endothelium, inducing a disseminated intravascular coagulation type of effect at a systemic level with local occlusion of tumor vessels. Tumor necrosis factor is directly toxic to vascular endothelial cells, causing the "third spacing" of plasma water and electrolytes into the extravascular spaces. It also induces the release

of interleukin-1, which may elicit the features of endotoxin poisoning: fever, hypotension, neutropenia, and thrombocytopenia (Beutler & Cerami, 1987).

Exposure to TNF activates macrophages to release cytotoxic factors, which mediate events leading up to hemorrhagic necrosis. The activated macrophages adhere to endothelial surfaces, enhancing their phagocytic activity. Within a few hours of administration, TNF induces hemorrhagic necrosis. The core of the tumor turns blue-black, owing to the extravasation of blood into the tumor, which may then slough off (Flick & Gifford, 1985).

Clinical Uses. The role of TNF in many phases of the immune response maintains a level of interest in its clinical role. The toxicity associated with TNF has prevented the administration of doses high enough to yield clinical responses with single-agent use of TNF

TABLE 23–8. *Side Effects of Tumor Necrosis Factor*

COMMON	UNCOMMON
Rigors	Hypotension
Fever	Peripheral vasoconstriction
Headache	Hypertension, tachycardia,
Local inflammation (at sub-	and mild chest discomfort
cutaneous injection site)	during rigors
Nausea and vomiting	Fatigue

(Table 23–8). Some promising results have been seen in intraperitoneal instillation and regional tumor perfusions with the agent, allowing higher levels of the agent at the tumor site and minimizing the systemic side effects (Holmlund, 1993). There is interest in studying TNF in combination with other treatment modalities for synergism and immunomodulary effects.

NURSING RESPONSIBILITIES

The nursing care of individuals undergoing biologic therapies offers a nursing challenge to provide comprehensive care. Other areas of nursing considerations include assessment of the immune response, administration, nursing management of side effects, and patient education and support (Irwin, 1987). The nurse must provide support and encouragement to the patient to continue with the therapy until beneficial results can be seen.

ASSESSMENT AND ADMINISTRATION

Biologics stimulate varied cytokine cascade responses. Responses induced by the different agents will vary depending on the dose, route, and schedule. There should be careful assessment of patients' clinical status prior to therapy with interferons and interleukins, since toxicities associated with these cytokines may be pronounced.

Biologics come in several subtypes and dilutions. The directions on package inserts for different agents should be followed carefully in the preparation of the correct dosage, concentration, route of administration, and procedure for reconstitution and maintenance of stability. Advise the patient not to change brands. Typically biologics must be stored in the refrigerator at 2° to 8° C and should not be frozen or shaken. Because these natural products contain no preservatives, a vial should be used only once and discarded. No other medication should be administered in the same syringe used for a biologic, since stability and compatibility are unknown.

Biologics do not possess vesicant properties, although phlebitis may result from prolonged intravenous infusions. Soreness and redness can occur at sites of subcutaneous or intramuscular injections. Data regarding handling of biologic agents are limited. The Oncology Nursing Society, in its 1995 edition of *Biological Response Modifiers Guidelines,* listed the following guidelines:

1. Reasonable caution to avoid direct skin contact and the generation of aerosols is advised with agents fused to chemotherapy molecules.
2. Immunoconjugated radioactive biologics should be handled according to the specific isotope used.
3. Health care facilities should periodically review the available literature, including manufacturer recommendations regarding handling, preparation, storage, administration, and disposal of biologic agents, to maintain related policies and procedures (1995, p. 7).

PATIENT SAFETY

Because biologic agents are high molecular weight proteins, they can potentially induce the production of host antibodies against themselves. Therefore the risk of hypersensitivity reactions exists. Resuscitation and intubation equipment should be readily available, as should emergency drugs such as parenteral corticosteroids, diphenhydramine, and epinephrine. Patients need to be closely observed for at least the first hour following administration of monoclonal antibodies. Assessments of vital signs and pulmonary status should be taken every 15 minutes, followed by assessments every hour for a period following completion of administration. The patient's response and communication with the primary physician about any possible allergic reaction such as hives, wheezing, urticaria, or rash should be carefully documented.

MANAGEMENT OF TOXICITIES

Contrary to original hopes that a natural therapy such as biologic agents would be nontoxic, they can induce significant toxicities. The severity of side effects ranges from the extremely mild and less common side effects of erythropoietin to the severe multiorgan toxicities of interleukin 2. However, the toxicities are dose-related, are generally mild to moderate severity, and are reversible with the cessation of administration. Tachyphylaxis is a term that refers to the tolerance to acute toxicities, such as fever and chills, that develops with time. With interferon, individuals develop a tolerance to the agent over the first few weeks and have a decreased response or tolerance to the agent. The long-term side effects, such as fatigue, accumulate over time. Specific toxicities for the various agents are outlined in Tables 23–4, 23–5, 23–7, and 23–8. The following review of the organ systems tends to omit the mild effects of the growth factors and outlines the toxicities seen with the monoclonal antibodies, interferons, and interleukins (Table 23–9).

Constitutional. The biologic agents each induce their own specific pattern of flulike symptoms ranging from the colony-stimulating factors having very mild effects (occasional low-grade fever) to the acute "flulike syndrome" consisting of severe chills, fever, malaise, myalgias, and headaches associated with interferons, interleukins, and tumor necrosis factor (Haeuber, 1989; Quesada, Talpaz, Rios, Kurzrodk, & Gutterman, 1986). This flulike syndrome is assumed to be caused by the action of cytokines on the hypothalamic temperature control center causing a release of prostaglandins (Haeuber, 1989, 1995).

TABLE 23–9. *Patients Receiving Biologic Response Modifiers: Risk Factors and Nursing Observations*

SYMPTOMS/ORGAN-SYSTEM SIDE EFFECTS	POTENTIAL RISK FACTORS	USUAL TIME FRAME	OBSERVATIONS
Constitutional Symptoms Headache Fever Chills Myalgias Flulike symptoms	Age Poor performance status	Acute	Observe for presence and severity of symptoms (acute symptoms generally abate with repeated dosing)
Fatigue Malaise Weakness	Age Poor performance status Malnutrition Anemia Other medications Inadequate social support system	Chronic	Monitor use of other medications (e.g., propranolol can contribute to fatigue) Monitor nutritional status (e.g., weight change) Monitor hematologic status
Cardiovascular	Cardiac history Unstable hypertension Dehydration Age	Acute and chronic	Observe orthostatic blood pressure changes with vital signs Monitor for potential cardiac symptoms
Neurologic	History of seizures History of mood swings, depression Age	Acute and chronic	Observe for cognitive and mood alterations Educate family to report subtle changes
Gastrointestinal	History of gastrointestinal disorders	Acute	Observe for symptoms
Hematologic	History of coagulation disorders Leukemia Multiple myeloma Bone marrow suppression	Chronic	Routinely monitor complete blood count, differential, platelets, prothrombin time, partial thromboplastin time
Renal/Metabolic	Renal disease	Acute and chronic	Routinely monitor blood urea nitrogen, creatinine, electrolytes Monitor for proteinuria in high-risk patients
Hepatic	History of ethly alcohol use Other hepatotoxic drugs Malnutrution Preexistent liver disease	Chronic	Obtain baseline liver function tests Routinely monitor lactose dehydrogenase, alkaline phosphatase, serum glutamic-oxaloacetic transaminase, serum glutamic-pyruvic transaminase, bilirubin Monitor nutritional status Monitor ethyl alcohol and other drug intake

(From Irwin, M. M. [1987]. Patients receiving biological response modifiers: Overview of nursing care. *Oncology Nursing Forum, 14*[Suppl. 6], 32–37. Reproduced by permission.)

Initially chills begin within hours after administration of the initial biologic dose. The severity ranges from a chilled sensation to severe teeth-chattering rigors accompanied by pallor due to peripheral vasoconstriction. The increased muscular activity associated with the shivers causes the body temperature to rise, along with the pulse rate and blood pressure, and results in generalized muscular aches. This clinical picture of fever and chills resembles the onset of sepsis. However, the predictable single temperature spike that is related to the timing of dose administration and that responds to the use of acetaminophen allows one to

closely observe the otherwise stable patient. If fever persists or is not responsive to acetaminophen, a full culture workup must be initiated.

The "flulike syndrome" subsides in 8 to 12 hours and can be managed with simple comfort measures. Tolerance develops within 2 to 4 weeks of treatment initiation. Acetaminophen is generally effective in controlling the fevers, which may peak at 39° to 40.5° C (102° to 105° F). The use of aspirin, nonsteroidal anti-inflammatory agents, or steroids to block this acute febrile reaction is generally avoided, because these drugs have effects upon the immune system (Witter et al., 1988). Hydration prior to and during treatment is important to avoid dehydration and hypotension (Haeuber, 1989). Blankets and warm beverages may comfort the patients; however, the use of morphine, demerol, or diazepam to lessen the severity of muscular contractions may be necessary for the most severe rigors that occur at the highest dose levels (Haeuber, 1989; Hood, 1988).

The day following the initial dose administration is usually free of fever, but a "washed out" feeling with muscular aches and fatigue may persist. Chronic, severe fatigue accumulates over the course of biologic therapy, with doses often needing to be reduced or postponed.

Central Nervous System. Problems with behavioral, cognitive, and affective functions were noted in the early 1980s with interferon trials. Up to 70 per cent of patients receiving interferon in initial dose-escalating trials have experienced dose-related central nervous system toxicities (Goldstein & Laszlo, 1986; Quesada et al., 1986). Adams, Quesada, and Gutterman (1984) suggest that a "diffuse toxic encephalopathy" is the cause for the disruption in frontal lobe function (Box 23–2). Interleukin 2 penetrates the blood-brain barrier and may cause a direct effect on neurologic function (Sarris et al., 1988). Other mechanisms for the effect of biotherapy agents on the central nervous system include the possible interaction with neuroendocrine hormones and neurotransmitters (Bender, 1994).

The side effects commonly seen with the biologics (excluding the growth factors) include confusion, depression, somnolence, fatigue, electroencephalogram changes with diffuse slowing as seen with enceph-

alopathies, and paresthesias. Patients may also note difficulty with concentration, reading, and calculations. At lower doses patients may note irritability, lack of patience, low motivation, and depression (Bender, 1994). Patients and family members should be forewarned of the potential for such behavioral changes and advised to report all changes promptly. Patients may forget appointments and become easily disoriented, requiring that patient safety issues be addressed with the family. Dose reduction or discontinuation along with psychiatric evaluation may be warranted.

Prior acknowledgement of potential neuropsychiatric side effects will facilitate early identification of changes and will help to alleviate fears that the changes are related to progressive worsening of the primary disease (Bender, 1994). Many of the neurologic changes are subtle, and patients tend to try to cover up these impairments, such that specific baseline and routine testing (e.g., serial sevens, Mini-mental state examination, Trail-making, etc.) and questioning of family members regarding the patient's status should be an important element in the assessment of patients (Bender, 1994; Hood, 1988). Although the neuropsychiatric effects of biologic therapies is well documented in the literature and commonly reported by patients, their occurrence must not be dismissed lightly. Attempted suicides were noted in multiple sclerosis patients receiving long-term interferon-β (Anonymous, 1993; Bender, 1994).

Gastrointestinal. Fewer than one third of patients experience mild nausea during the first week of treatment. This is a constant nausea, seldom accompanied by emesis, which is managed by the use of intermittent

---

Box 23–2. *Interferon: Neuropsychiatric Manifestations*

Adams, F., Quesada, J. R., & Gutterman, J. U. (1984). Neuropsychiatric manifestations of human leukocyte interferon therapy in patients with cancer. *Journal of the American Medical Association, 252,* 938–941.

This descriptive study was among the first to identify the intense fatigue-asthenia syndrome that accompanies human leukocyte interferon-α therapy as a manifestation of a complex neurotoxicity, with reversible impairment of some higher mental functions.

Ten patients with metastatic renal cell carcinoma (5 men and 5 women), aged 36 to 72 years (median = 54 years), were examined before, 1 week after, and 1 month after continuous, daily intramuscular doses of interferon. The assessment utilized a detailed, structured, clinical mental status examination that was supplemented by tests that were sensitive to neurodynamic and higher mental function alterations. Before interferon treatment, all 10 patients were found to be free of psychiatric illnesses or cognitive impairments.

Behavioral changes, manifested as reduced physical activity, were most pronounced in the first week of interferon therapy. Eight patients experienced psychomotor retardation, with slowing of spontaneous movements, speech, and thought. Symptoms of social withdrawal were also displayed. Complaints of decreased energy and disinclination to act or think were severe enough that some activities of eating, grooming, and daily living were ignored. Daily naps were necessary for all patients. Lack of drive and universal loss of libido were noted.

Cognitively fully oriented, all patients appeared duller, inattentive, and disinterested, with five patients complaining of memory and concentration difficulties. Half the patients exhibited speech blockage, with sentences interrupted by periods of silence and staring. Affectively, once interferon therapy started, the pretreatment anxiety of eight patients and the suicidal ideation of four patients ceased. Half of the patients became tearful, emotionally labile, or uncharacteristically irritable.

The sudden appearance and pronouncement of symptoms at the start of interferon therapy, with reversal following discontinuation, implies that they are drug-related. Metoclopramide (a dopamine antagonist) was found to reverse some of the neuropsychiatric effects of interferon. It was concluded that these side effects, expecially fatigue-asthenia, are manifestations of a complex, diffuse, toxic encephalopathy that interferes primarily with frontal lobe functions, especially those involved with planning, drive, and execution of activities.

oral antiemetics. Mild diarrhea is occasionally reported in the initial stages of therapy. More common gastrointestinal complaints include chronic taste alteration, early satiety, and cumulative anorexia (Mayer, Hetrick, Riggs, & Sherwin, 1984; Quesada et al., 1986). Decreased salivary flow may contribute to the occurrence of stomatitis, caries, and candidiasis, calling for good oral care.

Cardiovascular. The acute flulike syndrome with its associated rigors, tachycardia, cyanosis, and rapid breathing is very stressful for the patient with a history of cardiovascular problems. Sudden cardiac arrhythmias and myocardial infarctions are rare, but precautions are given against the use of high doses of biologics in individuals with a strong history of active cardiac disease and for the careful evaluation of the heart and electrocardiogram before the initiation of therapy.

Orthostatic hypotension is detected during patient monitoring, although many patients are unaware of it (Goldstein & Laszlo, 1986). Hypertensive medications may need to be lowered or discontinued during therapy. Mild hypotension is managed in most cases by encouraging intake of sufficient fluids and advising patients to avoid sudden changes in position. However, the fluid replacement for the leaky capillary syndrome associated with high doses of interleukin 2 can result in peripheral edema, ascites, and pulmonary interstitial edema, which may necessitate intubation.

Hematologic, Hepatic, and Renal. These organ toxicities are dose-related and disappear when treatment is discontinued or the dose is lowered. Mild decrease in granulocytes, platelets, and red cells is seen during therapy. Transient elevations in serum transaminase and bilirubin levels are seen to some degree.

As most of the biologics are cleared via the kidneys, patients with preexisting renal disease should be observed carefully. Mild proteinuria has been reported. More severe renal effects are noted with interleukin 2 including oliguria, proteinuria, and elevated serum creatinine and blood urea nitrogen levels. These also return to normal shortly after discontinuation of therapy.

Hypersensitivity. Evaluation of the patient's response and communication with the primary physician about any possible allergic reaction, such as hives, wheezing, urticaria, or rash, should be carefully documented. Allergic types of reactions such as generalized pruritus and urticaria and anaphylactic reactions occur rarely and are easily treated with corticosteroids, acetaminophen, and antihistamines (Dillman, 1994).

Integumentary. Subcutaneous injections may result in local site irritation. Minimal effects are seen with injections of the growth factors, whereas with subcutaneous administration of tumor necrosis factor inflammatory reactions, with erythema, induration, and blisters may occur. With the high-dose interleukin 2, a majority of patients develop diffuse erythema that may evolve into a pruritic desquamating rash.

PATIENT EDUCATION AND SUPPORT

Biotherapy is an innovative option about which the layperson has very little understanding. The role of advocate and interpreter are important for the nurse caring for patients on the initial studies with new agents when consent forms are presented and initial discussions take place.

The complex role of the immune system can best be explained through the use of multiple medias, including videotapes (Straw & Conrad, 1994). Charts, drawings, and printed materials about the immune system, the function of antibodies, and the role of clinical trials are useful information for the new patient. Patients need careful explanations, to educate them regarding both their treatment program and the unfamiliar terminology utilized with biological therapies. Clarification of misconceptions or preconceptions about the purpose and side effects of the prescribed biologic agent are needed to enable the patient to understand how to become an informed participant in the treatment program. Also, clear instruction regarding the pattern of potential side effects will alleviate the patient's and family's fears that the underlying disease is worsening.

Biologics possess varied characteristics, including different dosage and administration methods. Health care personnel who will be involved with patients receiving monoclonal antibodies need current information to enable them to provide appropriate care. The use of most biotherapy agents brings together multiple disciplines (tumor immunologist, pathologist, clinical chemist, radiation physicist, nuclear medicine, diagnostician, therapist, and nurse) to provide biotherapy to the patient with cancer (Goldenberg, 1994). A thorough assessment of the patient prior to the initiation of therapy will enable the health team member to recognize treatment-related side effects and to evaluate early and subtle changes in the patient's status (Yasko & Pelch, 1990).

When patients are able to receive their treatments in the home setting, they need to be taught to correctly self-administer the doses, including preparation of the injection, use of syringes, sterile technique, and proper administration of the injection with rotation of subcutaneous injection sites. Patients are also taught to recognize and report toxicities promptly to the health care team to prevent the development of more severe complications.

Patients should be closely monitored during the initial phase of treatment, especially elderly patients who are at increased risk of cardiac or neurologic toxicity. Providing self-care instructions, including use of acetaminophen, comfort measures, and hydration, will relieve many of the initial flulike symptoms. Administration of doses in the evening results in less fatigue (Abrams, McClamrock, & Foon, 1985; Bender, 1994). Reassurance that acute side effects will lessen as tachyphylaxis develops often encourages a patient to stick with the treatment plan for at least the first 2 to 4 weeks rather than drop out.

Suggestions to handle the chronic side effects, such as evening injections, frequent rest periods, energy conservation hints, good nutrition, mouth care, and use of calendars, notepads, and reminders during periods of confusion, will help patients to tolerate prolonged courses of therapy. Families should be encouraged to provide support and encouragement to help patients implement the suggestions. Advise patients and families to anticipate a degree of fatigue so that they will not be overly anxious that these symptoms signal the progression of their malignancy. Piper et al. (1989) discuss other interventions to combat the chronic fatigue of long-term therapy.

Nutritional counseling is important to help patients maintain their strength and to avoid muscle-wasting syndrome. Encourage patients to eat frequent nutritious snacks even if their appetite is diminished. Families should be forewarned to expect poor appetites. They can be given instructions regarding ways to support the patient nutritionally, through increased fluid intake, use of high caloric/high protein supplementation, and use of soft foods (Piper et al., 1989).

Quesada and colleagues (1986) summarize the necessary concerns of nurses who care for patients receiving interferon or other biologic therapy: "Close observation, attention to diet, careful instruction, and reassurance of the patient will avoid complications from the most severe side effects induced by interferon, thus helping to maintain the patient's performance status and quality of life" (p. 241).

REFERENCES

Abels, R. I. (1992). Use of recombinant human erythropoietin in patients who have cancer. *Seminars in Oncology, 19,* 29–35.

Abernathy, E. J. (1994). Biotechnology: Exploring the fourth modality of cancer treatment. *Quality of Life: A Nursing Challenge, 3*(2), 30–38.

Abrams, P. G., McClamrock, E., & Foon, K. A. (1985). Evening administration of alpha interferon. *New England Journal of Medicine, 312*(7), 443–444.

Adams, F., Quesada, J. R., & Gutterman, J. U. (1984). Neuropsychiatric manifestations of human leukocyte interferon therapy in patients with cancer. *Journal of the American Medical Association, 252,* 938–941.

Anonymous. (1993). FDA approved new drug bulletin. *RN, 56*(12), 47–50.

Applebaum, F. R. (1993). The application of hematopoietic colony stimulating factors (CSFs) in cancer management. In S. M. Hubbard, P. E. Greene, & M. T. Knobf (Eds.), *Current issues in cancer nursing practice updates* (pp. 1–13). Philadelphia: Lippincott.

Baldwin, G. C., Gasson, J. C., Kaufman, S. E., Quan, S. G., Williams, R. E., Avalos, B. R., Gazdan, A. F., Golde, D. W., & DiPersio, J. F. (1989). Nonhematopoietic tumor cells express functional GM-CSF receptors. *Blood, 73,* 1033–1037.

Baldwin, R. W., & Byers, V. S. (1987). Monoclonal antibody targeting of cytotoxic agents for cancer therapy. In V. S. Byers & R. W. Baldwin (Eds.), *Immunology of malignant diseases* (pp. 44–54). Lancaster, England: MTP Press.

Balmer, C. M. (1990). Clinical use of biologic response modifiers in cancer treatment: An overview. Part I. The Interferons. *DICP, The Annals of Pharmacotherapy, 24*(7–8), 761–768.

Bender, C. M. (1994). Cognitive dysfunction associated with biological response modifier therapy. *Oncology Nursing Forum, 21*(3), 515–523.

Beutler, B., & Cerami, A. (Feb. 12, 1987). Cachectin: More than a tumor necrosis factor. *New England Journal of Medicine, 316*(7), 379–385.

Beveridge, R. A., & Miller, J. A. (1993). Impact of colony stimulating factors on the practice of oncology. *Oncology, 7*(12), 43–48.

Biological response modifiers guidelines: Recommendations for nursing education and practice. (1995). Pittsburgh, PA: Oncology Nursing Society.

Bodey, G. P., Buckley, M. Sathe, Y. S., & Freireich, E. J. (1966). Quantitative relationships between circulating leukocytes and infection in patients with acute leukemia. *Annals of Internal Medicine, 64,* 328–340.

Burris, H. (1993). The future of cytokines. *Oncology, 7*(12), 55–60.

Bylinsky, G. (1985, November 25). Science scores a cancer breakthrough. *Fortune.*

Caligiuri, M. (1993). Low dose recombinant interleukin-2 therapy: Rationale and potential clinical applications. *Seminars in Oncology, 20*(6, Suppl. 9), 3–9.

Clark, J., & Longo, D. (1986). Biological response modifiers. *Mediguide to Oncology, 6*(2), 1–10.

Clark, J., & Longo, D. (1987). Interferons in cancer therapy. *Cancer: Updates, 4,* 1–16.

Coley, W. B. (1893). The treatment of malignant tumors by repeated innoculations of erysipelas: With a report of ten original cases. *American Journal of Medical Science, 105,* 487–511.

Crawford, J., Ozer, H., & Johnson, D. (1990). Prevention of chemotherapy induced febrile neutropenia in patients with small cell lung cancer: A randomized double-blind placebo-controlled trial. *Proceedings of American Society of Clinical Oncology, 9*(A884).

Crosier, P. S., & Clark, S. C. (1992). Basic biology of the hematopoietic growth factors. *Seminars in Oncology, 19,* 349–361.

Dillman, R. O. (1994). Antibodies as cytotoxic therapy. *Journal of Clinical Oncology, 12*(7), 1497–1515.

Dudjak, L. A., & Yasko, J. M. (1990). Biological response modifier therapy. In J. M. Yasko & L. A. Dudjak., (Eds.), *Biological response modifier therapy: Symptom management* (pp. 3–24). Pittsburgh, PA: Park Row.

Ehrlich, P. (1900). On immunity with special reference to cell life. *Proceedings of the Royal Society of London, 66,* 424–448.

Erslev, A. J. (1991). Erythropoietin. *New England Journal of Medicine, 324,* 1339–1344.

Estey, E. (1994). Use of colony stimulating factor in the treatment of acute myeloid leukemia. *Blood, 83*(8), 2015–2019.

Fisher, R. I. (1993). Introduction: Interleukin 2—Advances in clinical research and treatment. *Seminars in Oncology, 20*(6, suppl. 9), 1.

Flick, D. A., & Gifford, G. E. (1985). Tumor necrosis factor. In P. F. Torrence (Ed.), *Biological response modifiers: New approaches to disease intervention* (pp. 171–218). Orlando, FL: Academic Press.

Foon, K. (1993). The cytokine network. *Oncology, 7*(12), 11–16.

Foon, K., Bernhard, M., & Oldham, R. (1982). Monoclonal antibody therapy: assessment by animal tumor models. *Journal of Biological Response Modifiers, 1,* 277–304.

Gallucci, B. B. (1985). Selected concepts of cancer as a disease: From 1900 to oncogenes. *Oncology Nursing Forum, 12*(5), 69–78.

Goldenberg, D. M. (1994). New developments in monoclonal antibodies for cancer detection and therapy. *CA-A Cancer Journal for Clinicians, 44*(1), 47–64.

Goldstein, D., & Laszlo, J. (1986). Interferon therapy in cancer: From imaginon to interferon. *Cancer Research, 46,* 4315–4329.

Goodfield, J. (1984, April). Dr. Coley's toxins. *Science, 84,* 68–73.

Gresser, I., & Tovey, M. B. (1978, October). Antitumor effects of interferon. *Biochimica et Biophysica Acta, 516,* 231–247.

Gutterman, J. U. (1988). The role of interferons in the treatment of hematologic malignancies. *Seminars in Hematology, 25,* 3–8.

Haeuber, D. (1995). The flu-like syndrome. In P. T. Rieger (Ed.), *Biotherapy: A comprehensive overview* (pp. 243–258). Boston, MA: Jones & Bartlett.

Haeuber, D. (1989). Recent advances in the management of biotherapy-related side effects: Flu-like syndrome. *Oncology Nursing Forum, 16*(6, Suppl.), 35–41.

Haeuber, D. (1993). Therapeutic advances in chemotherapy related anemia. In D. Mayer (Ed.), *New therapies for the anemia of chemotherapy and hairy cell leukemia.* (pp. 5–10). Raritan, NJ: Ortho Biotech, Inc.

Haeuber, D., & Spross, J. A. (1991). Alterations in protective mechanisms: Hematopoiesis and bone marrow depression. In S. B. Baird, R. McCorkle, & M. Grant (Eds.), *Cancer nursing: A comprehensive textbook* (pp. 759–781). Philadelphia: W. B. Saunders Co.

Hansen, R. M., & Borden, E. C. (1992). Current status of interferons in the treatment of cancer. *Oncology-Williston Park, NY, 6*(11), 19–24.

Henry, D. (1992). Changing patterns of care in the management of anemia. *Seminars in Oncology, 19*(Suppl. 8), 3–7.

Herrmann, F., Schulz, G., Lindemann, A., Meyenburg, W., Oster, W., Kruwieh, D., & Mertelsmann, R. (1989). Hematopoietic responses in patients with advanced malignancy treated with recombinant human granulocyte-macrophage colony stimulating factor. *Journal of Clinical Oncology, 7,* 357–364.

Higgins, P. G. (1984). Interferons. *Journal of Clinical Pathology, 37,* 109–116.

Holmlund, J. T. (1993). Cytokines, (150–206). In H. M. Pinedo, D. L. Longo, & B. A. Chabner (Eds.), *Cancer chemotherapy & biological response modifiers: Annual 14.* Amsterdam: Elsevier Science.

Hood, L. E. (1988). Interferon: Getting in the way of viruses and tumors. *American Journal of Nursing, 87,* 459–465.

Hooks, J. J., & Detrick, B. (1985). Immunoregulatory functions of interferon. In P. F. Torrence (Ed.), *Biological response modifiers: New approaches to disease intervention* (pp. 57–75). Orlando, FL: Academic Press.

Hryniuk, W. M., Figueredo, A., & Goodyear, M. (1987). Applications of dose intensity to problems in chemotherapy of breast and colorectal cancer. *Seminars in Oncology, 14,* 3–11.

Irwin, M. M. (1987). Patients receiving biological response modifiers: Overview of nursing care. *Oncology Nursing Forum, 14*(6, Suppl.), 32–37.

Jakobsen, P. H. (1987). Human monoclonal antibodies—Still much to learn. *Leukemia, 1*(6), 521–523.

Jassak, P., & Sticklin, L. (1986). Interleukin 2: An overview. *Oncology Nursing Forum, 13*(6), 17–22.

Kirkwood, J. M., & Ernstoff, M. S. (1984). Interferons in the treatment of human cancer. *Journal of Clinical Oncology, 2*(4), 336–352.

Kohler, G., & Milstein, C. (1975). Continuous cultures of fused cells secreting antibody of predefined specificity. *Nature, 256,* 495–497.

Lindenmann, J. (1982). From interference to interferon: A brief historical introduction. In D. A. Tyrrell & D. C. Burke (Eds.), *Interferon: Twenty-five years on* (pp. 3–6). London: The Royal Society of London.

Lotze, M., Agarwala, S. S., & Kirkwood, J. M. (1994). The Sznol/Parkinson article reviewed. *Oncology, 8*(6), 67–71.

Lotze, M. T., Matory, Y. L., Rayner, A. A., Ettinghausen, S. E., Vetto, J. T., Seipp, C. A., & Rosenburg, S. A. (1986). Clinical effects and toxicity of interleukin-2 in patients with cancer. *Cancer, 58,* 2764–2772.

Mathe, G., & Amiel, J. (1969). Active immunotherapy for acute lymphoblastic leukemia. *Lancet, 1*(7597), 697–699.

Mayer, D., Hetrick, K., Riggs, C., & Sherwin, S. (1984). Weight loss in patients receiving recombinant leukocyte A interferon (IFLrA): A brief report. *Cancer Nursing, 6*(1), 53–56.

Melin, S. A., & Ozer, H. (1992). Biologic response modifiers: Principles of immunotherapy. In M. C. Perry (Ed.), *Chemotherapy source book* (pp. 144–164). Baltimore: Williams & Wilkins.

Metcalf, D. (1989). The molecular control of cell division, differentiation, commitment, and maturation in hematopoietic cells. *Nature, 339,* 27–30.

Miller, L., Smith, J., Urba, W., Gause, B., Janik, J., Korn, E., Garrison, L., Holcenburg, J., & Longo, D. (1993). A phase I study of an IL-3/GM-CSF fusion protein and high dose carboplatin in patients with advanced cancer. *Proceedings of the American Society of Clinical Oncology, 12,* 195.

Moldawer, N. P., & Figlin, R. A. (1995). The Interferons. In P. T. Rieger (Ed.), *Biotherapy: A comprehensive overview* (pp. 69–86). Boston: Jones & Bartlett.

Moldawer, N., & Murray, J. (1985). The clinical uses of monoclonal antibodies in cancer research. *Cancer Nursing, 8*(4), 207–213.

Morgan, A. C., & Foon, K. A. (1986). Monoclonal antibody therapy of cancer: Preclinical models and investigations in humans. In R. B. Herberman (Ed.), *Cancer immunology: Innovative approaches to therapy* (pp. 177–200). Boston: Martinus Nijhoff.

Morgan, P. A., Ruscetti, F. W., & Gallo, R. G. (1976). Selective in vitro growth of T-lymphocytes from normal human bone marrows. *Science, 193,* 1007–1008.

Nemunaitis, J. (1993). Role of GM-CSF and G-CSF in stem cell transplantation. *Oncology, 7*(12), 27–32.

Nemunaitis, J., Buckner, C. D., Applebaum, F. R., Higano, C. S., Mori, M., Bianco, J., Epstein, C., Lipani, J., Hansen, J., Storb, R., et al. (1991). Phase I/II trial of recombinant human granulocyte-macrophage colony-stimulating factor following allogeneic bone marrow transplantation. *Blood, 77*(9), 2065–2071.

Nemunaitis, J., Rabinowe, S. N., Singer, J. W., Bierman, P. J., Vose, J. M., Freedman, A. S., Onetto, N., Gillis, S., Oette, D., Gold, M. et al. (1991). Recombinant granulocyte-macrophage colony stimulating factor after autologous bone marrow transplantation in lymphoid cancer. *New England Journal of Medicine, 324,* 1773–1778.

Nienhuis, A. W., Donahue, R. E., Karisson, S., Clark, S. C., Agricola, B., Antinoff, N., Pierce, J. E., Turner, P., Anderson, W. F., & Nathan, D. G. (1987). Recombinant human granulocyte macrophage colony stimulating factor shortens period of neutropenia after autologous bone marrow transplantation in primate model. *Journal of Clinical Investigation, 80,* 573–577.

Oettgen, H. F., & Old, L. J. (1987). Tumor necrosis factor. In V. T. DeVita, Jr., S. Hellman, & S. A. Rosenberg (Eds.), *Important advances in oncology 1987* (pp. 105–127). Philadelphia: J. B. Lippincott.

Ohno, R., Tomonaga, M., Kobayashi, T., Kanamaru, A., Shirakawla, S., Masaoka, T., Omine, M., Or, H., Nomura, T., Sakai, Y., et al. (1990). Effect of granulocyte colony stimulating factor after intensive induction therapy in relapsed or refractory acute leukemia. *New England Journal of Medicine, 323,* 871–877.

Oldham, R. K. (1985). Biologicals for cancer treatment: Interferons. *Hospital Practice, 20,* 71–91.

Oldham, R. K. (1983). Monoclonal antibodies in cancer therapy. *Journal of Clinical Oncology, 1*(9), 582–590.

Oldham, R., & Smalley, R. (1983). Immunotherapy: The old and the new. *Journal of Biological Response Modifiers, 2,* 1–37.

Ortho Biotech, Inc. (1994). *Procrit for injection:* Package insert. Raritan, NJ: Author.

Paul, W. F. (1987). Interleukin 4/B cell stimulatory factor 1: One lymphokine, many functions. *FASEB Journal, 1,* 456–461.

Peters, W. P., Kurtzberg, J., Atwater, S., Borowitz, M., Gilbert, C., Rao, M., Currie, M., Shogan, J., Jones, R., Shpall, E. J., & Souza, L. (1988). Comparative effects of rHuG-CSF and rHuGM-CSF on hematopoietic reconstitution and granulocyte function following high dose chemotherapy and autologous bone marrow transplantation. *Blood, 72,* (Suppl. 1), 432.

Physicians' data query. (1994, Jan. 15). Bethesda, MD: National Library of Medicine.

Pimm, M. V. (1987). Immunoscintigraphy: Tumor detection with radiolabeled antibody monoclonal antibodies. In V. S. Byers & R. W. Baldwin (Eds.), *Immunology of malignant diseases* (pp. 21–43). Lancaster, England: MTP Press.

Piper, B. F., Rieger, P. T., Brophy, L., Haeuber, D., Hood, L. E., Lyver, A., & Sharp, E. (1989). Recent advances in the management of biotherapy-related side effects: Fatigue. *Oncology Nursing Forum, 16*(6, Suppl.) 27–34.

Pizzo, P. A., & Meyers, J. (1989). Infection in the cancer patient. Section 5. In V. T. DeVita, S. Hellman, & S. A. Rosenberg (Eds.). *Cancer principles & practice of oncology* (3rd ed., 2088–2133). Philadelphia: Lippincott.

Powles, R., Smith, C., Milan, S., Treleavan, J., Millar, J., McElwain, T., Gordon-Smith, E., Milliken, S., & Tiley, C. (1990). Human recombinant GM-CSF in allogeneic bone marrow transplantation for leukemia: Double blind, placebo controlled trial. *Lancet, 2,* 1417–1420.

Quesada, J. R., Talpaz, M., Rios, A., Kurzrodk, R., & Gutterman, J. U. (1986). Clinical toxicity of interferons in cancer patients: A review. *Journal of Clinical Oncology, 4*(2), 234–243.

Rieger, P. T. (1993). New dimensions of caring for chemotherapy related anemia. In *New therapies of the anemia of chemotherapy and hairy cell leukemia* (pp. 11–16). Raritan, NJ: Ortho Biotech, Inc.

Rieger, P. T., Weatherly, B., & Rumsey, L. A. (1993). Clinical update: Strategies for caring for the patient receiving IL-2 therapy. *Nursing Interventions in Oncology, 5,* 23–30.

Rosenberg, S. A. (1992). Kasnofsky Memorial Lecture: The immunotherapy and gene therapy of cancer. *Journal of Clinical Oncology, 11,* 661–670.

Rosenberg, S. A., Lotze, M. T., Muul, L. M., Leitman, S., Chang, A. E., Ettinghausen, S. E., Matory, Y. L., Skibber, J. M., Shiloni, E., Vetto, J. T., Seipp, C. A., Simpson, C., & Reichert, C. M. (1985). Observations on the systemic administration of autologous lymphokine-activated killer cells and recombinant interleukin-2 to patients with metastatic cancer. *New England Journal of Medicine, 313*(23), 1485–1494.

Rumsey, K. A., & Rieger, P. T. (Eds.). (1992). *Biological response modifiers: A self-instruction manual for health professionals.* Chicago: Precept.

Sarris, S. C., Rosenberg, S. A., Friedman, R. B., Rubin, J. T., Barba, D., & Oldfield, E. H. (1988). Penetration of recombinant interleukin-2 across the blood-cerebrospinal fluid barrier. *Journal of Neurosurgery, 69,* 29–34.

Shear, M. J., Turner, F. C., Perrault, A., & Shovelton, T. (1943). Chemical treatment of tumors. V. Isolation of the hemorrhage-producing fraction from Serratia marcescens (Bacillus prodigiosus) culture filtrate. *Journal of the National Cancer Institute, 4,* 81–97.

Simpson, C., Seipp, C. A., & Rosenberg, S. A. (1988). The current status and future applications of interleukin-2 and adoptive immunotherapy in cancer treatment. *Seminars in Oncology Nursing, 4*(2), 132–141.

Straw, L. J., & Conrad, K. J. (1994). Patient education resources related to biotherapy and the immune system. *Oncology Nursing Forum, 21*(7), 1223–1228.

St. Germain, D. (1992). Recombinant human erythropoietin: Pharmacology and clinical use. In *Treatment of cancer related anemias* (pp. 2–6). Raritan, NJ: Ortho Biotech, Inc.

Sznol, M., & Longo, D. L. (1993). Chemotherapy drug interactions with biological agents. *Seminars in Oncology, 20,* 80–93.

Sznol, M., & Parkinson, D. R. (1994). Clinical applications of IL-2. *Oncology, 8*(6), 61–65.

Sznol, M., Thurn, A., & Parkinson, D. R. (1993). Overview of interleukin-2 trials in patients with renal cell carcinoma. In E. A. Klein, R. M. Bukowski, & J. H. Finke (Eds.), *Renal cell carcinoma: Immunotherapy and cellular biology.* New York: Marcel Decker.

Terry, W., & Rosenberg, S. (Eds.). (1982). *Immunotherapy of human cancer.* New York: Excerpta Medica.

Thompson, J. A., Bianco, J., Benyunes, M., Neubaur, M., & Fefer, A. (1993). Pentoxifyllin and ciprofloxacin reduce the toxicity of IL-2 and LAK therapy./*Proceedings of the American Society of Clinical Oncology, 12,* 293.

Thor, A., Weeks, M. O., & Schlom, J. (1986). Monoclonal antibodies and breast cancer. *Seminars in Oncology, 13*(4), 393–401.

Traynor, B. (1992). The cytokine network. In International Society of Nurses in Cancer Care, *Proceedings of the seventh international conference on cancer nursing* (pp. 6–10). Vienna, Austria.

Trotta, P. (1986). Preclinical biology of alpha interferons. *Seminars in Oncology, 13*(3), 3–12.

Vilcek, J., Kelke, H. C., Jumming, L. E., & Yip, Y. K. (1985). Structure and function of human interferon gamma. In R. J. Ford (Ed.), *Mediators of cell growth and differentiation* (pp. 299–313). New York: Raven Press.

Weber, J., Yang, J. C., Topalain, S. L., Parkinson, D. R., Schwartzentruber, D. S., Ettinghausen, S. E., Gunn, H., Mixon, A., Kim, H., Cole, D. et al. (1993). Phase I trial of subcutaneous interleukin-6 in patients with advanced malignancies. *Journal of Clinical Oncology, 11,* 499–506.

Witter, F. R., Woods, A. S., Griffin, M. D., Smith, C. R., Nadler, P., Lietman, P. S. (1988). Effects of prednisone, aspirin, and acetaminophen on in vivo biologic response to interferon in humans. *Clinical Pharmacology and Therapeutics, 44,* 239–243.

Wordell, C. J. (1991). Biotechnology update. *Hospital Pharmacy, 26,* 897–900.

Wujcik, D. (1993). An odyssey into biologic therapy. *Oncology Nursing Forum, 20*(6), 879–887.

Yasko, J. M., & Pelch, K. A. (1990). Assessment of the patient receiving biological response modifier therapy. In J. M. Yasko & L. A. Dudjak (Eds.), *Biological response modifier therapy* (pp. 27–42). Park Row Press.

Zsebo, K. M., Wypych, J., Yuschenkoff, V. N., Lu, H., Hunt, P., Dukes, P. P., & Langley, K. E. (1988). Effects of hematopoietin 1 and interleukin 1 on early hematopoietic cells of the bone marrow. *Blood, 71,* 962–968.

The development of all malignant tumors among humans appears to have a genetic basis. Such a statement can easily be interpreted by the general public to mean that cancer is hereditary. The actual meaning of this statement is that internal and external forces influencing the genetic information of a normal cell can cause that cell to undergo malignant transformation and, over time, lead to the development of an overt malignancy (Bishop, 1982; Cooper, 1992). Thus cancer is "genetic"; however, at the present time relatively few cancers have proven to be hereditary.

With genetic involvement implicated in cancer development, it would seem logical to assume a role for gene therapy either in cancer treatment or as a preventative method to reduce the risk for specific cancers. Cancer prevention through gene therapy remains futuristic. Gene therapy as a primary or an adjunct cancer treatment modality has investigational status currently. Although response rates to date are limited, sufficient efficacy has been achieved to demonstrate probable future feasibility.

Nurses involved in the care of people and families with cancer need a working knowledge of genetic influences on cancer development and in cancer treatment. This chapter presents an overview of molecular genetics with specific reference to cancer development, rationale and techniques for gene therapy, and the role of oncology nurses in genetics counseling.

GENETICS AND CANCER

The controlling factors for any activity or function a cell performs are the genes. A gene is a limited segment of DNA that codes for a specific gene product (a protein). All cells make substances that are used for the normal "housekeeping" duties of the cell. In addition, some cells make at least one specific substance that leaves the cell and is either used by other cells or controls the activity of other cells. All of these substances are *proteins*, and the processes involved in making these proteins are termed *protein synthesis*. Protein synthesis involves the DNA (deoxyribose nucleic acid) and specific genes. The following paragraphs describing the molecular events surrounding protein synthesis appear originally in another book chapter by Workman, Kenner, and Hilse (1993).

MOLECULAR GENETICS

The nucleus of a cell holds the DNA, which contains the codes or patterns for construction of every protein made by every cell within the body. DNA is composed of two very long chains (strands) of interlocking nucleotides (Fig. 24–1). Each nucleotide is composed of a molecule of any one of the four bases shown in Figure 24–2. These bases are each attached to a five carbon sugar (a pentose arrangement called a "ribose") that is connected to a phosphate group. The phosphate groups actually provide the linkage between the individual bases so that long strands are formed (Fig. 24–3). Thus the phosphate connections are the actual "backbone" of the DNA strand.

In humans, DNA does not exist as a single strand. Instead, the DNA is double-stranded in an antiparallel arrangement. Relatively weak ionic forces hold the two strands in close proximity but not tightly bound

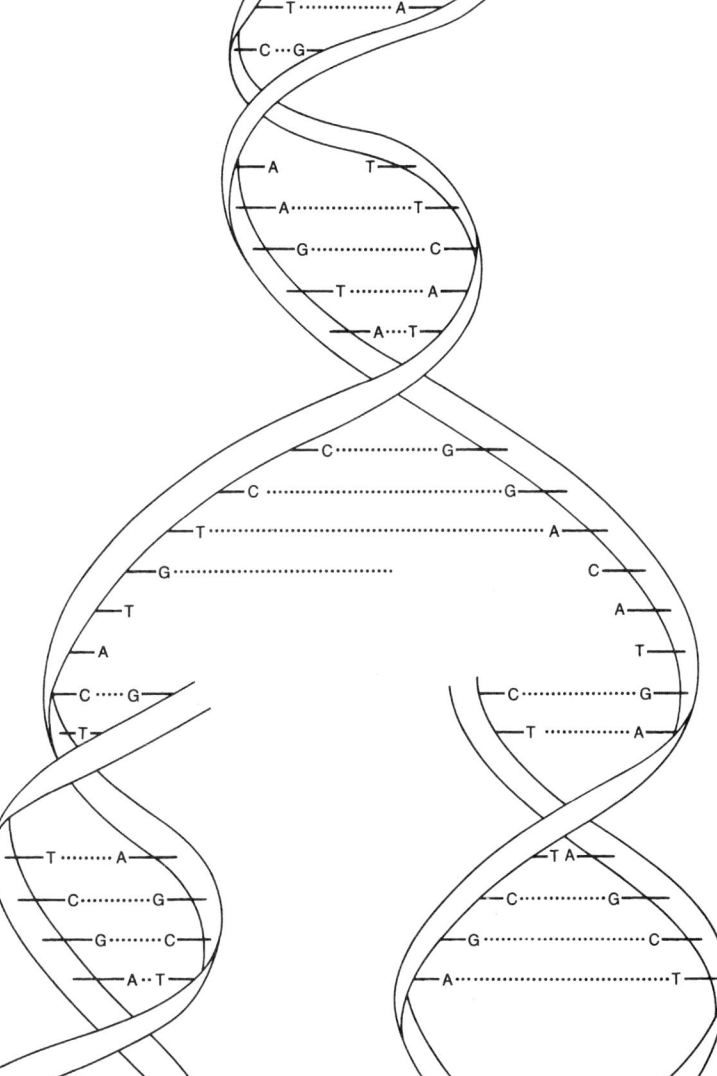

Figure 24–1. Double-stranded DNA. (Modified from Kenner, C., Bruggemeyer, A., & Gunderson, L. P. [1993]. *Comprehensive neonatal nursing: A physiologic approach.* Philadelphia: W.B. Saunders Co.)

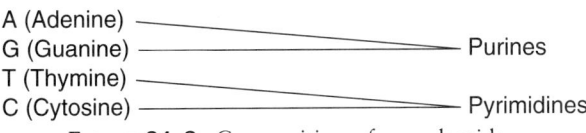

A (Adenine) —
G (Guanine) — → Purines
T (Thymine) —
C (Cytosine) — → Pyrimidines

Figure 24–2. Composition of a nucleotide.

together. The loose interaction between the two strands permits the strands to separate during critical steps in protein synthesis and in cell division.

The bases have a special and specific affinity for each other between the two strands. Adenine has an attraction for thymine and always pairs up with it (and vice versa), while guanine and cytosine have the same attraction for each other. Thus the two strands of DNA are lined up together, composed of interacting bases that form "base pairs." Because the bases are specific in their attractions, the two strands of DNA are "complementary" to each other in terms of their nucleotide sequence. Therefore, it is possible, if the sequence of one DNA strand is known, to be able to predict with accuracy the sequence of the complementary DNA strand.

$$
\begin{array}{cc}
5' & 3' \\
A & -- & T \\
C & -- & G \\
G & -- & C \\
T & -- & A \\
T & -- & A \\
A & -- & T \\
C & -- & G \\
T & -- & A \\
3' & 5'
\end{array}
$$

The double-stranded DNA remains in a loosely coiled helical arrangement throughout most of the cell's life span. At various times in the cell cycle the DNA becomes more tightly packed together (Fig. 24–4). This packing together involves further coiling of the DNA at well-regulated intervals around protein substances called "histones" so that the DNA at this stage has an appearance similar to that of beads on a string. The complex of DNA wound around each histone is called

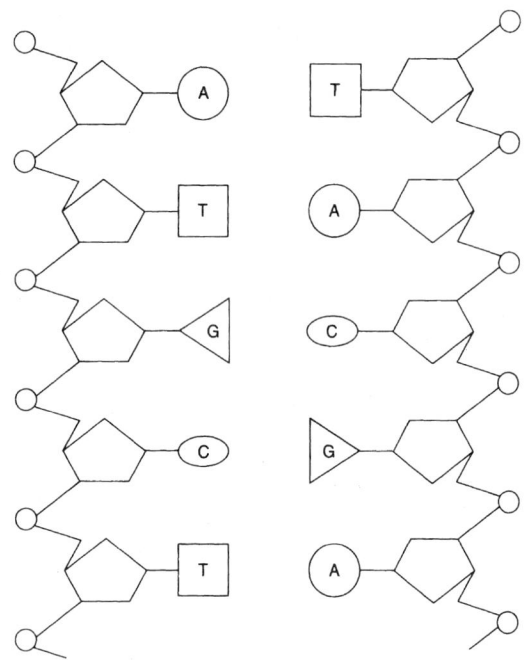

FIGURE 24–3. Close up of double-stranded DNA showing nucleotides with complementary bases, five-carbon sugars, and phosphate groups. (From Kenner, C., Bruggemeyer, A., & Gunderson, L. P. [1993]. *Comprehensive neonatal nursing: A physiologic approach.* Philadelphia: W.B. Saunders Co.)

a "nucleosome." During cell division, the DNA must become even more tightly packed together to form dense structures called *chromosomes.*

Protein Synthesis

All cells that make some protein have in the DNA the code for that protein, the actual *gene* for that protein. The unique DNA pattern (gene) for that specific protein is first converted into a piece of RNA (ribose nucleic acid). RNA is similar to DNA but instead of containing thymine (T), RNA contains uracil (U).

Proteins are formed by linking individual nitrogen units called "amino acids" together in a linear strand. There are 22 different amino acids. Each amino acid has a unique three-base code sequence, called a codon, that identifies the DNA and RNA pieces specific for that amino acid. Some amino acids have only one codon, whereas others have as many as four different but closely related codons. Examples of amino acid–specific codons are listed in Table 24–1.

The total number of amino acids in a specific protein and the exact order in which they are connected together help to determine the nature and activity of the protein. The actual making of protein is called protein synthesis. Figure 24–5 outlines the sequence of events central to protein synthesis and DNA synthesis.

When it is time for cells in a tissue to make a specific protein (for example, insulin), the cells must make the area of DNA that contains the amino acid codes (gene) for insulin loosen. The DNA in the region of the gene to be read loosens up and unwinds slightly from the histones. Once the appropriate area of DNA is unwound, the two strands are separated and held open by

a special enzyme complex. Next, a special RNA enzyme (RNA polymerase) binds to the gene area of the DNA and "reads" it. When the enzyme recognizes a "start" signal, it will move along the strand and synthesize a new strand of RNA complementary to the gene area of the DNA. When the enzyme reaches the end of the gene sequence, there will be a "stop" signal that tells the enzyme to stop making new RNA. This part of the protein synthesis process is called transcription because part of the DNA codes are being transcribed into a strand of RNA. The newly created RNA strand moves away from the gene area of the DNA. The DNA closes back together and assumes the normal helical formation.

The newly synthesized piece of RNA is called "messenger RNA" (mRNA or sometimes just the "message") because it contains the special coded pattern sequence for building the specific protein (in this case, insulin). After the mRNA has been transcribed from the gene areas of the DNA, it moves from the nucleus to the cytoplasm. In an active cell, the message becomes very busy here in conjunction with two other types of RNA. Many individual amino acids are stored inside the cytoplasm until the appropriate time and signal initiates a sequence of events that properly lines up and hooks together the correct amino acids to form a protein. This activity, known as translation, requires the interactions of additional substances called "ribosomes" (and these are made up of special types of ribosomal RNA) along with yet another type of RNA called "transfer RNA" (tRNA).

Transfer RNAs are adapter molecules that assist in bringing the correct amino acid into the lineup at the proper time (Fig. 24–6). Each tRNA can carry or hold only one amino acid at a time, and the tRNA has an "anticodon" that is complementary to that specific amino acid's codon. Therefore, because each tRNA can bind to only one of the 22 different amino acids, there must be at least 22 different types of tRNA.

In the cytoplasm, the ribosome attaches to the messenger RNA strand and begins to move along the strand, "reading" the strand as it moves along. When a three-base code is read and interpreted by the ribosome as a specific codon for one amino acid, the ribosome allows the tRNAs to come in and attempt to match their anticodons to the codon. When the correct tRNA matches up with the codon on the mRNA, the correct tRNA releases its amino acid and allows that amino acid to bind to the growing protein strand (Fig. 24–7). This process is repeated down the messenger RNA until all the correct amino acids are lined up and hooked together in the right order to make the specific protein.

Cells usually synthesize only the proteins needed directly by that cell or that are a part of that tissue's normal functions and do not synthesize other proteins. For example, while every human cell contains the gene for insulin, only the beta cells of the pancreas activate the gene for insulin and use it to synthesize the actual insulin protein. All other genes not essential to the beta cell's life or function remain in a repressed or unexpressed state.

Other genes were active in specific cells only during very limited times of development and should remain

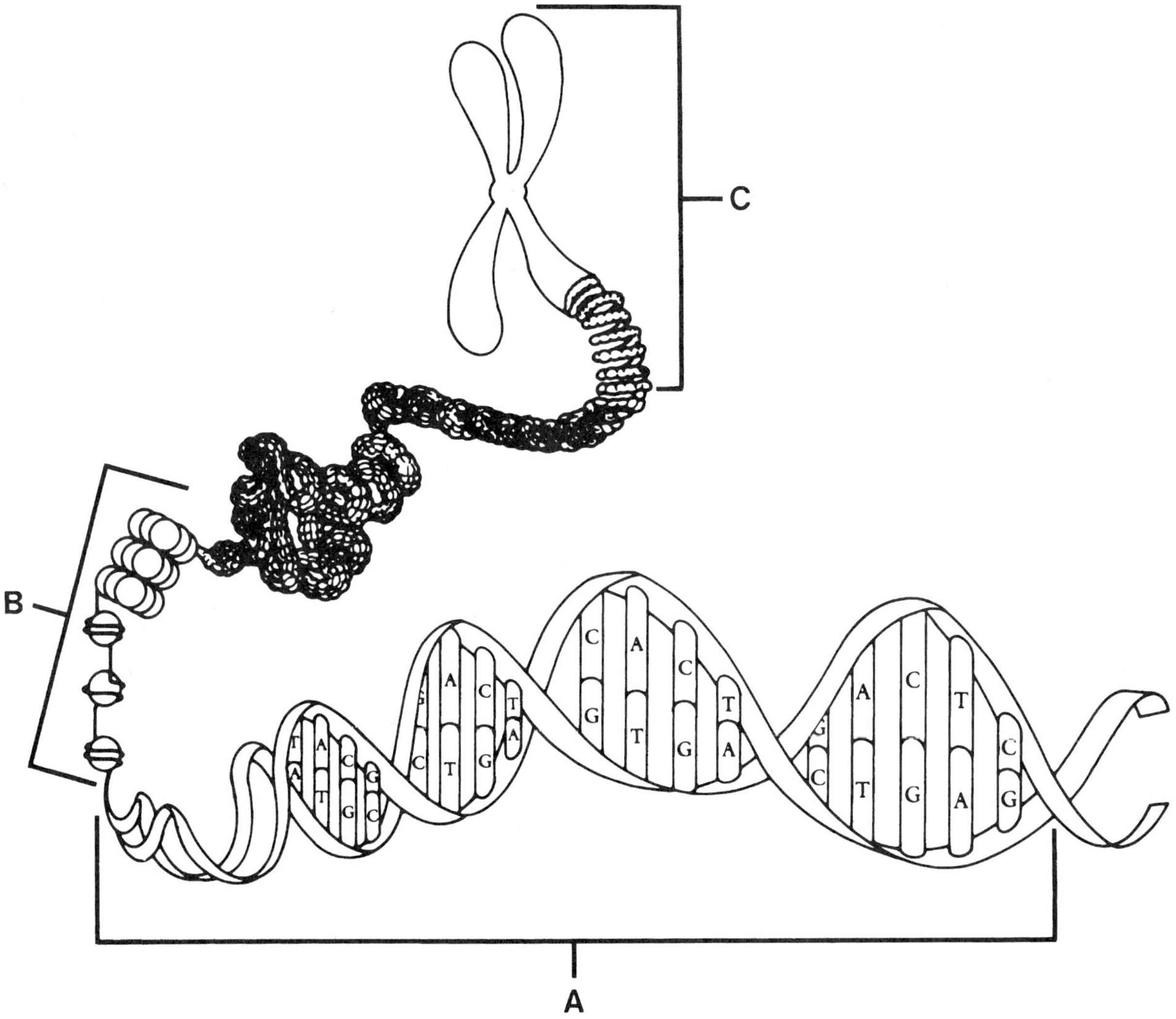

FIGURE 24–4. Schematic drawing of DNA changes through cell cycle. *A*, Structure of DNA in G_0, G_1, S, and G_2 phases of the cell cycle. The DNA is double-stranded and loosely coiled in a helical arrangement. *B*, At the end of the G_2 phase and in the early stages of the M phase, the DNA begins to coil more tightly and pack together. *C*, In the M phase, the DNA supercoils on itself to form definitive chromosome structures. (Reprinted by permission from p. 160 of *Human Heredity: Principles and Issues* by Cummings, M. R.; Copyright © 1988 by West Publishing Company. All rights reserved.)

TABLE 24–1. *Examples of Amino Acid RNA Codons*

AMINO ACID	RNA CODON
Alanine	GCU, GCC
Methionine	AUG
Phenylalanine	UUU, UUC
Serine	UCU, UCC, UCA, UCG
Tyrosine	UAU, UAC
Valine	GUU, GUC, GUA, GUG
"Start signal"	AUG
"Stop signals"	UAA, UAG, UGA

forever in a repressed state. For example, early in embryonic development, many specific genes were turned on and actively involved in making the embryo from conception up to approximately day eight after conception behave in the way that is normal for early embryos. Early embryonic behaviors or characteristics include rapid and continuous cell division, lack of specific morphology or functional capacity, lack of cell adhesiveness, large nuclear to cytoplasmic ratio, and an ability to migrate within the growing embryo.

After day eight in human development these early embryonic behaviors have to stop, and differentiation

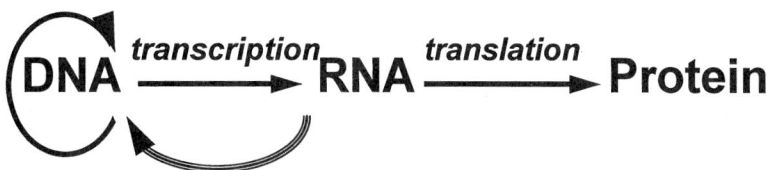

FIGURE 24–5. Sequence of events necessary for protein synthesis.

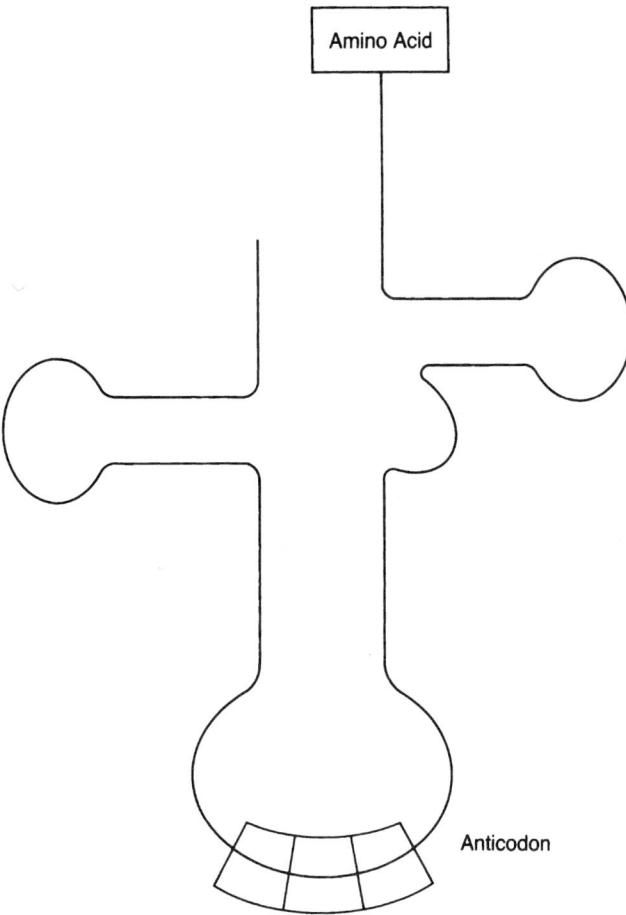

FIGURE 24–6. Transfer RNA (tRNA) molecule. (From Kenner, C., Bruggemeyer, A., & Gunderson, L. P. [1993]. *Comprehensive neonatal nursing: A physiologic approach.* Philadelphia: W.B. Saunders Co.)

must occur for normal development. The early embryonic genes must be turned off forever. This turning off of early embryonic genes is accomplished through the activity of special "repressor" genes that repress the activity of the early embryonic genes so that they can no longer be freely expressed. At the same time, other genes (different for each cell type) are selectively "turned on" or derepressed to assist the embryonic cells to develop and mature into the specific types of differentiated cells organized in appropriate patterns to form normal human beings. Repression of the early embryonic genes suppresses the synthesis of the proteins coded for by those genes.

CANCER DEVELOPMENT

As long as these early embryonic genes remain repressed, the mature cell behaves in the expected, normal way for its specific differentiated type. The normal differentiated cell contributes to the overall group effort necessary for healthy human function. Some cells stop expressing a normal appearance and behaviors and take on the appearance and activity of malignant cells. This process of changing from a normal cell to a cancer cell is called *malignant transformation* and occurs through carcinogenesis. The primary mechanism of carcinogenesis appears to be the derepression of early embryonic genes at an inappropriate time. Derepression of one or more of these genes causes an increase in the intracellular concentration of the gene product specified by the gene, eventually causing the cell to lose its normal appearance and function (normal phenotype) and to take on the appearance and characteristics of cancer cells (malignant phenotype) (Sandberg, 1990). Because the early embryonic developmental genes are capable of causing malignant trans-

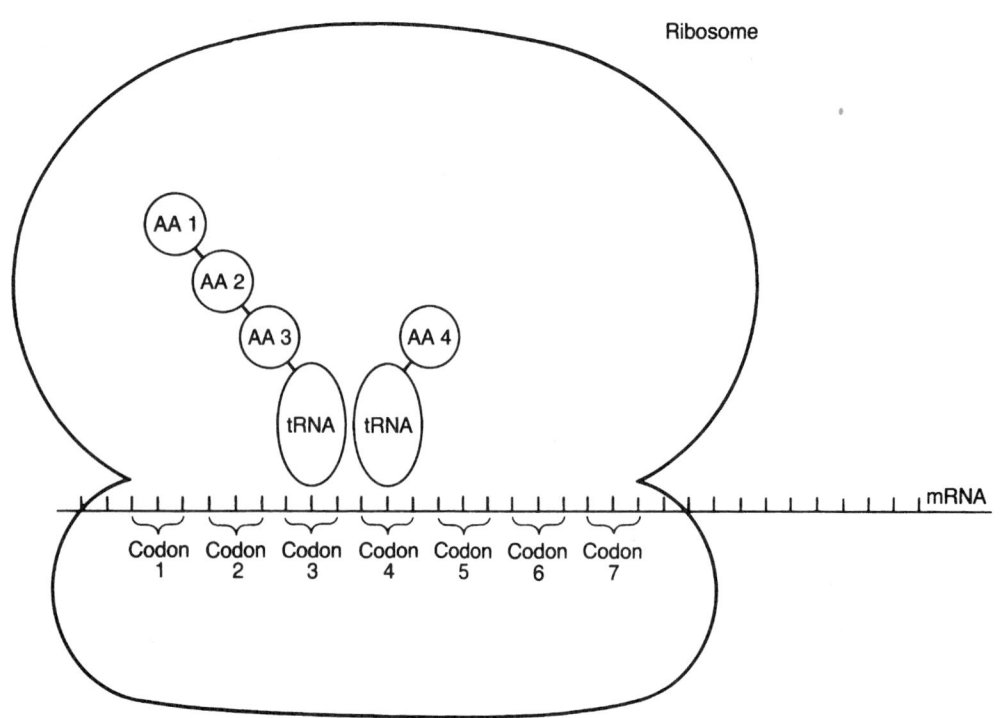

FIGURE 24–7. Ribosome and mRNA with growing amino acid chain. (From Kenner, C., Brueggemeyer, A., & Gunderson, L. P. [1993]. *Comprehensive neonatal nursing: A physiologic approach.* Philadelphia: W.B. Saunders Co.)

formation, they are referred to as proto-oncogenes in their repressed state and oncogenes when they are derepressed or activated (Bishop, 1985; Cooper, 1990; Weinberg, 1994; Yabro, 1992).

Carcinogenesis is a multistep process that initially involves exposure to an event or substance capable of altering the DNA of an affected cell (Fig. 24–8). Alteration of the DNA usually results in the mutation of one or more areas of the DNA directly or indirectly. Carcinogens (initiators) are known to cause malignant transformation at the cellular level through exertion of damaging effects on the cellular DNA that mutate gene expression and increase the synthesis of an oncogene protein. Thus many direct-acting carcinogens are mutagens, although the exact mechanism of mutagenesis varies with the specific carcinogenic agent. Some of the mutational mechanisms of chemical and physical carcinogens include DNA alkylation, demethylation of DNA proteins, base deletions/substitutions, and actual breaks in the DNA phosphate "backbone." These events cause errors in DNA expression through point mutations, frame-shift mutations, induction of "error-prone" DNA repair systems, inactivation of repressor genes, activation of oncogenes, and the inability of the cell to synthesize new DNA with high fidelity during cell division (Cooper, 1990). Any or all of these mechanisms can cause affected cells to change from expressing a normal phenotype to expressing a malignant phenotype.

An overt malignancy occurs when the initial phenotype transformation is enhanced or amplified by an increased ability of the cell to divide, an event called promotion. Usually the growth enhancement is the result of continuous exposure of the initiated (transformed) cell to a promoting agent. Promoting agents (promoters) enhance the mitotic activity of initiated (mutated) cells and contribute to the process of carcinogenesis through promotion of the DNA error created during initiation. Some endogenous hormones, especially steroid hormones, can serve as promoting agents, as can many exogenous substances.

GENE THERAPY

In theory, when a health problem is associated with a defect or absence of a single gene, it should be possible to "add a gene" and correct the problem. The concepts of genetic manipulation and gene therapy were first put forth in the 1950s, just after James Watson and Francis Crick first identified the general helical arrangement of DNA. However, because the true nature of DNA, its specific composition, and functional processes were unknown, gene therapy in the 1950s and 1960s was science fiction. In the 1970s molecular genetics techniques advanced to the point that individual components of DNA were identified and theories of activity were proposed. With technical refinement including cloning, the creation of "synthetic" genes, and the successful insertion of isolated specific genes into the genetic material of viruses and bacteria, the concept of gene therapy became less fiction and more science.

Adding a gene, literally splicing it into existing DNA, can now be done through a technique called *recombinant DNA technology*. Recombinant DNA technology such as that used to synthesize pure human insulin on a mass scale, is in a sense a type of gene therapy. In this case a synthetic human gene, identical to the natural human gene for insulin, is spliced or inserted into bacterial DNA to force the bacteria to synthesize the human form of the protein insulin. This artificially synthesized human protein is neither harmful nor beneficial to the bacterial host.

The processes involved in recombinant DNA technology with bacterial DNA have been used successfully in transferring genes into mammalian cells, both in cell culture and into animal models. Modification of these processes and techniques have been used to manipulate human genes with varying degrees of success. Human gene therapy for different problems and disorders can be permanent or temporary depending on the cell type that receives the gene as well as on the technique used to insert the gene.

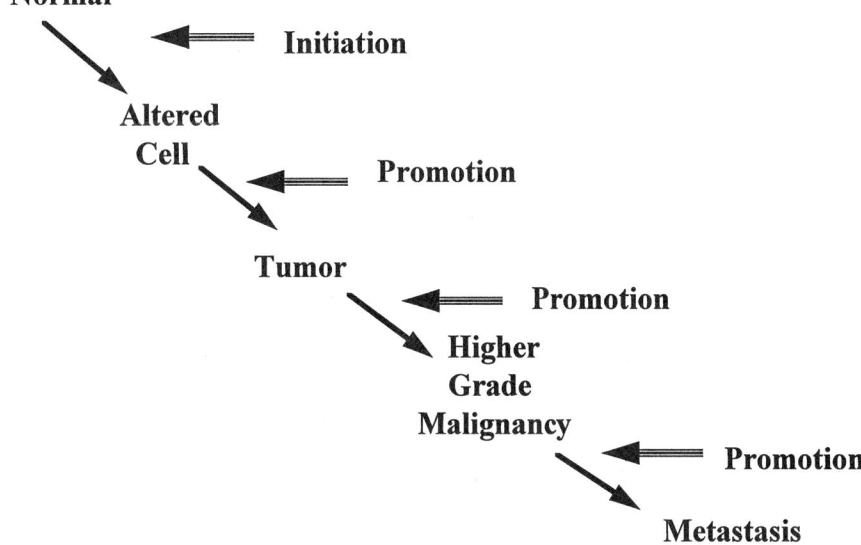

FIGURE 24–8. Steps involved in carcinogenesis. (Copyright 1994 M. Linda Workman. Reprinted with permission.)

PERMANENT GENE THERAPY

Permanent gene therapy involves inserting a gene into either germ line cells or some other cell type that will continue to reproduce throughout the person's life. This type of gene therapy involves inserting the gene into relatively small numbers of progenitor cells and then allowing those cells to propagate, continually passing on the inserted gene to all their progeny. The major impediments to permanent gene therapy in humans are (1) efficient gene delivery and appropriate insertion/integration into the genome, and (2) accessing the correct cell type to assure permanent gene expression.

Genes have been successfully inserted into mouse embryo cells and have remained active for the life of the mouse (Cohen-Haguenauer, 1994). In humans, manipulation of genes during embryonic life is neither feasible nor acceptable. Experimental studies on children and mature adults using bone marrow stem cells as recipients of additional or modified genes have shown some success.

TEMPORARY GENE THERAPY

Temporary gene therapy involves the transfer of a healthy or properly functioning gene into the more differentiated somatic cells of a person whose own gene is missing, defective, or not supplying enough of a specific product, or to change the behavior of one or more functions of that cell. For temporary gene therapy to be effective, the gene must be inserted into huge numbers of host cells. The major impediments to temporary gene therapy in humans are (1) efficient gene delivery and appropriate insertion/integration into the genome and (2) successfully inserting the gene into sufficient numbers of the target cell to obtain measurable gene expression.

Currently, investigational studies for cancer have demonstrated that this technique can be applied to living human beings. Lymphocytes have been taken from a person and grown for several weeks in cell culture. During culture, a special "marker gene" or "reporter gene" is added by the gene transduction method. The cells are then infused back into the person, and the distribution and activity of these genetically altered cells are monitored. So far, such cells have remained active for only 2 to 11 months.

GENE INSERTION/DELIVERY

One factor hampering widespread use of gene therapy is the problems surrounding gene insertion or delivery of the desired gene to the target cell population. Several systems of gene delivery have been developed, and all are successful to some extent; however, all current delivery systems have drawbacks that limit their general use. Variations of two major methods, gene transfection and gene transduction, form the basis of current gene delivery systems. Both systems couple a new gene (desired gene) to be inserted with a marker or reporter gene that when fully integrated into the genome will cause the host cell to demonstrate some observable difference so that the cells receiving gene therapy can be tracked (Noonan & Senner, 1994).

GENE TRANSFECTION

Gene transfection uses physical and chemical means to deliver and insert the new (desired or healthy) gene into target cells. This technique involves removing billions of targeted cells from the person for whom gene therapy is being attempted. These cells then are grown under artificial conditions in cell culture to expand the population and to ease access of the genomes of these cells to the new gene.

The new gene is synthetically multiplied many times so that huge numbers of copies of this pure new gene exist. When sufficient amounts of the gene have been generated and the target cell population has been greatly expanded, the cells are treated by physical or chemical means to alter the plasma membranes and permit the gene to enter the cells. Usually the genes and the membrane-altering chemicals are added to the cultures at the same time. This technique of gene delivery and insertion is the least complex; however, its efficiency of insertion is extremely poor. Only approximately one cell in 100,000 successfully takes up and inserts the new gene into the genome in such a way that expression of the new gene occurs (Verma, 1990). Therefore, although gene therapy by transfection is technically successful, it is not a feasible method of applying gene therapy to human malignant conditions.

GENE TRANSDUCTION

Gene transduction is a method of gene delivery with increased efficiency of new gene insertion into the genome. This method involves the use of a vector or carrier to penetrate the plasma membranes of the target cells and ensure new gene insertion into the genome. The most common vectors of the new genes are viruses, especially retroviruses. This technique takes advantage of the fact that when a virus infects a cell, the virus inserts its own genetic material into the DNA of the cell it is infecting. Retroviruses are most efficient at inserting their genetic material into the DNA of the infected cell.

Target cells are removed from the host and grown in cell culture in the same way as in gene transfection. Copies of the new gene are spliced into the genetic material (either DNA or RNA) of virus vectors. The viruses containing the new gene are then incubated with the target cells in culture and infect the target cells. After infection of the target cells has occurred, the infected host cells that have also undergone gene transduction are reintroduced into the host.

The efficiency of gene insertion by transduction ranges between 10 per cent and 30 per cent. The viruses most frequently used for this purpose are adenoviruses, adeno-associated viruses (AAV), human parvoviruses, vesicular stomatis virus (VSV), murine leukemia virus, feline leukemia virus (subgroup B), and Simian sarcoma-associated virus (Fairbairn, Cross, & Arrand, 1994). Major drawbacks of vector-mediated gene transduction are:

- the technique will only succeed in dividing cell populations;
- "foreign" or viral genes are present and may be expressed by the host cells;
- retroviruses are known to cause cancer in other species and are suspected of causing cancer in humans;
- gene insertion occurs randomly within the genome of the transduced cell, and the extra DNA may alter the function of surrounding normal genes.

GENE THERAPY FOR CANCER

Gene therapy for specific malignancies has been tested on a limited basis with small numbers of subjects. The approaches that have been tested against human tumors in preclinical and phase I and II clinical trials are those that (1) increase the susceptibility of tumor cells as a target, (2) increase the activity of specific immune reactive cells, and (3) are directly cell-damaging or cytotoxic. The results show promise for acceptance as an adjunct therapy in the future. More studies are needed to compare the efficacy of gene therapy (alone or in combination with more traditional therapies) with that of standard treatment modalities and to characterize short-term and long-term effects on noncancerous tissues.

GENE THERAPY TO INCREASE TUMOR CELL SUSCEPTIBILITY

Increasing tumor cell susceptibility through the use of gene therapy is an indirect rather than a direct method of achieving tumor cytotoxicity. Gene insertion into the tumor cells modifies the cells in such a way that either they are more easily recognized as targets by immunoreactive cells or the metabolism of the tumor cell is changed sufficiently to render it more susceptible to cell kill by other agents. Both of these two different but related approaches have been used to enhance the tumor cell–killing capability of other treatment modalities.

Altered Metabolism. One example of experimental gene insertion that increases the sensitivity of tumor cells to the cytotoxic effect of another agent but is not in itself directly cytotoxic is gene therapy of human brain tumors. In this instance, the gene for the herpes virus enzyme, thymidine kinase (TK), is transduced into brain tumor cells. It is this enzyme that renders the herpes virus sensitive to the cytotoxic effects of ganciclovir. Gene transduction with the TK gene allows brain tumor cells to express thymidine kinase and be susceptible to the killing effects of ganciclovir. Not only are the tumor cells that have been transduced likely to be killed by ganciclovir, so are the surrounding untransduced tumor cells. The additional sensitivity of untransduced nearby tumor cells is called the "bystander effect" (Culver, 1994).

Increased Immunogenicity. Another example of experimental gene therapy for cancer involves inserting into tumor cells a gene expressing an HLA (human leukocyte antigen) pattern different from the host into tumor tissue. Such an action increases the tumor cell's susceptibility to cytotoxic and cytolytic actions of specific and nonspecific immune reactive cells, thus making the tumor more "immunogenic." This type of gene therapy has shown some success with melanoma and renal cell carcinomas.

One experimental method to increase the immunogenicity of tumor cells makes use of nonviral vectors by surrounding the gene to be inserted within a liposome. Liposomes are spheric structures with an outer surface composed of the same types of phospholipids that form normal human plasma membranes. The core of a liposome is water-filled. Multiple copies of the gene to be transferred are placed in the water-filled centers of the liposomes, which are then injected into the tumor. Tumor cells ingest the liposomes by phagocytosis, incorporate the transferred gene into their genomes, and begin to express HLAs on the tumor cell surface different from the normal host cells' HLAs. The host's immune system cells then attack those cancer cells expressing the different HLAs.

GENE THERAPY TO INCREASE THE ACTIVITY OF IMMUNOREACTIVE CELLS

A person's own cytotoxic/cytolytic T-lymphocytes (CTLs), natural killer cells (NKs), tumor-infiltrating lymphocytes (TILs), and lymphokine activated killer cells (LAK cells) are capable of identifying and attacking tumor cells. This ability is increased in the presence of specific cytokines such as interleukin-2 (IL-2), especially when the cytokine is endogenous rather than exogenous. The earliest form of gene therapy for cancer to be attempted in living human beings exploits the immunosurveillance capability of certain leukocytes to enhance self-contained immunotherapy. In such cases the cells transduced with a new gene are the person's own immunoreactive cells rather than the tumor cells.

The general steps in gene therapy to increase the activity of immunoreactive cells begin with either plasma pheresis to remove immunoreactive cells from the person with cancer or setting up cultures of tumor tissue to remove immunoreactive cells (especially TILs) residing within tumor tissue. Once the immunoreactive cells have been isolated from the patient, they are grown in culture to increase their numbers and to provide easy access for gene insertion. After expansion in cell culture, the cells are transduced with gene-containing viral vectors. Genes that enhance the abilities of the immunoreactive cells to recognize tumor cells and induce tumor-directed cytotoxic action are inserted into the patient's cultured immunoreactive cells. Such genes include those for interleukin-2 and gamma interferon (Foa et al., 1994; Moritz, Wels, Mattern, & Groner, 1994; Rosenberg, 1992; Rosenberg et al., 1990). The transduced cells increase endogenous production of stimulatory cytokines.

When immunoreactive cells transduced with cytokine genes are infused back into the patient, the gene-transduced cells specifically attack the tumor cells much more aggressively than do the same immunoreactive cells that have not been transduced. The increased endogenous production of cytokines does not induce the same undesirable systemic side effects that administration of exogenous cytokines does. Immunoreactive cells that have been transduced with cytokine genes appear to remain functional for 6 months or longer after reinfusion into the patient.

CYTOTOXIC GENE THERAPY

Cytotoxic gene therapy for cancer during in vitro preclinical trials has been highly successful, and in vivo human testing is underway. This approach involves inserting genes that are cytolytic or cytotoxic directly into the tumor cells. The genes that have been demonstrated to induce cytotoxic actions when inserted into tumor cells are the genes for tumor necrosis factor (TNF), IL-6, and γ-interferon. When these substances are expressed by the transduced tumor cells, autocytolysis, cytostasis, and vascular damage occur to the tumor. IL-6 also tends to induce terminal differentiation of the tumor cells, changing their phenotype to a more normal appearance, possibly by suppressing tumor expression of an oncogene. In addition, all of these gene products, when expressed by tumor cells, increase the immunogenicity or recognition of the tumor cells by immune reactive cells (Porgador, Feldman, & Eisenbach, 1994).

FUTURE POTENTIAL FOR GENE THERAPY IN CANCER

Oncogene suppression in humans as a type of gene therapy for cancer remains a future goal of molecular geneticists and oncologists. At present, oncogene suppression has been successful in vitro using the transduction method to insert an "antisense" segment of DNA complementary to parts of an activated oncogene in colorectal tumor cells (Hamilton, 1993). The application of this technique to people with actual malignancies or those people who are at high risk for tumor development through oncogene activation awaits considerable testing and refinement (Lotzova, 1994).

The age of gene therapy for malignant conditions has only just dawned. Scientists are predicting that the impact of gene therapy on the health of people during the twenty-first century will be at least equivalent to the impact of antimicrobial agents on the health of people during the twentieth century (Blaese, Miller, Plautz, & Scriver, 1993). Areas under research in which we can expect future application of gene therapy for cancer include:

- Integrating genes capable of suppressing activated oncogenes into tumor cells.
- Conferring chemotherapy resistance to nonmalignant tissues through the integration of a gene that stimulates transduced normal cells to "pump out" specific chemotherapeutic agents.
- Correcting the expression of a mutated gene by inserting multiple copies of the normal version of the gene.
- Inserting more than one gene directly into tumor cells both to increase immunogenicity and to suppress oncogene activity.

GENETIC COUNSELING

OVERVIEW

Genetic counseling for people and families experiencing cancer is appropriate. The purpose of genetic counseling in such situations is to attempt to quantify personal risk with regard to specific cancer development or cancer recurrence for any one person within a family or kinship (Kelly, 1992). Counseling must consider genetic predisposition alone and in conjunction with environmental exposure to carcinogens and lifestyle influences as well as family history to provide any one person with an accurate assessment of risk for a given cancer over a lifetime. Such quantification permits people to make informed decisions regarding lifestyle changes, participation in early detection/screening procedures, prophylactic treatment, aggressiveness of therapy for actual cancer, follow-up testing, and reproductive options.

A confusing issue in considering the hereditary basis for development of some cancers is that of "familial" versus "hereditary." While both familial cancers and hereditary cancers probably involve transmission of altered genetic material, individual risk varies considerably. In addition, sporadic cancers not related to any hereditary basis also can occur among individuals who have a genetic predisposition for cancer. Geneticists estimate that approximately 66 per cent of all cancers are sporadic in origin, approximately 34 per cent of all cancers have a familial basis, and only 5 to 10 per cent of all cancers have an identifiable single gene pattern of inheritance (Biesecker et al., 1993). Although hereditary cancers are relatively rare, they may be the very ones that have the potential for the best outcome in terms of removal of known "at risk" tissue and early detection coupled with appropriate intervention (King, Rowell, & Love, 1993).

FAMILIAL CANCERS

Familial cancers are those that appear across and within generations of one family at a rate higher than can be explained by environmental exposure and general risk alone. Such familial cancers may be of all one type or of many different types of cancer. Familial cancers lack the identifiable and predictable pattern of inheritance associated with single gene disorders. Table 24–2 lists cancers that have a familial tendency as well

TABLE 24–2. *Potential Familial Cancers*

Breast cancer
Ovarian cancer
Colorectal cancer
Prostate cancer
Melanoma
Uterine cancer
Leukemia
Sarcomas
Primary brain tumors

as a sporadic occurrence. Current theories on the origins of familial cancers suggest that:

1. Expression of a familial cancer may require activation or mutation of more than one altered gene (polygenic effect);
2. Familial cancers may arise from one or more recessive genes, but their expression is increased under favorable environmental conditions (exposure to general or specific carcinogens);
3. Heritable alterations of certain regulatory genes, such as the p53 gene, may be permissive rather than causative of cancer.

Families with higher than normal rates of cancer development have undergone intense scrutiny to determine the combined influence of genetic and specific environmental factors. Such studies have led to the identification of several different "cancer family syndromes" (Table 24–3). The major syndromes are Li-Fraumeni Syndrome, Lynch Syndrome I, Lynch Syndrome II, Breast/Ovarian Syndrome, and the Multiple Endocrine Neoplasia Syndromes (MEN1, MEN2A, MEN2B).These syndromes share some features in common, even though different groupings of cancer types are manifested. The two most outstanding features are early age of disease onset and the likelihood of the cancer being present bilaterally. People with familial cancer tend to develop overt disease decades before the expected or average age of onset for that particular cancer. In addition, unlike sporadic cancer, for which the risk only increases with age, a person's risk for familial cancer tends to decrease with age. It is not unusual for individuals within a cancer family kinship to develop more than one primary tumor.

HEREDITARY CANCERS

Hereditary cancers are inherited as a single gene disorder, and patterns of inheritance are clearly predictable. Such cancers may be inherited as dominant or recessive genes and can be carried by autosomal chromosomes or sex chromosomes. Table 24–4 lists some known hereditary cancers. In addition to malignant tumors, a wide variety of benign tumors also appear to be hereditary.

In addition to an increased occurrence rate of a specific cancer type within a family, hereditary cancers usually occur at a very early age, many in childhood. Also, they are more often bilateral or found at sites remote from the organ of origin.

In spite of the greatly magnified risk that any one person may have for a hereditary cancer, survival rates appear longer than for the sporadic form of the same type of cancer. The proposed explanation is that when people are informed of this greatly increased risk, they have the option to increase their surveillance (thus finding the cancer at an early stage when it is more cur-

TABLE 24–3. *Cancer Family Syndromes*

SYNDROME	ASSOCIATED CANCERS
Li-Fraumeni	Breast carcinoma
	Primary central nervous sytem tumors
	Childhood sarcomas
	Adrenocortical tumors
	Leukemia
Lynch I	Colorectal
Lynch II	Colorectal
	Endometrium
	Melanoma
	Ovary
	Pancreas
	Prostate
	Skin
	Stomach
	Renal
	Breast
Breast/Ovarian Syndrome	Breast
	Ovary
Multiple Endocrine Neoplasia 1 (MEN1)	Parathyroid
	Pituitary
	Pancreas
Multiple Endocrine Neoplasia 2 (MEN2)	Thyroid
	Pheochromocytoma
	Parathyroid hyperplasia
Multiple Endocrine Neoplasia 2B* (MEN2B)	Thyroid medullary parafollicular
	Pheochromocytoma
	Mucosal
	Neuroma

* More lethal than MEN2A, earlier onset.

TABLE 24–4. *Hereditary Cancers*

CANCER TYPE	PROBABLE PATTERNS OF INHERITANCE
Breast cancer	Autosomal dominant
	X-linked recessive
Colorectal cancer	Autosomal dominant (familial polyposis coli) (Gardner's syndrome)
	Autosomal recessive
Dysplastic nevi—melanoma	Autosomal dominant
Retinoblastoma	Autosomal dominant
Wilm's tumor	Autosomal dominant
	Autosomal recessive
Ovarian carcinoma	Autosomal dominant
Multiple endocrine neoplasia I	Autosomal dominant
Anterior pituitary	
Parathyroid	
Pancreatic islet cell	
Thyroid	
Adrenal cortex	
Intestinal carcinoids	
Bronchial carcinoids	
Multiple endocrine neoplasia II	Autosomal dominant
Pheochromocytoma	
Medullary thyroid tumors	
Neurofibromas	
Neuroblastoma	Autosomal dominant
	Autosomal recessive
Renal cell carcinoma	Autosomal dominant

able), to undergo surgical prophylaxis (removal of at risk tissue), to alter lifestyle, or to attempt medical prophylaxis.

Role of the Oncology Nurse

Calculating individual risk for any one person is not a simple task. For example, the general risk for breast cancer among all women in North America is approximately 11 per cent (one in nine). This general risk is lower in women younger than aged 40 years and higher in women older than aged 60 years. The risk for breast cancer among women who are in families with hereditary breast cancer is 50 per cent. This risk decreases as the women age. However, the general risk for all breast cancers include the women with hereditary breast cancer and familial breast cancer. Therefore, the general risk for women who do not have family histories of either familial breast cancer or hereditary breast cancer is actually somewhat less than 11 per cent, whereas the risk for women who have positive family histories of both familial breast cancer and hereditary breast cancer may far exceed 50 per cent. Actual risk calculation is not within the realm of oncology nurses and should be left to the professionals who have sufficient specialty training in the field of genetic counseling. However, oncology nurses can and should play a major role in ensuring that people receive appropriate counseling (Kelly, 1993).

Identification of people who have or who are at risk for developing familial or hereditary cancers is a nursing responsibility (Fitzsimmons, Conway, Madsen, Lappe, & Coody, 1989). Nurses should be familiar with the basic risks involved with cancer family syndromes and heritable cancers. In addition, oncology nurses must provide their patients with accurate general information regarding cancer development, prevention, early detection, and treatment.

The nurse may be the health care professional who initially determines the need for genetic counseling for patients and families experiencing cancer. Whenever the oncology nurse interacts with people who either are diagnosed with cancer at an earlier than expected age or who have any close relatives with cancer, a detailed family history is obtained. Details include a graphed family history in the form of a pedigree (family health tree) and accurate information regarding specific cancer type as well as age at onset of anyone in the kinship with cancer (Beck et al., 1988). Many information and assessment tools are available for use in cases where cancer family syndromes are suspected (Kelly, 1992; Lippman, Bassford & Meyskens, 1992). Oncology nurses can clear a patient's confusion about cancer type and stress the importance of checking records. For example, some patients may give a history of a relative who died of a brain tumor when in reality the relative actually had breast cancer that metastasized to the brain.

It is important for patients to be referred to appropriate genetic counseling programs or centers. Nurses can assist in this process by first knowing what type of genetic services are available at their own institutions.

If cancer genetics are not included in local services, a certified genetic counselor should have listings of regional and nationwide resources.

REFERENCES

Beck, S., Breckenridge-Potterf, S., Walace, S., Ware, J., Asay, E., & Giles, R. (1988). The family high-risk program: Targeted cancer prevention. *Oncology Nursing Forum, 15*(3), 301–306.

Biesecker, B., Boehnke, M., Calzone, K., Markel, D., Garber, J., Collins, S., & Weber, B. (1993). Genetic counseling for families with inherited susceptibility to breast and ovarian cancer. *Journal of the American Medical Association, 269*(15), 1970–1973.

Bishop, J. (1982). Oncogenes. *Scientific American, 246*, 80–92.

Bishop, J. (1985). Proto-oncogenes, clues to the puzzle of purpose. *Nature, 316*, 483–485.

Blaese, R. M., Miller, A. D., Plautz, G. E., & Scriver, C. R. (1993). Gene therapy: Sci-fi no longer. *Patient Care, 27*(11), 24–42.

Cohen-Haguenauer, O. (1994). A review of current basic approaches to gene therapy. *Journal of Experimental and Clinical Hematology, 36*(Suppl I), S3–S9.

Cooper, G. (1990). *Oncogenes.* Boston: Jones & Bartlett Publishers.

Cooper, G. (1992). *Elements of human cancer.* Boston: Jones & Bartlett Publishers.

Culver, K. (1994). Clinical applications of gene therapy for cancer. *Clinical Chemistry, 40*(4), 510–512.

Fairbairn, L. J., Cross, M. A., & Arrand, J. R. (1994). Paterson symposium 1993—Gene therapy. *British Journal of Cancer, 69*(5), 972–975.

Fitzsimmons, T., Conway, T., Madsen, N., Lappe, J., & Coody, D. (1989). Hereditary cancer syndromes: Nursing's role in identification and education. *Oncology Nursing Forum, 16*(1), 87–94.

Foa, R., Guarini, A., Cignetti, A., Cronin, K., Rosenthal, F., & Gansbacher, B. (1994). Cytokine gene therapy: A new strategy for the management of cancer patients. *Natural Immunology, 13*(2-3), 65–75.

Hamilton, S. (1993). Therapeutic implications of molecular genetics. *Advances in Experimental Medicine and Biology, 339*, 297–301, 303–304.

Kelly, P. (1992). Breast cancer risk analysis: A genetic epidemiology service for families. *Journal of Genetic Counseling, 1*(2), 155–167.

Kelly, P. (1993). Breast cancer risk: The role of the nurse practitioner. *Nurse Practitioner Forum, 4*(2), 91–95.

King, M., Rowell, S., & Love, S. (1993). Inherited breast and ovarian cancer: What are the risks? What are the choices? *Journal of the American Medical Association, 269*(15), 1975–1980.

Lippman, S., Bassford, T., & Meyskens, F. (1992). A quantitatively scored cancer-risk assessment tool: Its development and use. *Journal of Cancer Education, 7*(1), 15–36.

Lotzova, E. (1994). Prospects and advances in gene therapy. *Natural Immunology, 13*(2-3), 63–64.

Moritz, D., Wels, W., Mattern, J., & Groner, B. (1994). Cytotoxic T lymphocytes with a grafted recognition specificity for ERBB2-expressing tumor cells. *Proceedings of the National Academy of Science, 91*, 4318–4322.

Noonan, N., & Senner, A. (1994). Gene therapy techniques in the treatment of adenosine deaminase-deficiency severe combined immune deficiency syndrome. *Journal of Perinatal and Neonatal Nursing, 7*(4), 65–78.

Porgador, A., Feldman, M., & Eisenbach, L. (1994). Immunotherapy of tumor metastasis via gene therapy. *Natural Immunology, 13*(2-3), 113–130.

Rosenberg, S. (1992). Gene therapy for cancer. *Journal of the American Medical Association, 268*(17), 2416–2419.

Rosenberg, S., Aebersold, P., Cornetta, K., Kasid, A., Morgan, P., Moen, R., Karson, E. P., Lotze, M., Yang, J., Topalian, S., Merino, M., Culver, K., Miller, D., Blaese, M., & Anderson, F. (1990). Gene transfer into humans—Immunotherapy of patients with advanced melanoma, using tumor-infiltrating lymphocytes modified by retroviral gene transduction. *New England Journal of Medicine, 323*(9), 570–578.

Sandberg, A. (1990). *The chromosomes in human cancer and leukemia.* (2nd ed). New York: Elsevier.

Verma, I. (1990). Gene therapy. *Scientific American, 263*(5), 68–72.

Weinberg, R. (1994). Oncogenes and tumor suppressor genes. *CA: A Cancer Journal for Clinicians, 44*(3), 160–170.

Workman, M. L., Kenner, C., & Hilse, M. (1993). Human genetics. In C. Kenner, A. Bruggemeyer, & L. P. Gunderson. *Comprehensive neonatal nursing: A physiologic perspective* (pp. 101–131). Philadelphia: W. B. Saunders Co.

Yarbro, J. (1992). Oncogenes and cancer suppressor genes. *Seminars in Oncology Nursing, 8*(1), 30–39.

SUGGESTED READINGS

Garber, J. E., Goldstein, A., Kantor, A., Dreyfus, M., & Fraumeni, J. (1991). A follow-up study of twenty-four families with Li-Fraumeni syndrome. *Cancer Research, 51*(22), 6094–6097.

Houlston, R., Murday, V., Harocopos, C., Williams, C., & Slack, W. (1990). Screening and genetic counseling for relatives of patients with colorectal cancer in a family cancer clinic. *British Medical Journal, 301,* 366–368.

Lynch, H., Watson, P., Smyrk, T., Lanspa, S., Boman, B., Boland, C. R., Lynch, J., Cavalieri, J., Leppert, M., White, R., Sidransky, D., & Vogelstein, B. (1992). Colon cancer genetics. *Cancer, 70*(5), 1302–1312.

Mitelman, F. (1994). Chromosomes, genes, and cancer. *CA: A Cancer Journal for Clinicians, 44*(3), 133–135.

Mulvihill, J., & Byrne, J. (1989). Genetic counseling of the cancer survivor. *Seminars in Oncology Nursing, 5*(1), 29–35.

Yeomans, A. (1990). Hereditary cancer syndromes: Implications for practice. *Dimensions in Oncology Nursing, 4*(3), 17–26.

Yoder, L. (1990). The epidemiology of ovarian cancer. *Oncology Nursing Forum, 17*(3), 411–415.

Implementation of Clinical Trials

Jean Jenkins • Gregory A. Curt

CLINICAL TRIALS DEVELOPMENT

Advances in cancer treatment have occurred largely because of the application of new knowledge gained in basic research in the clinical management of patients with cancer. The term *research* brings to mind the classic laboratory environment with its equipment, white-coated scientists, and experimental animals. This is the environment of basic research in which careful, systematic investigation leads to new ideas for patient treatment. Clinical trials are carefully controlled experiments aimed at using the smallest number of subjects to determine with statistical confidence the effectiveness of treatments and at the same time maintain patient safety. Information on the various kinds of clinical trials provides the background for defining the important role that nurses play in the scientific development of cancer care.

Whereas some clinical trials test new treatments, others investigate new ways of preventing cancer, screening patients for earlier diagnosis, and detecting the disease in its earliest stages with new imaging modalities such as magnetic resonance and positron emission (Gwyther, 1994). Studies are now monitoring the psychologic impact of cancer on patients and studying related changes in their quality of life (Guyatt, Feeny, & Patrick, 1993). Today's clinical trials are multifaceted, striving not only to improve survival rates of patients with cancer through testing of new therapies but also to determine the safest, most effective treatment available (Spilker, 1991).

OVERVIEW

Clinical research is the keystone of modern medicine. In the early 1900s, surgery was the only treatment available to patients with cancer, and few were cured. Local treatments such as surgical excision are inadequate for the 70 per cent of patients with solid tumors who have obvious or occult metastatic disease at the time of diagnosis. By the mid-1950s, options for treatment began to increase with the introduction of both radiotherapy (which improved local disease control) and anticancer chemotherapy. Chemotherapy offered effective treatment for patients with advanced malignancy for the first time.

The progress of cancer therapy has been steady. Although only 20 per cent of patients with cancer survived for 5 years (considered a cure) in the 1930s, improved surgical techniques and the developing field of radiotherapy cured 33 per cent of patients by the 1950s (DeVita et al., 1979). Further improvements in radiotherapy and the development of chemotherapy have improved the cure rate to 50 per cent. Overall, advances have been greatest for patients under the age of 65 years, for whom the 5-year survival rate reached 57.5 per cent in 1991 (National Cancer Institute[NCI], 1993b; Ries et al., 1994).

Clinical trials have made important contributions through the development of new drugs and through the pioneering of better overall treatments for patients with common cancers. These treatments include limb-sparing procedures for patients with sarcoma, limited surgery for patients with breast cancer, and effective adjuvant chemotherapy for those with lung, colon, and rectal cancers. Development of these treatments occurs through a series of preclinical and clinical investigations. The development of agents to be administered as therapy is used to discuss this process of investigation.

PRECLINICAL DRUG DEVELOPMENT

The first step in identifying a new cancer agent is screening or measuring a drug's antitumor activity in a cancer model system. During this phase the National Cancer Institute's (NCI's) computer systems scan the structures of approximately 40,000 new chemicals that are synthesized each year to select novel compounds for testing. Earlier this testing was done against mouse tumors, but for the past 4 years the NCI has screened drugs against a panel of human tumor cell lines that were derived from patients with cancer (Fig. 25–1). This system identifies novel structures that show specific activity against solid tumors of adults. The new screen is also particularly suited to natural products, such as those from marine organisms or plants, where the initial isolate may contain only a small amount of relatively impure material. Each year approximately 10,000 compounds are selected for testing, of which 10 will pass all the steps needed to reach their first use in patients in what is known as a phase I study (Hubbard, 1981). Although only one in perhaps 50,000 drugs screened will eventually be approved for marketing, all agents that are commercially available to cancer patients in the United States have undergone such testing (DeVita et al., 1979).

PHASES OF CLINICAL TRIALS

Once preclinical drug development has been completed, clinical trials progress through four phases of testing. These trials are identified as phases I, II, III, and IV. The purpose of the study, the study design, the monitoring required, and the role of the nurse are determined by the phase of the clinical research (Hubbard & Gross, 1994).

PHASE I

Phase I study is the first testing of new agents in humans. The purpose of phase I clinical trials is to establish the maximum tolerated dose of the agent in various schedules in humans. In addition, pharmacologic tests, how well the agent is absorbed, what blood levels are achieved, and how the drug is metabolized and eliminated by the body are important parts of phase I evaluation (Box 25–1).

Although all drugs entering phase I studies are selected carefully for their potential activity against cancer, certain constraints minimize the likelihood that the trials of these drugs will demonstrate a significant antitumor effect during this stage of development. For example, the initial dose must be as safe as possible to avoid possible overdosing. For this reason, the starting dose level of the agent is based on prior animal studies and is usually one tenth the maximum tolerated dose in mice (Hubbard, 1981). Doses are usually escalated via the Fibonacci search scheme (Table 25–1) (Buyse, Staquet, & Sylvester, 1984). This plan requires that three to five patients be treated at each dose level and evalu-

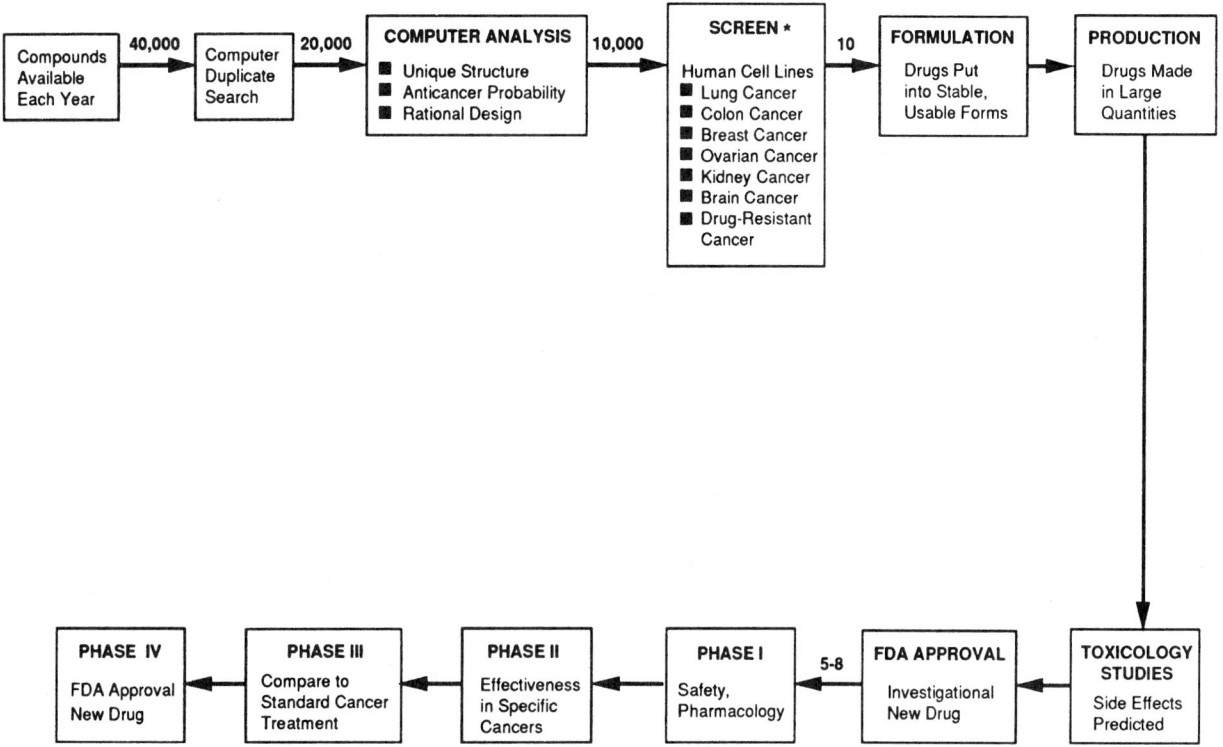

FIGURE 25–1. How a cancer drug is developed. *The new screening system using human cell lines replaces the mouse leukemia screen.

Box 25–1. *Phase I Study*

Budman, D. R., Igwemezie, L. N., Kaul, S., Behr, J., Lichtman, S., Schulman, P., Vinciguerra, V., Allen, S., Kolitz, J., Hock, K., O'Neill, K., Schacter, L., & Barbhaiya, R. H. (1994). Phase I evaluation of a water-soluble etoposide pro-drug, etoposide phosphate, given as a 5-minute infusion on days 1, 3, and 5 in patients with solid tumors. *Journal of Clinical Oncology, 12,* 1902–1909.

Sample: Thirty-six patients with solid tumors and a mean age of 63 years, performance status 0 to 1, white blood cell count > 4000, and platelet count > 100,000 with normal renal and hepatic function were studied. Doses evaluated in etoposide equivalents were 50, 75, 100, 125, 150, 175, and 200 mg/m^2/d. Etoposide in plasma and urine and etoposide phosphate in plasma were measured using high-pressure liquid chromatography (HPLC).

Measures: To determine the toxicities, maximal tolerated dose (MTD), and pharmacology of etoposide phosphate, a water-soluble etoposide derivative, administered as a 5-minute infusion on a schedule of days 1, 3, and 5, repeated every 21 days.

Findings: Grade 1 to 2 nausea, vomiting, alopecia, and fatigue were common. Leukopenia occurred at doses greater than 75 mg/m^2, with the nadir occurring between days 15 and 19 after treatment. All effects were reversible. The MTD due to neutropenia was determined to be between 175 and 200 mg/m^2/d. The conversion of etoposide phosphate to etoposide was not saturated at the dosages studied. Etoposide phosphate had peak plasma concentrations at 5 minutes, with a terminal half-life of 7 minutes. Etoposide reached peak concentrations at 7 to 8 minutes, with a terminal half-life of 6 to 9 hours.

Limitations: As in all phase I trials the recommended dose of drug must be verified in phase II studies, which will also give information about the clinical activity of the pro-drug. By its design the study cannot predict how the same doses of drug would be tolerated by patients who have either impaired liver or kidney function.

TABLE 25–1. *Fibonacci Search Scheme*

DRUG DOSE	PER CENT ABOVE PRECEDING LEVEL	NUMBER OF PATIENTS ENTERED
n (mg/m^2)	–	3
2 n	100	3
3.3 n	67	3
5 n	50	3
7 n	40	3
9 n	33	3
12 n	33	3
16 n	33	3

n = beginning dose.
(Modified from Buyse, M., Staquet, M., & Sylvester, R. [1984]. *Cancer clinical trials, methods, and practice.* New York: Oxford University Press. Reproduced by permission.)

ated for toxicity before advancing to the next level. Dose escalation occurs in smaller increments as the amount is increased because side effects are anticipated at higher dose levels. Approximately 15 to 20 patients are needed to complete a phase I study.

To minimize the number of phase I patients who receive subtherapeutic doses, new dosing regimens are currently under development (Collins, Zaharko, Dedrick, & Chabner, 1986). One of the most promising is to measure blood levels of the drug in animals that receive the optimal dose. These levels can then be compared with the drug blood levels in the first group of patients being tested. If these levels are far below those observed in the experimental animals, it may be possible to bypass some of the Fibonacci steps to reach the optimal dose in humans more quickly. How rapidly doses can be raised is determined by the therapeutic index of the agent in preclinical studies but may be either a geometric mean or a simple doubling of the

dose. Already this approach has been used successfully in several phase I studies including hexamethylene bisacetamide (HMBA), merbarone, pirozantrone, and iododoxorubicin with the result that fewer patients were needed to complete the trials and more were treated at safe and potentially therapeutic drug doses (Collins, Grieshaber, & Chabner, 1990). Different schedules for agent administration may be tested in phase I trials.

Only patients with malignant disease that is unresponsive to standard therapies or for which no standard therapy exists are eligible for phase I studies. Phase I trials are carefully controlled by the drug sponsor (whether the NCI or industry) and must be carried out by approved physicians at centers with expertise in this area. Before participation is allowed, approved physicians must meet certain criteria established by the Cancer Therapy Evaluation Program (CTEP) of the NCI and must be registered with CTEP. Phase I studies are frequently done by a single institution to maintain the highest level of safety and continuity of data (Cancer Therapy Evaluation Program, 1993).

For phase I studies sponsored by the NCI, principal investigators are required to submit current data biweekly. This requirement is needed to fulfill United States Food and Drug Administration (FDA) regulations. Phase I results are reviewed two times a year at a working group meeting during which all investigators report results and compare pharmacology, toxicities, and treatment responses.

Careful monitoring of phase I studies is essential in providing safety for the patient. A major nursing responsibility is the observation of toxic side effects. To facilitate this observation, a clinical brochure is available for each investigational agent developed by the NCI. This brochure provides information about the rationale for selecting the drug for clinical testing and the toxicity levels experienced in the animal studies. Anticipation of similar side effects in humans can allow early recognition of any potentially serious effect of the treatment. The first occurrence of any toxic reaction for phase I trials is reported by telephone to CTEP at 301-230-2330. Such information is used to collate details from diverse settings and to disseminate the information quickly to other investigators working with the drug. Any severe, life-threatening, or fatal event brought about by the new drug must also be reported by phone and later by letter (Cancer Therapy Evaluation Program, 1993).

Nurses frequently collect samples for pharmacokinetic monitoring of a patient on a phase I study. Timed blood samples are drawn to measure rates of drug absorption, metabolism, and excretion. The nurse coordinates or performs the timed studies to ensure both accuracy of the study and comfort of the patient.

The staff nurse contributes to the completeness of a phase I study through early recognition and management of the side effects of treatment. This information is then used to determine whether it is safe to escalate to the next higher drug dosage. Ethical concerns for patients in phase I studies include ensuring that informed consent has been given (discussed later) and emphasizing the patient's contribution to scientific knowledge regardless of the study's results. Patients eligible for phase I trials are often physically and emotionally debilitated and may need special attention to ensure that ethical considerations are addressed. For instance, a patient who is desperately ill may feel there is no other hope and may be easily persuaded to participate in research trials without understanding the total ramifications. Nurses can assist patients to consider the treatment alternatives but should be careful not to overstep a nurse's expertise. A case reported by Gargaro (1978) illustrates the right of the nurse to inform patients of nursing treatments available. The role of the nurse in relation to medical management issues is to be an advocate for the patient and, if questions still exist regarding treatment options, to be a liaison to the physician to insist that these questions of risks and alternative treatment options be clarified.

PHASE II

Phase I studies focus on the evaluation of drug toxicities and the determination of safe drug dosages to be used for testing in a phase II trial. Agents entered into phase II study are tested in humans with various types of cancer primarily to determine effectiveness against a given cancer. The most frequently tested tumors include those found in leukemia, lymphoma, and melanoma and in colon, lung, breast, ovarian, and brain cancers (DeVita, 1982). Additional information on toxicity may be determined, and more sophisticated pharmacology studies may also be performed. Many patients eligible for phase II clinical studies have had prior cancer treatment. Their disease may have progressed or become refractory to standard treatment. Patients must also have a tumor that is measurable so that the effectiveness of the agent against cancer can be determined.

Responses can then be graded as complete (all tumor regresses), partial (greater than 50 per cent regression), or minimal (less than 50 per cent regression). Pretreatment organ function must be normal, and life expectancy must be a sufficient amount of time for observation. Phase II studies usually require 18 to 30 patients to make a statistical determination about the effectiveness of the drug in specific human tumors (Simon, Wittes, & Ellenberg, 1985). The nurse can best contribute to the completeness of phase II studies by documenting benefits and side effects of the treatment. Patients must be eligible and able to be evaluated to ensure the accuracy of phase II data. The nurse may anticipate and prepare the patient for studies that monitor disease response. Knowledge of the means by which various cancers spread, effects of cancer therapy, and staging procedures required by the protocol will assist the nurse in preparing the patient for participation in phase II study (Box 25–2).

PHASE III

The purpose of phase III studies is to compare the effectiveness of an experimental drug or treatment with a standard regimen or treatment. A phase III study applies a more complex design than those of phase I and II studies, which describe a single treatment. Once activity of an agent in a specific tumor has been determined in a phase II study, a comparative phase III study is designed. A phase III study compares established therapy with a new therapy in terms of impact on overall survival, disease-free survival, and quality of life. Patients are stratified by a number of variables that may affect the outcome of the study (age, performance status, tumor grade, stage of disease). These stratifications assist in making the comparative groups equivalent so that valid conclusions can be drawn from study results. In phase III study, two equally effective treatments may be evaluated to determine whether one is less toxic and therefore preferable (Box 25–3).

Phase III study designs require large numbers of patients to allow comparisons. Unlike phase I and II trials, many phase III studies are multiinstitutional so that adequate numbers can be entered on a study in a timely manner. Patients considered eligible for phase III studies usually have had no prior treatment for cancer. To prevent bias, randomization is made to the standard treatment (control group) vs. the new treatment (Ellenberg & Eisenberger, 1985). Because of their size, phase III studies are the most costly and the most difficult to plan and implement. It is in this stage, however, that an improved treatment is discovered and becomes the standard of care. Objective criteria for measuring tumor response and study objectives (survival, disease-free survival) must be clearly defined.

The nursing role in phase III studies includes monitoring patient eligibility and protocol compliance, documenting therapeutic effects and toxicities, and providing continuity of care. Phase III observations may require that the patient make frequent long-term hospital visits to measure the effectiveness of treatment. Delineation of long-term effects of cancer treatment

---

Box 25–2. *Phase II Study*

Seewaldt, V., Greer, B., Cain, J., Figge, D., Tamimi, H., Brown, W., & Miller, S. (1994). Paclitaxel (Taxol) treatment for refractory ovarian cancer: Phase II clinical trial. *American Journal of Obstetrics and Gynecology, 170,* 1666–1670.

Sample: One hundred patients with ovarian cancer in whom three or more chemotherapy regimens had failed and who had demonstrated platinum resistance.

Measures: Paclitaxel was administered every 21 days at intravenous doses of 135 mg/m^2 over 24 hours with optional granulocyte colony-stimulating factor support. Patients were monitored for toxicities both hematologic and nonhematologic; CA 125 measurement day 22 each cycle; computed tomography (CT) scan every 3 weeks; and pelvic examination every 3 cycles.

Findings: One hundred patients were treated with a median of five cycles. Paclitaxel was generally well tolerated. Hematologic toxicity was moderate, affecting granulocytes more than platelets and red blood cells. Nine per cent of the patients experienced grade 3 to 4 nausea and vomiting; mild stomatitis was common as was alopecia; bowel perforation occurred in four patients; no patients had cardiac arrhythmias; and transient myalgias were common in one third of patients 24 to 48 hours after treatment. A 25 per cent response rate in patients with refractory ovarian cancer was observed, which was durable to six cycles. Six patients had a complete response.

Limitations: Extent of disease and number of prior therapies do affect the response of tumor to cytotoxic drugs. The response rate of 25 per cent is excellent but may not predict the overall usefulness of paclitaxel for treatment of ovarian cancer. Further studies will be needed to address whether this agent will be superior as a front-line agent, since this phase II study reports comparatively low toxicity and excellent potential as an effective agent in treating ovarian cancer.

Box 25–3. *Phase III Study*

Fisher, B., Costantino, J., Redmond, C., Fisher, E., Wickerham, L., Cronin, W., & other NSABP contributors. (1994). Endometrial cancer in tamoxifen-treated breast cancer patients: Findings from the national surgical adjuvant breast and bowel projects (NSABP) B-14. *Journal of the National Cancer Institute, 86,* 527–537.

Sample: Data were analyzed on 2843 patients with node-negative, estrogen receptor-positive, invasive breast cancer randomly assigned to placebo or tamoxifen (20 mg/d) and on 1220 tamoxifen-treated patients registered in the NSABP B-14 subsequent to randomization.

Measures: Follow-up information on women enrolled in these studies was crucial to the poststudy assessment of whether an increased risk of endometrial cancer was present in women treated with tamoxifen. Slides prepared from paraffin-embedded tissue blocks from patients reported to have developed endometrial cancer were reviewed by the NSABP Pathology Center. Specimens were masked so that the reviewer was unaware of the patient's treatment. Endometrial cancers were verified, graded, and staged.

Findings: Twenty-five cases of endometrial cancer were originally reported, one was reclassified after subsequent review. Two cases were in the placebo arm; 23 in the tamoxifen group. After review of annual hazard rate, cumulative hazard rate, and the National Cancer Institute's Surveillance, Epidemiology, and End Results (SEER) data, the authors conclude that risk of endometrial cancer increases following tamoxifen therapy but that net benefit greatly outweighs the risk. They conclude that tamoxifen treatment for breast cancer should continue.

Limitations: It is crucial to understand the quantitative information of risk vs. benefit of any therapeutic intervention. The extent of risk of endometrial cancer occurring as a result of tamoxifen therapy vs. the benefit achieved through tamoxifen reducing both breast cancer occurrence and relapse must be understood to determine the overall impact of such treatment.

Survival, impact on disease, and toxicity are all crucial pieces that an individual considers in selecting a prevention or treatment strategy for any illness.

---

may be a significant factor in the determination of the best therapy to offer to future patients.

PHASE IV

Phase IV studies are designed to integrate a new agent or treatment into a primary or proven plan. This additional study may elucidate data on the optimum use of the agent. At this stage of study, the drug is known to be effective but is not yet authorized for wide-scale commercial distribution. Long-term follow-up data are needed to show long-term efficacy and any development of other toxicities. Nurses caring for

patients receiving phase IV therapy must provide education and evaluate nursing interventions to decrease the morbidity associated with the regimen. Additionally, evaluation of drugs after their approval for clinical use has been proposed to provide ongoing scientific evaluation (Ray, Griffin, & Avorn, 1993).

RESOURCES FOR CLINICAL TRIALS

The NCI sponsors all the major phase I, II, and III cancer clinical trials in the United States. The CTEP is responsible for administration and coordination of the majority of the extramural clinical trials. These trials

TABLE 25–2. *National Cancer Institute Cooperative Clinical Trials Groups*

Multimodality Multidisease Groups
Cancer and Leukemia Group B (CALGB)
Children's Cancer Study Group (CCSG)
Eastern Cooperative Oncology Group (ECOG)
North Central Cancer Treatment Group (NCCTG)
Pediatric Oncology Group (POG)
Southwest Oncology Group (SWOG)

Multimodality Group Devoted to a Major Oncologic Disease or Modality Area
Brain Tumor Study Group (BTSG)
Gynecologic Oncology Group (GOG)
Intergroup Rhabdomyosarcoma Study Group (IRSG)
National Surgical Adjuvant Breast and Bowel Project (NSABP)
National Wilms' Tumor Study Group (NWTSG)
Radiation Therapy Oncology Group (RTOG)

Special Activities Groups
European Organization for Research on Treatment for Cancer (EORTC)—Operations and Statistical Office

are conducted by the NCI (1) through clinical or comprehensive cancer centers, (2) by cooperative study groups (Table 25–2), (3) through community clinical oncology programs, or (4) through specialized programs of research excellence (SPORES). Collaboration of the NCI and the pharmaceutical industry may occur at any step along the drug development process. The pharmaceutical industry is sponsoring an increasing proportion of all research on the effects of drugs.

The Clinical Oncology Program is the intramural treatment research arm of the NCI (NCI, 1992). Programs conducted at the Clinical Center, National Institutes of Health, focus on basic and clinical research in surgery, pharmacology, radiobiology, immunology, genetics, and molecular biology. Information about clinical trials in progress is available from The Physicians Data Query, which is a clinically oriented database that was developed to make current information on cancer treatment more widely available (Hubbard, Henney, & DeVita, 1987). The Physicians Data Query can be accessed directly by computer, by consulting a medical librarian with a connection to Medical Literature Analysis and Retrieval System (MEDLARS), or by telephoning 1-800-4-CANCER (Deininger, Collins, & Hubbard, 1989). NCI offers an information associates program that permits access to its vast network of oncology resources. Services can be reviewed through calling 1-800-NCI-7890. This service summarizes information on clinical protocols, available patient education materials, state-of-the-art cancer treatment, and physicians who are qualified to treat patients with cancer. Any patient who wishes to and who fits eligibility criteria can take part in a clinical trial. Any well-run clinical trial receives a careful review for scientific validity, humanitarian value, and patient safety to provide protection of human rights.

FEDERAL REGULATIONS OF CLINICAL TRIALS

All clinical trials in the United States must meet criteria established by the Department of Health and Human Services (DHHS) and the FDA (Levine, 1981).

Anyone receiving a grant from DHHS must file with the National Institutes of Health a statement of assurance of compliance with the DHHS regulations (Levine, 1986). The five general ethical norms required by these regulations for developing a clinical trial include a good research design, competent investigators, favorable balance of harm vs. risk benefit, informed consent, and equitable selection of subjects (Office of Science and Technology Policy, 1991).

The FDA is given the responsibility and authority by Congress for ensuring the safety of the public (Young, 1981). This governmental agency enforces the laws established by Congress that define the terms under which clinical work with experimental agents may proceed.

All clinical research is required by federal regulations to be reviewed at each participating institution by an institutional review board. Both the DHHS and the FDA have adopted policies designed to ensure the competent function of these boards. Projects must be reviewed by the institution's review board before protocol initiation and at least annually thereafter. The composition of an institutional review board includes physicians, scientists, lawyers, clergy, community members, and nurses. When these boards review pediatric protocols, persons who care for children should be members. The institutional review board affords protection for the investigator, the institution, and the patient through protocol review.

Federal interest in and oversight of clinical trials appear to be increasing. For example, in 1994 Congress passed legislation mandating that clinical studies recruit sufficient numbers of women and minorities into trials. The intent, of course, to make it possible to quantify the benefit that a new treatment will give in different subpopulations of the citizenry. How this law will be implemented is small studies, such as phase I and II trials, remains uncertain.

PROTOCOL COMPONENTS

A well-designed research trial has a written protocol, which is a clear, well-written plan of action (Cancer Therapy Evaluation Program, 1993). Components

TABLE 25–3. *Components of a Research Protocol*

COMPONENT	CRITERIA
Rationale for study	Objectives*
	Scientific data
	Patient selection
Treatment plan	Schedule, dose, route*
	Pharmaceutical information
	Expected toxicities*
Study parameters	Patient entry procedures
	Dose modifications
	Criteria for response
	Measurement parameters*
	Off-study criteria
	Records to keep
Statistical criteria	Method of analysis
	Numbers needed for study
	Expected duration of study
Bibliography	Contact persons*
	Informed consent

*To be included in informed consent document.
(Modified from Cancer Therapy Evaluation Program. [1993]. *Investigator's handbook*. Washington, DC: National Cancer Institute.)

TABLE 25–4. *Informed Consent**

Expected benefits from the study
Expected study participation duration
Alternative treatment options
Record confidentiality
Compensation for injury
Participation is voluntary
Withdrawal from the study is possible at any time

*All criteria marked in Table 25–3 with an asterisk (*), expressed in lay terms, are included here as well.
(Modified from Cancer Therapy Evaluation Program. [1993]. *Investigator's handbook*. Washington, DC: National Cancer Institute.)

of a research protocol are listed in Table 25–3. Clear definitions are essential in communicating the study findings. For multiinstitutional protocols, approval from each institution's review board is required. An essential component of a protocol proposal is the provision for informed consent (Tables 25–3 and 25–4). Information in the informed consent form is specific and must be communicated in lay terms to ensure patient understanding. Informed consent results in voluntary study participation or refusal (see "Informed Consent" section of this chapter).

APPROACHES TO ALLEVIATING OBSTACLES TO PERFORMING CLINICAL TRIALS

Participation in clinical trials is voluntary. Community physicians should engage in or support activities that will lead to improved patient care (Levine, 1986), and referrals to clinical trials should begin at the community level. Patients must be informed of the opportunity for study participation and the advantages of clinical trials. Feelings of hopelessness and fear of abandonment by the primary physician must be addressed so that the patient can hear the options and make an informed decision (Meisel & Roth, 1981).

A major obstacle to conducting clinical trials is the accrual of an adequate sample size to answer the study questions. Taylor, Maegolese, and Soskolne (1985) reported that some physicians did not enter patients in a specific National Surgical Adjuvant Project for Breast and Bowel Cancers (NSABP) randomized study because of concern that the doctor-patient relationship would be affected by the clinical trial (73 per cent), difficulty with obtaining informed consent (38 per cent), dislike for open discussion involving uncertainty (22 per cent), perceived difficulty in following procedures (9 per cent), and feelings of personal responsibility if the treatments were found to be unequal (8 per cent). The NCI is targeting several of these concerns by physicians in a campaign to publicize clinical trials to physicians and to the general public (Wittes & Friedman, 1988). Mechanisms such as video tapes to explain protocols and written materials for the lay person to describe clinical trials are being developed to address the patient's increased need for information.

Another obstacle is the attitude of the public toward participation in research. Patients may be reluctant to participate in a clinical trial because such experimentation makes them feel like a "guinea pig." A study by Cassileth, Lusk, Miller, and Hurwitz (1982) reported on a population of 295 subjects that included oncology patients, cardiology patients, and members of the general public (Box 25–4). Seventy-one per cent of the respondents felt that it is reasonable for patients to participate in clinical studies. Patients who participate in medical research are perceived to get the best medical care, to benefit others, and to broaden the base on which improved treatments could be developed. The NCI is making an effort to publicize the benefits of clinical trials and is working to make participation in clinical trials socially and medically acceptable for all patients and physicians (Gelber & Goldhirsch, 1989). Nurses can offer information to patients and families or direct them to appropriate resources for information about available treatments. This attention will help the patient and family consider all the benefits and risks of available treatments and make an informed decision about the best option.

The concern for protection of minors from exploitation is still another obstacle. Treating children in a clinical trial is a special challenge to the research nurse and physician. Children must be studied to make appropriate treatments available (American Academy of Pediatrics, 1977); indeed, many successful therapies have been pioneered in pediatric oncology. Many of the principles of cancer therapy were established initially in clinical trials involving children (Fletcher, Eyes, & Dorn, 1988). For example, the notion that combinations of drugs could be given in a cyclic fashion to allow for bone marrow nadir and recovery was first tested in childhood leukemias and only later was applied successfully to adults with lymphoma and solid tumors. Clinical trials involving children were the first

---

Box 25–4. *Public Attitudes Toward Research Participation*

Cassileth, B., Lusk, E., Miller, D., & Hurwitz, S. (1982). Attitudes toward clinical trials among patients and the public. *Journal of the American Medical Association, 248,* 968–970.

   Sample: Total population of 295 subjects, including 104 patients with cancer, 84 cardiology patients, and 107 members of the general public in Philadelphia, Pennsylvania.
   Measures: Self-report questionnaire of 10 multiple-choice questions and one open-ended item regarding opinions on the purpose and ethical status of contemporary clinical research.
   Findings: Seventy-one per cent of respondents believed that patients should serve as research subjects to make an important contribution to society. The majority felt that research would increase medical knowledge and help future patients and that any patient could participate. Respondents viewed clinical trials as important, ethical, and a means of attaining superior care.
   Limitations: Participants were being seen at a major university hospital and may view research differently from those in other settings. Additional public participants were selected from nonhealth, nonuniversity jobs but may not be a representative sample because selection for participation was not described. The majority of those responding in the study were white. It would be of interest to repeat a similar study in minority populations in which high incidences of cancer occur.

---

to establish that teams of surgeons, radiotherapists, and chemotherapists could work together to limit treatment effects without compromising care. These principles, first established in children with soft tissue sarcomas, were only later applied to adults with breast, bladder, and head and neck cancers. In addition, clinical trials involving children established the principles of supportive care for the febrile, neutropenic patient.

Emotional response by all involved with the child's care may interfere with the best individual treatment decision. The nurse can play a central role in helping families explore options and evaluate what is best for the child so that the family can make the most informed decision (Cogliano-Shutta, 1986).

NURSING RESPONSIBILITIES

Providing information to the patient and family is only one of many responsibilities of the nurse in a research setting as part of the research team. Nurses make significant contributions to the success of clinical investigations by implementing various roles. As part of the research team, each of these nurses will assume certain responsibilities, depending on the role being implemented (Table 25–5). The first role is that of a staff nurse. The staff nurse has varied levels of education and experience; administratively, he or she is under the head nurse of a unit or an outpatient area. A nurse who has developed additional skills and has pursued an advanced educational degree may become a clinical nurse specialist, a second role for the nurse in a research setting. The clinical nurse specialist role is that of a consultant, educator, researcher, and developer of advanced clinical practice skills. A clinical nurse specialist usually answers to the head nurse or director of the nursing service. A third role is that of the research nurse, who performs a variation of the staff nurse and clinical nurse specialist roles. The research nurse may or may not have an advanced educational degree, may work directly for physicians or nurses, and most often has advanced practice experience. The fourth role of a nurse in a research setting is that of data manager. Other types of persons can be hired to do the data retrieval and reporting often done by data managers;

these positions do not have to be filled by nurses. Data managers often report administratively to the principal investigators of the research study or to the research nurse.

ADVOCACY

Nurses can serve as advocates for patients considering participation in clinical trials. The nurse can be a liaison between the physician and the patient. The nurse identifies concerns, resolves conflicts, or assists as questions develop. Written information such as *What Are Clinical Trials All About?* (Davis, Nealon, & Stone, 1993) is available to patients to assist them in understanding what is involved in participating in clinical trials. This booklet and information about disease and treatment alternatives and clarification of unclear information can promote informed patient participation. Printed materials for English or Spanish persons can be obtained by calling the Cancer Information Service at 1-800-4-CANCER.

INFORMED CONSENT

Informed consent is a legal and ethical prerequisite for patient participation in clinical trials (see Table 25–4). The nurse is ideally situated to evaluate the patient's understanding of the study and to determine that the decision to participate has indeed been voluntary. The manner in which information is conveyed is important. Consideration of the patient's age, level of education, cultural background, or lack of knowledge may modify the process of obtaining informed consent.

There are always risks associated with experimental treatments (Chabner, Wittes, Hoth, & Hubbard, 1984). It is the responsibility of the principal investigator to develop a complete, clear consent form that states all possible risks known about the agents used in the study. The physician is responsible for seeing that the patient understands the available options, potential risks, and benefits of the treatment alternatives. The consent should be read by the patient, explained by the physician, and clarified by the nurse. Informed consent is a dynamic educative process and is often achieved

TABLE 25–5. *The Nurse in a Research Setting*

TYPE	ROLE	RESPONSIBILITIES
Staff nurse	Primary caregiver	Knowledge of preclinical information and rationale for basis of study
		Provision of patient care with optimal safety and comfort
		Clinical expertise with assessment skills that promote recognition of side effects
		Patient education
		Assistance with ensuring informed consent
		Patient advocacy
		Anticipation and documentation of treatment and disease effects
		Referral to appropriate resources
		Continuity of care and long-term follow-up
		Knowledge and application of ethical considerations
		Awareness of attitudes about research (self)
		Administration of treatment
Clinical nurse specialist	Consultant	Assessment of impact of medical research on nursing responsibilities
	Educator	Planning for implementation of research
	Advanced practice	Preparation and guidance of staff caring for patients
	Research	Education of staff about theory, rationale, and objectives of research
		Problem solving
		Patient and staff advocate
		Rapid dissemination of information on advances in practice and research
		Awareness of attitudes about research (self and staff)
Research nurse	Collaborator	Participate in study design and execution
	Liaison	Coordinate smooth implementation of study
		Assist clinical nurse specialist with education of staff and patients
		Develop teaching materials specific to protocol
		Pharmacokinetics
		Collaboration with all health care resources
		Liaison between patient and physician, nurse and physician relationships and concerns
		Awareness of attitudes about research (self and others)
		Liaison to drug companies and Cancer Therapy Evaluation Program
		Collection of patient data, review of medical records
		Monitor trends in side effects for early recognition of response to treatment
		Assist with data analysis and interpretation
		Advocate for patient and protocol
		Assist with summarizing of data for publication
Data manager	Management of research information	Design of data report forms
		Retrieval of patient information for summary
		Data entry onto forms or into computer for analysis
		Analysis of data

through oral and written explanations (Varricchio & Jassak, 1989). The informed consent must be signed by the patient and witnessed. The witness can only verify that the signature is that of the patient, not that the patient understands all that is written. Collaboration of the nurse with the rest of the health care team is essential to ensuring that an individual has knowingly consented to medical treatment.

MONITORING

The nurse in a research setting is also responsible for monitoring patients during the study. Depending on the role of the nurse, monitoring may include various kinds of assessment, planning, and documentation. For example, the research nurse and the clinical nurse specialist might review a protocol to monitor the impact of that study on nursing care. A proposed study might include a new method for delivery of

drugs, such as intraperitoneal administration that might require in-service demonstrations, changes in policies and procedures, and new equipment for protocol implementation. All nurses should be monitoring patients for how well the patient fits the eligibility criteria of the study. One of the goals of the principal investigator should be to maximize the number of patients who can be evaluated in the study. The nurse's roles may include preparing the patient for studies required to document protocol eligibility and ensuring protocol compliance.

Monitoring responsibilities also include assessing the side effects of treatment on a frequent basis to document the physical and psychologic responses of the patient. The staff nurse is often the first to notice unusual or expected symptoms and should report them to the research nurse or the principal investigator. Grading of toxicities such as nausea and vomiting (on a scale of 0 to 4, as in Table 25–6) promotes improved

TABLE 25–6. *Common Toxicity Criteria*

TOXICITY	GRADE 0	1	2	3	4
White blood cell count	≥ 4	3–3.9	2–2.9	1–1.9	< 1
Platelets	WNL	75–normal	50–74.9	25–49.9	< 25
Hemoglobin	WNL	10–normal	8–10	6.5–7.9	< 6.5
Granulocytes/bands	≥ 2	1.5–1.9	1–1.4	0.5–0.9	< 0.5
Lymphocytes	≥ 2	1.5–1.9	1–1.4	0.5–0.9	< 0.5
Hemorrhage (clinical)	None	Mild, no transfusion	Gross, 1–2 U transfusion per episode	Gross, 3–4 U transfusion per episode	Massive, > 4 U transfusion per episode
Infection	None	Mild	Moderate	Severe	Life-threatening
Nausea	None	Able to eat reasonable intake	Intake significantly decreased but can eat	No significant intake	–
Vomiting	None	1 episode in 24 hrs	2–5 episodes in 24 hrs	6–10 episodes in 24 hrs	> 10 episodes in 24 hrs or requiring parenteral support
Diarrhea	None	Increase of 2–3 stools per day over pre-Rx	Increase of 4–6 stools per day, nocturnal stools, or moderate cramping	Increase of 7–9 stools per day, incontinence, or severe cramping	Increase of ≥ 10 stools per day, grossly bloody diarrhea, or need for parenteral support
Stomatitis	None	Painless ulcers, erythema, or mild soreness	Painful erythema, edema, or ulcers but can eat	Painful erythema, edema, or ulcers and cannot eat	Requires parenteral or enteral support
Bilirubin	WNL	–	$< 1.5 \times N$	$1.5–3 \times N$	$> 3 \times N$
Transaminase (SGOT, SGPT)	WNL	$\leq 2.5 \times N$	$2.6–5 \times N$	$5.1–20 \times N$	$> 20 \times N$
Alkaline Phosphotase or 5'nucleotidase	WNL	$\leq 2.5 \times N$	$2.6–5 \times N$	$5.1–20 \times N$	$> 20 \times N$
Liver (clinical)	No change from baseline	–	–	Precoma	Hepatic coma
Creatinine	WNL	$< 1.5 \times N$	$1.5–3 \times N$	$3.1–6 \times N$	$> 6 \times N$
Proteinuria	No change	1+ or < 0.3 g% or < 3 g/L	2–3+ or 0.3–1 g% or 3–10 g/L	4+ or > 1 g% or > 10 g/L	Nephrotic syndrome
Hematuria	Negative	Micro only	Gross, no clots	Gross + clots	Requires transfusion
Alopecia	No loss	Mild hair loss	Pronounced or total hair loss	–	–
Pulmonary	None or no change	Asymptomatic, with abnormality in PFTs	Dyspnea on significant exertion	Dyspnea at normal level of activity	Dyspnea at rest
Cardiac dysrhythmias	None	Asymptomatic, transient, requiring no therapy	Recurrent or persistent, no therapy required	Requires treatment	Requires monitoring; hypotension, ventricular tachycardia, or fibrillation

WNL = within normal units; N = normal; PFT = pulmonary function test; CHF = congestive heart failure. (From Cancer Therapy Evaluation Program (1993). *Investigator's handbook*. Washington, DC: National Cancer Institute.)

Continued on following page.

TABLE 25–6. *Common Toxicity Criteria* Continued

Toxicity	Grade				
	0	1	2	3	4
Cardiac function	None	Asymptomatic, decline of resting ejection fraction by < 20% of baseline value	Asymptomatic, decline of resting ejection fraction by > 20% of baseline value	Mild CHF, responsive to therapy	Severe or refractory CHF
Cardiac—ischemia	None	Nonspecific T wave flattening	Asymptomatic, ST and T wave changes suggesting ischemia	Angina without evidence for infarction	Acute myocardial infarction
Cardiac—pericardial	None	Asymptomatic, effusion, no intervention required	Pericarditis (rub, chest pain, ECG changes)	Symptomatic effusion; drainage required	Tamponade; drainage urgently required
Hypertension	None or no change	Asymptomatic, transient increase by > 20 mm Hg (D) or to > 150/100 if previously WNL; no treatment required	Recurrent or persistent increase by > 20 mm Hg (D) or to > 150/100 if previously WNL; no treatment required	Requires therapy	Hypertensive crisis
Hypotension	None or no change	Changes requiring no therapy (including transient orthostatic hypotension)	Requires fluid replacement or other therapy but not hospitalization	Requires therapy and hospitalization; resolves within 48 hrs of stopping the agent	Requires therapy and hospitalization for > 48 hrs after stopping the agent
Neuro—sensory	None or no change	Mild paresthesias, loss of deep tendon reflexes	Mild or moderate objective sensory loss; moderate paresthesias	Severe objective sensory loss or paresthesias that interfere with function	—
Neuro—motor	None or no change	Subjective weakness; no objective findings	Mild objective weakness without significant impairment of function	Objective weakness with impairment of function	Paralysis
Neuro—cortical	None	Mild somnolence or agitation	Moderate somnolence or agitation	Severe somnolence, agitation, confusion, disorientation, or hallucinations	Coma, seizures, toxic psychosis
Neuro—cerebellar	None	Slight incoordination, dysdiadochokinesia	Intention tremor, dysmetria, slurred speech, nystagmus	Locomotor ataxia	Cerebellar necrosis
Neuro—mood	No change	Mild anxiety or depression	Moderate anxiety or depression	Severe anxiety or depression	Suicidal ideation
Neuro—headache	None	Mild	Moderate or severe but transient	Unrelenting and severe	—
Neuro—constipation	None or no change	Mild	Moderate	Severe	Ileus > 96 hrs
Neuro—hearing	None or no change	Asymptomatic, hearing loss on audiometry only	Tinnitus	Hearing loss interfering with function but correctable with hearing aid	Deafness not correctable

Table 25–6. *Common Toxicity Criteria* Continued

	GRADE				
TOXICITY	0	1	2	3	4
Neuro—vision	None or no change	–	–	Symptomatic sub-total loss of vision	Blindness
Skin	None or no change	Scattered macular or papular eruption or erythema that is asymptomatic	Scattered macular or papular eruption or erythema with pruritus or other associated eruption symptoms	Generalized symptomatic macular, papular, or vesicular	Exfoliative dermatitis or ulcerating dermatitis
Allergy	None	Transient rash, drug fever < 38° C (100.4° F)	Urticaria, drug fever = 38° C (100.4° F), mild bronchospasm	Serum sickness, bronchospasm; requires parenteral medications	Anaphylaxis
Fever in absence of infection	None	37.1–38° C 98.7–100.4° F	38.1–40° C 100.5–104° F	> 40° C > 104° F for < 24 hrs	> 40° C (104° F) for 24 hrs or fever accompanied by hypotension
Local	None	Pain	Pain and swelling, with inflammation or phlebitis	Ulceration	Plastic surgery indicated
Weight gain/loss	< 5%	5–9.9%	10–19.9%	> 20%	–
Hyperglycemia	< 116	116–160	161–250	251–500	> 500 or ketoacidosis
Hypoglycemia	> 64	55–64	40–54	30–39	< 30
Amylase	WNL	< 1.5 × N	1.5–2 × N	2.1–5 × N	> 5.1 × N
Hypercalcemia	< 10.6	10.6–11.5	11.6–12.5	12.6–13.5	≥ 13.5
Hypocalcemia	> 8.4	8.4–7.8	7.7–7	6.9–6.1	≤ 6
Hypomagnesemia	> 1.4	1.4–1.2	1.1–0.9	0.8–0.6	≤ 0.5
Fibrinogen	WNL	0.99–0.75 × N	0.74–0.5 × N	0.49–0.25 × N	≤ 0.24 × N
Prothrombin time	WNL	1.01–1.25 × N	1.26–1.5 × N	1.51–2 × N	> 2 × N
Partial thrombo-plastin time	WNL	1.01–1.66 × N	1.67–2.33 × N	2.34–3 × N	> 3 × N

Autologous Bone Marrow or Blood Stem Cell Support Studies Supplementary Toxicity Criteria
Grade 5   Death due to bacterial or fungal infection or hemorrhage associated with neutrophils < 500/μL or platelets < 10,000/μL more than 8 wk after marrow transplantation.
Grade 4   Neutrophils < 500/μL or platelets < 10,000/μL for a duration in excess of 8 wk.
Grade 3   Neutrophils < 500/μL or platelets < 10,000/μL for a duration of 4 to 8 wk.
Grade 2   Neutrophils < 500/μL or platelets < 10,000/μL for a duration up to 4 wk.
Grade 1   Neutropenia or thrombocytopenia, but neutrophils never < 500/μL and platelets never < 10,000/μL.
All other nonhematologic toxicities should be graded by the Common Toxicity Criteria.

recognition of trends in the study population. Laboratory tests seem to be one of the easiest side effects to quantify and monitor routinely. Monitoring of patients on clinical trials is critical to the accuracy of study results.

The importance of independent monitoring of a study through the process of site visiting is obvious from the recent allegations of misconduct in the entry of certain breast cancer patients in phase III NSABP tri-als (Davis, 1994). Although the number of patients involved was too small to alter the conclusion that lumpectomy and radiation is equivalent to mastectomy, the attention given to this issue was enormous and may impact public perceptions of clinical trials in a negative way. The National Institutes of Health are currently considering options on how independent review and monitoring of clinical trials in progress might be standardized.

DOCUMENTING

Side effects of cancer treatment are often noted by the staff nurse. Documentation on the patient's chart is critical to the evaluation of the experimental treatment. Toxicity is generally documented on a scale of 0 to 4, with 4 being the most severe (Vietti, 1980). Standardization of toxicity reporting allows a comparison of toxic effects of various regimens and an identification of unacceptable, intolerable, or life-threatening toxicities. Development of standard forms for reporting data promotes computer entry of data and easier analysis. Documentation should include type of toxicity, severity, when the toxicity occurred, and its duration.

DATA MANAGEMENT

Nurses in some institutions have assumed the added responsibility of abstracting data from charts. Data collection completed as soon as possible after it is generated ensures data accuracy, protocol compliance, and correction of procedural requirements while the study is in progress. Regular review of data is essential so that unsuspected toxicity or protocol infractions can be noted early. For multiinstitutional trials, procedures for ensuring the accuracy and safety of data reporting are implemented. Site visits for training may be required. Mechanisms for reporting problems and accessing information should be established. Nurses may assist in the collection and analysis of data and the publication of results.

NURSING RESEARCH

The nurse in a research setting has opportunities to collaborate as part of the research team, often as a coinvestigator. This role promotes the understanding of the research process and offers opportunities for incorporating nursing issues into medical protocols. Improvement of nursing care to patients may help decrease toxicities of treatment and thus promote greater use of medical research results in the community (Campbell & Chulay, 1990). Examples of research challenges and programs for nurses in the practice setting are provided by Hinshaw (1987). Nursing research may focus on symptom management such as pain management, nursing informatics that enhance patient care, or testing of interventions that strengthen an individual's personal resources in dealing with chronic illness.

COMMUNICATION

Education, support, administration of therapy, and prevention of toxicity for the patient with cancer require special skills and a trusting relationship between patient and nurse. Relationships with physicians involved in research are also based on effective communication, trust, and mutual respect. Collaboration in design, implementation, and follow-up of trials demonstrates recognition that nursing care, education, and research are critical to protocol results. Collaboration is a logical outgrowth when physicians and nurses have shared clinical goals and responsibilities (McEvoy, Cannon, & MacDermott, 1991).

Effective working relationships between the research (protocol) nurse and other staff nurses require good communication. Discussion among all health care providers of side effects noted may point out similarities or trends in patients on a specific protocol that should be reported to the investigator. Educational and emotional support for nurses during implementation of protocols that involve high toxicity or require technical skill is essential to maintaining adequate, safe care of patients and in preventing added stress. Stress can result in decreased quality of care and significant staff problems such as low morale, job dissatisfaction, and high turnover rates (Sarantos, 1988). Aggressive clinical trials may require considerable nursing support of patients, physicians, and other nurses.

IMPORTANCE OF CLINICAL TRIALS

Only a small percentage of cancer patients participate in clinical trials, although such trials often offer the best available cancer treatment (Gross, 1986). Indeed, less than 1 per cent of eligible cancer patients enter clinical studies. Currently 22,000 patients in the United States are being followed on clinical trials and 33,000 on cancer prevention and control protocols (M. McCabe, [CTEP] personal communication, November 2, 1994). Nurses can have an important role in increasing patient awareness of the advantages of clinical trials both for individuals in terms of improved care and for society through the advancement of the understanding of cancer and its treatment. The NCI is planning selected studies designed to enroll larger numbers of patients with the help of multidisciplines through specialized programs of research excellence. This mechanism has been established for breast, prostate, lung, and colorectal and pancreatic cancers. The goal is to expand the scientific network to facilitate rapid exchange of ideas and accelerate translational research (NCI, 1993a). Other trials that require more extensive data management and oversight will address the effectiveness of primary adjuvant treatment for patients with lung, head and neck, breast, colon, rectal, and bladder cancers. These trials will have considerable significance for more than 175,000 Americans each year and will be coordinated in national trial efforts through the NCI's cooperative group program.

PRIORITIES IN CANCER CARE

Broader use of clinical trials is one of the many approaches being used to meet the NCI's goal for the year 2000 of reducing cancer mortality by 50 per cent (National Institutes of Health, 1985). Priorities for future clinical trials will focus on immunology, drug resistance, vaccine development, genetics, and molecular biology. New drugs will continue to be developed. Transfer of research results to practice offers a continuing challenge to the nurse to be aware of the best treatment alternatives, the newer modes of therapy, and the effects of each on the patient.

SUMMARY

The process of research is a long, expensive, yet exciting road to advancement in the care of patients with cancer. The total time of bringing a treatment from initial screening to commercial availability can be as long as 14 years and can cost between $50 and $70 million (Gross, 1986). The NCI and the FDA are working to accelerate the availability of new drugs through revision of the regulatory process and improvement of participation in clinical trials (Kessler, 1989). As nursing participation in clinical trials increases, the nursing role as principal or coinvestigator in studies dealing with patients' responses to therapy will expand. There are many unknowns in research that challenge and stimulate nurses who want to become involved in caring for patients in clinical trials. As members of the research team, nurses can employ assessment, technical, psychosocial, and intellectual skills to advance and contribute to scientific knowledge and thus to overall quality patient care.

REFERENCES

American Academy of Pediatrics. (1977). Guidelines for the ethical conduct of studies to evaluate drugs in pediatric populations. *Pediatrics, 60,* 10-1-10.11.

Buyse, M., Staquet, M., & Sylvester, R. (1984). *Cancer clinical trial, methods, and practice.* New York: Oxford University Press.

Campbell, G., & Chulay, M. (1990). Establishing a clinical nursing research program. In J. Spicer & M. Robinson (Eds.), *Environmental management in critical care* (pp. 52–60). Baltimore: Williams & Wilkins.

Cancer Therapy Evaluation Program. (1993). *Investigator's handbook.* Washington, DC: National Cancer Institute.

Cassileth, B., Lusk, E., Miller, D., & Hurwitz, S. (1982). Attitudes toward clinical trials among patients and the public. *Journal of the American Medical Association, 248,* 968–970.

Chabner, B., Wittes, R., Hoth, D., & Hubbard, S. (1984). Investigational trials of anticancer drugs: Establishing safeguards for experimentation. *Public Health Reports, 99,* 355–360.

Cogliano-Shutta, N. (1986). Pediatric phase I clinical trials: Ethical issues and nursing considerations. *Oncology Nursing Forum, 13*(2), 29–32.

Collins, J., Grieshaber, C., & Chabner, B. (1990). Pharmacologically guided phase I clinical trials based on preclinical drug development. *Journal of the National Cancer Institute, 82,* 1321–1326.

Collins, J., Zaharko, D., Dedrick, R., & Chabner, B. (1986). Potential roles for preclinical pharmacology in phase I clinical trials. *Cancer Treatment Reports, 70,* 73–80.

Davis, N. (1994). The NSABP trials. *New England Journal of Medicine, 33,* 809.

Davis, S., Nealon, E., & Stone, J. (1993). Evaluation of the National Cancer Institute's Clinical Trials Booklet. *Monographs of the National Cancer Institute, 14,* 139–145.

Deininger, H., Collins, J., & Hubbard, S. (1989). Nurses and PDQ: What's in it for you? *Oncology Nursing Forum, 16,* 547–552.

DeVita, V. (1982). *Cancer treatment* (NIH Publication No. 82-1807). Washington, DC: U. S. Government Printing Office.

DeVita, V., Oliverio, V., Muggia, F., Wiernik, P., Ziegler, J., Goldin, A., Rubin D., Henney, J., & Shepartz, S. (1979).

The drug development and clinical trials programs of the Division of Cancer Treatment, National Cancer Institute. *Cancer Clinical Trials, 2,* 195–216.

Ellenberg, S., & Eisenberger, M. (1985). An efficient design for phase III studies of combination chemotherapies. *Cancer Treatment Reports, 69,* 1147–1152.

Fletcher, J., Eyes, J., & Dorn, L. (1988). Ethical consideration in pediatric oncology. In P. Pizzo & D. Poplack (Eds.), *Principles and practice of pediatric oncology* (pp. 309–320). Philadelphia: J. B. Lippincott Co.

Gargaro, W. (1978). Informed consent. *Cancer Nursing, 1,* 467–468.

Gelber, R., & Goldhirsch, A. (1989). Can a clinical trial be the treatment of choice for patients with cancer. *Journal of the National Cancer Institute, 80,* 886–887.

Gross, J. (1986). Clinical research in cancer chemotherapy. *Oncology Nursing Forum, 13,* 59–65.

Guyatt, G., Feeny, D., & Patrick, D. (1993). Measuring health-related quality of life. *Annals of Internal Medicine, 118,* 622–629.

Gwyther, S. (1994). Modern techniques in radiological imaging related to oncology. *Annals of Oncology, 5*(Suppl. 4), 3–7.

Hinshaw, A. (1987). Research challenges and programs for practice settings. *Journal of Nursing Administration, 17*(7,8), 20–26.

Hubbard, S. (1981). Chemotherapy and the cancer nurse. In L. Marino (Ed.), *Cancer nursing* (pp. 287–343). St. Louis: C. V. Mosby Co.

Hubbard, S., & Gross, J. (1994). Principles of clinical research. In B. Johnson & J. Gross (Eds.), *Handbook of oncology nursing* (pp. 195–218). New York: John Wiley & Sons.

Hubbard, S., Henney, J., & DeVita, V. (1987). A computer data base for information on cancer treatment. *New England Journal of Medicine, 316,* 315–318.

Kessler, D. (1989). The regulation of investigational drugs. *New England Journal of Medicine, 320,* 281–288.

Levine, R. (1981). *Ethics and regulations of clinical research.* Baltimore: Urban & Schwarzenberg.

Levine, R. (1986). Referral of patients with cancer for participation in randomized clinical trials: Ethical considerations. *CA: A Cancer Journal for Clinicians, 36,* 95–99.

McEvoy, M., Cannon, L., & MacDermott, M. (1991). The professional role for nurses in clinical trials. *Seminars in Oncology Nursing, 7,* 268–274.

Meisel, A., & Roth, L. (1981). What we do and do not know about informed consent. *Journal of the American Medical Association, 246,* 2473–2477.

National Cancer Institute. (1992). *92nd annual report of the Division of Cancer Treatment.* Washington, DC: Author.

National Cancer Institute. (1993a). *Budget estimate.* Washington, DC: Author.

National Cancer Institute. (1993b). *NCI fact book.* Washington, DC: Author.

National Institutes of Health. (1985). *NCI program 1983–84 directors report and annual plan 1986–1990* (NIH Publication No. 85-2765). Washington, DC: U.S. Government Printing Office.

Office of Science and Technology Policy. (1991). *Federal policy for the protection of human subjects; notices and rules.* In Federal Register (pp. 28002–28032). Vol. 56, 117.

Ray, W., Griffin, M., & Avorn, J. (1993). Evaluating drugs after their approval for clinical use. *New England Journal of Medicine, 329,* 2029–2032.

Reis, L., Miller, V., Hankey, B., Kosary, C., Harras, A., & Edwards, B. (Eds.). (1994). *SEER cancer statistics review 1973–1991 tables and graphs.* (NIH Publication No. 94-2789). Bethesda, MD: National Institutes of Health.

Sarantos, S. (1988). Innovations in psychosocial staff support: A model program for the marrow transplant nurse. *Seminars in Oncology Nursing, 4*(1), 69–73.

Simon, R., Wittes, R., & Ellenberg, S. (1985). Randomized phase II clinical trials. *Cancer Treatment Reports, 69,* 1375–1381.

Spilker, B. (1991). *Guide to clinical trials.* New York: Raven Press.

Taylor, K., Maegolese, R., & Soskolne, C. (1985). Physicians' reasons for not entering eligible patients in a randomized trial of surgery for breast cancer. *New England Journal of Medicine, 310,* 1363–1367.

Varricchio, C., & Jassak, P. (1989). Informed consent: An overview. *Seminars in Oncology Nursing, 5*(2), 95–98.

Vietti, T. (1980). Evaluation of toxicity: Clinical issues. *Cancer Treatment Reports, 64,* 457–461.

Wittes, R., & Friedman, M. R. (1988). Accrual to clinical trials. *Journal of the National Cancer Institute, 80,* 884–885.

Young, R. (1981). Role of the FDA in cancer therapy research. *Seminars in Oncology, 8,* 447–452.

Blood Component Therapy

Catherine A. Kefer • John Godwin • Patricia F. Jassak

The clinical practice of blood transfusion is a relatively new development of the latter half of the twentieth century. Practical problems of blood cell typing, cross-matching, development of blood anticoagulants, refrigeration, and storage in plastic were not solved until the 1950s and early 1960s. Today tens of millions of units are transfused every year, with approximately 14,500,000 total blood components transfused in the United States in 1985.

BLOOD PHYSIOLOGY: COMPOSITION AND FUNCTION

All blood cells are formed in the bone marrow by hematopoiesis (blood cell production). Blood is composed of plasma and the cellular elements—erythrocytes, platelets, and leukocytes—and is approximately 45 per cent cells and 55 per cent plasma. The average adult has from 4 to 5 L of blood. Blood is an organ with many different functions. The major functions of blood are to transport oxygen and absorbed nutrients to cells, transport waste products to kidneys, skin, and lungs, transport hormones from endocrine glands to other tissues, protect the body from life-threatening microorganisms, and also to regulate body temperature by heat transfer. The basic components of blood and their function are summarized in Table 26–1.

Blood transfusion may be considered the most frequent tissue transplant performed in medicine. Transfusion therapy plays an integral role in the comprehensive care of cancer patients and is one of the most important supportive care measures. Therefore, the oncology nurse should be familiar with all aspects of blood transfusion.

Advances in the use of blood components have improved the survival rate of cancer patients by contributing to the success of new cancer treatments associated with prolonged myelosuppression. One prominent example of the role of transfusion therapy is the rising use of bone marrow transplantation since the 1970s (Chapter 27). Another example is seen with improved responses in combination chemotherapy for chemosensitive tumors, and these advances have led to the search for even better results requiring increased dose intensity and supportive care with transfusion therapy.

This chapter reviews the principles of blood component therapy with particular attention to the cancer patient. Blood components and the technique of their administration are described. Practical points are illustrated with clinical examples and reference tables.

BASIC PRINCIPLES OF TRANSFUSION

There are a few basic things for the nurse to think about at the onset of each transfusion episode. Ask yourself two basic questions: What blood product is being transfused? Why is this product being given to my patient? Try to be more specific in your knowledge of the reason for transfusion than just low blood counts. For each blood component or product there are specific indications for the transfusion. These indications are often required by institutions to be present before a transfusion is begun. Tables listing the recommended indications for transfusion by product are shown (Table 26–2) (Beutler, 1993; Lundberg, 1994; Stehling, Luben, & Anderson, 1994). In some institutions practice guidelines have been developed for the

TABLE 26-1. *Description and Function of Blood Cells*

CELL	FUNCTION	LIFE SPAN
Erythrocyte (red blood cell)	Gas transport to & from tissue cells & lungs	120 days
Leukocytes (white blood cells)	Bodily defense mechanism	See specific cells
Lymphocyte	Humoral & cell-mediated immunity	Days or years, varies depending on cell
Monocytes	Phagocytosis	Months to years
Eosinophil	Phagocytosis; antibody-mediated defense against parasites, allergic reactions; recovery phase of infection.	11 days
Neutrophil	Phagocytosis; protects against infection, especially during early phase of infection	24 hr. or less
Basophil	Role in allergic & inflammatory reactions	11 days
Platelet (thrombocyte)	Hemostasis; normal coagulation & clot formation.	8–11 days
Plasma cells	Humoral immunity; cells committed to produce antibodies (IgG, IgA, IgM, etc.)	Few days to years

TABLE 26-2. *Indications for Transfusion by Blood Component*

BLOOD COMPONENT	INDICATION
Red cells (PRBCs)	Hemoglobin < 8.0 g/dl[a]
	Signs or symptoms of anemia
	Acute blood loss with signs or symptoms of anemia
Platelets	Prophylactic if platelets <10,000–20,000
	Signs or symptoms of bleeding and platelets <100,000
	Invasive procedure and platelets <50,000–75,000
Fresh frozen plasma	Bleeding and PT >1.5 × mid point nl range
	Massive transfusion of >1 blood vol (5 L)
	Reversal of Warfarin effect
	Congenital clotting factor deficiency
	Plasma exchange in thrombotic thrombocytopenic purpura

[a]Some authors recommend a lower threshold of 7.0 g/dl, especially in younger patients.

transfusion indications for each product and may be present as part of blood order form.

The most common cause underlying the need for transfusion in cancer patients is *bone marrow depression*. Bone marrow depression is a general term used to describe a decrease in blood cell production from the marrow. This is in contrast to the various causes of increased cell destruction (disseminated intravascular coagulation [DIC], immune reactions), loss (bleeding), or sequestration (splenomegaly). Bone marrow depression is manifest as a decrease in one or more blood cell lines, that is, anemia, thrombocytopenia, or granulocytopenia. There are three frequent causes of bone marrow depression in the cancer patient (1) the malignancy, (2) the therapy, or (3) a nutritional deficiency state. Specific terms for each of these types of bone marrow depression are malignancy-caused—(1) myelophthisis, a metastatic solid tumor or fibrosis infiltrating the bone marrow; therapy-caused—(2) myelosuppression, a chemo-therapy or radiation therapy-induced temporary reduction in the rapidly growing cells in the bone marrow; deficiency caused—(3) specific nutritional causes of bone marrow depression such as vitamin B_{12} and iron deficiency. Though these nutritional causes are rarely seen in the cancer patient, they should not be overlooked because they are easily reversible. Finally a primary marrow disorder, dysmyelopoiesis, which is a defect in the precursors of blood cells, can arise as a late sequelae to cancer chemotherapy or for unknown reasons in elderly patients.

From understanding the basic cause of bone marrow depression in the patient, some idea of the course and transfusion requirements can be determined. For example, in a patient with malignancy-caused depression—(1) myelophthisis, the strategy is to try and reverse the infiltration or fibrosis, if possible, while supporting the patient with transfusions. In therapy caused—(2) myelosuppression, the transfusion support given is expected to be temporary until the marrow recovers. In dysmyelopoiesis the patient will not recover normal marrow function unless the disorder is cured (e.g., by bone marrow transplant in patients who are eligible), and the usual strategy is to provide supportive transfusions on an indefinite basis.

Different transfusion requirements can be anticipated among malignancies due to the manifestations of the disease itself or the specific treatment strategies employed. The leukemic patient, for example, requires different blood component support than does the patient with a solid tumor. Solid tumors cause direct bone marrow depression much less frequently and require transfusions much less often than those in patients with leukemia. Different treatment strategies for the patient also result in different transfusion requirements. Leukemic patients are given chemotherapy despite the presence of severe cytopenias, but when severe cytopenias occur in patients with solid tumors the treatment regimen is usually adjusted by decreasing the dose or extending the length of the recovery period. This results in less severe marrow depression in solid tumor patients and a shorter duration of transfusion support due to myelosuppression.

The following are some don'ts to keep in mind when transfusing:

Do not transfuse platelets

1. to patients with immune thrombocytopenia purpura (ITP, unless there is life-threatening bleeding);
2. prophylactically with massive blood transfusion;
3. prophylactically following cardiopulmonary bypass.

Do not transfuse fresh frozen plasma (FFP)

1. for volume expansion or as a nutritional supplement;
2. prophylactically with massive blood transfusion or bypass graft.

SOURCES OF BLOOD COLLECTION

Blood components are available from three different donor sources: homologous, autologous, and directed (designated) donors (Widmann, 1985). Homologous blood is obtained from the general pool of volunteer donors and is currently the most common source of blood components for all patients. Autologous transfusion is the collection and reinfusion of a patient's own blood or blood components (Ereth, Oliver, & Santrach, 1994; Gerber, 1994). Directed or designated donor blood is when the recipient selects or recruits a specific donor to come for donation.

DONOR SELECTION AND SCREENING

When a potential blood donor is seen in a collection center, community drive, or hospital, based on criteria established by the FDA and the American Association of Blood Banks (Callery, 1991), two things are done to determine donor eligibility: (1) a prescreening interview and (2) screening health and blood tests. The interview includes extensive history-taking of each individual to determine risk factors for transmissable disease. Questions asked relate to donation history, past and present sexual relationships, drug history, and testing for human immunodeficiency virus (HIV) and hepatitis. Other pertinent factors are age, health status, and weight of at least 110 pounds. The screening examination includes standard blood pressure, pulse, temperature, and adequate hemoglobin determined by finger stick. Persons with a history of certain diseases, for example hepatitis, are permanently ineligible as candidates for donation. Individuals with known risk factors for transmissible disease (e.g., acquired immunodefi-

ciency syndrome [AIDS] or hepatitis) are removed from the donor pool. Today most centers allow the donors the option of indicating confidentially that their unit should be discarded without specifying a reason.

Directed (designated) donor programs have been established in response to the AIDS (Chapter 12) crisis and are actually mandated by law in some states. Directed donors are screened and tested for transmissible diseases and compatibility the same way as homologous units. When screening tests are positive, the units are discarded and the donor confidentially informed. If red cell incompatibility between the directed donor and the specified recipient is determined, and tests for transmissible disease are negative, the blood is released to the general donor pool.

Autologous transfusions are recommended to patients undergoing elective surgical procedures who can donate a number of units of blood during the month prior to the anticipated need. Autologous transfusions have dramatically increased since the recognition of the transmission of HIV from blood products (Harrison, 1994).

APHERESIS

Apheresis (or hemapheresis) is a method of blood collection in which whole blood is withdrawn, a desired component separated and retained, and the remainder of the blood returned to the donor. This process of separating or taking away can be identified by the different components (Table 26–3). Apheresis (or hemapheresis) is used to provide the cancer patient with selected blood components and in some cases to remove unwanted cellular or plasma elements. Apheresis cannot cure disease but can alleviate symptoms produced by the underlying disease. Apheresis is the general term used for procedures using machines with a centrifuge bowl (cell separator). These machines remove whole blood from the donor, separate it into cellular and plasma components (red blood cells [RBCs], white blood cells [WBCs], platelets, and plasma) by centrifugation based on the different densities of these components, and return the remaining blood to the donor. Technologic advances have allowed sophisticated in vivo cell separators that perform these separation tasks at the bedside. Complications of this procedure are listed in Table 26–4.

Leukapheresis is the removal and collection of leukocytes (WBCs) with the return of RBCs, plasma, and platelets to the donor. The specific cell product that is required for treating sepsis is the neutrophil, granulocyte. Therapeutic leukapheresis can be used in leu-

TABLE 26–3. *Apheresis Terminology*

COMPONENTS	PROCEDURE
White blood cells	Leukapheresis
Red blood cells	Erythrocytapheresis
Platelets	Plateletpheresis or thrombocytapheresis
Plasma	Plasmapheresis

TABLE 26–4. *Adverse Effects of Apheresis*

1. Citrate toxicity
2. Hematoma
3. Vasovagal reactions
4. Hypovolemia
5. Allergic reactions
6. Hemolysis
7. Air embolus
8. Depletion of clotting factors
9. Circulatory and respiratory distress
10. Transfusion-transmitted diseases
11. Lymphocyte loss
12. Depletion of proteins and immunoglobulins

kemic patients with very high white blood cell blast counts. These patients are at risk for leukostasis (leukocyte aggregates and thrombi may interfere with pulmonary and cerebral blood flow) of the central nervous system (CNS) and lungs. Lymphocytapheresis (removal of lymphocytes) is used as part of a specific cancer treatment to remove lymphocytes from the cancer patient that are then incubated in laboratory cultures with interleukin-2 to produce lymphokine-activated killer (LAK) cells.

Plateletpheresis or thrombocytapheresis is the removal or collection of platelets. They are harvested from whole blood, which results in 1 U of platelets. Therapeutic plateletpheresis can be used to treat patients who have abnormally elevated platelet counts with myeloproliferative disorders such as polycythemia vera. Clinical indications for transfusing platelets may be for bleeding caused by thrombocytopenia, a platelet count of 20 to 50 K, or <20 K without bleeding (Simon, 1994).

Plasmapheresis, or plasma exchange, is the removal and retention of the plasma with return of all cellular components to the patient. The purpose is to remove the offending agent in the plasma causing the clinical symptoms. Benefit of the procedure in diseases that involve malfunction of the immune system may be attributed to the removal of factors such as systemic lupus erythematous, factor VIII inhibitors, Waldenstrom's macroglobulinemia, and thrombotic thrombocytopenic purpura (TTP).

RED CELL COMPATIBILITY TESTING

The purpose of red cell compatibility testing is to prevent the destruction of the transfused cells, that is, to prevent a hemolytic transfusion reaction. To understand compatibility testing it is necessary to briefly review certain concepts of immunology.

BLOOD GROUP SYSTEMS

Over 400 different antigens are present on the human red blood cell surface. An antigen is a molecule that is recognized as foreign ("nonself") by the immune system. Simply put, an antigen distinguishes self from nonself. Families of these antigens with similar molecular characteristics and genetic properties form blood "groups" or, more properly, blood group systems. Antibodies are a family of proteins that have in common the ability to bind to antigens. *Antibodies recognize antigens as nonself.* Antigens react with sensitized monocytes and T cells, which stimulate B cells of the immune system to produce antibodies against the antigen.

Most of the blood groups have been detected serologically, that is, by detecting clumping (agglutination) of red cells by adding serum samples that contain antibodies that react with specific red cell antigens. Researchers would immunize animals to human or animal red cells and utilize animal sera to identify the antigens on the human red cell surface. From these efforts the complex red blood cell antigens that form blood groups have been individually identified. Such investigations were responsible for the discovery of the Rh system. "Rh" was the name given by Landsteiner and Wiener for the antibody made from sera from guinea pigs and rabbits immunized with red cells from Macacus mulata, the rhesus monkey (Landsteiner & Wiener, 1940). This "Rh" antibody reacted with most human red cells, 85 per cent, suggesting a similar antigen was present on the rhesus red cell and human red cell. Levine and Stetson independently reported an antibody in the sera of a mother who had a stillborn infant that appeared to recognize the same blood group antigen as "Rh" antibody. We now recognize the importance of Rh in hydrops fetalis and hemolytic disease of the newborn. Some blood group antigens are common to many people, and others are extremely rare. Examples of other blood groups include Kell, Lutheran, Rh, and P. Although the names may seem confusing at first, there is a systematic method of naming the red cell antigens (Box 26–1).

DISCOVERY OF THE ABO BLOOD GROUP SYSTEM

Early in the history of transfusion it was found that blood from an animal administered to man was rapidly hemolyzed, and the recipient became critically ill. The transfused red cells were recognized as foreign by the recipient. However, it was not understood why some attempts at transfusion from man to man were successful when others failed. In 1900 Karl Landsteiner clarified this by discovering that human red cells will react with the sera of some persons and not others. He described blood types that were different by virtue of the presence of different red cell antigens (Landsteiner, 1901). He recognized three different blood types, which he called A, B, and O (a fourth group, AB, was later added by Landsteiner's pupils). Landsteiner recognized that red cells contain either an A antigen, a B antigen, or neither (group O) and that serum contains antibodies to antigens not present on the individual's red cells (Table 26–5). We now know a great deal about the specific molecular characterization of the ABO blood group antigens and their genetics (Fig. 26–1).

Box 26–1. *Blood Group Terminology*

The naming of blood groups may seem arbitrary and complex, but there is a uniform system underlying the terminology. The real confusion lies in the terminology for the blood groups, which has historic origins and is dependent upon the discoverer for its name. There are FOUR components in each blood group system: (1) the blood group "family" name; (2) the gene responsible for synthesis; (3) the red cell surface antigen; (4) the antibodies made after immunization to the antigen.

In the table below are some common red cell blood group systems. Genes are written in italics, and their allele is usually a superscript. For example, a person can have the *K* (Big Kell gene) and a *k* (little Kell gene) and would have both K and k antigens on the red cell surface. Within each blood group family there are several possible genes.

Blood Group System	Antibody	Antigen	Gene
Kell	anti-K	K	*K*
Kidd	anti-Jk^a	Jk^a	*Jk^a*
P	anti-P$_1$	P$_1$	*P*
Duffy	anti-Fy4	Fy4	*Fy^4*

In the figure below the gene is seen encoding the message for the formation of the antigen that is on the mature red cell surface. Antibodies would be detected in certain patients exposed to red cells with these antigens if the patients did not have the antigen on their own red cells.

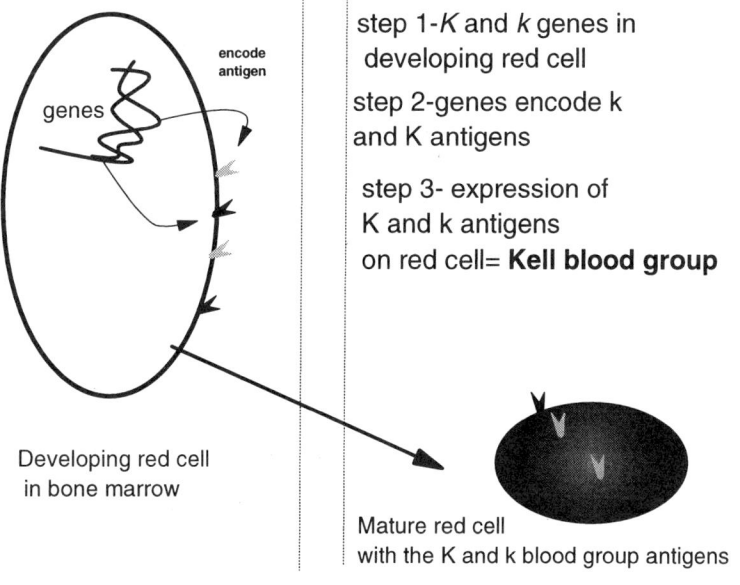

step 1-*K* and *k* genes in developing red cell

step 2-genes encode k and K antigens

step 3- expression of K and k antigens on red cell= **Kell blood group**

genes

encode antigen

Developing red cell in bone marrow

Mature red cell with the K and k blood group antigens

Table 26–5. *ABO Blood Group and Naturally Occurring Antibodies*

Red Cell Group	Frequency in Population (%) Whites	Blacks	Serum Antibody
A	40	27	anti-B
B	11	20	anti-A
AB	4	4	none
O	45	49	anti-A, anti-B

PRACTICAL ASPECTS OF RED CELL COMPATIBILITY TESTING

In view of the complex red cell antigen pattern on each individual's red cells, it would be difficult to match blood if all these antigens had to be typed. Instead of an exact match it is only necessary to match ABO and Rh groups and search for any antibodies in the recipient's serum that could react with the donor red cells. Although many different red cell antigens have been associated with hemolytic transfusion reactions in human populations, only a few are antigenic enough to commonly give rise to antibodies. Pretransfusion testing is designed to detect their presence. The "type and cross-match" order is a request for a specific series of four main pretransfusion tests (Table 26–6). The first step is to check the records for any previous transfusion. The second step is to determine the recipient's ABO and Rh blood cell type. The reason for this is that ABO mismatched (incompatible) blood is the most dangerous, as more than 95 per cent of recipients have naturally occurring anti-A or anti-B antibodies,

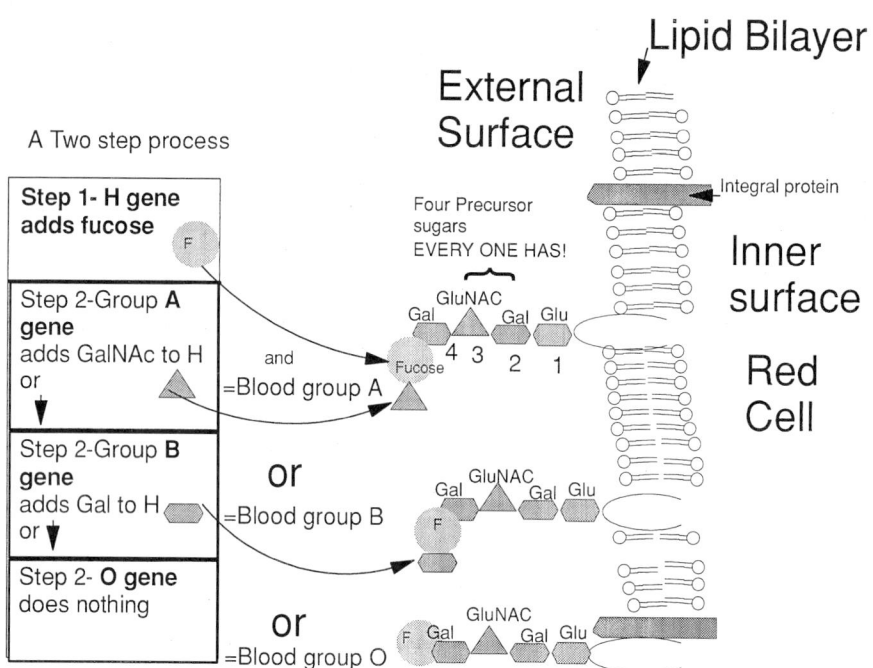

FIGURE 26-1. Red cell-ABO blood group antigens. ABO antigens are determined by specific carbohydrates placed on the developing red cell surface by enzymes coded from genes on chromosome 9. As seen in the figure above, a precursor sugar is present on all red cell and is formed by the H gene (step 1), which is inherited independently of the ABO group. The H gene is present in 99.99 per cent of humans. If it had not acted initially, the ABO genes could not act. The determination of the ABO antigens is then dependent upon which genes a person inherits. If the A gene is inherited, the sugar specific for A antigen is placed on the red cell. If the B gene is inherited, the sugar specific for the B antigen is placed. If both A and B genes are inherited, then both sugars are placed, and the AB blood type is formed. The B enzyme seems to place more B sugar antigens on the surface so the usual AB red cell has approximately 600,000 A sugar antigens and 720,000 B sugar antigens. The O gene is like a blank (termed-amorph) and does not code for any new sugar. Landsteiner thought that the O blood type had no antigen (thus the German word, ohne, for without). However, the H precursor is present in its unaltered form, and of course the O red cell has the highest concentration of H sugar antigens.

TABLE 26-6. *Type and Crossmatch*

STEP	PROCEDURE	RATIONALE
1	Evaluate previous records	Compare blood type & determine if prior alloantibody detected
2	Type blood—ABO, Rh group	ABO has naturally occurring antibodies; Rh important for female
3	Antibody screen	Determine if any "unexpected" or alloantibodies present
4	Crossmatch	React donor cells and recipient sera for compatibility

which can cause an immediate hemolytic reaction. Rh antibodies arise after exposure to the Rh antigen in Rh-negative persons. Exposure to Rh antigen can occur from prior pregnancies or transfusion. Rh-negative females of reproductive age should never receive Rh-positive blood, since the immune reaction could result in hemolytic disease of the newborn and possible fetal demise. The third step is the antibody screen. In this step a search is made for the other common antibodies

capable of causing a hemolytic reaction. The recipient's serum is tested for antibodies by reacting the serum with a standardized panel of red cells, all group O (to eliminate any ABO reactions), and these cells contain a representative mixture of the other common blood group antigens. A positive antibody screen means that the patient has antibodies to other blood group antigens such as Kell or Duffy. These antibodies are termed *alloantibodies* (from the word "allo" meaning other— these are antibodies to "other" persons' antigens) or "unexpected antibodies," and they usually occur when the patient has been exposed to blood via prior transfusion or pregnancy. Occasionally the presence of such alloantibodies may delay the availability of compatible blood. In some situations the pretransfusion testing is stopped after the first three steps, and this is commonly referred to as *type and screen or type and hold.* Donor units of the same ABO-Rh group are not reserved on the blood bank shelf in response to a type and screen. However, units can be made available rapidly upon request. The fourth step is testing of the donor red cells and recipient serum for direct compatibility. Compatible units are then reserved for a short period of time, usually 24 to 48 hours.

It is always preferable to administer blood of the same type. However, in emergencies or shortages, blood of other ABO groups can be given. It may seem

TABLE 26–7. *ABO Compatibility of Blood Components*

BLOOD COMPONENT	RECIPIENT BLOOD GROUP	DONOR SELECTION
Red cells	O	O only
	A	O, A
	B	O, B
	AB	AB, A, B, O
Fresh frozen plasma	O	O, A, B, AB
	A	A, AB
	B	B, AB
	AB	AB only
Platelet concentrate	O, A, B, AB	Any blood group may be used. Since large volume of plasma is given, it is preferable to use ABO compatible
Cryoprecipitate	O, A, B, AB	All ABO groups acceptable. Transfusion of cryoprecipitate may cause positive direct Coomb's for group A recipients, but rarely hemolysis

confusing, but it is easy to remember for red cells: group O recipients can only receive group O; for all others the same red cell type or group O is possible. Since group AB has both A and B antigens, these individuals can receive all types—group A, B, or O—for each blood group. Group A and group B recipients can receive group O. Group AB can receive either A or B red cells, although A is more commonly given due to its availability. Group O is not preferred for the AB patient because it is too valuable a resource for group O individuals. A summary of compatible products is seen in Table 26–7.

TISSUE COMPATIBILITY ANTIGENS (HLA)

Human leukocyte antigen (HLA) refers to the genetic system of antigens first detected on the surface of white blood cells and now known to be responsible for tissue compatibility. The tissue compatibility factors are surface antigens or cell receptors responsible for the recognition of tissues as self and the elimination of foreign tissues. Their importance to transfusion medicine is in the understanding of the immune destruction of transfused cells, especially platelets. The most common cause of failure of platelet rise after transfusion is immune platelet destruction due to the development of alloantibodies. This is similar to the problem described with red cells. However, the antibodies that cause the destruction of transfused platelets do not react against blood group antigens but against *tissue antigens*, that is, the HLA antigens (McLeod, 1980).

DESCRIPTION OF HLA ANTIGENS

The genes (loci) that code for tissue recognition or HLA antigens are referred to as the major histocompatibility complex (MHC) and reside on human chromosome 6. The HLA or MHC complex contains an estimated 35 to 40 different genes. These antigens are present on most of the cells in the body and in the blood are found on white cells and platelets, but not generally on red cells. As with red cell antigens, the HLA antigens can be identified serologically by react-

ing standard serum antibodies with the white cells (lymphocytes) of a patient.

The genes have been grouped into three families named class I, class II, and class III. Genes code for the class I antigens which are proteins that make up the cell surface antigens of classic transplantation recognition, termed HLA-A, HLA-B, and HLA-C. Class II genes encode antigens that are different from class I and have been found on certain immune cells but not all tissue cells as in class I. Class II antigens are found on monocytes, macrophages, and B lymphocytes. The class III genes code for a diverse family of proteins including complement molecules and tumor necrosis factor. Class III antigens are less directly involved in the immune response of tissue recognition. For each HLA gene family there are many different antigens possible. After each locus designation the specific gene is designated by a number. For example, the HLA-A locus codes for antigens called A1, A2, A43, and so on, and this would be written as HLA-A1, HLA-A43. HLA-B locus codes for B5 or Bw4 (the "w" indicates further definition and confirmation of the antigen is necessary), and these would be named HLA-B5, HLA-Bw4. HLA-C codes for Cw1 or Cw2, and so on, with many possible antigens for each gene. Each individual has two chromosomes with HLA gene loci coding for each of the A, B, and C antigens, and thus there are a total of six different antigens in each individual comprising the class I HLA-A,B,C antigens.

The HLA antigens are responsible for the development of antibodies that form after exposure blood components and cause destruction of platelets. Multiple transfusions expose the patient to numerous HLA antigens from the donors, and these are often recognized by the body as "foreign" antigens. In some patients an immune response occurs, and antibodies are produced to these HLA-A, HLA-B, and HLA-C antigens. When this occurs antibodies formed will destroy the transfused platelets (Lane, 1994). These antibodies are also termed "alloantibodies." Platelets contain small amounts of ABO antigens on their surface, but antibodies to red cell ABO antigens do not cause a significant amount of platelet destruction. The role of ABO mismatch of platelets causing a loss of platelets and poor response to transfusion is under

TABLE 26-8. *Strategies for Treating Patients with Platelet Alloantibodies (Refractory Responders)*

STRATEGY	RATIONALE
Single donor platelet unit (SDP); random, by apheresis	Platelets have one HLA type. May raise the platelet count in refractory responders if the recipient does not have antibodies to HLA antigens transfused
Single donor platelet unit; family, by apheresis	Sibling of the recipient may have nearly identical HLA type. Can raise platelet count in refractory responders. Parents and children are rarely suitable. They are haplo-identical (match one-half HLA type)
Single donor platelet unit HLA matched, by apheresis	Determine recipient's HLA-A, B, C, type (serologic testing). Donors obtained from a computer registry of known HLA types. Availability of service, expense, and rare recipient HLA types are drawbacks. Failure to respond suggests poor match or other cause for increased destruction
Autologous platelets	Recipient is apheresed and platelets stored. This requires special freezing of platelets, which is still experimental. Technique is not readily available
Immune interventions	High dose IV γ globulin (IgG) raises the platelet count in ITP patients but does not prevent alloantibody destruction of RD platelets. There is no current effective immune intervention

TABLE 26-9. *Failure of Adequate Platelet Transfusion Response*

MECHANISM	CLINICAL CONDITION
Platelet loss	Bleeding
	Fever
	Infection +/− fever
Sequestration	Splenomegaly
Immune destruction	Alloantibody
	Autoantibody

investigation. It is preferable to give ABO-compatible platelets as indicated in the discussion about red cell compatibility testing. When these HLA alloantibodies are present in a patient, there will often be a poor or no response to a platelet transfusion. Such a condition is called "refractory responder," and the causes for this state are listed in Table 26–8. Strategies for managing patients with platelet alloantibodies as a cause of refractory response are identified in Table 26–9 (Menitove, 1983).

CONSENT

Historically, most cases involving informed consent did not involve the use of transfusions. Informed consent was most frequently considered in invasive procedures when a bad outcome was involved and the patient or family claimed that they were not well informed of the possible risks involved. Moreover, if they had known what would happen, they would not have had the procedure or treatment. In these types of cases it was left to the patient to prove that disclosure was not given and that the physician held back pertinent information.

It was not until the 1980s and the arrival of transfusion-associated AIDS that informed consent became an issue in transfusion therapy. The *Doctrine of Informed Consent* addresses the issue of whether a patient (or donor) has agreed to undergo the procedure actually performed with full knowledge of the possible benefits and risks involved. This doctrine protects the patient (or donor) by requiring that information be provided in a manner *understandable* to the patient under circumstances that allow the patient to ask and receive answers to any questions or concerns he or she may have (Black's Law Dictionary, 1990; *Canterbury v. Spence*, 1972).

Informed consent developed reflecting the belief that individuals had the right to make their own decision, self-determination, and autonomy regarding their care. In 1974, Professor Capron stated the doctrine serves six functions that can benefit both the individual and society. The functions include (1) the promotion and protection of individual autonomy, (2) the protection of patients and subjects, (3) the prevention of fraud and duress, (4) the encouragement of self-scrutiny by health care practitioners, (5) the enhancement of rational decision making, and (6) increase public involvement (Capron, 1974).

Cases in the early twentieth century established the concept that a procedure performed without a patient's consent or in a patient who was given inadequate information was constituted as battery, or unlawful touching, and the failure to inform and obtain consent was constituted as negligence. In the 1972 landmark decision in *Canterbury v. Spence* the courts placed the duty upon the professional to warn of alternatives to treatment using the reasonable patient standard (patient-oriented standard of disclosure). The reasonable patient standard obligates the physician to provide the patient with information that a reasonable patient would have found important for making a decision on whether to agree to a course of therapy (*Canterbury v. Spence*, 1972).

The use of informed consent promotes autonomy as the highest value of personhood. Informed consent consists of two elements (1) *informed* refers to information given to the patient about a proposed procedure or treatment; and (2) *consent* refers to the patient's agreement to the procedure or treatment (Widmann, 1990). Emphasis in informed consent is placed more on informing than consenting. Language in the written informed consent document should be understandable to patients and should include risks and benefits, alternatives, autologous, directed donor, or no transfusions (Goodnough & Shuck, 1990).

Informing of risks and benefits for any procedure, whether it be for surgery, chemotherapy, or transfusions, is based on moral rights of individuals. Individual rights include a patient's moral right to self-determination through knowledge that health professionals provide regarding any procedure or treatment, that physicians have a moral duty to promote patient's autonomy, and that the need to establish trust in the relationship between the physician and the patient includes a fair and thorough discussion of the risks involved with the therapy (Leparc, 1991).

In *Kozup v. Georgetown University Hospital* (1990), an infant was brought into the hospital for treatment and died after contracting AIDS from a transfusion. In this case the parents claimed that they were not well informed about the potential harm of the transfusions and did not specifically agree to transfusions among other care given to their child. The District of Columbia Court ruled that their actions in bringing the child to the hospital and not objecting to transfusions at time of infusion amounted to implied consent. However, this issue of whether specific consent is required for transfusion and who should obtain such consent is still controversial. Although some states have statutes that regulate transfusions and informed consent, such as California where requirements have been established, many do not have statutes.

In a more recent case a Pennsylvania federal court decision expanded the doctrine of informed consent and applied it to cases involving blood transfusions. In this case the court held that a patient must be informed of all alternatives, options, risks of HIV, and the limitations of enzyme-linked immunosorbent assay (ELISA) for detecting HIV, along with the risks of false-negative results in the procedure (*Jones v. Philadelphia College of Osteopathic Medicine*, 1993).

Eisenstaedt, Glanz, Smith, and Derstine (1993) conducted a study that involved 92 hospitals in three state regions. These hospitals were surveyed to determine what their policy was for obtaining written informed consent for transfusions. The study then looked at what type of consent, if any, was used, its content, and who and when the consent was obtained. The results showed that of the 92 hospitals 81 responded, and only 50 required written informed consent. Some hospitals have separate consent forms, some use generic forms, and others include transfusions on their admission forms. Twenty-seven of 48 forms mentioned complications: hepatitis 80 per cent, HIV infection 46 per cent, nonhemolytic reactions 32 per cent, and hemolysis 25 per cent, and alternatives were mentioned on very few of the forms. Physicians had the responsibility for obtaining the consent in only 28 of 49 hospitals, and they were obtained usually the day or evening before surgery.

The American Association of Blood Banks (AABB) has endorsed the concept of seeking informed consent from transfusion recipients (Widman, 1990). The AABB believes that requiring a written informed consent for transfusions will improve communication between physicians and patients and also improve transfusion practice by physicians (Goodnough & Shuck, 1990; Kolins & Kolins, 1990). AABB recommendations include informing the patient of the risks, benefits, and alternatives of transfusions. When transfusions cannot be avoided due to the patient's condition, documentation should include the reason for transfusion (the underlying decision for transfusion) and laboratory values (Greve, 1991).

Certain criteria must be present for consent to be informed: first, the person(s) giving consent must fully comprehend the procedure to be performed, the risks involved, expected or desired outcomes, any complications or side effects and alternative therapies, including no therapy at all; and second, the consent must be given by one who has the legal capacity for giving such consent (i.e., competent adult, legal guardian, or representative for incompetent adult or child, emancipated-married minor, mature minor, parent, minor for the diagnosis and treatment of specific disease states or conditions, or court order).

As a result of federal court decisions, a separate informed consent form for blood transfusion should be used and must include, in detail, all risks, benefits, adverse reactions, and alternatives. Additionally, it is suggested that the physician obtain the informed consent.

BLOOD COMPONENTS AND THEIR ADMINISTRATION

Indications for transfusion include restoring blood volume, restoring oxygen-carrying capacity, replacing platelets, leukocytes, or plasma coagulation proteins, and providing exchange transfusion. Blood component therapy is the transfusion of a specific part of blood rather than whole blood and offers several advantages. First, it conserves precious resources: 1 U of donated whole blood provides several components. Dividing blood into components allows the tailoring of treatment for specific problems, for example, platelets for thrombocytopenia and packed red blood cells for anemia. Second, it provides an optimal method for patients who require numerous transfusions of a specific blood component. The most frequently used blood components in cancer therapy are packed red blood cells (PRBCs) and platelets (Plts). Other blood components are generally used for coagulation problems, for example, fresh-frozen plasma (FFP) for clotting factor deficiencies. Table 26–10 lists the most commonly used blood components and their characteristics. Key issues and responsibilities in the administration of blood

TABLE 26–10. *Blood Component Summary*

COMPONENT	INDICATION	VOLUME	INFUSION TIME	RESPONSE EXPECTED	POSSIBLE COMPLICATIONS
Red Cells					
PRBC	Blood loss; signs of anemia; Hgb <8g	250–350 ml	2–4 hrs	Increase Hgb 1g/dl per unit given	Hemolytic, febrile, allergic reactions; volume overload; hyperkalemia; Infections—HIV, hepatitis, CMV, other
Leukocyte-depleted PRBC & Platelets	Febrile reaction CMV (–) (under study to decrease CMV transmission)	250–350 ml	2–4 hrs	Same	Decrease febrile reactions; others same as PRBC & platelets
Irradiated PRBC & Platelets	Prevent GVHD	250–350 ml	2–4 hrs	Same	Same as PRBC & Platelets
Saline-washed PRBC	IgA deficiency; allergic reaction	200 ml	2–4 hrs	Same	Decrease febrile, allergic; others same as PRBC
Frozen PRBC	Rare blood type	200 ml	2–4 hrs	Same	Decrease febrile, allergic; others same as PRBC
Platelets					
Random-donor (RD)	<10,000–20,000 count; or bleeding or preoperative < 50,000	1 unit 30–50 ml (6 = 300 ml)	1 unit over 5–10 min	Increase 5000 per unit in 70 kg adult	Febrile, allergic reactions; alloantibodies; Infections—same as PRBC
Single donor (SD) not HLA-matched	Same; and alloantibodies	300 ml	30–60 min	Equal 6 RD = 30,000	Same; results in alloimmune variable
Single donor HLA-matched (SD-HLA)	Same and alloantibodies	300 ml	30–60 min	Same	Same; best choice for alloimmune
Granulocytes					
Single donor granulocytes	Sepsis with ANC <500 and failure to respond to antibiotics	400 ml	45–60 min	Hour rise in WBC	ARDS—especially with concomitant Amphotericin B, febrile, allergic reactions; volume overload; infections—HIV, hepatis, CMV, other
FFP					
FFP—homologous donor	Replace all coagulation factors—not for hemophilia or VWD	200–220 ml	30–60 min	1-unit increase coagulation factor by 3–5%	Febrile, allergic reactions; volume overload; rare hemolysis of recipient red cells; infections—HIV, hepatitis, CMV, other
Cyroprecipitate					
Cryohomologous donor	Hemophilia—FVIII deficiency; VWD; fibrinogen deficiency	10–15 ml (20 μ = 300 ml)	30–60 min	Variable FVIII and VWF averages are 100–200μ factor/per unit of cyro	Febrile, allergic reactions; volume overload; infections—HIV, hepatitis, CMV, other

component therapy are outlined in the nursing care plan (Table 26–11).

RED BLOOD CELLS

Packed red blood cells (PRBCs) are prepared from a unit of whole blood by removing 200 to 250 cc of plasma. Each unit of PRBCs still contains residual leukocytes, platelets, and plasma proteins, but the leukocytes and platelets become nonfunctional because of storage time and conditions (Synder, 1983; Widmann, 1985). PRBCs contain a portion of the anticoagulant-preservative used when drawing the whole blood. There are several ways in which red blood cells can be stored and prepared. These additive red blood cells are prepared by removing all plasma from a unit of whole blood and combining the additive solution with the cells. One anticoagulant-preservative solution is citrate phosphate dextrose with adenine (CPDA-1), which helps maintain viability of red blood cells (Har-

TABLE 26–11. *Nursing Care Plan—Transfusions*

Steps to providing safe transfusions:

1. Patient assessment
   - History
   - Education: signs/symptoms of reactions
   - Signed informed consent
2. Physician orders
3. Start IV line
   - 18- or 19-gauge needle
   - 0.9NS
   - Y-set blood tubing
   - 170 μm filter
4. Obtain blood product from blood bank
   - Proper identification: patient and blood product (2 persons to check)
   - Check compatibility: ABO type, Rh type & unit number
   - Check expiration date
   - Inspect blood for clots or discoloration
5. Take baseline vital signs
6. Start transfusion
   - 2 ml/min for the first 15 min.
   - Increase rate if no reactions (complete within 4 hours)
7. Take vital signs according to your policy, usually every 15 min × 1 hr, then every 30 min until transfusion completed
8. Watch for adverse reactions
9. Document vital information, including:
   - Who identified product
   - Product administered
   - Baseline vital signs
   - Time product started & completed
   - Accurate intake (product and fluids)
   - Patient response
   - Management of any adverse reactions
10. If inpatient, continue to monitor patient closely for any delayed reactions, and if outpatient, make sure patient knows who to contact in case of emergency

---

rison, 1994). Citrate is an anticoagulant, phosphate acts as a buffer, dextrose provides energy for red cell metabolism, and adenine serves as a source for ATP synthesis. PRBCs are stored at 1 to 6° C for a shelf life of 35 days (Coffland & Shelton, 1993). However, RBCs stored in CPDA-1 may not flow as well as whole blood and are difficult to administer rapidly. Other additive solutions are available and are more commonly used than CPDA-1. AS-1 contains adenine to maintain ATP, dextrose for glycolysis, mannitol to reduce hemolysis, and saline. AS-3 uses additional glucose in place of mannitol. These additive red blood cells extend the shelf life to 42 days and have flow similar to whole blood, making them easier to administer rapidly.

PRBCs vary in cost across the country, depending upon the donor source (e.g., regional blood center or hospital blood bank) and necessary routine processing. The technology required for specialized PRBC products increases their cost to two to three times.

Red cell transfusion in cancer patients should be based on clinical status rather than a predetermined hemoglobin value. Most patients experience symptoms of anemia with a hemoglobin less than 8 g, and this value is frequently used as a guideline for PRBC transfusions (Skillings, Sridhar, Wong, & Paddock, 1993; Stehling & Simon, 1994; Welch, Meehan & Goodnough, 1992). Patients may experience nonhemolytic, febrile reactions from red blood cell transfusions. These reactions are due to white blood cells (passenger leukocytes) in donor red blood cells (see complications discussed below). These reactions are common in patients who have had multiple pregnancies, prior transfusions, or organ transplantation. RBCs can be *washed, centrifuged,* or *filtered* to reduce the amounts of white cells present in the units. Washing the red blood cells is not efficient and expensive; they must also be used within 24 hours. Centrifugation is rarely used and reduces leukocytes up to only 85 per cent. A simpler method of leukocyte reduction is by the use of a microaggregate filter. These filters remove 99.9 per cent of the leukocytes from a unit of red blood cells and can be added externally to the infusion set during transfusion (Coffland & Shelton, 1993; Kao et al., 1995; Lane, 1994). Another method of washing red blood cells is the use of *frozen deglycerolized RBCs* (washing is used to remove glycerol). The use of these products depends upon availability, cost, and the severity of the patient's reaction.

PLATELETS

Platelet concentrates are one of the most important transfusion components for most patients with cancer and for patients undergoing a bone marrow transplant. In recent investigations, researchers have been able to identify growth factors that would stimulate platelet production, and several cytokines are being tested: IL-3, IL-6, and IL-11. At the present time these growth factors are still under clinical investigation, and platelet transfusions are the source of support for the thrombocytopenic cancer patient.

Platelets for transfusion come in two forms based on the source of the product. The first is a component derived from whole blood donation. Each individual platelet unit is prepared from 1 U of whole blood and stored in the blood bank. This product is often termed a random donor platelet unit (RD). A random donor unit of platelets has a volume of approximately 50 ml and contains varying amounts of residual leukocytes and red cells (Synder, 1983; Widmann, 1985). At the time of transfusion multiple units of random donor platelets are pooled as groups of six to eight by personnel from the blood bank. Once these units are pooled, they must be transfused within 4 hours (Harrison, 1994). The second product is obtained by apheresis. Platelets are obtained by placing the donor on a pheresis machine for 1 to 2 hours and collecting approximately 300 ml of platelet-enriched plasma (Table 26–9). This product is termed a single donor platelet (SD). HLA platelets are a special type of single donor platelet in which the donor and recipient are HLA-typed and -matched. Both RD and SD platelets can be stored for 5 days in a special "breathable" plastic at 20° to 24° C and are gently agitated on a rocker machine during storage.

In oncology, platelets are transfused as indicated by the patient's clinical condition (e.g., evidence of bleeding) and as prophylaxis to prevent bleeding. The standard platelet count number used for prophylactic transfusion is 20,000/mm (Beutler, 1993; Harovas & Anthony, 1993). HLA-matched platelets are a special product and are indicated when a patient has received multiple transfusions and has become "alloimmunized" and refractory to random donor platelets. Methods of reducing the risk of HLA alloimmunization from platelet transfusion include (1) limiting the number of transfusions or donors (i.e., single donor); (2) using leukocyte-depleted components (Table 26–9); and (3) using ultraviolet-B-irradiated platelets (Kao et al., 1995).

Random-donor platelet transfusion is expected to raise the platelet count by 5000/μL per unit transfused in a 70 kg patient. A single donor platelet transfusion should raise the platelet count by 30,000 to 60,000 μL (Coffland & Shelton, 1993). In the absence of normal platelet production, platelet transfusions are generally required every 3 days. Severe exogenous losses (e.g., hemorrhage or fever) will increase platelet transfusion requirements.

Monitoring the posttransfusion platelet count is critical in determining the outcome of a platelet transfusion. Often the patient's platelet count is determined on the next morning draw (referred to as a random count). Random counts may be adequate for stable patients but are not adequate in situations in which there is a question about the patient's response or when there is active bleeding. Failure of the random count to rise appropriately is an indication of excessive platelet destruction. A posttransfusion count should be obtained if the random count does not rise appropriately or there is active blood loss. The maximum platelet rise is seen approximately 15 minutes to 1 hour after transfusion. Counts taken 15 minutes to 1 hour after transfusion are a good indicator of the efficacy of the transfusion. A series of clinical examples illustrates these points (Table 26–12). In any thrombocytopenic patient the laboratory result should be verified when first reported. An artificial decrease in platelet count due to "clumping," or aggregation in the test tube, should be ruled out by visual inspection in the laboratory.

Common clinical causes for the failure of an appropriate rise in platelet count are found in Table 26–9. Immune destruction may be caused by the development of autoantibodies or alloantibodies. Autoantibodies are rarely identified in the cancer patient. When present, the patient usually presents with a history of preexisting thrombocytopenia, that is, ITP or drug-induced thrombocytopenia (Coffland & Shelton, 1993).

GRANULOCYTES

Granulocyte concentrates are prepared by leukapheresis of a single donor. Each concentrate contains WBCs, platelets, and red blood cells suspended in 200 to 400 ml of plasma. Granulocytes should ideally be transfused immediately after collection. If need be, they can be stored at room temperature up to 24 hours without agitation.

The use of granulocytes is controversial. Abrams and Disseroth (1985) suggest the use of granulocytes for patients who meet the following criteria: (1) a granulocyte count less than 500/mm^3, (2) early bone marrow recovery not expected, (3) documented gram-negative sepsis, (4) failure to show clinical improvement after the initiation of appropriate broad-spectrum antibiotic coverage, and (5) overall clinical setting and prognosis warranting the use of aggressive clinical supportive measures. Once initiated, granulocyte transfusions are given daily until bone marrow recovery or resolution of the identified clinical indication occurs (Strauss, 1994).

Preparing granulocytes is costly and requires expensive technology, close supervision, and 2 to 4 hours of the donor's time. Although studies have demonstrated the effectiveness of such treatments, the ratio of cost to

TABLE 26–12. *Clinical Examples of Platelet Transfusions*

EXAMPLE	PLATELET COUNTS	RESPONSE
70 kg leukemic patient. Day 15 of induction therapy. Afebrile. No bleeding. First platelet transfusion, 8 units of random donor (RD) platelets.	Pretransfusion: 10,000. Random count next AM draw post transfusion: 48,000 (12 hrs later)	Appropriate rise in platelet count (5000/U/kg). No evidence of excessive platelet destruction. Next transfusion monitored by random count.
70 kg female leukemic patient. Day 20 of therapy. Fever 38.5° C, possible pneumonia. 8 units RD platelets.	Pretransfusion: 20,000. Next AM draw after transfusion: 28,000	Failure of adequate response. This could be no platelet rise or rapid fall in transfused platelet. Need to assess count 1 hr after transfusion to determine cause.
70 kg female leukemic patient. Day 15. Afebrile. Heavy menstrual bleeding. 8 units RD platelet given	Pretransfusion: 15,000. Post transfusion: 12,000 (6 hrs later)	In setting of acute bleed, platelet loss is rapid. Need to determine the adequacy of rise with frequent counts at 1 hr post transfusion.
70 kg female leukemic patient. Day 20. Afebrile. No bleeding. 8 units RD platelets given.	Pretransfusion: 15,000. The last random count (8 hrs after transfusion) was 12,000. One hr post transfusion count now is 17,000	Refractory response to RD platelets. Search for causes listed in Table 26–9. Possible alloantibodies. Consider HLA typing of patient for HLA matched platelets.

benefit is high. Complications associated with the administration of granulocyte concentrates include pulmonary infiltrates, severe febrile reactions, and the transmission of viruses such as cytomegalovirus and hepatitis. In addition, the concomitant administration of granulocytes and amphotericin B has been reported to produce severe adverse pulmonary reactions (Strauss, 1994). A latter study failed to confirm this observation (Dana, Durie, White, & Huestis, 1981). In practice, the administration of amphotericin B and granulocytes should be separated by 4 to 6 hours, since either agent alone may cause a severe allergic reaction. Granulocyte transfusions in immunocompromised patients can cause graft-versus-host disease. The granulocyte product may be irradiated to kill lymphocytes to prevent this complication. This does not affect granulocyte function. It is unlikely that granulocyte transfusions will alter the clinical course of a neutropenic patient if recovery of bone marrow function is not expected (Strauss, 1994; Strauss et al., 1981).

PLASMA PRODUCTS

Plasma component products routinely available are (1) FFP and (2) cryoprecipitate (CRYO). These products are used in cancer patients to treat coagulopathies due to secondary disease states such as DIC or liver failure.

FFP is obtained by centrifugation of whole blood and rapid freezing of the plasma within 6 hours of collection and yields an average volume of 200 to 250 ml. If this single-donor unit is transfused immediately, it is called fresh plasma and contains all of the labile coagulation factors (II, VII, IX, and X). If the unit is not used, it may be frozen and stored up to 1 year at −30° C or below. FFP is outdated 12 months after it is donated. This blood component should be used to replace coagulation factors and not as a plasma expander or for fluid replacements. FFP is often indicated for replacement of multiple clotting factor deficiencies. All clotting factors are present in FFP, except fibrinogen, at an approximate concentration of 1 U of factor per milliliter of FFP. For adults, the average or usual replacement is 2 to 4 U of FFP every 6 hours. Transfusion of 2 U of FFP provides a replacement of roughly 6 to 10 per cent of the normal level of each clotting factor. Transfusion of large volumes of FFP is not appropriate for replacing an isolated clotting factor deficiency when an alternative product is available (Lundberg, 1994).

Cryoprecipitate is the only form of concentrated fibrinogen available. CRYO is prepared by thawing 1 U of FFP at 4° C and collecting the thick white precipitate that forms by centrifugation. It is stable for up to 1 year at −40° C. Each unit of CRYO has a volume of 10 to 15 ml and contains about 250 mg of fibrinogen, 80 to 120 U of Factor VIII:C (procoagulant activity), 40 to 70 per cent of Factor VIII:vWf (von Willebrand factor), and 20 to 30 per cent of Factor XIII (fibrin-stabilizing factor). CRYO is most often used to replace deficiencies of fibrinogen and Factor VIII. An average dose is 12 to 20 U of CRYO. The frequency of transfusion depends on the half-life of the specific factor replaced (Lundberg, 1994).

COMPLICATIONS OF TRANSFUSION

Transfusion of blood and blood components carries both risks and benefits to the recipient. A transfusion reaction can occur anytime during or after transfusion of blood or blood components. There are ways, however, of preventing or minimizing transfusion reaction by applying appropriate therapy. Of course the most important step to avoiding a serious transfusion reaction is proper recognition and identification. The adverse effects of transfusion can be characterized by the timing of their occurrence, *immediate (acute)* or *delayed,* and by the mechanism of the reaction, *immunologic* or *nonimmunologic* (Larison and Cook, 1994). The term "transfusion reaction" generally refers to the immediate immune reactions that occur (see below). Transfusion reactions are divided into immune and nonimmune and immediate and delayed. Table 26–13 lists immediate immune-mediated transfusion reactions, immediate nonimmune transfusion reactions, and delayed immune-mediated transfusion reactions. The table describes the signs and symptoms, management, and preventive measures to address each reaction (Callery, 1991; Harovas & Anthony, 1993; Heymann & Brewer, 1993; Larison & Cook, 1994; Spector, 1995).

The most frequent acute nonimmune complication of transfusion is congestive heart failure from volume overload. Bacterial contamination of the product is a rare complication. The most common delayed nonimmune reaction is the transmission of infection. Iron overload is another delayed reaction that is seen after many red cell transfusions (usually more than 100). The sections that follow discuss the immune and infectious complications of transfusion in greater detail.

COMPLICATIONS DUE TO IMMUNE MECHANISMS

The immediate transfusion reactions due to immunologic causes can be remembered by the acronym **NOFUN**—a**N**aphylaxis, hem**O**lysis, **F**ebrile, **U**rticaria, **N**oncardiogenic pulmonary edema.

Anaphylactic reactions are very rare. They are associated with IgA deficiency and occur in certain patients who develop antibodies to IgA. These reactions can occur after only a few milliliters of blood or plasma. They are characterized by the absence of fever and the presence of acute pulmonary symptoms such as cough and wheezing. Shock is common. Treatment is the same as for any anaphylactic reaction, but prevention should be the goal. Patients with hereditary or acquired immune deficiencies should be considered at risk.

Acute hemolytic reactions are the most dreaded but, fortunately, a rare complication of transfusion. They are almost always caused by red cell ABO incompatibility (Greenwalt, 1981). Errors in labeling the blood specimen or in identifying the component or patient are

TABLE 26–13. *Types of Transfusion Reactions*

TYPE	CAUSE	ONSET	SIGNS/SYMPTOMS	MANAGEMENT	PREVENTION
Acute hemolytic (rare)	ABO incompatibility	Usually during first 5–15 min, but may occur anytime during transfusion	Fever, chills Nausea Dyspnea, chest pain, back pain Hypotension Hemoglobinuria, oliguria Anemia Shock DIC, ARF	Stop transfusion Notify doctor & blood bank Send urine & blood specimen to blood bank Monitor I&O Keep vein open Vital signs as needed Documentation	Meticulously verify & document patient identification from sample collection to component infusion
Febrile, nonhemolytic (most common)	Sensitization to donor's WBCs, platelets or plasma	Immediately or within 6 hrs. after transfusion	Fever, chills Headache Nausea, vomiting Nonproductive cough Hypotension, chest pain, dyspnea Anxiety	Stop transfusion Notify doctor & blood bank Keep vein open Vital signs as needed	Leukocyte depleted components Premedicate with antipyretics
Allergic	Allergic reaction to plasma-soluble antigen contained in blood product	Anytime during the transfusion or within 1 hr after transfusion	Skin Rash (urticarial) Flushing Itching	Slow transfusion if mild Notify doctor & blood bank Vital signs as needed Do not restart if symptoms are severe	Treat prophylactically with antihistamines
Anaphylactic (rare)	Infusion of IgA proteins to IgA-deficient recipient who has developed IgA antibody	Immediately (after transfusion of only a few mls of blood)	Anxiety Urticaria Wheezing Tightness & pain in chest Dyphagia Cardiovascular collapse, shock Nausea, vomiting	Stop transfusion Keep vein open Notify doctor & blood bank Vital signs every 15 min & as needed Emergency equipment at bedside	Transfuse washed RBCs from which all plasma removed
Noncardiogenic pulmonary edema (NCPE)	Antileukocyte antibodies in donor or patient plasma, causing lung injury	Shortly after transfusion started	Chills Cough Fever Cyanosis Hypotension Increasing respiratory distress	Stop immediately Notify doctor & blood bank Monitor vital signs	If NCPE due to antileukocyte antibody, use leukocyte-poor components

DIC = disseminated intravascular coagulation; ARF = acute renal failure; I&O = intake and output; WBC = white blood cell; RBC = red blood cell; IVF = intravenous fluids; hgb = hemoglobin; hct = hematocrit; RUQ = right upper quadrant; LFT = liver function test.

the most common cause and result in the recipient's receiving the wrong blood product. The recipient may develop shock, DIC, or acute renal failure, any of which can be fatal. The severity of the reaction is in direct proportion to the amount of transfused incompatible blood and the elapsed time prior to appropriate intervention. Antibodies to blood group antigens other than the ABO system may cause an acute extravascular hemolytic reaction. Common offenders are antibodies to the blood groups Duffy and Kell. When these antibodies are not detected during initial antibody screen-ing, the transfusion of blood may result in an acute hemolytic reaction.

Febrile reactions (febrile nonhemolytic [FNH]) are the most common transfusion reactions, and they are usually immune-mediated (Dzieczkoski et al., 1995). These reactions are caused by antibodies in the recipient directed against antigens present on granulocytes, platelets, or lymphocytes in the transfused blood components. In platelet concentrates, these reactions may also be caused by cytokines in the plasma produced by the metabolism of white cells (Aye, Palmer, Giulivi, &

TABLE 26–13. *Types of Transfusion Reactions* Continued

TYPE	CAUSE	ONSET	SIGNS/SYMPTOMS	MANAGEMENT	PREVENTION
Bacterial contamination	Transfusion of contaminated blood components	Immediate or within about 30 min after transfusion	Rapid onset of: chills, fever vomiting diarrhea hypotension shock	Stop transfusion Notify doctor & blood bank Culture blood Send blood & blood bag to blood bank Antibiotics, IVFs, vasopressors, steroids as ordered	Collect, process, store, & transfuse blood products according to blood banking standards, Infuse within 4 hrs of starting Visual inspection of all products: color, clots or hemolysis
Circulatory overload	Fluid administered faster than the circulation can accommodate: TOO MUCH TOO FAST!	During transfusion	Cough Dyspnea, pulmonary congestion Headache Hypertension Tachycardia Distended neck veins Restlessness	Stop transfusion Keep vein open Fowler's position Notify doctor Administer O_2 & diuretics as ordered	Adjust fluid volume & rate based on patients size & clinical status Divide unit into smaller aliquots
Delayed hemolytic reaction (occurs in previous transfusion recipients or multiparous patients)	Incompatibility of RBC antigens other than ABO group	Days or weeks after transfusion	Decreasing hemoglobin Persistent low-grade fever Jaundice	Notify doctor & blood bank	Make sure patient is identified and tested properly
Alloimmunization	Immune system produces alloantibodies; prior exposure to donor blood components: antigenic RBCs	Days or weeks after transfusion	Slight fever Falling hgb & hct Severe platelet refractoriness with bleeding	Notify doctor & blood bank	Third-generation leukocyte filter Matching of RBC phenotypes to avoid sensitization
Posttransfusion purpura	Production of platelet alloantibody	7–14 days after transfusion	Thrombocytopenia platelet count <10,000/mm^3 Hematuria Melena Vaginal bleeding	Notify doctor & blood bank Test for antibodies	Corticosteroids, exchange transfusions, & plasmapheresis Thorough history
Transfusion-Associated Graft-Versus-Host Disease (TA-GVHD)	Transfused lymphocytes react against the recipient's tissue	Within 1–2 wks following blood cell transfusion	Fever, malaise Rash Nausea, vomiting Anorexia Bone marrow suppression Infection Pain RUQ Elevated LFT's	Monitor skin integrity, GI function, & bone marrow function Susceptible to infections & bleeding Emotional support Pain medication	Irradiation of blood products before transfusion reduces lymphocyte replication

Hashemi, 1995). The fever may occur early in the transfusion or even a few hours after the transfusion is complete. It is imperative that a thorough clinical evaluation of the patient be undertaken if fever occurs during blood transfusion. The leukopenic patient is at risk for infection, and this must be ruled out before fever can be attributed to a transfusion reaction. Fever can also be a sign of a hemolytic transfusion reaction, and the patient should be carefully observed until the cause is determined. Antipyretics and antihistamines are often given prior to transfusion in multiply transfused patients to prevent febrile reactions. Meperidine is extremely effective in relieving the shaking chills that can occur.

Urticarial reactions are thought to be due to antibodies against plasma proteins or soluble factors. These reactions are usually benign, and the transfusion is continued while the reaction is treated with antihistamines. As in the case of fever, urticaria can accompany a more severe reaction such as anaphylaxis or hemolysis. Such cases usually become evident, and the patient does not respond to antihistamines as in isolated urticaria.

Noncardiogenic pulmonary edema is also a rare complication of transfusion. The mechanism is not completely understood, but at least two triggers have been described. Antibodies in the donor product to leukocytes react with recipient white cells and cause leukoagglutination in pulmonary capillaries. In other cases complement is activated by the donor antibodies, and this causes recipient cells such as mast cells to release mediators that then cause leukoagglutination. When noncardiogenic pulmonary edema is suspected, the transfusion should be stopped immediately and supportive measures (some authors recommend steroids) instituted. A summary of the types of transfusion reactions, signs and symptoms, and clinical management is found in Table 26–13 (Callery, 1991; Harovas & Anthony, 1993; Heymann & Brewer, 1993; Larison & Cook, 1994; Spector, 1995).

Some transfusion reactions occur days after the transfusion and are dramatic reminders of what can go unrecognized. Table 26–13 lists these reactions and their cause and treatment. A brief discussion of delayed hemolytic transfusion reaction follows, since it is the most common of these rare complications.

A *delayed hemolytic transfusion reaction* is characterized by a drop in hemoglobin that may be gradual over days or sudden. The basic cause for this is an immune response with increasing antibody in the patient (recipient) after exposure to the transfused blood. The immune response may be a primary immunization (first exposure), the rise in antibodies is slow, and the hemolysis is gradual over 2 weeks after transfusion. In other patients the rise in antibodies is rapid and is felt to come from an anamnestic response (recalled memory immune response). This means that the recipient was already immunized, but when tested prior to transfusion the antibody titer was low so that the screening test results were negative. This is why a history of transfusion is important. Transfusion of blood into the patient results in a restimulation of the immune system, and the antibody titer rises after 7 to 10 days with sudden hemolysis. These patients generally have sudden fever, jaundice, and a marked drop in hemoglobin, but the reaction rarely causes renal problems or shock. The only means of preventing delayed hemolytic reactions is a thorough and accurate review of the patient's transfusion history (Vamvakus, Pineda, Reisner, Santrach, & Moore, 1995).

INFECTIOUS COMPLICATIONS

Several infectious diseases can be transmitted through transfusion. Although small, the possibility of transmitting one or more viruses continues to be one of the major complications (Table 26–14). The development of non-A, non-B hepatitis and AIDS are the greatest risks faced by the recipient of a transfusion. The risks of these complications are dramatically lower

TABLE 26–14. *Major Infection and Reaction Complications of Transfusion and Likelihood of Occurrence*

COMPLICATION	FREQUENCY PER TRANSFUSION
Infectious	
CMV	Common
Hepatitis C	1:2000
Hepatitis B	1:200,000
HIV	1:330,000 to 1:1,000,000
HTLV I/II	1:70,000 to 1:100,000
Immunologic	
Febrile reaction	1:50 to 1:100
Hemolytic transfusion reaction (delayed)	1:6000
Hemolytic transfusion reaction	1:600,000
Graft-versus-host reactions	Unknown; <1:1,000,000

since 1985 because of changes in blood testing and screening donor questions as well as the virtual elimination of paid donors from the general donor pool (Klapper & Goldfinger, 1992; Heymann & Brewer, 1993).

Hepatitis A is rarely transmissible by blood transfusion due to its short period of viremia and the absence of a carrier state. Mandatory testing for hepatitis B surface antigen (HBsAg) in blood products has significantly reduced the transmission of hepatitis B. However, testing of blood products for hepatitis B did not produce a decrease in the frequency of posttransfusion hepatitis. Subsequently, it was recognized that another virus, or group of viruses, was (were) capable of producing hepatitis after blood transfusion. The term non-A, non-B hepatitis refers to the infection caused by this virus(es). The majority of non-A, non-B hepatitis is now known to be due to the hepatitis C virus. In 1989 the virus was found in a chimpanzee infected with non-A, non-B hepatitis. It is an RNA virus and is entirely different from the DNA hepatitis B virus. After infection with hepatitis C, antibodies to the virus are made anti-hepatitis C antibody (anti-HCV). Routine screening of blood with anti-HCV began in the United States in May 1990. There appears to be at least one other virus causing non-A, non-B hepatitis, and this could now be considered non-A, non-B, non-C hepatitis (NANBNC). The incubation period of hepatitis C (the time from transfusion to the first rise in serum transaminase) is quite variable and varies from 2 weeks to 4 months. Jaundice is observed in only 20 per cent of patients and occurs about 1 to 4 weeks after the rise in serum transaminase. Thus many cases of transfusion hepatitis are "silent." Most patients who develop hepatitis C will have an abrupt increase in their serum transaminases followed by a gradual return to normal. Some patients will become chronic carriers of the virus, and some of these will subsequently develop cirrhosis. Currently, the most effective means of preventing hepatitis C is the use of volunteer blood and the rejection of blood products with elevated transaminase enzymes (a surrogate marker for hepatitis) or antibody to the gene products of hepatitis B virus.

The next infectious complication associated with transfusion is HIV and AIDS. HIV is probably one of the least frequent adverse outcomes of transfusion but remains of great concern for health care professionals and the community. Proper screening and testing, for example, ELISA and Western blot, has reduced the risk of contracting HIV from blood component transfusion. HIV is a lentivirus that causes chronic infection and grows slowly. Initial symptoms, which appear approximately 6 weeks after transfusion of an infected product, may be flulike acute illness. The mean incubation period between transfusion and diagnosis of AIDS is approximately 4.5 years with a range of 2 to 14 years. Once AIDS develops the patient has profound loss of the immune system characterized by opportunistic infections, malignancies, or both. The risk of AIDS from blood collected since testing was initiated in early 1985 is approximately 1:225,000 per unit (Dodd, 1994).

Another important infectious complication of transfusion is cytomegalovirus (CMV), which is a member of the herpes group of viruses. CMV is transmitted by viable leukocytes in the blood product. It is estimated that approximately 6 to 12 per cent of the blood products from the general donor pool are capable of transmitting CMV. The recipients at highest risk for complications of CMV infection are (1) immunocompromised patients, (2) the fetus in utero with primary CMV maternal infection, and (3) premature infants. Symptoms include mild fever, mild splenomegaly, and atypical serum lymphocytes. Complications in these recipients include CMV interstitial pneumonitis, birth defects, and death. There is no completely reliable way to prevent CMV infection, but donors who have anti-CMV IgM ("CMV-positive") are more likely to transmit infection. Therefore, in the high-risk settings outlined previously, "CMV-negative" blood is required. Most authorities would include all transplant recipients and leukemic patients who do not have anti-CMV in the high risk category (Heymann & Brewer, 1993; Dodd, 1994).

Use of leukocyte-depleted products may play a role in prevention of some transfusion-associated diseases, since transmission of these diseases are linked to leukocytes (Klapper & Goldfinger, 1992). Studies were conducted to determine whether use of leukocyte-depleted red cells (filtrated) and platelets (centrifugation) would prevent transfusion-associated CMV infection in patients with leukemia and lymphoma. In these groups of patients CMV infection did not develop in the 59 who received leukocyte-depleted components (Lane et al., 1992).

NURSING CONSIDERATIONS

Oncology nurses play a key role in the delivery of blood components to the cancer patient. Nurses must be knowledgeable about transfusion principles, indications for component use, product availability and its contents, the need for ABO-Rh compatibility, and potential transfusion reactions and complications. Administration guidelines for nurses to follow to en-

sure that oncology patients will receive blood components in a safe, efficient manner are identified in Table 26–10 (Harovas & Anthony, 1993).

Standard 170 μm blood filters are required for all blood components and factor concentrates to trap clots. Microaggregate filters have a pore size of 20 to 40 μm. The function of these filters is to remove leukocyte-platelet aggregates that form during blood storage. These filters have been used during massive transfusions and in clinical situations in which an increased risk of noncardiogenic pulmonary edema exists. It is not clear whether the presence of these leukocyte-platelet aggregates produces any direct harm to the patient. Leukocyte-poor filters are available for red blood cell and platelet component administration. These filters are used when a leukocyte-poor component is indicated.

The physician's order will specify the component and transfusion rate. All blood components should be infused within 4 hours after initiation. This decreases the risk of bacterial contamination and ensures component stability. The blood bank can divide the unit into two or more parts, dispensing one part at a time when clinically warranted. This allows a longer transfusion period without jeopardizing the blood component or increasing the patient's risk for adverse effects. Once the component is obtained, it must be used within 30 minutes or returned immediately to the blood bank for proper storage.

No medication should be added to blood at any time. Normal saline solution may be added for dilutional purposes, if needed. Other solutions, such as D5W, may destroy red blood cells, and lactated Ringer's solution may induce clot formation due to the presence of calcium. A large-gauge needle, 18- or 19-gauge, is recommended for peripheral blood administration, but if the patient has poor access routes, a 20-gauge needle may be used. Many oncology patients may have some type of venous access device, either an implanted port or a tunneled Silastic central catheter, providing a consistent access route. Blood administration through venous access devices requires adherence to the procedures established by the nurse's institution.

Blood components may be administered via infusion devices. However, the manufacturer or blood bank should be consulted to determine device capabilities, because hemolysis of red blood cells may occur with some models. Blood warmers—devices that warm the blood as it passes through are used for patients receiving massive amounts of blood over a short time and for patients who have cold agglutinins to prevent adverse reaction.

Thorough and accurate documentation is critical to the transfusion process. Many institutions require frequent monitoring of vital signs (e.g., every 15 minutes for 1 hour, then every 30 minutes until the transfusion is complete), although little clinical data exist to support this practice. Infuse blood components at 2 ml/min (not to exceed 30 ml) for the first 15 minutes, then increase to the appropriate rate if the patient does not have any signs of adverse reactions (other than allergic urticarial reaction) (Querin & Stahl, 1990).

Taylor, Wagner, and Kraus (1987) undertook a retrospective chart audit to determine when transfusion reactions occurred in relation to the vital sign monitoring. They found that fever and chills were the most common reactions reported, with reactions occurring from 30 minutes to 3 hours and 35 minutes from the onset of the transfusion. Recommendations included staying with the patient for the first 15 minutes or being readily available and seeing the patient every 5 minutes for the first 15 minutes, plus taking vital signs every 30 minutes and then every hour until the transfusion is completed. A flow sheet identifying assessment criteria to be monitored is helpful in establishing a consistent evaluation of transfusion therapy. Actual symptoms to be assessed, clinical data to be monitored, and the patient's response to therapy can be clearly identified and useful in planning nursing care.

Blood component therapy is essential in the supportive care of the patient with cancer. Patients and family will request information about the risks of transfusion therapy and participation in a designated donor program. Oncology nurses must have an adequate knowledge base to answer these questions. In addition, nurses must be familiar with their hospital's policies and procedures and be aware of available resources for their own educational needs. No transfusion should be considered routine. Each component administered requires strict adherence to guidelines throughout the transfusion process to provide optimal patient care.

SUMMARY AND FUTURE TRENDS

Knowledge of modern transfusion principles is essential for oncology nursing practice. Nurses are in an optimal position to provide education to the cancer patient and family regarding transfusion practice. The administration of blood products is a treatment directly provided to the patient and monitored almost exclusively by nurses.

New cancer treatments with biologic agents may prove to be effective and less toxic to bone marrow, thus reducing transfusion support requirements. Recombinant hormonal agents that stimulate hematopoietic cell production are being used in the clinical setting. These agents will allow cytotoxic therapy to be given with fewer and shorter intervals of bone marrow suppression. On the other hand, therapies such as high-dose chemotherapy with autologous bone marrow transplant require intensive blood component support. The oncology nurse must become familiar and knowledgeable with the principles of blood transfusion, including the purpose, administration, and reactions of each component.

REFERENCES

Abrams, R. A., & Deisseroth, A. (1985). Use of blood and blood products. In V. T. DeVita, S. Hellman, & S. A. Rosenberg (Eds.), *Cancer: Principles and practice of oncology* (pp. 1920–1940). Philadelphia: J. B. Lippincott.

Alter, M. J., Hadler, S. C., Judson, F. N., Mares, A., Alexander, W. J., Hu, P. Y., Miller, J. K., Moyer, L. A., Fields, H. A., Bradley, D. W., & Margolis, H. S. (1990). Risk factors for acute non-A, non-B hepatitis in the United States and association with hepatitis C virus infection. *Journal of the American Medical Association, 264* (17), 2231.

Anderson, K. C., & Braine, H. G. (1990). Specialized cell component therapy. *Seminars in Oncology Nursing, 6,* 140.

Aye, M. T., Palmer, D. S., Giulivi A., & Hashemi, S. (1995). Effect of filtration of platelet concentrates on the accumulation of cytokines and platelet release factors during storage. *Transfusion 35,* 117–124.

Beutler, E. (1993). Platelet transfusions: the 20,000/μL trigger. *Blood, 81*(6), 1411–1413.

Black's Law Dictionary. (1990). (6th ed., p. 779). St. Paul, MN: West Publishing Co.

Callery, M.F., Culhane, M. B., Francis, C. K., Harrington, P., Pavel, J. D., Snyder, E. L., Blair, J., McCurdy, P. R., Rogus, S. D., McDonald, M., & Pipp, M. (1991). National Blood Resource Education Program. Transfusion nursing: Trends and practices for the '90s: Building a safe community blood supply. *American Journal of Nursing, 91*(6), 51–52.

Canterbury v. Spence, 464 F.2d 772, (D.C. Cir. 1972). Certiorari denied, 409 U.S. 1064 (1973), 93 S.Ct. 560.

Capron, A. (1974). Informed consent in catastrophic disease research and treatment. *123 University of Pennsylvania Law Review 340,* 365–376.

Coffland, F. I., & Shelton, D. M. (1993). Blood component replacement therapy. *Critical Care Nursing Clinics of North America, 5*(3), 543–556.

Dana, B. W., Durie, B. G. M., White, R. F., & Huestis, D. W. (1981). Concomitant administration of granulocyte transfusions and amphotericin B in neutropenic patients: Absence of significant pulmonary toxicity. *Blood, 57*(1), 90–94.

Dodd, R. Y. (1994). Infectious complications of blood transfusion. *Annals of Hematology and Oncology, 2*(4), 280–287.

Dzieczkowski, J. S., Barrett, B. B., Nester, D., Campbell, M., Cook, J., Sugrue, M., Andersen, J. W., & Anderson, K. C. (1995). Characterization of reactions after exclusive transfusion of white cell-reduced cellular blood components. *Transfusion, 35,* 20–25.

Eisenstaedt, R. S., Glanz, K., Smith, D. G., & Derstine, T. (1993). Informed consent for blood transfusion: a regional hospital survey. *Transfusion, 33,* 558–561.

Ereth, M. H., Oliver, W. C., & Santrach, P. J. (1994). Perioperative interventions to decrease transfusion of allogeneic blood products. *Mayo Clinic Proceedings, 69,* 575–586.

Gerber, L. (1994). Autologous blood transfusion. *Journal of Intravenous Nursing, 17*(2), 67–69.

Goodnough, L. T., & Shuck, J. M. (1990). Risks, options, and informed consent for blood transfusion in elective surgery. *American Journal of Surgery, 159*(6), 602–609.

Greenwalt, T. J. (1981). Pathogenesis and management of hemolytic transfusion reactions. *Seminars in Hematology, 18,* 84–94.

Greve, P. A. (1991). Medical, ethical, and legal issues associated with HIV. *Journal of Intravenous Nursing, 14*(3), S30–S35.

Harovas, J., & Anthony, H. H. (1993). Your guide to trouble-free transfusions. *RN, 56*(11), 26–34.

Harrison, C. R. (1994). Technologic advances and future trends in blood banking. In D. M. Harmening (Ed.), *Modern blood banking and transfusion practices* (3rd ed., pp. 496–515). Philadelphia: F. A. Davis Co.

Heymann, S. J., & Brewer, T. F. (1993). The infectious risks of transfusions in the United States: A decision-analytic approach. *American Journal of Infection Control, 21,* 174–182.

Jones v. Philadelphia College of Osteopathic Medicine, 813 F. Supp. 1125 (E.D. Pa. 1993).

Kao, K. J., Mickel, M., Braine, H. G., Davis, K., Enright, H., Gernsheimer, T., Gillespie, M. J., Kickler, T. S., Lee, E. J., McCullough, J. J., McFarland, J. G., Nemo, G. J., Noyes, W. D., Schiffer, C. A., Sell, K., Slichter, S. J., Woodson, R. D., & the TRAP Study Group. (1995). White cell reduction in platelet concentrates and packed red cells by filtration: a multicenter clinical trial. *Transfusion, 35,* 13–19.

Klapper, E. B., & Goldfinger, D. (1992). Leukocyte-reduced blood components in transfusion medicine: current indications and prospects for the future. *Clinics in Laboratory Medicine, 12*(4), 711–721.

Kolins, F., & Kolins, M. D. (1990). Informed consent, risk, and blood transfusion. *Journal of Thoracic and Cardiovascular Surgery, 100,* 88–91.

Kozup v. Georgetown University Hospital, 663 F. Supp. 1048 (DC 1987); 851 F2d 437 (DC Cir 1988); 906 F2d 783 (DC Cir 1990).

Landsteiner, K. (1901). Uber agguluntinationserscheinungen normalen menschlichen blutes. *Klinische Wochenschrift, 14,* 1132–1145.

Landsteiner, K., & Wiener, A. S. (1940). An agglutinable factor in human blood recognized by immune sera for rhesus blood. *Proceedings of the Society for Experimental Biology (NY), 43,* 223.

Lane, T. A. (1994). Leukocyte reduction of cellular blood components: Effectiveness, benefits, quality control, and costs. *Archives of Pathology and Laboratory Medicine, 118,* 392–404.

Lane, T. A., Anderson, K. C., Goodnough, L. T., et al. (1992). Leukocyte reduction in blood component therapy. *Annals of Internal Medicine, 117,* 151–162

Larison, P. J., & Cook, L. O. (1994). Adverse effects of blood transfusion. In D. M. Harmening (Ed.), *Modern Blood Banking and Transfusion Practices* (3rd ed.). (pp. 351–374). Philadelphia: F. A. Davis Company.

Leparc, G. F. (1991). Informed consent for blood transfusion. *Journal of the Florida Medical Association, 78*(7), 423–425.

Lundberg, G. D. (Ed.). (1994). Practice parameter for the use of fresh-frozen plasma, cryoprecipitate, and platelets. *Journal of the American Medical Association, 271*(10), 777–781.

McLeod, B. C. (1980). Immunologic factors in reactions to blood transfusions. *Heart & Lung, 9*(4), 675–681.

Menitove, J. E. (1983). Platelet transfusion for alloimmunized patients. *Journal of Clinical Oncology, 2,* 587–609.

Querin, J. J., & Stahl, L. D. (1990). 12 simple steps for successful blood transfusions. *Nursing, 20*(10), 68–81.

Simon, T. L. (1994). The collection of platelets by apheresis procedures. *Transfusion Medicine Review, 8,* 132–145.

Skillings, J. R., Sridhar, F. G., Wong, C., & Paddock, L. (1993). The frequency of red cell transfusion for anemia in patients receiving chemotherapy. *American Journal of Clinical Oncology, 16*(1), 22–25.

Spector, D. (1995). Transfusion-associated graft-versus-host disease: An overview and two case reports. *Oncology Nursing Forum, 22*(1), 97–101.

Stehling, L., Luban, N. L. C., Anderson, K. C., Sayers, M. H., Long, A., Attar, S., Leitman, S. F., Gould, S. A., Kraskall, M. S., Goodnough, L. T., & Hines, D. M. (1994). Guidelines for blood utilization review. *Transfusion, 34*(5), 438–448.

Stehling, L., & Simon, T. L. (1994). The red blood cell transfusion trigger: Physiology and clinical studies. *Archives of Pathology and Laboratory Medicine, 118,* 429–434.

Strauss, R. G., Connett, J. E., Gale, R. P., Bloomfield, C. D., Herzig, G. P., McCullough, J., Maguire, L. C., Winston, D. J., Ho, W., Stump, D. C., Miller, W. V., & Keopke, J. A. (1981). A controlled trial of prophylactic granulocyte transfusions during initial induction chemotherapy for acute myclogensus leukemia. *The New England Journal of Medicine, 305*(11), 597–603.

Strauss, R. G. (1994). Granulocyte transfusion therapy for hem/onc patients. *Hem/Onc Annals, 2*(4), 304–309.

Synder, E. L. (Ed.). (1983). *Blood transfusion therapy: A physician's handbook.* Arlington, VA: American Association of Blood Banks.

Taylor, B. N., Wagner, P. L., & Kraus, C. L. (1987). Development of a standard for time-effective patient assessment during blood transfusion. *Journal of Nursing Quality Assurance, 1*(2), 66–71.

Vamvakus, E. C., Pineda, A. A., Reisner, R., Santrach, P. J., & Moore, S. B. (1995). The differentiation of delayed hemolytic and delayed serologic transfusion reactions: incidence and predictors of hemolysis. *Transfusion, 35,* 26–32.

Welch, H. G., Meehan, K. R., & Goodnough, L. T. (1992). Prudent strategies for elective red blood cell transfusion. *Annals of Internal Medicine, 116*(5), 393–402.

Widmann, F. K. (Ed.). (1985). *Technical manual.* Arlington, Virginia: American Association of Blood Banks.

Widmann, F. K. (1990). Informed consent for blood transfusion: Brief historical survey and summary of a conference. *Transfusion, 30,* 460–470.

Marrow Transplant and Peripheral Blood Stem Cell Transplantation

Rosemary Ford • Joanne McDonald • Karin J. Mitchell-Supplee • Barbara A. Jagels

HISTORIC PERSPECTIVE

The first marrow transplants in humans were conducted in the 1950s in patients with end-stage leukemia. These transplants were unsuccessful in that all the patients relapsed; however, the patients did show hematologic recovery. Extensive laboratory studies based on these early experiments were conducted during the next decade using mice and dogs. By the late 1960s several developments had offered encouragement to again try marrow transplant in humans, including advances in tissue typing, improved techniques for pheresis of blood products, and development of more effective and broad-spectrum antibiotics. Clinical trials resumed in the early 1970s using matched siblings, again with patients considered to be in the end stages of their disease (Box 27-1) (Thomas et al., 1977). Because of the success of these studies, protocols were initiated for patients earlier in their course of treatment, when their physical condition was better (Appelbaum, Fisher,

Thomas, & The Seattle Marrow Transplant Team, 1988).

Since the early 1970s, the number of long-term transplantation survivors has increased every year due to the expanding knowledge base of how to best treat these patients as well as improvements and increased availability in therapeutic agents. Several therapies have had particularly remarkable impact on patient survival including cyclosporine prophylaxis for graft-versus-host disease, antivirals acyclovir and ganciclovir, and the use of cytokines to enhance engraftment.

In the early 1980s, as the success of marrow transplant for hematologic malignancies was reported in the medical literature, numerous physicians and medical institutions initiated marrow transplant programs (Bortin & Rim, 1986). This trend increased in the late 1980s as transplants using a patient's own marrow became more widely utilized. Simultaneously, the National Marrow Donor Program was established in September 1987 to provide a registry of unrelated

---

Box 27–1. *The First Large-Scale Marrow Transplant Study*

Thomas, E. D., Buckner, C. D., Banaji, M., Clift, R. A., Fefer, A., Flournoy, N., Goodell, B. W., Hickman, R. O., Lerner, K. G., Neiman, P. E., Sale, G. E., Sanders, J. E., Singer, J., Stevens, M., Storb, R., & Weiden, P., (1977). One hundred patients with acute leukemia treated by chemotherapy, total body irradiation and allogeneic marrow transplantation. *Blood*, *49*, 511–533.

A milestone in the field was reached with the publication in 1977 of the results of bone marrow transplantation as a treatment for 100 patients with end-stage leukemia. In all 94 patients who lived long enough for engraftment to occur (21 days after transplantation) engraftment did not take place. This large-scale study compared various preparation regimens and reported the types and incidence of complications for which marrow transplant patients are at risk. Interstitial pneumonia was the cause of death in 34 patients, 50 patients developed moderate to severe graft-verses-host disease, and 31 patients had relapses.

The most remarkable finding, however, was the 13 patients alive without recurrent leukemia 1 to 4.5 years after transplantation. These patients would not have survived without the transplant. This was a major breakthrough in the field of oncology. From these encouraging early results, protocols were implemented for patients earlier in the course of their disease who were in better clinical condition to undergo the rigorous therapy required in marrow transplantation.

---

marrow donors as a resource to patients eligible for marrow transplant but without a family donor (Welte, 1994). At the same time, some centers entered patients onto protocols using family members with mismatched marrow. These trends offered marrow transplant as an option to an increasing number of patients. In addition, marrow transplantation is being considered as a treatment option for other types of malignancies, most notably solid tumors such as breast cancer.

Because of the intensive support required by patients undergoing marrow transplant, the cost of this therapy is high. Marrow transplant is often singled out as an example of high-technology/high-cost treatment. In response to the demand to lower costs, many centers are shifting as much care as possible to the ambulatory setting (Cavanaugh, 1994; Kelleher, 1994; Randolph, 1993). These programs are reporting success in maintaining quality while decreasing costs; however, there is concern regarding the ability of family caregivers to handle the increased responsibility (Peters, Ross, Vredenburgh, Hssein, & Rubin, 1994).

CURRENT CONTEXT OF MARROW TRANSPLANTATION

MARROW TRANSPLANT NURSING AS A SPECIALTY

As transplantation has become accepted on a wide scale in the medical community, nursing in this area has grown into a specialty requiring expertise in many established areas of nursing including oncology, critical care, ambulatory care, pediatrics, and psychosocial nursing. Transplant nursing can be characterized as provisional in nature in that nurses are continually redefining boundaries of practice, especially at the interface of psychosocial and biophysical therapeutics (Winters, Miller, Maracich, Compton, & Haberman, 1994).

There are obvious similarities between oncology nursing and marrow transplant nursing. Most patients who undergo transplantation have a malignant disease and the types of therapies and nursing approaches used with the patients often are the same as those used routinely with oncology patients. There are, however, some differences between the two specialties. First, although all marrow transplant patients have a life-threatening disease, not all have malignant disease. Second, whereas oncology nurses care for patients of all age groups, transplant patients tend to be a younger population with an average age of 35 years. Many transplant centers use a cutoff age of 50 years for acceptance into protocols. Third, all patients are on elective protocols. Marrow transplantation is almost always an experimental procedure and is the treatment of choice for only a small number of diseases. Fourth, whereas chemotherapy and irradiation doses are limited in the usual oncology setting because of marrow toxicity, supralethal doses of these therapies provide the basis of treatment in marrow transplant, creating maximum toxicities. Fifth, transplant patients may be treated far from their homes, away from established support systems. Finally, in addition to requiring the same knowledge base as oncology nurses, transplant nurses must know how to assess for unique complications such as veno-occlusive disease (VOD) and graft-versus-host disease, as well as side effects unique to marrow ablative therapy.

Effort has been made in several arenas to meet the professional needs of marrow transplant nurses. The Oncology Nursing Society created special interest groups (SIGs) within the Society's structure in 1990, and marrow transplant nurses were among the first and largest of the initial SIGs established. In addition, there are regional, national, and international networks of marrow transplant nurses who sponsor various activities, especially specific symposiums focusing on advanced nursing practice in caring for marrow transplant patients.

MARROW TRANSPLANT CONCEPTS

TREATMENT PURPOSE AND RATIONALE

The purpose of marrow transplantation is to treat otherwise fatal diseases due to malignant cells or nonfunctioning hematologic cells using a high dose regimen of chemotherapy, total body irradiation (TBI), or both. This treatment may be considered for patients with hematologic malignancies such as leukemias and lymphomas, hematologic disorders such as sickle cell anemia, certain types of solid tumors as well as diseases that result in a nonfunctioning bone marrow such as aplastic anemia and thalassemia. In oncologic diseases dose-response curves demonstrate that patients have significantly improved responses with larger doses of chemotherapy agents (Lin, Tierney, & Stadtmauer, 1993). In marrow transplantation much higher doses of chemotherapy and/or irradiation than that used in conventional treatment is used. The administration of this therapy immediately prior to transplantation is known as the preparative or conditioning regimen. Three major goals the conditioning regimen must achieve are (1) suppression of recipients' immune system so the donor marrow cells will not be rejected, (2) an antitumor effect if malignant disease is present, and (3) creation of a marrow space, that is, a microenvironment that will allow the new marrow to engraft.

PHYSIOLOGIC CONSEQUENCES OF MARROW TRANSPLANTATION

The consequence of the conditioning regimen on the immune and hematologic systems is a period of profound pancytopenia. The body's ability to produce blood cells such as erythrocytes, thrombocytes, and leukocytes is destroyed. Following transplantation the ability to replenish circulating blood cells does not return for weeks. During that time full blood product support with red cell and platelet transfusions are needed. Protecting the patient from infection with measures such as meticulous handwashing and the use of antibiotics is essential. Growth factors are administered in many treatment protocols to decrease the period of pancytopenia.

Several factors have an influence on how quickly the immune system becomes fully functional after transplant. Conditioning regimens that include irradiation may result in a slower lymphocyte recovery. Patients receiving autologous or syngeneic transplants tend to recover immune function more rapidly than patients receiving allogeneic transplants. And peripheral blood stem cell (PBSC) transplants engraft faster than bone marrow transplants, theoretically because the peripheral blood stem cell collection contains more developed and differentiated cells that require less time to mature. In general, the marrow is usually able to produce and release neutrophils into the peripheral circulation in 10 days to 3 weeks, and it may take a year or more

for a fully competent immune system to develop. By the end of the first year after transplant most patients have recovered the ability to produce antibodies to antigens.

The major complications seen in patients after transplantation are the result of the conditioning regimen (chemoirradiation) used to prepare for transplantation (Bearman et al., 1988), the lack of a functioning bone marrow, the replacement of the patient's immune system, or iatrogenic (the result of the therapies the patient received to treat other complications) (Table 27–1). The complications are rarely the result of the patient's original disease.

Figure 27–1 shows a visual representation of the time of onset of the most frequent complications and their peak time of occurrence; it also shows that the complications often occur simultaneously. There are important concepts to keep in mind in understanding the implication of these complications and the nursing care needed to assist patients in the months after transplantation (Ford & Ballard, 1988). One of these concepts is that the complications are interrelated (Fig. 27–2). One complication can cause or exacerbate another, or the treatment of one can cause or exacerbate another (Storb & Thomas, 1985). Or, the treatment of one complication may have to be modified or terminated because of the development of another complication and so the patient is at risk for the development of the complication originally being treated.

THERAPEUTIC GOALS

Following conditioning therapy the goal is to support the patient in three major ways: (1) to restore immune function by transplanting progenitor cells, also known as stem cells, from a donor, (2) to monitor and treat side effects and complications (Fig. 27–2), and (3) to assist the patient and family in coping throughout the transplant process.

RESTORATION OF IMMUNE AND HEMATOPOIETIC FUNCTION

Stem cells, the progenitor cells of the hematopoietic system, have the capacity to self-replicate as well as differentiate through several different cell development stages into cells that are committed to producing either erythrocytes, leukocytes, or platelets. The stem cells are capable of repopulating the bone marrow and entire hematopoietic system with new cells after conditioning therapy. Large numbers of stem cells are produced and stored in the bone marrow. Normally, relatively small numbers of stem cells are found in the peripheral blood circulation. An adequate number of stem cells for engraftment to take place can be obtained either by directly harvesting bone marrow or by mobilizing and then collecting stem cells from the peripheral circulation.

Transplants are called bone marrow transplants (BMT) when the stem cells are obtained from the bone

TABLE 27–1. *Causes of Acute and Chronic Complications*

CONDITIONING REGIMEN (CHEMOIRRADIATION THERAPIES)	LACK OF FUNCTIONING MARROW	REPLACEMENT OF IMMUNE SYSTEM	IATROGENIC COMPLICATIONS
Acute			
Nausea and vomiting	Hemorrhage	Acute GVHD	Renal failure
Diarrhea	Infections		Hypertension
Mucositis	Cytomegalovirus pneumonia		Electrolyte imbalance
Alopecia			
Lethargy			
Veno-occlusive disease			
Interstitial pneumonia			
Chronic			
Cataracts	Late infections	Chronic GVHD	
Sterility			
Delay or lack of puberty			

GVHD = Graft-versus-host disease.

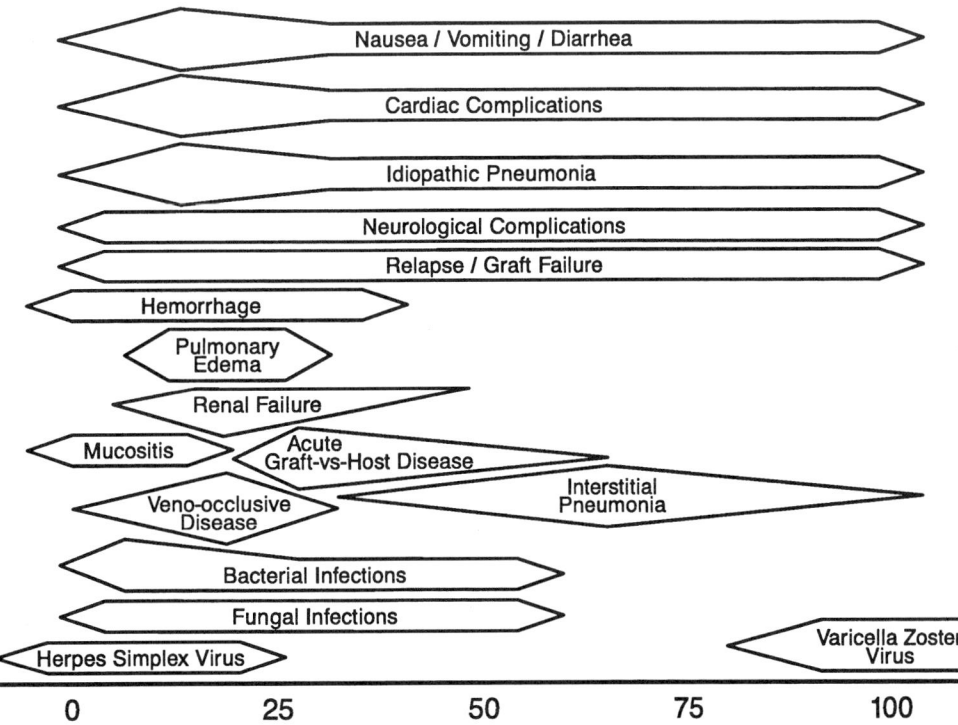

FIGURE 27–1. The approximate time of onset of the major acute complications after bone marrow transplantation. The peaks in the figures (when present) represent the peak incidence of each complication. (From Ford, R. C., & Ballard, B. [1988]. Acute complications after bone marrow transplantation. *Seminars in Oncology Nursing, 4,* 15–24. Reproduced by permission.)

marrow and peripheral blood stem cell (PBSC) or peripheral blood progenitor cell (PBPC) transplants when the stem cells are collected from the bloodstream.

TYPES OF MARROW TRANSPLANTS

The donor source of the stem cells determines the type of transplant. Figure 27–3 illustrates the usual schedules for each transplant type. The three transplant types are syngeneic, autologous, and allogeneic. In a syngeneic transplant the donor is the identical twin of the recipient.

In an autologous transplant the patient's own stem cells are collected, usually when the patient is in remission. The stem cells are sometimes treated in vitro with agents to remove any residual tumor cells. The cells are then cryopreserved (Kemshead et al., 1987; Linch & Burnett, 1986; Yeager et al., 1986). At a later date, the conditioning regimen is initiated followed by infusion of the previously collected cells.

In an allogeneic transplant the donor is a related or unrelated individual whose tissue type matches that of the recipient as closely as possible. If a suitable family member donor is not available, the search for a donor

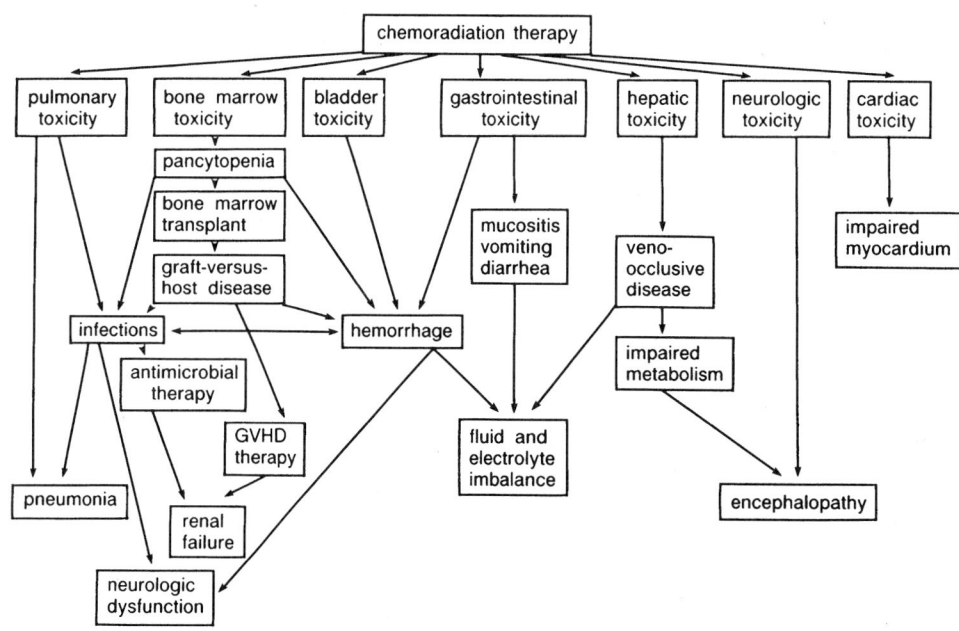

FIGURE 27–2. The interrelationships among the major acute bone marrow transplantation (BMT) complications, etiologies, and treatments. (From Ford, R. C., & Ballard, B. [1988]. Acute complications after bone marrow transplantation. *Seminars in Oncology Nursing, 4,* 15–24. Reproduced by permission.)

Autologous Marrow Transplant

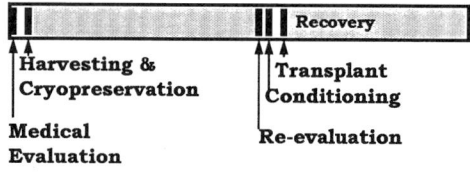

Allogeneic PBSC Transplant

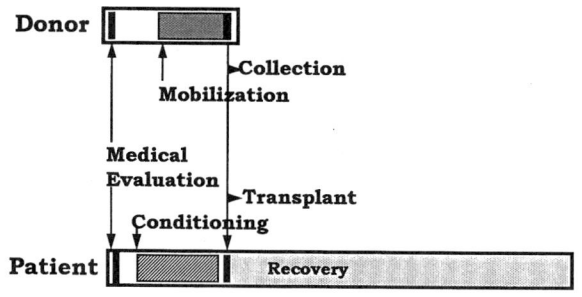

Autologous PBSC Transplant

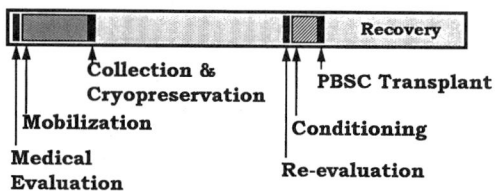

Allogeneic Marrow Transplant

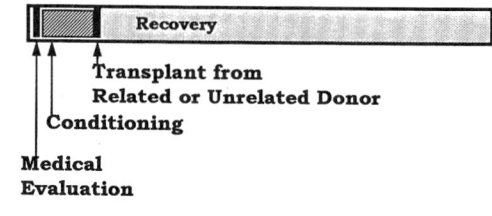

FIGURE 27–3. Schedules for autologous and allogeneic marrow transplants.

in the general population can be initiated through a bone marrow registry (Hansen, Anasetti, Petersdorf, Clift, & Martin, 1994). There is a National Marrow Donor Program in the United States and similar programs in England, Canada, Germany, and France. Donors with the same ethnic background as the patient are more likely to match.

It is preferable to use a related donor rather than an unrelated donor even if the human leukocyte antigens (HLA) match is identical in both cases. This is because the currently used HLA markers (see discussion below), although considered very important, are not the only markers of tissue compatibility (Christiansen et al., 1993). It is thought that other markers, currently unknown, must be present, since related transplants are associated with fewer complications than unrelated transplants. Transplants can be performed with HLA-mismatched cells if there are no other donors.

Each type of transplant has unique toxicities and complications. A complication unique to allogeneic transplantation is graft-versus-host disease (GVHD), and therapies used to prevent this disease increase the period of immunosuppression. Both autologous and syngeneic transplants have a higher relapse rate than allogeneic transplants, in which a possible "graft-versus-leukemia" effect has been hypothesized (Butturni, Bortin, & Gale, 1987; Weiden et al., 1981). Analysis of relapse rates suggests that the immunocompetent cells in the allogeneic graft eliminate residual host leukemia cells beyond the eradication of these cells by the conditioning regimen. It has also been noted that patients who develop GVHD have a lower incidence of recurrent leukemia (Sullivan et al., 1987).

TISSUE TYPING AND ABO COMPATIBILITY

To understand how the most appropriate donor is selected, an overview of the tissue typing process is necessary. The ABO system and the HLA (human leukocyte antigen) system are the two histocompatibility systems considered in matching donor to recipient. In searching for a marrow donor, the HLA are identified from blood drawn from the patient and all potential donors (Fig. 27-4). Two tests are used to determine HLA match. Through serotyping the class I antigens, HLA-A, B, and C are detected. The HLA-A, B, and C loci can be identified through a cytotoxic assay using anti-HLA antibodies. Until recently the class II antigen, HLA-D, was identified through mixed lymphocyte culture (MLC). Increasingly this test is being replaced by typing of HLA-DR/DQ alleles at the DNA level (van Leeuwen et al., 1994). This testing, known as oligonucleotide genotyping (OG), achieves more definitive matching because it is more highly sensitive and precise (Baxter-Lowe, Eckels, Casper, Hunter, & Gorski, 1991). OG involves a two-step process using new genetic technology: (1) amplification of HLA genes with the polymerase chain reaction (PCR), and (2) identification of specific sequences in the amplified products with a oligonucleotide probe.

The ABO blood antigens are also identified prior to transplant. A difference in ABO blood groups between

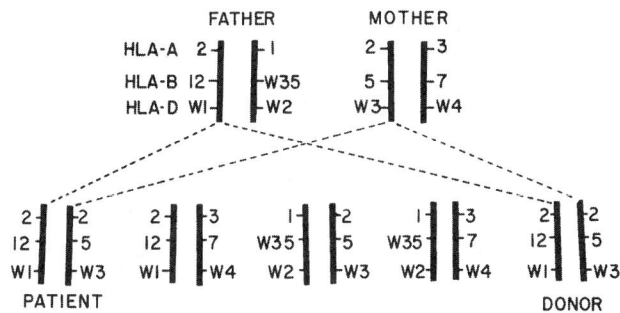

FIGURE 27-4. Example of the possible combinations of the human leukocyte antigen (HLA) region of chromosome 6 passed to a patient and siblings from the patient's parents. The patient and donor have inherited the same haplotypes and thus are HLA genotypically identical.

patient and donor will not interfere with donor selection; however, it does present unique clinical problems. The marrow may have to be depleted of red blood cells to prevent a hemolytic reaction caused by antibodies still circulating from the patient's original marrow. Usually the patient will undergo a plasma exchange to eliminate antibodies against the ABO group of the donor. The patient's plasma can be run through a column of synthetic antigens that attract and remove the ABO antibodies (Bensinger, 1984). The patient's own plasma is then returned missing only the ABO antibodies. After engraftment, the patient will become the ABO type of their donor.

DISEASES TREATED

A variety of both malignant and nonmalignant diseases can be treated with transplantation (Franco & Gould, 1994) (see Table 27-2). Allogeneic transplants are used for both malignant and nonmalignant diseases, although acute myelogenous leukemia (AML), acute lymphocytic leukemia (ALL), and chronic myelogenous leukemia (CML) are the most frequently treated diseases (Franco & Gould, 1994; Wujcik & Downs, 1992). Bortin and Horowitz (1992) report 16

TABLE 27-2. *Diseases Treated With Transplantation*

ACQUIRED DISEASES	GENETIC DISEASES
Aplastic anemia	Thallassemia
AML	Sickle cell disease
ALL	Combined
CML	immunodeficiency disease
Myelodysplastic disorders	Wiskott-Aldrich syndrome
Myeloproliferative disorders	Osteopetrosis
Multiple myeloma	Storage diseases
Lymphomas	White blood cell diseases
Hodgkins disease	Fanconi's anemia
Non-hodgkins lymphoma	
Solid tumors	
Breast cancer	
Germ-cell cancer	
Neuroblastoma	
AIDS	

per cent of allogeneic transplants were performed for aplastic anemia and other nonmalignant diseases. This number is increasing yearly.

Usually autologous transplants are used to treat malignant diseases (Wujcik & Downs, 1992). Although autologous transplants are used in the treatment of leukemias and lymphomas, this modality is being heavily explored for patients with solid tumors such as breast cancer, ovarian cancer, and germ-cell tumors (Crouch & Ross, 1994).

SURVIVAL RATES AFTER TRANSPLANTATION

Transplantation may offer the only hope for cure or an increased chance of survival in contrast with conventional therapy for the patient with cancer. For example, chemotherapy or chemoradiotherapy followed by marrow transplantation is the only known cure for patients with CML (Barnett, Eaves, & Eaves, 1994). Thomas et al. (1986) reported that patients with CML in chronic phase who receive an allogeneic transplant from a sibling have an 80 per cent disease-free survival at 2 years. This is compared with a similar group of patients with CML in chronic phase who have a 44 per cent survival with conventional treatment. Today survival rates of 80 to 90 per cent for patients with CML following transplant are not uncommon (Barnett, Eaves, & Eaves, 1994).

Many factors influence disease-free survival after transplantation (see Table 27–3). Nonmalignant states such as aplastic anemia, SCIDS, and thalassemia have long term survival rates ranging from 50 to 80 per cent compared with a malignant state such as AML, which ranges from 20 to 60 per cent long-term survival overall (Franco & Gould, 1994).

Success of transplantation also depends on the stage of the disease. For example, one center reported a 72 per cent 5-year survival for patients with breast cancer stage II following transplant compared with a 17 to 28 per cent for those with stage IV (Crouch &

TABLE 27–3. *Factors Influencing Disease-Free Survival Following Bone Marrow or PBSC Transplantation*

The disease treated
Disease stage
Phase (chronic, accelerated, blast)
Time since first diagnosed
Relapse
Remission
Previous therapy
Chemotherapy
Radiotherapy
Blood transfusions
Biologic response modifiers
Type of transplant
Preparative regimen
Purged vs. nonpurged marrow
Age
Medical status at time of transplant

Ross, 1994). Children with ALL who had been treated with autologous transplant and who had a remission greater than 48 months had an 80 to 90 per cent survival versus a 50 per cent survival for those with a shorter remission of 24 to 48 months (Ritz, Ramsay, & Kersey, 1994). In addition, previous therapy the patient received may affect the success of transplant. Previous chemotherapy, for example, may have decreased the functioning of vital organs such as heart or kidneys and make complications during transplant more likely. A patient with aplastic anemia who receives a blood transfusion prior to transplant has a much lower chance of long-term survival, and a patient with CML who receives a trial of α-interferon therapy may alter chances of survival by delaying transplantation (Barnett, Eaves, & Eaves, 1994).

Timing of transplant is important. Patients with AML transplanted in first remission have a higher survival rate (45 to 60 per cent) than do those treated in relapse (20 to 30 per cent) (Franco & Gould, 1994). Transplanting CML in chronic rather than accelerated or blast phase dramatically increases survival statistics.

The type of transplant, the specifics of the preparative conditioning regimen, as well as whether the marrow or PBSCs are manipulated, that is, purged or altered with newer genetic procedures, will have an impact on the success of transplant. For example, an allogeneic transplant for the patient with leukemia confers a "graft versus leukemia" effect as discussed previously. Selecting a conditioning regimen that results in the highest cell kill without lethal effects on vital organs is critical.

The clinical status of the patient when transplantation is initiated has a significant effect on complications and survival. Last, the likelihood of long-term disease-free survival decreases with age. However, despite lower survival statistics, transplantation can be a treatment option to patients in their fifth and sixth decades of life. In estimating survival rates for an individual patient, all of the influencing factors must be considered.

THE TRANSPLANTATION PROCESS

For patients, deciding to have a transplant is a significant event, not unlike embarking on a long, challenging journey. For health care providers the process is complex and demanding. As a guide, the transplant process has been separated into seven phases (see Table 27–4). The process begins when the patient considers treatment and concludes either when the patient has achieved optimal recovery or succumbs to transplant complications or disease recurrence. Each phase has its own purpose and character and its unique challenges and dangers. A description of each phase will include the goals of the phase, the experience of the patient and family, as well as psychologic and ethical issues. This is followed by medical treatment and management of complications.

PHASE 1: PLANNING AHEAD

DESCRIPTION

This phase begins when the patient first considers transplant as a treatment option. The goals of this phase are making the decision to accept transplantation, gaining access to treatment, and making preparations needed to initiate treatment. One of the most anxiety-provoking aspects of the pretransplant periods is in deciding whether to undertake the transplant at all. The patient is confronted with possible outcomes: (1) early death without transplantation, (2) death from the transplantation procedure, (3) later recurrence of disease after transplant, (4) survival with chronic complications and side effects, and (5) lifelong cure (Hare, Skinner, & Kliewer, 1989). The chances of surviving (see discussion under Survival Rates After Transplantation) may persuade a patient to avoid the risks and undergo conventional therapy, thereby giving up hope for a cure.

Patients and family members use information seeking as a way of coping with their threatening events and perceptions of uncertainty (Coxon, 1989; Derdiarian, 1986, 1987). Nurses assist in providing information and guiding the patient through the preparation for transplant (Downs, 1994). This may include patient teaching about the transplant therapy, directing a patient to resources, or allowing the patient to share feelings and concerns regarding the decision to undergo a transplant.

The patients' typical psychologic reactions unfold along with the activities of this phase. Many patients feel that making the decision to have a transplant marks a major turning point in their lives. They experience the elation and hope of achieving a cure. At the same time they may be denying the potential problems associated with transplant. Ambivalence and mild to severe anxiety is common at this stage (Wellisch & Wolcott, 1994). Feelings of uncertainty may linger even after the transplant decision has been made. These are all considered normal responses during this period.

Making arrangements to initiate treatment typically includes assessing financial coverage and resources, making plans for temporary relocation, selecting a family member or friend to act as a caregiver during treatment and recovery, and possibly completing special dental, nutrition, or fertility preparations. Depending on the type of transplant, a donor is selected and the mobilization, collection, and storage of marrow or peripheral blood stem cells is planned.

Allocation of resources is a major ethical issue faced by both the patient and the health care provider. Marrow transplantation has the potential to benefit many, but the resources to provide this high-cost treatment are scarce (Downs, 1994). After establishing eligibility for treatment, access to treatment may be based on financial criteria.

CHOOSING A TREATMENT CENTER

After the decision has been made to select bone marrow transplant as the treatment for disease, selecting a site for treatment becomes a priority. As many organizations that provide oncology therapy have entered the field of marrow transplantation, the selection of a transplant center has become a decision that can exacerbate apprehension and uncertainty for the patient and family (Wellisch & Wolcott, 1994). Generally there are four factors that affect a patient's decision to select a given center for transplant: the opinion of the referring physician, the geographic location of the nearest center, insurance reimbursement issues, and personal preference. As many hematologists and oncologists have received training in the field, an individual physician may develop a professional preference for treatment protocols offered at one cancer treatment center but not at another. Because transplant can mean an extended period of treatment, many patients wish to remain as close to home as possible to minimize disruption of family or work routines.

FINANCIAL ARRANGEMENTS

Patients and families often report that financial considerations are among the most significant stressors in preparing for transplant. The issue of insurance coverage

TABLE 27–4. *Transplant Phases*

TRANSPLANT PHASE	DEFINITION
Planning ahead	This phase begins with the patient considering transplant as a treatment option, selecting a treatment center and includes the preparation needed to initiate treatment.
Preparation	The patient arrives at the treatment center and begins the process of medical evaluation, orientation, informed consent, and preparation to start conditioning. Family members are educationally prepared to assume the caregiver role.
Conditioning	High-dose chemotherapy and/or radiotherapy is administered.
Transplant	Stem cells from previous marrow harvesting or PBSC collection are infused.
Waiting for engraftment	Close monitoring, supportive treatment and management of complications while waiting for signs the stem cells are engrafting.
Engraftment and early recovery	The phase after the first signs of engraftment when the patient is recovering immune and hematopoietic function. Close monitoring, supportive treatment and management of complications. Preparation for return to referring physician or center.
Long-term recovery	After discharge from the transplant center the referring physician assumes care of the patient. Management of possible late complications and re-establishing living patterns.

for the medical treatment aside, patients and families must often travel some distance to the transplant center. Upon arrival, there are housing expenses, deposits for utilities and phone, car rental, and unanticipated expenses. Patients most often must absorb the costs of maintaining two residences simultaneously. Eligibility for public assistance and the feasibility of fund-raising activities may be explored either before or during transplant. Social workers are very helpful in sorting out these options with patients and families (Kennedy, 1993).

ADVANCE DIRECTIVES

In many states, patients are encouraged to complete an "Advance Directive" such as "Durable Power of Attorney For Health Care" upon admission to the hospital. A living will is another example of an advance directive. Completing these documents enables a patient and family to specify a person who shall be legally responsible for making decisions about medical treatment should the patient become incapable of making decisions. For marrow transplant patients, this is an important point of discussion because the risk of disabling complications can be high. While social workers often assist the patient in completing this task, it is important for the physicians on the transplant team to be aware of the patient's wishes with regard to the use of life-prolonging measures.

SELECTING A CAREGIVER

Assistance with daily activities such as food preparation, laundry, bathing and grooming, and transportation to appointments requires the assistance of a full-time caregiver (generally a family member) whose time and energy is devoted entirely to the patient during the pretransplant, peritransplant, and posttransplant period. Because it is now possible for a patient to receive much of the transplant regimen outside of the hospital setting, the caregiver faces additional responsibilities. These may include dispensing oral medications and administering intravenous fluids, antibiotics, and antiviral agents via an infusion pump. Such therapy also requires the maintenance of a central venous catheter, with daily dressing changes and flushing. In addition, the caregiver must continually assess the patient in the home setting for fever, nausea or vomiting, diarrhea, or other changes that should be reported to the transplant team. Such sophisticated care can be delivered only by a responsible adult who has been educated by the transplant team to assume this role. Due to the complex nature of these activities, additional responsibilities for the caregiver (such as child care) should be minimized as much as possible.

DONOR SELECTION

Before a treatment regimen for allogeneic transplant can be chosen, a decision must be made regarding the selection of a donor. The odds of a patient matching a sibling are 1 in 4, resulting in only 35 to 40 per cent of patients having a matched sibling. Therefore, the search for a donor may be extended by typing parents, aunts, uncles, and cousins. If no match is found within the family, the search may lead to the National Marrow Donor Program (NMDP), which participates in a worldwide computer database containing the HLA typing of more than one million people (Welte, 1994). The decision to undertake a search for an unrelated donor is made in concert with the patient's primary physician and with a physician at the transplant center, who serves as a liaison between the patient and the National Marrow Donor Program. Enlisting a search for an unrelated donor is an expensive process costing $10,000 per identified match, while donor procurement or successful completion of donor work-up and harvest may cost $27,000 (National Marrow Donor Program, personal interview, October 1994). Because of this expense many patients are excluded from this opportunity due to lack of financial resources.

Currently, upwards of 50 per cent of those who initiate this search are fortunate enough to find an HLA-matched donor. While this is true for Caucasian patients, the numbers of matches found in the registry for African-American or Asian patients is much lower (Fig. 27–5). The National Marrow Donor Program is working to increase the number of donors available for this population. Once an unrelated donor has been identified, the individual is contacted, then undergoes counseling to confirm the potential donor's willingness to donate marrow. If the donor is agreeable, the patient is notified while the donor undergoes blood testing for viruses and a physical examination. When this is complete, a date for transplant may be set. Participation in the National Marrow Donor Program requires that the identity of the unrelated donor be kept confidential until 1 year after transplant to protect the privacy of the donor. A patient may be informed of the following details regarding the donor: age, sex, geographic location, ABO compatibility, and cytomegalovirus (CMV) status (NMDP, 1994).

PHASE 2: PREPARATION

DESCRIPTION

The patient's arrival at the treatment center marks the beginning of this phase. The goals are (1) medical evaluation, (2) orientation to the center and the transplant process, (3) completion of the informed consent process, (4) preparation of the family caregiver, and (5) establishing central venous access (Keller, 1994).

The patient undergoes a medical evaluation that confirms the treatment plan or protocol appropriate for the patient. As patients await test results, uncertainty and restlessness may be apparent. The approach to the patient and family must include sensitivity to the fears and anxieties that influence them (Hare et al., 1989). The treatment plan is outlined in detail for the patient including risks, potential complications, and anticipated duration of care. After the patient signs the consent forms, treatment can begin.

Despite the detailed information about the risks of the treatment, denial of potential problems is likely to persist (Wellisch & Wolcott, 1994). It is important to support hope throughout the transplant process (Ersek, 1992).

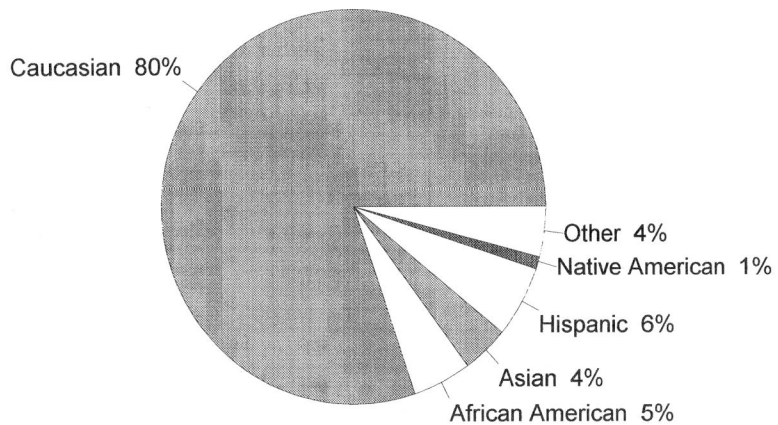

FIGURE 27–5. Donors registered with the U.S. National Marrow Donor Program (NMDP). As of July 1, 1993, 913,000 donors were registered. (Data from Hansen, J. A., Anasetti, C., Petersdorf, E., Clift, R. A., & Martin, P. J. [1994]. Marrow transplants from unrelated donors. *Transplantation Proceedings, 26,* 1710–1712.)

EVALUATION FOR TRANSPLANT

The evaluation or "work-up" may last from 2 to 10 days, depending on the number of tests that were performed prior to arrival, the complexity of the tests, and the clinical decisions that arise when all of the results are compiled. Patients with solid tumors (lymphomas, breast cancer, etc.) will be restaged utilizing the same type of diagnostic scan that was used in diagnosing the disease. Blood will be drawn to assess for hepatitis A, B, and C. The presence of hepatitis places the patient at increased risk for veno-occlusive disease and for acute hepatitis during the transplant process, and so may exclude a patient from transplant. Blood will also be drawn to look for antibodies against cytomegalovirus, the herpes simplex virus. The presence of these antibodies indicates that the patient may experience a reactivation of these viruses during the period of immunosuppression, so a regimen of prophylactic medications may be considered. A test to detect the human immunodeficiency virus (HIV) will be done on the patient and the donor. The presence of HIV is an exclusion for transplant, unless it is the primary diagnosis for treatment. Blood will be drawn from both the patient and donor for HLA testing to confirm that a match has been found. Blood will also be drawn to confirm the ABO type of the patient and donor. The patient will undergo pulmonary function testing, which will serve as a baseline should pulmonary compromise occur posttransplant.

Height, weight, and a baseline nutritional assessment should be done. The opportunity to counsel the patient regarding food and fluid intake during mucositis should be taken, in addition to a review of methods of coping with nausea and vomiting. Because the use of prophylactic antibiotics during the period of acute immunosuppression is widely accepted, the most likely cause of infection for the patient would be from the normal flora of the mouth and gastrointestinal tract. Therefore, prior to therapy, a thorough dental examination should be done to examine for dental caries, abscess, or periodontal disease, and dental treatment should be completed before the initiation of conditioning.

ESTABLISHING ELIGIBILITY

It is important to be aware that some patients who arrive at a transplant center will not meet eligibility criteria of transplant protocols at the completion of this workup process. Elevated liver function tests, whether caused by hepatitis or by the malignancy itself, place a patient in unacceptably high risk of liver failure (Shuhart & McDonald, 1994). Elevated creatinine and BUN levels may indicate renal failure (often caused by prior therapy), which contributes to renal failure during transplant and therefore to increased risk of mortality. The bone marrow donor may have medical problems that preclude him or her from donating. Furthermore, the malignancy itself may have progressed to the stage that any therapy is unlikely to prolong or improve survival.

INFORMED CONSENT

It is generally agreed that informed consent is a shared decision-making process between the patient and the health care provider (Downs, 1994). During this discussion, the physician should disclose the following: the nature and character of the proposed treatment, the anticipated results of the proposed treatment, the recognized possible alternative forms of treatment (including nontreatment), the serious possible risks or complications, and anticipated benefits of the treatment (Winters, Glass, & Sakurai, 1993). The goal of informed consent is to convey to the patient and family the genuine implications of test results and treatment plans. The nurse may serve as an intermediary in assessing the patient's comprehension of complex medical facts. The physician has the primary responsibility to obtain informed consent before treatment is initiated.

EDUCATION OF PATIENT AND CAREGIVER

The educational care plan needs to encompass the transplant process and all of its components (Walker,

Roethker, & Martin, 1994). The content of information desired by patients and caregivers includes (1) services and resources, (2) the patient's disease, (3) physiologic effects of marrow transplantation, (4) expectations of the caregiver role, and (5) how to manage care at home after transplant (Kristjanson & Ashcroft, 1994; McDonald, Stetz, Compton, & Strickland, 1994). A variety of educational strategies is required to meet both the learning needs and learning preferences of patients and family members. By having differing modes of instruction available during the appropriate transplant phase, the learning readiness and preference aspects of education are met. Information overload is minimized, and attention is given to individual ways of learning. Information guides to prepare patients for procedures such as peripheral blood stem cell (PBSC) collection or total body irradiation are an invaluable educational component (Dreifke & DeMeyer, 1992; Walker, Roethke, & Martin, 1994).

The period leading up to transplant is an important time for the caregiver to be prepared for the responsibilities that he or she will assume once therapy has begun. This preparation may include formal training in symptom management, medication administration, and the operation of an infusion pump. Written reference materials that enable the caregiver to decide whether a new symptom identified at home requires reporting, prompt care, or emergency care are provided. The goal of such a program is to assist the caregiver in maintaining a safe environment for the patient.

COLLECTION OF PERIPHERAL BLOOD STEM CELLS

Recent technology has adapted the technique of pheresis (which has been used for many years in kidney dialysis and granulocyte collection) to that of collecting pluripotent progenitor cells—also known as peripheral blood stem cells (Jassak & Riley, 1994) as an alternate to marrow harvest. This method of treatment is divided into three different stages: mobilization, collection and reinfusion. Mobilizing stem cells is achieved by administering growth factors, chemotherapy, or both (Walker et al., 1994). This causes the stem cells to leave the tissues they normally occupy and to circulate in the bloodstream (Wright, 1994). As a patient's white cell count begins to climb, the stem cells are collected using the pheresis machine (Hooper & Santas, 1993). An adequate quantity of cells are generally collected in one to four pheresis sessions. Occasionally a patient must undergo more than one cycle of mobilization to collect enough stem cells to proceed to transplant. Once pheresed, autologous stem cells are cryopreserved (frozen), whereas allogeneic stem cells are infused immediately following collection. Chemotherapy administered in this manner serves the dual purpose of stimulating the stem cells to circulate and reducing the tumor load. Once the patient has recovered from mobilization, conditioning for transplant can be initiated.

HARVEST OF STEM CELLS FROM BONE MARROW

Stem cells may also be collected through direct harvest of the bone marrow. A patient being evaluated for autologous transplant using this method must be in remission. When remission is confirmed, a marrow harvest is scheduled. For an allogeneic donor, a thorough physical examination is required before the harvest is scheduled to proceed.

Bone marrow harvest is a surgical procedure requiring general or spinal anesthesia. Multiple aspirations from the anterior and posterior iliac crests of the pelvic bone are performed (Fig. 27–6). The volume of marrow is determined by the size of the donor, with a pediatric donor usually yielding a volume of 300 ml and a male adult donor often yielding a volume of more than 1000 ml. The marrow is filtered for fat emboli and fragments of bone. If the marrow is to be used for an allogeneic transplant, the marrow is treated and reinfused within 24 hours of harvest. If the marrow is to be used for an autologous reinfusion, it is cryopreserved and stored until conditioning is complete.

PHASE 3: CONDITIONING

DESCRIPTION

During this phase high-dose chemotherapy, radiation therapy, or both are initiated. Patients are given medications to manage the side effects of the conditioning regimen. The goals of this phase are to (1) complete the conditioning therapy, (2) prevent and relieve the symptoms associated with this therapy, and (3) monitor the patient for the development of early complications.

According to Wellisch and Wolcott (1994) this is one of two phases in which patients experience the most severe psychologic responses. Patients report that persistent pain and psychologic distress occur during this phase (Gaston-Johansson, Franco, & Zimmerman, 1992). This is the point where the patient recognizes there is no going back after the chemotherapy and/or radiation begins. The patient's anxiety heightens and dependency needs escalate during this phase.

CONDITIONING REGIMENS

Chemotherapy is the major component of most conditioning regimens. During the first decade of marrow transplantation, cyclophosphamide was the mainstay chemotherapy. However, because patients continued to relapse, much research went into developing different combinations of agents. Research is currently being conducted to determine dosing, timing, and sequencing of a variety of chemotherapeutic drug combinations (Appelbaum, 1989; Bearman et al., 1988). Currently, the focus is on agents used in conventional treatment. These drugs, given in high doses that ablate marrow function, enable the greatest possibility of tumor kill (Peterson & Bearman, 1994). Agents that are currently being used include cyclophosphamide, dimethylbusulfan, cytarabine, etopi-

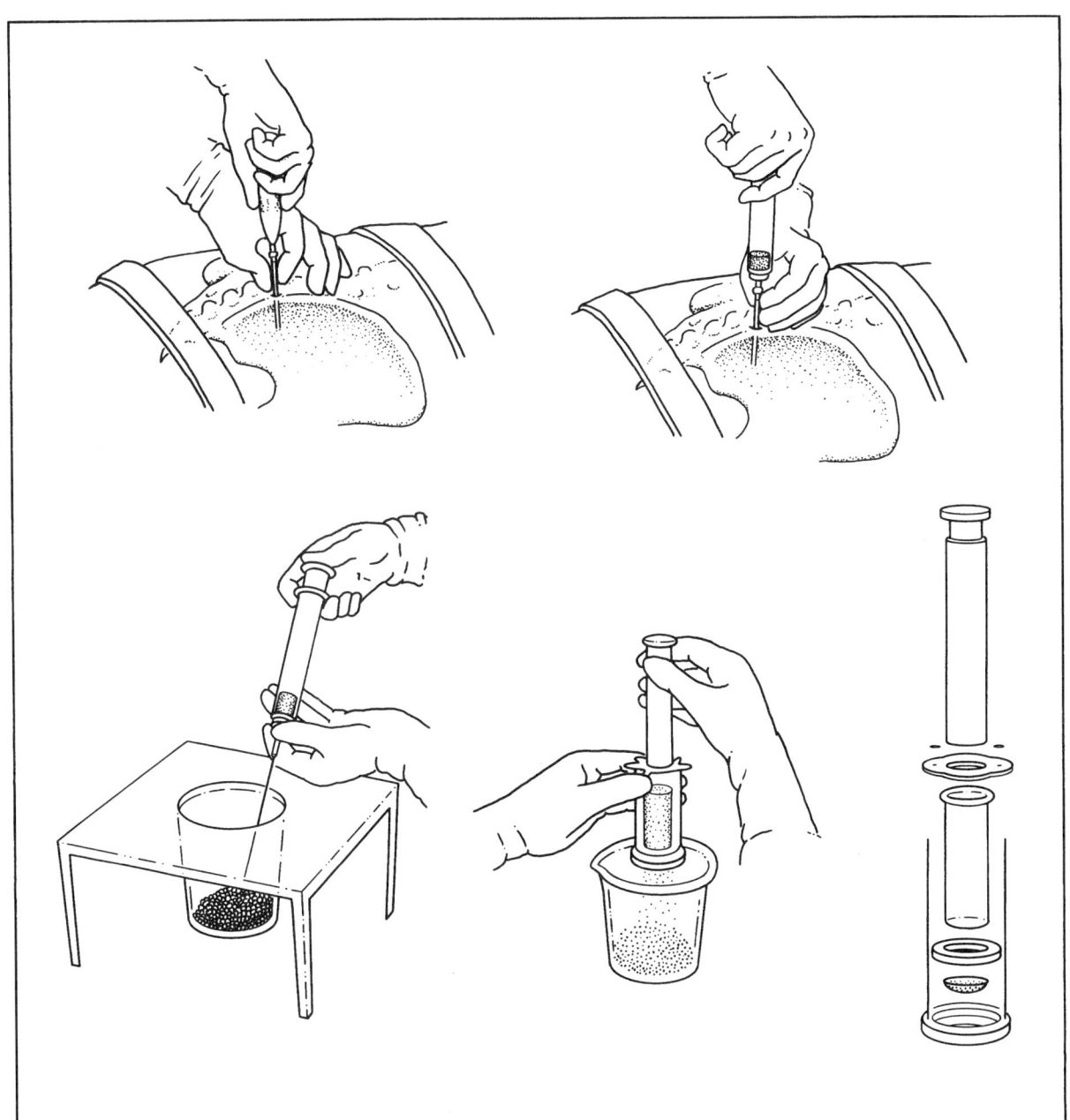

FIGURE 27–6. Sequence of steps in aspirations of marrow from donor. A large-bore needle is placed in the posterior illac crest, and multiple aspirations of 3 to 5 ml of marrow are performed. The marrow is placed in a collecting beaker, drawn up in a large syringe, and forced through a coarse metal grid to remove bone and fat particles. The marrow is then placed in a blood administration bag and administered through the patient's central venous catheter.

side, melphalan, thiotepa, cisplatin, bleomycin, 5-flurouracil and vincristine (Appelbaum, 1989; Jagannath et al., 1989; Kanfer et al, 1987; Riddell et al., 1988; Schmitz et al., 1988; Whedon, 1991).

Radiation continues to play a major role in transplantation. Initially, radiation was delivered in one large dose to the entire body. However, there was significant morbidity and subsequent mortality related to the single high dose. Based on the toxicity of single-dose, radiation dosing was changed to be given one time per day for 6 to 7 days (fractionated) (Peterson, Finn, & Bearman, 1994; Small, 1991). This schedule evolved to dosing multiple times per day for 3 to 4 days. Each change in the type of administration has allowed for higher total doses to be delivered with less side effects. For patients who have some major organ compromise before transplant, the fractionated irradiation causes significant toxicity. This led to the development of total lymphoid irradiation and total marrow irradiation in which major organs are shielded for the radiation (Whedon, 1991b). The goal of shielding is to eradicate disease while maintaining organ function. However, there is a risk that residual disease may remain in the shielded organs.

All patients experience side effects during the days of conditioning, including nausea, vomiting, diarrhea, and the beginning of mucositis. Other less common side effects are tumor lysis syndrome, hemorrhagic cystitis, and some drug-specific toxicities. The harmful impact of conditioning therapy is not limited to the immediate treatment period. Complications may occur weeks after transplant to as late as 3 to 10 years following the procedure. These late effects include the development of veno-occlusive disease, integumentary toxicities, capillary leak syndrome, secondary malignancies, cataracts, fibrotic pulmonary disease, cardiomyopathy, and various endocrine and neurologic complications.

CONDITIONING-RELATED COMPLICATIONS

Nausea, Vomiting, Diarrhea, Mucositis, and Anorexia. Gastrointestinal side effects are common during and following conditioning therapy. Levels of toxicity depend on the treatment combination (Peterson & Bearman, 1994). Nausea and vomiting are the initial side effects of the conditioning period. Irradiation typically produces less nausea and vomiting than high-dose chemotherapy (Shuhart & McDonald, 1994). Scheduled antiemetics given either orally or intravenously depending on the emetigenesis of the conditioning agents being utilized are recommended during this period. Because the antiemetics can cause profound sedation, nursing assessment and intervention needs to balance antiemetic relief with maintaining safety. Nursing can support and educate patients in utilizing a variety of coping mechanism such as visualization, distraction, and hypnosis to deal with the frustration of nausea and vomiting. Diarrhea occurs most notably during irradiation, and agents to slow motility are given to prevent significant fluid and electrolyte imbalances and to promote patient comfort (Vanacek, 1991).

Mucositis is a side effect that all transplant patients experience. Irradiation therapy causes more severe mucosal damage than regimens that include only chemotherapy (McDonald, Shulman, Sullivan, & Spencer, 1986). Mucositis begins around the day of transplant with dry mouth, sore throat, and thickening saliva (McDonald et al., 1986). Mucositis then progresses with increasing secretion of oral mucus and development of pain that often requires narcotic analgesia (McGuire et al., 1993). Infections often complicate the symptoms and bring added risk of hemorrhage. Mucositis can become severe enough that occlusion of the airway occurs and patients require intubation for oxygenation until the edema subsides. Frequent assessment of the oral cavity is a routine part of nursing care. In a multicenter survey it was found that there is no standard oral hygiene regimen for the prevention and treatment of mucositis. The agents most commonly utilized are normal saline solution and chlorohexidine rinses (Ezzone, Jolly, Reployle, Kapoor, & Totschka, 1993; Raybould et al., 1994). Tools that may be utilized include oral suction catheters and toothettes. Mucositis does not subside until the marrow graft starts to function and the new immune system begins to heal the tissue (McDonald et

al., 1986). Pain control varies on the extent of the mucositis. Agents may include topical anesthetics and intravenous narcotics (Peterson & Bearman, 1994). Patient-controlled analgesia pumps are especially effective in the control of pain. Recent studies have shown that with the use of growth factors, mucositis does not resolve any sooner (Peterson & Bearman, 1994). If oral pain and lesions persist after engraftment, oral infection or acute GVHD should be suspected (Kolbinson, Schubert, Flourney, & Truelove, 1988).

Anorexia is another common gastrointestinal side effect of conditioning therapy. Mucositis makes it difficult for many patients to maintain adequate oral intake. Many institutions currently utilize total parenteral nutrition (TPN) during this phase (Mawaji, Canten, Hartman, & McKinlay, 1992). However, with the emphasis on cost containment and the increased risk of sepsis in patients receiving TPN, dietitians are examining a variety of other ways to maintain nutritional intake. The nutrition options being examined range from intravenous hydration and a soft diet to tube feedings with enteral supplements.

Hemorrhagic Cystitis. Hemorrhagic cystitis is a complication of high-dose cyclophosphamide occurring in up to 13 per cent of patients (Peterson & Bearman, 1994). A metabolite of cyclophosphamide, acrolein, irritates the bladder lining and causes diffuse bleeding (Ballard, 1991). Hemorrhagic cystitis may be greater in regimens of busulfan and cytoxan than conditioning with cytoxan and total body irradiation (Peterson & Bearman, 1994). The goal is to prevent acrolein from having prolonged contact with the lining of the bladder. Preventive measures include intravenous hydration, at two times maintenance, along with continuous bladder irrigation via a three-way Foley catheter. Another intervention is the use of Mesna prophylactically during the infusion of cyclophosphamide. There are no data that delineate one treatment choice as better than the other at this time (Peterson & Bearman, 1994; Ballard, 1991; Lin et al., 1993). If hemorrhagic cystitis develops, the patient will have severe hematuria ranging from microscopic to frank blood, bladder spasms, and clots (Ballard, 1991). In severe cases treatment includes hydration, frequent platelet transfusions, continuous bladder irrigation with formaldehyde, or alum being added. A urology consult may be necessary for cauterization and removal of clots from the bladder via laparoscopy. Pain medications are necessary if the patient is having frequent spasms or is being irrigated manually through the urinary catheter.

Syndrome of Inappropriate Antidiuretic Hormone (SIADH). Cyclophosphamide may cause water retention via the syndrome of inappropriate antidiuretic hormone (SIADH) or may paradoxically cause significant dehydration by inducing nephrogenic diabetes insipidus (DI) (Wujcik et al., 1994). SIADH leads to weight gain, hyponatremia, and a decrease in the amount and an increase in the concentration of urine (Lin et al., 1993). This process begins 24 hours after the initial dose of cytoxan and typically resolves 48 hours after the last dose (Wujcik et al., 1994). Patients may be symptomatic or develop some pulmonary compromise if the fluid and electrolyte changes are rapid. Thorough nursing assessment of the patient's weight, lung sounds, and respiratory rate coupled with the monitoring of laboratory results are key to the process of early intervention. Medical therapy includes diuresis and variation of hydration (Lin et al., 1993; Wujcik et al., 1994). Diabetes insipidus, evidenced by dilute polyuria (potentially up to 10 L per day), occurs within 24 hours of the initial cytoxan dose and resolves once the blood levels of cytoxan decrease (Lin et al., 1993; Wujick et al., 1994). The medical therapy involves hydration replacement that is matched for the character and quantity of the fluid lost, typically hypotonic saline or dextrose (Lin et al., 1993; Wujcik et al., 1994). Frequent nursing assessment including volume and character of urine, orthostatic blood pressure, heart rate, weight changes, and review of laboratory results are necessary to manage the rapid changes in fluid and electrolyte balance that occur with DI.

Tumor Lysis Syndrome. Acute tumor lysis syndrome occurs when a large tumor load combined with high-dose conditioning therapy brings a rapid lysing of the tumor cells (Dietz & Flaherty, 1993). This results in the development of hyperkalemia, hyperphosphatemia, hyperuricemia, and hypocalcemia. Acute renal failure may also develop. Renal insufficiency and failure is prevented by aggressive hydration, alkalization of urine, and administration of allopurinal to decrease the uric acid levels (Dietz & Flaherty, 1993; Wujcik et al., 1994). Most institutions will place patients in relapse on allopurinal prior to initiating therapy to prevent TLS.

Veno-Occlusive Disease. Veno-occlusive disease is a disease of the liver, rarely seen in patient populations that do not receive high-dose chemoradiation therapy. It is a common conditioning toxicity occurring in 21 to 50 per cent of all patients (Wujcik et al., 1994; Shuhart & McDonald, 1994). Fifty per cent of the patients with VOD die with the liver disease as the primary or secondary cause of death (Lin et al., 1993). Patients at highest risk are those receiving a mismatched or unrelated transplant coupled with an intense conditioning regimen. Liver abnormalities prior to the initiation of conditioning therapy is the single most important factor in the development of veno-occlusive disease (Lin et al., 1993; Shuhart & McDonald, 1994; Wujcik et al., 1994). Many centers will postpone marrow transplant until the LFTs are within normal limits.

Veno-occlusive disease results from the synergistic effect of combination high-dose chemoradiation. Toxic damage to the venules leading out of the liver and subsequent fibrin deposition and debris collection results in impaired hepatic blood flow and occlusion (Lin et al., 1993; Shuhart & McDonald, 1994; Wujcik et al., 1994). Clinical manifestations include third spacing of fluid, abdominal distention from ascites, right upper quadrant pain, respiratory compromise, intravascular volume loss, elevated liver enzymes, and impaired hepatic function. With the loss of adequate liver function patients become jaundiced, develop signs and symptoms of encephalopathy, and have problems with coagulopathies (Ballard, 1991; Lin et al., 1993; Shuhart & McDonald, 1994; Wujcik et al., 1994).

VOD occurs within the first 3 weeks after transplantation (Ballard, 1991), although there are anecdotal reports of late VOD in autologous peripheral blood stem cell patients who receive stem cell mobilization less than 1 month prior to initiation of conditioning. This is a complication with insidious onset that requires astute nursing assessment. Keys to the care of these patients include monitoring of fluid and electrolyte balance, twice-daily weights and abdominal girths, adjustment of drug dosages based on hepatic and renal function, assessment for bleeding problems, daily integumentary evaluation and care, and assessment of neurologic status (Ballard, 1991).

There is currently no treatment for VOD. Research concerning anticoagulation with heparin and other coagulation breakdown agents is currently active in many centers. The use of low-dose dopamine has been discontinued because of complications with sodium excretion (Shuhart & McDonald, 1994).

Pulmonary Complications. Pulmonary complications continue to be a major cause of morbidity and mortality in marrow transplant patients. Idiopathic pneumonia syndrome (IPS) is described as diffuse lung injury occurring after marrow transplant for which an infectious etiology is not identified (Clark et al., 1993). Interstitial pneumonitis accounts for approximately 40 per cent of all transplant-related deaths in most large studies (Clark et al., 1993). Approximately 50 per cent of those deaths are the result of IPS (Clark et al., 1993).

IPS has been separated by allogeneic and autologous transplant (Clark et al., 1993). The incidence of IPS following allogeneic transplant is approximately 12 per cent (Clark et al., 1993). The clinical presentation includes dyspnea, nonproductive cough, hypoxemia, and diffuse radiographic infiltrates (Clark et al., 1993). Initial symptoms may range from incidental infiltrates to acute respiratory distress (Clark et al., 1993). Average onset is between days 42 and 49 posttransplant with an early peak within the first 2 weeks (Clark et al., 1993). There remains a low incidence thereafter through day 80 posttransplant (Clark et al., 1993). Within the first 28 days the majority of pneumonias are idiopathic, after which the percentage drops to approximately 20 (Clark et al., 1993).

The incidence of IPS following autologous transplant most likely results from pretransplant conditioning. In approximately 21 per cent of autologous patients, IPS presents as diffuse alveolar hemorrhage (DAH), with a presentation of nonproductive cough, dyspnea, tachypnea, rapid radiographic changes, and intraalveolar blood upon bronchoscopy (Clark et al., 1993; Robbins et al., 1989). With the addition of fevers and diffuse alveolar edema, up to 42 per cent of autologous patients may demonstrate DAH (Crawford & Meyers, 1991). DAH is associated with an age greater than 40 years, total body radiation as part of conditioning, treatment for solid tumors, high fevers, and renal insufficiency or failure (Clark et al., 1993). Onset may occur as early as the first 2 weeks following transplant (Crawford & Meyers, 1991).

Usual medical treatment for idiopathic pneumonias consists of high-dose steroids along with oxygen therapy (Crawford & Hackman, 1993; Chao, Duncan, Long, Horning, & Blume, 1991). As with other post-transplant complications, many research studies are in progress using steroids, cytokines, and various methods of mechanical ventilation to determine the best combination of treatment and support during this period. Researchers are also examining the combination of agents utilized in the conditioning phase to determine the drugs and/or radiation dose with the most tumor kill and least pulmonary toxicity (Peterson & Bearman, 1994). Nursing interventions consist of frequent assessment of breath sounds, assessment of oxygenation and respiratory pattern, and the patient's activity tolerance. Working with the patient to prevent atelectasis by maintaining good pulmonary toilet and encouraging ambulation facilitates gas exchange and enhances oxygenation (Shaffer & Wilson, 1990; Wikle, 1991).

Cardiac Complications. Cardiac complications are most commonly related to preexisting risk factors and conditioning-related toxicities (Shaffer & Wilson, 1990). Patients at higher risk are those who have previously received anthracyclines, cyclophosphamide, or chest radiation, patients with a history of mitral valve problems, and those with an ejection fraction of less than 50 per cent (Wikle, 1991). Many transplant centers will not offer therapy to patients with a cardiac ejection fraction less than 40 per cent. Severe cardiac toxicity occurs in 5 to 10 per cent of patients who receive cyclophosphamide in the conditioning regimen (Peterson & Bearman, 1994). Autologous transplant patients have a 40 per cent occurrence of cardiac complications, much higher than allogeneic or syngeneic transplant recipients (Wikle, 1991). Cardiac complications account for 10 per cent of all autologous transplant deaths (Wikle, 1991).

The damage caused by chemotherapeutic agents to the heart consists of a loss of myocardial fibers and necrosis of contraction bands. Damage related to these agents is usually irreversible and results in cardiomyopathy (Crawford, 1994; Shaffer & Wilson, 1990). Chemotherapy and radiation are associated with pericardial effusions, cardiac tamponade, and constrictive pericarditis (Shaffer & Wilson, 1990; Wikle, 1991). As with pulmonary complications, chemotherapy and radiation appear to have additive negative effect on the heart. Cardiac complications can occur within the first few weeks posttransplant or develop months later. Minor ECG changes, such as supraventricular dysrhythmias, may develop in up to 90 per cent of patients who have received cytoxan as a part of their preparative regimen (Crawford, 1994; Peterson & Bearman, 1994).

Thorough nursing assessment and knowledge of patients' history and risk factors are vital. Assessment for murmurs, friction rubs, pulsus paradoxus, changes in breath sounds, tachycardia or irregular heart rate, evaluation of fluid and electrolyte balance, weight changes and edema, adequate fever management, and balancing rest with activity are essential to aid prompt intervention if complications occur (Shaffer & Wilson, 1990; Wikle, 1991). Medical intervention includes diuresis,

drugs that enhance contractility, and supplemental oxygen (Peterson & Bearman, 1994).

Integumentary Complications. Integumentary toxicities are associated with high-dose conditioning therapies, especially those which include radiation, VP-16, and thiotepa (Lin et al., 1993). Most integumentary toxicities occur 1 to 2 weeks following the conditioning therapy. The insult is to the basal layer of the skin, and as new cells move upward toward the epidermal layer the damage becomes apparent. The degree of skin damage is variable and can be assessed only after the normal physiologic process of cell sluffing has occurred down to the layer of damage. Integumentary toxicity ranges from transient erythema and a localized rash requiring minimal intervention to excoriation, ulceration, and desquamation requiring the application of a biologic or synthetic graft. Moist areas such as the axillae and under the breasts and the groin are highly susceptible to toxic effects and should be assessed daily.

Nursing assessment and intervention are essential to prevent subsequent infections. Treatment is dependent on the grade of skin toxicity and is variable among transplant centers. Utilization of antibacterial/antifungal powders in moist areas to prevent breakdown and application of emollients to dry areas aid in the prevention of breakdown. Once excoriation has occurred, application of an antibacterial cream is dependent on the depth and diameter of the area. Use of high air loss beds aids in comfort and helps to absorb significant fluid loss, keeping the surface next to the patient dry. There is debate as to whether air loss therapy stimulates blood flow to areas of skin loss, aiding in granulation. Areas of desquamation are extremely painful, and patients may require analgesics during skin care and periodically during the day to maintain basic activities of daily living. Patients with greater than 30 per cent grade IV skin loss may require application of a graft. High mortality is associated with patients with greater than 60 per cent grade IV skin involvement.

PHASE 4: TRANSPLANT

DESCRIPTION

After the conditioning regimen is completed, the patient receives the infusion of bone marrow or peripheral blood stem cells. The goal is to administer the cells while monitoring the patient closely for any untoward reactions. Day zero, the day of transplant, is often celebrated as a special occasion by patients and family members. Some patients feel let down, asking, "Is this all there is to it?" (Wellish & Wolcott, 1994). Patients receiving allogeneic transplants may experience an indebtedness to or special bond with the donor.

INFUSION PROCEDURES

The actual infusion of marrow or PBSC is a relatively simple infusion into the patient's central venous catheter. The preparation, rate of infusion, and potential side effects depend on whether the marrow stem cells are "fresh," harvested or pheresed only a few hours before infusion, or if they are cryopreserved, or "frozen."

Fresh marrow or PBSC from allogeneic or syngeneic donors is infused as soon as available. The usual volume is 10 to 15 ml/kg of the recipient's body weight. With fresh marrow no premedications are necessary unless the patient has previously reacted to blood components. Filtration is not used unless there are clots or other obvious particulates. There are a number of potential side effects with fresh marrow or PBSC infusion, although many patients receive their infusing without complication. Volume overload must be monitored prior to and during the infusion (Whedon, 1991). Fat and particulates may result in microemboli with the patient complaining of chest pain, dyspnea, or sudden-onset cough. Patients may also experience acute or delayed hemolytic transfusion reactions.

Autologous marrow and PBSC are cyropreserved with dimethylsulfoxide (DMSO) as a preservative. This technique has two major complications. Renal failure may occur if the patient is not protected against red cell hemolysis. Second, a percentage of patients are sensitive to DMSO, which causes the release of histamine and affects cardiac conduction. Bradycardia (rarely heart block) and hypertension are potential problems 2 to 6 hours after infusion. Hydra-

tion should be administered to assure urine output of at least 2 to 3 ml/kg/hr.

PHASE 5: WAITING FOR ENGRAFTMENT

DESCRIPTION

In addition to watching for the first signs of engraftment, the patient continues to require careful monitoring and management of complications. The goals are (1) to support and protect the patient, and (2) to closely monitor the patient for complications and provide prompt treatment. Expert nursing care is required to detect early signs of complications (see Table 27–5). Routine nursing tasks such as taking vital signs, weights, and intake and output often offer the first clues to the development of a complication and must be performed by a professional staff well educated on the implications of their assessment (Ford & Ballard, 1988). A systematic method of assessment, providing for the patients' needs and at the same time encouraging the patients' involvement in their own care, are the key nursing implications during this phase (Mack, 1992). Pediatric patients should have their developmental levels determined before admission and have activities planned that are appropriate for their age and degree of illness (Kelleher, 1986).

TABLE 27–5. *Clinical Manifestations and Nursing Implications of Transplant Specific Acute Complications*

COMPLICATION	CLINICAL MANIFESTATION	NURSING IMPLICATIONS
Veno-occlusive disease	• Sudden weight gain, increase in bilirubin, SGOT, and alkaline phosphatase levels • Hepatomegaly • Ascites • Encephalopathy	• Exact assessment of fluid balances and therapy every 4–8 hours • Check weight twice daily • Measure abdominal girth daily • Postural blood pressure twice daily • Restrict fluids and sodium intake • Monitor narcotic usage in light of changed liver metabolism • Hemodynamic monitoring if indicated
Renal impairment	• Doubling of baseline serum creatinine • Decreased urine output • Decreased quality of urine	• Strict monitoring of intake and output • Check urine specific gravity every 4 hours • Monitor serum electrolytes • Obtain samples for urine electrolyte and sediment determinations • Monitor patient thirst • Postural blood pressure checks • Assess neck veins • Assess breath sounds • Assess peripheral edema • Monitor patient during dialysis
Graft-versus-host disease	*Initially:* • Maculopapular rash • Nausea and vomiting • Green watery diarrhea • Abdominal pain • Increased SGOT *May Progress to:* • Total body skin sloughing • Copious watery diarrhea • Progressive liver failure	• Daily skin assessment • Apply skin emollients • Daily assessment of stools for quantity, consistency, color and odor • Administer fluids to replace gastrointestinal losses • Administer narcotics as needed • Protect confused patient

Most patients experience the uncertainty of waiting for engraftment as stressful. Feeling defenseless and vulnerable are common experiences. Associated with the daily monitoring, medical procedures, and treatments is a feeling of loss of personal control of their life. Maintaining a sense of control is a major issue for patients (Northouse & Northouse, 1987). Anxiety reaches a peak and denial breaks down. Nurses have a major role in helping patients cope with the uncertainty and ambiguity of marrow transplantation and in fostering hope (Brack, LaClave, & Blix, 1988). Nurses can plan interventions that give the patient as much control as possible (Haberman, 1988). Fear of the unknown can be decreased through patient education about procedures and potential complications. Promoting physical activity throughout the transplant phases can help alleviate the effects of immobility and improve the patient's endurance, strength, and sense of well being (Sayre & Marcoux, 1992). Patients have said that it helps to talk with others, keep as active as possible, attend support groups, and engage in activities that allow them to take their mind off treatments temporarily. Some patients find that working out the details of their day such as timing of bathing, walks, and treatments helps them maintain control and gives structure to this period.

POTENTIAL COMPLICATIONS

During this phase the patient is at tremendous risk of several potentially fatal complications (Bearman et al., 1988). These complications are often insidious, with quick but subtle onsets.

Hemorrhage. Hemorrhage can occur any time after transplantation; however, it is most common within the first month while the patient is producing no or few megakaryocytes (Mawaji et al., 1992). Patients at increased risk for bleeding are those who have thrombocytopenia prior to transplant, leukemic patients receiving an autologous marrow/PBSC, and recipients of monoclonal antibody–purged marrow. Other factors that affect engraftment such as viral infection, coagulopathies from liver disease, graft-versus-host disease, and immunosuppressive therapy contribute to bleeding risk (Caudell & Whedon, 1991). Epistaxis is the most frequent site of bleeding (Ford & Ballard, 1988). Other sites of bleeding include oropharyngeal locations, gastrointestinal tract (Spencer, Shulman, Myerson, Thomas, & McDonald, 1986), genitourinary tract (Brugieres et al., 1989), cerebral sites, and any invasive procedure site (Mawaji et al., 1992). Women are at risk for significant blood loss if menses is not controlled (Mawaji et al., 1992). Provera is frequently prescribed during the preengraftment phase to suppress menses. Frequent assessment during the thrombocytopenic phase is imperative as signs of bleeding may be subtle, but significant.

Accessibility of blood products is essential (Osterwalder, Gratwohl, Reusser, Tichelli, & Speck, 1988; Wulff et al., 1983). Complete blood counts are frequently assessed to determine blood product therapy. Hematocrit values are generally kept above 26 per cent

and platelet levels at or above 20,000 per milliliter. All patients require platelet support during the preengraftment phase. Platelets from several randomly selected donors are used first. If the patient becomes refractory to pooled platelets, then platelets from a randomly selected single donor, community donor, or family donor are utilized (Press, Schaller, & Thomas, 1986). All blood products are irradiated to prevent T lymphocytes from blood donors from initiating a graft-versus-host response (Sullivan & Parkman, 1983; Weiden et al., 1981). Leukodepletion of red cells and platelets may be required to reduce the incidence of febrile reactions

Infections. Infections pose an enormous threat to these patients. There is no population of patients who are more immunosuppressed than marrow transplant patients in the days before engraftment. Infections caused by bacterial, fungal, or viral pathogens commonly occur alone or in combination in almost every transplant patient (Meyers & Thomas, 1988; Peterson et al., 1983; Winston, Gale, Meyer, Young, & the UCLA Bone Marrow Transplantation Group, 1979). Infections contribute to and often are the major cause of death in transplant patients (Peterson et al., 1983; Young, 1984). Early in transplant the patient is at greatest risk for gram-positive and gram-negative infections, candida, and to a lessor extent aspergilloses and herpes simplex (Caudell, 1991; Wingard, 1994). Once the neutrophil count has reached 500 ml, the major risks to the patient are general fungal infections, especially aspergillus, CMV, HSV, adenovirus, and gram-positive bacteria (Caudell & Whedon, 1991; Wingard, 1994). Finally, in the later engraftment period patients are at most risk for encapsulated bacterial infections, varicella zoster virus, and CMV (Caudell, 1991; Wingard, 1994).

Sites of infection will not resemble those of patients with intact immune systems because there is a lack of white blood cells to make pus and promote the inflammatory response (van der Meer, Guiot, van den Brock, & van Furth, 1984). Temperature elevation is the main parameter used to detect infection. However, in the BMT patient this can also be misleading because other factors, such as irradiation, GVHD, and drug or blood product administration can also elevate temperature (Ford & Ballard, 1988). Due to the suppression of inflammatory response related to steroid therapy, routine blood surveillance cultures should be done. Pan cultures should be obtained in patients suspected of being infected, although therapy is often started on a best-guess basis before culture susceptibility results are known.

Risk factors that increase the chance of developing an infection include prolonged granulocytopenia, GVHD, age of greater than 30 years, relapse at the time of transplant, and colonization before or early after transplantation (Caudell & Whedon, 1991; Meyers & Atkinson, 1983; van der Meer et al., 1984). Prevention of infection is a major focus of medical protocols on transplant units (Mooney, Reeves, & Larson, 1993). Handwashing is the major factor in the prevention of infection (Poe, Larson, McGuire, & Krumm, 1994). Washing for 15 seconds with soap and warm water before and after contact with the patient or the patient's environment should be the standard on every unit. All patients must be in private rooms with an air filtration system either in each individual room or on the unit itself (Ford & Ballard, 1988).

Some units are still maintaining a limited number of laminar air flow rooms. These rooms divide a single room in half, with one side being sterile. The patient enters the sterile side after skin decontamination and remains there until engraftment. All supplies, food, and medications entering the patient's side of the room are "low bacteria" or sterile (Caudell & Whedon, 1991).

Other prophylactic measures to prevent infections include administration of broad-spectrum oral or intravenous antibiotics, antivirals, and antifungals at the start of the transplant process (Burns, 1994; White, 1993; Wingard, 1994; Zaia, 1994). Fluconazole is the most recent antifungal agent to be used as a prophylactic measure. Research has demonstrated an impact on candidal infections but no impact on aspergillus-related infections. Fluconazole has been shown to decrease and delay the onset of colonization and also to decrease superficial and invasive infections (Wingard, 1994; White, 1993). Recently, studies have been completed that evaluated the prophylactic use of ganciclovir for CMV-positive patients. Due to ganciclovir-related neutropenia, which creates an increased risk for infection, and the expense of the agent, universal prophylaxis is no longer recommended (Zaia, 1994). CMV may be prevented in CMV-negative patients by the use of CMV-negative blood products (Zaia, 1994).

The development and wide use of colony-stimulating factors (CSF) has led to a number of benefits. Autologous marrow patients who have received either granulocyte-macrophage colony-stimulating factor (GM-CSF) or granulocyte colony-stimulating factor (G-CSF) have demonstrated accelerated marrow recovery, which has resulted in fewer infections, shorter hospital stays, and lower costs (Applebaum, 1993; Singer, Jack, & Neumunaitis, 1994). Both factors cause accelerated engraftment in the allogeneic marrow patient, but the clinical benefits have not as yet been clearly realized (Singer et al., 1994). Research has begun on a number of CSF, including IL-1 and IL-3, with the goal being the successful duplication of the results from G-CSF and GM-CSF studies (Applebaum, 1993).

Treatment of infection includes administration of appropriate antimicrobials, continued surveillance cultures, and close monitoring of patients for the development of further complications such as septic shock. Antimicrobial treatment is often limited by the patient's renal or hepatic function, which may prevent administration of optimal doses. More institutions are beginning to monitor patients for CMV antigenic reactivation to determine the institution of treatment with ganciclovir. The use of ganciclovir has greatly reduced the risk of developing CMV pneumonia or death related to CMV-IP from 70 per cent to 25 per cent (Zaia, 1994). A continuing area of controversy remains the treatment of patients with intravenous immunoglobulin to develop passive immunization with regard to CMV. Clinical trials at different institutions have mixed outcomes with a decreased incidence of CMV infection, but the effect on CMV-associated disease was variable (Zaia, 1994).

Neurologic Complications. Neurologic complications can occur after marrow transplantation as a result of previous chemotherapy and irradiation, conditioning therapy, infections, or as a consequence of therapies to control marrow transplant-related complications such as GVHD. Organ failure in other systems can lead to central nervous system dysfunction (Davis & Patchell, 1988).

Examples of neurologic infection are bacterial meningitis, fungal abscesses, septic emboli, or aneurysms (Meriney, 1991; Openshaw & Slatkin, 1994). Clinical presentation is typically an alteration in mental status and level of consciousness. Due to the restricted drug entry into the CNS through the blood-brain barrier, medical treatment results are variable based on the type of infection and the agent used to treat it.

Cerebrovascular complications occur in 6 to 28 per cent of marrow transplant patients (Meriney, 1991). Intracranial hemorrhages are most frequently associated with thrombocytopenia and are usually fatal (Openshaw & Slatkin, 1994). Ischemic strokes are most commonly associated with endocarditis or either infectious or nonbacterial thrombotic endocarditis (Openshaw & Slatkin, 1994).

Metabolic encephalopathy may be related to sepsis, sedative-hypnotic drugs, hepatic complications from veno-occlusive disease or GVHD, and renal complications. Signs and symptoms include confusion, decreased level of consciousness, and at an advanced stage, coma with extremity posturing (Openshaw & Slatkin, 1994).

Cyclosporin may cause mild tremulousness to coma (Furlong, 1993; Meriney, 1991). It also induces significant magnesium wasting, which may lead to seizures. During the administration of cyclophosphamide the fluid and electrolyte status of the patient must be closely monitored to prevent hyponatremia, which may lead to seizures. Corticosteriods are associated with mood changes and muscle weakness (Furlong, 1993; Meriney, 1991). Busulfan may cause seizures if appropriate prophylaxis with phenytoin is not initiated (Furlong, 1993; Meriney, 1991). Many of the antibiotics and antiviral agents have been associated with neurologic toxicities such as seizures and peripheral neuropathies (Meriney, 1991; Openshaw & Slatkin, 1994). Withdrawal of these agents to resolve the neurologic toxicities must be balanced with the prevention or treatment of the transplant-related complication (Meriney, 1991; Openshaw & Slatkin, 1994). Nursing assessment is vital to early diagnosis of any neurologic change, because many of the initial signs and symptoms are subtle changes in level of consciousness.

Renal Impairment or Failure. Renal impairment after transplantation is most often caused by medications initiated to prevent or treat other complications, the hypoperfusion related to veno-occlusive disease, or from the reaction to cell breakdown during the infusion of stem cells (King, Hoffart, & Murray, 1992; Mawaji et al., 1992; Peterson & Bearman, 1994; Shaffer &

Wilson, 1990; Wujcik et al., 1994). Roughly one half of all allogeneic transplant patients develop renal disease, as evidenced by a doubling of their serum creatinine levels (Peterson & Bearman, 1994). Risk factors for renal disease include infection and the subsequent therapies used, particularly amphotericin-B, having received cyclosporine, or having an intravascular volume deficit, a history of liver disease, or a mismatched transplant. Combinations of these factors are especially toxic (King et al., 1992; Mawaji et al., 1992; Peterson & Bearman, 1994; Shaffer & Wilson, 1990; Wujcik et al., 1994).

Prevention of renal disease focuses on frequent assessment of renal status through monitoring of serum creatinine levels and the amount and analysis of the patient's urine (Ford & Ballard, 1988). Attention needs to be focused on the daily fluid management of these patients to ensure adequate renal blood flow (King et al., 1992). Treatment of renal disease entails aggressive, frequent assessment of fluid and electrolyte status. At times this can be accomplished only through hemodynamic monitoring (O'Quin & Moravec, 1988). Monitoring for infections, bleeding, and urinary obstruction are also important in the total care of the patient with renal complications.

Nephrotoxic drugs should be decreased and ideally eliminated, although this is rarely possible (Shaffer & Wilson, 1990). Patients may require dialysis support until renal function returns. Mortality associated with dialyzed transplant patients is approximately 85 per cent; however, the cause of death is usually multiorgan failure (Ford & Ballard, 1988).

PHASE 6: ENGRAFTMENT AND EARLY RECOVERY

DESCRIPTION

Approximately 10 to 28 days after transplant, signs that the new bone marrow or stem cells are engrafting can be expected. As the new immune system is developing, the goal is to support the patient's recovery and to manage complications that may emerge, such as GVHD. The nurse continues to monitor the patient's physical and emotional responses closely and to coordinate the administration of treatments, whether the patient is in the inpatient or outpatient setting.

Most patients experience profound fatigue as they are recovering. They may find it difficult to focus on reading a book, watching television, or keeping up a conversation. It is important to encourage reasonable expectations of what is possible to accomplish. Balancing periods of rest with light exercise facilitates recovery and prevents the complications of bedrest.

Patients may feel frustrated because they want to get well and put this experience behind them as quickly as possible. Grief typically emerges in this phase and continues through the remaining transplant phases (Wellisch & Wolcott, 1994). The grief is in response to losses such as the decreased physical functioning and the dependence on others for care. A central role of the nurse is assisting the patient with coping during this time. Strategies found to be helpful by many patients include taking one day at a time and setting manageable goals to achieve each day.

As the patient recovers and no longer needs the intensive medical monitoring and nursing care, it is time to prepare for discharge from the center. Feelings of eager anticipation as well as separation anxiety are both common.

POTENTIAL COMPLICATIONS

Graft-versus-Host Disease. Graft-versus-host disease (GVHD) is unique to marrow transplant patients. GVHD is the recognition by the donor marrow that the host is "non-self." This recognition initiates a cascade of events that leads to tissue and target cell destruction (Press et al., 1986; Sullivan, 1994; Wujcik et al., 1994). There are three requirements for GVHD to occur:

1. An immunologically competent graft (fully functioning WBC, RBCs, and platelets) (Sullivan, 1994)
2. Host and donor disparity (not perfectly identical HLA as in identical twins) (Sullivan, 1994)
3. Ineffective host response (inability of recipient to respond to donor stem cell infusion due to lack of viable marrow) (Sullivan, 1994)

There are two types of GVHD: acute and chronic.

Major risk factors for acute GVHD include HLA mismatch, transplant from an unrelated donor, and age. Minor risks include prior donor pregnancies, infection, female to male transplants, and active malignancy (Sullivan, 1994; Wujcik et al., 1994).

In acute GVHD the pathophysiology consists of three phases: cognitive, activation, and effector. In the cognitive phase the role of the host tissue is the key factor. Chemotherapy, radiation, or infection cause an insult to the host tissue leading to epithelial and endothelial cell injury. These cells then release inflammatory cytokines such as interleukin-1 (IL-1) and tumor necrosis factor (TNF). IL-1 and TNF cause increased expression of host HLA proteins, which are the genetic identification components that the donor cells will recognize as "not-self."

In the second phase, activation, the T lymphocytes are the major component. The donor helper T cells recognize the host HLA as foreign and release the cytokines IL-2 and γ-interferon, which activate the donor mononuclear cells.

The final phase is the effector phase, in which cytokines released by the donor mononuclear cells cause the stimulation of a variety of cells (natural killer cells, macrophages, and cytotoxic T lymphocytes) that cause direct tissue injury. The cycle then begins again as the tissue injury caused by the stimulation of cells in the last phase causes the release of cytokines, and a loop is formed back to the first phase.

Acute GVHD may occur in any or all of the following three systems: the skin, the liver, and the gastrointestinal tract (Champlin & Gale, 1984; Press et al., 1986). Graft-versus-host disease can be fatal in any of the systems. Moderate to severe disease occurs in 20 to 45 per cent of HLA-matched allogeneic transplants, with 20 to 50 per cent of the patients dying of GVHD or related complications such as infection, hemorrhage, or liver disease (Press et al., 1986; Sullivan, 1994; Wujcik, Ballard & Camp-Sorrell, 1994).

The onset of GVHD coincides with engraftment. Diagnosis is difficult because the symptoms are hard to differentiate from lingering side effects of the conditioning regimen or other complications. Diagnosis is made on the basis of biopsy of the organ involved, laboratory data, and clinical observation (McDonald et al., 1986; Spencer et al., 1986; Storb & Thomas, 1985).

All therapies used for prevention or treatment of GVHD may have toxic side effects. Methotrexate has been administered in low doses to block the proliferation of T lymphocytes in response to HLA stimulus by the host (Caudell, 1991; Shaffer & Wilson, 1990; Wujcik et al., 1994). Cyclosporine is an immunosuppressive drug that inhibits the production of IL-2, thereby blocking the activation of T lymphocytes (Caudell, 1991; Shaffer & Wilson, 1990; Wujcik et al., 1994). Studies have shown that these two medications used in combination are more successful at preventing GVHD than either one alone (Caudell, 1991; Shaffer & Wilson, 1990; Sullivan, 1994). Prednisone has also been used for GVHD prophylaxis in combination with cyclosporin alone or cyclosporin and methotrexate (Sullivan, 1994; Wujcik & Downs, 1992). There is an increased infection risk associated with the administration of prednisone. Other types of therapies utilized to prevent GVHD are T-cell depletion from the marrow itself before infusion into the host and the use of intravenous immunoglobulins (Sullivan, 1994; Wujcik et al., 1994). Should GVHD occur despite prophylaxis, treatment includes increasing the dosage of cyclosporine and administering corticosteroids, monoclonal antibodies, and horse antithymocyte globulin (Martin et al., 1984; McDonald et al., 1986; Press et al., 1986). Clinical trials are currently underway on new therapies to prevent or treat GVHD such as trimetrexate, FK-506, rapamycin, thalidomide, and ultraviolet radiation (Sullivan, 1994).

The specific definition for chronic graft-versus-host disease varies. Some investigators consider it to be a late phase of acute GVHD due to minor antigen recognition (Sullivan, 1994), whereas other researchers consider it to be an autoimmune process (Caudell, 1991; Shaffer & Wilson, 1990; Sullivan, 1994). There is also loss of the function of the thymus by age or injury, which contributes to the lack of the body's ability to destroy T cells that do not recognize the body as self (Sullivan, 1994). The incidence of chronic GVHD in allogeneic patients alive greater than 150 days posttransplant is approximately 33 per cent in matched sibling transplants, 49 per cent in mismatched related transplants, and 64 per cent of unrelated matched transplants (Sullivan 1994). Major risk factors for C-GVHD include HLA mismatch, prior acute GVHD, and increasing patient age (Caudell, 1991; Shaffer & Wilson, 1990; Sullivan, 1994). Minor risks include an incomplete course of methotrexate, random cell transfusions, infection, and previous spleenectomy, although all minor risks are considered controversial (Sullivan, 1994). Chronic GVHD may occur from 80 days up to 2 years posttransplant.

Chronic GVHD affects multiple organ systems (Shaffer & Wilson, 1990). The clinical presentation of the integumentary system includes rough and scaly skin, pigmentation problems, premature graying, joint contractures, scleroderma, and loss of sweat glands (Caudell, 1991; Sullivan, 1994). Patients experience alopecia, and their nails grow slowly and are ridged. Hepatic complications include jaundice, bleeding and coagulopathy problems, and infection (Caudell, 1991; Sullivan, 1994). Patients with liver complications may need to remain on a low-fat diet. Ophthalmic problems are evidenced by grittiness, burning, and dry eyes (Caudell, 1991; Sullivan, 1994). Gastrointestinal manifestations include loss of taste, dental caries, anorexia, painful swallowing, nausea and vomiting, and weight loss (Caudell, 1991; Sullivan, 1994). Pulmonary complications include chronic sinusitis and obstructive lung disease (Caudell, 1991; Sullivan, 1994). Muscular weakness with repetitive motion may occur (Caudell, 1991; Sullivan, 1994). Gynecologic symptoms include vaginal dryness, inflammation, strictures, and painful intercourse (Caudell, 1991). The psychologic impact of the many and varied complications cannot be discounted, and the patient and family need significant support.

Prevention of C-GVHD includes prolonged immunosuppression, T cell depletion of the donor marrow, intravenous immunoglobulin, and other treatments for late infections (Sullivan, 1994). Treatment includes corticosteriods, antithymocyte globulin, thalidomide, and azathioprine (Caudell, 1991; Shaffer & Wilson, 1990; Sullivan, 1994). Long-term survival of patients with significant C-GVHD ranges from 26 to 42 per cent depending on the type and extent of the disease (Sullivan, 1994).

Graft Rejection. Graft rejection, the failure of the new marrow to engraft or the loss of engraftment after an initial period (Shaffer & Wilson, 1990), has become an increasing problem in recent years. Whereas in the early years of transplantation, the donors were always HLA-matched and the marrow was given to the patient without any manipulation, this is no longer the case. Current transplants using mismatched and unrelated donors along with depletion of T cells from the marrow to prevent GVHD has increased the incidence of graft rejection. Approximately 10 per cent of all marrow transplant patients fail to reconstitute their marrow, or they experience late hematopoietic failure (Singer & Neumunaitis, 1994; Applebaum, 1993). Use of recombinant growth factors has decreased the risk of permanent graft failure. In a recent study using GM-CSF, approximately 60 per cent of patients with graft failure responded to one or two courses of the agent with an increase of their absolute neutrophil count to greater than 500/ml within 14 days of starting therapy (Singer & Neumunaitis, 1994). Although no immediate platelet recovery was evident, most patients eventually became platelet-independent (Singer & Neumunaitis, 1994). Long-term survival previous to the use of growth factors was only 20 per cent compared with slightly less than 60 per cent with GM-CSF (Singer & Neumunaitis, 1994). Research continues to determine the best way to prevent graft rejection.

CAREGIVER ISSUES IN ASSISTING THE PATIENT'S RECOVERY

Family members are expected to play a major role in assisting the patient's recovery after transplant (Zabora, Smith, Baker, Wingard, & Curbow, 1992). Typically, family caregivers face the dilemma of deciding the appropriate level of patient dependence/independence, what is considered normal during recovery, what supportive resources, if any, to select, and how to balance the need for self-care with the demands of the caregiver role. Two major strategies nurses can use to assist caregivers are giving information and providing support (Northouse & Northouse, 1993). Information that is helpful includes discussing the typical feelings and physical symptoms experienced during each phase and options for dealing with commonly encountered home care scenarios. Supportive services include interpretation of the course of illness and anticipatory guidance, interpretation of illness to school-age children, cognitive processing of the meaning of illness, and referral to problem-focused services (Lewis, 1990). Caregivers can benefit from encouragement to engage in self-care practices as well as access to services that provide respite. Also, it is important to offer them the opportunity to discuss their concerns informally or provide referral to a support group or individual counseling.

PHASE 7: LONG-TERM RECOVERY

DESCRIPTION

The patient leaves the treatment center and begins to reestablish life patterns after transplant. Patients often become involved again in the quest for meaning in their lives (Steeves, 1992). The goals of this phase are to provide resources that help the patient reestablish previous activity and manage complications that may arise. This phase may take a year or longer. Late complications such as chronic GVHD, delayed growth and development, cataracts, or recurrence of disease may surface. Patients commonly experience slower energy return than anticipated. They may experience cognitive deficits, body image changes, and sexual problems. As the patient continues to recover from transplant, there are several issues that may affect the need for ongoing nursing assessment and intervention. When working with a patient posttransplant it is important to be aware of the type of immunosuppressive medication that the patient continues to take. This will influence the nature of patient teaching with regard to infection control and activity. It is also important to be aware of any medications that are used to treat complications, such as antibiotics for prophylaxis of pneumocystis pneumonia or insulin for serum glucose intolerance caused by prolonged use of corticosteroids. In some instances, patients may require intravenous fluids or medications in the home setting. Home-care nurses should be familiar with the management of central venous access devices and should work with the primary physician to determine whether the patient or caregiver can safely administer these items in the home setting.

Establishing new life patterns may include dealing with physical complications, decisions on when to return to work or school, and adjustments in relationships with spouse, family and friends (Box 27–2, Haberman & Bush, 1993). Grief over losses waxes and wanes and when severe can lead to depression (Eakes, 1993). The pathway to recovery varies depending on gender, marital status, age, and time since transplant (Curbow, Legro, Baker, Wingard, & Somerfield, 1993). For example, young single survivors may change their educational goals or career in reconstructing their lives. Married older survivors may turn inward to themselves or to other family members to establish a new life pathway.

Perhaps most important, the nurse may assist the patient in resuming a normal lifestyle while managing ongoing medical problems. Something as simple as devising a manageable schedule for intravenous fluids and medications or teaching different family members to serve as caregivers may provide the patient with the needed flexibility to pursue fulfilling activity. Throughout transplant the nurse employs strategies ultimately aimed at the patient's quality of life: being accessible,

---

BOX 27–2. *Quality of Life Evaluated in Long-Term Survivors of Bone Marrow Transplant*

Haberman, M., & Bush, N. (1993). Quality of life of adult long-term survivors of bone marrow transplantation: A qualitative analysis of narrative data. *Oncology Nursing Forum, 20*(10), 1545–1553.

Recently, clinicians and researchers alike have challenged the long-standing impression that survivors of bone marrow transplant (BMT) experience a less than optimal quality of life (QOL). Despite the accumulating evidence suggesting that most adult survivors adjust relatively well within 2 to 5 years after BMT, little is known about the growing population of recipients living well beyond 5 years. This paper reports the design and qualitative components of a large study that used a cross-sectional, descriptive, mailed survey design. The aim of the study was to document systematically how 125 adult survivors of BMT (6 to 18.4 years posttransplant) perceived the quality of their lives. An eight-item, open-ended questionnaire was used to gather information on the reestablishment of life after BMT, demands of recovery, coping strategies, limitations imposed by BMT, current health problems, QOL, and concerns for the future. Content analysis of the verbatim responses indicated the most long-term survivors, despite the persistence of lingering side effects, perceive themselves as cured and well, leading full and meaningful lives. Nursing therapeutics can focus on providing accurate and timely information about the known long-range complications of BMT. Further research is needed to examine the entire issue of social support following BMT and to identify the special care requirements of the recipients (5%) who reported poor physical and mental health.

providing education, suggesting coping strategies, and promoting the patient's participation in decision-making (Ferrell et al., 1992).

POTENTIAL COMPLICATIONS FOLLOWING TRANSPLANT

The intensive therapy delivered in the marrow transplant setting produces a unique set of complications that can linger long after transplant.

Infection. Up to 50 per cent of patients who are herpes simplex virus-positive may experience reactivation of the herpes zoster virus during the first year posttransplant (Locksley, Flourney, Sullivan, & Meyers, 1985). The infection, which is often referred to as "shingles," is painful and may cause scarring. It generally requires administration of intravenous antiviral medications to achieve remission (Nader & Arvin, 1994).

Pulmonary Complications. Patients with prior pulmonary problems are at greater risk of chronic pulmonary complications. Those who experience a reduction in pulmonary capacity are generally diagnosed with bronchiolitis obliterans, which is caused by an autoimmune response stimulated by GVHD. This condition is observed within 2 years of transplant and is characterized by diffuse necrotizing changes in the small airways. Symptoms such as shortness of breath and cyanosis may improve as the underlying GVHD is treated with immunosuppressive medications (Deeg, 1994).

Cataracts. Cataracts develop in 20 per cent of patients receiving fractioned irradiation and in 50 per cent of patients receiving single-dose irradiation. The range of time for cataract formation is 1 to 5 years after transplantation. Cataracts can be removed surgically with intraocular lens replacement (Buchsel, 1986).

Retarded Growth and Development in Children. Children who are prepubertal and receive conditioning with chemotherapy alone are likely to recover full gonadal function and are more likely to grow and experience a normal puberty (Sanders, Buckner, & Sullivan, 1988). Children who are prepubertal and receive TBI often experience a delay in the development of secondary sex characteristics (Sanders et al., 1988). Adolescents who are postpubertal at the time of transplant who receive chemotherapy alone generally do not experience gonadal failure. Those who receive TBI often require hormone replacement therapy to restore the development of secondary sex characteristics, growth, and sexual functioning (van der Wall, Nims, & Davies, 1988). Learning disabilities have been especially noted in children who receive prophylactic intrathecal MTX or Ara-C, which may produce leukoencelopathy that is irreversible (van der Wal et al., 1988). While deficiency of growth hormone is a problem in many of these children, relatively few children receive GH supplementation (Sanders, 1994).

Immune Reconstitution. Parkman (1994), in his study of immunological reconstitution, found the following. Total immune reconstitution of the marrow is affected by the degree of transfer of donor immunity, the return of normal T-and B-lymphocyte function, and the effects of acute and chronic graft-versus-host disease. When unmanipulated allogeneic marrow is transplanted there is the possibility that the donor T and B cells will contribute to the patients immune system. However, the impact is variable, so routine administration of intravenous immunoglobulin early posttransplant protects the patients from certain infections. B lymphocytes, measured by the level of various immunoglobulins, function in patients without chronic GVHD and return to normal in 8 to 9 months for IgG, 9 to 12 months for IgM, and 2 to 3 years for IgA. Function of T lymphocytes returns to normal in 4 to 6 months posttransplant in patients with unmanipulated marrow and no chronic graft-versus-host disease. Function of the T and B cells is delayed in patients with marrow that has been manipulated and those with chronic GVHD. Immunizations that result in prolonged antibody production can be effective only after the T lymphocytes have resumed normal function. Recommendations for patients without chronic GVHD are DPT at 3 to 6 months, inactivated polio at 6 to 12 months, and MMR at 1 to 2 years. In patients with chronic GVHD, only the DPT at 3 to 6 months is recommended until resolution of the disease process.

LIFE AFTER TRANSPLANT

Patients may experience a variety of emotions as they prepare to reenter work and family life following transplant. Many patients express their feelings in terms of loss, for example, the interruption in life plans, the inability to have children, difficulties with sexual functioning, physical disability, and psychologic loss (Curbow et al., 1993; Heiney, Neuberg, DeRosset, & Bergman, 1994). Others express emotions in the recovery theme, for example, psychologic gains, existential recovery, a redirected life, greater compassion for others, and improved family relations (Curbow et al., 1993). Despite the intensity of the bone marrow transplant experience, most patients demonstrate effective adjustment and an optimistic outlook for the future (Haberman & Bush, 1993).

FUTURE TRENDS

The field of marrow transplantation continues to undergo rapid change. Medical literature discusses the following areas as the focus of research and future directions.

New Indications. Marrow transplantation is currently being offered to most leukemic patients younger than aged 55 years, and it is felt that soon it will also become routine treatment for patients with lymphoma (Powles & Mehta, 1994). Depending to a large extent on issues of cost and reimbursement, marrow transplantation may be more widely utilized for solid tumors such as breast cancer and genetic disorders such as sickle cell anemia. Currently much attention is being given to the controversies regarding insurance companies not wanting to pay for transplants to treat solid tumors (Mahaney, 1994; Peters, 1994; Wynstra, 1994).

Extension of the Donor Pool. As the unrelated donor pools become larger, computerization will increase the likelihood of finding a donor in a timely manner. It is hoped there will be a single global electronic file.

Peripheral Blood Stem Cell Transplants. Peripheral blood pheresis may replace bone marrow aspiration as the stem cell source for autologous as well as allogeneic transplant (Shpall & Jones, 1994), providing advantages of no anesthesia, no postsurgical pain, and potentially less of a cost.

Gene Transfer. Retrovirus-mediated gene transfer followed by autologous transplant has the potential to cure genetic disorders or offer tumor-specific therapies as techniques improve (Cline, 1994).

Use of Cytokines. Research continues on how best to utilize growth factors in terms of use in combination, and timing within the transplant process (Wujcik, 1993).

GVHD Prophylaxis. New agents such as FK 506 may prove to be more effective and less toxic than current standard therapy. It has been theorized that if autologous transplant science evolves sufficiently extent, allogeneic transplants may not be necessary, and so graft versus host disease would cease to be an issue (Cline, 1994).

Infection. The magnitude of this problem is diminishing due to the improvements in antimicrobial therapy, and it is reasonable to assume that new classes of antiviral and antibacterial agents will continue to evolve (Cline, 1994).

Improved Antitumor Effect. Studies are currently being conducted utilizing IL-2 to enhance the antitumor effect of conditioning. There is also interest in manipulating allografts to eliminate GVHD while retaining an immunologic graft-versus-tumor effect. This may be disease-specific such as eliminating CD8 positive cells from allografts for chronic myelogenous leukemia.

Decrease Toxicity of Conditioning Regimens. This will be a priority in the future as conditioning regimens are manipulated to provide maximum tumor kill. Attention is being given to more tumor-selective chemotherapeutic agents, as well as trials utilizing pharmacologic agents to modify tissue injury (Cline, 1994).

In addition to advances in medicine, the future of the field of marrow transplantation will be greatly affected by allocation of resources. Cost containment will be a factor in decisions regarding therapies as well as patient care delivery systems. Regardless of the changes in therapies or treatment environments, nurses will need to respond to the shifting priorities in patient care. Patients need strong nursing support in terms of education, assessment, and administration of constantly evolving therapeutic interventions.

SUMMARY

Marrow transplantation has offered hope and cure to thousands of patients in the last decades. This success is due in large part to the dedicated nurses working in this specialty. The professional and personal re-

wards from making the transplantation experience as optimum for the patient and family as possible, regardless of the eventual outcome, are great for those nurses willing to take on the challenge.

REFERENCES

Appelbaum, F. R. (1989). Allogeneic marrow transplantation for malignancy: Current problems and prospects for improvement. In L. T. Magrath (Ed.), *New directions in cancer treatment* (pp. 143–165). Heidelberg, Germany: Springer-Verlag.

Appelbaum, F. R. (1993). The use of colony stimulating factors in marrow transplantation. *Cancer* (Suppl.) 72(11), 3387–3391.

Appelbaum, F. R., Fisher, L. D., Thomas, E. E., & the Seattle Marrow Transplant Team (1988). Chemotherapy versus marrow transplantation for adults with acute nonlymphocytic leukemia: A five-year follow up. *Blood, 72,* 179–184

Ballard, B (1991). Renal and hepatic complications. In M. B. Whedon (Ed.), *Bone marrow transplantation: Principles, practices and nursing insights* (pp. 240–261). Boston: Jones and Bartlett Publishers.

Barnett, M. J., Eaves, C. J., & Eaves, A. C (1994). Autografting in chronic myeloid leukemia. In S. J. Forman, K. G. Blume, & E. D. Thomas (Eds.), *Bone marrow transplantation* (pp. 743–753). Boston: Blackwell Scientific Publications

Baxter-Lowe, L. A., Eckels, D. D., Casper, A. J., Hunter, J. B., & Gorski, J (1991). Future directions in selection of donors for bone marrow transplantation: Role of oligonucleotide genotyping. *Transplantation Proceedings, 23,* 1699–1700.

Bearman, S. I., Appelbaum, F. R., Buckner, C. D., Peterson, F. B., Fisher, L. D., Clift, R. A., & Thomas, E. D. (1988). Regimen–related toxicity in patients undergoing bone marrow transplant. *Journal of Clinical Oncology, 6,* 1562–1568.

Bensinger, W. I. (1984). Selective removal of A and B isoagglutinins. In A. Pineda (Ed.), *Selective plasma component removal* (pp. 43–70). Mount Kisco, NY: Futura Publishing Co.

Bortin, M. M., & Howowitz, M. M. (1992). Increasing utilization of allogeneic bone marrow transplantation. Results of the 1988–1990 survey. *Annals of Internal Medicine, 6,* 505–512.

Bortin, M. M., & Rim, A. A (1986). Increasing utilization of bone marrow transplantation. *Transplantation, 43,* 229–234.

Bowden, R. A. (1994). Other viruses after marrow transplantation. In S. J. Forman, K. G. Blume, & E. D. Thomas (Eds.), *Bone marrow transplantation* (pp. 443–464). Boston: Blackwell Scientific Publications.

Brack, G., LaClave, L., & Blix, S. (1988). The psychological aspects of bone marrow transplant: A staff's perspective. *Cancer Nursing, 11,* 221–229.

Brugieres, L., Hartmann, O., Travagli, J. P., Benhammov, E., Pico, J. L., Valteau, D., Kalifa, C., Patte, C., Flamant, F., & Lemerle, J. (1989). Hemorrhagic cystitis following high-dose chemotherapy and bone marrow transplantation in children with malignancies: Incidence, clinical course, and outcome. *Journal of Clinical Oncology, 7,* 194–199.

Buchsel, P. C. (1986). Long term complications of allogeneic bone marrow transplant: Nursing implications. *Oncology Nursing Forum, 13(6),* 61–70.

Burns, W. H. (1994). Herpes simplex virus. In S. J. Forman, K. G. Blume, & E. D. Thomas (Eds.), *Bone marrow transplantation* (pp. 401–411). Boston: Blackwell Scientific Publications.

Butturni, A., Bortin, M. M., & Gale, R. P. (1987). Graft-versus-leukemia following bone marrow transplantation. *Bone Marrow Transplantation, 2,* 233–242.

Caudell, K. A. (1991). Graft-versus-host disease. In M. B. Whedon (Ed.), *Bone marrow transplantation: Principles, practice and nursing insights* (pp. 160–181). Boston: Jones and Bartlett Publishers

Caudell, K. A., & Whedon, M. B. (1991). Hematopoietic complications. In M. B. Whedon (Ed.), *Bone marrow transplantation: Principles, practice and nursing insights* (pp. 135–159). Boston: Jones and Bartlett Publishers.

Cavanaugh, C. A. (1994). Outpatient autologous bone marrow transplantation: A new frontier. *Quality of Life: Effects of Technology 3*(2), 25–29.

Champlin, R. E., & Gale, R. P. (1984). Role of bone marrow transplantation in the treatment of hematologic malignances and solid tumors. Critical review of syngeneic, autologous and allogeneic transplants. *Cancer Treatment Reports, 68,* 145–161.

Chao, N. J., Duncan, S. R., Long, G. D., Horning, S. J., Blume, K. G. (1991). Corticosteriod therapy for diffuse alveolar hemorrhage in autologous bone marrow transplant recipients. *Annals of Internal Medicine. 114*(2), 145–146.

Christiansen, F. T., Tay, G., Smith, L. K., Witt, C. S., Petersdorf, E. W., Bradley, B., & Dawkins, R. L. (1993). Histocompatibility matching for bone marrow transplantation. *Human Immunology, 38,* 42–51.

Clark, J., Hansen, J. A., Heitz, M. I., Parkman, R., Jensen, L., Peaoy, H. H. (1993). Idiopathic pneumonia syndrome after bone marrow transplantation. *American Review of Respiratory Disease, 147,* 1601–1606.

Cline, M. J. (1994). Bone marrow transplantation in the twenty-first century. In S. S. Forman, K. G. Blume, E. D. Thomas (Eds.), *Bone marrow transplantation* (pp. 919–927). Boston: Blackwell Scientific Publications.

Coxon, V. J. (1989). Subjective perceptions of the demands of hospitalization and anxiety in bone marrow transplant patients. Doctoral dissertation, University of Washington, 1–186.

Crawford, S. W. (1994). Critical care and respiratory failure. In S. J. Forman, K. G. Blume, & E. D. Thomas (Eds.), *Bone marrow transplantation* (pp. 513–526). Boston: Blackwell Scientific Publications.

Crawford, S. W., & Hackman, R. C. (1993). Clinical course of idiopathic pneumonia after bone marrow transplantation. *American Review of Respiratory Disease, 147,* 595–623.

Crawford, S. W., & Meyers, J. (1991). Respiratory disease in bone marrow transplant patients. In J. Shelhamer (Ed.), *Respiratory disease in the immunosuppressed host,* (pp. 1393–1400). St. Louis, MO: J. B. Lippincott

Crouch, M. A., & Ross, J. A. (1994). Current concept in autologous bone marrow transplantation. *Seminars in Oncology Nursing, 10,* 12–19.

Curbow, B., Legro, M. W., Baker, F., Wingard, J. R., & Somerfield, M. R. (1993). Loss and recovery themes of long-term survivors of bone marrow transplants. *Journal of Psychosocial Oncology, 10,* 1–20.

Davis, D. G., & Patchell, R. A. (1988). Neurologic complications of bone marrow transplantation. *Neurology Clinics, 6,* 377–387.

Deeg, H. J. (1994). Delayed complications after bone marrow transplantation. In S. J. Forman, K. G. Blume, & E. D. Thomas (Eds.), *Bone marrow transplantation* (pp. 538–544). Boston: Blackwell Scientific Publications.

Derdiarian, A. (1986). Informational needs of recently diagnosed cancer patients: A theoretical framework. Part I. *Cancer Nursing, 10,* 107–115.

Derdiarian, A. (1987). Informational needs of recently diagnosed cancer patients: Method and description. Part II. *Cancer Nursing, 10,* 156–163.

Dietz, K., & Flaherty, A. (1993). Oncologic emergencies. In S. L. Groenwald, et al. (Eds.), *Cancer nursing principles and practice* (3rd ed.), (pp. 801–839). Boston: Jones and Bartlett Publishers.

Downs, S. (1994). Ethical issues in bone marrow transplantation. *Seminars in Oncology Nursing, 10*(1), 58–63.

Dreifke, L., & DeMeyer, E. (1992). Information guide for patients receiving total body irradiation before bone marrow transplantation. *Cancer Nursing, 15,* 206–210.

Eakes, G. (1993). Chronic sorrow: A response to living with cancer. *Oncology Nursing Forum, 20*(9), 1327–1334.

Ersek, M. T. (1992). The process of maintaining hope in adults undergoing bone marrow transplantation for leukemia. *Oncology Nursing Forum, 19,* 883–889.

Ezzone, S., Jolly, D., Reployle, K., Kapoor, N., Totschka, P. (1993). Survey of oral hygiene regimens among bone marrow transplant centers. *Oncology Nursing Forum, 20*(9), 1375–1387.

Ferrell, B., Schmidt, G. M., Rhiner, M., Whitehead, C., Fonbuena, P., & Forman, S. J. (1992). The meaning of quality of life for bone marrow transplant survivors. Part 2. Improving quality of life for bone marrow transplant survivors. *Cancer Nursing, 15,* 247–253.

Ford, R. C., & Ballard, B. (1988). Acute complications after bone marrow transplantation. *Seminars in Oncology Nursing, 4,* 15–24.

Franco, T., & Gould, D. A. (1994). Allogeneic bone marrow transplantation. *Seminars in Oncology Nursing, 10,* 3–11.

Furlong, T. (1993). Neurologic complications of immunosuppressive cancer therapy. *Oncology Nursing Forum, 20,* 9.

Gaston-Johansson, F., Franco, T., & Zimmerman, L. (1992). Pain and psychological distress in patients undergoing autologous bone marrow transplantation. *Oncology Nursing Forum, 19,* 41–48.

Haberman, M. (1988). Psychosocial aspects of bone marrow transplant. *Seminars in Oncology Nursing, 4,* 55–59.

Haberman, M., & Bush, N. (1993). Quality of life of adult long-term survivors of bone marrow transplantation: A qualitative analysis of narrative data. *Oncology Nursing Forum, 20,* 1545–1553.

Hansen, J. A., Anasetti, C., Petersdorf, E., Clift, R. A., & Martin, P. J. (1994). Marrow transplants from unrelated donors. *Transplantation Proceedings, 26,* 1710–1712.

Hare, J., Skinner, D., & Kliewer, D. (1989). Family systems approach to pediatric bone marrow transplnatation. *Childrens Health Care, 18,* 30–36.

Heiney, S., Neuberg, R., DeRosset, M., Bergman, L. (1994). Aftermath of bone marrow transplant for parents of pediatric patients. A post-traumatic stress disorder. *Oncology Nursing Forum, 21*(5), 843–847.

Hooper, P. J., & Santas, E. J. (1993). Peripheral blood stem cell transplantation. *Oncology Nursing Forum, 20,* 1215–1221.

Jagannath, S., Armitage, J. O., Dicke, K. A., Tucker, S. L., Velasquez, W. S., Smith, K., Vaughan, W. P., Kessinger, A., Horwitz, L. J., Hagemeister, F. B., McLaughlin, P., Cabanill, F., & Spitzer, G. (1989). Prognostic factors for response and survival after high dose cyclosporine, carmustine and etiposide with autologous bone marrow transplantation for relapsed Hodgkin's disease. *Journal of Clinical Oncology, 7,* 179–185.

Jassak, P. F. & Riley, M. B. (1994). Autologous stem cell transplant. *Cancer Practice, 2,* 141–145.

Kanfer, E. J., Buckner, C. D., Fefer, A., Storb, R., Appelbaum, R. R., Hill, R. S., Amos, D., Doney, K. I. C., Clift, R. A., Shulman, H. M., McDonald, G. B., & Thomas, E. D. (1987). Allogeneic and syngeneic marrow transplantation following high dose dimethylbusulfan, cyclophosphamide and total body irradiation. *Bone Marrow Transplantation, 1,* 1–8.

Kelleher, J. (1986). Pediatric marrow transplantation. In M. J. Hockenberry & D. K. Coody (Eds.), *Pediatric hematology/oncology: Perspective on care* (pp. 347–363). St. Louis: C. V. Mosby Co.

Kelleher, J. (1994). Issues for designing marrow transplant programs. *Seminars in Oncology Nursing, 10,* 64–71.

Keller, C. (1994). Methods of drawing blood samples through central venous catheters in pediatric patients undergoing bone marrow transplant: Results of national survey. *Oncology Nursing Forum, 21*(5), 879–884.

Kemshead, J. T., Treleaven, J., Heath, L., Meara, A. O., Gee, A., & Vogelstad, J. (1987). Monoclonal antibodies and magnetic microspheres for the depletion of leukaemic cells from bone marrow harvested for autologous transplantation. *Bone Marrow Transplantation, 2,* 133–139.

Kennedy, V. (1993). The role of social work in bone marrow transplantation. *Journal of Psychosocial Oncology, 11*(1), 103–117.

King, C. R., Hoffart, N., & Murray, M. E. (1992). Acute renal failure in bone marrow transplantation. *Oncology Nursing Forum, 19*(9), 1327–1335.

Kolbinson, D. A., Schubert, M. M., Flournoy, N., & Truelove, E. L. (1988). Early oral changes following bone marrow transplantation. *Oral Surgery, Oral Medicine, Oral Pathology, 66,* 130–138.

Kristjanson, L. J., & Ashcroft, T. (1994). The family's cancer journey: A literature review. *Cancer Nursing, 17,* 1–17.

Lewis, F. M. (1990). Strengthening family supports: Cancer and the family. *Cancer, 65,* 752–759.

Lin, E. M., Tierney, D. K., & Stadtmauer, E. A. (1993). Autologous bone marrow transplantation: A review of the principles and complications. *Cancer Nursing, 16*(3), 204–213.

Linch, D. C., & Burnett, A. K. (1986). Clinical studies of ABMT in acute myeloid leukemia. *Clinics in Haematology (Autologous Bone Marrow Transplantation), 15,* 167–186.

Locksley, R. M., Flournoy, N., Sullivan, K. M., Meyers, J. D. (1985). Infection with varicella-zoster virus infections. *Bone Marrow Transplantation. 152,* 1152–1178.

Mack, C. H. (1992). Assessment of the autologous bone marrow transplant patient according to Orem's self care model. *Cancer Nursing, 15,* 429–436.

Mahaney, F. X. (1994). Bone marrow transplant for breast cancer: Some insurers pay, some insurers don't [news]. *Journal of the National Cancer Institute, 86*(6), 420–421.

Martin, P. J., Remlinger, K., Hansen, J. A., Storb, R., Thomas, E. D., & the Seattle Marrow Transplant Team (1984). Murine monoclonal anti-T cell antibodies for treatment of refractory acute graft-versus-host disease (GVHD). *Transplantation Proceedings, 16,* 1494–1495.

Mawaji, A., Canten, S., Hartman, J., McKinlay, M. (1992). Care of the bone marrow recipient: A nursing perspective, part II: Patient's response and complications. *Canadian Association of Critical Care Nurses, 3*(3), 13–17.

McDonald, G. B., Shulman, H. M., Sullivan, K. M., & Spencer, G. D. (1986). Intestinal and hepatic complications of human bone marrow transplantation. Parts I & II. *Gastroenterology, 90,* 460–477, 770–784.

McDonald, J., Stetz, K., Compton, K., & Strickland, J. (1994). *Informational needs of family members of bone marrow transplant patients.* Unpublished research. Fred Hutchinson Cancer Research Center.

McGuire, D., Altomante, V., Peterson, D., Windgard, J., Jones, R., Grochow, L. (1993). Patterns of mucositis and pain in patients receiving preparative chemotherapy and bone marrow transplantation. *Oncology Nursing Forum 20*(10), 1493–1502.

Meriney, D. K. (1991). Neurologic and neuromuscular complications of bone marrow transplantation. In M. B. Whedon (Ed.), *Bone marrow transplantation: Principles, practices and nursing insights* (pp. 262–279). Boston: Jones and Bartlett Publishers.

Meyers, J. D., & Atkinson, K. (1983). Infection in bone marrow transplantation. In D. G. Nathan (Ed.), *Bone marrow transplantation* (pp. 791–811). London: W. B. Saunders Co.

Meyers, J. D., & Thomas, E. D. (1988). Infection complicating bone marrow transplantation. In R. H. Rubin & L. S. Young (Eds.), *Clinical approach to infection in the immunocompromised host* (pp. 525–556). New York: Plenum Press.

Mooney, B. R., Reeves, S. A., & Larson, E. (1993). Infection control and bone marrow transplantation. *American Journal of Infection Control, 21*(3), 131–137.

Nader, S., & Arvin, A. M. (1994). Varicella zoster virus infections. In S. J. Forman, K. G. Blume, & E. D. Thomas (Eds.), *Bone marrow transplantation* (pp. 412–428). Boston: Blackwell Scientific Publications.

Northouse, L. & Northouse, H. (1993). Cancer and the family: Strategies to assist spouses. *Seminars in Oncology Nursing, 9,* 74–81.

Northouse, P. G., & Northouse, L. L. (1987). Communication and cancer: Issues confronting patients, health professionals, and family members. *Journal of Psychosocial Oncology, 5,* 17–46.

Openshaw, H., & Slatkin, N. E. (1994). Neurological complications of bone marrow transplantation. In S. J. Forman, K. G. Blume, & E. D. Thomas (Eds.), *Bone marrow transplantation* (pp. 402–496). Boston: Blackwell Scientific Publications.

O'Quin, T., & Moravec, C. (1988). The critical ill bone marrow transplant patient. *Seminars in Oncology Nursing, 4,* 25–30.

Osterwalder, B., Gratwohl, A., Reusser, P., Tichelli, A., & Speck, B. (1988). Hematologic support in patients undergoing allogeneic bone marrow transplantation. *Recent Results in Cancer Research, 108,* 44–52.

Parkman, R. (1994). Immunological reconsitution following bone marrow transplantation. In S. J. Forman, K. G. Blume, & E. D. Thomas (Eds.), *Bone marrow transplantation* (pp. 504–526). Boston: Blackwell Scientific Publications.

Peters, W. P. (1994). Variation in approval by insurance companies of coverage for autologous bone marrow transplantation for breast cancer. *New England Journal of Medicine, 330*(7), 473–477.

Peters, W. P., Ross, M., Vredenburgh, J. J., Hssein, A., Rubin, P. (1994). The use of intensive clinic support to permit outpatient autologous bone marrow transplantation for breast cancer. *Seminars in Oncology, 21*(4 suppl. 7), 25–31.

Peterson, F. B., & Bearman, S. I. (1994). Preparative regimens and their toxicity. In S. J. Forman, K. G. Blume, & E. D. Thomas (Eds.), *Bone marrow transplantation* (pp. 79–95). Boston: Blackwell Scientific Publications.

Peterson, P. K., McGlave, P., Ramsay, N. K. C., Rhame, F., Cohen, E., Perry, G. S., Goldman, A. I., & Kersey, J. (1983). A prospective study of infection diseases following bone marrow transplantation. Emergence of aspergillus and cytomegalovirus as the major causes of mortality. *Infection Control, 4,* 81–89.

Poe, S., Larson, E., McGuire, D., Krumm, S. (1994). A national survey of infection prevention practices on bone marrow transplant units. *Oncology Nursing Forum, 21*(10), 1687–1694.

Powles, R. L., and Mehta, J. (1994). The future of bone marrow transplantation. In K. Atkinson (Ed.), *Clinical bone marrow transplantation: A reference textbook* (pp. 736–740). New York: Cambridge University Press.

Press, O. W., Schaller, R. T., & Thomas, E. E. (1986). Bone marrow transplant complications. In L. H. Toledo-Pereyra (Ed.), *Complications of organ transplanation* (pp. 399–424). New York: Marcel Dekker.

Randolph, S. R. (1993). Home care of the bone marrow transplant recipient: High tech, high touch. *Home Healthcare Nurse, 11*(1), 24–28.

Raybould, T., Carpenter, A., Fervetti, G., Brown, A., Thomas, L., Heuslee, J. (1994). Emergence of gram-negative bacilli in the mouths of bone marrow transplant recipients using chlorheredine mouthrinse. *Oncology Nursing Forum, 21*(4), 691–695.

Riddell, S., Appelbaum, F. R., Buckner, C. D., Stewart, P., Clift, R., Sanders, J. E., Storb, R., Sullivan, K. M., & Thomas, E. D. (1988). High-dose cytarbine and total body irradiation with or without cyclosphosphamide as a preparative regimen for marrow transplantation for acute leukemia. *Journal of Clinical Oncology, 6*, 576–582.

Ritz, J., Ramsay, N. K., & Kersey, J. H. (1994). Autologous bone marrow transplantation for acute lymphoblastic leukemia. In S. J. Forman, K. G. Blume, & E. D. Thomas (Eds.), *Bone marrow transplantation* (pp. 731–742). Boston: Blackwell Scientific Publications.

Robbins, R. A., Linder, J., Stahl, M., Thompson, A, Hane, W., Kessinger, A., Armitage, J., Arneson, M., Woods, G., Vaughan, W., Rennard, S. (1989). Diffuse alveolar hemorrhage in autologous bone marrow transplant recipients. *The American Journal of Medicine, 87*, 511–578.

Sanders, J. E. (1994). Growth and development after bone marrow transplantation. In S. J. Forman, K. G. Blume, & E. D. Thomas (Eds.), *Bone marrow transplantation* (pp. 527–537). Boston: Blackwell Scientific Publications.

Sanders, J. E., Buckner, C. D., Sullivan, K. M., Doney, K., Applebaum, F., Witherspoon, R., Storlo, R., & Thomas, E. D. (1988). Growth and development in children after bone marrow transplantation. *Hormone Research, 30*, 92–97.

Sayre, R. S., & Marcoux, B. C. (1992). Exercise and autologous bone marrow transplant. *Clinical Management, 12*, 78–82.

Schmitz, N., Gassmann, W., Rister, M., Johannson, W., Suttorp, M., Brix, F., Holthuis, J. J. M., Heit, W., Hertenstein, B., Schaub, J., & Loffler, H. (1988). Fractionated total body irradiation and high dose VP16-213 followed by allogeneic bone marrow transplantation in advanced leukemias. *Blood, 72*, 1567–1573.

Shaffer, S., & Wison, J. (1990). Bone marrow transplantation: Critical care implications. *Critical Care Nursing Clinics of North America, 5*(3), 531–542.

Shpall, E. J. & Jones, R. B. (1994). In S. J. Forman, K. G. Blume, E. D. Thomas (Eds.), *Bone marrow transplantation* (pp. 913–918). Boston: Blackwell Scientific Publications.

Shuhart, M. C., McDonald, G. B. (1994). Gastrointestinal and hepatic complications following bone marrow transplant. In S. J. Forman, K. G. Blume, & E. D. Thomas (Eds.), *Bone marrow transplantation* (pp. 454–481). Boston: Blackwell Scientific Publications.

Singer, J. W., & Neumunaitis, J. (1994). Use of recombinant growth factors in bone marrow transplantation. In S. J. Forman, K. G. Blume, & E. D. Thomas (Eds.), *Bone marrow transplantation* (pp. 309–327). Boston: Blackwell Scientific Publications.

Small, V. (1991). Total body irradiation—An overview. *Canadian Journal of Medical Radiation Technology, 22*, 73–76.

Spencer, G. D., Shulman, H. M., Myerson, D., Thomas, E. D., & McDonald, G. B. (1986). Diffuse intestinal ulceration after marrow transplantation: A clinical pathological study of 13 patients. *Human Pathology, 17*, 621–633.

Steeves, R. H. (1992). Patients who have undergone bone marrow transplantation: Their quest for meaning. *Oncology Nursing Forum, 19*, 899–905.

Storb, R., & Thomas, E. D. (1985). Graft versus host disease in dog and man. The Seattle Experience. In G. Moller (Ed.), *Immunological reviews* No. 88 (pp. 215–238). Copenhagen: Munksgaard.

Sullivan, K. M. (1994). Graft-versus-host disease. In S. J. Forman, K. G. Blume, & E. D. Thomas (Eds.), *Bone marrow transplantation* (pp. 339–362). Boston: Blackwell Scientific Publications.

Sullivan, K. M., Fefer, A., Witherspoon, R., Storb, R., Buckner, C. D., Weiden, P., Schoch, G., & Thomas., E. D. (1987). Graft-versus-host disease to relapse of acute leukemia in man: Relationship of acute and chronic graft–versus–host disease to relapse of acute leukemia following allogeneic bone marrow transplantation. In R. L. Truitt, R. P. Gale, & M. M. Bortin (Eds.), *Cellular immunotherapy of cancer* (pp. 391–399). New York: Alan R. Lisa.

Sullivan, K. M., & Parkman, R. (1983). The pathophysiology and treatment of graft-versus-host disease. *Clinics in Haematology, 12*, 775–789.

Thomas, E. E., Buckner, C. C, Banaji, M., Clift, R. A., Fefer, A., Flournoy, N., Goodell, B. W., Hickman, R. O., Lerner, K. G., Neiman, P. E., Sale, G. E., Sanders, J. E., Singer, J., Stevens, M., Storb, R., & Weiden, P. L. (1977). One hundred patients with acute leukemia treated by chemotherapy, total body irradiation, and allogeneic marrow transplantation. *Blood, 49*, 511–533.

Thomas, E. D., Clift, R. A., Fefer, A., Appelbaum, F. R., Beatty, P., Bensinger, W. I., Buckner, C. D., Cheever, M. A., Deeg, H. J., Doney, K., Fournoy, N., Greenberg, P., Hansen, J. A., Martin, P., McGuffin, R., Ramberg, R., Sanders, J. E., Singer, J., Stewart, P., Storb, R., Sullivan, K., Weiden, P. L., & Witherspoon, R. (1986). Marrow transplantation for the treatment of chronic myelogous leukemia. *Annals of Internal Medicine, 104*, 155–163.

Vanacek, K. S. (1991). Gastrointestinal complications of bone marrow transplantation. In M. B. Whedon (Ed.), *Bone marrow transplantation: Principles, practice and nursing insights* (pp. 206–239). Boston: Jones and Bartlett Publishers.

van der Meer, J. W. M, Guiot, H. F L., van den Brock, P. J., & van Furth, R. (1984). Infections in bone marrow transplant recipients. *Seminars in Hematology, 21*, 123–138.

van der Wal, R., Nims J., Davies, B. (1988). Bone marrow transplantation in children. *Cancer Nursing, 11*(3), 132–143.

van Leeuwen, A., Oudshoorn, M., Schreuder, I., Giphart, M., Claas, F., & van Rood, J. J. (1993). Laboratory procedures used to select an unrelated HLA matched bone marrow donor. *Bone Marrow Transplantation, 11*(Suppl. 1), 13–16.

Walker, F., Roethke, S. K., & Martin, G. (1994). An overview of the rationale, process, and nursing implications of peripheral blood stem cell transplantation. *Cancer Nursing, 17*, 141–148.

Walker, F. E., Roethke, S. K., Sandman, V., Clark, K., & Martin, G. (1994). Guiding patients and their families through peripheral stem cell transplantation with the help of a teaching booklet. *Oncology Nursing Forum, 21*, 585–591.

Weiden, P. L., Zukerman, N., Hansen, J. A., Sale, G., Remlinger, K,. Beck, T. M., & Buckner, C. D. (1981). Fatal graft-versus-host disease in a patient with lymphoblastic leukemia following normal granulocyte transfusions. *Blood, 57*, 328–332.

Wellisch, D. K., & Wolcott, D. L. (1994). Psychological issues in bone marrow transplantation. In S. J. Forman, K. G. Blume, & E. D. Thomas (Eds.), *Bone marrow transplantation* (pp. 556–571). Boston: Blackwell Scientific Publications.

Welte, K. (1994). Matched unrelated transplants. *Seminars in Oncology Nursing, 10*(1), 20–27.

Whedon, M. B. (Ed.) (1991a). *Bone marrow transplanatation: Principles, practice, and nursing insights*. Boston: Jones and Bartlett Publishers, 1–462.

Whedon, M. B. (1991). Allogeneic bone marrow transplantation: Clinical indication, treatment process, and outcomes. In M. B. Whedon (Ed.), *Bone marrow transplantation: Principles, practice, and nursing insights* (pp. 20–48). Boston: Jones and Bartlett Publishers.

White, M. H. (1993). Antifungal prophylaxis. *Current Opinion in Infectious Disease, 6,* 737–743.

Wikle, T. J. (1991). Pulmonary and cardiac complications of bone marrow transplantation. In M. B. Whedon (Ed.), *Bone marrow transplantation: Principles, practice and nursing insights* (pp. 182–205). Boston: Jones and Bartlett Publishers.

Wingard, J. (1994). Prevention and treatment of bacterial and fungal infections. In S. J. Forman, K. G. Blume, & E. D. Thomas (Eds.), *Bone marrow transplantation* (pp. 363–375). Boston: Blackwell Scientific Publications.

Winters, G., Glass, E., Sakurai, C. (1993). Ethical issues in oncology nursing practice: An overview of topics and strategies. *Oncology Nursing Forum, 20*(10), 2 –34.

Winters, G., Miller, C., Maracich, L., Compton, K., & Haberman, M. R. (1994). Provisional practice: The nature of psychosocial bone marrow transplant nursing. *Oncology Nursing Forum, 21,* 1147–54.

Wright, D. (1994). Peripheral stem cell transplantation. *Medical-Surgical Nursing, 3*(1), 36–41.

Wujcik, D. (1993). An odyssey into biologic therapy. *Oncology Nursing Forum, 20*(6), 879–887.

Wujcik, D., Ballard, B., & Camp-Sorrell, D. (1994). Selected complications of allogeneic bone marrow transplantation. *Seminars in Oncology Nursing, 10*(1), 28–41.

Wujcik, D., & Downs, S. (1992). Bone marrow transplantation: Tissue and organ transplantation. *Critical Care Nursing Clinics of North America, 4,* 149–166.

Wulff, J. C., Santner, T. J., Storb, R., Banaji, M., Buckner, C. D., Clift, R., Stewart, P., Snaders, J., Slichter, S., & Thomas, E. D. (1983). Transfusion requirements after HLA-identical marrow transplantation in 82 patients with aplastic anemia. *Vox Sanguinis, 44,* 366–374.

Wynstra, N. A. (1994). Breast cancer. Selected legal issues. *Cancer, 74,* 491–511.

Yeager, A. M., Kaizer, H., Santos, G. W., Saral, R., Colvin, O. M., Stuart, R. K., Brainey, H. G., Burke, P. J., Ambinder, R. F., Burns, W. H., Fuller, D. J., David, J. M., Karp, J. E., May, W. S., Rowley, S. D., Sensenbrenner, L. L., Vogelsang, G. B., & Wingard J. R. (1986). Autologous bone marrow transplantation in patients with acute nonlymphocytic leukema using ex vivo marrow treatment with 4-hydroperoxycyclophosphamide. *New England Journal of Medicine, 315,* 141–148.

Young, L. S. (1984). An overview of infection in bone marrow transplant recipients. *Clinics in Haematology, 13,* 661–667.

Zabora, J. R., Smith, E. D., Baker, F., Wingard, J. R. & Curbow, B. (1992). The family: The other side of bone marrow transplantation. *Journal of Psychosocial Oncology, 10,* 35–46.

Zaia, J. (1994). Cytomegalovino infection. In S. J. Forman, K. G. Blume, & E. D. Thomas (Eds.), *Bone marrow transplantation* (pp. 376–403). Boston: Blackwell Scientific Publications.

CHAPTER
28

Alternative Cancer Therapies

Cynthia R. King

INTRODUCTION

Every year thousands of cancer patients in the United States use treatments outside of the mainstream of medicine. This occurrence may be attributed to the limited number of effective cancer treatments (this is especially true for advanced stages of cancer), treatments composed of multiple toxicities, and uncertain long-term survival. Recent studies demonstrate that alternative cancer treatments continue to flourish with the current health food industry and holistic health movement, rather than decline with advances in biomedicine (Cassileth, 1989; Cassileth et al., 1991; Furnham & Smith, 1988; Lerner & Kennedy, 1992). The use of unproven cancer practices has become a major public health issue.

Many different terms are used to describe alternative cancer therapies. Some of the most common include unconventional, unproven, unorthodox, questionable, quackery, and fraudulent. Surgery, radiation therapy, chemotherapy and biotherapy are considered conventional or orthodox treatments. Several terms (alternative, unproven, unconventional, and unorthodox) will be used interchangeably throughout the chapter.

Cancer is a disease in which questionable, often worthless, and frequently harmful therapies are popu-lar. The public spends a significant amount of money on these remedies despite the fact that 45 to 50 per cent of serious cancers diagnosed each year in the United States are curable (Curt, 1993; Miller & Howard-Ruben, 1983).

Alternative cancer therapies (ACTs) may vary greatly. Some are within legal mandates and ethical principles, whereas other practices rely on pharmacologic and biologic agents that are not approved within the U.S. legal system (U.S. Congress, 1990). The term alternative cancer therapy literally refers to any cancer therapy that is not approved by the United States Food and Drug Administration (FDA). These include therapies that lack scientific and/or clinical data demonstrating their effectiveness (U.S. Congress, 1990; Miller & Howard-Ruben, 1983).

The most common ACTs are based on a holistic philosophy. Most promoters of alternative methods perceive cancer as a clinical manifestation of an underlying systemic problem. Therefore, the clinical manifestation is treated rather than the cancer. Treatment involves lifestyle approaches. Self-care is a central theme underpinning the philosophy regarding many of these alternative methods of cancer care. Self-care provides the patient with a sense of control over the illness. Subsequently, patients may find these therapies appealing because human caring and psychologic support are routinely provided with these therapies (Holmes, 1992).

This chapter provides an overview and history of unproven cancer remedies as well as a description of four categories of unconventional practices. Clinical implications for the health care provider will be discussed.

OVERVIEW AND HISTORY

Medicine has made many major advances in public health; vaccinations and antibiotics have been successful in the prevention and treatment of life-threatening infectious diseases. As new clinical advances are made there is a greater need to distinguish between effective and ineffective cancer practices (U.S. Congress, 1990).

Unproven methods of cancer therapy have been promoted since 1748, when the House of Burgesses of the General Assembly of Virginia evaluated Mary Johnson's cure for cancer. The investigative panel included George Washington and James Madison. The remedy promoted by Johnson consisted of garden sorrel, bark celandine, persimmon bark, and spring water. Personal testimonies convinced the panel that this therapy cured cancer, and they awarded Mary Johnson 100 pounds to continue her cures (Guzley, 1992; Schaller & Carrol, 1976).

The hot/cold theory of disease gained favor in the early 1900s. At this time emetics and hot baths were promoted. By 1850 homeopathy prevailed. This was followed by naturopathy in the 1890s. Naturopathists believe that disease results from a violation of the natural laws of living, and remedies for disease involved diets, massages, and colonic irrigation (Cassileth, 1989). The 1890s brought early forms of osteopathy and chiropracty. Disease was viewed as resulting from a dislocation of spinal bones and could be corrected with spinal manipulation. The early quasi-medicines targeted at cancer appeared in pill and liquid forms in the 1900s. With the new electronic age in the 1920s came "energy" cancer cures and cosmic energy treatments.

The popularity of different ACTs has often paralleled advances in conventional clinical cancer medicine. In the 1940s and 1950s radiation therapy was beginning to improve control of disease. At this time unorthodox cancer remedies became device-oriented. Patients were treated with the oscilloclast (a device that "retuned" disharmonic electrons). Another device was the orgone energy accumulator. This looked like a telephone booth and was constructed of metal, wood, and asbestos board. This device was used to concentrate a visible and ubiquitous cosmic energy into depleted erythrocytes. In 1954 an injunction was issued against the owner of the orgone energy accumulator (Curt, 1993).

During the 1950s through the 1970s chemotherapy became an acceptable treatment for patients with advanced cancer. ACTs became quasi-medicines in pill or liquid form used to target cancer. Cures that were introduced included the Hoxsey treatment in extract, pill, and injection form; Krebiozen; and Laetrile. These agents will be discussed more thoroughly under types of therapies (Curt, 1993).

In 1987 the Office of Technology Assessment (OTA) was directed by the U.S. Congress to research ACTs and compile a report. The resultant report, entitled *Unconditional Cancer Treatments* (U.S. Congress, 1990), recommended that funding be available to study alternative therapies. The response to this study was the formation of the Office of Alternative Medicine housed within the National Institutes of Health in 1991. The office was developed to investigate and validate unconventional medical practices (Curt, 1993).

There have been two major shifts in the practice of unorthodox cancer treatment. The first involves a focus on biologic therapies. These include antineoplastons (proteins derived from urine) and immunoaugmentative therapy (claims to boost the immune response). The second change involves a shift back to unconventional methods that involve natural, holistic, diet-oriented regimens. The premise of these therapies is that cancer and other diseases are symptoms of metabolic imbalances rather than illnesses. Currently, cures involve lifestyle-oriented remedies rather than pills or liquids. The change to advocating lifestyle remedies avoids regulation by the FDA. Additionally, these treatments do not involve secret formulas but activities of daily living to be performed by the patient. Thus, these ACTs are less removed from conventional medicines. The lifestyle remedies advocated emphasize diet, lifestyle, environment, and the relationship of the psychosocial and the physical responses (Cassileth & Kleinbart, 1991; Curt, 1993) (Table 28–1).

FACTS

It is difficult to determine the exact amount spent on ACTs, but in 1984 the Subcommittee on Health and Long-term Care of the U.S. House of Representatives concluded that Americans spent $10 billion on unconventional remedies and specifically $4 to $5 billion on useless cancer treatments (*Quackery, a $10 billion scandal*, 1984). A study of inpatients at a large urban cancer center found that 13 per cent of the patients had used or were using unorthodox therapies in addition to therapy prescribed by their physicians (Cassileth, Lusk, Strouse, & Badenheimer, 1984). This represents a selected inpatient population at only one university referral center, but the findings are supported by information obtained from a study performed by the Division of Consumer Affairs of the Food and Drug administration in 1986. More than 6000 American households were surveyed. Fifteen per cent of all cancer patients surveyed had used one or more ACTs (Louis Harris Survey, 1987).

CREDENTIALS

The educational background of practitioners advertising ACTs vary from individuals with no education to physicians. Some of these physicians have degrees from reputable medical schools, and they may even hold prestigious academic positions. Other practitioners

TABLE 28–1. *Examples of Major Unorthodox Approaches Over Time*

ERA OF POPULARITY IN THE UNITED STATES	UNORTHODOX APPROACH	REFERENCE
1800–1850	*Thomsonianism* Belief: All disease results from one general cause (cold) and can be cured by one general remedy (heat). Opposed "mineral" drugs and the "tyranny" of doctors. Remedy: Emetics and hot baths.	Starr, 1982; Thompson, 1825; Thompsonian Record, 1832
1850–1900	*Homeopathy* Belief: Like cures like ("Law of Similia"); disease results from suppressed itch ("psora"). Remedy: More than 3000 different drugs, each a highly distilled organic or inorganic substance.	Gardner, 1957; Kaufman, 1971; Starr, 1982
1890–	*Naturopathy* Belief: Disease results not from external bacteria but from violation of the natural laws of living; drugs are harmful; "natural" products and activities cure. Remedy: Diets, massages, colonic irrigation.	Gardner, 1957; Kellog, 1923
1890–	*Early Osteopathy and Chiropracty* Belief: Mechanistic view of the body; disease caused by dislocation of bones in the spine. Rejected drugs and germ theory. Remedy: Spinal manipulation.	Gardner, 1957; Still, 1897
1900s	Tablet and ointment cancer cures by B. F. Bye, W. O. Bye, Buchanan, Chamlee, G. M. Curry, L. T. Leach (Cancerol), C. W. Mixer, E. H. Griffith (Radio-sulpho), F. W. Warner, R. Wells (Radol).	Cramp, 1912
1920s	"Energy" cancer cures by A. Abrams (radio wave cure), R. B. Brown (radio therapy), A. E. Kay (cosmic energy "vrilium"), D. Ghadiali (spectro-chrome light therapy); E. Cayce's psychic diagnoses and treatments.	Gardner, 1957
1940s	W. F. Koch's Glyoxylide.	American Cancer Society, 1964b; Janssen, 1979; Miller & Howard-Rubin, 1983
1950s	H. Hoxsey's cancer treatment.	American Cancer Society, 1964a; Janssen, 1979; Miller & Howard-Rubin, 1983
1960s	A. C. Ivy's Krebiozen.	American Cancer Society, 1962; Janssen, 1979; Miller & Howard-Rubin, 1983
1970s	Laetrile.	Markle & Petersen, 1980; Moertel et al., 1982
1980s	Metabolic therapies: diet, high colonics, vitamins and minerals, Simonton's imagery.	Cassileth et al., 1984 Simonton, 1982; Simonton et al., 1981
1990s	Psychologic and behavioral therapies: psychoneuroimmunology. Metabolic therapies: diet, high colonics, vitamins and minerals.	Curt, 1993; Engebretson & Wardell, 1993; Hauser, 1993; Holmes, 1992

have degrees in the basic sciences, nutrition, nursing, zoology, or veterinary medicine. Furthermore, some individuals may have training in other healing systems (e.g., chiropractic, naturopathy, or naprapathy). There are individuals who have received their degrees from correspondence schools or who may place letters behind their names that have no meaning. It is often difficult for the public to determine which practitioners are legitimate and which are not (Miller & Howard-Ruben, 1983).

SCIENTIFIC DATA

Proponents of ACTs rarely provide results of clinical trials in presentations or scientific journals. Instead these promoters generally use testimonials, case studies, pamphlets, audiovisuals, and books. ACTs tend to advertise in seminars, conventions, and publications aimed at the consumer (U.S. Congress, 1990).

INSURANCE COVERAGE

Insurance coverage for the Federal Medicare Program (for individuals aged 65 years and older) is limited only to care that is "reasonable and necessary." This generally means coverage for drugs that are approved by the Federal Drug Administration (FDA). Most private insurance companies have similar restrictions. The majority of insurance contracts have terms that exclude alternative therapies. These contracts may even specify particular therapies not covered (e.g., laetrile, immunoaugmentative therapy) (U.S. Congress, 1990).

ORGANIZATION EFFORTS RELATED TO ALTERNATIVE CANCER THERAPIES

During the past few decades there have been organizations created to advocate ACTs (e.g., National Health Federation, International Association of Cancer Victims and Friends, and the Committee for Freedom of Choice in Cancer Therapy). Unconventional cancer therapies have become a major focus for these organizations. There have been three significant regulatory bodies involved in researching and evaluating alternative methods of treatment. These organizations have included the federal government, the American Medical Association (AMA), and the American Cancer Society (ACS) (Miller & Howard-Ruben, 1983).

FEDERAL GOVERNMENT

Despite the 1906 Food and Drug Act, marketing of unorthodox methods continued. In 1910, the Supreme Court established a new ruling. This ruling, however, addressed only truthful labeling of drug ingredients. Promoters could still defraud patients and avoid prosecution by claiming the labeling was mistaken praise. President Taft remained concerned about the prevalence of unsound therapies and the possible dangers to the public. He urged the passage of legislation that would prevent false hopes for speedy cures by "mistaken praise" of worthless remedies (Curt, 1993; Guzley, 1992; Miller & Howard-Ruben, 1983). The Sherley Amendment was passed by Congress in response to Taft's concerns. This amendment made it a criminal offense to attribute false and fraudulent claims of therapeutic effectiveness to drugs. The Sherley Amendment also mandated that there be proof of a drug's safety and efficacy (Janssen, 1979). Because this act defined fraud as intentional deceit, patients could still be defrauded by claims made in ignorance or by mistake.

In 1938 a new food and drug law was passed that included several major changes. The need to prove fraud was eliminated. Simultaneously the need to prove safety was added. In 1962 drug controls mandating effectiveness and safety prior to the sale of a drug was established. Consequently, between 1962 and 1987 more than 7000 prescription medications were eliminated from the marketplace. These controls continued to be challenged by promoters of ACTs, but in 1973 the U.S Supreme Court upheld the FDAs program and associated laws (Curt, 1993; Miller & Howard-Ruben, 1983).

In the United States the Federal Food, Drug, and Cosmetic Act and other laws regulate the sale, manufacture, and marketing of medical products (Curt, 1993). Congress enacted laws believing the federal government has an interest in protecting the health of its citizens while also respecting their freedom of choice.

Medications and treatments must now be accepted by the FDA so that they may be marketed in the United States. Relevant laws and regulations address approval, labeling, advertising and marketing of pharmaceuticals and medical devices (U.S. Congress, 1990). Many of the unorthodox treatments involve drugs, devices, or biologics that remain unapproved by the FDA. In the United States the normal FDA approval for a new drug is a lengthy process—often many years. To avoid this lengthy FDA process many medications are researched and marketed in other countries. Each year thousands of Americans receive medications not approved for use in the United States by bringing these drugs back after traveling abroad. In 1988 the FDA Commissioner announced a new FDA policy. The FDA will now allow Americans to import medications from other countries in amounts up to a 3 month supply for personal use. This has increased the ease with which individuals can obtain ACTs from other countries (Pelton & Overholser, 1994).

The National Cancer Institute (NCI) is involved with alternative methods because it has a responsibility to educate the public about cancer. Several branches of the NCI supply information to the public about treatments. The Public Inquiries Office responds to written inquiries and questions from the National Institutes of Health (NIH). The Cancer Information Service is a telephone network composed of a national office and 25 regional offices. Information is available on a wide range of cancer-related topics. The statements describe the treatment, state the claims, summarize the evidence available to NCI, and draw a conclusion.

The situation in the United States is in contrast to an apparent openness to ACTs, which have had little to no testing in a number of European countries: Switzerland, Germany, England, and the Netherlands. Other countries do not require the extensive drug testing mandated by the United States. Thus, many of the treatments that are legally available in other countries are not available here (U.S. Congress, 1990).

AMERICAN MEDICAL ASSOCIATION

For many years the American Medical Association (AMA) was the chief leader of the medical community to attempt to eliminate alleged health fraud. It takes a less active role now. Many of the earlier activities of the AMA focused on cancer therapies. In 1962 the Committee on Quackery was formed to oppose the recognition of chiropractors as legitimate health care providers. In the mid-1970s four chiropractors brought suit against the AMA. After an 11-year lawsuit, the court decided in favor of the chiropractors. The Committee on Quackery was eliminated in 1975 (U.S. Congress, 1990).

The focus of the AMA shifted to prevent health fraud and educate professionals and the public as to the advantages and disadvantages of controversial therapies. This organization, however, refers many questions to other agencies such as NCI or the American Cancer Society (ACS) (U.S. Congress, 1990).

AMERICAN CANCER SOCIETY

The American Cancer Society has been a leader in defining the limits of orthodoxy in cancer treatment. It has developed an "Unproven Methods List," which is often utilized by health care professionals to counsel their patients about treatment and is available to the lay public. The list is also used by insurance companies to determine reimbursement (U.S. Congress, 1990).

By developing and circulating information about alternative treatment methods, the ACS has become a major influence in this area. The activities relating to ACTs are handled by the Committee on Unproven Methods of Cancer Management, which was started in 1954. The committee originally intended to provide information to physicians but now has expanded to provide information to the public. There are currently 25 to 30 individual statements on unproven methods of cancer management. All statements are being updated and they appear in *Ca: A Cancer Journal for Clinicians* (Pelton & Overholser, 1994).

ORGANIZATIONS PROMOTING ALTERNATIVE METHODS

Some of the most active organizations promoting ACTs include Cancer Control Society (CCS), International Association of Cancer Victors and Friends (IACVF), the National Health Federation (NHF), the Foundation for the Advancement in Cancer Therapies (FACT), and the American Quack Association (AQA). There are also some patient associations such as Immunoaugmentative Therapy Patient's Association (IATPA), Hans Nieper Foundation (HNF), and Friends of Dr. Revici. These organizations and groups actively promote and market alternative methods for cancer therapy (U.S. Congress, 1990).

COMMON CHARACTERISTICS OF ALTERNATIVE CANCER THERAPIES

Four specific characteristics are shared by most alternative cancer therapies. These characteristics include promise, pseudoscience, profit, and philosophy.

PROMISE

Practitioners of unorthodox cancer methods often exploit fear and promise painless nontoxic treatment with good results. The promoters promise patients that the results are as good as and often better than the results of conventional medical treatments and without adverse effects. Unfortunately, these promises are frequently not fulfilled (Danielson, Stewart, & Lippert, 1988; Duffy, 1975).

PSEUDOSCIENCE

Unconventional cancer therapies are often based on complex pseudoscientific theories that utilize scientific jargon. Yet, the promoters provide no scientific evidence in support of them. The one common element in the theories is use of a linear explanation of what causes cancer. All cancer is described as having one cause, and thus, one treatment can effect a cure. Even though the advocates of ACTs claim miraculous breakthroughs, they predominately present proof in anecdotal or case study form. Rarely do advocates of these methods participate in valid scientific studies that will subject their therapy to rigorous scrutiny. Social and political pressure has resulted in some questionable agents (e.g., laetrile, ascorbic acid) being examined scientifically. Results of these examinations have illustrated that there has been no significant benefit in terms of cure, improvement of symptoms, or extension of life span (Danielson et al., 1988; Moertel et al., 1978; Moertel, Fleming, Rubins, Kvols, & Tinker, 1982).

PROFIT

It is estimated that Americans spend $4 to 5 billion on ACTs each year. Profit can be a major motivation for promoters of a specific treatment. This was true in the case of laetrile. The entrepreneur who advocated laetrile was involved in the manufacturing and distribution of laetrile as well as all the related money-making services (Danielson et al., 1988).

PHILOSOPHY

Proponents of unorthodox therapies often have philosophic views that challenge conventional medicine. These individuals attempt to promote distrust of orthodox medicine by informing the patient that medical personnel are suppressing their new cure for cancer. In 1984 Cassileth and colleagues studied 356 cancer patients using alternative therapies and found that 50 per cent believed the government was denying them freedom of choice (Danielson et al., 1988; Duffy, 1975).

THE PATIENT'S CHOICE OF ALTERNATIVE THERAPIES

Originally it was thought individuals who sought ACTS did so out of ignorance. Individuals with cancer were considered to be victims (Cassileth & Kleinbart, 1991; Cobb, 1954; Duffy, 1975). Any individual who sought ACTs was considered to need factual, concrete information from organizations like ACS and the FDA to persuade them of the hazards of unconventional practices (Cassileth & Kleinbart, 1991; Olson, 1977). In essence these individuals were stereotyped as unsophisticated consumers who must be underprivileged, poor, or uneducated (Bruch, 1974; Cassileth & Kleinbart, 1991; Curt, 1993).

Research of oncology patients and of unconventional remedies has demonstrated that individuals utilizing ACTs are as or better educated than patients not utilizing these methods (Avina & Schneiderman, 1978; Bruch, 1974; Cassileth et al., 1984; Lupton, Najman, Payne, Sheehan, & Western, 1978; National Analysts, Inc., 1972; Wagenfeld, Vissing, Markle, & Petersen, 1979). In 1984 Cassileth and colleagues performed a study of 304 cancer inpatients compared with 356 cancer patients using alternative therapies alone or in combination with orthodox therapy. The investigators found that these patients were better educated ($p < 0.00001$) than those who used only conventional medical treatments. This is supported by a recent FDA telephone survey of 6000 American homes. Higher level of education was the single best predictor of whether the individual adopted an alternative therapy (Louis Harris Survey, 1987). The most educated patients were likely to select mental imagery as an alternative treatment. In part this may be a result of these unproven treatments requiring time, financial resources, and an educated questioning approach to illness. These same patients are often quite knowledgeable concerning orthodox cancer therapies as well. They may have already received several opinions and read relevant medical journals. The financial investment for travel, purchase of equipment, and special foods required by alternative treatments is more congruent with a middle to upper level of socioeconomic status.

Patients who tend to use ACTs often have a personal experience having known friends and neighbors who died of cancer, even though the medical community advertises that 50 per cent of people diagnosed with cancer are cured. There is a discrepancy then between what the medical profession portrays and the individual's personal experience. Patients begin to question the validity of conventional cancer statistics. This discrepancy creates uncertainty, and patients begin to seek alternative options. Realizing that there are toxic effects of orthodox cancer treatments, many hope that these ACTs will offer the same chance for cure and also be nontoxic. These are some of the reasons they turn to ACTs.

Patients may also react to perceived deficiencies in the traditional physician-patient relationship. In a study by Cassileth and colleagues (1984) patients remaining with conventional cancer therapies without use of unproven methods rated quality of relationship with their physician as higher (Danielson et al., 1988).

The literature cited patient's fears, previous negative experiences with conventional cancer treatment, excess media coverage of ACTs, and a search for a more holistic, supportive therapeutic environment as reasons for the use of ACTs (Barrett, 1978; Burkhalter, 1977; Howard-Ruben & Miller, 1984).

Currently the focus of ACTs is on self-care, which is what many patients want. They are seeking a more holistic method of care. Research has demonstrated that patients opting for alternative methods are intelligent and inquisitive and unlikely to be persuaded that a therapy is useless solely because the promoter lacks scientific credentials or has not conducted scientifically sound clinical trials. Individuals seeking alternative care may have had some conventional treatment prior to trying an unproven method. There are also some patients who continue orthodox medical treatments. Some patients may hide the fact they are pursuing unconventional therapies from their mainstream health care professional; others will confide in them. Overall there remains limited information to characterize reliably the reasons persons use ACTs. This is an area of future research for oncology nurses.

TYPES OF THERAPIES

The treatments that fall under alternative cancer therapies include a heterogenous group of practices. They vary in content, safety, effectiveness, and the types of practitioners administering them. Unfortunately, it is difficult to make general characterizations about these therapies. Positive or negative assessments regarding one therapy do not necessarily apply to another.

There are four general categories of ACTs: metabolic/nutritional, pharmacologic/biologic, machines and devices, and psychologic/behavioral. Some therapies are difficult to categorize as they include a variety of components, and thus, they are assigned categories based on the nature of the central element of the approach (U.S. Congress, 1990). A list of ACTs is provided in Table 28–2.

In a recent study conducted by ACS the most frequently used ACTs were psychologic/behavioral (50 per cent), certain diets (38 per cent), pharmacologic (33 per cent), and electronic (33 per cent) (Hauser, 1993).

METABOLIC/NUTRITIONAL THERAPIES

Metabolic therapies comprise a variety of alternative interventions. With these therapies cancer is seen as a symptom of an underlying metabolic imbalance. Metabolic therapists believe that cancer should be directed at cellular detoxification and restoration (Cassileth & Kleinbart, 1991; Curt, 1993; Gerson, 1977; Manner, DiSanti, & Michaelsen, 1978). These metabolic regimens vary by practitioner. They often consist of enzyme therapy, cellular therapy, dietary manipulation, vitamin treatment (especially laetrile and megavitamins), and detoxification by colonic cleansing. These remedies are available from clinics and practitioners in North America, Europe, and Mexico (Cassileth & Kleinbart, 1991; Curt, 1993).

The goals of metabolic therapies are to:

1. provide ideal nutrition
2. minimize the intake of carcinogens (eliminating smoking, decreasing alcohol intake, changing occupation)
3. help the patient develop a positive mental attitude
4. assist the body to eliminate toxic wastes
5. discourage the intake of any kind of drugs (Donsbach & Walker, 1981).

Metabolic interventions are not new. The theory is that metabolic imbalances caused the malignancy, and reversing the imbalance will cure the disease. In the early 1900s, Dr. Koch proposed that cancer could be treated by oxidizing toxic compounds generated in the body. Renewed interest in metabolic therapies has recently been reported (Curt, 1993).

Many clinics consider diet as an important component of metabolic interventions (e.g., East West Center for Macrobiotics and Kushi Foundation). Dr. Linus Pauling recommended, as an alternative therapy, that

TABLE 28–2. *List of Alternative Cancer Therapies*

Alkylating punch	Hett cancer serum
Alivizatos therapy	Hill hadley vaccine
Almonds	Hoxsey method
Aloe vera plant	Immunoaugmentative therapy (IAT)
Anti-cancer factor in clams	Iscador
Antineoplastons	Issels combination therapy
Asparagus oil	Kanfer Neuromuscular
Bacteria enema	KC-555
Bamfolin	Kelly malignancy index
Beard methods	Koch antitoxins
Biomedical detoxification therapy	Krebiozen
Bonifacia anticancer goat serum	Laetrile (amygdalin)
Cancer lipid concentrate	Lewis method
Carcin and neo-carcin	Livingston method
Carrot/Celery juice	Macrobiotic diet
Carzodelin	Makari intradermal test
CH-23	Manners metabolic method
Chamonils	Marijuana
Chaparral tea	Megadose vitamin therapy
Chase dietary method	Millet bread
Chelation	Millrue
C.N.T.	Miniburg system
Coffee enemas	MP virus
Collodarium and bichloracetic acid	Mucorhicin
Compound X	Multiple enzyme therapy
Contreras methods	Naessens serum
Cresson method	Nichols Escharotic method
Crofton immunization	Nieper
Cytec lung cancer screening	Olive oil
Diamond carbon compound	Oncone juice
D.M.S.O.	Orgone energy devices
Dotto electronic reactor	Oscilloclast
Drown Radio-Therapeutic instrument	Pap-check female testing
Ferguson plant products	Polonine
Fonti method	Psychic methods
Frances diet	Rand coupled fortified antigen (RCFA)
Fresh cell therapy	Revici cancer control
Frost method	Samuels endocrinotherapy
Ganner petroleum	Sander's Treatment
Germanium	Simonton method
Gerson method	Snake meat
Gibson method	Spears hygienic system
Glover serum	Staphylococcus phage lysate
Goat's milk	Sunflower seeds
Grape diet	Ultraviolet blood irradiation
Heat therapy	Wigmore program
Hemacytology index	Zen macrobiotic diet
Hendricks natural immunity therapy	

vitamin C might inhibit tumor cell invasion and metastasis. Most metabolic clinics offer combinations of diet, vitamin therapy, and detoxification (Curt, 1993).

MACROBIOTICS

One of the most popular health-oriented therapies in the world is the macrobiotic therapy. Macrobiotic diet and therapy are based on alternative concepts of physiology and illness. The proponents suggest there is a single red blood cell in the intestine that is considered the progenitor of all other cells and organs. The intake of food and fluids is balanced to counteract illness.

Macrobiotics, rooted in ancient oriental philosophy, was not developed as a treatment for cancer, but much of the recent literature markets it as a remedy for the prevention and treatment of cancer. A number of books have been written as testimonials to this approach, such as: *Confessions of a Kamikaze Cowboy* (Benedict, 1987) and *Recalled by Life* (Sattilaro & Monte, 1982). For these individuals macrobiotics is a philosophy and a way of life drawing on Japanese culture and Eastern philosophy (Arnold, 1984; U.S. Congress, 1990).

The introduction of macrobiotic therapy into the United States is attributed to George Ohsawa (the pen name for a Japanese teacher/physician). It is reported that he cured himself of cancer by changing his diet and lifestyle. For him, the cure for cancer involved returning to natural eating and drinking and combining this with the Zen Buddhist philosophy. This treatment is based on the theory of metabolic contamination, and the focus is on the need to cleanse and purify the body through special diets, internal irrigation, and/or spiritual attitude. He suggested that leukemia can be cured in 10 days by this method (Bowman, Kushner, Dawson, & Levin, 1984; Howard-Ruben & Miller, 1984; U.S. Congress, 1990). In 1971, serious nutritional deficiencies were found with this diet by the AMA Council on Foods and Nutrition, some of which were fatal. This diet was found to result in scurvy, anemia, hypocalcemia, hypoproteinism, emaciation due to starvation, and loss of kidney function in a number of cases. The publicity led to a strongly negative view of the regimen in the 1970s and 1980s (U.S. Congress, 1990).

In the 1970s Michio Kushi led a movement to change the content and focus of the macrobiotic therapy. He preserved elements of Ohsawa's philosophy while including a variety of broader and more complex components (U.S. Congress, 1990).

A macrobiotic diet (Table 28–3) is comprised of 50 per cent cooked whole grains, 20 to 30 per cent organically grown vegetables, and smaller quantities of soups, beans, and sea vegetables (seaweed). Fruits, white meats, and fish are allowed only in limited quantities. Foods to be avoided include meats, poultry, animal fat, eggs, dairy products, refined sugar, tropical fruits, and all artificially colored or preserved foods. The manner in which the food is cooked and prepared is stressed. Macrobiotics is not one single diet for every individual but a therapy that evaluates geographic variations, age, sex, and level of activity (Bowman et al., 1984; Pelton & Overholser, 1994).

TABLE 28–3. *Macrobiotic Dietary Guidelines*

CATEGORY	% OF DIET	EXAMPLES OF FOODS
Whole Grains	50-60	Brown rice, oats, barley, corn, rye, buckwheat, whole wheat
Vegetables	25-30	Prepare by saute, steam, boil, bake, pressure cook
Soups	5-10	1-2 bowls/day made from grains, beans, vegetables
Beans/Sea Vegetables	5-10	Seaweed is primary sea vegetable
Beverages		Fresh water, nonaromatic, nonstimulating herbal teas
Occasional Foods		Moderate amounts of white meat, fish, fresh fruits

Percentages refer to the volume of food consumed daily, not the weight.

TABLE 28–4. *Examples of Yin and Yang by Cancer Sites*

YIN	YANG	YIN & YANG
Skin	Colon	Lung
Stomach (upper)	Prostate	Stomach (lower)
Breast	Ovary	Uterus
Brain (outer)	Brain (inner)	Bladder/kidney
Mouth (except tongue)	Bone	Tongue
Leukemia	Rectum	Liver
Esophagus	Pancreas	Spleen

Macrobiotic therapy for cancer is approached from an Oriental perspective. The first step involves classifying the individual's cancer as "yin" (expansive), "yang" (contractive), or both depending upon the site of the primary tumor (Table 28–4). "Yin" and "yang" are antagonistic and complementary forces that create and balance all phenomena in the world. Tumors in the peripheral or upper parts of the body or in the hollow, expanded organs are described as yin (e.g., lymphoma, leukemia, Hodgkin's, tumors of the mouth), while tumors in the lower or deeper parts of the body or more compact organs are yang (e.g., colon, rectum, prostate, ovaries, pancreas). Foods are also classified as yin or yang energies. An excess of either yin or yang foods or both is thought to cause cancer. Thus, changes are made in a patient's diet, behavior, and exercise to rebalance their energy and obtain health (Bowman et al., 1984; U.S. Congress, 1990).

There is currently no evidence to support the use of macrobiotic therapy alone in the treatment of cancer. The Office of Technology Assessment (OTA) reviewed information regarding the efficacy of macrobiotics for cancer patients. The information provided was composed predominately of retrospective case review, two unpublished retrospective studies, and anecdotal reports. Due to serious flaws in the studies the data were inadequate to make an objective assessment. Additionally, the macrobiotic diet may be deficient in ascorbic acid and lacking in essential minerals, vitamins, and proteins and result in serious nutritional deficiencies. Some cancer patients may not get enough calories or proteins. Other difficulties that may arise are inability to locate some of the ethnic foods required by the diet, and time-consuming manner of preparing and cooking the food. The macrobiotic regimen involves time, effort, and a huge commitment (Arnold, 1984; Howard-Ruben & Miller, 1984; Pelton & Overholser, 1994; U.S. Congress, 1990).

GERSON THERAPY

This is one of the best known ACTs. Gerson developed his vegetarian diet to relieve his severe migraine headaches. Dr. Albert Schweitzer became Gerson's patient at age 75 years when he suffered from diabetes. Schweitzer underwent dietary treatment and was able to return to his work at an African hospital. Due to the prewar political climate in Germany in 1933, Gerson emigrated to New York City. It was at this time he applied his treatment to cancer (Pelton & Overholser, 1994).

In the 1950s Gerson's treatment was investigated by the ACS Committee on Unproven Methods of Cancer Management. They stated that they were unable to confirm that Gerson's therapy could cure cancer. In 1958 the Medical Society of the County of New York revoked Dr. Gerson's membership. He, however, continued to treat cancer patients until his death in 1959. In 1977 Charlotte Gerson Straus, Gerson's daughter, and Norman Fritz cofounded the Gerson Institute in California (Pelton & Overholser, 1994; U.S. Congress, 1990).

The aim of the therapy is to detoxify the body and restore electrolyte balance. Gerson believed the underlying problem was an impaired metabolism and that proper liver function was crucial to maintaining metabolic order. Cancer patients were seen as having impaired metabolism of fats, proteins, carbohydrates, vitamins, and minerals. Cancer patients must adhere to a strict vegetarian diet with fresh fruit and vegetable juices. The primary focus of this therapy is the restoration between cellular water and salt through potassium supplementation and avoidance of sodium intake. Gerson also recommended that protein be restricted for 6 to 8 weeks. Restricting protein causes the body to excrete even more sodium from the damaged cells. Protein restriction also stimulates the production of T lymphocytes and enhances immune functioning. Gerson developed this treatment over decades by using variations and combinations of foods and other agents. Initially, patients received coffee enemas every 3 to 4 hours to help stimulate the flow of bile and excrete wastes from the body. The diet then was supplemented by potassium, thyroid hormone, injectable crude liver extract, vitamin B12, and pancreatic enzymes. This therapy is time-consuming because it requires the juicing of fresh fruits and vegetables every hour, plus administering coffee enemas every 3 to 4 hours (Pelton & Overholser, 1994; U.S. Congress, 1990).

Potential adverse effects may result from the coffee enemas and use of raw calves liver juice. Coffee enemas have been associated with serious fluid and electrolyte imbalances—including death. Infection with *Camplyobacter fetus* may result from the ingestion of raw calves liver juice.

There have been several attempts since the 1940s by groups, organizations, or individuals to evaluate the effects of Gerson's regimen. In 1947 the NCI reviewed 10 case histories and found no convincing evidence of effectiveness. Then in 1959 the NCI reviewed another 50 cases and discovered that the basic clinical criteria for evaluating clinical effectiveness were not present (U.S. Congress, 1990).

PHARMACOLOGIC AND BIOLOGIC PRODUCTS

PHARMACOLOGIC AGENTS

For centuries herbs and medicine have been a part of ACTs. Four pharmacologic examples over the years have included the Koch Antitoxin therapy, Hoxsey Chemotherapy, Krebiozen, and Laetrile.

KOCH

A reagent, glyoxylide, was developed in 1919 by Dr. Koch to serve as an oxidation catalyst and body stimulant antagonist to cancer cells. The reagent was to enhance oxidative phosphorylation in cellular mitochondria. Chemical analyses of this potent drug revealed it contained only pure distilled water. The FDA prosecuted Dr. Koch. While this treatment remains unavailable in the U.S., it can still be obtained in Mexico (Howard-Ruben & Miller, 1984; Janssen, 1979).

HOXSEY CHEMOTHERAPY

Hoxsey developed a treatment to restore the body to its normal physiologic state. Hoxsey thought that healthy cells mutated and became cancerous if the body was in chemical imbalance. The remedy is based on Hoxsey's great-grandfather's remedy, which was used to cure a horse of cancer. The therapy involved taking a pink medicine and a black medicine. The pink medicine was potassium iodide and pepsin, while the black was cascara in an extract of licorice, red clover, burdock root, stillingia root, poke root, and the bark of the buckthorn and prickly ash. In the 1960s the federal court issued an injunction to stop sales of the Hoxsey treatment. Hoxsey was convicted of practicing medicine without a license after peddling his therapy from state to state. Hoxsey's therapy still remains available in Mexico (Curt, 1993; Donsbach & Walker, 1981; Guzley, 1992).

KREBIOZEN

This therapy was developed as an antihypertensive agent by Dr. Durovic and was popular in the 1950s and 1960s. The drug was supposedly derived by extracting the serum from horses injected with a pathogenic fungus, *Actinomyces bovis* (Curt, 1993). Of the 12 animals with tumors Dr. Durovic treated with the drug, seven were reported to have improvement of their disease (Durovic, 1961). These results were never reproduced. In 1963 the FDA analyzed samples of Krebiozen. Krebiozen was found to be creatinine, which is a simple organic acid widely distributed in muscle tissues and is not known to be an effective antitumor agent. In 1964 Durovic and the Krebiozen Research Foundation were indicted on 49 counts for violating the Food, Drug, and Cosmetic Act. Eventually the defendants were found innocent, but the interstate distribution of Krebiozen was stopped (Curt, 1993). Interest in Krebiozen waned after Durovic withdrew cash from the Foundation bank accounts and left for Switzerland.

LAETRILE

Laetrile continues to attract patients despite the U.S. government's efforts to prohibit its use. Laetrile has become the center of a struggle between the FDA and the supporters of laetrile. The FDA wants to protect the general public. The laetrile supporters view its use as a freedom of choice issue and accuse the government of conspiracy to suppress cures for cancer (Annas, 1980; Curt, 1993; Howard-Ruben & Miller, 1984).

Laetrile is the name used for a group of cyanogenic glucosides. These glucosides are isolated from a variety of natural sources including the pits of edible plant sources (plums, cloves, almonds, apricots, peaches). The main component of laetrile is called amygdalin. It was first used in cancer therapy by Dr. Ernest Krebs, Sr., in the 1920s. The compound was found to be too toxic for humans. Consequently, his son, Ernest Krebs, Jr., developed a purified product in the 1950s (Curt, 1993; Dorr & Pazxinos, 1978; Guzley, 1992; Howard-Ruben & Miller, 1984). Knowing that cancer cells abound with β-glucosidase, an enzyme, it was thought laetrile could cause this enzyme to release cyanide. Normal cells are spared during this process because they are low in this enzyme (Curt, 1993; Guzley, 1992).

In 1970 Krebs transformed cyanogenic glycosides into vitamin B_{17}. Laetrile could then be called a vitamin and Krebs could side-step the drug regulations of the FDA. The laetrile business was controlled by an entrepreneur named Andrew McNaughton who founded Bioenzymes International, Ltd. Laetrile was manufactured in Mexico and Canada. Because there was no evidence that laetrile was useful as an antitumor agent, the FDA began a series of actions against Krebs and the McNaughton Foundation. The Canadian FDA also prohibited distribution of laetrile in Canada. The FDA analysis of Mexican laetrile indicated that a 500 mg tablet often contained only 42 to 450 mg of amygdalin (Davignon, Trissel, & Kleinman, 1978). All of these activities only reinforced the belief that the government was attempting to suppress a useful therapy from the public. Thirty years and 70,000 patients later, laetrile was proven an ineffective anticancer agent (Moertel et al., 1978; Moertel et al., 1982).

From 1957 to 1977 the National Cancer Institute sponsored animal testing and found laetrile ineffective. In addition, oral laetrile was found to cause symptomatic cyanide toxicity and high blood levels of cyanide. Intravenous laetrile has also been shown to cause fever, rash, headache, hypotension, vomiting, diarrhea and motor disturbances (Howard-Ruben & Miller, 1984).

Some practitioners have combined laetrile with other metabolic therapies. Unfortunately, megadoses of vitamin C can cause the additional release of cyanide from laetrile and contribute to cyanide poisoning (Howard-Ruben & Miller, 1984).

BIOLOGIC AGENTS

Biologic therapies include vaccines and preparations from the patient's and/or animal blood or urine. Several examples include the Lewis Method, the Helt cancer serum, and the Rand vaccine. The Lewis method consists of injections of coupled tumor protein antigen (CTPA). The Helt cancer serum is of an unknown derivation. It contains *E. coli* and *streptococcus fecalis*.

The Rand vaccine was developed in 1966 and produced by injecting the blood of animals with material from human cancers. An application was submitted to the FDA. Their application was rejected because of heavy bacterial contamination of the vaccine that caused toxic effects in patients. The Rand vaccine resulted in accelerated growth of cancer in test results. The vaccine was last produced in 1967 (American Cancer Society, 1971).

IMMUNOAUGMENTATIVE THERAPY

A more recent biologic therapy has been immunoaugmentative therapy (IAT), which is alleged to bolster the immune system. This treatment was developed by Dr. Lawrence Burton, a biologist, and was first described by him while working in New York City in the 1960s. In 1973 he and Dr. Friedman opened the Immunology Research Foundation (IRF) in Great Neck, New York. At this time they submitted an application to the FDA for an Investigational New Drug permit. More information was requested by the FDA. These requests were not answered. Finally the application was withdrawn, and the center was established in the Bahamas in 1977 (Curt, 1993; Green, 1993; Howard-Ruben & Miller, 1984; Pelton & Overholser, 1994).

In 1978 a review committee of the Pan-American Health Organization recommended that the clinic be closed in the Bahamas. The Immunology Research Center, however, remained open to treat non-Bahamians. Finally in 1985 the Bahamian government forced Dr. Burton to close the clinic secondary to reported AIDs and hepatitis B viral contamination of his blood-derived products (Curt, 1993); however, the clinic was allowed to reopen in March 1986. The Bahamian government was convinced that adequate conditions had been met to eliminate the health hazards to the staff and clients (Green, 1993).

To receive the treatment at this center, patients must be referred by a physician. The first step involves a series of immunocompetence blood tests. These are analyzed to select the individual's treatment regimen. The actual therapy involves four immune serum protein fractions consisting of deblocking protein (DP), tumor antibody 1 (TA1), tumor antibody 2 (TA2), and tumor complement (TC). Promoters of this regimen claim that if these substances are used in the correct combination, they will restore the normal immune function in immunosuppressed cancer patients. Some or all of these serum protein fractions are given daily as subcutaneous injections. The length of therapy is uncertain. It ranges from weeks to months as patients must make follow-up visits for reevaluation or retuning of the immune system. The cost is more than $10,000 (Curt, 1993; Pelton & Overholser, 1994).

The components of the IAT treatment have been repeatedly analyzed. Each analysis of the reagents has demonstrated only diluted blood proteins. Albumin has been the major component of the reagents (Curt, Katterhager, & Mahaney, 1986). Repeatedly, the materials were shown to be contaminated with bacteria and hepatitis virus. An epidemic of abscesses has been reported at IAT injection sites (Curt, 1984). It appears that there is no scientific rationale for IAT. Patients appear to be treated with inert blood products that have been transmitting bacteria, hepatitis, and AIDs. The Bahamian clinic was closed in 1985, but Dr. Burton moved to develop clinics in Mexico.

ANTINEOPLASTONS

Antineoplaston treatment is an alternative therapy offered at the Burzynski Research Institute in Houston. In the 1960s Dr. Burzynski, a Polish biochemist, began advertising that medium-sized peptides normally present in the urine are able to control tumor growth. He called these chemicals antineoplastons. For the individual cancer patient the dosage of each antineoplaston fraction in serum and urine would be determined prior to treatment. This assists in the cancer diagnosis and evaluating the response to treatment (Liau, Szopa, Burzynski, & Burzynski, 1986; U.S. Congress, 1990). Generally the treatment requires 6 weeks to 1 year. Antineoplaston therapy may be given via a central venous catheter or in a newly available capsule form. Treatment starts with a small dose and increases gradually. It claims to be a nontoxic therapy and costs $45 per treatment. Complete responses have been claimed for lung, prostate, stomach, colon, breast, and bladder cancer (Burzynski & Kubove, 1987a; Burzynski & Kubove, 1987b; Burzynski, Kubove, & Burzynski, 1987; Curt, 1993). Confirmation of these results has not been achieved to date.

From 1974 to 1976 Burzynski received funding from NCI for research of gel filtration techniques to isolate peptides from urine. He did not receive a renewal for this grant in 1976. In 1983 he applied to the FDA for an Investigational New Drug (IND) to use antineoplastons in human subjects. The application was put on hold as there was not enough data submitted (U.S. Congress, 1990). In 1982, the Canadian ministry of Health made a site visit and found no evidence of therapeutic efficacy. Subsequently, they disallowed this remedy in Canada (Blackstein & Beasagel, 1982). No partial or complete responses were found in 1985 in a follow-up of 36 antineoplaston patients. In fact, 34 of 36 patients had died. The two survivors had already received prior curative conventional therapy.

MACHINES AND DEVICES

In the early part of this century mechanical devices were used to treat cancer. Individuals were fascinated with the machines. The oscilloclast was developed by Dr. Abrams, who considered cancer to be caused by disharmony in the electric oscillation of the body's electrons. The oscilloclast allegedly could detect the oscillations that were in disharmony and could adjust them. It eventually was made illegal (Milstead, Davis, & Dobelle, 1963; Miller & Howard-Ruben, 1983).

PSYCHOLOGIC AND BEHAVIORAL THERAPIES

A widely discussed topic in both the scientific and popular literature is the role of personal characteristics and behavior in the recovery from serious illness. Several popular books have been written on the role of emotions and behavior in recovery from illness: *Anatomy of an Illness* (Cousins, 1981) and *Love, Medicine, and Miracles* (Siegel, 1986). A variety of psycho-logic and behavioral methods are becoming key aspects of cancer treatment. The aim of most of these methods is to enhance quality of life. Some of these regimens are incorporated into mainstream medical treatments, whereas others are offered independently.

PSYCHONEUROIMMUNOLOGY

It has been suggested in the literature that some types of behavioral interventions that focus on reducing stress or promoting positive mental images in fact act by enhancing the immune system. Because the immune system is the primary defense system against diseases, the enhancement of the system is associated with reducing the susceptibility to cancer and/or improving the ability to fight cancer. Unfortunately the relationships among emotions, immunity, and disease are poorly understood. The relatively new field of psychoneuroimmunology (PNI) examines the interrelationships among personality, emotion, behavior, alterations in immune function, and neuroendocrinology. To date, PNI research has focused on correlations between psychosocial characteristics and biochemical measures of the immune system or between psychosocial characteristics and disease onset and progression. PNI has begun to assess techniques such as mental imagery, meditation, and self-regulation (e.g., hypnosis, biofeedback, and relaxation) (Ader, 1981, 1987; U.S. Congress, 1990).

LESHAN'S

One of the examples of unconventional psychotherapy is one-to-one psychotherapy developed by Lawrence LeShan. LeShan is a researcher and clinical psychologist. His research has focused on relationships among personality factors, traumatic life events, and onset and progression of cancer (U.S. Congress, 1990).

The premise of this method is that with psychotherapy, patients with metastatic disease may be able to increase the length and quality of life or possibly have tumor regression. The psychotherapeutic regimen is used to identify the self-healing ability of the patient. It is a process of self-examination and growth that delves deeply into the patients' past to discover the blocks that exist. He encourages patients to use the cancer as a "turning point" in their lives (LeShan, 1977, 1989; U.S. Congress, 1990).

To date, the reports of tumor regression have been entirely anecdotal.

MENTAL IMAGERY

In 1984 Cassileth and colleagues reported that 16 per cent of the patients used mental imagery as a means for curing malignant disease. Proponents suggest that psychologic therapies can influence the immune system and destroy cancer cells and, thus, counteract the malignant disease process. Mental imagery is considered to be a part of psychoneuroimmunology (Cassileth & Kleinbart, 1991; Howard-Ruben & Miller, 1984; Simonton, 1982; Simonton, Matthews-Simonton, & Creighton, 1981; Varan, 1989). Psychoneuroimmunology utilizes a variety of regimens to enhance immune function (Halvorsen & Vassand, 1987; Locke et al., 1984; Schleifer, Keller, Camerino, Thornton, & Stein,

1983; Stein, Keller, & Schleifer, 1985). Unfortunately, research to date has not proven that altered immune function affects cancer.

Simonton Method. The Simonton Method is one of the most popular psychologic and behavioral therapies utilized. It was developed by Dr. Carl O. Simonton and Stephanie Simonton-Atchley. It is a holistic approach to cancer treatment that was created to restore the physical, mental, and emotional balance of the individual. It emphasizes a strong connection between the mind and the body. They developed this method to motivate patients to produce a will to live. Patients utilize visual imagery and relaxation techniques to call on the body's defenses to attack their cancer. Mental imagery involves visualizing the destruction of malignant cells. It appears there are several positive outcomes of this method including promoting mastery over a situation, promoting relaxation, counteracting helplessness and hopelessness, decreasing fears, advocating continued conventional therapy, and assisting the patient to cope with the situation. There is, however, no scientific evidence that personality contributes to the growth of cancer, nor is there scientific evidence that imagery affects cancer (Howard-Ruben & Miller, 1984).

The techniques are simple and easily self-taught. Patients perform the techniques three times per day along with drawing analyses, exercising, counseling, and eating a sensible diet. This is not unsound, but is it of use? It remains relatively inexpensive and is easy to administer by oneself (Curt, 1993).

EVALUATION OF UNPROVEN THERAPIES

How should health care professionals evaluate alternative methods of cancer therapy? Herbert (1986b) suggests there are three principle ethical questions regarding alternative therapy:

1. Is it more effective than nothing?
2. Is it as safe as doing nothing?
3. If there is a question of safety, then is the balance between effectiveness and safety weighed for or against the patient?

If therapies fail to answer the above questions, then they should be considered experimental and not adequately tested (Herbert, 1986b).

Rigorous scientific method is the only way available for determining whether a therapy is effective or beneficial for cancer patients. Methodologically, evaluation methods for alternative treatments consisting of pharmacologic and biologic agents should be the same as those that have been utilized for conventional ones. Promoters of "middle ground therapies" (e.g., psychologic and behavioral and dietary) used with conventional treatment are the most interested in testing their methods but often feel the system is not supportive (U.S. Congress, 1990).

Multifaceted therapies that combine dietary, psychologic and behavioral aspects (e.g., Gerson's Therapy, Macrobiotics) and which intend to improve quality of life may require variations in conventional scientific methods, yet unbiased, scientific evaluation will still be required. It is essential that the evaluation be initiated by and be the responsibility of the practitioner(s) utilizing the ACT. Little is learned by testimonials and case reviews. Potential outcomes might include improvement in disease-free survival and quality of life.

In the 1990s there have been several attempts at evaluating the clinical efficacy of alternative cancer remedies. In 1991 Cassileth and colleagues studied 158 matched cohorts of patients with metastatic or recurrent colon cancer. One group received conventional medical care, while the other received autogenous immune-enhancing vaccine, vegetarian diet, and coffee enemas. Cassileth reports there was no difference in the two groups in terms of survival. However, the quality of life (QOL) was significantly better in the patients receiving only mainstream medical care. This contradicts the assumption that ACTs enhance QOL because of their emphasis on self-help and lack of toxicities associated with conventional treatments.

There is a need to increase the current knowledge base concerning:

1. characteristics and motivations of cancer patients seeking ACTs,
2. utilization studies to determine types and extent of alternative methods used in the U.S., and
3. incidence and potential adverse effects of ACTs.

It is only with further evaluation and scientific studies that health care professionals will be able to adequately evaluate the risks and benefits of each alternative method for treating cancer.

RISKS

Although some alternate practices are benign, many others are potentially harmful (Brown & Greenwood, 1987; Haman & Blackburn, 1986; Herbert, 1986a, 1987; Umstead, 1988). Alternative therapies lack the stringent controls that are in place in the current biomedical system. ACTs can cause severe morbidity and even death.

The risks associated with alternative cancer methods may take a variety of forms. They may involve the adverse effects resulting from delay or never receiving conventional medical treatment. In patients with advanced disease, alternative remedies may promote needless suffering if the patient does not receive symptom relief and appropriate palliative care. Some remedies provide false hope and prevent the patient and family from coping effectively with the progression of the illness. And last, the utilization of ACTs often involves travel, disruption in daily living, and significant expense (Braico, Humbert, & Terplan, 1979; Rynearson, 1974; U.S. Congress, 1990).

NURSING IMPLICATIONS

The business of alternative treatments is flourishing in the United States. Oncology nurses have a professional responsibility to oncology patients involved in alternative remedies. Their roles include educator, counselor, researcher, advocate, and provider of physical and psychologic care.

Nurses are generally the health care provider in closest contact with patients and families. The oncology nurse may play a crucial role in the patient's decision making process. As a patient advocate, the nurse must be sure the patient's values guide all treatment choices. If a patient decides to try an alternative therapy, then the nurse has a responsibility to respect the decision; yet, the nurse must also provide accurate information and protect the patient from exploitation, deception, and physical harm.

For several reasons it is essential that oncology nurses have knowledge regarding these unproven cancer therapies. These reasons include (1) epidemiologic—as more than 50 per cent of cancer patients currently utilize one or more of these methods, (2) social—an enormous amount of pressure is exerted on the patient by relatives, friends, and the media to seek alternative regimens, (3) economic—significant amounts of money are spent by patients on unorthodox therapies, and (4) scientific—health care professionals providing conventional treatments cannot ignore the existence of unproven methods. There is a need to collect and screen information about alternative remedies as a base for effective nurse-patient discussions (Hauser, 1993).

Other nursing interventions may include

1. establishing and maintaining open communication with the patient,
2. exploring the patient's fears and anxieties,
3. conveying empathy and acceptance,
4. clarifying misconceptions,
5. promoting patient autonomy,
6. maintaining a realistic attitude of hope.

A key strategy for oncology nurses is to initiate a discussion about unproven cancer therapies before the patients utilize them. Discussions may be initiated by utilizing a conversation opener such as: " A lot of people . . .", or "Some patients use . . .." These conversational openers are nonjudgmental and encourage the patient to share. During conversations with patients the nurse may also use open-ended questions and careful probing to facilitate discussions. It is also helpful to explain to the patients that they will hear about a variety of unconventional alternatives to standard treatment. Encourage the patient to discuss these alternative remedies at any time. If oncology nurses are able to demonstrate concern and openness then many patients will initiate discussions of alternative cancer practices.

Once the patients initiate a discussion, determine why they are interested in this unconventional practice. Explain why the treatment may not be effective. Have the patients bring copies of information provided by the practitioner. This allows the nurse to thoroughly assess the therapy. Explanations of the difference between testimonials and scientific evidence may help the patients evaluate the ACT.

Nurses must spend time and show concern during the discussion. Patients want information, to have hope, and to be heard. Unorthodox practitioners are often effective at providing time, encouragement, support, and cancer. Oncology nurses must take time out of their busy schedule to provide a sympathetic ear.

The nurse's behavior at the critical juncture when a patient is considering alternative therapies can be a positive or negative force. Oncology nurses should first determine what the patient and family know about the type of cancer, extent of disease, and purpose of current therapy. Clear and consistent, objective, concrete information is helpful. Additionally, nurses can propose that patients consider utilizing alternative methods in combination with, not in place of, conventional therapy. Nurses should also assess for psychologic factors that influence individuals to seek unproven methods (anxiety, feeling of helplessness). It is important for oncology nurses in all practice settings (e.g., office, hospital, home care) to be knowledgeable about the various ACTs available, including risks and benefits.

SUMMARY

Alternative cancer therapies continue to flourish in the U.S. Currently, they reflect the trend in holistic, self-care medicine. Health care professionals have the opportunity and obligation to help patients make informed health care choices. Patients need all the pertinent information before making a choice. Nurses need to serve as resources for patients. Conventional medical and nursing care should evaluate each new unproven cancer therapy and incorporate any reasonable component of this treatment into their practice.

REFERENCES

Ader, R. (Ed.). (1981). *Psychoneuroimmunology.* New York: Academic Press.

Ader, R. (1987). Clinical implications of psychoneuroimmunology. *Journal of Developmental and Behavioral Pediatrics, 6*(6), 357–358.

Aihara, H. (1985). *Basic macrobiotics.* New York: Japan Publishing.

American Cancer Society. (1971). *Unproven methods of cancer management.* New York: Author.

Annas, G. (1980). Laetrile: Should the dying patient decide? *Nursing Law and Ethics, 1*(7), 1–15.

Arnold, C. (1984). The macrobiotic diet: A question of nutrition. *Oncology Nursing Forum, 11*(3), 50–53.

Avina, R., & Schneiderman, L. (1978). Why patients choose homeopathy. *Western Journal of Medicine, 128,* 366–369.

Barrett, S. (1978). The health quack: Supersalesman of the seventies. *Archives of Internal Medicine, 138,* 1065–1066.

Benedict, D. (1987). *Confessions of a kamikazee cowboy.* North Hollywood, CA: Newcastle Publishing.

Blackstein, M. E., & Beasagel, D.E. (1982). *The treatment of cancer patients with antineoplastons and the Burzynski clinic in Houston, Texas.* Ontario: Report to the Ministry of Health.

Bowman, B., Kushner, R. F., Dawson, S. C., & Levin, B. (1984). Macrobiotic diets for cancer treatment and prevention. *Journal of Clinical Oncology, 2*(6), 702–711.

Braico, K., Humbert, J., & Terplan, K. (1979). Laetrile intoxication: Report of a fatal case. *New England Journal of Medicine, 300,* 238–240.

Brown, G. R., & Greenwood, J. K. (1987). Megavitamin toxicity. *Canadian Pharmaceutical Journal, 120,* 80–87.

Brown, N., & Stayman, S. (1984). *Macrobiotic miracle: How a Vermont family overcame cancer.* New York: Japan Publishing.

Bruch, H. (1974). The allure of food cults and nutrition quackery. *American Journal of Nursing, 73,* 928–930.

Burkhalter, P. K. (1977, March). Cancer quackery. *American Journal of Nursing, 77,* 451–453.

Burzynski, S. R., & Kubove, E. (1987a). Initial clinical study with antineoplaston A2 injections in cancer patients with five years' follow-up. *Drugs: Experimental and Clinical Research, 13*(Suppl. 1), 1–12.

Burzynski, S. R., & Kubove, E. (1987b). Phase I clinical studies of antineoplaston A3 injections. *Drugs: Experimental and Clinical Research, 13*(Suppl. 1), 17–29.

Burzynski, S. R., Kubove, E., & Burzynski, B. (1987). Phase I clinical studies of antineoplaston A injections. *Drugs: Experimental and Clinical Research, 13*(Suppl. 1), 37–43.

Cassileth, B. R. (1989). The social implications of questionable cancer therapies. *Cancer, 63,* 1247–1250.

Cassileth, B. R., & Kleinbart, J.M. (1991). Questionable cancer therapies. In S. B. Baird, R. McCorkle, & M. Grant (Eds). *Cancer Nursing: A Comprehensive Textbook* (pp. 415–423). Philadelphia: W.B. Saunders Co.

Cassileth, B. R., Lusk, E. J., Geurry, D., Blake, A. D., Walsh, W., Kascius, L., & Schultz, D. J. (1991). Survival and quality of life among patients receiving unproven as compared with conventional cancer therapy. *New England Journal of Medicine, 324*(17), 1180–1185.

Cassileth, B. R., Lusk, E. J., Strouse, T. B., & Badenheimer, B. A. (1984). Contemporary unorthodox treatments in cancer medicine: A study of patients, treatments and practitioners. *Annals of Internal Medicine, 101,* 105–112.

Cobb, B. (1954). Why do people detour to quacks? *Psychiatric Bulletin, 3,* 66–69.

Cousins, N. (1981). *Anatomy of an illness.* New York: Bantam Books.

Curt, G. A. (1984). Warning on immunoaugmentative therapy. *New England Journal of Medicine, 311,* 859.

Curt, G. A., Katterhager, G., & Mahaney, F. X. (1986). Immunoaugmentative therapy: A primer of the perils of unproven treatment. *JAMA, 255,* 505–507.

Danielson, K. J., Stewart, D. E., & Lippert, G. P. (1988). Unconventional cancer remedies. *Canadian Medical Association Journal, 138,* 1005–1011.

Davignon, P., Trissel, L. A., & Kleinman, L. M. (1978). Pharmaceutical assessment of amygdalin (laetrile products). *Cancer Treatment Reports, 62,* 99–104.

Donsbach, K. W., & Walker, M. (1981). *Metabolic cancer therapies.* Huntington Beach, CA: The International Institute of National Health Sciences, Inc.

Dorr, R., & Pazxinos, J. (1978). The current status of laetrile. *Annals of Internal Medicine, 89*(3), 389–397.

Duffy, P. H. (1975). Cancer quackery. *Arizona Medicine, 32,* 724–726.

Durovic, S. (1961). Cancer and krebiozen: A new concept in cancer. *Today Japan Orient West, 6,* 51–55.

Engebretson, J., & Wardell, D. (1993). A contemporary view of alternative healing modalities. *Nurse Practitioner,* 51–55.

Furnham, A., & Smith, C. (1988). Choosing alternate medicine: A comparison of the beliefs of patients visiting a general practitioner and a homeopath. *Social Science Medicine, 26,* 685–689.

Gerson, M. (1977). *A cancer therapy: Results of fifty cases.* Del Mar, CA: Totality Books.

Green, S. (1993). Immunoaugmentative therapy: An unproven cancer treatment. *Journal of the American Medical Association, 270*(14), 1719–1723.

Guzley, G. J. (1992). Alternative cancer treatment: Impact of unorthodox therapy on the patient with cancer. *Southern Medical Journal, 85*(5), 519–523.

Halvorsen, R., & Vassand, O. (1987). Effects of examination stress on some cellular immunity functions. *Journal of Psychosomatic Research, 31,* 693–701.

Haman, N. W., & Blackburn, J. L. (1986). *Herbs and health benefits and risks.* Winnipeg: Cantest Publishing.

Hauser, S. P. (1993). Unproven methods in cancer treatment. *Current Opinion in Oncology, 5*(4), 646–654.

Herbert, V. (1986a). Questionable cancer remedies. in A. I. Holleb (Ed.), *The American Cancer Society source book* (pp. 238–247). New York: American Cancer Society.

Herbert, V. (1986b). Unproven (questionable) dietary and nutritional methods cancer prevention and treatment. *Cancer, 58,* 1930–1941.

Holmes, S. (1992). Have alternative methods got a place in the treatment of cancer? *Journal of the Royal Society of Health,* 15–19.

Howard-Ruben, J., & Miller, N. J. (1984). Unproven methods of cancer management. Part II: Current trend and implications for patient care. *Oncology Nursing Forum, 11*(1), 67–73.

Janssen, W. F. (1979). Cancer quackery: The past in the present. *Seminars in Oncology, 6,* 526–536.

Lerner, I. J., & Kennedy. B. J. (1992). The prevalence of questionable methods of cancer treatment in the United States. *CA: A Cancer Journal for Clinicians, 42,* 181–191.

LeShan, L. L. (1977). *You can fight for your life. Emotional factors in the causation of cancer.* New York: M. Evans.

LeShan, L. L. (1989). *Cancer as a turning point.* New York: E.P. Dutton.

Liau, M. C., Szopa, M., Burzynski, B., & Burzynski, S. R. (1986). Quantitative assay of plasma and urinary peptides as an aid for the evaluation of cancer patients undergoing antineoplaston therapy. *Drugs and Experimental and Clinical Research, 13*(Suppl. 2), 61–70.

Locke, S. E., Kraus, L., Leserman, J., Hurst, M. W., Heisel, J. S., & Williams, R. M. (1984). Life change stress, psychiatric symptoms and natural killer cell activity. *Psychosomatic Medicine, 46,* 441–453.

Louis Harris Survey on the Use of Questionable Cancer Products. (1987). Food and Drug Administration. Division of Consumer Affairs.

Lupton, G., Najman, J., Payne, S., Sheehan, M., & Western, J. (1978). Demographic characteristics of patients presenting for chiropractic and related forms of treatment. *Community Health Studies, 1,* 51–56.

Manner, H. W., DiSanti, S. J., & Michaelsen, T. L. (1978). *The death of cancer.* Chicago: Advanced Century Publishing Corporation.

Miller, N. J., & Howard-Ruben, J. (1983). Unproven methods of cancer management. Part I: Background and historical perspectives. *Oncology Nursing Forum, 10*(4), 46–52.

Milstead, J. L., Davis, J. B., & Dobelle, M. (1963). Quackery in the medical device field. *Proceedings of the Second National Congress on Medical Quackery.*

Moertel, C. G., Ames, M. M., Kovach, J. S., Moyer, T. P., Rubin, J. R., & Tinker, J. H. (1978). A pharmacologic and toxicological study of amygdalin. *JAMA, 255,* 591–594.

Moertel, C. G., Fleming, T. R., Rubins, J., Kvols J. R., & Tinker, J. H. (1982). A phase II trial of amygdalin (laetrile) in human cancer. *New England Journal of Medicine, 306,* 201–206.

National Analysts, Inc. (1972). *A study of health practices and opinions.* Springfield, VA: U.S. Department of Commerce.

Olson, K.B. (1977). Drugs, cancer and charlatans. In J. Morton & G. J. Hill (Eds). *Clinical oncology* (pp. 182–191). Philadelphia: W.B. Saunders Co.

Pelton, R., & Overholser, L. (1994). *Alternatives in cancer therapy.* New York: A Fireside Book.

Quackery: A $10 billion scandal. Subcommittee on Health and Long-term Care of the Select Committee on Aging. House of Representatives. 98th Congress. 2nd session. 1984 (Committee publication 98–435).

Rynearson, E. (1974). Americans love hogwash. *Nutrition Review, 32*(Suppl. 1), 1–14.

Sattilaro, A., & Monte, T. J. (1982). *Recalled by life: The story of recovery from cancer.* Boston: Houghton-Mifflin Co.

Schaller, W., & Carrol, C. (1976). *Health quackery and the consumer.* Philadelphia: W.B. Saunders Co.

Schleifer, S. J., Keller, S. E., Camerino, M., Thornton, J. C., & Stein, M. (1983). Suppression of lymphocyte stimulation following bereavement. *Journal of the American Medical Association, 250*(3), 374–377.

Sherlock, P., & Rothschild, E. O. (1967). Scurvy produced by a zen macrobiotic diet. *Journal of American Medical Association, 199*(11), 794–798.

Siegel, B. (1986). *Love, medicine, and miracles.* New York: Harper-Collins.

Simonton, O. C. (1982). Unproven methods of cancer management. *CA: A Cancer Journal for Clinicians, 2,* 58–61.

Simonton, O. C., Matthews-Simonton, S., & Creighton, J. L. (1981). *Getting well again.* New York: Bantam Books.

Stein, M., Keller, S. E., & Schleifer, S. J. (1985). Stress and immunomodulation: The role of depression and neuroendocine function. *Journal of Immunology, 135,* (Suppl 0), 827–832.

Umstead, G. S. (1988). Unapproved drug therapies. Geriatrics, arthritis and cancer. *Journal of Pharmacy and Technology, 4,* 97–106.

U.S. Congress, Office of Technology Assessment (1990). *Unconventional cancer treatments,* OTA-H-405. Washington DC: U.S. Government Printing Office.

Varan, W. J. (1989). Imagery and immunity. *Holistic Living, 6,* 4.

Wagenfeld, M. O., Vissing, Y. M., Markle, G. E., & Peterson, J. C. (1979). Notes from the underground: Health attitudes and practices of participants in the Laetrile movement. *Social Science Medicine, 13A,* 483–485.

UNIT VI
EFFECTS OF COMMON ADULT CANCERS

CHAPTER

29

Breast Cancers

M. Tish Knobf

Carcinoma of the breast is the most common cancer and the leading cause of death among American women between the ages of 35 to 54 years. In 1995 in the United States an estimated 182,000 women will be diagnosed and 46,000 will die from this malignancy (Wingo, Tong, & Bolden, 1995).

Mortality rates have remained relatively constant over the past several decades, in contrast to a rising incidence rate (Fig. 29–1). Prior to 1980 incidence rose slightly, primarily in women 50 years of age or older. Since that time there has been a more dramatic rise in incidence, observed in both younger and older women (Kelsey & Horn-Ross, 1993). The increased use of screening mammography provides a partial, but not a full, explanation for the increased incidence. Support for the role of mammography in early detection is provided by the higher detection rates of smaller tumors and in situ disease during that time period (Miller, Feur, & Hankey, 1993; White, Lee, & Kristal, 1990). The role of other variables, specifically risk factors such as

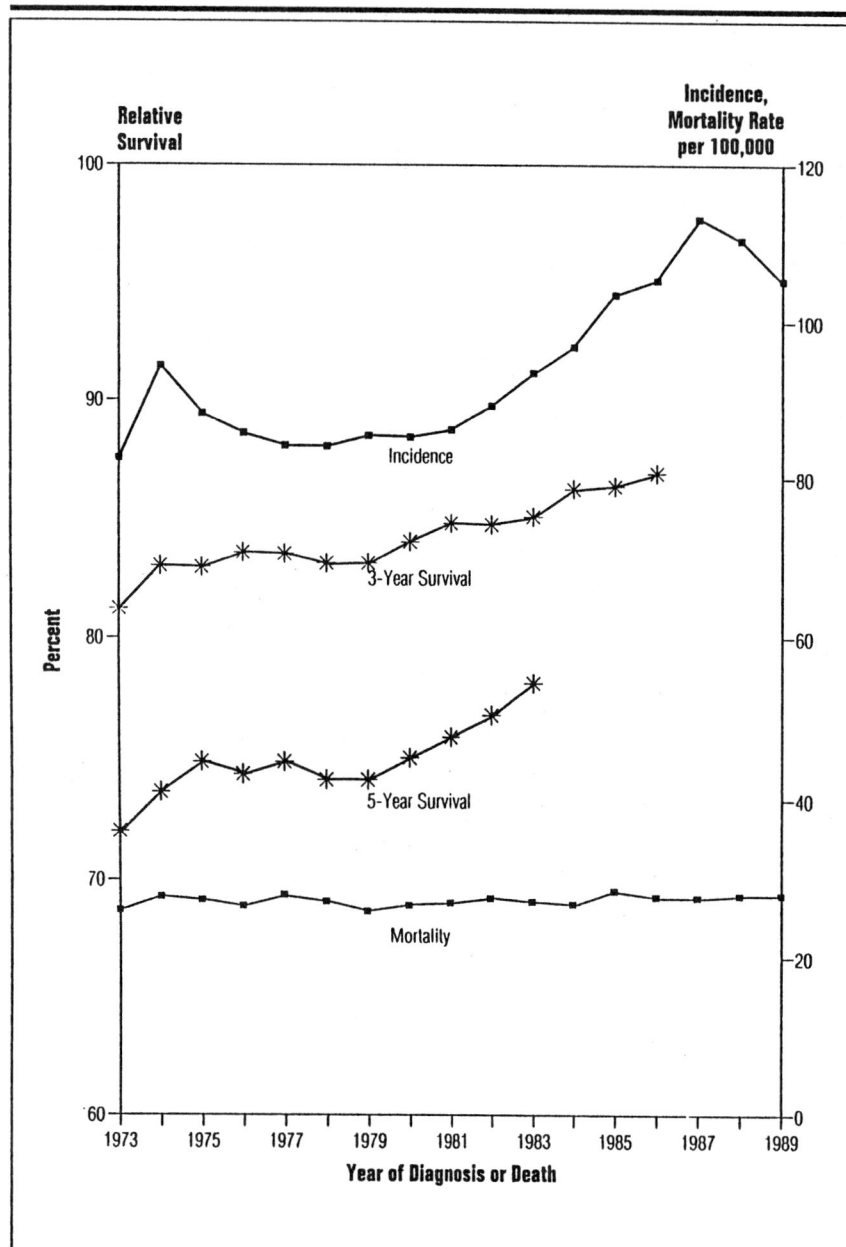

FIGURE 29–1. Invasive breast cancer incidence, relative survival, and mortality among women of all races and ages in the nine Surveillance, Epidemiology, and End Results (SEER) areas. Incidence and mortality rates are age-adjusted by the direct method to the 1970 U.S. standard population. (From Miller, B. A., Feur, E. J., & Hankey, B. F. [1993]. Recent incidence trends for breast cancer in women and the relevance of early detection: An update. *CA-A Journal for Clinicians, 43*, 27–41.)

reproductive pattern and hormone use, must be considered in evaluating the changes in incidence in various cohorts of women.

Overall survival rates for women diagnosed with breast cancer have improved. The improved survival outcome may partially explain the constancy of mortality rates (Sondik, 1994). While early detection appears to be associated with improved survival outcome, many other factors may also contribute, either independently or together. Advances in the understanding of biology and refinement in the predictive ability of prognostic factors have influenced treatment choices for women at different risk levels. Successful treatment strategies such as adjuvant therapy may reduce mortality but alone fail to explain survival differences among subsets of women who are diagnosed with this complex biologic disease.

EPIDEMIOLOGY AND ETIOLOGY

The incidence of breast cancer varies around the world. Incidence is highest in North America and northern Europe, intermediate in southern Europe and Latin America, and lowest in Asia and Africa. Recently, incidence rates in some Asian (e.g., Japan) and central European countries have risen. Also, incidence rates are known to change for the first- and second-generation descendants of low-risk geographic populations when they migrate to areas in which breast cancer is common. Environmental factors, lifestyle, and differences in known risk factors (e.g., reproductive patterns) can partially explain the variance of breast cancer risk observed throughout the world (Kelsey & Horn-Ross, 1993).

RISK FACTORS

Identification of risk factors for cancer is critical to determine individual risk, increase our knowledge about the cause of the disease, and promote preventive strategies to alter risk. Although a variety of risk factors for breast cancer have been identified (Table 29–1 and Table 29–2), it is critical to evaluate the weight and conclusive evidence for each. Female gender and age over 40 years are two definitive risk factors. In the United States an estimated one out of nine women (11

per cent risk) will develop breast cancer in her lifetime. This is the cumulative risk if a woman lives to 85 years of age (Fig. 29–2). Age-specific risk can be dramatically distinct from cumulative risk and critical for women's understanding of breast cancer risk and perception of their individual risk (Kelly, 1991).

In addition to age and gender, a personal or family history of breast cancer and use of reproductive hormones are established risk factors. A note of caution about risk factors must be made, however. Many women diagnosed with breast cancer do not have any risk factors; there is not a clearly established additive effect, and the evaluation of risk for any given factor varies significantly. Several other risk factors such as diet or benign breast disease are less well established as independent variables and subject to ongoing evaluation and research (Tables 29–1 and 29–2). Such factors must be carefully integrated into a comprehensive risk

TABLE 29–1. *Factors Associated with an Increased Risk of Breast Cancer*

RISK FACTOR	COMMENTS
Female gender	99% of breast cancers occur in women, 1% in men.
History of a previous breast cancer	The risk of developing a cancer in the opposite breast is five times greater than for the average population at risk.
Age > 40 yr	Incidence increases with age, peaks in the fifth decade, and then levels off somewhat.
Family history	Breast cancer risk increases with a maternal history, ranging from 15–30% lifetime risk (Kelly, 1991). The percent risk is dependent on several variables such as number of relatives, unilateral vs. bilateral cancer, and age at diagnosis (Colditz et al., 1993). Familial breast cancer is a distinct hereditary form of breast cancer associated with a much higher risk (≥ 50%) but occurs in a very small group of women, < 5% of those diagnosed (Smith, 1992).
Early menarche or late menopause or both	The risk of breast cancer rises as the interval between menarche and menopause increases; shortening the interval by castration reduces the lifetime risk about 50% if performed in women before age 40 yr (Kelsey, Gammon, & John, 1993).
Nulliparity	Full-term pregnancy at an early age offers a protective effect. Women who bear no children or bear their first child near or after age 30 have an increased risk. Evidence for effect or risk of multiparity is inconclusive.
First child born after 30 yr of age	
Ionizing radiation	Exposure to radiation due to nuclear war or accidents or multiple treatments with radiation (i.e., tuberculosis) are associated with an increased risk of breast cancer. The risk is dependent on dose and age at exposure, with young age associated with greatest risk (Hildreth, Shore, Dvoretsky, 1989; Miller et al., 1989). There is a long latent time with breast cancers diagnosed at predicted older ages, which may suggest involvement of other factors (e.g., hormones) in the development of the disease (John & Kelsey, 1994).
In situ breast carcinoma	Up to 50% of women diagnosed by biopsy with ductal carcinoma in situ (DCIS), if untreated, are at increased risk to develop invasive breast cancer within 15 years (Betsill, Rosen, Lieberman & Robbins, 1978; Page, DuPont, Rogers, & Landenberger, 1982; Rosen, Braun, & Kinne, 1980). The risk of invasive cancer after biopsy-proven lobular in situ (LCIS) has been reported in 8–30% of women over a 10 to 20 yr period following biopsy (Bodian, 1994).
Proliferative breast lesions	Women with noncancerous proliferative breast lesion have 1.9 times the risk of developing cancer than women with nonproliferative breast conditions (Dupont & Page, 1985). The risk increases significantly if the proliferative lesion is classified as atypical hyperplasia and there is a family history of breast cancer.
Nonproliferative breast conditions	Nonproliferative breast conditions have no associated breast cancer risk. Fibroadenoma, however, has been identified as a long-term risk factor. The degree of risk is influenced by specific histologic features of the lesion and presence of a family history (Dupont et al., 1994).

TABLE 29–2. *Factors Associated with Breast Cancer Risk: Inconclusive or Inconsistent Evidence for Increased Risk*

RISK FACTORS	COMMENTS
Oral contraceptives	There is no overall increase of risk of breast cancer for ever having used oral contraceptives when all ages of women are combined, although there appears to be a slight increased risk for subgroups of young women (< 45 years) with a history of prolonged use (Malone, Daling, & Weiss, 1993; Romieu, Berlin, & Colditz, 1990; Thomas, 1993b). Further study is recommended.
Exogenous hormones	Research findings do not support an overall risk of breast cancer for women who ever used post-menopausal estrogens, although some suggest a modest risk with prolonged use (> 10–15 years) (Brinton & Schairer, 1993; Henrich, 1992; Zumoff, 1993). Factors that affect the varied study results include duration of use, recency of use, latency, dosage, type of estrogen, regimen of use, route of administration, family history, presence of other known risk factors, and methodologic problems (Brinton & Schairer, 1993).
Dietary fat	The variation in breast cancer incidence world-wide suggested a possible relationship between fat intake and degree of breast cancer risk. Evidence does not support a strong association, but a weak association cannot be fully ruled out; further study is recommended (Holmberg et al., 1994; Howe, 1994; Willett & Hunter, 1994).
Alcohol intake	A weak association between alcohol intake and breast cancer risk is accepted and appears to be influenced by amount consumed and age (Holmberg et al., 1994; Willett & Hunter, 1994; Rosenberg, Metzger, & Palmer, 1994). Caution is suggested, however, related to compounding risk factors (e.g., socioeconomic status), inconsistent findings in reported studies, and methodologic problems (Roth, Levy, Shi, & Post, 1994).
Body weight	There are contradictory findings for obesity as a breast cancer risk factor. Some studies report an inverse relationship for premenopausal women (increased risk for lean weight), and many report an increased risk for obese postmenopausal women; most studies record weight close to diagnosis and fail to address important factors such as lifelong weight change and level of adiposity. Currently, there is little evidence to suggest obesity as an influencing factor for breast cancer risk (Ballard-Barbash, 1994).

assessment profile rather than identified as a single factor on which action is taken.

Race, socioeconomic status, religion, and residence have been identified as factors associated with breast cancer risk, specifically, white race, high socioeconomic status, Jewish religion, and urban residence (especially in the northeastern United States). These are not independent risk factors but are largely dependent on other risk factors such as reproductive history, lifestyle, or environmental influences (Kelsey & Horn-Ross, 1993). A realistic and objective assessment of risk must be maintained by health care professionals and provided in an accurate and clear manner to the public.

Despite identification of risk factors and advances in molecular biology and science, the exact cause for the development of breast cancer remains unknown. Epidemiologic data and clinical observations have led some to the hypothesis that a multistep process is responsible. A four-step process consisting of an initiation event, a promotional event, a transformation, and an early-to-late progression is suggested, which is consistent with current beliefs in cancer biology as described in Chapter 13.

BIOLOGY AND GENETICS

Proto-oncogenes and cellular oncogenes are important elements in the regulation and differentiation of cellular growth. Mutations or inappropriate expression of genes can result in uncontrolled growth and malignant transformation or progression. In breast cancer, numerous investigators have identified alterations in cellular proto-oncogenes that are thought to be related to the initiation or progression of breast cancer, which include ERBB2, HRAS, MYC, and WNT$_2$ (Callahan,

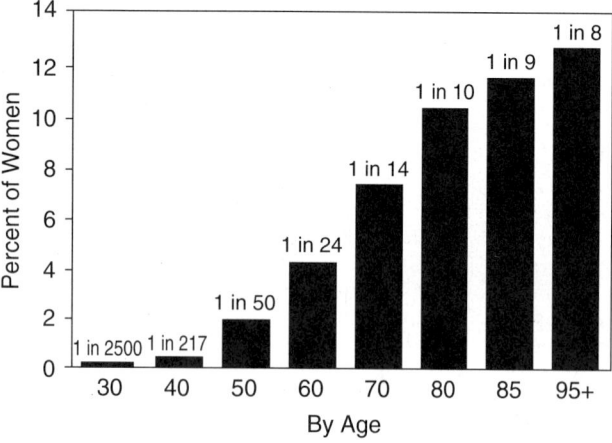

FIGURE 29–2. Probability of developing breast cancer by different ages. Each bar represents the per cent of women expected to develop breast cancer by the noted age. There is a 1 in 9 chance of developing breast cancer by age 85 years, and a 1 in 8 chance of developing breast cancer past age 90 years. (Prepared by the American Cancer Society from Incidence and mortality rates 1987–1988, Surveillance, Epidemiology, and End Results areas.)

1989; Harris, Morrow, & Bonadonna, 1993). Amplification of ERBB2 (also referred to as HER-2/*neu*), the most widely studied proto-oncogene, has been found in one fourth to one third of breast tumors and appears to be associated with nodal involvement (Slamon et al., 1989; Tandon, Clark, Chamness, Ullrich, & McGuire, 1989).

Continued interest in this proto-oncogene also comes from its similarity to the epidermal growth factor receptor (EGFR). We have learned that breast cancer cells are capable of stimulating their own growth with growth factors such as transforming growth factor (TGF) alpha and beta, insulin growth factors, and platelet-derived growth factors. Although the exact mechanism of each growth factor in the development and progression of breast cancer is not fully understood, the ongoing work in molecular biology provides continuous information that adds to our understanding of the biology of breast cancer. This knowledge is the basis for development of new therapeutic approaches, many of which will be directed at interference of genetic regulatory mechanisms.

BRCA1 SUSCEPTIBILITY GENE

A positive family history is a known risk factor for breast cancer. The increased risk among relatives in some families stimulated research to find a dominant gene to explain the familial or hereditary subset of breast cancer (Weber et al., 1994). A susceptibility gene for breast cancer was mapped to chromosome 17 in 1990 and isolated in 1994; it is now known as BRCA1 gene (Daly, 1994; Shattuck-Eidens et al., 1995). The described mutations for BRCA1 suggest that it is a tumor suppressor gene. Loss of suppressor function in these genes by mutations can lead to abnormal proliferation (Daly, 1994). BRCA1 gene has been found in tumors from familial and sporadic (no significant family history) breast cancer cases. Although familial cases only account for about 5 per cent of all breast cancer, the isolation of this gene is of great significance. The risk for familial breast cancer cases is estimated at 50 to 80 per cent. The ability to identify these women is an important advance and only one of the likely outcomes of the significance of the isolation and cloning of this gene (Weber et al., 1994).

BREAST CANCER RISK ASSESSMENT AND COUNSELING

Women in the general population are more aware of breast cancer now than ever before as a consequence of media attention but also the grass roots activity of breast cancer advocacy groups. The concern of the risk of developing breast cancer varies but generally higher in those with a family history. Women often perceive their risk inaccurately due to lack of information, lack of understanding of risk estimates, and lack of individual risk assessment and counseling (Kelly, 1991). Perception of risk is a critical factor to assess, since it may influence psychologic response and preventive screening behaviors. For the health care provider the first critical issue is defining the patient's risk, which should be part of a comprehensive risk counseling program (Table 29–3). Two important areas of assessment include family history and medical/reproductive history. These data can be used with a predictive risk model such as the commonly cited Claus or Gail models (Claus, Risch, & Thompson, 1990; Gail et al., 1989) to produce an individual risk estimate. These two models and other available prediction models differ in their advantages, disadvantages, and type of risk estimate produced (e.g., relative vs. cumulative) but offer clinicians a tool for estimating risk with a consistently defined method (Hoskins et al., 1995; Offit & Brown, 1994). Classifying risk based on family history is suggested to provide a framework for education, counseling, and screening recommendations for the individual woman: no family history, family history/moderate risk, family history/high risk (Hoskins et al., 1995). Women in the moderate-risk category may have a family history of one or two relatives, usually diagnosed in the older postmenopausal age group, and no evidence of ovarian cancer in the family. In contrast, the high-risk category is associated with multiple family members with breast cancer, often diagnosed before age 45 years, and may or may not be associated with a family history of ovarian cancer. This high-risk group represents an autosomal dominant pattern of inheritance and therefore is referred to as inherited, hereditary, genetic, or familial breast cancer (Smith, 1992; Daly, 1994).

Women in all risk categories should be assessed for current lifestyle (diet, exercise pattern), health behaviors (physical examinations, breast self-examination practice), and psychosocial factors (personality style, coping mechanisms, baseline emotional profile) to provide a foundation on which to base potential response to risk assessment, teaching, and supportive interventions. In addition, women should be assessed for their

TABLE 29–3. *Comprehensive Risk Counseling*

Assessment
Family history
Medical/reproductive history
Lifestyle
Health behaviors
Perception of breast cancer risk
Psychosocial factors

Information Giving
Breast cancer
Risk assessment
Genetics and cancer

Counseling
Explain predicted individual risk
Offer surveillance guidelines
Provide emotional support
Discuss preventive options, if appropriate
Encourage adherence to surveillance recommendations

knowledge of breast cancer, breast cancer risk, and risk assessment so that education can be tailored to meet the individual's information needs at an appropriate level for adequate comprehension. Counseling and screening recommendations are dependent on risk status. Screening guidelines, such as those proposed by the American Cancer Society, offer basic surveillance parameters for women with no family history. Alterations in those screening guidelines for women classified as moderate risk with a family history will depend on actual risk estimate and physician discretion.

Counseling of high-risk women carries significantly greater implications for the health care provider simply because of the reality of the substantial risk (> 80 per cent) of developing breast cancer. The psychologic response to such an increased risk for the individual and other family members, consideration of preventive options (such as prophylactic mastectomy or oophorectomy), recommended frequency and patient adherence to surveillance recommendations, insurance coverage, and current (and pending commercial availability of) genetic testing pose significant challenges. These challenges would be best confronted by experienced clinicians in basic genetic or breast cancer risk assessment rather than the primary care or generalist practitioners (Daly, 1994; Hoskins et al., 1995; Lynch, Lynch, Conway, & Severin, 1994; Smith, 1992; Stefanek, 1990).

Perceived susceptibility to breast cancer risk may relate to screening behaviors, and therefore it is important to help every woman identify her risk as accurately as possible. The influence of a family history of breast cancer on a woman's breast cancer screening behaviors is not fully known. Several reports suggest no difference in mammographic screening for women with or without a family history (Bondy, Vogel, Halabi, & Lustbader, 1992; Brigham, 1992; Kaplan, Weinberg, Small, & Herndon, 1991). Yet, women with a family history who perceive themselves at very high risk have been reported to be either hypervigilant or extremely reluctant (even incapacitated) to engage in screening practices (Baker, 1991; Easterling & Leventhal, 1989; Kash, Holland, Harper, & Miller, 1992). Low or moderate levels of anxiety, fear, and apprehension associated with risk may facilitate regular screening. But increased anxiety levels may result in greater psychologic distress, a decrease in recommended screening practices, and a potential need for counseling (Kash et al., 1992; Stefanek, 1990).

PREVENTION

Most of the prevention focus has been on secondary prevention (screening and early detection), with a small but growing interest in primary prevention, since many risk factors are associated with unknown, low, or modest elevations in risk and modification of those risk factors is not feasible in general or because of methodologic or economic factors. A good example of the challenge of primary prevention research is implementation of a low-fat diet in women at risk for diagnosis or recurrence of breast cancer. Despite early skepticism about feasibility, programmed education, support, and counseling with women has resulted in sustained reductions in dietary fat intake up to 1 to 2 years (Chlebowski et al., 1987; Holm, Nordevang, Ikkala, Hallstrom, & Callmer, 1990; Insull et al., 1990). However, skepticism about conduct and outcome of dietary prevention trials persists related to concerns of study design, methodology, cost, long-term compliance, and required duration of follow-up (Byar & Freedman, 1990; Mettlin, 1991).

The ability of micronutrients such as antioxidants and carotenoids to reduce breast cancer risk requires further study. Although there is some evidence suggestive of a benefit, evidence is not conclusive, and there are no data to support recommendations for supplemental vitamins at this time (Hunter & Willett, 1993; Hunter et al., 1993).

Prophylactic mastectomy has been considered as a preventive strategy, particularly for women at high risk, although recommendation for prophylactic surgery lacks consensus. One of the major concerns is the failure of surgery to remove all the breast tissue, even when optimal surgical techniques in performing total mastectomy are used (Hoskins et al., 1995). Thus, a woman has some level of protection against developing breast cancer, but prophylactic surgery does not completely eliminate the risk, which should be discussed in counseling women (Stefanek, 1990).

Chemoprevention with tamoxifen is the most widely known primary prevention strategy. Tamoxifen, a synthetic nonsteroidal antiestrogen with a reported low toxicity profile and demonstrated activity in breast cancer, was chosen for a pilot study of endocrine prevention of breast cancer in 1986 in the United Kingdom (Powles et al., 1989). Over a 2-year period with 200 women randomized to receive tamoxifen or placebo, mild toxicity was reported; this pilot study also suggested that a large multicenter trial was feasible, estimating a need for 10,000 women with a 10- to 15-year follow-up to detect a 25 per cent reduction in risk (Powles et al., 1989).

In 1992 the National Breast Cancer Trial began in 270 centers in the United States and Canada through the National Surgical Adjuvant Breast Program (NSABP) funded by the National Cancer Institute. The goal was to reduce the risk of breast cancer by 40 per cent in healthy women 60 years of age or older, who have an estimated risk of developing breast cancer of 1.7 per cent or more over 5 years (Varricchio & Johnson, 1993). Women 25 to 59 years of age who demonstrated a similar 1.7 per cent risk, using the Gail prediction risk model (Gail et al., 1989), were also eligible. The primary outcome of the trial was to reduce the incidence of invasive breast cancer, noninvasive cancer, and atypical hyperplasia; a secondary outcome was reduction in cardiovascular disease (Bush & Helzisouer, 1993). The premise for evaluating outcome is based on net benefit, that is, the difference between the predicted number of beneficial events (those prevented) and the number of detrimental events (those caused) in the group of women who received the tamoxifen treatment (Bush & Helzisouer, 1993). A sample of 16,000 women treated for 5 years with a 10-

to 15-year follow-up is required to evaluate outcome. Philosophic issues related to the trial are use of a drug with defined toxicity and how the net benefit effect is calculated (Bush & Helzisouer, 1993). Risks, especially those that were higher than originally reported or known at the initiation of the trial, for development of endometrial cancer raised serious concerns among the lay public and health professionals (Fugh-Berman & Epstein, 1992; Kedar et al., 1994; National Women's Health Network, 1994) and prompted the manufacturer to change the product brochure related to risk of uterine cancer (Milbauer, 1994) and NSABP to change the consent form for eligible women for the trial (Gould, Gates, & Miaskowski, 1994). Side effects such as hot flashes, depression, vaginal discharge, irregular menses, and ocular effects are not included in the net benefit equation, yet they do affect compliance (Bush & Helzisouer, 1993). While most side effects are transient, some such as hot flashes may persist over months; Mooney, Nail, Richtsmeier, and Ward (1994) reported side effects as the reason for an 18 per cent drop out rate among women taking the tamoxifen vs. a 6 per cent drop out rate among those taking placebo.

Without question, primary prevention of disease is far superior to secondary prevention, especially in a disease like cancer where mortality is a reality. The ultimate benefit of the tamoxifen prevention trial will need to stand the test of time over the next decade, with careful evaluation of the net benefit effect.

SCREENING

The goal of screening in breast cancer is to detect cancers at the earliest stage possible because the extent of tumor at diagnosis is correlated with survival. Women who have small tumors and no spread to the axillary lymph nodes have a very good long-term prognosis compared with those who have large tumors and axillary lymph nodes that test positive. Breast self-examination (BSE), clinical breast examination (CBE), and mammography are three methods of screening proposed by the American Cancer Society (Table 29–4). Education about the disease, the signs and symptoms, and the benefits of early detection is essential (see Chapter 17).

BREAST SELF-EXAMINATION

Self detection of a breast lump using BSE was recommended nearly 40 years ago, but the value is still questioned (McCool, 1994; Morra, 1985). Frequent BSE may be associated with earlier detection of tumors,

TABLE 29–4. *Screening for Breast Cancer*

METHOD	AGE	FREQUENCY
Physical examination by health care professional	20–40	Every 3 yr
	> 40	Annually
Breast self-examination	≥ 20	Monthly
Mammography	40–50	Every 1–2 yr
	> 50	Annually

but only 15 to 40 per cent of women perform monthly BSE (Brigham, 1992; Champion, 1989; Hailey & Bradford, 1991; Morra, 1985; Rutledge & Davis, 1988). Lack of confidence in the method, lack of comfort with this self-care activity, and older age are consistently reported to affect BSE practice (Champion, 1991; McCool, 1994; Stillman, 1977). Knowledge is correlated with intent to practice but not with adherence to monthly practice (Brigham, 1992; Champion, 1989). Individual teaching by the woman's health care provider influences the proficiency and the frequency of practice (Champion, 1989; Hailey & Bradford, 1991; Morra, 1985). Each woman should be taught BSE (Fig. 29–3) by her practitioner; a teaching program that includes support, reinforcement, and evaluation may further enhance the woman's confidence, knowledge, proficiency, and adherence to monthly BSE (Pool & Judkins, 1990).

CLINICAL BREAST EXAMINATION

The ultimate value of CBE by a health care provider as a single method of detection on outcome is unclear. Yet, combined with the limitations cited for BSE, the value of reinforcement of the importance of BSE by the practitioner, the potential to detect a tumor not evident on mammography, and the opportunity to educate and counsel women on preventive health care behaviors and breast cancer make arguments to support the recommendation for annual professional breast examinations (Brigham, 1992; Day & O'Rourke, 1990).

MAMMOGRAPHY

Mammography is an x-ray examination of the breast, which can be performed as a screening or diagnostic examination. The screening mammography is to detect occult breast cancer in asymptomatic women and thus reduce mortality. In review of studies conducted over the past three decades, screening mammography has reduced mortality by 20 to 30 per cent (Kerlikowske, Grady, Rubin, Sandrock, & Ernster, 1995; McLelland & Pisano, 1990; Mettlin & Smart, 1994). The goals of mammography are to produce optimal images and provide accurate interpretation at a low cost (McLelland & Pisano, 1990). The American College of Radiology (ACR) developed an accreditation program for mammography that sets minimum standards. In 1994 the Mammography Quality Standards Act was passed; the act requires all mammography facilities in the United States (except Veterans Health Administration facilities, which have their own standards) to be certified by the Food and Drug Administration (FDA). The Agency of Health Care Policy and Research (AHCPR) issued a Clinical Practice Guideline in 1994, accompanied by brief versions for the clinician (*Reference Guide for Clinicians*) and for consumers (*A Woman's Guide*). This guideline addresses quality-related activities of the mammography examination, responsibilities of the facility, personnel, information for health care providers, and adverse consequences or problems associated with mammography.

Screening mammography consists of two standard views of each breast. It is performed by a radiology

There are many good reasons for doing the breast self-exam (BSE) each month. One reason is that breast cancer is most easily treated and cured when it is found early. Another is that if you do BSE every month, it will increase your skill and confidence when doing the exam. When you get to know how your breasts normally feel, you will quickly be able to feel any change. Another reason, it is easy to do.

The best time to do BSE is about a week after your period, when breasts are not tender or swollen. If you do not hae regular periods or sometimes skip a month, do BSE on the same day every month.

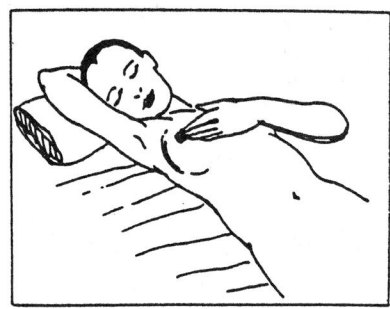

Remember: BSE could save your breast—and save your life. Most breast lumps are found by women themselves, but, in fact, most lumps in the breast are not cancer. Be safe, be sure.

1. Lie down and put a pillow under your right shoulder. Place your right arm behind your head.
2. Use the finger pads of your three middle fingers on your left hand to feel for lumps or thickening. Your finger pads are the top third of each finger.
3. Press firmly enough to know how your breast feels. If you're not sure how hard to press, ask your health care provider. Or try to copy the way your health care provider uses the finger pads during a breast exam. Learn what your breast feels like most of the time. A firm ridge in the lower curve of each breast is normal.
4. Move around the breast in a set way. You can choose either the circle (A), the up and down line (B), or the wedge (C). Do it the same way every time. It will help you to make sure that you've gone over the entire breast area, and to remember how your breast feels each month.
5. Now examine your left breast using right hand finger pads.
6. If you find any changes, see your doctor right away.

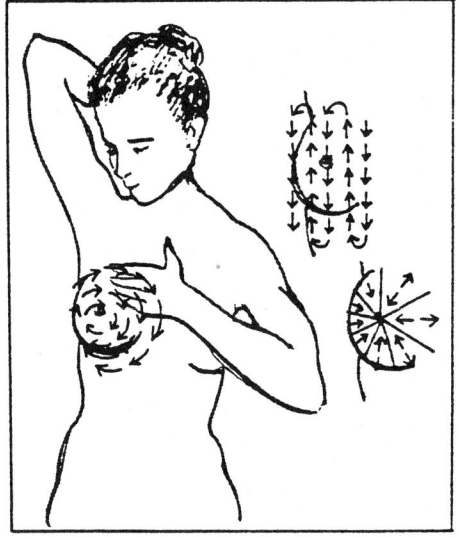

You might want to check your breasts while standing in front of a mirror right after you do your BSE each month. See if there are any changes in the way your breasts look: dimpling of the skin, or changes in the nipple, redness or swelling. You might also want to do an extra BSE while you're in the shower. Your soapy hands will glide over the wet skin making it easy to check how your breasts feel.

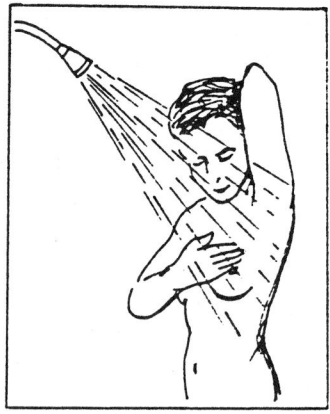

FIGURE 29–3. The nurse has an important role in teaching and promoting the regular practice of breast self-examination. These instructions describe the most commonly taught techniques. (From *How To Do Breast Self-Examination*. No. 2674. Atlanta, American Cancer Society.)

technologist using dedicated equipment (dedicated solely to the use for mammography examination), which is monitored regularly. Mammograms are interpreted by a qualified radiologist, and results should be communicated to the referring provider *and* to the screened woman as quickly as possible. Radiation exposure is approximately 0.05 rad per exposure (Paulus, 1987).

Screening mammography is significantly underutilized with less than 50 per cent of women over the age of 40 *ever* having had a mammogram (Breen & Kessler, 1994; Harris, Fletcher, et al., 1991; Lerman, Rimer,

Trock, Balshem, & Engstrom, 1990; Zapka, Hosmer, Costanza, Harris, & Stoddard, 1992). The percentage of women who have had a mammogram in the past year, which is used as an indicator of adherence to annual guidelines (Table 29–4) for women over 50 years of age is lower, in the range of 25 to 30 per cent (Lerman et al., 1990; Harris, et al., Fox, Murata, & Stein, 1991; Zapka et al., 1992).

The Year 2000 Goal of the National Cancer Institute (NCI) is to increase to 80 per cent the proportion of women ages 50 to 70 years who have annual mammography and clinical breast examination (Gregorio, Kegeles, Parker, & Benn, 1990). The challenges or barriers to meeting this goal are related to limitations of current research, system issues, the health care provider, and the woman as a consumer of preventive health care. The age of onset, age limit, and the interval for screening are known controversies, yet to be definitely resolved by current research (McLelland & Pisano, 1990). The controversy of age of onset is related to women between 40 and 49 years of age. Using reduction of mortality as the single evaluative outcome, some studies have reported no statistically significant reduction in mortality in this subgroup of women (Kerlikowske et al., 1995). The lack of mortality reduction from randomized trials provided the basis for NCI's change in screening guidelines from 40 to 50 years of age. Statistical power, subgroup analyses, and the fact that several of these screening trials demonstrated mortality reductions in younger women provide support to maintain screening recommendations for younger women (Kopans, 1994; Mettlin & Smart, 1994). In addition to randomized trials, the American Cancer Society (ACS) in review of guidelines also considered descriptive studies, trends in breast cancer incidence, large, nonrandomized study results (e.g., Breast Cancer Demonstration Project), and consideration of the fact that breast cancer is the leading cause of death in women aged 40 to 44 years (Mettlin & Smart, 1994). Age limit has risen as another issue and most trials have not included women over 74 years of age. In 1990 the Forum on Breast Cancer Screening in Older Women was convened with the purpose of examining scientific evidence and propose screening guidelines. A special issue of *The Journal of Gerontology* provides the Forum's recommendations (Table 29–5), supporting rationale, and background data (Costanza, 1992), yet controversies persist regarding interval of screening and upper age limit (Costanza, 1994). The primary system issues include access, convenience, and cost (Gregorio et al., 1990; Lerman et al., 1990; Rimer, Keintz, Kessler, Engstrom, & Rosan, 1989).

Health care provider barriers have been identified from a physician perspective. Physicians have been trained to treat disease with little or no emphasis on preventive health care; are uninformed or misinformed about ACR or ACS screening guidelines; have unreasonable expectations about mammography; and fail to recommend mammography especially to older, less well educated, low income women (Coll, O'Connor, Crabtree, & Besdine, 1989; McLelland & Pisano, 1990). Physician recommendation has repeatedly been identi-

TABLE 29–5. *The Forum Panel's Recommendations on Breast Cancer Screening in Older Women*

Clinical breast examination should be performed annually and mammography should be performed approximately every 2 yr for women aged 65–74 yr.

Clinical breast examination should be performed annually and mammography should be performed at regular intervals of approximately every 2 yr for women age 75 yr and older whose general health and life expectancy are good.

It is prudent to recommend that women age 65 yr and older perform monthly breast self-examination (BSE) to identify clinical lesions and seek professional care.

(*The Journals of Gerontology.* [1992]. [Special Issue]. 47, 5.)

fied as the *single most important determinant* in a woman's decision to get a mammogram (Coll et al., 1989; Fox et al., 1991; Gregorio et al., 1990; Henrich, Kornguth, Berg, & Schwartz, 1992; Lerman et al., 1990; Miller & Champion, 1993; Rimer et al., 1989; Wolosin, 1989;). Physician education, especially at the primary care provider level, is a critical component to current strategies aimed at meeting the Year 2000 Goal.

Factors associated with women who are least likely to participate in mammography screening include older age (especially over 65 years of age), low income, low educational level, minority groups, lack of or insufficient insurance coverage, and lack of a recommendation from a health care provider (Champion, 1989; Fox et al., 1991; Marshburn et al., 1994; McCool, 1994; Miller & Champion, 1993; Rimer et al., 1992). Risk of breast cancer rises with age, and yet screening participation is the lowest among women in the older age groups. Lack of perception of breast cancer as a major health concern, emphasis on disease treatment vs. preventive health care, lack of knowledge of the benefits of mammography, fear of discovering something serious, fear of procedural discomfort, single or widow status, and low or restricted income are reported factors that explain some of the underutilization by older women (Rimer et al., 1992; McCool, 1994).

Fear of discomfort and pain or actual painful experiences with mammography is an additional cited client barrier. Compression of the breast is an important part of the test for contrast, uniformity of breast tissue, and reduction of scatter radiation, all of which contribute to the quality and outcome of the mammographic examination. Baskin-Smith, Miaskowski, Dibble, and Nielson (1995) investigated procedural discomfort, with 23 per cent of women reporting uncomfortable or painful sensations. The AHCPR Clinical Practice Guideline highlights the importance of proper breast compression for quality mammography and recommends that the radiologic technologist advise the women about the importance of compression and when it will begin and gradually compress the breast to tolerance but not pain (U.S. Department of Health and Human Services [USDHHS], 1994). Some pain may be related to anxiety, and relaxation suggestions before and during the examination may be helpful (Nielson, Miaskowski, & Dibble, 1993; USDHHS, 1994).

Many successful strategies have been identified to improve the use of screening mammography, primarily targeted at primary care providers and women with low educational levels, low incomes, minority status, and high-risk related to age (Breen & Kessler, 1994). Community-based education programs (Forsythe, Fulton, Lane, Burg, & Krishna, 1992; McCoy et al., 1994); improving access such as evening and Saturday hours or use of mobile mammography vans (McCoy et al., 1994; Ressler, Rimer, Devine, Gatenby, & Engstrom, 1991; Rubin, Frank, Stanley, Bernreuter, & Han, 1990), low cost (Breen & Kessler, 1994; Gregorio et al., 1990; Rubin et al., 1990), scheduling reminders (Wolosin, 1990), and educating primary care providers about breast cancer risk with age, discussing the value of mammography screening, and promoting guidelines (Rimer et al., 1992) are feasible and successful interventions. Availability, accessibility, and acceptability are three key components identified in reaching medically underserved populations (McCoy et al., 1994) and must be sensitively tailored to meet the needs of the older, minority, and low-income groups of women (Brown & Williams, 1994; Freemen, Muth, & Kerner, 1995; Mack, McGrath, Pendleton, & Zieber, 1993).

BIOLOGIC CHARACTERISTICS

ANATOMY

The breast is a glandular organ, consisting of lobes, ducts, connective tissue, fat, a nipple, and an areola (Fig. 29–4). The entire organ is enclosed by fascia that separates the breast tissue and skin anteriorly and posteriorly by the chest wall muscles. The pectoralis major and minor muscles lie between the breast and rib cage. The axillary lymph nodes are the primary drainage site for the breast, followed by the internal mammary and supraclavicular nodes. The composition of the breast changes with age, primarily because of hormonal influences. Following maturation of the ducts and lobules after menarche, the breast is exposed to hormonal alterations (estrogen and progesterone) with each menstrual cycle. These changes affect the ducts, lobules, and breast tissue, which over time results in an increase in the percentage of fatty tissue.

STAGING

CLASSIFICATION OF TUMORS

Breast carcinomas arise primarily from epithelial cells, with the origin being either ductal or lobular. These carcinomas are invasive or noninvasive. The term *infiltrating* is synonymous with invasive and the term *in situ* with noninvasive. There are a variety of histopathologic types (Table 29–6), but invasive ductal carcinoma accounts for 70 to 80 per cent of all breast cancers (Beahrs, Henson, Hutter, & Kennedy, 1993). Lobular carcinomas account for 2 to 3 per cent of all invasive tumors and behave similarly to those of ductal origin.

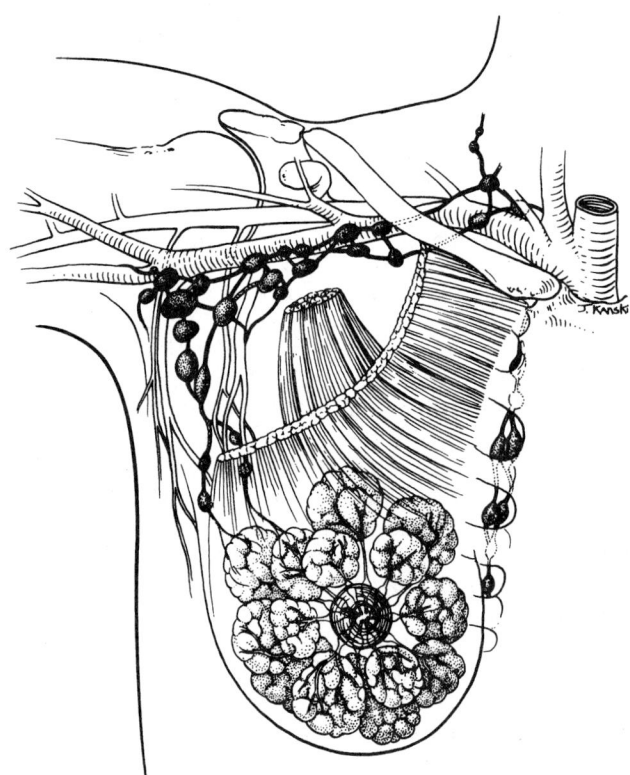

FIGURE 29–4. Anatomic figure at the breast. This schematic representation of the breast substance shows the lobules in the periphery of the ductal system, with the major ducts draining each portion of the periphery. The axillary drainage is primarily in a lateral fashion, first to the low axilla, then to the midaxilla at the lateral aspect of the axillary vein, and then to the apex of the axilla at the point where the axillary vein passes beneath the clavicle and becomes the subclavian vein. The apical axillary nodes then drain to the supraclavicular region. The medial and central aspect of the breast drains to the internal mammary lymph nodes through the pectoral musculature. (From Wilson, R. E. [1984]. Evaluation of a woman with a breast mass. In C. H. Pfeiffer & J. B. Mulliken [Eds.], *Caring for the patient with breast cancer* [p. 24]. Reston, VA: Reston Publishing Company. Reproduced by permission.)

Historically, the noninvasive carcinomas have represented less than 5 per cent of breast cancer that is diagnosed. However, the incidence of the detection of ductal carcinoma in situ has risen dramatically with the widespread use of screening mammography (Stomper & Margolin, 1994).

STAGE

Staging classifies patients clinically and pathologically according to the extent of disease. (Tables 29–7 and 29–8). This TNM system evaluates clinically the extent of cancer according to tumor size (T), axillary lymph node involvement (N), and presence or absence of metastases (M). The staging workup includes a complete history and physical examination, a hematologic and chemical blood profile, and a chest radiograph, mammogram, and baseline bone scan.

TABLE 29–6. *Histopathologic Types of Breast Carcinoma*

Carcinoma, NOS (not otherwise specified)

Ductal
Intraductal (in situ)
Invasive with predominant intraductal component
Invasive, NOS
Comedo
Inflammatory
Medullary with lymphocytic infiltrate
Mucinous (colloid)
Papillary
Scirrhous
Tubular
Other

Lobular
In situ
Invasive with predominant in situ component
Invasive

Nipple
Paget's disease, NOS
Paget's disease with intraductal carcinoma
Paget's disease with invasive ductal carcinoma
Undifferentiated carcinoma
Other

(Beahrs, O. H., Henson, D. E., Hutter, R. V., & Kennedy, B. J. [1993]. *Handbook for staging of cancer.* Philadelphia: J. B. Lippincott Co.)

Clinical staging guides the individual patient and physician in evaluating treatment options and provides data for comparison of therapies and outcomes in various stages of breast cancer. Because axillary lymph node status is the strongest prognostic factor, pathologic staging, particularly for the patient with locally resectable breast cancer, is required. Pathologic staging is a simple two-stage classification; stage I indicates no

TABLE 29–7. *TNM Classification of Breast Cancer*

T (tumor)	T0	No evidence of tumor
	Tis	In situ carcinoma
	T1	Tumor is 2 cm or less at greatest dimension
	T2	Tumor is less than 2 cm but not more than 5 cm at greatest dimension
	T3	Tumor is more than 5 cm at greatest dimension
	T4	Any size tumor with extension to chest wall or skin
N (nodes)	N0	No palpable homolateral axillary nodes
	N1	Movable homolateral axillary nodes
	N2	Homolateral axillary nodes that are considered to contain cancer and are fixed
	N3	Homolateral supraclavicular or infraclavicular nodes
M (metastatis)	M0	No evidence of distant metastases
	M1	Distant metastases

TABLE 29–8. *Staging of Breast Cancer*

Stage 0	Tis	N0	M0
Stage I	T1	N0	M0
Stage IIA	T0	N1	M0
	T1	N1	M0
	T2	N0	M0
Stage IIB	T2	N1	M0
	T3	N0	M0
Stage IIIA	T0	N2	M0
	T1	N2	M0
	T2	N2	M0
	T3	N1	M0
	T3	N2	M0
Stage IIIB	T4	Any N	M0
	Any T	N3	M0
Stage IV	Any T	Any N	M1

(Beahrs, O. H., Henson, D. E., Hutter, R. V., & Kennedy, B. J. [1993]. *Handbook for staging of cancer.* Philadelphia: J. B. Lippincott Co.)

axillary lymph node involvement, and stage II indicates nodal involvement. Because the extent of axillary nodal involvement is related to prognosis, stage II may be divided into categories of one to three, four to ten, and more than ten positive nodes, the last two categories being associated with a poor prognosis (Fig. 29–5).

PROGNOSTIC FACTORS

Axillary lymph node status remains the single most important predictor of recurrence and survival. Node-negative patients have a 70 to 75 per cent chance of being disease free at 10 years compared with only 20 to 25 per cent of node-positive patients, if no adjuvant therapy is received. Prognosis for node-positive patients worsens considerably as the number of nodes involved increases, even if adjuvant therapy is administered. Tumor size, histologic grading, steroid receptor status, and proliferative activity are established factors that have been related to prognosis (Table 29–9). Larger tumors and more undifferentiated tumors predict poorer survival.

Hormone receptors are cytoplasmic proteins, which in breast cancer act as receptors for estrogen and progesterone. These receptors are located on either the surface or the interior of the cell. Although the precise mechanism is unknown, once estrogen is bound to the receptor, a series of biologic steps occurs that allows a hormonal influence to alter the cell's activity. Patients are considered to be estrogen receptor (ER) or progesterone receptor (PR) positive or negative, based on the binding capacity. Values are expressed as femtomoles (fmol) of 3H-estradiol bound per milligram of cytosol protein, generally with less than 10 considered negative and more than 10 considered positive. Some values differ slightly, however, and the guidelines from specific laboratories and the method used to determine the ER and PR receptor value must be consulted for reference. ER-positive tumors have been associated with improved survival; in contrast, ER-negative tumors are associated with shorter survival outcomes. The contri-

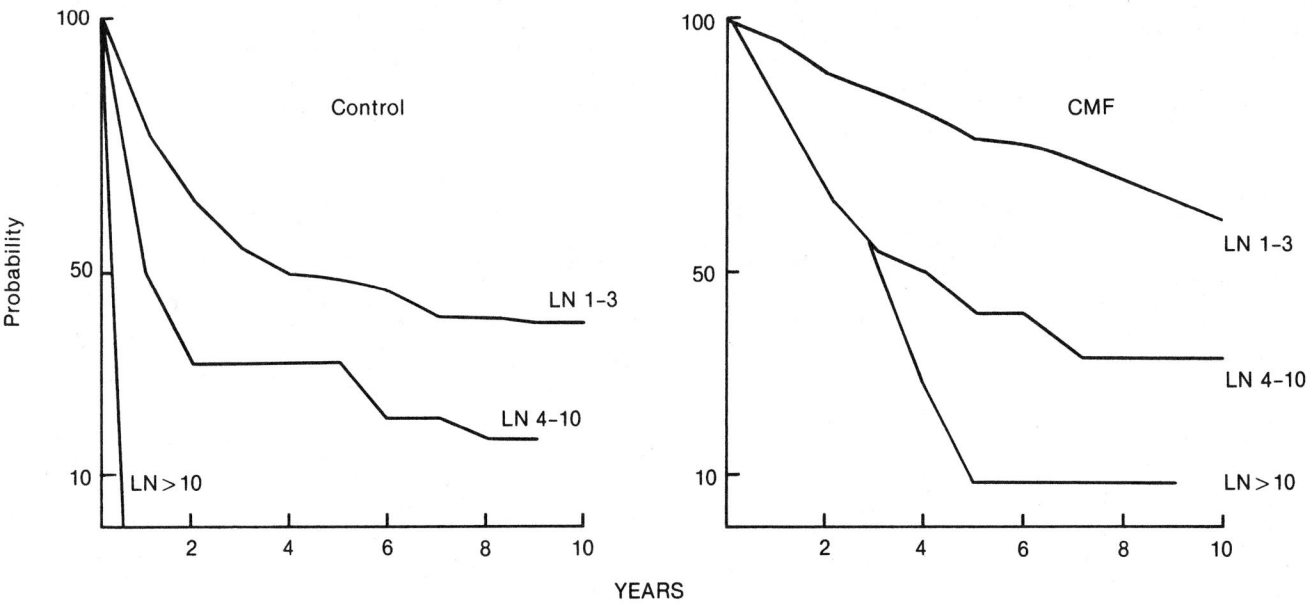

FIGURE 29–5. First cyclophosphamide, methotrexate, and fluorouracil (CMF) program (CMF = 12 cycles vs. control = no treatment): comparative relapse-free survival time in premenopausal women related to lymph node (LN) subsets. (From Bonadonna, G., Valagussa, P., Rossi, A., Tancini, G., Brambilla, C., Zambetti, M., & Veronesi, U. [1985]. Ten year experience with CMF-based adjuvant chemotherapy in resectable breast cancer. *Breast Cancer Research and Treatment, 5,* 95–115. Reproduced by permission.)

bution of progesterone receptor, differences in prognostic predictive value by nodal status (negative or positive), the small magnitude of prognostic survival predictiveness (< 10 per cent), and the strength of ER and PR predictability when combined with other prognostic factors raises concerns about the usefulness of hormone receptors as prognosticators (Mansour, Ravdin, & Dressler, 1994; Weiss & Kelstein, 1991). It is suggested that the major contribution of hormone receptor information is in treatment decision making, specifically predicting responsiveness to hormonal therapy (Ravdin, 1994; Weiss & Kelstein, 1991).

Proliferative activity has independent prognostic significance, but the value of ploidy (DNA content) is controversial. DNA flow cytometry is used to determine proliferative activity, the percentage of cells in S phase. Low proliferative activity (low percentage of cells in S phase) is associated with improved disease-free and overall survival. The prognostic value is compromised, however, by the lack of standardized measurement techniques and consensus of criteria for determining a cutoff of a positive test (Weiss & Kelstein, 1991). At present, the value of S phase as a prognostic indicator alone is not clear and best used in combination with other established prognostic factors.

Several other biologic factors have been investigated, suggesting their role in predicting recurrence and survival, but they await confirmation with continued study (Table 29–9). Oncogene expression, specifically over expression and amplification of HER-2/ *neu* oncogene, epidermal growth factor and angiogenesis have created the greatest excitement, not only for their potential predictive prognostic value but for the potential to select more appropriate therapy and design new target therapeutic approaches (Baselga & Mendelsohn, 1994; Rajkumar & Gullick, 1994; Ravdin, 1994; Tripathy & Benz, 1994; Weidner, Semple, Welch, & Folkman, 1991; Weiss & Kelstein, 1991).

Clinical decision making is challenged by the wealth of literature on existing and promising prognostic factors. The basic elements that impact on clinical decision making are shown in Figure 29–6, all of which may be influenced by prognostic factor information (Mansour et al., 1994). Clinical decision making is a dynamic and evolving process as new prognostic information emerges that directly influences treatment choices such as high-dose therapy for high-risk patients. Maintaining a holistic perspective on out-

TABLE 29–9. *Prognostic Factors in Breast Cancer*

Established
Axillary lymph node involvement
Tumor size
Histologic grade
Steroid receptor status
Proliferative activity

Controversial/Inconclusive
DNA ploidy

Promising: Further Study Needed
Angiogenesis
Cathepsin-D
Growth factors
Oncogene expression
Mutant p53 expression

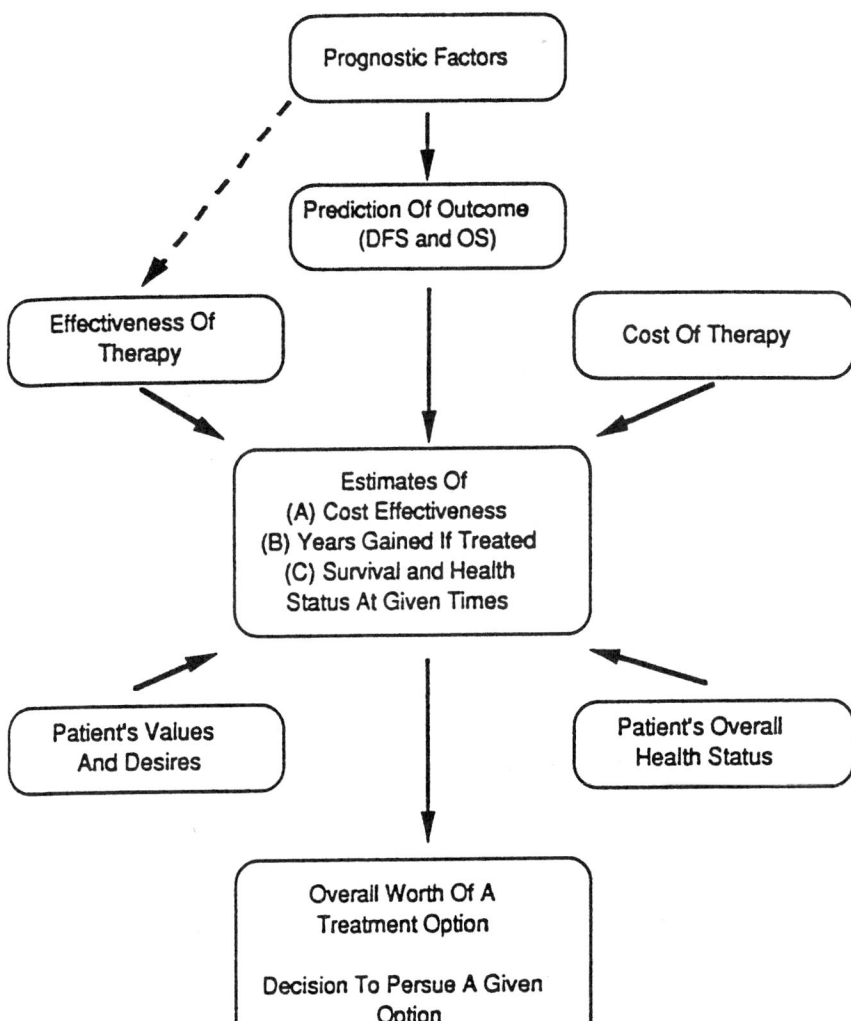

FIGURE 29–6. The use of prognostic factor information in modeling patient outcomes in clinical decision making. (From Mansour, E. G., Ravdin, P. M., & Dressler, L. [1994]. Prognostic factors in early breast carcinoma. *Cancer, 7,* 381–400.)

come, that is beyond survival statistics alone, is recommended (Fig. 29–6).

DIAGNOSTIC PHASE

CLINICAL SIGNS AND SYMPTOMS

The most common presenting symptom is a lump or thickening in the breast. More than 90 per cent of lumps are discovered by the woman herself, and only 20 to 25 per cent are malignant in nature. Nipple discharge, nipple retraction, scaly skin around the nipple, and skin changes (dimpling, "peau d'orange," or inflammation) are less frequently observed and are symptoms that are often associated with a more advanced stage of cancer.

Once a lump has been detected, a physical examination by a physician is recommended. A cyst, a benign tumor, and a malignant tumor are the possibilities for a palpable breast mass. If a cyst is suspected, needle aspiration may be attempted. If aspiration is successful, the lump will decrease in size significantly or will disappear, and the patient should have a follow-up visit. Ultrasonography, a noninvasive diagnostic test without

any radiation exposure, can distinguish between a fluid-filled cystic lump and a solid one. Ultrasonography is a valuable clinical tool that can aid in avoiding an invasive procedure such as a biopsy (Reynolds & Jackson, 1991). In women in the high-risk age group, mammography should also be performed. If a tumor is suspected, a mammogram and a biopsy should be scheduled. Mammography is the superior breast imaging tool; yet false-negative results have been reported as high as 10 per cent. Thus negative findings on a mammogram do not preclude a decision to perform a biopsy on a mass clinically suggestive of cancer (Winchester, 1990).

ABNORMAL MAMMOGRAPHY

The incidence of mammographic findings that are suggestive of cancer in asymptomatic women appears to be increasing, perhaps because of numbers of women obtaining mammograms, increasing low-cost mammography, mobile mammography vans that travel to communities, third-party reimbursement practices, and advances in technologic equipment. Mammographic findings that may indicate malignancy include asymmetry, clusters of microcalcifications, spicular masses, masses with a sunburst appearance, architectural distortion, and new density (Bassett & Gambhir, 1991). Further mammography evaluation may be indicated or a biopsy recommended based on degree of suspicion (Fig. 29–7).

NEEDLE LOCALIZATION AND STEREOTACTIC BIOPSY

For a mammography and a nonpalpable lesion suggestive of cancer, a localization procedure is indicated. The two major procedures are needle localization with surgical biopsy or a stereotactic fine-needle aspiration and/or biopsy. The needle localization biopsy procedure involves inserting a thin wire under mammographic guidance into the area of the breast prior to the surgical biopsy, surgical excision using the wire as a guide, and radiographic confirmation that the abnormal area identified on mammography was removed

(Senofsky, Davies, Olson, Skully, & Olshen 1990). This procedure is collaboratively performed with the radiologist and surgeon and often takes place in two separate environments. Patients require information on the specific procedures, sequencing, duration, timing, and predicted outcome (Habegger & Ellerhorst-Ryan, 1988).

Stereotactic fine-needle aspiration (SFNA) or stereotactic core-needle biopsy (SCNB) is an x-ray–guided method for localizing and sampling nonpalpable breast lesions that have been identified as suggestive of cancer on mammography (Schmidt, 1994). The procedure involves the patient lying prone on a specifically designed table, which has an opening through which the breast is suspended. The breast is immobilized with equipment similar to the compression plates for a routine mammography, which have coordinates allowing for exact identification of the position of the suspected lesion. It is indicated primarily for lesions that appear to be of low to intermediate risk on mammography and is reported to have comparable sensitivity to surgi-

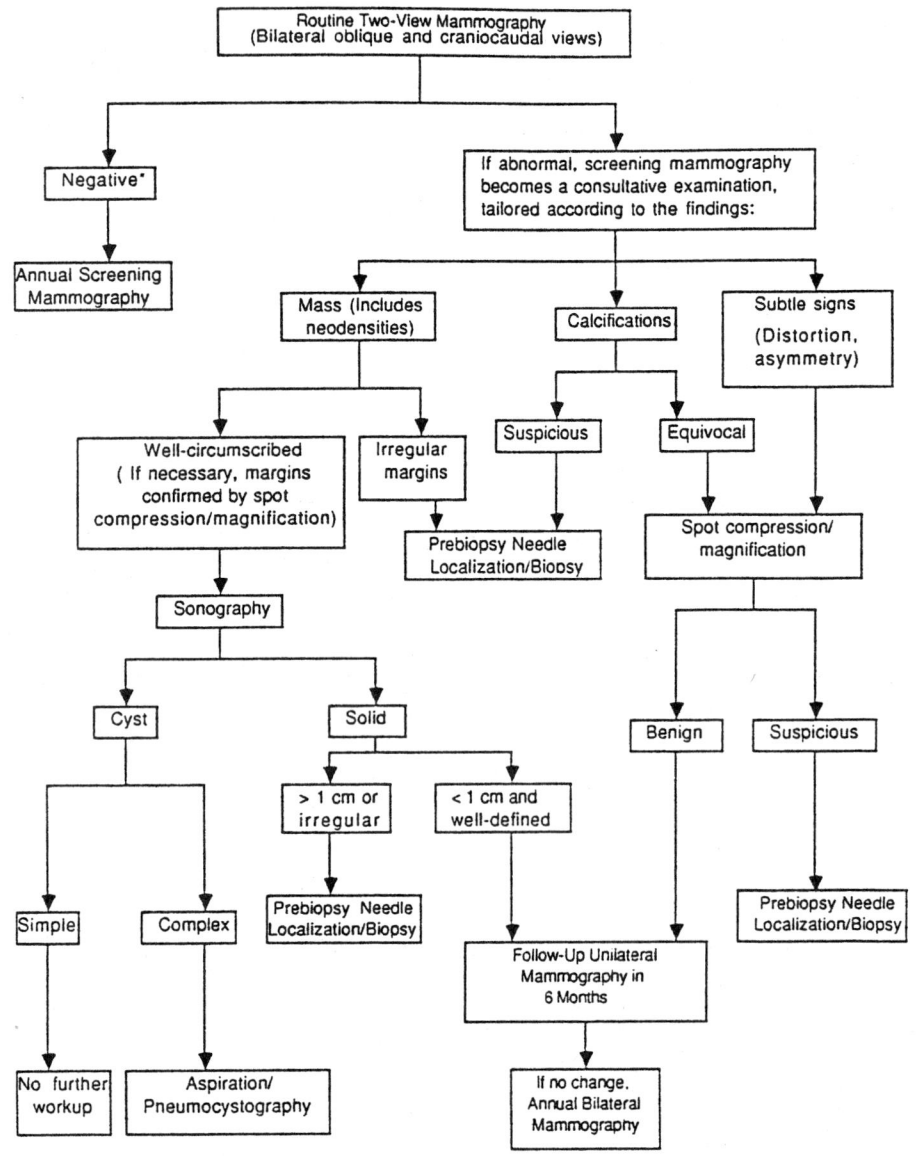

FIGURE 29–7. Algorithm for screening mammography for asymptomatic women. (From Bassett, L. W., & Gambhir, S. [1991]. Breast imaging for the 1990's. *Seminars in Oncology, 18*[2], 80–86.)

cal biopsy (Schmidt, 1994). Limitations associated with SFNA are similar to those associated with FNA in its inability to diagnose invasive cancer and specifically identify benign breast conditions. The emergence of an instrument to perform core biopsies with the stereotactic procedure has expanded the enthusiasm and use of this approach. But problems exist with SCNB, including sampling from women with small breasts, sampling superficial lesions, and presence of microcalcifications on mammography (Schmidt, 1994). Many clusters of microcalcifications that are suggestive of cancer represent ductal carcinoma in situ. A stereotactic procedure is not the diagnostic method of choice in many centers for microcalcifications that are suggestive of cancer, and in those centers that support the procedure, the patient may be referred afterward for a definitive surgical biopsy. As with any other technologic advance, nurses must become knowledgeable about the procedure to provide anticipatory guidance and education to the woman and her family.

PALPABLE BREAST MASS

Approaches to diagnosing a palpable breast mass include fine-needle aspiration, core-needle biopsy, and incisional or excisional biopsies. Fine-needle aspiration is an established method (Fig. 29–8) to diagnose breast lesions. The success is dependent on the skill of the person performing the procedure and expertise of the cytopathologist in the interpretation of the smears (Ljung et al., 1994). Cytologic diagnosis cannot distinguish noninvasive from invasive carcinoma; thus if a positive cytologic result is reported, a tissue biopsy is required (Wilson, 1984). A core-needle biopsy allows the surgeon to obtain a core of tissue that is ample for diagnostic examination but may not be sufficient for hormone receptor assays, depending on the method used. This approach, however, is not recommended for small resectable tumors and is generally reserved for patients with large breast masses, for whom treatment options would be limited. Excisional biopsy is recommended whenever possible, particularly for early-stage breast cancer, in which options for treatment are defined. The goal is to remove the entire tumor mass with an area of surrounding normal tissue.

NURSING PRACTICE: BIOPSY AND DIAGNOSIS

Recognizing that only two out of every ten lumps discovered are malignant does not alleviate a woman's distress (Shaw, Wilson, & O'Brien, 1994). Emotional support and education are major nursing interventions. Anxiety is the predominant emotional response prior to biopsy and between biopsy and diagnosis (Benedict, Williams, & Baron, 1994; Scott, 1983). A thorough explanation of the test should be given and supplemented by written materials. For invasive procedures, patients must know where to report, which health care professional will be involved, how the procedure will be performed, and how long it will take. They also should be informed about the need for anesthesia, predictable

side effects, follow-up care, and when the results will be available. Nurses in ambulatory health care settings are challenged with meeting patients' needs. Providing educational materials, coordinating the various health care team and department members toward a unified approach in delivery, and evaluating the type of care are system issues that nurses can facilitate. Information and support are critical interventions. Barrere (1992) suggests five techniques of goal-directed communication: rephrasing, personalizing, gentle confrontation, refocusing, and facilitation. This approach focuses discussion, aids in identifying individual concerns, and provides the foundation for information and guidance before and after biopsy.

Following biopsy predictable side effects and follow-up care should be specific to the type of biopsy performed, the surgeon's technique, and the complexity of the surgical procedure. General guidelines following a breast biopsy include the following: (1) expect mild to moderate discomfort, for which pain relief measures will be prescribed; (2) wear a supportive bra for 24 hours to enhance comfort; (3) avoid strenuous arm activity for the first few days; (4) expect sutures, if present, to be removed in 5 to 7 days and anticipate that the area will be ecchymotic and tender with gradual dissolution (Wiley, 1981). Indentation at the biopsy site will fill in with fat in a month or two, and significant alterations are rare if incisions follow recommended guidelines according to location of the mass (Fig. 29–9A and B).

Following diagnosis, the nurse continues to provide information and support, expanding the focus to help the patient, spouse, and family process the information to optimize their coping strategies and facilitate decision making (McHugh, Christman, & Johnson, 1982; Messerli, Garamedi, & Romano, 1980).

NONINVASIVE BREAST CANCER: DUCTAL CARCINOMA IN SITU AND LOBULAR CARCINOMA IN SITU

Intraductal or ductal carcinoma in situ (DCIS) was previously observed in 0.8 to 5 per cent of all breast cancers, typically as a palpable lesion. Today, DCIS represents 20 to 30 per cent of all breast cancers detected mammographically (Fowble, 1991; Frykberg & Bland, 1994; Stomper & Margolin, 1994). Intraductal carcinoma is characterized by multicentricity but is restricted primarily to the ipsilateral breast (Betsill, Rosen, Lieberman, & Robbins, 1978; Carter & Smith, 1977); occult invasive cancer has been observed in 6 to 21 per cent of breast specimens (Carter & Smith, 1977; Lagios, Westdahl, Margolin, & Rose, 1982). The biologic behavior of intraductal tumors ranges from benign lesions to ones consistent with invasive cancer (Stomper & Margolin, 1994). Up to 40 per cent of women treated with excision alone for DCIS may develop an invasive cancer over a 10-year period (Betsill et al., 1978; Page, DuPont, Rogers, & Landenberger, 1982).

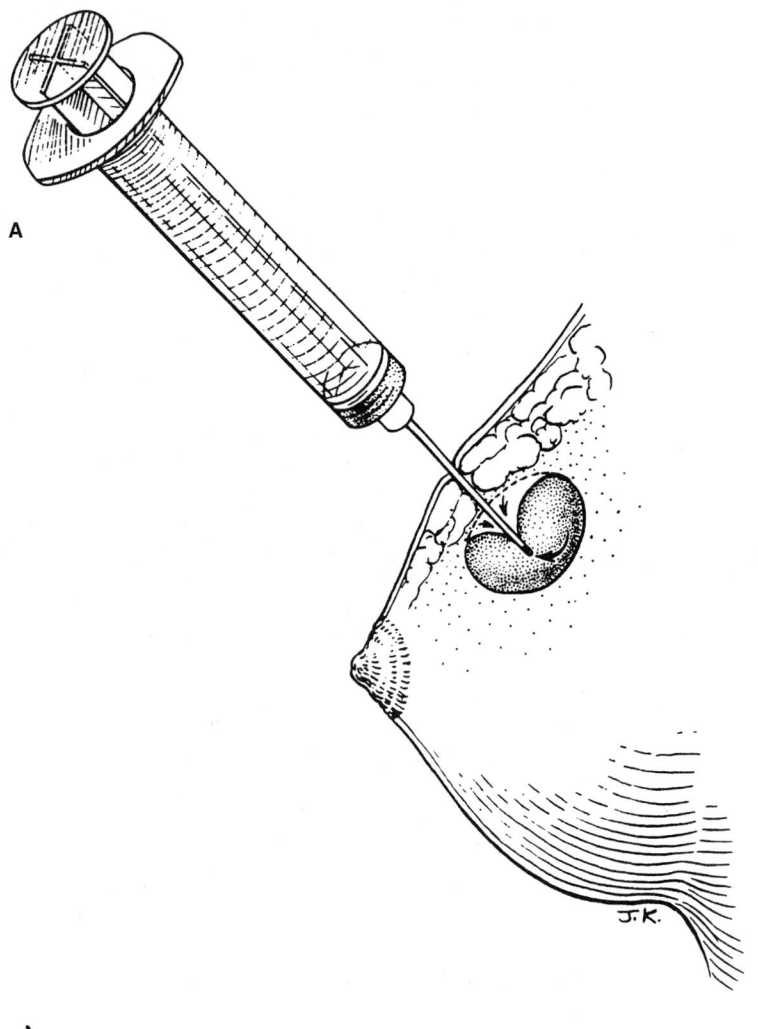

A

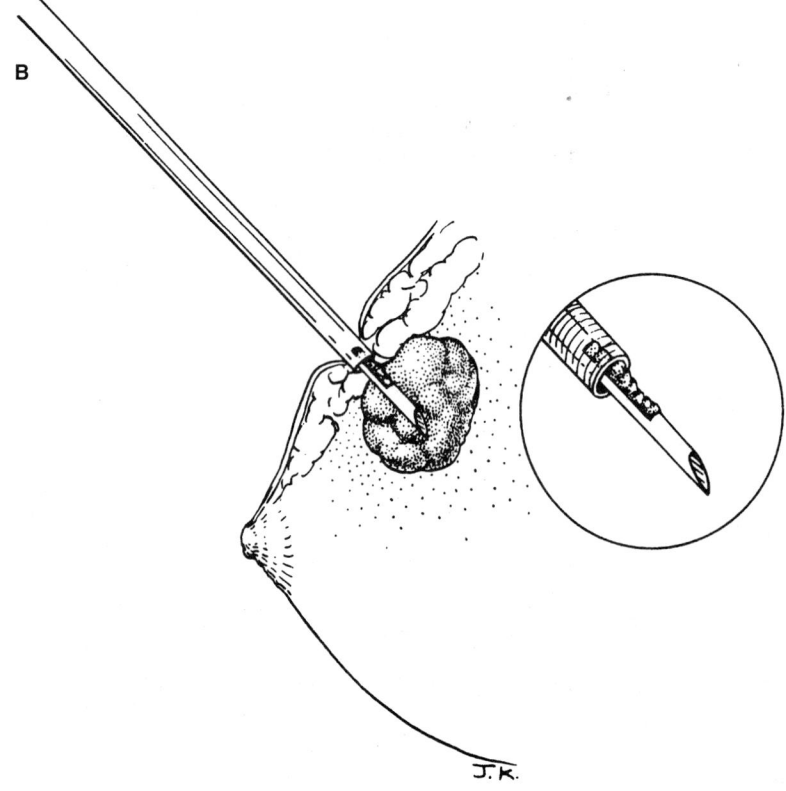

B

FIGURE 29–8. A, Fine-needle aspiration of a breast mass. **B,** A core-needle biopsy with a TruCut needle. (From Wilson, R. E., & Kroehl, S. A. [1984]. Diagnosis. In C. H. Pfeiffer & J. B. Mulliken (Eds.), *Caring for the patient with breast cancer* [pp. 21–40]. Reston, VA: Prentice Hall.)

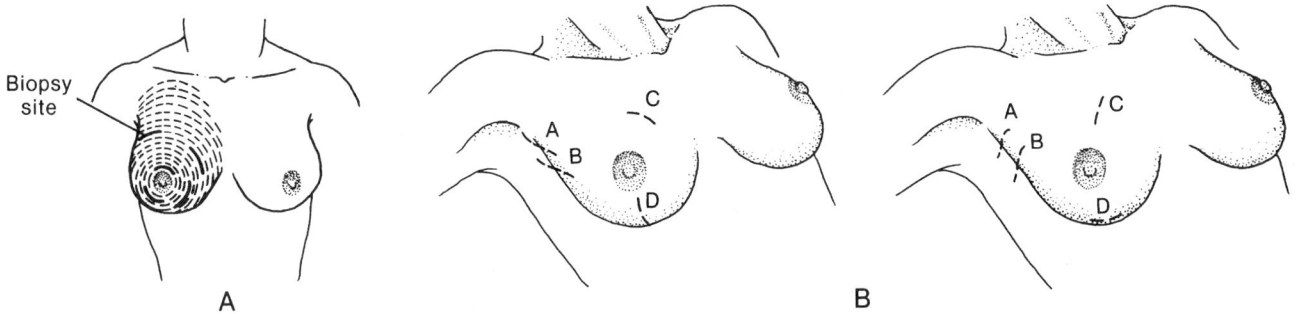

FIGURE 29–9. Recommended biopsy sites of the breast. **A,** Curvilinear (Langer's) lines, showing ideal incision placement for optimal cosmetic result. **B,** Examples of incision for peripheral malignant lesions. *(Left)* Recommended. *(Right)* Poor. (From Kinne, D. W., & Kopans, D. B. [1987]. Physical examination and mammography in the diagnosis of breast diseases. In J. R. Harris, S. Hellman, I. C. Henderson, & D. W. Kinne [Eds.], *Breast diseases* [pp. 54–85]. Philadelphia: J. B. Lippincott Co. Reproduced by permission.)

At present, there is no consensus for defining the optimal treatment of intraductal carcinoma. Mastectomy has been the traditional treatment of choice related to the observed frequency of multicentric disease, presence of occult foci of invasive cancer, and ipsilateral recurrence (Fowble, 1991). Wide excision and radiotherapy is an alternative, but concerns about within-breast recurrence (which may be invasive carcinoma) and sparse research suggest careful patient selection and caution. Patients who have diffuse microcalcifications, multifocal areas of calcifications, or clinical evidence of multicentric disease should *not* be considered candidates for conservative surgery (Fowble, 1991). The presence of the histologic subtype, comedocarcinoma, is controversial as a contraindication but has been associated with increased risk of recurrence following wide excision and radiation (Silverstein et al., 1990). Prebiopsy and postbiopsy mammograms, assessment of margins, and identification of the extent of intraductal disease are important factors in considering treatment alternatives. Mastectomy should be recommended to any patients with positive or unknown margins following excision or residual microcalcifications on mammography because of the increased risk of recurrence. Wide excision alone may be an alternative for selected patients such as those with small tumors present only on mammography, those with diploid tumors or papillary or micropapillary subtypes, those who have breasts that are easily examined clinically and who are informed of the risk and have no other risk factors (Lagios et al., 1982; Fowble, 1991). Concern remains, however, about ipsilateral recurrence; Fisher et al., (1993) reported significant reduction in recurrence at 5 years in the ipsilateral breast in women who received radiation after wide excision versus excision alone.

Axillary dissection is another treatment-related issue. Since the incidence of positive nodes is less than 5 per cent, it is generally not recommended unless there is a question of an invasive component (Fowble, 1991).

Lobular carcinoma in situ (LCIS) represents 1 to 6 per cent of all breast cancers and is less common than DCIS (Fowble, 1991). It occurs in premenopausal women and is characterized by multicentricity, a generally less aggressive natural history, and better survival rates (Carter & Smith, 1977; Frykberg, Santiago, Betsill, & O'Brien, 1987). The risk of developing an invasive cancer occurs in a minority of patients but not until 15 or more years have passed. LCIS is almost always an incidental finding on a pathology report and is often undetected by mammography (Senofsky et al., 1986). Pathologic interpretation and clinical applicability are controversial (Frykberg et al., 1987). Treatment is controversial and includes unilateral mastectomy with or without a contralateral breast biopsy, bilateral mastectomy, or excision with close follow-up (Fowble, 1991). With bilateral mastectomy, the cure rate is 100 per cent, but this solution is perceived as overtreatment by many. Support has increased for conservative approaches because of the natural history and the good prognosis if subsequent disease develops and is detected early.

The incidence of in situ carcinomas restricts the average physician's experience, perhaps with the exception of those at large university or cancer centers. Therefore, treatment decisions will likely be controversial and subject to discussions and case presentations, and patients should be encouraged to enter clinical trials, if available. The patient's role in decision making for the treatment of in situ carcinomas is stressful because many women have difficulty understanding that the treatment options are the same as those for truly invasive cancer. Nurses in the ambulatory care setting are a resource for information, questions, clarification of issues, reassurance, and support.

PRIMARY TREATMENT AND DECISION MAKING

INFORMATION AND DECISION MAKING

Women diagnosed with breast cancer in the 1990s have more opportunity for being informed consumers and participants in the treatment decision-making process than ever before. Consumer-oriented attitudes toward health care, women's ability to voice concerns in today's society, breast cancer advocacy groups, and media attention to breast cancer have played a role in heightening the average woman's awareness of the disease. They have also had a significant impact on the role of the physician from one who controls the information and decision making to one of a legally responsible provider of information and participant in the treatment decision-making process. In the United States, laws have been passed in 18 states related to disclosure of information on treatment alternatives for breast cancer (Nayfield, Bongiovanni, Alciati, Fischer, & Bergner, 1994). Informed consent, physician behavior in the patient-physician relationship, and medical information related to the treatment are generic components to these statutes, but the impact in daily clinical practice is unknown. What is known is that informational needs and information-seeking behavior vary considerably among women who are newly diagnosed with breast cancer, and the decision-making process is exceedingly complex (Knobf, 1994b).

Women desire information about breast cancer and its treatment, but not all women will be active information seekers. Older age, emotional response to the diagnosis, perceived vulnerability, physician authority figure, and female gender are factors that may partially explain why many women do not come prepared with

questions and why it is difficult for women to ask questions. Information seeking can be a learned skill, however, and nurses are the key health care providers who can teach and support women in the process of informational exchange over time. Disclosure of basic information on breast cancer treatment is a critical first step for nurses and physicians but insufficient as a single intervention. To meet the patient's informational and supportive needs, the nurse must help the patient process the information, encourage and guide development of questions, clarify information, encourage participation of family or significant others, provide information on the expected outcome related to physical, psychologic, familial, social, and functional aspects of one's life, and assure the patient and family that the nurse is accessible and available (Cantril, 1991; Hilton, 1993; Hughes, 1993a, 1993b; Kalinowski, 1991; Knobf, 1990).

Decision making is a very complex process influenced by multiple variables (Fig. 29–10). Although there seems to be an accepted philosophy that all women desire participation in the decision-making process for breast cancer treatment, it is not a universal reality. Variations in patient preferences for desired level of participation, physician support for patient involvement, and physician behavior in the process challenge the promoted model of collaborative patient-

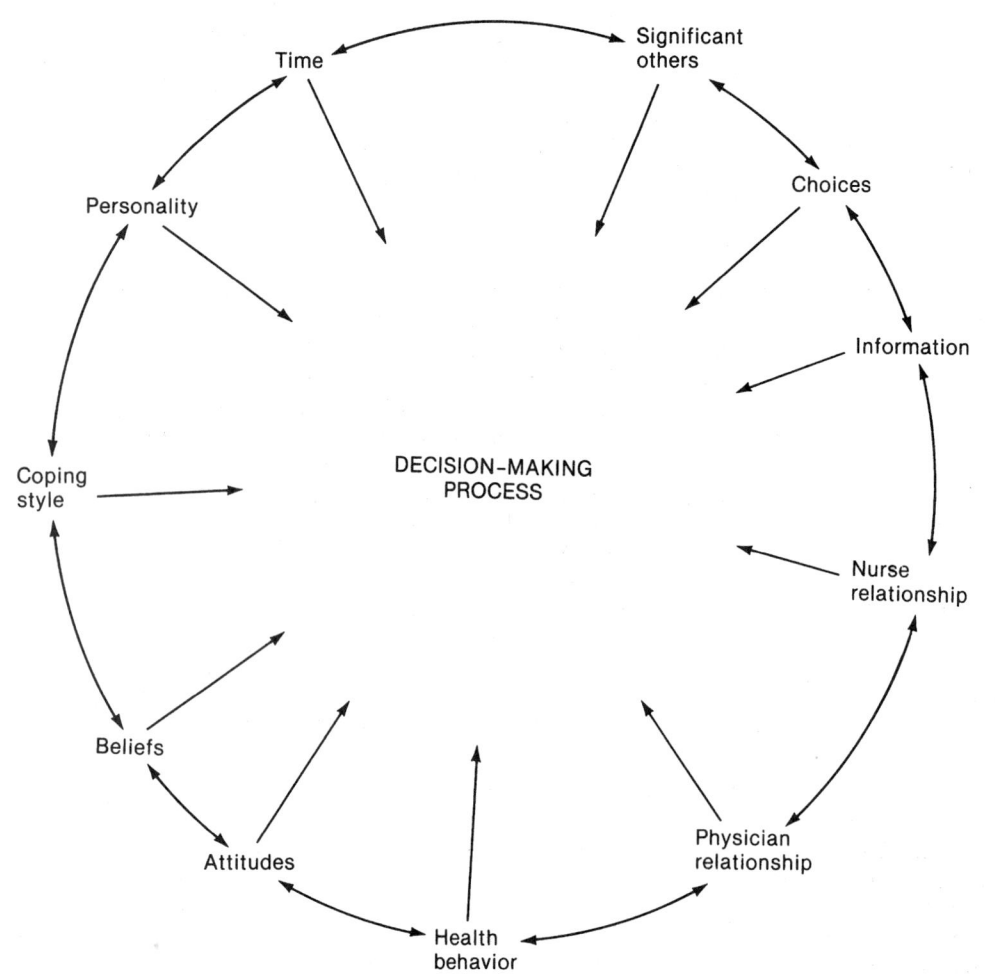

FIGURE 29–10. Variables influencing decision making in breast cancer therapy.

physician decision making (Degner & Russell, 1988; Degner & Sloan, 1992; Pasacreta, McCorkle, & Margolis, 1991). Three roles have been identified for patient preferences in decision making that can generally be described as active, passive, or collaborative (Hack, Degner, & Dyck, 1994; Neufeld, Degner, & Dick, 1993; Pierce, 1993). The active role is associated with the patient having full control. In the passive role the physician has full control. Preference for the physician to make the decision has been reported by 35 to 65 per cent of cancer patients, although shared decision making appears to be the most common desired preference (Cassileth, Zupkis, Sutton-Smith, & March, 1980; Degner & Sloan, 1992; Pierce, 1993).

Pierce (1993) interviewed women diagnosed with early-stage breast cancer prior to their decision about treatment (Box 29–1). Three decision styles emerged from the data: deferrer (41 per cent), delayer (44 per cent), and deliberator (15 per cent). The deferrer type followed the physician's recommendation, made a relatively quick and conflict-free decision, and were older. The delayer type weighed the options but made a decision as soon as a difference was noted, which was associated with a relatively uncomplicated decision-making process. The deliberator type made a decision only after all information was processed, which was associated with considerable time, resources (patient and health care providers), energy, and psychologic distress. This research gives us some insight into our daily clinical practice and may help us in determining patient needs and allocating our resources. Women who desire a very active role in treatment decision making also desire detailed and comprehensive information (Hack, Degner, & Dyck, 1994). In practice, these are the women who will utilize nurses as resources for information and support and may consume considerable time. Neufeld, Degner, and Dick (1993) provide a creative approach to identify women's preferences for decision-making participation (Fig. 29–11) through use of decision-making cards in the initial nursing assessment of the new patient's visit. The authors describe the nurse's role in providing decisional support as encompassing information, guiding the processing of information, developing questions, and providing support during and after the consultative visit. The woman's previous experience with cancer, demographic profile (e.g., age, marital status, educational level), and personal characteristics, such as personality traits, marital satisfaction, coping patterns and self concept, are additional factors to consider in providing decisional support to the patient and family (Knobf, 1994a; Valanis & Rumpler, 1985). Assessment of the informational needs, decision-making style, and personal data of the individual woman can help plan for allocation of nursing resources within a typical busy ambulatory setting, yet maintain the supportive role as patient advocates (Ganz, 1992; Langer & Hassey-Dow, 1994).

LOCAL REGIONAL CONTROL

The goal of surgery for stages I and II breast cancer is to control local regional disease. Surgical approaches have been modified as new theories of breast cancer have evolved and as radical surgery has failed to alter mortality rates. The theory in the early 1900s on which radical surgery was based proposed that breast cancer metastasized in an orderly sequence from the breast to lymph nodes to distant sites. In the last decade, major advances in the understanding of the biology of cancer have occurred. Heterogeneity, genetic instability of cancer cells, tumor burden, and intrinsic drug resistance support the observation that breast cancer is a systemic disease, which means that micrometastases could be present at the initial presentation with or without nodal involvement (Bonadonna & Valagussa, 1985; Goldie, 1983). Consequently, current efforts focus on achieving optimal local regional control and identifying prognostic factors that discriminate patients likely to harbor micrometastases (Harris, Lippman, Veronessi, & Willett, 1992a).

The primary treatment options for resectable breast cancer are modified radical mastectomy (with or without breast reconstruction) and breast conservation surgery with radiotherapy. The modified radical mastectomy is synonymous with total mastectomy and axillary lymph node dissection; it includes removing the breast and lymph nodes and preserving the pectoralis major muscle with or without preservation of the pectoralis minor muscle.

Breast-preserving surgery combined with radiotherapy involves removing the tumor along with some adjacent normal tissue (referred to as lumpectomy, tylectomy, local excision, partial mastectomy, wide excision, segmental mastectomy, or tumorectomy),

---

BOX 29–1. *Decision Styles for Breast Cancer Treatment*

Pierce, P. F. (1993). Deciding on breast cancer treatment: A description of decision behavior. *Nursing Research, 42,* 22–28.

Purpose: To describe the naturally occurring and unaided decision making of women facing treatment for early-stage breast cancer and to provide empirical grounding to develop a conceptual framework for more structured research.

Sample: 48 female subjects diagnosed with early-stage breast cancer.

Method: Open-ended semistructured interview conducted after diagnosis but before subjects had made a treatment decision.

Findings: Five empirical indicators of decision-making behavior were identified: perceived salience of alternatives, decision conflict, information seeking, risk awareness, and deliberation. These indicators discriminated subjects into one of three decision styles: deferrer, delayer, or deliberator.

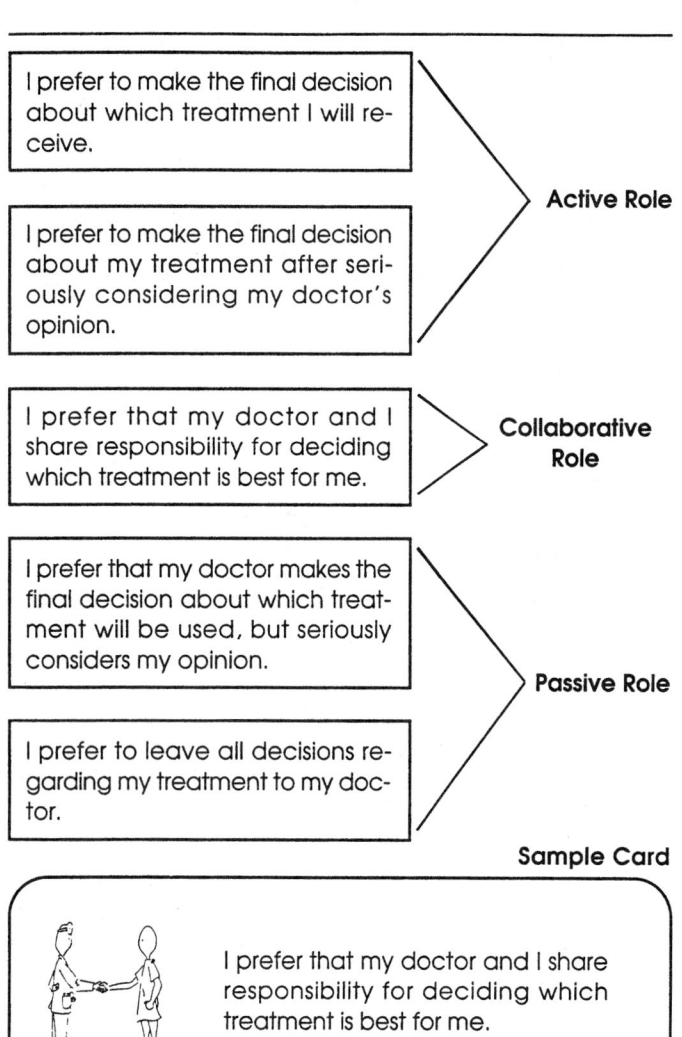

FIGURE 29-11. Statements to help patients identify their desired level of participation in decision making. (From Neufeld, K. R., Degner, K. F., & Dick, J. A. [1993]. A nursing intervention strategy to foster patient involvement in treatment decision. *Oncology Nursing Forum, 20*[4], 631–635.)

axillary node dissection, and radiotherapy for about 6 weeks. Radiotherapy is delivered to the entire breast and the tumor bed area with external electron beam boost and is an essential treatment component, particularly in the reduction of local recurrence risk (Box 29-2). Axillary lymph node dissection provides important prognostic information, guides selection of adjuvant therapy, and simplifies delivery of radiotherapy (Harris, Lippman, Veronesi, & Willett, 1992a). Axillary lymph nodes are divided into three levels (Fig. 29-12). Level I is tissue between the latissimus dorsi muscle and the lateral border of the pectoralis minor muscle; level II is tissue from the lateral border of the latissimus dorsi to the lateral and medial borders of the pectoralis minor muscle, with clearing of the axillary vein; and level III is tissue between the medial border of the pectoralis minor and Halsted's ligament (Danforth et al., 1986; Kinne, 1987). *Axillary sampling* is a vague, imprecise term that does not define boundaries and should not be used (Fisher & Wolmark, 1986; Kinne, 1987).

Excision of the axillary contents from levels I and II is recommended to achieve adequate nodal dissection for prognostic information and local disease control (Danforth et al., 1986; Fisher & Wolmark, 1986). The future role of axillary dissection may change with the widespread use of systemic adjuvant therapy, but currently it provides the information on which to base adjuvant therapy recommendations by degree of nodal risk (Harris et al., 1993).

CONSERVATIVE SURGERY AND MASTECTOMY

Conservative breast surgery with irradiation (CBS/RT) for women with small tumors (< 4–5 cm) is equivalent to mastectomy for local control and survival (Fisher, Redmond, Poisson et al., 1989; Jacobson et al., 1995; Veronesi et al., 1981). Although there is agreement on equivalency of survival outcome, there are several factors influencing the treatment decision beyond

---

Box 29-2. *Primary Therapy for Breast Cancer*

Fisher, B., Redmond, C., Poisson, R., Margolese, R., Wolmark, N., Wickerham, L., Fisher, E., Deutsch, M., Caplan, R., Pilch, Y., Glass, A., Shibata, H., Lerner, H., Terz, S., & Sidorovich, L. (1989). Eight-year results of a randomized clinical trial comparing total mastectomy and lumpectomy with or without irradiation in the treatment of breast cancer. *New England Journal of Medicine, 320,* 822–828.

Sample: 1855 women with stage I or II breast cancer randomized to groups of total mastectomy (n = 590), lumpectomy (n = 636), or lumpectomy and irradiation (n = 629).

Findings: No significant differences were found in the rates of disease-free, distant-disease-free, and overall survival among the three treatment groups. However, there was a significantly greater increase in the incidence of ipsilateral breast recurrences for women who underwent only lumpectomy when compared with those who had lumpectomy followed by irradiation. The investigators conclude that these data continue to support breast conservation approaches in the treatment of stages I and II breast cancer but note that irradiation reduces the local tumor recurrence risk in patients treated with lumpectomy.

---

the woman's personal choice. Absolute contraindications to CBS/RT include presence of multicentric disease, prior radiation to the chest area, first or second trimester pregnancy, and a history of collagen vascular disease (McCormick, 1994; Winchester & Cox, 1992). Breast size, central location of the tumor, large tumors, access to radiation therapy center, geographic location, and pulmonary compromise are additional factors that may be considered as relative contraindications or determinants of radiation as a less optimal choice. A small breast or central location may compromise cosmetic outcome. Large breasts influence the homogeneity of radiation dose delivered, and the expertise of the radiation therapist and use of the appropriate radiation equipment are critical components in determining whether radiation is an available option. Geographic location is a definite influencing factor. Breast conservation occurs more often in urban areas, large hospitals, hospitals with on-site radiation centers, and in the New England, mid-Atlantic, and Pacific areas of the country (Farrow, Hunt, & Samet, 1992; Nattinger, Gotlieb, Veum, Yahnke, & Goodwin, 1992; Osteen, Steele, Menck, & Winchester, 1992).

The decision for primary treatment should include deliberation of multiple factors by the health care providers and the patient: long-term survival, local recurrence, treatment procedure, patient preference, posttreatment recovery, complications and risks, and impact on quality of life (Knobf, 1994c). Expectations of the different treatments and recovery are important in the decision-making process for many women. In a sample of 69 women who chose CBS/RT, Cawley and Cappello (1990) reported that 26 per cent stated preoperative information was unsatisfactory and devoid or lacking in information about axillary dissection, need for arm rehabilitation, and radiotherapy. Similarly, Cantril (1991) reported that side effects of treatment options, recovery, and complications were not uniformly explained. Although poor recall may explain some of these results (Hughes, 1993a), inadequate discussion of the advantages and disadvantages of each treatment option beyond survival statistics is a clinical reality, especially in settings where there are no nurses as patient advocates.

If one assumes that a woman has been adequately informed about each treatment option and no absolute contraindications exist, individual patient variables will affect patient choice. Preservation of body integrity and concern over appearance are two reasons provided by women for the choice of CBS/RT over mastectomy (Leinster, Ashcroft, Slade, & Dewey, 1989; Owens, Ashcroft, Leinster, & Slade, 1987; Ward, Heidrich, & Wolberg, 1989; Wolberg, Romsaas, Tanner, & Malec, 1989). Younger age was frequently cited in the past as influencing a radiotherapy choice, but research and clinical practice have challenged age as a variable. Preservation of the breast has been identified as an important outcome of CBS/RT, and as a result some physicians cite it as the preferred treatment choice; yet mastectomy remains the choice for many women, influenced by such factors as their desire to get rid of the cancer or concerns about the efficacy and side effects of radiation (Ward et al., 1989). Table 29-10 provides an overview of treatment options, side effects, and complications.

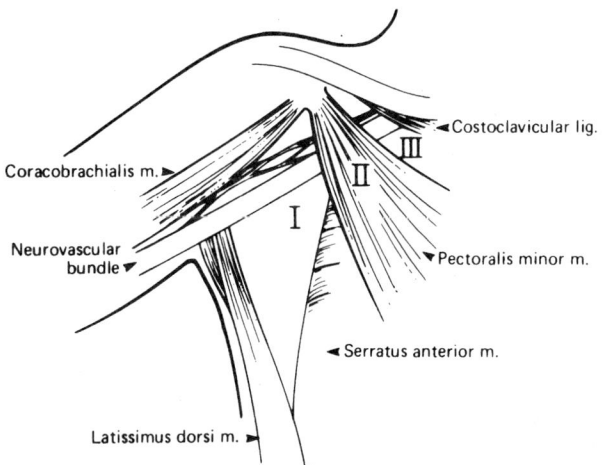

FIGURE 29-12. Levels of axillary lymph nodes. (From deMoss, E. et al. [1983]. Complete axillary lymph node dissection before radiotherapy for primary breast cancer. In J. R. Harris, S. Hellman, & W. Silen [Eds.], *Conservative management of breast cancer* [p. 166]. New York: J. B. Lippincott Co. Reproduced by permission.)

TABLE 29-10. *Treatment Options, Side Effects, Complications, and Patient Issues*

PROCEDURE	DESCRIPTION OF PROCEDURE	SURGICAL SETTING	SIDE EFFECTS	POTENTIAL SHORT-TERM COMPLICATIONS	POTENTIAL LONG-TERM COMPLICATIONS	PATIENT ISSUES
Modified radical mastectomy	Removal of breast, preservation of pectoralis muscle, axillary dissection	Hospital stay 1–2 days	Chest wall tightness, phantom breast sensations, arm swelling, sensory changes	Skin flap necrosis, seroma, hematoma, infection	Muscle atrophy, muscle weakness, lymphedema	Loss of breast, incision, body image, need for prosthesis, impaired arm mobility
Breast conservation surgery with radiation therapy	Wide excision of tumor, axillary dissection, radiation therapy	One-day surgery or hospital stay of 1–2 days; Radiation 5 days a week for 6–7 wk	Breast soreness, breast edema, skin reactions, arm swelling, sensory changes (surgery—arm; radiation—breast), fatigue	Moist desquamation, hematoma, seroma, infection	Fibrosis, rib fractures, lymphedema, myositis, pneumonitis	Prolonged treatment, impaired arm mobility, change in texture and sensitivity of breast
Reconstruction—implant	Implantation of prosthesis under musculofascial layer of chest wall	Immediate: hospital stay 1–3 days Delayed: Ambulatory surgery	Discomfort (greater than mastectomy alone due to elevation and stretching of muscles)	Skin flap necrosis, wound separation, seroma, hematoma, infection	Capsular contractions, loss of implant, ? risks of silicone implants	Body image, prolonged physician visits (expander implants), opposite breast (desire for additional procedures)
Reconstruction—flap procedures	A musculocutaneous or free flap transposed to chest wall area	Hospital stay 3–5 days	Pain related to two surgical sites and extension of the surgery	Infection, seroma, hematoma, flap necrosis		Prolonged postoperative recovery

(Adapted from Knobf, M. T. [1994c]. Treatment options for early stage breast cancer. *Medsurg Nursing, 3*(4), 249–257.)

NURSING PRACTICE

The goal of nursing care is to promote physical and psychologic recovery, which is similar in women regardless of choice of mastectomy or conservative surgery with radiotherapy (Ganz, Schag, Polinsky, Heinrich, & Flack, 1987; Ganz, Schag, Lee, Polinsky, & Tan, 1992). Initially, it was hypothesized that breast conservation surgery with radiotherapy would provide a superior cosmetic and psychologic outcome, related to preserving the breast. Psychologic adjustment is similar whether women chose breast conservation or mastectomy (Table 29–11), despite variations in methodology, design, or selected variables in published studies (Fallowfield, 1990; Kiebert, deHaes, & van de Velde, 1991). The psychologic distress appears primarily related to the diagnosis of cancer, not the loss of the breast. Breast conservation surgery with radiotherapy is associated with a more intact body image, with patients reporting fewer negative feelings about themselves nude, no changes in perceived attractiveness, less difficulty with clothing, and generally a more positive body image than women who have mastectomy (Beckman, Johansen, Richardt, & Bilchert-Toft, 1983; Ganz et al., 1987; Ganz et al., 1992; Kemeny, Wellisch, & Schain, 1988; Lasry et al., 1987; Omne-Ponten, Holmberg, & Sjöden, 1994; Sanger & Reznikoff, 1981; Schain, d'Angelo, Dunn, Lichter, & Pierce, 1994; Steinberg, Juliano, & Wise, 1985). Physical recovery and quality of life issues such as social or role functions are equally similar between treatment groups (Ganz et al., 1987; Ganz et al., 1992; Knobf, 1990).

The postoperative period should focus on meeting the patient's basic needs (Table 29–12). Written information to supplement verbal teaching is strongly recommended, especially since most hospital stays today are short. Discharge instructions can facilitate self-care at home and have the potential to decrease anxiety levels (Table 29–13). Communication among the surgeon, nurses (from inpatient, ambulatory, and home care settings), and other involved health care providers is essential to the patient's rehabilitation. Volunteer programs, such as the American Cancer Society's Reach to Recovery Program, have been challenged to revise their program structures to meet the changing needs of women newly diagnosed with breast cancer (Rinehart, 1994; Willits, 1994). Such adjunct volunteer support with coordination of the nurse in the ambulatory setting can facilitate recovery and rehabilitation in today's changing health care environment with limited resources.

BREAST SURGERY: SEQUELAE AND COMPLICATIONS

The majority of physical complaints associated with breast surgery relate to the axillary lymph node dissection, which is a technically difficult part of the surgical procedure. Problems specific to breast removal are integrated into the discussion of sequelae following axillary lymph node dissection. Seroma, hematoma, infection, nerve injury, muscle atrophy, arm swelling, and impaired shoulder function are potential complications of dissecting the axillary nodes. Seroma is a fluid accumulation in the operative site with an observed incidence of 4.2 to 32 per cent (Aitken & Minton, 1983; Lotze, Duncan, Gerber, Woltering, & Rosenberg, 1981; Martinez & Clarke, 1984; Say & Donegan, 1974). Major preventive strategies are the placement of continuous closed suction drains and the suturing of skin flaps to deep structures (Aitken & Minton, 1983). Initiation of early range of motion exercises (postoperative day 1) has been shown to increase the amount and duration of drainage. Delay of 7 to 10 days for initiation of physical rehabilitative exercises did not alter range of motion function when evaluated at 3 and 6 months; therefore it is recommended that active motion exercises be delayed for at least 1 week (Lotze et al., 1981).

The guideline for removal of closed continuous suction drains is based on amount of drainage, generally 25 to 30 ml per 24 hours (Aitken & Minton, 1983; Lotze et al., 1981). Drainage from the chest wall tubes subsides rather soon, but axillary drainage may persist for 7 to 14 days. In a clinical analysis of 88 patients with breast cancer who had axillary dissection with or without breast removal, drains remained in place for an average of 10.7 days (McKhann & Knobf, 1985). Seromas occurred in 15 per cent of patients regardless of the average number of days the drain had been in place, the preceding 24-hour drainage, the number of nodes removed at surgery, and the surgical techniques used. Treatment of seroma is aspiration; if fluid accumulation persists after several taps, placement of a Penrose drain and prescription of a course of antibiotics is recommended.

Sensory changes secondary to trauma to the nerves or transection of the nerves occur in patients with axillary dissection and mastectomy. Although surgeons attempt to keep as many nerves intact as possible, trauma may result in muscular atrophy and sensory changes (Table 29–14). The subjective complaints include numbness, weakness, increased skin sensitivity, itching, heaviness, "pins and needles," and stiffness, all of which may change in character and persist for 12 to 18 months (Maunsell, Brisson, & Deschênes, 1993; Nail, Jones, Giuffre, & Johnson, 1984). Once initial recovery is achieved from surgery, sensory changes are the most frequent chronic complaint of patients for the first year and sometimes longer. Patients need continual reassurance and confirmation that the recovery process is gradual, although for some, full sensation to the area may not return. In addition, women who have mastectomy may experience phantom breast sensations with or without pain (Lierman, 1988).

Lymphedema has been reported in 6.7 to 70 per cent of patients, occurring as early as 2 months after surgery and up to 15 to 20 years later (Aitken & Minton, 1983; Brennan, 1992; Markowski, Wilcox, &

Helm, 1981; Stillwell, 1969; Treves, 1957). The major risk factor is removal of the axillary lymph nodes. Therefore patients who have conservative breast surgery (excision and axillary dissection) have the same risk as those who have mastectomy (Norby, 1990). If no further aggravating factors are present, such as infection, trauma, or radiation, and if sufficient collateral pathways develop, adequate lymphatic drainage will be maintained. But the patient *always* remains at risk because of the surgical interruption of the lymph vessels (Brennan, 1992).

To determine if any stasis is present, the arm is measured 5 to 10 cm above and below the olecranon process and compared with the opposite side (Aitken & Minton, 1983; Markowski et al., 1981). Lymphedema is defined as the difference between one extremity and its opposite of 1 to 1.5 cm; it is categorized as mild if the difference is 3 cm, moderate if it is 3 to 5 cm, and severe if it is greater than 5 cm. Mild lymphedema may not be observed clinically, yet it is a warning sign for increased risk. Patients should be asked if they notice a difference between the two extremities (fit of clothes, heaviness), and measurements should be taken periodically and documented in the record. Once lymphedema occurs, management is aimed at prevention of further lymph accumulation. Elevation, mild exercise, massage, salt restriction, avoidance of local heat and trauma, and elastic support are basic interventions. A patient should be measured for an elastic support sleeve when the swelling is at a minimal level and should be reevaluated every 2 to 3 months for a replacement (Zeissler, Rose, & Nelson, 1972). For moderate to severe lymphedema, an intermittent sequential pneumatic compression is recommended (Brennan, 1992). Patients must have realistic expectations of the amount of benefit from such an intervention, and they may require ongoing support to cope with this chronic problem. Functional impairment and disturbance in psychosocial adjustment have been reported in women with arm swelling secondary to breast cancer surgery (Tobin, Lacey, Meyer, & Mortimer, 1993). A multidisciplinary team approach or at least consultation with other disciplines such as physical therapy, occupational therapy, social work, and psychology will enhance the evaluation, management, and support for the woman with lymphedema.

RADIOTHERAPY: SEQUELAE AND COMPLICATIONS

Long-term toxicity such as fibrosis, rib fractures, pneumonitis, pericarditis, and myositis occurs in less than 2 per cent of patients (Clarke, Martinez, & Cox, 1983; Fowble, Solin, & Schultz, 1991). Short-term side effects, however, are much more common. In two early retrospective investigations (Schain et al., 1983; Shannon-Bodnar & Flynn, 1987), breast soreness, breast tenderness, arm swelling, pain, and fatigue were reported by more than half the women questioned. Trying to discriminate accurately which symptoms are related to irradiation and which are specifically related to surgery is challenging, and to the patient it is irrelevant.

Text continued on page 575.

TABLE 29–11. Comparison of Psychosocial Responses in Women According to Treatment for Breast Cancer: Mastectomy (M) vs. Conservative Breast Surgery with Radiation (S/RI)

Author	Subjects M	Subjects S/RT	Time from Surgery	Body Image	Overall Psychologic Adjustment	Sexual Adjustment	Marital Relationship	Chemotherapy	Comments
Sanger & Reznikoff, 1981	20	20	Range = 2–52 mo; S/RT $\bar{x}$ = 15 mo; M $\bar{x}$ = 16 mo	M patients had a greater change in body satisfaction.	Similar	Not studied	Similar	Not mentioned	Retrospective study; subjects were matched pairs.
Beckman, Johansen, Richardt, & Bilchert-Toft, 1983	11	11	6–12 mo	S/RT patients reported better body image; M patients had greater problem with nakedness.	Not studied	Earlier resumption of sexual relations in S/RT patient group	Not studied	No	Subjects were matched pairs; uncertainty and fear of the future similar in both groups.
Schain et al., 1983	20	18	Range = 2–20 mo; S/RT $\bar{x}$ 11.5 mo; M $\bar{x}$ = 11 mo	M patients had a greater negative reaction to their body nude.	Similar	Similar	Similar	50% M 39% S/RT	Retrospective; mailed questionnaire (97% response rate).
Cohen, Wellisch, Christiansen, & Giuliano, 1984	28	15	Not given	Similar in measure of self-concept.	Similar (POMS)	Not studied	Similar (Dyadic Adjustment Scale)	Not given	
Steinberg, Juliano, & Wise, 1985	46	21	Range = 5–43 mo; S/RT $\bar{x}$ = 14.5 mo; M $\bar{x}$ = 15.8 mo	M patients reported feeling less attractive & less feminine and had greater concerns about appearance and clothes.	Similar	Somewhat less for M vs. S/RT patients	Not studied	45% M 43% S/RT	Retrospective; subjects were matched pairs; of subjects receiving chemotherapy, 66–80% were receiving treatment at time of study.
Taylor et al., 1985	40	26	Range = 2–60 mo; $\bar{x}$ = 25.5 mo	M patients had greater concern about disfigurement related to loss of breast.	S/RT patients better adjusted	Greater decline in affectional and sexual relations in M patients	Not studied	23% receiving chemotherapy at time of study	Retrospective; 9/40 M patient had a radical procedure.
deHaas & Welvaart, 1985	18	21	11 mo; M $\bar{x}$ = 11.8 mo; S/RT $\bar{x}$ = 10.7 mo	Significantly greater negative attitude among M patients.	Similar	Similar	Similar	Not given	Retrospective, mailed questionnaire (95% response rate).

Study	N		Time since treatment	Body image	Emotional distress	Sexual functioning	Marital adjustment	Reproductive/other	Comments
Bartelink, van Dam, & van Dongen, 1985	58	114	2 yr	Significantly more positive body image among S/RT patients.	Not studied	Report by M patients of feeling more sexually inhibited than S/RT patients	Not Studied	Yes, but %'s not provided	All M patients had radical M performed.
Baider, Rizel, Kaplan & DeNour, 1986	32	32	S/RT $\bar{x}$ = 17.2 mo; M $\bar{x}$ = 21.2 mo	Not studied.	Similar	Not studied	Not studied	Not provided, but stated no patients were in active treatment at time of study	Subjects were matched for age, time since operation, and postoperative treatment; husbands also studied and no differences in adjustment found.
Fallowfield, Baum, Maquire, 1986	53	48	Range = 4–32 mo; S/RT $\bar{x}$ = 15.2 mo; M $\bar{x}$ = 16.7 mo	Not addressed.	Similar	Similar	Not studied	1% M, 8% S/RT	34/53 M patients received postoperative radiation; retrospective.
Lasry et al., 1987	43*	36*	$\bar{x}$ = 3.5 yr	M patients reported less satisfaction with body image and increased fear of not being sexually attractive	Similar, although slight increase in depressive symptoms in S/RT group	Not studied	Not studied	Yes, but no specific information	*Total sample of 123 included 44 women who underwent lumpectomy only; retrospective.
Kemeny, Wellisch, & Schain, 1988	27*	11*	Range = 6–48 mo; $\bar{x}$ = 18 mo	S/RT patients reported a more positive body and sexual image.	Similar, but S/RT patients reported less emotional distress	Similar	Not studied	57% M, 53% lumpectomy	*Total sample of 52 included 14 patients who had lumpectomy and axillary dissection alone; questionnaire, retrospective.
Meyer & Aspergren, 1989	30	28	5 yr	M patients reported less leisure time activities related to body exposure; and disagreeable to be naked in front of spouse.	Similar	Similar	Similar	Not reported	Interviews.

Continued on following page.

TABLE 29–11. *Comparison of Psychosocial Responses in Women According to Treatment for Breast Cancer: Mastectomy (M) vs. Conservative Breast Surgery with Radiation (S/RT)* Continued

Author	Subjects M S/RT	Time from Surgery	Body Image	Overall Psychologic Adjustment	Sexual Adjustment	Marital Relationship	Chemotherapy	Comments
Holmberg, Omne-Ponten, Burns, Adami, & Bergstrom, 1989	62 37	Two time points; 4 and 13 mo	Not studied.	More disturbances in overall adjustment in M patients	Reported disturbances in adjustment to sexual relationship among S/RT patients	Not studied	6.5% M 0% S/RT	No statistically significant differences reported, only trends favoring improved adjustment in women with surgery and radiotherapy.
Leinster, Ashcroft, Slade, & Dewey, 1989	Total sample = 45	0, 3 and 12 mo	Body satisfaction was similar in both groups; M patients were all offered reconstruction option.	Similar decrease in anxiety for all groups over time; no differences between patients for depression	Not studied	Similar	Not reported	Concern about appearance was greater for S/RT and M patients who chose reconstruction; no differences in self-esteem, ability to socialize, or feelings of femininity between M and S/RT patients.
Wolberg, Romsaas, Tanner, & Malec, 1989	78 41	0, 4 or 8 and 16 mo	Not studied.	Similar over time	Higher score on general sexual experience at 16-mo follow-up, for S/RT patients	Similar	Some patients received chemotherapy but not specified	Preoperatively, patients who elected lumpectomy with radiation reported higher values for breast appearance than M patients; second assessment (4 or 8 mo) was based on completion of all radiation or chemotherapy.

Ganz, Schag, Lee, Polinsky, & Tan, 1992	57	52	1, 3, 6, and 12 mo	M patients reported more difficulty with clothing and body image; but body image scores improved in both groups over time.	Similar with improvement in both groups over the year	Similar	Similar	25% M 31% S/RT	Prospective study; no difference in global rehabilitation or quality of life; increase in mood disturbance in S/RT patients at 1 mo (not statistically significant).
Omne-Ponten, Holmberg, & Sjoden, 1994	40	26	Range = 5.8–8.1 yr median = 6 yr	M patients reported more problems with nakedness and perceived attractiveness.	Similar	Not studied	Not studied		
Schain, d'Angelo, Dunn, Lichter, & Pierce, 1994	66	76	0, 6, 12 and 24 mo	M patients were more distressed by their nude appearance.	Similar throughout 24-mo assessment	More reported concerns about sexual relations among M patients; difference diminished over 24 mo	Not studied	42% M 41% S/RT	Prospective; no differences over time between groups for fear of recurrence; psychologic adjustment scores for both groups similar to referent populations.

TABLE 29–12. *Nursing Care for the Woman with Breast Cancer*

Patient with Axillary Node Dissection

Physical

Begin exercises 24 hrs after surgery. Demonstrate limited exercises involving the hand, wrist, and elbow such as squeezing a ball, flexing fingers, touching hand to shoulder, and circular wrist motions.

Communicate with the surgeon about further exercise, considering factors of wound healing, status of suture line, and drainage. Identify the time to begin further exercise, usually about 1 wk later or after the drains and sutures are removed.

Demonstrate range of motion exercises for upper extremity and shoulder. Encourage normal (preoperative) use of arm following drain removal.

Stress the importance of continuing range of motion exercises of arm and shoulder on a daily basis for at least the first 6 mo. Suggest arm elevation for at least 30 min at a time if inactivity is prolonged.

Discuss the potential complications of infection and edema.

Review with the patient methods of preventing infection:

Avoid breaks in the skin (wear gloves when gardening, thimble when sewing, electric razor for shaving axilla; avoid trauma to cuticles and injections in that arm).

If a break in the skin occurs, wash with soap and water and cover. Call the physician for any signs of warmth, swelling, or redness in the area.

Avoid constriction of circulation in that arm such as tight sleeves, snug fitting wrist jewelry, or carrying very heavy objects for prolonged periods of time. Strenuous exercise or use of the arm should be interrupted at 20-min intervals.

Avoid burns. Suggest tanning gradually in the sun and use of sun screens; use of oven mitts to prevent stove burns.

Discuss initial care of the axilla such as avoiding depilatory creams, strong deodorants, and shaving under the arm. Advise the patient to check with the nurse and physician at follow-up visits for guidelines on when it is safe to resume shaving the axilla and using deodorants.

Identify when the sutures will be removed.

Discuss with the patient that numbness around the incision and arm is common. Describe changes in sensation in arm and axilla over time and explain why this happens.

Early Detection

Discuss with the patient the importance of breast self-examination and provide a pamphlet demonstrating the method.

Psychosocial

Diagnosis of cancer/extent of disease

Allow the patient to verbalize her feelings about the diagnosis, fears, and concerns.

Incorporate the spouse or significant other in care and communication as much as possible.

Discuss with the physician the pathology of the axillary nodes.

Identify when the patient may be expected to learn the results.

Identify the patient's perception and significance of the pathology of the axillary nodes.

Assess the patient's response and need for support and information.

Suggest readings for the patient on breast cancer, if desired.

Volunteer visitation programs

Identify what types of volunteer visitation programs are available through your institution, American Cancer Society or local advocacy groups for women with breast cancer.

Discuss the opportunity to have a volunteer visit with the patient.

Sexual Relationship

Identify that sexual relationship, specifically intercourse, may be resumed at any time, as desired.

Postmastectomy Patient

Physical

Discuss with the patient that slight redness around the surgical site sutures and some tightness and swelling in the area are normal.

If dressings over the incision are still required, discuss how often they should be changed, the procedure, and what supplies are to be used.

Describe the healing process over time.

If discomfort remains, identify where it exists and the degree. Describe relief measures such as pain medication and relaxation techniques.

Cosmesis

Demonstrate the use of the temporary prosthesis and bra extender. Explain the "lightness" of the temporary prosthesis and need to secure well in her bra. Assure the patient that this will not be a problem with the heavier permanent form.

Discuss with the patient that it is best to wait a few weeks to be fitted for a permanent breast form. This will allow resolution of any postoperative swelling and incisional healing.

Assure the patient that very few to no changes will be needed in her present wardrobe.

Consider referral to supportive programs, such as Look Good, Feel Better (American Cancer Society).

Psychosocial

Discuss the mastectomy with the patient. Encourage the patient to express her feelings and concerns about the loss of the breast, the incision, and relationship with spouse or significant other.

Identify with the patient sources of support for her over the next few months, such as spouse, family, friends, clergy, social worker or support groups.

Sexual Relationships

Discuss with the patient that initially a soft pillow or the temporary prosthesis in a comfortable bra may provide padding to alleviate any fear of discomfort during sexual relations and to avoid confrontation of the surgical area.

(Adapted from Knobf, M. T. [1985]. Primary breast cancer: Physical consequences and rehabilitation. *Seminars in Oncology Nursing 1,* 214–224. Reproduced by permission.)

TABLE 29–13. *Patient Discharge Instructions Following Breast Cancer Surgery*

Dressings
Incision
There will be a dry gauze dressing over the incision when you leave the hospital. It is not necessary to change this dressing until you return to see the doctor.
Drain site
A small dry dressing will be around the site where the drain is placed. Often there is some leakage of fluid around the drain. Check the gauze dressing for drainage and change if soiled. Some leakage is normal, but if the dressing becomes soaked more than once a day, call your doctor.

Drains
Your nurse has shown you how to empty the reservoir from your drain and how to measure the volume of drainage. You should empty the drain twice a day and record the measurements.
Drains are generally removed when drainage is about 30 ml in 24 hrs.
Drains are often removed at the same time as the stitches, generally 7 to 10 days after surgery.

Bathing
Sponge baths or tub baths, making certain that the area of the drain and incision stay dry, are permitted. You may shower after the stitches and drains are removed.

Hand and Arm Care
You can begin using your arm for normal activities such as eating or combing your hair. Exercises involving the wrist, hand, and elbow such as flexing your fingers, circular wrist motions, and touching hand to shoulder are very good. More strenuous exercises can usually be resumed after the drains have been removed.

Comfort
Some discomfort or mild pain is expected following surgery, but within 4 to 5 days, most women have no need for medication or require something only at bedtime.
Numbness in the area of the surgery and along the inner side of the arm from the armpit to the elbow occurs in virtually all patients. It is a result of injury to the nerves that provide sensation to the skin in those areas. Women have described sensations such as heaviness, pain, tingling, burning, and "pins and needles." These sensations change over the months and usually resolve by 1 yr.

Support and Information
Pamphlets on exercises, hand and arm care, and general facts about breast cancer are available from your nurse or the local American Cancer Society or Cancer Information Service (1-800-4-CANCER).

Based on a pilot study by Teeple (1987), Knobf (1994a) conducted a prospective investigation to describe the occurrence, severity, and pattern of symptoms during and after primary breast irradiation. A Symptom Profile Tool adapted from King, Nail, Kreamer, Strohl, and Johnson (1985) and the Profile of Mood States (POMS) (McNair, Lorr, & Droppleman, 1971) were administered to a convenience sample of 30 women every week during radiation and monthly for 3 months after irradiation was completed. Psychologic status as measured by the POMS remained relatively constant over time, except for the subscale of fatigue. The most common symptoms reported were fatigue, skin changes, sleep alterations, and sensation changes in the breast. Fatigue was reported at every time point (Fig. 29–13), but the highest incidence occurred during weeks 3 to 6 with improvement in the 3 months after therapy. These data are consistent with other published research that report fatigue as the most common side effect during the second half of the radiation treatment course with gradual improvement over the months following treatment (Barrere, Trotta, & Foster, 1993; Graydon, 1994; Greenberg, Sawicka, Eisenthal, & Ross, 1992). Sensation changes in the breast were reported by more than 50 per cent of subjects (Knobf, 1994a) and were described as pain, twinges, or burning (Fig. 29–14).

TABLE 29–14. *Nerves Involved in Breast Cancer Surgery*

NERVE	INNERVATION	POTENTIAL INJURY
Intercostobrachial	Axilla/upper arm	Numbness in axilla and upper arm and diminished sweat production
Anterior thoracic—medial	Lower half of pectoralis major Pectoralis minor	Muscle atrophy
Anterior thoracic—lateral	Upper half of pectoralis major	Muscle atrophy
Posterior thoracic	Serratus anterior	Increased prominence of scapula tip ("winged scapula deformity")
Thoracodorsal	Latissimus dorsi	Weakness in adduction and internal rotation

(From Knobf, M. T. [1985]. Primary breast cancer: Physical consequences and rehabilitation. *Seminars in Oncology Nursing, 1,* 214–224. Reproduced by permission.)

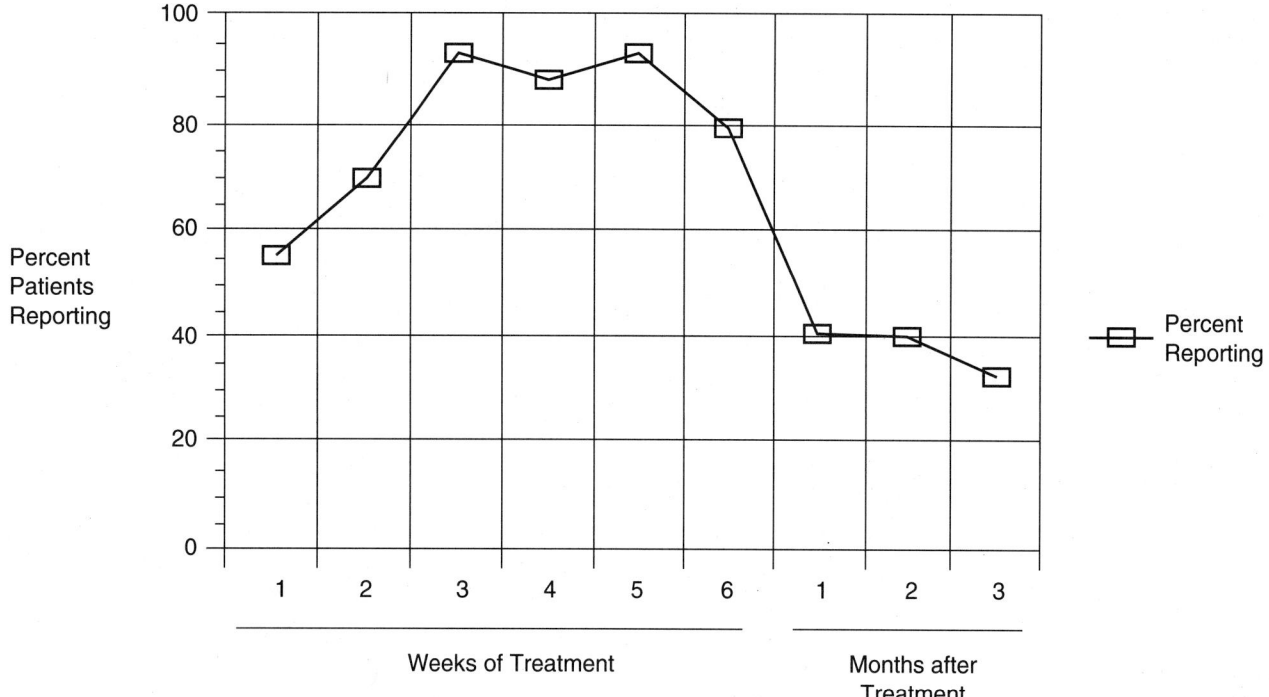

FIGURE 29–13. Incidence of fatigue before and after radiation for breast cancer.

Although these complaints were common, they were not very distressful to the women. On a Likert scale from 1 to 5 (1 = no distress, 5 = great distress), the mean distress score ranged from 1.3 to 2.1. Skin changes were reported at all time points, but most common during weeks 3 to 6 of treatment and described as red, itchy, or dry. Sleep alterations were reported by 39 to 64 per cent of subjects throughout the study period with very little variation over time. Other symptoms reported included breast swelling, arm swelling, and problems with arm mobility. Overall, subjects reported some distressing physical symptoms, especially in the middle to the end of treatment, but no significant psychologic distress. The knowledge of the pattern and

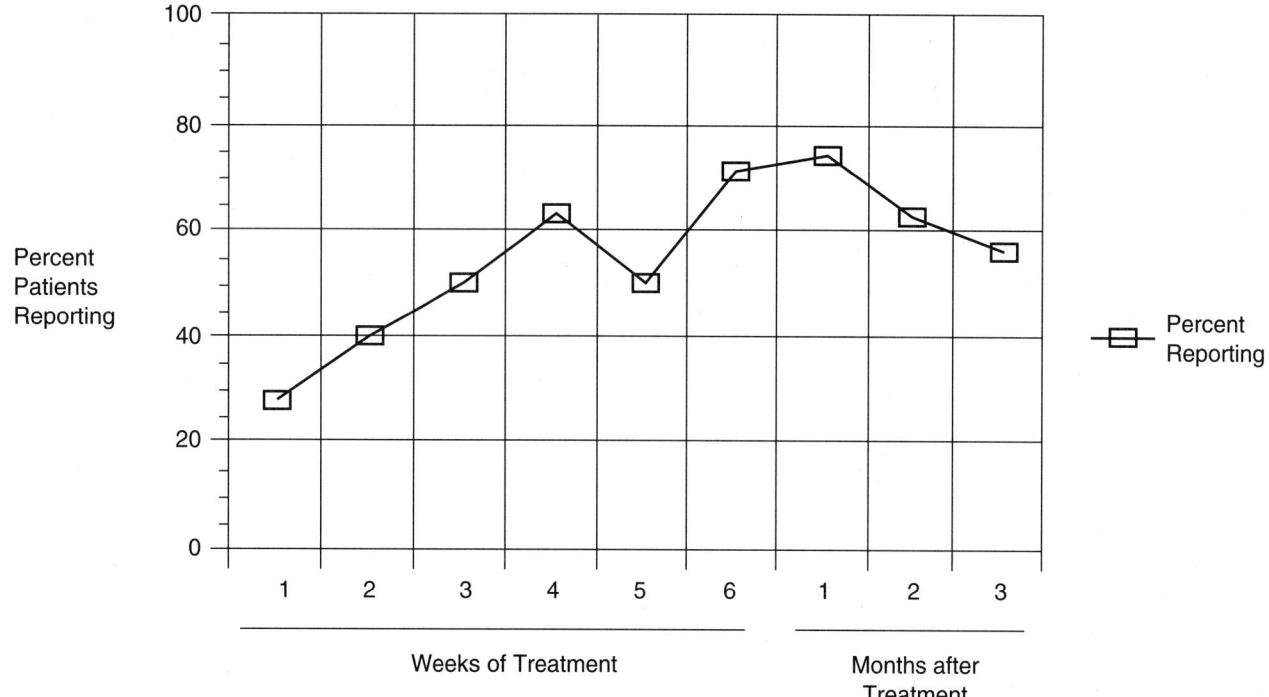

FIGURE 29–14. Incidence of sensation changes in the breast.

severity of symptoms over time adds to our ability to specifically prepare patients for the experience (Table 29–15) and, as our research base grows, will direct assessments and guiding patients in self-care activities.

BREAST RECONSTRUCTION

Breast reconstruction has gradually been integrated into primary breast cancer treatment. The goal of breast reconstruction is to provide symmetry and preserve or restore the woman's body image. Although the goal of symmetry is technically feasible for the majority of women, the patient's self-concept, motivation, choice of procedure, and expectations for reconstruction will influence satisfaction with outcome and incorporation of the reconstructed breast into the woman's body image. For women choosing mastectomy or having mastectomy recommended as primary treatment, breast

reconstruction should be discussed prior to definitive surgery. Controversies about the timing, specifically arguments against immediate procedures, appear to have been based largely on clinical judgment and personal preference rather than on research or clinical data (Frazier & Noone, 1985). Simultaneous or immediate reconstruction does not alter recurrence or survival rates, does not interfere with adjuvant therapy (Bostwick, 1990; Johansen et al., 1989; Noone et al., 1994; Russell, Collins, Holmes, & Smith, 1990), and may improve psychologic and sexual adjustment (Johansen et al., 1989; Schain, Wellisch, 1985; Stevens et al., 1984; Wellisch, Schain, Noone, & Little, 1985).

Factors to consider in evaluating breast reconstruction options with patients include self-concept, motivation, expectations, general health status, previous irradiation, prior surgery (related to a potential donor site), muscle innervation (for delayed procedures), the

---

TABLE 29–15. *Patient Guidelines for Breast Irradiation*

General Information
There will be several persons involved in your care: physician, nurse, technologist, physicist, and receptionist. You will see your doctor and nurse once a week. If you have questions or a problem arises, notify them sooner.
The schedule is daily visits Monday through Friday for about 6 wk. Appointments can be made to accommodate your work schedule or other activities.

Treatments
The first visit will include special x-rays films (called simulation) of the chest area. Your skin will be marked to outline the treatment area. A common way to mark is with Castaderm, a purple indelible ink. It is important that these marks are not removed during the treatment course.
The treatments are invisible, silent, painless, and have no odor. Machines may make a whirring or clicking sound, which is normal.
You will be alone in the room during the actual treatment, which may vary from 1 to 3 min. The entire procedure may take longer if positioning is required by the staff. You will be monitored constantly even while you are alone in the room.
There are three to five areas that may receive treatment. These areas, also called fields include different sides of the breast, around the collarbone, center of the chest, and under the arm.
The usual position is with your hand behind your head. This may cause slight discomfort during your first few treatments due to your surgery. To ease the discomfort, continue your arm exercises, and if necessary take medication 1 hr before treatment.

Possible Reactions and Care Measures
Side effects are usually minimal and do not appear until the second or third week of treatment. The most common are feeling tired and skin changes. Report any changes to your nurse and doctor.
If you feel tired, you may find it helpful to plan an afternoon nap or an early bedtime.
You may be more comfortable during treatment if you wear a loose-fitting bra.
It is best to avoid perfumes, soaps, or any other such substances on the area being treated.
You may shower, but use warm water. Be careful not to remove the markings if Castaderm was used (wash but do not use soap and scrub the area; rinse and gently pat dry).
Your breast may become swollen, and the area around your incision may become firm. These are expected reactions and will subside over time.
Wearing soft, light clothing may help reduce irritation of your skin. A cotton T-shirt may be more comfortable than a bra and very helpful to protect your clothing from the Castaderm markings.
Your skin may become pink, swollen, dry, or itchy during the second or third week of treatment. Report these changes to your nurse. A cream or light sprinkling of cornstarch on the area may help the itching. Lotions that are gentle and soothing include Nivea, Eucerin, Aquaphor, and Lubriderm.
Occasionally, the skin may blister. Report this to your nurse or physician so that he or she can monitor you and suggest the best treatment. Skin changes will generally go away within 1 to 3 wk.
If the area under your arm is treated, the hair and sweat glands will likely be affected. This means that hair may not regrow there, and you may not perspire. This may be for a short time or may last for long periods of time.
To avoid further skin irritation, cover the treated area when you go into the sun. Also, avoid heating pads, hot water bottles, or ice packs to the area.
Your skin may appear tan after the treatment is completed and remain that way for some time. Your skin may also be somewhat more sensitive for a short time. Remember, we are only talking about the skin in the areas being treated. Care for the rest of your body and skin in your usual way.

(Data from Heery, M. [1984]. Unpublished patient teaching pamphlet. Yale University School of Nursing.)

contralateral breast, skin tone, and length of predicted recovery (Knobf & Stahl, 1991). Loss of the breast has a significant impact on body image and self-concept. Women who strongly integrate physical attractiveness and appearance into their self-concept will most likely experience a greater impact on body image with loss of the breast than will other women (Goldberg, Stolzman, & Goldberg, 1984). Concern about appearance and fears about an altered feminine body image are reported patient factors influencing choice of an immediate vs. a delayed procedure (Leinster et al., 1989; Ward et al., 1989). The option of a choice not only for the type of procedure but also for the timing of the reconstruction may influence the woman's adjustment and outcome (Margolis, Goodman, & Rubin, 1989; Noone, Murphy, Spear, & Little, 1985; Rowland, Holland, Chaglassian, & Kinne, 1993; Schain et al., 1985; Wellisch et al., 1985).

Reconstruction Methods

Creating the contours of a natural-looking breast remains a challenge for the reconstructive surgeon, although advances in technology and plastic surgery have improved the cosmetic outcomes of the procedures (Bostwick, 1990). This is a critical factor in choosing a procedure that best meets the patient's desires and expectations. There are two basic methods of breast reconstruction: prosthetic implant and a flap procedure using autologous tissue, muscle, and skin from a donor site.

Implantation of a Prosthesis

Implantation of a prosthesis under the musculofascial layer of the chest wall (Fig. 29–15) has historically been the most common reconstructive approach. This procedure has a low complication rate and a short recovery and can be easily performed as an immediate procedure. Permanent prostheses are either filled with silicone gel or saline with a silicone outer covering. Tissue expanders are implants with saline sacs that are partially filled and designed to be gradually filled with saline by serial injections over time. These implants can be temporary (requiring removal and replacement with a permanent implant later) or permanent. Criteria for implant reconstruction include sufficient skin, adequate subcutaneous tissue, and an innervated pectoralis muscle. The cosmetic outcome of implant reconstruction is a breast mound, which does achieve the goal of symmetry when the woman is wearing a bra. Therefore, it is important to evaluate the contralateral breast and discuss in light of the patient's expectations. Tissue expansion improves outcome, but achieving a natural breast contour remains a primary challenge with implant reconstruction. Options for procedures on the opposite breast to maximize symmetry may be considered such as mastoplexy for a sagging or drooping breast, reduction mammoplasty for a large breast, or augmentation mammoplasty for a small contralateral breast.

The purpose of tissue expanders is to gradually stretch the skin and tissues of the chest wall over time, which has both short- and long-term benefits. Postoper-

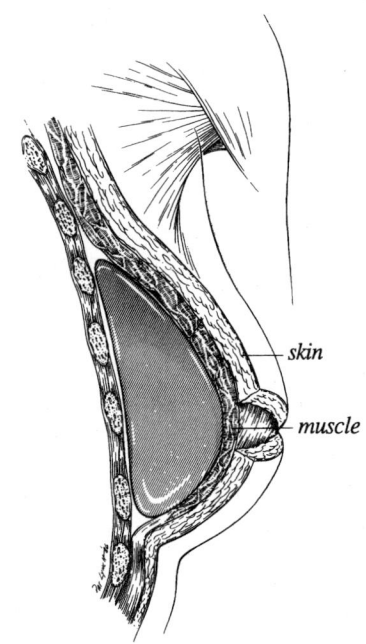

Figure 29–15. Silicone breast implant under muscle and skin. (From Knobf, M. T., & Stahl, R. (1991). Reconstructive surgery in primary breast cancer treatment. *Seminars in Oncology Nursing, 7*(3), 200–206.)

atively, there is less tension on the wound, thereby reducing risks of flap necrosis. Long-term, the gradual changes in the skin may result in a more natural-looking breast mound. Tissue expanders can be placed at the time of mastectomy or any time thereafter. Initially the expander contains 100 to 200 ml of saline. Within a few weeks following implantation, saline is injected subcutaneously into a port that is attached to the implant every 1 to 3 weeks (d'Angelo & Gorrell, 1989). The amount of saline injection varies from 30 to 100 ml and is dependent on patient tolerance and the time goal for expansion. This process continues until a state of over-inflation is reached, about 200 ml more than the desired volume. This overinflation maximizes the tissue stretch, thereby maximizing the cosmetic outcome of a softer more natural-looking breast mound. Many women complain of mild to moderate levels of discomfort associated with the expansion injections; the discomfort is successfully managed with over the counter analgesics (Knobf & Stahl, 1991). The entire procedure for full expansion can take up to 6 months, and women may require encouragement and emotional support (d'Angelo & Gorrell, 1989; Goin & Goin, 1988).

Discharge instructions (Table 29–16) for the patient are similar whether the patient has an immediate procedure or a delayed procedure (Knobf & Stahl, 1987; Pfeiffer & Mullikne, 1984). Complications (seroma, hematoma, skin necrosis, delayed wound healing, leakage, migration, cellulitis, failure of tissue expander to inflate, and capsular contractions) occur in less than 10 per cent of patients, and the risk of capsular contractions has been reduced by changes in the linings of the prostheses. Due to the decreased risk because of material improvements and concern about leakage or rup-

TABLE 29-16. *Discharge Guidelines for Patients With Implant Breast Reconstruction*

Incision
A small gauze dressing over the incision should be changed once a day. Small amounts of clear odorless fluid or slightly blood-tinged drainage is common. Sutures, if present, will be removed 1 to 2 wk after surgery by your physician.

Drains
Drainage tubes may be present if your reconstruction was performed at the same time as your mastectomy.

Bathing
Sponge baths or tub baths are permitted, keeping the incision dry. Once the sutures are removed, showers are permitted, and the incisional area should be washed gently. Once the incision begins healing, application of vitamin E oil or cream, cocoa butter, or aloe-based cream will moisturize the area and may enhance the healing process.

Comfort
Because the surgery involves operating on muscle, there will be some pain and discomfort. You will be given a pain medication to take at home that will keep you comfortable.

Daily Activities
General household activities and mild exercise, such as walking, are permitted. Strenuous exercise, heavy lifting, and extreme stretching should be avoided for 4 to 6 wk to allow time for the muscle over the implant to heal. Driving a car may be resumed in 1 to 2 wk. When in a car, the seat belt should always be worn to protect the reconstructed breast in case of an abrupt stop. Sexual relations can be resumed after you leave the hospital. However, avoid heavy pressure on the reconstructed breast for 4 to 6 weeks, which includes not sleeping on your stomach.

Return to Work
The type of job you have dictates when you can return to work. If no strenuous activity is required, you may return as early as 1 week after surgery. But as with the exercise restriction, it is recommended to wait 4 to 6 wk if your job involves heavy physical activity.

Care of the Reconstructed Breast
Bra
Immediate reconstruction: Delay wearing a bra for several weeks to optimize blood supply to the muscle and skin. A very soft, stretchy bra with no wires could be worn if needed for a special occasion.
Delayed reconstruction: Begin wearing a bra immediately and for 24 hrs a day for 2 wk. The bra should be slightly supportive without seams.
Sun
Use a number 15 sunscreen if you are exposed to the sun. The blood supply of the skin over the implant has been interrupted by surgery and may be more vulnerable to sun exposure and burning.

---

ture of the implant, massage exercises are no longer routinely recommended to the patient. Adjustment of the woman to the implant requires time, and the role of the nurse in the ambulatory setting is critical in the assessment and support of the woman. For patients with tissue expanders, asymmetry is expected until expansion reaches full capacity and suggestions for clothing and provision of support is important. For patients with permanent implants, the initial cosmetic outcome of a firm round breast mound may not match the expectations. Women require reinforcement and support over the next several months as the tissues soften and settle before symmetry and satisfaction can be evaluated (Knobf & Stahl, 1991).

The controversies over the safety of silicone implants have changed the use and interest in implant reconstruction methods. Claims that systemic exposure to silicone resulted in the development of autoimmune diseases raised the issue of risk of leakage from implants and or rupture of the implant. In 1991 the FDA issued a regulation requiring manufacturers of silicone-filled breast implants to submit scientific data to demonstrate the safety and efficacy of the product. In 1992 the FDA restricted the use of silicone implants to clinical trials and women who had a medical need, such as reconstruction for breast cancer (Kessler, 1992). Allowing selected groups to continue with implants while risks were being evaluated, the lack of evidence for association with autoimmune disease, and the general guideline to retain implants already placed resulted in great controversy related to the FDA action (Angell, 1992, 1994; Kessler, 1992). The continued lack of association with autoimmune diseases (Gabriel et al., 1994) has not changed the public acceptance that breast implants cause connective tissues diseases (Angell, 1994). Multi-million dollar settlements by the manufacturers have resulted, with some considering bankruptcy. Silicone is widely used in the food, beverage, and cosmetic industry and in many medical products and in medical technology (Fisher, 1992). Silicone is ubiquitous, and biologic exposure to anyone in society is a reality. The risk of greater exposure from leakage or rupture from a breast implant remains unknown and awaits critical analysis of further data (Angell, 1994). Nurses must be aware of the controversies for women currently with implants and for those who are considering reconstruction. Most of the saline implants have silicone outer coverings, but thus far the controversy and risk is focused on the gel filling, not linings or coverings, which are also used in many other medical products.

FLAP RECONSTRUCTION
Pedical musculocutaneous and free flap reconstructive methods transpose skin, fat, and muscle to the

chest wall. The musculocutaneous flaps consists of the muscle with its blood supply, whereas the free flaps are performed using a microvascular technique to reestablish blood supply at the recipient site (Reese, 1990). The latissimus dorsi musculocutaneous flap (LDMF) uses skin, fat, and muscle from the upper back, which is tunneled over to the chest wall. This type of flap may be useful in women with small breasts, otherwise an implant is required to achieve symmetry. Disadvantages of the LDMF include a visible scar on the back and possible upper extremity weakness.

The transverse rectus abdominis muscle (TRAM) flap uses the rectus abdominis muscle with associated fat, skin, and blood supply, commonly referred to as the "tummy tuck." The advantages include a relatively hidden abdominal scar, removal of excess abdominal tissue, and a relatively natural-looking ptotic breast (Bostwick, 1990). Disadvantages of the pedical flap procedures include prolonged operative time, hospitalization (3 to 6 days), and a recovery of 3 to 6 weeks. Postoperative complications of flap necrosis and loss can be minimized by careful selection of patients. Contraindications for flap reconstruction include obesity, older age (> 65 years), compromised pulmonary function, and factors that influence microcirculation such as caffeine, nicotine, and diabetes mellitus (Bostwick, 1990).

Free flap reconstructive procedures involve transfer of the skin and muscle using a microvascular technique to establish the blood supply at the recipient site. The rectus abdominis, lateral thigh, or gluteal muscle are possible donor sites. The availability of an experienced plastic surgeon is essential to consider this type of reconstruction method. Flap viability, a critical outcome, is dependent on the microsurgical anastomosis of the vessels, which is very time consuming (operative time 5 to 8 hours) and technically complex (Giomuso & Suster, 1994). And postoperatively, maintenance of blood flow is equally critical. Flap viability is assessed by color, temperature, tissue turgor, capillary refill, and arterial blood flow (Giomuso & Suster, 1994; Reese, 1990). Color should be compared to the donor site; pale, mottled, or purplish color of the flap indicates altered perfusion. Immediately postoperatively, the flap may be slightly cooler than surrounding tissues (Hutcheson, 1986) but should soon feel warm to touch (Giomuso & Suster, 1994). The tissue should not appear tense or tight, which might indicate venous congestion and compromise. Capillary refill is a critical assessment parameter, and a well-perfused flap will blanch for 1 to 3 seconds (Giomuso & Suster, 1994). In addition, some institutions may use ultrasonic or laser Doppler imaging to monitor blood flow. Any changes in assessment parameters should be reported immediately to the surgeon; a tool such as a flowsheet with parameters and timings of assessments may enhance early detection of a compromised flap (Giomuso & Suster, 1994). Discharge planning must include directions to avoid anything that may cause vascular constriction such as smoking, caffeine, or exposure to extreme temperatures, as well as expectations for resuming activities involving use of the donor muscle site.

NIPPLE-AREOLA COMPLEX

Some women may desire further procedures such as nipple reconstruction to enhance cosmetic outcome or symmetry. Donor site or available skin at the site may be used, and outcome (symmetry, color match, size, and shape) should be assessed after 2 to 3 months of healing (Knobf & Stahl, 1991). Intradermal tatooing may be used to achieve optimal pigmentation (Spear, Convit, & Little, 1989), and any of these procedures are easily performed in the ambulatory setting.

ADJUVANT SYSTEMIC THERAPY

The pioneering efforts for randomized clinical trials of adjuvant therapy of breast cancer by Bonadonna et al., (1976) from the Milan Cancer Institute and Fisher, Slack, Katrych, and Wolmark (1975) from the National Surgical Adjuvant Breast Project (NSABP) were based on the conceptualization of breast cancer as a systemic disease, and these reports provided preliminary evidence of the efficacy of adjuvant therapy. These early efforts provided an international stimulus for hundreds of trials with chemotherapy and hormonal therapy in attempts to reduce recurrence and mortality in women with breast cancer. Now 20 years later, adjuvant therapy trials have demonstrated that chemotherapy and hormone therapy reduce mortality and recurrence (Bonadonna, Valagussa, Moliterni, Zambetti, & Brambilla, 1995; Early Breast Cancer Trialists' Collaborative Groups, 1992a, 1992b; Henderson, 1994), but the evolution and results of these trials have raised many more questions about efficacy related to subsets of patients, risk-benefit ratio, dose intensity, timing and sequencing, and optimal drug regimen (Bonadonna et al., 1991; Harris, Lippman, Veronessi, & Willett, 1992b; Henderson, 1987). In an international review of 133 randomized trials, the Early Breast Cancer Trialists' Group addressed 5- and 10-year outcomes and concluded that adjuvant polychemotherapy and use of tamoxifen reduce mortality and recurrence of breast cancer (Box 29-3). The results of this metaanalysis, however, need careful interpretation, particularly for subsets of patients, as well as maintaining a perspective of the benefits and limitations of analysis of combined data (Harris et al., 1992b). Treatment of patients with node-positive vs. node-negative breast cancer, chemotherapy alone, hormone therapy alone, chemoendocrine regimens, anthracycline-containing regimens, age, ovarian castration, dose intensity, high-dose therapy with stem cell or autologous bone marrow transplant rescue, and sequencing adjuvant therapy with primary radiotherapy are everyday practice issues and questions for clinical trials, many of which are in progress.

NODE-POSITIVE BREAST CANCER: ADJUVANT CHEMOTHERAPY

Nodal status continues to be the most important prognostic factor (see Fig. 29-5) and has dramatically influenced the outcome of adjuvant therapy and design of trials. Women with more than four affected axillary lymph nodes are at significantly greater risk for relapse

---

Box 29–3. *Adjuvant Therapy for Primary Breast Cancer*

Early Breast Cancer Trialists' Collaborative Group (1992). Systemic treatment of early breast cancer by hormonal, cytotoxic or immunotherapy: 133 randomized trials involving 31,000 recurrences and 24,000 deaths among 75,000 women. *Lancet, 339*(8784), 2–15; (8785), 71–85.

Purpose: Metaanalysis of recurrence and mortality from randomized trials of systemic adjuvant treatment.
Findings:
- Adjuvant tamoxifen therapy resulted in a 25 per cent reduction in recurrence and a 17 per cent reduction in mortality (p < 0.00001).
- Tamoxifen therapy reduced the risk of developing contralateral breast cancer by 39 per cent (p < 0.00001).
- Long-term tamoxifen therapy is significantly more effective than shorter tamoxifen regimens.
- Polychemotherapy reduced recurrence by 28 per cent and mortality by 16 per cent (p < 0.00001).
- Polychemotherapy is significantly better than single-agent chemotherapy.
- Short-term chemotherapy (e.g., 6 months) is as good as long-term therapy (e.g., 12 months).
- Chemotherapy plus tamoxifen therapy is better in reducing recurrence and mortality in women ages 50 to 69 years than chemotherapy alone (p < 0.00001).
- Chemotherapy plus tamoxifen therapy is better in reducing recurrence of disease than tamoxifen therapy alone in women ages 50 to 69 years (p < 0.00001).

---

and death from breast cancer and receive less benefit from conventional adjuvant therapy regimens. The efficacy of polychemotherapy is greatest in premenopausal women with one to three nodes positive (Bonadonna, Valagussa et al., 1995). Age or menopausal status is also a critical factor in evaluating adjuvant therapy outcome. After 20 years of follow-up in patients who received cyclophosphamide (Cytoxan), methotrexate, and fluorouracil (CMF), 47 per cent of premenopausal patients were alive vs. 22 per cent of postmenopausal women. Similarly, if the international overview data (Box 29–3) is assessed by age, polychemotherapy reduced risk of recurrence by 36 per cent in women under 50 years of age vs. 24 per cent reduction for women over 50 years, and reduction in the risk of death is 24 per cent for younger vs. only 13 per cent for older women (Harris et al., 1992b). There is not yet a definitive answer to the question of polychemotherapy in postmenopausal women. Biologic differences related to the hormonal status and drug dosing are two plausible explanations. Bonadonna, Valagussa et al. (1995) have maintained the importance of optimal drug dosing on outcome (Fig. 29–16). In a comparison of three dosing regimens for cyclophosphamide, doxorubicin, and fluorouracil (CAF), Wood et al. (1994) reported significantly improved disease-free and overall survival in premenopausal and postmenopausal women who received either the moderate or higher dosing regimens. These data support the importance of optimal dosing of drugs for maximum clinical benefit (DeVita, 1986), which should not be confused with the separate question of high-dose therapy with rescue.

The prognosis of women with more than four nodes positive is poor (see Fig. 29–5), and this patient subset has been the focus of clinical trials. The addition of doxorubicin to adjuvant regimens, sequencing of drugs, chemoendocrine combinations, and high-dose therapy with rescue arose from the data in attempt to improve survival in high-risk patients. Once the shorter duration of chemotherapy (e.g., 6 months) was known to be equivalent to longer courses (Henderson, Gel-

man, Harris, & Canellos, 1986) and data on adjuvant therapy identified specific subsets of patients who had little or no benefit from CMF alone, the inclusion of doxorubicin (Adriamycin) was logically obvious with its known efficacy in metastatic disease (Buzzoni, Bonadonna, Valagussa, & Zambetti, 1991; Fisher, Brown, Dimitrov et al., 1990). As the role of doxorubicin became established in adjuvant therapy in clinical practice, additional strategies to improve outcome of high-risk patients, such as sequential drug administration, were being evaluated in clinical trials. A sequential regimen of four courses of doxorubicin followed by eight courses of CMF in women with more than three positive results was compared with an alternating regimen (two courses of CMF alternated with one course of doxorubicin for a total of 12 courses). At 10 years the sequential regimen was superior to the alternating schedule with a reported relapse-free survival of 42 per cent vs. 28 per cent, and overall survival was 58 per cent vs. 44 per cent (Bonadonna, Zambetti, & Valagussa, 1995). Researchers continue to strive to improve survival outcome, as demonstrated by the sequential doxorubicin/CMF over CMF study in women with 4 to 10 positive nodes (Table 29–17), yet significant tumor burden at diagnosis (e.g., > 10 positive nodes) continues to challenge our treatment strategies.

NODE-NEGATIVE BREAST CANCER: ADJUVANT CHEMOTHERAPY

Although node-negative patients represent a better prognostic group, 25 to 30 per cent will eventually relapse by 10 years and die of their disease. Efforts have focused on identifying subsets of higher risk patients within the node-negative group who may benefit from adjuvant therapy. Negative estrogen receptors, large tumors, and high proliferative activity are suggestive of an increased risk of recurrence. Four trials initiated in the 1980s (Milan IV [Zambetti, Valagussa, & Bonadonna, 1992], NSABP B-13 [Fisher, Redmond, Dimitrov et al.,

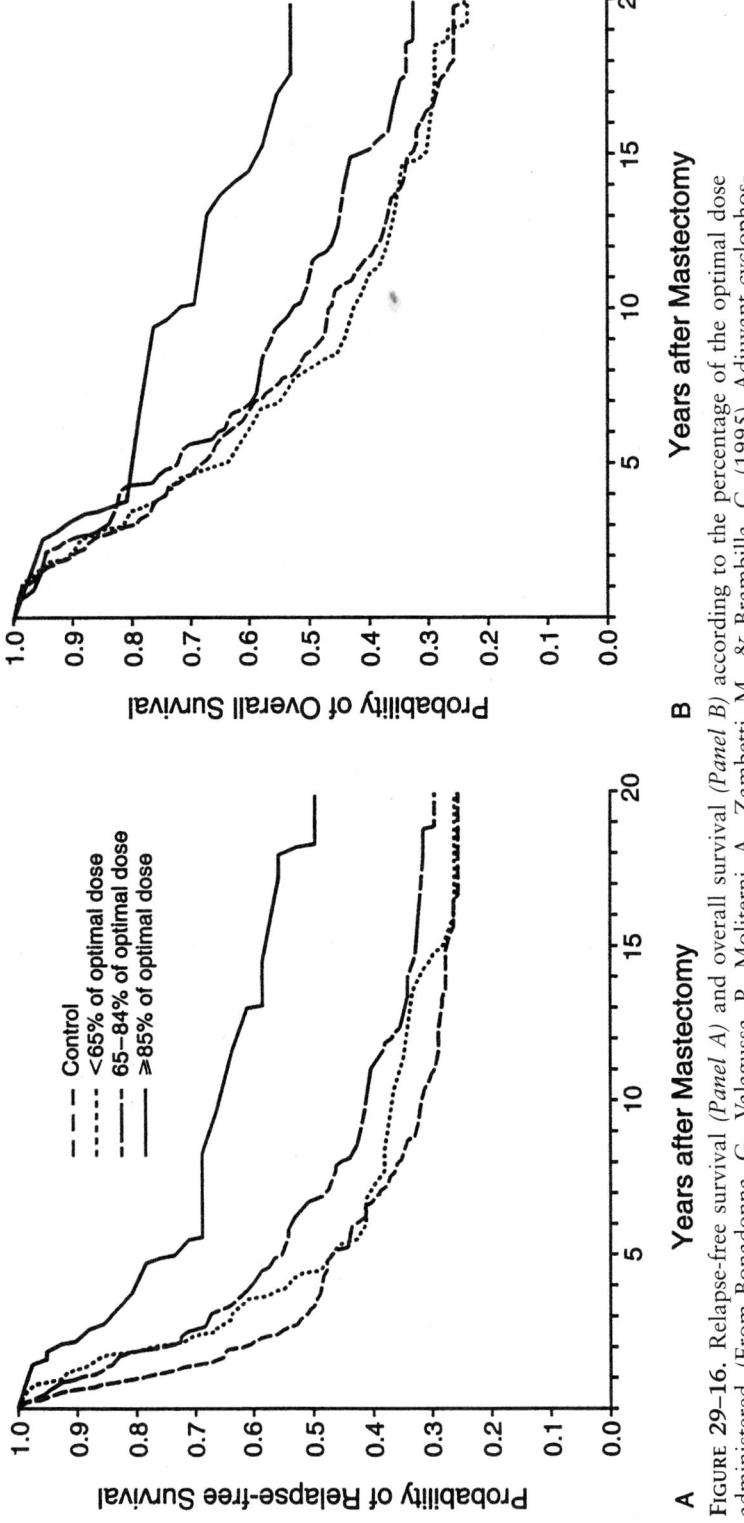

A   Years after Mastectomy

B   Years after Mastectomy

FIGURE 29–16. Relapse-free survival *(Panel A)* and overall survival *(Panel B)* according to the percentage of the optimal dose administered. (From Bonadonna, G., Valagussa, P., Moliterni, A., Zambetti, M., & Brambilla, C. (1995). Adjuvant cyclophosphamide, methotrexate and fluorouracil in node-positive breast cancer: The results of 20 years of follow-up. Reprinted by permission of *The New England Journal of Medicine, 332*(14), 901–906. Copyright 1995, Massachusetts Medical Society.)

TABLE 29–17. *Comparison of 10-Year Results of CMF Adjuvant Therapy Sequential Adriamycin/CMF Therapy in High-Risk Breast Cancer*

NODAL GROUP/TREATMENT	% OF 10-YEAR RELAPSE-FREE SURVIVAL	% OF OVERALL 10-YEAR SURVIVAL
4–10 Positive Nodes		
CMF*	34%	44%
A/CMF**	47%	64%
> 10 Positive Nodes		
CMF*	11%	44%
A/CMF**	29%	41%

A/CMF = doxorubicin (Adriamycin)/cyclophosphamide (Cytoxan), methotrexate, and fluorouracil;
  CMF = cyclophosphamide (Cytoxan), methotrexate, and fluorouracil.
  *Bonadonna, Rossi, & Valagussa, 1985.
  **Bonadonna, Zambetti, & Valagussa, 1995.

1989], Intergroup 001 [Mansour et al., 1994], and Ludwig V [Goldhirsch, Castiglione, & Gelber, 1992]) compared chemotherapy to no treatment in node-negative patients and demonstrated survival benefit for those women treated (Table 29–18). In a review of these trials and the overview analysis including node-negative subgroups of women, Davidson and Abeloff (1992) concluded that women with node-negative breast cancer benefit from adjuvant therapy regardless of age. The risk of recurrence within the node-negative group varies, and we have not yet been able to finely discriminate by degree of risk. Thus, the degree of benefit and risk associated with adjuvant therapy becomes difficult to quantify and challenges the decision-making process for both the physician and patient. Identification and further refinement of the predictive value of specific prognostic factors will guide selection of patients. In the interim it is critical that patients receive accurate information about the risk of recurrence, potential benefit of adjuvant therapy, and short- and long-term risks associated with therapy.

ADJUVANT ENDOCRINE THERAPY

Adjuvant endocrine therapy regained its status in the 1970s with the availability of the antiestrogen, tamoxifen, and the discovery of steroid receptors. Adjuvant tamoxifen reduces recurrence and mortality with the greatest effect observed in postmenopausal women (Pritchard, 1987; Early Breast Cancer Trialists' Groups, 1992a, 1992b). When the international overview data (Box 29–3) were assessed by age for endocrine therapy, tamoxifen therapy reduced recurrence 29 per cent in women over 50 years of age vs. only 12 per cent for younger women; similarly a 20 per cent reduction in risk of death was reported for those women over 50 years of age vs. 6 per cent in women younger than 50 years (Harris et al., 1992b). Some investigators have reported that response is related to the quantity of receptor levels (Fisher et al., 1983; Fisher, Constantino, Redmond et al., 1989; Rose et al., 1985; Rutqvist et al., 1987) while others have reported response to be independent of age, menopausal status, or receptor content (NATO, 1988). There is no question that tamoxifen improves relapse-free survival significantly in node-positive postmenopausal women with an associated improvement in overall survival. The degree of effect of adjuvant tamoxifen alone in node-negative and premenopausal subgroups with breast cancer continues to be defined as clinical trials mature and results are published.

TABLE 29–18. *Adjuvant Systemic Therapy Trials with No Treatment Control Arm in Node-Negative Breast Cancer*

STUDY	ELIGIBILITY	THERAPY DRUGS	THERAPY DURATION	MEDIAN FOLLOW-UP	SURVIVAL BENEFIT DISEASE-FREE	SURVIVAL BENEFIT OVERALL
Milan IV	ER neg	CMF	9 mo	8 yr	p = 0.0002	p = 0.005
NSABP B-13	ER neg	MF	12 mo	5 yr	p = 0.0007	p = 0.09
Intergroup 0011	ER neg and/or T ≥ 3 cm	CMFP	6 mo	4.5 yr	p < 0.0001	p = 0.31
Ludwig V	Any ≤ 65 yr	CMF	1 mo	5 yr	p = 0.02	p = 0.31

C = cyclophosphamide; M = methotrexate; F = 5-fluorouracil; P = prednisone; T = tamoxifen; ER = estrogen receptor; neg = negative; pos = positive.
(Adapted from Davidson, N. E., & Abeloff, M. [1992]. Adjuvant systemic therapy from node negative breast cancer. In V. T. DeVita, S. Hellman, S. A. Rosenberg (Eds.), *PPO updates* [pp. 1–13]. Philadelphia: J. B. Lippincott Co.)

Adjuvant castration predated adjuvant systemic therapy by several decades. Henderson (1987) provides a concise historical overview of oophorectomy following mastectomy in premenopausal women, beginning some 40 years ago. The ovaries were either removed or irradiated, but a definite survival advantage could not be determined. Lack of complete data on axillary lymph nodes and no data on receptor status limited interpretation of these early trials. Interest was rekindled with observed responses to tamoxifen and suggestions of chemotherapy response being related to ovarian ablation in premenopausal women. Although amenorrhea in premenopausal women following adjuvant therapy has not been associated with improved survival outcomes, the possibility of a dual action of direct cytotoxic effect and endocrine effect remains (Bonadonna et al., 1991). The Scottish Cancer Trials Breast Cancer Group (1993) randomized premenopausal women to ovarian ablation (surgical or radiation) or CMF with prednisone and reported no differences in survival. There was a significant interaction, however, between estrogen receptor (ER) content and treatment. Ovarian ablation was associated with an improved survival in women with higher ER concentrations, and in contrast CMF chemotherapy was associated with better outcomes for women with lower ER concentrations. The authors conclude that ovarian ablation and chemotherapy may affect different tumor types and that ER data are critical to future studies, especially those evaluating chemoendocrine therapy in premenopausal patients.

The outcome for chemoendocrine approaches in the adjuvant setting remains controversial. Node-positive, ER-positive postmenopausal women may (Fisher, Redmond, Poisson et al., 1990; Pearson et al., 1989) or may not (Boccardo et al., 1990; Rivkin et al., 1990) benefit from combining chemotherapy with tamoxifen when compared to tamoxifen alone. Multiple trials to evaluate chemoendocrine adjuvant therapies in premenopausal and postmenopausal women are ongoing. Publication of results must await adequate follow-up, especially related to duration of tamoxifen therapy, so that interpretation of the data in evaluation of risks and benefits (survival and quality of life issues) is useful to clinical decision making.

TIMING AND SEQUENCING OF ADJUVANT THERAPY

In routine clinical practice, adjuvant therapy is initiated within 4 to 6 weeks after primary surgery. This time frame is based on concepts of tumor biology, including genetic mutations, development of resistant cells, and tumor cell burden, although the optimal time to begin chemotherapy is unknown. A major unresolved clinical practice issue is the optimal combination of adjuvant therapy with primary radiation. The goals of combining the administration of these therapies are to minimize failure (local and systemic disease) and to avoid interactions that would influence the treatment effect, complications, and cosmetic outcome (Recht,

Harris, & Come, 1994). Surgical techniques, radiotherapy treatment (e.g., equipment, daily dose, field arrangements), chemotherapy (e.g., dose, duration, drugs used), and timing of the modalities are the major variables that may affect recurrence and complications of primary breast cancer treatment. Although all variables have importance, the interval between treatments receives focused attention because of the associated risks for local recurrence and systemic relapse. Major concerns include local recurrence with delays in radiotherapy and systemic relapse for delays in initiation of chemotherapy. Clinical data suggest no risk of local recurrence if radiotherapy is delayed up to 8 weeks; however, the risks of delaying chemotherapy are less clear and clinical trials are ongoing to answer these questions (Recht, Harris, & Come, 1994). Concurrent administration of therapy resolves the delay problem and may provide a synergistic tumor effect, yet it has several disadvantages. These include increased marrow suppression, acute skin reactions, delays or dose reductions secondary to side effects, increased risk of subacute side effects (e.g., pneumonitis) or chronic risks (e.g., cardiotoxicity), and impact on cosmetic outcome (Recht, Harris, & Come, 1994). The impact on the woman's functional status and overall quality of life has not been addressed. Concurrent administration of chemotherapy is feasible, with the exception of doxorubicin, which is not recommended because of the risks of cardiotoxicity (Lippman et al., 1986; Recht, Harris, & Come, 1994). Sequential therapy is associated with less toxicity than concurrent therapy, but the optimal sequencing remains undetermined (Fowble, 1994; McCormick & Norton, 1994). The approach of radiotherapy followed by chemotherapy vs. chemotherapy followed by radiotherapy may be influenced by the local vs. systemic risk of the individual patient, the physician's interpretation of the data, an institutional consensus or protocol, or a combination of these factors. Critical to nursing practice is knowledge of the predicted toxicity when radiation and chemotherapy are combined with a careful ongoing assessment of the patient and communication with our colleagues across settings during treatment.

CURRENT AND FUTURE ADJUVANT THERAPY TRIALS

Chemoendocrine therapy is a major focus of current trials, although dose intensity and the value of doxorubicin in node-negative women with breast cancer are also being addressed (Goldhirsch et al., 1994; Osborne, 1994; Pritchard, 1994; Wood, 1994). Future proposed directions include sequencing of single-agent with combination chemotherapy, use of paclitaxel (Taxol), ovarian ablation compared to tamoxifen therapy, and evaluation of synthetic retinoids. In addition, several groups have identified evaluation of hormone replacement therapy for women who are experiencing menopausal symptoms from chemotherapy or tamoxifen therapy (Goldhirsch et al., 1994; Osborne, 1994; Wood, 1994). The uterine cancer risk with tamoxifen therapy, lack of data of the incidence of menopausal symptoms in women with breast cancer across age groups, lack of or sparse data on the impact on quality of life of women who experience menopausal symptoms, and fears of women toward hormone replacement therapy related to cancer risk are significant issues for hormone replacement therapy. As patient advocates, nurses must be cognizant of the risks, benefits, and controversies about hormone replacement therapy, especially in a woman with breast cancer.

TOXICITY

The incidence, frequency, and severity of side effects associated with adjuvant therapy are influenced by the specific drugs, drug regimens, combination therapy, endocrine therapy, and duration of treatment. A wide variety of established side effects and complications have been reported such as nausea, vomiting, anorexia, taste changes, hair loss, insomnia, fatigue, weight change, mucositis, constipation, diarrhea, conjunctivitis, amenorrhea, menopausal symptoms, and thromboembolic events. Less well-established side effects are emerging (e.g., postchemotherapy rheumatism [Loprinzi, Duffy, & Ingle, 1993]) as more women are treated and as quality of life becomes a more integrated treatment outcome. Psychologic symptoms such as depressed mood and anxiety are reported by women during and after adjuvant therapy, but it is difficult to determine the exact cause. Depressed mood may reflect a composite response to the diagnosis and treatment or be directly related to systemic therapy, such as use of tamoxifen (Cathart et al., 1993). Anxiety may similarly be related to the total experience or fear of intravenous needles, nausea, vomiting, or hair loss or as a response to completion of treatment (Greene, Nail, Fieler, Dudgeon, & Jones, 1994; Lenox, 1995; Ward, Viergutz, Tormey, deMuth, & Paulen, 1992). Regardless of origin, physical and psychologic distress is common in women with breast cancer who receive adjuvant systemic therapy.

Symptoms and Symptom Distress

Knowledge of the existence and incidence of physical or psychologic symptoms is essential. But knowledge of incidence of symptoms alone may be insufficient. The severity or distress associated with side effects as perceived by the individual is critical in understanding predictable patient responses to adjuvant therapy and designing interventions. In an early study with 78 patients who received adjuvant therapy with CMF (with or without prednisone), mild physical distress, mild to moderate psychologic distress, minimal lifestyle changes, and significant weight gain were reported by subjects (Knobf, 1986). The mild severity rating of symptoms by women in this study was unexpected yet confirmed by Ehlke (1988). Fatigue, insomnia, and nausea were rated as the most distressful side effects in both studies. A more recent prospective investigation assessed patients 2 and 5 days after the first two chemotherapy cycles, either with cyclophosphamide (Cytoxan), methotrexate, and fluorouracil (CMF); cyclophosphamide (Cytoxan), mitoxantrone (Novantrone), and fluorouracil (CNF); or cyclophosphamide (Cytoxan), doxorubicin (Adriamycin), and fluorouracil (CAF) (Greene et al., 1994). Fatigue, nausea, anorexia, taste change, and headache were the five most frequent side effects reported, with severity ratings of 1.1 to 3.8 on a 5-point scale (1 = not at all severe, 5 = extremely severe). The CAF drug regimen was associated with more severe nausea and more disruption in ability of women to complete their activities of daily living. In a pilot study with 14 women with breast cancer receiving adjuvant therapy assessed before treatment and at 3, 6, and 9 months, symptom distress was highest during treatment for symptoms of insomnia, fatigue, weight change, and hair loss ($p < .05$) (Lenox, 1995).

Fatigue

Fatigue, insomnia, and nausea appear universal regardless of drug regimen or study design (Greene et al., 1994; Ehlke, 1988; Knobf, 1986; Mock, Burke, & Creaton, 1993; Piper et al., 1993). Fatigue occurs in the majority of women and has been described as whole body tiredness, anxiety, tired legs, wanting to lie down, forgetfulness, and eye strain (Piper, Friedman, Hartigan, Post, & Smith, 1989). Severity ratings for fatigue for women receiving CMF regimens range from 1.6 to 2.6 on a 5-point scale (Ehlke, 1988; Greene et al., 1994; Knobf, 1986) and averaged 4.5 (10 point visual analog scale) during treatment (Lenox, 1995), indicating mild to moderate levels of distress.

Weight Gain

Differences in reporting of other symptoms such as hair loss, weight change, menopausal symptoms, or psychologic responses relate to a variety of factors such as study design, methodology, research questions, drug regimens, duration of therapy, when the study was conducted, and patient characteristics. Weight gain is one example. Average weight gains of 4 kg were reported in the 1980s for women receiving adjuvant regimens (Bonadonna et al., 1985; Heasman, Sutherland, Campbell, Elhakim, & Boyd, 1985; Knobf, 1986; Knobf, Mullen, Xistris, & Moritz, 1983; Subramanian, Raich, & Walker, 1981). Increased appetite, decreased activity, increased caloric intake, mild nausea, mood changes, and decreased estradiol levels have been associated with weight gain (Foltz, 1985; Grindel, Cahill, & Walker, 1989; Heasman et al., 1985; Knobf, 1986; Mukhopadhyay & Larkin, 1986). Premenopausal status, concurrent use of steroids, and longer treatment duration were associated with a greater total amount of weight gained (Foltz, 1985; Heasman et al., 1985; Knobf, 1986). Most of these reports reflect adjuvant treatment of 12 to 18 months vs. the common 6-month treatment plan of today, and the predominant therapy was CMF with oral cyclophosphamide. Thus, a shorter duration of therapy results in less weight gain, since weight gain was continuous during the time of treatment (Knobf et al., 1983); changes in therapy such as use of intravenous cyclophosphamide in CMF regimens or replacing methotrexate with doxorubicin have eliminated weight gain as a potential side effect for many women. Mild nausea associated with oral CMF continues to be associated with weight changes (Lenox, 1995). Although nausea is only one explanation for weight gain, it is somewhat predictive of the risk and consequent distress from weight gain in this patient population. Nutritional counseling and aerobic exercise are identified interventions to minimize the risk of weight gain and associated distress (Winningham & MacVicar, 1988; Winningham, MacVicar, Bondoc, Anderson, & Minton, 1989).

MENOPAUSAL SYMPTOMS

Menopausal symptoms are associated with chemotherapy drug-induced ovarian failure and with hormonal therapy. The majority of women 40 years of age or older who receive adjuvant chemotherapy can be expected to develop some degree of ovarian failure that is progressive with drug cycles and unlikely reversible (Bianco et al., 1991; Fisher, Sherman, & Rockette, 1979; Goldhirsch, Gelber, & Castiglione, 1990; Mehta, Beattie, & DasGupta, 1991; Reyno, Levine, Skingley, Arnold, & AbuZahra, 1992; Rose & Davis, 1980; Samaan, deAsis, Buzdar, & Blumenstein, 1978). Associated menopausal symptoms of hot flashes, sweats, headaches, vaginal dryness, dyspareunia, menstrual irregularities, and amenorrhea have been reported as toxicity data from clinical trials, nursing research, or clinical literature, although these data are limited in scope and specificity (Aikin, 1994; Chamorro, 1991; Feldman, 1989; Fisher, Constantino, Redmond et al., 1989; Hull, 1993; Love, Leventhal, Easterling, & Nerenz, 1989; Tarpy & Rothwell 1983). Preliminary data on the outcome of menopausal symptoms suggest that symptoms disrupt routine activities, interfere with sleep and rest, and may affect the quality and frequency of the patient's sexual relationship (Chapman, 1982; Derogotis, 1980; Knobf, 1986; Ringer, 1983; Schover, 1991; Young-McCaughan, personal communiation, 1995). Adjuvant endocrine therapy with tamoxifen is also associated with menopausal symptoms of hot flashes, menstrual irregularities, vaginal discharge, fatigue, nausea, and headache (Fisher, Constantino et al., 1989; Mooney et al., 1994). It is evident in clinical practice that a proportion of women have significant distress related to menopausal symptoms, but little is known about the actual incidence and scope of the problem. Successful symptom management has been limited by the contraindication to estrogen replacement therapy, although that contraindication has more recently been challenged (Cobleigh et al., 1994; Wile, Opfell, & Margileth, 1993). Estrogen replacement therapy in women with breast cancer remains highly controversial. The major symptoms for which women seek help are hot flashes and night sweats, both of which can significantly interfere with sleep and vaginal dryness (Knobf, in press). A variety of nonestrogen drugs have been considered for relief of vasomotor symptoms (Young, Kumar, & Goldzieher, 1990). Progestins and clonidine have been relatively successful in relieving hot flashes but are also associated with their own side effects (Clayden, Bell, & Pollard, 1974; Loprinzi et al., 1994; Nagamani, Kelver, & Smith, 1987; Plowman, 1988). Ergotamine (Bellergal) has been frequently used and has efficacy, but due to the potential addictive risk and availability of safer alternatives, it is *not* recommended for practice (Walsh & Schiff, 1990). Clinically, diphenhydramine (Benadryl) at bedtime has been used in attempts to minimize sleep deprivation from hot flashes and sweats; vitamin E has some suggested benefit, particularly in women with mild vasomotor symptoms, although there is no research to support its use at this time. Vaginal dryness can be managed with water-soluble lubricants or newer lubricants such as Replens or Astroglide, which are available over the counter. Nurse researchers have begun investigations of the experience of menopausal symptoms in women with breast cancer but await completion and publication. In the interim, careful and sensitive assessment of symptoms and assessment for interference of routine activities (e.g., sleep, sexual relationship) are critical to develop interventions to minimize distress.

PRIMARY CHEMOTHERAPY AND LOCALLY ADVANCED BREAST CANCER

Locally advanced breast cancer represents stage III disease, defined either by tumor size ($\geq$ T3) or by inflammatory breast carcinoma. An estimated 10 to 30 per cent of patients will present with locally advanced noninflammatory breast cancer. Historically, the treatment strategy was surgery followed by radiation and chemotherapy and was associated with a high incidence of local and distant failure and a poor 5-year survival rate. Today, the accepted strategy for treating noninflammatory locally advanced breast cancer is induction (also referred to as primary or neoadjuvant) chemotherapy followed by surgery or radiation or adjuvant therapy (Bonadonna, 1989; Hortobagyi, 1994). Traditional outcome measures have been response to chemotherapy, local and distant relapse, and survival. More recently, other benefits to primary chemotherapy include use of response to chemotherapy as an in vivo chemosensitivity assay, downstaging of the tumor (which allows for breast conservation instead of mastectomy), and assessment of morphologic and biologic characteristics of the tumor (Bonadonna, 1989; Hortobagyi, 1994; Rasbridge et al., 1994). This approach has also been extended to selected stage II patients, those with tumors measuring more than 3 cm. Primary chemotherapy has achieved significant responses in women with primary breast tumor, allowing for a breast conservation alternative to mastectomy, and the combination of primary chemotherapy followed by surgery, radiation, or adjuvant therapy has improved outcome (Bonadonna et al., 1990; Calais et al., 1994; Jacquillat et al., 1990; Swain et al., 1987; Valagussa, Zambetti, & Bonadonna, 1990). Initial tumor size is an important predictor of response to chemotherapy (Bonadonna, 1989; Calais et al., 1994) and for survival. Ten-year survival for women with tumors less than 5 cm was 48 per cent in contrast to a 20 per cent survival for women with tumors measuring 5 to 10 cm and 4 per cent survival for women with tumors more than 10 cm at presentation (Valagussa et al., 1990). Response of the primary tumor to chemotherapy, downstaging of the primary tumor, feasibility, and improved outcome for combination therapy approaches to locally advanced breast cancer have been demonstrated. The optimal chemotherapy (drugs, dose, number of courses) to achieve maximum tumor response with primary chemotherapy, the need for or optimal sequencing of surgery, radiation, and adjuvant therapy following primary chemotherapy, and the ultimate survival benefit remain as unanswered questions at this time (Ahern, Barraclough, Bosch, Langlands, & Boyages, 1994; DeVita, 1990; Harris et al., 1993; Hortobagyi, 1994). Although improved survival is the ultimate goal of patients and health care providers, toxicity and complications of more aggressive approaches (Sauter et al., 1993) are important outcome variables to monitor for an accurate risk-benefit analysis of locally advanced breast cancer therapy.

Inflammatory breast cancer is a highly aggressive form of breast cancer, characterized by diffuse erythema and edema (peau d'orange) of the skin with or without a palpable breast mass. Combined modality therapy with induction chemotherapy, surgery, radiation, and maintenance chemotherapy has dramatically changed outcome; 5-year survival rates now range from 30 to 70 per cent, and about one third of patients may be expected to live beyond 10 years (Fowble & Glover, 1991; Hortobagyi, 1994). Similar to locally advanced breast cancer therapy for women with large tumors, current research strategies include developing more effective systemic induction treatments to improve the primary tumor response and identification of prognostic factors to identify patient subsets and direct treatment choices (Fowble & Glover, 1991).

HIGH-DOSE THERAPY

High-dose therapy producing high-peak plasma drug levels has evolved over time as a major research focus in breast cancer treatment. The purpose is to improve tumor response and survival. Patients with advanced disease were treated in the early studies, primarily focused on the feasibility of administering high doses of drugs (Ayash, 1994). The next generation of studies used multiple drugs based on therapeutic synergy such as combinations of cyclophosphamide, carmustine, and cisplatin (Stadtmauer, 1991). Once dose ranges and toxicity were established (Table 29–19), the next group of studies evaluated induction chemotherapy followed by high-dose therapy (Ayash et al., 1994; Vaughn, Reed, Edwards, & Kessinger, 1994). It appears that the combined approach of induction chemotherapy followed by consolidation with high-dose therapy can improve survival in approximately 15 to 25 per cent of patients with metastatic breast cancer (Ayash, 1994; Livingston, 1994). Those patients with chemoresponsive disease will be more likely to benefit in contrast to those patients with advanced refractory disease, who are least likely to benefit from this therapeutic approach. The next group of trials addressed induction and consolidation with high-dose therapy followed by local treatment and its efficacy in poor-prognosis patients—those with high-risk stage II disease (> 10 nodes positive) and stage III disease (deGraaf et al., 1994; Kotasek, Sage, Dale, Norman, Bolton, 1994; Livingston, 1994; Marks et al., 1994; Razis et al., 1994; Somlo et al., 1994). Current trials continue to address optimal drug combinations and schedules, efficacy of autologous bone marrow vs. peripheral stem cell support or a combination of the two, single vs. multiple consolidations with high-dose therapy, optimal role and schedule for granulocyte colony-stimulating factor (GCSF), and toxicity. The most commonly used drugs include carmustine, carboplatin, cisplatin, cyclophosphamide, etoposide, melphalan, and thiotepa at various high-dose levels dependent on the protocol.

TABLE 29–19. *Characteristics of Agents Used in High-Dose Therapy*

AGENT	CONVENTIONAL DOSE (MG/M²)	MAXIMUM DOSE WITHOUT ABMT (MG/M²)	MAXIMUM DOSE WITH ABMT (MG/M²)	DOSE ESCALATION	LIMITING TOXICITY
Cyclophosphamide	1000	8000	8000	8	Cardiac
Melphalan	40	140	225	6	Mucositis
Thiotepa	40	180	1135	28	Mucositis
Cisplatin	100	200	200	2	Renal
Carmustine	200	600	1200	6	Hepatic
Busulfan	1.5 mg/kg	6 mg/kg	16 mg/kg	10	Hepatic
Ifosfamide	8000	18,000	18,000	2.25	Renal
Carboplatin	400	1600	2000	5	Hepatic
Etoposide	300	2700	3000	10	Mucositis
Radiation	150 cGy	300 cGy	1500 cGy	10	Lung

ABMT = autologous bone marrow transplant.
(From Stadtmauer, E. A. [1991]. Bone marrow transplantation for breast cancer. In B. Fowble, R. L. Goodman, J. H. Glick & E. K. Rosato [Eds.], *Breast cancer treatment* [pp. 489–506]. St. Louis: Mosby-Year Book.)

Acute toxicity is well established (see Chapter 27), but long-term toxicity is yet to be fully defined. Concerns about major organ system toxicity from high-dose therapy are realistic (Patz, Peters, & Goodman, 1994; Stemmer, Stears, Burton, Jones, & Simon, 1994). Acute assessment skills are needed to identify, sometimes subtle, changes, which may indicate serious toxicity. Inherent in the need for assessment skills and optimal management of side effects and toxicity is an adequate, experienced nursing staff to care for these complex patients, as care continues to move into the ambulatory care setting (Buschel, 1995; Peters et al., 1994).

METASTATIC DISEASE

Approximately 50 per cent of women with breast cancer will develop metastatic disease (Greenberg, 1991). The greatest risk of relapse in breast cancer occurs within the first 2 to 3 years after diagnosis. Although 90 per cent of those who relapse do so by the fifth year, recurrences have been observed as long as 20 to 25 years later. Bone is the most common site of relapse (40 to 60 per cent), followed by lung (15 to 20 per cent), pleura (10 to 14 per cent), soft tissue (7 to 15 per cent), and liver (5 to 15 per cent) (Canellos, 1987). The mainstay of treatment for metastatic disease is hormone and cytotoxic therapy. Indications for surgery and radiotherapy are limited, with the most common being palliative radiotherapy for symptomatic bone metastases (Petrek, 1987). Selection of treatment is influenced by menopausal status, receptor content, specific metastatic site or sites, and aggressiveness of the tumor.

ENDOCRINE THERAPY

Clinical criteria for selection of hormone therapy include a relatively long disease-free interval (> 2 years), slow-growing or indolent disease, bone and soft tissue metastatic sites, and hormone-responsive tumors (Haller, Fox, and Schuchter, 1991). Hormonal manipulation has been used for decades in the treatment of breast cancer, but not until the discovery of hormone receptors could the selection of patients for hormone responsiveness be determined. ER-negative patients rarely respond, yet a response rate of 50 to 60 per cent may be achieved with ER-positive patients. Average responses last 12 to 18 months, and response rates are related to the quantity of receptor protein. Clinical experience indicates that postmenopausal patients respond more often than premenopausal patients; bone and soft tissue are the most responsive metastatic sites; and patients who respond to one hormonal therapy will likely respond to another.

Treatments. Approaches to inhibit breast cancer growth with endocrine therapy are either ablative or additive (Fig. 29–17). The surgical ablative therapies are gradually being replaced by systemic endocrine therapies such as antiestrogens, progestins, aminoglutethimide, and luteininzing hormone–releasing hormone (LH-RH) analogs (Table 29–20).

The nonsteroidal antiestrogen, tamoxifen, is the most widely used hormone therapy for breast cancer

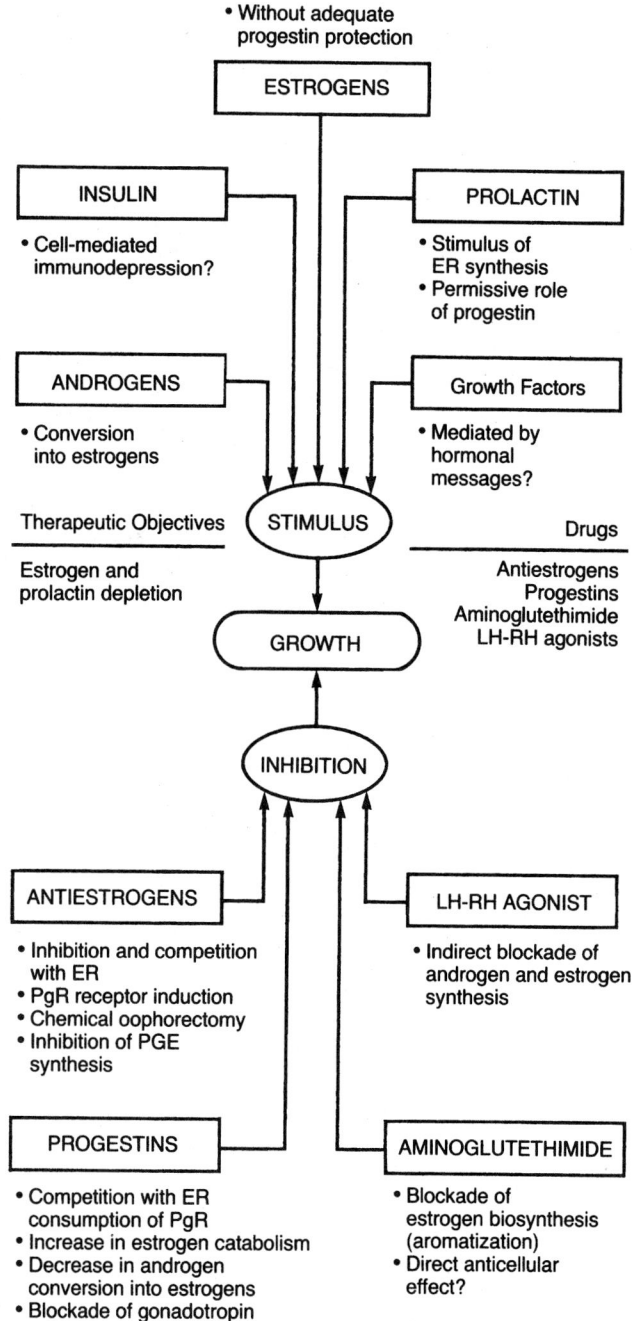

FIGURE 29–17. Endocrine correlations in breast cancer. ER, estrogen receptor; LH-RH, luteinizing hormone–releasing hormone; PgR, progesterone receptor; PGE, prostaglandin E. (From Robustelli della Cuna, G. [1988]. Principles of endocrine therapy. In G. Bonadonna & G. Robustelli della Cuna [Eds.], *Handbook of medical oncology,* [3rd ed. pp. 255–271]. Milan: Masson Publishers. Reproduced by permission.)

and is the treatment of choice for ER-positive postmenopausal women. It is primarily an estrogen antagonist but also has weak estrogenic properties. Response is similar to endocrine therapy in general, with an overall response rate of 34 per cent; but response rates as high as 78 per cent have been reported in hormone-responsive tumors (Haller et al., 1991).

TABLE 29–20. *Hormonal Therapies for Metastatic Breast Cancer*

OPTIONS	FAVORABLE	UNFAVORABLE
Tamoxifen	Effective in premenopausal and postmenopausal women	Minimal toxic effects, including hot flashes, amenorrhea, mild nausea
Progestins	Effective in premenopausal and postmenopausal women As effective as tamoxifen Effective in tamoxifen failures	Toxicity includes weight gain and fluid retention
Androgens	Effective in premenopausal and postmenopausal women	Masculinizing effects
Aminoglutethimide	Effective in postmenopausal women or in women after oophorectomy	Initial toxicities include lethargy, skin rash Usually require additional glucocorticoid therapy
Luteinizing hormone–releasing hormone (LH-RH) analogs	Effective in premenopausal women	Menopausal symptoms including hot flashes, amenorrhea
Glucocorticoids	May have additive effects with tamoxifen or oophorectomy	Toxicities include cushingoid effects
Oophorectomy	Equally effective as tamoxifen Effective in premenopausal patients	Requires surgery or radiation therapy; hot flashes, amenorrhea

(From Haller, D. G., Fox, K. R., & Schuchter, L. M. (1991). Metastatic breast cancer. In B. Fowble, R. H. Goodman, J. H. Glick, & E. F. Rosato (Eds.), *Breast cancer treatment* (pg. 413). St. Louis: Mosby-Year Book.)

Progestins have similar response rates in the 30 to 40 per cent range. The two most common progestins and doses are megestrol acetate (Megace, 160 mg daily) and medroxyprogesterone acetate (Provera, Depo-Provera, 400 to 600 mg daily). Progestins are associated with few side effects, but the associated weight gain and fluid retention, which are very common, may be quite distressful to the individual patient.

Aminoglutethimide blocks adrenal steroid synthesis. The adrenal gland is a major source of estrogen in the postmenopausal woman, and aminoglutethimide, in essence, produces a medical adrenalectomy. The overall response rate is in the range of 35 per cent. Because of the complex feedback mechanisms in the endocrine system, a steroid replacement is recommended, usually hydrocortisone 40 mg/d in physiologically divided doses. Side effects are common during the first 6 weeks of therapy but usually diminish thereafter and include lethargy (35 to 41 per cent), maculopapular skin rash (< 30 per cent), dizziness (20 per cent), ataxia (10 per cent), and mild hypertension (5 per cent) (Harris et al., 1993). Aminoglutethimide is generally used in postmenopausal women but may be considered as second-line hormonal therapy in premenopausal women previously responsive to oophorectomy or tamoxifen therapy (Haller et al., 1991).

The LH-RH analogs represent the newest hormonal agents in breast cancer treatment and include leuprolide (Lupron), buserelin, and goserelin (Zoladex). These agents inhibit ovarian function primarily through inhibition of LH and follicle-stimulating hormone (FSH) and are associated with response rates in the range of 40 to 45 per cent (Bajetta et al., 1994; Greenberg, 1991). In essence, a medical oophorectomy results, and trials comparing LH-RH analogs with or without tamoxifen therapy vs. oophorectomy in pre-menopausal patients with metastatic breast cancer are being conducted.

Combining hormonal agents has potential therapeutic advantage, and it is hypothesized that increases in side effects or toxicity are unanticipated. Combination hormone therapy has gained enthusiasm in breast cancer treatment but remains investigational at the present time. Prediction of outcomes related to response rate, durability of response, incidence of side effects, and patient symptom distress await the results of clinical trials.

Response to endocrine therapy is associated with prolonged survival. Whether the observed prolonged survival is due to multiple therapeutic responses to endocrine therapy or to the presence of less-aggressive disease is unknown.

CHEMOTHERAPY

Only a few clinical predictors exist for response to chemotherapy. A good performance status, a long disease-free survival, and an absence of liver metastases are favorable factors, whereas pretreatment weight loss, extensive disease, anemia, and prior chemotherapy or radiotherapy are associated with a poorer response rate and prognosis (George & Hoogstraten, 1978; Swenerton et al., 1979). Hundreds of studies of chemotherapy in advanced breast cancer have been conducted and several conclusions can be drawn (Haller et al., 1991; Harris, et al., 1993). Combination chemotherapy is superior to single-agent therapy, producing an average response rate of 50 per cent, with a median duration of response ranging from 6 to 12 months. Doxorubicin (Adriamycin) can increase the response rates by 10 to 20 per cent. Complete responders are very uncommon and are not associated with a significantly prolonged survival. The average survival time following metastatic disease is 18 to 36 months. The combination of chemotherapy and hormone therapy may increase the response rate, but generally is not associated with an increased duration of response or survival.

Multiple drugs are active in breast cancer and used routinely in clinical practice. The most standard combinations are few and include cyclophosphamide, methotrexate, and fluorouracil (CMF) and cyclophosphamide, doxorubicin (Adriamycin), and fluorouracil (CAF) (Norton, 1994). Multiple combinations of drugs have been studied, however, and are available as first-line or second-line therapy (Fischer, Knobf, & Durivage, 1993; Norton, 1994). Once patients relapse, response rates diminish for subsequent treatments, generally in low ranges of 20 to 30 per cent (Abrams, Moore, & Friedman, 1994; Porkka, Blomqvist, Rissanen, Elomma, & Pyrhonen, 1994).

Side effects and interventions are reviewed in Chapter 21. Predictable side effects are related primarily to single-agent therapy and must be weighed carefully according to dose, duration, and scheduling when combining one drug with another. Increasing the database for predictable toxicity of combination chemotherapy regimens is needed to improve patient preparation and to plan interventions.

NEW DRUGS

Innovative strategies to improve response rates have included using established drugs in new ways, but these strategies have generally not altered the outcome in metastatic breast cancer. Thus, identification and incorporation of new drugs into breast cancer treatment is an important research agenda. The taxines, paclitaxel and docetaxel, represent newer agents, now widely studied with demonstrated activity in breast cancer. In a nonheavily pretreated patient, paclitaxel has reported response rates of more than 50 per cent and is now being evaluated in phase III trials for its role against and with other chemotherapeutic agents (Abrams, Moore, & Friedman, 1994). Phase II trials with vinorelbine, edatrexate, and losoxantrone have sufficient reported activity in women with advanced breast cancer to also proceed to phase III trials. The next several years will provide data on other new compounds being evaluated such as topoisomerase-I inhibitors and the role of monoclonal antibodies, gene therapy, and growth factor inhibitors in the management of breast cancer (Abrams, Moore, & Friedman, 1994).

Management of Advanced Disease. Multiple clinical problems are associated with advanced breast cancer, the nature and severity of which are determined by the site of metastasis and extent of disease. In a seminal study by McCorkle (1973), 64 women with advanced breast cancer were followed to identify nursing needs. Four classes of metastatic sites were identified (bone, chest and soft tissue, brain, viscera), and nursing care was described based on the most common subjective symptoms. Despite the more than 20-year span since publication of this article and advances in treatment,

the clinical issues remain strikingly similar to the current practice such as pain control, wound management, respiratory compromise, self-care needs, elimination, dyspnea, and gastrointestinal toxicity of drug therapy. The importance of the nurse's knowledge of symptoms related to complications and site of disease is highlighted by the quote "nursing care is based on what is happening to the patient at any given time" (McCorkle, 1973, p. 1034). This knowledge predicts patients at risk and directs assessment and plan of care. The basic principles of the nursing interventions described by McCorkle (1973) remain applicable to today's practice. Nursing research in symptom management over the past 20 years has made significant contributions to care. Yet many challenges remain in managing disease-related complications of advanced breast cancer such as pathologic fractures, liver metastases, pleural effusions, spinal cord compression, and local chest wall recurrences. These disease-related clinical problems, as well as treatment-induced side effects and toxicity, are detailed in other chapters of this book.

MALE BREAST CANCER

Breast cancer in men is uncommon, representing less than 1 per cent of all cancers in males. Its natural history is similar to that of women, with a major exception of age of onset. Men are most commonly diagnosed between the ages of 60 and 70 years, and they present with a slightly more advanced stage of disease and a proportionally higher percent of estrogen-positive tumors as compared with women (Kinne & Hakes, 1991; Lartigau, el-Jabbour, Dubray, & Dische, 1994; Ouriel, Lotze, & Hinshaw, 1984; Thomas, 1993a). The majority of men present with a firm, painless subareolar mass and are diagnosed with infiltrating ductal carcinoma. Primary treatment is modified radical mastectomy, and postoperative radiation may be recommended to improve local disease control, particularly recommended in patients with large tumors and close surgical margins. As in women with breast cancer, the major prognostic factors are tumor size and axillary node involvement. Recommendations for adjuvant therapy have largely been extrapolated from the data on women and based on risk of relapse (Harris et al., 1993). Tamoxifen has been commonly used as adjuvant therapy. In a small study with 24 men receiving adjuvant tamoxifen therapy, decreased libido, weight gain, hot flashes, mood alterations, depression, insomnia, and deep vein thrombosis were reported side effects, with 21 per cent terminating therapy because of side effects (Anelli, Anelli, Tran, Lebwohl, & Borgen, 1994). While there may be a benefit of tamoxifen replacing orchiectomy, it is important to assess these patients for side effects and symptom distress.

Systemic treatment for metastatic disease is primarily hormonal because of the predominance of hormonally positive tumors in men. Response rates exceeding 50 per cent have been reported for first-line endocrine therapy, with decreasing responses observed for second- and third-line hormonal therapies (Bezwoda, Hesdorffer, & Dansey, 1987; Kinne & Hakes, 1991). Chemotherapy has been used, again based on regimens successful in women, but data on responsiveness are sparse. The limited data on chemotherapy effect are largely related to the choice of hormone therapies as first- and second-line treatments.

PSYCHOLOGIC REACTIONS TO SURVIVORSHIP

Psychosocial research in breast cancer has a dynamic history influenced by improved survival rates, new treatments, evolving emphasis on quality of life, and issues for survivors. The primary focus on the individual woman's response has also shifted over time to the response of the spouse and the family. Early clinical articles and research on the psychologic impact and adaptation to breast cancer focused on response to mastectomy and included postoperative adjustment, impact on body image, quality of the marital/sexual relationship, available support, and psychologic reactions such as anxiety, depression, and fear of recurrence (Asken, 1975; Carroll, 1981; Holland & Mastrovito, 1980; Jamison, Wellisch, & Pasnau, 1978; Morris, 1979; Morris, Greer, & White, 1977; Northouse, 1981; Quint, 1963; Thomas, 1978). With the onset of reports of the efficacy of adjuvant therapy in the mid to late 1970s (Bonadonna et al., 1976), the focus on psychologic response shifted from mastectomy to adjuvant therapy. At the same time, a more broad research perspective emerged, including the social, functional, marital, lifestyle, and role function aspects of the woman's life, as well as response of the spouse (Grandstaff, 1976; Knobf, 1986; Maguire, 1981; Maguire, Tait, & Brooke, 1980; Meyerowtiz, Sparks, & Spears, 1979; Sabo, Brown, & Smith, 1986; Silberfarb & Mauer, 1980; Wellisch, Jamison, & Pasnau, 1978).

PARTNER RESPONSE

The 1980s highlighted the significance of the impact of breast cancer on the spouse. Fear of death, uncertainty, emotional distress, impact of lifestyle, and role changes were also experienced by the spouse, and the stress of the cancer influenced the couple's communication patterns (Gates, 1980; Gotay, 1984; Oberst & James, 1985; Sabo et al., 1986; Wellisch et al., 1978). The importance of the spouse and the family of women with breast cancer followed the emerging research on families with cancer (Lewis, 1986). In the past decade (1986 to 1995), 12 studies addressing the response of women and their spouses have been published (Table 29–21). The phase of the illness on the family's response and adjustment has been identified as important (Lewandowski & Jones, 1988; Sales, 1991). In the review of the studies presented in Table 29–21, the first 2 years since diagnosis is the time frame of all but one study (Germino, Fife, & Funk, 1995). The study by Given and Given (1992) included newly diagnosed (within 1 year) women and women with recurrent diseases, but the authors presented separate, as well as comparison, data.

There were some similar findings for psychologic adjustment across the 12 studies (Table 29–21). Mild psychologic distress or few problems were reported during the first 2 years for the majority of subjects (Hannum, Geise-Davis, Harding, & Hatfield, 1991; Northouse & Swain, 1987; Northouse, 1989b). A subset of patients and spouses, however, have been identified who adjust less well, as evidenced by more psychologic distress, anxiety, and depression (Ell, Nishimoto, Mantell, & Hamovitch, 1988; Germino et al., 1995; Given & Given, 1992; Northouse, 1989b). Universal concerns related to survival were reported by patients and spouses alike, specifically identified as living with uncertainty, fear of dying, and facing the diagnosis (Germino et al., 1995; Hilton, 1993; Northouse, 1989a). Lifestyle changes and balancing demands of everyday life were secondary concerns but became more significant over time (Hilton, 1993; Northouse, 1989b). Although many similar reactions were evident between the patient and spouse, some differences also emerged. Patients focused more on themselves, reported more difficulty with adjustment in family relations (Germino et al., 1995), and reported more alterations in role function 1 and 18 months after surgery than their partners (Northouse, 1989b). Husbands focused on the patient but also on themselves—but as related to their relationship (Germino et al., 1995)— and were more concerned about their wife's coping in the early phase than any lifestyle changes (Northouse, 1989b). These findings have significant practice implications. Assessment should include the spouse, as well as the patient, and supportive interventions should be designed to meet individual needs but also the needs of the couple. The spouse as the major support is often a well-established assumption, but these research findings suggest that the spouse also needs support. Communication difficulties are not uncommon, and may in part relate to the husband's suppression of feelings in attempts to protect his wife's emotional well-being (Gates, 1980; Sabo et al., 1986; Vess et al., 1988). Assessment and interventions to improve communication patterns or provide resources to meet the individual communication needs for each partner (e.g., support group for women with breast cancer) are important nursing interventions.

FAMILY RESPONSE

The importance of the family of patients with cancer in clinical practice is known, but they very often are perceived as the supporters and caregivers. Much has been written about support of caregivers when the patient has terminal stages of disease, but research suggests that the impact of cancer on the family is significant regardless of stage of disease or caregiver role (Lewis, 1986). In research with families of women with breast cancer, the affect on children has been assessed including children's concerns about their mother's illness (Lewis, Ellison, & Woods, 1985) and the relationship between mothers and their children following the cancer diagnosis (Lichtman, Taylor, & Wood, 1984). The developmental age of the child and family stage

Text continued on page 597.

TABLE 29–21. *Studies Addressing the Response of Women and Their Families to Breast Cancer Diagnosis*

Author	Purpose	Sample	Method	Unit of Analysis	Analytic Method	Findings
Baider, Rizel, Kaplan, & DeNour, 1986	To gather information about adjustment of women with breast cancer who had lumpectomy or mastectomy	64 patients, 41 partners, 21 couples	1. Speilberger State Trait Anxiety Scale 2. Beck Depression Rating Scale 3. Psychologic Adjustment to Illness Scale 4. Sharan's Sentence Completion Test 5. Family Environment Scale	Patient, partner	Descriptive mean scores; t-tests	1. Patients: The only significant difference between patients by treatment was on family perception; mastectomy patients reported more cohesion and less conflict ($p = 0.03$). 2. Husbands of lumpectomy patients had somewhat higher anxiety scores and husbands of mastectomy patients reported more family cohesion ($p = 0.05$). 3. Couples: Psychologic adjustment was similar. Anxiety and depression scores were similar for husbands and wives in the lumpectomy group, but mastectomy patients were significantly more anxious than their husbands ($p = 0.05$) and more depressed ($p = 0.02$). No differences were found between husbands or wives of either group on family perception.
Ell, Nishimoto, Mantell, & Hamovitch, 1988	To extend knowledge on psychologic adaptation of family members of patients with cancer	143 patients and significant others	Two-phase design (T1 = 3–6 since diagnosis and T2 = 6 mo later) 1. Self-report of symptoms 2. Role-Rand Health 3. Social support-modified interview schedule for social interaction 4. Five-item personal sense of control 5. Mental Health Inventory	Patient, partner	Descriptive mean scores; t-tests; multiple regression	1. There was a decline in mental health ($p = 0.01$) and personal well-being ($p < 0.001$) and an increase in distress ($p = 0.001$) over time. 2. Initial psychologic status was the most important predictor of psychologic adaptation ($p < 0.001$), followed by education and routine change of significant other ($p < 0.05$). 3. Subjects with declining mental health scores over time also reported decreases in social integration, presence of physical symptoms, and increases in reported stress levels that were unrelated to the patient's physical condition or role limitation.

Study	Purpose	Sample	Instruments	Unit of analysis	Analysis	Findings
Hannum, Giese-Davis, Harding, & Hatfield, 1991	To gather information on coping strategies of patients with breast cancer and their husbands	22 patients and husbands	1. Individual structured interview 2. Locke Wallace Marital Adjustment Scale 3. FACES 4. SCL-90 5. Health Symptom Checklist 6. Friendship Scale 7. Philosophy Marriage Scale 8. Couple Interactional Behavior (video)	Patient, partner, couple	Descriptive mean scores; correlations; multiple regression	1. Psychologic distress: generally low reported distress but a moderate negative correlation observed between husbands' and wives' overall distress scores. 2. Couples reported high level of marital satisfaction; psychologic distress scores of both husbands and wives were more strongly related to each other's cohesion scores (FACES) than their own scores. 3. Wives' psychologic distress was more related to their husbands' behavior and reported cohesion of their relationship ($p < 0.01$) than their own. 4. Husbands' psychologic distress was related to their denial (as reported by wife), observed confronting behavior, and wife's self-reported optimism ($p < 0.01$).
Hilton, 1993	To study family adjustment to breast cancer over the first year since diagnosis	35 patients and their partners; 12 families for all time points	Qualitative longitudinal Problem Centered Coping and Marital Dyad Interview Guide	Couple	Grounded theory; constant comparative analysis of content	Three themes based on problems, concerns, and challenges faced by dyads: (1) taking care of the cancer (facing diagnosis, tests, uncertainty); (2) family patterns (communication, emotional distress, managing household); (3) other issues (managing overload, health concerns of family, current life issues); The first theme predominated throughout all time periods.
Northouse & Swain, 1987	To examine psychosocial adjustment of mastectomy patients and husbands	50 mastectomy patients and husbands	Two-phase design (hospital and 1 mo later) 1. Interview 2. Affect Balance Scale 3. Psychologic Adjustment Mental Illness Scale 4. Brief Symptom Inventory	Patient, partner	Descriptive mean scores; t-tests ANOVA	1. The pattern of mood for patients and husbands was similar, improved over time, and was more positive at T2 than T1 ($p = 0.0001$). 2. Patients and husbands reported similar levels of distress, which remained unchanged over time ($p = 0.08$). 3. Patients significantly differed from husbands on overall role adjustment at T2 ($p < 0.0001$).

Continued on following page.

TABLE 29-21. *Studies Addressing the Response of Women and Their Families to Breast Cancer Diagnosis* Continued

AUTHOR	PURPOSE	SAMPLE	METHOD	UNIT OF ANALYSIS	ANALYTIC METHOD	FINDINGS
Northouse, 1988	To assess relationship between social support and adjustment to mastectomy	As Northouse & Swain	As Northouse & Swain, 1987 and 5. Social Support Questionnaire	Patient, partner	Descriptive mean scores; t-tests correlation ANOVA multiple regression	1. Patients with higher levels of support had fewer psychologic adjustment problems (p = 0.0001) and the same was true for husbands (p = 0.03). 2. No relationship was found between size of support network and adjustment for patients and husbands. 3. At T1, there was no difference in perceived support from spouse and family by patient or partner (p = 0.49, 0.26). At T2, patients reported greater perceived support than husbands from friends, nurses, and physicians (p = 0.01).
Northouse, 1989a	To describe psychosocial adjustment and concerns of newly diagnosed breast cancer patients and husbands	50 mastectomy patients and husbands	Two-phase design (hospital and 1 mo after); structured interview format	Patient, partner, couple	Content analysis	1. At T1 and T2, primary concern was survival for patient and partner. T1 secondary concern for *patient* = lifestyle changes, for *partner* = wife's coping ability. T2 secondary concern *for both* = lifestyle changes. 2. Mastectomy site: By T2, 98% of husbands viewed the incision. 72% of patients perceived their husband's reactions as positive, and 76% of husbands reported no difficulty viewing the surgical incision. 3. Both patients and husbands reported that emotional support was the major factor that helped them to cope.
Northouse, 1989b	To assess ongoing psychosocial adjustment to breast cancer for patients and husband	50 mastectomy patients and husbands	Three-phase design: hospital, 1 and 18 mo later 1. Interview 2. Affect Balance Scale 3. Psychological Adjustment to Illness Scale 4. Brief Symptom Inventory	Patient, partner	Descriptive mean scores; ANOVA	1. Mild psychologic distress was reported by most subjects although moderate to severe distress was reported by 35% of patients and 24% of husbands. 2. Mood: Patients' and husbands' scores were similar; better at T2 and T3. 3. Psychologic distress: No significant differences between patients and husbands, but remained unchanged over time.

Study	Purpose	Sample	Design/Measures	Unit	Analysis	Findings
						4. Alterations in role for patients was greatest at T2 but also reported at T3.
Given & Given, 1992	To assess psychosocial status of patients and families with new and recurrent breast cancer	49 patients and caregivers	Two-phase design (T1 = diagnosis, T2 = 6 mo later) 1. CES-D depression 2. Symptom Distress Scale 3. For caregiver: hours care; impact schedule; impact health; family assistance for care	Patient, partner	Descriptive mean scores; regression	1. Depression was slightly higher in newly diagnosed vs. recurrent patients at T1 and decreased in both groups by T2. Increases in reported depression by caregivers were higher at T2 for both groups but highest for those with recurrent disease. 2. Impact on health and schedule were greater for caregivers of recurrent patients at both time points measured.
Lewis, Hammond, & Woods, 1993	To test an explanatory model of family functioning with newly diagnosed breast cancer	40 patients and partners (who had school-aged children)	1. SES 2. Support-network size 3. Dyadic Adjustment Scale 4. Family Peer Relationship 5. F COPES 6. CES-D 7. FACES IV 8. Norbeck Social Support	Patient, partner	Descriptive mean scores: regression path analysis	1. There was a similar pattern between patients and spouses. 2. The number of illness demands predicted the level of depressed mood and marital adjustment. 3. Families with better marital adjustment or who used introspective coping behavior reported better family functioning. 4. Social support predicted only the patient's depressed mood but was not predictive of family functioning. 5. The patient's level of marital adjustment directly affected the quality of the parent-child relationship. In contrast, family coping influenced the father-child relationship. Better coping resulted in better quality of exchange between father and child and better reported child social competencies.

Continued on following page.

TABLE 29-21. **Studies Addressing the Response of Women and Their Families to Breast Cancer Diagnosis** Continued

AUTHOR	PURPOSE	SAMPLE	METHOD	UNIT OF ANALYSIS	ANALYTIC METHOD	FINDINGS
Germino, Fife, & Funk, 1995	To identify the meaning and significance of the cancer illness on the partner relationship	50 patients and their partners; within 6 mo of diagnosis	Semistructured interview; qualitative	Patient-partner comparison	Not stated, part of a larger study	1. Patients' primary focus was on themselves: future and trajectory of illness 2. Partners focused equally on concerns about patient and themselves, particularly intimacy and relationship. 3. Most common concern of the dyad: uncertainty of future and balancing demands of daily living.
Germino, Fife, & Funk, 1995	To identify the meaning and significance of the cancer illness on the partner relationship	412 patients and 175 partners; all phases of illness	1. Self-report measure: meaning of illness 2. Profile of Mood States 3. Psychologic Adjustment to Illness Scale 4. Dyadic Adjustment Scale	Patient, partner	Descriptive mean scores; t-tests correlations	1. No difference in mean scores for meaning of illness. 2. Patients were more anxious and depressed ($p < 0.05$) and had more difficulty with adjustment in family relations ($p < 0.05$). 3. Correlations: *Patients* = A more positive illness meaning was correlated with a more positive emotional response, greater sense of control, and overall adjustment ($p < 0.05$). *Partners* = A more positive illness meaning was correlated with better partner communication and sexual adjustment ($p < 0.05$).

appears to influence response and impact on role function, with families of school-aged children or younger experiencing the greatest alterations (Vess, Moreland, & Schwebel, 1985). Lewis, Hammond, and Woods (1993) tested an explanatory model of family functioning with newly diagnosed breast cancer patients (Table 29–21). Family functioning was positively influenced by better marital adjustment or use of introspective coping behaviors or both. The number of illness demands predicted the level of depressed mood and marital adjustment. The demands of illness as perceived by the patient and spouse appear to be an important variable in family functioning and one that nurses might begin to incorporate into their assessments (Loveys & Kaich, 1991; Zahlis & Shands, 1991, 1993). Care of the woman with breast cancer occurs primarily in the outpatient setting. The reality of the demands of care for the nurse such as high-patient volume, complex treatments, and symptom management challenges our efficiency and skills to secure comprehensive assessments and provide optimal physical and psychosocial care to the patient and family. Yet the research presented compels us to meet these daily challenges. And we must maintain an acute awareness of the influence of current therapies on patient response, symptom distress, demands of illness, and impact on families. The universal use of adjuvant therapy has influenced the incidence of premature menopause with associated menopausal symptoms, and the impact of those symptoms on the marital relationship has yet to be defined. Dose-intensive drug regimens and high-dose therapy with hematopoietic rescue as adjuvant therapy for high-risk breast cancer create significantly different demands of illness than the known standard adjuvant regimens. Such examples of treatment changes may dramatically affect family adjustment to breast cancer, as identified thus far in the literature. Research cannot keep pace with the reality of dynamic clinical practice with new treatments and toxicities but can provide the frameworks for assessment and design of interventions that serve as a foundation for nursing care (Lewis et al., 1993).

QUALITY OF LIFE

Quality of life is a multidimensional construct defined by a variety of dimensions such as psychologic, physical, social, spiritual, functional, and economic. Research with one or more of these dimensions as outcomes can be conceptualized as relating to the patient's quality of life. An early study with women with breast cancer after radical mastectomy by Schottenfeld and Robbins (1970) investigated quality of survival using return to normal activities and performance status as outcome variables. They reported that 57 per cent of women resumed normal daily activities within 1 to 3 months, 26 per cent within 4 to 6 months, and 16 per cent took longer than 6 months. Woods and Earp (1978) studied quality of survival 4 years after mastectomy as defined by symptoms of depression and sexual adaptation. The effect of demographics, surgical complications, and social support on these two variables

were also investigated. The major findings included persistent physical complaints; women with more physical complaints had more depressive symptoms; and social support buffered the depressive symptoms associated with physical complaints, but only if there were minimal symptoms. The majority of women reported no change and were satisfied with their sexual relationship.

Researchers also began to address the quality of life in women with advanced breast cancer. Evaluation of the effect of treatment demonstrated that treatment response was correlated with improved scores on a variety of quality of life indicators, despite some transient decreases within the first 3 days following chemotherapy (Coates et al., 1987; Priestman & Baum, 1976).

The initiation of adjuvant therapy in the late 1970s shifted the focus from rehabilitation after breast surgery to the quality of life with systemic therapy in women free of disease but at risk for recurrence. Meyerowitz, Watkins, and Spears (1983) interviewed 50 women receiving adjuvant CMF, with 60 per cent of subjects reporting physical symptoms as a major disruptive factor; social activity and work-related activity was affected in more than 75 per cent of women; 23 per cent reported changes in marital and family life; and 94 per cent of all women reported that such changes experienced were emotionally upsetting. The importance of quality of life as an outcome measure in cancer treatment has grown and now is commonly incorporated into clinical trials for breast cancer (Hayden et al., 1993; Levine et al., 1988). Quality of life is also a dynamic construct, and longitudinal studies with women with breast cancer will help capture changes over time and direct our interventions and use of resources more appropriately (Lenox, 1995). One example is the continuation of physical symptoms over time related to surgery (Ferrans, 1994; Polinsky, 1994; Woods & Earp, 1978). Persistent swelling, numbness, pain, stiffness, and weakness reported in women 2 to 4 years after surgery (Polinsky, 1994; Woods & Earp, 1978) is an important finding related to nursing practice. Do we continue to assess for symptoms of lymphedema and arm function over time? What is the pattern of symptoms and symptom distress related to these surgical complications? How effective are the currently employed interventions to prevent or minimize lymphedema complications? Answers to these questions might help us more accurately assess the impact of breast surgery on the woman's quality of life over time.

SURVIVORSHIP

Long-term survival in women with breast cancer has been a more recent focus related to quality of life. The survivorship experience has been explored from a variety of perspectives. Wyatt, Kurtz, and Liken (1993) conducted focus group interviews with women 5 or more years since diagnosis of breast cancer. Four themes emerged: (1) integrating the disease into current life, (2) change in relationship with others, (3) restructuring life's perspective, and (4) unresolved issues. Carter (1993) interviewed 25 women more than 5 years after diagnosis and described phases of the survival process: diagnosis, confronting mortality, reprioritizing, coming to terms, moving on, and flashing back. These phases sometimes occurred simultaneously and were reported by women as nonlinear. Fredette (1995) interviewed 14 women more than 5 years after diagnosis and described coping mechanisms such as work, spirituality, information seeking, and taking control. The author also addressed the impact of cancer, which was characterized by increased concern for others, reprioritizing, increased assertiveness, and change in distress over small matters. Ferrans (1994) mailed questionnaires to women with breast cancer and reported on 61 women who were more than 2 years past diagnosis and treatment. The most significant conclusion of this study was that women get on with living following breast cancer treatment, although some still suffer physical symptoms and the psychologic concern of recurrence persists. There are strong similarities among the results of these four cited studies: breast cancer becomes integrated into the woman's life; priorities in life are reevaluated; susceptibility to recurrence persists; a sensitivity appears to develop to help or be concerned about others; and women seem to develop strength from the experience that influences their life perceptions and actions. These findings appear to confirm clinical experience yet are limited by the characteristics and sample sizes of the studies described. Therefore, the picture of a strong, independent, reprioritized breast cancer survivor who is moving on with her life may represent many but certainly not all women. We are thus challenged to provide ongoing assessment to identify those women who adjust less well or who may be compromised by physical symptoms, lack of support, or other stressors. This is a formidable challenge related to the volume of patients in ambulatory settings, the available nursing resources, and the reality of the needs of patients who are in active treatment or who have active disease.

Breast cancer is a complex and increasingly challenging disease for the patient, the family, health care providers, and researchers. Nurses have a critical role in advocacy, clinical care, and research as we move into the next century of increasing breast cancer incidence, prevention and control strategies, and new and innovative therapeutic approaches.

REFERENCES

Abrams, J. S., Moore, T. D., & Friedman, M. (1994). New chemotherapeutic agents for breast cancer. *Cancer, 74*(3), 1164–1176.

Ahern, V., Barraclough, B., Bosch, C., Langlands, A., & Boyages, J. (1994). Locally advanced breast cancer defining an optimum treatment regimen. *International Journal of Radiation, Oncology, Biology, and Physics, 28*(4), 867–875.

Aikin, J. L. (1994). Menopausal symptoms resulting from cancer therapies: Helping women cope. *Oncology Nursing Forum, 21*(2), 381.

Aitken, D. R., & Minton, J. P. (1983). Complications associated with mastectomy. *Surgical Clinics of North America, 63*, 1331–1362.

Anelli, R. G., Anelli, A., Tran, K. H., Lebwohl, D. E., & Borgen, P. I. (1994). Tamoxifen administration is associated with a high rate of treatment limiting symptoms in male breast cancer patients. *Cancer, 74*(1), 74–77.

Angell, M. (1992). Breast implants—protection or paternalism. *New England Journal of Medicine, 326*,(25), 1695–1696.

Angell, M. (1994). Do breast implants cause systemic disease? Science in the courtroom. *New England Journal of Medicine, 330*(24), 1748–1749.

Asken, M. J. (1975). Psychoemotional aspects of mastectomy: A review of recent literature. *American Journal of Psychiatry, 132*(1), 56–59.

Ayash, L. J. (1994). High dose chemotherapy with autologous stem cell support for the treatment of metastatic breast cancer. *Cancer, 74*(1), 532–535.

Ayash, L. J., Elias, A., Wheeler, C., Reich, E., Schwartz, G., Mazanet, R., Tepler, I., Warren, D., Lynch, C., & Gonin, R. (1994). Double dose-intensive chemotherapy with autologous marrow and peripheral-blood progenitor-cell support for metastatic breast cancer: A feasibility study. *Journal of Clinical Oncology, 12*(1), 37–44.

Baider, L., Rizel, S., Kaplan DeNour, A. (1986). Comparison of couples' adjustment to lumpectomy and mastectomy. *General Hospital Psychiatry, 8*, 251–257.

Bajetta, E., Zilembo, N., Buzzoni, R., Celio, L., Zampino, M. G., Colleoni, M., Oriana, S., Attili, A., Sacchini, V., & Martinetti, A. (1994). Goserelin in premenopausal advanced breast cancer: Clinical and endocrine evaluation of responsive patients. *Oncology, 51*(3), 262–269.

Baker, N. C. (1991). *Relative risk: Living with a family history of breast cancer*. New York: Viking.

Ballard-Barbash, R. (1994). Anthropometry and breast cancer. *Cancer, 74*(3), 1090–1100.

Barrere, C. C. (1992). Breast biopsy support program: Collaboration between oncology clinical nurse specialist and the ambulatory surgery nurse. *Oncology Nursing Forum, 19*(9), 1375–1379.

Barrere, C., Trotta, P., & Foster, J. (1993). The experience of fatigue in women undergoing radiation therapy for early stage breast cancer. *Oncology Nursing Forum, 20*(2), 335.

Bartelink, H., van Dam, F., & van Dongen, J. (1985). Psychological effects of breast conserving therapy in comparison with radical mastectomy. *International Journal of Radiation, Oncology, Biology, and Physics, 11*, 381–385.

Baselga, J., & Mendelsohn, J. (1994). The epidermal growth factor receptor as a target for therapy in breast carcinoma. *Breast Cancer Research and Treatment, 29*(1), 127–138.

Baskin-Smith, J., Miaskowski, C., Dibble, S., & Nielsen, B. B. (1995). Perceptions of the mammography experience. *Cancer Nursing, 18*(1), 47–52.

Bassett, L. W., & Gambhir, S. (1991). Breast imaging for the 1990's. *Seminars in Oncology, 18*(2), 80–86.

Beahrs, O. H., Henson, D. E., Hutter, R. V., & Kennedy, B. J. (1993). *Handbook for staging of cancer*. Philadelphia: J. B. Lippincott Co.

Beckman, J., Johansen, L., Richardt, C., & Bilchert-Toft, M. (1983). Psychological reactions in younger women operated on for breast cancer. *Danish Medical Bulletin, 30*, 10–13.

Benedict, S., Williams, R. D., & Baron, P. L. (1994). Recalled anxiety: From discovery to diagnosis of a benign breast mass. *Oncology Nursing Forum, 21*(10), 1723–1727.

Betsill, W. L., Rosen, P. P., Lieberman, P. H., & Robbins, G. F. (1978). Intraductal carcinoma. *JAMA, 239*, 1863–1867.

Bezwoda, W., Hesdorffer, D., & Dansey, R. (1987). Breast cancer in men. Clinical features, hormone receptor status and response to therapy. *Cancer, 60,* 1337–1340.

Bianco, A. R., DelMastro, L., Gallo, C., Perrone, F., Matano, E., Pagliarulo, C., & DePlacido, S. (1991). Prognostic role of amenorrhea induced by adjuvant chemotherapy in premenopausal patients with early breast cancer. *British Journal of Cancer, 63,* 799–803.

Boccardo, F., Rubagotti, A., Bruzzi, P., Cappellini, M., Isola, G., Nenci, J., Piffanelli, A., Scanni, A., Sismondi, P., Santi, L., Genta, F., Saccani, F., Sassi, M., Malacarne, P., Donati, D., Farris, A., Castagnetta, L., DiCarlo, A., Traina, A., Galletto, L., Smeriere, F., & Buzzi, F. (1990). Chemotherapy versus tamoxifen versus chemotherapy plus tamoxifen in node-positive, estrogen receptor-positive breast cancer patients: Results of a multicentric Italian study. *Journal of Clinical Oncology, 8,* 1310–1320.

Bodian, C. A. (1994). Benign breast diseases, carcinoma in situ and breast cancer risk. *Epidemiologic Reviews, 15*(1), 177–187.

Bonadonna, G. (1989). Conceptual and practical advances in the management of breast cancer. The Karnofsky Memorial Lecture. *Journal of Clinical Oncology, 7,* 1380–1397.

Bonadonna, G., Brusamolino, E., Valagussa, P., Rossi, A., Brugnatelli, L., Brambilla, C., DeLena, M., Tancini, G., Bajetta, E., Musumeci, R., & Veronessi, U. (1976). Combination chemotherapy as an adjuvant treatment in operable breast cancer. *New England Journal of Medicine, 294,* 405–410.

Bonadonna, G., Rossi, A., & Valagussa, P. (1985). Adjuvant CMF chemotherapy in operable breast cancer: Ten years later. *World Journal of Surgery, 9,* 707–713.

Bonadonna, G., & Valagussa, P. (1985). Adjuvant systemic therapy for resectable breast cancer. *Journal of Clinical Oncology, 3,* 259–275.

Bonadonna, G., Valagussa, P., Brambilla, C., Ferrari, L., Lusni, A., Guco, M., Bartoli, C., Coopmans de Yoldi, C., Zucali, R., & Valagussa, P. (1990). Primary chemotherapy to avoid mastectomy in tumors with diameters of three centimeters or more. *Journal of the National Cancer Institute, 82*(19), 1539–1545.

Bonadonna, G., Valagussa, P., Brambilla, C., Moliterni, A., Zambetti, M., & Ferrari, L. (1991). Adjuvant and neoadjuvant treatment of breast cancer with chemotherapy and/or endocrine therapy. *Seminars in Oncology, 18*(6), 515–524.

Bonadonna, G., Valagussa, P., Moliterni, A., Zambetti, M., & Brambilla, C. (1995). Adjuvant cyclophosphamide methotrexate and fluorouracil in node-positive breast cancer: The results of 20 years of follow-up. *New England Journal of Medicine, 332*(14), 901–906.

Bonadonna, G., Valagussa, P., Rossi, A., Tancini, G., Brambilla, C., Zambetti, M., & Veronessi, U. (1985). Ten year experience with CMF-based adjuvant chemotherapy in resectable breast cancer. *Breast Cancer Research and Treatment, 5,* 95–115.

Bonadonna, G., Zambetti, M., & Valagussa, P. (1995). Sequential or alternating doxorubicin and CMF regimens in breast cancer with more than three positive nodes. *JAMA, 273*(7), 542–547.

Bondy, M. L., Vogel, V. G., Halabi, S., & Lustbader, E. D. (1992). Identification of women at increased risk for breast cancer in a population-based screening program. *Cancer Epidemiology Biomarkers and Prevention, 1,* 143–147.

Bostwick, J. (1990). Breast reconstruction after mastectomy. *Cancer, 66,* 1402–1411.

Breen, N., & Kessler, L. (1994). Changes in the use of screening mammography: Evidence from the 1987 and 1990 National Health Interview Survey. *American Journal of Public Health, 84*(1), 62–67.

Brennan, M. J. (1992). Lymphedema following the surgical treatment of breast cancer: A review of pathophysiology and treatment. *Journal of Pain and Symptom Management, 7*(2), 41–47.

Brigham, M. W. (1992). *Women and breast cancer: Variables influencing health behavior and perceptions of the disease.* Unpublished master's thesis, Yale University School of Nursing, New Haven, CT.

Brinton, L. A., & Schairer, C. (1993). Estrogen replacement therapy and breast cancer risk. *Epidemiologic Review, 15*(1), 66–79.

Brown, L. W., & Williams, R. D. (1994). Culturally sensitive breast cancer screening programs for older black women. *Nurse Practitioner, 19*(3), 21, 25–26, 31.

Buschel, P., (1995). Peripheral stem cell transplantation. In S. Hubbard, M. Knobf, & M. Goodman (Eds.), *Oncology nursing* (pp. 1–14). Philadelphia: J. B. Lippincott Co.

Bush, T. L. & Helzisouer, K. J. (1993). Tamoxifen for the primary prevention of breast cancer: A review and critique of the concept and trial. *Epidemiologic Reviews, 15,* 233–243.

Buzzoni, R., Bonadonna, G., Valagussa, P., & Zambetti, M. (1991). Adjuvant chemotherapy with doxorubicin plus cyclophosphamide, methotrexate, and fluorouracil in the treatment of resectable breast cancer with more than three positive axillary nodes. *Journal of Clinical Oncology, 9,* 2134–2140.

Byar, D. P., & Freedman, L. S. (1990). The importance and nature of cancer prevention trials. *Seminars in Oncology, 17,* 413–424.

Calais, G., Berger, C., Descamps, P., Chapet, S., Reynaud-Bougnoux, A., Body, G., Bougnoux, P., Larsac, J., & Lefloch., O. (1994). Conservative treatment feasibility with induction chemotherapy, surgery and radiotherapy for patients with breast carcinoma larger than 3 cm. *Cancer, 74*(4), 1283–1288.

Callahan, R. (1989). Genetic alterations in primary breast cancer. *Breast Cancer Research and Treatment, 13,* 191–203.

Canellos, G. P. (1987). Selection of therapy. In J. R. Harris, S. Hellman, I. C. Henderson, & D. W. Kinne (Eds.), *Breast diseases* (pp. 385–391). Philadelphia: J. B. Lippincott Co.

Cantril, C. (1991). Informational needs of women with early stage breast cancer [Abstract]. *Oncology Nursing Forum, 18,* 347.

Carroll, R. M. (1981). The impact of mastectomy on body image. *Oncology Nursing Forum, 8*(4), 29–32.

Carter, B. J. (1993). Long term survivors of breast cancer. *Cancer Nursing, 18*(1), 35–46.

Carter, D., & Smith, R. I. (1977). Carcinoma in situ of the breast. *Cancer, 40,* 1189–1193.

Cassileth, B. R., Zupkis, R. V., Sutton-Smith, K., & March, V. (1980). Information and participation preferences among cancer patients. *Annals of Internal Medicine, 92,* 832–836.

Cathart, C. K., Jones, S. E., Pumroy, C. S., Peters, G. N., Knox, S. M., & Cheek, J. H. (1993). Clinical recognition and management of depression in node negative breast cancer patients treated with tamoxifen. *Breast Cancer Research and Treatment, 27*(3), 277–281.

Cawley, M., & Cappello, C. (1990). Informational and psychosocial needs of women choosing conservative surgery/primary radiation for early stage breast cancer. *Cancer Nursing, 13,* 90–94.

Chamorro, T. (1991). Gonadal and reproductive sequelae of cancer therapy. In S. M. Hubbard, P. M. Greene, & M. T. Knobf (Eds.), *Current issues in cancer nursing practice* (pp. 1–15). Philadelphia: J. B. Lippincott Co.

Champion, V. L. (1989). Effect of knowledge, teaching method, confidence and social influence on breast self examination behavior. *IMAGE, 21,* 76–80.

Champion, V. L. (1991). The relationship of selected variables to breast cancer detection behaviors in women 35 and older. *Oncology Nursing Forum, 18*(4), 733–739.

Chapman, R. M. (1982). Effect of cytotoxic therapy on sexuality and gonadal function. *Seminars in Oncology, 9,* 84–94.

Chlebowski, R. T., Nixon, D. W., Blackburn, G. L., Jochimsen, P., Scanlon, E. F., Insell, W., Buzzard, M., Elashoff, R., Butrum, R., & Wynder, E. (1987). A breast cancer nutrition adjuvant study (NAS): Protocol design and initial patient adherence. *Breast Cancer Research and Treatment, 10,* 21–29.

Chrysogelos, S. A., & Dickson, R. B. (1994). EGF receptor expression, regulation and function in breast cancer. *Breast Cancer Research and Treatment, 29*(1), 29–40.

Clarke, D., Martinez, A., & Cox, R. S. (1983). Analysis of cosmetic results and complications in patients with stage I and II breast cancer treated by biopsy and radiation. *International Journal of Radiation Oncology, Biology, and Physics, 9,* 1807–1813.

Claus, E. B., Risch, N., & Thompson, W. D. (1990). Age of onset as an indicator of familial risk of breast cancer. *American Journal of Epidemiology, 131,* 961–972.

Clayden, J. R., Bell, J. W., & Pollard, P. (1974). Menopausal flushing: Double-blind trial of a non-hormonal medication. *British Medical Journal, 1,* 409–412.

Coates, A., Gebski, V., Stat, M., Bishop, J. F., Jeal, P. N., Woods, R. L., Snyder, R., Tattersall, M. H., Byrne, M., Harvey, V., Gill, G., Simpson, J., Drummond, R., Browne, J., van Voyyrn, T., Cooten, R., & Forbes, J. (1987). Improving the quality of life during chemotherapy for advanced breast cancer. *New England Journal of Medicine, 317,* 1490–1495.

Cobleigh, M. A., Berris, R. E., Bush, T., Davidson, N. E., Robert, N. J., Sparano, J. A., Tormey, D. C., & Wood, W. C. (1994). Estrogen replacement therapy in breast cancer survivors. *JAMA, 272*(7), 540–545.

Cohen, R. S., Wellisch, D. K., Christiansen, A., & Giuliano, A. E. (1984). Effect of mastectomy and lumpectomy on dimensions of mood, self concept impairment and marital satisfaction [Abstract]. *Proceedings of the American Society of Clinical Oncology, 3,* 72.

Colditz, G. A., Willett, W. C., Hanks, D. J., Stampfer, M. J., Manson, J. E., Hennekens, C. H., Rosner, B. A., & Spiezer, F. E. (1993). Family history, age and risk of breast cancer. *JAMA, 270*(3), 338–343.

Coll, P. O., O'Connor, P. J., Crabtree, B. F., & Besdine, R. W. (1989). Effect of age, education and physician advice on utilization of screening mammography. *Journal of the American Geriatric Society, 37,* 957–962.

Cooper, R. G., Holland, J. F., & Gidewell, O. (1979). Adjuvant chemotherapy of breast cancer. *Cancer, 44,* 793–798.

Costanza, M. E. (1992). Breast cancer screening in older women: An overview. *Journal of Gerontology, 47,* 1–3.

Costanza, M. E. (1994). Issues in breast cancer screening in older women. *Cancer, 74,* (Suppl. 7), 2009–2015.

Daly, M. B. (1994). New perspectives in breast cancer: The genetic revolution. In S. M. Hubbard, P. E. Greene, & M. T. Knobf (Eds.), *Oncology Nursing* (pp. *1*(6), 1–10). Philadelphia: J. B. Lippincott Co.

Danforth, D. N., Findlay, P. A., McDonald, H. D., Lippman, M. E., Reichart, C. M., d'Angelo, T., et al. (1986). Complete axillary node dissection for stage I & II carcinoma of the breast. *Journal of Clinical Oncology, 4,* 655–662.

d'Angelo, T. M., & Gorrell, C. R. (1989). Breast reconstruction using tissue expanders. *Oncology Nursing Forum, 16,* 23–27.

Davidson, N. E., & Abeloff, M. D. (1992). Adjuvant systemic therapy for node-negative breast cancer. *PPO Updates, 6*(7), 1–13.

Day, D. J., & O'Rourke, M. G. (1990). The diagnosis of breast cancer: A clinical and mammographic comparison. *Medical Journal of Australia, 152,* 635–639.

Degner, L. F., & Russell, C. A. (1988). Preferences for treatment control among adults with cancer. *Research Nursing and Health, 11,* 367–374.

Degner, L. F., & Sloan, J. A. (1992). Decision making during serious illness: What role do patients really want to plan? *Journal of Clinical Epidemiology, 45,* 941–950.

deGraaf, H., Willemse, P. H., deVries, E. G., Siejfer, D. T., Mulder, P. O., vander Graaf, W. T., Smit, C. T., van der Ploeg, E., Dolsma, W. V., & Mulder, N. H. (1994). Intensive chemotherapy with autologous bone marrow transfusion as primary treatment in women with breast cancer and more than five involved axillary lymph nodes. *European Journal of Cancer, 30*(2), 150–153.

deHaas, J., & Walveert, K. (1985). Quality of life after breast cancer surgery. *Journal of Surgical Oncology, 28,* 1231–1237.

Derogotis, L. R. (1980). Breast and gyn cancers. *Frontiers in Radiation Therapy and Oncology, 14,* 1–11.

DeVita, V. T. (1986). Dose response is alive and well. *Journal of Clinical Oncology, 4*(8), 1157–1158.

DeVita, V. T. (1990). Primary chemotherapy can avoid mastectomy, but there is more to it than that. *Journal of the National Cancer Institute, 82*(19), 1522–1523.

Dupont, W. D., & Page, D. L. (1985). Risk factors for breast cancer in women with proliferative breast disease. *New England Journal of Medicine, 312,* 145–151.

Dupont, W. D., Page, D. L., Parl, F. F., Vnencak-Jones, C. I., Plummer, W. D., Rados, M. S., & Schuyler, P. A. (1994). Long term risk of breast cancer in women with fibroedema. *New England Journal of Medicine, 331,* 101–105.

Early Breast Cancer Trialists' Collaborative Groups. (1992a). Systemic treatment of early breast cancer by hormonal, cytotoxic or immune therapy, Part I. *Lancet, 339*(8784), 1–5.

Early Breast Cancer Trialists' Collaborative Group. (1992b). Systemic treatment of early breast cancer by hormonal, cytotoxic or immune therapy, Part II. *Lancet, 339*(8785), 71–85.

Easterling, D. V., & Leventhal, H. (1989). Contribution of concrete cognition to emotion: Neutral symptoms as elicitors of worry about cancer. *Journal of Applied Psychology, 74,* 787–796.

Ehlke, G. A. (1988). Symptom distress in breast cancer patients receiving chemotherapy in the out-patient setting. *Oncology Nursing Forum, 15,* 343–346.

Ell, K., Nishimoto, R., Mantell, J., & Hamovitch, M. (1988). Longitudinal analysis of psychological adaptation among family members of patients with cancer. *Journal of Psychosomatic Medicine, 32*(4/5), 429–438.

Fallowfield, L. J. (1990). Psychosocial adjustment after treatment for early stage breast cancer. *Oncology, 4*(4), 89–98.

Fallowfield, L. J., Baum, M., & Maquire, P. (1986). Effects of breast conservation on psychiatric morbidity associated with the diagnosis and treatment of early breast cancer. *British Medical Journal, 293,* 1331–1334.

Farrow, D. C., Hunt, W. C., & Samet, J. M. (1992). Geographic variation in the treatment of localized breast cancer. *New England Journal of Medicine, 326,* 1097–1103.

Feldman, J. E. (1989). Ovarian failure and cancer treatment: Incidence and interventions for the premenopausal women. *Oncology Nursing Forum, 16,* 651–657.

Ferrans, C. E. (1994). Quality of life through the eyes of survivors of breast cancer. *Oncology Nursing Forum, 21*(10), 1645–1651.

Fischer, D., Knobf, M. T., & Durivage, H. (1993). *The cancer chemotherapy handbook* (4th ed.). St. Louis: Mosby-Year Book.

Fisher, B. (1983). Relation of estrogen and/or progesterone receptor content of breast cancer to patient outcome following adjuvant chemotherapy. *Breast Cancer Research and Treatment, 3,* 355–364.

Fisher, B., Brown, A. M., Dimitrov, N. V., et al. (1990). Two months of doxorubicin-cyclophosphamide with and without interval reinduction therapy compared with 6 months of cyclophosphamide, methotrexate, and fluorouracil in positive-node breast cancer patients with tamoxifen-non-responsive tumors: Results from the National Surgical Adjuvant Breast and Bowel Project B-15. *Journal of Clinical Oncology, 8,* 1483–1496.

Fisher, B., Constantino, J., Redmond, C., Fisher, E., Margolese, R., Dimitrov, N., Wolmark, N., Wickerham, D. L., Deutsch, M., Ore, L., Mamounas, E., Poller, W., & Kavanaugh, M. (1993). Lumpectomy compared with lumpectomy and radiation therapy for the treatment of intraductal breast cancer. *New England Journal of Medicine, 328*(22), 1581–1586.

Fisher, B., Costantino, J., Redmond, C., Poisson, R., Bowman, D., Couture, J., Dimitrov, N., Wolmark, N., Wickerham, D. L., Fisher, E., Margolese, R., Robidoux, A., Shibata, H., Terz, J., Paterson, A. H. G., Feldman, M. I., Farrar, W., Evans, J., Lickley, H. L., & Ketner, M. (1989). A randomized clinical trial evaluating tamoxifen in the treatment of patients with node-negative breast cancer who have estrogen-receptor-positive tumors. *New England Journal of Medicine, 320,* 479–484.

Fisher, B., Redmond, C., Brown, A., Wickerham, L., Wolmark, N., Allegra, J., Escher, G., Lippman, M., Savlov, E., Wittliff, J., & Fisher, E. R. (1983). Influence of tumor estrogen and progesterone levels on the response to tamoxifen and chemotherapy in primary breast cancer. *Journal of Clinical Oncology, 1,* 227–241.

Fisher, B., Redmond, C., Dimitrov, N. V., Bowman, D., Legault-Poisson, S., Wickerham, L., Wolmark, N., Fisher, E., Margolese, R., Sutherland, C., Glass, A., Foster, R., Caplan, R., et al. (1989). A randomized clinical trial evaluating sequential methotrexate and fluorouracil in the treatment of patients with node-negative breast cancer who have estrogen-receptor-negative tumors. *New England Journal of Medicine, 320,* 473–478.

Fisher, B., Redmond, C., Poisson, S., Dimitrov, N., Margolese, R., Bowman, D., Glass, A., Robidoux, A., Wickerham, D., Wolmark, N., & Jochimsen, P. (1990). Increased benefit from addition of Adriamycin and cyclophosphamide (AC) to tamoxifen (TAM, T) for positive node TAM-response postmenopausal breast cancer patients: Results from NSABP B-16. *Proceedings of the American Society of Clinical Oncology, 9,* 20.

Fisher, B., Redmond, C., Poisson, R., Margolese, R., Wolmark, N., Wickerham, L., Fisher, E., Deutsch, M., Caplan, R., Pilch, Y., Glass, A., Shibata, H., Lerner, H., Terz, S., & Sidorovich, L. (1989). Eight-year results of a randomized clinical trial comparing total mastectomy and lumpectomy with or without irradiation in the treatment of breast cancer. *New England Journal of Medicine, 320,* 822–828.

Fisher, B., Sherman, B., & Rockette, H. (1979). L-Phenylalanine-mustard (L-PAM) in the management of premenopausal patients with primary breast cancer. *Cancer, 44,* 847–857.

Fisher, B., Slack, N., Katrych, D., & Wolmark, N. (1975). Ten year follow up results of patients with carcinoma of the breast in a cooperative clinical trial evaluating surgical adjuvant chemotherapy. *Surgery, Gynecology and Obstetrics, 140,* 528–531.

Fisher, B., & Wolmark, N. (1986). Conservative surgery: The American experience. *Seminars in Oncology, 13,* 425–433.

Fisher, J. C. (1992). The silicone controversy: When will science prevail? *New England Journal of Medicine, 326*(25), 1696–1697.

Foltz, A. (1985). Weight gain among stage II breast cancer patients: A study of five factors. *Oncology Nursing Forum, 12,* 21–26.

Forsythe, M. D., Fulton, D. L., Lane, D. S., Burg, M. A., & Krishna, M. (1992). Changes in knowledge, attitudes and behavior of women participating in a community outreach education program on breast cancer screening. *Patient Education and Counseling, 19,* 241–250.

Fowble, B. (1991). In situ breast cancer. In B. Fowble, R. L. Goodman, J. H. Glick, & E. F. Rosato (Eds.), *Breast cancer treatment* (pp. 325–344). St. Louis: Mosby-Year Book.

Fowble, B. (1994). The Recht/Harris/Come article reviewed. *Oncology, 8*(3) 30–32.

Fowble, B., & Glover, D. (1991). Locally advanced breast cancer. In B. Fowble, R. L. Goodman, J. H. Glick, & E. F. Rosato (Eds.), *Breast cancer treatment* (pp. 345–372). St. Louis: Mosby-Year Book.

Fowble, B., Solin, L. J., & Schultz, D. J. (1991). Conservative surgery and radiation for early breast cancer. In B. Fowble, R. L. Goodman, J. H. Glick, & E. F. Rosato (Eds.), *Breast cancer treatment* (pp. 105–149). St. Louis: Mosby-Year Book.

Fox, S. A., Murata, P. J., & Stein, M. A. (1991). The impact of physician compliance on screening mammography for older women. *Archives of Internal Medicine, 15,* 50–56.

Frazier, T. G., & Noone, R. B. (1985). An objective analysis of immediate simultaneous reconstruction in the treatment of primary carcinoma of the breast. *Cancer, 55,* 1202–1205.

Fredette, S. L. (1995). Breast cancer survivors: Concerns and coping. *Cancer Nursing, 18*(1), 35–46.

Freeman, H. P., Muth, B. J., & Kerner, J. F. (1995). Expanding access to cancer screening and clinical follow-up among the medically underserved. *Cancer Practice, 3*(1), 19–30.

Frykberg, E. R., & Bland, K. I. (1994). Overview of the biology and management of ductal carcinoma in situ of the breast. *Cancer, 74*(Suppl. 1), 350–361.

Frykberg, E. R., Santiago, F., Betskill, W. L., & O'Brien, P. H. (1987). Lobular carcinoma in situ of the breast. *Surgery, Gynecology and Obstetrics, 164,* 285–301.

Fugh-Berman, A., & Epstein, S. (1992). Should healthy women take tamoxifen? *New England Journal of Medicine, 327,* 1596.

Gabriel, S. E., O'Fallon, M., Kurland, L. T., Beard, C. M., Woods, J. E., & Melton, L. J. (1994). Risk of connective-tissue diseases and other disorders after breast implantation. *New England Journal of Medicine, 330*(24), 1697–1702.

Gail, M. H., Brinton, L. A., Beyar, D. P., Corle, D. K., Green, S. G., Schairer, C., & Mulvihill, J. J. (1989). Projecting individualized probabilities of developing breast cancer for white females who are being examined annually. *Journal of the National Cancer Institute, 81,* 1879–1888.

Ganz, P. A. (1992). Advocating for the woman with breast cancer. *CA: A Cancer Journal for Clinicians, 45*(2), 114–126.

Ganz, P. A., Schag, A. C., Lee, J. J., Polinsky, M. L., & Tan, S. (1992). Breast conservation versus mastectomy. Is there a difference in psychological adjustment or quality of life in the year after surgery? *Cancer, 69,* 1792–1738.

Ganz, P. A., Schag, A. C., Polinsky, M. K., Heinrich, R. L., & Flack, V. F. (1987). Rehabilitation needs and breast cancer: The first month after primary therapy. *Breast Cancer Research and Treatment, 10,* 243–253.

Gates, C. C. (1980). Husbands of mastectomy patients. *Patient Counseling and Health Education, 2*(1), 38–41.

George, S. L., & Hoogstraten, B. (1978). Prognostic factors in the initial response to therapy by patients with advanced breast cancer. *Journal of the National Cancer Institute, 60,* 731–736.

Germino, B. B., Fife, B. L., & Funk, S. G. (1995). Cancer and the partner relationship: What is its meaning? *Seminars in Oncology Nursing, 11*(1), 43–50.

Giomuso, C. B., & Suster, V. (1994). Free-flap breast reconstruction. *Medsurg Nursing, 3*(1), 9–24.

Given, B., & Given, C. W. (1992). Patient and family caregiver reaction to new and recurrent breast cancer. *Journal of the American Medical Women's Association, 47*(5), 201–207.

Goin, M. K., & Goin, M. J. (1988). Growing pains: The psychological experience of breast reconstruction with tissue expansion. *Annals of Plastic Surgery, 21,* 217–222.

Goldberg, P., Stolzman, M., Goldberg, H. M. (1984). Psychological considerations in breast reconstruction. *Annals of Plastic Surgery, 13,* 39–43.

Goldhirsch, A., Castiglione, M., & Gelber, R. D. (1992). A single perioperative adjuvant chemotherapy course for node-negative breast cancer: Five-year results of trial V. *Journal of the National Cancer Institute Monographs, 11,* 89.

Goldhirsch, A., Gelber, R. D., & Castiglione, M. (1990). The magnitude of endocrine effects of adjuvant chemotherapy of premenopausal breast cancer patients. *Annals of Oncology, 1,* 183–188.

Goldhirsch, A., Gelber, R. D., Castiglione, M., Price, K. N., Rudenstam, C., Lindtner, J., Collins, J., Senn, H., Brunner, K. W., Galligioni, E., Cavalli, F., Gudgen, A., Cortes-tunes, H., Tattersall, M., Marini, G., Byrne, M., Snyder, R., Forbes, J. F., Humay, C., & Cooks, A. (1994). Present and future projects of the International Breast Cancer Study Group. *Cancer, 74,* 1139–1149.

Goldie, J. H. (1983). Drug resistance and cancer chemotherapy strategy in breast cancer. *Breast Cancer Research and Treatment, 3,* 129–136.

Gotay, C. C. (1984). The experience of cancer during the early and advanced stages: The views of patients and their mates. *Social Science Medicine, 18*(7), 605–613.

Gould, K., Gates, M. L., & Miaskowski, C. (1994). Breast cancer prevention: A summary of the chemoprevention trial with taxomifen. *Oncology Nursing Forum, 21,* 835–840.

Grandstaff, N. W. (1976). The impact of breast cancer on the family. In J. M. Vaeth (Ed.), *Frontiers of radiation therapy and oncology* (pp. 146–156). Basel, Switzerland: Karger Publishers.

Graydon, J. E. (1994). Women with breast cancer: Their quality of life following course of radiation therapy. *Journal of Advanced Nursing, 19*(4), 617–622.

Greenberg, D. B., Sawicka, J., Eisenthal, S., & Ross, D. (1992). Fatigue syndrome due to localized radiation. *Journal of Pain Symptom Management, 7,* 38–45.

Greenberg, E. J. (1991). The treatment of metastatic breast cancer. *CA: A Cancer Journal for Clinicians, 41*(4), 242–256.

Greene, D., Nail, L. M., Fieler, V. K., Dudgeon, D., & Jones, L. S. (1994). A comparison of patient reported side effects among three chemotherapy regimens for breast cancer. *Cancer Practice, 2*(1), 57–62.

Gregorio, D. I., Kegeles, S., Parker, C., & Benn, S. (1990). Encouraging screening mammograms. *Connecticut Medicine, 54*(7), 370–373.

Grindel, C. G., Cahill, C. A., & Walker, M. (1989). Food intake of women with breast cancer during the first six months of chemotherapy. *Oncology Nursing Forum, 16,* 401–407.

Habegger, D., & Ellerhorst-Ryan, J. M. (1988). Needle localization of non-palpable breast lesions. *Oncology Nursing Forum, 15,* 192–194.

Hack, T. F., Degner, L. F., & Dyck, D. G. (1995). Relationship between preferences for decisional control and illness information among women with breast cancer: A quantitative and qualitative analysis. *Social Science and Medicine, 39*(2), 279–289.

Hailey, B. J., & Bradford, A. C. (1991). Breast self examination and mammography among university staff and faculty. *Women and Health, 17*(3), 59–77.

Haller, D. G., Fox, K. R., & Schuchter, L. M. (1991). Metastatic breast cancer. In B. Fowble, R. H. Goodman, J. H. Glick & E. F. Rosato, (Eds.), *Breast cancer treatment,* (pp. 403–456). St. Louis: Mosby-Year Book.

Hannum, J. W., Giese-Davis, J., Harding, K., & Hatfield, A. K. (1991). Effects of individual and marital variables on coping with cancer. *Journal of Psychosocial Oncology, 9*(2), 1–20.

Harris, J. R., Lippman, M. E., Veronessi, U., & Willett, W. (1992a). Breast cancer (second of three parts), *New England Journal of Medicine, 327*(6), 390–398.

Harris, J. R., Lippman, M. E., Veronessi, U., & Willett, W. (1992b). Breast cancer (third of three parts). *New England Journal of Medicine, 327*(7), 473–480.

Harris, J. R., Morrow, M., & Bonadonna, G. (1993). Cancer of the breast. In V. T. DeVita, S. Hellman, & S. A. Rosenberg (Eds.), *Cancer: Principles and practice* (4th ed., 1264–1332). Philadelphia: J. B. Lippincott.

Harris, R. P., Fletcher, S. W., Gonzalez, J. J., Lannin, D. R., Degnan, D., Earp, J., & Clark, R. (1991). Mammography and age: Are we targeting the wrong women? *Cancer, 67,* 2010–2014.

Hayden, K. A., Moinpur, C. M., Metch, B., Feige, P., O'Bryan, R. M., Green, S., & Osborne, C. K. (1993). Pitfalls in quality-of-life assessment: Lessons from a Southwest Oncology Groups Breast Cancer Clinical Trial. *Oncology Nursing Forum, 20*(9), 1415–1419.

Heasman, K. Z., Sutherland, H. J., Campbell, J. A., Elhakim, T., & Boyd, N. F. (1985). Weight gain during adjuvant chemotherapy for breast cancer. *Breast Cancer Research and Treatment, 5,* 195–200.

Henderson, I. C. (1994). Adjuvant systemic therapy for early breast cancer. *Cancer, 74* (Suppl. 1), 401–409.

Henderson, I. C. (1987). Adjuvant systemic therapy of early breast cancer. In J. R. Harris, S. Hellman, I. C. Henderson, & D. W. Kinne (Eds.), *Breast diseases* (pp. 398–428). Philadelphia: J. B. Lippincott Co.

Henderson, I. C., Gelman, R. S., Harris, J. R., & Canellos, G. P. (1986). Duration of therapy in adjuvant chemotherapy. *NCI Monographs, 1,* 95–98.

Henrich, J. B. (1992). The postmenopausal estrogen/breast cancer controversy. *JAMA, 28*(14), 1900–1902.

Henrich, J. G., Kornguth, D. J., Berg, A. T., & Schwartz, G. E. (1992). Psychosocial factors and mammography use. *Journal of Women's Health, 1*(2), 123–129.

Hildreth, N. G., Shore, R. E., & Dvoretsky, P. M. (1989). The risk of breast cancer after irradiation of the thymus in infancy. *New England Journal of Medicine, 321,* 1281–1284.

Hilton, A. B. (1993). Issues, problems and challenges for families coping with breast cancer. *Seminars in Oncology Nursing, 9*(2), 88–100.

Holland, J. C., & Mastrovito, R. (1980). Psychologic adaptation to breast cancer. *Cancer, 46*(4), 1045–1052.

Holm, L., Nordevange, E., Ikkala, E., Hallstrom, L., & Callmer, E. (1990). Dietary intervention as adjuvant therapy in breast cancer patients: A feasibility study. *Breast Cancer Research and Treatment, 16,* 103–109.

Holmberg, L., Ohlander, E. M., Byers, T., Zack, M., Wolk, A., Bergstrom, R., Bergkist, L., Thurfjell, E., Bruce, A., & Adami, H. O. (1994). Diet and breast cancer risk. Results of a population-based case control study in Sweden. *Archives of Internal Medicine, 154*(16), 1805–1811.

Holmberg, L., Omne-Ponten, M., Burns, T., Adami, H. O., & Bergstrom, R. (1989). Psychosocial adjustment after mastectomy and breast-conserving treatment. *Cancer, 64,* 969–974.

Hortobagyi, G. N. (1994). Multidisciplinary management of advanced primary and metastatic breast cancer. *Cancer, 74*(1), 416–423.

Hoskins, K. F., Stopfer, J. E., Calzone, K. A., Merajver, S. D., Rebbeck, T. R., Garber, J. E., & Weber, B. (1995). Assessment and counseling for women with a family history of breast cancer. *JAMA, 273*(7), 577–585.

Howe, G. R. (1994). Dietary fat and breast cancer risks. *Cancer, 74*(Suppl. 3), 1078–1084.

Hughes, K. K. (1993a). Decision making by patients with breast cancer: The role of information in treatment selection. *Oncology Nursing Forum, 20,* 623–628.

Hughes, K. K. (1993b). Psychosocial and functional status of breast cancer patients. *Cancer Nursing, 18,* 222–229.

Hull, M. (1993). Breast cancer experiences of premenopausal women [Abstract]. *Oncology Nursing Forum, 20,* 36.

Hunter, D. J., Manson, J. E., Colditz, G. A., Stampfer, M. J., Rosner, B., Hennekens, C. H., Speizer, F. E., & Willett, W. (1993). A prospective study of the intake of vitamins C, E, and A and the risk of breast cancer. *New England Journal of Medicine, 329,* 234–240.

Hunter, D. J., & Willett, W. C. (1993). Diet, body size, and breast cancer. *Epidemiologic Reviews, 15,* 110–132.

Hutcheson, H. A. (1986). TAIF: New option for breast reconstruction. *Nursing, 86*(16), 51–53.

Insull, W., Henderson, M. M., Prentice, R. L., Thompson, D. J., Clifford, C., Goldman, S., Gorbach, S., Moskowitz, M., Thompson, R., & Woods, M. (1990). Results of a randomized feasibility study of a low fat diet. *Archives of Internal Medicine, 150,* 421–427.

Jacobson, J. A., Danforth, D. N., Cowan, K. H., d'Angelo, T., Steinberg, S. M., Pierce, L., Lippman, M. E., Lichter, A. S., Glatstein, E., & Okunieff, P. (1995). Ten-year results of a comparison of conservation with mastectomy in the treatment of stage I and II breast cancer. *New England Journal of Medicine, 322*(14), 907–911.

Jacquillat, C., Weil, M., Baillet, F., Borel, C., Auclerc, G., de Maublanc, M. A., Housset, M., Forget, G., Thill, L., Soubrane, C., Khayat, D. (1990). Results of neoadjuvant chemotherapy and radiation in the breast-conserving treatment of 250 patients with all stages of infiltrative breast cancer. *Cancer, 66,* 119–129.

Jamison, K. R., Wellisch, D. K., & Pasnau, R. O. (1978). Psychosocial aspects of mastectomy: I. The women's perspective. *American Journal of Psychiatry, 135*(4), 432–436.

John, E. M., & Kelsey, J. L. (1994). Radiation and other environmental exposures and breast cancer. *Epidemiologic Reviews, 15*(1), 157–162.

Johansen, C. H., vanHeerdan, J. A., Donahue, J. H., Martin, J. K., Jackson, I. T., & Ilstrup, D. M. (1989). Oncological aspects of immediate reconstruction following mastectomy for malignancy. *Archives of Surgery, 124,* 819–824.

Kalinowski, B. H. (1991). Local therapy for breast cancer: Treatment choices and decision making. *Seminars in Oncology Nursing, 7,* 187–193.

Kaplan, K. M., Weinberg, G. B., Small, A., & Herndon, J. L. (1991). Breast cancer screening among relatives of women with breast cancer. *American Journal of Public Health, 81,* 1174–1179.

Kash, K. M., Holland, J. C., Halper, M. S., & Miller, O. J. (1992). Psychological distress and surveillance behaviors of women with a family history of breast cancer. *Journal of the National Cancer Institute, 84,* 24–30.

Kedar, R. P., Bourne, T. H., Powles, T. J., Collins, W. D., Ashley, S. E., Cosgrove, D. O., & Campbell, S. (1994). Effects of tamoxifen on uterus and ovaries of post menopausal women in a randomised breast cancer prevention trial. *Lancet, 343,* 1318–1321.

Kelly, P. T. (1991). *Understanding breast cancer risk.* Philadelphia: Temple University Press.

Kelsey, J. L., Gammon, M. D., & John, E. M. (1993). Reproductive factors and breast cancer. *Epidemiologic Reviews, 15*(1), 36–47.

Kelsey, J. L., & Horn-Ross, P. L. (1993). Breast cancer: Magnitude of the problem and descriptive epidemiology. *Epidemiologic Reviews, 15*(1), 7–16.

Kemeny, M. M., Wellisch, D. K., & Schain, W. S. (1988). Psychosocial outcomes in a randomized surgical trial for treatment of primary breast cancer. *Cancer, 62,* 1231–1237.

Kerlikowske, K., Grady, D., Rubin, S. M., Sandrock, C., & Ernster, V. L. (1995). Efficacy of screening mammography. *JAMA, 273*(2), 149–154.

Kessler, D. A. (1992). The basis of the FDA's decision on breast implants. *New England Journal of Medicine, 326*(25), 1713–1715.

Kiebert, G. M., deHaes, J. C., & van de Velde, C. J. (1991). The impact of breast-conserving treatment and mastectomy on the quality of life of early stage breast cancer patients: A review. *Journal of Clinical Oncology, 9,* 1059–1070.

King, K., Nail, L., Kreamer, K., Strohl, R., & Johnson, J. E. (1985). Patients descriptions of the experience of receiving radiation therapy. *Oncology Nursing Forum, 12,* 55–61.

Kinne, D. W. (1987). Primary treatment of breast cancer surgery. In J. R. Harris, S. Hellman, I. C. Henderson & D. W. Kinne (Eds.), *Breast diseases* (pp. 259–284). Philadelphia: J. B. Lippincott Co.

Kinne, D., & Hakes, T. (1991). Male breast cancer. In J. Harris, S. Hellman, I. C. Henderson & D. Kinne (Eds.), *Breast diseases*, (2nd ed., pp. 782–790). Philadelphia: J. B. Lippincott Co.

Knobf, M. T. (1986). Physical and psychological distress associated with adjuvant chemotherapy in women with breast cancer. *Journal of Clinical Oncology, 4,* 678–684.

Knobf, M. T. (1990). Symptoms and rehabilitation needs of patients with early breast cancer during primary therapy. *Cancer, 66,* 1392–1401.

Knobf, M. T. (1994a). Symptoms associated with primary radiotherapy for breast cancer [Abstract]. *Proceeding of the Third American Cancer Society Nursing Research Conference.* Newport Beach, CA: American Cancer Society.

Knobf, M. T. (1994b). Decision-making for primary breast cancer treatment. *Medsurg Nursing, 3*(3), 169–174, 180.

Knobf, M. T. (1994c). Treatment options for early stage breast cancer. *Medsurg Nursing, 3*(4), 249–328.

Knobf, M. T. (in press). Menopausal symptoms associated with breast cancer treatment. In K. Hassey Dow (Ed.), *Contemporary issues in breast cancer.* Boston: Jones & Bartlett.

Knobf, M. T., Mullen, J., Xistris, D., & Moritz, D. A. (1983). Weight gain in women with breast cancer on adjuvant chemotherapy. *Oncology Nursing Forum, 10,* 28–33.

Knobf, M. T., & Stahl, R. (1987). *Breast reconstruction. What to do after an implant.* New Haven, CT: Yale Cancer Center.

Knobf, M. T., & Stahl, R. (1991). Reconstructive surgery in primary breast cancer treatment. *Seminars in Oncology Nursing, 7*(3), 200–206.

Kopans, D. B. (1994). Screening for breast cancer and mortality reduction among women 40–49 years of age. *Cancer, 74,* (Suppl. 1), 311–322.

Kotasek, D., Sage, R. E., Dale, B. M., Norman, J. E., & Bolton, A. (1994). Dose intensive therapy with autologous blood stem cell transplantation in breast cancer. *Australian and New Zealand Journal of Medicine, 24*(3), 288–295.

Lagios, M. D., Westdahl, P. R., Margolini, F. R., & Rose, M. R. (1982). Duct carcinoma in situ. *Cancer, 53,* 700–704.

Langer, A. S., & Hassey-Dow, K. (1994). The breast cancer advocacy movement and nursing. In S. M. Hubbard, P. E. Greene & M. T. Knobf (Eds.), *Oncology Nursing* pp. *1*(3), 1–13. Philadelphia: J. B. Lippincott Co.

Lartigau, E., el-Jabbour, J. N., Dubray, D., & Dische, S. (1994). Male breast carcinoma: A single centre report of clinical parameters. *Clinical Oncology 6*(3), 162–166.

Lasry, J. M., Margolese, R. G., Poisson, R., Shibata, H., Fleischer, D., Lafleur, D., Legault, S., & Tallefer, S. (1987). Depression and body image following mastectomy and lumpectomy. *Journal of Chronic Disease, 40,* 529–534.

Leinster, S. J., Ashcroft, J. J., Slade, P. D., & Dewey, M. E. (1989). Mastectomy versus conservative surgery: Psychosocial effects of the patient's choice of treatment. *Journal of Psychosocial Oncology, 7*(1/2), 179–192.

Lenox, R. W. (1995). *Adjuvant therapy for breast cancer: A longitudinal quality of life study.* Unpublished master's thesis, Yale University School of Nursing, New Haven, CT.

Lerman, C., Rimer, B., Trock, B., Balshem, A., & Engstrom, P. F. (1990). Factors associated with repeat adherence to breast cancer screening. *Preventive Medicine, 19,* 279–290.

Levine, M. N., Guyatt, G. H., Gest, M., DePauw, S., Goodyear, M. D., Hryniuk, W., Arnold, A., Findlay, B., Skillings, J. R., Bramwell, V. H., Levine, L., Bush, H., Abu-Zahra, H., & Kotalik, J. (1988). Quality of life in stage II breast cancer: An instrument for clinical trials. *Journal of Clinical Oncology, 6,* 1798–1810.

Lewandowski, W., & Jones, S. L. (1988). The family with cancer. *Cancer Nursing, 11*(6), 313–321.

Lewis, F. M. (1986). The impact of cancer on the family: A critical analysis of the research literature. *Patient Education and Counseling, 8,* 269–289.

Lewis, F. M., Ellison, E. S., & Woods, N. F. (1985). The impact of breast cancer on the family. *Seminars in Oncology Nursing, 1*(3), 206–213.

Lewis, F. M., & Hammond, M. A. (1992). Psychosocial adjustment of the family to breast cancer: A longitudinal analysis. *Journal of the American Medical Women's Association, 47*(5), 194–200.

Lewis, F. M., Hammond, M. A., & Woods, N. F. (1993). The family's functioning with newly diagnosed breast cancer in the mother: The development of an explanatory model. *Journal of Behavioral Medicine, 16*(4), 351–370.

Lichtman, R. R., Taylor, S. E., & Wood, J. V. (1984). Relation with children after breast cancer: the mother-daughter relationship at risk. *Journal of Psychosocial Oncology, 2,* 1–19.

Lierman, L. M. (1988). Phantom breast experiences after mastectomy. *Oncology Nursing Forum, 15,* 41–44.

Lippman, M. E., Sorace, R. A., Bagly, C., Danforth, D. W., Lichter, A., & Wesley, M. (1986). Treatment of locally advanced breast cancer using primary induction chemotherapy with hormonal synchronization followed by radiation with or without debulking surgery. *NCI Monographs, 1,* 153–159.

Livingston, R. B. (1994). Dose intensity and high dose therapy. Two different concepts. *Cancer, 74*(3), 1177–1183.

Ljung, B., Chew, K., Deng, G., Matsumura, K., Waldman, F., & Smith, H. (1994). Fine needle aspiration techniques for the characterization of breast cancers. *Cancer, 74,* 1000–1005.

Loprinzi, C. L., Duffy, J., & Ingle, J. N. (1993). Post chemotherapy rheumatism. *Journal of Clinical Oncology, 11,* 768–770.

Loprinzi, C. L., Michalak, C., Quella, S. K., O'Fallon, J. R., Hatfield, A. K., & Oesterling, J. E. (1994). Placebo controlled clinical trial of megestrol acetate (MA) in ameliorating hot flashes in both men and women: A North Central Cancer Treatment Group Study. *Proceedings of the American Society of Clinical Oncology, 13,* 432.

Lotze, M. T., Duncan, M. A., Gerber, L. H., Woltering, E. A., & Rosenberg, S. A. (1981). Early vs. delayed shoulder motion following axillary dissection. *Annals of Surgery, 193,* 288–295.

Love, R. R., Leventhal, H., Easterling, D. V., & Nerenz, D. R. (1989). Side effects and emotional distress during cancer chemotherapy. *Cancer, 63,* 604–612.

Loveys, B. J., & Kaich, K. (1991). Breast cancer: Demands of illness. *Oncology Nursing Forum, 18*(1), 75–80.

Lynch, H. T., Lynch, J., Conway, T., & Severin, M. (1994). Psychological aspects of monitoring high risk women for breast cancer. *Cancer, 74* (Suppl. 3), 1184–1192.

Mack, E., McGrath, T., Pendleton, D., & Zieber, N. A. (1993). Reaching poor populations with cancer prevention and early detection programs. *Cancer Practice, 1*(1), 35–39.

Maguire, P. (1981). The repercussions of mastectomy on the family. *International Journal of Family Psychiatry, 1,* 485–503.

Maguire, G. P., Tait, A., & Brooke, M. (1980). Psychiatric morbidity and physical toxicity associated with adjuvant chemotherapy after mastectomy. *British Medical Journal, 281,* 1179–1180.

Malone, K. E., Daling, J. R., & Weiss, N. S. (1993). Oral contraceptives in relation to breast cancer. *Epidemiologic Reviews, 15*(1), 80–97.

Mansour, E. G., Ravdin, P. M., & Dressler, L. (1994). Prognostic factors in early breast carcinoma. *Cancer, 74,* 381–400.

Margolis, G. J., Goodman, R. L., & Rubin, A., (1989). Psychological factors in the choice of treatment for breast cancer. *Psychosomatics, 30,* 192–197.

Margolis, G. J., Goodman, R. L., & Rubin, A. (1990). Psychological effects of breast conserving cancer treatment and mastectomy. *Psychosomatics, 31,* 33–39.

Markowski, J., Wilcox, J. P., & Helm, P. A. (1981). Lymphedema incidence after postmastectomy therapy. *Archives of Physical Medicine and Rehabilitation, 62,* 449–452.

Marks, L. B., Rosner, G. L., Prosnitz, L. R., Ross, M., Vredenburgh, J. J., & Peters, W. P. (1994). The impact of conventional plus high dose chemotherapy with autologous bone marrow transplantation on hematologic toxicity during subsequent local-regional radiotherapy for breast cancer. *Cancer, 74*(11), 2964–2971.

Marshburn, J., Bradham, D. D., Studnicki, J., Nemec, L., Luther, S., & Clark, R. A. (1994). Mass mammography screening. *Cancer Practice, 2*(2), 146–153.

Martinez, A. A., & Clarke, D. (1984). Treatment results, cosmesis and complications in stage I and II breast cancer patients treated by excisional biopsy and irradiation. In F. C. Ames, G. R. Blumenschein, & E. D. Montague (Eds.), *Current controversies in breast cancer* (pp. 369–381). Austin: University of Texas Press.

Maunsell, E., Brisson, J. & Deschénes, L. (1993). Arm problems and psychological distress after surgery for breast cancer. *Canadian Journal of Surgery, 36,* 315–320.

McCool, W. F. (1994). Barriers to breast cancer screening in older women. *Journal Nurse-Midwifery, 39*(5), 283–299.

McCorkle, M. R. (1973). Coping with physical symptoms in metastatic breast cancer. *American Journal of Nursing, 73*(6), 1034–1038.

McCormick, B. (1994). Selection criteria for breast conservation. The impact of young and old age and collagen vascular disease. *Cancer, 74*(Suppl. 1), 430–435.

McCormick, B., & Norton, L. (1994). The Recht/Harris/Come article reviewed. *Oncology, 8*(3), 32 & 37.

McCoy, C. B., Smith, S. A., Metsch, L. R., Anwyl, R. S., Correa, R., Bankston, L., & Zavertnik, J. J. (1994). Breast cancer screening of the medically underserved. *Cancer Practice, 2*(4), 267–274.

McHugh, N. G., Christman, N. J., & Johnson, J. (1982). Preparatory information: What helps and why. *American Journal of Nursing, 82,* 78–82.

McKhann, C. F., & Knobf, M. T. Unpublished data. (1985). Department of Surgery, Yale University School of Medicine.

McLelland, R., & Pisano, E. D. (1990). Issues in mammography. *Cancer, 66,* 1341–1344.

McNair, D. M., Lorr, M., & Droppleman, L. K. (1971). *Manual profile of mood states.* San Diego: Educational and Industrial Testing Service.

Mehta, R. R., Beattie, C. W., & DasGupta, T. K. (1991). Endocrine profile in breast cancer patients receiving adjuvant chemotherapy. *Breast Cancer Research and Treatment, 20,* 125–134.

Messerli, M. L., Garamedi, C., & Romano, J. (1980). Breast cancer: Information as a technique of crisis intervention. *American Journal of Orthopsychiatry, 50,* 728–731.

Mettlin, C. (1991). Research in cancer prevention and detection. In S. M. Hubbard, P. Greene, M. T. Knobf (Eds.), *Current issues in cancer nursing practice* (pp. 1–10). Philadelphia: J. B. Lippincott Co.

Mettlin, C., & Smart, C. R. (1994). Breast cancer detection guidelines for women aged 40 to 49 years: Rationale for the American Cancer Society reaffirmation of recommendations. *CA: A Cancer Journal for Clinicians, 44*(4), 248–255.

Meyer, L., & Aspergen, K. (1989). Long term psychological sequelae of mastectomy and breast conserving treatment for breast cancer. *Acta Oncology, 28,* 13–18.

Meyerowitz, B. E., Sparks, F. C., & Spears, I. K. (1979). Adjuvant chemotherapy for breast carcinoma: Psychosocial implications. *Cancer, 43,* 1613–1618.

Meyerowitz, B. E., Watkins, I. K., & Sparks, F. C. (1983). Quality of life for breast cancer patients receiving adjuvant chemotherapy. *American Journal of Nursing, 2,* 232–235.

Milbauer, A. J. (1994). An open letter to ONS members: Prescribing information for Nolvadex changes. *Oncology Nursing Forum, 21*(5), 815–816.

Miller, A. B., Howe, G. R., Sherman, G. J., Lindsay, J. P., Martin, S. A., Yaffe, J., Dinner, P. J., Risch, H. A., & Preston, D. L. (1989). Mortality from breast cancer after irradiation during fluoroscopic examinations in patients being treated for tuberculosis. *New England Journal of Medicine, 321:*1285–1289.

Miller, A. M., & Champion, V. L. (1993). Mammography in women ≥ 50 years of age. *Cancer Nursing, 16*(4), 260–269.

Miller, B. A., Feur, E. J., & Hankey, B. F. (1993). Recent incidence trends for breast cancer in women and the relevance of early detection: An update. *CA: A Cancer Journal for Clinicians, 43,* 27–41.

Mock, V., Burke, M. B., & Creaton, E. (1993). A nursing rehabilitation program for breast cancer patients receiving adjuvant chemotherapy. *Oncology Nursing Forum, 20*(2), 336.

Mooney, K., Nail, L., Richtsmeier, J., & Ward, J. (1994). Symptom and symptom distress associated with taking tamoxifen as chemo prevention for breast cancer. *Proceedings of the American Cancer Society Third Nursing Research Conference.* Atlanta: American Cancer Society.

Morra, M. E. (1985). Breast self-examination today: An overview of its use and value. *Seminars in Oncology Nursing, 1*(3), 170–175.

Morris, T. (1979). Psychological adjustment to mastectomy. *Cancer Treatment Reviews, 6*(1), 41–61.

Morris, T., Greer, H. S., & White, P. (1977). Psychological and social adjustment to mastectomy. A two-year follow-up study. *Cancer, 40,* 2381–2387.

Mukhopadhyay, M. G., & Larkin, S. (1986). Weight gain in cancer patients on chemotherapy. *Proceedings of the American Society for Clinical Oncology, 5,* 254 (Abstract No. 992).

Nagamani, M., Kelver, M., & Smith, E. R. (1987). Treatment of menopausal hot flashes with transdermal administration of clonidine. *American Journal of Obstetrics and Gynecology, 156,* 581–565.

Nail, L., Jones, L. S., Giuffre, M., & Johnson, J. E. (1984). Sensations after mastectomy. *American Journal of Nursing '84, 9,* 1121–1124.

National Women's Health Network. (1994). A tamoxifen alert becomes a tamoxifen crisis. (June newsletter.)

Nattinger, A. B., Gottlieb, M. S., Veum, J., Yahnke, D., & Goodwin, J. S. (1992). Geographic variation in the use of breast-conserving treatment for breast cancer. *New England Journal of Medicine, 326,* 1102–1107.

Nayfield, S. G., Bongiovanni, G. C., Alciati, M. H., Fischer, R. A., & Bergner, L. (1994). Statutory requirements for disclosure for breast cancer treatment alternatives. *Journal of the National Cancer Institute, 86*(16), 1202–1208.

Neufeld, K. R., Degner, L. F., & Dick, J. A. (1993). A nursing intervention strategy to foster patient involvement in treatment decision. *Oncology Nursing Forum, 20,* 631–635.

Nielsen, B., Miaskowski, C., & Dibble, S. (1993). Pain with mammography: Fact or fiction? *Oncology Nursing Forum, 20*(4), 639–642.

Nolvadex Adjuvant Trial Organization. (1988). Controlled trial of tamoxifen as single adjuvant agent in the management of early breast cancer. Analysis at eight years. *British Journal of Cancer, 57,* 608–611.

Noone, R. B., Frazier, T. G., Noone, G. C., Blanchet, N. P., Murphy, J. B., & Rose, D. (1994). Recurrence of breast carcinoma following immediate reconstruction: A 13 year review. *Plastic and Reconstructive Surgery, 93*(1), 96–106.

Noone, R. B., Murphy, J. B., Spear, S. L., & Little, J. W. (1985). A six year experience with immediate reconstruction after mastectomy for cancer. *Plastic and Reconstructive Surgery, 76,* 258–269.

Norby, P. (1990). Rehabilitation after conservative breast cancer surgery: Management of lymphedema and limited range of motion. *Oncology Nursing Forum, 17*(Suppl. 2), 209.

Northouse, L. L. (1981). Mastectomy patients and the fear of cancer recurrence. *Cancer Nursing, 4*(3), 213–220.

Northhouse, L. L. (1988). Social support in patient's and husband's adjustment to breast cancer. *Nursing Research, 37*(2), 91–95.

Northouse, L. L. (1989a). The impact of breast cancer on patients and husbands. *Cancer Nursing, 12*(5), 276–284.

Northouse, L. L. (1989b). A longitudinal study of the adjustment of patients and husbands to breast cancer. *Oncology Nursing Forum, 16*(4), 511–516.

Northouse, L. L., & Swain, M. A. (1987). Adjustment of patients and husbands to the initial impact of breast cancer. *Nursing Research, 36*(4), 221–225.

Norton, L. (1994). Salvage chemotherapy of breast cancer. *Seminars in Oncology, 21*(Suppl. 4), 19–24.

Oberst, M. T., & James, R. H. (1985). Going home: patient and spouse adjustment following cancer surgery. *Topics in Clinical Nursing, 7,* 46–57.

Offit, K., & Brown, K. (1994). Quantitative risk counseling for familial cancer: A resource for clinical oncologists. *Journal of Clinical Oncology, 12,* 1724–1736.

Omne-Ponten, M., Holmberg, L., & Sjoden, P. O. (1994). Psychosocial adjustment among women with breast cancer stages I and II: Six year follow-up of consecutive patients. *Journal of Clinical Oncology, 12*(8), 1778–1782.

Osborne, K. C. (1994). Current trials and future directions of the Southwest Oncology Group Breast Cancer Committee. *Cancer, 74,* 1135–1138.

Osteen, R. T., Steele, G. D., Menck, H. R., & Winchester, D. P. (1992). Regional differences in surgical management of breast cancer. *CA: A Cancer Journal for Clinicians, 42,* 39–43.

Ouriel, K., Lotze, M. T., & Hinshaw, J. R. (1984). Prognostic factors of carcinoma of the male breast. *Surgery, Gynecology and Obstetrics, 159,* 373–376.

Owens, R. G., Ashcroft, J. J., Leinster, S. J., & Slade, P. D. (1987). Informal decision analysis with breast cancer patients: An aid to psychological preparation for surgery. *Journal of Psychosocial Oncology, 5*(2), 23–33.

Page, D. L., DuPont, W. D., Rogers, L. W., & Landenberger, M. (1982). Intraductal carcinoma of the breast: Follow-up after biopsy only. *Cancer, 49,* 751–758.

Pasacreta, J., McCorkle, R., & Margolis, G. (1991). Psychosocial aspects of breast cancer. In B. Fowble, R. Goodman, J. Glick & E. Rosato (Eds.), *Breast cancer treatment* (pp. 551–570). St. Louis: Mosby-Year Book.

Patz, E. F., Peters, W. P., & Goodman, P. C. (1994). Pulmonary drug toxicity following high-dose chemotherapy with autologous bone marrow transplantation: CT findings in 20 cases. *Journal of Thoracic Imaging, 9*(2), 129–134.

Paulus, D. D. (1987). Imaging in breast cancer. *CA: A Cancer Journal for Clinicians, 37*(3), 133–150.

Pearson, O. H., Hubay, C. A., Gordon, N. H., Marshall, J. S., Crowe, J. P., Arafah, B. M., & McQuire, W. (1989). Endocrine versus endocrine plus five-drug chemotherapy in postmenopausal women with stage II estrogen receptor-positive breast cancer. *Cancer, 64,* 1819–1823.

Peters, W. P., Ross, M., Vredenburgh, J. J., Hussein, A., Rubin, P., Dukelow, K., Cavanaugh, C., Beauvais, R., & Kaprzak, S. (1994). The use of intensive clinic support to permit outpatient autologous bone marrow transplantation for breast cancer. *Seminars in Oncology, 21*(Suppl. 4), 25–31.

Petrek, J. A. (1987). Surgery for metastatic disease. In J. R. Harris, S. Hellman, I. C. Henderson, & D. W. Kinne (Eds.), *Breast diseases* (pp. 391–394). Philadelphia: J. B. Lippincott Co.

Pfeiffer, C. H., & Mullikne, J. B. (1984). Caring for the patient with breast cancer. Reston, VA: Reston Publishing.

Pierce, P. (1993). Deciding on breast cancer treatment: A description of decision behavior. *Nursing Research, 42,* 22–28.

Pike, M. C., Spiar, D. J., Dahmoush, L., & Press, M. F. (1993). Estrogens, progestins, normal breast cell proliferation, and breast cancer risk. *Epidemiologic Reviews, 15*(1), 17–35.

Piper, B., Friedman, L., Hartigan, K., Post, B., & Smith, J. (1989). Fatigue patterns over time in women receiving CMF chemotherapy for breast cancer. *Oncology Nursing Society, 16* (Suppl.), 217 (Abstract No. 355).

Piper, B. F., Lindsey, A. M., Dodd, M. J., Ferketich, S., MacVicar, M., & Paul, S. (1993). Patterns and predictors of chronic fatigue in women receiving six cycles of adjuvant chemotherapy for breast cancer [Abstract]. *Oncology Nursing Forum, 20*(2), 342.

Plowman, P. N. (1988). Treatment of menopausal symptoms in breast cancer patients. *Lancet, 2*(8603), 164.

Polinsky, M. L. (1994). Functional status of long term breast cancer survivors: Demonstrating chronicity. *Health and Social Work, 19*(3), 165–173.

Pool, K. N., & Judkins, A. F. (1990). A health investment that may save your life. *Cancer Nursing, 13*(6), 329–334.

Porkka, K., Blomqvist, C., Rissanen, P., Elomma, I., & Pyrhonen, S. (1994). Salvage therapies in women who fail first line treatment with fluorouracil, epirubicin and cyclophosphamide for advanced breast cancer. *Journal of Clinical Oncology, 12*(8), 1639–1647.

Powles, T. J., Hardy, J. R., Ashley, S. E., Cosgrove, D., Davey, J. B., Dowsett, M., MacKinna, A., Nash, A. G., Rundle, S. K., Sinnett, D., Tillyer, C. R., & Treleaven, J. G. (1989). Chemo prevention of breast cancer. *Breast Cancer Research and Treatment, 14,* 23–31.

Priestman, T. J., & Baum, M. (1976). Evaluation of quality of life in patients receiving treatment for advanced breast cancer. *Lancet, 1,* 1899–900.

Pritchard, K. I. (1987). Current status of adjuvant endocrine therapy for resectable breast cancer. *Seminars in Oncology, 14,* 23–33.

Pritchard, K. I. (1994). Clinical coopertive trials of the National Cancer Institute of Canada Clinical Trials Group Breast Cancer Site Group. *Cancer, 74,* 1150–1155.

Quint, J. C. (1963). The impact of mastectomy. *American Journal of Nursing, 63*(11), 88–93.

Rajkumar, T., & Gullick, W. J. (1994). The type I growth factor receptors in human breast cancer. *Breast Cancer Research and Treatment, 29*(1), 3–9.

Rasbridge, S. A., Gillett, C. E., Seymour, A. M., Patel, K., Richards, M. A., Rubens, R. D., Millis, R. R. (1994). The effects of chemotherapy on morphology, cellular proliferation, apoptosis and oncoprotein expression in primary breast cancer. *British Journal of Cancer, 70*(2), 335–341.

Ravdin, P. M. (1994). A practical view of prognostic factors for staging adjuvant treatment planning and as baseline studies for possible future therapy. *Hematology-Oncology Clinics of North America, 8*(1), 197–211.

Razis, E. D., Samonis, G., Cook P., Beer, M., Mittelman, A., Lake, D. E., Feldman, E. J., Puccio, C., & Ahmed, T. (1994). TMJ: A well tolerated high-dose regimen for the adjuvant chemotherapy of high risk breast cancer. *Journal of Medicine, 25*, 241–250.

Recht, A., Harris, J. R., & Come, S. E. (1994). Sequencing of irradiation and chemotherapy for early-stage breast cancer. *Oncology, 8*(3), 19–30.

Reese, J. L. (1990). Nursing interventions for wound healing in plastic and reconstructive surgery. *Nursing Clinics of North America, 25*, 223–233.

Ressler, H., Rimer, B., Devine, P. J., Gatenby, R. A., & Engstrom, P. F. (1991). Corporate-sponsored breast cancer screening at the work site: Results of a statewide program. *Radiology, 179*, 107–110.

Reyno, L. M., Levine, M. N., Skingley, P., Arnold, A., & AbuZara, H. (1992). Chemotherapy induced amenorrhea in a randomized trial of adjuvant chemotherapy duration in breast cancer. *European Journal of Cancer, 29A*, 21–23.

Reynolds, H. E., & Jackson, V. P. (1991). The role of ultrasound in breast imaging. *Applied Radiology, 11*, 55–59.

Rimer, B. K., Keintz, M. K., Kessler, H. B., Engstrom, P. F., & Rosan, J. R. (1989). Why women resist screening mammography: Patient related barriers. *Radiology, 172*, 243, 246.

Rimer, B. K., Resch, N., King, E., Ross, E., Leman, C., Bryce, A., Kessler, H., & Engstrom, P. F. (1992). Multistrategy health education program to increase mammography use among women ages 65 and older. *Public Health Reports, 107*(4), 369–380.

Rinehart, M. E. (1994). The "Reach to Recovery" program. *Cancer, 74* (Suppl. 1), 372–375.

Ringer, K. E. (1983). *Coping with chemotherapy.* Ann Arbor: UMI Research.

Rivkin, S., Green, S., Metch, B., Cruz, A., McDivitt, R., Knight, W., Glick, J., & Osborne, K. (1990). Adjuvant combination chemotherapy (CMFVP) vs tamoxifen (Tam) vs CMFVP + TAM for postmenopausal women with ER + operable breast cancer and positive axillary lymph nodes: An Intergroup study [abstract]. *Proceedings of the American Society of Clinical Oncology, 9*, 24.

Romieu, I., Berlin, J. A., & Colditz, G. (1990). Oral contraceptives and breast cancer. *Cancer, 66*, 2253–2263.

Rose, C., Mouridsen, H. T., Thorpe, S. M., Anderson, J., Bilchert-Toft, M., & Anderson, K. W. (1985). Anti-estrogen treatment of postmenopausal breast cancer patients with high risk of recurrence: 72 months of life table analysis and steroid hormone receptor status. *World Journal of Surgery, 9*, 765–774.

Rose, D. P., & Davis, T. E. (1980). Effects of adjuvant chemohormonal therapy on the ovarian and adrenal function of breast cancer patients. *Cancer Research, 40*, 4043–4047.

Rosen, P. O., Braun, D. W., & Kinne, D. E. (1980). The clinical significance of preinvasive breast carcinoma. *Cancer, 46*, 919–925.

Rosenberg, L., Metzger, L. S., & Palmer, J. R. (1993). Alcohol consumption and risk of breast cancer: A review of epidemiological evidence. *Epidemiologic Reviews, 15*(1), 133–144.

Rowland, J. H., Holland, J. C., Chaglassian, T., & Kinne, D. (1993). Psychological response to breast reconstruction: Expectations for and impact on postmastectomy functioning. *Psychosomatics, 34*(3), 241–250.

Rubin, E., Frank, M. S., Stanley, R. J., Bernreuter, W. K., & Han, S. Y. (1990). Patient initiated mobile mammography. *Southern Medical Journal, 83*(2), 178–184.

Russell, I. S., Collins, J. P., Holmes, A. D., & Smith, J. A. (1990). The use of tissue expansion for immediate reconstruction after mastectomy. *Medical Journal of Australia, 152*, 632–635.

Rutledge, D. N., & Davis, G. T. (1988). Breast self-examination in compliance and the health belief model. *Oncology Nursing Forum, 15*, 175–179.

Rutqvist, L. E., Cedermark, B., Glas, U., Johansson, H., Nordenskjold, B., Skoog., L., Somell, A., Theve, T., Friberg, S., & Askergen, J. (1987). The Stockholm trial on adjuvant tamoxifen in early breast cancer. Correlation between estrogen receptor level and treatment effect. *Breast Cancer Research and Treatment, 10*, 255–266.

Sabo, D., Brown, J., & Smith, C. (1986). The male role and mastectomy: Support groups and men's adjustment. *Journal of Psychosocial Oncology, 4*(1/2), 19–31.

Sales, E. (1991). Psychosocial impact of the phase of cancer on the family: An updated review. *Journal of Psychosocial Oncology, 9*(4), 1–18.

Samaan, N. A., deAsis, D. W., Buzdar, A. U., & Blumenstein, G. R. (1978). Pituitary-ovarian function in breast cancer patients on adjuvant chemoimmunotherapy. *Cancer, 41*, 2084–2087.

Sanger, C. K., & Reznikoff, M. (1981). A comparison of the psychological effects of breast saving procedures with modified radical mastectomy. *Cancer, 48*, 2341–2346.

Sauter, E. R., Eisenberg, B. L., Hoffman, J. P., Ottery, F. D., Boraas, M. C., Goldstein, L. J., Solin, L. J. (1993). Post mastectomy morbidity after combination preoperative irradiation and chemotherapy for locally advanced breast cancer. *World Journal of Surgery, 17*(2), 237–241.

Say, C. C., & Donegan, W. (1974). A biostatistical evaluation of complications from mastectomy. *Surgery, Gynecology and Obstetrics, 138*, 370–376.

Schain, W. S., d'Angelo, T., Dunn, M. E., Lichter, N. S., & Pierce, L. J. (1994). Mastectomy versus conservative surgery and radiation therapy. *Cancer, 73*, 1221–1228.

Schain, W. S., Edwards, B. K., Gottell, C., Moss, E. V., Lippman, M. E., Gerber, L., & Lichter, A. S. (1983). Psychosocial and physical outcomes of primary breast cancer therapy: Mastectomy vs. excisional biopsy and irradiation. *Breast Cancer Research and Treatment, 3*, 377–382.

Schain, W. S., Wellisch, D. K., Pasnau, R. O., & Landsverk, J. (1985). The sooner the better: A study of psychological factors in women undergoing immediate versus delayed breast reconstruction. *American Journal of Psychology, 142*, 40–46.

Schmidt, R. A. (1994). Stereotactic breast biopsy. *CA: A Cancer Journal for Clinicians, 44*(3), 172–191.

Schottenfeld, D., & Robbins, G. F. (1970). Quality of survival among patients who have had radical mastectomy. *Cancer, 28*(5), 650–654.

Schover, L. R. (1991). The impact of breast cancer on sexuality, body image and intimate relationships. *CA: A Cancer Journal for Clinicians, 41,* 112–120.

Scott, D. (1983). Anxiety, critical thinking, and information processing during and after breast biopsy. *Nursing Research, 32,* 24–28.

Scottish Cancer Trial. (1987). Adjuvant tamoxifen in the management of operable breast cancer: The Scottish trial—report from the Breast Cancer Trials Committee. *Lancet, 2,* 171–175.

Scottish Cancer Trials Breast Cancer Group. (1993). Adjuvant ovarian ablation versus CMF chemotherapy in premenopausal women with pathological stage II breast carcinoma: The Scottish trial. *Lancet, 341*(8856), 1293–1298.

Senofsky, G. M., Davies, R. J., Olson, L., Skully, P., & Olshen, R. (1990). The predictive value of needle localization mammographically assisted biopsy of the breast. *Surgery, Gynecology and Obstetrics, 171*(5), 361–365.

Senofsky, G. M., Wanebo, H. J., Wilhelm, M. L., Pope, T. L., Fechner, R. E., & Kaiser, D. L. (1986). Has monitoring the contralateral breast improved the prognosis in patients treated for primary breast cancer? *Cancer, 57,* 597–602.

Shannon-Bodner, R. M., & Flynn, K. T. (1987). Symptom distress of women treated with conservative surgery and primary radiation therapy for carcinoma of the breast. *Oncology Nursing Forum, 14* (Suppl.), Abstract No. 234.

Shattuck-Eidens, D., McClure, M., Simard, J., Labrie, F., Narod, S., Couch, F., Hoskins, K., Weber, B., Castilla, L., Erdos, M., Brody, L., Friedman, L., Ostermeyer, E., Szabo, C., King, M., Jhanwar, S., Offit, K., Norton, L., Gilwski, T., Lubin, M., Osborne, M., Black, D., Boyd, M., Steel, M., Ingles, S., Haile, R., Lindblom, A., Olsson, H., Borg, A., Bishop, T., Soloman, E., Radice, P., Spatti, G., Gayther, S., Ponder, B., Warren, W., Stratton, M., Liu, Q., Fujimura, F., Lewis, C., Skolnick, M., & Goldgar, D. (1995). A collaborative survey of 80 mutations in the BRCA1 breast and ovarian cancer susceptibility gene: Implications for presymptomatic testing and screening. *JAMA, 273*(7), 535–541.

Shaw, C. R., Wilson, S. A., & O'Brien, M. E. (1994). Information needs prior to breast biopsy. *Clinical Nursing Research, 3*(2), 119–131.

Silberfarb, P. M., & Mauer, L. H. (1980). Psychosocial aspects of disease: Functional status of breast cancer patients during different treatment regimens. *American Journal of Psychiatry, 17*(4), 450–455.

Silverstein, M., Waisman, J. R., Gamagami, P., Gierson, E. D., Colburn, W. J., Rosser, R. J., Gordon, P. S., Lewinsky, B. S., & Fingerhut, A. (1990). Intraductal carcinoma of the breast (208 cases). *Cancer, 66*(1), 102–108.

Slamon, D. J., Godolphin, W., Jones, L. A., Holt, J. A., Wong, S. G., Keith, D. E., Levin, W. J., Stuart, S. G., Udove, J., Ullrich, A., & Press, M. F. (1989). Studies of HER-2/*neu* proto-oncogene in human breast and ovarian cancer. *Science, 244,* 707–712.

Smith, P. E. (1992). Familial breast and ovarian cancers. *Seminars in Oncology Nursing, 8*(4), 258–264.

Somlo, G., Doroshow, J. H., Forman, S. J., Leong, L. A., Margolin, K. A., Morgan, R. J., Raschko, J. W., Alman, S. A., Ahn, C., & Sniecinski, I. (1994). High dose cisplatin, etoposide and cyclophosphamide with autologous stem cell reinfusion in patients with responsive metastatic or high risk primary breast cancer. *Cancer, 73*(1), 125–134.

Sondik, E. J. (1994). Breast cancer trends: Incidence, mortality and survival. *Cancer, 74*(Suppl. 3), 995–999.

Spear, S. L., Conuit, R., & Little, J. W. (1989). Intradermal tattoo as an adjunct to nipple areola reconstruction. *Plastic and Reconstructive Surgery, 83,* 907–911.

Stadtmauer, E. A. (1991). Bone marrow transplantation for breast cancer. In B. Fowble, R. L. Goodman, J. H. Glick, & E. F. Rosato (Eds.), *Breast cancer treatment* (pp. 489–506). St. Louis: Mosby-Year Book.

Stefanek, M. E. (1990). Counseling women at high risk for breast cancer. *Oncology, 4*(1), 27–37.

Steinberg, M. D., Juliano, M. A., & Wise, L. (1985). Psychological outcome of lumpectomy versus mastectomy in the treatment of breast cancer. *American Journal of Psychiatry, 142,* 34–39.

Stemmer, S. M., Stears, J. C., Burton, B. S., Jones, R. B., & Simon, J. H. (1994). White matter changes in patients with breast cancer treated with high dose chemotherapy and autologous bone marrow support. *American Journal of Neuroradiology, 15*(7), 1267–1273.

Stevens, L. A., McGrath, M. H., Druss, R. C., Kister, S. J., Gump, F. E., & Forde, K. A. (1984). The psychological impact of immediate breast reconstruction for women with early breast cancer. *Plastic and Reconstructive Surgery, 73,* 619–628.

Stillman, M. J. (1977). Women's health beliefs about breast cancer and breast self-examination. *Nursing Research, 26,* 121–127.

Stillwell, G. K. (1969). Treatment of postmastectomy lymphedema. *Modern Treatment, 6,* 396–412.

Stomper, P. C., & Margolin, F. R. (1994). Ductal carcinoma in situ: The mammographer's perspective. *American Journal Roentgenology, 162*(3), 585–591.

Subramanian, V. P., Raich, P. C., & Walker, B. K. (1981). Weight gain in breast cancer patients undergoing chemotherapy. *Breast Cancer Research and Treatment, 1,* Abstract No. 170.

Swain, S. M., Sorace, R. A., Bagley, C. S., Danforth, D. H., Bader, J., Wesley, M. N., Steinberg, S. M., & Lippman, M. E. (1987). Neoadjuvant chemotherapy in combined modality approach of locally advanced non-metastic breast cancer. *Cancer Research, 47,* 3889–3894.

Swenerton, K. D., Legha, S. S., Smith, T., Hortobagyi, G. N., Gehan, E. A., Yap, H., Guttermne, J. U., & Blumenschein, G. R. (1979). Prognostic factors in metastatic breast cancer treated with combination chemotherapy. *Cancer Research, 39,* 1552–1562.

Tandon, A. K., Clark, G. M., Chamness, G. C., Ullrich, A., & McGuire, W. L. (1989). HER-2/*neu* oncogene protein and prognosis in breast cancer. *Journal of Clinical Oncology, 7,* 1120–1128.

Tarpy, C., & Rothwell, S. (1983). Menses and related menopausal symptomatology of the breast cancer patient on chemotherapy. *Proceedings of the Oncology Nursing Society,* Abstract No. 15, p. 50.

Taylor, S. E., Lichtman, R. R., Wood, J. V., Bluming, A. Z., Dosik, G. M., & Leibowitz, R. L. (1985). Illness-related and treatment-related factors in psychological adjustment to breast cancer. *Cancer, 55,* 2506–2513.

Teeple, C. (1987). *Symptoms associated with primary radiation therapy for breast cancer: The six week experience.* Unpublished master's thesis, Yale University School of Nursing, New Haven, CT.

Thomas, D. B. (1993a). Breast cancer in men. *Epidemiologic Reviews, 15*(1), 220–231.

Thomas, D. B. (1993b). Oral contraceptives and breast cancer. *Journal of the National Cancer Institute, 85*(5), 359–364.

Thomas, S. G. (1978). Breast cancer: The psychosocial issues. *Cancer Nursing, 1*, 53–60.

Tobin, M. P., Lacey, H. J., Meyer, L., & Mortimer, P. S. (1993). The psychological morbidity of breast cancer-related arm swelling: Psychological morbidity of lymphedema. *Cancer, 72*(1), 3248–3253.

Treves, N. (1957). Lymphedema after radical mastectomy. *Cancer, 10*, 444–459.

Tripathy, D., & Benz, C. (1994). Growth factors and their receptors. *Hematology-Oncology Clinics of North America, 8*(1), 29–50.

U.S. Department of Health and Human Services. (1994). *Clinical Practice Guideline. Quality Determinants of Mammography* (AHCPR Publication No. 95-0632, pp. 23–24). Rockville, MD: Author.

Valagussa, P., Zambetti, M., & Bonadonna, G. (1990). Prognostic factors in locally advanced noninflammatory breast cancer. Long term results following primary chemotherapy. *Breast Cancer Research and Treatment, 15*, 137–147.

Valanis, B. G., & Rumpler, C. H. (1985). Helping women choose breast cancer treatment alternatives. *Cancer Nursing, 8*, 167–175.

Varricchio, C. G., & Johnson, K. A. (1993). The use of tamoxifen in the prevention and treatment of breast cancer. In S. M. Hubbard, P. Greene & M. T. Knobf, (Eds.), *Current issues in cancer nursing practice* (pp. 1–10). Philadelphia: J. B. Lippincott.

Vaughn, W. P., Reed, E. C., Edwards, B., & Kessinger, A. (1994). High-dose cyclophosphamide, thiotepa and hydroxyurea with autologous hematopoietic stem cell rescue: An effective consolidation chemotherapy regimen for early metastatic breast cancer. *Bone Marrow Transplantation, 13*(5), 619–624.

Veronesi, U., Saccozzi, R., DelVecchio, M., Banfi, A., Clemente, C., & Delena, M. (1981). Comparing radical mastectomy and quadrantectomy, axillary dissection and radiotherapy in patients with small cancers of the breast. *New England Journal of Medicine, 305*, 6–11.

Vess, J. D., Moreland, J. R., & Schwebel, A. I. (1985). An empirical assessment of the effects of cancer on family role functioning. *Journal of Psychosocial Oncology, 3*(1), 1–16.

Vess, J. D., Moreland, J. R., Schwebel, A. I., & Kraut, E. (1988). Psychosocial needs of cancer patients: Learning from patients and their spouses. *Journal of Psychosocial Oncology, 6*(1-2), 31–51.

Vogel, V. G., Graves, D. S., Coody, D. K., Winn, R. J., & Peters, G. N. (1990). Breast screening compliance following a statewide low-cost mammography project. *Cancer Detection and Prevention, 14*, 573–576.

Vogel, V. G., Graves, D. S., Vernon, S. W., Lord, J. A., Winn, R. J., & Peters, G. N. (1990). Mammographic screening of women with increased risk of breast cancer. *Cancer, 66*, 1613–1620.

Walsh, B., & Schiff, I. (1990). Vasomotor flushes. *New York Academy of Sciences, 592*, 346–356.

Ward, S., Heidrich, S., & Wolberg, W. (1989). Factors women take into account when deciding upon type of surgery for breast cancer. *Cancer Nursing, 12*, 344–351.

Ward, S. E., Viergutz, G., Tormey, D., deMuth, J., & Paulen, A. (1992). Patients' reactions to completion of adjuvant breast cancer therapy. *Nursing Research, 41*(6), 362–366.

Warren, B., & Pohl, J. M. (1990). Cancer screening practices of nurse practitioners. *Cancer Nursing, 13*(3), 143–151.

Weber, B. L., Abel, K., Brody, L. C., Flejter, W. L., Chandrasekharappa, S. C., Couch, F. J., Merajver, S. D., & Collings, F. S. (1994). Familial breast cancer. *Cancer, 74*(3), 1013–1020.

Weidner, N., Folleman, J., Pozza, F., Bevilacqua, P., Allred, E. N., Moore, D. H., Meli, S., & Gasparini, G. (1992). Tumor androgenesis: A new significant and independent prognostic indicator in early stage breast carcinoma. *Journal of the National Cancer Institute, 84*(24), 1875–1887.

Weidner, N., Semple, J. P., Welch, W. R., & Folkman, J. (1991). Tumor angiogenesis and metastases: Correlation in invasive breast carcinoma. *New England Journal of Medicine, 324*(1), 1–8.

Weiss, M. C., & Kelstein, M. L. (1991). Biologic markers of breast cancer prognosis. In B., Fowble, R. L. Goodman, J. H. Glick, & E. F. Rosato (Eds.), *Breast cancer treatment* (pp. 209–242). St. Louis: Mosby-Year Book.

Wellisch, D. (1981). Family relationships of the mastectomy patient: Interactions with the spouse and children. *Israeli Journal of Medical Science, 17*, 993–996.

Wellisch, D. K., Jamison, K. R., & Pasnau, R. O. (1978). Psychosocial aspects of mastectomy II. The man's perspective. *American Journal of Psychiatry, 135*, 543–546.

Wellisch, D. K., Schain, W. S., Noone, R. B., & Little, J. W. (1985). Psychosocial correlates of immediate versus delayed reconstruction of the breast. *Plastic and Reconstructive Surgery, 76*, 713–718.

White, E., Lee, C. Y., & Kristal, A. R. (1990). Evaluation of the increase in breast cancer incidence in relation to mammography use. *Journal of the National Cancer Institute, 82*, 1546–1552.

Wile, A. G., Opfell, R. W., & Margileth, D. A. (1993). Hormone replacement therapy in previously treated breast cancer patients. *American Journal of Surgery, 165*, 372–375.

Wiley, R. R. (1981). Postbiopsy care. *American Journal of Nursing '81, 9*, 1660–1662.

Willett, W. C., & Hunter, D. J. (1994). Prospective studies of diet and breast cancer. *Cancer, 74* (Suppl. 3), 1085–1089.

Willits, M. J. (1994). Role of "Reach to Recovery" in breast cancer. *Cancer, 74* (Suppl. 7), 2172–2173.

Wilson, R. E. (1984). Evaluation of the woman with a breast mass. In C. H. Pfeiffer & J. B. Mulliken (Eds.), *Caring for the patient with breast cancer* (pp. 21–35). Reston, VA: Reston Publishing.

Winchester, D. P. (1990). Evaluation and management of breast abnormalities. *Cancer, 66*, 1245–1347.

Winchester, D. P., & Cox, J. D. (1992). Standards for breast conservation treatment. *CA: A Cancer Journal for Clinicians, 42*, 134–162.

Wingo, P. A., Tong, T., & Bolden, S. (1995). Cancer statistics, 1995. *CA: A Cancer Journal for Clinicians, 45*, 8–30.

Winningham, M. L., & MacVicar, M. G. (1988). The effect of aerobic exercise on patient reports of nausea. *Oncology Nursing Forum, 15*, 447–450.

Winningham, M. L., MacVicar, M. G., Bondoc, M., Anderson, J. I., & Minton, J. P. (1989). Effect of aerobic exercise on body weight and composition in patients with breast cancer on adjuvant chemotherapy. *Oncology Nursing Forum, 16*, 683–689.

Wolberg, W. H., Romsaas, E. P., Tanner, M. A., & Malec, J. F. (1989). Psychosexual adaptation to breast cancer surgery. *Cancer, 63*, 1645–1655.

Wolosin, R. J. (1989). The experience of screening mammography. *Journal of Family Practice, 29*(5), 499–502.

Wolosin, R. J. (1990). Effect of appointment scheduling and reminder postcards on adherence to mammography recommendations. *Journal of Family Practice, 30*(5), 542–547.

Wood, W. C. (1994). Current trials and future directions of the Eastern Cooperative Oncology Group Breast Cancer Committee. *Cancer, 74,* 1132–1134.

Wood, W. C., Budman, D. R., Korzun, A. H., Cooper, M. R., Younger, J., Hart, R. D., Moore, A., Ellerton, J. A., Norton, L., Ferree, C. R., Ballow, A. C., Frei, T., & Henderson, I. C. (1994). Dose and dose intensity of adjuvant chemotherapy for stage II, node positive breast carcinoma. *New England Journal of Medicine, 330*(8), 1253–1259.

Woods, N. F., & Earp, J. L. (1978). Women with cured breast cancer. *Nursing Research, 27*(5), 279–285.

Wyatt, G., Kurtz, M. E., & Liken, M. (1993). Breast cancer survivors: An exploration of quality of life issues. *Cancer Nursing, 16*(6), 440–448.

Young, R. L., Kumar, N. S., & Goldzieher, J. W. (1990). Management of menopause when estrogen cannot be used. *Drugs, 40,* 220–230.

Zahlis, E. H., & Shands, M. E. (1991). Breast cancer: Demands of the illness on the patient's partner. *Journal of Psychosocial Oncology, 9*(1), 75–93.

Zahlis, E. H., & Shands, M. E. (1993). The impact of breast cancer on the partner 18 months after diagnosis. *Seminars in Oncology Nursing, 9*(2), 83–87.

Zambetti, M., Valagussa, P., & Bonadonna, G. (1992). Eight-year results with adjuvant intravenous CMF in node-negative (N-) and estrogen receptor-negative (ER-) breast cancer. *Proceedings of the American Society of Clinical Oncology, 11,* 61.

Zapka, J. G., Hosmer, D., Costanza, M. E., Harris, D. R., & Stoddard, A. (1992). Changes in mammography use: Economic, need and service factors. *American Journal of Public Health, 82*(10), 1345–1351.

Zeissler, R. H., Rose, G. B., & Nelson, P. A. (1972). Postmastectomy lymphedema: Late results of treatment in 385 patients. *Archives of Physical Medicine and Rehabilitation, 53,* 159–166.

Zumoff, B. (1993). Biological and endocrinological insights into the possible breast cancer risk from menopausal estrogen replacement therapy. *Steroids, 58,* 196–204.

Lung Cancer

Ada M. Lindsey • Linda Sarna

Lung cancer, incidence and mortality, has increased more than any other single cancer in the past 20 years and has masked the declining incidence of other cancers (Garfinkle & Silverberg, 1991). An estimated 172,000 new cases of lung cancer (72,000 in women), and 153,000 lung cancer deaths (59,000 deaths in women) were projected for 1994 (Ries et al., 1994). Mortality rates for lung cancer are similar to incidence rates because early diagnosis is infrequent and treatment for advanced disease is ineffective, resulting in overall poor survival. The current 5-year survival rate for all stages of lung cancer is 10 to 13 per cent (Boring, Squires, Tong, & Montgomery, 1994; Rubin, 1991). Since 1987, lung cancer has been the leading cause of cancer deaths in the United States in both men and women. A very large majority of the lung cancers occur in smokers. In one of the longest ongoing studies investigating the relationship of tobacco to mortality, risk of lung cancer for current smokers was 15 times that of nonsmokers (increasing to 25 times the risk for heavy smokers), and decreasing to four times the risk for former smokers (Doll, Peto, Wheatley, Gray, & Sutherland, 1994). However, only 10 to 13 per cent of cigarette smokers develop lung cancer (Haque, 1991; Peto et al., 1994). Lung cancer and other smoking-related causes of death eventually kill 50 per cent of all smokers; these other causes remove some smokers prematurely from risk of developing lung cancer (Peto, Lopez, Boreham, Thun, & Heath, 1994). In addition to exposure to smoking and other carcinogenic agents, there is some evidence suggesting a genetic predisposition to the development of lung cancer (Haque, 1991; Hinson & Perry, 1993).

There are two major classifications of bronchogenic carcinoma: small-cell lung cancer (SCLC) and non-small-cell lung cancer (non-SCLC). The non-SCLCs are further classified as squamous cell or epidermoid lung cancer, adenocarcinoma, and large-cell carcinoma. The ratio of incidence of non-SCLC to SCLC is 3 to 1. In the United States, the incidence of adenocarcinoma has increased, and that of squamous cell carcinoma has decreased (Reyes, Chua, & Aranha, 1987; Valaitis, Warren, & Gamble, 1981). The increase is occurring in both men and women, but women have a propensity for developing adenocarcinoma (Choi, Grillo, & Huberman, 1986). Thus the increased incidence of lung cancer in women partially accounts for the change in relative frequency of adenocarcinoma.

RISK FACTORS AND INCIDENCE

The primary risk factor in the development of bronchogenic carcinoma is longer total exposure to cigarette smoking (including number of cigarettes smoked, age when smoking began, duration of smoking, and tar and nicotine content of cigarettes smoked) (Table 30–1) (Garfinkle & Silverberg, 1991; Loeb, Ernster, Warner, Abbotts, & Laszio, 1984; Stayner & Wegman, 1983). The population at greatest risk for developing lung cancer currently is older male smokers; this may change with the increase in female smokers.

Data available suggest that in addition to cigarette smoking and exposure to second hand smoke, industrial and environmental pollutants are risk factors for lung cancer development. Other carcinogenic

TABLE 30–1. *Risk Factors in Development of Lung Cancer*

Cigarette smoking
Second hand smoke
Industrial and environmental pollutants
    Asbestos
    Ionizing radiation
    Hydrocarbons
    Metals (e.g., nickel, silver, chromium)
    Chloromethyl ethers

substances associated with increased risk include asbestos, ionizing radiation, hydrocarbons, chromium, and nickel (Filderman, Shaw, & Matthay, 1986; Frank, 1982). Asbestos exposure in cigarette smokers increases the risk of lung cancer 80 to 90 times (Craighead & Mossman, 1982). Older men and women who have been smoking at least a pack of cigarettes a day for most of their lives and men and women who have been exposed to cigarette smoking and occupational or environmental carcinogens are at risk for developing lung cancer. These individuals remain at risk even after the exposure is removed because the development of lung cancer is a long-term process.

A smoker's risk of developing lung cancer decreases from a sixteenfold to about a fivefold increase approximately 5 years after cessation of smoking and in 15 years approaches the risk of developing lung cancer for those who have never smoked (Doll & Hill, 1964; Halpern, Gillespie, & Warner, 1993; U. S. Department of Health and Human Services, 1990). Thus following cessation of smoking, the risk of developing lung cancer progressively decreases for 10 to 15 years. The role of passive smoking in the development of lung cancer in nonsmokers was studied by pooling data from three large investigations. The risk was greater for older women whose husbands were heavy smokers: the histologic types of cancer that occurred were squamous and small-cell carcinomas (Dalager et al., 1986). Recently the Environmental Protection Agency recog-

nized the role of passive smoking in lung cancer development (U.S. Environmental Protection Agency, 1992). An additional 3000 lung cancer deaths occur each year in nonsmokers due to second hand smoke.

The rates of lung cancer are higher among those who consume alcohol and those in the lower socioeconomic groups. Because cigarette smoking and alcohol consumption are associated with greater risk for development of (lung) cancer, Marino and Levy (1986) proposed health promotion as a requisite for primary cancer prevention in pediatric practice.

Considerable interest has been shown in the role of diet in the prevention of cancer and the inhibition of tumor growth. Although some specific dietary constituents have been associated with some cancers, very little evidence supports any dietary constituent as having a preventive role in lung cancer development (Colditz, Stampfer, & Willett, 1987). Refer to Chapter 16 on chemoprevention for additional information. Refer to Chapter 12 for more detail on the causes of cancer.

GENDER AND LUNG CANCER

Historically, lung cancer was not considered a high-risk cancer for women. Over the past 20 years, lung cancer rates among women have soared, primarily due to the aftermath of increased smoking prevalence among women (Table 30–2). Since 1973, age-specific mortality in women aged 65 years and older has increased over 200 per cent (58.2 in 1973 to 181.7 per 100,000 in 1991) (Ries et al., 1994). Increases have been less dramatic among men; however, the prevalence among men is greater (Fig. 30–1 and Table 30–3). The lag in decreasing smoking prevalence among women as compared with men suggests continued tobacco-related morbidity and mortality among women in decades to come (Novotny et al., 1990). Based on current analysis of smoking and mortality, tobacco-related mortality for women in the United States will exceed that of men after the turn of the century (Peto, Lopez, Boreham, Thun, & Heath, 1992).

TABLE 30–2. *Increases in Lung Cancer Incidence Rates per 100,000 by Gender, Age, and Race, 1973–1991*

	1973–1974	1990–1991	% CHANGE
Female	19.1	41.6	118.0
0–54 yrs	6.6	8.3	25.9
55–64 yrs	68.6	139.9	103.9
≥ 65 yrs	75.8	223.7	195.2
White	18.8	42.4	125.7
Black	21.3	47.7	124.2
Male	73.9	80.3	8.7
0–54 yrs	14.6	11.5	–21.0
55–64 yrs	228.3	236.8	3.7
≥ 65 yrs	417.0	499.3	19.7
White	73.1	78.8	7.9
Black	103.7	120.1	15.8

(From Ries, L. A. G., Miller, B. A., Hankey, B. F., Kosary, C. L., Harras, A., & Edwards, B. K. [Eds.]. [1994]. *SEER cancer statistics review, 1973–1991: Tables and graphs* [NIH Publication No. 94–2789]. Bethesda, MD: National Cancer Institute.)

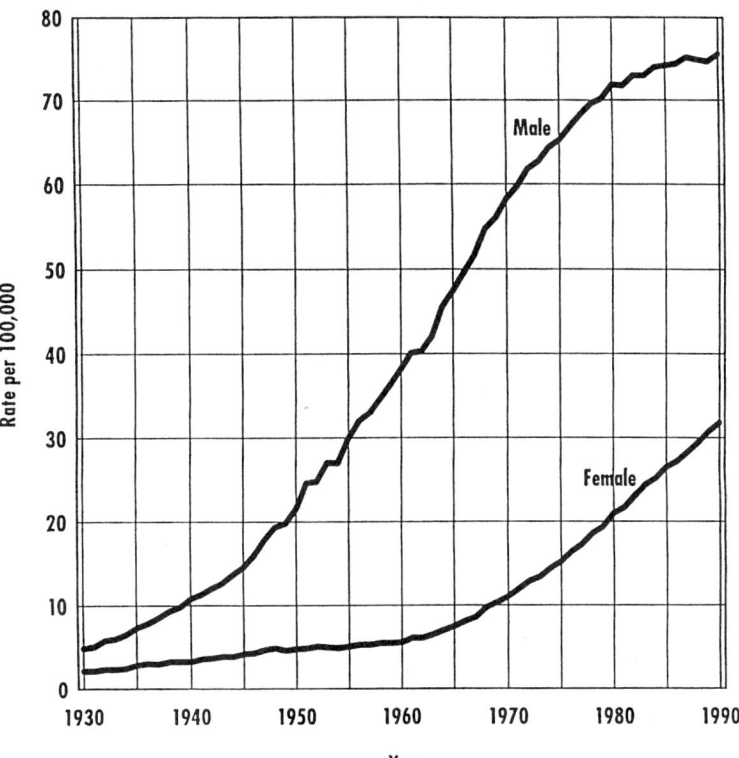

FIGURE 30–1. United States lung cancer trends, adjusted for age to U.S. 1970 population. The American Cancer Society lung cancer rate for non-smoking males is 6 per 100,000 and for non-smoking females is 4 per 100,000. (From Peto, R., Lopez, A. D., Boreman, J., Thun, M., & Heath, C. Jr. [1994]. Mortality from smoking in developed countries: Indirect estimates from national vital statistics. New York: Oxford University Press.)

Lung cancer, as the number one cause of cancer-related death among women, is clearly an issue of concern for women's health (Gritz, 1993; Sarna, 1995a).

There are some important differences in lung cancer among men and women. Women may be diagnosed at a younger age and with a shorter smoking history (Harris, Zang, Anderson, & Wynder, 1993; McDuffie, Klaassen, & Dosman, 1991; Scheinok, Engler, Robertson, Hutter, & Henson, 1989). There is evidence that women who smoke may be even more vulnerable to the risks of lung cancer than male smokers with a two- to threefold increase in relative risk (Risch et al., 1993). Symptom presentation also may be different. For example, chronic bronchitis prior to lung cancer was more frequently reported by women (McDuffie et al., 1991).

Additional factors have been associated with increased lung cancer risk in nonsmoking women. Exposure to environmental tobacco smoke (ETS) is an important risk factor for lung cancer, accounting for 20 per cent of lung cancer cases. Risks may be higher for women exposed to passive smoking during childhood and adolescence (Stockwell et al., 1992). Preexisting lung disease, independent of smoking, also has been identified as a factor for increased risk of lung cancer, particularly for adenocarcinoma (Alavanja, Brownson,

TABLE 30–3. *Changes in Lung Cancer Mortality Rates per 100,000 by Gender, Age, and Race, 1973–1991*

	1973–1974	1990–1991	% CHANGE
Female	13.8	31.9	131.5
0–54 yrs	4.5	5.7	27.5
55–64 yrs	48.5	102.6	111.3
≥ 65 yrs	58.2	181.7	212.5
White	13.8	32.4	134.2
Black	13.9	32.0	129.7
Male	63.3	75.0	18.6
0–54 yrs	12.4	9.8	−21.5
55–64 yrs	198.8	215.8	8.6
≥ 65 yrs	354.4	479.7	35.4
White	62.4	73.0	17.1
Black	76.8	106.2	38.2

(From Ries, L. A. G., Miller, B. A., Hankey, B. F., Kosary, C. L., Harras, A., & Edwards, B. K. [Eds.]. [1994]. *SEER cancer statistics review, 1973–1991: Tables and graphs* [NIH Publication No. 94–2789]. Bethesda, MD: National Cancer Institute.)

Boice, & Hock, 1992; Osann, 1991). Saturated fat intake has been proposed as a lung cancer promotor and has been associated with a sixfold increase among women with highest fat consumption and an eleven-fold increase for adenocarcinoma (Alavanja, Brown, Swanson, & Brownson, 1993); vegetable intake and carotene may offer a protective effect for nonsmoking women (Candelora, Stockwell, Armstrong, & Pinkham, 1992). Family history of malignancies also has been associated with increased risk of lung cancer; however this may be due to both increased smoking prevalence and exposure to ETS (Osann, 1991; Sellers, Potter, & Folsom, 1991). Nonsmoking women who have been exposed to asbestos, pesticides (occupational exposure), and who work in the dry cleaning industry (with exposure to chemicals and solvents) are at higher risk for lung cancer (Brownson, Alavanja, & Chang, 1993). Residential radon, as well as occupational exposure, may be an additional risk factor for lung cancer, affecting nonsmoking women of younger age (Pershagen, Liang, Hrubec, Svensson, & Boice, 1992).

Although the biology of lung cancer appears to be similar for both sexes, some histologic differences are apparent. The incidence of small-cell lung cancer (strongly associated with smoking) over the past 19 years has increased 181.1 per cent in women as compared with a 40.9 per cent increase in men (Ries et al., 1994). Similarly, women have experienced a 107.1 per cent increase in non-small-cell lung cancer as compared with 4.5 per cent in men. Mesothelioma has increased among both men (40 per cent) and women (20 per cent) in the past 20 years (Devesa et al., 1995).

Relative survival for both small-cell and non-small-cell lung cancers is slightly better in females at all stages of disease (Ferguson, Skosey, Hoffman, & Golomb, 1990; Ries et al., 1994). The 5-year relative survival rate is currently 16.2 per cent for women and 12.1 per cent for men. Significantly longer postoperative survival has been noted in women with non-small-cell lung cancers (Mitsudomi et al., 1989).

AGE AND LUNG CANCER

Only a minority of lung cancers (13.4 per cent) are diagnosed before 55 years of age (Ries et al., 1994). However, this percentage may increase as smoking initiation begins at an earlier age among adolescents, resulting in cases occurring at a younger age. Currently, lung cancer continues to increase in older men and women; 61 per cent of all cases are in those 65 years of age or older with 36.7 per cent of the diagnoses occurring between age 65 and 74 (Ries et al., 1994). The median age for diagnosis is age 68; almost two thirds (64.9 per cent) of all lung cancer deaths are in those 65 years of age and older (Ries et al., 1994). Increases in small-cell lung cancer for older adults (139.7 per cent) are almost three times greater than the increases in non-small-cell lung cancer (44.6 per cent).

Five-year relative survival decreases as age increases at diagnosis for both non-small-cell lung cancer (12.9 per cent of those 65 years or older vs. 16.8 per cent of those 55 to 64 years of age), and small-cell lung cancer

(3.6 per cent of those 65 years or older vs. 5.9 per cent of those 55 to 64 years of age) (Ries et al., 1994). There has been some evidence that lung cancer may be more localized at diagnosis and grow at a slower rate in older age groups as compared with middle-age groups (Teeter, Holmes, & McFarlane, 1987). Older smokers diagnosed with lung cancer may be more likely to suffer other physical symptoms, which will compound the alleviation of symptom distress due to disease and treatment (Colsher et al., 1990; Pierce, 1990).

RACE, SOCIOECONOMIC STATUS, AND LUNG CANCER

In a low-income population, knowledge about the link between smoking and lung cancer was lower among women, African-Americans, those with less education, those who are older, and current smokers (Brownson et al., 1992). Lung cancer rates differ by geographic location largely due to smoking prevalence. States with the highest average annual age-adjusted cancer mortality rate from lung cancer include Kentucky, Louisiana, Nevada, Arkansas, and West Virginia (Ries et al., 1994). Lower socioeconomic status and less education are both predictors for increased smoking prevalence and increased risk for lung cancer (Pierce, Fiore, Novotony, Hatziandreu, & Davis, 1989a, 1989b). Smoking prevalence differs by ethnicity; Native Americans and Alaskan natives (38.7 per cent smoking prevalence) have the highest smoking prevalence at highest risk for lung cancer (Bartecchi, McKenzie, & Schrier, 1994). Hispanic women have the lowest rate (15.5 per cent) (Centers for Disease Control, 1994). Increased smoking among African-American men (32.4 per cent) is substantially higher than that among African-American women (21.0 per cent), white women (24.0 per cent), and white men (27.0 per cent). The increase in lung cancer incidence for African-American men over the past 20 years (15.8 per cent) is 8 per cent higher than for white men (7.9 per cent) (Ries et al., 1994). Overall increases in lung cancer mortality are slightly greater in white women (134.2 per cent) than in black women (129.7 per cent). Lung cancer death rates among some Asian American populations (Cambodian and Thai) are higher than among whites (Dumbauld, McCullough, & Sutocky, 1994).

Disadvantaged circumstances and poverty situations are associated with increased smoking prevalence for men and women and place them at subsequent increased risk for lung cancer (Centers for Disease Control, 1994; Pugh, Power, Goldblatt, & Arber, 1991). Current data suggest that African-American teens may be less likely to smoke than white teens and that this difference is widening (Nelson et al., 1995). This may reverse the trend in higher lung cancer mortality among blacks (Garfinkle & Silverberg, 1991).

PRIMARY PREVENTION

An estimated 3 million people will die annually of tobacco-related diseases by the year 2025, many due to lung cancer (Peto et al., 1994; Peto et al., 1992). The tragedy of lung cancer is that it is one of the few cancers where a major causative factor, smoking, is known, and the majority of cases are preventable (McGinnis & Foege, 1993). An important barrier to preventive action is the misleading delay from increased smoking in the 1940s and the current high prevalence of lung cancer cases (Peto et al., 1994). Regardless of age, smokers have a rate of mortality approximately twice that of nonsmokers, resulting in an overall loss of 8 years of life for smokers. In adults aged 35 to 69 years, an average of 22 years are lost to premature death from smoking (Peto et al., 1994).

Cigarette smoking is the major factor in the dramatic increase in lung cancer in women and has become an international concern (Chollat-Traquet, 1992; Devesa et al., 1995). In undeveloped countries, the epidemic is just beginning, with expected upward spiraling of lung cancer cases in the next century (Peto et al., 1992). Gender differences with unsuccessful smoking cessation have been attributed to increased risk for lung cancer among women (U. S. Surgeon General, 1980). A higher proportion of women as compared with men has been projected to be smokers by the year 2000 and subsequently will be at increased risk for morbidity and mortality from lung cancer (Pierce, Fiore, Novotony, Hatziandreu, & Davis, 1989b). Data from the Lung Health Study, which investigated the efficacy of a structured smoking cessation program, support previously reported findings that women have more difficulty quitting, particularly if they have less than a high school education and live with other smokers (Bjornson et al., 1995). The Oncology Nursing Society's recognition of the importance for involvement in tobacco control activities is emphasized by adoption of a recent resolution that supports nursing tobacco control activities in practice, education, and research (Sarna & Brown, 1995).

Because very few persons begin smoking after they reach adulthood and because of the long lag time from exposure to tobacco and development of lung cancer, prevention of lung cancer is largely dependent on prevention of adolescents from smoking. Mortality from tobacco-related disease is inversely related to age of initiation of smoking, particularly before age 15 (Kawachi et al., 1993). Teenagers are the primary source for the recruitment of new smokers and thus should be an important target group for the prevention of lung cancer (Elders, Perry, Eriksen, & Giovino, 1994). The current slowing of the rate of decline among teen smokers is a cause for serious concern for future morbidity, especially for future lung cancer, and a focus for health advocacy (Nelson et al., 1995; Pierce et al., 1994). School and community-based nursing interventions focused on health promotion have been suggested to decrease uptake among young women (Dumas, 1992).

Nursing interventions are pivotal to dealing with nicotine withdrawal symptoms, preventing relapse, and ultimately reducing the risk of lung cancer among the 46 million Americans who currently smoke (Centers for Disease Control, 1994; Nett & Obrigewitch, 1993; Taylor, Houston-Miller, Killen, & DeBusk, 1990; Wew-

ers, Bowen, Stanislaw, & Desimone, 1994). The degree of decreased risk of cancer mortality for smokers varies across studies but it does not approach the risk for nonsmokers until at least 10 to 14 years after cessation (Kawachi et al., 1993). The inclusion of smoking status as part of traditional vital signs is one intervention that has been associated with a significant increase in the identification of smokers and in the amount of information given to patients to encourage them to stop smoking (Fiore et al., 1995). Weight gain is a greater concern for women who are attempting to stop smoking than it is for men and a discussion of it should be included as part of any intervention plan (Pirie, Murray, & Luepker, 1991). Patients who stop smoking at an older age may still reduce their risk of lung cancer (Halpern, Gillespie, & Warner, 1993; Orleans, Jepson, Resch, & Rimer, 1994; U.S. Department of Health and Human Services, 1990).

Few smoking cessation intervention studies have been reported in those with lung cancer (Gritz, 1991). Continued smoking has been suggested by some (Richardson et al., 1993), but not all, (Bergman & Sorenson, 1988) to increase the risk of recurrence. The diagnosis of lung cancer may be an opportunity for smoking cessation interventions for both the patient and family (Sarna, 1995b). Smoking cessation and relapse prevention should be a component of any rehabilitation program of patients with curable lung cancer. Smoking cessation, however, is not included in current self-help materials for patients with lung cancer (Cox, Carr, & Lee, 1992). The majority of smokers with curable lung cancer have been reported to stop smoking after diagnosis; however, relapse can continue to be a problem (Gritz, Nisenbaum, Elashoff, & Holmes, 1991; Knudsen, Schulman, van den Hoek, & Fowler, 1985). Women smokers with lung cancer were more likely to quit than men (Gritz et al., 1991). Despite acknowledging smoking as one cause of lung cancer, patients may not change their smoking behavior (Berckman & Austin, 1993).

The benefits of smoking cessation after diagnosis with advanced disease are less clear. It is not known whether smoking cessation is associated with increased emotional distress and withdrawal symptoms, which may decrease quality of life (Rienzo, 1993). One of the negative consequences of continued smoking in the face of progressive lung cancer may be escalating weight loss and functional decline (Brown, 1993). Findings from the Sarna, Lindsey, Dean, Brecht, and McCorkle (1994) study (Box 30–1) suggest that weight loss may be an important factor in increased symptom distress and functional decline. Continued smoking may exacerbate weight loss during treatment (Larson, Lindsey, Dodd, Brecht, & Packer, 1993) as well as during palliative care. The effects of smoking cessation in this vulnerable population necessitate further study.

HISTOLOGIC TYPES

The postulated histogenesis of lung cancer is that normal respiratory epithelium becomes metaplastic, then dysplastic, and ultimately malignant (Haque,

---

Box 30–1. *The Impact of Weight Change in Lung Cancer*

Sarna, L., Lindsey, A. M., Dean, H., Brecht, M. L., & McCorkle, R. (1994). Weight change and lung cancer: Relationships with symptom distress, functional status, and smoking. *Research in Nursing & Health, 17,* 371–379.

Purpose: To describe pattern of weight change and to explore the relationships of symptom distress, functional status, and smoking status.

Sample: Sixty patients with progressive lung cancer; followed every 2 months, beginning 2 months after diagnosis.

Procedures: Weight was measured on a calibrated scale every 2 months beginning 2 months after diagnosis over a 6-month time period. Symptom distress (measured by the Symptom Distress Scale) and functional status (measured by the Enforced Social Dependency Scale) were measured at each time period. Smoking status was available at the time of diagnosis only.

Major Findings:
- Weight loss of 10 per cent or more occurred in 35 per cent of subjects; 37 per cent lost weight at three or more time periods.
- Differences in patterns of weight loss over time by smoking status were evident, with smokers having an average loss at each time interval.
- Weight loss was related to decline in functional status at three time periods and was correlated with subsequent increased symptom distress at three time periods. Subjects who received chemotherapy (50 per cent) or smoked (25 per cent) predicted 28 per cent of the variance in weight loss from Time 1 to 5.

1991). Evidence suggests that lung cancer cells arise from a bronchial precursor cell with the different histologic types occurring as a result of the differentiation pathways. Histologically, bronchial carcinomas are classified into two large groups, small-cell lung cancer (SCLC) and non-small-cell lung cancer (NSCLC). Mixtures of histologic types also can occur (e.g., adeno, squamous carcinomas) (Table 30–4). Lung cancer is not a single disease; the different histopathologic types determine the resulting pathology and prognosis and also the selection of treatment.

In addition to histologic classification, tumors may be characterized as endocrine- or non-endocrine-producing and by the biologic marker or markers expressed. The histologic cell type, degree of differentiation, and paraneoplastic expression are related to prognosis.

SMALL-CELL LUNG CANCER

Approximately 20 to 25 per cent of lung cancers are histologically classified as small-cell carcinoma. This type of cancer and squamous cell cancer are most frequently linked with cigarette smoking (Hinson & Perry, 1993). Approximately 80 per cent of these tumors are located centrally and submucosally. Small-cell cancer is the most aggressive type of lung cancer; it spreads rapidly to submucosal vessels and regional lymph nodes (Hinson & Perry, 1993; Yesner & Carter, 1982). Thus at the time of diagnosis, more than 50 per cent of the

patients have extensive metastatic disease, 23 per cent have regional involvement, and 7 per cent have localized disease (Ries et al, 1994). Owing to the frequent occurrence of micrometastases, SCLC is considered to be a systemic disease at diagnosis (Hande & Des Prez, 1982; Haque, 1991; Hinson & Perry, 1993). A survival rate of more than 1 year is more likely for those with limited disease. Prognosis and survival remain poor even in the few patients with SCLC who present with limited disease and have had surgical resection. Five-year survival for those with localized disease is 17 per cent, 9 per cent for regional disease, and 2 per cent for distant metastases (Ries et al, 1994). The failure of curative resection results from the presence of undetectable, subclinical metastases. Although SCLC cells are quite sensitive to irradiation, failure with radiation therapy also occurs due to the presence of occult metastases. Thus considering that SCLC is usually disseminated at the time of diagnosis, chemotherapy is usually the first treatment of choice. Although the response to treatment with multiple agents is high initially, the duration of the response is short (6 to 8 months). Because of the frequent central location of the tumor, compression of the bronchial lumen may occur. The occurrence of paraneoplastic syndromes is more frequent with this tumor type (Carr, 1981; Hansen & Pedersen, 1986; Haque, 1991; Hinson & Perry, 1993; Lindsey, Piper, & Carrieri, 1981). Examples of paraneoplastic syndromes that occur with SCLC include Cushing's syndrome (ectopic production of adrenocorticotropin hormone by malignant lung tissue that stimulates excess production of adrenal gland glucocorticoids) and syndrome of inappropriate antidiuretic hormone secretion (ectopic production of antidiuretic hormone by malignant lung tissue) (see "Clinical Manifestations").

NON-SMALL-CELL LUNG CANCERS

Non-small-cell lung cancers represent three (squamous cell, adenocarcinoma, large-cell carcinoma) of

TABLE 30–4. *Histologic Types of Lung Cancer*

HISTOLOGIC CELL TYPE	PERCENTAGE OF LUNG CANCERS
Small-cell	20–25
Non-small-cell	
Squamous cell	30–40
Adenocarcinoma	33–50
Large-cell carcinoma	5–15

the four histologic groups of lung cancer; 70 to 80 per cent of the lung cancers can be classified into these three subgroups. If these tumors are localized, surgery is the treatment of choice; however, in only a small percentage of the cases (10 to 15 per cent) are the tumors considered to be surgically resectable at the time of diagnosis. The 5-year survival rate for those with localized disease is almost 50 per cent (Ries et al., 1994). Because most patients with lung cancer have disseminated disease at the time of diagnosis, chemotherapy is used as the major treatment modality.

SQUAMOUS CELL CARCINOMA

Squamous cell carcinoma currently represents about 30 to 40 per cent of all lung cancers (Haque, 1991; Martini, 1993). The majority of these tumors also occur centrally but are seen anywhere in the lung. Because of the central location and the tendency for local invasion, bronchial obstruction does occur. There is also a tendency for ulceration and bleeding with squamous cell carcinoma. This type of cancer is much more frequent in males; approximately 90 per cent of the cases are seen in men. Early metastases are less common than is invasion of local structures (Bone & Balk, 1982). This histologic type is more prone to cavitation. Squamous cell carcinoma occurs in areas in which the bronchial epithelium has been chronically damaged (Gazdar, Carney, & Minna, 1983; Yesner & Carter, 1982).

Patients may present with obstructive atelectasis, pneumonitis, and/or hemoptysis (Filderman & Matthay, 1985). The tumor may also impinge on other thoracic structures such as the mediastinum, chest wall, ribs, or diaphragm. An inflammatory response and an early positive sputum cytologic evaluation are common findings; these sometimes are observed before changes appear in the chest radiograph (Woolner, Fontana, & Cortese, 1984; Yesner & Carter, 1982).

ADENOCARCINOMA

Adenocarcinoma is now the most common type of lung cancer in some geographic areas. This increase in incidence is attributable in part to the increased incidence of lung cancer in women and in part to changes in histologic criteria for diagnosis. Adenocarcinoma represents about 33 per cent of all bronchogenic cancers (Valaitis et al., 1981; Haque, 1991). Others have reported the proportion of adenocarcinomas to be as high as 50 per cent in the United States (Martini, 1993). It is the most common type of lung cancer in women and in nonsmokers. Bronchoalveolar carcinoma is a subset of adenocarcinoma, which is generally more indolent but tends to spread diffusely through both lungs. These tumors frequently are small and occur peripherally. Adenocarcinoma is seen in areas of previous pulmonary damage with fibrosis, or it may arise from bronchial glands or peripheral mucosa. As a result of its origin, mucin production is frequent (Mathews, McKay, & Lukeman, 1983). Adenocarcinoma is most often detected by a routine chest radiograph; at the time of diagnosis, patients frequently are asymptomatic (Mathews et al., 1983; Haque, 1991).

However, adenocarcinoma has a tendency toward early metastasis, and approximately 40 per cent of patients are considered to have unresectable tumor at the time of diagnosis. Due to the more common peripheral location of this tumor type, an early positive sputum cytologic finding is rare.

LARGE-CELL CARCINOMA

Large-cell carcinomas are extremely undifferentiated forms of other types of lung cancer. Less than 5 to 15 per cent of lung tumors are categorized as large-cell carcinoma (Haque, 1991; Martini, 1993). Because tumors with unclear differentiation may be classified as large-cell carcinoma, this percentage may be an overestimate of the actual incidence. Usually they are large, bulky, peripheral tumors, and they can occur in any part of the lung. They are known to mimic other types of lung cancer. Early invasion of the mediastinum and central nervous system occurs.

OTHER HISTOLOGIC TYPES OF LUNG CANCER

The remaining lung cancers, about 5 per cent, are classified as relatively uncommon types, such as carcinoid tumors and mucoepidermoid lung cancer. Mixed histologic types of lung cancer have been found on examination of tumor specimens. Recent evidence supports the idea that all types of lung tumors may have a common stem cell origin. Mixed-cell tumors are thought to be the result of the secondary development of different cell types (Yesner & Carter, 1982). Some tumors may undergo differentiation, for example, small cell to adenocarcinoma or squamous cell lung cancer (Carney, 1986).

CLINICAL MANIFESTATIONS

The presenting clinical manifestations for lung cancer diagnosis are diverse because they may be due to one or more of the following: the primary tumor; metastatic involvement, either local or distant; or systemic, paraneoplastic expression (Table 30–5). Some patients who are asymptomatic are diagnosed with lung cancer following a routine chest radiograph. Approximately 15 per cent of those with lung cancer are asymptomatic at diagnosis (Filderman & Matthay, 1985).

Clinical manifestations caused by local involvement of proximal airways include coughing, hemoptysis, dyspnea, and vague chest pain. Coughing occurs as a symptom of lung cancer in about 40 per cent of cases; however, it may also be due to the chronic bronchitis frequently seen in those with a history of cigarette smoking. A change in an existing cough should be determined. Infection may occur if clearance of mucous secretions from airways is impaired. In lung cancer, a developing cough or a change in cough may be the result of a central airway obstruction or a bronchial mucosal ulceration.

In more than half the cases, hemoptysis is the initial symptom of lung cancer. Dyspnea also commonly

TABLE 30–5. *Clinical Manifestations of Lung Cancer by Extent of Involvement*

LOCAL	REGIONAL	DISTANT	SYSTEMIC
Cough	Hoarseness	Bone pain	Anorexia
Dyspnea	Pleural effusion	CNS changes	Cachexia
Hemoptysis	Dyspnea	Hypertrophic pulmonary osteoarthropathy	Fatigue
Wheezing	Pericardial involvement		Weight loss
Pain	Elevated diaphragm		Paraneoplastic syndromes
	Horner's syndrome		
	Pancoast's syndrome		
	Superior vena cava obstruction		

occurs and is associated with increased coughing and sputum production. Dyspnea may be the result of atelectasis distal to the tumor. Dyspnea is a subjective symptom defined as difficult, uncomfortable breathing. Dyspnea may occur at any point along the disease continuum; it may be present at diagnosis or may begin later with advancing disease. Obstructive tumors, pleural effusions, pneumonitis, and cachexia are among the factors contributing to dyspnea. In a study of 30 lung cancer patients experiencing dyspnea. Brown, Carrieri, Janson-Bjerklie, and Dodd (1986) reported that these patients had significant dyspnea and felt extreme fatigue. Over an 8-week period, their activity decreased significantly due to progressive weakness associated with disease progression. Foote, Sexton, and Pawlik (1986) described nursing therapies that may be useful in ameliorating the discomforts of dyspnea. These include relaxation, planning for activity, body positioning, and instruction in breathing techniques.

Lung cancer can occlude airways and invade or compress blood vessels. Wheezing, usually localized unilaterally, is due to airway obstruction from the tumor, but wheezing is an infrequent complaint. Most commonly, lung cancer involves the central airways; only about 20 per cent occurs in the periphery. Frequently patients present with atelectasis.

Weight loss is a clinical feature characteristic of lung cancer. At the time of diagnosis, weight loss for the preceding 6 months is an important factor in determining prognosis. The survival time of patients who have sustained a 5 per cent weight loss is significantly shorter than that of patients who have not experienced a weight loss (Chlebowski, Heber, & Block, 1983; Costa et al., 1981; DeWys et al., 1980). In one large study, 57 per cent of the SCLC patients and 61 per cent of the non-SCLC patients had experienced weight loss in the preceding 6 months; the median survival time of those who presented with weight loss was approximately 2 months less than that of those who presented without weight loss (DeWys et al., 1980). Decreased dietary intake was shown to account for weight loss during chemotherapy for SCLC patients (Lindsey & Piper, 1985). A case study of a patient with SCLC who showed progressive weight loss is reported by Lindsey, Piper, and Stotts (1982). Weight loss as one component of cancer cachexia is described elsewhere (Lindsey, 1986a, 1986b; Lindsey et al., 1982).

As many as 40 per cent of patients present with chest pain described as being a nonspecific, dull inter-mittent ache that is on the same side as the tumor (Spiro, 1984). Chest pain associated with a rib or pleuritic pain is indicative of metastatic disease. Pancoast's tumor, which grows in the apex of the lung, may cause shoulder pain (described later).

Extension of the tumor to the pleural surface of the lung may result in a pleural effusion. Often, the amount of the effusion is large; unless treatment yields significant tumor regression, the fluid rapidly reaccumulates following removal of the fluid.

At the time of diagnosis, the majority of lung cancer patients have either regional or distant metastases and will seek health care for symptoms occurring as a result of the metastases. An example is hoarseness. It occurs secondary to involvement of the left recurrent laryngeal nerve at the left hilum.

A potentially life-threatening syndrome occurs with superior vena cava obstruction, and it requires treatment. Patients most commonly present with edema of the face, neck, and upper torso (nipples and above), appearance of collateral venous circulation on upper body, and increased jugular venous pressure (Sculier et al., 1986). The syndrome occurs secondary to peritracheal lymphadenopathy and results in compression of the great veins that drain the head and upper trunk. It is seen more often in patients with SCLC; it occurs in approximately 7 to 12 per cent of the cases. Because of the anatomic location of the superior vena cava, the preponderance is in those with tumors in the right lung. The symptoms include severe headache occurring with cough, blackouts after bending or on rising, dyspnea, and dysphagia. General facial puffiness and periorbital edema may occur. Emergency treatment directed at relieving the edema is required. Diuretics and dexamethasone have been used, but treatment of the tumor by radiation, chemotherapy, or both may be the most useful.

Cancer occurring in the lung apex (superior sulcus) may invade the brachial nerve roots; this extension is associated with brachial neuritis. Pancoast described the syndrome associated with tumors involving the superior (apical) sulcus. Patients present with pain, wasting of muscles of the hand, and Horner's syndrome. If the eighth cervical and first thoracic segments of the sympathetic nerve trunk are involved, symptoms indicating Horner's syndrome are observed (Cohen, 1982). These include a small pupil, partial ptosis of the eyelid, enophthalmos, and ipsilateral absence of thermal sweating on the face.

Tumor extension through the pericardium results in pericarditis and abnormalities in cardiac rhythm. Cardiac output may be diminished if the tumor causes a pericardial effusion.

Local spread of lung cancer occurs initially in the hilar glands and usually is present at diagnosis. Metastatic involvement of peritracheal and subcarinal nodes is evident at diagnosis in a third or more of the patients, and spread to supraclavicular lymph nodes and deep cervical chain nodes is observed in about 20 per cent of the patients. Metastatic involvement results in symptomatic disease. Older patients at diagnosis have less incidence of metastatic disease, and a significant decrease in frequency of metastatic disease has been reported in studies of elderly lung cancer patients (Ershler, Socinski, & Greene, 1982; Suen, Lau, & Yermakov, 1974).

Evidence of systemic disease or the distant effects of lung cancer include lymph node, bone, liver, and central nervous system metastases and paraneoplastic phenomena. Neurologic involvement from intracerebral metastases may be the presenting pathology for lung cancer; complaints may be varied and include headache, unsteadiness or difficulty in walking, seizures, changes in mental status, and personality changes.

Some patients present with bone pain; the ribs, vertebrae, humerus, and femoral bones are those with the most frequent occurrence of metastases. Pathologic fractures may be the presenting symptom. Bone marrow involvement occurs in 25 to 50 per cent of cases of SCLC (Carney & Minna, 1982; Muss, Jackson, Richard, White, & Cooper, 1984) (see also Chapter 15).

Symptoms of hepatic metastases occur later; only a few patients newly diagnosed with lung cancer have indications of liver involvement. The usual changes include an increasingly firm, irregular, enlarged liver. If the metastases are small and isolated, liver function tests will remain in the normal range. Jaundice and anorexia may occur. Early liver involvement may be observed more commonly in those with SCLC of the bronchus.

Ectopic hormone secretion has been associated with lung cancer. Some patients present with endocrine-related pathologies such as Cushing's syndrome that result from increased ectopic secretion of adrenocorticotropic hormone from the lung tumor. This syndrome occurs in about 5 per cent of the cases of SCLC. A case study of an SCLC patient presenting with Cushing's syndrome as a result of ectopic production of adrenocorticotropic hormone has been reported by Lindsey and colleagues (1981). Another endocrine-related syndrome seen particularly in patients with SCLC that results from ectopic hormone production by the tumor is the syndrome of inappropriate antidiuretic hormone secretion (SIADH). It occurs in 5 to 10 per cent of the cases of SCLC. These patients present with high urine osmolality, low serum sodium, and plasma osmolality reflecting a retention of fluid; they may show confusion, lethargy, or other mental disturbances. The presence of SIADH is associated with a poor prognosis. Hypercalcemia may occur as a result of ectopic secretion of parathyroid hormone from squamous cell lung cancer. Hypercalcemia usually occurs in association with a large tumor mass. These paraneoplastic syndromes are most commonly seen with SCLC but do occur with other lung cancers (Carr, 1981; Neal, Kosinski, Cohen, & Orenstein, 1986).

Clubbing of the fingers occurs in up to a third of the cases of lung cancer; it is observed more frequently in patients with squamous cell tumors.

An osteitis may occur during the course of lung cancer. The distal parts of the radius, ulna, tibia, and fibula are the most frequently involved bones. Swelling, erythema, and tenderness occur with the symmetric proliferation of subperiosteal tissue of the wrists and ankle joints. This condition is referred to as hypertrophic pulmonary osteoarthropathy. It is seen more frequently with squamous cell carcinoma.

Benedict (1989) conducted a study designed to determine the incidence of suffering associated with lung cancer. Only 10 per cent of her sample of 30 adults with primary pulmonary malignancies reported no suffering, whereas 50 per cent indicated "very much" suffering. There was a statistically significant difference in the amount of suffering associated with psychologic aspects between those with known metastatic disease and those with no known metastatic disease. Disability, pain, anxiety, changed daily activities, and weakness and fatigue were reported as the sources of greatest suffering. The suffering associated with physical aspects was found to be greater than that reported for psychologic and for interactional aspects of the lung cancer experience. Sarna recently studied correlates of symptom distress in women with lung cancer (Box 30–2) (Sarna, 1993). In self-reporting on the McCorkle Symptom Distress Scale, fatigue, frequent pain, and insomnia were the most frequent distressing symptoms.

These findings have implications for nursing care. First, it is important to recognize the high incidence of suffering experienced by lung cancer patients and the fact that more suffering is associated with the physical aspects of the disease. If the sources of greatest suffering are made explicit, such as from disability, pain, or weakness and fatigue, the nurse can provide suggestions or nursing actions for the patient and family that may alleviate or ameliorate the sources of suffering. For example, the nurse can discuss and arrange for analgesic administration that allows the patient to be functional but also relieves the pain.

In addition to detection of symptoms of lung cancer and assessment and surveillance of the progression or regression of these symptoms, the nurse has a major responsibility for assisting the patient with symptom management. Examples include suggesting that the patient limit activity; assisting the patient with essential activity when pain and dyspnea are most severe; providing for nutritional intake when the patient is most comfortable; and providing small amounts of high-calorie, high-protein food frequently when anorexia is present. Provision of oxygen and instruction in breathing techniques may be required. Nursing care is based on the specific clinical manifestations that the patient experiences, and these include a range from local to systemic manifestations.

BOX 30–2. *Symptom Distress and Lung Cancer*

Sarna, L. (1993). Correlates of symptom distress in women with lung cancer. *Cancer Practice, 1*, 21–28.

Purpose: To explore and describe symptom distress and its correlates experienced by women with lung cancer.
Sample: Convenience sample of 69 women with primary or recurrent lung cancer. The majority had non-small-cell lung cancer, were not currently receiving treatment, and had lived with lung cancer for more than 1 year.
Procedures: Subjects completed self reports of their symptom distress (measured with the McCorkle Symptom Distress Scale) and quality of life (measured by the CARES-SF).
Major Findings:
- Fatigue, frequent pain, and insomnia were the most frequent distressing symptoms. Sixty-one per cent had two or more distressing symptoms.
- Concurrent respiratory disease, recurrent lung cancer, low income, and previous chemotherapy were associated with higher levels of symptom distress. Symptom distress was strongly correlated to lower quality of life and lower functional status.

SCREENING

Early detection through large screening programs has shown only very limited success in reducing mortality. In the Mayo Lung Project, 9211 male smokers who were older than 45 years of age were followed from 1972 to 1982 (Woolner et al., 1981). The control group had an annual chest radiograph, and a sputum specimen was collected for cytologic study; the close surveillance group had the same screening every 4 months. At the time of the report (1982), 78 in the control group and 109 in the close surveillance group were diagnosed with lung cancer. The great majority were diagnosed by chest radiograph. Despite the screening effort, only about half were determined to have operable disease at the time of diagnosis. The conclusion from this long-term screening project is that the detection of new cases of lung cancer is low compared with the expense involved.

Results of a large cooperative screening project (National Cancer Institute Cooperative Early Lung Cancer Detection Programs) indicated that chest radiographs and sputum cytologic evaluations were both useful (Melamed et al., 1984). The central squamous cell cancers were detected by cytologic studies, whereas the peripheral large-cell carcinomas and adenocarcinomas were detected by chest radiographs. Less than 10 per cent of the cancers were detected simultaneously by both screening procedures.

For detection of lung cancer on radiograph, the tumor must be in the range of 1 cm in diameter. This size requires 30 doublings, by which time metastases may have occurred (Geddes, 1979). Thus early detection of lung cancer by chest radiographic screening is unlikely. At 40 doublings, the tumor burden usually results in death (Bone & Balk, 1982).

Regular annual screening procedures have not been shown to be cost-effective for early detection of lung cancer (Flehinger et al., 1984; Fontana et al., 1984; Frost et al., 1984). That is, there has been no real benefit in terms of long-term survival. Improvement in early diagnosis in some circumstances has been reported (Bechtel, Kelley, Petty, Patz, & Saccomanno, 1994). Based on their study of patients with roentgeno-graphically occult cancer, Bechtel and colleagues suggest use of sputum cytologic testing for case finding, particularly for those who are at greater risk because of heavy smoking or occupation (Bechtel et al., 1994). Thus screening for lung cancer may be more efficacious for those with high-risk factors, but to date mass radiologic and cytologic screening for lung cancer is not recommended.

TUMOR MARKERS

Production of some hormones, antigens, and proteins have been found to be associated with some tumors. In some cases they serve as tumor markers and are useful in monitoring tumor response to therapy or in relapse. For example, carcinoembryonic antigen (CEA) concentration has been shown to correlate well with the extent of NSCLC tumor and with metastatic disease. Neuron-specific enolase (NSE) is a tumor marker for SCLC and for all neuroendocrine tumors; it can be used for monitoring tumor response.

The production of ectopic hormones by some lung cancers has been reported for years; however, no marker has yet been identified that can be used for screening for lung cancer (Hansen & Pedersen, 1986; Lindsey et al., 1981). A number of tumor markers have been measured in serum specimens from SCLC patients; these include adrenocorticotropic hormone, antidiuretic hormone, oxytocin, carcinoembryonic antigen, and calcitonin. Patients with SCLC have higher levels of ectopic hormone and other peptides than do patients with other histologic types of lung cancer. Levels of two enzymes, neuron-specific enolase and creatine kinase BB, have been found to be elevated in patients with untreated SCLC (Akoun, Scarna, Milleron, Benichoun, & Herman, 1985; Carney et al., 1984; Johnson et al., 1984). Studies reporting incidence of ectopic hormone and other peptide production in SCLC patients are reviewed elsewhere (Hansen & Pedersen, 1986). Measurement of tumor markers in the cerebral spinal fluid of lung cancer patients with the derivation of a ratio of cerebral spinal fluid and plasma concentrations has been suggested as a potential means for determining the presence of brain metastases. As yet, tumor markers have not been effective for use in screening and early detection of lung cancer.

CYTOGENETICS

Much new information about carcinogenesis is being accumulated with the use of cytogenetic and molecular genetic techniques (Mitelman, 1994). Investigators are studying the dominant oncogenes and the recessive tumor suppressor genes. The work on genetic aberrations has important relevance for diagnosis, prognosis and ultimately to the design of more specific therapies. Chromosomal changes have been found in solid tumors from epithelial origin such as adenocarcinoma of the lung, but the changes are complex and probably reflect a process of genetic changes which leads to the malignant transformation (Sandberg, 1994). Roth has reported the presence of transforming growth factor alpha, dominant oncogenes, HER-2/erb B2 and K-ras, and abnormalities of the tumor suppressor gene, p53, in human NSCLC cells (Roth, 1992). Others have found little or no expression of HER-2 in SCLC. Increased expression of this protein in lung cancer patients also has been associated with poor prognosis (Kern, Schwark, & Nordberg, 1990). Findings of K-ras oncogene mutation in lung adenocarcinoma is associated with poor prognosis (Roth, 1992; Rodenhuis & Slebos, 1990). K-ras mutation is found in about 30 per cent of that tumor type in smokers but not in nonsmokers (Rodenhuis & Slebos, 1990). Mutation of the tumor suppressor p53 gene is often found in human lung cancers—more than 50 per cent; mutation of this gene also occurs commonly in other human cancers (Roth, 1990). Progress in cancer cytogenetics has been reviewed recently (Sandberg, 1994; Weinberg, 1994). This work certainly holds promise for better understanding and possible control of carcinogenesis and to the creation of gene specific therapies.

DIAGNOSIS

Diagnostic techniques include the use of chest radio-graphs, sputum cytologic evaluations, fiberoptic bronchoscopy and transthoracic needle aspiration biopsy to obtain tissue specimens, and computed tomographic (CT) scans (Hinson & Perry, 1993; Loke, Matthay, & Ieda, 1982; Martini, 1993; Rubin, 1991). Very few lung tumors are detected in an occult stage. The diagnosis of lung cancer must be histologically or cytologically confirmed from tissue or sputum specimens, respectively. Centrally located tumors have a higher percentage of positive sputum cytologic evaluations than do peripherally located tumors. For the most accurate diagnostic results, a series of three or four sputum specimens should be collected and subjected to cytologic examination. Bronchoscopy is also useful in diagnosing centrally located tumors. Bronchoscopy done with a fiberoptic instrument passed through a nostril or mouth is a common diagnostic procedure. It is used for visualization of the tracheobronchial tree, including access to upper lobes, and for obtaining

bronchial biopsy specimens and brushings. Tumor tissue can also be obtained through the use of bronchial needle aspiration technique. Transthoracic needle biopsies are most useful for diagnosing the more peripherally located tumors and for obtaining pleural and mediastinal tissue (Wang & Terry, 1983). Because pneumothorax is a complication of transthoracic needle biopsies, observation for this problem is critical. A thoracotomy or mediastinoscopy may be necessary for tissue diagnosis. Thoroscopy may be useful for diagnosis when there is pleural involvement.

Computed tomography is an important adjunct to chest radiographs in the diagnosis of lung cancer; it is particularly useful in evaluating the mediastinal and hilar lymph node involvement and the extent of disease (Heitzman, 1986; Hinson & Perry, 1993). It is most helpful in the staging of bronchogenic carcinoma, for example, in the identification of metastases in the central nervous system, abdominal nodes, adrenal and liver metastases, or other extrapulmonary sites. Computed tomography and radiographs are also used in evaluating the response to therapy. The use of CT in lung cancer diagnosis and management is reviewed elsewhere (Heitzman, 1986). Magnetic resonance imaging and experimental positron emission tomography also have been used. The most sensitive imaging technique for detecting bone metastases is the radionuclide bone scan (Hinson & Perry, 1993; Waxman, 1986). Bone metastases are seen at diagnosis for approximately 40 per cent of the patients with SCLC but only 10 per cent of those with non-SCLC.

The nurse should describe the specifically ordered diagnostic procedures to the patient and family; this description should include what will occur and what the patient is to do. Again, assessment and surveillance for recovery or complications following the specific procedures are the nurse's responsibility.

STAGING

Staging follows the diagnosis and histologic classification of lung cancer. Extensive efforts have been directed to accurate staging of lung cancer because selection of treatment and subsequent survival are predicated on accurate assessment of the extent of tumor involvement. There is a high correlation between tumor metastases and prognostic survival.

For non-SCLCs, the TNM (tumor, node, metastasis) classification developed by the American Joint Committee on Cancer Staging for Lung Cancer is used for staging (Table 30–6). The T number reflects the extent of the primary tumor, the N number reflects the absence or presence of lymph node (hilar or mediastinal) involvement, and the M number reflects the existence of distant metastases. Stage I refers to cases where the tumor is confined to the lung with no metastases. Stage II reflects involvement of hilar or peribronchial lymph nodes. Stage III disease includes locally advanced tumors with metastases to mediastinal or cervical lymph nodes or tumors that have extended to the chest wall, diaphragm, mediastinium, or carina. The distinction between IIIA and IIIB has important prognostic and clinical implica-

TABLE 30–6. *Staging for Lung Carcinoma*

AJCC/UICC Stage Grouping

Occult Carcinoma	TX	N0	M0
Stage 0	Tis	N0	M0
Stage I	T1	N0	M0
	T2	N0	M0
Stage II	T1	N1	M0
	T2	N1	M0
Stage IIIA	T1	N2	M0
	T2	N2	M0
	T3	N0	M0
	T3	N1	M0
	T3	N2	M0
Stage IIIB	Any T	N3	M0
	T4	Any N	M0
Stage IV	Any T	Any N	M1

Definitions:

Primary Tumor (T)

TX Primary tumor cannot be assessed, or tumor proven by presence of malignant cells in sputum or bronchial washings but not visualized by imaging or bronchoscopy

TO No evidence of primary tumor

Tis Carcinoma in situ

T1 Tumor 3 cm or less in greatest dimension, surrounded by lung or visceral pleura, without bronchoscopic evidence of invasion more proximal than the lobar bronchus* (i.e., not in the main bronchus)

T2 Tumor with any of the following features of size or extent: more than 3 cm in greatest dimension; involves main bronchus, 2 cm or more distal to the carina; invades the visceral pleura; or associated with atelectasis or obstructive pneumonitis which extends to the hilar region but does not involve the entire lung

T3 Tumor of any size that directly invades any of the following: chest wall (including superior sulcus tumors), diaphragm, mediastinal pleura, parietal pericardium; or tumor in the main bronchus less than 2 cm distal to the carina*, but without involvement of the carina; or associated atelectasis or obstructive pneumonitis of the entire lung

T4 Tumor of any size that invades any of the following: mediastinum, heart, great vessels, trachea, esophagus, vertebral body, carina; or tumor with a malignant pleural effusion**

*Note: *The uncommon superficial tumor of any size with its invasive component limited to the bronchial wall, which may extend proximal to the main bronchus, is also classified T1.*

**Note: *Most pleural effusions associated with lung cancer are due to tumor. However, there are a few patients in whom multiple cytopathologic examinations of pleural fluid are negative for tumor. In these cases, fluid is non-bloody and is not an exudate. When these elements and clinical judgment dictate that the effusion is not related to the tumor, the effusion should be excluded as a staging element and the patient should be staged T1, T2, or T3.*

Regional Lymph Nodes (N)

The regional lymph nodes are the intrathoracic, scalene, and supraclavicular nodes.

NX Regional lymph nodes cannot be assessed

N0 No regional lymph node metastasis

N1 Metastasis in ipsilateral peribronchial and/or ipsilateral hilar lymph nodes, including direct extension

N2 Metastasis in ipsilateral mediastinal and/or subcarinal lymph node(s)

N3 Metastasis in contralateral mediastinal, contralateral hilar, ipsilateral, or contralateral scalene or supraclavicular lymph node(s)

Distant Metastasis (M)

MX Presence of distant metastasis cannot be assessed

M0 No distant metastasis

M1 Distant metastasis

(Reprinted with permission from American Cancer Society, Inc.)

tions. Stage IV refers to cases with distant metastatic involvement.

For SCLC, the limited or extensive classifications are used more frequently for staging than the TNM system. Limited classification refers to tumors that are confined to the ipsilateral hemithorax; extensive classification refers to tumors that have spread beyond the ipsilateral hemithorax and adjacent lymph nodes. The

limited or extensive categories are more useful for SCLC because with the rapid extrathoracic spread of small-cell lung tumors, most would be classified as stage III at diagnosis. The prognosis for those classified as stage I or II is also poor due to the undetected micrometastases (Filderman et al., 1986). SCLC is generally viewed as being disseminated at diagnosis (Hinson & Perry, 1993). In staging for SCLC, bone marrow aspiration and biopsy may be performed because bone marrow involvement has been commonly observed (Muss et al., 1984).

For more accurate staging of lung cancer, CT scans are used. Direct tumor extension into mediastinal, pleural, or other structures is better identified with CT scans; for example, metastatic disease in the adrenal gland can be detected. Mediastinoscopy is frequently used prior to thorocotomy to ensure resectability. A tissue sample is obtained to determine if mediastinal involvement is inflammatory or malignant. Using a mediastinoscopy, the presence or absence of mediastinal (paratrachael and subaortic) lymph node involvement is used to determine resectability for lung cancer. Generally, a poor prognosis is associated with positive mediastinal nodes (Spiro, 1984). More extensive information about staging procedures is reviewed elsewhere (Bone & Balk, 1982; Feinstein & Wells, 1982; Filderman et al., 1986; Mountain, 1986; Tisi et al., 1983).

TNM staging is important for NSCLC because treatment choice and effectiveness vary with tumor extent and location of involvement. Those with stage I with no metastases have the best prognosis. Stage II includes those with T1 or T2 tumors with intrapulmonary and/or hilar lymph node metastasis. Stage III has been divided into IIIA and IIIB groups, designating those considered to have operable disease (IIIA) and those considered to have inoperable disease (IIIB) because of more extensive extrapulmonary involvement, such as spread to the contralateral lymph nodes (mediastinal, hilar, supraclavicular, or scalene) or pleural effusion. Those with distant metastases are classified as stage IV.

The specific histologic cell type and the degree of differentiation are related to prognosis. Generally, those diagnosed with squamous cell carcinoma have a better prognosis than those with other types of lung cancer. Prognosis is associated not only with type of lung tumor but also with location and size of tumor, extent of spread, and absence of complications such as pleural effusion or paraneoplastic syndrome.

The prognosis for those with a small (< 3.0 cm) peripheral tumor is better than for those with larger or more centrally located tumors (Mountain, 1983). The 5-year survival rate for those with distant metastases at diagnosis is approximately 2 per cent, for those with regional involvement is 16 per cent, and for those with localized disease is 50 per cent (Rics et al., 1994). Performance status and weight also have been shown to be predictors of survival (DeWys et al., 1980; Feinstein & Wells, 1982).

TREATMENT

The management of lung cancer depends on the histologic cell type, the extent and pattern of invasion and spread and the patient's physical condition. When possible, surgery is the primary treatment of NSCLC and chemotherapy is the most frequently used treatment of SCLC. Some small peripheral SCLC tumors also may be surgically cured. Generally, the treatment of lung cancer is not terribly effective. There is no really effective therapy for lung cancer patients with disseminated disease.

SURGERY

If the mediastinal nodes are determined to be disease-free, then surgery is usually the initial procedure. Functional or performance status is also considered in determining treatment. Surgery may be the choice of treatment when there is no evidence of metastatic spread beyond the ipsilateral hemithorax and when other patient characteristics, such as respiratory, cardiac, and cerebral status, are determined to be satisfactory for a favorable surgical outcome.

Patients with SCLC generally are not candidates for surgery because of the extent of disease at diagnosis. Surgery is the choice of treatment for patients with stage I or II non-SCLC. For small peripheral tumor removal, segmental or wedge resections can be used to preserve lung tissue, but lobectomy or pneumonectomy is the more usual approach for more centrally located tumors (Ginsberg, 1989; Hinson & Perry, 1993; Martini, 1993). In addition to removal of lung tissue, lymph node dissection is done systematically to determine if there is mediastinal or hilar lymph node involvement (Hinson & Perry, 1993). The choice of procedure depends on location, size, and extent of tumor spread. Those being considered for surgical resection should have a forced expiratory volume in 1 second (FEV_1) greater than 2 L and a predicted postpulmonary resection FEV_1 of 800 ml or greater (Olsen, Block, & Tobias, 1984). This value is necessary to ensure adequate respiratory function following surgery, that is, to prevent respiratory insufficiency.

Before surgery, the nurse may have to assist the patient with airway clearance measures to improve ventilatory capacity. Examples of these measures are to teach the patient coughing and deep breathing techniques, to assist with postural drainage, or to provide for inhalation of aerosol solutions. Smoking cessation may be advised before surgery. If infection is present, antibiotic administration will be prescribed. Nursing actions include explanations about the surgical procedure and about what is expected after surgery. Postoperatively, the patient is likely to have mechanical ventilatory assistance for a short time, but positive pressure ventilation is discontinued to prevent or minimize stress to sutured tissues. Following extubation, coughing and deep breathing exercises are necessary; splinting the incision will help decrease the pain, as will timing the exercises with analgesic administration. The patient should be positioned to facilitate lung expansion.

Nursing care depends on the surgical procedure used. For example, with a lobectomy, chest tubes with a closed drainage system may be used, whereas following a pneumonectomy, chest tubes will be clamped to allow filling of the thoracic cavity to prevent mediastinal shift. Thus it is critical that the nurse knows what procedure has been done and understands the underlying physiologic alterations to determine the appropriate specific nursing actions.

Survival rate decreases as size of tumor increases. Thus for those with more extensive disease, the evidence of increased survival rate with surgery is more controversial. With incomplete resection, in those with locally advanced stage IIIA lung cancer, 5-year survival is limited. Surgery for stage IIIA non-small-cell lung cancer is used; however, the value may be limited (Bains, 1991; Watanabe, Shimiyu, Oda et al., 1991). Five-year survival rates vary from 14 to 30 per cent. While these are regionally advanced tumors and may be resectable, frequently micrometastases are present and thus long-term survival following resection has remained poor. This has led to the trials of short-term preoperative chemotherapy (neoadjuvant therapy) followed by surgery for Stage IIIA and IIIB. Since the presence of micrometastases and distant metastases influences long-term survival in these patients, the induction chemotherapy prior to surgery has shown some promise in prolonging survival, but further study is needed. In addition to induction therapy, use of chemotherapy and radiation therapy following surgery also in some cases has enhanced survival of this group. With surgical resection alone, survival rates range from 20 to 40 months (Roth et al., 1994). Because at the time of diagnosis, those with SCLC frequently have extensive intrathoracic disease and evidence of extrathoracic disease, surgical resection is not generally a choice (Baker et al., 1987).

Surgical resection is used when there is chest wall involvement if all involved tissue can be removed (Martini, 1993). With complete resection of tumor, a 40 per cent 5-year survival rate has been reported for a group of patients with chest wall invasion (McCaughan, Martini, Bains, & McCormack, 1985). Survival of those without complete tumor resection or those with unresectable tumors was 2.5 years or less. Radiation therapy is used for those with unresectable chest wall tumors. Surgical resection may be done for other than curative purposes; for example, tumor excision can prevent invasion of the chest wall or involvement of ribs and intercostal spaces, which can result in severe pain. Surgery may be used in conjunction with adjuvant radiation therapy or in combination with chemotherapy or with chemotherapy alone.

Pulmonary resection may not be possible for those who have coexisting chronic lung disease or compromised pulmonary function. For example, the elderly may have diminished pulmonary function. Wedge resection may be used as an alternative to lobectomy in poor-risk patients or sleeve resection as an alternate to a pneumonectomy.

From a review of prognostic factors for patients with inoperable lung cancer, the initial Karnofsky performance score, the extent of disease, and the weight loss in the preceding 6 months were the most important prognostic factors (Stanley, 1980).

NEOADJUVANT THERAPY

More recently preoperative administration of two to three courses of chemotherapy has been tried to decrease the size of the tumor and local and distant metastasis. Use of preoperative chemotherapy for this purpose is referred to as neoadjuvant therapy. Also, if preoperative tumor response occurs, the surgery may then be followed by administration of the same chemotherapy regimen. Generally neoadjuvant therapy

is used for patients with stage IIIA NSCLC. Different trials have used different drug combinations, for example, cyclophosphamide, adriamycin and cisplatin, or cisplatin and 5-fluorouracil, or mitomycin, vinblastine, and platinum; some trials also have included radiation (Patterson, 1991). Preoperative chemotherapy and radiation therapy have been shown to improve resectability. However, unlike the improvement in survival rate being demonstrated with the use of preoperative (neoadjuvant) chemotherapy, the survival benefit of using preoperative radiation has not been shown to be significant (Cox, 1986; Patterson, 1991). Prior to the use of neoadjuvant therapy in the locally advanced stage IIIA (N2) bronchogenic carcinoma, radiation therapy alone had been the standard therapy.

One recent study compared the effectiveness of three courses of preoperative chemotherapy plus surgery with that of surgery alone in 60 patients with stage IIIA non-small-cell lung cancer (Rosell et al., 1994). The preoperative chemotherapy group received IV mitomycin (a bolus dose of 6 mg/m^2 of body surface area), ifosfamide (a 3-hour administration 3g/m^2 with mesna), and cisplatin (over 1 hour 50 mg/m^2) at three 3-week intervals followed by surgery in 4 to 5 weeks. Approximately 4 weeks after surgery both the preoperative chemotherapy and the surgery alone groups were subjected to mediastinal radiation. A significant difference in the median period of survival and median period of disease-free survival between the two groups was found. The median period of survival was 26 months and the median period of disease-free survival was 20 months for the preoperative chemotherapy group, in comparison with 8 months and 5 months, respectively, for the surgery only group. The preoperative chemotherapy group also had a lower rate of recurrence (56 per cent) than did the surgery only group (74 per cent). The majority of the subjects had squamous cell carcinoma. The investigators concluded that for patients with stage IIIA non-small-cell lung cancer, preoperative chemotherapy with mitomycin, ifosfamide, and cisplatin increases the median survival. Similar findings have been reported by other investigators (Martini et al., 1993; Murren, Buzaid, & Hait, 1991; Weiden & Piantadosi, 1991).

Another recent study compared the effectiveness of preoperative chemotherapy plus surgery with surgery alone for patients with resectable stage IIIA non-small-cell lung cancer (Roth et al., 1994). Three 28-day cycles of IV cyclophosphamide (500 mg/m^2 of body surface area), etoposide (100 mg/m^2), and cisplatin (100 mg/m^2) were used. A greater number of subjects in this study than in the Rosell et al. study had adenocarcinoma. The researchers also reported the effectiveness of preoperative chemotherapy in increasing the median survival and disease-free survival rates in comparison with the rates observed in the surgery alone group. While use of preoperative chemotherapy prolongs the total treatment, results of this study and those of other studies make induction chemotherapy for patients with resectable stage IIIA non-small-cell cancer the standard treatment. However, because different chemotherapy agents have been used in these studies, final recommendation of which combination of agents is most effective remains to be answered. Trials using chemotherapy and radiation therapy preoperatively are continuing.

RADIATION THERAPY

Radiation therapy is rarely curative for lung cancer, although a small percentage of patients survive 5 years following therapy. Initially, complete regression is seen in about half of those undergoing radiation therapy; however, there is a high incidence of local recurrence. The failure of radiation may be due to the presence of radio-resistant hypoxic tumor cells. Despite the local effectiveness of the radiation, the survival rate remains low because of distant metastatic involvement.

Radiation is more successful for those with small, peripheral, non-SCLC tumors with no evidence of metastases (Hande & Des Prez, 1982; Hoffman, Albain, Bitran, & Golomb, 1984; Perez et al., 1987). Patients with limited squamous cell carcinoma are those for whom radiation therapy has been the most effective. Although SCLC is quite sensitive to radiation, chemotherapy is the first treatment of choice because of the high frequency of extrathoracic metastatic disease with this type of lung cancer. (Pignon et al., 1992; Seifter & Ihde, 1988). Primarily radiation is used for patients with unresectable tumors, for those with regional lymph node involvement, and for those with direct invasion of other thoracic structures. For increased effectiveness of the therapy, the patient should be able to tolerate a 6- to 7-week course of therapy.

Radiation therapy has also been used preoperatively and postoperatively, but the benefit at those times remains controversial (Filderman & Matthay, 1985). Following tumor resection, radiation therapy may be prescribed for patients who have tumor cells at tissue margins (Hande & Des Prez, 1982). Radiation may be preferable for those who have resectable tumors but who may not be able to tolerate surgery.

Radiotherapy may be used for palliation of symptoms that result from compression or infiltration of intrathoracic structures by the tumor. For example, it has been shown to improve atelectasis resulting from lung cancer. It is also employed for palliation in chest wall invasion and for relief of bone pain, intractable cough, dyspnea, and hemoptysis. Radiation is used to treat complications such as bronchial obstruction, superior vena cava syndrome, and rib invasion; it is also used prophylactically for possible central nervous system involvement (Cox, 1981).

Prophylactic brain irradiation has been used for those with adenocarcinoma of the lung, but there is no evidence of increased duration of survival (Filderman & Matthay, 1985). Evidence supports the use of prophylactic cranial irradiation for those SCLC patients who show complete remission. This prophylaxis is important because cerebral metastases can occur with relapse of SCLC. Radiation is also employed in the treatment of metastatic central nervous system involvement (Carney & Minna, 1982; Greco & Oldham, 1979). Prophylactic cranial irradiation has been shown to decrease incidence of cerebral metastases and to improve survival, but this improvement has not been statistically significant (Blechen, 1984). Thus, controversy exists about the role of prophylactic cranial irradiation; some suggest that since there is no real survival benefit and brain metastases have been shown to respond to chemotherapy, cranial radiation should be used only when brain metastases occur (Kristensen, Kristjansen, & Hansen, 1992). Brain metastases are a common site for recurrence, particularly for resected adenocarcinoma. About one third of the patients with resected NSCLC have recurrence with brain metastases (Martini, 1993). A much higher incidence of brain metastases is found on autopsy of patients with lung cancer than of patients with other types of cancer. If brain metastases are not treated, the median survival is less than 3 months. Initial treatment is generally use of high-dose corticosteroid to reduce edema followed in several days by whole-brain radiation therapy. If there is a single isolated brain metastasis, surgery may be the treatment of choice (Burt et al., 1992). Following removal of a brain metastasis, whole-brain irradiation is recommended. Cranial irradiation is important when brain lesions are found, but its use prophylactically remains controversial.

Contraindications for the use of curative irradiation include inadequate respiratory reserve, pleural effusion, distant metastases, large tumor, weight loss greater than 4.5 kg, and a Karnofsky performance status of less than 70. These contraindications are similar to those that also exclude surgery as the choice of treatment.

Complications from radiation therapy increase as the dose increases and as the extent of normal tissue included in the field increases. For example, the incidence of fibrosis has been shown to increase with increased dose (Van Houtte, Piron, Lustman-Marechal, Osteaux, & Henry, 1980). Pulmonary fibrosis can result from permanent damage to the alveolar endothelium, and the extent of fibrosis is related to the amount of tissue irradiated. Some patients will experience dyspnea as a later consequence of this radiation-induced pulmonary fibrosis. Most patients usually have pulmonary fibrosis following chest radiation therapy but are asymptomatic. One complication that occurs 1 to 3 months after chest irradiation is pneumonitis; the patient experiences dyspnea and a nonproductive cough. Corticosteroids may be used for symptomatic relief, although the efficacy of this treatment is debatable; recovery usually occurs within a few weeks. Because of their effect on respiratory function, pneumonitis and fibrosis can influence the patient's quality of life (Wickham, 1986). If they are severe, respiratory complications may result in death.

Other complications are radiation-induced myelitis that occurs when protection of the spinal cord has been inadequate and pericarditis that results from inclusion of the heart in the irradiated field. Following postradiation dysphagia, long-term effects may be observed in the esophagus. Toxicities resulting from therapy have been described in detail elsewhere (Wickham, 1986).

Nurses have a role in explaining the use of radiation therapy and in helping the patient minimize the side effects, such as anorexia, nausea, and fatigue. Because the therapy requires long-term, almost daily treatment, it is important for the nurse to help the patient adhere to the scheduled therapy. The nurse also needs to be alert for clinical manifestations of the complications associated with radiation and to participate in the therapeutic management of the specific complication. It is important to understand that these complications may occur some time after radiation therapy has been completed.

CHEMOTHERAPY

Because local and distant metastases frequently are present at the time of lung cancer diagnosis, chemotherapy often is treatment of choice, particularly for SCLC. Reviews of the effectiveness of chemotherapy in the treatment of SCLC and non-SCLC are reported elsewhere (Greco, Johnson, Hainsworth, & Wolff, 1985; Klastersky & Sculier, 1985; Livingston, 1986; Zinreich, Baker, Ettinger, & Arder, 1984). The drugs most commonly used alone or in some combination for treatment of non-SCLC are carboplatin, velban, cisplatin, etoposide (VP-16-213), mitomycin, and vindesine. Newer agents include taxol and navelbine. An increase in survival time after using these agents is not yet well demonstrated. Most of the drugs in the chemotherapeutic regimen are associated with considerable side effects (morbidity). Good performance status, female sex, and an age of 70 years or older were found to be good predictors of outcome in a large group of patients with extensive-stage NSCLC (Albain, Crowley, LeBlanc, & Livingston, 1991). Use of cisplatin also was a predictor of improved outcome in this group.

Chemotherapy is the main treatment for SCLC. Chemotherapy is less effective for non-SCLCs, except that survival time has been observed to lengthen with the use of cisplatin. Small-cell lung cancer is more sensitive to chemotherapy than are non-SCLCs; however, the response occurs for only a short time, and relapse is frequent. Chemotherapy, with combination regimens, has been somewhat effective in both limited and extensive small-cell disease; there are reports of 50 per cent complete response rates for limited disease and 30 per cent for extensive disease (Hinson & Perry, 1993). Regimens that contain etoposide have been found to be more effective than the commonly used cyclophosphamide, doxorubicin, and vincristine (CAV) regimen (Ihde, 1992). Other agents used for treating SCLC are carboplatin, cisplatin, lomustine, ifosfamide methotrexate, taxol, vinblastine, and vindesine (Hinson & Perry, 1993). The other commonly used regimens are doxorubicin, cyclophosphamide and etoposide (ACE), and with cisplatin (PACE), and etoposide and cisplatin (EP) (Ihde, 1992). Generally there is an initial response rate but prolonged survival occurs only in 2 to 12 per cent of the SCLC patients because the rate of local relapse is high. For patients with limited disease, the median survival time is approximately 10 to 12 months (Carney & Minna, 1982); for those with extensive disease, it is

even less—approximately 8 to 9 months (Hoffman et al., 1984). Factors found to be associated with a more favorable long-term response to chemotherapy include a good performance status, less than a 5 per cent loss of usual body weight, maintenance of physical activity during therapy, and no liver or bone metastases (Finkelstein, Ettinger, & Ruckdeschel, 1986).

Tumor resistance to the drugs occurs; in new trials, attempts are being made to include non-cross-reactive agents to delay tumor resistance. Sequencing different drug combinations is another strategy to delay drug resistance; however, failure occurs with the emergence of drug-resistant cells. Little evidence suggests that a truly non-cross-resistant drug regimen has been identified for successful therapy for SCLC (Livingston, 1986).

Stem cell transfusion has been used to reestablish hematopoiesis when severe myelosuppression is a result of therapy. Monoclonal antibodies to SCLC can be used for in vitro removal of tumor cells from bone marrow for autologous transplantation but is experimental (Okabe, Kaizu, Fujisawa, Watanabe, & Takaku, 1985).

The major nursing care associated with chemotherapy frequently includes administration of the prescribed agents, assisting the patient in managing the side effects experienced, assessing for signs and symptoms of toxicities specific to the agents used, and monitoring patient responses. Again, as is true for radiation therapy, the nurse can play a role in helping the patient understand the principles of the therapy and the necessity for completing the prescribed treatment protocol.

COMBINATION THERAPY

Some investigators have shown improved complete response rates and survival using combination radiation therapy of the primary limited small-cell tumor along with chemotherapy (Choi et al., 1987; Perry et al., 1987). Response rates in the elderly being treated for SCLC are similar to the responses of others (Clamon, Audeh, & Pinnick, 1982). Surgery is not considered to be curative in patients with SCLC; thus if surgery is used in treatment of SCLC, postoperative chemotherapy and radiation therapy also are used. Preoperative neoadjuvant therapy is being tried in patients with SCLC, but survival benefits remain undetermined. Chemotherapy and radiation therapy administered concomitantly, as a split course, or sequentially also are used in treatment of SCLC. Cisplatin is a radiation sensitizer and thus may enhance tumor cell destruction when combination therapies are used.

The success of surgical adjuvant therapies for non-SCLC patients has been reviewed (Holmes, 1986). Almost 50 per cent of the patients with NSCLC have mediastinal metastasis (Martini, 1993). These patients with N2 disease are treated with surgery and radiation or chemotherapy. If the nodes are enlarged and visible on chest x-ray, surgery may not be of benefit. When the contralateral hilum or mediastinal lymph nodes are involved, surgery generally is not indicated. Patients with stage IIIB lung cancer are treated with irradiation or chemotherapy or a combination because the extent of their disease generally precludes a complete or successful surgical resection. For those non-SCLC patients whose disease is considered inoperable, combined radiation therapy for control of locoregional involvement and chemotherapy for control of distant metastases are used. However, survival rates have not improved greatly; systemic recurrence remains a problem. Response rates to chemotherapy for those with advanced non-SCLC range from 25 to 40 per cent; for those whose disease is limited to the thorax, the response rates are 50 to 70 per cent. New active non-cross-resistant drugs need to be developed.

The most common first site of recurrence in patients treated for adenocarcinoma and large-cell undifferentiated carcinoma is extrapulmonary, usually the brain (Holmes, 1986). The most common first site of recurrence for squamous cell carcinoma is local; postoperative radiation therapy results in decreased incidence of local recurrence in patients with squamous cell cancer but has not been shown to prolong survival significantly (Holmes, 1986). Regardless of the small successes achieved with therapies, deaths from lung cancer result from the presence of distant metastases in most cases.

IMMUNOTHERAPY

Lung cancer is an immunosuppressive disease; that is, some lung cancer patients have a depressed immune response, and lymphocytes that have infiltrated the tumor have depressed activity (Holmes, 1986). These immune system defects may contribute to the rapid disease progression. In a study of anorexia and immune response in patients with SCLC, the only patient who was alive 1 year after diagnosis remained responsive to two out of three skin test antigens (Lindsey & Piper, 1986). Despite attempts of treatment with immunotherapy, evidence remains controversial. Improvement in duration of survival after treatment with nonspecific immunoadjuvants has not been shown to occur (see Chapter 23 on biologic response modifiers for more detail).

Although monoclonal antibodies (MoAbs) have been made in response to lung cancer antigens, the antigenic and biologic heterogeneity of SCLC in particular results in the lack of antibody specificity and thus limits the utility of this approach for treatment (Carney, 1986). Monoclonal antibodies were used to demonstrate the presence of SCLC cells in bone marrow specimens that had been considered to be tumor-free and to demonstrate bone marrow metastases in patients who had been determined clinically to have limited disease (Bernal & Speak, 1984). These antibodies have potential value in the preparation of bone marrow for autologous transplantation, because specific MoAbs lyse the SCLC cells that are present in the ex vivo bone marrow. The concept is that the creation of specific MoAbs or other biologic response modifiers has the potential to eliminate any residual microscopic drug-resistant cells; until these cells are eradicated, therapy remains ineffective in improving survival rates.

Over the past 2 decades, little change has occurred in the survival rates for new lung cancer patients.

OTHER THERAPIES

Photodynamic therapy (PDT) has been tried as an alternative to surgery in patients with small endobronchial lung cancers (Edell & Cortese, 1987; Imamura et al., 1994). Tumors can be localized with fiberoptic bronchoscopic procedures, and a radiosensitizer such as a hematoporphyrin derivative is used for the photodynamic therapy. Good response rates have been reported with use of this therapy with early small tumors. PDT is used when surgery is contraindicated. Other experimental techniques for these lesions include laser therapy and radiation implants.

Chemoprevention trials are being conducted in attempts to prevent development of lung cancer and the development of second primary tumors in patients with NSCLC (Benner, Lippman & Hong, 1995). Compounds with vitamin A-like activity, the retinoids, are being used in chemoprevention trials. For example, Pastorino et al. (1993) found a beneficial effect of retinyl palmitate following surgical resection of NSCLC over 1 year of observation. A long-term multi-institutional study is examining the effects of low-dose isotretinoin on development of second primary tumors in patients treated with surgical resection of stage I NSCLC. The treatment will be carried out for 3 years with a subsequent 4-year follow-up (Benner, Lippman, & Hong, 1995). Other chemoprevention trials are aimed at preventing lung cancer. However a recent clinical trial suggested an increase in lung cancer with a dietary intervention of vitamin E and beta carotene in smokers (The Alpha-Tocopherol, Beta Carotene Cancer Prevention Study Group, 1996). Considering the poor prognosis associated with lung cancer, smoking prevention, smoking cessation, and decreased exposure to environmental tobacco smoke are the best approaches to disease prevention; chemoprevention may also be a promising approach to disease control (The Alpha-Tocopherol, Beta Carotene Cancer Prevention Study Group, 1994; Dumbauld et al., 1994; Centers for Disease Control, 1994).

QUALITY OF LIFE, SYMPTOM DISTRESS, AND LUNG CANCER

Because of the significant mortality rate and the minimal effectiveness of current treatment for advanced lung cancer, the impact of lung cancer on quality of life has been the object of considerable discussion and study, particularly as part of clinical trials. The issue of the benefits of treatment for advanced disease has been controversial, with some (e.g., Fayers, Bleehen, Girling, & Stephens, 1991; Geddes et al., 1990) suggesting poor quality of life in those undergoing treatment, and others (Bergman & Sorenson, 1987) suggesting important benefits of treatment. Without treatment, the median survival of patients with lung cancer is less than 6 months, and most do not survive a year following diagnosis (Martini, 1993). Poor quality of life has been reported to be a predictor of shorter survival in lung cancer (Ganz, Lee & Siau, 1991; Kaasa, Mastekaasa, & Lund, 1989; Kukull, McCorkle, & Driever, 1986). Attempts to develop lung cancer–specific quality of life measures also are underway (Hollen, Gralla, Kris, & Potanovich, 1993; Hopwood, Stephens, & Machin, 1994). Symptom distress is a critical component of quality of life for persons with lung cancer and is an important foci for nursing intervention. Recent reviews of quality of life research and lung cancer emphasize the strong relationship to symptom distress (Bernhard & Ganz, 1991a, 1991b; Fergusson & Cull, 1991; Sarna, 1993). Distressing symptoms prevalent during the course of advanced lung cancer include fatigue, functional decline, pain, dyspnea, cough, weight loss, anorexia, insomnia, and difficulties with concentration (Blesch et al., 1991; Geddes et al., 1990; Sarna, 1994; Wilkie, Keefe, Dodd, & Copp, 1992). An experimental nursing home care intervention program for persons with lung cancer was associated with less symptom distress and prolonged functional ability as compared with those receiving standard care (McCorkle et al., 1989).

High levels of emotional distress (both anxiety and depression) have been reported in patients with lung cancer (Hopwood & Thatcher, 1990). Weisman and Worden's (1977) classic study of emotional distress in persons with cancer identified lung cancer as a diagnosis associated with the most symptoms, the most emotional distress, and the greatest overall concerns as compared with other cancer patients. Emotional and symptom distress of persons with lung cancer can profoundly impact family caregiving needs as well (McCorkle & Wilkerson, 1991).

Studies have examined other psychosocial and physiologic factors experienced by patients and their families during the diagnosis and treatment of lung cancer (Germino & McCorkle, 1985; Driever & McCorkle, 1984; Cooper, 1984; Larson et al., 1993; Sarna et al., 1994; Lindsey, Larson, Sarna, & Brown, 1993). For example, refer to Box 30–1, which summarizes a study that examined the relationships of weight change, symptom distress, and functional status in 60 patients with progressive lung cancer. In this longitudinal study, weight loss was found to be related to decline in functional status and increased symptom distress. The reported findings from many studies reflect a range of variables that have the potential to influence the quality of life of individuals with lung cancer. These findings also have implications for directing nursing care.

SUMMARY

In those who have no metastatic spread, non-SCLCs are potentially curable by surgery but are relatively resistant to chemotherapy and radiation. For those with SCLC, surgery is relatively ineffective due to the frequent existence of metastatic disease, but the tumor cells are responsive to radiation and chemotherapy. At the time of diagnosis, only about 20 per cent of lung cancer patients have localized tumor.

For those whose tumors do not respond to treatment, therapy is changed, and if the tumor remains unresponsive after different therapeutic regimens have been used, therapy may be withheld.

For some lung cancer patients with extensive disease, supportive care with antibiotics, analgesics, and bronchodilators may be the treatment of choice. For some, quality of life may be increased with symptom management rather than with aggressive anticancer therapy.

REFERENCES

Akoun, G. M., Scarna, H. M., Milleron, B. H., Benichoun, M. R., & Herman, D. P. (1985). Serum neuron-specific enolase: A marker for disease extent and response to therapy for small cell lung cancer. *Chest, 87,* 39.

Alavanja, M. C. R, Brown, C. C., Swanson, C., & Brownson, R. C. (1993). Saturated fat intake and lung cancer risk among nonsmoking women in Missouri. *Journal of the National Cancer Institute, 85,* 1906–1916.

Alavanja, M. C. R, Brownson, R. C., Boice, J. D., & Hock, E. (1992). Preexisting lung disease and lung cancer among nonsmoking women. *American Journal of Epidemiology, 136,* 623–632.

Albain, K. S., Crowley, J. J., LeBlanc, M., & Livingston, R. B. (1991). Survival determinants in extensive-stage non-small cell lung cancer: The Southwest Oncology Group experience. *Journal of Clinical Oncology, 9*(9), 1618–1626.

The Alpha-Tocopherol, Beta Carotene Cancer Prevention Study Group. (1994). The effect of vitamin E and beta carotene on the incidence of lung cancer and other cancers in male smokers. *New England Journal of Medicine, 330,* 1029–1035.

Bains, M. S. (1991). Surgical treatment of lung cancer. *Chest, 100,* 826–837.

Baker, R. R., Ettinger, D. S., Ruckdeschel, J. D., Eggleston, J. C., McKneally, M. F., Abeloff, M. D., Woll, J., & Adelstein, D. J. (1987). The role of surgery in the management of selected patients with small-cell carcinoma of the lung. *Journal of Clinical Oncology, 5,* 697–702.

Bartecchi, C. E., McKenzie, T. D., & Schrier, R. W. (1994). The human costs of tobacco use. Part I. *New England Journal of Medicine, 330,* 907–912.

Bechtel, J. J., Kelley, W. R., Petty, T. L., Patz, D. S., & Saccomanno, G. (1994). Outcome of 51 patients with roentgenographically occult lung cancer detected by sputum cytologic testing: A community hospital program. *Archives of Internal Medicine, 154,* 975–980.

Benedict, S. (1989). The suffering associated with lung cancer. *Cancer Nursing, 12,* 34–40.

Benner, S. E., Lippman, S. M., & Hong, W. K. (1995). Current status of retinoid chemoprevention of lung cancer. *Oncology, 9,* 205–210.

Berckman, K. L., & Austin, J. K. (1993). Causal attribution, perceived control, and adjustment in patients with lung cancer. *Oncology Nursing Forum, 20,* 23–30.

Bergman, B., & Sorenson, S. (1987). Return to work among patients with small cell lung cancer. *European Journal of Respiratory Diseases, 70,* 49–53.

Bergman, B., & Sorenson, S. (1988). Smoking and effect of chemotherapy in small cell lung cancer. *European Respiratory Journal, 1,* 932–937.

Bernal, S., & Speak, J. A. (1984). Membrane antigen in small cell carcinoma of the lung defined by monoclonal antibody SMI. *Cancer Research, 44,* 266–270.

Bernhard, J., & Ganz, P. A. (1991a). Psychosocial issues in lung cancer patients (Part 1). *Chest, 99,* 216–223.

Bernhard, J., & Ganz, P. A. (1991b). Psychosocial issues in lung cancer patients (Part 2). *Chest, 99*, 2480–2485.

Bjornson, W., Rand, C., Connett, J. E., Lindgren, P., Nides, M., Pope, F., Buist, A. S., Hoppe-Ryan, C., & O'Hara, P. for The Lung Health Study Research Group (1995). Gender differences in smoking cessation after 3 years in the Lung Health Study. *American Journal of Public Health, 85*, 223–230.

Blechen, N. M. (1984). Management of small cell cancer: Radio therapy. In W. Duncan (Ed.), *Recent results in cancer research: Lung cancer* (pp. 65–78). New York: Springer-Verlag.

Blesch, K. S., Paice, J. A., Wickham, R., Horte, N., Schnoor, D. K., Purl, S., Rehwalt, M., Kopp, P. L., Manson, S., Coveny, S. B., McHale, M., & Cahill, M. (1991). Correlates of fatigue in people with breast or lung cancer. *Oncology Nursing, 18*, 81–87.

Bone, R. C., & Balk, R. (1982). Staging of bronchogenic carcinoma. *Chest, 82*, 473–480.

Boring, C. C., Squires, T. S., Tong, T., & Montgomery, S. (1994). Cancer statistics, 1994. *CA-A Cancer Journal for Clinicians, 44*, 7–26.

Brown, J. (1993). Gender, age, usual weight, and tobacco use as predictors of weight loss in patients with lung cancer. *Oncology Nursing Forum, 20*, 466–472.

Brown, M. L., Carrieri, V. L., Janson-Bjerklie, S., & Dodd, M. J. (1986). Lung cancer and dyspnea: The patient's perception. *Oncology Nursing Forum, 13*(5), 19–24.

Brownson, R. C., Alavanja, M. C. R., & Chang, J. C. (1993). Occupational risk factors for lung cancer among non-smoking women: a case-control study in Missouri (United States). *Cancer Causes and Control, 4*, 449–454.

Brownson, R. C., Jackson-Thompson, J., Wilkerson, J. C., Davis, J. R., Owens, N. W., & Fisher, E. B. (1992). Demographic and socioeconomic differences in beliefs about the health effects of smoking. *American Journal of Public Health, 82*, 99–103.

Burt, M., Wronski, M., Arbit, E., et al. (1992). Resection of brain metastases from non-small cell lung carcinoma: Results of therapy. *Journal of Thoracic Cardiovascular Surgery, 103*, 399–410.

Candelora, E. C., Stockwell, H. G., Armstrong, A. W., & Pinkham, P. A. (1992). Dietary intake and risk of lung cancer in women who never smoked. *Nutrition & Cancer, 17*, 263–270.

Carney, D. N. (1986). Recent advances in the biology of small cell lung cancer. *Chest, 89*(4 Suppl.), 253S–257S.

Carney, D. N., & Minna, J. D. (1982). Small cell cancer of the lung. *Clinics in Chest Medicine, 3*, 389–398.

Carney, D. N., Zweig, M. H., Ihde, D. C., Cohen, M. H., Makuch, R. W., & Gazdor, A. F. (1984). Elevated serum creatine kinase BB levels in patients with small cell lung cancer. *Cancer Research, 44*, 5399–5403.

Carr, D. T. (1981). Malignant lung disease. *Hospital Practice, 17*, 97–115.

Centers for Disease Control (1994). Cigarette smoking among adults—United States, 1993. *Morbidity and Mortality Weekly Report, 43*, 925–930.

Chlebowski, R. T., Heber, D., & Block, J. B. (1983). Lung cancer cachexia. In F. A. Greco (Ed.), *Biology and management of lung cancer* (pp. 125–142). Boston: Martinus Nijhoff Publishers.

Choi, N. C., Carey, R. W., Kaufman, S. D., Grillo, H. C., Younger, J., & Wilkins, E. W. (1987). Small cell carcinoma of the lung. *Cancer, 59*, 6–14.

Choi, N. C., Grillo, H. C., & Huberman, M. S. (1986). Cancer of the lung. In B. Cody (Ed.), *Cancer manual* (pp. 166–177). Boston: American Cancer Society Massachusetts Division, Inc.

Chollat-Traquet, C. (1992). *Women and tobacco.* Geneva: World Health Organization.

Clamon, G. C., Audeh, M. W., & Pinnick, S. (1982). Small cell lung carcinoma in the elderly. *Journal of American Geriatric Society, 30*, 299–302.

Cohen, M. H. (1982). Natural history of lung cancer. *Clinics in Chest Medicine, 3*, 229–241.

Colditz, G. A., Stampfer, M. J., & Willett, W. C. (1987). Diet and lung cancer: A review of the epidemiologic evidence in humans. *Archives of Internal Medicine, 147*, 157–160.

Colsher, P. L., Wallace, R. B., Pomrehn, P. R., LaCroix, A. Z., Cornoni-Huntley, J., Blazer, D., Scherr, P. A., Berkman, L., & Hennekens, C. H. (1990). Demographic and health characteristics of elderly smokers: results from established populations for epidemiologic studies of the elderly. *American Journal of Preventive Medicine, 6*, 61–70.

Cooper, E. T. (1984, August). A pilot study on the effects of the diagnosis of lung cancer on family relationships. *Cancer Nursing, 7*, 301–308.

Costa, G., Lane, W. W., Vincent, R. G., Siebold, J. A., Aragon, M., & Bewley, P. T. (1981). Weight loss and cachexia in lung cancer. *Nutrition and Cancer, 2*, 98–103.

Cox, B. G., Carr, D. C., & Lee, R. E. (1992). *Living with lung cancer, a guide for patients and their families* (3rd ed.). Gainesville, FL: Triad Publishing Company.

Cox, J. D. (1981). The role of radiation therapy for carcinoma of the lung. *Yale Journal of Biology and Medicine, 54*, 195–200.

Cox, J. D. (1986). Non-small cell lung cancer: Role of radiation therapy. *Chest, 89*(Suppl), 284S–288S.

Craighead, J. E., & Mossman, B. T. (1982). The pathogenesis of asbestos-related diseases. *New England Journal of Medicine, 306*, 1446–1455.

Dalager, N. A., Pickle, L. W., Mason, T. J., Correa, P., Fontham, E., Stemhagan, A., Buffler, P. A., Ziegler, R. G., & Fraumeni, J. F. (1986). The relation of passive smoking to lung cancer. *Cancer Research, 46*, 4808–4811.

Devesa, S. S., Blot, W. J., Stone, B. J., Miller, B. A., Tarone, R. E., & Fraumeni Jr, J. F. (1995). Recent cancer trends in the United States. *Journal of the National Cancer Institute, 87*, 175–182.

DeWys, W. D., Begg, C., Lavin, P. T., Band, R. P., Bennett, M. J., Bertino, R. J., Cohen, H. M., Douglas, Jr., O. H., Engstrom, F. P., Ezdinli, Z. E., Horton, J., Johnson, J. G., Moertel, G. C., Oken, M. M., Perlia, C., Rosenbaum, C., Silverstein, N. M., Skeel, T. R., Sponzo, W. R., & Tormey, C. D. (1980). Prognostic effect of weight loss prior to chemotherapy in cancer patients. *American Journal of Medicine, 69*, 491–497.

Doll, R., & Hill, A. B. (1964). Mortality in relation to smoking: Ten year observations of British doctors. *British Medical Journal, 1*, 1399–1410.

Doll, R., Peto, R., Wheatley, K. Gray, R., & Sutherland, I. (1994). Mortality in relation to smoking: 40 years' observations on male British doctors. *British Medical Journal, 390*, 901–911.

Driever, M. J., & McCorkle, R. (1984, June). Patient concerns at 3 and 6 months postdiagnosis. *Cancer Nursing, 7*, 235–241.

Dumas, L. (1992). Lung cancer in women: Rising epidemic, preventable disease. *Nursing Clinics of North America: Women's Health, 27*, 859–869.

Dumbauld, S., McCullough, J. A., & Sutocky, J. W. (1994). *Analysis of health indicators in California's Minority Populations.* Minority Health Information Improvement Project No. 180M-5-92. Sacramento, California.

Edell, E. S., & Cortese, D. A. (1987). Bronchoscopic phototherapy with hematoporphyria derivative for treatment of localized bronchogenic carcinoma: A five-year experience, *Mayo Clinic Proceedings, 62,* 8–14.

Elders, M. J., Perry, C. L., Eriksen, M. P., & Giovino, G. A. (1994). The report of the Surgeon General: Preventing tobacco use among young people. *American Journal of Public Health, 84,* 543–547.

Ershler, W. B., Socinski, M. A., & Greene, C. J. (1982). Bronchogenic cancer, metastases, and aging. *Journal of the American Geriatric Society, 31,* 673–676.

Fayers, P. M., Bleehen, N. M., Girling, D. J., & Stephens, R. J. (1991). Assessment of quality of life in small-cell lung cancer using a Daily Diary Card developed by the Medical Research Council Lung Cancer Working Party. *British Journal of Cancer, 64,* 299–306.

Feinstein, A. R., & Wells, C. K. (1982). Lung cancer staging: A critical evaluation. *Clinics in Chest Medicine, 3,* 291–305.

Ferguson, M. K., Skosey, C., Hoffman, P. C., & Golomb, H. M. (1990). Sex-associated differences in presentation and survival in patients with lung cancer. *Journal of Clinical Oncology, 8,* 1402–1407.

Fergusson, R. J., & Cull, A. (1991). Quality of life measurement for patients undergoing treatment for lung cancer. *Thorax, 46,* 671–675.

Filderman, A. E., & Matthay, R. A. (1985, November/December). Update on lung cancer. *Respiratory Therapy, 15(6),* 21–31.

Filderman, A. E., Shaw, C., & Matthay, R. A. (1986). Lung cancer in the elderly. *Clinics in Geriatric Medicine, 2,* 363–383.

Finkelstein, D. M., Ettinger, D. S., & Ruckdeschel, J. C. (1986). Long-term survivors in metastatic non-small cell lung cancer. *Journal of Clinical Oncology, 4,* 702–709.

Fiore, M. C., Jorenby, D. E., Schensky, A. E., Smith, S. S., Bauer, R. R., & Baker, T. B. (1995). Smoking status as the new vital sign: effect on assessment and intervention in patients who smoke. *Mayo Clinics Proceedings, 70,* 2029–2213.

Flehinger, B. J., Melamed, M. R., Zaman, M. B., Heelan, T., Perchick, B. W., & Martini, N. (1984). Early lung cancer detection: Results of the initial (prevalence) radiologic and cytologic screening in the Memorial Sloan Kettering study. *American Review of Respiratory Disease, 130,* 555–560.

Fontana, R. S., Sanderson, D. R., Taylor, W. F., Woolner, B. L., Miller, E. W., Muhm, R. J., & Uhlenhopp, A. M. (1984). Early lung cancer detection: Results of the initial (prevalence) radiologic and cytologic screening in the Mayo Clinic Study. *American Review of Respiratory Disease, 130,* 561–565.

Foote, M., Sexton, D. L., & Pawlik, L. (1986). Dyspnea: A distressing sensation in lung cancer. *Oncology Nursing Forum, 13(5),* 25–31.

Frank, A. L. (1982). The epidemiology and etiology of lung cancer. *Clinics in Chest Medicine, 3,* 219–228.

Frost, J. K., Ball, W. C., Levin, M. L., Tockman, S. M., Baker, R. R., Carter, D., Eggleston, C. J., Erazan, Y., Gupta, K. P., Khouri, F. N., Marsh, R. B., & Stitik, P. F. (1984). Early lung cancer detection: Results of the initial (prevalence) radiologic and cytologic screening in the Johns Hopkins Study. *American Review of Respiratory Disease, 130,* 549–554.

Ganz, P. A., Lee, J. J., & Siau, J. (1991). Quality of life assessment: An independent prognostic variable for survival in lung cancer. *Cancer, 67,* 3131–3135.

Garfinkle, L., & Silverberg, E. (1991). Lung cancer and smoking trends in the United States over the past 25 years. *CA-A Cancer Journal for Clinicians, 41,* 137–145.

Gazdar, A. F., Carney, D. N., & Minna, J. D. (1983). The biology of non-small cell lung cancer. *Seminars in Oncology, 10,* 3–19.

Geddes, D. M. (1979). The natural history of lung cancer: A review based on rates of tumour growth. *British Journal of Diseases of the Chest, 73,* 1–17.

Geddes, D. M., Dones, L., Hill, E., Law, K., Harper, P. G., Spiro, S. G., Tobias, J. S., & Souhami, R. L. (1990). Quality of life during chemotherapy for small cell lung cancer: Assessment and use of a daily diary card in a randomized trial. *European Journal of Cancer, 26,* 484–492.

Germino, B., & McCorkle, R. (1985). Acknowledged awareness of life-threatening illness. *International Journal of Nursing Studies, 22,* 33–44.

Ginsberg, R. J. (1989). Limited resection in the treatment of stage I non-small cell lung cancer: An overview. *Chest 96(Suppl.)* 505–515.

Greco, F. A., Johnson, D. H., Hainsworth, J. D., & Wolff, S. N. (1985). Chemotherapy of small cell lung cancer. *Seminars in Oncology, 12(4, Suppl. 6),* 31–37.

Greco, F. A., & Oldham, R. K. (1979). Small-cell lung cancer. *New England Journal of Medicine, 301,* 355–358.

Gritz, E. R. (1991). Smoking and smoking cessation in cancer patients. *British Journal of Addiction, 86,* 549–554.

Gritz, E. R. (1993). Lung cancer: Now, more than ever, a feminist issue. *CA-A Cancer Journal for Clinicians, 43,* 197–199.

Gritz, E. R., Nisenbaum, R., Elashoff, R., & Holmes, E. C. (1991). Smoking behavior following diagnosis in patients with stage I non-small cell lung cancer. *Cancer Causes Control, 2,* 105–112.

Halpern, M. T., Gillespie, B. W., & Warner, K. E. (1993). Patterns of absolute risk of lung cancer mortality in former smokers. *Journal of the National Cancer Institute, 68,* 395–399.

Hande, K. R., & Des Prez, R. M. (1982). Chemotherapy and radiation therapy for non-small cell lung carcinoma. *Clinics in Chest Medicine, 3,* 399–414.

Hansen, M., & Pedersen, A. G. (1986). Tumor markers in patients with lung cancer. *Chest, 89(4 Suppl.),* 219S–224S.

Haque, A. K. (1991). Pathology of carcinoma of lung: An update on current concepts. *Journal of Thoracic Imaging, 7(1),* 9–20.

Harris, R. E., Zang, E. A., Anderson, J. I., & Wynder, E. L. (1993). Race and sex differences in lung cancer risk associated with cigarette smoking. *International Journal of Epidemiology, 22,* 592–599.

Heitzman, E. R. (1986). The role of computed tomography in the diagnosis and management of lung cancer. *Chest, 89(4 Suppl.),* 237S–241S.

Hinson, J. A., & Perry, M. C. (1993). Small cell lung cancer. *CA-A Cancer Journal for Clinicians, 43,* 216–225.

Hoffman, P. C., Albain, K. S., Bitran, J. D., & Golomb, M. H. (1984). Current concepts in small cell carcinoma of the lung. *CA-A Cancer Journal for Clinicians, 34,* 269–281.

Hollen, P. J., Gralla, R. J., Kris, M. G., & Potanovich, L. M. (1993). Quality of life assessment in individuals with lung cancer: Testing the Lung Cancer Symptom Scale (LCSS). *European Journal of Cancer, 29A,* S51–S38.

Holmes, E. C. (1986). Surgical adjuvant therapy of non-small cell lung cancer. *Chest, 89(4 Suppl.),* 295S–300S.

Hopwood, P., Stephens, R. J., & Machin, D. for the MRC Lung Cancer Working Party. (1994). Approaches to the analysis of quality of life data: experiences gained from a Medical research council lung cancer working party palliative chemotherapy trial. *Quality of Life Research, 3,* 339–352.

Hopwood, P., & Thatcher, N. (1990). Preliminary experience with quality of life evaluation in patients with lung cancer. *Oncology Williston Park, 4,* 158–162.

Ihde, D. C. (1992). Chemotherapy of lung cancer. *New England Journal of Medicine, 327,* 1434–1441.

Imamura, S., Kusunoki, Y., Takifuji, N., Kudo, S., Matsui, K., Masuda, N., Takada, M., Negoro, S., Ryu, S., & Fukuoka, M. (1994). Photodynamic therapy and/or external beam radiation therapy for roentgenologically occult lung cancer. *Cancer, 73*(6), 1608–1614.

Johnson, D. H., Marangos, P. J., Forbes, J. T., Hainsworth, J. D., Welch, V. R., Hande, K. R., & Greco, A. F. (1984). Potential utility of serum neuron-specific enolase levels in small cell carcinoma of the lung. *Cancer Research, 44,* 5409.

Kaasa, S., Mastekaasa, A., & Lund, E. (1989). Prognostic factors for patients with inoperable non-small cell lung cancer, limited disease. The importance of patients' subjective experience of disease and psychosocial well-being. *Radiotherapy and Oncology, 15,* 235–242.

Kawachi, I., Colditz, G. A., Stampfer, M. J., Willet, W. C., Manson, J. A. E., Rosner, B., Hunter, D. J., Hennekens, C. H., & Speizer, J. E. (1993). Smoking cessation in relation to total mortality rates in women. A prospective cohort study. *Annals of Internal Medicine, 119,* 992–1000.

Kern, J. A., Schwark, D. A., & Nordberg, J. E. (1990). p185—neu expression in human lung adenocarcinomas predicts shortened survival. *Cancer Research, 50,* 5184–5191.

Klastersky, J., & Sculier, J. P. (1985). Chemotherapy of non-small cell lung cancer. *Seminars in Oncology, 12*(4, Suppl. 6), 38–48.

Knudsen, N., Schulman, S., van den Hoek, J., & Fowler, R. (1985). Insights on how to quit smoking: a survey of patients with lung cancer. *Cancer Nursing, 8,* 145–150.

Kristensen, C. A., Kristjansen, P. E., & Hansen, H. H. (1992). Systemic chemotherapy of brain metastases from small-cell lung cancer: A review. *Journal of Clinical Oncology, 10,* 1498–1502.

Kukull, W. A., McCorkle, R., & Driever, M. (1986). Symptom distress, psychosocial variables, and lung cancer survival. *Journal of Psychosocial Oncology, 4,* 91–104.

Larson, P. J., Lindsey, A. M., Dodd, M. J., Brecht, M. L., & Packer, A. (1993). Influence of age on problems experienced by patients with lung cancer undergoing radiation therapy. *Oncology Nursing Forum, 20,* 473–480.

Lindsey, A. M. (1986a). Cachexia. In V. Carrieri, A. M. Lindsey, & C. West (Eds.), *Pathophysiological phenomena in nursing: Human responses to illness* (pp. 122–136). Philadelphia: W. B. Saunders Co.

Lindsey, A. M. (1986b). Cancer cachexia: Effects of the disease and its treatment. *Seminars in Oncology Nursing, 2,* 19–29.

Lindsey, A. M., Larson, P. J., Sarna, L., & Brown, J. K. (1993). The lung cancer experience: Comparison of variables and findings across three studies. *Oncology Nursing Forum, 20,* 490–493.

Lindsey, A. M., & Piper, B. F. (1985). Anorexia and weight loss: Indicators of cachexia in small cell lung cancer. *Nutrition and Cancer, 7*(1 & 2), 65–76.

Lindsey, A. M., & Piper, B. F. (1986). Anorexia, serum zinc, and immunologic response in small cell lung cancer patients receiving chemotherapy and prophylactic cranial radiation. *Nutrition and Cancer, 8,* 231–238.

Lindsey, A. M., Piper, B. F., & Carrieri, V. L. (1981). Malignant cells and ectopic hormone production. *Oncology Nursing Forum, 8,* 13–15.

Lindsey, A. M., Piper, B. F., & Stotts, N. (1982). The phenomenon of cancer cachexia: A review. *Oncology Nursing Forum, 9*(2), 38–42.

Livingston, R. B. (1986). Current chemotherapy of small cell lung cancer. *Chest, 89*(4 Suppl.), 258S–263S.

Loeb, L. A., Ernster, V. L., Warner, K. E., Abbotts, J., & Laszio, J. (1984). Smoking and lung cancer: An overview. *Cancer Research, 44,* 5940–5958.

Loke, J., Matthay, R. A., & Ieda, S. (1982). Techniques for diagnosing lung cancer. *Clinics in Chest Medicine, 3,* 321–329.

Marino, L. B., & Levy, S. M. (1986). Primary and secondary prevention of cancer in children and adolescents: Current status and issues. *Pediatric Clinics of North America, 33,* 975–993.

Martini, N. (1993). Operable lung cancer. *CA-A Cancer Journal for Clinicians, 43,* 201–214.

Martini, N., Kris, M. G., Flehinger, B. J., Gralla, R. J., Bains, M. S., Burt, M. E., Heelan, R., McCormick, P. M., Pisters, K. M. W., Rigas, J. R., Rusch, V. W., & Ginsberg, R. J. (1993). Preoperative chemotherapy for stage IIIa (N2) lung cancer: The Sloan-Kettering experience with 136 patients. *Annals of Thoracic Surgery, 55,* 1365–1374.

Mathews, M. J., McKay, B., & Lukeman, J. (1983). The pathology of non-small cell carcinoma of the lung. *Seminars in Oncology, 10,* 34–55.

McCaughan, B. C., Martini, N., Bains, M. S., & McCormack, P. M. (1985). Chest wall invasion of carcinoma of the lung: Therapeutic and prognostic implications. *Journal of Thoracic Cardiovascular Surgery, 89,* 836–841.

McCorkle, R., Benoliel, J. Q., Donaldson, G., Georgiadou, F., Moinpour, C., & Goodell, B. (1989). A randomized clinical trial of home nursing care for lung cancer patients. *Cancer, 64,* 199–206.

McCorkle, R. & Wilkerson, K. (1991) *Home care needs of cancer patients and their caregivers.* Final Report. National Center for Nursing Research, NR01914.

McDuffie, H. H., Klaassen, D. J., & Dosman, J. A. (1991). Men, women and primary lung cancer—a Saskatchewan personal interview study. *Journal of Clinical Epidemiology, 44,* 537–544.

McGinnis, J. M., & Foege, W. H. (1993). Actual causes of death in the United States. *Journal of the American Medical Association, 2,* 2207–2212.

Melamed, M. R., Flehinger, B. J., Zaman, M. B., Heelan, R. T., Perchick, W. A., & Martini, N. (1984). Screening for early cancer. *Chest, 86,* 44–53.

Mitsudomi, T., Tateishi, M., Oka, T., Yano, T., Ishida, T., & Sugimachi, K. (1989). Longer survival after resection of non-small cell lung cancer in Japanese women. *Annals of Thoracic Surgery, 48,* 639–642.

Mountain, C. F. (1983). Therapy of stage I and stage II non-small cell lung cancer. *Seminars in Oncology, 10,* 71–80.

Mountain, C. F. (1986). New international staging system for lung cancer. *Chest, 89*(4 Suppl.), 225S–233S.

Murren, J. R., Buzaid, A. C., & Hait, W. N. (1991). Critical analysis of neoadjuvant therapy for stage IIIa non-small cell lung cancer. *American Review of Respiratory Disease, 143,* 889–894.

Muss, H. B., Jackson, D. V., Jr., Richards, F., White, D. R., & Cooper, M. R. (1984). Bone marrow evaluation in small cell lung cancer. *American Journal of Clinical Oncology, 6,* 59–63.

Neal, M. H., Kosinski, R., Cohen, P., & Orenstein, J. M. (1986). Atypical endocrine tumors of the lung. *Human Pathology, 17,* 1264–1277.

Nelson, D. E., Giovino, G. A., Shopland, D. R., Mowery, P. D., Mills, S. L., & Eriksen, M. P. (1995). Trends in cigarette smoking among U.S. adolescents, 1974–1991. *American Journal of Public Health, 85,* 34–38.

Nett, L. M., & Obrigewitch, R. (1993). Nicotine dependency treatment: a role for the nurse practitioner. *Nurse Practitioner Forum, 4,* 37–42.

Novotny, T. E., Fiore, M. C., Hatziandreu, E. J., Giovino, G. A., Mills, S. L., & Pierce, J. P. (1990) Trends in smoking by age and sex, United States, 1974–1987: The implications for disease impact. *Preventive Medicine, 19,* 552–561.

Okabe, T., Kaizu, T., Fujisawa, M., Watanabe, J., & Takaku, F. (1985). Clinical application of monoclonal antibodies to small cell lung cancer. *Japanese Journal of Medicine, 24,* 250–256.

Olsen, G. N., Block, A. J., & Tobias, J. A. (1984). Prediction of postpneumonectomy pulmonary function using quantitative macroaggregate lung scanning. *Chest, 66,* 13–16.

Orleans, C. T., Jepson, C., Resch, N., & Rimer, B. K. (1994). Quitting motives and barriers among older smokers. *Cancer, 74*(Suppl. 7), 2055–2061.

Osann, K. E. (1991). Lung cancer in women: The importance of smoking, family history of cancer, and medical history of respiratory disease. *Cancer Research, 51,* 4893–4897.

Pastorino, R., Infante, M., Maioli, M., et al. (1993). Adjuvant treatment of stage I lung cancer with high-dose vitamin A. *Journal of Clinical Oncology, 11,* 1216–1222.

Patterson, G. A. (1991). Neoadjuvant therapy of lung cancer. *Chest, 100*(3), 845–846.

Perez, C. A., Pajak, T. F., Rubin, P., Simpson, J. R., Mohiuddin, M., Brady, L. W., Perez-Tamayo, R., & Rotman, M. (1987). Long-term observations of the patterns of failure in patients with unresectable non-oat cell carcinoma of the lung treated with definitive radiotherapy. *Cancer, 59,* 1874–1881.

Perry, M. C., Eaton, W. L., Propert, K. J., Ware, J. H., Zimmer, B., Chahinian, A. P., Skarin, A., Carey, R. W., Kreisman, H., Faulkner, C., Comis, R., & Green, M. R. (1987). Chemotherapy with or without radiation therapy in limited small-cell carcinoma of the lung. *New England Journal of Medicine, 316,* 912–918.

Pershagen, G., Liang, Z. H., Hrubec, Z., Svensson, C., & Boice, J. D. (1992) Residential radon exposure and lung cancer in Swedish women. *Health Physics, 63,* 179–186.

Peto, R., Lopez, A. D., Boreham, J., Thun, M., & Heath Jr, C. (1992). Mortality from tobacco in developed countries: Indirect estimation from national vital statistics. *Lancet, 339,* 1268–1278.

Peto, R., Lopez, A. D., Boreham, J., Thun, M., & Heath Jr, C. (1994). *Mortality from smoking in developed countries, 1950–2000: Indirect estimates from national vital statistics.* New York: Oxford University Press.

Pierce, J. P. (1990). Trends in smoking by age and sex, United States, 1974–87: The implications for disease impact. *Preventive Medicine, 19,* 552–561.

Pierce, J. P., Fiore, M. C., Novotny, T. E., Hatziandreu, E. J., & Davis, R. M. (1989a). Trends in cigarette smoking in the United States: Educational differences are increasing. *Journal of the American Medical Association, 261,* 56–60.

Pierce, J. P., Fiore, M. C., Novotny, T. E., Hatziandreu, E. J., & Davis, R. M. (1989b). Trends in cigarette smoking in the United States: Projections to the year 2000. *Journal of the American Medical Association, 261,* 61–65.

Pierce, J. P., Lee, L., & Gilpin, E. A. (1994). Smoking initiation by adolescent girls, 1944 through 1988. *Journal of the American Medical Association, 271,* 608–611.

Pignon, J. P., Arriagada, R., Ihde, D. C., et al. (1992). A meta-analysis of thoracic radiotherapy for small cell lung cancer. *New England Journal of Medicine, 327,* 1618–1624.

Pirie, P. L., Murray, D. M., & Luepker, R. V. (1991). Gender differences in cigarette smoking and quitting in a cohort of young adults. *American Journal of Public Health, 81,* 324–327.

Pugh, H., Power, C., Goldblatt, P., & Arber, S. (1991). Women's lung cancer mortality, socio-economic status and changing smoking patterns. *Social Science and Medicine, 32,* 1105–1110.

Reyes, C. V., Chua, D., & Aranha, G. V. (1987). Changing incidence of adenocarcinoma of the lung: A brief review. *Journal of Surgical Oncology, 35,* 50–51.

Richardson, G. E., Tucker, M. A., Venzon, D. J., Linnolla, R. I., Phelps, R., Phares, J. C., Edison, M., Ihde, D. C., & Johnson, B. E. (1993). Smoking cessation significantly reduces the risk of second primary cancer in long-term cancer-free survivors of small-cell lung cancer (SCLC). *Proceedings of ASCO, 12,* 326.

Rienzo, P. G. (1993). *Nursing care of the person who smokes.* New York: Springer Publishing Company, Inc.

Ries, L. A. G., Miller, B. A., Hankey, B. F., Kosary, C. L., Harras, A., & Edwards, B. K. (Eds). (1994). *SEER cancer statistics review, 1973–1991: Tables and graphs* [NIH Publication No. 94-2789]. Bethesda, MD: National Cancer Institute.

Risch, H. A., Howe, G. R., Jain, M., Burch, J. D., Holowaty, E. J., & Miller, A. B. (1993). Are female smokers at higher risk for lung cancer than male smokers. *American Journal of Epidemiology, 138,* 281–293.

Rodenhuis, S., & Slebos, R. J. C. (1990). The ras oncogenes in human lung cancer. *American Review of Respiratory Diseases, 142,* 527–530.

Rosell, R., Gomez-Codina, J., Camps, C. Maestre, J., Padille, J., Cantó, A., Mate, J. L., Li, S., Roig, J., Olazabal, A., Canela, M., Ariza, A., Skacel, Z., Morera-Prat, J., & Abad, A. (1994). A randomized trial comparing preoperative chemotherapy plus surgery with surgery alone in patients with non-small cell lung cancer. *New England Journal of Medicine, 330*(3), 153–158.

Roth, J. A. (1992). Molecular surgery for cancer. *Archives of Surgery, 127,* 1298–1302.

Roth, J. A., Fossella, F., Komaki, R., Ryan, M. B., Putnam Jr., J. B., Lee, J. S., Dhingra, H., DeCaro, L., Chasen, M., McGavran, M., Atkinson, E. N., & Hong, W. K. (1994). A randomized trial comparing perioperative chemotherapy and surgery with surgery alone in resectable stage IIIA non-small cell lung cancer. *Journal of the National Cancer Institute, 86*(9), 673–680.

Rubin, S. A. (1991). Lung cancer: Past, present & future. *Journal of Thoracic Imaging, 7*(1), 1–8.

Sandberg, A. A. (1994). Cancer cytogenetics for clinicians. *CA-A Cancer Journal for Clinicians, 44,* 136–159.

Sarna, L. (1993). Women with lung cancer: Impact on quality of life. *Quality of Life Research, 2,* 13–22.

Sarna, L. (1994). Correlates of symptom distress. *Cancer Practice, 1,* 21–28.

Sarna, L. (1995a). Lung cancer: The overlooked womens' health priority. *Cancer Practice, 3,* 13–18.

Sarna, L. (1995b). Smoking behaviors of women after diagnosis with lung cancer. *Image, 27,* 35–41.

Sarna, L. & Brown, J. (1995). Tobacco prevention and cessation in oncology nursing practice, education, and research. *Oncology Nursing Forum, 22,* 256–257.

Sarna, L., Lindsey, A. M., Dean, H., Brecht, M. L., & McCorkle, R. (1994). Weight change and lung cancer: Relationships with symptom distress, functional status, and smoking. *Research in Nursing & Health, 17,* 371–379.

Scheinok, P. A., Engler, P. E., Robertson, P. D., Hutter, R. V. P., & Henson, D. E. (1989). Lung cancer: Difference in age at diagnosis between men and women. *New Jersey Medicine, 86,* 951–957.

Sculier, J. P., Evans, W. K., Feld, R., De Boer, G., Payne, D. G., Shepherd, F. A., Pringle, J. F., Yeoh, J. L., Quirt, I. C., Curtis, J. E., & Herman, J. G. (1986). Superior venal caval obstruction syndrome in small cell lung cancer. *Cancer, 57,* 847–851.

Seifter, E. J., & Ihde, D. C. (1988). Therapy of small cell lung cancer: A perspective on two decades of clinical research. *Seminars in Oncology, 15,* 278–299.

Sellers, T. A., Potter, J. D., & Folsom, A. R. (1991). Association of incident lung cancer with family history of female reproductive cancers: The Iowa Women's Health Study. *Genetic Epidemiology, 8,* 199–208.

Spiro, S. G. (1984). Diagnosis and staging. In W. Duncan (Ed.), *Recent results in cancer research: Lung cancer* (pp. 16–29). New York: Springer-Verlag.

Stanley, K. E. (1980). Prognostic factors for survival in patients with inoperable lung cancer. *Journal of the National Cancer Institute, 65,* 2532.

Stayner, L. T., & Wegman, D. H. (1983). Smoking, occupation, and histopathology of lung cancer: A case control study with the use of the Third National Cancer Survey. *Journal of the National Cancer Institute, 70,* 421–426.

Stockwell, H. G., Goldman, A. L., Lyman, G. H., Noss, C. I., Armstrong, A. W., Pinkham, P. A., Candelora, E. C., & Brusa, M. R. (1992). Environmental tobacco smoke and lung cancer risk in nonsmoking women. *Journal of the National Cancer Institute, 84,* 1417–1422.

Suen, K. C., Lau, L. L., & Yermakov, V. (1974). Cancer and old age: An autopsy study of 3535 patients over 65 years old. *Cancer, 33,* 1164–1168.

Taylor, C. B., Houston-Miller, N., Killen, J. D., & DeBusk, R. F. (1990). Smoking cessation after acute myocardial infarction: Effects of a nurse-managed intervention. *Annals of Internal Medicine, 113,* 118–123.

Teeter, S. M., Holmes, F. F., & McFarlane, M. J. (1987). Lung carcinoma in the elderly population: Influence of histology on the inverse relationship of stage to age. *Cancer, 60,* 1331–1336.

Tisi, G. M., Friedman, P. J., Peters, R. M., Pearson, G., Carr, D., Lee, R. E., & Selaury, O. (1983). Clinical staging of primary lung cancer. *American Review of Respiratory Disease, 127,* 659–664.

U.S. Department of Health and Human Services. (1980). *The health consequences of smoking for women: A report of the surgeon general.* Washington, DC: U.S. Department of Health and Human Services.

U.S. Department of Health and Human Services. (1990). *The health benefits of smoking cessation,* U.S. Department of Health and Human Services Public Health Service, Centers for Disease Control. Center for Chronic Disease Prevention and Health Promotion, Office on Smoking and Health. DHHS Publication No. (CDC) 90-8416.

U.S. Environmental Protection Agency. (1992). *Respiratory health effects of passive smoking.* Washington, DC: United States Environmental Protection Agency, Office of Research and Development, Office of Health and Environmental Assessment, Office of Air and Radiation. EPA/600/6-90/006F.

Valaitis, J., Warren, S., & Gamble, D. (1981). Increasing incidence of adenocarcinoma of the lung. *Cancer, 47,* 1042–1046.

Van Houtte, P., Piron, A., Lustman-Marechal, J., Osteaux, M., & Henry, J. (1980). Computed axial tomography (CAT) contribution for dosimetry and treatment evaluation in lung cancer. *International Journal of Radiation Oncology, Biology, Physics, 6,* 995–1000.

Wang, K. P., & Terry, P. B. (1983). Transbronchial needle aspiration in the diagnosis and staging of bronchogenic carcinoma. *American Review of Respiratory Disease, 127,* 344–347.

Watanabe, Y., Shimizu, J., Oda, M., Hayashi, Y., Watanabe, S., Talsuzaura, Y., Iwa, T., Suzuki, M., & Takashima, T. (1991). Aggressive surgical intervention in N2 non-small cell cancer of the lung. *Annals of Thoracic Surgery, 51,* 253–261.

Waxman, A. D. (1986). The role of nuclear medicine in pulmonary neoplastic processes. *Seminars in Nuclear Medicine, 41,* 285–295.

Weiden, P. L., & Piantadosi, S. (1991). Preoperative chemotherapy (cisplatin and fluorouracil) and radiation therapy in stage III non-small cell lung cancer: A phase II study of the Lung Cancer Study Group. *Journal of the National Cancer Institute, 83,* 266–273.

Weinberg, R. A. (1994). Oncogenes and tumor suppressor genes. *CA-A Cancer Journal for Clinicians, 44,* 160–170.

Weisman, A. D., & Worden, J. W. (1977). The existential plight in cancer: Significance of the first 100 days. *International Journal of Psychiatry and Medicine, 1976–1977, 7,* 1–15.

Wewers, M. E., Bowen, J. M., Stanislaw, A. E., & Desimone, V. B. (1994). A nurse-delivered smoking cessation intervention among hospitalized postoperative patients—influence of a smoking-related diagnosis: A pilot study. *Heart & Lung, 23,* 151–156.

Wickham, R. (1986). Pulmonary toxicity secondary to cancer treatment. *Oncology Nursing Forum, 13*(5), 69–76.

Wilkie, D. J., Keefe, F. J., Dodd, M. J., & Copp, L. (1992). Behavior of patients with lung cancer: description and associations with oncologic and pain variables. *Pain, 51,* 231–240.

Woolner, L. B., Fontana, R. S., & Cortese, D. A. (1984). Roentgenographically occult lung cancer: Pathologic findings and frequency of multicentricity during a 10-year period. *Mayo Clinic Proceedings, 59,* 453–466.

Woolner, L. B., Fontana, R. S., Sanderson, D. R., Miller, E. W., Muhm, R. J., Taylor, F. W., & Uhlenhopp, A. M. (1981). Mayo lung project. *Mayo Clinic Proceedings, 56,* 544–547.

Yesner, R., & Carter, D. (1982). Pathology of carcinoma of the lung. *Clinics in Chest Medicine, 3,* 257–289.

Zinreich, E. S., Baker, R. R., Ettinger, D. S., & Arder, S. E. (1984). New frontiers in the treatment of lung cancer. *CRC Critical Reviews in Oncology/Hematology, 3,* 279–308.

Gastric and Related Cancers

Faith D. Ottery • Marianne McLaughlin-Hagan

The gastrointestinal (GI) tract accounts for the largest number of malignancies of any one body system. This is not particularly surprising considering the direct exposure (topically or via portal vein) to potential carcinogens. This, combined with internal location and the expansile nature of the GI tract, leads to late discovery and poor prognosis. Screening techniques are cost-effective only in high-risk populations and then only in the upper and lower aspects of the tract, that is, esophageal and colorectal. Distribution of cancers by site and prognosis varies dramatically by geographic location worldwide. Although epidemiologic information will be discussed, in this chapter emphasis will be placed on aspects of oncologic care in the United States. The common sites and incidence in the United States are identified in Figure 31–1.

CANCER OF THE ESOPHAGUS

DEFINITION AND INCIDENCE

The incidence of cancer of the esophagus has increased slightly in the United States during the past several years. For 1995, a total of 12,100 new cases were predicted to be diagnosed (Wingo, Tong, & Bolden, 1995). Esophageal cancer is more common in males than females, occurs most frequently in the fifth and sixth decades, and in the United States is generally associated with a poor prognostic outcome. Overall 5-year survival rates are generally less than 10 per cent (Hoebler & Irwin, 1992).

EPIDEMIOLOGY AND ETIOLOGY

Esophageal cancer has been noted to occur with significant geographic variation in incidence. For example, specific areas in China and Iran are associated with very high incidences, actually allowing for the possibility of successful screening programs that are not feasible in the United States due to the relatively low incidence of esophageal cancer. In central Asia, there has been noted to be a specific "esophageal cancer belt" (Frank-Stromborg, 1989). In the United States, there are reports of significantly higher incidence of esophageal cancer in African-American versus caucasian males (Ellis, Levitan, & Lo, 1992).

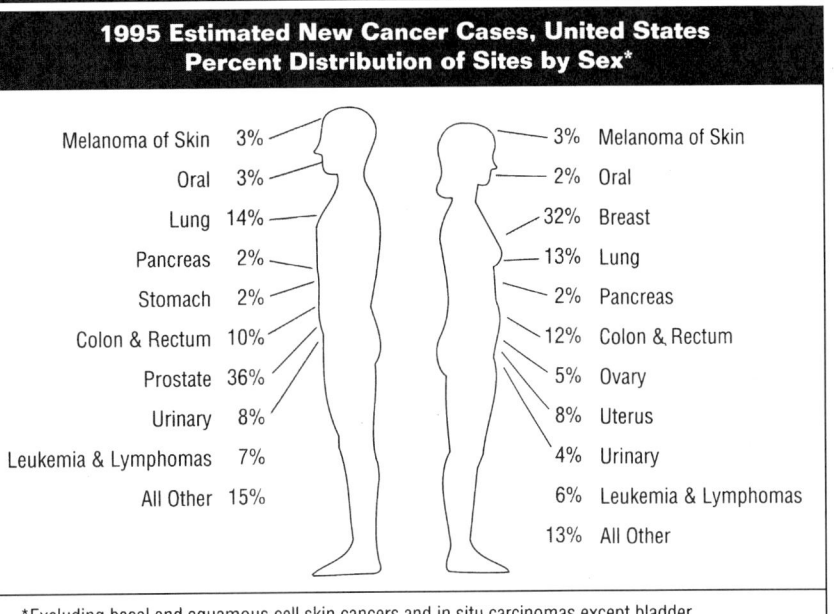

FIGURE 31–1. Estimated cancer incidence by site and sex, 1995. (From Wingo, P. A., Tong, T., & Bolden, S. [1995]. Cancer Statistics, 1995. *CA: A Cancer Journal for Clinicians*, 45(1), 8–30. Reproduced by permission.)

There have been a number of correlations made between various medical conditions and development of cancer of the esophagus. These include achalasia, Plummer-Vinson syndrome, Barrett's esophagus, and tylosis (Ellis, Levitan, & Lo, 1992).

Other risk factors include chronic alcohol consumption, tobacco smoking, and distant history of severe lye ingestion. Correlation with dietary factors include deficiencies in specific vitamins, including vitamin A, beta-carotene, and vitamin C, and diets high in nitrosamines (Fox & Kandi, 1984).

BIOLOGY AND NATURAL HISTORY

Esophageal cancer is classified according to histology (Table 31–1). Two thirds of esophageal cancers will be squamous in type, with the cells arising from the surface epithelium in both the upper and lower esophagus. Adenocarcinoma of the esophagus is being increasingly diagnosed in the United States and is often felt to be associated with the presence of Barrett's esophagus (Lerut et al., 1994).

Cancer of the esophagus is staged using the TNM system (Table 31–2). Staging is based on tumor size, nodal involvement, invasion into adjacent structures, and distant metastases. Treatment options are broadly based on staging criteria. More aggressive treatment in general will be warranted for early, noninvasive disease, whereas a palliative approach is usually taken in more advanced disease.

SIGNS AND SYMPTOMS

The most frequent presenting complaint or symptom in patients with esophageal carcinoma is dysphagia. Severity of the dysphagia can range from difficulty with solid foods to inability to take even liquids orally. Patients, therefore, often present with weight loss and may have regurgitation of foods that lodge above the area of constriction or tumor. Patients may also have symptoms of odynophagia (pain on swallowing). Reflux symptoms may be seen in the context of the patient with Barrett's esophagus.

With progressive disease and late diagnosis, the presenting symptoms may include chronic cough due either to aspiration of retained esophageal contents or tracheal involvement due to local invasion, hoarseness suggesting laryngeal nerve involvement/paralysis, and pain radiating to the patient's back if the tumor has invaded adjacent structures.

DIAGNOSIS

Diagnosis of esophageal cancer is usually made after the patient has presented with symptomatology. In general there are no standard screening procedures in the general population in the United States. In very high-risk populations, as in China and Iran, as well as in patients in the United States who have previously had at least one primary malignancy of the upper aerodigestive tract (including head and neck primaries and squamous cell carcinoma of the lung), brush cytology with endoscopy has been successful in diagnosing esophageal cancer at an earlier stage. The association of esophageal cancer and Barrett's esophagus continues to be somewhat controversial, as is the screening protocol with endoscopy in this specific patient population (Robertson, Mayberry, Nicholson, James, & Atkinson, 1988).

Diagnosis is made most frequently based on endoscopic evaluation with (1) visualization of tumor, (2) multiple biopsies in suspicious areas or in areas of chronic Barrett's esophagus, and (3) brush cytology. Endoscopic ultrasound is increasingly being used in a number of centers to determine the extent and depth of local involvement. Bronchoscopy is also an important component of staging.

TABLE 31–1. *Malignant Esophageal Tumors*

Epithelial Tumors
  Squamous cell carcinoma
    Well differentiated
    Moderately differentiated
    Poorly differentiated
  Variants of squamous cell carcinoma
    Spindle cell carcinoma
    Pseudosarcoma and carcinosarcoma
    Verrucous carcinoma
    In situ carcinoma
  Adenocarcinoma
    Adenoacanthoma
  Adenoid cystic carcinoma (cylindroma)
  Mucoepidermoid carcinoma
  Adenosquamous carcinoma
  Carcinoid
  Undifferentiated carcinoma
    Oat cell carcinoma

Nonepithelial Tumors
  Leiomyosarcomas
  Malignant melanoma
  Myoblastoma
  Choriocarcinoma
  Rhabdomyosarcoma

(Data from Rosenberg, J. C., Schwade, J. G., & Vaitkevicius, V. [1982]. Cancer of the esophagus. In V. T. DeVita, S. Hellman, & S. A. Rosenberg [Eds.], *Cancer: Principles and practice of oncology* [p. 505]. Philadelphia: J. B. Lippincott Co.)

TABLE 31–2. *TNM Staging for Esophageal Cancer*

Primary Tumor (T)
  T0   No demonstrable tumor
  TIS Carcinoma in situ
  T1   Tumor involves 5 cm or less of esophageal length with no obstruction or complete circumferential involvement or extraesophageal spread
  T2   Tumor involves more than 5 cm of esophagus and produces obstruction with circumferential involvement of the esophagus but no extraesophageal spread
  T3   Tumor with extension outside the esophagus involving mediastinal structures

Regional Lymph Nodes (N)
  Cervical esophagus (cervical and supraclavicular lymph nodes)
  N0   No nodal involvement
  N1   Unilateral involvement (moveable)
  N2   Bilateral involvement (moveable)
  N3   Fixed nodes
  Thoracic esophagus (nodes in the thorax, not those of the cervical supraclavicular or abdominal areas)
  N0   No nodal involvement
  N1   Nodal involvement

Distant Metastases
  M0   No metastases
  M1   Distant metastases. Cancer of thoracic esophagus with cervical, supraclavicular, or abdominal lymph node involvement is classified as M1

(Data from Rosenberg, J. C., Schwade, J. G., & Vaitkevicius, V. [1982]. Cancer of the esophagus. In V. T. DeVita, S. Hellman, & S. A. Rosenberg [Eds.], *Cancer: Principles and practice of oncology* [p. 509]. Philadelphia: J. B. Lippincott Co.)

Computed tomography is useful in determining local extent of the tumor as well as in determining distant disease including lung, liver, and regional adenopathy.

Differential diagnosis of esophageal cancer includes abnormalities of both benign and malignant etiologies. Benign causes of symptoms that may mimic esophageal cancer include symptoms from benign strictures (corrosives, reflux, scleroderma) motility disorders, and diverticulae. Malignant diagnoses obviously include primary esophageal carcinoma, but on occasion patients present with an area of local involvement of the bronchoesophageal complex, and the primary site is difficult to clarify. Annular carcinomas may be mistaken for benign strictures, especially if most of the growth is extramural. Benign papillomas, polyps, and granulomatous masses can be distinguished from early carcinoma only on histologic examination.

TREATMENT

Therapeutic approaches are generally categorized as either curative or palliative in intent. Curative approaches may include either single or combined modality options.

Surgical intervention with curative intent generally includes an esophagogastrectomy. The approach to esophageal resection can include thoracotomy or abdominal approach with a so-called "blunt esophagectomy." Options for reconstruction of a conduit from the upper esophagus to the intestinal tract can include mobilization of the stomach for a "gastric pull-up" into the thoracic cavity, a gastric tube fashioned from the greater curvature of the stomach, or interpositions of colon or jejunum.

Chemotherapy in combination with radiation therapy may be used either preoperatively (known as neoadjuvant or protoadjuvant therapy) or postoperatively (adjuvant). The intent of the neoadjuvant approach is to improve local control and to reduce tumor burden at the time of resection. Additionally, combined modality therapy of radiation therapy with a radio-sensitizing chemotherapeutic regimen has shown some success, primarily for local control. Maintenance of adequate nutritional status will be discussed below under nursing management and in greater detail in Chapter 51.

If palliation is the therapeutic goal, treatment is aimed primarily at symptom management and improvement in quality of life. The use of esophageal stents to maintain patency is not associated with any long-term success and is often associated with limited life expectancy. Use of endoscopic laser therapy has been associated with some success in terms of palliation. Placement of a feeding tube (including endoscopic, radiologic, open surgical or laparoscopic gastrostomy, or jejunostomy tube) may be able to prevent progressive nutritional deterioration if performed in appropriately chosen patients, but the other components of the patient's quality of life also need to be thoughtfully considered in the palliative therapy in esophageal cancer.

NURSING ISSUES

Components of nursing management need to be based on the treatment plan chosen or being considered. Preoperative nutritional status needs to be addressed in a manner outlined in Figure 31–2. This is especially important in patients who are to undergo surgical resection. Postoperatively, malnourished patients (especially if they have received preoperative radiation therapy) will be at increased risk of anastomotic leak and fistula formation. The placement of a feeding tube at the time of esophagectomy should be considered an important component of the decision making process intraoperatively if the patient has pre-existing nutritional deficit. Pulmonary toilet is a particular concern in these patients if a thoracotomy was performed. Patients with gastric pull-up reconstruction need to eat or be fed in an upright position and remain in this position for at least 30 minutes after each meal. Semiupright in bed is not adequate because this will increase intraabdominal pressure and increase reflux into the newly reconstructed conduit with increased risk of aspiration. Additionally, having the patient walk a few minutes after eating may also be helpful in decreasing risk of aspiration.

Patients receiving radiation therapy and chemotherapy need to be monitored aggressively for esophagitis, especially with candidal involvement. This latter is especially important in the nutritionally compromised patient with or without history of antibiotic use (e.g., during neutropenia). Symptom management including issues of pain control, nausea, mucositis, and constipation improve quality of life and may potentially contribute to maintenance of adequate nutritional intake.

Overall the nurse needs to understand the potential side effects of therapy and anatomic changes of specific surgical approaches of resection and reconstruction. Nursing management should, therefore, be directed as provision of symptom relief and maintenance of the several aspects of patient quality of life. These considerations must be made regardless of whether the therapeutic intent is curative or palliative.

GASTRIC CARCINOMA

DEFINITION AND INCIDENCE

Gastric malignancy can include adenocarcinoma, sarcoma, and lymphoma. The term gastric cancer refers only to the adenocarcinoma histology. Similar to other GI malignancies, incidence of stomach cancer varies globally. The incidence in the United States has steadily decreased over the past 60 years. As of data from 1988 to 1991, the United States had the lowest rate of cancer deaths per 100,000 internationally (Boring et al., 1994). In 1930, death rates in the United States were approximately 30 per 100,000, compared with 7.5 in the recent report (Boring et al., 1994). In comparison, the highest rates per 100,000 include Costa Rico with 77.5, Japan 50.4, China 48.3, and Ecuador 46.1.

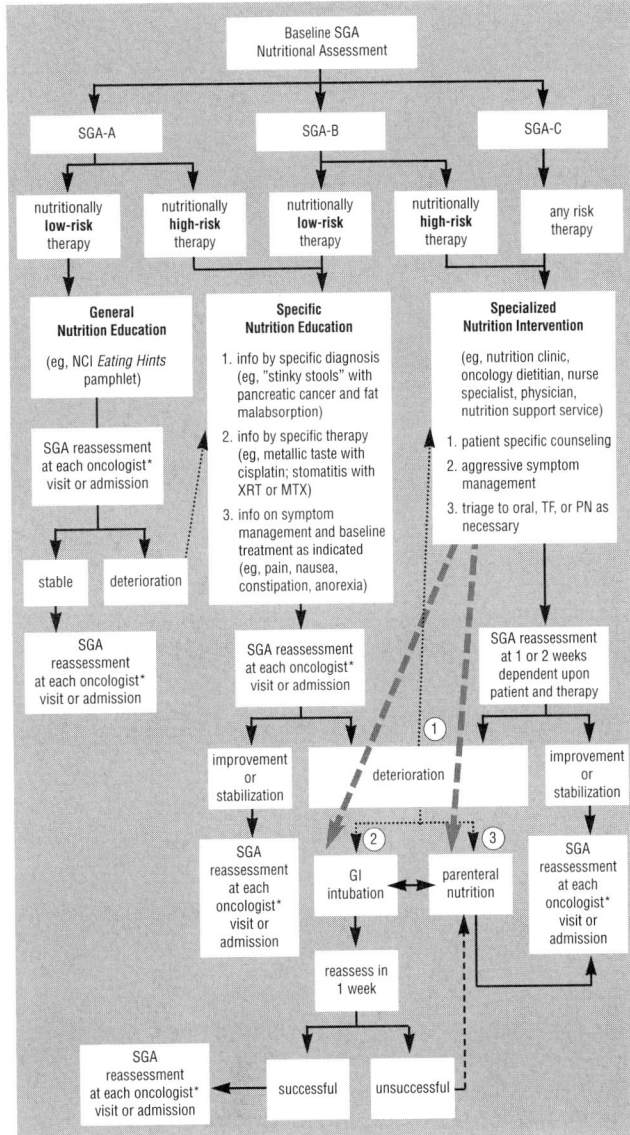

FIGURE 31–2. Algorithm of optimal nutritional intervention is based on the Patient-Generated Subjective Global Assessment (Table 31–5). Once the PG-SGA stage is determined, the approach is based on whether the antineoplastic therapy has known risk for nutritional deterioration (e.g., nausea, vomiting, mucositis). XRT = radiation therapy; MTX = methotrexate; TF = tube feeding; PN = parenteral nutrition.

Unless otherwise specified, the discussion below will describe American statistics and biologic behavior.

The peak age for gastric cancer is 55 to 65 years (Burn & Welbourne, 1975), with a male to female ratio of approximately 3:2. In general, survival statistics are better for females (Waterhouse, 1984).

EPIDEMIOLOGY AND ETIOLOGY

As noted, international incidence data vary significantly. In general, survival is determined by the extent of disease at time of diagnosis and anatomic location. Localized carcinoma of the distal stomach offers cure in nearly 50 per cent. Unfortunately, in the United States this accounts for only a small percent of the gastric diagnoses, with regional and distant disease present in 80 to 90 per cent. Data on survival reflect the differences in stage at diagnosis.

Gastric cancer has been associated etiologically with a number of factors including heredity, diet, methods of food preservation, socioeconomic status, exposure to carcinogens as in dust in coal mines and pottery and chronic use of H_2 blockers, and colonization with *Heliobacter pylori* (Hwang, Dwyer, & Russell, 1994). Use of refrigeration with decreased use of salting as means of food preservation has been implicated in the decrease in gastric cancer in the United States. Additionally, presence of nitroso compounds with inadequate antioxidant protection has also been offered as potentially playing a role. These all may contribute to the wide variation in incidences and death rates internationally. Other etiologic hypotheses that have been offered include a decrease in gastric atrophy in American adults (Hill, 1984).

BIOLOGY AND NATURAL HISTORY

Classification of gastric carcinoma includes components of both gross and microscopic pathologic evaluation. Grossly, gastric cancers are subdivided into fungating or polypoid, ulcerating, superficial spreading, and diffusely spreading (the so-called linitis plastica or leather-bottle stomach). Histologic classification impacts prognosis and includes intestinal, pylorocardial (antral), signet ring cell, and anaplastic.

Staging of gastric carcinoma at diagnosis significantly impacts prognosis. TNM staging is dependent on the degree of penetration of the gastric wall, presence of microscopic perforation, and invasion into adjacent structures (Table 31–3). Pathologic lymph node status may determine both regional (N) and distant metastatic (M) staging, depending on the location of the nodes included in the surgical resection. Positive nodes implicating distant metastatic disease include retropancreatic, hepatoduodenal, aortic, portal, retroperitoneal, and mesenteric. N staging involves the distance of 3 cm from the edge of the primary tumor and along specific gastric drainage patterns (Beahrs, Henson, Hutter, & Kennedy, 1993). Survival based on staging is summarized in Table 31–4.

SIGNS AND SYMPTOMS

Early gastric cancer may be asymptomatic or may be associated with nonspecific, vague abdominal discomfort. Gross presentation as described above may be associated with differences in presenting complaints. In most studies of presenting complaints, the common presentation is nondescript abdominal discomfort and vague GI symptoms, often initially felt to be related to ulcer disease. The role of *H. pylori,* is increasingly recognized as playing a role in peptic ulcer disease as well as gastric cancer (Hwang et al., 1994). Patients with depressed or ulcerated lesions tend to present with abdominal pain (Biasco et al., 1987). Additional symptoms seen in gastric cancer patients include anorexia, nausea and/or vomiting, fullness or early satiety, associated weight loss, and postprandial dyspepsia (including belching, regurgitation, and pain).

DIAGNOSIS

Differential diagnosis in gastric cancer includes both benign and malignant disease processes. Benign etiologies of gastric pathology include peptic ulcer disease, gastritis, benign polyps, and pseudolymphoma. Malignancy includes adenocarcinoma, sarcoma, lymphoma, and metastatic disease.

Diagnostic evaluation includes both endoscopic and radiologic evaluation, with endoscopy offering the greatest benefit because of its ability to confirm histologically and cytologically the presence of malignant cells. Use of barium study in early gastric diagnosis is much less sensitive and specific but may be part of the initial workup of diffuse GI complaints. Radiologic evaluation including chest radiograph, computed tomography (CT), magnetic resonance imaging (MRI), and nucleotide scans are used primarily in preoperative staging for distant disease. Laboratory/biochemical evaluations do not routinely contribute to diagnosis.

TABLE 31–3. *Stage Grouping of Stomach Cancer and TNM Classification*

STAGE	TUMOR	NODE	METASTASIS
I	T1	N0	M0
II	T2	N0	M0
	T3	N0	M0
III	T1, T2, T3	N1, N2	M1
	T1, T2, T3 (Resectable for cure)		
	T4 (Resectable for cure)	Any N	M0
IV	T1, T2, T3 (Not resectable for cure)	N3	M0
	T4 (Not resectable for cure)	Any N	M0
	Any T	Any N	M1

(Data from Morton, J. M., Poulter, C. A., & Pandya, K. J. [1983]. Alimentary tract cancer. In P. Rubin, R. F. Bakemeier, & S. K. Krackov [Eds.], *Clinical oncology—a multidisciplinary approach* [p. 160]. New York: American Cancer Society.)

TABLE 31–4. *Gastric Survival Data*

STAGE	5-YEAR SURVIVAL
0 (in-situ)	> 90%
I	52%–85% for distal cancers 10%–15% for proximal
II	> 20% for distal
III	17% for distal
IV	< 5%

TREATMENT

Surgical resection with partial or complete gastrectomy and lymphadenectomy is generally the treatment of choice in stage 0 through II disease. Patients with stage III disease who are resectable should be offered this option. Neoadjuvant therapy with radiation and various chemotherapeutic modalities may play a role in nonresectable, locally advanced stage III patients in an effort to convert them to resectable. The success of surgical resection with high cure rates has long been reported in Japan and has been confirmed in an American series (Green, O'Toole, Slonim, Wang, & Weg, 1988). Surgical resection options in patients with stage I include radical distal subtotal gastrectomy, proximal subtotal gastrectomy, or total gastrectomy. Stage II patients standardly undergo surgical resection (radical subtotal, proximal subtotal, or total gastrectomy) with extended lymphadenectomy. Reports of improved survival with extended lymphadenectomy have been published. Use of adjuvant chemotherapy, radiation therapy, or both are under clinical evaluation. Patients with stage III disease should be resected, if possible, and should be considered for clinical trial therapy.

Palliative treatment options for stage IV gastric cancer can include palliative resection, endoscopic resection to open a gastric outlet obstruction, and palliative chemotherapy. Surgical resection offers the opportunity to prevent the sequelae of progressive disease with bleeding and obstruction. Use of aggressive preoperative chemotherapy (e.g., etoposide, doxorubicin, and cisplatin) has been reported to impact resectability but is associated with severe toxicity, and such options must be considered in the context of quality of life.

Radiation therapy can play a role at various steps in gastric cancer treatment and includes external beam (preoperative and postoperative) as well as intraoperative therapy. Use is generally multimodality with chemotherapy and surgery. Combined treatment may use protocols with 5-fluorouracil with or without nitrosourea (CCNU), and the so-called FAM regimen (5-fluorouracil, Adriamycin, and mitomycin C) or FAP 5-fluorouracil, Adriamycin, and cisplatin).

NURSING ISSUES

As with other GI malignancies, nutrition is of significant importance in terms of quality of life and potential therapy complications, especially surgical. The algorithm in Figure 31–2 summarizes a proactive approach for the health care team. The issue of maintenance of nutritional status is important at each step of the patient's course. Placement of enteral feeding tubes may be an option for postoperative support, especially in a patient with baseline nutritional deficit. A modification of the Subjective Global Assessment (SGA) of nutritional status has been developed, which helps triage patients into appropriate proactive nutritional intervention (Table 31–5). This allows the addressing of nutritional issues in high-risk patients at an early stage rather than waiting until end-stage progressive malnutrition has resulted. Postoperative nutritional status can be compromised in a significant number of patients (up to 80 percent at 1 year postoperatively). This nutritional deficit may include GI symptoms related to gastric reconstruction (e.g., gastroenterostomy, esophagoenterostomy) and may include the need for pancreatic enzymes in patients with symptoms of fat malabsorption (malodorous stools, diarrhea, bloating). This latter can occur in up to 25 per cent of patients, depending on the type of reconstruction. Use of pancreatic enzymes is a therapeutic modality that can be quite successful in improving nutritional status but is often overlooked unless good questioning for symptoms of malabsorption is carried out by the clinician.

Additional nursing management issues include adequate pain management and discussions with the patient and his or her support system in terms of lifestyle changes with the cancer diagnosis, possible changes in eating habits, and the impact of aggressive therapy in the face of advanced disease. Early changes in ability to eat adequately postoperatively are not universal and tend to improve over time.

SMALL BOWEL MALIGNANCY

DEFINITION AND INCIDENCE

Cancer of the small bowel is relatively rare. Of all new cancer cases for 1995 in the United States, primary small bowel malignancy is estimated to account for approximately 0.04 of all cancers or 2 per cent of gastrointestinal tract malignancies (Wingo et al, 1995). Similarly, it will account for 0.02 per cent of overall cancer deaths. The term small bowel includes duodenum, jejunum, and ileum and comprises 98 per cent of intestinal surface and 90 per cent of the length of the bowel (Gabos, Berkel, Band, Robson, & Whittaker, 1993).

Theories for the disparate rareness of small bowel versus large bowel primary malignancies include liquid consistency of small bowel contents, faster transit times, less mucosal exposure time to potential toxins or carcinogens, and lower bacterial counts with decreased bacterial production of carcinogens. Additionally, protection may be afforded by alkaline pH and high concentrations of the enzymes benzopyrene hydroxylase and diamine oxidase, active in detoxifying certain carcinogens. There is also greater immunosurveillance provided by mucosal production and higher concentration of IgA (Gabos et al., 1993; Viamonte & Viamonte, 1992).

In addition to primary malignancies, the small bowel may be a site for metastatic disease arising from the uterus, cervix, lung, breast, kidney, urinary bladder, ovary, and skin (Viamonte & Viamonte, 1992).

EPIDEMIOLOGY AND ETIOLOGY

The first case of small bowel malignancy was diagnosed in 1746, with greater than 35 different histologic types of small bowel tumors subsequently described. Interestingly, benign tumors of the small bowel are relatively common, occurring at a rate of 1 in 127 in necropsy series (Mason & Sabiston, 1986). These are generally asymptomatic compared with primary or metastatic lesions, which are symptomatic in 75 to 80 per cent of cases. Unfortunately, these small bowel can-

TABLE 31–5. *Oncology Patient Generated Subjective Global Assessment of Nutritional Status*

A. HISTORY

1. weight change

   I weigh _____ (about) pounds

   A year ago I weighed about _____ pounds

   Six months ago I weighed about _____ pounds

   During the past two weeks my weight has
   _____ decreased

   _____ not changed

   _____ increased

2. I would rate my food intake
   during the past month as
   (compared to my normal)
   _____ no change

   _____ changed
   _____ more than usual
   _____ less than usual
   _____ taking little solid food
   _____ taking <u>only</u> liquids
   _____ taking <u>only</u> nutritional supplements
   _____ really taking in very little of anything

3. Over the past two weeks I have had the
   following problems that kept me from
   eating enough (check all that apply)
   _____ no problems eating
   _____ no appetite, just do not feel like eating
   _____ nausea
   _____ vomiting
   _____ diarrhea
   _____ constipation
   _____ mouth sores
   _____ dry mouth
   _____ pain
   _____ things taste funny or have no taste
   _____ smells bother me
   _____ other: _____

4. Over the past month I would
   rate my activity as generally
   _____ 0=normal, no limitations

   _____ 1=not my normal self, but able
   to be up and about with fairly
   normal activities

   _____ 2=not feeling up to most things
   but in bed less than half the day

   _____ 3=able to do little activity & I spend
   most of the day in bed or chair

   _____ 4=pretty much bedridden
   (rarely out of bed)

The remainder of the form will be filled out by your doctor, nurse, therapist. Thank you.

5. Disease and its relation to nutritional requirements
   Primary diagnosis _____   Stage _____
   Metabolic stress:
   _____ none   _____ low   _____ moderate   _____ high

B. PHYSICAL (for each trait specify: 0=normal 1+=mild 2+=moderate 3+=severe)
   _____ loss of subcutaneous fat (triceps, chest)   _____ muscle wasting (quadriceps, deltoid)
   _____ ankle edema   _____ sacral edema   _____ ascites

C. SGA rating (select one)
   _____ A = well nourished
   _____ B = moderately (or suspected of being) malnourished
   _____ C = severely malnourished

(Modified from Detsky, A. S. et al. [1987]. *Journal of Parenteral and Enteral Nutrition, 11,* 8–13. From Ottery, F. D. [1995]. Supportive nutrition to prevent cachexia and improve quality of life. *Seminars in Oncology, 22* [Suppl. 3], 98–111.)

cers are insidious in development and are often diagnosed at late stages.

Leiomyomata are the most common benign small bowel tumors, with adenocarcinomas and carcinoids being the most common primary small bowel malignancies. It has been suggested that the epidemiology of adenocarcinomas of the small bowel is similar to that of large bowel, despite the markedly different incidence rates (Neugut & Santos, 1993). Their rates co-vary in different countries, and they both appear to have adenomatous polyps as precursor lesions. Additionally, patients with familial adenomatous polyposis have multiple adenomatous polyps in both large and small

bowel, with concomitant increased risk of adenocarcinomas in each of these regions (Sellner, 1990).

Concepts of etiology of malignancies of the small bowel are relatively speculative. There are rare hereditary syndromes such as neurofibromatosis, juvenile familial polyposis, Peutz-Jeghers, Cronkhite-Canada and Gardner's syndromes, and other generalized gastrointestinal polyposis syndromes. Hereditary nonpolyposis colon cancer (HNPCC), another heritable disorder, has been associated with adenocarcinoma of the ileum and distal jejunum (Lynch et al., 1989). Crohn's disease has variably been reported as being associated with increased risk of small bowel malignancy, especially in the ileum (Lashner, 1992; Munkholm, Langholz, Davidsen, & Binder, 1993). Crohn's disease has been significantly associated with small bowel cancer with increased risk in patients with jejunal disease, hazardous occupational exposures (halogenated aromatic compounds, aliphatic amines, asbestos, and others) and prolonged (greater than 6 months) use of 6-mercaptopurine therapy (Lashner, 1992).

BIOLOGY AND NATURAL HISTORY

Adenocarcinomas account for approximately 40 per cent of primary small bowel malignancies, with one third located in the duodenum and jejunum. The remaining primary malignancies include carcinoid tumors, lymphomas, and leiomyosarcomas. As noted above, the basis of small and large bowel adenocarcinomas may be similar in arising from adenomatous polyps (Neugut & Santos, 1993; Sellner, 1990). Often this association with the adenomatous component is not as obvious in the small as in the large bowel because of the rather later diagnosis as well as the lack of screening tools such as endoscopy used in the lower gastrointestinal tract. Shared common genetic defects as well as environmental exposures may explain the association of small and large bowel cancers in polyposis states. Nitroso compounds, either consumed or created endogenously, as well as degradation of bile acids may contribute to this small bowel risk.

SIGNS AND SYMPTOMS

Primary tumors generally are asymptomatic in early stages, unless located at strategic positions, for example, at the ampulla of Vater, where jaundice may be the basis of presentation. Metastatic lesions may present with obstruction or bleeding. Metastatic melanoma to the gastrointestinal tract may often present emergently with bleeding or anemia, obstruction, abdominal pain, intestinal perforation, and acute GI bleed (Ihde & Coit, 1991).

DIFFERENTIAL DIAGNOSIS AND DIAGNOSTIC EVALUATION

Differentiation is generally not an issue in terms of benign and malignant lesions, based on the generally asymptomatic versus symptomatic nature of the two. Biopsy at time of presentation with surgical treatment is usually the basis of diagnosis, with two primary exceptions, carcinoid with elevated levels of urinary 5-hydroxyindoleacetic acid and with known diagnosis or history of lymphoma. Lymphomatous involvement of the small bowel may present with symptoms of malabsorption.

Evaluation is based mainly on the presenting symptom, for example, GI bleed, obstruction, jaundice.

TREATMENT

Management generally is based on local excision or management of the acute presenting problem. If the lesion is a periampullary one, a Whipple procedure (pancreatogastroduodenectomy) may be indicated with loco/regional disease only. If the diagnosis is carcinoid or lymphoma, treatment may include chemotherapy or multimodality therapy.

NURSING ISSUES

Given the rarity of the lesions, there are no specific issues from a nursing standpoint that can be specifically addressed. However, if lymphomatous involvement of the small bowel is diagnosed, the management of the nutritional complications may be the overriding issue.

PANCREATIC MALIGNANCY

DEFINITION AND INCIDENCE

Pancreatic cancer is the fourth leading cause of adult cancer mortality (Evans, Rich, Byrd, & Ames, 1991). This cancer comprises 3 per cent of the annual incidence of malignancy in the United States and accounts for 5 per cent of U. S. cancer deaths (Mohiuddin et al., 1994). The incidence of carcinoma of the pancreas has steadily increased over the past few years; however, the cure rate remains low at less than 2 per cent at 5 years (Mohiuddin et al., 1994). Overall, pancreatic malignancies include two major categories—those of exocrine and endocrine etiologies.

EPIDEMIOLOGY AND ETIOLOGY

The cause of pancreatic carcinoma remains unclear. However, there has been a degree of correlation to various associated factors. These include cigarette smoking, coffee consumption, and fat intake (Steel, Osteen, Winchester, Murphy, & Menck, 1994). However, no positive conclusions have been made. This type of cancer has not been linked to a particular disease state such as preexisting pancreatitis or diabetes mellitus (DM). With respect to diabetes, a patient may have been diagnosed with DM just prior to the diagnosis of the pancreatic malignancy with carcinoma found coincidentally during the diabetic workup.

Comparing male to female ratios, there is an essentially equal ratio. This equalization of the gender ratio is felt possibly to be related to the increased use of tobacco by females in recent years. Correlation with onset of the disease relative to age demonstrates that peak incidence is the seventh decade with 82 per cent of patients being diagnosed between 50 and 80 years of age (Gary, Crook, & Cohen, 1972). Potential impact of ethnic origin in terms of development of pancreatic malignancy may be demonstrated in the United States in that African-Americans have a five times greater incidence than Japanese Americans or Hispanic Americans from Puerto Rico (Fonthan, Corrisa, & Cohen, 1984). Unfortunately, since the cause of pancreatic cancer still remains a mystery, no factors can be linked to a specific population who would be at risk for developing this disease.

BIOLOGY AND NATURAL HISTORY

Pancreatic carcinoma is classified according to histology. Ductal adenocarcinomas account for 80 per cent of pancreatic malignancies and are more common in the head of the pancreas (66 per cent) than in the body or tail (33 per cent). Classification of pancreatic malignancy is summarized in Table 31–6. Staging using the TNM system is found in Table 31–7.

TABLE 31–6. *Histologic Classification of Pancreatic Carcinoma*

TYPE	PERCENTAGE OF PATIENTS
Duct cell adenocarcinoma	75
Giant cell carcinoma	4
Adenosquamous carcinoma	4
Mucinous cystadenocarcinoma	1
Acinar cell adenocarcinoma	1
Others	15

(Data from Macdonald, J., Gunderson, L., & Cohn, I., Jr. [1982]. Cancer of the pancreas. In V. T. DeVita, S. Hellman, & S. A. Rosenberg [Eds.], *Cancer: Principles and practice of oncology* [p. 564]. Philadelphia: J. B. Lippincott Co.)

SIGNS AND SYMPTOMS

Symptoms of pancreatic cancer are often insidious, and the tumor frequently invades adjacent structures early in the patient's course. Therefore, resection is possible in less than 10 per cent of patients. Jaundice may be the presenting symptom or basis for the patient seeking medical care (Sarr & Cameron, 1984). Other symptoms may be nonspecific and include pain, weight loss, anorexia, nausea, and vomiting. Additionally, symptoms may be related to the site or histology of the tumor. In terms of location, those found in the tail of the pancreas may be silent for a longer period of time with insidious progressive growth and advanced disease at time of diagnosis. Specifically, metastatic disease is often found at presentation, and symptoms related to tumor invasion include abdominal mass, weight loss/weakness, ascites, and pain. When the tumor arises in the head of the pancreas, jaundice occurs in 80 to 90 per cent of cases (Saltzburg & Foley, 1989). Tumor invasion may cause pain in 60 to 90 per cent of patients. When the body of the pancreas is involved, the patient may experience significant back pain, often worse in recumbency. This is the basis for the patient often finding relief in an upright position, including the finding that patients may sleep in a sitting or fetal-type rather than a supine position.

In addition to diabetes and its associated acute complications, other hormonally mediated symptoms can be seen in endocrine or islet cell tumors. Specifically, glucagonoma is associated with hyperglycemia, gastrinoma with ulcer disease, etc. Management may often include pharmacologic management of symptoms.

Symptoms of patients who have pancreatic cancer (adenocarcinoma) or who are undergoing therapy (e.g., radiation therapy) may include exocrine pancreatic insufficiency and fat malabsorption. Signs and symptoms associated with this condition include particularly malodorous bowel movements, bloating, floating stools, or diarrhea. Patients may also note an oily appearance surrounding the stool in the toilet. This malabsorption combined with anorexia leads to the progressive inanition (wasting syndrome or cachexia) that is often seen in patients with progressive pancreatic cancer. Unfortunately, in the general case, the symptoms of pancreatic cancer are often nonspecific, leading to delayed diagnosis in the majority of patients.

DIAGNOSIS

Specific diagnostic evaluation is generally based on the presenting symptomatology. Because pancreatic carcinoma causes vague, nonspecific symptoms, the diagnostic workup is initiated with the least invasive studies, proceeding on to more invasive modalities if the diagnosis is not conclusive.

TABLE 31–7. *Staging of Pancreatic Cancer*

T	**Primary Tumor**			
	T0	Primary tumor cannot be assessed		
	T1	Tumor limited to the pancreas		
		T1a	Tumor 2 cm or less in greatest diameter	
		T1b	Tumor more than 2 cm in greatest diameter	
	T2	Tumor extends directly to any of the following: duodenum, bile duct, or peripancreatic tissues		
	T3	Tumor extends directly to any of the following: stomach, spleen, colon, or adjacent large vessels		
	TX	Primary tumor cannot be assessed		
N	**Regional Lymph Node Involvement**			
	N0	Regional nodes not involved		
	N1	Regional nodes involved		
	NX	Regional node involvement not assessed or not recorded		
M	**Distant Metastasis**			
	M0	No distant metastasis		
	M1	Distant metastatic involvement		
	MX	Distant metastatic involvement not assessed or not recorded		
	Stage I	T1	N0	M0
		T2	N0	M0
	Stage II	T3	N0	M0
	Stage III	Any T	N1	M0
	Stage IV	Any T	Any N	M1

(From Beahrs, O. H., Henson, D. E., Hutter, R. V. P., & Kennedy, B. J. [Eds.]. [1993]. *Handbook for staging of cancer from the manual for staging of cancer.* Philadelphia: J. B. Lippincott Co.)

Differential diagnoses include both benign and malignant disease. Benign causes generally include pancreatitis of several etiologies and pancreatic pseudocyst. Malignancy is usually primary in nature, but metastatic disease from sites such as breast and thyroid has been reported. CT scan is frequently helpful in the diagnosis and staging of pancreatic cancer. This scan can demonstrate the size of the primary tumor, invasion of adjacent structures including stomach, colon, and vascular structures, presence of lymphadenopathy, and liver metastases. Doppler ultrasound and angiography may be useful in detecting vascular invasion. Additionally, they may aid in determination of surgical resectability. Both CT scan and ultrasound can be used to direct needle biopsy to establish cytologic diagnosis of malignancy. Use of MRI is generally not the primary evaluative scan but may also be included. In terms of cost-effectiveness and additional information gained, MRI may not add previously unknown information.

Endoscopic retrograde cholangiopancreatography (ERCP) may also aid in diagnosis of malignancy. This approach is relatively invasive but does allow the endoscopist to directly visualize the ampulla of Vater and duodenum, and may allow contract evaluation of the pancreatico-biliary duct system. Pancreatic secretions are obtained for cytologic evaluation, and direct biopsy of periampullary or intraductal lesions may be obtained. Transhepatic cholangiography may occasionally be helpful if ERCP is not possible.

Occasionally, because of the vagueness of the symptoms, patients may undergo evaluation by barium swallow and small bowel follow-through study, which may lead to suspicion of cancer due to extrinsic compression. Also, relative or complete gastric outlet obstruction can be diagnosed in this manner, leading to further evaluation as described above. Rarely, the diagnosis may be due to lower gastrointestinal symptoms (e.g., obstruction or bleeding) due to colonic invasion.

Laparoscopy increasingly is being used for diagnosis of pancreatic cancer. In addition, the procedure, if performed prior to exploratory laparotomy, may save the patient from undergoing an open procedure if evidence of peritoneal disease or other intraabdominal findings that may preclude surgery for cure is discovered.

It is important in the workup of the patient with suspected pancreatic malignancy to confirm the diagnosis as expeditiously as possible. However, no one specific study will consistently lead to diagnosis, and the clinician may need to approach confirmation of malignancy from several approaches.

Laboratory determinations may include cytologic evaluations as above, as well as biomarkers including serum CA19-9 and CEA. Recent reporting of the use of repetitive DNA fragments in secretions may also be a possible diagnostic option in the future, especially in situations with tumor in a patient with concomitant pancreatitis. Patients with symptoms that are hormonally mediated may also be diagnosed with biochemical evaluations including serum glucagon, vasoactive peptide (VIP), or others.

TREATMENT

Surgical resection, if possible, is still the best option for cure. Treatment options are included in Table 31–8. Few patients are candidates for curative resection at presentation due to advanced disease at the time of diagnosis as previously discussed. If a patient is deemed a candidate for surgery, the options include pancreaticoduodenectomy (Whipple procedure), distal pancreatectomy (with resection of involved adjacent organs, if necessary), or occasionally total pancreatectomy. The latter tends to be favored by specific surgeons but generally has not been shown to be better than the other options. Total pancreatectomy affects the patient significantly in terms of severe endocrine and exocrine insufficiency, with marked changes in lifestyle for the patient. Again, the extent of the pancreatic resection is dependent on the location and degree of the tumor involvement. Postoperative symptoms of dumping and nutritional complications may be helped by the preservation of the pylorus compared with the historically performed Whipple procedure (Grace, Pitt, & Longmire, 1990). The extensiveness of the lymphadenectomy also varies somewhat by surgeon and country (United States versus Japan). When all patients who are candidates for potential curative surgery are considered, the extensiveness of the surgery (as long as margins are negative at time of surgery) does not consistently affect overall survival of approximately 5 per cent at 5 years.

Increasing use of the neoadjuvant approach with multimodality therapy preoperatively to convert a patient from being nonresectable to resectable has been used in pancreatic cancer, in a manner similar to several other sites such as esophagus or head and neck primaries. The approach for pancreas generally uses radiation with a radio-sensitizing chemotherapy regimen such as 5-fluorouracil and mitomycin C. The nutritional complications of this type of regimen may be particularly difficult for the patient as discussed below.

When a palliative approach is used for symptomatic control and improvement in quality of life, biliary bypass with or without gastric bypass may be carried out. Procedures such as choledochojejunostomy and cholecystojejunostomy may provide patients with palliation of biliary or gastric obstruction or prevention of such symptoms with progressive disease. Gastric outlet obstruction is treated or prevented with a gastroenterostomy. The combined procedures of biliary and gastric bypass have been termed a "double bypass" procedure for pancreatic cancer. If a patient is not deemed to be a surgical candidate, biliary decompression can be carried out utilizing either an endoscopic or percutaneous (e.g., transhepatic) approach.

The surgical management of patients with pancreatic cancer requires careful preoperative evaluation to determine the extent of disease. Additionally, thoughtful consideration must be given in determination of which surgical or palliative procedure will best provide the patient an acceptable quality of life.

The roles of radiation and chemotherapy with or without surgical resection have been reviewed. If the cancer is deemed resectable and surgical intervention is

TABLE 31–8. *Comparison of Types of Pancreatic Resections for Malignancy*

	PANCREATICODUODENECTOMY (WHIPPLE)	TOTAL PANCREATECTOMY	REGIONAL PANCREATECTOMY	DISTAL PANCREATECTOMY
Indications	Periampullary or small carcinoma of head	Large carcinoma of head or diffuse carcinoma	Carcinoma involving portal system	Carcinoma localized to body or tail
Tissues removed	Head of pancreas Duodenum Gastric antrum Bile duct Gallbladder	Whole pancreas Duodenum Gastric antrum Bile duct Gallbladder Spleen Peripancreatic nodes	Whole pancreas Duodenum Gastric antrum Bile duct Gallbladder Spleen Peripancreatic, celiac mesenteric nodes	Distal pancreas Spleen
Anastomoses	Choledochojejunostomy Gastrojejunostomy Pancreaticojejunostomy	Choledochojejunostomy Gastrojejunostomy	Choledochojejunostomy Gastrojejunostomy Portal vein	None
Potential advantages	Pancreatic remnant may prevent diabetes and malabsorption	Excision of pancreas may remove multifocal tumor. Complete peripancreatic nodal dissection. No pancreaticojejunostomy	Wide excision may remove microscopic residual tumor. Complete regional nodal dissection. No pancreaticojejunostomy	Pancreatic remnant may prevent diabetes and malabsorption. No pancreaticojejunostomy
Potential disadvantages	Limited resection may leave residual tumor. Pancreaticojejunostomy may fail	Diabetes and malabsorption result	Diabetes and malabsorption result. Technically complex Venous anastomosis may fail.	Limited resection may leave residual tumor.

(From Sinclair, W. F., Kinsella, T. J., Mayer, R. J. [1985]. Cancer of the pancreas. In V. T. DeVita, S. Hellman, & S. A. Rosenberg, [Eds.], *Cancer: Principles and practice of oncology* [2nd ed., pp. 691–739.] Philadelphia: J. B. Lippincott.)

planned, combined modality therapy has been demonstrated to be associated with increased survival (Willet, Lewandiowski, Waishaw, Efird, & Compton, 1993). Utilization of this approach may theoretically decrease the risk of systemic dissemination during the operative procedure and increase the possibility of curative resection. Again, when used in a neoadjuvant setting, this generally involves chemotherapy being used as a radiosensitizer. Intraoperative radiation therapy has also been used.

The use of palliative chemotherapy and radiation therapy in combination or alone has not been defined. However, for symptom relief and increasing quality of life, these may be included as a component of the treatment options offered to a patient. Combined radiation therapy and chemotherapy in the context of surgery with curative intent has demonstrated the possibility of improved survival time in highly selected patients. Once again, consideration of quality of life needs to be determined if aggressive treatment modalities are to be considered.

Hormonal or biologic response modifiers are not generally considered major options of therapy for patients.

NURSING ISSUES

The focus of nursing management will be dependent on the type and aggressiveness of treatment. Patients undergoing combined modality therapy will need intervention related to symptomatology induced by the tumor or the treatment plan. These include adequate treatment of nausea, vomiting, pain, mucositis, and pancreatic insufficiency. Of primary nursing consideration in these patients are the overall symptoms that lead a patient to seek medical attention. In addition to those listed, the systemic effects of anorexia, progressive weight loss, and decrease in performance status need to be addressed proactively, especially in the context of neoadjuvant therapy where the plan is for surgical resection after up-front chemotherapy and radiation therapy.

An algorithm of nutritional approaches in patients with pancreatic as well as other GI malignancies is found in Figure 31–2. Briefly, nutritional intervention is generally necessary from time of diagnosis, since approximately 26 per cent of patients with pancreatic cancer may present with weight loss, which will be further exacerbated with single or multimodality therapy. The most important components of this nutritional intervention include education of the patient and family concerning appropriate symptom management as it affects adequate nutritional intake. Additionally, practical issues of defining calorie and protein goals for the patient as well as specific issues of oral intervention are important for success. Use of pancreatic enzymes will often allow a patient to take in a normal amount of dietary fat to help maintain body composition and performance status. The option of fat restriction to decrease risk of fat malabsorption is generally counterproductive in a patient who has progressive inanition, cachexia, or both. Beyond proactive symptom management and oral intervention, more aggressive supportive nutrition may be indicated with use of enteral or short-course parenteral nutrition.

Pain management is of primary importance in these patients in terms of quality of life, compliance with and tolerance of therapeutic modalities, as well as its affect on nutritional intake. Additional issues of nutrition care in oncology patients is found in Chapter 51.

Overall, nursing management will require ongoing assessment of the patient, including psychosocial variables, and support systems to identify those problems that can be effectively addressed to affect quality of life and therapeutic success. Early intervention will provide patients with comfort and will allow patients to actively participate with treatment.

HEPATOCELLULAR CARCINOMA

DEFINITION AND INCIDENCE

Primary liver cancer (hepatocellular carcinoma or HCC) is among the top 10 most common cancers internationally and worldwide accounts for between 0.25 and 1 million new cases per year. HCC is a sex-linked disease with significantly higher frequency in males (London, 1981). Higher prevalence of HCC is generally observed in those countries (South Africa) or races (Chinese) where the highest incidence of cirrhosis is observed. In the United States, the incidence is relatively low compared with a number of international sites, but is increasing, potentially related both to risk factors and immigration patterns. In 1995, estimated new cases of liver and biliary passage malignancies included 18,500 (compared with 15,800 in 1993) and cancer deaths at these sites of 14,200 (compared with 12,600) (Boring, Squires, & Tong, 1993; Wingo et al., 1995).

Hepatocellular carcinoma (HCC) is one of the most common malignancies worldwide and accounts for approximately 2 per cent of all cancers. It has, intriguingly, been called "Nature's model tumor" (Johnson, 1993). In common with several other epithelial gastrointestinal neoplasms, it occurs in a chronically injured organ—the cirrhotic liver. It has strong epidemiologic links with chronic viral infections (hepatitis B and C), and there is also epidemiologic evidence to link it with an extraordinarily strong dietary carcinogen, aflatoxin. Not only are there abundant data on these major mechanisms of carcinogenesis, but the tumor is also present in nearly epidemic proportions in some countries. Furthermore, all the putative etiologic factors have profound practical applications: the cirrhosis limits surgical resection and complicates serologic and radiologic diagnosis. The viral hepatitis is, in the case of hepatitis B virus, preventable by vaccination, and aflatoxin exposure is potentially controllable.

EPIDEMIOLOGY AND ETIOLOGY

Approximately 80 per cent of hepatocellular carcinoma has been attributed to the hepatitis B virus. Particularly high-risk areas include China, where liver cancer ranks third in men and fourth in women as cause of death. In China, hepatocellular carcinoma is the most common malignancy in those aged 15 to 34 years (Zhou, DeTolla, Custer, & London, 1987). Additionally, in the United States, cirrhosis is also a significant risk factor, with up to 50 per cent of patients with hepatocellular carcinoma having cirrhosis. The change in these data with immigration patterns from high-risk countries may decrease this impact of cirrhosis over time. Recommendation for use of hepatitis vaccination in children is being offered as an intriguing way to prevent the development of a well-defined and internationally significant health problem with significant international cost savings and impact on morbidity and cancer mortality.

Other etiologic factors related to hepatocellular carcinoma include intestinal parasites, hemochromatosis, and presence of carcinogens in food (e.g., aflatoxin mycotoxin from the fungus *Aspergillus flavus* in moldy peanuts) (Adams, Poulter, & Pandya, 1983). Associations with steroid use (androgens and oral contraceptives) and primary liver cancer have also been reported (Prentice, 1991).

BIOLOGY AND NATURAL HISTORY

Approximately 90 per cent of primary liver cancer is HCC. The remaining 10 per cent includes cholangiocarcinoma in approximately 7 per cent and uncommon tumors such as hepatoblastoma, angiosarcoma, and sarcoma. Several different histologic patterns have been described, but classification can be simplified into subtypes of trabecular and undifferentiated tumors. Additionally, two other subtypes include fibrolamellar carcinoma (presentation in younger adults, with better resectability, prognosis, and survival rate than the more common HCC) and sclerosing HCC, which is actually a type of cholangiocarcinoma that may secrete mucus but not bile. The latter may be associated with hypercalcemia.

In general, hepatocellular carcinoma advances by direct extension within and around the liver and by direct invasion of venous and lymphatic channels.

α-fetoprotein (AFP) is a major tumor marker associated with hepatocellular carcinoma and is elevated in over 70 per cent of patients with the disease, particularly in Asia (Waldmann & McIntire, 1974; Wanebo & Vezeridis, 1993).

Evaluation of prognostic factors (Ellis, Demers, & Roh, 1992) in hepatic malignancy in resected specimens have included DNA content, which has shown aneuploidy in 50 per cent. This has been significantly correlated with tumor size, the presence of vascular invasion or intrahepatic metastases, and poorer overall survival. Prognostic factors in unresectable cases of hepatocellular carcinoma include Karnofsky performance score of less than 80, ascites, bilirubin greater than 1.5 mg/dl, serum glutamic-oxaloacetic transaminase > 35, alkaline phosphatase > 95, and α-fetoprotein positivity (Wanebo & Vezeridis, 1993).

Factors predictive for intrahepatic recurrence following resection include tumor size > 5 cm, number of tumors (> 3), presence of cancer cell infiltration of the tumor's fibrous capsule, portal involvement by tumor, and the stage of the tumor (Wanebo & Vezeridis, 1993).

SIGNS AND SYMPTOMS

Most patients present with right upper quadrant pain and weight loss. Although the pain is generally dull in nature, it can be sharp and may frequently radiate to the right shoulder (Wanebo & Vezeridis, 1993). Fatigue, anorexia, and weight loss are common, and unexplained fever may be present. Because of the hepatomegaly, there may be early satiety, a feeling of constant fullness, and vague abdominal complaints. The latter may also be contributed to by fat malabsorption and bloating. Jaundice may be noted at various points in the general course dependent on the location and size of the tumor and the underlying health of the remaining liver (i.e., cirrhotic or noncirrhotic). The findings of firm nodular hepatomegaly, arterial bruit, and hepatic rub strongly suggest advanced HCC. In early stages, hepatomegaly may be the only finding on physical examination.

DIFFERENTIAL DIAGNOSIS

Differential diagnosis includes primary versus secondary malignancy (i.e., metastatic disease) versus benign disease. Benign liver lesions that can mimic malignancy in terms of presentation with a mass in the liver include adenomas and focal nodular hyperplasia, both of which have been associated with oral contraceptive use, and angiomas (which are often found on CT scan for vague symptoms or for evaluation of an entirely different problem). Generalized hepatomegaly is also a finding with diffuse metastatic disease from a number of primary sites. Occasionally, liver metastases may be the first presentation of malignancy from primary disease at other sites.

DIAGNOSTIC EVALUATION

Ultrasound is inexpensive and versatile in detecting small lesions in the liver, usually hypoechoic in nature. In high-risk patients with chronic hepatitis B virus or cirrhosis, ultrasound and AFP monitoring may lead to earlier diagnosis. Ultrasonography is also useful in directing fine-needle aspiration biopsy for cytology. Additionally, intraoperative ultrasound (IOU) is useful in detecting additional lesions that may not be identified by other imaging modalities. IOU has a sensitivity of 96 to 98 per cent and may also allow visualization of intrahepatic vessels. CT scan and MRI may delineate extent and anatomic location, with MRI also useful in distinguishing HCC from angiomatous cysts and regenerating nodules of cirrhosis. Dynamic CT scan can also be helpful. Patients who are considered surgical candidates need, in general, to have preoperative hepatic angiography, to provide information about tumor extent and vascular status, and to evaluate the vascular distribution of the liver if nonresectional therapy is required.

The use of tumor markers (AFP) has been discussed above and may be helpful in a patient who has a known diagnosis or history of malignancy that may need to be considered in the differential diagnosis.

TREATMENT

Potential treatment options for hepatocellular carcinoma are summarized in Table 31–9. In general, surgical resection is the best option for cure (Ellis et al., 1992); however, the majority of patients presenting with HCC are not resectable at diagnosis. In a series using an extremely aggressive surgical approach (including as-needed vascular reconstruction for portal vein thrombus, inferior vena cava tumor thrombus, resection or ethanol injection of daughter nodules in both lobes, or resection in patients with tumor recurrence), the authors were able to obtain a 91 per cent resectability compared with the 20 per cent rate of other Japanese series (Ozawa et al., 1991). With this aggressive approach, 1-, 2-, and 3-year survival rates were 70 per cent, 60 per cent, and 35 per cent, respectively. For resection in general, improved survival is noted with the following: (1) age between 30 and 50 years, (2) absence of coexisting liver disease, (3) fibrolamellar carcinoma, (4) solitary tumor, (5) unilobar

---

TABLE 31–9. *Potential Treatment Options for Hepatocellular Carcinoma (HCC)*

Resectable Lesions
Hepatic resection (with or without adjuvant chemotherapy on clinical trial basis)

Recurrent HCC Confined to Liver
Hepatic resection
Transcatheter arterial embolization (TAE)
Percutaneous ethanol injection (PEI)

Recurrent HCC with Hepatic and Extrahepatic Disease
Transcatheter arterial embolization or percutaneous ethanol injection (with or without chemotherapy on clinical trial basis)

Unresectable HCC Due to Size or Number of Lesions
Transcatheter arterial embolization
Orthotopic liver transplantation

Unresectable HCC Due to Location of Tumor or Underlying Cirrhosis
Orthotopic liver transplantation
Percutaneous ethanol injection
Transcatheter arterial embolization (if mild to moderate cirrhosis)

(From Ellis L. M., Demers M. L., & Roh M. S. [1992]. Current strategies for the treatment of hepatocellular carcinoma. *Current Opinion in Oncology, 4,* 741–751.)

tumor, (6) absence of vascular invasion, (7) portal vein thrombosis, (8) extrahepatic spread, and (9) surgery with the intent to cure.

Earlier treatment options are possible when screening AFP monitoring in high-risk patients directs the use of CT scan or ultrasound to detect early HCC.

Surgical options have also included total hepatectomy and orthotopic liver transplantation (OLT) for otherwise unresectable HCC. Also, the treatment of HCC may be incidental when such a lesion is found in the resected liver when performed for end-stage liver insufficiency. Two-year survival data from the University of Cincinnati was 30 per cent (including 365 patients with "usual hepatoma or HCC"), with the majority (84 per cent) of recurrences occurring within 2 years (Penn, 1991). However, the 2-year survival for patients without recurrence was just under 50 per cent. In patients with incidental diagnoses of HCC, the 2- and 5-year survival rates were 57 per cent. Fibrolamellar hepatoma had a 2- and 5-year survival of 60 per cent and 55 per cent. Similar results have been found at other institutions. Favorable prognostic factors include tumor size < 5 cm in diameter, single tumor, no vascular invasion, no lymph node metastases, presence of a pseudocapsule, circumscribed tumor, absence of margin invasion, and unilobar involvement.

Nonsurgical therapy includes systemic chemotherapy as well as other innovative methods of palliation (Carr, Iwatsuki, Starzl, Selby, & Madariaga, 1993; Luporini, Labianca, & Pancera, 1993; Moore & Pazdur, 1993). No given chemotherapeutic regimen has shown significant promise, and this approach is generally associated with significant toxicity. In general, systemic chemotherapy for HCC should be carried out in the context of clinical trials.

Innovative palliative therapy includes options of percutaneous transcatheter arterial embolization (TAE) (Ellis, Demers, & Roh, 1992). This is based on the observation that hepatic tumors derive their blood supply from the hepatic artery, whereas the liver vascularity is predominantly from the portal vein (in noncirrhotics). Embolization can be carried out with or without gelatin sponge, iodized oil or cisplatin, fluorodeoxiuridene or doxorubicin, or mitomycin-C microcapsules. This technique has also been used for recurrent HCC after initial resection.

Radiation may be used palliatively, but use of external beam radiation is limited because of hepatic radiotoxicity. Brachytherapy is rarely used, but hepatic artery infusion of radioisotopes (^{131}I and ^{90}Y) have been studied. ^{131}I is associated with less toxicity and can be delivered to the tumor in the form of hepatic artery infusion of labeled Lipiodol, with an objective response rate of 40 per cent (Raoul et al., 1992).

An additional nonsurgical option for palliation also includes percutaneous ethanol injection (PEI), although it has also been used by some investigators with curative intent. PEI can also be used in combination with TAE (Livraghi et al., 1992; Shiina, Tagawa, Unuma, & Terano, 1990).

NURSING ISSUES

Due to the potential extensiveness of the surgical resection, especially in the hands of an aggressive surgeon, patients may need significant nursing intervention. This includes attention to pain, respiratory care, and fluid management during the initial postoperative period. Additionally, attention to mental status changes that may be associated with liver insufficiency in a patient with cirrhosis is important in the nursing management of the patient with HCC. As the patient is over the initial postoperative stress period, attention to nutrition and activity are particularly important if the patient has had significant preoperative anorexia and weight loss. This combination of attentions is important in preventing several potential postoperative complications, including decubiti.

Decompressive tubes as well as percutaneous or surgically placed transhepatic biliary stents will often be used, and the patient and family/caregiver need to have adequate teaching prior to discharge concerning tube care as well as potential complications, their presentations, and how the complications should be addressed. Additionally, management of ascites through Tenckhoff tubes or via peritoneal-venous shunts is an important aspect of patient education.

Pain may well be a major issue with progressive disease and is an important aspect of supportive care.

Chronic active hepatitis, a precursor of hepatocellular carcinoma, can be prevented by use of the hepatitis B vaccine and must be considered by nursing staff as part of the prudent care of patients (Centers for Disease Control, 1990). While universal precautions must be carried out with all patient secretions, the viral dose necessary to infect a health care worker, for example, through a needle puncture or body fluid splash, is much less than that for infection with the human immunodeficiency virus (HIV) and more importantly is preventable through vaccination.

BILIARY MALIGNANCY

DEFINITION AND INCIDENCE

Cancer of the biliary tract includes the gallbladder and the bile ducts from the canals of Hering to the ampulla of Vater. In general, the prognosis is poor, and overall survival is usually less than 1 year. Histologically, more than 95 per cent of biliary tract cancers are adenocarcinomas. Various synonyms for biliary ductal carcinoma have included cholangiocarcinoma, cholangiocellular carcinoma, bile duct carcinoma, and adenocarcinoma of the liver.

Carcinoma of the gallbladder was described more than 200 years ago, and it has been noted that overall, little has changed in this disease since then. This is due to the generally late presentation due to nonspecific initial complaints. In less than 9 per cent of patients with gallbladder cancer is the diagnosis made preoperatively. It is usually a finding at the time of cholecystectomy for presumed cholecystitis or cholelithiasis. Although primary carcinoma of the gallbladder is relatively rare, it is the most common malignancy of the biliary tract and the fifth most common gastrointestinal cancer diagnosed in the United States. Annual incidence of gallbladder cancer is approximately 2.5 per 100,000 population and is found in 1 to 3 per cent of cholecystectomy specimens. Incidence peak is in the elderly, and it is more commonly diagnosed in females. Carcinoma of the gallbladder has a significant ethnic variability in the United States, with this being the most frequently identified malignancy at postmortem examination of southwestern American Indians (where greater than 90 to 95 per cent of women of this group have gallstones).

Biliary ductal carcinoma has an autopsy frequency of approximately 0.1 to 0.5 per cent in the United States and occurs in approximately 0.5 per cent of biliary tree operations. Overall survival at 5 years with surgical management is 5 to 8 per cent. In general, men and women are equally affected, with diagnosis possible between the ages 20 and 80 years, with an average age of 60. However, an increase in younger adults has been recently noted (Way, 1991). Ulcerative colitis may be a common associated condition, and biliary duct cancer may develop after long-standing sclerosing cholangitis. Tumors involving the bifurcation of the common hepatic duct are known as Klatskin tumors.

Survival in both gallbladder and biliary ductal carcinoma is optimized with a multidisciplinary approach (Kraybill et al., 1994).

EPIDEMIOLOGY AND ETIOLOGY

Gallbladder. Several predisposing conditions have been linked with gallbladder carcinoma, but the exact etiology remains unknown (Wanebo & Vezeridis, 1993). There is an association with cholelithiasis, with three fourths of patients with carcinoma of the gallbladder having gallstones (although less than 1 per cent of patients with gallstones develop gallbladder cancer). The size of the stones correlate with risk (Diehl, 1983). The association has recently been suggested to be related to common risk factors rather than cause and effect. Calcification of the gallbladder (known as porcelain gallbladder) is a significant risk and when noted is considered an indication for prophylactic cholecystectomy. Risk of carcinoma of the gallbladder is increased sixfold in typhoid carriers compared with the general population.

Biliary Duct. Ulcerative colitis and primary sclerosing cholangitis are considered predisposing conditions for carcinoma of the bile ducts. The relative risk for individuals with ulcerative colitis is approximately 31.3 times that of the general population. Hepatobiliary fibropolycystic disease, which includes choledochal cyst, is also associated with increased risk for cancer development. In general, gallstone disease has historically been considered a risk factor, but that continues to be reconsidered (Rossi, Heiss, Beckmann, & Braasch, 1985). However, the association question may be related to the differences between gallstone composition between the United States and Asia, which may contribute to different risk profiles. Less common con-

ditions that predispose to bile duct carcinoma include portal bacteremia (specifically recurrent pyogenic cholangitis), typhoid infections, viral infections, secondary bile acid formation (e.g., lithocholic acid) and copper overload. Patients with liver fluke infection (*Clonorchis sinensis* and *Opisthochis viverrini*) have an elevated risk for development of cholangiocarcinoma. Primary sclerosing cholangitis and congenital bile duct cysts represent the conditions at highest risk of biliary duct carcinoma development.

BIOLOGY AND NATURAL HISTORY

Grossly, cholangiocarcinoma or biliary duct carcinoma are to be divided into massive, multinodular, and diffuse types. In general, the tumor appears as a large, gray-white, firm mass with infiltrative margins and smaller satellite nodules arising in a noncirrhotic liver. Major duct involvement may cause obstruction and consequent cholestasis, occasionally followed by abscess formation. Vein invasion is less frequent than in HCC.

Histologically, biliary duct carcinoma is an adenocarcinoma. Rare variants with squamous differentiation have been reported. It has been suggested that there is no certain way of establishing the identity of primary duct cancer in the liver, as metastases from the pancreas and other sites may look similar. The differential diagnosis between primary biliary duct carcinoma and metastatic adenocarcinoma is made possible only by demonstrating (1) in situ carcinoma in the ducts near the tumor, (2) modulation from bile duct to parenchymal liver cells, and (3) ductal plate configuration within the tumor.

SIGNS AND SYMPTOMS

Presentation of biliary tract carcinoma is one of gradual onset of jaundice or pruritis. Whereas acute onset of biliary obstruction is associated with fever, chills, and biliary colic, these are not seen with the gradual onset of biliary malignancy. Except for deep discomfort in the right upper quadrant, the patient generally feels fairly well. Bilirubinuria is present early, and light-colored stools are common. Progressive weight loss is often seen secondary to progressively severe anorexia. Physical examination reveals icterus. Hepatomegaly is common, and if obstruction is not relieved, the liver may become cirrhotic with development of splenomegaly, ascites, or bleeding varices. If the common hepatic duct is obstructed, the gallbladder distends and can be felt with palpation (not the tumor itself), whereas patients with tumors of the hepatic duct do not develop distended/palpable gallbladders.

With gallbladder carcinoma, the most common presenting complaint is right upper quadrant pain, similar to previous episodes of biliary colic but more persistent. Obstruction of the cystic duct by tumor may precipitate an attack of acute cholecystitis. Others may present with obstructive jaundice and occasionally cholangitis due to secondary involvement of the common duct.

DIFFERENTIAL DIAGNOSIS

Obviously for gallbladder carcinoma, the differential diagnosis includes cholelithiasis or cholecystitis. For biliary tract cancers in general, the differential diagnosis includes causes of extrahepatic and intrahepatic cholestatic jaundice, including choledocholithiasis (common bile duct stones), liver involvement with primary (usual HCC or fibrolamellar carcinoma) or metastatic cancer, hepatitis, and chronic pancreatitis. Additionally, periampullary carcinoma (arising in the duodenum near the ampulla of Vater) may be included in the differential diagnosis.

DIAGNOSTIC EVALUATION

Diagnostic evaluation is similar to that discussed under hepatocellular carcinoma. Endoscopic retrogradecholangiopancreatography (ERCP) is an additional diagnostic modality that is useful in biliary duct carcinoma in terms of visualization of the ductal abnormality directly or via contrast injected into the pancreatico-biliary ductal system. The procedure also allows direct biopsy of a visualized lesion as well as evaluation of bile for cytology and tumor markers.

TREATMENT

Kraybill et al. (1994) have stressed the importance of a multidisciplinary approach to therapy of biliary tract cancers. The majority of patients present with jaundice, with an increasing number of patients undergoing palliative treatment with percutaneously and endoscopically placed stents. Prognosis in biliary tract tumors is generally poor, with median survival in a number of studies in the range of 11 months, with no difference between males and females nor between patients with gallbladder and biliary duct carcinomas.

Improved prognosis compared with the general patient population has been seen in patients with gallbladder cancer who underwent resection. The extent of resection is a matter of discussion, but it has been recommended that lymph node dissection of the porta hepatis along with resection of the gallbladder and wedge of liver from the gallbladder bed may result in improved survival. Additionally, extensive resection, including major hepatectomy and pancreacticoduodenectomy, has been offered as potentially appropriate in selected patients with advanced gallbladder carcinoma with a result of prolonged survival (Tsukada et al., 1994). In general, surgical treatment is most successful when negative margins can be obtained, usually possible only in early or incidental diagnoses.

Survival trends toward improvement in patients with surgically negative margins who received RT have been seen. Additionally, patients who receive $\geq$ 4000 cGy have better survival than those receiving < 4000 cGy (Kraybill et al., 1994).

Combined modality therapy may be an option (Minsky et al, 1990)—including laparotomy and biopsy or subtotal resection or ERCP or percutaneous transhepatic cholangiography (PTC) and biliary drainage; 5000 cGy to the tumor bed and primary nodal area followed by a 1500 cGy boost to the tumor bed; and chemotherapy consisting of 5-fluorouracil and mitomycin-C given at the beginning of each radiation therapy treatment course. Overall 5-year survival with this regimen was 50 per cent, with mean survival of 32 months and median of 16 months. However, at this point the use of chemotherapy in the disease is generally rare and limited to specific centers.

NURSING ISSUES

Approaches of nursing management in biliary tract malignancies are similar to those of hepatocellular carcinoma.

REFERENCES

Adams, J. T., Poulter, C. A., & Pandya, K. J. (1983). Cancer of the major digestive glands: Pancreas, liver, bile ducts, gallbladder. In P. Rubin, R. F. Bakemeier, & S. K. Krackov (Eds.), *Clinical oncology—a multidisciplinary approach* (pp. 178–190). New York: American Cancer Society.

Beahrs, O. H., Henson, D. E., Hutter, R. V. P., & Kennedy, B. J. (Eds) (1993). *Handbook for staging of cancer from the manual for staging of cancer* (4th ed.). Philadelphia: J. B. Lippincott Co.

Biasco, G., Paganelli, G. M., Azzaroni, D., Grigioni, W. F., Merighi, S. M., Stoja, R., Villanacci, V., Rusticali, A. G., Cuoco, D. L., Caporale, V., & Barbara, L. (1987). Early gastric cancer in Italy. *Digestive Diseases and Sciences, 12,* 113–120.

Boring, C. C., Squires, T. S., & Tong, T. (1993). Cancer statistics, 1993. *CA: A Cancer Journal for Clinicians, 43,* 7–26.

Boring, C. C., Squires, T. S., Tong, T., & Montgomery, S. (1994). Cancer statistics, 1994. *CA: A Cancer Journal for Clinicians, 44,* 7–26.

Burn, I. A., & Welbourn, R. B. (1975). Cancer of the Stomach. In R. Smith (Ed.), *Gastric surgery: Surgery forum* (pp. 121–148). Boston: Butterworths.

Carr, B. I., Iwatsuki, S., Starzl, T. E., Selby, R., & Madariaga, J. (1993). Regional cancer chemotherapy for advanced stage hepatocellular carcinoma. *Journal of Surgical Oncology Supplement, 3,* 100–103.

Centers for Disease Control. (1990). Protection against viral hepatitis: Recommendations of the Immunization Practices Advisory Committee (ACIP). *Morbidity Mortality Weekly Report, 39,* 1–23.

Detsky, A. S., McLaughlin, J. R., Baker, J. P., Johnston, N., Whittaker, S., Mendelson, R. A., & Jeejeebhoy, K. N. (1987). *Journal of Parenteral and Enteral Nutrition, 11,* 8–13.

Diehl, A. K. (1983). Gallstone size and risk of gallbladder cancer. *Journal of the American Medical Association, 250,* 2323–2326.

Ellis, F., Levitan, N., & Lo, T. (1992). In A. Holleb, D. Fink, & G. Murphy (Eds.), *American Cancer Society textbook of clinical oncology* (pp 254–262) Atlanta: American Cancer Society.

Ellis, L. M., Demers, M. L., & Roh, M. S. (1992). Current strategies for the treatment of hepatocellular carcinoma. *Current Opinion in Oncology, 4,* 741–751.

Ellis, P., & Cunningham, D. (1994). The management of carcinomas of the upper gastrointestinal tract. *British Medical Journal, 26,* 834–838.

Evans, D. B., Rich, T. A., Byrd, D. R., & Ames, F. (1991). Adenocarcinoma of the pancreas: Current management of resectable and locally advanced disease. *Southern Medical Journal 84,* 566–570.

Fonthan, R., Corrisa, P., & Cohen, I. (1984). Epidemiology of cancer of the pancreas. In I. M. Howard, G. I. Jordon, & H. A. Reber (Eds.), *Surgical diseases of the pancreas* (pp. 613–626). Philadelphia: Lea and Febiger.

Fox, H., & Kandi, A. (1984). The vulnerable esophagus, riboflavin deficiency and squamous cell dysplasia of the skin and the esophagus. *Journal of the National Cancer Institute, 72,* 941–943.

Frank-Stromborg, M. (1989). The epidemiology and primary prevention of gastric and esophageal cancer. A worldwide perspective. *Cancer Nursing, 12,* 53–64.

Gabos, S., Berkel, J., Band, P., Robson, D., & Whittaker, H. (1993). Small bowel cancer in western Canada. *International Journal of Epidemiology, 22,* 198–206.

Gary, L. W., Crook, J. N., & Cohn, D. (1972). Carcinoma of the pancreas. Proceedings of the Seventh National Cancer Conference, 503–510.

Grace, P. A., Pitt, H. A., & Longmire, W. P. (1990). Pylorus preserving pancreacticoduodenectomy: an overview. *British Journal of Surgery, 77,* 968–974.

Green, P. H., O'Toole, K. M., Slonim, D., Wang, T., & Weg, A. (1988). Increasing incidence and excellent survival of patients with early gastric cancer: Experience in a United States medical center. *American Medical Journal, 85,* 658–661.

Hill, M. J. (1984). Aetiology of gastric cancer. *Clinics in Oncology, 3,* 237–249.

Hoebler, L., & Irwin, M. (1992). Gastrointestinal tract cancer: Current knowledge, medical treatment, and nursing management. *Oncology Nursing Forum, 14,* 1403.

Hwang, H., Dwyer, J., & Russell, R. M. (1994). Diet, *Helicobacter pylori* infection, food preservation, and gastric cancer risk: Are there new roles for preventative factors? *Nutrition Reviews, 52,* 75–83.

Ihde, J. K., & Coit, D. G. (1991). Melanoma metastatic to stomach, small bowel or colon. *American Journal of Surgery, 162,* 208–211.

Johnson, P. J. (1993). Hepatitis, viruses, cirrhosis, and liver cancer. *Journal of Surgical Oncology Supplement, 3,* 28–33.

Kraybill, W. G., Lee, H., Pucus, J., Ramachandran, G., Lopez, M. J., Kucik, N., & Myerson, R. J. (1994). Multidisciplinary treatment of biliary tract cancers. *Journal of Surgical Oncology, 55,* 239–245.

Lashner, B. A. (1992). Risk factors for small bowel cancer in Crohn's disease. *Digestive Diseases and Sciences, 37,* 1179–1184.

Lerut, T., Coosemans, W., Van Raemdonck, D., Dillemans, B., DeLeyn, P., Marnette, J. M., & Geboes, K. (1994). Surgical treatment of Barrett's carcinoma: Correlations between morphologic findings and prognosis. *Journal of Thoracic & Cardiovascular Surgery, 107,* 1059–1066.

Livraghi, T., Bolondi, L., Lazzaroni, S., Marin, G., Morabito, A., Rapaccini, G. L., Salmi, A., & Torzilli, G. (1992). Percutaneous ethanol injection in the treatment of hepatocellular carcinoma in cirrhosis. *Cancer, 69,* 925–929.

London, W. T. (1981). Primary hepatocellular carcinoma. *Human Pathology, 12,* 1085–1097.

Luporini, G., Labianca, R., & Pancera, G. (1993). Medical treatment of hepatocellular carcinoma. *Journal of Surgical Oncology Supplement, 3,* 115–118.

Lynch, H. P., Smyrk, T. C., Lynch, P. M. Lanpsa, S. J., Boman, B. M., Ens, J., Lynch, J. S., Strayhorn, P., Carmody, T., & Cristofaro, G. (1989). Adenocarcinoma of the small bowel in Lynch syndrome II. *Cancer, 64,* 2178–2183.

Macdonald, J., Gunderson, L., & Cohn, I., Jr. (1982). Cancer of the pancreas. In V. T. DeVita, S. Hellman, & S. A. Rosenberg (Eds.), *Cancer: Principles and practice of oncology* (pp. 563–589). Philadelphia: J. B. Lippincott Co.

Mason, A. R., & Sabiston, D. C. (1986). Textbook of surgery (13th ed., pp. 868–873). Philadelphia: W. B. Saunders Co.

Minsky, B. D., Wesson, M. F., Armstrong, J. G. et al. (1990). Combined modality therapy of extrahepatic biliary system cancer. *International Journal of Radiation Oncology, Biology, Physics, 18,* 1157–1163.

Mohiuddin, M., Rosato, F., Schuricht, A., Barbot, D., Biermann, W., & Canctor, R. (1994). Carcinoma of the pancreas—the Jefferson experience. 1975–1988. *European Journal of Surgical Oncology, 20,* 13–20.

Moore, D., & Pazdur, R. (1993). Systemic therapies for unresectable primary hepatic tumors. *Journal of Surgical Oncology Supplement, 3,* 112–114.

Morton, J. M., Poulter, C. A., & Pandya, K. J. (1983). Alimentary tract cancer. In P. Rubin, R. F. Bakemeier, & S. K. Krackov (Eds.), *Clinical oncology—a multidisciplinary approach* (pp. 154–176). New York: American Cancer Society.

Munkholm, P., Langholz, E., Davidsen, M., & Binder, V. (1993). Intestinal cancer risk and mortality in patients with Crohn's disease. *Gastroenterology, 105,* 1716–1723.

Neugut, A. I., & Santos, J. (1993). The association between cancers of the small and large bowel. *Cancer Epidemiology, Biomarkers, & Prevention, 2,* 551–553.

Ottery, F. D. (1995). Supportive nutrition to prevent cachexia and improve quality of life. *Seminars in Oncology, 22* (Suppl. 3), 98–111.

Ozawa, K., Takayasu, T., Kumada, K., Yomaoka, Y., Tanaka, K., Kobatashi, N., Inamoto, T., Shimahara, Y., Mori, K., Honda, K., & Asonuma, K. (1991). Experience with 225 hepatic resections for hepatocellular carcinoma over a 4-year period. *American Journal of Surgery, 161,* 677–682.

Penn, I. (1991). Hepatic transplantation for primary and metastatic cancer of the liver. *Surgery, 110,* 726–735.

Prentice, R. L. (1991). Epidemiologic data on exogenous hormones and hepatocellular carcinoma and selected other cancers. *Preventive Medicine, 20,* 38–46.

Raoul, J., Bretagne, J. F., Pariente, E. A., Boyer, J., Paris, J. C., Michel, H., Bourguet, P., Victor, G., Therain, F., Lejeune, J. J., Lemaire, B., Collet, H., Duvauferrier, R., Puech, J. L., Viala, J. F., L'Hoste, P., Poisonnier, M., & Guiry, P. (1992). Internal radiation therapy for hepatocellular carcinoma results of a French multicenter phase II trial of transarterial infection of Iodine 131-labeled Lipiodol. *Cancer, 69,* 346–352.

Robertson, C. S., Mayberry, J. F., Nicholson, D. A., James, P. D., & Atkinson, M. (1988). Value of endoscopic surveillance in the detection of neoplastic changes in Barrett's esophagus. *British Journal of Surgery, 75,* 760–763.

Rosenberg, J. C., Schwade, J. G., & Vaitkevicius, V. (1982). Cancer of the esophagus. In V. T. DeVita, S. Hellman, & S. A. Rosenberg (Eds.), *Cancer: Principles and practice of oncology* (pp. 499–533). Philadelphia: J. B. Lippincott Co.

Rossi, R. L., Heiss, F. W., Beckmann, C. F., & Braasch, J. W. (1985). Management of cancer of the bile duct. *Surgical Clinics of North America, 65,* 59–78.

Saltzburg, D., & Foley, K. (1989). Management of pain in pancreatic cancer. *Surgical Clinics of North America, 69,* 629–649.

Sarr, M., & Cameron, J. (1984). Surgical palliation of unresectable carcinoma of the pancreas. *World Journal of Surgery, 8,* 906–918.

Sellner, F. (1990). Investigations on the significance of the adenoma-carcinoma sequence in the small bowel. *Cancer, 66,* 702–715.

Shiina, S., Tagawa, K., Unuma, T., & Terano, A. (1990). Percutaneous ethanol injection therapy for the treatment of hepatocellular carcinoma. *American Journal of Roentgenology, 154,* 946–951.

Steele, G. D., Osteen, R. T., Winchester, D. P., Murphy, G. P., & Menck, H. R. (1994). Clinical highlights from the National Cancer Data Base: 1994. *CA: Cancer Journal for Clinicians, 44,* 71–80.

Tsukada, K., Yoshida, K., Aono, T., Koyama, S., Shirai, Y., Uchida, K., & Muto, T. (1994). Major hepatectomy and pancreatoduodenectomy for advanced carcinoma of the biliary tract. *British Medical Journal, 81,* 108–110.

Viamonte, M., & Viamonte, M. (1992). Primary squamous-cell carcinoma of the small bowel: Report of a case. *Diseases of the Colon and Rectum, 35,* 806–809.

Waldmann, T. A., & McIntire, K. R. (1974). The use of radioimmunoassay for alpha-fetoprotein in the diagnosis of malignancy. *Cancer, 34,* 1510–1515.

Wanebo, H. J., & Vezeridis, M. P. (1993). Hepatoma. *Journal of Surgical Oncology, 3,* 40–45.

Wanebo, H. J., & Vezeridis, M. P. (1993). Carcinoma of the gallbladder. *Journal of Surgical Oncology Supplement, 3,* 134–139.

Waterhouse, J. A. H. (1984). Epidemiology of stomach cancer. *Clinics in Oncology, 3,* 221–236.

Way, L. W. (1991). Biliary tract. In L. W. Way (Ed.), *Current surgical diagnosis and treatment* (p. 550). Norwalk, CT: Appleton & Lange.

Willet, C., Lewandiowski, K., Waishaw, A., Efird, J., & Comptom, C. (1993). Resection margins in carcinoma of the head of the pancreas. *Annals of Surgery, 217,* 144–148.

Wingo, P. A., Tong, T., & Bolden, S. (1995). Cancer Statistics, 1995. *CA: A Cancer Journal for Clinicians 45,* 8–30.

Zhou, X., DeTolla, L., Custer, R. P., & London, W. T. (1987). Iron, ferritin, hepatitis B surface and core antigens in the livers of Chinese patients with hepatocellular carcinoma. *Cancer, 59,* 1430–1437.

Colorectal Cancer

Sara C. Gold • Charlene Sakurai

DEFINITION AND INCIDENCE

Colorectal cancer is the second leading cause of death due to cancer in the United States. Approximately 138,200 new cases will be diagnosed in 1995 (70,700 male and 76,500 female), and greater than 55,300 deaths will occur from this disease (27,200 male and 28,100 female) (Wingo, Tong, & Bolden, 1995). The majority of cases of colorectal cancer are still seen in persons over the age of 50 years; however, in the high-risk population (family history of colorectal disease, familial syndromes), diagnosis is frequently made at a much earlier age. Early diagnosis offers a fairly good survival—92% for colon and 85% for rectal cancer—(American Cancer Society, 1995), but survival rates drop drastically for advanced and metastatic disease. The overall 5-year survival for colorectal cancer as a whole is between 51 and 54 per cent (Cohen, Minsky, & Schilsky, 1993).

EPIDEMIOLOGY AND ETIOLOGY

In the United States the mortality rate of colorectal cancer is second only to that of lung cancer. Geographically, the incidence of colorectal cancer is higher in the Western world and lowest in third world countries (Doughty, 1986) related primarily to a diet high in saturated fats and refined carbohydrates but low in fiber, vitamins (especially C, D, and E), and calcium (Cohen, Minsky, & Schilsky, 1993; Willett, Stampfer, Colditz, Rosner, & Speizer, 1990). High calorie consumption and the resultant increase in body weight have also been associated with an increased risk of colorectal cancer (Winawer, 1991). Studies are showing that as populations emigrate to other areas and adapt dietary

customs and habits as well as other societal practices, the incidence of colorectal cancer changes, suggesting that both diet and environment are significant factors in the development of this disease (Willett et al., 1990). For example, those who immigrated from Scotland, an area at high risk for colon cancer, to Australia exhibit a decreased incidence, and therefore decreased risk, of the disease (McMichael et al., 1980). And a classic study comparing Japanese living in Japan, Hawaii, and the mainland United States (Haenszel & Kurihara, 1968) found that those living in Japan had the highest incidence of gastric cancer, while mainland residents had the highest incidence of colorectal cancer. Interestingly, the increase is with distal, left-sided cancer (Trock, Lanza, & Greenwald, 1990).

Because the Western diet is high in refined carbohydrates but low in fiber, transit through the colon is slow, and as a result, the extended presence of bile acids may result in carcinogenic effects on the bowel tissue (Hill, Drasar, & Williams, 1975). In addition, the method of cooking, especially grilling over hot coals or frying, may be a contributory factor to the development of colon cancer (Schiffman, 1990). Rectal cancer, which is more prevalent in the male population, has been associated with alcohol consumption (Kune & Vitetta, 1992).

Genetic and familial predisposition to the development of colorectal cancer has been widely examined. Familial adenomatous polyposis, Gardner's syndrome, inflammatory bowel disease, ulcerative colitis, diverticulosis, hemorrhoids, as well as a family history of colon cancer and familial colorectal cancer syndrome are significant factors in the etiology of colon cancer. Villous adenomas are reported to be up to 10 times more likely to be cancerous than polyps (Cohen, Minsky, & Schilsky, 1993). It is thought that those with inflammatory bowel disease have a 30-fold increase in risk, depending upon the area and extent of involvement. Additionally, those with a history of breast, endometrial, or ovarian cancers appear to have an increased risk (Weisburger, 1991).

Adenomatous polyps, particularly familial adenomatous polyposis, are considered precursor lesions, based upon established criteria involving size, rapidity of growth, and extent of dysplasia. Any polyp greater than 2 cm is considered to be at high risk (DeCosse, Tsioulias, & Jacobson, 1994; Konsker, 1992).

Risk factors for the development of rectal cancer are not specifically known but are believed to be different from those of ascending and transverse colon cancers (Weisburger, 1991).

PREVENTION

Primary prevention of colorectal cancer addresses those risks that a person or population can minimize or control. It involves both the identification of risks or causative factors and the effort to modify or eliminate them. Diet has been the main focus of primary prevention for years. Identification of the role of fiber and cruciferous vegetables (broccoli, cabbage, brussels sprouts, etc.) in preventing the development of colorectal cancer was a significant step.

Secondary prevention efforts focus on those at high risk for developing colorectal cancer, involving both identification of individuals and appropriate intervention strategies. This includes those with precancerous conditions, hereditary syndromes, and family history.

Chemoprevention is a fairly new strategy for decreasing both the development and incidence of colorectal cancer primarily in those populations most at risk (Winn & Levin, 1989). The purpose of these studies is threefold: to address those agents that might interfere with carcinogen formation, those agents that could increase the rate of detoxification of carcinogens, and those agents that might inhibit or prevent the development of colorectal cancer (Levin, 1992). Chemoprevention studies (Table 32-1) are currently under way, evaluating the roles of antioxidants, calcium carbonate,

TABLE 32-1. *Chemoprevention Trials*

AGENT	POPULATION
Wheat bran—13.5 or 2 g/day	Prior adenoma of colon
Calcium carbonate—3 or 5 g/day (high risk); 1200 mg/day (prior adenoma)	High-risk patients; prior adenoma of colon
Aspirin—80 or 325 mg/day	History of neoplastic polyp(s)
Sulindac—150 mg bid	Familial adenanomatous polyps; prior adenoma of colon
Ascorbic acid—1 g/day	Prior adenoma of colon
β-carotene—30–180 mg/day	Previous colon cancer

(Adapted from Szarka, C. E., Grana, G., & Engstrom, P. [1994]. Chemoprevention of cancer. *Current Problems in Cancer, 18,* 63.)

β carotene, aspirin, suldinac, wheat bran, and even garlic (Szarka, Grana, & Engstrom, 1994).

BIOLOGY, PATHOPHYSIOLOGY, AND NATURAL HISTORY

The development of cancer, carcinogenesis, is an involved multistage process during which normal cells in the gut are somehow transformed into something different—abnormal, premalignant, or frank cancer. This process has been called the adenoma-carcinoma sequence or the dysplastic-carcinoma sequence (Lewin, Riddell, & Weinstein, 1992). To better understand the progression of colorectal cancer, one must consider the process of carcinogenesis in the context of the anatomy of the bowel wall and the vasculature supplying the entire area (Fig. 32–1 *A* & *B*).

The bowel consists of four layers: the mucosal layer, the submucosal layer, the muscularis, and finally the serosal layer. The normally rapid and continual sloughing and regeneration of tissue/cells occurs in the mucosal layer. This turnover takes place primarily in the Crypts of Lieberkuhn. This may be moderated by a genetic mutation in the APC (adenomatous polyposis coli) gene or any one of the other four genes that have been identified with colon cancer: *ras*, p53 suppressor gene, MCC (mutated in colon cancer), and DCC (deleted in colon cancer). Changes or inactivation of p53 genes have also been associated with other solid tumors such as lung and breast (Boland, 1993; Markowitz, 1992), and lack of expression of p53 (Fig. 32–2) may predict a poor outcome in colorectal cancer (Nathanson et al., 1994).

As the new cells start to differentiate, they tend to rise to the top of the crypt, leaving the more undifferentiated cells in the lower layers (Doughty, 1986). As cells change, become abnormal, or become frankly malignant, the normal process of differentiation is affected and, in some cases, eliminated. This initial process takes place within the mucosal layer. Over time, the process will descend or progress into successive layers of the bowel. Traditional staging systems follow these processes very closely and are based primarily upon the depth of invasion rather than the size of the lesion.

As changes advance through all four layers of the bowel, lymphatic invasion may occur, and nodes may or may not be enlarged and frankly palpable. There is little correlation between gross appearance of the nodes at surgery and the amount of microscopic invasion present (Lewin et al., 1992).

In colon cancer, normal lymphatic flow is through the lymphatic channels along major arteries. If tumors lie between two major vascular pedicles, lymphatic flow may drain in either or both directions (Cohen, Minsky, & Schilsky, 1993). Rectal cancers tend to spread in an orderly and predictable fashion. Disease metastasizes to the lymph nodes at the level of the primary tumor and continues into the chains above it (Gabriel, Dukes, & Bussey, 1935). The risk for lymph node metastases rises with increasing tumor grade (Dukes & Bussey, 1958).

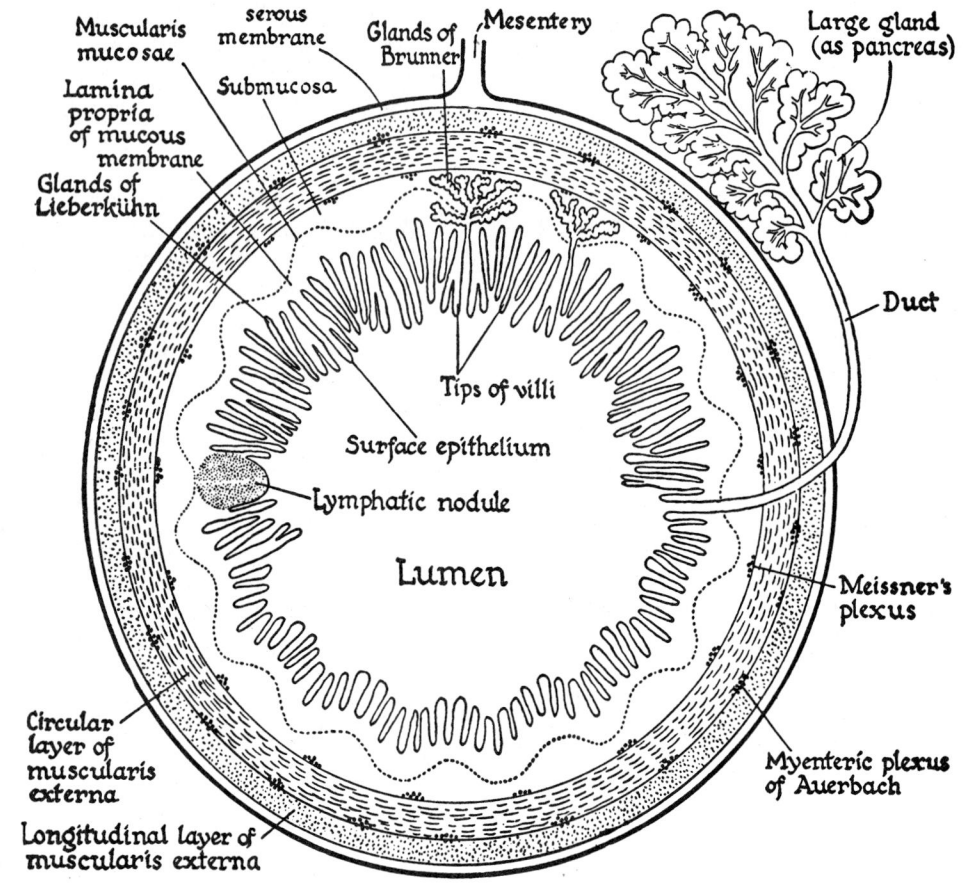

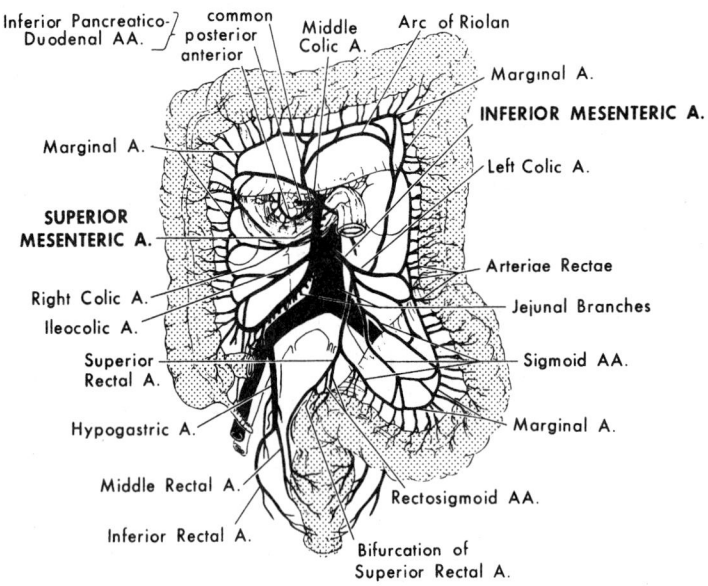

FIGURE 32–1. Schematic diagram of a cross section of the intestinal tract. (**A**, From Bloom, W. N., & Fawcett, D. W. [1968]. *A textbook of histology.* New York: Chapman & Hall. **B**, from Sleisenger, M. H., & Fordtran, J. S. [Eds]. [1989]. *Gastrointestinal disease: Pathophysiology, diagnosis, management* [p. 1903]. Philadelphia: W.B. Saunders Co.)

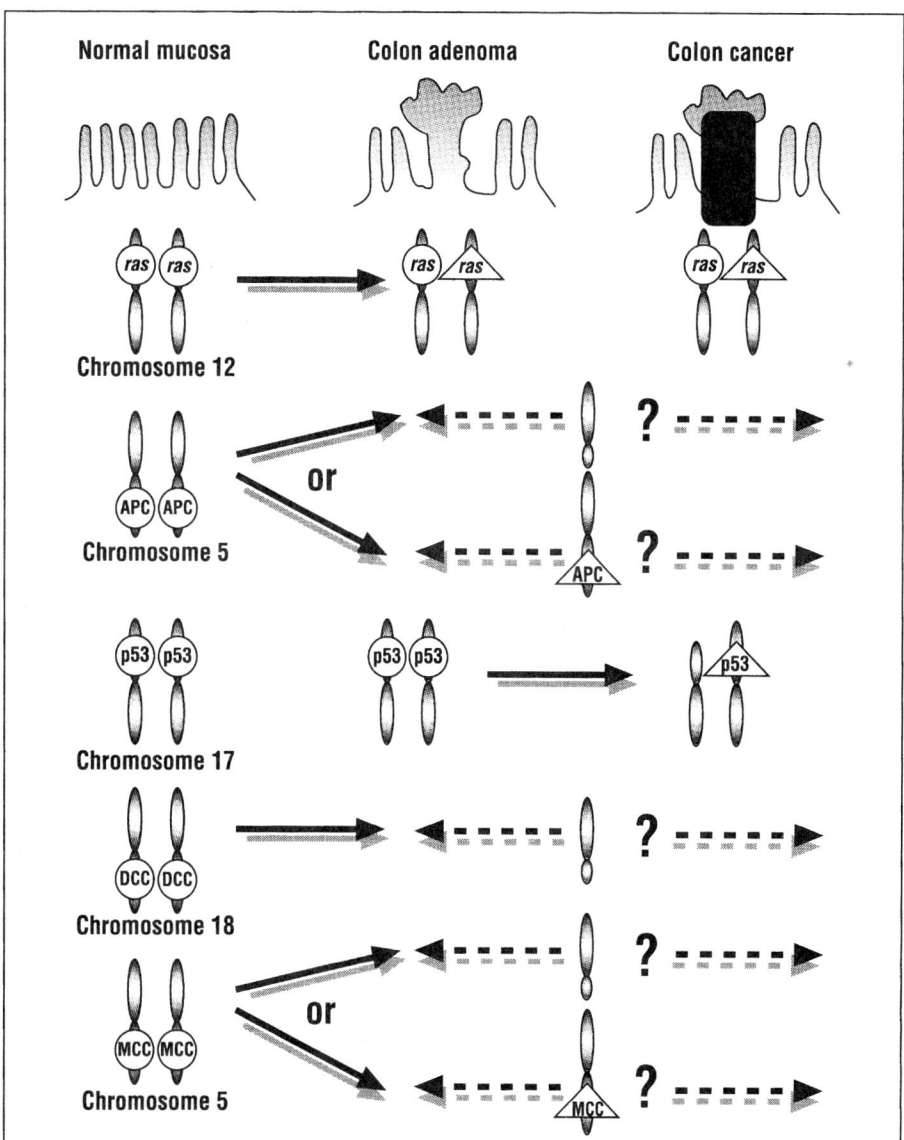

FIGURE 32–2. Genetic changes are shown for each of five target genes. The circles designate wild-type genes. The triangles represent mutant genes. Deleted genes are designated by the presence of an empty chromosome. Changes characteristic of a given stage lesion are shown under the lesion. The broken lines indicate when a given change may occur during several different stages. Solid lines represent the transition from normal to altered genes. When known, the fate of both copies of a gene is indicated. Question marks are used when the fate of one copy of a gene is not yet known. (From Markowitz, S. (1992). Molecular biology of colon cancer. *Cancer: Concept to Clinic, 1,* 5–10.)

Hematogenous spread occurs primarily to the liver followed by metastasis to the lung. Major venous drainage of the area happens via a dual system: blood from the superior hemorrhoidal veins enters the portal system to the liver, whereas blood from the middle and inferior hemorrhoidal veins reaches the vena cava to get to the lungs. Rare bony metastases to the sacrum and vertebral bodies may occur through the vertebral venous plexus (Batson, 1940).

Simultaneously, gradual cytologic changes occur allowing each malignancy to take on unique histologic characteristics, such as Signet-ring or mucinous. Colorectal tumor configuration may grossly appear as fungating, ulcerating, stenosing, or constricting. The major histologic type of large-bowel cancer is adenocarcinoma, which accounts for 90 to 95 per cent of all tumors (Spjut, 1984). Malignant intestinal tumors have been classified by the World Health Organization. These histologic classifications are presented in Table 32–2.

Following local invasion of the mucosa, a colorectal tumor may continue to grow in several directions. It usually protrudes into the lumen first and spreads in a transverse manner. This leads to circumferential growth and subsequent constriction of the bowel (Dukes, 1932). An additional pattern of local spread is perineural invasion, or spread along the perineural spaces (Seefield & Bargen, 1943).

TABLE 32–2. *Histologic Classification of Malignant Intestinal Tumors*

Adenocarcinoma	Adenosquamous carcinoma
Mucinous adenocarcinoma	Undifferentiated carcinoma
Signet ring carcinoma	Unclassified carcinoma
Squamous cell carcinoma	

(Data from World Health Organization. [1978]. *International histologic classification of tumors,* Nos. 1–20. Geneva: Author.)

SCREENING

Both the American Cancer Society and the National Cancer Institute have adopted guidelines for screening subjects for colorectal cancer. Because the incidence and mortality rates are greatest in the population 40 to 50 years or older, screening is directed primarily toward this population, as well as those at high risk. Studies have shown that early detection provides a substantial survival benefit; 90 per cent in Dukes' A compared with 5 per cent in Dukes' D. Table 32–3 describes some of the screening tools and the benefits/rationale of each. It must be noted that occult blood screening, although the most common mechanism used, is very controversial; however, it meets the criteria of safe, simple, available, and inexpensive.

As tissue becomes more abnormal, alterations in biochemical markers and other substances may be detected (Fitzsimmons & Fales, 1993). Abnormal levels of CEA (carcinoembryonic antigen) and other tumor markers in the peripheral blood have traditionally been used not only to indicate the presence of a malignancy but also as a potential indicator of prognosis. Although CEA is not routinely used as a screening test, over time CEA has proven to be a nonspecific marker for colorectal cancer and may be elevated to high normal levels in smokers. If the level is elevated prior to treatment and falls to normal levels postoperatively, then it is accepted as an indicator of tumor burden and may be monitored as an indicator of recurrence.

CEA is a glycoprotein found normally in secretions throughout the gastrointestinal and biliary tract, in cord blood, and in the large intestine in embryos. Normal CEA is <2.5 for nonsmokers and <5.0 ng/ml for smokers (Chernecky, Krech, & Berger, 1993) and has a short half-life. Elevated levels will return to normal about 4 to 6 weeks postoperatively if there is no other precipitating factor such as smoking, liver dysfunction, or biliary obstruction (Posner & Mayer, 1994).

AFP (α-fetoprotein) is a marker primarily elevated in liver abnormalities, primarily hepatoma. It may, however, be produced by hepatocarcinoma cells and thus indicate metastasis of colorectal cancer to the liver. Normal AFP is <8.5 ng/ml (Chernecky et al., 1993).

CA (cancer antigen) 19-9 was originally picked up by a monoclonal antibody. Its epitope is present in biliary tract tissue. Although this marker may be elevated with colorectal malignancies, it is more specific for cancers of the pancreas (Posner & Mayer, 1994). Normal CA 19-9 is <37 U/ml (Chernecky et al., 1993). It has been suggested that CA 19-9 should be followed in patients with advanced disease (Kouri, Nordling, Kuusela, & Pyrhönen, 1993).

Among the difficulties faced by the proponents of screening, compliance and false-positive or false-negative results are issues. When screening an asymptomatic population, a question that must be asked is whether a particular screening mechanism detects cancers early enough to be of benefit, and is it cost-effective (Shapiro, 1992). At this point, there is no mechanism that meets all of the criteria.

CLINICAL FEATURES AND DIAGNOSIS

In recent decades, the site distribution of colorectal cancer has changed significantly. At present, 38 per cent of the tumors occur proximally (ascending, transverse, and descending colon), whereas 62 per cent are located distally (sigmoid colon and rectum). Previously, the site distribution was 22 per cent proximal and 78 per cent distal (Beart, 1991). The reason for this apparent shift in tumor location remains unclear. A trend toward smaller tumors and less frequent lymph node involvement of distal lesions has also been noted (Corman, 1993a). This trend possibly reflects an improvement in early detection techniques.

The signs and symptoms of colorectal cancer depend on the location of the tumor. The right (ascending) side of the colon receives up to 1 L of content from the ileum daily. This material is largely water, and this is the portion of the colon in which absorption of fluids and electrolytes takes place. Lesions in this area are frequently

TABLE 32–3. *Screening for Colorectal Cancer*

SCREENING MECHANISM	BENEFITS/DRAWBACKS
Digital rectal examination	Inexpensive; easy to perform; little discomfort; although limited to only a few centimeters, it will allow detection of low rectal and anal lesions.
Fecal occult blood	Inexpensive; easy to perform; no discomfort; available to large population; poor screening tool for early cancers, especially adenomas which rarely bleed. False-negatives may be obtained if: patient is taking large amounts of vitamin C, the concentration of stool hemoglobin is low, or there is intermittent bleeding. All positive results should be followed up with additional diagnostic tests (Cohen, Minsky, & Schilsky, 1993).
Flexible sigmoidoscopy	Easily performed; moderate discomfort; visualization of rectal and sigmoid areas— up to 60 cm— (where approximately 50% of all colorectal cancers arise); if positive or suspicious findings, colonoscopy should be performed; provides biopsy access.
Colonoscopy	Fairly easily performed; moderate discomfort; visualization into transverse colon. Should be used only in high-risk population.
American Cancer Society guidelines for screening	Flexible sigmoidoscopy: Age 50 and over; every 3–5 years. Fecal occult blood: Age 50 and over; yearly. Digital rectal exam: Age 40 and over; yearly.

slow-growing, and because symptoms are nonspecific and insidious, the tumor is more advanced at the time of diagnosis. Tumors of the right colon tend to present with vague discomfort to dull abdominal pain, some nausea, weight loss, and some bleeding and anemia. The pain and discomfort are sometimes initially thought to be related to ulcers or even cholecystitis. As the disease advances, a palpable tumor may be felt. This is more easily palpated in the transverse colon.

Tumors of the left or descending colon, sigmoid, and rectum present more frequently with obstructive type symptoms, primarily because this portion of the colon is narrower and has less liquid in the stool. Common complaints include increased gas pain, rectal bleeding and bloody stools, change in stool caliber and frequency, tenesmus and the sensation of incomplete evacuation, constipation and increased use of laxatives, or even diarrhea. A classic indication of colorectal cancer is increased mucus in the stool; mucousy diarrhea may occur.

Rectal cancers are more frequently associated with rectal pain, bright red blood in the stool, and a sensation of rectal pressure. If the tumor extends into the anus, irritation and pruritis may also be present.

Classic signs of advanced disease include obstruction, perforation, ascites and the associated distention and feeling of abdominal fullness, as well as accelerated anorexia and weight loss.

A high index of suspicion is necessary for the diagnosis of colorectal cancer, and the cause for all associated symptoms should be explored. Typical diagnostic tests include those used as screening modalities, that is, occult blood, tumor markers, and digital rectal examination. However, additional testing may be indicated to adequately assess the presence and extent of the disease. Table 32–4 illustrates indications and rationale for typical diagnostic modalities.

STAGING AND PROGNOSTIC FACTORS

The process for staging colorectal cancer is generally complicated and has evolved over the last 50 years with disagreement still present among authors. Most authors agree that stage of cancer is the most important prognostic factor for survival or recurrence after potentially curative surgery. Stage of cancer is determined by the depth of penetration through the bowel wall and presence and number of positive lymph nodes.

Dukes' classification of colorectal cancer was the first practical system devised. It classified rectal tumors from A to C, with stage A indicating penetration into

TABLE 32–4. *Diagnostic Tests for Colorectal Cancer*

TEST	DESCRIPTION AND RATIONALE
Medical history	The importance of a complete and probing history, including all risk factors, family history, and seemingly unrelated and subtle symptoms cannot be minimized.
Double-contrast barium enema	The "traditional" BE is associated with a high percentage of false negatives. In a double-contrast study, high concentration (90%–100%) barium is instilled up to the splenic flexure. Then air is added to distend the colon. The patient is turned and repositioned in order to coat the entire area (Laufer, 1985). More diagnostic with air contrast; will detect a high percentage of lesions >5 mm diameter. Assesses patency and shape of bowel.
	Disadvantage: rectal cancers may be missed with this procedure (Cohen, Minsky, & Schilsky, 1993).
Flexible sigmoidoscopy	Although this procedure may not be used for routine screening in certain populations, it is considered an important adjunct to other screening modalities if not done recently. Visualization and removal/biopsy of polyps is easily accomplished. 60–65 cm of colon can be examined.
Fiberoptic colonoscopy	Allows visualization of the right side of the colon; however, splenic and hepatic flexures may be missed or seen with difficulty. For those with known colorectal cancer this procedure may be used to look for synchronous lesions.
Radioimmunoscintigraphy	Use of a monoclonal antibody (mAb) to bind with colorectal cancer cells or antigens. mAb's are radiolabeled with a substance, i.e., iodine-125, for easy detection. May be useful for radio-immunoguided surgery, delineating optimal margins, metastatic lesions, lymphatic invasion, etc.
Intrarectal or transrectal ultrasound	Used to assess the degree of tumor penetration and lymphatic involvement in the rectum, bladder or vagina.
Magnetic resonance imaging (MRI)	This procedure is more useful in assessing recurrence (75%–80% accuracy). The advantage of this procedure is the ability to assess differences in soft tissues and their relaxation times, which differs between normal and diseased tissues, and also between different diseases in the same tissue (Kressel & Thickman, 1985).
Computed tomography (CT) of the abdomen or pelvis	A radiographic scan useful to evaluate liver and periaortic nodes. It may be done with or without contrast. Colorectal metastases to the liver may remain hidden in a liver that is grossly normal at the time of surgery. Baseline CT is common and is more accurate than the MRI.
Tumor markers	Overall sensitivity with the primary lesion is about 40%. It may be lower with a Duke's A lesion.

but not through the bowel wall, stage B indicating penetration through the bowel wall, and stage C indicating involvement of lymph nodes, regardless of the extent of bowel wall penetration. This system was valuable because of its simplicity and prognostic accuracy. It has been modified to reflect finer levels of penetration and nodal metastases and has been extended to include the colon (Gabriel et al., 1935).

In 1954, Astler and Coller initiated a staging system that allowed separation of wall penetration and nodal status. Gunderson and Sosin (1974) modified the Astler-Coller staging system by subdividing T3 tumors into those with microscopic and gross penetration of tumor through the bowel wall. The Gastrointestinal Tumor Study Group (GITSG) (1985) included the number of positive nodes in its classification system. TNM systems adopted by the American Joint Committee on Cancer (AJCC) and the Union International Contra le Cancer (UICC) also took into consideration the number of positive nodes. These two systems further classify positive lymph nodes by stratifying them 1 to 3 vs. 4 or more.

Although the issue of which staging system to use remains unresolved, authors conclude that the number of positive lymph nodes remains the most important prognostic factor. Another important prognostic factor is the depth of serosal penetration by the tumor. The AJCC/UICC and GITSG staging systems utilize this information, whereas the Astler-Coller system incorporates microscopic and gross extension of tumor

through the bowel wall. In spite of this, Cohen, Minsky, and Schilsky (1993) recommend use of the AJCC/UICC TNM system for staging patients and reporting results. Table 32–5 and Figure 32–3 outline the most widely used systems for staging colorectal cancer: the Dukes', the modified Astler-Coller, and the TNM/UICC. Stage grouping and TNM classification of colon and rectal cancer can be reviewed in Table 32–6.

There are several prognostic indicators that can be assessed in colorectal cancer patients. These include age, presence of risk factors, clinical presentation, tumor markers, degree of differentiation, ploidy, stage of disease, and genetic mutations. Table 32-7 elucidates the prognostic indicators by presenting the clinical factor, description, and clinical significance. Several studies and clinical trials indicate a favorable prognosis for stage I and II colon cancer and stage I rectal cancer (NIH Consensus Conference, 1990). In contrast, the prognosis for patients with more advanced stages is poor. Colon and rectal cancer have distinct differences in natural history and patterns of recurrence; therefore separate consideration of adjuvant approaches for these cancers is appropriate.

TREATMENT

The treatment modality of choice for colorectal cancer is surgical resection. Extent of the resection depends on tumor location, vascular supply, and distribution of the lymph nodes in the region. Surgical

---

TABLE **32–5.** *1987 AJCC/UICC Staging Classification of Colorectal Cancer*

Primary Tumor (T)
TX   Primary tumor cannot be assessed
T0   No evidence of tumor in resected specimen (prior polypectomy or fulguration)
Tis   Carcinoma in situ
T1   Invades submucosa
T2   Invade muscularis propria
T3–T4 Depends on whether serosa is present
    Serosa present:
    T3   Invades through muscularis propria into
        Subserosa
        Serosa (but not through)
        Pericolic fat within the leaves of the mesentery
    T4   Invades through serosa into free peritoneal cavity
        or through serosa into a contiguous organ
    No serosa (distal two thirds rectum, posterior left or right colon):
    T3   Invades through muscularis propria
    T4   Invades other organs (vagina, prostate, ureter, kidney)

Regional Lymph Nodes (N)
NX   Nodes cannot be assessed (e.g., local excision only)
N0   No regional node metastases
N1   1–3 positive nodes
N2   4 or more positive nodes
N3   Central nodes positive

Distant Metastases (M)
MX Presence of distant metastases cannot be assessed
M0 No distant metastases
M1 Distant metastases present

Dukes Staging System Correlated With TNM
Dukes' A = T1N0M0
          T2N0M0
Dukes' B = T3N0M0
          T4N0M0
Dukes' C = T(any)N1M0, T(any)N2M0
Dukes' C2 = T(any)N3M0
Dukes' D = T(any)N(any)M1

Modified Astler-Coller (MAC) System Correlated With TNM
MAC A = T1N0M0
MAC B1 = T2N0M0
MAC B2 = T3N0M0, T4N0M0
MAC B3 = T4N0M0
MAC C1 = T2N1M0, T2N2M0
MAC C2 = T3N1M0, T3N2M0
            T4N1M0, T4N2M0
MAC C3 = T4N1M0, T4N2M0

Note: In all pathologic staging systems, particularly those applied to rectal cancer, the abbreviations (m) and (g) may be used: (m) denotes microscopic transmural penetration; (g) or (m + g) denotes transmural penetration visible on gross inspection and confirmed microscopically. (Modified from American Joint Committee on Cancer. [1988]. *Manual for staging of cancer* [3rd ed.]. Philadelphia: J.B. Lippincott; and from Union International Contre le Cancer. [1987]. *TNM classification of malignant tumors* [4th ed.]. Geneva: UICC.)

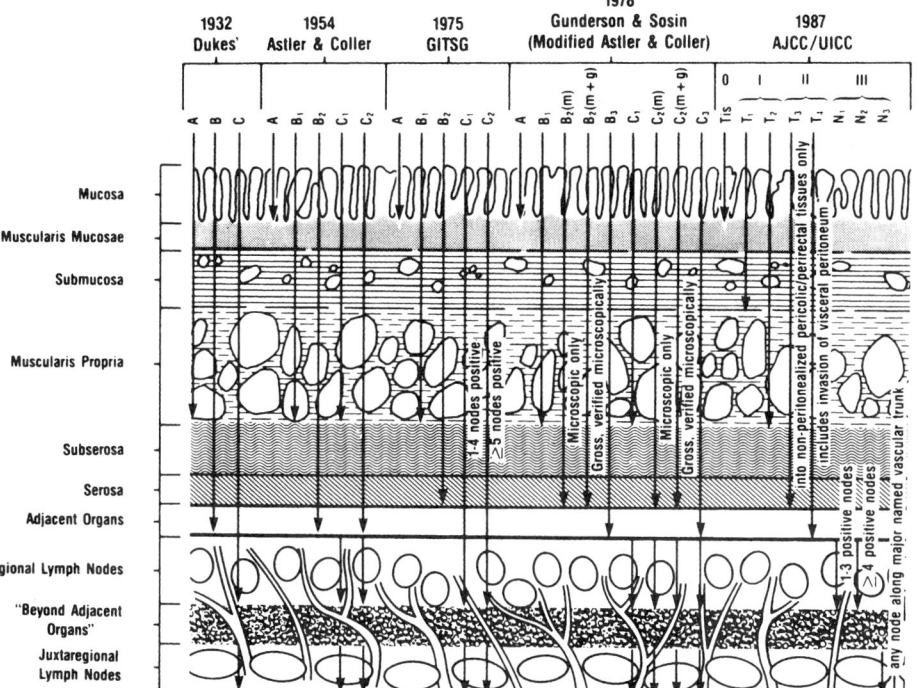

FIGURE 32–3. Comparison of various pathologic staging systems. (From Cohen, A. M., Minsky, B. D., & Schilsky, R. L. [1993]. Colon cancer. In V. T. Devita, S. Hellman, & S. A. Rosenberg (Eds.), *Cancer: Principles and practice of oncology* (4th ed., pp. 929–977). Philadelphia: J. B. Lippincott Co.)

treatment of colon cancer requires excision of normal tissue proximal and distal to the tumor, with adequate lateral margins if indicated. While most resections include a margin of 2 to 5 cm on either side of the tumor, wider resections may be required to achieve necessary ligation of the arterial blood supply (Fengler & Pearl, 1994; Smith, 1992). Almost all of these cancers can be treated without a permanent or even a temporary colostomy.

For patients with rectal cancer, the associated treatment is colostomy. This concern may lead to delay in seeking medical care. Actually, fewer than one third of

TABLE 32–6. *Stage Grouping of Colon and Rectal Cancers and TNM Classification*

STAGE	TUMOR	NODE	METASTASIS
Colon Cancer			
I	T1	N0	M0
IB	T2	N0	M0
II	T3, T4	N0	M0
III	Any T	N1	M0
IV	Any T	N4	M0
	Any T	Any N	M1
Rectal Cancer			
IA	T1	N0	M0
IB	T2	N0	M0
II	T3, T4	N0	M0
III	Any T	N1	M0
IV	Any T	N4	M0
	Any T	Any N	M1

(Data from Morton, J. M., Poulter, C. A., & Pandya, K. J. [1983]. Alimentary tract cancer. In P. Rubin, R. F. Bakeemeir, & S. K. Krackov [Eds.], *Clinical oncology—a multidisciplinary approach* [p. 170]. New York: American Cancer Society.)

patients with rectal cancer require permanent colostomy (Cohen, Minsky, & Friedman, 1993). There are sphincter-preserving procedures available that allow better quality of life without jeopardizing cure rates. Studies are being planned to investigate distal rectum irrigation as part of these procedures to minimize the risk of suture-line recurrence (Corman, 1993b). Results of the primary surgical approaches for both colon and rectal cancer can be improved with adjuvant radiation therapy and chemotherapy.

COLON CANCER

SURGERY

The 5-year survival rates after surgical resection for colon cancer appear to have improved in recent years (Cohen, Minsky, & Schilsky, 1993). Reports also indicate that patients with more than five positive lymph nodes have a poor prognosis regardless of how radical the surgery is. Appropriate application of surgical technique for colon cancer includes en bloc resection of the tumor and segments of major arterial and venous supply to the tumor. Resection of the mesentery associated with primary lymphatic drainage of the colon segment is also part of the en bloc technique. Prior to removal of the primary tumor, the lymphovascular pedicle may be ligated (no-touch technique) to prevent vascular spread of the cancer (Fengler & Pearl, 1994; Wiggers, Jeekel, & Arends, 1988). General guidelines for the appropriate operative resection of colon cancers involving the major locations are illustrated in Figures 32–4 and 32–5.

RADIATION THERAPY

Radiotherapy for the treatment of colon cancer has a limited adjuvant role. Colon cancer can be resected

TABLE 32-7. *Prognostic Indicators*

Clinical Factor	Description	Clinical Significance
Age	The average incidence is in the 40–50 year and over range.	Over 90% incidence in population over 50 years. A poorer prognosis is reported in patients under age 40 yrs, possibly due to more rapid progression of the disease (Hoerner, 1958; Cohen, Minsky, & Schilsky, 1993). Data show women have a better prognosis.
Presence of risk factors	Inflammatory syndromes; polyposis; genetic predisposition; history of colon cancer or other malignancy.	The natural history and progression in these patients with inflammatory disease is different and may develop in more than one site from the beginning (Winawer, 1991).
Clinical presentation	Bleeding, melena, pain, weight loss, obstruction, perforation. Duration and intensity of symptoms must be considered.	The extent of tumor penetration into or through the wall of the colon may point toward peritoneal seeding and implantation and poorer survival.
Tumor markers	CEA, AFP, CA 19-9.	Elevation of markers preoperatively may offer a way to track recurrence post-operatively. Future marker elevations, and related treatment, may not offer any long-term survival advantage, nor should they be based on tumor markers alone (Fritsche, 1993).
Degree of differentiation (grade)	This factor must be considered together with the stage, or depth/extent of invasion; neither factor stands alone as a prognostic indicator.	Well-differentiated tumors are related to a better prognosis than those that are poorly differentiated.
Ploidy	Ploidy refers to the amount of DNA in the cell, especially during cell division. Diploid cells have a pair of each chromosome; aneuploid cells show abnormal amounts of DNA.	Aneuploid cells are on a spectrum of less well differentiated to undifferentiated. Prognosis is poorer as cells become and appear more abnormal (Cavaliere et al., 1994). Ploidy will not stand alone as a prognostic indicator.
Extent of tumor invasion (stage)	Duke's and other staging classifications.	Size of tumor, per se, seems to have no detrimental impact on survival. Vascular invasion increases with higher stage and grade in rectal cancers and may be responsible for lower survival (Minsky, Mies, & Rich, 1988).
Lymph node involvement	The risk of nodal involvement increases as the tumor grade advances. The traditional approach is the higher the grade, the more lymph nodes will be involved. Size of nodes is not prognostic.	Increased node involvement is indicative of increased potential for systemic or distant metastases. There is agreement that the number of positive nodes is the most significant prognostic consideration.
Genetic mutations	Deletion of p53 suppressor gene, presence or absence of DCC.	One study shows a better survival in Dukes' B and C patients if p53 was not deleted (Kern et al., 1991).

without much concern for extent of the surgery and adequacy of margins. This disease tends to recur in the peritoneal cavity, the liver, or in distant sites, with only isolated local failure. The treatment technique for colon cancer may involve therapy to the whole pelvis and a boost to the tumor bed, the draining lymphatics, or both (Rostock, Zajac, & Gallagher, 1992). There are dose limits of radiotherapy to the pelvis related to tissue tolerance of surrounding organs and structures in the treatment field. For patients with residual tumor, 45 to 60 Gy (4500 to 6000 rads) is usually administered over a period of 5 to 6 weeks (Corman, 1993a). There is some evidence to suggest that this reduces the likeli-

hood of local recurrence and improves survival rates. However, it would be useful to reserve this therapy for a selected subgroup of patients who would not only benefit from postoperative radiation but would also benefit if chemotherapy was added (Hampton, 1993).

CHEMOTHERAPY

Systemic chemotherapy is the dominant adjuvant modality for colon cancer at this time. It is usually administered after primary surgical resection for those patients at high risk for tumor recurrence (stage II, III, and/or Dukes' B, C). Some clinical trial data demonstrate benefit for patients who receive their chemother-

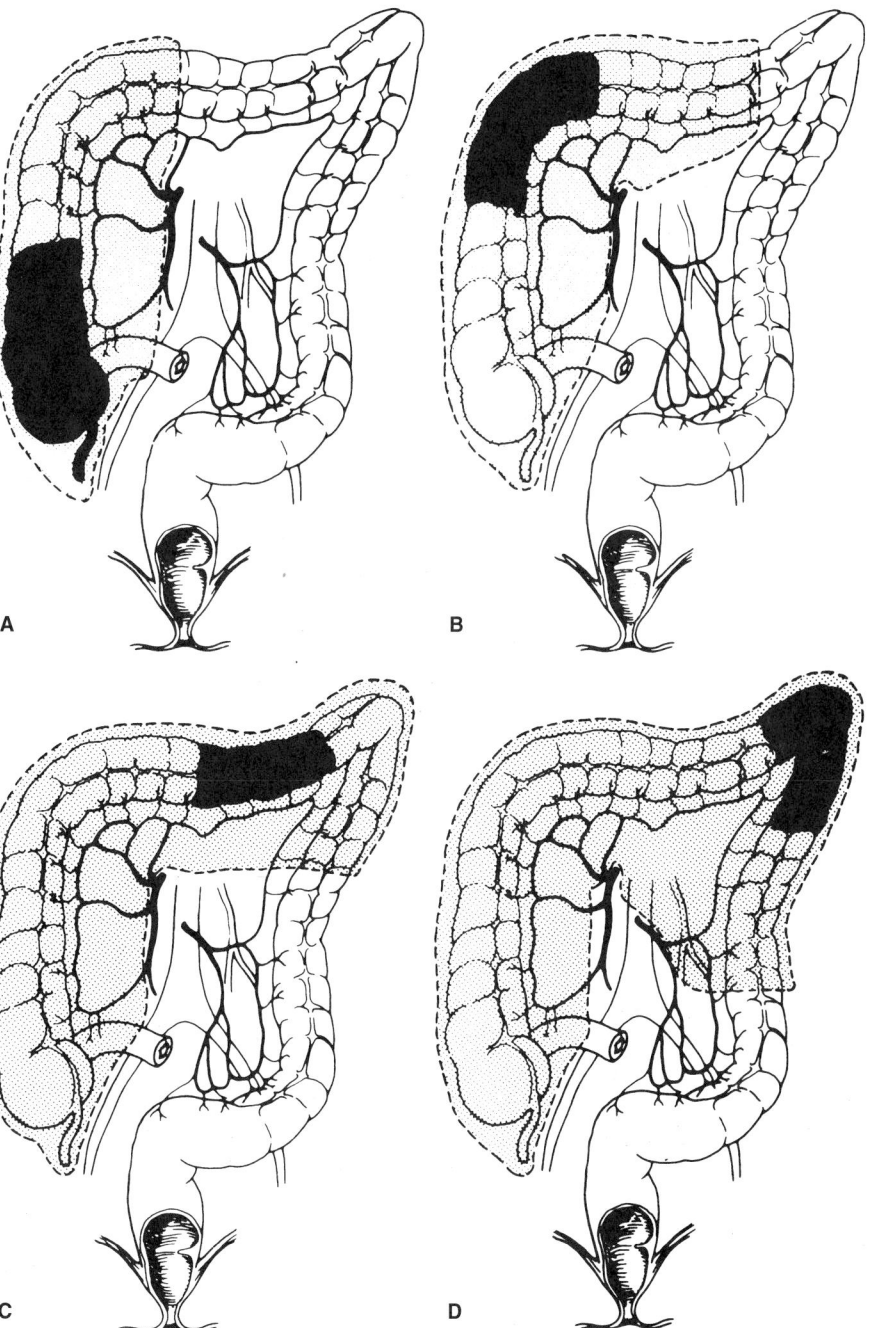

FIGURE 32–4. Surgical resection for ascending and transfer colon cancers. **A,** Surgical resection for a cecal or ascending colon cancer. **B,** Surgical resection for a cancer at the hepatic flexure. **C,** Preferable surgical resection for cancer for the transverse colon. A segmental resection may be appropriate in poor-risk patients. **D,** Preferred extensive resection for cancer at the splenic flexure. (Modified from Enker, W.E. [1978]. Surgical treatment of large bowel cancer. In W.E. Enker (Ed.). *Cancer of the colon and rectum.* [pp 73–106]. Chicago: Yearbook.)

apy within 6 weeks of surgery (NIH Consensus Conference, 1990). Unfortunately, the general perception is that chemotherapy for colon cancer remains ineffective because it appears resistant to most antineoplastic agents. Results from various studies have indicated limited response or improved survival for those with advanced lesions or metastatic disease (Kemeny, Lokich, Anderson, & Ahlgren, 1993). In the 1960's, fluorodeoxyuridine (FUDR) and fluorouracil (5-FU) were given as adjuvant agents for varying periods following surgery with a wide range of dosage schedules. These clinical trials demonstrated antitumor activity but not with convincing statistical significance.

5-FU as a chemotherapeutic drug continues to be the most researched single agent. It has been used to treat different stages of the disease with various dosage schedules. The traditional method and schedule of administration is a bolus injection over 5 to 10 minutes repeated daily for 5 days at 5-week intervals or a weekly regimen. Several clinical trials suggest a response rate of approximately 10 per cent to the single-agent bolus administration (Kemeny et al., 1993). A single-agent bolus injection of 5-FU results in limited tumor kill because of the drug's short plasma half-life and the slow growth of colon cancer cells. These findings have provided the scientific rationale for investi-

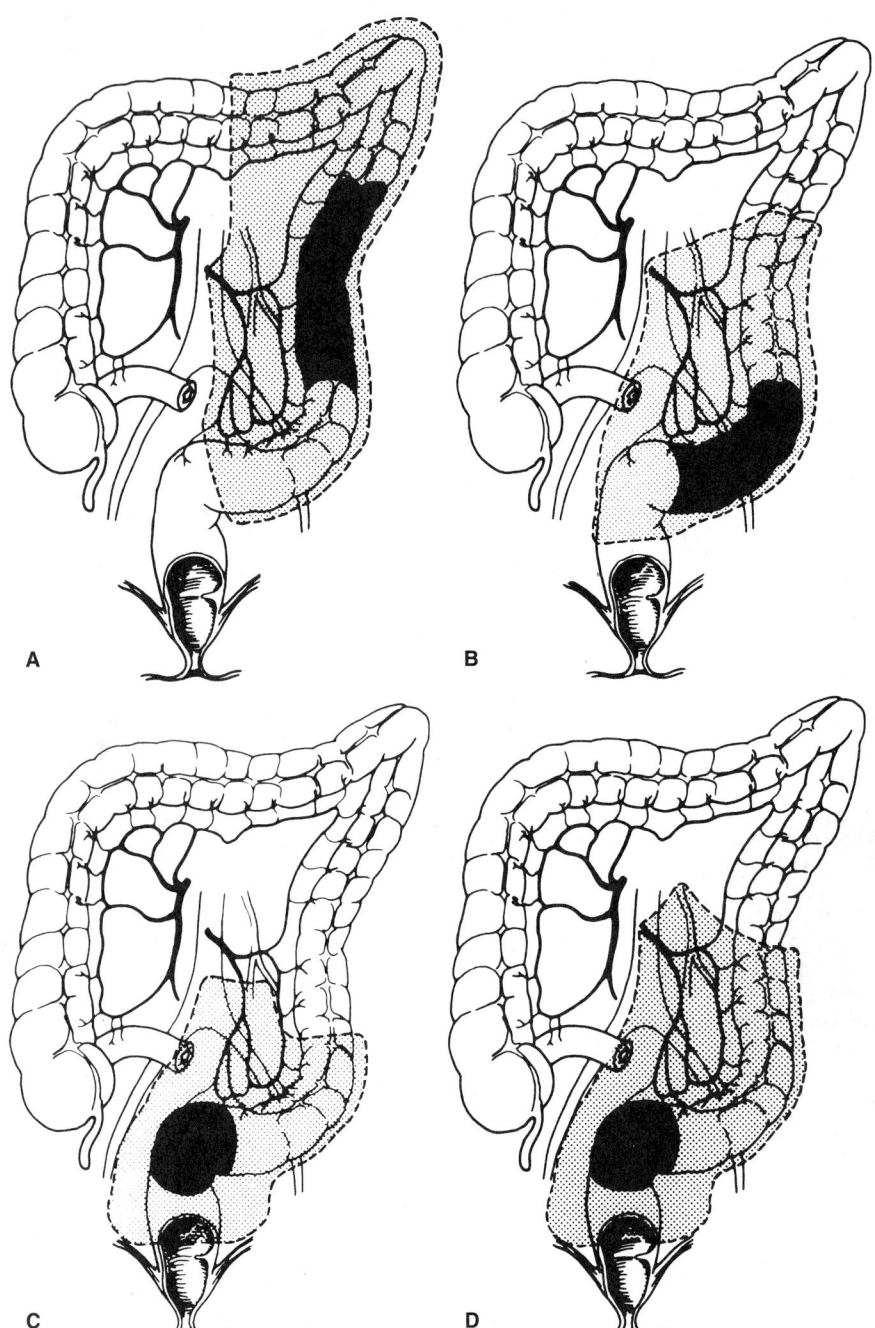

FIGURE 32–5. Surgical resection for distal colon cancer. **A,** Surgical resection for a descending colon cancer. **B,** Preferred surgical procedure for cancer of the middle and proximal sigmoid colon. In poor-risk patients the inferior mesenteric artery and the left colic artery may be preserved. **C,** Surgical resection for cancer of the rectosigmoid. **D,** A more radical surgical resection for cancer of the rectosigmoid. (Modified from Enker, W.E. [1978]. Surgical treatment of large bowel cancer. In W.E. Enker (Ed.). *Cancer of the colon and rectum.* [pp. 73–106]. Chicago: Yearbook.)

gating 5-FU administered by continuous infusion (Drewinko & Yang, 1985). Clinical trials using a continuous infusion schedule have shown response rates in the 30 to 35 per cent range. In studies of prolonged-infusion 5-FU vs. bolus dose, the survival difference was not statistically significant (Kemeny et al., 1993). Ongoing trials are needed to define the role of infusion therapy vs. bolus dose of 5-FU in colon cancer.

The utilization of combination chemotherapy has also been tried for the treatment of colon disease. Various studies have been done with 5-FU in combination with methotrexate, methyl-CCNU, vincristine, and levamisole. Although it was believed that combination chemotherapy should improve response rates, to this

date evidence has been lacking. To improve combination chemotherapy, the concept has been expanded to include biochemical modulation. This may be defined as the use of a pharmacologic agent to increase the biologic effect of a second drug by enhancing its antitumor activity. Major clinical success for biochemical modulation has been achieved with the use of 5-FU and leucovorin (Kemeny et al., 1993). Response rates have been reported to be from 20 to 45 per cent, but there have not been significant differences in the length of survival.

Other agents such as biologic response modifiers (BRMs) have also been evaluated for their effectiveness. Studies with α-interferon, interleukin-2, monoclonal antibodies, and BCG also document no improvement in long-term survival (Macdonald & Axelrod, 1992).

Recognition that the liver is the most common site of metastases is the basis for adjuvant hepatic intraarterial chemotherapy. Colon cancer cells that metastasize to the liver obtain most of their blood supply from the hepatic artery. Hepatic arterial administration of chemotherapy permits direct application of the agent resulting in high concentrations with little systemic exposure (Corman, 1993a). Both 5-FU and FUDR have been infused intraarterially with high response rates of 50 to 60 per cent, but again the survival benefits have not been revealed (Kemeny et al., 1993). The high response rates suggest that further study of this technique in combination with effective systemic therapy should be considered. Toxicity of this treatment can be significant and includes chemical hepatitis, catheter thrombosis, and hemorrhage, which presents a challenge to the physician and nurse.

Following intraarterial infusion of chemotherapy, chemoembolization procedures have been attempted. This procedure involves the injection of chemotherapeutic agents (adriamycin, mitomycin, and cisplatin) to the tumor site through the hepatic catheter. Injection of these agents creates a blockage or embolic event that inhibits blood flow to the tumor (Lyster, Benson, Vogelzang, & Talamonti, 1993). The chemotherapy then destroys hepatic cells as it leaks out, infiltrating tumor cells and normal hepatic cells. Most patients experience side effects that include nausea, vomiting, fever, transient encephalopathy, pain, ascites, edema, and potential infection (Lynes, 1993). Results from studies utilizing this procedure still need to be evaluated.

RECTAL CANCER

SURGERY

Three fourths of patients with node-negative rectal cancer are cured by radical surgery (Cohen, Minsky, & Friedman, 1993). Few patients whose rectal cancers have spread to regional lymph nodes are cured by surgery. When discussing surgical resection for rectal cancer, the rectum is considered in three distinct sections. These sections are in relation to the anal verge: upper third, middle third, and lower third. The rectum is approximately 15 cm in length; therefore each section roughly correlates with 5-cm intervals. Figure 32–6 illustrates division of the rectum into the three distinct areas. Selection of surgical procedure for rectal tumors is based on the location of the tumor and consideration for sphincter preservation and continuity of the bowel.

Tumors located in the upper third of the rectum are treated essentially the same as proximal colon cancers. These tumors are removed with an anterior or low anterior resection. For tumors in the middle third of the rectum, abdominoperineal resection with permanent colostomy was the operation of choice. Recently, it has been shown that this procedure does not yield superior results to those achieved with sphincter-saving surgery (Enker, Paty, Minsky, & Cohen, 1992; Williams, 1984). Restoration of intestinal continuity by low anterior resection should be possible in patients with cancers 6 to 11 cm from the anal verge.

Most cancers in the lower 5 cm of the rectum require abdominoperineal resection with permanent colostomy. However, there is a trend to attempt sphincter-saving approaches for certain patients with lower third rectal cancer (Enker et al., 1992; Fengler & Pearl, 1994). These approaches include abdominosacral resection of tumor and resection with a coloanal anastomosis (Corman, 1993b). Other approaches involve local treatment such as transanal excision, fulguration, and endocavity radiation (Cohen, Minsky, & Friedman, 1993). Appropriate selection criteria for sphincter-saving approaches, whether they are surgery, cauterization, or radiation, must be determined and followed.

In addition to location, there are several other factors that determine the choice of operation for rectal cancer. The surgical margins, tumor's degree of differentiation, tumor DNA content, presence of metastatic disease, and the patient's age, gender, and physical condition are considered when selecting a surgical

FIGURE 32–6. Division of the rectum into upper, middle, and lower thirds. (From Cohen, A. M., Minsky, B. D., & Friedman, M. A. [1993]. Rectal cancer. In V. T. Devita, S. Hellman, & S. A. Rosenberg (Eds), *Cancer: Principles and practice of oncology* (pp. 978–1004). Philadelphia: J. B. Lippincott Co.)

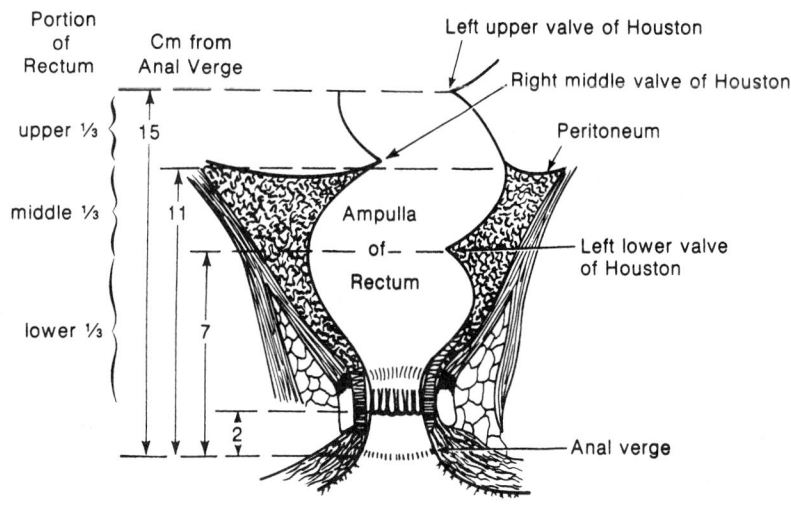

approach (Corman, 1993b). Other conditions that might contraindicate colostomy (e. g., blindness, severe arthritis, mental incapacity) are also contemplated prior to a decision being made about surgical intervention. However, no matter what decision is reached regarding sphincter preservation, the surgeon's goal should ultimately be cure for the patient. While quality of life remains a major concern, there will be some patients who require an abdominoperineal resection and permanent colostomy.

Abdominoperineal Resection (APR). The abdominoperineal resection has been the standard surgical procedure for tumors approximately 8 cm from the anal verge. This procedure involves a synchronous transabdominal and perineal approach to resecting the tumor and creating an external ostomy. Extent of the APR procedure can be seen illustrated in Figure 32–7. Malignant tumor and rectum are excised while the remaining sigmoid colon is brought out through the abdomen and a colostomy is created in the left iliac fossa. It is a procedure associated with high morbidity rates (55 to 61 per cent) and requires psychologic and social adjustment to a permanent colostomy (Corman, 1993b).

There are various complications from the procedure. They include injury to the ureters and trauma to the bladder during surgery that results in urinary dysfunction. The abdominal and perineal wounds may become infected. Intestinal obstruction and stomal complications have been noted as well. Sexual dysfunction, especially in males, occurs because of the extensive pelvic resection and subsequent nerve damage. Traditionally, the perineal wound was left open to heal by granulation. Now in most patients the pelvic fat and skin can be closed primarily, with greatly improved recovery (Cohen, Minsky, & Friedman, 1993).

Low Anterior Resection (LAR). A low anterior resection (LAR) will be the surgical approach selected for tumors lying in the distal sigmoid and upper rectum (6 to 11 cm from the anal verge). This approach allows resection of tumor abdominally and the creation of a very low anastomosis in the pelvis (Griffin, Knight, & Whitaker, 1990). Most surgeons choose to restore bowel integrity with an end-to-end anastomosis constructed with staples. The development of CEEA (circular end-to-end anatosmosis) staplers has allowed the surgeon to create these low anastomoses and thus avoid permanent colostomy while maintaining margins free of tumor. Figure 32–8 illustrates how the stapling instrument is inserted through the anus, the ends of the bowel are approximated, and the instrument fires staples, making the anastomosis complete.

Sphincter-saving treatment of rectal cancer is not without complications. The LAR may result in impaired bowel function, because the normal rectal reservoir is replaced with a less capacious proximal colon. Frequent bowel action, incontinence of fecal material, and poor control of gas are experienced by the majority of patients. These bowel management difficulties usually resolve 6 to 12 months following surgery, and in the meantime patients can regulate themselves by some diet controls (Nakahara, Itoh, &

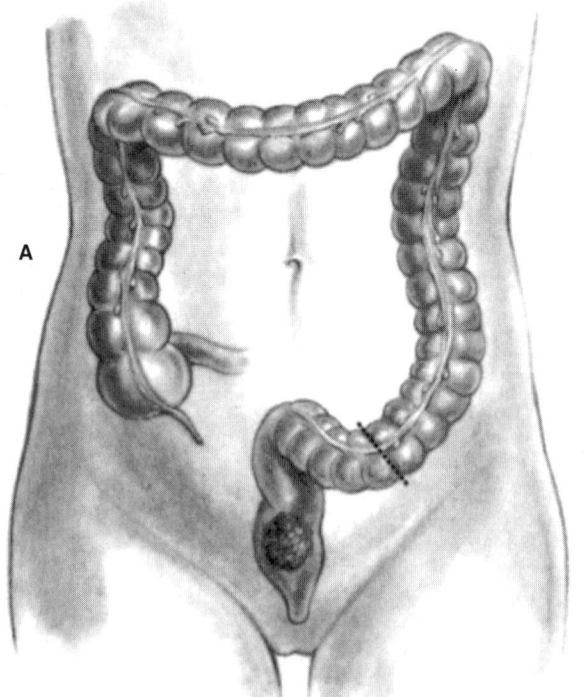 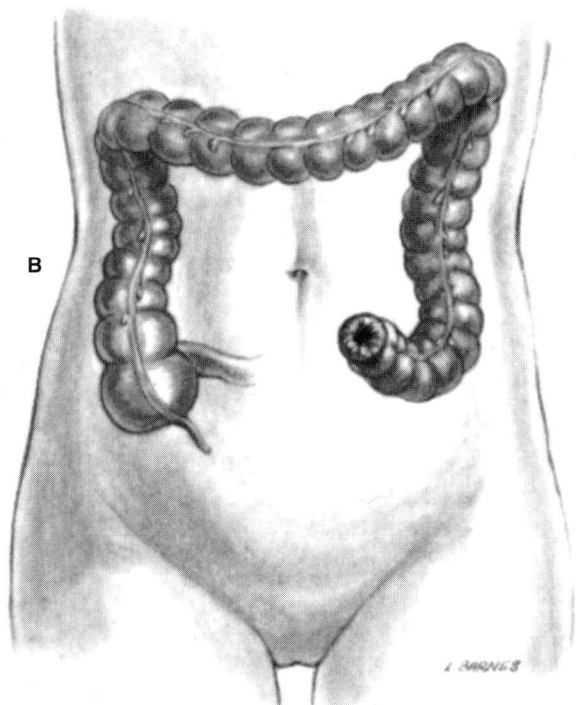

FIGURE 32–7. Carcinoma of the rectum. **A,** Extent of removal in classical abdominoperineal resection. **B,** The sigmoid colostomy is created in the left iliac fossa. (From Corman, M. L. (1993). Carcinoma of the rectum. In *Colon and rectal surgery* (pp. 596–720). Philadelphia: J. B. Lippincott Co. Illustrated by Lois Barnes.)

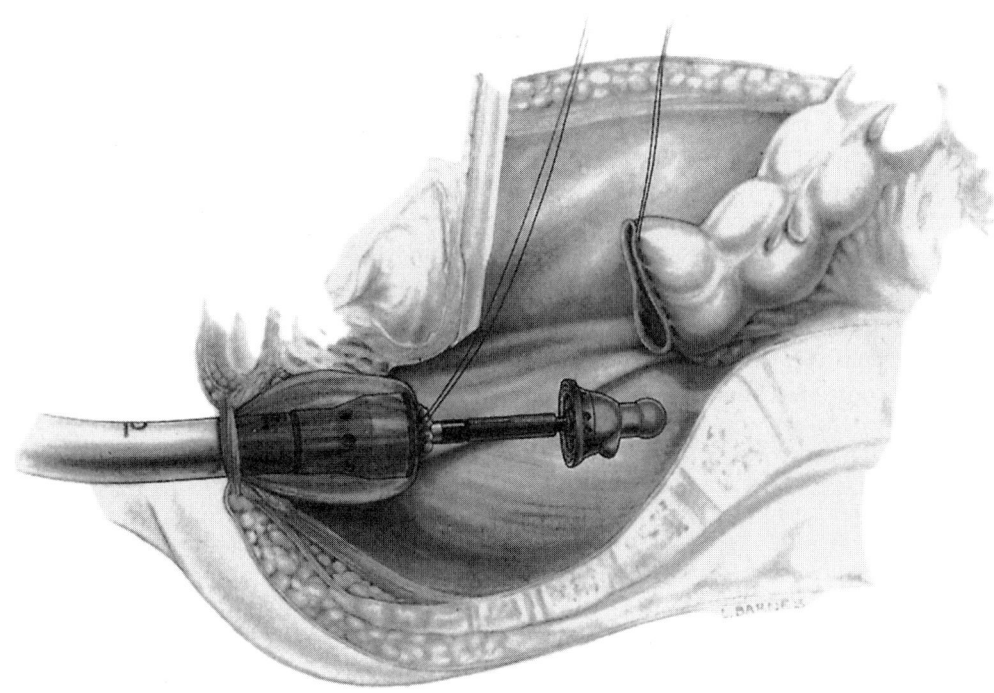

A

FIGURE 32–8. **A,** Circular stapled anastomosis instrument is inserted through the anus and the distal purse-string secured. **B,** Circular stapled anastomosis. Proximal and distal purse-string sutures are secured. **C,** Circular stapled anastomosis. The instrument is fired after the ends of the bowel have been approximated. (From Corman, M. L. [1993]. Carcinoma of the rectum. In *Colon and rectal surgery.* [pp. 596–720]. Philadelphia: J.B. Lippincott Co. Illustrated by Lois Barnes.)

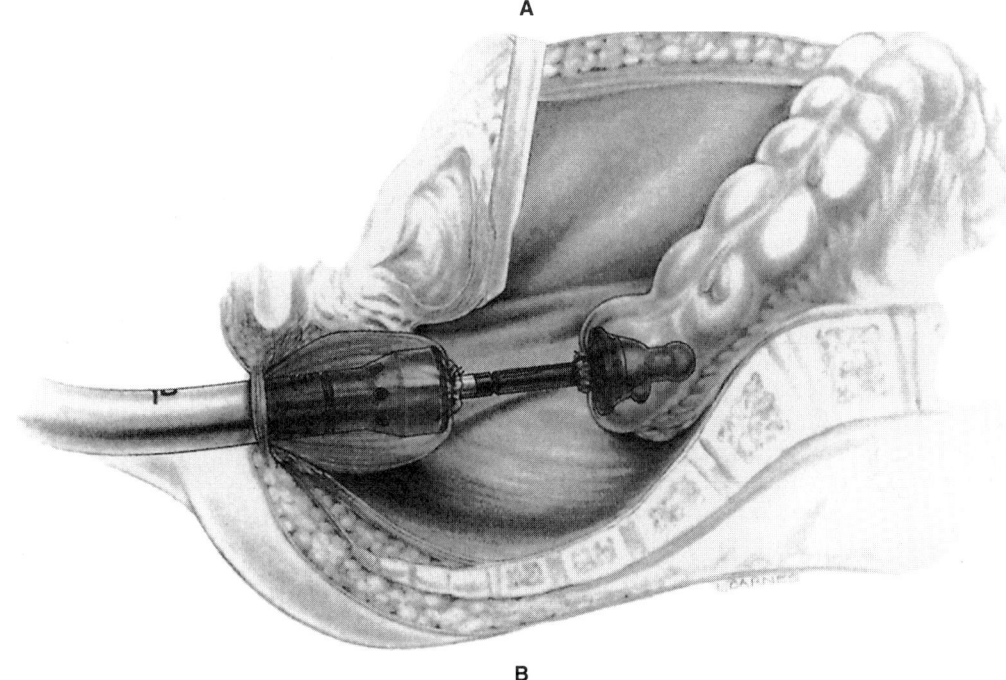

B

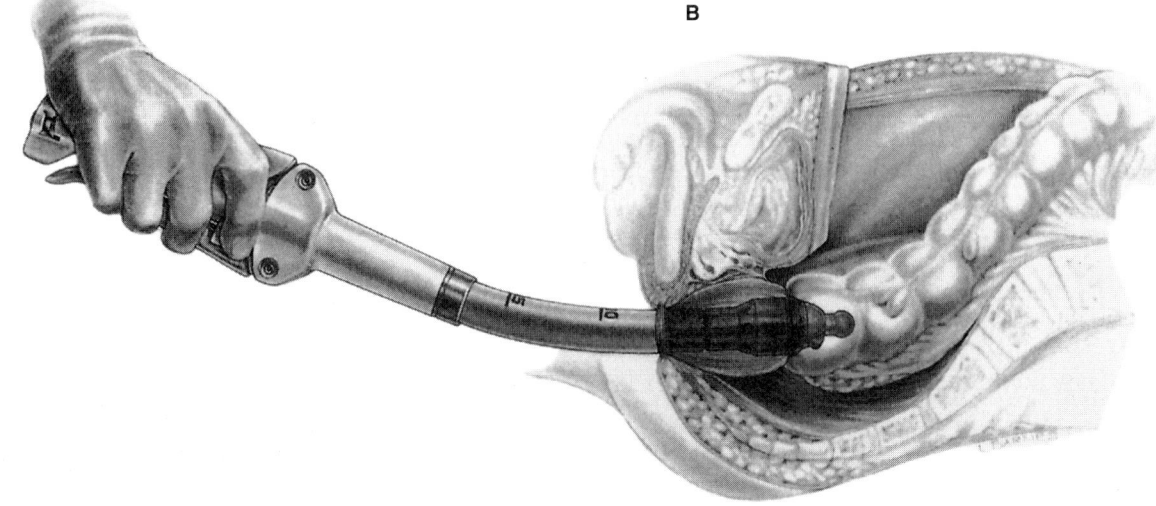

C

Mibu, 1988). Other postoperative complications associated with the LAR include problems with the anastomosis. There may be anastomotic bleeding, obstruction of the anastomosis, or anastomotic leakage with subsequent fecal fistula. Later complications that occur are the rare incidence of a pelvic abscess and the possibility of stricture of the anastomosis.

RADIATION THERAPY

Endocavity irradiation is used as an alternative to surgery for potentially curable lesions. A special device with high-intensity radiation is inserted through a large-diameter proctoscope and placed directly against the lesion. The effective area is approximately 3 cm in diameter, with absorption of the x-rays essentially limited to a depth of 2 cm (Papillon, 1984). Treatment schedules are three to five insertions every 6 to 7 weeks for a total dose of 2000 to 3000 cGy. This form of irradiation can be administered on an outpatient basis with minimal complications, such as mild proctitis and occasional bleeding. Noninfiltrating lesions that are accessible, smaller than 5 cm in size, and less than 12 cm from the anal verge are most appropriate for this therapy (Papillon, 1982).

The use of external beam radiation therapy in the treatment of rectal cancers has received considerable attention in recent years. To improve mortality rates, adjuvant use of radiation therapy preoperatively and postoperatively has been investigated. Preoperative treatment should decrease the volume of primary tumor, reduce the viability of tumor cells, and lower the number of positive lymph nodes. These effects of treatment may allow the surgeon to perform a sphincter-conserving procedure that would not otherwise be possible and lessen the chance of local recurrence without compromising cure rate (Stockholm Rectal Cancer Study Group, 1990). It is recommended that approximately 45 Gy should be delivered over 5 or 6 weeks followed by resection (with or without anastomosis) 6 to 8 weeks later (Corman, 1993b). Initial studies suggested that preoperative treatment resulted in better survival rates and decreased incidence of local recurrence. These conclusions have not been well supported, but there is little question that the technique is of benefit for the management of "unresectable tumors" (Mendenhall, Bland, & Pfaff, 1987).

Postoperative radiation therapy offers a distinct advantage in that the extent of the patient's disease has been determined. Individuals whose tumor has penetrated the bowel wall and who have positive lymph nodes are most likely to have local recurrence following resection. These patients are the best candidates for postoperative radiation therapy, and treatment should start no sooner than 1 month following surgery (to avoid problems with wound healing) or later than 2 months (to limit the likelihood of spread). The dosage to the tumor bed should be approximately 60 Gy (Corman, 1993b). Local recurrence is decreased by the radiation therapy, but distant metastasis remains a problem. Studies are currently being reviewed to determine whether survival rates are altered (Rostock et al., 1992). Investigators are also evaluating the use of radiation therapy following local resection of rectal cancer as a curative procedure (Summers, Mendenhall, & Copeland, 1992). In either case, the significant complications of radiotherapy should be considered before embarking on a treatment plan. Urinary tract infections, diarrhea, small-bowel injury, and skin and wound breakdown are complications that may occur. They should be contemplated along with other factors such as the age of the patient and the quality of life expected.

Intraoperative radiotherapy (IORT) is a technique by which a resectable lesion is removed and the remaining cancer cells are sterilized at the time of the operation. This technique is an alternative for a select number of individuals with localized tumor, tumor accessible to treatment field and in an area where normal tissue can be displaced, and a potentially curable tumor that cannot be controlled by surgery alone (Gunderson, Shipley, & Suit, 1982). In some cases a "booster dose" of external beam radiation therapy is combined with the intraoperative dose to provide for more local control (Rostock et al., 1992).

Palliative radiation therapy can be effective in treating the symptoms of metastatic rectal cancer. The symptoms of pain and bleeding from advanced rectal tumors are controlled. Symptoms of metastasis to the liver, bone, and brain are also managed.

CHEMOTHERAPY

In resected rectal cancer there is significant risk of symptomatic local-regional failure as the first sign of recurrence. The reason for this appears to be related to anatomic constraints in obtaining wide margins. Thus, aggressive adjuvant chemotherapy with 5-FU and methyl-CCNU should be considered for the higher stage patients with rectal cancer (Krook et al., 1991). However, the long-term effects of increased risk for secondary leukemia and renal toxicity associated with methyl-CCNU should be evaluated before therapy is initiated. More clinical trials will be planned for studying this recommended regimen.

NURSING CARE OF THE COLORECTAL CANCER PATIENT

The nursing care of patients who have been treated for a colorectal malignancy has shifted focus over the last several years. Decreased mortality and morbidity following surgical resection has occurred because of improvements in preoperative preparation of the patient and enhanced surgical and anesthesia techniques. For more detailed discussion of surgery-related information, see Chapter 19, Surgical Oncology. Transfusion of blood, blood products, and antibiotics for the management of sepsis has also contributed to the overall recovery of patients.

As mentioned earlier, the CEEA staplers have permitted surgeons to perform bowel resections with anastomosis for most colorectal tumors. This has resulted in the decreased need for creation of temporary and permanent colostomies. Table 32–8 presents a detailed

TABLE 32–8. *Colon Resection (Hemicolectomy)**

NURSING DIAGNOSES/ DEFINING CHARACTERISTICS	NURSING INTERVENTIONS/RATIONALES	EXPECTED OUTCOMES
Preoperative or Intraoperative Anxiety *Related to:* Impending surgery Impending pathology results Possibility of ostomy Preoperative preparation **Defining Characterestics** Nervous appearance Trembling Hand wringing Multiple questions/lack of questions Increased BP, pulse, and respiratory rate	**Ongoing Assessment** • Assess knowledge and understanding of impending surgery. • Assess degree of anxiety. **Therapeutic Interventions** • Arrange for visit from operating room personnel. *Preoperative visit promotes confidence in operating room staff.* • Provide information about intraoperative care. *Knowledge of what to expect may relieve some anxiety.* • Document and communicate patient's concerns to others involved in care (i. e., recovery room personnel). • Inform patient that significant other will be allowed to wait with patient in preanesthesia care unit. • Maintain a quiet operating room environment. *Noise, traffic, hurried movements increase anxiety level.* • Remain with patient before and during induction of anesthesia. *Having someone close by at critical moment is very reassuring.*	Anxiety will be managed.
Intraoperative Potential for Injury *Related to:* Urinary catheterization Lithotomy position during 5- to 6-hr procedure (pelvis higher than head) **Defining Characteristics** Cloudy, foul-smelling urine Positive urine cultures Frequency, urgency, burning after catheter removal Pain in extremities Numbness, tingling of extremities Swelling of legs	**Ongoing Assessment** • Monitor catheterization procedure to ensure asepsis. • Assess patient's body alignment throughout procedure to: *Provide optimum access and exposure to operative site. Sustain circulatory and respiratory function. Guard against joint damage, muscle stretch, and strain.* **Therapeutic Interventions** • Position and tape urinary catheter securely *to prevent disconnection, traction, or kinking.* • Adjust and pad stirrups *to ensure symmetrical position and minimize pressure and venous pooling.* • Adjust arm boards properly *to prevent hyperextension, abduction, and damage to brachial plexus;* cover arms, hands, and fingers with drawsheet *for additional protection.* • Wrap each of lower extremities with ace bandage *(lessens pooling and may prevent thrombosis formation).* • Raise and lower patient's legs simultaneously and slowly, supporting foot and knee. *Any change in body position affects hemodynamics; slow movements allow gradual circulation adjustment.* • Apply straps snugly across foot and lower leg *to keep leg in place.* • Remind surgical team not to lean on arms or legs during procedure.	Risk of injury during operation is reduced.
Potential Ineffective Thermoregulation *Related to:* Use of anesthetic agents	**Ongoing Assessment** • Monitor temperature throughout procedure. • Monitor vital signs. • Send specimen for ABGs and electrolyte analysis.	Appropriate body temperature will be maintained.

*Removal of the lower sigmoid or rectosigmoid portion of the rectum through a low midline incision in the abdomen. Continuity is established by an end-to-end anastomosis of the proximal colon and the rectum by sutures or a circular stapling device. This procedure is used to treat adenocarcinoma and polyposis of colon and/or rectum.

(From Gulanick, M., et al. [1990]. *Nursing care plans: Nursing diagnosis and intervention* [pp. 304–307]. St. Louis: Mosby. Originated by Jacqueline Monao, RN and Sharon Canariato, RN, BSN.)

Continued on following page.

nursing care plan for patients undergoing colon resection. Routine prophylactic use of nasogastric tubes following colon segment anastomosis is now being discouraged (Corman, 1993a). Primary closure of the perineal surgical wound has eliminated some of the "chronic drainage" problems associated with the APR (Cohen, Minsky, & Friedman, 1993). Both of these

technique changes have added to the quality of life for colorectal cancer patients.

If the colorectal cancer patient needs a colostomy because of tumor biology or anastomotic difficulties, there are nursing issues to consider. These patients should have expert preoperative and postoperative teaching. The colostomy site should be selected and

TABLE 32–8. *Colon Resection (Hemicolectomy)* * Continued

NURSING DIAGNOSES/ DEFINING CHARACTERISTICS	NURSING INTERVENTIONS/RATIONALES	EXPECTED OUTCOMES
Cool OR environment Exposure during preparation Prolonged visceral exposure Family history of hyperthermia during induction **Defining Characteristics** *Hypothermia:* Decreased baseline temperature Decreased BP Arrhythmia Abnormal ABGs and electrolytes Postoperative shivering Skin pale and cold *Hyperthermia:* Increased baseline temperature Tachycardia Acidosis Electrolyte imbalance Hyperventilation Arrhythmia Muscular vesiculation	**Therapeutic Interventions** *To prevent hypothermia:* • Place a blanket-size aquamatic K pad on operating room bed; set to appropriate temperature before patient's arrival. *Device raises, lowers, or maintains body temperature through heat conduction or cold transfer between blanket and patient.* • Maintain adequate room temperature until draping completed. • Cover patient with warm blankets until ready for skin preparation and immediately after sterile drape removal *(allows minimal exposure and loss of body heat).* • Use warm irrigation and warm moist sponges to cover exposed abdominal organs *(warms circulating blood in abdominal cavity).* • Consult anesthesiologist about use of humidified air delivered via ventilator and warm IV solution via warmers. *To treat hyperthermia:* • Set aquamatic machine to desired temperature. • Assist anesthesiologist to discontinue anesthesia and administer emergency drugs. *This is a life-threatening complication of anesthesia that can be triggered by commonly used anesthetic agents (succinylcholine and halothane).* • Remove IV from warmer: hang cold IV fluids. • Place ice packs around patient. • Prepare for iced gastric lavage. • Assist surgical team to complete procedure as quickly as possible.	
Potential Fluid Volume Deficit *Related to:* Blood loss in surgery Blood loss after surgery **Defining Characteristics** *Intraoperative:* Decreased blood pressure Increased heart rate Decreased central venous pressure Decreasing Hct *Postoperative:* As above, plus Saturated dressings Large amount of blood from NG or other tubes Decreased urine output Restlessness Confusion	**Ongoing Assessment** *Intraoperative:* • Assess vital signs throughout procedure. *Early detection of symptoms will enable surgical team to institute treatment, prevent shock.* • Monitor and record I & O during procedure *to replace blood loss accurately.* • Observe for signs/symptoms of transfusion reaction if blood administered. *Postoperative:* • Assess vital signs per institution's postoperative protocol. • Monitor abdominal dressing for excess drainage. • Monitor Hb and Hct. • Monitor changes in LOC, differentiating changes related to hypovolemia/anesthesia. **Therapeutic Interventions** • Check availability of blood; have half sent to the operating room. Blood must be *accessible for immediate transfusion.* • Inform anesthesiologist of blood loss through sponges, suction, and drapes *to ensure appropriate fluid replacement.* • Administer IV fluids and/or blood/blood components as ordered. *Most patients can tolerate 500 ml to 1 L blood loss without difficulty. Blood replacement is necessary if blood loss exceeds this amount. Albumin, dextran, hydroxyethyl starch, and electrolyte solution can be used instead of blood.* • Report laboratory results to physician *so correct replacement of blood, fluid and electrolyte can be maintained.* • Administer O_2 if blood loss after procedure.	Normal fluid volume will be maintained.

TABLE 32–8. *Colon Resection (Hemicolectomy)** Continued

NURSING DIAGNOSES/ DEFINING CHARACTERISTICS	NURSING INTERVENTIONS/RATIONALES	EXPECTED OUTCOMES
Potential Infection *Related to:* Length of procedure, tissue exposure Leakage of bowel contents intraoperatively Insertion of circular staple gun through rectum to abdominal cavity Incomplete line of staples Postoperative wound contamination Incomplete suturing caused by staple gun malfunction or misfiring **Defining Characteristics** Incisional redness Swelling, pain Foul-smelling wound drainage Fever Positive wound culture Elevated white blood count History of difficult anastomosis	**Ongoing Assessment** *Intraoperative:* • Assess aseptic technique throughout procedure. *Aseptic techniques exclude microorganisms in environment, prevent them from reaching operative wound, prevent infection, facilitate wound healing.* *Postoperative:* • Assess wound for redness, drainage, pain, swelling, or dehiscence. • Culture suspicious drainage. • Monitor temperature. • Monitor WBC. **Therapeutic Interventions** *Intraoperative:* • Clean and disinfect skin area of and around proposed incision site. • Shave operative site only as necessary and immediately before surgery. *Abraded, injured skin is very conducive to cutaneous bacteria proliferation, increasing chance of infection.* • Correct breaks in technique when observed. *Sterile members of surgical team not always aware of violations of asepsis while concentrating on the operative field.* • Irrigate and suction around rectum *to remove retained fluid from enema to keep rectosigmoid free of fluid and fecal material and prevent leakage into abdominal cavity.* • Keep instruments contacting GI mucosa separate from other instrument; remove entirely from field after anastomosis. • *Ensure availability and function of stapling devices by:* Having all sizes available at outset of procedure. Reviewing function of instrument with team. Assisting with use at appropriate time. • Have GI suture material ready *in case stapling is unsatisfactory.* • Irrigating abdominal wound with water to check for bubbles *(indicate anastomotic leak).* *Postoperative:* • Use aseptic technique for dressing changes. • Administer antibiotics and antipyretics as ordered. • If stoma present, isolate fecal drainage by maintaining good skin seal.	Risk of infection will be reduced.
Postoperative Pain *Related to:* Surgical incision Endotracheal intubation for anesthesia administration Tubes/drains present **Defining Characteristics** Report of incisional pain Verbalization of sore throat Grimacing Reluctance to move, cough, or take deep breaths Protection of tubes/drains	**Ongoing Assessment** • Assess pain: Location Intensity Duration Precipitating factors Quality • Assess degree to which pain interferes with ability to turn, cough, and deep breathe. **Therapeutic Interventions** • Anticipate need for analgesia *to prevent peak pain periods.* • Provide oral hygiene, lozenges, and throat spray *to ease sore throat.* • Teach patient to use hands or pillows to splint incision when deep breathing, coughing, or changing positon. • Consider/recommend use of patient-controlled analgesia (PCA). • Secure all tubes/drains *to minimize movement and subsequent pain.*	Pain will be relieved.

Continued on following page.

TABLE 32–8. *Colon Resection (Hemicolectomy)** Continued

NURSING DIAGNOSES/ DEFINING CHARACTERISTICS	NURSING INTERVENTIONS/RATIONALES	EXPECTED OUTCOMES
Altered Bowel Elimination: Postoperative Ileus *Related to:* General anesthesia Manipulation of bowel **Defining Characteristics** Silent abdomen on auscultation No stooling Report of bloated feeling	**Ongoing Assessment** • Assess for bowel sounds every shift. • Note passage of first flatus, stool. *Postoperative ileus usually resolves within 96 hr after surgery.* **Therapeutic Interventions** • Maintain NPO status until bowel sounds return. • Ensure patency of NG tube *to keep stomach empty.* • Encourage/assist with ambulation *to hasten resolution of ileus.* • Assist patient with initial food/fluid selection *to minimize gaseous distention.* • Inform patient that stool pattern, consistency, frequency may not return to preoperative status, *depending on portion/length of colon resected.*	Bowel elimination will return to normal.
Altered Nutrition: Less Than Body Requirements *Related to:* Increased metabolic demands (stress of surgery) NPO Primary diagnosis Fever **Defining Characteristics** Weight loss Poor wound healing Low serum albumin Low energy level Low Hb, Hct	**Ongoing Assessment** • Assess postoperative weight; compare to preoperative weight. • Remain cognizant of length of NPO status. • Monitor vital signs, especially temperature. **Therapeutic Interventions** • Administer IV fluids as ordered: *1 L of 5% dextrose provides approximately 200 calories, which may achieve protein sparing for short time.* • If evidence of poor nutritional status and ileus has not resolved, consider peripheral or central hyperalimentation *to maintain anabolic state.* • Administer antipyretics *to control fever; for each 1°C above normal body temperature, metabolic need for calories increases by 7%.* • Plan activities *to allow adequate rest.*	Adequate nutrition will be maintained.
Knowledge Deficit *Related to:* Lack of previous experience with colon surgery Need for home management **Defining Characteristics** Multiple questions Lack of questions Inability to provide self-care upon discharge	**Ongoing Assessment** • Assess readiness and ability to learn. • Determine diet, activity, and wound care needs. **Therapeutic Interventions** • Teach patient/significant other the following: Importance of well-balanced diet based on food tolerances *to promote continued healing.* Bowel activity will stabilize over 6-8 wk (*normal time to adapt to shortened bowel)* Importance of prescribed wound care Need for follow-up appointments Signs/symptoms to report: fever, loss of appetite, abdominal pain, change in appearance of wound, significant change in bowel elimination Need for gradual return to preoperative activity level • Allow for return demonstration of wound care. • Document teaching done and patient's responses.	Patient/significant other will verbalize and/or demonstrate home care.

new stoma managed with consultation from an enterostomal nurse (Hampton, 1993). Patients should be referred to support groups for assistance with the psychologic and social adjustments necessary (Dobkin & Broadwell, 1986). Table 32–9 indicates a comprehensive care plan for patients needing creation of a fecal ostomy.

In addition, the increased utilization of adjuvant radiation and chemotherapy therapy has introduced new nursing care issues. The management of colorectal cancer patients receiving more intensive doses of radiotherapy and chemotherapy presents great challenges. Each of these adjuvant therapies brings with it an entire set of side effects and toxicities. Antineoplastic

TABLE 32–9. *Fecal Ostomy (Colostomy; Ileostomy; Fecal Diversion; Stoma)* *

NURSING DIAGNOSES/ DEFINING CHARACTERISTICS	NURSING INTERVENTIONS/RATIONALES	EXPECTED OUTCOMES
Preoperative Knowledge Deficit *Related to:* Lack of previous similar experience Need for additional information **Defining Characteristics** Verbalized need for information Verbalized misinformation/misconceptions	**Ongoing Assessment** • Assess previous surgical experience. • Inquire as to information from surgeon about ostomy formation (i.e., purpose, site). • Ascertain (from chart, physician) whether stoma permanent or temporary. **Therapeutic Interventions** • Reinforce and re-explain proposed procedure. • Answer questions directly and honestly. • Use diagrams, pictures, and AV equipment to explain: Anatomy, physiology of GI tract Pathophysiology necessitating ostomy Proposed location of stoma • Explain need for pouch in terms of loss of sphincter. • Show patient actual pouch or one similar to his/hers. • Allow patient to wear pouch preoperatively. *Stoma site selection is facilitated by observing adhesive faceplate in situ.*	Patient will understand alteration in normal GI anatomy or physiology requiring surgical creation of the ostomy and understand that loss of spincter will likely necessitate wearing a pouch.
Fear *Related to:* Proposed creation of ostomy Previous contact with poorly rehabilitated ostomate **Defining Characteristics** Verbal expression of concern/anxiety Tense facial expression Restlessness Multiple questions Lack of questions	**Ongoing Assessment** • Assess patient's level of anxiety; note nonverbal signs. • Elicit from patient (or other source) normal coping strategies. **Therapeutic Interventions** • Ask patient to describe in detail what is causing fear/anxiety. • Correct misconceptions; fill in knowledge gaps. • Offer visit from rehabilitated ostomate. *Often, contact with another individual who has "been there" is more beneficial in decreasing fear/anxiety than factual information.*	Level of anxiety will be decreased or manageable.
Anticipatory Grief *Related to:* Proposed loss of fecal continence Anticipated loss of function, love, job, body image **Defining Characteristics** Crying Rage Questioning Bargaining with self, God, health care professionals Withdrawal from usual relationships	**Ongoing Assessment** • Recognize the signs of anticipatory grief (see Defining Characteristics). • Assess perceived loss of: Life Function Social status Love Control Other **Therapeutic Interventions** • Encourage patient to verbalize feelings. • Assure patient such grief is real, expected, and appropriate. *Anticipatory grief facilitates postoperative grieving; and often follows patterns similar to actual grief patterns.*	Anticipatory grief will be recognized and facilitated.

*A surgical procedure that results in an opening into small or large intestine for the purpose of diverting the fecal stream past an area of obstruction or disease, protecting a distal surgical anastomosis, or providing an outlet for stool in the absence of a functioning intact rectum.
(From Gulanick, M., et al. [1990]. *Nursing care plans: Nursing diagnosis and intervention* [pp. 311–314]. St. Louis: Mosby. Originated by Audrey Klopp, RN, PhD, ET and Nola D. Johnson, RN.)   *Continued on following page.*

agents cause bone marrow suppression with resulting side effects of leukopenia, thrombocytopenia and anemia. Radiation therapy for these cancers produces gastrointestinal changes such as nausea, vomiting, stomati-tis, strictures, ulcers, and radiation-induced skin reactions. See specific chapters in Unit VIII for more detailed information on management of these patient care issues.

TABLE 32–9. *Fecal Ostomy (Colostomy; Ileostomy; Fecal Diversion; Stoma)* * Continued

NURSING DIAGNOSES/ DEFINING CHARACTERISTICS	NURSING INTERVENTIONS/RATIONALES	EXPECTED OUTCOMES
Altered Bowel Elimination *Related to:* Preoperative preparation for surgery	**Ongoing Assessment** • Assess preparedness of bowel for surgery; clear/near-clear returns on enemas. *Postoperative complications are decreased when surgical area properly emptied and cleansed.* • Observe for weakness, bradycardia, perianal discomfort.	Bowel will be sufficiently prepared for surgical procedure.
Defining Characteristics Orders for dietary restriction, cathartics, cleansing enemas	**Therapeutic Interventions** • Carry out necessary bowel preparation. • Explain necessity of bowel preparation. • Provide privacy during evacuation. • Allow rest periods between enemas.	
Potential Toileting Self Care Deficit *Related to:* Presence of stoma Presence of pouch	**Ongoing Assessment** • Assess abdominal surface for presence of: Old scars Bony prominences Skin folds Contour Visibility to patient	Potential for self-care deficit will be decreased.
Defining Characteristics Presence of old abdominal scars Presence of bony prominences on anterior abdominal surface Presence of skinfolds over abdomen Extreme obesity Pendulous breasts	**Therapeutic Interventions** • Indelibly mark proposed stoma site in area: Patient can easily see Patient can easily reach Scars, bony prominences, skinfolds are avoided Hip flexion does not change contour *Stoma location is a key factor in self-care. A poorly located stoma can delay/preclude self-care abilities.* • Note usual sites for stoma: *Ileostomy: lower right quadrant.* *Ascending colostomy: right upper or lower quadrant.* *Transverse colostomy: midwaist or just below midwaist.* *Descending and sigmoid colostomies: lower left quadrant.* • If possible, have patient wear pouch over proposed site; evaluate effectiveness 12-24 hr after applying pouch.	
Postoperative Alteration in Bowel Elimination *Related to:* Surgical diversion of fecal stream	**Ongoing Assessment** • Assess stoma every 4h postoperatively for: Color Shape Size Presence of supportive device (rod, catheter) Function (flatus, stool) Drainage that is not stool	Bowel function via stoma will return within 8 hr (ileostomy) or 1-4 days (colostomy).
Defining Characteristics Structural or functional absence of anal sphincter Presence of stoma	**Therapeutic Interventions** • Apply pouch to stoma as soon as possible postoperatively *to protect other surgical sites from fecal contamination and protect peristomal skin.* • Notify physician if stoma appears dusky or blue. *Stoma (a piece of intestine) should be pink, moist, indicating good perfusion and adequate venous drainage.*	
Body Image Disturbance *Related to:* Presence of stoma; loss of fecal continence	**Ongoing Assessment** • Assess perception of change in body structure and function. • Assess perceived impact of change. *Assigned importance of body part or importance major factor in impact.* • Note verbal references to stoma, altered bowel eliminaton.	Feelings about altered bowel function, stoma, and changes in self-concept will be acknowledged.

TABLE 32–9. *Fecal Ostomy (Colostomy; Ileostomy; Fecal Diversion; Stoma)* * Continued

NURSING DIAGNOSES/ DEFINING CHARACTERISTICS	NURSING INTERVENTIONS/RATIONALES	EXPECTED OUTCOMES
Defining Characteristics Verbalized feelings about stoma and altered bowel elimination Refusal to discuss, acknowledge, touch, or care for stoma, pouch	**Therapeutic Interventions** • Acknowledge appropriateness of emotional response to perceived change in body structure and function. *Because control of elimination is skill/task of early childhood and socially private function, loss of control precipitates body image change and possible self-concept change.* • Assist patient in looking at, touching, and caring for stoma when ready. • Reoffer visit from rehabilitated ostomate.	
Knowledge Deficit: Ostomy Self-Care *Related to:* Presence of new stoma Lack of similar experience **Defining Characteristics** Demonstrated inability to empty and change pouch Verbalized need for information about diet, odor, activity, hygiene, clothing, interpersonal relationships, equipment purchase, financial concerns	**Ongoing Assessment** • Assess: Ability to empty and change pouch Ability to care for peristomal skin and identify problems, potential problems Appropriateness in seeking assistance Knowledge of: Diet Activity Hygiene Clothing Interpersonal relationships Equipment purchase Financial reimbursement for ostomy equipment **Therapeutic Interventions** • Build on information given preoperatively. • Plan and share teaching plan with patient. • Begin psychomotor teaching during first and subsequent applications of pouch. • Gradually transfer responsibility for pouch emptying and changing to patient. • Allow at least one opportunity for supervised return demonstration of pouch change before discharge. *Ostomy care requires both cognitive and psychomotor skills. Postoperatively, learning ability may be decreased requiring repetition and opportunity of return demonstrations.* • Instruct patient on the following: Diet: *For ileostomy:* balanced diet; special care in chewing high-fiber foods (popcorn, peanuts, coconut, vegetables, string beans, olives); increased fluid intake during hot weather, vigorous exercise. *For colostomy:* balanced diet; no foods specifically contraindicated; certain foods (eggs, fish, green leafy vegetables, carbonated beverages) may increase flatus and fecal odor. Odor control: best achieved by eliminating odor-causing foods from diet, oral agents, deodorant available. Activity: should not be restricted because of stoma or pouch; direct forceful blows to stoma should be prevented.	Patient will be capable of ostomy self-care on discharge.
Pain *Related to:* Surgical incision(s) **Defining Characteristics** Facial mask of pain Verbal complaints of pain	**Ongoing Assessment** • Assess level of comfort. • Elicit from patient possible sources of discomfort/recommendations for relief. **Therapeutic Interventions** • Institute pain relief measures, incorporating patient's suggestions when possible. *Patients who have undergone abdominal-perineal resection have both abdominal and perineal incisions and may need additional assistance achieving adequate pain relief.*	Pain will be reduced.

Continued on following page.

Table 32–9. *Fecal Ostomy (Colostomy; Ileostomy; Fecal Diversion; Stoma)** Continued

NURSING DIAGNOSES/ DEFINING CHARACTERISTICS	NURSING INTERVENTIONS/RATIONALES	EXPECTED OUTCOMES
Inability to turn, cough, deep breathe, get out of bed Decreased concentration		

REFERENCES

American Cancer Society. (1995). *Cancer facts and figures.* Atlanta, GA: Author.

American Joint Committee on Cancer. (1988). *Manual for staging of cancer* (3rd ed.). Philadelphia: J. B. Lippincott Co.

Astler, V. B., & Coller, F. A. (1954). The prognostic significance of direct extension of carcinoma of the colon and rectum. *Annals of Surgery, 139,* 846–851.

Batson, O. V. (1940). The function of the vertebral veins and their role in the spread of metastases. *Annals of Surgery, 112,* 138–149.

Beart, R. W. Jr. (1991). Colorectal cancer. In A. I. Holleb, D. J. Fink, & G. P. Murphy (Eds.), *American Cancer Society textbook of clinical oncology* (pp. 213–218). Atlanta, GA: The American Cancer Society, Inc.

Bloom, W. N., & Fawcett, D. W. (1968). *A textbook of histology.* Phildelphia: W. B. Saunders Co.

Boland, C. R. (1993). The biology of colorectal cancer. Implications for pretreatment and follow-up management. *Cancer, 71*(Suppl. 12), 4180–4186.

Cavaliere, F., Guadagni, F., D'Agnano, I., Casaldi, V., Sciarretta, F., Spila, A., & Cosimelli, M. (1994). Biologic and clinical correlations among ploidy, cell kinetics, and the tumor-associated glycoprotein-72 tissue expression in colorectal cancer. Preliminary findings. *Diseases of the Colon and Rectum, 37*(Suppl. 2), S24–S29.

Chernecky, C. C., Krech, R. L., & Berger, B. J. (1993). *Laboratory tests and diagnostic procedures.* Philadelphia, PA: W. B. Saunders Co.

Cohen, A. M., Minsky, B. D., & Friedman, M. A. (1993). Rectal cancer. In V. T. DeVita, S. Hellman, & S. A. Rosenberg (Eds.), *Cancer: Principles and practice of oncology* (4th ed., pp. 978–1004). Philadelphia: J. B. Lippincott Co.

Cohen, A. M., Minsky, B. D., & Schilsky, R. L. (1993). Colon cancer. In V. T. DeVita, S. Hellman, & S. A. Rosenberg (Eds.), *Cancer: Principles and practice of oncology* (4th ed., pp. 929–977). Philadelphia: J. B. Lippincott Co.

Corman, M. L. (1993a). Carcinoma of the colon. In *Colon and rectal surgery* (pp. 487–595). Philadelphia: J. B. Lippincott Co.

Corman, M. L. (1993b). Carcinoma of the rectum. In *Colon and rectal surgery* (pp. 596–720). Philadelphia: J. B. Lippincott Co.

DeCosse, J. J., Tsioulias, G. J., & Jacobson, J. S. (1994). Colorectal cancer: Detection, treatment, and rehabilitation. *CA A Cancer Journal for Clinicians, 44*(1), 27–42.

Dobkin, K. A., & Broadwell, B. C. (1986). Nursing considerations for the patient undergoing colostomy surgery. *Seminars in Oncology Nursing, 2,* 249–256.

Doughty, D. B. (1986). Colorectal cancer: Etiology and pathophysiology. *Seminars in Oncology Nursing, 2,* 235–241.

Drewinko, B., & Yang, L. Y. (1985). Cellular basis for the inefficiency of 5-fluorouracil in human colon carcinoma. *Cancer Treatment Reports, 69,* 1391–1398.

Dukes, C. E. (1932). The classification of cancer of the rectum. *Journal of Pathology, 35,* 323–332.

Dukes, C. E., & Bussey, H. J. R. (1958). The spread of rectal cancer and its effect on prognosis. *British Journal of Cancer, 12,* 309–320.

Enker, W. E., Paty, P. B., Minsky, B. D., & Cohen, A. M. (1992). Restorative or preservative operations in the treatment of rectal cancer. *Surgical Oncology Clinics of North America, 1,* 57–70.

Fengler, S. A., & Pearl, R. K. (1994). Technical considerations in the surgical treatment of colon and rectal cancer. *Seminars in Surgical Oncology, 10,* 200–207.

Fitzsimmons, M. L., & Fales, L. (1993). Colon cancer prevention update. *Seminars in Oncology Nursing, 9,* 163–168.

Fritsche, H. A. (1993). Serum tumor markers for patient monitoring: a case-oriented approach illustrated with carcinoembryonic antigen. *Clinical Chemistry, 39,* 2431–2434.

Gabriel, W. B., Dukes, C., & Bussey, H. J. R. (1935). Lymphatic spread in cancer of the rectum. *British Journal of Surgery, 23,* 395–413.

Gastrointestinal Tumor Study Group. (1985). Prolongation of the disease-free interval in surgically treated rectal carcinoma. *New England Journal of Medicine, 312,* 1465–1472.

Griffin, F. D., Knight, C. D., & Whitaker, J. M. (1990). The double stapling technique for low anterior resection: Results, modifications, and observations. *Annals in Surgery, 211,* 745–752.

Gulanic, M., Klopp, A., Galanes, S., Gradishar, D., & Puzas, M. K. (1990). *Nursing care plans: Nursing diagnosis & intervention* (pp. 304–314). St. Louis: The C. V. Mosby Company.

Gunderson, L. L., & Sosin, H. (1974). Areas of failure found at reoperation (second or symptomatic look) following "curative surgery" for adenocarcinoma of the rectum: Clinicopathologic correlation and implications for adjuvant therapy. *Cancer, 34,* 1278–1292.

Gunderson, L. L., Shipley, W. V., & Suit, H. (1982). Intraoperative irradiation: A pilot study combining external beam photons with "boost" dose intraoperative electrons. *Cancer, 49,* 2259–2266.

Haenszel, W., & Kurihara, M. (1968). Studies of Japanese migrants: 1. Mortality from cancer and other diseases among Japanese in the United States. *Journal of the National Cancer Institute, 40,* 43–68.

Hampton, B. (1993). Gastrointestinal cancer: Colon, rectum, and anus. In S. L. Groenwald (Ed.), *Cancer nursing: Principles and practices* (pp. 544–557). Boston: Jones & Bartlett Publishers, Inc.

Hill, M. J., Drasar, B. S., & Williams, R. E. D. (1975). Fecal bile acid and clostridia in patients with cancer of the large bowel. *Lancet, 1,* 535–539.

Hoerner, M. T. (1958). Carcinoma of the colon and rectum in persons under twenty years of age. *American Journal of Surgery, 96,* 47–53.

International Union Against Cancer. (1987). *TNM classification of malignant tumors* (4th ed.). Berlin: Springer Verlag.

Kemeny, N., Lokich, J. J., Anderson, N., & Ahlgren, J. D. (1993). Recent advances in the treatment of advanced colorectal cancer. *Cancer, 71,* 9–18.

Kern, S., Fearon, E., Tersmete, K., Enterline, J., Leppert, M., Nakamura, Y., White, R., Vogelstein, B., & Hamilton, S. (1991). Allelic loss in colorectal cancer. *Journal of the American Medical Association, 261,* 3099–3103.

Konsker, K. A. (1992). Familial adenamatous polyposis: Case report and review of extracolonic manifestations. *Mount Sinai Journal of Medicine, 59*(1), 85–91.

Kouri, M., Nordling, S., Kuusela, P., & Pyrhönen, S. (1993). Poor prognosis associated with elevated CA 19-9 level in advancd colorectal carcinoma, independent of DNA ploidy or SPF. *European Journal of Cancer, 29A,* 1691–1969.

Kressel, H. Y., & Thickman, D. I. (1985). Magnetic resonance imaging. In J. E. Berk (Ed.), *Bockus gastroenterology* (4th ed., pp. 552–563). Philadelphia: W. B. Saunders Co.

Krook, J. E., Moertel, C. G., Gunderson, L. L., et al. (1991). Surgical adjuvant therapy for high-risk rectal carcinoma. *The New England Journal of Medicine, 324,* 709–715.

Kune, G.A., & Vitetta, L. (1992). Alcohol consumption and the etiology of colorectal cancer: a review of the scientific evidence from 1957 to 1991. *Nutrition and Cancer, 18*(2), 97–111.

Laufer, I. (1985). Barium contrast examinations. In J. E. Berk (Ed.), *Bockus gastroenterolgy* (4th ed., pp. 456–469). Philadelphia: W. B. Saunders Co.

Levin, B. (1992). Chemoprevention of colon cancer: Rationale and biologic basis. *Cancer Concept to Clinic, 1*(2), 24–28.

Lewin, K. J., Riddell, R. H., & Weinstein, W. M. (1992). *Gastrointestinal pathology and its clinical implications* (pp. 1256–1306). New York: Igaku-Shoin.

Lynes, A. C. (1993). Percutaneous hepatic arterial chemotherapy and chemoembolization. *Cancer Nursing, 16,* 283–287.

Lyster, M. T., Benson III, A. B., Vogelzang, R., & Talamonti, M. (1993). Chemoembolization: Alternative for hepatic tumors. *Contemporary Oncology, August,* 17–26.

Macdonald, J. S., & Axelrod, R. (1992). Adjuvant therapy of colon and rectal cancer. In J. D. Ahlgren & J. S. Macdonald, (Eds.), *Gastrointestinal oncology* (pp. 383–395). Philadelphia: J. B. Lippincott Co.

Markowitz, S. (1992). Molecular biology of colon cancer. *Cancer-Concept to Clinic, 1,* 5–10.

McMichael, A. J., McCall, M. G., Hartshorne, J. M., et al. (1980). Patterns of gastrointestinal cancer in European migrants to Australia: The role of dietary change. *International Journal of Cancer, 25,* 431–437.

Mendenhall, W. M., Bland, K. T., & Pfaff., W. (1987). Initially unresectable rectal adenocarcinoma treated with pre-

operative irradiation and surgery. *Annals of Surgery, 205,* 41.

Minsky, B. D., Mies, C., & Rich, T. A. (1988). Potentially curative surgery of colon cancer. The influence of blood vessel invasion. *Journal of Clinical Oncology, 6,* 119–127.

Morton, J. M., Poulter, C. A., & Pandya, K. J. (1983). Alimentary tract cancer. In P. Rubin, R. F. Bakeemeir, & S. K. Krackov (Eds.), *Clinical oncology—a multidisciplinary approach* (pp. 154–176). New York: American Cancer Society.

Nakahara, S., Itoh, H., & Mibu, R. (1988). Clinical and manometric evaluation of anorectal function following low anterior resection with low anastomotic line using an EEATM stapler for rectal cancer. *Diseases of the Colon and Rectum, 31,* 762.

Nathanson, S. D., Linden, M. D., Tender, P., Zarbo, R. J., Jacobsen, G., & Nelson, J. T. (1994). Relationship among p53, stage, and prognosis of large bowel cancer. *Diseases of the Colon and Rectum, 37,* 527–534.

NIH Consensus Conference. (1990). Adjuvant therapy for patients with colon and rectal cancer. *Journal of the American Medical Association, 264,* 1444–1450.

Papillon, J. (1984). New prospects in the conservative treatment of rectal cancer. *Diseases of the Colon and Rectum, 27,* 695.

Papillon, J. (1982). *Rectal and anal cancers.* Berlin: Springer-Verlag.

Posner, M. R., & Mayer, R. J. (1994). The use of serologic tumor markers in gastrointestinal malignancies. *Hematology/Oncology Clinics of North America, 8,* 533–541.

Rostock, R. A., Zajac, A. J., & Gallagher, M. J. (1992). Radiation therapy in the treatment of colorectal cancer. In J. D. Ahlgren & J. S. Macdonald (Eds.), *Gastrointestinal oncology* (pp. 359–381). Philadelphia: J. B. Lippincott Co.

Schiffman, M. F. (1990). Re: fried foods and the risk of colon cancer. *American Journal of Epidemiology, 131,* 376–378.

Seefeld, P., & Bargen, J. A. (1943). The spread of carcinoma of the rectum: Invasion of lymphatics, veins and nerves. *Annals of Surgery, 118,* 76–90.

Shapiro, S. (1992). Goals of screening. *Cancer, 70,* 1252–1258.

Sleisenger, M. H., & Fordtran, J. S. (Eds). (1989). *Gastrointestinal disease: Pathophysiology, diagnosis, management.* Philadelphia: W. B. Saunders Co.

Smith, L. (1992). Colorectal cancer: Surgical approach. In J. D. Ahlgren & J. S. Macdonald (Eds.), *Gastrointestinal oncology* (pp. 299–377). Philadelphia: J. B. Lippincott Co.

Spjut, H. J. (1984). Pathology of neoplasms. In J.S. Spratt (Ed.), *Neoplasms of the colon, rectum, and anus: Mucosal and epithelial* (pp. 159–204). Philadelphia: W. B. Saunders Co.

Stockholm Rectal Cancer Study Group. (1990). Preoperative short-term radiation therapy in operative rectal carcinoma. *Cancer, 66,* 49.

Summers, G. E., Mendenhall, W. M., & Copeland, E. M. (1992). Update on the University of Florida experience with local excision and postoperative radiation therapy. *Surgical Oncology Clinics of North America, 1,* 125–130.

Szarka, C.E., Grana, G., & Engstrom, P. (1994). Chemoprevention of cancer. *Current Problems in Cancer, 18*(1).

Trock, B., Lanza, E., & Greenwald, P. (1990). Dietary fiber, vegetables, and colon cancer: Critical review and meta-analysis of the epidemiologic evidence. *Journal of the National Cancer Institute, 82,* 650–681.

Weisburger, J. H. (1991). Causes, relevant mechanisms, and prevention of large bowel cancer. *Seminars in Oncology, 18*(4), 316–336.

Wiggers, T., Jeekel, J., & Arends, J. W. (1988). No-touch isolation technique in colon cancer: A controlled prospective trial. *British Journal of Surgery, 75,* 409–415.

Willett, W. C., Stampfer, M. J., Colditz, G., Rosner, B., & Speizer, F. (1990). Relation of meat, fat, and fiber intake to the risk of colon cancer in a prospective study among women. *The New England Journal of Medicine, 323,* 1664–1672.

Williams, N. S. (1984). The rationale of preservation of the anal sphincter in patients with low rectal cancer. *British Journal of Surgery, 71,* 575–581.

Winawer, S. J. (1991). Diagnosis and prevention of GI malignancies. *Seminars in Oncology, 18(1)* (Suppl. 1), 7–16.

Wingo, P.A., Tong, T., & Bolden, S. (1995). Cancer statistics, 1995. *CA A Cancer Journal for Clinicians. 45*(1):8–30.

Winn, R.J., & Levin, B. (1989). Chemoprevention of colon cancer. *Hematology/Oncology Clinics of North America, 3*(1), 65–73.

World Health Organization. (1978). *International histologic classification of tumors,* Nos. 1–20. Geneva: Author.

33

Genitourinary Cancers

Connie J. Leek • Wanda Sebastian • Mark H. Kawachi • Liz Sullivan

Cancers of the prostate, kidney, and bladder are common in adults. Testicular cancer, although uncommon, is important to discuss because it is the most common cancer in young men between 25 and 30 years of age. Figure 33–1 shows the tumor sites and routes of metastases in men.

PROSTATIC CANCER

DEFINITION AND INCIDENCE

The prostate is a small, firm organ made up of glands and musculature enclosed in a fibrous capsule through which the urethra passes as it exits the bladder. Its consistency is similar to the tip of the nose with an inverted triangular shape and a groove dividing the gland into four anatomic zones. It is a secondary sex organ whose only known function is its contribution to seminal fluid. Figure 33–2 illustrates the anatomic relationships of the prostate.

Prostate cancer accounts for approximately 20 per cent of all cancers in men and 10 per cent of all cancer deaths (Silverberg & Lubera, 1989). Between 1980 and 1990, prostate cancer incidence rates increased 50 per cent largely due to improved detection. Prostate cancer is now the second leading cause of cancer death in men (American Cancer Society [ACS], 1994a).

EPIDEMIOLOGY AND ETIOLOGY

The peak incidence of prostatic cancer is in men between 60 and 70 years of age, and it is found incidentally on routine autopsy examination in most men older than 70 years of age. The highest rate of prostatic cancer in the world is among African-Americans; the lowest incidence is found among Japanese men. In fact, prostate cancer incidence rates are 30 per cent higher for African-American men than white men (ACS, 1994a).

Four major factors are hypothesized to contribute to the causation of prostatic cancer: age, infectious agents, endocrine factors, and familial factors. Age is the most important variable yet described. Prostatic cancer in men under 40 years old is rare. African-American men in Los Angeles, for example, have a one in four risk of developing clinically significant prostatic cancer by 85 years of age (Ross, Paganini-Hill, & Henderson, 1988b).

Although they are not completely understood, hormonal interactions seem to play a role in the development of prostate cancer. Also, abnormal estrogen and androgen metabolite levels have been detected in patients with either prostate cancer or hyperplasia of the prostate (Maxwell, 1993). For example, prostatic cancer does not develop in eunuchs, and many cases of metastatic disease respond to hormonal manipulation (Perez, Ihde, Fair, & Labrie, 1985). Furthermore, although prostatic cancer is difficult to induce in animal models, subcutaneous testosterone alone can produce this cancer in rats (Noble, 1980). Familial factors might also be implicated, since prostate cancer has been noted to cluster within certain families. In fact, patients with a brother or father with prostate cancer are four times more likely to be diagnosed before the age of 65 (Maxwell, 1993).

BIOLOGY AND NATURAL HISTORY

Prostatic cancers are almost always adenocarcinomas, which vary in differentiation and appearance. As of January 1993, the TMN staging system is consid-

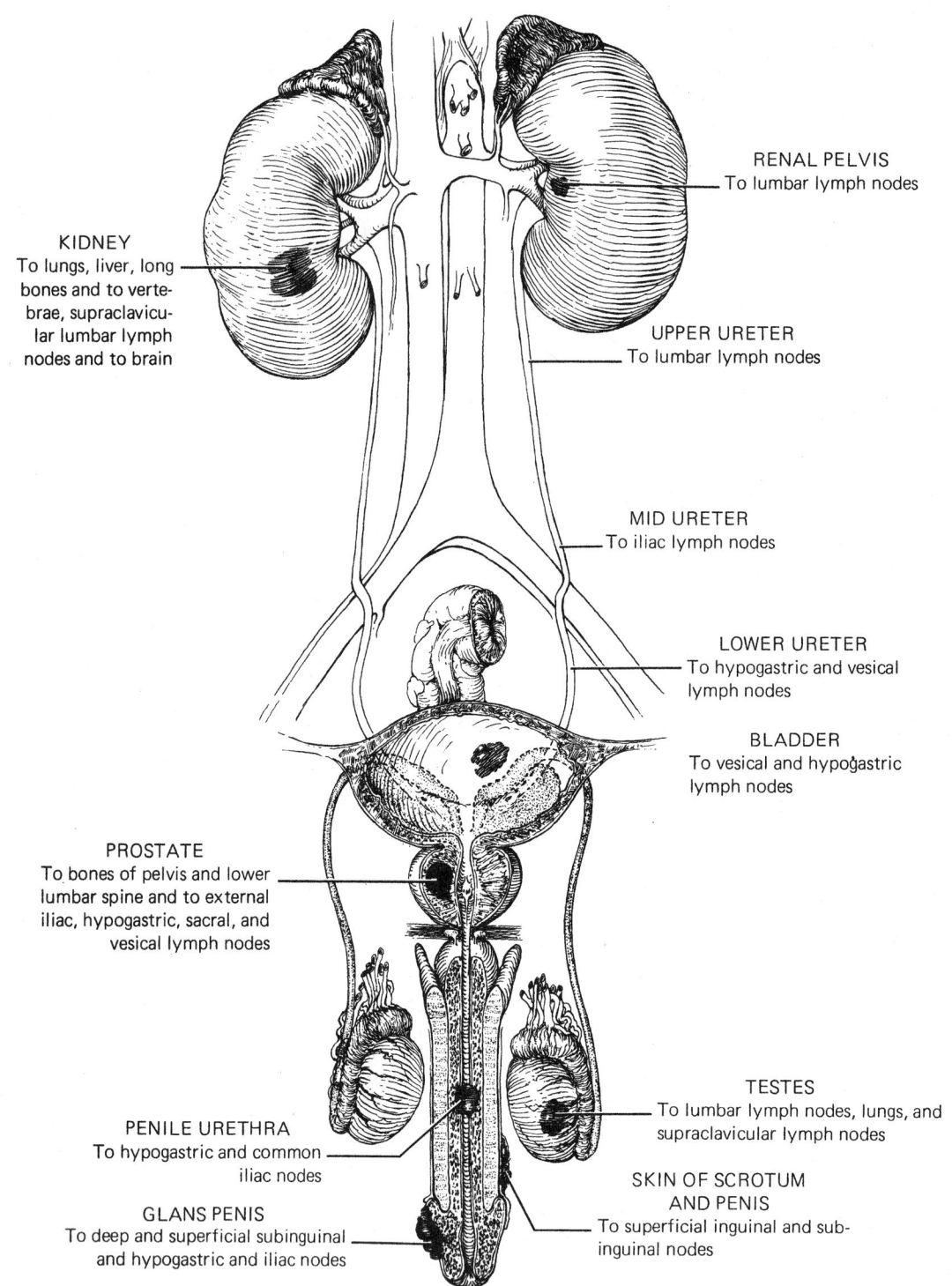

RENAL PELVIS
To lumbar lymph nodes

KIDNEY
To lungs, liver, long
bones and to verte-
brae, supraclavicu-
lar lumbar lymph
nodes and to brain

UPPER URETER
To lumbar lymph nodes

MID URETER
To iliac lymph nodes

LOWER URETER
To hypogastric and vesical
lymph nodes

BLADDER
To vesical and hypogastric
lymph nodes

PROSTATE
To bones of pelvis and lower
lumbar spine and to external
iliac, hypogastric, sacral, and
vesical lymph nodes

TESTES
To lumbar lymph nodes, lungs, and
supraclavicular lymph nodes

SKIN OF SCROTUM
AND PENIS
To superficial inguinal and sub-
inguinal nodes

PENILE URETHRA
To hypogastric and common
iliac nodes

GLANS PENIS
To deep and superficial subinguinal
and hypogastric and iliac nodes

FIGURE 33–1. Sites of tumor origin and metastases in the male. (From Smith, D. R. (1981). Tumors of the genitourinary tract. In D. R. Smith [Ed.]. *General urology* [10th ed., p. 272]. Los Altos, CA: Lange. Reproduced by permission.)

ered mandatory for the classification of all cancers in hospitals evaluated by the American Joint Commission on Cancer. However, the American Urological Association continues to use an A, B, C, D system (Fig. 33–3).

Also used today is the Gleason classification. This is a system of histopathologic grading based on the glandular pattern of the tumor at relatively low magnification. Combining clinical staging and histopathologic

grading helps predict the biologic potential of prostate cancer (Gleason, Mellinger, & the Veteran's Administration Cooperative Urological Research Group, 1974; Kramer, Spahr, Brendler, Glenn, & Paulson, 1980; Layfield et al., 1984).

Local spread to the seminal vesicles and the bladder is common. Prostatic cancer also disseminates hematogenously to the bones and rarely to the lungs

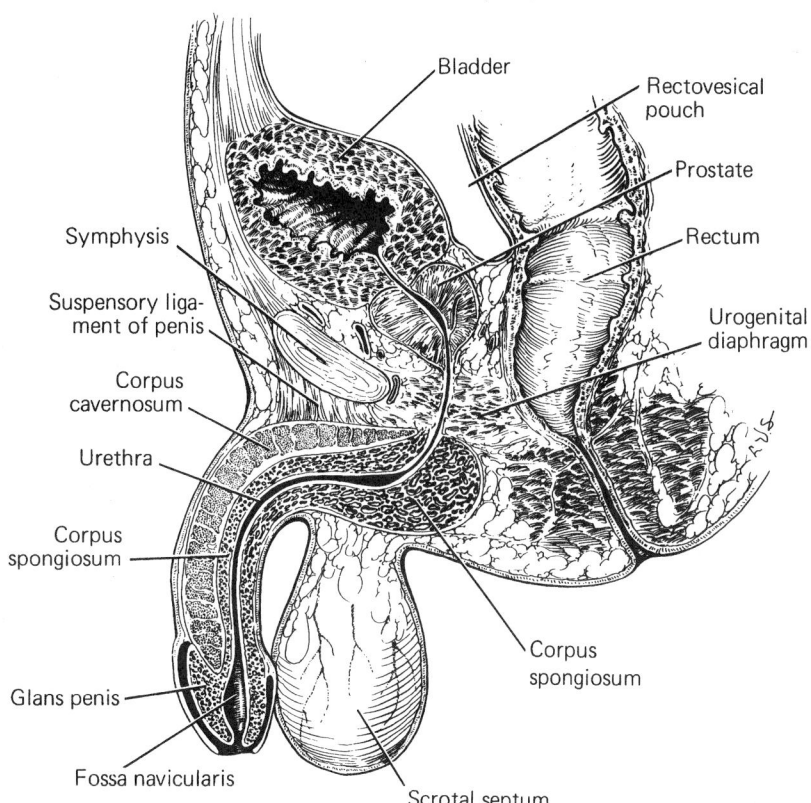

FIGURE 33–2. Relations of the bladder, prostate seminal vesicles, penis, urethra, and scrotal contents. (From Smith, D. R. [1981]. Tumors of the genitourinary tract. In D. R. Smith [Ed.]. *General urology* [10th ed., p. 9]. Los Altos, CA: Lange. Reproduced by permission.)

and liver. The disease spreads via the lymphatics to the pelvic lymph nodes, then to the periaortic nodes, and occasionally to the supraclavicular nodes. In fact, as many as one third of the men with early disease (stage B and low-volume stage C) have evidence of metastases to the pelvic lymph nodes (Waisman & Mott, 1978).

In the last 2 decades, the survival rates for prostatic cancer have increased significantly (Silverberg & Lubera, 1989). Five-year survival after prostatectomy for stage A is 88 to 91 per cent, and for stage B, 73 to 81 per cent (Middleton, Smith, Melzer, & Hamilton, 1986). Survival rates for advanced cancer are much less encouraging (Kramer et al., 1980).

Presenting Signs and Symptoms. On rectal examination the gland normally feels rubbery. In early cancer it will feel like a nonraised, firm nodule that may have a sharp edge. However, less than 10 per cent of prostate cancers detected on routine examinations are discovered early enough for potential cure. Unfortunately, there are no real symptoms in early-stage disease, and small tumors are easily missed. Later tumors might be detected as a hard lump on rectal examination or as an unexpected finding during histologic examination of transurethral resection specimens.

Urinary disorders such as frequency, hematuria, hesitancy starting stream, dysuria, and obstruction are common presenting symptoms. A frequent symptom of late disease is bone pain related to metastasis. See Table 33–1 for a list of common symptoms.

Differential Diagnosis. The urinary tract symptoms of benign prostatic hypertrophy closely resemble cancer. Because only 50 per cent of prostatic nodules are malignant tumors, it is imperative to establish a tissue diagnosis. This is most commonly done by needle aspiration or biopsy (Layfield et al., 1984). A hardened area felt on rectal examination could also be the result of prostatitis, tuberculosis, fibrous benign prostatic hypertrophy (BPH), or prostatic calculi.

Determination of serum prostatic acid phosphatase by either biochemical or radioimmunologic assay should be included in the prostatic cancer workup. More than 80 per cent of men with stage D disease have an increased serum acid phosphatase level (McCullough, 1988). A bone scan and an excretory urogram (intravenous pyelogram, or IVP) are also usually performed. A controversy currently exists regarding the availability of various screening techniques such as digital rectal examination (DRE), prostatic-specific antigen (PSA), and transrectal ultrasonography (TRUS). The current recommendation according to the American Cancer Society is that every man over 40 should have DRE yearly and that men over 50 should have an annual PSA (ACS, 1994a). Table 33–2 clearly illustrates the advantages and disadvantages of the various screening tests currently available for prostate cancer.

Because the sudden discovery of prostatic cancer may take the asymptomatic patient and his family by complete surprise, nursing interventions should focus on education and emotional support. Helping the patient and family to understand the implications of his treatment options—for example, possible impotence or incontinence—is a significant challenge.

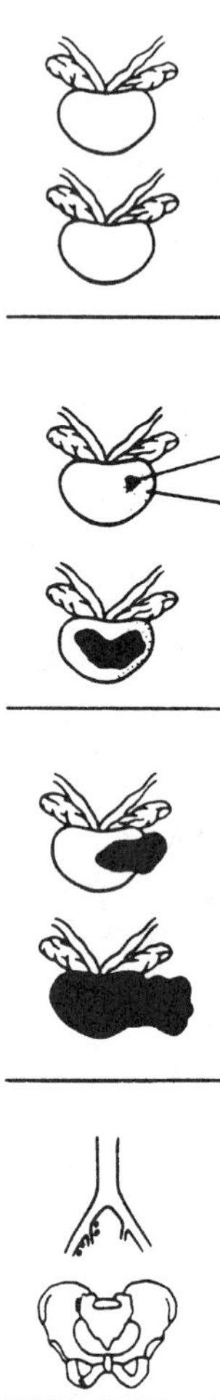

Staging System		Extent of Disease	Proportion of Patients at Diagnosis*
TNM[1]	AUS[2]		
T_1	A	**Incidental histological finding of cancer; prostate normal to palpation**	29.3%
T_{1a}	A_1	Single focal area of well-differentiated tumor	
T_{1b}	A_2	Multiple areas of cancer in the gland or cancer is poorly differentiated	
T_2	B	**Tumor palpable but confined to prostate**	37.7%
T_{2a} T_{2b}	B_1	Single nodule <2 cm in diameter	
T_{2c}	B_2	Multiple nodules or single nodule >2 cm in diameter. Both lobes involved	
T_3	C	**Tumor is localized to periprostatic area**	12.5%
T_{3a}	C_1	No involvement of seminal vesicles and tumor <70 gm	
T_{3c}	C_2	Involvement of seminal vesicles and tumor <70 gm	
T_4	D	**Advanced disease**	20.6%
N+	D_1	Pelvic node metastases or ureteral obstruction	
M+	D_2	Distant metastases	

*Data from 1990   [1]TNM Staging System, [2]American Urological Staging System

FIGURE 33-3. Staging of prostate cancer comparing the TNM Staging System with the American Urological Staging System (AUS). (From Maxwell, M. [1993]. Cancer of the prostate. *Seminars in Oncology Nursing,* 9(4), 237–251. Data from Mettlin, C., Jones, G., Murphy, G. P. [1993]. Trends in prostate cancer in the United States, 1974–1990: Observations from the patient care evaluation studies of the American College of Surgeons Commission on Cancer. *CA-A Cancer Journal for Clinicians, 43,* 83–91.)

TREATMENT

Surgery. A radical prostatectomy is utilized for the extirpation of prostate cancer (Paulson, Lin, Hinshaw, Stephani, & the Uro-Oncology Research Group, 1982; Walsh, 1992). It is the surgical removal of the entire prostate, including the true prostate capsule, the seminal vesicles, and the attached portion of the vas deferens. It can be done with or without a pelvic lymph node dissection. The radical prostatectomy is indicated for stage T1 and T2, N0 M0 disease. The perineal and retropubic approaches are used. See Figures 33–4 and 33–5 for greater detail.

Transurethral resection of the prostate (TURP) also plays a role in treatment. Although it is not used for curative intent, it can be helpful in treating obstructive symptoms in advanced cancer. It may also reveal an unsuspected cancer when used to treat BPH (T1A and T1B disease).

Complications of radical prostatectomy include infection and bleeding (short term) and incontinence and impotence (long term) (Walsh, 1992). Impotence following radical prostatectomy is the result of autonomic nerve damage posterior lateral to the prostate (Andriole, 1993; Walsh, 1992). The Walsh modification of the retropubic prostatectomy (nerve-sparing prostatectomy) carefully preserves the autonomic nerves and has demonstrated impressive potency preservation rates (Andriole, 1993; Walsh, 1992).

Nursing implications involve initially exploring preoperative concerns regarding sexual competence. People in general may hold certain prejudices concerning sexuality in the older adult, which the nurse should avoid. Teaching should be geared to the role of the prostate in sexual activity and alleviating misconceptions that all sexual activity is over (Heinrich-Rynning, 1987). The reader is referred to Chapter 62 for an in-depth discussion of sexuality.

Immediate postoperative nursing responsibilities include maintaining catheter presence and patency, preventing urinary tract infection, and administering antispasmodics to decrease the discomfort caused by bladder spasms (Lind, 1987). Interestingly, clot retention after radical prostatectomy is less of a problem than it is after simple prostatectomy.

Radiotherapy. Radiotherapy has been used for curative, adjunctive, and palliative treatment of

TABLE 33–1. *Assessment of the Patient with Suspected Carcinoma of the Prostate*

Subjective Indicators

Early disease:
Obstructive	Irritative
symptoms	symptoms
Hesitancy	Urgency
Intermittency	Sensation of
Weak, forceless	incomplete
urinary stream	voiding
Straining to void	Dysuria
Postvoid dribbling	Incontinence
Nocturia	

Advanced disease: Lumbosacral back pain (which may radiate to hips or down legs)
Migratory bone pain

Objective Indicators

Early disease: On DRE, nonraised, firm nodule(s) with sharp edge, also may be induration, asymmetry

Advanced disease: On DRE, hard and stone-like nodule(s), may be induration
Weight loss
Hematuria (if spread to the bladder or urethra)
Anemia

Laboratory Indicators

Early disease: Elevated PSA
Positive transrectal ultrasonography
MRI (with endorectal coil)

Advanced disease: Same as above, plus the following:
Tumor markers positive (Acid phosphatase, PSA at higher levels)
Bone scan: if negative, pelvic CT or MRI to evaluate pelvic nodes
Chest x-ray
Renal function studies

CT = computed tomography; MRI = magnetic resonance imaging; DRE = digital rectal examination; PSA = prostate-specific antigen.
(From Maxwell, M. [1993]. Cancer of the prostate. *Seminars in Oncology Nursing, 9*[4], 237–251.)

TABLE 33–2. *Advantages and Disadvantages of Screening Tests for Prostate Cancer*

	ADVANTAGES	DISADVANTAGES
Digital rectal examination (DRE)	Inexpensive Specific	Misses 40% of cancers Subjective—dependent on operator performance
Prostate-specific antigen (PSA)	Objective Inexpensive Sensitive Better patient acceptance	Nonspecific false-positive from benign prostatic diseases Misses up to 30% of localized tumors Uncertainty as to cutoff points
Transrectal ultrasonography (TRUS)	Can detect small lesions out of range of DRE Provides guidance for biopsies	Subjective—dependent on operator performance Can fail to detect 30% of lesions False-positives may occur from inflammation Requires special equipment and operator training Expensive Time-consuming

DRE = digital rectal examination.
(From Maxwell, M. [1993]. Cancer of the prostate. *Seminars in Oncology Nursing, 9*[4], 237–251.)

prostate cancer. Various methods of delivering the necessary radiation to the prostate are currently being utilized (Gibbons et al., 1986; Hanks, 1991; Paulson, 1988a; Paulson et al., 1982; Schellhammer, 1994). External beam (photon, neutron, and proton) and interstitial seed (Ir, I, Au) have their proponents (Schellhammer, 1994). As prostate cancer is relatively radioresistant, all treatments must deliver high doses of radiation to be effective (Schellhammer, 1994). Few controlled clinical trials have been performed validating the efficacy of radiotherapy. An earlier Veterans Administration study reported a higher relapse rate in patients treated with radiotherapy (Babaian, Zagars, & Ayala, 1990; Hanks, 1991; Paulson, 1988a; Robertson & Paulson, 1991; Schellhammer, 1994).

Adjunctive radiotherapy may be used in conjunction with surgery. Postoperative radiotherapy for localized disease is of equivocal benefit (Brawer, 1992; Freeman et al., 1993; Gibbons et al., 1986; Meier, Mark, St. Royal, Tran, Colburn, & Parker, 1992; Stein, DeKernion, Dorey, & Smith, 1992). Studies are currently underway to quantitate this benefit. Preoperative

radiotherapy is of little benefit with extensive local disease.

Palliative radiotherapy is primarily for symptomatic metastatic disease (especially to bone) (Bolger et al., 1993; Porter & McEwan, 1993; Porter et al., 1993). Spot, high-dose, short-course external beam radiation to specific painful metastatic sites can be very helpful. For multiple painful sites of bone metastasis, a newer form of "systemic" radiotherapy, Strontium-89, has proven beneficial (Bolger et al., 1993; Porter & McEwan, 1993; Porter et al., 1993).

Radiation-induced cystitis usually occurs during the first 2 to 3 weeks of therapy. Education by the nurse would include encouraging the patient to drink at least 2 L of fluid per day and explaining the benefits of antispasmodics and analgesics in decreasing the discomfort.

Nursing care of the patient with afterloading interstitial implants (^{192}Ir) should be done quickly to reduce radiation exposure to the nursing personnel; however, seed implants pose minimal risk. Provided that the patient's urine is promptly disposed of, there is no risk to others from ^{125}I radiation because this isotope's

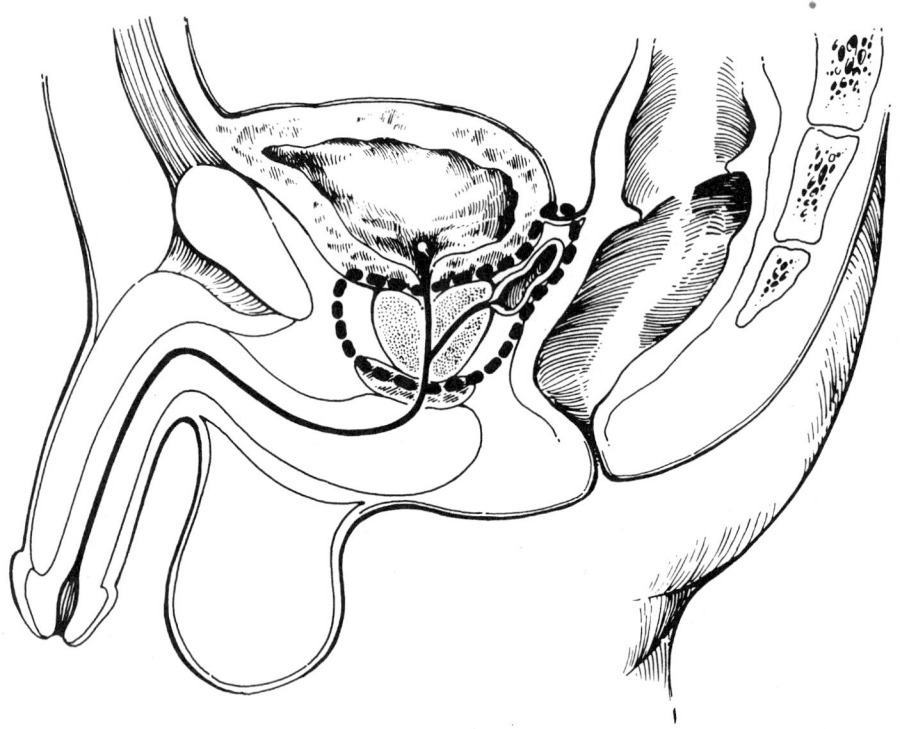

Figure 33–4. Surgical boundaries of a radical prostatectomy. (From Swanson, D. [1981]. Cancer of the bladder and prostate: The impact of therapy on sexual function. In A. von Eschenbach & D. Rodriguez [Eds.]. *Sexual rehabilitation of the urologic cancer patient* [p. 93]. Boston: G. K. Hall, Reproduced by permission.)

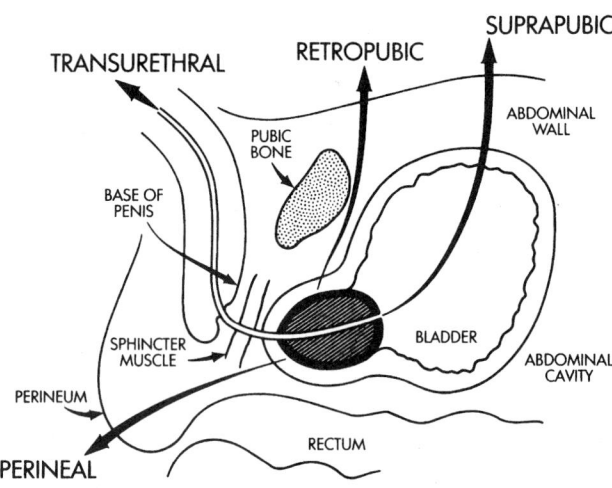

Figure 33–5. Surgical approaches to prostatectomy. (From Henrich-Rynning, T. [1987]. Prostatic cancer treatments and their effects on sexual functioning. *Oncology Nursing Forum, 14*[6], 39. Reproduced by permission.)

decay is by β emission. Patients are understandably concerned about radiation exposure, and every attempt should be made to provide reassurance for them and their families.

Chemotherapy. Chemotherapy plays a limited role in the treatment of advanced, hormonally unresponsive prostatic cancer (Dawson, 1993; Labrie, Belanger, Simard, Labrie, & Dupont, 1993; McLeod, Crawford, Blumenstein, & Eisenberger, 1992). Both single-agent and combination protocols have been attempted (Dawson, 1993; McLeod et al., 1992). Agents tested include cyclophosphamide, methotrexate, doxorubicin, 5-fluorouracil, cisplatin, vincristine, VP-16, prednisone, mel-

phalan, and estramustine (Dawson, 1993; McLeod et al., 1992). Suramin (a growth factor antagonist) has shown early promise but may be of only marginal long-term value (Dawson, 1993; Eisengerger et al., 1993; McLeod et al., 1992).

Hormonal Manipulation. Hormonal treatment of adenocarcinoma of the prostate is based on the assumption that prostatic carcinoma cells are to some degree androgen-dependent (Paulson, 1988b). Diminishing androgen availability or utilization will theoretically retard tumor growth (Rowland, Mitchell, Bihrle, Kahnoski, & Piser, 1987). Although this treatment is primarily indicated for patients with metastatic disease, it may also be considered for patients with localized cancer as well.

Current methods of hormone manipulation include (1) orchiectomy, (2) administration of estrogens, (3) administration of leutinizing hormone-releasing hormone (LH-RH) agonists, (4) administration of anti-androgens, (5) adrenalectomy, and (6) hypophysectomy (Dawson, 1993; Drago et al.,1983; Labrie et al, 1983; McConnell, 1991; McLeod et al., 1992).

Bilateral orchiectomy is the most definitive means of ablating the vast majority of circulating testosterone (Rohl & Beuke, 1992; McLeod et al., 1992). The subepididymal technique may be utilized to avoid the psychologic impact of castration (Gleen, 1990). Diethylstilbestrol (DES) was at one time the mainstay of medical therapy for arresting testicular production of testosterone. Significant side effects (thromboembolic disease and congestive heart failure) along with the development of newer, less potentially harmful medications have supplanted the use of DES (Dawson, 1993; Labrie et al., 1993). LH-RH agonists are currently enjoying tremendous popularity. By clinically inducing pituitary down regulation of LH production, the testicular stimulation to produce testosterone is abolished.

Drugs that affect the action of testosterone within the prostate cancer cell include cytoplasmic-receptor binding drugs (e. g., flutamide) and 5 α-reductase inhibitors (e. g., finesteride). Although somewhat controversial, each drug may potentiate the effect of hormone ablative therapy.

Persistent androgen stimulation from weak adrenal androgen production (androsterone, dehydroepiandrosterone) may be suppressed by a surgical or medical adrenalectomy (aminoglutethemide) (Dawson, 1993; Drago et al., 1983; Labrie et al., 1993; McLeod et al., 1992). Hypophepectomy (surgical removal of the pituitary) ablates both testicular and adrenal productions of androgens, but it is rarely used because of profound endocrine side effects.

The most significant nursing implications related to hormonal manipulation include patient teaching regarding the side effects of DES, particularly sodium retention, the potential for cardiac complications, and feminization effects (Lind & Nakao, 1987).

Recurrence and Palliative Treatment. Many prostatic cancers are advanced at the time of diagnosis or will advance during treatment (Dawson et al., 1992). Bone metastases to the vertebra, pelvis, femur, or ribs are very common. As curative treatments are not available, pain management is often an issue.

Endocrine manipulation (testosterone ablation) is the usual palliative treatment (Dawson, 1993; Dawson et al., 1992; Labrie et al., 1993; McLeod et al., 1992). Hormone resistance ultimately develops in this group.

Nursing management for patients with recurrent disease focuses on providing for pain relief, teaching the patient how to manage the side effects of hormonal therapy, and offering emotional support.

Patient Teaching Highlight. Throughout the various therapies for prostate cancer, alteration in sexual functioning can occur. Since sexuality is certainly a significant issue, patient teaching in this area is a priority (American Nurses Association and Oncology Nursing Society, 1987). Table 33–3 identifies changes in sexual functioning associated with specific therapies. See Chapter 62 for nursing interventions related to sexual functioning.

TABLE 33–3. *Current Therapies for Prostatic Neoplasm and Potential Side Effects on Sexual Functioning*

TREATMENT MODALITY	POTENTIAL SIDE EFFECTS that AFFECT SEXUALITY	NURSING INTERVENTIONS	CONCURRENT CHANGES ASSOCIATED WITH AGING
Surgery			**Physical Changes**
Perineal	Physiologic erectile dysfunction related to interruption of vasculature and innervation	Discuss alternate expressions of sexuality with patient and partner	Slower to achieve erections Slower to ejaculate Longer resolution phase/ refractory period
Retropubic and suprapubic	Psychologic erectile dysfunction related to fears or knowledge deficit and	Teaching, support, and referrals as indicated	Reduced force of ejaculation Reduced orgasmic sensation Diminished intensity and
Transurethral	Retrograde ejaculation related to bladder neck trauma	Teaching: "dry" ejaculation does not prevent a sexual relationship	duration of the localized vasocongestive processes Decreased fluid production Emotional changes
Radiation Therapy			
External beam	Temporary or permanent physiologic erectile dysfunction related to vascular or nerve damage Fatigue, diarrhea, cystitis, ejaculatory disturbances	Teaching, support Function may or may not return; may not even be impaired Reinforce positive attitude, alternate expressions of sexuality, manage symptoms	Many losses experienced: May involve significant or sexual partner, social status, financial status, roles Cultural devaluation
Seed implant	Less impact on impotence than external beam	Teaching, support	
Hormone Manipulation			
Orchiectomy	Decreased libido/sex drive related to decreased circulating testosterone Gynecomastia	Alternate expressions, mood enhancement, psychologic support	
Estrogen therapy and analogues	Decreased orgasmic experience erectile dysfunction	Gynecomastia is preventable with pre-irradiation of tissue	
Chemotherapy			
	Nausea, vomiting, fatigue other chemo side effects such as nervous system damage, body image change, and malaise	Symptom management Nursing support	

(Adapted with permission from Heinrich-Rynning, T. [1987]. Prostatic cancer treatments and their effects on sexual functioning. *Oncology Nursing Forum, 14*[6], 37–41.)

BLADDER CANCER

DEFINITION AND INCIDENCE

In the United States bladder cancer accounts for approximately 6 per cent of cancers in men and 2 per cent of all cancers in women. In 1994, the estimated new cases of bladder cancer in men is projected to be 38,000 and 13,200 in women. The total estimated deaths in men is 7000 and in women 3600 (American Cancer Society, 1994b). The greatest number appear on the mucosal lining of the bladder. The incidence of bladder cancer is four times greater in men than in women, and higher in the Caucasian population than in the African-American population (American Cancer Society, 1994b). Bladder cancer is a disease of the older population, with the peak seen in the seventh decade (Fair, Fuks, & Scher, 1993).

EPIDEMIOLOGY AND ETIOLOGY

Bladder cancer is more typically seen in urban areas. Geographic location accounts for a tenfold difference in incidence rates, with highest rates seen in North America, Scandinavia, and western Europe. In contrast, lower incidences are seen in Asia and eastern Europe (Pack, 1993).

Environmental factors associated with increased bladder cancer risk include occupational chemical exposure (aniline dye workers, truck drivers, and workers exposed to dye, rubber, leather, paint, aromatic amines, aluminum, and organic chemicals), cigarette smoking, chronic urinary tract infection history, chronic analgesic use, exposure to cytotoxic drugs, and radiation (Hossan & Striegel, 1993).

BIOLOGY AND NATURAL HISTORY

Most bladder cancers in the United States are transitional cell carcinomas (95 per cent) arising from the transitional epithelium of the mucosal lining. Within the classification of transitional cell carcinoma are the subdivisions of carcinoma in situ (confined to urothe-

lial lining), papillary noninfiltrating or infiltrating (tend to recur), and solid tumors. Less frequent types of bladder cancer include squamous cell (~5 per cent), adenocarcinomas (~1 per cent), and sarcomas (~3 per cent) (Sarosdy, 1993).

The most common staging systems used in the United States are the Jewett-Strong-Marshall System and the TNM (tumor, nodes, and metastases) system developed by Union International Contra Cancer (UICC) and the American Joint Committee on Cancer Staging. Both of these staging systems define the extent of disease by the depth of tumor infiltration, the presence or absence of nodal involvement, and the presence or absence of distant metastases. See Table 33–4 for a compilation of these systems.

If detected early, the five-year survival rate is 91 per cent, with regional disease 46 per cent and distant metastases 9 per cent (American Cancer Society, 1944b).

Presenting Signs and Symptoms. Gross hematuria is the most common presenting symptom. The hematuria is not necessarily associated with pain in 80 per cent of the patients presenting. Other symptoms include irritability of the bladder (dysuria, frequency, or urgency). Symptoms associated with large tumor growth may also be present. These symptoms may include edematous lower extremities, bowel habit changes, or flank, rectal, or pelvic pain.

Differential Diagnosis. In the evaluation of any patient with gross hematuria, an intravenous pyelogram (IVP) can help evaluate a suspected bladder tumor by possibly showing the tumor itself or by showing evidence of ureteral obstruction. Cystoscopy provides not only tumor visualization but also an opportunity to perform a biopsy and palpate the tumor. Urine cytology can help in the evaluation of those patients who have hematuria and are suspected of having a malignancy (Lieskovsky, Ahlering, & Skinner, 1988).

Nursing implications at the time of diagnosis include patient and family teaching about what to

TABLE 33–4. *Bladder Cancer Staging*

1946 JEWETT-STRONG	1952 JEWETT	1952 MARSHALL		1974, TNM CLINICAL	PATHOLOGICAL
		0	No tumor definitive specimen	T0	P0
			Carcinoma-in-situ	TIS	PIS
			Papillary tumor s̄ invasion		
A	A	A	Invasion lamina propria	T1	P1
B	B1	B1	Superficial	T2	P2
	B2	B2	Deep — Muscle invasion	T3A	
C	C	C	Invasion perivesical fat	T3B	P3
			Invasion contiguous viscera	T4A-B	P4
		D1	Pelvic nodes		N1-3
			Distant metastasis		M1
		D2	Nodes above aortic bifurcation		N4

(From deKernion, J. Bladder Cancer. In C. Haskell [Ed.], *Cancer treatment* [2nd ed., p. 371]. Philadelphia: W. B. Saunders Co.)

expect from the diagnostic tests. For example, patients may be anesthetized for cystoscopy. Following the procedure, patients are advised to drink plenty of fluids and to expect some hematuria. As another example, it is useful to know that urine cytology specimens are more reliable if they are not obtained as the first voided specimen of the day. If the specimens are not sent immediately for analysis, the urine should be refrigerated. A further nursing role involves clarifying test results for the patient and family. If cancer is found, they will need assistance in understanding their treatment options. It must be emphasized here that if cystectomy is indicated, choosing a setting for treatment with access to an enterostomal therapist is extremely important. The patient's future adjustment to treatment and his or her quality of life very well might depend on interactions with an enterostomal therapist.

TREATMENT

Surgery. Surgical therapy depends on the clinical stage of the tumor (Droller, 1993). For tumors that are confined to the mucosa or submucosa (0 to A) every effort is made to preserve the bladder. Therapy of these superficial lesions is generally transurethral resection or intravesical chemotherapy (e.g., Bacillus Calmette-Guérin [BCG]). More advanced (invasive) disease (stage B to C) is best managed by radical cystectomy and urinary diversion. The rare exception to this is when the lesion is solitary and located in the dome of the bladder, and specimens from random mucosal biopsies remote from the tumor are normal. In this case, a partial cystectomy can be considered. A thorough bilateral pelvic lymph node dissection should always be conducted for both diagnostic and therapeutic benefit

(Klein, 1992). Figure 33–6 and Figure 33–7 depict the appropriate surgical boundaries for men and women, respectively.

The method of urinary diversion associated with radical cystectomy may be an intestinal conduit (e.g., ileal, jejunal, or colonic), a continent urinary reservoir to the skin (e.g., Kock pouch or Indiana pouch), or an orthotopic neo-bladder (e.g., Hemi-kock or ileo-colonic neo-bladder). The conduits are relatively simple to construct and potentially minimize complications, but they require external urinary collection (Fig. 33–8) (Razor, 1993). The continent reservoirs are dry and inconspicuous and are of large capacity, but they are technically more difficult and time-consuming to create (Ahlering, Weinberg, & Razor, 1991; Freiha, 1990; Razor, 1993; Rowland et al., 1987; Skinner, Lieskovsky, & Boyd, 1988a; Studer, Ackermann, Casanova, & Zingg, 1988; Thuroff, Alken, Riedmiller, Jacobi, & Hofenfellner, 1988). The orthotopic neo-bladders require the most surgical expertise but allow the patient to volitionally void per urethra in the normal fashion (generally offered to male patients only) (Springer, Turner, & Studer, 1994; Thuroff et al., 1988).

A wide variety of techniques are available for the construction of continent urinary diversions, utilizing small or large bowel segments in their construction. The limits of this section do not allow comprehensive discussion of all available techniques, and readers are referred to specific texts on each method. Figures 33–9 and 33–10 depict one type of continent diversion (described by Kock) utilizing only ileum in its construction.

Ureterosigmoidostomy, a procedure in which the ureters are implanted into the sigmoid colon and urine

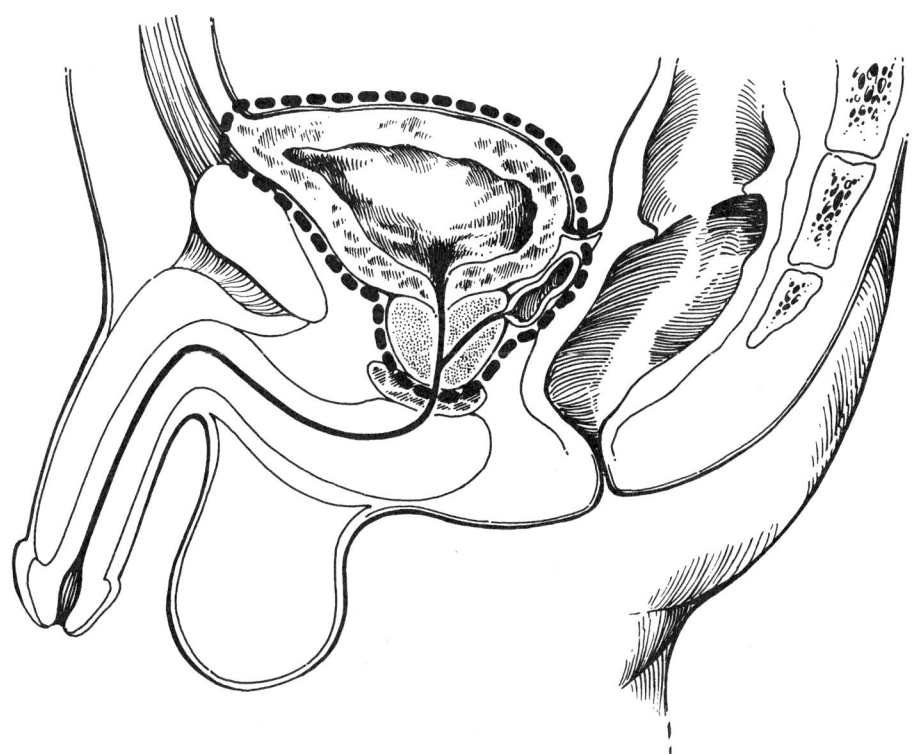

FIGURE 33–6. Surgical boundaries of a radical cystectomy in a man. (From Swanson, D. [1981]. Cancer of the bladder and prostate: The impact of therapy on sexual function. In A. von Eschenbach & D. Rodriguez [Eds.]. *Sexual rehabilitation of the urologic cancer patient* [p. 102]. Boston: G. K. Hall. Reproduced by permission.)

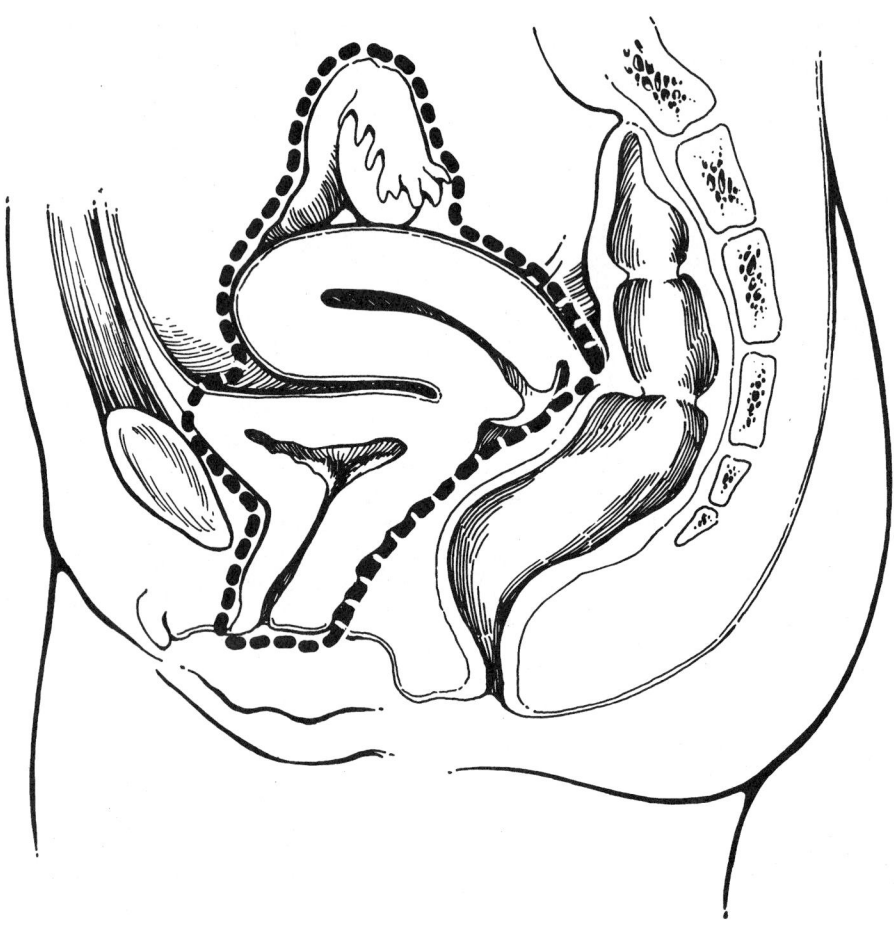

FIGURE 33-7. Surgical boundaries of a radical cystectomy in a woman. (From Swanson, D. [1981]. Cancer of the bladder and prostate: The impact of therapy on sexual function. In A. von Eschenbach & D. Rodriguez [Eds.] *Sexual rehabilitation of the urologic cancer patient* [p. 103]. Boston: G. K. Hall. Reproduced by permission.)

is then excreted through the rectum, is rarely done today.

Nursing Implications. Potential problems occurring in the first month after creation of an ileal conduit include wound infections, enteric fistulas, urine leaks, ureteral obstruction, bowel obstruction, and pelvic abscesses (Boyd, Lieskovsky, & Skinner, 1988). Late complications include stomal stenosis, peristomal hernias, chronic pyelonephritis, ureteroileal obstruction, intestinal obstruction, calculi, and metabolic problems with hyperchloremic acidosis.

Unlike a fecal diversion, the urinary diversion should produce urine from the time of surgery, and a urinary appliance is needed. Ideally, a urinary stoma should protrude 1.25 to 2 cm (0.5 to 0.75 inch) above the skin to allow the urine to drain into the aperture of an appliance (Lind & Nakao, 1987).

The color of the stoma should be checked frequently in the early postoperative period. Normal color is deep pink to dark red. A dusky appearance could indicate stoma necrosis.

Because the intestine normally produces mucus, mucus will be present in all urinary diversions that use bowel segments. Excessive mucus can, on occasion, clog the urinary appliance. Increasing fluid intake to 3 L per day will help.

Skin care and the pouching of the stoma are important nursing considerations. Several excellent sources describe these techniques (Broadwell & Jackson, 1982;

Lind & Nakao, 1987; Watt, 1986). Patient and family teaching is essential; it should begin early in the preoperative period and should be continually reinforced postoperatively. Concepts that should be emphasized include leakage prevention to protect peristomal skin, comfort and ease in handling the various pieces of equipment, early identification of kidney infections, and resources to call on when at home. Body image and sexuality issues should also be addressed. Postoperative teaching should not begin until the patient's physical discomfort has subsided and the physiologic state has stabilized. Enterostomal therapists are skilled specialists in technical matters and help the patient and family learn that a normal life is possible with an ileal conduit.

Complications after radical cystectomy with placement of a continent ileal reservoir, such as a Kock or Indiana pouch, include incontinence, difficult catheterization, urinary reflux, obstruction, bacteriuria, electrolyte imbalances, or absorptive deficits (Montie, MacGregor, Fazio, & Lavery, 1986).

Immediate postoperative nursing concerns for the patient who has had a Kock pouch include checking the stoma for ischemia and irrigating the Medina tube with normal saline solution to wash out both clots and mucus, which might plug the pouch (Lind & Nakao, 1987; Montie et al., 1986). Three to 4 weeks after the operation, when the Medina tube is removed, the nurse will teach the patient to perform self-catheterizations,

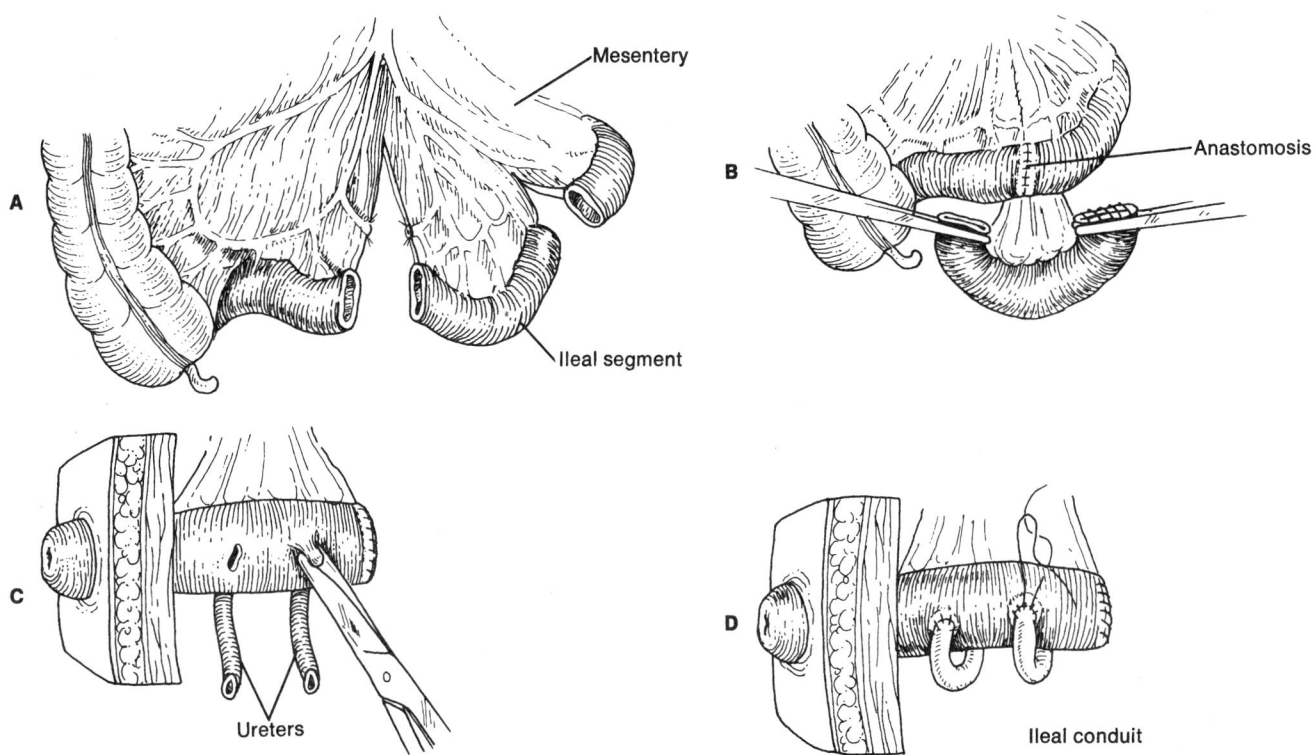

FIGURE 33–8. Ileal conduit. **A.** A segment of ileum is isolated from the gastrointestinal tract with its mesenteric blood flow. **B.** The gastrointestinal tract is reanastomosed. One end is sutured closed, and the other end will be used to form an abdominal stoma. **C.** The ureters, which are located retroperitoneally, are brought into the abdominal cavity. Incisions are made in the conduit for ureteral implantation. **D.** The abdominal stoma is matured, and the ureters are anastomosed to the ileum segment in an end-to-side fashion. (From Broadwell, D. C., & Jackson, B. S. [1982]. A primer: Definitions and surgical techniques. In D. C. Broadwell & B. S. Jackson [Eds.], *Principles of ostomy care* [p. 93]. St. Louis: C. V. Mosby Co. Reproduced by permission.)

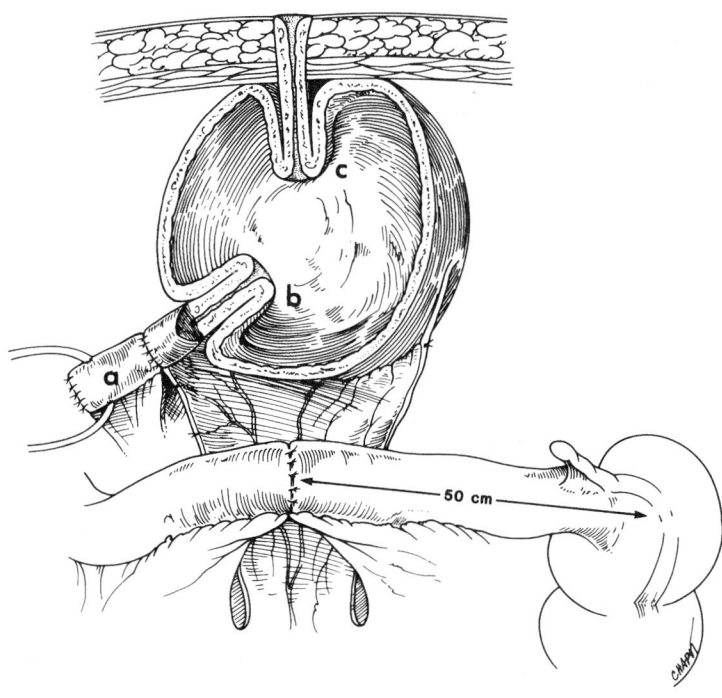

FIGURE 33–9. The continent ileal reservoir. *(a)* The original ileal conduit with implanted ureters. *(b)* The reflux-preventing nipple valve. *(c)* The continence-maintaining nipple valve. (From Gerber, A. [1983]. The Kock continent ileal reservoir for supravesical urinary diversion. *American Journal of Surgery, 146,* 16. Reproduced by permission.)

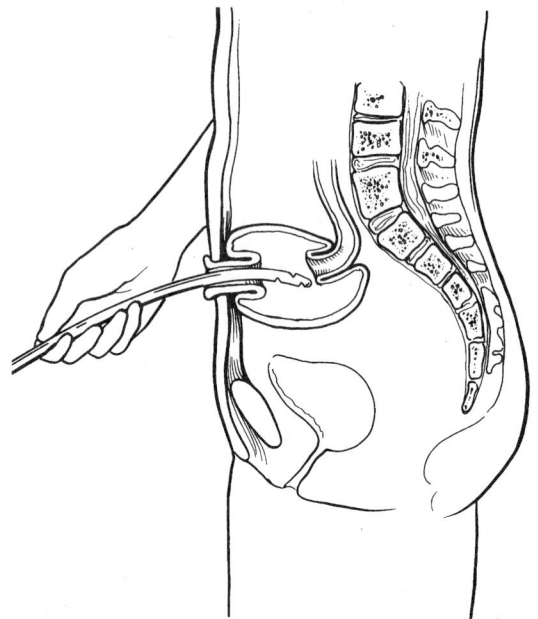

FIGURE 33–10. Emptying the continent ileal reservoir. (From Monhe., J. E., MacGregor, P. S., Fazio, V. W., & Lavery, I. [1986]. Continent ileal reservoir [Kock pouch]. *Urology Clinics of North America, 13,* 254. Reproduced by permission.)

first every 2 to 3 hours and then every 4 to 6 hours during the day and once at night (Lind & Nakao, 1987; Skinner, Boyd, & Lieskovsky, 1984). Figure 33–10 shows the method of emptying the pouch. With a continent ileal reservoir, there is no need for an external appliance, and intubation of the pouch can duplicate normal bladder function.

A radical cystectomy with urinary diversion affects many aspects of sexual function. The cause of erectile dysfunction after radical cystectomy is similar to that associated with radical prostatectomy for prostatic cancer. However, patients can still achieve orgasm (Schover, von Eschenbach, Smith, & Gónzalez, 1984). Because the prostate and seminal vesicles are removed, men experience dry orgasms without emission of semen but still have normal muscle contractions (Schover, Evans, & von Eschenbach, 1986). Women may experience some physiologic problems during intercourse as a result of a shortened vagina. The reader is referred to Chapter 62 for further information on sexual counseling.

Radiation Therapy. Radiation therapy plays a limited role in the treatment of bladder cancer. Definitive radiotherapy in bladder cancer is generally reserved for patients who are not candidates for surgery (Skinner & Lieskovsky, 1988b). Radiation therapy for curative intent has only marginal (15 per cent) efficacy (Freiha, 1990). However, outside the United States, invasive bladder cancer is frequently treated primarily by radiotherapy (Duncan & Quilty, 1986).

Neo-adjuvant preoperative (e.g., 1600 to 2000 Gy) radiation therapy was previously advocated to decrease the possibility of tumor spread during surgery but is no longer deemed necessary (Freiha, 1990). Postoperative radiation following intraoperative tumor spillage may be beneficial.

Laser surgery to treat superficial and invasive disease has been attempted. Neodymium YAG has shown the ability to eradicate selected B1 and B2 lesions (Smith, 1986).

Complications of radiotherapy include radiation enteritis or colitis and skin reactions. See Chapter 20 for a discussion of nursing care of radiation complications.

Chemotherapy. Intravesical and systemic chemotherapy are currently used depending on the stage of the bladder cancer under treatment.

For superficial, low-grade disease, the goal of intravesical chemotherapy (direct instillation of drugs into the bladder) is twofold. It may be used to treat known superficial lesions or more commonly to diminish the recurrence rate following transurethral resection of superficial lesions. BCG has the greatest efficacy and is currently the drug most commonly used (Lum & Torti, 1991). The mechanism of action is not fully understood. Nursing implications include assessment of lower urinary tract irritative symptoms, handling precautions while the BCG is being instilled, disposal precautions, and teaching the patient to recognize and report symptoms of hematuria, fever, lethargy, and malaise.

Thiotepa, mitomycin C, and doxorubicin (Adriamycin) have also been used (Herr, 1987; Smith, Chisholm, Newsom, & Hargreave, 1986).

Systemic chemotherapy (single agent and combination programs) has been advocated for extensive local disease as a method of downstaging prior to surgical extirpation and also for organ preservation in the presence of invasive disease (Herr et al., 1990). Both techniques are still considered investigational at this time and should only be used in carefully selected patients.

Nursing implications include assessment of myelosuppression symptomology and chemical cystitis (thiotepa, mitomycin C), rash occurring on the palms or genitalia (mitomycin C), and patient teaching regarding symptom recognition and reporting (Hossan & Streigel, 1993).

Recurrence and Palliative Treatment. Superficial bladder cancer recurrences are common and are best managed by repeated transurethral resection. Frequent recurrence may be inhibited by intravesical chemotherapy. Invasive bladder tumors spread rapidly to the regional lymph nodes and by direct extension into the adjacent structures. About 50 per cent of patients with high-stage, high-grade tumor will have relapses after definitive treatment (Skinner et al., 1991).

Combination chemotherapy is the treatment of choice for metastatic bladder cancer (Ahmed, Yagoda, & Needles, 1985). The most effective combination of drugs includes methotrexate, vincristine, adriamycin, and cisplatin (MVAC) (Skinner et al., 1991; Sternberg et al., 1988). Modifications of this regimen would take into consideration the specific side effects of each drug. Nursing management of the side effects of high doses of cisplatin and doxorubicin is challenging. Nausea and vomiting, renal toxicity, ototoxicity, myelosuppression, and the potential for extravasation all must be considered. See Chapters 21 and 22 for a more in-depth discussion of these side effects and their nursing implications.

TESTICULAR CANCER

DEFINITION AND INCIDENCE

Testicular cancer is a disease of the testes that arises from embryonal tissue. This germ tissue provides the root for the term "germ cell" or "germinal," which describe most testicular cancers. This disease usually occurs in only one testis; 2 to 3 per cent occur bilaterally either simultaneously or successively (Richie, 1993a). Testicular cancer occurs in approximately 1 per cent of American men each year, and it is estimated that 7100 new cases of testis cancer will be diagnosed in 1995 (Wingo Tong, & Bolden, 1995). Although it can occur at any age, cancer of the testis occurs primarily in young men between the ages of 15 and 34 (National Cancer Institute, 1988). Because these men are so young, they are very concerned with sexuality and reproductive issues. Fortunately, progress in treatment has contributed to successful outcomes and high cure rates (National Cancer Institute, 1990). Testicular cancer is potentially curable and has a 5-year survival rate of approximately 90 per cent (Brock et al., 1993).

EPIDEMIOLOGY AND ETIOLOGY

Testicular cancer is the leading cause of cancer in American men between the ages of 20 and 34 (National Cancer Institute, 1990). Cancer of the testes is also seen in men over age 60. In the United States, cancer of the testes is much more common among white men than African-American men and less common among Hispanics, American Indians, and Asians. Approximately 0.2 per cent of American men will develop testicular cancer during their lifetime (Richie, 1993a).

The actual cause(s) of testicular cancer is unknown at this time, although there are some known risk factors. One such factor, cryptorchidism, the failure of one or both testes to descend into the scrotal sac, occurs in 10 per cent of the patients who develop cancer of the testis (National Cancer Institute, 1990). Other abnormalities have been linked to cancer of the testicles. These include chromosomal abnormalities such as Klinefelter's syndrome, as well as abnormalities in the prenatal development of the reproductive tract (National Cancer Institute, 1990). These abnormalities include gonadal aplasia and varying forms of hermaphroditism. Additionally, there may also be some relationship to infectious diseases or scrotal injuries, but these have not been confirmed to date (National Cancer Institute, 1990). At one time it was believed that exposure to DES prior to birth was a contributing factor, but studies have not shown that exposure to DES increases the risk of testicular cancer (National Cancer Institute, 1990).

BIOLOGY AND NATURAL HISTORY

Ninety-five per cent of testicular tumors arise from the germ cell (Richie, 1993a). These germ cell cancers are usually malignant and can be classified as seminomas or nonseminomas. These types differ both in their tendency to spread and their reaction to treatment. Less than 5 per cent of testicular tumors arise from stromal tissue, primarily Leydig cell and Sertoli cell tumors (Skarin, 1991). Table 33–5 provides additional details about these tumors.

Many tumors, however, are mixed and contain several distinct elements. There are several staging systems used for cancer of the testis. Two of the most common (Richie, 1988) are described in Table 33–6. A TNM system is also used (Table 33–7).

Patients usually have a painless swelling in one gonad, which is described as a lump or hardness and sometimes a heaviness or dull aching in the scrotum or lower abdomen (Richie, 1993a). Although the mass is usually irregular and hard, a smooth mass should be evaluated promptly.

Once there is a palpable nodule within the testis, local involvement or metastasis can occur either lymphatically or via the hematogenous route. More than half the patients with nonseminomatous tumor have disseminated disease at first presentation. Direct invasion of the inguinal or retroperitoneal lymph nodes may also occur. Metastasis to the lungs, bone, or liver may occur via hematogenous spread. Generally, germ cell tumors have a high growth rate. Survival time is related to the stage at presentation and the amount of tumor burden present (Richie, 1993a).

Acute pain is present in about 10 per cent of patients (Richie, 1993a). In 10 per cent of patients, pre-

TABLE 33–5. *Primary Tumors of the Testis*

HISTOLOGIC CLASSIFICATION	CHARACTERISTICS
Germinal Neoplasms	95% of total
Seminomas	Most common type; 30–40% of all testicular tumors; slow growing
Typical (classic)	85% of all seminomas
Anaplastic	10% of all seminomas
Spermatocytic	10% of all seminomas
Nonseminomatous	More aggressive than seminomas; 60–70% of patients with non-seminomas at diagnosis have lymph node spread
Embryonal carcinoma	Highly malignant; 20–25% of all testicular tumors
Choriocarcinoma	Secretes chorionic gonadotropin (Garnic et al., 1990); 1–3% of all nonseminomatous
Teratoma	5–10% of all nonseminomatous
Yolk sac tumor	Most common testicular tumor of infants and children. In adults, may be responsible for production of α-fetoprotein (AFP)
Nongerminal Neoplasms	5% of total

TABLE 33–6. *Staging of Testicular Tumors*

Walter Reed General Hospital*	Skinner†
IA: Confined to testis; no clinical or radiographic evidence of spread	A: Same, but includes no positive nodes on node dissection
IB: Same as IA, but at lymph node dissection metastases to iliac or para-aortic lymph nodes are found	B: Disease below diaphragm, normal mediastinum, normal chest radiograph
II: Disease below diaphragm, with no spread to visceral organs: clinical or radiographic evidence of metastases to para-aortic, femoral, inguinal, and iliac lymph nodes	B1: < 6 positive nodes that are well encapsulated and show no extension into retroperitoneal fat
II+: Palpable abdominal	B2: > 6 positive nodes that are encapsulated and may or may not show extension into retroperitoneal fat; any node > 2 cm
	B3: Bulky, palpable mass (≥ 5 cm) abdominal mass (> 5 cm)
III: Disease above diaphragm or spread to body organs (clinical radiograph)	C: Metastases above diaphragm or liver involvement

*From Maier, J. E., & Sulak, M. H. (1973). Proceedings: Radiation therapy in malignant testis tumors. II. Carcinoma. *Cancer, 32,* 1212–1216.

†From Skinner, D. G. (1969). Non-seminomatous testis tumors: A plan of management based on 96 patients to improve survival in all stages by combined therapeutic modalities. *Journal of Urology, 115,* 65–69.

(From Richie, J. [1988]. Diagnosis and staging of testicular cancer. In D. G. Skinner & G. Lieskovsky [Eds.], *Diagnosis and management of genitourinary cancer* [p. 501]. Philadelphia: W. B. Saunders Co. Reproduced by permission.)

TABLE 33–7. *TNM Staging of Testicular Tumors*

Primary Tumor (T)

TX	Minimal requirements cannot be met (in the absence of orchiectomy, TX must be used)
T0	No evidence of primary tumor
T1	Tumor limited to body of the testis
T2	Tumor extends beyond the tunica albuginea
T3	Involvement of the rete testis or epididymis
T4A	Invasion of the spermatic cord
T4B	Invasion of the scrotal wall

Nodal Involvement (N)

NX	Minimum requirements cannot be met
N0	No evidence of involvement of regional lymph nodes
N1	Involvement of a single homolateral regional lymph node, which, if inguinal, is mobile
N2	Involvement of contralateral or bilateral or multiple regional lymph nodes, which, if inguinal, are mobile
N3	Palpable abdominal mass present or fixed inguinal lymph nodes
N4	Involvement of juxtaregional nodes

Distant Metastasis (M)

MX	Not assessed
M0	No (known) distant metastasis
M1	Distant metastasis present

(From Beahrs, O. H., & Myers, M. H. [Eds.]. [1983]. *Manual for staging of cancer* [2nd ed. p. 166–167]. Philadelphia: J. B. Lippincott Co. Reproduced by permission.)

senting symptoms may be due to metastasis and may include a neck mass, respiratory symptoms, GI disturbance, or lumbar back pain.

Survival from testicular cancer has improved dramatically in recent years. The overall 5-year survival is 89 per cent in whites and 78 per cent in African-Americans (Silverberg & Lubera, 1989). Patients with early-stage seminomas treated by radiotherapy experience a 5-year survival of more than 90 per cent (Graham & Bagshaw, 1983). The cumulative survival rate for stage II disease is 69 per cent (Smith, 1988). In later stages the prognosis is not as favorable.

Stage I nonseminomatous tumors have a reported 5-year survival of 99 per cent; stage II has a survival of 95 per cent (Fraley, Narayan, Vogelzang, Kennedy, & Lange, 1985). Patients with disseminated nonseminomatous tumors have a long-term survival of approximately 70 per cent (Einhorn, 1988).

Presenting Signs and Symptoms. Two thirds of patients have a history of painless enlargement of the testes. Other symptoms include a dragging sensation in the scrotum and rarely a painful mass due to intratesticular bleeding. Symptoms related to spread of the disease include abdominal fullness, lower extremity edema, lumbar pain, and abdominal or supraclavicular pain caused by enlarged lymph nodes. Gynecomastia can occur due to high levels of chorionic gonadotrophin (Keller, Sahasrabudhe, & McCune, 1993).

Differential Diagnosis. Epididymitis and hydrocele both occasionally mimic the symptoms of testis cancer. The differential diagnosis usually includes testicular torsion, epididymitis, or epididymal orchitis. Hydrocele, hernias, hematomas, or spermatoceles might also mimic testicular tumors (Richie, 1993a). According to Richie, "in any patient with a solid, firm intratesticular mass within the tunica albuginea, testicular cancer must be the considered diagnosis until proven otherwise" (Richie, 1993a, p. 157).

Ultrasonography is helpful as an imaging study, as it can demonstrate whether a mass is intratesticular or extratesticular. It is in the patients with intratesticular tumors that testicular cancer must be the diagnosis until proven otherwise (Richie, 1993a). Table 33–8 lists the procedures commonly used to diagnose testicular cancer.

The laboratory studies determining AFP and hCG-β are used as preoperative tumor markers, and because they reflect the clinical course of the disease, they are very important in the staging of testicular cancer (Horwich & Peckham, 1986; Johnson, Swanson & von Eschenbach, 1987).

Elevated serum AFP levels are never seen in men with *pure* seminomas and therefore help to indicate the

TABLE 33–8. *Procedures Used to Diagnose Testicular Cancer*

Manual palpation of testes and surrounding structures
Radical inguinal orchiectomy (as biopsy)
Radiologic techniques
    Chest radiograph (for lung metastases)
    Computed tomographic (CT) scan of chest (detects lung metastases)
    Abdominal and pelvic CT scan (detects retro-peritoneal nodes)
    Excretory urogram
Laboratory studies
    Serum α-fetaprotein (AFP)
    Serum human chorionic gonadotropin-β subunit (hCG-β)

presence of a nonseminomatous testicular tumor. Because liver damage can also produce elevated AFP levels, hepatotoxicity from chemotherapy or radiotherapy should be ruled out.

About 50 to 60 per cent of patients with nonseminomatous testicular tumors will have an elevated hCG-β level, and occasionally patients with pure seminomas will also have elevated levels of hCG (Richie, 1988). hCG is normally produced only in pregnant women.

Nursing implications regarding detection of testicular cancer should include educating the public about testicular self-examination (TSE) (American Cancer Society, 1988). A 1986 report stated that a moderate percentage of professional men had knowledge of TSE but that very few practiced it. Nurses need to participate in teaching individuals about testicular cancer and the importance of performing TSE on a regular basis.

Patient and family education is another important nursing function. Young, otherwise healthy young men with testicular cancer need help in understanding their treatment and its sequelae. They especially need help with their sexuality and body image concerns. The psychosocial dynamics may also be complex. Independent young adults are often forced to be dependent again on their parents. Nurses can help both the young men and their parents to adjust to the situation.

The diagnostic procedures to be completed may add to the many concerns that the patient might have at this time. After assessing the knowledge level and the patient's desire for information, adequate explanations about specific tests and their significance should be given to the patient. Pertinent questions should be addressed to allay fears and anxieties. Preoperative teaching such as coughing and deep breathing, ambulation, and pain management should begin when initial arrangements are made for the surgery.

TREATMENT FOR SEMINOMATOUS TUMORS

Surgery. High radical inguinal orchiectomy, in which the testis, the epididymis, a portion of the vas deferens, and portions of the gonadal lymphatics and blood supply are removed, is routinely done as a diagnostic step and therapeutic modality.

The orchiectomy has no defined adverse effect on sexual potency or fertility in the otherwise normal patient, as the remaining testicle is still functional. Studies, however, have shown that many testis cancer patients have lower sperm counts even before any treatment is instituted (Lange, Chang, & Fraley, 1987).

Radiotherapy. Seminomas are extremely radiosensitive. Radiation therapy to the retroperitoneum is the treatment of choice for stages A, B, and B2 disease. Although more advanced disease (e.g., B3, C) has been treated in the past with additional radiation therapy to the mediastinum and supraclavicular areas, chemotherapy is currently the preferred treatment for these patients.

Complications associated with pelvic irradiation include fatigue, diarrhea, and possible azoospermia. The seminiferous tubules are extremely sensitive to radiation, and damage may result from as little as 8 to 50 cGy.

Nursing implications include teaching the patient and family to manage the side effects of radiotherapy and providing information on sexuality issues. Common side effects include nausea, vomiting, diarrhea, myelosuppression, and azoospermia. The mild nausea and vomiting can be controlled with antiemetics. Myelosuppression is usually mild and lasts about 4 to 6 weeks.

Chemotherapy. Seminomas are also chemosensitive. Patients with advanced seminoma (stage B3 and C) are candidates for chemotherapy with or without radiation therapy to the pelvis. Most protocols use a combination of cisplatin, etoposide, and bleomycin (Wettlaufer, 1990). Because this protocol is essentially the same for nonseminomatous testicular cancers, the reader is referred to that section for complications and nursing implications.

TREATMENT FOR NONSEMINOMATOUS TUMORS

Surgery. As presented in the discussion of seminomatous tumors, high radical inguinal orchiectomy is both diagnostic and therapeutic. The role of retroperitoneal lymph node dissection in the treatment of nonseminomatous germ cell testicular tumors (NSGCTT) is quite controversial (Herr, Toner, Geller, & Bosi, 1991). Prior to effective chemotherapy, the principal treatments for NSGCTT were surgery and radiation, neither of which were effective for advanced disease. Today, with the availability of more effective chemotherapy, the emphasis has shifted to the reduction in treatment morbidity.

Advocates of retroperitoneal lymph node dissection (RPLND) believe that this procedure facilitates accurate clinical staging and may obviate the need for potentially toxic chemotherapy in selected patients (Fraley et al., 1985). Others find that the benefit would only affect a few patients and that many would be subjected to the risks and side effects of this procedure unnecessarily (Bihrle, Donohue, & Foster, 1988; Richie, 1993b).

Improvements in the understanding of retroperitoneal anatomy and the specific retroperitoneal lymph node regions at highest risk for metastatic involvement have allowed for nerve-sparing lymph node dissections and subsequent preservation of ejaculatory function, potentially allowing more patients to appreciate its benefits (Donohue, Foster, Rowland, Bihrle, Jones, & Geier, 1990; Foster & Donohue, 1993a, 1993b).

Nursing implications after RPLND include observation for infection and bleeding immediately after the operation and later patient education regarding sexuality.

Radiotherapy. Because nonseminomatous germ cell tumors are relatively radioresistant, radiotherapy is not routinely used in the United States to treat these tumors.

Chemotherapy. The identification of effective chemotherapeutic agents has been the single most important factor in the astounding overall cure rates with NSGCTT. In 1974, studies were begun at Indiana University using a combination of cisplatin, vinblastine, and bleomycin (PVB). The remarkable results have revolutionized the treatment of testicular cancer. Cure rates for all stages of testicular cancer now exceed 85 per cent.

However, the PVB regimen is highly toxic. Nausea, vomiting, leukopenia, sepsis, and cisplatin-induced nephrotoxicity are common. Raynaud's phenomenon is also a long-term side effect associated with vinblastine therapy.

An improvement in this regimen is the substitution of etoposide for vinblastine. The efficacy of cisplatin, etoposide, and bleomycin (PEB) combination therapy matches the previous PVB combination but diminishes the toxic side effects (Williams & Einhorn, 1982). PEB now represents the standard for testicular cancer chemotherapy. Although other forms of combination chemotherapy (e.g., vinblastine, actinomycin D, cyclophosphamide and cisplatin, the VAB regimen) have been tried, none has shown the overall efficacy of PEB.

Because the majority of patients with NSGCTT are being cured of their malignancy, the focus has turned to diminishing long-term side effects. As side effects are often dose-related, efforts are underway to minimize the amount of chemotherapy rendered without sacrificing the therapeutic benefit.

Nursing implications for those men treated with chemotherapy are specifically related to the significant side effects of the PVB and the VAB regimens. See Chapters 21 and 22 for nursing management of the side effects of cisplatin, bleomycin, vinblastine, actinomycin D, and cyclophosphamide.

Sexuality is also an important nursing concern. These young men are concerned with issues of fertility and sexual potency. Education, information about sperm banking, and emotional support are critical to this patient population.

Recurrence and Palliative Treatment. Testicular cancer spreads to the retroperitoneal lymph nodes, to the lungs, and rarely to the brain and liver (Ghosn et al., 1988).

In tumors that have been refractory to the PEB regimen, the substitution of ifosfamide for bleomycin (a dose-limited drug) may be beneficial (Goldiner & Schweizer, 1979). The etoposide (VP-16), ifosfamide, cisplatin (VIP) protocol has "salvaged" some patients after PEB failure (Ghosn et al., 1988). Of additional current interest is the use of extremely high-dose cisplatin-based combination chemotherapy with autologous bone marrow rescue. It is too soon to state the actual therapeutic value of this form of treatment.

Nursing implications for late-stage disease are directed primarily toward relieving the side effects associated with chemotherapy. Emotional support for the patients and families is also very important. This disease affects primarily young men, and the family might include wife, small children, and siblings as well as parents. Concern for all of the members of the family will be an important nursing consideration.

CANCER OF THE KIDNEY

DEFINITION AND INCIDENCE

In 1994 the estimated new cases of kidney and other urinary organ cancer (excludes bladder, prostate, and testicular) in males was 17,000 and in females 10,600. The estimated death rate in males was 6800 and was 4500 in females (American Cancer Society, 1994b). Kidney cancer is not a common cancer and accounts for only about 2 per cent of all cancers. Renal cell cancer, which occurs in the parenchyma of the kidney, is also known as renal adenocarcinoma, renal cell carcinoma, cancer of the kidney, and hypernephroma. Renal cell cancer accounts for 85 per cent of all kidney tumors and is the only type of kidney cancer discussed in this chapter.

EPIDEMIOLOGY AND ETIOLOGY

There is a 2-to-1 male predominance in kidney cancer. This disease occurs mostly in persons aged 50 to 70 years of age (Linehan, Shipley, & Parkinson, 1993).

The rate of renal cell cancer is highest in Scandinavian countries, parts of France, and the United States. Lowest incidence rates are found in Latin America and Asia (Pack, 1993).

Etiologic relevant factors in the development of kidney cancer include exposure to petrochemical products, smoking of tobacco products, chewing tobacco, obesity, and high dietary fat intake. An autosomal-dominant disorder called Von Hippel-Lindau disease suggests an inherited susceptibility to kidney cancer. Bilateral kidney involvement results from this disorder, with identical abnormalities observed in both kidneys (Davis, 1993).

BIOLOGY AND NATURAL HISTORY

The most common type of kidney cancer is renal cell adenocarcinoma, accounting for 75 per cent of all kidney cancers. Three different subtypes arise from the epithelium of the distal portion of the proximal renal tubule. These subtypes are (1) clear cell (hypernephroma), (2) granular cell, and (3) spindle or sarcomatoid variant. Transitional cell carcinoma commonly occurs in the renal pelvis but is also seen in the kidney (Davis, 1993). Table 33–9 describes the staging system for cancer of the kidney.

Presenting Signs and Symptoms. Gross hematuria is the most common presenting symptom in approximately 56 per cent of patients with renal cell cancer. Pain, described as a dull, aching flank pain, is present

TABLE 33–9. *TNM Staging for Renal Cancer*

CLASSIFICATION	CRITERIA
T1	Small tumor (< 2.5 cm) no enlargement of kidney
T2	Large tumor (> 2.5 cm) cortex not broken
T3	Perinephric or hilar extension Venous involvement
T4	Extension to neighboring organs
N1	Single homolateral regional (< 2cm)
N2	Contra- or bilateral/multiple regional
N3	Fixed regional
N4	Juxtaregional
M0	No metastasis
M1	Distant metastasis

STAGE	GROUPING			5-YEAR SURVIVAL RATE
Stage I	T1	N0	M0	75%
Stage II	T2	N0	M0	60%
Stage III	T3	N0	M0	40%
Stage IV	T4	N0	M0	5%
	Any T	N1,2,3,4	M0	
	Any T	Any N	M1	

(From Tobias, J., & Williams, C. J. [1991]. *Cancer slide atlas—gynaecological cancer/genitourinary cancer* [Vol. 5, p. 151]. London: Gower Medical Publishing.)

in approximately 38 per cent of cases, and finally, a palpable abdominal mass can also be noted on presentation in 36 per cent of cases (Keller et al., 1993). It is rare for these three symptoms, the "classic triad," to appear simultaneously (10 per cent of cases) (Sarosdy, 1993). A wide variety of other vague symptoms also are seen, including fever, weight loss, anemia, and hypercalcemia, which occur infrequently.

Differential Diagnosis. The differential diagnosis is that of a renal mass, most commonly renal cysts and renal tumors. Diagnosis is usually made radiographically because of the variety of presenting symptoms and nonspecific laboratory findings. The advent of renal ultrasound and CT scanning has greatly simplified making the distinction between simple cysts and renal cancer. In many cases, renal angiography is no longer necessary. Tests used in the diagnosis and staging of renal cell cancer include the following: kidneys, ureters, bladder radiograph (KUB), excretory urogram (IVP), nephrotomogram, renal sonogram, renal CT scan, and renal angiogram.

The role of magnetic resonance imaging (MRI) is not yet determined. It does not appear to be better than CT in identifying regional or metastatic disease (Paulson, 1987).

Nursing implications involve education about the nature of the diagnostic tests. Allaying misunderstandings about the implications of losing a kidney might also be important.

TREATMENT

Surgery. Radical nephrectomy is the treatment of choice for localized renal cell cancer including malig-

nancies with tumor extension into the renal vein and vena cava. The radical nephrectomy includes removal of the kidney, the ipsilateral adrenal gland, and the perinephric fat.

Regional retroperitoneal lymph node dissection is often routinely performed during a radical nephrectomy, although there are no solid data supporting its use in improving survival (Skinner et al., 1988a).

Nursing implications during the immediate postoperative period include pain management and prevention of postoperative complications. Pain can be quite severe after nephrectomy. As a result of the position on the operating table, the patient experiences not only incisional pain but also muscular strain. Use of moist heat, massage, and pillows to support the back while the patient is lying on his or her side can provide relief.

Postoperative nursing interventions include prevention of atelectasis and pneumonia, monitoring renal function of the remaining kidney, anticipating paralytic ileus, monitoring for bleeding, and preventing infection at the incision site.

Radiotherapy. Most renal cell tumors are radioresistant. Although various trials have utilized preoperative or postoperative radiotherapy, neither has demonstrated any long-term benefit. Currently there is no definite role for the use of radiation therapy in the treatment of the primary renal malignancy itself (Paulson, 1987).

Chemotherapy. There is no effective chemotherapy for renal cell carcinoma. Hormonal therapy (e.g., tamoxifen) has also demonstrated little efficacy.

Immunotherapy. As traditional treatment of disseminated disease (chemotherapy and radiotherapy) is ineffective for renal cell cancer, immunotherapy has been explored as a possible treatment modality. Interferon (IFN) and interleukins (IL-2) are cytokines that have been studied to date. Cytokines are proteins elaborated by cells in response to antigenic stimulation, that affect other cells. IFN has an overall response rate of 16 per cent (Belldegrun, Figlin, Danella, & deKernion, 1992). IL-2 is produced by T lymphocytes and stimulates sensitive lymphocytes to become lymphokine activated killer (LAK) cells. Response has been 18 per cent (Belldegrun et al., 1992). In combination, IFN/IL-2 regimens have resulted in response rate of up to 31 per cent (Belldegrun et al., 1992). The passive transfer of immunotherapy (adoptive immunotherapy) to the tumor-bearing host has been explored utilizing tumor-infiltrating lymphocytes (TIL) (Belldegrun et al., 1992). Although early results of TIL therapy were quite impressive, the overall response rate does not vary greatly from the results of IFN or IL-2 treatment (Belldegrun et al., 1992).

While the side effects of IFN and TIL therapy are manageable, the side effects of IL-2 therapy have been very serious indeed, including but not limited to malaise, fever, hepatic dysfunction, thrombocytopenia, somnolence, disorientation, pulmonary edema, respiratory distress, and even myocardial infarction (Belldegrun et al., 1992).

Nursing implications associated with this experimental therapy include extensive patient education and support and intensive monitoring of the severe side effects, such as hypotension, fever, hepatic dysfunction, thrombocytopenia, and disorientation or somnolence.

The prognosis for patients with metastatic renal cell cancer may be brightening through the use of innovative forms of immunotherapy.

Recurrence and Palliative Treatment. Over 30 per cent of patients have metastases at the time of initial diagnosis. Lung, bone, brain, and liver are common sites of metastasis.

Nephrectomy for palliation is done infrequently. Anecdotal reports of metastatic disease regression after treatment are captivating but inconclusive (Skinner, Pritchett, Lieskovsky, Boyd, & Stiles, 1989). Although local bleeding, pain, and fever can be managed by nephrectomy, other less invasive techniques (angiographic infarction) and conservative observation are currently preferred (Elson, 1994).

Chemotherapy has no great impact on metastatic renal cell cancer (Belldegrun et al., 1992).

Hormonal therapy including tamoxifin, provera, and megace have few side effects but are not very effective and thus of little import at this time.

Radiation therapy for localized symptomatic metastasis (e.g., bone) is quite beneficial for palliation but does not change the overall prognosis.

Immunotherapy as described above is promising and is currently our greatest hope in the treatment of metastatic renal cell cancer.

SUMMARY

Cancers of the genitourinary system affect patients, particularly men, of all ages. Depending upon the primary site, treatment is quite varied; patient outcomes are directly related to histology and stage of disease at the time of diagnosis, treatment utilized, and patient education provided by the nurse. Testicular cancer in particular has been one of the true cancer treatment success stories of this decade. Progress has also been made with the treatment of bladder and prostate cancer. Successful treatment for renal cell cancer continues to elude the health care profession.

Genitourinary cancers represent an area in which the nurse plays a crucial role in terms of patient education related to screening and early detection. This should be done for patients of all ages. Patient education continues to be a critical component of any treatment or maintenance regimen (radiotherapy, chemotherapy, surgery) and is certainly a critical element of postoperative care. Because these patients cross the life span continuum, issues are specific to disease and treatment being considered/conducted. The nursing management challenges offered by these patients are many and unique. The outcomes are equally rewarding to nurses.

REFERENCES

Ahlering, T. E., Weinberg, A. C., & Razor, B. (1991). Modified Indiana pouch. *The Journal of Urology, 145,* 1156–1158.

Ahmed, T., Yagoda, A., & Needles, B. (1985). Vinblastine and methotrexate for advanced bladder cancer. *Journal of Urology, 133,* 602–604.

American Cancer Society. (1988). *Facts on testicular cancer.* Atlanta: American Cancer Society.

American Cancer Society. (1994a). *Facts & figures-1994.* Atlanta: American Cancer Society.

American Cancer Society. (1994b). Estimated new cancer cases and deaths, United States - 1994. In *Cancer facts & figures - 1994* (pp. 6 & 16). Atlanta: American Cancer Society.

American Nurses' Association and Oncology Nursing Society. (1987). *Standards of oncology nursing practice.* Kansas City, MO: American Nurses' Association.

Andriole, G. L. (1993). Nerve-sparing radical retropubic prostatectomy patient selection and technique. *AUA update series,* Vol. 12, Lesson 13. Houston: American Urological Association, Office of Education.

Babaian, R. J., Zagars, G. K., & Ayala, A. G. (1990). Radiation therapy of stage C prostate cancer: Significance of gleason grade to survival. *Seminars in Urology, 8*(4), 225–231.

Belldegrun, A., Figlin, R., Danella, J., & deKernion, J. (1992). Immunotherapy for renal cell carcinoma. *Seminars in Urology, 10*(1), 23–27.

Bihrle, R., Donohue, J. P., & Foster, R. S. (1988). Complications of retroperitoneal lymph node dissection. *Urologic Clinics of North America, 15*(2), 237–242.

Bolger, J. J., Dearnaley, D. P., Kirk, D., Lewington, V. J., Mason, M. D., Quilty, P. M., Reed, N. S. E., Russell, J. M., Yardley, J., & Members of the UK Metastron Investigators' Group (1993). Strontium-89 (metastron) versus external beam radiotherapy in patients with painful bone metastases secondary to prostatic cancer: Preliminary report of a multicenter trial. *Seminars in Oncology, 20*(3) (Suppl. 2), 32–33.

Boyd, S. D., Lieskovsky, G., & Skinner, D. G. (1988). Cutaneous urinary diversion in the cancer patient. In D. G. Skinner & G. Leiskovsky (Eds.), *Diagnosis and management of genitourinary cancer* (pp. 634–648). Philadelphia: W. B. Saunders Co.

Brawer, M. K. (1992). The role of radiotherapy following radical prostatectomy. In H. Lepor & R. K. Lawson (Eds.), *Therapy for genitourinary cancer* (pp. 41–51). Boston: Kluwer Academic Publishers.

Broadwell, D. C., & Jackson, B. S. (Eds.). (1982). *Principles of ostomy care.* St. Louis: C. V. Mosby Co.

Brock, D., Fox, S., Gosling, G., Haney, L., Kneebone, P., Nagy, C., & Qualitza, B. (1993). Testicular cancer. *Seminars in Oncology Nursing, 9*(4), 224–236.

Davis, M. (1993). Renal cell carcinoma. *Seminars in Oncology Nursing, 9*(4), 267–271.

Dawson, N. A. (1993). Treatment of progressive metastatic prostate cancer. *Oncology, 7*(5), 17–29.

Dawson, N. A., Wilding, G., Weiss, R. B., McCleod, D. G., Linehan, W. M., Frank, J. A., Jacob, J., & Gelman, E. P. (1992). *Cancer, 69,* 213–218.

deKernion, J. Bladder cancer. In C. Haskell (Ed.), *Cancer treatment* (2nd ed., p. 371). Philadelphia: W. B. Saunders Co.

Donohue, J. P., Foster, R. S., Rowland, R. G., Bihrle, R., Jones, J., & Geier, G. (1990). *The Journal of Urology, 144,* 287–292.

Drago, J. R., Santen, R. J., Lipton, A., Worgul, T. J., Harvey, H. A., Boucher, A., Manni, A., & Rohner, T. J. (1983). Clinical effect of aminoglutethimide, medical adrenalectomy in treatment of 43 patients with advanced prostatic carcinoma. *Cancer, 53,* 1447–1450.

Droller, M. J. (1993). Bladder cancer, Part II. *1993 Monographs in Urology, 14*(4), 53–65.

Duncan, W., & Quilty, P. M. (1986). The results of a series of 963 patients with transitional cell carcinoma of the urinary bladder primarily treated by radical megavoltage x-ray therapy. *Radiotherapy and Oncology, 7,* 299–310.

Einhorn, L. H. (1988). Chemotherapy of disseminated testicular cancer. In D. G. Skinner & G. Lieskovsky (Eds.), *Diagnosis and management of genitourinary cancer* (pp. 526–531). Philadelphia: W. B. Saunders Co.

Eisengerger, M. A., Reyno, L. M., Jodrell, D. I, Sinibaldi, V. J., Tkaczuk, K. H., Sridhara, R., Zuhowski, E. G., Lowitt, M. H., Jacobs, S. C., & Egorin, M. J. (1993). Suramin, an active drug for prostate cancer: Interim observations in a phase I trial. *Journal of the National Cancer Institute, 85*(8), 611–621.

Elson, P. J. (1994). Identifying prognostic factors in metastaic renal cell carcinoma. *The Kidney Cancer Journal, 1*(2), 1–17.

Fair, W., Fuks, Z., & Scher, H. (1993). Cancer of the bladder. In V. T. DeVita, S. Hellman, & S. A. Rosenberg (Eds.), *Cancer: Principles & practice of oncology* (4th ed., pp. 1052–1054). Philadelphia: J. B. Lippincott Co.

Foster, R. S., & Donohue, J. P. (1993a). Nerve-sparing retroperitoneal lymphadenectomy. *Urologic Clinics of North America, 20*(1), 117–125.

Foster, R. S., & Donohue, J. P. (1993b). Nerve-sparing RPLND. *AUA update series*, Vol. 12, Lesson 15. Houston: American Urological Association, Office of Education.

Fraley, E. E., Narayan, P., Vogelzang, N. J., Kennedy, B. J., & Lange, P. (1985). Surgical treatment of patients with stages I and II nonseminomatous testicular cancer. *Journal of Urology, 134*, 70–73.

Freeman, J. A., Lieskovsky, G., Cook, D. W., Petrovich, Z., Chen, S-C, Groshen, S., & Skinner, D. G. (1993). Radical retropubic prostatectomy and postoperative adjuvant radiation for pathologic stage C (PCN0) prostate cancer from 1976 to 1989: Intermediate findings. *The Journal of Urology, 149*, 1029–1034.

Freiha, F. S. (1990). Treatment options for patients with invasive bladder cancer. *Monographs in Urology, 11*(3), 34–47.

Garnick, M. B., Krane, R. J., Scully, R. E., & Weber, E. T. (1990). Cancer of the testes. In R. T. Osteen, B. Cody, & P. E. Rosenthal (Eds.), *Cancer Manual* (pp. 304–314). Boston: American Cancer Society.

Ghosn, M., Droz, J. P., Theodore, C., Pico, J. L., Baume, D., Spielmann, M., Ostronoff, M., Moran, A., Salloum, E., Kramar, A., & Hayat, M. (1988). Salvage chemotherapy in refractory germ cell tumors with etoposide (AP-16) plus ifosfamide plus high-dose cisplatin. *Cancer, 62*, 24–27.

Gibbons, R. P., Cole, B. S., Richardson, R. G., Correa, R. J., Brannen, G. E., Mason, J. T., Taylor, W. J., & Hafermann, M. D. (1986). Adjuvant radiotherapy following radical prostatectomy: Results and complications. *Journal of Urology, 135*, 65–68.

Gleason, D. F., Mellinger, G. T., & the Veteran's Administration Cooperative Urological Research Group. (1974). Prediction of prognosis for prostatic adenocarcinoma by combined histological grading and staging. *Journal of Urology, 111*, 58–64.

Gleen, J. F. (1990). Subepididymal orchiectomy: The acceptable alternative. *The Journal of Urology, 144*, 942–944.

Goldiner, P. L., & Schweizer O. (1979). The hazards of anesthesia and surgery in bleomycin-treated patients. *Seminars in Oncology, 6*(1), 121–124.

Graham, L. D., & Bagshaw, M. (1983). Treatment of testicular germinomas. In D. G. Skinner (Ed.), *Urological cancer* (pp. 281–300). New York: Grune & Stratton, Inc.

Hanks, G. E. (1991). Radiotherapy or surgery for prostate cancer? Ten and fifteen-year results of external beam therapy. *Acta Oncologica, 30*(2), 231–237.

Heinrich-Rynning, T. (1987). Prostatic cancer treatments and their effects on sexual functioning. *Oncology Nursing Forum, 14*(6), 37–41.

Herr, H. W., Whitmore, W. F., Morse, M. J., Sogani, P. C., Russo, P., & Fair, W. R. (1990). Neoadjuvant chemotherapy in invasive bladder cancer: the evolving role of surgery. *The Journal of Urology, 144*, 1083–1088.

Herr, W. H., Toner, G. C., Geller, N. L., & Bosi, G. J. (1991). Patient selection for retroperitoneal lymph node dissection after chemotherapy for nonseminomatous germ cell tumors. *European Journal of Urology, 19*, 1–5.

Horwich, A., & Peckham, M. J. (1986). Transient tumor marker elevation following chemotherapy for germ cell tumors of the testis. *Cancer Treatment Reports, 70*, 1329–1331.

Hossan, E., & Striegel, A. (1993). Carcinoma of the bladder. *Seminars in Oncology Nursing, 9*(4), 252–266.

Johnson, D. E., Swanson, D. A., & von Eschenbach, A. C. (1987). Tumors of the genitourinary tract. In E. A. Tanagho, & J. W. McAnich (Eds.), *Smith's general urology* (12th ed., pp. 330–434). San Mateo, CA: Appleton & Lange.

Keller, J. W., Sahasrabudhe, D. M., & McCune, C. S. (1993). Urologic and male genital cancers. In P. Rubin, S. McDonald, & R. Qazi (Eds.), *Clinical oncology: A multidisciplinary approach for physicians and students* (7th ed., pp. 419–425, 442–453). Philadelphia: W. B. Saunders Co.

Klein, E. A. (1992). Options in the surgical treatment of bladder cancer. *Journal of Enterostomal Therapy Nursing, 19*, 122–125.

Kramer, S. A., Spahr, J., Brendler, C., Glenn, J., & Paulson, D. F. (1980). Experience with Gleason's histopathologic grading in prostatic cancer. *Journal of Urology, 124*, 223–225.

Labrie, F., Belanger, A., Simard, J., Labrie, C., & Dupont, A. (1993). Combination therapy for prostate cancer. *Cancer, 71*, 1059–1067.

Lange, P. H., Chang, W. Y. & Fraley, E. E. (1987). Fertility issues in the therapy of nonseminomatous testicular tumors. *Urologic Clinics of North America, 14*(4), 731–747.

Layfield, L. J., Mukamel, E., Hilborne, L. H., Hannah, J. B., Glasgow, B. J., Ljung, B., & deKernion, J. B. (1984). Cytological grading of prostatic aspiration biopsy: A comparison with the Gleason grading system. *Journal of Urology, 138*, 798–800.

Lieskovsky, G., Ahlering, T., & Skinner, D. G. (1988). Diagnosis and staging of bladder cancer. In D. G. Skinner & G. Lieskovsky (Eds.), *Diagnosis and management of genitourinary cancer* (pp. 264–280). Philadelphia: W. B. Saunders Co.

Lind, J. (1987). Prostate cancer. In C. R. Ziegfeld (Ed.), *Core curriculum for oncology nursing* (pp. 129–136). Philadelphia: W. B. Saunders Co.

Lind, J., & Nakao, S. L. (1987). Urologic and male genital malignancies. In S. Groenwald (Ed.), *Cancer nursing principles and practice* (pp. 700–745). Boston: Jones & Bartlett.

Linehan, W. M., Shipley, W., & Parkinson, D. R. (1993). Cancer of the kidney and ureter. In V. T. DeVita, S. Hellman, & S. A. Rosenberg (Eds.), *Cancer: Principles & practice of oncology* (4th ed., pp. 1023–1029). Philadelphia: J. B. Lippincott Co.

Lum, B. L., & Torti, F. M. (1991). Adjuvant intravesical pharmacotherapy for superficial bladder cancer. *Journal of the National Cancer Institute, 83*(10), 682–694.

Maxwell, M. (1993). Cancer of the prostate. *Seminars in Oncology Nursing, 9*(4), 237–251.

McConnell, J. D. (1991). Physiologic basis of endocrine therapy for prostatic cancer. *Urologic Clinics of North America, 18*(1), 1–11.

McCullogh, D. L. (1988). Diagnosis and staging of prostatic cancer. In D. G. Skinner & G. Lieskovsky (Eds.), *Diagnosis and management of genitourinary cancer* (pp. 405–416). Philadelphia: W. B. Saunders Co.

McLeod, D. G., Crawford, E. D., Blumenstein, B. A., & Eisenberger, M. A. (1992). Controversies in the treatment of metastatic prostate cancer. *Cancer, 70,* 324–328.

Meier, R., Mark, R., St. Royal, L., Tran, L., Colburn G., & Parker, R. (1992). Postoperative radiation therapy after radical prostatectomy for prostate carcinoma. *Cancer, 70*(7), 1960–1966.

Middleton, R. G., Smith, J. A., Melzer, R. B., & Hamilton, P. E. (1986). Patient survival and local recurrence rate following radical prostatectomy for prostatic carcinoma. *Journal of Urology, 136,* 422–424.

Montie, J. E., MacGregor, P. S., Fazio, V. W., & Lavery, I. (1986). Continent ileal reservoir (Kock pouch). *Urology Clinics of North America, 13,* 251–260.

National Cancer Institute. (1988). *What you need to know about testicular cancer* (NIH Publication No. 88-1565). Bethesda, MD: Author.

National Cancer Institute. (1990). *Testicular cancer* (NIH Publication No. 90-654, p. 3). Bethesda, MD: Author.

Noble, R. (1980). Production of Nb rat carcinoma of the dorsal prostate and response of estrogen-dependent transplant to sex hormones and tamoxifen. *Cancer Research, 40,* 3547–3550.

Pack, R. (1993). Descriptive epidemiology of genitourinary cancers. *Seminars in Oncology Nursing, 9*(4) 220–223.

Paulson, D. F. (1987). Treatment strategies in renal carcinoma. *Seminars in Nephrology, 7,* 140–151.

Paulson, D. F. (1988a). Randomized series of treatment with surgery versus radiation for prostate adenocarcinoma. *National Cancer Institute Monograph, 7,* 127–131.

Paulson, D. F. (1988b). Role of endocrine therapy in the management of prostatic cancer. In D. G. Skinner & G. Lieskovsky (Eds.), *Diagnosis and management of genitourinary cancer* (pp. 464–472). Philadelphia: W. B. Saunders Co.

Paulson, D. F., Lin, G. H., Hinshaw, W., Stephani, S., & the Uro-Oncology Research Group. (1982). Radical surgery vs. radiotherapy for adenocarcinoma of the prostate. *Journal of Urology, 128,* 502–504.

Perez, C. A., Ihde, D. C., Fair, W. R., & Labrie, F. (1985). Cancer of the prostate. In V. T. DeVita, Jr., S. Hellman, & S. A. Rosenberg (Eds.), *Cancer: Principles and practice of oncology* (2nd ed., pp. 929–960). Philadelphia: J. B. Lippincott Co.

Porter, A. T., & McEwan, A. J. B. (1993). Strontium-89 as an adjuvant to external beam radiation improves pain relief and delays disease progression in advanced prostate cancer: Results of a randomized, controlled trial. *Seminars in Oncology, 20*(3, Suppl. 2), 38–43.

Porter, A. T., McEwan, A. J. B., Powe, J. E., Reid, R., McGowan, D. G., Lukka, H., Sathyanarayana, J. R., Yakemchuk, V. N., Thomas, G. M., Erlich, L. E., Crook, J., Gulenchyn, K. Y., Hong, K. E., Wesolowski, C. & Yardley, J. (1993). Results of a randomized phase-III trial to evaluate the efficacy of strontium-89 adjuvant to local field external beam irradiation in the management of endocrine resistant metastatic prostate cancer. *International Journal of Radiation Oncology, Biology and Physics, 25,* 805–813.

Razor, B. R. (1993). Continent urinary reservoirs. *Seminars in Oncology Nursing, 9*(4), 272–285.

Richie, J. (1988). Diagnosis and staging of testicular cancer. In D. G. Skinner & G. Lieskovsky (Eds.), *Diagnosis and management of genitourinary cancer* (pp. 498–507). Philadelphia: W. B. Saunders Co.

Richie, J. P. (1993a). Detection and treatment of testicular cancer. *CA: A Cancer Journal for Clinicians, 43,* 151–175.

Richie, J. P. (1993b). Complications of retroperitoneal lymph node dissection. *AUA update series,* Vol. 12, Lesson 16. Houston: American Urological Association, Office of Education.

Robertson, C. N., & Paulson, D. F. (1991). Radical surgery versus radiation therapy in early prostatic carcinoma. *Acta Oncologica, 30*(2), 239–242.

Rohl, H. F., & Beuke, H-P. (1992). Effect of orchidectomy on serum concentrations with testosterone and dihydrotestosterone in patients with prostatic cancer. *Scandinavian Journal of Urology and Nephrology, 26,* 11–14.

Ross, R. K. Paganini-Hill, A., & Henderson, B. E. (1988b). Epidemiology of prostate cancer. In D. G. Skinner & G. Lieskovsky (Eds.), *Diagnosis and management of genitourinary cancer* (pp. 40–45). Philadelphia: W. B. Saunders Co.

Rowland, R. G., Mitchell, M. E., Bihrle, R., Kahnoski, R. J., & Piser, J. E. (1987). Indiana continent urinary reservoir. *The Journal of Urology, 137,* 1136–1139.

Sarosdy, M. (1993). Genitourinary cancer. In G. R. Weiss (Ed.), *Clinical Oncology* (pp. 180–185). Norwalk, CT: Appleton & Lange.

Schellhammer, P. F. (1994). Radiation therapy for localized prostate cancer: What has been and still remains to be learned. *Monographs in Urology, 15*(5), 78–92.

Schover, L. R., Evans, R., & von Eschenbach, A. C. (1986). Sexual rehabilitation and male radical cystectomy. *Journal of Urology, 136,* 1015–1017.

Schover, L. R., von Eschenbach, A. C., Smith, D. B., & Gonzalez, J. (1984). Sexual rehabilitation of urologic cancer patients: A practical approach. *Cancer, 34,* 66–68.

Silverberg, E., & Lubera, J. (1989). Cancer statistics, 1989. *CA: A Cancer Journal for Clinicians, 39,* 3–20.

Skarin, A. T. (1991). Testicular cancer. In A. T. Skarin (Ed.), *Atlas of diagnostic oncology* (pp. 4.30–4.38). Philadelphia: J. B. Lippincott Co.

Skinner, D. G., Boyd, S. D., & Lieskovsky, G. (1984). Clinical experience with the Kock continent ileal reservoir for urinary diversion. *Journal of Urology, 132,* 1101–1107.

Skinner, D. G., Daniels, J. R., Russell, C. A., Lieskovsky, G., Boyd, S. D., Nichols, P., Kern, W., Sakamoto, J., Krailo, M., & Groshen, S. (1991). The role of adjuvant chemotherapy following cystectomy for invasive bladder cancer: A prospective comparative trial. *The Journal of Urology, 145,* 459–467.

Skinner, D. G., & Lieskovsky, G. (1988b). Management of invasive and high grade bladder cancer. In D. G. Skinner & G. Lieskovsky (Eds.), *Diagnosis and management of genitourinary cancer* (pp. 684–703). Philadelphia: W. B. Saunders Co.

Skinner, D. G., Lieskovsky, G., & Boyd, S. D. (1988a). Continent urinary diversion: A 5 1/2-year experience. *Annals of Surgery, 208*(3), 337–344.

Skinner, D. G., Pritchett, T. R., Lieskovsky, G., Boyd, S. D., & Stiles, Q. R. (1989). Vena cava involvement by renal cell carcinoma: Surgical resection provides meaningful long-term survival. *Annals of Surgery, 210*(3), 387–394.

Smith, J. A. (1986). Treatment of invasive bladder cancer with a neodymium:YAG laser. *Journal of Urology, 135,* 55–57.

Smith, R. A. E., Chisholm, G. D., Newsom, J. E., & Hargreave, T. B. (1986). Superficial bladder cancer: Intravesical chemotherapy and tumor progression to muscle invasion or metastases. *British Journal of Urology, 58,* 659–663.

Smith, R. B. (1988). Testicular seminoma. In D. G. Skinner & G. Lieskovsky (Eds.), *Diagnosis and management of genitourinary cancer* (pp. 508–515). Philadelphia: W. B. Saunders Co.

Springer, J. P., Turner, W. H., & Studer, U. E. (1994). Continent urinary diversion: how to select the best procedure. *Urology International, July,* 9–11.

Stein, A. V. I., DeKernion, J. B., Dorey, F., & Smith, R. B. (1992). Adjuvant radiotherapy in patients post-radical prostatectomy with tumor extending through capsule or positive seminal vesicles. *Urology, 39*(1), 59–62.

Sternberg, C. N., Yagoda, A., Scher, H. I., Watson, R. C., Herr, H. W., Morse, M. J., Sogani, P. C., Vaughan, E. D., Bander, N., Weiselberg, L. R., Geller, N., Hollander, P. S., Lipperman, R., Fair, W. R., & Whitmore, W. F. (1988). M-VAC (methotrexate, vinblastine, doxorubicin and cisplatin) for advanced transitional cell carcinoma of the urothelium. *The Journal of Urology, 139,* 461–469.

Studer, U. E., Ackermann, D., Casanova, G. A., & Zingg, E. J. (1988). A newer form of bladder substitute based on historical perspectives. *Seminars in Urology, 6*(1), 57–65.

Thuroff, J. W., Alken, P., Riedmiller, H., Jacobi, G. H., & Hohenfellner, R. (1988). 100 cases of mainz pouch: continuing experience and evolution. *The Journal of Urology, 140,* 283–288.

Tobias, J., & Williams, C. (1991). *Cancer slide atlas—gynaecological cancer/genitourinary cancer* (Vol. 5, p. 151). London: Gower Medical Publishing.

Waisman, J., & Mott, L. J. (1978). Pathology of neoplasms of the prostate gland. In D. G. Skinner & J. B. deKernion (Eds.), *Genitourinary cancer* (pp. 310–343). Philadelphia: W. B. Saunders Co.

Walsh, P. C. (1992). Radical retropubic prostatectomy. In P. C. Walsh, A. B. Retig, T. A. Stamey, & E. D. Vaugn, Jr. (Eds.), *Campbell's urology* (6th ed., pp. 2865–2886). Philadelphia: W. B. Saunders.

Watt, R. C. (1986). Nursing management of a patient with a urinary diversion. *Seminars in Oncology Nursing, 2,* 265–269.

Wettlaufer, J. N. (1990). The management of advanced seminoma. *AUA update series,* Vol. 9, Lesson 11. Houston: American Urological Association, Office of Education.

Williams, S. D., & Einhorn, L. H. (1982). Etoposide salvage therapy for refractory germ cell tumors: an update. *Cancer Treatment Reviews, June:* Suppl. 9, 67–71.

Wingo, P. A., Tong, T., & Bolden, S. (1995). Cancer statistics, 1995. *CA: A Cancer Journal for Clinicians, 45*(1), 12.

Gynecologic Cancers

Marie Steenberg De Stefano • Katrina Bertin-Matson

CARCINOMA OF THE UTERINE CERVIX

INCIDENCE

In the United States, the incidence of cervical cancer has declined 70 per cent over 30 years. This decline is largely due to improved screening techniques and earlier detection. In 1993 cervical cancer ranked ninth in incidence and last as a cause of cancer death in women (American Cancer Society, 1993). DiSaia and Creasman (1993a) report 500,000 women worldwide will be diagnosed with the disease this year, and approximately half will die of their disease. Invasive cervical cancer has been termed a "poor woman's disease," as it is more prevalent in underdeveloped countries where screening programs and health education is often lacking.

The incidence of cervical cancer is highest among Native American Indians. For this group, cervical cancer ranks first in cancer incidence, whereas with white women, cervical cancer ranks fourth in incidence (Yoder & Rubin, 1992). Incidence rates for African-Americans and Hispanics are approximately twice that of those for whites. Hispanics and African-Americans are more likely to be diagnosed at a more advanced stage than whites (Boring, Squires, & Heath, 1992).

EPIDEMIOLOGY

The cause of cervical cancer is unknown. Cervical cancer is associated with several risk factors including multiple sex partners, exposure to partners with multiple partners, exposure to sexually transmitted diseases, coitus at an early age, immunosuppressive states such as human immunodeficiency virus (HIV), and cigarette smoking. Cervical cancer is rare in celibate groups and has often been referred to as a sexual disease (DiSaia & Creasman, 1993a).

Factors that were earlier thought to play a role in the development of cervical cancer have recently been discounted in the medical literature. These factors include multiple pregnancies, uncircumcised male partner, douching, and exposure to smegma (Alexander, 1973). Current research is being focused on the role of viral agents, exposure to passive cigarette smoke, nutrition, and immunosuppressive therapy in the development of cervical cancer (Graham, 1993). Table 34–1 summarizes risk factors related to cervical cancer.

ETIOLOGY

Various etiologic factors have received attention over the past years, including exposure to smegma, trichomonas species, and sperm. These factors have been discounted. The herpes simplex virus-type 2 (HSV-2) has been studied as an etiologic factor, but there remains a controversy whether the virus is the cause or development of cervical cancer is related to lifestyle characteristics. Many studies involving HSV-2 found no difference in prevalence between patients and controls (Vonka et al., 1984; Wright & Richart, 1992). Most investigators do not consider HSV-2 a primary factor in the development of cervical cancer (DiSaia & Creasman, 1993a).

Attention has been given to the role of the human papillomavirus (HPV) as an etiologic factor in the development of cervical cancer. Over 60 different types of HPV have been identified. HPV types 16 and 18 are found commonly in women with cervical cancer. HPV has been isolated in approximately 80 to 100 per cent of cervical intraepithelial lesions (Graham, 1993). The presence of HPV in the young population is increasing. Women with abnormal Papanicolaou smears (Pap smears) should be questioned regarding known exposure to condylomata acuminata and treated accordingly. The use of barrier contraception can help reduce the risk of HPV spread.

Cervical cancer is largely a preventable disease due to its long preinvasive state, availability of improved screening measures, and the availability of effective treatment measures for early lesions. For these reasons, young women must be educated in the importance of regular Pap smears and measures to decrease their risk of contracting the disease. In Swaffield's study (1989), 90 per cent of the women who died of cervical cancer had never had a Pap smear. McMullin (1992) concludes because women are marrying later in life, and divorce and remarriage is common in today's society, large numbers of women have more than one sexual partner in their lifetime. This should be thought of as a societal norm rather than a stigma associated with a risk for contracting cervical cancer.

BIOLOGY AND HISTORY

Cervical intraepithelial neoplasia (CIN), often referred to as cervical dysplasia, is represented by the development of abnormal cervical tissue. The degree of neoplasia corresponds with the amount of squamous epithelial cells replaced by atypical cells and the degree of cellular abnormality (Fig. 34–1). CIN I represents an involvement of one third of the thickness of the epithelium; CIN II represents up to two thirds involvement; CIN III represents two thirds to full-thickness involvement of the cervix (Nolte & Hanjani, 1990). CIN is detected by a Pap smear and confirmed by colposcopic examination and biopsy. Preinvasive disease is usually asymptomatic. Studies have shown the transition time from CIN to invasive cervical cancer is 8 to 20 years,

---

TABLE 34–1. *Risk Factors Associated with Cancer of the Uterine Cervix*

Female Factors
- Sexual history including intercourse at an early age and multiple sex partners
- Exposure to cigarette smoke
- Immunosuppressive states such as HIV
- Human papillomavirus
- DES exposure

Male Factors
- Sexual history
- Addiction to cigarettes
- Carcinogen from environment
- Human papillomavirus
- Former lover with history of cervical cancer

Questionable Factors
- Herpes simplex virus
- Low socioeconomic status
- Hormones (oral contraceptives, pregnancy)
- Nutritional implication

(Data from Graham, 1993; Nolte & Hanjani, 1990; McMullin, 1992.)

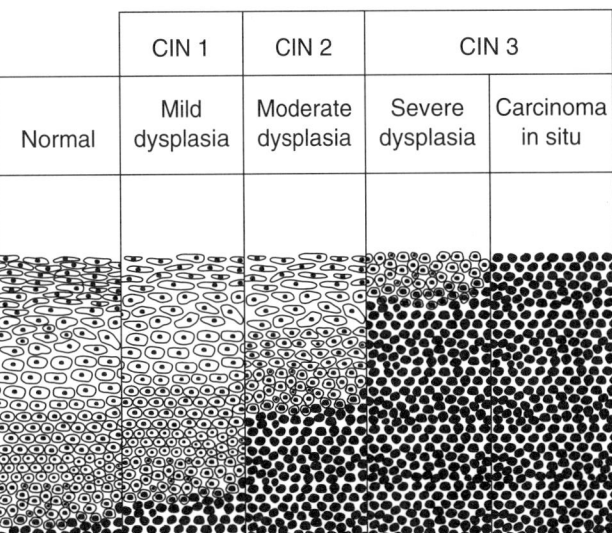

	CIN 1	CIN 2	CIN 3	
Normal	Mild dysplasia	Moderate dysplasia	Severe dysplasia	Carcinoma in situ

FIGURE 34–1. Schematic representation of CIN. (Reprinted with permission from Nolte, S., & Hanjani, P. [1990]. Intraepithelial neoplasia of the lower genital tract. *Seminars in Oncology Nursing*, 6[3], 181–189.)

although some patients present with the disease much faster (DiSaia & Creasman, 1993a).

Symptoms of invasive cervical carcinoma may include watery blood-tinged vaginal discharge appearing most commonly postcoitus. As the lesions progress, bleeding may occur more frequently. Symptoms of advanced disease are indicative of metastasis and may include leg and flank pain, dysuria, and lower extremity edema (DiSaia & Creasman, 1993b).

The International Federation of Gynecology and Obstetrics (FIGO) staging system is used to classify the different stages of invasive cervical cancer (Table 34–2). Approximately 85 to 90 per cent of cervical cancers are of the squamous cell type. There are three typical lesion types associated with squamous cell type:

1. Endophytic lesion—located within the endocervical canal. The cervix appears normal but feels hard to touch.
2. Exophytic lesions—the most common cervical lesions. These lesions resemble a cauliflower, are friable, and bleed easily.
3. Ulcerative lesions—appear necrotic. They take over the cervix and upper vagina and are often associated with infection (DiSaia & Creasman, 1993b).

Adenocarcinomas represent approximately 15 per cent of all cervical cancers. Adenocarcinomas arise from the mucous-secreting glands of the endocervix. These lesions are bulky and expand the cervical canal to create a barrel-shaped effect. Due to their position in the cervix, they often go undetected for quite some time. Adenocarcinomas are associated with higher rates of metastasis and treatment failure.

PROGNOSIS

The FIGO annual report on cervical cancer indicates cure rates from 1979 to 1981 to be 75.7 per cent for stage I (DiSaia & Creasman, 1993b). The 5-year survival rates for stage II and stage III disease involving multimodal treatment modalities were 54.6 to 30.65 per cent. (Survival rates from radiation or surgery alone range from 60 to 90 per cent.) Factors associated with a poorer prognosis include histologic type of the tumor, the size of the tumor, and extension outside the cervix. Approximately 35 per cent of patients with cervical cancer experience persistent or recurrent disease (Thompson, 1990). Persistent and recurrent cervical cancer is discouraging, with 1-year survival rates reported at 10 to 15 per cent (DiSaia & Creasman, 1993b).

THE PAPANICOLAOU SMEAR

The Pap smear is a screening test utilized to detect cervical lesions. It has evolved into one of the most cost-effective screening tests devised, allowing hundreds of thousands of women to have precancerous cervical lesions detected for early intervention. The American Cancer Society recommends that all women who are or have been sexually active or have reached the age of 18 years should have an annual Pap smear and pelvic examination. After a woman has three or more consecutive negative annual examination results,

---

TABLE 34–2. *FIGO Staging System for Cancer of the Cervix Uteri*

Preinvasive Carcinoma

Stage 0	Carcinoma in situ, intraepithelial carcinoma (Cases of stage 0 should not be included in any therapeutic statistics)

Invasive Carcinoma

Stage I	The carcinoma is strictly confined to the cervix (extension to the corpus should be disregarded)
Stage IA	Preclinical carcinomas of the cervix, that is, those diagnosed only by microscopy
Stage IA^1	Minimal microscopically evident stromal invasion
Stage IA^2	Lesions detected microscopically that can be measured. The upper limit of the measurement should not show a depth of invasion of more than 5 mm taken from the base of the epithelium, either surface or glandular, from which it originates, and a second dimension, the horizontal spread, must not exceed 7 mm. Larger lesions should be staged as IB
Stage IB	Lesions of greater dimensions than stage IA^2 whether seen clinically or not. Preformed space involvement should not alter the staging but should be specifically recorded so as to determine whether it should affect treatment decisions in the future
Stage II	The carcinoma extends beyond the cervix but has not extended onto the pelvic wall. The carcinoma involves the vagina, but not the lower third
Stage IIA	No obvious parametrial involvement
Stage IIB	Obvious parametrial involvement
Stage III	The carcinoma has extended onto the pelvic wall. On rectal examination, there is no cancer-free space between the tumor and the pelvic wall. The tumor involves the lower third of the vagina. All cases with hydronephrosis or nonfunctioning kidney
Stage IIIA	No extension onto the pelvic wall
Stage IIIB	Extension onto the pelvic wall or hydronephrosis (or both) or nonfunctioning kidney
Stage IV	The carcinoma has extended beyond the true pelvis or has clinically involved the mucosa of the bladder or rectum. A bullous edema as such does not permit a case to be allotted to stage IV
Stage IVA	Spread of growth to adjacent organs
Stage IVB	Spread to distant organs

(Data from Gynecology Oncology Group Pathology Manual [Unpublished].)

the Pap smear may be performed less frequently at the discretion of her physician (American Cancer Society, 1993). Cervical cancer can be a problem in elderly women. Mandelblatt, Gopaul, and Wistreich (1986) report that 25 per cent of all cervical cancers occur in women over the age of 65 years. Therefore, screening should continue throughout a woman's lifetime.

The high false-negative rates from Pap smears have intensified efforts to improve the system for obtaining and evaluating smears as well as for reporting the findings. The Bethesda Classification System for reporting cervical and vaginal cytology was an effort to standardize terminology in reporting smears. The system also identifies smears that cannot be evaluated due to an inadequate cellular count (Lundberg, 1989). An inadequate report allows the clinician to repeat the smear rather than assume all is well when it is not.

To achieve optimal results, it is important the procedure is done in a systematic and precise manner (Fig. 34–2). Koss (1989) recommends the cervical sample include cells from the ectocervix, the squamocolumnar junction, and the endocervix. Lack of endocervical cells

will produce an unsatisfactory reading. The procedure of securing cells includes utilizing a cytobrush to brush the cells from the endocervical area. A spatula is used to gently scrape epithelial cells from the squamocolumnar junction. The cells are rubbed onto a slide and fixed immediately.

The patient is instructed on vaginal rest for 24 to 48 hours prior to the examination. The use of vaginal creams and jellies, sexual intercourse, and douching can produce abnormalities in the Pap smear results. The smear is postponed if the patient is menstruating.

CERVICAL INTRAEPITHELIAL NEOPLASIA

DIAGNOSIS

A definitive diagnosis of cervical intraepithelial neoplasia and invasive cervical cancer requires histologic examination of the lesion. The use of multiple diagnostic techniques prevents the risk of missing invasive cancer. The Pap smear, endocervical curettage (ECC), and biopsy are the recommended diagnostic tests needed to confirm CIN or cervical cancer.

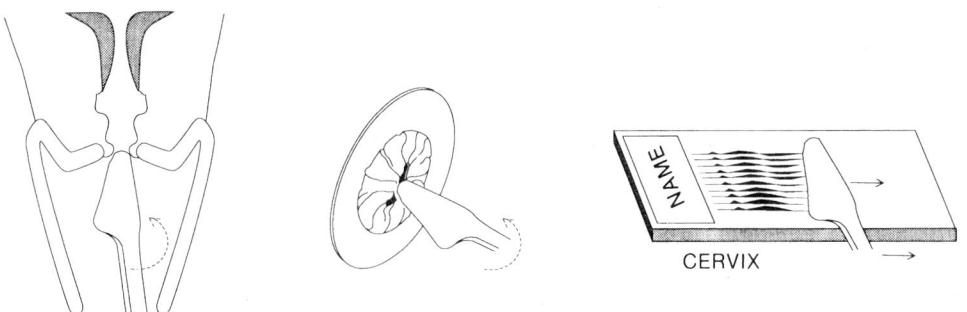

Sample the squamocolumnar junction using the heart-shaped end of a cervical spatula, rotating it 360 degrees. Apply a thin smear to the slide and immerse in fixative.

FIGURE 34–2. The Papanicolaou procedure. (Courtesy of P. Townsend, graphic artist.)

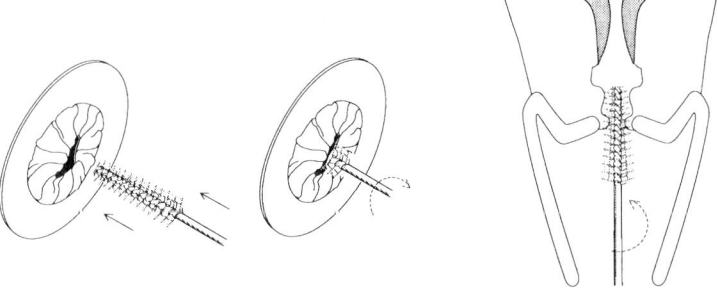

Sample the endocervix by gently inserting a Cytobrush (Hollywood, FL) dipped in saline, until only the bristles closest to the handle are exposed. Rotate one-quarter to one-half turn. Remove.

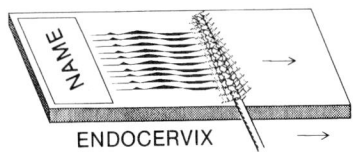

Prepare the slide by rolling and twisting the brush with moderate pressure across the slide.

Colposcopy. Colposcopy gained recognition in the 1970's for evaluating abnormal cells identified with the Pap smear. The transformation zone is the area evaluated by colposcopy. A 2 to 3 per cent acetic acid solution is applied to the cervix to remove mucous and to provide better visualization of abnormalities. The examiner visualizes the entire transformation zone of the cervix with a magnifying instrument called the colposcope. The presence of white patches with or without unusual vessel patterns indicates probable CIN. A biopsy is taken of the site to confirm histology (Nolte & Hanjani, 1990).

DiSaia and Creasman (1993a) believe an endocervical curettage (ECC) should be performed on all nonpregnant patients at time of colposcopy. An ECC provides the clinician with objective proof of the absence of disease in the endocervical canal. During curettage, the entire cervical canal is scraped with a spatula. The debris is examined for malignant cells by the laboratory. After the ECC, punch biopsies are performed through visualization of the colposcope. Silver nitrate may be applied to the biopsy sites to prevent bleeding. Figure 34-3 represents an algorithm for examination and treatment of a patient with an abnormal Pap smear.

A small amount of pink vaginal spotting is normal. Patients may experience mild cramping when undergoing an ECC and punch biopsies. Postprocedural instructions include vaginal rest for 2 weeks.

Cone Biopsy. Cone biopsy or cold knife conization is a diagnostic technique indicated if the ECC is positive, if invasive cancer has not been ruled out, or if there is a discrepancy between the Pap smear results and biopsy results. Conization may be employed for the treatment of CIN in patients who wish to preserve fertility and is contraindicated for use in pregnant patients due to the increased vascularization of the pelvic region during pregnancy.

A cone biopsy is preformed utilizing a colposcope for visualization. An iodine solution is applied to the cervix to stain the region. A cone-shaped biopsy is excised with the apex of the cone containing part of the external os. The biopsy site is sutured, and vaginal packing may be placed to prevent bleeding.

Conization requires intravenous sedation or anesthesia depending on the biopsy size. The procedure is commonly performed in an outpatient setting by a trained nurse colposcopist or physician. Adverse side effects occur infrequently but may include postoperative hemorrhage, infection, cervical stenosis, and cervical incompetency leading to infertility (DiSaia & Creasman, 1993a). Vaginal spotting is common after conization. The patient is instructed on vaginal rest for 4 to 6 weeks. Figure 34-4 represents cone biopsy for endocervical disease.

MANAGEMENT

There are many treatment options available for the patient with CIN. The choice of treatment depends on several factors including the patient's age, skill of practitioner, and desire to maintain fertility. The goal of treatment is to eradicate the transformation zone at the squamocolumnar junction of the cervix. Table 34-3 lists treatment options for CIN.

Electrocautery. Electrocautery has been effective in the treatment of CIN. Success rates range from 100 per cent in CIN I and CIN II and 87 per cent in CIN III (Ortiz, Newtown, & Tsai, 1973). The procedure is painful relative to the amount of tissue burned; therefore anesthesia is used. These factors have made other treatment options more popular.

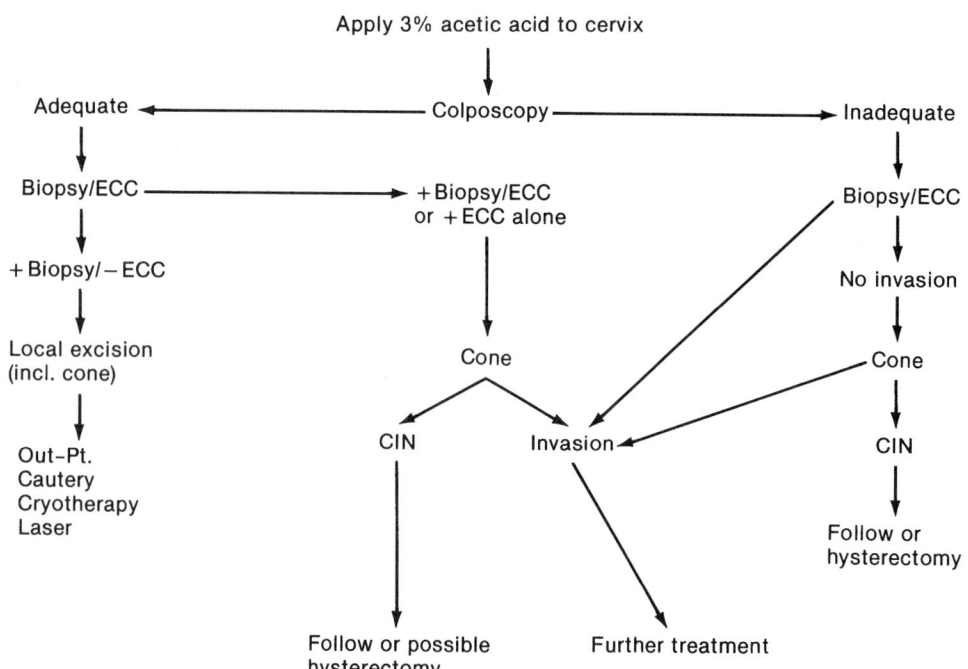

FIGURE 34-3. Algorithm for examination and treatment of a patient with the abnormal Papanicolaou smear. (Adapted by permission from DiSaia, P. J., & Creasman, W. T. [1993]. *Clinical gynecologic oncology* [4th ed.]. St. Louis: Mosby.)

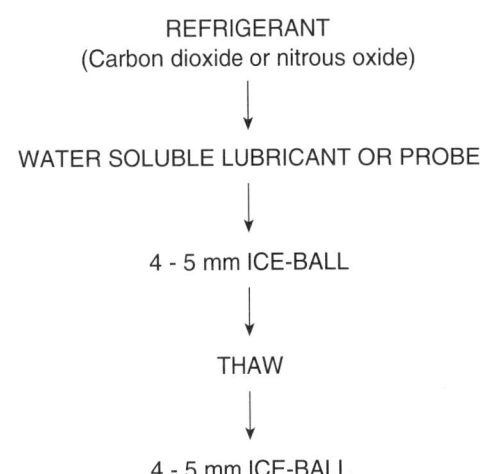

FIGURE **34–5**. Cryosurgery procedure. (Data from DiSaia, P. J., & Creasman, W. T. [1993a]. Preinvasive disease of the cervix. In *Clinical gynecologic oncology* [4th ed., pp. 1–36]. St. Louis: Mosby Year Book.)

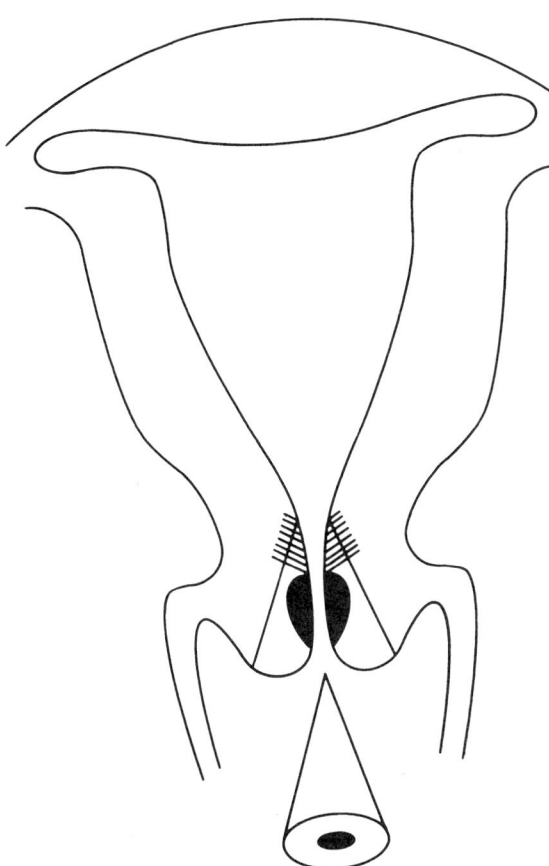

FIGURE **34–4**. Endocervical cone biopsy. (Reproduced by permission from DiSaia, P. J., & Creasman, W. T. [1993]. *Clinical gynecologic oncology* [4th ed.]. St. Louis: Mosby.)

Cryosurgery. Cryosurgery is a popular treatment option for CIN. The procedure is relatively painless, performed in the outpatient setting, and less costly than electrocautery. The procedure is associated with a high success rate and fewer adverse side effects. Cryosurgery is contraindicated in pregnancy and is best performed 1 week after menses. Figure 34–5 outlines the procedure for cryosurgery.

The refrigerant used during cryosurgery is carbon dioxide or nitrous oxide. The probe utilized should cover the entire lesion. A water-soluble lubricant is applied over the probe for better conduction. DiSaia and Creasman (1993a) recommend a double freezing process whereby a 4 to 5 mm ice ball is required. The cervix is allowed to thaw and is refrozen utilizing the

same technique. A watery discharge is common for 10 to 14 days. The patient is instructed in vaginal rest until the discharge has subsided. A repeat Pap smear is performed at 4 months. If the results are positive it is probably related to the healing process, and the Pap smear should be repeated in a month.

Laser Surgery. The term laser represents "light amplification by stimulated emission of radiation" (DiSaia & Creasman, 1993a). The tissue is destroyed by vaporization created by a carbon dioxide beam. The procedure may be carried out in a physician's office and is associated with cramping. Laser surgery is slightly more painful than cryosurgery and takes more time to perform. The advantage of laser surgery is its ability to treat the transformation zone only, sparing surrounding tissue. The major adverse effect is bleeding, although spotting is more common. Vaginal rest is advised for 4 weeks postprocedure.

Loop Electrosurgical Excision Procedure (LEEP). The LEEP procedure is gaining popularity in the treatment of CIN. During colposcopy, the transformation zone is excised using a low-voltage diathermy loop with the patient under local anesthesia. Care should be taken not to touch the vaginal wall with the loop. Table 34–4 outlines the LEEP procedure.

TABLE **34–3**. *Treatment Options for Cervical Intraepithelia Neoplasia (CIN)*

Observation	Laser surgery
Excision	LEEP
Electrocautery	Conization
Cryosurgery	Hysterectomy

(Data from DiSaia, P. J., & Creasman, W. T. [1993a]. Preinvasive disease of the cervix. In *Clinical gynecologic oncology* [4th ed., pp 1–36]. St. Louis: Mosby Year Book.)

TABLE **34–4**. *LEEP Procedure*

1. Cervix colposcopied and the lesion is outlined.
2. Patient grounded with pad return electrode.
3. Inject anesthetic around excision site.
4. Turn on machine and set cut/blend to 25–50 watts (the larger the loop the higher voltage needed).
5. Set coagulation to 60 watts for ball electrode use.
6. Excise lesion utilizing the LEEP.
7. Coagulate base of cone even if no apparent bleeding.
8. Place ferric subsulfate paste on base.

(Reprinted with permission. DiSaia, P. J., & Creasman, W. T. [1993]. Preinvasive disease of the cervix. In *Clinical gynecologic oncology*. [4th ed., pp. 1–36]. St. Louis: Mosby Year Book.)

The advantages of the LEEP procedure are many. The procedure is done in the outpatient setting, and side effects are minimal. Because tissue is available for study, diagnosis and therapy are completed at the same time. Hemorrhage occurs in 1 to 2 per cent of patients studied (DiSaia & Creasman, 1993a).

Hysterectomy. For patients presenting with CIN who are not interested in preserving fertility, a hysterectomy may be an option. Although hysterectomy is considered definitive treatment for CIN, the patients must be followed the same as those patients receiving outpatient treatment. Recurrence of invasive cervical cancer has been noted in a very small percentage of women who have undergone a hysterectomy for preinvasive disease.

MICROINVASIVE CARCINOMA OF THE CERVIX

The term "microinvasive carcinoma of the cervix" was defined by the Society of Gynecologic Oncology in 1973 as a lesion in which neoplastic epithelium invades the stroma from the basement membrane to a depth of 3 mm and in which there is no vascular or lymphatic involvement.

MANAGEMENT

DiSaia and Creasman (1993a) advocate conization of the cervix or simple hysterectomy as appropriate therapy for lesions up to 3 mm in depth. Because there is a greater risk of lymphatic and vascular involvement, lesions between 3 mm and 5 mm are best treated with a radical hysterectomy.

CARCINOMA OF THE CERVIX

DIAGNOSIS AND STAGING

The patient with carcinoma of the cervix usually presents with a thin, watery, vaginal discharge. Intermittent postcoital spotting is a frequent complaint. As the tumor grows, the bleeding episodes become more frequent and intense. Advanced symptoms may include pelvic, abdominal, back, or flank pain resulting from tumor invasion to the pelvic sidewall and sciatic nerve. Lower extremity edema may occur due to lymphatic compression; rectal and ureteral bleeding indicate bowel and bladder involvement. Anorexia and anemia are also common concerns (Thompson, 1990). Hemorrhage and uremia are predictive of a preterminal state.

The definitive diagnosis of cervical cancer requires histologic examination of a tissue sample. The histologic diagnosis and clinical stage are determined by an examination with the patient under anesthesia (EUA). Radiographic tests assist with the diagnostic process and may include cystoscopy, sigmoidoscopy, chest x-ray, intravenous pyelogram, and lymphangiogram (Thompson, 1990). Nursing interventions include reducing the patient's anxiety during the diagnostic period and patient education regarding diagnostic tests and procedures.

MANAGEMENT

The principle of treatment for cervical cancer involves eradicating the local disease and any potential lymph node spread. The two main treatment modalities for cervical cancer are surgery and radiation therapy. Surgical therapy is limited to patients with stage I and IIA disease who have cancer either confined to the cervix or with extension beyond the cervix but not to the pelvic sidewall. Radiation is the most common treatment modality because it can be used to treat all stages of the disease. Both radiation and surgery offer similar cure rates for stage IB and IIA disease. The advantage of surgery over radiation is the shorter treatment time, preservation of ovarian function, and limited sexual morbidity with greater patient acceptance. Radiation therapy can cause permanent damage to healthy tissue, resulting in chronic adverse effects. Bulky adenocarcinomas of the cervix are treated with multimodality radiation and surgery.

Surgery. The trend in the surgical management of cervical cancer is toward less radical surgical procedures for earlier disease. The Rutledge classification of hysterectomy was devised in the 1970's to assist the surgeon with tailoring the patient's treatment (Piver, Rutledge, & Smith, 1974). The hysterectomy procedure is broken down into five classes from least radical (class I) to most radical (class IV).

A simple, total, or extrafascial hysterectomy (class I) involves the removal of the uterus and cervix but not the adjacent structures. A class I hysterectomy is performed primarily for CIN and microinvasive cervical carcinoma. The modified radical hysterectomy (class II) is the removal of more paracervical tissue, the upper one third of the vagina, and pelvic lymph nodes. Pertinent vessels and nerves are preserved. A class II hysterectomy is indicated in the treatment of microinvasive carcinomas with stromal invasion and postirradiation recurrences. Radical hysterectomy (class III) is the treatment of choice for patients with stage I or stage II disease. The procedure involves the removal of the uterus supporting ligaments, upper third of the vagina, parametruim, and pelvic and iliac lymph nodes. The ovaries may be preserved in the young patient, since ovarian metastasis is rare. A class IV hysterectomy involves the removal of the ureter or bladder when recurrent cancer is present. This has value in a selected population when pelvic exenteration is unnecessary or refused by the patient (DiSaia & Creasman, 1993b).

Complications. The major adverse consequence of radical surgery is bladder dysfunction. The extent of dysfunction is related to the amount of surgical tissue dissected and is manifested in the patient experiencing a loss of the sense to void (Thompson, 1990). The Crede' maneuver is helpful in emptying the bladder and involves bending over while voiding (Lamb, 1985). Most patients recover totally from the sensory and motor loss. Occasionally, the patient may require intermittent self-catheterization.

Lymphocyst or seroma formation may occur after lymphadenectomy due to the pooling of lymph fluid or serous drainage. Percutaneous suction drains are utilized to reduce the risk of this complication. If the collection is large enough, surgery may be warranted to evacuate the cyst. Percutaneous evacuation is associated with a high infection rate.

Pulmonary embolism is a risk especially in obese patients and those with a history of varicosities and thrombolytic problems and is associated with high mortality. Subcutaneous heparin may be used in the high-risk population postoperatively. Sequential compression stockings have proven helpful in the prevention of postoperative thrombosis and should be applied until the patient is ambulatory. Chapter 19 provides the reader with a description of care of the surgical oncology patient.

Radiation Therapy. Radiation therapy may be utilized for all stages of cervical cancer and is associated with high cure rates for early disease. Radiation is a viable treatment option for patients with more advanced disease who cannot withstand radical surgery. The treatment involves a combination of external beam to the pelvis to treat the lymph nodes and intracavitary therapy to treat central disease. External radiation is usually administered over a 4- to 6-week period, and the dose delivered is between 4000 and 5000 cGy (DiSaia & Creasman, 1993b).

Brachytherapy. Brachytherapy is the use of intracavitary radiation sources to treat cancer. The goal of brachytherapy is to administer larger doses of radiation directly to the tumor. Cesium-137 or radium-226 are the common isotopes used in doses of 15,000 to 20,000 cGy. The isotopes are administered into the vaginal area by means of a Fletcher-Suit consisting of a tandem and colpostats (Fig. 34–6). The isotope remains in the patient for approximately 3 days with two applications 2 to 3 weeks apart. The Fletcher-Suit is placed in the operating room with the patient under intravenous sedation. The isotope is "loaded" after the

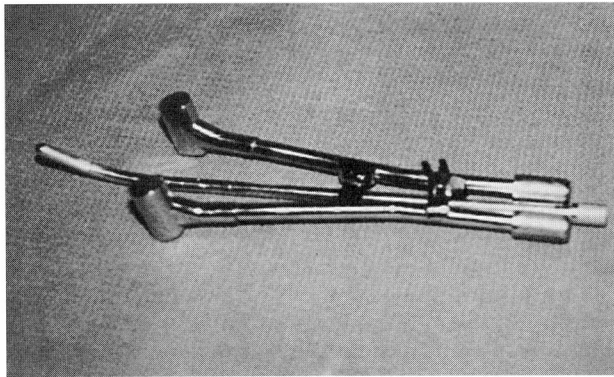

FIGURE 34–6. Fletcher-Suit system with tandem and colpostats.

patient returns to her hospital room. The patient is radioactive while the isotope is in place. After the source is removed, little or no radiation is emitted from the patient. Nursing care should be limited to 30 minutes or less per shift. Refer to Table 34–5 for nursing care of the patient receiving brachytherapy.

Interstitial radiation is of value in the treatment of cancer of the cervical stump or in advanced cancer where accurate placement of intracavitary radiation is not possible. Iridium-192 is commonly used and is administered via multiple needle implants attached to a vaginal template (Fig. 34–7).

The role of neoadjuvant chemoradiation is being explored. Despite the advances of chemotherapy as a treatment modality, chemotherapy has limited use in the treatment of cervical cancers. Randomized studies support the use of concomitant chemoradiation for the treatment of locally advanced cervical cancer but do

---

TABLE 34–5. *Nursing Management of the Patient Receiving Brachytherapy*

Lack of Knowledge Related to Brachytherapy
- Instruct patient and family in the following:
  - Absolute bedrest is maintained until cylinder is removed
  - The patient may roll side to side. Assist patient in log rolling every 2 hours
  - Notify nursing of the urge to defecate, abdominal pain, changes in the position of the cylinder, sense of bladder fullness
  - No pregnant visitors or visitors under age 18
  - Visitors to stay at least 6 feet from the bed, and limit visitation time to less than 3 hours per day
  - Nursing care is limited to 30 minutes per 24-hour period per staff member
  - Encourage patient to bring diversional activities from home, such as books, puzzles

Potential for Injury Related to Cesium Implant
- Assign patient to private room
- Elevate head of bed 30–50 degrees, per physician order
- Assess and document vaginal discharge every 8 hours until implant is removed
- Maintain Foley catheter until cylinder is removed
- Assess and document level of comfort secondary to prescribed immobility and constipation
- Maintain low-residue diet and administer "anti-diarrhea medications" per physician order
- Assess bowel status and skin integrity every shift and document changes
- After cesium, cylinder, and Foley are removed:
  - Assist patient out of bed
  - Administer fleets enema and douche, per physician order
  - Assess and document patient's ability to void prior to discharge

(Data from the University of Pennsylvania Medical Center. [1995]. Clinical practice guidelines: Nursing management of the patient receiving brachytherapy. In *Nursing practice manual* [Vol. 4D]. Philadelphia: Author.)

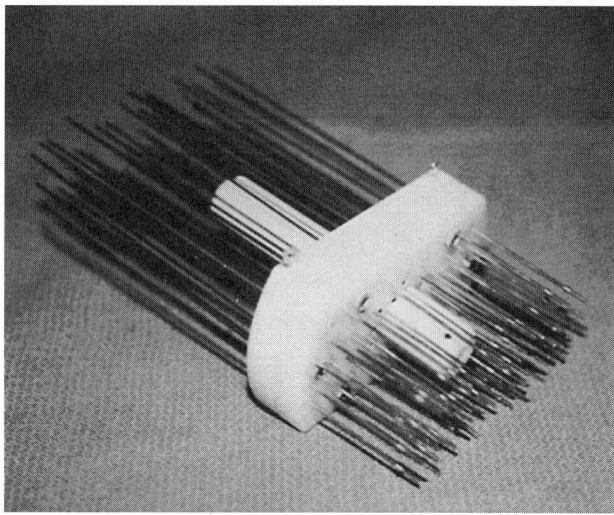

FIGURE 34–7. Vaginal template with needles and obturator for interstitial implant.

TABLE 34–6. *Percentage Involvement of Common Metastatic Sites of Patients Treated with Cervical Cancers*

Site	%
Liver	16%
Lung	14%
Vertebra	9.2%
Large bowel	7.2%

(Data from Henriksen, E. [1949]. Lymphatic spread of carcinoma of the cervix and body of the uterus: Study of 420 necropsies. *American Journal of Obstetrics and Gynecology, 58,* 924–942.)

not support the use of neoadjuvant chemoradiation (Rose, 1994). Several agents have been tested, most with platinum-based compounds. Further studies must be implemented to determine whether this technique offers long-term improved outcomes.

Complications. Complications of radiation therapy can be classified as acute or latent. Acute complications are the result of damage to the epithelium of the bowel, bladder, and other mucosa. Symptoms may include diarrhea, nausea, vomiting, cramping, dysuria, and bleeding from the mucosal lining. A respite from the radiation for a short time may be required.

Latent complications are rare but may include fistula formation, bowel obstruction, perforation, vaginal stenosis, and radiation necrosis. Vaginal dialators are often prescribed for 2 weeks after therapy to prevent vaginal stricture. Nursing care involves patient instruction on vaginal care after pelvic irradiation. The patient is instructed to encourage her partner to wear a condom to prevent irritation from sperm. The patient should refrain from sexual intercourse if vaginal irritation is present. Chapter 20 provides the reader with a complete description of the care of the patient receiving radiation.

RECURRENT CARCINOMA OF THE CERVIX

Mortality rates of cervical cancer have dropped drastically over the year due to improved screening measures and early detection. Despite this improvement in statistics, DiSaia and Creasman (1993b) estimate that approximately 35 per cent of patients with invasive cervical cancer will experience recurrence following therapy. Table 34–6 lists the common metastatic sites of treated patients with cervical cancer and the percentage of involvement. The clinical presentation of recurrent disease is often insidious, with the patient experiencing a loss of appetite and weight loss. Ureteral obstruction is a common clinical presentation. Other signs and symptoms of recurrent cervical cancer include leg edema, thigh, buttock, or pelvic pain, serosanguineous vaginal drainage, lymph node enlargement, cough, hemoptysis, and chest pain (DiSaia & Creasman, 1993b).

MANAGEMENT

Persistent or recurrent cervical cancer is associated with a 1-year survival rate of approximately 10 to 15 per cent (DiSaia & Creasman, 1993b). Most recurrences are treated with palliative management. Radiation of recurrent disease outside the original treatment field will offer symptomatic relief. Responses to the use of chemotherapy for recurrent cervical carcinoma are varied with median response rates of only 3 to 7 months. Ureteral obstructions can be surgically treated. Patients who have never received radiation therapy for treatment of their cervical cancer are candidates for urinary conduit, whereby the surgeon anastomoses both ureters into a loop of the ileum or creates a continent pouch from the bowel. When previous irradiation has occurred, the physician may opt for palliative management of the recurrent disease. Pain management and progressive cachexia are a challenge to the health care team. A surgically placed nephrostomy tube will reverse uremia but will not necessarily add to the quality of life of these patients. Without ureteral decompression, the patient will most likely die of uremia; with decompression, the patient will most likely experience problems of pain and bleeding as the cancer progresses.

PELVIC EXENTERATION

Pelvic exenteration is a radical surgical procedure with curative intent performed on a select group of patients with recurrent cervical cancer. Exenterative surgery is performed on those patients who have no demonstrated metastasis outside the pelvis. The selected individual must demonstrate the ability to withstand the radical nature of the procedure. A total exenteration includes the removal of the rectum, distal sigmoid colon, urinary bladder, distal portion of the ureters, all pelvic reproductive organs, dissection of the pelvic lymph nodes and internal iliac vessels, and excision of the entire pelvic floor, including the pelvic peritoneum, levator muscles, and perineum (McKenzie, 1988). In select cases, an anterior exenteration or posterior exenteration may be appropriate with preservation of either the bladder or rectosigmoid. There exists the risk of incomplete resection with the latter two procedures.

Prior to exenterative surgery, the patient must withstand a rigorous preoperative workup including routine preoperative tests, additional biopsies, and radiographic studies to rule out distant metastasis. Table 34–7 lists the procedures utilized in the evaluation for pelvic exenteration. Metastasis outside the pelvis is a contraindication for a pelvic exenteration. Symptoms of unilateral leg edema, sciatic pain, and ureteral obstruction are indicative of unresectable disease in the pelvis (DiSaia & Creasman, 1993b). All three symptoms must be present before halting exenterative surgery. If the patient fails any of the preoperative tests, the procedure is not performed. Other factors that may be a contraindication for pelvic exenteration include advanced age, obesity, and psychologic status of the patient.

The exenterative procedure begins with exploratory laparotomy which allows direct visualization of the pelvic and abdominal cavity. Tissue biopsy and lymph node sampling occurs. The exenterative procedure is halted if the frozen section of the periaortic lymph nodes are positive. A neovagina may be created at time of surgery utilizing a split-thickness skin graft, myocutaneous grafts, or piece of bowel. Figure 34–8 represents visualization of pelvic exenteration procedures.

Complications related to pelvic exenteration surgery are numerous. The long-term morbidity associated with exenterative surgery is largely related to urinary diversion and sepsis. The nursing care of patients experiencing pelvic exenteration is complex and starts at the preoperative phase with emotional support and comprehensive patient education regarding the procedure, recovery phase, and care of ostomies. Astute physical assessment skills of the clinician are paramount. Body image and sexuality issues are a predominant concern of these patients. Involving the patient's significant other is important in assisting the patient and family unit with postoperative adjustment. Women undergoing exenterative surgery and their partners often require extensive counseling in the postdischarge phase not only in the area of sexuality but also to facilitate adjustment to the physical and emotional impact of this surgery. The patient is best served utilizing a collaborative health care team approach. Table 34–8 outlines the nursing care involved with pelvic exenteration.

SURVIVAL

Survival rates of patients experiencing pelvic exenteration surgery vary and depend largely on the patient selection criteria used. Five-year survival rates range from 20 to 60 per cent (DiSaia & Creasman, 1993b).

Fistula. A fistula is defined as an abnormal tract that occurs between two areas of the body that do not normally communicate with each other. They are named after the body parts they connect. Fistula formation occurs frequently in gynecologic cancer due to many factors including recurrent tumor, incidental enterotomy at the time of surgery, anastomotic dehiscence after surgical bypass for intestinal obstruction, intraoperative disruption of blood flow to pelvic structures, and tissue damage from previous irradiation (Boarini, Bryant, & Irrgang, 1986).

The three most common fistulas are rectovaginal, vesicovaginal, and enterocutaneous types. They can be classified as high-output fistulas that produce greater than 500 cc of fluid per 24-hour period, low-output producing less than 500 cc of fluid per 24-hour period, and minimal output, producing less than 100 cc of fluid per 24-hour period. The nursing care of fistulas is challenging. Skin breakdown, electrolyte imbalances, odor, and body image issues are common problems.

ADENOCARCINOMA OF THE UTERINE CORPUS

INCIDENCE

Corpus cancer, also called endometrial carcinoma, has been increasing over the past 20 years. Since 1972, cancer of the endometrium has been the most common gynecologic cancer. It is the most common site of invasive cancer of the female genital tract. The American Cancer Society estimated 31,000 new cases in 1994, representing 7 per cent of all cancers in women. This places endometrial adenocarcinoma as the fourth most common cancer in females, ranking behind breast, lung, and colon cancers. In the United States this lesion is seen over twice as frequently as carcinoma of the cervix, excluding carcinoma in situ (Boring et al., 1994).

The incidence of endometrial carcinoma varies from nation to nation, with the highest being the United States and the lowest being India and Japan (Mahboube, Eyler, & Wynder, 1982). The accuracy of statistics, however, can be questioned due to possible misdiagnoses of hyperplasia and inaccuracies in data collection, that is, separating out cervical cancer and uterine sarcomas.

Influencing the prominence of endometrial cancer is the increased availability of medical care, prolonged life expectancy, earlier diagnosis, a broadening of criteria for the diagnosis of endometrial carcinoma, and unknown environmental factors (Greenblatt & Stoddard, 1978).

TABLE **34–7.** *Evaluation for Pelvic Exenteration Procedure*

- Chest film
- Computed tomography scan of abdomen and pelvis with intravenous contrast
- Creatinine clearance
- Liver function tests
- Complete hematologic workup
- Lymphangiogram*
- Bone scan*
- Liver scan*
- Scalene node biopsy*
- Exploratory laparotomy
- Psychologic evaluation

---

* As needed.
(Data from DiSaia, P. J. & Creasman, W. P. [1993]. *Clinical gynecology oncology* [4th ed.]. St. Louis: C. V. Mosby Co.)

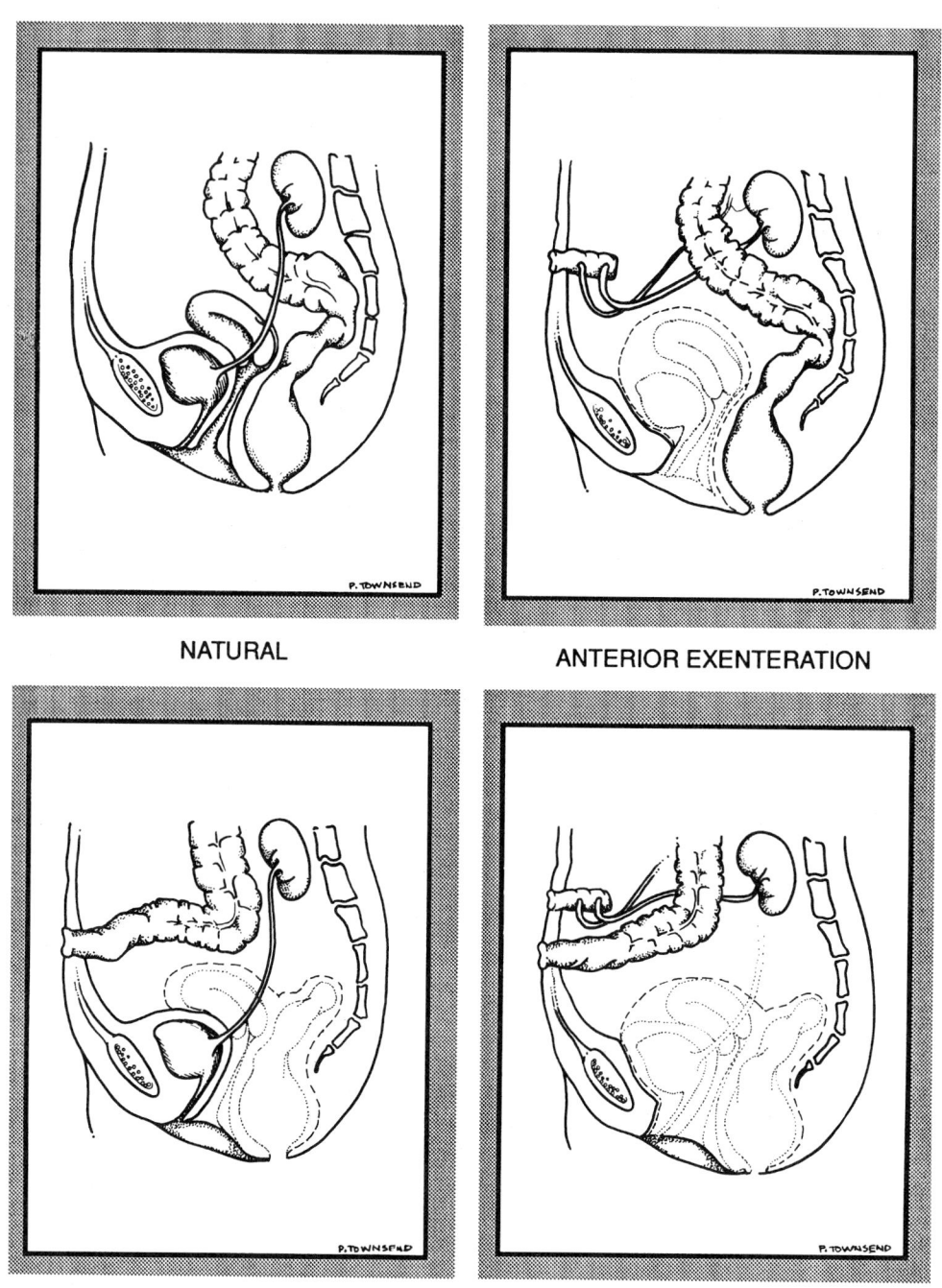

NATURAL

ANTERIOR EXENTERATION

POSTERIOR EXENTERATION

TOTAL EXENTERATION

FIGURE 34–8. Pelvic exenteration procedures. (Courtesy of P. Townsend, graphic artist.)

EPIDEMIOLOGY AND ETIOLOGY

Although cancer of the endometrium is increasing in younger women, it is primarily a disease of postmenopausal patients, with only 25 per cent occurring in premenopausal women and only 5 per cent in patients younger than 40 years (Hoskins, Perez, & Young, 1992). The incidence appears to decline over the age of 70 years (Bond, 1986).

Investigations into the etiology of adenocarcinoma of endometrial carcinoma indicate that obesity, nulliparity, late onset of menopause, diabetes mellitus, and hypertension are frequently correlated with this disease

(Park, Grigsby, Muss, & Norris, 1992). Table 34–9 lists risk factors associated with endometrial cancer. Although the actual cause is unknown, at least two different mechanisms have been implicated. One mechanism involves a spontaneous carcinoma, which arises in a background of atrophic or inert endometrial cells. The second mechanism begins with endometrial hyperplasia and progresses to carcinoma.

Women with a history of exposure to unopposed estrogen have a higher incidence of endometrial carcinoma, whether the estrogen is endogenous or exogenous. Table 34–10 lists symptoms associated with

TABLE **34–8.** *Nursing Management of the Patient Undergoing Pelvic Exenteration*

Potential for Alterations in Skin Integrity Related to Myocutaneous Graft Sites
- Promote bedrest for 48 hours, then gradually increase activity.
- Maintain pneumatic compression stockings until patient is fully ambulatory, then switch to TED stockings.
- Assess flap for signs and symptoms of good vascularization/viability. Report abnormalities.
- Assess flap for signs and symptoms of infection and report immediately.
- Monitor amount and type of vaginal drainage postoperatively. Report large output volumes.
- Utilize pillows, rolled towels for positioning between legs for comfort.
- Avoid knee gatch.
- Assist patient with ROM exercises.
- Refer to physical therapy if appropriate.

Potential for Sexual Dysfunction Related to Neovagina Stricture
- Instruct patient in use of vaginal dialator.
- Discuss sexual alternatives with patient and partner, i.e., masturbation, oral-genital stimulation, the importance of touch, erotica stimulation (Chapter 62).
- Avoid sexual intercourse until flap is fully healed (approximately 6 to 8 weeks).
- Utilize water-soluble vaginal lubricant when resuming sexual intercourse.
- Encourage verbalization of feelings.
- Refer to sexual counseling if appropriate.

Potential for Alteration in Body Image Related to Ostomies, Incisions, Neovagina
- Establish rapport with patient and family.
- Provide continuity of care.
- Involve patient in care, i.e., dressing changes, monitoring incisions and ostomies.
- Encourage patient to visualize ostomies early in postoperative phase.
- Instruct patient and family in ostomy care.
- Supply patient with address/telephone number of local chapter of United Ostomy Association.
- Arrange visit with Ostomate if appropriate.
- Refer patient to ET nurse.

(Data from the University of Pennsylvania Medical Center. [1995]. Clinical practice guidelines: Nursing management of the patient undergoing pelvic exenteration. In *Nursing practice manual* [Vol. 4D]. Philadelphia: Author.)

unopposed estrogen stimulation. It has also been suggested that consumption of diets high in animal fats may also play an etiologic role.

In postmenopausal women, endogenous estrogens rise because of peripheral aromatization of adrenal androstenedione into estrone, the most prevalent postmenopausal estrogen. This occurs primarily in adipose cells. These levels increase in obese patients and those with hepatic disease. Prolonged stimulation of the endometrium by this unopposed estrogen increases the risk of endometrial cancer. Estrone, which serves as a promoter, is considered a carcinogen; however, the exact mechanism of action remains unknown.

Exogenous estrogens are administered primarily for hormonal replacement therapy in postmenopausal women. These estrogens may also play a role in the development of endometrial cancer through direct stimulation of the endometrium. Not all cases of endometrial cancer can be explained by the unopposed estrogen theory. Endometrial cancer has arisen in ovulatory patients, and not all tumors show hormone receptors. Bokhman (1985) found that 35 per cent of his patients had no hormonal abnormalities.

TABLE **34–9.** *Risk for Endometrial Carcinoma*

CHARACTERISTIC	INCREASED RISK
Complex atypical hyperplasia	29×
Obesity	Depends on pounds overweight
>30 pounds	3×
>50 pounds	10×
Nulliparous	2×
Late menopause	2.4×
Bloody menopause	4×
Diabetes mellitus	2.8×
Hypertension	1.5×
Unopposed estrogen	9.5×

(Reprinted with permission from Hoskins, W. J., Perez, C. A., & Young, R. C. [1992]. *Principles and practice of gynecologic oncology.* Philadelphia: J. B. Lippincott Co.)

TABLE **34–10.** *Symptoms of Unopposed Estrogen Stimulation*

1. Early menarche
2. Premature menopause
3. Excessively heavy menses
4. Menses after age 50
5. Idiopathic sterility
6. Hyperplasia and endometrial polyps
7. More than one spontaneous abortion
8. Polycystic disease of the breast

(Data from Nagell, J. R., & Barber, H. R. [1982]. *Modern concepts of gynecologic oncology.* Boston: John Wright–PSG, Inc.)

TABLE 34–11. *Progression of Endometrial Hyperplasia*

TYPES OF ENDOMETRIAL HYPERPLASIA	% PROGRESSING TO CANCER
Cystic hyperplasia (cystic without atypia) minimal malignant potential	1
Adenomatous hyperplasia (complex adenomatous without atypia) considered precancerous	3
Simple (cystic with atypia)	8
Complex (adenomatous with atypia) further divided into mild, moderate and severe (considered carcinoma in situ—often treated as cancer)	29

(Data from DiSaia, P. J., & Creasman, W. T. [1989]. *Clinical gynecologic oncology* [3rd ed.]. St. Louis: C. V. Mosby Co.; and Hoskins, W. J., Perez, C. A., & Young, R. C. [1992]. *Principles and practice of gynecologic oncology*. Philadelphia: J. B. Lippincott Co.)

BIOLOGY AND NATURAL HISTORY

Endometrial Hyperplasia. Hyperplasia of the endometrium is somewhat analogous to cervical intraepithelial neoplasia. Endometrial hyperplasia, if untreated, proceeds along a continuum of increasing abnormality, progressing to adenocarcinoma of the endometrium (Table 34–11).

Histopathology. The endometrium is composed of a glandular and a stromal component. Either or both of these may undergo cellular transformation, giving rise to a variety of tumors. Endometroid adenocarcinoma, the most common form of endometrial carcinoma, comprises 75 to 80 per cent of the cases and involves a malignant transformation of the glandular epithelium associated with a benign stroma.

Adenoacanthoma, a mixed form of adenocarcinoma with a benign squamous element, represents 20 per cent of endometrial adenocarcinomas and behaves similarly to the pure adenocarcinoma. Adenosquamous carcinoma contains both malignant adenocarcinoma and malignant squamous elements. These three types account for approximately 88 per cent of histologic patterns identified (DiSaia & Creasman, 1989). Less frequently found tumors are the clear cell, undifferentiated carcinoma, secretory squamous, and mixed cell type (Table 34–12). In addition to cell type, tumor grade is an important variable, varying from well dif-

ferentiated (low grade) to undifferentiated (high grade). Regardless of the cell type, patients with higher grade tumors are associated with an increased potential for myometrial invasion and for lymph node metastases (Hoskins et al., 1992).

PROGNOSIS

Prognosis is affected by age, race, and endocrine status, as well as by the presence or absence of specific uterine and extrauterine risk factors (Connelly, Albershasky, & Christopherson, 1982). Uterine risk factors include histologic type, tumor volume, distance of the lesion from the internal cervical os, histologic differentiation, myometrial invasion, and vascular space invasion. Extrauterine factors include adnexal metastasis, lymph node involvement, intraperitoneal spread, and peritoneal cytology (Table 34–13).

Cell type may be determined by a dilatation and curettage. However, for accuracy in determining the grade and other prognostic factors, FIGO defines endometrial cancer as a surgically staged disease.

STAGING

Signs and symptoms of endometrial cancer vary from patient to patient (Table 34–14). Histologic confirmation is necessary for diagnosis. Endometrial biopsies, although uncomfortable, can be performed on an

TABLE 34–12. *Classifications of Endometrial Carcinoma*

1. Endometrioid adenocarcinoma
   A. Papillary
   B. Secretory
   C. Ciliated cell
   D. Adenocarcinoma with benign-appearing squamous epithelium (adenoacanthoma)
2. Mucinous
3. Serous
4. Clear cell
5. Squamous
6. Undifferentiated
7. Mixed types
8. Miscellaneous
9. Metastatic

(Data from Mann, W. J. [1991]. The etiology and epidemiology of uterine adenocarcinoma. In G. R. Blackledge, et al. [Eds.], *Textbook of gynecologic oncology* [pp. 198–210]. Philadelphia: W. B. Saunders Co.)

TABLE 34–13. *Prognostic Factors in Endometrial Carcinoma*

UTERINE FACTORS	EXTRAUTERINE FACTORS
Histologic type	Adnexal metastases
Histologic differentiation	Lymph node involvement
	Pelvic nodes
	Aortic nodes
Tumor volume	Intraperitoneal spread
Distance from lesion to internal cervical os	Positive peritoneal cytology
Myometrial invasion	
Vascular space invasion	

(Data from Connelly, P. J., Albershasky, R. C., & Christopherson, W. W. [1982]. Carcinoma of the endometrium. *Obstetrics and Gynecology, 59,* 569; and Shen, Y. L., & Wang, E. Y. [1990]. *Endometrial carcinoma.* Beijing: The People's Publishing House, Berlin: Springer Verlag.)

TABLE 34–14. *Signs and Symptoms of Endometrial Cancer*

1. Abnormal uterine bleeding
2. Irregular menses in perimenopausal women
3. Regular menstruating after 50 years of age
4. Watery, pussy, or blood-stained vaginal discharge
5. Suprapubic discomfort
6. Lower abdominal or lumbosacral pain

(Data from Mattingly, R. F. [1985]. Malignant tumors of the uterus. In R. F. Mattingly & J. D. Thompson [Eds.], *Telinde's operative gynecology* [6th ed.]. Philadelphia: J. B. Lippincott.)

outpatient basis in the physician's office. Explanation of this procedure is a nursing responsibility. The patient should be advised to take a non-narcotic analgesic such as acetaminophen, ibuprofen, or aspirin, unless contraindicated, prior to the procedure. The patient should be advised of the possibility of vaginal discharge for 24 to 48 hours postbiopsy. If the discharge becomes heavy or continues past 2 or 3 days, the patient should be advised to contact the physician. Any preinvasive abnormality would necessitate further evaluation with a fractional dilatation and curettage (Table 34–15), EUA, and possibly a cone biopsy. These procedures are performed on an outpatient basis with the patient under general anesthesia. Nursing responsibilities include preoperative instructions (nothing by mouth) and postoperative instructions (control of bleeding, drainage, cramping, or pain).

When a histologic diagnosis is confirmed, a diagnostic and clinical workup should be performed (Table 34–16). In 1988 the FIGO revised the staging recommendations for endometrial cancer (Table 34–17). Surgical staging includes grouping according to degree of differentiation (FIGO, 1989).

TREATMENT

Of all female pelvic malignancies, endometrial cancer seems to have more advocates for different treatment regimens than any other. Surgery, consisting of a total abdominal hysterectomy and bilateral salpingo-oophorectomy (TAH-BSO), is generally accepted as the standard of treatment for tumors clinically confined to the uterus. However, preoperative and postoperative radiation and chemotherapy have been used.

The current treatment trend is to avoid preoperative chemotherapy and radiation therapy and to surgically stage all patients. This is due to improved preoperative, intraoperative, and postoperative care and provides the clinician with more accurate information about tumor

TABLE 34–15. *Components of a Fractional Dilatation and Curettage (D&C)*

1. Endocervical curettage—to determine cervical involvement
2. Uterine sounding
3. Cervical dilatation
4. Endometrial curettage

TABLE 34–16. *Pretreatment Evaluation of the Endometrial Cancer Patient*

1. Complete history and physical exam, including pelvic, rectal, and rectovaginal examination, dilation and curettage, and endocervical curettage
2. Routine preoperative blood studies, clotting values, and blood sugars
3. Chest radiograph
4. EKG
5. Intravenous pyelogram or renal scan
6. Sigmoidoscopy and/or barium enema, if indicated
7. Brain, liver, and bone scan, if indicated

(Data from Berek, J. S., & Hacker, N. F. [1989]. *Practical gynecologic oncology* [pp. 441–468]. Baltimore: Williams & Wilkins; and DiSaia, P. J., & Creasman, W. T. [1989]. *Clinical gynecologic oncology* [3rd ed.]. St. Louis: C. V. Mosby Co.)

spread. The use of postoperative radiation therapy is then reserved for patients with poor prognostic indicators (Table 34–18). Hormonal and chemotherapies have not been shown to increase survival in early stages (Hoskins et al., 1992).

If a patient's medical illness or condition prevents the performance of surgical staging, the patient may be treated with radiation alone. This would include external beams, intracavitary implants, or a combination of both.

Nursing implications would include patient education regarding the treatment plan, symptom management, and follow-up care.

Recurrence. Endometrial carcinoma recurs locally either inside the vaginal vault or above the upper vagina. For patients with isolated vaginal vault recurrence, irradiation is the preferred treatment. For patients with metastatic disease, progestin therapy is used. Single-agent and combination chemotherapy regimens are used for patients with disseminated endometrial cancer.

TABLE 34–17. *FIGO Staging of Endometrial Carcinoma*

Stages and Characteristics

IA	Tumor limited to endometrium
IB	Invasion to < ½ myometrium
IC	Invasion to > ½ myometrium
IIA	Endocervical glandular involvement only
IIB	Cervical stromal invasion
IIIA	Tumor invades serosa or adnexa or positive peritoneal cytology
IIIB	Vaginal metastases
IIIC	Metastases to pelvic or paraaortic lymph nodes
IVA	Tumor invasion bladder and/or bowel mucosa
IVB	Distant metastases including intraabdominal and/or inguinal lymph node

Group and Degree of Differentiation

G1	5% or less of a nonsquamous solid growth pattern
G2	6%–50% of a nonsquamous solid growth pattern
G3	More than 50% of a nonsquamous solid growth pattern

TABLE 34–18. *Treatment of Endometrial Carcinoma*

STAGE	SURGERY	POSTOPERATIVE TREATMENT
IA, G1, G2	TAH-BSO, peritoneal cytology	Phosphorus-32—if positive cytology (questionable)

IA, G3
  IB, IC (all grades)
  IIA, IIB (all grades)
  IIIA (positive cytology)
	TAH-BSO, peritoneal cytology, pelvic and paraaortic lymphadenectomy	Whole pelvic radiation 4000–5000 cGy irradiation of vaginal cuff 5000–7000 cGy (vaginal cuff implant)

IIIA, IIIB, IIIC (all grades) IVA, IVB (all grades)	TAH-BSO, peritoneal cytology, pelvic and paraaortic lymphadenectomy	Vaginal cuff radiation, pelvic radiation, abdominal radiation (intraabdominal spread), paraaortic radiation plus aortic nodes

(Data from Hoskins, W. J., Perez, C. A., & Young, R. C. [1992]. *Principles and practice of gynecologic oncology.* Philadelphia: J. B. Lippincott Co.)

Hormonal Therapy. Progestins have been found to be valuable, particularly in patients with recurrent disease. Approximately 25 per cent of all patients with recurrent disease have shown a response to progestin therapy. The dose and route of administration do not appear to be related to response. Well-differentiated tumors have been shown to respond better than moderately or poorly differentiated lesions.

Chemotherapy. Single-agent or combination chemotherapy may be used for advanced and recurrent disease. Response rate depends on prior treatment, performance status, extent of disease, and the criteria used for evaluation.

The most active single agents are doxorubicin and cisplatin. Combination therapy includes regimens using cyclophosphamide, doxorubicin, and cisplatin; doxorubicin and cisplatin; or cyclophosphamide and doxorubicin.

Treatment with chemotherapy is palliative, with short response and survival times. Cytotoxic agents should be reserved for endocrine therapy failure.

UTERINE SARCOMAS

Uterine sarcomas are rare mesodermal tumors that account for approximately 3 per cent of all uterine cancers. They are characterized by rapid clinical progression and a poor overall prognosis. These tumors can be divided into two types, pure and mixed. Pure tumors are composed of a single cell type, and mixed tumors contain more than one cell type. Uterine sarcomas can also be classified on the basis of their origin, the endometrium, the myometrium, or nonspecific connective tissues such as blood vessels or nerves.

Two problems exist in the pathologic interpretation of uterine sarcomas. The first is to establish malignancy potential and the second is to define the predominant cell type.

Patient symptoms relate to the origin of the tumor. Tumors of endometrial origin cause abnormal bleeding, vaginal discharge, dysuria, and weight loss. Tumors of myometrial origin cause pelvic pain and present as an asymptomatic pelvic mass.

Prognosis relates not only to the size of the tumor but to the cell type, stage, depth of myometrial invasion, and presence of lymph node metastasis. The FIGO system for endometrial carcinoma is used for surgical staging. Patients with endometrial stromal sarcoma appear to have more control of local disease and a higher cure rate. Leiomyosarcoma, of myometrial origin, has an unfavorable prognosis because of early spread to distant organs. Tumors that contain heterologous elements, elements foreign to the uterus such as cartilage, striated muscle, or bone, are usually associated with a poor prognosis.

The overall survival suggest that no single modality is curative. However, experience with this heterogenous group of tumors is limited; hence no standardized protocols are available. Refer to DeSaia and Creasman's book (1993) for additional information.

OVARIAN CANCER

INCIDENCE

It is estimated that in 1994 there will be 24,000 new cases of ovarian cancer diagnosed in the United States, and 13,600 women will die of the disease. Ovarian cancer is the fifth leading cause of cancer death among women in the United States, and the disease claims more lives each year than all other gynecologic cancers combined. A woman's lifetime risk of developing the disease is estimated to be one in 70. Women with a family history of ovarian cancer may have as high as a 50 per cent chance of developing the disease during their lifetime (Steele, Osteen, Winchester, Murphy, & Menck, 1994).

EPIDEMIOLOGY AND ETIOLOGY

Malignant ovarian neoplasms can occur at any age. Germ cell tumors of the ovary are seen most commonly in females younger than 20 years. Epithelial ovarian cancers are the most common ovarian cancer seen in women over the age of 50 years in the United States. Age-specific rates for ovarian cancer rise steadily to age 77 and then drop off. The greatest number of cases is found in women between 60 and 64 years of age (Barber, 1993).

The etiology of ovarian cancer is unknown. Many factors have been implicated in the development of the disease. Ovarian cancer is more prevalent in industrialized countries, which suggests environmental factors related to industry may be a major contributing factor. The highest rates are in northern and western Europe and North America. An interesting exception to this is Japan, where rates for the disease are lowest in the world. This trend may suggest the causes are related to the immediate environment such as cultural customs or food preferences (DiSaia & Creasman, 1993c).

Studies have suggested that pregnancy and the use of oral contraceptives act as a protective mechanism towards the development of ovarian cancer. When ovulation is suppressed, gonadotropin levels are low, suggesting the development of ovarian cancer may be a result of repeatedly high levels of gonadotropin acting on the ovary. Fathalla (1972) suggested the "incessant ovulation theory," stating that continuous ovulation causes repeated trauma to the ovary, leading to the development of ovarian cancer. In support of these two theories, studies have demonstrated that nulliparous, low-parity women have a higher incidence of ovarian cancer.

A small subset of reported ovarian cancer cases is thought to have a genetic link. In families in which ovarian cancer exists in two or more first-degree relatives, there is a threefold increase in risk of developing the disease (Eriksson & Walczak, 1990). There also exists breast/ovarian cancer syndrome and colon/ovarian cancer syndrome clustering in extended pedigrees (Lynch, Conway, & Lynch, 1990).

Other factors thought to play a role in the development of ovarian cancer include exposure to industrial products such as talc and asbestos, higher socioeco-nomic status, celibacy, type A blood, history of breast cancer, high-fat diet, and the mumps virus. Although various factors leading to the development of ovarian cancer have been identified, there has been no etiology identified to date.

BIOLOGY AND NATURAL HISTORY

The ovaries can give rise to various primary tumors including germ cell tumors and stromal and epithelium tumors. Table 34–19 provides the reader with a histologic classification of ovarian tumors. The epithelial type is the most common, accounting for 85 per cent of all malignant ovarian tumors, and most commonly occurring in woman after age 40 years (DiSaia, 1987). Stromal tumors are uncommon, and germ cell tumors are most common in young women under the age of 20 years.

The high mortality rate associated with ovarian cancer is not due to the biologic aggressiveness of the disease but to the anatomic position of the ovaries. The positioning of the ovaries allows silent growth and spread of the disease through the peritoneum and to distant organs by direct extension or through lymphatic channels. Although ovarian cancer generally remains confined to the peritoneum, distant metastasis to the liver and lungs may occur. Ovarian cancer is first diagnosed in stage III or stage IV in 60 to 70 per cent of cases. In these patients, the 5-year survival rate is less than 20 per cent. Barber (1993) identifies a triad of clinical findings which should arouse suspicion of ovarian cancer.

TABLE **34–19.** *Derivation of Ovarian Neoplasms and Age Group Affected*

First developmental stage: coelomic epithelium cells. Most prevalent over 50 years of age; 80% of tumors.
    Serous tumor
    Mucinous tumor
    Endometrioid tumor
    Mesonephroid (clear cell) tumor
    Brenner tumor
    Undifferentiated carcinoma
    Carcinosarcoma and mixed mesodermal tumor
Second developmental stage: arrival of germ cells and proliferation of coelomic epithelium and mesenchyme. Most prevalent before 20 years of age.
    Teratoma
        Mature teratoma (dermoid cyst)
        Immature teratoma
    Dysgerminoma
    Embryonal carcinoma
    Endodermal sinus tumor
    Choriocarcinoma
    Gonadoblastoma
Third developmental stage: ovary divided into cortex and medulla.
    Granulosa-theca cell tumors
    Sertoli-Leydig tumors
    Gynandroblastoma
    Lipid cell tumors
Fourth developmental stage: development of cortex and involution of medulla.
    Fibroma
    Lymphoma
    Sarcoma

(Adapted from DiSaia, P. J. & Creasman, W. T. [1989]. *Clinical gynecologic oncology* [3rd ed.]. St. Louis: C. V. Mosby Co.)

- Woman in the high-risk age group (> 40 years of age).
- History of ovarian dysfunction.
- Vague gastrointestinal symptoms such as dyspepsia, indigestion, and gas with abdominal distention.

Borderline Malignant Epithelial Neoplasms

Borderline malignant ovarian cancers are histologically between benign tumors and invasive tumors. They account for 10 to 20 per cent of all ovarian tumors. The class of borderline ovarian tumors consists most commonly of serous and mucinous tumors. These tumors are treated conservatively with surgery (Barber, 1993). If metastasis is found, these patients should be treated as if they present with advanced disease. Survival rates are 95 per cent for stage I borderline neoplasms. Approximately 25 per cent of patients develop recurrent lesions 20 to 50 years after initial diagnosis (DiSaia & Creasman, 1993c).

Prognosis

Long-term survival rates for ovarian cancer are based on important prognostic factors such as tumor histology, staging, and residual disease after debulking surgery. Survival rates vary with the stage of the disease—50 to 70 per cent in stage I disease and less than 5 per cent for stage IV (Table 34–20).

Early Detection/Diagnosis

Routine pelvic examination detects only one cancer for every 10,000 examinations. An ovarian mass is not palpable until it reaches approximately 15 cm (Barber, 1993). Although with limitations, the pelvic examination remains an important vehicle by which to detect ovarian masses. Any palpable mass in a woman who is 3 years or more postmenopausal should suggest a malignancy. There exists several causes of ovarian enlargement; some are benign. Table 34–21 lists the different nonmalignant ovarian masses. A benign mass is characterized as a smooth-walled, mobile, unilateral cyst less than 8 cm in size. A malignant mass is solid, irregular, fixed, and occurs bilaterally.

A variety of screening tests have been investigated for use in the high-risk population. These tests include the use of ultrasonography, radiography, serum tumor

TABLE 34–20. *Five-Year Survival Rates for Epithelial Ovarian Cancer*

Stage	Per Cent
IA	70
IB	64
IC	50
IIA	52
IIB OR IIC	42
III	13
IV	4

(Adapted from DiSaia, P. J., & Creasman, W. T. [1989]. *Clinical gynecologic oncology* [3rd ed.]. St. Louis: C. V. Mosby Co.)

TABLE 34–21. *Non-malignant Ovarian Masses*

Cysts
Germinal inclusion cyst
Follicular cyst
Corpus luteum cyst
Pregnancy luteoma
Theca lutein cyst
Sclerocystic ovaries

Cystic Tumors from Epithelium
Serous cystoma
Endometrioma
Mucinous cystoma
Mixed forms

Tumors from Stroma of Epithelium
Fibroma, adenofibroma
Brenner tumor

Tumors from Germ Cells
Dermoid (benign cystic teratoma)

(Adapted from DiSaia, P. J., & Creasman, W. T. [1989]. *Clinical gynecologic oncology* [3rd ed.]. St. Louis: C. V. Mosby Co.)

markers, immunologic markers, and cytologic studies. Although helpful in screening for high-risk populations, definitive diagnosis of ovarian cancer can be made only by biopsy at time of exploratory surgery.

Ultrasonography is helpful in detecting masses of the ovary but lacks specificity in distinguishing between malignant and benign masses. The use of serum antibodies such as CA-125 has been investigated (Jacobs & Bast, 1989). These antigens have been found to correlate with the stage of cancer and the amount of residual disease. Unfortunately, CA-125 levels are often elevated in other physiologic states and therefore are not considered a sensitive and specific test for detection of ovarian cancer. Runowicz (1992) reports the cost of ultrasonography and CA-125 as screening tools far outweighs their benefit in accurately detecting ovarian cancer in the general population.

As a primary means of prevention, nurses should obtain a thorough family history to identify women at risk for developing ovarian cancer. It is important to elicit a family history of breast, colon, and ovarian cancer. Some women report a family member with a history of "stomach cancer." These patients should be advised to obtain family history documents that will more definitively described the relative's disease.

The conservative approach to manage a woman with familial risk consists of an annual pelvic examination, assay for CA-125, and transvaginal ultrasonography. Woman at risk should understand that these tests cannot predict the development of ovarian cancer. In the high-risk premenopausal group, birth control pills are recommended until pregnancy is desired. Prophylactic oophorectomy is a viable recommendation for high-risk women with family histories including two or more first-degree relatives with ovarian cancer (Piver, Baker, Piedmont, & Sandecki, 1991). These women should be counseled that prophylactic oophorectomy does not offer absolute protection against the disease, as peritoneal carcinoma has been reported after prophylactic oophorectomy (Chen, Schooley, & Flam, 1985).

SIGNS AND SYMPTOMS

Ovarian cancer has been referred to as "the silent killer." The majority of women with ovarian cancer have no symptoms for long periods of time. Symptoms of ovarian cancer (Table 34–22) are often vague and include abdominal discomfort, pelvic pressure, urinary frequency or constipation, dyspepsia, and other digestive symptoms that may be attributed to life changes rather than a physiologic state. In advanced disease, the patient will present with symptoms related to the presence of metastasis, such as nausea and vomiting, anorexia, and abdominal distention.

TABLE 34–22. *Most Frequent Presenting Symptoms of Ovarian Carcinoma*

- Abdominal swelling
- Pelvic pressure
- Changes in bowel and/or bladder functioning
- Dyspepsia

(Data from DiSaia, P. J., & Creasman, W. T. [1993c]. Epithelial ovarian cancer. In *Clinical gynecologic oncology* [4th ed., pp. 333–425]. St. Louis: Mosby Year Book.)

Detection occurs when the mass is large enough to palpate or when the patient presents with ascites. Unfortunately, these symptoms represent advancing disease. Any woman over 40 years of age presenting with the aforementioned symptoms or with a palpable ovarian mass requires a more thorough investigation of the symptoms. The diagnostic preoperative workup for ovarian cancer involves a complete surgical workup and may include proctosigmoidoscopy and gastrointestinal series. Paracentesis is not recommended as a diagnostic test. Paracentesis may cause the spillage of tumor and seeding along the needle pathway.

STAGING

The diagnosis of ovarian cancer requires an exploratory laparotomy with histologic staging of the tumor. Table 34–23 shows the FIGO staging system for cancer of the ovary. Treatment response depends on the stage and grade of the tumor as well as on the amount of residual disease after the staging laparotomy is performed.

TREATMENT
Surgery
Borderline Malignant Epithelial Neoplasms. Premenopausal patients with borderline malignant epithelial neoplasms who desire preservation of ovarian func-

---

TABLE 34–23. *FIGO Staging System for Cancer of the Ovary*

Based on findings at clinical examination or surgical exploration, or both. The histology is to be considered in the staging, as is cytology as far as effusions are concerned. It is desirable that a biopsy be taken from suspicious areas outside the pelvis.

STAGE I	Growth limited to the ovaries.
STAGE IA	Growth limited to one ovary; no ascites. No tumor on the external surface; capsule intact.
STAGE IB	Growth limited to both ovaries; no ascites. No tumor on the external surfaces; capsules intact.
STAGE IC*	Tumor either stage IA or IB but with tumor on surface of one or both ovaries; or with capsule ruptured; or with ascites present containing malignant cells or with positive peritoneal washings.
STAGE II	Growth involving one or both ovaries with pelvic extension.
STAGE IIA	Extension or metastases, or both, to the uterus or tubes (or both).
STAGE IIB	Extension to other pelvic tissues.
STAGE IIC*	Tumor either stage IIA or IIB, but with tumor on surface of one or both ovaries; or with capsule(s) ruptured; or with ascites present containing malignant cells or with positive peritoneal washings.
STAGE III	Tumor involving one or both ovaries with peritoneal implants outside the pelvis or positive retroperitoneal or inguinal nodes. Superficial liver metastasis equals stage III. Tumor is limited to the true pelvis but with histologically proved malignant extension to small bowel or omentum.
STAGE IIIA	Tumor grossly limited to the true pelvis with negative nodes but with histologically confirmed microscopic seeding of abdominal peritoneal surfaces.
STAGE IIIB	Tumor of one or both ovaries with histologically confirmed implants of abdominal peritoneal surfaces none exceeding 2 cm in diameter. Nodes are negative.
STAGE IIIC	Abdominal implants greater than 2 cm in diameter or positive retroperitoneal or inguinal nodes, or both.
STAGE IV	Growth involving one or both ovaries with distant metastases. If pleural effusion is present, there must be positive cytology to allot a case to stage IV. Parenchymal liver metastasis equals stage IV.

---

*To evaluate the impact on prognosis of the different criteria for allotting cases to stage IC or IIC, it would be of value to know (1) if rupture of the capsule was (a) spontaneous or (b) caused by the surgeon, or (2) if the source of malignant cells detected was (a) peritoneal washings or (b) ascites.

(Data from Gynecology Oncology Group pathology manual [unpublished].)

tion may be treated with a unilateral oophorectomy. Biopsy of the remaining ovary is controversial, as infertility may result with multiple biopsies. Studies have demonstrated the 5-year survival rate of unilateral oophorectomy is comparable to that of patients in whom both ovaries were removed. In a study performed by Lim-Tan, Cajigas, and Scully (1988) 8 per cent of patients studied had recurrences 2 to 18 years later, all with confined disease to the remaining ovary. Nursing interventions include instruction regarding the risk of recurrence and the importance of close follow-up for the rest of their lives. The remaining ovary and the uterus are removed at the completion of childbearing. Adjuvant treatment such as radiation or chemotherapy are not warranted in borderline disease.

Epithelial Ovarian Cancer. The surgical procedure performed for epithelial ovarian cancer is relatively the same regardless of the stage or grade. The staging laparotomy is carried out to determine the extent of the disease and to examine the pattern of disease. A longitudinal midline incision is made from the pubis symphysis to above the umbilicus. Ascitic fluid or pelvic washings are performed to examine cytology. There is an examination and palpation of all peritoneal surfaces, including inspection of the liver, intestines, and diaphragm. A total abdominal hysterectomy (TAH) and bilateral salpingo-oophorectomy (BSO) are performed with omentectomy. Multiple pelvic biopsies are collected, and pelvic paraaortic lymph node sampling occurs. Debulking or cytoreductive surgery is performed. Any nodule larger than 1 cm is removed (Eriksson & Walczak, 1990). Figure 34–9 summarizes treatment modalities for stage I to IV epithelial ovarian carcinoma.

Radiation Therapy. The role of radioactive isotopes in the management of ovarian cancer has not been established. The use of external beam therapy has decreased with the advent of aggressive chemotherapeutic regimes. Special problems related to ovarian cancer and the ineffectiveness of radiation therapy include the diverse spread pattern of the disease, the tumor burden is usually large, there exists variability of radiosensitivity, and radiation dosage is restricted by neighboring organs (DiSaia & Creasman, 1993c). Additionally, the use of external beam to the abdomen causes varying dose-limiting side effects such as nausea, vomiting, diarrhea, and intestinal obstruction.

The use of P32 intraperitoneally is more common in stage II or stage III ovarian cancer with little or no residual disease. P32 is administered via an abdominal port-a-catheter or Tenckoff catheter. The patient is instructed to change position frequently to facilitate dispersion of the isotope. Although the radioactive source emitted from P32 is of relatively low potential, the patient requires a private room, and appropriate radiation precautions should be maintained.

Chemotherapy. Systemic chemotherapy is an active anticancer therapy against epithelial ovarian cancer. Response rates have been variable regarding the use of single agents versus combination chemotherapy. Active drugs used as single agents include cisplatin, carboplatin, Taxol, ifosfamide, adriamycin, hexamthylme-

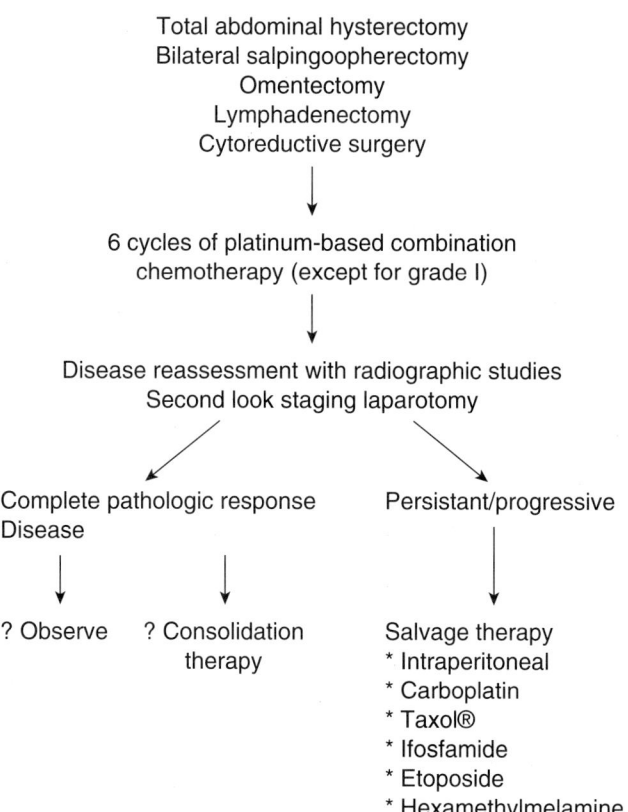

FIGURE 34–9. Treatment algorithm for Stage I to IV epithelial ovarian carcinoma.

lamine, doxorubicin, methotrexate, and 5FU. Cisplatin alone or in combination with cytoxan or doxirubicin is considered the most effective agent for the treatment of ovarian cancer with response rates as high as 90 per cent and complete response rates at 40 to 50 per cent (DiSaia & Creasman, 1993c).

Carboplatin, a cisplatin analog, is frequently utilized to treat ovarian cancer. It acts similarly as cisplatin with limited toxic side effects. Carboplatin responds favorably in patients who have had responses to cisplatin-based chemotherapeutic regimes and who cannot tolerate further treatment with cisplatin due to toxic side effects such as neurotoxicity or nephrotoxicity.

One of the most talked about new drugs in the treatment of ovarian cancer is Taxol. Taxol is a plant derivative from the Western Yew tree and is proving to be the most active agent since cisplatin. The overall response rate in phase II trials in previously treated patients is 30 per cent (McGuire, Rowinsky & Rosenheim, 1989). Studies regarding the use of Taxol as a single agent or in combination with cisplatin continue to prove promising. The utilization of intraperitoneal Taxol is being explored as well.

RECURRENCE

Second-Look Laparotomy. A second-look laparotomy is performed in many centers to determine the extent of disease after anticancer treatment. The second-look laparotomy allows the surgeon to explore the patient, remove any residual disease, and devise a new treatment plan for the patient. Barber (1993) states the most important use of a second-look surgery is the decision of whether to continue therapy. The second-look laparotomy procedure is identical to the initial surgical staging procedure performed at the time of diagnosis. Multiple biopsies, are taken, and visual exploration of the pelvic cavity occurs.

Controversy exists regarding the value of second-look laparotomies. Some physicians believe that if a patient has received first-line therapy utilizing cisplatin, they have received the best chance at controlling their disease and second-look surgery will not affect prognosis favorably. Freidman and Weiss (1990) report second-look laparotomies have not been shown to influence patient survival and therefore should be performed in research settings only where "salvage" therapies and research protocols can be made available to the patient. Second-look laparotomies provide the physician with important information on which to base further treatment judgments. Additionally, many patients are anxious and request an accurate account of their disease status prior to making decisions regarding further treatment. For these reasons, second-look laparotomies are valuable. Barber (1993) considers the surgery of value if it is possible to control or reduce the tumor burden at the time of the procedure.

If disease is present at time of second-look surgery, the patient is switched to an alternative treatment such as second-line chemotherapy consisting most frequently of Taxol or carboplatin regiments or intraperitoneal chemotherapy.

INVESTIGATIONAL APPROACHES

Bone Marrow Transplant. Autologous bone marrow transplantation is being utilized in select patients with minimal residual disease and those who have demonstrated response to chemotherapy (McGuire & Rowinsky, 1991). The morbidity of bone marrow transplantation is high. Stem cell transplantation is an alternative to autologous transplantation and is currently being investigated. Refer to Chapter 27 for a complete description of bone marrow transplantation.

Immunotherapy. The use of immunotherapy is being investigated. Systemically administered interferons have demonstrated little activity in the treatment of ovarian cancer. Runowicz (1992) reports intraperitoneal administration of interferon, γ-interferon, lymphocyte-activated killer cell (LAK), and interleukin-2 has demonstrated some response both systemically and intraperitoneally. Investigation is being done in the use of monoclonal antibodies as transporters of anticancer therapies and also for diagnostic purposes. Further studies are warranted in immunologic therapy. Refer to Chapter 23 for a complete description of immunotherapy.

INTRAPERITONEAL CHEMOTHERAPY

Intraperitoneal chemotherapy offers an alternative to second-line chemotherapy and is appropriately used in patients with minimal residual disease after second-look laparotomy. Intraperitoneal administration allows the direct instillation of a chemotherapeutic agent into the peritoneal cavity. The principle supporting the effectiveness of intraperitoneal administration is that high concentration of drugs can be administered directly onto surfaces of the tumor.

The administration of intraperitoneal chemotherapy requires the use of a catheter inserted into the peritoneal cavity. Tenckoff catheters or implantable port-a-catheters are commonly used for instillation of the drug (Fig. 34–10). The chemotherapy is infused directly into the peritoneal cavity via the catheter. The patient is asked to change position frequently to facilitate the dispersion of drug along all peritoneal surfaces. In most protocols, the drug is left in the peritoneal cavity for absorption. Systemic absorption levels are moderate; therefore side effects related to chemotherapy administration may occur.

Drugs commonly utilized for intraperitoneal administration in ovarian cancer include cisplatin, Taxol, carboplatin, 5-FU, Ara-C, etoposide, melphalan, and doxorubicin. The response rates for intraperitoneal chemotherapy range from 20 to 40 per cent (Runowicz, 1992). Cisplatin appears to be the most reactive drug. Other combinations such as cisplatin and etoposide have shown significant activity (Howell et al., 1990). Intraperitoneal chemotherapy is not suitable for use in patients with disease outside the pelvis and those with extensive intraperitoneal adhesions.

Complications of intraperitoneal chemotherapy include the formation of adhesions from the sclerosing effects of the chemotherapy, extravasation of the drug around the catheter, peritonitis, fibrin sheath formation at the proximal tip of the peritoneal catheter, and catheter infection. Care must be taken to infuse peritoneal fluid at body temperature to prevent abdominal contractions and discomfort.

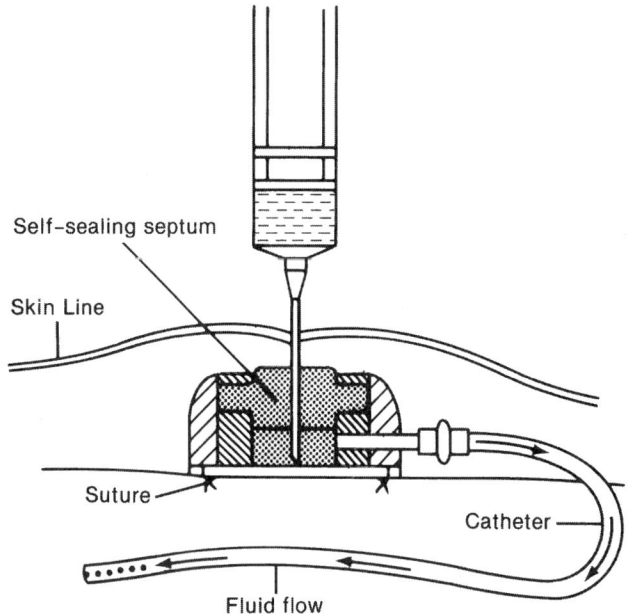

FIGURE 34–10. Port-a-Cath implanted peritoneal access device. (Courtesy of Port-a-Cath, Piscataway, NJ.)

Nursing implications include skill in caring for the peritoneal catheter of choice, knowledge of the procedure, warming the peritoneal fluids to body temperature prior to administration, instructing the patient on the procedure, and encouraging the patient to wear loose-fitting clothing, as abdominal distention is prevalent for 48 hours. The nurse should offer unconditional support to patients undergoing intraperitoneal chemotherapy, as it is associated with discomfort and body image issues related to the presence of the catheter and distended abdomen. Table 34–24 outlines the nursing care of a patient receiving intraperitoneal chemotherapy.

HORMONES

Hormonal manipulation in the treatment of ovarian cancer continues to be explored. Progestins, gonadotropin-releasing hormones, and tamoxifen have been utilized with varying results. Studies involving the use of progestins report response rates of about 10 to 15 per cent (Slotman & Rao, 1988). Tamoxifen's role appears to be limited to a small population of patients. Investigators report stabilization of disease with an increase in survival for responders (Hatch, Bucham, Blessing, & Creasman, 1991). The studies involving the use of gonadotropin-releasing hormones require further investigation utilizing larger sample sizes to document its role in the treatment of ovarian cancer.

TERMINAL MANAGEMENT

Recurrent ovarian cancer is a treatment challenge. Barber (1993) explains a balance must be struck between doing too much and doing too little. The focus of treatment for advanced disease should be on the alleviation of symptoms and maintaining quality of life. Most symptoms arise from the intestinal area and lungs due to tumor compression and infiltration. The abdomen is commonly distended.

MALIGNANT EFFUSIONS

Malignant effusions including abdominal ascites and pleural effusions are common in advanced ovarian cancer and can be effectively managed using chemotherapy 90 per cent of the time (DiSaia & Creasman, 1993c). Ascites is the accumulation of fluid in the abdomen. The cause is unknown but may be related to an irritant effect of the tumor on normal serous membranes or lymphatic or venous obstruction. In those patients who demonstrate a poor response to chemotherapy, paracentesis is a viable option.

Pleural effusions are yet another medical challenge in ovarian cancer. Pleural effusions are caused by tumor studding on the diaphragmatic surfaces and venous congestion related to tumor compression. DiSaia and Creasman (1993c) report one third of patients with ascites will present with pleural effusions. Chemotherapy agents such as nitrogen mustard or tetracycline

---

TABLE 34–24. *Nursing Management of the Patient Receiving Intraperitoneal Chemotherapy*

Talk of Knowledge Related to Intraperitoneal Chemotherapy
- Review anatomic location of the catheter
- Review catheter care
- Discuss intraperitoneal procedure
- Discuss potential side effects of intraperitoneal chemotherapy:
  - expansion of abdomen
  - peritonitis
  - extravasation
  - infection
  - nausea/vomiting
  - diarrhea/constipation
  - dislodgement of catheter
  - clotting of IP port
  - shortness of breath
  - lightheadedness
  - drug-related side effects

Potential for Alteration in Comfort Related to Abdominal Distention
- Encourage patient to wear loose-fitting clothes
- Teach relaxation techniques and assist patient with exercises
- Medicate patient with antianxiety agent and/or analgesic as needed per physician order
- Warm all intraperitoneal fluid to 37° C with heating pad
- Infuse intraperitoneal fluid slowly
- Assist patient with changing position to dispense fluids
- Small frequent feedings are better tolerated
- Allow patient to verbalize feelings

Potential for Injury Related to Intraperitoneal Chemotherapy (Intraperitoneal Catheter Problems, Peritonitis, Infection)
- Intraperitoneal Port-a-Cath is accessed utilizing sterile technique with a non-coring Huber needle
- Dress Port-a-Cath site with sterile dressing and secure tubing to abdomen
- Assess intraperitoneal catheter site every half-hour during the infusion for edema, pain, redness, sloughing. Stop infusion immediately if any of these symptoms occur
- After the infusion is complete, flush the catheter with 5 ccs of saline and 5 ccs of heparin solution. Be aware that bi-directional flow (blood return) is not obtainable from abdominal intraperitoneal catheters. If there is fluid return, it should be clear or straw colored; there should be no blood in the fluid

(Adapted from The University of Pennsylvania Medical Center [1993]. *Clinical practice guideline: Management of the patient receiving intraperitoneal chemotherapy. Nursing policy and procedure manual* [Ravdin 9 Unit Manual] and Swenson, R. K., & Eriksson, J. H. [1986]. Nursing management of intraperitoneal chemotherapy. *Oncology Nursing Forum, 13*(5), 33–39.)

injected into the pleural cavity may control pleural effusions by their sclerosing effect.

Nursing care of patients experiencing end-stage ovarian cancer is focused on providing comfort measures. This includes positioning the patient to facilitate improved respiration and comfort, the assessment and management of pain, and providing emotional support. Table 34–25 summarizes the nursing care of a patient with end-stage ovarian cancer.

CANCER OF THE VAGINA

Cancer of the vagina accounts for less than 2 per cent of all gynecologic malignancies. Most cancers occur in the vagina by direct spread or metastasis from the cervix, endometrium, bladder, vulva, rectum, or sigmoid. Primary carcinoma of the vagina is rare. Cancer of the vagina occurs most frequently in women in their sixth and seventh decades (Baker, 1991). Vaginal clear-cell adenocarcinoma is an unusual tumor occurring primarily among young women between 17 and 21 years of age (median 19 years).

EPIDEMIOLOGY AND ETIOLOGY

Squamous cell carcinoma is the most common vaginal cancer, although adenocarcinomas, melanomas, and sarcomas are also seen. Sarcomas occasionally follow radiotherapy for cervical cancer. There is no clear epidemiologic predisposing factor to invasive squamous cell carcinoma of the vagina. In Brinton's 1990 study of 41 women, several potential risk factors were identified: low socioeconomic level, vaginal trauma, vaginal discharge or irritation, early hysterectomy, previous abnormal PAP smear, and history of genital warts. Irradiation has also been suggested as a possible cause of primary squamous cell carcinoma of the vagina (Baker, 1991).

Among pelvic malignancies, only primary tumors of the fallopian tube are less common. There has been a decrease in the incidence of primary vaginal carcinomas, possibly because of early detection of cervical cytology or because of more rigid diagnostic criteria.

DES-RELATED CANCER OF THE VAGINA

Clear-cell adenocarcinoma of the vagina is linked to the treatment of women with diethylstilbestrol (DES)

TABLE **34–25.** *Nursing Management of the Patient with End-Stage Ovarian Cancer*

Potential for Alteration in Coping Related to Disease Prognosis
- Assess patient and familial support systems
- Assess patient's and family's level of understanding regarding the patient's condition
- Provide patient and family with accurate information regarding patient's condition
- Provide patient and family with emotional support and opportunity to express feelings
- Arrange Hospice/Home Care if appropriate
- Refer patient and family to community support resources if indicated

Alteration in Nutritional Status Related to Gastrointestinal Tumor Compression
- Assess nutritional intake
- Monitor weight loss
- Encourage small, frequent meals
- Encourage patient to sit in upright position when eating and for 30 minutes after meal to facilitate digestion
- Maintain nasogastric tube if warranted (gastrostomy tube or jejunostomy tube placement is appropriate in chronic obstructions)

Alteration in Fluid Volume: Excess Related to Ascites and/or Pleural Effusions
- Assess abdomen for fluid wave
  - Percuss for dullness
  - Auscultate for absence of bowel sounds
  - Measure abdominal girth
- Auscultate lung sounds for rales
- Monitor patient's weight, presence of edema, intake and output
- Encourage patient to raise head of bed at least 45° to facilitate respirations and comfort
- Prepare patient for paracentesis/thoracentesis. Assist with procedure
- Maintain dry dressing over paracentesis/thoracentesis site. A drainage pouch may be applied over site if excessive drainage is an issue
- Promote increase in fluid intake

Alteration in Respiratory Status Related to Recurrent Pleural Effusions
- Prepare patient for chest tube insertion
- Administer analgesics as ordered
- Assist with insertion
- Dress tube site with sterile, occlusive dressing
- Monitor chest tube output
- Prepare patient for pleurodesis (installation of sclerosing agent into the pleural space)
- Administer analgesic prior to pleurodesis
- Rotate patient to dispense the sclerosing agent

(Data from Herberth, L., & Gosnell, D. [1987]. Nursing diagnosis for oncology practice. *Cancer Nursing, 10,* 41–51; and Rosetti, A. C. [1985]. Nursing care of patients treated with intrapleural tetracycline for control of malignant pleural effusion. *Cancer Nursing, 8,* 103–109.)

during pregnancy. An association was found between the risk of developing vaginal cancer and the time of first exposure to DES. The risk was greatest for those exposed during the first 16 weeks in utero and declined for those exposed at 17 weeks or later. Data about the epidemiology and clinical manifestations of this disease have been gathered since 1971 through the formation of a registry.

BIOLOGY AND NATURAL HISTORY

Squamous Cell Carcinoma. Vaginal cancers occur most commonly in older women and are located on the posterior wall of the upper third of the vagina. Tumors originating in the vagina may spread to involve the cervix or vulva. If biopsies of the cervix or vulva are positive at the time of the diagnosis, the tumor is not considered a primary vaginal lesion. Vaginal tumors frequently spread to surrounding tissues due to the absence of anatomic barriers.

Frequently preceding or in conjunction with invasive cancer are areas of dysplasia or in situ disease (Table 34–26) called vaginal intraepithelial neoplasia (VAIN). There is no certainty that this condition will advance to vaginal cancer, but it should be monitored by the clinician.

In addition to possible viral etiology, patients with prior radiation for cervical cancer may be at increased risk for a second pelvic neoplasm.

Histologically, squamous cell carcinomas of the vagina are similar to squamous tumors in other sites.

Clear-Cell Adenocarcinoma (CCA). Clear-cell adenocarcinoma of the vagina, associated with diethylstilbestrol exposure in utero, represents 6 to 7 per cent of vaginal carcinoma. In contrast to squamous cell carcinoma, vaginal clear-cell carcinoma usually involves the exocervix, anterior wall, and upper third of the vagina. Clear-cell carcinoma has no unusual clinical features, although adenosis, a benign cellular change, is found in 97 per cent of women with vaginal CCA (Hoskins et al., 1992). Adenosis is characterized by the presence of red, velvety, grapelike clusters in the vagina. Adenosis is progressively covered with metaplastic squamous epithelium as the individual matures, and it may disappear completely.

DIAGNOSIS AND STAGING

Abnormal vaginal bleeding is the presenting symptom in 50 to 75 per cent of patients with vaginal cancer (Hoskins et al., 1992). This may occur as dysfunctional bleeding or postcoital spotting (Table 34–27). Other presenting symptoms may include urinary frequency or retention and pelvic pain, which occurs more with advanced disease.

The diagnosis of carcinoma of the vagina is often missed on the first examination. This is particularly true if the lesion is small and in the lower two thirds of the vagina. A biopsy of the lesion can be performed in the office for a definitive diagnosis. Careful inspection along with a diagnostic workup by a gynecologist remains the most productive diagnostic technique for cancer of the vagina (Table 34–28). Large lesions may be detected by visual examination.

Staging is best performed by a gynecologist and a radiation oncologist with the patient under general anesthesia. Multiple biopsies of the vagina should be taken due to the multifocal nature of dysplasia. Multiple biopsies of the cervix should be taken to rule out cervical cancers. Although biopsies can be obtained without anesthesia, regional or general anesthesia will allow for wider biopsies for better histologic analysis. Patients are then staged using the FIGO guidelines (Table 34–29). Due to the aggressive behavior of tumors with parametrial involvement, a proposal has been made that the FIGO subdivide stage II into IIA, subvaginal infiltration, and IIB, parametrial infiltration.

The extent of lymph node involvement varies according to the stage and location of the primary tumor. Since the lymphatic system of the vagina is so complex, any of the nodal groups may be involved regardless of the location of the tumor. Metastases to

TABLE 34–27. *Signs and Symptoms of Vaginal Cancer*

1. Painless vaginal bleeding
2. Abnormal vaginal discharge
3. Bladder pain
4. Frequency of micturition
5. Pelvic pain

TABLE 34–28. *Workups for Vaginal Cancer*

Diagnostic
1. Thorough history (teratogenic exposure, fertility problems, spontaneous abortions)
2. Physical examination
   A. Speculum examination
   B. Lugol's staining of the entire area
   C. Cervical and vaginal Papanicolaou smears
   D. Colposcopy with Schillers test
   E. Examination and palpation of the entire vagina and cervix
   F. Biopsy of suspicious nodules or vaginal abnormalities

Metastatic
1. Cystoscopy
2. Proctosigmoidoscopy
3. Chest x-ray
4. Barium enema and IVP, if indicated
5. Computed tomography
6. Magnetic resonance imaging

(Data from Hoskins, W. J., Perez, C. A., & Young, R. C. [1992]. *Principles and practice of gynecologic oncology.* Philadelphia: J. B. Lippincott Co.)

TABLE 34–26. *Classifications of Vaginal Dysplasia*

Vaginal intra-epithelial neoplasia (VAIN)	
VAIN I	Mild dysplasia
VAIN II	Moderate dysplasia
VAIN III	Severe dysplasia
Carcinoma in situ	

(Data from DiSaia, P. J., & Creasman, W. T. [1989]. *Clinical gynecologic oncology* [3rd ed.]. St. Louis: C. V. Mosby Co.)

TABLE 34–29. *Clinical Staging of Malignant Cancer of the Vagina: FIGO System*

Stage 0	Carcinoma in situ, intraepithelial carcinoma
Stage I	The carcinoma is confined to the vaginal wall
Stage II	The carcinoma has involved the subvaginal tissue but has not extended onto the pelvic wall
Stage IIA*	The tumor has subvaginal infiltration
Stage IIB*	The tumor has parametrial infiltration
Stage III	The carcinoma has extended onto the pelvic wall
Stage IV	The carcinoma has extended beyond the true pelvis or has involved the mucosa of the bladder or rectum

*Proposed subdivision.
(Data from Hoskins, W. J., Perez, C. A., & Young, R. C. [1992]. *Principles and practice of gynecologic oncology*. Philadelphia: J. B. Lippincott Co.)

the lungs and supraclavicular nodes may occur in patients with more advanced disease.

PROGNOSIS

The clinical stage of the disease, reflecting the depth of tumor penetration into the vaginal wall or surrounding tissue, is the most significant factor influencing prognosis. The gross appearance of the lesion, age of the patient, and extent of mucosal involvement are no longer believed to have an impact on prognosis.

Overall survival varies from stage to stage and from study to study. The average 5-year survival for squamous cell carcinoma is about 42 per cent (Berek & Hacker, 1989). The overall 5-year survival for clear-cell carcinoma is approaching 80 per cent.

Patients with sarcoma and melanoma have a poor prognosis. This is due to a high incidence of both local failure and distant metastases.

GENERAL MANAGEMENT

Squamous Cell Carcinoma. Radiation therapy is the preferred treatment for most carcinomas of the vagina. Treatment of the patient is complex, requiring individualization based on age, degree of sexual activity, and patient preference. For most patients, maintaining a functional vagina is an important factor in treatment decisions.

Treatment is usually started with about 5000 cGy of external irradiation to shrink the primary tumor and the pelvic lymph nodes. If the lower one third of the vagina is involved, a radical inguinal node dissection is done prior to radiation to prevent early lymph node invasion. Intracavitary treatment follows. If the cervix has been previously removed, a vaginal cylinder application may be used. If the lesion is thicker than 0.5 cm, interstitial radiation may be used alone or in conjunction with intracavitary radiation.

Clear-Cell Adenocarcinoma. Surgery for vaginal clear-cell adenocarcinoma requires removal of most of the vagina with reconstructive surgery. After the sampling of paraaortic lymph nodes, a radical hysterectomy and lymph node dissection are performed to encompass the entire area. Efforts are made to preserve

the ovaries if possible, due to the young age of the patients. This disease tends to metastasize early, necessitating this aggressive surgical procedure. Patients with positive lymph nodes or more extensive lesions receive external radiation (Perez, Gersell, Hoskins, & McGuire, 1992).

RECURRENCE

Squamous Cell Carcinoma. Recurrence of squamous cell carcinoma usually occurs within 2 years. Recurrent or persistent squamous cell carcinoma can be effectively treated with surgery, or irradiation can be used for local failure. The surgical procedure may range from wide local excision to total pelvic exenteration. Distant metastases are rare.

Radiation therapy should originally be planned carefully with reevaluation of the patient during the course of therapy. This allows for alterations in the treatment as indicated to produce optimal results.

Clear-Cell Adenocarcinoma. Distant metastases are more common with this type of vaginal cancer, which tends to make it more difficult to control. A higher incidence of local and regional recurrence is associated with local surgical excision of small primary tumors (Berek & Hacker, 1989). Surgery and radiation have sometimes been effective. There are no published data on first-line chemotherapy for clear-cell carcinoma of the vagina and only scattered reports for salvage therapy. This is partially due to the low incidence of this type of cancer.

VULVAR CARCINOMA

Neoplasia of the vulva is rare, accounting for 4 to 5 per cent of all gynecologic cancers. Vulvar cancer is the fourth most common gynecologic cancer. This disorder, which is extremely rare before adolescence, is most common between the ages of 50 and 70 years, although 15 per cent of patients are under 40 years of age and have extensive vulvar epithelial neoplasia (DiSaia & Creasman, 1989). The etiology of vulvar cancer is not clear and is probably multifactorial. Like cervical cancer, vulvar malignancies may be preceded by vulvar intraepithelial neoplasia, which may then transform to vulvar cancer. Vulvar cancer is most commonly found in patients who are obese, hypertensive, and diabetic. Smoking has recently been implicated, along with a history of another genital tract malignancy. Other diseases known to be associated with vulvar cancer include chronic granulomatous venereal diseases, particularly lymphogranuloma venereum, granuloma inguinale, and syphilis.

There is a strong association between vulvar cancer and herpes simplex virus type 2, human papillomavirus particles, and capsid antigens (Hacker, Eifel, McGuire, & Wilkinson, 1992).

The immune status of the woman is also an important factor. Immunosuppressed women are at an increased risk of developing vulvar neoplasms.

BIOLOGY AND NATURAL HISTORY

Most vulvar malignancies arise within the squamous epithelium, most commonly on the labia minora, clitoris, fourchette, perineal body, or medial aspects of the labia majora. Other tumor sites include the inguinal gluteal folds, extreme lateral labia majora, or pubis area. Squamous cell cancers account for 68 per cent of vulvar tumors, with 14 per cent being squamous cell carcinoma in situ. Other vulvar tumors are malignant melanoma, 8 per cent; Pagets disease, 6 per cent; basal cell carcinoma, 2 per cent; and the other malignant cells, the remaining 2 per cent including adenocarcinoma of the Bartholin gland and sarcoma.

Vulvar cancer is usually relatively indolent, extending slowly and metastasizing fairly late. Vulvar cancer spreads by direct extension to adjacent structures, lymphatic embolization to regional lymph nodes, and hematogenous spread to distant sites including the lungs, liver, and bone. Lymphatic metastases may occur early in the disease starting in the inguinal lymph nodes.

Vulvar Dystrophies and Intraepithelial Neoplasia. The most common precursor of malignancy is squamous cell carcinoma in situ, although other vulvar lesions have been implicated (Table 34–30). Basal cell hyperplasia have been associated with basal cell carcinoma. There is presently no known precursor of malignant melanoma. Table 34–31 contains a description of various dystrophies.

Invasive Vulvar Carcinoma. Vulvar tumors are most frequently located in the labia majora and minora. The lesions are usually raised and may be fleshy, ulcerated, leukoplakia, or warty in appearance. Only about 5 per cent are multifocal.

Since this is predominantly a disease of the elderly and these women tend to be reluctant to seek professional advice for burning or itching, a large percentage are diagnosed with advanced lesions.

DIAGNOSIS AND STAGING

Since a screening test for VIN is not available, symptomatology and biopsies are extremely important. Seventy-five per cent of patients present with one or more symptoms, the most frequent being pruritus (Table 34–32). Clinical examinations should include complete vulvar surveillance even in the absence of symptoms. Patients may present with a vulvar "bumpiness," indicating a need for further workup.

On the cutaneous surface, VIN III lesions are usually white, lichenified, or hyperkeratotic and are frequently hyperpigmented. Lesions on the mucous membranes can be erythematous or gray, some resembling

TABLE 34–30. *Classifications of Vulvar Dysplasia*

Vulvar intraepithelial neoplasia (VIN)	
VIN I	Mild dysplasia
VIN II	Moderate dysplasia
VIN III	Severe dysplasia
	Carcinoma in situ
	Pagets disease

(From Knapstein, P. G., diRe, F., DiSaia, P., Haller, U., & Stein, B.- U. [1991]. *Malignancies of the vulva.* New York: Thieme Medical Publishers Inc.)

TABLE 34–31. *Superficial Appearance of Premalignant Vulvar Diseases*

Hyperplastic dystrophies	Small or extensive lesions, with white patches, redness, fissures, scars, and frequent excoriation
Lichen scleroses	Parchment-like, rough skin surface, or diffuse, macular, pale, or wet. Edema, destroyed hair follicles, ulceration and erosion of skin
Mixed dystrophy	Discrete circumscribed areas of hyperplastic dystrophy and Lichen scleroses
Paget's disease	Moist, reddish lesions
Cellular atypia	No gross external changes. Superficial, red to pink, velvety eczematoid lesion with pruritus
VIN lesions	Single or multiple, hyperpigmented, pink, white, gray red or a combination, ulceration and bleeding occurs if irritated

(Data from Knapstein, P. G., diRe, F., DiSaia, P., Haller, U., & Stein, B. - U. [1991]. *Malignancies of the vulva.* New York: Thieme Medical Publishers Inc.)

condylomata. A wedge biopsy or excisional biopsy for smaller lesions should be done on any vulvar abnormality. A biopsy should also be done of any confluent mass or warts to exclude squamous cell carcinoma. The patient should also have a colposcopy of the cervix, vagina, and vulva prior to treatment to rule out invasive lesions at other sites.

In 1989 a surgical staging system for vulvar carcinomas was approved by the FIGO (Table 34–33). Surgical staging recognizes the importance of the lymph node status as a prognostic indicator and recognizes the inadequacy of palpation to determine metastatic disease. The depth of invasion is also important and is measured by the distance from the most superficial dermal papilla adjacent to the tumor to the deepest focus of invasion.

PROGNOSIS

Lesion size, depth of invasion, histologic type of the primary tumor, as well as lymphatic and vascular invasion are all closely related to the prognosis of vulvar cancer. Survival has been directly correlated with the pathologic status of the inguinal nodes. The 5-year survival rate is 85 per cent with negative nodes and 50 per cent with positive nodes (Hoskins et al., 1992). Exten-

TABLE 34–32. *Signs and Symptoms of Vulvar Carcinoma*

1. Visible tumor	5. Vaginal discharge
2. Pruritus	6. Dysuria
3. Pain	7. Precursor lesion
4. Bleeding	

TABLE 34–33. *FIGO (1989) Staging of Vulvar Carcinoma*

Stage 0	Carcinoma in situ; intraepithelial carcinoma
Stage I	Tumor confined to the vulva or perineum; 2 cm or less in greatest dimension; no nodal metastasis
Stage II	Tumor confined to the vulva or perineum; more than 2 cm in greatest dimension; no nodal metastasis
Stage III	Tumor of any size extending to the urethra, vagina, anus, or perineum but without grossly positive lymph nodes
Stage IVA	Lesions involving mucosa of the rectum, bladder, or urethra or involving the pelvic bone
Stage IVB	All cases with pelvic or distant metastases including pelvic lymph nodes

(Modified from Hoskins, W. J., Perez, C. A., & Young, R. C. [1992]. *Principles and practice of gynecologic oncology.* Philadelphia: J. B. Lippincott Co.)

sion of the primary tumor to the urethra, vagina, and anal area is indicative of a worse prognosis.

TREATMENT

Premalignant Intraepithelial Neoplasias and Dystrophies. The focus of therapy is the local destruction of the involved portion of the skin. The therapy that is chosen depends on the age of the patient, size of the lesions, multiplicity of foci, involvement of adjacent organs, prospects for success, and wishes of the patient. Procedures include simple vulvectomy, skinning vulvectomy, local excision, laser therapy, cryosurgery, 5 fluorouracil (local), 2,4 dinebrochlorobenzene, or bleomycin (local).

Surgical excisions should include large margins of healthy tissue. Local excisions are suitable for small foci. The therapeutic and cosmetic results need to be discussed with the patient prior to any treatment along with advantages and disadvantages (Table 34–34).

Early Invasive Squamous Cell Carcinoma of the Vulva. The goals of vulvar cancer treatment include preservation of as much sexual function as possible, provision of the best cosmetic result possible, and cure of the disease. This has led toward a more conservative resection of the primary lesion, sparing as much of the vulva as possible. The determining factor for treatment is not based on the depth of invasion but on the age

and status of the remaining vulvar tissue. If an isolated lesion is on an otherwise healthy vulva, a radical local excision is done. If the vulvar tumor arises in the presence of vulvar dystrophy or vulvar intraepithelial neoplasia, a radical vulvectomy or a radical excision with appropriate treatment of the remaining vulva is indicated. Since the risk of local recurrence is not decreased by a radical vulvectomy for an isolated lesion in an otherwise normal vulva, a radical local vulvar excision should be considered the treatment of choice. An ipsilateral inguinal femoral lymphadenectomy should be performed in all patients with greater than 1 mm of stromal invasion. Mortality is high when there is a delayed diagnosis of groin node metastases (see Table 34–35 and Table 34–36 for treatment of vulvar carcinoma).

Invasive Squamous Cell Carcinoma of the Vulva. The current treatment of choice for invasive carcinoma of the vulva is a radical vulvectomy and bilateral dissection of both the inguinal and femoral nodes. This can be accomplished by two different surgical approaches. The butterfly or trapezoid is used for larger, more involved lesions. The separate incision approach uses three incisions, one for the radical vulvectomy and one for each groin node dissection. The results are equally satisfactory with either procedure.

The major complications of either procedure are groin wound infection, necrosis, and breakdown. Other complications include urinary tract infection, seromas in the femoral triangle, deep venous thrombosis, pulmonary embolism, hemorrhage, osteitis pubis, and femoral nerve injury. Late complications include chronic leg edema, cellulitis, urinary stress incontinence, introital stenosis, femoral hernia, recto-vaginal or recto-perineal fistulas, and pubic osteomyelitis.

There is considerable variation in patient reactions to radical surgery. Each patient should be treated as an individual and counseled about the body image alteration. Patients need to be reminded that sexual functioning is possible, as well as childbearing, if the patient is young.

RECURRENCE

Local recurrence can usually be treated by further wide surgical excision. The surgery can be done alone or in combination with radiation therapy. Recurrence of vulvar cancer correlates most closely with the number of positive lymph nodes. Patients with three or

TABLE 34–34. *Alternative Treatment Methods for Premalignant Vulvar Lesions*

THERAPY	ADVANTAGES	DISADVANTAGES
Topical 5-fluorouracil	Good cosmetic results	Pain, long healing process, poor patient compliance
Destructive cautery	Excellent cosmetic results	Necrotic ulcer may develop
Laser	Preserves the anatomy and function of the area	Requires anesthesia, painful procedure
Cryosurgery	Preserves the anatomy	Pain
Simple vulvectomy	Overtreatment	Mutilating procedure
Skinning vulvectomy	Good cosmetic result	Requires anesthesia, painful procedure

(Data from Knapstein, P. G., diRe, F., DiSaia, P., Haller, U., & Seven, B. - U. [1991]. *Malignancies of the vulva.* New York: Thieme Medical Publishers, Inc.)

TABLE **34–35.** *Treatment of Squamous Cell Carcinoma of the Vulva by Stage*

Early Vulvar Cancer T1 N0–N1 Healthy remaining vulva	Radical local excision (adjuvant irradiation for 2 or more positive ipsilateral groin nodes)
Early Vulvar Cancer T1 N0–N1 Widespread VIN or vulvar dystrophy (older patient)	Radical vulvectomy
Early Vulvar Cancer T1 N0–N1 Widespread VIN or vulvar dystrophy (young patient)	Radical local excision, local excision of VIN, topical steroid therapy for dystrophy
Early Vulvar Cancer Clitoral lesion (young patient)	Radiation therapy, repeat biopsy in 6–8 weeks
T2 N0–N1 T3 N0–N1	Radical vulvectomy and bilateral inguinal-femoral lymphadenectomy or modified radical vulvectomy and bilateral inguinal-femoral lymphadectomy or radical local excision
T2 N2–N3 T3 or T4	Removal of all enlarged groin nodes, full pelvic and groin irradiation or if no metastatic disease in removed nodes, a full groin dissection
Locally advanced disease	Pelvic exenteration and radical vulvectomy and bilateral groin dissection or intracavitary radiation therapy and external irradiation and subsequent surgery or preoperative radiation therapy and radical vulvectomy with or without concurrent chemotherapy

(Data from Hoskins, W. J., Perez, C. A., & Young, R. C. [1992]. *Principles and practice of gynecologic oncology.* Philadelphia: J. B. Lippincott Co.)

more positive lymph nodes have a higher incidence of recurrence (Hoskins et al., 1992).

GESTATIONAL TROPHOBLASTIC DISEASE

Gestational trophoblastic disease (GTD) encompasses a continuum of tumors that arise during pregnancy in the fetal chorion. These tumors include complete and partial hydatidiform moles, invasive moles, gestational choriocarcinoma, and placenta-site trophoblastic tumors. Molar pregnancies have some malignant potential and are at increased risk for developing gestational choriocarcinoma.

Partial moles are associated with a fetus, cord or amniotic membranes. Most have chromosomal abnormalities and a low rate of malignant degeneration. Complete moles are not associated with a fetus, cord or amniotic membrane and have a 46XX chromosomal pattern. The complete mole has been shown to develop malignant degeneration.

Historical epidemiology of GTD is difficult because of early studies combining complete hydatidiform moles, partial moles and malignant gestational trophoblastic disease. Older studies were also based on live birth rates, not including rates of induced abortions. Current studies, however, show differences in the epidemiology of hydatidiform moles and gestational choriocarcinoma, as well as the differences and similarities in their risk factors (Table 34–37).

DIAGNOSIS AND STAGING OF BENIGN GESTATIONAL TROPHOBLASTIC DISEASE

Neoplasia and Hydatidiform Mole. The symptoms of a hydatidiform mole vary based on whether the mole is a complete mole or a partial mole (Table 34–38). Patients presenting with any abnormalities throughout pregnancy, but particularly in the first

TABLE **34–36.** *Treatment for Various Types of Vulvar Disease*

TYPE OF DISEASE	TREATMENT
Vulvar melanoma	
Less then 2 mm of invasion	Radical local excision
Greater than 2 mm of invasion	En bloc resection and regional nodes
Bartholin gland carcinoma	Radical vulvectomy, bilateral groin and pelvic node dissection
Paget's disease of vulva	Wide local excision
Other adenocarcinomas	Radical vulvectomy, bilateral groin dissection and postoperative radiation
Basal cell	Radical local excision without lymph node dissection
Verrucous carcinoma	Radical local excision
Leiomyosarcomas	Radical local excision
Rhabdomyosarcomas	Chemotherapy, radiation therapy, less radical surgery
Other vulvar malignancies	Physician and patient preference after evaluation

(Data from Hoskins, W. J., Perez, C. A., & Young, R. C. [1992]. *Prinicples and practice of gynecologic oncology.* Philadelphia: J. B. Lippincott Co.)

TABLE 34–37. *Risk Factors Associated with Hydatidiform Moles and Gestational Choriocarcinoma*

RISK FACTOR	HYDATIDIFORM MOLE	GESTATIONAL CHORIOCARCINOMA
Non-white	Increased risk	Increased risk
Pregnancy >40	Increased risk	Increased risk
Pregnancy <15	Increased risk	Increased risk
Paternal age over 45	Increased risk	Not studied
Prior hydatidiform mole	Increased risk	Increased risk
History of therapeutic abortion	Increased risk	————
History of spontaneous abortion	Increased risk	Increased risk
Below normal level of estrogen	Not studied	Increased risk
Low carotene intake	Increased risk	Not studied

(Data from Soper, J. T., Hammond, C. B., & Lewis, J. L. [1992]. Gestational trophoblastic disease. In W. J. Hoskins, C. A. Perez, & R. C. Young [Eds.], *Principles and practice of gynecologic oncology* [pp. 795–825]. Philadelphia: J. B. Lippincott Co.)

trimester, should be considered at risk for a molar pregnancy or postmolar GTD. The nurse should be aware of the different types of moles as well as presenting signs and symptoms. Follow-up of human chorionic gonadotropin (hCG) levels is an important factor in patient follow-up after molar pregnancies.

Diagnoses consist of a careful history and physical examination, high-resolution ultrasound, and quantitative hCG. A histologic confirmation and grading of the hydatidiform mole is done after evacuation.

Certain patients are at risk for developing malignant disease after evacuation (Table 34–39). The risk increases for patients over 40 years of age or those with one or more high-risk factors.

DIAGNOSIS AND STAGING OF GESTATIONAL TROPHOBLASTIC NEOPLASIA

Patients with GTD clinically present with irregular vaginal bleeding, theca lutein cysts, asymmetric enlargement of the uterus, and persistent elevation of serum hCG titers. The tumor may perforate the myometrium, causing intraperitoneal bleeding, or it may erode into uterine vessels, causing vaginal hemorrhage.

An uncommon but important variant of the GTN is the placental-site-trophoblastic tumor. Contrary to the GTN, these tumors produce small amounts of hCG and tend to remain confined to the uterus, metastasizing late in their course (Berkowitz & Goldstein, 1989).

Patients with plateauing or elevated hCG titer after molar evacuation should immediately be evaluated for malignant GTN (Table 34–40). Staging is done in accordance with the FIGO staging system (Table 34–41), or clinical classification by dividing patients into nonmetastatic, metastatic, low risk with a good prognosis, and high risk with a poor prognosis (Hammond, Haney, & Currie, 1980). The clinical classification system is the most frequently used in the United States to determine treatment and report results (Table 34–42).

MANAGEMENT OF HYDATIDIFORM MOLE

The management of complete and partial hydatidiform moles is the same. The primary management of both includes a surgical evacuation of the uterus by suction dilatation and curettage. A simple hysterectomy may be performed if the patient does not desire further pregnancies. Surveillance of serum hCG titer is an important follow-up process until normal hCG levels are present for 6 months (see Table 34–43 for complete follow-up). Patients are recommended to use oral contraceptives to prevent pregnancy during this time.

TABLE 34–38. *Comparison of Complete and Partial Hydatidiform Moles*

PARAMETER	COMPLETE MOLE	PARTIAL MOLE
Uterine size	Markedly enlarged or top normal	Normal to small
Bleeding	May be heavy	Usually light
Usual preoperative diagnosis	Complete mole	Missed abortion
Vesicles	Markedly hydropic, large	Small, scanty
Tissue volume	Moderate to marked	Low, scanty
Ultrasound picture	Homogeneously ectogenic with varying cystic sizes	Variable gestational sac with increased transverse diameter; cystic irregularities in tissues around sac
Serum HCG	Usually very high (>100,000)	Usually low (<50,000)
Trophoblastic proliferation	May be marked	Usually low
Fetal features	Virtually absent	Varying but present; intact fetus possible
Cytogenetics	XX, all paternal origin	XXY, paternal, maternal origin
Malignant sequelae	XX, all paternal origin. Relatively high (10–30%)	XXY, paternal, maternal origin. Relatively low (4–10%)

(Reprinted with permission from Blackledge, G. R. P., Jordan, J. A., & Shingleton, H. M. [1991]. *Textbook of gynecologic oncology*. Philadelphia: W. B. Saunders Co.)

TABLE 34–39. *Risk Factors for Developing GTN After Hydatidiform Mole*

Delayed postevacuation bleeding
Theca lutein cysts
Large-sized uterus at diagnosis
Enlarged ovaries and or uterus
Previous hydatidiform mole
Advanced maternal age
High initial hCG (>100,000)
Complete mole type

(Data from DiSaia, P. J., & Creasman, W. T. [1989]. *Clinical gynecologic oncology* [3rd ed.]. St. Louis: C. V. Mosby Co.; and Blackledge, G. R. P., Jordan, J. A., & Shingleton, H. M. [1991]. *Textbook of gynecologic oncology*. Philadelphia: W. B. Saunders Co.)

Further treatment with chemotherapy would be necessary after a plateau or rise in serial hCG values for three consecutive weeks or in patients found to have metastatic disease.

MANAGEMENT OF MALIGNANT GTD

The clinical staging classification system is a system that looks at more than the extent of the tumor. This is a system based on risk factors that have a direct effect on the prognosis of the patient. There are three categories derived from this system: nonmetastatic, low-risk metastatic, which has a good prognosis, and high-risk metastatic, which has a poor prognosis. This system allows patients to be identified early so as to initiate appropriate treatment immediately.

Nonmetastatic Disease. Treatment of nonmetastatic trophoblastic disease is almost 100 per cent curable after primary treatment. Methotrexate with citrovorum rescue is the most effective therapy with dactinomycin added, if needed. For resistant disease a patient may require combination therapy or a hysterectomy.

Low-Risk/Good-Prognosis Metastatic Trophoblastic Disease. Therapy is almost 100 per cent curable for this category of patient. The recommended treatment is similar to that of nonmetastatic disease. Methotrexate or dactinomycin are used as the initial therapy, with the alternate being saved for salvage therapy. Hysterectomy may be performed as the treatment of choice in patients no longer desiring childbearing (Soper, Hammond, & Lewis, 1992)

High-Risk/Poor-Prognosis Metastatic Trophoblastic Disease. Patients with metastatic trophoblastic disease

TABLE 34–40. *Workup for Patients with Gestational Trophoblastic Disease*

1. Complete history and physical, including pelvic exam
2. CAT scan of pelvis, lungs, and brain
3. Total CAT scan if indicated
4. Repeat pelvic ultrasound
5. Laboratory studies to include hematologic profile
6. IVP
7. hCG levels
8. Thyroid function test

TABLE 34–41. *FIGO Staging For Gestational Trophoblastic Disease*

Stage I.	Disease confined to the uterus
Stage II.	Disease confined to the uterus and pelvis
Stage III.	Lung metastasis present
Stage IV.	Disease metastatic to other sites

with one or more risk factors benefit from initial multiagent chemotherapy rather than single-agent therapy. These patients must be treated intensively if remission is to be achieved. Overall successful treatment of the patient ranges from 63 to 80 per cent (Soper et al., 1992).

Current therapy consists of methotrexate, dactinomycin, and chlorambucil or cyclophosphamide, each given over 5 days and repeated every 14 to 21 days. Patients being treated with chemotherapy should be monitored at least weekly with serum hCG (Table 34–44). Concurrent brain or liver irradiation is given for metastatic disease. Patients with high-risk metastatic trophoblastic disease who fail primary chemotherapy have a very poor prognosis.

RECURRENCE

Recurrence is defined as an elevation of hCG levels or the appearance of new metastases after remission, without a subsequent pregnancy. Recurrence occurs in less than 5 per cent of patients with low-risk metastatic disease and in 20 per cent of those with high-risk disease. The risk of recurrence is the greatest in the first year after completion of therapy. For this reason some physicians recommend one to four additional cycles of chemotherapy for patients after normal hCG levels depending on the patient's risk factors.

TABLE 34–42. *Clinical Classification of Gestational Trophoblastic Disease*

Nonmetastatic
Persistent hydatidiform mole
No evidence outside of the uterus
Choriocarcinoma destruen
Choriocarcinoma

Metastatic Disease
Good prognosis/low risk
  low hCG level < 40,000 m.i.u./ml
  short duration < 4 months
  no liver or brain metastasis
  no antecedent term pregnancy
  no prior chemotherapy
Poor prognosis/high risk
  hCG > 40,000 m.i.u./ml.
  long duration > 4 month since last pregnancy
  liver or brain metastasis
  prior chemotherapy
  disease following pregnancy

(Data from Soper, J. T., Hammond, C. B., & Lewis, J. L. [1992]. Gestational trophoblastic disease. In W. J. Hoskins, C. A. Perez, & R. C. Young [Eds.], *Principles and practice of gynecologic oncology* [pp. 795–825]. Philadelphia: J. B. Lippincott Co.)

TABLE 34–43. *Postevacuation Monitoring of Hydatidiform Mole*

1. Baseline hCG level within 48 hours after evacuation
2. hCG weekly until normal
3. hCG every 1–2 months for 6 months after hCG is normal
4. Pelvic exam every 2 weeks until hCG is less than 1000 m.i.u./ml
5. Chest x-ray monthly until hCG is less than 1000 m.i.u./ml

(Data from Soper, J. T., Hammond, C. B., & Lewis, J. L. [1992]. Gestational trophoblastic disease. In W. J. Hoskins, C. A. Perez, & R. C. Young [Eds.], *Principles and practice of gynecologic oncology* [pp. 795–825]. Philadelphia: J. B. Lippincott Co.)

TABLE 34–44. *Follow-up for Gestational Trophoblastic Neoplasia*

1. Chemotherapy as indicated until three normal weekly hCG levels have been obtained
2. Give 1 to 4 courses of chemotherapy after reaching normal hCG levels
3. Serial hCG values every 2 weeks for 3 months
4. hCG values at least monthly for the first year after the completion of the first 3-month follow-up
5. Contraception for 1 year

(Data from Soper, J. T., Hammond, C. B., & Lewis, J. L. [1992]. Gestational trophoblastic disease. In W. J. Hoskins, C. A. Perez, & R. C. Young [Eds.], *Principles and practic of gynecologic onoclogy* [pp. 795–825]. Philadelphia: J. B. Lippincott Co.)

SUMMARY

Gynecologic oncology is a rapidly changing field. In a time of educated consumers, emphasis is placed on individualization of treatments. These treatments address not only the physical aspect of cancer but also the psychosocial needs and concerns of the patient. With clinical practices changing on an almost daily basis, it is important for health care providers to not only be current with new treatments but also to be sensitized to the concerns and needs of the whole woman.

REFERENCES

Alexander, E. (1973). Possible etiologies of cancer of the cervix other than herpes virus. *Cancer Research, 33,* 1485–1496.

American Cancer Society. (1993). *American Cancer Society facts and figures: 1993.* Atlanta, GA: American Cancer Society.

Baker, V. V. (1991). *The etiology and epidemiology of vulvar and vaginal neoplasms.* In G. R. Blackledge, J. A. Jordan, & H. M. Shingleton (Eds.), *Textbook of gynecologic oncology* (pp. 383–389). Philadelphia: W. B. Saunders Co.

Barber, H. (1993). *Ovarian carcinoma: Etiology, diagnosis and treatment* (3rd ed.). New York: Springer-Verlag.

Berek, J. S., & Hacker, N. F. (1989). *Practical gynecologic oncology.* Baltimore: Williams & Wilkins.

Berkowitz, R. S., & Goldstein, D. P. (1989). Gestational trophoblastic neoplasia. In J. S. Berek & N. F. Hacker (Eds.), *Practical gynecologic oncology* (pp. 441–468). Baltimore: Williams & Wilkins.

Blackledge, G. R. P., Jordan, J. A., & Shingleton, H. M. (1991). *Textbook of gynecologic oncology.* Philadelphia: W. B. Saunders Co.

Boarini, J. H., Bryant, R. A., & Irrgang, S. J. (1986). Fistula management. *Seminars in Oncology Nursing, 2,* 287–292.

Bokhman, J. V. (1985). Two pathogenetic types of endometrial carcinoma. *Gynecologic Oncology, 15,* 10–17.

Bond, A. P. (1986). Carcinoma of the endometrium: changing trends in etiology and management. *British Journal of Clinical Practice, 40,* 157–164.

Boring, C. C., Squires, T. S., & Heath, C. W. (1992). Cancer statistics for African Americans. *CA: Cancer Journal for Americans, 42,* 7–17.

Brinton, L. A., Nasca, P. C., Mallin, K., Schairer, C., Rosenthal, J., Rothenberg, R., Yordan, E. Jr., & Richart, R. M. (1990). Case-control study of in situ and invasive carcinoma of the vagina. *Gynecology Oncology, 38,* 49.

Chen, R. T., Schooley, J. L., & Flam, M. S. (1985). Peritoneal carcinomatosis after prophylactic oophorectomy in familial ovarian syndrome. *Obstetrics and Gynecology, 66,* 935–945.

Connelly P. J., Albershasky, R. C., & Christopherson, W. W. (1982). Carcinoma of the endometrium. *Obstetrics and Gynecology, 59,* 569.

DiSaia, P. J. (1987). Diagnosis and management of ovarian cancer. *Hospital Practice,* 235–250.

DiSaia, P. J., & Creasman, W. T. (1989). *Clinical gynecologic oncology* (3rd ed.). St. Louis: C. V. Mosby Co.

DiSaia, P. J., & Creasman, W. T. (1993a). Preinvasive disease of the cervix. In *Clinical gynecologic oncology* (4th. ed., pp. 1–36). St. Louis: Mosby Year Book.

DiSaia, P. J., & Creasman, W. T. (1993b). Invasive cervical cancer. In *Clinical gynecologic oncology* (4th ed., pp. 58–125). St. Louis: Mosby Year Book.

DiSaia, P. J., & Creasman, W. T. (1993c). Epithelial ovarian cancer. In *Clinical gynecologic oncology* (4th ed., pp. 333–425.) St. Louis: Mosby Year Book.

DiSaia, P. J., & Creasman, W. T. (1993d). Germ cell, stromal and other ovarian tumors. In *Clinical gynecologic oncology* (4th ed., pp. 426–457). St. Louis: Mosby Year Book.

Eriksson, J. H., & Walczak, J. R. (1990). Ovarian cancer. *Seminars in Oncology Nursing, 6*(3), 214–227.

Fathalla, M. F. (1972). Factors in the causation and incidence of ovarian cancer. *Obstetrics and Gynecology Survey, 27,* 751.

Freidman, J. B., & Weiss, N. S. (1990). Second thoughts about second look laparotomy in advanced ovarian cancer. *New England Journal of Medicine, 322,* 1079.

Graham, C. A. (1993). Cervix cancer prevention and detection update. *Seminars in Oncology Nursing, 9*(3), 155–162.

Greenblatt, R. B., & Stoddard, L. D. (1978). The estrogen-cancer controversy. *Journal of the American Geriatric Society, 26,* 1–8.

Hacker, N. F., Eifel, P., McQuire, W., & Wilkinson, E. J. (1992). Vulva. In W. J. Hoskins, C. A. Perez, & R. C. Young (Eds.), *Principles and practice of gynecologic oncology* (pp. 537–566). Philadelphia: J. B. Lippincott Co.

Hammond, C. B., Haney, A. F., & Currie, J. L. (1980). The role of operation in the current therapy of gestational trophoblastic disease. *American Journal of Obstetrics and Gynecology, 136,* 844–858.

Hatch, K. D., Bucham, J. B., Blessing, J. A., & Creasman, W. T. (1991). Responsiveness of patients with advanced ovarian carcinoma to tomoxifen: A gynecologic oncology group study of second line therapy in 105 patients. *Cancer, 68,* 269–271.

Henrickson, E. (1949). Lymphatic spread of carcinoma of the cervix and body of the uterus: Study of 420 necropsies.

American Journal of Obstetrics and Gynecology, 58, 924–942.

Herberth, L., & Gosnell, D. (1987). Nursing diagnosis for oncology practice. *Cancer Nursing, 10,* 41–51.

Hoskins, W. J., Perez, C. A., & Young, R. C. (1992). *Principles and practice of gynecologic oncology.* Philadelphia: J. B. Lippincott Co.

Howell, S. B., Kirmani, S., & Lucas, A. (1990). A phase II trial of intraperitoneal cisplatin and etopoide for primary treatment of ovarian cancer. *Journal of Clinical Oncology, 8,* 137.

International Federation of Gynecology and Obstetrics (FIGO). (1989). Corpus cancer staging. *International Journal of Gynecology and Obstetrics. 28,* 190.

Jacobs, I., & Bast, R. C. (1989). The CA 125 tumor-associated antigen: A review of the literature. *Human Reproduction, 4,* 1–12.

Knapstein, P. G., diRe, F., DiSaia, P., Haller, U., & Stein, B. - U. (1991). *Malignancies of the vulva.* New York: Thieme Medical Publishers, Inc.

Koss, L. (1989). The papanicolaou test for cervical cancer detection: A triumph and a tragedy. *Journal of the American Medical Association, 261(5),* 737–743.

Lamb, M. A. (1985). Sexual dysfunction in the gynecologic oncology patient. *Seminars in Oncology Nursing, 1,* 9–17.

Lim-Tan, S. R., Cajigas, H. E., & Scully, R. E. (1988). Ovarian cystectomy for serous borderline tumors: A follow-up study of 35 cases. *Obstetrics and Gynecology, 72,* 775.

Lundberg, G. (1989). The bethesda system for reporting cervical/vaginal cytological diagnosis. *Journal of the American Medical Association, 267(7),* 931–934.

Lynch, H. T., Conway, T., & Lynch, J. (1990). Hereditary ovarian cancer. In F. Sharp, W. P. Mason, R. E. Leake (Eds.), *Ovarian cancer: Biological and therapeutic challenges* (pp. 7–19). London: Chapman & Hall Medical.

Mahboube, E., Eyler, N., & Wynder, E. L. (1982). Epidemiology of cancer of the endometrium. *Clinical Obstetrics and Gynecology, 25,* 5–18.

Mandelblatt, J., Gopaul, F. W. P., & Wistreich, M. (1986). Gynecological care of elderly women. *Journal of the American Medical Association, 3,* 367–371.

Mann, W. J. (1991). The etiology and epidemiology of uterine adenocarcinoma. In G. R. Blackledge, J. A. Jordan, & H. M. Shing Leton (Eds.), *Textbook of gynecologic oncology* (pp. 198–210), Philadelphia: W. B. Saunders Co.

Mattingly, R. F. (1985). Malignant tumors of the uterus. In R. F. Mattingly, J. D. Thompson (Eds.), *Telinde's operative gynecology* (6th ed., pp. 845–876) Philadelphia: J. B. Lippincott.

McGuire, W. P., & Rowinsky, E. K. (1991). Old drugs revisited, new drugs, and experimental approaches in ovarian cancer therapy. *Seminars in Oncology Nursing, 18,* 225–269.

McGuire, W. P., Rowinski, E. K., & Rosenheim, N. E. (1989). Taxol: A unique antineoplastic agent with significant activity in advanced ovarian epithelial neoplasms. *Annals of Internal Medicine, 111,* 273.

McKenzie, F. (1988). Sexuality after total pelvic exenteration. *Nursing Times, 84,* 27–29.

McMullin, M. (1992). Holistic care of the patient with cervical cancer. *Nursing Clinics of North America, 27(4),* 847–858.

Nagell, J. R., & Barber, H. R. (1982). *Modern concepts of gynecologic oncology.* Boston: John Wright—PSG Inc.

Nolte, S., & Hanjani, P. (1990). Intraepithelial neoplasia of the lower genital tract. *Seminars in Oncology Nursing, 6(3),* 181–189.

Ortiz, R., Newtown, M., & Bai, A. (1973). Electrocautery treatment of cervical intraepithelial neoplasia. *Obstetrics and Gynecology, 41,* 113–116.

Park, R. C., Grigsby, P. W., Muss, H. B., & Norris, H. J. (1992). Corpus: epithelial tumors. In W. J. Hoskins, C. A. Perez, & R. C. Young (Eds.), *Principles and practice of gynecologic oncology* (pp. 663–693). Philadelphia: J. B. Lippincott Co.

Perez, C. A., Gersell, D. J., Hoskins, W. J., & McGuire, W. P. III (1992). Vagina. In W. J. Hoskins, C. A. Perez, & R. C. Young (Eds.), *Principles and practice of gynecologic oncology* (pp. 567–590). Philadelphia: J. B. Lippincott Co.

Piver, M. S., Baker, T. R., Piedmont, M., & Sandecki, A. M. (1991). Epidemiology and etiology of ovarian cancer. *Seminars in Oncology Nursing, 18,* 177–185.

Piver, M. S., Rutledge, F. N., & Smith, P. J. (1974). Five classes of extended hysterectomy of women with cervical cancers. *Obstetrics and Gynecology, 44,* 265.

Rose, P. (1994). Locally advanced cervical carcinoma: The role of chemoradiation. *Seminars in Oncology, 21(1),* 47–53.

Rossetti, A. C. (1985). Nursing care of patients treated with intrapleural tetracycline for control of malignant pleural effusion. *Cancer Nursing, 8,* 103–109.

Runowicz, C. (1992). Advances in the screening and treatment of ovarian cancer. *CA: Cancer Journal for Clinicians, 42(6),* 327–349.

Shen, Y. L., & Wang, E. Y. (1990). *Endometrial carcinoma.* Beijing: The Peoples Medical Publishing House, & Berlin: Springer Verlag.

Slotman, B. J., & Roa, B. R. (1988). Ovarian cancer: Etiology, diagnosis, prognosis, surgery, radiotherapy, chemotherapy, and endocrine therapy. *Anticancer Research, 8,* 417–434.

Soper, J. T., Hammond, C. B., & Lewis, J. L. (1992). Gestational trophoblastic disease. In W. J. Hoskins, C. A. Perez, & R. C. Young (Eds.), *Principles and practice of gynecologic oncology* (pp. 795–825). Philadelphia: J. B. Lippincott Co.

Steele, G., Osteen, R., Winchester, D., Murphy, G., & Menck, H. (1994). Clinical highlights from the national cancer data base: 1994. *CA: A Cancer Journal for Clinicians, 44(2),* 78.

Swaffield, L. (1989). Wasted lives. *Nursing Times, 85,* 22–23.

Swenson, R. K., & Erikson, J. H. (1986). Nursing management of intraperitoneal chemotherapy. *Oncology Nursing Forum, 13(5),* 33–39.

Thompson, L. (1990). Cancer of the cervix. *Seminars in Oncology Nursing, 6(3),* 190–197.

University of Pennsylvania Medical Center. (1995). Clinical practice guidelines: Nursing management of the patient receiving brachytherapy. In *Nursing practice manual* (Vol. 4D). Philadelphia: Author.

Vonka, V., Kanka, J., Hirsch, I., Zavadova, H., Krcmar, M., Suchankova, A., Rezacova, D., Broucek, J., Press, M., Domorazkova, E., Svoboda, B., Havrankova, A., & Jelinek, J. (1984). Propective study on the relationship between cervical neoplasia and herpes simplex type II virus. Herpes simplex type II antibody present in serum taken at enrollment. *International Journal of Cancer, 33,* 61–66.

Wright, T. C., & Richart, K. M. (1992). *Pathogenesis and diagnosis of preinvasive lesions of the lower genital tract.* In W. J. Hoskins, C. A. Perez, & R. D. Young (Eds.), *Principles and practice of gynecologic oncology.* Philadelphia: J. B. Lippincott.

Yoder, L., & Rubin, M. (1992). The epidemiology of cervical cancer and its precursors. *Oncology Nursing Forum, 19(3),* 485–493.

Hodgkin's Disease and Non-Hodgkin's Lymphomas

Colette Carson

Cancers that originate in the lymphatic tissue are collectively referred to as malignant lymphomas. Because of the function of the lymphocyte in the immune system, these neoplasms are often referred to as immunologic cancers and are often confused with hematopoietic malignancies such as leukemias. Blood cells that originate in the bone marrow are called hematopoietic cells; those that originate in the thymus and lymphatic tissue are called lymphoid cells. In general, when the bone marrow and peripheral blood are major sites of involvement, the neoplasm is classified as a leukemia (see Chapter 36); likewise malignancies that originate in the lymphatic tissue are called lymphomas.

The lymphomas consist of two major subtypes: Hodgkin's disease and non-Hodgkin's lymphomas. In 1932, Thomas Hodgkin first described a disease that was characterized by progressive enlargement of the lymph nodes. Many years later, Hodgkin's disease became distinct from other lymphomas when the giant Reed-Sternberg cell was recognized in some lymphomas and not in others. The differentiation resulted in the classification of Hodgkin's disease, which is characterized by the presence of Reed-Sternberg cells, and non-Hodgkin's lymphomas, which are characterized by an absence of Reed-Sternberg cells. Although both diseases have some similarities, they are distinctly different in cellular origin, pattern of spread, and response to treat-

ment. They are addressed separately with references to similarities and differences throughout the text.

The clinical manifestation of each of these malignancies presents an array of symptoms that require nursing intervention. It is the purpose of this chapter to describe the disease process and treatment, identify nursing issues, and refer the reader to specific chapters for a more in-depth review of nursing measures.

HODGKIN'S DISEASE

OVERVIEW

The treatment for Hodgkin's disease and the survival rate have improved dramatically in the past 2 decades. More than 75 per cent of all newly diagnosed patients with adult Hodgkin's disease are curable. National mortality is falling more rapidly for adult Hodgkin's disease than for any other malignancy. Much of this success is largely due to the ability to understand the disease process and to technicologic advances in radiotherapy and complex chemotherapeutic methods.

According to the American Cancer Society (1994) there will be an estimated 7900 new cases of Hodgkin's disease in 1994. This number represents approximately 1 per cent of all cancers; therefore in actuality Hodgkin's disease is not a common disease. Hodgkin's disease may develop at any age, from early childhood to advanced old age. A bimodal curve of age incidence is found, with a peak in the United States in the mid to late 20s and a second peak after age 50 years. The young adult group is composed equally of men and women, and the predominant disease is the nodular sclerosis subtype. Among the older patients, men exceed women. Survival and disease-free survival decrease as age increases. The overall incidence is lower in economically underdeveloped countries, with more cases occurring proportionally at older ages. There is also a difference in the distribution of subtypes (American Cancer Society, 1994; DeVita, Hellman, & Rosenberg, 1985).

ETIOLOGY

The etiology of Hodgkin's disease is unknown, though many theories have been explored. Several peculiar characteristics of Hodgkin's disease have implicated viral, possibly genetic, and environmental factors.

Findings suggest that an infectious process, possibly viral, may be involved. Long-standing observations have indicated the defective T cell function and persistent immune defect in patients with Hodgkin's disease. Similarities have also been noted between patients with Hodgkin's disease and graft-vs.-host disease. The auto-immune response could be indicative of a virus and lack of T cell response. Other studies have indicated an increased risk of Hodgkin's disease with history of infectious mononucleosis. An etiologic association of Hodgkin's disease with Epstein-Barr virus (EBV) is of interest. A proportion of biopsy specimens have demonstrated EBV DNA, and it is not known whether EBV plays a direct role in the pathogenesis of Hodgkin's disease. Other inconclusive observations include a higher than expected incidence in the discussion on siblings of the same sex and an increased risk of Hodgkin's disease with higher economic and educational status (DeVita et al., 1985; Haskell & Parker, 1985).

Studies presenting results that contradict the viral contagious bias have indicated that although siblings have demonstrated higher risk for contracting Hodgkin's disease, it is very rare to observe this pattern with marital partners. In addition, health professionals caring for patients with Hodgkin's disease have not shown an increased incidence (Haskell & Parker, 1985). Despite interesting findings, it is not known what causes the disease or what is required to prevent it.

ORIGIN AND SPREAD

Although information is inconclusive regarding the cause of Hodgkin's disease, there has been greater understanding of the tumor's clinical behavior, including its pattern of spread and prognostic indications such as histologic type and extent of disease.

In the 1960s and 1970s a large number of patients at clinical research centers underwent very careful clinical evaluations and laparotomies, which precisely identified the extent of abdominal disease. Important information regarding the origin and spread of disease resulted from these studies.

It appears that Hodgkin's disease arises as a single focal area, beginning in lymph nodes in more than 90 per cent of patients. In the early stages, the disease remains confined to lymph nodes for a variable period, making diagnosis sometimes difficult until multiple nodes are involved. In the majority of cases, Hodgkin's disease spreads in predictable patterns from the original site to lymph nodes in other areas. Disease usually spreads to adjacent lymph nodes. This orderly pattern of contiguous spread is most evident in nodular sclerosing Hodgkin's disease (Kaplan, 1981; Rosenberg, 1986). For example, a lesion that originates in the mediastinum will first spread to nodes in the lower neck and then to nodes in the upper retroperitoneal area. Figure 35–1 represents the orderly pattern of contiguous lymphoid spread characterized in Hodgkin's disease (Rosenberg, 1986).

There are exceptions. Other histologic types may also spread contiguously, but some lesions first noted in the cervical region skip the mediastium and spread to retroperitoneal nodes without causing intrathoracic disease. It is suggested that spread occurs by retrograde flow in the thoracic duct. It is also possible that disease begins in the retroperitoneum but does not become evident until it spreads to the cervical nodes.

Disease spreads to extranodal areas by direct extension; for example, it spreads from hilar lymph nodes to lungs—a vascular invasion—which then results in hematologenous dissemination. When the spleen becomes involved, it is usually evidence of hematologic dissemination and raises the possibility of liver and bone marrow involvement. Conversely, no evidence of splenic disease would suggest an absence of hematogenous dissemination to other organs. By this predictable pattern of spread, the spleen represents the final lymph node area of involvement before hematologous dissemination occurs. Therefore, the most important fact influencing both staging and treatment is that Hodgkin's disease is a unifocal disease that usually spreads in a contiguous manner (DeVita, 1982; Haskell & Parker, 1985; Lacher, 1985; Rapaport, 1987).

HISTOPATHOLOGIC CLASSIFICATION

Hodgkin's disease differs histologically from that of other lymphomas. In Hodgkin's disease, the diagnostic cell—the Reed-Sternberg cell—rarely predominates on a biopsy section and sometimes is difficult to find. Most of the tumor mass is usually composed of lymphocytes, histiocytes, granulocytes, plasma cells, and fibroblasts, presumed not to be neoplastic. The Reed-Sternberg cell is multinucleated, and each nuclei contains a giant nucleolus. Mononuclear cells with neoplastic features are also evident and are sometimes referred to as Hodgkin's cells or pre-Sternberg cells. These cells alone may not be distinctive enough to diagnose Hodgkin's disease without the presence of Reed-Sternberg cells (Rapaport, 1987).

According to the Rye Classification, which was developed in the 1960s and widely used, Hodgkin's diseases is divided into four categories. The histopathology reflects the host resistance and subsequently prog-

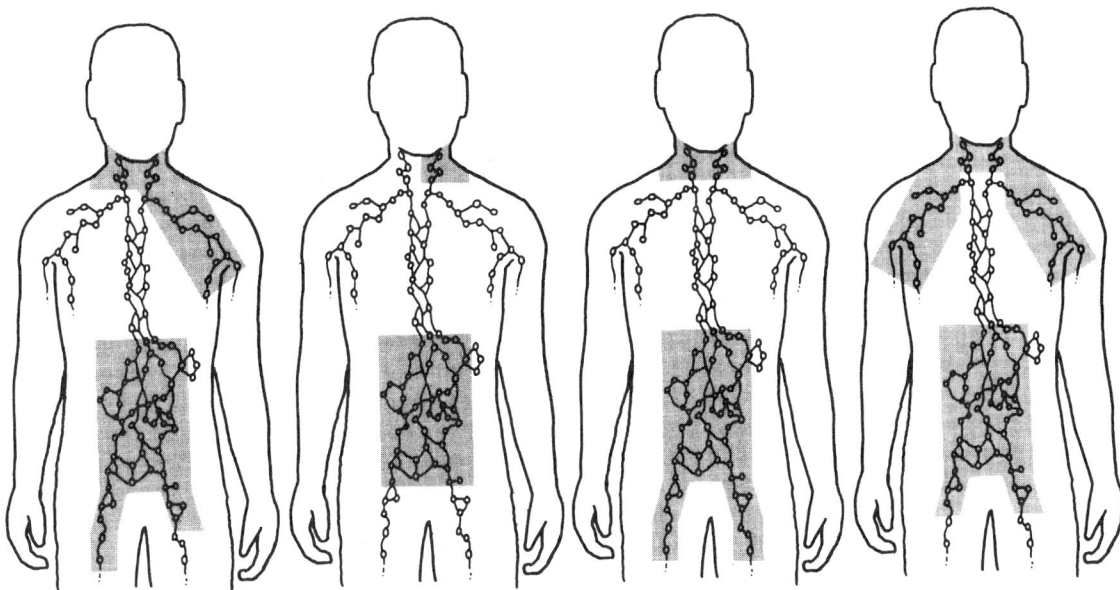

FIGURE 35–1. Orderly pattern of contiguous lymphoid spread in Hodgkin's disease. (From Rosenberg, S. A. [1986]. Hodgkin's disease: No stage beyond cure. *Hospital Practice, 21*[8], 91–98, 101–108. Reproduced by permission.)

nosis, which proceeds from favorable to less favorable. The four categories are listed in Table 35–1.

The first and last subgroups are the least common. The lymphocyte-predominant subgroup has a good prognosis and is most commonly found in young males with localized cervical node involvement; the lymphocyte-depleted subgroup has the least favorable prognosis; biopsy indicates an increased number of Reed-Sternberg cells and breakdown of normal cellular components. Lymphocyte depletion is indicative of a breakdown in host resistance. The two more common subtypes, nodular sclerosis and mixed cellularity, fall between lymphocyte predominance and lymphocyte depletion in degree of neoplastic cells and prognosis.

The nodular sclerosis subtype is most often seen in younger patients and twice as frequently in women than in men. Because these large, so-called lacunar cells are so predominant, it is sometimes impossible to find Reed-Sternberg cells. All subtypes except the nodular

sclerosis subtype may develop into a less favorable subtype (Haskell & Parker, 1985; Rapaport, 1987).

As prognostic indicators, the histologic subtypes have lost much of their predictive value as therapy has improved. Other more important prognostic factors include volume and site of disease, extent of disease spread, presence of systemic symptoms, age, and sex.

CLINICAL PRESENTATION

One characteristic symptom of Hodgkin's disease generally is progressive, painless, "rubbery" lymph node enlargement, usually localized in the neck region in 60 to 80 per cent of cases (DeVita et al., 1985). Most patients are asymptomatic, but 40 per cent of patients may have associated "B" symptoms of fever, night sweats, and unexplained weight loss. Occasionally a patient is diagnosed after a mediastinal mass is discovered on routine chest film or after a persistent

TABLE 35–1. *Rye Classification of Hodgkin's Disease*

SUBGROUP	MAJOR HISTOLOGIC FEATURES	APPROXIMATE FREQUENCY (%)
Lymphocyte predominance	Abundant normal-appearing lymphocytes with or without benign histiocytes; occasionally nodular, rare Reed-Sternberg cells	2–10
Nodular sclerosis	Nodules of lymphoid tissue separated by bands of collagen; numerous variants of Reed-Sternberg cells	40–80
Mixed cellularity	Pleomorphic infiltrate of eosinophils, plasma cells, histiocytes, and lymphocytes, with numerous Reed-Sternberg cells	20–40
Lymphocyte depletion	Paucity of lymphocytes with numerous Reed-Sternberg cells, diffuse fibrosis and necrosis	2–15

(Adapted from Rosenberg, S. A. [1986]. Hodgkin's disease: No stage beyond cure. *Hospital Practice, 21*[8], 91–98, 101–108.)

cough provokes a visit to a physician. When disease originates in the retroperitoneal area, it may be accompanied with prolonged fever. Rarely, a patient may present with complaints indicative of an extranodal lesion, for example, gastrointestinal (GI) bleeding or pain due to obstruction. Compared with non-Hodgkin's lymphoma the lymph node disease in Hodgkin's disease is usually centripedal and axial in nature, with cervical, supraclavicular, and mediastinal presentation being common.

Other disorders presenting with similar characteristics are infectious mononucleosis, acquired immunodeficiency syndrome (AIDS), or other infectious inflammations.

DIAGNOSIS AND STAGING

The initial evaluation of Hodgkin's disease requires an adequate surgical specimen for the histologic diagnosis. Needle biopsy is not adequate for diagnosis, as insufficient tissue is obtained to exclude other disease and to subclassify the disease. An excisional lymph node is required to fully appreciate the architecture of the lymphoma. A detailed clinical history that establishes the presence or absence of systemic symptoms including fever, night sweats, and weight loss is required. A complete physical examination includes an examination of all lymph node chains, including Waldeyers ring, and determination of abdominal involvement such as that of the liver and spleen. Specific laboratory and radiologic procedures are listed in Table 35–2.

EXTENT OF DISEASE

The primary purpose of the staging workup is to identify the anatomic extent of the disease to determine the most effective therapy. The extent or stage of disease strongly influences the choice of treatment and must be carefully determined in each patient. This process is referred to as staging. *Clinical staging* usually refers to all procedures except a staging laporatomy. *Pathologic staging* refers to findings indicated from staging laporatomy.

After the initial staging workup is completed, the extent of the disease is staged by a widely used system called the Ann Arbor Staging Classification of Hodgkin's Disease (Table 35–3). As Hodgkin's disease appears to spread contiguously from one lymph node to the next, the staging system is anatomically based. The Ann Arbor staging system was originated in 1971 but was recently modified in 1989 in Cotswald, England (Table 35–3). Cotswald modifications address the location, bulk, and number of anatomic regions. Staging must be defined as CS for clinical stage or PS for pathologic stage. The Ann Arbor system divides Hodgkin's disease into four stages based on the extent of disease involvement. Stages range from a single node or region of involvement (stage I) to diffuse disseminated involvement (stage IV). In the first three stages, extranodal involvement is delineated using the subscript *E*, meaning direct extension rather than that of hematologic dissemination, as in stage IV. Additionally,

TABLE 35–2. *Laboratory and Radiologic Procedures Used in Determining the Extent of Disease in Hodgkin's Disease*

STUDY OR PROCEDURE	FUNCTION
Laboratory Studies	
CBC, platelet count, ESR	Evidence of peripheral blood involvement
Liver function tests, particularly serum alkaline phosphatase	Hepatic involvement
Urinalysis and renal function tests	Proteinuria
Radiographic Studies	
For thoracic disease: Chest radiographs, posteroanterior and lateral; whole lung tomograms (if abnormal chest radiograph)	Visualizes mediastinal masses, hilar and paratracheal lymphadenopathy
For abdominal disease: CT scan of the abdomen	Can visualize lymph node enlargement in areas not seen on lymphangiogram; visualizes tumor nodules in spleen and liver
Bilateral lower lymphangiogram (dye injected into lymphatic channels in both feet)	Internal structural changes in a node from Hodgkin's disease may be evident on lymphangiogram but not on a CT scan because the node may not be large enough
Intravenous pyelogram	
Bilateral bone marrow biopsy	To obtain histologic report of marrow. Sometimes omitted in young patients with early disease I and II with favorable histologic results on lymph node biopsy

CBC = complete blood count; ESR = erythrocyte sedimentation rate; CT = computed tomography.

all stages are given the letter *A* to indicate the absence of systemic symptoms or the letter *B* to indicate the presence of systemic symptoms. Patients with *B* symptoms have presence of unexplained fever, night sweats, or weight loss of more than 10 per cent of body weight in the past 6 months. Presence of B symptoms indicate a less favorable prognosis. At diagnosis, about 10 to 15 per cent of patients will have disease limited to a single lymph node (stage I), and another 10 to 15 per cent of patients will have extranodal disease or bone marrow involvement (stage IV). About 70 to 80 per cent of patients will be at stage II or III at presentation (Lister et al., 1989; Mouch et al., 1990).

LAPAROTOMY

The routine use of staging laporatomy has resulted in an understanding of the natural spread of Hodgkin's disease. A number of investigators are questioning the routine application of staging laparotomies in Hodgkin's disease. The laporatomy entails multiple

TABLE 35–3. *Ann Arbor Staging System for Hodgkin's Disease and Non-Hodgkin's Lymphoma*

Stage I
Involvement of a single lymph node region or lymphoid structure (e.g., spleen, thymus, Waldeyer's ring)

Stage II
Involvement of two or more lymph node regions on the same side of the diaphragm

Stage III
Involvement of lymph node regions or structures on both sides of the diaphragm

Stage IV
Involvement of extranodal site(s) beyond that designated "E"

For All Stages
A: No symptoms
B: Fever (> 38°C), drenching sweats, weight loss (> 10% body weight over 6 months)

For Stages I to III
E: Involvement of a single, extranodal site contiguous or proximal to known nodal site

Cotswold Modifications

(i) Suffix "X" to designate bulky disease as > ⅓ widening of the mediastinum or > 10 cm maximum dimension of nodal mass

(ii) The number of anatomical regions involved should be indicated by a subscript (e.g., II3)

(iii) Stage III may be subdivided into:
III1: with or without splenic, hilar, celiac, or portal nodes
III2: with para-aortic, iliac, mesenteric nodes

(iv) Staging should be identified as clinical stage (CS) or pathologic stage (PS)

(v) A new category of response to therapy, unconfirmed/uncertain complete remission (CR[U]) be introduced because of the persistent radiologic abnormalities of uncertain significance

---

lymph node biopsies, wedge and needle biopsies of the liver, and a spleenectomy. Laparotomies increase the accuracy of staging patients with Hodgkin's disease beyond that achieved by clinical methods. There is no question that the use of laporotomies in research treatment centers has provided important information on the origin and spread of Hodgkin's disease. It provides the most precise evaluation of intraabdominal disease. The controversy rests on the issues of whether—and if so, when—to perform surgical staging laporotomies.

Multiple studies have shown that laporatomy will alter the clinical stage in about one fourth to one third of patients, of whom one third will be downstaged and about one third will be upstaged (Aragon de la Cruz et al., 1989; Taylor, Kaplan, & Nelsen, 1985; Wobbles, 1994). The procedure should be performed only if the information obtained will potentially change the course of treatment and not just the stage of the disease (Bonadonna, Valagussa, & Santoro, 1986).

Staging laparotomies are usually restricted to patients in whom radiotherapy alone will be used for treatment. Patients with a clinical stage of IIIB or IV Hodgkin's disease require chemotherapy and therefore would not be candidates for a staging laparotomy. Similarly, patients with a clinical stage of IB, IIB, or IIA with mediastinal involvement generally require chemotherapy and radiotherapy (combined modality) and would not be candidates for laparotomy. Therefore, candidates eligible for staging laparotomy given no medical contraindications are patients with clini-

cal stages of IA, IIA without mediastinal involvement, and IIIA Hodgkin's disease (Ultmann & Bitran, 1989). Because the clinical staging process is not always absolute, some claim advantages to doing staging laparotomies on all patients who are not clearly in stage IV.

Disadvantages of doing a staging laparotomy include the risk of morbidity (0.7 per cent) and operative mortality (0.7 per cent) that is associated with the surgical procedure. Complications include postsplenectomy sepsis and late bowel obstructions associated with radiation therapy (Schimpff et al., 1975). Infection is always a possibility and is confounded by the immunosuppressive effects of radiation therapy, chemotherapy, and energy from the disease itself. To decrease the risk of pneumococcal pneumonia, a prophylactic pneumococcal vaccine is sometimes given before a planned splenectomy (Ultmann & Bitran, 1989).

PROGNOSIS

Many factors influence the prognosis of Hodgkin's disease in an individual patient. Although current treatment has resulted in a dramatic increase in survival, some patients still respond poorly. Many factors contribute to a favorable or a less favorable prognosis (Table 35–4).

The prognosis of Hodgkin's disease is dependent on several variables, including the histologic classification, as it reflects host resistance and therefore the prognosis.

TABLE 35–4. *Variables in the Prognosis of Hodgkin's Disease*

FAVORABLE	LESS FAVORABLE
Clinical Factors	
Young age	Older age (over 60)
Stages IA, IIA, III1A	Bulky mediastinal disease
	Stage III2B or IVA or B
	B symptoms
	Male sex
Histologic Factors	
Lymphocyte predominance	Lymphocyte depletion
Few Reed-Sternberg cells	Many Reed-Sternberg cells

(Data from Rapaport, S. I. [1987]. *Introduction to hematology* [2nd ed.]. Philadelphia: J. B. Lippincott.)

The extent and volume of disease at diagnosis—less being better—are equally important influential prognostic variables. An elevated erythrocyte sedimentation rate and the number of extranodal sites also affect prognosis. Other factors include age, older age being associated with decreased host resistance and decreased tolerance to aggressive therapy; and gender, women having a better prognosis than men, which is associated with the proclivity for young women to have nodular sclerosing Hodgkin's disease. The nodular sclerosis subtype inherently has less dissemination to extranodal sites. The presence of systemic B symptoms is associated with a less favorable prognosis (Rapaport, 1987, Weinshel & Peterson, 1993).

TREATMENT

The goal of management of Hodgkin's disease is cure. The success of the treatment for Hodgkin's disease has improved dramatically over the past 20 years. Several factors have contributed to this success. They include the following:

- The orderly process by which the disease spreads and the ability to stage the disease clinically and pathologically.
- Modern megavoltage techniques in radiation therapy, which allow beam direction to specific sites but shield normal tissue to prevent unnecessary damage. Consequently, tumoricidal doses of radiation can be administered, thus eradicating disease.
- Combination chemotherapy (e.g., mechlorethamine [Mustargen], vincristine [Oncovin], procarbazine, and prednisone [MOPP], doxorubicin [Adriamycin], bleomycin, vinblastine, and dacarbazine [ABVD]), which is curative in many patients with disseminated disease.

Treatment of Hodgkin's disease is based, for the most part, on the stage of disease rather than on the histologic type. Various forms of treatment include radiation therapy, combination chemotherapy, and combined methods, which include both radiation therapy and chemotherapy prescribed at different intervals.

The basic goal of radiation therapy is the eradication of all tumor in a specific tissue volume or in all sites of disease. Radiation fields used in treating Hodgkin's disease are shown in Figure 35–2. Hodgkin's disease is very radiosensitive, and it has been documented that eradication of tumor is proportional to the dose of radiation administered. Thus the therapeutic objective is to give the maximum dose possible to eradicate disease without compromising normal tissue (Kaplan, 1981).

Patients with stage IA or IIA disease can obtain a complete response following either involved field or subtotal nodal irradiation. It has not been determined whether radiation limited to involved fields results in a decrease in long-term survival as compared with "extended field" or "total nodal" irradiation. The last two techniques eradicate suspected disease as well as known disease. Ten-year survival ranges from 90 per cent to 76 per cent, respectively (Willet et al., 1987b).

Patients with stage IB or IIB disease have a higher rate of relapse after radiation therapy than patients with stage IA or IIA disease. Furthermore, patients with large mediastinal masses also demonstrate a higher relapse rate after treatment. Therefore, treatment of early-stage disease with B symptoms is often combination chemotherapy. The focus of treatment investigation in these patients has been to compare radiotherapy alone with combined modality (XRT and chemotherapy). This is in contrast to studies done in advanced disease that compare chemotherapy alone with combined modality (Biti et al., 1992, Longo et al., 1991).

Patients with stage IIIA disease present a more controversial therapeutic group. There are several approaches to treatment for these patients. There seems to be a general consensus that radiation therapy alone results in an unacceptably high rate of relapse. There are differing opinions on whether combined modality should be used as a first approach to treatment or only after radiation therapy alone and combination chemotherapy alone have failed to be effective. There are several prognostic variables within these patients with stage IIIA disease that influence whether a more aggressive approach such as combined modality should be the treatment course over combination chemotherapy. These variables include splenic involvement with more than five nodules; IIIa disease with a large mediastinal mass, III2a disease with paraaortic/iliac involvement, and clinical stage IIIa (rather than pathologic) disease. To some extent all these factors represent more extensive disease requiring more intensive therapy (Greenberger, Mauch, Canellow, & Larson, 1989; Hoppe, Cox, Rosenberg, & Kaplan, 1982). The majority of patients with stage IIIA disease fall into these categories. Some recommend that the remaining patients with less disease be treated with radiotherapy alone and while those with more disease are treated with combination chemotherapy or combined modality (Prosnitz, 1992; Willet et al., 1987a). Though optimum treatment is not clear preliminary evidence would now support combination chemotherapy for initial management in selected patients though others suggest combined modality may be superior (Crowther et al., 1984; Brizel et al., 1990; Pronitz & Robert, 1992; Straus, 1986;

Urba & Longo, 1992). Ultimately the decision will be influenced by the toxicities of the treatment available.

In patients with advanced disease, defined as stage IIIA with five or more nodules in the spleen, stage IIIB, or stage IVA or IVB, combination chemotherapy is clearly the treatment of choice. Various regimens have

been evaluated over the years, with cures using chemotherapy alone ranging from 25 to 60 per cent in advanced disease (Rosenberg, 1986). The first successful combination of drugs—the well-known and widely used MOPP regimen—was developed by DeVita and colleagues in 1964 at the National Cancer Institute (NCI). The combination of mechlorethamine, vincristine (Oncovin), procarbazine, and prednisone regimen is given in 28-day cycles, with 2 weeks of treatment and 2 weeks of recovery period. This combination of drugs is administered for at least six courses, or two courses beyond evidence of disease for consolidation. The results of the NCI experience after a 20-year study demonstrated that 84 per cent of patients treated with MOPP had a complete remission, 66 per cent remained disease-free for 10 years, and overall disease-free survival was 54 per cent at 15 years (DeVita, 1982).

Over the years, a number of modifications of the MOPP regimen have been introduced, as well as the concept of non-cross-resistant combinations of chemotherapy. These combinations support the Goldie-Goldman hypothesis that the earlier the tumor is exposed to all potential therapeutic methods, the better the chance of avoiding refractoriness to treatment, which is the greatest obstacle to cure (Goldie, Goldman, & Guaduskus, 1982).

The best and most studied is the ABVD combination of drugs doxorubicin (Adriamycin), bleomycin, vinblastine, and dacarbazine, developed by Bonadonna and colleagues in Milan. ABVD has the advantage of efficacy without showing evidence of the sterility and secondary malignancies found in patients receiving MOPP (Bonadonna, Santoro, Simonetta, & Valagussa, 1988). Many clinical trials are ongoing comparing ABVD and MOPP as primary treatment or ABVD/MOPP or alternating the two drug regimens or variations and thus providing a non-cross-resistant regimen. Cooperative group studies have found that ABVD alone or alternating with MOPP is more superior to MOPP alone (Bonadonna et al., 1986; DeVita & Hubbard, 1993). Radiation therapy is also used to reduce sites of initial disease or to consolidate bulky disease. Other combinations are being studied with the intent of reducing the toxicities of the current regimens (Straus, 1986; Urba & Longo, 1992). Table 35–5 lists the various chemotherapeutic agents used in the treatment of Hodgkin's disease (Bonadonna et al., 1988).

The success of chemotherapy, like that of radiation therapy, is dependent on the dosage and timing of the drug. Reduction of the dose or dose rate by 20 per cent can totally abolish the curative effect of combination chemotherapy (DeVita, 1982). Because of some of the severe side effects from the most successful regimes (MOPP, ABVD), patients may request dose and schedule changes to avoid disruption in their lifestyles. It is extremely important for the oncology nurse to explain to the patient that such alterations will decrease the effectiveness of treatment and ultimately may lead to the loss of life. The importance of symptom management is critical throughout the treatment phase to provide the support necessary for the patient to accept and tolerate life-saving therapy.

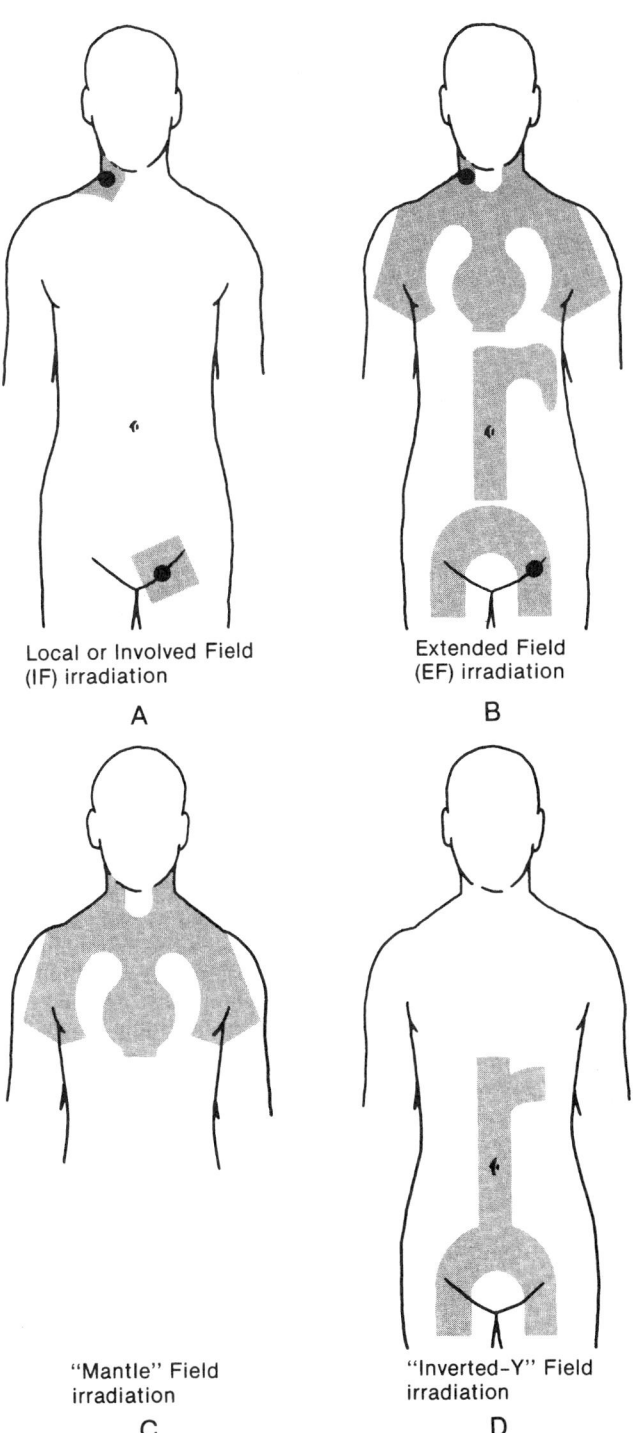

Local or Involved Field
(IF) irradiation

A

Extended Field
(EF) irradiation

B

"Mantle" Field
irradiation

C

"Inverted-Y" Field
irradiation

D

FIGURE 35–2. Radiation fields in the treatment of Hodgkin's disease. (From Haskell, C. M., & Parker, R. G. [1985]. Hodgkin's disease. In C. Haskell, *Cancer treatment* [2nd ed., pp. 758–788]. Philadelphia: W. B. Saunders Co. Reproduced by permission.)

TABLE 35–5. *Chemotherapy Regimens for Hodgkin's Disease*

REGIMEN	DOSAGE	REGIMEN	DOSAGE
MOPP		**B-CAVe**	
Mechlorethamine	6 mg/m², IV, days 1 and 8	Bleomycin	5.0 units/m², IV, days 1, 28, 35
Vincristine	1.4 mg/m², IV, days 1 and 8	CCNU	100 mg/m², PO, day 1
	(maximum 2.0 mg)	Doxorubicin	60 mg/m², IV, day 1
Procarbazine	100 mg/m², PO, days 1 to 14	Vinblastine	5 mg/m², IV, day 1
Prednisone	40 mg/m², PO, days 1 to 14	Cycles repeated every 6 weeks (if blood counts permit)	
	(cycles 1 and 4 only)	to a total of 9 cycles.	
Cycles repeated every 4 weeks.		**LOPP**	
COPP		Clorambucil	6 mg/m² PO, days 1 to 14
Cyclophosphamide	600 mg/m², IV, days 1 and 8	Vincristine	1.4 mg/m² IV, days 1 and 8
Vincristine	1.4 mg/m², IV, days 1 and 8	Procarbazine	100 mg/m² PO, days 1 to 14
	(maximum 2.0 mg)	Prednisone	40 mg/m² PO, days 1 to 14
Procarbazine	100 mg/m², PO, days 1 to 14	**ChlVPP**	
Prednisone	40 mg/m², PO, days 1 to 14	Clorambucil	6 mg/m² PO, days 1 to 14
	(cycles 1 and 4 only)	Vinblastine	6 mg/m² IV, days 1 and 8
Cycles repeated every 4 weeks, as described for MOPP.		Procarbazine	100 mg/m² PO, days 1 to 14
MVPP		Prednisone	40 mg/m² PO, days 1 to 14
Mechlorethamine	6 mg/m², IV, days 1 and 8	**MOPP/ABVD**	
Vinblastine	6 mg/m², IV, days 1 and 8	Alternating months of MOPP and ABVD	
Procarbazine	100 mg/m², PO, days 1 to 14	**MOPP/SBV hybrid**	
Prednisone	40 mg/m², PO, days 1 to 14	Nitrogen mustard	6 mg/m² IV, day 1
Drug administration during a 42-day cycle with 4		Vincristine	1.4 mg/m² IV, day 1
weeks of rest.		Procarbazine	100 mg/m² PO, days 1 to 7
ABVD		Prednisone	40 mg/m² PO, days 1 to 14
Doxorubicin	25 mg/m², IV, every 2 weeks	Doxorubicin	35 mg/m² IV, day 8
Bleomycin	10 units/m², IV, every 2 weeks	Bleomycin	10 mg/m² IV, day 8
Vinblastine	6 mg/m², IV, every 2 weeks	Vinblastine	6 mg/m² IV, day 8
Dacarbazine	375 mg/m², IV, every 2 weeks	Each cycle lasts 28 days.	
Maximum total cumulative dose of doxorubicin 450			
mg/m² and 450 units bleomycin.			
Dosage of drugs reduced for bone marrow suppression.			

IV = intravenously; PO = orally.

SIDE EFFECTS

The most commonly used chemotherapy regimes, MOPP and ABVD, cause nausea and vomiting. Anticipatory nausea and vomiting are not unusual and should be prevented. In one study of patients with Hodgkin's disease, conditioned responses were usually firmly developed by the fourth or fifth course of treatment (Devlin, Maguire, Phillips, Crowther, & Chambers, 1987; Devlin, Maguire, Phillips, & Crowther, 1987). Early recognition and avoidance of anticipatory nausea and vomiting are the most effective nursing interventions. Regular nausea and vomiting require skilled nursing prevention and intervention and are discussed in Chapter 51. Other side effects such as hair loss are related to administration of individual drugs and are discussed in Chapter 22. It is extremely important to assist the patient in controlling these difficult side effects to maintain optimal curative doses.

Fatigue and lack of energy during treatment and at 1 year after treatment have been reported in several studies of patients with Hodgkin's disease and are identified as major factors in coping with disease. Preparing the patient for this ongoing problem may help to reduce anxiety (Fobair et al., 1986). Nursing research

in this area will hopefully provide outcomes for intervention in the future.

Patients receiving radiation to the chest experience sore throats, difficulty swallowing, nausea, and vomiting. The nutritional status of the patient may be compromised owing to difficulties in eating and lack of appetite. Radiation to the abdominal and pelvic areas can cause the patient discomfort from diarrhea, which then leads to fluid and electrolyte loss. Good skin care is essential, because a common side effect in radiation therapy is skin desquamation. Measures for nursing intervention are addressed in Chapter 20.

COMPLICATIONS OF TREATMENT

As the response to treatment for Hodgkin's disease has improved and many adults are being cured, attention is focusing on defining and minimizing the early and late complications of therapy. Significant and even life-threatening treatment consequences are seen more than 10 years postdiagnosis. These late complications are due to the results of chemotherapy and radiotherapy treatment regimens and to underlying immunologic deficits of the disease and treatment. As the number of long-term cancer survivors increases, the late consequences will also increase, creating a need for education and counseling before complications occur. Figure 35–3 shows when common complications of Hodgkin's disease are most likely to occur (Morgan, 1994).

HYPOTHYROIDISM

Late complications of high-dose irradiation include chronic hypothyroidism. Hypothyroidism is most common in patients receiving radiation to the cervical nodes or mantle area and can be expected to occur in 60 to 70 per cent of patients (Golde & Koeffler, 1985). Grave's disease and thyroid cancer can also occur. The risk of these late complications persist for more than 25 years after patients have received radiation. A thyroid-stimulating hormone (TSH) level should be followed periodically after treatment to evaluate for thyroid hormone replacement.

STERILITY

MOPP chemotherapy is known to cause sterility. Several studies have indicated that fertility may still be possible for some young patients treated for Hodgkin's disease (teens to early 20s). Little suppression of fertility occurs in young women; suppression is greater in men receiving MOPP (DeVita, 1982; Horning, Hoppe, & Kaplan, 1981). Men receiving MOPP and mechlorethamine, vinblastine, procarbazine, and prednisone (MVPP) chemotherapy show evidence of permanent azoospermia, testicular atrophy, and elevated follicle-stimulating hormone after one or two cycles of treatment. Before treatment, men should be given the opportunity to store sperm, though many male patients with Hodgkin's disease have impaired spermatogenesis prior to receiving any treatment. ABVD is less toxic to the male gonad, and appears to spare long term testicular and ovarian function; therefore if fertility is of major concern, ABVD may be the better choice of therapy.

Women receiving MOPP chemotherapy have associated ovarian failure after six cycles of MOPP. Alternat-ing MOPP and ABVD reduces the number of MOPP cycles and therefore the risk of sterility. Even after intensive treatment with combination chemotherapy for Hodgkin's disease, women have become pregnant and delivered normal children. A woman undergoing a staging laparotomy should have an oophoropexy in case subsequent radiation affects the abdomen or pelvic area. Radiation therapy can result in the loss of ovarian function even with these precautions in 30 to 70 per cent of patients receiving pelvic irradiation (Cooley & Cobb, 1986; Horning et al., 1981).

SECONDARY MALIGNANCIES

Secondary malignancies are probably the most distressing late effect of curative therapy for Hodgkin's disease. They can be both solid tumors or leukemias.

Patients treated with chemotherapy (especially MOPP) and radiation therapy (combined modality) are at greater risk for late-onset acute leukemia and non-Hodgkin's lymphoma, but the incidence is rare after radiation alone. The quantity of the alkalating agent and the extent of the irradiation field strongly correlate with increased risk (Kaldor et al., 1990; Van der Velden et al., 1988). These risks mandate the physician making a careful assessment before recommending combined modality therapy for stage IIIA disease and limiting treatment to one therapy or the other in early disease.

Irradiation also increases the risk of second solid tumors. These include mostly lung cancers, though sarcomas, melanomas, and tumors of the breast and stomach are also included (Tucker, 1988). Due to the increased risk of lung cancer, patients should be advised to avoid smoking. The use of bleomycin-containing combination chemotherapy, especially after radiation to the mantle site, can result in an increase of pulmonary toxicity (Horning et al., 1994). There is also concern over the increased risk of breast cancer in women who have received mantle irradiation. These solid tumors appear to be directly related to radiation

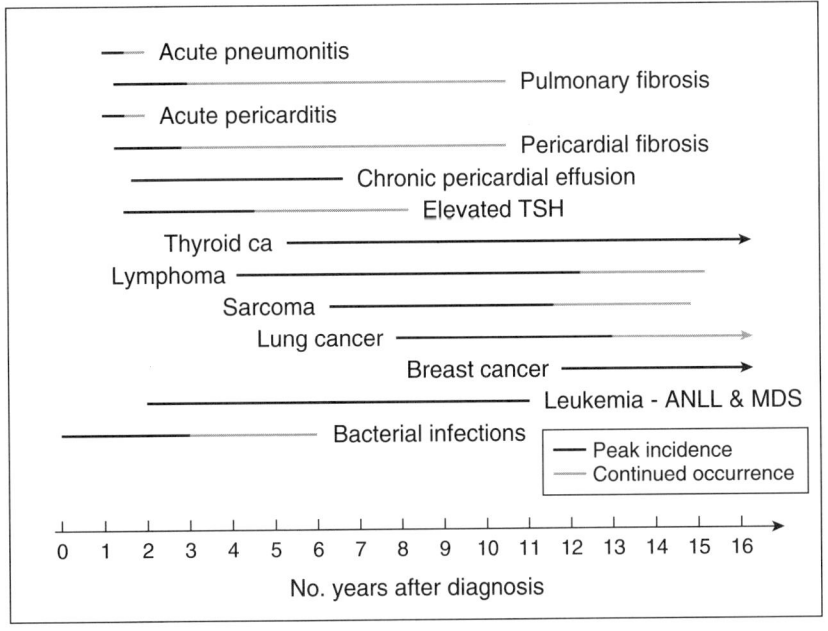

FIGURE 35–3. Hodgkin's disease treatment complications. Selected complications in patients after remission following therapy for Hodgkins disease. TSH = thyroid stimulation hormone; Ca = cancer; ANLL = acute nonlymphocytic leukemia; MDS = myelodysplastic syndrome. (Adapted from Bookman, M. A., Longo, D. L., & Young, R. C. [1988]. Late complications of curative treatment of Hodgkin's disease. *Journal of the American Medical Association, 260,* 680.)

and are not significantly affected by additional exposure to chemotherapy (Hancock, Tucker, & Hoppe, 1993; Kennedy et al., 1992).

NON-HODGKIN'S LYMPHOMAS

OVERVIEW

Non-Hodgkin's lymphomas are a heterogeneous group of malignant neoplasms that originate in the lymphoid compartment of the immune system. It has long been recognized that they possess a wide and often bewildering spectrum of clinical and biologic behavior from indolent to very aggressive. As previously mentioned, the boundaries that separate non-Hodgkin's lymphomas from other diseases, for example, lymphocytic leukemia and lymphocyte-predominant Hodgkin's disease, are often difficult to determine. Non-Hodgkin's lymphomas can be defined as malignancies of the lymphatic tissue, with the exception of Hodgkin's disease, acute and chronic lymphoid leukemias, multiple myeloma, Waldenstrom's macroglobulinemia, and hairy cell leukemia (Haskell & Parker, 1985).

In the United States, non-Hodgkin's lymphomas occur three times as often as Hodgkin's disease. The American Cancer Society (1994) estimates that approximately 45,000 new cases and 21,000 deaths will occur in 1995. For reasons that are not understood, the incidence of lymphoma is increasing yearly, especially in patients with autoimmune deficiencies (e.g., AIDS). The peak age incidence is higher than that for Hodgkin's disease, with about 25 per cent of cases occurring between the ages of 50 and 59 years and the greatest risk occurring between the ages of 60 and 69 years, with males predominating.

ETIOLOGY

The cause of non-Hodgkin's lymphoma remains unknown, although several theories have been postulated. A number of lymphomas have been associated with chromosome translocations and rearrangement of proto-oncogenes (e.g., bcl-2, c-myc). These changes may be important to the etiology and progression of the disease. In addition, certain viruses and the competence of the immune system play a role in some lymphomas.

Current data suggest an etiologic role for the HTLV 1 in some adult T cell lymphomas. This virus has been strongly associated with adult T cell malignancies in the Caribbean, parts of South Africa, and southwestern Japan. The HTLV 1 infection has also been found in patients with AIDS and subsequent lymphomas.

Burkitt's lymphoma, which is confined almost exclusively to Africa, is associated with the presence of the Epstein-Barr virus, a lymphotropic herpes virus. The precise role of this virus is unknown.

Compared with the general population, individuals with congenital and acquired immunodeficiencies (e.g., AIDS) and those receiving immunosuppressive treatment are at increased risk for developing non-Hodgkin's lymphoma. Inheritable immunodeficient states include Wiskott-Aldrich syndrome and Bloom's syndrome.

Non-Hodgkin's lymphoma is 45 to 100 times more common among organ transplant patients (particularly renal), with lymphomas accounting for 29 per cent of cancers in these patients receiving immunosuppressive therapy (Sarna & Kagan, 1985a; Ultmann & Jacobs, 1985). Other patients predisposed to non-Hodgkin's lymphoma are those with autoimmune diseases, such as rheumatoid arthritis and systemic lupus erythematosus.

As mentioned, chromosomal abnormalities have also been linked with both immunodeficiency and lymphoma. Genetic abnormalities of chromosome 14 are recognized in many follicular lymphomas and in Burkitt's disease.

PATHOPHYSIOLOGY

To understand the different lymphomas and to appreciate the lymphoma classification systems, it is helpful to review the process of lymphocyte maturation. Lymphomas, for the most part, are the malignant counterpart of the maturing lymphocyte. Therefore, different lymphomas are related to different maturational phases of the lymphocyte. In the process of lymphocytic maturation, the early lymphocyte continues to mature in a predictable manner into an immunocompetent lymphocyte. In non-Hodgkin's lymphoma, an abnormal proliferation of neoplastic cells occurs that resembles a phase or site of maturation. Instead of progressing to the next phase, the cells remain fixed at one phase of development and continue to proliferate. These neoplastic cells may also take on functional characteristics and activities of their normal counterparts. It is possible to predict some of the clinical manifestations of non-Hodgkin's lymphoma based on characteristics of the predominant cell (or normal cell counterpart). The neoplastic cells often retain the surface of their cell of origin. Therefore, it is also possible to group these cells according to surface markers or phenotypic properties (Foon, Schroff, & Gale, 1982).

Lymphocytes consist of two functional classes of cells in the immune system: the T lymphocyte, which is involved in regulation of antibody synthesis and cellular immune processes, and the B lymphocyte, which contributes to the humoral immune response that requires antigen sensitization by antigen. In considering the nature of each lymphoma, it is helpful to visualize the specific site of lymphocytic maturation that is related to each neoplastic entity. Figure 35–4 illustrates lymphoid maturation and theoretic sites for development of non-Hodgkin's lymphomas. The lymphoid stem cell is programmed via the bone marrow to become a T cell or B cell precursor, respectively. B cell maturation occurs in the follicles of the lymph node after exposure to an antigen. B cells can be divided into four cytologic types that represent different stages of maturation and that contribute to the new classification system: (1) small cleaved, (2) large cleaved, (3) small noncleaved, and (4) large noncleaved. In some lymphoma classification systems, lymphomas are given names that are based on characteristics of their location in the activation process, for example, small cleaved cell lymphoma. The majority of lymphomas,

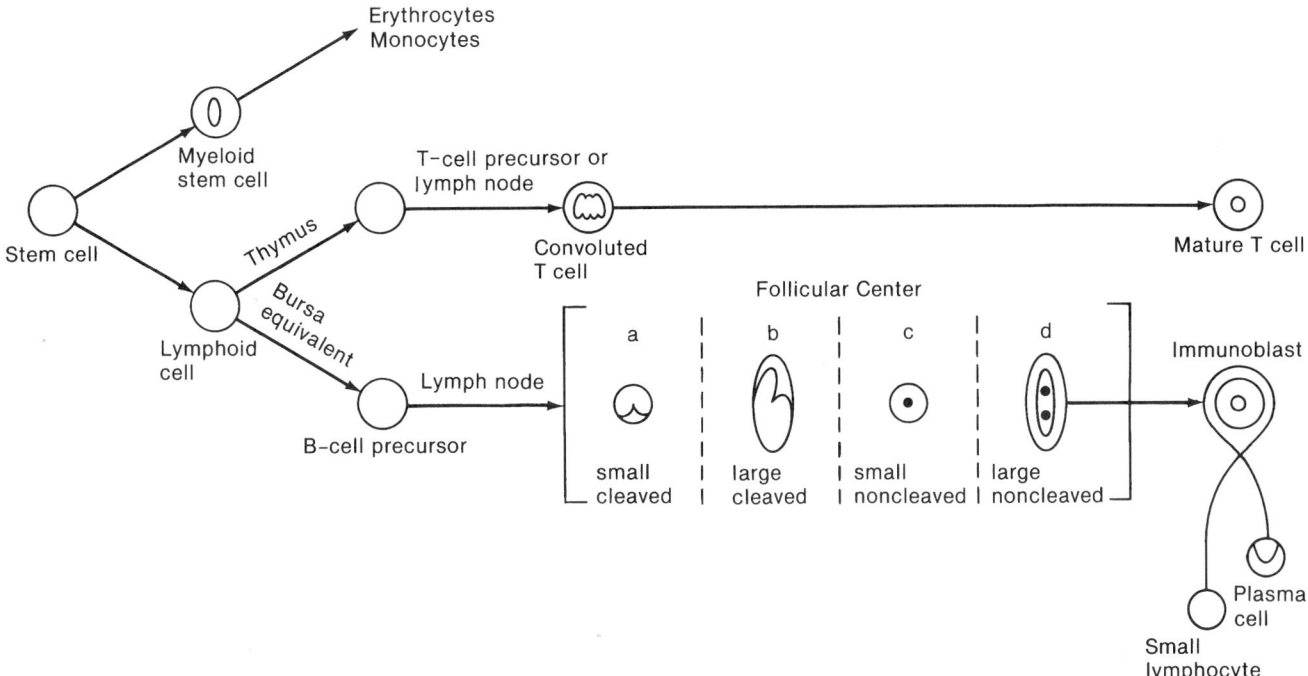

FIGURE 35–4. Maturation of the lymphocyte.

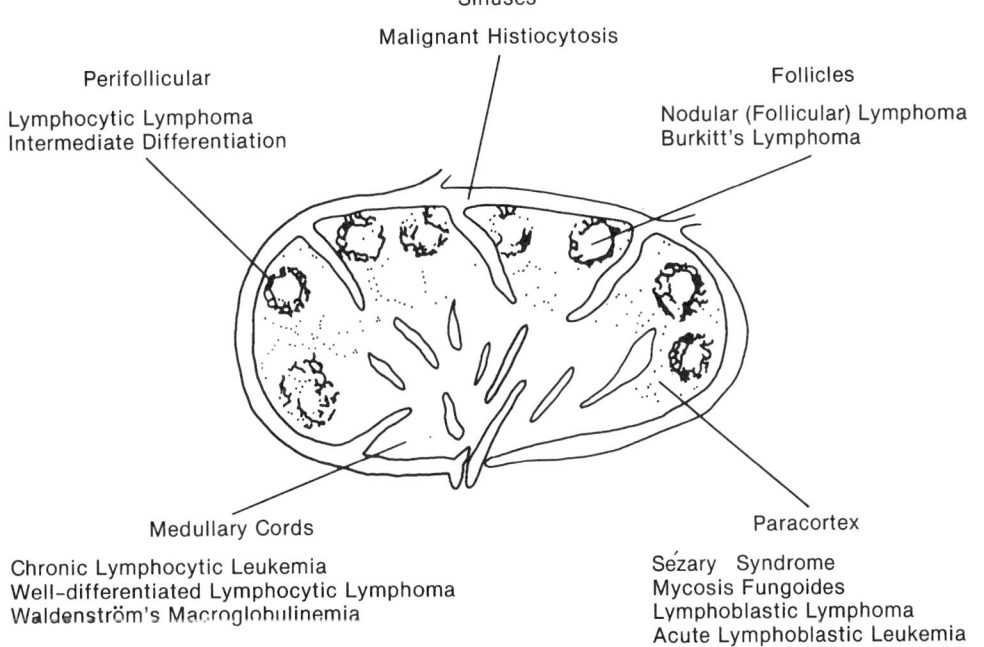

FIGURE 35–5. Lymph node. Non-Hodgkin's lymphomas according to functional anatomy. (From Mann, R. B., Jaffe, E. S., & Bernard, C. W. [1972]. Malignant lymphomas—a conceptual understanding of morphological diversity. *American Journal of Pathology, 94,* 103–191. Reproduced by permission.)

approximately 70 per cent, are B cell lymphomas. Lymphoid malignancies of T cell origin are less common, consisting of approximately 20 to 30 per cent of lymphomas (Jaffe, 1986).

CELLULAR ORIGIN

The cells of the immune system have different locations in the peripheral lymph nodes. Because lymphoma cells often retain certain characteristics of their cell of origin, it is often possible to relate tumors to their function and anatomic properties. Figure 35–5 depicts the normal lymph node architecture and areas in which malignancies may arise. Normal lymph nodes include B cells, T cells, and histiocytes. Approximately 10 per cent of lymphomas are of unknown origin, and less than 1 per cent are from true histiocytes.

Clinical correlations have been established that recognize the more indolent nature of nodular architecture and small cleaved lymphocytic cytologic characteristics and the more aggressive nature of diffuse architecture and large-cell characteristics.

CLASSIFICATION OF NON-HODGKIN'S LYMPHOMAS

The many different categorization systems for non-Hodgkin's lymphomas have led to controversy and confusion and have made interpretation of treatment difficult for many practitioners. In the 1960s the Rapaport classification system was the most widely used system in the United States. This system describes the histopathologic classification of non-Hodgkin's lymphoma. Although this system correlates well with clinical observations, it has many scientific inaccuracies as it gives little insight into the pathophysiology involved. For example, the histiocytic lymphomas are not derived from histiocytes but from transformed lymphocytes. In the 1970s other systems such as the Lukes-Collins attempted to incorporate immunologic concepts into classification. To act as a link between different classification systems the National Cancer Institute's International Cooperative Study (1982) developed the Working Formulation of non-Hodgkin's lymphoma. In the working formulation, tumors are divided into low-, intermediate-, and high-grade lymphomas, depending on the activity of the specific lymphoma. Lymphomas listed under each category are defined by histologic, anatomic, and immunomorphic characteristics (National Cancer Institute, 1982). After introduction of the working formulation in 1982, many centers have

developed their own variations of classifications of non-Hodgkin's lymphoma to correct for the deficiencies of the working formulation and other classifications and to accommodate the new lymphoma entities. For example, two new entities of low-grade lymphoma include mantle cell lymphoma, which refers to intermediate (differentiation) lymphocytic lymphomas of either mantle zone or diffuse type, and mucosa-associated lymphoid tissue (MALT) lymphomas, which typically involve extranodal tissue (GI tract, thyroid, breast, and skin) (Pugh, 1993). The Working Formulation and the Rapaport classification system are shown in Table 35–6. Whenever possible, a pathologist should be consulted prior to biopsy, and tissue should be frozen for special studies. In terms of prognostic and therapeutic value, the importance of new diagnostic techniques such as cell surface markers, immunoglobular, and T cell receptor gene rearrangement is not yet clear.

Most clinical protocols divide lymphomas into two broad categories: (1) indolent, or low-grade, and (2) aggressive, or intermediate- and high-grade. Patients with low-grade non-Hodgkin's lymphoma usually have a relatively long survival with or without aggressive treatment. Tumors can be controlled with chemotherapy, but they are rarely cured. High-grade tumors may result in death for the patient within 1 or 2 years, but paradoxically, with aggressive treatment, certain subsets of patients can be cured. Manifestations of specific lymphomas are addressed in a following section.

CLINICAL PRESENTATION

The clinical presentation of patients with non-Hodgkin's lymphoma is similar to that of Hodgkin's

TABLE 35–6. *Classification of Malignant Non-Hodgkin's Lymphomas*

WORKING FORMULATION FOR CLASSIFICATION OF NON-HODGKIN'S LYMPHOMAS FOR CLINICAL USAGE	RAPAPORT CLASSIFICATION EQUIVALENT
Low Grade	
Small lymphocytic	Diffuse well-differentiated lymphocytic (DWDL)
Follicular, small cleaved cell	Nodular poorly differentiated lymphocytic (NPDL)
Follicular, mixed small cleaved cell	Nodular mixed lymphoma (NML)
Intermediate Grade	
Follicular, predominantly large cell	Nodular histiocytic lymphoma (NHL)
Diffuse, small cleaved cell	Diffuse poorly differentiated lymphoma (DPDL)
Diffuse, mixed small and large cell	Diffuse mixed lymphocytic-histiocytic (DML)
Diffuse large cell	Diffuse histiocytic lymphoma (DHL)
High Grade	
Large cell, immunoblastic	Diffuse histiocytic lymphoma (DHL)
Large cell, lymphoblastic	Lymphoblastic, convoluted or nonconvoluted
Small noncleaved cell	Undifferentiated, Burkitt's and non-Burkitt's diffuse undifferentiated lymphoma (DUL)
Miscellaneous	
Composite	
Mycosis fungoides	
Histiocytic	
Extramedullary plasmacytoma	
Unclassifiable	

(Modified from the National Cancer Institute-sponsored study of the classifications of non-Hodgkin's lymphomas. [1982]. *Cancer, 49,* 2112–2135.)

disease and various other disorders involving the lymph system. Because palpable nodes are often found on normal individuals, differential diagnosis is dependent on size, shape, feel, and location of lymph nodes. Differences in clinical features of Hodgkin's disease and non-Hodgkin's lymphoma are noted in Table 35–7. The most frequent clinical presentation in Hodgkin's disease and non-Hodgkin's lymphoma is painless superficial lymphadenopathy. A history of waxing and waning lymphadenopathy over a period of months is not unusual. Except for an awareness of lymph node enlargement, patients with lymphadenopathy are generally asymptomatic.

Systemic symptoms (fever, weight loss, night sweats) may be present but are more frequently seen in Hodgkin's disease and do not have as strong an association with poor prognosis as they do in Hodgkin's disease. Nodal involvement in Hodgkin's disease is typically axial (cervical, mediastinal, and paraaortic), whereas primary involvement of mesenteric nodes or extranodal sites, such as bone, gastrointestinal tract, and brain, is rare. In contrast, non-Hodgkin's lymphoma is commonly more extensive, most often stage III or stage IV disease at diagnosis (DeVita et al., 1985). Non-Hodgkin's lymphoma frequently involves lymphoid sites such as epitrochlear nodes and Waldeyer's tonsillar ring. Localized disease is uncommon; extranodal disease, bone marrow infiltration, and bulky disease are often characteristic features. Truly localized disease is rare, appearing in approximately 10 per cent of patients who present with non-Hodgkin's lymphoma (DeVita et al., 1985).

MANIFESTATIONS OF SPECIFIC LYMPHOMAS

LOW-GRADE LYMPHOMA

Lymphomas that exhibit a nodular type of histologic pattern display a more indolent behavior pattern than those possessing a diffuse histologic and therefore more aggressive nature. Low-grade lymphomas, according to the Working Formulation, consist of small lymphocytic lymphomas and follicular lymphomas, both small cleaved cell and mixed small cleaved cell. Nearly all low-grade lymphomas are neoplasms of mature B-cell origin. However, a number of T cell lymphomas are considered to be low-grade. The terms

good risk, indolent, favorable, and low-grade as categorizing lymphomas are often used synonymously, although even in these subgroups there is a degree of clinical heterogeneity. These lymphomas are characterized by considerably longer survival, but various treatment approaches have failed to yield permanent cures.

Most often, patients with low-grade lymphomas present with widespread disease. Because of the indolent nature of the disease, patients remain asymptomatic, and therefore the disease remains unnoticed. By the time the patient is diagnosed, the low-grade lymphomas show wide dissemination of disease to lymph nodes, bone marrow, and occasionally the liver. Mediastinal lymph node involvement is less common than in Hodgkin's disease, but abdominal lymphadenopathy may be evident and is far more common in non-Hodgkin's lymphoma than in Hodgkin's disease.

Spontaneous regression of disease has been observed in various subtypes of lymphoma (Horning & Rosenberg, 1984). It has occurred in approximately 5 to 15 per cent of low-grade lymphomas and may occur in previously untreated patients or in patients who have relapsed after treatment. Duration can last longer than a year or can be indefinite. Though exciting when it occurs, the cause of spontaneous regression is unknown.

Histologic conversion over time from a low grade to a higher, more aggressive grade is also evident in low-grade lymphomas. Progression is from nodular to diffuse and from small to large cell (Acker et al., 1987). Progression can occur as early as 6 months after an original diagnosis of low-grade lymphoma at biopsy (Hubbard et al., 1982). The most common progression is from nodular, poorly differentiated lymphoma (NPDL, Rapaport, 1987) or follicular small cleaved cell lymphomas (working formulation) to more aggressive lymphoma. In a Stanford study, the risk of conversion has been estimated to be approximately 60 per cent. Histologic conversion has occurred in patients who have had prior treatment as well as in patients who have had no prior treatment (Horning & Rosenberg, 1984). Therefore, additional biopsy specimens are often examined if the disease progresses, the disease progression changes rate, or the disease resists treatment so that the treatment can be directed at the new histologic pattern. Patients may also present with divergent histologic patterns at the initial staging evaluation.

TABLE 35–7. *Clinical Differences in Hodgkin's Disease and Non-Hodgkin's Lymphoma*

CHARACTERISTIC	HODGKIN'S DISEASE	NON-HODGKIN'S LYMPHOMA
Nodes	Contiguous spread	Noncontiguous
Extranodal disease	Uncommon	More common involvement of gastrointestinal tract, testes, bone marrow
Site of disease	Mediastinal involvement common in 50% of patients	Mediastinal involvement less common (20%)
	Bone marrow involvement uncommon	Bone marrow involvement common
	Liver involvement uncommon	Liver involvement common
Extent of disease	Often localized	Rarely localized (10%)
B symptoms	Common (40%)	Uncommon (20%)

(Adapted from DeVita, V. T., Jr., Hellman, S., & Rosenberg, S. A. [1985]. *Cancer: Principles and practice of oncology* [2nd ed.]. Philadelphia: J. B. Lippincott Co.)

In a study conducted at the NCI, of a total of 101 patients who had multiple tissue sites biopsied, 18 patients had a nodular pattern in one site and a diffuse pattern in another (Hubbard et al., 1982). In addition, diffuse involvement as well as areas of nodularity may occasionally be evident in a single biopsy specimen.

Although the picture regarding low-grade lymphomas initially appears optimistic, the disease responds poorly over time to most treatments. Clinical morbidity and life-threatening problems are related to increasing tumor bulk. Eventually symptoms include fever, night sweats, weight loss, and infection. Bone marrow involvement and renal and hepatic dysfunction are manifested in widespread disease.

AGGRESSIVE NON-HODGKIN'S LYMPHOMAS

Patients with aggressive lymphomas exhibit a large cell or mixed histologic pattern. Before the improvement of combination chemotherapy, complete remissions for patients with intermediate and high-grade lymphomas were rare, with median survival for diffuse histology rarely over a year. This was attributed to the fact that most patients presented with advanced-stage disease with a rapidly growing tumor. Typically aggressive lymphomas exhibit high fraction tumor growth with rapid doubling times. Paradoxically, these aggressive lymphomas respond better to chemotherapy and therefore present with a greater potential for cure than most low-grade, indolent lymphomas. Salvage therapy after relapse results in few and short-term remissions, though many combinations of drugs, radiation therapy, and biologic response modifiers have allowed greater potential for cure.

DIAGNOSIS AND STAGING

Since the prognosis and treatment are influenced by histopathology, obtaining a careful review of biopsy specimens by a pathologist who is experienced in diagnosing lymphomas is extremely important. Special studies require special preparation of tissue; therefore a pathologist should be consulted prior to the biopsy.

Once a histopathologic diagnosis is established by lymph node biopsy, further clinical evaluation is needed to determine the sites and extent of disease involvement. This process, referred to as *staging,* is necessary to plan effective treatment methods and to establish parameters to follow the patient's response to therapy. It is also helpful in predicting the clinical course and prognosis of the specific lymphoma.

Studies useful for the clinical evaluation of non-Hodgkin's lymphoma are listed in Table 35–8. The extent of clinical examination is based on the histologic findings and the type of treatment expected for a specific lymphoma. For example, if a patient has a positive bone marrow biopsy result and therefore stage IV disease, other invasive tests are not necessary. Patients are required at a minimum to have a history and physical examination, a complete blood count, chest radiograph, screening chemistries, a urinalysis, an abdominal computed tomographic (CT) scan, and a bone marrow examination.

Several factors indicate the need for a bone marrow aspirate early in the evaluation process. In patients with low-grade lymphomas, 50 to 95 per cent have bone marrow involvement at presentation, which establishes stage IV disease (Ultmann & Jacobs, 1985). Patients with intermediate or high-grade lymphomas are less likely to have marrow involvement, with the exception of those who have lymphoblastic lymphomas. Because of the importance of a thorough bone marrow examination, it is recommended that core biopsies be obtained from each posterior iliac crest.

Computed tomography is very useful in patients with non-Hodgkin's lymphoma for assessing any abnormalities observed after baseline studies. A chest CT scan is required for patients with evident abnormalities on chest radiograph. Because extranodal presentations are more common in non-Hodgkin's lymphoma, the abdominal CT scan is valuable because it visualizes nodal and extranodal disease, picking up enlarged nodes greater than 2 cm. The CT scan can visualize the size but not the architecture of the node. It is used to evaluate the upper abdominal, mesenteric, splenic, and hepatic lymph nodes, all of which are commonly involved nodes in non-Hodgkin's lymphoma. In addition, the abdominal CT scan demonstrates hepatic and splenic enlargement and a potential emergency— hydronephrosis. The CT scans are useful in stages III and IV disease to provide a baseline for later evaluation of complete response from therapy (Clouse et al., 1985).

In contrast, the lymphangiogram provides a very accurate evaluation of lower abdominal involvement such as the lower aortic, iliac, and retroperitoneal lymph nodes. This test is used in clinical stages I and II disease, after all other noninvasive evaluations have been negative, to verify early-stage disease. The importance of verifying early-stage disease is optimum, because cure can be achieved with treatment of local radiation therapy. A lymphangiogram is not recommended for patients with large mediastinal involvement, pulmonary disease, or extensive retroperitoneal involvement. These restrictions limit the use of this test in non-Hodgkin's lymphoma, which typically affects the older patient with bulky disease.

For the majority of patients, accurate assessment of extent of disease and subsequent treatment can be made based on the results of the previously mentioned tests. A staging laparotomy is not utilized in non-Hodgkin's lymphoma because, in contrast to Hodgkin's disease, the majority of non-Hodgkin's lymphoma patients present with disease below the diaphragm and do not require further staging workup. Therefore laparotomy, if used, is reserved for the few patients with clinical stage Ie and IIe disease in whom evidence of abdominal involvement would change the course of treatment from radiation therapy to combination chemotherapy.

The Ann Arbor Staging Classification for Hodgkin's disease (Table 35–3) is also used for staging non-Hodgkin's lymphoma but has some deficiencies in its use in non-Hodgkin's lymphomas. This staging system does not account for facts such as histology, bulk of

TABLE 35–8. *Studies Useful in the Clinical Evaluation of Lymphoma*

STUDY	INDICATION	USEFULNESS
Complete blood count (including differential and platelet count)	All patients	Direct evidence for peripheral blood involvement Indirect evidence for bone marrow involvement or immune hemolytic anemia
Erythrocyte sedimentation rate (ESR)	All patients	Nonspecific; baseline data for subsequent follow-up
Urinalysis	All patients	Screen for proteinuria
Routine chemistries (including calcium and uric acid)	All patients	Hypercalcemia, hyperuricemia, elevated lactate dehydrogenase, electrolyte abnormalities, and acidosis may reflect complications of lymphoma
Liver function tests	All patients	If abnormal, may suggest hepatic involvement
Kidney function tests	All patients	If abnormal, may suggest direct renal parenchymal involvement, hydronephrosis due to retroperitoneal lymphadenopathy; may be secondary to hypercalcemia, hyperuricemia, or paraproteinemia
Serum protein electrophoresis (SPEP)	All patients	Detection of paraprotein
Serum immunoelectrophoresis with quantitation	All patients with an abnormal SPEP	Identification and quantitation of the paraprotein
Chest x-ray (CXR)	All patients	Screen for mediastinal, hilar, and paratracheal lymphadenopathy, and parenchymal involvement
Bone marrow aspirate and four bone core biopsies	All patients	Documents bone marrow involvement (pathologic stage IV disease)
Lumbar puncture with cytology	Diffuse histiocytic lymphoma with a positive result on a bone marrow scan Lymphoblastic lymphoma Undifferentiated lymphoma Any histology with an unexplained alteration in mental status	Documents central nervous system involvement
Abdominal/pelvic computed tomographic (CT) scan	All patients	Evaluates lymph node enlargement in the porta hepatis, splenic hilum, para-aortic region, mesentery, and retroperitoneum; liver and splenic involvement, presence or absence of hydronephrosis
Chest CT scan	All patients with an abnormal CXR	Further evaluation of suspected lymphadenopathy, mediastinal masses, or parenchymal disease
Intravenous pyelogram	All patients with a renal abnormality on CT scan	Further evaluation of renal abnormalities; however, this procedure may be contraindicated in the presence of paraproteinemia or renal failure due to hypercalcemia or hyperuricemia
Gallium scan	Patients with intermediate and high-grade lymphomas	Sensitivity varies with histology and location of disease. It is most sensitive for diffuse histiocytic lymphoma above the diaphragm*
Bone scan	All patients	Baseline data; all abnormal areas must be evaluated by a radiologic examination*
Liver-spleen scan	All patients	Baseline data; may suggest hepatic or splenic involvement*
Lymphangiogram	Patients with clinical stage I and II disease above the diaphragm with a negative abdominal/pelvic CT scan in whom the discovery of abdominal disease would alter treatment	Detects abnormalities in lymph node architecture in the lower para-aortic, retroperitoneal, and iliac lymph nodes. Provides a guide for the surgeon if a staging laparotomy is performed; any abnormal lymph node must be removed if the laparotomy is to be considered adequate*

*If any abnormalities are found, they require biopsy confirmation before changing the treatment based on these studies. When abnormal, these are useful parameters for following a patient's response to therapy.
(From Ultmann, J. E., & Jacobs, R. H. [1965]. The non-Hodgkin's lymphomas. *CA: A Cancer Journal for Clinicians, 35,* 36.)

disease (Table 35–3), and site of disease such as extranodal involvement, all important prognostic indicators in non-Hodgkin's lymphoma. The Cotswald additions, which address bulk and site of disease, make this system much more useful for staging lymphoma.

TREATMENT

The treatment of malignant non-Hodgkin's lymphoma is a rapidly evolving area with the continuous introduction of new drugs, drug regimens, and other therapeutic methods such as autologous bone marrow transplantation, monoclonal antibodies, and biologic response modifiers. Radiation alone is a limited option that is used for early-stage disease. Chemotherapy or combined modality represent the most common treatment, because most patients present with late-stage disease. The most appropriate management of widespread lymphoma remains controversial. In designing a treatment program for an individual patient, the health care team must take into account the patient's age and general health, the extent of lymphoma, and the histologic subtype. Chemotherapy regimens have evolved over the past several years with different combinations of non-cross-resistant drugs now being utilized for optimum benefit. Because the goal is cure, especially with the aggressive lymphomas, regimens are often vigorous and cause side effects such as nausea, vomiting, hair loss, and infection. Nursing support is crucial throughout the treatment phase to clarify questions regarding therapeutic regimens and to assist the patient in preventing and managing side effects.

INDOLENT LYMPHOMAS—LOW GRADE

Various treatment approaches have failed to demonstrate durable remissions in low-grade lymphomas, although these lymphomas are characterized by a relatively long survival. Indolent lymphomas have demonstrated a high sensitivity to a wide range of chemotherapeutic agents (with complete remissions from 60 to 70 per cent), but the duration of remissions is short (between 17 and 24 months). Unfortunately, at 4 years, 80 per cent of patients initially treated have relapsed. At 5 years the survival rate is greater than 70 per cent but at 10 years is less than 30 per cent (Young, 1987).

Treatment of patients with low-grade lymphomas is controversial. Owing to the failure of current therapeutic approaches of chemotherapy or radiation therapy to "cure" indolent lymphomas, many physicians advocate observing the patient and initiating therapy when symptoms require intervention. Following this policy of watchful waiting, 50 per cent of patients will avoid treatment for more than 1 to 3 years, 10 per cent will avoid treatment for longer than 5 years, and approximately 30 per cent will have partial spontaneous regression of disease that may be prolonged but not permanent (Connors, Fisher, & Armitage, 1989; Gattiker, Wiltshaw, & Galton, 1981). Stanford, NCI, and other institutions have conducted randomized trials comparing observation with combination chemotherapy followed by total nodal irradiation. Although early treatment has demonstrated longer remissions, long-term survival appears to be equal. At present, there are no convincing data to suggest that early, more aggressive treatments have any survival benefit, although clinical trials are ongoing.

Once the decision is made to treat a low-grade lymphoma, the most widely used approach is chemotherapy. The most common chemotherapeutic agents used to treat low-grade lymphomas are listed in Table 35–9. Again, there is controversy over whether palliation of symptoms or complete remission should be the primary goal of therapy. For the less than 10 per cent of patients with stage I and II disease, involved field radiation therapy is the treatment of choice. Prognosis is good for these patients, with an expected 50 to 80 per cent chance of disease-free survival exceeding 10 to 20 years with some variation by site and age (Connors et al., 1989). For stage III and IV disease chemotherapy approaches have included therapy with single alkalating agents such as chlorambucil and cyclophosphamide or one of several combination regimens (e.g., CVP, COPP, CHOP). Combination regimens yield slightly higher complete remission rates than single alkalating agents, but the ranges overlap considerably. It is apparent there is no single regimen that is clearly best.

There have been developments with new agents for relapse low-grade lymphoma that have a unique mechanism of action. The most promising agents are the purine analogs (fludarabine, CdA), ADA inhibitors (DCF), topoisomerase I inhibitors (campathothecin-11, topotecan, 9-amino-campatothecin), and the taxanes (Taxol, Taxotere). Nevertheless, the experience with any of these agents has been limited, making it difficult to accurately estimate response rates, response duration, and impact on survival (Cheson, 1993).

AGGRESSIVE LYMPHOMAS

The aggressive lymphomas are considered to be intermediate or high-grade lymphomas as defined by the working formulation, except for lymphoblastic lymphoma and Burkitt's lymphoma. The probability of remaining free of disease after 10 years is currently better for patients with diffuse aggressive lymphomas than for those with indolent lymphomas. In the last decade, a major change in the prognosis of aggressive lymphomas has evolved with the advancement of chemotherapeutic regimens. Chemotherapy regimens are listed in Table 35–10.

Early lymphoma studies in the 1970s introduced the first combination chemotherapy regimen: Cyclophosphamide, vincristine, and prednisone (CVP or Cop). This combination regimen was reported by DeVita (1982) after successfully employing the MOPP regimen in Hodgkin's disease. If complete remission was not obtained after three cycles of these drugs, cure was not considered likely. Such partial response is considered to represent resistance, and therefore further chemotherapy would not be effective. Survival plateaus were achieved in approximately 30 per cent of patients (Connors et al., 1989). More recently, the use of combination-chemotherapy regimens containing doxorubicin (e.g., CHOP) yielded very high cure rates (in excess of 75 per cent) in patients with stage I and non-bulky stage II diffuse aggressive non-Hodgkin's lym-

TABLE 35-9. *Therapy in Advanced Low-Grade Lymphomas*

REGIMEN	DOSAGE*
Defer therapy/careful observation	—
Single-Agent Chemotherapy	
Cyclophosphamide or	1.5-2.5 mg/kg/day (orally)
chlorambucil	0.1-0.2 mg/kg/day (orally)
(continue therapy until CR is achieved and for 2 years as maintenance therapy)	
Prednisone	30-50 mg/kg/day (orally) × 4 weeks
(optional: may be started with a single drug)	
Fludarabine	25 mg/m^2 day for 5 days every 3 to 4 weeks
2-Chlorodeoxyeadenosine	0.1 mg/kg/day for 5 to 7 days continuous infusion
2'-Deoxycoformycin	5 mg/m^2/day for 3 days every 3 weeks
Combination Chemotherapy	
CVP	
Cyclophosphamide	400 mg/m^2 (orally) days 1-5
Vincristine	1.4 mg/m^2 (maximum 2.0 mg) day 1
Prednisone	100 mg/m^2 (orally) days 1-5
(repeat every 21 to 28 days until CR; CVP × four cycles as consolidation followed by CVP every 3 months as maintenance for a total of 2 years)	
COPP	
Cyclophosphamide	600 mg/m^2 days 1 and 8
Vincristine	1.4 mg/m^2 (maximum 2.0 mg) days 1and 8
Procarbazine	100 mg/m^2 (orally) days 1-14
Prednisone	40 mg/m^2 (orally) days 1-14
(repeat every 21 days)	
CHOP	
Cyclophosphamide	750 mg/m^2 day 1
Doxorubicin	50 mg/m^2 day 1
Vincristine	1.4 mg/m^2 (maximum 2.0 mg) day 1
Prednisone	100 mg (orally) days 1 to 5
(repeat every 21-28 days)	
Whole-Body Irradiation	
30 rad per week for a total of 150 rad	
Boost irradiation to all initial sites of involvement, mantle or minimantle, Waldeyer region, whole abdomen, and pelvis; 2000 rad in 2-3 weeks in each field	
Combined Modality	
CVP + total lymphoid irradiation (TLI)	
CVP, as above, for three cycles followed by TLI including 4400 rad to Waldeyer's ring, mantle, and inverted-Y; 3000 rad to whole abdomen	
CVP is given again for three or more cycles until CR is achieved; the dose of cyclophosphamide is reduced to 300 mg/m^2 (orally) days 1 to 5	
CHOP + irradiation	
Phase I: CHOP is given every 28 days as above for four cycles, except prednisone is given for 8 days	
Phase II: 150 rad total body irradiation for extensive disease, or 3500 rad local irradiation for local disease	
Phase III: CHOP for four cycles every 8 weeks	

*Drug is given intravenously unless otherwise stated. CR = complete remission.
(Adapted from Ultmann, J. E., & Jacobs, R. H. [1985]. The non-Hodgkin's lymphomas. *CA: A Cancer Journal for Clinicians, 35,* 66–87; Cheson, B. D. [1993]. New chemotherapeutic agents for the treatment of low-grade Non-Hodgkin's lymphomas. *Seminars in Oncology, 20* [5, Suppl. 5], 96–110.)

phoma (Armitage, 1993b). CHOP therapy remains one of the most frequently used regimens.

Several institutions developed second- and third-generation treatment programs that utilized a combination of six to eight chemotherapy drugs. Owing to the aggressive nature of the non-Hodgkin's lymphomas, the goal was to give more drugs in less time through marrow-sparing non-cross-resistant drugs (Table 35–10) (Goldie et al., 1982; Skarin, 1986). The best known regimens include COP-BLAM III, MACOP-B,

ProMACE-CytaBOM and M-BAEOD. Some regimens add mid-cycle chemotherapy: chemotherapy is interspersed between the main cycle because disease regresses quickly, but often it regrows before the next cycle of chemotherapy begins. These regimens have produced complete remission in approximately 80 per cent of patients with aggressive large-cell lymphomas (Coleman et al., 1987). These results are especially significant because the response rate includes patients with previously described poor prognostic factors such

TABLE 35–10. *Chemotherapy Regimens for Non-Hodgkin's Lymphoma—Aggressive*

REGIMEN	DRUGS	DOSAGE (MG/M^2)	DAYS OF TREATMENT	FREQUENCY
1. C-MOPP	Cyclophosphamide	650 IV	1 and 8	q 28 days
	Vincristine (Oncovin*)	1.4 IV	1 and 8	
	Procarbazine	100 PO	1 to 14	
	Prednisone	40 PO	1 to 14	
2. CHOP	Cyclophosphamide	750 IV	1	q 21 days
	Doxorubicin (Adriamycin†)	50 IV	1	
	Vincristine (Oncovin*)	1.4 IV	1 and 5	
	Prednisone	100 PO	1 to 5	
3. CHOP-LEO	Cyclophosphamide	750 IV	1	q 21 days
	Doxorubicin (Adriamycin†)	50 IV	1	
	Vincristine (Oncovin*)	1.4 IV	1 and 5	
	Prednisone	100 PO	1 to 5	
	Bleomycin	4 IV	1 and 5	
4. BCVP	Carmustine (BCNU)	60 IV	1	q 21 days
	Cyclophosphamide	1000 IV	1	
	Vincristine (Oncovin*)	1.4 IV	1	
	Prednisone	100 PO	1 to 15	
5. BACOP	Cyclophosphamide	650 IV	1 and 8	q 28 days
	Doxorubicin (Adriamycin†)	25 IV	1 and 8	
	Vincristine (Oncovin*)	1.4 IV	1 and 8	
	Bleomycin	5 IV	15 and 21	
	Prednisone	60 PO	15 to 28	
6. COMLA	Cyclophosphamide	1500 IV	1	q 21 days
	Vincristine (Oncovin*)	1.5 IV	1, 8, and 15	
	Methotrexate	120 IV	22, then weekly × 7	
	Leucovorin	25 PO	q 6 hr × 4, 24 hr after MTX	
	Cytosine arabinoside	300 IV	22, then weekly × 7	q 21 days
7. m-BACOD	Methotrexate	200 IV	8 and 15; LV 10 mg/m^2 po q6h × 8; 9 and 16	
	Bleomycin	4 IV	1	
	Doxorubicin (Adriamycin†)	45 IV	1	
	Cyclophosphamide	600 IV	1	
	Vincristine (Oncovin*)	1.0 IV	1	
	Dexamethasone	6 PO	1 to 5	
8. PROMACE-MOPP (flexitherapy)	Cyclophosphamide	650 IV	1 and 8	q 28 days
	Doxorubicin (Adriamycin†)	25 IV	1 and 8	
	Epipodophyllotoxin (VP-16-213)	120 IV	1 and 8	
	Prednisone	60 PO	1 to 14	
	Methotrexate	1500 IV	14 (LV 50 mg/m^2 q6h × 5 day 15)	
	Standard MOPP		after remission	q 28 days
9. COP-BLAM-I	Cyclophosphamide	400 IV	1	
	Vincristine (Oncovin*)	1 IV	1	
	Prednisone	40 PO	1 to 10	q 21 days
	Bleomycin	15 IV (total)	14	
	Doxorubicin (Adriamycin†)	40 IV	1	
	Procarbazine (Matulane)	100 PO	1 to 10	
10. ACOMLA	Doxorubicin (Adriamycin†)	40 IV	1	
	Cyclophosphamide	1000 IV	1	
	Vincristine (Oncovin*)	2 IV total	1, 8, 15	q 3 months
	Methotrexate	120 IV	22, 29, 35, 43, 50, 57, 64, 71	
	Leucovorin	25 PO total	24 hrs after MTX, q6h × 6	
	Ara-C	300 IV	1 hr after MTX on same days	
11. Pro-MACE (day 1) Cytaboma (day 8)	ProMace	see above	1 (no MTX)	
	Cytarabine	300 IV	8	q 21 days
	Bleomycin	5 IV	8	
	Methotrexate	120 IV	8	
	Leucovorin	25 PO	9 q6h × 4, 24 hrs after MTX	

TABLE 35–10. *Chemotherapy Regimens for Non-Hodgkin's Lymphoma—Aggressive*   Continued

REGIMEN	DRUGS	DOSAGE (MG/M^2)	DAYS OF TREATMENT	FREQUENCY
12. COP-BLAM-III	Cyclophosphamide	350 IV (Escalate to 500)	1 and 22	
	Vincristine (Oncovin*)	1 IV	1 to 2; 22 to 23 (cont. IV infusion)	q 6 weeks
	Prednisone	40 IV	1 to 5; 22 to 27	
	Bleomycin	7.5 IV	1 (IV push) 1 to 5; 22 to 23 (cont. IV infusion)	
	Doxorubicin (Adriamycin†)	35 IV (Escalate to 50)	1 and 22	
	Procarbazine (Matulane)	100 PO	1 to 5; 22 to 27	
13. MACOP-B	Methotrexate	400 IV	Weeks 2, 6, 10	
	Doxorubicin (Adriamycin†)	50 IV	Weeks 1, 3, 5, 7, 9, 11	
	Cyclophosphamide	350 IV	Weeks 1, 3, 5, 7, 9, 11	
	Vincristine (Oncovin*)	1.4 IV	Weeks 2, 4, 6, 8, 10, 12	
	Bleomycin	10U IV	Weeks 4, 8, 12	
	Prednisone	75 PO	Daily, dose tapered over the last 15 days	
	Co-trimoxazole	2 tablets PO	Twice daily throughout	

*Manufactured by Eli Lilly and Company, Indianapolis, IN.
†Manufactured by Adria Laboratories, Columbus, OH.
IV=intravenously; LV=leucovorin; MTX=methotrexate; PO=orally.
(From Skarin, A. T. [1986]. Diffuse aggressive lymphomas: A curable subset of non-Hodgkin's lymphomas. *Seminars in Oncology, 13*[4], 10–25.)

as bulky abdominal disease. It is important to treat the patient with as full a dose as possible, because the most important factor affecting outcome is dose intensity (Armitage, 1993b; Coleman et al., 1987; DeVita, Hubbard, Young, & Longo, 1988; Goldie et al., 1982; Gordon et al., 1992; Skarin, 1986). The intensity of treatment can be increased by the use of hematopoietic growth factors to allow an increased dose or shortened treatment intervals. Patients are treated to a documented complete response as determined by prior staging. Those patients in subsets requiring prophylactic central nervous treatment or who have bulky disease may also require consolidated radiotherapy.

Patient selection for these regimens is important for disease characteristics and patient tolerance. Age appears to be a limiting factor, with drug toxicity being more formidable in patients older than 50 years of age.

THERAPY FOR PATIENTS WITH HIV-RELATED LYMPHOMA

Non-Hodgkin's lymphomas frequently occur in patients with human immunodeficiency virus (HIV) infection. They are usually B cell lymphomas and large-cell or small noncleaved-cell subtype and frequently occur in extranodal sites that are unusual, such as the brain. Patients diagnosed with acquired immunodeficiency syndrome (AIDS) on the basis of opportunistic infections tolerate treatment poorly, and their survival may be aggravated by aggressive chemotherapy. HIV-positive patients with non-Hodgkin's lymphoma and no opportunistic infections often respond to therapy,

and a subgroup can be cured of their lymphoma. Although their long-term prognosis remains poor because of the HIV infection, there is agreement that the survival rate and quality of life are improved. There remains controversy in the choice of treatment for these patients; some advocate aggressive treatment while others have found success with less intensive therapy (Levine, 1990; Levine et al., 1991).

BONE MARROW TRANSPLANTATION

Bone marrow transplantation has become a widely applied therapy for the treatment of patients with lymphoma. Transplantation has been utilized for patients who have failed primary treatment, have advance disease, or as a part of primary treatment. In the 1980s bone marrow transplantation became widely applied for the treatment of aggressive lymphoma; however, in the 1990s bone marrow transplantation remains controversial in indolent low-grade lymphoma (Armitage, 1993a). Bone marrow transplantation is just now beginning to be studied in patients with low-grade lymphoma. Long-term follow-up is needed to find the eventual cure rate. It has not been extensively studied because of the long history of the disease, the high frequency of bone marrow involvement, and the relatively old age of the patients at presentation. Bone marrow transplantation is only available to a minority of patients who relapse, since it cannot be used by most elderly patients because of poor tolerance and unacceptable high treatment-related deaths. There has been an increase in the number of clinical trials for low-grade lymphoma, as a 10-year median survival is not viewed as favorable by a younger patient. Questions that are being raised in the application of bone marrow transplantation include the timing of the therapy (i.e., as part of the initial treatment or after relapse) and the best source of hematopoietic rescue. These and other questions will be the focus of future clinical trials (Armitage 1993b).

EXPERIMENTAL TRIALS

Although the use of high-dose chemotherapy with bone marrow transplantation has shown promise in low-grade or refractory and relapsed high-grade lymphomas, not all patients derive long-term benefit from this treatment. As a result, new therapeutic approaches are being evaluated, including the use of immunotherapy. This alternative to conventional chemotherapy involves the use of monoclonal antibodies (MoAbs) alone or combined with radioactive material. Advantages to testing MoAbs in lymphoma include the disease's accessibility to the vascular system and presence of surface antigens with restricted expression (Czuczman & Scheinberg, 1992).

Monoclonal antibody (MoAb) therapy alone represents one experimental therapeutic option as a potentially nontoxic approach for the treatment of lymphoma. It has shown ability to mediate cytotoxicity on antibody-dependent cells. It recognizes and binds to a tumor-associated antigen on over 90 per cent of lymphoma cells. In ongoing phase I/II clinical trials the genetically engineered antibody appears to be safe and well tolerated with mild to moderate reactions that are generally limited to the duration of the infusion. A subsequent form of immunotherapy with more toxicity is radioimmunotherapy, radioactively labeled MoAbs utilizing radionuclides such as yttrium 90, iodine 125, bismuth 212, and others. In general, radioimmunotherapy trials demonstrate increased response rates compared with unlabeled-MoAb trials because of the relative radiosensitivity of lymphoid cells (Czuczman et al., 1992). By using MoAbs conjugated to radionuclides that generate long path-length radiation, a field effect is created, allowing the radiation to kill antigen-negative tumor cell variants and tumor cells that are unreachable by antibody. Their drawback is significant increase in hematologic toxicity compared with unconjugated MoAb therapy. However, the number of clinical trials is expanding due to the encouraging results brought about by better antibodies and radionuclides and more effective labeling techniques.

The evolution of these therapeutic measures and others have marked significant advances for non-Hodgkin's lymphoma leading to improved rates of remission and overall survival. The current increase in the knowledge of the disease should lead the way to more effective and better targeted treatment strategies.

SIDE EFFECTS

Studies have suggested a strong relationship between the side effects of disease and treatment and the patient's psychologic morbidity (Devlin, Maguire, Phillips, & Crowther, 1987; Devlin, Maguire, Phillips, Crowther, & Chambers, 1987). The strain of coping with side effects as well as the fear that cancer is spreading result in varying degrees of anxiety and depression. The oncology nurse can provide support by educating the patient about potential physical and psychologic side effects of treatment (Fobair et al., 1986).

The intensity of treatment regimens for aggressive lymphomas results in potential side effects and toxicities. Side effects have included substantial hematologic and mucosal difficulty, such as infection and mucositis (Coleman et al., 1987). Nursing observation for signs and symptoms of infection is critical. Mucositis remains a continual problem, because many patients remain neutropenic throughout treatment. Nursing interventions regarding good and safe oral hygiene and preventative measures are discussed in Chapter 52. Hair loss should be anticipated with the treatment of regimens including doxorubicin and cyclophophamide. Patient education is important before therapy to allow sufficient time to make choices such as obtaining a wig or other alternatives. Potential body image concerns requires nursing observation and intervention (see Chapter 61).

Major toxicities resulting from chemotherapy include pulmonary, related to bleomycin, and severe neuropathy, either gastrointestinal or peripheral, as a result of vincristine therapy.

ONCOLOGIC EMERGENCIES

Patients with progressive lymphoma are at risk for several oncologic emergencies such as superior vena cava syndrome in patients with mediastinal masses, spinal cord compression from tumor growth, and tumor lysis syndrome as a result of the rapid breakdown of cells from aggressive chemotherapy. Patients with central nervous system involvement are at risk of intracranial pressure. Oncologic emergencies are discussed extensively in Chapter 66.

Patients with gastric lymphomas have a high incidence of perforation with treatment, particularly with bulky disease. Often these patients will undergo a debulking procedure before receiving chemotherapy, such as a subtotal gastrectomy, and in some cases a total gastrectomy. When treating a patient with known gastric involvement, it is important to educate the patient about the signs and symptoms of perforation and the urgency of reporting this emergency (Jacobs, 1988).

PRIMARY CENTRAL NERVOUS SYSTEM (CNS) LYMPHOMA

Primary CNS lymphoma is rising in incidence in both the AIDS and non-AIDS population. This non-Hodgkin's lymphoma is usually restricted to the central nervous system and presents as a brain tumor. Other areas of involvement include the eyes and spinal cord. Because systemic lymphoma is not present, comprehensive staging procedures are not warranted, though a neurologic staging workup is essential. Formerly the disease was rare, but there has been a threefold rise in incidence in immunocompetent patients. It is most common in patients with AIDs, of whom as many as 6 per cent develop CNS lymphoma during their illness.

Because of the diffuse nature of CNS lymphomas, aggressive surgical measures or gross removal of the tumor is of no benefit. In contrast, radiation therapy significantly improves median survival to approximately 15 months in non-AIDs patients but to 2 to 5 months in AIDs patients. To reduce late neurologic effects from cranial radiotherapy, combination chemotherapy with radiotherapy trials are ongoing and are showing some prolonged survival (DeAngelos, 1995).

CUTANEOUS T CELL LYMPHOMA— MYCOSIS FUNGOIDES

Mycosis fungoides is a rare cutaneous lymphoma of the T lymphocyte. In the United States, this malignant skin disease affects only 400 to 600 patients per year, ranging from 45 to 69 years of age at diagnosis. First described by French physician Alibert in 1806, the name *mycosis fungoides* resulted from the mushroom-like appearance of the tumors. Though indolent in nature, with a median survival of 8 to 10 years, systemic spread to peripheral blood, lymph nodes, and other organs is common. The prognosis is highly dependent on the stage of disease, which is determined by the type of skin lesions, peripheral blood, lymph node, and visceral involvement (Sarna & Kagan, 1985b; Winkler & Bunn, 1983).

The cause of mycosis fungoides is not known but has been correlated with factors such as exposure to chemicals, family history of Hodgkin's disease and lymphoma, and defects in host immune surveillance. The disease often appears superficially with a variety of skin lesions.

Three clinical stages have been identified: (1) premyotic or erythematous, (2) plaque, and (3) the tumor. The first stage is characterized by a general itching and superficial skin eruptions of varying sizes (Stabb, 1980). At this early stage the disease can be confused easily with other skin disorders, such as psoriasis and dermatitis. The lesions may wax and wane and spontaneously disappear and reappear. These lesions usually appear approximately 6 years before most patients are diagnosed. Usually the relentless itching and fear of contagion lead the patient to seek diagnosis (Winkler & Bunn, 1983). The premyotic stage may last from several months to 10 years.

The plaque stage of mycosis fungoides is an aggravated symptom and causes great discomfort. This stage is characterized by an irregular thickening of the skin, with raised and irregularly shaped plaques, which may be accompanied by palpable lymph nodes. Lesions are no longer transitory and may lead to painful fissures of the palms and soles. Scalp involvement may result in alopecia. Itching may become an annoying symptom, especially if it was present in the premyotic phase (Hallowach, McFadden, & Supik, 1984; Sarna & Kagan, 1985b; Stabb, 1980).

The tumor stage is characterized by mass lesions, which can appear in previously normal skin, in plaques, or previous mycotic lesions. They may appear anywhere but are most often in the face and body folds such as the axillae, groin, cubital folds, neck, and breasts (Winkler & Bunn, 1983). The most frequent cause of death with cutaneous T-cell lymphoma is infection followed by progressive dissemination.

Treatment for mycosis fungoides includes topical as well as systemic chemotherapy, radiation therapy, biologic response modifiers, and supportive care. Patients respond better with early treatment, but at present there is no cure.

Innovative nursing care is required for the patient with mycosis fungoides, which includes skin care, infection control, and nutritional support. Comfort measures are necessary for pruritus and pain relief. The psychosocial impact of this disease, including the insult to body image and self-esteem, presents multifaceted challenges for nursing intervention.

PROBLEMS ASSOCIATED WITH SURVIVORSHIP

The successful treatment of the lymphomas has resulted in cure for many patients and progressively longer lives for others. Studies of patients with Hodgkin's disease and non-Hodgkin's lymphoma have identified several physiologic and psychologic difficulties of long-term survival.

Lack of energy or tiredness is a common complaint often accompanied by depression. In a study of patients with Hodgkin's disease, 37 per cent of patients complained that energy had not adequately returned. For others, it took 12 to 18 months following treatment for energy to return (Fobair et al., 1986). Loss of libido and problems with infertility from chemotherapy may cause major physical, mental health, and lifestyle complications for survivors of Hodgkin's disease. Impairment or disturbance of short-term memory may be a short- or long-term effect. Anxiety and the fear of relapse and further treatment are also problems but appear to decrease as the patient lives longer free of disease (Devlin, Maguire, Phillips, & Crowther, 1987; Devlin, Maguire, Phillips, Crowther, & Chambers, 1987; Fobair et al., 1986).

The failure of some patients to return to work or to resume normal activities years after treatment is cause for early intervention. Those returning to work often experience job discrimination or difficulties at work. Career interruptions and insurance-related problems are common (Kornblith, 1992). Marital difficulties and an increase in divorce among survivors of Hodgkin's disease have been attributed to role changes, stress of treatment, and anger at the well spouse. Educating the patient about potential psychosocial difficulties during treatment and recovery is a suggested intervention to decrease the impact of these difficulties once they occur (Fobair et al., 1986). As patients continue to live longer, the problems associated with survivorship are a continual challenge. Long-term comprehensive care is important, and the oncology nurse plays a key role in assessing and preventing patient difficulties to ensure quality of life.

REFERENCES

Acker, B., Hoppe, R. T., Cooby, T. V., Cox, R. S., Kaplan, H. S., & Rosenberg, S. A. (1987). Histologic conversion in the non-Hodgkin's lymphomas. *Journal of Clinical Oncology, 1*(1), 11–16.

American Cancer Society. (1994). Cancer statistics, 1994. *Ca–A Cancer Journal for Clinicians, 44* (1).

Aragon de la Cruz, G., Cardenes, H., Otero, J., et al. (1989). Individual risk of abdominal disease in patients with stages I and II supradiaphragmatic Hodgkin's disease: A rule index based on 341 laparotomized patients. *Cancer, 63,* 1799–1803.

Armitage, J. O. (1993). Bone marrow transplantation for indolent lymphomas. *Seminars in Oncology, 20* (Suppl. 5), 136–141.

Armitage, J. O. (1993). Treatment of non-Hodgkin's lymphoma. *New England Journal of Medicine, 328,* (14), 1023–1030.

Biti, G. P., Cimino, G., Cartoni, C., et al. (1992). Extended-field radiotherapy is superior to MOPP chemotherapy for the treatment of pathologic stage I-IIA Hodgkin's disease: Eight-year update of an Italian prospective randomized study. *Journal of Clinical Oncology, 10*(3), 378–382.

Bonadonna, G., Santoro, A., Simonetta, V., & Valagussa, P. (1988). Treatment strategies for Hodgkin's disease. *Seminars in Hematology, 25*(2), 51–57.

Bonadonna, G., Valagussa, P., & Santoro, A. (1986). Alternating non-cross-resistant combination chemotherapy or MOPP in stage IV Hodgkin's disease: A report of 8 year results. *Annals of Internal Medicine, 104,* 739–736.

Bookman, M. A., Longo, D. L., & Young, R. C. (1988). Late complications of curative treatment of Hodgkin's disease. *Journal of the American Medical Association, 260,* 680.

Brizel, D. M., Winer, E. P., Pronitz, L. R. et al. (1990). Improved survival in advanced Hodgkin's disease with the use of combined modality therapy. *International Journal of Radiation Oncology, 19,* 535–542.

Cheson, B. D. (1993). New chemotherapeutic agents for the treatment of low-grade non-Hodgkin's lymphomas. *Seminars in Oncology, 20*(Suppl. 5), 96–110.

Clouse, M., Harrison, D., Grassi, C. J., Costello, P., Edwards, S. S., & Wheeler, H. (1985). Lymphangiography, ultrasonography, and computed tomography in Hodgkin's disease and non-Hodgkin's lymphoma. *The Journal of Computed Tomography, 9*(1), 1–7.

Coleman, M., Gerstein, G., Topilow, A., Lebowicz, J., Berhardt, B., Chiarieri, D., Silver, R., & Pasmantier, M. W. (1987). Advances in chemotherapy for large cell lymphoma. *Seminars in Hematology, 24*(2), 8–20.

Connors, J. M., Fisher, R. I., & Armitage, J. O. (1989). Decision making in the treatment of malignant lymphoma. *American Society of Hematology Educational Session* (pp. 41–45). Atlanta.

Cooley, M., & Cobb, S. C. (1986). Sexual and reproductive issues for women with Hodgkin's disease. I. Overview of issues. *Cancer Nursing, 9*(4), 188–193.

Crowther, D., Wagstaff, J., Deakin, D., et al. (1984). A randomized study comparing chemotherapy alone with chemotherapy followed by radiotherapy in patients with pathologically staged IIIA Hodgkin's disease. *Journal of Clinical Oncology, 2*(8), 892–897.

Czuczman, M. S., Scheinberg, D. A. (1992). Monoclonal antibody therapy for NHL. *Contemporary Oncology, 2*(7), 45–50.

DeAngelos, L. (1995). Current management of primary central nervous system lymphoma. *Oncology, 9* (1), 63–75.

DeVita, V. T., (1982). Hodgkin's disease: Conference summary and future directions. *Cancer Treatment Reports, 66*(4), 1045–1055.

DeVita, V. T., Hellman, S., & Rosenberg, S. A. (1985). *Cancer: Principles and practice of oncology* (2nd ed., pp. 1696–1741). Philadelphia: J. B. Lippincott.

DeVita, V. T., & Hubbard, S. M. (1993). Hodgkin's disease. *New England Journal of Medicine, 328*(8), 560–565.

DeVita, V., Hubbard, S., Young, R., & Longo, D. (1988). The role of chemotherapy in diffuse aggressive lymphoma. *Seminars in Hematology, 25*(2), 2–10.

Devlin, J., Maquire, P., Phillips, P., & Crowther, D. (1987). Psychological problems associated with diagnosis and treatment of lymphomas. II. Prospective study. *British Medical Journal, 295,* 955–957.

Devlin, J., Maquire, P., Phillips, P., Crowther, D., & Chambers, H. (1987). Psychological problems associated with diagnosis and treatment of lymphomas. I. Retrospective study. *British Medical Journal, 295,* 953–954.

Fobair, P., Hoppe, R. T., Bloom, J., Cox, R., Varghese, A., & Spiegel, D. (1986). Psychosocial problems among survivors of Hodgkin's disease. *Journal of Clinical Oncology, 4*(5), 805–813.

Foon, K. A., Schroff, R. W., & Gale, R. P. (1982). Surface markers on leukemia and lymphoma cells: Recent advances. *Blood, 60*(1), 1–19.

Gattiker, H. H., Wiltshaw, E., & Galton, A. G. (1981). Spontaneous regression in non-Hodgkin's lymphoma. *Cancer, 45,* 2627–2632.

Golde, D. W., & Koeffler, H. P. (1985). Hodgkin's disease and lymphomas. In C. Haskell (Ed.), *Cancer treatment* (2nd ed.). Philadelphia: W. B. Saunders Co.

Goldie, J. H., Goldman, A. J., & Guaduskus, G. A. (1982). Rationale for the use of alternating non-cross resistant chemotherapy. *Cancer Treatment Reports, 66,* 39.

Gordon, L. I., Harrington, D., Andersen, J., et al. (1992). Comparison of a second-generation combination chemotherapeutic regimen (m-BACOD) with a standard regimen (CHOP) for advanced diffuse non-Hodgkin's lymphoma. *New England Journal of Medicine, 327*(19), 1342–1349.

Greenberger, J., Mauch, P., Canellow, G., & Larson, R. (1989). Controversies in Hodgkin's disease. *American Society of Hematology Educational Session.* (pp. 34–40), Atlanta.

Hallowach, S., McFadden, M. E., & Supik, K. (1984). Mycosis fungoides: A nursing perspective. *Oncology Nursing Forum, 11*(1), 20–34.

Hancock, S. L., Tucker, M. A., & Hoppe, R. T. (1993). Breast cancer after treatment of Hodgkin's disease. *Journal of the National Cancer Institute, 85*(1), 25–31.

Haskell, C. M., & Parker, R. G. (1985). Hodgkins disease. In C. Haskell (Ed.), *Cancer treatment* (pp. 758–788). Philadelphia: W. B. Saunders Co.

Hoppe, R. T., Cox, R. S., Rosenberg, S. A., & Kaplan, H. S. (1982). Prognostic factors in pathologic stage 3 Hodgkin's disease. *Cancer Treatment Reports, 66,* 743–749.

Horning, S. J., Adhikari, A., Rizk, N. et al. (1994). Effect of Hodgkin's disease on pulmonary function: Results of a prospective study. *Journal of Clinical Oncology, 12*(2), 297–305.

Horning, S. J., Hoppe, R. T., & Kaplan, H. S. (1981). Female reproductive potential after treatment for Hodgkin's disease. *New England Journal of Medicine, 304*(23), 1377–1382.

Horning, S. J., & Rosenberg, S. A. (1984). The natural history of initially untreated low-grade non-Hodgkin's lymphoma. *New England Journal of Medicine, 311*(23), 1471–1475.

Hubbard, S. M., Chabner, B. A., DeVita, V. T., et al. (1982). Histologic progression in non-Hodgkin's lymphoma. *Blood, 59*, 258–264.

Jacobs, C. (1988). Lymphomas: Diagnosis, staging and principles of treatment. In *Oncology nursing: A national conference on today's clinical issues.* San Francisco.

Jaffe, E. S. (1986). Relationship of classification to biologic behavior of non-Hodgkin's lymphomas. *Seminars in Oncology, 13*(4), 3–9.

Kaldor, J. M., Day, N. E., Clarke, E. A., et al. (1990). Leukemia following Hodgkin's disease. *New England Journal of Medicine, 322*(1), 7–13.

Kaplan, H. S. (1981). Hodgkin's disease: Biology, treatment, prognosis. *Blood, 57*, 813–822.

Kennedy, B. J. V., Peterson, V., et al. (1992). Survival in Hodgkin's disease by stage and age. *Medical and Pediatric Oncology, 20*(2), 100–104.

Kornblith, A. B., Anderson, J., Celia, D. F., et al. (1992). Hodgkin's disease survivors at increased risk for problems in psychosocial adaptation. *Cancer, 70*, 2214.

Lacher, M. J. (1985). Hodgkin's disease: Historical perspective, current status, and future directions. *Ca–A Cancer Journal for Clinicians, 35*(2), 88–94.

Levine, A. M. (1990). Lymphoma in acquired immunodeficiency syndrome. *Seminars in Oncology, 17*, 104–112.

Levine, A. M., Sullivan-Halley, J., Pike, M. C., et al. (1991). Human immunodeficiency virus-related lymphoma: Prognostic factors predictive of survival. *Cancer, 68*, 2466–2472.

Lister, T. A., Crowther, D., Sutcliffe, S. B., et al. (1989). Report of a committee convened to discuss the evaluation and staging of patients with Hodgkin's disease: Cotswolds meeting. *Journal of Clinical Oncology, 7*(11), 1630–1636.

Longo, D. L., Glatstein, E., Duffey, P. L., et al. (1991). Radiation therapy versus combination chemotherapy in the treatment of early-stage Hodgkin's disease: Seven-year results of a prospective randomized trial. *Journal of Clinical Oncology, 9*(6), 906–917.

Longo, D. L., Glatstein, E., Duffey, P. L., et al. (1989). Treatment of localized aggressive lymphomas with combination chemotherapy followed by involved-field radiation therapy. *Journal of Clinical Oncology, 7*(9), 1295–1302.

Mann, R. B., Jaffe, E. S., & Bernard, C. W. (1992). Malignant lymphomas—a conceptual understanding of morphological diversity. *American Journal of Pathology, 94*, 103–192.

Morgan, E. (1994). Recognizing late effect in Hodgkin's disease survivors. *Contemporary Oncology, 4*(1), 50–60.

Mouch, P., Larson, D., Osteen, R., et. al. (1990). Prognostic factors for positive surgical staging in patients with Hodgkin's disease. *Journal of Clinical Oncology, 8*(2), 257–265.

National Cancer Institute sponsored study of classifications of non-Hodgkin's lymphomas. (1982). Summary and description of a working formulation for clinical usage. The non-Hodgkins lymphoma classification project. *Cancer, 49*(10), 2112–2135.

Paryane, S., Hoppe, R. T., Burke, J. S., Sneed, P., Dawley, D., Cos, R. S., Rosenberg, S. A., & Kaplan, H. S. (1983). Extralymphatic involvement in diffuse non-Hodgkin's lymphoma. *Journal of Clinical Oncology, 1*(11), 682–687.

Prosnitz, P., & Robert, K. (1992). Combined chemotherapy and radiation therapy for Hodgkin's disease. *Oncology,* 113–128.

Pugh, W. C. (1993). Is the working formulation adequate for the classification of the low grade lymphomas? *Leukemia and Lymphoma, 10*(Suppl.), 1–8.

Rapaport, S. I. (1987). *Introduction to hematology* (2nd ed.). Philadelphia: J. B. Lippincott.

Rosenberg, S. A. (1986). Hodgkin's disease: No stage beyond cure. *Hospital Practice, August,* 91–108.

Sarna, G. P., & Kagan, R. A. (1985a). Non-Hodgkin's lymphomas. In C. Haskell, (Ed.), *Cancer treatment* (pp. 789–828). Philadelphia: W. B. Saunders Co.

Sarna, G. P., & Kagan, R. A. (1985b). Mycosis fungoides. In C. Haskell, (Ed.), *Cancer treatment* (pp. 829–845). Philadelphia: W. B. Saunders Co.

Schimpff, S. C., O'Connell, M. J., Greene, W. H., et al. (1975). Infections in 92 splenectomized patients with Hodgkin's disease: A clinical review. *American Journal of Medicine, 59*(5), 695–701.

Skarin, A. T. (1986). Diffuse aggressive lymphomas: A curable subset of non-Hodgkin's lymphomas. *Seminars in Oncology, 13*(4), 10–25.

Stabb, M. A. (1980). Mycosis fungoides: A rare cutaneous malignant lymphoma with multifaceted nursing challenges. *Cancer Nursing, February,* 17–25.

Straus, D. J. (1986). Strategies in treatment of Hodgkin's disease. *Seminars in Oncology, 13*(4), 26–23.

Takvorian, T. (1987). Autologous bone marrow transplantation for non-Hodgkin's lymphoma. *Advances in Oncology, 3*(2), 27–30.

Taylor, M. A., Kaplan, H. S., & Nelsen, T. S. (1985). Staging laparotomy with splenectomy for Hodgkin's disease: The Stanford experience. *World Journal of Surgery, 9*, 449– 460.

Tucker, M. A., Coleman, C. N., Cox, R. S. et al. (1988). Risk of second cancers after treatment for Hodgkin's disease. *New England Journal of Medicine, 318*(2), 76–81.

Ultmann, J. E., & Bitran, J. D. (1989). Current recommendations for the staging and restaging of lymphoma. *Current Opinions in Oncology, 1*(1), 17–22.

Urba, W. J., & Longo, D. L. (1992). Hodgkin's disease. *New England Journal of Medicine, 326*(10), 678–687.

Ultmann, J. E., & Jacobs, R. H. (1985). The non-Hodgkin's lymphomas. *Ca–A Cancer Journal for Clinicians, 35*(2), 66–87.

Van der Velden, J. W., van Putten, W. L., Guinee, V. F., et al. (1988). Subsequent development of acute non-lymphocytic leukemia in patients treated for Hodgkin's disease. *International Journal of Cancer, 42*(2), 252–255.

Weinshel, E. L., & Peterson, B. (1993). Hodgkin's disease. *CA-A Cancer Journal for Clinicians, 43*(6), 325–342.

Willet, C. G., Linggood, R. M., Meyer, J., Orlow, E., Linfors, K., Doppke, M. S., & Aisenberg, A. D. (1987a). Results of treatment of stage 3A Hodgkin's disease. *Cancer, 59*(1), 27–30.

Willett, C. G., Linggood, R. M., Meyer, J., Orlow, B. A., Lindfors, K., Doppke, M. S., & Aisenberg, A. C. (1987b). Results of treatment of stage IA and IIA Hodgkin's disease. *Cancer, 59*, 1107–1111.

Winkler, C. F., & Bunn, P. A. (1983). Cutaneous T-cell lymphoma: A review. *CRC Critical Reviews in Oncology/Hematology, 1*(1), 49–92.

Young, R. C. (1987). Combination chemotherapy in advanced non-Hodgkin's lymphoma. *Advances in Oncology, 3*(2), 20–26.

CHAPTER

36

Leukemia

Mary E. Callaghan

The hematopoietic malignancies are diseases in which there is a proliferation of malignant cells that derive originally from the bone marrow, thymus, and lymphatic tissue. Blood cells that originate in the bone marrow are called hematopoietic cells; those that originate in the thymus and lymphatic tissue are called lymphoid cells. In general, when the bone marrow and peripheral blood are major sites of involvement, the neoplasm is classified as a leukemia. Neoplasms that originate in the lymphatic tissue are collectively referred to as malignant lymphomas. Lymphoid cells differ from hematopoietic cells in both anatomic distribution and function; therefore, their neoplastic proliferation is usually distinguishable. Occasionally, differentiating between a leukemia and a lymphoma may be difficult. The distinction between non-Hodgkin's lymphoma and lymphocytic leukemia becomes blurred when a lymphoma infiltrates the bone marrow or results in large numbers of malignant lymphocytes entering the peripheral blood from tissues other than the bone marrow.

Hematologic malignancies meet immunologic criteria that describe their development as a malignant process. Malignant proliferation of hematopoietic and lymphoid cells is usually marked by monoclonality, that is, cells arising as a single clone, whereas normal tissues are composed of a mixture of cells. Wherever the malignant clone proliferates—lymphoid tissues, bone marrow, extranodal organs, or all of these—it has the advantage of replacing normal cell lines (Rapaport, 1987). In both leukemia and non-Hodgkin's lymphomas, the proliferating cell often takes the characteristics of a normal cell in a specific phase of maturation. Instead of progressing to the next stage of development, the cell becomes fixed and continues to proliferate in its immature phase. The names of specific leukemia and lymphoma subtypes (e.g., acute myeloid leukemia, small cleaved cell lymphomas) often represent the description of the normal cellular counterpart in a particular maturational phase. Figure 36–1 reviews the hematopoietic progenitor cell development.

The clinical manifestations of specific hematologic malignancies present an array of symptoms that require nursing intervention. It is the purpose of this chapter to describe the disease process and treatment, identify nursing issues, and refer the reader to specific chapters for a more in-depth review of nursing measures.

LEUKEMIAS

The leukemias are classified along with lymphomas, multiple myeloma, and Waldenström's macroglobulinemia as hematologic malignancies. The common characteristic of all the leukemias is an "unregulated proliferation in the bone marrow of a cell of hematopoietic origin" (Rapaport, 1987). The malignant cell has a growth advantage over normal cells and replaces the normal elements in all areas of hematopoietic bone marrow.

The leukemias are described by the particular cell type of origin. Most originate in the white blood cell lines, but occasionally they can begin in the megakaryocyte line or the erythroid line.

The leukemias are classified on the basis of their cellular differentiation. The acute leukemias describe disease in which differentiation is very minimal, with early forms of cells or blasts being the cell type. The chronic leukemias describe diseases in which the malignant cells have some degree of differentiation. The following discussion describes the major leukemias and their treatment in the adult population.

ACUTE LEUKEMIAS

Acute leukemias arise from the alteration and clonal reproduction of hematopoietic progenitor cells into the populations of poorly differentiated malignant cells. The acute leukemias have been broadly classified as either lymphoid leukemia or myeloid leukemia.

In differentiating between lymphoid and myeloid leukemia, the classification system relies on morphol-

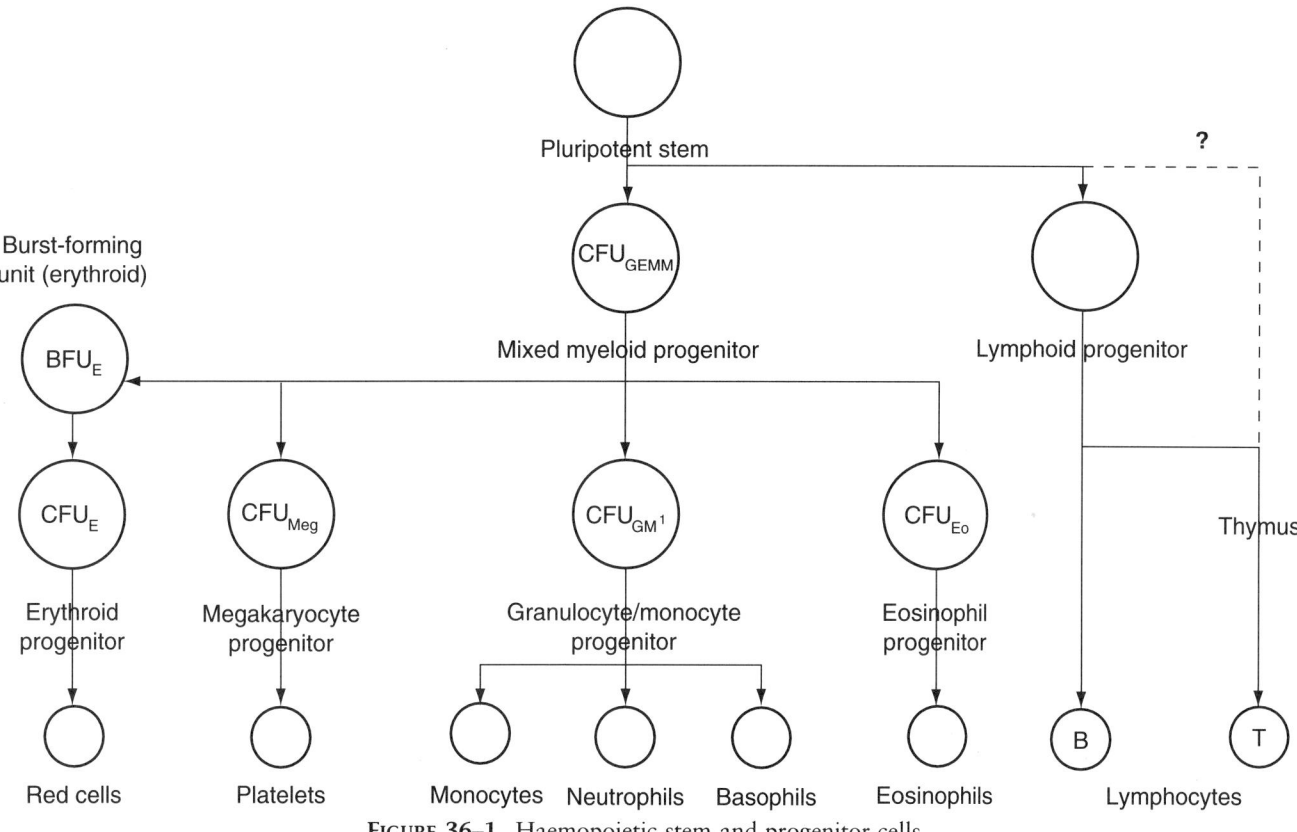

FIGURE 36–1. Haemopoietic stem and progenitor cells.

ogy and cytochemistry. With newer technology, electron microscopy with cytochemical and immunohistochemical stains is utilized to supplement the morphologic classification. Table 36–1 describes common stains utilized in acute leukemia classification.

ACUTE LYMPHOBLASTIC LEUKEMIA

Overview. Acute lymphoblastic leukemia (ALL) is a hematologic malignancy of uncontrolled proliferation and accumulation of immature lymphocytes and their

TABLE 36–1. *Cytochemical and Immunohistochemical Stains Used for the Classification of Acute Leukemia*

Myeloperoxidase (MPO), an enzyme found in the primary (azurophilic) granules of cells of the granulocytic and monocytic series, is vital for distinguishing lymphoid from myeloid leukemia. The granules are stained a dark blue to dark brown color when free oxygen liberated by the peroxidase reacts to change a benzidine dye from its clear to colored state.

Nonspecific esterase (NSE), prominent in monocytes and their precursors, employs a-naphthyl butyrate (ANB) or a-naphthyl acetate following pretreatment with sodium fluoride (ANA-F) as substrates for the enzymatic cleavage of the naphthyl group, which is then reacted with a diazo dye. Although staining is prominent in the monocytic series, there can be weak staining in some ALL cases, and in some cases of AML, M3 (APL).

Periodic acid-Schiff reaction (PAS) depends on the liberation of carbohydrate radicals, which are oxidized to aldehydes and then reacted with Schiff reagent. Positivity in hematopoietic cells usually denotes glycogen, which is prominent in malignant erythroid precursors (blush- and block-positive). Granules can also be seen in some lymphoid and some myeloid leukemias.

Sudan Black B (BB) stains the phospholipids of monocytes and granulocytes but is not as specific as MPO in distinguishing lymphoid from myeloid leukemia (1.6% of ALL cases have 5% or greater SBB positivity).

Naphthol AS-D chloracetate esterase (NASD), found in granulocytic precursors, cleaves the naphthyl group, which combines with a diazonium salt to give an azo dye. This enzyme can be absent in very early granulocytic differentiation and is therefore not as sensitive as MPO.

Terminal deoxynucleotidyl transferase (TdT), detected by immunofluorescence or immunoperoxidase techniques, is a nuclear enzyme that allows for template-independent addition of deoxynucleotides onto DNA chains. Although not specific for non-B-cell ALL (10% of AML have greater than 10% TdT-positive cells), it is considered a valuable marker for immature lymphoid neoplasms (i.e., lymphoblastic lymphoma and ALL).

(From Hirsch-Ginsberg, C., Huh, Y. O., Kagan, J., Liang, J. C., & Stass, S. A. [1993]. Advances in the diagnosis of acute leukemia. *Hematology Oncology Clinics of North America, 7* [1], 1–46. Used with permission.)

progenitors (Henderson, 1983). Although ALL is the most common childhood malignancy, it accounts for only 20 per cent of adult leukemias (Henderson & Han, 1986). This discussion reviews current thoughts about adult ALL.

Etiology. The exact etiology of ALL is unknown, but several factors have been implicated. These factors include radiation, chemicals and drugs, viruses, and genetic abnormalities.

Certain genetic disorders, for example, Down's syndrome, ataxia, and telangiectasia, are associated with an increased risk of developing ALL in children (Berenson, Zigelboim, & Gale, 1985). In adults, the evidence for this etiologic factor is less clear-cut. In one study, chromosomal abnormalities were identified in approximately 66 per cent of patients with ALL (Bloomfield et al., 1983). The data in this study suggest that chromosomal abnormalities influence prognosis in adults with ALL, but no evidence regarding a causal factor has been documented.

The survivors of the atomic bomb have shown an increased incidence of both ALL and acute myelogenous leukemia (AML), probably due to the effects of ionizing radiation. The increased incidence of leukemia with exposure to high levels of ionizing radiation is well established, but studies attempting to link low-level radiation to the development of adult leukemia have not shown such an association (Berenson et al., 1985).

The documentation linking the exposure to chemicals to the increased incidence of developing leukemia is stronger for AML than for ALL. Benzene exposure has been reported as increasing the incidence of ALL, as well as that of AML (Berenson et al., 1985). After treatment with chemotherapy, the development of leukemia has been reported as a result of the therapy; the leukemia that develops is usually AML, although ALL has been reported.

Exogenous retroviruses (RNA tumor viruses) are known to cause leukemia and lymphoma in chickens, cats, cows, and primates (Jacobs & Gale, 1986). In humans the identification of human T cell leukemia/lymphoma virus (HTLV) has been demonstrated in patients with T cell lymphoproliferative malignancies (Blayney et al., 1983; Bloomfield et al., 1983). Although viruses have been identified in some patients with ALL, the cause of most cases is undetermined.

Despite the research and technologic advances, the cause of ALL in most patients will be unknown. Evidence supports a multifactorial approach to its development, yet most patients may never have a factor that is associated with the development of ALL.

Nurses can help dispel false information and educate patients and their families regarding what is currently known about etiologic factors when the patient begins to ask "Why me?"

Classification. Two classification systems have been developed that describe the types of ALL. The first is based on the morphologic description of the disease and is called the French-American-British classification system (FAB). The FAB classification recognizes three types of lymphoblasts: L_1, L_2, and L_3 (Table 36–2). In childhood ALL, 85 per cent of patients have L_1 mor-

TABLE 36–2. *FAB Classification of Acute Lymphoblastic Leukemia (ALL)*

ALL-L_1: MPO-negative, with small cells predominating. Cells have a high N/C ratio (scant amount of cytoplasm), regular nuclear border, and inconspicuous nucleoli. TdT is usually positive.

ALL-L_2: MPO-negative, heterogeneous population often with larger blasts. The cells have a low N/C ratio (moderate amount of cytoplasm), with irregular nuclear border and prominent nucleoli. TdT is usually positive.

ALL-L_3: (Burkitt type) MPO-negative, homogeneous population of large blasts. The cells have a moderate amount of deeply basophilic cytoplasm and prominent cytoplasmic vacuolation. The nuclei are regular with one or more prominent nucleoli. The blasts are TdT-negative and may be associated with t(2;8), t(8;14), or t(8;22) chromosomal abnormalities.

MPO = myeloperoxidase; N/C = nuclear to cytoplasmic ratio; TdT = terminal deoxynucleotidyl transferase.
(From Hirsch-Ginsberg, C., Huh, Y. O., Kagan, J., Liang, J. C., & Stass, S. A. [1993]. Advances in the diagnosis of acute leukemia. *Hematology Oncology Clinics of North America,* 7 [1], 1–46. Used with permission.)

phology with relatively few having L_2 or L_3. In adult ALL, L_1 and L_2 are common, with a preponderance of L_2. L_3 morphology represents a small percentage of patients with ALL (Hoelzer & Gale, 1987). L_3 subtype is morphologically identical to the malignant cells in Burkitt's lymphoma (Devine & Larson, 1994).

There has been controversy surrounding the use of the FAB classification and its ability to thoroughly describe the heterogeneous ALL population as well as to determine prognostic variables. Another classification has been developed that is being utilized with some success.

This approach to the classification of ALL is based on immune properties of the leukemia cells and is called immunophenotyping (Bennett et al., 1976). The subtypes include the common T, B, or null cell ALL. The subtypes are based on the detection on the cell surface of one of the following: the common ALL antigen (CALLA), T cell antigens or immunoglobulin molecules, or B cell markers (Bennett et al., 1976). The null-cell type has none of the cell surface features. An immunologic/morphologic classification is listed in Table 36–3 (Devine & Larson, 1994). Table 36–3 illustrates the ALL subtypes and the response of each subtype to the immunologic cell markers.

Prognostic variables in adult ALL have been studied, although less frequently than those in childhood ALL, to identify patients in high-risk groups. Investigations correlating the FAB classification with prognosis have produced contradictory results (Hoelzer & Gale, 1987).

Data from studies evaluating prognosis utilizing the immunologic classification indicate that adults with T cell ALL have the best prognosis, those with common ALL have an intermediate prognosis, and those with null cell ALL have a slightly inferior prognosis. There are recent data that a subset of T cell ALL with early T cell lineage responds poorly to treatment (Huh et al.,

TABLE 36–3. *Immunologic/Morphologic Classification of Acute Lymphoblastic Leukemia Cell Markers*

CATEGORY	TdT	Ia	CD19	CD10	CIg	SIg	CD7	CD2	FAB MORPHOLOGY
B-Lineage									
Early B-Precursor ALL	+	+	+	−	−	−			L_1, L_2
Common ALL	+	+	+	+	−	−			L_1, L_2
Pre-B ALL	+	+	+	+	+	−			L_1
B-ALL	−	+	+	±	−	+			L_3
T-Lineage									
Early T-Precursor ALL	+						+	−	L_1, L_2
T-ALL	+						+	+	L_1, L_2

ALL = acute lymphoblastic leukemia; TdT = terminal deoxynucleotidyl transferase; CIg = cytoplasmic immunoglobulin; SIg = surface immunoglobulin; FAB = French-American-British Classification; Ia = immunoglobulin a.

(From Devine, S. M., & Larson, R. A. [1994]. Acute leukemia in adults: Development in diagnosis and treatment. *Cancer, 44*[6], 326–352. Copyright © 1994 Wiley-Liss. Reprinted by permission of Wiley-Liss, a division of John Wiley and Sons, Inc.)

1990). Patients with B-cell ALL have the least favorable prognosis (Hoelzer & Gale, 1987).

Cytogenetic abnormalities including inversions, insertions, translocations, and deletions are normally only associated with certain leukemias (Hirsch-Ginsberg, Huh, Kagan, Liang, & Stass, 1993). T cell ALL is associated with a number of translocations such as t(7;9) (q34;q34), t(7;9) (q34;q34,3), t(8;14) (q24;q11) (Hirsch-Ginsberg et al., 1993). About 35 per cent of adult ALL has the Philadelphia chromosome (Devine & Larson, 1994). Philadelphia-positive (Ph+) ALL is usually classified as having an FAB L_2 morphology but may occasionally be L_1. The Philadelphia chromosome is found in about one third of adult ALL. The presence of Philadelphia chromosome is associated with B lineage and carries a poor prognosis (Lesting & Hooberman, 1993). Although Philadelphia-positive ALL response to initial chemotherapy is not different from that of Philadelphia-negative ALL, the short duration of response leads to the poor prognosis.

Other factors are reported to influence negatively the remission rates. These include male sex, initial presentation with central nervous system (CNS) leukemia, high white blood count on presentation, older age, time to achieve complete response, immunologic subtypes (pre-pre-B-ALL, pre-T-ALL, mixed or hybrid leukemias), and presence of a mediastinal mass (Bernard et al., 1978; Hirsch-Ginsberg et al., 1993). These factors have been reported to influence a poorer prognosis but do not always confirm a poor prognosis. A 1980 study reported that the only significant prognostic finding in its group was that patients presenting with a white blood count greater than 35×10^9/L had a lower probability of surviving 3 years (Amadori et al., 1983).

Studies investigating prognostic variables originate in various centers, and conclusions drawn must not be taken as definitive predictors of outcomes in individual patients. Patients are individuals with unique diseases that may respond very differently to similar treatment regimens.

Clinical Features. The clinical features of acute leukemia are outlined in Table 36–4 (Henderson, 1983). The classic clinical features of fatigue, fever, bruising, and pallor are manifestations of failure of normal bone marrow. Malaise, lethargy, weight loss, fever, and night sweats may be present but are usually not severe. Most patients have these symptoms less than 3 months (Henderson, 1983). Common laboratory findings include leukocytosis with immature blasts or cells, anemia, thrombocytopenia, and bone marrow packed with poorly differentiated lymphoid blast cells. The peripheral leukocyte count can range from 1000 to 400,000/mm³. Although more commonly seen in patients with chronic myelogenous leukemia (CML) blast crisis and AML, intravascular clumping of leukemia cells may occur in patients with blast counts in excess of 100,000/mm³ (Berenson et al., 1985).

Other clinical features associated with ALL are lymph node enlargement, hepatic or splenic enlargement, meningeal leukemia, bone or joint pain, genitourinary manifestations including hematuria, cystitis, pyelonephritis, priapism, renal failure, hyperuricemia, uric acid nephropathy, and testicular involvement (Henderson, 1983). These symptoms are related to leukemic infiltration of extramedullary lymphatic tissue.

Infections are common in patients presenting with disease and as a cause of death. Acute lymphoblastic leukemia causes marked impairment in the host defense system (Berenson et al., 1985). There is a marked reduction in the number of phagocytic leukocytes and an impairment in ability to mobilize against infection. Patients with ALL show a decreased response to mutagen, have reduced delayed hypersensitivity reactions, and often have low levels of immunoglobulins at diagnosis (Berenson et al., 1985). Diagnosis is based on morphologic and cytochemical analysis of bone marrow.

Treatment. The treatment of ALL is generally divided into two phases termed *remission induction therapy* and *postremission therapy*. The purpose of induction chemotherapy is to eradicate all detectable leukemic cells, induce a remission, and restore normal bone marrow function. Postremission therapy usually consists of central nervous system prophylaxis, consolidation-intensification chemotherapy, and maintenance chemotherapy. The goal of postremission therapy is to eradicate undetectable leukemic cells and thereby prevent a relapse.

The terminology utilized in describing postremission therapy can be confusing. Consolidation-intensifi-

TABLE 36–4. *Clinical Features of Acute Leukemia Related to Pathophysiology*

SYMPTOMS	SIGNS	LABORATORY ABNORMALITIES	CAUSE
Fatigue, weakness	Pallor, lethargy, weakness	Anemia, hypocalcemia, hypercalcemia, hypomagnesemia	Marrow failure, release of cellular ions and metabolites
Weight loss	Weight loss		Reduced food intake, anemia, hepatosplenomegaly, increased catabolism
Bleeding in skin, mucous membranes, gums, or gastrointestinal or genitourinary tracts	Purpura, gum oozing or hypertrophy, hematuria, melena	Thrombocytopenia, hypofibrinogenemia, reduced factors V or VIII, increased fibrin split products	Marrow failure, DIC
Infection of skin, throat, gums, or respiratory or urinary tracts	Fever, chills, tissue infiltrates, pyoderma gangrenosum	Granulocytopenia; radiographic evidence of pneumonia, sinusitis, and the like; positive cultures	Marrow failure, granulocytopenia, immunodeficiency
Headache, nausea, vomiting, blurred vision, cranial nerve dysfunction	Papilledema, cranial nerve palsy, meningeal irritation	Spinal fluid pleocytosis, reduced CSF sugar, increased CSF protein	Meningeal, CNS, or nerve infiltration, compression, or both
Bone pain and tenderness	Increased bone tenderness	Periosteal elevation, bone destruction by x-rays, abnormal bone marrow, pressure fibrosis	Local leukemic infiltration
Abdominal fullness, anorexia	Hepatosplenomegaly, abdominal tenderness	Hyperfibrinogenemia, elevated SGOT or SGPT, alkaline phosphatase	Infiltration of abdominal viscera
Enlarged lymph nodes or tumor masses	Enlarged lymph nodes or masses in node areas, skin, breast, or testes	Abnormal liver or spleen biopsy results, abnormal bone scan results	Local tumor growth or infiltration
Oliguria	Oliguria	Concentrated urine, elevated BUN, elevated uric acid	Dehydration, uric acid nephropathy, DIC
Obstipation	Abdominal fullness, tenderness	Abnormal results for scans or radiographic contrast studies	Local infiltration or obstruction, calcium/magnesium imbalance

DIC = disseminated intravascular coagulation; CSF = cerebrospinal fluid; SGOT = serum glutamic-oxaloacetic transaminase; SGPT = serum glutamic-pyruvic transaminase; BUN = blood urea nitrogen; CNS = central nervous system.
(From Henderson, E. S. [1983]. Acute leukemias—general considerations in hematology. In W. J. Williams, E. Beutler, A. J. Erslev, & M. A. Lichtman [Eds.], *Hematology* [p. 221]. New York: McGraw-Hill Book Co. Used with permission.)

cation chemotherapy usually refers to therapy given after remission has been achieved and restoration of normal bone marrow has occurred. This therapy can involve high-dose chemotherapy, use of new agents to help prevent drug resistance, or, less often, readministration of the induction regimen (Hoelzer & Gale, 1987). Maintenance follows consolidation and involves less intensive therapy.

Remission Induction Therapy. Specific drugs utilized in the treatment of adult ALL have been reviewed elsewhere (Hoelzer, 1993). At present, most remission induction regimens include vincristine, prednisone, an anthracycline, and L-asparginase. Cytoxan is included in most adult regimens because studies have shown that it improves the continuous complete response (CR) rate and the survival for the subtype, T-ALL (Schiffer, Larson, & Bloomfiels for the CALGB, 1991). Cytarabine (ara-C) is another drug added to most adult ALL regimens because of its enhancement in the remission induction (Rohatiner et al., 1990).

Currently in clinical trials is the investigation of drugs previously utilized in relapsed or refractory ALL, such as etoposide, teniposide, m-amsacrine, mitoxantrone, idarubicin, and also high-dose ara-C and high-dose methotrexate (Berman et al., 1991).

The goals of the remission induction trials are to obtain a high CR rate and a prolonged leukemia-free survival. To reach these goals, AML-type induction regimens have been investigated. In one pilot study, selected young adult ALL patients (15 to 35 years old) received the AML regimen TAD (thioguanine, ara-C, and daunorubicin) with vincristine, prednisone, and L-asparginase. This combination resulted in a CR rate of 91 per cent, but the median remission duration was 15 months (Hoelzer, 1993).

In another trial, high-dose ara-C and mitoxantrone were utilized obtaining a 95 per cent CR rate, but leukemia-free survival is not yet analyzed (Arlin et al., 1991). Therefore, the trials for induction therapy will continue to evolve with the introduction of new agents and escalating doses in an attempt to obtain higher CR rates and longer leukemia-free survival.

In general, current chemotherapy regimens utilizing an anthracycline, usually daunomycin, can achieve 70 to 80 per cent remission rates. With optimal postremission therapy, 3- to 5-year actuarial leukemia-free survival has been achieved in 20 to 35 per cent of unselected patients (Hoelzer, 1993). Table 36–5 lists the variety of regimens utilized in the therapy of ALL. Evaluation of treatment benefit is difficult because of

TABLE 36–5. *Results of Chemotherapy for Adult Acute Lymphoblastic Leukemia in Recent Large Studies (Exceeding 100 Patients)*

Group/Author	Year	Number of Patients	Median Age (yrs)	Induction	Consolidation	Complete Remission (%)	MRD (mo)	LFS (%) at ≥ 5 yrs
SWOG/Hussein et al.	1989	168	28	V, P, Ad, C, A, V, P, C	MTX, ara-C, TG	68	23	30
MD Anderson/Kantarjian et al.	1990	105	30	V, Ad, Dex, C, V, P	MTX, A, Ad, HdAC,	84	22	34
GIMEMA/Mandelli et al.	1990	358	31	V, P, A, D	V, IdM, IdAC, P	79	19	25
MSKCC/Clarkson et al.	1990	199		V, P, [D, A, Ad, C]	ara-C, TG, A, V, P, MTX, C, BCNU	82	28	33
GMALL (01/81)/Hoelzer et al.	1992	368	25	V, P, A, D, C ara-C, MTX, MP	V, Dex, Ad ara-C, C, TG	74	24	35
GMALL (02/84)/Hoelzer, et al.	1992	562	28	V, P, A, D, C ara-C, MTX, MP VM26, ara-C	V, Dex, Ad ara-C, C, TG	75	27	41
EORTC/Stryckmans et al.	1991	106	27	V, P, Ad (HdAC]	A, C [M, TG, AC]	74		39
GATLA/Lluesma Gonalons et al.	1991	145		V, P, D, A, C, ara-C, MP	Ad, V, Dex, A, ara-C, C, MP	78	28	34
CALGB/Ellison et al.	1991	277	33	V, P, A, D	[AC, D], MTX, MP	64	21	29
FGTALL/Fiére et al.	1990	467		V, P, D, C	Ad, ara-C, A	76		39
JALSG/Tomonaga et al.	1991	117	38	V, P, D, A, C	VP16, mitox, +	81	(4 yr)	27
SWEDEN/Smedmyr et al.	1991	113	38	V, P, A, D, C	V, D, VP-16, ara-C, P	77	(3 yr) (4 yr) HR 37	LR60
Totals		2985				75*	24*	34*

V = vincristine; P = prednisone; A = *L*-asparaginase; D = daunorubicin; MTX = methotrexate; MP = mercaptopurine; BCNU = carmustine; ara-C = cytarabine; Ad = doxorubicin; TG = thioguanine; C = cyclophosphamide; Dex = dexamethasone; HdM = high-dose methotrexate; IdM = intermediate-dose methotrexate; HdAC = high-dose ara-C; IdAC = intermediate-dose ara-C; VM26 = teniposide; VP16 = etoposide; SWOG = Southwest Oncology Group; MDACC = MD Anderson Cancer Center; GIMEMA = Gruppo Italiano Malattie Ematologiche Maligne Adupo; MSKCC = Memorial Sloan-Kettering Cancer Center; GMALL = German Multicenter trials in adult ALL; EORTC = European Organization for Research and Treatment of Cancer; GATLA = Argentine Group for Treatment of Acute Leukemia; CALGB = Cancer and Leukemia Group B; FGTALL = French Group for Treatment of Adult Acute Lymphoblastic Leukemia; JALSG = Japan Adult Leukemia Study Group; SWEDEN = Swedish ALL Group; MRD = median remission duration; LFS = probability of leukemia-free survival; LR = low risk; HR = high risk.
*Weighted mean.
(From Hoelzer, D. [1993]. Therapy of the newly diagnosed adult with acute lymphoblastic leukemia. *Hematology Oncology Clinics of North America,* 7[1], 139–160. Used with permission.)

the varying treatment regimens and the diversity of prognostic variables.

Central Nervous System Prophylaxis. In adult ALL, the CNS relapse rate without specific CNS therapy is 21 to 50 per cent (Kantajian, et al., 1988). In childhood ALL, the role of CNS prophylaxis in prolonging survival is well documented (Berenson et al., 1985). In adult ALL, the usefulness of central nervous system prophylaxis in prolonging survival has been difficult to document. In general, most treatment regimens in adult ALL include intrathecal methotrexate with or without central nervous system irradiation, and systemic high-dose chemotherapy with high-dose methotrexate or high-dose cytosine arabinoside (ara-C) so that sufficient doses will cross the blood-brain barrier to achieve sufficient cerebrospinal fluid (CSF) levels (Hoelzer, 1993).

Postremission Therapy

Consolidation Therapy. The use of a variety of regimens in consolidation therapy indicates that consolidation therapy improves the leukemia-free survival rate. The drugs utilized consist of standard doses of a variety of drugs including ara-C, daunorubicin, methotrexate, vincristine, dexamethasone, Adriamycin, thioguanine, and Cytoxan.

The use of high-dose ara-C in consolidation especially for high-risk patients has been demonstrated in Table 36–6 (Devine & Larson, 1994).

Maintenance Therapy. In childhood ALL, the use of maintenance therapy has been a favorable approach in the design of therapy that has been utilized in the adult ALL population. There are contrasting data indicating that the use of maintenance therapy may or may not be necessary if consolidation with the induction therapy is utilized (Mandelli, Annino, & Giona, 1990). Hoelzer reviews the results of trials without maintenance therapy (Hoelzer, 1993). The leukemia-free 2-year survival in the reviewed studies was 18 to 35 per cent.

It will be important that future trials identify which subtypes, if any, of ALL will benefit from maintenance therapy.

Relapsed and Resistant Leukemia. Hoelzer and Gale (1987) have reviewed the experimental drugs utilized in patients who have relapsed and resistant ALL. The most active regimens appear to be moderate- to high-dose methotrexate with Leucovorin or folinic acid rescue, the combination of teniposide and cytarabine, and high-dose cytarabine in combination with amsacrine or an anthracycline.

Limited studies utilizing immunotherapy have not shown convincing benefit to patients. Studies utilizing monoclonal antibodies are in progress, but no complete responses have been reported (Hoelzer & Gale, 1987).

Bone Marrow Transplantation. Christiansen (1993) has reviewed the data evaluating bone marrow transplantation (BMT) in adult ALL. In patients with advanced disease, the 2- to 4-year survival rate is 10 to 20 per cent. Patients in first or second remission have a 2- to 4-year survival rate of 30 to 50 per cent. These statistics are utilizing allogeneic transplants and vary in different studies.

Autologous bone marrow transplantation in adult ALL has been performed. Disease-free survival of approximately 20 per cent in 2 years is reported in individuals with ALL in second or third remission (Champlin & Gale, 1987). The value of autologous transplantation in ALL remains an area for further critical investigation.

Nursing Care. The mainstay in the treatment of ALL is effective elimination of leukemic cells in the bone marrow by chemotherapeutic agents. The resultant pancytopenia is a nursing challenge. Nursing care of patients receiving treatment for ALL requires an integrated knowledge of blood component therapy; of management of infection in immunosuppressed patients; of management of patients experiencing alteration in elimination, alteration in skin integrity, alteration in protective mechanisms, alteration in comfort, and alteration in nutritional status; and of the psychosocial problems of facing a life-threatening illness. Refer to Unit VIII for elaboration of these specific nursing interventions.

TABLE 36–6. *High-Dose ARA-C for High-Risk Adult Acute Lymphoblastic Leukemia Patients*

Investigator/Year	Number of Patients in Complete Remission (CR)	Risk Features	Treatment	Median Remission/ Duration (mo)	Continuous Complete Remission/ Leukemia-Free Survival
Rohatiner et al. (1990)	20	High WBC, T-, B-, null-ALL	V, Ad, A, P HdAC 2 g/m² × 12*	34	49%, 5 yr
GMALL/Hoelzer et al. (1992)	81	High WBC, late CR null-ALL, Ph⁺?	HdAC 3 g/m² × 8† mitox	21	43%, 4 yr
MDACC/Kantarjian et al. (1990)	63	High WBC, late CR B-ALL, Ph⁺, CNS	HdAC 3 g/m² × 6†	13	< 30%, 3 yr

*Induction.
†Consolidation.
V = vincristine; Ad = doxorubicin; A = *L*-asparaginase; P = prednisone; HdAC = high-dose cytarabine; mitox = mitoxantrone.
(From Hoelzer, D. [1993]. Therapy of the newly diagnosed adult with acute lymphoblastic leukemia. *Hematology Oncology Clinics of North America,* 7[1], 139–160. Used with permission.)

ACUTE MYELOGENOUS LEUKEMIA

Overview. Acute myelogenous leukemia (AML) or acute non-lymphocytic leukemia (ANLL) is a group of diseases in which an abnormal hematologic stem cell gives rise to a monoclonal population of myeloid cells whose ability to differentiate beyond early forms is impaired (Rai & Montserrat, 1987). These abnormal cells have a growth advantage, and therefore blasts and other early forms eventually replace the normal hematopoietic marrow cells. This disease is characterized by a proliferation and accumulation of malignant myeloblasts or other immature myeloid cells. The cell lines that can be affected by the malignancy are the granulocytic, monocytic, erythroid, and megakaryocyte.

Etiology. The exact etiology of AML is unknown. Like ALL, several factors have been implicated. These factors include radiation, chemicals and drugs, viruses, and genetic abnormalities.

Acute myelogenous leukemia occurs with increased frequency in several congenital disorders including Down syndrome, Klinefelter's syndrome, Fanconi's anemia, osteogenesis imperfecta, and Wiskott-Aldrich syndrome (Bloomfield et al., 1983).

The effects of ionizing radiation on the survivors of the atomic bomb are well documented with the increased incidence of leukemia, especially AML (Cronkite, Maloney, & Bond, 1960; Graham, 1960; Heysel et al., 1960). Exposure to chemicals has been associated with an increased incidence of AML. The association of benzene exposure and AML has been noted (Vigliani & Sart, 1964). Chloramphenicol, phenylbutazone, alkylating agents, procarbazine, and the nitrosoureas are the drugs most commonly associated with the development of AML, although the association is identified in few patients (Vigliani & Sart, 1964).

A relationship between RNA viruses and myeloid leukemias in animals has been found, but viral cancer in humans has not been identified (Blayney et al., 1983). An interest in cellular oncogenes has been evident. Cellular oncogenes are closely related to RNA tumor viruses called viral oncogenes (Blattner et al., 1983). The cellular oncogenes have been found near sites of chromosomal rearrangements common in AML, but there is no evidence yet that the oncogenes are directly involved in the development of AML.

Classification. The FAB classification is a widely accepted classification system for AML. This system is based on the morphologic description of the malignant cell line involved. Table 36–7 describes this classification (Rapaport, 1987). Acute myelogenous leukemia with granulocyte differentiation includes acute undifferentiated leukemia (M1), acute myelogenous leukemia (M2) with maturation to or beyond promyelocyte stage, and acute progranulocytic leukemia (M3). The M4, M5, and M6 types of AML show varying cell types as indicated in the table and are less common than the previously described types. M0 is a form of AML in which the myeloid differentiation is minimal, and the diagnosis requires the use of immunohis-

tochemical staining (Bennett et al., 1991). Cytogenic studies are being utilized to further classify different types of AML, and surface marker analysis is being used to characterize cell types of very early blast forms (Rapaport, 1987).

Clinical Features. The clinical presentation of patients with AML usually reflects the degree of replacement of normal bone marrow by leukemic cells. Table 36–4 summarizes the various symptoms associated with acute leukemia. Zigelboim, Foon, and Gale (1985) estimate that 20 per cent of patients present with symptoms of anemia, pallor, weakness, and fatigue. The median age of patients at presentation is 60 years.

Bleeding is another important manifestation of this disease. Twenty to 50 per cent of patients with AML will have moderately severe thrombocytopenia at the time of diagnosis. The severe thrombocytopenia is usually related to decreased platelet production or increased consumption of cells from infection, hypersplenism, and, rarely, disseminated intravascular coagulation. Patients with acute promyelocytic leukemia (M3 or APL) can have additional coagulation abnormalities (Gale & Foon, 1986). These coagulation abnormalities include hypofibrinogenemia, abnormal factors V and VII, increased fibrin degradation products, and circulating anticoagulants. These abnormalities present unique challenges in the induction phase of a patient with acute promyelocytic leukemia.

The treatment for APL or M3 leukemia is currently being modified. This type of AML has a high rate of complete remission, and many are cured, although there is an increased rate of morbidity during induction related to the coagulopathies. ALL-trans-retinoic acid (TRA) induces the leukemia cells in APL to differentiate into mature granulocytes and thus establish a complete remission (Frankel, 1993). The optimal treatment regimen utilizing TRA is currently being investigated. TRA with other agents or biologics may improve the long-term disease-free survival in patients with APL.

Twenty-five per cent of patients with AML at diagnosis will present with a serious infection (Devine & Larson, 1994). Because of myeloid leukemic involvement, the neutrophils are decreased and can function abnormally. Bacterial infections are most common, but fungal, viral, and protozoal infections can occur.

Patients will also present with physical complaints that reflect the infiltration of normal tissues with leukemic cells. Bone or joint pain can indicate infiltration of the bone marrow. Hepatomegaly, splenomegaly, and lymph node enlargement have been reported in 10 to 60 per cent of patients. Renal abnormalities may occur as a result of direct infiltration; gout from increased uric acid and gastrointestinal symptoms, including distention, satiety, and obstipation as a result of organ infiltration, are reported (Zigelboim et al., 1985).

Skin lesions can occur. The most common skin lesions are petechiae related to thrombocytopenia. Leukemic skin infiltrates are uncommon but can be found in patients with monocytic and myelomonocytic

TABLE 36–7. *French-American-British Classification of Acute Myeloid Leukemia*

FAB SUBTYPE	MORPHOLOGIC AND CYTOCHEMICAL FEATURES	FREQUENCY (%)
M0	Large, agranular myeloblasts, sometimes resembling lymphoblasts of FAB subtype L_2. Stain negative for myeloperoxidase and Sudan black. Express CD13 or CD33 antigens on cell surface.	2–3
M1	Acute myeloblastic leukemia without maturation: Large, poorly differentiated myeloblasts represent 90% or more of the nonerythroid cells. At least 3% of the myeloblasts stain positive for myeloperoxidase.	20
M2	Acute myeloblastic leukemia with maturation: Between 30% and 89% of the nonerythroid cells are myeloblasts having abundant cytoplasm with moderate to many granules. Auer rods are often visible.	25–30
M3	Leukemia cells usually contain heavy azurophilic granulation. Nuclear size varies greatly. Nuclei are often bilobed or kidney-shaped. Some cells contain bundles of Auer rods. Leukemia cells stain strongly positive for myeloperoxidase. There is a microgranular variant.	8–15
M4	Myeloblasts, promyelocytes, myelocytes, and other granulocytic precursors make up over 30% of the nonerythroid cells but do not exceed 80%. Monocytic cells account for up to 20% of the nonerythroid cells. Nonspecific esterase and chloroacetate stains are often positive. Auer rods may be present.	20–25
M4Eo	Myelomonoblasts with cytochemically and morphologically abnormal eosinophils.	5
M5	Monoblasts, promonocytes, or monocytes make up 80% or more of the nonerythroid cells. In one subtype (M5a), 80% or more of all the monocytic cells are monoblasts. In the well-differentiated subtype (M5b), less than 80% are monoblasts. Naphthol AS-D acetate positivity is extinguished by sodium fluoride.	
M6	Greater than 50% of the nucleated marrow cells are erythroid. Erythroblasts are usually strongly positive for the periodic acid-Schiff reaction. Myeloblasts represent 30% or more of the nonerythroid cells.	5
M7	Large and small megakaryoblasts with high nuclear/cytoplasm ratio. Cytoplasm is pale and agranular. Standard cytochemical stains not definitive. Platelet peroxidase and platelet-specific antibodies often positive.	1–2

(From Devine, S., & Larson, R. [1994]. Acute leukemia in adults: Development in diagnosis and treatment. *Cancer, 44*[6], 326–352. Copyright © 1994 Wiley-Liss. Reprinted by permission of Wiley-Liss, a division of John Wiley and Sons, Inc.)

leukemia, relapsed or resistant leukemia, and high white blood cell counts (Rapaport, 1987). In addition to skin infiltrates, patients with monocytic leukemia can have hypertrophied gums, oral ulcers, palpable spleen, anorectal ulcerations, and central nervous system involvement (Rapaport, 1987).

Central nervous system involvement in AML is uncommon but is primarily seen in patients with monocytic (M2) and myelomonocytic leukemia (Zigelboim et al., 1985). When patients experience headaches, diplopia, changes in mental status, cranial nerve palsies, and papilledema, central nervous system involvement is suspected.

Acute myelogenous leukemia is diagnosed by bone marrow aspiration and evidence from biopsy specimens. One classic feature of AML is the presence of Auer rods on the leukemic blast (Graham, 1960). The other method of distinguishing myeloblasts from lymphoblasts is to use a histochemical stain that demonstrates peroxidase activity (Henderson, 1983). More recently, monoclonal antibodies have been used to identify some types of AML, but these need further development (Ball et al., 1991; Griffin et al., 1986).

Prognostic variables have been investigated in an attempt to identify patients who will respond favorably to therapy. Gale and Foon (1987) have summarized the pretreatment variables that may influence treatment outcomes. In general, older age, previous cancer, previous therapy, and specific chromosomal abnormalities are variables that are associated with unfavorable prognosis. A favorable prognosis is associated with patients in the younger age group, with the presence of Auer rods, and with a shorter time between treatment and complete remission. With cytogenetic analysis, specific chromosomal abnormalities are also associated with a favorable prognosis (Table 36–8) (Devine & Larson, 1994).

In acute leukemia, it is not uncommon to find cytogenetic abnormalities. Prior to the initiation of induction therapy for AML, it is a general practice to obtain cytogenetic analysis to obtain information regarding prognostic factors that will influence postremission therapy.

Treatment. The goal of induction therapy in AML is to achieve hematologic remission. Hematologic remission is generally defined as the reduction of leukemia cells to undetectable levels (i.e., from about 10^{12} to less than 10^8 to 10^9 leukemic cells remaining); restoration of bone marrow function, including normalization of hemoglobin, granulocytes, and platelets; resolution of hepatosplenomegaly; and return to a normal performance status (Gale & Foon, 1987).

Various drug regimens have been utilized in the treatment of AML. Table 36–9 lists the various multichemotherapy drug regimens (Devine & Larson, 1994). In general, most centers use cytarabine (100 to 200 mg/m^2/day) for 7 days by continuous infusion and 3 days of daunorubicin (Griffin et al., 1986). In patients younger than 60 years, daunorubicin doses range from 45 to 75 mg/m^2/day. In patients older than 60 years, lower doses of daunorubicin are sometimes given because of the toxicity at higher doses. Addition of other drugs to this regimen has not improved the results sufficiently to be statistically significant.

TABLE 36–8. *Cytogenetic Subsets in Acute Myeloid Leukemia*

KARYOTYPE	COMPLETE REMISSION RATE	REMISSION DURATION	TREATMENT APPROACH
t(8;21)	High	Long	Standard induction and consolidation with chemotherapy alone.
inv(16)(p13q22) or t(16;16), t(15;17)	High	Intermediate to long	Standard induction with an anthracycline. Intensive consolidation chemotherapy with high-dose cytarabine. Transretinoic acid prior to chemotherapy for t(15;17) to be tested.
t(9;11)	High	Short	Standard induction. Consider bone marrow transplantation in first remission for most t(9;11) patients.
del(5q), +13, +8, inv(3), del(12p)	Low	Short	New induction regimens, including use of growth factors during chemotherapy or modulators of drug resistance. Consider bone marrow transplantation in first complete remission.

(Adapted with permission from Bloomfield, C. D., Hoelzer, D. F., Schiffer, & C. A. [1991]. Acute leukemia: Recent advances in management. In American Society of Hematology, *Educational session booklet*. Denver, CO: American Society of Hematology 33rd Annual Meeting; from Devine, S. M., & Larson, R. A. [1994]. Acute leukemia in adults: Development in diagnosis and treatment. *Cancer, 44*[6], 326–352. Copyright © 1994 Wiley-Liss. Reprinted by permission of Wiley-Liss, a division of John Wiley and Sons, Inc.)

Investigation for more effective and potentially less toxic regimens have led to trials evaluating standard-dose ara-C to high-dose ara-C and the use of other potentially active drugs. The results from two randomized studies, one from the Australian Leukemia Study Group and one from the Southwest Oncology Group (SWOG), suggest that the use of high-dose ara-C (1 to 3 g/m² q 12 hours × 8 to 12 doses) in substitution of standard ara-C offered no benefit during induction for patients with newly diagnosed AML (Bishop et al., 1992).

An array of drugs including mitoxantrone, amsacrine, and idarubicin have been found to be active in relapsed or refractory leukemia. Randomized trials utilizing these drugs have demonstrated an equivalent CR rate when compared with standard induction drugs (Stone & Mayer, 1993).

Idarubicin is thought to be a potential substitute for daunomycin. Consequently, there are randomized trials evaluating the efficacy of idarubicin versus daunorubicin when administered in combination with ara-C (Berman et al., 1991; Vogler et al., 1992; Wiernik et al., 1992). These studies indicate that there is a trend that idarubicin may be more beneficial in obtaining a CR than daunorubicin, but more investigation needs to be accomplished before idarubicin becomes included in the standard therapy.

It is not unusual for patients to undergo two induction courses to obtain a remission. The drugs used at the second induction may be the same ones used during the first induction, or the regimen may be different. Once remission has been achieved, the goal becomes one of preventing relapse. If no further therapy is given, recurrence of leukemia occurs in a majority of

TABLE 36–9. *Remission-Induction Chemotherapy Regimens for Acute Myeloid Leukemia*

DRUGS	DOSE	COMMENT
1. Cytarabine	100 mg/m² daily as a continuous infusion for 7 days	"Standard" induction regimen resulting in about 60%–80% remission rate and acceptable toxicity in patients younger than 60 years.
Daunorubicin	45 mg/m² intravenous push on each of the first 3 days of treatment	
2. Cytarabine	3 g/m² twice daily for a total of 12 doses	Yields a 90% remission rate. However, substantial toxicity in patients older than 40 years precludes postremission therapy in a substantial proportion of patients.
Daunorubicin	45 mg/m² intravenous push for 3 days following cytarabine	
3. Cytarabine	100 mg/m² daily as a continuous infusion for 7 days	Has produced a greater remission rate (88% versus 70%) compared with cytarabine/daunorubicin in younger patients. Appears superior to daunorubicin in patients with hyperleukocytosis. Overall survival not clearly superior to "standard" regimen.
Idarubicin	13 mg/m² intravenous push on each of the first 3 days of treatment	
4. Cytarabine	100 mg/m² daily as a continuous infusion for 7 days	Remission rate similar to "standard" induction regimen. Remission duration significantly improved but overall survival comparable to "standard" regimen. May prolong survival in patients younger than 55 years but at expense of increased toxicity.
Daunorubicin	50 mg/m² intravenous push on each of first 3 days of treatment	
Etoposide	75 mg/m² daily as a continuous infusion for 7 days	

(From Devine, S., & Larson, R. [1994]. Acute leukemia in adults: Development in diagnosis and treatment. *Cancer, 44*[6], 326–352. Copyright © 1994 Wiley-Liss. Reprinted by permission of Wiley-Liss, a division of John Wiley and Sons, Inc.)

patients. It is believed that recurrence is related to the presence of residual leukemic cells that are undetectable by current methods. The approach to preventing relapse is to administer chemotherapy to the patient in remission (Gale & Foon, 1987).

Postremission Therapy. Various protocols have been employed in the chemotherapy of postremission AML. Gale and Foon (1987) reviewed these protocols, stating that most contained two to six additional cycles of ara-C and 6-thioguanine with or without daunomycin. They found that occasionally other drugs were used alone or in combination. These drugs included 5-azacytidine, amsacrine, methotrexate, prednisone, vincristine, cyclophosphamide (Cytoxan), doxorubicin (Adriamycin), and carmustine.

The investigation into finding the most effective postremission therapy has led to several protocols utilizing high-dose chemotherapy. CALGB trials evaluating patients in first remission were randomized to receive consolidation with four courses of high-dose ara-C (3 g/m^2/day for six doses) versus intermediate-dose ara-C (400 mg/m^2/day) versus standard-dose ara-C (100 mg/m^2/day) (Mayer et al., 1994). The results indicated that patients in the high-dose and intermediate-dose regimens who were under 40 years of age had significant longer remission and survival. For patients between 40 and 60 years of age, the high-dose regimen was superior. For patients older than 60, the three arms were equivalent.

Another regimen currently being investigated is high-dose Cytoxan (50 mg/kg) and VP-16 (3600 mg/m^2) without bone marrow transplant for high-risk and relapse leukemias. This regimen has produced about 30 per cent remission rates in patients who have relapsed after initial therapy (Brown et al., 1990). Studies are continuing to determine the role of this therapy for leukemia.

Because of the various reports, results, and uncontrolled data, most centers administer one to three cycles of chemotherapy to patients in remission. These chemotherapy regimens usually consist of the same drugs used to obtain remission or new drugs to prevent multidrug resistance. Once sustained remission has been accomplished, the question of continued chemotherapy in the form of maintenance therapy can be addressed.

The efficacy of maintenance therapy has been reviewed by Gale and Foon (1987). In general, studies have shown little or no benefit in continuing therapy 1 to 3 years after remission. Most centers currently do not utilize maintenance therapy in the treatment of AML.

Most patients relapse within 1 to 2 years. Remission can be achieved in 25 to 50 per cent of patients with resistant or recurrent leukemia. The drugs that have been utilized are summarized in Table 36–10 (Gale & Foon, 1987).

Although remission in resistant or relapsed leukemia may occur, the duration of remission is short. Remission of more than 1 year occurs in less than 10 per cent of responding patients (Gale & Foon, 1987). Given these small numbers, the use of BMT is often considered (see Chapter 27).

Before the advent of chemotherapy, the median survival for patients with AML was 3 months (Tivey, 1954). Within current drug regimens, remission occurs in 60 to 80 per cent of patients, and prolonged remission is 33 to 42 per cent several years after the diagnosis (Gale & Foon, 1987). The median duration of remission has been reported to be 9 to 16 months, with some reports of 20 to 40 per cent of patients in remission for 2 years or more (Gale & Foon, 1987).

Bone Marrow Transplantation. Bone marrow transplantation has been utilized in the treatment of AML. Several centers utilizing allogeneic transplants report continuous disease-free survival of 45 to 57 per cent at 2 to 5 years after transplantation (Santos, 1989). These figures have led some investigators to recommend that allogeneic BMT be the treatment of choice for patients under the age of 50 who have a suitable donor. This recommendation remains controversial, however, because in more recent trials with high-dose ara-C, intensive chemotherapy regimens have shown survival curves similar to allogeneic transplant. Studies continue to ascertain the role of BMT in patients in first remission.

Autologous BMT is currently being investigated at various centers. Initial results in studies of autologous transplant in first remission AML suggests that a long-term leukemia-free survival can be achieved for a select group of patients. The role of autologous transplant in first remission AML requires critical study before it can be routinely recommended (Ball & Ryloka, 1993). Autologous BMT in relapsed AML is generally recommended in patients who have good performance status and are under the age of 60 (Ball & Ryloka, 1993).

Clinical trials investigating the methods of marrow purging and the role of peripheral stem cells are provoking newer approaches (see also Chapters 26 and 27).

Nursing Care. Nursing care of patients with AML can be very challenging. The goal of therapy is to achieve remission. To accomplish this means that bone

TABLE 36–10. *Useful Drugs in Resistant Acute Myelogenous Leukemia**

Cytarabine + daunorubicin[†]
High-dose cytarabine + *L*-asparaginase
High-dose cytarabine + daunorubicin
High-dose cytarabine + amsacrine
Amsacrine ± other drugs
Mitoxantrone
Aclarubicin
Cytarabine analogues
Harringintonine
High-dose methotrexate + *L*-asparaginase
Epipodophyllotoxins
2,5-Piperazinedione
Zinostatin

---

*Drugs are ranked in estimated order of efficacy.
[†]In patients who are receiving limited therapy or who are off therapy for prolonged periods.
(From Gale, R. P., & Foon, K. A. [1987]. Therapy of acute myelogenous leukemia. *Seminars in Hematology, 24,* 40–54.)

marrow hypoplasia and pancytopenia will occur. Nursing care is critical during the recovery period of bone marrow after chemotherapy.

The newer regimens utilizing high-dose chemotherapy offer newer challenges for oncology nurses. With total white blood cell counts below 500 and platelet counts below 20,000, life-threatening infection and bleeding are common problems. Nursing assessment and intervention are critical components in the care of patients with these problems. Knowledge of the administration and side effects of chemotherapy agents, as well as the administration of blood components, is important for nursing intervention. Other chapters in this text address issues that will help prepare nurses to care for a patient with AML.

CHRONIC LYMPHOCYTIC LEUKEMIA

Overview. Chronic lymphocytic leukemia (CLL) is a hematologic malignancy characterized by proliferation and accumulation of relatively mature-looking but immunologically ineffective lymphocytes. It is the most common leukemia in Western countries, accounting for about 30 per cent of all leukemia cases (Gale & Foon, 1986). It is extremely rare in the Orient.

Chronic lymphocytic leukemia generally occurs in older individuals (median age is 60), although occasionally it can develop in young adults and even children. It occurs twice as often in males as in females.

Etiology and Pathologic Expression. The exact etiology of CLL is unknown, but various factors seem to be important. Unlike other hematologic malignancies, there is no increased incidence following exposure to alkylator therapy or radiation. Chronic lymphocytic leukemia has been the most common type of leukemia associated with familial leukemia (Rundles, 1982). Although CLL has a propensity to occur in closely related individuals, there is no definite pattern of inheritance. Extra chromosomes have been found in some CLL patients (most notably trisomy 12 in 30 per cent of CLL patients), but no chromosome abnormality has yet been identified as specific for CLL. Approximately 50 per cent of patients will have chromosomal abnormalities that remain unchanged through the disease course (Juliusson et al., 1990). Other specific chromosomal abnormalities that would be characteristic of CLL have *not* been found (Whang-Peng & Knutsen, 1980).

In CLL, the malignant transformation occurs most frequently in the B lymphocyte, with a small proportion occurring in T lymphocytes (Foon & Gale, 1987). In the United States, 95 per cent of the malignant transformation occurs in the B lymphocyte, while the T cell transformation predominates in Asia (Morrison, 1994). The most common immunoglobulin expressed in B cell CLL is IgM. These cells exhibit various B cell antigens such as CD19, CD20, CD21, CD23, and CD24 (International Workshop on Chronic Lymphocytic Leukemia, 1989). (The International Workshop on CLL defined the diagnostic criteria demonstrated in Table 36–11.) The malignant cells have a long life and a low proliferative capability and tend to be immunologically dysfunctional.

In general, patients' first symptoms of the disease are fatigue and reduced exercise tolerance, enlargement of superficial lymph nodes, or splenomegaly (Rundles, 1982). In many patients, the signs and symptoms have occurred gradually so that a specific date of onset is unknown. In about a quarter of the patients, the diagnosis is discovered by accident, in a routine examination, during which enlarged lymph nodes, splenomegaly, or abnormal blood counts are found (Morrison, 1994; Rundles, 1982).

Classification. Two types of staging systems have been utilized to describe CLL. The Rai system categorizes patients into five stages on the basis of the lymphocyte count and the presence or absence of lymphadenopathy, splenomegaly, hepatomegaly, anemia, and thrombocytopenia (Rai et al., 1975). Table 36–12 summarizes the Rai system. Stage 0 represents patients at low risk, stages I to II patients are at intermediate risk, and stages III and IV patients are considered to be at high risk.

The Binet system categorizes patients into three groups. Table 36–13 describes this schema (Binet et al., 1981). The prognosis for patients with stage A disease

---

TABLE 36–11. *Minimum Requirements for the Diagnosis of Chronic Lymphocytic Leukemia*

Absolute peripheral blood lymphocytosis with mature lymphocytes, which is sustained for ≥ 4 weeks, with no other identifiable cause:
  Absolute lymphocyte count > 10×10^9/L with either marrow involvement or a B cell phenotype
                          OR
  Absolute lymphocyte count > 5.0×10^9/L with both marrow involvement and a B cell phenotype
Hypercellular or normocellular bone marrow with ≥ 30% mature lymphocytes
Peripheral blood lymphocyte phenotype
  B cell lineage with expression of low-density surface immunoglobulin with either kappa or lambda light chain*
  CD5[+], CD2[–], CD3[–][†]
  Rosette formation with mouse red blood cells[‡]
Mature lymphocytes with < 55% atypical mature or immature lymphoid cells

*Normal peripheral blood lymphocytes express high-density surface immunoglobulin.
[†]A small number of CD5[+] B cells are normally present in lymph nodes and are increased following allogeneic bone marrow transplant, in patients with rheumatoid arthritis, and in fetal and early postnatal life.
[‡]A marker of mature B cells.
(From Morrison, V. A. [1994]. Chronic leukemias. *Cancer, 44*[6], 353–377. Copyright © 1994 Wiley-Liss. Reprinted by permission of Wiley-Liss, a division of John Wiley and Sons, Inc.)

TABLE 36–12. *Rai Clinical Staging System for Chronic Lymphocytic Leukemia*

STAGE	FINDINGS AT DIAGNOSIS
0	Lymphocytes in blood 15,000 × 100^9/L or higher, and 40% or more lymphocytes in marrow
I	Above plus enlarged lymph nodes
II	Above plus splenomegaly, hepatomegaly, or both
III	Above plus anemia (Hb < 11 g/dL)
IV	Above plus thrombocytopenia (platelets < 100,000/μl)

(Data from Rai, K. R., Sawitsky, A., Cronkite, E. P., Chanana, A., Levy, R. N., & Pasternak, B. S. [1975]. Clinical staging of chronic lymphocytic leukemia. *Blood, 46,* 219–234. Used with permission.)

equals that of the general population; for patients with stage B disease, median survival is approximately 7 years; and for patients with stage C disease, median survival is less than 2 years.

Other staging systems have been introduced in the literature, but most clinicians utilize either the Rai or the Binet system. The limitation of these staging systems is that they cannot predict for some patients in the low- and intermediate-risk groups (Binet's A and B and Rai's 0, I, and II) who will have an indolent course and good prognosis and those patients in the group whose disease is aggressive and progresses rapidly (Rai & Montserrat, 1987).

Natural History. During the early phase of CLL, no treatment is given. Patients are usually asymptomatic, but as time goes on, fatigue and reduced exercise tolerance may worsen. Lymph nodes gradually increase in size with new lymph nodes becoming involved. The spleen enlarges, and hepatomegaly may develop. Lymph tissue may grow in unusual areas, such as the scalp, orbit, subconjunctiva, pharynx, pleura, lung parenchyma, walls of the gastrointestinal tract, liver, prostate, and gonads. Obstructive jaundice can occur from periportal infiltration, and, very rarely, congestive heart failure can occur as a result of myocardial infiltration (Morrison, 1994; Rundles, 1982).

As the CLL becomes more aggressive and advanced, patients may experience severe fatigue; recurrent or persistent infection with fevers, pallor, edema, or thrombophlebitis from nodal obstruction; and increasing back tenderness and pain (Rundles, 1982).

The absolute lymphocyte count in CLL ranges from 10 to 150 × 10^3/μl, but counts up to 1000 × 10^3/μl can

occur in patients who are untreated. The abnormal lymphocytes in CLL are smaller than the lymphoblasts and myeloblasts of acute leukemia; therefore, the incidence of thrombotic and embolic complications is small (Rundles, 1982).

As the tumor burden of lymphoid tissue increases, the proportion of normal marrow precursors decreases until eventually only lymphocytes remain in the marrow (Rundles, 1982). It is not unusual for the differential white blood cell count of these patients to contain 90 to 100 per cent lymphocytes with only a few of the other types of white blood cells in the peripheral blood. As replacement of the marrow with lymphocytes occurs, granulocytopenia, thrombocytopenia, and anemia occur and can be mild to severe. Most patients will die of the complications related to pancytopenia.

Treatment. The treatment of CLL varies depending on the stage of disease. In general, no data suggest that treatment of patients with elevated leukocyte counts and lymphadenopathy prolongs survival. In one study, patients with stages I and II, or A, were given chlorambucil alone, chlorambucil with prednisone, or no treatment (Shapiro, Shustic, Anderson, & Sawitsky, 1984). No advantage in survival was shown in any group. In general, when patients experience organomegaly or cytopenias, treatment is then initiated (Table 36–14). Several treatment modalities have been utilized in the treatment of CLL.

Chemotherapy. The chemotherapy used in the treatment of CLL is either a single-agent or a multiagent regimen. The initial treatment for patients who require intervention is usually chlorambucil or cyclophosphamide with or without prednisone.

Chlorambucil is the most common drug. The usual dose is 0.1 to 0.2 mg/kg/day until the disease is controlled or toxicity is experienced; then the dose is reduced. Pulse therapy is given in a dose of 0.4 to 1.0 mg/kg once every 2 to 4 weeks. A response rate of 60 per cent is common using chlorambucil, with 10 to 20 per cent complete remission reported (Foon & Gale, 1987). Pulse therapy is utilized because it is reported to cause less hematologic toxicity (Knospe, Lolb, & Huguley, 1974).

Cyclophosphamide is reported to be as effective as chlorambucil (Huguley, 1977). It is often administered to patients who are unresponsive to chlorambucil. The usual dose is 2 to 3 mg/kg/day or 20 mg/kg every 2 to 3 weeks.

Corticosteroids are utilized to control the increase in leukocytic count and to treat the immune-mediated

TABLE 36–13. *Binet Staging System for Chronic Lymphocytic Leukemia*

STAGE	CLINICAL CHARACTERISTICS	PERCENT OF PATIENTS	MEDIAN SURVIVAL (YEARS)
A	Hemoglobin ≥ 10 g/dl, platelet count ≥ 100 × 10^9/L, and < 3 lymphoid sites involved*	60	> 9
B	Hemoglobin ≥ 10 g/dl, platelet count ≥ 100 × 10^9/L, and ≥ 3 lymphoid sites involved	30	5
C	Hemoglobin < 10 g/dl or platelet count < 100 × 10^9/L, or both	10	2

*Lymphoid sites include cervical (including Waldeyer's ring), axillary, and inguinal lymph nodes, spleen, and liver.
(From Morrison, V. A. [1994]. Chronic leukemias. *Cancer, 44*[6], 353–377. Copyright © 1994 Wiley-Liss. Reprinted by permission of Wiley-Liss, a division of John Wiley and Sons, Inc.)

TABLE 36-14. *Indications for Initiation of Therapy for Patients with Chronic Lymphocytic Leukemia*

Progressive systemic symptoms (fever, night sweats, weight loss)

Progressive bone marrow failure (anemia, thrombocytopenia)

Autoimmune thrombocytopenia, granulocytopenia, or hemolytic anemia

Massive splenomegaly

Bulky lymphoid disease

Progressive leukocytosis

Increased frequency of bacterial, fungal, and viral infections

---

(From Morrison, V. A. [1994]. Chronic leukemias. *Cancer, 44*[6], 353–377. Copyright © 1994 Wiley-Liss. Reprinted by permission of Wiley-Liss, a division of John Wiley and Sons, Inc.)

hemolytic anemia and thrombocytopenia (Livingston & Carter, 1970). Prednisone is given as 20 to 60 mg/m² body surface area. Corticosteroids are not prescribed alone in the treatment of CLL.

In patients with advanced disease, combination chemotherapy with cyclophosphamide (Cytoxan), vincristine, and prednisone (CVP) has been used, as has cyclophosphamide, hydroxydaunorubicin (Adriamycin), vincristine (Oncovin), and prednisone (CHOP) (Huguley, 1977; Livingston & Carter, 1970). In reported data, the response rate and time to progression and survival were similar between CVP or CHOP and chlorambucil (French Cooperative Group on Chronic Lymphocytic Leukemia, 1990; Chevret et al., 1992).

Several new drug therapies have been investigated in the therapy of relapsed CLL. Fludarabine 25 mg/m²/day for 5 days every 4 weeks has resulted in response rates of up to 60 per cent in previously treated patients with a median duration of remission of 21 months (Keating et al., 1989). In current trials, fludarabine is being evaluated in combination with other standard chemotherapy agents (Binet et al., 1993). Thus, fludarabine is a choice for treatment for previously treated patients, but its role of first-line therapy is yet to be evaluated.

Another drug that has shown antilymphocytic activity is 2-chlorodeoxyadenosine (2-CdA). This drug has been given as a monthly infusion of 0.1 mg/kg/day for 7 days by continuous infusion (Piro, Carrera, Beutler, & Carson, 1988). Response rates of up to 55 per cent in patients with relapsed or refractory disease have been reported. The use of this drug in combination with chlorambucil and its use in fludarabine-resistant patients is being investigated.

Pentostatin (2'-deoxycoformycin) has shown activity in controlling lymphoid malignancies, including CLL. Initial studies utilizing this drug identified considerable toxicities, although current studies testing pentostatin at low-dose levels indicate toxicities have been reduced (Grever et al., 1985).

In summary, patients who develop organomegaly or cytopenia are initially treated with single-agent chemotherapy. As the disease progresses, multiagent chemotherapy is utilized to control the disease. Investigations continue to find drugs that are more effective in the treatment of CLL.

Biologic Response Modifiers. The role of monoclonal antibodies is being investigated in the treatment of CLL. Treatment with T-101 monoclonal antibody, anti-CD5 monoclonal antibody, or a similar antibody has shown some activity or response in patients with CLL, but these studies are in the early phases of investigation (Clendeninn et al., 1993; Foon et al., 1983).

Another approach utilizing monoclonal antibodies is the development of antiidiotype monoclonal antibodies. These antibodies are "tailor-made" specifically for an individual patient's tumor cells (Foon & Gale, 1986). CAMPATH-1H, an antibody directed against a lymphocyte antigen, is in phase I and II clinical trials (Clendeninn et al., 1993).

Interferon, another biologic response modifier, has been studied in patients with CLL (Figlin, 1989; Foon et al., 1985). Although reported responses from the initial trials have been low in numbers, interferon's activity in combination with alkylating agents and as maintenance therapy continues to be investigated in patients with CLL (Figlin, 1989).

Splenectomy. The benefits of splenectomy in patients with CLL have been debated over the years. Today splenectomy is used in selected patients with hemolytic anemia, thrombocytopenia, pancytopenia, and painful splenomegaly (Foon & Gale, 1986). Only in these unusual cases is splenectomy recommended.

Radiotherapy. The primary role of radiation therapy in CLL is one of palliation and symptom control. Radiation therapy is generally used to treat enlarged lymph nodes, painful bony lesions, or massive splenomegaly that is resistant to chemotherapy (Rundles, 1982). Splenic radiation has also been utilized to treat painful splenomegaly, progressive lymphocytosis, anemia, and thrombocytopenia (Byhardti, Brace, & Wiernic, 1975).

Leukapheresis. When the number of circulating white blood cells is great enough to produce vascular thrombosis or embolism in patients who are unresponsive to chemotherapy, removal of the lymphocytes by pheresis has been utilized (Curtis, Hersh, & Freirich, 1972). Leukapheresis does not treat the disease and, therefore, when discontinued, the problem of increasing white blood cells continues. Routine use of leukapheresis is probably not justified but in selected patients may be beneficial for a period of time.

Systemic Complications of CLL. Table 36-15 identifies the complications experienced by patients who have CLL (Henderson & Han, 1986). These complications usually occur as the disease advances and becomes refractory to therapy.

Nursing Care. Nursing care of patients with CLL begins with the initial diagnosis. Patient and family education about the disease and its treatment is an important area in which nurses can intervene. Questions and issues related to treatment versus no treatment will have to be clarified for patients. Nurses can assist the medical team in identifying and clarifying questions.

TABLE 36–15. *Systemic Complications in Chronic Lymphocytic Leukemia and Their Management*

CONDITION	MANAGEMENT
Hypogammaglobuline-mia and recurrent infections	Gammaglobulin (intramuscularly) Gammaglobulin (intravenously) Appropriate antibiotics
Immune-mediated ane-mia; thrombocytope-nia and neutropenia	Prednisone Immunosuppressive agents Splenectomy Gammaglobulin (intravenously)
Hyperviscosity syn-drome (rare)	Plasmapheresis Prednisone Chemotherapy
Hyperuricemia (rare)	Hydration Allopurinol
Hypercalcemia (very rare)	Hydration Diuretics Prednisone Calcitonin

(Data from Henderson, E. S., & Han, T. [1986]. Current therapy of acute and chronic leukemia in adults. *CA: A Cancer Journal for Clinicians, 36*, 322–350.)

As the disease progresses, education related to the treatment and the side effects of treatment must be undertaken with patients and families. As patients experience the symptoms of the disease and the complications associated with CLL, nursing care becomes an integral part of the treatment.

Bone marrow replacement with ineffective lymphocytes results in neutropenia, thrombocytopenia, and anemia. Chapter 53 provides nursing interventions for these problems.

Infiltration of bone and other organs with lymphocytes will cause the patient pain. Chapters 57 and 58 discuss comfort measures nurses can provide.

Hemolytic anemia associated with CLL requires the nurse to have expertise in blood component therapy. Patient education and support are important, because some patients may require weekly transfusions. Other complications associated with CLL—hyperviscosity syndrome, hyperuricemia, and hypercalcemia—although uncommon, are challenging to the nursing and medical team.

Patients with CLL can live long lives. As the disease progresses, quality of life issues become important. Toward the end of their lives, many patients spend increasing time in hospitals with recurrent infections and bleeding and are dependent on blood transfusions. Emotional support of patients and families during times of crisis are important in nursing care.

CHRONIC MYELOGENOUS LEUKEMIA

Overview. Chronic myelogenous leukemia (CML) accounts for approximately 20 to 30 per cent of the adult leukemias. It is a relatively rare disease in children. The peak incidence of CML has been in the fourth decade of life but has been found to be shifting to a later age. This leukemia occurs more frequently in men than in women (Rundles, 1982).

Etiology. Exposure to radiation has been implicated in the development of CML. The exposure of the Japanese in Hiroshima and Nagasaki during the atomic bomb explosions demonstrated the leukopenic effects of single-dose radiation (Cronkite et al., 1960). After a 3-year latency period, the yearly incidence of leukemia in survivors gradually increased to its maximum by 7 years and then began to fall. Yet at 14 years, the rate still exceeded the national average for incidence of CML in the general population. The most common leukemias among the survivors were CML and AML (Heysel et al., 1960). Other evidence associating radiation exposures with development of CML was demonstrated in patients with ankylosing spondylitis who were treated with radiotherapy in Great Britain (Graham, 1960).

Although radiation exposure can be an etiologic factor, very few patients with CML are exposed to unusual amounts of radiation. Approximately one person in 15 or 20 who develops the disease has had unusual exposure to any form of radiation or chemicals (Rundles, 1982). Any chemical capable of damaging hematopoietic stem cells is potentially leukopenic, although identification of causative agents can be difficult. The chemical that has clearly been identified as one that increased the incidence of myelogenous leukemia in humans is benzene associated with heavy occupational exposure (Vigliani & Sart, 1964).

In most cases, the etiology of CML is unknown. Nurses can educate as well as allay the fears of patients who look for something that they may have done to cause this disease.

Biologic Manifestations. Chronic myelogenous leukemia is a hematologic malignancy that results from the development of an abnormal hematopoietic stem cell that gives rise to offspring that have the Philadelphia chromosome (Rundles, 1982). With the development of cytogenetic studies and the enzyme marker G-6-PD (glucose-6-phosphate dehydrogenase), it has been established that CML is a clonal disorder resulting from the malignant transformation of a pluripotent hematopoietic stem cell (Rapaport, 1987).

The chromosome abnormality, found in 90 to 95 per cent of patients, is thought to be a key element in the steps of the malignant transformation. These chromosomal rearrangements are associated with translocation and activation of cellular oncogenes (Champlin, 1986). The presence of the BCR-ABL fusion gene has been identified as playing a role in the transformation of the malignant cell (Morrison, 1994).

The transformed malignant stem cell in CML shows a marked increase in proliferation of marrow granulocytic and occasionally megakaryocytic progenitor and precursor cells (Rundles, 1982). The marrow cells with increased proliferation seem to have a growth advantage and to overproduce in the marrow itself, replacing normal myeloid cells and expanding into the peripheral blood. Thus, large numbers of immature and mature granulocytic cells accumulate in the blood. With further expansion into the peripheral blood, the malignant cells proliferate in the spleen, replacing the normal lymphoid elements of that organ, and accumulate in the sinusoids of the liver (Rapaport, 1987). This extramedullary proliferation results in enlargement of both the spleen and the liver. It is believed that the increase in myeloid production is not due to an accelerated proliferation of cells but to a massive expansion in the cells that are committed to myeloid production.

Diagnosis. The diagnosis of CML is based on sustained granulocytosis, which is usually associated with splenomegaly, a low leukocyte alkaline phosphatase (LAP score), and the presence of the Ph^1 chromosome. Myeloid cells at all stages of differentiation are found in the peripheral blood, and they appear to be normal in morphology. Platelet counts are usually normal or slightly depressed. A bone marrow aspiration is obtained for cytogenic studies to confirm the presence of the Ph^1 chromosome (Champlin, 1986), or the BCL-ABL fusion gene (Morrison, 1994). Chemical abnormalities associated with CML include hyperuricemia, low LAP score, increase in vitamin B_{12} levels, increase in lactate dehydrogenase, and increase in K^+ (Rundles, 1982).

Clinical Phases. Chronic myelogenous leukemia is characterized by three phases: chronic, accelerated, and acute or blastic phase. During the chronic phase, there is an overproduction of relatively normal granulocytes that respond to treatment. At diagnosis, patients will experience malaise, fatigue, lack of exercise tolerance, and weight loss (Rundles, 1982). Splenomegaly is common, and there are 20 per cent or less immature myeloid cells in the peripheral blood and 30 per cent or less in the bone marrow. As the disease progresses, aching in the bones that contain red blood cell marrow is present, as well as tenderness in the lower half of the sternum, and discomfort and fullness in the upper abdomen, indicating hepatosplenomegaly.

The symptoms usually subside with treatment, and patients may be asymptomatic during these periods for from 1 to 4 years. After this period, the signs and symptoms gradually become worse and less responsive to treatment.

The accelerated phase is characterized by progressive symptoms and resistance to chemotherapy. Systemic symptoms (fever, night sweats, weight loss), increasing hepatosplenomegaly, lymphadenopathy, and extramedullary leukemia are common manifestations (Champlin, 1986). The blood counts that were so responsive to therapy during the chronic phase now become unresponsive.

The acute phase or blastic phase is highlighted by a significant increase in the blast count and further progression of anemia, thrombocytopenia, or myelofibrosis (Champlin, 1986). Extramedullary leukemia with tumors or diffuse infiltration involving skin, mucous membranes, lymph nodes, orbit, pleurisy, synovia, extradural tissues, peripheral nerves, and meninges occurs in approximately 40 per cent of patients. Most patients will develop the acute or blast crisis phase in which the disease now resembles acute leukemia (Keating et al., 1989). Approximately 5 to 10 per cent of patients move from a chronic phase, in which the disease seems to be controlled, to a sudden acute or blast crisis phase (Canellos, 1990; Rundles, 1982).

During this phase, the manifestations of CML resemble those of acute leukemia. The cells no longer differentiate to mature granulocytes, and maturation arrest occurs at the blast or promyelocyte stage of maturation. The blast crisis generally occurs in one of two forms: myeloid and lymphoid. Approximately 60 per cent of patients will develop a myeloblastic acute leukemia, 20 per cent will develop a lymphoblastic leukemia, 15 per cent will develop an undifferentiated acute leukemia, and the remaining 5 per cent will have abnormalities in megakaryocytes, erythroid, or progranulocytic cell lines (Morrison, 1994). To determine the appropriate treatment, it is important to determine whether the blast crisis is of lymphoid or myeloid origin.

Treatment. The purpose of treating CML is to control the white blood cell count and to relieve symptoms. The growth of malignant cells is controlled by chemotherapeutic agents, the two most common being busulfan and hydroxyurea. Busulfan is given in pulses for several weeks and then is discontinued after white blood cell counts return to normal. The usual dosage is 1 to 4 mg/day until normal results are achieved. During the busulfan treatment, peripheral blood counts must be monitored to prevent life-threatening pancytopenia. After prolonged use of busulfan, pulmonary fibrosis, skin pigmentation, hypogonadism, or a muscle-wasting syndrome with features of Addison's disease may develop (Haut, Abbott, Wintrobe, & Cartwright, 1961; Morrison, 1994).

Hydroxyurea, which must be given daily, is another commonly used drug that effectively suppresses myelopoiesis. It provides more erratic control of the leukemia and requires monitoring of blood counts every week. The most common dosage is 500 mg to 2 g/day (Kennedy, 1972).

The chemotherapy drugs control the growth of the malignant cells but do not eradicate the disease. Patients who achieve normal white blood cell counts continue to have Ph^1 chromosome-positive cells in their bone marrow (Champlin, 1986). Chemotherapy relieves the symptoms of the disease, but no single drug has been shown to delay the development of a blast crisis or to prolong survival.

Combination chemotherapy has been attempted in patients with CML. It has resulted in significant toxicity and has provided no convincing evidence that the duration of the chronic phase is prolonged or that the probability of survival is improved (Cunningham et al., 1979).

Interferon is beginning to be evaluated for the treatment of CML and to be shown to have a direct antiproliferative effect on the malignant clone. In initial studies, interferon has been effective in controlling granulocytosis and thrombocytosis in CML (Talpaz, 1987). Interferon α-2a 5×10^6 U/m²/day resulted in a response rate of 55 to 75 per cent with a median time to response of 3.4 months (Ozer, 1988). The duration of complete hematologic response is reported up to 41 months. Longer follow-up in patients treated with interferon is needed to determine duration of remissions and the effect on overall survival. The effectiveness of interferon with other agents will need further study to determine its role in the treatment of CML (Ozer et al., 1992).

Splenectomy has been suggested as a potential treatment of CML. In general, splenectomy has not proved to be beneficial in prolonging the chronic phase or the patient's survival (Italian Cooperative Group on Chronic Myeloid Leukemia, 1984). In patients with painful splenomegaly, anemia produced by hypersplenism, or severe thrombocytopenia, splenectomy may be considered. The decision to do a splenectomy in a patient with CML is difficult to make because of the complications from the operation and the propensity of these patients to develop extreme thrombocytosis after the operation (Champlin, 1986).

The prognosis for patients in the acute phase is poor. Once patients have entered the acute phase, survival without treatment may be limited to 2 to 6 months.

Patients who present with the acute lymphocytic leukemia-type crisis are treated with ALL standard therapy: vincristine and prednisone. At least one half of these patients will respond to this therapy with complete remission that can last from 2 to 18 months, utilizing aggressive induction or cyclic reinduction therapy (Janossy et al., 1979; Morrison, 1994).

Patients who present with the acute myelogenous leukemia-type crisis do not respond to vincristine and prednisone, nor do they respond to the type of therapy utilized for acute myelogenous leukemia. Only 20 to 30 per cent achieve a remission with this intensive chemotherapy, and their remissions are brief (Cunningham et al., 1979; Morrison, 1994).

Bone Marrow Transplantation. In the past several years, bone marrow transplantation (BMT) has been utilized to treat CML. Approximately 65 per cent of patients in the chronic phase who received syngeneic transplants and 20 per cent who were treated in blast crisis have achieved complete remission (Champlin, 1986). Allogeneic transplantation has yielded a complete remission rate of 63 per cent in the chronic phase and 12 per cent in the acute phase (Champlin, 1986). The 5-year disease-free survival is 50 to 60 per cent for patients transplanted in chronic phase, 30 per cent for patients transplanted in accelerated phase, and 10 to 20 per cent for patients transplanted in acute phase (Thomas et al., 1986). Younger patients tolerate this procedure better than do older patients. Most centers do not perform transplant operations on patients older than 50 years. Autologous BMT is being evaluated in CML with the best results in patients transplanted in the chronic phase (McGlave et al., 1990). The role of autologous BMT and the treatment of marrow ex vivo is under continued study.

Nursing Care. Nursing care of patients with CML revolves around the education and treatment of patients and family members. During the chronic phase, educating the patient and family about the dis-

ease, the initial treatment, and the role of BMT is important. As the disease progresses and as patients develop more symptoms, nursing care will address alteration in protective mechanisms, nutritional status, and comfort and other areas, depending on the manifestations of disease progression (see Unit VIII).

HAIRY CELL LEUKEMIA

Overview. Hairy cell leukemia is described as a lymphoproliferative disease similar to CLL (Golde & Koeffler, 1985). It is usually seen in patients older than 30 years of age, with the median age in the early 50s. The ratio of males to females is 5:1. It represents 2 per cent of all leukemias (Cawley, Burns, & Hayhoe, 1980).

Etiology. The etiology of hairy cell leukemia is unknown. Little information is available on environmental factors associated with this disease, although rare cases are associated with human T cell lymphotropic virus II infection (Jacobs, 1986; Foon & Gale, 1987).

Clinical Features. Hairy cell leukemia is considered primarily a B lymphocyte disorder. The term *hairy* describes the projections on the abnormal lymphocyte that are characteristic of the disease (Golde & Koeffler, 1985). Hairy cells must be present in the bone marrow for the diagnosis. Approximately 50 per cent of a patient's bone marrow cannot be aspirated. Other sites involved include the liver, spleen, and lymph nodes.

Patients may be asymptomatic, but they usually present with symptoms caused by splenomegaly, pancytopenia, or infection (Golomb, Catovsky, & Golde, 1978). Splenomegaly is present in 80 to 90 per cent of patients, whereas the presence of lymphadenopathy is unusual (Golde & Koeffler, 1985; Golomb et al., 1978). Weight loss, fever, and night sweats are not common (Bennett, Vardiman, & Golomb, 1986). Patients may experience moderate to severe pancytopenia (Golde & Koeffler, 1985). Stages of hairy cell leukemia are listed in Table 36–16.

TABLE 36–16. *Clinical Staging for Hairy Cell Leukemia*

STAGE	HEMOGLOBIN (G/DL)	SPLEEN SIZE*
I	> 12.0 or	≤ 10
	> 8.5	< 4
II	> 12.0 or	> 10
	8.5–12.0 or	4–10
	< 8.5	< 4
III	8.5–12.0 or	> 10
	< 8.5	≥ 4

*Related to centimeters from upper costal margin.
(From Morrison, V. A. [1994]. Chronic leukemias. *Cancer, 44*[6], 353–377. Copyright © 1994 Wiley-Liss. Reprinted by permission of Wiley-Liss, a division of John Wiley and Sons, Inc.)

Splenectomy Treatment. When patients become symptomatic, treatment for hairy cell leukemia is initiated. Splenectomy is usually the first treatment. The cytopenias related to the splenic sequestration are improved by splenectomy, although not completely in most cases. Splenectomy is usually beneficial to all patients, but approximately half will require further therapy at a later date (Golomb & Vardiman, 1978).

Chemotherapy. Hairy cell leukemia progresses in two different forms. One, in which the bone marrow is replaced by hairy cells, causes pancytopenia. In the other, the disease appears with an increasing white blood cell count and resembles a leukemia (Golomb et al., 1978). Usually chemotherapy is required for both forms of disease.

Various drug regimens have been utilized with varying effects: chlorambucil as a single agent, and multi-agent regimens that contained rubidazone, ara-C, cyclophosphamide, and high-dose methotrexate and leucovorin rescue have been used (Golomb et al., 1978).

Studies of 2′-deoxycoformycin (Pentostatin) have shown that complete bone marrow remission can be achieved and may be long-lasting (Urba et al., 1989). A complete response has been reported in 60 to 90 per cent of patients. The average duration of therapy is 6 months with treatment continued for one to two cycles after a complete response is documented (Spiers et al., 1987). The most frequently used regimens are 5 mg/m^2/day for 3 days each month; 5 mg/m^2/day for 2 days every 2 weeks; 4 mg/m^2/week for 3 weeks every 8 weeks; or 4 mg/m^2/day every 2 weeks (Spiers et al., 1987). The major toxicities are fever and infection in 15 to 40 per cent of patients. Other side effects include nausea, vomiting, diarrhea, lethargy, conjunctivitis, and hepatitis (Morrison, 1994).

2-Chlorodeoxyadenosine (2-CdA) is a new lymphocyte-selective, antineoplastic drug that has been approved by the Food and Drug Administration for the treatment of hairy cell leukemia. A study by Piro, Carrera, Carson, and Beutler (1990) indicates that 2-CdA has become an effective therapy for hairy cell leukemia. In 12 patients treated with 2-CdA, 11 patients obtained complete remission, the longest remission being 3.8 years. The reported complete response rate of 2-CdA is 78 to 92 per cent with a prolonged duration (Estey et al., 1992). Common dose schedules are 0.1 mg/kg/day for 7 days by continuous infusion or 4 mg/m^2/day for 7 days by continuous infusion. Most patients require only one or two cycles of therapy. Studies are ongoing to develop routes and schedules of administration.

In the past, the treatment of choice had been the interferons, however, 2-CdA now has become the most effective therapy. Interferon has shown high response rates in large numbers of patients. The length of response to the interferons is now being investigated. Approximately 80 per cent of patients treated with interferon-α achieve beneficial clinical responses, but there are few complete responders (< 10 per cent) (Figlin, 1989).

Radiation Therapy. Radiation therapy provides symptomatic relief of bone pain. In hairy cell leukemia, bone involvement can occur that causes lytic bone lesions in rare cases (Jacobs, 1986; Lembersky, Ratain, & Golomb, 1988). Bilateral hip joint involvement with pain and necrosis of the joint is the most common symptom (Jacobs, 1986). Radiation therapy to local areas of involvement can provide symptomatic relief of pain and radiographic changes of lytic bone lesions.

Nursing Care. Some patients with hairy cell leukemia have a very indolent course with little nursing intervention required. Others require nursing care similar to that performed for CLL, depending on presenting symptoms. Infection is a major cause of death; therefore, alteration in protective mechanisms is an important problem. Alteration in comfort because of splenomegaly or bone lesions will be another area for nursing interventions. As pancytopenia develops, nursing skills related to blood component therapy and administration of chemotherapeutic agents will be necessary. Therapy administration requires patient instruction on delivery as well as side effects to be expected. As with the other leukemias, nursing care will be an integral part of the team approach.

REFERENCES

Amadori, S., Meloni, G., Baccarini, M., Haanen, C., Willemze, R., Corbelli, G., Drenthe-Schonk, A., Lopes Cardozo, P., Tura, S., & Mandelli, F. (1983). Long-term survival in adolescent and adult lymphoblastic leukemia. *Cancer, 52,* 30–34.

Arlin, Z., Feldman, E., Ahmed, T., Cook, P., Mittleman, A., Puccio, C., Chun, H., Helson, L., & Baskind. (1991). After 25 years with vincristine/prednisone (V/P) have we found a better induction therapy for acute lymphoblastic leukemia (ALL)? *Blood, 78*(Suppl. 1), 447a.

Ball, E. D., Davis, R. B., Griffin, J. D., Mayer, R. J., Davey, F. R., Arthur, D. C., Wurster-Hill, D., Noll, W., Allen, S. L., & Elghetany, M. T. (1991). Prognostic value of lymphocyte surface markers in acute myeloid leukemia. *Blood, 77,* 2242–2250.

Ball, E. D., Ryloka, W. B. (1993). Autologous bone marrow transplantation for adult acute leukemia. *Hematology/Oncology Clinics of North America, 7*(1), 201–231.

Bennett, J. M., Catovsky, D., Daniel, M., et al. (1976). Proposals for the classification of the acute leukemias. *British Journal of Haematology, 33,* 451.

Bennett, J. M., Catovsky, D., Daniel, M. T., Flandrin, G., Galton, D. A., Gralniek, H. R., & Sultan, C. (1991). Proposal for the recognition of minimally differentiated acute myeloid leukemia (AML-M$_0$). *British Journal of Haematology, 78,* 325–329.

Bennett, C., Vardiman, J., & Golomb, H. (1986). Disseminated atypical myobacterial infection in patients with hairy cell leukemia. *American Journal of Medicine, 80,* 891–896.

Berenson, J., Zigelboim, J., & Gale, R. (1985). Acute lymphoblastic leukemia. In C. Haskell (Ed.), *Cancer treatment* (2nd ed., pp. 706–721). Philadelphia: W. B. Saunders Co.

Berman, E., Hudis, C., Offit, K., Jhanwar, S., Chaganti, R. S., Wong, G., Weiss, M., Gee, T., Bertino, J., & Clarkson, B. (1991). Therapy of adult acute lymphocytic leukemia (ALL). *Haematologica, 76*(Suppl. 45), 106.

Binet, J. L., Auquier, A., Dighiero, G., Chastang, C., Piguet, H., Goasguen, J., Vaugier, G., Potron, G., Colona, P., Oberling, E., Thomas, M., Tchernia, G., Jacquillat, C.,

Boivin, P., Lesty, C., Duault, M. T., Monconduit, M., Belabbes, S., & Gremy, F. (1981). A new prognostic classification of chronic lymphocytic leukemia derived from multivariable survival analyses. *Cancer, 48,* 198–206.

Binet, J. L., Chastang, C., Chevret, S., Dighiero, G., Maloum, K., Travade, P., & the French Cooperative Group on CLL. (1993). Comparison of fludarabine (FDB), CAP, and CHOP in advanced previously untreated chronic lymphocytic leukemia (CLL). Preliminary results of a randomized clinical trial [Abstract]. *Blood, 82*(Suppl. 1), 223.

Bishop, J. F., Young, G. A., Szer, J., Matthews, J. P., & the Australian Leukemia Study Group. (1992). Randomized trial of high-dose cytosine arabinoside (ara-C) combination in induction of acute myeloid leukemia (AML). *Proceedings of the American Society of Clinical Oncologists, 11,* 260.

Blayney, D. W., Jaffe, E. S., Blattner, W. A., Cossman, J., Robert-Guroff, M., Longo, D. L., Bunn, P. A., Jr., & Gallo, R. C. (1983). The human T-cell leukemia/lymphoma virus associated with American adult T-cell leukemia/lymphoma. *Blood 62,* 401–405.

Bloomfield, C. D., Hoelzer, D. F., & Schiffer, C. A. (1991). Acute leukemia: Recent advances in management. In American Society of Hematology, *Educational session booklet.* American Society of Hematology 33rd Annual Meeting, Denver, CO.

Bloomfield, C. D., Rowley, J. D., Goldman, A. I., Lawler, S. D., Walker, L. M., & Mitelman, F. (1983). For the third international workshop on chromosomal abnormalities and their clinical significance in acute lymphoblastic leukemia. *Cancer Research, 43,* 868–873.

Borjum, A. (1968). Separation of leukocytes from blood and bone marrow. *Scandinavian Journal of Clinical and Laboratory Investigation, 21*(Suppl. 97), 77–89.

Brown, R. A., Herzig, S. N., Wolff, D., Frei-Lalr, L., Piniero, L., Bolwell, B. S., Lowder, J. N., Harden, E. A., Hande, K. R., & Herzig, G. P. (1990). High-dose etoposide and cyclophosphamide without bone marrow transplantation for resistant hematologic malignancy. *Blood, 76*(3), 437–479.

Byhardti, R. W., Brace, W. C., & Wiernic, P. H. (1975). The role of splenic irradiation in chronic lymphocytic leukemia. *Cancer, 35,* 1621–1625.

Canellos, G. P. (1990). Clinical characteristics of the blast phase of chronic granulocytic leukemia. *Hematology/Oncology Clinics of North America, 4,* 359–367.

Cawley, J. C., Burns, G. F., & Hayhoe, F. G. J. (1980). *Hairy cell leukaemia* (p. 1080). Berlin: Springer-Verlag.

Champlin, R. E. (1986). Chronic myelogenous leukemia in leukemia therapy. In R. P. Gale (Ed.), *Leukemia therapy* (p. 148). Boston: Blackwell Scientific Publications.

Champlin, R. E., & Gale, R. P. (1987). Bone marrow transplantation for acute leukemia: Recent advances and comparison with alternative therapies. *Seminars in Hematology, 24,* 55–67.

Chevret, S., Trevade, P., Chastang, C., Fenaux, P., Dighiero, G., Binet, J. L., & the French Cooperative Group on CLL. (1992). The CHOP polychemotherapy in stage B chronic lymphocytic leukemia (CLL): Interim results of a controlled clinical trial on 287 patients [Abstract]. *Proceedings of the American Society of Clinical Oncologists, 11,* 267.

Christiansen, N. P. (1993). Allogeneic bone marrow transplantation for the treatment of adult acute leukemia. *Hematology/Oncology Clinics of North America, 7*(1), 177–200.

Clarkson, B., Gaynor, J., Little, C., Berman, E., Kempin, S., Andreeff, M., Gulati, S., Cunningham, I., & Gee, T. (1990). Importance of long-term follow-up in evaluating treatment regimens for adults with acute lymphoblastic leukemia. *Haematology and Blood Transfusions, 33,* 397–408.

Clendeninn, N. J., Nethersell, A. B. W., Scott, J. E., & Offenhauser, K. O. (1993). Early safety and efficacy results using CAMPATH™-1H (CP-1H), a humanized antilymphocytic monoclonal antibody (MAB) in non-Hodgkin's lymphoma and chronic lymphocytic leukemia (CLL) [Abstract]. *Proceedings of the American Society of Clinical Oncologists, 12,* 378.

Cronkite, E. P., Maloney, W. C., & Bond, V. P. (1960). Radiation leukogenesis: An analysis of the problem. *American Journal of Medicine, 28,* 673.

Cunningham, I., Gee, T., Dowling, M., Chaganti, R., Bailey, R., Hopfan, S., Bowden, L., Turnbull, A., Knapper, W., & Clarkson, B. (1979). Results of treatment of Ph^I + chronic myelogenous leukemia with an intensive treatment regimen (L-5 protocol). *Blood, 53,* 375–393.

Curtis, J. E., Hersh, E. M., & Freirich, E. M. (1972). Leukopheresis therapy of chronic lymphocytic leukemia. *Blood, 39,* 163.

Devine, S. M., & Larson, R. A. (1994). Acute leukemia in adults: Recent developments in diagnosis and treatment. *CA: A Cancer Journal for Clinicians, 44*(6), 326–352.

Ellison, R. R., Mick, R., Cuttner, J., Schiffer, C. A., Silver, R. T., Henderson, E. S., Woliver, T., Royston, I., Davey, F. R., Glicksman, A. S., Bloomfield, C. D., & Holland, J. F. (1991). The effects of postinduction intensification treatment with cytarabine and daunorubicin in adult acute lymphocytic leukemia: A prospective randomized clinical trial by Cancer and Leukemia Group B. *Journal of Clinical Oncology, 9,* 2002–2015.

Estey, E. H., Kurzrock, R., Kantarjian, H. M., O'Brien, S. M., McCredie, K. B., Beran, M., Koller, C., Keating, M. J., Hirsch-Ginsberg, C., Huh, Y. O., Stass, S., & Freireich, E. J. (1992). Treatment of hairy cell leukemia with 2-chlorodeoxyadenosine (2-CdA). *Blood, 79,* 882–887.

Fiére, D., Gisselbrecht, C., Witz, F., & Maupas, J. (1990). Comparison of chemotherapy, autologous and allogeneic transplantation as postinduction regimen in adult acute lymphoblastic leukemia: A preliminary multicenter study. In R. P. Gale & D. Hoelzer (Eds.), *Acute lymphoblastic leukemia* (pp. 285–292). New York: Alan R. Liss.

Figlin, R. A. (1989). Biotherapy in clinical practice. *Seminars in Hematology, 26*(3, Suppl. 3), 15–24.

Foon, K. A., Bottina, G. D., Abrams, P. G., Fer, M. F., Longo, D. L., Schoenberger, C. S., & Oldham, R. K. (1985). A phase II trial of recombinant leukocyte α-interferon for patients with advanced chronic lymphocytic leukemia. *American Journal of Medicine, 78,* 216–220.

Foon, K. A., & Gale, R. P. (1987). Staging and therapy of chronic lymphocytic leukemia. *Seminars in Hematology, 24,* 264–274.

Foon, K. A., & Gale, R. P. (1986). Chronic lymphocytic leukemia. In R. P. Gale (Ed.), *Leukemia therapy* (p. 165). Boston: Blackwell Scientific Publications.

Foon, K. A., Schroff, R. W., Mayer, D., Sherwin, S. A., Oldham, R. K., Bunn, P. A., & Hsu, S. (1983). Monoclonal antibody therapy of chronic lymphocytic leukemia and cutaneous T-cell lymphoma: Preliminary observations. In B. E. Boss, R. E. Langman, I. S. Trowbridge, & R. Dulbecco (Eds.), *Monoclonal antibodies and cancer* (pp. 38–53). New York: Academic Press.

Frankel, S. R. (1993). Acute promyelocytic leukemia: New insights into diagnosis and therapy. *Hematology/Oncology Clinics of North America, 7*(1), 109–138.

French Cooperative Group on Chronic Lymphocytic

Leukemia (1990). A randomized clinical trial of chlorambucil versus COP in stage B chronic lymphocytic leukemia. *Blood, 75,* 1422–1425.

Gale, R. P., & Foon, K. A. (1986). Acute myelogenous leukemia. In R. P. Gale (Ed.), *Leukemia therapy* (pp. 99–145). Boston: Blackwell Scientific Publications.

Gale, R. P., & Foon, K. A. (1987). Therapy of acute myelogenous leukemia. *Seminars in Hematology, 24,* 40–54.

Golde, D. W., & Koeffler, H. P. (1985). Hairy cell leukemia. In C. Haskell (Ed.), *Cancer treatment* (2nd ed.). Philadelphia: W. B. Saunders Co.

Golomb, H. M., Catovsky, D., & Golde, D. W. (1978). Hairy cell leukemia. A clinical review based on 71 cases. *Annals of Internal Medicine, 89*(1), 677–683.

Golomb, H. M., & Vardiman, J. W. (1978). Response to splenectomy in 65 patients with hairy cell leukemia: An evaluation of spleen weight and bone marrow involvement. *Blood, 61,* 349–352.

Graham, D. C. (1960). Leukemia following x-ray therapy for ankylosing spondylitis. *Archives of Internal Medicine, 105,* 51.

Grever, M. R., Leiby, J. M., Krant, E. H., Wilson, H. W., Niedhart, J. A., Wall, R. L., & Bacerzak, S. P., (1985). Low-dose deoxycoformycin in lymphoid malignancy. *Journal of Clinical Oncology, 3,* 1196.

Griffin, J. D., Davis, R., Nelson, D. A., Davey, F. R., Mayer, R. J., Schiffer, C., McIntyre, O. R., & Bloomfield, C. D. (1986). Use of surface marker analysis to predict outcome of adult acute myeloblastic leukemia. *Blood, 68,* 1232–1241.

Haut, A., Abbott, W. S., Wintrobe, M. M., & Cartwright, G. E. (1961). Busulfan in the treatment of chronic myelocytic leukemia: The effect of long-term intermittent therapy. *Blood, 117,* 1–19.

Henderson, E. S. (1983). Acute leukemias—general considerations in hematology. In W. J. Williams, E. Beutler, A. J. Erslev, & M. A. Lichtman (Eds.), *Hematology* (p. 221). New York: McGraw-Hill Book Co.

Henderson, E. S., & Han, T. (1986). Current therapy of acute and chronic leukemia in adults. *CA: A Cancer Journal for Clinicians, 36,* 322–350.

Heysel, R., Britt, A. M., Woodbury, L. A., Nishimura, E. T., Ghase, T., Hoshino, T., & Yamasaki, M. (1960). Leukemia in Hiroshima atomic bomb survivors. *Blood, 15,* 313.

Hirsch-Ginsberg, C., Huh, Y. O., Kagan, J., Liang, J. C., & Stass, S. A. Advances in the diagnosis of acute leukemia. *Hematology/Oncology Clinics of North America, 7*(1), 1–46.

Hoelzer, D. (1993) Therapy of the newly diagnosed adult with acute lymphoblastic leukemia. *Hematology/Oncology Clinics of North America, 7*(1), 139–160.

Hoelzer, D., & Gale, R. O. (1987). Acute lymphoblastic leukemia in adults. Recent progress, future direction. *Seminars in Hematology, 24,* 27–34.

Hoelzer, D., Thiel, E., Loffler, H., Maschmeyer, G., Volkers, B., Ludwig, W. D., Buchner, T., Freund, M., Heil, G., & Hiddemann, W. (1992). The German multicenter trials for treatment of acute lymphoblastic leukemia in adults. *Leukemia, 6*(Suppl. 2), 175–177.

Huguley, C. M., Jr. (1977). Treatment of chronic lymphocytic leukemia. *Cancer Treatment Reviews, 4,* 261–273.

Huh, Y. O., Kantarjian, H., Childs, C. C., Reuben, J., & McCredie, K. (1990). Classification of adult lymphoblastic leukemia by immunophenotype. *Blood, 76,* 282.

Hussein, K. K., Dahlberg, S., Head, D., Waddell, C. C., Dabich, L., Weick, J. K., Morrison, J. H., Metz, E., Saiki, J. H., Riukin, S. E., Grever, M. R., & Boldt, D. (1989). Treatment of acute lymphoblastic leukemia in adults with intensive induction, consolidation, and maintenance chemotherapy. *Blood,* 73, 57–63.

International Workshop on Chronic Lymphocytic Leukemia (1989). Chronic lymphocytic leukemia: Recommendations for diagnosis, staging and response criteria. *Annals of Internal Medicine, 110,* 236–238.

Italian Cooperative Group on Chronic Myeloid Leukemia (1984). Results of a prospective study of early splenectomy in chronic myeloid leukemia. *Cancer, 54,* 333–338.

Jacobs, A. (1986) Hairy cell leukemia. In R. P. Gale (Ed.), *Leukemia therapy.* Boston: Blackwell Scientific Publications.

Jacobs, A. D., & Gale, R. P. (1986). Acute lymphoblastic leukemia in adults. In R. P. Gale (Ed.), *Leukemia therapy* (pp. 71–98). Boston: Blackwell Scientific Publications.

Jacquillat, C., Weil, M., Auclerc, M. F., Chastang, C., Flandrin, G., Israel, V., Schaison, G., Degos, L., Boiron, M. & Bernard, J. (1978). Prognosis and treatment of acute lymphoblastic leukemia. *Cancer Chemotherapy and Pharmacology, 1,* 113–122.

Janossy, G., Woodruff, R. K., Pippard, M. J., Prentice, G., Hoffbrand, A. V., Paxton, A., Lister, T. A., Bunch, C., & Greaves, M. F. (1979). Relation of *"lymphoid"* phenotype and response to chemotherapy incorporating vincristine, prednisone in the acute phase of Ph[1]-positive leukemia. *Cancer, 43,* 426–434.

Juliusson, G., Oscier, D. G., Fitchett, M., Ross, F. M., Stockdill, G., Mackie, M. J., Parker, A. C., Castoldi, G. L., Guneo, A., & Knuutila, S. (1990). Prognostic subgroups in B-cell chronic lymphocytic leukemia defined by specific chromosomal abnormalities. *New England Journal of Medicine, 323,* 720–724.

Kantarjian, H. M., Walters, R. S., Keating, M. J., Smith, T. L., O'Brien, S., Estey, E. H., Huh, Y. O., Spinolo, J., Dicke, K., & Barlogie, B. (1990). Results of the vincristine, doxorubicin and dexamethasone regimen in adults with standard- and high-risk acute lymphocytic leukemia. *Journal of Clinical Oncology, 8,* 994–1004.

Kantarjian, H. M., Walters, R. S., Smith, T. L., Keating, M. J., Barlogie, B., McCredie, K. B., & Freireich, E. J. (1988). Identification of risk groups for development of central nervous system leukemia in adults with adult lymphocytic leukemia. *Blood, 72,* 1784–1789.

Keating, M. J., Kantarjian, H., Talpaz, M., Radman, J., Koller, C., Barlogie, B., Velasquez, W., Plunkett, H., Freirich, E. J., & McCredie, K. B. (1989). Fludarabine: A new agent with major activity against chronic lymphocytic leukemia. *Blood, 74,* 19–25.

Kennedy, B. J. (1972). Hydroxyurea therapy in chronic myelogenous leukemia. *Cancer, 29,* 1052–1056.

Knospe, W. H., Lolb, V., Jr., & Huguley, C. M., Jr. (1974). Biweekly chlorambucil treatment of chronic lymphocytic leukemia. *Cancer, 33,* 555–562.

Lembersky, B. C., Ratain, M. J., & Golomb, H. M. (1988). Skeletal complications in hairy cell leukemia: Diagnosis and therapy. *Journal of Clinical Oncology, 6,* 1280–1284.

Lestingi, T., & Hooberman, A. (1993) Philadelphia chromosome-positive acute lymphoblastic leukemia. *Hematology/Oncology Clinics of North America, 7*(1), 161–175.

Livingston, R. B., & Carter, S. K. (Eds.). (1970). Prednisone and prednisolone. In *Single agents in cancer chemotherapy* (pp. 337–358). New York: IFF/Preview Data.

Lluesma-Gonalons, M., Pavlovsky, S., Santarelli, M. T., Eppinger-Helf, M., Dorticos-Bavea, E., Carnot, J., & Corrado, C. (1991). Improved results of an intensified therapy in adult acute lymphoblastic leukemia. *Annals of Oncology, 2,* 33–39.

Mandelli, F., Annino, L., & Giona, F. (1990). GIMEMA ALL0183: A multicenter study on adult acute lymphoblastic leukemia in Italy. In R. P. Gale & D. Hoelzer (Eds.), *Acute lymphoblastic leukemia* (pp. 205–220). New York: Alan R. Liss.

Maxam, A. M., & Gilbert, W. (1980). Sequencing end-labeled DNA with base-specific chemical cleavage. *Methods in Enzymology, 65*, 499–560.

Mayer, R. J., Davis, R. B., Schiffer, C. A., Berg, D. T., Powell, B. L., Schulman, P., Omura, G. A., Moore, J. O., McIntyre, O. R., & Frei, E. (1994). Intensive postremission chemotherapy in adults with acute myeloid leukemia. *New England Journal of Medicine, 331*, 896–903.

McGlave, P. B., Arthur, D., Miller, W. J., Lasky, L., & Kersey, J. (1990). Autologous transplantation for CML using marrow-treated *ex vivo* with recombinant human interferon-gamma. *Bone Marrow Transplant, 6*, 115–120.

Morrison, V. A. (1994). Chronic leukemias. *Cancer, 44*(6), 353–377.

Ozer, H. (1988). Biotherapy of chronic myelogenous leukemia with interferon. *Seminars in Hematology, 15*(Suppl. 5), 14–20.

Ozer, H., George, S. L., Pettenati, M., Wurster-Hill, D., Bloomfield, C. D., Arthur, D., Rao, K., Powell, B., Gottlieb, A., Peterson, B., Rai, K., & Schiffer, C. (1992). Subcutaneous α-interferon (α-IFN) in untreated chronic phase Philadelphia chromosome-positive (Ph+) chronic myelogenous leukemia (CML) [Abstract]. *Blood, 80*(Suppl. 1), 358a.

Piro, L., Carrera, C., Beutler, E., & Carson, D. (1988) 2-chlorodeoxyadenosine: An effective new agent for the treatment of chronic lymphocytic leukemia. *Blood, 72*, 1069–1073.

Piro, L. D., Carrera, C. J., Carson, D. J., & Beutler, E. (1990). Lasting remissions in hairy cell leukemia induced by a single infusion of 2-chlorodeoxyadenosine. *New England Journal of Medicine, 322*, 1117–1121.

Rai, K. R., & Montserrat, E. (1987). Prognostic factors in chronic lymphatic leukemia. *Seminars in Hematology, 24*, 252–256.

Rai, K. R., Sawitsky, A., Cronkite, E. P., Chanana, A., Levy, R. N., & Pasternak, B. S. (1975). Clinical staging of chronic lymphocytic leukemia. *Blood, 46*, 219–234.

Rapaport, S. I. (1987). *Introduction to hematology.* Philadelphia: J. B. Lippincott Co.

Rohatiner, A. Z. S., Bassan, R., Battista, R., Barnett, M. J., Gregory, W., Lim, J., Arness, J., Oza, A., Barbui, T., & Horton, M. (1990). High-dose cytosine arabinoside in the initial treatment of adults with acute lymphoblastic leukemia. *British Journal of Cancer, 62*, 454–458.

Rundles, R. W. (1982). Chronic myelogenous leukemia. In W. J. Williams, E. Beutler, A. J. Erslev, & M. A. Licheman (Eds.), *Hematology* (pp. 196–214) New York: McGraw-Hill Book Co.

Rundles, R. W. (1982). Chronic lymphocytic leukemia. In W. J. Williams, E. Beutler, A. J. Erslev, & M. A. Licheman (Eds.), *Hematology* (p. 983). New York: McGraw-Hill Book Co.

Santos, G. (1989). Marrow transplantation in acute nonlymphocytic leukemia. *Blood, 75*, 901–908.

Schiffer, C. A., Larson, R. A., & Bloomfiels, C. D. for the CALGB (1991). Cancer and leukemia group B (CALGB) studies in acute lymphocytic leukemia (ALL). *Haematologica, 76*(Suppl. 4), 106.

Shapiro, L., Shustic, C., Anderson, K., & Sawitsky, A.

(1984). Intermittent chlorambucil in chronic lymphocytic leukemia: A randomized trial of treatment versus observation in early stage of disease [Abstract]. *Proceedings of the American Society of Clinical Oncology, 3*, 191.

Smedmyr, B., Simonsson, B., Bjorkholm, M., Carneskog, J., Gahrton, G., Grimfors, G., Hast, R., Jarnmark, M., Killander, A., & Kimby, E. (1991). Treatment of adult acute lymphoblastic and indifferentiated (ALL/AVL) leukemia according to a national protocol in Sweden. *Haematologica, 76*(Suppl. 4), 107.

Spiers, A. S., Moore, D., Cassileth, P. A., Harrington, D. P., Cummings, F. J., Neiman, R. S., Bennett, J. M., & O'Connell, M. J. (1987). Remissions in hairy cell leukemia with pentostatin (2′-deoxycoformycin). *New England Journal of Medicine, 316*, 825–830.

Stone, R. M., & Mayer, R. J. (1993) Treatment of the newly diagnosed adult with *de novo* acute myeloid leukemia. *Hematology/Oncology Clinics of North America, 7*(1), 47–64.

Stryckmans, P., de Witte, T. H., Fillet G., Marie, J. P., Peetermans, M., Hayat, M., Labar, B., Jaksic, B., Roozendaal, K., & Suciu, S. (1991). Treatment of adult acute lymphoblastic leukemia: ALL-2 and ALL-3 EORTC studies. *Haematologica, 76*(Suppl. 4), 109.

Talpaz, M., McCredie, K. B., Trujillo, J., Kantarjian, H. M., Keating, M. J., & Guttermen, J. (1987). Clinical investigation of human α-interferon in chronic myelogenous leukemia. *Blood, 69*, 1280–1288.

Thomas, E. D., Clift, R. A., Fefer, A., Appelbaum, F. R., Beatty, P., Bensinger, W. I., Buckner, C. D., Cheever, M. A., Deeg, H. J., & Doney, K. (1986). Marrow transplantation for the treatment of chronic myelogenous leukemia. *Annals of Internal Medicine, 104*, 155–163.

Tivey, H. (1954). The natural history of untreated acute leukemia. *Annals of the New York Academy of Science, 60*, 322.

Tomonaga, M., Omine, M., Morishima, Y., Hirano, M., Dohi, H., Imai, K., Hiraoka, A., Asoh, N., Tsubaki, K., & Ohshima, T. (1991). Individualized induction therapy followed by intensive consolidation and maintenance including asparaginase in adult ALL: JALSG-ALL87 study. *Haematologica, 76*(Suppl. 4), 68.

Urba, W., Baseler, M., Kopp, W., Steis, R., Clark, J., Smith, I. J., Coggin, D., & Longo, D. (1989). Deoxycoformycin-induced immunosuppression in patients with hairy cell leukemia. *Blood, 73*, 38–46.

Vigliani, E. C., & Sart, G. (1964). Benzene and leukemia. *New England Journal of Medicine, 271*, 872.

Vogler, W. R., Velez-Garcia, E., Weiner, R. S., Flaum, M. A., Bartolucci, A. A., Omura, G. A., Gerber, M. C., & Banks, P. L. C. (1992). A phase III trial comparing idarubicin and daunorubicin in combination with cytarabine in acute myelogenous leukemia: A southeastern cancer study group study. *Journal of Clinical Oncology, 10*, 1103–1111.

Whang-Peng, J., & Knutsen, T. (1980). Lymphocytic leukemias, acute and chronic. *Clinical Hematology, 9*, 87.

Wiernik, P. H., Banks, P. L. C., Case, D. C., Jr., Arlin, Z. A., Periman, P. O., Todd, M. B., Ritch, P. S., Enck, R. E., & Weitberg, A. B. (1992). Cytarabine plus idarubicin or daunorubicin as induction and consolidation therapy for previously untreated adult patients with acute myeloid leukemia. *Blood, 79*, 313.

Zigelboim, J., Foon, K., & Gale, R. (1985). Acute myelogenous leukemia. In C. Haskell (Ed.), *Cancer treatment* (pp. 694–706). Philadelphia: W. B. Saunders Co.

Head and Neck Cancers

Jean L. Reese

The new cases of head and neck cancers in 1994 is expected to reach 42,100. In 1990 head and neck cancers accounted for 4.5 per cent of the nearly 400,000 cases collected by the National Cancer Data Base (NCDB) (Steele, Winchester, Menck, & Murphy, 1993) (Table 37–1). This small percentage belies the multiple and severe challenges to the physical, psychologic, and social well-being of those afflicted. Cancerous processes in the paranasal sinuses, nasal and oral cavities, salivary glands, pharynx, and larynx can affect speech, appearance, eating, and breathing. Any one or a combination of these altered functions makes psychosocial adjustment difficult. In addition, the person with head and neck cancer often bears concomitant health problems associated with aging, malnutrition, smoking, and alcohol abuse.

Environmental factors and personal habits are often closely associated with the development of cancer in the head and neck region. Although squamous cell carcinomas constitute the majority of tumors in this region, the biologic behavior of this cell type varies considerably from site to site. A difference of even a few cen-

timeters within the same site of the same tumor type can result in a different natural history (Harnsburger & Dillon, 1987). Location, stage of development on discovery, and treatment alternatives all influence survival rates.

TRENDS

Head and neck cancer is increasing among women, the elderly, and African-Americans. Social habits changed considerably after World War II, and women are now smoking cigarettes and drinking alcoholic beverages to greater extents. Head and neck cancer among women, like lung cancer, is likely to continue increasing.

A comparison of the estimated incidence of cancer in men and women in the years 1984 and 1994 shows an increase in all head and neck sites except the lip (Table 37–1). Males had a 5 per cent increase while the females gained 15 per cent. Males historically have had a higher ratio compared with females, but the gap continues to narrow. Using the figures from the NCDB, the

TABLE 37–1. *Comparison of Estimated New Head and Neck Cancer Cases and Deaths by Sex in 1984 and 1994 in the U.S.*

SITES	TOTAL		MALES		FEMALES	
Oral	29600	(7925)	19800	(5150)	9800	(2775)
Oral	*27500*	*(9350)*	*18700*	*(6400)*	*8800*	*(2950)*
Lip	3300	(75)	2800	(50)	500	(25)
Lip	*4900*	*(175)*	*4200*	*(150)*	*700*	*(25)*
Tongue	6000	(1750)	3800	(1100)	2200	(650)
Tongue	*4900*	*(2050)*	*3200*	*(1400)*	*1700*	*(650)*
Mouth	11100	(2100)	6600	(1200)	4500	(900)
Mouth	*9800*	*(2825)*	*5800*	*(1850)*	*4000*	*(975)*
Pharynx	9200	(4000)	6600	(2800)	2600	(1200)
Pharynx	*7900*	*(4300)*	*5500*	*(3000)*	*2400*	*(1300)*
Larynx	12500	(3800)	9800	(3000)	2700	(800)
Larynx	*11100*	*(3750)*	*9300*	*(3100)*	*1800*	*(650)*

Italics = 1984 data; ( ) = number of deaths.
(Data from Silverberg, E. [1984]. Cancer statistics, 1984. *Ca-A Cancer Journal for Clinicians,* 34[1], 14–15, and *Cancer facts & figures*-1994. American Cancer Society.)

male:female ratio is now close to 2.4:1. McGuirt reported a ratio of 3:1 in 1979 and, in 1983, a ratio of 2:1 from a series of newly diagnosed patients from the tobacco growing states. This series forecasted the narrow margin between the sexes that we see today.

Thirty-year trends reported by Boring, Squires, and Heath (1992) showed that African-Americans had a 70 per cent and 110 per cent increase in oral and laryngeal cancers, respectively. Because this trend applied only to those blacks who were economically depressed, the authors surmised the differences between African-Americans and whites were a consequence of cultural factors, not a racial predisposition. When rates were adjusted for income and education, African-Americans actually had a rate lower than whites. Still, African-Americans as a whole have higher incidence rates, a later stage at diagnosis, and worse survival rates than whites.

Survival rates for whites with oral and pharyngeal cancers fluctuate around 55 per cent since 1974, while survival rate in African-American cancer patients has dropped from 36 per cent to 33 per cent (Boring, Squires, Tong, & Montgomery, 1994).

Since the data on smoking tobacco and its relationship to lung cancer have become common knowledge, some smokers have switched to smokeless tobacco to satisfy the need for nicotine. The number of pounds of snuff manufactured in the United States had doubled by 1991 to 54.4 million pounds in 20 years (Wray & Mc-Quirt, 1993).

Alarming is the nearly 20 per cent prevalence rate of smokeless tobacco use in boys and a 1.4 per cent usage rate in girls (MMWR, 1989). What happens after long-term use of smokeless tobacco has been firmly established by Wray and McQuirt (1993) in their report of elderly women who used smokeless tobacco for 40 years or more. Seventy-eight per cent of the women who presented with oral carcinoma were snuff users. Young snuff users are candidates for future oral cancer patient populations.

More than 50 per cent of all cancers occur in persons over 65 years old. This percentage holds, with slight variation in different sites, for the elderly who have cancers of the head and neck (Baranovsky & Myers, 1986). The numbers of these cancers will more than likely increase because of the larger numbers of people who will be aging in the next decades. Of 758 patients observed in a London clinic between the years 1975 and 1981, 57 per cent were 61 years of age and older (Lampe, Lampe, & Skillings, 1986). Carcinomas in this group most frequently developed in the buccal mucosa, hard palate, soft palate, and tongue. In addition, the 56 per cent 5-year survival rate for the over-61 age group compared unfavorably with the 79 per cent survival rate among patients aged 40 years or less.

Studies about the interrelationship of patient, tumor, and treatment factors on prognosis are appearing more frequently in the literature. Researchers realized that although patients had the same disease stage and treatment, outcomes differed for individual patients. Selecting a tailored treatment scheme for each patient will hopefully lead to better outcomes. With this in mind, more studies are being analyzed using regression and variate analyses to isolate prognostic factors.

ORAL CAVITY AND PHARYNX

DEFINITION

Oral cavity cancer occurs in the lips, oral tongue, floor of the mouth, buccal mucosa, upper and lower gingiva, retromolar trigone, and hard palate (Fig. 37–1).

The pharynx, composed of the nasopharynx, oropharynx, and hypopharynx, extends from the base of the skull superiorly to the level of the esophagus inferiorly. The soft palate forms the floor and anterior wall of the nasopharynx. The eustachian tube orifice and the adenoids are located in the nasopharynx. The extensive submucosal capillary lymphatic plexus present in the nasopharynx leads to frequent metastasis from this region to the neck. The oropharynx includes

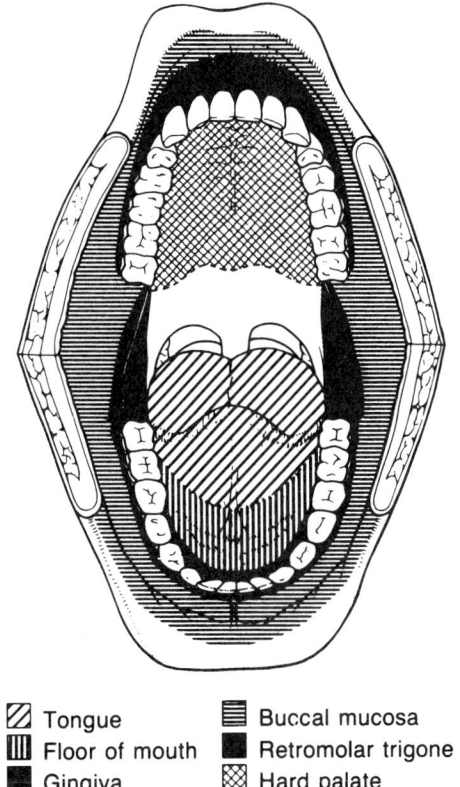

Symbol	Site	Symbol	Site
▨	Tongue	▤	Buccal mucosa
▥	Floor of mouth	■	Retromolar trigone
◼	Gingiva	▨	Hard palate

FIGURE 37–1. Anatomic sites within the oral cavity. (From Shah, J. P., Shemen, L. J., & Strong, E. W. [1987]. Buccal mucosa, alveolus, retromolar trigone, floor of mouth, hard palate, and tongue tumors. In S. E. Thawley & W. R. Panje [Eds.], *Comprehensive management of head and neck tumors* [Vol. 1, p. 552]. Philadelphia: W. B. Saunders Co. Reproduced by permission.)

the base of the tongue, the tonsillar area, the soft palate, and the posterior pharyngeal wall. The base of the tongue is bounded by the circumvallate papillae anteriorly, by the epiglottis posteriorly, and by the glossopharyngeal sulcus laterally. The hypopharynx extends from the level of the hyoid bone to the lower border of the cricoid cartilage, where the esophagus begins. The pharyngeal walls, pyriform sinus, and postcricoid area make up the hypopharynx (Kornblut, 1987; Mahboubi & Sayed, 1982) (Fig. 37–2).

INCIDENCE, MORTALITY, AND SURVIVAL RATES

CANCER OF THE MOUTH AND PHARYNX

The estimated incidence rate for cancers of the oral cavity and the pharynx are 16.6 per 100,000 for males and 6.4 per 100,000 for females in the United States with the estimated death rates at 4.7 per 100,000 and 1.7 per 100,000 respectively (SEER program) (Table 37–2). While the estimated number of new cases has increased for both sexes, the number of estimated deaths has decreased compared with 1984 figures. Close to 8000 deaths are expected in 1994 from cancer in this anatomic region (Table 37–1). Death rates from oral carcinomas range from 1.7 to 14.5 per 100,000 in Europe (La Vecchia, Francesch, Levi, Lucchini, & Negri, 1993).

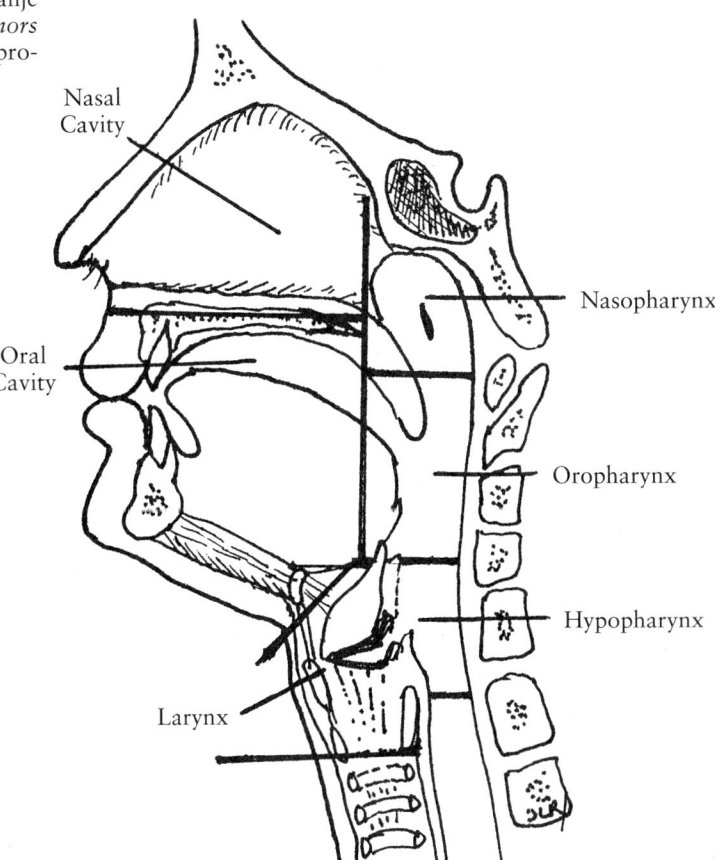

FIGURE 37–2. Anatomic regions of the head and neck.

TABLE 37–2. *Incidence and Mortality Rates (1985 to 1989) for Oral Cavity and Pharyngeal Cancer by Age, Sex, and Race**

AGE AT DIAGNOSIS	ALL RACES			AFRICAN-AMERICANS			WHITES		
	TOTAL	M	F	TOTAL	M	F	TOTAL	M	F
All ages	11.0	16.6	6.4	14.2	23.9	6.7	10.7	16.1	6.4
	(3.1)	(4.7)	(1.7)	(5.2)	(9.4)	(2.3)	(2.8)	(4.3)	(1.7)
Under 65	7.0	10.3	3.9	11.6	18.9	5.5	6.6	9.6	3.8
	(1.7)	(2.6)	(0.9)	(4.0)	(6.9)	(1.6)	(1.5)	(2.2)	(0.8)
65 & over	47.1	73.7	28.7	38.2	69.5	17.6	48.2	75.2	29.8
	(15.4)	(24.2)	(9.5)	(17.4)	(31.6)	(8.3)	(15.3)	(23.6)	(9.6)

*SEER program. Rates are per 100,000 and age-adjusted to 1970 U.S. standard population.
( ) = mortality rates.
(Data from *Cancer Statistics Review, 1973–1989*, National Cancer Institute, NIH Publication No. 92-2789, pp. xix, 4, 5.)

More than 90 per cent of all oral and pharyngeal cancers occur in people over 45 years old (Mahboubi & Sayed, 1982). An exception arises with nasopharyngeal carcinomas, of which 15 to 20 per cent appear in persons under 30 years old (Cassisi, 1987). Nasopharyngeal cancer (NPC) incidence is very low in most of the world (0.5-2/100,000) except in southern China and Hong Kong, where rates range from 25 to 50 per 100,000. The interplay between environmental and genetic factors may explain this variation. Tumors occur at a rate of less than 1 per 100,000 among European and North American caucasians (Liebowitz, 1994). In the late 1940s, incidence rates for mouth and pharynx cancers increased with each decade of age. Most recently, however, these rates show a different pattern, with the peak incidence occurring in the 65- to 69-year age group (see Table 37–3). Mortality rates increased from the early 1950s to mid-1980s for white women with a decrease for white men in the same time period (Devesa et al., 1987). Incidence and mortality figures show a dramatic increase for those at 65 and older for both sexes, either African-American or white. Interest-ingly, African-Americans, aged 65 years and older, of both sexes, have a lower incidence rate than same-aged whites. Older African-American males, however, have a higher death rate than do the older white males. Those African-Americans younger than 65 years have higher incidence and death rates than do the same-aged whites (Table 37–2).

The incidence of oral cancers varies widely internationally. Oral cancer accounts for no more than 5 per cent of all cancers in Western countries but represents almost 50 per cent of all cancers in some parts of India (Mahboubi & Sayed, 1982). The age-adjusted death rate for men is above 10 per 100,000 in Hong Kong, France, Singapore, the Bahamas, Puerto Rico, and Hungary. Hong Kong has the highest death rate for women at 6.6 per 100,000, followed by Singapore, Kuwait, Panama, and Puerto Rico. The United States ranked thirteenth (men) and eleventh (women) in death rate from oral cancers in 1980–1981 (Silverberg, 1983).

Untreated oral cavity cancers have resulted in mortality rates of 50 per cent at 13 months and 75 per cent

TABLE 37–3. *Selected Age-Specific Average Annual Incidence Rates for Head and Neck Cancers per 100,000 White Men (M) and Women (F) in Five Geographic Areas in the United States*

CANCER TYPE		AGE RANGES						
		35–39	45–49	55–59	65–69	75–79	85+	AA
Mouth and pharynx	F (1947–1950)	0.7	4.5	10.4	16.0	12.8	27.3	3.4
tumors (other	F (1983–1984)	1.0	4.8	17.4	28.1	19.9	18.9	5.3
than larynx or	M (1947–1950)	2.5	6.2	25.8	51.5	77.3	113.0	12.5
salivary glands)	M (1983–1984)	2.6	14.7	45.5	66.1	56.3	50.6	13.5
Larynx	F (1947–1950)	—	1.2	1.9	1.8	2.2	—	0.5
	F (1983–1984)	0.6	2.3	4.9	7.3	5.4	2.1	1.5
	M (1947–1950)	0.9	4.6	20.6	21.3	26.5	14.6	5.6
	M (1983–1984)	0.9	6.5	28.5	46.8	44.3	30.2	9.0
Salivary glands	F (1947–1950)	0.7	2.9	5.2	7.1	6.2	4.8	1.9
	F (1983–1984)	0.8	1.0	1.7	1.9	2.4	3.7	0.8
	M (1947–1950)	2.0	0.9	4.1	5.5	18.4	18.2	1.8
	M (1983–1984)	0.4	0.8	1.7	3.7	6.5	12.9	1.0

AA, average annual age-adjusted (1970 standard) incidence rates per 100,000 population.
(Data from Devesa, S. S., Silverman, D. T., Young, J. L., Jr., Pollack, E. S., Brown, C. C., Horm, J. W., Percy, C. L., Myers, M. H., McKay, F. W., & Fraumeni, J. F., Jr. [1987]. Cancer incidence and mortality trends among whites in the United States, 1947–1984. *Journal of the National Cancer Institute, 79*, 748, 752.)

at 20 months (Shimkin, 1951). Jones (1994) reported a crude median survival rate of 7 months after diagnosis for untreated patients. Survival rates vary depending on the site of cancer in the mouth, with the malignant gradient increasing as the site of the cancer moves posteriorly in the oral cavity. Thus cancer of the lip has the best survival rate (85 to 95 per cent) when compared with other oral structures (Hosal, Onerci, Kaya, & Turan, 1992). The buccal mucosa tumors have the next best 5-year survival rate, ranging between 50 and 70 per cent. Cancers in other areas of the mouth for early stages (I & II) tend to congregate around a 50 to 80 per cent range. Stage IV survival rates drop precipitously to a range of 17 to 35 per cent (Jones, 1994). Shah, Shemen, and Strong (1987) compared data from four surveys of patients who had cancer of the oral cavity. A greater percentage of oral tongue and floor of the mouth cancers were diagnosed at stage I than either cancers of the buccal mucosa or palate. Five-year survival rates for all four sites treated at stage I were well above 70 per cent, with floor of the mouth cancers registering nearly 90 per cent survival. When diagnosed at stage IV, floor of the mouth cancers had, after 5 years, a survival rate of 32 per cent, compared with less than 20 per cent for the other three sites. Although cancers of the oral cavity of stage T_1 hold an optimistic outlook when treated, early diagnosis is not commonplace (Sisson, 1985). One half of the oral cancers, when diagnosed, are associated with lymphadenopathy (Mashberg & Samit, 1989). Jones's (1994) study of 524 patients with oral cavity malignancies showed, using multivariate analysis, that the significant prognostic factors were the T and N stages. In addition, well-differentiated tumors showed a slightly better survival rate than poorly differentiated tumors. The crude 5-year survival rate for treated patients was 40 per cent. See Table 37–4 for TNM categories of head and neck cancers.

CANCER OF THE TONGUE

In 1995, 5550 new cases and 1870 deaths from cancer of the tongue were estimated (*Cancer facts & figures*, 1995). Patients younger than 40 years, who rarely present with tongue carcinoma, tend to have poor overall treatment results despite an earlier stage of presentation than patients in the fifth and sixth decades of life (Sarkaria & Harari, 1994). Survival rates also drop with nodal disease regardless of the T designation. T1 and T2 tumors together without nodal disease show a 58.5 to 90 per cent survival rate, while those with nodal disease have a 15 to 33 per cent survival rate. T3/T4 tumors show very limited survival regardless of nodal status (Mitchell & Crighton, 1993). The lateral border of the middle third of the tongue is the most common site for cancers; the dorsum, tip, and ventral surfaces are the least common sites (Batsakis, 1987). About 75 per cent of the cancers occur in the mobile portion of the tongue, and the remainder originate in the posterior third of the tongue.

FLOOR OF THE MOUTH CARCINOMAS

Floor of the mouth carcinomas are nearly as common as those occurring in the tongue. Originating in the midline or next to the frenulum, lesions can extend into the tongue via the ventral surface and to the anterior mandible before detection. Metastasis to the cervical lymph nodes occurs in 35 to 70 per cent of the cases but develops later in the disease process than does metastasis from cancer of the tongue (Batsakis, 1987).

CARCINOMA OF THE PALATE

Carcinoma of the palate is usually of salivary gland origin and is rare. Ten-year disease free survival ranges from 55 to 80 per cent. Adenoid cystic carcinomas often recur many years after initial treatment (Kovalic & Simpson, 1993). It occurs most frequently in men in their sixties. The tumors are usually ulcerated, are surrounded by leukoplakia, and have indistinct borders. The size of the tumor has more bearing on outcome than does location on the hard palate (Batsakis, 1987).

SIGNS AND SYMPTOMS

ORAL CAVITY CARCINOMAS

A painless mass present for varying periods of time, persistent ulceration, difficulty wearing dentures, local or referred pain to the jaw or ear, and blood-tinged sputum are common complaints with oral cavity carcinomas. Later complaints include dysphagia, difficulty chewing, or changes in articulation. Some lesions may be discovered during a dental examination. In other cases, patients first note a mass in the neck (Kornblut, 1987).

Cancer of the tongue metastasizes more frequently to the cervical lymph nodes than does any other primary intraoral site (Batsakis, 1987). Kornblut (1987) cautioned that almost all tongue lesions are much more extensive than what is usually apparent. This extensiveness is confirmed by the 40 per cent cervical node involvement on initial presentation. Up to 20 per cent of the nodal involvement may be bilateral, reflecting the pattern of lymphatic drainage in the region. Tumors often are visually apparent or palpable at presentation; other manifestations include local pain and dysphagia (Kornblut, 1987).

Mashberg and Samit (1989) emphasize that mucosal erythroplasia rather than leukoplakia is the earliest visual sign of oral and pharyngeal carcinomas. In addition, if mucosal redness or inflammation persists for more than 14 days in the high-risk areas (floor of the mouth, ventrolateral tongue, and soft palate) without obvious cause, the area should be biopsied (Mashberg & Samit, 1989).

Dysplastic lesions from the use of snuff tend to be reversible with cessation of snuff use (Axéll, 1993). The mucosal change, coined "snuff dipper's lesion," looks wrinkled or folded with or without the color change of yellowish to brown.

NASOPHARYNGEAL CANCERS (NPC)

Malignant tumors in the nasopharyngeal area overwhelmingly arise in epidermoid tissue with endemic distribution among specific ethnic groups (Fandi, Altun, Azli, Armand, & Cvitkovic, 1994). Presenting symptoms are vague and variable. A painless enlarged

TABLE 37–4. *Definitions of TNM Categories for Head and Neck Cancer Sites*

Primary Tumor
TX Primary tumor cannot be assessed
T0 No evidence of primary tumor
Tis Carcinoma in situ

Lip and Oral Cavity
T1 Tumor 2 cm or less in greatest dimension
T2 Tumor more than 2 cm but not more than 4 cm in greatest dimension
T3 Tumor more than 4 cm in greatest dimension
T4 (lip) Tumor invades adjacent structures (e.g., through cortical bone, tongue, skin of neck)
T4 (oral cavity) Tumor invades adjacent structures (e.g., through cortical bone, into deep [extrinsic] muscle of tongue, maxillary sinus, skin)

Pharynx (Including Base of Tongue, Soft Palate, and Uvula)
Oropharynx
T1 Tumor 2 cm or less in greatest dimension
T2 Tumor more than 2 cm but not more than 4 cm in greatest dimension
T3 Tumor more than 4 cm in greatest dimension
T4 Tumor invades adjacent structures (e.g., through cortical bone, soft tissues of neck, deep [extrinsic] muscle of tongue)
Nasopharynx
T1 Tumor limited to one subsite of nasopharynx
T2 Tumor invades more than one subsite of nasopharynx
T3 Tumor invades nasal cavity and/or oropharynx
T4 Tumor invades skull and/or cranial nerve(s)
Hypopharynx
T1 Tumor limited to one subsite of hypopharynx
T2 Tumor invades more than one subsite of hypopharynx or an adjacent site, without fixation of hemilarynx
T3 Tumor invades more than one subsite of hypopharynx or an adjacent site, with fixation of hemilarynx
T4 Tumor invades adjacent structures (e.g., cartilage or soft tissues of neck)

Larynx
Supraglottis
T1 Tumor limited to one subsite of the supraglottis with normal vocal cord mobility
T2 Tumor invades more than one subsite of the supraglottis or glottis, with normal vocal cord mobility
T3 Tumor limited to the larynx with vocal cord fixation and/or invades the postcricoid area, medial wall of the pyriform sinus, or preepiglottic tissues
T4 Tumor invades through the thyroid cartilage and/or extends to other tissues beyond the larynx (e.g., to the oropharynx or soft tissues of the neck)
Glottis
T1 Tumor limited to the vocal cord(s) (may involve anterior or posterior commissures) with normal mobility
　T1a Tumor limited to one vocal cord
　T1b Tumor involves both vocal cords
T2 Tumor extends to the supraglottis and/or subglottis, and/or with impaired vocal cord mobility
T3 Tumor limited to the larynx with vocal cord fixation
T4 Tumor invades through the thyroid cartilage and/or extends to other tissues beyond the larynx (e.g., to the oropharynx or soft tissues of the neck)

Subglottis
T1 Tumor limited to the subglottis
T2 Tumor extends to the vocal cord(s) with normal or impaired mobility
T3 Tumor limited to the larynx with vocal cord fixation
T4 Tumor invades through the cricoid or thyroid cartilage and/or extends to other tissues beyond the larynx (e.g., to the oropharynx or soft tissues of the neck)

Maxillary Sinus
T1 Tumor limited to the antral mucosa with no erosion or destruction of bone
T2 Tumor with erosion or destruction of the infrastructure (see anatomic division, above), including the hard palate and/or the middle nasal meatus
T3 Tumor invades any of the following: skin of cheek, posterior wall of maxillary sinus, floor or medial wall of orbit, anterior ethmoid sinus
T4 Tumor invades orbital contents and/or any of the following: cribriform plate, posterior ethmoid or sphenoid sinuses, nasopharynx, soft palate, pterygomaxillary or temporal fossae, or base of skull

Regional Lymph Nodes (N)
NX Regional lymph nodes cannot be assessed
N0 No regional lymph node metastasis
N1 Metastasis in a single ipsilateral lymph node, 3 cm or less in greatest dimension
N2 Metastasis in a single ipsilateral lymph node, more than 3 cm but not more than 6 cm in greatest dimension; or in multiple ipsilateral lymph nodes, none more than 6 cm in greatest dimension; or in bilateral or contralateral lymph nodes, none more than 6 cm in greatest dimension
　N2a Metastasis in a single ipsilateral lymph node more than 3 cm but not more than 6 cm in greatest dimension
　N2b Metastasis in multiple ipsilateral lymph nodes, none more than 6 cm in greatest dimension
　N2c Metastasis in bilateral or contralateral lymph nodes, none more than 6 cm in greatest dimension
N3 Metastasis in a lymph node more than 6 cm in greatest dimension

Distant Metastasis (M)
MX Presence of distant metastasis cannot be assessed
M0 No distant metastasis
M1 Distant metastasis

Stage Grouping

Stage 0	Tis	N0	M0
Stage I	T1	N0	M0
Stage II	T2	N0	M0
Stage III	T3	N0	M0
	T1	N1	M0
	T2	N1	M0
	T3	N1	M0
Stage IV	T4	N0	M0
	T4	N1	M0
	Any T	N2	M0
	Any T	N3	M0
	Any T	Any N	M1

(Adapted from Beahrs, O. H., Henson, D. E., Hutter, R. V. P., & Kennedy, B. J. [Eds.]. [1992]. *Manual for Staging of Cancer* [4th ed.]. American Joint Committee on Cancer. Philadelphia: J. B. Lippincott Co. Reproduced by permission.)

neck node is a common first indicator of tumor presence. Nasal discharge (sometimes bloody), nasal stuffiness, and hypernasal speech are other indicators. Spread of the tumor can produce unilateral conductive hearing loss, atypical facial pain, and paresthesias, diplopia, trismus, nasal regurgitation, tongue paralysis, and shoulder weakness (Panje, 1987).

Presentation without extension beyond the nasopharynx and clinically involved neck nodes accounts for only 9 per cent of cases. Cranial nerve palsies indicate advanced disease. Invasion of the parapharyngeal space is a common occurrence (Lee, Poon, & Foo, 1992). The drainage from the nasopharyngeal lymphatic vessels to the internal jugular vein, posterior cervical chains, and retropharyngeal chains often results in bilateral node involvement (Fandi et al., 1994).

OROPHARYNGEAL CANCERS

The tumors in the oropharyngeal area arise in the soft palate, tonsil, base of the tongue, and pharyngeal wall. The most frequent subsites of cancer in the oropharynx are the tonsillar region and the base of the tongue.

Cancers of the oropharynx tend to be highly metastatic, aggressive, and undifferentiated. The majority of these cancers are beyond the T_1 designation when first seen (Batsakis, 1987). Tumors of the base of the tongue frequently occur without ulceration. Weiland (1987) postulated that tumor spread relates to the mobile nature of the tongue, which "milks" tumor cells into the lymphatic channels. Signs and symptoms are dysphagia, pain on swallowing, and possible nodal disease.

HYPOPHARYNGEAL CANCERS

Hypopharyngeal cancers occur most frequently in men in their sixth and seventh decades of life. The pyriform sinus is most commonly involved, with moderately to poorly differentiated squamous cell carcinoma accounting for most of the cancers (Weber & Manzione, 1986). The common presenting symptoms include a sore throat and neck mass. Localized pain with swallowing and referred pain to the ear are also typical (Marks, 1987). Weight loss and dysphagia occur with enlargement of the tumor (Thawley & Sessions, 1987). See Table 37–4 for staging of pharyngeal tumors.

RISK FACTORS

Persons in the lower socioeconomic groups have a higher incidence of oral and pharyngeal cancers. Unskilled workers have a higher risk rate than professionals, perhaps reflecting exposure to more irritating substances in the environment (Wynder & Stellman, 1977).

Tobacco is strongly associated with oral and pharyngeal cancers. Most geographic differences in oral cancer are due to tobacco and alcohol consumption, and this cancer explains over three quarters of approximately 20,000 deaths in Europe each year (La Vecchio et al., 1993). In other parts of the world, notably in India, Asia, and Melanesia, betel quids are associated with a high incidence of oral carcinoma. Betel quids contain areca nut, betel leaf, tobacco, slaked lime, and variety of spices (Thomas & Kearsly, 1993). Chewing "pan," a mixture of betel leaf (a climbing pepper), areca (or betel) nut, lime (calcium hydroxide), and catechu, is common in India where oral carcinomas abound (Muir, 1967). The effect of tobacco is multiplied by the ingestion of alcohol (Flanders & Rothman, 1982). Also, data from the study by Mashberg, Garfinkel, and Harris (1981) suggest alcohol has an independent role in the development of oral cancer.

The different types of smokeless tobacco have shown different degrees of change on the oral mucosa. Loose snuff rather than portion-package snuff had the greatest effect on the oral mucosa in a study of 252 Swedish users of moist snuff (Andersson & Axéll, 1989). In the same study a stepwise logistic regression showed that placement of the quid in one place, longer hours of daily use, more grams used each day, more years of snuff use, and older age influenced the severity of mucosal changes.

Other identified risk factors include poor nutrition and poor oral hygiene (Silverberg & Lubera, 1989). Previously, physical irritation was believed to be associated with oral carcinoma development. Currently, the evidence suggests that chronic oral irritation has little influence on the development of squamous cancers. The oral sites receiving the most trauma (tip of tongue, gingiva, cheeks, and hard palate) are those with the lowest incidence of squamous cell cancers. As mentioned earlier, the three intraoral areas that most frequently show squamous cell carcinoma are the floor of the mouth, the ventrolateral tongue, and the soft palate complex (Mashberg & Samit, 1989).

Nutrition-based studies reveal an association with the incidence of oral cancer. In a case-controlled study conducted in China, total carotene intake, intake from fruits and vegetables, and vitamin C were inversely related to the risk of oral cancer, while millet and corn bread raised the risk (Zheng, Boyle, et al., 1993). Similarly, a European study showed a significant protective effect from vegetable and fruit ingestion (LaVecchia et al., 1993).

Boot and shoe manufacturers and repairers have exhibited an increased incidence of buccal cavity cancer owing to exposure to noxious substances in their work. In addition, cotton, wool, and asphalt workers have had a higher than expected incidence for mouth and pharyngeal cancers (Saracci, 1985). Sun exposure has long been associated with the development of lower lip cancer in outdoor workers.

Leukoplakia, a relatively common mucosal disorder, becomes malignant in about 5 to 6 per cent of the cases. Although leukoplakia appears most commonly on commissures, progression of leukoplakia to a malignant lesion occurs most frequently on the tongue (Banoczy, 1977).

The relationship of the Epstein-Barr virus (EBV) to NPC is well established with immunoglobulin (IgG)- and IGA-related responses (Fandi et al., 1994). In fact, the viral capsid antigen (VCA-IgA) was the most important predictor for the development of NPC in a study by Zheng, Christensson, & Drettner (1993). Environmental factors such as eating salt-preserved food items and genetic susceptibility with a human leukocyte antigen and potential tumor suppressor genes located on chromosome 3 are other risk factors (Liebowitz, 1994).

DIAGNOSIS

Locating the site of the tumor is of great importance for exact staging. The site determines the pattern of lymphatic drainage, which, in turn, affects surgical and radiation treatments and prognosis.

Needle and simple open biopsies are common methods of determining tissue histology. The use of toluidine blue to differentiate the margins of squamous cell carcinoma is helpful with leukoplakia or erythroplasia (Peterson, Overholser, Bergman, & Beckerman, 1986). Routine radiographs of the area serve initially to localize a suspected lesion, whereas chest radiographs rule out lung metastasis. Computed tomography (CT) shows soft tissue densities as well as bony structures, muscles, fascial planes, opacification, and enlarged lymph nodes (Peterson et al., 1986; Weber & Manzione, 1986). Magnetic resonance imaging (MRI) is superior for soft tissue delineation.

MEDICAL TREATMENT

SURGERY AND RADIATION

The choice between radiation or surgery as the initial treatment hinges on many factors. Tumor location and volume, patterns of spread, and the impact of treatment on function, rehabilitation, and cosmesis are a few of the considerations (Parsons & Million, 1987).

Cancer of the Oral Cavity. With lip lesions, irradiation or local excision is used. Neck dissection is performed for metastatic disease or for high risk of tumor spread. Cancers of the lower gingiva that are less than 3 cm require wide local excision with radiation. Initial surgical treatment produces better results than does radiation (Parsons & Million, 1987). Tumors over 3 cm are treated with radical excision, radical neck dissection, and postoperative radiation (Elias, 1986).

Most T1 and T2 tumors can be excised through the open mouth, especially mobile tongue lesions. Larger infiltrated lesions require more exposure. The depth of tongue tumors is hard to assess, and these tumors sometimes require splitting the mandible (mandibular swing or mandibulotomy-midline or lateral) for accessing the borders of the lesion. The location of the osteotomy, outside the area of irradiation is to avoid malunion or nonunion. Advances in mandibular plates has increased the stabilization of the mandible (Wenig, 1994).

Irradiation of T1 and T2 tumors is an effective management. Treatment often entails external beam irradiation to the primary tumor and first level of lymph nodes and an extra boost with brachytherapy or an intraoral cone. Radiation therapy avoids an operation

with mortality rates of 1 to 2 per cent. In addition, fewer functional and cosmetic defects occur than with surgery (Sweeney, Haraf, Vokes, Dougherty, & Weichselbaum, 1994).

Advanced lesions of the oral cavity require a composite resection, otherwise known as the Commando procedure. A wide resection, segmental mandibulectomy and neck dissection compose the cornerstone of surgical treatment for these tumors. An alteration to this procedure is a partial manibulectomy, which maintains the continuity of the jaw. The primary tumor and neck dissection are removed en bloc, usually through the neck incision (Wenig, 1994).

A review of survival rates of tonsillar carcinoma by Foote et al. (1994) shows wide-ranging results (0 to 75 per cent) for mostly stage III and IV tumors. Treatments varied from surgery or radiation, or in combination with differing sequences. Foote and associates recommended postoperative adjuvant irradiation for resected stage III or IV squamous cell carcinoma (SCC). Ipsilateral nodal metastasis is a significant risk with tonsillar SCC. Two recent studies showed overall 5-year survival rates of 52.5 per cent (Kajanti, Holsti, & Mantyla, 1992) and 78 per cent (Foote et al., 1994) for tonsillar cancer.

In a comparison of irradiation effectiveness with tonsillar and base of the tongue carcinoma, the overall 3-year survival rate was 57 per cent and 38 per cent, respectively. Reported local control rates are higher at 65 per cent and at around 50 per cent for the same sites (Mak-Kregar et al., 1993).

Cancer of the Nasopharynx. Nasopharyngeal tumors are treated by irradiation because surgical removal is nearly impossible and bilateral metastases develop early. However, some extensive surgical procedures are being initiated with an infratemporal fossa or transparotid approach (Panje, 1987). Radiation therapy, with advanced techniques can achieve high (80 to 100 per cent) percentages of local control with T1 and T2 tumors, while local control for T3 and T4 ranges from 44 to 90 per cent (Harrison & Pfister, 1991). Survival rates range from 31 to 85 per cent. Recurrence is also treatable by intracavitary radiation, and excision of nodes can be an effective salvage option. Cisplatin, adriamycin, epirubicin, bleomycin, and methotrexate are single-agent drugs that have shown to be active against NPC. In addition, studies show NPC to be sensitive to preirradiation chemotherapy. The purpose of adding chemotherapy to irradiation therapy is to increase locoregional control and decrease systemic dissemination, particularly for patients with bulky tumors or massive adenopathy. Responses with interferon are equivocal (Fandi et al, 1994).

Cancer of the Oropharynx. Radiation therapy is the treatment of choice for early lesions of the tonsillar region. Methods to ease the effects of radiation xerostomia include using angled photon beams, electrons, and interstitial implants. T3 tonsillar tumors may be treated in various combinations of irradiation and surgery. Surgery may be used for salvage of radiation therapy failure, or irradiation may be given preoperatively or postoperatively (Sweeney et al., 1994). Treatment choices for T4 lesions follow much the same pattern but with reduced survival rates.

The base of the tongue is in an inaccessible location and rich in lymphatics, which results in patients presenting with palpable nodes. Radiotherapy, using external beam and occasional interstitial irradiation, is the usual choice of treatment.

With recent advances in surgical techniques several approaches are used: intraoral for small lesions, the rare mandibular resection, the common mandibulotomy, and the unconventional transhyoid, which sometimes eliminates the need for flap reconstruction (Wenig, 1994).

Flap reconstruction has revolutionized the approach to the tissue deficits left by tumor removal. The reliable and well-vascularized attached or free flaps often avoid the complications of bony reconstruction and the poor quality of radiated tissue (Wenig, 1994). An attached flap is myocutaneous tissue with or without bone with its blood supply connected to its origin. Examples of muscles used are the pectoralis major, trapezius, platysma, and latissimus dorsi. A free flap contains different types of tissue with its vessels dissected free and anastomosed to the recipient site vessels. Examples of tissue selected for free flaps are vascularized osseofascial, sensate fasciocutaneous, and motor-innervated musculocutaneous. Sites from which composite flaps (the addition of bone) are taken includes the internal oblique-iliac crest, fibula, radius, and scapula (Wenig, 1994). Selection of the type of flap warrants several considerations. For example, repair of glossectomy defects using motor-innervated musculocutaneous tissue provides volume and rapid healing. Rectus abdominis or latissimus dorsi flaps fit these criteria (Urken, Moscoso, Lawson, & Billar, 1994).

Cancer of the Hypopharynx. Cancers in this region are often late presenters requiring a combination of surgery and radiotherapy. Radiation therapy can be used alone for early lesions (Sweeney et al., 1994). Surgical ablation of tumor in this deep-lying area requires extensive excision and repair. A relatively new technique, CO_2 laser microsurgery, gives a bloodless field to more precisely identify tumor borders and retain as much function as possible (Wenig, 1994).

The choice of a neck dissection depends on the risk or presence of lymph node metastasis. Figure 37–3 and Table 37–5 describe and show the different levels of neck dissections.

Chemotherapy

For patients with newly diagnosed early-stage or localized advanced squamous cell carcinoma of the head and neck (SCCHN), the standard local treatment is surgery, radiation, or both. Local failure rate after surgery, radiotherapy, or both is frequently more than 50 per cent for stages T3, T4, and N1 to N3. In addition, without clinical evidence, 30 to 50 per cent of the neck dissections show lymph node involvement (Stupp, Weichselbaum, and Vokes, 1994). These generally disappointing results for the current stage III and IV therapies led to testing of other treatments, most notably chemotherapy. Chemotherapy is now considered a standard treatment option given the two following conditions: (1) distant metastatic disease in newly presenting or relapsed patients, and (2) local recurrent disease where salvage or palliation is not feasible (Browman & Cronin, 1994).

Stupp et al. (1994) summarized the results of chemotherapeutic effectiveness in treating head and neck cancers. (1) The few studies that have shown increased survival have used concomittant chemoradiotherapy. (2) Several chemotherapy induction studies have shown a reduction in distant metastasis and in-

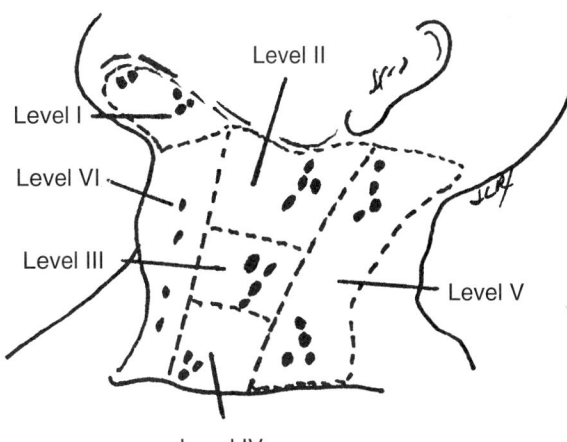

FIGURE 37–3. Levels of neck dissections with cervical lymph nodes. I = submental and submandibular; II = upper jugular; III = mid jugular; IV = lower jugular; V = posterior triangular; VI = anterior compartment-midline.

TABLE 37–5. *Types of Neck Dissections and Levels Involved*

Radical neck dissection
Levels I-V lymph node removal with cranial nerve XI (CNXI), internal jugular vein (IJV), and sternocleidomastoid muscle (SCM) removal.

Extended radical neck dissection
Removal of additional lymph groups or nonlymphatic structures in addition to the radical procedure.

Modified radical neck dissection
Levels I-V lymph node removal with one or more nonlymphatic structures (CNXI, IJV, or SCM).

Selective neck dissection
Preservation of one or more lymph node groups without removal of nonlymphatic structures.
   Supraomohyoid = Levels I, II, & III lymph node removal.
   Lateral = Levels II, III, & IV node removal.
   Posterolateral = Levels II, III, IV, & V lymph node removal.
   Anterior compartment = Level VI lymph node removal.

(Adapted from Robbins, K. T. [Ed.]. [1991]. *Pocket guide to neck dissection classification and TNM staging of head and neck cancer.* American Academy of Otolaryngology-Head and Neck Surgery Foundation, Inc. Alexandria, VA: Reproduced by permission.)

creased laryngeal preservation without reduction in overall survival. (3) Several studies using a variety of drugs and schedules along with concommitant radiotherapy have reduced local recurrence rates. The authors conclude that continued trials are necessary before chemotherapy can be considered a standard therapy in head and neck cancer.

The disappointing therapeutic effects of cytotoxic drugs caused other factors to be researched. Problematic is the differing responses to cytotoxic agents by patients who have similar degrees of disease and clinical features. Ensley & Maciorowski (1994) stress that success of research strategies "will require the identification...of mechanisms that underlie response and resistance to cytotoxic therapy" (p. 309). DNA diploid and aneuploid tumors have shown different behavior patterns. DNA diploid tumors tend to recur less in contrast to the aneuploid tumors. The aneuploid tumors, however, are more sensitive to cisplatinum-based chemotherapy (Ensley & Maciorowski, 1994).

Another factor that has drawn attention for head and neck cancer investigation is the p53 tumor marker. While Frank and associates (1994) concluded that p53 lacked significance as an indicator of survival, Field et al. (1991) found that an elevated p53 correlated with heavy smoking, indicating a genetic link.

Chemoprevention. In patients who are cured by standard treatments the threat of second primary tumors remains. The risk for the occurrence of second primary tumors (annual rate of 5 to 7 per cent) becomes the major cause of late cancer death. The concept of field cancerization, which proposes that an entire area of epithelium is at risk to develop malignancies because of exposure to carcinogens, applies to the upper aerodigestive tract. Attention is directed to premalignant lesions. Results of some studies suggest that retinoids, carotenoids, and α-tocopherol can reverse oral leukoplakia (Huber, Lippman, & Hong, 1994).

NASAL CAVITY AND PARANASAL SINUSES

DEFINITION

The nasal cavity connects laterally with the maxillary sinuses and superiorly with the frontal, ethmoid, and sphenoid sinuses. The nasal epithelium is interspersed with mucus-secreting glands and islands of squamous epithelium (Batsakis, 1979; Redmond, Sass, & Roush, 1982). The nasal passageway acts as a sieve, warmer, and humidifier for the inhaled air. The paranasal sinuses supply additional mucus to the nasal cavity (Rice & Stanley, 1987).

INCIDENCE, MORTALITY, AND SURVIVAL RATES

The annual adjusted incidence rates of sinonasal cancers (SNC) is 0.8 for men and 0.5 for women per 100,000 in the United States. According to the Third National Cancer Survey Incident Cases, the cancers occur most frequently in the internal nose and maxillary sinus, followed by the ethmoid sinus. Women have more cancers of the internal nose, whereas men have a greater proportion of maxillary sinus cancers (Redmond et al., 1982). Several studies have found up to 80 per cent of sinus cancers originating in the maxilla (Batsakis, 1979). Squamous cell carcinoma (SCC) is the most frequent neoplasm (80 to 90 per cent) in both the nose and sinus. Adenocarcinoma (7 to 15 per cent), transitional cell carcinoma, and sarcoma follow in decreasing order (Batsakis, 1979). Adenocarcinomas predominate in the ethmoid sinus, have a low frequency of metastatic spread, and occur more commonly before age 65 years. SCC develops more frequently in people over 65 years old (Klintenberg, Olofsson, Hellquist, & Sokjer, 1984).

Five-year relative survival rates for localized lesions are about double those of regional spread. The vast majority of tumors present at T3 and T4 (Stern et al., 1993). Five-year survival rates for these stages range from 35 to 46 per cent (Rosen et al., 1993). Local recurrence is the most common cause of failure, with 30 to 40 per cent of recurrences developing in the nasal cavity and ethmoidal-sphenoid complex. Kraus et al. (1992) reported that involvement of the dura, brain, nasopharynx, or sphenoid sinus foretold a poor prognosis from ethmoid sinus cancers. Survival rates for maxillary sinus SCC hover around 50 per cent regardless of treatment modality. The factor that predicts locoregional control and survival is the presence or development of regional disease (Stern et al., 1993). Treatment with radiation alone for unresectable lesions results in a 12 to 19 per cent 5-year survival rate. Malignant tumors of the paranasal sinuses involve the orbit and sinus wall in 60 per cent of the cases, of which 45 per cent will require exenteration (Conley & Baker, 1979).

RISK FACTORS

Data abstracted from the Registrar General in 1958, 1961, and 1971 for male workers in England and Wales consistently showed that the unskilled possessed a higher standardized mortality rate for sinonasal cancer than other classes of workers, particularly in the most recent 20 years (Fraumeni, 1978; Redmond et al., 1982). Luce et al. (1992) in France found that risk for adenocarcinomas of the sinonasal region was significantly increased for people who worked with wood, for example, cabinetmakers and carpenters. Significant risk for SCC, on the other hand, emerged for bakers, pastry cooks, and grain millers. Female textile workers showed increased risk for each cell type. The risk for SNC in farm workers was elevated for both sexes. Other environmental factors associated with SNC are bootmaking and shoemaking, nickel refining, chromium, paints, lacquers, glues, formaldehyde, wool dust, mustard gas, nitrosamines, and radium (Luce et al., 1992; Redmond et al., 1982). Because of the low incidence rate of sinonasal cancers in the general population, even a small increase in a group exposed to these substances is sufficient to constitute increased risk (Redmond et al., 1982).

SIGNS AND SYMPTOMS

Tumors arising from the paranasal sinuses are usually asymptomatic, and diagnosis occurs late in the disease progression, making successful treatment difficult. Moreover, symptoms may be present for several months before a definitive diagnosis is made, and bone destruction is likely to have occurred (Wang, 1983). Symptoms are often mistaken for upper respiratory infections or inflammation of the sinuses (Rice & Stanley, 1987). Stuffy noses, epistaxis, unilateral nasal obstruction, headaches, and facial pains appear months before other symptoms create suspicion. Facial deformation, orbital and dental displacement, cranial nerve involvement, and bone destruction herald advanced disease (Pearson, 1987). Tumors arising in the ethmoid sinus may cause a dull retro-orbital headache along with less common proptosis, diplopia, anosmia, and broadening of the nasal dorsum (Kraus et al., 1992). The staging for carcinoma of the sinuses is not as well established as that for other head and neck tumors. Definitions of tumor categories of maxillary sinus involvement are given in Table 37–4.

DIAGNOSIS

Knowing the extent of the tumor is paramount for determining treatment. This determination is based on a history and on direct and indirect examination of nasal cavity and nasopharynx. Computed tomographic scans and magnetic resonance imaging aid detection of bony and soft tissue changes.

MEDICAL TREATMENT

SURGERY AND RADIATION

Radiation or surgical removal or both is employed, depending on the extent of the tumor (Wang, 1983). Surgical intervention with irradiation has produced better results than irradiation alone. Survival rates have ranged from 29 to 48 per cent for combined therapies, compared with 10 to 34 per cent for irradiation alone (Tong, 1986).

The results of one recent study (Bjork-Eriksson, Mercke, Petruson, & Ekholm, 1992) shows promise with chemotherapy, preoperative irradiation, and limited surgery. The treatment plan avoided irradiation side effects of blindness, dry or painful eye, and brain necrosis while limiting surgical mutilation or cosmetic interference. Ten patients out of 12 were alive without evidence of disease after 27 months.

Surgical procedures may leave the patient with a severe facial deformity requiring specially made prosthetic devices to cover cavities and aid swallowing and articulation. These devices need to be skillfully made to minimize detection without hindering removal and reinsertion.

Craniofacial surgery has increased as an option to remove tumors involving the base of the skull. The team approach, incorporating head and neck surgeons, neurosurgeons, microvascular surgeons, radiologists, anesthesiologists, and prosthodontists, has helped to advance this therapy (Schramm, 1987). En bloc tumor resection from the base of the skull is now possible. Postoperative complications such as cerebrospinal fluid leak (the most common), meningitis, and flap failure are not uncommon due to the tumor site and extension (Irish et al., 1994). The patient and family must understand the potential dangers, expected functional ability, and possible complications. The sequelae, depending on the surgical approach and anatomic position of the tumor, may include loss of smell, loss of vision, numbness of the face, temporary facial paralysis, and facial deformities.

SALIVARY GLANDS

DEFINITION

The salivary glands are divided into the major glands, comprising the parotid, submandibular, and sublingual glands, and the minor salivary glands, found in the mucous membrane throughout the upper aerodigestive tract.

The triangularly shaped parotid gland extends from the zygomatic arch to below the mandible and from the sternocleidomastoid to the midportion of the masseter muscle. This gland lies deeply behind the ascending ramus of the mandible, anterior to the external auditory canal and mastoid process. The lobes of the parotid are distinguished on the basis of their location vis á vis the facial nerve. The portion of the gland overlying the facial nerve (80 per cent) is considered superficial, and that portion lying under the facial nerve (20 per cent) is called deep. The parotid or Stensen's duct penetrates the buccinator muscle from the anterior portion of the parotid and exits at the level of the second maxillary molar. The transverse facial artery (from the external carotid) and vein often run parallel to the duct (Johns & Kaplan, 1987).

The auriculotemporal nerve, arising from the mandibular branch of the trigeminal, supplies parasympathetic secretomotor innervation to the parotid. After parotidectomy, redness and sweating may occur over the distribution of this nerve after eating. This phenomenon, known as Frey's syndrome, results from faulty regeneration of the secretory nerve fibers to the sweat glands in the skin (Johns, 1980).

The submandibular gland lies within the space formed by the digastric muscle bellies, the inferior border of the mandible, the mylohyoid muscle, the hypoglossus muscle, and the genioglossus muscle. The marginal mandibular, lingual, and hypoglossal nerves traverse this area. The sublingual glands lie within the anterior floor of the mouth above the mylohyoid muscle and are in close proximity to the lingual and hypoglossal nerves. The minor salivary glands are scattered throughout the oral cavity and pharynx.

INCIDENCE, MORTALITY, AND SURVIVAL RATES

Malignant tumors of the major salivary glands are rare, the incidence rate being 0.8 to 1.0 per 100,000 for the years 1983 and 1984. Higher incidence rates occur in the older age groups in both sexes (see Table 37–3). Mortality during this same time frame was less than 1.0 per 200,000, slightly less than that during the three previous decades (Devesa et al., 1987). The parotid gland accounts for approximately 80 per cent of salivary gland neoplasms with about 20 to 30 per cent of the parotid tumors being malignant. Tumors of the submandibular and minor salivary glands are rare with adenoid cystic carcinoma being the most common tumor arising from the minor salivary glands (Garden et al., 1994). However, 60 to 88 per cent of those that do develop are malignant (Johns & Goldsmith, 1989a).

As with other cancers of the head and neck, the type of tumor, location, and extent of disease have a major effect on the outcome. Five-year survival rates differ widely between low-grade (96 per cent) and high-grade (51 per cent) tumors, as well as between staging levels (Spiro, 1985). Undifferentiated tumors record the worst survival rates for the parotid gland—30 to 44 per cent at 5 years and 22 to 25 per cent at 10 years (Johns, 1980).

RISK FACTORS

Occurrence of salivary gland tumors is associated with prior radiation exposure in the head and neck region. Persons living in or near Hiroshima have shown a 2.6 times higher incidence of salivary gland tumors than those not exposed to radiation from the atomic bomb (Takeichi, Hirose, & Yamamoto, 1976).

SIGNS AND SYMPTOMS

Malignant salivary neoplasms often appear as well-demarcated, localized, firm masses. A painful, large, firm preauricular mass with complete facial nerve paralysis is the classic picture of advanced malignant parotid tumor. However, pain is not necessarily an indication of malignancy (Johns & Goldsmith, 1989a). Most submandibular and minor salivary gland malignancies are manifested clinically as enlarging masses that may be tender or painful. If the tumor invades the lingual or hypoglossal nerves in the submandibular triangle, clumsiness of the tongue and loss of sensation may ensue (Boles, 1985).

DIAGNOSIS

Parotid tumors present a diagnostic problem because of their notorious heterogeneity. More than 20 categories of epithelial tumors exist with variations within some categories (Fechner, 1985).

Needle aspiration biopsy is viewed favorably as a diagnostic method. Johns and Kaplan (1987) state that the routine sialograms, radionuclide images, and ultrasonograms are not helpful in determining diagnosis and

rarely alter therapeutic approaches. Open biopsy is used to make a diagnosis when other methods have failed and to plan palliative radiation or chemotherapy (Johns & Kaplan, 1987).

MEDICAL TREATMENT

SURGERY AND RADIATION

A parotid tumor less than 4 cm in size can be removed by a subtotal parotidectomy that preserves the facial nerve (Spiro, 1985). Conversely, large stage III tumors require a radical parotidectomy with facial nerve sacrifice. Facial nerve repair with an autogenous nerve graft is accomplished at the time of surgery, and regional flaps are used to cover extensive resection. Large high-grade tumors are associated with limited survival, regardless of how radical a surgical procedure is performed (Spiro, 1985). Salivary glands were previously thought to be radiation-resistant. Current indications for irradiation include high-grade T1 and T2 tumors, all T3 and T4 tumors, positive regional nodes, recurrence, deep lobe cancers, residual disease, and tumor next to facial nerve (Garden et al., 1994; Johns & Goldsmith, 1989b). Most reports show the advantage of combined surgery and postoperative irradiation for advanced disease (Garden et al., 1994; Johns & Goldsmith, 1989b).

LARYNX

DEFINITION

The larynx extends from the superior tip of the epiglottis (anterior surface included) to the inferior margin of the cricoid cartilage. The larynx is divided into three regions—supraglottic, glottic, and subglottic (Fig. 37–4). Embryologically, the glottis develops from paired structures that fuse at the anterior commissure; this line of fusion serves to retard the spread of tumors. The absence of midline divisions in the supraglottis and subglottis allows tumors in these areas to spread circumferentially. In addition, anatomic structures that separate the supraglottis from the glottis and the subglottis from the glottis prevent extraglottic tumors from immediate extension into the glottis. Consequently, hoarseness develops later in the course of the disease, making early detection less frequent (van Nostrand, 1987). The supraglottis includes the epiglottis, aryepiglottic folds, ventricular folds (false vocal cords), ventricles, and arytenoids without their vocal extensions.

INCIDENCE, MORTALITY, AND SURVIVAL RATES

The 1994 estimated new laryngeal cancer cases numbers 12,500 with deaths estimated at 3800 (Table 37–1). The age-adjusted rates (per 100,000) for new cases of laryngeal cancer in the period from 1985 to 1989 were 8.3 and 1.7 for the males and females, respectively. Cancer of the larynx occurs in every country, with men consistently having a higher incidence rate

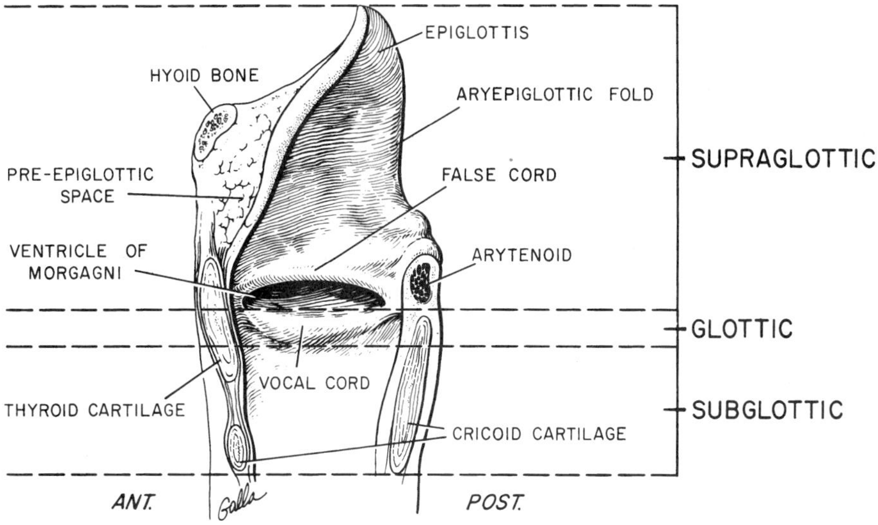

FIGURE 37–4. Diagram showing anatomic subdivision of the larynx into supraglottic, glottic, and subglottic. (From Wang, C. C. [1987]. Radiation therapy of laryngeal tumors: Curative radiation therapy. In S. E. Thawley & W. R. Panje [Eds.], *Comprehensive management of head and neck tumors* [Vol. 1, p. 906]. Philadelphia: W. B. Saunders Co. Reproduced by permission.)

than women. The higher incidence rate for African-Americans continues at 7.1 compared with whites, who have a rate of 4.6.

Thirty-year laryngeal cancer death rate trends (1958 to 1960 and 1988 to 1990) show an 87 per cent increase for females and a 6 per cent decrease for males (*Cancer facts and figures,* 1995). Both African-Americans and whites who are 65 years and older have more than a sevenfold and fivefold increase, respectively, in incidence compared with those under age 65 years of their own race. Death rates by age parallel the incidence rates. When compared with the younger members of their own race, older whites have a greater increase in death rates than do the older African-Americans (Table 37–6).

Overall laryngeal cancer survival rates have remained steady at 68 per cent for whites and have been slowly decreasing for African-Americans to a 54 per cent level since 1977 (Boring et al., 1992). The survival rates drop significantly between the stages of T2 and T3. T1 survival rates range from 95 to 99 per cent. T2 rates range from 76 to 97 per cent, T3 rates range from 40 to 85 per cent, and T4 rates range from 30 to 54 per cent (Mendenhall, Parsons, Stringer, Cassisi, & Million, 1990; Silver & Moisa, 1990). Reported rates vary given the type of treatment, sample number, staging ac-

curacy, and end point analysis (Terhaard et al., 1992). Without treatment, 90 per cent of persons afflicted with cancer of the larynx die within 3 years (Shimkin, 1951). Most tumor recurrence takes place within 3 years after treatment (Simpson, Robertson, & Lamont, 1993).

The most frequent abnormalities (90 per cent) arise from the squamous cell. The nonsquamous carcinomas make up no more than 1 per cent of all epithelial malignancies of the larynx. (Batsakis, Luna, & El-Naggar, 1992). Other cell types are verrucous carcinoma, carcinosarcoma, adenocarcinoma, lymphoma, and sarcoma. The squamous cell abnormality that will most likely become cancerous is keratosis with atypia (Romm, 1986).

RISK FACTORS

Laryngeal cancer, as with most other head and neck cancers, is closely associated with smoking and alcohol consumption. Using data from the Third National Cancer survey, Flanders and Rothman (1982) found a moderate synergy between alcohol and tobacco, with the resulting risk being approximately 50 per cent greater than if the effects of the two were simply additive. Smoking is associated with the development of squamous cell carcinoma in all portions of the larynx. In ad-

TABLE 37–6. *Incidence and Mortality Rate (1985–1989) for Laryngeal Cancer by Age, Sex, and Race**

AGE AT DIAGNOSIS	ALL RACES			AFRICAN-AMERICANS			WHITES		
	TOTAL	M	F	TOTAL	M	F	TOTAL	M	F
All ages	4.6	8.3	1.7	7.1	13.1	2.6	4.6	8.2	1.7
	(1.2)	(2.5)	(0.5)	(2.7)	(5.4)	(0.8)	(1.2)	(2.3)	(0.4)
Under 65	2.9	4.7	1.2	5.0	8.3	2.2	2.8	4.6	1.1
	(0.7)	(1.2	(0.3)	(1.8)	(3.3)	(0.6)	(0.6)	(1.0)	(0.2)
65 & older	20.5	40.7	6.4	26.6	57.3	6.0	20.6	40.9	6.7
	(7.2)	(14.7)	(2.3)	(11.0)	(24.2)	(2.6)	(6.9)	(14.0)	(2.3)

*SEER program. Rates are per 100,000 and age-adjusted to 1970 U.S. standard population.
( ) = mortality rates.
(Data from *Cancer statistics review 1973–1989*, National Cancer Institute, NIH Publication No. 92-2789, pp. xii, 4 & 5.)

dition, the type of cigarette smoked has a bearing on the incidence (De Stephani, Oreggia, Rivero, & Fierro, 1992; Wynder & Hoffman, 1982; Wynder & Stellman, 1977). Increased incidence of laryngeal cancer also occurs among persons who work with asbestos and wood. Communities in which paper, chemicals, or petroleum are manufactured show a higher incidence of laryngeal cancer (Cowles, 1983). Templar (1987) concluded that there is not enough evidence to link therapeutic radiation with increased occurrence of laryngeal tumors. Decreased amounts of vitamins A and C in the diet have been associated with increased risks of laryngeal cancer (Graham, Mettlin, & Marshall, 1981).

SIGNS AND SYMPTOMS

Persons who become hoarse see, on the average, three physicians in an attempt to identify the cause, and as many as 8 months can elapse before a diagnosis of laryngeal cancer is made. Any hoarseness that persists longer than 2 weeks should be evaluated by a physician skilled in throat examination techniques (Griffith, Meeker, & McMahan, 1979).

In a review of 85 patients with laryngeal cancer, 81 presented with hoarseness as the symptom of longest duration, while the four remaining presented with sore throat, stridor, hemoptysis, or otalgia. The mean duration of hoarseness was 8.4 months with a range of 1 to 48 months. A duration of hoarseness for 10.9 months placed 23 patients at the T3 stage (Reddy, Vinayak, Jefferis, & Wallace, 1993).

Symptoms depend on location, size, and degree of invasion (Table 37–7). If the tumor develops on a vocal fold, intermittent hoarseness appears early in the course of the disease, and the tumor can be diagnosed at stage I. Conversely, a tumor arising subglottically may progress to stage III before definitive symptoms appear. Supraglottic and subglottic tumors may be asympto-

matic until the vocal folds are involved or a suspicious node arises in the neck. A mild persistent sore throat may be the only indication of a stage II supraglottic tumor. At stage IV, symptoms become very similar regardless of the original tumor site: pain radiating to the ear, dysphagia, dyspnea, neck mass, and odynophagia (Templar, 1987). Otalgia can be referred from the tumor around the ninth and tenth cranial nerves (Jacobs, Goffinet, & Fee, 1990). Otalgia has been significantly related to the clinical presence of lymph nodes (Manni et al., 1992). Palpation of all the outer surfaces of the laryngeal skeleton is important to detect masses. Table 37–4 contains the definition of T categories for laryngeal tumors.

DIAGNOSIS

The diagnostic workup includes viewing the larynx with a mirror (indirect laryngoscopy), a flexible fiberoptic endoscope, or a laryngoscope—or all three. Radiographic studies, xerography, MRI, and CT add other dimensions to the diagnostic process.

MEDICAL TREATMENT

SURGERY AND RADIATION

Early glottic lesions constitute about 4.7 per cent of all laryngeal carcinomas (Fein et al., 1993). Early glottic lesions present a continuum from microscopic in situ to carcinomas involving both vocal cords without cord fixation. The most prognostically important sign is the mobility of the vocal cord.

Treatment options for this spectrum of early disease include transoral excision, open laryngeal procedures, and external beam radiotherapy (Thomas, Olsen, Neel, DeSanto, & Suman, 1994). All three modalities have demonstrated primary cure rates greater than 85 per cent with secondary salvage rates greater than 90 per cent (Myers, Wagner, & Johnson, 1994).

TABLE 37–7. *Signs and Symptoms of Cancer of the Larynx*

STAGE	SUPRAGLOTTIC	GLOTTIC	SUBGLOTTIC
I	Sensation of local irritation or no symptoms	Hoarseness if on mobile vocal fold	No symptoms
II	Sore throat, mild, persistent Hoarseness if vocal fold involved	Hoarseness Irritation of throat	Mild sensation of irritation or no symptoms
III	Sore throat, localized Hoarseness is probable Odynophagia Single neck mass, 3 cm on same side as other symptoms	Voice reduced to stage whisper Neck mass (possible)	Hoarseness if vocal folds are invaded Dyspnea if tumor is bulky
IV	Pain radiating to ear Hoarseness Odynophagia Neck mass Dysphagia Dyspnea	Pain radiating to ear Severe hoarseness Odynophagia Unilateral or bilateral nodes (probable) Dyspnea Cough	Pain referred to ear Neck mass Odynophagia Dysphagia Dyspnea

(From Templer, J. [1987]. Clinical evaluation of the larynx. In S. E. Thawley & W. R. Panje [Eds.], *Comprehensive management of head and neck tumors* [Vol. 1, p. 876]. Philadelphia: W. B. Saunders Co. Reproduced by permission.)

Transoral excision involves tumor removal by endoscopic laser resection or vocal cord stripping. Open laryngeal procedures include laryngofissure with cordectomy, frontolateral partial laryngectomy (anterior commissure technique), and hemilaryngectomy. Radiation doses vary from 4200 cGy to 6600 cGy. Of three types of treatment, the transoral excision is the most cost-effective (Myers et al., 1994).

A literature review by Fein and associates (1993) showed local control rates for glottic carcinoma in situ after primary treatment with radiotherapy, laser resection, and vocal cord stripping to be 84, 68, and 66 per cent, and quality of voice preservation 93, 100, and 88 per cent, respectively.

The cure for the Stage I vocal cord lesion is excellent because of the easily diagnosed early symptoms and confinement of the cancers to a rigid box with few lymphatics. Less than 1 per cent of these patients present with cervical metastasis (Ossoff & Matar, 1988). Also, local control is better for T2 tumors with vocal cord mobility than those with reduced vocal cord mobility (Slevin, Vasanthan, & Dougal, 1993). Vocal fixation, clinically evident cervical node metastasis, or both separate early stages (I and II) from the later stages (III and IV) (Silver & Moisa, 1990).

In most centers, radiotherapy represents the initial treatment for T1 and T2 lesions with surgery reserved for salvage of irradiation failures. The expected advantages of radiotherapy over surgical intervention are the better quality of voice, a major surgery is avoided, and it is less costly. During radiotherapy for T1 and T2 glottic tumors, patients will experience a transient worsening of the voice, dry desquamation of the treatment field skin, and a sore throat (Mendenhall et al., 1990).

Generally, treatment of T3 and T4 glottic lesions combines total laryngectomy with postoperative irradiation. This treatment also holds true for supraglottic lesions that involve the glottis (Silver & Moisa, 1990). The usual time period for starting postoperative irradiation is within 6 weeks, which tends to reduce local and regional recurrence compared with a longer time interval (Ampil, Buechter, Baiirnsfather, Shockley, 1993).

Irradiation as initial treatment for selected advanced laryngeal tumors usually produces a sore throat, loss of taste, and variable xerostomia because of the increased dosage and location of the irradiated field (Mendenhall et al., 1990). The survival rates for T3N0 tumors treated with radiotherapy have been reported to be equivalent to those achieved by initial laryngectomy (Guiney, Smith, Hughes, & Narayan, 1992). Although early stage T_1 supraglottic lesions can be treated with irradiation, if radiotherapy fails, a total laryngectomy must be performed (Kirchner & Owen, 1977). Postoperative complications include fistula formation and wound infections (Sheman & Spiro, 1986).

A supraglottic laryngectomy, while preserving the voice, invites aspiration. A total laryngectomy, on the other hand, avoids the problem of aspiration but requires a major adjustment in communication. Persons can learn to communicate by means of esophageal speech, artificial larynges, or voice buttons placed in a primary tracheoesophageal fistula.

NURSING MANAGEMENT

PREVENTION

The high correlation of smoking and alcohol consumption with head and neck cancer demands unrelenting education of the public and individual discouragement of usage by health professionals—who themselves do not smoke or abuse alcohol. In my opinion, the most potent deterrent to smoking and alcohol abuse for young people is a significant adult who does not smoke or abuse alcohol.

The nurse can operate in the prevention arena at several levels: contacting government representatives to condemn the political and economic advantages that the tobacco industry enjoys, supporting local or national groups that are trying to invoke laws curbing usage of addictive substances, and presenting educational programs in elementary and secondary schools as well as in the community at large. The opportunities to inform patients of the risks and to give information on where help can be obtained abound in the clinical setting. Of particular value is the nurse who has experienced withdrawal and can interact with a patient on a level unavailable to nurses who have not endured that process.

The newly diagnosed patients tend to be more receptive to changing their personal habits because of perceived vulnerability and knowing the results of that habit (Schleper, 1989). Teaching patients oral self-examination skills empowers them to improve their health status. Knowledge of the symptoms arising from cancerous lesions alerts patients to changes that otherwise may be discounted.

DETECTION

The higher incidence of cancer in older adults than in middle-aged adults requires the nurse who works with the elderly to be aware of the signs and symptoms of head and neck cancer. Institution of regular assessments for residents of extended care facilities may be successful in spotting early lesions during the quiet progression of head and neck tumors. Inspection of the oral cavity is of particular significance because asymptomatic cancerous lesions remain undetected. Mashberg and Samit (1989) describe these lesions as characterized by "innocuous-appearing red inflammatory or erythroplastic mucosal changes, …|the| lesions are less than 2 cm in diameter; are predominantly red, with or without a white component; and are smooth, granular, or minimally elevated." Schleper (1989) compiled a list of signs and symptoms related to specific structures of the head and neck (Table 37–8).

PATIENT PREPARATION FOR TREATMENT

Treatment methods include surgery, radiation, and chemotherapy (see Chapter 20 for nursing care related to irradiation). Surgical intervention for head and neck tumors ranges from minor to extremely complex. Preparation and continuing support of the patient to

TABLE 37–8. *Site-Specific Head and Neck Assessment and Symptoms*

Direct and Indirect Assessment	Signs and Symptoms

Larynx (Indirect assessment)
Supraglottis
  Epiglottis
  Aryepiglottic folds
  Arytenoid cartilages
  False vocal folds
Glottis
  True vocal folds
  Commissures
Subglottis
  Area below true vocal folds to inferior border of cricoid
    cartilage
  Rare site of tumor occurrence
	Inquire about:
	Supraglottis
	  Voice change—absence of higher pitched voice tones
	  Throat pain
	  Dysphagia, odynophagia
	  Referred otalgia
	  Stridor or dyspnea
	  Cervical adenopathy
	    Upper jugular
	    Mid jugular
	Glottis
	  Persistent hoarseness (hallmark symptom)
	  Sore throat
	  Stridor or dyspnea
	Subglottis
	  Same as glottis

Hypopharynx (Indirect assessment)
Absent thyroid cartilage crepitus when moving laryngeal
  framework over the cervical spine
	Inquire about:
	Throat pain
	Referred ear pain
	Dysphagia
	Cervical adenopathy
	  Upper jugular
	  Mid jugular

Cervical esophagus (Indirect assessment) "Silent area"	**Inquire about:** Dysphagia Recent unexplained weight loss of 10 lb or more Hemoptysis Regurgitation

Cervical lymphatics
Superior horizontal group
  Facing patient, palpate this U-shaped group of nodes:
    Preauricular and parotid
    Submandibular and submaxillary
    Submental
    Postauricular and mastoid
    Occipital
Vertical nodes
  Jugular chain (anterior to sternocleidomastoid muscle;
    palpate standing behind patient)
    Subdigastric and jugulodigastric
    Mid jugular
    Low jugular
  Posterior cervical or spinal accessory chain (anterior to
    trapezius; posterior to sternocleidomastoid)
  Check motor function of cranial nerve XI
Inferior horizontal nodes
  Supraclavicular (often indicative of distant metastasis)
	Palpate for:
	Nodes >1 cm
	Firm to hard consistency
	Limited mobility or fixed
	Spherical, matted, or poorly defined
	Nontender
	Subdigastric nodes: most common site for metastasis

Major salivary glands
Parotid
Submandibular
Sublingual
	Observe for:
	Mass over gland
	  With pain
	  Without pain
	Facial palsy
	Note swelling of duct openings in oral cavity

Assess symmetry of: Face Neck	**Inspect for:** Asymmetry or masses Deficits of cranial nerve VII Jugular distention

Inspect skin surfaces of:
Face
  Scalp
  Skinfolds
Neck
	Inspect for:
	Persistent ulcerations
	Pink, red, or white elevated lesions with a waxy appearance,
	  telangiectasias, and central umbilication or ulceration
	Inspect pigmented lesions for changes in color, size, shape,
	  surface, or elevation

TABLE 37–8. *Site-Specific Head and Neck Assessment and Symptoms* Continued

DIRECT AND INDIRECT ASSESSMENT	SIGNS AND SYMPTOMS
Nasal cavity, paranasal sinuses (indirect assessment of sinuses)—these tumors are often misdiagnosed	Inquire and observe for:
Frontal sinus	Asymmetry, pain or numbness over involved sinus, cheeks, upper alveolar ridge
Palpate under supraorbital margin	Proptosis, diplopia, epiphora, headaches
Ethmoid, maxillary	Unilateral nasal obstruction, bleeding, discharge, anosmia
Palpate infraorbital margin	In oral cavity: unexplained loosening of upper molars, upper denture, or upper partial plate.
Palpate under the inferior border of the maxilla and zygoma	
Assess motor functions of cranial nerves:	
III, IV, VI	
Sensory function of cranial nerve V	
Inspect nasal cavity for:	
Symmetry	
Discharge or odor	
Lesions or color changes	
Patency	
Optional: cranial nerve I	
Nasopharynx (Indirect assessment): "Silent" area. Symptoms are noted later than for other head and neck sites	Inquire and observe for:
Inspect tympanic membranes for:	Unilateral nasal obstruction
Bulging	Epistaxis or blood in postnasal drip
Retraction	Ear symptoms or the stopped-up ear
Fluid	Nasal voice quality
Intactness	Cervical adenopathy:
Color changes or lesions	Posterior cervical
Inspect nasal cavity (as above)	Jugular chain
Inspect soft palate for:	
Symmetry	
Oral cavity, oropharynx	Observe especially in the U-shaped area previously described for the following:
Inspect and palpate:	Painless color changes
Lips, buccal and labial mucosa	Erythroplasia
Gums, teeth (if present), or alveolar ridges	Leukoplakia
Retromolar trigones	Pigment changes
Hard and soft palates	Persistent ulcerations
Dorsal, ventral, lateral surfaces of oral tongue	Mass or thickening
(Check motor function of cranial nerves V, XII)	Unilateral or specific sore throat
Floor of mouth	Referred otalgia
Tonsillar fossae and pillars	Dysphagia, odynophagia
Base of tongue (mirror examination)	Pain, numbness, or tingling
Oropharyngeal wall: check motor functions of cranial nerves IX, X	Trismus, deficits of cranial nerves IX, X, or XII
	Cervical adenopathy
	Subdigastric
	Submandibular

(From Schleper, J. R. [1989]. Prevention, detection, and diagnosis of head and neck cancers. *Seminars in Oncology Nursing, 5,* 144–145. Reproduced by permission.)

meet this challenge on a day-to-day basis falls to the nurse.

PREOPERATIVE CARE

Sigler (1988) puts the nurse's preoperative assessment into perspective when she advises gaining some insight into the basic lifestyle of the patient. Areas to probe are usual daily activities, eating habits, living arrangements, and availability of the support of significant others. From this information, likely problems can be addressed. Explanations about incisions, tubes, alterations in airway, swallowing, or speech and changes in appearance must be given in terms and in ways the patient can understand.

POSTOPERATIVE CARE

Airway Management. Airway management for patients with surgery of the oral cavity or pharynx entails keeping the temporary tracheostomy patent. Instillation of sterile saline solution in small amounts (2 to 5 ml) stimulates coughing and allows easier expulsion of thick mucus. Suctioning with sterile equipment may be done as often as every hour depending on the amount of mucus produced. As the patient becomes more ambulatory, the ability to cough up secretions increases and the need for suctioning decreases. Humidification, by ultrasonic nebulization or oxygen mist, provides an essential element in liquefying secretions in the early postoperative period.

Usually plastic disposable cuffed tracheostomy tubes are used to prevent aspiration of oral secretions until the patient gains control of swallowing. I agree with Sigler's preference (1989) to release the cuff around the tracheostomy tube every shift to remove secretions that have collected above the cuff. The amount of tension the cuff exerts on the tracheal wall can be controlled by checking the amount of pressure in the cuff's bladder using a sphygmomanometer, 10 ml syringe, and stopcock.

The inner cannula holds the key to maintenance of a patent airway. It can be removed, without risking the loss of the airway, if it suddenly becomes plugged. Disposable versus reusable inner cannulas have been shown to save time in the cleansing procedure with no difference in the infection rate (Wagner & Sigler, 1988). After the need for a cuffed tracheostomy tube passes, it is replaced by a metal tracheostomy tube.

Corking of the tracheostomy tube allows evaluation of the patient's ability to breathe through the upper aerodigestive tract before removing the tube. If the patient has an adequate airway through the aerodigestive tract and can clear secretions through the mouth, the tracheostomy tube is removed. The tracheostomy incision closes without suturing by applying an airtight pressure dressing over it. The patient is instructed to press fingers over the dressing when coughing to prevent air flow from separating the incision.

If a total laryngectomy is performed, the sequence of events varies slightly with respect to the type of airway device used after the cuffed disposable plastic tube is removed. A plastic stent may be placed in the tracheal stoma to reduce contraction of the stomal opening.

Complications, such as fistula formation, may require reinsertion of a cuffed plastic tracheostomy tube. The cuffed tracheostomy tube prevents secretions from draining into the lungs and also provides a seal for mechanical hyperinflation of the lungs.

Regional Flap Management. The success of reconstructive surgery of the head and neck using a flap rests on the viability of that flap. The use of myocutaneous and free flaps revolutionized the surgical treatment of head and neck cancers. After surgery, the nurse's responsibility centers on maintaining flap viability (Reese, 1990). Because the myocutaneous flap crosses the neck to its destination or the anastomosing vessels for the free flap are in the neck region, all constricting items around the neck are avoided, such as gown ties, humidification mask cords, and tracheostomy ties. Plastic cuffed tracheostomy tubes may be held in place with sutures rather than ties the first few days after the operation. Humidification delivery by T-piece rather than mask obviates the use of an elastic band encircling the neck. The position of the patient's head can create external compression on the vessel pedicles (Urken et al., 1994). Changes in the temperature and color of a flap need to be reported immediately to the surgeon.

The blood flow in free flaps may be monitored with Doppler ultrasound. Loss of the Doppler signal indicates the need for immediate wound evaluation and possible exploration (Sigler, 1988). The donor site of the free flap requires observation also. If a radial free flap included bone, the arm will have a circumferential immobilizer. Checking blood flow signs and sensation in the fingers and keeping the arm elevated avoids problems caused by edema. The lower extremity with a fibular graft also requires elevation.

Neck dissection includes dermal lifting to expose the underlying structures and requires either pressure dressing or drain placement. The dermis must adhere to the underlying structures to reestablish its blood supply. Functioning drains help prevent the occurrence of hematomas or seromas. Drains are attached to collecting devices and are removed when the daily output becomes scant. In addition to measuring the drain output, the nurse observes the color of the drainage. If it becomes milky rather than reddish, chyle is leaking owing to accidental severance of a lymphatic duct during surgery.

Neck dissection incisions often leak serous fluid, which is removed with hydrogen peroxide followed by normal saline solution and sometimes ointment application. Draining material and its crusting around the tracheostomy stoma require gentle cleansing and application of a tracheostomy bib to absorb secretions. Zinc oxide ointment may be applied on the skin below the tracheostomy stoma for protection from secretions; however, the value of this action has not been established under controlled circumstances.

Communication. The patient with a tracheostomy is without a voice. The patient's call light or some other communication device must always be within reach. Labeling the public address apparatus with the room numbers of patients who cannot speak reminds nurses to tell the patient by public address that they will respond immediately when a call comes in. Paper and pen, flash cards, and pictorial boards are examples of ways in which the patient can let the nursing staff know what is needed. After removal of the tracheostomy tube, the patient may have difficulty with articulation as a result of the oral cavity or pharyngeal surgery. Listening and verifying the communication are essential nurse behaviors to gain the confidence of the patient.

For the patient who has had a total laryngectomy, the loss of voice is permanent. For those persons who have had hemilaryngectomies or supraglottic laryngectomies, the removal of the tracheostomy tube allows return of the voice, albeit somewhat altered from its original timbre. Loss of the voice results in an inability to sing, whistle, make quick verbal retorts, laugh, or change voice inflections. The voice conveys much more than words; it holds emotions—joy, pain, anger, fear, delight. This revelation of self to the world is gone for the laryngectomee. Replacements, such as with esophageal speech, the voice button, or the artificial larynges, give the laryngectomee a means to communicate, but they lack the expressiveness of the "normal" voice. Yet it is not unusual for an individual with a laryngectomy to overcome this handicap and continue a lifestyle with style.

Camouflaging the stoma may be important to some laryngectomees. Bibs, ascots, lace collars, or shirts with a tie provide cover for appearance in public and prevent inhalation of small particles. The laryngectomee must unlearn some reflexes: covering the mouth when coughing, blowing on liquids to cool them, and blowing the nose. Other restrictions include prohibition of swimming or fishing from a boat. As the integration of this change occurs within the self, the patient may develop depression, especially if alternative forms of communication are difficult and if talking was a major way of meeting emotional needs.

Nutrition. Nutrition can be a problem preoperatively as well as postoperatively for the head and neck cancer patient. Preoperatively, patients often suffer from deficient intake owing to alcoholism or dysphagia. Postoperatively, a patient may have insufficient intake because of swallowing difficulties and aspiration (Box 37–1). This is particularly true of patients who have had surgery that interferes with the changing positions of the upper areodigestive tract structures that control swallowing (Logemann, 1989).

The process of swallowing encompasses four phases: oral preparation and the oral, pharyngeal, and esophageal phases. The functions of any one of these phases or combinations thereof can be altered with surgery. Drooling, pocketing of food in the lateral sulcus, and losing food into the pharynx while chewing are examples of swallowing problems (Logemann, 1989). Procedures that are used to help with swallowing include postural changes and alterations in food consistencies, exercises to strengthen muscles and increase jaw range of motion, and exercises with specific instructions to change the coordination of the swallow (Logemann, 1989). (See Chapter 51 for nutritional needs of the cancer patient.) Patients will frequently have a feeding tube in place while the areodigestive surgical site is healing. The administration of formula can produce abdominal discomforts such as fullness, cramping, nausea, and vomiting. Diarrhea accompanies tube feedings regularly. Reese et al. (in review) found that formulas with fiber reduced the risk of diarrhea in male head and neck surgical cancer patients.

Psychosocial Aspects. Persons who have cancer of the head and neck often have a history of alcoholism and, with it, lack of close personal relationships, unstable work histories, and dysfunctional family interactions. Characteristics of dependence, inability to change habits, and poor adaptive coping skills make adjustment to the disfigurement and dysfunction from the treatment methods especially difficult (Dropkin, 1989). Other factors that impede adjustment are isolation, fear of rejection, negative changes in family interaction, and the patient's dependence on physical appearance for self-concept.

The alterations in appearance and function of speech, swallowing, or breathing require self-image adjustments and learning of self-care tasks. Dropkin (1989) postulates that the increase in performance of tasks occurs between postoperative days 4 and 5 because of the interaction between staff and the teaching of new tasks, which decrease the patient's initial anxiety about interaction with others. Task performance by the patient was interpreted as acceptance of the physical change and usually preceded social affiliative behaviors (see Chapter 61 for discussion of alterations in body image).

Box 37–1. *Altered Swallowing Processes*

Logemann, J. A. (1985). Aspiration in head and neck surgical patients. *Annals of Otology, Rhinology, Laryngology, 94,* 373–376.

One of the major problems occurring after surgical removal of aerodigestive tract cancer is aspiration with swallowing. This study identified what sequence of the swallowing process is altered with several types of surgical treatments for cancer of the aerodigestive tract that result in aspiration.

A total of 30 patients were studied, of whom 16 had partial laryngectomies, 13 had surgically treated oral cancer, and one had a resection of the posterior pharyngeal wall. Of the 16 patients with partial laryngectomy, 5 had hemilaryngectomies and 11 had supraglottic laryngectomies.

A videofluorographic examination using three consistencies of barium and two views yielded information to appraise the swallowing sequence. The patients with hemilaryngectomies had normal oral control of the bolus during the oral stages of the swallow and a normal swallowing reflex. The problems occurred in the laryngeal adduction and reduced pharyngeal peristalsis phases. The patients with supraglottic laryngectomies showed aspiration before, during, and after the swallow. Most prevalent problems were reduced vocal fold adduction and reduced laryngeal elevation. For the oral cancer patient groups, different deglutition problems occurred depending on the site of the resection. Those patients with anterior composite resection showed only oral disorders. All of them aspirated before the swallow because of reduced tongue control and because part of the bolus entered the pharynx before swallowing was begun. The lateral composite patients showed either a delayed swallowing reflex, reduced tongue control, or reduced pharyngeal peristalsis. Eight patients showed a combination of problems.

The information about the effect of food consistency showed that there is no single best food consistency that aids swallowing for dysphagic patients. The food consistency should be matched with the physiology of each patient's swallow.

The author strongly recommends that a modified barium swallow be the method used to attain the correct information about the physiology of a patient's swallowing, because this uses a small amount of food and keeps the radiographic tube focused on the oral cavity and pharynx for 10 to 30 seconds after the swallow. Identifying the cause of aspiration in the head and neck cancer patient results in application of the correct management technique for improved swallowing.

If the family interaction is dysfunctional, a spouse or significant other can hinder the progress of the patient in accepting physical changes and taking care of physical needs. Trying to alter long-standing interaction patterns during the short hospitalization period is unrealistic. Giving information about what to expect, both physically and psychologically; listening to concerns and giving direction; and including significant others in home care planning will—it is hoped—provide some stability for the patient and family. The quality of life for head and neck cancer patients is a relatively new research interest. The retention of as much function as possible in the areas of cosmesis, speech, and eating while maintaining survival rates has always been a concern. The potential effects of treatment on these functions are frequently considered as a part of treatment planning and selection (Logemann, 1994). However, the physical and psychosocial aftermath from the patients' perspective has been missing (Morris, 1994).

Not all patients who have major head and neck surgery are alcoholics or have dependency needs. Many travel through the grieving process without unusual aberrations and retain their self-esteem despite physical changes. The team approach, with nurses coordinating the work of social workers, pastors, dietitian, speech therapists, physical therapists, and surgeons for physical and psychosocial support of the patient, increases the probability of a better life adjustment to the treatment outcomes.

REFERENCES

Ampil, F. L., Buechter, K. J., Baiirnsfather, L.E., & Shockley, W. W. (1993). Timing and dosage of postoperative radiotherapy for squamous cell carcinoma of the upper aerodigestive tract. *Journal of Oral Maxillofacial Surgery, 51*(11), 1194–1197.

Andersson, G., & Axéll, T. E. (1989). Clinical appearance of lesions associated with the use of loose and portion-bag packaged Swedish moist snuff: A comparative study. *Journal of Oral Pathology Medicine, 18*(1), 2–7.

Austen, D. F. (1982). Larynx. In D. Schottenfeld & J. F. Fraumeni (Eds.), *Cancer epidemiology and prevention* (pp. 554–563). Philadelphia: W. B. Saunders Co.

Axéll, T. E. (1993). Oral mucosal changes related to smokeless tobacco usage: Research findings in Scandinavia. *Oral Oncology, European Journal of Cancer, 29B*(4), 299–302.

Banoczy, J. (1977). Follow-up studies in oral leukoplakia. *Journal of Maxillofacial Surgery, 5,* 69–75.

Baranovsky, A., & Myers, M. H. (1986). Cancer incidence and survival in patients 65 years of age and older. *CA: A Cancer Journal for Clinicians, 36,* 26–41.

Batsakis, J. G. (1979). Cancer of the nasal cavity and the paranasal sinuses. In J. G. Batsakis (Ed.), *Tumors of the head and neck* (2nd ed., pp. 177–178). Baltimore: Williams & Wilkins.

Batsakis, J. G. (1987). Pathology of tumors of the oral cavity. In S. E. Thawley & W. R. Panje (Eds.), *Comprehensive management of head and neck tumors* (Vol. 1, pp. 480–515). Philadelphia: W. B. Saunders Co.

Batsakis, J. G., Luna, M. A., & El-Naggar, A. (1992). Nonsquamous carcinomas of the larynx. *Annals of Otology Rhinology Laryngology, 101*(12), 1024–1026.

Beahrs, O. H., Henson, D. E., Hutter, R. V. P., & Kennedy, B. J. (Eds.). (1992). *Manual for Staging of Cancer* (4th ed.), American Joint Committee on Cancer. Philadelphia: J. B. Lippincott Co.

Bjork-Eriksson, T., Mercke, C., Petruson, B., & Ekholm, S. (1992). Potential impact on tumor control and organ preservation with cisplatin and 5-fluorouracil for patients with advanced tumors of the paranasal sinuses and nasal fossa: A prospective pilot study. *Cancer, 70*(11), 2615–2620.

Boles, R. (1985). Carcinoma of the submandibular minor salivary glands. In P. B. Chretien, M. E. Johns, D. P. Shedd, E. W. Strong, & P. H. Ward (Eds.), *Head and neck cancer* (Vol. 1, pp. 225–227). Proceedings of the International Conference, Baltimore, 1984. St. Louis: C. V. Mosby Co.

Boring, C. C., Squires, T. S., Tong, T., & Montgomery, S. (1994). Cancer statistics, 1994. *Ca-A Cancer Journal for Clinicians, 44*(1), 7–26.

Boring, C. C., Squires, T. S., & Heath, C. W. (1992). Cancer statistics for African Americans. *Ca-A Cancer Journal for Clinicians, 42*(1), 7–17.

Browman, G. P., & Cronin, L. (1994). Standard chemotherapy in squamous cell head and neck cancer: What we have learned from randomized trials. *Seminars in Oncology, 21*(3), 311–319.

Cancer facts and figures—1995 (1995). Atlanta: American Cancer Society, Inc.

Cancer statistics review, 1973—1989. National Cancer Institute, NIH Publication No. 92-2789, pp. xix, 4 & 5.

Cassisi, N. J. (1987). Clinical evaluation of pharyngeal tumors. In S. E. Thawley & W. R. Panje (Eds.), *Comprehensive management of head and neck tumors* (pp. 614–629). Philadelphia: W. B. Saunders Co.

Centers for Disease Control and Prevention, (1989). Tobacco use among high school students—United States, 1990. *Morbidity, Mortality, Weekly Reports, 40,* 617–619.

Conley, J., & Baker, D. L. (1979). Management of the eye socket in cancer of the paranasal sinuses. *Archives of Otolaryngology, 105,* 702–705.

Cowles, S. R. (1983). Cancer of the larynx: Occupational and environmental association. *Southern Medical Journal, 76,* 894–898.

De Stephani, E., Oreggia, F., Rivero, S., & Fierro, L. (1992). Hand-rolled cigarette smoking and risk of cancer of the mouth, pharynx and larynx. *Cancer, 70*(3), 679–682.

Devesa, S. S., Silverman, D. T., Young, J. L., Jr., Pollack, E. S., Brown, C. C., Horm, J. W., Percy, C. L., Myers, M. H., McKay, F. W., & Fraumeni, J. F., Jr. (1987). Cancer incidence and mortality trends among whites in the United States, 1947–1984. *Journal of the National Cancer Institute, 79,* 701–770.

Dropkin, M. J. (1989). Coping with disfigurement and dysfunction after head and neck cancer surgery: A conceptual framework. *Seminars in Oncology Nursing, 5,* 213–219.

Elias, E. G. (1986). Surgical management of head and neck neoplasia. In D. E. Peterson, E. G. Elias, & S. T. Sonis (Eds.), *Head and neck management of the cancer patient* (pp. 255–274). Boston: Martinus Nijhoff.

Ensley, J. F., & Maciorowski, Z. (1994). Clinical applications of DNA content parameters in patients with squamous cell carcinomas of the head and neck. *Seminars in Oncology, 21*(3), 330–339.

Fandi, A., Altun, M., Azli, N., Armand, J. P., & Cvitkovic, E. (1994). Nasopharyngeal cancer: Epidemiology, staging, and treatment. *Seminars in Oncology, 21*(3), 382–397.

Fein, D. A., Mendenhall, W. M., Parsons, J. T., Stringer, S. P., Cassisi, N. J., & Million, R. R. (1993). Carcinoma *in situ* of the glottic larynx: The role of radiotherapy. *International Journal of Radiation Oncology Biology Physics, 27*(2), 379–384.

Fechner, R. E. (1985). Diagnosis of salivary gland neoplasms. In P. B. Chretien, M. E. Johns, D. P. Shedd, E. W. Strong, &

P. H. Ward (Eds.), *Head and neck cancer* (Vol. 1, pp. 219–222). Proceedings of the International Conference, Baltimore, 1984. St. Louis: C. V. Mosby Co.

Field, J. K., Spandidos, D. A., Malliri, A., Gosney, J. R., Yiagnisis, M., & Stell, P. M. (1991). Elevated P53 expression correlates with a history of heavy smoking in squamous cell carcinoma of the head and neck. *British Journal of Cancer, 64*(3), 573–577.

Flanders, W. D., & Rothman, K. J. (1982). Interaction of alcohol and tobacco in laryngeal cancer. *American Journal of Epidemiology, 115,* 371–379.

Foote, R. L., Schild, S. E., Thompson, W. M., Buskirk, S. J., Olsen, K. D., Stanley, R. J., Kunselman, S. J., Schaid, D. J., & Grill, J. P. (1994). Tonsil cancer: Patterns of failure after surgery alone and surgery combined with postoperative radiation therapy. *Cancer, 73*(10), 2638–2647.

Frank, J. L., Bur, M. E., Garb, J. L., Kay, S., Ware, J. L., Sismanis, A., & Neifeld, J. P. (1994). p53 tumor suppressor oncogene expression in squamous cell carcinoma of the hypopharynx. *Cancer, 73*(1), 181–186.

Fraumeni, J. F., Jr. (1978). Geographic distribution of the head and neck cancers in the United States. *Laryngoscope* (Suppl. No. 8)*88,* 40–43.

Garden, A. S., Weber, R. S., Ang, K. K. Morrison, W. H., Matre, J., & Peters, L. J. (1994). Postoperative radiation therapy for malignant tumors of minor salivary glands: Outcome and patterns of failure. *Cancer, 73*(10), 2563–2569.

Graham, S., Mettlin, C., & Marshall, J. (1981). Dietary factors in the epidemiology of cancer of the larynx. *American Journal of Epidemiology, 113,* 675–680.

Griffith, G. L., Meeker, W. R., & McMahan, A. (1979). Management of carcinoma of the larynx. *Journal of the Kentucky Medical Association, 77,* 169.

Guiney, M., Smith, J., Hughes, P., & Narayan, K. (1992). Radiation therapy of glottic carcinoma: Peter MacCallum Cancer Institute experience. *Australia, New Zealand Journal of Surgery, 62*(8), 622–627.

Harnsburger, H. C., & Dillon, W. P. (1987). Imaging tumors of the central nervous system and extracranial head and neck. *CA: A Cancer Journal for Clinicans, 37,* 225–245.

Harrison, L. B., & Pfister, D. G. (1991). Chemotherapy as part of the initial treatment for nasopharyngeal cancer. *Oncology, 5*(2), 67–70.

Hosal, I. N., Onerci, M., Kaya, S., & Turan, E. (1992). Squamous cell carcinoma of the lower lip. *American Journal of Otolaryngology, 13*(6), 363–365.

Huber, M. H., Lippman, S. M., & Hong, W. K. (1994). Chemoprevention of head and neck cancer. *Seminars in Oncology, 21*(3), 366–375.

Irish, J. C., Gullane, P. J., Gentili, F., Freeman, J., Boyd, J. B., Brown, D., & Rutka, J. (1994). Tumors of the skull base: Outcome and survival analysis of 77 cases. *Head & Neck, 16*(1), 3–10.

Jacobs, C. D., Goffinet, D. R., Fee, W. E., Jr. (1990). Head and neck squamous cancers. In C. M. Haskell (Ed.), *Current problems in cancer* (Vol. 14, no. 1, pp. 9–16). Chicago: Yearbook Medical Publishers.

Johns, M. E. (1980). Parotid cancer: A rational basis for treatment. *Head and Neck Surgery, 3,* 132–141.

Johns, M. E., & Goldsmith, M. M. (1989a). Current management of salivary gland tumors (Part 1). *Oncology, 3*(2), 47–56.

Johns, M. E., & Goldsmith, M. M. (1989b). Current management of salivary gland tumors (Part 2). *Oncology, 3*(3), 85–91.

Johns, M. E., & Kaplan, M. J. (1987). Surgical therapy of tumors of the salivary glands. In S. E. Thawley & W. R. Panje (Eds.). *Comprehensive management of head and neck tumors* (pp. 1104–1138). Philadelphia: W. B. Saunders Co.

Jones, A. S. (1994). Prognosis in mouth cancer: Tumour factors. *Oral Oncology, European Journal of Cancer, 30B*(1), 8–15.

Kajanti, M. J., Holsti, L. R., & Mantyla, M. M. (1992). Postoperative radiotherapy of squamous cell carcinoma of the tonsil: Factors influencing survival and time to recurrence. *Acta Oncologica, 31*(1), 49–52.

Kirchner, J. A., & Owen, J. R. (1977). Five hundred cancers of the larynx and pyriform sinus. *Laryngoscope, 87,* 1288–1303.

Klintenberg, C., Olofsson, J., Hellquist, H., & Sokjer, H. (1984). Adenocarcinoma of the ethmoid sinuses. *Cancer, 54,* 482–488.

Kornblut, A. D. (1987). Clinical evaluation of tumors of the oral cavity. In S. E. Thawley & W.R. Panje (Eds.), *Comprehensive management of head and neck tumors* (pp. 460–479). Philadelphia: W. B. Saunders Co.

Kovalic, J. J., & Simpson, J. R. (1993). Carcinoma of the hard palate. *Journal of Otolaryngology, 22*(2), 118–120.

Kraus, D. H., Sterman, B. M., Levine, H. L., Wood, B. G., Tucker, H. M., & Lavertu, P. (1992). Factors influencing survival in ethmoid sinus cancer. *Archives of Otolaryngology Head Neck Surgery, 118*(4), 367–372.

Lampe, H. B., Lampe, K. M., & Skillings, J. (1986). Head and neck cancer in the elderly. *Journal of Otolaryngology, 15,* 235–238.

La Vecchia, C., Franceschi, S., Levi, F., Lucchini, F., & Negri, E. (1993). Diet and human oral carcinoma in Europe. *Oral Oncology, European Journal of Cancer, 29B*(1), 17–22.

Lee, A. W. M., Poon, Y. F., Foo, W. (1992). Retrospective analysis of 5037 patients with nasopharyngeal carcinoma treated during 1976–1985: Overall survival and patterns of failure. *International Journal of Radiation Oncology Biology Physics, 23,* 261–270.

Liebowitz, D. (1994). Nasopharyngeal carcinoma: The Epstein-Barr virus association. *Seminars in Oncology, 21*(3), 376–381.

Logemann, J. (1994). Rehabilitation of the head and neck cancer patient. *Seminars in Oncology, 21*(3), 359–365.

Logemann, J. A. (1989). Swallowing and communication rehabilitation. *Seminars in Oncology Nursing, 5,* 205–212.

Luce, D., Leclerc, A., Morcet, J., Casal-Lareo, A., Gerin, M., Brugere, J., Haguenoer, J., & Goldberg, M. (1992). Occupational risk factors for sinonasal cancer: A case-control study in France. *American Journal of Industrial Medicine, 21*(2), 163–175.

Mahboubi, E., & Sayed, G. B. (1982). Oral cavity and pharynx. In D. Schottenfeld & J. F. Fraumeni, Jr. (Eds.), *Cancer epidemiology and prevention* (pp. 583–595). Philadelphia: W. B. Saunders Co.

Mak-Kregar, S., Baris, G., Lebesque, J. V., Balm, A. J. M., Hart, A. A. M., Hilgers, F. J. M. (1993). Radiotherapy of tonsillar and base of the tongue carcinoma. Prediction of local control. *Oral Oncology, European Journal of Cancer, 29B*(2), 119–125.

Manni, J. J., Terhaard, C. H. J., de Boer, M. F., Croll, G. A., Hilgers, F. J. M., Annyas, A. A., van der Metj, A., & Hordijk, G. J. (1992). Prognostics factors for survival in patients with T$_3$ laryngeal carcinoma. *The American Journal of Surgery, 164*(6), 682–687.

Marks, J. E. (1987). Treatment of tumors of the hypopharynx: Radiation therapy. In S. E. Thawley & W. R. Panje (Eds.), *Comprehensive management of head and neck tumors* (pp. 756–774). Philadelphia: W. B. Saunders Co.

Mashberg, A., Garfinkel, L., & Harris, S. (1981). Alcohol as a primary risk factor in oral squamous carcinoma. *CA: A Cancer Journal for Clinicians, 31,* 146–155.

Mashberg, A., & Samit, A. M. (1989). Early detection, diagnosis, and management of oral and oropharyngeal cancer. *CA: A Cancer Journal for Clinicians, 39,* 67–88.

McGuirt, W. F. (1979). Complications of radical neck dissection: A survey of 788 patients. *Head and Neck Surgery, 1,* 481–487.

McGuirt, W. F. (1983). Head and neck cancer in women—a changing profile. *Laryngoscop, 93,* 106–107.

Mendenhall, W. M., Parsons, J. T., Stringer, S. P., Cassisi, N. J., & Million, R. R. (1990). The role of radiation therapy in laryngeal cancer. *Ca: A Cancer Journal for Clinicians, 40*(3), 150–165.

Mitchell, R., & Crighton, L. E. (1993). The management of patients with carcinoma of the tongue. *British Journal of Oral and Maxillofacial Surgeons, 31*(5), 304–308.

Morris, J. (1994). Widening perspectives: Quality of life as a measure of outcome in the treatment of patients with cancers of the head and neck. *Oral Oncology, European Journal of Cancer, 30B*(1), 29–31.

Muir, C. S. (1967). The oral cavity. In R. W. Raven & F. J. C. Roe (Eds.), *The prevention of cancer* (pp. 71–77). London: Butterworths.

Myers, E. N., Wagner, R. L., & Johnson, J. T. (1994). Microlaryngoscopic surgery for T1 glottic lesions: A cost-effective option. *Annals of Otology Rhinology Laryngology, 103*(1), 28–30.

Ossoff, R. H., & Matar, S. A. (1988). The advantages of laser treatment of tumors of the larynx. *Oncology, 2*(9), 58–60.

Panje, W. R. (1987). Treatment of tumors of the nasopharynx: Surgical therapy. In S. E. Thawley & W. R. Panje (Eds.), *Comprehensive management of head and neck tumors* (Vol. 1, pp. 662–683). Philadelphia: W. B. Saunders Co.

Parsons, J. T., & Million, R. R. (1987). Radiation therapy of tumors of the oral cavity. In S. E. Thawley & W. R. Panje (Eds.), *Comprehensive management of head and neck tumors* (Vol. 1, pp. 516–535). Philadelphia: W. B. Saunders Co.

Pearson, B. W. (1987). Surgical therapy of the nasal cavity and paranasal sinuses. In S. E. Thawley & W. R. Panje (Eds.), *Comprehensive management of head and neck tumors* (Vol. 1, pp. 353–367). Philadelphia: W. B. Saunders Co.

Peterson, D. E., Overholser, C. D., Jr., Bergman, S. A., & Beckerman, T. (1986). Initial detection and evaluation: Intraoral neoplasms. In D. E. Peterson, E. G. Elias, & S. T. Sonis (Eds.), *Head and neck management of the cancer patient* (pp. 163–177). Boston: Martinus Nijhoff.

Reddy, K. T. V., Vinayak, B. C., Jefferis, A. F., & Wallace, M. (1993). Primary radiotherapy for treating all laryngeal cancer: A district hospital experience. *The Journal of Laryngology and Otology, 107*(5), 434–436.

Redmond, C. K., Sass, R. E., & Roush, G. C. (1982). Nasal cavity and paranasal sinuses. In D. Schottenfeld & J. F. Fraumeni, Jr. (Eds.), *Cancer epidemiology and prevention* (pp. 519–535). Philadelphia: W. B. Saunders Co.

Reese, J. L. (1990). Nursing interventions for wound healing in plastic and reconstructive surgery. *Nursing Clinics of North America, 25*(1), 223–233.

Reese, J. L., Clearman, B., Colwill, M., Dawson, C., Hanrahan, K., & Means, M. E. (in review). Diarrhea associated with nasogastric tube feedings. *Oncology Nursing Forum.*

Rice, D. H., & Stanley, R. B., Jr. (1987). Surgical therapy of nasal cavity, ethmoid sinus, and maxillary sinus tumors. In S. E. Thawley & W. R. Panje (Eds.), *Comprehensive management of head and neck tumors* (pp. 368–389). Philadelphia: W. B. Saunders Co.

Robbins, K. T. (Ed.). (1991). *Pocket guide to neck dissection classification and TNM staging of head and neck cancer.* Alexandria, VA: American Academy of Otolaryngology-Head and Neck Surgery Foundation, Inc.

Romm, S. (1986). Cancer of the larynx. Current concepts of diagnosis and treatment. *Surgical Clinics of North America, 66,* 109–118.

Rosen, A., Vokes, E. E., Scher, N., Haraf, D., Weichselbaum, R. R., & Panje, W. R. (1993). Locoregionally advance paranasal sinus carcinoma: Favorable survival with multimodality therapy. *Archives Otolaryngology Head Neck Surgery, 119*(7), 743–746.

Saracci, R. (1985). Occupation. In M. P. Vessey & M. Gray (Eds.), *Cancer risks and prevention* (pp. 99–118). Oxford: Oxford University Press.

Sarkaria, J. N., & Harari, P. M. (1994). Oral tongue cancer in young adults less than 40 years of age: Rationale for aggressive therapy. *Head & Neck, 16*(2), 107–111.

Schleper, J. R. (1989). Prevention, detection, and diagnosis of head and neck cancers. *Seminars in Oncology Nursing, 5,* 139–149.

Schramm, V. L., Jr. (1987). Craniofacial surgery for sinus tumors. In S. E. Thawley & W. R. Panje (Eds.), *Comprehensive management of head and neck tumors* (Vol. 1, pp. 390–407). Philadelphia: W. B. Saunders Co.

Shah, J. P., Shemen, L. J., & Strong, E. W. (1987). Buccal mucosa, alveolus, retromolar trigone, floor of mouth, hard palate, and tongue tumors. In S. E. Thawley & W. R. Panje (Eds.), *Comprehensive management of head and neck tumors* (Vol. 1, pp. 551–563). Philadelphia: W. B. Saunders Co.

Sheman, L. J., & Spiro, R. H. (1986). Complications following laryngectomy. *Head and Neck Surgery, 8,* 185–191.

Shimkin, M. B. (1951). Duration of life in untreated cancer. *Cancer, 4,* 1–8.

Sigler, B. A. (1988). Nursing care of the head and neck cancer patient. *Oncology, 2*(12), 49–53.

Sigler, B. A. (1989). Nursing care of patients with laryngeal cancer. *Seminars in Oncology Nursing, 5,* 160–165.

Silver, C. E., & Moisa, I. I. (1990). The role of surgery in the treatment of laryngeal cancer. *Ca-A Cancer Journal for Clinicians, 40*(3), 134–149.

Silverberg, E. (1984). Cancer Statistics, 1984. *Ca-A Cancer Journal for Clinicians, 34*(1), 14–15.

Silverberg, E. (1983). Cancer Statistics, 1983. *CA: A Cancer Journal for Clinicians, 33,* 17.

Silverberg, E., & Lubera, J. (1986). Cancer Statistics, 1986. *CA: A Cancer Journal for Clinicians, 36,* 20.

Silverberg, E., & Lubera, J. (1987). Cancer Statistics, 1987. *CA: A Cancer Journal for Clinicians, 37,* 3–19.

Silverberg, E., & Lubera, J. (1989). Cancer Statistics, 1989. *CA: A Cancer Journal for Clinicians, 39,* 3–20.

Simpson, D., Robertson, A. G., & Lamont, D., 1993. A comparison of radiotherapy and surgery as primary treatment in the management of T3N0M0 glottic tumours. *The Journal of Laryngology and Otology, 107*(10), 912–915.

Sisson, G. A. (1985). Cancer of the oral cavity. In P. B. Chretien, M. E. Johns, D. P. Shedd, E. W. Strong, & P. H. Ward (Eds.), *Head and neck cancer* (Vol. 1, pp. 168–169). Proceedings of the International Conference, Baltimore, 1984. St. Louis: C. V. Mosby Co.

Slevin, N. J., Vasanthan, S., & Dougal, M. (1993). Relative clinical influence of tumor dose versus dose per fraction on the occurrence of late normal tissue morbidity following larynx radiotherapy. *International Journal of Radiation Oncology Biology Physics, 25*(1), 23–28.

Spiro, R. H. (1985). Tumors of the parotid gland. In P. B. Chretien, M. E. Johns, D. P. Shedd, E. W. Strong, & P. H. Ward (Eds.), *Head and neck cancer* (Vol. 1, p. 223). Proceedings of the International Conference, Baltimore, 1984. St. Louis: C. V. Mosby Co.

Steele, G. D., Jr., Winchester, D. P., Menck, H. R., & Murphy, G. P. (1993). Clinical highlights from the National Cancer Data Base: 1993. *Ca-A Cancer Journal for Clinicians, 43*(2), 71–82.

Stern, S. J., Goepfert, H., Clayman, G., Byers, R., Ang, K. K., El-

Naggar, A. K., & Wolf, P. (1993). *Archives of Otolaryngology Head Neck Surgery, 119*(9), 964–969.

Stupp, R., Weichselbaum, R. R., & Vokes, E. E. (1994). Combined modality therapy of head and neck cancer. *Seminars in Oncology, 21*(3), 349–258.

Sweeney, P., Haraf, D. J., Vokes, E., Dougherty, M., & Weichselbaum, R. R. (1994). Radiation therapy in head and neck cancer: Indications and limitations. *Seminars in Oncology, 21*(3), 296–303.

Takeichi, N., Hirose, F., & Yamamoto, H. (1976). Salivary gland tumors in atomic bomb survivors, Hiroshima, Japan. I. Epidemiologic observations. *Cancer, 38*, 2462–2468.

Templer, J. (1987). Clinical evaluation of the larynx. In S. E. Thawley & W. R. Panje (Eds.), *Comprehensive management of head and neck tumors* (Vol. 1, pp. 868–886). Philadelphia: W. B. Saunders Co.

Terhaard, C. H. J., Hordjik, G. J., van den Broek, P., de Jong, P. C., Snow, G. B., Hilgers, F. J. M., Annyas, A. A., Tjho-Hesling, R. E., & de Jong, J. M. A. (1992). T3 laryngeal cancer: A retrospective study of the Dutch Head and Neck Oncology Cooperative Group: Study design and general results. *Clinical Otolaryngology, 17*(5), 393–402.

Thawley, S. E., & Sessions, D. G. (1987). Surgical therapy of hypopharyngeal tumors. In S. E. Thawley & W. R. Panje (Eds.), *Comprehensive management of head and neck tumors* (Vol. 1, pp. 774–812). Philadelphia: W. B. Saunders Co.

Thomas, J. V., Olsen, K. D., Neel III, H. B., DeSanto, L. W., & Suman, V. J. (1994). Early glottic carcinoma treated with open laryngeal procedures. *Archives of Otolaryngology Head & Neck Surgery, 120*(3), 264–268.

Thomas, S., & Kearsly, J. (1993). Betel quid and oral cancer: A review. *Oral Oncology, European Journal of Cancer, 29B*(4), 251–255.

Tong, D. Y. (1986). Radiotherapeutic management of head and neck neoplasia. In D. E. Peterson, E. G. Elias, & S. T. Sonis (Eds.), *Head and neck management of the cancer patient* (pp. 275–297). Boston: Martinus Nijhoff.

Urken, M. L. Moscoso, J. F., Lawson, & Billar, H. F. (1994). A systemic approach to functional reconstruction of the oral cavity following partial and total glossectomy. *Archives Otolaryngology Head Neck Surgery, 120*(6), 589–601.

van Nostrand, A. W. P. (1987). Pathology of laryngeal tumors. In S. E. Thawley & W. R. Panje (Eds.), *Comprehensive management of head and neck tumors* (Vol. 1, pp. 887–905). Philadelphia: W. B. Saunders Co.

Wagner, R. L., & Sigler, B. (1988). The efficacy of a disposable inner cannula in tracheostomy associated with head and neck surgery. *Society of Otorhinolaryngology Head Neck Nursing, 6*(2), 13–17.

Wang, C. C. (1983). *Radiation therapy for head and neck neoplasms: Indications, techniques and results* (pp. 213–221). Boston: John Wright, PSG Inc.

Weber, A. L., & Manzione, J. V. (1986). Diagnostic radiology for head and neck neoplasms with emphasis on computerized tomography. In D. E. Peterson, E. G. Elias, & S. T. Sonis (Eds.), *Head and neck management of the cancer patient* (pp. 191–199). Boston: Martinus Nijhoff.

Weiland, L. H. (1987). Pathology of pharyngeal tumors. In S. E. Thawley & W. R. Panje (Eds.), *Comprehensive management of head and neck tumors* (Vol. 1, pp. 630–648). Philadelphia: W. B. Saunders Co.

Wenig, B. (1994). The role of surgery in head and neck cancer: Standard care and new horizons. *Seminars in Oncology, 21*(3), 289–295.

Wray, A., & McGuirt, F. (1993). Smokeless tobacco usage associated with oral carcinoma. *Archives of Otolaryngology, Head Neck Surgery, 119*(9), 929–933.

Wynder, E. L., & Hoffman, D. (1982). Tobacco. In D. Schottenfeld & J. F. Fraumeni (Eds.), *Cancer epidemiology and prevention* (pp. 277–292). Philadelphia: W. B. Saunders Co.

Wynder, E. L., & Stellman, S. D. (1977). Comparative epidemiology of tobacco related cancer. *Cancer Research, 37*, 4608–4622.

Zheng, T., Boyle, P., Willet, W. C., Hu, H., Dan, J., Evstifeeva, T. V., Niu, S., & MacMahon, B. (1993). A case-control study of oral cancer in Beijing, People's Republic of China. Associations with nutrient intakes, foods and food groups. *Oral Oncology, European Journal of Cancer, 29B*(1), 45–55.

Zheng, X., Christensson, B., & Drettner, B. (1993). Studies on etiological factors of nasopharyngeal carcinoma. *Acta Otolaryngology* (Stockholm), *113*(3), 455–457.

CHAPTER
38

Endocrine Cancers

Bonny Libbey Johnson

Endocrine tumors as a group are relatively rare, and oncology nurses have only limited chances to care for patients with these cancers. However, the care of these patients is challenging, and the details of the natural history and treatment for each tumor type remain fascinating and complex. The clinical behavior of the endocrine tumors ranges from the most indolent to the most virulent. The disease presentation is highly variable and frequently combines tumor symptoms with unusual endocrine syndromes. Knowledge of the pathophysiologic processes involved guides the history and physical assessment and provides a scientific basis for educating patients about their disease and its management.

Advances in the treatment of endocrine tumors have generally been slow. Randomized clinical trials to evaluate new treatment approaches and studies to identify characteristics of the diseases and prognostic variables are difficult to conduct because of the rarity of these tumors and the resultant inadequate patient accrual. Current research focuses on the use of endocrine tumor markers for both diagnostic and therapeutic purposes as well as the role of immunomodulation in treatment regimens.

THYROID CANCERS

INCIDENCE

Although they account for 90 percent of endocrine cancers, thyroid neoplasms account for just over 1 per cent of all cancers and approximately 0.2 per cent of cancer deaths (Wingo, Tong, & Bolden, 1995). Incidence is higher in women than in men by a ratio of almost 3:1, and the majority of cases occur in people between the ages of 25 and 65 years (Norton, Levin & Jensen, 1993, Wingo et al., 1995).

RISK FACTORS

Radiation exposure to the head and neck area, especially in infancy and childhood, is a well-documented etiologic factor for thyroid cancers (Favis et al., 1976; Refetoff et al., 1975; Schneider et al., 1985; Wilson, Platz, & Block, 1970). Before the 1950s, there was a widespread practice of treating benign diseases, such as tonsillitis, sinusitis, and acne, with radiation. In 1950, the first reports of postirradiation thyroid carcinoma in children raised the possibility of irradiation as an etiologic factor (Duffy & Fitzgerald, 1950) (Box

38–1). Risk is dose-dependent; however, at a total dose of 2000 cGy, the risk begins to decline (Norton et al., 1993). There is an inverse relationship between risk for thyroid cancer and age at the time of exposure, with children under the age of 10 years at greatest risk (Ron et al., 1987). Generally a latency period of 5 to 10 years elapses after exposure before thyroid tumors develop, but an increased risk for development of these cancers persists for at least 35 years in exposed subjects (Schneider et al., 1985). In contrast, no relationship has been established between the use of radioactive iodine (^{131}I) therapy for Graves disease and the development of thyroid cancer (Holm, Dahlquist, Israelsson, & Lundell, 1980).

An association may exist between chronic stimulation of secretion of thyroid-stimulating hormone (TSH) secondary to severe iodide restriction or partial thyroid gland resection and the development of well-differentiated thyroid tumors (Williams, 1979).

Medullary thyroid cancer (MTC) is transmitted genetically as an autosomal-dominant trait in approximately 25 per cent of cases as part of multiple endocrine neoplasia (MEN) syndrome (Alexander & Norton, 1991; Saad et al., 1984).

PROGNOSTIC FACTORS

Important prognostic factors include histologic type, age, and extent of disease at the time of diagnosis, with histologic features being the greatest determinant of overall survival (Kerr et al., 1986). Patients with papillary carcinoma, those under 50 years of age, and those with limited disease have the most favorable prognosis. A symptom cluster of dysphonia, dysphagia, and dyspnea appears to confer a worse prognosis and probably reflects locally invasive disease (Kerr et al., 1986). In medullary thyroid carcinoma, gender has also been identified as a prognostic factor, with women having a significantly better prognosis (Schroder et al., 1988).

CLASSIFICATION AND STAGING

Malignant thyroid neoplasms have been divided into four major types, although other rarer forms of primary thyroid cancer (e.g., sarcoma, lymphoma) make up approximately 5 per cent of the total. The histologic classification of the major types of thyroid carcinomas is given in Table 38–1. The American Joint Committee on Cancer has incorporated histologic type and age in its most recent staging system of thyroid cancer because of the prognostic significance of these factors (Table 38–2) (Beahrs, Henson, Hutter, & Myers, 1992).

BIOLOGY AND NATURAL HISTORY

Papillary and follicular carcinomas are well differentiated cancers that closely resemble their tissue of origin within the thyroid gland (Table 38–1). These tumors generally follow an indolent clinical course even in the presence of nodal involvement or distant metastases, whereas the anaplastic (undifferentiated) types behave more aggressively and are associated with severe morbidity secondary to rapid invasion of contiguous structures (Leeper, 1985). Undifferentiated, or anaplastic carcinomas, do not resemble thyroid tissue and are nonfunctioning, and death frequently occurs within months of diagnosis (Demeter, DeJong, Lawrence, & Paloyan, 1991). A histologic progression from well- to poorly differentiated carcinoma has been suspected in cases in which there is a sudden change in the rate of growth in a known papillary adenocarcinoma (Mazzaferri, Young, Oertel, Kemmerer, & Page, 1977). This may reflect end-stage behavior in the natural history of that tumor.

Medullary carcinoma of the thyroid (MCT) originates from thyroid parafollicular C cells and varies in its clinical behavior due to the secretion of calcitonin as well as other active hormones (Philippe, 1992). The majority of patients show an indolent course, but those patients with the familial form that occurs with MEN

BOX 38–1. *Cancer of the Thyroid in Children*

Duffy, B. J., & Fitzgerald, P. J. (1950). Cancer of the thyroid in children: A report of 28 cases. *Journal of Clinical Endocrinology, 10,* 1296–1308.

Sample: Twenty eight children between the ages of 4 and 18 years with carcinoma of the thyroid.

Purpose of Study: These authors analyzed the records of all patients in the above sample for the purposes of (1) examining the tumor characteristics and biologic behavior of cancer of the thyroid in children, (2) identifying possible etiologic factors, and (3) emphasizing the importance of including thyroid cancer in the differential diagnosis of tumors of the neck in children.

Results: The most significant finding of this study was that 9 of 28 patients who developed thyroid cancer had been treated with external radiation for "enlargement of the thymus." Twenty-six of 28 patients had cervical lymph node involvement at diagnosis; 23 of 28 patients had well-differentiated thyroid cancers; and the age of onset correlated with puberty in 25 cases.

Discussion: In addition to providing descriptive information pertaining to histology, progression of disease, and treatment of thyroid cancer in this sample, Duffy and Fitzgerald were the first investigators to examine the relationship between external irradiation of the head and neck and the development of thyroid cancer. Although the authors were reluctant, at that time, to propose a cause-and-effect relationship between these irradiation practices and the development of cancer, their studies raised questions prompting further analysis of cases of childhood thyroid cancer and, ultimately, identified head and neck irradiation during childhood as a definitive etiologic factor.

TABLE 38–1. *Major Malignant Tumors of the Thyroid*

TYPE	INCIDENCE	DISTINGUISHING CHARACTERISTICS	PATTERN OF METASTASES	PROGNOSIS
Papillary	Most common type in United States; totals 50%–60% of thyroid tumors; mean age is 42 years; women > men	Indolent, slow growth; can be aggressive in older patients; usually multifocal; may be bilateral	50% metastasize; tends to spread locally, usually to cervical and mediastinal nodes	Even with metastases, prognosis is excellent; younger patients have poorer prognosis; many patients have normal life span with no symptoms
Follicular	Represents 18%–25% of thyroid cancers; peak age range is 50–60 years; affects more men than women at an older age	Occurs more in iodine-deficient areas; often presents as solitary nodule that is encapsulated; fine-needle aspiration (FNA) cannot distinguish between benign and malignant follicular cells; Hurthle cell tumors are subgroup	Nodal spread; tends to adhere to trachea, skin, muscle, and great vessels, which then causes symptoms such as dysphagia; spread is usually by bloodstream or direct extension of a locally invasive tumor	Small, localized tumors have good prognosis; stage is valid prognostic factor; capsular or vascular invasion has poor prognosis
Medullary (solid)	Approximately 5%–10% of thyroid cancers; peak age range is 50–60 years; equal numbers of men and women	Familial in 20% of cases; found in both lobes of thyroid, with multiple endocrine neoplasia (MEN) vs one lobe with sporadic MTC type; secretes calcitonin; is associated with increased carcino-embryonic antigen (CEA), endocrine disorders, and pheochromocytoma	Invades surrounding structures; spreads by blood and lymphatic systems; tends to metastasize early	50% 10-year survival; high cure rate if no palpable tumor; familial type has better prognosis
Anaplastic	10%–18% of thyroid cancers; highest incidence between 60 and 80 years of age; women outnumber men	Highly aggressive, lethal tumor; sometimes divided into spindle, giant, and small cell disease	Widespread early; all considered stage IV regardless of extent; invades neck structures	Nearly 0% 2-year survival

(Reprinted with permission from Baker, K. H., & Feldman, J. E. [1993]. Thyroid cancer: A review. *Oncology Nursing Forum, 20,* 96.)

IIB (Table 38–3) have a particularly aggressive form of the disease (Norton et al., 1993; Saad et al., 1984).

CLINICAL MANIFESTATIONS

On physical examination of the head and neck, the thyroid is inspected and palpated for symmetry and masses, and the neck is examined for adenopathy (Baker & Feldman, 1993). The gland should also be assessed for tenderness, enlargement, and fixation. Frequently, an asymptomatic mass discovered incidentally by the patient or on routine physical examination is the first indication of disease. A preexisting, painless thyroid nodule that changes rapidly as well as any nodule larger than 4 cm raises the suspicion of a malignant process. A fixed nodule, local cervical adenopathy, and associated symptoms such as dysphonia, dysphagia, or airway obstruction are suggestive of later stages of disease (Wool, 1993).

Anaplastic masses are more likely to have symptoms indicative of local invasion or compression: hoarseness, dysphagia, stridor, and referred ear pain (Leeper, 1985). Symptoms of hormonal imbalance may be present if tumor growth has resulted in actual destruction of the thyroid gland or if the tumor itself is producing excess thyroid hormone. A severe, watery diarrhea syndrome is seen in approximately 25 per cent of cases of MCT with an increased incidence in advanced disease (Saad et al., 1984).

TABLE 38–2. *Staging Classification of Thyroid Cancer*

Papillary or Follicular Thyroid Cancer

Stage I	Patients < 45 years of age Any T, Any N, M0 Patients ≥ 45 years of age T1, N0, M0
Stage II	Patients < 45 years of age Any T, Any N, M1 Patients ≥ 45 years of age T2, N0, M0 T3, N0, M0
Stage III	Patients ≥ 45 years of age T4, N0, M0 Any T, N1, M1
Stage IV	Patients ≥ 45 years of age Any T, Any N, M1

Medullary Thyroid Cancer

Stage I	T1, N0, M0
Stage II	T2–4, N0, M0
Stage III	Any T, N1, M0
Stage IV	Any T, Any N, M1

Undifferentiated Thyroid Cancer
All cases are Stage IV

Stage IV	Any T, Any N, Any M

Definition of TNM
Primary Tumor (T)
TX: Primary tumor cannot be assessed
T0: No evidence of primary tumor
T1: Tumor 1 cm or less in greatest dimension limited to the thyroid
T2: Tumor more than 1 cm but not more than 4 cm in greatest dimension limited to the thyroid
T3: Tumor more than 4 cm in greatest dimension limited to the thyroid
T4: Tumor of any size extending beyond the thyroid capsule

Regional Lymph Nodes (N)
N: Regional lymph nodes cannot be assessed
N0: No regional lymph node metastasis
N1: Regional lymph node metastasis
   N1a: Metastasis in ipsilateral cervical lymph node(s)
   N1b: Metastasis in bilateral, midline, or contralateral cervical or mediastinal lymph node(s)

Distant Metastasis (M)
MX: Presence of distant metastasis cannot be assessed
M0: No distant metastasis
M1: Distant metastasis

Note: All categories may be subdivided into (A) solitary tumor and (B) multifocal tumor (the largest determines the classification).
(From Beahrs, O. H., Henson, D. E., Hutter, R. V. P, & Myers, M. H. [Eds.]. [1992]. *Manual for staging of cancer* [4th ed., pp. 53–54. Philadelphia: J. B. Lippincott Co. Reproduced by permission.)

DIAGNOSTIC EVALUATION

Although the incidence of thyroid nodules is common, the development of cancer within a nodule is relatively uncommon. Diagnosis remains difficult due to the nonspecific nature of the tests used to evaluate nodules. Signs of thyroid hormone excess or deficiency may be present; however, most patients with thyroid cancer have normal levels of TSH, triiodothyronin (T3), and thyroxine (T4) (Norton et al., 1993). Thyroid scan will determine whether the lesion is "hot" (functional), "cold," or "warm," but biopsy is necessary to make a diagnosis of cancer; while malignant tumors are generally "cold," both "hot" and "warm" nodules may also be malignant.

The fine-needle aspiration biopsy (FNAB) becomes a first-line diagnostic tool in the evaluation of thyroid nodules (Friedman, Toriumi, & Mafee, 1988; Wool, 1993). It is the only method that can differentiate benign from malignant nodules with a high degree of accuracy. Fine-needle aspiration is performed by introducing a 22-gauge needle into the nodule and aspirating tissue for cytologic examination. Fine-needle aspiration has a reported false-negative rate of 0.3 to 10 per cent and a false-positive rate of 0 to 2.5 per cent (Frable, 1986). Results are classified as follows: class 0 (insufficient material), class 1 (benign), class 2 (suspicious), and class 3 (frankly malignant) (Wool, 1993). In a series of 848 patients undergoing FNAB, 78 per cent had benign nodules, 20 per cent were suspicious, and 12 per cent had a malignancy (Hamburger, 1987). Fine-needle aspiration cytology has resulted in fewer patients undergoing unnecessary surgery and more definitive diagnoses of malignant thyroid nodules. A cutting needle biopsy is preferred if the nodule is >4 cm or when lymphoma is suspected (Norton et al., 1993).

Radionuclide scanning is indicated when fine-needle aspiration is inadequate, the findings reveal benign changes, or the thyroid is diffusely enlarged (Friedman et al., 1988). Scans provide useful clinical information regarding the functional status of a nodule but lack specificity in differentiating malignant from benign tissue. Functional nodules are those that produce and secrete thyroid hormones. They are called "hot" nodules because the radioactive isotope is concentrated in the nodule and appears as an area of increased uptake on the scan. Because most malignant nodules produce lower amounts of thyroid hormones than normal thyroid tissue, they appear "cold" on scan. Technetium-99m is the preferred agent for initial thyroid scanning. A follow-up scan with radioactive iodine may be performed to confirm a true functional or "hot" nodule noted on a technetium-99m scan (Friedman et al., 1988).

Ultrasonography is used to measure the size of a thyroid lesion and to determine whether other nodules or local adenopathy exists; however, it cannot differentiate a benign lesion from a malignant tumor (Norton et al., 1993). Other purposes include evaluating changes in the size of thyroid nodules after thyroxine-suppressive therapy, guiding fine-needle aspiration, and detecting recurrent disease. Both magnetic resonance imaging (MRI) and computed tomography (CT) scans provide information for treatment planning by delineating the extent of disease within the thyroid and surrounding structures (Friedman et al., 1988).

Thyroid function studies are nondiagnostic for cancer. Only the measurement of serum calcitonin may be helpful in confirming a diagnosis of MCT, since MCT is a tumor of calcitonin-secreting cells. This test is used as a tumor marker for the detection and postoperative management of patients with MCT (Norton et al., 1993). Recently, plasma levels of calcitonin gene-re-

TABLE 38–3. *Multiple Endocrine Neoplasia (MEN) Syndromes*

CHARACTERISTIC	MEN-I	MEN-IIA	MEN-IIB
Medullary thyroid carcinoma	Absent	Present in all cases (indolent)	Present in all cases (more virulent)
Parathyroid hyperplasia	Present in 80%–90%	Present	Rare
Pancreatic involvement	Present in 80%–90%	Absent	Absent
Pituitary involvement	Present	Absent	Absent
Pheochromocytoma	Absent	Present	Present
Adrenal cortex tumors	Present	Absent	Absent
Other thyroid tumors	Present	Absent	Absent
Common presenting signs and symptoms	Hypercalcemia kidney stones, peptic ulcers, hypoglycemia, headache; Zollinger-Ellison syndrome in 20% of cases	Symptoms of hypertension: headache, dizziness	Signs of MTC: mucosal neuromas, bony abnormality, puffy eyes, prominent jaw

lated peptide have been used to diagnose MCT as well as determine the presence of metastases (Carter, Taylor, Kao, & Heath, 1991).

TREATMENT

Surgery. Surgery is recommended as initial therapy for all thyroid cancers, but the extent of the surgery and postoperative treatment vary and continue to be areas of controversy among clinicians (Leeper, 1985; McConahey, Hay, Woolner, vanHeerden, & Taylor, 1986, Norton et al., 1993). Rational selection of a therapeutic approach should take into consideration age, histologic type, and extent of disease as they relate to prognosis.

Although total lobectomy may be an acceptable procedure in papillary carcinoma when the lesion is less than 2 cm and confined to one lobe, there is a high probability that microscopic foci exists in the contralateral lobe. Therefore, many clinicians suggest at least a near-total or a total thyroidectomy in all well-differentiated and medullary cancers of the thyroid because of the much higher incidence of recurrence in patients treated with less radical surgery and the relative safety of the procedure when performed by experienced surgeons (Norton et al., 1993). Lateral lymph node dissection is recommended for patients with clinical lymphadenopathy or positive preoperative thyroid scan.

Nursing management requires an awareness of the potential complications that can occur. Postoperatively, patients should be observed for signs of tetany, because hypoparathyroidism occurs in 6 to 8 per cent of patients (Mazzaferri et al., 1977; McConahey et al., 1986). If some parathyroid tissue has been preserved or transplanted to local muscle tissue, normal function

will gradually return. In the interim, however, hypocalcemia may occur, and patients should be monitored with daily serum calcium levels and close observation for Chvostek's sign (tingling or twitching around the mouth or face), Trousseau's phenomenon (muscle spasms), as well as other symptoms of hypocalcemia (Baker & Feldman, 1993). The likelihood of permanent hypoparathyroidism is significantly higher in patients undergoing total thyroidectomy, and these patients may require lifelong administration of calcium and vitamin D replacement.

Bilateral damage to the recurrent laryngeal nerves during surgery results in permanent vocal cord paralysis in less than 2 per cent of cases and occurs more frequently in patients undergoing second resection for residual disease (McConahey et al., 1986, Herranz-Gonzalez, Gavilan, Marinez-Vidal, & Gavilan, 1991). With near-total thyroidectomy, the nerve on one side may be salvaged, and resulting hoarseness will be temporary.

Unless a patient has experienced respiratory distress due to extensive local disease, airway complications generally are a transient intraoperative and early postoperative management problem. However, nurses should be alert to the possibility of respiratory obstruction, which can result from (1) recurrent laryngeal nerve damage, which can cause vocal cord spasms, (2) tracheal compression from hemorrhage, (3) local edema, or (4) tetany (Baker & Feldman, 1993).

Patients should be monitored for 12 to 24 hours after surgery for hemorrhage. Excessive bleeding can be assessed by checking the back of the surgical dressing under the neck and shoulders. The patient is kept in semi-Fowlers position, and humidified oxygen is provided. Respiratory distress, a sensation of choking, hoarseness, or dysphagia may indicate bleeding into and compression of adjacent structures. An emergency tracheostomy set should be kept at the bedside.

Because of the loss of endocrine function after all or part of the thyroid gland is removed, most patients are given thyroid replacement to prevent hypothyroidism. Levothyroxine (Synthroid) is the most commonly used preparation.

Radiation Therapy. Starting about 4 to 6 weeks after surgery, ^{131}I therapy is used for the ablation of thyroid remnants. ^{131}I is also used for the treatment of known residual or metastatic disease outside the confines of the thyroid (Greenfield, 1987). For ^{131}I therapy to exert its antitumor effect, the tumor must be sufficiently well differentiated to concentrate and retain the radioisotope. Thus, ablation and treatment with ^{131}I is not indicated in medullary or undifferentiated thyroid cancers, which are unable to concentrate and retain this radioisotope (Table 38-1). ^{131}I treatment is indicated following surgery for patients with tumors 2 to 4 cm in size, for patients whose tumors are >4 cm with direct invasion of local structures, or for patients with distant metastases (Norton et al., 1993).

The purpose of ^{131}I ablation is to destroy any remaining ^{131}I-concentrating tissues in the thyroid bed and create a hypothyroid state that stimulates increased secretion of TSH (Freitas, Gross, Ripley, & Shapiro, 1985). This prepares the patient for ^{131}I therapy by promoting uptake of ^{131}I in remaining tumor deposits and metastatic foci. Exogenous administration of bovine TSH may be required if residual tumor is secreting enough thyroid hormone to suppress endogenous TSH (Blahd, 1985). It should be used cautiously because of the high incidence of hypersensitivity reactions with repeated doses.

In contrast to ^{131}I ablation, in which a relatively fixed dose of radioactive iodine is given, optimal ^{131}I therapy requires dosimetry calculations to deliver the maximally tolerated dose with minimal toxicity (Freitas et al., 1985). Systemic effects include nausea and vomiting, inflammation of the salivary glands, bone marrow suppression, and, rarely, pulmonary radiation fibrosis and leukemia (Freitas et al., 1985). Treatment doses are given at 4- to 6-month intervals until there is no evidence of functioning tumor on whole-body imaging studies (Leeper, 1985). Thyroid hormone replacement is restarted immediately after therapy to permanently suppress TSH, which may act as a growth stimulus for thyroid follicular cells (Greenfield, 1987).

Patients generally require inpatient admission for administration of ^{131}I owing to the higher doses given for therapy. Radiation precaution procedures are instituted and may vary among hospitals, but sample guidelines are listed in Table 38-4 (Greenfield, 1987). Refer to Chapter 20 for other considerations relating to brachytherapy.

External irradiation can be used with or without ^{131}I for patients with inoperable, residual, or metastatic differentiated thyroid cancers. With this approach, local control of residual disease has been reported in tumors with poor ^{131}I uptake (Tubiana et al., 1985). Treatment of anaplastic carcinomas with ^{131}I and exter-

nal irradiation has not been effective due to the radioresistance of this type of thyroid neoplasm, but a study combining a hyperfractionated radiation therapy schedule with low-dose doxorubicin as a radiosensitizer for hypoxic, radioresistant tumor cells has yielded excellent results with local control (Kim & Leeper, 1983; Tennvall et al., 1990). External radiation may also be used to palliate pain due to bone metastases.

Chemotherapy. To date, the role of chemotherapy in the treatment of advanced thyroid cancer has been limited to palliation in patients with locally uncontrolled or widely metastatic disease (Norton et al., 1993). Only doxorubicin has demonstrated any significant antitumor activity, with response rates of 38 per cent (Ahuja & Ernst, 1987).

ADRENAL CANCER: ADRENOCORTICAL CARCINOMA

Adrenal neoplasms can arise from tissue within the cortex or medulla of the gland. Because of the physiologic diversity of these two areas, adrenocortical and adrenal medullary tumors are discussed separately.

INCIDENCE

Malignant tumors of the adrenal cortex are extremely rare, accounting for 1 to 2 cases per million per year (DeAtkine & Dunnick, 1991; Norton et al., 1993). The average age at presentation is 40 to 50 years, but tumors are found in all age groups, including children (Norton et al., 1993). Sex distribution is equal, but women have a higher incidence of functional tumors (Cohn, Gottesman, & Brennan, 1986; DeAtkine & Dunnick, 1991; Luton et al., 1990). Bilateral involvement is uncommon, and tumor more often involves the left adrenal than the right (DeAtkine & Dunnick, 1991). There are no definitive etiologic factors for adrenocortical cancers.

BIOLOGY AND NATURAL HISTORY

Adrenocortical carcinomas are aggressive tumors, usually large, and frequently metastatic at the time of diagnosis (Cohn et al., 1986; Decker & Kuehner, 1991). This is due in part to the anatomic protection afforded the adrenal glands within the abdominal cavity, which prevents early detection. Most patients present with stage III or IV disease; local spread is common, with tumor extending to the kidneys, liver, vena cava, pancreas, and diaphragm (Norton et al., 1993). In addition, functional tumors or tumors that secrete steroid hormones (cortisol, aldosterone, progesterone, testosterone, and estradiol) are common, occurring in approximately 80 per cent of patients at diagnosis (Luton et al., 1990).

Overall, survival ranges from 1 to 5 years, with a median 5-year survival of 16 to 30 per cent despite surgery, chemotherapy, or radiation therapy (Decker & Kuehner, 1991). Histologic grade and number of mitotic figures appear to be the most significant determinants of survival, with poorly differentiated adrenocortical carcinoma carrying the poorest prognosis (Weiss, Medeiros, & Vickery, 1989).

TABLE 38–4. *Guidelines for Patients Receiving Iodine-131(^{131}I)*

Planning
Order ^{131}I at least 48 hours in advance. Schedule patient for hospital admission.

Room Preparation
Charcoal filters in room air system and exhaust vent in hallway.
Must cover with plastic bags: telephone, food table, basin faucet handles, nurse call set.
Disposable mats next to bed, commode, and shower.
Seat liners for commode.
Two radiation waste containers in room (laundry and foods or paper).

Patient Preparation
Instruct patient on how to replace and dispose of covers and mats.
Instruct patient to keep outside door closed and bathroom door open at all times.
Obtain vital signs and blood and urine samples before ^{131}I administration.

Administration
Patient must wear hospital gown with a "chuck" around neck and in lap.
Personnel administering ^{131}I should wear gown, gloves, and mask.
Vial containing ^{131}I should be vented in nuclear medicine hood to allow any volatile ^{131}I to escape just before administration.
Patient is to sit on side of bed in front of ^{131}I in lead vial on covered table.
Instruct patient to open vial with T-bar, insert drinking straw, put small amount of water in vial (running it down the straw so it does not splash).
Swish and then swallow several cups of water to rinse ^{131}I from oral cavity.
Do not remove straw from vial; bend it over and carefully place lead cap on.

Initial Survey
Within 15 minutes, measure the radiation exposure rate at 1 m from the midline of patient's abdomen in both anteroposterior and lateral directions. Calculate the average. Patient may be released when same readings show less than 30 mCi of ^{131}I—usually about 48 to 72 hours after 100 mCi was given, but highly variable.
Posted on room door must be room diagram showing safety shields position, inventory-survey form with initial activity and exposure rate, nursing instructions, and decontaminating form.
Do not collect urine unless lead container is available and there is specific reason.

Safety
Nursing recommendations: No pregnant nurses should care for patients receiving ^{131}I. Nurses should not be assigned to care for more than one radioactive patient a month. At 30 mCi ^{131}I discharge, exposure rate is 100 cGy/hour at 25 cm.
Visiting is discouraged: limit to ½ hour/day/visitor; no children under 18 years or pregnant women. Visitors should wear gown, gloves, and mask and sit in a designated chair across the room. If they come close to patient, they should sit behind a lead shield.
Patients should wear hospital gown, not personal clothing (^{131}I is found in breath, sweat), and should leave bed only to go to bathroom or to a designated chair.
Patient should drink copious amounts of water to speed release of unused radioactive agent, shower frequently, and flush toilet several times after each use. Men should urinate seated.
No personal items should be used except those to be disposed of at discharge.
After discharge: sleep alone for 3 days. Do not hold children closely for 3 days.

(From Greenfield, L. D., & Luk, K. H. [1992]. Thyroid tumors. In C. A. Perez & L. W. Brady [Eds.], *Principles and practice of radiation oncology* [2nd. ed., p. 1381]. Philadelphia: J. B. Lippincott Co. Reproduced by permission.)

CLASSIFICATION AND STAGING

Clinically, adrenocortical carcinomas can be classified as functional (hormone-producing) or nonfunctional, with the vast majority being functional and producing excess androgen, estrogen, or cortisol. The staging classification for adrenocortical carcinoma discriminates between disease confined to the adrenal and locally invasive or metastatic disease and is described in Table 38–5.

CLINICAL PRESENTATION

Patients with *nonfunctional* adrenocortical tumors present with symptoms related to local pressure, necrosis, or hemorrhage secondary to an enlarging intraabdominal mass (Cohn et al., 1986). Most nonfunctional tumors are benign; however, careful evaluation may reveal some steroid hormone secretion.

Because the adrenal cortex produces glucocorticoids and mineralocorticoids, patients with *functional* tumors will have symptoms and clinical findings related to hypersecretion of these hormones. Other physical findings result from extensive tumor and include abdominal pain, weight loss, bone pain due to metastases, and fatigue (Decker & Kuehner, 1991). Characteristic symptoms of adrenal endocrine syndromes are listed in Table 38–6. The most common presentation of functional tumor is Cushing's syndrome, resulting from hypercortisolism. The excessive secretion of these steroid hormones may affect every body system, and each patient may present with a unique combination of

TABLE 38–5. *Staging of Adrenocortical Carcinoma*

STAGE	TNM	DESCRIPTION
I	T1, N0, M0	Tumor less than 5 cm without local invasion of nodal or distant metastases
II	T2, N0, M0	Same as Stage I except the tumor is greater than 5 cm
III	T1–2, N1, M0 or T3, N0, M0	Tumor with local invasion or positive lymph nodes
IV	T1–4, N0–1, M1 or T3–4, N1, M0	Tumor with local invasion and positive lymph nodes or distant invasion

TNM Definitions

T1	Tumor less than or equal to 5 cm
T2	Tumor greater than 5 cm
T3	Tumor outside adrenal in fat
T4	Tumor invading adjacent organs
N0	No positive lymph nodes
N1	Positive lymph nodes
M0	No distant metastases
M1	Distant metastases

(Adapted with permission from Norton, J. A., Levin, B., & Jensen, R. T. [1993]. Cancer of the endocrine system. In V. T. DeVita, Jr., S. Hellman, & S. A. Rosenberg [Eds.], *Cancer: Principles and practice of oncology* [4th ed., p. 1361]. Philadelphia: J. B. Lippincott Co.)

signs and symptoms. Virilization may accompany Cushing's syndrome. Conn's syndrome, resulting from hypersecretion of aldosterone, is rare, accounting for 2 per cent of all carcinomas (Norton et al., 1993).

DIAGNOSTIC EVALUATION

Although clinical presentation alone may be suggestive of an adrenal neoplasm, studies of adrenocortical function are important to confirm the presence of excess hormone production. Patients with adrenocortical carcinoma commonly excrete large amounts of 17-ketosteroids if excessive glucocorticoid or sex steroid production is occurring (Samaan & Hickey, 1987). CT scan is invaluable in localizing the tumor and for further staging the disease by delineating nodal involvement or metastases (DeAtkine & Dunnick, 1991; Thompson & Cheung, 1987). Reports regarding the ability of MRI to discriminate benign adenomas from adrenocortical carcinomas and pheochromocytomas will increase the use of this diagnostic tool and may ultimately improve the early detection of asymptomatic adrenal masses (Chang, Glazer, Lee, Ling, & Heiken, 1987; Doppman et al., 1987, Norton et al., 1993).

TREATMENT

Surgery. Surgery is the primary and only potentially curative treatment for all adrenal tumors. Complete resection of tumor may not always be possible because of invasion into adjacent vital structures, but maximal debulking should be undertaken to alleviate symptoms, decrease the amount of cortisol-secreting tissue, and optimize the effectiveness of postoperative systemic therapy (Norton et al., 1993). Surgical treatment can be curative for stage I tumors, and resection of recurrent or metastatic disease is not curative but may slightly prolong survival.

Corticosteroids are administered in high doses preoperatively to prevent acute adrenal insufficiency during surgery and are continued for at least 24 hours after the operation. Patients undergoing bilateral adrenalectomy will require lifelong replacement therapy. A suggested outline for patient teaching is listed in Table 38–7. In patients who have had only unilateral adrenalectomy, replacement doses of steroids will be rapidly tapered and discontinued as function of the contralateral adrenal gland returns (Norton et al., 1993).

After adrenalectomy, patients require intensive monitoring because of the potential for Addisonian crisis, serious fluid and electrolyte disturbances, and hypoglycemia (Cassmeyer, 1987). Poor wound healing and infection can be a major postoperative complication because of the immunosuppressive effects of corticosteroid therapy. Strict aseptic technique should be maintained for wound care.

TABLE 38–6. *Clinical Manifestations of Adrenocortical Hormone Excess*

HORMONE	SYNDROME	CLINICAL MANIFESTATIONS
Aldosterone	Conn's syndrome (aldosteronism)	Hypernatremia, hypokalemia, hypertension, neuromuscular weakness, paresthesias, EKG and renal function changes
Cortisol (ACTH)	Cushing's syndrome	Acid-base imbalance, obesity, hypertension, osteoporosis, hyperglycemia, psychosis, excessive bruising, renal calculi
Sex hormones (testosterone, estrogen, and progesterone)	Virilization (in women)	Male pattern baldness, hirsutism, deepening voice, breast atrophy, decreased libido, oligomenorrhea
	Feminization (in men)	Gynecomastia, breast tenderness, testicular atrophy, decreased libido

TABLE 38–7. *Topic Outline for Patients Needing Replacement Doses of Corticosteroids*

Function of Adrenal Glands
Secretion of corticosteroids
Action of glucocorticoids and mineralocorticoids in body

Medication Regimen
Ingestion with meals or snacks
Glucocorticoids
⅔ dose at 8:00 AM
⅓ dose at 4:00 PM
Mineralocorticoids: Full dose at 8:00 AM
Technique for parenteral administration if unable to retain oral form of drugs
Rationale for carrying drugs on person at all times.

Complications
Signs and symptoms of adrenal insufficiency: anorexia, nausea and vomiting, fatigue, weakness, dehydration, mental status changes, increased pulse and respiratory rate, dizziness
Signs and symptoms of excessive drug therapy: rapid weight gain, round face, edema, hypertension
Effects of stressors on daily corticosteroid requirements
Ability of corticosteroids to mask infection
Purpose and method of obtaining a Medic Alert bracelet or necklace
Indications of contacting a physician

Chemotherapy. Although prolonged tumor regression has been reported in isolated patients treated with mitotane (*o,p′*-DDD) (Jarabak & Rice, 1981), responses are generally of short duration and do not significantly affect length of survival (Luton et al., 1990). The drug is poorly tolerated at high doses, causing significant lethargy, muscle weakness, and gastrointestinal toxicity. Patient tolerance has been improved with doses of 2 to 6g per day in divided doses, increasing to maximum tolerance (Norton et al., 1993). Blood levels of *o,p′*-DDD are measured to ensure levels of at least 14 mcg/ml; levels below this level are not considered therapeutic (Van Slooten, Moolner, Van Seters, & Smeenk, 1990). Because of its postulated mechanism of action in necrosing segments of the adrenal cortex, corticosteroid replacement is necessary during therapy (Thompson & Cheung, 1987).

Although cytotoxic chemotherapy has not been shown to be effective, promising areas of research include regimens with cisplatin and etoposide or mitotane and streptozotocin (Norton et al., 1993). Suramin has been used in phase I studies against metastatic adrenocortical carcinoma, because it may antagonize the ability of such growth factors as epidermal growth factor and transforming growth factor-β to stimulate tumor growth (LaRocca et al., 1990). Because the prognosis for this tumor is poor, and the incidence is low, the use of systemic therapy in the adjuvant setting is advocated within the context of a clinical trial (Norton et al., 1993).

Radiation Therapy. The role of irradiation in the management of adrenocortical carcinoma is limited to the palliation of metastatic bone pain, with no prolongation of survival. Radiation has shown little effect in controlling bulky residual disease (Decker & Kuehner, 1991).

ADRENAL CANCER: PHEOCHROMOCYTOMA

INCIDENCE

Pheochromocytoma is a rare catecholamine-secreting tumor that occurs predominantly in middle age and is slightly more common among women (Daly & Landsberg, 1992). Approximately 10 per cent of pheochromocytomas are malignant, and they differ from benign cases only in their invasive and metastatic behavior (Samaan, Hickey, & Shutts, 1988). Bilateral occurrence is rare. Ninety per cent of cases arise from chromaffin cells of the adrenal medullary tissue; the remaining cases are termed *paragangliomas* and are detected in ectopic sites of catecholamine-secreting tissues (Daly & Landsberg, 1992, Samaan et al., 1988). It is a rare tumor, occurring in <1 per 100,000 person-years, and develops idiopathically or, in 10 per cent of cases, is inherited as part of an MEN syndrome (Daly & Landsberg, 1992).

CLINICAL PRESENTATION

Diagnosis is difficult, since presenting signs and symptoms may resemble other medical conditions (Table 38–8). They result from excess secretion of epinephrine and norepinephrine and include hypertension (either episodic or sustained), excessive perspiration, headache, nervousness, palpitations, nausea, vomiting, abdominal or chest pain, blurred vision, and syncope. Pheochromocytoma can produce other hormones as well, including ACTH, causing Cushing's syndrome. Somatostatin, calcitonin, oxytocin, and vasopressin may also be secreted but seldom cause symptoms (Norton et al., 1993).

TABLE 38–8: *Medical Conditions Resembling*
Pheochromocytoma

Abdominal catastrophe
Anxiety, or other psychiatric disorders
Aortic dissection
Cerebral infarction or hemorrhage
Cocaine or other sympathomimetic drug use
Diabetes (non-insulin-dependent)
Malignant hyperthermia
Menopause
Migraine headache
Myocardial infarction
Pulmonary edema
Renal vascular hypertension
Sepsis
Seizure disorder
Thyrotoxicosis
Toxemia of pregnancy

DIAGNOSTIC EVALUATION

Elevated levels of catecholamines can be documented with measurement of 24-hour urine samples for catecholamines (vanillylmandelic acid [VMA], metanephrines) and can aid in confirming the diagnosis (Hanson, Feldman, Beam, Leight, & Coleman, 1991). In addition, norepinephrine and epinephrine and their metabolites may be measured in the blood or urine (Norton et al., 1993). The clonidine suppression test has become one of the most definitive tests for pheochromocytoma. In the absence of a pheochromocytoma, clonidine taken orally will result in suppression of epinephrine and norepinephrine; in cases of pheochromocytoma, these hormones will not be suppressed (Norton et al., 1993).

Once abnormal urinary test results have been documented, localization of the adrenal tumor and ectopic or metastatic disease is done with noninvasive radiologic procedures such as CT or ^{131}I-metaiodobenzylguanidine (MIBG) scan (Bravo & Gifford, 1984). The MIBG scan uses an agent that mimics norepinephrine and is taken up by catecholamine-producing cells, thereby localizing both adrenal and extraadrenal pheochromocytomas (Sisson et al., 1981).

TREATMENT

Surgery. Aggressive surgical resection of all accessible disease and metastases is indicated for malignant pheochromocytoma, although it may not be possible to remove all active (functional) tissue (Hull, 1986; Norton et al., 1993). Patients are routinely given α-adrenergic blocking agents after a definitive diagnosis is made to minimize the potential for uncontrolled release of catecholamines during localization procedures and surgery (Hull, 1986). Myocardial damage may be present at the time of surgery as a result of prolonged exposure to epinephrine and norepinephrine, thereby placing the patient at a higher intraoperative risk for cardiovascular complications (Hull, 1986; Sardesai, Mourant, Sivathandon, Farrow, & Givvons, 1990).

After removal of the tumor, rigorous monitoring is required because profound shock can develop owing to the dramatic decrease in circulating catecholamine levels (Bravo & Gifford, 1984). Adequate volume replacement is of paramount importance.

After surgery, patients with malignant pheochromocytoma are maintained on α- and β-adrenergic blocking agents and α-methyl-paratyrosine, which reduces the production of catecholamines indefinitely, to prevent recurrence of symptoms (Hull, 1986).

Systemic Treatment. Systemic therapy for malignant pheochromocytoma includes ^{131}I-MIBG treatment as well as chemotherapy (Norton et al., 1993). For a pheochromocytoma to concentrate and retain ^{131}I-MIBG, it must consist of sufficiently well-differentiated chromaffin cells and have an active neuronal pump mechanism; in the case of malignant disease, the cells are often poorly differentiated and do not take up enough ^{131}I-MIBG to have an antitumor effect. While some responses to this treatment are reported, no complete responses have been achieved (Krempf et al., 1991). Active chemotherapy agents include streptozotocin and combination regimens with cyclophosphamide, vincristine, and dacarbazine (Averbuch et al., 1988, Norton et al., 1993).

Radiation Therapy. Painful bone metastases may respond to external radiation therapy. In general, however, radiation is not used in the treatment of pheochromocytoma.

PITUITARY TUMORS

INCIDENCE

Pituitary tumors account for approximately 10 per cent of symptomatic intracranial neoplasms. They are found in all age groups but most commonly in middle-aged and older patients, with both sexes being affected equally (Kovacs & Horvath, 1987).

BIOLOGY

The majority of pituitary tumors are adenomas, slow-growing, benign neoplasms arising from adenohypophyseal cells in the anterior pituitary and are confined to the sella turcica. Some, however rare, are pituitary carcimonas, which exhibit more aggressive, invasive behavior and metastasize to brain, subarachnoid space, or distant sites (Kovacs & Horvath, 1987; Scheithauer, Kovacs, Laws, & Randall, 1986). The etiology is unknown.

CLASSIFICATION

Adenomas arise from cells in the anterior lobe of the pituitary gland, and early classification schemes were based on the chemical staining properties of tumor cells. This classification was of little value because of the lack of correlation between staining characteristics, level of cellular differentiation, and hormone content (Scheithauer et al., 1986). More sophisticated laboratory techniques have permitted a more functional categorization of pituitary adenomas, which are now classified primarily according to their morphology and endocrinologic activity, and as endocrine-active (approximately 80 per cent) or endocrine-inactive (Scheithauer et al., 1986). In one large series, the major hormones secreted by pituitary adenomas were prolactin (52 per cent), growth hormone (GH) (27 per cent), adrenocorticotropic hormone (ACTH) (20 per cent), and TSH (0.3 per cent) (Wilson, 1983); follicle-stimulating hormone (FSH), and luteinizing hormone (LH) are rare. Tumors are frequently named according to the hormone secreted (e.g., prolactinomas, GH-secreting adenomas).

Pituitary adenomas are also classified according to size. Microadenomas are tumors smaller than 10 mm in diameter, and macroadenomas are larger (Ciric, 1985). Microadenomas are associated with a better overall prognosis, because generally they are confined to the sella turcica and are easily resectable (Scheithauer et al., 1986).

CLINICAL PRESENTATION

The signs and symptoms of pituitary adenomas reflect the specific hormone produced by the tumor and the compression effects of the tumor mass (Piziak & Gilliland, 1993). Headache occurs in approximately 20 per cent of patients with pituitary tumors (Levin, Gutin, & Leibel, 1993). Symptoms related to hormone secretion may be subtle and insidious.

Prolactin-secreting tumors are by far the most common pituitary adenoma (Levin et al., 1993; Piziak & Gilliland, 1993). These tumors cause clinical symptoms of amenorrhea and galactorrhea in women, detected most easily in premenopausal women. Early detection is not as likely in nonmenstruating women, and presenting symptoms in this group are generally from the compressive effect of the expanding tumor (Dollar & Blackwell, 1986). In men, hyperprolactinemia causes diminished libido or impotence. Infertility may result for either sex.

Overproduction of growth hormone (GH) over time results in acromegaly (pituitary gigantism in children); clinical manifestations include alterations in facial features (broadening of the jaw) and enlargement of hands and feet. Systemic effects are nonspecific: lethargy, headache, and paresthesias. Late effects include weight gain, hypertension, cardiomegaly, and glucose intolerance (Piziak & Gilliland, 1993).

Cushing's disease is caused by hypersecretion of ACTH. The most common cause of Cushing's disease is a pituitary tumor (Piziak & Gilliland, 1993). Common clinical findings include obesity, hirsutism, muscle weakness and wasting, abdominal striae, acne, prominent dorsocervical fat pad, and easy bruising. Glucose intolerance and hypertension also occur (Piziak & Gilliland, 1993).

LH-, FSH-, and TSH-secreting adenomas are rare. The major sign of gonadotropin hypersecretion is infertility due to the disruption in cyclic hormonal release. Signs of hypogonadism result despite high circulating levels of hormone because of disruption of the normal cyclic hormone secretion. TSH hypersecretion causes signs of hyperthyroidism: tremor, tachycardia, weight loss, muscle wasting, and a small goiter. Symptoms include weakness, fatigue, and irritability.

One quarter of pituitary tumors are nonsecretory, and in both cases, widespread endocrine abnormalities result from loss of pituitary hormonal action on target organs throughout the body. The clinical effects of hypopituitarism attributable to destruction of normal anterior pituitary tissue or impairment of the hypothalamic-pituitary axis are listed in Table 38–9.

Because of its strategic location within the skull, the mass effect of a growing pituitary neoplasm can cause headache compression of surrounding critical structures, including the optic chiasm, hypothalamus, and cranial nerves. Patients with involvement of the optic nerves or chiasm may experience loss of visual acuity or visual field defects (Levin et al., 1993, Piziak & Gilliland, 1993).

DIAGNOSTIC EVALUATION

The first step in evaluating a patient with a suspected pituitary tumor includes endocrinologic testing to determine whether hypersecretion of any of the pituitary hormones is present. Laboratory documentation of elevated hormone levels aids in confirming the diagnosis of a functional pituitary adenoma and provides baseline information for assessing response to subsequent therapy (Ciric, 1985).

Radiologic diagnostic tests provide additional information on the structure of both functional and nonfunctional tumors. The most useful techniques in delineating tumor size and extension outside the confines of the gland are CT and MRI. MRI is the most sensitive tool for providing definition of the pituitary and surrounding structures as well as consistency and density of the tumor and normal pituitary tissue (Maroldo, Dillon, & Wilson, 1992). In patients with macroadenomas, carotid angiography may also be indicated to further delineate the surrounding vasculature (Kaufman, Kaufman, Arafah, Roessman, & Selman, 1987).

TREATMENT

Surgery. Selection of a treatment method is contingent on the size and extent of the tumor. Surgery is the single most effective treatment for pituitary microadenomas and results in long-term local control for approximately 85 per cent of patients (Chun, Masko, & Hetelekidis, 1988). For endocrine-active and -inactive macroadenomas, surgery is also the treatment of choice even when total resection is not possible; debulking procedures resolve visual impairment and normalize hormone hypersecretion (Comtois et al., 1992). Partially resected nonfunctional tumors may be cured with adjuvant radiotherapy, whereas functional tumors require complete resection (Levin et al., 1993).

With few exceptions, the transsphenoidal approach (access through the mouth into the sphenoid sinus and up into the sella turcica) has largely replaced the transfrontal technique (craniotomy), which provided better visualization of the area but was associated with higher morbidity and mortality (Laws, 1987, Levin et al., 1993). Whenever possible, salvage of nor-

TABLE 38–9. *Clinical Effects of Hypopituitarism*

HORMONE	TARGET TISSUE	CLINICAL EFFECTS
ACTH	Adrenal cortex	Postural hypotension; impaired tolerance of stress (trauma, surgery); shock
Prolactin, FSH, LH	Gonads	Gonadal atrophy; loss of reproductive function; decreased gonadal hormones
TSH	Thyroid	Hypothyroidism (fatigue, slow or slurred speech, bradycardia, decreased reflexes, cold intolerance)
GH	Bones, muscles, organs	Decreased bone growth, lethargy, hypoglycemia

ACTH = Adrenocorticotropic hormone; FSH = follicle-stimulating hormone; LH = luteinizing hormone; TSH = thyroid-stimulating hormone; GH = growth hormone.

mal pituitary tissue is desirable to avoid panhypopituitarism.

The most common complications of surgery are diabetes insipidus (DI), cerebrospinal fluid (CSF) leak, and meningitis. Diabetes insipidus is observed in 30 to 50 per cent of patients (Laws, 1982), but even in completely hypophysectomized patients, it is usually temporary because the hypothalamus assumes the secretory function of the pituitary in releasing antidiuretic hormone (ADH). In the immediate postoperative period, patients will have extremely dilute urine, and adequate fluid replacement is essential to prevent hypovolemia.

Because the dura is disrupted during entry into the sella turcica, CSF can drain from the wound site. Activities that increase intracranial pressure, such as coughing, sneezing, and bending over, are to be avoided to minimize the possibility of CSF leakage (Cassmeyer, 1987). Patients should be assessed for persistent postnasal drip and constant swallowing. Any drainage noted should be tested for glucose, because CSF differs from normal nasal drainage in that CSF contains glucose.

Aseptic technique is essential during wound care because of the increased risk of meningitis in patients after intracranial surgery. The suture line is located within the oral cavity if the transsphenoidal approach has been used. The mouth can be rinsed with normal saline solution and cleansed with a Toothette or cotton swab. Regular toothbrushing is contraindicated until healing occurs because of the possibility of disrupting the suture line (Cassmeyer, 1987).

Radiation Therapy. External irradiation is frequently used in conjunction with surgery to decrease the incidence of local recurrence (Chun et al., 1988). It can be given immediately after surgery or as salvage therapy after recurrence. By employing a combined approach, local control can be achieved in almost 95 per cent of patients (Chun et al., 1988; Levin et al., 1993).

Radiation therapy is rarely used as the sole treatment modality for hypersecreting tumors, since maximal response to therapy may be delayed for months to years (Halberg & Sheline, 1987).

Chemotherapy. Traditional cytotoxic chemotherapy has been of limited usefulness because of difficulties in administering concentrations of drug high enough to cross the blood-brain barrier without causing prohibitive toxicity (Levin et al., 1993). Instead, the focus has been on pharmacologic manipulation of pituitary hormone secretion.

Bromocriptine, a dopamine agonist, is effective in temporarily reducing levels of prolactin. However, bromocriptine is not considered curative when used alone; the drug must be continued indefinitely, because discontinuation can result in rapid regrowth of the tumor (Dollar & Blackwell, 1986). Considerable controversy surrounds the use of this agent, but several studies now support short-term (4 to 6 weeks) preoperative treatment with bromocriptine for prolactinomas to reduce tumor size and increase resectability, or as adjuvant treatment during radiation therapy (Bevan et al., 1987; Hubbard, Scheithauer, Abboud, & Laws, 1987; Levin et al., 1993). Long-term treatment may hinder surgical resection because of the development of tumor necrosis and fibrosis.

A long-acting somatostatin analog, octreotide (SMS 201—995), shows promise in the preoperative treatment of GH-producing macroadenomas by suppressing GH hypersecretion (Barkan et al., 1988). Maximal tumor reduction occurs after 8 to 12 weeks of therapy, and GH levels remain within the normal range in 80 per cent of patients postoperatively (Barkan et al., 1988).

PARATHYROID TUMORS

INCIDENCE

Parathyroid adenoma is the most common cause of primary hyperparathyroidism (83 per cent); parathyroid carcinoma is extremely rare, accounting for only 1 per cent of all cases of primary hyperparathyroidism (Shane & Bilezidian, 1982; Norton et al., 1993). A history of irradiation to the head and neck is associated with primary hyperparathyroidism (Norton et al., 1993; Shane & Bilezidian, 1982). A history of irradiation to the head and neck is associated with the development of hyperparathyroidism due to adenoma (Hickey et al., 1991). Men and women are equally affected with parathyroid hyperplasia, and a parathyroid tumor can occur as part of an MEN I or II syndrome. Distinguishing characteristics are summarized in Table 38–10.

BIOLOGY AND NATURAL HISTORY

Parathyroid carcinoma is slow-growing but can metastasize late in the course of disease to regional nodes, lung, bone, and liver (Norton et al., 1993). Death generally occurs as a result of the renal and cardiac effects of prolonged hypercalcemia (McCance, Kenny, Sloan, Russell, & Hadden, 1987). First-year survival appears to be less than 50 per cent; less than 35 per cent of patients survive 10 years (Schantz & Castleman, 1973; Shane & Bilezidian, 1982).

CLINICAL PRESENTATION

Clinical manifestations of parathyroid carcinoma result from the effect of parathyroid hormone (PTH) on the kidneys, bone, gastrointestinal tract, and neuromuscular system. Serum calcium and PTH levels are significantly more elevated in parathyroid carcinoma than for parathyroid adenoma (Shortell, Andrus, Phillips, & Schwartz, 1991). Hypersecretion of PTH results in hypercalcemia and leads to the development of renal calculi, demineralization of bone, gastrointestinal disturbances, pancreatitis, muscle weakness, and lethargy. A neck mass can be palpated in 30 to 50 per cent of patients (Schantz & Castleman, 1973; Shane & Bilezidian, 1982).

TREATMENT

Surgery. Surgical removal of the carcinoma is indicated in all cases, although 30 to 65 per cent of patients will have recurrent disease even after apparent complete resection of the tumor (Schantz & Castleman, 1973). At the time of operation, complete resection of disease is recommended, including ipsilateral thyroid lobectomy and lymph node dissection if involved by tumor (Shortell et al, 1991, Norton et al, 1993). Because of the indolent nature of this tumor, patients with recurrent tumor who have symptoms of hypercalcemia can obtain long-term palliation with additional surgery (Flye & Brennan, 1981).

Chemotherapy or Radiation Therapy. Experience with chemotherapy in the management of metastatic disease is limited. These treatment methods do not appear to affect survival, although responses have been reported using dacarbazine and 5-fluorouracil and cyclophosphamide in combination, or dacarbazine alone (Bukowski, Sheelar, Cunningham, & Esselstyn, 1984; Shane & Bilezidian, 1982). Radiation therapy has not proved to be effective for treatment of primary or metastatic lesions (Norton et al., 1993).

Symptom management is the focus of treatment for patients with bone pain and hypercalcemia. Pharmacologic agents that block PTH or lower serum calcium level are employed for palliation of symptoms. Calcitonin, diphosphonates, and mithramycin have been used with limited success for short-term management of hypercalcemia. The role of a parathyroid hormone antagonist is currently being explored (Rosenblatt, 1986). Gallium nitrate (Warrell et al, 1988) and etidronate (Singer, Ritch, Lad, & Ringinberg, 1991) may be more useful in the management of chronic hypercalcemia. However, antitumor treatment remains the most effective way to control the hypercalcemia of parathyroid carcinoma.

MULTIPLE ENDOCRINE NEOPLASIAS

Hyperplasia or neoplasia of endocrine cells can occur in a single site or involve several different endocrine glands or tissues. The term *multiple endocrine neoplasia* has been used to describe constellations of endocrine abnormalities occurring in families and involving the pituitary gland, parathyroid glands, and the pancreas (Norton et al., 1993). Three distinct MEN syndromes have been described (Table 38–3).

Patients who have any tumor identified as a component of one of the MEN syndromes should be evaluated for the presence of other tumors. The MEN syndromes

TABLE 38–10. *Differentiation Between Parathyroid Adenoma and Carcinoma*

FACTOR	PARATHYROID ADENOMA	PARATHYROID CARCINOMA
Etiology	Associated with previous radiation to head/neck	?Familial pattern
Frequency	Cause of primary parathyroid hyperplasia in 83% cases	Cause of primary parathyroid hyperplasia in 1% of cases
Physical findings	Urinary calculi, bone pain, elevated alkaline phosphatase	Palpable neck mass, vocal cord paralysis
Serum calcium	12 mg/dl	14 mg/dl
Serum PTH	Elevated	Markedly elevated
Treatment	Excision of gland	Resection of gland with ipsilateral thyroid lobe and suspicious lymph nodes
Recurrence rate	1%	> 50%
5-Year survival	100%	29%–44%

are transmitted genetically in an autosomal-dominant fashion. Consequently, it has been recommended that screening of all family members in an affected kindred be done in an effort to increase the early detection of lesions in asymptomatic persons (Norton et al., 1993). While most of the tumors are adenomas, early diagnosis is necessary to control symptoms related to functional endocrine tumors and because some pancreatic tumors may be malignant.

Although each component of MEN syndromes is treated independently, patients with more than one tumor at the time of diagnosis will need to have decisions made regarding which tumor to treat first. Survival to adulthood is rare (Norton et al., 1993).

APUDOMAS

OVERVIEW

Tumors arising from APUD cells, which share the common biochemical characteristics for *a*mine *p*recursor *u*ptake and *d*ecarboxylation (APUD), were first described by Pearse (1977). The APUD concept provides a framework for relating a variety of hormonally active tumors arising in diverse organs, such as the pituitary gland, peripheral autonomic ganglia, adrenal medulla, gastrointestinal tract, pancreas, lung, gonads, and thymus glands (Philippe, 1992). The incidence of APUD-derived gastrointestinal and pancreatic endocrine tumors is extremely rare, but a brief discussion of carcinoid tumor is warranted, because increased detection of this tumor has been made possible with advances in radioimmunoassay techniques and because it provides an example of the varied presentation and behavior of an apudoma.

CARCINOID TUMORS

Carcinoid tumors are examples of APUD neoplasms and occur most frequently within the gastrointestinal tract, especially the appendix, small intestine, rectum, and main bronchus (Godwin, 1975). They are slow-growing tumors that are difficult to identify histologically, as they resemble pancreatic endocrine tumors and adenocarcinoma. Diagnosis is confirmed by endocrine tumor markers, such as chromogranin A and neuron-specific enolase (McLeod, Few, & Shapiro, 1993; Norton et al., 1993). Earlier diagnosis has resulted in a marked increase in carcinoids of the bronchus possibly due to ability to distinguish these tumors from small-cell lung cancer or adenocarcinoma with the use of tumor marker staining techniques (Vinik, McLeod, Fig, Shapiro, Lloyd, & Cho, 1989). Metastatic spread of carcinoid is uncommon, occurring in approximately 20 per cent of cases; however, if the tumor is >2 cm at diagnosis, metastases are common (Godwin, 1975; Moertel, 1987).

Clinical Presentation. Patients are frequently asymptomatic until the disease is advanced, and the median time from symptoms to diagnosis is 2 to 20 years (Moertel, 1987; Norton et al., 1993). The most common presenting signs of carcinoid tumors are

related to small bowel obstruction, such as abdominal pain or bleeding; more commonly the disease is diagnosed incidentally by endoscopy or chest x-ray.

The malignant carcinoid syndrome (MCS), an indication of advanced disease, is a constellation of symptoms caused by the secretion of hormones by the tumor, specifically serotonin and its metabolite, urinary 5-hydroxyindolacetic acid (5-HIAA) (Norton et al., 1993). The syndrome is manifested by facial flushing, diarrhea, valvular heart disease, wheezing, and facial telangiectasia. The etiology of flushing is unclear but in some cases may be related to histamine release or vasoactive peptides or tachykinins such as neuropeptide K (NPK) or substance P(SP) (Reubi, 1993). Serotonin production results in diarrhea because of increased motility and fat malabsorption. Carcinoid crisis refers to a potentially life-threatening manifestation of MCS, when the symptoms are particularly intense, and cardiac arrhythmia with alterations in blood pressure occur (Kvols et al., 1986; Moertel, 1987).

Clinical Evaluation. Diagnosis using routine endoscopic or scanning techniques has proved inadequate in localizing carcinoid tumors due to their small size and ubiquitous location. ^{123}I-MIBG or ^{131}I-MIBG scans, together with CT scans, are recommended (Norton et al., 1993). Since these tumors have receptors for the hormone, somatostatin, ^{123}I-labeled octreotide, a synthetic somatostatin analog, is reported to localize carcinoid tumors (Kubota et al., 1994; Lamberts, Reubin, & Krenning, 1992). Urinary serotonin and 5-HIAA levels are used to confirm the carcinoid syndrome and as markers for tumor response or symptomatic treatment.

Treatment. Surgical resection is indicated for most carcinoid tumors, but the extent of the surgical procedure required varies according to location and size of the primary tumor. Tumors larger than 2 cm require more radical surgery, because they routinely metastasize (Moertel, 1987).

Several approaches have been employed for palliation of MCS symptoms in patients with unresectable disease. Octreotide, a somatostatin analog, is effective as an antitumor agent as well as in relieving symptoms of carcinoid syndrome and carcinoid crisis (Kvols et al., 1986; Moertel, 1987). Cyproheptadine (Periactin) has been effective in controlling diarrhea related to MCS (Moertel, 1987). Patients are advised to use bronchodilators if necessary and to avoid foods that precipitate flushing (e.g., cheese or alcohol) and stress or excessive exercise (Norton et al., 1993).

In general, cytotoxic chemotherapy is not recommended with metastatic carcinoid tumors. Multiple agents have been investigated, but response rates have been low and of short duration and therefore do not appear to justify the significant toxicity associated with their administration (Moertel, 1987). Hepatic artery occlusion (via ligation or embolization), which is aimed at decreasing oxygenation of tumor in the liver, thereby causing cell death, has been somewhat successful in transiently relieving symptoms (Moertel, 1987; Odurney & Birch, 1985). Interferon α may be effective as an antitumor agent, as its use has resulted in prolonged survival of patients with metastatic carcinoid over patients treated with chemotherapy or chemotherapy plus interferon (Oberg & Erickson, 1991).

Metastatic disease portends poor survival, and the chance of finding metastases is directly related to the size of the primary tumor. Five-year survival depends on the site and extent of disease and varies from 18 per cent (distant metastases) to 99 per cent (localized disease) (Godwin, 1975; Norton et al., 1993).

SUMMARY

Technologic advances as well as epidemiologic studies have provided new information regarding specific characteristics of many of the endocrine neoplasms. This knowledge is translating into new approaches for (1) modifying the hormonal effects of these tumors within the body, (2) identifying persons at risk for the development of endocrine tumors, and (3) improving early detection with laboratory and radiologic techniques. Nurses caring for patients with endocrine cancers must keep abreast of the advances in this field to educate patients and provide knowledgable care.

ACKNOWLEDGMENT. The author wishes to acknowledge and thank Michele G. Donehower for permission to revise her chapter from the first edition of this textbook.

REFERENCES

Ahuja, S., & Ernst, H. (1987). Chemotherapy of thyroid cancer. *Journal of Endocrinology Investigation, 10,* 303–310.

Alexander, J. R., & Norton, J. A. (1991). Biology and management of medullary thyroid carcinoma of the parafollicular cells. In J. Robbins (Moderator). Thyroid cancer: A lethal endocrine neoplasm. *Annals of Internal Medicine, 115,* 133–147.

Averbuch, S. D. (1992). Endocrine tumors. In: H. M. Pinedo, D. Longo, & B. A. Chabner (Eds.), *Cancer Chemotherapy and Biological Response Modifier Annual* (pp. 493–507). New York: Elsevier Science Publishers.

Averbuch, S., Steakley, C. S., Young, R. C., Gelmann, E. P., Goldstein, D. S., Stull, R., & Keiser, H. R. (1988). Malignant pheochromocytoma: Effective treatment with a combination of cyclophosphamide, vincristine, and dacarbazine. *Annals of Internal Medicine, 109,* 267–273.

Baker, K. H., & Feldman, J. E. (1993) Thyroid cancer: A review. *Oncology Nursing Forum, 20,* 95–104.

Barkan, A. M., Lloyd, R. V., Chandler, W. F., Hatfield, M. K., Gebarshi, S. S., Kelch, R. P., & Beitins, I. Z. (1988). Preoperative treatment of acromegaly with long-acting somatostatin analog SMS 201–995: Shrinkage of invasive pituitary macroadenomas and improved surgical remission rate. *Journal of Clinical Endocrinology and Metabolism, 67,* 1040–1048.

Beahrs, O. H., Henson, D. E., Hutter, R. V. P., & Myers, M. H. (Eds.) (1992). *Manual for staging of cancer* (4th ed., pp. 53–55). Philadelphia: J. B. Lippincott Co.

Bevan, J. S., Adams, C. B. T., Burke, C. W., Morton, K. E., Molyneux, A. J., Moore, R. A., & Esiri, M. M. (1987). Factors in the outcome of transsphenoidal surgery for prolactinoma and non-functioning pituitary tumors, including pre-operative bromocriptine therapy. *Clinical Endocrinology, 26,* 541–556.

Blahd, W. H. (1985). Treatment of thyroid cancer. *Comprehensive Therapy, 11*(9), 26–32.

Bravo, E. L., & Gifford, R. W. (1984). Pheochromocytoma: Diagnosis, localization and management. *New England Journal of Medicine, 311,* 1298–1303.

Bukowski, R. M., Sheelar, L., Cunningham, J., & Esselstyn, C. (1984). Successful combination chemotherapy for metastatic parathyroid carcinoma. *Archives of Internal Medicine, 144,* 399–402.

Carter, W. B., Taylor, R. L., Kao, P. C., & Heath, H. (1991). Determination of plasma calcitonin-gene related peptide concentration by a new immunochemiluminometric assay in normal persons and patients with medullary thyroid carcinoma and other neuroendocrine tumors. *Journal of Clinical Endocrinology and Metabolism, 72,* 327–325.

Cassmeyer, V. L. (1987). Interventions for persons with problems of the endocrine system: Pituitary, thyroid, parathyroid, and adrenal glands. In W. J. Phipps, B. C. Long, & N. F. Woods (Eds.), *Medical-surgical nursing: Concepts and clinical practice* (3rd ed., pp. 549–600). St. Louis: C. V. Mosby Co.

Chang, A., Glazer, H. S., Lee, J. K. T., Ling, D., & Heiken, J. P. (1987). Adrenal gland: MR imaging. *Radiology, 163,* 123–128.

Chun, M., Masko, G. B., & Hetelekidis, S. (1988). Radiotherapy in the treatment of pituitary adenomas. *International Journal of Radiation Oncology, Biology, Physics, 15,* 305–309.

Ciric, I. (1985). Pituitary tumors. *Neurology Clinics, 3,* 751–766.

Cohn, K., Gottesman, L., & Brennan, M. (1986). Adrenocortical carcinoma. *Surgery, 100,* 1170–1177.

Comtois, R., Beauregard, H., Somma, M., Serri, O., Aris-Jilwas, N., & Hardy, J. (1991) The clinical and endocrine outcome to transsphenoidal microsurgery of nonsecreting pituitary adenomas. *Cancer, 68,* 860–866.

Daly, P. A., & Landsberg, L. (1992). Phaeochromocytoma: Diagnosis and management. *Bailliere's Clinical Endocrinology and Metabolism, 6,* 143–166.

DeAtkine, A. B., & Dunnick, N. R. (1991). The adrenal glands. *Seminars in Oncology, 18,* 131–139.

Decker, R. A., & Kuehner, M. E. (1991). Adrenocortical carcinoma. *American Surgeon, 57,* 502–513.

Demeter, J. G., DeJong, S. A., Lawrence, A. M., & Paloyan, E. (1991). Anaplastic thyroid carcinoma: risk factors and outcome. *Surgery, 110,* 956–963.

Dollar, J. R., & Blackwell, R. E. (1986). Diagnosis and management of prolactinomas. *Cancer and Metastases Review, 5,* 125–138.

Doppman, J. L., Reinig, J. W., Dwyer, A. J., Frank, J. P., Norton, J., Loriaux, L., & Keiser, H. (1987). Differentiation of adrenal masses by magnetic resonance imaging. *Surgery, 102,* 1018–1025.

Duffy, B. J., & Fitzgerald, P. J. (1950). Cancer of the thyroid in children: A report of 28 cases. *Journal of Clinical Endocrinology, 10,* 1296–1308.

Favus, M. J., Schneider, A. B., Stachura, M. E., Arnold, J. E., Ryo, V. Y., Pinsky, S. M., Colman, M., Arnold, M. J., & Frohman, L. A. (1976). Thyroid cancer occurring as a late consequence of head and neck irradiation: Evaluation of 1056 patients. *New England Journal of Medicine, 294,* 1019–1025.

Flye, M. W., & Brennan, M. F. (1981). Surgical resection of metastatic parathyroid carcinoma. *Annals of Surgery, 193,* 425–435.

Frable, W. J. (1986). The treatment of thyroid cancer: The role of fine needle aspiration. *Archives of Otolaryngology—Head and Neck Surgery, 112,* 1200–1203.

Freitas, J. E., Gross, M. D., Ripley, S., & Shapiro, B. (1985). Radionuclide diagnosis and therapy of thyroid cancer: Current status report. *Seminars in Nuclear Medicine, 15,* 106–131.

Friedman, M., Toriumi, D. M., & Mafee, M. F. (1988). Diagnostic imaging techniques in thyroid cancer. *American Journal of Surgery, 155,* 215–223.

Godwin, D. J. (1975). Carcinoid tumors: An analysis of 2837 cases. *Cancer, 36,* 560–569.

Greenfield, L. D. (1987). Thyroid tumors. In C. A. Perez & L. W. Brady (Eds.), *Principles and practice of radiation oncology* (pp. 1126–1156). Philadelphia: J. B. Lippincott Co.

Halberg, F. J., & Sheline, G. E. (1987). Radiotherapy of pituitary tumors. *Endocrinology and Metabolism Clinics, 16,* 667–683.

Hamburger, J. I. (1987) Consistency of sequential needle biopsy findings for thyroid management implications. *Archives of Internal Medicine, 147,* 97–99.

Hanson, M. W., Feldman, J. M., Beam, D. A., Leight, G. S., & Coleman, E. (1991) Iodine [131]-labeled metaiodobenzylguanidine scintigraphy and biochemical analyses in suspected pheochromocytoma. *Archives of Internal Medicine, 151,* 1397–1402.

Herranz-Gonzalez, J., Gavilan, J., Marinez-Vidal, J., & Gavilan, C. (1991). Complications following thyroid surgery. *Archives of Otolaryngology—Head and Neck Surgery, 117,* 516–518.

Hickey, R. C., Jung, P. A., Merrell, R., Ordonez, N., & Samaan, N. A. (1991). Parathyroid adenoma in a cancer center patient population. *American Journal of Surgery, 161,* 439–432.

Holm, L. E., Dahlquist, I., Israelsson, A., & Lundell, G. (1980). Malignant thyroid tumors after iodine—131 therapy. *New England Journal of Medicine, 303,* 188–191.

Hubbard, J. L., Scheithauer, B. W., Abboud, C. F., & Laws, E. L., Jr. (1987). Prolactin secreting adenomas: The preoperative response to bromocriptine treatment and surgical outcome. *Journal of Neurosurgery, 67,* 816–821.

Hull, C. J. (1986). Phaeochromocytoma: Diagnosis, preoperative preparation and anesthetic management. *British Journal of Anesthesiology, 58,* 1453–1468.

Jarabak, J., & Rice, K. (1981). Metastatic adrenal cortical carcinoma: Prolonged regression with mitotane therapy. *Journal of the American Medical Association, 246,* 1706–1707.

Kaufman, B., Kaufman, B. A., Arafah, B. M., Roessmann, V., & Selman, W. R. (1987). Large pituitary gland adenomas evaluated with magnetic resonance imaging. *Neurosurgery, 21,* 540–546.

Kerr, D. J., Burt, A. D., Boyle, P., MacFarlane, G. J., Storer, A. M., & Brewin, T. B. (1986). Prognostic factors in thyroid tumors. *British Journal of Cancer, 54,* 475–482.

Kim, J. H., & Leeper, R. D. (1983). Treatment of anaplastic giant and spindle cell carcinoma of the thyroid gland with combination Adriamycin and radiation therapy: A new approach. *Cancer, 52,* 954–957.

Kovacs, K., & Horvath, E. (1987). Pathology of pituitary tumors. *Endocrinology and Metabolism Clinics, 16,* 667–683.

Krempf, M., Lumbroso, J., Mornex, R., et al. (1991). Use of [131]Imiodobenzylguanidine in the treatment of malignant pheochromocytoma. *Journal of Clinical Endocrinology and Metabolism, 72,* 455–461.

Kubota, A., Yamada, Y., Kagimoto, S., Shimatsu, A., Imamura, M., Tsuda, K., Imura, H., Seino, S., & Seino, Y. (1994). Identification of somatostatin receptor subtypes and an implication for the efficacy of somatostatin analogue SMS 201–995 in treatment of human endocrine tumors. *Journal of Clinical Investigation, 93,* 1321–1325.

Kvols, L. K., Moertel, C. G., O'Connell, M. J., Schutt, A. J., Rubin, J., & Hahn, R. G. (1986). Treatment of the malignant carcinoid syndrome: Evaluation of a long-acting somatostatin analog. *New England Journal of Medicine, 315,* 663–666.

Lamberts, S. W., Reubi, J. C., & Krenning, E. P. (1992) Somatostatin receptor imaging in the diagnosis and treatment of neuroendocrine tumors. *Journal of Steroid Biochemistry & Molecular Biology, 43,* 185–188.

LaRocca, R. V., Stein, C. A., Danesi, R., Jamis Dow, D. A., Weiss, G. H., & Myers, C. E. (1990). Suramin in adrenal cancer: Modulation of steroid hormone production, cytotoxicity in vitro and clinical antitumor effect. *Journal of Clinical Endocrinology and Metabolism, 71,* 497–504.

Laws, E. R., Jr. (1982). Complications of transsphenoidal microsurgery for pituitary adenomas. In M. Brock (Ed.), *Modern neurosurgery* (Vol. 1, pp. 181–191). New York: Springer-Verlag.

Laws, E. R., Jr. (1987). Pituitary surgery. *Endocrinology and Metabolism Clinics, 16,* 647–665.

Leeper, R. D. (1985). Thyroid cancer. *Medical Clinics of North America, 69,* 1079–1096.

Levin, V. A., Gutin, P. H., & Leibel, L. (1993). Neoplasms of the central nervous system. In V. T. DeVita, Jr., S. Hellman, & S. A. Rosenberg (Eds.), *Cancer: Principles and practice of oncology* (4th ed., pp. 1723–1724). Philadelphia: J. B. Lippincott Co.

Luton, J. P., Cerdas, S., Billaud, L., et al. (1990). Clinical features of adrenocortical carcinoma, prognostic factors, and the effect of mitotane therapy. *New England Journal of Medicine, 322,* 1195–1201.

Maroldo, T. V., Dillon, W. P., Wilson, C. B. (1992). Advances in diagnostic techniques of pituitary tumors and prolactinomas. *Current Opinions in Oncology, 4,* 105–115.

Mazzaferri, E. L., Young, R. L., Oertel, J. E., Kemmerer, W. T., & Page, C. P. (1977). Papillary thyroid carcinoma: The impact of therapy in 576 patients. *Medicine, 56,* 171–196.

McCance, D. R., Kenny, B. D., Sloan, J. M., Russell, C. F. J., & Hadden, D. R. (1987). Parathyroid carcinoma: A review. *Journal of the Royal Society of Medicine, 80,* 505–509.

McConahey, W. M., Hay, I. D., Woolner, L. B., vanHeerden, J. A., & Taylor, W. F. (1986). Papillary thyroid cancer treated at the Mayo Clinic, 1946 through 1970: Initial manifestations, pathologic findings, therapy, and outcome. *Mayo Clinic Proceedings, 61,* 978–996.

McLeod, M. K., Few, J. W., Jr., & Shapiro, B. (1993). Diagnostic advances in APUDomas and other endocrine tumors: imaging and localization. *Seminars in Surgical Oncology, 9,* 399–432.

Moertel, C. G. (1987). An odyssey in the land of small tumors. *Journal of Clinical Oncology, 5,* 1503–1522.

Norton, J. A., Levin, B., & Jensen, R. T. (1993). Cancer of the endocrine system. In V. T. Devita, Jr., S. Hellman, & S. A. Rosenberg (Eds.), *Cancer: Principles and practice of oncology* (4th ed., pp. 1333–1435). Philadelphia: J. B. Lippincott Co.

Oberg, K., Erickson, B. (1991). The role of interferons in the management of carcinoid tumors. *Acta Oncologica, 30,* 519–522.

Odurney, A., & Birch, S. J. (1985). Hepatic arterial embolization in patients with metastatic carcinoid tumors. *Clinical Radiology, 36,* 597–602.

Pearse, A. G. E. (1977). The diffuse neuroendocrine system and the APUD concept: Related endocrine peptides in brain, intestine, pituitary, placenta, and anuran cutaneous glands. *Medical Biology, 55,* 115–125.

Philippe, J. (1992). APUDomas: acute complications and their medical management. *Bailliere's Clinical Endocrinology and Metabolism, 6,* 217–228.

Piziak, V. K., & Gilliland, P. F. (1993) Pituitary tumors: look for early signs and symptoms. *Emergency Medicine, May,* 125–132.

Refetoff, S., Harrison, J., Karanfilski, B. T., Kaplan, E. L., DeGroot, L. J., & Bekerman, C. (1975). Continuing occurrence of thyroid carcinoma after irradiation to the neck in infancy and childhood. *New England Journal of Medicine, 292,* 171–175.

Reubi, J. (1993). The role of peptides and their receptors as tumor markers. *Endocrinology and Metabolism Clinics of North America, 22,* 917–939.

Ron, E., Kleinerman, R. A., Boice, J. D. Jr., LiVolsi, V. A., Flannery, J. T., & Fraumeni, J. F. Jr. (1987). A population-based case-control study of thyroid cancer. *Journal of the National Cancer Institute, 79,* 1–12.

Rosenblatt, M. (1986). Peptide hormone antagonists that are effective in vivo: Lessons from parathyroid hormone. *New England Journal of Medicine, 315,* 1004–1011.

Saad, M. F., Ordinez, N. E., Rashid, R. K., Guido, J. J., Hill, C. S., Hickey, R. C., & Samaan, N. A. (1984). Medullary carcinoma of the thyroid: A study of the clinical features and prognostic factors in 161 patients. *Medicine, 63,* 319–342.

Samaan, N. A., & Hickey, R. C. (1987). Adrenocortical carcinoma. *Seminars in Oncology, 14,* 292–296.

Samaan, N. A., Hickey, R. C., & Shutts, P. E. (1988). Diagnosis, localization, and management of pheochromocytoma: Pitfalls and follow-up in 41 patients. *Cancer, 62,* 2451–2460.

Sardesai, S. H., Mourant, A. J., Sivathandon, Y., Farrow, R., & Givvons, D. O. (1990). Phaeochromocytoma and catecholamine induced cardiomyopathy presenting as heart failure. *British Heart Journal, 63,* 234–237.

Schantz, A., & Castleman, B. (1973). Parathyroid carcinoma: A study of 70 cases. *Cancer, 31,* 600–605.

Scheithauer, B. W., Kovacs, K., Laws, E. R., Jr., & Randall R. V. (1986). Pathology of invasive pituitary tumors with special reference to functional classification. *Journal of Neurosurgery, 65,* 733–744.

Schneider, A. B., Shore-Freedman, E., Ryo, U. Y., Bekerman, C., Favus, M., & Pinsky, S. M. (1985). Radiation-induced tumors of the head and neck following childhood irradiation. *Medicine, 64,* 1–15.

Schroder, S., Bocker, W., Baisch, H., Burk, C. G., Arps, H., Meiners, I., Kastendieck, H., Heitz, P. V., & Kloppel, G. (1988). Prognostic factors in medullary thyroid carcinomas: Survival in relation to age, sex, stage, histology, immunocytochemistry, and DNA content. *Cancer, 61,* 806–816.

Shane, E., & Bilezidian, J. P. (1982). Parathyroid carcinoma: A review of 62 patients. *Endocrine Reviews, 3,* 218–226.

Shortell, C. K., Andrus, C. H., Phillips, C. E., & Schwartz, S. I. (1991). Carcinoma of the parathyroid gland: A 30-year experience. *Surgery, 110,* 704–708.

Singer, F. R., Ritch, P. S., Lad, T. E., & Ringinberg, Q. S. (1991). Treatment of hypercalcemia of malignancy with intravenous etidronate. *Archives of Internal Medicine, 151,* 471–476.

Sisson, J. C., Frager, M. S., Valk, T. W., Gross, M. D., Swanson, D. P., Wieland, D. M., Tobes, M. C., Bierwaltes, W. H., & Thompson, N. W. (1981). Scintigraphic localization of pheochromocytoma. *New England Journal of Medicine, 305,* 12–17.

Tennvall, J., Tallroth, E., El Hassan, Aa., Lundell, G., Akerman, M., Biorklund, A., Blomgren, H., Lohagen, T., & Wallin, G. (1990). Anaplastic thyroid carcinoma: Doxorubicin, hyperfractionated radiotherapy and surgery. *Acta Oncologica, 29,* 1025–1028.

Thompson, N. W., & Cheung, P. S. (1987). Diagnosis and treatment of functioning and nonfunctioning adrenocortical neoplasms including incidentalomas. *Surgical Clinics of North America, 67,* 423–436.

Tubiana, M., Haddad, E., Schlumberger, M., Hill, C., Rougier, P., & Sarrazin, D. (1985). External radiotherapy in thyroid cancers. *Cancer, 55*(Suppl. 9), 2062–2071.

Van Slooten, H., Moolner, A. J., Van Seters, A. P., & Smeenk, D. (1990). The treatment of adrenocortical carcinoma with o,p'DDD: Prognostic implications of serum level monitoring. *European Journal of Clinical Oncology, 20,* 47–53.

Vinik, A. J., McLeod, M. K., Fig, L. M., Shapiro, B., Lloyd, R. V., & Cho, K. (1989). Clinical features, diagnosis, and localization of carcinoid tumors and their management. *Gastroenterology Clinics of North America, 18,* 865–896.

Warrell, R. P., Jr., Israel, R., Frisone, M., Snyder, T., Gaynor, J. J., & Bockman, R. S. (1988). Gallium nitrate for acute treatment of cancer-related hypercalcemia in a randomized double-blind comparison to calcitonin. *Annals of Internal Medicine, 108,* 669–674.

Weiss, L. M., Medeiros, L. J., & Vickery, A. L. (1989). Pathologic features of prognostic significance in adrenocortical carcinoma. *American Journal of Surgical Pathology, 13,* 202–206.

Williams, E. D. (1979). The aetiology of thyroid tumors. *Clinics in Endocrinology and Metabolism, 8,* 193–207.

Wilson, C. B. (1983). Surgical management of endocrine-active pituitary adenomas. In M. D. Walker (Ed.), *Oncology of the nervous system.* Boston: Martinus-Nijoff.

Wilson, S. M., Platz, C., & Block, G. M. (1970). Thyroid carcinoma after irradiation: Characteristics and treatment. *Archives of Surgery, 100,* 330–337.

Wingo, P. A., Tong, T., Bolden, S. (1995). Cancer Statistics, 1995. *CA: A Cancer Journal for Clinicians, 45,* 8–30.

Wool, M. S. (1993). Thyroid nodules: The place of fine-needle aspiration biopsy in management. *Postgraduate Medicine, 94*(1), 111–122.

Soft Tissue Sarcomas and Bone Cancers

Stephanie Chang

SOFT TISSUE SARCOMAS

Soft tissue sarcomas (STS) are uncommon neoplasms, constituting less than 1 per cent of all malignancies (American Cancer Society, 1995). These relatively rare primary malignant tumors are characterized by their diverse histologic appearance, biologic behavior, and anatomic locations. Over the past 2 decades there has been significant progress made in the recognition and treatment of soft tissue sarcomas. Management has centered on an improved understanding of the biology and natural history of these tumors, as well as new imaging techniques, newer treatment regimens, and innovative surgical procedures (Eilber et al., 1990; Rosenthal, Terek, & Lane, 1993).

EPIDEMIOLOGY AND ETIOLOGY

Soft tissue sarcomas have an annual age-adjusted incidence rate of two per 100,000 (Rosier & Constine, 1993). In the United States it is estimated that 6000 new cases will be diagnosed in 1995 with approximately 3600 deaths (American Cancer Society, 1995). It is more common in children than in adults, constituting 6.5 per cent of all neoplasms and ranking fifth as a cause of death in children below the age of 15 years (Rosier & Constine, 1993).

Very little is known about the etiology of these tumors. Hereditary factors are thought to play a part in some instances. Genetically linked diseases such as multiple neurofibromatosis, tuberous sclerosis, Werner's syndrome, intestinal polyposis, Gardner's syndrome, and basal cell nevus syndrome have been associated with soft tissue sarcomas. Occasionally, soft tissue sarcomas have developed in old scars (Rosier & Constine, 1993; Storm, 1994).

In addition, there are some soft tissue sarcomas that are linked to exogenous factors such as radiation therapy. Fibrosarcomas have developed in individuals who have received prior irradiation for benign conditions such as tuberculosis of the skin or thyroid disease. Postirradiation sarcomas also occur following high-dose cytotoxic treatment for other types of cancer, generally with a latent period from 5 to 15 years (Antman, Eilber, & Shiu, 1989; Rosier & Constine, 1993).

Chemicals such as asbestos are associated with mesothelioma and polyvinyl chloride, arsenic, and hemochromatosis with angiosarcoma of the liver. Dioxin (Agent Orange) exposure has been associated with the development of soft tissue sarcomas (Antman et al., 1989; Storm, 1994).

Identification of a sarcoma virus has been well documented in animal species but not conclusively in humans. Circulating immune complexes have been described in individuals with sarcoma and their relatives (Eilber et al., 1990).

Lymphangiosarcomas have developed in individuals with chronic lymphedema status-post-radical mastectomy. Neurofibrosarcomas or malignant schwannomas have occurred in patients with von Recklinghausen's disease (Rosier & Constine, 1993).

The majority of patients who present with soft tissue sarcomas have a history of trauma. Current studies have indicated that trauma has never been proven as a cause in the development of these tumors (Antman et al., 1989; Rosier & Constine, 1993).

BIOLOGIC PROPERTIES

Soft tissue sarcomas arise from the mesenchymal connective tissues, constituting greater than 50 per cent of total body weight. Their distinction from carcinomas is based on their origin from connective rather than epithelial tissues. Connective tissues arise from the mesoderm and include tendons, fibrous tissue, adipose tissue, blood vessels, striated and smooth muscles, fascia, and other supporting tissues located between the skin and visceral organs. Consequently, soft tissue sarcomas are classified according to their tissue of origin (Rosier & Constine, 1993; Storm, 1994).

Initially, soft tissue sarcomas grow centrifugally and form a pseudocapsule of fibrous connective tissue around the lesion. This capsule is formed as a host reaction to the neoplasm and consists of compressed normal tissue cells, inflammatory cells, and newly formed blood vessels at the expanding border of the growing sarcoma. The reactive zone at the periphery of the pseudocapsule usually contains microscopic malignant cells. It is clear from several histologic studies of these tumors that there is no true tumor capsule, even though it may appear to be totally encapsulated (Eilber et al., 1990; Peabody & Simon, 1993; Rosier & Constine, 1993).

Soft tissue sarcomas can develop in almost any anatomic site but most commonly occur in the lower extremities. These tumors are notorious for their propensity for local recurrence after simple surgical excision. This may be due to microscopic extensions of the tumor, which are often considerable distances from the visible tumor site (Eilber, 1990; Peabody & Simon, 1993).

Metastases usually occurs by hematogenous spread or local invasion into surrounding tissues by the tumor. Regional lymph node involvement is extremely rare but is seen in 8 to 10 per cent of patients with rhabdomyosarcoma or synovial cell sarcoma. The lung is the most common site of metastatic spread and may be seen in about 10 per cent of musculoskeletal neoplasms at the time of diagnosis (Peabody & Simon, 1993). Approximately 70 per cent of patients who die of soft tissue sarcomas do so because of either an uncontrolled primary or metastatic disease confined to the lung (Eilber, 1990). Rarely, distant nonpulmonary metastases are found in bone and other soft tissues (Peabody & Simon, 1993).

Presenting symptoms vary due to the anatomic location of the tumor. Peripheral neuralgia, paralysis, or edema can occur because of compression of nerves or vascular structures. Tumor involvement of visceral functions may obstruct bowel, ureters, or mediastinal structures (Eilber, 1990; Rosier & Constine, 1993).

CLASSIFICATION AND STAGING

HISTOPATHOLOGY

Soft tissue sarcomas are classified histologically and named according to the tissues they most resemble. Although there are several histologic subtypes, the two most common subtypes are liposarcoma and malignant fibrous histiocytoma. Other histologic subtypes are leiomyosarcoma, fibrosarcoma, rhabdomyosarcoma, synovial sarcoma, angiosarcoma, hemangiopericytoma, alveolar soft-part sarcoma, and epitheliod sarcoma (Tables 39–1 & 39–2) (Karakousis & Perez, 1994).

There are more than 30 different histologic subtypes of soft tissue sarcomas. This has made it difficult to determine the difference between some nonmalignant soft tissue tumors and true neoplastic lesions. Certain tumors may exhibit histologic characteristics of malignancy such as high cellularity, mitotic activity, infiltrative spread, and rapid growth (Angervall & Kindblom, 1993).

Electron microscopy and immunohistochemical staining methods are currently being utilized to further clarify various subtypes of soft tissue sarcomas. Elec-

TABLE 39–1. *Histologic Types of Soft Tissue Sarcomas*

CLASSIFICATION	SUBTYPE
Fibrous tissue	Fibrosarcoma
Adipose tissue	Liposarcoma—well differentiated, myxoid, pleomorphic
Smooth muscle	Leiomyosarcoma
Striated muscle	Rhabdomyosarcoma—alveolar, pleomorphic, embryonal
Vascular origin	Angiosarcoma
	Lymphangiosarcoma
	Malignant hemangiopericytoma
Synovial tissue	Synovial sarcoma
Mesothelioma	Malignant mesothelioma
Neurogenic origin	Neurogenic sarcoma (malignant schwannoma)
Histiocytic origin	Malignant fibrous histiocytoma
	Giant cell tumor of soft tissue
Cartilaginous origin	Extraskeletal chondrosarcoma (chordoid sarcoma)
Uncertain origin	Dermatofibrosarcoma protuberans
	Epithelioid sarcoma
	Clear cell sarcoma
	Kaposi's sarcoma
	Alveolar soft part sarcoma
	Ewing's sarcoma in soft tissue

TABLE 39–2. *Relative Incidence of Histologic Types of Soft Tissue Sarcomas*

TYPE	RANGE OF INCIDENCE (%)	AVERAGE (%)
Unclassified	5.6–36.4*	11.2
Liposarcoma	11.5–33.9	19.2
Rhabdomyosarcoma	2.9–30.0	12.8
Synovialsarcoma	0.8–19.5	12.8
Neurofibrosarcoma	3.2–19.3*	5.0
Fibrosarcoma	3.6–44.0	22.6
Angiosarcoma	0.3–4.8*	1.6
Leiomyosarcoma	2.4–11.4*	4.9
Mesenchymoma	0.3–0.9*	0.1
Malignant fibrous histiocytoma	1.0–22.8*	8.5
Other	1.7–13.5*	6.3

"Range of Incidence" column is a composite of the incidence of several researchers. Total number of cases = 4226.

*Signifies that at least one researcher found an incidence of 0%. In these cases the second lowest incidence reported is used in place of the lowest.

(From Rosier, R. N. & Constine, L. S. [1993]. Soft tissue sarcoma. In R. N. Rosier [Ed.], *Clinical oncology*. Philadelphia: W. B. Saunders Co.)

TABLE 39–3. *TNM Classification and Stage Grouping of Soft Tissue Sarcomas*

T1	Tumor 5 cm or less
T2	Tumor greater than 5 cm
N1	Regional lymph node metastasis
G1	Well differentiated
G2	Moderately well differentiated
G3–4	Poorly differentiated, undifferentiated
M1	Distant metastasis

T = tumor; N = node; M = Metastasis; G = grade.

TABLE 39–4. *Stage Grouping of Soft Tissue Sarcomas*

Stage IA	G1	T1	N0	M0
Stage IB	G1	T2	N0	M0
Stage IIA	G2	T1	N0	M0
Stage IIB	G2	T2	N0	M0
Stage IIIA	G3–4	T1	N0	M0
Stage IIIB	G3–4	T2	N0	M0
Stage IVA	Any G	Any T	N1	M0
Stage IVB	Any G	Any T	Any N	M1

(Adapted from Peabody, T. D., & Simon, M. A. [1993]. Principles of staging of soft-tissue sarcomas. *Clinical Orthopedics and Related Research, 289,* 19–31.)

TABLE 39–5. *Prognostic Factors for Soft Tissue Sarcomas*

Grade	Low grade better than high grade
Size	Smaller is better
Location	Extremity better than nonextremity
Lymphatic metastasis	Absence is better
DNA Ploidy?	Diploid may be better; data limited to high-grade sarcoma

(Adapted from Karakousis, C. P., & Perez, R. P. [1994]. Soft tissue sarcomas in adults. *CA-A Cancer Journal for Clinicians, 44(4),* 200–209. Reproduced by permission.)

tron microscopy is not only beneficial in determining histogenetic type but also aids in assessing cellular changes associated with nuclear pleomorphism, mitotic activity including abnormal mitosis, degree of cellularity, cellular growth patterns, and presence of necrosis and hemorrhages (Angervall & Kindblom, 1993; Eilber, 1990; Karakousis & Perez, 1994). Immunohistochemical stains are utilized to identify specific cellular proteins that are found in most soft tissue sarcomas. Vimentin is one of these proteins as well as keratin, myoglobin, actin, desmin, and factor 8 (Eilber, 1990). Chromosome rearrangements and cytogenetic abnormalities were of diagnostic value in establishing a definitive diagnosis in 25 per cent of cases in which routine microscopy was unable to clearly identify the tissue of origin (Rosier & Constine, 1993).

STAGING

For adult soft-tissue sarcomas, two staging systems are currently used. They are the American Joint Committee on Cancer (AJCC) staging system and the International TNM (tumor-node-metastases) staging classification. The AJCC staging system is based on grade, size, and evidence of dissemination (Table 39–3). The TNM staging system also includes a G category that represents tumor grade (Table 39–4). A panel of the AJCC is currently reviewing and revising the TNM staging system for soft tissue (Eilber, 1990; Karakousis & Perez, 1994).

The most important prognostic indicator in soft tissue sarcomas is the grade of the tumor. The grade of a tumor is a measure of its aggressiveness or tendency to metastasize. Other prognostic factors include size and extent, location, and the presence or absence of metastases (Table 39–5). The extent of the tumor as well as its size directly influence survival. The risk of local recurrence and distant metastases is greater for large vs. small tumors. Tumors 5 cm or less in diameter have a better prognosis. Extremity sarcomas generally have a better prognosis than nonextremity tumors. In the future, DNA proliferative indexes and the presence or absence of certain oncogenes or other karyotypic markers may assist in a more accurate assessment of biologic aggressiveness (Karakousis & Perez, 1994; Peabody & Simon, 1993; Rosenthal et al., 1993).

CLINICAL PRESENTATION

The majority of soft tissue sarcomas develop in the lower extremities. Most patients present with complaints of swelling and pain in the affected extremity. The average delay in seeking medical attention is approximately 4 months (Karakousis & Perez, 1994). Part of the delay is that many patients attribute the swelling to a minor injury. Those who seek medical attention may have been told that the growth is "benign" and consequently seek no further medical care. Other local signs may include peripheral neuralgia, paralysis, or edema if the tumor is compressing nerves or vascular structures (Rosier & Constine, 1993).

Most lesions tend to be large (> 5 cm) and may not be easily palpated depending on where they are located anatomically. Pelvic sarcomas may cause extremity edema or pain in the distribution of the femoral or sciatic nerve or cause obstruction to other visceral organs, which may interfere with bowel, ureters, bladder, or mediastinal structures (Karakousis & Perez, 1994; Rosier & Constine, 1993).

HISTOLOGIC SUBTYPES

LIPOSARCOMA

This tumor is the second most common soft tissue sarcoma, accounting for approximately 10 per cent of all cases. It occurs almost exclusively in adults and arises from malignant lipoblasts. Liposarcomas rarely derive from a preexisting lipoma. These neoplasms are found most often in the thigh or retroperitoneum. Recent cytogenetic analysis has revealed a consistent translocation between chromosomes 12 and 16 (Springfield, 1993).

Liposarcomas tend to be large tumors compared with other soft tissue sarcomas. Most patients present with a painless mass or complain of only a mild, dull ache. The mass is not associated with signs of inflammation, tenderness, or pulsation. The majority of cases reported occur in patients between 40 and 60 years of age. Males are affected more commonly than females. The lung is the most common site of metastases, but liposarcomas, unlike other soft tissue sarcomas, have a propensity to metastasize to the retroperitoneum, mediastinum, and bone (Springfield, 1993).

Surgical resection is the treatment of choice with or without preoperative and postoperative irradiation. Currently, no evidence exists to indicate that adjuvant chemotherapy is effective, but trials are ongoing to evaluate different treatment regimens for those patients with metastatic disease or those who are at high risk of developing metastases (Springfield, 1993).

MALIGNANT FIBROUS HISTIOCYTOMA

This tumor arises from histiocytes and is found most commonly in the thigh but can present anywhere in the body. More recently, a number of soft tissue sarcomas, once called liposarcoma or adult rhabdomyosarcoma, have been reclassified as malignant fibrous histiocytoma (MFH) (Springfield, 1993). This neoplasm accounts for 8 to 10 per cent of all nonrhabdomyosarcomas (NRSTS) in the pediatric population and can occur at any age and at any site. MFH has a higher rate of occurrence in males between the ages of 40 and 60 years. In patients who develop radiation-induced sarcomas, MFH is one of the most common diagnoses (Wexler & Helman, 1994).

Surgical resection is the treatment of choice. The benefit of adjuvant chemotherapy in patients with completely and grossly resected high-grade tumors is still unproven, but there are clinical trials currently evaluating this as well as postoperative irradiation and chemoradiotherapy regimens for nonresectable and metastatic tumors (Wexler & Helman, 1994).

RHABDOMYOSARCOMAS

This malignant tumor arises from skeletal muscle and is the third most common neoplasm in children. Nearly 50 per cent of rhabdomyosarcoma (RMS) cases are diagnosed in children 5 years of age or younger. It is slightly more common in males than females (about 1.3 to 1.4 times more common) (Wexler & Helman, 1994).

The two major histologic subtypes of RMS are embryonal and alveolar. The most common type is embryonal, and it occurs most often in young children. The most frequent site of origin is the head and neck, and these tumors rarely spread to the lymph nodes. Alveolar RMS occurs in both children and young adults. This is a very aggressive tumor with a high potential for metastases and therefore carries a poor prognosis (Wexler & Helman, 1994).

The primary aim of therapy focuses on achievement of both local control and eradication of metastases. A multimodality approach is used with surgical intervention, "risk-based" chemotherapy, and radiation therapy.

LEIOMYOSARCOMA

This rare malignant tumor arises from smooth muscle and can arise in a variety of visceral sites, including the retroperitoneum, vascular tissue, peripheral soft tissue, and gastrointestinal tract (Wexler & Helman, 1994). This soft tissue sarcoma has a poor prognosis due to its early metastatic spread (Enterline, 1981). Leiomyosarcoma is an extremely uncommon tumor in children, accounting for less than 2 per cent of nonrhabdomyosarcoma soft tissue sarcomas (Wexler & Helman, 1994).

SYNOVIAL SARCOMA

Synovial sarcomas arise from primitive mesenchymal cells and occur most frequently in the vicinity of ligaments, tendons, bursae, and joints. Sixty per cent of these lesions involve the lower extremities of individuals under the age of 40 years. Published 5-year survival figures vary from 40 to 50 per cent (Rosier & Constine, 1993).

Histologically, they are subclassified as monophasic or biphasic and occur with equal incidence. The biphasic subtypes have a better prognosis due to their differentiation and low mitotic rate. Synovial sarcomas have various growth rates, and metastases is usually to the lungs and occasionally to the regional lymph nodes. The prognosis is also more favorable in children than in adults and in more distal and smaller lesions (Cagle et al., 1987; Rosier & Constine, 1993).

The majority of patients will have pain or tenderness for 1 to 18 months prior to the appearance of a mass. Occasionally a patient will present with only a mass. Twelve months is the average duration a patient will wait before seeking medical assistance (Rosier & Constine, 1993).

HEMANGIOENDOTHELIOMA AND ANGIOSARCOMA

These rare neoplasms are derived from vascular endothelial cells and compose less than 1 per cent of sarcomas. Hemangioendothelioma is a low-grade malignant tumor with an indolent growth pattern. Metastasis occurs in about 10 to 15 per cent of reported cases. Angiosarcoma represents a high-grade tumor that metastasizes early via the hematogenous route and occurs most frequently in the skin, breast, and liver (Machleder, 1990; Rosier & Constine, 1993).

Vascular sarcomas generally present with an asymptomatic mass. High-grade lesions such as cutaneous angiosarcomas may present with one or more small reddish or purplish nodules that grow gradually. Other manifestations may be warmth, venous distension in overlying skin, and occasionally a pulsation over the area of the mass (Machleder, 1990; Rosier & Constine, 1993).

KAPOSI'S SARCOMA

This malignant lesion arises in blood vessels. Prior to the epidemic of AIDS in the United States, Kaposi's sarcoma occurred primarily in Jewish and Italian men over 65 years of age. Since 1978 there have been increasing numbers of cases that are associated with AIDS, and today this is the leading cause of Kaposi's sarcoma (Rosier & Constine, 1993).

Initially, Kaposi's sarcoma commonly presents as a raised purplish nodule or plaque on the lower distal extremities. As the disease progresses, more nodules appear, involving both the skin and viscera. When edema of the surrounding skin occurs, this indicates a sign of advanced disease. Survival in patients without AIDS is approximately 8 years. For those individuals with AIDS the prognosis is significantly worse (Rosier & Constine, 1993).

LYMPHANGIOSARCOMA

This tumor is of lymphatic vascular origin and arises most commonly in patients with long-standing lymph stasis, lymphedema, or both. Lymphangiosarcoma occurs most frequently in women with postmastectomy edema of the arm. The average age of onset is 62 years, and the frequency of occurrence is less than 1 per cent of women who develop postmastectomy lymphedema (Machleder, 1990; Rosier & Constine, 1993).

The development of an ecchymotic area in the affected upper extremity is usually the first clinical sign, and this can develop from as early as 5 years to as late as 25 years following radical mastectomy. Metastasis is common, and the median survival for patients has been reported to be 1.33 years (Machleder, 1990; Rosier & Constine, 1993).

MALIGNANT PERIPHERAL NERVE SHEATH TUMORS

Malignant schwannoma, neurogenic sarcoma, neurofibrosarcoma, and malignant neurilemmoma are all categorized as malignant peripheral nerve sheath tumors. These neoplasms can occur at any age but are uncommon in the first 2 decades of life. The brachial plexus, sciatic, medial, and spinal nerves are most commonly affected. Although they are rare, these tumors tend to be high-grade and locally invasive. Common sites of metastases are the lungs and bones. Approximately, 25 to 35 per cent occur in individuals with von Recklinghausen's disease (neurofibromatosis). Surgical intervention is the only option for definitive treatment (Antman et al., 1989; Wexler & Helman, 1994).

BONE CANCERS

Primary malignant bone tumors represent only 0.2 per cent of all primary cancers in the United States today (American Cancer Society, 1995). In the past 2 decades tremendous strides have been made in the management of these tumors. Improvements and advances in orthopedics, surgery, bioengineering, radiograph imaging, radiotherapy, chemotherapy, pathology, and a standardized surgical staging system have all contributed to the improvement and increased survival of individuals with these neoplasms (Malawer, Link, & Donaldson, 1989; Rosier, Boros, & Konski, 1993).

EPIDEMIOLOGY AND ETIOLOGY

Approximately 2070 new cases occur in the United States annually (American Cancer Society, 1995). The incidence is highest during adolescence, with a rate of three per 100,000, yet it composes only 3.2 per cent of childhood malignancies before the age of 15 years. The incidence falls to 0.2 per 100,000 between the ages of 30 to 35 years. A steady climb ensues after this, and by the age of 60 years, the incidence equals that of adolescence (Rosier et al., 1993). Males account for 1100 of the annual reported cases, and females are slightly less with an annual incidence of 970. The annual death rate is approximately 1380 (American Cancer Society, 1995).

Osteosarcoma and Ewing's sarcoma are the two most common bone tumors. Other bone tumors include fibrosarcoma, chondrosarcoma, and liposarcoma as seen in Table 39–6 (Malawer et al., 1989).

TABLE 39–6. *Classification of Malignant Bone Tumors*

HISTOLOGIC TYPE	SUBTYPE
Chondrogenic	Primary chondrosarcoma
	Secondary chondrosarcoma
	Dedifferentiated chondrosarcoma
	Mesenchymal chondrosarcoma
Osteogenic	Osteosarcoma
	Parosteal osteosarcoma
Fibrosarcoma	
Unknown origin	Ewing's tumor
	Malignant giant cell tumor
	Adamantinoma
Notochordal	Chordoma
Vascular	Hemangioendothelioma
	Hemangiopericytoma
Lipogenic	Liposarcoma

There are multiple etiologic factors that have been implicated in certain types of primary bone cancers. Radiation has been linked to the formation of osteogenic sarcomas, chondrosarcomas, and fibrosarcomas. Postirradiation sarcomas characteristically occur in the previously irradiated fields and are seen more frequently when high doses of radiation have been utilized. The median time from radiation therapy to the occurrence of postirradiation sarcoma is between 10 and 11 years, although cases have been reported as early as 4 years and as late as 25 years. The most common sites of these postirradiation sarcomas include the sternum, sternoclavicular joint, cervical and thoracic spine, and the pelvis (Rosen et al., 1990a; Rosier et al., 1993).

Prolonged growth or overstimulated metabolism as seen with long-standing Paget's disease is another etiologic factor associated with the development of osteosarcoma and giant cell tumors. The incidence of osteogenic sarcoma in this population is 1000 times greater than in the normal population and is almost always highly malignant. The pelvis and proximal femur are the most common sites of Paget-induced osteosarcoma. Other disorders associated with bone tumors due to metabolic stimulation include hyperparathyroidism (osteosarcoma), chronic osteomyelitis (osteosarcoma), old bone infarcts (malignant fibrous histiocytoma), and fracture callus (Rosen et al., 1990a; Rosier et al., 1993).

Rapid skeletal growth in children may account for the development of primary skeletal neoplasms. The most common site of bone sarcomas is in the distal femur and proximal tibia, the two areas with the most active growth plates (Rosier et al., 1993).

There is a rare form of osteogenic sarcoma that arises in patients with familial or bilateral retinoblastoma. Familial retinoblastoma is a bilateral congenital disease in which radiation therapy is used as part of the treatment. It has been noted that in patients with this disease the incidence of osteogenic sarcoma in the irradiated site (usually maxilla) is 1000 times greater than that in the normal population. Patients with familial retinoblastoma also have an incidence 500 times that of the normal population of developing osteogenic sarcoma at distant sites, such as the distal femur. Chromosomal abnormalities have been noted in this group, particularly deletions in chromosome 13. Another chromosomal abnormality, an 11:22 translocation, has been identified in Ewing's sarcoma (Rosen et al., 1990b).

The role of infectious agents, such as a sarcoma virus, has been well documented in other species but not conclusively in humans. It is generally felt that there is no one single cause but rather a combination of etiologic factors that promote the growth of these tumors (Rosier et al., 1993).

BIOLOGIC PROPERTIES

Primary bone tumors are categorized by their biologic behavior, which is identified as their ability to grow and extend beyond their natural barriers. Some malignant bone tumors have a slow, indolent growth pattern and a low incidence of metastases. Others exhibit aggressive and destructive behavior and are associated with a high incidence of metastases (Enneking & Conrad, 1989).

Specific anatomic barriers of bone cancers include the pseudocapsule, which consists of bone or fibrous tissue around the lesion. This is seen most frequently at the periphery of the tumor where the cells are least mature. The reactive zone forms between the pseudocapsule and the surrounding normal bone. It is formed by reactive bone or fibrous tissue and neovascular and inflammatory tissues. Tumors frequently break through the pseudocapsule and invade the reactive zone to form noncontiguous satellite lesions. These satellite lesions are called "skip metastases" and are usually associated with a poor prognosis (Enneking & Conrad, 1989; Meyer & Malawer, 1991).

There are three mechanisms associated with the growth and extension of bone tumors. These include the compression of normal tissue by the malignant lesion, resorption of normal bone by reactive osteoclasts, and direct destruction of normal tissue. In general, bone sarcomas take the path of least resistance. Most benign bone tumors are unicompartmental; they remain confined and may expand the bone in which they arose. Malignant bone tumors are bicompartmental; they destroy the overlying cortex and extend and invade the adjacent soft tissue (Malawer et al., 1989).

CLASSIFICATION AND STAGING

HISTOPATHOLOGY

Bone tumors are classified histologically by the cell or tissue type from which they originate. Bone consists of cartilaginous, osteoid, fibrous tissue, reticuloendothelial, and vascular. Cartilage tumors are lesions in which cartilage is produced. Chondrosarcoma is the most common malignant cartilage tumor. Osteoid tumors are lesions in which the stroma produces osteoid. Osteosarcoma are the most common primary malignant tumors of the bone. Other primary malignant bone tumors include fibrosarcoma, Ewing's sarcoma, and giant cell tumors (Malawer et al., 1989; Rosier et al., 1993).

The tumor's mitotic activity, degree of cellular differentiation, and/or degree of tissue necrosis determines the "histologic grade" and biologic activity of the tumor. Assessment of the histologic type and grade is the key to identification and appropriate treatment of these specific neoplasms (Enneking & Conrad, 1989).

High-grade sarcomas have a poorly defined reactive zone and appear to have little or no pseudoencapsulation. They rapidly invade and extend beyond this zone to adjacent tissues. Satellite nodules may occur in normal appearing tissue, which is distant from the primary tumor. These nodules are skip metastases (Enneking & Conrad, 1989; Malawer et al., 1989).

Low-grade sarcomas have a slower growth pattern and tend to invade local tissue, yet have a low risk of metastases. They have a thick reactive zone that forms a pseudocapsule around the lesion. These tumors are usually asymptomatic, appearing as slowly growing masses (Malawer et al., 1989; Enneking & Conrad, 1989).

STAGING

In 1980, the Musculoskeletal Tumor Society (MSTS) adopted a Surgical Staging System (SSS) for bone sarcomas (Table 39–7). It is based on the GTM (grade, location, metastases) classification and compartmental localization of the tumor. The histologic grade (G) of the tumor determines whether it is low-grade (G1) or high-grade (G2). The location (T) represents the site and the compartmental location of the tumor, which may be intracompartmental (T1) or extracompartmental (T2). A compartment is an anatomic space delineated by natural barriers to tumor extension. Involvement of more than one compartment leads to placement in a higher surgical stage and correlates with poorer prognosis. Metastases (M1) of bone tumors carries a poor prognosis whether there is regional lymphatic involvement or distant metastases. Both indicate wide dissemination of the disease (Heare, Enneking, & Heare 1989; Malawer et al., 1989; Rosier et al., 1993).

Heare et al. (1989) developed the SSS to assist in surgical planning and assessment. The stages of malignant lesions are designated by the Roman numerals I, II, and III. They are further subdivided into A (intracompartmental) and B (extracompartmental) and are summarized in Table 39–7 (Heare et al., 1989; Malawer et al., 1989).

CLINICAL PRESENTATION

Generally, patients present with pain in the area of the lesion. This is due to the stretching of the periosteum by the tumor. The intensity of the pain may be worse at night and does not tend to increase with physical activity. In more advanced lesions soft tissue swelling may be noted. Occasionally, a patient may present with a pathologic fracture of the involved bone. If the lesion is near a joint, an effusion or stiffness may

occur. Systemic symptoms such as weight loss, fever, malaise, or night sweats are uncommon for most bone sarcomas with the exception of Ewing's sarcoma or patients who present with multiple metastases (Rosier et al., 1993).

HISTOLOGIC SUBTYPES

OSTEOSARCOMA

Clinical Characteristics. Classic osteosarcoma (osteogenic sarcoma) is a high-grade, malignant, spindle-cell tumor arising within the bone. It is the most common primary malignant bone tumor, accounting for approximately 20 per cent of all reported cases (Klein, Kenan, & Lewis, 1989). Most osteosarcoma are the classic variety, but there are subclassifications as well (Table 39–6). It typically occurs during childhood and adolescence with a peak incidence between the ages of 10 and 20 years. Its peak incidence in females is 13.5 years and in males, 14.5 years, corresponding to the peak adolescent growth spurt in each gender. Males are affected more frequently than females by a ratio of 1:6 to 1:0. There are approximately 1.7 cases per million reported in the United States annually. In patients older than 40 years, it is usually associated with a pre-existent condition, such as Paget's disease, irradiated bones, hereditary exostosis, or polyostotic fibrous dysplasia (Klein et al., 1989; Malawer et al., 1989; Rosen et al., 1990a).

The most common site of involvement is the knee area (50 per cent), particularly the distal femur, followed by the proximal tibia and the proximal humerus (25 per cent). Other less common sites are the distal radius, proximal femur, and pelvis. In general, 80 to 90 per cent of osteosarcomas occur in the metaphysis of long bones (Enneking & Conrad, 1989; Malawer et al., 1989; Rosen et al., 1990a).

At the time of diagnosis, most patients will have stage IIB lesions, while 20 per cent will present with skip metastases. Due to its high propensity for distant hematogenous spread, 10 per cent of patients with osteosarcoma will have developed clinically detectable pulmonary or lymph node metastases, and over 80 per cent will have micrometastases. Although lymph node metastases does occur, it is extremely rare because bones lack a lymphatic system. Laboratory studies are seldom helpful, with the exception of serum alkaline phosphatase levels, which are elevated in 45 to 50 per cent of these patients. This laboratory study cannot be utilized for diagnostic purposes, because it can be elevated in association with other skeletal diseases (Enneking & Conrad, 1989; Malawer et al., 1989; Meyer & Malawer, 1991).

Radiographic Characteristics. Radiographically, the bone involved in osteosarcoma may be sclerotic, lytic, or show a mixed response. Other characteristics include early cortical destruction, poorly defined margins, and a periosteal reaction that may appear as a triangular area of bone known as "Codman's triangle" or a "sunburst" pattern produced by spicules of neoplastic bone (Enneking & Conrad, 1989; Klein et al., 1989; Rosier et al., 1993).

TABLE 39–7. *Staging System for Malignant Bone Tumors*

STAGE		GRADE	SITE	METASTASIS
IA	Low-grade, intracompartmental	G1	T1	M0
IB	Low-grade, extracompartmental	G1	T2	M0
IIA	High-grade, intracompartmental	G2	T1	M0
IIB	High-grade, extracompartmental	G2	T2	M0
IIIA	Low- or high-grade, intracompartmental with metastases	G1–2	T1	M1
IIIB	Low- or high-grade, extracompartmental with metastases	G1–2	T2	M1

(Adapted from Enneking, W. F. [1989]. Common bone tumors. *Clinical Symposia, 41*(3), 2–32. Reproduced by permission.)

The current treatment of choice for osteogenic sarcomas is surgery combined with chemotherapy. Prior to the addition of chemotherapy, the 5-year survival rate for patients with surgery alone or a combination of surgery and radiation was between 10 and 20 per cent. Today, with combined chemotherapy and surgery, the survival rate is 60 to 80 per cent (Eilber et al., 1987; Rosen et al., 1990a; Rosier et al., 1993).

EWING'S SARCOMA

Clinical Characteristics. Ewing's sarcoma is a highly malignant bone tumor and is classified as a small round tumor that originates from the nonmesenchymal elements of the bone marrow. It usually occurs in the midshaft or diaphysis of flat and long bones.

Histologically, the tumor consists of sheets of cells that are round and have small round nuclei. In most cases the tumor extends beyond the confines of the cortex and may be solid or semiliquid. There is no capsule surrounding the lesion, and it is common to find areas of necrosis and hemorrhage at the tumor site. Ewing's sarcoma occurs commonly in the second decade of life and affects males about twice as frequently as females. It is a relatively uncommon tumor in persons above the age of 30 years and below the age of 10 years and composes 6 per cent of all primary malignant bone lesions. It is extremely rare in the African-American population and occurs only at 1/11 the frequency seen in other racial populations (Enneking & Conrad, 1989; Pritchard, 1989; Rosen et al., 1990b).

This primary malignant bone lesion occurs most frequently in the femoral diaphysis, followed by the skull, pelvis, ilium, tibia, humerus, fibula, and ribs. Tumors in the pelvis pose an especially difficult challenge in treatment. By the time they are clinically detectable, the tumor is usually very large, thus making surgical resection difficult.

Patients usually present with progressive pain and swelling at the tumor site. Some patients experience symptoms for several months before seeking medical aid. Other common manifestations include a low-grade fever or flulike symptoms such as malaise, weakness, and fatigue. Occasionally, patients may experience weight loss, lethargy, anemia, leukocytosis, and an elevated erythrocyte sedimentation rate. The presence of pulmonary metastases at time of initial diagnosis has been reported in 14 to 35 per cent of patients. Other sites of metastases include the bones (primarily the skull) and regional lymph nodes. Metastatic disease most commonly presents as multiple or "showers" of metastatic lesions versus a solitary mass (Enneking & Conrad, 1989; Nirenberg & Bridgewater, 1986; Pritchard, 1989; Rosen et al., 1990b).

Radiographic Characteristics. Radiographically, Ewing's sarcoma appears as a mottled or moth-eaten lesion with diffuse bone involvement. Lytic destruction is the most common finding due to reactive new bone formation that produces dense areas. There may be multiple layers of subperiosteal reactive new bone, which radiographically gives this neoplasm an "onion-skin" appearance. The formation of this new bone is the result of periosteal reaction to the tumor tissue that has invaded the cortex (Enneking & Conrad, 1989; Nirenberg & Bridgewater, 1989).

Current treatment recommendations include a multimodality approach utilizing radiation, chemotherapy, and surgery. Ewing's sarcoma is extremely radiosensitive and chemosensitive. Originally, surgery was advocated only for large bulky tumors due to their high local recurrence rate. Currently, surgery is recommended for a majority of these tumors, since local recurrence is being seen even with small, localized extremity tumors treated with megavoltage radiation. Amputation is rarely done, since most patients are able to undergo limb salvage surgery. The estimated 5-year survival rates range from 54 to 74 per cent (Rosen et al., 1990b; Pritchard, 1989).

CHONDROSARCOMA

Clinical Characteristics. Classic chondrosarcoma is the second most common primary spindle-cell tumor of bone and is characterized by the formation of cartilage by tumor cells. Several variants of this tumor type have been identified (Table 39–6). The classic chondrosarcomas are central (arising within a bone) or peripheral (arising from the surface of a bone). Seventy-six per cent of these neoplasms arise centrally. Fifty per cent of all chondrosarcomas occur in persons older than 40 years of age. Only 3.8 per cent occur in patients younger than 20 years. Males are affected twice as often as females (Enneking & Conrad, 1989; Greenspan, 1989; Malawer et al., 1989).

Chondrosarcomas occur most frequently in the pelvis (31 per cent), femur (21 per cent), and shoulder girdle (13 per cent). They are the most common malignant tumors of the sternum and scapula (Malawer et al., 1989).

Initial clinical presentation of patients with chondrosarcoma varies. Peripheral tumors may become quite large without causing pain, and local symptoms occur due to mechanical irritation of the lesion. Pelvic chondrosarcomas are often large and may be painless or present with referred pain to the back or thigh. Sciatica may also occur due to sacral plexus irritation. Other associated symptoms include urinary abnormalities from bladder neck involvement or unilateral edema due to iliac vein obstruction. Central chondrosarcomas present with a persistent, dull, aching pain similar to that of arthritis. Pain is an ominous sign of a central cartilage lesion, because it indicates active tumor growth. The majority of chondrosarcomas are either grade I or II. Metastases will occur in 15 to 40 per cent of moderate-grade lesions, whereas high-grade lesions have a 75 per cent rate of dissemination (Greenspan, 1989; Malawer et al., 1989).

Radiographic Characteristics. Central chondrosarcomas have two distinct radiologic patterns. One appears as a small, well-defined lytic lesion with a sclerotic border and comma-shaped calcifications surrounding it. The second type has no sclerotic border and is difficult to localize. Endosteal scalloping is the key sign indicating that the lesion is malignant. Peripheral chondrosarcomas are much easier to identify radiographically. They appear as a large, calcified mass protruding from bone (Enneking & Conrad, 1989; Greenspan, 1989; Malawer et al., 1989).

Surgical resection with limb-sparing procedures is the primary treatment intervention for chondrosarcomas. The majority of these tumors tend to be low-grade and slow-growing, thus making surgical intervention a viable option for long-term survival. Neither adjuvant chemotherapy nor radiation therapy has proven to be effective in the treatment of this disease (Enneking & Conrad, 1989; Greenspan, 1989; Malawer et al., 1989).

FIBROSARCOMA

Clinical Characteristics. Fibrosarcoma accounts for less than 4 per cent of all primary malignant bone tumors and is most often seen in adolescents and middle-aged adults. It is characterized by interlacing bundles of collagen fibers that resemble a "herringbone" pattern. These malignant lesions may be either central or cortical (periosteal) (Malawer et al., 1989).

The long bones are most affected, particularly the femur and the tibia, but 15 per cent of tumors are found in the bones of the head and neck. The histologic grade is a good indicator of metastatic potential. Late metastases do occur, and 10-year and 15-year survival rates vary. In general, the prognosis is better for periosteal (cortical) versus central lesions. Patients generally present with pain and swelling of the affected area (Malawer et al., 1989).

Radiographic Characteristics. Radiographically, chondrosarcoma reveals a radiolucent lesion of the metaphyseal area. This appearance closely correlates with the histologic grade of the tumor. Low-grade tumors are well defined and usually remain within the bone. High-grade tumors have poorly defined margins with a "moth-eaten" pattern signifying bone destruction (Enneking & Conrad, 1989; Malawer et al., 1989).

Surgical management is the optimal treatment for fibrosarcomas. Excision with a wide margin is indicated for stage IA lesions, whereas stage IIB lesions require radical or wide resections with adjuvant chemotherapy or radiation therapy. The prognosis is guarded for stage II tumors, and the reported 5-year survival rate is 21.8 per cent (Enneking & Conrad, 1989).

CLINICAL STAGING

The evaluation of a patient with a suspected primary malignant bone tumor or soft tissue sarcoma involves a multidisciplinary approach by the health care team. The evaluation begins with a thorough medical history and physical examination. The individual's age, site and size of the lesion, presenting symptoms, occupation, and the presence of associated risk factors such as Paget's disease of the bone (osteosarcoma) or neurofibromatosis (neurofibrosarcoma) are identified. Selected laboratory studies and radiographs are obtained. Based on the results of these tests, further staging studies may be initiated to determine histologic diagnosis, local extent, and regional or distant spread (Enneking & Conrad, 1989).

Diagnostic Imaging. Although a biopsy will be necessary to determine the histopathology of a tumor, both the local and distant extent of the tumor must first be determined by radiographic staging. The purpose of this is twofold. The first is to obtain information regarding probable diagnosis, and the second is to define the anatomic extent of the tumor. Surgical manipulation of the lesion prior to adequate staging studies will make interpretation of the study results more difficult. If the plain radiographs suggest an aggressive or malignant tumor, further staging studies should be performed prior to the biopsy (Heare et al., 1989; Peabody & Simon, 1993).

The first study obtained in most instances is the plain radiograph (Table 39-8). Plain radiographs give the most general diagnostic information about the tumor. This study is of lesser value in the evaluation of soft tissue sarcomas than it is in primary bone sarcomas, but it still remains an important component of clinical staging. Plain radiographs are able to demonstrate the bone involved, the extent and pattern of destruction, and the amount of reactive bone formed (Heare et al., 1989; Peabody & Simon, 1993; Rosier et al., 1993).

Bone scintigraphy (bone scans) is utilized to estimate the extent of local intramedullary involvement of the tumor and to screen for the presence of distant metastases. Bone scans also play an important role in the posttreatment follow-up of many primary and metastatic tumors (Peabody & Simon, 1993; Heare et al., 1989).

Computed tomography (CT) is used to delineate intraosseous and extraosseous extension of the tumor. CT scanning is the most sensitive technique to detect pulmonary metastases, which occurs frequently with both soft tissue and primary bone sarcomas.

Magnetic resonance imaging (MRI) is now accepted as the primary imaging method for estimating tumor extension within the marrow space and with respect to muscle groups, subcutaneous fat, joints, and major neovascular structures around the tumor. MRI is the single most valuable imaging study in the evaluation of the local extent of soft tissue sarcomas. This is essential in planning surgical biopsy or treatment (Murphy, 1991; Rosier et al., 1993).

TABLE 39–8. *Imaging Techniques for Evaluation of Primary Bone and Soft Tissue Sarcomas*

Radiography	Initial staging technique for primary bone tumors. Identifies bone involved, extent and type of destruction, and amount of reactive bone formed.
Bone scan	Essential to evaluate for presence of bone lesions, extent of local intraosseous involvement, activity of tumor, and skeletal metastases.
Computed tomography	Determines intraosseous and extraosseous extension of tumor and presence of matrix or cortical penetration. Essential in identifying surgical options (i.e., limb-sparing surgery).
Magnetic resonance imaging	Most accurate to determine extent of soft tissue involvement. Mainly used with soft tissue rather than bone tumors.
Angiography	Seldom useful except to serve as a vascular road map for surgery.

Currently, the use of thallium scintigraphy in the evaluation of musculoskeletal tumors is under investigation. The role of this technique may prove useful for measuring the effect of preoperative adjuvant treatment if a baseline study is obtained (Peabody & Simon, 1993).

Angiography is no longer used as frequently in delineating the location of major vessels surrounding the primary tumor due to the increasing use of CT with contrast or MRI. Both these imaging techniques provide this information. However, in pelvic lesions, angiography is still useful in defining the location of major vessels in relationship to the tumor (Rosier & Constine, 1993; Rosier et al., 1993).

Biopsy. The biopsy is a critical part of the overall management of patients with soft-tissue and bone sarcomas. It should be performed only after all imaging studies have been completed. Information obtained from these diagnostic studies will help determine not only the type of biopsy to be performed but also its location (Shives, 1993).

The biopsy is necessary for specific histologic diagnosis and pathologic grading of the tumor. Tissue for diagnosis may be obtained by closed (fine-needle aspiration or trocar) or open (incisional or excisional) biopsy. Currently, no consensus exists as to which is the preferred method.

The location of the biopsy incision is critical. One of the most common causes for amputation is a poorly placed biopsy in which local tumor contamination occurs. The incision for biopsy should be placed so that it can be excised en bloc at the time of the definitive surgical procedure. It is recommended that the biopsy be done by the same surgeon or surgical team who will perform the surgery (Meyer & Malawer, 1991; Shives, 1993).

To document the importance of biopsy technique, Mankin, Lange, and Spannier (1982) performed an extensive analysis of complications caused by inappropriate biopsy methods; the complications include the following.

1. The incidence of significant problems in patient management was 20 per cent.
2. The incidence of wound healing complications after biopsy was 20 per cent.
3. Eight per cent of biopsies produced a significant adverse effect on prognosis.
4. Five per cent of biopsies significantly contributed to an unnecessary amputation.
5. Errors in diagnosis leading to inadequate treatment occurred twice as often when the biopsy was done in a community hospital before referral, as opposed to when the biopsy was done after referral to an oncology center (Shives, 1993).

TREATMENT MANAGEMENT

SURGERY

Surgical management in conjunction with other treatment modalities is indicated for a majority of primary bone and soft tissue sarcomas. Surgery was the first treatment modality applied to these tumors and remains an essential element in the treatment management of these patients.

Until the early 1970's amputation had been the standard method of ablation of the primary tumor. Local control was achieved in most cases by cross-bone amputations or disarticulations, yet only 20 per cent of patients survived for 5 years or longer. This indicated that about 80 per cent of patients most likely had systemic microscopic disease at the time of initial diagnosis (Klein et al., 1989).

In the early to mid-1980's multiple research studies supported the validity of the limb salvage protocol for high-grade sarcomas. This limb-sparing procedure resulted in excellent local control of tumor and a high salvage rate of functional limbs. This surgical approach in conjunction with chemotherapy, radiation therapy, or both has proven to be as successful for long-term survival as that of amputation utilizing the same adjuvant therapies. Approximately 90 per cent of all sarcomas are salvageable (Antman et al., 1989, Piasecki, 1991; Simon, 1991).

The surgical approach is determined by the tumor location and histology. The general process of a limb-sparing technique, which avoids amputation while achieving adequate disease control, consists of tumor excision, bone reconstruction, and soft tissue and muscle coverage. If there is no evidence of distant metastases, the excision must be wide or radical to achieve tumor-free margins. The excision of the sarcoma must be en bloc. This technique involves wide excision of surrounding normal tissue, removal of entire muscle bundles at points of origin and insertion, and resection of involved bone as well as vascular structures. A whole block or "compartment" is surgically removed. A margin of at least 5 to 7 cm above and below the limit of tumor activity is necessary to ensure complete tumor removal (Bowden & Booher, 1958; Frieden et al., 1993; Hockenberry & Lane, 1988; Rosier et al., 1993).

Orthopaedic oncologists have developed new techniques of limb reconstruction to assist in the success of limb-sparing surgery with the development of custom prosthetic implants, bone grafts, allografts, or free vascularized tissue transfers to reestablish skeletal continuity and vascularity. In cases involving resection of all or parts of joints, arthrodesis with segmental allografts or custom prosthetic joint replacements can be used.

In previous years amputation was believed to be the procedure of choice for most patients with soft tissue and bone sarcomas. This surgical procedure continues to be a definitive treatment option for many individuals in whom a limb-sparing resection would not be feasible. Contraindications to receiving a limb-sparing surgery include: (1) major neurovascular involvement, (2) pathologic fractures, (3) inappropriate biopsy sites, (4) infection, (5) immature skeletal age, and (6) extensive muscle involvement (Klein et al., 1989; Meyer & Malawer, 1991).

CHEMOTHERAPY

SOFT TISSUE SARCOMAS

Currently, there are many chemotherapeutic regimens used in the United States and throughout the world. It is difficult to evaluate chemoresponsiveness, because so few clinical trials have been run in a randomized, stratified manner based on tumor grade and histology. Therefore, it has been difficult to provide accurate assessment of the benefits of chemotherapy for soft tissue sarcomas.

The modest response rates achieved with single-agent or combination chemotherapy for advanced or metastatic disease have been disappointing. The role of adjuvant chemotherapy remains controversial. Currently, the association of anthracyclines and ifosfamide combined with or without dacarbazine represents the treatment of choice for advanced soft tissue sarcomas (Santoro & Bonadonna, 1993). This observation is highly supported by the preliminary results of both the ongoing European Organization on Research and Treatment of Cancer (EORTC) trial group as well as the Milan Cancer Institute. Both have demonstrated a 45 per cent response rate using this regimen (Santoro & Bonadonna, 1993). The majority of papers currently published have analyzed the results of this regimen and conclude that the response rate was generally superior to other treatment regimens, but the ifosfamide-containing regimens do not provide an increased survival advantage compared with doxorubicin alone. Doxorubicin still remains the most active single agent for soft tissue sarcomas, yielding a response rate of 26 (15 to 34) per cent (Eilber et al., 1988). Several doxorubicin analogs such as epirubicin, pirarubicin, carminomycin, and azotomnycin also have demonstrated similar activity and are now being incorporated into combination regimens (Santoro & Bonadonna, 1993; Elias, 1993).

Preliminary results of phase II studies using cisplatin showed very little activity in soft tissue sarcomas, but it is currently being reinvestigated because of the significant response observed in pediatric bone sarcomas (Elias, 1993).

Phase I and II trials are evaluating the efficacy of standard and high-dose methotrexate as well as some of the investigational methotrexate analogs (trimetrexate, edatrexate). Actinomycin-D, etoposide, and vincristine are quite active in the the treatment of pediatric sarcomas, but they have shown very little activity in their adult counterparts (Elias, 1993; Mertens & Bramwell, 1993).

The biologic response modifiers such as interleukin-2, interferon, lymphokine activated cells, and tumor necrosis factor have not demonstrated any activity in the treatment of these neoplasms (Elias, 1993).

The role of adjuvant chemotherapy in the treatment of soft tissue sarcomas has not been clearly established. Local therapy has improved dramatically over the last 10 years, leading to enhanced local control and function. Systemic therapy still remains relatively ineffective and has not been shown to affect long-term survival.

PRIMARY BONE SARCOMAS

Survival results for osteosarcoma and Ewing's sarcoma have steadily improved with the development of increasingly effective systemic chemotherapeutic regimens. Dose intensity of specific cytotoxic agents, such as high-dose methotrexate, has led to a marked increase in survival (Santoro & Bonadonna, 1993).

Doxorubicin, cisplatin, and high-dose methotrexate with leucovorin rescue are the most effective single agents in the primary treatment for metastatic unresectable osteosarcoma. Combination chemotherapy regimens include the addition of bleomycin, cyclophosphamide, and dactinomycin (BCD) to high-dose methotrexate and doxorubicin (Rosier, et al., 1993; Santoro & Bonadonna, 1993).

Combination chemotherapy is currently being used in both the preoperative as well as postoperative settings for localized primary osteosarcoma. Study results clearly demonstrate that chemotherapy plays a significant role in prolonging disease-free survival. At the University of California, Los Angeles, a prospective randomized trial compared patients who received postoperative adjuvant chemotherapy and those who received no adjuvant treatment. Chemotherapy consisted of vincristine, high-dose methotrexate/leucovorin rescue, doxorubicin, and BCD. At a median follow-up of 2 years, the chemotherapy arm had a greater disease-free survival (DFS) of 55 per cent vs. 20 per cent and an overall survival of 80 per cent vs. 48 per cent. A second prospective randomized study, the Multi-Institutional Osteosarcoma Study, showed similar results (Rosen et al., 1990a; Rosier et al., 1993).

Preoperative or neoadjuvant chemotherapy is the newest approach for treatment of primary osteosarcomas. Neoadjuvant therapy begins after the initial biopsy of the tumor and utilizes the same combination chemotherapy regimen as the postoperative course. This approach, unlike postoperative therapy, avoids any delay in systemic treatment. Neoadjuvant chemotherapy can shrink the primary tumor, better define the surgical margins, and markedly decrease the vascularity of the tumor prior to surgery (Rosen et al., 1990a; Rosier et al., 1993).

At the time of surgery, chemoresponsiveness of the tumor is assessed according to the percentage of tumor necrosis in the resected specimen (Table 39–9). Postoperatively, the patients with greater than 90 per cent necrosis were continued on the same regimen they had received preoperatively. Utilizing this approach, Rosen

TABLE 39–9. *Histologic Grading of the Effect of Preoperative Chemotherapy on Primary Osteosarcoma*

GRADE	EFFECT
I	Little or no effect identified
II	Areas of acellular tumor osteoid, necrotic, or fibrotic material due to the effect of chemotherapy, with areas of histologically viable tumor
III	Predominant areas of acellular tumor osteoid, necrotic, or fibrotic material due to the effect of chemotherapy with only scattered foci of histologically visible viable tumor cells
IV	No histologic evidence of viable tumor identified within the entire specimen

(Adapted from Malawer, M. [1987]. Sarcomas of bone. In V. T. DeVita, S. Hellman, & S. A. Rosenberg (Eds.), *Cancer: principles and practice of oncology* [pp. 1418–1468]. Philadelphia: J. B. Lippincott Co.)

et al. (1990a) treated 49 patients. Forty-eight (98 per cent) of these patients were disease-free at 7 to 51 months of follow-up. Twenty-nine patients had less than 90 per cent necrosis of their tumor, so the postoperative chemotherapy regimen was changed from high-dose methotrexate to cisplatin. Twenty-seven (93 per cent) of these patients were disease-free at 6 to 29 months of follow-up (Rosier et al., 1993).

Multiple studies support Rosen's results (Rosier et al., 1993). The results in these studies suggest that response to neoadjuvant therapy can be used to identify those patients who will have an excellent prognosis. Further studies are underway to determine the necessity and the frequency of postoperative chemotherapy if an individual has obtained a complete histologic response to preoperative chemotherapy (Rosen et al., 1990a).

Etoposide has recently been added to neoadjuvant regimens (cyclophosphamide, cisplatin, and doxorubicin) for osteosarcoma. Cassano, Graham-Pole, and Dickson (1991) have demonstrated a response rate of 88 per cent. Though these reported findings are preliminary, they do suggest that full-dose etoposide will probably represent a new effective drug in the primary treatment of localized and metastatic osteosarcoma (Santoro & Bonadonna, 1993).

The overall 5-year survival for Ewing's sarcoma following local treatment with surgery or radiation therapy is less than 15 per cent. Chemotherapy has been shown to be effective in improving survival. Most patients receive a four-drug regimen consisting of cyclophosphamide, doxorubicin, dactinomycin, and vincristine (VACA). Cyclophosphamide is currently the most effective cytotoxic agent utilized in the treatment of Ewing's sarcoma, followed by doxorubicin (Pritchard, 1989; Rosen et al., 1990b; Rosier et al., 1993). Rosen et al. (1990) treated 20 patients with adjuvant VACA. Fifteen of 20 patients had no evidence of recurrent disease at a median follow-up of 46 months. LeMevel, Hoerni, and Durant (1979) treated 23 patients with VAC and procarbazine or dactinomycin. The estimated disease-free survival was 56 per cent at 3 years (Rosier et al., 1993). Ifosfamide has demonstrated activity in Ewing's sarcoma and is currently being used in randomized trials comparing the efficacy of high-dose cyclophosphamide with that of ifosfamide (Pritchard, 1989; Rosen et al., 1990).

Ewing's sarcoma may be improved by the addition of surgery following preoperative chemotherapy and radiation. As with osteosarcoma, the tumor specimen is assessed for tumor necrosis. Those patients with less than 90 per cent tumor necrosis had only a 30 per cent survival, whereas patients with 90 per cent or greater tumor necrosis had an 80 per cent disease-free survival at 4 years (Rosen et al., 1990b). The utilization of surgical intervention following preoperative chemotherapy and radiation therapy can, as in the case of osteosarcoma, predict the success of therapy in curing the patient.

RADIATION THERAPY

SOFT TISSUE SARCOMAS
Radiation therapy when utilized alone is of marginal value in the treatment of soft tissue sarcomas. Occasionally, it is used in patients who have inoperable tumors or have metastatic or advanced recurrent disease. It is typically employed as an adjuvant for local tumor control and can be administered either preoperatively or postoperatively. Postoperative irradiation is the approach most commonly used, because it will not alter the histology of the tumor specimen (Eilber, 1990; Rosier & Constine, 1993).

Interstitial implantation is a technique that is currently under investigation. Following an en bloc local excision, plastic tubes are inserted and sewn into the tumor bed. Afterloading with iridium-192 seeds or iodine-125 is done 5 to 6 days following surgery. Nonrandomized studies using this technique showed a local recurrence rate of 18 per cent (Eilber, 1990; Rosier & Constine, 1993).

PRIMARY BONE SARCOMAS
Radiation therapy has limited effect on osteosarcoma, chondrosarcoma, and fibrosarcoma. Bone tumors are thought to be radioresistant because they contain a significant hypoxic fraction or they have a high capacity to repair radiation damage (Rosier et al., 1993). Radiation has been used alone, preoperatively, or postoperatively in the treatment of osteosarcoma when patients are unable to undergo definitive surgical resection.

Radiation therapy plays an important role in the treatment of Ewing's sarcoma due the radiosensitivity of this bone malignancy. Radiation therapy given with preoperative chemotherapy helps to prevent the development of tumor resistance to the cytotoxic agents during the preoperative period. It also assists in managing the primary tumor before surgical resection is undertaken. In certain instances bilateral pulmonary irradiation can be curative for patients who present with pulmonary metastases following systemic chemotherapy (Eilber, 1990).

Presently, radiation therapy continues to be used almost exclusively for plasma cell tumors, metastatic tumors, and reticulum cell sarcomas. Future trends include the possible use of neutron therapy for primary bone tumors.

SUMMARY

Great strides have been made in the past decade with the addition of combination chemotherapy, radiation therapy, new surgical techniques, and the addition of new and improved imaging technology. Survival has improved and hopefully will continue to improve as more collaborative research is implemented and data collected to address newer advances in the fields of radiation therapy, chemotherapy, surgery, and the growing field of cytogenetics.

REFERENCES

American Cancer Society. (1995). *Cancer statistics, 1995. CA: A Cancer Journal for Clinicians, 45*(1).

Angervall, L., & Kindblom, L. G. (1993). Principles for pathologic-anatomic diagnosis and classification of soft-tissue sarcomas. *Clinical Orthopaedics and Related Research, 289,* 9–18.

Antman, K. H., Eilber, F. R., & Shiu, M. H. (1989). Soft tissue sarcomas: Current trends in diagnosis and management. In C. M. Haskell (Ed.), *Current problems in cancer.* Chicago: Year Book Medical Publishers, Inc.

Bowden, L., & Booher, R. J. (1958). The principles and technique of resection of soft parts for sarcoma. *Surgery, 44*(6), 963–977.

Cagle, L. A., et al. (1987). Histologic features relating to prognosis in synovial sarcoma. *Cancer, 59,* 1810–1814.

Cassano, W., Graham-Pole, J., & Dickson, N. (1991). Etoposide, cyclophosphamide, cisplatin, and doxorubicin as neoadjuvant chemotherapy for osteosarcoma. *Cancer, 68,* 1899.

Eilber, F. R., (1990). Soft tissue sarcomas. In C. M. Haskell (Ed.), *Cancer treatment.* Philadelphia: W. B. Saunders Co.

Eilber, F. R., et al. (1984). Limb salvage for skeletal and soft tissue sarcomas. *Cancer, 53*(6), 2579–2584.

Eilber, F. R., et al. (1987). Adjuvant chemotherapy for osteosarcoma: A randomized prospective trial. *Journal of Clinical Oncology, 5*(1), 21–26.

Eilber, F. R., et al. (1988). A randomized prospective trial using postoperative adjuvant chemotherapy (adriamycin) in high-grade extremity soft-tissue sarcoma. *American Journal of Clinical Oncology, 11*(1), 39–45.

Eilber, F. R., et al. (1990). Progress in the recognition and treatment of soft tissue sarcomas. *Cancer, 67*(4), 1169–1176.

Elias, A. D. (1993). Chemotherapy for soft-tissue sarcomas. *Clinical Orthopaedics and Related Research, 289,* 94–105.

Enneking, W. F., & Conrad, E. U. (1989). Common bone tumors. *Clinical Symposia, 41*(3), 2–32.

Enterline, H. (1981). Histopathology of sarcomas. *Seminars in Oncology, 8,* 133–135.

Frieden, R. A., et al. (1993). Assessment of patient function after limb-sparing surgery. *Archives Physical Medicine and Rehabilitation, 74,* 38–43.

Greenspan, A. (1989). Malignant chondroblastic lesions. *Orthopedic Clinics of North America, 20*(3), 358–365.

Heare, T. C., Enneking, W. F., & Heare, M. M. (1989). Staging techniques and biopsy of bone tumors. *Orthopedic Clinics of North America, 20*(3), 273–285.

Hockenberry, M. J., & Lane, B. (1988). Limb salvage procedures in children with osteosarcoma. *Cancer Nursing, 11*(1), 2–8.

Karakousis, C. P., & Perez, R. P. (1994). Soft tissue sarcomas in adults. *CA: A Cancer Journal for Clinicians, 44*(4), 200–209.

Klein, M. J., Kenan, S., & Lewis, M. M. (1989). Osteosarcoma—clinical and pathological considerations. *Orthopedic Clinics of North America, 20*(3), 327–345.

LeMevel, B. P., Hoerni, D., & Duranto, O. (1979). EORTC/GTO adjuvant chemotherapy program for primary Ewing's sarcoma: Results at 5 years. *Recent results. Cancer Research, 68,* 52–59.

Machleder, H. I. (1990). Vascular sarcomas. In C. M. Haskell (Ed.), *Cancer treatment.* Philadelphia: W. B. Saunders Co.

Malawer, M. M., Link, M. P., & Donaldson, S. S. (1989). Sarcomas of the bone. In V. T. Devita, S. Hellman, & S. A. Rosenberg, (Eds.), *Cancer: Principles and practice of oncology.* (3rd ed.). Philadelphia: J. B. Lippincott.

Mankin, H. J., Lange, T. A., & Spannier, S. S. (1982). The hazards of biopsy in patients with malignant primary bone and soft tissue sarcomas. *Journal of Bone and Joint Surgery, 64A,* 1121.

Mertens, W. C., & Bramwell, V. H. (1993). Adjuvant chemotherapy in the treatment of soft-tissue sarcoma. *Clinical Orthopaedics and Related Research, 289,* 81–93.

Meyer, W. H., & Malawer, M. M. (1991). Osteosarcoma. Clinical features and evolving surgical and chemotherapeutic strategies. *Pediatric Clinics of North America, 38*(2), 317–343.

Murphy, W. A. (1991). Imaging bone tumors in the 1990s. *Cancer, 67*(4), 1169–1176.

Nirenberg, A., & Bridgewater, C. (1986). Malignancies in adolescents. *Seminars in Oncology Nursing, 2*(2), 75–83.

Peabody, T. D., & Simon M. A. (1993). Principles of staging of soft-tissue sarcomas. *Clinical Orthopaedics and Related Research, 289,* 19–31.

Piasecki, P. A. (1991). The nursing role in limb salvage surgery. *Orthopedic Nursing, 26*(1), 33–41.

Pritchard, D. J. (1989). Small round cell tumors. *Orthopedic Clinics of North America 20*(3), 367–372.

Rosen, G., et al. (1990b). Ewing's sarcoma. In C. M. Haskell (Ed.), *Cancer treatment.* Philadelphia: W. B. Saunders Co.

Rosen, G., et al. (1990a). Osteogenic sarcoma. In C. M. Haskell (Ed.), *Cancer treatment.* Philadelphia: W. B. Saunders Co.

Rosenthal, H. G., Terek, R. M., & Lane, J. M. (1993). Management of extremity soft-tissue sarcomas. *Clinical Orthopaedics and Related Research, 289,* 66–72.

Rosier, R. N., Boros, L., & Konski, A. (1993). Bone tumors. In R. N. Rosier (Ed.), *Clinical oncology.* Philadelphia: W. B. Saunders Co.

Rosier, R. N., & Constine, L. S. (1993). Soft tissue sarcoma. In R. N. Rosier (Ed.), *Clinical oncology.* Philadelphia: W. B. Saunders Co.

Santoro, A. & Bonadonna, G. (1993). Soft tissue and bone sarcomas. In H. M. Pinedo, D. L. Longo & B. A. Chabner, (Eds.), *Cancer chemotherapy and biologic response modifiers, annual 14.* Elsevier Science Publishers B. V.

Shives, T. C. (1993). Biopsy of soft-tissue tumors. *Clinical Orthopaedics and Related Research, 289,* 32–35.

Simon, M. (1991). Limb salvage for osteosarcoma in the 1980s. *Clinical Orthopaedics and Related Research, 270,* 264–269.

Springfield, D. (1993). Liposarcoma. *Clinical Orthopaedics and Related Research, 289,* 50–57.

Storm, H. H. (1994). Cancers of the soft tissues. *Cancer Surveys, 19/20,* 197–217.

Wexler, H. L., & Helman, L. J. (1994). Pediatric soft tissue sarcomas. *CA: A Cancer Journal for Clinicians, 44*(4), 211–243.

Central Nervous System Tumors

Vivian R. Sheidler • *Jennifer Dunn Bucholtz*

INCIDENCE/PREVALENCE

Central nervous system (CNS) malignancies include primary, metastatic, and spinal cord tumors. American Cancer Society statistics for primary CNS tumors are an estimated 17,200 new cases and 13,300 deaths in 1995. CNS tumors are the tenth leading cause of death for all cancer sites (Wingo, Tong, & Bolden, 1995). They account for 1.3 per cent of all diagnosed cancers and 2 per cent of all deaths from cancer. Except for meningiomas, they are more common in men than women. The United States, Sweden, and Israel have the highest average age-adjusted incidence of primary brain tumors at a rate of 8 to 10 per 100,000 (Radhakrishnan, Bohnen, & Kurland, 1994). CNS tumors are the most common solid tumor in children, and they are the second leading cause of death in children under aged 15 years. They are more common in whites than in other ethnic groups (Fan & Pezeshkpour, 1992; Wingo et al., 1995).

EPIDEMIOLOGY

Several reports indicate an increasing incidence of primary brain tumors in the elderly (Davis, Ahlbom, Hoel, & Percy, 1991; Desmeules, Mikkelsen, & Mao, 1992; Greig, Ries, Yancik, & Rapoport, 1990). Although the reasons for this increase are unknown, improvements in diagnostic imaging and environmental factors have been proposed as possible explanations.

Familial and genetic disorders such as neurofibromatosis and Li-Fraumeni syndrome (Black, 1991), environmental factors such as exposure to ionizing radiation, and exposure to certain industrial chemicals have been associated with primary brain tumors (Wrensch, Bondy, Wrencke, & Yost, 1993). Even though cellular telephones are widely available, there

have been no studies to link the occurrence of brain tumors with the use of cellular phones. The epidemiologic evidence for environmental risk factors for primary malignant brain tumors is summarized in Table 40–1.

Although primary brain tumors are not considered hereditary cancers, they have been reported in families. Grossman, Osman, Hruban, and Piantadosi (1995) described 127 cases from 59 families of gliomas reported to The National Familial Brain Tumor Registry. They reported 30 parent-child, 27 sibling-sibling, and nine husband-wife cases of histologically confirmed primary malignant brain tumors. These data suggest environmental rather than genetic factors may contribute to the etiology of brain tumors.

BRAIN TUMOR CLASSIFICATIONS

BENIGN PRIMARY CNS TUMORS

Approximately 50 per cent of primary brain tumors are benign and can be successfully treated (Black, 1991). Meningiomas and pituitary adenomas, the most common benign tumors, account for 30 per cent of all primary CNS tumors. Meningiomas are more common in women, and they can enlarge during pregnancy because of hormonal changes. They are treated primarily with surgery, but they can also be treated with radiation therapy for residual and recurrent disease. A study with the investigational agent RU-486, an antiprogesterone agent, is in progress through the Eastern Cooperative Oncology Group. Depending on size and location, meningiomas can also be observed. A change in size or neurologic function usually prompts active therapeutic approaches.

TABLE **40–1.** *Summary of Evidence for Environmental Risk Factors for Primary Malignant Brain Tumors*

	EPIDEMIOLOGIC FINDINGS		
FACTOR	ADULTS	CHILDREN	METHODOLOGIC ISSUES AND COMMENTS[a]
Viral infection			Pertinent exposure time period
SV 40		+[b]	Prenatal versus postnatal exposure
Chicken pox—prenatal		+	Sample size, one study
Toxoplasma gondii infection	+	+	One study
Medications			
Anti-convulsants	Mixed[c]		Use may be early symptom of brain cancer
Barbiturates—prenatal		−[d]	
Antinausea meds—prenatal		Mixed	
Head injuries	Mixed +[e]		Recall and publication bias, most findings not significant
Occupational & industrial chemicals			Pertinent exposure time period, many potential carcinogens
N-nitroso compounds	+		Indirect exposure assessment, confounders
Synthetic rubber production	+		
Vinyl chloride	+		
Petroleum refining/petrochemical production	Mixed		Study designs, diagnostic sensitivity bias
Pesticides	Mixed		Pertinent chemicals, confounders
Formaldehyde	Mixed		Diagnostic sensitivity
Parental exposures		Mixed	Prenatal versus postnatal exposures
Dietary N-nitroso compounds	Mixed +	Mixed +	Pertinent exposure time period, confounders
Hair dyes and sprays	Mixed		Two studies
Smoking	−		Active versus passive smoking
Maternal		−	Two studies
Alcohol	−		Some positive findngs for specific beverages
Maternal		Mixed	Two studies
Ionizing radiation			
Therapeutic	+	+	
Prenatal exposures		Mixed +	
Diagnostic/dental		Mixed	
Industrial	Mixed +		Confounders, multiple causes
Parental		Mixed	
Extremely-low-frequency electromagnetic fields			Questionable biologic plausibility
Residential wire-codes		+	Pertinent exposures, confounders
Occupational	Mixed +		Pertinent exposures, confounders

[a]These are caveats and unresolved issues; almost all the factors studied suffer from problems of accurate exposure definition and classification.
[b]+ = preponderence of studies show a positive association.
[c]Mixed = both positive and negative studies.
[d]− = most studies show a negative association.
[e]Mixed + = there are more positive than negative studies.
(Reprinted with permission from Wrensch, M., Bondy, M. L., Wiencke, J., & Yost, M. [1993]. Environmental risk factors for primary malignant brain tumors: A review. *Journal of Neuro-Oncology, 17,* 47–64.)

MALIGNANT PRIMARY CNS TUMORS

Malignant CNS tumors are classified as either metastatic or primary in origin. Primary malignant brain tumors comprise a diverse group of cancers with more than 100 histologic classifications and grades (Burger, Scheithauer, & Vogel, 1991). The most common primary CNS tumors are gliomas. Gliomas are further classified as astrocytomas, oligodendrogliomas, ependymomas, and medulloblastomas. Astrocytomas and oligodendrogliomas are more common in adults, and ependymomas and medulloblastomas are more common in children.

Many grading systems exist for classifying astrocytomas. The most common one used today uses three tiers: (1) astrocytomas (grades I and II), (2) anaplastic astrocytoma (grade III), and (3) glioblas-

toma multiforme (grade IV) (Bruner, 1994; Burger et al., 1985). Although lower grade astrocytomas carry a better prognosis and have in the past sometimes been called "benign," they are, in fact, classified as malignancies. Anaplastic astrocytomas and glioblastoma multiforme are commonly called high-grade astrocytomas.

Average survival for the most common benign and malignant brain tumors is shown in Figure 40–1. Anaplastic astrocytomas and glioblastoma multiforme have a 2- and 1-year survival, respectively. Although there have been reports of patients with high-grade astrocytomas living longer than 1 to 2 years (Chandler, Prados, Malec, & Wilson, 1993; Salcman, Scholtz, Kaplan, & Kulik, 1994), these tumors almost always recur after initial treatment with either single or combination approaches.

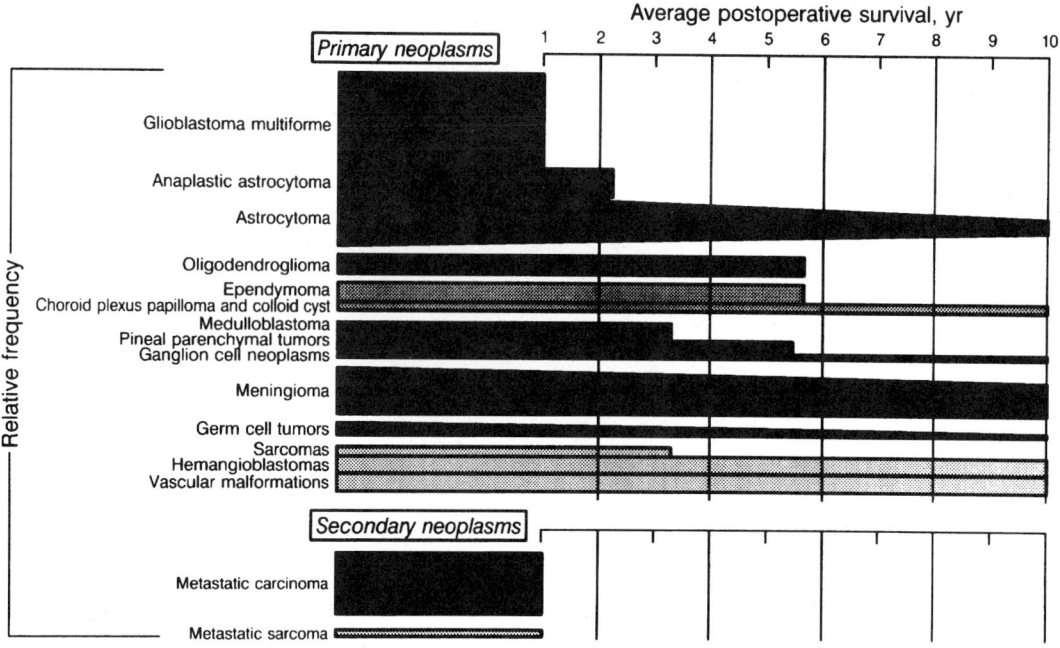

FIGURE 40–1. Central nervous system tumors: incidence and survival rates. Primary and metastatic tumefactions of the brain are represented here. Their relative incidences and average postoperative survivals are indicated, respectively, by the width and length of the individual arms. (Reprinted with permission from Burger, P. C., Scheithauer, B. W., & Vogel, F. S. [1991]. *Surgical pathology of the nervous system and its coverings* [3rd ed, p. 195]. New York: Churchill Livingstone, Inc.)

Multiple factors influence prognosis and survival in adults with brain tumors. Age, histologic grade, and Karnofsky performance status are the most significant prognostic indicators for survival in astrocytomas (Burger et al., 1985; Levin et al., 1990; Shapiro et al., 1989). Selected prognostic factors for astrocytomas and meningiomas are presented in Table 40–2.

CLINICAL PRESENTATION

SIGNS AND SYMPTOMS

Although adults with brain tumors can have many clinical problems, the presenting signs and symptoms are often from local disturbances or from increasing intracranial pressure. Local problems include tumor, edema, and seizures. Increasing intracranial pressure is caused by tumor, edema, and obstruction of cerebral spinal fluid (CSF) flow.

The focal sequelae and disturbance or destruction of normal brain tissue occur from tumor invasion, infiltration, and compression. The specific signs and symptoms are related to the location, size, and type of tumor, as well as the degree of edema and CSF obstruction. Figure 40–2 shows the brain anatomy with correlating signs and symptoms of tumors. A tumor must grow to a certain size to cause compression and neurologic symptoms. Aggressive, fast-growing tumors may lead to signs or symptoms in a matter of weeks or months, but slower growing tumors, such as a benign pituitary tumor, may take years to cause symptoms. The most common presenting signs identified in a national patterns of care study for brain tumor patients were (1) progressive neurologic function loss (68 per

cent), (2) headache (54 per cent), and (3) seizures (26 per cent) (Mahaley, Mettlin, Natarajen, Laws, & Peace, 1989). Presenting signs and symptoms may differ not only by tumor type and location but also by age group (Newton, 1994). The most common symptoms of primary brain tumors in adults over 65 years are subtle personality changes, unilateral weakness, headaches, and aphasia (Zachariah, Zachariah, Wang, & Balducci, 1992). Younger persons, especially those who are ultimately diagnosed with an oligodendroglioma, more commonly present with seizures. Adults experiencing seizures without recent head trauma or a history of epilepsy should undergo a workup for a possible intracranial lesion. In addition, individuals who experience headaches, especially with any combined abnormal neurologic finding, including nausea or vomiting, should be suspected for a possible CNS lesion (Forsyth & Posner, 1993).

CLINICAL NEUROLOGIC EXAMINATION

Clinical examination of a person suspected of having a CNS tumor should include a thorough history, physical, and neurologic examination. Family members and significant others can provide useful information regarding a subtle change in a person's cognitive function, and they may help unravel the progressive course of the individual's symptoms. In some cases, due to a compromised neurologic condition, the family must act as the primary historian for the patient. An initial neurologic examination not only elicits signs and symptoms of possible neurologic dysfunction but also establishes a baseline and foundation for the person's response to prescribed treatments and the progression of disease.

TABLE **40–2.** *Prognostic Factors of Astrocytomas and Meningiomas*

	ASTROCYTOMAS		MENINGIOMAS	
FACTOR	FAVORABLE	UNFAVORABLE	FAVORABLE	UNFAVORABLE
Patient age[+]	<40	≥40	<60	>70
Neurologic status	Near normal	Impaired	Normal	Impaired
Seizures	Present	Absent	Present	Absent
Increased intracranial pressure	Absent	Present	Absent	Present
Extent of resection	Complete	Incomplete	Complete	Incomplete
Grade of tumor[+]	1,2	3,4	*	*
Karnofsky performance status[+]	≥70	<70	*	*
Atypical histologic features	*	*	Absent	Present

[+]Most significant prognostic factors for gliomas.
*Not applicable.
(Modified with permission from Laws, E. R., & Thapar K. [1993]. Brain tumors. *Ca- A Cancer Journal for Clinicians, 43*, 263–271.)

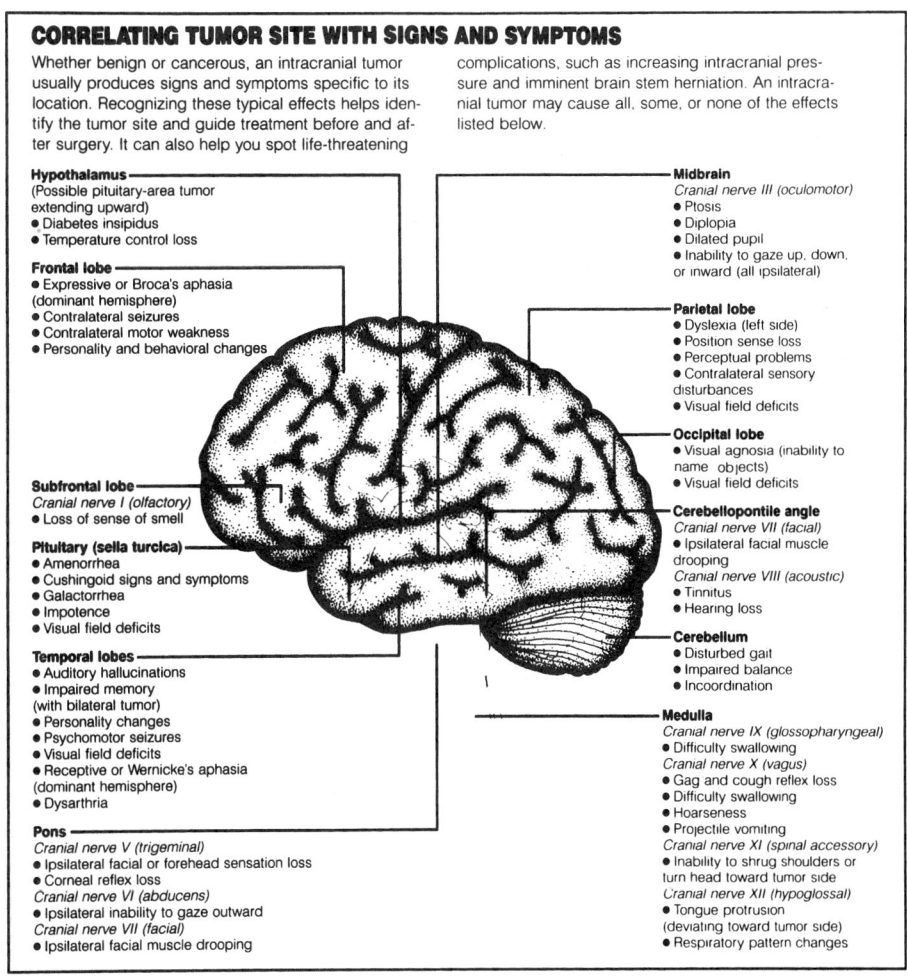

FIGURE **40–2.** Brain anatomy with correlating signs and symptoms. (Reprinted with permission from *Nursing 90,* 32F.)

DIAGNOSTIC TESTS

In the past 20 years numerous changes and improvements in the diagnosis of brain tumors have taken place (Ramsey, 1994). Non-invasive techniques of computerized tomography (CT) and magnetic resonance imaging (MRI) have revolutionized neuroimaging. Diagnostic tests such as EEG, radionuclide brain scan, arteriogram, and plain skull x-ray are now reserved for limited, clinical use. Information about neurodiagnostic tests is summarized in Table 40–3. Intravenous contrast agents significantly enhance the quality and clinical value of neuroimages of brain tumors. Normal brain tissue with an intact blood-brain barrier (BBB) does not show an uptake of contrast, but tumor vasculature that alters the BBB allows contrast agents to permeate brain tumors and be clearly demar-

TABLE 40–3. *Information Regarding Neurodiagnostic Tests*

Test	Purpose	Patient Experience	Approximate Time Required	Potential Risks	Comments
Computerized tomography (CT)	Detect brain, spine abnormalities, including masses, edema	Lie on narrow table, head inside large donut-shaped ring; IV contrast usually given	30 minutes (brain) 45 minutes (spine)	Allergic reaction to IV contrast agent	• Uses ionizing radiation • Useful in evaluating bony abnormalities of skull • IV contrast reactions can be mild to severe, including anaphylaxis; requires informed consent • 3–D pictures using special computers
Magnetic resonance imaging (MRI)	Detect brain, spine abnormalities, including edema, & nature/extent of tumor blood flow	Lie on thin table inside large magnet; claustrophobic feeling; loud noises from magnet, sounds like galloping, drilling; some scanners play music, videotapes; IV contrast usually given	45–60 min (brain) 2–3 hrs (total spine)	Anxiety, claustrophobia	• Preferred method of neuroimaging • More expensive than CT • Sedation/antianxiety medicines may be required • Does not use ionizing radiation • Reactions to IV contrast gadolinium rare • Not used for patients with metal foreign bodies, pacemakers • More sensitive than CT for detecting multiple brain mets, posterior fossa & spinal lesions • Open scanners may give lower quality images • Patient weight limit 300 lbs for most scanners • MR angiography fast replacing need for traditional invasive angiogram
Positron emission tomography (PET)	Measures regional brain metabolism, & cerebral blood flow; may show difference between radiation necrosis & recurrent tumors	Lie on narrow table; patient wears customized mask; head in special holder; IV and/or arterial line required	2 hrs	Arterial line complications	• Limited availability • Uses positron-emitting radionuclides; thymidine and glucose common radiotracers • Insurance reimbusement a problem
Single photon emission computed tomography (SPECT)	Attempts to show difference between radiation necrosis & recurrent tumors; differentiate lymphoma from non-neoplastic masses in AIDS patients	IV radionuclide used; patient scanned on traditional nuclear medicine-like table	May be scanned at set time after radionuclide given, similar to bone scan		• Uses conventional radiotracers • More available & less expensive than PET

are commonly used for malignant brain lesions. A summary of the common treatments for many brain tumors is listed in Table 40–4.

SURGERY

Surgery is the initial treatment for primary brain tumors. Although the intent of surgery is complete removal of the tumor, this goal is difficult to accomplish because of the infiltrating nature of certain tumors.

The decision to perform a stereotactic biopsy vs. an open craniotomy is based on the tumor location, patient status, the anticipated results, and the potential risks. In general, if the risks are minimal, a cytoreductive craniotomy is preferred to a stereotactic biopsy.

Surgical debulking of primary brain tumors accomplishes many goals. It provides definitive pathology, relieves tumor mass effect, lowers intracranial pressure, may improve neurological deficits, may prolong life, and provides extra space in the brain to allow for possible side effects from treatment (Newton, 1994). With improvements in neurosurgical anesthesia, microsurgical techniques aided by sophisticated intraoperative neuroimaging, and improved resection tools, modern neurosurgery has become more efficient. Complications from neurosurgery have decreased (Black, 1991). The fatality rate from brain surgery is fairly low. Potential risks from surgery include herniation, hemorrhage, and brain injury. Potential complications indirectly related to the surgery include pulmonary embolism, deep vein thrombosis, postoperative hematomas, wound flap infection, cerebral spinal fluid leak or fistula, aseptic meningitis, and cranial nerve injury (Wilson, 1994).

Preoperatively, patients receive glucocorticoids and a prophylactic anticonvulsant. They use a special antiseptic shampoo to clean the hair and scalp. Postoperatively, patients will be in a neurointensive care suite for 24 to 48 hours. They receive steroids and are on fluid restrictions to prevent cerebral edema. Nurses monitor patient's neurologic status to alert the medical team of any acute surgical complications. A postoperative scan is performed to provide a baseline scan showing the tumor resection and to identify possible surgical complications.

RADIATION THERAPY

Radiation therapy plays a major role in the standard treatment of benign and malignant primary brain tumors. It can be used alone or in combination with other treatments for curative intent, control of tumor growth, and palliation of neurologic complications.

The radiation dose, fractionation schedule, and amount of brain tissue treated depend on a patient's tumor histology, grade, location, radioresponsiveness, the intent of therapy, as well as individual patient variables. Brain lesions that are unlikely to infiltrate beyond set borders, such as meningiomas, pituitary adenomas, and acoustic neuromas, are usually treated with narrow margins of normal brain tissue surrounding the tumor. High-grade astrocytomas, which are more infiltrative with less discrete borders, may be treated with larger radiation therapy fields to encom-

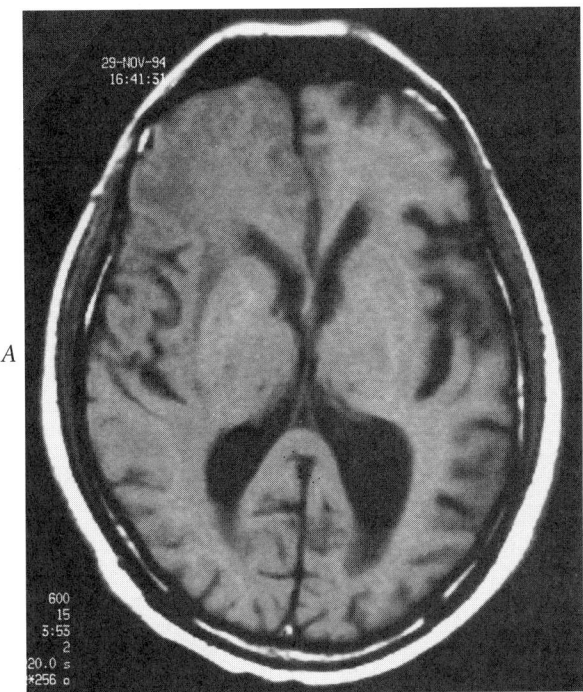

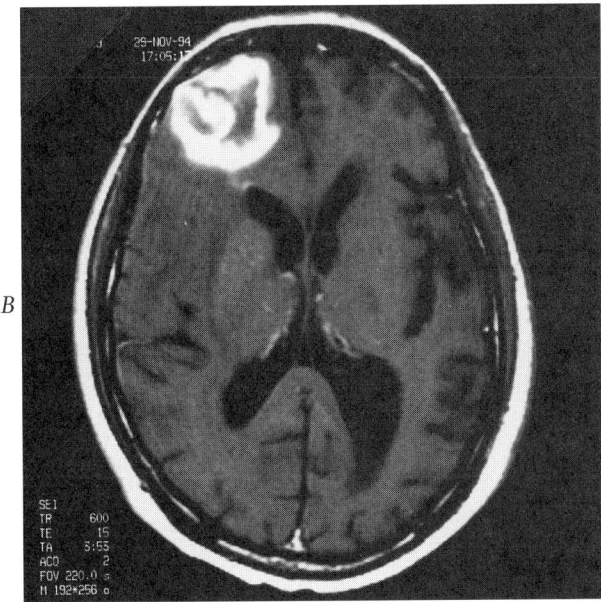

FIGURE 40–3. MRI scan. **A,** without gadolinum, **B,** with gadolinum. (Courtesy of Department of Radiology, Johns Hopkins Hospital, Baltimore, MD.)

cated on CT and MRI. The benefit of contrast agents is illustrated in Figure 40–3.

TREATMENTS FOR CNS TUMORS

Similar to progress in the imaging of brain tumors, advances in the treatment of these tumors have also been made. Although surgery is the usual treatment for many brain tumors, especially those of benign pathology, multimodal approaches with surgery, radiation therapy, chemotherapy, and experimental treatments

TABLE 40–4. *Usual Treatment Options for Common Adult Primary Brain Tumors*

TUMOR TYPE	SURGERY	CONVENTIONAL RADIATION THERAPY	CONVENTIONAL CHEMOTHERAPY
Astrocytoma			
Low-grade	Yes	Yes	No
High-grade	Yes	Yes	Yes
Ependymoma			
Low-grade	Yes	Yes	No
High-grade	Yes	Yes	Sometimes
Oligodendroglioma			
Low-grade	Yes	Yes	No
Anaplastic	Yes	Yes	Yes
Medulloblastoma			
Low-risk	Yes	Yes	No
High-risk	Yes	Yes	Yes
Germ cell			
Germinoma	Yes	Yes	Yes
Other	Yes	Yes	No
Pineal			
Pineocytoma	Yes	Yes	No
Pineoblastoma	Yes	Yes	Yes
Primary CNS lymphoma	Sometimes	Yes	Yes
Meningioma	Yes	Sometimes	No
Pituitary adenoma	Yes	Sometimes	No

(Adapted with permission from Lesser, G. J., & Grossman, S. A. [1993]. The chemotherapy of adult primary brain tumors. *Cancer Treatment Reviews, 19,* 270.)

pass surrounding edema. Whole-brain radiation therapy is no longer recommended for high-grade astrocytomas, as it increases morbidity and does not improve survival (Leibel & Sheline, 1987). It is universally accepted that radiation therapy prolongs survival in patients with high-grade astrocytomas (Kristiansen et al., 1981; Walker et al., 1978); however, controversy remains concerning the timing of radiation therapy for low-grade astrocytomas (Cairncross & Laperriere, 1989; Recht, Lew, & Smith, 1992).

Similar to technologic improvements in neurosurgery, significant advances have occurred in standard and innovative radiation therapy modalities. Since radiation therapy aims to destroy tumor cells while sparing normal cells from damage, these advances have centered on improving the precision of the radiation therapy planning and delivery. Technical improvements in conventional brain irradiation include (1) three-dimensional treatment planning systems using integrated CT or MRI, (2) multileaf collimators to improve beam shaping, and (3) portal imaging systems that confirm treatment fields on a daily basis (Laperriere & Bernstein, 1994).

Techniques such as interstitial brachytherapy, stereotactic radiosurgery, and proton beam particle delivery attempt to increase the dose of radiation and to improve the focused delivery of the radiation dose to a brain tumor with improved normal tissue sparing. Information specific to these techniques is listed in Table 40–5.

Side Effects of Brain Radiation Therapy. Since the normal cells of the adult brain do not actively divide, patients tolerate the therapy quite well. Most patients will not experience significant acute morbidity with a dose of 6000 centiGray (cGy) in conventional fraction

doses of 180 to 200 cGy given five times a week (Levin, Gutin, & Leibel, 1993). Potential side effects can be grouped into acute effects (during the course of therapy); early-delayed effects (occurring within a few weeks to 3 months after therapy); and delayed, long-term effects (occurring months to years after radiation therapy). The side effects of CNS radiation therapy are listed in Table 40–6.

CHEMOTHERAPY

Astro-glial tumors, primary CNS lymphoma, and leptomeningeal metastases are treated with chemotherapy. Chemotherapy is used in conjunction with surgery and radiation as initial treatment and at the time of recurrence. Nearly every drug active in systemic tumors, either alone or in combination, has been evaluated in primary CNS tumors (Lesser & Grossman, 1994; Mahaley, 1991). Despite efforts to treat these tumors, advances have been slow because of a paucity of active agents, a small number of well-controlled, prospective clinical trials, and the absence of uniform response criteria (Fine, 1994).

The BBB is disrupted in patients with primary brain tumors. For chemotherapy to be effective, it penetrates an already altered BBB. As a result of vascular abnormalities, higher concentrations of chemotherapy may be effectively delivered to the central portion of the tumor (Lesser & Grossman, 1994). Lipid solubility and molecular weight are two major factors that affect the passage of chemotherapy across the BBB (Grossman & Tuma, 1993).

The role of chemotherapy in the treatment of primary CNS tumors has been extensively reviewed (Lesser & Grossman, 1994; Moynihan & Grossman,

TABLE **40–5.** *Specialized Radiation Therapy Techniques Used for Brain Tumors*

TECHNIQUE	EXAMPLES OF TUMORS TREATED	DESCRIPTION	COMMENTS
Interstitial brachytherapy	High-grade astrocytomas	Stereotactic placement of temporary (Iridium-192) or permanent (Iodine-125) radioactive seeds directly into tumor tissue	• Used for recurrent tumors after standard therapies or with standard therapies as radiation boost • Allows higher radiation dose rate than standard radiation therapy • Tumors must be small & discrete • Necrosis is major side effect; may require surgery • May be combined with interstitial hyperthermia
Stereotactic radiosurgery	Benign lesions • arteriovenous malformations • acoustic neuromas • pituitary tumors • meningiomas Malignant lesions • brain metastases • high-grade astrocytomas	Precise delivery of radiation to small, well-defined lesion; uses one, high-dose radiation fraction with minimal dose to adjacent brain tissue	• Requires special equipment ("gamma knife—cobalt machine; modified linear accelerator or high energy particle beam machine) • Requires specialized computer planning and patient immobilization in stereotactic head ring frame that is screwed into skull • Minimal side effects; usually no alopecia unless lesion close to scalp • Sub-acute cerebral edema, necrosis up to 2 yrs post-treatment
Stereotactic radiotherapy	Benign tumors Astrocytomas—low- & high-grade	Same as radiosurgery, but given in multiple fractions	• Uses radiosurgery techniques to decrease radiation to normal cells • Small & well-defined tumors • Uses noninvasive head masks or relocatable frames for treatment set-up
Photodynamic therapy (investigational)	Recurrent high-grade astrocytomas	Photosensitizing drug followed by activated light treatment	• May require stereotactic implantation of optical fibers to deliver light source • Side effects—headache & neurologic deterioration

Continued on following page.

1994). The nitrosoureas, procarbazine, and cisplatin are the most commonly used chemotherapeutic agents for the treatment of malignant gliomas. These drugs are able to penetrate the BBB. BCNU is used as part of initial therapy with surgery and radiation therapy (Levin et al., 1990; Walker et al., 1980) and for treatment at the time of recurrence. Response rates of 10 to 40 per cent have been reported with BCNU in patients with recurrent gliomas (Fine et al., 1993). BCNU has been given intravenously (intermittent bolus and continuous infusion) and intraarterially in many schedules and doses. An example of a common intravenous schedule is 240 mg/m^2 every 6 weeks.

Combination chemotherapy regimens have been used in patients with gliomas. Cisplatin and BCNU (Grossman et al., 1992; Yung, Janus, Maor, & Feun, 1992), cyclophosphamide and vincristine (Longee et al., 1990), as well as a combination of eight drugs (Rozental et al., 1989) have been used to treat high-grade astrocytomas. Another commonly used regimen for gliomas is PCV. This therapy is procarbazine on days 8 to 21, CCNU on day 1, and vincristine on days 8 and 29 (Cairncross et al., 1994; Levin et al., 1990).

The combination of surgery, radiation therapy, and chemotherapy has not produced durable, long-term responses in patients with high-grade astrocytomas. As

TABLE 40–5. *Specialized Radiation Therapy Techniques Used for Brain Tumors* Continued

TECHNIQUE	EXAMPLES OF TUMORS TREATED	DESCRIPTION	COMMENTS
Particle therapy (protons, neutrons, helium ions)	Skull-based tumors (chordomas), AVM's, meningiomas	High-energy particles delivered by special machines, usually cyclotron	• Limited availability • Improved tumor coverage, less normal tissue dose since particles delivered at desired depth in finite pathway without exit beam • Improved survival in skull-based tumors compared to standard photon treatment
Boron neutron capture therapy (investigational)	High-grade astrocytomas	IV administration of boron-containing chemical, followed by neutron beam treatment. When boron atoms in cancer cells capture neurons, they become unstable & fission into cell-destroying fragments	• Clinical trials underway • Early trials in US in 1960s, disappointing results; different compound used today • Boron compound does not concentrate in normal brain tissue
Radiosensitizers (investigational)	High-grade astrocytomas	Administration of chemicals that preferentially increase lethal effects of radiation to cells compared to normal cells. Given in combination with radiation therapy	• Radiosensitizers include halogenated pyrimidines—BUDR (IV or IA), IUDR; hydroxyurea, cisplatin

(Data from Gutin, et al., 1993; Edwards, Stupperich, & Welsh, 1991; Brada, 1991; Wilson, Larson, & Gutin, 1992; Krause, et al., 1991; Souhami, et al., 1991; Bleehan & Ford, 1993; Goffman, et. al., 1992; Sneed, Larson, & Gutin, 1994.)

a result, experimental approaches are often presented to patients as potential first-line therapy as well as at the time of recurrence. Taylor (1994) summarized phase II trials of standard drugs (e.g., cisplatin and etoposide) and experimental drugs (AZQ and temozolomide). Examples of experimental approaches that have not produced a significant impact on survival are intraarterial administration of BCNU and high-dose chemotherapy with autologous bone marrow transplantation (Fine & Antman, 1992; Shapiro et al., 1992).

Some experimental approaches include changes in schedule or doses of existing FDA-approved drugs. For example, Grossman et al. (1992) have used 72-hour simultaneous continuous infusions of BCNU and cisplatin followed by standard radiation. Fetell et al. (1994) have used 96-hour infusions of Taxol, also followed by standard radiation in patients with newly diagnosed gliomas. In an attempt to treat gliomas with local rather than systemic therapy, Brem et al. (1995) have demonstrated safety and efficacy of implantable biodegradable BCNU polymers for patients with recurrent gliomas.

Other techniques under investigation for primary brain tumors include blood-brain barrier disruption-chemotherapy (Gummerlock & Neuwelt, 1994), immunotherapy with interferon and interleukins (Jaeckle, 1994), and gene therapy with herpes simplex thymidine kinase gene (Culver & Van Gilder, 1994). The goal of these new, experimental therapies is to discover better treatments for patients with poor-prognosis malignant brain tumors.

BRAIN METASTASES

Brain metastases are the most common neurologic complication of systemic cancer, occurring in 24 per cent of patients (DeAngelis, 1994; Patchell, 1991). The incidence of brain metastases (100,000 per year in the United States) far exceeds the incidence of primary brain tumors (Lesser & Grossman, 1993b). The primary solid tumors that commonly spread to the brain are lung, breast, colon, renal, and melanoma. Eighty per cent of the metastatic lesions occur in the cerebral hemispheres, 17 per cent in the cerebellum, and 3 per cent in the basal ganglia or brainstem (Lesser & Grossman, 1993b). Spread may be hematogenous from primary or metastatic foci in the lungs. Similar to patients with primary brain tumors, patients who have metastatic brain lesions present with alteration in cognitive function (75 per cent), seizures (15 to 20 per cent), and a "strokelike" picture (5 per cent) (DeAngelis, 1994). Patients may have multiple or solitary brain metastasis. About 50 per cent of patients have solitary lesions (DeAngelis, 1994).

Although most patients with brain metastasis die within 6 months of progressive, systemic disease, some patients have a better prognosis. Those who have solitary lesions, Karnofsky performance status of >70 per cent, age <60 years, primary tumor in remission, and metastases confined to the brain benefit by aggressive, definitive treatment (Wharam, 1993). This treatment includes surgical resection of the solitary lesion, followed by radiation. One series reported a 29 per cent five year survival rate in patients treated in this manner

TABLE 40–6. *Side Effects of Radiation Therapy to the Brain*

SIDE EFFECT	COMMENTS
Acute	
Cerebral edema	May occur early in course of treatment; headache, nausea, vomiting, neurologic changes
	Treated with glucocorticoids, usually dexamethasone
Fatigue	Variable amount; increased if patients receiving concomitant chemotherapy
Alopecia	Hair loss limited to areas transited by beam
	May take 3–6 months after treatment to regrow
	No known preventative measure once threshold dose received
Skin reactions—scalp	Erythema, dry desquamation common; moist desquamation rare
	Symptoms more pronounced at skin folds (behind ears, forehead)
	May be more enhanced by chemotherapy & head immobilization devices
Subacute	
Radiation somnolence syndrome	Can occur 6–12 weeks after treatment; lasts up to 2 weeks
	Symptoms—excessive sleepiness, lethargy, exacerbation of previous neurologic deficits
	Possible etiology—temporary demyelination of certain brain cells or radiation changes in capillary permeability
	Can be symptomatically treated with glucocorticoids
Long Term	
Radiation necrosis	Occurs in 4%–9% of patients
	Increased incidence with high doses
	Difficult to distinguish from recurrent tumor on CT/MRI
	May require surgical treatment
White matter changes	Present on CT/MRI, but patient asymptomatic
Cognitive changes	Evidence for cognitive changes in young children treated during brain development
	Few prospective studies
	Data show both normal cognitive function & cognitive decline
	Cognitive function assessment should use neuropsychologic instruments, in addition to Karnofsky & IQ
	Cognitive change in adults—memory deficits most often reported
	Tumor, surgery, & chemotherapy may also be responsible for cognitive changes
Decreased hormone production	Occurs in 40%–50% of patients treated for pituitary tumors
	Develops slowly over several years
	Requires follow-up with endocrinologist
	All hormones replaceable with medications
Radiation-induced neoplasms	Rare; may take years to develop

(Data from Hoffman, Levin, & Wilson, 1979; Delattre et al., 1988; Levin et al., 1993; Moore et al., 1991; Meadows et al., 1981; Imperato, Paleologos, & Vick, 1990; Maire et al., 1987; Hochberg & Slotnick, 1980; Kleinberg, Wallner, & Malkin, 1993; Armstrong et al., 1993; Archibald et al., 1994; Blevins & Wand, 1993; Bucholtz, 1992.)

(Wharam, 1993). In recent years, stereotactic radiosurgery followed by external beam radiation has replaced surgical resection for those lesions inaccessible or for patients who are medically inoperable.

A combination of whole-brain radiation therapy and steroids is the most effective palliative treatment of brain metastases, with symptomatic relief achieved in 70 to 90 per cent of patients and survival extended for 3 to 6 months (Coia, 1992). The usual radiation therapy dose for patients with a prognosis of greater than 1 year is 3000 to 5000 cGy in 180 to 200 cGy fractions. This schedule is given to reduce side effects. For patients with progressive systemic disease, the radiation therapy can be delivered in 10, 300 cGy fractions. Different fractionations and total doses have produced similar results (Buckner, 1992).

Chemotherapy has a limited role in the treatment of brain metastases, but it may be used in patients whose primary tumor is sensitive to chemotherapy.

LEPTOMENINGEAL METASTASES

Leptomeningeal metastases occur as a result of multifocal seeding of the leptomeninges by tumor cells. This neurologic complication of systemic cancer occurs in 10 to 20 per cent of patients with solid tumors (Flowers & Yung, 1993; Grossman & Tuma, 1993). Patients may present with headaches, mental status changes, low back pain, radiculopathy, cranial neuropathy, and incontinence. Some patients will be asymptomatic, and a diagnosis will be made as a result of incidental findings on MRI. Neuroimaging, a neurologic examination, and a lumbar puncture are part of the evaluation for leptomeningeal disease. Cerebrospinal fluid (CSF) is usually abnormal, with elevations in opening pressure and protein, and reductions in glucose. Patient may require more than one lumbar puncture to obtain a positive CSF cytology.

The goals of treatment for leptomeningeal metastases are to improve or stabilize neurologic function and prolong life. The median survival without treatment is 4 to 6 weeks. Standard treatment for leptomeningeal metastases includes radiation to bulk disease, intrathecal chemotherapy with methotrexate, thiotepa, or cytarabine, and treatment of systemic disease (Grossman & Tuma, 1993). An Ommaya reservoir is often used to deliver intrathecal chemotherapy.

SPINAL CORD TUMORS

Spinal cord tumors compose a small percentage of CNS malignancies. The overall incidence is approximately 15 per cent of that of brain tumors (Levin, Gutin, & Leibel, 1993). Extradural metastatic spinal axis tumors are more common than primary spinal tumors. The most common intradural, extramedullary (within the dura, outside the cord) spinal tumors are Schwannomas and meningiomas (Preston-Martin, 1990). The most common intradural, intramedullary (within the cord itself) spinal tumors are astrocytomas and ependymomas (Levin et al., 1993).These tumors are evenly distributed along the spinal axis, even though some tumors such as meningiomas have a predisposition to arise from specific areas.

Symptoms from primary spinal cord tumors are produced locally and distally. Local presentation refers to the tumor's location along the spinal axis, and distal reflects motor and sensory involvement. Thus, clinical manifestations will depend upon the location of the lesion. For example, patients who present with a tumor originating in the cervical spine may report ipsilateral arm weakness and decreased pain and temperature sensation. Patients who present with a lumbosacral spine tumor, however, may report inguinal pain and impotence.

Surgery with curative intent is the primary treatment for spinal cord tumors. Patients whose tumors cannot be completely resected would receive radiation therapy at doses of 50 to 55 Gy. Some patients may benefit from proton beam radiation over conventional radiation. Even though controlled trials with chemotherapy have not been conducted, the drugs that are used to treat intracranial tumors may work against spinal cord tumors.

PROBLEMS UNIQUE TO PATIENTS WITH BRAIN TUMORS

Although any cancer diagnosis can be devastating, a brain tumor diagnosis carries with it many unique and profound differences. Health care providers need to understand these differences to anticipate problems and meet the needs of the patient and the family.

A brain tumor may impair cognitive and sensory functions, communication skills, and mobility. These impairments can occur at the time of diagnosis or develop at any time during the illness. If these problems occur at the time of diagnosis, they may or may not improve with treatment. Depending on a patient's symptoms, activities of daily living such as eating, bathing, and toileting can become arduous tasks. Safety issues become paramount as often a patient cannot be left alone.

Depending on the degree of cognitive impairment, the question of mental competence is often raised. If patients have expressive or receptive aphasia or short-term memory deficits, they may not be able to give informed consent for treatment or procedures. These decisions then become the responsibility of family members.

All of these contribute to patients' unexpected and sometimes sudden dependence on their family. One of the first major limits to a patients' independence relates to restrictions on driving a car. Depending upon where they live, patients may not drive for 3 months to 2 years after having a seizure. Some states also require periodic medical updates after the requisite seizure-free period (Epilepsy Foundation of America, 1992). If patients are unable to drive, they must rely on family or friends for transportation for everyday activities, as well as transportation to receive treatment for the tumor.

The financial impact of a brain tumor diagnosis can be dramatic. If the patients worked outside the home, they suddenly may not be able to continue full-time or even part-time employment. Similarly, if a spouse or family member provided a major source of income, then that individual may also have to make adjustments in a work schedule to take care of the patient. Limitations to income as well as the costs associated with brain tumor treatments can devastate a family. Clearly, problems associated with a brain tumor and its treatment threaten quality of life (Mackworth, Fobair, & Prados, 1992). Living with a malignant brain tumor has been described as an "emotional roller coaster" of uncertainty with many losses experienced over varying lengths of time (Newton & Mateo, 1994; Amato, 1991).

These losses are caused not only by the tumor but also from problems with treatments, side effects of medications, and other conditions related to the tumor. For example, thromboembolic disease is a common, tumor-related problem (Norris & Grossman, 1994). Another major problem most patients experience is side effects from glucocorticoids. Patients take steroids for months, and some patients may need them for the remainder of their lives to control edema. Dexamethasone can cause many side effects, but significant weakness from a proximal myopathy is one of the more distressing ones. Patients often have difficulty rising from a sitting or lying position and with walking. The problems with weakness and mobility are compounded further if a patient has gained weight as a result of a steroid-induced increase in appetite.

For controlling seizures and for monitoring toxicities of antineoplastic treatment, patients need to have blood drawn frequently. Chemotherapy alters the metabolism of certain anticonvulsants, thus placing the patient at risk for seizures (Grossman, Sheidler, & Gilbert, 1989; Schwandt, 1994). Patients also have frequent neuroimaging studies to evaluate the response to treatment and disease status. Interpretation of CT's and MRI's may be difficult because the images are affected by postradiation changes and adjustments in steroid dose.

Wegmann (1991) describes supportive care for patients with malignant brain tumors and their families. This support is needed throughout the trajectory of the illness. Community resources exist to meet some of the unique needs of patients and families. These include local support groups and the American Brain Tumor Association. This organization has educational material that is available free of charge for patients and families (1-800-886-2282).

SUMMARY

Central nervous system tumors comprise a variety of benign and malignant diseases. The goals of treatment are for cure, control, or palliation. These goals are accomplished with a combination of surgery, radiation, and chemotherapy. A primary brain tumor diagnosis can have devastating effects on the patient and family. Nurses and physicians need to pay careful attention to tumor- and treatment-related problems and toxicities. Future research efforts are focused on improving long-term survival with acceptable toxicity profiles.

REFERENCES

Amato, C. A. (1991). Malignant glioma: Coping with a devastating illness. *Journal of Neuroscience Nursing, 23,* 20–22.

Archibald, Y. M., Lunn, D., Ruttan, L. A., McDonald, M. D., DelMaestro, F., Barr, H. W. K., Pexman, J. H., Fisher, B. J., Gaspar, L. E., & Cairncross, J. G. (1994). Cognitive functioning in long-term survivors of high grade glioma. *Journal of Neurosurgery, 80,* 247–253.

Armstrong, C., Mollman, J., Corn, B.W., Alavi, J., & Grossman, M. (1993). Effects of radiation therapy on adult brain behavior: Evidence for a rebound phenomenon in a phase I trial. *Neurology, 43,* 1961–1965.

Black, P. M. (1991). Brain tumors (Parts I & II). *New England Journal of Medicine, 324,* 1471–1476, 1555–1564.

Bleehan, N. M., & Ford, J. M. (1993). Radiotherapy, hyperthermia, and photodynamic therapy for central nervous system tumors. *Current Opinion in Oncology, 5,* 458–463.

Blevins, L. S., & Wand, G. S. (1993). Pituitary adenomas. In R. T. Johnson, J. W. Griffin & B. C. Decker (Eds.), *Current therapy in neurologic disease* (pp.231–235). St. Louis: Mosby Year Book, Inc.

Brada, M. (1991). Radiosurgery for brain tumors. *European Journal of Cancer, 27,* 1545–1548.

Brem, H., Piantadosi, S., Burger, P. C., Walker, M., Selker, R., Vick, N. A., Black, K., Sisti, M., Brem, S., Mohn, G., Muller, P., Morawetz, R., & Schold, S. C. for the Polymer-Brain Tumor Treatment Group. (1995). Intraoperative controlled delivery of chemotherapy by biodegradable polymers: Safety and effectiveness for recurrent gliomas evaluated by a prospective, multi-institutional, placebo-controlled clinical trial. *Lancet, 345* (8956), 1008–1012.

Bruner J. M. (1994). Neuropathology of malignant gliomas. *Seminars in Oncology, 21,* 126–138.

Bucholtz, J. (1992). Radiation carcinogenesis. In K. H. Dow & L. J. Hilderley (Eds.), *Nursing care in radiation oncology* (pp.342–357). Philadelphia, PA: W. B. Saunders Co.

Buckner, J. (1992). Surgery, radiation therapy, and chemotherapy for metastatic tumors to the brain. *Current Opinion in Oncology, 4,* 518–524.

Burger, P. C., Scheithauer, B. W., & Vogel, F. S. (1991). *Surgical pathology of the nervous system and its coverings* (3rd ed.). New York: Churchill Livingstone, Inc.

Burger, P. C., Vogel S., Green S. B., & Strike, T. A. (1985). Glioblastoma multiforme and anaplastic astrocytoma. Pathologic criteria and prognostic implications. *Cancer, 56,* 1106–1111.

Cairncross, J. G., & Laperriere, N. J. (1989). Low grade glioma: To treat or not to treat? *Archives of Neurology, 46,* 1238–1239.

Cairncross G., Macdonald, D., Ludwin, S, Lee, D., Cascino, T., Buckner, J., Fulton, D., Dropcho, E., Steward, D., Schold, C., Wainman, N., & Eisenhauer, E. for the National Cancer Institute of Canada Clinical Trials Group. (1994). Chemotherapy for anaplastic oligodendroglioma. *Journal of Clinical Oncology, 12,* 2013–2021.

Chandler, K., Prados, M. D., Malec, M., & Wilson, C. B. (1993). Long term survivors in patients with glioblastoma multiforme. *Neurosurgery, 32,* 716–720.

Coia, L. R. (1992). The role of radiation therapy in the treatment of brain metastases. *International Journal of Radiation Oncology, Biology, and Physics, 23,* 229–238.

Culver, K. W., & Van Gilder, J. (1994). Gene therapy for the treatment of malignant brain tumors with in vivo tumor transduction with the herpes simplex thymidine kinase gene/ganciclovir system. *Human Gene Therapy, 5,* 343–379.

Davis, D. L., Ahlbom, A., Hoel, D., & Percy, C. (1991). Is brain cancer mortality increasing in industrial countries. *American Journal of Industrial Medicine, 19,* 421–431.

DeAngelis, L. M. (1994). Management of brain metastases. *Cancer Investigation, 12,* 156–165.

Delattre, J. Y., Rosenblum, M. K., Thaler, H. T., Mandell, L., Shapiro, W. R., & Posner, J. B. (1988). A model of radiation myelography in the rat: Pathology, regional capillary permeability changes and treatment with dexamethasone. *Brain, 111,* 1319–1336.

Desmeules, M., Mikkelsen, T., & Mao, Y. (1992). Increasing incidence of primary malignant brain tumors: influence of diagnostic methods. *Journal of the National Cancer Institute, 84,* 442–445.

Edwards, D. K., Stupperich, T. K., & Welsh, D. (1991). Hyperthermia treatment for malignant brain tumors: nursing management during therapy. *Journal of Neuroscience Nursing, 23,* 34–38.

Epilepsy Foundation of America. (1992). *Driving and epilepsy.* Landover, Maryland.

Fan, K. J., & Pezeshkpour G. H. (1992). Ethnic distributions of primary central nervous system tumors in Washington D.C. 1971–85. *Journal of the American Medical Association, 84,* 858–863.

Fetell, M. R., Grossman, S. A., Balmaceda, C., Leu, J. G., Erlanger, B. F., Rowinsky, E., Khandji, A. G., Yue, N., & Zeltzman, M. (1994). Clinical and pharmacologic study of pre-irradiation taxol administered as a 96 hour infusion in adults with newly diagnosed glioblastoma multiforme. *Proceedings of the American Society of Clinical Oncology, 13,* 179.

Fine, H. A. (1994). The basis for current treatment recommendations for malignant gliomas. *Journal of Neuro-Oncology, 20,* 111–120.

Fine, H. A., & Antman, K. H. (1992). High dose chemotherapy with autologous bone marrow transplantation in the treatment of high grade astrocytomas in adults: therapeutic rationale and clinical experience. *Bone Marrow Transplantation, 10,* 315–321.

Fine, H. A., Dear, K. B. G., Loeffler, J. S., Black, P. M., & Canellos, G. P. (1993). Meta-analysis of radiation therapy with and without adjuvant chemotherapy for malignant gliomas in adults. *Cancer, 71,* 2585–2597.

Flowers A., Yung, W. K. A. (1993). Carcinomatous meningitis and acute cord compression by tumor. In R. T. Johnson & J. W. Griffin (Eds.), *Current therapy in neurologic disease* (4th ed., pp. 227–230). St. Louis: Mosby–Year Book, Inc.

Forsyth, P. A., & Posner, J. B. (1993). Headaches in patients with brain tumors: A study of 111 patients. *Neurology, 43,* 1678–1683.

Goffman, T. E., Dachowski, L. J., Bobo, H., Oldfield, E. H., Steinberg, S. M., Cook, J., Mitchell, J. B., Katz, D., Smith, R., & Glatstein, E. (1992). Long term follow-up on National Cancer Institute phase I/II study of glioblastoma multiforme treated with iododeoxyuridine and hyperfractionated radiation. *Journal of Clinical Oncology, 10,* 264–268.

Greig, N. H., Ries, L. G., Yancik, R., & Rapoport, S. I. (1990). Increasing annual incidence of primary malignant brain tumors in the elderly. *Journal of the National Cancer Institute, 82,* 1621–1624.

Grossman, S. A., Osman, M., Hruban R. H., & Piantadosi, S. (1995). Familial gliomas: The potential role of environmental exposures. *Proceedings of the American Society of Clinical Oncology, 14,* 149.

Grossman, S. A., Sheidler, V. R., & Gilbert, M. R. (1989). Decreased phenytoin levels in patients receiving chemotherapy. *American Journal of Medicine, 87,* 505–510.

Grossman, S. A, & Tuma, R. (1993). Chemotherapy for central nervous system malignancies. In J. E. Niederhuber (Ed.), *Current therapy in oncology* (pp.546–550). St. Louis: Mosby–Year Book, Inc.

Grossman, S. A., Wharam, M., Sheidler, V, Zeltzman, M., Zinreich, J., Moynihan, T., Gibert, M., & Ahn, G. (1992). BCNU/Cisplatin (B/C) followed by radiation in poor-prognosis patients with high grade astrocytomas (HGA). *Proceedings of the American Society of Clinical Oncology, 11,* 149.

Gummerlock, M. K., & Neuwelt, E. A. (1994). Chemotherapy of brain tumors: Innovative approaches. In R. A. Morantz, & J. W. Walsh (Eds.), *Brain tumors: A comprehensive text* (pp. 763–778). New York, NY: Marcel Dekker, Inc.

Gutin, P. H., Shrieve, D. C., Larson, D. A., & Sneed, P. (1993). Interstitial brachytherapy and hyperthermia for malignant gliomas. *Journal of Neuro-Oncology, 17,* 161–166.

Hochberg, F. H., & Slotnick, B. (1980). Neuropsychologic impairment in astrocytoma survivors. *Neurology, 30,* 172–177.

Hoffman, W. F., Levin, V. A., & Wilson, C. B. (1979). Evaluation of malignant glioma patients during the postirradiation period. *Journal of Neurosurgery, 50,* 624–628.

Imperato, J. P., Paleologos, N. A., & Vick, N. A. (1990). Effects of treatment on long-term survivors with malignant astrocytomas. *Annals of Neurology, 28,* 818–822.

Jaeckle, K. A. (1994). Immunotherapy of malignant gliomas. *Seminars in Oncology, 21,* 249–259.

Kleinberg, L., Wallner, K., & Malkin, M. G. (1993). Good performance status of long-term disease-free survivors of intracranial gliomas. *International Journal of Radiation Oncology Biology and Physics, 26,* 129–133.

Krause, E. A., Lamb, S., Ham, B., Larson, D. A., & Gutin, P. H. (1991). Radiosurgery: A nursing perspective. *Journal of Neuroscience Nursing, 23,* 24–27.

Kristiansen, K., Hagan, S., Kollevold, T., Torvik, A., Holme, I., Nesbakken, R., Hatlevoll, R., Lindgren, M., Brun, A., Lindgren, S., Notter, G., Anderson, A. P., & Elgen, K. (1981). Combined modality therapy of operative astrocytomas grade III and IV: Confirmation of the value of postoperative irradiation and lack of potentiation of bleomycin on survival time. A prospective multicenter trial of the Scandinavian Glioblastoma Study Group. *Cancer, 47,* 649–652.

Laperriere, N. J., & Bernstein, M. (1994). Radiotherapy for brain tumors. *Ca-A Cancer Journal for Clinicians, 44,* 96–108.

Laws, E. R., & Thapar K.(1993). Brain tumors. *Ca- A Cancer Journal for Clinicians, 43,* 263–271.

Leibel, S. A., & Sheline, G. E. (1987). Radiation therapy for neoplasms of the brain. *Journal of Neurosurgery, 66,* 1–22.

Lesser, G. J., & Grossman, S. A. (1993a). The chemotherapy of adult primary brain tumors. *Cancer Treatment Reviews, 19,* 261–281.

Lesser, G. J., & Grossman, S. A. (1993b). Metastatic cancer to the brain and spinal cord. In J. E. Niederhuber (Ed.), *Current therapy in oncology* (pp.224–230). St. Louis: Mosby–Year Book, Inc.

Lesser, G. J., & Grossman S. (1994). The chemotherapy of high-grade astrocytomas. *Seminars in Oncology, 21,* 220–235.

Levin, V. A., Gutin, P. H., & Leibel, S. A. (1993). Neoplasms of the central nervous system. In V. T. DeVita, S. Hellman, & S. A. Rosenberg (Eds.), *Cancer: Principles and practice* (pp.1679–1737). Philadelphia, PA: J. B. Lippincott.

Levin, V. A., Silver, P., Hannigan, J., Wara, W. M., Gutin, P. H., Davis, R. L., & Wilson, C. B. (1990). Superiority of postradiotherapy adjuvant chemotherapy with CCNU, procarbazine, and vincristine (PCV) over BCNU for anaplastic gliomas: NCOG 6G61 final report. *International Journal of Radiation Oncology Biology and Physics, 18,* 321–324.

Longee, D. C., Friedman, H. S., Albright, R. E., Burger, P. C., Oakes, W. J., Moore, J. O., & Schold, S. C. (1990). Treatment of patients with recurrent gliomas with cyclophosphamide and vincristine. *Journal of Neurosurgery, 72,* 583–588.

Mackworth, N., Fobair, P., & Prados, M. D. (1992). Quality of life self-reports from 200 brain tumor patients: Comparison with Karnofsky performance scores. *Journal of Neuro-Oncology, 14,* 243–253.

Mahaley, M. S. (1991). Neuro-oncology index and review. *Journal of Neuro-Oncology, 11,* 85–147.

Mahaley, M. S., Mettlin, C., Natarajen, N., Laws, E. R. Jr., & Peace, B. B. (1989). National survey of patterns of care for brain tumor patients. *Journal of Neurosurgery, 71,* 826–836.

Maire, J. P. L., Coudin, P., Guerin, J., & Caudry, M. (1987). Neuropsychologic impairment in adults with brain tumors. *American Journal of Clinical Oncology, 10,* 156–162.

Meadows, A. T., Gordon, J., Massari, D. J., Littman, P., Fergusson, J., & Moss, K. (1981). Declines in IQ scores and cognitive dysfunction in children with acute lymphocytic leukaemia treated with cranial irradiation. *Lancet, 2,* 1015–1018.

Moore, I. M., Kramer, J. H., Wara, W., Halberg, F., & Ablin, A. R. (1991). Cognitive function in children with leukemia. *Cancer, 68,* 1913–1917.

Moynihan, T. J., & Grossman, S. A. (1994). The role of chemotherapy in the treatment of primary tumors of the central nervous system. *Cancer Investigation, 12,* 88–97.

Newton, C., & Mateo, M. A., (1994). Uncertainty: Strategies for patients with brain tumor and their family. *Cancer Nursing, 17,* 137–140.

Newton, H. B. (1994). Primary brain tumors: Review of etiology, diagnosis and treatment. *American Family Physician, 49,* 787–797.

Norris, L. K., & Grossman, S. A. (1994). Treatment of thromboembolic complications in patients with brain tumors. *Journal of Neuro-Oncology, 22,* 127–137

Patchell, R. A. (1991). Brain metastases. *Neurologic Clinics, 9,* 817–824.

Preston-Martin, S. (1990). Descriptive epidemiology of primary tumors of the spinal cord and spinal meninges in Los Angeles County, 1972–1985. *Neuroepidemiology, 9,* 106–111.

Radhakrishnan, K., Bohnen, N. I., & Kurland, L. T. (1994). Epidemiology of brain tumors. In R. A. Morantz, & J. W. Walsh (Eds.), *Brain tumors: A comprehensive text* (pp. 1–18). New York: Marcel Dekker, Inc.

Ramsey, R. G. (1994). The order of neuroradiologic procedures. In R. G. Ramsey (Ed.), *Neuroradiology* (pp. 1–19). Philadelphia: W. B. Saunders Co.

Recht, L. D., Lew, R., & Smith, T. W. (1992). Suspected low grade glioma: Is deferring treatment safe? *Annals of Neurology, 31,* 431–436.

Rozental, J. M., Robins, H. I., Finlay, J., Healy, B., Levin, A. B., Steeves, R. A., Kohler, P. C., Schutta, H. S., & Trump, D. L. (1989). Eight-drugs-in-one-day: Chemotherapy administered before and after radiotherapy to adult patients with malignant gliomas. *Cancer, 63,* 2475–2481.

Salcman, M., Scholtz, H., Kaplan, R. S., & Kulik, S. (1994). Long term survival in patients with malignant astrocytoma. *Neurosurgery, 34,* 213–220.

Schwandt, R. E. (1994). Selected aspects of phenytoin therapy in oncology practice. *Cancer Control: Journal of the Moffitt Cancer Center, 1,* 150–155.

Shapiro, W. R., Green, S. B., Burger, P. C., Selker, R. G., VanGilder, J. C., Robertson, J. T., Mealey, J. Jr., Ransohoff, J., & Mahaley, M. S. (1992). A randomized comparison of intra-arterial versus intravenous BCNU, with or without intravenous 5-fluorouracil for newly diagnosed patients with malignant glioma. *Journal of Neurosurgery, 76,* 772–781.

Shapiro, W. R., Green, S. B., Burger, P. C., Mahley, M. S. Jr., Selker, R. G., VanGilder, J. C., Robertson, J. T., Ransohoff, J., Mealey, J. Jr., & Strike, T. A. (1989). Randomized trial of three chemotherapy regimens and two radiotherapy regimens in postoperative treatment of malignant gliomas. *Journal of Neurosurgery, 71,* 1–9.

Sneed, P. K., Larson, D. A., & Gutin, P. H. (1994). Brachytherapy and hyperthermia for malignant gliomas with radiation therapy. *Seminars in Oncology, 21,* 186–197.

Souhami, L., Olivier, A., Podgorsak, E. B., Villemure, J. G., Pla, M., & Sadikot, A. F. (1991). Fractionated stereotactic radiation therapy for intracranial tumors. *Cancer, 68,* 2101–2108.

Taylor, S. A. (1994). New agents in the treatment of primary brain tumors. *Journal of Neuro-Oncology, 20,* 141–153.

Walker, M. D., Alexander, E., Hunt, W. E., MacCarty, C. S., Mahaley, M. S. Jr., Mealey, J. Jr., Norrell, H. A., Owens, G., Ransohoff, J., Wilson, C. B., Gehan, E. A., & Strike, T. A. (1978). Evaluation of BCNU and/or radiotherapy in the treatment of anaplastic gliomas. *Journal of Neurosurgery, 49,* 333–343.

Walker, M. D., Green, S. B., Byar, D. P., Alexander, E. Jr., Batzdorf, U., Brooks, W. H., Hunt, W. E., MacCarty, C. S., Mahaley, M. S. Jr., Mealey, J. Jr., Owens, G., Ransohoff, J. II, Robertson, J. T., Shapiro, W. R., Smith, K. R. Jr., Wilson, C. B., & Strike, T. A. (1980). Randomized comparison of radiotherapy and nitrosoureas for the treatment of malignant glioma after surgery. *New England Journal of Medicine, 303,* 1323–1329.

Wegmann, J. (1991). CNS tumors: Supportive management of the patient and family. *Oncology, 5,* 109–113.

Wharam, M. D. (1993). Brain tumors: Radiation therapy. In J. E. Niederhuber (Ed.), *Current therapy in oncology* (pp. 542–550). St. Louis: Mosby–Year Book.

Will history repeat for boron capture therapy? (1994). *Science, 265,* 468–469.

Wilson, C. B. (1994). General considerations. In M. L. J. Apuzzo (Ed.), *Brain surgery: Complication avoidance and management* (pp.177–185). New York: Churchill Livingstone.

Wilson, C. B., Larson, D. A., & Gutin, P. H. (1992). Radiosurgery: A new application? *Journal of Clinical Oncology, 10,* 1373–1374.

Wingo, P. A., Tong, T., & Bolden, S. (1995). Cancer statistics 1995. *CA- A Cancer Journal for Clinicians, 45,* 8–30.

Wrensch, M., Bondy, M. L., Wrencke, J., & Yost, M. (1993). Environmental risk factors for primary malignant brain tumors: A review. *Journal of Neuro-Oncology, 17,* 47–64.

Yung, W. K. A., Janus, T. J., Maor, M., & Feun, L. G. (1992). Adjuvant chemotherapy with carmustine and cisplatin for patients with malignant gliomas. *Journal of Neuro-Oncology, 12,* 131–135.

Zachariah, S. B., Zachariah, B., Wang, T., & Balducci, L. (1992). Primary brain tumors in the older patient: An annotated review. *Journal of the American Geriatrics Society, 40,* 1265–1271.

Multiple Myeloma

Ann M. Collins-Hattery

Multiple myeloma is one of a group of related disorders arising from plasma cells. It is the most malignant of the plasma cell dyscrasias. Multiple myeloma is characterized by an uncontrolled proliferation and accumulation of immunoglobulin-secreting plasmocytes that are derived from B-lymphocytes. Typically one specific immunoglobulin (i.e., IgA, IgD, IgE, IgG, or IgM) is cloned and produced in mass quantities in multiple myeloma. Clinically, multiple myeloma may present itself as destruction of bone, infiltration of bone marrow, presence of immunoglobulin in the urine or serum, or even symptoms of renal failure (Salmon & Cassady, 1993). Malignant plasma cells appear to replicate relatively slowly with a doubling time in the range of 2 to 4 months. It is likely that the malignant transformation of plasma cells actually occurs approximately 4 to 6 years prior to any clinical signs or symptoms (Barton Cook, 1990).

EPIDEMIOLOGY

Multiple myeloma accounts for about 10 to 15 per cent of all hematologic malignancies (Niesvizky, Siegel, & Michaeli, 1993) and 1 per cent of overall malignancies in the United States (Salmon & Cassady, 1993). The incidence of multiple myeloma has been steadily increasing, and it is estimated that there will be 12,700 new cases diagnosed in the United States this year. The incidence in males is slightly higher than that of females in all races, and there is a significantly higher incidence in African-Americans than whites (National Cancer Institute [NCI], 1994). The incidence of multiple myeloma in both African-Americans and whites increases with age. Although the disease has been reported in young adults and children, the median age at onset in the United States is 68 for men and 70 for women (Reidel & Pottern, 1992). Five year survival has shown significant improvement in the past 20 years for whites. There has been no significant improvement in five year survival observed in African-Americans (American Cancer Society, 1994).

ETIOLOGY

The causes of multiple myeloma are largely unknown; however, a number of factors have been implicated in the pathogenesis. Multiple myeloma, as discussed above, is more prevalent in African-Americans than whites in the United States. This suggests there may be a genetic component that predisposes persons to developing multiple myeloma, although environmental influences could also be responsible for the difference.

Environmental or occupational factors have been examined in multiple myeloma. The strongest risks of myeloma have been associated with agriculture, radiation exposure, food processing, and exposure to certain chemicals. An association between farming and multiple myeloma has been reported. Eriksson and Karlsson (1992) documented exposure to some domestic farm animals (cattle, horses, and goats) and to two individual pesticides (phenoxyacetic acids and DDT) as specific risk factors. Other studies, however, have failed to support this link (Brown, Burmeister, Everett, & Blair, 1993; Brown, Everett, Burmeister, & Blair, 1992; Heineman et al., 1992).

Chronic exposure to low-level radiation may increase the risk of myeloma as much as six times with the disease developing up to 20 years after the exposure (McIntyre, 1985). Diagnostic x-rays have been implicated in the development of myeloma. An increased risk for multiple myeloma was found among those patients who were frequently exposed to diagnostic x-rays, the relative risk increasing with the number of x-rays performed (Boice et al., 1991).

The incidence of myeloma is significantly increased in a number of occupations, for example, road and railroad workers, precision metalworkers, and workers in the transportation and communication industries. Risk increased significantly with duration of employment in production of synthetic yarns, plastic packaging, and miscellaneous chemical compounds, production of structural metal and stationary tanks, auto body factories, electrical plants, and retail sale of paint. A fivefold risk has been documented in persons with exposure to vinyl chloride for 5 or more years (Heineman et al., 1992).

The use of hair-coloring products containing mutagenic and carcinogenic chemicals has also been implicated with the development of multiple myeloma. Researchers have found a significant risk that is greatest among those using hair dyes at least once a month for a year or more (Brown et al., 1992).

Immune-stimulating conditions have been investigated as potential risk factors in myeloma. A significant positive correlation exists between chronic bacterial infections, inflammatory conditions (particularly eczema and inflammatory musculoskeletal conditions), and the development of myeloma. The incidence of myeloma increases with the number of inflammatory conditions, the length of time from onset of the inflammatory condition, and the number of bacterial diseases (Bourguet & Logue, 1993; Doody et al., 1992; Gramenzi, et al., 1991).

In culture, myeloma cells secrete a number of lymphokines: interleukins-1, -5, and -6 and tumor necrosis factors α and β (or lymphotoxin). Myeloma cells also have receptors for IL-5 and IL-6 on their surfaces, which may suggest that IL-5 and IL-6 play a role in the pathogenesis and proliferation of myeloma cells (Barlogic, Epstein, Salvanayagam, & Alexanian, 1989; Lichtenstein, Berenson, Norman, Chang, & Carlilr, 1989; Fattori et al., 1994). IL-6 has been shown to prevent programmed cell death; this may be its mechanism of action in multiple myeloma (Niesvizky et al., 1993). Other studies have not supported IL-6 as a major growth factor in multiple myeloma but have noted, instead, a negative correlation between IL-6 levels and multiple myeloma tumor burden. They have found that patients with high levels of IL-6 production defined a subgroup of patients with low tumor burden. Conversely, patients with high proliferative indexes had significantly lower levels of IL-6 than those patients with low proliferative indexes (Ballester et al., 1994).

BIOLOGY AND NATURAL HISTORY

NORMAL IMMUNE RESPONSE

Immunoglobulins are the building blocks of antibodies. They are produced by plasma cells in response to the invasion of antigens. In the normal immune response, *specific* immunoglobulins are produced and secreted in response to *specific* antigens. Each antibody molecule is composed of two identical heavy chains and two identical light chains. These chains all have constant, unchanging regions that account for the appearance and classifications of the immunoglobulins. They likewise have variable regions that change to accommodate the specific antigen and bind it. As antibodies are cloned in response to antigens, they are produced as complete molecules with the production of heavy and light chains being in balance (Salmon & Cassady, 1993). In a matter of minutes a single activated plasma cell can produce thousands of immunoglobulins, which come together to form antibody molecules specific to the invading antigen.

There are five classes of immunoglobulins, IgA, IgD, IgE, IgG, and IgM, and each plays a specific and vital role in the combat against infection (Table 41–1). IgA has an integral function in the body's first line of defense. It is the principal immunoglobulin in tears, saliva, respiratory tract secretions, and gastrointestinal secretions. IgD is found in much lower quantities than IgA and is referred to as a trace immunoglobulin. The main function of IgD is to bind with the antigen on the cell's surface and stimulate further B-lymphocyte production and differentiation. IgE, also a trace immunoglobulin, is often elevated in response to allergic responses, asthma, and parasitic infections. IgE binds to receptors on basophils and mast cells and may stimulate these cells to secrete vasoactive substances as part of the allergic response. IgG is the immunoglobulin found in greatest quantity in the serum, followed by IgA and IgM. IgG is the only immunoglobulin that can cross the placenta and is responsible for passive immunity in newborns. There are four subclassifications of IgG, IgG 1–4, each having slightly different characteristics and roles. IgM is the first immunoglobulin produced in response to antigenic invasion. It is also the first immunoglobulin produced in infants (Barton Cook, 1990; Bubley & Schnipper, 1991).

PATHOPHYSIOLOGY OF MULTIPLE MYELOMA

In multiple myeloma it appears that malignant plasma cells have replaced normal functioning B lymphocytes or B cells. Severe B-cell deficiencies are seen in virtually all myeloma patients (Pilarski, Mant, Ruether, & Belch, 1984). In some patients, the B cells that are present are functionally abnormal and are unable to mature normally (Pilarski, Ruether, & Mant, 1985). Because B cells are the precursors for immunoglobulin-secreting plasma cells, these deficiencies or abnormalities account for the lack of humoral response seen in patients with multiple myeloma. The malignant plasma

TABLE 41–1. *Functions of Immunoglobulins*

IMMUNOGLOBULIN CLASS	FUNCTIONS
IgA	First line of defense, present in tears, saliva, respiratory secretions, gastrointestinal secretions
IgD	Trace immunoglobulin; binds with cell surface antigen and stimulates B cell production and differentiation
IgE	Trace immunoglobulin; binds to receptors on basophils and mast cells; may stimulate secretion of vasoactive substances in allergic response
IgG 4 subclassifications IgG-1 through 4	Found in greatest quantity; crosses placenta, responsible for passive immunity in newborns
IgM	Produced first in response to antigenic invasion; first Ig produced in infants

cells massively overproduce one particular type of immunoglobulin, while the production of normal immunoglobulins is suppressed, compounding the humoral immune response deficit.

Multiple myeloma is classified according to the immunoglobulin clone that is being overproduced. This specific immunoglobulin is known as the monoclonal component or M-component. Detection of a significant amount of M-component or "M-spike" is made by serum protein electrophoresis (SPEP) and is of major diagnostic significance in plasma cell dyscrasias. An overproduction in any one of the immunoglobulins will cause a monoclonal spike to occur. The exact immunoglobulin responsible for the spike is determined through serum immunoelectrophoresis (SIEP). Multiple myeloma is associated with M-components IgA, IgD, IgE, or IgG. Monoclonal spike in IgM is associated with another plasma dyscrasia, Waldenstom's Macroglobulinemia.

Unlike the normal cloning of antibodies in response to antigenic stimulation, in the malignant cloning process the synthesis of light chains and heavy chains often becomes unbalanced, and light chains are produced in excess. Because of their low molecular weight, light chains are normally filtered by the glomeruli. Some are reabsorbed and broken down by the renal tubules and are partially excreted in the urine. These urinary light chains are called Bence Jones proteins. Substantial quantities of Bence Jones proteins provide significant diagnostic information (Salmon, 1973).

DIAGNOSIS AND STAGING

PRESENTING SIGNS AND SYMPTOMS

The signs and symptoms of multiple myeloma are varied and result from the products secreted by the myeloma cells themselves. These symptoms may be hormonal, immunologic, or physicochemical in nature and tend to correlate in severity with the tumor burden.

Multiple myeloma is most often diagnosed in advanced stages due to the prolonged prodromal period during which the disease is developing but the patient is asymptomatic (Salmon & Cassady, 1993).

The most common presenting symptom is bone pain. Pathologic fractures, spinal cord compression, hypercalcemia, renal failure, pancytopenia, and recurrent bacterial infections all complicate the clinical course of multiple myeloma (Sheridan, 1993).

DIFFERENTIAL DIAGNOSIS

Accurate diagnosis of myeloma is dependent on a combination of morphologic findings, radiographic studies, and an extensive laboratory workup (Table 41–2). Elevated serum protein levels on a chemistry profile may be the first finding noted. An M-spike on serum or urine protein electrophoresis (Fig. 41–1) along with a bone marrow biopsy showing increased (>10 per cent), abnormal, immature plasma cells in the marrow can confirm the diagnosis. It is noteworthy that approximately 25 per cent of patients at presentation do not have an M-protein that can be detected by SPEP. Most of these patients do, however, have excessive light-chain in their urine, which can be detected by urine electrophoresis or immunoelectrophoresis. When

TABLE 41–2. *Diagnostic Work-up of Multiple Myeloma*

SOURCE	DIAGNOSTIC STUDY
Hematologic studies	Bone marrow aspirate
	Complete blood count
	Platelet count
	Reticulocyte count
	Bleeding time
	Partial thromboplastin time (PTT), prothrombin time (PT)
	Direct Coombs' test
Blood chemistry studies	BUN
	Creatinine clearance
	Serum calcium
	Serum uric acid
	Serum protein electrophoresis (SPEP)
	Quantitative immunoglobulins
	LDH
	β-2 microglobulin
	Serum viscosity
	Immunoelectrophoresis (IEP)
Urine studies	Quantitative 24 hr urine protein
	Urine protein electrophoresis
	Urine immunoelectrophoresis (if indicated)
Radiographic and imaging studies	Skeletal survey (including skull, long bones, and chest x-rays)
	Computed tomography (CT), magnetic resonance imaging (MRI) of spine (if indicated)

(From Schrier, S. L.: Multiple myeloma and related serum protein disorders. Scientific American Medicine, Dale D. C., Federman, D. D., Eds. Section 5, Subsection IX. c 1995 Scientific American, Inc. All rights reserved.)

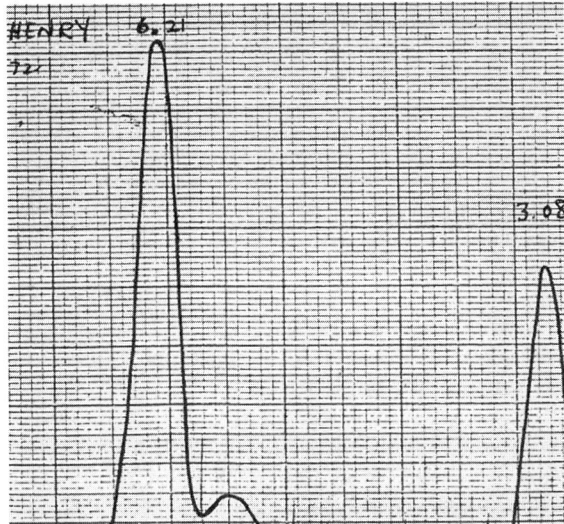

FIGURE 41–1. Serum protein electrophoresis showing classic monoclonal spike. (Courtesy of Marvin J. Stone, M.D., Sammons Cancer Center, Baylor University Medical Center, Dallas, Texas.)

TABLE 41–3. *Durie and Salmon Proposed Staging System for Multiple Myeloma*

STAGE	CLINICAL DETERMINANTS
Stage I	All of the following: Hemoglobulin > 10 mg/dl Serum calcium (corrected) < 12 mg/dl Normal bone structure on x-rays or solitary bone lesion only M-component production values: IgG < 5 g/dl IgA < 3 g/dl Urine light chain excretion < 4g/24 hrs Low measured myeloma cell mass (< 0.6)
Stage II	Intermediate measured myeloma cell mass (0.6–1.2) Criteria that fits neither stage I or III
Stage III	Any one or more of the following: Hemoglobulin < 8.5 mg/dl Serum calcium (corrected) > 12 mg/dl Advanced lytic bone lesion on x-rays M-component production values: IgG > 7 g/dl IgA > 5 g/dl Urine light chain excretion > 12g/24 hrs High measured myeloma cell mass (> 1.2)

(From V. T. DeVita, S. Hellman, & S. A. Rosenberg [Eds.], *Cancer: Principles and practice of oncology* [4th ed., p. 1995]. (c) 1993 Table 56–4. Data from *Cancer* 1975, 36, 1192–1201.)

multiple myeloma is suspected, a normal SPEP does not rule out the diagnosis (Rubenstein & Federman, 1990).

Osteolytic lesions may or may not be present but are useful in confirming the diagnosis. Radiography is still the technique of choice for evaluating skeletal lesions, particularly when cost is a factor. Computed tomography (CT) scans and magnetic resonance imaging (MRI) provide far more information in evaluating vertebral lesions and their potential effects on the spinal cord. Radioisotope bone scans are of no value in multiple myeloma because they are sensitive only in detecting osteoblastic lesions, and the vast majority of bony lesions associated with multiple myeloma are osteolytic (Salmon & Cassady, 1993).

The diagnostic workup provides information about the extent of organ involvement and prognosis. The presence of renal failure, elevated β-2 microglobulin levels, and LDH levels at diagnosis are all considered negative prognostic findings. An elevated β-2 microglobulin level indicates a large malignant cell mass, renal impairment, or both. A highly elevated LDH is predictive of an aggressive, lymphoma-like disease (Barlogie, Smallwood, Smith, & Alexanian, 1989; Kyle, 1990; Simonsson, et al., 1988).

STAGING

The information used in diagnosing myeloma has also been used to construct a staging system. Durie and Salmon (1975) proposed a staging system in which multiple myeloma is divided into three groups based on tumor burden: stage I (low tumor burden), stage II (intermediate), and stage III (high) (Table 41–3). Staging in multiple myeloma is used for more accurate comparison of study groups and to encourage better initial assessment of the patient.

CLINICAL MANIFESTATIONS AND SEQUELAE

BONE INVOLVEMENT

Myeloma cells are thought to secrete osteoclast-activating factors (OAF). OAF are cytokines that stimulate the proliferation and activation of osteoclasts, which cause bone destruction and resorption. It is not surprising then that bone pain is the most common presenting symptom in multiple myeloma (Sheridan, 1993). Sixty-eight to 80 per cent of individuals with multiple myeloma have painful lytic bone lesions at the time of diagnosis (Mundy & Bertolini, 1986). Without treatment these lytic lesions progress to pathologic fractures and, depending on location, neurologic deficits. The bone lesions seen in patients with multiple myeloma can be in the form of single lytic lesions, multiple lytic lesions, giving the bones a "Swiss cheese" appearance (Fig. 41–2), or, more rarely, the lesions may be of a blastic nature.

The most common areas of involvement are the thoracic and lumbar vertebrae. These lesions often result in spinal cord compression, so early detection and treatment is critical in preserving neurologic integrity. The ribs, skull, pelvis, and long bones are also frequently involved (Sheridan, 1993).

HYPERCALCEMIA

At any one time 99 per cent of the body's calcium is contained in the bones and teeth. The remaining 1 per cent is the circulating or serum calcium and is kept in

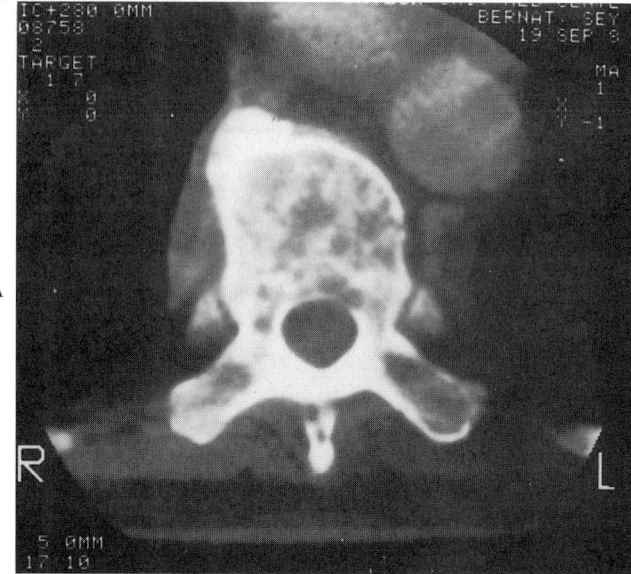

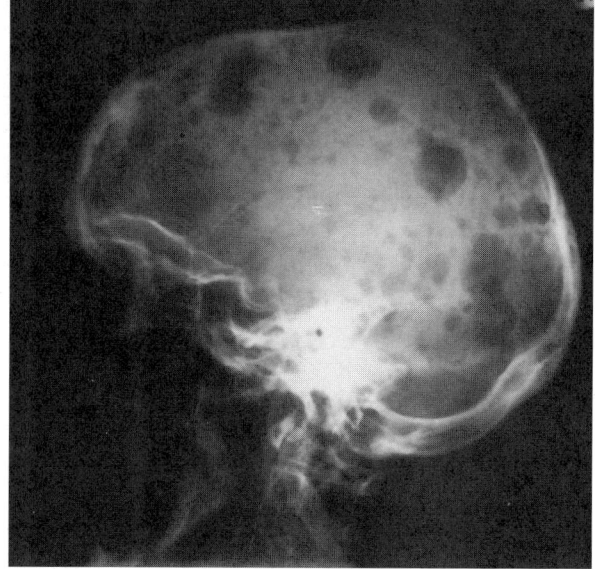

FIGURE 41–2. Vertebral body (**A**) and skull (**B**) x-rays showing osteolytic bone lesions characteristic of multiple myeloma. (Courtesy of Marvin J. Stone, M.D., Sammons Cancer Center, Baylor University Medical Center, Dallas, Texas.)

check by a number of homeostatic mechanisms. The bone destruction and resorption associated with multiple myeloma releases large amounts of calcium into the serum at such a pace that the normal homeostatic measures are unable to keep up and the serum calcium rises. Signs and symptoms of hypercalcemia include lethargy progressing to somnolence, nausea, constipation, polydipsia, polyuria, and hyporeflexia. Untreated hypercalcemia can result in renal failure due to precipitation of calcium salts in the tubules or renal interstitium. This results in diminished glomerular filtration and creates a vicious cycle of rising calcium levels and increased renal damage (Rubenstein & Federman, 1990).

RENAL FAILURE

Renal insufficiency progressing to renal failure has a number of contributing events in persons with multiple myeloma. The principal cause of renal failure in this population is the deposition of light chains in the tubules, but hypercalcemia, hyperuricemia, plasma cell infiltration, amyloid deposits, pyelonephritis, and hyperviscosity all can result in renal impairment.

It is likely that Bence Jones proteins are toxic to the tubules. They are characteristically present as dense casts of light chains in the renal tubules. These casts impair glomerular filtration and reabsorption and result in destruction of the tubular epithelium, inflammation and fibrosis of the renal interstitium, and tubular degeneration. This condition is referred to as "myeloma kidney" (Hamblin, 1986). Large amounts of Bence Jones proteins in the urine in conjunction with dehydration with a low urine pH increases the risk of precipitation of proteins in the renal tubule. The possible coprecipitation with calcium further exacerbates the acute renal failure (Sheridan, 1993).

Amyloid is an accumulation of insoluble fibrin-like proteins in various tissues that are a precipitant of a reaction between the myeloma protein and tissue polysaccharides (Barton Cook, 1990; Glenner, 1980; Sheridan, 1993). Approximately 10 to 30 per cent of myeloma patients develop amyloid deposits. These deposits can occur in the tubular basement membranes, renal vasculature, or the glomerulus, all of which will have significant effects on the renal function. Additionally amyloid deposits have been found in the blood vessels, heart, gastrointestinal tract, skin, and major organs (Glenner, 1980).

Pyelonephritis is often present in patients with multiple myeloma. Tubular obstruction resulting in diminished kidney function compounded by the lack of normal immunoglobulins sets the stage for the development of pyelonephritis.

Renal insufficiency is present in approximately 29 per cent of patients with multiple myeloma at diagnosis (Oken, 1984). Renal failure at the time of diagnosis has a negative impact on overall survival (Cherng, Asal, Kuebler, Lee, & Solanki, 1991; Oken, 1984).

BONE MARROW INVOLVEMENT

Because plasma cells reside in the bone marrow, myeloma infiltration of the bone marrow results in suppression of the normal bone marrow components with subsequent anemia, thrombocytopenia, and leukopenia. The marrow can become so packed with myeloma cells that plasmablasts appear in the circulating blood. This excess of plasma cells in the marrow may also contribute to bone pain as a presenting symptom (Sheridan, 1993). Hypoplasia of normal bone marrow components with resultant pancytopenia is also seen relatively frequently in the absence of total myeloma infiltration of the marrow (Bartl et al., 1982).

HYPERVISCOSITY

Hyperviscosity is most common with IgM myeloma (Waldenstrom's Macroglobulinemia). IgA myeloma and IgG myeloma, specifically IgG3 and IgG4, may occasionally result in hyperviscosity syndrome as well (McGrath & Penny, 1976; Somer, 1987). It occurs as a result of a high concentration of the abnormal protein (paraprotein) in the serum, increasing the blood viscosity. It can also occur if the paraprotein interacts with red blood cells, causing extensive aggregation of erythrocytes. Hyperviscosity leads to widespread circulatory disturbances leading to obstruction of the microscopic vasculature. Initial clinical signs of hyperviscosity include headache, visual disturbances, irritability, drowsiness, and confusion. Additionally, obstruction of blood flow in the kidneys may occur, increasing the risk of renal failure. Plasmapheresis is the treatment of choice for hyperviscosity syndrome (McGrath & Penny, 1976).

INFECTION

Infection is the leading cause of death in persons with multiple myeloma. The primary sites for infection are the respiratory and urinary tracts (Jacobson & Zolla-Pazner, 1986). As discussed previously, a number of factors contribute to the increased susceptibility to bacterial infections seen in the patient with multiple myeloma. Initially, there is a lack of response to antigenic invasion due to the decrease in B lymphocytes (B cells). As the marrow becomes packed with myeloma cells, the production of other bone marrow components, namely the granulocytes, is suppressed. Paglieroni, Caggiano, and MacKenzie (1992) suggest that certain immune defects may actually be involved in the development of myeloma and are not simply a consequence of the malignancy. This immune defect is thought to be due to immunosuppressive CD5-positive B cells that may be present prior to the development of myeloma. Once treatment is initiated, the immunosuppressive properties of the chemotherapeutic agents furthers the risk of infection.

TREATMENT

There is no known cure for multiple myeloma. Treatment is aimed at eradication of symptoms, prolonged survival, and enhanced quality of life.

CHEMOTHERAPY

Because multiple myeloma is a disseminated disease, systemic cytotoxic therapy is the treatment of choice. However, treatment of patients with asymptomatic, indolent, or stage I multiple myeloma has not demonstrated an advantage in survival. Exposing these individuals to the risks of chemotherapy unnecessarily is considered inappropriate. These patients are usually followed until disease progression can be documented. Treatment is usually reserved for symptomatic patients or those in whom a doubling in the M-component has occurred in less than a year. Symptoms or signs that warrant treatment include development of bone pain, spinal cord compression, hypercalcemia, renal failure, or severe suppression of bone marrow functions (Salmon & Cassady, 1993). Patients who have severe pancytopenia and a bone marrow packed with myeloma cells should undergo therapy promptly, but the therapy must be carefully monitored because it may intensify and further prolong the pancytopenia and potentially lead to death (Rubenstein & Federman, 1990).

PHASES OF TREATMENT

Multiple myeloma appears to follow a fairly predictable sequence of events. Initially, the disease is sensitive to the cytotoxic effects of the drugs in most patients. This drug-sensitive phase is usually followed by a plateau phase during which the tumor burden is reduced and appears to be stable during maintained or unmaintained remission. Eventually the neoplasm becomes drug-resistant to conventional antineoplastic drugs (Durie, Russell & Salmon, 1980; Salmon, 1973). The effects of chemosensitizers such as verapamil for reversing multidrug resistance in multiple myeloma continue to be studied with some success (Salmon et al., 1991).

TREATMENT REGIMENS

Melphalan (L-PAM, Alkeran), an alkylating agent, and prednisone, a corticosteroid, are still considered the gold standard in first-line therapy for myeloma (Bubley & Schnipper, 1991; Rubenstein & Federman, 1990; Salmon & Cassady, 1993). These drugs are usually given in intermittent cycles, are easy to administer on an outpatient basis, and the clinical responses are frequently good (30 to 60 per cent) (Oken, 1994). Melphalan plus prednisone shows an increased response rate over melphalan alone but does not affect long-term survival. Additionally, the prednisone decreases bone resorption, which could be advantageous in the prevention of pathologic fractures and hypercalcemia (Barton Cook, 1990). However, treatment failure usually occurs within 2 years, and the 5-year survival is low. Cyclophosphamide (Cytoxan) is another alkylating agent that may be instituted in the face of drug resistance to melphalan. It may also be administered orally.

Combinations of alkylating agents may produce a higher response rate and more prompt palliation, but the survival is the same as with treatment with melphalan and prednisone. The combination of IFN-α 2 with multiple alkylating agents appears to prolong the plateau phase but does not prolong survival (Kyle, 1993; Niesvizky et al., 1993).

Several studies have shown that the use of more aggressive combination chemotherapeutic regimens such as vincristine, doxorubicin (Adriamycin), and dexamethasone (VAD) produces improved response rates (84 per cent) and median survival (44 months) (Niesvizky et al., 1993; Samson et al., 1989). Adam (1993) and Boccadoro et al. (1991) have reported that although there may be an increased response rate, there is no difference in survival with the more aggressive regimens.

The main side effects of the melphalan/prednisone regimen are bone marrow suppression and renal toxicity. Blood counts must be closely monitored, particularly in older patients. Patients should be cautioned about the dangers of infection and bleeding. Those patients taking cyclophosphamide should be encouraged to drink fluids to avoid possible hemorrhagic cystitis. When allopurinol is administered concurrently with cyclophosphamide, bone marrow suppression may be intensified (Salmon & Cassady, 1993).

With more intensive therapy comes greater drug toxicity. Knowledge of the expected side effects as well as potential adverse reactions is imperative in caring for this patient population. Marked bone marrow suppression, cardiotoxicity, and neurotoxicity are potential problems. Due to its cardiotoxic properties, the maximum lifetime dose of doxorubicin should not exceed 450 mg/M2. The cumulative dose must be recorded with each treatment cycle to ensure that this maximum dose is not exceeded. Baseline cardiac ejection fractions should be obtained on all patients prior to initiation of doxorubicin-containing therapy.

The neurotoxicity associated with vincristine may present as paresthesias of the hands and feet or constipation that can progress to a paralytic ileus. For that reason the dosage must be reduced with the onset of neurologic symptoms.

Both doxorubicin and vincristine are vesicant drugs and present risks when administered by peripheral intravenous administration. Venous access devices should be considered prior to the initiation of therapy for these agents.

Corticosteroids have significant side effects. Insulin-dependent hyperglycemia, fluid and sodium retention, difficulty sleeping, dyspepsia, duodenal ulcers, and steroid psychosis are all possible toxicities and may require reduction in dosage. Mild arthralgias the day after the drug is discontinued are also common. Patients should be instructed to take steroids with meals or a glass of milk.

About 15 to 20 per cent of patients with myeloma will be resistant to all forms of drug therapy at the time of presentation. Patients with multiple myeloma who have a response to therapy can expect a median survival of approximately 40 months, much of it pain-free and in good health. Approximately 2 per cent of patients survive for 10 years or longer after diagnosis (Kyle, 1983; Salmon & Cassady, 1993). Studies continue on effective second-line therapy for relapsed multiple myeloma.

BONE MARROW TRANSPLANTATION

Bone marrow transplantation has been explored as a treatment option for myeloma. Only about 5 to 10 per cent of myeloma patients are appropriate for allogeneic bone marrow transplantation due to age restrictions and matched donor availability. The main advantage of allogeneic transplantation is that the graft contains no tumor cells that can subsequently produce a relapse. Autologous bone marrow transplantation is applicable for more patients, because the age limit is higher and a matched donor is not necessary. However,

there are two main problems with using autologous marrow. First, the eradication of myeloma cells from the patient may not be possible even with high doses of chemotherapy and radiation. Second, the harvested and infused autologous marrow may be contaminated with myeloma cells and result in relapse (Kyle, 1993).

Autologous peripheral blood stem cell (PBSC) transplantation may be another option. Tribalto et al. (1993) used this option in patients with multiple myeloma with a 46 per cent complete response and 71 per cent overall response rate. The patient was initially treated with two cycles of VAD followed by high-dose cyclophosphamide plus granulocyte-colony-stimulating factor (G-CSF). After the peripheral blood stem cells are harvested, the patient is treated with melphalan and busulfan followed by G-CSF. Maintenance therapy was interferon α2. Although no long-term progression-free survival data are yet available, PBSC transplantation may be a feasible option with low toxicity.

RADIATION THERAPY

Radiation therapy is used primarily for palliative treatment of bone lesions in persons with myeloma. Localized radiotherapy is the immediate therapy for vertebral involvement that threatens the spinal cord as well as lesions of the long bones to prevent pathologic fractures. Multiple myeloma is highly radiosensitive, and treatment is usually rapidly effective in alleviating the pain associated with these lesions (Salmon & Cassady, 1993). Patients and their families should be instructed on the side effects of radiation therapy specific to the treatment field.

IMMUNOTHERAPY

The interferons have the ability to inhibit viral replication, influence protein synthesis, and stimulate antiproliferative effects and the immune response (Roth & Foon, 1987). Interferon-α (IFN-alpha) is known to have activity in myeloma and has been widely studied for its effects on the proliferation and function of various tumor cells. There are ongoing studies with IFN-α used either in combination with alkylating agents or as a single agent to prolong the plateau phase in patients in partial remission. Although the exact mechanism of action is unknown, IFN-α has proven to be of some benefit in multiple myeloma. The most beneficial strategy for administration is not yet established (Brouet, 1994; Simonsson et al., 1988; Urabe, 1994).

The employment of monoclonal antibodies is another area being studied. When chemotherapy is not particularly rewarding, treatment with passive antibody against a known surface marker on the malignant plasma cell is, in theory, the ideal alternative. Monoclonal antibodies (MoAbs) have been described that recognize plasma cells. The CD38 antigen is known to be present on most malignant plasma cells and appears to be the best target for MoAbs attack. The CD38 antigen, however, is also present on natural killer (NK) cells, which mediate antibody-dependent cellular cytotoxicity and may help the body fight cancer and the progenitor cells of hematopoiesis. The point in question then is whether the MoAbs will affect these cells as well. It appears, at least in vitro, that there is only a minor reduction in cellular cytotoxicity and no effect in the growth of progenitor cells (Stevenson et al., 1991).

NURSING CARE

Because of the shift in health care away from the inpatient setting, most of the care and treatment of patients with multiple myeloma is delivered in the outpatient and home setting. Therefore, instead of giving "hands-on" care, much of what we do for this population is in the form of education and referrals. We provide the patient and family with the information they need to care for themselves. The focus of most patient teaching is centered around symptom management and prevention of complications. This requires a good understanding of the etiology and sequelae of multiple myeloma as well as the early signs and symptoms of problems that can develop.

Nursing diagnoses for this patient population focus on a number of actual and potential responses. Alteration in comfort, alteration in renal function, potential for alteration in mobility, potential for injury, potential for fluid and electrolyte imbalance, activity intolerance, and alteration in elimination pattern are common responses to myeloma and its treatment. Psychosociologic responses such as depression, anxiety, role changes, sleep disturbances, and limited resources are also common. Teaching the patient and family about these potential and actual responses and their etiologies as well as their prevention and management is an integral part of the role of the nurse in caring for patients with myeloma.

PAIN MANAGEMENT

Pain is the most frequent presenting symptom in myeloma patients. The pain, which can be acute or chronic in nature, is due to osteolytic bone lesions causing compression fractures of long bones and the axial skeleton. Thorough, ongoing assessment and communication is necessary in providing adequate pain management. Often the symptoms accompanying chronic pain are very dissimilar to those of acute pain, and many of the physiologic indicators are not present. Acute pain is of short duration (less than 6 months) and is usually the result of a trauma of some sort such as pathologic fracture. Typically acute pain is accompanied by elevations in heart and respiratory rate and blood pressure. Chronic pain, on the other hand, often lasts longer than 6 months, may not be attributable to any specific insult, and commonly has few if any physiologic manifestations (McCaffrey & Beebe, 1989).

Back pain is the most common sign of impending spinal cord compression. It may be radicular in nature, usually is accompanied by localized tenderness over the vertebral body involved, is not relieved by position changes, and increases with Valsalva. Back pain in this patient population should never be ignored. It is an early sign, and early diagnosis of cord compression can make the difference in the ultimate functional state of the patient (see Chapter 66). The characteristics of back pain should be included in all patient and family teaching.

Interventions for managing pain include pharmacologic management with narcotics and nonnarcotic analgesics, and nonpharmacologic interventions such as distraction, visualization, relaxation techniques, and cutaneous stimulation. Most nonpharmacologic interventions work best as an adjunct to pharmacologic management. Pain is depressing, anxiety-provoking, and leads to a reduction in activity. Relieving cancer pain effectively facilitates ambulation and activity, relieves distressing psychologic symptoms, and restores dignity and quality of life in patients with cancer (Paice, 1991).

MOBILITY PROBLEMS

Spinal cord compression and pathologic fractures, both of which arise from osteolytic lesions, are primary causes of impaired mobility. Pain, as mentioned above, is a major contributor to immobility as well. It is important that bedrest is avoided in persons with myeloma, because it leads to increased mobilization of calcium and predisposes to the development of pneumonia and urinary tract infection, which are major causes of death among multiple myeloma patients. A progressive exercise program should be instituted to increase muscle tone and reduce bone resorption.

POTENTIAL FOR INJURY

The patient with multiple myeloma is at risk of injury from infection due to neutropenia, bleeding due to thrombocytopenia, weakness, and activity intolerance due to anemia secondary to either the myelomatous marrow or the chemotherapy. Infection is the leading cause of death in myeloma patients due to the decrease in humoral immunity and myelomatous infiltration of the bone marrow. Upper respiratory and urinary tracts are the most common sites of infection. It is important that patients and their families are educated regarding signs and symptoms of infection and notifying the physician immediately should these symptoms arise.

Patients with hyperviscosity syndrome or hypercalcemia are at risk for injury secondary to confusional states that may accompany them. The signs and symptoms of hypercalcemia should be routinely included in the patient and family teaching, reinforcing that early intervention can minimize complications (Sheridan, 1993). Providing information on maintaining a safe environment, dealing with patients in a reassuring manner, and explaining the etiology of the symptoms to family members may alleviate some of the anxiety that accompanies confusional states.

POTENTIAL FOR FLUID AND ELECTROLYTE IMBALANCE

Fluid and electrolyte disturbances can arise from renal insufficiency or failure. Adequate fluid intake consisting of 2 to 3 L per day can potentially prevent kidney damage from Bence-Jones proteins and elevated levels of calcium and uric acid (Barton Cook, 1990). Patients and families must be instructed on the importance of taking allopurinol as part of the chemotherapy regimen to prevent kidney damage from hyperuricemia.

ACTIVITY INTOLERANCE

Pain, anemia, weakness, and depression all contribute to activity intolerance in the person with myeloma. The fatigue and weakness associated with anemia may require the patient to alter his or her lifestyle. In contrast, however, if the anemia has developed insidiously, the patient may have a seriously low hemoglobin without being overtly handicapped. Maintaining as close to normal activities as possible is important in maintaining self-esteem, independence, and a sense of control. Teaching the patient and family about managing activity intolerance should include planning for frequent rest periods, grouping activities, using assistive devices as necessary, and progressively increasing activity as tolerated. Transfusions may be necessary to treat the anemia.

ALTERATION IN ELIMINATION PATTERN

Constipation may develop in myeloma patients due to the use of narcotics, decreased physical activity, and dehydration. The patient and family should be instructed that vincristine-containing chemotherapy regimens often cause constipation, which can progress to paralytic ileus if not treated. Again, it is important to stress that early intervention can minimize complications (Sheridan, 1993). Patients taking vincristine should make note of their normal bowel routine so that they can recognize deviations. Increasing fluid intake and taking laxatives as necessary should be included in the teaching plan.

Urinary hesitancy or precipitancy may be prodromal signs of cord compression, usually in the company of back pain. Patients and families should be alerted to these signs as early indicators.

SUMMARY

Multiple myeloma is a disease characterized by both acute and chronic episodes. Delivering care to these patients can be challenging, particularly in our current health care environment where the thrust of care is being delivered in the outpatient or home setting. In large part symptom management takes place over the telephone or through brief interactions in the office or clinic setting. Nurses caring for these patients must be well versed on the potential problems that persons with myeloma may face. Knowing the right questions to ask the patient to gain critical information and educating the patient and family about these critical elements may make the difference in the patient's ultimate functional capacity and quality of life. Coping with the changes in lifestyle and roles imposed by this illness is difficult for many patients. Providing emotional support and information on local support groups is an invaluable service the oncology nurse provides.

Although the 5-year survival rate has shown significant overall improvement during the past 20 years, research is ongoing with regard to risk factors and therapy for multiple myeloma. Technologic advances being integrated into practice, the impact of growth factors, and other biologicals may change the future of the disease.

REFERENCES

Adam, Z. (1993). Initial treatment of multiple myeloma (Review Abstract). *Vnitrni Lekarstvi, 39*(12), 1199–1204.

American Cancer Society. (1994). *Cancer facts and figures—1994* (pp. 18–19). Atlanta: American Cancer Society.

Ballester, O. F., Moscinski, L. C., Luman, G. H., Chaney, J. V., Saba, H. I., Spiers, A. S., & Klein, C. (1994). High levels of interleukin-6 are associated with low tumor burden and low growth fraction in multiple myeloma. *Blood, 83*(7), 1903–1908.

Barlogie, B., Epstein, J., Selvanayagam, P., & Alexanian, R. (1989). Plasma cell myeloma: New biological insights and advances in therapy. *Blood, 73*(4), 865–879.

Barlogie, B., Smallwood, L., Smith, T., & Alexanian, R. (1989). High serum levels of lactic dehydrogenase identify a high-grade lymphoma-like myeloma. *Annals of Internal Medicine, 110*(7), 521–525.

Bartl, R., Frisch, B., Brukhardt, R., Fateh-Mogahadam, A., Mahl, G., Giester, P., Sund, M., & Kettner, G. (1982). Bone marrow histology in myeloma: Its importance in diagnosis, prognosis, classification and staging. *British Journal of Haematology, 51*(3), 361–375.

Barton Cook, M. (1990). Multiple myeloma. In S. L. Groenwald, M. Hansen Frogge, M. Goodman, & C. Henke Yarbro (Eds.), *Cancer nursing principles and practice* (2nd ed., pp. 990–998). Boston: Jones and Bartlett.

Boccadoro, M., Marmont, F., Tribalto, M., Avvisati, G., Andriani, A., Barbui, T., Cantonetti, M., Carotenuto, M., Comotti, B., Dammacco, F. et al. (1991). Multiple myeloma: VCMP/VBAP alternating combination chemotherapy is not superior to melphalan and prednisone even in high-risk patients. *Journal of Clinical Oncology, 9*(3), 444–448.

Boice, J. D., Jr., Morin, M. M., Glass, A. G., Friedman, G. D., Stovall, M., Hoover, R. N., & Fraumeni, J. F., Jr. (1991). Diagnostic x-rays and the risk of leukemia, lymphoma, and multiple myeloma. *Journal of the American Medical Association, 265*(10), 1290–1294.

Bourguet, C. C., & Logue, E. E. (1993). Antigenic stimulation and multiple myeloma: A prospective study. *Cancer, 72*(7), 2148–2154.

Brouet, J. C. (1994). Interferon therapy in multiple myeloma [Review]. *Nouvelle Revue Francaise D'Hematologie, 36*(Suppl.1), S37–S38.

Brown, L. M., Burmeister, L. F., Everett, G. C., & Blair, A. (1993). Pesticide exposures and multiple myeloma in Iowa men. *Cancer Causes & Control, 4*(2), 153–156.

Brown, L. M., Everett, G. C., Burmeister, L. F., & Blair, A. (1992). Hair dye use and multiple myeloma in white men. *American Journal of Public Health, 82*(12), 1673–1674.

Bubley, G. J., & Schnipper, L. E. (1991). Multiple myeloma. In A. I. Holleb (Ed.), *American Cancer Society textbook of clinical oncology* (pp. 397–409). Atlanta, GA: American Cancer Society.

Cherng, N. C., Asal, N. R., Kuebler, J. P., Lee, E. T., & Solanki, D. (1991). Prognostic factors in multiple myeloma. *Cancer 67*(12), 3150–3156.

Doody, M. M., Linet, M. S., Glass, A. G., Friedman, G. D., Pottern, L. M., Boice, J. D., Jr., & Fraumeni, J. F., Jr.

(1992). Leukemia, lymphoma, and multiple myeloma following selected medical conditions. *Cancer Causes & Control, 3*(5), 449–456.

Durie, B. G. M., Russell, D. H., & Salmon, S. E. (1980). Reappraisal of plateau phase in myeloma. *Lancet, 2*(8185), 65–68.

Durie, B. G. M., & Salmon, S. E. (1975). A clinical staging system for multiple myeloma: Correlation of measured myeloma cell mass with presenting clinical features, response to treatment and survival. *Cancer, 36*(3), 842–854.

Eriksson, M., & Karlsson, M. (1992). Occupational and other environmental factors and multiple myeloma: a population based case-control study. *British Journal of Industrial Medicine, 49*(2), 95–103.

Fattori, E., Della Rocca, C. I., Dosta, P., Giorgio, M., Dente, B., Pozzi, L., & Ciliberto, G. (1994). Development of progressive kidney damage and myeloma kidney in interleukin-6 transgenic mice. *Blood, 83*(9), 2570–2579.

Glenner, G. G. (1980). Amyloid deposits and amyloidosis: The B-fibrilloses (Part 1). *New England Journal of Medicine 302*(23), 1283–1292.

Gramenzi, A., Buttino, I., D'Avanzo, B., Negri, E., Franceschi, S., & La Vecchia, C. (1991). Medical history and the risk of multiple myeloma [Abstract]. *British Journal of Cancer, 63*(5), 769–772.

Hamblin, T. J. (1986). The kidney in myeloma [Editorial]. *British Medical Journal of Clinical Research, 292*(6512), 2–3.

Heineman, E. F., Olsen, J. H., Pottern, L. M., Gomez, M., Raffn, E., & Blair, A. (1992). Occupational risk factors for multiple myeloma among Danish men. *Cancer Causes & Control, 3*(6), 555–568.

Jacobson, D. R., & Zolla-Pazner, S. (1986). Immunosuppression and infection in multiple myeloma. *Seminars in Oncology, 13*(3), 282–290.

Kyle, R. A. (1983). Long-term survival in multiple myeloma. *New England Journal of Medicine, 308*(6), 314–316.

Kyle, R. A. (1990). Multiple myeloma: An update on diagnosis and management [Review abstract]. *Acta Oncologica, 29*(1), 1–8.

Kyle, R. A. (1993). Newer approaches to the management of multiple myeloma. *Cancer, 72*(Suppl. 11), 3489–3494.

Lichtenstein, A., Berenson, J., Norman, D., Chang, M. P., & Carlilr, A. (1989). Production of cytokines by bone marrow cells obtained from patients with multiple myeloma. *Blood, 74*(4), 1266–1273.

McCaffrey, M., & Beebe, A. (1989). *Pain: clinical manual for nursing practice*. St. Louis, MO: The C. V. Mosby Co.

McGrath, M. A., & Penny, R. (1976). Paraproteinemia: blood hyperviscosity and clinical manifestations. *Journal of Clinical Investigation 58*(5), 1155–1162.

McIntyre, O. R. (1985). Myeloma. In P. Calabresi, P. Schein, & S. A. Rosenberg (Eds.), *Medical oncology: Basic principles and clinical management of cancer*. New York: MacMillan.

Mundy, G. R., & Bertolini, D. R. (1986). Bone destruction and hypercalcemia in plasma cell myeloma. *Seminars in Oncology 13*(3), 291–299.

Niesvizky, R., Siegel, D., & Michaeli, J. (1993). Biology and treatment of multiple myeloma. *Blood Reviews, 7*(1), 24–33.

Oken, M. M. (1984). Multiple myeloma. *Medical Clinics of North America, 68*(3), 757–787.

Oken, M. M. (1994). Standard treatment of multiple myeloma [Review abstract]. *Mayo Clinic Proceedings, 69*(8), 781–786.

Paglieroni, T., Caggiano, V., & MacKenzie, M. (1992). Abnormalities in immune regulation precede the development of multiple myeloma. *American Journal of Hematology, 40*(1), 51–55.

Paice, J. A. (1991). Unraveling the mystery of pain. *Oncology Nursing Forum, 18*(5), 843–849.

Pilarski, L. M., Mant, M. J., Ruether, B. A., & Belch, A. (1984). Severe deficiency of B lymphocytes in peripheral blood from multiple myeloma patients. *Journal of Clinical Investigation, 74*(4), 1301–1306.

Pilarski, L. M., Ruether, B. A., & Mant, M. J. (1985). Abnormal function of B lymphocytes from peripheral blood of multiple myeloma patients: lack of correlation between the number of cells potentially able to secrete immunoglobulin M and serum immunoglobulin M levels. *Journal of Clinical Investigation, 75*(6), 2024–2029.

Riedel, D. A., & Pottern, L. M. (1992). The epidemiology of multiple myeloma [Review]. *Hematology—Oncology Clinics of North America, 6*(2), 225–247.

Roth, M. S., & Foon, K. A. (1987). Biotherapy with interferon in hematologic malignancies. *Oncology Nursing Forum, 14*(Suppl. 6), 16–22.

Rubenstein, E., & Federman, D. D. (Eds.). (1990). Plasma cell myeloma and related serum protein disorders. In *Scientific American Medicine*. New York: Scientific American.

Salmon, S. E. (1973). Immunoglobulin synthesis and tumor kinetics of multiple myeloma. *Seminars in Hematology, 10*(2), 135–144.

Salmon, S. E., & Cassady, J. R. (1993). Plasma cell neoplasms. In V. T. DeVita, S. Hellman, & S. A. Rosenberg (Eds.), *Cancer: Principles and practice* (4th ed., pp. 1984–2016). Philadelphia: J. B. Lippincott.

Salmon, S. E., Dalton, W. S., Grogan, T. M., Plezia, P., Lehnert, M., Roe, D. J., & Miller, T. P. (1991). Multidrug-resistant myeloma: Laboratory and clinical effects of verapamil as a chemosensitizer. *Blood, 78*(1), 44–50.

Samson, D., Gaminara, E., Newland, A., Van de Pette, J., Kearney, J., McCarthy, D., Joyner, M., Aston, L., Mitchell, T., Hamon, M., Barrett, A., & Evans, M. (1989). Infusion of vincristine and doxorubicin with oral dexamethasone as first-line therapy for multiple myeloma. *Lancet, 2*(8668), 882–885.

Sheridan, C. A. (1993). Multiple myeloma. In S. L. Groenwald (Ed.), *Cancer nursing principles and practice* (3rd ed., pp. 1229–1237). Boston: Jones and Bartlett.

Simonsson, B., Kallander, C. F. R., Brenning, G., Killander, A., Gronowitz, J. S., & Bergstrom, R. (1988). Biochemical markers in multiple myeloma: a multivariate analysis. *British Journal of Haematology, 69*(3), 47–53.

Somer, T. (1987). Rheology of paraproteinaemias and the plasma hyperviscosity syndrome [Abstract]. *Baillieres Clinical Haematology, 1*(3), 695–723.

Stevenson, F. K., Bell, A. J., Cusack, R., Hamblin, T. J., Slade, C. J., Spellerberg, M. B., & Stevenson, G. T. (1991). Preliminary studies for an immunotherapeutic approach to the treatment of human myeloma using chimeric anti-CD38 antibody. *Blood, 77*(5), 1071–1079.

Tribalto, M., Papa, G., Coppetelli, U., Adorno, G., Caravita, T., Dentamaro, T., Rainone, A., Avvisati, G., La Verde, G., Leone, G., et al. (1993). Treatment of multiple myeloma with autologous blood stem cell transplantation: Preliminary results of an Italian multicentric pilot study [Abstract]. *International Journal of Artificial Organs, 16*(Suppl. 5), 51–56.

Urabe, A. (1994). Interferons for the treatment of hematological malignancies [Review]. *Oncology, 51*(2), 137–141.

Unknown Primary Malignancies

Mary E. Cooley

UNKNOWN PRIMARY MALIGNANCIES

The past decade has brought about major changes in the diagnosis and treatment of unknown primary malignancies (UKPM). Until recently, little evidence has occurred to suggest that aggressive treatment is beneficial in this population. Thus the primary focus has been to provide supportive care. Recent studies, however, suggest that up to 40 per cent of patients have highly responsive malignancies, and effective local and systemic treatments are now possible (Hainsworth & Greco, 1993b). For nurses to provide optimal care, up-to-date knowledge about the diagnosis and treatment of UKPM is essential. This chapter provides an overview of UKPM, discusses medical aspects of care, and identifies subsets of patients who have a favorable prognosis. The unique aspects of providing care to this population will be highlighted.

INCIDENCE AND DEFINITION

A UKPM is defined as a biopsy-proven malignancy whose origin remains unknown despite a complete history, physical examination, basic laboratory studies, stool for occult blood, chest radiograph, and appropriate imaging studies (Sporn & Greenberg, 1990).

UKPM are the eighth most common form of malignancies and account for approximately 5 to 10 per cent of all cancers (Greco & Hainsworth, 1993). Recorded incidence of UKPM may be underestimated. Often times, the UKPM may be recorded in tumor registry and epidemiologic data as a known primary site based on inconclusive information or the best clinical guess (Steckel & Kagan, 1991).

EPIDEMIOLOGY

The typical age of onset for UKPM is between 40 to 80 years with a median of 60 years (Diggs, 1989). Although there is near equal distribution between the sexes, there is a slight increase in the incidence in men (Gaber et al, 1983).

Individuals often present with widespread metastasis and the primary site of malignancy is rarely identified. A study by Nystrom et al. (1977) clearly illustrates the difficulty of finding a primary site of malignancy. Two hundred sixty-four patients with UKPM in their study underwent extensive radiologic workup. Only 30 patients had primary cancer sites identified prior to death. Furthermore, 130 patients underwent necropsy, and a primary cancer site was identified in only 22 patients. Pancreas, lung, and gastrointestinal (liver, colon, and gastric) were the primary sites most frequently identified.

BIOLOGIC CHARACTERISTICS

Although UKPM appear to be a heterogeneous group with many different primary tumor sites, they share several common biologic characteristics: (1) they usually present with rapid and widespread metastasis when compared with known primary malignancy sites; (2) the pattern of metastasis in UKPM tends to be atypical and cannot be used to predict the source of the primary malignancy; and (3) less common malignancies compose a disproportionate share of UKPM. For example, the incidence of pancreatic carcinoma in the general population is 2 per cent, whereas in UKPM it has been identified in 20 per cent of patients (Hainsworth & Greco, 1993a; Nystrom et al., 1977).

Authors have postulated reasons for the inability to locate the primary malignancy in UKPM. These reasons include: (1) spontaneous regression of the malignancy; (2) destruction of the primary site by the immune system but an inability to contain the metastasis; (3) surgical excision of the primary site; (4) nondetection because the primary site is small; and (5) obscured primary site because of extensive metastasis or an atypical pattern of metastasis (Holmes & Fouts, 1970; Perchalski, Hall, & DeWar, 1992).

NATURAL HISTORY

The natural history of UKPM is dismal. Despite the fact that most individuals seek care within 12 weeks of the initial signs and symptoms of the disease, most present with widespread metastasis and poor performance status (Leonard & Nystrom, 1993). The overall prognosis is grim with an expected survival of 2 to 9 months. The 5-year survival rate is reported to be 3.5 per cent (Greco & Hainsworth, 1992; Gunthrie, 1989).

Although the majority of patients do not benefit from cancer-directed treatment, advances in the last decade have identified subsets of patients who may benefit from palliative therapy and a few who are candidates for potentially curative therapy (see Table 42–1). Careful evaluation is essential to identify this group of individuals (Hainsworth & Greco, 1993b).

MEDICAL ASPECTS OF CARE

PRESENTING SIGNS AND SYMPTOMS

Unfortunately, there are no early signs or symptoms for UKPM. Typically, patients present with metastatic disease, and the signs and symptoms vary according to the presenting site of disease. The most common presenting sites are lymph nodes, liver, bone, lung, and brain (Nystrom et al., 1977). Constitutional symptoms are common at diagnosis and include anorexia, weight loss, and fatigue (Hainsworth & Greco, 1993b).

DIAGNOSTIC EVALUATION

The diagnostic evaluation is guided by two major goals. The first goal is to identify patients who may benefit from effective local or systemic therapy. The second goal is to identify local complications, such as bowel obstruction, that may benefit from palliative treatment (Gaber et al, 1983).

The first step in the diagnostic workup is to perform a complete history, physical examination, basic laboratory, and radiographic studies. The history should include prior tobacco and alcohol use, occupational exposure, family history of cancer, and any prior tumor removal such as warts, moles, or polyps (Diggs, 1989; Leonard & Nystrom, 1993). A thorough review of systems is useful in identifying constitutional symptoms and their severity along with any additional diagnostic clues. The physical examination includes the integument, thyroid, mucus membranes, breasts, testicles, pelvis, prostate, and rectum. Basic laboratory tests include complete blood count, chemistry panel, liver function tests, creatinine, urinalysis, and guaiac stool for occult blood. Routine radiographic studies include a chest radiograph and an abdominal computed tomography (CT) scan (Leonard & Nystrom, 1993; McMillan, Levine, & Stephens, 1982). Further diagnostic studies may be ordered based on information from the history and physical examination. Specific clinical presentations may warrant further studies (see Table 42–1). For the vast majority of patients, however, given the absence of specific abnormalities, an exhaustive search for the primary site of malignancy is not indicated (Gaber et al, 1983; Nystrom, Weiner, Meshnik-Wolfe, Bateman, & Viola, 1979).

The second step in conducting the diagnostic evaluation is to acquire tissue for pathologic examination. Histologic definition of the UKPM plays a major role in determining further diagnostic studies and subsequent treatment. For example, identification of an adenocarcinoma in an elderly man with skeletal metastasis provides evidence to suspect prostate cancer. Thus, prostate-specific antigen stain of the biopsy tissue is recommended. Appropriate acquisition and processing of the biopsy specimen are essential (Mackay & Ordonez, 1993). Biopsy of the most accessible lesion is recommended. Although fine needle aspiration can be done, open biopsy is preferable. The latter method provides a larger specimen and enables the pathologist to better evaluate histologic features and provide more material for special studies that may be required (Hainsworth & Greco, 1993b).

Four methods are used to examine the tissue obtained from UKPM: light microscopy, immunoperoxidase staining, electron microscopy, and genetic analysis.

Light microscopy is used to examine the biopsy tissue and identifies one of four histologies: poorly differentiated malignant neoplasm (PDMN), poorly differentiated carcinoma (PDC), adenocarcinoma (AC), or squamous cell carcinoma (SCC) (Greco & Hainsworth, 1993). This method of examination is readily accessible and is inexpensive. It is the preferred method of obtaining the initial histologic diagnosis, but there are limitations to its use. Light microscopy does not provide a specific diagnosis in the case of PDMN and PDC (Hainsworth & Greco, 1993b; Mackay & Ordonez, 1993). Since these diagnoses may include treatment-responsive malignancies, it is important to pursue further pathologic studies.

Immunoperoxidase staining is a method of pathologic examination that has developed over the last decade and has improved the care of patients with UKPM. This technique is often used to identify lymphoma, melanoma, sarcoma and specific carcinomas (see Table 42–2) (Hainsworth & Greco, 1993b; Mackay & Ordonez, 1993). Monoclonal or polyclonal antibodies directed at specific cell components or products such as enzymes, normal tissue components, hormones, and hormone receptors and oncofetal antigens are used to help classify neoplasms that cannot be identified by using light microscopy alone. Although widely available, immunoperoxidase staining carries certain limitations. Since the reagents used are not tumor-specific, definitive

TABLE 42–1. *Carcinoma of Unknown Primary Site—Recommended Evaluation and Therapy of Subsets*

HISTOPATHOLOGY	CLINICAL EVALUATION	SPECIAL PATHOLOGIC STUDIES	SUBSETS WITH RESPONSIVE TUMORS	THERAPY	PROGNOSIS
Adenocarcinoma (well differentiated or moderately differentiated)	CT scan of abdomen Men: serum PSA Women: mammograms Additional studies to evaluate signs, symptoms	Men: PSA stain Women: ER, PR	1. Women, axillary node metastasis 2. Women, peritoneal carcinomatosis 3. Men, blastic bone metastases or high serum PSA or (+) tumor PSA staining	Treat as primary breast cancer Surgical cytoreduction + chemotherapy effective in ovarian cancer Hormonal therapy for prostate cancer	Poor for entire group (median survival = 4 months) Better for special therapeutic subgroups
Poorly differentiated carcinoma, poorly differentiated adenocarcinoma	CT abdomen, chest Serum HCG, AFP Additional studies to evaluate signs, symptoms	Immunoperoxidase staining Electron microscopy	1. Neuroendocrine tumors 2. Tumor location in mediastinum, retroperitoneum, lymph nodes	Cisplatin-based therapy Cisplatin/etoposide ± bleomycin	High response rate 10% to 20% cured with therapy
Squamous carcinoma	Cervical presentation: direct laryngoscopy, nasopharyngoscopy, fiberoptic bronchoscopy Inguinal presentation: pelvic, rectal examinations, anoscopy		1. Cervical adenopathy (high or midcervical) 2. Inguinal adenopathy	Neck dissection and/or radiation therapy Inguinal dissection and/or radiation therapy	5-year survival rate of 25% to 50% Potential long-term survival

CT = Computed tomography; *ER* = Estrogen receptor; *HCG* = Human chorionic gonadotropin; *PSA* = Prostate-specific antigen; *PR* = Progesterone receptor; *AFP* = Alpha/fetoprotein.
(From Greco, F., & Hainsworth, J. [1992]. Tumors of unknown origin. *Cancer, 42,* 96–115. Reprinted with permission.)

diagnosis cannot be made on the basis of immunoperoxidase staining alone; the pathologist must correlate the histologic appearance from light microscopy with the immunoperoxidase staining. This requires considerable technical expertise to accurately interpret the results and may lead to variation of interpretation between pathologists (Hainsworth & Greco, 1993b).

Electron microscopy is a useful technique to help define tumor lineage when light microscopy and immunoperoxidase staining fail to provide a definite diagnosis. Identification of specific ultrastructural features of poorly differentiated neoplasms help to distinguish lymphoma from carcinoma and to detect sarcomas, neuroendocrine neoplasms, adenocarcinoma, and squamous cell carcinoma. There are limitations associated with the use of electron microscopy. It requires a special tissue fixation technique, it is relatively expensive, and it is not readily available (Greco & Hainsworth, 1993).

Genetic analysis is a technique with broadened clinical applicability. Although chromosomal abnormalities have been best studied in hematopoietic neoplasms, recent evidence suggests chromosomal abnormalities have a role in nonlymphoid tissues. Genetic analysis can reliably distinguish lymphomas from carcinomas if other studies fail to provide a definite diagnosis (Arnold et al., 1983). In addition, chromosome rearrangements associated with peripheral neuroepitheliomas, Ewing's sarcoma, and testicular and extragonadal germ cell neoplasms can be identified (Mukherjee et al., 1991; Turc-Carel, Philip, Berger, Philip, & Lenoir, 1983; Whang-Peng et al., 1984). A study by Motzer et al. (1991) identified the clinical utility of genetic analysis as a diagnostic tool that helped to predict response to antineoplastic therapy in midline UKPM (see Box 42–1). It is possible that genetic analysis techniques will have greater applications in the future (Ilson, Motzer, Rodriquez, Chaganti, & Bosh, 1993).

TABLE 42–2. *Immunoperoxidase Staining for the Differential Diagnosis of Poorly Differential Tumors*

TUMOR	COMPONENT DETECTABLE BY IMMUNOSTAINING
Lymphoma	Leukocyte common antigen
Carcinoma	Cytokeratin
Specific carcinomas	
Prostate carcinoma	Prostate-specific antigen
Follicular thyroid carcinoma	Thyroglobulin
Medullary thyroid carcinoma	Calcitonin
Neuroendocrine carcinoma	Neuron-specific enolase, chromogranin
Germ cell tumors	Chorionic gonadotropin, α-fetoprotein
Melanoma	5-100 protein, HMB-45 antigen, vimention
Specific sarcomas	
Rhabdomyosarcoma	Desmin
Angiosarcoma	Factor VIII antigen

(From Hainsworth, J., & Greco, F. [1993b]. Treatment of patients with cancer of an unknown primary site. *New England Journal of Medicine, 329,* 257–263. Reprinted by permission of the *New England Journal of Medicine.*)

HISTOLOGIC SUBGROUPS OF UNKNOWN PRIMARY MALIGNANCIES

Rapid identification of favorable prognostic groups and histology are key to successful treatment of UKPM. There are four major histologies in UKPM occurring in varying frequencies: adenocarcinoma (AC), poorly differentiated carcinoma (PDC), poorly differentiated malignant neoplasm (PDMN), and squamous cell carcinoma (SCC) (see Table 42–3).

ADENOCARCINOMA

AC is the most common histology identified in UKPM. Patients are typically elderly, present with metastasis at various sites, and often have poor performance status at time of diagnosis. The clinical course of disease is dominated by symptoms related to the sites of metastasis. The most common sites for metastasis are lung, liver, and bone (Greco & Hainsworth, 1993). The primary site of malignancy is rarely identified (Nystrom et al., 1977). Overall, patients have a poor prognosis. However, clinical subsets of patients with a more favorable prognosis have been identified and include women with peritoneal carcinomatosis, women with axillary lymph node metastasis, and men with skeletal metastasis.

Light microscopy is used to identify AC. Immunoperoxidase staining may be useful in identifying subsets of patients with either breast or prostate cancer. Mammograms in women and serum prostate-specific antigen in men are additional studies that are recommended in this population (Greco & Hainsworth, 1993).

The treatment of AC in UKPM differs according to the clinical presentation. Although the majority of pa-

tients are not candidates for aggressive therapy, the identification of several favorable prognostic groups has created the option for palliative treatment and even potentially curative treatment in some individuals (Muggia & Baranda, 1993; Sporn & Greenberg, 1993). The clinical management of the various subsets of patients differ, and, therefore, therapeutic considerations will be discussed separately.

Peritoneal Carcinomatosis. Peritoneal carcinomatosis is a favorable prognostic group within AC that has been identified in elderly women. The median age at presentation is 60 years. Typical presenting signs and symptoms are abdominal pain and distention, pelvic mass, and ascites. Some patients may have pleural effusions, liver metastasis, or lymphadenopathy (Strnad et al., 1989). Anecdotal reports first identified this entity as a distinct group that responded favorably to treatment for ovarian cancer in the 1980s (Chen & Flam, 1986). Since that time, larger studies have confirmed substantial responses. Strnad et al. (1989) performed a retrospective analysis of 18 patients to define the clinical features and results of systemic treatment for women with peritoneal carcinomatosis. Patients were treated with standard regimens for advanced ovarian cancer. All patients had a surgical laparotomy and debulking procedure. Of these patients, 16 received cisplatin-based chemotherapy. Results demonstrated a median survival of 23 months. Five patients had complete responses, and three patients remained disease-free up to 77 months after diagnosis. Given these promising results, current recommendations are to treat these women as if they had advanced ovarian cancer. Aggressive surgical cytoreduction followed by cisplatin-based combination chemotherapy is the suggested treatment (Greco & Hainsworth, 1993).

Axillary Lymph Node Metastasis in Women. Although axillary lymph node metastasis can represent a wide spectrum of diagnostic possibilities, biopsy-proven AC in women is most likely an occult breast cancer. Axillary lymph node metastasis as a presenting site for breast cancer is a well-documented entity. As early as 1907 this phenomena was described by Halsed (Halsed, 1907). The presenting signs and symptoms are a painless axillary mass and, in some cases, discharge from the nipples. In one series, 60 per cent of women had no evidence of a breast mass on physical examination of the breast (Ashikari, Rosen, Urban, & Senoo, 1976). Similarly, another study identified that mammograms detected a breast primary in only 47 per cent of patients (Patel, Nemoto, Rosner, Dao, & Pickren, 1981). All of the women in this series presented with an axillary lymph node as the single source of metastasis and had a mastectomy as the primary treatment. Subsequently, 44 per cent of the patients who had a negative mammogram prior to surgery were found to have a breast primary upon pathologic examination. The majority of these primaries were of microscopic size. Hence, it is important to recognize while mammograms, if positive or suspicious, may lead to a primary tumor in some patients, when negative, a breast primary cannot be excluded as the source of malignancy.

Box 42–1. *Genetic Analysis as an Aide in Diagnosis of Midline Carcinomas of Unknown Origin*

Motzer, R., Rodriquez, E., Reuter, V., Samaniege, F., Dmitrovsky, E., Bajorin, D., Pfister, D., Parsa, R., Chaganti, S., & Bosl, G. (1991). Genetic analysis as an aide in diagnosis for patients with midline carcinoma of uncertain histologies. *Journal of National Cancer Institute, 83,* 341–346.

Purpose: Establish the utility of genetic analysis as an aide in the histologic diagnosis of midline carcinomas of uncertain histology.

Sample: Biopsy tissue from nine patients with carcinomas of uncertain histology were evaluated for genetic abnormalities associated with malignancy. Of these patients, eight had poorly differentiated carcinoma involving primarily midline structures, and one had a diagnosis of seminoma with atypical clinical features.

Methods:
- All patients were evaluated and treated at Memorial Sloan-Kettering Cancer Center. Seven patients were chosen in a retrospective manner. Two patients were treated in an ongoing prospective trial for patients with midline carcinoma of uncertain histology.
- Cytogenetic and southern blot analyses were done on biopsy tissue. The same biopsy tissue that was used for light microscopy, immunoperoxidase staining, and electron microscopy to make the diagnosis of carcinoma of uncertain histology was used for the genetic analysis.

Results:
- Six of eight patients had diagnoses established with the use of genetic analysis.
- Four of eight patients with poorly differentiated carcinoma had abnormalities of chromosome 12 consistent with the diagnosis of germ cell tumor.
- Three of the four patients with a diagnosis of germ cell tumor established by genetic analysis obtained a complete response to cisplatin-based chemotherapy.
- One patient was diagnosed with neuroepithelioma.
- The one patient with seminoma and atypical clinical features was diagnosed with Non-Hodgkin's lymphoma.

Conclusions:
- Genetic analysis proved to be a useful diagnostic tool in patients with midline carcinomas of unknown histology.
- Results suggest a relationship between specific genetic changes and the action of antineoplastic agents.

Because there are few instances of symptoms and signs that suggest breast cancer such as a palpable breast mass, nipple retraction, or a positive mammogram, the histologic diagnosis is a critical factor in deciding about future treatment. It is absolutely essential that provisions are made to perform estrogen and progesterone receptor testing on all axillary node tissue. Elevated receptor levels suggest the presence of breast cancer. Immunoperoxidase staining and electron microscopy should be available in the event of poorly differentiated tissue. Mammograms are recommended in all women who present with an axillary lymph node metastases identified to be an AC. Other diagnostic testing such as bone scans and computed tomography scans are ordered based upon the presence of symptoms. An extensive diagnostic workup to identify a primary site is not recommended (Patel et al., 1981).

TABLE 42–3. *Frequency of Various Histologies in UKPM*

HISTOLOGY	FREQUENCY
Adenocarcinoma	60%
Poorly differentiated carcinoma/poorly differentiated adenocarcinoma	30%
Poorly differentiated malignant neoplasm	5%
Squamous cell carcinoma	5%

(Data from Hainsworth, J., & Greco, F. [1993b]. Treatment of patients with cancer of an unknown primary site. *New England Journal of Medicine, 329,* 257–263.)

Once the diagnosis of AC is confirmed, modified radical mastectomy is recommended because women with the axillary node as the single site of metastasis are believed to have stage II breast cancer. Curative therapy is thus possible. Although data documenting the efficacy of systemic chemotherapy is lacking for this population, Hainsworth and Greco (1993b) suggest the addition of systemic chemotherapy or hormonal therapy. The 5-year survival rate is 79 per cent (Greco & Hainsworth, 1993). Women who have metastatic sites in addition to the axillary lymph node may also have breast cancer. Palliative therapy for metastatic breast cancer is recommended (Greco & Hainsworth, 1993).

Skeletal Metastasis in Men. Elderly men who present with metastatic AC may have prostate cancer. Osteoblastic bone metastasis and pelvic adenopathy are the most common clinical presentations. Atypical patterns of metastasis can occur and include lung, mediastinal adenopathy, and/or upper abdominal lymphadenopathy (Greco & Hainsworth, 1993).

Diagnostic tests to confirm prostate cancer include serum prostate-specific antigen and immunoperoxidase staining of the biopsy material. Effective palliative therapy is available for advanced prostate cancer. Hormonal treatment can provide remissions in 70 per cent of patients. The duration of this response varies from several months to several years (Kozlowski, Ellis, & Grayhack, 1991).

Empiric Chemotherapy for Adenocarcinoma UKPM. Most patients who present with AC UKPM do not fall into one of the three favorable prognostic categories. In these situations empiric chemotherapy may be considered for selected individuals. Candidates may be considered for treatment if a good performance status is present. Those who are symptomatic from the sites of metastasis may also be considered. Response rates for these individuals have not been promising. 5-Fluorouracil (5-FU) is the only drug that has been adequately studied as a single agent. Response rates range from 0 to 16 per cent with a median survival of 3.5 months (Sporn & Greenberg, 1990). Combination treatment with 5-FU, doxorubicin, and mitomycin (FAM) is another commonly studied regimen. Reported response rates range from 7 to 37 per cent with median survival 5 to 15 months (Sporn & Greenberg, 1993).

In light of the modest response rates, short median survival times, and the lack of long-term survivors, supportive therapy alone may be a reasonable option for patients. A discussion that focuses on the risks versus benefits of therapy and special consideration toward quality of life is warranted.

POORLY DIFFERENTIATED CARCINOMA/ POORLY DIFFERENTIATED ADENOCARCINOMA

Poorly differentiated carcinoma of unknown primary site accounts for 20 per cent of UKPM. An additional 10 per cent of patients have poorly differentiated adenocarcinoma (Hainsworth & Greco, 1993b). Evidence accumulated during the last 15 years reveals that these UKPM histologies are similar and often respond to treatment with chemotherapy. Recent studies have elucidated the presence of subsets within this category that are highly responsive to treatment and include extragonadal germ cell and neuroendocrine malignancies (Hainsworth, Johnson, & Greco, 1992; Hainsworth, Johnson, & Greco, 1988). These patients usually present with rapid progression of symptoms and have objective evidence of rapid tumor growth. The most common sites of involvement are the mediastinum, retroperitoneum, and peripheral lymph nodes. The median age at presentation is between 40 and 50 years. Clinical characteristics that predict response to treatment have been identified and include: (1) the presence of retroperitoneum or peripheral lymph nodes as the predominant site of tumor location ($p = 0.001$); (2) one or two sites of metastasis ($p = 0.001$); and (3) no smoking history ($p = 0.025$) (Hainsworth et al., 1992).

Recent advances in pathologic diagnostic techniques have played a major role in advancing knowledge about PDC. Light microscopy techniques classify the histology but cannot provide a more specific diagnosis. Hainsworth, Wright, Johnson, Davis, and Greco (1991) evaluated the clinical utility of immunoperoxidase staining in the tissue obtained from 87 patients. Results indicated that immunoperoxidase staining confirmed the diagnosis of PDC in 56 per cent of patients, identified the presence of melanoma (9 per cent), lymphoma (5 per cent), prostate (1 per cent), and yolk sac (1 per cent) carcinoma, and identified a group of patients who may benefit from electron microscopy studies. Electron microscopy was found to identify the presence of neurosecretory granules in 10 per cent of patients, thus confirming a neuroendocrine-type UKPM. Genetic analysis has been found to be useful in

identifying germ cell tumors and in predicting response to antineoplastic therapy (see Box 42–1) (Motzer et al., 1991). Additional diagnostic studies are recommended in this population and include a CT scan of the chest and abdomen and serum testing for HCG and AFP. The elevation of these tumor markers suggests the presence of extragonadal germ cell tumor (Greco & Hainsworth, 1993).

Advances in treatment for PDC have also occurred. Hainsworth et al. (1992) reviewed the results of their 12-year experience in treating patients with PDC and PDA (see Box 42–2). Two-hundred twenty patients were treated with cisplatin-based combination therapy. Overall, 63 per cent of patients had objective responses to therapy, 26 per cent had a complete response, and 36 per cent had a partial response. The median survival for the entire group was 12 months, with an actuarial 12-year survival rate of 16 per cent. Given the high response rate to treatment, current recommendations suggest that patients with PDC and PDA should receive a trial of combination therapy, the majority of which was cisplatin-based. Patients should receive at least two cycles of chemotherapy, and then tumor response should be ascertained. If treatment response occurs, a total of four cycles of chemotherapy should be administered. There is no evidence that more than four cycles provide added benefit (Greco & Hainsworth, 1993).

Atypical germ cell and neuroendocrine neoplasms have been identified as two highly responsive subsets within PDC and PDA. Early anecdotal reports suggested that extragonadal germ cell cancer syndrome, a type of atypical germ cell neoplasm, was a highly treatable, poorly differentiated malignancy that occurred predominantly in young men with mediastinal tumors (Richardson et al., 1981). Since that time, studies have confirmed high response rates to chemotherapy. Hainsworth et al. (1992) analyzed a group of 34 men with clinical features highly suggestive of extragondal germ cell tumors for response to cisplatin-based combination chemotherapy and long-term survival. Results revealed 85 per cent responded to treatment, with 50 per cent having a complete response. Twenty-nine per cent of patients remained disease-free 12 years after completion of treatment.

Hainsworth et al. (1988) described 29 patients with neuroendocrine tumors of unknown origin and evaluated their response to treatment with either combination chemotherapy or local treatment modalities for those patients with tumor at only one site.

Twenty-five of 29 patients received combination chemotherapy. The majority of these patients received cisplatin-based chemotherapy. Twenty-three of the patients were evaluable. There was an overall response rate of 78 per cent (N = 18); six patients obtained a complete response, an additional 12 patients had a partial response, and five patients had no response to treatment. Ten per cent of the patients remained disease-free for more than 24 months after completing therapy. Four patients had local treatment (surgery or radiation therapy). All four patients are alive and free of disease up to 12 months after completion of therapy.

Box 42–2. *Cisplatin Based Combination Chemotherapy Treatment*

Hainsworth, J., Johnson, D., & Greco, F. (1992). Cisplatin based combination chemotherapy in the treatment of poorly differentiated carcinoma and poorly differentiated adenocarcinoma of unknown primary site: Results of a 12 year experience. *Journal of Clinical Oncology, 10,* 912–922.

Purpose:
1. Identify clinical characteristics of patients with PDC/PDA.
2. Evaluate patients with PDC/PDA response to treatment with cisplatin-based chemotherapy.
3. Identify factors that affect prognosis in PDC/PDA.
Sample: All patients (220) with the histologic diagnosis of PDC or PDA of UKPM evaluated at Vanderbilt Medical Center between February 1978 and December 1989.
Methods: All patients had history and physical examination, routine laboratory tests, CXRs, HCG, and AFP pretreatment. Further studies were done as clinically indicated. All patients were treated with cisplatin-based chemotherapy. Patients received two courses of treatment at 3-week intervals and then were evaluated for response. Patients who demonstrated evidence of response to chemotherapy treatment completed four cycles. If patients did not have objective response to two cycles of chemotherapy, they were removed from treatment.
Results:
1. Clinical characteristics of the group included median age 39 years, men outnumbered women 3 to 1, and 74 per cent had metastasis in two or more sites.
2. Treatment results: 63 per cent of the group had objective response; 26 per cent had complete response; 36 per cent had partial response; 16 per cent are disease-free at a median of 61 months after treatment. Actuarial 10-year survival is 16 per cent.
3. Favorable prognostic factors: Predominant tumor location in the retroperitoneum or peripheral lymph nodes; tumor limited to one or two sites of metastasis; no prior cigarette use; younger age.
Conclusions: Potentially curative therapy is available for patients with PDC/PDA. Patients should receive a trial of cisplatin-based chemotherapy.

POORLY DIFFERENTIATED MALIGNANT NEOPLASMS

The diagnosis of PDMN is made by the pathologist when light microscopy techniques are unable to distinguish a more specific category of neoplasm. Clinically, these patients often have rapidly growing masses. Lymphadenopathy is common, but other sites such as gastrointestinal, sinuses, bone, and skin may be involved. Constitutional symptoms may include fever, weight loss, and night sweats. Laboratory tests often reveal anemia, hyperuricemia, and elevated LDH (Gunthrie, 1989).

A more precise diagnosis is important in this population since many have neoplasms that are highly responsive to treatment. Immunoperoxidase staining, electron microscopy, and genetic analysis are pathologic studies that are particularly helpful in narrowing the diagnoses. Immunoperoxidase staining can help answer several important questions. First and most important, common leukocyte antigen stain can differentiate lymphoma from carcinoma (Warnke et al., 1983). Other staining techniques can suggest melanoma, sarcoma, germ cell, neuroendocrine, or prostate cancer (see Table 42–2). If immunoperoxidase staining is inconclusive, electron microscopy or genetic analysis can be used to further identify the tumor lineage.

Non-Hodgkins lymphoma (NHL) has been identified through immunoperoxidase staining techniques to be the most common malignancy in PDMN (Gatter et al., 1984; Horning, Carrier, Rouse, Warnke, & Michie, 1989). These tumors are potentially curable with combination chemotherapy. Horning et al. (1989) evaluated the response of 35 PDMN patients who presented with histologically unclassified neoplasms that expressed common leukocyte antigen upon immunoperoxidase staining and compared their response and survival with those of a concurrent group of 107 patients who presented with a typical histologic NHL. Results of the study demonstrated that response to chemotherapy and overall survival were similar in both groups. In the atypical histologic group, 65 per cent of patients were alive, and of these patients, 45 per cent were free of progressive disease. This study underscores the importance of rapid identification of patients with PDMN who are highly responsive to treatment with combination chemotherapy.

SQUAMOUS CELL CARCINOMA

The incidence of squamous cell carcinoma in UKPM is 5 per cent (Greco & Hainsworth, 1993). The clinical groups included here are cervical and supraclavicular adenopathy and inguinal adenopathy. Effective treatment is available for many of the subsets.

Cervical and Supraclavicular Adenopathy. Squamous cell carcinoma involving the cervical and supraclavicular nodes most often presents in older men. The median age at presentation is 55 years. Risk factors associated with developing this syndrome are excessive tobacco and alcohol use (Greco & Hainsworth, 1992).

Typically, patients present with a solitary, unilateral, and painless mass. The site of the node may give clues as to the origin of the primary site. In general, metastatic nodes that are found in the upper two thirds of the cervical region will originate in the head and neck area. The most common sites of head and neck primaries includes nasopharynx, mid base of tongue, pyriform sinuses, and tonsils. The lower cervical or supraclavicle lymph nodes most often suggest the lung as the primary site of malignancy (Perchalski et al., 1992; deBraud & Al-Sarraf, 1993).

Cytologic diagnosis of squamous cell carcinoma is easily accomplished with fine needle aspiration (FNA). Seventy-six to 96 per cent of patients can be diagnosed in this manner; therefore, open biopsy is reserved for those in whom the FNA is nondiagnostic (deBraud & Al-Sarraf, 1993). Further diagnostic workup is indicated for this population. Patients with upper and mid-cervical nodes should undergo an aggressive evaluation to help identify a head and neck primary. Suggested diagnostic studies include direct laryngoscopy, nasopharyngoscopy, and a magnetic resonance imaging study of the sinuses and neck. In the case of lower cervical or supraclavicular adenopathy, additional workup should exclude the possibility of a lung primary. Suggested studies include CT scan of the chest and bronchoscopy if chest radiograph or CT scan of the chest are abnormal (Greco & Hainsworth, 1993; deBraud & Al-Sarraf, 1993).

Treatment options vary depending on the size and location of the lymph nodes. There are two major prognostic groups for upper and mid-cervical adenopathy: those with N1 disease and those with N2/N3 disease. The overall 5-year survival rates for both groups range from 30 to 50 per cent (Hainsworth & Greco, 1993b). N1 disease has a better prognosis than N2/N3 disease. Local treatment, surgery, radiation therapy, or a combination is recommended for N1 disease. The local recurrence rate is higher in patients who receive surgery alone (20 to 40 per cent) when compared with that of those receiving radiation therapy (5 to 10 per cent). The recommended treatment field in radiation encompasses the nasopharynx, hypopharynx, and oropharynx. Radiation therapy carries significant morbidity, and therefore, an aggressive search for the primary tumor site is recommended before embarking upon empiric treatment (Marcialvega et al., 1990).

Combined modality treatment (surgery and radiation therapy) is recommended for patients with N2/N3 and for those who have unfavorable signs for N1 (multiple nodes, extracapsular invasion, or both) (deBraud & Al-Sarraf, 1993). Because patients with N3 disease generally fare much worse than those with N1 or N2 disease, the addition of chemotherapy has shown promising results in clinical trials (deBraud, Heilburn, & Ahmad, 1989). Further studies are needed to more clearly define the role of chemotherapy in the treatment of N3 disease.

Given that the most likely source of a primary tumor site in lower cervical and supraclavicular adenopathy is lung, these patients tend to do worse than those with upper and mid-cervical adenopathy. If the search for a lung primary is negative, aggressive local therapy (surgery, radiation, or both) is recommended. Long-term survival is possible in those treated with local therapy and ranges between 10 and 15 per cent (Greco & Hainsworth, 1993).

Inguinal Adenopathy. Squamous cell carcinoma of the inguinal nodes is uncommon and most often signals a primary site of malignancy in the genital or anorectal area. Therefore, an extensive diagnostic workup should be done to identify a primary site of malignancy. The workup should include physical examination of the vulva, vagina, and cervix in women and the penis in men. Digital examination and anoscopy should be done in both sexes (Greco & Hainsworth, 1993).

Treatment will vary depending on the identified site of malignancy. Curative therapy is possible for locally advanced genital or anorectal cancers. In the absence of an identified primary site, surgical resection with or without radiation therapy is the recommended treatment. Long-term survival is possible after local therapy and ranges between 30 and 50 per cent (Greco & Hainsworth, 1993).

NURSING ASPECTS OF CARE

UKPM are a diverse group of malignancies. The nursing implications of providing care to this population are broad, and specific interventions must be individualized based on the histologic type of UKPM, options for treatment, and overall goals for care. Symptom management, psychosocial care, and patient education are general categories of care, however, that should be considered for all patients (Yeomans & Washington, 1991).

Symptom management is the cornerstone of providing nursing care to this population. It is appropriate for patients who are receiving supportive care as well as for those who are receiving aggressive therapy. Patients with UKPM often present with a myriad of symptoms that must be managed appropriately to promote quality of life. Pain management is an especially important aspect of care. Other symptoms such as dyspnea, decreased appetite, weight loss, fatigue, nausea, and bowel problems are a few examples of symptoms that may need to be addressed (Billings, 1985; Yeomans & Washington, 1991). In the event of aggressive cisplatin-based combination chemotherapy, adequate control of symptoms is essential for individuals to tolerate potentially curative therapies. Prevention of nausea, interventions to minimize renal impairment, and monitoring of myelosuppression associated with chemotherapy are a few examples of appropriate symptom care (Cooley, Davis, & Abrahm, 1994).

The diagnosis of UKPM carries unique implications for psychosocial care. It is often difficult for patients diagnosed with an unknown primary malignancy to understand that an extensive diagnostic workup may not help uncover the source of the primary tumor site. A common misunderstanding expressed by patients is that finding the primary site may make their tumors more treatable (Yeomans & Washington, 1991). Therefore, patients may request that additional diagnostic studies be done in an attempt to find the primary site of malignancy. In addition, patients may seek care from multiple health care providers in an attempt to establish a primary site of malignancy.

A second unique problem for most patients with UKPM is the advanced nature of their disease at diagnosis. Because the median survival is so short, patients may not have the time needed to make psychosocial adjustments to terminal illness. Therefore, it is essential for health care providers to target specific interventions to assist patients in dealing with the implications of their disease. Open and honest communication is the first step in building a trusting relationship. The physician shares the information, plan, and prognosis. The nurse should be present, if possible, to provide follow-up and reinforce the information provided by the physician. The nurse can help clarify information or help secure additional information from the physician, if needed. Adequate time for ongoing discussion about the disease, treatment, and prognosis are essential in this population, and the nurse should incorporate this into the plan of care.

Common emotional responses to the diagnosis of cancer are denial, anxiety, fear, depression, withdrawal, acceptance, resignation, and anger (Scanlon, 1989). Often times, the emotional response, especially anxiety and fear, may be more pronounced in patients with UKPM. Ongoing assessment of emotional responses can identify individuals who may benefit from further interventions. It is important to recognize that the individual is part of a family system and the family should be included in the assessment and care provided. The use of a multidisciplinary team is especially helpful in managing the complex psychosocial needs of this population. Nurses are in an ideal position to identify unmet needs and to coordinate the health care services (social work, pastoral care, psychologists, community health) that may be needed by patients and their families (Benoliel & McCorkle, 1978; Tornberg, Burns-McGrath, & Benoliel, 1984).

An important aspect of care in UKPM is ascertaining the individual's wishes for advanced directives. A discussion about advanced directives gives patients the opportunity to share their concerns and wishes for life-sustaining treatment in the event of terminal illness and often provides patients with a sense of control. Studies have demonstrated that the majority of patients think about this issue and would like to discuss options for care with their health care providers; however, many are not given this opportunity (Emanuel, Barry, & Stoeckle, 1991; Lo, McLeod, & Saika, 1986). Diamond (1992) provides an excellent discussion about the oncology nurse's role in advanced directives and suggests that questions regarding this issue be integrated as a routine part of the admission assessment.

Providing patients with the information they need to make decisions regarding their future care is important. Educational interventions can help decrease anxiety and depression and increase one's sense of control (Yeomans & Washington, 1991). Several authors have identified necessary components of a teaching plan for patients with advanced cancer. The major areas of care that should be addressed include facts related to the disease process, proposed treatment, schedule of appointments, management of side effects associated with treatment or the disease, normalcy of feelings, and emotional responses to the cancer diagnosis. The teaching plan should be individualized so that patients are given small amounts of information in a manner that

they can easily understand. Information may have to be repeated at frequent intervals, because anxiety is often a problem (Hagopian, 1993).

Nursing management of patients with UKPM is diverse and multifacted. Although new treatment modalities have been identified as useful in certain favorable prognostic groups, palliative care remains the mainstay of care in UKPM. Through appropriate symptom management, psychosocial care, and patient education, nurses can help promote adjustment to the disease and improve quality of life.

REFERENCES

Arnold, A., Cossman, J., Bakhshi, A., Jaffe, E., Waidmann, T., & Korsmeyler, S. (1983). Immunoglobulin-gene rearrangements as unique clonal markers in human lymphoid neoplasms. *New England Journal of Medicine, 309*, 1593–1599.

Ashikari, R., Rosen, P., Urban, J., & Senoo, T. (1976). Breast cancer presenting as an axillary mass. *Annals of Surgery, 183*, 415–417.

Benoliel, J., & McCorkle, R. (1978). A holistic approach to terminal illness. *Cancer Nursing, 1*, 143–149.

Billings, J. (1985). *Outpatient management of advanced cancer: Symptom control, support and hospice in the home*. Philadelphia: J. B. Lippincott Co.

Chen, K., & Flam, M. (1986). Peritoneal papillary serious carcinoma with long term survival. *Cancer, 58* 1371–1373.

Cooley, M., Davis, L., & Abrahm, J. (1994). Cisplatin: A clinical review. Part II: Assessment and management of side effects. *Cancer Nursing, 17*, 283–293.

deBraud, F., & Al-Sarraf, L. (1993). Diagnosis and management of squamous cell carcinoma of unknown primary tumor site of the neck. *Seminars in Oncology, 20*, 273–278.

deBraud, F., Heilburn, L., & Ahmad, K. (1989). Carcinoma of unknown primary metastatic to the neck: Advantage of an aggressive treatment. *Cancer, 54*, 510–515.

Diamond, E. (1992). The oncology nurse's role in patient advanced directives. *Oncology Nursing Forum, 19*, 891–898.

Diggs, C. (1989). Cancer of unknown primary site: Deciding how far to carry evaluation. *Postgraduate Medicine, 86*, 186–191.

Emanuel, L., Barry, M., & Stoeckle, J. (1991). Advanced directives for medical care: A case for greater use. *New England Journal of Medicine, 324*, 889–895.

Gaber, A., Rice, P., Eaton, C., Pietraffitta, J., Spatz, E., & Deckers, P. (1983). Metastatic malignant disease of unknown origin. *American Journal of Surgery, 145*, 493–497.

Gatter, K., Alcock, C., Heryet, A., Pulford, K., Heyberman, E., Taylor-Papadimitriou, J., Stein, H., & Mason, D. (1984). The differential diagnosis of routinely processed anaplastic tumors using monoclonal antibodies. *American Journal of Clinical Pathology, 82*, 33–43.

Greco, F., & Hainsworth, J. (1993). Cancer of unknown primary site. In V. Devita, S. Hellman, & S. Rosenberg, (Eds.), *Cancer: Principles and practice of oncology* (4th ed., pp. 2072–2092). Philadelphia: J. B. Lippincott Co.

Greco, F., & Hainsworth, J. (1992). Tumors of unknown origin. *Cancer, 42*, 96–115.

Gunthrie, T. (1989). Treatable carcinoma of unknown origin. *Journal of Medical Science, 289*, 74–78.

Hagopian, G. (1993). Cognitive strategies used in adapting to a cancer diagnosis. *Oncology Nursing Forum, 20*, 759–763.

Hainsworth, J., & Greco, F. (1993a). Introduction: Unknown primary tumor. *Seminars in Oncology, 20*, 205.

Hainsworth, J., & Greco, F. (1993b). Treatment of patients with cancer of an unknown primary site. *New England Journal of Medicine, 329*, 257–263.

Hainsworth, J., Johnson, D., & Greco, F. (1988). Poorly differentiated neuroendocrine carcinoma of unknown primary site: A newly recognized clinicopathologic entity. *Annals of Internal Medicine, 109,* 364–372.

Hainsworth, J., Johnson, D., & Greco, F. (1992). Cisplatin based combination chemotherapy in the treatment of poorly differentiated carcinoma and poorly differentiated adenocarcinoma of unknown primary site: Results of a 12 year experience. *Journal of Clinical Oncology, 10,* 912–922.

Hainsworth, J., Wright, E., Johnson, D., Davis, B., & Greco, F. (1991). Poorly differentiated carcinoma of unknown primary site: Clinical usefulness of immunoperoxidase staining. *Journal of Clinical Oncology, 9,* 1931–1938.

Halsed, W. (1907). Results of radical operations for cure of carcinoma of the breast. *Annals of Surgery, 46,* 1.

Holmes, F., & Fouts, T. (1970). Metastatic cancer of unknown primary site. *Cancer, 26,* 816–820.

Horning, S., Carrier, E., Rouse, R., Warnke, R., & Michie, S. (1989). Lymphomas presenting as histologically unclassified neoplasms: Characteristics and response to treatment. *Journal of Clinical Oncology, 7,* 1281–1287.

Ilson, D., Motzer, R., Rodriquez, E., Chaganti, R., & Bosl, G. (1993). Genetic analysis in the diagnosis of neoplasms of unknown primary tumor site. *Seminars in Oncology, 20,* 229–237.

Kozlowski, J., Ellis, W., & Grayhack, J. (1991). Advanced prostatic carcinoma: Early versus late endocrine therapy. *Urologic Clinics of North America, 18,* 15–24.

Leonard, R., & Nystom, J. (1993). Diagnostic evaluation of patients with carcinoma of unknown tumor site. *Seminars in Oncology, 20,* 244–250.

Lo, B., McLeod, G., & Saika, G. (1986). Patients attitudes toward discussing life sustaining treatment. *Archives of Internal Medicine, 146,* 1613–1615.

Mackay, B., & Ordonez, N. (1993). Pathological evaluation of neoplasms with unknown primary tumor site. *Seminars in Oncology, 20,* 206–228.

Marcialvega, V., Cardenes, H., Perez, C., Devineni, V., Simpson, J., Fredrickson, J., Sessions, D., Spector, G., & Thawley, S. (1990). Cervical metastases from unknown primaries: Radiotherapeutic management and appearance of subsequent primaries. *International Journal of Radiation Oncology Biologic Physics, 19,* 919–928.

McMillan, J., Levin, E., & Stephens, R. (1982). Computed tomography in the evaluation of metastatic adenocarcinoma from an unknown primary site. *Radiology, 143,* 143–146.

Motzer, R., Rodriquez, E., Reuter, V., Samaniego, F., Dmitrovsky, E., Bajorin, D., Pfister, D., Parsa, N., Chaganti, S., & Bosl, G. (1991). Genetic analysis as an aid in diagnosis for patients with midline carcinomas of uncertain histologies. *Journal of the National Cancer Institute, 83,* 341–346.

Muggia, F., & Baranda, J. (1993). Management of peritoneal carcinomatosis of unknown primary tumor site. *Seminars in Oncology, 20,* 268–272.

Mukherjee, A., Murty, V., Rodriquez, E., Reuter, V., Bosl, G., & Chaganti, R. (1991). Detection and analysis of origin of i(12 p): A diagnostic marker of human male germ cell tumors, by fluorescence in situ hybridization. *Genes, Chromosomes & Cancer, 3,* 300–307.

Nystrom, J., Weiner, J., Heffelfinger-Juttner, J., Irwin, L., Bateman, J., & Meshnik-Wolfe, R. (1977). Metastatic and histologic presentations in unknown primary cancer. *Seminars in Oncology, 4,* 53–58.

Nystrom, J., Weiner, J., Meshnik-Wolfe, R., Bateman, J., & Viola, M. (1979). Identifying the primary site in metastatic cancer of unknown origin: Inadequacy of roentgenographic procedures. *Journal of the American Medical Association, 241,* 381–383.

Patel, J., Nemoto, T., Rosner, D., Dao, T., & Pickren, J. (1981). Axillary lymph node metastasis from an occult breast cancer. *Cancer, 47,* 2923–2927.

Perchalski, J., Hall, K., & Dewar, M. (1992). Metastasis of unknown origin. *Primary Care, 19,* 747–757.

Richardson, R., Schoumacher, R., Fer, M., Hande, K., Forbes, J., Oldham, R., & Greco, F. (1981). The unrecognized extragonadal germ cell cancer syndrome. *Annals of Internal Medicine, 94,* 181–186.

Scanlon, C. (1989). Creating a vision of hope: The challenge of palliative care. *Oncology Nursing Forum, 16,* 491–498.

Sporn, J., & Greenberg, B. (1990). Empirical chemotherapy in patients with carcinoma of unknown primary site. *American Journal of Medicine, 88,* 49–55.

Sporn, J., & Greenberg, B. (1993). Empiric chemotherapy for adenocarcinoma of unknown primary tumor site. *Seminars in Oncology, 20,* 261–267.

Steckel, K., & Kagan, R. (1991). Metastatic tumors of unknown origin. *Cancer, 67,* 1242–1244.

Strnad, C., Grosh, W., Baxter, J., Burnett, L., Jones, H., Greco, F., & Hawsworth, J. (1989). Peritoneal carcinomatosis of unknown primary site in women: A distinctive subset of adenocarcinoma. *Annals of Internal Medicine, 111,* 213–217.

Tornberg, M., Burns-McGrath, B., & Benoliel, J. (1984). Oncology transition services: Partnerships of nurses and families. *Cancer Nursing, 7,* 131–138.

Turc-Carel, C., Philip, I., Berger, M., Philip, T., & Lenoir, G. (1983). Chromosomal translocations in Ewing's sarcoma. *New England Journal of Medicine, 309,* 497–498.

Warnke, R., Gatter, K., Falini, B., Hildreth, P., Woolston, R., Pulford, K., Cordell, J., Cohen, B., DeWolfe-Peters, C., & Mason, D. (1983). Diagnosis of human lymphoma with monoclonal antileukocyte antibodies. *New England Journal of Medicine, 309,* 1275–1281.

Whang-Peng, J., Triche, T., Knutsen, T., Miser, J., Douglass, E., & Isreal, M. (1984). Chromosome translocation in peripheral neuroepithelioma. *New England Journal of Medicine, 311,* 584–585.

Yeomans, A., & Washington, J. (1991). Occult primary malignancies. *Oncology Nursing Forum, 18,* 539–544.

Alice J. Longman

Skin cancers are estimated to develop in more than 700,000 people annually and lead all other cancers in the rate of increase (American Cancer Society, 1994). Directly visible and easily accessible, skin cancers offer a unique opportunity for early detection, early diagnosis, early treatment, and cure.

DEFINITION AND INCIDENCE

The vast majority of skin cancers are highly curable basal cell carcinomas and squamous cell carcinomas. The most serious skin cancer is malignant melanoma, which affects about 32,000 men and women each year. Since 1973, the incidence rate of malignant melanoma has increased at the rate of 4 per cent each year (American Cancer Society, 1994). In 1994, an additional 10,000 invasive nonmelanoma skin cancers will occur, mostly sarcomas, including Kaposi's sarcoma. Skin cancers account for an estimated 9200 deaths per year; 6900 from malignant melanoma and 2300 from other skin cancers (American Cancer Society, 1994). Those deaths from other skin cancers, in particular squamous cell carcinomas, are usually the result of metastases to the proximal lymph nodes and to distant organs such as the lungs, brain, and bone. Skin cancer is not only a public health problem; it is also a rapidly worsening one.

SKIN STRUCTURE AND CARCINOGENESIS

The sun or, more precisely, ultraviolet radiation from the sun is the major etiologic factor in the development of skin cancers. Exposure to the sun and ultraviolet radiation has a cumulative effect; thus the signs of skin cancer appear years after the exposure (Loescher & Booth, 1990; Longman, 1992; Stewart, 1987).

The epidermis is the outer layer of the skin, and the entire layer is replaced every 15 to 30 days (Stewart, 1987). Fibrous protein keratin, the end product of the maturing epidermal cells that make up the stratum corneum, is found in the epidermis. Keratin's thickness in the stratum corneum varies, offering the greatest protection in areas such as the palms of the hands and the soles of the feet. Keratinocytes undergo changes in shape, structure, and composition as they are gradually pushed toward the surface in a continuing process.

The inner layer of the epidermis, the stratum basilis, has basal keratinocytes. Interspersed within the basal cells are melanocytes, which synthesize the pigment melanin. Melanin, a brownish-black pigment, protects the epidermis and the superficial dermal vasculature. It does this by simultaneously activating previously synthesized melanin to produce tanning and activating the melanin production cycle to create delayed tanning. Pigment is nature's sunscreen, and the more a person has, the greater the protection he or she has from the sun (Stewart, 1987; Vargo, 1991).

Basal cell carcinoma and squamous cell carcinoma are named for the cells from which they develop. Basal cells lie in the lowest part of the epidermis, which is the outermost layer of the skin (see Fig. 43–1). Most of the epidermis is composed of squamous cells. Keratinocytes reach the stratum spinosum or "prickle cell" layer and become elongated and flat. Within these cells, squamous cell carcinoma begins (see Fig. 43–2). Malignant melanoma arises from pigment cells (see Fig. 43–3).

Several age-related changes occur in the skin. The outer layer or the stratum corneum flattens and thins with age (Berliner, 1986a). Chemicals are able to pass through more easily. As subcutaneous fat decreases,

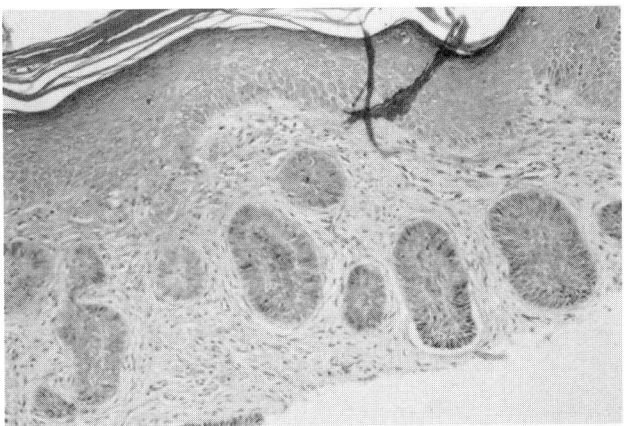

FIGURE 43–1. Basal cell carcinoma. (Courtesy of Libby Edwards, MD.)

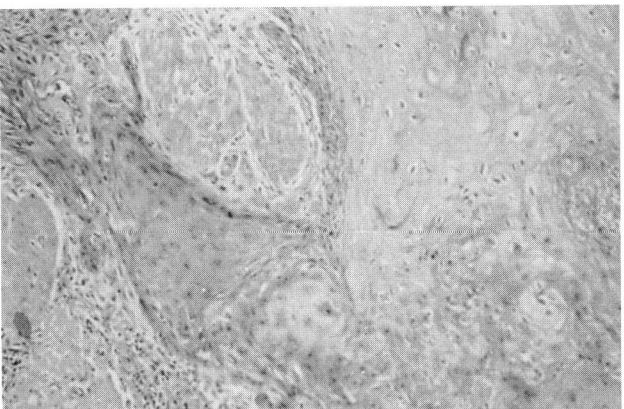

FIGURE 43–2. Squamous cell carcinoma. (Courtesy of Libby Edwards, MD.)

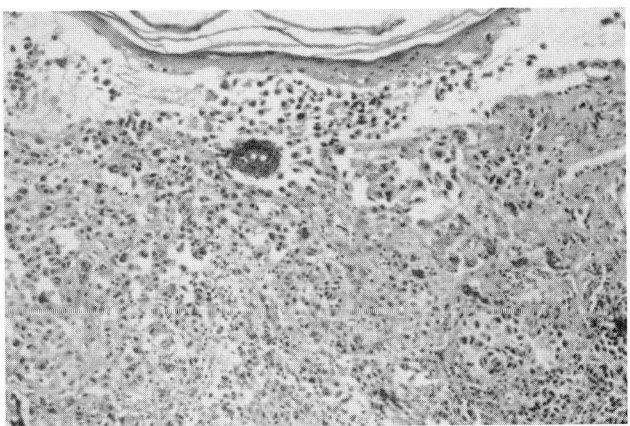

FIGURE 43–3. Malignant melanoma. (Courtesy of Libby Edwards, MD.)

skin elasticity, shape, and support are lost. The collagen fibers stiffen, and glutamic acid and lysine needed for elastin formation decrease. Wrinkles and sagging skin result. Changes in melanin production that occur account for changes in skin and hair color (Berliner, 1986b).

A spectrum of radiant electromagnetic energy called ultraviolet radiation is produced by the sun. Ultraviolet light is of the greatest photobiologic importance and is divided into wavelengths known as A, B, and C (Stewart, 1987). The wavelengths emanating from the sun range from 200 nm to more than 18,000 nm (Stewart, 1987). The skin is damaged by ultraviolet radiation in the 200 to 400 nm range. Longer waves (320 nm to 400 nm) are known as ultraviolet A or UV-A; rays falling in a shorter range (290 nm to 320 nm) are ultraviolet B, or UV-B; and the shortest waves (200 nm to 290 nm) are ultraviolet C, or UV-C (Stewart, 1987). The worst damage to the skin in the form of short-term erythema and carcinogenesis following long-term exposure is attributed to UV-B. Ultraviolet C rays are largely filtered by the ozone layer in the stratosphere (Lawler & Schreiber, 1989; Stewart, 1987).

The skin responds to ultraviolet light by becoming reddened. The UV-A rays stimulate the cells to produce melanin. Other nearby cells begin dividing and making their way to the surface, carrying the melanin with them. Ultraviolet B rays dilate the blood vessels lying near the skin's surface. The reddening phase of sunburn is caused by the increased circulation of the blood to these injured vessels. Ultraviolet light continues to thicken and break down the network of supportive collagen and elastic fibers in the dermis (Bargoil & Erdman, 1993).

NONMELANOMA SKIN CANCERS

Basal cell carcinoma is the most common form of skin cancer (Vargo, 1991). The actual incidence of basal cell carcinoma may be higher than reported, as it may be treated as a problem of little consequence. The inability of the basal cells to mature into keratinocytes is the cellular defect characterizing basal cell carcinoma. Areas of the body that receive the greatest exposure to sunlight are the most common sites for basal carcinoma (see Table 43–1).

Basal cell carcinoma is classified according to clinical and histologic differences (Vargo, 1991). The four major classifications are nodulo-ulcerative, superficial, pigmented, and morphea-like (Loescher & Booth, 1990; Longman, 1992; Vargo, 1991). Nodulo-ulcerative basal cell carcinoma begins as a small, firm, well-demarcated, dome-shaped papule. It is characterized by (1) an elevated lesion, (2) an umbilicated, ulcerated cen-

TABLE 43–1. *Common Sites of Nonmelanoma Skin Cancers*

TYPE OF SKIN CANCER	COMMON SITES
Nodular basal cell	Face, head, neck
Superficial basal cell	Trunk, extremities
Pigmented basal cell	Face, head, neck
Morphea-like basal cell	Head, neck
Squamous cell	Head, forehead, nose, border of lips, back of hands

ter with raised margins, and (3) a moderate firmness to the touch. The lesion has a pearly or waxy gleam (Fig. 43–4, see Color Plate I). Superficial basal cell carcinoma appears as a superficial, sharply marginated plaque with a raised, pearly, threadlike border. The center is usually crusted, scaly, and erythematous. There are often multiple lesions, and they frequently appear on the trunk of the body. Irregular local extension is the principal problem of management. Pigmented basal cell carcinoma may be nodular or superficial. There is melanin in the epidermis and dermis and in the lesion itself. The lesion has a brown, black, or blue color. There is a shiny, pearly border with well-defined margins and telangiectases. Morphea-like basal cell carcinoma is the rarest type. The lesion has fingerlike projections of fibroepitheliomatous strands of tumor. There is a flat or depressed scarlike plaque that is pale yellow or white. Nodularity, ulceration, and bleeding may occur.

Squamous cell carcinoma is the predominant skin cancer in skin exposed to ionizing radiation, carcinogenic chemicals, or trauma (see Table 43–1). Actinic keratosis is implicated in the development of squamous cell carcinoma and is considered a premalignant state. Bowen's disease is also considered in situ squamous cell carcinoma.

The appearance of squamous cell carcinoma varies from an elevated, erythematous, nodular mass with varying amounts of scaling or crusting to an ulcerative lesion or fungating mass (Loescher & Booth, 1990; Longman, 1992; Vargo, 1991). In contrast to basal cell carcinomas, squamous cell carcinomas are opaque (Fig. 43–5, see Color Plate I). Squamous cell carcinomas have the potential for metastases to regional and distant sites.

MALIGNANT MELANOMA

Malignant melanoma is potentially the most lethal of the skin cancers and appears on all areas of the skin (see Table 43–2). Melanomas arise from melanocytes, which are cells specializing in the biosynthesis and transport of melanin, and more often than not from a nevus or mole (Fig. 43–6, see Color Plate II). Nevi or moles are aggregates of melanocytes that are present at birth (Lawler, 1991; Lawler & Schreiber, 1989).

EPIDEMIOLOGY

Several epidemiologic factors are important in the prevention, detection, and early diagnosis of malignant melanoma. The incidence and mortality rates of malignant melanoma have risen dramatically in the last several decades. Evidence suggests that the development of malignant melanoma is related to ultraviolet radiation. Precursor lesions include dysplastic nevi that may be familial (B-K moles) or nonfamilial (sporadic dysplastic nevi) and pigmented congenital nevi covering large areas of the body (Lawler, 1991; Lawler & Schreiber, 1989). It is important that differentiation be made between normal moles and dysplastic nevi (see Table 43–3).

TABLE 43–2. *Common Sites of Malignant Melanoma*

TYPE OF MELANOMA	COMMON SITES
Lentigo maligna	Face, neck, trunk, dorsum of hands
Superficial spreading	Backs of men, legs of women
Nodular	Head, neck, trunk
Acral-lentiginous	Palms of hands, soles of feet, nail beds, mucous membranes

Ninety per cent of melanomas arise in the skin, with the rest developing in the eye and the mucous membranes of the mouth and anus. The prognosis is good if the lesion is localized and thin. Prognosis depends on several features of the primary tumor: (1) depth of invasion, (2) anatomic site, (3) thickness, (4) presence or absence of tumor ulceration, and (5) growth pattern (Lawler, 1991; Loescher & Booth, 1990; Longman, 1992). Another factor is the sex of the person with melanoma, because steroid hormones may affect the etiology and behavior of the lesion.

CLASSIFICATION OF CUTANEOUS MELANOMAS

Cutaneous melanomas are classified as follows.

1. *Lentigo maligna melanoma.* This type of melanoma is the slowest growing and least aggressive. It most often occurs on a premalignant lesion. The lesion is tan with shades of brown and dark areas.
2. *Superficial spreading melanoma.* This is the most common type of melanoma and usually arises in a preexisting nevus. It develops as a slower growing, pigmented, macular lesion and often has red, blue, or white areas.
3. *Nodular melanoma.* This type of melanoma is extremely aggressive and metastasizes rapidly unless treated early. There is a raised, dome-shaped, blue-black or red nodule.

TABLE 43–3. *Comparison of Normal Moles and Dysplastic Nevi*

FEATURE	NORMAL MOLES	DYSPLASTIC NEVI
Color	Usually one shade of tan or brown	Variation in color; speckles of tan, brown, or black
Shape	Round or oval	Irregular or hazy
Diameter	Usually less than 5 mm	Usually more than 5 mm
Border	Sharp and well defined	Irregular or hazy
Location	Sun-exposed skin	Most common on sun-exposed skin; occur anywhere on body

4. *Acral-lentiginous melanoma.* This variety develops as a pigmented lesion on the palms of the hands, on the soles of the feet, and under the nails. It is commonly seen in African-Americans, Hispanics, and Orientals. There are variegated shades of blue and black (Lawler, 1991; Loescher & Booth, 1990; Longman, 1992).

The characteristic features of early malignant melanoma are similar. They can be remembered by thinking of A B C D: A for Asymmetry, B for Border irregularity, C for Color variegation, and D for Diameter (Friedman, Rigel, Silverman, Kopf, & Vossaert, 1991). Early lesions tend to grow asymmetrically. As the melanocytes in early melanoma extend horizontally within the epidermis in an uncontrolled fashion, the borderline of early lesions is irregular and exhibits characteristic notching or scalloping. Early lesions appear as flat and pigmented with various tones of brown. Layering of melanin is uneven, which results in color variegation. The diameter is usually greater than 6 mm. The earlier the diagnosis of malignant melanoma is made, the higher the survival rate is (Friedman et al., 1991).

RISK FACTORS ASSOCIATED WITH NONMELANOMA SKIN CANCERS

Ultraviolet radiation from sunlight (UV-B spectral range, 290 to 320 nm range) is the major risk factor in the development of skin cancers. The increase in the incidence of skin cancers among whites can be attributed in part to changes in lifestyles with subsequent changes in clothing styles, ideas about sunbathing and tanning, and alterations in the ozone layer of the atmosphere (Frank-Stromborg, 1986a, 1986b; Lawler & Schreiber, 1989). Thus prolonged exposure to ultraviolet radiation from the sun is the major exogenous factor in the development of nonmelanoma skin cancers and melanoma.

Other exogenous factors related to the development of squamous cell carcinomas in particular are exposure to ionizing radiation, to chemical carcinogens, and to petroleum including coal, tar, pitch, and creosote preparations. Radiologists and uranium miners are at occupational risk for skin cancer, as are individuals who received small repeated doses of radiation for the treatment of acne. Chemical carcinogens include arsenicals in agriculture sprays, psoralens for the treatment of psoriasis, and fumes and burns from molten metals. A history of repeated trauma or chronic infections such as topical ulcers or burns resulting in scarification also predisposes an individual to skin cancer (Longman, 1992; Vargo, 1991).

Endogenous factors in the development of skin cancers include fair or freckled complexion, red, blonde, or light brown hair, light-colored eyes, xeroderma pigmentosum or albinism, and immunodeficiency or suppression. Those at risk for immunodeficiency or suppression include individuals who have received renal or heart transplants and those with lymphoproliferative carcinomas (Loescher, 1993; Longman, 1992; Tokar, Fraser, & Bale, 1992; White, 1986b).

Premalignant states or lesions have been described as placing persons at risk for squamous cell carcinoma and are as follows.

1. *Actinic and senile keratosis.* These lesions are usually found on sun-exposed skin such as the head, neck, hands, and arms. The lesions are slightly elevated, well circumscribed, and reddened with a rough or scaly surface. Malignant transformation is slow and rare.
2. *Seborrheic keratosis.* The lesion is benign, brownish, sharp in delineation, flat, and can arise from indolent warts. Malignant transformation is rare.
3. *Arsenic keratosis.* The lesions appear as hard corn-like areas on the palms of the hand or the soles of the feet and appear to be surrounded by warts. Associated skin surfaces may be diffusely pigmented. Malignant transformation is rare.
4. *Bowen's disease.* The lesion may appear on any part of the body as a single, slightly raised papule that gradually increases in size. It is superficial and red and eventually crusts but does not heal completely. This lesion is referred to as squamous cell carcinoma in situ (Vargo, 1991; White, 1986b).

RISK FACTORS FOR MALIGNANT MELANOMA

Exposure to ultraviolet radiation is thought to be the major risk factor for malignant melanoma (Friedman et al., 1991; Lawler & Schreiber, 1989). Evidence indicates that the incidence of melanoma is highest in areas receiving the greatest sunlight exposure, such as the "sunbelt" states. There is also speculation that malignant melanoma may be due to intense, intermittent exposure to ultraviolet radiation rather than prolonged exposure. Other factors increasing the risk of developing malignant melanoma are family history of the disease, presence of melanocytic nevi, light complexion, history of sunburns, and susceptible age (Friedman et al., 1991; Lawler & Schreiber, 1989).

Two types of acquired nevi are also implicated in the development of malignant melanoma: commonly acquired nevi, which rarely become malignant, and dysplastic nevi, which sometimes become malignant (Fraser, Hartge, & Tucker, 1991; Tokar et al., 1992). Common acquired nevi are aggregates of melanoncytes, which become most noticeable during the middle years. White adults have approximately 25 to 40 commonly acquired nevi, mainly located on skin above the waist. These moles are small (less than 5 mm), round, and uniformly tan or brown. Dysplastic nevi occur as a result of atypical cell development in the melanocytes. They are often larger than 5 mm, irregular in shape, and mixtures of tan, brown, black, and red or pink (Fig. 43–7, see Color Plate II). They occur most commonly on the back but do appear on the scalp, breasts, and buttocks. Dysplastic nevus syndrome is a precancerous mole pattern and is confirmed when irregular, variably pigmented moles appear. Dysplasia is verified by biopsy specimens (Tokar et al., 1992). Two subtypes of dysplastic nevus syndrome have been described: the familial variant and the sporadic variant. The familial variant affects persons who may or may not have melanoma but have a family history for dysplastic nevi, malignant melanoma, or both. Those individuals who may or may not have melanoma and have no family history of dysplastic nevi, melanoma, or both are included in the sporadic subtype (Tokar et al., 1992).

NURSING IMPLICATIONS

Oncology nurses have unique opportunities to expand public awareness of the long-term effects of sun exposure on the skin. Formal and informal activities have been described in the literature (Entrekin & McMillan, 1993; Kelly, 1991; White & Spitz, 1993). Knowledge about exposure of the skin to sunlight, different types of skin, and systematic and periodic skin assessment is important if nurses are to make an impact on the prevention and early detection of skin cancers (see Box 43–1).

ASSESSMENT OF SKIN EXPOSURE

Several factors are important in assessing the impact of exposure to sunlight on skin. These include the time of day during exposure, geographic area, altitude and weather conditions, time of year, and length of exposure(s) (Fraser et al., 1989; Loescher, 1993). Ultraviolet rays are more direct from 10:00 AM to 2:00 PM, and caution should be exercised during this time of day. On a cloudy day, roughly 70 to 80 per cent of the UV-B rays penetrate the clouds and reach the earth. Various surfaces such as snow, water, and sand reflect the sun's rays. Additionally, there are more direct rays from May to October. Certain areas of the world receive sun all year long; in the United States areas roughly south of a horizontal line from North Carolina to southern California are affected. Those who live or vacation in higher altitudes should be alerted to the fact that there is less atmosphere to filter out the UV-B rays. In tropical areas, more UV-B rays reach the earth. Thus caution should be exercised in relation to sun exposure in these areas.

SKIN TYPES AND SUN PROTECTION

A person's skin type is determined by genetic history and pigmentation and erythema histories (Lawler & Schreiber, 1989; Longman, 1992). Six sun reaction types have been described (see Table 43–4). Knowledge of an individual's skin type determines both natural protection and response to the sun. The minimal erythema dose or the amount of time unprotected skin can be exposed to sunlight before reddening occurs is useful in determining sun protection factor needs. The development of sunscreens and sunblocks has made it possible to decrease solar damage to the skin (see Table 43–5). Recommendations for the use of sunscreens include the use of commercial sunscreens with a sun protection factor of greater than 10, for example, Presun

---

BOX 43–1. *Nurses' Knowledge, Beliefs, and Practices Related to Cancer Prevention and Detection*

Entrekin, N. M., & McMillan, S. C. (1993). Nurses' knowledge, beliefs, and practices related to cancer prevention and detection. *Cancer Nursing, 16,* 431–439.

Purpose: The purpose of this study was to assess the needs of nurses in six areas of cancer prevention and early detection to concentrate future programming resources in areas of greatest need. The areas assessed were breast, lung, colorectal, prostate, gynecologic, and skin cancers.

Sample: A stratified purposive sample of 7000 nurses was sought from eight districts of Florida based on the population in each district; responses from 2348 were usable. Nurses were from all types of settings and from urban and rural areas. Years of experience ranged from less than 2 years to more than 15 years. Numerous positions were reported with staff nurses or general duty nurses being predominant. Twenty-three per cent reported themselves as oncology nurses, and eight per cent were oncology certified nurses.

Measures: Six alternate forms of a survey instrument developed by the investigators were used to assess the knowledge base, beliefs, and practices of nurses related to six areas of prevention and detection. Each respondent completed a questionnaire on one specific type of cancer. The instruments' content was based on published American Cancer Society guidelines for cancer prevention and detection. Part I asked for demographic information, and Part II asked for what percentage of clients nurses offered specific information on screening related to a particular cancer. Basic knowledge was tested by using three or four multiple choice items. Part III addressed attitudes about accountability for cancer prevention and detection and satisfaction with participation in these activities. A five-point rating scale was used to assess attitudes. Optical scanner forms were used for the answers. Data were analyzed using the statistical package called Crunch, and frequencies, percentages, and means were reported.

Findings: Four research questions were addressed by this study. Results from the knowledge section indicated that nurses knew the most about prostate, colorectal, and breast cancer. Nurses knew the most about the early warning signs of skin and prostate cancer. Results revealed that nurses seldom practiced prevention and early detection measures with clients. The third area assessed was accountability and satisfaction with activities related to prevention and detection; the results indicated that nurses took responsibility for their activities. The fourth area dealt with the reasons nurses were not able to address prevention and detection measures. Two reasons were cited: one was not enough time and the other was lack of information.

Nursing Implications: There is a necessity for nurses to be better educated about the activities related to prevention and detection and to assume responsibility for these activities.

TABLE 43–4. *Skin Types and Skin Reactions*

SKIN TYPE	SKIN REACTIONS
1	Burns easily and severely; tans little or not at all
2	Burns easily and severely; tans minimally or lightly
3	Burns moderately; tans approximately average
4	Burns minimally; tans easily
5	Burns rarely; tans easily and substantially
6	Never burns; tans profusely

TABLE 43–5. *Guide to Sun Protection*

DEGREE OF PROTECTION	SUN PROTECTION FACTOR	EXAMPLES OF SUNSCREENS
Minimal sun protection	2 to 4	Coppertone Dark Tanning
Moderate sun protection	4 to 6	Sea & Ski Golden Tan
Extra sun protection	6 to 8	Maxafil
Maximal sun protection	8 to 15	PreSun 8
Ultra sun protection	15 or more	Sundown 15 Ultra Protection

and Pabanol; the use of commercial sunblocks that have the active ingredients of titanium dioxide, zinc oxide, talc, iron oxide, and kaolin; and the reapplication of sunscreen every 2 to 3 hours during long sun exposure. For those taking thiazides, sulfonamides, or other photosensitizing drugs, sunscreens containing benzophenones are recommended.

EXAMINATION OF THE SKIN

Complete and thorough examination of the skin is important and is to be encouraged if early detection is to become a reality (Berwick, Bolognia, Heer, & Fine, 1991; Friedman et al., 1991). The examination should be systematic and done annually by physicians or nurses. Self-examination of the skin should be performed monthly in a well-lighted area. The following procedure is recommended:

1. Inspect and palpate all accessible skin surfaces including smooth skin, skin folds, mucosal surfaces, and epidermal appendages.
2. Assess preexisting lesions of the skin such as moles, freckles, warts, birthmarks, and scars.
3. Inspect the scalp and entire hairline and palpate the scalp.
4. Inspect the face, lips, and neck, including the posterior neck and postauricular areas.
5. Inspect and palpate all surfaces of the upper extremities.
6. Inspect and palpate the skin of the back, buttocks, and back of legs.
7. Inspect the external genitalia. In women, the skin fold of the labia and perineum should be separated

to adequately view the surfaces. Men should inspect all sides of the penis and scrotal sac.
8. Inspect and palpate the anterior surfaces of the legs and feet.
9. Inspect and palpate all hairy surfaces, including those beneath axillary, thoracic, and pubic hair.
10. Note characteristics of normal moles.

With practice, skin self-examination can be accomplished quickly and easily. Guidelines are available from the American Cancer Society, the National Cancer Institute, the American Academy of Dermatology, and the Skin Cancer Foundation.

CLINICAL FEATURES, DIAGNOSIS, AND PROGNOSIS

Because most skin cancers are highly visible on the exposed surfaces of the body, early signs can be detected readily. Early signs of nonmelanoma skin cancers are: (1) a sore that does not heal, (2) a persistent lump or swelling, and (3) changes in skin markings. These changes in skin markings are related to size, color, surface, shape, surrounding skin, sensation, and elevation (Longman, 1992; Vargo, 1991). A confirmed tissue diagnosis is essential to definitive treatment. With adequate treatment, basal cell carcinoma is highly curable (90 to 95 per cent). Squamous cell carcinoma is also highly curable (75 to 80 per cent), but the recurrence of lesions is the major complication. The tumor may metastasize to the lymph nodes.

The characteristic clinical features of malignant melanoma are related to changes in skin markings. These include changes in color, size, shape, elevation, surface, surrounding skin, sensation, and consistency (see Table 43–6). Although there is variegation in color change, red, black, or both are the most significant. Enlargement of the mole with concurrent changes in surface and shape is noteworthy. If the mole is already black, there may be a new raised area, which creates a high index of suspicion for malignant melanoma (Lawler, 1991; Longman, 1992). The appearance of new moles is also of critical importance. The association between thickness of the lesion and survival is strong. Those who have thin (less than 0.76 mm) melanoma lesions have a high cure rate (95 to 100 per cent) following removal of the melanoma. Thus the most important prognostic feature of malignant melanoma is the size of the lesion at the time of its removal. Special considerations associated with malignant melanoma are primary melanoma of the eye, primary mucosal melanoma, local advanced disease, and metastasis to the brain (Lawler, 1991; Loescher & Booth, 1990).

TREATMENT OF NONMELANOMA SKIN CANCERS

The goal of treatment for nonmelanoma skin cancers is to eradicate the tumor and yet attain an acceptable cosmetic result. Definitive treatment depends on the location and size of the lesion, exact histologic type,

TABLE 43–6. *Danger Signs of Malignant Melanoma*

Change in Color
Especially multiple shades of dark brown or black; red, white, and blue; spread of color from the edge of the lesion into surrounding skin
Change in Size
Especially sudden or continuous enlargement
Change in Shape
Especially development of irregular margins
Change in Elevation
Especially sudden elevation of a previously macular pigmented lesion
Change in Surface
Especially scaliness, erosion, oozing, crusting, ulceration, bleeding
Change in Surrounding Skin
Especially redness, swelling, satellite pigmentations
Change in Sensation
Especially itching, tenderness, pain
Change in Consistency
Especially softening or friability

(From Friedman, R. J., Rigel, D. D., Silverman, M. K., Kopf, A. W., & Vossaert, K. A. (1991). Malignant melanoma in the 1990s: The continued importance of early detection and the role of physician examination and self-examination of the skin. *CA-A Cancer Journal for Clinicians, 41,* 201–226.)

possible extension into nearby structures, previous treatment, and age and general condition of the patient (Loescher & Booth, 1990; Longman, 1992; Vargo, 1991).

An accurate histologic diagnosis is achieved by (1) excisional biopsy with 0.5 to 1.0 cm margins if the lesion is small, and (2) incisional biopsy, including a 1.0 cm margin for larger lesions. These procedures give adequate specimens with margins in all directions. Often, an excisional biopsy is considered definitive treatment (Loescher & Booth, 1990; Vargo, 1991).

Surgery for nonmelanoma skin cancers is indicated if the lesion is large and invades bone or cartilage. Planning must be done for acceptable cosmetic results, which can include a skin graft or flap (Loescher & Booth, 1990; Vargo, 1991). Curettage and electrodesiccation are used for small, superficial, recurrent lesions. Mohs' microscopic surgery or chemosurgery is available in select tumors. The procedure is useful if the tumor margins are difficult to determine or if the lesion has reappeared. The technique involves horizontal shaving and staining of tissues in thin layers (Loescher & Booth, 1990). Mohs' surgery is most often used for cancers in high-risk areas such as the nose and nasolabial folds, the medial canthus, and preauricular and postauricular locations. Cryosurgery using thermocouples is another method of surgical treatment.

Radiation therapy is used in the treatment of nonmelanoma skin cancers when inadequate tumor margins are shown. In a location such as the eyelids, radiation therapy might be the treatment of choice, as surgical excision could involve extensive reconstructive surgery. A highly fractionated schedule (4500 rad/3 weeks in 200 rad daily fractions) with attention to shielding offers excellent results. If bone and cartilage are involved, radiation may be combined with surgery.

Treatment of premalignant actinic keratosis is topical 5-fluorouracil (5-FU). Shielding exposed areas from repeated sun exposure is a first step. Topical applications of 5-FU are also used in the treatment of multiple keratotic lesions. Therapy usually lasts for at least 2.5 months, and healing usually occurs within 2 weeks of cessation of treatment. For unusual recurrent skin cancers that are no longer manageable by surgery, radiation, or both, various agents have been used through arterial infusion, local injection, and topical application. Although these agents are not curative, difficult lesions may be controllable for periods of time. Investigational studies for the treatment of nonmelanoma skin cancers have shown promising results. Intralesional interferon shows encouraging results (Vargo, 1991). Vitamin A or retinoic acid has been suggested as a chemopreventive agent (Loescher, 1993).

TREATMENT OF MALIGNANT MELANOMA

Most malignant melanomas are thought to have two growth phases, radial and vertical. Early melanocytic hyperplasia occurs at the epidermal-dermal junction and is characterized by horizontal growth. As the tumor becomes aggressive, it grows vertically, and it is this vertical growth that is thought to define the prognosis.

To describe the level of invasion of the melanoma as well as maximum tumor thickness, two parameters of microstaging are used (Lawler, 1991; Loescher & Booth, 1990; Longman, 1992). These two parameters are Clark's level and Breslow's level or measurement. Clark categorized malignant melanoma into five histologic levels that measure the amount of vertical growth. The first two levels involve the epidermis, the third level involves the basal cell layer, the papillary dermis, or both, the fourth level involves the reticular dermis, and the fifth level involves the subcutaneous tissue. However, skin thickness varies in different individuals and in different sites (Lawler, 1991; Loescher & Booth, 1990; Longman, 1992).

Breslow modified Clark's system to measure the vertical thickness of the melanoma in millimeters. The measurement is made from the top of the granular cell layer of the tumor to the deepest level of invasion. The range is from 0.10 mm to more than 4 mm (Lawler, 1991; Loescher & Booth, 1990; Longman, 1992).

There are currently several staging systems in use for malignant melanoma. The original system consists of three stages: (1) local disease (stage I), (2) regional nodal disease (stage II), and (3) disseminated disease (stage III). There is also the modified three-stage system, the MD Anderson Hospital Staging System, and the International Union Against Cancer (UICC) staging system. Increasingly, a four-stage system developed by the American Joint Committee on Cancer (AJCC) is being used. The system includes tumor thickness, level of invasion, and nodal involvement (see Table 43–7). It is hoped that the system will provide a more useful classification system of malignant melanoma (Balch, 1992).

TABLE 43–7. *Four-Stage System for Melanoma: AJCC*

STAGE	CRITERIA	TNM
IA	Localized melanoma, <0.75 mm, or level II*	(T1, N0, M0)
IB	Localized melanoma, 0.76 mm to 1.5 mm, or level III*	(T2, N0, M0)
IIA	Localized melanoma, 1.5 mm to 4 mm, or level IV*	(T3, N0, M0)
IIB	Localized melanoma, >4.0 mm, or level V*	(T4, N0, M0)
III	Limited nodal metastases involving only one regional lymph node basin, or <5 intransit metastases, but without nodal metastases	(Any T, N1, M0)
IV	Advanced regional metastases, or any patient with distant metastases	(Any T, any N, M1 or M2)

* When the thickness and level of invasion criteria do not coincide within a T classification, thickness should take precedence.
(From Ketcham, A. S., & Balch, C. M. [1985]. Classification and staging systems. In Balch, C. M., & Milton, G.W. [Eds.]. *Cutaneous melanoma: Clinical management and treatment results worldwide* [p. 55]. Philadelphia: J. B. Lippincott.)

Surgical excision is the mainstay of treatment for malignant melanoma. The treatment may be divided into the problems of biopsy, definitive excision, and reconstruction of the defect (Holmstrom, 1992). The diagnosis of malignant melanoma is made by an excisional biopsy, and the technique requires removal of full thickness of skin and some underlying subcutaneous fat (Loescher & Booth, 1990). Margins of 0.5 cm to 1 cm are adequate for thin lesions (Lawler, 1991). For lesions greater than 0.76 mm, margins of 1 cm to 3 cm are recommended. Large borders frequently require split-thickness grafting. Nodal dissection is advocated but remains controversial. Symptoms caused by intestinal obstruction, neurologic defects, pain, or chronic ulceration of skin nodules may be relieved by surgical resection. Surgery is also used for the palliative management of a solitary metastatic lesion. The prognosis of disseminated disease is generally poor.

The usefulness of adjuvant chemotherapy remains questionable. The most consistently active drug has been dacarbazine with response rates of 14 per cent to 30 per cent. Side effects are dose limiting. The nitrosoureas have shown some activity with response rates of 10 per cent to 18 per cent (Loescher & Booth, 1990). A variety of agents have been used and continue to be tested in clinical trials (Lawler, 1991). These include the vinca alkaloids, mephalan, cisplatin, and procarbazine. A controversial therapy is hyperthermic regional perfusion or isolated limb perfusion (Lawler, 1991). Large doses of drugs can be delivered, and melphalan (L-PAM) is the most commonly used drug. For those with metastatic melanoma, high-dose chemotherapy followed by autologous bone marrow transplant has been used. The agents that have been used are nitrogen mustard, melphalan, and carmustine. Further studies are needed to evaluate the effectiveness of this therapy.

The effectiveness of radiation therapy for the treatment of recurrent or metastatic melanoma remains questionable, as melanoma has been regarded as a radioresistant tumor. It is most effective when tumor volume is low and when a high dose per fewer fractions radiation level is used. Radiation therapy may be used for elderly patients whose lesions are not suited for surgery and for symptomatic metastases. To reduce pain and prevent pathologic fractures subsequent to bone lesions, radiation therapy is most effective.

Hormonal therapy for malignant melanoma is under investigation, as a relationship may exist between hormones and melanoma. Estrogen and progesterone receptors have been found in melanoma cells. Tamoxifen and diethylstilbestrol are two of the agents that have demonstrated some response (Lawler, 1991; Loescher & Booth, 1990).

Biotherapy or immunotherapy is being investigated in the adjuvant treatment of malignant melanoma. One of the first agents used was Calmette-Guerin bacillus; however, the treatment is now considered to have little effect. Agents being investigated are interferons, interleukins, tumor necrosis factors, monoclonal antibodies, and retinoids. The use of these agents requires further study, as no drug or combination of drugs is effective (Lawler, 1991; Loescher & Booth, 1990) (see Box 43–2).

PROGNOSIS

Skin cancers offer a unique opportunity for early detection, early diagnosis, early treatment, and cure. For basal cell carcinoma, the cure rates are equally high for either surgery or radiation therapy. Although its metastatic ability is poor, basal cell carcinoma can create extensive local spread. Acceptable cosmetic results are achieved with full-thickness skin grafts.

For squamous cell carcinoma, the recurrence of the lesion is the major complication. Surgery and radiation therapy have equally high cure rates. Follow-up visits two to four times a year are recommended.

Malignant melanoma is the most serious skin cancer, and the most important prognostic feature is the size of the lesion at the time of diagnosis and treatment. The survival rate is correlated with the depth of invasion and location of the lesion. However, the difficult and unpredictable problem of hematogenous dissemination has not been solved.

SUMMARY

Perhaps the greatest contributions nursing can make are those related to the prevention and early detection of skin cancers. Attention to the cultural implications is most important (Olsen & Frank-Stromborg, 1993). By encouraging individuals to become "sun aware," skin cancers can be recognized early (see Box

---

BOX 43–2. *Cutaneous Melanoma: Prognosis and Treatment Results Worldwide*

Balch, C. M. (1992). Cutaneous melanoma: Prognosis and treatment results worldwide. *Seminars in Surgical Oncology, 8,* 400–414.

Introduction: This report was the first metanalysis of melanoma from 14 treatment centers worldwide. It consisted of 15,798 patients with localized melanoma and 2116 stage III patients with nodal metastases. The centers contributed data in a standardized format to enable a more accurate comparison of the data.

Epidemiologic Features of Melanoma: The reporting centers had different climate conditions, latitude of residence, and mixture of ethnic groups. From the analysis it was clear that people around the world were diagnosed at an earlier stage of disease and with thinner melanomas. The analysis verified the fact that melanoma occurred predominantly in white persons. In those centers reporting data on dark-skinned persons, most of the lesions were on the feet and were thicker lesions.

Staging Systems: The three-stage classification system was discussed and the limitations noted. The new staging system developed by the American Joint Committee on Cancer was discussed. The point made was that this four-stage system provides a more useful and practical classification system for clinicians.

Prognostic Factors: For all centers, the overall prognosis for stage I and II patients was good, with an average survival rate of 79 per cent for all centers. A prognostic factors analysis for stage I and II melanoma using a multivariate analysis technique was performed by eight centers. The most significant predictive variables were (1) tumor thickness, (2) ulceration, (3) site, (4) sex, and (5) growth pattern. Six of the centers ranked ulceration among the first three most dominant factors. The site of the melanoma was a relatively more important factor for predicting the outcome of the disease. Data regarding stage III disease were compiled for 13 of the centers. Men were more likely to have stage III melanomas with thicker and more ulcerated lesions. For stage IV patients, the number and site of metastases were found to be the most dominant features.

Summary: This analysis showed consistent results from center to center despite the heterogeneity of the patient populations. Also, there continues to be significant diversity in melanoma.

43–3). Young adults in particular should be educated about the cumulative effects of prolonged sun exposure (Lawler & Schreiber, 1989; White, 1986a). The avoidance of tanning salons and sunlamps cannot be overemphasized. For older persons, the risks of skin cancers should be carefully explained. Individuals who are identified as being at high risk for malignant melanoma can reduce their chances of developing the disease with appropriate teaching and support. Skin self-examination should be taught and the procedure

verified on contacts with clients in whatever setting they are seen.

The nonmetastatic behavior of basal cell carcinoma can be carefully explained, particularly to older patients. The need for follow-up, however, must be reinforced. For those individuals with squamous cell carcinoma, periodic examinations must be conducted to evaluate the sites for potential recurrence.

For those individuals with malignant melanoma follow-up is crucial. Early and prompt treatment of reoc-

---

BOX 43–3. *Arizona Sun Awareness Project*

Southern Arizona receives one of the highest intensities of ultraviolet radiation in the United States. The sun is a mixed blessing, and people in southern Arizona are at risk for developing skin cancer because of the high sun intensity, latitude (32 N), altitude (2410 feet) and skies that are clear for more than 190 days.

The high intensity of ultraviolet radiation in southern Arizona has been confirmed with the use of a Robertson-Berger Sunburn Meter (one of 21 in the United States) under the auspices of the National Oceanic and Atmospheric Administration, which is studying ozone concentration. The meter detects solar ultraviolet radiation below 33 nm (UV-B), the response varying with decreasing wavelengths. The data produced by the meter have been termed the sunburn unit (SBU). The SBU is equal to a minimal erythema dose or the amount of UV-B radiation that will produce redness 24 hours after exposure.

The Robertson-Berger Sunburn meter at the Arizona Health Sciences Center prints the sun intensity data on paper tape every 30 minutes. The sun intensity index is reported to local newspapers and to the television stations for the weather news reports.

A sample report follows.

Sun Intensity Prediction (predictions are for untanned Caucasians, assuming no clouds)

Minutes in sun today to redden skin

Time	Minutes	Time	Minutes
9 AM	60	1 PM	19
10 AM	39	2 PM	23
11 AM	26	3 PM	31
Noon	21	4 PM	60

Data from Arizona Sun Awareness Project, University of Arizona Cancer Center.

currence is of the utmost importance. There should be an open and optimistic approach in discussing feelings and attitudes about the impact of a life-threatening illness. The nursing profession is in a unique position to deal with the public health problem of skin cancers.

REFERENCES

American Cancer Society. (1994). *Cancer facts and figures-1994.* Atlanta: Author.

Balch, C. M. (1992). Cutaneous melanoma: Prognosis and treatment results worldwide. *Seminars in Surgical Oncology, 8,* 400–414.

Bargoil, S. C., & Erdman, L. K. (1993). Safe tan: An oxymoron. *Cancer Nursing, 16,* 139–144.

Berliner, H. (1986a). Aging skin. *American Journal of Nursing, 86,* 1138–1141.

Berliner, H. (1986b). Aging skin: Part two. *American Journal of Nursing, 86,* 1259–1261.

Berwick, M., Bolognia, J. L., Heer, C., & Fine, J. A. (1991). The role of the nurse in skin cancer prevention, screening, and early detection. *Seminars in Oncology Nursing, 7,* 64–71.

Entrekin, N. M., & McMillan, S. C. (1993). Nurses' knowledge, beliefs, and practices related to cancer prevention and detection. *Cancer Nursing, 16,* 431–439.

Frank-Stromborg, M. (1986a). The role of the nurse in early detection of cancer: Population sixty-six years of age and older. *Oncology Nursing Forum, 13,* 66–74.

Frank-Stromborg, M. (1986b). The role of the nurse in cancer detection and screening. *Seminars in Oncology Nursing, 2,* 191–199.

Fraser, M. C., Hartge, P., & Tucker, M. A. (1991). Melanoma and nonmelanoma skin cancer: Epidemiology and risk factors. *Seminars in Oncology Nursing, 7,* 2–12.

Friedman, R. J., Rigel, D. S., Silverman, M. K., Kopf, A. W., & Vossaert, K. A. (1991). Malignant melanoma in the 1990s: The continued importance of early detection and the role of physician examination and self-examination of the skin. *CA-A Cancer Journal for Clinicians, 41,* 201–226.

Holmstrom, H. (1992). Surgical management of primary melanoma. *Seminars in Surgical Oncology, 8,* 366–369.

Kelly, P. P. (1991). Skin cancer and melanoma awareness campaign. *Oncology Nursing Forum, 18,* 927–931.

Lawler, P. E. (1991). Cutaneous malignant melanoma. *Seminars in Oncology Nursing, 7,* 26–35.

Lawler, P. E., & Schreiber, S. (1989). Cutaneous malignant melanoma: Nursing's role in prevention and early detection. *Oncology Nursing Forum, 16,* 345–352.

Loescher, L. J. (1993). Skin cancer prevention and detection update. *Seminars in Oncology Nursing, 9,* 184–187.

Loescher, L. J., & Booth, A. (1990). Skin cancer. In S. L. Groenwald, M. H. Frogge, M. Goodman, & C. H. Yarbro (Eds.), *Cancer nursing: Principles and practice* (2nd ed., pp. 999–1014). Boston: Jones & Bartlett Publishers, Inc.

Longman, A. (1992). Skin cancer. In J. Clark & R. McGee, (Eds.). *Core curriculum for oncology nursing* (2nd ed., pp. 488–498). Philadelphia: W. B. Saunders Co.

Olsen, S. J., & Frank-Stromborg, M. (1993). Cancer prevention and early detection in ethnically diverse populations. *Seminars in Oncology Nursing, 9,* 198–209.

Stewart, D. S. (1987). Indoor tanning: The nurse's role in preventing skin damage. *Cancer Nursing, 10,* 93–99.

Tokar, I. P., Fraser, M. C., & Bale, S. J. (1992). Genodermatoses with profound malignant potential. *Seminars in Oncology Nursing, 8,* 272–280.

Vargo, N. L. (1991). Basal and squamous cell carcinomas: An overview. *Seminars in Oncology Nursing, 7,* 13–25.

White, L. N. (1986a). Cancer prevention and detection: From twenty to sixty-five years of age. *Oncology Nursing Forum, 13,* 59–64.

White, L. N. (1986b). Cancer risk assessment. *Seminars in Oncology Nursing, 11,* 184–190.

White, L. N., & Spitz, M. R. (1993). Cancer risk and early detection assessment. *Seminars in Oncology Nursing, 9,* 188–197.

AIDS and the Spectrum of HIV Disease

Christine Grady • Bill Barrick

The acquired immunodeficiency syndrome (AIDS), resulting from infection with human immunodeficiency virus (HIV), is characterized by infections and neoplasms that are the consequence of profound immunodeficiency. AIDS represents only one end of the spectrum of HIV disease; it is the most advanced stage in a continuum of clinical and immunologic consequences of HIV infection. AIDS was first recognized in the United States in 1981. By the mid-1980s the virus had spread throughout the world as a global pandemic. Over time, it is inevitable that nurses all over the world and in all types of settings will become involved in the care of patients with HIV disease. The purpose of this chapter is to provide an overview of HIV disease for the practicing nurse. It is incumbent upon all nurses whose skills will be required by HIV-infected patients to keep pace with a rapidly evolving scientific and clinical discipline.

DEFINITION

The definition of AIDS has taken several forms for various purposes, and some confusion has arisen when these definitions are applied incorrectly. We will present both the AIDS surveillance definition and the clinical definition separately; application of a surveillance definition for purposes of clinical management may not be appropriate or useful.

The Centers for Disease Control (CDC) has revised the *surveillance* definition (also called *reporting* definition) of AIDS several times since the syndrome was first identified in 1981. Surveillance definitions detail the conditions when case information should be forwarded to agencies that collect epidemiologic data about disease (e.g., the CDC and state public health agencies). The first CDC surveillance definition defined AIDS as the documented presence of a disease that was (at least) moderately predictive of a profound immunologic defect in the absence of any other known cause for such a defect. Examples of these diseases included Kaposi's sarcoma and *Pneumocystis carinii* pneumonia, the first two clinical manifestations of HIV infection noted in the literature (CDC, 1981). With identification of the etiologic agent, development of antibody and virus testing, and advances in the understanding of the epidemiology and clinical manifestations of HIV infection, the CDC revised the surveillance definition of AIDS first in 1984, again in 1987, and again in 1992 to its current form (CDC, 1992). The surveillance definition of AIDS now includes positive and confirmed testing for anti-HIV antibody and either or both of the following: (1) the presence of specific infections or neoplasms that are associated with HIV infection (see Table 44–1), and (2) the presence of a profound CD4+ lymphopenia ($\leq$200 μL). This surveillance definition places the population in one of three epidemiologic groupings: (1) not infected, (2) infected but without features of disease, and (3) infected with features of disease. This characterization is inadequate for deciding how best to treat patients.

A clinical definition of AIDS has been somewhat elusive. Clinical definitions are used to stage and treat persons with infection or disease. Several staging schemes for HIV infection and AIDS have been presented in the literature and are in use at various institutions nationally. The most widely used are the Centers for Disease Control and Prevention classification system (CDC, 1992) and the Walter Reed HIV-1 Staging

TABLE 44–1. *Conditions Included in the 1993 AIDS Surveillance Definition*

Candidiasis of bronchi, trachea, lungs, or esophagus
Cervical cancer, invasive
Coccidiomycosis, disseminated or extrapulmonary
Crypotococcosis, extrapulmonary
Cryptosporidiosis, chronic intestinal (>1 month duration)
Cytomegalovirus disease (other than liver, spleen, or nodes)
Cytomegalovirus retinitis (with loss of vision)
Encephalopathy, HIV-related
Herpes simplex: chronic ulcer(s) or bronchitis, pneumonitis or esophagitis
Histoplasmosis, disseminated or extrapulmonary
Isosporiasis, chronic intestinal
Kaposi's sarcoma
Lymphoma, Burkitt's (or equivalent), immunoblastic (or equivalent), or primary CNS
Mycobacterium avium complex or *M. kansasii*, disseminated or extrapulmonary
Mycobacterium tuberculosis, any site (pulmonary or extrapulmonary)
Pneumocystis carinii pneumonia
Pneumonia, recurrent
Progressive multifocal leukoencephalopathy
Salmonella septicemia, recurrent
Toxoplasmosis of brain
Wasting syndrome due to HIV

TABLE 44–2. *Categories of CD4+ Lymphocyte Counts and Percentages with Interventions*

CD4+ T Cell Count/ml	CD4+ Percentage	Primary Interventions
≥600	≥29	Education. Monitor CD4+ lymphocyte counts every 6 months.
599–200	28–14	Monitor CD4+ lymphocyte counts every 3 months. Begin antiretroviral therapy if count <500/μl.
<200	<14	Begin primary prophylaxis for *Pneumocystis carinii* pneumonia. Monitor CD4+ lymphocyte counts as desired.

(From El-Sadr, W., Oleske, J. M., Agins, B. D., et al. [1994]. *Evaluation and management of early HIV infection. Clinical practice guideline no. 7.* AHCPR Pub. No. 94-0572. Rockville, MD: Agency for Health Care Policy and Research, Public Health Service, U.S. Department of Health and Human Services.)

Criteria (Redfield, Wright, & Tramont, 1986). Both classification systems are complex and awkward, and more work will be needed to develop a useful and easily understandable staging scheme. Most clinicians stage by CD4+ lymphocyte count and percentage (of total lymphocyte count) as shown in Table 44–2 (El-Sadr et al., 1994).

SCOPE

More than 400,000 cases of AIDS have been reported in the United States (CDC surveillance data 1994) and more than 1,000,000 cases have been reported worldwide (WHO, 1994). Estimates of the number of HIV infections range from 1.0 to 2.5 million in the U.S. and as many as 17 million worldwide. HIV infection has occurred in nine groups: (1) recipients of blood from infected donors; (2) hemophiliacs who received contaminated factor VIII before 1985; (3) men who have penile-rectal intercourse with infected men; (4) women who have penile-vaginal or penile-rectal intercourse with infected men; (5) men who have penile-vaginal intercourse with infected women; (6) intravenous drug users who share needles with infected individuals; (7) children born to infected mothers; (8) children breastfed from infected mothers; and (9) health care workers with occupational exposures (primarily inoculations) to infected blood.

Men are the most frequently infected persons in the United States and the developed world. In the developing world, the proportions of men and women have been approximately equal from the outset. The World Health Organization (WHO) predicts that by the year

2000 up to 40 million people will be infected worldwide, and the number of new infections globally among men and women will be equal (WHO, 1994). Rising rates of infection in women also mean higher rates in the number of children born with HIV infection. To date, the WHO estimates that more than 1 million children in the world have been infected with HIV through mother-to-child transmission. These children generally develop AIDS more rapidly than adults and often die before the age of 5 years. This chapter will focus solely on adults with HIV disease.

The U.S. population of persons with AIDS represents all ethnic groups with whites predominating numerically. However, when factoring the frequency of AIDS in each ethnic group against the representation of that ethnic group as a proportion of the U.S. population, African-American and Spanish-speaking groups show a disproportionately higher frequency of disease.

Testing of donated blood and the use of autologous blood donations have resulted in a virtually safe blood bank in the developed world, where infection by transfusion is now almost nonexistent. Infection by transfusion is still common in countries where testing of donated blood is not done.

TRANSMISSION

HIV-1 has been recovered from the blood, ejaculate, vaginal secretions, and other body fluids and tissues of infected persons and is transmitted by inoculation. The proven routes of transmission of HIV include: (1) contaminated blood products, (2) rectal intercourse, (3) vaginal intercourse, (4) contaminated needles shared by intravenous drug users, (5) organ transplant and insemination from infected donors, (6) prenatal and perinatal exposures for infants, (7) penetrating occupational injuries (e.g., needlesticks), (8) contaminated breast milk, and (9) ejaculate in the mouth.

While the nature of transmission of this bloodborne pathogen in groups exposed to blood (i.e., recipients of blood or blood products, injection drug users [IDUs], or health care workers with percutaneous injuries) is evident, the exact mode of sexual transmission is less clear. Hence, uncertainty persists in the community regarding which sexual behaviors are risky and which are not. Although a number of published case findings suggested oral transmission routes associated with fellatio (Rozenbaum, Gharakhanian, Cardon, Duval, & Coulaud, 1988; Lifson et al., 1990), large prospective epidemiologic studies have shown that HIV is transmitted sexually by penile-vaginal and penile-rectal routes, with little definitive evidence of oral transmission (Detels et al., 1989; Kingsley et al., 1987; Schechter et al., 1986). However, ejaculate or preejaculate in the mouth does have a potential risk and should not be considered "safer sex."

ETIOLOGY

The causative agent of AIDS is the human immunodeficiency virus (HIV). The virus was identified in 1983 and was shown to be causally related to AIDS in 1984. HIV belongs to the family retroviridae, subfamily lentivirus (Melnick, 1994; Palker & Riggs, 1994). Retroviruses are RNA viruses and contain an enzyme called reverse transcriptase (RT) that mediates the conversion of viral RNA to proviral DNA. The provirus integrates into the genome of the host cell and may remain latent for the life of the cell or transcribe messenger and genomic RNA to form new virus (Fauci, 1988).

INFECTION AND IMMUNOPATHOGENESIS

Although the course of HIV disease is quite variable, the typical pattern involves acute or primary infection, usually followed by a lengthy period of relative wellness (sometimes referred to as "clinical latency") that may last for years. During this period of few or no clinical symptoms there continues to be a gradual but inexorable decline in immune function in the vast majority of patients. The advanced stage of HIV disease, AIDS, is one of profound immunodeficiency and clinically apparent and ultimately fatal disease. The common denominator of HIV immunodeficiency is a significant depletion of CD4+ T cells. The mechanisms of destruction of the immune system are complex and not fully understood but likely result from both infection (virus-mediated cytopathicity) and specific and nonspecific immune responses to the infection.

HIV INFECTION OF THE IMMUNE SYSTEM

HIV infects human cells that express a CD4 surface molecule. These are predominantly CD4+ T lymphocytes (helper T cells) but also include some cells of the monocyte/macrophage group, dendritic cells, Langerhans's cells, microglial cells, and both thymic and bone marrow precursor cells (Fauci, 1988; Fauci & Lane,

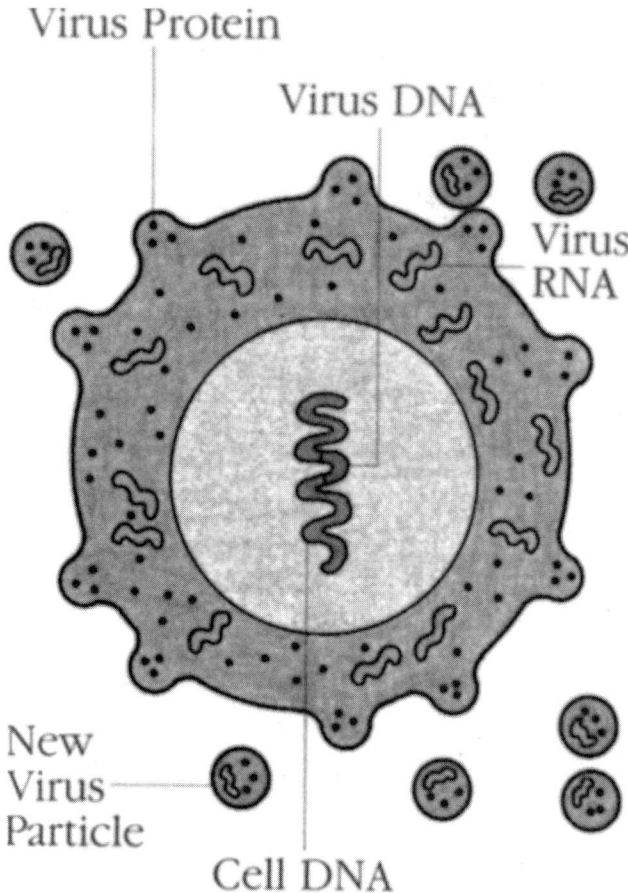

FIGURE 44–1. AIDS virus budding from infected T cell. (From U.S. Department of Health and Human Services [1988]. *Understanding the immune system*, NIH Publication No. 88-529.)

1994; Vlahov, 1989). The envelope gp120 of HIV binds avidly and specifically to the CD4 molecule, which acts as a receptor on the host cell (Fauci, 1988). The bound virus then fuses with the cell membrane and is uncoated, and HIV genomic RNA enters the cell (Ho, Pomerantz, & Kaplan, 1987). Once inside the cell, the retroviral RNA is reverse-transcribed into DNA by the polymerase reverse transcriptase (RT). The viral DNA integrates into the cellular genome in the nucleus as "provirus" (Rosenberg & Fauci, 1989). Under certain circumstances DNA may remain unintegrated in the cell cytoplasm. Chronic low-level replication of HIV may follow, although some infected cells remain latent (i.e., no HIV expression). Activation of an infected cell causes accelerated HIV replication. The cell remains infected for its lifetime and throughout the processes of normal cell division generates progeny cells that also contain proviral DNA (Fauci, 1988; Ho et al., 1987) (see Fig. 44–1).

CD4 CELL DEPLETION

The immunopathogenic mechanisms of HIV probably involve both direct and indirect means by which the virus causes progressive dysfunction and depletion of the CD4+ T cell repertoire (Pantaleo, Graziosi, & Fauci, 1993). A cell may remain infected with little or no viral expression for a variable length of time, usually years (Pantaleo et al., 1993). Ultimately, the infected cell will be destroyed through a number of mechanisms, which may include destruction of the cell wall by newly synthesized budding virus, accumulation of unintegrated viral DNA, inhibition of cellular protein synthesis, syncytia formation, apoptosis (a kind of programmed cell death), and other mechanisms (Fauci & Lane, 1994; Fauci, Schnittman, Poli, Koenig, & Pantaleo, 1991). Probably as important are immune-mediated mechanisms of cell destruction (Fauci, 1993). *Uninfected* cells may also be destroyed through syncytia formation or apoptosis (Pantaleo et al., 1993). Syncytia are formed when viral proteins expressed on the surface of an infected cell allow it to fuse to the cell membranes of uninfected cells, forming a multinucleated giant cell. Uninfected CD4+ and possibly CD8+ T cells and B cells may also be destroyed through apoptosis (Pantaleo et al., 1993). Apoptosis is likely a reflection of the state of heightened cellular activation in HIV disease. Over time the CD4 + T cell population is steadily depleted.

Besides a decline in the *number* of CD4+ lymphocytes, HIV infection causes abnormalities in the *function* of T cells, B cells, and macrophages. Many of these abnormalities are detectable before clinical symptoms of HIV disease appear (Lane, et al., 1985), and the degree of dysfunction increases as the disease progresses (Fauci & Lane, 1994). Perhaps the most important T cell functional defect is the loss of memory cell response to specific antigen (such as tetanus toxoid) (Lane et al., 1985). A CD4+ T cell that is unresponsive to specific antigen cannot perform its normal function of inducing or regulating an immune response. Abnormalities in other components of the immune response are at least in part a consequence of this CD4+ T cell defect (Rosenberg & Fauci, 1989). The B cell hyperactivity characteristic of HIV disease is due in part to faulty regulation by HIV-infected CD4+ T cells. Hypergammaglobulinemia and circulating immune complexes are a result of this heightened B cell activity. Despite high levels of circulating immunoglobulin, specific antibody response to antigen is impaired, most likely contributing to the frequent bacterial infections seen in advanced HIV disease (Fauci & Lane, 1994). Macrophage function is also deficient in HIV infection, and this contributes to the susceptibility to certain parasitic and other intracellular infections. Additionally, infected macrophages may release tissue-damaging cytokines into surrounding tissues (such as in the brain) and may serve as an important reservoir for HIV infection (Fauci & Lane, 1994; Meltzer et al., 1990). Although HIV-specific CD8+ cytolytic T cells are evident early in infection, their functional capability is lost as the disease progresses (Fauci & Lane, 1994.

The progressive deficiencies in CD4+ T lymphocytes are the primary feature of the immunodeficiency that eventually leads to clinical disease. When the CD4+ T cell count falls below a certain level (>200 cells per μL), the infected individual is at high risk of developing a variety of opportunistic diseases and other AIDS-defining illnesses.

IMMUNE RESPONSE TO HIV

An impressive and appropriate humoral and cell-mediated immune response to HIV usually occurs during primary HIV infection following initial exposure to virus. The vast majority of infected individuals produce detectable antibody to most of the major viral proteins (gp120, gp160, gp41, and p24) within 3 to 12 weeks after exposure (Zunich & Lane, 1991). Strong cytotoxic activity against HIV has also been demonstrated in vitro (Zunich & Lane, 1991). Initially the immune responses suppress HIV replication and markedly decrease measurable plasma viremia. Unfortunately, the immune response ultimately proves to be ineffective in suppressing virus replication, since the vast majority of infected individuals go on to develop clinical disease. In fact, the chronic activation of the immune system in response to HIV probably has an overall negative effect by providing an environment for viral replication (virus spreads rapidly among activated cells) and by the inappropriate production of inflammatory cytokines (such as TNF-α) that can enhance viral expression (Fauci, 1993).

DIAGNOSTIC METHODS OF MEASURING INFECTION AND IMMUNE FUNCTION

Tests that detect the presence and activity of HIV provide critical information to clinicians and researchers and serve to keep the nation's blood supply safe. The most commonly employed tests used to detect HIV actually measure antibody to the virus. A person found to definitively have antibody to HIV is considered infected and infectious. Laboratory evidence for HIV, usually in the form of a positive antibody test, is part of the CDC surveillance case definition for AIDS (CDC, 1992). The CDC recommends that HIV antibody testing always be done with the individual's informed consent and with pretest and posttest counseling (CDC, 1988). The most widely used antibody test to detect HIV is an enzyme-linked immunosorbent assay (ELISHA or EIA), which was initially developed for screening blood before transfusion. The HIV ELISA is a very sensitive test, and the predictive value depends on the seroprevalence in the population being tested (Grady & Vogel, 1993; Saag, 1992). Its specificity is highest in populations with high seroprevalence. Because of the sensitivity of the assay and the possibility of false-positives, it is recommended that a positive or reactive ELISA be repeated and then confirmed by a more specific antibody test (CDC, 1989). The most widely used confirmatory test for HIV antibody is the Western blot analysis. Unlike the ELISA, which detects antibody to the whole virus, the Western blot identifies antibodies to the individual structural components of the virus. The Western blot is considered positive if bands are found that correspond to two or more of the

TABLE 44–3. *Diagnostic Tests for HIV Detection and Disease Monitoring*

HIV Antibody Tests	Tests for Virus	Immune Function and Disease Progression
ELISA/EIA Western blot analysis Immunofluorescence	p24 antigen assay co-culture of peripheral blood mononuclear cells* plasma viremia as determined by culture, RT-PCR, quantitative competitive PCR or branched DNA assays* DNA-PCR or RNA-PCR to determine viral burden or replication*	CBC with differential CD4+ lymphocyte count and percentage Total immunoglobulins In vitro tests of lymphocyte and monocyte function Intradermal skin testing β-2-microglobulin Neopterin

*Used for research purposes.

gp120/160, gp41, or p24 components of HIV (Davey & Lane, 1990).

Direct determination of the presence and quantity of virus has been more of a challenge. Tests used to detect virus are primarily used in research laboratories and to evaluate the effectiveness of investigational antiviral therapies. The sensitivity of the p24 antigen capture assay, which measures serum p24, ranges from as low as 4 per cent in asymptomatic seropositive individuals to about 70 per cent in patients with AIDS (Harry, Jennings, Yee, & Carlson, 1989). Early in HIV infection there is a sudden rise in the level of p24 antigen. As the individual forms functional HIV (anti-p24) antibody, the level of measurable serum p24 drops. It has recently been shown that the initial burst of virus seeds multiple lymph nodes. Considerable amounts of virus and persistent viral replication are detected in the lymph nodes and other lymphoid organs during the time viral antigen is low or undetectable in serum and the infected person is clinically well (Pantaleo et al., 1993). As HIV disease progresses, p24 antigen again becomes measurable in the serum. Spikes in p24 titers or new detection of p24 antigen in an individual who was previously p24 antigen negative may be an important indication of the need to initiate or change therapy, since persons with measurable p24 antigen progress to clinical disease or AIDS faster than those with no detectable p24 antigen (Fauci & Lane, 1994). Direct culture of virus from either plasma or peripheral blood cells is also possible, although cumbersome. Cultures are maintained for a 28-day period, during which time reverse transcriptase or p24 antigen is measured in culture supernatant and cultures are observed for syncytia formation (Davey & Lane, 1990). Polymerase chain reaction (PCR) is a highly sensitive procedure by which the genetic material of a cell is amplified multiple times to detect HIV proviral DNA or RNA. Recently, standard RT-PCR, quantitative competitive PCR, and branched DNA assays have been used to quantify viral load (Dewar et al., 1994). These tests, originally used for only research purposes, have been recently used to make patient decisions about the initiation or changing of antiretroviral therapy. PCR is also useful for studying viral sequence diversity and resistance to antiretrovirals (Fauci & Lane, 1994). Newer tests such as in situ PCR to detect and quantify proviral and replicating virus are currently being investigated.

In addition, laboratory tests that evaluate immune function or serve as surrogate markers of disease progression are important in the evaluation and monitoring of HIV disease (see Table 44–3). An *immune profile* is a group of tests that can be used to monitor the degree of immunodeficiency and thereby help to predict clinical events and determine appropriate therapies. An immune profile usually includes a complete blood cell count (CBC) with white blood cell differentiation, number and percentage of CD4+ T4 lymphocytes, quantitative immunoglobulins, *in vitro* tests of lymphocyte and monocyte function, and sometimes intradermal skin testing with common antigens. CBC and differential may be normal in early HIV disease and show a pronounced lymphopenia in advanced HIV disease. Quantification of CD4+ T cells correlates best with clinical course and is therefore currently accepted as the most reliable indicator of progression of HIV disease. The gradual depletion of CD4+ T lymphocytes can leave persons with advanced HIV disease with as few as 5 to 10 CD4+ T cells per μL or 1 to 2 per cent of their lymphocyte pool (normal range 600 to 1200 cells per μL and ≥40 per cent). Total immunoglobulin levels, especially of IgG, are usually elevated in HIV infection. *In vitro* tests usually indicate abnormalities in the function of both lymphocytes and monocytes (see above). Intradermal skin testing with common antigens reveals a high frequency of anergy (no response), especially in advanced disease. Studies have shown that two other markers, β-2-microglobulin and serum neopterin, can correlate with clinical stage of HIV disease (Davey & Lane, 1990; Hofman et al., 1990). Because both are nonspecific markers of immune activation, CD4+ cell counts are believed to be better indicators of disease progression (Davey & Lane, 1990; Saag, 1992). In fact, frequently the only test used for clinical decision making is the CD4+ T cell count; however, some of these other tests will likely become more reliable, available, and useful in the next few years (Saag, 1992).

CLINICAL SPECTRUM OF HIV DISEASE

The clinical spectrum of HIV disease is broad and variable. The majority of infected persons experience an acute syndrome associated with primary infection.

This is usually followed by an extended period of relative wellness (mean time approximately 10 years) with few or no clinical symptoms. Finally, increasingly complex clinical symptoms and secondary opportunistic diseases invariably occur in advanced disease. During each phase of HIV disease, individual needs for clinical assessment and management should be evaluated. The nurse's role in assessment and treatment is critical, and therefore thorough information about the clinical and immunologic processes at each stage of HIV disease is essential to HIV nursing practice.

PRIMARY INFECTION

The majority of HIV-infected individuals (50 to 70 per cent) experience an acute syndrome about 3 to 6 weeks after infection with HIV that gradually subsides in a week or two as an immune response develops and seroconversion occurs (Fauci & Lane, 1994). This acute syndrome varies in severity and may include fever, pharyngitis with oral ulcerations, lymphadenopathy, headache, arthralgias/myalgias, lethargy and malaise, anorexia, nausea, vomiting, and diarrhea. Less commonly meningitis, encephalitis, and maculopapular rash may be seen (Tindall, Imrie, Donovan, Penny, & Cooper, 1992). Most individuals recover spontaneously. The number of CD4+ T cells often drops dramatically during this period but usually rebounds to near normal levels.

EARLY HIV DISEASE

Following primary HIV infection, most infected individuals experience an extended period during which time clinical symptoms are few or nonexistent. This has often been referred to as the asymptomatic or clinically latent stage. It is critical that during this time individuals have access to comprehensive primary care and periodic evaluation of their immune status. According to guidelines recently developed by the Agency for Health Care Policy and Research (AHCPR, 1994), evaluation should begin with a complete medical, sexual, and substance abuse history, a thorough physical examination, CD4+ T cell determination, and screening for *M. tuberculosis* and syphilis. Periodic clinical monitoring should include complete oral and eye examinations. Monitoring of CD4+ T cell count should be done every 6 months, and antiretroviral treatment and prophylaxis of *Pneumocystis carinii* pneumonia should be initiated when appropriate (see Fig. 44–2). Although symptoms during this period may not be severe or persistent enough to be classified as AIDS-defining constitutional disease, symptoms such as fatigue and depression are quite common and can interfere with daily activities and life quality.

CONSTITUTIONAL SYMPTOMS AND SIGNS

As time goes on and immune function continues to decline, infected individuals begin to experience more persistent and severe symptoms. Patients may experience fatigue, anorexia, weight loss, diarrhea, and night sweats with or without fever. Some of these symptoms are associated with minor or occult opportunistic diseases, while others are believed to be a direct effect of HIV infection. One common finding is generalized lymphadenopathy (lymph nodes >1 cm in two or more extrainguinal sites for more than 3 months). HIV lymphadenopathy in which lymph nodes are discrete and moveable is generally distinguishable from lymphadenopathy associated with Kaposi's sarcoma or lymphoma by the absence of other systemic signs and symptoms (i.e., fever, weight loss). Oral candidiasis (thrush), hairy leukoplakia, and aphthous ulcers are common early clinical findings in progressing HIV disease. Thrush responds well to treatment with local antifungal agents. If symptoms or discomfort are reported with hairy leukoplakia or aphthous ulcers, symptomatic treatment should be initiated. Thrombocytopenia has been seen in some patients as an early manifestation of HIV. Thrombocytopenia may be picked up as an incidental finding on CBC or can present as bleeding of the gums, petechiae of the extremities, or easy bruisability. When other causes of thrombocytopenia are ruled out, HIV-associated thrombocytopenia usually responds well to treatment with the antiretroviral drug Zidovudine. Sometimes intravenous immunoglobulins or corticosteroids are needed. In the past, signs and symptoms such as unexplained weight loss, diarrhea, night sweats, and fever were included under a broad category previously referred to as AIDS-Related Complex (ARC). Many of these symptoms are now being diagnosed as specific opportunistic infections; therefore, a thorough workup of unexplained signs and symptoms is always in order.

AIDS-DEFINING ILLNESSES

In advanced HIV disease, when immune function has been significantly compromised (CD4+ T cells of <200 per mm), secondary opportunistic diseases, which include opportunistic infections and neoplasms, begin to appear. Many of these diseases are AIDS-defining according to the CDC surveillance definition of AIDS. These diseases are described in Table 44–4 with notes on intervention and outcome (Drew, Buhles, & Erlich, 1992; Gallant, Moore, & Chaisson, 1994; Jacobson, 1992; Kaplan & Northfelt, 1992; Saah et al., 1994; Sarosi, 1992; Stansell & Sande, 1992; Ungvarski, 1992; Worley & Price, 1992). Opportunistic infections (OIs) are caused by a variety of primarily ubiquitous pathogens that rarely cause disease in persons with intact immune systems. Although effective treatments have been developed for several OIs, most require chronic therapy or secondary prophylaxis to prevent recurrence (see Table 44–4). Because of severe immunodeficiency, people with AIDS often experience more than one OI concurrently, infection in multiple body organs or systems, disseminated infections that are severe and difficult to treat, or a combination. HIV-related malignancies tend to be aggressive, resulting in significant morbidity and mortality. While cutaneous Ka-

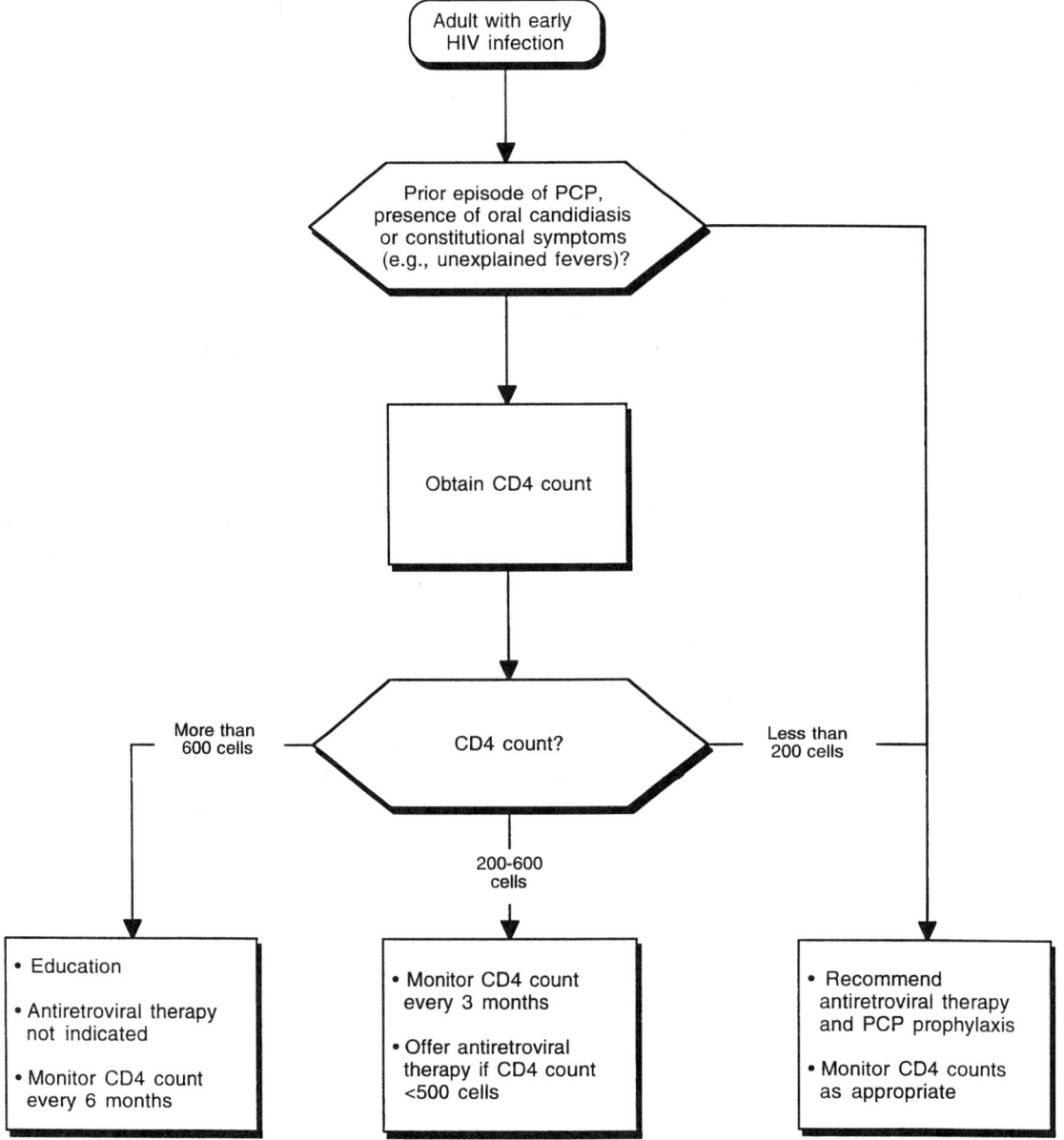

FIGURE 44–2. Evaluation for initiation of antiretroviral therapy and PCP prophylaxis. (Adapted from Agency for Health Care Policy and Research [1994]. *Evaluation and management of early HIV infection.* AHCPR Publication No. 94-0572.)

posi's sarcoma responds to treatment, especially in those with more intact immune systems, lymphomas seen in HIV-infected individuals are usually more resistant to therapy. The incidence of allergic reactions to and intolerance of antimicrobial drugs are also very high in HIV-infected individuals (Ungvarski, 1992). Multisystem disease and complex treatment regimens present a genuine nursing challenge.

OTHER CLINICAL PROBLEMS

Besides its impact on the immune system, which leads to susceptibility to opportunistic disease, HIV also appears to directly affect other organ systems such as the neurologic, gastrointestinal (GI), renal, endocrine, dermatologic, and cardiac systems. In addition

to HIV encephalopathy or AIDS dementia complex (ADC) (as described in Table 44–4), peripheral neuropathies and vacuolar myelopathy are found in HIV-infected persons (Worley & Price, 1992). The GI tract is a major target for HIV disease, with the etiology likely to be multifactorial. GI dysfunction may be caused by OIs, neoplasms, and the adverse effects of medications, but when these are ruled out, there appears to exist an HIV enteropathy of uncertain etiology (Cello, 1992). HIV-associated nephropathy has been described and occurs primarily in intravenous drug-using African-American males (O'Regan, Russo, LaPointe, & Rousseau, 1990). A range of endocrinopathies, including pituitary, thyroid, and adrenal, have been documented in HIV disease. Although most of the endocrine pathology is associated

TABLE 44-4. Clinical Manifestations in Advanced HIV Disease

CLASS	PROBLEM	CD4 COUNT	DIAGNOSTICS	SIGNS/SYMPTOMS	MEDICAL AND NURSING MANAGEMENT
AIDS defining not otherwise classified	AIDS dementia complex (ADC)	☐ Undetermined ☒ <50 ☒ 50–100 ☐ 101–200 ☐ >200	Neuropsychiatric testing; imaging; culture and cytology of the CSF to rule out other causes.	Global, nonfocal cognitive, motor, or behavioral changes consistent with encephalitis or encephalopathy that may progress to vegetative state requiring total care.	Conventional dose antiretroviral therapy (ART), usually zidovudine or didanosine or both. High-dose ART is currently investigational. Palliative care: pain management, sedation as needed, advancing to total care. Safety management. Skin care. Management of other symptoms as appropriate. **Outcome** Prognosis is usually poor and death following a vegetative state occurs within weeks or months.
AIDS defining not otherwise classified	Wasting syndrome	☐ Undetermined ☒ <50 ☒ 50–100 ☐ 101–200 ☐ >200	Clinical observation; nutritional assessment to include anthropometrics and diet; diagnostic testing, imaging, culture, and cytology to rule out other causes.	Weight loss in excess of 10% of baseline and including either chronic diarrhea, anorexia, or weakness and fever.	Management of nausea, vomiting and diarrhea. Nutritional counseling and individualized plans for nutrition. Management of emotional problems associated with changing body image and decreased energy. Megestrol to enhance appetite and intake. Merinol for nausea and weight loss. Some community providers are trying testosterone by injection or transdermal patch. **Outcome** Highly variable and dependent on individual response to intervention. Median survival in one study was 16 months.
Neoplasm	Cervical cancer	☒ Undetermined ☐ <50 ☐ 50–100 ☐ 101–200 ☐ >200	Pelvic examination; cytology by Papanicolaou smear (PAP); colposcopy with biopsy followed by conization as required to establish the diagnosis.	Pain, discharge and bleeding may be associated with later stage disease but early disease is rarely symptomatic.	Surgery, radiation, and chemotherapy as appropriate to tumor staging. Management of symptoms associated with treatment. Management of alterations in coping. **Outcome** Variable and based on individual response to treatment.
Neoplasm	Kaposi's sarcoma	☐ Undetermined ☒ <50 ☒ 50–100 ☒ 101–200 ☒ >200	Clinical examination; endoscopic examination; histology.	Cutaneous: palpable, firm, hyperpigmented, irregular non-painful lesions or nodules. Visceral: site-dependent and may include pain, fluid retention, anasarca, cough and dyspnea, dysphagia and odynophagia, bleeding.	Radiation for discretely localized lesions. Antineoplastics or interferon-α for generalized disease. Management of pain, skin integrity, emotional distress, and other symptoms associated with site and severity. **Outcome** Dependent on site, severity, and CD4+ lymphocyte count. Median survival in one study was 18 months.
Neoplasm	Non-Hodgkin's lymphoma, CNS	☐ Undetermined ☒ <50 ☐ 50–100 ☐ 101–200 ☐ >200	Clinical examination; biopsy and histology.	Headache, confusion, seizures and focal neurologic deficits.	Irradiation and combination chemotherapy. Management of pain, cognitive or motor changes including confusion and seizure, emotional distress, patient safety from injury (especially falls), and side effects of chemotherapy. **Outcome** Relapse is common and prognosis poor. Median survival in several studies for all NHL was between 2 and 5 months.

Continued on following page.

TABLE 44–4. *Clinical Manifestations in Advanced HIV Disease* Continued

CLASS	PROBLEM	CD4 COUNT	DIAGNOSTICS	SIGNS/SYMPTOMS	MEDICAL AND NURSING MANAGEMENT
Neoplasm	Non-Hodgkin's lymphoma, not CNS	□ Undetermined ☒ <50 ☒ 50–100 ☒ 101–200 ☒ >200	Clinical examination; histology.	Site-dependent, can occur almost anywhere.	Irradiation and combination chemotherapy. Management of pain, fever, emotional distress, side effects of chemotherapy, and other symptoms associated with site and severity. **Outcome** Relapse is common and prognosis variable. Survival depends largely on site, morphologic subtype, and CD4+ lymphocyte count. Median survival in several studies was 4 to 7 months.
OI: Bacterial	*Mycobacterium avium intracellulare (Mycobacterium avium* complex [MAI or MAC])	□ Undetermined ☒ <50 ☒ 50–100 □ 101–200 □ >200	Cultures of blood, bone marrow or other body fluids.	Fever, malaise, weight loss, night sweats, increased alkaline phosphatase.	Clarithromycin or azithromycin for documented disease, often in combination with one or more other antimycobacterial drugs. Rifabutin approved for prophylaxis; clarithromycin and azithromycin (investigational) are in wide community use. Management of fever, nutrition, fatigue, safety (especially falls), and other symptoms associated with severity and duration of infection. **Outcome** Response to antibiotics is variable. Median survival in one study was 10.44 months (MACs). More time will be required to determine if recently approved agents will extend survival.
OI: Bacterial	*Mycobacterium tuberculosis* (MTB)	□ Undetermined ☒ <50 ☒ 50–100 ☒ 101–200 ☒ >200	Intradermal antigen testing (PPD), chest x-ray, and culture.	Productive cough, fever, weight loss, and other constitutional symptoms. Although pulmonary TB is most common, high frequency of extrapulmonary TB is seen in HIV infection and disease.	Particulate mask protection is indicated for patient-contact personnel during period of infectiousness. Initial treatment includes isoniazid (INH), rifampin, pyrizinamide +/- ethambutol. In areas where multidrug-resistant tuberculosis (MDR-TB) has been documented, multidrug regimens must be individualized. Management of respiratory distress, cough and fever. Management of other symptoms associated with extrapulmonary infection. **Outcome** Depends most of all on compliance with medication regimens. Survival post INH-sensitive MTB is better than survival post MDR-TB.
OI: Fungal	Coccidioidomycosis	□ Undetermined ☒ <50 ☒ 50–100 ☒ 101–200 □ >200	Culture, serology or biopsy; sometimes requiring several iterations to recover; critical to differentiate from *Pneumocystis carinii* pneumonia.	Presentation is very similar to *Pneumocystis carinii* pneumonia. Shortness of breath, fever and anorexia. Symptoms are variable and early disease may present with subtle and ambiguous signs and symptoms.	Amphotericin-B or fluconazole for treatment and fluconazole for secondary prophylaxis. Management of shortness of breath, fever and anorexia. **Outcome** Disseminates rapidly untreated, prognosis fair with current treatment regimens.

Type	Disease	CD4 Count	Clinical Presentation	Diagnosis	Management / Outcome
OI: Fungal	Cryptococcosis	☐ Undetermined ☒ <50 ☒ 50–100 ☐ 101–200 ☐ >200	Headache, fever, mental status changes, other nonfocal neurologic deficits. May disseminate to almost any organ system with signs and symptoms dependent on site.	India ink test of cerebral-spinal fluid; cryptococcal antigen in CSF, urine, and blood.	Primary treatment by induction with amphotericin-B and maintenance with fluconazole. Secondary prophylaxis with fluconazole. Primary prophylaxis with fluconazole is successful but remains controversial. Management of headache, cognitive changes including confusion, patient safety (especially falls) and side effects of therapy with amphotericin-B. **Outcome** Median survival is 13.2 months (MACs) and may improve with more current therapy.
OI: Fungal	Esophageal candidiasis	☐ Undetermined ☒ <50 ☒ 50–100 ☒ 101–200 ☐ >200	Retrosternal pain or burning, dysphagia, odynophagia, anorexia, taste changes. Esophageal candidiasis may be preceded by less severe candidial infections including but not limited to oral and vaginal sites. Conventional anti-fungal therapy is standard of care.	Esophageal examination; KOH-prep; histology.	Ketoconazole, fluconazole or itraconazole may be used for treatment. Use of fluconazole or itraconazole for secondary prophylaxis is becoming increasingly controversial because of issues of compliance, resistance, drug interactions and ease of diagnosis and treatment. Management of pain and emotional distress. Optimization of diet for weight maintenance and comfort. **Outcome** Response to treatment is variable and probably dependent on the degree of immune compromise and resistance to drugs. Median survival in one study was 15.84 months.
OI: Fungal	Histoplasmosis	☐ Undetermined ☒ <50 ☒ 50–100 ☒ 101–200 ☐ >200	Fever, wasting, and shortness of breath, sometimes progressing rapidly to a septic shock-like picture. Disseminated intravascular coagulation (DIC) is often seen in severe cases.	Serodiagnosis by histoplasma polysaccharide antigen is highly reliable but currently available through only one laboratory; culture and histology; bone marrow examination.	Amphotericin-B for acute treatment or induction followed by itraconazole for maintenance and secondary prophylaxis. Management of symptoms associated with amphotericin-B. Management of fever, wasting, respiratory symptoms, and other symptoms of dissemination. **Outcome** Generally responds to antifungal therapy, although duration of treatment may be extensive.
OI: Protozoal	Cryptosporidiosis	☐ Undetermined ☒ <50 ☒ 50–100 ☐ 101–200 ☐ >200	Severe diarrhea up to 50 times per day. Abdominal cramping, dehydration, weight loss, biliary obstruction, nausea/vomiting, fever, and electrolyte imbalance.	Modified acid fast bacillus (AFB) stain or IFA on stool (must be specially requested in most hospitals); immunofluorescent assay may also be used.	No effective treatment has been documented. Paramomycin has shown limited efficacy in a small series of patients. Azithromycin is currently investigational but failures have been reported. Management of dysnutrition and hypovolemia with antidiarrheals and hydration. Management of emotional consequences of changing body image, decreased energy, and compromises in personal hygiene. **Outcome** Median survival in one study was 22.92 months.

Continued on following page.

TABLE 44–4. *Clinical Manifestations in Advanced HIV Disease* Continued

CLASS	PROBLEM	CD4 COUNT	DIAGNOSTICS	SIGNS/SYMPTOMS	MEDICAL AND NURSING MANAGEMENT
OI: Protozoal	Microsporidio-sis	☐ Undetermined ☒ <50 ☐ 50–100 ☐ 101–200 ☐ >200	Electron microscopy of bowel biopsy or stool smear.	Severe diarrhea up to 50 times per day. Abdominal cramping, dehydration, weight loss, nausea/vomiting, fever, and electrolyte imbalance.	Albendazole and atovaquone are currently investigational. Management of dysnutrition and hypovolemia with antidiarrheals and hydration. Management of emotional consequences of changing body image, decreased energy, and compromises in personal hygiene. **Outcome** Undetermined but probably similar to cryptosporidiosis.
OI: Protozoal	*Pneumocystis carinii* pneumonia (PCP)	☐ Undetermined ☒ <50 ☒ 50–100 ☒ 101–200 ☐ >200	Sputum and bronchoalveolar lavage stain.	Fevers, shortness of breath, and nonproductive cough.	Primary therapy with trimethoprim-sulfamethoxazole (TMP-Sulfa) or pentamidine isethionate. Trimethoprim/dapsone may be used in mild cases. Addition of steroids is recommended for more severe cases. TMP-Sulfa is used for both primary and secondary prophylaxis. Dapsone or aerosolized pentamidine isethionate (via Respigard II delivery system) may be used for prophylaxis if TMP/Sulfa is not tolerated. Combination prophylaxis with dapsone and pyrimethamine may also provide protection against toxoplasmosis. Management of fever and respiratory symptoms. **Outcome** Median survival in one study was 18.6 months.
OI: Protozoal	Toxoplasmosis	☐ Undetermined ☒ <50 ☐ 50–100 ☐ 101–200 ☐ >200	CT or MRI to establish presumptive diagnosis; biopsy and histology to confirm.	Fever, headache, confusion, focal deficits, seizures.	Pyrimethamine and sulfadiazine with leucovorin, or clindamycin and pyrimethamine with leucovorin usually follows characteristic CT or MRI findings. Secondary prophylaxis with same drugs. Management of fever, headache, altered mental status, and other neurologic symptoms. **Outcome** Median survival in one study was 10.44 months.
OI: Viral	CMV, other sites distinct from retinitis	☐ Undetermined ☒ <50 ☐ 50–100 ☐ 101–200 ☐ >200	Cytology of biopsied specimens.	Esophagitis, colitis, adrenalitis, pneumonitis, encephalitis, or hepatitis.	Ganciclovir or foscarnet for primary treatment and secondary prophylaxis. Primary prophylaxis with oral ganciclovir is investigational. Management of symptoms associated with site and severity.

Category	Condition	CD4 count	Diagnosis	Symptoms	Treatment / Outcome
OI: Viral	CMV retinitis	□ Undetermined ☒ <50 □ 50–100 □ 101–200 □ >200	Physical findings on ophthalmologic examination.	Visual cuts or blurred vision.	Ganciclovir or foscarnet for primary treatment and secondary prophylaxis. Primary prophylaxis with oral ganciclovir is investigational. Ganciclovir implants (investigational). **Outcome** Prognosis poor possibly due to coexisting morbidities. Extension arrested in 50% of cases. Any vision loss is generally permanent. Relapses occur even on secondary prophylaxis. Median survival in one study was 9.72 months.
OI: Viral	Herpes simplex—persistent	□ Undetermined ☒ <50 ☒ 50–100 □ 101–200 ☒ >200	Characteristic lesions; culture of surface scrapings or biopsy.	Painful erythematous sometimes vesicular oral, genital, rectal, or disseminated cutaneous lesions.	Acyclovir for acute treatment and secondary prophylaxis. Primary prophylaxis with acyclovir is increasingly common but not validated by clinical study. Foscarnet is indicated in strains with proven resistance to acyclovir. Management of pain. Wound care and maintenance of personal hygiene. Management of emotional problems associated with changing body image. **Outcome** Acyclovir sensitive strains usually resolve completely. Acyclovir resistant strains require treatment with foscarnet with greater than 90% resolution.
OI: Viral	Progressive multifocal leukoencephalopathy (PML)	□ Undetermined □ <50 ☒ 50–100 □ 101–200 □ >200	Biopsy.	Focal neurologic deficits, and headache.	No treatment of proven efficacy. Management of symptoms as they arise. **Outcome** Prognosis poor, usually seen in end-stage disease.
OI: Viral	Varicella zoster; cutaneous, disseminated	□ Undetermined □ <50 ☒ 50–100 ☒ 101–200 ☒ >200 ×	Examination; culture.	Cutaneous: dermatomal distribution of painful vesicular lesions. VZV may rarely disseminate to lung, liver, and CNS.	Acyclovir for acute treatment. Secondary prophylaxis may be used if episodes are frequent and painful. Foscarnet is indicated in strains with proven resistance to acyclovir. Management of pain. Skin care and maintenance of personal hygiene. Management of emotional problems associated with changing body image. **Outcome** Cutaneous: depends on response to treatment, generally good outcome.

with OIs or neoplasms, some has occurred early in HIV disease (Stansell, 1992). Cardiac disease is an infrequent clinical problem in HIV; however, abnormalities have been found in the majority of patients either at autopsy or by invasive exploration (Acierno, 1989). If effective therapy for noncardiac disease continues to improve, cardiac disease, particularly myocarditis and myopathy, may become more prevalent (Stansell, 1992). Dermatologic problems such as psoriasis, various rashes, and dry skin are also quite common and are usually first recognized by the nurse.

MANAGEMENT OF HIV INFECTION

Scientific information about the nature, life cycle, and pathogenesis of HIV has provided a valuable foundation for the development of appropriate therapies and vaccines. Medical treatment of a person with HIV disease involves several critical strategies including specific antiretroviral and other antimicrobial therapy, prophylaxis, treatment of symptoms, counseling, education, and emotional and social support. A major management priority is prevention, early detection, and adequate treatment of the opportunistic diseases and symptoms that arise throughout the course of HIV, especially in advanced disease. Current treatment research is focusing on finding better antiretroviral drugs, prophylaxes, and therapies for OIs as well as finding effective ways of restoring or reconstituting the damaged immune system.

TREATMENT AND PROPHYLAXIS OF OPPORTUNISTIC INFECTIONS

Improved methods of preventing and treating opportunistic infections as well as earlier detection have contributed to enhanced survival and quality of life for persons with HIV disease. Recommended treatment for OIs is found in Table 44–4.

Prophylaxis for *Pneumocystis carinii* pneumonia (PCP) is recommended for anyone with fewer than 200 CD4+ T cells per µL (AHCPR, 1994); trimethoprim-sulfamethoxazole is the preferred regimen (see Table 44–4). For those who cannot tolerate trimethoprim-sulfa, alternatives include aerosolized pentamidine, clindamycin, and atovaquone. Isoniazid (INH) prophylaxis is recommended for any HIV-infected person with a positive PPD skin test. Primary prophylaxis for MAI with Clarithromycin or Azithromycin is increasingly being used, although this approach is still investigational. Primary prophylaxes for toxoplasmosis, cryptococcosis, candidiasis, and cytomegalovirus infections are currently under investigation.

Secondary prophylaxis, the prevention of recurrence of infection, is recommended for almost all HIV-related OIs (see Table 44–4). Without chronic therapy, recurrence of infection is quite common.

Community and research health professionals are increasingly concerned by the possibility that current and future prophylaxis regimens may induce resistant forms of microbes. Because of this concern published recommendations for prophylactic regimens will likely change over time. Until more is known, many providers will individualize prophylaxis based on this and other concerns.

Because of the multitude of medications that may be recommended for an HIV-infected person, especially in advanced disease, careful monitoring for side effects and drug interactions is crucial. Educating the individual about the proper administration of medications and possible side effects to be aware of as well as periodic review of the same is an important part of nursing care.

ANTIRETROVIRAL THERAPY

Suppression of HIV with antiretroviral drugs is important in enhancing the quality and length of a person's life. Currently there are four FDA-approved antiretrovirals for the treatment of HIV infection: Zidovudine (ZDV, formerly azidothymidine or AZT), Didanosine (ddI), Zalcitabine (ddC), and Stavudine (D4T). All four are nucleoside analogues that act by inhibiting viral reverse transcriptase and terminating the formation of the DNA chain. Although there are still questions about the most appropriate time to start antiretroviral therapy and the optimal dose, current recommendations for initiating therapy are based on immune status, specifically CD4+ T cell count. Antiviral therapy should be deferred for asymptomatic HIV-infected persons with greater than 500 CD4+ T cells per µL (El-Sadr et al., 1994; Sande, Carpenter, Cobbs, Holmes, & Sanford, 1993). Zidovudine (500 mg divided daily dose) should be considered for asymptomatic persons with 200 to 500 CD4+ T cells and is recommended for anyone with symptoms and fewer than 500 CD4+ T cells (Sande et al., 1993). Decisions about initiation of therapy should be made after a thorough provider-patient discussion of the risks and the benefits for that individual. The nucleoside analogues may have several adverse effects (see Table 44–5), and the problem of microbial resistance has been increasingly recognized. Persons who do not tolerate ZDV or who demonstrate progression of dis-

TABLE 44–5. *Antiretroviral Drugs and Their Adverse Effects*

ANTIRETROVIRAL DRUG	ADVERSE EFFECTS
Zidovudine (ZDV), formerly AZT or azidothymidine	Granulocytopenia, anemia, macrocytosis, nausea, headache, confusion, myopathy, anorexia, fatigue, hepatitis (rare), nail discoloration
Didanosine (ddI)	Peripheral neuropathy, pancreatitis (potentially fatal), nausea, diarrhea, confusion
Zalcitabine (ddC)	Peripheral neuropathy, stomatitis, aphthous ulcers, rash, thrombocytopenia, pancreatitis (rare)
Stavudine (D4T)	Peripheral neuropathy, elevated transaminase

ease on ZDV should be offered other antiretroviral therapies either as monotherapy or combination therapy (Sande et al., 1993).

Several other antiretroviral agents (e.g., protease inhibitors, non-nucleoside RT inhibitors), many with different mechanisms of action than those of the nucleoside analogues, are currently under investigation, with the hope that a more effective, less susceptible to resistance, and less toxic treatment can further improve quality of life and survival (Hirsh & D'Aquila, 1993).

NURSING MANAGEMENT

Nursing management of the HIV-infected patient can be at once difficult, challenging, frustrating, satisfying, and rewarding. The presentation of unusually complex physical and psychosocial problems and needs require that nurses caring for HIV-infected persons be well informed, competent, and compassionate.

Nurses have an important role in educating and counseling persons about HIV and how to protect themselves from HIV infection. Risk-reductive counseling should occur in a number of health care and educational settings. Once a person is infected, proper attention to a patient's needs requires a thorough understanding of the spectrum of HIV disease and also a careful assessment of the individual. In addition to a complete medical and psychologic history and physical examination, nurses must be able to obtain with sensitivity adequate information about current and past substance abuse and sexual practices. Expert symptom management, management of complex therapeutic regimens, and provision of appropriate support and education to patients and their families throughout the course of disease presumes that the nurse has a solid grounding in the pathophysiology, clinical manifestations, and management of HIV disease. Because there is currently no cure for HIV disease, the emphasis of nursing care is on reducing the burden of symptoms and improving quality of life. Nurses help individuals learn how to maintain their optimal level of health, and to protect others from infection. Since HIV disease can ultimately involve every organ system, a multiplicity of nursing diagnoses and interventions may be pertinent. Especially important in the care of people with advanced HIV disease are attention to neurologic, respiratory, nutritional, dermatologic, and psychosocial problems. Information found in Unit VIII of this book will be useful in the nursing care of the person with HIV disease.

Additionally, nurses must understand the nature and mechanisms of HIV disease and how to protect themselves from occupationally acquired infection to fulfill their professional obligations well and without undue anxiety. Occupationally acquired HIV infection has been well documented. The risk, calculated from pooled data from several prospective studies of health care workers exposed by percutaneous injuries to HIV contaminated needles or sharps, is 0.31 per cent (31 transmissions per 10,000 percutaneous injuries with HIV-contaminated blood) (Henderson, 1994). Compared with the occupational risk of acquiring infection

with another serious bloodborne pathogen, hepatitis B virus (HBV) (risk of transmission per percutaneous injury = 27 to 43 per cent) (Henderson, 1994), the risk of HIV infection by needlestick injury is remarkably low. The implementation of universal precautions, recommended by the CDC in 1987 and regulated by the Occupational Safety and Health Agency (OSHA) since 1991, further reduces the risk of infection with bloodborne pathogens in the health care setting. Although it is incumbent upon each health care professional to understand and consistently implement universal precautions, studies have shown that this is not always occurring (Courington, Patterson, & Howard, 1991).

THE FUTURE OF HIV SCIENCE AND NURSING

Our understanding of HIV disease has gradually developed from the hope that HIV infection would be treatable (and resolvable) by a single pharmacologic agent, to the realization that HIV/AIDS is a chronic disease that requires elaborate and sophisticated pharmacologic regimens to treat and that there is no cure in the foreseeable future. This understanding places HIV/AIDS conceptually much closer to certain cancers than to most other infectious diseases. We now have the responsibility of educating our patients and the public about HIV disease as a chronic disease requiring combination treatment over the lifetime.

As of this writing, the research community has produced four approved antiretroviral drugs with at least some activity against HIV (see above), and several more are in clinical trials. Even though the efficacy of these drugs is limited, it is important to better learn how to utilize them to their maximal advantage, alone or in combination. Community practice needs better and more direct ways of answering questions about an individual's response to drug(s) and how to combine the available drugs in optimal regimens *on an individual patient basis.*

Quick, available, reliable, and affordable assays are needed to determine viral burden and resistance to drugs. With a greater understanding of viral burden and immunopathogenesis, and with answers to questions of viral sensitivity and resistance, practitioners can treat *individual* patients with antiretrovirals more effectively. With more reliable predictors of disease progression and more effective means of prophylaxes, both primary and secondary, significant clinical morbidity can be delayed or more readily abated. With the early and appropriate use of effective strategies of managing the myriad symptoms found in HIV disease, the quality of life of infected individuals will be enhanced.

REFERENCES

Acierno, L. (1989). Cardiac complications in AIDS. *Journal of the American College of Cardiology, 13,* 1144–1154.

Cello, J. (1992). Gastrointestinal tract manifestations of AIDS. In M. Sande & P. Volberding (Eds.), *The medical management of AIDS* (3rd ed., pp. 176–192). Philadelphia: W. B. Saunders Co.

Centers for Disease Control. (1981). Follow up on Kaposi's sarcoma and *Pneumocystis carinii* pneumonia. *Morbidity and Mortality Weekly Report, 30,* 409–410.

Centers for Disease Control. (1988). Update: Serologic testing for antibody to HIV. *Morbidity and Mortality Weekly Report, 36* 833–840.

Centers for Disease Control. (1989). Interpretation and use of the western blot assay for serodiagnosis of HIV-1. *Morbidity and Mortality Weekly Report, 38*(5-7), 1–7.

Centers for Disease Control. (1992). 1993 Revised classification system for HIV infection and expanded surveillance case definition for AIDS among adolescents and adults. *Morbidity and Mortality Weekly Report, 41*(RR-17), 1–19.

Courington, K., Patterson, S., & Howard, R. (1991). Universal precautions are not universally followed. *Archives of Surgery 26,* 93–96.

Davey, R., & Lane, H. (1990). Laboratory methods in the diagnosis and prognostic staging of infection with the human immunodeficiency virus type 1. *Review of Infectious Diseases, 12,* 912–930.

Detels, R., English, P., Visscher, B., Jacobson, L., Kingsley, L., Chmiel, J., Dudley, J., Eldred, L., & Ginzburg, H. (1989). Seroconversion, sexual activity, and condom use among 2915 HIV seronegative men followed for up to 2 years. *Journal of Acquired Immunodeficiency Syndromes, 2,* 77–83.

Dewar, R., Highbarger, H., Sarmiento, M., Todd, J., Vasudevachari, M., Davey, R., Kovacs, J., Salzman, N., Lane, H., & Urdea, M. (1994). Application of branched DNA signal amplification to monitor HIV-1 burden in human plasma. *The Journal of Infectious Diseases, 170,* 1172–1179.

Drew, W., Buhles, W., & Erlich, K. (1992). Management of herpes virus infections (CMV, HSV, ZVZ). In M. Sande & P. Volberding (Eds.), *The medical management of AIDS* (3rd ed., pp. 359–382). Philadelphia: W. B. Saunders Co.

El-Sadr, W., Oleske, J., Agins, B., et al. *Evaluation and management of early HIV infection. Clinical practice guideline No. 7.* AHCPR Pub. No. 94-0572. Rockville, MD: Agency for Health Care Policy and Research, Public Health Service, U.S. Department of Health and Human Services.

Fauci, A. (1988). The human immunodeficiency virus: Infectivity and mechanisms of pathogenesis. *Science, 239,* 617–622.

Fauci, A. (1993). Multifactorial nature of human immunodeficiency virus disease: Implications for therapy. *Science, 262,* 1011–1018.

Fauci, A., Schnittman, S., Poli, G., Koenig, S., & Pantaleo, G. (1991). Immunopathogenic mechanisms in human immunodeficiency virus infection. *Annals of Internal Medicine, 114,* 678–693.

Fauci, H., & Lane, H. (1994). Human immunodeficiency virus (HIV) disease. In K. Isselbacher, E. Braunwald, G. Wilson, J. Martin, A. Fauci, & D. Kasper (Eds.), *Harrison's principles of internal medicine* (pp. 1566–1618). New York: McGraw Hill.

Gallant, J., Moore, R., & Chaisson, R. (1994). Prophylaxes for opportunistic infections in patients with HIV infection. *Annals of Internal Medicine, 120,* 932–944.

Grady, C., & Vogel, S. (1993). Laboratory methods for diagnosing and monitoring HIV infection. *Journal of the Association of Nurses in AIDS Care, 4,* 11–21.

Harry, D., Jennings, M., Yee, J., & Carlson, J. (1989). Antigen detection for human immunodeficiency virus. *Clinical Microbiology Reviews, 2*(3), 241–249.

Henderson, D. (1994). HIV-1 in the Health Care Setting. In J. Mandell, R. Douglas, & J. Bennett (Eds.). *Principles and practices of infectious diseases* (pp. 62–86). New York: J. Wiley & Sons.

Hirsch, M., & D'Aquila, R. (1993). Therapy for human immunodeficiency virus infection. *New England Journal of Medicine, 328,* 1686–1689.

Ho, D., Pomerantz, R., & Kaplan, J. (1987). Pathogenesis of infection with HIV. *New England Journal of Medicine, 317,* 278–286.

Hofman, B., Wang, Y., Cumberland, W., Detels, R., Bozorgmehri, M., & Fahey, J. (1990). Serum beta-2 microglobulin increases in HIV infection: Relation to seroconversion, CD4 T cell fall, and prognosis. *AIDS, 4,* 207–214.

Jacobson, M. (1992). Mycobacterial diseases: Tuberculosis and disseminated *Mycobacterium avium* complex infection. In M. Sande & P. Volberding (Eds.), *The medical management of AIDS* (3rd ed., pp. 284–296). Philadelphia: W. B. Saunders Co.

Kaplan, L., & Northfelt, D. (1992). Malignancies associated with AIDS. In M. Sande & P. Volberding (Eds.), *The medical management of AIDS* (3rd ed., pp. 399–429). Philadelphia: W. B. Saunders Co.

Kingsley, L., Kaslow, R., Rinaldo, C., Detre, K., Odaka, N., VanRaden, M., Detels, R., Polk, B., Chmeil, J., Kelsey, S., Ostrow, D., & Visscher, B. (1987). Risk factors for seroconversion to human immunodeficiency virus among male homosexuals. *The Lancet, 8529,* 345–348.

Lane, H., Depper, J., Greene, W., Whalen, G., Waldman, T., & Fauci, A. (1985). Qualitative analysis of immune function in patients with the acquired immunodeficiency syndrome: Evidence for a selective defect in soluble antigen recognition. *New England Journal of Medicine, 313,* 79–84.

Lifson, A., O'Malley, P., Hessol, N., Buchbinder, S., Cannon, L., & Rutherford, G. (1990). HIV seroconversion in two homosexual men after receptive oral intercourse with ejaculation: Implications for counseling concerning safe sexual practices. *American Journal of Public Health, 80*(12), 1509–1511.

Melnick, J. (1994). Taxonomy of viruses. In A. Balows & W. Hausler (Eds.), *Manual of clinical microbiology* (5th ed., pp. 811–817). Washington, DC: American Society for Microbiology.

Meltzer, M., Skillman, D., Hoover, D., Hanson, B., Turpin, J., Kalter, C., & Gendelman, H. (1990). Macrophages and the human immunodeficiency virus. *Immunology Today, 11,* 217–223.

O'Regan, S., Russo, P., LaPointe, N., & Rousseau, E. (1990). AIDS and the urinary tract. *Journal of Acquired Immunodeficiency Syndromes, 3,* 244–251.

Palker, T., & Riggs, E. (1994). Retroviruses. In J. Lederberg (Ed.), *Encyclopedia of microbiology* (pp. 545–553). London: Academic Press, Inc.

Pantaleo, G., Graziosi, C., & Fauci, A. (1993). New concepts in the immunopathogenesis of human immunodeficiency virus infection. *New England Journal of Medicine, 328,* 327–335.

Redfield, R., Wright, D., & Tramont, E. (1986). The Walter Reed Staging classification for HTLV-III/LAV infection. *New England Journal of Medicine, 314,* 131–132.

Rosenberg, Z., & Fauci, A. (1989). The immunopathogenic mechanisms of HIV infection. *Advances in Immunology, 47,* 377–431.

Rozenbaum, W., Gharakhanian, S., Cardon, B., Duval, E., & Coulaud, J. (1988). HIV transmission by oral sex. *The Lancet, 8599,* 1395.

Saag, M. (1992). AIDS testing: Now and in the future. In M. Sande & P. Volberding (Eds.), *The medical management of AIDS* (3rd ed., pp. 33–53). Philadelphia: W. B. Saunders Co.

Saah, A., Hoover, D., He, Y., Kingsley, L., Phair, J., & the Multicenter AIDS Cohort Study. (1994). Factors influencing survival after AIDS: Report from the Multicenter AIDS Cohort Study (MACS). *Journal of Acquired Immunodeficiency Syndromes, 7,* 287–295.

Sande, M., Carpenter, C., Cobbs, G., Holmes, K., & Sanford, J. (1993). Antiretroviral therapy for adult HIV-infected patients: Recommendations from a State-of-the-Art conference. *Journal of the American Medical Association, 270,* 2583–2589.

Sarosi, G. (1992). Endemic mycoses in HIV infection. In M. Sande & P. Volberding (Eds.), *The medical management of AIDS* (3rd ed., pp. 311–318). Philadelphia: W. B. Saunders Co.

Schecter, M., Boyko, W., Douglas, B., Willoughby, B., McLeod, A., Maynard, M., Craib, K., & O'Shaughnessy, M. (1986). The Vancouver lymphadenopathy-AIDS study. HIV seroconversion in a cohort of homosexual men. *Canadian Medical Association Journal, 135,* 1355–1360.

Stansell, J. (1992). Cardiac, endocrine, and renal complications of HIV infection. In M. Sande & P. Volberding (Eds.), *The medical management of AIDS* (3rd ed., pp. 247–257). Philadelphia: W. B. Saunders Co.

Stansell, J., & Sande, M. (1992). Cryptococcal infection in AIDS. In M. Sande & P. Volberding (Eds.), *The medical management of AIDS* (3rd ed., pp. 297–310). Philadelphia: W. B. Saunders Co.

Tindall, B., Imrie, A., Donovan, B., Penny, R., & Cooper, D. (1992). Primary HIV infection. In M. Sande & P. Volberding (Eds.), *The medical management of AIDS* (3rd ed., pp. 67–86). Philadelphia: W. B. Saunders Co.

Ungvarski, P. (1992). Clinical manifestations of AIDS. In J. Flaskerud & P. Ungvarski (Eds.), *HIV/AIDS: A guide to nursing care* (pp. 54–145). Philadelphia: W. B. Saunders Co.

Vlahov, D. (1989). AIDS: Overview, immunology, virology, and informational needs. *Seminars in Oncology Nursing, 5,* 227–235.

World Health Organization (WHO) Global Programme on AIDS. (1994). *The HIV/AIDS pandemic: 1994 overview.* Geneva: WHO.

Worley, J., & Price, R. (1992). Management of neurologic complications of HIV-1 infection and AIDS. In M. Sande & P. Volberding (Eds.), *The medical management of AIDS* (3rd. ed., pp. 193–217). Philadelphia: W. B. Saunders Co.

Zunich, K., & Lane, H. (1991). Immunologic abnormalities in HIV infection. *Hematology/Oncology Clinics of North America, 5,* 215–228.

CHAPTER

45

My Story: Responding to Severe Cervical Dysplasia

Judith M. Saunders

This is the story of my experience with severe cervical dysplasia: what led me to seek evaluation for frequent menstrual periods, the subsequent diagnosis, and the successful treatment. I encountered some unexpected obstacles over the past 10 years in monitoring my health and making sure that any reoccurrence would be found and treated promptly. Diagnosis and treatment of my cervical dysplasia could be written in a brief paragraph of a chart entry, but my story as a person experiencing this frightening diagnosis requires more than a paragraph written in the depersonalized language of clinical notations.

ENDING THE PROCRASTINATION

It's 1994, 10 years after I received my diagnosis of severe cervical dysplasia. Digging in the dirt, getting the ground ready to plant, sometimes yields a garden of thoughts and memories more than it yields marigolds or tomatoes. I have been thinking about that time of fear and anxiety when I first learned my diagnosis. As I loosened the soil and mixed in the compost, I tried to remember why it was 10 years ago that I decided to see someone about having menstrual periods every other week. I had been having periods every other week for 2 to 3 years, not all the time, but often, and hadn't really checked them out. I had told myself often enough that this was probably the beginning of my menopause. I remember a variety of circumstances that came together as barriers to my making an appointment with a doctor: my regular gynecologist had retired, I was busy with a new job, I moved to a new city and state, and my long-term relationship was beginning to unravel. I stopped digging when I remembered so vividly how I had carried this sense of unease around with me for

those 2 to 3 years while I found ways to deliberately avoid a medical workup. I had minimized the extent of my abnormal periods in framing the descriptive language that I used in describing my frequent menstrual periods: occasional extra periods, but normal in amount, length, etc. But why did I stop my self-pretense and seek an appointment? I couldn't remember, so I shifted my thinking from why I sought that appointment to the larger context of my life at that time.

I began my postdoctoral fellowship in psychosocial oncology in the fall of 1984 at the School of Nursing, University of Washington, Seattle. Prior to that I had taught in the Midwest during the breakup of a 20-year relationship. I remembered my excitement of newness and adventure: a new career direction, a lifestyle of being single, and a new city. Seattle had cooperated with my high spirits since my arrival by presenting weather characterized by a record-breaking stream of sunlight to mark the days instead of the customary dampness and grey.

I remember now, and in the remembering, can understand why the reason was so elusive. I was seeking a dramatic event that broke through my denial and fragile complacency. Instead of one event, there was an altered personal readiness coupled with a simple fortuitous event. The fortuitous event: in one of my many walks to explore the campus, I walked by the Student Health Office and they were open. I went in to explore their services and scheduled an appointment to be seen by a nurse practitioner in a couple of weeks. My personal readiness came partly from feeling less vulnerable as I was exploring new directions. It also came from a value of "getting more honest with myself." If I were to move closer to oncology as a specialty, then I had to be willing to face my own personal shadows with cancer. It was the unspoken cancer, not menopause, that frightened me and that had constricted my movements.

Now I wonder how much we ever know of the timing of our patients' readiness for exploring their health problems formally. I didn't have to be an expert nurse in oncology to know that I behaved foolishly in postponing a comprehensive exploration of my every-other-week menstrual periods. If I had discussed my frequent menstrual periods with my friends, they would have nudged me to check this out sooner, but I wasn't ready. Fortunately, I didn't pay a high price for my own avoidance, as have many other women. As a nurse, I have urged my patients to have their physician or nurse evaluate their symptoms promptly when those symptoms are clear danger signals for cancer. As I reflect on these interactions with patients, I remember how often I learned about their danger signals casually—often sandwiched in the middle of a seemingly unrelated discussion. Now I make a mental note to myself to consider this topic for research in the future, so I can learn more about the process of deciding to have symptoms formally evaluated.

BEGINNING THE DIAGNOSTIC PROCESS

Most of my health care had been in the American tradition of illness care, in which I scheduled appointments with my physician when some problem prompted a physical assessment. In my pattern of health care coverage, I had always seen a private physician, and none of them employed nurse-practitioners (NP). I sat in the student health waiting room after completing the usual, very routine history forms and realized how out of place I felt. University students are not usually 44 years old, and the few others in the waiting room reflected the more typical students who were in their twenties.

The NP called me in and her manner quickly put me at ease. She reviewed the history form with me and asked for more information about my menstrual periods and my history of a breast biopsy (negative, but with precancerous tissue) several years earlier. I liked her immediately. She treated me as a partner in this health history and examination and readily explained her concerns and her findings. After the physical examination was completed without the NP finding any obvious problems, she advised me to see a gynecologist to check out the frequent periods. She explained that I should have this consultation because of my age and the endurance of the symptom, regardless of what the PAP smear results might be.

I asked her to refer me to a gynecologist who would not have a problem with my being a lesbian. I chose the physician the NP described as very competent (they all were), honest and open with patients, would not have a problem with my being a lesbian, and whose practice was within walking distance of my apartment. By the time the PAP smear results came back as normal, I had already scheduled an appointment with Dr. K for the next month.

Dr. K's extensive history-taking and further laboratory tests gave no support to my own personal hypothesis that I was entering menopause, but she cautioned that the prodromal signs and symptoms of menopause were not well understood or defined. I told her I was a lesbian, and although I lived alone, I was sexually active within a relationship. Dr. K immediately modified her history-taking to eliminate assessment of my use of birth control devises. She clearly was comfortable and nonjudgmental. I breathed a sigh of relief. My own personal experiences with physicians and nurses disapproving of my homosexuality were only occasional, but the stakes were higher this time, and I wanted a medical care experience without the extra "baggage" of a negative attitude toward me as a lesbian.

Dr. K repeated the PAP smear; this time the results came back as "atypical, Class II, endocervical origin. Recommend repeating in 3-4 months."[1] I was puzzled about why the results of this PAP smear were so different from those of the PAP smear completed only a month earlier.[2] Although I was uneasy that Dr. K recommended scheduling a dilatation and curettage (D&C) now instead of waiting the recommended 3 months to repeat the PAP smear, I also welcomed a more definitive and accurate procedure. I knew that a probable explanation of the altered menstrual pattern was cervical polyps and welcomed the possibility that the D&C might correct the problem at the same time the diagnosis was clarified.

I was anxious about the approaching D&C and didn't enjoy hearing everyone's personal nightmare about their own experiences, such as "I didn't get my energy back for six months" or "I had cramps for 3 weeks and couldn't concentrate at work." My anxiety was more diffuse than what the D&C would reveal as the cause of my frequent menstrual periods, and this lack of focus for my anxiety made it easy for me to return to my uneasy complacency. I arranged for a long weekend so the D&C could be scheduled on a Friday, and I was confident that I could return to work and studies Monday with little disruption.

Seattle is a city of hills, and the hills have both proper names and nicknames. I lived adjacent to "Pill Hill," named because it housed several major hospitals and a whole nexus of medical resources. I was scheduled to be at the outpatient surgery area early, and I knew I would be calmed by walking the short mile to the hospital. The morning was dark and very cold, and I had to concentrate on staying upright and not succumbing to falling from the many patches of ice. That walk provided me with the last moment of calm I knew until I lost count as the anesthesiologist induced the "calm" of general anesthesia.

---

[1]Clinical findings in quotations or indented have been taken from my copy of D. K's files that she gave me when I returned to Los Angeles in 1986.

[2]Dr. K reported PAP smear reports often were inaccurate from that laboratory. I called the NP in student health to report this and she and the other staff subsequently changed laboratories.

The hospital was a well respected, large medical center where many physicians in private practice admitted patients; few were patients at this hospital if their expenses weren't covered through private insurance. The outpatient area was full of light and comfortable chairs and gave a feeling of spaciousness and affluence. I wasn't quite certain what to do, and the directions I received from the receptionist were vague. Most other patients were accompanied, so they had someone to help with clarifying vague directions. I learned that this process, like many others, is not designed for the alone patient.

Eventually, I completed all the preoperative instructions, put my clothes and belongings in the dressing room locker, and entered the suite of operating rooms. I met the nurses who were putting the finishing touches on the equipment and supplies in the operating room, talked briefly with the anesthesiologist, and received preoperative medicine. I dozed some and awakened when I realized I had grown cold. One of the nurses noticed my shivering and brought me a blanket from the warmer. I felt bathed in comfort. It soon became apparent that Dr. K had neither arrived nor called. The staff called Dr. K's home and were assured that she had left home. My surgery was already an hour behind schedule, so I was taken to the recovery room where I dozed while waiting.

Soon, I heard Dr. K's familiar voice arouse me from my light sleep. She explained that she had been in a minor car accident en route, but everything was ready now and we could proceed. I told her that I didn't want a physician operating on me who was shaken up from a car accident. She laughed, gave me more details about the accident, and convinced me easily that she was not physically injured and was recovered enough from the accident's emotional stress to proceed safely.

I heard muffled voices in the recovery room and realized, in my haze, that the surgery was over. Dr. K appeared to let me know all had proceeded routinely and that she would have the pathology report back within a couple of days. I was surprised to learn that I had to take a taxi home, instead of walking, because I had a general anesthetic. Looking back, I realize my judgment was very impaired if I ever expected to walk a mile of up-and-down terrain after my D&C and general anesthesia. I can only wonder at my ability to minimize effects of experiences that arouse my anxiety.

ENCOUNTERING MY CONFUSION, FEAR, AND INDIGNATION

I lived alone and didn't know very many people in Seattle yet. I had refused offers of out-of-state friends to come stay with me after surgery and was grateful for my privacy during that weekend. I had prepared for my miniconvalesce by cooking in advance and freezing meals. I also had bought paper plates and plastic utensils, so that taking care of myself was easy. I slept and slept and slept. And I talked on the phone a lot to let family and friends know that I was fine.

I don't remember when I learned about the confusion surrounding the pathology report from the D&C. Dr. K's dictated note and the histology report reflect this confusion (see Box 45–1 for her note in the clinical chart). Not only the severity of the dysplasia was in question, but exactly where the dysplasia was located was also obscure. I was confused. Dr. K was also confused and a bit embarrassed. I appreciated her honesty.

Trying to sort out the diagnostic confusion led to a colposcopy where Dr. K found a small, but obvious and distinct lesion at the 1 o'clock position on my cervix. The biopsy of this lesion was definitive: "Pathology report. Specimen A. ECC B. 1 o'clock cervical biopsy. Findings from the biopsy was focally severe cervical dysplasia." What still wasn't totally clear was whether this lesion accounted for the dysplastic tissue identified in the D&C. Dr. K arranged for a three-way consultation with herself, an oncologist, and a pathologist. Armed with all the clinical and laboratory data, the three physicians discussed the data back and forth. Dr. K needed to make sure that the lesion she had seen on my cervix accounted for the severely dysplastic tissue; she was a little concerned that she might treat one site only to overlook another site that accounted for the dysplastic tissue identified in the D&C. She also wanted a second opinion about which treatment approach (conization, laser, cryosurgery, etc.) to recommend, and treatment approaches typically take into account age, desire for children, availability of tissue to confirm diagnosis, etc.

Box 45–1. *Excerpt from Clinical Chart*

Notes from Fractional D&C. Pt is a 44 yo nulligravida female, who has had irregular menses over the last several years. She noticed the 1st episode of every other week flow about 2-3 years ago, but didn't seek medical advice until recently. Flow on 9/13, 10/1, 10/12, 11/6, 11/22. Denies Sx of menopause. D&C unremarkable.

Histology: Found a polyp composed of endometrial stroma with tubal metaplasia noted focally. No evidence of malignancy. Findings: A.) endocervical curretings: Fragments of dysplastic squamous epithelium. B.) Endometrial curretings: endometrial/lower uterine segment polyp with focal adenomatous change and tubal metaplasia. Fragments were too small to allow an accurate assessment of the degree of severity of the dysplasia.

RESPONDING TO THE DIAGNOSIS OF SEVERE DYSPLASIA

I guess I should have been grateful that my diagnosis was one that usually responded to local treatment and had an encouraging prognosis. I couldn't focus on that rational response; I was reeling from surprise and outrage. I wasn't at all upset with the confusion that troubled Dr. K. I responded to the diagnosis of severe dysplasia.

Using one of my customary coping strategies, I turned to the literature to learn more about severe cervical dysplasia. I found confusion about the terminology in the literature: severe dysplasia, carcinoma in situ, cervical intraepithelial neoplasia (CIN II or III), preinvasive disease, etc.

I found that the identified risk factors discussed in the literature didn't fit me at all. I kept returning to the literature to review the risk factors, as though a new reading might change the list and make more sense to me. I still could find only one risk factor that applied to me: history of smoking, and I had quit smoking several years earlier. I had no history of Human Papilloma Virus, herpes simplex virus type 2, or any sexually transmitted disease, became sexually active rather late in life, had few sexual partners, and had always lived a middle-class lifestyle. I knew that under my confusion and indignation was fear, and this fear fluttered in and out of my awareness. Mostly, I didn't deal very openly with that fear. I also learned for the first time that severe dysplasia was now being classified as a sexually transmitted disease, and I was both angry and embarrassed.

HAVING LASER SURGERY

Dr. K and the consulting physicians believed the evidence pointed to severe dysplasia in only one site and that it would be safe to treat that site locally. The idea of laser surgery appealed to me for a number of reasons. I knew that many risks (infection, bleeding) were reduced with laser surgery, as compared with conization (See Unit V for discussion of treatments). I hated the sluggish after-effects of general anesthesia following the D&C, and I told Dr. K that I wanted to use a hypnosis tape for this surgery instead of a general anesthetic. She was skeptical and cautioned that I could be injured during the procedure if I wasn't perfectly still while she was using the laser. She agreed to let me use a hypnosis tape but recommended that an anesthesiologist be present during the laser surgery as a precaution.

Two and a half months after the D&C, I walked to the hospital once again, and this time I knew my way around and didn't feel so strange and out of place. Dr. K arrived on time for this surgery, and I adjusted my earphones so I could hear the tape comfortably. A major advantage to using the tape was that I was aware of what was going on and could answer questions or respond to directions as needed. The anesthesiologist was curious, supportive, and nonintrusive. Although the whole procedure was very brief, I felt the three of us were a team working together. Instead of the recovery room rituals, Dr. K and I had a cup of tea together in the recovery room, where I stayed a half-hour or so and then I walked home.

After the surgery, a friend came from Los Angeles to stay the weekend. This time, I was more eager to have someone there to talk things over with than I was to have privacy. The second night after surgery, I woke up around 2 AM. Immediately I knew something was wrong but couldn't figure out what it was. I felt wet. I got up and realized that I was bleeding. Before this, I had only been spotting occasionally. I was really scared. My friend tried to talk me into calling Dr. K, but I wanted to wait because I knew I hadn't lost much blood yet. I felt I wasn't in any danger yet. The bleeding gradually slowed down. Dr. K later figured out that my regular period had started, and this period dislodged the clot from the laser surgery. That was the only scary event in the otherwise routine recovery from laser surgery.

MONITORING CERVICAL DYSPLASIA OVER TIME

I followed the routine regimen of PAP smears, colposcopy examination, and pelvic examinations at the intervals that Dr. K recommended for the rest of that year. I was very clear that I no longer trusted PAP smears to accurately detect problems early. I knew I wouldn't feel safe if I relied on PAP smears alone, so I became determined to have annual colposcopy examinations as long as they were appropriate (while I was still menstruating or using hormone replacement therapy).

I was involved in several research projects in the postdoctoral fellowship program, and time passed quickly. As the second year of the postdoctoral program arrived, it brought the distressing news that I was no longer covered for health insurance as a part of the postdoctoral fellowship. I started exploring different systems (private insurance and health maintenance organizations [HMOs]) and their costs for health care, and found, like so many other Americans, that major obstacles existed for those trying to access health care coverage privately. first, I found that I couldn't afford even the cheapest plan if I had to pay the full cost myself. Student health coverage was limited in scope and was not intended to meet all health care needs. Second, any problems that might emerge from the severe cervical dysplasia would be excluded from coverage for varying lengths of time in all the plans. I was discouraged. I had taken health insurance for granted. While I couldn't afford to pay for insurance, I couldn't afford not to have the coverage. I couldn't understand how health insurance could be covered under the fellowship one year, and not the next year. My personal health insurance coverage crisis was averted when the faculty decided they would continue to include health insurance coverage for fellows, despite the strain on the budget.

During that second year, I developed one more cervical lesion, but the biopsy results were negative. Over the next 3 years I developed typical symptoms of menopause—symptoms that did not include increased frequency of menstrual periods. I decided to use replacement hormone therapy, partly so I could continue to use a monitoring program that included annual colposcopy examinations.

After completing my fellowship, I returned to the Los Angeles area and continued with an insurance plan, through work, that allowed me to select my own physician for medical care. A change in my employment status once again led me to consider a less expensive health care plan. I grumbled to myself that America doesn't offer health care plans—only illness care plans. Eventually I changed my health plan to an HMO. Economics decreed this change, and I was not confident that I could receive comprehensive monitoring through an HMO. I quickly realized that I had to be assertive about the type of care that I needed. I was assigned to a family practice physician who seemed competent and sensitive. She agreed that using an annual colposcopy examination to monitor cervical dysplasia was warranted but explained that a gynecologist would make that final decision. She referred me to the gynecology department, but the first gynecologist that I saw didn't do colposcopies. I scheduled an appointment with a different gynecologist who somewhat reluctantly agreed that he would use a colposcopic examination, not just PAP smears, for my annual examinations.

Because of my lack of confidence in the health care I received through my HMO gynecology services, I volunteered to be a participant in a multisite trial, the Postmenopausal Estrogen/Progestin Interventions (PEPI). I was pleased that large-scale studies were finally being directed toward issues that concerned women. I also was aware that I ask patients to participate in my nursing research, and I should give energy back by participating as a volunteer in appropriate research as a study participant. I was attracted to this study also because of the extensive clinical and laboratory monitoring that was integral to the study. This 3-year study provided me with a check-and-balance system for monitoring my gynecologic health status.

I was randomized to the estrogen-only arm of this study, and after a year on the study, I developed endometrial hyperplasia. This time, I wasn't so scared. I knew what triggered the hyperplasia (estrogen without progesterone) and was confident that 3 months of Provera therapy would likely resolve the problem, and it did.

LOOKING BACK AND MAKING SENSE OUT OF MY EXPERIENCE

As a nurse, I often try to identify and manage barriers that keep patients from seeking medical care they need. My search to identify those barriers often has not been as successful as I would like. When I do find barriers, however, such as lack of transportation or lack of awareness of available resources, I know that finding workable solutions is more likely. In looking back, though, the more productive question was, "what caused me to seek medical care—to end the avoidance?" I am struck that the positive forces that led me to seek care were only tangentially related to the barriers that had kept me from seeking medical care. Perhaps nurses would be more successful in helping people seek needed treatment if we understood as much about forces that pull patients toward medical care as we do about forces that keep patients away from medical care.

Understanding the personal factors was, and is, an important dimension in my experience with cervical dysplasia. I quickly learned how important contextual issues were when I was faced with loss of insurance coverage through my postdoctoral traineeship. Regardless of my personal motivation or health status, I could not have afforded health insurance without my employer's economic subsidy of a major portion of the cost. The social-economic context of my experience was just as real a problem as was the cervical dysplasia.

I was fortunate to have health care providers—both the NP and the gynecologist—who regarded me as a partner in my health care. They sought my views and respected my concerns. The hospital, on the other hand, seemed interested in processing large numbers of people. There were inadequate directions for patients and their families in the outpatient processing area and they seemed to have no interest in addressing problems that arose. I was fortunate that I read and spoke English and that I knew which questions to ask. Once I entered the operating and recovery room suites, the focus shifted back to me as an individual, and my needs were addressed promptly and effectively.

The hardest issue for me to make sense about continues to be the confusion about the terminology of my diagnosis. I have been guided by the adage, "if it isn't invasive, it isn't cancer." I learned in cancer cell biology classes about the controversy surrounding in situ cancers: "are they cancers or not?" I could never sort out whether severe cervical dysplasia is synonymous with in situ cervical cancer. While the terminology hasn't altered my recovery or my continued monitoring, the words used in labeling a condition do make a difference. If it didn't, so much time and energy wouldn't be placed in choosing an effective and accurate labeling system. I never quite know how to complete a history form that asks if I have a history of cancer. When I read articles about cancer survivorship, I don't quite feel they are speaking to me and my experiences. I feel vulnerable from having three separate episodes of precancerous experiences and grateful that the dysplasia was successfully treated and that I have no lasting effects of the treatment.

MAKING RECOMMENDATIONS OUT OF MY EXPERIENCES

In looking back and making sense out of my personal experiences with severe cervical dysplasia, I have identified a few recommendations for nurses.

1. Nurses should study the positive forces that help patients initiate and maintain actions that help them meet their health care needs.

2. Nurses have an important and informed voice to call for a national health plan that establishes policy and procedures for universal health care access for all Americans. Our practice has to attend to patients, their families, and appropriate contextual issues that frame the illness experience.

3. Nurses should assess their practice settings to determine whether adequate information and directions are available to the patient who is new to their setting. This assessment will be more effective if they try to determine information needs of a diverse cross-section of the population they serve. I should be able to go to an outpatient surgery appointment alone, if I choose, and receive clear and adequate directions from staff.

4. When nurses and physicians, in the manner of their interactions with me, made me feel like a person who was a functioning member of the team, I felt cared for and respected. I would encourage nurses to attend to the manner of their interactions, not just to providing accurate instructions and information.

5. The objective data does not always provide the most effective clue for what concerns patients. In this experience, I knew that my diagnosis had an excellent prognosis with local treatment. My being upset was out of proportion to that objective data. I would encourage nurses to look beyond the objective reality in trying to understand the patient's response to the illness and its treatment. Only in understanding the patient's perspective—what matters to her or him—can the nurse implement interventions that address the particular concerns of a specific patient.

6. It may seem small and silly, but one of the most memorable and helpful nursing interventions was the nurse who after noticing my shivering in the operating room, gave me a warm blanket. To me, it was a critical and caring behavior, and one that often goes unnoticed.

46

Surviving Breast Cancer

Ruth McCorkle

SOMETHING WAS WRONG

I had just finished packing for a trip to Michigan to consult with colleagues about our research study on home care. It was late, and I was showering before going to bed. I was shaving my underarms and quickly examined my breasts as I did routinely when bathing. As I rinsed my left armpit, my fingers slid across my breast over a small lump. I dried myself, dressed, and went to bed. The next day as I was sitting on the plane, I remembered the lump and quickly went to the bathroom to check my breast again. It was still there. I asked myself, how can this be happening? I knew right away that there was something wrong and that I had to find out if it was serious. As soon as the plane landed, I called my physician's office and asked if I could see her as soon as I returned the following week. I asked her to schedule a mammogram and a consult with a surgeon. Her response was "Ruth, aren't you putting the cart before the horse?"—but she agreed to have her receptionist make the appointments. I returned prior to the weekend, and my appointment was scheduled for Tuesday; Monday was a national holiday. After my internist agreed that the lump needed to be evaluated, I arrived in radiology for my mammogram. As I sat, I thought about some of my own patients who had been in similar situations. Then I heard my name called, approached the desk, and handed the clerk the order for my x-ray examination. As she reached to take it from me, she looked me straight in the eyes and said "Good luck." I cannot tell you how much it meant to have someone connect with me; someone who knew I was going through an incredibly frightening experience—an experience that I was soon to learn would change my life as I had always lived it.

The mammogram was not easy and not obviously abnormal. My lump was located in the tail of my breast near the axilla and was not readily identifiable on x-ray examination. The technician took three times as many views of the breast as she would have with routine orders. The radiologist finally felt he had captured an adequate number of angles, but no mass was obvious, only a slight indication of a few calcium deposits. Several hours later I saw the surgeon after he had completed his operating room schedule. He was a coinvestigator on my research study, and I had complete trust in him. He aspirated the lump in the clinic and was able to tell me within 15 minutes that the cells were malignant. He scheduled an appointment with the medical oncologist and the radiation therapist for me to discuss treatment options the next day. The official laboratory test of the aspiration would take 2 days. While I waited for the report, I had a workup to rule out metastatic disease, including a thorough physical examinaton, complete laboratory assays, a bone scan, and chest x-ray examination. I was not frightened about the word "cancer," but I was frightened about the stage of my disease.

THE DECISION

As a clinician, I have always been concerned about patients being urged to make irreversible decisions under time-limited constraints. I have talked with many women about the advantages and disadvantages of various treatment choices for breast cancer. My medical oncologist was the most direct with his opinion, telling me what I "should do." There was no doubt whatsoever in his mind that I should have breast conservation surgery with chemotherapy and radiation. I had concerns about radiation. I am very athletic and love sports. I was worried that radiation might affect my endurance to run and play softball. I was assured that the side effects were minimal and that the latest radiation equipment reduces potential problems.

I was ambivalent about the type of surgery to have. I felt I was betraying the women who had elected to have mastectomies if I had a lumpectomy. Somehow, it didn't seem right that I was to keep my breast. My internist listened to me and told me I could have a two-step procedure, where the lump and node dissection could be done in the initial surgery and a mastectomy could be scheduled at a later date. The surgeon allowed me to decide up until the final moment before being anesthetized when I was lying on the operating room table. I remain ambivalent about my decision today.

TELLING OTHERS

There are people who need to know if you have cancer, especially if the diagnosis has a direct impact on their lives. The challenge is deciding how and when to communicate to others. As soon as I realized I had a lump, I called my parents to tell them I had discovered it and was scheduled to have tests. Once the diagnosis was confirmed through the needle aspiration, I knew they had to be told the gravity of the situation. I did not feel I could handle their anxiety and questions myself, so I asked my medical oncologist to call them. In hindsight, this was a terrific idea because I knew that they would think that I would not tell them the complete truth.

I had to tell my family and my children; David was 8 and Amanda was 9. I knew how important it was to be honest with them, and yet I did not want to alarm them unnecessarily. I said, "I have a small tumor in my breast and I am going to have it removed and then I am going to be okay." I remember they did not say much, but they were particularly attentive to me and gave me many hugs that week. Amanda took a beautiful pink ribbon, marked X's and O's for hugs and kisses on it, signed her name, and gave it to me. I still have it.

Next, I had to tell my dean at the School of Nursing and the co-director of our Oncology Graduate Program. Everyone was wonderful to me. The dean allowed me to continue to work as much as I wanted, but my coworkers really assumed my work responsibility and did the bulk of what needed to be done. I communicated to my friends by writing to them. I included all their names on the letter, so they were aware of who else knew. Once people were initially informed, it was easier to talk further about the cancer with them. It was particularly hard to verbalize about cancer to those people who didn't know about my illness when I met them face-to-face. Often their reaction was one of shock and disbelief that "one of our own in cancer care had been stricken." It was hard to respond to people during this time, but I understood it was a reaction of love and a threat to my colleagues' potential vulnerability.

THE TREATMENT

The surgery was uneventful, except I seemed to have more pain postoperatively than I remember other patients experiencing. I was discharged with two drains and a packet of written instructions about exercises and wound care. I never read them, not because I did not need to know what I was supposed to do, but because I could not focus on reading. My head just was not in a place where I could concentrate and be attentive.

As with a number of patients, when I returned to the surgical clinic to have my drains removed, the area under my incision in the axilla had to be aspirated. The stitches were removed, and the doctor finally told me I could take a shower. I was encouraged to exercise the arm and to return to the clinic if I had any problems; otherwise I was released for follow-up care to the medical oncologist.

My first visit to the chemotherapy clinic was horrendous. The walk from the parking lot was long and tiring. I went to the registration desk to check in, and the receptionist handed me a form to take to the next desk. I later found out that this was a form for billing. At the second desk, a receptionist took that form and gave me another form, which was the physician's order for blood work. She said, "Put that paper in the slot over there," and walked away. I turned, but couldn't see a slot. I walked over to where she indicated the slot to be by tilting her head as she spoke and saw other similar papers around the corner in a slot on the other side of the wall. I put my paper in front. Immediately, one of the patients sitting shouted, "Put it in the back, we were here before you." About 15 minutes later, a technician drew my blood and told me to have a seat in the waiting room. Several minutes later I heard someone shout, "Get on the scale." I ignored the command and continued to look through a magazine I had brought with me. Suddenly, the receptionist who had handed me the order for my blood studies said, "I told you to get on the scale." I looked up and said, "Are you talking to me?" She said, "Yes, the scales are back here," as she pointed to the partition. I was exhausted and eager to lie down. I finally met with the oncologist, and he reviewed the plan for my schedule of chemotherapy. I quickly learned that I needed to bring someone with me to navigate me through the clinic and to remember what was said.

The oncologist wanted to start the chemotherapy protocol as soon as possible. I had plans to take the kids to Disney World that spring and wanted to keep my commitment to them. The oncologist agreed to space my chemotherapy so we could make the trip. My first treatment was a week later. I received CMF—Cytoxan, Methotrexate, and 5FU.

CHEMOTHERAPY TREATMENT

I was very confident about my decision to have chemotherapy. I immediately called Tish Knobf at Yale University to discuss my options. (See Chapter 29 for a complete discussion of breast cancer.) I was interested in the longest length of survival with minimal reduction to quality of life. I learned quickly that there were many advantages to having a background in cancer care, because I was knowledgeable about the terminology used, the different options for drug administration, and the range of pharmacologic agents to prevent or reduce potential side effects. Similarly, there were disadvantages in being recognized as an oncology expert. It was not easy to be treated in the cancer center where I worked. At times, I felt that the nurses who administered the chemotherapy were intimidated by questions. They assumed that I was knowledgeable about my cancer and what to expect. They always asked how I was doing, but they never asked directly if I had any problems.

I received eight cycles of chemotherapy and never had the same nurse administer my drugs in consecutive cycles. Each time I was asked which arm I wanted the intravenous therapy in and the amount of antiemetic drug and dose of cortisone I preferred. Each time I would use my energies to tell them that I couldn't have any injections in my left arm and that whatever drugs I received last time seemed okay, but I really couldn't remember. It would have been such a relief if the nurse had documented the procedure and it could have been referred to by the next nurse. The nurse could have reviewed the previous procedure but not have the expectation that I would direct the care, since I assumed there was no previous documentation about the procedure on the outpatient chart.

In retrospect, I believe the experience of treating me was quite stressful for the nurses. Many of them knew or worked with me as students or colleagues in a variety of capacities before any diagnosis was made. The role changes that ensued when I began treatment as well as my being a symbol of their own vulnerability proved difficult at times. The experience underscored the need for structured support for oncology staff.

As the nurse administered the drug, she often reviewed in detail the side effects and related what to expect that day and in the weeks to come. Let me assure you, I rarely heard what was said. It was like someone moving her lips yet making no sound. It was extremely helpful to have someone accompany me during subsequent treatments. I didn't need to listen to the nurse; I trusted the person with me to remember what was said and used my energy just to get through the treatment. I decided to purchase a wig after my first treatment, before my hair fell out.

RADIATION THERAPY

On one level, radiation is impersonal and cold, and yet, on another level, the daily contact over 6 weeks affords unique opportunities to form lasting relationships with both staff and patients. The simulation procedure where my treatment was calculated and fitted to my chest felt like a seamstress fitting me for a perfectly calibrated suit of armor. I lay on the hard table for more than 2 hours while three specialists measured me, permanently marked the boundaries of their measurements with pinpoint tattoos, and conferred with each other about "the field." They touched my breast, my chest, and my underarm without saying a word. Finally, I was instructed to put my patient gown on and sent to the area where the "mold" to stabilize my arm in position was made. The material to make the mold was warm (almost hot) before it hardened. The warmth against my body was a great relief from the coldness and hardness of the table.

Of course, the purpose of this "crude" method of "precision" was to ensure that the same area on my body was irradiated in the same way each time. I was assigned a machine and allowed to select a time to receive my treatment each day, Monday through Friday. My first treatment started the following day. I found that what worked best for me was to come to my office mid-morning, work 2 hours, have lunch, get my treatment at 1:00 PM, return to my office for about an hour, then go home for a nap. My skin became irritated but never ulcerated. A light, cool shower on my chest often would feel very soothing.

The hardest part of the radiation therapy was the length of time my arm had to remain in a forced position, immobilized by the "mold," to receive the treatment. The arm was placed at a right angle and extended to about 140 degrees away from the side of my body. Although the actual treatment was limited to only a few minutes, the positioning remained painful throughout the treatments, often bringing tears to my eyes. Only once my machine was "down," meaning that the machine had to be serviced, and an additional day was added to the schedule. I was fortunate that the machine stayed "healthy" for me. Often, I would carry on a conversation with the machine while I was lying on the table. I knew I was dependent upon the machine to complete my radiation therapy.

MANAGING SIDE EFFECTS

The primary purpose of the multimodal treatment approach was to remove my breast cancer and eradicate any potential remaining cancer cells in my body. I experienced side effects associated with all these treatments: surgery, radiation, and chemotherapy. Some of the side effects were potentiated by a cumulative effect of radiation and chemotherapy given during the same time period.

Postsurgically I had difficulty regaining the mobility and range of motion in my left arm after the node dissection, even with a structured program of exercise. In hindsight, I think if I had been encouraged to take pain medication to assist me, my recovery would have been sooner and more complete. The nurses in the chemotherapy unit were vigilant about preparing me for common side effects associated with drugs: nausea, vomiting, alopecia, and signs of infection.

The administration of antiemetics with the chemotherapy was excellent for controlling vomiting, which I rarely experienced. I did, however, experience episodes of nausea. Nausea always came as a surprise. I would be hungry and wanted to eat, and I'd sit down to start a meal and a wave of stomach distress would occur. I'd have to push myself back from the food and actually leave the table. This was difficult for me and my family. Preparing meals and eating together were important times for me and my immediate and extended families to be together. My chemotherapy regimen extended for more than $6\frac{1}{2}$ months, covering a number of holidays and family gatherings. On one or two occasions, I tried to prevent the nausea prophylactically, but the medication would often make me drowsy and I abandoned trying to prevent it. I found it difficult throughout my chemotherapy to prepare meals for others and pack lunches for my school-aged children.

As I said earlier, I bought a wig prior to beginning chemotherapy. My goal was to match the color, style and texture of my own hair. I was fortunate because I could afford to purchase a good quality wig. A number of resources in Philadelphia specialize in assisting both adults and children with wigs, turbans, and other beauty aids to enhance appearance. I lost all my hair, including my eyebrows. I actually lost all the hair on my body. One benefit was not having to shave my legs.

I often didn't wear my wig in the privacy of my home, but I wore a cap. My head would get cold during the seasonal changes. I never realized the protective role my hair served until I lost it. Psychologically, my hair loss didn't seem to bother me, mainly because I knew it was temporary.

After I completed my radiation therapy and continued with my chemotherapy, problems started with the fourth cycle. The fifth cycle was delayed because my blood counts dropped and didn't recover as projected. During that time, I had a crisis with a fever and chills that required antibiotics. Immediate response to signs of infection was essential. It was not easy to recognize the seriousness of these symptoms of infection when I was so fatigued. My previous response to warning signs prior to cancer was to wait a while before calling the doctor, but when your blood counts are neutropenic, delay can be life-threatening. It was particularly helpful to have someone available to validate that my symptoms warranted immediate attention. With antibiotics, my symptoms improved within a few hours and the infection was controlled. The problem was a simple bladder infection.

The ability to concentrate, read, and write was particularly troublesome during my treatment and did not improve much between chemotherapy cycles. In my professional position, I was required to write numerous reports, articles, speeches, and grants. The etiology of lack of concentration is difficult to understand. Some believe it is related to drug effects, fatigue, emotional reactions to illness, or a combination of those factors. I made "to do" lists and it helped to some degree, but the best solution was to recognize my limitations and to delegate tasks to others.

The most overwhelming side effect I experienced was fatigue. I was emotionally drained and physically unable to do the things I wanted and was accustomed to doing. I would go to bed tired and not wake up rested. Scheduling activities with structured rest periods helped. Energy levels increased in between chemotherapy treatments, but my fatigue eventually reached its peak level at the completion of the chemotherapy treatment. It took months to recover and feel rested. I think a good indication of when fatigue will resolve is to expect it to take 1 month of fatigue for every month of treatment. I also went to an internist who specializes in nutrition; he prescribed a vitamin program that I continue today.

AREAS WHERE HELP WAS NEEDED

Throughout my treatment, I needed assistance in household activities, particularly in meal preparation, laundry, and light house cleaning. I arranged to have someone to assist my family for 6 months. I also needed help with transportation. On the days I received chemotherapy, it was impossible to drive home alone. In addition, I had little energy to walk long distances from the parking lot to the treatment center.

Another major area of help needed was assistance with problem-solving. Throughout the course of my illness, problems occurred that needed evaluating. It was not only the problems related to the treatment effects and their consequences, but a host of other problems related to day-to-day living. For example, I had to decide how many after-school activities my children would participate in if they were dependent on me for transportation or whether other arrangements could be made on a temporary basis. I also had to decide to be relieved of many of my work responsibilities. The illness gave me a legitimate reason to let go and concentrate on getting well.

At first, it was not easy for me to acknowledge that there were many areas where I needed help. For a variety of reasons, I believe it is particularly difficult for nurses to ask for and accept help. There is no question that the love and outpouring of support and help from others was at the core of what got me through the treatment experience. It was important for me to struggle with my problems to some degree before I realized that it would be easier with help.

LATE EFFECTS THAT REQUIRE LIFESTYLE CHANGES

I was grateful that my cancer could be treated, but I had residual and permanent effects from the treatment that I've had to learn to live with. Specific late effects required changes in my lifestyle. The first was the lymphedema that developed in my left arm. I first became aware of my arm becoming heavy and my ring and watch on my left hand becoming tight about 7 months after the completion of the radiation. This coincided with the first anniversary of my diagnosis, and I reported my concerns to my medical oncologist, who minimized them. He told me that the edema was not enough to measure and he assured me that it would not increase. At my next 3-month follow-up appointment with my oncologist, I requested a referral to physical therapy. The therapist measured my arm and documented that I had lymphedema. She reviewed my arm exercises, I demonstrated my techniques, and she reenforced specific skills she wanted me to do daily.

I also pursued obtaining a Jobst sleeve at the same time. I had to convince my physician to order these additional treatments. When I visited the Jobst office, I tried their pneumatic pump. They had arrangements where I could rent the pump on a monthly basis. Again, I had to return to my physician for an order to use the pump. I was fortunate because my health insurance partially paid for these services.

Over the next 2 months, my lymphedema remained stable. I used the pump faithfully every evening for 45 minutes, executed daily exercises in the morning, and wore a pressure sleeve throughout the day.

At the annual Oncology Nursing Society meeting in May 1991, I attended the Lymphedema Special Interest group and also attended a roundtable on lymphedema. It was there that I learned about the Breast Cancer Physical Therapy Clinic owned and operated by a physical therapist, Linda Miller. At the clinic, Linda assessed my upper body, evaluated the treatments that I had tried, and established a 10-week management program to strengthen and maintain my total body. The program consisted of aerobic and stretching exercises, heat, massage, and weights. The program also consisted of the daily use of a pneumatic pump, but one that was sequential. Within 3 weeks, I had lost an inch in circumference of my arm.

I remain on a maintenance exercise program with the use of a Jugo sleeve. I've been able to minimize the edema with this regime and forgo the use of the pump. I found the fabric the Jobst sleeve was made of to be too restrictive. After having it on all day, my skin was irritated. The material of the Jugo sleeve is very elastic and flexible. The sleeves come in preset sizes, so the cost is less because they do not have to be custom-made. However, to purchase one, I still needed a physician's order.

Another symptom I experienced that accompanied the lymphedema was the presence of a quarter-inch band that started in my axilla and descended down the medial aspect of my arm to the tip of my thumb and followed to the end of my first finger. This band felt like a piano string and was associated with discomfort. The band lasted for about 6 months but gradually disappeared as I received treatment for my lymphedema.

It took over 2 years to regain strength in my arm, although it remains weaker than prior to surgery. I also think it's natural to protect the arm from movement if it's not the dominant side. The presence of lymphedema added to the delay of my fully using my arm. I found I couldn't lift packages that I was accustomed to lifting. I couldn't open heavy doors of buildings with my left arm. I couldn't wear my watch on my left wrist. I couldn't carry my briefcase on my left shoulder. I have learned to accommodate. It took struggling to do these activities for me to realize that if I attempt to do things that strain my arm, my lymphedema becomes worse. It often means that I have to ask for help or delay doing something until I have sufficient help so I don't have to lift things myself. These latter behaviors have been difficult for me to come to terms with, but I have come to the realization that the protection of my arm is a priority because the potential permanent damage is too costly.

Another difficult thing I had to adjust to was the frequent inquiries as to why I wear a pressure sleeve. Often people will ask me if I have carpal tunnel syndrome. I had to decide if I wanted people to know why I was wearing the sleeve or whether to give a simple answer, such as that I had sprained my arm. I now generally tell people that I have had surgery and my lymph nodes were removed.

Two other problems that I experienced were weight gain and hot flashes. The weight I gained required me to purchase clothes two sizes larger than I had previously worn. Over the first few years after my cancer treatment, I had resolved to accept my new size, but gradually I've realized that I can lose some of the weight even if I can't resume my pretreatment weight. I've been able to find a balance in maintaining my weight with a structured exercise program and low-fat diet.

The hot flashes were induced by the chemotherapy, and initially my oncologist recommended I take vitamin E twice a day and eliminate caffeine. Both of these recommendations have helped to some degree, and the hot flashes have lessened over the last year.

MONITORING ONE'S OWN HEALTH

Initially, I felt discounted and discouraged. I knew my arm and hand were swollen, and I couldn't get anyone to acknowledge that it was a problem. For more than 6 months, I searched for someone to listen and work with me to identify a regimen that I could adopt to fit my personal and professional life. Once I realized that other women have lymphedema, I felt I was not alone. As a patient at The Breast Cancer Physical Therapy Clinic, I realized that I had to take charge of monitoring my own health and evaluating my lifestyle behaviors. Taking charge had a positive impact on my emotional status. I found that I was able to make a difference in how I felt on a daily basis.

As I said earlier, I searched for answers to manage my lymphedema. Generally, physicians didn't want to talk with me about it because they felt I was blaming them. But in fact, what I really wanted to know was their views on what causes it and what successes they've had with treating it. I wanted to know if it's reversible. I also found that, in general, a physical therapist who specialized in breast cancer and who treated my entire body, not just my arm, was the most skilled and knowledgeable resource. Her approach was to make me responsible for the management of my own health by recommending a regimen to be followed at least 4 or 5 days a week. She taught me that I needed to change my behavior and to adopt a management plan that could become a part of my everyday life. It's knowing what makes the edema worse and what makes it better, and avoiding or at least minimizing the things that make it worse.

RECOMMENDATIONS FOR IMPROVEMENT OF PRACTICE

Women who find a lump in their breast need to pursue a diagnostic workup to determine if the lump is malignant. There is no question in my mind that my cancer was curable because it was found early. It is not uncommon for someone who has a lump to want to be reassured that it's not serious, but false reassurance is too high a price to pay if in fact the lump is cancerous.

Patients need information, but nurses need to be selective in the timing and amount of content of their teachings. Some patients cannot handle too much information at one time, and they reach a point where they are no longer able to attend to what is said or comprehend its meaning. Individual differences are vitally important to assess with regard to these matters.

Health care professionals need to listen to the problems patients perceive as distressing to them. It was humiliating to have my physician tell me that my lymphedema was nonexistent. It was a problem for me, and I needed someone to acknowledge that I was distressed about it.

Women who perceive they have lymphedema need to see a health provider who will work with them to develop a comprehensive program that includes a variety of treatments. It is not enough to treat the arm by itself. Be persistent and continue to search for a management program that provides relief, personal control, and satisfaction.

Cancer is a disease that can present an opportunity to confront values and priorities in life. As Ganz (1990) states, rehabilitation is an important component of cancer care. I recognized early in my treatment that I needed assistance with my continuing care needs. Patients may need assistance in recognizing their need for help and to be directed to resources for assistance with their problems. Nurses need to follow-up with patient problems to see if they have been resolved. If problems continue, alternative strategies need to be pursued.

Fiore (1979), a psychologist, described his experience with cancer as including secondary gains. I used my experience with cancer to improve my life and re-order my priorities. Making decisions about what was happening to me and the support I received from others had a positive influence on my life, enhancing the quality of my living. Equally important, nurses need to explore with patients whether cancer has had a positive impact on their lives and to assist in helping them strive to fulfill their goals.

REFERENCES

Fiore, N. (1979). Fighting cancer—one patient's perspective. *New England Journal of Medicine, 300,* 384–389.

Ganz, P. A. (1990). Current issues in cancer rehabilitation. *Cancer, 65,* 742–751.

47

Living with the Consequences of a Spouse's Cancer

Margaret McLean Heitkemper

THE DIAGNOSIS
TREATMENT AND STAGING

RECOMMENDATIONS

In the early summer of 1981 my husband, David, was diagnosed with testicular cancer. It was the beginning of a challenging period for us as we faced the immediate consequences of the diagnosis and subsequent treatment. In addition, there were the challenges of living with the long-term consequences of cancer such as the fear of recurrence and infertility.

THE DIAGNOSIS

We were living in Chicago at the time of the diagnosis. David was teaching in a metropolitan Chicago high school while I was finishing my doctoral degree at the University of Illinois Medical Center. It was June, and the school year was over for David. I had committed to a faculty position in Seattle, and David was planning to leave in July to job- and house-hunt. I would follow as soon as my dissertation was completed. Since we both had grown up in Washington state and most of our family lived there, it was a dream come true for both of us to return.

In 1981, we had been married 8 years and were anxious to start a family. Due to education and training goals, we had put off starting a family for several years. Although we were anticipating a lot of change ahead, the timing seemed right for both of us. But as the winter and spring months went by, we were unable to conceive. Finally, we consulted an infertility specialist. In addition to several tests for me, a sperm count was needed. The results of this test indicated a low sperm count, and David was referred to a urologist.

Although there seemed to be no urgency, David opted to see the urologist before leaving for Seattle. His insurance coverage would end in June, and it seemed efficient to seek medical care in case additional tests were needed. The day of the appointment was memorable. Due to a delay in the physician's schedule we waited more than 4 hours for this relatively routine visit. During that period we talked about rescheduling the appointment or delaying until we returned to Seattle. But in the end, we waited.

It was a fast appointment. During the physical examination a small lump was found in the right scrotum.

The urologist was blunt. The tumor was cancerous. The only questions were the cell type and the degree of spread. There was no time to think about a second opinion and no need for a biopsy—testicular tumors are rarely benign. A blood sample was obtained for the potential presence of tumor markers such as HCG. It was a Wednesday and David was scheduled for surgery on Friday.

We were stunned by the diagnosis. There had been no warning signs, no illness, no symptoms of nausea or pain, no signs of weight loss—all the stereotypical signs and symptoms one associates with cancer. David was in the "prime" of his life and feeling great.

TREATMENT AND STAGING

Between that Wednesday and the day of surgery, there was little time to dwell on the meaning of the illness. We had no family in Chicago, and we greatly missed their support during this stressful period. In the previous year, David had lost his mother to metastatic breast cancer. She died within 10 months of the initial diagnosis. Thus, his personal experience with cancer had been the worst. Although a nurse, I knew little about testicular cancer. My specialty area was geriatrics. As a new graduate registered nurse in 1973, I had cared for a young man who eventually died from testicular cancer. There were few treatment options at that time. I remembered vividly the devastating effect of his illness on his wife and family.

We looked for causes or explanations. We wondered about the risk factors for testicular cancer and which ones he might have had. There had been no history of cryptorchism (undescended testicle) or trauma. There was a positive family history for breast and prostate cancer on his mother's side, but the link to testicular cancer had not been determined. David was 36 years old at the time, a year older than the magical age range for testicular cancer. For 2 years during the Vietnam War David had served on an aircraft carrier, and we thought about potential exposure to chemicals or other potential environmental factors. There was no answer to the question of why.

One of the concerns we had during this initial period was finances. Due to the fact that it was early June, we were able to request that his medical insurance be converted to a private policy so that subsequent treatment ahead would be covered. This helped allay our anxieties about the immediate costs of the treatment. If the diagnosis had been made 3 weeks later, we would have had no insurance coverage.

The surgery, a unilateral orchiectomy, was uneventful in its course. Within 24 hours David was home. After the surgery, the urologist was unable to tell us about the extent of the cancer. We had to wait for the histology report regarding cell type and additional diagnostic tests to determine regional or metastatic involvement, which would be done during the next 2 weeks. These included an intravenous pyelogram, lymphangiogram, abdominal CT scan, and chest tomography. Everything considered, this was the hardest 2 weeks we ever experienced. The not knowing and assuming the worst made the days drag. The lack of family and additional support made this period particularly difficult.

After all the test results were in, we met with the urologist. It was unbelievably good news. There appeared to be no overt signs of metastasis. It was one of those few cases of testicular cancer in which the tumor had not spread, not even to the regional lymph. Although these tests could not rule out micrometastasis, there appeared to be no gross lesions. Another piece of good news was the histology report. The cell type was seminoma with no additional cell types. We were told the prognosis was better because this cell type is sensitive to radiation. The final good news was that tumor markers were all negative.

The next appointment was with the oncologic radiologist to schedule the radiation therapy. The radiation treatment, directed at the abdominal lymph, would last for 3 weeks. During this period David suffered from mild nausea and lost weight, but compared with the rigors of chemotherapy, which was used at that time to treat other forms of testicular cancer, it was a relatively easy period. The possibility of a good prognosis buoyed our spirits during this time.

During this period of time, the long-term consequences of the disease began to come to the forefront. Initially we had been focused on the life-threatening nature of the problem and potential discomfort of the treatment. Once these issues had been addressed, we began to think and talk about the implications for the family we had hoped to have. Looking back, it was unfortunate that none of the health professionals with whom we came into contact on a daily or weekly basis talked to us about our desire to have children. We had questions. Even during the hospitalization no one mentioned the potential impact of the surgery or treatment on fertility. Immediately after his discharge from the hospital, David confided in me that his cancer must be very serious, because none of the nurses who cared for him mentioned the nature of his surgery to him. This showed me that the failure to talk with patients about their physical health problems can leave them with the wrong impression.

In one respect our infertility had been a blessing. Without the initial low sperm count, David would not have seen a urologist, and his testicular cancer would likely have metastasized prior to diagnosis. But during this time, it seemed that cancer and its treatment would add to our struggles to start a family. We knew little about infertility treatments.

As a nurse I knew the importance of open communication regarding cancer and its treatment and prognosis. However, as a wife this was more difficult because I foremost wanted to be positive and supportive. David and I were able to discuss it openly and to make plans. Our discussions helped David share his feelings and concerns with his brothers and sisters, who had already experienced cancer within the family.

After the radiation treatment, we resumed our original plans to relocate. David returned to Seattle in August, and I joined him in late September. David continued to see a local urologist every 3 to 4 months for a year, then every 6 months until the 5-year anniversary of his diagnosis. At first, finding an appropriate physician was difficult because of variations in treatment protocols and insurance coverage. Some of the information we were told in Chicago did not match what we were told in Seattle. This added to our stress. With respect to health care, it would have been ideal to have stayed within the same health care system for the duration of the treatment. It was stressful to switch providers, particularly when there were differences in the treatment philosophies.

We also resumed our plans to start a family. We were counseled to wait for 1 to 2 years because of the potential for radiation scatter. However, we were not optimistic that even after that period of time that we would be able to have a biologic child. We began our exploration into the adoption options. Most startling and distressing to us was that many of the in-country adoption programs that we consulted would not consider us because of David's positive and recent history of cancer.

On the suggestion of a friend we began to explore options available through international adoptions. These agencies required a physical examination and a physician's opinion regarding potential for long-term survival. With both of these positive, we were able to successfully adopt two children over a 5-year period. Both of our daughters were born in Korea. Our oldest was 3 months of age at the time of adoption, and our youngest was $10\frac{1}{2}$ months of age. They are now 12 and 7 years old. In a way, David's tumor was a blessing to us again. Without his tumor, we would not have had the joy and pleasure of raising the two most beautiful girls in the world.

Although there are always concerns, even following a successful treatment of cancer, they have faded over the years. For several years, it was the threat of recurrence, and even now there is the potential long-term negative effects of the radiation treatment. Regular annual checkups do much to allay these anxieties.

RECOMMENDATIONS

In the past 14 years since David's diagnosis and treatment, there have been many advances in the treatment and management of testicular cancer. Tumor types that were considered more difficult to treat in 1981 are now "treatable." Testicular cancer remains one of the most curable forms of cancer. The survival rate is most optimistic in those patients like David, whose tumors are found early. Testicular self-examination would seem to be an important tool in the early detection of cancer. After his diagnosis David admitted to having felt a small lump in his scrotum 2 months prior to his physician's visit. He thought it was not serious and that it would go away. As health care practitioners we need to educate patients on how to monitor their bodies and when to seek health care.

There are also more options available to couples regarding family planning. Sperm can be collected prior to surgery and treatment and banked for later use. Low sperm counts can be enhanced by specific procedures. More expensive options, frequently not covered by health insurance, include artificial insemination and various in vitro procedures. All of these options need to be discussed with the family in an open fashion early in the process. In addition, the success and failure rates of various procedures need to be fully presented so families can evaluate their options and make informed decisions. Nurses can potentially provide this counseling to couples throughout all stages of the illness.

Recovering from the Experience of a Family Member's Illness and Death*

Marilyn Frank-Stromborg

These are my reflections as my husband's sister underwent the rigors of autologous bone marrow transplant (ABMT) for breast cancer. Throughout the experience, my husband (a physician) and I found that while we were both health professionals, we were also family members who had emotions that fluctuated from day to day. These included denial, anger, depression, grief, sadness, confusion, and hope. Furthermore, we found that our roles—"health professional versus family member"—alternated daily and sometimes hourly.

THE BEGINNING

My sister-in-law, Christine Smith, received a diagnosis of breast cancer in January 1989. At that time, she was a healthy 39-year-old mother of three school-aged children (aged 7, 10, and 12 years) and regularly practiced breast self-examination (BSE). She had had a negative baseline mammogram 4 years previously. Immediately after discovering the lump during BSE, she saw her gynecologist, who confirmed the presence of a mass and ordered an ultrasound of the breasts. When she tearfully called me about the lump and the confirmation by ultrasound and told us that a breast biopsy was needed, my immediate response was to cite all the statistics about the high number of nonmalignant lesions found with biopsy, her lack of risk factors for breast cancer, her health-promoting lifestyle, and the fact that she practiced regular BSE. All this was designed to decrease her anxiety as well as mine and to instill a sense of hopefulness about the future for both of us.

---

*This chapter is dedicated to my sister-in-law Chris Smith, 1949–1990, who was beloved by everyone who knew her.

Much of the material in this chapter appeared in Frank-Stromborg, M. (1990). Autologous bone marrow transplant: Personal reflections. *Innovations in Oncology Nursing*, 6(4), 1, 9–12.

THE DIAGNOSTIC PHASE

The initial biopsy revealed that the lesion was malignant and that it was a lymph node located in the breast, an unusual occurrence. Because my nursing specialty was oncology, I became the "designated information seeker." Information-seeking activities on my part included calling Physician's Data Query, doing a MEDLINE literature review at the university library, calling professional colleagues who specialized in breast cancer, as well as contacting those in the area to obtain the names of physicians (surgeons and medical oncologists) they would recommend. It quickly became evident that in the treatment of breast cancer there was a divergence of opinion and no one "right" approach. This made our role as health professionals even more difficult, because we could not advocate one approach or drug protocol with absolute certainty. Unfortunately, having choices may also contribute to a sense of guilt later, that if a cure isn't achieved, then the wrong choice was made. Our final decisions were made based on our literature review, discussions with professional colleagues, and the recommendations of physicians whom we all trusted. Ultimately, an oncologist known as a breast cancer specialist in a large teaching hospital was chosen as the primary physician, as was a surgical oncologist from the same institution. A modified radical mastectomy was performed; five lymph nodes were positive (three out of four axillary nodes, a lymph node in the pectoral muscles, and the original biopsy node).

POSTMASTECTOMY TREATMENT

The initial appointment, several days after discharge from the hospital, with the medical oncologist to discuss the proposed treatment plan went well, until autologous bone marrow transplant (ABMT) was mentioned as a treatment procedure that was being used elsewhere. I can remember thinking that this suggestion was premature and that I would be hard-pressed to recommend it. All the horror stories I had heard about it came to mind, and I quickly dismissed the possibility. Two weeks after surgery, four courses of chemotherapy with Adriamycin and cyclophosphamide were initiated, which were scheduled for every 3 weeks. Complications included (1) low blood counts that necessitated rescheduling treatments to every 4 weeks, and (2) hospitalization for 1 week for a generalized infection and treatment with intravenous antibiotics. The expected side effects of hair loss, loss of appetite, taste changes, nausea, heartburn, and sleep disturbances occurred and prevented any of us from denying that she had cancer. The role that I assumed during much of the initial discussions with oncologists in the early treatment phases was to act as both an interpreter and a forecaster. I found that I was asked to (1) translate the discussions we had with health care professionals into understandable and useable information, (2) explain what should be expected in the near future and how to deal with these future events, and (3) reassure everyone that what was happening was a normal occurrence.

My sister-in-law's psychologic reaction to the cancer and its treatments was extremely positive. She read as much as she could, sought out other women who had breast cancer to find out what to expect, and attended "Y-Me" meetings. She eagerly read all the patient education booklets, books, and professional articles that I sent her and many times managed the side effects of treatment herself, basing her self-care strategies on what she had learned from these materials.

Following chemotherapy, radiation to the chest wall and axilla was initiated. Radiation treatments were administered 5 days a week for 7 weeks. As with chemotherapy, she experienced radiation side effects (i.e., a dramatic skin reaction) that caused a disruption in the treatment schedule. Treatment delays had a markedly depressing effect, because she was anxious to finish all cancer treatments as projected and put the experience behind her. The most difficult things for my sister-in-law to cope with throughout the two treatments were (1) the suddenness of the diagnosis, (2) the fact that she felt so healthy at the time of the diagnosis, (3) the severity of the treatments that were designed to cure her disease, and (4) the uncertainty about treatment outcomes and anxiety about the possibility of dying and about what would happen to her three children. I found that the themes of suddenness of the diagnosis, feeling healthy yet being told she was sick, and severity of the treatments were continually repeated in her conversations with me as well as with her husband, mother, other family members, and friends. The possibility of not being successfully cured was rarely discussed by anyone and was clearly a taboo subject for others to raise. But it was like an ever-present shadow in all our conversations.

By early fall all cancer treatments were completed, and the first 3-month follow-up physical examination/laboratory tests showed that all measured parameters were normal. The same positive results were found in the December follow-up visit, and a long-awaited trip to Hawaii was planned for February. Everything seemed wonderful to all of us at this point: completion of her cancer treatments, positive follow-up visits, the resumption of all her usual activities, and the fact that she felt both physically and mentally "great."

METASTATIC SPREAD OF THE CANCER

Following the vacation to Hawaii, however, the prognosis changed overnight from optimism to absolute despair. During the March follow-up visit abnormal liver enzymes were found, and a CAT scan of the liver was ordered. My husband and I attempted to decrease everyone's anxiety by pointing out all the other diagnoses that might cause abnormal results, urging optimism until the CAT scan results were known. Unfortunately, the results showed metastatic involvement of more than half the liver, and bone x-ray examinations found involvement in the femur. The primary oncologists started conventional chemotherapy with different drugs and discussed the limited options that were available. Again, the ABMT option was raised for consideration. And once again as the "designated information seeker," I began to search for information. What had been unthinkable less than a year ago suddenly held out the only hope for my sister-in-law. Information gathered from the research literature and from personal contacts with health professionals involved in bone marrow transplantation was conflicting and did not give definitive answers on the success of this procedure. My husband and I discussed the pros and cons of ABMT with the family but emphasized that the ultimate decision rested with my sister-in-law. With no hesitation, she stated that she wanted to undergo the procedure. The next week was spent gathering records, visiting various BMT units in the area, and interviewing the physicians who were in charge of each unit. The major considerations for selecting where to have the transplant done were nurse-patient ratio, location of the hospital, visiting regulations in terms of family and children, and reputation of the physician. Once the ultimate decision was made, chemotherapy with 5-fluorouracil, methotrexate, and leucovorin was continued to reduce the tumor burden, diethylstilbestrol was added, and her response was monitored. In a short period of time (four treatments), liver enzymes were in the normal range, and the physician felt more optimistic about my sister-in-law's candidacy for ABMT. After the CAT scan showed that the tumor had shrunk more than 75 per cent and a biopsy of the bone marrow was normal, the procedure was scheduled for early May.

One of the questions that my relatives and friends asked frequently was, "What do other cancer patients do who don't have relatives or friends with a medical background to help find out the information necessary to make informed decisions?" We discussed the possibility of every hospital assigning one nurse who would be with the patient throughout the disease trajectory.

He or she would do all the things that I had been doing for my family: be an information-seeker, interpreter of medical information, forecaster of expected events, and cheerleader during rough periods. I also assisted my family with formulating questions they needed to ask to make informed decisions and to clarify the meaning of unexpected events.

THE TRANSPLANT

In preparation for the transplant, I talked with as many people in the "business" as possible and actually memorized all the success stories that I heard. I also found that there was a tendency on the part of others to focus on the positive cases and skip over those who did poorly. I'm sure that I was nonverbally communicating that I wanted to hear about those who did well rather than those who didn't. I would relay all this positive information to the family and thus further convince all of us that the treatment was bound to work.

The day after the bone marrow harvesting, the intravenous chemotherapy conditioning was started. Because the previous hospitalization for a generalized infection had proved to be traumatic, we promised to spend nights with her during the transplant. While receiving the chemotherapy over the next 5 days, Chris would doze in and out of a sleepy state. She was alert enough to get up for the frequent bathroom trips due to the hydration necessary with cisplatin but would then drift back into a sleepy state. The first day of chemotherapy was uneventful, and it seemed it would be a "piece of cake." However, that evening she began vomiting and was unable to hold down anything she ate or drank from then on. It was interesting that in later conversations she had no recollection of that week, the vomiting, or any discomfort experienced due to the antiemetics she was receiving. Nonetheless, it was a very difficult time for all of us to see her so uncomfortable and sick. The family member who spent the night with her got little or no sleep because of her frequent trips to the bathroom or the hourly visits by the night nurse to change intravenous bags, check the intravenous line, or take vital signs. We coordinated who would stay with her each night, trying to keep the nights her husband stayed to a minimum. As the days wore on, the stress of traveling long distances to the hospital and of trying to continue meeting our own work commitments, in conjunction with sleep deprivation from spending the night at the hospital, took its toll on all of us. At home, tempers became short, and I found I was easily moved to tears. My brother-in-law had the most difficult time because he was trying to maintain a large legal practice as well as be the primary caretaker for their three children, while still traveling to the hospital every day to spend time with his wife and be as supportive as possible. The help of other relatives, neighbors, and friends was absolutely invaluable in terms of assisting him with the care of their three children. By the end of the hospitalization, he seemed to have aged 10 years.

Six days after the chemotherapy was initially administered, a central line was inserted, and the next day

the bone marrow was infused. The evening the bone marrow was infused my husband was spending the night with Chris. Many jokes were made about the strong garlic smell he experienced all night, and it helped cheer up my sister-in-law.

Seeing her sitting in her tiny room wearing a mask, with all the intravenous bags of antibiotics, hyperalimentation lipids and blood products, and with her bald head, it was very hard to keep in mind that in time she would leave the hospital, let alone ever be healthy again. As she limped toward the bathroom due to the pain of the infected bone marrow aspiration sites, pushing her intravenous pump and all the intravenous bags, I marveled at the strength of human beings to cope with the discomforts necessary to achieve a cure. For me, this was the most difficult and depressing time of the whole experience. I just couldn't visualize that she would eventually leave and, in time, be healthy. During this period we all made a very conscious effort to remain optimistic, keep conversations cheerful, and bring different humorous videotapes when we stayed at night. I deliberately steered away from asking any probing questions that might make her sad. However, by day 12 postinfusion, everyone was discouraged and beginning to wonder if her blood values would ever start to rise.

I found that the most important roles we played during her hospitalization were those of cheerleaders as well as information-seekers. The one thing that helped me the most was hearing professional colleagues say that everything that was happening was "normal" for someone going through ABMT and that she was right on target in terms of blood values and so on. I found these types of positive comments extremely reassuring and quickly passed them on to the family. Nurses need to keep in mind the very important role family members play in helping to keep the patient's spirits up and purposely include the provision of psychosocial support for these family members.

GOING HOME

Finally, on day 13 postinfusion (more than 3 weeks of hospitalization), the physician announced that my sister-in-law might be able to go home in 4 days: intravenous bags running, bone marrow site infections, low blood counts, and all. I don't think that I've ever heard such wonderful, spirit-lifting news in my life. There were concerns about handling her care at home, but we were assured that a home care nurse would visit daily to monitor things initially. An end to this ordeal was finally visible. As it turned out, her counts didn't go up to an acceptable level for going home until more than a week later. Every day things would improve a little: counts slowly went up, infection sites slowly healed, and her appetite slowly improved. However, just the thought that the end was near and she would be able to go home to her children was enough to keep all of us cheerful and full of hope.

Three weeks after she was discharged and able to go home, all the complications and side effects had ceased, and her counts were within the normal range. Life was slowly settling into a routine again, and it was absolutely wonderful for all of us. Initially it was a little difficult letting go of our involvement. We offered to visit and help her and continued to advise her that she really needed to "take it easy and rest." However, my sister-in-law made it very clear that she wanted to return to a normal existence as soon as possible, and she did not want to be treated as an "ill person."

About a month after the ABMT, the lab results and scans indicated that metastatic disease was still present in the liver and that the tumor was continuing to grow. Many tears were shed by all of us at this news. Of everything that has happened in the past year, this was the most difficult news to hear because it clearly indicated that a cure was not going to be achieved. My sister-in-law once again started receiving chemotherapy as an outpatient. She insisted on living the best she could with her cancer and keeping up her daily routine. In my opinion, her quality of life was excellent. She had an active social life, was involved in her children's activities, jogged or played an hour of tennis each day, and always had a smile and a cheerful attitude. My role during this period of time was clearly that of a concerned family member who did whatever I could to facilitate her wish to continue to live each day to its fullest until that was no longer a reality.

DYING

During early November, my husband had to go out-of-state for training with the Air National Guard for several weeks. Chris usually talked with him daily to tell him how she was getting along. During his absence, Chris called to report on her progress. She started commenting on how large she was getting around the waist. I minimized these reports and commented that it probably just seemed that way to her. Toward the end of the time my husband was out-of-state, my oldest son went to visit his aunt for the day. He came back visibly disturbed from his visit with his aunt. I made some comment about his foul mood, and he yelled back that his aunt looked like she was 9 months pregnant and didn't I realize that she was dying. This hit me like a bolt of lightning, since I had obviously been in a total state of denial about her premature deterioration.

The day my husband arrived home, we went together to visit my sister-in-law. The closer we got to her home, the slower he drove. Unconsciously he didn't want to confront the reality of what was happening to his sister. When we walked into her home, we were shocked by her appearance. She literally looked like she was 9 months pregnant. We all cried, realizing that the end was near. There was comfort in being able to function as a health professional. I called several hospices and arranged to have the hospice coordinator visit her in the coming week. My husband called his colleagues to get the name of an oncologist in the local hospital who could see his sister and evaluate "tapping" some of the fluid to make her more comfortable. Chris's mother, my mother-in-law, was very upset that we were making these plans, since she was convinced that the new chemotherapy would help and would save her daughter.

Later that day, I went shopping to get my sister-in-law underwear and decorative tops that she could wear to accommodate her increased abdominal growth. My saddest experience was buying these clothes at a maternity shop. The salesperson asked me who I was shopping for and I said my sister-in-law. She asked me how many months pregnant she was and I mumbled she was just about due.

When I returned from shopping, I helped put my sister-in-law to bed. Before going upstairs, she commented that she had been inundated with phone calls from friends. She looked at me and said, "I must be dying." All I could do is sadly move my head in agreement. At that moment, all the training that I had as a health professional in terms of therapeutic communication was for naught. I was simply a grieving relative who was attempting to cope with my sister-in-law's impending death.

As Thanksgiving approached, we felt that Chris would not be able to make our annual family gathering at her house. We agreed that I would do the cooking, since my sister-in-law was spending most of the day sleeping.

Two days later I answered the phone, and it was my sister-in-law speaking in a clear, upbeat manner. When I inquired about what had happened to make her sound so alert, she said she had stopped taking the antiemetic medication because it was making her sleepy and drowsy. Like a miracle, she was her old self again and it lifted my spirits and rekindled unrealistic expectations about her prognosis. She was feeling great and insisted on making the Thanksgiving dinner. This was the last phone call I had with her.

THE DEATH WATCH

Late that night, we got a call from my brother-in-law that they were going to the hospital since my sister-in-law was vomiting blood. My husband and I rushed to the hospital in Chicago and would remain there for the next week while Chris died. She was transferred from the emergency room to medical intensive care. She was vomiting blood clots the size of basketballs and was in intensive pain. A phone call was made to bring her three children to the hospital as soon as possible for her to say good-bye. She was sedated for gastroscopy to determine the site of the profuse bleeding. The gastroscopy revealed that the tumor had gone through the gastric wall and that the bleeding was successfully stopped. My husband stayed for this procedure and assumed the role of a relative who was a health professional. He conversed with the oncologist and gastroenterologist about her prognosis and the family's wish to provide palliative care. Once she was alert from the procedure, she asked for pain medication, and it was obvious she was in severe discomfort. A morphine drip was started to try and make her more comfortable.

About this time, her three children arrived at the hospital, and we left the room for Chris to have time alone with them to say good-bye. My mother-in-law went with my older son to the cemetery to select Chris's burial plot. All of us faced the inevitability of her death in our own way.

Chris was moved to a small room on the general medical-surgical floor and remained there for a week until she died. Chris was heavily sedated throughout the week it took her to die. Shortly after she was moved to the general floor, an alert nurse noted that Chris had a distended bladder. Catherization obtained a tremendous amount of urine. I felt very guilty that neither myself nor my husband had thought about this. We also realized that her severe back pain may have been due to the extensively distended bladder. Since she was sedated and not able to communicate, I raised the issue of decreasing her pain medication so she could talk. Maybe the severe back pain was due to the distended bladder and not the extensive disease? I felt so helpless.

My husband reassured me that she had disease-related pain and it was essential to keep her medication level high enough to keep her as comfortable as possible. My desire to have her talk to us was a reluctance to lose the vibrant, loving human being that was Chris. The oncologist came into the room and discussed with the family what approach they wanted to take and assured us that maximum pain control would be given to Chris. He impressed all of us with his caring attitude and desire to make her death as easy as possible. We elected to provide a morphine drip at this time and not artificial nutrition.

The week spent with her and waiting for her death was a blur. We all slept in the room or hospital waiting room; usually her husband would sleep in the chair next to her, I would sleep on the floor of the room, and my husband would sleep in the waiting room. She slowly fell into a deeper coma. Since she was receiving only a slow MS drip and nothing by mouth, mouth care became as issue. I attempted to do mouth care throughout the day and night and would assist the nurses in bathing and positioning her. I taught the other family members to give her mouth care and assist in periodic repositioning. Being able to provide her physical care gave all us enormous comfort.

Since we were aware that hearing was the last sensation to stop functioning, we talked to her throughout the day. We told her the date, time, how the weather was outside of the hospital, and how much we loved her. During the first days of the week, she attempted to talk to us, but it was unintelligible. With time, she was unable to even make guttural sounds.

The most difficult time for all of us was the last day when she was drowning in her own secretions, and she labored to take even the shallowest of breaths. Her husband had to leave the room during the several hours, when she was visibly drowning, and my husband and I sat and held her hands. During the last hour of her life, the cyanosis of the fingers deepened and climbed from her hands towards her body. Finally, she no longer had the strength to breath and stopped. We stood around the bed sobbing. Slowly blood started pouring out of her mouth and nose. This was very disturbing to all of us. The nurse started to clean Chris and suggested we step outside for a moment until she was finished. The family returned to say good-bye.

SUMMARY

In retrospect we were able to function in the role of health care professionals throughout much of my sister-in-law's illness. Specifically our roles involved information-gathering, guiding her through the health care system, cutting red tape, interpreting what was happening, providing patient education, and being optimistic cheerleaders. Towards the end of her illness, the only role we were able to assume was that of grieving relatives. We were grieving relatives who provided emotional support to her and needed emotional support ourselves. It was clear to us that as Chris was dying we needed health professionals who were knowledgeable about managing the symptoms of dying. The health professionals who were involved in her care assumed that we knew more than we did about this area. If you are involved in providing care to a health professional or a member of their family, treat them like you would any other family in terms of the patient-family education, family support, and medical attention that you provide. In retrospect, Chris's death rattle may have been limited if additional drugs other than morphine had been used. It is difficult to know for sure, since she obviously hemorrhaged at the end.

Other health professionals going through this type of experience need to realize that at some point in the illness, the role of close relative will overpower the role of health professional. Towards the end of her illness, we lost all objectivity, denied the reality of her illness, and clung to the unrealistic hope that even though the cancer was widespread, she would continue to enlighten our lives.

Our knowledge of the "system" enabled us to navigate Chris through the system and to see that she had every survival opportunity that was available. Unfortunately, most patients don't have their own "navigator" to traverse the system, answer the questions that arise once they go home, and provide patient education as well as fill in the patient education gaps.

When A Colleague Has Cancer

Judith K. Much • Susan B. Baird

When a colleague has cancer, we can be struck in a variety of ways. We respond in part from our professional base, drawing from our experience and knowledge. We may jump immediately to thinking about what we know in dealing with this particular type of cancer, about staging, treatment, and prognosis. Patients we have known in similar situations come to mind, and we think about their disease course, wondering how things will be for our colleague. We may think about where the colleague will be treated and by whom, recognizing the pros and cons of a professional being treated within their own facility.

We respond in part from our collegial base, thinking about how this person's disease will affect the facility and the person's role within the facility. Regardless of how close we may actually be to this person, we will have questions about the meaning of this person's disease and treatment to their department and to specific projects or responsibilities. If this is a colleague we work with regularly, we may begin to wonder who will take on some of these roles. How will others be affected? It may be that no immediate changes are needed. Alternatively, work schedules may need to be adjusted, reporting relationships may need to be temporarily reassigned, or perhaps plans need to be initiated to cover indefinitely.

Finally, we are affected personally. We have each experienced this in our own way. When a good friend was diagnosed with cancer, one of us remembers going through all the usual grief reactions: anger, fear, denial, bargaining, depression. Judie felt these not only for her friend but also for herself. The situation left her feeling extremely vulnerable. Her reaction also influenced the manner in which she could relate to her friend and colleague. Many oncology nurses find it particularly difficult when their colleagues are diagnosed with cancer, more difficult than other life-threatening diseases. After all, shouldn't these people have some sort of "credit" or "immunity" for the commitment they have made to helping others? Such thoughts may not make sense intellectually, but some variation of this thinking is common. And, we are angry—especially if the outcome doesn't look positive.

This chapter briefly tells the story of three colleagues and their cancer experience. It is written from the perspective of colleague, not caregiver, and highlights the range of experiences that commonly accompany such situations. The summaries are not intended to convey all aspects of their illness or care but rather to highlight points of common concern to coworkers and associates. All three have died of their cancers, but that is just coincidence. The main issues we want to convey surface when colleagues are living with their cancers as well. The recollections are followed by a discussion of common issues that arise when a colleague has cancer and by recommendations for how those issues may be addressed within the boundaries of a therapeutic relationship.

ROB

The night log in the nursing department contained a brief notation that Dr. Rob had been admitted during the night for abdominal pain and gastrointestinal (GI) bleeding. He had been a hematologist in the cancer center's medical oncology department for a number of years and had recently left the center to serve as director of the cancer program at a community hospital. Rob was well known throughout the center and universally liked and respected. News of his admission spread quickly throughout the center with staff reassuring one another that it made sense for Rob to come directly to the center, expediently admitted by a long-time colleague and thus avoiding a middle-of-the-night emergency room experience. As the day shift activities began, word quickly spread that Rob's problem was not a minor one, nor a benign one. Speculation began tempered by reminders that Rob was young and healthy.

Bits and pieces of test results were seized upon and deliberated as people sought information. As information became available, his treatment team consulted with one another and with experts at other centers to explore all avenues of possible treatment. In our small facility, information spreads very quickly. Rob himself did not discourage the spread of information. As he walked the halls he routinely stopped to talk with his colleagues and asked their opinions. When there were positive moments, the staff morale picked up. Likewise, when news was bad, a pall seemed to hang over the entire staff. The diagnosis of angiosarcoma was made, and the effect of this diagnosis on all members of the staff was readily apparent.

From the very beginning, the desire for information seemed insatiable. Our medical record is primarily a paper one, so this provided for at least some limitations on information access. Results reporting, however, is computerized and easily accessible to a wide variety of individuals. Early in his first hospital stay, the system was adjusted to close access to Rob's results.

During the months of Rob's illness, he had several hospital admissions at our center as well as some specialized treatment at another center in the city. Initially it was hard to see Rob's family members coming and going. Most staff had never met his wife, children, or parents, yet seeing them made us all aware of this whole part of Rob's life with which most of the staff had no connection. No one was sure just how Rob and his family could deal with the many people in the facility who wanted to express their caring. Attempting to meet Rob's wishes and tolerance regarding visits from staff members became a task for the unit leadership.

A number of people experienced stress related to Rob's care. Decisions were made about who would head the treatment team. Physicians especially close to Rob had to determine their role, deciding when and how to proceed with care planning. A senior fellow became the primary physician, a role he fulfilled beautifully and for which we are all grateful. This allowed Rob's chief colleague and friend to have input into treatment decisions but sufficient distance to focus on his role of friend and family support. Certainly the nurses who cared for Rob found it difficult to see his condition deteriorate, but this was countered by their ability "to do" in a very tangible way. Those who had no direct role often felt at a loss, not knowing how to express their caring. The nurse who had worked in a close, collaborative relationship with Rob in his practice at our center had her own distress and needed support. When Rob had left the center, careful arrangements were made to transfer the care of Rob's patients. Now when patients asked the nurse about Rob, she had to deal with responding appropriately while dealing with her own emotions.

There were difficult aspects of Rob's care during the course of his disease, and these were addressed as they arose. Nonetheless, it was hard to watch the physical deterioration, to know of Rob's pain, to feel helpless to change the course of his disease, and to accept that cancer would take one of our own. Continuity of care was facilitated by admitting Rob to the same unit each admission, a small unit where the nurses could easily become familiar with Rob's needs and desires. It is impossible to predict the extent to which this planning allowed Rob to be a patient in the way that worked best for him. Certainly it was his choice to be at home as much as possible and to receive care through the center's hospice. Both in the hospital and at home, Rob seemed to exert his preferences among providers and to express his needs.

Rob presided over his last few months in ways similar to the running of his practice. He was very clear about how colleagues could assist him, and one could only assume he was aware of the need for the many of us who were close to him to contribute to this last part of his life. For example, Rob would ask me (Judie) to take him to another nurses' station when the unit on which he was staying was slow in providing him with his lab results. He also explained one day how difficult it was to discuss his death with his young son and daughter. I asked if I could bring in a book I had used previously in explaining death to children. Rob and his wife allowed me to feel I contributed a small but important part of his care by utilizing that book in discussions with the kids. Finally, Rob also knew when to say good-bye. One by one he walked with us, shared quiet moments with us, and clearly said his good-byes. Rob's last days were spent at home with his family. Center physicians and the hospice director provided needed care.

At both Rob's funeral service and at a center memorial service, staff had opportunities to express their grief. There was an opportunity to thank those who had contributed in tangible ways to his care. Without anyone actually saying so, it seemed to ease our loss by knowing that Rob had chosen to be cared for at the center that had been his professional home and where he had so many close contacts.

ROSE

Rose was a cancer survivor. At age 15 she had been diagnosed with Hodgkin's disease and was treated with both chemotherapy and radiation. As a respiratory therapist at our cancer center, Rose used her experience to help current and former cancer patients. She was currently serving as president of our Survivors Association and had been quoted in a center publication as saying, "I can't describe the bond I feel when I see all these people together and realize they've gone through the same things I did. They've taught me so much, and they're so helpful" (Tobin, 1995). Rose always had a big smile to share as well. Just about 1½ years after she married another respiratory therapist in the department, Rose began to have some distressing physical symptoms. An adrenal mass was detected and believed initially to be a dysfunctional adrenal or other benign condition. On surgery, adrenal cancer was diagnosed, and Rose was out of work for several months. Several coworkers kept in regular touch with Rose, visiting her at home and encouraging communication and activity when Rose exhibited signs of depression.

When Rose returned to work part time, staff noted obvious changes in her physical appearance but were reluctant to address their concerns directly to Rose. Instead, questions about her condition were relayed to her coworkers. People were pleased she was able to return to work and expressed those thoughts directly, but there was a continual undercurrent of concern. Again, the need for information seemed insatiable.

About 2 weeks after Rose returned to work, she asked her supervisor to accompany her to the car as she left for the day. The supervisor came back to find that Rose had left some work undone, a most unusual occurrence. She had not recorded a pulse oxymetry reading on one unit. She had not responded to a stat arterial blood gas request on another. Her supervisor followed up with Rose at home; clearly Rose was too ill to be at work. She called out sick for the next several days. Her condition deteriorated during these days, and she was admitted to the center with a severely depleted potassium level and high cortisol levels. She spent the next month in the hospital, in the intensive care unit, and on one of the patient units.

Coworkers had many issues of concern. They expressed anger that a diagnosis had not been made sooner when, they felt, treatment options might have been greater or more effective. They had real difficulty with her appearance and the changes in her affect. Frequently she would not respond to visitors, sometimes she would not answer direct questions, and her depression seemed very deep. Colleagues seemed to have some preconceived expectations of how other colleagues should respond in terms of visiting or otherwise keeping contact. When these expectations were not met, there was obvious anger.

Several different plans were developed for Rose's care following hospitalization. Clearly she was too debilitated to be alone. A final decision was made for her to be admitted to a long-term care facility. Some staff members seemed to have difficulty with this family decision; it was almost as though they felt they were abandoning Rose. There was unspoken yet acknowledged knowledge that most would not see Rose alive again. Approximately 1 week later, Rose had a rapid deterioration. Close colleagues were able to make a final visit and to provide support for her husband and family. Many attended her services and shared in the general sadness that spread throughout the center. It was commonly felt that, at age 42, Rose's death was far too premature, her disease course too rapid. It could have been them. The uncertainties of life and the apparent randomness of its tragedies had struck too close to home.

GRACEANN

Graceann had been complaining about this vague abdominal pain for several weeks. Now even walking up one flight of stairs meant having to sit for several minutes before the pain would subside enough for her to continue her activities. She had just taken a new position with the American Nurses Association. She was to go to Kansas City for a week of orientation. Her main concern was how she would get from the hotel to the office, a block and a half away. She saw the gastroenterologist who had treated her for an ulcer a few years before. Tests took forever! She scheduled an appointment with the physician and then would wait a week or so for the scheduled test, then another wait for a visit followed by another wait for a test. Her nurse friends and colleagues grew tremendously impatient. We knew she needed a CAT scan; why wasn't it happening?

Graceann had experienced some very difficult times the year or so before this episode of pain. She had completed her doctorate at Catholic University but was not approved for tenure at George Mason University, a very deep trauma. She had taken a position in AIDS education that turned out to be a poor fit. The position she accepted in the ANA Certification Corporation seemed tailor-made. It would allow her to continue to live in her condominium in the Washington area where she had a wide circle of friends and colleagues. Things were definitely looking up!

During this bout of pain, she was seen by a fellow at the Lombardi Cancer Center for a routine visit, part of a breast prevention program she had been on for several years at NIH. When Dr. M. left NIH for Georgetown, Graceann continued in the study with him. The fellow found several supraclavicular nodes and wanted them biopsied. Graceann asked me (Susan) to be with her when she went for the results. Both Dr. M. and the fellow were present when they told Graceann that they had found metastatic pancreatic cancer. It was inoperable. They recommended port placement and chemotherapy. Graceann was clearly overwhelmed. "Well, you knew it would be bad news." Dr. M. responded perfunctorily. Friend, nurse, or colleague, to this very minute I can still feel my rage at that comment. It was not meant, I believe, to come across in such a callous fashion, but they are words Graceann never forgot. And neither did I. They were clearly not helpful.

Graceann had been diagnosed with a thymoma in 1966 and had undergone surgery and radiation. Doctors would later argue that it was probably not a thymoma but rather Hodgkin's disease, but whatever, it was cancer, and it affected her early adult years. In writing of that early experience, Graceann related, "I always said to myself that I can handle anything that is said to me. I also remind myself that if I went through a cancer experience at the age of 24 I can go through anything" (Ehlke, 1978). During the course of her second cancer, she referred often to that early experience.

I was Graceann's friend, and it is difficult to separate the friend role from the colleague role here. I want to focus on how Graceann's wide circle of nurse friends and colleagues took part in her care and her life in the months that followed. In her earlier experience Graceann had noted that, ". . . having a positive experience with a disease such as cancer necessitates much support from colleagues, friends, and family. I am grateful that I received such support" (Ehlke, 1978).

The way people came together for Graceann was truly amazing, albeit a little crazy-making at times.

Graceann lived alone. She made the difficult decision early in the course of her disease to remain in her home and not to return to her native home, Hawaii. This decision was difficult for her father and stepmother, but they were supportive. From day 1, Graceann made her own decisions. She would continue to be treated at Lombardi Cancer Center, but she grilled the fellow about just how long he would be around, telling him that she had no intention of being left at a critical time. He assured her he would be present throughout this illness and that Dr. M. would also remain active in her case. In the days I spent with her immediately following her diagnosis, she made several things very clear to me. She would not be forced to eat. If she didn't want to eat, she would not, and she did not want to be badgered about it. She was clear that her greatest fear was pain. She feared pain more than anything and made me promise I would let everyone, everywhere know she could not tolerate pain. Graceann made an early decision that she would not return to work. Her family helped make that financially feasible.

Immediate planning needed to be accomplished to meet Graceann's needs. She lived in Virginia; I lived in Philadelphia. Relying heavily on two other colleagues, Joan and Mary, we organized a team approach to meeting Graceann's needs. I took care of Graceann's medical and financial needs. Early on she wanted things settled legally, giving me medical power of attorney. Her family supported this decision. During the week Mary, a George Mason colleague, arranged for a coworker to check on Graceann each day and run any errands or provide simple services at home. Joan arranged transportation to and from appointments, calling on other colleagues to do so. She also arranged for food when Graceann's family visited. One colleague took Graceann for her chemotherapy each Friday morning. I would arrive Friday evening, take over the chemotherapy infusion monitoring, give her Ondansetron, and disconnect the infusion pump. Another colleague would pick up the pump on Sunday and return it to Georgetown.

Whenever things got too disconcerted, we held a Sunday morning team meeting. Graceann, Joan, Mary, and I would discuss upcoming needs and how they would be met. There were more than enough colleagues volunteering their help, but it did take coordination. Graceann wanted to see some of her colleagues and friends from out-of-town. Several of these people came for a week at a time, giving them private time with Graceann to visit and reminisce and yet participating in her day-to-day care. Each seemed to find some new food that Graceann would eat, at least for a day or so, or help her organize some other aspect of her care. These were very special times.

Pain was a major problem from the beginning. Graceann had trouble retaining oral medications and would get confused about what to take when. Sometimes she seemed to take too little and sometimes too much. Here her physician suggested trying an analgesic patch. The results were outstanding! She had a great deal of confidence in the patch, she had far less worry about pain, and there was improved quality in her life as she knew her pain was under control. Those of us who saw what a difference the patch made for Graceann were extremely grateful for this decision. It was difficult for us to hear from others not involved in her care that going to the patch "this early" was not a good idea, that it was too expensive, too difficult to control, and so on. There is much to be said for individualizing care, and for Graceann, the analgesic patch was probably the greatest asset.

At one of our Sunday team meetings, Graceann seemed restless and not interested in planning for her care. "I don't know what I'm going to do with all the salmon I have in the freezer. I just don't like thinking about you people eating it all when I'm gone." she said. That was the beginning of planning a party. Graceann got out her recipe box, set the menu, and assigned her favorite dishes to different colleagues. She made out the guest list and set a date. It was a rare moment of animation and lightness. Many colleagues had a role in the party, and it was a huge success. The videotape was treasured throughout the rest of her life.

As care became more demanding, my weekend visits and those of her colleagues were not enough. Someone was needed to put order to her routine and to give her more of a sense of security as she began to get fearful in the night. Her stepmother, Peggy, came from Hawaii to keep house. All of us remain grateful to Peggy for this wonderful gift to Graceann. Later on, more help was needed, and practical nurses came on board. They started with her during one hospitalization and went home with her and stayed on. During that particular hospital visit, Graceann was confused and agitated. She had a threatened cord compression and needed to wear a neck brace, which she would not keep in place. She had an unbelievable number of visitors, each with a different idea of how her care should proceed. I received a call from the nursing unit that we had to set some limits and separate care providers from friends. We had to let the unit manage her actual care. This was communicated to all, and no further problems arose.

Graceann's illness lasted slightly less than 8 months. Several aspects went very well—we respected her desires, even when they were not our own. Some colleagues felt she should have kept working longer, but most of us respected Graceann's decision. After all, she really knew more about herself and her cancer than we did. Overall, her oncology colleagues and her nononcology nursing colleagues worked well together in exchanging information and in providing tangible help. We found people ready to respond to any request from laundry to errands. Graceann listened to the advice of others and then responding in her characteristic way, taking on what she agreed with and ignoring the rest. She was always grateful for everything that was done for her, and the caring of others lifted her tremendously.

Few people will be able to live their final months as Graceann did, surrounded by colleagues and having special moments with each of them. The support of her family, both in presence and financially, made many things possible. Having nursing help in the home kept Graceann's hospitalizations to only two. Graceann loved her home and her cat and was more at ease there than anywhere. It was a loving experience in which we used our cancer and nursing experience in the best possible way. We all had a chance to give of ourselves, to be part of her journey and to accept that it was time for her to let go. And, we were there for each other in our loss of our friend, colleague, teacher, and professional acquaintance.

ISSUES COMMONLY ENCOUNTERED

BOUNDARIES

The goal of interactions that we, as professionals, have with our patients, is to empower them through establishing a therapeutic relationship. Therapeutic relationships have been defined by Barnsteiner and Gillis-Donovan (1990) as those that are respectful of both personal and professional boundaries, provide for a caring and well-defined relationship between nurse, patient, and family, and promote the patient and family's control over the health care situation in which they are found. Our interactions and relationships with those who are ill and also happen to be our friends and colleagues are deserving of the same careful and deliberate care.

Barnsteiner and Gillis-Donovan define "boundaries" in this context to mean "where self leaves off and another person begins" (p. 226). Boundaries can be characterized as being clear (well defined), aloof (separate and distinct), or having too much relatedness (diffuse). In the oncology setting, we often struggle with maintaining clear boundaries. Repeat admissions, patients the same age with similar life circumstances, or reminiscences of family members may all complicate the therapeutic relationship and cause boundaries to become blurred or enmeshed. When a colleague has cancer, similar problems may arise, not only for the same, but also for slightly different reasons.

CARE DIRECTION

There are difficulties inherent in directing the care of a colleague. If the individual is your friend or close colleague, it may be difficult to be objective enough to direct the care and help to make decisions. We may and often do feel the need to be involved. The goal of care is to support or empower the individual to make his or her own decisions, not to make decisions for them. There may be more than one colleague who wants to direct care or be a caregiver. There may not be enough "jobs," or it may not be possible to accommodate all who would like to do the caring.

CONFIDENTIALITY

Computerization of medical record information can be both a blessing and burden when trying to keep private the information on colleagues. Information should be available on a need-to-know, not want-to-know basis. When a well-known colleague is hospitalized, their "celebrity" status should not overshadow or preclude their right to privacy. When a colleague is admitted to his or her "own" institution, information needs accelerate. Gossip surrounds the case. One can ask if it is better that facts be shared or simply gossip and rumor. Immunity from wanting to know the medical information to arrive at your own evaluation of how he or she is doing is very hard to come by. This "need" to know and evaluate is helpful in providing perceived control when we are feeling vulnerable.

FEELINGS

Anger. A colleague who is sick and may be dying may express anger at you, just as any other patient may direct their anger. It feels much different when you receive this from a colleague. We may be less likely to even think about the anger we may feel toward him or her. Anger also arises in those who want to be involved in care but are not. Disagreement among family members of a colleague may feel uncomfortable, especially if the family member then relays this disagreement to another member of the staff.

Jealousy. A well-known colleague is emergently admitted with an unexpected diagnosis of cancer. All nursing units want to care for him. All friends, who are also all professionals, want to be involved. The physician and his or her family pick the unit with private rooms, and one particular friend may be chosen for the care. Colleagues may feel jealousy because one unit or caregiver was chosen over others. This is not an unusual feeling in the caregiver role. It is similar to "who owns the patient?"

COLLEAGUES, FRIENDS, AND CAREGIVERS

It may be difficult to be both friend/colleague and caregiver. Often we wonder whether we must give up one role for another. For example, we must give up the professional role if we are to act as a friend. It is important to separate the roles. The answer is a personal one. It is difficult to put your grief on hold to maintain your objectivity needed to direct care or be a professional caregiver. This may make your colleague feel better, but it is unfair to you. Roles may change at different points along the disease continuum.

Caring for a colleague who has cancer leaves us feeling a special vulnerability that few other patients can bestow upon us. Here lies one of us—someone who has been devoted to taking care of others with cancer—who has been struck with the disease. There is no justice, and we are alone with our own fear. It can happen to any of us. It has and it will—and we know it.

SPECIAL CARE

Ever notice what kind of treatment VIPs or the patients whom staff members "really like" receive? Our professional instinct tells us that all of our patients should receive the same level of care. But, as humans, we tend to give good care to all and *really* good care to those we really care for, or for whom it "pays" to care in a special way. Certainly our friends receive special treatment. We go the "extra mile." We volunteer to "special" them. We make house calls. We give "special care" to these, our "special" patients. This may become problematic to us if we find or feel we are giving someone else less care to have more time to care for our colleague. Alternately, we may be resentful if we perceive our colleague is not getting the amount or level of care we would like to have him or her receive.

RECOMMENDATIONS

INDIVIDUAL

There are approaches that may be useful in situations where colleagues are patients. It may be helpful to remember that we have our own feelings and issues related to life-threatening disease and that these can cause interference over our outcomes and responses when we are caring for those we work with and/or care about. It is generally useful to pick a role. . . any role, but be clear about which role you pick, and then do it. It may be best to function in the role of a friend and leave caregiving to others. This might make you more emotionally and physically present for your colleague. You may be a welcome change from the parade of caregivers in your colleague's life. If you want to be the caregiver, be sure to assess where you stop and your colleague starts. Being clear about roles doesn't mean there is less angst or pain involved in the relationship, but it may help you clarify whose needs are to be met and why. Sometimes both roles can be juggled successfully, but it may be helpful to seek feedback from others on how that is going.

Communicate with the patient and family members. Find out what your colleague needs or wants from you. Are the expectations reasonable? Facilitate empowerment of the patient and family. Make sure that there is room for the family in the care and that the collegial presence is not overwhelming. Talk it out prior to the time it becomes a problem, and respect the needs of the colleague and family as being primary.

Finally, support each other. All of us feel hopeless and want desperately to "fix it" or do something when a colleague has cancer. We will each grieve in our own way, but we will each feel a sense of loss, regardless of the outcome of the disease process. For the one with cancer, the loss of privacy and professional stature must be tremendous. Fear may replace rational thought processes. Often, the one with cancer continues to be the one supporting others, a tremendous gift to those who receive it, but nonetheless exhausting to the individual. To those colleagues who are not involved in the direct care of the colleague, there may be tremendous longing to *do something* and anxiety in not knowing what to do or where to fit in. Again, speaking to either the individual or family members may shed light on what we may be able to contribute, for example, books, baby-sitting, knitting caps, contributing to meals, etc. It may be that our presence alone, which feels wanting many times, may be the greatest need. Once a need is made known by the colleague and family, it should be communicated throughout the organization so that any one who wishes to can contribute and feel useful in that way. Helping everyone "fit" or be useful is a gift in itself.

INSTITUTIONAL

When a colleague known throughout an institution has cancer, it affects the entire institution. It feels like any other type of tragedy that besets a family. We know through our practice that cancer is a disease that affects families, not just individual patients. When a colleague has cancer, the "institutional family" experiences it. The institutional grieving process is a reflection of the individuals grieving within it. First there is institutional shock, disbelief, and anger. Tempers may flare as individuals struggle to comprehend what has occurred. What appears to be gossip abounds, as individuals need to repeat the story as they know it, over and over. Doing so helps what has happened to become real.

Individuals also struggle for meaning in the face of tragedy. As we feel increasingly vulnerable, we look for blame. Did our colleague ignore warning signs? Was lifestyle such that cancer risk was increased? Surely, we would have recognized earlier or changed our habits before it got to this stage. When the reality of the situation is at full impact, we look at the information we have at hand, through the computers or medical records or through word of mouth, and then we do what in our profession is second nature: we determine in our own mind what the prognosis is. When caring for patients, this can be a helpful exercise in knowing what may occur in the future. When the patient is a colleague, this information frequently puts us into instant anticipatory grief. This friend, this colleague who has meant something in our professional lives will be changed or will no longer be there. Because of this phenomenon and our struggle to continue, whole institutions can grieve and effectively bury the individual long before the actual treatment or death occurs. This is tragic for all involved, for when the individual leaves the institution or dies, real mourning must happen, and the "institution" may have little tolerance for that if mourning has already occurred. Anticipatory grief can also rob the colleague of much-needed hope and support if all that is seen in the eyes of those caring is, "Poor Joe, can't he see this is a futile effort?"

Communication is the hallmark of recommendations for grieving institutions. The individual with cancer must have a say in what information is to be presented to the institution as a whole. Based upon the wishes of that person, support must be given to those who do or do not get information. A representative or group of colleagues can talk to the patient or family to determine what might be the most useful yet unintrusive way that individuals can be involved. The institution must be tolerant of the needs of all concerned and must take time to support and talk about the vulnerability felt by cancer institution members when cancer strikes their own. Individuals within the institution must be allowed to express their discomfort at not knowing everything they might wish to know, yet support for the family who wishes some normalcy in confidentiality must be maintained. Caution in communicating anticipatory grief should be exercised to have hope preserved for as long as possible or necessary. Gossip must be discouraged, but understanding about the need to reinforce what is real is encouraged. Various support needs must be identified and addressed. For instance, there will be one group who may need support because of direct involvement in the individual's care. Another group needing support includes those who want to be involved in care but are not. Still a third group includes the remaining individuals who have had a collegial relationship with the individual but who cannot or do not wish to provide care.

If the colleague with cancer dies, it is important to recognize the loss that the institution as a whole has sustained. There should be some institutional recognition of this fact, through either a service, flying the flag at half staff, etc. A group project such as a memorial lectureship, scholarship, or special planting are ways to keep the spirit of the individual alive. The important point is that when the loss is recognized as being a loss to the entire institution, permission is given for the institution and the individuals within it to grieve.

REFERENCES

Barnsteiner, J. H., Gillis-Donovan, J. (1990) Being related and separate: A standard for therapeutic relationships. *American Journal of Maternal Child Nursing, 15*(4), 223–228.

Ehlke, G. A. (1978) From the inside looking out . . . a personal experience with cancer. In P. K. Burkholter & D. L. Donley (Eds.), *Dynamics of oncology nursing* (pp. 3, 17). New York: McGraw-Hill Book Co.

Tobin, S. (Ed). (1995). In memoriam: Rose Brown O'Connell. *In Touch, A Newsletter of the Fox Chase Cancer Center* (p. 8). Philadelphia: Spring.

My Mother's Struggle with Endometrial Cancer: Coping from a Distance

Patricia E. Greene

It was a chilly morning in January 1985. I arrived at my desk at the National Office of the American Cancer Society, which was then in New York City. A message was waiting; my mother had called to say that she was in the community hospital, in the town 80 miles from the retirement village where my parents had lived for 5 years.

She had been admitted 2 days earlier but had not wanted to alarm me until she had an explanation for her sudden vaginal hemorrhage. The explanation had come in the form of a pathology report from a fractional dilation and curettage. She had clear-cell carcinoma of the endometrium. Diagnosis in hand, the gynecologist managing her care was ready to move forward with treatment. He had initiated a referral to the radiation therapy department at the teaching hospital in town. Mother was scheduled for a pretreatment consultation the next afternoon.

CANCER COMES AS A SHOCK, NO MATTER HOW WELL YOU ARE PREPARED

Cancer is a common diagnosis in my mother's family, so I had long lived with a low-grade fear that Mother would develop some form of cancer. At the time of her call, I had been working in the field of cancer for 15 years. I thought I knew the disease well.

During those horrible moments when Mother described the events of the previous few days, I realized that my fears had come true. I was not surprised that her cell type indicated one of the variants of endometrial cancer carrying the poorest prognosis. I was very surprised at the realization that I did not know as much about cancer as I thought. Those many years as a clinical nurse specialist in pediatric oncology left me ill-pre-pared. In this situation, I was not a skilled oncology nurse caring for someone's child with cancer. I was a child whose mother had cancer.

GETTING A SECOND OPINION: MORE COMPLICATED THAN "IF YOU WISH"

At the time of Mother's diagnosis I was married to a medical oncologist. With the *American Cancer Society Textbook of Clinical Oncology* in hand, I called him away from a busy clinic to discuss treatment options. I learned that there were two opposing schools of thought about the treatment of choice for endometrial cancer. The prevailing view favored surgery first, for tumor debulking and definitive staging, followed by radiation therapy. At a few centers, however, radiation therapy was used first. Mother was clearly at one of those centers. After several phone calls to other experts—both at my husband's hospital and around the country—we opted for surgery first.

Thinking things were now well in hand, I booked the first flight out of New York the next day. While I was en route, my husband was talking by phone to Mother's local physician, requesting that he perform the surgery first.

On arrival at the airport, I called my husband from the pay phone. His phone call to the local physician had not gone well. He perceived that the local doctor had been decidedly insulting and unprofessional. He did not agree with our treatment choice.

My husband had made arrangements for Mother to be transferred to his hospital in New York City for surgery the following week. My job was to break this news to the radiation therapists and to gather pathology slides and radiographic films to take back to New York.

By the time I got to Mother's side, she was already on the examining table in the radiation therapy department. I asked the attending physician and the resident assigned to her case to step outside for a moment. I explained that we preferred surgery as the first-line treatment. They protested, cordially. They explained why they thought our choice was ill-advised but agreed to treat her postoperatively, if we wished.

Mother and my father returned with me to New York City. Surgery went well. Mother recovered easily, for a 78-year-old woman. The nurses and physicians at the New York facility were skilled and caring. We even had a few laughs when the junior physician obtaining consent for the hysterectomy cautioned Mother that, after the surgery, she would no longer be able to have children. The bad news was that the tumor had deeply invaded the myometrium, adding to the signs that we could expect a poor prognosis.

In about a month, Mother returned to her home. We made arrangements for her care to be transferred back to the GYN Oncology department at the teaching hospital. Her treatment plan called for a 5-week course of external beam therapy, followed by brachytherapy. She came under the care of the same resident. He quickly made it clear that he had not forgiven us for our disputing his treatment plan. Each time he examined Mother, he asked her if she was experiencing any side effects from the treatment. When she reported that she was not, he would reply, "Well, you're lucky. You know we expect you to have more trouble than our other patients because your family insisted on going against our recommendations." So, even though Mother was tolerating the treatments well, needless emotional pain was being inflicted on her. She would call from home, crying and exclaiming that a sick person should not be subjected to such rudeness. I agreed. I offered to call the attending physician and put a stop to it. She pleaded with me not to. My intervention had brought this suffering, and she feared that more intervention would lead to more retribution.

All this was not lost on me. I began to doubt our rights to seek a second opinion and select a treatment plan that differed from the original proposal. I felt guilty for having intervened in the first place. I had already made enough trouble for Mother. I dared not add to her difficulties by reporting this inappropriate behavior.

I still think of this experience when I talk with patients about seeking a second opinion, "if they wish." I learned, the hard way, how easy it is to be intimidated in the process.

MAKING THE BEST OF THE GOOD TIMES

Mother completed her treatment in June 1985. Fatigue was a significant problem for the duration of her illness, but gradually, she increased her activity somewhat. Fortunately, my parents had traveled extensively in the years following their retirement and had been to all the places on their "must see" list. They were content to make short trips, to enjoy special moments with the family.

In November 1985, my nephew, Randy, was playing forward for Vanderbilt's varsity basketball team. Being positioned behind Will Purdue, still playing with the Chicago Bulls, limited Randy's time on the court, but it didn't dampen our spirits as Vanderbilt fans and our enthusiasm for following the team's progress. My father listened to the games when he could pick them up on the radio, and my sister, Janet, kept everyone supplied with newspaper clippings and team promotional materials, including photos of the celebrity grandson.

In March 1986 Janet and her husband took my parents for a weekend trip to Callaway Gardens, near Atlanta. The azaleas and dogwoods were in full bloom. They enjoyed the time together, as well as nature's splendor.

In May, my parents had the opportunity to attend the 1986 graduation ceremony at my college of nursing where I received the first Outstanding Alumnus Award bestowed by the college. Fifteen years earlier, both of my parents had missed my own graduation. Mother had fallen accidentally the night before the ceremony. As I was walking down the aisle—the only member of my family to graduate from college, at that time—Mother was in the operating room, undergoing a nephrectomy to stop bleeding resulting from the fall. The Outstanding Alumnus Award presentation gave us an unexpected second chance. I gave a small speech. My head was reeling, because just 24 hours earlier, I had received the first Oncology Nursing Society Excellence in Oncology Nursing Education Award at the Oncology Nursing Society's Congress in Los Angeles. It was a very exciting and rewarding time in my life, and my parents were proud and pleased to be a part of it. All of us knew that we had to capture and hold these moment's tightly. Mother's time—and ours with her—was running out.

THINGS ALWAYS GET WORST AT THE WORST POSSIBLE TIME

Around the first of August 1986, I returned from an out-of-town trip to the phone call I had been dreading. Mother had the classic signs and symptoms of an abdominal obstruction. She was planning to wait and see if her symptoms would pass.

I knew the symptoms would not pass. I placed a call to her attending gynecologic oncologist. Mother was completely obstructed and failed to respond to medical interventions. After a week of nasogastric tubes and intravenous fluids, she was scheduled for surgery.

I arrived from New York just in time to see her off to surgery. The surgeons were able to temporarily bypass the obstruction, but they found extensive intra-abdominal disease. Her postoperative recovery was stormy.

I felt torn. I was serving as Chair of the Nursing Education Project of the International Union Against Cancer (UICC) in Geneva. My responsibilities as chair included running the nursing conference held within the UICC quadrennial congress in Budapest, Hungary, and I was scheduled to leave for Budapest just 2 weeks later. I had done all of the planning for the conference, including selecting the agenda, inviting the speakers, and negotiating the details with the local organizers in Budapest. I did not feel I could turn the responsibility for the conference over to someone else at the last minute.

As time went by and Mother did not pull out of postoperative complications, I realized that I would have to leave the country, with her in a precarious state. Communication with the Hungarian conference organizers had been very difficult, so I knew it would be difficult to keep in touch, even by telephone. I felt terribly torn between my responsibility to follow through with my commitment to the UICC and my need to stay with my family in a time of crisis.

ENCIRCLED BY CARING AND CLINICAL EXPERTISE

As I prepared to leave, my good friend Genevieve Foley, then Director of Pediatric and Surgical Nursing at Memorial Sloan-Kettering Cancer Center in New York, proposed a solution. She would step into the role as nurse daughter. Each day she phoned my mother and her nurse to answer my parent's questions and to get a status report from the nurse. Gen called my sister, Janet, in Nashville each evening with a report. Before my sister went to sleep, she would call me in Budapest. With the time difference, her late-night call was an early morning call for me, routing through the sparse Hungarian telephone network before it became clogged with the business-day calls.

The system worked like a charm. Gen was better than a substitute. She was a knowledgeable surgical nurse, much more at home with the issues confronting Mother than I was. One day Gen demonstrated that you can do a physical assessment by telephone. She detected that Mother was short of breath and experiencing a shaking chill. Her careful questions elicited a classic picture of septic shock. Unfortunately, Gen also got a picture of a busy inpatient unit. The nurses had not been in to check Mother in several hours.

Gen called the nurses' station and put in a request for an immediate evaluation. Sure enough, it was determined that Mother had developed an overwhelming infection. Intravenous antibiotics were started immediately.

Gen reinstated and sustained the chain of communication and protection that I broke when I left the country. We were all completely reassured by her presence and caring. We were amazed that she could be so present from such a distance.

LEARNING FIRST-HAND THE VALUE OF SOCIAL SUPPORT SYSTEMS

Eventually Mother's condition stabilized sufficiently for her to be discharged. Unable to eat, she was confined by fatigue and diarrhea for several weeks. She left the house only to travel to the oncology clinic for fol-

low-up appointments. During this period, the beautiful, supportive environment of a retirement village came into clear focus for me. I learned that friends and neighbors visited regularly, bringing food that appealed to Mother and dishes for my father. The village services included an ambulatory clinic as well as a nursing home. The physician's assistant in the clinic kept in constant touch, even making home visits when Mother did not feel well enough to go to the clinic.

I continued to use my long-distance network of experts. Mother was given a referral for home-care nursing through a service based in the near-by town—a prospect that raised, then dashed, my hopes. A nurse came to visit, once. Mother was not on intravenous fluids and did not need dressing changes. Failing to find a high-technology nursing need to address, the nurse was at a loss for what to offer.

I spoke with her by phone and talked about a general nursing care assessment, including nutrition, activity, comfort, skin condition—the usual. I felt like I was speaking in a foreign language. This was clearly not an approach to care embraced by this home care service. They either followed a doctor's order for skilled care, or there was no need for a home care nurse.

I shared my disappointment with Ruth McCorkle, who came to the rescue. Again, she proved that good nursing care can be delivered by phone. She conducted a long-distance nursing history and assessment, then developed a plan for activities we could undertake to deal with the immediate problems and plan for the future as a family. She was able to put issues into perspective in a way that I could not, caught up in my own personal struggle as a family member.

The local Division of the American Cancer Society was marvelous. When Mother was receiving outpatient radiation therapy, my parents were overwhelmed by a daily, 80-mile one-way trip to the treatment center. The Society stepped in and offered to provide housing, free-of-charge, at a motel near the hospital. All the arrangements were made by the American Cancer Society. All Mother and Dad had to do was show up and give their name. A room was waiting for them.

The impact of having someone step in and take care of a problem was profound. Cost was not the real concern; the burden was having yet another problem to solve. As soon as therapy was completed, my parents made a donation to the Society that more than repaid the cost of housing. My Dad even volunteered to be a neighborhood coordinator for the annual fund-raising appeal.

The American Cancer Society continued to help. When Mother became confined to bed, the Society arranged for loaned home-care equipment. The Division Director of Service and Rehabilitation called my parents from time to time, just to see if there was anything else they needed. That ongoing contact made such a difference.

Ironically, I am now head of the Patient Services Department in the National Home Office of the American Cancer Society. I struggle with the fact that many of our Divisions are having to reduce or eliminate direct financial assistance due to increasing demands in an environment of limited resources. On one hand, I know that the Society cannot meet the overwhelming needs for assistance with direct and indirect costs of cancer care. On the other hand, I remember clearly what a difference it made to have someone step in and solve a problem at a time of stress.

The trip to Budapest provided a lifetime benefit: I met Margo McCaffery, world-renowned expert in cancer pain management. The UICC conference schedule always includes a free day in the middle of the week. The free day was the same day that I learned about Mother's septic shock. Margo spent the day with me, reassuring me and distracting me when there was no more that I could do. She offered to consult at any time in the future.

At one point in the progression of the cancer, Mother developed thoracic pain. As is so often the case, Meperidine was prescribed. I didn't think this was the best approach, so I called Margo for advice. We talked about the limitations of Meperidine and the benefits of a long-acting oral morphine. Before we could get a prescription for MS Contin, the pain disappeared. Fortunately, pain was not a problem again, but knowing Margo was there to back me up was a constant source of security.

Mother's condition worsened, so Janet and I took turns, with one of us spending every other week at home. I was fortunate that my career was unfolding in an environment that valued family support in the cancer experience. Dr. Arthur Holleb, my supervisor, picked up the loose ends as I juggled family and work responsibilities for several months.

In February, Janet arrived to find that, during the week that Mother and Dad were on their own, conditions had crossed the line of manageability. The constant demands for care had taken a tremendous toll on my father, and he was no longer able to bear the burden alone. On a Saturday morning, my sister called Barbara Bradley, the Director of Nursing in the village nursing home, to ask for help. Barbara's reply was, "We've been expecting to hear from you and we are ready to help. We'll be right over." Within 5 minutes, two nurses and an assistant from the nursing home drove into the driveway to help Mother prepare for admission to the nursing home. They gave her the special observation room next to the nurse's station and reassured us that she would be able to stay in that room as long as she needed.

I often reflect on what a blessing it was to be able to make that transition so easily, with the help of caring and skilled nursing staff. Mother presented several nursing challenges that were new for the staff. Each time she needed something new, Barbara would come in, night or day, to do a personal nursing assessment and develop policies and procedures for the staff to follow. I was in constant contact with Barbara and the other members of the nursing staff. They involved me in decision-making.

My beloved cat, Jessica, had been on loan to Mother and Dad, to keep Mother company while she spent so much time in bed. The nurses allowed Jessica to visit and sit on Mother's bed in the nursing home.

With great patience, they concealed their fear and resentment when Jessica hissed and scratched when they tried to care for Mother.

Six weeks after Mother was admitted to the nursing home, she died of pneumonia or aspiration. We weren't really sure of the exact cause of her death, though surely it was a result of the cancer, which took not only my mother, but over time, her three siblings.

I was scheduled to arrive the next day, so Dad was alone when she died. Barbara came in at midnight and stayed with him until he was ready to go home. We felt so grateful for the consistent excellence in nursing care Mother and the whole family received at the end of her life. I wished I could be with her throughout her illness, but I could not. In retrospect, her care was better than I could have provided alone. The input of others who formed my network of support countered my lack of knowledge and experience as well as my clouded perspective. With their help, we overcame many of the problems Mother encountered.

LESSONS LEARNED

As I reflect on my experience, I realize that there are some things I would do differently and some things I would do again. One thing I did immediately. I communicated clearly to my father that I want to know immediately when he enters the health care system for a problem. We had a chance to try this out when, at the age of 83 years, he had an elevated PSA level and prostate nodularity was detected.

His initial referral was to a private urologist in town who had diagnosed and treated several other men from the village in their eighties. I intervened and made an appointment to see the urologic oncology group at the teaching hospital. They ruled out prostate cancer and focused their attention on treating his benign prostatic hyperplasia. We'll never know, but I suspect that we might have gone down the road of radiation therapy if we had foregone the opportunity to be involved in decision-making from the start.

If I could relive the experience, I would not allow myself to become intimidated by a negative reaction to a second opinion. I would deal with the problem directly and professionally. I would confront the resident about his inappropriate behavior and discuss the issue with the attending physician. If I had done what I knew was right, I could have solved the problem. We could all have been spared unnecessary disappointment and frustration.

BRING THE DISAPPOINTMENTS TO CLOSURE

Having my mother punished for my attempts to assure the best medical care was a disappointment I carried for many years. I didn't realize how much I was troubled by it until about 6 years after her death. I got a phone call from a very kind attending physician in the radiation therapy department where Mother had been treated. He was conducting a retrospective chart review for a research study. He wanted to know the date of

Mother's death and my impressions of any evidence of treatment complications she had experienced prior to her death.

I did my best to answer his questions, then asked him about the purpose of his study. He told me that the Gynecologic Oncology Group had recently initiated a protocol for the treatment of endometrial cancer that mandated surgery as first-line treatment. He indicated that he knew, from notes in the chart, of the controversy surrounding our treatment decisions. He acknowledged that his institution was one of the few remaining centers still recommending radiation therapy first.

At last, under the pressure of the cooperative group, the center was seeking data to support their opinion. I told him of our experience and of the feelings that had weighed on me for so long. He apologized and assured me that the current treatment team was more sensitive and responsive to patients' needs. Why? Largely because nurse practitioners had been brought on staff, and the resident we had come to know had departed.

One mistake I have made again. After Mother died, I realized that we had become so focused on her illness that we were not paying attention to my father's health. Right before our unseeing eyes, he had become severely debilitated, worn out by the demands of chronic illness and his grief. He recovered slowly, but eventually regained his strength and spirit.

Three years after Mother died, when Dad was 83, he married Sue, a delightful woman. They were very happy together for 3 years. Then Sue developed end-stage renal failure and died after 6 months of relentless illness. Again, my father was the primary caregiver, and again we focused all of our attention on Sue's illness. Again he lost weight and became very debilitated. Now, at 88, he is living alone and is in remarkably good physical health. Most elderly men are not as resourceful and resilient. I was given a third chance. I won't make the same mistake again.

I will continue to ask for help from my friends and colleagues and accept it graciously. As an oncology nurse, I have a built-in network of the most knowledgeable and caring people on earth. I will always reach out to that network, and hopefully I can be a part of a caring network for others in need. I also know that I am vulnerable. My knowledge, my experience, and my contacts help me cope with an illness crisis, but they do not protect me or my family from oversights, errors in judgement, or disappointments in health care delivery. One thing is certain: I have few, if any, surviving illusions about the cancer experience, both as a professional and as a family member.

UNIT VIII
MANAGEMENT OF MAJOR CLINICAL NURSING PROBLEMS

CHAPTER

51

Alterations in Nutrition

Marcia Grant • Mary E. Ropka

Alterations in nutritional status associated with the cancerous disease itself as well as with the antitumor treatments are common in cancer patients. Although weight gain has been reported in a small select subpopulation of cancer patients, mainly breast cancer patients undergoing adjuvant therapy (Knobf, 1985), the majority of cancer patients with alterations in nutritional status experience anorexia, weight loss, cachexia, and malnutrition (Heber, 1989). Malnutrition ranges from 31 per cent to 87 per cent depending on the tumor type (DeWys et al., 1980). Eighty per cent

of terminally ill patients are malnourished (Bruera & MacDonald, 1988). Such nutritional alterations further compromise the patient's health when they cause disease and therapy complications or intolerances (Holroyde & Reichard, 1986). The potential life-threatening nature of this sequence of events is exemplified by serious secondary infections or an inability to complete essential cancer treatment. Approximately two thirds of those patients who die from cancer experience anorexia and weight loss before death (DeWys et al., 1980; Morrison, 1976).

SIGNIFICANCE OF NUTRITIONAL ALTERATIONS

Weight loss is an important clinical composite indicator of nutritional status. A loss of weight ≥ 10 per cent is a clinically significant weight loss (ASPEN, 1993; Gottschlich, Matarese, & Shronts, 1993). Although such a significant weight loss may not in and of itself be dangerous, complications can occur when the weight loss is coupled with any other major stress, such as trauma, surgery, fever, or infection (Blackburn & Harvey, 1980). A maximum of 7 days of severely decreased nutrient intake is the limit most clinicians set before beginning nutritional interventions (ASPEN, 1993).

Anorexia and cachexia can lead to compromised immune status as manifested by decreased macrophage mobilization, depressed lymphocyte function, and impaired phagocytosis (Shils, 1979). In such a compromised state, the patient is vulnerable to infections that may be life-threatening. When the nutritional state is corrected, the immune state may also be reversed, improving the patient's response to disease and therapy (Kaminski, Nasr, Moss, Berger, & Sriran, 1982).

If anorexia and a subsequent malnutrition occur during cancer therapy, the response to medical and surgical therapies may be suboptimal (ASPEN, 1993). For example, radiation therapy for patients who lose significant amounts of weight may be discontinued before an adequate tumoricidal dose of radiation is administered (Copeland, Souchon, MacFadyen, Rapp, & Dudrick, 1977). Surgical patients with recent substantial weight loss may experience impaired wound healing (Ruberg, 1984). When the surgical procedure involves extensive resection of soft tissue, as with radical neck dissection, wound healing complications may occur (Copeland et al., 1975). For patients receiving selected antitumor chemotherapy, nutritional compromise frequently occurs secondary to other treatment-associated side effects such as nausea, vomiting, and mucosal ulcerations. These side effects can be dose-limiting, thus decreasing the amount of chemotherapy that was administered to levels below therapeutic doses (Costa & Donaldson, 1979).

The most devastating nutritional consequence associated with cancer is cachexia, a profound systemic abnormality in host metabolism that is characterized by weakness, wasting, general depletion, redistribution of host components, hormonal aberrations, and progressive failure in vital function (Costa, 1977; Lindsey, Piper, & Stotts, 1982). Cachexia is a common occurrence in progressive malignancy and is seen in as many as two thirds of terminally ill cancer patients (Morrison, 1976). The prevalence of protein-calorie malnutrition in hospitalized cancer patients was examined by Nixon and colleagues (1980). Findings revealed a nearly universal occurrence of protein-calorie malnutrition, characterized by loss of adipose tissue, lean body mass, and skeletal muscle that varied unpredictably in extent among patients with various cancers.

Nutritional alterations that occur in patients with cancer can lead to complications that interfere with patient progress and treatment. These alterations are found in a variety of patients who have cancer and may appear early in the course of the disease. Early recognition and aggressive management of these nutritional alterations is an important component of patient care.

PHYSIOLOGIC FEATURES OF NUTRITION

Provision of adequate nutrition at the cellular level involves a number of processes, including ingestion of food, digestion, absorption, elimination, and metabolism. Each of these processes provides critical components in the chain of events that maintains cellular nutrition. Digestion and absorption occur throughout the gastrointestinal tract. Accessory organs such as the liver and pancreas provide substances critical to both digestion and metabolism.

INGESTION

In health, control of food ingestion includes physiologic, psychologic, and sociocultural factors (Fig. 51–1). A functional gastrointestinal tract is essential.

PHYSIOLOGIC FACTORS

Physiologic factors include central and peripheral components. The central components are located in the central nervous system and function as a central integrating and ingestion-controlling center (DeWys, Costa, & Henkin, 1981). For example, the glucostatic hypothalamic dual center hypothesis predicts a central nervous system component with two centers: (1) the feeding center, which activates feeding, and (2) the satiety center, which inhibits feeding behavior. It has been hypothesized that the source of stimulation for these centers is the blood glucose level (Mayer, 1955). Peripheral components include a system of sensors for taste and smell in the oronasal region (Rolls, 1981); a system of sensors that is primarily volumetric in the upper gastrointestinal tract (Davis & Campbell, 1973); and a system of sensors (for example, in the liver) that is responsive to changes in metabolites and hormones in the blood (DeWys et al., 1981).

Long-term controls over feeding behavior have also been identified and include the lipostatic theory, also known as the set point theory (Friedman & Stricker, 1976). According to this theory, when fat reserves are depleted, the satiety signal is decreased, and an increase in feeding behavior occurs. The thermostatic theory proposes a relationship between body temperature and feeding as demonstrated by studies of cold-stressed rats who eat more and engage in more activity so as to generate heat through increased metabolism (Spector, Brobeck, & Hamilton, 1968). Another long-term control theory proposes a relationship between levels of circulating amino acids and food intake. In one study, animals reduced their intake of food when their diet was low or devoid of a single amino acid or when there was an excess of one amino acid (Mellinkoff, Frankland, & Boyle, 1956).

Experimental studies have been conducted to test the physiologic factors of the system for maintaining

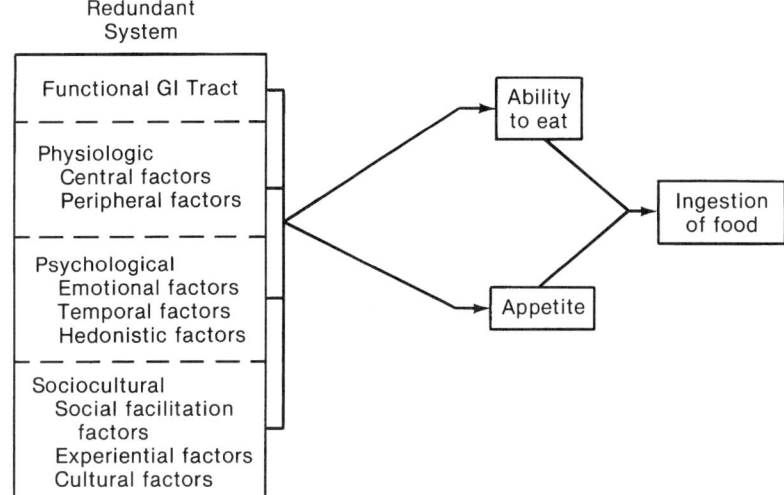

FIGURE 51–1. Food intake model. *GI* = gastrointestinal.

dietary intake, but specific relationships between factors are not yet known. The system appears to be a multifactorial one, with no hierarchy yet described.

PSYCHOLOGIC FACTORS

Psychologic factors are influential in the control of dietary intake as well. Emotional states such as depression and anxiety have been known to result in decreased dietary intake (Beck, 1972). Stress has been associated with both decreases and increases in dietary intake, whereas other factors, such as time of day, have been associated with the initiation of feeding activity (Wooley et al., 1975). Another factor associated with food intake is the pleasure of good meals enjoyed in an ambient atmosphere (Wooley et al., 1975).

SOCIOCULTURAL FACTORS

Sociocultural factors are influential in determining the environment for eating, the companions with whom people eat, and the specific types of foods that are prepared and eaten (Wooley et al., 1975).

The psychologic and sociocultural factors influencing dietary intake have not been studied as extensively as the physiologic factors. The extent of the potential impact of each on feeding behavior is not yet known, nor is the influence of the combination of physiologic, psychologic, and sociocultural factors.

In summary, the system for maintaining dietary intake appears to be one with built-in redundance. That is, multiple factors initiate feeding behavior, but absence of one does not involve a breakdown in the system stimulating food intake. Thus, an integrated approach to studying the phenomenon of eating disorders is needed. The projected outcome of maintaining adequate food intake is normal nutritional status (Fig. 51–2). The healthy animal eats to stay alive and functional. For humans, however, ingestion of food is heavily intertwined with social and pleasurable events. Ingestion of food not only is necessary for normal human growth and development but also provides pleasure and adds to the quality of life.

DIGESTION

The mouth, esophagus, stomach, small intestine, and large intestine form the major anatomic structures of the gastrointestinal tract. Normal oral status is reviewed in Chapter 52. The esophagus is a muscular, collapsible tube through which ingested food passes to the stomach. Although digestion begins in the mouth, it occurs primarily in the stomach and the small intestine. Other organs, namely the liver, gallbladder, and pancreas, facilitate digestion by secretion of enzymes and hormones. Enzymes contained in oral, gastric, and intestinal secretions initiate and aid the breakdown of ingested complex food substances into simpler components that are more readily absorbed, such as glucose, fatty acids, and amino acids.

ABSORPTION

Absorption of digested food occurs predominantly in the small intestine. The intestinal rugae with their microscopic villi provide a large absorptive surface through which the end products of digestion can be absorbed into the bloodstream and the lymphatics. Substances required immediately by cells move directly from the bloodstream into the cellular structures. In contrast, excess substances such as simple sugars are primarily stored as glycogen in the liver, whereas fatty acids are deposited in fat cells located in various parts of the body. Some amino acids are deaminized in the liver, with the rest remaining in the bloodstream for use as needed by various body cells.

METABOLISM

Metabolism is the process by which energy is provided to drive the various vital body and cellular functions. This energy is provided as the digestive end products are used by various cells. Energy is used by cells to build tissue and secrete substances. The basal metabolic rate (BMR) is defined as the amount of heat produced

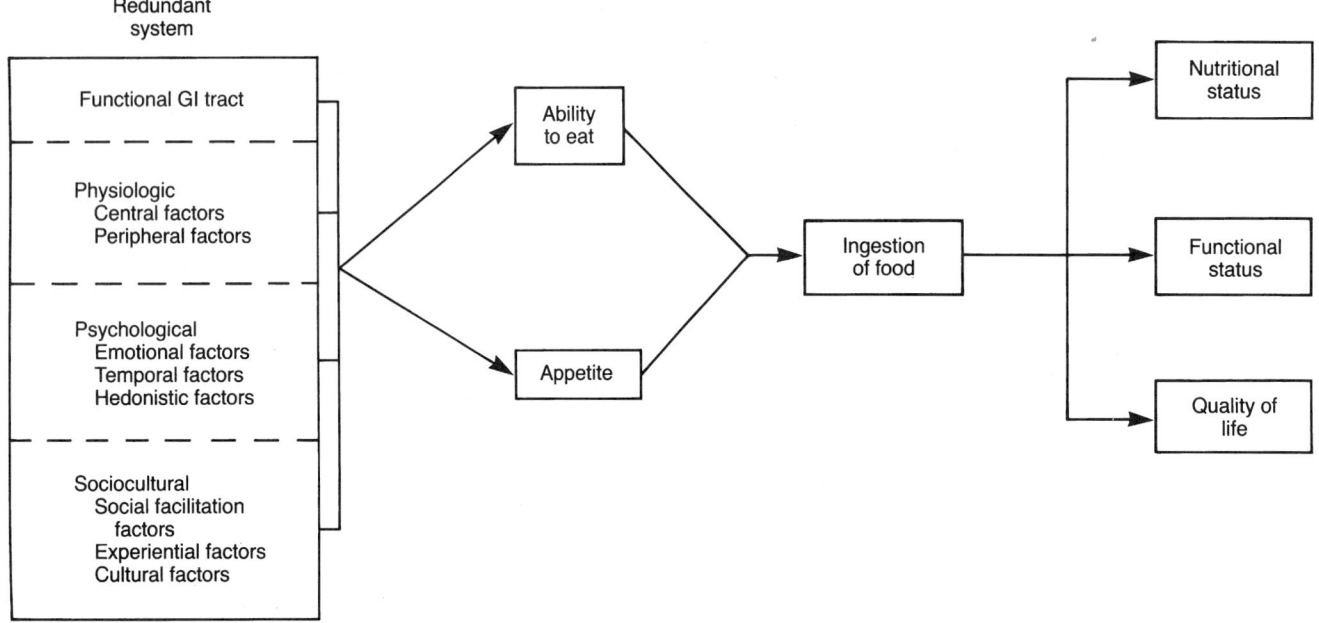

FIGURE 51–2. Impact of maintaining an adequate food intake.

by the body 14 to 18 hours after the last meal in a room approximately at 22.5° C with the body at complete rest (Frohse, Brodel, & Schlossberg, 1985). This rate equals the energy requirements needed by the body for maintenance of vital functions, such as circulation, respiratory and digestive activities, and muscle tone.

OCCURRENCE OF NUTRITIONAL DEPLETION IN CANCER AND DURING CANCER TREATMENT

Factors influential in the occurrence of nutritional depletion in cancer patients may be divided into gastrointestinal dysfunction, central nervous system disturbances, peripheral factors, and psychosocial factors. Frequently several factors are involved simultaneously.

DYSFUNCTIONAL GASTROINTESTINAL TRACT

Diminished dietary intake in cancer patients is related to abnormalities of digestion and absorption in the gastrointestinal tract. Two potential processes may occur. The first involves tumors that impinge directly on the gastrointestinal tract and accessory organs, such as the liver, and thus interfere with the normal movement of food through the gastrointestinal tract and with the digestion of food and absorption of digestive end products. The second involves changes within the gastrointestinal tract that are associated with malnutrition.

Tumors that arise in or impinge on the gastrointestinal tract may directly affect nutritional status by interfering with the ingestion, digestion, or absorption of food. Tumors located at different anatomic locations affect nutritional status differently. For example, the

difficulty resulting from tumors of the head and neck is primarily one of mechanical interference with food intake and chewing that results in decreased food ingestion (Lawrence, 1979).

Tumors of the stomach may affect nutritional status by interfering mechanically with normal gastric function and by causing intragastric losses of blood and protein-rich fluid (Lawrence, 1979). Gastrectomy is the treatment of choice for most of the gastric cancers. Following gastrectomy, carbohydrate and protein digestion remain relatively intact as long as eating patterns are altered (small, frequent meals), but malabsorption of fat can occur (Lawrence, 1979). Although primary tumors of the small intestine are rare, metastases from other sites are not uncommon. Mechanical obstruction can occur. Loss of blood and protein-rich fluids into the intestinal lumen can result in severe nutritional depletion (Dickerson, 1983).

Tumors of the liver and the pancreas result in deficiencies in digestive enzymes and hormones, resulting in malabsorption of fat, protein, carbohydrates, vitamins, and minerals (Dickerson, 1983). Anorexia is a frequent complaint in patients with pancreatic cancer and leads to progressive weight loss (Lawrence, 1979).

When the malnourished state is present for a sufficiently long period of time to cause changes in the small intestinal lining, a vicious cycle of further depletion may occur. The migrating cells of the intestinal villi are shed into the intestinal lining, carrying with them enzymes used in the digestion of food (Moog, 1981). When a malnourished state persists, changes in this lining occur that include decreases in numbers of villi and result in reduction of available intestinal enzymes so that malabsorption occurs (Dickerson, 1983). This is frequently referred to clinically as the smooth bowel syndrome.

In summary, when tumors involve the gastrointestinal tract and other digestive accessory organs, interference with the mechanical aspects of digestion and with the absorption of digestive end products occurs, which can lead to nutritional depletion. A malnourished state further compromises nutritional status of the patient with gastrointestinal pathology.

CENTRAL NERVOUS SYSTEM DISTURBANCES

Evidence has been found that links nutritional depletion with disturbances in the central nervous system. One mechanism involves the hypothesis that as brain tryptophan levels increase, serotonin synthesis increases. Because high levels of brain serotonin can cause anorexia (Krause, Humphrey, von Meyenfeldt, James, & Fischer, 1981), patients with cancer may experience anorexia when increased levels of tryptophan are present. Increased levels of tryptophan and brain serotonin have been demonstrated in tumor-bearing rats (Krause et al., 1981; Nichols, Maickel, & Yim, 1983; Wesdorf, Krause, & von Meyenfeldt, 1983). Tryptophan may be secreted by tumor tissue, but this has not been demonstrated. Other causes of central nervous system-related anorexia include the occurrence of distressing symptoms such as nausea, vomiting, and pain (Bernstein, 1986). Decreased food intake and chronic nausea are the two main manifestations of cachexia (Bruera, 1992).

Early satiety is yet another general symptom that leads to decreased gastric emptying, slow peristalsis, and complaints of feeling of fullness. Several factors may be present at any one time, making it difficult to identify a clear cause for nutritional depletion.

PERIPHERAL FACTORS

Peripheral factors originating in the oral-gustatory system have also been implicated in decreased intake experienced by cancer patients. Such disturbances include stomatitis or mucositis, xerostomia, taste and smell changes, and learned food aversions. Abnormalities of taste and smell have been observed in a variety of populations of patients with cancer. DeWys and Walters (1975) studied 50 patients with metastatic cancer who ranged in age from 16 to 79 years (median, 57 years). Decreased taste sensation was reported by 25 of the patients, and aversion to meat was reported by 16 of the patients. Patients with reported abnormal taste demonstrated increased incidence of weight loss.

In contrast, another study of taste thresholds in patients with esophageal cancer did not reveal the same pattern of taste changes (Kamath, Mams, Lad, Kohrs, & McGuire, 1983). Twelve patients with cancer were compared with a control group matched for age as well as for smoking and alcohol consumption. No significant difference in taste threshold changes was demonstrated. However, comparison with another control group of healthy nonsmokers showed marked differences. Thus,

taste changes may be related to smoking and alcohol consumption, rather than to the existence of cancer.

Bernstein (1982) hypothesized that tumor growth may suppress appetite indirectly by causing learned food aversions. These aversions are learned because they are associated with unpleasant internal symptoms and ultimately result in decreased dietary intake. This hypothesis was first identified in Bernstein's studies of children and adults, followed by studies using an experimental animal model (Bernstein & Bernstein, 1981). Bernstein (1986) views these food aversions as a likely contributing factor to the occurrence of anorexia in patients with cancer who undergo cancer chemotherapy.

In 1982, Johnston, Keane, and Prudo reported a study involving 31 patients receiving 6 weeks of primary radiation therapy for localized head and neck cancers. Patients whose mean age was 58 years, with a range of 40 to 79 years, rated each one of the following symptoms on separate 10 cm visual analogue scales, once a week during therapy and at 3 months and 6 months after therapy: ability to smell, dysgeusia, dysphagia for solids or liquids, appetite, fatigue, xerostomia, mouth or throat pain, and skin irritation. Twenty of the 31 patients (68 per cent) lost more than 5 per cent of their original weight within 1 month of completing treatment. Weight losses ranged from 5.4 to 18.9 per cent. Some patients continued to lose weight up to 6 months after treatment. Analysis revealed that the symptom scores were worse for patients who lost more than 5 per cent of their pretreatment weight within the first 4 weeks of radiation therapy. Each symptom became more severe during the treatment period. Xerostomia and dysphagia continued to increase up to the end of treatment and persisted for up to 6 months, whereas other symptoms decreased by the first follow-up visit at 3 months.

Mossman and Henkin (1978) conducted a series of studies focusing on taste, smell, and salivary and appetite changes in patients undergoing radiation therapy. A descriptive study of 27 patients with various cancers of the head and neck was composed of two study groups (Mossman & Henkin, 1978). In the first group ($n = 9$), all patients were tested 1 year after completion of radiation therapy. All had persistent taste changes, six reported anorexia, and five had xerostomia. In the second group of subjects ($n = 18$), one had taste changes before radiation therapy, and three had anorexia before radiation therapy. During and after therapy, 12 of the 18 patients experienced taste loss, and 9 of the 18 patients experienced anorexia. Not all patients with taste changes experienced anorexia; however, all except one patient with anorexia experienced taste changes. Taste changes started 3 weeks after radiation therapy began; bitter and salt tastes showed the earliest and greatest impairment, and sweet taste the least.

Dental problems may occur in a variety of cancer populations but can be particularly important when found in patients already experiencing eating problems. Dental problems lead to nutritional disorders because they frequently result in patients' limiting their dietary selections, especially to diets low in protein and total calories.

CHANGES IN METABOLIC REQUIREMENTS

If decreased food intake alone accounted for the nutritional depletion frequently observed in patients with cancer, provision of excess calories should reverse the depletion. Although such an approach is sometimes successful, a large number of patients with cancer lose weight out of proportion to their intake. Provision of adequate calories by oral, enteral, or parenteral routes does not change median survival rates of patients with advanced cancer (Heber, Byerley et al., 1986; Heber, Chlebowski, Meguid, & McAndrew, 1986). Abnormalities in energy expenditure and in glucose and fat metabolism are hypothesized as additional factors that influence nutritional depletion in cancer patients (Heber, Chlebowski et al., 1986; Rothkopf, 1990).

Although improvement in measurements of energy expenditure via metabolic bedside carts has resulted in more data about patients with cancer, measurement of metabolic expenditure has not yielded any information that can account for observed weight losses. Both heterogeneous and homogeneous populations of patients with cancer have been studied, with equivocal results (Bozzetti, Pagnoni, & Del Vecchio, 1980; Dempsey et al., 1984). Some patients appear to be hypermetabolic, some have findings within normal limits, and some are hypometabolic. Comparisons with factors such as location of disease, extent of disease, and age have not revealed significant differences among these groups.

ALTERATIONS IN CARBOHYDRATE AND FAT METABOLISM

Marked changes in the metabolism of carbohydrate and fat have been demonstrated in patients with cancer.

ALTERATIONS IN CARBOHYDRATE METABOLISM

Abnormalities in glucose metabolism include increased glucose turnover and oxidation, lack of the adaptive starvation response, glucose intolerance, impaired insulin sensitivity, increased gluconeogenesis, and abnormal glucose oxidation (Rothkopf, 1990). In the context of these abnormalities, the tumor cells remain metabolically hyperactive at the expense of the host (Rothkopf, 1990). These abnormalities indicate the need to approach clinical management by limiting glucose calories to those needed for the glucose-dependent body tissues: central nervous system, blood cells, and scar tissue.

ALTERATIONS IN FAT METABOLISM

Alterations in fat or lipid metabolism have also been demonstrated. Fatty acid oxidation is a dominant energy source for cancer patients. Enhanced lipid mo-bilization and utilization have been demonstrated (Heber, Chlebowski et al., 1986). Clinical management recommendations include providing 40 to 50 per cent of caloric requirements by administration of lipids (Rothkopf, 1990).

In summary, one explanation of the nutritional depletion that occurs in patients with cancer focuses on alterations in energy expenditure and in carbohydrate and fat metabolism (Kurzer & Meguid, 1986; Lundholm, 1986). Findings demonstrate abnormalities, but patterns are not consistent and the degree of abnormality demonstrated does not account for the extent of weight loss that occurs in most patients (Kaempfer & Lindsey, 1986). It appears that although alterations in energy expenditure and carbohydrate and fat metabolism may account for some of the nutritional depletion seen in patients with cancer, decreases in dietary intake continue to play a major role in the continued and profound weight loss observed.

PSYCHOSOCIAL FACTORS INFLUENCING NUTRITIONAL DEPLETION

A number of psychosocial factors are thought to be associated with nutritional depletion in cancer patients (Gorter, 1991; Spaulding, 1989). Depression in cancer patients is associated with a loss of appetite and fatigue. Psychologic distress, such as anxiety and fear, may decrease oral intake. Weakness and fatigue are common during cancer treatment, and lead to loss of appetite and a lack of interest in eating.

Social factors related to nutritional depletion include cultural differences reflected in choices of food during hospitalization, absence of usual eating companions, and the inability to consume usual foods. For example, if the normal diet includes spicy, highly seasoned foods and the patient is undergoing treatment that leads to a sore, inflamed mouth, these foods are no longer tolerated.

Examination of factors influencing dietary intake and feeding behavior reveals a multifactorial, redundant model, composed of physiologic, psychologic, and sociocultural factors (Novin & VanderWeele, 1977; Toates, 1981). Interference with one of the factors may produce a temporary decrease in dietary intake, whereas interference with several of the factors over a period of time could result in devastating nutritional problems (Grijalva & Lindholm, 1982).

In patients with cancer, diverse physiologic and psychosocial factors influence food intake by decreasing dietary intake and increasing metabolic need. To prevent serious nutritional depletion, early and consistent interventions for the precipitating problems are needed. Plans to help patients, especially those undergoing active treatment, must be comprehensive and individualized. One approach to the initiation of such a plan is to identify the major factors present and then plan interventions specific to each factor. The foundation needed to manage these problems is a thorough nutritional assessment.

ASSESSMENT AND MANAGEMENT OF NUTRITIONAL PROBLEMS

NUTRITIONAL ABNORMALITIES IN THE PERSON WITH CANCER

Nutritional abnormalities in patients with cancer occur as a result of the tumor itself or as a consequence of the effects of various cancer treatment methods, including surgery, chemotherapy, radiation therapy, and immunotherapy, used alone or in combination.

DEFINITION

Malnutrition, or nutritional depletion, occurs when provision of energy and nutrients is inadequate to sustain the functioning of all physiologic systems. Protein-calorie malnutrition has received the most attention, although deficiencies of many individual nutrients (including fluids and electrolytes, vitamins, minerals, and trace elements) have also been described. In addition to deficits, excesses of nutrients must also be considered in this age of macrobiotic diets, megavitamin therapy, and other nutritional fads.

Although much is written about malnutrition, the term is frequently not defined. *Malnutrition, or macronutrient deficiency(ies),* commonly observed in some patients with cancer may be categorized as adult marasmus (chronic depletion of muscle and fat), acute visceral attrition (kwashiorkor-like), or a combination of the two (protein-calorie malnutrition). Malnutrition occurs when intake of nutrients is inadequate, in terms of either quantity or quality, to meet metabolic needs.

The term *protein-calorie malnutrition,* also called *protein-energy malnutrition,* includes a wide spectrum of general nutritional conditions that range clinically from almost undetectable symptoms to frank starvation and kwashiorkor (Viteri & Torun, 1988). Protein-energy malnutrition results from a protracted period in which the patient fails to ingest or receive adequate amounts of energy and protein, resulting in a combination of marasmus and kwashiorkor (Holman, 1987). *Marasmus* occurs as a result of prolonged inadequate intake of energy sources during (metabolically) unstressed starvation. Marasmus is characterized by gradual wasting of body fat and skeletal muscle mass, with preservation of visceral proteins (serum albumin, transferrin, and prealbumin) and immunocompetence. The marasmic individual has minimal nutritional reserves and tolerates repeated or prolonged stress poorly (Grant, Custer, & Thurlow, 1981). *Kwashiorkor* is the term used for another type of malnutrition that occurs as a result of stressed starvation and an inadequate intake of protein relative to energy. Kwashiorkor is characterized by preserved anthropometric measurements, especially fat stores; low visceral protein levels (serum albumin, transferrin, and prealbumin); and measures that reflect impaired immunologic function, specifically impaired cell-mediated immunity. In addition, muscle wasting may occur after prolonged catabolic conditions. The person suffering from kwashiorkor may not appear overly thin because of the presence of edema. Frequently the patient with cancer experiences a combination of the two. Combined marasmus-kwashiorkor is characterized by skeletal muscle wasting; depletion of fat stores; low serum visceral protein concentrations, such as serum albumin and transferrin; and impaired immunocompetence. Persons with the combined form are at greatest risk of serious morbidity and mortality if nutritional support is not provided.

CAUSES OF MALNUTRITION

Nutritional abnormalities that occur in the person with cancer can result from the tumor itself; from the various methods of antitumor therapy, such as surgery, radiation therapy, chemotherapy, and immunotherapy; or from the combined effects of both.

The degree of malnutrition that occurs is influenced by the anatomic site of the tumor; the extent of disease; and duration, amount, and combination of antitumor therapy. The frequency with which malnutrition is reported varies, but it tends to occur more commonly with tumors at certain sites, specifically tumors of the head and neck, central nervous system, gastrointestinal tract, and lung. In addition, highly malignant lymphomas also are frequently accompanied by malnutrition (Ollenschlager, Konkol, & Modder, 1988). Subsequent development of malnutrition can impair the digestive and absorptive abilities of the gastrointestinal tract, especially as a result of mucosal atrophy that further compromises the bowel's absorptive function and as a result of dysfunction of major organ systems such as the liver.

Surgery. Surgery is performed with both curative and palliative intent. Surgery itself can affect the development of malnutrition because of the usually expected increased metabolic demands that result from perioperative catabolism. Surgery is at times associated with undesirable prolonged periods (7 days for hospitalized patients) of inadequate nutritional intake resulting from preoperative diagnostic workups, surgery itself and its requisite healing period, or surgical complications (ASPEN Guidelines for the Use of Parenteral and Enteral Nutrition in Adult and Pediatric Patients, 1993). In addition, radical resection of specific anatomic sites is likely to impair the patient's ability to ingest, digest, or absorb nutrients, resulting in chronic nutritional consequences. These anatomic sites include the head and neck region and the gastrointestinal tract, specifically radical resection of the oropharyngeal area; esophagectomy; gastrectomy; intestinal resection of the jejunum, ileum, and bowel; or pancreatectomy.

Radiation Therapy. Although radiation therapy has desired therapeutic effects in that it kills tumor cells, it also causes changes in or destruction of normal cells. Radiation therapy, particularly of the oral cavity, pharynx, esophagus, abdomen, and pelvis is likely to result in impaired nutrition owing to decreased ability to ingest, digest, or absorb nutrients. Furthermore, this type of therapy contributes to symptoms such as anorexia, nausea and vomiting, mucositis, xerostomia, and fatigue that make it more difficult for people to eat. Radiation therapy factors that are reported to affect the development of nutritional problems include (1) the part of the body in the radiation field, (2) the intensity of the radiation tumor dose, (3) the time period over which radiation therapy is delivered, (4) the volume of tissue that receives radiation therapy, (5) the nutritional status of the patient when he or she begins radiation therapy, (6) the sensitivity of the tissue to radiation, and (7) the person's general physical and psychologic status before treatment. Side effects and complications of radiation therapy may be fairly immediate, beginning as early as within 2 to 4 weeks after initiating radiation therapy or 6 weeks after completing radiation therapy. Late effects of radiation therapy may be extensive and irreversible, occurring years after the culmination of radiation therapy.

Chemotherapy. Antitumor chemotherapy contributes to the development of malnutrition by interfering with the person's ability to ingest nutrients due to taste change, sore mouth, or nausea, or excessive loss from vomiting or diarrhea. As with radiation therapy, chemotherapy is therapeutic in that it kills tumor cells but it also can cause side effects and toxicities, such as taste changes, nausea, vomiting, stomatitis, anorexia, and diarrhea, which interfere with intake.

NUTRITIONAL ASSESSMENT IN CANCER

Nutritional assessment is performed to determine a person's nutritional status or the degree to which his or her need for nutrients and energy is being met by present intake. Detection of protein-energy malnutrition has received the most attention, particularly among hospitalized patients. However, it is also important to consider vitamins, minerals, trace elements, fats, and electrolytes. In addition to deficits, nutrient excesses are potential problems, largely through supplementation rather than food sources.

GOALS OF NUTRITIONAL ASSESSMENT

Nutritional assessment can be performed for a number of reasons, including to: (1) screen for persons with cancer who are *at high risk* for developing nutritional problems; (2) identify those patients with *existing* nutritional abnormalities; (3) determine nutritional *requirements* so that appropriate nutritional interventions can be prescribed; and (4) follow *responses* to nutritional therapies. Determination of which specific nutritional assessment methods are most appropriate must be made to match the goal or goals of the nutritional assessment. The assessment goals above that are most relevant for clinical purposes can be summarized either as (1) approaches to evaluate current nutritional status or (2) approaches to prescribe treatment and follow response to nutritional intervention.

METHODS OF NUTRITIONAL ASSESSMENT

Unfortunately, no simple direct method or single datum has been identified by which the nutritional status of a person can be accurately established. Instead, measures that are thought to indirectly reflect nutritional status are used. It is difficult to determine which of these single measures or combinations of measurements is most accurate because of the absence of a "gold standard" by which malnutrition can be determined and used for comparison. Judgments regarding the presence or absence of malnutrition and the degree to which it exists are usually based on the comparison of a patient's results to standard values. The Metropolitan Height-Weight Tables can be used for weight. Those published by Frisancho and developed from cross-sectional data collected by the NHANES I and NHANES II surveys can be used for multiple anthropometric measures. Finally, many of the potential measures thought to indirectly reflect nutritional status are useful for research and epidemiologic purposes but are not practical or effective for making clinical judgments about individual patients.

Individual Assessment Measures. Trends in nutritional assessment have gone full circle since the 1970s, when protein-energy malnutrition in hospitalized patients was first widely recognized. For many years before that time, nutritional assessment involved primarily "clinical judgment" based on the history and physical examination obtained by the health professional. In the 1970s, a number of investigators proposed more technical and quantitative methods for nutritional assessment that were believed to reflect nutritional status indirectly. They can be categorized into five main areas: (1) biochemical, (2) immune function, (3) body composition, (4) dietary intake, and (5) clinical observation.

Biochemical laboratory measures proposed to reflect nutritional status include serum albumin, transferrin, prealbumin, and retinol binding protein levels; nitrogen balance studies; and creatinine-height index.

Measures of *immune function* associated with nutritional status include anergy panels reflecting cell-mediated immunity, and total lymphocyte counts. Particularly in the patient with cancer, alterations in immune function may result from the disease or its treatment rather than from nutritional factors. This can confuse the evaluation.

Body composition measurements involve skinfold (SF) measures obtained anthropometrically at various anatomic sites, midarm muscle circumference (MAMC), and body weight (WT). Body weight can be considered (1) as an isolated measure; (2) in relation to height (weight for height or Body Mass Index); or (3) in comparison to ideal body weight (percentage IBW), to usual body weight (percentage UBW) for that person, or to weight prior to illness (percentage weight change). Anthropometric measures are interpreted by comparing each to an appropriate table to determine percentile, which is then categorized in terms of degree of malnutrition based on percentile range (ASPEN, 1993).

Dietary evaluation can include both an assessment of what the person actually eats and drinks as well as an evaluation of knowledge about nutrition (Ireton-Jones & Hasse, 1992). A number of approaches for assessing dietary intake can be employed such as: 24-hour recall; food frequency questionnaires; complete dietary histories; direct observation of food intake; or evaluation by the basic four food groups, dietary goals, or recommended dietary allowances (RDA). A comprehensive dietary history estimates whether the diet is sufficient, determines food preferences, evaluates current and previous dietary patterns, and provides information on social and economic factors influencing the person's ability to obtain and prepare food. A simple diet history provides a rough idea of the adequacy of intake by reviewing meal patterns, extent of "empty" calories consumed, and amount and type of snack foods and oral nutritional supplements. Asking the patient with cancer to maintain a diary of all intake for a limited period of time can be helpful in assessing what he or she is actually eating and also can provide motivation for the patient.

Finally, *clinical observation* involves evaluation of the person's physical condition; consideration of psychosocial factors, including the ability to obtain and prepare food; determination of socioeconomic status, including ability to afford food; review of current medications (including vitamins and mineral supplements); and information regarding comorbidity or other current health problems that can influence nutritional status.

Reduced Assessment Schemes. Instead of using all of these potential measures related to nutritional status, some investigators have attempted to develop reduced schemes or combinations of nutritional assessment measures that could be useful clinically. Because of the absence of a "gold standard" by which to establish malnutrition, the measures included in these reduced combinations have not been judged in terms of their ability to predict malnutrition per se. Instead they have been judged by their ability to predict surrogate outcomes that are both associated with malnutrition and more easily determined, such as occurrence of surgical complications like delayed wound healing and infection, differences in tolerance of or response to antitumor therapy, or shorter survival. This is appropriate because the clinician is, after all, ultimately interested in what happens to the patient. The clinician wants to identify correctly which nutritional changes make a difference in outcomes meaningful to the patient. The clinician also wants to find those persons in whom nutritional intervention is indicated and for whom it will improve clinical outcomes.

One example of a reduced assessment scheme is the Prognostic Nutrition Index (PNI), developed by Buzby, Mullen, Matthews, Hobbs, and Rosata (1980). The PNI is a statistical model developed to predict surgical morbidity and mortality from four selected nutritional parameters measured preoperatively. This method is not appropriate for following response to nutritional intervention, nor is it a useful predictor for metabolically stressed patients. The PNI is calculated by the following formula: PNI = 158 − 16.60 (serum albumin level in grams [g] per deciliter [dl] − 0.78 (triceps skinfold thickness in millimeters [mm]) − 0.20 (serum transferrin level in deciliters [dl]) − 5.8 (cutaneous delayed hypersensitivity reaction to mumps virus, streptokinase-streptodornase, or *Candida*). The cutaneous delayed hypersensitivity skin tests were graded as 0 (nonreactive), 1 (< 5 mm induration), or 2 (≥ 5 mm induration). The investigators suggest that patients with a PNI of less than 40 per cent are at low risk for

complications; a PNI of 40 to 49 per cent indicates intermediate risk; and a PNI ≥ 50 per cent reveals the high-risk category. Although this system was developed in patients undergoing gastrointestinal surgery, it has been evaluated in patients with other tumors, including those of the head and neck, who were also surgical candidates (Hooley, Levine, Flores, Wheeler, & Steiger, 1983). Patients assigned to the PNI high-risk category were far more likely to experience greater complications at a higher rate than those in the other PNI categories (Buzby et al., 1980; Goodwin & Torres, 1984; Hooley et al., 1983; Muller, Keller, Brenner, Walter, & Holzmuller, 1986).

GENERAL MANAGEMENT OF NUTRITIONAL PROBLEMS

Two important considerations in approaching the management of nutritional alterations in the patient with cancer include: (1) when does nutritional status make a difference in terms of clinical outcomes? and (2) who benefits from nutritional intervention, or when does nutritional intervention make a difference in clinical outcomes? For a number of years, it was assumed that aggressive nutritional intervention would be good for every patient with cancer who was actively undergoing antitumor therapy. It is important to take a careful look at the answers to the foregoing questions both because of increasingly limited resources for patient care and because nutritional interventions themselves are not always benign or without risk or cost.

Ollenschlager and colleagues (1988) state two general indications for intensive nutritional therapy. The first indication is *apparent malnutrition*, characterized by current body weight less than 90 per cent of IBW, weight loss greater than 10 per cent over 6 months or 5 per cent within 1 month, or serum albumin levels less than 3.5 g/100 ml. The second indication is *imminent malnutrition*, characterized by inadequate spontaneous oral intake less than 60 per cent of predicted nutrient requirements for more than 1 week, administration of intensive antineoplastic therapy, or sepsis. Other sources offer similar guidelines (ASPEN, 1993; Bloch, 1991; DeChicco, & Matarese, 1992; Ireton-Jones & Hasse, 1992; Kelly, 1993).

The second important consideration in approaching the management of nutritional alterations in persons with cancer involves determining which patients will actually benefit from nutritional intervention. This question has been considered regarding the administration of total parenteral nutrition (TPN) to patients with cancer who are receiving chemotherapy or radiation therapy or to cancer patients undergoing surgery. Appropriate evaluation of the potential efficacy of nutritional intervention should consider the degree of malnutrition that exists prior to treatment. Although it is generally agreed that nutritional supplementation does not improve morbidity and mortality of well-nourished individuals, it has not been clearly demonstrated that nutritional therapy generally enhances patient outcomes even when malnutrition is indeed present. Preoperative or postoperative nutritional therapy, or both, resulted in improved complication or mortality rates in some studies when the nutritional intervention was limited to those patients who were "significantly malnourished" (Maillet, 1987).

Evidence for the efficacy of nutritional support by TPN in decreasing radiation therapy- or chemotherapy-associated morbidity and mortality is weak (American College of Physicians, 1989; Bloch, 1994). The American College of Physicians' (ACP) Clinical Efficacy Assessment Project was conducted to evaluate and provide information about the safety and efficacy of diagnostic and therapeutic methods and medical practices. A position paper resulting from this project was issued reflecting state-of-the-art knowledge obtained by a meta-analysis of 11 prospective, controlled, randomized trials of perioperative TPN. The individual studies included end points of iatrogenic complications from the TPN itself, complications from major surgery, and death. Only one of the original studies showed a statistically significant reduction in complications or fatality rates for patients treated with perioperative TPN. The authors of this position paper concluded that even though nutritional supplementation did not benefit those who were well nourished, it was possible that perioperative TPN may be helpful for three subgroups: (1) patients who are severely malnourished before undergoing major surgery; (2) patients who are well nourished before surgery but who develop complications that are expected to result in a prolonged period of ileus or inadequate nutritional intake; and (3) patients who are well nourished before undergoing surgery that usually results in prolonged periods of inadequate nutritional intake even if complications do not occur (Detsky, Baker, O'Rourke, & Goel, 1987). These conclusions are further supported by the American Society of Parenteral and Enteral Nutrition (ASPEN) guidelines (1993) for use of parenteral and enteral nutrition in adult and pediatric patients.

A similar ACP Clinical Efficacy Assessment Project (American College of Physicians, 1989) position paper addressed the evidence regarding efficacy of nutritional supplementation by TPN to decrease morbidity and mortality during chemotherapy or combined chemotherapy and radiation therapy. A meta-analysis approach was used to pool the results of 12 prospective controlled randomized clinical trials whose outcomes included overall survival, short-term survival, tumor response, and treatment toxicity (McGeer, Detsky, & O'Rourke, 1990). This study recommended that the routine use of TPN for patients receiving chemotherapy should be strongly discouraged. The authors suggested that TPN may not be as detrimental to persons who were already malnourished, but the overall rate of complications from the TPN itself was indeed troubling.

Klein and Koretz (1994) reviewed published prospective, randomized, controlled trials evaluating clinically important end points, including morbidity, mortality, and duration of hospitalization. Overall they were unable to demonstrate any clinical efficacy in providing nutrition support for most cancer patients and

therefore recommended that guidelines for cancer patients parallel those for patients with benign disease. However, these conclusions are based on the pooling of studies whose shortcomings may influence the ability to find differences, such as low statistical power; heterogeneous patient populations; diverse composition, timing, and duration of nutrients; variable anticancer therapies; poor quality reporting; and failure to evaluate alternative end points that may be effected by nutritional therapy. In spite of those limitations, their specific conclusions are summarized as follows.

1. Perioperative parenteral nutrition is not clinically beneficial to most patients treated surgically.
2. Parenteral nutrition for at least 7 days before surgery may decrease postoperative complications slightly, with potentially greater benefits in those severely malnourished.
3. Enteral nutrition before surgery in "malnourished" patients may decrease postoperative complications, assuming gastrointestinal complications do not preclude it.
4. Neither parenteral or enteral nutrition improves outcomes for patients receiving chemotherapy or radiation therapy.
5. Parenteral nutrition is associated with more infections in patients receiving chemotherapy.
6. Parenteral nutrition given after bone marrow transplant may increase long-term survival (> 6 months) and improve tumor relapse, even though it does not improve short-term survival and is associated with more infections.
7. Enteral nutrition given along with peripherally infused nutrients can meet nutritional requirements for most bone marrow transplant patients. Nutrition intervention should, whenever possible, be given in conjunction with oncologic therapy (ASPEN, 1993).

DETERMINING ENERGY AND PROTEIN NEEDS

Once it has been established that a patient requires nutritional intervention, the prescription must be based on individualized estimates of energy and protein requirements. Overfeeding of carbohydrates may produce respiratory distress in patients with marginal pulmonary reserve, may produce hepatic steatosis, or hyperglycemia (Bloch, 1991; Kelly, 1993). Inadequate provision of substrates may lead to suboptimal nitrogen retention and loss of lean body mass.

Energy Requirements. One pretreatment expectation is the estimation of energy requirements to provide a nutritional regimen that replaces burned fuel and prevents loss of tissue mass. The goal in the metabolically stressed or catabolic patient is to maintain energy stores, whereas in the metabolically unstressed patient it is to replete existing deficits (Rombeau, Caldwell, Forlaw, & Guenter, 1989). This is accomplished by estimating total caloric requirements on the basis of sex, height, weight, age, and disease state, or by measuring oxygen consumption and determining actual metabolic requirements. The precise metabolic effect of the presence of a tumor is still controversial, although resting metabolism is not consistently elevated in cancer patients. Some studies report differences in energy expenditure, including hypermetabolism and hypometabolism, and some report no changes (ASPEN, 1990; Knox et al., 1983).

Energy expenditure estimates that provide a basis for calculating caloric requirements can be obtained either by indirect calorimetry or by use of the Harris-Benedict formula (Harris & Benedict, 1979) to estimate basal energy expenditure. A third approach is utilization of a simple "kilocalorie per kilogram formula" to meet estimated calorie needs.

Indirect calorimetry actually measures calorie requirements based on energy expenditure. With indirect calorimetry, heat production (estimated energy expenditure) is calculated by measuring oxygen consumption and carbon dioxide production during respiratory gas exchange. Although metabolic carts are available for bedside measurement, this method is impractical for routine clinical use and finds its primary application in research or critical care or when precise energy prescriptions are indicated (McClave & Snider, 1992). A specific indirect calorimetry measurement must be combined with other information to determine the degree of and need for nutrition support, as well as the composition of nutrients that should be provided (Kinney, 1992).

The Harris-Benedict formula differs slightly according to the patient's sex. For men, the basal energy expenditure (BEE) is calculated as follows:

$$BEE \text{ (men)} = 66.47 + (13.75) \text{ (weight in kg)} + (5.00) \text{ (height in cm)} - (6.76) \text{ (age in years)}$$

For women, the BEE is calculated using the Harris-Benedict formula as follows:

$$BEE \text{ (women)} = 655.1 + (9.56) \text{ (weight in kg)} + (1.85) \text{ (height in cm)} - (4.68) \text{ (age in years)}$$

The BEE, also known as basal metabolic rate (BMR), can then be multiplied by an adjustment factor that reflects either activity level or metabolic stress level, or both, to determine an estimate of total energy needs. Factors for activity suggested by Long, Schaffel, Geiger, Schiller, and Blackmore (1979) are 1.2 for persons who are on bed rest and 1.3 for hospitalized but ambulatory patients. Injury factors are 1.2 for minor surgery, 1.2 to 1.7 for acute-phase septic patients who are normotensive, 0.5 for acute-phase septic patients who are hypotensive, and 1.0 for septic patients during the recovery phase (Rombeau et al., 1989). Activity factors suggested by Bloch (p 291-2, Table 25.3) are 1.3 to 1.5 for weight maintenance and 1.5 for weight gain. In addition, the metabolic rate is elevated by fever, during which energy expenditure increases approximately 7 per cent for every degree of temperature above normal measured on the Fahrenheit scale or 13 per cent per degree of temperature elevation measured on the Celsius scale (Kinney & Roe, 1962; Kinney, 1992; Wilmore, 1977).

The third method of estimating energy needs is the kilocalorie per kilogram method which is by far the easiest method to use in the clinical setting. Daily calorie needs are determined by multiplying the current weight in kilograms by the suggested estimated kilocalorie levels. The suggested kilocalorie per kilogram levels vary slightly depending on the source, but are basically very similar. Recommendations for meeting calorie requirements are measured in total calories per kilogram of body weight per day. *Nutrition Support Dietetics: Core Curriculum* (Gottschlich, Matarese, & Shronts, 1993) suggests the following: 20 to 25 kcal/kg for nonambulatory or sedentary patients; 30 to 35 kcal/kg for slightly hypermetabolic patients or for weight gain/anabolism; 35 kcal/kg for hypermetabolic or severely stressed patients or those with significant malabsorption. In addition, carbohydrate modules, fat modules, or both are often helpful to achieve calorie levels.

Protein Requirements. Requisite amounts of protein can be estimated from energy expenditure, such as from the Harris-Benedict formula. Nitrogen is used as a marker for protein, so that the two terms are used essentially interchangeably. When the calculated energy expenditure is used to form the basis of the protein requirement calculation, the suggested ratio of nitrogen in grams to calories is 1:200 to 300 for maintenance and 1:150 for repletion (Blackburn, Bistrian, & Miani, 1976). Alternatively, the actual mathematical conversion is 6.25 g of protein per 1 g of nitrogen (Rombeau et al., 1989). The recommended daily allowance (RDA) for protein is 0.8 g of protein/kg of body weight/day in the healthy adult. To formulate nutritional support recommendations to meet protein requirements, the following is recommended: (1) 0.8 to 1.0 g/kg for normal maintenance; or (2) 1.5 to 2.5 g/kg for patients with cancer if protein demands are obviously elevated, as with hypermetabolism or extreme wasting (Bloch, 1991, p. 220). Generally, 15 to 20 per cent of the daily caloric intake should come from protein sources. About 300 nonprotein calories are needed for optimal utilization of 1 g of nitrogen in the normal individual.

Nitrogen balance studies provide a means for verifying whether nitrogen intake is in balance with metabolic demands. They reflect the adequacy of protein supplied to maintain lean body mass. Nitrogen balance studies are useful both to determine a baseline index of protein status and as a measure of net changes in total body protein mass. Eighty-five to 90 per cent of nitrogen is lost through urinary excretion of urea. In addition, a small constant amount is lost through the skin and feces. Nitrogen balance is calculated by the following formula:

$$\frac{\text{protein intake (g)}}{6.25} - (24 \text{ hr urinary urea nitrogen [g]} + \text{obligatory nitrogen losses})$$

The left part of this formula, protein intake in grams divided by 6.25, represents nitrogen intake in grams. The obligatory nitrogen losses through skin and feces that appear in the right-hand side of the equation range from 2 to 4 g/day. Nitrogen balance studies can be particularly helpful when used intermittently to evaluate the protein intake of the critically ill patient receiving enteral or parenteral nutritional support. During treatment or recovery from illness, the daily goal for anabolism is a positive nitrogen balance of 2 to 4 g. A negative balance is indicative of catabolism. Nitrogen balance cannot be accurately interpreted when creatinine clearance is less than 50 ml/min.

Patients with preexisting malnutrition of more than 5 days' duration who are taking little by mouth are candidates for nutritional support. Those with normal nutritional status and inadequate oral intake can forego nutritional support for a longer period, but after 7 to 10 days nutritional intervention will be necessary. Once the decision is made that a patient with cancer requires nutritional therapy, one of the first considerations is deciding what route should be used to deliver it. In general, the rule that guides this decision is, "If the gut works, use it." Nutritional repletion is more successful when delivered enterally than parenterally. In addition, the use of TPN involves a fairly high risk of complications and is expensive and relatively complicated to deliver.

Regardless of the route by which nutritional support is administered, assessment of the nutrition knowledge of the individual patient and his or her caregiver is essential. This includes understanding of the importance of adequate nutrition in maintaining or restoring health, knowing about proper dietary selection, and knowing how to manage cancer or treatment symptoms that potentially interfere with receiving adequate nutrition.

INCREASING ORAL INTAKE

Although the symptoms that result from the cancer or its treatment perhaps do not obviously appear to be directly related to nutrition, their management is very important because of the impact that these symptoms or side effects—such as pain, nausea, vomiting, dysphagia, odynophagia, taste changes, xerostomia, fatigue, respiratory distress, diarrhea, constipation, or depression and anxiety—can have on limiting the patient's ability to obtain, prepare, and receive adequate nutrition. This is especially true of nutrition by the oral route. Oral feeding is the preferred approach as long the patient is able to chew, swallow, and digest food. Mechanical adjustments can be made by grinding or pureeing food when the patient has chewing or swallowing limitations. Nutritional content or consistency may be modified for dietary intake.

General measures that can help maintain adequate nutritional status involve (1) good oral hygiene; (2) moistening of the mouth with nonharmful agents; (3) careful dental evaluation to assess and correct gum disease, missing teeth, caries, poorly fitting dentures, and stomatitis; and (4) encouraging physical activity and exercise at an appropriate level for the patient.

Instruction regarding the importance of a high-protein, high-calorie intake is an essential beginning (Box 51–1). Involving the patient and family in planning or providing meals and snacks that are appealing may increase the likelihood that the patient will be able to consume more. Food preparation and presentation can also influence the ability to eat. Avoiding spicy or acidic foods and beverages and foods served at hot temperatures minimizes discomfort from stomatitis and oral lesions. Altering food texture may make it easier to chew or swallow when mastication or deglutition problems are present. When xerostomia (dry mouth) is a problem, serving foods with juices, liquids, gravies, or other sources of moisture may help. However, this comfort measure must be balanced with the need to avoid consumption of liquids or other foods that are devoid of nutritional value, sometimes referred to as consuming "empty calories." Nutritional approaches to decreasing diarrhea are discussed separately later in this chapter. Decreasing portions and increasing the frequency of eating by serving small, frequent meals, six or more times per day, instead of three large meals may be more effective for the person who has difficulty eating, especially in the presence of anorexia. In addition,

---

BOX 51–1. *Increasing Oral Intake in Cancer Patients*

Grant, M., Padilla, G. V., & Rhiner, M. (1991). Patterns of anorexia in cancer patients. *Proceedings of the American Cancer Society First National Nursing Research Conference*, Publication No. 71-25M-3332-03 PE, American Cancer Society.

A quasiexperimental study of 41 patients with head and neck cancer was conducted to test the effects of a structured teaching program aimed at increasing oral intake during radiation therapy. Subjects were randomized to (1) an experimental group whose members were given individualized dietary caloric and protein intake requirements; an audiovisual program of usual diet intake problems occurring during therapy and the related self-care; a handout of the program contents; and a book, *Eating Hints*, published by the National Cancer Institute that contained recommendations for dietary intake and nutritious recipes or (2) a control group whose members received the usual care. A 3-day diet intake history was taken weekly during the study. For experimental patients, analysis of food intake, comparing it with recommended dietary intake, was conducted, and the information obtained was relayed to the patient to encourage adjustments in the diet as needed. Analysis included the impact of the program on anorexia, adequacy of oral intake, nutritional status including weight changes, functional status, and quality of life.

Results revealed that the experimental group had a possible vulnerability to nutritional problems during radiation therapy because of a history of significantly greater weight loss before treatment. Three experimental trends were (1) lower appetite scores, (2) higher caloric and protein intake, and (3) weight loss comparable with that in the control group.

The experimental group maintained dietary intake at a level higher than that of the control group despite the loss of appetite and ability to eat. It would appear that cancer and cancer treatment affect oral intake during radiation therapy, and a nutritional counseling program can be used to encourage increased oral intake.

when the ability to consume adequate amounts through normal dietary approaches is significantly limited, the use of oral enteral supplements becomes essential. In reality, supplements may then become the major source of nutrition, and the usual dietary intake of food and beverage becomes the "supplement."

Pharmacologic approaches to anorexia and cachexia involve medications that control symptoms interfering with oral intake and medications that stimulate appetite. Control of nausea should be implemented with appropriate pharmacologic interventions (See below under nausea and vomiting.) Early satiety and the slowing of gastric emptying can be controlled with metoclopramide (Table 51–1). Corticosteroids have been found to give cancer patients an increased sense of well-being and ultimately, increased appetite (Bruera, Roca, Cedaro, Carraro, & Chacon, 1985). Progesterone derivatives, namely megestrol acetate, have been tested in a number of studies and found effective in increasing appetite, weight gain, food intake, and quality of life (Spaulding, 1989; Tchekmedyian, 1993). Cannabinoids have been used to enhance mood and enhance appetite (Nelson, Walsh, & Sheehan, 1994). Results have shown some promise and a need for dose escalation studies. As more information on clinical effects is gained, increased use of a variety of pharmacologic interventions for anorexia is expected (Table 51–1).

NUTRITIONAL SUPPLEMENTS

Decisions regarding what supplements to use for enteral feeding, including feedings given as oral supplements or by tube to meet individual requirements, are based on many factors that are both nutritional and practical. Nutritional supplements may be prepared at home, prepared institutionally, or purchased commercially. Commercially prepared products are advantageous in that they are convenient and their nutritional composition is known and standardized. When the gastrointestinal system is functioning well, intact formulas are given. When digestive or absorptive problems are evident, hydrolyzed formulas are given.

Enteral feeding formula products are classified as: (1) standard; (2) milk-based oral supplements; (3) fiber-containing/blenderized; (4) high-nitrogen; (5) predigested/elemental; (6) concentrated; and (7) modular feedings (ASPEN, 1993). Standard products contain intact macronutrients and are similar in composition to the standard American diet. They usually contain 1 kcal/ml. Standard products, such as Isocal and Osmolite, are indicated for the individual with a fully functional gastrointestinal tract. Milk-based oral supplements, such as Carnation Instant Breakfast and Meritene, are similar to milkshakes and also contain intact nutrients. Fiber-containing/blenderized products, such as Compleat, Enrich, and Jevity, contain fiber from natural food sources or from added soy polysaccharide. They are indicated when problems with bowel function exist. High-nitrogen products, such as Osmolite HN, Sustacal, and Travasorb HN, contain intact macronutrients, but greater than 15 per cent of the total calories are delivered as protein. These products are indicated in individuals who are malnourished, catabolic, or have AIDS. Predigested/elemental products contain hydrolyzed macronutrients, are hyperosmolar (> 450 mOsm/kg), and are generally low in total fat (< 10 per cent) or may contain 30 per cent of calories as fat with < 50 per cent from long-chain triglycerides. Examples of elemental products include Reabilan, Vital/High Nitrogen, and Vivonex T.E.N. They are useful with a partially functioning gastrointestinal tract, when individuals have received nothing by mouth for more than 7 days, or to allow bowel rest. Concentrated products contain intact macronutrients and are similar in composition to the typical American diet. They are especially useful when restricted fluid intake is required. Isocal HCN and Magnacal are two examples.

Modular feedings contain specific nutrient sources that can be added to liquid feedings. They may be carbohydrates and electrolytes (Polycose, Moducal, Sumacal); medium-chain triglycerides (MCT oil); protein (Casec, Propec, or Nutrisource Protein); fat sources; vitamins; or minerals.

ENTERAL NUTRITION

When provision of nutrition is inadequate by normal dietary intake because patients either cannot eat or will not eat but the gastrointestinal tract is functioning normally, the administration of nutritional support by enteral feedings as oral supplements or by tube is preferable to the parenteral route. Enteral nutrition promotes more efficient utilization of nutrients and better preservation of intestinal functioning than adminis-

TABLE 51–1. *Pharmacological Interventions for Anorexia*

MEDICATION	CLASSIFICATION	PROPOSED ACTION
Megestrol acetate	Oral synthetic progesterone	May inhibit tumor necrosis factor Increases weight gain of fat and body cell mass
Pentoxifylline	Methylxanthene derivative	Inhibits the production of tumor necrosis factor
Metoclopramide	Anti-emetic gastrointestinal stimulant	Increases gastric emptying Useful for patients with early satiety and delayed gastric emptying
Cannabinoids	Marijuana derivative	Seems to increase appetite and act as an antiemetic High doses may lead to dizziness and somnolence
Dexamethasone Prednisolone	Corticosteroids	Appetite stimulating and increases well being

(From Grant, M., & Rivera, L. M. (in press). Anorexia, cachexia, and dysphagia. *Seminars in Oncology Nursing.*)

tration by the parenteral route (Goodwin & Wilmore, 1988). If the gastrointestinal tract is functioning, it is preferable that it be used because making use of this route is less expensive, has a lower potential for complications, and is generally easier to manage.

Indications for nasoenteric tube feeding are summarized in Table 51–2 (Feldman, 1988). Nasoenteric feedings are appropriate for treatment that is expected to be short-term (less than 4 to 6 weeks) or as a temporary measure prior to placement of a long-term feeding tube (DeChocco & Materese, 1992). Nasoenteric tube feedings are contraindicated when complete or incomplete gastric or intestinal obstruction is present, severe gastroesophageal reflux is a problem, or paralytic ileus occurs.

Enteral administration can be by bolus, intermittently by gravity drip or pump, or continuously by infusion pump. Bolus feedings are much easier to provide as long as they are tolerated well and do not cause symptoms such as nausea, vomiting, discomfort, or diarrhea. Bolus feedings refer to the rapid delivery of 4 to 6 ounces into the stomach. These may begin by introducing 50 to 100 ml of isotonic or slightly hypotonic formula every 3 hours, increasing by 50 ml every one or two feedings up to a maximum of 250 to 300 ml every 3 to 4 hours. This is then followed by an increase to full-strength solution.

When enteral feedings must be administered by pump instead of by bolus to minimize symptoms, administration of the enteral feedings entirely during the night or intermittently throughout any part of the day or night may be less disruptive to the patient's other activities, including simple ambulation. Enteral nutrition can be provided in any setting, including the home.

A number of anatomic locations are possible for insertion of tubes for enteral feedings, including, but not limited to, (1) nasogastric intubation, (2) a gastrostomy tube placed surgically through the abdominal wall, (3) an endoscopically placed percutaneous endoscopically guided gastrostomy (PEG) tube, or (4) cervical feeding esophagostomy or pharyngostomy. Occa-

sionally, an enteral feeding tube called a jejunostomy is inserted into the small intestine, in which case bolus feedings are not tolerated and a continuous infusion pump must be used. The development of pliable, small-caliber feeding tubes and defined-formula diets and modular products has increased the tolerance and attractiveness of enteral feeding as opposed to parenteral routes. It is usually preferable to use the smallest tube that the feeding will flow through. Tube sizes, which range from 5 to 12 "French," vary with the type of product used, for example, 5 to 6 with protein hydrolysates, 7 to 10 for protein isolates, and 8 to 12 for intact proteins. Because proteins are the largest molecule given by tube, tube size is influenced by type of protein.

Selection of enteral feeding products depends on the mode of administration, the patient's underlying nutritional difficulty, the route and rate of administration, product osmolarity, and nutrient content of the feedings. Adults should receive 30 to 60 cc of free water per kg daily to meet daily fluid requirements.

Persons receiving enteral nutrition should be monitored for commonly occurring side effects or complications, including nausea and vomiting, diarrhea, constipation, aspiration, over- or underhydration, and metabolic complications. Daily monitoring of the following should be performed: weight, intake and output, bowel function, electrolytes, blood urea nitrogen, and blood glucose until stable. Weekly evaluation should include electrolytes, nitrogen balance, and nutritional indicators.

PARENTERAL NUTRITION

Utilization of the parenteral route for administering nutritional support is the least preferable. Enteral approaches are preferred, regardless of whether they are delivered in the home or the institutional setting because of the increased risk with parenteral nutrition of mechanical, metabolic, or septic complications; greater expense; and potential complexity in managing parenteral administration, especially by nonprofessionals. If the gastrointestinal tract is functioning, it is always the route of choice for administration. Parenteral feeding is used when the gastrointestinal tract is inaccessible, not functioning, or needs rest, or when it is functioning but is not capable of absorbing sufficient nutrients to meet metabolic requirements. Specific cancer-related conditions include massive small bowel resection, radiation enteritis, intractable vomiting or diarrhea. Parenteral nutrition is inappropriate when nutritional therapy is expected to be required for less than 5 days or when a poor prognosis does not warrant aggressive nutritional intervention (DeChocco & Matrese, 1992). Studies comparing the efficacy of enteral nutrition routes as compared to parenteral have found no difference. In the cancer patient, TPN is an adjunctive therapy and should not be administered in the absence of antitumor therapy (Sax & Souba, 1993). As a supportive therapy, it should not be administered to improve the outcome of disease. Conclusive evidence that TPN benefits length of survival, treatment tolerance, treatment toxicity, or tumor response does not

TABLE 51–2. *Indications for Nasoenteric Tube Feeding*

Severe protein or calorie malnutrition
Anorexia
Fractures or neoplasms of head and neck preventing oral intake
Neurologic or psychiatric disorders, preventing oral intake
Coma or depressed mental state
Serious illness with very high metabolic requirements (burns)
Enterocutaneous fistulas
Short bowel syndrome
Bowel preparation for surgery in seriously ill or malnourished patients
Crohn's disease
Type I glycogen storage disease
Chemotherapy or radiotherapy
Renal or hepatic failure

(From Feldman, E. B. [1988]. *Essentials of clinical nutrition.* Philadelphia: F. A. Davis. Reproduced by permission.)

exist (Bloch, 1991). It may be helpful in allowing delivery of complete antitumor therapy regimens.

Parenteral nutritional support can be administered either peripherally or through a central line. Peripheral Parenteral Nutrition (PPN), also called Peripheral Vein Nutrition, is indicated when intravenous administration of nutrient solutions with low osmolality is planned for limited periods of time. PPN is used most effectively for weight maintenance in nonhypermetabolic patients (BEE less than 1800 kcal/day), for maintenance before initiating central parenteral feeding, or for supplementing enteral feedings. It also is used to limit protein breakdown in stable postoperative patients whose oral intake is expected to return to adequate levels within 10 days (Goodwin & Wilmore, 1988). Type of access and route of delivery are usually determined according to length of therapy.

Cancer-specific indications for TPN include inability to absorb nutrients; undergoing high-dose chemotherapy, radiation, and bone marrow transplants; severe malnutrition with a nonfunctional gastrointestinal tract; severely catabolic patient with or without malnutrition when the gastrointestinal tract is not usable within 5 to 7 days; or undergoing major surgery. TPN is not appropriate when other feeding approaches can be used, the need is for less than 5 days, or if aggressive nutritional support is not desired by the patient or family (ASPEN, 1993).

TPN is administered through a central vein and provides all nutritional needs. All essential nutrients, including water, energy, protein in the form of essential amino acids, essential fatty acids, minerals, electrolytes, trace minerals, and vitamins, must be provided by TPN. Adult TPN solutions are generally 40 to 70 per cent dextrose. Amino acids, given to provide a positive nitrogen balance, are selected based on disease considerations. Calories and essential fatty acids are provided by lipids. Essential fatty acid deficiency (EFAD) is prevented by giving approximately to 4 to 10 per cent of kilocalories from lipids, administered periodically (a couple of times per week) or during one shift a day. Twenty per cent fat emulsion provides 2.0 kcal/ml or 1000 kcal per 500 cc bottle, whereas 10 per cent fat emulsion yields 1.1 kcal/ml or 550 kcal per 500 cc bottle.

Solutions infused through a peripheral vein are usually reserved for short-term parenteral nutrition of less than 7 to 10 days when severe malnutrition is not present. The total concentrations of glucose, amino acids, and electrolytes determine the osmolarity of the infusate.

Administration of parenteral nutrition through a long-term venous access device requires placement of a central venous line into the subclavian vein or an alternative anatomic site that can tolerate high-volume, high-osmolality infusions. Permanent catheters that are tunneled, such as Hickman, Broviac, or Groshong catheters, may be inserted to provide access to the subclavian vein. Peripherally inserted central catheters (PICC) are an option for administering intravenous nutrition centrally. Triple-lumen catheters may be inserted when the central line is required for administration of medications, such as antitumor or antimicrobial chemotherapy.

Administration of nutrition support through a central line requires the use of an infusion pump. Selected drugs, such as vasopressors, antiarrhythmics, heparin, insulin, oxytocin (Pitocin), and various chemotherapeutic agents, may also be administered using these pumps. Infusion pumps are electronic devices that deliver fluid at a relatively constant, preset flow rate. Three types of infusion pumps are (1) peristaltic, (2) piston syringe, or (3) piston cylinder cassette pumps. Peristaltic pumps work by applying an external force to the tubing of the intravenous administration set. Accuracy of peristaltic pumps depends on a number of factors: speed of the rotor, length of the tubing segment between rollers, amount of deformation of the tubing with use, and internal diameter of the tubing. The second type of piston syringe pump involves a prefilled syringe that delivers fluid at a constant rate by a pump motor that drives the syringe plunger. These pumps are usually used when small amounts of fluid are to be delivered. In the third type, the piston cylinder cassette pump, a small-volume syringe located in the line between the bottle and the patient alternately fills by positive pressure and expels its contents. Meticulous central venous catheter care, which is usually provided by the nurse, is essential to prevent catheter-related infectious complications, especially in the immunocompromised cancer patient. In addition, the central catheter should not be used for administration of blood products or for blood sampling. "Piggybacking" medications through the catheter should be avoided.

SPECIAL PROBLEMS ASSOCIATED WITH NUTRITIONAL DEPLETION

EARLY SATIETY

DEFINITION

Early satiety is experienced as a feeling of fullness shortly after beginning to ingest a meal. It may be caused by tumor directly impinging on the upper gastrointestinal tract and decreasing the size of the meal that can be ingested. Other causes of early satiety are delayed gastric emptying and decreased peristalsis. Early satiety frequently is absent at breakfast, mild at lunch, and severe by dinnertime.

MANAGEMENT

Interventions for early satiety include providing the largest proportion of required calories and protein for breakfast, when early satiety is minimal. Frequent small meals may allow for ingestion of adequate calories and protein. "Empty calorie" foods, such as diet drinks, coffee, and tea, should be avoided, especially at mealtimes. Ideally, every mouthful ingested should provide the maximum calories and protein possible. Use of nutritional supplements for patients suffering from early satiety is recommended. Pharmacologic management involves metaclopramide, which increases gastric emptying, relieving the feeling of fullness.

NAUSEA AND VOMITING

DEFINITION

Nausea and vomiting are common symptoms experienced by cancer patients. Associated causes include radiation to the brain or the total body, fluid and electrolyte imbalances, chemotherapy or analgesic side effects, uremia, intestinal obstruction, brain and hepatic metastases, infections, and septicemia (Donaldson, 1984; Eyre & Ward, 1984; Reuben & Mor, 1986).

Nausea is an extremely uncomfortable sensation experienced in the back of the throat and epigastrium, which generally ends with vomiting. It may be accompanied by pallor, cold clammy skin, increased salivation, faintness, tachycardia, and diarrhea. Frequently, decreased gastric activity accompanies nausea.

Vomiting is an involuntary reflex by which the contents of the stomach and the intestine are expelled. Vomiting is immediately preceded by widespread autonomic stimulation resulting in tachypnea, copious salivation, dilation of the pupils, sweating, pallor, and rapid heartbeat (Nord & Sodeman, 1985).

Several types of vomiting occur in cancer patients. When associated with the administration of chemotherapy, vomiting varies, depending on the emetic potential of the medications administered (Table 51–3). Anticipatory nausea and vomiting (ANV) is a learned phenomenon that is stimulated by something that occurs in association with the true stimulant. Learned stimuli include thoughts, sights, tastes, and odors related to the treatment. Because ANV is a learned response, it occurs after the first chemotherapeutic dose has been administered. Occurrence of ANV may increase with each successive cycle of chemotherapy. Vomiting also occurs in association with radiation therapy, obstructions, infections, and intestinal inflammatory diseases.

PATHOPHYSIOLOGIC MECHANISMS

Nausea and vomiting occur after stimulation of a complex reflex coordinated by the vomiting center in the medullary lateral reticular formation (Sallan & Cronin, 1985). Neurologic stimulation may occur in one or more of several pathways. Pathways most frequently involved in cancer patients include the chemoreceptor trigger zone, which responds to circulating levels of chemicals; the vagal visceral afferents, which respond to gastrointestinal pathology; the sympathetic visceral afferents, which respond to hollow organ pathology; and the cerebral cortex and limbic system, which respond to stimuli from the senses, anxiety, pain, and increases in intracranial pressure (Yasko, 1985). Mediation of stimuli is carried out by a variety of neurotransmitters, such as acetylcholine, dopamine, and serotonin.

MANAGEMENT

Clinical assessment of nausea and vomiting begins with a description of the patterns of occurrence and severity. As the patient moves from the potential for nausea and vomiting to the occurrence of moderate and severe symptoms, the assessment changes (Table 51–4). Interventions for nausea and vomiting include both pharmacologic and nonpharmacologic approaches (Grant, 1987a). Medications used to prevent and control these symptoms differ and depend on the cause and severity of the symptoms. Selection of the most appropriate antiemetic regimen is related to the different mechanisms involved. The classes of medications used and their mechanisms of action, side effects, and specific examples are given in Table 51–5. Combination antiemetic therapy is used to tailor control of nausea and vomiting with a particular chemotherapeutic regimen. Nonpharmacologic approaches include dietary interventions and behavioral interventions. These are summarized in Table 51–6.

Helping patients to control and manage the distress associated with nausea and vomiting is a challenging area of oncology nursing. Improvements in both pharmacologic and nonpharmacologic interventions have provided the oncology nurse with a beginning understanding of how to provide skilled nursing care for these problems. Continued testing and refinement of this care are needed to support the patient and improve the quality of life in this vulnerable population.

TASTE AND SMELL CHANGES

DEFINITION

Changes in taste and smell have been documented in studies of both humans and animals with cancer. Even though mechanisms for development of these

TABLE 51–3. *Emetic Potential of Common Chemotherapeutic Agents*

MILD/RARE	MODERATE	SEVERE AND COMMON
Asparaginase	Actinomycin	Carmustine
Busulfan	Cyclophosphamide	Cisplatin
Bleomycin	Daunorubicin	Cyclophosphamide*
Chlorambucil	Doxorubicin	Dacarbazine
Cytarabine	Methotrexate	Hydroxyurea*
Diethylstilbestrol	Mitomycin	Lomustine
Dromostanolone		Mechlorethamine
Etoposide		Methotrexate*
Floxuridine		Mitotane
Fluorouracil		Nitrogen mustard
Leuprolide		Pipobroman
Medroxy-		Plicamycin
progesterone		Procarbazine
acetate		Streptozocin
Megestrol		Uracil mustard
Melphalan		
Mercaptopurine		
Polyestradiol		
Tamoxifen		
Testolactone		
Thioguanine		
Thio-TEPA		
Vinblastine		
Vincristine		

*High dose.
(From Grant, M. [1987b]. Nausea, vomiting and anorexia. *Seminars in Oncology Nursing, 3,* 277–286.)

TABLE 51–4. *Nursing Care Plan for the Patient with Potential Nausea and Vomiting*

ASSESSMENT	EXPECTED OUTCOMES	INTERVENTIONS
Determine whether patient or family expects nausea and vomiting (N&V)	Expectations of patient or family are realistic	Determine whether patient has a high potential for N&V related to the disease present and the treatment Teach patient or family what to expect regarding N&V
Determine what the patient or family believes about the occurrence of N&V	Myths about the occurrence of N&V need to be corrected	Describe the causes of N&V and its relationship to disease and treatment
Determine what coping patterns patient usually uses to manage stress and discomfort	Patient manages to cope effectively with N&V	Identify previous successful coping behaviors; encourage patient to use these behaviors to manage N&V
Determine the potential for N&V depending on the treatment or stage of disease	Prevent or minimize N&V	Administer antiemetic agents as prescribed to prevent occurrence; institute nonpharmacologic measures
Identify patterns of occurrence, amount of distress, and effectiveness of interventions	Provide the most effective management of N&V	Evaluate effectiveness of interventions, revising approaches to provide the most effective relief of N&V and the associated distresses
Evaluate dietary intake	Maintain nutritional status	Provide for oral intake during times of least N&V; have patient avoid foods high in fat Provide frequent small meals
Identify environment most conducive to eating	Maintain adequate nutritional intake	Avoid areas with strong odors; provide a clean, pleasant environment for meals

abnormalities have been studied extensively, many questions persist. Taste abnormalities may involve the development of a taste aversion, learned taste preferences, or changes in taste acuity. Development of taste and smell changes in cancer patients may be associated with administration of chemotherapy, radiation therapy, or tumor growth. For example, the occurrence of side effects such as nausea and vomiting with administration of specific chemotherapeutic agents can result in aversions to foods ingested during the course of therapy. Aversions may be stronger and may occur more quickly if new or novel foods are ingested (Bernstein, 1982). Aversions may disappear on completion of the therapy and when tumor growth has been stopped.

Common taste changes include aversions to meat and meat products, increased tolerance for sweet substances, and avoidance of foods taken during the time immediately surrounding treatment. Variations occur with individual patients.

MANAGEMENT

Interventions for taste and smell changes generally are individualized to the specific patient. However, some general guidelines are recommended. Protein sources should be derived from bland protein foods, such as milk and milk products, fish, and chicken. Beef and pork tend to taste bitter and should be avoided. When the "sweet" threshold is elevated, foods that ordinarily are considered too sweet will be acceptable. Some patients add additional sugar to sweeten foods more; other patients have reported a decrease in sweet threshold and develop an intolerance for anything

sweet. For these patients, complex carbohydrates can be substituted to meet needed energy and carbohydrate requirements.

If supplements are used, a taste test is advised. The patient can then select the supplement that tastes best. To avoid developing specific taste intolerances, favorite foods should be avoided during periods of nausea and vomiting. Also, substituted food, such as supplements introduced during radiation therapy, may become the target for development of taste aversions. If supplements are required, switching supplements may prove to be more successful for the patient.

MOOD CHANGES

DEFINITION

Changes in moods are common in cancer patients. Depression and anxiety may occur before the diagnosis is confirmed, after the diagnosis is made, during treatment, and at the time of recurrences. These mood states tend to be accompanied by decreases in food intake. Careful monitoring of the type and timing of dietary intake is an initial step in evaluating the seriousness of the mood on food intake.

MANAGEMENT

Improving the environment for eating and providing familiar foods and familiar settings can be used to make meals more appealing. Presence of friends or family members during mealtimes also makes the atmosphere more pleasant and homelike for the patient. Disruptive interactions with family members

TABLE 51–5. *Antiemetics Used for Nausea and Vomiting in Cancer Patients*

Pharmacologic Effects	Side Effects and Toxicities	Comments	Examples (Including Routes and Common Dosages)
Anticholinergics Depress vestibular stimuli Suppress emetic center	Sedation	Effective in nausea and vomiting due to motion sickness	Scopolamine transdermal
Antihistamines Depress cerebral cortex Depress vestibular stimuli Inhibit histamine-mediated stimuli	Drowsiness (frequently a desired effect) Anticholinergic effects at high doses	Most effective in nausea and vomiting due to motion sickness Used primarily in combination antiemetic regimens	Diphenhydramine: PO, IM, IV, 25–50 mg
Barbiturates Depress CNS	Respiratory depression Somnolence	Action potentiated when administered with phenothiazines Used primarily in combination antiemetic regimens	Pentobarbital: PO, 100 mg Secobarbital: PO, IV, 100 mg
Benzodiazepines Depress CNS Produce amnesic effects	Sedation	Sedation effects may compromise older patients and those with known respiratory difficulty Amnesic effects considered an advantage Used in combination antiemetic regimens	Lorazepam: IV, 0.05 mg/kg Diazepam: PO, 5 mg; IM, 2.5 mg
Benzoquinolizines Suppress CTZ Anxiolytic Anticholinergic activity	Sedation Hypersensitivity Rare hypotension	Clinical trials report controversial results on efficacy	Benzquinamide: IM, IV, 25–50 mg Trimethobenzamide: PO, 250 mg; IV, 200 mg
Butyrophenones Suppress CTZ Block dopamine-mediated stimuli Decrease vestibular stimuli Anxiolytic	Hypertension Extrapyramidal effects Sedation and somnolence Agitation and restlessness	Side effects partly controlled with diphenhydramine Tolerance develops after repeated doses	Haloperidol: PO, IM, 2–5 mg; IV, 2 mg Droperidol: IM, IV, 1–3 mg

Classification / Mechanism of action	Side effects	Comments	Agents and dosages
Cannabinoids Anticholinergic activity Other unknown	Extrapyramidal effects, including ataxia, hallucinations, dysphoria, hypertension, euphoria, frank psychosis Somnolence	Side effects fewer in younger patients or experienced user Abuse potential	Marijuana cigarettes Delta-9-tetrahydrocannabinol: PO, 5–15 mg/M^2 Levonantradol: PO, 0.05–1.5 mg
Phenothiazines Suppress CTZ Block dopamine-mediated stimuli Depress emetic center Inhibit autonomic effects via the vagus nerve	Faintness, nasal stuffiness, dry mouth, palpitations, orthostatic hypotension, constipation Hypersensitivity Extrapyramidal effects Jaundice, blood dyscrasias	Diphenhydramine used for side effects Good for mild nausea Causes sedation	Prochlorperazine: PO, IM, IV, 10 mg; rectal, 25 mg Thiethylperazine: PO, IM, IV, rectal, 10 mg Chlorpromazine: PO, IM, IV, rectal, 12.5–50 mg Promethazine: PO, IM, IV, rectal, 25 mg
Serotonin Antagonists Block serotonin binding in wall of gut	Headaches, diarrhea, constipation, fever, transient increases in SGOT/SGPT Headache, asthenia, somnolence, diarrhea, fever, constipation	Effective for highly, moderately high, or moderately emetagenic chemotherapy Dose reduction to match chemotherapy agents not recommended	Ondansetron: IV 0.15 mg every 4 hrs × 3 doses or 32 mg prechemotherapy × 1 dose PO 8 mg TID × 3 days Granisetron: IV 10 mcg/kg over 5 min within 30 min of chemotherapy
Steroids Possible prostaglandin inhibition	Lethargy Weakness Generalized swelling	Used primarily in combination antiemetic regimens	Dexamethazone: PO, 4–10 mg; IM, IV, 10–20 mg Methylprednisone: IV, 250 mg
Substituted Benzamides Suppress CTZ Block dopamine-mediated stimuli Anticholinergic activity	Extrapyramidal effects such as anxiety, restlessness, dystonia	Side effects decreased in patients under 40 Side effects partly controlled with diphenhydramine	Metoclopramide: IV, 1–3 mg/kg

CNS = central nervous system; CTZ = Chemotactic trigger zone; SGOT/SGPT = serum glutamic oxaloacetic transaminase/serum glutamic pyruvic transaminase.
(From Grant, M. [1987b]. Nausea, vomiting and anorexia. *Seminars in Oncology Nursing, 3,* 277–286.)

TABLE 51–6. *Nonpharmacologic Interventions for Nausea and Vomiting*

Nutrition Interventions

Adjust time of eating to coordinate with periods of least nausea and vomiting

Avoid foods that precipitate nausea and vomiting (e.g., foods high in fat content, spicy foods, or foods patient associates with nausea and vomiting)

Provide foods that are bland, easily digestible, and still nutritious (e.g., crackers, baked and boiled foods, sodas, mild fruits and vegetables)

Use nutritional supplements to provide maximum calories and protein with a minimum of intake

Avoid favorite foods during periods of nausea and vomiting to avoid developing aversions to these foods

Provide small meals, pleasant environment, and good company during mealtimes

Behavior Interventions

Use distraction to decrease distress during periods of nausea and vomiting (e.g., music, television, radio)

Teach the patient behavior techniques (e.g., hypnosis, guided imagery, biofeedback, and progressive muscle relaxation)

should be avoided, and the nurse may need to ask family members to leave if such a situation arises. Providing rest before mealtime may help the patient be better prepared for eating. A positive and supportive approach helps the depressed or anxious patient to ingest adequate calories and protein. Pharmacologic intervention includes administration of corticosteroids.

DYSPHAGIA

DEFINITION

Problems with swallowing can pose a severe threat to maintaining adequate nutritional status. *Dysphagia* is a term used to identify inability or difficulty swallowing (as opposed to the term *odynophagia*, which refers to painful swallowing [Greenberger, 1986]). It is most commonly associated with neurologic or structural damage. Dysphagia is particularly likely to occur as a result of the local effects of tumors of the head and neck or the esophagus, or secondary to treatment, especially with radiation therapy or surgical resection. Surgical excision of structures important to swallowing, such as the tongue, the soft or bony palate, the supraglottic larynx, or the esophagus, is particularly likely to result in dysphagia.

Twenty-nine muscles and six cranial nerves working together are required to perform a successful swallow. Types of dysphagia relate to the three phases of swallowing—oral preparatory and oral, pharyngeal, and esophageal. *Transfer dysphagia* refers to problems in the delivery of a bolus of food or fluid from the mouth into the esophagus, involving dysfunction of the mouth or tongue, pharynx, or hypopharynx. Transfer dysphagia frequently results from neuromuscular incoordination of these areas. It may also be caused by carcinoma of the mouth, tongue, or hypopharyngeal region. Cricopharyngeal dysfunction is another common cause

of transfer dysphagia. *Transport dysphagia* is an esophageal problem in which transport of the bolus down the body of the esophagus is altered. The presence of an extrinsic or intrinsic lesion, such as a tumor or stricture, obstructing the esophageal lumen can cause transport dysphagia. Weak, absent, or disorganized peristaltic activity of the esophagus is another source of transport dysphagia. Finally, *delivery dysphagia*, or problems with bolus entry into the stomach, also can occur. Benign or malignant obstructing lesions, such as tumors or strictures, or lower esophageal sphincter dysfunction can produce this problem.

MANAGEMENT

Thorough assessment of potential or existing problems with dysphagia is an important first step, in addition to evaluation of the patient's current nutritional status. Signs and symptoms to observe for and report include (1) choking when swallowing liquids or solids; (2) drooling, regurgitation, or retention of food accompanying swallowing of liquids or solids; (3) food sticking in the pharynx or esophagus; (4) pain or discomfort when swallowing liquids or solids; (5) weakness of lips, tongue, or jaw; (6) lesions in the oral cavity; (7) cough before, during, or after a swallow; (8) voice changes; or (9) aspiration.

Some relatively simple interventions help minimize or eliminate dysphagia (Grady, Farnen, Ascheman, Passman, & Palazola, 1985; Schmitz, 1990). The patient should sit with his or her head elevated at least 45 degrees while eating or drinking and should maintain that upright position for 15 to 30 minutes after finishing. The head may be held forward or to one side.

Dietary accommodations may be part of the treatment, including appropriate liquid as well as solid consistency. Modification of solids may include stiff gelled, gelled, strained, pureed, and ground foods that are soft or regular in consistency. Liquids when needed can be thickened with a variety of products, including strained foods, rice cereal, potato flakes, and cornstarch. Special products that thicken liquids without altering their taste include Thick-It and Frutex. Cold foods trigger a swallow more easily than hot foods. Six to eight frequent, small feedings are more desirable than three big meals. Milk products should be avoided if mucus is copious. When aspiration is feared or likely, suction apparatus should be readily available. When the oral musculature is defective, bites should make use of the strong side of the mouth. If propelling the bolus to the posterior part of the tongue is a problem, food should be placed on the posterior part of the tongue with a syringe or long-handled spoon.

The following swallowing exercise or technique is helpful to prevent aspiration: (1) flex the neck; (2) inhale; (3) place a small amount of food on the tongue; (4) consciously hold the breath while swallowing; (5) exhale and gently cough or clear the throat; and (6) wait at least 30 seconds between swallows.

Dysphagia involving the oral musculature may be improved by providing semisolid foods (puddings, canned fruit, mashed potatoes) when chewing is impaired; by consuming thin, pureed foods; or by placing food on the posterior part of the tongue with a long-handled spoon (DeLisa, Miller, Melnick, Mikulic, & Gerber, 1985; Donoghue, 1988). Dysphagia involving the pharyngeal phase of swallowing may be minimized by alternating solids and liquids, making postural changes, or performing the swallowing exercises described earlier. Esophageal dysphagia may require use of food supplements or ultimately enteral nutritional support.

MALABSORPTION AND DIARRHEA

DEFINITION

Expressed functionally, diarrhea is too much of a too-loose or liquid stool. Tremendous variation exists as to what different people consider to be "normal" in terms of their usual bowel function. A change in bowel habits is implicit in the identification of diarrhea as a problem for the patient with cancer. Clinically, significant alterations in stool frequency, fluidity, or abnormal constituents herald diarrhea; however, stool weight greater than 300 g on the usual Western diet is an operational definition of diarrhea (Greenberger, 1986).

PATHOPHYSIOLOGIC MECHANISMS

Understanding of the potential pathophysiologic mechanisms of diarrhea is essential to its identification and management. Diarrhea can be classified according to one of three predominant mechanisms—secretory, osmotic, or mixed. Table 51–7 summarizes information regarding the three classifications of diarrhea mechanisms in terms of (1) actual pathophysiologic mechanism, (2) characteristics of the diarrhea and its fluid composition, and (3) cancer-related examples.

Etiology. Diarrhea that is specific to the person with cancer can result either from the tumor itself or from its treatment. Examples of conditions causing diarrhea that are directly tumor-related include carcinoma of the pancreas (osmotic, from inadequate digestive enzymes); carcinoid syndrome (secretory, from serotonin or prostaglandins); villous adenoma (secretory, from unidentified secretagogue); medullary carcinoma of the thyroid (secretory, from calcitonin or prostaglandins); tumors producing vasoactive intestinal peptide (VIP) (secretory, from VIP); and Zollinger-Ellison syndrome (secretory, from gastrin). Tumors that infiltrate the small or large intestine (osmotic from decreased absorption of solutes) can alter the digestive or absorptive functions that normally occur in the gastrointestinal tract so that diarrhea results.

Each of the modalities employed in cancer treatment—surgical resection, chemotherapy, radiation therapy to fields including the gastrointestinal tract, or immunotherapy—potentially involves anatomic or physiologic alterations that can lead to diarrhea (Culhane, 1983). When these treatments are used in combination, the results can be compounded. Medications that are used to treat side effects of antitumor therapy, such as antacids, antibiotics, or colchicine, can also secondarily cause diarrhea. Lactose intolerance, occurring temporarily from radiation therapy or chemotherapy or permanently from surgical resection, can also cause diarrhea. Increased stress or anxiety can produce increased gastric motility that then results in diarrhea. Malnutrition itself can contribute to the occurrence of diarrhea as a result of decreased functioning absorptive surface in the intestine. Finally, supplemental feedings

TABLE 51–7. *Pathophysiologic Mechanisms of Diarrhea*

TYPE OF DIARRHEA	MECHANISM	CHARACTERISTICS AND COMPOSITION	CANCER-RELATED EXAMPLES
Osmotic	Unabsorbable or poorly absorbable solute in gastrointestinal tract	24-hr stool volume usually < 1 L Stool volume decreases when fasting Potassium lost in excess of sodium Net effect is water and potassium depletion rather than electrolyte depletion Stool pH acidic < 7	Lactose intolerance Cathartics Postgastrectomy
Secretory	Increased secretory activity of gastrointestinal tract (absorption may be normal); also from inhibition of electrolyte and water absorption	24-hr stool volume usually > 1 L (large stool volume) Stool volume does not decrease when fasting Sodium lost in excess of potassium Net effect is electrolyte depletion Stool pH neutral, 7	Non-beta islet cell tumors of pancreas Zollinger-Ellison syndrome Villous adenoma Medullary carcinoma of thyroid
Mixed	Hypermotility states involve increased rate of transit; osmotic effect of ingested solutes occurs from rapid intestinal transit and diminished net absorption	Variable	Cholinergic medication Carcinoid syndrome

(Adapted from Greenberger, N. J. [1986.] *Gastrointestinal disorders: A Pathophysiologic Approach* [3rd ed.]. Chicago: Year Book Medical Publishers.)

with products whose osmolality is high can cause an osmotic diarrhea.

MANAGEMENT

Thoughtful evaluation to determine the cause of the diarrhea, as well as confirmation of it as a problem, provides a firm foundation for planning interventions for the cancer patient (Davis, 1985). A careful and thorough history that includes review of signs and symptoms, medications, dietary and nutritional status, usual patterns of elimination, prior surgeries, and concurrent medical conditions is essential. Management may emphasize, but is not limited to, dietary and pharmacologic measures. Treatment of underlying conditions, such as pancreatic insufficiency, hyperthyroidism, or diabetes mellitus, is essential when they are thought to play a significant role.

Assessment should include consideration of (1) ability to care for oneself, including food acquisition and preparation; (2) activity and exercise tolerance; (3) gastrointestinal discomfort; (4) family and support systems; (5) sources of stress and anxiety; (6) usual patterns of elimination; (7) pattern of diarrhea (onset, duration, amount, appearance, frequency); (8) associated symptoms (cramping, flatus, abdominal distention); (9) possibility of partial fecal obstruction; (10) nutritional status and requirements, including fluid and electrolyte balance; (11) dietary patterns; (12) sleep-rest patterns and level of fatigue; (13) perineal-perianal skin integrity; and (14) effect on usual lifestyle (Ropka, 1985).

Interventions should be developed that (1) are based on information acquired from the assessment and (2) are appropriate for both the etiology and pathophysiologic mechanism of the diarrhea. Providing the patients with appropriate information is particularly important if they are to manage the problems as independently as possible.

Pharmacologic agents for control of diarrhea, such as Kaopectate (Upjohn), Lomotil (Searle), Immodium, low-dose codeine, or bulk-forming agents should be administered as directed. Patients should be cautioned to observe for side effects or toxicities of these medications and should be advised about what to report to their health care provider. Many antacids contain substances that work osmotically, such as magnesium. When antacids are required on a regular basis, their selection should include consideration of bowel status, avoiding antacids that contain magnesium if diarrhea is a concurrent problem.

Nutritional and dietary considerations are important in the management of diarrhea, both to decrease the occurrence of diarrhea and to ensure adequate nutritional status. They include the following: (1) eat low-residue foods that are high in protein and calories; (2) attempt small, frequent snacks rather than three large meals per day; (3) avoid foods that irritate or stimulate the gastrointestinal tract; (4) avoid extreme temperatures in foods or beverages; (5) eliminate foods that are highly spiced or greasy; (6) ensure adequate intake of uncarbonated fluids (2 to 3 quarts per day), best served at room temperature; (7) eliminate lactose-containing foods and beverages to prevent lactose intolerance; (8) utilize nutritional supplements to increase calorie and protein intake; (9) consider a liquid diet or enteral nutritional support if diarrhea becomes severe.

Local and systemic measures that will increase comfort are essential. Heat may be applied to the abdomen to relieve the discomfort of cramping. Substances that protect skin and mucous membranes and promote healing, such as A & D ointment, Desitin, or Nupercainal, can be applied to the perirectal area. Local anesthetics, such as Tucks, may be used around the rectum. Sitz baths may provide further comfort. The rectal area and perineum should be gently and thoroughly cleaned, followed by careful drying after each bowel movement. Anal or rectal stimulation should be avoided.

CONSTIPATION

DEFINITION

The occurrence of constipation is common in cancer patients. Prevention of this symptom by active management in vulnerable patients is of utmost importance. Constipation occurs when the stool becomes hard, dry, and difficult to pass, or when bowel movements are so infrequent that patients experience abdominal discomfort.

ETIOLOGY

Constipation in the cancer patient may occur as a result of decreased motility of the gastrointestinal tract, metabolic changes such as hypocalcemia, inadequate food intake, decreased exercise, and medications such as narcotics and vinca alkaloids. The environment of the cancer patient may have an effect on the occurrence of constipation because of hospital admission, the need for using a bedpan, a lack of privacy, and a change in normal daily routines.

MANAGEMENT

Management of constipation begins with a thorough assessment of the patient via a comprehensive history and physical examination. Evaluation should include a review of medications, diet, and liquid intake. Symptoms to look for include a distended abdomen with palpable colon, abdominal discomfort, hypoactive bowel sounds, and a history of no bowel movement for more than 2 days despite oral intake of food. A small amount of diarrhea may also be present, and hard stool may be palpable in the rectum.

Nutritional and dietary considerations effective in the treatment of constipation include increasing fluid intake to more than six glasses of water per day and increasing the fiber content of the diet. When pain medications are ordered, they should be accompanied by increased fluids, increased fiber, and specific medications such as Peri-Colace or Doxidan (Brooks, 1978; Portenoy, 1987). If fecal impaction is present, manual evacuation may be needed and can be preceded by a stool softener.

Patients and their families need to be educated to monitor bowel movements, maintain fluid intake, increase fiber sources, and avoid constipating foods such as dairy products and fried foods. The best approach to constipation is to identify a potential problem and vigorously implement approaches to prevent both constipation and impaction.

SUMMARY

Alterations in nutrition are common in cancer patients. They may occur at any stage of disease but are most common during treatment and when tumors are extensive. Anorexia and cachexia are frequently present in terminally ill patients. Skillful and creative nursing care is essential in individualizing approaches to maintaining patients' nutritional status.

REFERENCES

American College of Physicians. (1989). Parenteral nutrition in patients receiving cancer chemotherapy. *Annals of Internal Medicine, 110,* 734–735.

A.S.P.E.N. Board of Directors. (1993). Guidelines for the use of parenteral and enteral nutrition in adult and pediatric patients. *Journal of Parenteral and Enteral Nutrition, 17* (Suppl. 4) 1SA–52SA.

Beck, A. (1972). *Depression: Causes and treatment.* Philadelphia: University of Pennsylvania Press.

Bernstein, I. L. (1982). Physiological and psychological mechanisms of cancer anorexia. *Cancer Research, 42,* 7155–7205.

Bernstein, I. L. (1986). Etiology of anorexia in cancer. *Cancer, 58*(Suppl. 8), 1881–1886.

Bernstein, I. L., & Bernstein, I. D. (1981). Learned food aversions and cancer anorexia. *Cancer Treatment Reports, 65*(Suppl. 5), 43–47.

Blackburn, G. L., Bistrian, B. R., & Miani, B. S. (1976). Nutritional and metabolic assessment of the hospitalized patient. *Surgical Clinics of North America, 56,* 1192–1225.

Blackburn, G. L., & Harvey, K. B. (1980). Clinical nutritional assessment of the hospitalized patient. In P. J. Garry (Ed.), *Human nutrition: Clinical and biochemical aspects* (pp. 15–26). Washington, DC: American Association for Clinical Chemistry.

Bloch, A. S. (Ed.). (1991). *Nutrition management of the cancer patient.* Rockville, MD: ASPEN Publishers.

Bloch, A. S. (1994). Feeding the cancer patient: Where have we come from, where are we going? *Nutrition in Clinical Practice, 9,* 87–89.

Bozzetti, F., Pagnoni, A. M., & Del Vecchio, M. (1980). Excessive caloric expenditure as a cause of malnutrition in patients with cancer. *Surgery, Gynecology, and Obstetrics, 150,* 229–234.

Brooks, F. (1978). *Gastrointestinal pathophysiology.* New York: Oxford University Press.

Bruera, E. (1992). Clinical management of anorexia and cachexia in patients with advanced cancer. *Oncology, 49*(Suppl. 2), 35–42.

Bruera, E., & MacDonald, R. N. (1988). Nutrition in cancer patients: An update and review of our experience. *Journal of Pain and Symptom Management, 3,* 133–140.

Bruera, E., Roca, E., Cedaro, L., Carraro, S., & Chacor, R. (1985). Action of oral methylprednisone in terminal cancer patients: A prospective randomized double-blind study. *Cancer Treatment Reports, 69,* 751–754.

Buzby, G. P., Mullen, J. L., Matthews, D. C., Hobbs, C. L., & Rosata, E. F. (1980). Prognostic nutrition index in gastrointestinal surgery. *American Journal of Surgery, 139,* 160–167.

Copeland, E. M., Souchon, E. A., MacFadyen, V. V., Rapp, M. A., & Dudrick, S. J. (1977). Intravenous hyperalimentation as an adjunct to radiation therapy. *Cancer, 39,* 609–616.

Costa, G. (1977). Cachexia, the metabolic component of neoplastic diseases. *Cancer Research, 37,* 2327–2336.

Costa, G., & Donaldson, S. S. (1979). Current concepts in cancer: Effects of cancer and cancer treatment on the nutrition of the host. *New England Journal of Medicine, 300,* 1417–1474.

Culhane, B. (1983). Diarrhea. In J. M. Yasko (Ed.), *Guidelines for cancer care: Symptom management* (pp. 188–197). Reston, VA: Reston Publishing.

Davis, J. D., & Campbell, C. S. (1973). Peripheral control of meal size in the rat: Effect of sham feeding on meal size and drinking rats. *Journal of Comparative and Physiological Psychology, 83,* 379–387.

Davis, M. (1985). Bowel elimination, alterations in: Diarrhea. In J. C. McNally, J. C. Stair, & E. T. Somerville (Eds.), *Guidelines for cancer nursing practice* (pp. 239–242). Orlando, FL: Grune & Stratton, Inc.

DeChocco, R. S., & Matarese, L. (1992). Selection of nutrition support regimens. *Nutrition in Clinical Practice, 7,* 239–245.

DeLisa, J. A., Miller, R. M., Melnick, R. R., Mikulic, M. A., & Gerber, L. H. (1985). Rehabilitation of the cancer patient: Nutrition and glutition. In V. T. DeVita, Jr., S. Hellman, & S. A. Rosenberg (Eds.), *Cancer: Principles and practice of oncology* (2nd ed., pp. 2168–2169). Philadelphia: J. B. Lippincott Co.

Dempsey, D. T., Feurer, I. D., Knox, L. S., Crosby, L. O., Buzby, G. P., & Mullen, J. L. (1984). Energy expenditure in malnourished gastrointestinal cancer patients. *Cancer, 53,* 1265–1273.

Detsky, A. S., Baker, J. P., O'Rourke, D., & Goel, V. (1987). Perioperative parental nutrition: A meta-analysis. *Annals of Internal Medicine, 107,* 195–203.

DeWys, W. D., Begg, C., Lavin, P. T., Band, P. R., Bennett, J. M., Bertino, J. R., Cohen, M. H., Douglass, H. O., Engstrom, P. F., Ezdinli, E. Z., Horton, J., Johnson, C., Silverstein, N. M., Skeel, R. T., Sponzo, R. W., & Tormey, D. C. (1980). Prognostic effect of weight loss prior to chemotherapy in cancer patients. *American Journal of Medicine, 69,* 491–497.

DeWys, W. D., Costa, G., & Henkin, R. (1981). Clinical parameters related to anorexia. *Cancer Treatment Reports, 65*(Suppl. 5), 49–52.

DeWys, W. D., & Walters, K. (1975). Abnormalities of taste sensation in cancer patients. *Cancer, 36,* 1888–1896.

Dickerson, J. W. T. (1983). Nutrition of the cancer patient. In H. H. Draper (Ed.), *Advances in nutritional research* (pp. 105–131). New York: Plenum Press.

Donaldson, S. S. (1984). Nutritional support as an adjunct to radiation therapy. *Journal of Parenteral and Enteral Nutrition, 8,* 302–310.

Donoghue, M. (1988). Dysphagia. In S. B. Baird (Ed.), *Decision making in oncology nursing* (pp. 96–97). Toronto: B. C. Decker.

Eyre, H., & Ward, J. H. (1984). Control of cancer chemotherapy-induced nausea and vomiting. *Cancer, 54,* 2642–2648.

Feldman, E. B. (1988). *Essentials of clinical nutrition.* Philadelphia: F. A. Davis.

Friedman, M. I., & Stricker, E. M. (1976). The physiological psychology of hunger: A physiological perspective. *Psychological Review, 83,* 409–424.

Frohse, F., Brodel, M., & Schlossberg, L. (1985). *Atlas of human anatomy* (pp. 62–67). New York: Barnes and Noble.

Goodwin, C. W., & Wilmore, D. W. (1988). Enteral and parenteral nutrition. In Paige, D. M., Jacobson, H. N., Owen, G. M., Sherwin, R., Solomons, N., & Young, V. R. (Eds.), *Clinical nutrition* (2nd ed, pp. 476–503). St. Louis: C. V. Mosby Co.

Goodwin, W. J., & Torres, J. (1984). The value of the Prognostic Nutritional Index in the management of patients with advanced carcinoma of the head and neck. *Head and Neck Surgery, 6*, 932–937.

Gorter, R. (1991). Management of anorexia-cachexia associated with cancer and HIV disease. *Oncology, 5*(Suppl.), 13–17.

Gottschlich, M. M., Matarese, L. E., & Shronts, E. P. (Eds.) (1993). *Nutrition support dietetics: Core curriculum.* (2nd ed.). Silver Spring, MD: ASPEN.

Grady, R. P., Farnen, J., Ascheman, P., Passman, B., & Palazola, S. M. (1985). Nutrition, alteration in: Less than body requirements related to dysphagia. In J. C. McNally, J. C. Stair, & E. T. Somerville (Eds.), *Guidelines for cancer nursing practice* (pp. 239–242). Orlando, FL: Grune & Stratton, Inc.

Grant, J. P., Custer, P. B., & Thurlow, J. (1981). Current techniques of nutritional assessment. *Surgical Clinics of North America, 61*, 437–463.

Grant, M. (1987a). Nausea and vomiting. In Nursing Management of Common Problems. *Proceedings of the Fifth National Conference on Cancer Nursing*, American Cancer Society, September, pp. 16–24.

Grant, M. (1987b). Nausea, vomiting, and anorexia. *Seminars in Oncology Nursing, 3*, 277–286.

Grant, M., Padilla, G. V., & Rhiner, M. (1991). Patterns of anorexia in cancer patients. *Proceedings of the American Cancer Society First National Nursing Research Conference*, Publication No. 71-25M-3332-03PE, American Cancer Society.

Grant, M., & Rivera, L. M. (in press). Anorexia, cachexia, and dysphagia. *Seminars in Oncology Nursing.*

Greenberger, N. J. (1986). *Gastrointestinal disorders: A pathophysiologic approach* (3rd ed.). Chicago: Year Book Medical Publishers.

Grijalva, C. V., & Lindholm, E. (1982). The role of the autonomic nervous system in hypothalamic feeding syndromes. *Appetite, 3*, 111–124.

Harris, J. A., & Benedict, F. G. (1979). *Biometric studies of basal metabolism in man.* Publication No. 279. Washington, DC: Carnegie Institute of Washington.

Heber, D. (1989). Metabolic pathology of cancer malnutrition. *Nutrition, 5*, 135–137.

Heber, D., Byerley, L. O., Chi, J., Grosvenor, M., Bergmon, R. N., Coleman, M., & Chlebowski, R. (1986). Pathophysiology of malnutrition in the adult cancer patient. *Cancer, 58*, 1867–1873.

Heber, D., Chlebowski, R. T., Meguid, M., & McAndrew, P. (1986). Malnutrition in cancer: Mechanisms and therapy. *Nutrition International, 2*, 184–187.

Holman, S. R. (1987). *Essentials of nutrition for the health professions.* Philadelphia: J. B. Lippincott Co.

Holroyde, C. P., & Reichard, G. A. (1986). General metabolic abnormalities in cancer patients: Anorexia and cachexia. *Surgical Clinics of North America, 66*, 947–956.

Hooley, R., Levine, H., Flores, T. C., Wheeler, T., & Steiger, E. (1983). Predicting postoperative head and neck complications using nutritional assessment: The Prognostic Nutritional Index. *Archives of Otolaryngology, 109*, 83–85.

Ireton-Jones, C. S., & Hasse, J. M. (1992). Comprehensive nutritional assessment: The dietician's contribution to the team effort. *Nutrition, 8*, 75–81.

Johnston, C. A., Keane, T. J., & Prudo, S. M. (1982). Weight loss in patients receiving radical radiation therapy for head and neck cancer: A prospective study. *Journal of Parenteral and Enteral Nutrition, 6*, 399–402.

Kaempfer, S. H., & Lindsey, A. M. (1986). Energy expenditure in cancer: A review. *Cancer Nursing, 9*, 194–199.

Kamath, S., Mams, P. B., Lad, T. E., Kohrs, M. B., & McGuire, W. P. (1983). Taste thresholds of patients with cancer of the esophagus. *Cancer, 52*, 386–389.

Kaminski, M. V., Nasr, N. J., Moss, A. J., Berger, R. L., & Sriran, K. (1982). Nutritional status, immunity and survival in neoplastic disease. *Nutritional Support Services, 2*, 7–13.

Kelly, K. G. (1993). Advances in perioperative nutritional support regimens. *Medical Clinics of North America, 77*(2), 465–475.

Kinney, J. (1992). Indirect calorimetry: The search for clinical relevance. *Nutrition in Clinical Practice, 7*(5), 203–206.

Kinney, J. M., & Roe, C. F. (1962). Caloric equivalent of fever. I. Patterns of postoperative response. *Annals of Surgery, 156*, 610–622.

Klein, S., & Koretz, R. L. (1994). Nutrition support in patients with cancer: What do the data really show? *Nutrition in Clinical Practice, 7*, 203–206.

Knobf, M. K. P. (1985). Weight gain and adjuvant chemotherapy. *Oncology Nursing Forum, 12*(6); 13–22.

Knox, L. S., Crosby, L. O., Feurer, I. D., Buzby, G. P., Miller, C. L., & Mullen, J. L. (1983). Energy expenditure in malnourished cancer patients. *Annals of Surgery, 197*, 152–162.

Krause, R., Humphrey, C., von Meyenfeldt, M., James, H., & Fischer, J. E. (1981). A central mechanism for anorexia in cancer: A hypothesis. *Cancer Treatment Reports, 65*, 15–21.

Kurzer, M., & Meguid, M. M. (1986). Cancer and protein metabolism. *Surgical Clinics of North America, 66*, 969–1001.

Lawrence, W., Jr. (1979). Effects of cancer on nutrition. *Cancer, 43*(Suppl.), 2020–2029.

Lindsey, A. M., Piper, B. F., & Stotts, N. A. (1982). The phenomenon of cancer cachexia: A review. *Oncology Nursing Forum, 9*(2), 38–42.

Long, C. L., Schaffel, N., Geiger, J. W., Schiller, W. R., & Blackmore, W. S. (1979). Metabolic response to injury and illness: Estimation of energy and protein needs from indirect calorimetry and nitrogen balance. *Journal of Parenteral and Enteral Nutrition, 3*, 452–456.

Lundholm, K. G. (1986). Body compositional changes in cancer patients. *Surgical Clinics of North America, 66*, 1013–1023.

Maillet, J. O. (1987). The cancer patient. In C. E. Lange (Ed.), *Nutritional support in critical care* (pp. 243–264). Rockville, MD: Aspen.

Mayer, J. (1955). Regulation of energy intake and body weight. The glucostatic theory and the lipostatic hypothesis. *Annals of the New York Academy of Sciences, 63*, 15–43.

McClave, S. A., & Snider, H. L. (1992). Use of indirect calorimetry in clinical nutrition. *Nutrition in Clinical Practice, 9*, 207–221.

McGeer, A. J., Detsky, A. S., & O'Rourke, K. (1990). Parenteral nutrition in cancer patients undergoing chemotherapy: A meta-analysis. *Nutrition, 6*, 233–240.

Mellinkoff, S. M., Frankland, D., & Boyle, D. (1956). Relationship between serum amino acid concentration and fluctuations in appetite. *Journal of Applied Physiology, 8*, 535–538.

Moog, F. (1981). The lining of the small intestine. *Scientific American, 245*(5), 154–203.

Morrison, S. D. (1976). Theoretical review: Control of food

intake in cancer cachexia: A challenge and a tool. *Physiology and Behavior, 17,* 705–614.

Mossman, K. L., & Henkin, R. I. (1978). Radiation-induced changes in taste acuity in cancer patients. *International Journal of Radiation Oncology, Biology, Physics, 4,* 663–670.

Muller, J. M., Keller, H. W., Brenner, U., Walter, M., & Holzmuller, W. (1986). Indications and effects of preoperative parenteral nutrition. *World Journal of Surgery, 10,* 53–63.

Nelson, K. A., Walsh, D., & Sheehan, F. A. (1994). The cancer anorexia-cachexia syndrome. *Journal of Clinical Oncology, 12*(1), 213–225.

Nichols, M., Maickel, R. P., & Yim, G. K. W. (1983). Increased central serotonergic activity associated with nocturnal anorexia induced by Walker 256 carcinoma. *Life Sciences, 32,* 1819–1825.

Nixon, D. W., Heymsfield, S. B., Cohen, A. E., Kutner, M. H., Ansley, J., Lawson, D. H., & Rudman, D. (1980). Protein-calorie undernutrition in hospitalized cancer patients. *American Journal of Medicine, 68,* 683–690.

Nord, H. J., & Sodeman, W. A. (1985). The stomach. In W. A. Sodeman, & T. M. Sodeman (Eds.), *Sodeman's pathologic physiology: Mechanisms of disease* (pp. 787–791). Philadelphia, W. B. Saunders Co.

Novin, D., & VanderWeele, D. A. (1977). Visceral involvement in feeding: There is more to regulation than the hypothalamus. *Progress in Psychological and Physiological Psychology, 7,* 193–241.

Ollenschlager, G., Konkol, K., & Modder, B. (1988). Indications for and results of nutritional therapy in cancer patients. *Recent Results in Cancer Research, 108,* 172–184.

Portenoy, R. K. (1987). Constipation in the cancer patient: Causes and management. *Medical Clinics of North America, 71,* 303–311.

Reuben, D. B., & Mor, F. (1986). Nausea and vomiting in terminal cancer patients. *Archives of Internal Medicine, 146,* 2021–2023.

Rolls, E. T. (1981). Central nervous system mechanism related to feeding and appetite. *British Medical Bulletin, 37,* 131–134.

Rombeau, J. L., Caldwell, M. D., Forlaw, L., & Guenter, P. A. (1989). *Atlas of nutritional support techniques* (p. 54). Boston: Little, Brown & Co.

Ropka, M. E. (1985). Nutrition. In B. L. Johnson & J. Gross (Eds.), *Handbook of oncology nursing* (pp. 185–227). New York: John Wiley.

Rothkopf, M. (1990). Fuel utilization in neoplastic disease: Implications for the use of nutritional support in cancer patients. *Nutrition, 6*(Suppl. 4), 14S–16S.

Ruberg, R. L. (1984). Role of nutrition in wound healing. *Surgical Clinics of North America, 64,* 705–714.

Sallan, S. E., & Cronin, C. M. (1985). Nausea and vomiting. In V. T. DeVita, Jr., S. Hellman, & S. A. Rosenberg (Eds.), *Cancer: Principles and practice of oncology* (pp. 2008–2013). Philadelphia: J. B. Lippincott Co.

Sax, H. C., & Souba, W. W. (1993). Enteral and parenteral feedings. Guidelines and recommendations. *Medical Clinics of North America, 77*(4), 863–880.

Schmitz, J. (1990). Dysphagia. In D. J. Gines. (Ed.), *Nutrition management in rehabilitation.* Rockville, MD: ASPEN Publishers.

Shils, M. E. (1979). Principles of nutritional therapy. *Cancer, 143,* 2093–2102.

Spaulding, M. (1989). Recent studies of anorexia and appetite stimulation in the cancer patient. *Oncology, 3*(Suppl.), 17–23.

Spector, N. H., Brobeck, J. R., & Hamilton, C. L. (1968). Feeding and core temperature in albino rats: Changes induced by preoptic heating and cooling. *Science, 161,* 286–288.

Tchekmedyian, N. S. (1993). Treatment of anorexia with megestrol acetate. *Nutrition in Clinical Practice, 8,* 115–118.

Toates, F. M. (1981). The control of ingestive behavior by internal and external stimuli—a theoretical review. *Appetite, 2,* 35–50.

Viteri, F. E., & Torun, B. (1988). Protein-energy malnutrition. In D. M. Paige, H. N. Jacobson, G. M. Owen, R. Sherwin, N. Solomons, & V. R. Young (Eds.), *Clinical nutrition* (2nd ed., pp. 531–546). St. Louis: C. V. Mosby Co.

Wesdorf, R. L. C., Krause, R., & von Meyenfeldt, M. F. (1983). Cancer cachexia and its nutritional implications. *British Journal of Medicine, 70,* 352–355.

Wilmore, D. W. (1977). *Metabolic management of the critically ill.* New York: Plenum.

Wooley, O. W., Bartoshuk, L. M., Cubanac, M. J. C., Ferstl, R., Gutezeit, G. W. R., McFarland, D. J., Oetting, M., Pudel, V. E., Rodin, J., & Simmons, F. J. (1975). Psychological aspects of feeding: Group report. In T. Silverstone (Ed.), *Appetite and food intake: Report of the Dahlem Workshop on Appetite and Food Intake* (pp. 285–312). Berlin: Abakon Verlagsyesellschoft.

Yasko, J. M. (1985). Holistic management of nausea and vomiting caused by chemotherapy. *Topics in Clinical Nursing, 7,* 26–38.

Alterations in Oral Status

Ryan R. Iwamoto

Approximately 400,000 episodes of oral complications occur in persons with cancer each year (National Institutes of Health, 1989). Damage to the oral mucosa is often inevitable with cancer treatments or as a result of the disease itself. The pain and discomfort that accompany this side effect are frequently considered to be major problems for persons with cancer (Daeffler, 1980a). Oral hygiene measures may not prevent the damage caused by the local tissue effect of radiation therapy or the inhibition of cell replication due to chemotherapy (Daeffler, 1981). However, when oral care is provided systematically, infections and further damage to the oral mucosa can be prevented (Beck, 1979).

ANATOMY AND PHYSIOLOGY OF THE MOUTH

The mouth is composed of the lips, buccal mucosa, gingiva, teeth, hard and soft palates, and tongue (Fig. 52–1). The epithelium of the oral mucosa is made up of stratified squamous cells. These cells have a high turnover rate of approximately 10 to 14 days, making them extremely vulnerable to the effects of cancer treatments such as radiation therapy and chemotherapy. In comparison, the turnover rate of the epithelial cells of the skin is approximately 4 weeks. There are three types of oral mucosa. (1) The lining mucosa is a nonkeratinized epithelium that covers the labial and buccal regions, the soft palate, and the ventral side of the tongue. (2) The masticatory mucosa, which covers the gingiva and hard palate, is a keratinized epithelium. (3) The specialized mucosa, which contains the taste buds, lines various areas of the oral cavity.

The mucosa normally appears moist, soft, and pink. The oral mucosa serves as the first line of defense against infection and humidifies air as it is inhaled. The oral mucosa also facilitates ion exchange of sodium, potassium, chloride, and bicarbonate. Three pairs of salivary glands as well as other glands in the mouth normally keep the mucous membranes moist and lubricate food for chewing and swallowing. The salivary glands also secrete the digestive enzymes ptyalin and amylase. The tongue is used for speech, chewing, and swallowing.

Taste buds are located on the tongue as well as on the soft palate, glossopalatine arch, and posterior wall of the pharynx. The primary taste sensations are sweet, sour, salty, and bitter. An individual can perceive many different tastes that result from a combination of the different primary sensations.

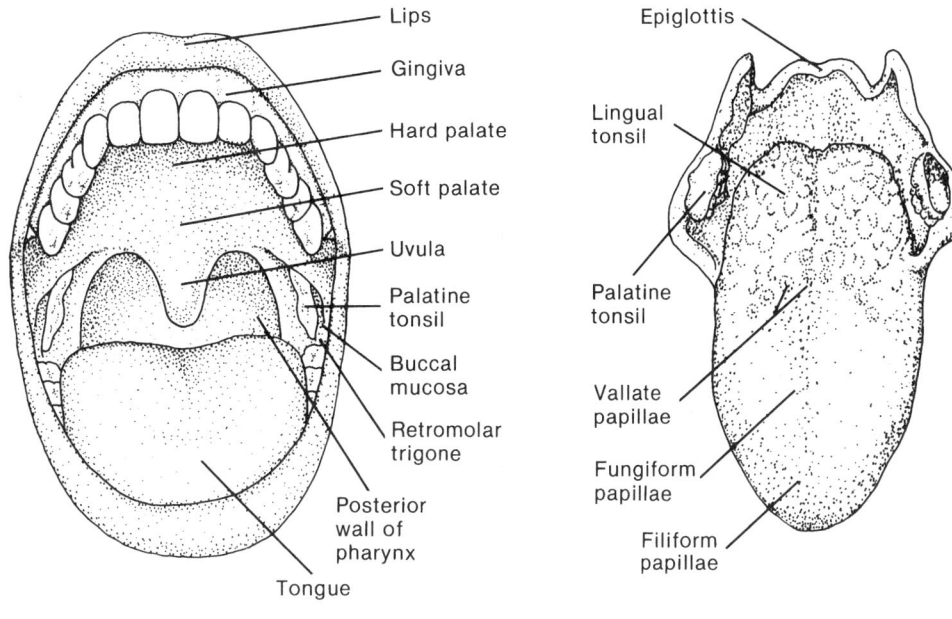

FIGURE 52–1. Anatomy of the mouth.

ORAL CAVITY

SURFACE OF TONGUE

STRESSORS IN THE ORAL CAVITY

GENERAL STRESSORS

There are many stressors in the oral cavity. Routine oral hygiene measures such as brushing and flossing can cause trauma to the tissues, which results in transient bacteremia (McElroy, 1984). DeWalt and Haines (1969) evaluated the effect of specific stressors on normal oral mucosa. The stressors studied included oral breathing, continuous nasal oxygen, intermittent mechanical suction, and absence of oral intake. The subject in this investigation was studied for 5 hours. After 1 hour, significant changes in the mouth were seen. These changes included xerostomia, taste alterations, pain, enlargement of the tongue papillae, edema, and hyperemia of the oral mucosa.

Habitual poor oral hygiene and the consumption of tobacco and alcohol can damage the oral mucosa. When mouth care is neglected, plaque, calculus, and debris collect around the teeth, causing irritation of the gingiva. This irritation develops into an inflammatory response, and the gingiva separates from the teeth and forms pockets. Debris and bacteria collect in these pockets and result in increased inflammation and proliferation of bacteria (Daeffler, 1980a; Hickey, Toth, & Lindquist, 1982).

In persons with cancer, alterations in the oral status occur as a result of the disease, the treatment, or both (Fig. 52–2). Infiltration of the oral and pharyngeal mucosa by leukemias or lymphomas can cause gingival and tonsillar enlargement and inflammation (Barrett, 1984b). Pain and bleeding of mucosal tissues are frequently experienced.

Nutritional deficiencies can cause thinning of the oral mucosa, inflammation of the tongue, and decreased ability to repair tissues. Many factors lead to nutritional deficits in persons with cancer. The incidence of anorexia and cachexia is well documented. Chapter 51 describes the nutritional alterations associated with cancer and its treatment. Nausea and vomiting from the treatment or the disease, gastrointestinal obstructions and malabsorption, fatigue, and depression are often experienced by persons with cancer and can lead to nutritional deficiencies. In addition, the oral complications as a result of cancer or its treatment can further prevent the person from eating and drinking adequately.

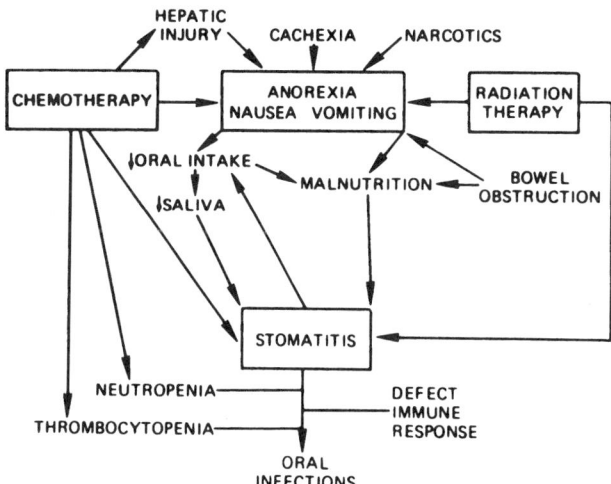

FIGURE 52–2. Interrelationships of factors contributing to alterations of oral status in persons with cancer. (From Daeffler, R. [1980]. Oral hygiene measures for patients with cancer. I. *Cancer Nursing, 3,* 348. Reproduced by permission.)

CHEMOTHERAPY

The nonspecific effects of chemotherapy on highly proliferating cells can result in alterations of the oral mucosa (Barrett, 1984b; Carl, 1993; Peterson & Sonis, 1982). The antitumor antibiotics, such as dactinomycin, daunorubicin, doxorubicin, and bleomycin, as well as the antimetabolites 5-fluorouracil and methotrexate, are known for their toxic effects on the oral mucosa. A number of abnormalities occur (Table 52–1).

STOMATITIS

Stomatitis (also called mucositis) is a generalized inflammation of the oral mucosa that may range from mild erythema to severe ulceration. Approximately 40 per cent of persons receiving chemotherapy will develop some form of stomatitis (Peterson & Sonis, 1982). Chemotherapy interferes with cell production and maturation. Therefore, the basal cell layers of the oral mucosa are inhibited from replacing the superficial epithelium. The mucosa atrophies, which results in an inflammatory response—stomatitis (DeGregorio, Lee, & Ries, 1982). The development of stomatitis is varied and can occur on any mucosal surface, although ulceration usually occurs on nonkeratinized surfaces (Barrett, 1987; Hickey et al., 1982; Lindquist, Hickey, & Drane, 1978; Peterson & Sonis, 1982). Within 5 to 7 days of drug administration, changes in the oral mucosa are seen and may persist for 4 to 10 days (Daeffler, 1980a; Ostchega, 1980; Poland, 1991). Initially, the oral mucosa may have a slight burning sensation and erythema. This reaction may spontaneously resolve or progress to superficial epithelial desquamation, severe ulceration and pain, glossal edema, and secondary infections (Barrett, 1984b; Beck, 1979; Ketron, 1984). In addition, any minor, local trauma can disrupt the remaining thin layer of mucosa, leading to further inflammation and ulceration.

These changes in oral status that result from chemotherapy correlate with the timing of myelosuppression (Hickey et al., 1982; Poland, 1991). Oral toxicity is observed 3 to 5 days before the initial drop in leukocyte counts following chemotherapy. The oral symptoms reach their most severe form before the peripheral granulocyte nadir. Subsequently, a complete resolution of stomatitis is found to occur 3 to 5 days before the full recovery of granulocyte counts.

Predisposing factors for stomatitis include poor oral hygiene, dental caries, improperly fitting dental prostheses, gingival diseases, chronic low-grade mouth infections, smoking and alcohol habits, and older age, which is accompanied by decreased salivary flow rates and mucosal atrophy (Daeffler, 1980a). A significant relationship has been noted between the presence of dental plaque and stomatitis (Lindquist et al., 1978).

People with dental plaque who are receiving chemotherapy develop significantly more stomatitis for longer periods of time than people without dental plaque. Stomatitis is graded according to level of severity, as shown in Table 52–2 and Figure 52–3 (see Color Plate III) (Barrett, 1984b; Hickey et al., 1982; Hyland, 1986; Lindquist et al., 1978).

A descriptive, longitudinal study by McGuire et al. (1993) described the incidence and patterns of mucositis and pain in 47 patients undergoing bone marrow transplantation. These patients received a conditioning regimen of high-dose chemotherapy without total body irradiation. Mucositis began approximately 3 days after transplant, lasted 9.5 days, and resolved by 12.6 days posttransplant. Patient reports of pain did not necessarily correspond with the severity of mucositis; patients with severe mucositis did not always report significantly more pain than those with mild mucositis.

In a retrospective chart review, Zerbe, Parkerson, Ortlieb, and Spitzer (1992) studied the pattern of oral mucositis in 20 bone marrow transplant patients with moderate to severe mucositis who received a conditioning regimen of either total body irradiation or busulfan in combination with cyclophosphamide and etoposide. Mucosal changes began about 2 days before transplant, peaked at about 8 days, and returned to baseline about 20 to 25 days after transplant. Patients who received total body irradiation experienced more severe oral mucositis and required additional days of parenteral nutrition than those who received busulfan.

INFECTIONS

The symptoms of oral infections frequently mimic or coexist with stomatitis, making early diagnosis difficult. When a person is immunocompromised, the appearance of the infection may be atypical (Poland, 1991). Chemotherapy inhibits the primary and secondary immune responses to antigens. This immune deficiency combined with chemotherapy-induced leukopenia results in increased incidence of infections. The infections are usually those of gram-negative opportunistic bacteria, such as *Pseudomonas* and *Klebsiella*, *Enterobacter*, *Escherichia coli*, and the fungus *Candida* (Minah et al., 1986). Persistent local oral infections can be transferred to the esophagus and stomach, become invasive, and lead to septicemia and death (Daeffler, 1980a; DePaola, Peterson, Leupold, & Overholser, 1983; Hickey et al., 1982).

The two normal host defenses against gram-negative bacteria that are weakened by chemotherapy and antibiotics are a lessening of oral secretions and an alteration of the interbacterial inhibition of normal oral flora. As a result, oral bacteria increase in number and pathogenicity. An in vitro study demonstrated that resident flora and gram-positive organisms were inhibited by chemotherapeutic agents to a greater degree than nonresident and gram-negative organisms (Harchar, 1981). Because chemotherapeutic agents diffuse into the oral tissues, the drugs may have a direct effect on the oral flora. Gram-positive infections may appear as dry, brownish-yellow, purulent, circular eruptions. Gram-negative infections appear as creamy white, glis-

TABLE 52–1. **Oral Complications of Chemotherapy**

Stomatitis	Xerostomia
Infections	Neuropathy
Bleeding	Taste changes

TABLE 52–2. *Nursing Care Plan for a Patient with Stomatitis*

ASSESSMENT	INTERVENTIONS	EXPECTED OUTCOMES
Nursing Diagnosis: Alteration in Oral Mucous Membrane		
Grade 0		
No stomatitis. Mucosa is moist, pink, and soft. No ulceration or lesions. No discomfort in mouth.	Instruct the client to stop smoking and reduce the intake of alcoholic beverages.	Minimization of mouth irritation.
	After each meal and at bedtime, brush teeth with dentifrice and floss (except during periods of thrombocytopenia and neutropenia).	Cleansing of oral cavity.
	A plaque-disclosing dye can be helpful in identifying plaque to be removed by brushing or flossing. If client is edentulous, frequent oral irrigations should be performed.	
Grade I		
Mild stomatitis. Whitish gingival area observable, or client mentions slight burning sensation or discomfort in oral cavity.	Every 2 hr, provide normal saline rinses. Brush teeth after meals and at bedtime using dentifrice if not irritating.	Cleansing of oral cavity.
	Floss at least once a day (except during periods of thrombocytopenia and neutropenia).	
	Use an ice massage to the web between the thumb and index finger of the hand on the same side as the painful area in the mouth.	Reported to be an effective measure to reduce pain (see Box 48–2), possibly because of the intense peripheral stimulation that activates the brainstem inhibitory fibers (Howard-Ruben, 1984).
	Provide a soft, bland diet.	Less irritation to the oral tissues as result of a soft diet.
Grade II		
Moderate stomatitis. Moderate erythema, shallow ulcerations, or white patches present. Client complains of pain but can continue to eat, drink, and swallow.	Every 1 to 2 hr, provide normal saline rinses. Brush teeth after meals and at bedtime using dentifrice if not irritating. Use Toothettes if toothbrushing is not tolerated. Floss once a day if tolerated (except during periods of thrombocytopenia and neutropenia).	Providing maximum oral care with least mucosal trauma.
	Topical anesthetics may be used if needed.	Decrease in pain.
	Provide a soft, bland diet, especially cool foods. A dietitian can help plan meals to meet the nutritional needs of the client.	Increase in comfort while eating and minimization of mucosal trauma. (Cool foods are better tolerated.)
Grade III		
Severe stomatitis. Severe erythema, full thickness ulceration, mucosal necrosis, bleeding, white patches present. Client complains of severe pain and is unable to eat, drink, or swallow.	Every 1 to 2 hr, provide normal saline rinses. Toothbrushing and flossing may not be tolerated, so Toothette or gauze-wrapped finger is used to remove debris and plaque. Oral irrigations gently cleanse the mouth.	Providing maximum oral care with least mucosal trauma.
	An interim dental prosthesis to protect ulcerated mucosa and provide a surface for chewing has been described (DePaola, 1983). It is worn while eating and at night while sleeping.	Prosthesis allows for immediate comfort and function.
	Topical anesthetics and systemic analgesics may be used as needed.	Pain reduction.
	Topical thrombin may be used.	Topical thrombin may stop oral bleeding.
	Tube feeding or parenteral nutrition may be needed.	Nutritional status of client will be maintained.

Note: Following resolution of stomatitis, clients should again brush their teeth after each meal and at bedtime and floss once a day.

tening, nonpurulent ulcers (Clinical Practice Committee, 1982; Goodman & Stoner, 1985). These lesions are usually painful.

Candida is a common organism found in the mouth (Poland, 1991). Candidiasis tends to occur in persons who have received intensive chemotherapy, have experienced long periods of leukopenia and increased incidence of stomatitis, and have received broad-spectrum antimicrobial therapy, steroid medications, or both (DeGregorio et al., 1982; Epstein, 1989). Manifestations and symptoms of candidiasis vary (Table 52–3). *Candida* usually appears as irregular, white plaques with multiple dome elevations, involves localized or large areas of the oral mucosa, and is usually preceded by stomatitis. These plaques may be scraped off, leaving a raw, excoriated mucosal surface (Poland, 1991). Persons may notice a "dry," burning sensation or tenderness in their mouths that is unrelated to xerostomia (Cheater, 1985). *Candida* can be difficult to isolate and identify. Persons with oropharyngeal candidiasis are at significant risk of developing esophageal and systemic candidiasis.

Many studies have evaluated prophylaxis and treatment of candidiasis. Oral nystatin has not shown prophylactic efficacy against the incidence of localized or systemic candidiasis (Barrett, 1984a; DeGregorio et al., 1982). In addition, nystatin's ability to eliminate colonized *Candida* from the oropharynx is questionable (Barrett, 1984a). The use of topical and systemic amphotericin B has been reported to be effective in preventing and treating candidiasis (de Vries-Hospers, Mulder, Sleijfer, & Van Saene, 1982; DeGregorio et al., 1982). Ketoconazole was not significantly more or less effective than amphotericin B in preventing yeast colonization in neutropenic persons (Donnelly et al., 1984). However, prophylaxis tended to fail in persons treated with ketoconazole alone. Absorption of ketoconazole is dependent on gastric acidity. Therefore, antacids and medications that affect gastric secretions should be taken at least 2 hours after ketoconazole. Both ketoconazole and fluconazole are effective in treating oral, pharyngeal, and esophageal candidiasis.

Clotrimazole has been found to be effective in the treatment of oral candidiasis and may prevent the development of esophageal candidiasis (Quintiliani, Owens, Quercia, Klimek, & Nightingale, 1984; Shechtman, Funaro, Robin, Bottone, & Cuttner, 1984). Hepatotoxicity can occur with these medications and

require liver function monitoring in vulnerable persons. Chlorhexidine mouth rinses have also shown some effectiveness in modifying candidiasis (Weisdorf et al., 1989).

Reactivation of herpes simplex virus involving the lip is the most common cause of viral infections (Poland, 1991). Herpetic stomatitis has a wide range of manifestations and severity (Barrett, 1984b; National Institutes of Health, 1989). Clusters of vesicles or lesions may appear within the oral cavity and extend over the lips. These vesicles can rupture and progress to ulcerative lesions. The person frequently experiences pain (Daeffler, 1981). The antiviral agent acyclovir is used for prophylaxis and treatment of oral herpes simplex infections (Barrett, 1984b).

The myelosuppressive and mucosal effects of chemotherapy can result in an acute exacerbation of preexisting periodontal disease (Peterson & Sonis, 1982; Williams, Peterson, & Overholser, 1982). Periodontal disease, which includes gingivitis and periodontitis, is an extremely prevalent chronic inflammatory disease of the supporting structures of the teeth (Carl, 1993; Hickey et al., 1982; Peterson & Sonis, 1982). A tenfold increase of bacterial and fungal organisms is seen with periodontitis (McElroy, 1984). The signs and symptoms of acute periodontal exacerbation are localized tenderness to palpation, temperatures higher than 38.3° C, and slight trismus (Williams et al., 1982). However, during periods of leukopenia, oral infections may develop without these symptoms (Daeffler, 1980a).

The simple act of chewing can introduce thousands of potential pathogens into the bloodstream around diseased periodontal tissues (McElroy, 1984). Chronic infections of dental pulp may become sources of systemic infection during myelosuppression (Peterson & Sonis, 1982). Although optimal therapy for pulp infection is controversial, elimination of the source of infection by tooth extraction or pulp extirpation may often be the treatment of choice. Tooth extractions performed during myelosuppression are managed carefully with antibiotic prophylaxis and platelet transfusions to minimize complications (Peterson & Sonis, 1982).

People with dentures are susceptible to infection while receiving chemotherapy. Although removing the dentures during chemotherapy can lead to decreases in self-esteem, chewing ability, and nutritional intake, a poorly fitting denture can lead to inflammation, ulceration, and secondary infections (DePaola et al., 1983).

BLEEDING

Bleeding in the oral mucosa often occurs as a result of thrombocytopenia. The oral cavity may demonstrate an early warning of severe thrombocytopenia, because oral petechiae often precede skin bruising (Barrett, 1984b). The person experiences oozing of blood in the mouth, which causes intermittent blood clots to form and break away (Ostchega, 1980). These blood clots may be aspirated and cause choking. Prolonged and spontaneous bleeding occurs mainly in the gingival interdental areas and can increase the person's susceptibility to infection. Spontaneous gingival bleeding can

---

TABLE 52–3. *Clinical Manifestations of Candidiasis*

Pseudomembranous (thrush)
White plaques on mucosa that can be wiped off
Atrophic
Erythema with few, if any, white plaques. May be accompanied by angular cheilitis
Hyperplastic
Leukoplakia-like plaques that cannot be removed as a result of invasion into epithelium

(Data from Epstein, J. B. [1989]. Oral and pharyngeal candidiasis. *Postgraduate Medicine, 85,* 257–269.)

occur when the platelet count falls below 15,000/mm^3; it tends to be more severe in persons with preexisting periodontal disease or poor oral hygiene (Carl, 1980; Peterson & Sonis, 1982). Petechiae and hematoma formation in the oral mucosa can occur when the platelet count falls below 20,000/mm^3.

XEROSTOMIA

Xerostomia related to chemotherapy has been reported (Carl, 1993; Peterson & Sonis, 1982). Doxorubicin hydrochloride has been noted for causing xerostomia by diminishing salivary gland activity (Ostchega, 1980). On examination, the oral membranes appear dry and atrophic. In severe cases of xerostomia, the tongue becomes heavily furred, and the oral mucosa and lips become cracked and painful. Xerostomia also occurs as a result of other medications taken by persons with cancer (Cheater, 1985). These classes of medications include phenothiazines, tricyclic antidepressants, antihistamines, anticholinergics, and antispasmodics. Xerostomia is temporary and is treated palliatively with saliva substitutes.

NEUROPATHY

Chemotherapy-induced neuropathy may affect the oral cavity (DePaola et al., 1983; Peterson & Sonis, 1982). The symptoms mimic those of odontogenic or periodontal origin. Vincristine sulfate has been reported to cause neuropathy of the trigeminal and facial nerves, which manifests as jaw pain, circumoral paresthesias, and weakness of the facial muscles (Carl, 1980).

TASTE CHANGES

An unpleasant taste in the mouth has been reported anecdotally while cyclophosphamide is being administered or immediately following the infusion of the drug. Eating or smelling plain, white, soft mints during and after the infusion has been reported to be helpful in masking or eliminating the bad taste (Pehanrich, 1983).

RADIATION THERAPY

Radiation therapy to the head and neck region causes several alterations in the oral cavity (Table 52–4). A study evaluating nutritional compromise in 10 patients related to side effects of head and neck irradiation found that subjects lost between 1.3 to 7.5 per cent of their initial body weight during the course of therapy (Iwamoto, 1981). Although muscle mass was maintained, fat stores were lost. The subjects who had an adequate amount of energy stores tended to be younger and to experience less stomatitis in spite of a decreased caloric intake and weight loss than did the subjects who were older and more nutritionally depleted. Taste changes were reported by 42 per cent of the subjects, and decreases in salivary flow rates were noted in 80 per cent of the subjects. The subjects who had adequate energy stores received a higher radiation dosage before their lowest salivary flow rate was reached; recovery to 80 per cent of their initial salivary flow rate was quicker for them than for the subjects who were nutritionally depleted.

STOMATITIS

Radiation-induced stomatitis occurs as a result of hyperemia and edema of the mucosa, which can lead to the formation of ulcers. These ulcers can appear after the oral cavity has received 1000 cGy (1 to 2 weeks). The early changes in the mucosa occur as a result of the effect of radiation on the fine vasculature of the tissues, which leads to vascular congestion and increased capillary permeability (Beumer, Curtis, & Harrison, 1979). In some instances, the mucosa becomes whitish, and then a pseudomembrane gradually forms (Fig. 52–4, see Color Plate III). This membrane can slough off, leaving a reddish and friable underlying epithelium with ulcer formation. At 2500 cGy the entire mucosa may become involved (Carl, 1993). Severe stomatitis occurs with treatment of tumors of the nasopharynx, soft palate, floor of the mouth, and retromolar area. The severity of the reaction depends on the area and volume treated, the radiation dose, and the individual. Persons who have a compromised oral mucosa as a result of alcoholism and who continue to consume alcohol and tobacco will have the most severe mucosal changes (Beumer et al., 1979; Miller, Vergo, & Feldman, 1981). With high doses of radiation to the head and neck area, chronic ulcers may form.

The peak of symptoms occurs at 6000 to 7000 cGy and may persist for 2 to 3 weeks after the completion of therapy (Beumer et al., 1979; Carl, 1993). Mucosal reactions as a result of radiation therapy are frequently hastened or enhanced with concomitant chemotherapy (Hilderley, 1986). An increased mucosal reaction can also occur as a result of scatter radiation from large metallic tooth restorations to adjacent areas. The radiation oncologist may place an acrylic oral stent or a piece of gauze between the mucosa and tooth during treatment to minimize this reaction (Jones & Hafermann, 1986). In addition, a rest from radiation treatment is sometimes needed to allow the tissues to heal.

Edema of the buccal mucosa, submental, and submandibular areas of the mouth and tongue can occur. As a result, persons receiving head and neck irradiation may have difficulty with the fit of their dental prostheses, impaired salivary control, and speech problems. The acute symptoms of radiation-induced stomatitis resolve within a few weeks after treatment is completed. However, long-term mucosal effects may occur and may include a thinned, overlying epithelium as a result of decreased keratinization and a less vascular and more fibrotic submucosa (Bersani & Carl, 1983; Beumer et al., 1979).

TABLE 52–4. *Oral Complications of Radiation Therapy*

Stomatitis	Infections
Taste changes	Osteoradionecrosis
Xerostomia	Trismus
Caries formation	

TASTE CHANGES

Taste changes as a result of head and neck irradiation often occur. These changes can affect each of the primary taste sensations and may involve partial or complete loss of taste (Conger, 1973). The decrease in all tastes has been termed *mouth-blindness* (McCarthy-Leventhal, 1959). In addition, unpleasant tastes are sometimes evident. An increased sensitivity for bitter tastes and a decreased sensitivity for sweet tastes are commonly noted. Changes in bitter and salty tastes can occur by the second week of radiation therapy and become a chronic problem (Mossman & Henkin, 1978). A "burnt" or "bad" taste is noted by some people. As a result, these people find the taste of coffee and chocolate very unpleasant.

Degeneration and atrophy of the taste buds as well as damage to the microvilli of the taste cells are noted at 1000 cGy and can continue until the end of treatment (Beumer et al., 1979; Sullivan & Fleming, 1986). Although some return of taste may occur several months after treatment, some taste changes are permanent (Lowe, 1986). Mossman, Shatzman, and Chencharick (1982) reported that impairment of taste and salivary function persisted in some persons for up to 7 years after radiation therapy. The most commonly affected tastes were salty and bitter, and the least affected were sweet and sour. The presence of saliva may play an important role in regaining normal taste acuity.

XEROSTOMIA

Xerostomia, or a decrease in saliva production, occurs when a dose range of 1000 to 2000 cGy is reached (Carl, 1993; Iwamoto, 1981). Saliva is important for taste as well as for chemical digestion. People with xerostomia have difficulty with speech, chewing, and swallowing. Increased friction with removable oral prostheses and problems with retention of the prostheses are also noted. The serous acinar cells of the parotid glands are more affected than the mucinous acinar cells. Therefore, the saliva flow rate decreases, and the saliva becomes viscous and ropey and adheres to the oral mucosa. Xerostomia is initially worse at night (especially in mouth breathers) and better during the day but eventually becomes a more persistent problem as treatment continues. The severity and chronicity of xerostomia is related to the type and dose of radiation, the area treated, and the age of the person. When the retromolar trigone, tonsils, soft palate, and nasopharynx are treated, severe xerostomia occurs. If the parotid and submandibular glands are within the treatment field, salivary gland function almost completely ceases (Carl, 1993). The parotid gland is less affected when the floor of the mouth and the base of the tongue are treated with radiation therapy, and a progressive increase in saliva output can be noted 1 to 2 years after treatment (Beumer et al., 1979).

Xerostomia seldom reverses completely and remains a chronic problem in people who receive a cumulative dose of greater than 4000 cGy to the head and neck region. Although some persons have a subjective improvement in xerostomia, there usually is no measurable change (Dreizen, Brown, Daly, & Drane, 1977). Some improvement is noted in younger persons who are treated in the head and neck region for Hodgkin's disease (Carl, 1980, 1993).

CARIES

When xerostomia occurs, the pH of the saliva is lowered, and the saliva no longer acts as a buffering and lubricating agent. Therefore, an increase in caries formation is observed, and periodontal breakdown occurs (Carl, 1980). This breakdown starts as a diffuse demineralization and can lead to progressive tooth decay with lessened capacity for repair and regeneration of the periodontium.

Caries occur first in the cervical areas of teeth, close to and below the margins of the gingiva (Carl, 1980). Teeth are at risk for caries if they lie within the treatment field. If the nasopharynx and posterior soft palate are being treated, the teeth in these areas are especially vulnerable to caries development. A rampant form of caries occurs secondary to xerostomia (Dreizen et al., 1977). In addition, a shift in the oral flora composition to increased numbers of cariogenic bacteria occurs. This shift is long-lasting and is seen up to 4 years after therapy (Beumer et al., 1979).

INFECTIONS

Stomatitis, xerostomia, poor oral hygiene, broken teeth, faulty restorations, and periodontal disease contribute to persistent oral infections in persons with head and neck cancer (Lowe, 1986). Oral candidiasis frequently occurs during radiation therapy to the head and neck region. The tongue, buccal mucosa, and mucosal surfaces beneath dentures are prime sites for infection (Beumer et al., 1979). In addition, an increase in enteric bacteria is observed in the mouth as a result of xerostomia and increased age (Bernhoft & Skaug, 1985).

OSTEORADIONECROSIS

All persons who receive head and neck irradiation are susceptible to osteoradionecrosis. The potential for osteoradionecrosis lasts a lifetime and can be evident several months to years after therapy is completed (Levin & Ferris, 1980). Poor oral hygiene and continued use of mouth irritants such as alcohol and tobacco are major contributing factors in the development of osteoradionecrosis (Dreizen et al., 1977). Osteoradionecrosis is progressive and irreversible and occurs more frequently in the mandible than in the maxilla, because the blood supply in the mandible is less profuse than it is in the maxilla (Wescott, 1985). The marrow becomes acellular and avascular, with increased fibrosis and fatty degeneration. Therefore, the bone structure is unable to respond to trauma or infection (Beumer et al., 1979). These changes are subclinical effects that are neither felt immediately by the patient nor seen on clinical examination. However, with severe osteoradionecrosis, the person experiences pain, trismus, fistula formation, and pathologic fractures with loss of tissue and bone (Carl, 1980).

PLATE I

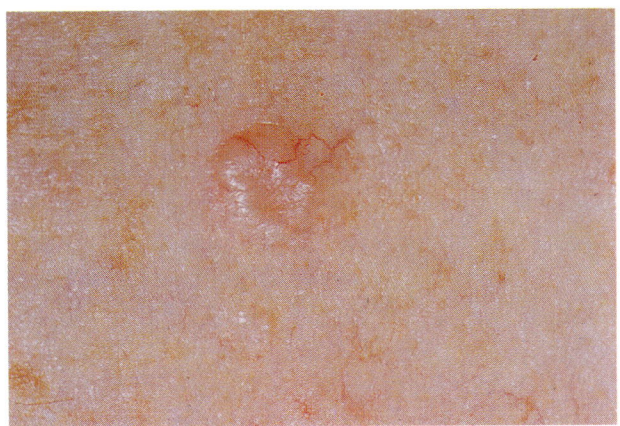

FIGURE 43–4. Basal cell carcinoma. (Courtesy of Anna Graham, M.D.)

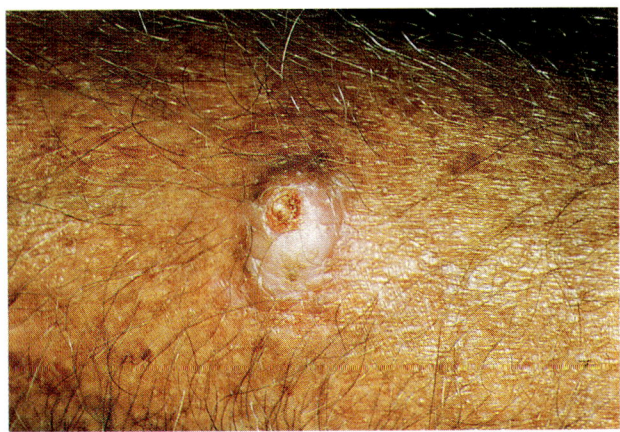

FIGURE 43–5. Squamous cell carcinoma. (Courtesy of Anna Graham, M.D.)

PLATE II

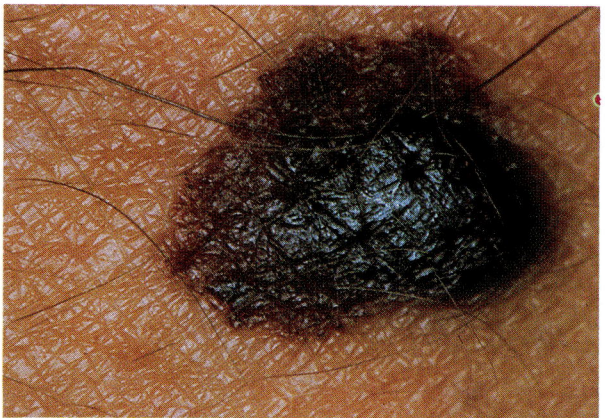

FIGURE 43–6. Malignant melanoma. (Courtesy of Anna Graham, M.D.)

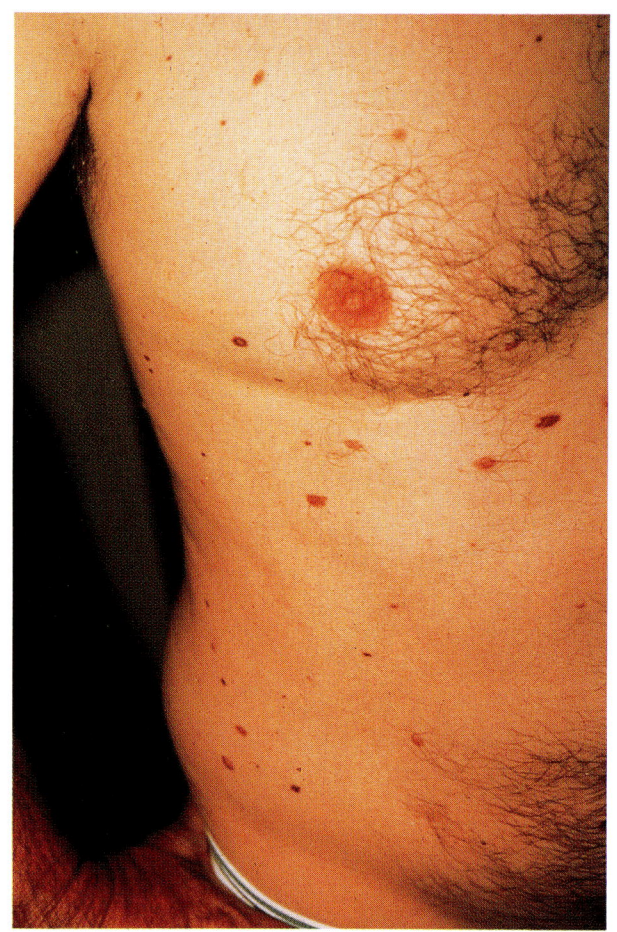

FIGURE 43–7. Dysplastic nevi. (Courtesy of Libby Edwards, M.D.)

Plate III

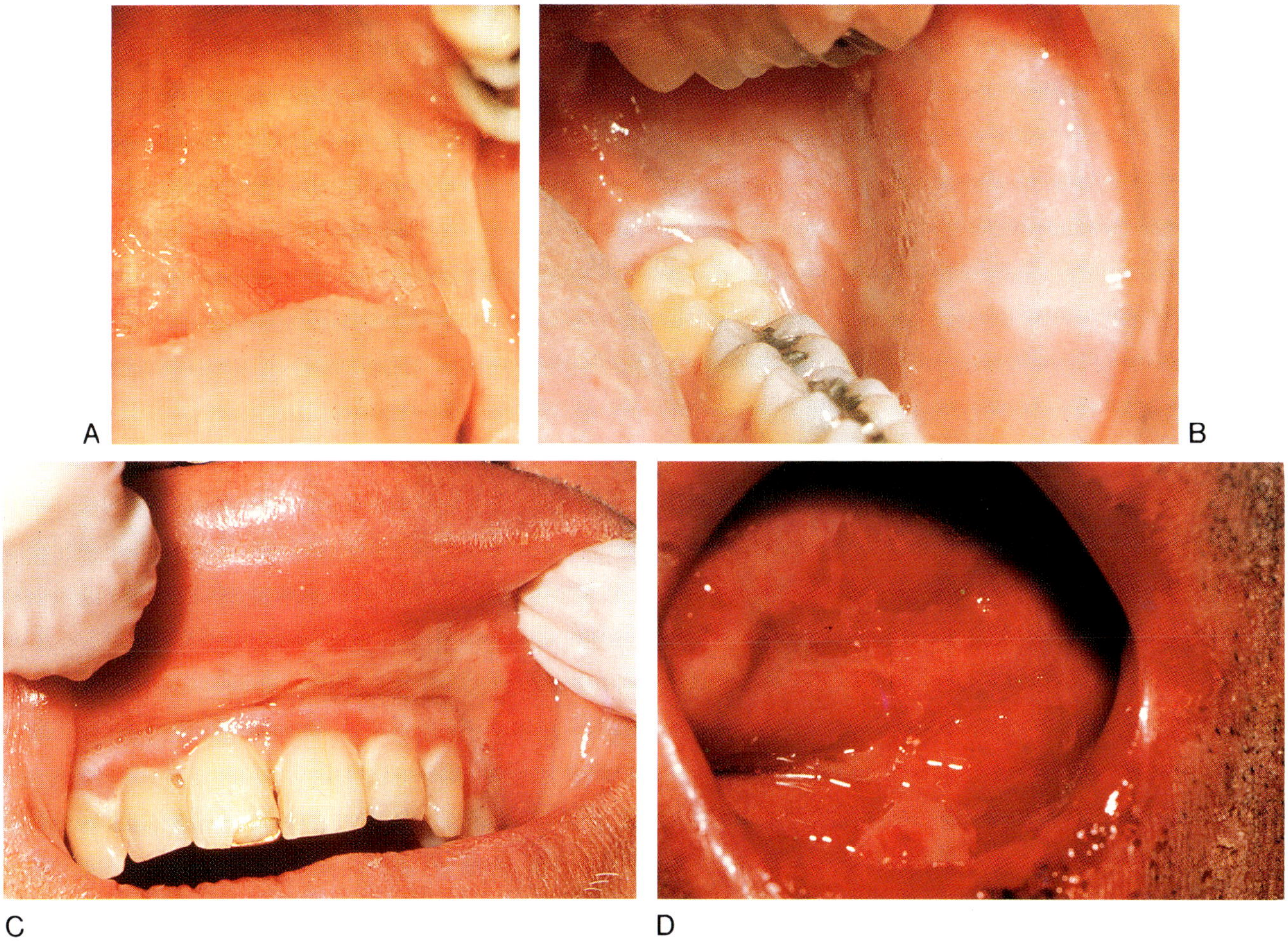

Figure 52–3. Examples of stomatitis. *A*, grade 0; *B*, grade I; *C*, grade II; *D*, grade III. (Courtesy of Mark M. Schubert, D.D.S., M.S.D., Oral Medicine Oncology Support Services, School of Dentistry, University of Washington, Seattle.)

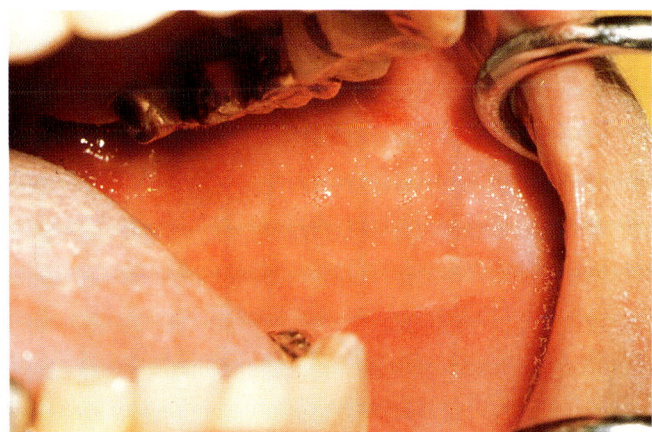

Figure 52–4. Pseudomembrane formation on buccal mucosa as a result of radiation therapy. (Courtesy of Mark M. Schubert, D.D.S., M.S.D., Oral Medicine Oncology Support Services, School of Dentistry, University of Washington, Seattle.)

PLATE IV

Category	Voice	Swallow	Lips	Tongue	Saliva	Mucous membranes	Gingiva	Teeth, Dentures, or denture bearing area
Tools for Assessment	Auditory assessment	Observation	Visual/palpatory	Visual/palpatory	Tongue blade	Visual assessment	Tongue blade and visual assessment	Visual assessment
Methods of Measurement	Converse with patient	Ask patient to swallow. To test gag reflex, gently place blade on back of tongue and depress	Observe and feel tissue	Feel and observe appearance of tissue	Insert blade into mouth, touching the center of the tongue and the floor of the mouth	Observe appearance of tissue	Gently press tissue with tip of blade	Observe appearance of teeth or denture bearing area
1 *Numerical and descriptive rating*	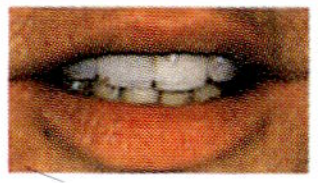 Normal	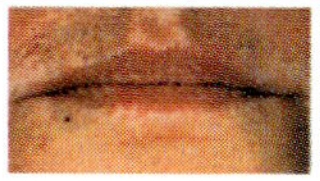 Normal swallow	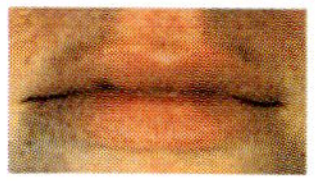 Smooth and pink and moist	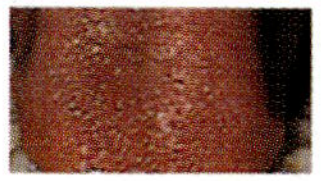 Pink and moist and papillae present	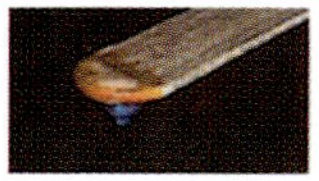 Watery	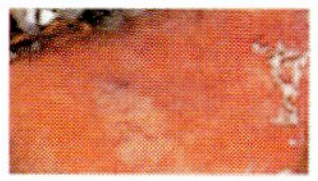 Pink and moist	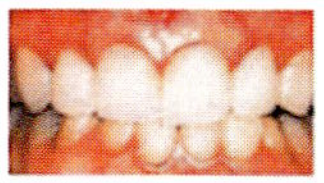 Pink and stippled and firm	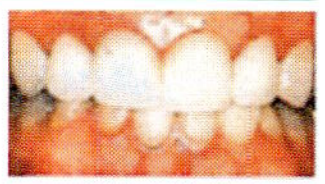 Clean and no debris
2	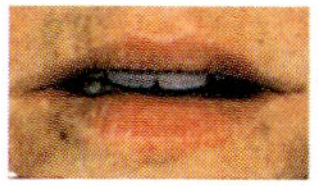 Deeper or raspy	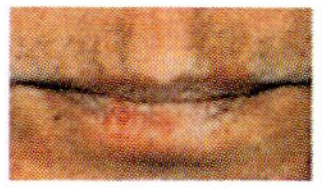 Some pain on swallow	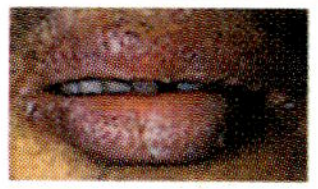 Dry or cracked	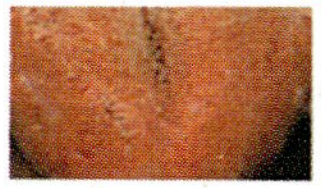 Coated or loss of papillae with shiny appearance with or without redness	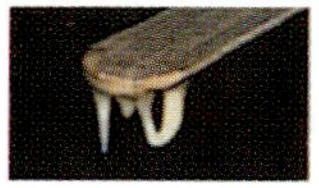 Thick or ropy	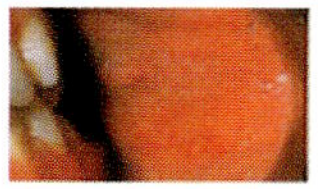 Reddened or coated (increased whiteness) without ulcerations	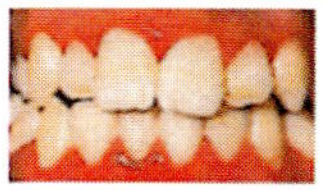 Edematous with or without redness	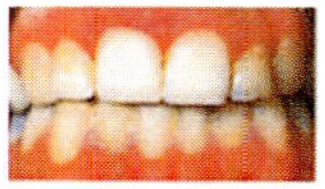 Plaque or debris in localized areas (between teeth if present)
3	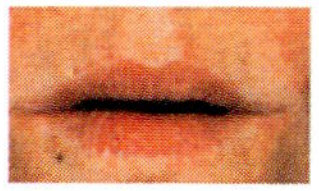 Difficulty talking or painful	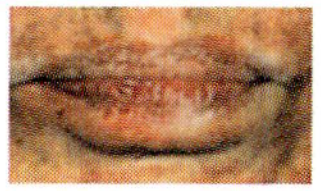 Unable to swallow	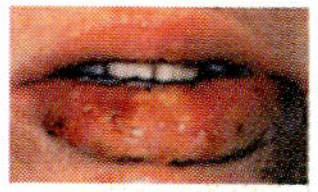 Ulcerated or bleeding	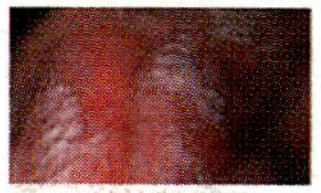 Blistered or cracked	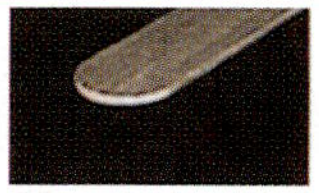 Absent	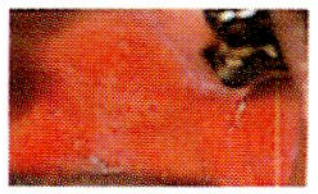 Ulcerations with or without bleeding	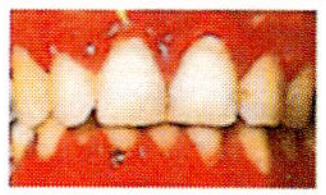 Spontaneous bleeding or bleeding with pressure	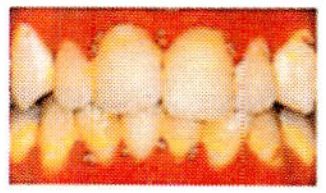 Plaque or debris generalized along gum line or denture bearing area

FIGURE 52–5. The oral assessment guide. (From June Eilers, R.N., M.S.N. et al., University of Nebraska Medical Center, Omaha, 2-84, rev. 5-84, 4-85, 11-85, and Halbrand, Inc., Willoughby, OH. Reproduced by permission.)

Osteoradionecrosis tends to occur in persons who have chronic and advanced periodontal disease and is frequently preceded by periodontal infections associated with teeth within the treatment field (Carl, 1980). Prior to starting radiation therapy, the dentist provides cleaning of the teeth and treatment of any periodontal disease. If at all possible, the teeth are retained. However, to avoid potential complications, partial or full-tooth extractions are done for people who are unmotivated or unable to perform oral hygiene or who have unrestorable teeth (Carl, 1980; Miller et al., 1981; Ritchie, Brown, Guerra, & Mason, 1985; Wescott, 1985). Extractions and restorations are completed 10 to 14 days before the start of radiation therapy to allow for healing (Lane & Forgay, 1981; Wescott, 1985).

Following head and neck irradiation, trauma in the oral cavity, such as extraction of teeth, oral surgery, and denture irritation, must be avoided (Miller et al., 1981). Tooth extraction or periodontal surgery can be the precipitating event leading to tissue breakdown. When osteoradionecrosis occurs, treatment involves gentle debridement with salt and soda rinses, antibiotic packs, and systemic antibiotic therapy. Hyperbaric oxygen has been used alone and in combination with surgery to improve tissue healing (Mansfield, Sanders, Heimbach, & Marx, 1981; Ritchie et al., 1985; Wescott, 1985).

TRISMUS

Trismus is a disturbance due to myositis of the muscles of mastication and occurs with unpredictable frequency and severity. As a result of fibrosis, trismus can become a chronic problem (Miller et al., 1981). The mouth opening may be restricted to 10 to 15 mm, which impairs chewing and oral access. Trismus occurs when the temporomandibular joint and masticatory muscles are within the treatment field. This treatment field is used for tumors in the nasopharynx, retromolar areas, and posterior palate. Trismus tends to be more severe when surgery and radiation therapy are combined (Bersani & Carl, 1983; Beumer et al., 1979).

Treatment for trismus involves the repetition of jaw exercises and the use of dynamic bite openers, which can increase the mouth opening by 10 to 15 mm. Early exercising of the mandible can lessen the severity of trismus in persons at high risk for this problem (Beumer et al., 1979). Exercises help to decrease fibrosis of the muscles and increase the mouth opening (Table 52–5). The sudden onset of trismus over several days to weeks may indicate tumor invasion into the muscles of the jaw and requires an evaluation (Rosenberg, 1991).

SURGERY

Surgery to the head and neck region disrupts the oral mucosa when the tumor and surrounding structures are removed. Complications may develop during and after surgery. Indications for oral surgery include fractures, hemorrhage, and orofacial abscesses. For the

TABLE 52–5. *Exercises for Trismus*

1. Open mouth as wide as possible 20 times in succession three times a day.
2. Place heels of both hands under jaw, push up with hands while stretching mouth open. The pressure provides resistance to the mandible as it opens and thereby strengthens the muscles.
3. Place middle and index finger on mandibular teeth and thumb on maxillary teeth. Use fingers in twisting motion to pry the mouth open. Hold open as wide as possible for 2 seconds, then relax. Repeat 10 times with the right hand and then repeat with the left hand. Repeat the entire sequence 4 times a day.

(Data from Ritchie, J. R., Brown, J. R., Guerra, L. R., & Mason, G. [1985]. Dental care for the irradiated cancer patient. *Quintessence International*, 16, 837–842; Sullivan, M. D., & Fleming, T. J. [1986]. Oral care for the radiotherapy-treated head and neck cancer patient. *Dental Hygiene*, 60, 112–114.)

person who requires oral surgery for infectious complications during myelosuppression, careful planning during the preoperative, intraoperative, and postoperative periods can avert complications. Difficulty with speech, chewing, and swallowing are common problems after hemimandibulectomy or glossectomy. If the muscles of mastication have been surgically manipulated, fibrosis may occur, leading to trismus.

ORAL CARE

Systematic performance of oral care is most effective in minimizing the destructive effects of cancer therapy on oral mucosa (Box 52–1) (Beck, 1979; Carl, 1993; Dudjak, 1985). The process of providing oral care itself improves the general condition of the mouth (Van Drimmelen & Rollins, 1969). Passos and Brand (1966) found that improved oral conditions were evident the longer oral care was provided. Regardless of the agent used, oral status improved when the person resumed oral feedings.

The purpose of oral care is to provide a comfortable and functional mouth, which is necessary for nutrition and communication, and to prevent infections (Daeffler, 1981). This is accomplished by keeping the oral mucosa and lips clean, soft, moist, and intact. As a result, the reservoir of pathogens in the mouth is reduced. Irritants that could further damage the oral mucosa are minimized to prevent hemorrhage, periodontal disease, and caries. Oral pain and discomfort are relieved to enhance oral intake, and the oral cavity is kept aesthetically clean and fresh (Daeffler, 1981; Hickey et al., 1982; McElroy, 1984).

Hickey et al. (1982) described other benefits of oral care, including minimizing treatment delays, decreasing length of hospitalization as a result of lessened complications, decreasing cost, and reducing staff time needed to manage complications.

Hart and Rasmussen (1982) reported that although most nurses identified the need to prevent stomatitis to maintain comfort and nutrition and to minimize infec-

---

Box 52–1. *Systematic Oral Care Protocol Improves Oral Status After Chemotherapy*

Beck, S. (1979). Impact of systematic oral care protocol on stomatitis after chemotherapy. *Cancer Nursing, 2,* 185–199.

A systematic oral care protocol was evaluated to determine its efficacy in minimizing or preventing stomatitis in patients who had recently received chemotherapy. Parameters included general physical condition, condition of the oral tissues, and oral perceptions. This protocol included a thorough inspection and assessment of the mouth, with specific interventions being dependent on the condition of the tissues.

The control group of patients ($n = 25$) was evaluated every other day for a 25-day period. Twenty-two treated patients were then similarly evaluated for another 25-day period.

The condition of the oral tissues in the treated patients was better than that in the control group ($p < 0.01$). The incidence of oral infections was 32 per cent in the treated group as compared with 48 per cent in the control group.

Interestingly, in spite of the poor condition of the oral tissues in the control group, the perceptions of control group patients were not significantly different from those of the patients in the treated group. This finding reinforces the need for a nursing assessment of the oral tissues to detect changes early and provide prompt interventions. Patients may not complain until the stomatitis is severe.

---

tions, there was a lack of consistency in the assessment and provision of care.

In comparing two oral care protocols on the incidence of stomatitis in patients with hematologic malignancies receiving high-dose chemotherapy alone or with radiation, Kenny (1990) found that patient compliance with oral care improved with reinforcement of oral care instruction and nursing assessments. Similarly, Dudjak (1987) found that systematic performance of oral care with consistency in both person and frequency of reinforcement promoted patient compliance with oral care protocols. The use of a quality improvement approach demonstrated beneficial effects of minimizing the occurrence of stomatitis (Box 52–2) (Graham, Pecoraro, Ventura & Meyer, 1993).

ASSESSMENT

Oral care starts with assessment. Consideration of the type of cancer, its location and treatment, as well as the person's age and medical condition will identify those at risk for developing oral complications (Poland, 1991; Sonis & Clark, 1991). By carefully and systematically inspecting the person's mouth, the nurse can detect alterations in oral status and provide early interventions. An individualized assessment is needed, because perceptions and symptoms vary greatly from person to person (Daeffler, 1981). This assessment includes an initial history, which evaluates oral hygiene habits (flossing and brushing), history of gingivitis, use and fit of oral prosthesis or dentures, other sources of irritation and infection, and previous complications with cancer therapy. The initial assessment should be done before the start of treatment (Beck, 1979; Hyland, 1986; Ostchega, 1980; Williams et al., 1982). An examination of the oral cavity is necessary at least daily once treatment has started and twice a day during periods of myelosuppression (Barrett, 1984b; Beck, 1979; Ostchega, 1980). Observations and changes in oral status should be recorded.

The equipment used in an examination includes gloves, pen-sized flashlight, and tongue blades. All mucosal surfaces within the oral cavity should be examined: hard and soft palates, buccal mucosa, dorsal and ventral surfaces of the tongue, gingiva, lips, and tonsillar fossa. Moisture, color, and texture of the mucosa and debris in the oral cavity are assessed during the examination (Beck, 1979; Schweiger, Lang, & Schweiger, 1980). Teeth are evaluated for color, shine, and debris. The amount of saliva as well as the perception of changes in taste, voice, and comfort are noted.

Several assessment tools have been published (Table 52–6). The Oral Assessment Guide (OAG), as described by Eilers, Berger, and Petersen (1988), was developed to help standardize the assessment of the mouth, voice, and swallowing ability. Based on clinical

---

Box 52–2. *Quality Assessment and Improvement Approach Reduces Incidence of Stomatitis*

Graham, K. M., Pecoraro, D. A., Ventura, M., & Meyer, C. C. (1993). Reducing the incidence of stomatitis using a quality assessment and improvement approach. *Cancer Nursing, 16,* 117–122.

A quality assessment and improvement approach was utilized to reduce the incidence of chemotherapy-induced stomatitis. Review of patient records revealed inconsistent documentation of pretreatment chemotherapy teaching and reinforcement of this teaching during subsequent courses of therapy. In addition, when stomatitis occurred, the oral care provided by nurses varied from patient to patient.

A unit-based oral care protocol was established that included a baseline prechemotherapy assessment and teaching, stomatitis treatment protocol, and follow-up care with reinforcement of teaching. A nursing care monitor was utilized to document compliance with this protocol. Over 21 months, 1017 chemotherapy treatment cycles were administered. The oral care protocol was utilized with each treatment cycle. Consistent use of the unit's oral care protocol demonstrated a decreased incidence of stomatitis.

TABLE 52–6. *Oral Assessment Tools and Methods*

SOURCE	TOOLS AND METHODS
Ginsberg, 1961	Description of oral assessment
Passos & Brand, 1966	Guide for numeric rating of the condition of the mouth
Van Drimmelen & Rollins, 1969	Guide for numeric rating of the condition of the mouth (adapted from Passos & Brand, 1966)
DeWalt, 1975	Schematic presentation of dependent variables, tools for data collection, methods of measurement, and ratings
Beck, 1979	Oral exam guide; oral perception guide
Schweiger, Lang, & Schweiger, 1980	Oral assessment
Ostchega, 1980	A guide to assessing and treating chemotherapy's oral complications
Daeffler, 1981	Process standard for oral care
Allbright, 1984	Description of specific problems and suggested interventions
Goodman & Stoner, 1985	Assessment
Eilers, Berger, & Petersen, 1988	Oral assessment guide
Western Consortium for Cancer Nursing Research (WCCNR), 1991	WCCNR Staging System for stomatitis

TABLE 52–7. *Western Consortium for Cancer Nursing Research Staging System for Stomatitis*

Healthy Status
The mouth appears healthy. The color is normal pink. There are no lesions present. There is no bleeding. The mucosa is moist. There is no edema or infection present. There are no oral limitations to eating or drinking. The patient experiences no oral discomfort.

Stage 1
The mouth has evidence of slightly increased redness in one or more areas. There are 1 to 4 lesions (may be small ulcers or canker sores) somewhere in the oral cavity. The mucosa may appear to be thinning in several areas. There is no bleeding or infection present. The mucosa is moist. There is mild edema in one to several areas. The patient tends to avoid harsh, hot, or spicy foods because the mouth is sensitive to such irritation. The patient experiences mild discomfort that may be described as burning sensation.

Stage 2
There is moderate increase in redness throughout most of the mucosal surfaces. There are more than 4 lesions (may be ulcers, canker sores) somewhere in oral cavity, but they still are discretely separate and not coalescing with adjacent lesions. The mucosa tends to bleed upon probing or manipulating. The mucosa appears slightly drier than normal. The saliva may be slightly thicker than normal. Most areas are moderately edematous. There may be evidence suggesting that infection is present in the mouth manifested by white or yellow patches. The patient is unable to eat except for very bland soft foods but is able to drink liquids that are not hot, spicy, or acidic. The patient experiences moderate continual pain and requires intermittent (usually topical) analgesics.

Stage 3
The oral mucosa is severely red throughout all of the oral cavity. There are multiple confluent ulcers that may be to the point of total denudation of the oral cavity. Bleeding is occurring spontaneously without any particular stimulation. There is marked xerostomia. Edema is severe throughout the entire mouth. There are white, yellow, or purulent patches present in the mouth suggesting infection. The patient is unable to eat or drink or even to swallow own saliva. With persuasion, the patient may be able to take oral medications. The patient has severe constant pain requiring systemic analgesia.

(Reprinted by permission from Western Consortium for Cancer Nursing Research. [1991]. Development of a staging system for chemotherapy-induced stomatitis. *Cancer Nursing, 14,* 11.)

experience, expert panel review, and review of other oral assessment tools, the OAG defines three levels of descriptors for each of eight categories (Fig. 52–5, see Color Plate IV). High reliability of 0.912 among raters was established by registered nurses who were trained in the use of the tool.

A pilot study using the OAG with 20 subjects who were undergoing bone marrow transplantation concluded that the tool was useful in quantifying changes in the oral cavities of these patients. There was a high level of compliance by nurses using the tool. The OAG is used to communicate changes in the oral cavity and to determine and plan interventions.

Another tool, the Western Consortium for Cancer Nursing Research (WCCNR) Staging System, was developed to measure the progressive severity of chemotherapy-induced stomatitis (Table 52–7) (WCCNR, 1991). This tool utilizes observable and functional data in evaluating overall oral status.

An examination by a dentist is important before the start of cancer therapy (Cacchillo, Barker, & Barker, 1993; Hickey et al., 1982; Ketron, 1984; Lowe, 1986; National Institutes of Health, 1989). The dentist performs a clinical examination to evaluate the condition of the teeth and surrounding structures, identify possible foci of infection, and correct oral and dental problems (Carl, 1993; Lowe, 1986). The dentist also evaluates whether teeth should be extracted before starting radiation therapy to the head and neck region. The dentist is able to perform initial dental prophylaxis:

scaling to remove tartar, and polishing of teeth (Lowe, 1986; Williams et al., 1982).

The correlation between the presence of dental plaque and the development of stomatitis during chemotherapy is high. Lindquist et al. (1978) found that people who received dental scaling and prophylaxis as well as oral hygiene instructions before chemotherapy experienced less stomatitis with shorter duration of symptoms than did those who had oral hygiene instructions but did not receive dental scaling. Dental prophylaxis also decreased the incidence of oral infections (Hickey et al., 1982). There was no increase in the systemic sequelae (fever and bacteremia) as a result of oral and dental care, and no correlation was seen between the severity and duration of stomatitis and the dose of chemotherapy. Therefore, dental care before chemotherapy can help to reduce the incidence of oral complications.

For the person about to start head and neck irradiation, the dentist can provide initial fluoride therapy and instruct the person on the procedure for daily fluoride applications (Lowe, 1986). Oral radiographs are not contraindicated before, during, or after radiation therapy. When a full series of radiographs is done, no area of the mouth receives a dose of more than 1 cGy (Levin & Ferris, 1980).

Careful assessment of denture use is necessary to reduce the oral complications that can occur in the edentulous person (Bernhoft & Skaug, 1985). The denture wearer's mouth is inspected for signs of irritation. Dentures also need to be evaluated for stability, retention, and occlusion (DePaola et al., 1983). Unstable or unretentive dentures can cause tissue irritation or ulceration. Xerostomia may also cause problems with denture retention. Almost all persons with dentures report that their dentures do not seem to fit so well shortly after chemotherapy has started or on withdrawal of chemotherapy (DePaola et al., 1983). The cause of this phenomenon is unknown. However, if they are used with care, well-fitted and tolerated dentures do not have to be temporarily discontinued (Bernhoft & Skaug, 1985). After cancer therapy, denture construction for edentulous persons should be delayed until epithelialization is complete (DePaola et al., 1983).

INTERVENTION

The performance of oral care is extremely important. The frequency of oral care is determined by the medical condition of the person and the status of the oral tissues. Table 52–2 describes the nursing care for a patient with stomatitis. Oral care should be done at least after each meal and at bedtime. In addition, oral care before meals helps to freshen the mouth and stimulate the appetite (Beck, 1979). For those patients who have mild stomatitis (grade I), care is given at least every 2 hours. For those with moderate-to-severe stomatitis (grades II and III), oral care should be done at least every 1 to 2 hours (Lane & Forgay, 1981). Unfortunately, when oral pain occurs, the person may be unwilling to perform mouth care and decrease the frequency and quality of oral care. As a result, more oral pain and dysphagia occurs (Poland, 1991). There is great variation in how oral care is provided (Holmes, 1991). Ezzone, Jolly, Replogle, Kapoor, and Tutschkan (1993) surveyed the oral care regimens of 73 bone marrow transplantation centers and found few similarities. Utilizing the Oral Assessment Guide, Armstrong (1994) proposed an oral care protocol for persons receiving a bone marrow transplant (Table 52–8). Beck (1979) reported that systematic care minimized oral complications in persons receiving chemotherapy regardless of their hydration status. DeWalt (1975) demonstrated that although daily improvement in oral tissues is seen with oral care, the tissue responses to oral care are not cumulative over a

TABLE 52–8. *Oral Care Protocol*

Brushing
The teeth should be brushed with a fluoride-containing dentrifice using the Bass technique.
A soft-bristled toothbrush should be used.
Rinsing
After brushing, the mouth should be rinsed with sterile normal saline solution.
Lubricant
Apply petroleum jelly to the lips as necessary to prevent drying.

OAG ≤ 8. Goal: prevention of stomatitis. To be performed every 8 h while awake and as required.
OAG = 8–10. Goal: management of mild stomatitis. To be performed at least every 4 h while awake.
OAG > 10. Goal: management of moderate-severe stomatitis. To be performed every 1–2 h.

OAG = Oral Assessment Guide.
(Reprinted by permission from Armstrong, T. S. [1994]. Stomatitis in the bone marrow transplant patient: an overview and proposed oral care protocol. *Cancer Nursing, 17,* 407.)

long period of time. Further, omission of oral care for 2 to 6 hours can nullify the past benefits of care (DeWalt, 1975; Ginsberg, 1961). Ginsberg (1961) studied the oral care of persons in acute renal failure. In that study, all mouth care equipment or procedures improved oral status, and complications were avoided when mouth care was provided at specified intervals and was specific to the person's individual needs.

While a person is undergoing cancer therapy, meticulous denture cleansing habits are needed (DePaola, 1983). Daily mechanical cleansing with a denture brush and an antimicrobial detergent such as chlorhexidine gluconate should be performed. Soft liners may be used to improve the stability of dentures. These liners are changed daily to minimize microbial growth. Dentures should be removed while sleeping and at other times to allow the mucosa to rest. Dentures should be soaked overnight, and the oral mucosa may be rinsed with chlorhexidine gluconate (Bernhoft & Skaug, 1985). If a person is unable to wear dentures because of pain, stomatitis, or bleeding, the dentures should be stored in a denture cup that contains a solution of Efferdent (Warner-Lambert Co., Morris Plains, NJ), Kleenite (Richardson-Vicks, Inc., Wilton, CT), or water (Cunningham, 1984). This solution should be changed daily. Before placing the dentures in the mouth, it is important to rinse the dentures well with water.

Cunningham (1984) cautions against the use of dentures that are in poor repair or are more than 5 years old. In addition, if the neutrophil count is less than or equal to 1000, the platelet count is less than or equal to 50,000, and no other pathology is present, the prostheses should be worn only for meals.

INSTRUMENTS FOR ORAL CARE

Various instruments are used in oral care to help remove debris and stimulate the gingiva. Periodontal disease is prevented by removing plaque from teeth. Plaque is best removed with toothbrushing and flossing (Beck, 1979; Williams et al., 1982). A small, soft, nylon-bristled toothbrush effectively removes debris and stimulates gingival tissue. The Bass technique of brushing used in combination with flossing is the most effective method in minimizing the accumulation of plaque (Carl, 1993). The toothbrush is held at a 45-degree angle at the junction of the gingival margin and teeth and is moved in short, horizontal strokes. The teeth should be brushed for at least 3 to 4 min (Bersani & Carl, 1983). Unwaxed dental floss is used once a day in conjunction with tooth brushing to remove dental plaque and debris (Ostchega, 1980). Although toothbrushing and flossing are the most effective means of removing debris and plaque, they are contraindicated during periods of severe stomatitis, neutropenia, and thrombocytopenia (platelet count less than 20,000) because of the potential for bleeding, bacteremia, fungemia, and septicemia (Daeffler, 1981; Williams et al., 1982).

During periods of thrombocytopenia and neutropenia, Toothettes are more appropriate to use. Toothettes are sponge-tipped applicators that are less traumatic to gingival tissues but are also less effective than a toothbrush in removing plaque and debris (Daeffler, 1981). Toothettes are useful for stimulating gingival tissue. Unflavored Toothettes are recommended because the flavoring and dentifrice that is sometimes applied to the Toothette can further irritate the mucosa. For severe discomfort, a piece of gauze wrapped around the finger is useful and less painful to remove debris (Allbright, 1984; Williams et al., 1982).

A gavage bag or gravity drip container with tubing is sometimes used to gently remove crusts and debris from the mouth. A red rubber-tipped catheter can be connected to the tubing to facilitate irrigation. A 500-ml normal saline intravenous solution bag with tubing attached to an 18-gauge angiocatheter can also be used to gently irrigate the mouth (Mosco, 1986). A bulb syringe can serve the same purpose (Daeffler, 1980b).

The power spray or Water Pik (Teledyne Water Pik, Fort Collins, CO) used at a low-pressure setting is helpful in removing debris. Hickey et al. (1982) reported that although water lavage did not alter the duration and severity of stomatitis, it did decrease oral debris and saliva viscosity and gave the person a sense of cleanliness. However, some question exists about whether such a power spray causes a transient septicemia (Daeffler, 1981). An atomizer may be used for mouth care (Pegram, 1983). A small portable air compressor is connected to an atomizer with a long nozzle tip. The atomizer is filled with normal saline or other solution and delivers a fine mist to the oral tissues without damaging them. People report a soothing effect on dry, inflamed, and ulcerated tissues. Suction equipment should be available for people who are at risk for aspiration.

AGENTS FOR ORAL CARE

The ideal mouthwash removes debris and moistens and softens the mucosa. The different agents used in oral care have three main purposes: to clean and remove debris, to lubricate and moisturize the oral mucosa, and to control pain (Table 52–9). Combination solutions are available that incorporate two or three different agents to provide more comprehensive oral care. Passos and Brand (1966) described the optimal oral hygiene measure as one that mechanically or chemically cleans the oral cavity without altering the properties and functioning of the mouth. In addition, this oral hygiene measure would leave the mucosa moist and lubricated.

CLEANSING AGENTS

Cleansing agents provide mechanical or chemical washing action that removes loose debris and softens and removes mucous crusts. Normal saline acts as a palliative agent to aid granulation (Carter, 1992; Daeffler, 1980b). Saline is economical, readily available, and least damaging of the agents. A normal saline solution can be made with 1 teaspoon of salt mixed in 1 L of water. Daeffler (1980b) suggests the use of normal saline for persons with leukemia because it is not irritating or harmful to the mucosa. Sterile saline is used if the person is neutropenic or if ulcers are present. However, normal saline does not effectively remove hardened mucus, debris, or crusts.

Sodium bicarbonate is used as a cleansing agent and helps to decrease odor and relieve pain (Daeffler, 1980b). This agent also helps to buffer acidity in the mouth and dissolve mucin (Cheater, 1985). Sodium bicarbonate may be used after meals for general care and every 2 hours when ulcerations are present (Barrett, 1984b). A combination mouthwash of "salt and soda" is described in the literature (Daeffler, 1980b; Ritchie et al., 1985; Sullivan & Fleming, 1986; Wescott, 1985). Salt and sodium bicarbonate in a 1:1 ratio is mixed in warm water ($\frac{1}{2}$ to 1 teaspoon of each in a L of water) and used every 3 to 4 hours. This mouthwash is able to clean and lubricate tissues and provide moderate local pain control (Daeffler, 1980b).

Hydrogen peroxide is a germicidal solution that is used for its mechanical cleansing, debriding, and effervescence (Daeffler, 1980b; Lowe, 1986). Passos and Brand (1966) evaluated the use of milk of magnesia, aromatic mouth wash, and hydrogen peroxide for oral care of persons who had had surgery. Although there was no significant difference in the efficacy of the three agents, hydrogen peroxide maintained and improved mouth conditions in some patients. However, since hydrogen peroxide can also break down tissue and damage exposed bone, caution must be used when ulcers or fresh granulation surfaces are present (Daeffler, 1980b; Passos & Brand, 1966). It is also irritating to the tongue and buccal mucosa. Elongation of the filiform and foliate papillae of the tongue has been noted (Tombes, 1987). The elongated papillae serve as an excellent matrix for candidiasis. Therefore, hydrogen peroxide should be used with caution (Sciubba, 1991).

The efficacy and safety of long-term use of hydrogen peroxide has also been questioned (Amigoni, Johnson, & Kalkwarf, 1987; Weitzman, Weitberg, Niederman, & Stossel, 1984). Cells are damaged when they are

TABLE 52–9. *Agents for Oral Care*

AGENTS	COMMENTS
Cleansing	
Normal saline	Economical, available, least irritating
Sodium bicarbonate	Decreases odors, buffers acidity, dissolves mucin
Hydrogen peroxide	Germicidal, mechanical cleansing, debriding. Use diluted solution and follow with normal saline or water rinse. Aspiration precautions with foaming action
Commercial mouthwashes	Avoid mouthwashes containing alcohol, oils, astringents, antiseptics, and flavorings
Chlorhexidine gluconate	Antimicrobial: decreases dental plaque and gingival inflammation. Bitter taste, tooth staining
Lubricating	
Saliva substitutes	Decreases pain, dryness; protects mucosa
Lemon-glycerin	Mouth irritant, decalcifies teeth
Water-soluble lubricant, lanolin	Lip emollient; if petrolatum used, avoid aspirating
Pain Control	
Coating	
Kaopectate, milk of magnesia, Orabase	Covers ulcerated mucosa; temporary pain relief; may dry mucosa
Sucralfate	Binds to exposed mucosa for pain relief and protection
Hydroxypropyl cellulose film former (Zilactin)	Binds to oral mucosa forming protective coating; transient stinging with gel application
Vitamin E	Anecdotal reports of pain control; heals stomatitis
Topical Anesthetic	
Lidocaine viscous	Transient pain relief; interferes with gag reflex when swallowed
Dyclonine hydrochloride	Transient pain relief; useful in persons with xerostomia; aspiration precautions if swallowed
Cocaine solution	Transient pain relief; monitor central nervous system effects; tachycardia
Combination mouthwashes	Usually contains nonsteroidal anti-inflammatory agent in addition to topical anesthetic
Systemic	
Narcotic medications	For severe pain; taken 30–60 min before meals and as needed
Nonsteroidal anti-inflammatory agents	
Other	
Topical thrombin	To control minor bleeding
Fluoride	To prevent caries; apply to debris-free teeth after thorough mouth care
Allopurinol	To minimize chemotherapy-induced stomatitis
Antibiotic mouthwashes	For prophylaxis and treatment of oral infections such as candidiasis and gram-negative opportunistic organisms

exposed to a high concentration of oxidants. With long-term use, peroxide may function as a co-carcinogen (Weitzman et al., 1984). Caution must be observed when a person has a compromised cough reflex be-cause of the foaming action of hydrogen peroxide. The person who is unable to cough may have a problem with aspirating the foam (Daeffler, 1980b). Fungal adherence may be increased with the use of hydrogen peroxide (Tombes, 1987). Superinfections may occur as the normal oral flora balance is disturbed. In some people, oral use of hydrogen peroxide also causes nausea and subjective feelings of thirst and dryness of the mouth.

Hydrogen peroxide 3 per cent should be used only if mechanical cleansing action is essential and should be diluted to one-fourth strength (Daeffler, 1980b; Goodman & Stoner, 1985; Lowe, 1986). Use of hydrogen peroxide must be followed with a normal saline or water rinse. Suction equipment should be readily available for people who are unable to tolerate the foaming action of this agent.

Hogan (1983) found that a refrigerated solution of hydrogen peroxide provided a numbing anesthetic effect. She suggests that the cold solution can cause vasoconstriction and help stop bleeding secondary to severe stomatitis, thrombocytopenia, or both. The preference for half-strength hydrogen peroxide versus baking soda and water has been evaluated in persons receiving head and neck irradiation (Dudjak, 1985, 1987). These investigators found that half-strength hydrogen peroxide was less irritating to use than baking soda and water.

Commercial mouthwashes should be avoided because they often contain oils, astringents, and antiseptics. These can lead to drying, irritation, erythema, ulceration, and epithelial sloughing (Bersani & Carl, 1983; Cheater, 1985; Daeffler, 1980b; Sullivan & Fleming, 1986).

Chlorhexidine is an antimicrobial agent used to help decrease dental plaque and gingival inflammation. Investigations of the prophylactic use of chlorhexidine gluconate in preventing or decreasing oral complications have had conflicting results. In a double-blind, placebo-controlled study, McGaw and Belch (1985) found the mouth rinse provided good control of plaque and gingival inflammation with decreased severity and duration of mucositis in 16 leukemic patients undergoing remission-induction therapy. In contrast, Weisdorf et al. (1989) in a double-blind, placebo-controlled trial of chlorhexidine gluconate in bone marrow transplant recipients (*n* = 100) found trends toward improved oral hygiene in the treated group but no significant difference in mucositis. Raybould et al. (1994) reviewed case reports of immunosuppressed patients who used chlorhexidine. Although opportunistic gram-negative bacteria oral infections occurred in the patients receiving chlorhexidine, the benefits of this agent's antifungal properties outweighed that risk of bacterial infection. In patients with a compromised oral mucosa, chlorhexidine can be used as an oral hygiene "bridge" until brushing and flossing can be resumed (Poland, 1991). Transient staining of teeth and a mild burning sensation with the use of chlorhexidine have been reported. Using viscous lidocaine with the chlorhexidine can minimize the burning sensation (Rowan, 1992).

LUBRICATING AGENTS

Lubricating agents such as saliva substitutes contain methyl cellulose. Some saliva substitutes contain ptyalin, a salivary enzyme, and fluoride to prevent caries (Beumer et al., 1979). These lubricating agents help to decrease oral discomfort and buffer the hyperacidity that occurs with xerostomia (Bernhoft & Skaug, 1985; Cheater, 1985). Saliva substitutes lubricate and protect the denture-supporting tissues and increase bonding of the prosthesis to the mucosa.

Lemon-glycerin solutions and swabs have been studied for their use as oral care agents (Daeffler, 1980b; Van Drimmelen & Rollins, 1969; Wiley, 1969). Glycerin has a drying effect as it absorbs water and irritates the mucosa. The acidity of the lemon can decalcify teeth, reduce the buffering capacity of saliva, and be painful on broken mucosal surfaces (Wiley, 1969). Therefore, lemon-glycerin swabs should be avoided.

Moi-Stir (Kingswood Laboratories, Inc., Carmel, IN) is one type of saliva substitute that was compared with lemon-glycerin swabs for effect on oral status in a study by Poland (1987). The subjects tended to prefer Moi-Stir over lemon glycerin, and on examination, the measures of oral status (dryness, etc.) improved with Moi-Stir and worsened with lemon glycerin.

A thin layer of water-soluble lubricant or lanolin applied to sore, dry, and cracked lips helps to lubricate and soften them. These agents prevent evaporation and drying. If petrolatum is used, caution must be taken against aspirating the lubricant (Daeffler, 1980b).

PAIN CONTROL AGENTS

Pain control agents are categorized by their function: coating agents, topical anesthetic agents, and systemic analgesics.

Coating Agents. Kaopectate (Upjohn Co., Kalamazoo, MI), milk of magnesia, and Orabase (Colgate-Hoyt Laboratories, Canton, MA) help to coat painful mucosal areas. The pectin in Kaopectate coats the denuded areas of the mucosa to prevent further irritation. Milk of magnesia has been used to coat the

mucosa and is reported to decrease acidity, dissolve mucin, and stimulate saliva production (Cheater, 1985; Daeffler, 1980b). Milk of magnesia also exerts an osmotic effect, can dry the mucosa, and should not be used if a person has xerostomia. Orabase is a protective paste that is composed of gelatin, pectin, and carboxymethyl cellulose in a hydrocarbon gel. This odorless and tasteless paste is applied to ulcerations and provides temporary relief of pain (Daeffler, 1980b).

Sucralfate suspension is a compound of sulfated sucrose and aluminum hydroxide that has been used for gastric and duodenal ulcers. This agent forms an adhesive substance that binds to exposed mucosa and forms a protective barrier that promotes healing of ulcerated tissues. Anecdotal reports of the use of sucralfate suspension for chemotherapy-induced oral stomatitis described mouth ulcers that were healed within 2 to 3 days of use, enabling tolerance of oral nutrition (Ferraro & Mattern, 1984; Shenep et al., 1988; Wilkes, 1986). A randomized, double-blind study of 48 children and adolescents who received remission-induction chemotherapy for leukemia revealed that subjects who used sucralfate reported less oral pain than those who used placebo (58 per cent and 25 per cent, respectively, reported no discomfort; *p* = 0.06). Observers also noted more moderate to severe mucositis in the placebo group (38 per cent) than in the treated group (12 per cent). However, there was no difference in the maximal subjective and objective mucositis scores. In addition, the incidence of infection was similar in both groups. The investigators did not find objective evidence of healing or lessening of stomatitis in the treated group. Sucralfate suspension has also been found to be helpful in reducing oral pain associated with radiation-induced stomatitis (Epstein & Wong, 1994).

Hydroxypropyl cellulose film former (Zilactin, Zila Pharmaceuticals, Phoenix, AZ) binds to oral mucosal surfaces, which provides a protective coating and leads to pain relief. With application of the gel, there is a transient stinging sensation as the gel dries and forms a film. Investigators have found this product protects areas of ulcerations from irritation associated with food intake (Rodu & Russell, 1988).

The use of vitamin E has been reported anecdotally to be beneficial in controlling pain and promoting healing of oral stomatitis (Hogan, 1984; Oncology Staff Nurses, 1982).

Topical Anesthetic Agents. Topical anesthetic agents numb the oral mucosa. Lidocaine viscous is frequently used 15 to 20 minutes before meals to provide comfort during meals. The anesthetic effect is brief, and some people find the taste of lidocaine unpleasant (Daeffler, 1980b). If swallowed, lidocaine viscous may also interfere with the pharyngeal stage of swallowing (Daeffler, 1981). Dyclonine hydrochloride has been reported to be an effective topical anesthetic agent that is especially effective for people with xerostomia (Daeffler, 1980b; Lowe, 1986). This agent takes 10 minutes before onset of effects and lasts for approximately 1 hour.

Gentzsch (1983) described the use of a dilute solution of cocaine to control pain associated with stomatitis. People used this solution every 2 to 3 hours around the clock and had a significant reduction in oral pain without tachycardia, central nervous system effects, or alterations in taste.

Combination mouthwashes of topical anesthetics, diphenhydramine, and milk of magnesia or Kaopectate have been reported (Beck, 1979; Carter, 1986; Hilderley, 1986; Wescott, 1985). A nonsteroidal antiinflammatory agent is frequently included in the mouthwash to decrease inflammation and provide topical as well as systemic (peripheral) relief of pain (Beck, 1979).

Innovative strategies to administer these agents have been reported. Carter (1986) described administering 5 ml of a mixture of equal parts of dyclonine hydrochloride and diphenhydramine over crushed ice in a 30-ml medicine cup. The person sips this mixture 30 minutes before meals and as needed. The analgesia that is provided with the agents is enhanced by the cold temperature of the solution.

Anesthetic sprays may provide topical relief of pain. However, caution must be used in administering these sprays because of the damage that can be done to inflamed mucosa (Daeffler, 1981).

Systemic Analgesic Agents. Systemic analgesics may sometimes be necessary for severe oral discomfort and should be taken about 30 to 60 minutes before meals. These analgesics include nonsteroidal antiinflammatory agents as well as narcotic medications (Schubert & Newton, 1987).

OTHER AGENTS

A variety of other agents are used to control oral complications such as bleeding, caries, and infections. Topical thrombin has been described in the literature for controlling minor, persistent oral bleeding (Barrett, 1984b; Carl, 1993; Peterson & Sonis, 1982; Preston, 1983). The medication is applied with a cotton-tipped applicator or gauze to the affected area every 4 hours and as needed. Bleeding is stopped with as few as two applications (Peterson & Sonis, 1982).

Daily fluoride treatments are important to prevent caries when xerostomia occurs as the result of radiation therapy to the head and neck region. Fluoride acts by incorporating into the enamel and dentin, thereby remineralizing the teeth and preventing caries formation (Beumer et al., 1979; Lowe, 1986). In addition, fluoride may inhibit plaque formation and decrease the number of cariogenic organisms in the mouth (Lowe, 1986). Dreizen et al. (1977) reported that in a 3-year follow-up study, fluoride was effective in protecting high-risk persons who received head and neck irradiation from developing xerostomia-related caries regardless of the sucrose content of their diet. They found that oral hygiene alone was not adequate to prevent dental decay. Caries occurred and progressed rapidly in persons not using fluoride. In addition, when fluoride was added to the oral hygiene program for these persons, ongoing caries were stopped, and new developments were prevented.

A 1 per cent sodium fluoride or 0.4 per cent stannous fluoride gel is used. For people with good oral hygiene practices and minimal xerostomia, the fluoride gel or special toothpaste may be applied on the teeth with a toothbrush (Carl, 1993; Sullivan & Fleming, 1986). For others, custom-made fluoride carriers or trays are used. The gel is placed within the trays, which are then fitted over the teeth. The trays remain on the teeth for 5 to 10 minutes and then are removed (Sullivan & Fleming, 1986; Wescott, 1985). The person may expectorate the excess fluoride but may not eat, drink, or rinse his or her mouth for 30 minutes following the fluoride application. To be effective, the fluoride treatment needs to be done on debris-free teeth following thorough mouth care (Carl, 1980, 1993; Dreizen et al., 1977; Lowe, 1986; Sullivan & Fleming, 1986). If tooth decay occurs in spite of the daily use of fluoride, the fluoride treatments are then applied twice a day (Ritchie et al., 1985). For persons who have xerostomia as a result of irradiation to the head and neck region, the fluoride treatments need to be continued indefinitely to prevent caries (Sullivan & Fleming, 1986; Wescott, 1985).

Allopurinol mouth rinses have been shown to minimize chemotherapy-induced stomatitis (Clark & Slevin, 1985; Porter, Moroni & Natasi, 1994). Because the medication is diluted and spit out after use, there are minimal systemic effects. One interesting effect of using allopurinol mouth rinse was a reported improvement in taste alterations in two patients studied.

Antibiotic mouthwashes are used to prevent and treat oral infections due to *Candida* species and gram-negative opportunistic organisms. Frequently, antiinflammatory agents and antihistamines are used in combination with antibiotic mouth rinses to provide symptomatic relief of the infection.

CLIENT NEEDS AND NURSING INTERVENTIONS

STOMATITIS

Assess the person's willingness and competence to perform mouth care. Instruct the client to stop smoking and reduce the intake of alcoholic beverages to minimize mouth irritation. Interventions for stomatitis vary depending upon the degree of tissue damage. See Table 52–2 for a description of the levels or grades of stomatitis and the related nursing interventions. A randomized trial was conducted to evaluate the difference between a 30-minute and a 60-minute application of ice chips in the mouth to prevent stomatitis associated with 5-fluorouracil chemotherapy (Rocke et al., 1993). Subjects (N = 178) placed ice chips in their mouths 5 minutes before initiation of the chemotherapy and continuously swished the ice in their mouths for 30 or 60 minutes. The study revealed that 30 minutes was as effective as 60 minutes in minimizing the incidence of stomatitis.

LEUKEMIC INFILTRATION OF GINGIVAL TISSUES

Nursing interventions are palliative. Frequent warm saline rinses five to six times a day will help to keep the mouth clean until the oral cavity and blood counts improve (Bersani & Carl, 1983). Dietary modifications to a soft, bland diet may be necessary if chewing is difficult. If hemorrhage occurs, utilize nursing interventions for bleeding that are listed in the following section.

BLEEDING

Monitor platelet counts. For persons who have thrombocytopenia, the risk of bleeding in the oral cavity is always present. Provide systematic mouth care. Utilize bleeding precautions by reducing or eliminating mouth irritants such as ill-fitting dentures or retainers. These dental prostheses should be removed at least 8 hours daily. Orthodontic bands and wires are also mechanical irritants and can traumatize the oral mucosa and precipitate periodontal infections (Carl, 1993). Although plaque control is important to maintain a healthy gingiva, toothbrushing and flossing should be discontinued if the platelet count falls below 20,000/mm^3. A Toothette or gauze-wrapped finger may be useful to remove debris and plaque from teeth surfaces.

If active bleeding occurs, gently irrigate the oral cavity with normal saline to identify the areas that are bleeding. A periodontal dressing pack may be applied to exert pressure to the bleeding site (Carl, 1980; Wescott, 1985). Bleeding usually stops within a few minutes. During this time, the person should not smoke or suck on straws, because the clot can be dislodged. A soft diet should be provided to reduce the trauma of chewing. Topical thrombin may be helpful to stop persistent, mild bleeding.

If thrombocytopenia is anticipated during the course of therapy, a dentist should examine the person before starting therapy and between courses of treatment to evaluate oral status, eliminate sharp or rough tooth margins, modify ill-fitting dentures, and provide dental prophylaxis and scaling (Barrett, 1984b; Hickey et al., 1982).

INFECTIONS

Intensive oral hygiene before and after myelosuppressive therapy has been found to be helpful in preventing infections (Peterson & Sonis, 1982). Monitor neutrophil counts; anticipate complications as the neutrophil count decreases. Inspect the mouth twice a day for local signs of an infection: erythema, pain, plaque formation, and candidiasis. Observe for systemic effects such as fever, increased pulse, and malaise. Culture suspicious mouth lesions to determine whether the lesion is an infection or a treatment-related reaction (Poland, 1991). Administer antibiotics as prescribed. If an oral fungal infection develops in a person who wears dentures, the dentures should be removed during the administration of topical antibiotics (Barrett, 1984b). Continue with mouth care and maintain cleanliness of instruments used in the mouth.

TASTE CHANGES

Assess changes in taste perception. Assess which foods have altered or disagreeable tastes and which foods taste the same. It is important to remember that "taste" is influenced by many factors, including color and smell of food, emotional state of the person, and learned responses (Gallucci & Iwamoto, 1981). Modification of these factors can improve the appetite. Adding herbs, seasonings, sauces, or sugar can improve the taste of foods and enhance their palatability. Varying the temperatures of food and presenting foods with different textures can be helpful. Marinating and cooking meats in sweet sauces help to disguise the unpleasant tastes many people experience (Strohl, 1984). Cold cooked chicken, eggs, mild-flavored fish, and cheeses are frequently preferred over meats as sources of protein. Some people have reported that certain foods have little taste or may taste odd but that sweet and sour-flavored foods are palatable. Sweet and sour salad dressings have been used to enhance the flavor of foods other than salads (Strohl, 1984). The senses of taste and smell are closely interrelated. With cancer therapy, the sense of smell is frequently less affected than that of taste. Some people have found that sniffing food before placing it in their mouths gives them a "taste" of the food. Mouth care before and after meals is especially important to refresh and clear the mouth of residual tastes. Since taste changes can last for several years after the course of treatment is completed, assessment for taste alterations and their effect on nutritional status should be done with each follow-up visit (Strohl, 1983).

XEROSTOMIA

Saliva substitutes are convenient, although temporary, palliative measures to relieve xerostomia. Approximately 2 ml of the solution will provide some relief. Sugarless gum or mints can help to stimulate saliva production in persons with low salivary flow rates (Cartwright & Facciponti, 1992; Cheater, 1985; Lowe, 1986; Sullivan & Fleming, 1986). Increasing fluid intake can help relieve dryness and moisten the mouth. People frequently carry containers of water, iced tea, or other liquids to use as needed. For people with xerostomia without oral inflammation or pain, carbonated drinks such as cider or apple juice with soda or lemonade can be especially enjoyable. Some find sucking on ice chips helpful. Eating fresh fruits such as melons or grapes is well tolerated. Dry foods and foods that require an increased amount of saliva for chewing should be avoided. Foods need to be softened or moistened with gravy to make swallowing easier. Fluids should accompany meals and snacks. Mouth care itself stimulates saliva flow and should be performed before and after meals. Evaluate medications for anticholinergic side effects, which diminish saliva flow. Lip care needs to be provided with an emollient.

Papain, the proteolytic enzyme found in papayas and used in meat tenderizers, may assist in dissolving and breaking up thick, ropey oral secretions (Larsen, 1982). Eating fresh papayas or drinking papaya juice may be recommended before meals. Papain can also be purchased over the counter. The patient holds a solution of $\frac{1}{2}$ teaspoon papain in 10 ml of water in the mouth for about 10 minutes before meals. An alternative method is to swab the oral cavity with meat tenderizer before meals.

When a person experiences xerostomia, sleeping can be difficult because of mucosal dryness. Using a humidifier in the bedroom can help promote comfort and sleep (Ladd, 1991).

A major consequence of xerostomia is dental caries. The gingival areas and crevices need to be kept free of debris and plaque to prevent dental decay and periodontal disease (Carl, 1980). Mouth care with toothbrushing and flossing and daily use of fluoride should be maintained (Cacchillo et al., 1993; Dreizen et al., 1977). Follow-up appointments with the dentist every 2 to 3 months are important for an evaluation of oral care, fluoride use, prosthesis fit, periodontal disease, and osteoradionecrosis.

Pilocarpine, a parasympathomimetic agent, has been found to be effective in improving saliva production in persons who have received head and neck irradiation (Johnson et al., 1993; LeVeque, et al., 1993; Rieke et al., 1995). The most common side effect is transient sweating that occurs 20 to 60 minutes after taking a dose of pilocarpine.

SUMMARY

Alterations in the mouth as a result of cancer or its treatment can result in pain, increased susceptibility to serious infection, and compromised nutritional status. Nurses are in a vital position to assess high-risk persons for early symptoms and provide care to prevent or minimize these problems. Teach the patient and the family about oral complications that may occur as a result of cancer therapy. Instruct the patient on ways to examine the mouth, what signs and symptoms to monitor and report, and how to perform mouth care. Emphasize the importance of regular and systematic mouth care to prevent or minimize oral complications. With consistent application of oral care, further damage to the oral mucosa can be prevented, pain can be relieved or minimized, and tolerance and response to treatment can be improved.

REFERENCES

Allbright, A. (1984). Oral care for the cancer chemotherapy patient. *Nursing Times, 80,* 40–42.

Amigoni, N. A., Johnson, G. K., & Kalkwarf, K. L. (1987). The use of sodium bicarbonate and hydrogen peroxide in periodontal therapy: A review. *Journal of the American Dental Association, 114,* 217–221.

Armstrong, T. S. (1994). Stomatitis in the bone marrow transplant patient: an overview and proposed oral care protocol. *Cancer Nursing, 17,* 403–410.

Barrett, A. P. (1984a). Evaluation of nystatin in prevention and elimination of oropharyngeal *Candida* in immunosuppressed patients. *Oral Surgery, 58,* 148–151.

Barrett, A. P. (1984b). Oral mucosal complications in cancer chemotherapy. *Australia and New Zealand Journal of Medicine, 14,* 7–12.

Barrett, A. P. (1987). Clinical characteristics and mechanisms involved in chemotherapy-induced oral ulceration. *Oral Surgery, Oral Medicine, Oral Pathology, 63,* 424–428.

Beck, S. (1979). Impact of a systematic oral care protocol on stomatitis after chemotherapy. *Cancer Nursing, 2,* 185–199.

Bernhoft, C-H., & Skaug, N. (1985). Oral findings in irradiated edentulous patients. *International Journal of Oral Surgery, 14,* 416–427.

Bersani, G., & Carl, W. (1983). Oral care for cancer patients. *American Journal of Nursing, 83,* 533–536.

Beumer, J., Curtis, T., & Harrison, R. E. (1979). Radiation therapy of the oral cavity: Sequelae and management, Part I. *Head and Neck Surgery, 1,* 301–312.

Cacchillo, D., Barker, G. J., & Barker, B. F. (1993). Late effects of head and neck radiation therapy and patient/dentist compliance with recommended dental care. *Specialty Care Dentistry, 13,* 159–162.

Carl, W. (1980). Dental management of head and neck cancer patients. *Journal of Surgical Oncology, 15,* 265–281.

Carl, W. (1993). Local radiation and systemic chemotherapy: preventing and managing the oral complications. *Journal of the American Dental Association, 124,* 119–123.

Carter, L. W. (1992). Alternatives to unwaxed floss and peroxide rinses recommended. *Oncology Nursing Forum, 19,* 939–940.

Carter, P. (1986). Pain relief for mucositis. *Oncology Nursing Forum, 13,* 88.

Cartwright, F., & Facciponti C. (1992). Educational guide improves management of xerostomia. *Oncology Nursing Forum, 19,* 941.

Cheater, F. (1985). Xerostomia in malignant disease. *Nursing Mirror, 161,* 25–27.

Clark, P. I., & Slevin, M. L. (1985). Allopurinol mouthwashes and 5-fluorouracil induced oral toxicity. *European Journal of Surgical Oncology, 11,* 267–268.

Clinical Practice Committee. (1982). Guidelines for nursing care of patients with altered protective mechanisms. *Oncology Nursing Forum, 9*(1), 68–73.

Conger, A. (1973). Loss and recovery of taste acuity in patients irradiated to the oral cavity. *Radiation Research, 53,* 338–347.

Cunningham, M. (1984). Dental prosthetics: Physical and microbial insults. *Oncology Nursing Forum, 11,* 78.

Daeffler, R. (1980a). Oral hygiene measures for patients with cancer. I. *Cancer Nursing, 3,* 347–356.

Daeffler, R. (1980b). Oral hygiene measures for patients with cancer. II. *Cancer Nursing, 3,* 427–432.

Daeffler, R. (1981). Oral hygiene measures for patients with cancer. III. *Cancer Nursing, 4,* 29–35.

DeGregorio, M. W., Lee, W. M. F., & Ries, C. A. (1982). *Candida* infections in patients with acute leukemia: Ineffectiveness of nystatin prophylaxis and relationship between oropharyngeal and systemic candidiasis. *Cancer, 50,* 2780–2784.

DePaola, L. G. (1983). The use of an interim protective prosthesis during cancer chemotherapy. *Journal of Prosthetic Dentistry, 49,* 527–528.

DePaola, L. G., Peterson, D. E., Leupold, R. J., & Overholser, C. D. (1983). Prosthodontic considerations for patients undergoing cancer chemotherapy. *Journal of the American Dental Association, 107,* 48–51.

de Vries-Hospers, H. G., Mulder, N. H., Sleijfer, D. T., & Van Saene, H. K. F. (1982). The effect of amphotericin B lozenges on the presence and number of *Candida* cells in the oropharynx of neutropenic leukemia patients. *Infection, 10,* 71–75.

DeWalt, E. M. (1975). Effect of timed hygienic measures on oral mucosa in a group of elderly subjects. *Nursing Research, 24,* 104–108.

DeWalt, E. M., & Haines, A. K. (1969). The effects of specified stressors on healthy oral mucosa. *Nursing Research, 18,* 22–27.

Donnelly, J. P., Starke, I. D., Galton, D. A. G., Catovsky, D., Goldman, J. M., & Darrell, J. H. (1984). Oral ketoconazole and amphotericin B for the prevention of yeast colonization in patients with acute leukemia. *Journal of Hospital Infection, 5,* 83–91.

Dreizen, S., Brown, L. R., Daly, T. E., & Drane, J. B. (1977). Prevention of xerostomia-related dental caries in irradiated cancer patients. *Journal of Dental Research, 56,* 99–104.

Dudjak, L. A. (1985). The effects of two oral care protocols on mucositis due to head and neck radiation. *Oncology Nursing Forum, 12*(Suppl.); Abstract No. 194.

Dudjak, L. A. (1987). Mouth care for mucositis due to radiation therapy. *Cancer Nursing, 10* (3), 131–140.

Eilers, J., Berger, A. M., & Petersen, M. C. (1988). Development, testing and application of the oral assessment guide. *Oncology Nursing Forum, 15,* 325–330.

Epstein, J. B. (1989). Oral and pharyngeal candidiasis. *Postgraduate Medicine, 85,* 257–269.

Epstein, J. B., & Wong, F. L. (1994). The efficacy of sucralfate suspension in the prevention of oral mucositis due to radiation therapy. *International Journal of Radiation Oncology, Biology and Physics, 28,* 693–698.

Ezzone, S., Jolly, D., Replogle, K., Kapoor, N., & Tutschka, P. J. (1993). Survey of oral hygiene regimens among bone marrow transplant centers. *Oncology Nursing Forum, 20,* 1375–1381.

Ferraro, J. M., & Mattern, J. Q. A. (1984). Sucralfate suspension for stomatitis. *Drug Intelligence and Clinical Pharmacy, 18,* 153.

Gallucci, B. B., & Iwamoto, R. R. (1981). *Taste alterations in patients with cancer.* Nursing Care of the Cancer Patient with Nutritional Problems: Report of the Ross Oncology Nursing Round Table, pp. 40–46.

Gentzsch, P. (1983). Control of pain associated with stomatitis. *Oncology Nursing Forum, 10,* 78.

Ginsberg, M. K. (1961). A study of oral hygiene nursing care. *American Journal of Nursing, 61,* 67–69.

Goodman, M. S., & Stoner, C. (1985). Mucous membrane integrity, impairment of: Stomatitis. In J. C. McNally, J. C. Stair, & E. T. Somerville, (Eds.), *Guidelines for cancer nursing practice* (pp. 178–182). Orlando: Grune & Stratton, Inc.

Graham, K. M., Pecoraro, D. A., Ventura, M. & Meyer, C. C. (1993). Reducing the incidence of stomatitis using a quality assessment and improvement approach. *Cancer Nursing, 16,* 117–122.

Harchar, M. A. J. (1981). *The effect of five chemotherapeutic agents and nystatin on normal oral and skin flora and on common pathogenic organisms.* Unpublished master's thesis, University of Washington, Seattle, WA.

Hart, C. N., & Rasmussen, D. (1982). Patient care evaluation: A comparison of current practice and nursing literature for oral care of persons receiving chemotherapy. *Oncology Nursing Forum, 9,* 22–27.

Hickey, A. J., Toth, B. B., & Lindquist, S. B. (1982). Effect of intravenous hyperalimentation and oral care on the development of oral stomatitis during cancer chemotherapy. *Journal of Prosthetic Dentistry, 47,* 188–193.

Hilderley, L. (1986). Relieving radiation esophagitis. *Oncology Nursing Forum, 13,* 71.

Hogan, C. (1983). Oral hygiene. *Oncology Nursing Forum, 10,* 69.

Hogan, C. (1984). Vitamin E for stomatitis. *Oncology Nursing Forum, 11,* 69.

Holmes, S. (1991). The oral complications of specific anticancer therapy. *International Journal of Nursing Studies, 28,* 343–360.

Hyland, S. (1986). Selecting a tool for measuring stomatitis. *Oncology Nursing Forum, 13,* 119–120.

Iwamoto, R. R. (1981). *The nutritional status of patients with head and neck cancer receiving radiation therapy.* Unpublished master's thesis, University of Washington, Seattle, WA.

Johnson, J. T., Ferretti, G. A., Nethery, W. J., Valdez, I. H., Fox, P. C., Ng, D., Muscoplat, C. C., & Gallagher, S. C. (1993). Oral pilocarpine for post-irradiation xerostomia in patients with head and neck cancer. *New England Journal of Medicine, 329,* 390–395.

Jones, D., & Hafermann, M. D. (1986). A radiolucent bite-block apparatus. *International Journal of Radiation Oncology, Biology and Physics, 13,* 129.

Kenny, S. A. (1990). Effect of two oral care protocols on the incidence of stomatitis in hematology patients. *Cancer Nursing, 13,* 345–353.

Ketron, F. R. (1984). Chemotherapy: Oral hygiene measures for resulting stomatitis. *Journal of Tennessee Dental Association, 64,* 36–38.

Ladd, L. (1991). The dry mouth dilemma. *Oncology Nursing Forum, 18,* 785–786.

Lane, B., & Forgay, M. (1981). Upgrading your oral hygiene protocol for the patient with cancer. *The Canadian Nurse, 77,* 27–29.

Larsen, G. L. (1982). Rehabilitation for the patient with head and neck cancer. *American Journal of Nursing, 82,* 119–122.

LeVeque, F. G., Montgomery, M., Potter, D., Zimmer, M. B., Rieke, J. W., Steiger, B. W., Gallagher, S., & Muscoplat, C. C. (1993). A multicenter, randomized, double-blind, placebo-controlled, dose-titration study of oral pilocarpine for treatment of radiation-induced xerostomia in head and neck cancer patients. *Journal of Clinical Oncology, 11*(6), 1124–1131.

Levin, A. C., & Ferris, G. M. (1980). The treatment of post-radiation therapy patients. *Florida Dental Journal, 51,* 41–44.

Lindquist, S. F., Hickey, A. J., & Drane, J. B. (1978). Effect of oral hygiene on stomatitis in patients receiving cancer chemotherapy. *Journal of Prosthetic Dentistry, 40,* 312–314.

Lowe, O. (1986). Pretreatment dental assessment and management of patients undergoing head and neck irradiation. *Clinical Preventive Dentistry, 8,* 24–30.

Mansfield, M. J., Sanders, D. W., Heimbach, R. D., & Marx, R. E. (1981). Hyperbaric oxygen as an adjunct in the treatment of osteoradionecrosis of the mandible. *Journal of Oral Surgery, 39,* 585–589.

McCarthy-Leventhal, E. (1959). Post-radiation mouth blindness. *Lancet, 2,* 1138–1139.

McElroy, T. H. (1984). Infection in the patient receiving chemotherapy for cancer. Oral considerations. *Journal of the American Dental Association, 109,* 454–456.

McGaw, W. T., & Belch, A. (1985). Oral complications of acute leukemia: Prophylactic impact of a chlorhexidine mouth rinse regimen. *Oral Surgery, Oral Medicine, and Oral Pathology, 60,* 275–280.

McGuire, D. B., Altomonte, V., Peterson, D. E., Wingard, J. R., Jones, R. J., & Grochow, L. B. (1993). Patterns of mucositis and pain in patients receiving preparative chemotherapy and bone marrow transplantation. *Oncology Nursing Forum, 20,* 1493–1502.

Miller, E. C., Vergo, T. J., & Feldman, M. I. (1981). Dental management of patients undergoing radiation therapy for cancer of the head and neck. *The Compendium of Continuing Education, 2,* 350–356.

Minah, G. G., Rednor, J. L., Peterson, D. E., Overholser, C. D., DePaola, L. G., & Suzuki, J. B. (1986). Oral succession of gram-negative bacilli in myelosuppressed cancer patients. *Journal of Clinical Microbiology, 24,* 210–213.

Mosco, M. (1986). Oral irrigation tips. *Oncology Nursing Forum, 13,* 88.

Mossman, K., Shatzman, A., & Chencharick, J. (1982). Long-term effects of radiotherapy on taste and salivary function in man. *International Journal of Radiation Oncology, Biology and Physics, 8,* 991–997.

Mossman, K. L., & Henkin, R. T. (1978). Radiation-induced changes in taste acuity in cancer patients. *International Journal of Radiation Oncology, Biology and Physics, 4,* 663–670.

National Institutes of Health. (1989). Oral complications of cancer therapies: Diagnosis, prevention, and treatment. *Consensus Development Conference Statement, 7*(7), 1–11.

Oncology Staff Nurses. (1982). Stomatitis treatment. *Oncology Nursing Forum, 9*(4), 65.

Ostchega, Y. (1980). Preventing and treating cancer chemotherapy's oral complications. *Nursing '80, 10,* 47–52.

Passos, J. Y., & Brand, L. M. (1966). Effects of agents used for oral hygiene. *Nursing Research, 15,* 196–202.

Pegram, S. (1983). Atomizer helps mouth care. *Oncology Nursing Forum, 10,* 59.

Pehanrich, M. (1983). A tip for the taste buds . . . . *Oncology Nursing Forum, 10,* 60.

Peterson, D. E., & Sonis, S. T. (1982). Oral complications of cancer chemotherapy: Present status and future studies. *Cancer Treatment Reports, 66,* 1251–1256.

Poland, J. M. (1987). Comparing Moi-stir to lemon-glycerin swabs. *American Journal of Nursing, 87,* 422–424.

Poland, J. (1991). Prevention and treatment of oral complications in the cancer patient. *Oncology, 5,* 45–50.

Porter, C., Moroni, M., & Nastasi, G. (1994). Allopurinol mouthwashes in the treatment of 5-fluorouracil-induced stomatitis. *American Journal of Clinical Oncology, 17,* 246–247.

Preston, F. A. (1983). Management of oral bleeding caused by thrombocytopenia. *Oncology Nursing Forum, 10,* 59.

Quintiliani, R., Owens, N. J., Quercia, R. A., Klimek, J. J., & Nightingale, C. H. (1984). Treatment and prevention of oropharyngeal candidiasis. *American Journal of Medicine, 76,* 44–48.

Raybould, T. P., Carpenter, A. D., Ferretti, G. A., Brown, A. T., Lillich, T. T., & Henslee, J. (1994). Emergence of gram-negative bacilli in the mouths of bone marrow transplant recipients using chlorhexidine mouthrinse. *Oncology Nursing Forum, 21,* 691–696.

Rieke, J. W., Hafermann, M. D., Johnson, J. T., LeVeque, F. G., Iwamoto, R., Steiger, B. W., Muscoplat, C. C. & Gallagher, S. (1995). Oral pilocarpine for radiation-induced xerostomia: integrated efficacy and safety results from two prospective randomized clinical trials. *International Journal of Radiation Oncology, Biology and Physics, 31,* 661–669.

Ritchie, J. R., Brown, J. R., Guerra, L. R., & Mason, G. (1985). Dental care for the irradiated cancer patient. *Quintessence International, 16,* 837–842.

Rocke, L. K., Loprinzi, C. L., Lee, J. K., Kunselman, S. J., Iverson R. K., Finck, G., Lifsey, D., Glaw, K. C., Stevens, B. A., Hatfield, A. K., Vaught, N. L., Bartel, J. & Pierson, N. (1993). A randomized clinical trial of two different durations of oral cryotherapy for prevention of 5-fluorouracil-related stomatitis. *Cancer, 72,* 2234–2238.

Rodu, B., & Russell, C. M. (1988). Performance of a hydroxypropyl cellulose film former in normal and ulcerated oral mucosa. *Oral Surgery, Oral Medicine, Oral Pathology, 65,* 699–703.

Rosenberg, S. W. (1991). The article reviewed: prevention and treatment of oral complications in the cancer patient. *Oncology, 5,* 57.

Rowan, C. (1992). Peridex® decreases oral mucositis. *Oncology Nursing Forum, 19,* 939.

Schubert, M. M., & Newton, R. E. (1987). The use of benzydamine HCl for the management of cancer therapy-induced mucositis: Preliminary report of a multicentre study. *International Journal of Tissue Reactions, 9,* 99–103.

Schweiger, J. L., Lang, J. W., & Schweiger, J. W. (1980). Oral assessment. How to do it. *American Journal of Nursing, 80,* 654–657.

Sciubba, J. J. (1991). The article reviewed: Prevention and treatment of oral complications in the cancer patient. *Oncology, 5,* 52.

Shechtman, L. B., Funaro, L., Robin, T., Bottone, E. J., & Cuttner, J. (1984). Clotrimazole treatment of oral candidiasis in patients with neoplastic disease. *American Journal of Medicine, 76,* 91–94.

Shenep, J. L., Kalwinsky, D. K., Hutson, P. R., George, S. L., Dodge, R. K., Blankenship, K. R., & Thornton, D. (1988). Efficacy of oral sucralfate suspension in prevention and treatment of chemotherapy-induced mucositis. *Journal of Pediatrics, 113,* 758–763.

Sonis, S., & Clark, J. (1991). Prevention and management of oral mucositis induced by antineoplastic therapy. *Oncology, 5,* 11–18.

Strohl, R. (1983). Taste sensations after radiation therapy. *Oncology Nursing Forum, 10,* 80.

Strohl, R. (1984). Understanding taste changes. *Oncology Nursing Forum, 11,* 81–84.

Sullivan, M. D., & Fleming, T. J. (1986). Oral care for the radiotherapy-treated head and neck cancer patient. *Dental Hygiene, 60,* 112–114.

Tombes, M. E. (1987). *The effects of hydrogen peroxide rinses on normal oral mucosa.* Unpublished master's thesis, University of Washington, Seattle, WA.

Van Drimmelen, J., & Rollins, H. F. (1969). Evaluation of a commonly used oral hygiene agent. *Nursing Research, 18,* 327–332.

Weisdorf, D. J., Bostrom, B., Raether, D., Mattingly, M., Walker, P., Pihlstrom, B., Ferrieri, P., Haake, R., Goldman, A., Woods, W., Ramsay, N. K. C., & Kersey, J. H. (1989). Oropharyngeal mucositis complicating bone marrow transplantation: Prognostic factors and the effect of chlorhexidine mouth rinses. *Bone Marrow Transplantation, 4,* 89–95.

Weitzman, S. A., Weitberg, A. B., Niederman, R., & Stossel, T. P. (1984). Chronic treatment with hydrogen peroxide: Is it safe? *Journal of Periodontology, 55,* 510–511.

Wescott, W. B. (1985). Dental management of patients being treated for oral cancer. *CDA Journal, 13,* 42–47.

Western Consortium for Cancer Nursing Research. (1991). Development of a staging system for chemotherapy-induced stomatitis. *Cancer Nursing, 14,* 6–12.

Wiley, S. B. (1969). Why glycerol and lemon juice? *American Journal of Nursing, 69,* 342–344.

Wilkes, G. M. (1986). Sucralfate suspension for mucositis. *Oncology Nursing Forum, 13,* 71–72.

Williams, L. T., Peterson, D. E., & Overholser, C. D. (1982). Acute peridontal infection in myelosuppressed oncology patients: Evaluation and nursing care. *Cancer Nursing, 5,* 465–467.

Zerbe, M. B., Parkerson, S. G., Ortlieb, M. L., & Spitzer, T. (1992). Relationships between oral mucositis and treatment variables in bone marrow transplant patients. *Cancer Nursing, 15,* 196–205.

Infection is a common occurrence in patients with cancer as a result of the underlying disease, treatment for the disease, or prolonged hospitalization. Infection is defined as the process by which microbes enter a susceptible site in the body and multiply, resulting in disease (Clark, Landis, & McGee, 1987). The type of infection likely to occur in patients with cancer is fairly predictable, and therefore, infections are potentially preventable and often treatable.

This chapter describes normal host defense mechanisms, such as skin and mucous membranes, the pathophysiologic effects caused by cancer, cancer treatments or other factors, nursing assessment, care of persons who are at risk for or have cancer-related infection, and preventive measures shown to be useful in reducing infections in patients with neoplastic disease.

HOST DEFENSE MECHANISMS

SKIN AND MUCOUS MEMBRANES

The skin is the body's largest organ and the first line of defense against invading organisms. The skin is continuous with mucous membranes at external openings of the digestive, respiratory, and urogenital organ systems. Skin and mucous membrane integrity are at risk in patients with cancer due to the effects of chemotherapy, radiotherapy, surgery, and invasive diagnostic procedures and devices. Skin lesions or ulcerations secondary to tumor, alterations in tissue integrity throughout the gastrointestinal tract, the development of oral mucosal lesions from treatments, and inadequate nutrition are just a few examples of the way can-

cer and its treatment disrupts the defensive barrier provided by the skin and mucous membranes.

BONE MARROW

The hematologic system contains blood and sites where blood is produced and stored including the bone marrow, spleen, and lymphoid tissues. Bone marrow is the principal site for production of blood cells. From birth until about the age of 4 years, most bones are involved in hematopoiesis. By the age of 18 years, much of the marrow has been replaced by fat cells, so that hematopoietic marrow is found only in the vertebrae, ribs, skull, pelvis, and proximal epiphyses of the femur and humerus. The distribution of active bone marrow in adults is illustrated in Figure 53–1. In the elderly, the proportion of fatty marrow increases so that only half of the ribs and sternum are sites of hematopoiesis.

Physiologic function of bone marrow depends on a number of factors, including the availability of selected micronutrients, a specialized microenvironment, normal stem cell function, regulation by specific hematopoietic and other hormones, and feedback inhibition from cell production (Gordon & Barrett, 1985). The reticular cells and stroma, which contain macrophages and fat cells, provide a hematopoietic inductive microenvironment (HIM), which is essential to blood cell production. The exact nature of HIM in humans is unclear. The marrow is also richly innervated, suggesting one mechanism by which the marrow may be activated on demand. These nerves may influence blood flow in the marrow and cellular release by

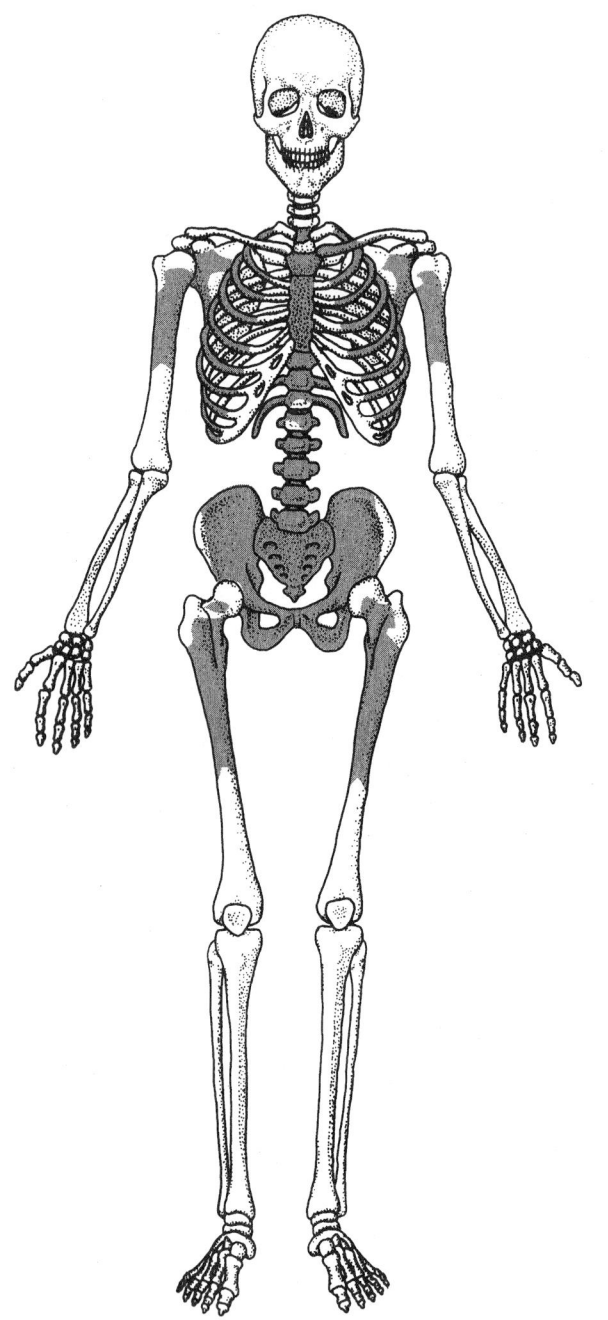

FIGURE 53–1. Distribution of active bone marrow in a normal adult. The shaded portion represents the area of active marrow.

responding to changes in intramedullary pressure and to extramedullary influences.

SPLEEN

The spleen contains both lymphoid and reticuloendothelial components. The spleen is an "early responder" to infection. It is a site of antibody and opsonin activity (opsonins prepare foreign material for phagocytosis). Other functions include phagocytosis, storage of platelets (20 to 30 per cent of the total platelet

mass), iron metabolism, and mechanical filtration of cellular and noncellular debris.

LYMPHOID TISSUE

Lymph nodes are collections of lymphocytes, plasma cells, and macrophages existing in chains along the course of large blood vessels throughout the body. They drain regional tissue and empty into large, efferent lymph channels, clearing foreign material from the blood. Solitary lymph nodules found in certain parts of the body (such as the Peyer's patches of the ileum) produce a local response to antigen (any substance introduced into an organism that will elicit an immune response).

NORMAL HEMATOPOIETIC PROCESSES

Normal hematopoiesis results in the production of white cells, platelets, and red cells, and the processes of proliferation, differentiation, and maturation are mediated by various humoral factors. Predominant among these are the expanding set of hematopoietic growth factors, also known as colony-stimulating factors (CSFs) or naturally occurring glycoproteins. Figure 53–2 provides a schematic of marrow cell kinetics that illustrates the continuum of proliferation and differentiation of stem cells and the factors that mediate the process.

The stem cell is the foundation of bone marrow hematopoiesis. Pluripotential stem cells, the youngest and most "primitive" of stem cells purified to homogeneity thus far, are capable of extensive, possibly lifelong self-renewal and of differentiation to all cell lineages, both myeloid and lymphoid (Whetton & Dexter, 1993). This concept of self-renewal (or stem cell immortality) is important when the effects of cancer treatment on bone marrow and people's ability to recover bone marrow function after cytotoxic treatment are considered. One explanation of this concept hypothesizes a "stem cell niche," in which one daughter cell remains in a regulatory framework of cells, retaining its capacity for self-renewal. The other daughter cell leaves the niche to enter the HIM of the marrow. On being exposed to the various influences in HIM, including growth factors, this daughter cell is induced to divide further and gradually loses its capacity of self-renewal as it proceeds to differentiate (Graham & Pragnell, 1992).

Multipotential stem cells are characterized by limited self-renewal capability. These cells, like pluripotential stem cells, are not irreversibly committed to a single cell lineage but are more differentiated than pluripotential stem cells. The best example of a multipotential stem cell is the CFU-GEMM (Fig. 53–2). (The term colony-forming unit [CFU] or colony-forming cell [CFC] preceeding the name of a cell line describes a specific stem cell or progenitor cell.) CFU-GEMM is capable of differentiating to a more mature progenitor cell in any one

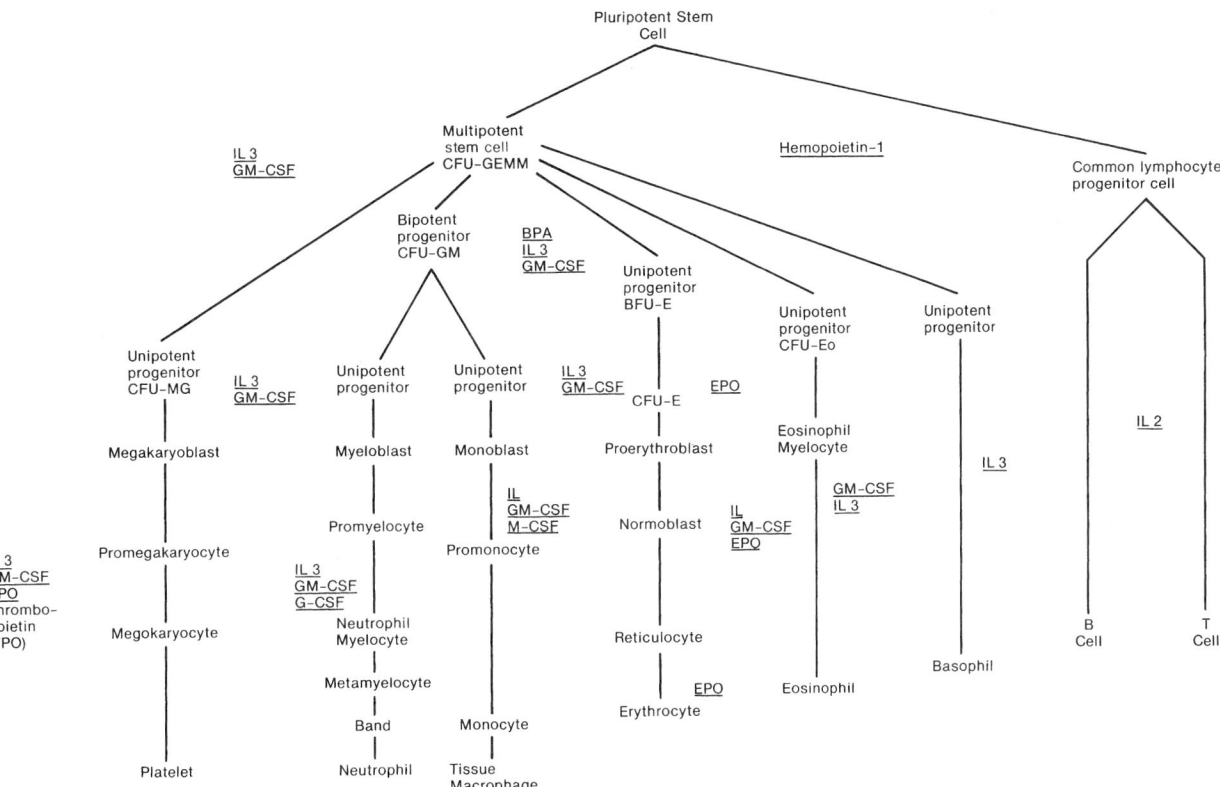

FIGURE 53–2. Schematic of marrow cell kinetics, proliferation, and differentiation. Factors mediating cell differentiation are italicized. CFU = colony-forming unit; GEMM = *g*ranulocyte, *e*rythroid, *m*onocyte, *m*egakaryocyte; Eo = eosinophil; CSF = *c*olony-stimulating *f*actor; IL = interleukin; G-CSF = granulocyte colony-stimulating factor; GM-CSF = granulocyte-macrophage colony-stimulating factor; M-CSF = macrophage colony-stimulating factor; BPA = burst-promoting activity; EPO = Erythropoietin; BFU-E = burst-forming unit-erythroid; CFU-E = colony-forming unit-erythroid; CFU-GM = colony-forming unit-granulocyte-monocyte.

of the following cell lines: granulocyte, erythroid, monocyte, or megakaryocyte. These cells provide offspring that are better differentiated and more responsive to poietins. Bipotential cells are progenitor cells capable of limited self-renewal and of differentiation to two cell lines. Unipotential cells are progenitor cells capable of limited self-renewal and of differentiation to one cell line (e.g., CFC-Eo [eosinophil]; CFC-Mk [megakaryocyte]). The progeny of these various progenitor cells are termed precursor cells and are incapable of self-renewal, and they are morphologically recognizable as members of a single cell line.

Another important element in the process of normal hematopoiesis is a set of growth factors termed colony stimulating factors (CSFs). These are highly specific proteins or cytokines that stimulate progenitor and precursor cells to differentiate and mature. Hematopoiesis is dependent on their presence. As with other cytokines, CSFs act on target cells via receptors on cell membranes. Numerous types of CSFs have been identified. Some, such as multi-CSF, interleukin 2 (IL-2), and granulocyte-macrophage-CSF (GM-CSF), affect more than one cell line. Others, such as granulocyte-CSF (G-CSF) and erythropoietin, are specific to a particular cell line or a group of precursor cells.

LEUKOPOIESIS

Leukopoiesis or granulopoiesis refers to the development, differentiation, and maturation of white blood cells (WBCs). The major function of WBCs is to defend the host against infection. White blood cells are divided into two main groups: *granulocytes* (polymorphonuclear leukocytes) consisting of neutrophils, eosinophils, and basophils, and *agranulocytes* (mononuclear leukocytes) consisting of lymphocytes and monocytes-precursors of macrophages. These cells and their functions, except for lymphocytes, which will be discussed in more detail later, are listed in Table 53–1. Table 53–2 shows the total white blood cell count, as well as the differential white cell count, that is used to identify the five types of leukocytes in the peripheral blood. This test gives the health care provider clues to the patient's current clinical status. For example, an increase in circulating neutrophils (neutrophilia) is usually due to increased output from the bone marrow in response to bacterial infections, inflammation and necrosis of tissues, or to acute hemorrhage.

WBCs are responsible for both cell-mediated immunity (CMI) and humoral immunity (HI). Cell-mediated immunity refers to immune defenses that rely on a

TABLE 53–1. *Functions of Granulocytes and Monocytes*

CELL TYPE	FUNCTION
Granulocyte	
Neutrophil	Phagocytosis, random locomotion, chemotaxis, killing microorganisms, pus formation, lysosome production
Basophil	Releases histamine, heparin, and enzymes in acute inflammation; may prevent clot formation and growth
Eosinophil	Phagocytosis and elaboration of enzymes in allergic reactions; may contribute to fibrin clot digestion; detoxify foreign protein
Monocytes-macrophages	
Blood (free)	Phagocytosis of microorganisms, tumors, cellular debris
Tissue (fixed; also called histiocytes)	Phagocytosis of microorganisms, tumor, cellular and noncellular debris; mediate lymphocyte antibody activity; filtration of particles

direct cellular activity (e.g., phagocytosis by a neutrophil). Humoral immunity refers to immune defenses that rely on an indirect cellular activity (e.g., the production of antibody by B lymphocytes).

The production and release of granulocytes and monocytes is mediated by various hemopoietic-negative and -positive regulators acting in concert to provide a mechanism for rapid, reversible, and specific proliferative responses to changes in the demand for these cells (Axelrod, 1990). Little is known about how hemopoietic-negative regulators work, but the positive regulators, or CSFs, have been studied longer and are influenced by the presence of infection and inflammation and by exercise, stress, and glucocorticoids. The interaction between infection and the increased production of neutrophils has not been clearly defined. It seems to involve a feedback loop in which the presence of endotoxins and other bacterial by-products causes increased production and release of CSFs by macrophages and endothelial cells, which in turn leads to the proliferation and release of neutrophils from the bone marrow. In addition, another humoral agent, neutrophil-releasing factor, has been postulated. There is probably a negative arm of the feedback loop in which the presence of mature neutrophils causes certain subpopulations of monocytes to release prostaglandin E (PgE), which has an inhibitory effect on the neutrophil

population. Various populations of lymphocytes, such as natural killer (NK) cells, are also involved in this process.

The multipotential progenitors of granulocytes are granulocyte, erythroid, monocyte, megakaryocyte (GEMM-CFC), or granulocyte-monocyte colony-forming cells (GM-CFC). During proliferation, these cells divide and differentiate to myeloblasts, promyelocytes, and myelocytes. As these cells mature they become metamyelocytes, bands, and finally, neutrophils, basophils, or eosinophils. Neutrophils are the first line of defense against infection. They constitute 50 to 70 per cent of the total WBC count (Table 53–2). Immature neutrophils are referred to as bands (0 to 5 per cent of the total neutrophil count) or segmental forms (50 to 65 per cent of the total neutrophil count) because of the nature of their nuclei. "Left shift" is a term used to describe an increase in the percentage of neutrophils and bands (immature neutrophils) in response to infection. When an infection occurs, the level of circulating neutrophils increases through the processes described above.

In addition to their presence in the marrow, granulocytes exist in the bloodstream as a circulating pool, where they have a half-life of about 6 to 8 hours. (Granulocytes have a half-life of 7 to 14 days in the tissues.) They are quite mobile and can be attracted to the site of

TABLE 53–2. *Values for White Blood Cells and the Differential*

CELL TYPE	Normal Range*	
	RELATIVE VALUE (%)	ABSOLUTE VALUE (CELLS/MM³)
Total white blood count	100	500–10,000
Granulocytes		
Neutrophils (Total)	50–70	2500–7000
Segments	50–65	2500–6500
Bands	0–5	0–500
Eosinophils	1–4	100–400
Basophils	0.5–1.0	50–100
Agranulocytes		
Lymphocytes	25–45	1500–4000
Monocytes	2–6	100–500

*Normal values vary slightly depending on laboratory equipment.
(Adapted by permission from McFarland, M. B., & Grant, M. M. [1994]. *Nursing implications of laboratory tests* [3rd ed.]. Albany, NY: Delmar Publishers. Copyright 1994.)

infection by a process called chemotaxis. Once there, granulocytes are capable of becoming attached to vessel endothelial cells (marginating) and can enter the tissues by diapedesis. This process allows the cells, portions of which are momentarily constricted, to squeeze through pores in blood vessels. In cancer patients, depressed neutrophil counts are often associated with cancer therapies or infiltration of bone marrow by cancer.

Less is known about basophils than about the other granulocytes. They are not phagocytic. The granules in the basophils are related to the granules in mast cells, and therefore, these two cell lines are usually considered together. In fact, debate continues on whether basophils are precursors of mast cells. Mast cells, located outside many capillaries in the body, play a role in allergies, anaphylactic shock, and regulation of blood flow. Elevations of basophils are associated with some cancers, with postsplenectomy states, and with estrogen use. However, their numbers seem unaffected by infection. Basophils constitute up to 0.5 to 1 per cent of the total WBC (Table 53–2). Eosinophils detoxify foreign protein. They control the effects of mast cells and neutralize the products of mast cells. Eosinophils account for 1 to 4 per cent of the total WBC (Table 53–2).

Monocytes (Table 53–1) act as mechanical barriers against organisms and play a role, previously described, in the neutrophil feedback loop. Fixed monocytes (macrophages) are found in the spleen, lymph nodes, bone marrow, liver capsule, and adrenals. In addition to their phagocytic activities, macrophages influence antibody synthesis by lymphocytes. They are sensitive to steroids, and elevations in their numbers occur in persons with chronic infections, in those recovering from infection, and in those with neutropenia.

LYMPHOPOIESIS

Lymphopoiesis is the term used to describe the process for lymphocyte maturation. Although the development of lymphocytes occurs separately from that of other blood cell lineages, research indicates that like other cell lines, the lymphoid line has its origin in the pluripotential stem cells discussed above. At some point soon after the initial division of the pluripotential stem cell into daughter cells, the lymphoid line follows a separate course, influenced by some of the same CSFs (e.g., interleukin 3 [IL-3] or multi-CSF) as well as by different ones (IL-2).

Development of lymphocytes depends on the migration of bone marrow precursors to specialized sites in the mononuclear phagocyte system (MPS) (formerly termed the reticuloendothelial system or RES), where further proliferation and differentiation occur. This sequence is illustrated in Figure 53–2. The lymphocyte stem cell gives rise to at least two types of cells: the T lymphocytes (T cells), which mature under the influence of thymic endothelium (a thymopoietin has been postulated), and the B lymphocytes (B cells), which differentiate and mature in the MPS in response to a postulated B cell growth factor.

Each of these cell groups performs a variety of functions (Table 53–3). Their primary role is to enable the

TABLE 53–3. *Functions of Lymphocytes*

CELL	FUNCTION
Lymphocytes	
B cells (humoral immunity)	Complement fixation
Plasma cell	Antibody production
Memory cell	"Remembers" antigen
T cells (cellular immunity)	
Null cells (natural killer and killer cells)	Produce lymphokins; destroy cells directly or indirectly
Helper cells	Medicate antibody production by B cells; promote T cell activity
Suppressor cells	Diminish B cell and possibly T cell activity; mediate both cellular and humoral immunity
Memory cells	Recognize and respond to previously encountered antigens

immune system to distinguish self from nonself or foreign antigens, and to respond to foreign antigens. These cells are responsible for the "memory" of the immune system, so that when exposed to the same antigen in the future, a quicker response can be mounted. T cells have both regulator and effector functions in the immune system. T cells are the primary effectors of CMI and immunoregulation. They mediate delayed cutaneous hypersensitivity reactions and transplant rejection. They seem to orchestrate the overall immune response to specific antigen as well as provide immunosurveillance against cancer. T cells protect against fungi and viruses and respond to bacterial diseases that have an insidious onset.

Lymphocytes are mobile and long-lived. Their life span may be measured in terms of years. They recirculate by passing from the thoracic duct into the bloodstream, which carries the cells to the lymph nodes. Lymphocytes can also be transported to lymph nodes through lymphatic drainage. Lymphocytes constitute 25 to 45 per cent of the total WBC count. Elevations in their numbers are seen in viral infections. Lymphopenia is often associated with the acquired immunodeficiency syndrome (AIDS).

PATHOPHYSIOLOGIC EFFECTS OF CANCER AND CANCER THERAPY ON INFECTION

As a compromised host, the patient with cancer is at risk for developing infection as a result of altered or deficient defense mechanisms (Wujcik, 1993). In addition to marrow replacement by tumor, the patient often experiences bone marrow toxicity from chemotherapy, radiation therapy, and surgery. When caring for persons with cancer, the nurse needs to be alert to these and other factors, such as nutrition and age, that may predispose patients to infection. The best predictor of infection in patients with cancer is the presence of neutropenia. Neutropenia is defined as an absolute neutrophil count (ANC) of less than 1000 cells/mm³ (Table 53–4). The ANC indicates the number of cells capable of fighting infection by phagocytosis. An ANC less than 1000 cells/mm³ increases the patient's risk for acquiring an infection. The longer the duration of neutropenia and/or the lower the ANC, the higher the risk is for life-threatening infection (Table 53–5).

TUMOR EFFECTS

Cancer may cause infection directly or indirectly. Invasion and replacement of the bone marrow by tumor is called myelophthisis. Cancer cells compete with normal hematopoietic cells for nutrients and destroy hematopoietic cells. Granulocytopenia and impaired NK cell activity may result (Beck, 1985; Sarzotti, Baron, & Klimpel, 1987). Acute leukemias infiltrate the marrow, creating pancytopenia, which places the patient at risk for multiple complications from bone marrow depression (BMD).

Cancer can cause infection or alter immune regulation whether or not bone marrow invasion occurs (Robinson & Donowitz, 1992). With cancer there is a decrease in T cell proliferation in response to mitogens, antigens, allogeneic major histocompatibility complex (MHC) molecules, syngeneic MHC molecules, and a reduction in the percentage of CD4+ T cells (Walker, Burger & Elgert, 1994). Cancer alters macrophage functions during T cell proliferation and decreases expression of MHC class II molecules. Many functional alterations are associated with tumor-induced changes in cytokine synthesis and responsiveness, and these changes result in the failure of the immune system to mount an effective attack when challenged.

CHEMOTHERAPY

The treatment most often associated with hematologic toxicity and bone marrow suppression is chemotherapy. The degree to which a patient experiences bone marrow suppression after chemotherapy depends on the agent(s) used; dosage, schedules, and routes of administration; previous antineoplastic treatment; concomitant adjuvant therapy; and other factors such as age, nutritional status, tumor type, and stage of disease.

The hematologic toxicity of chemotherapy varies widely. Acute chemotherapy-induced myelosuppression is usually caused by the destruction of the proliferating progenitors (e.g., CFU-GM, BFU-E) of mature cells. As progenitor cells are destroyed, preexisting mature cells are removed at the end of their natural cycles, and the nadir or lowest point of a person's blood cell count occurs. The incidence of granulocytopenia is due to the relatively brief life cycle of neutrophils.

Antineoplastic agents that are phase-specific are myelosuppressive because of their impact on proliferating progenitor cells, which are in active phases when drugs are administered, but do not destroy cells in the resting phase. Agents that are phase-nonspecific destroy cells in the resting phase and can have a delayed, prolonged, and cumulative myelosuppressive effect. This is a consequence of the damage they do to nonproliferating stem cells, which are essential in the marrow response to a challenge such as chemotherapy. The relative degrees of myelosuppression of specific agents are listed in Table 53–6.

A new approach to the problem of BMD involves the administration of CSFs or hematopoietic growth factors. The most commonly used CSFs are granulocyte colony-stimulating factor (G-CSF) and granulocyte-macrophage colony-stimulating factor (GM-CSF). These naturally occurring glycoprotein hormone-like substances stimulate one or more of the cell lines in the hematopoietic system, inducing proliferation and differentiation. Although their presence in the body has been known for some time, advances in genetic engineering have allowed them to be produced in "industrial" quantities and have led to clinical use of these agents.

Studies have documented that G-CSF enhances neutrophil recovery after various chemotherapy regimens, including those that are anthracycline- or platinum-based (Hollingshead & Goa, 1991). As a consequence of improved white cell counts, a reduction in the number of infectious episodes and fewer days of hospitalization and antibiotic treatment have been observed (Peters et al., 1993).

TABLE 53–4. *Calculation of Absolute Neutrophil Count (ANC)*

Total white blood cell count = 1600 m³
Differential: 41% polymorphonuclear leukocytes (or segments)
       14% bands
       38% lymphocytes
        0% eosinophils
        0% basophils
        7% monocytes

$$ANC = \text{total WBC} \frac{\times (\% \text{ polymorphonuclear leukocytes [or segments]} + \% \text{ bands})}{100}$$

$$ANC = 1600 \frac{\times (41 + 14)}{100}$$

$$ANC = 880$$

TABLE 53–5. *Risk of Bacterial Infection Associated with Granulocytopenia*

Absolute Granulocyte Count	Risk of Bacterial Infection
1500–2000 per mm^3	Not significant
> 1000 per mm^3	Minimal
> 500 per mm^3	Moderate
< 500 per mm^3	Severe

(From Brandt, B. [1984]. A nursing protocol for the client with neutropenia. *Oncology Nursing Forum, 11*[2], 24–28. Reproduced by permission.)

Clinical experience with GM-CSF has documented accelerated recovery of peripheral neutrophil counts after bone marrow transplantation, and results of placebo-controlled randomized trials correlate this with reduced infectious episodes and shortened length of hospitalization in patients with lymphoid malignancies (Grant & Heel, 1992).

In 1991, the Food and Drug Administration approved the use of both G-CSF and GM-CSF. G-CSF is indicated for the purpose of reducing the incidence of infection, as manifested by febrile neutropenia in patients with nonmyeloid malignancies receiving myelosuppressive anticancer drugs. GM-CSF has been approved for acceleration of myeloid recovery in patients undergoing autologous bone marrow transplantation for non-Hodgkin's lymphoma, acute lymphoblastic leukemia, and Hodgkin's disease. Side effects appear to be limited to mild to moderately severe bone pain that generally responds to analgesia and may resolve with continued use. Discontinuing treatment results in resolution of the discomfort.

The American Society of Clinical Oncology convened an expert panel to review the results of clinical data documenting the activity of CSFs. A clinical practice guideline was published in 1994 with the following recommendations:

Primary CSF Administration:

1. The expected incidence of chemotherapy-induced febrile neutropenia is ≥ 40 per cent.
2. Increased risk for developing chemotherapy-induced infectious complications due to:
   a. Preexisting neutropenia due to disease
   b. Extensive prior chemotherapy
   c. Previous irradiation to the pelvis or other areas containing large amounts of bone marrow
   d. History of febrile neutropenia while receiving earlier chemotherapy of similar or lesser dose intensity
   e. Conditions potentially increasing the risk of serious infection (i.e., open wounds).

Secondary CSF Administration:

1. If febrile neutropenia has not occurred, use of CSFs may be considered if prolonged neutropenia is causing excessive dose reduction or delay in chemotherapy (American Society of Clinical Oncology, 1994).

RADIOTHERAPY

The effects of radiotherapy on bone marrow and immunity are similar to those of chemotherapy. The immediate effects include neutropenia and thrombocytopenia increasing patient susceptibility to infections and hemorrhage and may interfere with treatment out-

TABLE 53–6. *Drug Class or Compound and Degree and Duration of Myelosuppression*

Drug or Drug Class	Degree of Suppression*	Nadir of Myelosuppression (Days)	Duration of Marrow Recovery (Days)
Anthracycline	III	8–13	21–24
Vinca alkaloids	I–II	4–8	7–21
Mustard alkylator			
Nitrogen mustard	III	7–14	28
Antifolates	III	7–14	14–21
Antipyrimidines	III	7–14	22–24
Antipurines	II	7–14	14–21
Podophyllotoxins	II	8–14	22–28
Alkylators	II	10–21	18–40
Nitrosoureas	III	28–60	35–85
Miscellaneous†			
Busulfan	III	11–30	24–54
Cisplatin	I	14	21
Dacarbazine	III	21–28	28–35
Hydroxyurea	II	7	14–21
Mithramycin	I	5–10	10–18
Mitomycin	II	28–42	42–56
Procarbazine	II	25–36	35–60
Razoxane (ICRF)	II	11–16	12–25

*I = mild; II = moderate; III = severe (based on common dose schedules).
†Agents differing from their class of compounds.
(From Hoagland, H. [1982]. Hematologic complications of cancer chemotherapy. *Seminars in Oncology, 9,* 95–102. Reproduced by permission.)

comes (Tubiana, Carde, & Frindel, 1993). Additionally, long-term effects include a depletion in the stem cell pool that reduces the ability of the bone marrow to react to an insult (Croizat, Frindel, & Tubiana, 1979).

Several factors in a radiotherapy treatment regimen determine the degree of risk for BMD. Although total radiation dosage and fractionation schedule are important, the most significant factor is the volume of productive marrow in the treatment field (Fig. 53–1). The volumes of bone marrow in several typical fields are listed in Table 53–7. In addition, radiation to sites that include major blood vessels and lymphatic channels is toxic to lymphocytes. For this reason, mediastinal radiotherapy can be more immunosuppressive than radiotherapy to other sites.

Radiotherapy is not as destructive to progenitor cells as chemotherapy, but it is much more damaging to cells in the G_o phase. Therefore, radiotherapy has a greater impact on pluripotential stem cells. Except for total nodal or total body irradiation, radiotherapy does not usually cause the nadirs in blood counts that are seen with chemotherapy. This is because radiation treatment is usually a local therapy that leaves substantial amounts of marrow intact; this marrow is able to compensate for the damage caused to the irradiated marrow (unless compromised by prior radiotherapy or prior chemotherapy).

Irradiated marrow recovers through a twofold process: (1) migration of stem cells from unirradiated bone marrow to the treated area and (2) conversion of mesenchymal cells in the haversian canal of the cortex of irradiated bone into actively proliferating cells (Rubin & Scarantino, 1978). An intact marrow stroma is vital to maintaining a suitable environment for stem cell seeding and hematopoiesis. However, unlike chemotherapy, radiotherapy has a clear, negative effect on stromal elements, causing disruption of the sinusoidal architecture, fibrosis, and necrosis (Fliedner, Northdurft, & Clavo, 1986). It is estimated that radiation doses above 8-Gy, without an accompanying bone marrow transplant, prevent bone marrow regeneration (Baranov, Selidovkin, Butturini, & Gale, 1994). However, there is clinical evidence in both animals and humans to suggest that even with very high doses of total body radiation, some stem cells survive (Schattenberg et al., 1989; Schuening et al., 1989).

The destruction of the bone marrow microenvironment and the fact that radiotherapy is most damaging to the pluripotential stem cell pool that is not actively proliferating account for the potential long-term effects of this therapy. Residual effects include hypoplasia or aplasia of certain marrow segments and a propensity to develop various myelodysplastic syndromes. As a result, the patient receiving radiotherapy may be relatively intolerant of further antineoplastic therapy such as chemotherapy. The peripheral blood counts, although providing essential data to determine the timing and scheduling of chemotherapy and the type of supportive care a patient requires, are unreliable indicators either of the functional status of the bone marrow or of its ability to tolerate additional antineoplastic therapy (Fliedner et al., 1986; Schofield, 1986). It is apparent that the volume of bone marrow irradiated is as important in determining future treatment tolerance as is the therapeutic dose.

The precise effects of radiotherapy on lymphocytes have not been determined, but it is agreed that in radiation-induced lymphopenia the T cell subset is particularly affected (DuBois & Serrou, 1981). Delayed-hypersensitivity immune responses are more depressed than antibody responses to antigen. Evidence of continued immunosuppression persists for 6 months to 2 years after treatment (Blomgren et al., 1981; McLaren et al., 1981; Wara, Wara, & Amman, 1981). It should be noted that although research has repeatedly confirmed these immunosuppressive effects, a clear link between the effects of radiotherapy on the immune system and clinical effects such as increased susceptibility to infection has not been established (Davies, Wallis, & Peckham, 1981; Tubiana, Arriagada, & Sarrazin, 1986).

SURGERY

The phenomenon of immunosuppression resulting from surgery was first reported by Fielding and Wells (1974). Since then many studies have reported that a major surgical procedure not only suppresses immunity but also results in enhancement of tumor growth and spread. While the mechanism for postsurgical immune suppression is not clear, the most likely causes include endogenous mediators of immunodepression, exoge-

TABLE 53–7. *Estimated Percentage of Bone Marrow Volume in Selected Radiation Treatment Fields*

DISEASE	RADIOTHERAPY TECHNIQUE	PERCENTAGE OF MARROW IN FIELD
Hodgkin's disease	Total nodal irradiation	60–70
	Extended field	40–50
	Segmental field	20–25
Non-Hodgkin's	Total body irradiation	100
	Extended field	40–50
Leukemias	Cranial and spinal	25–40
Breast cancer	Chest wall	15–20
Pancreatic cancer	Abdominal	14–20

(Reprinted by permission of the publisher from Ruben, P., & Scarantino, C. [1978]. The bone marrow organ: The critical structure in radiation-drug interactions. *International Journal of Radiation Oncology, Biology, and Physics, 4,* 3–23. Copyright 1978 by Elsevier Science Inc.)

nous administration of immune suppressive drugs, or both (Colacchio, Yeager, & Hildebrandt, 1994).

Suppression of both cellular and humoral immunity can be detected within hours of a surgical procedure (Holch, Grob, Fierz, Glinz, & Geroulanos, 1989). In mice, NK cell cytotoxicity decreased following amputation and remained abnormally low for the first 12 postoperative days (Pollock & Roth, 1989). In humans, NK cell cytotoxicity has been found to be significantly depressed after major surgery (Lukomska, Olszewski, Engeset, & Kolstad, 1983). A transient severe lymphopenia may be detected in the immediate postoperative period, with complete recovery of immune function taking from 10 days to a month (Virella & Fudenberg, 1982).

A surgical procedure exposes the patient to an increased risk of infection as a result of barrier breakdown caused by the incision and hospital-acquired microorganisms. Given the possible effects of a depressed immune response from surgery, the patient is at an increased risk for infection, septicemia, and increased mortality. Because surgery is a common intervention in cancer patients, it is important to be aware of potential surgically induced immunosuppression during the postoperative period and of the prolonged recovery time that may be needed for cancer patients to return to a normal immunologic state.

BIOTHERAPY

Biotherapy, or the use of biologic response modifiers (BRMs), has now been established as the fourth modality of cancer treatment. These agents, including CSFs, interferons (IFNs), tumor necrosis factor (TNF), monoclonal antibodies (MAB), and interleukins, exert potentially therapeutic effects through several possible mechanisms: (1) exerting a direct antitumor effect, (2) restoring, augmenting, or otherwise modulating the patient's immune system, and (3) demonstrating other biologic effects, such as interference with tumor cells' ability to metastasize (Abernathy, 1987).

Considering that the mechanism of action of BRMs is to modulate the immune system, the potential for hematologic toxicity is apparent. In fact, in those agents with which there is the most experience (IFNs and IL-2), hematologic toxicities have been identified. Abundant evidence exists that IFN therapy causes a reversible fall in WBCs, and with continued treatment a patient may experience leukopenia, anemia, and thrombocytopenia (Moldawer & Figlin, 1994). The WBC counts may drop 40 to 60 per cent but return to normal when therapy is discontinued. However, IFN-induced leukopenia has not translated into an increase in infections among patients experiencing this toxicity (Moldawer & Figlin, 1994). In addition, granulocytopenia is rarely dose-limiting. With IL-2, leukopenia is also possible, but once treatment has been discontinued, a marked rebound lymphocytosis occurs (Sharp, 1994).

The mechanisms by which the BRMs cause their hematologic effects continue to be the subject of speculation. Some authorities maintain that the pattern of hematologic toxicity of IFN indicates a sequestration process, in which the release of blood components from the bone marrow is blocked (Kirkwood & Ernstoff, 1984; Scott, 1983). In addition, results of some in vitro studies indicate that the proliferation of hematopoietic progenitor cells (GM-CFC, BFU-E, GEMM-CFC) is inhibited by exposure to IFN (Contino, Testa, & Dexter, 1986). Given the complexity of these systems, there is undoubtedly more than one mechanism of action. These reports suggest that nurses should monitor hematologic status of patients undergoing BRM therapy.

AGING

A reduction in cell-mediated and humoral immune responses and an increased response to autologous antigens have been observed in elderly patients (Makinodan, James, Inamizu, & Chang, 1984; Weksler, 1983). The susceptibility of major tissues of the immune system to aging indicates that the elderly may not be able to mount an effective resistance against infection.

The most active research regarding aging and hematopoietic function has focused on changes in the immune system. Although there are some contradictory conclusions, aging seems to be accompanied by defects in delayed hypersensitivity response and in cytotoxic T cell generation, as well as by diminished quality and quantity of antibody responses to antigen (Weksler, Hausman, & Schwab, 1984). Many of the changes that occur seem to be related to alterations in T lymphocyte function. This may be an outcome of involution of the thymus and decreased thymic hormone production. One result of changing T cell function is a diminished production of the lymphokine IL-2, which is necessary for amplification of the effector cells' response to antigen (Thoman, 1985; Trofatter, 1986). There may also be a disruption in the ratio of T helper or T suppressor cells, which could account in part for the increased numbers of autoantibodies found in the elderly (Weksler et al., 1984). The most important conclusion is that aging may be a factor in the inability of a patient's hematopoietic system to withstand the stress of cancer and its treatment.

NUTRITION

Nutritional status is a critical factor in determining immunocompetence. A relationship exists between nutrition and immunity. Cell-mediated immunity is profoundly affected by protein-calorie malnutrition (Chandra, 1980). Instrumental in the regulation and differentiation of T cells, the thymus gland atrophies and is replaced by fibrofatty tissue in the malnourished patient. Lymphoid organs have the highest rate of cell proliferation, regulate lymphoid cellular activity, and are extremely susceptible to nutritional deficiencies.

Research suggests that dietary factors, such as inadequate intake of vitamins and minerals, may profoundly affect the immune system (Lahita et al., 1984). Vitamin A and B_6 deficiencies affect the production and function of both the T and B cells, while iron deficiency impairs the function of both the T cell and neutrophil. Zinc deficiency also affects the function of the thymus and cellular immunity, particularly helper and cytotoxic cells.

Inadequate nutrition adversely influences the immune system's ability to recognize and destroy antigens. Without a competent immune system, the patient is at risk for severe infection. Malnourished patients have a higher incidence of morbidity and mortality and are more prone to opportunistic infections than patients receiving adequate nutrition.

SUMMARY

Nurses need to be aware of the effects cancer, cancer treatments, and other factors have on the immune system to anticipate the potential for infection. Armed with this information, nurses will be better able to assess and provide appropriate interventions for patients who are highly susceptible to infection.

NURSING ASSESSMENT OF THE CANCER PATIENT WITH INFECTION OR AT RISK FOR INFECTION

BMD is a common occurrence following cytotoxic therapy such as chemotherapy or radiation therapy. New and aggressive treatment modalities such as high-dose chemotherapy, intensive radiotherapy-chemotherapy combinations, conditioning regimens before bone marrow transplantation, as well as bone marrow transplantation can lead to severe and prolonged bone marrow depression. Cytotoxic therapies do not selectively attack only malignant cells. These therapies cause destruction of the proliferating progenitor cells that produce mature white blood cells, red blood cells, and platelets. The stem cell population is often unable to repopulate itself quickly enough to prevent a potentially fatal infection (Schofield, 1986).

Neutropenia is the most significant factor contributing to infection, morbidity, and mortality in the immunocompromised patient. Neutropenia delays treatment and causes dose reduction in patients receiving chemotherapy, potentially leading to less than optimal treatment. Neutropenia can also result in hospitalization, increased medical costs, lost wages, and compromised quality of life. This section will discuss the various factors that influence an oncology patient's risk for infection as well as the strategies to prevent, minimize, and treat infections.

Patients with an ANC of less than 1000 cells/mm^3 are at increased risk for serious infection (Bodey, Buckley, Sathe, & Freireich, 1966; Bodey, Rodriguez, McCredie, & Freireich, 1976). The risk for infection escalates rapidly as the ANC falls below 500 cells/mm^3. Bodey and colleagues (1966) identified that the frequency of infection ranges from 10 per cent (at 1000 cells/mm^3) to 28 per cent (with 100 cells/mm^3). Table 53–5 shows the risk of infection related to degree of neutropenia. The patient's risk of infection increases with prolonged neutropenia.

Other factors that influence the cancer patient's risk for infection include (1) the age of the patient (older patients have less cellular marrow with more fat spaces, and possible aplasia); (2) the presence of chronic disease; (3) the nutritional status of the patient (a greater negative nitrogen balance, with its associated loss of weight, decreases the patient's tolerance to treatment); (4) the degree of bone marrow reserve in relation to the amount of tumor involvement; (5) the degree of host compromise by previous chemotherapy or radiation therapy; (6) the presence of compromised host defenses such as occurs with in-dwelling catheters, surgery, and other invasive procedures that disrupt skin integrity; and (7) colonization with potential pathogens (Creaven & Mihich, 1977; Dewys et al., 1980).

Prevention of infection is a high priority in the immunocompromised patient. Thus, nurses caring for patients receiving cytotoxic therapies must provide baseline and ongoing assessment of patients who are at risk or potentially at risk for infection. Nurses need to manage the patient's care to decrease the risk for morbidity and mortality by avoiding damage to host defenses, bolstering host defenses, preventing acquisition of new organisms or potential pathogens, suppressing colonizing organisms, and providing appropriate care, as well as patient and family education (Brandt, 1990; Pizzo, 1989; Rostad, 1990).

ASSESSMENT

Because infection is the leading cause of morbidity and mortality in cancer patients, early detection is essential, particularly in the patient with neutropenia. Fever remains the most reliable indicator of infection in the neutropenic patient. Therefore, infection should always be considered in the neutropenic patient with a fever. An undetected, untreated infection can end in death for the febrile cancer patient with neutropenia (Pizzo & Young, 1985). An elevated temperature in the neutropenic patient must be reported immediately to the physician. While infection is the most likely cause of fever in the neutropenic patient, other causes may include medications such as amphotericin B or interleukins, transfusion therapy, cell lysis, and the cancer itself.

The absence of sufficient, functional neutrophils in the neutropenic patient may prevent the development of the classic signs and symptoms of infection such as erythema, edema, pain, and purulence. Subtle clues indicative of infection in these patients should lead the nurse to explore further the possibility of infection. For example, anorectal pain in the presence of neutropenia may be the first sign of a perirectal infection. In fact, in the neutropenic patient, this sign may precede objective findings by 2 to 10 days. A periodontal infection initially manifested only by a report of oral pain or discomfort may evolve into a serious infection. Table 53–8 shows common clinical manifestations of infection in neutropenic patients.

Infection in immunocompromised patients may be caused by bacteria, viruses, protozoa, or fungi. Table

TABLE 53–8. *The Influence of Neutropenia on the Clinical Manifestations of Infection*

SITE OF INFECTION	COMMON SIGNS AND SYMPTOMS OF INFECTION IN THE PATIENT WITH NEUTROPENIA	LESS COMMON SIGNS AND SYMPTOMS OF INFECTION IN THE PATIENT WITH NEUTROPENIA
Pharyngitis/stomatitis	Fever, pain Erythema	Exudate, cervical adenopathy
Skin (includes anorectal and intertriginous areas)	Fever	Ulceration, fissure
	Erythema	Regional lymph node enlargement and tenderness
	Pain	Local heat and swelling
Pneumonia	Fever, tachypnea, dyspnea	Cough
	Infiltration evident on chest x-ray (after first 1–3 days of infection)	Sputum production Pulmonary consolidation (absent in 50%–60% of patients with neutropenia)
Urinary tract	Fever	Dysuria Frequency Urgency Pyuria Flank pain

(From Brandt, B. [1990]. Nursing protocol for the patient with neutropenia. *Oncology Nursing Forum, 17* [Suppl. 1], 9–15. Adapted from Schimff, S. [1977]. Therapy of infection in patients with granulocytopenia. *Medical Clinics of North America, 61,* 1103.)

53–9 shows infections commonly seen in cancer patients including pathogens and their sources, common sites for infection, and treatments. Although immunocompromised patients often become infected with their own endogenous organisms, hospitalization and inpatient procedures increase the patient's risk for acquiring a nosocomial or hospital-acquired infection. Careful handwashing is an important means of reducing the acquisition of and colonization by new organisms from the environment (Larson, 1989; Larson, McGinley, Grove, Leyden, & Talbot, 1986; Pizzo, 1989). Research has shown that the hands of health care providers are the most important means by which nosocomial infections are transmitted to patients (Gould, 1991).

Assessment of the neutropenic patient includes a system-oriented history and physical examination that focus on the patient's risk for infection. The assessment can be performed in relation to body systems (Table 53–10). Because granulocytes have a short half-life of 6 to 8 hours in the bloodstream, the nurse should also calculate the ANC in the neutropenic patient on a daily basis (Table 53–4).

Changes in health care delivery from the inpatient to the outpatient setting often place the responsibility for infection assessment and care on patients and their family members. They must learn to use infection control practices in environments that may be less than optimal. However, the nurse can help patients and family members improvise with the available resources to maintain and promote hygienic practices and infection control techniques. It is important to teach patients and family members to have a high index of suspicion for infection when changes in the patient's condition occur and to report these changes to the physician or nurse. Patients and their family members must understand

that a timely response to fever can mean the difference between life and death and that infections, if discovered early, can be effectively treated without adverse complications.

The importance of patient and family education cannot be overemphasized. Family members should be involved in teaching sessions, because patients undergoing active therapy may be too ill or too stressed to absorb or process information that is provided. Written information or instructions are useful. Table 53–11 provides information related to prevention and early detection of infection that should be provided to cancer patients and their families/caregivers.

MANAGEMENT OF THE NEUTROPENIC PATIENT WITH INFECTION

While fever in the nonneutropenic patient can be evaluated and treated according to general medical principles, the urgency with which fever in the presence of neutropenia must be addressed cannot be overemphasized. Medical therapy of infection in the neutropenic patient consists primarily of antibiotics and supportive therapy. A decision tree that illustrates the usual medical approach to the febrile neutropenic patient is provided in Figure 53–3.

Pizzo and Young (1985) have recommended that institutional criteria and policies should be established and closely followed to minimize infection-related morbidity. Their recommendations follow.

1. Any patient with a granulocyte count less than 1000 cells/mm^3 who has a single temperature elevation above 38.3° C or two or more elevations above 38° C will have a fever workup. The fever workup generally includes two sets of preantibiotic

TABLE 53–9. *Infections in Cancer Patients and Usual Therapy*

PATHOGEN	SOURCES	COMMON SITES	PRESENTATION	TREATMENT
Bacteria				
Pseudomonas	Multiple	Wounds	Purulence	AG ± AP, Ceph3,
		GI tract	Enterocolitis	Imipenem
		GU tract	UTI	
		Lung	Pneumonia	Aztreonam
		Blood	Sepsis	Ciprofloxacin
Klebsiella	Multiple	Lung	Pneumonia	Ceph3
		GU tract	UTI	Imipenem
		Blood	Sepsis	Aztreonam, FQ
Escherichia coli	Multiple	GI tract	Enterocolitis	AG
		GU tract	UTI	AP
		Wounds	Purulence	Ceph3
		Blood	Sepsis	Imipenem, Aztreonam, FQ
Staphylococci				
S. aureus	Multiple	Lung	Pneumonia	PRSP
		GI tract	Enterocolitis	Vancomycin (MRSA)
		Wounds	Purulence	
		Blood	Sepsis	
Coagulase negative	Normal flora	Catheters	Sepsis	Vancomycin
		Prosthetic devices	Meningitis	
Fungi				
Candida	Normal flora	GI tract	Thrush,	Topical AF
		GU tract	Esophagitis	Amphotericin B
		Blood	Hepatitis, UTI,	Fluconazole
			vaginitis, sepsia	Intraconazole
Cryptococcus	Soil, pigeon feces	Lung	Pneumonia	Amphotericin B +
		CNS	Meningitis	5-fluorocytosine
				Fluconazole
Aspergillus	Soil, air, building materials	Lung	Pneumonia	Amphotericin B ± 5-fluorocytosine or rifampin
				Intraconazole
Viruses				
Herpes simplex type 1	Mucosa, person-to-person transmission	GI tract	Stomatitis,	Acyclovir
		GU tract	Esophagitis, vaginitis,	Foscarnet
		Skin	Vesicles	
		CNS	Encephalitis	
Varicella-zoster	Respiratory tract, person-to-person transmission	Lung	Shingles	Acclovir
		Skin	Pneumonia	Foscarnet
		CNS	Disseminated	Famciclovir
				Steroids
Cytomegalovirus	Respiratory secretions, blood	Lung	Pneumonia	Gancyclovir
		GI Tract	Enterocolitis, esophagitis	Foscarnet
		CNS	Encephalitis	
Parasites				
Pneumocystis	Unknown	Lung	Pneumonia	SXT
				Pyrimethamine, Atovaquene
				Trimetrexate + folinic acid
				Primaquine + clindamycin
Toxoplasma	Cat feces	Disseminated	Encephalitis	Pyrimethamine +
	Raw meat		Myocarditis	sulfadiazine
	Blood		Pneumonia	Spiramycin
			Ocular	

GI = gastrointestinal; GU = genitourinary; CNS = central nervous system; UTI = urinary tract infection; AG = aminoglycoside (amikacin, tobramycin, netilmicin, gentamicin); AP = antipseudomonal penicillin (ticarcillin, piperacillin, mezlocillin); Ceph3 = 3rd generation cephalosporin (ceftazidime, cefoperazone, ceftriaxone, etc.); PRSP = pencillinase-resistant penicillin (nafcillin, oxacillin, methicillin, clozacillin, didoxacillin); MRSA = methicillin-resistant *S. aureus;* FQ = fluoroquinofone (ciprofloxacin, ofloxacin, norfloxacin [UTI only]); SXT = trimethoprim/sulfamethoxazole; AF = topical antifungals (nystatin, clostrimazole).

(From Ellerhorst-Ryan, J. M. [1985]. Complications of the myeloproliferative system; Infection and sepsis. *Seminars in Oncology Nursing, I,* 244–250. Reproduced and updated by permission.)

TABLE 53–10. *Assessment of the Patient with Potential or Actual Risk for Infection*

General Condition
Age, fatigue, malaise
History of allergies
History of prior chemotherapy, radiation therapy, or other immunosuppressive therapies such as steroid use
Chronic diseases
History of febrile neutropenia and associated symptoms
Nutritional status
Functional status—problems with immobility
Tobacco use—cigarettes, pipe, cigars, oral
Recreational drug use
Alcohol use
Prescribed and over-the-counter medication use
Baseline and ongoing vital signs—blood pressure, heart rate, respiratory rate, and temperature

Skin and Mucous Membranes
Thorough inspection of all skin surfaces with special attention to axilla, perineum (particularly the anorectal area), and under breasts. Inspect skin for color, vascularity, bleeding, lesions, edema, moist areas, excoriation, irritation, erythema. General condition of hair and nails, pressure areas, swelling, pain, tenderness, biopsy or surgical sites, wounds, enlarged lymph nodes, catheters, or other devices
Inspect the oral cavity including lips, tongue, mucous membranes, gingiva, teeth, and throat—color, moisture, bleeding, ulcerations, lesions, exudate, mucositis, stomatitis, placque, swelling, pain, tenderness, taste changes, amount and character of saliva, ability to swallow, changes in voice, dental caries, patient's routine for oral hygiene
History of past or present skin disorders or problems with the mucous membranes

Head, Eyes, Ears, Nose
Pain, tenderness, exudate, crusting, enlarged lymph nodes

Cardiopulmonary
Respiratory rate and pattern, breath sounds (presence/absence, adventitious sounds), quantity and characteristics of sputum, shortness of breath, use of accessory muscles, dysphagia, diminished gag reflex, tachycardia, blood pressure

Gastrointestinal
Pain, diarrhea, bowel sounds, character and frequency of bowel movements, constipation, rectal bleeding, hemorrhoids, change in bowel habits, sexual practices, erythema, ulceration

Genitourinary
Dysuria, frequency, urgency, hematuria, pruritus, pain, vaginal or penile discharge, vaginal bleeding, burning, lesions, ulcerations, characteristics of urine

Central Nervous System
Cognition, level of consciousness, personality, behavior

Musculoskeletal
Tenderness, pain, loss of function

TABLE 53–11. *Content for Patient and Family Education on the Prevention and Early Detection of Infection*

Susceptibility to infection
Impact of treatment regimen on the immune system
Functions of white blood cells (WBCs)
Expected time of WBC nadir
Infection transmission
Prevention of exposure to communicable or infectious diseases
Temperature-taking
Reportable signs and symptoms
Accessing health care system—how and who to contact—with reportable signs and symptoms, questions, and concerns
Basic handwashing practices
Hygienic practices (skin, oral, sexual) that minimize growth and transmission of organisms
Inspection of high-risk areas for signs of infection
Care of vascular access devices and other invasive devices
Monitoring for superinfection when on antibiotics
Health-promoting practices such as diet, sleep, exercise, stress reduction techniques
Risk reduction such as avoidance of raw milk products, undercooked meats, and raw fruits and vegetables; avoidance of crowds, young children, and ill persons; and proper handling of food and storage

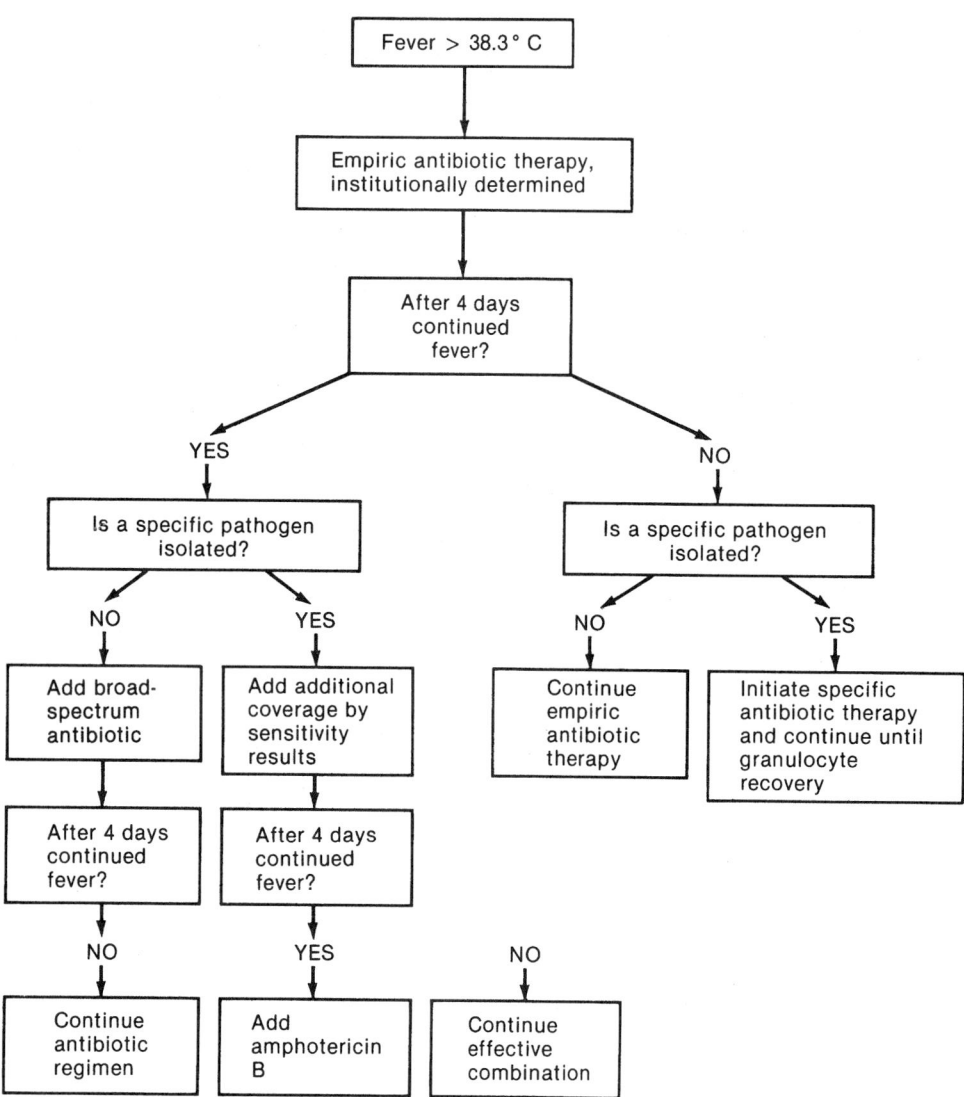

FIGURE 53-3. Example of antibiotic management for fevers in the neutropenic patient.

blood cultures, chest x-ray, and cultures of sputum, urine, wound, and other accessible sites suggestive of infection. If blood is drawn for culture from a vascular access device or in-dwelling silastic catheter, additional blood for cultures should be obtained from a peripheral vein.

2. Once the fever workup is completed, a regimen of empiric antibiotics is usually begun without waiting for culture results.

3. Once culture and sensitivity test results are known, therapy can be adjusted to treat the identified organisms.

Nursing care for the neutropenic patient is directed at preventing cross-infection and controlling colonization with exogenous organisms. The following practices should be observed: (1) meticulous handwashing by *all* persons entering the room as well as the patient (gloves are not a substitute for handwashing); (2) a private room; (3) a low-bacteria diet that does not include raw fruits and vegetables; (4) no fresh flowers or plants in the patient's room; (5) no persons with a draining

wound, infection, or communicable disease should enter the patient's room to either provide care or to visit; (6) invasive procedures should be avoided whenever possible including use of indwelling urinary catheters, rectal examinations, and rectal temperatures; and (7) educate the patient, family, and health care providers regarding precautions and required practices and rationale.

Granulocyte transfusions are rarely used in treatment of the neutropenic patient. Their efficacy in prophylaxis has not been established; therapeutically, they seem to improve survival in patients with prolonged, severe neutropenia (< 500 cells/mm^3 for longer than 30 days). Donor availability is also a limiting factor.

Other practices that have been considered controversial in the treatment of infection in neutropenic patients include use of a totally protected environment and of oral nonabsorbable antibiotics. These modalities have been studied to see whether risk and severity of infection can be reduced (Pizzo, 1989). Results suggest that these measures, which are quite expensive and may cause discomfort for the patient, should be used only in patients undergoing high-risk therapies, such as high-dose chemotherapy or bone marrow transplantation.

Although antipyretics are often used, at least one investigator recommends against using antipyretics when temperature is below 105° F in the patient with neutropenia (Cunha, 1985). Fever maximizes host defenses by several mechanisms: (1) inhibition or destruction of microorganisms; (2) diminishing certain trace elements, which further inhibits replication of microorganisms; (3) increased production of antiviral interferons; and (4) increased mobility and phagocytosis of polymorphonuclear leukocytes. Cunha (1985) identifies three situations in which physicians might consider antipyretics in the febrile patient with neutropenia: (1) if the patient is particularly uncomfortable; (2) if the temperature is 105° F or above; and (3) if the patient has serious cardiopulmonary disease that may be exacerbated by the fever. Prolonged fever in persons with limited ability to ingest food and fluid may increase the risk of metabolic complications from dehydration and malnourishment.

CSFs lessen the risk for treatment-induced neutropenia, thereby reducing the patient's risk for infections. CSFs such as granulocyte-macrophage colony-stimulating factor and granulocyte colony-stimulating factor reduce the incidence, severity, and duration of neutropenia. CSFs promote the volume and speed of cell production, enhance their survival, and stimulate their functional activities.

SUMMARY

This chapter has described the physiology of hematopoiesis as it relates to infection, cancer-related pathophysiology of the immune system, as well as nursing assessment and interventions. Complications of infection may be life-threatening. Astute nursing care involving early identification of risk factors, preventive interventions, patient education, early detection and reporting of signs and symptoms of infection, and supportive care during infectious complications can make the difference between life or death for the neutropenic patient.

REFERENCES

Abernathy, E. (1987). Biotherapy: An introductory overview. *Oncology Nursing Forum, 14*(Suppl.), 13–15.

American Society of Clinical Oncology. (1994). Recommendations for the use of hematopoietic colony-stimulating factors: Evidence-based, clinical practice guidelines. *Journal of Clinical Oncology, 12*, 2471–2508.

Axelrod, A. A. (1990). Some hemopoietic negative regulators. *Experimental Hematology, 18*, 143–150.

Baranov, E. B., Selidovkin, G. D., Butturini, A., & Gale, R. P. (1994). Hematological recovery after 10-Gy acute total body Radiation. *Blood, 83*(2), 596–599.

Beck, W. S. (1985). Normocytic anemias. In W. S. Beck (Ed.), *Hematology* (pp. 43–57). Cambridge, MA: MIT Press.

Blomgren, H., Baral, E., Jarstrand, C., Petrini, B., Strender, L. E., Wallgren, A., & Wasserman, J. (1981). Effect of external radiation therapy on the peripheral lymphocyte subpopulation. In J.B. DuBois, B. Serrou, & C. Rosenfeld

(Eds.), *Immunopharmacologic effects of radiation therapy* (pp. 299–319). New York: Raven Press.

Bodey, G. P., Buckley, M., Sathe, Y. S., & Freireich, E. J. (1966). Quantitative relationship between circulating leukocytes and infection in patients with acute leukemia. *Annals of Internal Medicine, 64*, 328–340.

Bodey, G. P., Rodriguez, V., McCredie, K. B., & Freireich, E. J. (1976). Neutropenia and infection following cancer chemotherapy. *International Journal of Radiation Oncology, Biology, and Physics, 1*, 301–304.

Brandt, B. (1990). Nursing protocol for the patient with neutropenia. *Oncology Nursing Forum, 17*(Suppl. 1), 9–15.

Chandra, R. (1980). Cell-mediated immunity in nutritional imbalance. *Federal Proceedings, 39*, 3088–3092.

Clark, J., Landis, L., & McGee, R. (1987). Nursing management of outcomes of disease, psychological response, treatment, and complications. In C. R. Ziegfeld (Ed.), *Core curriculum for oncology nursing* (pp. 271–319). Philadelphia: W. B. Saunders Co.

Colacchio, T. A., Yeager, M. P., & Hildebrandt, L. W. (1994). Perioperative immunomodulation in cancer surgery. *American Journal of Surgery, 167*, 174–179.

Contino, L. H., Testa, N. G., & Dexter, T. M. (1986). The myelosuppressive effect of recombinant interferon (gamma) in short-term and long-term marrow cultures. *British Journal of Haematology, 63*, 517–524.

Creaven, P. J., & Mihich, E. (1977). The clinical toxicity of anticancer drugs and its prediction. *Seminars in Oncology, 4*, 147–163.

Croizat, H., Frindel, E., & Tubiana, M. (1979). Long term radiation effects on the bone marrow stem cells of C3H mice. *International Journal of Radiation Biology, 36*, 91–99.

Cunha, B. A. (1985). Significance of fever in the immuno-compromised host. *Medical Clinics of North America, 20*, 163–170.

Davies, A. J. S., Wallis, V. J., & Peckman, M. J. (1981). Suppression of the immune response by ionizing radiation. In J. B. DuBois, B. Serrou, & C. Rosenfeld (Eds.), *Immunopharmacologic effects of radiation therapy* (pp. 275–299). New York: Raven Press.

Dewys, W. D., Begg, C., Lavin, P. T., et al. (1980). Prognostic effect of weight loss prior to chemotherapy in patients. *American Journal of Medicine, 69*, 491–497.

DuBois, J. B., & Serrou, B. (1981). Effects of ionizing radiation on cell-mediated immunity cancer patients. In J. B. DuBois, B. Serrou, & C. Rosenfeld (Eds.), *Immunopharmacologic effects of radiation therapy* (pp. 275–299). New York: Raven Press.

Fielding, L. P., & Wells, B. W. (1974). Survival after primary and after staged resection for large bowel obstruction caused by cancer. *British Journal of Surgery, 61*, 16–18.

Fliedner, T. M., Northdurft, W., & Clavo, W. (1986). The development of radiation late effects to the bone marrow after single and chronic exposure. *International Journal of Radiation Biology, 49*, 35–46.

Gordon, M., & Barrett, A. (1985). *Bone marrow disorders: The biological basis of clinical problems*. Oxford: Blackwell Scientific Publishers.

Gould, D. (1991). Nurse's hands as vectors of hospital-acquired infections: A review. *Journal of Advanced Nursing, 16*, 1216–1225.

Graham, G. J., & Pragnell, I. B. (1992). The hemopoietic stem cell: Properties and control mechanisms. *Cell Biology, 3*, 423–434.

Grant, S. M., & Heel, R. C. (1992). Recombinant granulocyte-macrophage colony-stimulating factor (rGM-CSF): A review of its pharmacological properties and prospective role in the management of myelosupression. *Drugs, 43,* 516–560.

Holch, M. W., Grob, P. J., Fierz, W., Glinz, W., & Geroulanos, S. (1989). Graduation of immunosuppression after surgery or severe trauma. *Second Vienna shock forum* (pp. 491–494). New York: Alan R. Liss, Inc.

Hollingshead, L. M., & Goa, K. L. (1991). Recombinant granulocyte colony-stimulating factor (rG-CSF): A review of its pharmacological properties and prospective role in neutropenic conditions. *Drugs, 42,* 300–330.

Kirkwood, J., & Ernstoff, M. (1984). Interferons in the treatment of human cancer. *Journal of Clinical Oncology, 2,* 336.

Lahita, R., Levy, J., Weksler, M., Perrie, B., Hausman, P., & Schwab, R. (1984). Effects of sex hormones, nutrition and aging on the immune response. In D. Stites, J. Stobo, H. Fudenberg, & J. Wells (Eds.), *Basic and clinical immunology* (5th ed., pp. 288–311). Los Altos, CA: Lange Medical.

Larson, E. (1989). Infection control. *Annual Review of Nursing Research, 7,* 95–113.

Larson, E., McGinley, K., Grove, G., Leyden, J., & Talbot, G. (1986). Physiologic, microbiologic, and seasonal effects of handwashing on the skin of health care personnel. *American Journal of Infection Control, 14,* 51–59.

Lukomska, B., Olszewski, W. L., Engeset, A., & Kolstad, P. (1983). The effect of surgery and chemotherapy on blood NK cell activity in patients with ovarian cancer. *Cancer, 51,* 465–469.

Makinodan, T., James, S. J., Inamizu, T., & Chang, M. P. (1984). Immunologic basis for susceptibility to infection in the aged. *Gerontology, 30,* 278–289.

McLaren, J. R., Olkowski, Z., Skeen, M., McConnell, F., Benigno, B., Mansour, K., Nixon, D., Shah, N., & Ells, R. (1981). Responses of immune parameters to irradiation of patients with head and neck, bronchogenic, and uterine cervical cancers and to subsequent immunotherapy. In J. B. DuBois, B. Serrou, & C. Rosenfeld (Eds.), *Immunopharmacologic effects of radiation therapy* (pp. 253–274). New York: Raven Press.

Moldawer, N. P., & Figlin, R. A. (1994). The interferons. In P. T. Rieger (Ed.), *Biotherapy: A comprehensive overview* (pp. 69–92). Boston: Jones and Bartlett.

Peters, W. P., Rosner, G., Ross, M., Vredenburgh, J., Meisenberg, B., & Gilbert, J. (1993). Comparative effects of GM-CSF and G-CSF on priming peripheral blood progenitor cells, for use with autologous bone marrow after high-dose chemotherapy. *Blood, 81,* 1709–1719.

Pizzo, P. (1989). Combating infections in neutropenic patients. *Hospital Practice 24,* 93–110.

Pizzo, P. A. (1989). Considerations for the prevention of infectious complications in patients with cancer. *Reviews of Infectious Diseases, 11*(Suppl. 7), 51551–51563.

Pizzo, P. A., & Young, R. C. (1985). Infections in the cancer patient. In V. T. DeVita, Jr., S. Hellman, & S. A. Rosenberg (Eds.), *Cancer: Principles and practice of oncology* (pp. 1963–1998). Philadelphia: J. B. Lippincott, Co.

Pollack, R. E., & Roth, J. A. (1989). Cancer induced immunosuppression: Implications for therapy? *Seminars in Surgical Oncology, 51,* 414–419.

Robinson, B. E., & Donowitz, G. R. (1992). Infections in patients with cancer: Host defenses and the immune compromised state. In A. R. Moosa, S. C. Schmiff, & M. C. Robson (Eds.), *Comprehensive textbook of oncology* (pp. 1733–1730). Philadelphia: Williams & Wilkins.

Rostad, M. E. (1990). Management of myelosuppression in the patient with cancer. *Oncology Nursing Forum, 17*(Suppl. 1), 4–8.

Rubin, P., & Scarantino, C. W. (1978). The bone marrow organ: The critical structure in radiation-drug interaction. *International Journal of Radiation Oncology, Biology, and Physics, 4,* 3–23.

Sarzotti, M., Baron, S., & Klimpel, G. R. (1987). EL-4 metastases in spleen and bone marrow suppress the NK activity generated in these organs. *International Journal of Cancer, 39,* 118–125.

Schattenberg, A., DeWitte, T., Salden, M., Vet, J., VanDijk, B., Smeets, D., Hoogenhout, J., & Haanen, C. (1989). Mixed hematopoietic chimerism after allogeneic transplantation with lymphocytic-depleted bone marrow is not associated with higher incidence of relapse. *Blood, 73,* 1367.

Schofield, R. (1986). Assessment of cytotoxic injury to bone marrow. *British Journal of Cancer, 53*(Suppl. VII), 115–125.

Schuening, F. G., Strob, R., Goehle, S., Graham, T. C., Appelbaum, F. R., Hackman, R., & Souza, L. M. (1989). Effect of recombinant human granulocyte colony-stimulating factor on hematopoiesis of normal dogs and on hematopoietic recovery after otherwise lethal total body irradiation. *Blood, 74,* 1308.

Scott, G. M. (1983). The toxic effects of interferon in man. In I. Gressor (Ed.), *Interferon* (pp. 85–114). London: Academic Press.

Sharp, E. (1994). The interleukins. In P. T. Rieger (Ed.), *Biotherapy: A comprehensive overview* (pp. 93–111). Boston: Jones and Bartlett.

Thoman, M. L. (1985). Role of interleukin-2 in the age-related impairment of immune function. *Journal of the American Geriatrics Society, 33,* 781–787.

Trofatter, K. E. (1986). Immune responses and aging. *Clinical Obstetrics and Gynecology, 29,* 384–396.

Tubiana M., Arriagada, R., & Sarrazin, D. (1986). Human cancer natural history, radiation-induced immunodepression and postoperative radiation therapy. *International Journal of Radiation Oncology, Biology, and Physics, 12,* 477–485.

Tubiana, M., Carde, P., & Frindel, E. (1993). Ways of minimizing hematopoietic damage induced by radiation and cytostatic drugs-the possible role of inhibitors. *Radiotherapy & Oncology, 29,* 1–17.

Virella, G., & Fudenberg, H. (1982). Secondary immunodeficiencies. In J. Tmomey, (Ed.), *The pathophysiology of human immunologic disorders* (pp. 91–124), Baltimore: Urban & Schwarzenberg.

Walker, T. M., Burger, C. J., & Elgert, K. D. (1994). Tumor growth alters T cell and macrophage production of and responsiveness to GM-CSF: Partial dysregulation through interleukin-10. *Cellular Immunology, 154,* 342–357.

Wara, W., Wara, D., & Amman, A. J. (1981). Immunosuppression and reconstruction after radiation therapy. In J. B. DuBois, B. Serrou, & C. Rosenfeld (Eds.), *Immunopharmacologic effects of radiation therapy* (pp. 219–229). New York: Raven Press.

Weksler, M. (1983). The senescence of the immune system. *Hospital Practice, 16*(10), 53–64.

Weksler, M. E., Hausman, P. B., & Schwab, R. (1984). Effects of aging on the immune response. In D. P. Stites, J. D. Stobo, H. H. Fudenberg, & J. V. Wells (Eds.), *Basic and clinical immunology* (pp. 302–310). Los Altos, CA: Lange Medical Publications.

Whetton, A. D., & Dexter, T. M. (1993). Influence of growth factors and substrates on differentiation of hemopoietic stem cells. *Current Opinion in Cell Biology, 5,* 1044–1049.

Wujcik, D. (1993). Infection control in oncology patients. *Nursing Clinics of North America, 28,* 639–650.

Abnormalities in Hemostasis and Hemorrhage

Esther Muscari Lin • Sandra Mitchell Beddar

Alterations of hemostasis, including thrombosis and bleeding, are commonplace and sometimes fatal complications of many neoplastic diseases, their therapy, or both. In an era in which cancer patients receive aggressive treatments and experience prolonged survival, there is a greater opportunity for these complications to develop. Nurses play a key role in the prevention and earliest detection of alterations in hemostasis and in the assessment and management of patients experiencing these complications. To address the problems of thrombosis or hemorrhage in the patient with cancer the nurse requires a thorough understanding of the physiology of hematopoeisis, hemostasis, and coagulation.

This chapter provides an overview of the problems of hemostasis and bleeding in the patient with cancer. Current concepts of hematopoiesis, normal and abnormal coagulation, and cancer treatment that interferes with hemostasis are presented. Clinical manifestations and laboratory findings associated with abnormal hemostasis and bleeding are discussed with an emphasis on prevention, assessment, and management.

BLOOD COMPOSITION AND PHYSIOLOGY

Blood is a unique tissue that is pumped through the vascular system by the heart. Circulating blood is composed of cellular elements suspended in an aqueous solution of salts and proteins. The cellular elements consist of red cells (erythrocytes), white cells (leukocytes), and platelets (thrombocytes). The fluid component of blood is known as plasma and contains water as well as substances such as plasma proteins, blood clotting factors, antibodies, nutrients, metabolic endproducts, and inorganic solutes of mineral electrolytes and salts (Griffin, 1986).

Blood serves a number of functions that are summarized in Table 54–1. In particular, it serves as a transport medium for oxygen and other substances necessary for the metabolism of cells and works to maintain vascular system integrity. The platelets along with the coagulation system (a variety of plasma proteins, chemicals, and other substances that circulate in the bloodstream in an inactive form) cooperate in this endeavour. The coagulation system is composed of a series of plasma proteins that interact to convert fibrinogen to fibrin, thus producing gelatinous plugs for sealing breaks and leaks in the vasculature.

A system of proteins complementary to the coagulation proteins inhibits the coagulation system. It prevents the whole circulation from clotting up at once, and it also breaks down formed clots when they are no longer needed. This system is called the fibrinolytic system. The components and interactions of the coagulation and fibrinolytic systems are described in greater detail below.

TABLE 54–1. *Functions of the Blood*

1. Transportation of oxygen from the lungs to the cells and carbon dioxide from the tissues to the lungs for excretion
2. Transportation of absorbed nutrients from the gastrointestinal tract to the cells
3. Transportation of metabolic wastes from the cells to the liver, kidneys, lungs, and skin for excretion
4. Distribution of hormones, enzymes, and other endogenous substances needed to regulate numerous physiologic processes in the body
5. Protection of the individual against foreign substances through the action of white blood cells, lymphocytes, and complement proteins
6. Protection of the individual against excessive blood loss through coagulation
7. Maintenance of fluid, electrolyte, and acid-base imbalance

HEMATOPOIESIS

Of the many body cells, blood cells are among those with the highest rate of self-renewal or turnover. The life span of neutrophils, eosinophils, and basophils is approximately 6 hours, the life span of platelets approximately 8 to 10 days, and the life span of erythrocytes approximately 120 days. Hematopoiesis is the term used to describe the process of proliferation, differentiation, and maturation of blood cells. The high turnover rate of blood cells is in part geared to the capacity to respond to the stress of blood loss and infection.

The organs of hematopoeisis include the bone marrow, spleen, and lymphoid tissues. The liver, marrow, and spleen are the blood-forming organs in the fetus. After birth this function is limited largely to the bone marrow (Erslev & Lichtman, 1990). In young children, the long bones, ribs, sternum, skull, pelvis, vertebrae, and sometimes spleen and liver are involved. In adults, the vertebrae, ribs, sternum, skull, proximal epiphyses of long bones, pelvis, and spleen are the major sites of blood cell production. In adulthood, fatty tissue replaces some of the areas of previous hematopoietic activity in the bone marrow.

Except for the early portion of fetal life, the bone marrow is the site of production for most blood cells. As shown in Figure 54–1, the ultimate source of blood cells is the pluripotent hematopoietic stem cell. This cell is present in small numbers in the bone marrow and in the peripheral blood. The pluripotent stem cell is capable of self-replication and is uncommitted, meaning that it can differentiate into an erythroid, granulocytic, thrombocytic, or lymphoid cell line. Studies suggest that these pluripotent stem cells give rise to progressively more committed progenitors that differ from stem cells in that they lack the capacity for self-renewal (Quesenberry, 1990; Rothstein, 1993). The most pluripotential of these is the colony-forming unit-GEMM, from which are derived fully committed precursors for erythrocytes, granulocytes, macrophages, and megakaryocytes (Rothstein, 1993).

The next stage in cell development is the committed or unipotential stem cell. These cells have little or no self-replicating capacity and are capable of differentiating into only one cell line. Each cell line has its own specific unipotential stem cell, one for lymphocytes, one for granulocytes and macrophages, one for erythrocytes, and one for platelets.

In the bone marrow, blood cells develop in sinuses lined with endothelial cells and fibroblasts. The endothelium, fibroblasts, and abundant fat cells constitute what is termed the stroma of the bone marrow. Normal bone marrow function depends upon intact marrow architecture, the availability of key nutrients including iron, folic acid, and vitamin B_{12}, and regulatory hormones such as erythropoietin, the colony-stimulating factors (CSFs), and interleukins. At any point in time the hematopoietic cells found in the bone marrow include a small pluripotential stem cell compartment, a large compartment of proliferating cells of committed lineage, and a large compartment of postmitotic maturing cells.

Unipotential stem cells are in the active cell cycle in the bone marrow but require one or more CSFs to stimulate their development and maturation into more mature blood cells. CSFs are hematopoietic hormones that stimulate stem cell differentiation and enhance maturation (Quesenberry, 1990).

Although there is evidence that stem cells circulate in the peripheral blood (Quesenberry, 1990), it is primarily the completely mature blood cells that leave the bone marrow and can be observed in the peripheral blood. Erythrocytes and platelets that are released from the bone marrow live out their life spans in the blood. Phagocytes enter the tissues and do not return to the blood. However, lymphocytes represent an exception to this pattern and do not necessarily follow a unidirectional development from mitotic stem cells to mature cells. Rather, lymphocytes can vacillate between actively dividing cells and dormant memory cells. These dormant memory cells are capable of actively growing and dividing again, resuming this capacity and the capacity to produce antibodies when presented with an antigen (see Chapter 14, Principles of Immunology). Lymphocytes move back and forth between the bone marrow, the blood and lymph circulations, and the tissues. Several papers and texts provide excellent reviews of hematopoeisis including those of Alkire and Collingwood (1990), Babior and Stossel (1990), Goodnough et al., (1993), Griffin (1986), Guyton (1991), Lee, Bithell, Foerster, Athens, and Lukens (1993), and Williams, Beutler, Erslev, and Lichtman (1990).

The smallest of the formed elements of the blood are the platelets. Platelets are disk-shaped anucleate fragments released from a giant cell called the megakaryocyte. It takes roughly 5 days for a committed stem cell to produce a mass of new platelets (Babior & Stossel, 1990). After platelets leave the marrow, they are taken up by the spleen. Platelets move freely between the spleen and the circulating platelet pool. At any time, approximately 70 per cent of platelets are circulating, and about 30 per cent are localized in the spleen. Platelets have a life span of approximately 10 days before disappearing from the circulation. Aging as

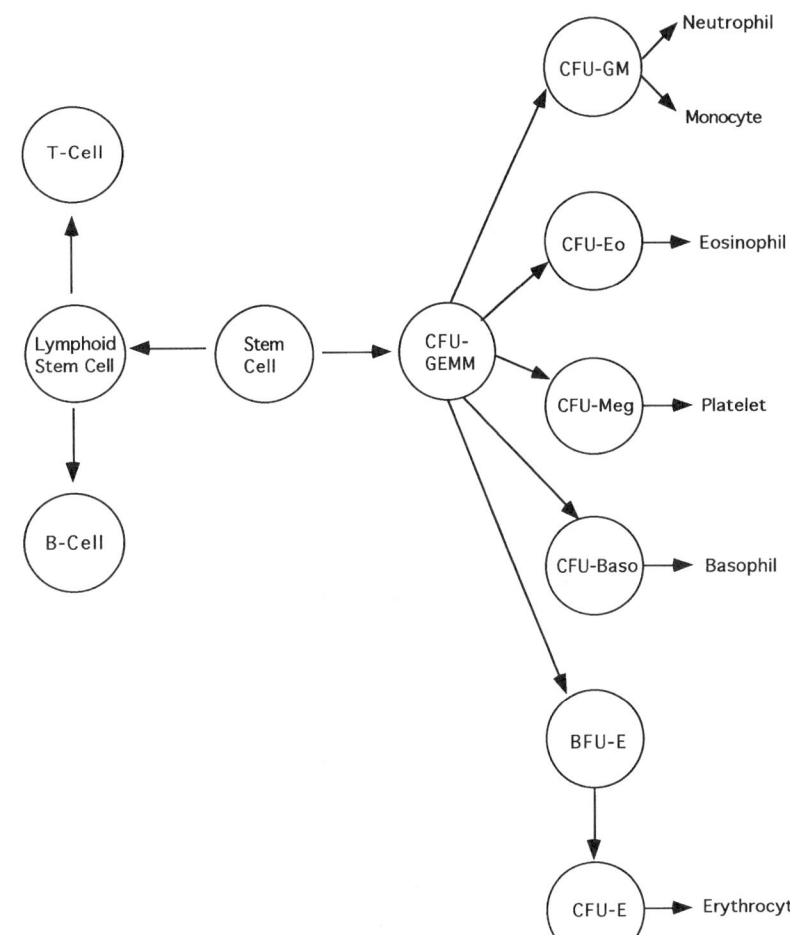

FIGURE 54–1. Hematopoietic stem cell differentiation and maturation.

they circulate, the platelets shrink in size and lose functional capacity, until they are removed from the blood.

In the circulation, platelets normally travel separately, showing little tendency to interact with each other or with the endothelial cells that form the capillaries and line the walls of larger blood vessels. When tissues are damaged, however, the platelets are exposed to platelet-activating agents that are released at the site of injury. This contact with activating agents initiates a series of events, the final outcome of which is the formation of clot composed of thousands of platelets fused into a single mass. Platelets form a hemostatic plug, helping to stop the flow of blood from a damaged blood vessel, and are a source of adenosine diphosphate (ADP), catecholamines, platelet factor-3, and several other substances that are essential in reactions of the coagulation system plasma proteins.

NORMAL HEMOSTASIS AND COAGULATION

Hemostasis is the process whereby breaks in the vasculature are rapidly repaired while the blood is maintained in a fluid state through clot dissolution known as fibrinolysis. In human beings, normal hemostasis and coagulation is the result of four interrelated phenomena: (1) various reactions of the blood vessels, (2) the formation of a platelet plug, (3) the formation of fibrin, the end result of the process of the coagulation system, and (4) clot dissolution through fibrinolytic mechanisms. Detailed reviews of the physiology of each of these phases may be found in a number of texts including those of Coleman, Hirsch, Marder, and Salzman (1994), Thorup (1987), Corriveau (1988), and Bithell (1987).

The normal vascular endothelium maintains blood fluidity by inhibiting blood coagulation and platelet aggregation and promoting fibrinolysis. It also provides a protective barrier that separates the platelets and plasma factors from highly reactive elements contained in the deeper layers of the vessel wall. These highly reactive elements include collagen and von Willebrand factor, which promote platelet adhesion and tissue-activating factor that triggers blood coagulation.

When the blood vessel is cut or injured, it constricts, thereby diverting blood from the site of injury. At the same time, platelets adhere to the injured area, especially where collagen is exposed. This first step is called platelet adhesion and is dependent upon the presence of von Willebrand factor and a platelet surface receptor site. Within seconds of adhesion, the platelet swells and releases a number of substances that attract other platelets and affect clotting, inflammation, and repair at a site of injury. The substances released include calcium, serotonin, adrenaline, ADP, thromboxane, platelet factor-3, and various other procoagulant factors. It is suggested that some of the chemicals released are responsible for the continued vasoconstriction that occurs at the site of injury. The ADP released by the platelets causes them to become very sticky and to adhere to each other. With each wave of platelet adhesion and release, more platelets are attracted to the site, resulting in a growing aggregate. It is this sequence of events that leads to the formation of a platelet mass at the site of tissue injury large enough to plug the injured vessel.

Formation of a stable clot requires that a soluble protein called fibrinogen be converted to an insoluble protein, fibrin. This is accomplished through a series of events diagrammed in Figure 54–2. As illustrated, the clotting cascade is a series of transformations that are interlinked in a sequential manner such that each activated factor converts the factor next in line into its active form. The clotting cascade can be activated via two possible pathways: the extrinsic pathway and the intrinsic pathway. The extrinsic pathway is activated by tissue thromboplastin released from injured cells including endothelial and smooth muscle cells. The intrinsic pathway is activated following injury to the blood vessel when blood comes in contact with exposed endothelial collagen. Both pathways merge into the common pathway, which leads to the conversion of fibrinogen into fibrin via the enzyme thrombin.

The series of reactions that forms the clot is balanced by a series of reactions that limits the size of the clot and later dissolves it. Therefore in the normal

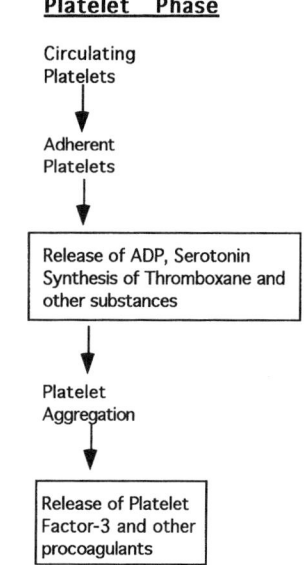

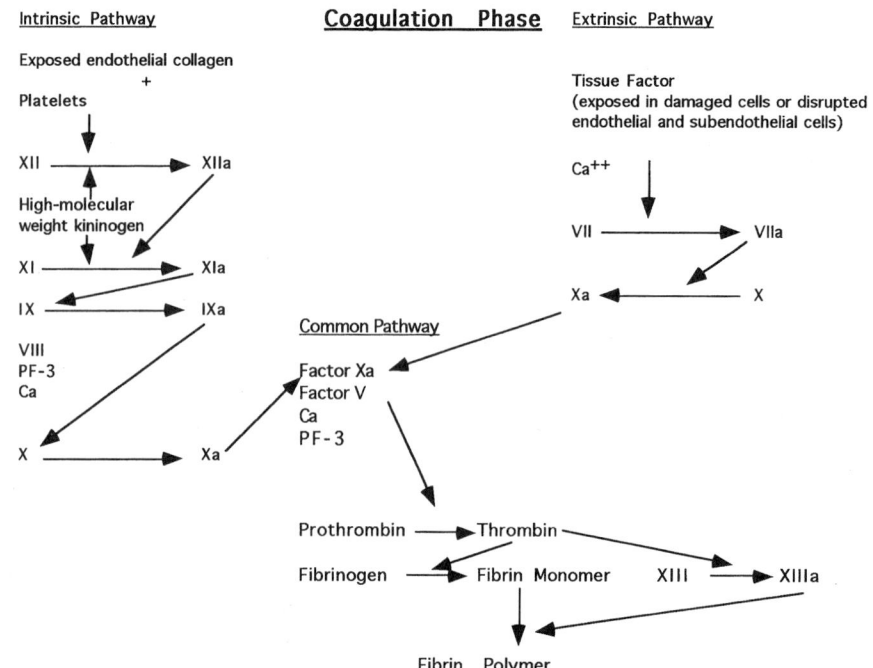

FIGURE 54–2. Stages of the hemostatic and coagulation process.

physiologic state, clot dissolution or fibrinolysis occurs in conjunction with clot formation. The process of fibrinolysis is depicted in Figure 54–3. Plasminogen, the precursor of plasmin, is found in the plasma and attaches to the fibrin as it is forming the clot. Tissue plasminogen activator is released by the endothelial cells damaged by the blood vessel injury. Tissue plasminogen activator catalyses the conversion of plasminogen to plasmin. Plasmin breaks down the clot, and the fibrin fragments are removed by the reticuloendothelial system.

When fibrin is broken down by fibrinolysis, fibrin degradation products (FDPs) or fibrin split products (FSPs) are produced. As these fragments circulate, they themselves interfere with the formation of fibrin, and they also coat the platelets, decreasing the platelet's adhesive ability.

The entire hemostatic process involving endothelial cells and platelets, clotting factors, and adhesive proteins and inhibitory mechanisms of clotting, fibrinolysis, and platelet aggregation serves to promote the right balance and location of hemostasis and recovery. This process can be considered as a system of checks and balances allowing a rapid and efficient hemostatic response to bleeding but preventing the development of thrombosis distant from the site of injury or persisting beyond the time of its physiologic need. Disturbances in any portion of this intricate process can produce an imbalance, resulting in a hemorrhagic or thrombotic clinical disorder.

PATHOPHYSIOLOGY OF ALTERED HEMOSTASIS

There are four pathophysiologic alterations that occur in the hemostatic system in patients with cancer. They are (1) platelet alterations, including thrombocytopenia, and altered platelet aggregation and activation, (2) abnormal activation of the coagulation system, (3) abnormal activation of the fibrinolytic system, and (4) altered quantities of clotting factors, anti-clotting factors, or both (Bick, 1992; Nand & Messmore, 1990; Schwartzberg & Holbert, 1988).

PLATELET ABNORMALITIES

Platelet abnormalities may be categorized as quantitative (an abnormal quantity of platelets) or qualitative (abnormalities in the functional ability and quality).

QUANTITATIVE DYSFUNCTION

An abnormally low number of platelets, thrombocytopenia, is defined as less than 100,000 platelets per mm^3. It is the most common and easily recognizable platelet disorder and is characterized by an increased risk of bleeding. Thrombocytopenia in the patient with cancer can result from decreased production, defective maturation, increased destruction, massive platelet consumption/loss, and platelet sequestration. The risk of serious bleeding increases as the platelet level falls. The risk of spontaneous bleeding occurs when the level falls below 20,000 platelets per mm^3 (Burke, Wilkes, Berg, & Bean, 1991).

Chemotherapy is the most common reason for inadequate platelet synthesis, destroying the immature, proliferating precursors in the bone marrow—the megakaryocytes. Since platelet life span is approximately 10 days once released into the circulation, the destructive effects of chemotherapy are not seen for approximately 7 to 14 days after drug administration, when all the circulating cells have died naturally and there are no replacements from the bone marrow.

Myelosuppression, resulting in thrombocytopenia, is seen more commonly now in patients with solid tumors as a result of the more intensive treatment approaches, which may include combinations of myelosuppressive drugs, and combined modality approaches with chemotherapy and radiation therapy. In addition, bone marrow involvement by tumor cells may lead to lower pretreatment platelet counts and decreased marrow reserves following treatment.

Radiation therapy usually does not interfere in bone marrow function unless 25 per cent or more of the active bone marrow is within the treatment field (Yasko, 1982). Sites of active hematopoiesis in the adult include the pelvis, vertebrae, skull, ribs, sternum, and long bones. Bone marrow suppression tends to be seen if more than one area of the body is being irradiated at one time, as is the case with radiation treatment for lymphoma and with craniospinal radiation. Bone marrow suppression is also more severe when chemotherapy and radiation therapy are delivered in combined protocols. Radiation therapy does not alter the survival of circulating platelets, and the observation that platelet counts do not begin to fall until at least 5 days after radiation exposure suggests that the more mature megakaryocyte precursors are not damaged by radiation exposure (Seifter & Bell, 1983).

Bacterial and viral infection can also contribute to myelosuppression and thus thrombocytopenia in the

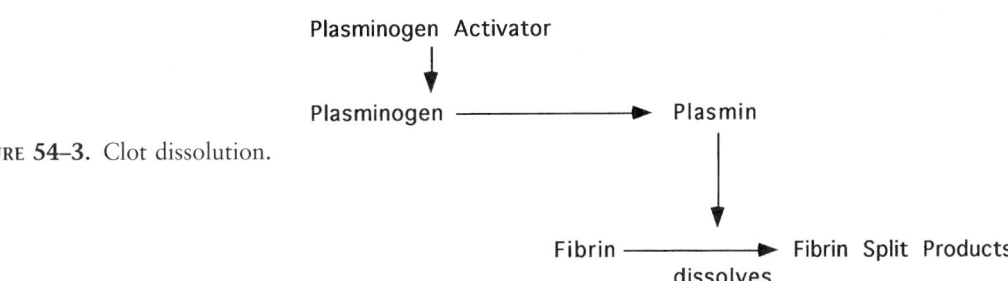

FIGURE 54–3. Clot dissolution.

immunosuppressed cancer patient (Seifter & Bell, 1983). Both bacterial and viral septicemia can result in reduced platelet survival, possibly through immune destruction of circulating platelets (Schwartzberg & Holbert, 1988). The combination of sepsis and active bleeding in the cancer patient continues to be a major cause of morbidity and mortality (Bodensteiner, Tilzer, Adams, & Bayer, 1992).

Defective Platelet Maturation. Myeloproliferative disorders such as myelodysplasia and leukemia are characterized by defective platelet maturation. This results in an insufficient release of mature platelets from the bone marrow, thus producing thrombocytopenia.

Immune Destruction of Platelets. In immune thrombocytopenic purpura (ITP), the patient develops autoantibodies, which bind to platelet membrane antigens, mediating the rapid destruction in the spleen and liver of antibody-coated cells (Nugent, 1993). The presence of antiplatelet antibodies has also been associated with lymphomas, chronic lymphocytic leukemia, acute leukemia, and multiple myeloma. ITP can also develop in patients with cancer as a result of drugs such as phenytoin, thiazides, acetaminophen, erythromycin, penicillin, spironolactone, and sulphonamides (Marcus, 1992), as well as secondary to viral infection or following exposure to blood products (Nugent, 1993).

Consumption. Rapid platelet consumption can be seen whenever extensive clotting occurs. In the patient with cancer, the body can consume massive numbers of platelets in an attempt to stop hemorrhage or during times of fever and sepsis (Seifter & Bell, 1983). Conditions of increased coagulation such as disseminated intravascular coagulation, thrombotic thrombocytopenic purpura (TTP), and microangiopathic hemolytic anemia can also result in rapid platelet utilization.

Platelet Sequestration. Splenic sequestration is the primary cause of disordered platelet distribution and may occur in patients with lymphoma or the acute and chronic leukemias. While the normal spleen may sequester 30 per cent of the circulating platelets, hypersplenism may deplete 90 per cent of the pool. The bone marrow responds to the resultant thrombocytopenia by increasing platelet production; however, this compensatory response only produces more platelets to be sequestered. Splenectomy may be required if splenic rupture or infarction is imminent. Thrombocytosis may follow splenectomy due to maintenance of the accelerated thrombopoiesis.

QUALITATIVE DYSFUNCTION

Neoplastic Causes of Platelet Dysfunction. Myeloproliferative syndromes such as polycythemia vera, myelofibrosis, hairy cell leukemia, and the acute and chronic leukemias result in the production of dysfunctional platelets. Paraproteins secreted in patients with multiple myeloma and lymphomas can coat the surface of platelets or can neutralize von Willebrand factor, resulting in abnormal platelet function (Glaspy, 1992). In addition, cancer cells have been reported to secrete prostacyclin, which impairs platelet function locally.

Drugs. A number of medications commonly used in cancer care have also been shown to induce platelet dysfunction (Kempin, 1991; Seifter & Bell, 1983). These are listed in Table 54–2.

ABNORMAL ACTIVATION OF THE COAGULATION SYSTEM

There is evidence that tumor cells directly or indirectly cause the release of a number of substances that activate the coagulation system (Patterson & Ringenberg, 1990). For example, there is evidence that tissue thromboplastin, which directly initiates the extrinsic pathway of the coagulation cascade, is released by leukemia cells as well as lymphoma cells, adenocarcinomas, and osteogenic sarcomas (Nand & Messmore, 1990). In addition, increased production of tissue thromboplastin by host macrophages has been demonstrated in response to tumor cell invasion. Materials rich in tissue thromboplastin may be released directly into the bloodstream during surgical manipulation of neoplastic and normal tissues and after construction of a peritovenous shunt for malignant ascites (Schwartzberg & Holbert, 1988).

Some tumors also secrete procoagulant substances that can directly activate factor X, thus bypassing the intrinsic and extrinsic pathways and proceeding

TABLE 54–2. *Medications Which May Induce Platelet Dysfunction*

Antimicrobials
Penicillin, carbenicillin, ticarcillin, piperacillin
Cephalosporins
Pentamidine
Amphotericin-B

Antiinflammatory agents
Aspirin
Nonsteroidal antiinflammatory drugs, e.g., Ibuprofen, Naprosyn

Chemotherapy
Actinomycin D
Cyclophosphamide
Daunorubicin
Melphalan
Mithramycin
Mitomycin
Vincristine

Miscellaneous
Phenothiazines
Antidepressants

Selected Nonprescription Products Containing Aspirin
Alka-Seltzer
Aspergum
Coricidin
Doan's Pills
Midol
Pepto-Bismol
Sine-Off Medicine Tablets
Vanquish

directly to the common pathway. For example, factor X activators have been found to be secreted by tumors of the lung, breast, colon, kidney, and vagina, as well as the leukemias (Nand & Messmore, 1990). Adenocarcinomas produce mucin, which has also demonstrated an ability to activate factor X.

Tumor necrosis factor causes a rise in biochemical markers of coagulability and is potentially an important mediator in the hypercoagulability of patients with cancer (Luzzatto & Schaefer, 1990). Tumor necrosis factor is able to dramatically enhance the procoagulant properties of cultured vascular endothelial cells by increasing their tissue thromboplastin activity and to suppress the fibrinolytic activity of cultured vascular endothelial cells (Bick, 1992a). Increased levels of tumor necrosis factor can occur in as many as 50 per cent of cancer patients with active disease (Patterson, 1990).

ABNORMAL ACTIVATION OF THE FIBRINOLYTIC SYSTEM

The fibrinolytic system is abnormally activated in patients with cancer via tumor cell release of plasminogen activator, as well as circulating FDP in patients with disseminated intravascular coagulation (DIC) (Nand & Messmore, 1990; Patterson & Ringenberg, 1990). Cancers of the breast, thyroid, colon, stomach, and the leukemias (particularly AML) can secrete a plasminogen activator substance that results in abnormal clot breakdown and an increased risk of bleeding. Abnormal anticoagulant proteins are produced by a wide variety of tumors including tumors of the lung, breast, and myeloma (Bick, 1992), and they can lead to enhanced fibrinolysis by interfering with the clotting mechanism directly. Fibrin degradation products (FDP), which circulate in patients experiencing a low-grade or chronic disseminated intravascular coagulation, also result in anticoagulation.

ALTERED CLOTTING FACTORS AND ANTICLOTTING FACTOR PRODUCTION

Clotting Factors. Abnormal clotting factor levels can result from liver impairment or specific disease states. Extensive liver involvement from metastatic disease or from other causes such as viral hepatitis or hepatotoxic chemotherapeutic agents may depress the synthesis of clotting factors produced in the liver, including vitamin K. Liver disease can result in the production of dysfunctional clotting proteins and may also impair the clearance of substances such as fibrin degradation products, either of which will result in poor clot formation. Various cancers associated with acquired factor deficiencies include factor X deficiency with thymoma and factor XIII deficiency with chronic myelomonocytic and chronic granulocytic leukemia (Rossle & Ostermann, 1990).

The development of antibodies to one or more of the coagulation factors have been described both in lymphoproliferative disease and in solid tumors. Also, paraproteins secreted by plasma cells in patients with multiple myeloma may surround the coagulation factors and prevent their normal interaction in the coagulation cascade.

Certain chemotherapeutic agents can affect the production of coagulation factors. L-asparaginase alters protein synthesis in the liver and leads to decreased production of factors V and VIII (Ey & Goodnight, 1990) as well as production of a functionally abnormal fibrinogen. Evidence also suggests that L-asparaginase may cause an abnormally rapid clearance of plasma fibrinogen from the circulation (Bick, 1992a). The net result is a decrease in effective plasma fibrinogen levels and clotting factors, which may predispose the patient to bleeding. Other chemotherapeutic drugs that affect coagulation include Actinomycin D, which causes decreased absorption of vitamin K from the gastrointestinal tract, and the anthracyclines, Doxorubicin and Daunorubicin, which have been reported to cause primary fibrinogenolysis (Dutcher, 1987).

Vitamin K is required by the liver in the synthesis of several clotting factors, and vitamin K deficiency can result in impaired synthesis of prothrombin as well as coagulation factors II, VII, IX, and X. A deficiency of vitamin K may result from malabsorption, from the alteration of small bowel flora secondary to treatment with chemotherapy or broad-spectrum antibiotics, or from malnutrition. Replacement with vitamin K can reverse this state within 12 to 48 hours.

Anticlotting Factors. Antithrombin III and protein C are the two major natural anticoagulants produced by the liver. Antithrombin III is the main inhibitor of thrombin, and protein C is a potent inhibitor of activated factors V and VIII. Hepatic synthesis of these anticoagulants is decreased following administration of L-asparaginase (Homans, Rybak, Baghini et al., 1987) and in the setting of metastatic cancer (Bick, 1992a; Nand, Fisher, Slagia, & Fisher, 1987; Rodeghiero, Mannucci, & Vigano, 1984).

CLINICAL MANIFESTATIONS OF ALTERED HEMOSTASIS IN THE CANCER PATIENT

The hemostatic balance is significantly altered by the presence of a malignant tumor. Laboratory evidence of some abnormality of hemostasis is detectable in 50 per cent of patients with cancer and in up to 95 per cent of those patients with metastatic disease (Bick, 1978; Nand et al., 1987; Nand & Messmore, 1990; Prins, Lensig, & Hirsch, 1994). Both the disease itself and the treatment of cancer serve as stimuli for a number of complex interactions involving hemostatic mechanisms. Changes in hemostasis secondary to cancer or its treatment are multifaceted, and the development of clinically significant thrombosis or hemorrhage in cancer patients often represents the expression of many changes in hemostasis (Bick, 1992). The alterations seen include thrombocytosis, thrombocytopenia, elevated fibrin degradation products, prolonged bleeding times, and elevated or depressed levels of clotting factors. This rather variable picture appears to be the end product of a state in which both the coagulation pathway as well as the fibrinolytic pathway are activated, leading to either thrombosis or hemorrhage, depending upon the dominant pathway (Schwartzberg & Holdbert, 1988).

THROMBOSIS

The association between cancer and thrombosis, first described in 1865 by Armand Trousseau, has been confirmed in subsequent observations (Kies & Kwaan, 1982; Seifter & Bell, 1983). The general incidence of thrombosis in malignancy is about 15 per cent but may be higher in specific tumors such as pancreatic carcinoma, where this may be seen in more than 50 per cent of patients (Bick, 1978). While virtually every tumor type has been associated with thrombotic complications, the highest prevalence of both single and successive episodes of thrombosis is noted in patients with cancers of the gastrointestinal tract, male or female genitourinary tract, lung, melanoma, lymphosarcoma, myeloma, lymphoma, Hodgkin's disease, or leukemia (Bick, 1992; Glaspy, 1992; Ratnoff, 1989). Arterial thrombi are less common than venous.

An episode of thrombosis may precede clinical recognition of malignancy by weeks or months (Aderka, Brown, Zelikovski, & Pinkhas, 1986; Goldhaber, Burning, & Hennekens, 1987; Prins et al., 1994; Schaefer, 1985). Controversy exists regarding pursuing a cancer workup for an episode of thrombophlebitis, particularly at an unusual site, since the contrary view exists that deep vein thrombosis or pulmonary embolism carries no increased risk of neoplasm (Goldberg et al., 1987; Gore, Appelbaum, Green, Dexter, & Dalen, 1982; Griffin et al., 1987).

While the association between malignancy and hypercoagulability has led to the description of a myriad of hemostatic system abnormalities in patients with cancer, the pathogenesis of thrombosis associated with neoplasm is only vaguely understood. Some of the laboratory indicators of increased coagulability observed in patients with cancer include shortening of partial thromboplastin time (PTT) and bleeding time, elevated plasma levels of fibrinogen, factors V, VIII, IX, and XI, and thrombocytosis (Elby, 1993).

Hypercoagulability in cancer patients may arise from platelet abnormalities including both thrombocytosis and increased platelet adhesion (Gerson & Lazarus, 1989). Increased platelet adhesion appears to be a uniform abnormality in a variety of solid tumors (Bick, 1992; Nand & Messmore, 1990), and thrombocytosis occurs commonly in tumors of the pancreas, lung, gastrointestinal tract, ovary, breast, and myeloproliferative syndromes (Elby, 1993).

Ratnoff (1989) suggests that thrombosis occurs when clot-promoting agents enter the bloodstream and initiate the clotting process. Factor X may be directly activated by mucin, an agent produced by many tumors. In pancreatic carcinoma, the release of systemic trypsin triggers intravascular coagulation events (Bick, 1992a; Bick & Kunkel, 1992). In other cases, necrosis of tumor cells may release intracellular tissue thromboplastin into the bloodstream.

Another alteration that may increase the likelihood of thrombosis in patients with tumors is an increase in the plasma titer of substances that inhibit tissue plasminogen activator, a change that might impair fibrinolysis (Ruiz et al., 1989). Substances have also been obtained from various animal and human tumors that can directly aggregate platelets. It is postulated that this can lead to clot formation on the vascular subendothelium, resulting in hemostatic activation.

A variety of clinical situations that commonly occur in cancer care can also place the patient at greater risk for thrombosis. These include vascular stasis secondary to pressure from the tumor or immobility, surgery, treatment with hormones or chemotherapeutic agents, and sepsis. Localized thrombophlebitis may also be the result of invasion of veins by neoplastic tissue.

CLINICAL EXAMPLES OF THROMBOSIS

Central Venous Catheters. Thrombosis within and around the catheter is a recognized complication of these devices as platelets and fibrin can deposit on these foreign bodies. The rate of thrombotic complications of these devices is not clearly established, but rates between 4 and 12 per cent have been reported (Ross, et al., 1984). The rates of catheter-related thrombosis in patients with solid tumors may be higher than in those with hematologic malignancies. Incomplete vascular occlusion may be clinically silent. Occlusion of the catheter may be an important clue to the presence of an underlying thrombus, which can progress to complete occlusion of the subclavian vein. Some patients will also go on to develop superior vena cava syndrome or pulmonary emboli.

Hyperviscosity. Another factor contributing to thrombotic events in patients with malignancies is increased viscosity, resulting in stasis, which in turn fosters coagulation (Patterson, Caldwell, & Doll, 1990). The hyperviscosity syndrome may result from markedly elevated cell numbers, as in polycythemia vera, thrombocythemia or leukemia, or from high levels of paraproteins (Gerson & Lazarus, 1989). If blood flow is significantly impeded by increased viscosity, then organ dysfunction, including thrombosis or infarction results as a consequence of impaired capillary circulation. The clinical symptoms of hyperviscosity are generally manifested as neurologic and pulmonary dysfunction (Gerson & Lazarus, 1989). Neurologic symptoms include reduced visual acuity, blurred vision, papilledema, tinnitus, headache, dizziness, ataxia, stupor and coma, and intracranial hemorrhage. Pulmonary symptoms include tachypnea, dyspnea, and hypoxia.

Chemotherapy-induced Thrombosis. While some coagulation abnormalities tend to normalize following initiation of therapy for the particular malignancy (Bick, 1992), considerable data now exist that thromboembolic complications may also result from cancer chemotherapy. This has been recognized with

Hodgkins disease, breast and prostate cancers (Rogers, Murgo, Fontana, & Raich, 1988; Weiss, Tormey, Holland, & Weinberg, 1981). Women with breast cancer receiving cytotoxic regimens containing cyclophosphamide, methotrexate, and 5FU appear to be at increased risk for developing thromboses. While the pathophysiologic basis for the thrombogenicity of chemotherapy in breast cancer patients is not well understood, possible explanations include impairment of vitamin K metabolism, decreased synthesis of the anticoagulants protein C and protein S by the liver, and initiation of intravascular coagulation (Jennis & Bauer, 1993). Thrombotic complications involving both the extremities and the central nervous system have also been attributed to L-asparaginase therapy (Luzzatto & Schafer, 1990). A thrombotic microangiopathy has also been described as a complication of chemotherapy with cisplatin, bleomycin, vinca alkaloids, and mitomycin (Jackson, Rose, & Graff, 1984). The clinical picture includes renal failure, microangiopathic hemolytic anemia, and usually thrombocytopenia. The mechanism of thrombosis associated with chemotherapy remains unclear but may include deficient liver synthesis of some of the naturally occurring anticoagulant proteins. In addition, a number of the cytotoxic drugs cause vascular fibrosis and endothelial cell damage, which may then trigger the coagulation cascade (Patterson & Ringenberg, 1990).

Thrombotic Thrombocytopenia Purpura (TTP) and Microangiopathic Hemolytic Anemia. Thrombotic thrombocytopenia purpura and microangiopathic hemolytic anemia are syndromes in which small clots of platelets and thrombin form in blood vessels. These clots lodge in the arteries and arterioles throughout the body and produce symptoms of hemolysis, renal insufficiency, and thrombocytopenia. TTP differs from ITP or immune thrombocytopenic purpura, described earlier. While both produce thrombocytopenia, TTP produces thrombocytopenia through increased consumption of platelets with disseminated formation of clots. ITP produces thrombocytopenia through immune-mediated destruction of platelets. Both TTP and microangiopathic hemolytic anemia have been associated with a variety of malignancies including breast, GI, lung, prostate, and pancreas (Rosove & Schwartz, 1990), and bacterial and viral infection (Bell, 1993), and have been reported to occur in some cancer patients following treatment with cytotoxic agents (Bell, 1993; Rosen, 1992) and following bone marrow transplantation (Catani et al., 1993) in association with both graft versus host disease and in association with the use of Cyclosporin A (Kroll & McCarthy, 1994; Rosen, 1992). While the etiology of the syndrome is unknown, Rosove & Schwartz (1990) suggest that the pathophysiology most likely involves intravascular coagulation, tumor emboli, and endothelial damage, caused by immune complexes.

Nonbacterial Thrombotic Endocarditis (NBTE). Nonbacterial thrombotic endocarditis is a thrombotic syndrome in which sterile vegetations composed of platelet and fibrin are deposited on the valves of the heart. While this syndrome is generally uncommon, with an overall incidence of about 0.3 per cent (Biller et al., 1982), the incidence of this syndrome is highest in patients with adenocarcinomas and lung cancer. The diagnosis of this syndrome can often be confirmed only on autopsy, since less than 50 per cent of patients have audible cardiac murmurs, and small lesions may not be identified by echocardiography. The possibility of nonbacterial thrombotic endocarditis should be considered in all cancer patients who develop an acute cerebral embolism. The major clinical manifestations are due to emboli from the vegetations on the heart valves, rather from valvular dysfunction itself. Emboli are often released and lodge in the spleen, kidney, and extremities, where they can produce organ dysfunction, ischemia and gangrene of limbs, and cerebrovascular accidents. The most significant morbidity arises from emboli to the central nervous system and coronary arteries.

Nursing Implications. Knowledge of the incidence and pathophysiology of thrombotic complications in the patient with cancer can assist the nurse in anticipating this potential complication and facilitate interventions for prevention and early detection as well as prompt treatment and patient and family education (Ellenberger, Haas, & Cundiff, 1993; Levine & Hirsch, 1990; Naschitz, Yeshurum, & Lev, 1993). Table 54–3 outlines the signs and symptoms, evaluation, and management of several thrombotic complications that may occur in the patient with cancer.

HEMORRHAGE

Disease-related Thrombocytopenia. Thrombocytopenia is an intrinsic component of the disease process of hematologic malignancies, particularly of acute leukemia. Chapter 35 discusses the pathology and consequences of leukemia in terms of its effects on bone marrow function. Replacement and crowding out of the normal bone marrow elements decreases the number of platelet precursors. Although a patient with leukemia can be supported with platelet transfusions for a limited time, eradicating the disease offers the only chance for restoring normal platelet production through repopulation of the bone marrow with normal platelet progenitor cells.

Bleeding can be a presenting sign at diagnosis, a complication of treatment, or a consequence of prolonged thrombocytopenia in the patient with either an acute or chronic leukemia or a myelodysplastic syndrome (Aderka, Praff, Santo, Weinberger, & Pinkhas, 1986; Collins, 1990; Ey & Goodnight, 1990; Sheridan, 1990; Yeomans & Harle, 1990). Abnormal progenitor cell differentiation and maturation in each disease results in a qualitative or quantitative platelet abnormality, or both, at some point in the disease process.

In many cases, the first clinical sign leading to a diagnosis of leukemia is spontaneous bleeding or bleeding following an invasive procedure inadvertently performed when the patient is asymptomatic but has moderate thrombocytopenia. Treatment of the underlying disease is essential. Unlike patients with solid tumors, patients with leukemia usually have a markedly dimin-

TABLE 54–3. *Evaluation and Management of Selected Thrombotic Complications in the Patient With Cancer*

COMPLICATION	SIGNS AND SYMPTOMS	ASSESSMENT AND EVALUATION	NURSING IMPLICATIONS	MEDICAL RESPONSE
Thrombosis	• Sharp, constant, well-localized pain • Feeling of fullness in the skin • Slight increase in the skin color and/or temperature • Edema and accentuated venous patterning of the affected limb	• Physical examination findings may be nonspecific • Doppler ultrasound of the affected limb(s) • Venogram of the affected limb(s) may be needed to confirm diagnosis	• Elastic stockings and the avoidance of activities/postures that promote venous stasis may reduce the occurrence. • Assess and monitor for side effects to the circulatory system or client's skin from stockings. • Heat, elevation, and rest since superficial venous thrombosis may respond to local therapy. • Monitor for signs and symptoms of bleeding if receiving anticoagulants.	• Treatment of tumor • Warfarin or heparin therapy • Antiplatelet medications, i.e., Aspirin 600 mg P.O. bid, Dipyridamole 500 mg P.O. qid • Inferior vena cava filter
Pulmonary embolus	• Sharp, pleuritic pain • Dyspnea • Hemoptysis • Apprehension • Augmented pulmonic component of second heart sound	• Arterial blood gas analysis • EKG • Chest x-ray • V-Q scan if EKG and chest x-ray are normal • Pulmonary angiogram may be needed to confirm diagnosis	• Frequent assessment and documentation of vital signs, arterial blood gases, and oxygen saturations. • Contact physician as soon as possible if decreased mental status or worsening oxygen saturation. • Assist positioning of patient in high-Fowlers with oxygen therapy. • Frequent oral care and skin care when oxygen is in use. • Monitor for signs and symptoms of bleeding if receiving anticoagulants.	• Heparin therapy • Possible thrombolytic therapy • Oxygen • Morphine sulfate for comfort
Thrombotic thrombocytopenia purpura (TTP)	• Anemia • Thrombocytopenia • Fluctuating neurologic signs (e.g., headache, seizures, pareses, dysphasia, obtundation, or visual disturbances) • Fever • Abdominal pain • Bruising/bleeding	Evaluation is directed toward excluding other causes for these symptoms: • CBC: increased reticulocyte count, and increased circulating nucleated RBCs • Peripheral blood smear: fragmented erythrocytes • Coagulation studies (PT, PTT, fibrinogen levels are usually normal) • Serum chemistries: increased LDH, increased indirect bilirubin • Urinalysis: hematuria, proteinuria • Infection workup • Neurologic evaluation • Abdominal evaluation	• Administration of fresh-frozen plasma and blood products as needed. • Monitor urine and blood for glucose if the patient is receiving glucocorticoids.	• Plasmapheresis with fresh-frozen plasma • Vincristine or Azathioprine may be used for refractory TTP • Glucocorticoids

ished capacity to produce platelets due both to the disease process and to the subsequent chemotherapy, which produces marrow hypoplasia lasting several weeks.

The potential for bleeding and the degree of thrombocytopenia is greater in the early period of diagnosis and treatment with acute leukemia. As remission is achieved and the body rehabilitates after intensive treatment, the incidence of bleeding diminishes (Aderka et al., 1986; Ey & Goodnight, 1990). For the patient with a chronic form of leukemia, bleeding may not be an issue until later disease stages.

Nursing Implications. Assessment of thrombocytopenia begins with an evaluation of the peripheral blood and bone marrow aspirate. One must first determine whether it is a problem of decreased platelet production within the bone marrow or increased platelet destruction in the peripheral blood. A review of the patient's history identifies insults to the marrow such as previous chemotherapy and radiation therapy where the treatment fields included areas of active bone marrow. The patient's current medication profile should also be reviewed to identify any medications that may cause marrow suppression or which may cause quantitative or qualitative platelet defects. A physical examination is aimed at identifying any bleeding sites or signs of internal or occult bleeding.

Patients and their families need instruction regarding the relationship between the circulating platelet count and the risk of bleeding. As the platelet level decreases, education needs to be very specific regarding which activities patients should avoid to minimize the risk of bleeding. Emphasis should also be placed on teaching the patient and family the signs and symptoms of bleeding. The frequency of patient assessments and reinforcement of education should intensify as patient's platelet levels drop (Rostad, 1991). Table 54–4 outlines problems and nursing interventions in the patient with thrombocytopenia.

Leukostasis. Leukostasis in the lung and brain associated with pulmonary and intracranial hemorrhages is a complication that can occur in the presence of a circulating leukocyte count greater than 100,000. Leukocyte counts in excess of 100,000 can occur with AML, ALL, and with the blast crisis of CML. These complications contribute to increased morbidity and mortality. The pathophysiology of leukostasis is not clear; however, Lichtman and Rowe (1982) and Rossle and Ostermann (1990) suggest that leukemic blast cells are large and relatively deformed, thereby producing stasis and impeding microcirculation. Impaired blood flow, stasis, and the high oxygen consumption of blast cells result in hypoxemia, which causes vascular endothelial damage. When this occurs in the central nervous system, particularly in the setting of concommittant thrombocytopenia and coagulation abnormalities, catastrophic hemorrhage can result (Lichtman & Rowe, 1982; Rossle & Ostermann, 1990).

Disseminated Intravascular Coagulation. Disseminated intravascular coagulation is the coagulopathy most frequently associated with malignancy. It is reported to occur in as many as 15 per cent of patients with malignancy (Belt, Leite, Haas & Stephens, 1978). Resulting from a generalized activation of the coagulation system, the consequences of DIC are consumption of clotting factors, among them fibrinogen and platelets, and, secondarily, initiation of the fibrinolytic pathway. Fibrinogen and fibrin are broken down by fibrinolysis, resulting in the appearance of FDPs or FSPs. As these fragments circulate, they themselves interfere with the formation of fibrin, and they also coat the platelets, thus decreasing the platelet's adhesive ability. The result is continued anticoagulation along with the process of fibrinolysis. These processes bring about generalized and often catastrophic bleeding as well as evidence of both gross and microscopic thrombosis (Colman & Rubin, 1990).

DIC has been reported as a complication of many neoplastic disorders but is most likely to occur in carcinoma of the prostate, lung, breast, and gastrointestinal tract, in melanoma, and in leukemia, particularly acute promyelocytic leukemia (Bick, 1992; Lankiewicz & Bell, 1993; Rosen, 1992; Sack, Levin, & Bell, 1977). Tumor-associated initiators of the clotting process in DIC can include mucin secretion (which directly activates factor X) and the release into the bloodstream of tissue thromboplastin-like tumor products (which interact with factor VII and result in the formation of thrombin) (Brain et al., 1970; Gralnick & Abrell, 1973).

Both an acute and a more chronic pattern of DIC may be seen in association with malignancy. Acute forms of DIC are likely to present with minor bleeding from mucosal or cutaneous surfaces, or extensive life-threatening hemorrhage involving visceral sites. Patients with acute DIC may also demonstrate hypercoagulability and can manifest deep venous thrombosis, disseminated thrombosis in the vasculature of major organs, or nonbacterial thrombotic endocarditis. More common in patients are chronic forms of DIC. Many such patients are asymptomatic, and laboratory data often show only modest reductions in fibrinogen and platelet count, elevated FDPs, and minimal changes in the PT or PTT. The laboratory picture commonly associated with DIC is presented in Table 54–5.

TTP-induced Hemorrhage. Rapid consumption of platelets and clotting factors resulting in hemorrhage may be seen whenever extensive widespread clotting occurs, particularly in the setting of the cancer patient who has decreased production of either platelets or clotting factors. The body can consume massive amounts of both platelet and clotting factors in an attempt to stop hemorrhage. Conditions of increased coagulation may occur with DIC, TTP, and microangiopathic hemolytic anemia, resulting in bleeding because of rapid platelet and clotting factor depletion.

LABORATORY EVALUATION OF THE PATIENT WITH ALTERED HEMOSTASIS

Several blood studies may be done to assess all parts of the blood-clotting mechanism. The results of

TABLE 54–4. *Patient Problems and Nursing Interventions for the Myelosuppressed Patient With Cancer: Thrombocytopenia*

KNOWLEDGE DEFICIT	POTENTIAL FOR INJURY
Level I Potential/Mild (Platelet Count 50,000-100,000/mm³) Instruct the client* on: <ul><li>Relation of platelets and bleeding</li><li>Occurrence of thrombocytopenia after treatment</li><li>Signs and symptoms of bleeding</li><li>Measures to prevent/manage bleeding episodes</li></ul>	<ul><li>Obtain the past and present treatment history; identify occurrences of thrombocytopenia</li><li>Monitor the CBC and platelet count with each visit</li><li>Conduct a physical assessment at each visit to detect signs of bleeding</li><li>Assess oral cavity, sclera, excretions, skin, vital signs, and neurologic status</li><li>Implement preventive measures:<ul><li>Soft toothbrush, no flossing, and nonastringent mouthwash</li><li>Fluids and high-fiber diet to prevent constipation</li><li>Avoid IM injections and rectal medications, examinations, or temperatures</li><li>Minimize invasive procedures whenever possible (e.g., IVs, bladder catheterization)</li><li>Avoid drugs that interfere with platelet function (e.g., ASA)</li><li>Use only an electric razor when shaving</li><li>Avoid contact sports and activities that predispose to injury</li><li>Instruct women to use sanitary napkins for menstrual flow and not tampons. Use water-soluble lubricant prior to sexual intercourse</li></ul></li></ul>
Level II: Moderately Severe (Platelet Count 20,000-50,000/mm³) Level I plus: <ul><li>Inform the client of moderately low platelet count and increased risk of bleeding</li><li>Inform the client of risks associated with platelet transfusion</li></ul>	Level I plus: <ul><li>Assess for the presence of factors that further compromise platelet function (e.g., fever, sepsis)</li><li>Conduct a physical assessment daily to detect signs of bleeding (more frequently if signs of bleeding are noted)</li><li>Implement measures to control nausea and vomiting</li><li>Assist the patient with ambulation/getting up if required</li><li>Provide a safe physical environment free of hazards that might lead to injury</li><li>Arrange for platelet donation</li><li>Control bleeding episodes by applying pressure to site, ice packs, and topical thrombin if prescribed</li><li>Administer platelets as prescribed</li><li>Assess effects of platelet transfusion and other interventions</li><li>Monitor posttransfusion platelet counts</li><li>Estimate blood loss (e.g., volume, number of tissues/pads saturated)</li></ul>
Level III: Severe (Platelet Count ≤ 20,000/mm³) Levels I and II plus: <ul><li>Inform the client of seriousness of problem and the need for frequent assessment/immediate intervention.</li></ul>	Levels I and II plus: <ul><li>Assess the patient for signs of bleeding every 8 hours or more frequently if bleeding episodes have occurred</li><li>Have IV access available at all times</li><li>Monitor for the immediate availability of donor platelets</li><li>Be prepared for a medical emergency if significant blood loss occurs</li></ul>

*Client = patient, family, significant other person. CBC = complete blood count; IM = intramuscular; IV = intravenous; ASA = acetylsalicylic acid (aspirin).

(From Rostad, M. E. [1991]. Current strategies for managing myelosuppression in patients with cancer. *Oncology Nursing Forum, 18* (Suppl.), 7–15.)

TABLE 54–5. *Typical Laboratory Profile in DIC*

LABORATORY TEST	TREND EXPECTED IN PATIENT WITH DIC
Prothrombin time	Prolonged
Partial thrombo-plastin time	Prolonged
Thrombin time	Prolonged
Fibrinogen level	Decreased
Platelet count	Decreased
Fibrinogen/fibrin degradation products	Increased
D-Dimers	Elevated
Hemoglobin and hematocrit	May be decreased with active bleeding

these laboratory tests are considered in conjunction with the patient's clinical manifestations and history. Table 54–6 lists the major tests of hemostasis and coagulation, the hemostatic mechanisms assessed by each test, and selected causes of a deviation from normal.

In planning care for the patient at risk for or experiencing bleeding, a number of additional factors should be considered since they can increase the risk of bleeding. These include tumor invasion of blood vessels, altered mucosal integrity, esophagitis, infection, episodes of fever, or sepsis which may contribute to increased platelet consumption, invasive procedures, and any concommitant coagulopathies.

TISSUE EROSION AND ULCERATION

Neoplastic growth can cause bleeding when blood vessels are invaded by growing tumor or when mucosal surfaces become ulcerated secondary to tumor erosion. The bleeding that results can range from microscopic, scant amounts to gross hemorrhage. The amount of bleeding is determined by the blood vessel(s) involved, the patient's platelet and coagulation status, and the integrity of surrounding mucosa and tissue. Previously irradiated tissue can become fibrotic or friable, predisposing it to damage with even minimal trauma.

Small Bowel Cancer. The second, most common sign of small bowel cancers on presentation is bleeding into the stool, occurring in 20 to 50 per cent of cases (Ashley & Wells, 1988). Blood loss is usually minimal but can result in microcytic, hypochromic anemia because of the chronic nature of the bleeding. Hemorrhage occurrence varies among malignant small bowel lesions, is more common with leiomyosarcomas than adenocarcinomas, and is rare with carcinoid tumors (Ashley & Wells, 1988).

Colon Cancer. Lesions in the duodenum result in obvious signs of jaundice and chronic bleeding, whereas signs and symptoms of jejunal and ileal lesions are more vague. Bleeding and blood loss are common symptoms of colon cancer, since this disease presents as red blood mixed with stool when the bleeding is acute or as melena if the tumor is located on the right side. Bleeding tends to be from tumor erosion into the mucosa. Iron deficiency anemia may be present in the patient who has been experiencing chronic, occult loss (Cohen, Minsky & Shilsky, 1993).

Esophageal Cancer. Clinical presentation is similar for all esophageal cancer cell types. Although the majority of presenting signs and symptoms reflect subjective feelings of a "lump" or "difficulty swallowing," bleeding from the tumor can occur. Hematemesis, melena, or hemoptysis tend to occur with more advanced lesions (Skinner & Belsey, 1988).

Exsanguination in the patient with esophageal cancer occurs when tumor erosion into the aorta occurs. Cilley, Strodel, and Peterson (1989) showed on autopsy that 12 per cent of patients with esophageal cancer died from exsanguination due to tumor erosion into the thoracic aorta. There are often no prewarning signs other than the fact that the tumor is advanced and unresponsive to further therapy. Patients die quickly, since it takes only minutes for a patient's total blood supply to be depleted (Roth, Putnam, Lichter, & Forastiere, 1993; Skinner & Belsey, 1988). Intense, supportive education to family members is a means of preparing the family for a possible hemorrhagic terminal event.

Head and Neck Cancer. Minor bleeding can occur with tumors of the oral cavity, and as the lesions advance, bleeding often increases. Intermittent bleeding or blood-streaked saliva is associated with irritation of the tumor caused by chewing or from close proximity of the tumor to the patient's teeth (Schantz, Harrison & Hong, 1993).

Tumors of the hypopharynx are characterized by blood-streaked saliva rather than frank blood. A mass in the nasopharynx may lead to hemorrhage if it enlarges rapidly (Stimson et al., 1993).

Carotid artery erosion and rupture has a high mortality rate and an incidence rate of 3 to 4 per cent (Lesage, 1986). It is a devastating experience to witness and a physical challenge to care for. Arterial erosion is a consequence of a number of mechanisms: poor wound healing, exposure of the artery to the atmosphere, tumor growth and invasion, previous radiation/chemotherapy treatment, and infection (Morris & Holland, 1993; McDonnell, 1994).

During head and neck dissections, the outermost layer of the artery carrying 80 per cent of the blood supply to the remaining artery layers can dry out when exposed to the atmosphere during surgery or if there is wound dehiscence. As a result, blood supply to the other layers is compromised, and the result is that layers of the arterial wall progressively become destroyed (McDonnell, 1994).

Previous irradiation is the greatest risk factor associated with a carotid erosion. Radiation therapy alters the carotid arterial layers; tissue healing in surgical wounds is affected as well as that associated with tumor invasion causing tissue breakdown. Blood flow is decreased by 50 per cent after 3000 cGy and by 70 per cent after 9000 cGy, predisposing the arterial wall to invasion and injury (Lesage, 1986). See Table 54–7 for risk factors predisposing a patient to carotid artery rupture.

TABLE 54–6. *Major Laboratory Tests of Hemostasis and Coagulation*

TEST	NORMAL VALUE	NORMAL MECHANISM MEASURED	CAUSES OF DEVIATION FROM NORMAL
Platelet count	150,000–400,000	Number of platelets in the peripheral blood.	ITP, bone marrow suppression, bone marrow involvement with tumor, vitamin B_{12} deficiency, folic acid deficiency, infection, loss through hemorrhage
Bleeding time	Depends on test methodology used	Measures the amount of time bleeding occurs from a small incision in the skin. Assesses the adequacy and functional capacity of platelets and the ability of blood vessels to constrict.	Prolonged with low platelet count, with platelet dysfunction, and with ingestion of aspirin
Partial thromboplastin time (PTT)/Activated partial thromboplastin time (aPTT)	PTT: 16–25 seconds aPTT: 30–45 seconds	Used to detect abnormalities of all plasma clotting factors except factor VII, factor XIII, and platelets. Often used to monitor heparin therapy.	Prolonged in the presence of high levels of FDP, decreased clotting factors, liver disease, DIC, aspirin therapy, vitamin K deficiency, and in the presence of heparin.
Prothrombin time (PT)	Approximately 12–14 seconds; reported values must be related to a control	Identifies defects in the extrinsic clotting mechanism by reflecting the activity of factor V, factor VII, and factor X as well as fibrinogen and prothrombin.	Prolonged in the presence of high levels of FDP, decreased clotting factors, liver disease, DIC, aspirin therapy, vitamin K deficiency, and in the presence of coumadin.
Thrombin time	10–15 seconds	Measures time required for a fibrin clot to form when thrombin is added to plasma. Because this test artificially bypasses stages I and II of the coagulation process, deficits due to abnormal fibrinogen can be detected.	Prolonged in the presence of decreased levels of plasma fibrinogen, a defect or alteration in the structure of fibrinogen, with liver disease, and in the presence of FDP or heparin
Platelet aggregation	Visible in less than 5 minutes	Ability of platelets to aggregate or clump together.	Altered in the presence of high levels of FDP, aspirin, with medications which alter platelet function
Fibrinogen level	160–300 mg/100 ml	Assesses the amount of fibrinogen present in the plasma.	Decreased with consumption of fibrinogen, fibrinogenolysis, decreased fibrinogen synthesis with liver disease
Fibrin/fibrinogen degradation products (FDPs)	Less than 10 mg/ml	FDPs are partially digested fragments that result from the lysis of fibrin or fibrinogen by plasmin; FDPs have an anticoagulant effect and inhibit blood clotting when they circulate in large quantities.	Increased with fibrinogen/fibrin destruction by plasmin, conditions associated with extensive intravascular clotting, e.g., DIC
D-Dimers	Less than 200 ng/ml	D-Dimers are produced in the breakdown of cross-linked or stable fibrin. Cross-linked fibrin occurs with the formation of a stable clot. Therefore, D-Dimer levels are a more sensitive measure than the FDP of the breakdown of stable clots versus the breakdown of both soluble fibrinogen and insoluble fibrin.	Increased in conditions associated with extensive intravascular clotting, e.g., DIC, TTP

Timing of a rupture is unpredictable, so nursing interventions are preventive in nature. Occasionally a rupture may be signaled by the patient reporting a pressure in his or her chest. Education is aimed at preparing the patient and family for a possibly horrifying event. It also means reassuring the patient that care will be provided and learning how aggressive the interventions should be. Preparation for the physical demands of a carotid rupture include relieving discomfort and distress during the event as well as anticipating what equipment will be necessary for arterial end ligation, if that is the goal (McDonnell, 1994). See Table 54–8 for a nursing protocol regarding management of carotid artery rupture.

Mucous Membranes. Mucositis/stomatitis in response to antineoplastic therapy places the patient at risk for bleeding from the mucosa. Since the mucosa can become denuded and friable by the epithelial changes that occur in response to treatment, the protective barrier weakens. The mucosa can also be altered by leukemic infiltrates, graft-versus-host disease, and superimposed infections. The risk of bleeding increases

TABLE 54–7. *Risk Factors Predisposing to Carotid Artery Rupture*

- Prior irradiation to neck region
- Irradiation to neck region within 2 months of surgery
- Salivary fistula
- Skin flap necrosis
- Localized bacterial infection
- Vertical incision line over the carotid
- Over 50 years of age
- Poor nutritional status
- Diabetes
- Atherosclerosis
- Tumor growth

with each insult and alteration to the mucosa (Daeffler, 1994; Greifzu, Radjeski & Winnick, 1990; Holmes, 1991; Shaffer, 1994.)

Thrombocytopenia increases the likelihood of bleeding as well as the total blood lost. Trauma or irritation can result in hemorrhagic complications. Thrombocytopenia in isolation of other risk factors does not cause spontaneous mucosal oozing or diffuse bleeding. But the combination of a prolonged PT and thrombocytopenia do tend to result in more severe bleeding (Chu, Shivshanker, Stroehlein, & Nelson, 1983).

Mucous membrane hypersensitivity in the oral cavity is manifested by spontaneous as well as traumatic bleeding. Teeth brushing, flossing, rinsing with mouthwash or irrigation, as well as chewing are significant irritants that may initiate hemorrhagic events. It is common to have marked gingival bleeding. Although soft blood clots form in response to intermittent bleeding, they are easily abraded, and significant blood loss can occur. Bleeding and hemorrhagic tendency increase with oral infection, preexisting periodontal disease, leukemic cell infiltration of the gums, and mucosal dryness from mouth breathing, oxygen therapy, and xerostomia (Holmes, 1991).

SITES AND SOURCES OF BLEEDING

GASTROINTESTINAL TRACT

Since the mucous membranes line the entire gastrointestinal (GI) tract, bleeding can occur anywhere along the tract from mouth to anus. The GI tract is prone to bleeding, since the mucosa is often altered and the vasculature is close to the mucosal surface. Mucosal ulceration at almost any point along the GI tract could lead to arterial erosion and bleeding (Shelton, 1993). GI bleeding in the cancer patient can occur because of a bleeding disorder or coagulopathy, or from gastritis (ulcers), esophageal varices, Mallory-Weiss tears, esophagitis, and gastrointestinal lymphomas (Baker, 1993; Morris & Holland, 1993; Shivshanker, Chu, Stroehlein, & Nelson, 1983; Stellato & Shenk, 1989). Potentiating factors for GI pathology and bleeding include chronicity of disease, use of NSAIDs, anticoagulation, corticosteroids, alcohol abuse, malnutrition, and concurrent stresses such as sepsis, hepatitis, and organ failure (Morris & Holland, 1993; Shivshanker et al., 1983). Lesions that bleed tend to be unifocal, whereas diffuse mucosal bleeding from more than one site is associated with a platelet count less than 40,000/mm^3 (Chu et al., 1983).

Gastritis. Shivshanker et al. (1983) documented a 32 per cent incidence of benign gastritis in cancer patients who had experienced a 2 g drop in hemoglobin. This finding was comparable with a similar study performed 10 years earlier (Lightdale, Kurtz, Boyle, Sherlock, & Winawer, 1973). Twenty-six per cent of the patients (N = 133) that Shivshanker's (1983) team studied were found to have gastric or duodenal ulcers that were not infectious or malignant in etiology. This was the most common cause of bleeding in the population of cancer patients studied.

Gastritis ulcerations are controversial in their cause. In the patient experiencing cancer, the GI mucosa can be altered by possible insult from infection, chemother-

TABLE 54–8. *Nursing Protocol for the Aggressive Management of Carotid Artery Rupture*

FACTOR	INTERVENTION
Airway maintenance	Inflate cuff of tracheostomy or laryngectomy tube to prevent aspiration of blood
	Insert oral airway if patient does not have a tracheostomy
	Suction aspirated blood
	Administer oxygen
Minimizing blood loss	Position patient in Trendelenburg's position to minimize cerebral hypoxia
	Determine site of bleeding
	Apply digital pressure with gauze or dressing material to the bleeding site
	Notify caregivers of the emergency situation
Stabilization of cardiovascular status	Maintain rapid infusion of IV fluids
	Initiate blood-product transfusion
	Monitor vital signs
Comfort	Reassure patient and family that everything is being done
	Act in a calm, organized manner
	Administer analgesics as prescribed

(From McDonnell, K. K. [1994]. Leukostasis. In J. Gross & B. L. Johnson [Eds.], *Handbook of oncology nursing* [2nd ed., pp. 756–763]. ©1994. Boston: Jones and Bartlett Publishers. Reprinted with permission.)

apy or radiation-induced mucositis, hyperacidity from increased acid secretion due to stress or corticosteroids, or concurrent physical stressors. The thickness of the mucosa and GI barrier erodes and continues to erode with repeated exposure to damaging causes. As the mucosal barrier wears away, acid backwashes, leading to gastric erosion (Shelton, 1993; Wallach & Kurtz, 1992). Depending upon the location of the erosion and the number of sites, blood loss occurs.

Esophagitis. In the immunocompromised patient, esophagitis is manifested by fever, retrosternal burning chest pain, nausea, emesis, odynophagia, and/or bleeding. Pathogens causing esophagitis in the immunocompromised population can be viral (cytomegalovirus [CMV] and herpes simplex virus [HSV]), fungal (*Candida* or *Aspergillus*), or bacterial (McDonald, Sharma, Hackman, Meyers, & Thomas, 1985; Walsh, Belitsos, & Hamilton, 1986). Organisms identified through oral examination and culture do not necessarily correlate with the invading esophageal organism; therefore endoscopic biopsy is necessary for pathologic confirmation (McDonald et al., 1985).

McDonald et al. (1985) identified esophageal infections as causes of esophagitis in 46 per cent of bone marrow transplant patients studied. Of those studied (N = 39), CMV and HSV infections occurred with equal incidence. Fungal infections tended to occur much later than viral infections following BMT. All had similar signs and symptoms. Hematemesis was correlated with patients having a platelet count less than 50,000/mm³. The most common endoscopic finding were diffuse, shallow erosions in the distal half of the esophagus.

Mallory-Weiss Syndrome. Mallory-Weiss syndrome is characterized by violent vomiting leading to acute hemorrhage from a tear in the mucosal layer on the gastric side of the esophagogastric junction. For a spontaneous rupture to occur in the patient with a normal esophagus, precipitating conditions are needed. The conditions include a full stomach, nausea, violent vomiting, and temporary obstruction in the esophagus most likely caused by an acute reflex spasm. The conditions are then simultaneously accompanied by a sudden, explosive increase in esophageal intraluminal pressure to rupture the organ. Although uncommon, it is a life-threatening event that may require emergency surgery (Skinner & Belsey, 1988).

Gastrointestinal Hemorrhage

GI hemorrhage (1000 cc blood loss) is manifested as hematemesis (vomiting of bright red or coffee ground blood), melena (black, tarry stools), or hematochezia (red blood per rectum) (Shelton, 1993). As blood remains in the GI tract and mixes with gastric acid, it darkens and can range in color from dark red to black stool or coffee ground emesis. Patients may complain of abdominal discomfort, and in the event of a massive bleed, a sense of impending doom. Correlating any invasive interventions or physical stresses along with the color and consistency of a bleed assists in identifying site and insult.

Signs and Symptoms. Upper GI tract, esophageal, and stomach bleeds can be characterized by hematemesis, maroon stool, and abdominal pain. Lower GI tract, large bowel, and rectal bleeding are reflected in melena, painless, occult, or obvious blood in the stool (Labovich, 1994; Shelton, 1993). Thorough physical assessment is conducted upon initial patient contact and should be conducted frequently to diagnose change. Each assessment finding should be reviewed within the context of previous findings, interventions, and occurrences (Miaskowski, 1985).

Diagnosis. In patients with upper GI bleeding, endoscopy is useful in identifying the precise site and etiology of the bleeding. Although bleeding can stop spontaneously, there can be as high as an 80 per cent incidence of recurrent bleeding (Wara, 1985). An abdominopelvic CT scan is the best evaluation for hemorrhage into the free abdominal cavity, liver, or retroperitoneum (Baker, 1993).

Nursing and Medical Implications. Preventive care includes antacids, sucralfate, and H₂-receptor antagonist therapy, especially in the physically stressed patient or the patient receiving corticosteroids (Roubein & Levin, 1993). Conservative management of bleeding includes volume replacement, coagulopathy, correction of nasogastric drainage to low intermittent suction, ice lavage or ice enema, blood product support, and gut rest. Care is taken to minimize injury to the gastric mucosa and to avoid abrading newly formed clots. Blood product replacement for the patient experiencing GI hemorrhage is determined by volume lost and presence of coagulopathy. Blood contains coagulation proteins and calcium, which need to be monitored and replenished along with red blood cells and platelets (Labovich, 1994).

More aggressive attempts to control bleeding without surgery in nonvariceal upper gastrointestinal hemorrhage include electrocoagulation, heater probe, laser treatment, or injection sclerosis therapy. These are equally effective in controlling actively bleeding lesions in the gastroduodenal areas in as many as 95 per cent of patients and decrease rates of further bleeding (Cook, Guyatt, Salena, & Laine, 1992; Hui, Ng, Lok, Lai, Lau & Lam, 1991; Waring, Sanowski, Sawyer, Woods, & Foutch, 1991).

Angiography is utilized to locate and treat lesions located in the small bowel or colon. Agents capable of vessel occlusion such as gelfoam can be instilled via the same catheter with varying degrees of success (Baker, 1993). The expertise of the angiographer is critical to patient outcomes since ongoing decisions are made regarding the patient's ability to sustain a dye load and the lengthy time needed for studying the major vessels—inferior mesenteric artery, superior mesenteric artery, and celiac axis (Baker, 1993; Hui et al., 1991).

Surgical interventions are chosen when less invasive alternatives are unsuccessful or inappropriate because of the patients' physical status. Surgery is indicated to control free intraperitoneal bleeding in the abdominal cavity or from the spleen, liver, or aorta (Baker, 1993).

URINARY TRACT

Frank bleeding is a presenting sign of kidney, urethral, and prostate cancer. It is also the result of metastatic invasion into the urinary tract by gynecologic, colon, or pelvic cancers (Russo, 1993).

Etiology. Hemorrhagic cystitis is inflammation of the bladder leading to ulceration and bleeding. Its causes are either viral in nature, secondary to radiation therapy, or due to toxic metabolites from antineoplastic drugs. Hemorrhagic cystitis can be acute, occurring during the antineoplastic drug administration or shortly afterward. It can also be delayed, occurring long after therapy has been completed. Delayed hemorrhagic cystitis is most common in patients receiving long-term oral cyclophosphamide. Bleeding can range from microscopic to frank, gross amounts requiring transfusion. It is difficult to predict which patients will experience hemorrhagic cystitis (DeVries & Freiha, 1990; Levine & Richie, 1989; Russo, 1993).

Twenty one per cent of patients receiving curative radiation therapy to the pelvic area and bladder (gynecologic, genitourinary, and rectal cancers) experience bladder complications, with very few experiencing bladder hemorrhage (Dean & Lytton, 1978; Parsons, 1986). Following radiation therapy to the pelvis, small blood vessels along the bladder mucosa become friable and can rupture spontaneously. Serious hemorrhage can result. There is a direct relationship between the dose of radiation and the incidence of cystitis (Dean & Lytton, 1978).

The bone marrow transplant population has been cited as experiencing viral causes of hemorrhagic cystitis (Ambinder et al., 1986; Rice, Bishop, Apperley, & Gardner, 1985). Ambinder et al. (1986) identified Adenovirus type II in less than 10 per cent of bone marrow recipients over a 7-year period in weekly urine virology surveillance cultures. Rice et al. (1985) identified BK virus in the urine of bone marrow transplant patients during investigation of hemorrhagic cystitis causes. Both groups of clinicians noted that preventative measures for hemorrhagic cystitis had been instituted.

Signs and Symptoms. Hematuria can be divided into different categories of bleeding severity. Mild hematuria characterized by microscopic or small amounts of bleeding does not affect the hematocrit and can be easily controlled. Moderate hematuria is characterized by blood loss requiring 6 units or less of packed red blood cell transfusions over several days, whereas severe hematuria requires transfusions greater than 6 units and is refractory to simple irrigations, installations, or drug therapy (DeVries & Freiha, 1990).

Difficulty passing urine, or the urgency to void, can be attributed to clots in the bladder. Cramping, frequent discomfort, and occasional burning may also accompany hemorrhagic cystitis (Levine & Richie, 1989; Russo, 1993). Severe pubic pain and flank pain can be reported when bladder hemorrhage is massive and urinary clot retention occurs (Russo, 1993).

Nursing and Medical Implications. Acrolein is the by-product of cyclophosphamide and ifosfamide that damages the urothelium when coming in contact with the mucosa. In an attempt to minimize the contact acrolein has with the bladder mucosa, intravenous hydration sometimes in combination with bladder irrigation is administered. Diluting the urinary acrolein has resulted in decreased incidence and severity of hemorrhagic events (DeVries & Freiha, 1990; Levine & Richie, 1989).

Mesna is a uroprotective agent administered in conjunction with cyclophosphamide. This drug binds to acrolein, neutralizing it and preventing it from damaging the bladder mucosa. There is negligible if any toxicity from the drug (DeVries & Freiha, 1990).

In the event of hematuria, hydration rates and bladder irrigation rates are increased to whatever rate will clear the urine of blood. Hydration and general supportive care in combination with drug cessation are usually sufficient in managing the hemorrhagic cystitis caused by antineoplastic therapy. If lavage and clearance of clots is not successful, aminocaproic acid (EACA) can stabilize bleeding or intravesicular instillation of alum, or silver nitrate should be attempted before resorting to formalin therapy or surgical procedures (DeVries & Freiha, 1990; Russo, 1993). EACA can result in existing clots becoming more dense and tenacious, making it difficult for clots to pass in the urine or through the urinary catheter.

Close monitoring of the lavage is necessary to maintain an appropriate hydration rate to clear the fluid/urine of blood and clots. Monitoring the hemoglobin and hematocrit assists in quantifying blood loss and determining how many replacement units are needed. Carefully documenting and determining actual urine output is necessary to avoid fluid overload or to identify cyclophosphamide-induced syndrome of inappropriate antidiuretic hormone (Levine & Richie, 1989).

PULMONARY SYSTEM

Etiology. Hemoptysis frequently occurs in patients with neoplastic disease. The incidence of occurrence varies depending upon the initiating insult and the patient population (Albelda, Talbot, Gerson, Miller, & Cassileth, 1985). Lung parenchyma can become necrotic because of a fungal infection or tumor invasion, which in turn can lead to bleeding.

Aspergillus fumigatus is the commonly identified pathogen seen in fungal pneumonia. It has a reported incidence of 20 to 30 per cent in patients with acute leukemia (Rolston & Bodey, 1993). The aspergillus pathogens are airborne and are inhaled and deposited in either the lungs or paranasal sinuses. Pulmonary aspergillosis is divided into classic invasive aspergillosis and chronic necrotizing aspergillosis. The "classic" group affects the severely immunocompromised patient population, whereas the chronic disease occurs in normal or marginally immunocompromised patients (Pai, Blinkhorn & Tomashefski, 1994).

Clinical Presentation. Typical manifestation of pulmonary aspergillosis is fever that is unresponsive to antibacterial antibiotic regimens and occasionally accompanied by sudden onset of pleuritic chest pain, pleural rub, and hemoptysis (Rolston & Bodey, 1993). Chest radiography can depict noncharacteristic pulmonary infiltrates, lobar pneumonia, or the "air crescent" sign, which is a relatively specific appearance of lung cavitation(s) (Pai et al., 1994). Four to 16 per cent of patients with invasive aspergillosis have lung cavitations (Pai et al., 1994). The percentage of cavities that are radiographically demonstrable reportedly rises with bone marrow recovery and granulocytopenia resolution. Patients with granulocytopenia may not have the ability to reveal cavitations on chest radiograph (Albelda et al., 1985). This is important to recognize, since suspicion of an aspergillosis needs to be high even without radiographic evidence. CT of the chest can provide visibility in the granulocytopenic patient and may be a good alternative when there is suspicion of an aspergillosis.

Pulmonary aspergillosis invades blood vessels and lung parenchyma with mycotic thrombi, acute necrotizing inflammation, and infarction. The cavitation or "lung ball" most commonly seen on chest radiograph is necrotic lung parenchyma separated from viable lung tissue and is not a mycetoma (fungal ball) (Albelda et al., 1985; Pai et al., 1994). Cavitation formation provokes release of proteolytic enzymes by neutrophils that destroy lung parenchyma around the periphery of the infection.

Hemoptysis and fatal pulmonary hemorrhage is associated with the lung cavitations. Although hemoptysis can result from newly forming or organizing cavities and in distant lung sites, the risk of massive hemoptysis is greatest when a newly formed necrotic cavity is located near the hilum (Pai et al., 1994). Although thrombocytopenia certainly increases a patient's risk of bleeding, Albelda et al. (1985) noted an average platelet count of 205,000/mm^3 in 38 episodes of hemoptysis experienced by 10 patients. The particular point of emphasis was that granulocytes played an important role in cavity formation, which subsequently led to hemorrhagic episodes. Massive hemoptysis did not occur in patients who were granulocytopenic, despite severe thrombocytopenia.

Diagnosis. Since signs and symptoms of pulmonary infections are vague, accurate premortem diagnosis can be difficult. A number of studies have reported an episode(s) of bleeding prior to massive fatal pulmonary events (Albelda et al., 1985, Pai et al., 1994; Panos, Barr, Walsh, & Silverman, 1988). In Albelda et al.'s study (1985) these "signal" bleeds were observed 1 to 2 days following cavity formation, which was closely associated with granulocyte recovery.

Tumor invasion of the lung leading to hemorrhage is associated with necrotic squamous cell carcinoma. Tumor cells invade vascular structures, leading to ischemia and vascular necrosis (Panos et al., 1988). Bronchiogenic carcinoma is the most common cause of massive hemoptysis for patients over the age of 40 years. The rationale behind hemoptysis associated with neoplastic diseases is similar to the necrosis and cavitation process that occurs with aspergillosis (Morris & Holland, 1993; Panos et al., 1988).

Nursing and Medical Implications. Vigilant assessment and monitoring of the recovering immunocompromised patient who has been persistently febrile with radiographic changes must occur for patients to have any chance of survival. Assessment of breath sounds, use of accessory muscles, and sputum production as well as vital signs, orientation, and oxygenation is the baseline approach in caring for the patient at risk of pulmonary hemorrhage. Lower than baseline pulse oximetry measurements and percussion of dullness alert the nurse to hemorrhage. Since brisk bleeding can fill the lungs rapidly, every 5 minutes auscultation is indicated (Belcaster, 1993).

Oxygen, fluid, and blood product administration assist in maintaining circulatory volume while diagnosis and interventions are implemented. Conservative management consists of vessel tamponade with a balloon catheter, ice-saline lavage, or bronchial arteriography. Bronchoscopy assists in locating the site and determining the cause of bleeding. Surgical resection in the patient with uncontrolled hemorrhage provides a better chance of survival than conservative, nonsurgical management (Morris & Holland, 1993). Surgical excision of cavitary lesions in patients who are clinically capable may be the only preventive measure, since platelet transfusions and Amphotericin B are insufficient in preventing pulmonary hemorrhage (Albelda et al., 1985; Pai et al., 1994; Panos et al., 1988).

Upon first indication of hemoptysis or cavitary lesions, blood should be made available in the blood bank in conjunction with pulmonary medicine and thoracic surgery consultations in preparation of an emergency. Supplemental oxygen, raising the head of the bed to high Fowlers position, and/or positioning the patient on the affected side reduces the risk of aspiration and maximizes lung inflation on the unaffected side. Intubation and mechanical ventilation may be indicated in attempts to maintain oxygenation and to assist suctioning. Chronic cavities that persist also should be considered for excision, since they serve as reservoirs for reinfection, especially when the patient becomes granulocytopenic again (Pai et al., 1994; Rolston & Bodey, 1993).

CENTRAL NERVOUS SYSTEM

Etiology. Despite the risk of intracerebral, subarachnoid, or intraventricular hemorrhage in the patient with cancer, very little is reported in the literature. Central nervous system hemorrhage has been associated with intracranial metastasis from melanoma, choriocarcinoma, bronchogenic carcinoma, and bleeding disorders or coagulopathy (Klein, 1985). The leukemias may produce a scenario of subacute basal meningitis from hemorrhage, possibly due to severe thrombocytopenia or secondary to leukocytosis (McDonnell, 1994; Pryse-Phillips & Murray, 1982). Intracranial hemorrhage is the most common and most lethal manifestation of leukostasis (McDonnell, 1994). Intracranial pressure (ICP) will increase if significant intracranial bleeding occurs, since the skull forms an essentially closed container and cannot accommodate increased volume (Hickey, 1992; St. Clair & Bove, 1987).

Clinical Presentation. As ICP rises, cerebral blood flow is decreased due to the pressure on cerebral vessels. As blood flow decreases, brain ischemia occurs, and metabolic waste products of carbon dioxide and lactic acid accumulate, increasing the blood volume and worsening the cerebral edema secondary to vasodilation. These physiologic changes are reflected in alterations in level of consciousness, unequal pupillary reactions, decreased motor strength and function, changing vital signs with widening pulse pressure, seizures, and new onset of nausea and vomiting (Hickey, 1992; St. Clair & Bove, 1987).

Nursing Implications. Neurologic assessment performed meticulously and on a frequent basis can detect subtle changes before the patient's condition becomes serious (St. Clair & Bove, 1987). Transient "pressure signs" are associated with transient elevations in ICP and cerebral hypoxia, lasting only a few minutes. It is important to document frequently and compare with previous symptoms to identify this transient trend. The transient signs include decreased level of consciousness, pupillary abnormalities, visual disturbances, motor dysfunction, headache, aphasia, changes in respiratory pattern, and vital sign changes (Hickey, 1992). The symptom of headache is not as common as sometimes thought and can actually be a late sign of ICP (Hickey, 1992).

In caring for the patient with increased ICP, it is critical to avoid actions that can increase ICP. ICP can increase from suctioning, turning the patient and causing hip flexion, as well as extending and flexing the patient's head. Valsalva's maneuver, vomiting, constipation, coughing, painful procedures, emotionally upsetting stimuli, and clustering of patient care activities also need to be avoided (Boortz-Marx, 1985; Hickey, 1992; St. Clair & Bove, 1987). Patients require constant observation during times of confusion to prevent falls and head injury. Restraints should be avoided if possible, as well as the use of Trendelenburg, since both can increase ICP. Patients need to be well oxygenated to avoid hypoxia and subsequent cerebral edema.

INVASIVE PROCEDURES

Most invasive procedures carry the risk of bleeding. Invasive procedures range from diagnostic tests to palliative and curative interventions. Patients with cancer experience this broad range of procedures and interventions numerous times throughout the course of their illness. The risk of bleeding is obviously correlated with the procedure being performed. Yet, that risk rises greatly if the patient has any one of the conditions previously discussed, i.e., sepsis, thrombocytopenia, coagulation abnormalities.

Central Venous Access Devices. Long-term central venous access devices (VAD) should be chosen for their appropriateness to the patient's anticipated plan of therapy. An implanted port may not be appropriate for the patient who is expected to have prolonged periods of thrombocytopenia. Accessing and reaccessing the implanted device requires needle puncture through the skin. Repeated skin pricks in the patient with chronically low platelet count can lead to bleeding, hematoma formation, and possible catheter pocket infection requiring removal (Cedermark & Swedborg, 1989; Wickham, 1990; Wickham, Purl, & Welker, 1992). Foresight and anticipation of therapy side effects should guide catheter choice.

Therapeutic procedures such as catheter line placement, biopsy, or surgery require a predetermined level of platelets. Holbrook and Palmer (1993) found a statistically significant increase in bleeding complications in placement of tunnelled venous access catheters in patients with platelet counts less than $50,000/mm^3$. Placement technique, cutdown or percutaneous, did not affect complications, with similar types and rates of bleeding complications occurring in both groups.

The practitioner performing a procedure usually requests platelet transfusions prior to the procedure in patients with counts below $50,000/mm^3$, followed by a postplatelet count. Some practitioners, depending upon the procedure, will in addition transfuse the patient while the procedure is being done.

CARE OF THE BLEEDING PATIENT

Assessment and care begin with an awareness that the patient is at risk for bleeding. The health history points out particular factors that could be contributing to the risk of bleeding: prolonged thrombocytopenia, history of altered mucosal integrity from stomatitis/mucositis, and recent antineoplastic therapy. Factors altering platelet function or prolonging bleeding time such as fever, sepsis, medications, and paraproteinemia need to be recognized for anticipation of bleeding risk (Alexander, 1987).

Questions that elicit color, consistency, frequency, and initiating events assist in identifying bleeding. Skin examination for petechiae, hematomas, scleral hemorrhage, and oozing cuts indicates thrombocytopenia. Examining nailbeds for pallor and delayed capillary refill may suggest anemia secondary to blood loss (Alexander, 1987; Mayer, 1988).

SIGNS AND SYMPTOMS OF BLOOD LOSS

Signs and symptoms of hemorrhage are related to volume status and tissue perfusion and can range from dizziness and weakness to hypotensive shock (Shelton, 1993). Hemodynamic changes may be seen earlier in the patient experiencing rapid bleeding or who is elderly, anemic, and has baseline cardiovascular or pulmonary problems than in the patient whose body can easily compensate (McAdams & McClure, 1986). Table 54–9 contains signs and symptoms of response and compensation to blood loss organized by body systems (McAdams & McClure, 1986; Burns, 1990). Inquiring into experiences of dizziness, increasing fatigue (more than normal), inability to climb the steps without dyspnea on exertion, or reports of shortness of breath prompt further inquiry and diagnostic testing into the potential for blood loss.

TABLE 54–9. *Body Systems Responses to Blood Loss/Hypovolemia*

SYSTEM	PRIMARY RESPONSE	SIGNS/SYMPTOMS	COMPENSATORY RESPONSE
Cardiac	↓BP 2° ↓ Strokevolume ↓ 2° R sided return	Orthostatic vital signs Hypotension Dizziness CVP Syncope Dysrhythmia	↑ Heart rate Eventually bradycardia
Respiratory	↓ pO^2	SOB DOE Tachypnea Upright body position	Tachypnea
Genitourinary	↓ Blood flow ↓ Glomerular filtration rate Activation of renin-angiotensin cycle	↓ Urine output ↑ Specific gravity Oliguria Anuria BUN ↑ Creatinine	Further vasoconstriction in order to shunt blood to vital organs
Gastrointestinal	Vasoconstriction ↓ Blood flow	Nausea Abdominal cramps Diarrhea	Persistent vasoconstriction
Integumentary	Vasoconstriction	Pale, cool, clammy skin Sluggish capillary refill Cyanotic	Persistent vasoconstriction
Central nervous system	Cerebral hypoxia	Confusion Lethargy Stupor	

SOB = shortness of breath; CVP = central venous pressure; BP = blood pressure; R = right; DOE = dyspnea on exertion; BUN = blood urea nitrogen.

Reviewing the complete blood count should be done in comparison to previous counts. Red blood cells have an approximate life span of 30 days. For the patient whose marrow is hypocellular, with few erythrocyte precursors, it may be normal to see the hematocrit drifting down. Precipitous drops in the hematocrit in short time spans suggest blood loss.

NURSING CARE

Nursing care is critical in the bleeding patient, with priority placed on maintaining volume and tissue perfusion and preventing circulatory collapse. Interventions as listed in Table 54–10 occur simultaneously.

Occult bleeding is blood loss detectable through testing rather than the naked eye and can be detected in the urine, stool, or emesis. Bleeding and hemorrhage are often used interchangably, yet hemorrhage suggests a large quantity of bleeding or lost blood volume, which can be quantified. Decreases in hemoglobin and hematocrit are used to quantify amount lost, and treatment methods depend upon location and whether the bleeding is microscopic, moderate, or severe. Conservative interventions usually focus on stopping the bleeding at the source. Localized care interventions are reviewed in Table 54–11. Once bleeding reaches the point of requiring transfusions and controlling the bleeding is unsuccessful with conservative measures, more aggressive, systemic interventions are considered.

PLATELET THERAPY

Appropriate platelet transfusion therapy is defined as transfusion of only what is necessary to meet a patient's needs (Bodensteiner et al., 1992). In the past, prophylactic transfusions were generally administered when patients' platelet levels fell below a certain level, commonly 20,000/mm^3 (Aderka, Praff, Santo, Weinberger, & Pinkhas, 1986; Fuller, 1990). This approach, although modified to meet individual institution's policies, is presently being questioned since there are indications that patients receiving prophylactic platelets versus those receiving therapeutic platelets reflect no difference in survival, number of remissions, or bleeding deaths (Bodensteiner et al., 1992; Heyman & Schiffer, 1990). There is an increasing trend towards transfusing platelets in response to bleeding, rather than at a predetermined level (Aderka, Praff et al., 1986; Fuller, 1990).

In addition to platelet prophylaxis, avoidance of factors that can lead to bleeding or worsen the risk of bleeding is routine in thrombocytopenic nursing protocols (Alexander, 1987). Institution restrictions specify which interventions should be avoided in the thrombocytopenic patient as well as which activities patients should avoid. Patients are often instructed to avoid or modify activities that can vary from self-care habits to sexual intercourse. Recommendations are usually made in the context of a platelet count less than or greater

TABLE 54-10. *Nursing and Medical Response to the Patient With Active Bleeding*

ACTIVITY	OCCURRENCE
Vital signs assessment/bedside documentation	Frequent, Constant
Intravenous fluids	
Normal saline	
Colloids	
Blood product transfusions	As needed to keep pace with volume and clotting factors lost
Packed red blood cells	As needed to keep platelet level as high as possible or greater
Fresh-frozen plasma	than 50,000/mm^3
Cryoprecipitate	
Vitamin K	
Platelets	
Pharmacologic therapy	Continuous infusion
Epsilon aminocaproic acid	
Vasopressin	
Desmopressin acetate	
Diagnostic studies	Initially and as indicated
Endoscopy	
Angiography	
CT scan	
Surgery	
Invasive, aggressive interventions	As indicated, dependent upon patient physical status
Angiography	
Endoscopy	
Surgery	
Mechanical ventilation	
Nasogastric tube	
Sengsten-Blackemore tube	
Complete blood count	As indicated by blood loss as frequently as every 2 hours
(hematocrit, hemoglobin, platelet levels)	
Coagulation studies	

than 50,000/mm^3, and in some cases there may not be research to support the recommendation. As the threshold for prophylactic transfusion decreases and the initiative to transfuse changes to active bleeding, then patient instructions will also change.

Platelet products are either randomly collected, pooled platelets or single-donor platelets obtained via a cell separator from one individual (Erickson, 1990; Fuller, 1990; Ho, 1990). One unit of whole blood yields one unit of platelets; therefore, numerous units of blood are necessary to collect sufficient platelets. Success of a platelet transfusion is determined by the increment obtained following transfusion. In the best circumstances, one unit of platelet concentrate is anticipated to cause a minimum rise in platelet count of 7000/mm^3. Six units of platelets are usually transfused at one time (Schwartzberg & Holbert, 1988). In the oncology population, a platelet increase between 10,000/mm^3 to 30,000 shortly following the transfusion is adequate. Twenty-four-hour posttransfusion counts should range between 5000/mm^3 and 15,000/mm^3 (Fuller, 1990). Ten-minute posttransfusion increments are as sufficient as 1-hour counts (O'Connell, Lee, & Schiffer, 1988).

Platelet Refractoriness. Thirty to 70 per cent of multitransfused patients develop platelet refractoriness (Bodensteiner et al., 1992). Alloimmunization is characterized by a consistent inability to achieve satisfactory increments from platelets transfused and can be divided into immune and nonimmune causes. In nonimmune alloimmunization the immediate posttransfusion increment is in the normal range, but the survival at 24 hours is abnormally low. Reviewing the early and late platelet increments helps differentiate between immune and nonimmune causes of platelet refractoriness (Table 54-12). Factors that interfere with platelet recovery after transfusion such as fever, sepsis, and spleen sequestration need to first be ruled out when assessing for alloimmunization.

HLA alloimmunization is a sensitization to HLA or non-HLA antigens on donor platelets. Alloimmunization does not depend on the number of exposures or transfusions, since some patients develop alloimmunization after only a few exposures and others never do (Nugent, 1992; Schiffer & Wade, 1987). The rate of alloimmunization is influenced by underlying disease and the patient's immune responsiveness and competence (Nugent, 1992). Antiplatelet antibodies rapidly bind and clear transfused platelets from the peripheral blood. Upon suspicion of immune mechanisms, antibodies directed against allogeneic platelet antigens can be tested for and their specificity identified (Benson et al., 1993).

Attempts to prevent platelet refractoriness include transfusion of apheresis platelets and leukopoor platelets. The majority of attempts focus on depleting leukocytes from the platelet product, thereby prevent-

TABLE 54–11. *Local Care Methods of Bleeding Cessation*

NAME	INDICATION	ACTION
Pressure dressing	Oozing skin and wound sites	"Pinches" off blood in order for platelets to surround vessel and create a plug
Potassium aluminum sulfate (Alum)	Viral or antineoplastic induced hemorrhagic cystitis	An astringent that acts by protein precipitation over the bleeding surface administered via three-way Foley catheter
Microfibrillar collagen hemostat (Avitene)	Topical oozing or bleeding site, i.e., uncontrolled epistaxis, bleeding gums	Powdery substance that adheres to moist surfaces resulting in platelet adherence and thrombi formation "blood coagulator"
Absorbable gelating sponge (Gelfoam)	Capillary oozing and bleeding in highly vascular areas that are difficult to suture	A sponge capable of absorbing many times its weight in blood Provides an absorbable matrix into which a clot forms and granulation tissue grows Not to be removed since it liquefies in 2–5 days
Laser therapy/photocoagulation	Upper GI bleeds that can be located on endoscopy Nonarterial bleeds Vascular lesions Linear gastritis Ulcers	The energy of the monochromatic light emitted by way of fiberoptic probe through an endoscope causes tissue necrosis and coagulation of the bleeding site

ing or delaying HLA alloimmunization. This is achieved through leukocyte-depletion filters that are attached to the standard blood administration set and have an efficiency close to 100 per cent (Benson et al., 1993; Erickson, 1990; Fuller, 1990; Nugent, 1992). Additional advantages of leukocyte-depleting filters are seen in Table 54–13.

Supportive care of the patient with an alloimmunization is a challenge. Cross-match-compatible platelets and HLA-matched platelets are the main options for achieving standard platelet increments. Cross-matching procedures determine the presence of antiplatelet antibodies and identify cross-match-compatible platelet components (Benson et al., 1993) HLA testing of the patient requires a white blood cell count

of 2000 with 10 to 15 per cent lymphocytes and no circulating blast cells. Unfortunately, many patients presenting with a hematologic malignancy have insufficient blood counts, and HLA matching is not possible until their white count returns to normal (Benson et al., 1993). Therefore, cross-matching a blood bank's platelet inventory with a patient's serum may be the only option. Continued use of random-donor platelets is a waste in the patient with proven alloimmunization, since they will be ineffective (Schiffer & Wade, 1987).

Intravenous immunoglobulin (IVIG) is successful in treating autoantibody-mediated thrombocytopenia but is controversial in modulating the platelet response in refractory patients. Success tends to occur more when administered with HLA-matched, single-donor platelets rather than random donor products (Nugent, 1992). IVIG is often considered when a patient is experiencing active bleeding in the face of poor responses to histocompatible platelets. In patients who do respond to IVIG, the benefit is transient, only lasting a short time. The decision to use the drug needs to be carefully weighed in light of expense ($5000 for a 5-day course). Therapies that have been used unsuccessfully in the treatment of alloimmunization include high-dose corticosteroids, splenectomy, plasma exchange, and leuko-

TABLE 54–12. *Immune vs. Nonimmune Causes of Small or Nonexistent Platelet Increments*

IMMUNE	NONIMMUNE
HLA alloimmunization	Fever
Platelet-specific antibodies	Sepsis
	DIC
	Active capillary oozing or bleeding
	Spleen sequestration
	Amphotericin B
	Antibiotics such as Carbenicillin, Ticarcillin, Penicillin G

DIC = disseminated intravascular coagulation.

TABLE 54–13. *Advantages of Leukocyte-Depleting Filters*

- ↓ Risk of febrile, nonhemolytic transfusion reactions
- ↓ Risk of leukocyte-transmitted diseases such as CMV
- ↓ Risk/delayed onset of HLA alloimmunization

cyte-reduced platelets (Bensinger, Buckner, & Clift, 1986; Hogge, Dutcher, & Aisner, 1984).

Drug Therapy

Epsilon Aminocaproic Acid (EACA). EACA acts as an inhibitor of fibrinolysis by inhibiting plasminogen activator substance; insufficient plasmin is available to dissolve clots (Benson et al., 1993; Fuller, 1990; Shannon & Wilson, 1992). Although its use is not labeled for control of excessive hematuria or upper GI bleeding and theoretically seems limited, it has been used in these circumstances, with a maximum response seen in 8 to 12 hours of drug institution (Benson et al., 1993; DeVries & Freiha, 1990; Shannon & Wilson, 1992). In the BMT population studied by Benson et al. (1993), EACA was used more successfully in the allogeneic population, with gastrointestinal bleeding the primary site, without complication. Thrombotic complications are the major risk of this intervention, and Schiffer and Wade (1987) warn that widespread thrombosis is a particular risk for patients who are febrile, infected, or possibly experiencing DIC secondary to tumor lysis. Signs of arm or leg pain/swelling, positive Homan's sign, chest pain, or dyspnea should alert the nurse to a possible thrombotic event.

Vasopressin. Vasopressin has been used to control upper GI bleeding (Burns & Martin, 1990; Wallach & Kurtz, 1992). Vasopressin is a posterior pituitary antidiuretic hormone that reduces portal pressure thus reducing blood flow to splanchnic, coronary, GI, pancreatic, skin, and muscular systems. Its use in the control of massive GI hemorrhage tends to occur in emergency situations when other options are unsuccessful or inappropriate (Burns & Martin, 1990; Shannon & Wilson, 1992; Shelton, 1993). Vasopressin can be administered intravenously or directly into the bleeding artery when the vessel is located by angiography (Shelton, 1993; Wallach & Kurtz, 1992). Treatment with vasopressin is short-term with a maximum of 72 hours in attempt to avoid the risk of an ischemic event. Combination of vasopressin with nitroglycerin results in reversal of the detrimental effects of the vasopressin and even some enhancement of the beneficial effects (Burns & Martin, 1990).

Negative side effects of vasopressin include abdominal cramping, nausea, the feeling of urgency and need to move the bowels, occasional diarrhea, bradyarrhythmias, angina, and a decreased cardiac output. Peripheral vasoconstriction is experienced as confusion, headaches, cool extremities with cyanosis, hypertension, and lightheadedness. In addition to documentation of side effect onset and severity, patient education and reassurance is necessary, since side effects can be very uncomfortable. Assessment for ischemic events, including cardiac, intestinal, and intracerebral, is crucial for early identification and drug cessation (Burns & Martin, 1990; Wallach & Kurtz, 1992).

Desmopressin (DDAVP). DDAVP, a synthetic analog of vasopressin, is also an antidiuretic with vasopressor activity. It produces a dose-related increase in factor VII and von Willebrand's factor, which is neces-sary for platelet adhesion. DDAVP may temporarily improve platelet function in patients with dysfunction by promoting adhesion. It can be administered intravenously or subcutaneously for short periods of time. Caution during administration is warranted since hypertension, acute myocardial infarction, and stroke have followed its use, particularly in the older patient (Ey & Goodnight, 1990; Shannon & Wilson, 1992).

Replacement Therapy

In addition to transfusions and the interventions outlined in Table 54–10, replacement therapy is tailored to the patient's losses and coagulation status. In the setting of acute hemorrhage, priority is to keep pace with blood loss (Schwartzberg & Holbert, 1988). Indications for platelet transfusions other than prophylaxis are active bleeding and any diagnostic or invasive procedures.

Fresh-frozen Plasma (FFP). FFP contains the clotting factors necessary for coagulation. Cryoprecipitate is a portion of FFP that is rich in factor VII, fibrinogen, and fibronectin. Indications for these products are active bleeding in which the clotting factors are being consumed, DIC, and any of the clotting disorders (Erickson, 1990; Schwartzberg & Holbert, 1988).

Packed Red Blood Cells (PRBCs). PRBCs are used to replace lost blood volume. In addition to being prescribed for myelosuppressed patients with hematocrit levels less than 25 to 30 per cent or hemoglobin levels below 10 g/dl, PRBCs are transfused in bleeding emergencies at a rate that keeps pace with the loss. Each unit of PRBC raises the hematocrit by 3 points and the hemoglobin by 1 g/dl (Erickson, 1990; Goodman, 1989).

Transfusion Complications

In addition to complications of transfusion therapy as outlined in Table 54–14, disease transmission remains a serious concern. CMV, Epstein-Barr (EBV), HIV, hepatitis-C, and bacteria from preparative contamination can be transmitted to the recipient. Prevention of disease transmission is attempted by testing for the CMV virus and infusing only EBV- and CMV-negative products to patients with impaired immune function and who are tested negative for those viruses (Freedman et al., 1990). Screening for hepatitis A and B as well as HIV infections is also a preventive measure, although there is no screening for non-A, non-B hepatitis and patients who have been exposed to the HIV virus but have not yet developed antibodies. Although the risks of disease transmission exist, meticulous screening, handling, and administration procedures keep the risk small.

Transfusion complications tend to be managed according to institutional policies. In general, suspicion of a transfusion reaction usually leads to infusion cessation and physical assessment of the signs and symptoms being experienced by the patient. In collaboration with the physician, decisions are made as to how to proceed and whether to complete a transfusion workup.

TABLE 54–14. *Managing Transfusion Reactions*

	REACTION	SIGNS AND SYMPTOMS	TREATMENT	PREVENTION
Immediate febrile	Recipient's antibodies directed against donor antigens on leukocytes, platelets, or in plasma	Fever: Chills, rigors; headache; flank pain	Stop transfusion immediately and notify physician Symptomatic relief with acetaminophen, diphenhydramine, or demerol	Premedicate with acetaminophen, diphenhydramine, and possibly steroids Use leukocyte-poor or washed blood products
Allergic	Recipient reacts to allergin in donor's blood Many signs and symptoms due to activation of complement by antigen-antibody complex	Possibly fever; flushing, itching; wheels, hives; may progress to anaphylactic reaction; wheezing; laryngeal edema	Stop transfusion immediately Administer antihistamines Possibly give epinephrine for wheezing or anaphylactic reaction	Give antihistamines as premedication to persons with history of allergic reactions Monitor patient closely for first 5 minutes of transfusion
Hemolytic	Due to ABO-incompatible blood Intradonor incompatibility multiple transfusions	Chills: shaking; fever; anxiety, headache; chest pain; flank pain; nausea/vomiting; abnormal bleeding; hemoglobinuria; oliguria; dyspnea; may progress to signs of shock and/or renal failure	Stop blood transfusion immediately and notify physician Maintain NS IV line Monitor blood pressure for shock Treat hypotension with IVFs and dopamine Administer furosemide to increase renal blood flow Monitor urine output 100 ml/hr Observe for signs of hemorrhage resulting from DIC Posttransfusion blood sample and urine sample to lab for evaluation	Proper identification of donor and recipient blood types before transfusion with one other nurse or physician Transfuse blood slowly first 15–20 minutes

ANEMIA SECONDARY TO BLOOD LOSS

The hematocrit, or packed cell volume, is the percentage of the total blood volume occupied by red blood cells, erythrocytes. Hemoglobin is the oxygen-carrying capacity of the blood. Therefore, anemia results when there is a decrease of blood, resulting in decreased circulating erythrocytes.

Symptoms of anemia relate directly to the diminished oxygenating capacity and include dyspnea on exertion, fatigue, light-headedness, dizziness, and irritability (Maxwell, 1984). As the blood loss continues or worsens without sufficient replacement, the anemia signs and symptoms progress to syncope, tachycardia, tachypnea, hypotension, and tissue hypoxia.

Rostad (1991) identifies three problems patients and families encounter: knowledge deficit, potential for injury, and activity intolerance. Patients and families need to know that fatigue, dizziness, and a lack of energy to continue their daily activities can in many situations be directly correlated with their anemia. Patients need to be instructed how to modify their schedules to maximize their energy and strength with

out placing themselves at risk for harm. Table 54–15 reviews patient problems associated with anemia and the nursing responsibilities.

Treatment of anemia due to blood loss in the patient with cancer is straightforward: PRBC transfusions. A hematocrit value of 25 to 30 per cent or a hemoglobin less than 10 g/dL in adults usually results in a two- to three-unit transfusion (Rostad, 1991). Patients who are experiencing bleeding will be transfused to maintain a stable hematocrit and hemoglobin while efforts are made to treat the cause.

HEMATOPOIETIC GROWTH FACTORS

The recent availability of hematopoietic growth factors or CSFs is decreasing the severity of side effects patients are experiencing from the myelosuppressive effects of chemotherapy (Haeuber & DiJulio, 1989). Success has mainly been centered on decreasing the intensity and duration of neutropenia by increasing the proliferation and maturation of neutrophils with granulocyte colony stimulating factor (G-CSF) and granulocyte-macrophage colony stimulating factor (GM-CSF) (Vadhan-Raj, 1989). The development of thrombopoi

TABLE 54–14. *Managing Transfusion Reactions* Continued

	REACTION	SIGNS AND SYMPTOMS	TREATMENT	PREVENTION
Bacterial contamination	Usually caused by gram-negative organisms which can survive cold; species of pseudomonas	High fever; abdominal cramps; vomiting; diarrhea; shock; renal failure	Stop transfusion Broad-spectrum antibiotics Vasopressor Steroids Dopamine	Observe blood before transfusion for gas, clots, and dark purple color Maintain sterile technique when administering blood products
Circulatory overload	Due to rapid infusion of blood or transfusion of excessive quantity	Dyspnea; chest tightness; elevated blood pressure; dry cough; rales; distended neck veins; pulmonary edema on chest radiograph	Stop transfusion Place patient in semi-Fowler's position Possibly administer oxygen Administer diuretics	Transfuse blood slowly Avoid use of whole blood
Air emboli	May occur if blood infused under pressure	Sudden shortness of breath; sharp chest pain; anxiety; coughing; decreased blood pressure	Place patient on left side Administer 100% oxygen Treat shock if it develops	Observe for air in tubing when infusing under pressure Stop transfusion if air observed, and clamp tubing
Citrate toxicity	Occurs when citrate treated blood is infused rapidly. Citrate binds calcium	Cardiac arrhythmias; nausea/vomiting; hypokalemia; alkalosis; decreased blood pressure	Slow transfusion or discontinue, depending on severity of reaction Worse reaction in hypothermia patients and patients with ↑ K + May give calcium gluconate	Infuse blood slowly Monitor K^+ and Ca^{++} Use blood less than 2 weeks old if many units to be given
Hypothermia	Due to rapid infusion of large amounts of cold blood Decreases myocardial temperature	Ventricular fibrillation; decreased blood pressure; cardiac arrest if core temperature < 30°C; shaking chills	Stop transfusion until patient can be warmed Obtain ECG	Warm blood to 35°–37°C
Delayed hemolytic	Results from patient sensitization to red blood cell antigen not in ABO system Sensitization occurs with pregnancy or previous transfusions	May be asymptomatic; first reaction may take weeks; will show continued anemia; possibly hemoglobinuria; possibly increased bilirubin and direct Coomb's test; possibly fever; second exposure occurs in 1–5 days	Treat fever if present	Continue to update patient's antibody file

NS = normal saline; IVF = intravenous fluid; DIC = disseminated intravascular coagulation; ECG = electrocardiogram.
(Freedman, S., Haisfield, M. E., McGuire D. B., Morell, L., Paulaitis, L., & Wohlganger, J. [1990]. Nursing considerations in the administration of blood component therapy. *Seminars in Oncology Nursing, 6,* 155–162.)

etin (TSF) and interleukin-3 as hormones that stimulate both proliferation and maturation of hematopoietic precursor cells in a similar manner as the other hemopoietic regulators is exciting.

TSF is a hormone released into the circulation in response to a decrease in the number, mass, and/or function of platelets. It acts principally on megakaryocytes to increase platelet production (Breton-Gorius, Levin, Nurden, & Williams, 1990). An impressive characteristic of TSF is its ability to increase platelet numbers to previously unattainable levels (Metcalf, 1994).

In addition to stimulating proliferation and differentiation of hematopoietic precursor cells, mature myeloid cell function is enhanced, and it appears to be a more potent stimulator of megakaryocytopoiesis than G-CSF, GM-CSF, and macrophage colony stimulating factor (M-CSF). It also stimulates erythroid progenitor cells, resulting in increased reticulocyte counts (Ganser et al., 1991; Hoelzer, Seipelt, & Ganser, 1991). The increase in both megakaryocytic and erythrocytic cells supports the belief that these two cell lines may share a common precursor (McDonald & Sullivan, 1993). There is also the possibility that IL-3's effect on hematopoietic progenitors and precursor cells might be enhanced by IL-6, since IL-3 administration is accompanied by increases in plasma IL-6 levels. IL-6 is known to be a potent megakaryocyte maturation factor (Hoffman, 1993).

TABLE 54–15. *Patient Problems and Nursing Interventions for the Myelosuppressed Patient With Cancer: Anemia*

KNOWLEDGE DEFICIT	POTENTIAL FOR INJURY	ACTIVITY INTOLERANCE
Level I: Standard Care Instruct the client* on relation of: • RBCs, hemoglobin, and availability of oxygen as required for normal body tissue function • Occurrence of anemia after treatment • Signs and Symptoms of rapid onset	• Monitor lab data, especially CBC • Obtain the treatment history, past and present. Identify any occurrence of anemia. Conduct a physical assessment—looking for signs of anemia (pallor, bleeding, etc.) • Protect the patient from sources of infection • Provide a nutritious diet	• Note the signs and symptoms of fatigue, shortness of breath, tachycardia on exertion, and/or dizziness
Level II: Mild/Moderate (Hemoglobin 8–12 g/dl) Level I plus: • Emphasize the importance of adjusting lifestyle so that anemia can be better tolerated • Outline the importance of preventing secondary problems related to tissue hypoxia: infection, tissue breakdown, and/or blood loss	Level I plus: • Check vital signs frequently • Observe for frank or occult bleeding • Administer iron supplements as prescribed • Maintain integrity of skin and mucous membrane • Provide a diet high in protein, vitamins, and iron • Arrange for home health nursing follow-up as required by health status and medical needs	Level I plus: • Adjust ADL to match energy level • Provide frequent rest periods; shorter periods of work • Provide small, frequent meals to save strength • Assist patient in getting up—ambulating • Maintain safe physical surroundings
Level III: Severe (Hemoglobin ≤ 7.5 g/dl) Levels I and II plus: • Inform the client of interventions necessary to reverse anemia and to reduce risk of secondary complications • Inform the client of hazards, risks, and benefits of blood transfusion	Levels I and II plus: • Report bleeding • Administer blood transfusion as prescribed • Administer oxygen to prevent tissue hypoxia and decrease cardiac workload • Provide oral care • Turn the patient; provide skin care • Assess/arrange for home health nursing follow-up	Levels I and II plus • Enforce rest periods; plan physical activity based on individual tolerance level • Provide range-of-motion exercises to limit residual disabilities if anemia persists • Gradually increase activity under supervision as the problem resolves

*Client = patient, family, significant other person. RBCs = red blood cells; CBC = complete blood count; ADL = activities of daily living.
(Rostad, M. E. [1991]. Current strategies for managing myelosuppression in patients with cancer. *Oncology Nursing Forum, 18*[Suppl.], 7–15.)

Recombinant human IL-3 (rHuIL-3) exerts its main action at the level of multipotent and committed hematopoietic progenitor cells and not at the level of the multipotent and lineage-committed progenitor cells in the bone marrow (Ganser et al., 1990; Hoelzer et al., 1991). The target stem cell level aimed at by rHuIL-3 is evident in that mobilization of cells from the bone marrow after administration of rHuIL-3 does not occur immediately as is suggested with G-CSF and GM-CSF. The difference is also seen in that there are longer lasting effects from IL-3 than the other CSFs because of the level of stimulation (Ganser et al., 1990).

Platelet proliferation and side effects appear to be dose-related, with both responses diminishing with dose reductions (Ganser, 1993; Hoelzer et al., 1991). rHuIL-3 can be administered subcutaneously or intravenously, with more frequent and severe adverse reactions occurring in patients receiving intravenous administration (Nemunaitis, Appelbaum, & Singer et al., 1993). The most common toxicity is fever, with as many as 70% of patients experiencing a temperature, usually during the first few days of drug administration. Other common side effects include headache, stiff neck, facial flushing, chills, bone pain, and mild, local erythema at the injection site (Hoelzer et al., 1991; Nemunaitis et al., 1993). These adverse reactions and toxicities are similar to those experienced with other CSF administration.

Nursing Implications. Close monitoring of patient reactions to rHuIL-3 is in accordance with the nursing activities for other CSFs and biologic response modifiers. Symptom management can be anticipated and planned for, since patients will eventually be most likely self-administering the drug. Patients need to understand the "normality" of the side effects and feel free to clarify their experiences with their caregivers.

SUMMARY

Comprehension of hematopoiesis, clotting cascade mechanisms, and colony-stimulating factors is tedious but crucial for an in-depth knowledge base about hemostasis. This knowledge provides the basis from which nurses can not only understand what is occurring in the patients for whom they are caring, but more important, can anticipate patient needs, potential problems, and any necessary interventions. Proactively caring for the cancer patient with any type of coagulopathy or bleeding complication provides the patient with a high level of care and a better chance of survival.

REFERENCES

Aderka, D., Brown, A., Zelikovski, A., & Pinkhas, J. (1986). Idiopathic deep vein thrombosis in an apparently healthy patient as a premonitory sign of occult cancer. *Cancer, 57,* 1846–1849.

Aderka, D., Praff, G., Santo, M., Weinberger, A., & Pinkhas, J. (1986). Bleeding due to thrombocytopenia in acute leukemias and reevaluation of the prophylactic platelet transfusion policy. *American Journal of the Medical Sciences, 291,* 147–151.

Albeda, S. M., Talbot, G. H., Gerson, S. L., Miller, W. T., & Cassileth, P. A. (1985). Pulmonary cavitation and massive hemoptysis in invasive pulmonary aspergillosis. *American Review of Respiratory Diseases, 131,* 115–120.

Alexander, E. J. (1987). Injury, potential for, related to thrombocytopenia. In J. C. McNally, E. T. Somerville, C. Miaskowski & M. Rostad (Eds.), *Guidelines for oncology nursing practice* (pp. 203–207). Kansas City, KS: American Nurses' Association & Oncology Nursing Society.

Alkire, K., & Collingwood, J. (1990). Physiology of blood and bone marrow. *Seminars in Oncology Nursing, 6(2),* 99–108.

Ambinder, R. F., Burns, W., Forman, M., Charache, P., Arthur, R., Beschorner, W., Santos, G., & Saral, R. (1986). Hemorrhagic cystitis associated with adenovirus infection in bone marrow transplantation. *Archives of Internal Medicine, 146,* 1400–1401.

Ashley, W. A., & Wells, S. A. (1988). Tumors of the small intestine. *Seminars in Oncology, 15,* 116–128.

Babior, B., & Stossel, T. (1990). *Hematology: A pathophysiological approach.* New York: Churchill Livingstone.

Baker, A. R. (1993). Surgical emergencies. In V. T. DeVita, S. Hellman, S. Rosenberg (Eds.), *Cancer: Principles and practices of oncology* (Vol. 2, 4th cd., pp. 2141–2158). Philadelphia: J. B. Lippincott Co.

Belcaster, A. (1993). Responding to pulmonary hemorrhage. *Nursing 93, 23,* 23.

Bell, W. (1993). Thrombotic thrombocytopenia purpura-hemolytic uremic syndrome. In W. Bell (Ed.), *Hematologic and oncologic emergencies* (pp. 177–196). New York: Churchill Livingstone.

Belt, R. J., Leite, C., Haas, C. D., & Stephens, R. L. (1978). Incidence of hemorrhagic complications in patients with cancer. *Journal of the American Medical Association, 239,* 2571–2574.

Bensinger, W. I., Buckner, C. D., & Clift, R. A. (1986). Plasma exchange for platelet alloimmunization. *Transplantation, 41,* 602–605.

Benson, K., Fields, K., Heimenz, J., Zorsky, P., Ballester, O., Perkins, J., & Elfenbein, G. (1993). The platelet-refractory

bone marrow transplant patient: prophylaxis and treatment of bleeding. *Seminars in Oncology, 20*(Suppl.), 102–109.

Bick, R. (1978). Alterations of hemostasis associated with malignancy: Etiology, pathophysiology, diagnosis and management. *Seminars in Thrombosis and Hemostasis, 5,* 1–26.

Bick, R. (1992). Coagulation abnormalities in malignancy: A review. *Seminars in Thrombosis and Hemostasis, 18(4),* 353–372.

Bick, R. (1992a). Alterations of hemostasis in malignancy. In R. Bick, J. Bennett, R. Brynes, M. Cline, L. Kass, G. Murano, & P. Ward (Eds.), *Disorders of thrombosis and hemostasis: Clinical and laboratory practice* (pp. 1583–1602). Chicago: ASCP Press.

Bick, R., & Kunkel, L. (1992). Disseminated intravascular coagulation. *International Journal of Hematology, 55,* 1–26.

Biller, J., Challa, V., Toole, J., et al. (1982). Nonbacterial thrombotic endocarditis: A neurological perspective of clinicopathologic correlations in 99 patients. *Archives of Neurology, 39,* 95–98.

Bithell, T. C. (1987). Normal hemostasis and coagulation. In O. Thorup (Ed.), *Fundamentals of clinical hematology* (5th ed., pp. 126–162). Philadelphia: W. B. Saunders Co.

Bodensteiner, D. C., Tilzer, L. L., Adams, M. E., & Bayer, W. L. (1992). Use of blood components in cancer patients with bleeding. *Hematology Oncology Clinics of North America, 6,* 1375–1392.

Boortz-Marx, R. (1985). Factors affecting intracranial pressure: A descriptive study. *Journal of Neurosurgical Nursing, 17,* 89–94.

Brain, M., Azzopardi, J., Baker, L., Pineo, G., Roberts, P., & Dacie, J. (1970). Microangiopathic hemolytic anemia and mucin-forming adenocarcinoma. *British Journal of Hematology, 18,* 183–193.

Breton-Gorius, J., Levin, J., Nurden, A., & Williams, N. (1990). Role of thrombopoietin in controlling blood platelet production. *Progress in Clinical and Biological Research, 356,* 219–227.

Burke, M. B., Wilkes, G. M., Berg, D., & Bean, C. K. (1991). Potential toxicities and nursing management. In M. B. Burke, G. M. Wilkes, D. Berg, & C. K. Bean (Eds.), *Cancer chemotherapy: A nursing process approach* (pp. 49–138). Boston: Jones and Bartlett.

Burns, E. R. (1990). When to suspect a bleeding disorder. *Emergency Medicine, 22,* 67–70.

Burns, S. M., & Martin, M. J. (1990). VP/NTG therapy in the patient with variceal bleeding. *Critical Care Nurse, 10,* 42–49.

Catani, L., Gugliotta, L., Belmonte, M., Vianelli, N., Gherlinzoni, T., Miggiano, M., Belardinelli, A., Rosti, G., Calori, E., Bandini, G., & Tura, S. (1993). Hypercoagulability in patients undergoing autologous or allogeneic bone marrow transplantation for hematological malignancies. *Bone Marrow Transplantation, 12,* 253–259.

Chu, D. Z., Shivshanker, K., Stroehlein, J. R., & Nelson, R. S. (1983). Thrombocytopenia and gastrointestinal hemorrhage in the cancer patient: prevalence of unmasked lesions. *Gastrointestinal Endoscopy, 29,* 269–272.

Cilley, R. E., Strodel, W. E., & Peterson, R. O. (1989). Cause of death in carcinoma of the esophagus. *The American Journal of Gastroenterology, 84,* 147–149.

Cohen, A. M., Minsky, B. D., & Schilsky, R. L. (1993). Colon cancer. In V. T. DeVita, S. Hellman, & S. A. Rosenberg (Eds.), *Cancer: Principles and practices of oncology* (Vol. 1, 4th ed., pp. 929–977). Philadelphia: J. B. Lippincott Co.

Coleman, R., Hirsch, J., Marder, V., & Salzman, E. (1994). *Hemostasis and thrombosis.* Philadelphia: J. B. Lippincott.

Collins, P. M. (1990). Diagnosis and treatment of chronic leukemia. *Seminars in Oncology Nursing, 6,* 31–43.

Colman, R., & Rubin, R. (1990). Disseminated intravascular coagulation due to malignancy. *Seminars in Oncology, 17*(2), 172–186.

Cook, D. J., Guyatt, G. H., Salena, B. J., & Laine, L. A. (1992). Endoscopic therapy for acute nonvariceal upper gastrointestinal hemorrhage: A meta-analysis. *Gastroenterology, 102,* 139–148.

Corriveau, D. (1988). Major elements of hemostasis. In D. Corriveau & G. Fritsma (Eds.), *Hemostasis and thrombosis in the clinical laboratory* (pp. 1–33). Philadelphia: J. B. Lippincott.

Daeffler, R. J. (1994). Mucous membranes. In J. Gross & B. L. Johnson (Eds.), *Handbook of oncology nursing* (2nd ed.) (pp. 399–421). Boston: Jones and Bartlett.

Dean, R., & Lytton, B. (1978). Urologic complications of pelvic irradiation. *Journal of Urology, 119,* 64–67.

DeVries, C. R., & Freiha, F. S. (1990). Hemorrhagic cystitis: A review. *The Journal of Urology, 143,* 1–9.

Dutcher, J. (1987). Bleeding and coagulopathy. In J. Dutcher & P. Wiernik (Eds.), *Handbook of hematology and oncologic emergencies* (pp. 123–138). New York: Plenum Press.

Elby, C. (1993). A review of the hypercoagulable state. *Hematology-Oncology Clinics of North America, 7*(6), 1121–1141.

Ellenberger, B., Haas, L., & Cundiff, L. (1993). Thrombotic thrombocytopenic purpura: Nursing during the acute phase. *Dimensions of Critical Care Nursing, 12*(2), 58–65.

Erickson, J. (1990). Blood support for the myelosuppressed patient. *Seminars in Oncology Nursing, 6*(1), 61–66.

Erslev, A., & Lichtman, M. (1990). Structure and function of the marrow. In W. Williams, E. Beutler, A. Erslev, & M. Lichtman (Eds.), *Hematology* (4th ed., pp. 129–147). New York: McGraw-Hill Publishing Co.

Ey, F., & Goodnight, S. (1990). Bleeding disorders in cancer. *Seminars in Oncology, 17*(2), 187–197.

Freedman, S., Haisfield, M. E., McGuire, D. B., Morell, L., Paulaitis, L., & Wohlganger, J. (1990). Nursing considerations in the administration of blood component therapy. *Seminars in Oncology Nursing, 6,* 155–162.

Fuller, A. K. (1990). Platelet transfusion therapy for thrombocytopenia. *Seminars in Oncology Nursing, 6,* 123–128.

Ganser, A. (1993). Clinical results with recombinant human interleukin-3. *Cancer Investigation, 11,* 212–218.

Ganser, A., Lindemann, A., Seipelt, G., Ottmann, O. G., Herrmann, F., Eder, M., Frisch, J., Schulz, G., Mertelsmann, R., & Hoelzer, D. (1991). Clinical effects of recombinant human interleukin-3. *American Journal of Clinical Oncology, 14*(Suppl.), 51–63.

Ganser, A., Lindemann, A., Seipelt , G., Ottmann, O. G., Herrmann, F., Eder, M., Frisch, J., Schulz, G., Mertelsmann, R., & Hoelzer, D. (1990). Effects of recombinant human interleukin-3 in patients with normal hematopoiesis and in patients with bone marrow failure. *Blood, 76,* 666–676.

Gerson, S., & Lazarus, H. (1989). Hematopoietic emergencies. *Seminars in Oncology, 16*(6), 532–542.

Glaspy, J. (1992). Hemostatic abnormalities in multiple myeloma and related disorders. *Hematology-Oncology Clinics of North America, 6*(6), 1301–1313.

Goldberg, R., Seneff, M., Gore, J., Anderson, F., Greene, H., Wheeler, H., & Dalen, J. (1987). Occult cancer in patients with acute pulmonary embolism. *Archives of Internal Medicine, 147,* 251–253.

Goldhaber, S., Burning, J., & Hennekens, C. (1987). Cancer and venous thromboembolism. *Archives of Internal Medicine, 147,* 216–217.

Goodman, M. (1989). Managing the side effects of chemotherapy. *Seminars in Oncology Nursing, 5,* 29–52.

Gore, J., Appelbaum, J., Greene, J., Dexter, L., & Dalen, J. E. (1982). Occult cancer in patients with acute pulmonary embolism. *Annals of Internal Medicine, 96,* 556–560.

Goudnough, L., Anderson, K., Kurtz, S., Lane, T., Pisciotto, P., Sayers, H., & Silberstein, L. (1993). Indications and guidelines for the use of hematopoietic growth factors. *Transfusion, 33,* 944–959.

Gralnick, H., & Abrell, E. (1973). Studies of the procoagulant and fibrinolytic activity of promyelocytes in acute promyelocytic leukemia. *British Journal of Hematology, 24,* 89–99.

Greifzu, S., Radjeski, D., & Winnick, B. (1990). Oral care is part of cancer care. *RN,* 43–46.

Griffin, J. (1986). *Hematology and immunology: Concepts for nursing.* Norwalk, CT: Appleton-Century Crofts.

Griffin, M., Stanson, A., Brown, M., Hauser, M., O'Fallon, W., Anderson, H., Kazmier, F., & Melton, L. (1987). Deep venous thrombosis and pulmonary embolism: Risk of subsequent malignant neoplasms. *Archives of Internal Medicine, 147,* 1907–1911.

Guyton, A. C. (1991). *Textbook of Medical Physiology* (8th Ed.). Philadelphia: W. B. Saunders Co.

Hall, P., Cedermark, B., & Swedborg, J. (1989). Implantable catheter system for long-term intravenous chemotherapy. *Journal of Surgical Oncology, 41,* 39–41.

Haeuber, D., & DiJulio, J. E. (1989). Hemopoietic colony stimulating factors: An overview. *Oncology Nursing Forum, 16,* 247–255.

Heyman, M., & Schiffer, C. (1990). Platelet transfusion therapy for the cancer patient. *Seminars in Oncology, 17*(2), 198–209.

Hickey, J. V. (1992). Increased intracranial pressure. In J. V. Hickey (Ed.), *Neurological and neurosurgical nursing* (3rd ed., pp. 249–288). Philadelphia: J. B. Lippincott.

Ho, W. (1990). Transfusion and apheresis of blood cells. In C. Haskell (Ed.), *Cancer treatment* (3rd ed., pp. 862–866). Philadelphia: W. B. Saunders Co.

Hoelzer, D., Seipelt, G., & Ganser, A. (1991). Interleukin 3 alone and in combination with GM-CSF in the treatment of patients with neoplastic disease. *Seminars in Hematology, 28,* 17–24.

Hoffman, R. (1993). Interleukin-3: A potentially useful agent for treating chemotherapy-related thrombocytopenia. *Journal of Clinical Oncology, 11,* 2057–2060.

Hogge, D. E., Dutcher, J. P., & Aisner, J. (1984). The ineffectiveness of random donor platelet transfusion in splenectomized, alloimmunized recipients. *Blood, 64,* 253–256.

Holbrook, G. R., & Palmer, M. (1993). Tunnelled venous access in the thrombocytopenic patient: Percutaneous vs. cutdown. *Proceedings of the Annual Meeting of the American Society of Clinical Oncologists, 12,* 1472.

Holmes, S. B. (1991). The oral complications of specific anticancer therapy. *International Journal of Nursing Studies, 28,* 343–360.

Homans, A. C., Rybak, M. E., Baglini, R., Tiarks, C., Steiner, M., & Forman, E. N. (1987). Effect of L-asparaginase on coagulation and platelet function in children with leukemia. *Journal of Clinical Oncology, 5,* 811–817.

Hui, W. M., Ng, M. M., Lok, A. S., Lau, Y. N., & Lam, S. K. (1991). A randomized comparative study of laser photocoagulation, heater probe, and bipolar electrocoagulation in the treatment of actively bleeding ulcers. *Gastrointestinal Endoscopy, 37,* 299–304.

Jackson, A., Rose, B., & Graff, L. (1984). Thrombotic microangiopathy and renal failure associated with antineoplastic chemotherapy. *Annals of Internal Medicine, 101,* 41–44.

Jennis, A., & Bauer, K. (1993). Coagulopathic complications of cancer. In J. Holland, E. Frei, R. Bast, D. Kufe, D. Morton, & R. Weichselbaum (Eds.), *Cancer medicine* (3rd Ed.). Philadelphia: Lea & Febiger.

Kempin, S. (1991). Disorders of hemostasis. In J. Groeger (Ed.), *Critical care of the cancer patient* (2nd ed., pp. 103–139). St. Louis: Mosby Year Book.

Kies, M. S., & Kwaan, H. C. (1982). Thromboembolism in cancer patients. In H. C. Kwaan & E. J. Bowie (Eds.), *Thrombosis* (pp. 175–184). Philadelphia: W. B. Saunders Co.

Klein, P. W. (1985). Neurologic emergencies in oncology. *Seminars in Oncology Nursing, 1,* 278–284.

Kroll, M., & McCarthy, P. L. (1994). Hemostatic complications of bone marrow transplantation. In J. Loscalzo & A. Schafer (Eds.), *Thrombosis and hemorrhage* (pp. 1039–1050). Boston: Blackwell Scientific Publications.

Labovich, T. M. (1994). Selected complications in the patient with cancer and spinal cord compression, malignant bowel obstruction, malignant ascites, and gastrointestinal bleeding. *Seminars in Oncology Nursing, 10,* 189–197.

Lankiewicz, M., & Bell, W. (1993). Disseminated intravascular coagulation. In W. Bell (Ed.), *Hematologic and oncologic emergencies* (pp. 105–124). New York: Churchill Livingstone.

Lee, G., Bithell, T., Foerster, J., Athens, J., & Lukens, J. (1993). *Wintrobe's clinical hematology* (9th ed.). Philadelphia: Lea & Febiger.

Lesage, C. (1986). Carotid artery rupture: prediction, prevention, and preparation. *Cancer Nursing, 9,* 1–7.

Levine, L. A., & Richie, J. P. (1989). Urological complications of cyclophosphamide. *The Journal of Urology, 141,* 1063–1069.

Levine, M., & Hirsh, J. (1990). The diagnosis and treatment of thrombosis in the cancer patient. *Seminars in Oncology, 17*(2), 160–171.

Lichtman, M., & Rowe, J. (1982). Hyperleukocytic leukemias: rheological, clinical, and therapeutic considerations. *Blood, 60,* 279–283.

Lightdale, C. J., Kurtz, R. C., Boyle, C. C., Sherlock, P., & Winawer, S. J. (1973). Cancer and upper gastrointestinal tract hemorrhage. *Journal of the American Medical Association, 226,* 139–141.

Luzzatto, G., & Schaefer, A. (1990). The prethrombotic state in cancer. *Seminars in Oncology, 17*(2), 147–159.

Marcus, A. J. (1992). Hemorrhagic disorders: Abnormalities of platelet and vascular function. In J. B. Wyngaarden & L. H. Smith (Eds.), *Cecil textbook of medicine* (pp. 979–992). Philadelphia: W. B. Saunders Co.

Maxwell, M. B. (1984). When the cancer patient becomes anemic. *Cancer Nursing, 7,* 321–326.

Mayer, D. K. (1988). Gastrointestinal bleeding. In S. Baird (Ed.), *Decision making in oncology nursing* (pp. 108–109). Philadelphia: B. C. Decker, Inc.

McAdams, R. C., & McClure, K. (1986). Hypovolemia: When to suspect it. *RN, 49,* 34–37.

McDonald, G. B., Sharma, P., Hackman, R. C., Meyers, J. D., & Thomas, E. D. (1985). Esophageal infections in immunosuppressed patients after marrow transplantation. *Gastroenterology, 88,* 1111–1117.

McDonald, T. P., & Sullivan, P. S. (1993). Megakaryocytic and erythrocytic cell lines share a common precursor cell. *Experimental Hematology, 21,* 1316–1320.

McDonnell, K. K. (1994). Infiltrative emergencies. In J. Gross & B. L. Johnson (Eds.), *Handbook of oncology nursing* (2nd ed., pp. 745–755). Boston: Jones and Bartlett.

McDonnell, K. K. (1994). Leukostasis. In J. Gross & B. L.

Johnson (Eds.), *Handbook of oncology nursing* (2nd ed., pp. 756–763). Boston: Jones and Bartlett.

Metcalf, D. (1994). Thrombopoietin—at last. *Nature, 369,* 519–520.

Miaskowski, C. A. (1985). Assessment of the acutely ill cancer patient. *Seminars in Oncology Nursing, 1,* 230–236.

Morris, J. C., & Holland, J. F. (1993). Oncologic emergencies. In J. F. Holland, E. Frei, R. Bast, D. Kufe, D. Morton, & R. Weichselbaum (Eds.), *Cancer medicine* (pp. 2442–2465). Philadelphia: Lea & Febiger.

Nand, S., Fisher, S., Salgia, R., & Fisher, R. (1987). Hemostatic abnormalities in untreated cancer: Incidence and correlation with thrombotic and hemorrhagic complications. *Journal of Clinical Oncology, 5,* 1998–2003.

Nand, S., & Messmore, H. (1990). Hemostasis in malignancy. *American Journal of Hematology, 35,* 45–55.

Naschitz, J., Yeshurum, D., & Lev, L. (1993). Thromboembolism in cancer: Changing trends. *Cancer, 71*(4), 1384–1390.

Neumanaitis, J., Appelbaum, F. R., Singer, J. W., Lilleby, K., Wolff, S., Greer, J. P., Bierman, P., Resta, D., Campion, M., Levitt, D., Zeigler, Z., Rosenfeld, C., Shadduck, R. K., & Buckner, C. D. (1993). Phase I trial with recombinant human interleukin-3 in patients with lymphoma undergoing autologous bone marrow transplantation. *Blood, 82,* 3273–3278.

Nugent, D. (1993). Immune thrombocytopenic purpura. In W. Bell (Ed.), *Hematologic and oncologic emergencies.* (pp. 83–103). New York: Churchill Livingstone.

Nugent, D. J. (1992). Alloimmunization to platelet antigens. *Seminars in Hematology, 29,* 83–88.

O'Connell, B., Lee, E. J., & Schiffer, C. A. (1988). The value of 10-minute posttransfusion platelet counts. *Transfusion, 28,* 66–67.

Pai, U., Blinkhorn, R. J., & Tomashefski, J. F. (1994). Invasive cavitary pulmonary aspergillosis in patients with cancer: A clinicopathologic study. *Human Pathology, 25,* 293–303.

Panos, R. J., Barr, L. F., Walsh, T. J., & Silverman, H. J. (1988). Factors associated with fatal hemoptysis in cancer patients. *Chest, 94,* 1008–1013.

Parsons, C. L. (1986). Successful management of radiation cystitis with sodium pentosanpolysulfate. *The Journal of Urology, 136,* 813–814.

Patterson, W. (1990). Coagulation and cancer: An overview. *Seminars in Oncology, 17*(2), 137–139.

Patterson, W., Caldwell, C., & Doll, D. (1990). Hyperviscosity syndromes and coagulopathies. *Seminars in Oncology, 17*(2), 210–216.

Patterson, W., & Ringenberg, S. (1990). The pathophysiology of thrombosis in cancer. *Seminars in Oncology, 17*(2), 140–146.

Perkins, J., & Elfenbein, G. (1993). The platelet-refractory bone marrow transplant patient: Prophylaxis and treatment of bleeding. *Seminars in Oncology, 20*(5, Suppl. 6), 102–109.

Prins, M., Lensig, A., & Hirsch, J. (1994). Idiopathic deep venous thrombosis: Is a search for malignant disease justified? *Archives of Internal Medicine, 154,* 1310–1312.

Pryse-Phillips, W., & Murray, T. J. (1982). Neoplastic disease. In W. Pryse-Phillips & T. J. Murray (Eds.), *Essential neurology* (2nd ed., pp. 501–526). Garden City, NJ: Medical Examination Publishers.

Quesenberry, P. (1990). Hematopoietic stem cells, progenitor cells and growth factors. In W. Williams, E. Beutler, A. Erslev, & M. Lichtman (Eds.), *Hematology* (4th ed., pp. 129–147). New York: McGraw Hill Publishing.

Ratnoff, O. (1989). Hemostatic emergencies in malignancy. *Seminars in Oncology, 16*(6), 561–571.

Rice, S. J., Bishop, J. A., Apperley, J., & Gardner, S. D. (1985). BK virus as cause of hemorrhagic cystitis after bone marrow transplantation. *The Lancet, 11,* 844–845.

Rodeghiero, F., Mannucci, P., & Vigano, P. (1984). Liver dysfunction rather than intravascular coagulation is the main cause of low protein C and AT-III in acute leukemia. *Blood, 63,* 965–969.

Rogers, J., Murgo, A., Fontana, J., & Raich, P. (1988). Chemotherapy for breast cancer decreases plasma protein C and protein S. *Journal of Clinical Oncology, 6,* 276–281.

Rolston, K. V., & Bodey, G. P. (1993). Infections in patients with cancer. In J. F. Holland, E. Frei, R. C. Blast, D. W. Kufe, D. L. Morton, & R. R. Weichselbaum (Eds.), *Cancer medicine* (pp. 2416–2441). Philadelphia: Lea & Febiger.

Rosen, P. (1992). Bleeding problems in the cancer patient. *Hematology-Oncology Clinics of North America, 6(6),* 1315–1328.

Rosove, M., & Schwartz, G. (1990). Hematologic complications of cancer and its treatment. In C. Haskell (Ed.), *Cancer treatment* (3rd ed., pp. 850–861). Philadelphia: W. B. Saunders Co.

Ross, A., Griffith, C., Anderson, J., et al. (1984). Thromboembolic complications with silicone elastomer subclavian catheters. *The Journal of Parenteral and Enteral Nutrition, 6,* 61.

Rossle, A., & Ostermann, H. (1990). What's new in the causes of hemorrhage in acute myelogenous leukemia? *Pathology in Research and Practice, 186,* 415–420.

Rostad, M. E. (1991). Current strategies for managing myelosuppression in patients with cancer. *Oncology Nursing Forum, 18*(Supp.), 7–15.

Roth, J. A., Putnam, J. B., Lichter, A. S., & Forastiere, A. A. (1993). Cancer of the esophagus. In V. T. DeVita, S. Hellman, S. A. Rosenberg (Eds.), *Cancer: Principles and practices of oncology* (Vol. 1, 4th ed., pp. 776–817). Philadelphia: J. B. Lippincott Co.

Rothstein, G. (1993). Origin and development of the blood and blood forming tissues. In G. Lee, T. Bithell, J. Foerster, J. Athens & J. Lukens (Eds.), *Wintrobe's clinical hematology* (9th ed., pp. 41–78). Philadelphia: Lea & Febiger.

Rubein, L. D., & Levin, B. (1993). Gastrointestinal complications. In J. F. Holland, E. Frei, R. C. Blast, D. W. Kufe, D. L. Morton & R. R. Weichselbaum (Eds.), *Cancer medicine* (pp. 2370–2381). Philadelphia: Lea & Febiger.

Ruiz, M., Marugan, I., Estelles, A., Navarro, I., Espana, F., Alberola, V., San Juan, L., Aznar, J., & Garcia-Conde, J. (1989). The influence of chemotherapy in plasma coagulation and fibrinolytic systems on lung cancer patients. *Cancer, 63,* 643–648.

Russo, P. (1993). Urologic emergencies. In V. T. DeVita, S. Hellman, S. A. Rosenberg (Eds.), *Cancer: Principles and practices of oncology* (Vol. 2, 4th ed., pp. 2159–2169). Philadelphia: J. B. Lippincott Co.

Sack, G., Levin, J., & Bell, W. (1977). Trousseau's syndrome and other manifestations of chronic disseminated coagulopathy in patients with neoplasms: Clinical, pathophysiologic, and therapeutic features. *Medicine, 56,* 1–37.

Schaefer, A. (1985). The hypercoagulable states. *Annals of Internal Medicine, 102,* 814–828.

Schantz, S. P., Harrison, L. B., & Hong, W. K. (1993). Tumors of the nasal cavity and paranasal sinuses, nasopharynx, oral cavity, and oropharynx. In V. T. DeVita, S. Hellman, & S. A. Rosenberg (Eds.), *Cancer: Principles and practices of oncology* (Vol. 1, 4th ed., pp. 574–630). Philadelphia: J. B. Lippincott Co.

Schiffer, C., & Wade, J. (1987). Supportive care: Issues in the use of blood products and treatment of infection. *Seminars in Oncology, 14*(4), 454–467.

Schwartzberg, L., & Holbert, J. (1988). Hemorrhagic and thrombotic abnormalities of cancer. *Critical Care Clinics, 4*(1), 107–128.

Seifter, E., & Bell, W. (1983). Coagulation abnormalities in patients with cancer. *Clinics in Oncology, 2*(3), 657–704.

Shaffer, S. (1994). Protective mechanisms. In S. E. Otto (Ed.), *Oncology nursing* (2nd ed., pp. 698–719). St. Louis: Mosby.

Shannon, M. T., & Wilson, B. A. (1992). *Drugs and nursing implications* (7th ed.). Norwalk, CT: Appleton & Lange.

Shelton, B. K. (1993). Gastrointestinal bleeding. In J. E. Wright & B. K. Shelton (Eds.), *Critical care nursing* (pp. 873–886). Boston: Jones and Bartlett.

Sheridan, C. A. (1990). Uncommon leukemias: Implications for clinical practice. *Seminars in Oncology Nursing, 6,* 44–49.

Shivshanker, K., Chu, D. Z. J., Stroehlein, J. R., & Nelson, R. S. (1983). Gastrointestinal hemorrhage in the cancer patient. *Gastrointestinal Endoscopy, 29,* 273–275.

Skinner, D. B., & Belsey, R. H. (1988). Esophageal malignancies: Incidence, etiology, presentation, and diagnosis. In D. B. Skinner & R. H. Belsey (Eds.), *Management of esophageal disease* (pp. 728–735). Philadelphia: W. B. Saunders Co.

St. Clair, K. M., & Bove, L. A. (1987). What you can do to prevent increased ICP. *Nursing Life, 7,* 49–56.

Stellato, T. A., & Shenk, R. R. (1989). Gastrointestinal emergencies in the oncology patient. *Seminars in Oncology, 16,* 521–531.

Thorup, O. (1987). *Fundamentals of clinical hematology* (5th ed.). Philadelphia: W. B. Saunders Co.

Vadhan-Raj, S. (1989). Clinical applications of colony stimulating factors. *Oncology Nursing Forum, 16*(Suppl.), 21–26.

Wallach, C. B., & Kurtz, R. C. (1992). Gastrointestinal problems. In J. S. Groeger (Ed.), *Critical care of the cancer patient* (2nd ed., pp. 165–191). St. Louis: Mosby.

Walsh, T. J., Belitsos, N. J., & Hamilton, S. R. (1986). Bacterial esophagitis in immunocompromised patients. *Archives of Internal Medicine, 146,* 1345–1348.

Wara, P. (1985). Endoscopic prediction of major rebleeding: A prospective study of stigmata of hemorrhage in bleeding ulcer. *Gastroenterology, 88,* 1209–1214.

Waring, J. P., Sanowski, R. A., Sawyer, R. L., Woods, C. A., & Foutch, P. G. (1991). A randomized comparison of multipolar electrocoagulation and injection sclerosis for the treatment of bleeding peptic ulcer. *Gastrointestinal Endoscopy, 37,* 295–298.

Weiss, R., Tormey, D., Holland, J., & Weinberg, V. (1981). Venous thrombosis during multimodal treatment of primary breast carcinoma. *Cancer Treatment Reports, 65,* 677–679.

Wickham, R., Purl, S., & Welker, D. (1992). Long-term central venous catheters: Issues for care. *Seminars in Oncology Nursing, 8,* 133–147.

Wickham, R. S. (1990). Advances in venous access devices and nursing management strategies. *Advances in Oncology Nursing, 25,* 345–364.

Williams, W., Beutler, E., Erslev, A., & Lichtman, M. (1990). Structure and function of hemopoietic organs. *Hematology* (4th ed., pp. 37–47). New York: McGraw-Hill Publishing.

Yasko, J. M. (1982). Bone marrow depression. In J. M. Yasko (Ed.), *Care of the client receiving external radiation therapy* (p. 202). Reston, VA: Reston Publishing Co.

Yeomans, A. C., & Harle, M. T. (1990). Myelodysoplastic syndromes. *Seminars in Oncology Nursing, 6,* 9–16.

Gayle Giboney Page

The nature of pain has been described in many ways. The International Association for the Study of Pain (IASP) defines pain as "an unpleasant sensory and emotional experience associated with actual or potential tissue damage, or described in terms of such damage" (Bonica, 1979, p. 250). This definition is widely accepted, but our understanding of the multidimensional nature of pain has expanded exponentially since the IASP definition was drafted. While this definition is not incorrect, it is perhaps incomplete. It is now known that there are psychologic and cognitive aspects to the pain experience, both of which have been shown to significantly affect the phenomenon of the pain experience. From a clinical nursing perspective, McCaffery attributes the knowledge of the pain experience to the individual experiencing the pain: "pain is whatever the experiencing person says it is, existing whenever he says it does" (1979, p. 11).

This section on the physiology of pain will highlight what is known about the transmission of pain impulses from the periphery to the central nervous system (CNS), how the CNS might be perpetuating the sensation of pain after the painful stimulus is no longer present, mechanisms of pain inhibition, neuropathic pain, and a brief summary of the psychologic and cognitive contributions to the pain experience. The particular issues related to the pain of cancer will be introduced.

With the publication of the Gate Control Theory by Melzack and Wall (1965), our understanding regarding the physiology of pain has exploded. The Gate Control Theory continues to be acknowledged as the major conceptualization of pain mechanisms despite not being accurate in some details. This theory was seminal in promoting the emergence of a new field, the neurophysiology of pain. We now know something of the peripheral fiber types and characteristics that initiate nociceptive impulses and which tracts transmit these impulses up the spinal cord and through the brain stem and medulla up to the thalamus, where the various cognitive and emotional interpretations of the impulse are directed to their respective sites in the higher centers of the brain. We know something of what occurs at the site of tissue damage and the transmitters involved. We are learning how injury brings about change in both the peripheral and central nervous system. By no means do we have a "complete" understanding of these phenomena, but our knowledge about pain mechanisms is expanding at a very rapid pace.

Pain is different from other somatosensations. It is not merely a stimulus that is converted to simple signals in nerve fibers for information transfer to the central nervous system. If this were the case, treatment would be easy: simply interrupt this process (Woolf, 1991). This simple analysis may serve for some very specific acute pain experiences but is inadequate for most clinical pain syndromes.

An important distinction must be made between pain and nociception before the discussion regarding pain physiology can begin. Nociception is used to denote the transmission of nervous impulses from the periphery to the brain. It is observable and recordable using available neurophysiologic measurement techniques. Pain, on the other hand, is an individual experience. It includes the cognitive, emotional, and psychologic awareness of the individual. Pain is not directly observable by anyone other than the individual who is experiencing it.

THE PERIPHERAL AND NEURAL MECHANISMS OF PAIN

The anatomy and physiology of two different "types" of pain will be reviewed in this section: acute nociceptor-mediated pain in the absence of obvious tissue damage and the peripheral and central mechanisms associated with tissue damage.

PERIPHERAL AND NEURAL MECHANISMS OF PAIN IN THE ABSENCE OF TISSUE DAMAGE

Several characteristics are distinctive of pain in the absence of tissue damage. Typically, the pain stimulus is highly localized such as a pinch, a chemical irritant, or mild abrasion. This pain serves as a warning signal to the organism and is associated with a withdrawal reflex. The classic example is touching a hot stove; only after one's hand is withdrawn from the surface of the stove does one become aware that the stove was hot. This withdrawal reflex, which occurs at the level of the spinal cord, transpires before the brain has had a chance to interpret the nervous impulse transmission into an awareness that the stove is hot. The pain threshold for initiating this type of response is distinctively high, and the vigor of the response to the pain stimulus correlates with the intensity of the stimulus. That is, one would be expected to respond with a more vigorous withdrawal from touching a very hot stove than from touching a stove that is only moderately hot.

AT THE PERIPHERY

Nociception begins with the stimulation of the sensory units (free nerve endings) in the skin referred to as the primary afferents. It is important to note that under normal circumstances, the primary afferents that transmit nociceptive impulses are not spontaneously active; that is, they are quiescent unless stimulated. The magnitude of the activity in the primary afferent is proportional to the intensity of the stimulus: a larger stimulus results in greater activity. Once activated, the nociceptive impulse is transmitted by various fiber types to the spinal cord. The particular fiber type depends upon whether the stimulus is mechanical, thermal, or chemical (Payne, 1987; Yaksh, 1993).

There are two cutaneous fiber types that respond to noxious mechanical, thermal, and chemical stimuli

(Table 55–1). The A delta (δ) fiber, a lightly myelinated nerve fiber, responds almost exclusively to mechanical stimulation. Because these fibers are myelinated, they conduct impulses very quickly. Aδ receptors have a very high threshold for activation that has been shown to be many times greater than the threshold for non-nociceptive mechanoreceptors. It has been shown that the activation of a single fiber is sufficient to cause pain and is described as a sharp, stinging pain (Payne, 1987).

The C fiber is an unmyelinated polymodal nociceptor that responds to noxious mechanical, thermal, and chemical stimuli. Given its lack of myelination, the conduction velocity of the C fiber is much slower than the Aδ fiber. The threshold for mechanical activation of C fibers is greater than that of the Aδ fibers. C fiber activation is associated with dull, burning, or aching pain.

The differences in the transmission velocities of the Aδ and C fibers can be illustrated by the experiences of "first pain" and "second pain" that occur after an intense and painful event, for example, stubbing your toe. Within a second or two of the unfortunate incident, you realize you have stubbed your toe and that it is hurting some; this is the phenomenon of "first pain." The impulse initiated by the very fast conducting myelinated Aδ fiber is responsible for transmitting this first awareness of the sharp pain in your toe to your brain. Just when you realize you have stubbed your toe and that it is going to hurt something awful, a second wave of pain arrives. The slow-conducting, unmyelinated C fiber is responsible for the ongoing aching pain in your toe that lasts for some time.

IN THE SPINAL CORD

The primary afferents transmit impulses to the spinal cord, entering at the dorsal horn through dorsal root entry zone (Yaksh, 1993). Several things happen after the nervous transmission arrives in the spinal cord. First, there is an activation of the flexor motor neurons resulting in the flexion withdrawal reflex, the pulling away from the source of pain. Second, sympathetic preganglionic neurons at the spinal and supraspinal levels are activated, resulting in two sequelae: (1) a general autonomic response manifested by an increase in the individual's heart rate and blood pressure; and (2) a segmental response that causes changes in local blood flow, piloerection, and sweating. Finally, there is the generation of the sensation of pain and associated pain behav-

TABLE 55–1. *Afferent Fiber Types That Are Capable of Transmitting Pain Impulses from Free Nerve Endings in the Skin to the Secondary Neuron in the Dorsal Horn*

AFFERENT FIBER	CHARACTERISTICS	SENSATION
Aδ	Myelinated, conduction velocity is 5-50m/second	Mechanical
Aβ	Myelinated, conduction velocity is 30-70m/second	Touch, deep tissue pressure, joint movement
C polymodal	Unmyelinated, conduction velocity is 0.6-2.0m/second	Mechanical, thermal, chemical

iors, such as a coordinated effort to escape the pain and vocalizations.

Upon entering the spinal cord at the dorsal root, the pain impulse ascends one to two segments in Lissauer's tract, then synapses with the secondary neuron at the dorsal horn. The dorsal horn contains six laminae, the first of which is the marginal zone, the most dorsal of the six. Laminae II and III constitute the substantia gelatinosa, an important site where non-nociceptive and nociceptive input are integrated. The Aδ fibers synapse with secondary neurons at lamina I and the ventral portion of laminae II and III, and C fibers synapse with secondary neurons primarily in lamina II (Fig. 55–1) (Guyton, 1991). The axons of the secondary neuron decussate (cross) the midline at the white commissure and ascend to the thalamus via the anterolateral pathway (Fig. 55–2) (Guyton, 1991).

A second class of neurons, wide dynamic range (WDR) neurons, also receive input from primary afferents in the dorsal horn. The WDR neurons are located in laminae IV and V and receive input from both nociceptive and non-nociceptive afferents including Aβ (low threshold and nonpainful in normal states), Aδ and C (high threshold) afferents. The activity of WDR neurons increases with the intensity of the stimulus. Additionally, WDR neurons exhibit complex cutaneous receptive fields that overlap. Typically, WDR neurons respond most vigorously to transmissions from afferents within the cutaneous segments they innervate and with progressively less vigor as the distance between primary afferent and the innervating axon increases.

FROM THE MIDBRAIN UP

The axons of the secondary neurons terminate at several locations in the thalamus (including the ventral posterior lateral nucleus and the intralaminar nuclei) and synapse with tertiary neurons, which in turn project to the somatosensory cortex, the limbic system, and the cerebral cortex (Guyton, 1991). The sensory-discriminative aspects of pain, stimulus location, and intensity and their perception are processed in the somatosensory cortex. The limbic system and the cerebral cortex process arousal as well as the affective and emotional components of pain such as suffering (Payne, 1987).

PERIPHERAL AND NEURAL MECHANISMS OF PAIN IN THE PRESENCE OF TISSUE DAMAGE

When tissue damage occurs, the complexity of both the peripheral and central mechanisms increase a great deal. The body's local response to tissue destruction includes the release of a host of chemicals, all of which contribute to peripheral sensitization and in turn, changes in the CNS.

Several additional characteristics of the pain associated with tissue damage have been summarized by Woolf (1989). Pain may occur in the absence of a clear stimulus. A good example is postoperative pain; it just hurts, even without doing anything other than lying in bed, motionless. Pain may also occur in response to a stimulus that would not normally be a painful one (allodynia). Both allodynia and hyperalgesia, an exaggerated or prolonged response to a painful stimulus, occur after a burn. Simply touching or bumping the site of the burn results in pain (allodynia), and the pain might be excruciating and unrelenting if one is so unlucky as to scrape it (hyperalgesia).

THE LOCAL ENVIRONMENT

There are a number of chemical changes that occur at the peripheral terminals after tissue damage. The secretion of factors such as histamine, kinins, and other peptides can directly activate free nerve endings and produce pain. Table 55–2 lists some of these factors and their contribution to pain resulting from tissue damage. In general, these factors facilitate afferent input by lowering the nociceptive threshold and facilitating the response of C and Aδ fibers. The pain-producing power of these factors is believed to be proportional to their local concentration, a higher local concentration resulting in greater tenderness and pain.

The observable local response to tissue damage, brought about by the chemical factors listed in Table 55–2, is characterized by two phenomena at the site of injury: redness, due to local arterial dilation, and swelling from an increase in capillary permeability. These two responses result in an increase in the excitability of both the polymodal nociceptors (C fibers) and the high threshold mechanoreceptors (Aδ fibers), sensitization. Once these nerve fibers are sensitized, a previously nonpainful stimulus becomes a painful one.

Somatically, there are two zones of hyperalgesia. The zone of primary hyperalgesia immediately surrounds the area of tissue damage and is characterized by an increased sensitivity to thermal and mechanical stimulation. The zone of secondary hyperalgesia is

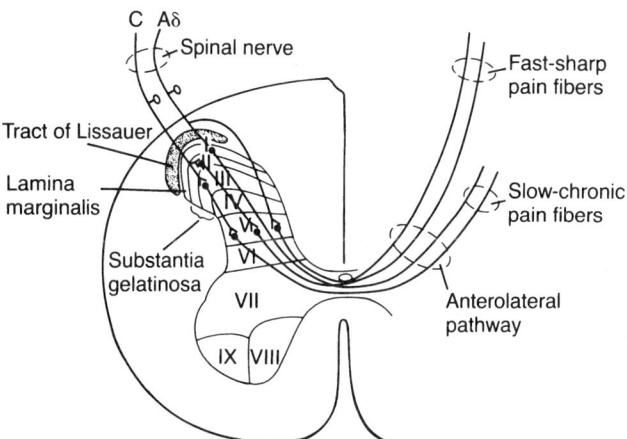

FIGURE 55–1. Laminae of the dorsal horn and illustration of the transmission of acute-sharp (first) and slow-chronic (second) pain impulses from the periphery (via Aδ and C fibers) through the tract of Lissauer, synapsing with the secondary neuron, then ascending the anterolateral spinal pathway. (From Guyton, A. [1991]. *Textbook of medical physiology* [8th ed.]. Philadelphia: W. B. Saunders Co.)

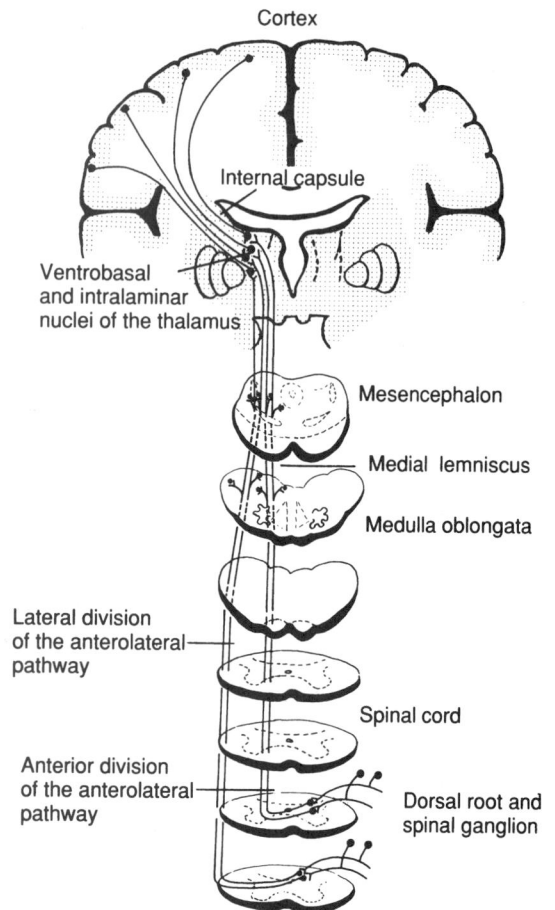

FIGURE 55–2. The anterior and lateral divisions of the antero-lateral pathway. (From Guyton, A. [1991]. *Textbook of medical physiology* [8th ed.]. Philadelphia: W. B. Saunders Co.)

located in the uninjured tissue surrounding that of the primary. The hyperalgesic response of this secondary zone is limited to mechanosensitivity. The fact that no studies have been able to document changes in the nociceptors of the area implies that there is a central nervous system component to secondary hyperalgesias (Woolf, 1991).

CENTRAL MECHANISMS OF PAIN FACILITATION

A phenomenon referred to as afferent barrage was first discussed in the literature in 1984 when Wall and Woolf found in rats that a prolonged excitation of the flexion (withdrawal) reflex resulted when deep muscle fibers were stimulated electrically (Wall & Woolf, 1984). The implication of this finding was that deep tissue damaging stimuli resulted in a continuing barrage of nervous activity in the spinal cord long after the stimulus was withdrawn, thus explaining a possible central mechanism for the continuing pain associated with damage of the deep tissues. Later, it was found that a relatively small amount of morphine administered before the stimulus was initiated would completely block the occurrence of the afferent barrage

resulting from electrical stimulation of the deep muscle. If, on the other hand, morphine was administered after the electrical stimulus, it took a tenfold greater dose to suppress the nervous excitability once it had been established (Woolf & Wall, 1986). Additionally, as the input increases (i.e., with continuing stimulation as from a prolonged surgery), the dose of analgesia required to overcome the nervous activity also increases, whether the analgesia is from a narcotic medication or some endogenous inhibitory transmitter. These studies are seminal in providing the research foundation for the belief that so-called "pre-emptive analgesia" does a better job of relieving surgical pain. Many clinical studies striving to support this hypothesis have been conducted recently, and evidence does appear to support that the preincisional administration of an analgesic medication is better at relieving the pain of surgery and reduces the requirement for postoperative analgesic medications.

Indeed, Richmond, Bromley, and Woolf (1993), in a randomized double-blind study, found that individuals receiving morphine before their abdominal surgery commenced used less morphine (via patient controlled analgesia [PCA]) compared with individuals receiving the same amount of morphine administered after closure of the peritoneum. Further, pain sensitivity around the wound was reduced in the preoperative morphine group compared with the postperitoneal closure group. The findings of Katz et al. (1992) were of a similar nature, using preincisional versus postincisional epidural fentanyl. Compared with the postincisional group, the preincisional group indicated significantly less pain on a visual analog scale and used significantly less morphine via PCA postoperatively.

The plasticity of the CNS is now believed to be responsible for the transformation of a situation wherein not only are nociceptors (Aδ and C fibers) driving the nervous system to produce pain, but Aβ afferents are producing pain sensations as well. Under normal circumstances, Aβ fibers are low threshold afferents sensitive to tactile, deep tissue pressure, and joint movement (Table 55–1). In the case of this phenomenon, the WDR neuron, the dorsal horn neuron that normally receives input from A and C fibers, begins to respond in an exaggerated way to Aβ input. In essence, stimuli that would not produce pain in a normal situation become painful once central sensitization has been established; thus, even light touch becomes pain-producing, evoking the withdrawal reflex (Woolf, 1991; Yaksh, 1993).

It has been learned that this phenomenon of central sensitization, wind-up, also possesses two particular mechanisms of perpetuation. First is the peripheral release of chemical factors as described previously and summarized in Table 55–2. The second is the glutamate receptor (an excitatory amino acid) in the dorsal horn neuron, N-methyl-D-aspartate acid (NMDA), that prolongs the duration of synaptic potentials. This NMDA receptor extends the time during which the neuron is responsive to the summation of nervous impulses, thus enhancing its excitability and pain response to "nonnoxious" stimulation (Woolf, 1991; Yaksh, 1993).

TABLE 55–2. *Chemical Factors Released Peripherally in Response to Tissue Damage and Their Contribution to Pain States*

CHEMICAL	ORIGIN	ACTIONS
Histamine	Granules of mast cells, basophils, and platelets	Stimulate free nerve endings and evoke vasodilatation.
Serotonin (5-HT)	Granules of mast cells and platelets	Stimulate free nerve endings and evoke vasodilatation.
Lipidic acids (e.g., prostaglandins)	Synthesized in the arachidonic acid cascade	Sensitize free nerve endings and increase capillary permeability.
Kinins (e.g., bradykinin)	Released by physical trauma	Powerful activator of free nerve endings.
Cytokines (e.g., IL-1)	Released as a function of immune activity	Induce hypersensitivity reactions.
Primary afferent peptides (e.g., calcitonin gene-related peptide [CGRP] and substance P [sP])	Released from the peripheral terminals of C fibers	Role for pain transmission uncertain, but when these peptides are released by antidromic nerve stimulation, local cutaneous vasodilatation and plasma extravasation occur in the region innervated by that sensory nerve.

The clinical implications for this wind-up phenomenon are profound. These findings provide a rationale for attempting to prevent the initiation of central sensitization (e.g., use of regional anesthesia before incision for surgery). If central sensitization cannot be prevented, as is the case in trauma, once it is recognized, it should be understood that treatments directed at preventing nociceptor action at the periphery will likely be inadequate. Once the nervous system is in this abnormal state, it can be driven by low threshold afferents (e.g., touch and movement). This implies that treatment of both the periphery and central nervous system is necessary to interrupt wind-up. Additionally, greater than normal doses of narcotic may be necessary given the findings of Woolf and Wall (1986). This explanation of events is applicable to the clinical arena in the case of an individual who has been experiencing uncontrolled and intensifying pain for a time and also supports the too frequent observation that repeated doses of narcotic are necessary to overcome such pain.

PAIN INHIBITION

Portions of the brain appear to serve a natural pain-inhibitory function. This phenomenon was first described virtually simultaneously by three different groups who showed that noxious or fear-provoking stimuli in animals produces a state of decreased responsiveness to pain, stress-induced analgesia (SIA). These findings suggest that stress is an important trigger for activating endogenous analgesia-producing substrates (Akil, Madden, Patrick, & Barchas, 1976; Hayes, Bennett, Newlon, & Mayer, 1976, Rosecrans & Chance, 1976). Subsequently, SIA has been demonstrated in a wide variety of animals, including humans, and can be elicited by a wide range of stressors.

The type of analgesia that results from a stressful experience may be non-opioid or opioid in nature, or a combination of both. Opioid analgesia is commonly defined as a condition that can be eliminated by opioid antagonists such as naloxone and naltrexone and as manifesting tolerance with repetition and cross-toler-

ance to morphine. Just as repeated doses of morphine result in a less effective analgesia for severe pain and physical tolerance, animals become less responsive to the analgesic effects of a repeated stressful event. Cross-tolerance to morphine indicates that despite never having received a dose of morphine, an animal that has developed a tolerance to the analgesic effects of stress-induced releases of endogenous opioids is also tolerant to the analgesic effects of morphine. The implication of these findings is that SIA and morphine both activate the same opioid system of pain inhibition. Alternatively, a non-opioid form of stress-induced analgesia is commonly suggested if opiate antagonists fail to block the SIA.

The electrical stimulation of certain areas of the brain also is known to induce analgesia, a phenomenon termed stimulation-produced analgesia (SPA). Of interest is that the characteristics of stress-induced analgesia have been found to share many features with SPA. For example, both SPA and SIA have been shown to be mediated by both opioid and non-opioid systems. While electrical stimulation of some brain sites (e.g., the ventral periaqueductal gray matter [PAG]) produce an analgesia that meets all three of the previously mentioned opioid criteria, stimulation of other sites results in a non-opioid analgesia (e.g., the rostral PAG) (Cannon, Prieto, Lee, & Liebeskind, 1982).

Endogenous opioids are likely mediators of pain inhibition. High concentrations of opiate receptors and opiate peptides have been found in the same areas of the CNS that have been shown to be involved in pain inhibition, the PAG, the nucleus raphe magnus and neighboring reticular nuclei, as well as in the spinal cord. The activation of these descending pathways from the brain stem to the spinal cord modulate afferent impulses in the dorsal horn at Laminae I, II, and IV.

There are three recognized opiate receptor types, mu (μ), delta (δ), and kappa (K). Opiate drugs bind with opiate receptors in the CNS to exert their analgesic effects. Opioids produce a dose-dependent suppression of nociceptive activity in the WDR neurons and thus reduce pain intensity. For example, morphine largely binds with μ receptors located in both the brain and spinal cord (Yaksh & Malmberg, 1994).

NEUROPATHIC PAIN

Nerve injury, whether a complete sectioning or a partial injury, may trigger bizarre and uncontrollable sensations. Wall (1991) lists the characteristics of neuropathic pains (p. 632):

1. Some pains are ongoing and little influenced by peripheral stimuli.
2. Some pains are lancinating spontaneous stabs.
3. Some pains are provoked by normally innocuous stimuli (allodynia).
4. All pains except trigeminal neuralgia are associated with hypesthesia.
5. Provoked pains require summation by prolongation, movement, and repetition of the stimulus.
6. Some pain states appear immediately after nerve injury, others after delays.

Provoked pains are not usually evoked by a single brief innocuous stimulus; however, repeated minor sensations such as rhythmic tapping can produce excruciating pain that peaks in severity after tens of seconds. The individual might sense the beginning of the pain and stop the stimulus, but the pain would continue to get worse, despite having stopped the stimulus. An example is the Tinel sign, where tapping over the site of a neuroma produces an intense radiating pain.

"An injured nerve does not behave like a severed telephone cable, either letting through its message or not letting it through" (Devor 1991, p. 620). It appears that neuropathic pain results from a large number of pathophysiologic mechanisms existing in isolation or combination, and at the periphery or centrally.

PERIPHERAL MECHANISMS

Changes in the nerve fiber's ability to transmit impulses occur with injury. Ectopic discharges may be produced by the proximal stump of the nerve, local patches of demyelination along the axon, and the dorsal root ganglion. The distal portion of the nerve, now separated from the soma, degenerates. The molecular products produced in the body of the dorsal root ganglion now travel toward the nonexistent or damaged sensory ending and dam up the injury site. Now, without the regulatory processes that normally control the excitability of nerve endings, these pooled molecular products likely produce abnormal sensations, including pain.

Other phenomena that might stimulate ectopic neural sites are mechanical stimulation, evidenced by a Tinel sign, nerve constriction, ischemia, anoxia, inflammatory mediators such as prostaglandins, cold, and circulating and locally released catecholamines. Unlike normal afferents, these ectopic neural sites are capable of autonomous firing; once triggered, a site might continue to fire for hours. This phenomenon is referred to as neuropathic aftersensation. Often after an intense burst, the site will become refractory (unresponsive) to stimulation for a time (Bennett, 1994; Devor, 1991).

Further, there is a phenomenon referred to as cross-excitation in which injured or diseased neurons promote the firing of neighboring neurons, or non-nociceptive afferents may activate nociceptive afferents. Several types of "crosstalk" have been described. Chemical crosstalk refers to the excitation of sensory neurons resulting from noradrenaline release from sympathetic neurons; in turn, the firing of the sensory neurons is interpreted by the brain as pain. Ephaptic crosstalk refers to the coupling of axons such that impulses in one sensory or motor neuron drive impulses in a second neuron, a communication between non-nociceptive and nociceptive fibers. Finally, there is crossed afterdischarge in which a group of neurons engage the repetitive firing of their neighbors. Crossed afterdischarge is different from ephaptic crosstalk, because it is characterized by groups of neurons driving their neighbors rather than the one-to-one coupling of ephaptic crosstalk (Devor, 1991; Portenoy, 1992).

CENTRAL MECHANISMS

Despite the fact that the initial insult is in the periphery, abnormalities of neural processing develop in both the peripheral and central nervous systems. The central nervous system receives impulses and interprets them "literally" as if the impulse was originating in the normal tissue that was served by the nerve before injury (Wall, 1991). The afferent barrage associated with repeated peripheral impulses brings about chemical changes in the dorsal horn cells (convergent cells) such that they are now responsive to input from the innocuous stimulation of nociceptive cells; thus, nociceptive specific fibers (Aδ and C fibers) become sensitive to innocuous stimuli, transmitting pain messages in response to a gentle stimulus (allodynia). These changes in the CNS are believed to involve NMDA receptors at the spinal cord, and research in this area is moving at a feverish pace (Bennett, 1994; Wall, 1991). It has been shown in animals that giving an NMDA antagonist blocks the initiation of this wind-up phenomenon. Early indicators of the effectiveness of such drugs in humans is encouraging (Abram, 1993; Bennett, 1994).

Changes in populations of what are thought to be inhibitory neurons in the brain and spinal cord may cause a toxicity that kills or results in irreparable damage to the neuron. If this is the case, then there would be permanent changes in how sensations are processed in the CNS. This hypothesis is consistent with the difficulty in both the long-standing nature of neuropathic pain and its relief (Bennett, 1994).

Based upon what is known currently about neuropathic pain, there are several reasons for the great variability among individuals suffering from neuropathic pain states. One source of variability is how the neural pacemaker site in the periphery responds to injury. Different nerves and different axon types respond in various ways to injury, and further, the degree of injury affects their response. Postinjury stimuli vary at the site, and given that sympathetic tone may affect spontaneous activity at the injured stump of a neuron, differences in the systemic and local catecholamine levels affect how the nerve and axon will respond to any postinjury stimuli present. Additionally, there are inherent individual differences in whether an ectopic neural discharge will even develop after nerve injury; not everyone will experience neuropathic pain after surgery or some other insult (Devor, 1991). Finally, it is possible that individual variation in the participation of descending systems of pain inhibition also affect the experience of neuropathic pain (Wall, 1991).

A USEFUL MODEL FOR CATEGORIZING NEUROPATHIC PAIN

DEAFFERENTATION PAIN

It is believed that an alteration in somatosensory processing results from damage to an afferent pathway at any point upon its ascending path. Most syndromes of deafferentation pain are well defined and might be precipitated by such insults as peripheral or central lesions, surgical incision, trauma, or cancer. In many cases the deafferentation pains spread over time, incorporating a larger area of painful sensations. It is also believed that lesions in afferent pathways may affect descending systems of pain inhibition.

Common intervention efforts include attempts to isolate the painful part by administering nerve blocks. Typically, these efforts do not provide long-term relief. This clinical finding provides strong evidence that an alteration in central somatosensory processing is the underlying pathology (Portenoy, 1989).

SYMPATHETICALLY MAINTAINED PAIN

This categorization of neuropathic pain has come about only recently and refers to a rather diverse group of neuropathic pains. The disorders composing this category, including reflex sympathetic dystrophy (RSD) and causalgia, share several features. Typically, this type of neuropathic pain begins with some kind of injury with a simultaneous manifestation of pain, local autonomic dysregulation such as edema, vasomotor disturbances, and abnormal sweating. There may be trophic changes in the area as well.

The pathophysiology of sympathetically maintained pain has been a major focus of both animal and human research, and no clear answers have emerged. It is believed that both peripheral and central mechanisms play a role in these disorders. One likely mechanism, which has been demonstrated in animals, is the formation of ephapses between nociceptors and sympathetic nerves after injury. In this case, local catecholamine release excites neighboring nociceptors, resulting in the sensation of pain. A number of hypotheses are under investigation (Portenoy, 1989).

PERIPHERAL NEUROPATHIC PAIN

This category is used to designate the neuropathic pains from which individuals gain permanent relief after a peripheral intervention. It is believed that neuroma formation after nerve injury plays a significant role in the development of peripheral neuropathic pain. This rather simplistic explanation does fail to acknowledge the profound central changes that occur with the barrage of impulses arising from a damaged nerve; however, this designation has proven to be useful clinically (Portenoy, 1989).

THE PATHOPHYSIOLOGY OF CANCER PAIN

Cancer contributes to the experience of pain from three essential origins: the tumor itself, the hormones it secretes, and the generation of neurogenic pain. The tumor is a source of mechanical stimulation by virtue of its ability to infiltrate, compress, and distend or stretch the anatomic structures surrounding it. The pain emanating from thoracic or abdominal tumors might be described as deep, squeezing, and a feeling of pressure that is poorly localized. The encroachment of such tumors on the autonomic nervous system may be associated with nausea, vomiting, and diaphoresis. Pain may also be referred to cutaneous sites either near the site of origin or at a remote site. Pain resulting from neoplastic involvement of the bone is the most prevalent pain syndrome among individuals with cancer. Metastasis to the bone may result in infiltration of the periosteum, and descriptions of pain might include an aching or gnawing sensation that tends to be well localized (Payne, 1987; Portenoy, 1992).

Neurogenic pain in cancer patients is a consequence of peripheral or central nervous system damage. Sources for such damage include tumor encroachment on peripheral nerves, in the spinal cord, or in the brain; trauma to the peripheral or spinal nerves from surgery; and chemical and radiation injury resulting from treatments. As is the case in individuals not suffering from cancer, the sympathetic nervous system is believed to play a role in neurogenic pain states in cancer patients (Payne, 1987).

Certainly, surgical procedures may bring about a chronic neuropathic pain state. Amputation of a limb may result in stump pain related to localized neuroma formation or phantom limb pain, regarded as a deafferentation-type neuropathic pain. This phantom pain may also be experienced by individuals losing other body parts such as the breast. Postmastectomy pain may follow any surgical procedure involving the breast and may occur as late as 1 year or more after surgery (Portenoy, 1992).

Hormone-secreting cells in the tumor constitutes the third essential origin of cancer pain. Just as normal endocrine cells respond to various stimulatory agents, tumor cells with similar capabilities release such factors as bradykinin, serotonin, histamine, and prostaglandins, all of which are capable of facilitating pain processing (Yaksh, 1993).

PSYCHOLOGIC DISTRESS AND SUFFERING

The relationships between the psyche and the experience of cancer pain are very complex, evidenced by a very large literature exploring the many aspects of this dynamic. A thorough review of this extremely important issue is beyond the scope of this section. It should be noted, however, that belief systems, mood states and traits, and coping resources and processes have been shown to affect any individual's pain experience. Further, a diagnosis of cancer, an illness often perceived as life-threatening, likely brings about concerns of future debilitation, pain, and suffering (Breitbart, Passik, & Rosenfeld, 1994; Portenoy, 1992). Given that the experience of pain and the overlay of life experiences are entirely individual, it is vital that such considerations are made as each person with the pain of cancer is touched by health care practitioners.

REFERENCES

Abram, S. (1993). Advances in chronic pain management since gate control (1992 Bonica Lecture). *Regional Anesthesia, 18,* 66–81.

Akil, H., Madden, J., Patrick, R., & Barchas, J. (1976). Stress-induced increase in endogenous opiate peptides: Concurrent analgesia and its partial reversal by naloxone. In H. Kosterlitz (Ed.), *Opiates and endogenous opioid peptides* (pp. 63–70). Amsterdam: Elsevier.

Bennett, G. (1994). Chronic pain due to peripheral nerve damage: An overview. In H. Fields & J. Liebeskind (Eds.), *Progress in pain research and management* (Vol. 1, pp. 51–59). Seattle: IASP Press.

Bonica J. J. (1979). The need for a taxonomy. *Pain, 6,* 247–252.

Breitbart, W., Passik, S., & Rosenfeld, B. (1994). Psychiatric and psychosocial aspects of cancer pain. In P. Wall & R. Melzack (Eds.), *Textbook of pain* (3rd ed., pp. 825–859). Edinburgh: Churchill Livingstone.

Cannon, J., Prieto, G., Lee, A., & Liebeskind, J. (1982). Evidence for opioid and nonopioid forms of stimulation-produced analgesia in the rat. *Brain Research, 243,* 315–321.

Devor, M. (1991). Neuropathic pain and injured nerve: Peripheral mechanisms. *British Medical Bulletin, 47,* 619–630.

Guyton, A. (1991). *Textbook of medical physiology* (8th ed.). Philadelphia: W. B. Saunders Co.

Hayes, R., Bennett, F., Newlon, P., & Mayer, D. (1976). Analgesic effects of certain noxious and stressful manipulations in the rat. *Society for Neuroscience Abstracts, 2,* 1350.

Katz, J., Kavanagh, B., Sandler, A., Nierenberg, H., Boylan, J., Friedlander, M., & Shaw, B. (1992). Preemptive analgesia. *Anesthesiology, 77,* 439–446.

McCaffery, M. (1979). *Nursing management of the patient with pain* (2nd ed.). Philadelphia: J. B. Lippincott Company.

Melzack, R., & Wall, P. (1965). Pain mechanisms: A new theory. *Science, 150,* 971–979.

Payne, R. (1987). Anatomy, physiology, and neuropharmacology of cancer pain. *Medical Clinics of North America, 71,* 153–167.

Portenoy, R. (1989). Mechanisms of clinical pain: Observations and speculations. *Neurologic Clinics, 7,* 205–230.

Portenoy, R. (1992). Cancer pain: Pathophysiology and syndromes. *The Lancet, 339,* 1026–1031.

Richmond, C., Bromley, L., & Woolf, C. (1993). Preoperative morphine pre-empts postoperative pain. *The Lancet, 342,* 73–75.

Rosecrans, J., & Chance, W. (1976). Emotionally induced antinociception. *Society for Neuroscience Abstracts, 2,* 919.

Wall, P. (1991). Neuropathic pain and injured nerve: Central mechanisms. *British Medical Bulletin, 47,* 631–643.

Wall, P., & Woolf, C. (1984). Muscle but not cutaneous C-afferent input produces prolonged increases in the excitability of the flexion reflex in the rat. *Journal of Physiology, 356,* 443–458.

Woolf, C. (1989). Recent advances in the pathophysiology of acute pain. *British Journal of Anaesthesia, 63,* 139–146.

Woolf, C. (1991). Generation of acute pain: Central mechanisms. *British Medical Bulletin, 47,* 523–533.

Woolf, C., & Wall, P. (1986). Morphine-sensitive and morphine-insensitive actions of C-fiber input on the rat spinal cord. *Neuroscience Letters, 64,* 221–225.

Yaksh, T. (1993). New horizons in our understanding of the spinal physiology and pharmacology of pain processing. *Seminars in Oncology, 20,* 6–18.

Yaksh, T., & Malmberg, A. (1994). Interaction of spinal modulatory receptor systems. In H. Fields & J. Liebeskind (Eds.), *Progress in pain research and management* (Vol. 1, pp. 151–171). Seattle: IASP Press.

56

Pain Assessment

Lynne M. Rivera • Margo McCaffery

Cancer pain can be managed effectively through relatively simple means in up to 90 per cent of the 8 million Americans who have cancer or a history of cancer. Unfortunately, pain associated with cancer is frequently undertreated (Management of Cancer Pain Guideline Panel, 1994a).

Pain assessment and its management are fundamental in providing nursing care to patients with cancer. However, despite current pain management knowledge and the availability of highly effective therapeutic pain management strategies, pain remains a significant problem for individuals with cancer. It affects between 50 to 70 per cent of patients in the early stages of the disease and 60 to 90 per cent of patients in the later stages (Bonica, Ventafridda, & Twycross, 1990; Coyle, Adelhardt, Foley, & Portenoy, 1990; Daut & Cleeland, 1982; Johanson, 1991; Portenoy et al., 1992; Twycross & Fairfield, 1982; Ventafridda, Ripamonti, et al., 1990). In the United States, it is estimated that 1.1 million people experience cancer related pain annually (Bonica et al., 1990). However, in reviewing these statistics, the nurse must be aware that most prevalence studies were carried out within large inpatient cancer centers. Therefore, these statistics may only be the tip of the iceberg, excluding those cancer patients with pain who are cared for in small community hospitals or at home.

These statistics must also be considered in relation to the impact that pain has on the person experiencing it. Historically, many patients have not only suffered pain needlessly, they may also have been harmed by their unrelieved pain. Pain has been associated with increased hospital stays (Grant & Ferrell, 1992) and an increased incidence of complications following surgery (Acute Pain Management Guideline Panel, 1992d). In fact, pain may inhibit the immune system and even enhance tumor growth (Liebeskind, 1991).

Pain can be incapacitating and interfere with physical functioning and social interaction and has been associated with psychologic distress (Cleeland, 1984; Portenoy et al, 1992; Massie & Holland, 1987; Ventafridda, De Conno, Ripamonti, Gamba, & Tamburini, 1990). Ineffective pain assessment and its management has also been shown to precipitate patients' distress for the burden they cause family members providing care, as well as frustration and exhaustion (Ferrell, Johnston Taylor, Grant, Fowler, & Corbisiero, 1993). Uncontrolled pain can also influence the family's ability to care for a loved one, make family members wish for an early death, and cause them feelings of helplessness, hopelessness, frustration, and anger (Ferrell, Rhiner, Cohen, & Grant, 1991).

Nurses spend more time with patients with pain than any other member of the health care team. In the palliative care setting, nurses are recognized as the cornerstone of pain relief. In 1986, a consensus development conference on pain, sponsored by the National Institutes of Health (NIH), identified that the nurse's role is the key link in facilitating communication between the patient, the health care team, and the family (Engber, 1986). It is increasingly apparent that nurses will play an equally important role in the relief of pain in acute care settings (McCaffery, 1990).

The undertreatment of pain has been apparent for over 2 decades and continues to be a problem today (Cleeland, 1991; Donovan, Dillon, & McGuire, 1987; Marks & Sachar, 1973; Paice, Mahon, & Faut-Callahan, 1991; Van Roenn, Cleeland, Gonin, Hatfield, & Pandya, 1993). Nurses and other health care professionals in their educational preparation continue to be taught very little about pain management. A survey of NLN-accredited baccalaureate nursing programs revealed that 48 per cent spent 4 hours or less on pain content (Graffam, 1990). Another survey revealed that only 13 per cent of graduating baccalaureate student nurses thought that cancer pain management should be taught as part of the nursing school curriculum (Sheehan, Webb, Bower, & Einsporn, 1992). In light of these dismal reports, the inclusion of cancer pain management content in the basic education of nurses and physicians is recommended by the Oncology Nursing Society (ONS) (Spross, McGuire, & Schmitt, 1991), the World Health Organization (WHO) (1990), the American Society of Clinical Oncology (ASCO) (ASCO Ad Hoc Committee on Cancer Pain, 1992), the American Cancer Society (ACS) (ACS Professors of Clinical Oncology, 1993), the International Association for the Study of Pain (1993), and more recently the California Board of Registered Nurses (1994).

The focus of this chapter is to provide nurses with the knowledge needed to adequately assess pain in adults including those who pose special challenges to pain assessment such as the elderly, as well as a discussion of the barriers that affect adequate pain assessment. The authors acknowledge that adequate pain assessment and its management require the nurse to have an understanding of pain pathophysiology, the ability to identify and evaluate pain syndromes, and an understanding of various pain management strategies including pharmacologic and nondrug therapies. These topics are found in Chapters 55, 57, and 58 contained in this text.

CLINICAL PRACTICE GUIDELINES: ESTABLISHING STANDARDS OF CARE FOR PAIN ASSESSMENT

In recent years, several professional organizations have convened committees or expert panels to develop clinical practice guidelines for the assessment and management of pain. For example, the federally mandated Agency for Health Care Policy and Research (AHCPR) has developed guidelines as well as patient education materials for the management of acute pain (Acute Pain Management Guideline Panel, 1992a, 1992b, 1992c, 1992d) and cancer pain (Management of Cancer Pain Guideline Panel, 1994a, 1994b, 1994c). The AHCPR guideline for cancer pain was developed by an expert panel through a comprehensive scientific review of 19 databases, 9600 citations, and 625 research studies. Its expert panel met six times over 2 years, wrote 17 drafts (two of which were peer-reviewed), and had the guideline field tested in various clinical sites. This expert panel was assisted by 486 consultants, peer reviewers, and site testers, as well as a panel staff.

Several organizations have also developed guidelines that can be used in clinical settings to establish a common base of knowledge and to assist in the development of standards of care related to pain assessment and pain management. Table 56–1 provides information on how to order some of these guidelines. The World Health Organization (WHO) (1990) has developed guidelines for the control of cancer pain. The Oncology Nursing Society (ONS) (Spross et al., 1991) has developed cancer pain management guidelines that

include professional and educational guidelines as well as administrative responsibilities in pain management. The American Pain Society (1992) has developed guidelines for the management of acute pain and cancer pain. In addition, the Joint Commission on Accreditation of Healthcare Organizations (JCAHO) (JCAHO, 1994) recently published a standard of care for patient education that emphasizes appropriate pain management for all patients.

In the international arena, Australia's National Health and Medical Research Council (NHMRC) (NHMRC, 1988) has published information and recommendations for the care of patients with severe acute pain. In 1989, the Canadian Cancer Society convened the Cancer 2000 Task Force with an Expert Panel on Palliative Care. The Expert Panel made recommendations for patients receiving palliative care (Canadian Cancer Society, 1991; Palliative Care 2000, 1992). In addition, undergraduate curriculum guidelines have been distributed to all medical schools, medical students, and to Canada's national licensing body for physicians as well as others (MacDonald, Mount, Boston, & Scott, 1993).

MISCONCEPTIONS THAT HAMPER THE ASSESSMENT OF PAIN IN PATIENTS WITH CANCER

Pain assessment begins with the patient's report of pain. The Agency for Health Care Policy and Research (AHCPR) has stated, "The mainstay of pain assessment is the patient's self-report" (Management of Cancer Pain Guideline Panel, 1994a, p. 3). The AHCPR charges health care professionals to "believe the patient and family in their reports of pain and what relieves it" (Management of Cancer Pain Guideline Panel, 1994c, p. 2). In addition, the American Pain Society (1992) states, "The clinician must accept the patient's report of pain" (p. 2). Health care providers have a professional responsibility to accept and respect the patient's report of pain and to proceed with appropriate assessment and treatment.

When the patient's report of pain is accepted as fact, then the assessment and treatment of pain are much simpler. This results in the prevention of needless suffering, avoidance of missing the diagnosis, and avoidance of an adversarial relationship between the health care provider and the patient or family. However, in reality the patient's report of pain is not always believed, patients do not always report their pain, and physicians and nurses do not always have the knowledge needed to adequately assess and treat the patient's pain.

Pain assessment is hampered by several factors including patient, physician, and nurse barriers; educational issues related to the patient, family, and health care professionals; the need for cancer pain research; and regulatory barriers. This is not an exhaustive list. There are many other barriers and misconceptions that also adversely influence the appropriate assessment and management of cancer-related pain.

TABLE 56–1. *Information for Ordering Clinical Practice Guidelines*

American Pain Society
- American Pain Society. (1992). *Principles of analgesic use in the treatment of acute pain and cancer pain* (3rd ed.).Skokie, IL: American Pain Society.
  Charge: Members—$3; non-members—$5
    American Pain Society
    5700 Old Orchard Road, First Floor
    Skokie, IL 60077-1057
    Phone: (708) 966-5595
- American Pain Society Quality Assurance Guidelines
  Max, M. (1990). *American Pain Society quality assurance standards for relief of acute pain and cancer pain.* In M. R. Bond, J. E. Charlton, & C. J. Wolfe (Eds.), *Proceedings of the VI World Congress on pain.* (pp. 186-189). Amsterdam, The Netherlands: Elsevier.

Agency for Health Care Policy and Research—Cancer Pain Guideline
- *Clinical practice guideline: Management of cancer pain.* AHCPR Publication No. 94-0592.
- *Management of cancer pain: Adults. Quick reference guide for clinicians.* AHCPR Publication No. 94-0593.
- *Managing cancer pain. Patient guide.* AHCPR Publication No. 94-0595.
- *Drug charts (NSAIDs, opioids) and pain assessment scale.* AHCPR Publication No. 92-0086.
    AHCPR Clearinghouse
    P.O. Box 8547
    Silver Spring, MD 20907
    Phone: (800) 358-9295
    No charge.

American Society of Clinical Oncology (ASCO)
- For a fee the organization provides educational materials related to cancer pain.
- Papers and slides presented at the 1993 ASCO Meeting.
    435 N Michigan Avenue, Suite 1717
    Chicago, IL 60611
    Charge $130.00
- Ad Hoc Committee on Cancer Pain of the American Society of Clinical Oncology. (1992). Cancer pain assessment and treatment curriculum guidelines. *Journal of Clinical Oncology, 10,* 1976–1982.

Canadian Cancer Society Report to Cancer 2000 Task Force by Expert Panel on Palliative Care
- Cancer 2000 Documents
    c/o Canadian Cancer Society
    10 Alcorn Avenue
    Toronto, Ontario M4V 3B1, Canada

Oncology Nursing Society
- *Oncology Nursing Society Position Paper on Cancer Pain.* (1991). ID number PPOP9101.
    Oncology Nursing Society
    Department 1889
    Pittsburgh, PA 15278-1889
    Charge: ONS members $6.00
                Non-members $7.00

SUBJECTIVITY VERSUS OBJECTIVITY

What is pain? Whose pain is it? McCaffery (1968) has proposed a definition for pain in the clinical setting, "Pain is whatever the experiencing person says it is, existing whenever the experiencing person says it does" (p. 95). Thus, health care providers and family members must acknowledge the patient's report of pain and respond positively to relieve that pain.

The authors acknowledge that there are situations in which patients deny pain and other situations in which patients are unable to communicate their pain. Pain assessment in these vulnerable patients will be addressed later in this chapter.

Often, pain is inadequately assessed because health care professionals identify themselves as the authority about the existence and nature of the patient's pain sensation. This promotes a situation in which the professional caregiver conveys to the patient that his or her report of pain is not accepted, which amounts to accusing the patient of lying! Because the sensation of pain is completely subjective, the patient is the only authority about his pain. Therefore, adequate pain assessment and its management depend on accepting and acting on the patient's report of pain.

One reason for a reluctance to believe the patient's report of pain is fear of being fooled. The malingerer is defined as a person who says that pain is present when it is not. This person fakes pain or pretends to have pain, usually to avoid or gain something. The malingerer does not feel pain but tries to make others believe that the pain is real. In fact, there are very few malingerers (Hendler, 1984; Leavitt & Sweet, 1986; Reesor & Craig, 1988; Social Security Administration, 1986). However, sometimes patients are erroneously labeled as malingerers if the cause of their pain cannot be identified, when their pain cannot be relieved, or when their symptoms are vague.

Malingering cannot be confused with psychogenic pain or secondary gain. Psychogenic pain is rare, but when it occurs the pain may be as severe as any other type of pain with a physical origin. Patients with pain who receive secondary gain may also have a very painful condition and hurt as much as they say they do. Secondary gain is defined as any practical or emotional advantages that result from having pain, especially financial compensation and preferential treatment. This patient has pain but uses it to his or her advantage.

Since pain is subjective and cannot be proved or disproved, health care professionals must deal with the fact that the patient may lie about pain. While this is probably rare, it certainly may occur. However, by responding positively to all patients' reports of pain the health care professional ensures that all patients with pain will receive care.

Unfortunately, research has shown that nurses do not always accept the patient's report of pain. In one survey, nurses (N = 78) were asked how they identified whether a patient was experiencing pain. Less then 75 per cent reported that they first asked the patient (Dalton, 1989). In another survey, nurses (N = 443) ranked the patient's verbal report of pain as fifth on a list of seven indicators of pain (Jacox, 1979). Current research has also shown that even when a patient reports his or her pain using a pain rating scale, some nurses record a different number in the patient's medical record based on *their* personal opinion of the patient's pain intensity (McCaffery & Ferrell, 1991).

Another factor influencing inadequate pain assessment is the health care professional's need to deal with a symptom that can be measured objectively. A truly objective means of measuring pain intensity does not exist. There is no laboratory report or measurement device for objectively assessing the patient's pain. The only scientific tool for measuring the intensity of pain is the patient's self-report.

ACUTE PAIN MODEL VERSUS ADAPTATION

The observation of behavior and use of vital signs should not be used instead of the patient's self-report (Acute Pain Management Guideline Panel, 1992b). Visible signs, either physiologic or behavioral, cannot be used to verify the existence of pain nor its intensity in the patient who can perform a self-report. The lack of pain expression does not indicate that the patient's pain does not exist! Even with severe pain, the patient may have periods of minimal pain or no signs of pain. Both physiologic and behavioral adaptation occur. The pain may be intense, but the vigor of the patient's responses to it may decrease.

Figure 56–1 provides a comparison of the acute pain model versus adaptation. In the acute pain model, certain signs of pain will occur with the sudden onset of severe pain. Physiologically, the patient may have an increased blood pressure, increased heart rate, increased respiratory rate, dilated pupils, pallor, or profuse perspiration. Behaviorally, the patient may talk incessantly about the pain, cry, moan, have tense skeletal muscles, or rub the painful site. However, the acute pain model exists only for a short time, with physiologic or behavioral responses sometimes lasting only minutes or seconds. In the patient with chronic cancer pain, the health care provider must not be fooled by the lack of objective signs. This "may prompt the inexperienced caregiver to say that the patient does not 'look' like he or she is in pain" (APS, 1992, p. 3).

A survey of 456 nurses revealed that over half the nurses did not know that the patient's report of pain should be recorded in the nursing assessment of pain intensity regardless of the patient's behavior (McCaffery & Ferrell, 1991). They were more willing to accept the pain rating reported by a grimacing patient than from one who was smiling. In a similar study conducted in Australia, nurses (N = 517) were again more willing to accept a report of pain from a grimacing patient than from a smiling patient (McCaffery & Ferrell, 1994). For the smiling patient, approximately half the nurse respondents recorded a lower pain rating than was stated by the patient. Research has also shown that some nurses fail to record the patient's report of severe pain when his or her vital signs are not elevated (McCaffery & Ferrell, 1992).

The adaptation response does not necessarily indicate that the patient's pain has decreased in intensity. The body seeks physiologic equilibrium. Behaviorally the patient also adapts. Behavioral adaptation may occur because the patient senses the value of being a "good patient," wants to avoid being a "sissy," or because the patient is simply exhausted from the pain. Sleep cannot be equated with a lack of pain.

Jacox (1979) interviewed 102 adult patients with various types of acute and chronic pain. Seventy per cent reported that they did not discuss their pain with others or reported ambivalence about their pain. Sixty-six per cent reported that they tried to remain calm and not show their pain. In a survey of 53 patients with chronic cancer pain, laughing was rated as the most effective means for coping with their pain (Fritz, 1988). In a study of 13 patients with advanced cancer, patients reported that behaviors they used to control their pain included sleeping, watching television, or visiting with family and friends (Wilkie, Lovejoy, Dodd, & Tesler, 1988). These studies show that behavior cannot be used instead of self-report as a means of assessing the patient's pain.

KNOWN PHYSICAL CAUSE VERSUS UNKNOWN PHYSICAL CAUSE

The study of pain is a new science. Therefore, it is foolish to expect that the cause of pain will always be identifiable. Yet, it is not unusual to hear a health care professional say, "There's no reason for the patient to hurt," suggesting that they cannot believe the pain until they know the cause of it. They erroneously think, "If there's pain, there's a cause. If there's a cause, we can find it. If we can't find the cause, there's no pain."

When the physical cause of pain is not known, it is tempting to focus on the patient's emotional responses

RESPONSE TO
ACUTE PAIN

OVER TIME, SOMETIMES WITHIN
SECONDS, RESPONSES TO PAIN
CHANGE AND MAY BE DUE TO:

ADAPTATION

(observable signs of
discomfort)

(decrease in observable signs
although pain intensity
unchanged)

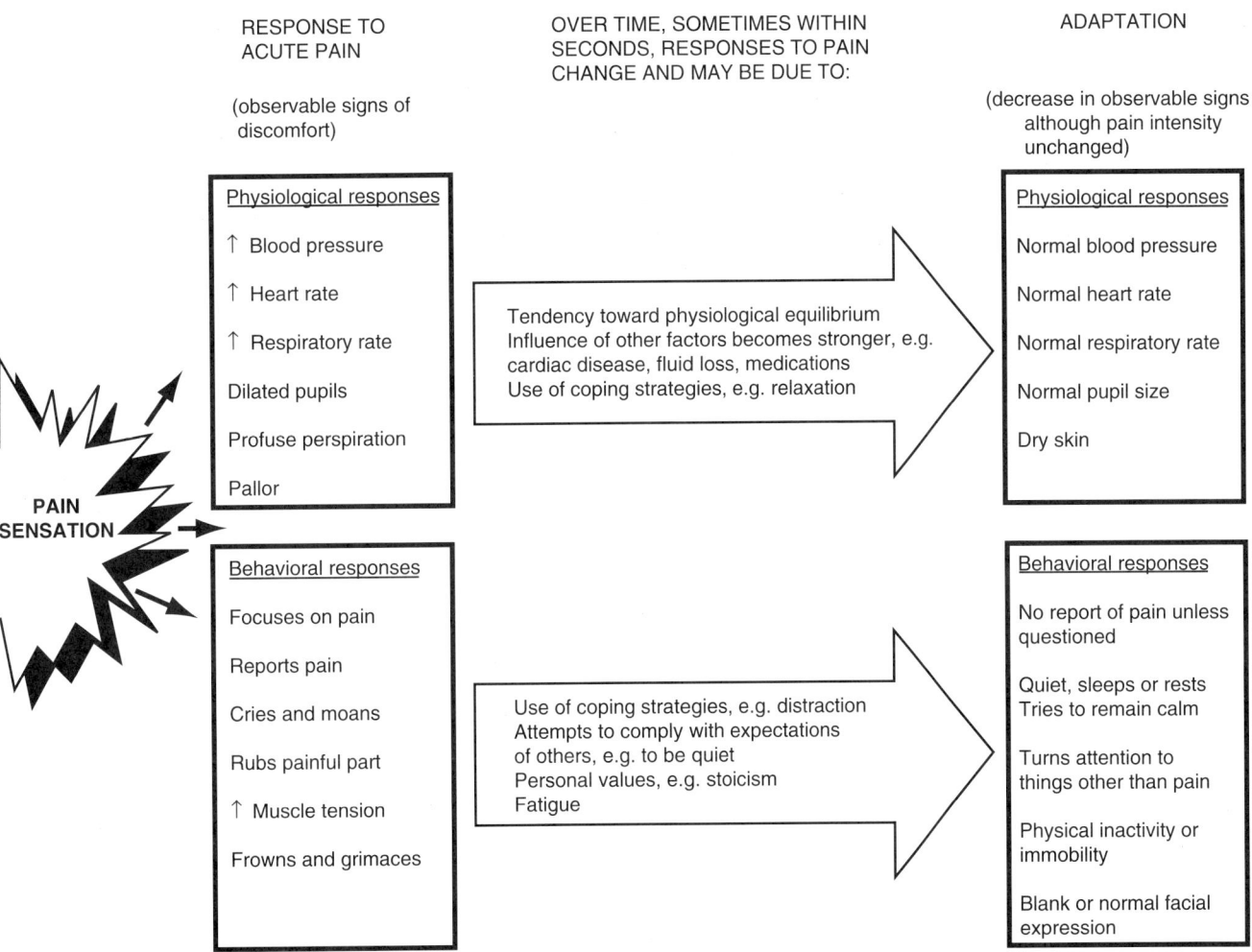

FIGURE 56–1. The acute pain model versus adaptation. (Adapted from Smeltzer, S. C. & Bare, B. G. [1992]. *Brunner & Suddarth's textbook of medical-surgical nursing* [7th ed.], Philadelphia: J. B. Lippincott.)

as the cause of the pain. The clinician may discount the pain and say that the patient is "merely upset," suggesting that pain is a displaced symptom of psychologic disturbance. However, research on whether anxiety or depression cause or increase the intensity of pain is inconclusive (Ahles, Blanchard, & Ruckdeschel, 1983; McGuire, 1987). For example, a study of cancer patients identified that depressed patients did not report more intense pain than did those patients who were not depressed (Cleeland, 1984a). Depression did not alter their reports of pain intensity. However, depression did influence their perception of their quality of life. What we do know is that pain almost always results in some anxiety or depression. Therefore, when a patient reports pain and is also anxious or depressed, the most logical approach is to first assume that pain is causing the emotional responses and attempt to relieve the pain with an analgesic as opposed to assuming that the pain is caused by the anxiety or depression.

Another misconception related to the cause of pain is the belief that treating pain of unknown origin will mask important diagnostic information. However, pain can be assessed and relieved while diagnostic proce-

dures are conducted. The American Pain Society (1992) acknowledges that while establishing a diagnosis is a priority, the symptomatic treatment of the patient's pain should be provided while the workup is proceeding. The APS stresses that a comfortable patient is more likely to be able to cooperate with the diagnostic workup.

Even when the cause of pain is known, health care providers should not become complacent in treating all patients alike who have similar physical causes of pain. Variations in pathology and differences in pain duration and intensity among patients do exist. For example, many health care providers expect that postoperative pain will subside rapidly over the first 3 days and be negligible by the fourth day. However, research does not support this assumption. In a study of 88 patients on a general surgical unit, 31 per cent reported pain that persisted beyond the fourth postoperative day (Melzack, Abbott, Zackon, Mulder, & Davis, 1987). The pain was often related to the patient being older or to complications such as infection. These patients typically received inadequate pain control because less potent analgesics were being given.

PERSONAL VALUES VERSUS PROFESSIONAL RESPONSIBILITY

The personal values and beliefs of health care professionals influence pain assessment and its management. As health care professionals, we engage in the care of patients with a dual frame of reference. As human beings, we have values and preferences that determine how well we like other people. We disapprove of or like certain characteristics or behaviors. We are also better able to relate to or identify with those who are most like ourselves. However, as health care professionals, we are responsible for rendering care to patients without biases.

Vigilance is essential if we wish to render care without biases. Research suggests biases may go into hiding but may adversely affect the care we provide for patients with pain. Do we know when our biases are showing? Apparently, not always. Consider the following current research findings.

The patient's physical appearance may affect care. One study revealed that physicians infer more pain in unattractive patients and those who express pain (e.g., facial expression) than they do in attractive patients and those who do not express pain (Hadjistavropoulos, Ross, & von Baeyer, 1990).

Gender may affect care. Workups by physicians in response to five common complaints, including back pain, headache, and chest pain, were found to be significantly more extensive for men than for women (Armitage, Schneiderman, & Bass, 1979). In a study of cancer patients, inadequate pain management was more likely in females than in males (Cleeland et al., 1994).

Race or culture may also affect care. A survey of University of California at Los Angeles emergency department physicians revealed that Hispanic patients were twice as likely as non-Hispanic whites to receive *no* analgesia (Todd, Samaroo, & Hoffman, 1993). At centers treating predominantly minorities, cancer patients were found to be three times more likely to have inadequate pain management (Cleeland et al., 1994).

Sometimes, we are aware of our biases and try to keep them from adversely affecting our care. For example, one survey asked nurses about assessments and analgesic choices for a patient described as a risk taker, consumer of alcohol, and unemployed and for a patient described as typically middle-class (McCaffery, Ferrell, & O'Neil-Page, 1992). The nurses said that they themselves would provide the same care for both patients, but they believed that their colleagues would treat the patients differently, tending to disbelieve and undertreat the "irresponsible" patient. Nurses revealed that they did not want personal values to interfere with their quality of care, but they needed assistance, for example, permission to say they do not like a certain patient and discussion about how to prevent this from interfering with care.

While it is not uncommon for health care professionals and the lay public as well to judge others by one's own personal values, it is not a professional prerogative to use these same methods when providing care to patients with pain. Because the sensation of pain is subjective, health care professionals may be tempted to rely on personal biases and judgments to determine the truthfulness of a patient's report of pain. However, biases and personal judgments are a disservice to the patient and adversely affect care.

ADDICTION: LABEL VERSUS DIAGNOSIS

The longer a patient is on opioids the more concerned nurses become about addiction (McCaffery & Ferrell, 1994). Unfortunately, nurses do not know what does and what does not happen as the length of time on opioids increases. Patients who take opioids several times daily for more than 1 month develop tolerance and physical dependence, but data suggest that the risk of iatrogenic addiction is rare (APS, 1992). In a prospective study of 11,882 hospitalized medical patients who received at least one opioid, the risk of addiction was reported to be less than 1 per cent (Porter & Jick, 1980). Another study examined the incidence of addiction in over 10,000 hospitalized burn patients cared for in burn facilities across the United States (Perry & Heidrich, 1982). Study results indicated that no patients developed iatrogenic addiction despite long-term use of opioids. Two other studies of over 500 patients on heroin (taken by mouth or intramuscularly) for pain control, some for weeks or months, found that no patients developed iatrogenic addiction (Twycross, 1974; Twycross & Wald, 1976). These data negate the erroneous information provided by the lay media and in many professional textbooks (Ferrell, McCaffery, & Rhiner, 1992).

The term "addict" has negative connotations and should be used only when there is strong evidence of addictive behaviors (APS, 1992). Therefore, it is important to be knowledgeable about the terms "opioid addiction," "physical dependence," and "tolerance" (Table 56–2). Each of these conditions is a separate entity with a different treatment. Any one may occur alone, any two may occur together, or all three can occur at the same time. It is highly unlikely that addiction/psychologic dependence will develop in patients without drug abuse histories who use opioids for acute pain (Porter & Jick, 1980). Vallerand provides an excellent discussion about the similarities and differences between street addicts and patients with pain (Vallerand, 1994).

If the patient is diagnosed as chemically dependent, the patient is entitled to the same quality of pain management as any other patient. Many health care professionals have the misconception that individuals with a chemical dependence are irresponsible and weak-willed and therefore should not receive opioids for pain relief. This unethical position infers that the health care provider *can* provide pain relief and has the resources to do so but *chooses not to* because the care provider does not believe that the patient deserves pain relief. Chemical dependency is a serious health care problem,

TABLE 56–2. *Definitions of Terminology*

TERM	UNDERLYING MECHANISM	TREATMENT
Opioid addiction: Psychologic dependence. Pattern of compulsive drug use characterized by continued craving for an opioid and the need to use the opioid for effects other than pain relief (or for a nonmedical reason).	Psychologic, biochemical, social.	Ongoing rehabilitation program to cope with tendency to relapse due to psychologic dependence.
Physical dependence: Occurrence of withdrawal symptoms when the opioid is suddenly stopped or an antagonist is given.	Physiologic changes related to repeated administration.	Increase dose or decrease dose interval; more drug required.
Tolerance: Decrease in one or more effects of the opioid such as decreased analgesia, sedation, or respiratory depression.	Physiologic changes related to repeated administration.	Gradual withdrawal of the opioid, e.g., decrease by 10% per day over 10-day period.

and the patient with an addiction deserves pain assessment and pain relief.

PAIN RELIEF FROM PLACEBOS

A placebo is defined as any medical treatment or nursing care that produces an effect in a patient because of its implicit or explicit intent and not because of its specific nature or therapeutic properties (McCaffery & Beebe, 1989). The American Pain Society (1992) and the AHCPR (Management of Cancer Pain Guideline Panel, 1994a) cancer pain guideline emphatically state that there is no justifiable use for placebos in the assessment or treatment of pain. Unfortunately, placebos are still used occasionally in a deceptive manner, and health care professionals may be tempted to discredit a patient's report of pain if the patient reports pain relief after receiving a placebo. However, there is no evidence in the literature to justify the use of placebos to determine the presence or absence of pain or to determine whether pain has a physical or psychogenic origin.

Research has shown that a minimum of one third of all people with a known physical cause for pain such as abdominal surgery or cancer-related pain report adequate pain relief from a placebo (Goodwin, Goodwin, & Vogel, 1979; Lasagna, Mosteller, von Felsinger, & Beecher, 1954). Although the exact mechanism underlying the placebo effect is not understood, it does have a physiologic basis, possibly involving an increase in endorphins (Grevert, Albert, & Goldstein, 1983; Levine, Gordon, & Fields, 1978).

The nurse who receives a physician's order to give a placebo must be aware of the ethical and legal issues related to carrying out the order. Giving a placebo usually requires that the nurse lie to the patient about what medication he or she is receiving. This can destroy the nurse-patient relationship and foster a venue for distrust. Fox (1994) discusses the steps she took to initiate policy change related to placebo use within her institution. To support her case, Fox contacted nurses and attorneys throughout the United States and used the American Nurses Association's *Code for Nurses* (1985), the American Medical Association's opinions on "Informed Consent" and "Patient Information," (Fox, 1994) and the JCAHO's standards of care (1994).

NURSING ASSESSMENT OF PAIN

Pain is recognized as a nursing diagnosis. The care of patients with pain is best accomplished by a team approach. Thus, the nursing assessment is combined with assessments by other members of the health care team, such as the physician. This forms the basis for an overall plan of care for the patient.

Acceptance of the patient's report of pain and acknowledgement of the influence pain can have on the patient and family are critical to performing a thorough pain assessment. Knowledge about the basic anatomy and physiology causing pain as well as an awareness of common pain syndromes, multiple sites of pain, and profiles of patients with cancer-related pain is a necessary foundation for conducting the nursing assessment for the patient with pain. However, it is important to remember that pain not only reflects tissue damage but is also a complex state influenced by other factors such as age, sex, culture, environment, and psychologic variables. These factors must all be considered when conducting a thorough pain assessment.

A variety of tools are available for assessing pain. While there is unquestionable value in a thorough, comprehensive, detailed assessment of pain, there is also the reality that time and resources limit what can be achieved in most clinical areas. For practical reasons, this chapter offers assessment tools that are currently recognized as valuable but are also reasonably quick and easy to use. These tools may lack the detail desired in certain situations, and the clinician is encouraged to refer to the AHCPR cancer pain guideline (Management of Cancer Pain Guideline Panel, 1994a) and other resources to revise and to add to these tools as necessary to benefit individual patients.

The following tools are presented.

- Initial pain assessment tools, for example, "Brief Pain Inventory (Short Form)" and "Barriers Questionnaire."
- Pain rating scales currently used in clinical practice, for example, simple descriptive and numeric scales and faces.
- Tools for ongoing assessment, for example, pain control record and daily pain diary.

INITIAL PAIN ASSESSMENT TOOLS

An initial pain assessment tool that has been used extensively in the care of the patient with chronic cancer pain is the "Brief Pain Inventory (Short Form)" (Figure 56–2) developed at the University of Wisconsin-Madison. This tool provides brief information related to the past and current status of pain as well as its impact on quality of life. The tool may be duplicated for use in the clinical setting.

Following are the components of the tool.

- Questions 1 and 2 ask the patients whether they have pain other than "everyday types of pain" and to identify on a body chart the location of their pain including where it hurts.
- Questions 3 to 6 ask the patients to identify the intensity of their pain at several points in time—the *worst pain* and the *least pain* in the past 24 hours, the *average* pain, and the pain *right now*. This information provides the health care provider with an overall picture of the patient's pain intensity. Clinical experience has shown that often patients do not report their pain because they do not have pain at the time they are asked. These four questions prevent this situation from occurring.
- Questions 7 and 8 elicit information about the treatments or medications that the patients are using for their pain and how much relief the patients have received in the past 24 hours using these treatments or medications.
- Question 9 asks the patients to identify how their pain in the past 24 hours has interfered with various aspects of their functional status and quality of life including general activity, mood, walking ability, normal work (outside the home and housework), relations with others, sleep, and enjoyment of life.

The initial assessment should be implemented with each new report of pain and should be used for each type of pain identified by the patient. Assessment is ongoing and should include an assessment of the pain relief plan. On a regular basis, it is important that nurses and other health care professionals ask patients whether they have pain. The patients may not tell the health care provider that they (the patients) are having pain unless they are asked. The nurse may also find it necessary to reassure patients who are reluctant to report their pain that there are many safe and effective ways to relieve pain. The patients' report of pain is the primary source of assessment.

A companion to the "Brief Pain Inventory (Short Form)" is a nine-item "Barriers Questionnaire" (Table 56–3). Using a 6-point scale with 0 (do not agree at all) to 5 (agree very much), respondents are asked to rate the extent to which they agree with each item. The questionnaire can be administered to both patients and family members. It identifies concerns that patients and their family members have that may contribute to the patient's and family's hesitancy to report pain or to follow the pain treatment plan (Ward et al., 1993). Research using the "Barriers Questionnaire" has shown that high levels of concern are related to high levels of pain. Patients may be reluctant to report their pain for several reasons including concerns about addiction (top of the list); increased pain means increased disease; side effects such as constipation and nausea; fear of injections; tolerance—wanting to save medicine until it is really needed; distracting the physician from curing the disease; "good" patients avoid talking about their pain; and pain is inevitable (Ward & Gatwood, 1994; Ward et al., 1993). Nurses can assist these patients in reducing their concerns about reporting pain and using analgesics by initiating discussion about their concerns *before* pain occurs. It may be helpful to explain addiction, tolerance, and physical dependence and discuss the management of side effects. The authors have found it helpful to include the family in these discussions.

PAIN RATING SCALES

For patients who are able to provide a self-report of pain, the following instruments are most commonly used. (Table 56–4).

- Simple descriptive or word descriptor scales, for example, none, mild, moderate, severe, very severe.
- 0–10 or 0–5 or 0–100 Numeric Pain Intensity Scales.
- Faces.

In choosing an assessment tool, it is important to select one that can be understood and used effectively by the patient. It is often helpful to combine numbers and word descriptors. The same pain rating scale should be used consistently, and the type of tool used should be recorded in the patient's medical record. The nurse and physician should teach the patient and family members to use pain rating scales both in the inpatient and outpatient settings to promote continuity of the pain management plan. The AHCPR has developed a patient education pamphlet that can be used for this purpose (Acute Pain Management Guideline Panel, 1992a; Management of Cancer Pain Guideline Panel, 1994b). Table 56–5 provides information that should be taught to the patient and his or her family about pain assessment and using a pain rating scale.

It is important that pain rating scales be used to set a *goal* for pain relief. The nurse should identify the patient's goal for pain control (as scores on a pain scale) and document it in the medical record (Management of Cancer Pain Guideline Panel, 1994a).

In a recent study conducted at the University of Wisconsin Hospitals and Clinics, 217 adults were surveyed (Ward & Gordon, 1994). Eighty-four per cent reported that the importance of pain management was

Brief Pain Inventory (Short Form)

Study ID# _____   Hospital# _____

Do not write above this line

Date ____/____/____   Time: _____

Name: _____ _____ _____
           Last   First   Middle Initial

1) Throughout our lives, most of us have had pain from time to time (such as minor headaches, sprains, and toothaches). Have you had pain other than these everyday kinds of pain today?   1. Yes   2. No

2) On the diagram, shade in the areas where you feel pain. Put an X on the area that hurts the most.

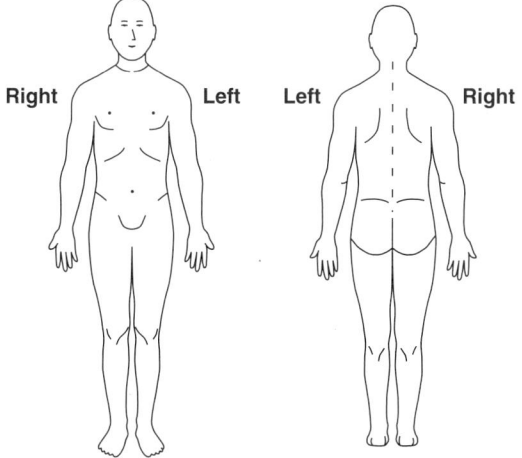

Right   Left   Left   Right

3) Please rate your pain by circling the one number that best describes your pain at its **worst** in the past 24 hours.
   0   1   2   3   4   5   6   7   8   9   10
   No   Pain as bad as
   pain   you can imagine

4) Please rate your pain by circling the one number that best describes your pain at its **least** in the past 24 hours.
   0   1   2   3   4   5   6   7   8   9   10
   No   Pain as bad as
   pain   you can imagine

5) Please rate your pain by circling the one number that best describes your pain on the **average**.
   0   1   2   3   4   5   6   7   8   9   10
   No   Pain as bad as
   pain   you can imagine

6) Please rate your pain by circling the one number that tells how much pain you have **right now.**
   0   1   2   3   4   5   6   7   8   9   10
   No   Pain as bad as
   pain   you can imagine

7) What treatments or medications are you receiving for your pain?

   _____

8) In the past 24 hours, how much relief have pain treatments or medications provided? Please circle the one percentage that most shows how much relief you have received.
   0% 10% 20% 30% 40% 50% 60% 70% 80% 90% 100%
   No   Complete
   relief   relief

9) Circle the one number that describes how, during the past 24 hours, **pain has interfered** with your:

   A. General activity
   0   1   2   3   4   5   6   7   8   9   10
   Does not   Completely
   interfere   interferes

   B. Mood
   0   1   2   3   4   5   6   7   8   9   10
   Does not   Completely
   interfere   interferes

   C. Walking ability
   0   1   2   3   4   5   6   7   8   9   10
   Does not   Completely
   interfere   interferes

   D. Normal work (includes both work outside the home and housework)
   0   1   2   3   4   5   6   7   8   9   10
   Does not   Completely
   interfere   interferes

   E. Relations with other people
   0   1   2   3   4   5   6   7   8   9   10
   Does not   Completely
   interfere   interferes

   F. Sleep
   0   1   2   3   4   5   6   7   8   9   10
   Does not   Completely
   interfere   interferes

   G. Enjoyment of life
   0   1   2   3   4   5   6   7   8   9   10
   Does not   Completely
   interfere   interferes

FIGURE 56–2. The initial pain assessment using the brief pain inventory. (From Pain Research Group. Department of Neurology, University of Wisconsin-Madison.)

discussed with them, and 90 to 95 per cent of them were satisfied with how their pain was managed.

However, research has identified that there is little relationship between pain severity and patient satisfaction with pain relief measures (Miaskowski, Nichols, Brody, & Synold, 1994; Ward & Gordon, 1994). Of

interest was that even patients with severe pain were very satisfied with the pain management they received from their health care providers. Satisfaction was related to whether their care providers had communicated to them that pain management was a high priority in the delivery of care.

TABLE 56–3. *Barriers Questionnaire*

We are interested in learning more about what you think about treatment of pain. Some of the questions may seem similar to other ones, but please answer all of the questions. For each of the items below, please *circle the number* (0, 1, 2, 3, 4, or 5) that comes closest to *how much you agree* with that item.

1. Pain medicine cannot really control pain.
  0   1   2   3   4   5
  Do not agree at all   Agree very much
2. People get addicted to pain medicine easily.
  0   1   2   3   4   5
  Do not agree at all   Agree very much
3. Good patients avoid talking about pain.
  0   1   2   3   4   5
  Do not agree at all   Agree very much
4. I do not want to bother the nurse—she is busy with other patients.
  0   1   2   3   4   5
  Do not agree at all   Agree very much
5. It is easier to put up with pain than with the side effects that come from pain medicine.
  0   1   2   3   4   5
  Do not agree at all   Agree very much
6. Pain medicine should be saved in case the pain gets worse.
  0   1   2   3   4   5
  Do not agree at all   Agree very much
7. Pain builds character—it is good for you.
  0   1   2   3   4   5
  Do not agree at all   Agree very much
8. Complaining about pain will distract my doctor from his primary responsibility—curing my illness.
  0   1   2   3   4   5
  Do not agree at all   Agree very much
9. Patients should expect to have pain; it is part of almost every hospitalization.
  0   1   2   3   4   5
  Do not agree at all   Agree very much

(From Gordon, D. B., & Ward, S. E. [1995]. Correcting patient misconceptions about pain. *American Journal of Nursing, 95*[7], 43–45.)

The nurse should recognize that patients do not know how much pain relief can be expected. Unless they are told otherwise, patients have low expectations about pain relief. If they do not believe nurses and physicians are able to provide pain relief, then they are satisfied when told that pain relief is important, whether pain relief is actually achieved. Patients who are reluctant to report pain should be taught that there are many safe and effective ways to relieve pain (Management of Cancer Pain Guideline Panel, 1994a).

TOOLS FOR ONGOING ASSESSMENT

The nurse should encourage the patient and family to keep a record of pain ratings to evaluate the methods used for pain relief. Pain ratings are recorded for the patient at rest and with activity. Pain ratings are compared with the pain rating goal that is satisfactory for the patient. If the pain ratings are above the goal, interventions are indicated.

Tools that may be used by the patient at home include a pain control record (Fig. 56–3) or a daily pain diary (Fig. 56–4). These tools can be used to provide information that can be shared with the physician and nurse during follow-up visits. These tools not only assist the physician and nurse in evaluating the patient's pain and the effectiveness of the pain relief measures used but also empower the patient and provide the patient with information and documentation of the progress or lack of progress that is being made with the pain relief plan. Patients should also be taught to report changes in their pain so that reassessment and changes in treatment can be implemented.

In the inpatient setting, a pain flow sheet can be used. In research on cancer patients using a pain flow sheet similar to Figure 56–5, construct validity was supported by results that indicated that both pain intensity and sedation level were significantly less in patients with whom the flow sheet was used compared with those patients in whom no flow sheet was used (Faries, Mills, Goldsmith, Phillips, & Orr, 1991; McMillan, Williams, Chatfield, & Camp, 1988).

In the patient who is opioid-naive it is necessary to monitor sedation level (see sedation scale at the bottom of Fig. 56–5) and to record vital signs. However, this is usually not necessary with the opioid-tolerant patient (Pasero & McCaffery, 1994). Opioid-induced respiratory depression is uncommon in patients receiving long-term opioid therapy, because they develop tolerance to the respiratory depressant effects of these agents (Management of Cancer Pain Guideline Panel, 1994a). Far more common is the subacute overdose that manifests slowly (hours to days) as somnolence and respiratory depression. The method for managing the subacute overdose is to withhold one or two doses, then reduce the previous dose by 25 per cent (Management of Cancer Pain Guideline Panel, 1994a).

SPECIAL CHALLENGES IN PAIN ASSESSMENT

There are several groups at risk for underassessment and undertreatment of their pain. These groups include nonverbal patients, patients with impaired communication, patients who deny pain, and the elderly. Other adults at risk include those who have cognitive impairment, severe emotional disturbance, dementia, and delirium; who are psychotic or frail; the oldest-old (>85 years); those who speak a different language and whose educational or cultural background is significantly different from that of the health care team (Acute Pain Management Guideline Panel, 1992d). Other patients include those who have an altered level of consciousness (the lack of consciousness does not necessarily mean lack of pain); who have an endotracheal tube; or who have received a neuromuscular blocking agent such as pancuronium (which does not alter sensitivity to pain). Health care professionals should have a high degree of suspicion for pain in these individuals.

TABLE 56–4. *Examples of Pain Rating Scales*

I. Numeric Pain Intensity Scale

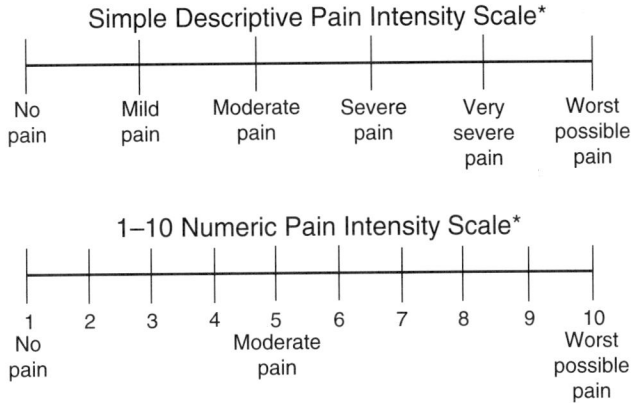

Simple Descriptive Pain Intensity Scale*

| No pain | Mild pain | Moderate pain | Severe pain | Very severe pain | Worst possible pain |

1–10 Numeric Pain Intensity Scale*

1 No pain   2   3   4   5 Moderate pain   6   7   8   9   10 Worst possible pain

*If used as a graphic rating scale, a 10-cm baseline is recommended

The numeric pain intensity scale can be verbally explained to the patient instead of actually showing the patient the scale. It should be explained in the following way.
• "On a scale of 0 to 10 with 0 = no pain and 10 = the worst possible pain, how would you rate your pain?"

II. Faces Rating Scale

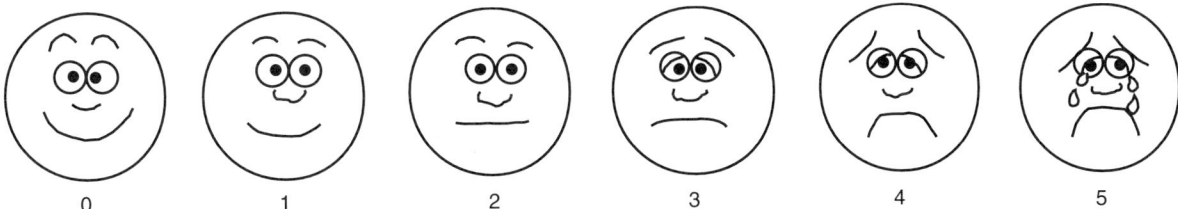

0   1   2   3   4   5

• Recommended for persons aged 3 years and older.
• Explain to the person that each face is a person who feels happy because he has no pain (hurt or whatever word the person uses) or feels sad because he has some or a lot of pain.
• Point to an appropriate face and state, "This face . . ."
   • Face 0—"is very happy because he doesn't hurt at all."
   • Face 1—"hurts just a little bit."
   • Face 2—"hurts a little more."
   • Face 3—"hurts even more."
   • Face 4—"hurts a whole lot."
   • Face 5—"hurts as much as you can imagine, although you don't have to be crying, to feel this bad."
• Ask the person to choose the face that best describes how he is feeling. Be specific about which pain (e.g., "shot" or incision) and what time (e.g., now? earlier today?).

(Part I from Acute Pain Management Guideline Panel. [1992c]. *Acute pain management in infants, children, and adolescents: Operative and medical procedures. Quick reference guide for clinicians.* ACHPR Pub. No. 92-0020. Rockville, MD: ACHPR, Public Health Service, U.S. Department of Health and Human Services. Part II from Wong, D. L. [1995]. *Whaley & Wong's nursing care of infants and children* (5th ed., p. 1085). St. Louis: C. V. Mosby.)

In a sample of 24 ICU patients, 63 per cent recalled moderate to severe pain (Puntillo, 1990). Those who could not talk (80 per cent had an endotracheal tube) described numerous behaviors they used in an attempt to communicate their pain such as signaling with their eyes and moving legs up and down.

When the nurse encounters patients who are unable or unwilling to report pain, the following clues may be used to alert the health care team to the possibility that the patient has pain.

• Presence of pathology known to cause pain, for example, bone metastases.
• Reports by family/friends.

• Patient behaviors, for example, moaning, frowning, or grimacing.
• Changes in vital signs must be used with extreme care because "they are neither sensitive nor specific as indicators of pain" (Acute Pain Management Guideline Panel, 1992c, p. 7).

When the patient's self-report of pain is available, it is always the mainstay of assessment. However, when patient's behaviors or known pathology suggests the existence of pain but the patient denies pain or refuses analgesics, it is important for the nurse to explore the possible reasons for his or her refusal. Information from the "Barriers Questionnaire" is often helpful. In

TABLE 56–5. *Use of Pain Rating Scales: Patient/Family Education*

- Explain the primary purposes of a pain rating scale. Show the patient/family the scale.
  Provides quick, consistent communication between patient and caregivers including the nurse and physician. Emphasize that the patient must volunteer information. Although caregivers will ask about the pain regularly, they do not know when the patient has pain.
  Helps establish pain relief satisfactory to the patient.
- Explain the specific pain rating scale, e.g., 0 to 10 with 0 = no pain and 10 = the worst possible pain. When a numeric scale is used, verify that the patient can count up to the number used. If the patient does not understand whatever scale is "standard" in that clinical setting, select another scale.
- Discuss the definition of the word "pain," e.g., that pain is a fairly localized bodily or physical discomfort that may have various characteristics such as aching, pulling, tightness, burning, or pricking; and that pain may be mild to severe. If the patient, e.g., child, prefers some other term such as "hurt" use that word.
- To verify that the patient understands how the word pain (or other word preferred by the patient) is used, ask the patient to give examples of pain he or she has experienced. If the patient is already in pain, use the present situation as the example.
- Ask the patient to practice using the pain rating scale by rating his or her present painful experiences or those he or she remembers.
- Ask the patient what pain rating would be acceptable or satisfactory to him or her. This helps set a realistic, initial goal. Zero pain is not always possible. Once the initial goal is achieved, the possibility of better pain relief can be considered. Emphasize to the patient that satisfactory pain relief is a level of pain that is not distressing and one that enables the patient to sleep, eat, and perform other required or desired physical activities.

the patient who deliberately denies pain, possible reasons for denying pain may be fear of injections, fear of addiction, desire to protect his or her family, or lack of trust. Some patients inadvertently deny pain because they do not understand the term "pain"—it may be helpful to ask whether the patient is experiencing any achiness, burning, or soreness. The patient may lose the ability to identify the existence of pain—the patient may have been "in pain too long to know." In some instances, the patient really thinks others know about the pain without the patient having to tell them.

When self-report is not available, the nurse must use the following hierarchy of assessment measures. Assessment strategies in noncommunicating patients include the following.

- Ask the patient's family or other close caregiver whether they think the patient has pain and why. A pain rating guess by a family member is useful.
- Medicate the noncommunicating patient who undergoes a procedure that would be painful for others.
- Systematically observe (using a flow sheet) possible pain and comfort behaviors related to vocalizations, facial expressions, body movements, behavior/activity changes, or automatic responses.
- Use a trial dose of analgesic, observing behavior before and after.
- For intubated ICU patients, offer writing materials, use a pain rating scale, and supplement morphine with nondrug pain relief measures (Puntillo, 1990).
- Continue opioids and other analgesics in the terminally ill patient who loses consciousness to ensure that death is as painless and peaceful as possible.

It is often necessary to reassure nurses caring for the terminally ill, unconscious patient that continuation of opioids is a logical continuation of the goal to keep the patient comfortable while he or she is alive and that this is not euthanasia. Even when the patient no longer responds to painful stimuli, he or she may still feel pain. A recent report of a patient who became comatose illustrates this point (Stephens, 1994). A ter-

minally ill patient with metastatic cancer and severe pain, especially with positioning, required "large" doses of intravenous morphine every 3 hours. The patient gradually became unresponsive to voices and did not grimace with positioning. The morphine was discontinued. Three days later, the patient awakened and reported hearing voices during her coma. She also reported suffering such intense pain that she prayed that the tumor would sever her nerves.

Continuing opioids when the dying patient who has had pain is no longer able to communicate has long been recommended. In 1985, Levy said, "When patients are no longer able to verbally communicate whether they are in pain or not, the best approach is to assume that their cancer is still painful and to continue them on their regular medications . . . a therapeutic narcotic level should be maintained . . . continued narcotics simply assure that the death will be as peaceful and painless as possible" (pp. 397–398). The intent is to bring comfort, not to hasten death.

The American Nurses Association assures nurses that continuation of opioids is ethical. The ANA's "Position Statement on Promotion of Comfort and Relief of Pain in Dying Patients" (1991) states that, "Nurses should not hesitate to use full and effective doses of pain medication for the proper management of pain in the dying patient. The increasing titration of medication to achieve adequate symptom control, even at the expense of life, thus, hastening death secondarily, is ethically justified" (p. 1).

Further, as discussed earlier in this chapter, patients on long-term opioid therapy become opioid-tolerant so that respiratory depression is very unlikely (APS, 1992). The clinician's fears that continuing opioids will contribute to the patient's death are usually unfounded. A study by Grond, Zech, Schug, Lynch, & Lehmann (1991) illustrates this point. Four hundred one terminally ill patients with cancer-related pain were treated according to the WHO guidelines and followed until death. Analgesics were the mainstay of therapy. The last pain rating before death revealed that only 3 per

Pain Control Record

You can use a chart like this to rate your pain and to keep a record of how well the medicine is working. Write the information in the chart. Use the pain intensity scale to rate your pain before and after you take the medicine.

Pain Intensity Scale

| 0 | 1 | 2 | 3 | 4 | 5 | 6 | 7 | 8 | 9 | 10 |

| No pain | | | | Medium pain | | | | | Worst pain |

Date	Time	Pain intensity scale rating.	Medicine I took.	Pain intensity scale rating 1 hour after taking the medicine.	What I was doing when I felt the pain.
1/3/94	2:35	6	*two aspirin tablets*	3	*Sitting at my desk and reading.*

The authors strongly suggest that the patient's goal for pain relief be documented on the form.

FIGURE 56–3. Pain control record. (From Management of Cancer Pain Guideline Panel. [1994]. *Clinical practice guideline: Patient guide. Managing cancer pain* (pp. 18–19). AHCPR Pub. No. 94-0593. Rockville, MD: Agency for Health Care Policy and Research, Public Health Service, U.S. Department of Health and Human Services.)

cent of the patients experienced severe or very severe pain. The highest recorded doses were 540 mg/day parenterally. None of the patients demonstrated signs of respiratory depression.

According to the National Center of Health Statistics, in the United States by the year 2020, it is estimated that individuals aged 65 years or older will total approximately 51 million (or 17 per cent of the total U.S. population) (Havlik & Suzman, 1987). Pain is a significant problem and a common symptom associated with many disorders experienced by the elderly. Although pain is often considered an expected outcome

of growing old (Ferrell, Ferrell, & Osterweil, 1990; Forman & Stratton, 1991), it is not an inevitable part of aging. Thus, its presence necessitates assessment, diagnosis, and intervention similar to the pain experienced in any other age group.

A misconception that affects pain assessment in the elderly is that pain perception or sensitivity to pain decreases with age. Research has shown that older postoperative patients have less analgesic medication prescribed and administered (Faherty & Grier, 1984). In a recent study of 56 men 60 years of age and older undergoing major elective surgery, nurses administered

Daily Pain Diary

Name _____   Date _____

Pain rating scale used _____   Pain rating goal satisfactory to patient ____

Time	Pain rating scale	Medication type & amount taken	Other pain relief measures tried or anything that influences your pain	Major activity being done: lying sitting standing/walking
12 MIDNIGHT				
1 AM				
2				
3				
4				
5				
6				
7				
8				
9				
10				
11				
noon 12				
1				
2				
3				
4				
5				
6				
7				
8				
9				
10				
11				

Comments: _____

_____

_____

FIGURE 56–4. Daily pain diary. (From McCaffery, M., & Beebe, A. [1989]. Pain assessment. *Pain: Clinical manual for nursing practice.* St. Louis, MO: C. V. Mosby.)

Patient _____   Date _____

*Pain rating scale used _____   Pain rating satisfactory to patient: _____

Purpose: To evaluate the safety and effectiveness of the analgesic(s).

Analgesic(s) prescribed: _____   _____-

Time	Pain rating	Analgesic	R	P	BP	Level of Seda-tion**	Other†	Plan & comments

* Pain rating scale: A number of different scales may be used. Indicate which scale is used and use the same one each time. Example: 0 to 10 (0 = no pain, 10 = worst possible pain).

**Example of sedation scale: S = sleep; 1 = awake & alert; 2 = occasionally drowsy, easy to arouse; 3 = frequently drowsy, arousable, drifts off to sleep during conversation; 4 = somnolent, minimal or no response to stimuli. If opioid induced, at level 3 decrease or discontinue opioid; at level 4, discontinue opioid and consider naloxone.

† Possibilities for other columns: bowel function, physical activities, nausea/vomiting, other pain relief measures. Identify side effects of greatest concern to patient, family, physician, nurses.

FIGURE 56–5. Pain flow sheet. (Adapted from McCaffery, M., & Beebe, A. [1989]. *Pain: Clinical manual for nursing practice* St. Louis, MO: C. V. Mosby.)

about one fourth of what the patients could receive on the first postoperative day, and 16 patients received no parenteral postoperative medication (Short, Burnett, Egbert, & Parks, 1990). In another study assessing pain in elderly postoperative patients, the researchers found that mental status diminished after surgery (Duggleby & Lander, 1994). A major predictor of mental status decline was found to be pain and not analgesic intake. The researchers also identified that fatigue was often reported by study subjects and may have played a role in mental status assessment.

Currently, pain assessment tools specifically developed for use in the elderly are lacking. Therefore, the elderly patient with pain requires special consideration in performing a pain assessment. Physiologic, psychologic, and cultural changes that occur with aging may influence the patient's report of pain (Fordyce, 1978). The elderly may exhibit hearing loss or visual impairment that can complicate pain assessment. Therefore, it is important to ensure that the patient uses whatever aids (e.g., eye glasses or hearing aid) he or she requires for seeing or hearing. For the older adult, the nurse should also consider using larger assessment tools with larger lettering.

Some older adults may not use the word "pain," so their pain may go unreported and therefore, untreated. The nurse should use other terms when assessing the elderly patient's pain such as "discomfort," "achiness," "soreness," "hurt," "pressure," or "burning." The elderly patient may not report mild to moderate pain in an effort to be stoic or in relation to their pioneer spirit, exposure to the prohibition, and tendency to be a passive recipient of health care. Older adults may underreport their pain because of depression or a feeling of unworthiness or they may think that their health care providers *know* they have pain, or that the pain cannot be relieved. Thus, the nurse must be especially careful to ask elderly patients if they have pain.

SUMMARY

Pain assessment is an important component of providing care to the patient with cancer. It is the foundation for the appropriate and effective management of the patient's report of pain. Pain assessment is carried out by all members of the health care team. Many pain assessment tools are easily and quickly administered. The nurse plays an important role in providing comfort for the cancer patient with pain.

REFERENCES

Acute Pain Management Guideline Panel. (1992a). *Acute pain management: A patient's guide.* AHCPR Pub. No. 92-0019. Rockville, MD: Agency for Health Care Policy and Research, Public Health Service, U.S. Department of Health and Human Services.

Acute Pain Management Guideline Panel. (1992b). *Acute pain management in adults: Operative procedures. Quick reference guide for clinicians.* AHCPR Pub. No. 92-0019. Rockville, MD: Agency for Health Care Policy and Research, Public Health Service, U.S. Department of Health and Human Services.

Acute Pain Management Guideline Panel. (1992c). *Acute pain management in infants, children, and adolescents: Operative and medical procedures. Quick reference guide for clinicians.* AHCPR Pub. No. 92-0020. Rockville, MD: Agency for Health Care Policy and Research, Public Health Service, U.S. Department of Health and Human Services.

Acute Pain Management Guideline Panel. (1992d). *Acute pain management: Operative or medical procedures and trauma. Clinical practice guideline.* AHCPR Pub. No. 92-0032. Rockville, MD: Agency for Health Care Policy and Research, Public Health Service, U.S. Department of Health and Human Services.

Ahles, T. A., Blanchard, E. B., & Ruckdeschel, J. C. (1983). The multidimensional nature of cancer-related pain. *Pain, 17,* 277–288.

American Cancer Society Professors of Clinical Oncology. (1993). *Cancer curriculum guidelines for medical students.* Atlanta: American Cancer Society.

American Nurses' Association. (1985). *Code for nurses with interpretive statements.* Kansas City, MO: American Nurses' Association.

American Nurses' Association. (1991). Position statement on promotion of comfort and relief of pain in dying patients. Washington, DC: American Nurses' Association.

American Pain Society. (1992). *Principles of analgesic use in the treatment of acute pain and cancer pain.* (3rd ed.). Skokie, IL: American Pain Society.

American Society of Clinical Oncology Ad Hoc Committee on Cancer Pain. (1992). Cancer pain assessment and treatment curriculum guidelines. *Journal of Clinical Oncology, 10*(12), 1976–1982.

Armitage, K. J, Schneiderman, L. J., & Bass, R. A. (1979). Response of physicians to medical complaints in men and women. *Journal of the American Medical Association, 241*(20), 2186–2187.

Bonica, J. J., Ventafridda, V., & Twycross, R. G. (1990). Cancer pain. In J. J. Bonica (Ed.), *The management of cancer pain.* (pp. 400–460). Philadelphia: Lea & Febiger.

California Board of Registered Nurses. (1994). Curriculum guidelines for pain management. Sacramento, CA: Author.

Canadian Cancer Society. (1991). *Report to Cancer 2000 Task Force by expert panel on palliative care.* Toronto: Canadian Cancer Society.

Cleeland, C. (1991). Research in cancer pain: What we know and what we need to know. *Cancer, 67,* 823–827.

Cleeland, C. S. (1984). The impact of pain on the patient with cancer. *Cancer, 54,* 2635–2641.

Cleeland, C. S., Gonin, R., Hatfield, A. K., Edmonson, J. H., Blum, R. H., Stewart, J. A., & Pandya, K. J. (1994). Pain and its treatment in outpatients with metastatic cancer. *New England Journal of Medicine, 330,* 592–596.

Coyle, N., Adelhardt, J., Foley, K. M., & Portenoy, R. K. (1990). Character of terminal illness in the advanced cancer patient: Pain and other symptoms during the last four weeks of life. *Journal of Pain and Symptom Management, 5,* 83–93.

Dalton, J. (1989). Nurses' perceptions of their pain assessment skills, pain management practices, and attitudes toward pain. *Oncology Nursing Forum, 16,* 225–231.

Daut, R. L., & Cleeland, C. S. (1982). The prevalence and severity of pain in cancer. *Cancer, 50*(9), 1913–1918.

Donovan, M., Dillon, P., & McGuire, L. (1987). Incidence and characteristics of pain in a sample of medical-surgical inpatients. *Pain, 30*(1), 69–78.

Duggleby, W., & Lander, J. (1994). Cognitive status and postoperative pain: Older adults. *Journal of Pain and Symptom Management, 9*(1), 19–27.

Engber, D. (1986). Report on the NIH consensus development conference on pain. *Journal of Pain and Symptom Management, 1,* 165–167.

Faherty, B. S., & Grier, M. R. (1984). Analgesic medication for elderly people post-surgery. *Nursing Research, 33,* 369–372.

Faries, J. E., Mills, D. S., Goldsmith, K. W., Phillips, K. D., & Orr, J. (1991). Systematic pain records and their impact on pain control. *Cancer Nursing, 14*(6), 306–313.

Ferrell, B., McCaffery, M., & Rhiner, M. (1992). Pain and addiction: An urgent need for change in the nursing curriculum. *Journal of Pain and Symptom Management, 7*(2), 48–55.

Ferrell, B. A., Ferrell, B. R., & Osterweil, D. (1990). Pain in the nursing home. *Journal of the American Geriatrics Society, 38*(4), 409–414.

Ferrell, B. R., Johnston Taylor, E., Grant, M., Fowler, M., & Corbisiero, R. (1993). Pain management at home: Struggle, comfort, and mission. *Cancer Nursing, 16*(3), 169–178.

Ferrell, B. R., Rhiner, M., Cohen, M. Z., & Grant, M. (1991). Pain as a metaphor for illness. Part I: Impact of cancer pain on the family. *Oncology Nursing Forum, 18*(8), 1303–1309.

Fordyce, W. E. (1978). Evaluating and managing chronic pain. *Geriatrics, 33,* 59–62.

Forman, W. B., & Stratton, M. (1991). Current approaches to chronic pain in older patients. *Geriatrics, 46*(7), 47–52.

Fox, A. E. (1994). Confronting the use of placebos for pain. *American Journal of Nursing, September,* 42–46.

Fritz, D. J. (1988). Noninvasive pain control methods used by cancer outpatients [Abstract]. *Oncology Nursing Forum,* (Suppl.), 108.

Goodwin, J. S,, Goodwin, J. M., & Vogel, A. A. (1979). Knowledge and use of placebos by house officers and nurses. *Annals of Internal Medicine, 91,* 106–110.

Gordon, D. B., & Ward, S. E. (1995). Correcting patient misconceptions about pain. *American Journal of Nursing, 95*(7), 43–45.

Graffam, S. (1990). Pain content in the curriculum: A survey. *Nurse Educator, 15,* 20–23.

Grant, M. M., & Ferrell, B. R. (1992). Is pain adequately controlled in patients with cancer? *Oncology Nurse Bulletin, May,* 9–11.

Grevert, P., Albert, L. H., & Goldstein, A. (1983). Partial antagonism of placebo analgesia by naloxone. *Pain, 16,* 129–143.

Grond, S., Zech, D., Schug, S. A., Lynch, J., & Lehmann, K. A. (1991). Validation of the World Health Organization guidelines for cancer pain the last days and hours of life. *Journal of Pain and Symptom Management, 6*(7), 411–422.

Hadjistavropoulos, H. D., Ross, M. A., & von Baeyer, C. L. (1990). Are physicians' ratings of pain affected by patients' physical attractiveness? *Social Science and Medicine, 31*(1), 69–72.

Havlik, R. H., & Suzman, R. (1987). Health status—mortality. In R. H. Havlik, B. M. Liu, M. G. Kovar, R. Suzman, J. J. Feldman, T. Harris, & J. VanNorstrand (Eds.), *Health statistics on older persons, United States, 1986. Vital and Health Statistics* (pp. 5–15). Series 3, No. 25. DHHS Publication No. (PHS) 87-1409. Public Health Service, Washington D.C.: U.S. Government Printing Office.

Hendler, N. (1984). Depression caused by chronic pain. *Journal of Clinical Psychiatry, 45,* 30–38.

International Association for the Study of Pain. (1993). Pain curriculum for basic nursing education. *IASP Newsletter, September/October,* 4–6.

Jacox, A. (1979). Assessing pain. *American Journal of Nursing, 79,* 865–900.

Johanson, G. A. (1991). Symptom character and prevalence during cancer patients' last days of life. *American Journal of Hospice and Palliative Care, 8*(2), 6–8,18.

Joint Commission on Accreditation of Healthcare Organizations. (1994). *Accreditation manual for hospitals.* Oak Brook Terrace, IL: JCAHO.

Lasagna, L., Mosteller, F., von Felsinger, J. M., & Beecher, H. K. (1954). A study of the placebo response. *American Journal of Medicine, 16,* 770–779.

Leavitt, F., & Sweet, J. J. (1986). Characteristics and frequency of malingering among patients with low back pain. *Pain, 25,* 357–364.

Levine, J. D, Gordon, N. C., & Fields, H. (1978). The mechanism of placebo analgesia. *Lancet, 2,* 654–657.

Levy, M. (1985). Pain management in advanced cancer. *Seminars in Oncology, 12,* 394–410.

Liebeskind, J. C. (1991). Pain can kill. *Pain, 44,* 3–4.

MacDonald, N., Mount, B., Boston, W., & Scott, J. F. (1993). The Canadian palliative care undergraduate curriculum. *Journal of Cancer Education, 8*(3), 197–201.

Management of Cancer Pain Guideline Panel. (1994a). *Clinical practice guideline: Management of cancer pain.* AHCPR Pub. No. 94-0592. Rockville, MD: Agency for Health Care Policy and Research, Public Health Service, U. S. Department of Health and Human Services.

Management of Cancer Pain Guideline Panel. (1994b). *Clinical practice guideline: Patient guide. Managing cancer pain.* AHCPR Pub. No. 94-0593. Rockville, MD: Agency for Health Care Policy and Research, Public Health Service, U. S. Department of Health and Human Services.

Management of Cancer Pain Guideline Panel. (1994c). *Clinical practice guideline: Quick reference guide. Management of cancer pain: Adults.* AHCPR Pub. No. 94-0595. Rockville, MD: Agency for Health Care Policy and Research, Public Health Service, U. S. Department of Health and Human Services.

Marks, R. M., & Sachar, E. J. (1973). Undertreatment of medical inpatients with narcotic analgesics. *Annals of Internal Medicine, 78,* 173–181.

Massie, M. J., & Holland, J. C. (1987). The cancer patient with pain: Psychiatric complications and their management. *Medical Journal of North America, 71,* 243–258.

McCaffery, M. (1968). *Nursing practice theories related to cognition, bodily pain, and man-environment interactions.* Los Angeles: University of California at Los Angeles.

McCaffery, M. (1990). Pain management: Nurses lead the way to new priorities. *American Journal of Nursing, October,* 45–50.

McCaffery, M., & Beebe, A. (1989). Pain assessment. *Pain: Clinical manual for nursing practice.* St. Louis, MO: C. V. Mosby.

McCaffery, M., & Ferrell, B. (1991). How would you respond to these patients in pain? *Nursing 91, 21,* 34–37.

McCaffery, M., & Ferrell, B. R. (1992). How vital are vital signs? *Nursing 92, 22,* 42–46.

McCaffery, M., & Ferrell, B. R. (1994). Nurses' assessment of pain intensity and choice of analgesic dose. *Contemporary Nurse, 3*(2), 68–74.

McCaffery, M., Ferrell, B. R., & O'Neil-Page, E. (1992). Does life-style affect your pain-control decisions? *Nursing 92, April,* 58–61.

McGuire, D. B. (1987). Cancer-related pain: A multidimensional approach. *Dissertation Abstracts International, 48,* 705.

McMillan, S. C., Williams, F. A., Chatfield, R., & Camp, L. D. (1988). A validity and reliability study of two tools for assessing and managing pain. *Oncology Nursing Forum, 15,* 735–741.

Melzack, F., Abbott, V., Zackon, W., Mulder, D. S., & Davis, M. W. L. (1987). Pain on a surgical ward: A survey of the duration and intensity of pain and the effectiveness of medication. *Pain, 29,* 67–72.

Miaskowski, C., Nichols, R., Brody, R., & Synold, T. (1994). Assessment of patient satisfaction utilizing the American Pain Society's quality assurance standards on acute and cancer-related pain. *Journal of Pain and Symptom Management, 9*(1), 5–11.

National Health and Medical Research Council. (1988). Management of severe pain. Canberra, Australia: Australian Government Publishing Service.

Paice, J., Mahon, S. M., & Faut-Callahan, M. (1991). Factors associated with adequate pain control in hospitalized postsurgical patients diagnosed with cancer. *Cancer Nursing, 14*(6), 298–305.

Palliative Care 2000. (1992). Expert panel report to Cancer 2000 Task Force. *Journal of Palliative Care, 8*[entire issue].

Pasero, C. L., & McCaffery, M. (1994). Avoiding opioid-induced respiratory depression. *American Journal of Nursing, 94*(4), 25–30.

Perry, S., & Heidrich, G. (1982). Management of pain during debridement: A survey of U.S. burn units. *Pain, 13,* 267–280.

Portenoy R. K., Miransky J., Thaler H. T., Hornung, J., Bianchi, C., Cibas-Kong, I., Feldhamer, E., Lewis, F., Matamoros, I., Sugar, M. Z., Olivieri, A. P., Kemeny, N. E., & Foley, K. M. (1992). Pain in ambulatory patients with lung or colon cancer: Prevalence, characteristics, and effect. *Cancer, 70,* 1616–1624.

Porter, J., & Jick, H. (1980). Addiction rare in patients treated with narcotics [letter]. *New England Journal of Medicine, 302,* 123.

Puntillo, K. A. (1990). Pain experiences of intensive care unit patients. *Heart and Lung, 19*(5), 526–533.

Reesor, K. A., & Craig, K. D. (1988). Medically incongruent chronic back pain: Physical limitations, suffering, and ineffective coping. *Pain, 32,* 35–45.

Sheehan, D. K., Webb, A., Bower, D., & Einsporn, R. (1992). Level of cancer pain knowledge among baccalaureate student nurses. *Journal of Pain and Symptom Management, 7,* 478–484.

Short, L. M., Burnett, M. L., Egbert, A. M., & Parks, L. H. (1990). Medicating the postoperative elderly: How do nurses make their decisions? *Journal of Gerontological Nursing, 16*(7), 12–17.

Social Security Administration. (1986). *Report to the commission on the evaluation of pain.* Washington, DC: U.S. Government Printing Office.

Spross, J. A., McGuire, D. B., & Schmitt, R. M. (1991). Oncology Nursing Society position paper on cancer pain. Pittsburgh, PA: Oncology Nursing Press.

Stephens, S. T. (1994). A promise to Billie. *Nursing 94, April,* 96.

Todd, K. H., Samaroo, N., & Hoffman, J. R. (1993). Ethnicity as a risk factor for inadequate emergency department analgesia. *Journal of the American Medical Association, 269*(12), 1537–1539.

Twycross, R. G. (1974). Clinical experience with diamorphine in advanced malignant disease. *International Journal of Clinical Pharmacology, 9,* 184–198.

Twycross, R. G., & Fairfield, S. (1982). Pain in far-advanced cancer. *Pain, 14,* 303–310.

Twycross, R. G., & Wald, S. J. (1976). Long-term use of diamorphine in advanced cancer. In J. J. Bonica, & D. Albe-Fessard (Eds.), *Advances in pain research and therapy* (Vol. 1., pp. 653–661). New York: Raven Press.

Vallerand, A. H. (1994). Street addicts and patients with pain: Similarities and differences. *Clinical Nurse Specialist, 8*(1), 11–15.

Van Roenn, J. H., Cleeland, C. S., Gonin, R., Hatfield, A. K., & Pandya, K. J. (1993). Physician's attitudes and practice in cancer pain management: A survey from the Eastern Cooperative Oncology Group. *Annals of Internal Medicine, 119,* 121–126.

Ventafridda, V., De Conno, F., Ripamonti C., Gamba, A., & Tamburini, M. (1990). Quality-of-life assessment during a palliative care programme. *Annals of Oncology, 1,* 415–420.

Ventafridda, V., Ripamonti, C., De Conno, F., et al. (1990). Symptom prevalence and control during cancer patients' last days of life. *Journal of Palliative Care, 6,* 7–11.

Ward, S., & Gatwood, J. (1994). Concerns about reporting pain and using analgesics: A comparison of persons with and without cancer. *Cancer Nursing, 17*(3), 200–206.

Ward, S. E., Goldberg, N., Miller-McCauley, V., Mueller, C., Nolan, A., Pawlik Plank, D., Robbins, A., Stormoen, D., & Weisman, D. (1993). Patient-related barriers to management of cancer pain. *Pain, 52,* 319–324.

Ward, S. E., & Gordon, D. (1994). Application of the American Pain Society quality assurance standards. *Pain, 56,* 299–306.

Wilkie, D., Lovejoy, N., Dodd, M., & Tesler, M. (1988). Cancer pain control behaviors: Description and correlation with pain intensity. *Oncology Nursing Forum, 15*(6), 723–731.

World Health Organization. (1990). *Cancer pain relief and palliative care.* Report of a WHO expert committee [WHO Technical Report Series. 804]. Geneva, Switzerland: World Health Organization.

Pharmacologic Management of Cancer Pain

Nessa Coyle • Russell K. Portenoy

Inadequate knowledge of analgesic pharmacotherapy is one of the most commonly cited reasons for the undertreatment of cancer pain. Because of the frequency of pain in the cancer population, developing expertise in the use of analgesic drugs is integral to oncology nursing (Ferrell, Eberts, McCaffery, & Grant, 1991).

Over a decade ago, an expert committee convened by the the Cancer Unit of the World Health Organization (WHO) developed a three-step "analgesic ladder" approach to the selection of drugs for the treatment of cancer pain. Drug selection was guided by severity of pain (Fig. 57–1). When such an approach is combined with appropriate dosing, approximately 70 to 90 per cent of cancer patients can have their pain adequately controlled (Grond, Zech, Schug, Lynch, & Lehman, 1991; Jorgensen, Mortensen, Jensen, & Eriksen, 1990; Schug, Zech et al., 1990; Takeda, 1986; Ventafridda, Tamburini, Caracenia, DeConno, & Naldi, 1987; World Health Organization, 1986, 1990). This three-step approach has gained wide acceptance throughout the world and was most recently endorsed in the Agency for Health Care Policy and Research clinical practice guideline for the management of cancer pain (AHCPR, 1994).

Using the "analgesic ladder" as a framework, this chapter will provide basic information about the use of

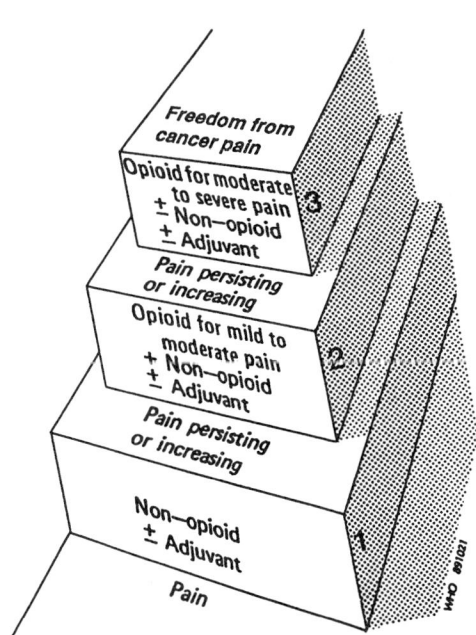

FIGURE 57–1. WHO analgesic ladder. (Reproduced by permission from *Cancer pain relief and palliative care: Report of a WHO Expert Committee*. Geneva, World Health Organization, 1990 [Technical Report Series, No 804], Fig. 1.)

drugs to manage cancer pain. Three categories of analgesic drugs will be discussed: nonopioids, opioids, and adjuvant analgesics. Included in the discussion will be the rationale for drug selection, dose titration, routes of administration, and side effect management.

NONSTEROIDAL ANTIINFLAMMATORY DRUGS

The nonsteroidal antiinflammatory drugs (NSAIDs) used in step one of the "analgesic ladder" are analgesic, antipyretic, and antiinflammatory. NSAIDs are most effective in treating mild to moderate pain when an inflammatory component is present. In the cancer population, they are frequently used in combination with an opioid in step two and step three of the "analgesic ladder." Acetaminophen, although lacking in significant antiinflammatory effects, is often classified with the NSAIDs and is also helpful in managing pain in this group of patients.

Unlike the opioid drugs, the NSAIDs have a ceiling effect (a dose beyond which added analgesia is not obtained). These drugs do not produce tolerance or physical dependence. They are not associated with psychologic dependence (addiction).

DRUGS USED IN STEP ONE OF THE "ANALGESIC LADDER": ACETAMINOPHEN AND THE NSAIDs

ACETAMINOPHEN

Analgesic effects produced by this drug appear to result primarily from a central mechanism (Piletta, Porchet, & Dayer, 1991). Acetaminophen has fewer adverse effects than the NSAIDs. Gastrointestinal toxicity is rare, and there are no adverse effects on platelet function or cross-reactivity in patients with aspirin hypersensitivity. Hepatic toxicity can occur, however, and patients with chronic alcoholism and liver disease can develop severe hepatotoxicity even when the drug is taken in usual therapeutic doses (Seeff, Cuccherini, Zimmerman, Alder, & Benjamin, 1986).

NSAIDs

The NSAIDs comprise many subclasses, all of which inhibit prostaglandin synthetase (Table 57–1). A peripheral site of action is assumed, but there is evidence that these drugs also exert central effects (Vane, 1971; Willer, DeBroucker, Bussel, Robi-Brami, & Harrowyn, 1989). Nurses must be alert for potential adverse effects relevant to the cancer patient, including those affecting the hematologic, gastrointestinal, renal, and central nervous systems.

Hematologic Effects. Single doses of aspirin above 40 mg irreversably inhibit platelet aggregation (normal platelet function is expressed only by those platelets produced after cessation of aspirin therapy) (Sunshine & Olson, 1994). Consequently, aspirin may prolong bleeding for many days after administration ceases. Because of this interference with platelet function, patients who are to undergo surgery should be specifically asked whether they have injested aspirin during the past 48

hours. In contrast, other NSAIDs produce reversible platelet aggregation inhibition. These drugs render the patient more susceptible to bleeding only for the period during which the drug circulates in the blood.

A bleeding diathesis of any cause is a strong relative contraindication to the use of these drugs. The nonacetylated salicylates such as choline magnesium trisalicylate, a less widely known antiinflammatory drug, do not change bleeding time and, on this basis, may be relatively safer in patients at risk for bleeding (Sunshine & Olson, 1994). The improved safety profile of these drugs has not been confirmed, however.

Gastrointestinal Effects. NSAIDs inhibit gastrointestinal prostaglandins that protect the gastrointestinal mucosa. This may result in dyspepsia, peptic erosions, or ulcerations. People with previous ulcer disease and the elderly appear to be most susceptable (Roth, 1988). Aspirin appears to produce more of these gastrointestinal adverse effects than other NSAIDs. Chronic administration of ketorolac is also not recommended due to a relatively high risk of adverse gastrointestinal effects (DiPalma, 1991; Kenny, 1990; Saxen, 1992).

Renal Effects. NSAIDs can cause renal insufficiency and significant nephrotoxicity by several mechanisms (Cooper & Bennett, 1987). Acute reversible renal insufficiency may occur and is thought to be be the result of the blockade of intrarenal vasodilatory prostaglandins. Patients at increased risk include the elderly and those with congestive heart failure, chronic renal insufficiency, cirrhosis with ascites, and intravascular volume depletion. Patients receiving diuretics may also be at relatively high risk. NSAIDs can also affect tubular function, including renal handling of potassium, sodium, and water. Hyponatremia can be related to renal salt wasting or to an enhanced action of diuretic hormone. Finally, NSAIDs can cause the insidious development of chronic renal failure. This risk necessitates periodic monitoring of renal function during long-term use of these drugs.

Central Nervous System Effects. Tinnitus, deafness, headache, and dizziness, well-known manifestations of salicylate toxicity, can also be side effects of other NSAIDs (Goodwin & Regan, 1982). These effects typically disappear after dose reduction.

Other Adverse Effects Associated with Aspirin. Two subgroups of aspirin-sensitive patients have been reported. One subgroup develops a respiratory reaction with rhinitis, asthma, or nasal polyps. A second subgroup develops urticaria, wheals, angioedema, and hypotension (Clissold, 1986; Szczeklik, 1986). These hypersensitivities usually occur within minutes of injestion, and almost always within an hour. Patients who are sensitive to aspirin may also develop sensitivities to the other NSAIDs. A history of aspirin intolerance is therefore a contraindication to use drugs within this category.

PRINCIPLES OF ADMINISTRATION OF THE NSAIDs

DRUG SELECTION

A careful medical and pain history provides the nurse with information about potential benefits and risks for a patient about to receive a NSAID. An anal-

TABLE 57–1. *Nonsteroidal Antiinflammatory Drugs**

CHEMICAL CLASS	GENERIC NAME	HALF-LIFE (H)	DOSING SCHEDULE	RECOMMENDED STARTING DOSE** (MG)	MAXIMUM DOSE RECOMMENDED (MG/DAY)	COMMENTS
p-aminophenol derivatives	Acetaminophen	3–4	q 4–6 h	650	6000	Overdosage produces hepatic toxicity. No GI or platelet toxicity.
Salicylates	Aspirin	3–12	q 4–6 h	650	6000	Standard for comparison. May not be as well tolerated as some of the newer NSAIDs.
	Diflunisal	8–12	q 12 h	500	1500	Less GI toxicity than aspirin.
	Choline magnesium trisalicylate	8–12	q 12 h	500–1000	4000	Minimal GI toxicity. No effect on platelet aggregation.
	Salsalate	8–12	q 12 h	500–1000	4000	
Proprionic acids	Ibuprofen	3–4	q 6 h	400	4200	Available as a sus-suspension.
	Naproxen	1–3	q 12 h	250	1500	
	Fenoprofen	2–3	q 6 h	200	3200	
	Ketoprofen	2–3	q 6 h	25	300	
	Flurbiprofen	5–6	q 12 h	100	300	
	Oxaprozin	40	q 24 h	600	1800	
Acetic acids	Indomethacin	4–5	q 8 h	25	200	Higher incidence of GI and CNS side effects than proprionic acid. Available in slow-release preparations.
	Tolmetin	1	q 8 h	200	2000	
	Sulindac	14	q 12 h	150	400	
	Diclofenac	2	q 8 h	25	200	
	Ketorolac	4–7	q 6 h	***	150 day 1, 120 day 2 and after (parenteral) 40 (oral).	Experience limited to acute pain. Efficacy and safety with chronic use to be determined. Long term use not recommended.
Oxicams	Piroxicam	45	q 24 h	20	40	
Fenamates	Mefenamic acid	2	q 6 h	250	1000	
Pyranocarboxylic acids	Etodolac	7	q 8 h	200	1200	
Naphtyl alkanones	Nabumetone	22–30	q 12 h	500	2000	

*Table based on clinical experience of the authors and a variety of published sources.
**Starting dose should be one half to two thirds recommended dose in the elderly, those on multiple drug or those with renal insufficiency.
***30–60 load, then 15–30 q 6 h (parenteral), 10 q 6 h (oral).
q = every; h = hour.
(Reproduced by permission from Coyle, N., Cherny, N. I., & Portenoy, R. K. [1995]. Pharmacologic management of cancer pain. In D. B. McGuire, C. H. Yarbro, & B. R. Ferrell [Eds.], *Cancer pain management* [2nd ed., pp. 91–92]. © 1995 Boston: Jones & Bartlett Publishers. Reprinted with permission.)

gesic history should illuminate the patient's prior exposure to the NSAIDs, including frequency of administration and both analgesic effects and adverse effects. Information regarding the timing interval of other analgesics is important so that a prescribed NSAID regimen fits in with the patients total analgesic plan. For example, if a patient is on an 8- or 12-hour dosing regimen of a controlled-release morphine preparation, an NSAID with a similar dosing profile would be appropriate (refer to Table 57–1). This may improve compliance. Although around-the-clock (ATC) dosing regimens are the mode of choice for most cancer patients with chronic pain, an "as needed" schedule is appropriate in some cases. For "as needed" dosing, the use of acetaminophen or an NSAID with a short half-life, such as aspirin or ibuprofen, might be appropriate.

CHOICE OF A STARTING DOSE AND DOSE TITRATION

The NSAID is combined with an opioid drug in step 2 and 3 of the "analgesic ladder." Monitoring of the patient's satisfaction and presence of side effects must be ongoing. Doses are often started at the lower end of the recommended scale, then increased if needed (Table 57–1). Based on clinical experience and customary use, maximal doses of 1.5 to 2 times the standard recommended dose are suggested as a prudent limit (Cherny & Portenoy, 1994). There is great variability in patient response to different NSAIDs. Patients who are maintained at doses above the standard dose require close monitoring, including a test for occult fecal blood, urinalysis, and evaluation of blood urea nitrogen and creatinine every few months or when appropriate.

Although several weeks are needed to evaluate the efficacy of a dose when NSAIDs are used in the treatment of grossly inflammatory conditions such as arthritis, clinical observation suggests a shorter period, usually a week, is adequate for the same purpose in a patient with cancer pain. Table 57–2 provides guidelines to the nurse for the selection and use of NSAIDs in the management of cancer pain.

GASTROPROTECTIVE THERAPIES DURING NSAID THERAPY

The occurrence of gastric ulcers in patients receiving chronic NSAID therapy has been demonstrated to be reduced by coadministration of misoprostol. Those patients with a relatively high risk for developing ulcers, including those with a history of peptic ulcer disease, advanced age, and concurrent corticosteroid use, should be considered for this therapy. Patients who cannot tolerate misoprostol and are candidates for gastroprotective therapy should be considered for an alternative approach; the combination of an H$_2$ blocker and sucralfate is a well-tolerated empiric alternative.

OPIOID ANALGESICS

Opioid analgesics are the mainstay of cancer pain treatment. These drugs are used for moderate to severe pain in step 2 and step 3 of the "analgesic ladder." They are frequently used in combination with an NSAID. Opioids produce their analgesic effects by binding to the μ, δ and κ receptors in the central nervous system (Jaffe & Martin, 1990). The various compounds can be divided into agonists, agonist-antagonist, and antagonist classes based on their interactions with these receptor subtypes. The agonist-antagonist analgesics can be further subdivided into mixed agonist-antagonists and partial agonists.

The morphine-like pure agonist drugs such as morphine, hydromorphone, oxymorphone, oxycodone, levorphanol, methadone, and fentanyl are most commonly used in the management of cancer pain. These drugs appear to have no ceiling effect to analgesia, but adverse effects such as sedation, confusion, nausea and vomiting, or respiratory depression impose a limit to

TABLE 57–2. *Nursing Guidelines for Selection and Use of Acetaminophen and NSAIDs in the Management of Cancer Pain*

1. Avoid NSAIDs, if possible, in patients with gastroduodenopathy, bleeding diathesis, renal insufficiency, hypertension, severe encephalopathy and cardiac failure; avoid acetaminophen in patients with severe liver disease.
2. If NSAIDs strongly indicated in patients with relative contraindications (except severe liver disease), consider acetaminophen; if antiinflammatory effects wanted, consider choline magnesium trisalicylate or salsalate.
3. Consider individual differences (note prior treatment outcomes) and patient preference.
4. Be aware of available routes of administration (e.g., oral, rectal, intravenous).
5. Begin with a low dose and adjust weekly if dose escalation is needed.
6. Increase dose until adequate analgesia occurs, ceiling dose is identified, or maximal recommended dose is reached.
7. Be aware that several weeks may be necessary to fully assess efficacy.
8. If the patient is being treated in step 1 of the "analgesic ladder" and fails to receive "satisfactory" pain relief, step 2 of the ladder should be instituted.

(Adapted from Coyle, N., Cherny, N. I., Portenoy, R. K. [1995]. Pharmacologic management of cancer pain. In D. B. McGuire, C. H. Yarbro, & B. R. Ferrell [Eds.], *Cancer pain management* [2nd ed., pp. 91–92]. © 1995. Boston: Jones & Bartlett Publishers. Reprinted with permission.)

useful dose escalation. Dose escalation is governed by the balance between pain relief and intolerable and unmanageable side effects (Cherny & Portenoy, 1994). This balance can be determined only by ongoing assessment and documentation of the effects and side effects produced by the opioid.

Morphine is the prototype opioid agonist. The WHO has placed oral morphine on the essential drug list and has requested that it be made available throughout the world for cancer pain relief (World Health Organization, 1986). The controlled-release relief morphine preparations provide analgesia with a duration of 8 to 12 hours and allow the patient respite from frequent dosing. Patients with severe pain should be initially titrated on immediate-release morphine, and once stabilized, converted to the controlled-release preparation. To manage "breakthrough" pain or "incident" pain, immediate-release morphine should be made available to all patients receiving controlled-release preparations.

Information regarding an active metabolite of morphine, morphine-6-glucuronide (M-6-G), may influence its clinical use. M-6-G binds to opioid receptors and may produce opioid effects (Osborne, Joel, & Slevin, 1986; Paul, Standifer, Inturrisi, & Pasternak, 1989). Patients with impaired renal function may accumulate M-6-G, which can result in signs of opioid toxicity (Osborne et al., 1986; Portenoy et al., 1991; Portenoy, Thaler, Inturrisi, Friedlander-Klar, & Foley, 1992; Sawe, Dahlstrom, Pazlow, & Rane, 1981; Sawe, Svensson, & Odar-Cedarlof, 1985). Nurses must be aware of a patient's renal status when administering morphine and use caution in patients with renal insufficiency.

Hydromorphone and oxycodone are short half-life opioids that may be very useful alternatives to morphine. Hydromorphone can be administered by the oral or parenteral routes and is available in a concentrated parenteral dosage form of 10 mg/ml. Neither hydromorphone or oxycodone are currently available in controlled-release preparations. In the United States, both these drugs are used in step 3 of the "analgesic ladder."

Methadone is another useful drug for cancer pain, but clinical experience suggests that it is more difficult to administer than other morphine-like opioids because of its long half-life, which averages 24 hours (range 13 hours to over 100 hours) (Plummer, Gourlay, Cherry, & Cousins, 1988), and a discrepancy between drug half-life and duration of analgesic effect. Patients are at increased risk for drug accumulation and subsequent toxicity when treatment is initiated, the dose is increased, or multiple organ failure develops (Inturrisi, Colburn, Kauko, Houde, & Foley, 1987; Inturrisi, Portenoy, Max, Colburn, & Foley, 1990). Because of this risk, methadone is considered a "second-line" drug in the treatment of cancer pain. Nursing knowledge of the long half-life of methadone has a special relevance for the nurse if severe respiratory depression develops and the use of naloxone is required. Because of the short half-life of naloxone in comparison with methadone, either repeated doses or an infusion of naloxone may be required to prevent recurrence of respiratory depression as the effects of naloxone decline and the methadone rebinds to the opioid binding sites.

The risk of delayed toxicity from methadone accumulation can be reduced if the initial period of dosing is accomplished with "as needed" administration (Cherny & Portenoy, 1994; Fainsinger, Schoeller, & Bruera, 1993). When a steady state has been approached, a fixed dosing schedule of every 4 to 6 hours can be substituted. An opioid with a short half-life such as morphine or hydromorphone should be used for supplementary or "rescue" dosing.

Meperidine is not a drug of choice for chronic cancer pain. Meperidine has an active metabolite, normeperidine, that is twice as potent as a convulsant and one-half as potent as an analgesic as its parent compound. The half-life of normeperidine is three to four times that of meperidine, and accumulation of the metabolite with repetitive dosing can result in central nervous system excitability characterized by tremor, multifocal myoclonus and seizures (Inturrisi & Umans, 1986). Naloxone does not reverse meperidine-induced seizures and potentially could precipitate seizures by blocking the depressant effects of meperidine and allowing the convulsant effects of normeperidine to become manifest. If naloxone is given, it should be diluted and slowly titrated while seizure precautions are taken.

The agonist-antagonist opioids include the mixed-agonist antagonists pentazocine, butorphanol, nalbuphine, and dezocine, and the partial agonist buprenorphine. All these drugs play a minor role in cancer pain management (Foley, 1985). Their pharmacology is characterized by a ceiling effect for analgesia and the ability to precipitate withdrawal in patients who are physically dependent on morphine-like drugs. The incidence of psychotomimetic effects (agitation, dysphoria, confusion) from the mixed agonist-antagonist is greater than that of the pure agonists (morphine-like drugs).

The opioid antagonist drugs include naloxone and naltrexone. These drugs also bind to opioid receptors but block the effect of morphine-like agonists.

PLACEBO DRUGS

A placebo is an intervention designed to simulate medical therapy but not believed by the investigator or clinician to be a specific therapy for the target condition (Turner, Deyo, Loeser, Vonkorff, & Fordyce, 1994). Placebo drugs have no place in the management of cancer pain, except with full patient consent during a clinical drug trial. Pain relief after administration of a placebo drug does not indicate that the pain is psychogenic or that the patient is a malingerer; it means only that the patient is a placebo-responder (Turner, Deyo, Loeser, Vonkorff, & Fordyce, 1994; Wall, 1994). Factors that influence the placebo response include expectations of treatment effects, positive attitude towards the provider and towards the treatment, high anxiety levels, high degree of compliance with all medical treatments, and a clinician who is warm, empathic, and has a positive attitude towards the patient and treatment (Turner et al., 1994). The use of a placebo is not informative and has the potential to greatly undermine the basic nurse/patient therapeutic relationship, a relationship based on truth-telling and trust.

PRINCIPLES OF ADMINISTRATION OF OPIOIDS

Numerous factors, both patient-related and drug-related, must be considered in the selection of an appropriate opioid for a patient. The opioid should be compatible with the patient's pain severity, age, dosing requirements, underlying illness, and metabolic state. For the younger adult without any major organ dysfunction, any of the available agonist opioids could be selected within the framework of step 2 and 3 of the "analgesic ladder." For example, a patient with moderate pain might be treated initially with a combination product containing acetaminophen plus codeine or acetaminophen plus oxycodone, whereas a patient with more severe pain might be treated with morphine. Selection of an opioid that is available as a controlled-release formulation (such as morphine) is an important consideration for some patients. For the elderly or those who have major organ dysfunction, an opioid with a short half-life, such as morphine, hydromorphone, or oxycodone, is preferable. Patients with renal impairment may accumulate the active metabolites of morphine, and this drug should be used cautiously in such patients, with close monitoring for signs of toxicity.

The potential for additive side effects and serious toxicities from drug combinations must be recognized by the nurse each time a new drug is added or deleted from a patient's regimen. For example, the tricyclic antidepressants, such as amitriptyline, may both increase the plasma concentration of morphine and produce additive side effects such as somnolence (Ventafridda et al., 1990). The sedative effects of an opioid may also add to numerous other centrally acting drugs, such as anxiolytics and neuroleptics.

Sequential trials of opioid drugs may be needed to find the most favorable balance between pain relief and adverse effects (Galer, Coyle, Pasternak, & Portenoy, 1992). The sequential administration of opioid drug trials requires knowledge of the relative potencies among opioid drugs (Table 57–3).

Selecting a Route and Dosing Intervals

Opioids should be administered by the least invasive and safest route capable of providing adequate analgesia (AHCPR, 1994). Clinical experience indicates that most patients can use the oral route throughout most of the course of their illness. However, many patients become unable to use this route, and the nurses must be skilled in selecting among the alternative routes to meet the needs of a particular patient (Coyle, Adelhardt, Foley, & Portenoy, 1990). The most commonly used alternative routes include rectal (Hanning, 1990; Kaiko et al., 1989), sublingual (Hirsch, 1984; Weinberg et al., 1988), transdermal (Adams, Cruz, Deachman, & Zamora, 1989; Calis, Kohler, & Corso, 1992; Miser et al., 1989; Varvel, Shafer, Hwang, Coen, & Stanski, 1989), subcutaneous (Bruera et al., 1991; Coyle, Cherny, & Portenoy, 1994; Moulin et al., 1992; Storey, Hill, St. Louis, & Tarker, 1990; Swanson, Smith, Burlich, New, & Shiffman, 1989), intravenous (Portenoy, 1987), and epidural (Arner, Rawal, & Gustafsson, 1988; Cousins & Plummer, 1991; Hardy & Wells, 1990; Moulin, Inturrisi, & Foley, 1986; Yaksh, 1981). Table 57–4 reviews the alternate routes of opioid administration, patient selection criteria, and advantages and disadvantages of each.

Patient-controlled-analgesia (PCA) is a technique that usually refers to parenteral drug administration in which the patient controls a pump that delivers analgesics according to parameters set by the nurse and physician. These parameters include concentration of the drug and time interval between doses. Frequently, the patient has a baseline subcutaneous (Bruera, 1988; Coyle et al., 1994; Moulin et al., 1992; Moulin, Kreeft, Wang, & Bouquillon, 1991), or intravenous infusion (Portenoy, 1987) to which PCA is added and acts essentially as a provision for supplemental "rescue" doses (Portenoy & Hagen, 1990). Use of a PCA device may be helpful for patients who require parenterel opioids (Chapman, 1989; Citron et al., 1992; Kerr et al., 1988; Marlowe, Engstrom, & White, 1989). A switch in route of drug administration, like a change from one opioid to another, requires consideration of relative potency to avoid overdosing or underdosing (Table 57–3). The equianalgesic dose table provides a guide to dose selection when these changes are made. The calculated equianalgesic dose is usually reduced 25 to 50

per cent when switching drugs to account for incomplete cross tolerance (Cherny & Portenoy, 1994). Based on clinical observation, a larger reduction is often used when switching to methadone. The problems associated with switching the route of drug administration can be minimized by accomplishing this in a step-by-step manner (e.g., slowly reducing the parenteral dose and increasing the oral dose over a 1- to 2-day period). Another approach is to place the patient on a fixed dosing schedule using the new route and to make provisions for supplementary or "rescue" doses every 1 to 2 hours.

Patients with continuous or frequent pain generally benefit from scheduled ATC dosing to prevent pain from reoccurring (Cherny & Portenoy 1994; AHCPR, 1994; American Pain Society, 1992; World Health Organization, 1986, 1990). A "rescue" dose is offered on a "prn" basis and provides a means to treat pain that breaks through the fixed analgesic schedule. The drug used for the supplemental dose is usually the same as that administered on a regular basis (Cherny & Portenoy, 1994). An alternative short half-life drug is recommended when using methadone or transdermal fentanyl. Clinical experience suggests that the rescue dose should be calculated as about 25 to 50 per cent of the hourly dose, or 5 to 15 per cent of the 24-hour baseline dose (Cherny & Portenoy, 1994). For example, a patient receiving 60 mg of a controlled-release oral morphine preparation every 12 hours should have a rescue or supplementary dose of 10 to 15 mg of immediate-release morphine available on a 1- to 2-hour basis.

Choice of a Starting Dose and Dose Titration

A patient who is relatively opioid-naive should generally begin treatment at an opioid dose equivalent to 5 to 10 mg of parenteral morphine every 4 hours (Cherny & Portenoy, 1994). Titration of the opioid dose is usually necessary at the start of pain therapy and at different points during the disease course. At all times, inadequate relief should be addressed through gradual dose escalation until relief is reported or intolerable and unmanageable side effects occur. Integration of ATC dosing with supplemental "rescue" doses provides a rational stepwise approach to dose escalation that is applicable to all routes of drug administration. Patients who require more than 4 to 6 "rescue" doses per day should generally undergo escalation of the baseline dose. In all cases, escalation of the baseline dose should be accompanied by a proportionate increase in the "rescue" dose so that the size of the supplemental dose remains a constant percentage of the fixed dose. Nursing assessment of the patient's pattern of pain and response to the "rescue" dose is essential for dose titration. Table 57–5 summarizes the basic principles in the use of opioid drugs to manage cancer pain.

Tolerance, Physical Dependence and Addiction

Tolerance is a poorly understood phenomenon characterized by the need for increasing doses to main-

TABLE 57–3. *Equianalgesic Dose Table: Relative Potencies, Half-lives, and Duration of Action of Commonly Used Opioid Drugs.* *

DRUG	HALF-LIFE (H)	EQUIANALGESIC INTRAMUSCULAR DOSE (MG)	INTRAMUSCULAR/ ORAL POTENCY (MG)	STARTING ORAL DOSE RANGE (MG)	COMMENT
Morphine-like Agonists					
Morphine	2–3	10	3 (repeated dose)	15–30	Standard of comparison for opioid analgesics. Multiple routes of administration. Controlled release available. M6G accumulation in patients with renal failure. Lower doses for the elderly.
Hydromorphone	2–3	1.5	5	4–8	Useful alternative for morphine. No known active metabolite. Multiple routes available.
Methadone	15–190	10	2	5–10	May accumulate with repetitive dosing.
Levorphanol	12–15	2	2	2–4	May accumulate with repetitive dosing.
Meperidine	2–3	75	4	Not recom-mended	CNS excitatory toxic metabolite, normeperidine. Contraindicated for repetitive dosing, for patients with renal failure, or receiving MAO inhibitors.
Fentanyl	7–14	—	—	—	Short half-life when used acutely. Parenteral use via infusion. Clinical experience suggests 2mg morphine sulfate/hr = 100 μg transdermal patch. Patches available to deliver 25, 50, 75, 100 μg/hr.
Oxycodone	2–3	15	2	5–10	Available in liquid or tablet preparation. Also in combination with a nonopioid.
Codeine	2–3	130	1.5	30–60	Used orally for less severe pain. Usually combined with a nonopioid.
Propoxyphene	2–3	—	—	65–130	Usually combined with nonopioid. Norpropoxyphene accumulates, with renal impairment may cause seizures.
Hydrocodone	4	—	—	5–10	Usually combined with nonopioid.
Mixed Agonist Antagonists					
Pentazocine		60	3	—	May cause psychomimetic effects. May precipitate withdrawal in opioid-dependent patients.
Nalbuphine		10	—	—	Not available orally, incidence of psychomimetic effects less than with pentazocine. May precipitate withdrawal in opioid-dependent patients.
Butorphanol		2	—	—	Not available orally. May precipitate withdrawal in opioid-dependent patients.
Dezocine	2	10	—	—	Not available orally. May precipitate withdrawal in opioid-dependent patients.
Partial Agonist					
Buprenorphine		0.4	—	—	Not available orally. May precipitate withdrawal in opioid-dependent patients.

*Table based on clinical experience of the authors and a variety of published sources.
(Reproduced with permission from Coyle, N., Cherny, N. I., & Portenoy, R. K. [1995]. Pharmacologic management of cancer pain. In D. B. McGuire, C. H. Yarbro, & B. R. Ferrell [Eds.], *Cancer pain management* [2nd ed., pp. 101–102]. © 1995 Boston: Jones & Bartlett Publishers. Reprinted with permission.)

tain the same drug effect. Large surveys of cancer patients suggest that tolerance alone is seldom the reason for dose escalation. Usually, the need for dose escalation occurs in the setting of increasing pain associated with progressive disease (Kanner & Foley, 1981; Coyle, Adelhardt, & Foley, 1988; Foley, 1989a, 1991). This observation, integrated with the knowledge that there is no "ceiling" effect to the opioid drugs, implies the following: (1) concern about tolerance to analgesic effects should not impede the use of opioids early in the course of the disease, and (2) worsening pain in a patient on a stable dose of opioids is assumed to be evidence of disease progression until proved otherwise.

Physical dependence is an altered physiologic state that occurs in patients who use opioids on a long-term basis. If the drug is stopped abruptly or an antagonist is given, the patient exhibits signs of withdrawal. Signs of opioid withdrawal include anxiety, alternating hot flashes and cold chills, salivation, lacrimation, rhinorrhea, diaphoresis, piloerection, nausea, vomiting, abdominal cramping, and insomnia. The time frame of the withdrawal syndrome depends on the half-life of the drug. For example, abstinence from drugs with a short half-life, such as morphine or hydromorphone, may occur within 6 to 12 hours of stopping the drug and be most severe after 24 to 72 hours. After withdrawal of drugs with a long half-life, such as methadone or levorphanol, the symptoms may not occur for a day or longer. Gradual reduction of the opioid dose in the physically dependent patient who no longer has pain will prevent the withdrawal syndrome.

The use of an antagonist, such as naloxone, in the physically dependent patient will precipitate acute withdrawal symptoms unless carefully titrated. If a drug overdose is suspected in a patient who has received opioids for more than a few days, a dilute solution of naloxone should be used (0.4 mg in 10 ml of normal saline solution) (American Pain Society, 1992). This may be administered in 1 ml bolus injections every 2 minutes until the patient becomes responsive. As the half-life of naloxone is considerably shorter than that of the majority of opioid drugs, an intravenous infusion of naloxone, carefully titrated to respirations and level of pain, may be the safest approach once the patient has become stable.

TABLE 57–4. *Commonly Used Routes of Drug Administration*

ROUTE	PATIENT SELECTION CRITERIA	ADVANTAGES	DISADVANTAGES	COMMENTS
Oral (PO)	Route of choice Mild to severe pain Most common reasons for oral route failure: Amount given not sufficient for severity of pain Equianalgesic ratios not adhered to when switching from parenteral to oral route Parenteral to oral change made too quickly Drug administered at intervals too long for time action curve of the drug	Most acceptable to patients Simple Noninvasive Longer duration of effect than parenteral route Controlled-release preparations of morphine available and can be given at 8- to 12-hr intervals Preparations available in liquid form	Onset of action slower than parenteral route Absorption affected by stomach emptying time, presence of food, gastrointestinal mobility	Patients with gastrointestinal disease may not absorb the analgesic and may need an alternate route
Sublingual, Buccal, Rectal	Unable to tolerate oral route (e.g., nausea, vomiting) Unable to swallow (e.g., head & neck cancer, esophageal disease)	Avoids need for repeated injections Easy to administer	Unpalatable taste (sublingual and buccal) Limited drugs available for sublingual and buccal routes Rectal route unacceptable to some patients Tissue irritation (rectal) Onset of action similar to oral (rectal)	Hypodermic, tablets, and oral solutions have been used as sublingual and buccal preparations with varying effect Opioids available in suppository form are morphine, hydromorphone (Dilaudid), and oxymorphone (Numorphan) Suppositories contraindicated in patients with a platelet count of 50 or below

(Reproduced with permission from Coyle, N., Cherny, N. I., & Portenoy, R. K. [1995]. Pharmacologic management of cancer pain. In D. B. McGuire, C. H. Yarbro, & B. R. Ferrell [Eds.], *Cancer pain management* [2nd ed., pp. 101–102]. © 1995 Boston: Jones & Bartlett Publishers. Reprinted with permission.)

TABLE 57–4. *Commonly Used Routes of Drug Administration* Continued

ROUTE	PATIENT SELECTION CRITERIA	ADVANTAGES	DISADVANTAGES	COMMENTS
Transdermal	Inability to use the oral route Stable pain Occasionally need to improve patient compliance with opioid therapy	No need for SC or IV access Long duration of action, 48–72 hrs Provides continuous administration of an opioid	Need alternate route for "rescue" medication Relatively slow onset of action Adverse effects continue after patch removed Fentanyl only opioid available by this route	Short half-life opioid recommended for "breakthrough" pain Difficult to titrate rapidly Serum concentration falls 50% in about 24 hrs If naloxone indicated, may need an infusion
Subcutaneous (SC) Intermittent Infusion	Moderate to severe pain Unable to tolerate the oral route Variable or uncertain PO absorption	Intravenous access not required Subcutaneous route can be continuous or intermittent Onset of action more rapid than oral route Family can learn administration techniques, both continuous infusion and intermittent injections	Absorption variable depending on muscle, fat, and blood supply Peaks and troughs unless continuous SC infusion Duration of action shorter than oral route (intermittent SC) Patient may be dependent on others to administer the analgesic on time (intermittent SC) Milligram dose of drug may be limited by volume requirement.	Intermittent injections contraindicated in patients with a platelet count of 50 or below Methadone should not be used for continuous SC infusions as it is a tissue irritant Continuous SC infusion is the method of choice in an obstructed patient being cared for at home A variety of portable pumps are available for continuous SC infusion use
Intravenous (IV) Bolus Infusion	Severe pain (rapid control needed) Dying patient with rapidly escalating pain Postoperative period Children unable to take oral medications Alternative routes ineffective	Bioavailability 100% Rapid onset of action (10–15 min) Can be given by bolus or continuous infusion Variety of access ports available Milligram dose of drug administered not limited by volume requirement	Need for IV access Short duration of effect with bolus "Bolus" effect with intermittent injections Hospital constraints (e.g., nurses not permitted to administer IV opioid bolus)	IV opioids do not guarantee adequate pain relief

Continued on following page.

Addiction is defined as a pattern of compulsive drug use characterized by a continued craving for an opioid and loss of control (psychologic dependence) and continued use despite harm to the user or others. Addiction is rare in patients who are receiving opioids for cancer pain (Porter & Jick, 1980), but concern about this outcome is a reason for undertreatment (Cleeland, 1989; Foley, 1989a; Hill & Fields, 1989; Jaffe, 1989; Jaffe & Martin, 1990; Morgan, 1989; Schuster, 1989). In the setting of poorly relieved pain, "aberrant" drug-seeking behavior such as "clock watching" requires careful assessment. For the most part, this signifies inadequate pain relief. The term "pseudoaddiction" has been used to describe drug-seeking behavior reminiscent of addiction that occurs in the setting of inade-

quate pain relief and is eliminated by improved analgesia (Weissman & Haddox, 1989). The risk of compromising the patient's physical and psychologic functioning through inadequate pain management is great, and a well-informed oncology nurse is the patient's best advocate in these situations.

A group of patients who are at high risk for having their pain undertreated because of fear of addiction are those with a history of drug abuse who develop cancer pain. Within this category, three subgroups of patients can be identified: those who are actively using street drugs, those who are in methadone maintenance programs, and those who have not abused drugs for many years (Foley, 1985). Patients in the first subgroup strain the resources of the most sophisticated pain manage-

TABLE 57–4. *Commonly Used Routes of Drug Administration* Continued

ROUTE	PATIENT SELECTION CRITERIA	ADVANTAGES	DISADVANTAGES	COMMENTS
Epidural (ED) and Intrathecal (IT)	Pain mid-chest preferable or midline sacral or perineal Unable to tolerate side effects of opioids by other routes	Selective activation of spinal opiod receptors so that analgesia may be achieved with fewer side effects Smaller dose of opioid required than when given by alternate route	Adverse effects can be similar to those after systemic administration Onset of analgesia may occur later than IV route (30–60 min with morphine) Respiratory depression from morphine can occur both early (after 1–2 hr) and late (after 6–25 hr) Adverse effects include facial pruritis and urinary retention (15%)	Epidural opioids are administered by intermittent injection, continuous infusions, or both (the family can be taught to do this) Intrathecal opioids are usually administered via an implanted catheter and subcutaneous resevoir by continuous infusion A patient who is tolerant to opioids by the oral or parenteral route will also be tolerant to opioids by the IT or ED route To determine the dose for IT morphine: Administer via lumbar puncture 0.5–1.0 mg IT for each 10 mg IM q4h given systemically Titrate slowly for adequate pain relief (assessed as 50% pain relief over 8 hrs) This dose provides the basis for calculating the initial morphine infusion. Clinical experience indicates this should be 2–3 times the bolus dose of morphine delivered over the next 24 hrs If the initial infusion rate provides inadequate analgesia, the dose can be increased by 50% to 100% (CSF elimination half-life of morphine is about 2 hrs. It takes 8 to 10 hrs to reach steady state. Therefore, it is important to assess the effect of each infusion rate over at least a 24 hr period before dose escalation

TABLE 57–5. *Nursing Guidelines for the Use of Opioids in Chronic Cancer Pain*

1. Select a drug from step 2 or step 3 of the "analgesic ladder" appropriate to the patient's level of pain and analgesic history.
2. Take into consideration patient's age, metabolic state, presence of major organ failure (renal, hepatic, or respiratory), and presence of coexisting disease.
3. Consider pharmacologic issues (e.g., potential accumulation of metabolites and effects of concurrent drugs and possible interactions).
4. Know the drug class (e.g., agonist, agonist/antagonist), duration of analgesic effects, and pharmacokinetic properties.
5. Be knowledgeable about the various drug formulations available (e.g., controlled-release or immediate-release).
6. Be aware of the available routes of drug administration (e.g., oral, rectal, transdermal, subcutaneous, and intravenous) and equianalgesic doses among drugs and between routes.
7. Select the least invasive route appropriate to the patients needs.
8. Consider patient compliance, convenience, ease for home management, and cost.
9. Administer the analgesic(s) on a regular basis. Make sure supplemental or "rescue" doses are available.
10. Use drug combinations, if appropriate, to provide added analgesia (e.g., NSAIDs and adjuvants).
11. Avoid drug combinations that increase sedation without enhancing analgesia (e.g., most phenothiazines).
12. Anticipate and treat side effects.
13. Prevent precipitating an acute withdrawal syndrome in the patient who is physically dependent on an opioid drug (e.g., dilute naloxone, 0.4:10 ml of saline if needed to reverse respiratory depression; taper opioids if the patient is painfree).
14. Systematically evaluate effectiveness of analgesic regimen (amount of relief, duration of relief, frequency of breakthrough pain, number and pattern of supplementary or "rescue" doses used in a 24-hour period, presence of side effects, and satisfaction with mode of therapy).
15. Teach the patient and family the principles of analgesic use. Include the clinical significance of tolerance, physical dependence, and psychologic dependence.

(Adapted from Coyle, N., Cherny, N. I., & Portenoy, R. K. [1995]. Pharmacologic management of cancer pain. In D. B. McGuire, C. H. Yarbro, & B. R. Ferrell [Eds.], *Cancer pain management* [2nd ed., p. 99]. © 1995 Boston: Jones & Bartlett Publishers. Reprinted with permission.)

ment team and require tight controls during opioid therapy. One oncology nurse should be identified as the individual to coordinate care, and one physician should be identified as the individual to write all analgesic prescriptions. It must be recognized that these patients may experience severe pain like any other cancer patient but may well require larger doses of opioids because of tolerance. Patients in methadone maintenance programs and those who have not used drugs for many years usually only present a problem of undertreatment. Patients in methadone maintenance programs may require relatively larger doses of opioids to control pain. This is tolerance, not drug abuse. Staff may have concerns about administering opioid drugs to those with a history of drug abuse. The validity of such concerns must be addressed by knowledgeable professionals (Passik, 1993).

Overall, oncology nurses play a major role in educating their colleagues as well as patients and families that the risk of addiction is extremely small when patients are receiving opioids for cancer pain.

OPIOID SIDE EFFECTS AND THEIR MANAGEMENT

Constipation. Constipation is the most frequently encountered side effect experienced during opioid therapy (Foley & Inturrisi, 1987; Inturrisi, 1989; Sykes, 1991; Walsh, 1990). Opioid binding to peripheral receptors in the gut prolongs colonic transit time by increasing segmental contractions and decreasing propulsive peristalsis. Central opioid receptors are also thought to be involved in colonic transit and the urge to defecate (Kaufman et al., 1988; Rogers & Cerda, 1989). Tolerance may develop very slowly, if at all, to these opioid effects. Because the likelihood of constipation is so great for the cancer patient on chronic opioid therapy,

especially those who are elderly, immobile, debilitated or have abdomial disease, laxative medications are frequently prescribed in a preemptive manner (Cherny & Portenoy, 1994). Table 57–6 outlines a nursing approach to the assessment and management of constipation in the patient receiving chronic opioid therapy.

Sedation. Some level of sedation is experienced by many patients at the initiation of opioid therapy and during significant dose escalation. Patients usually develop tolerance to this effect in days to weeks. Should sedation persist, however, careful evaluation by the nurse is needed. Confounding factors such as other sedating drugs, metabolic disturbances, and sleep deprivation must be identified. Nursing evaluation and management of persistant sedation in the cancer patient receiving opioid therapy is outlined in Table 57–7. Management steps include elimination of nonessential drugs with central nervous system depressant effects, reduction of the opioid dose if feasible, changing to an alternative opioid, and, if necessary, adding a psychostimulant such as dextroamphetamine, methylphenidate, or pemoline (Bruera, Brenneis, Paterson, & MacDonald, 1989; Bruera, Chadwick, Brenneis, Hanson, & MacDonald, 1987; Forrest, Brown, & Brown, 1977).

Respiratory Depression. Fear of respiratory depression is a frequently cited concern among medical and nursing staff when initiating opioid therapy or when rapidly increasing opioid drugs to control pain in a debilitated cancer patient and is a major reason for inadequate cancer pain management. Respiratory depression appears to be mediated by a specific opioid receptor subtype (mu2) in the medulla (Ling, Spiegel, Lockhart, & Pasternak, 1985). It is important for the oncology nurse to recognize that clinically significant respiratory depression is always accompanied by other signs of cen-

TABLE 57–6. *Nursing Guidelines in Assessment and Management of Constipation in the Patient Receiving Chronic Opioid Therapy*

1. Identify "normal" bowel pattern for individual patient.
2. Identify present bowel pattern and how it varies from the patient's norm.
3. Identify factors that may be contributing to the patient's constipation and address those that are treatable:
   - Drugs (e.g., opioids or tricyclics).
   - Inactivity.
   - Generalized weakness (e.g., unable to get to the toilet).
   - Lack of privacy when toileting.
   - Dehydration, fever.
   - Poor diet (lack of bulk and fiber).
   - Metabolic (e.g., hypercalcemia, hypokalemia).
4. Disimpact patient if necessary.
5. Establish a bowel management program appropriate to the patient and level of debility
   - Anticipate daily oral laxatives will be needed by most patients receiving ATC opioids.
   - Consider combination of stool softener with drug that increases peristalsis as a first-line management approach (e.g., docusate plus senna).
   - Use bulk agent to supplement fiber in the diet if appropriate; avoid in severly debilitated patients and those with partial bowel obstruction. May increase flatulance, distension, bloating, and abdominal pain in patients with intraabdominal disease.
   - Have "backup" agents available for episodes of refractory constipation (e.g., lactulose, magnesium citrate, rectal suppository, enema).
6. In patients with persistant refractory constipation consider use of:
   - A prokinetic agent to improve colonic transit (e.g., cisapride or metaclopramide).
   - Oral administration of naloxone to produce "bowel withdrawal" without concurrent systemic withdrawal. Treatment should always incorporate dose escalation (e.g., starting at a dose 0.8 mg daily, and doubling the dose every 2 to 3 days until a favorable response or signs of withdrawal occur).

(Adapted from Coyle, N., Cherny, N. I., & Portenoy, R. K. [1995]. Pharmacologic management of cancer pain. In D. B. McGuire, C. H. Yarbro, & B. R. Ferrell [Eds.], *Cancer pain management* [2nd ed., p. 112]. © 1995 Boston: Jones & Bartlett Publishers. Reprinted with permission.)

tral nervous system (CNS) depression, such as sedation and mental clouding, and is unusual in the patient receiving chronic opioid therapy unless other contributing factors are present. Pain antagonizes CNS depression, and respiratory effects are unlikely to occur in the presence of severe pain. With repeated administration of an opioid, tolerance develops rapidly to the respiratory depressant effects of the drug. Rare patients have been known to tolerate in excess of the equivalent of 35 g of morphine per 24 hours to control pain without becoming respiratory depressed (Coyle et al., 1990). Unwarranted concerns about respiratory depression should not interfere with appropriate upward titration of opioid drugs to pain relief or the onset of intolerable and unmanageable side effects. However, opioid-induced respiratory depression can occur if pain is suddenly eliminated (e.g., after a neurolytic or neuroablative procedure) and the opioid is not reduced.

Confusion. Like sedation, cognitive impairment is common after initiation of opioid therapy or dose escalation (Bruera, Macmillan, Hanson, & MacDonald, 1989). Patients may express this as "feeling hazy" or 'not as sharp as before." Patients should be reassured that these effects are transient in most patients and last from a few days to a week or two. Persistant confusion attributable to opioids alone is uncommon. Potential causes for persistant confusion include electrolyte disorders, neoplastic involvement of the CNS, sepsis, vital

TABLE 57–7. *Nursing Guidelines to Assessment and Management of Persistant Sedation in the Patient Receiving Chronic Opioid Therapy*

1. Evaluate potential disease or treatment-related causes for patient's persistant sedation, including sleep deprivation.
2. Eliminate nonessential central nervous system depressant medication.
3. If analgesia is satisfactory, reduce opioid dose by 25%.
4. If analgesia is unsatisfactory, or dose reduction is not viable, consider switching to an alternate opioid, especially if the present opioid is one with a long half-life.
5. Consider addition of a NSAID or adjuvant analgesic that may allow reduction in opioid dose without compromise to analgesia.
6. If sedation persists:
   - Consider addition of a psychostimulant.
   - Consider change to the intraspinal route to allow dose reduction.
   - Consider use of an anesthetic or neurosurgical approach.

(Adapted from Coyle, N., Cherny, N. I., & Portenoy, R. K. [1995]. Pharmacologic management of cancer pain. In D. B. McGuire, C. H. Yarbro, & B. R. Ferrell [Eds.], *Cancer pain management* [2nd ed., p. 110]. © 1995 Boston: Jones & Bartlett Publishers. Reprinted with permission.)

organ failure, and hypoxia (Bruera, Chadwick, Weinlick, & MacDonald, 1987; Breitbart & Holland, 1988). Table 57–8 guides the nurse in the evaluation and management of persistant confusion in the cancer patient receiving opioid therapy.

Nausea and Vomiting. Nausea and vomiting are not uncommon at the start of opioid therapy (Campora et al., 1991; Walsh, 1990). Tolerance to this effect typically develops within weeks. Both peripheral and central mechanisms are thought to be involved. Opioids stimulate the medullary chemoreceptor trigger zone and increase vestibular sensitivity. Direct effects on the gastrointestinal tract include increased gastric antral tone, diminished motility, and delayed gastric emptying (Rogers & Cerda, 1989). Constipation may also be a contributing factor. Establishing the pattern of nausea may clarify the etiology of the symptom and guide management approaches. Frequently, a combination of cognitive and pharmacologic approaches are used, depending on the pattern of the nausea and assumed underlying mechanism. Cognitive techniques might include relaxation training with focused breathing, guided imagery, and distraction. For nausea associated with early satiety and bloating, which can be features of delayed gastric emptying, metoclopramide is often the initial pharmacologic approach. If vertigo or movement-induced nausea are the predominant features, the patient may benefit from an antivertigenous drug, such as scopolamine (in patch form) or meclizine. Other options include trials of alternative opioids or treatment with an antihistamine (e.g., hydroxyzine or diphenhydramine), neuroleptic (e.g., haloperidol or chlorpromazine), benzodiazepine (e.g., lorazepam), or steroid (e.g., dexamethasone). The role of the serotonin antagonists (e.g., odansetron) has not been established in opioid-induced nausea and vomiting.

Multifocal Myoclonus. Mild and infrequent multifocal myoclonus can occur with all opioids but is most prominent with meperidine, presumably due to metabolite accumulation. The effect is dose-related, and the mechanism is unclear. If the myoclonus is pronounced and distressing to the patient, the opioid may be switched, a benzodiazepine (e.g., clonazepam) may be added (Eisele, Grigsby, & Dea, 1992), or the use of intraspinal opioids or neurolytic techniques might be considered.

Urinary Retention. Urinary retention can occasionally occur in patients receiving opioid drugs. Opioids increase smooth muscle tone and infrequently cause bladder spasm or an increase in spincter tone. The latter may lead to urinary retention (Jaffe & Martin, 1990). Tolerance can develop rapidly, but catheterization may be needed for a short period.

ADJUVANT ANALGESICS

"Adjuvant analgesics" are those drugs that have a primary indication other than pain but are analgesic in some painful conditions (Walsh, 1990a). These drugs can be used at any step of the "analgesic ladder." Adjuvant analgesics can be classified into three broad groups: multipurpose adjuvant analgesics; adjuvant analgesics used predominently for neuropathic pain, and adjuvant analgesics used for bone pain. Table 57–9 provides a guide to the commonly used adjuvant drugs. As a general principle, low initial doses and dose titration is suggested.

MULTIPURPOSE ADJUVANT ANALGESICS

CORTICOSTEROIDS

Corticosteroids are used both chronically in the advanced cancer patient and acutely in the patient with a pain flare (Cherny & Portenoy, 1994; Ettinger & Portenoy, 1988). The use of steroids can be particularly helpful in patients with metastatic bone pain and patients with neuropathic pain associated with infiltration or compression by tumor. Pain relief is assumed to be associated with antiiflammatory and antiedema effects.

NEUROLEPTICS

Methotrimeprazine has an analgesic effect similar to that of morphine in the nontolerant patient (Montilla, Frederick, & Cass, 1963; Oliver, 1985). The sedative, anxiolytic, antiemetic effects of this drug can be very helpful for the far-advanced cancer patient who is confined to bed. Sedative effects as well as the potential for significant hypotension, however, limit its use in the more active individual. The analgesic effects of other neuroleptic drugs have not been confirmed, and their role in cancer pain management is limited. Patients receiving neuroleptic drugs must be monitored for early signs of extrapyramidal effects, including akithisia, parkinsonism, acute dystonic reaction, and tardive dyskinesia. If the patient is benefiting from the neu-

TABLE 57–8. *Nursing Guidelines to the Assessment and Management of Confusion in the Patient Receiving Chronic Opioid Therapy*

1. Evaluate potential disease or treatment-related causes for the patient's confusion, include sleep deprivation. Treat underlying cause wherever possible.
2. Review patient's drug therapy. Eliminate nonessential centrally acting medications.
3. If analgesia is satisfactory, reduce opioids by 25%; reassess.
4. If analgesia is unsatisfactory or confusion persists, consider switching to an alternate opioid. Select one with a short half-life.
5. Consider trial of a neuroleptic (e.g., haloperidol).
6. Consider use of anaesthetic or neurosurgical technique to allow for opioid reduction.

(Adapted from Coyle, N., Cherny, N. I., & Portenoy, R. K. [1995]. Pharmacologic management of cancer pain. In D. B. McGuire, C. H. Yarbro, & B. R. Ferrell [Eds.], *Cancer pain management* [2nd ed., p. 111]. © 1995 Boston: Jones & Bartlett Publishers. Reprinted with permission.)

TABLE 57–9. *Commonly Used Adjuvant Analgesics**

CLASS	INDICATION	PREFERRED DRUGS	DOSING SCHEDULE	STARTING DOSE (MG/DAY)	USUAL DAILY DOSE (MG/DAY)	COMMENT
Antidepressants	Continuous neuropathic pain. Pain complicated by depression or insomnia	Amitriptyline Doxepin Imipramine Desipramine Nortriptyline Paroxetine	qhs	10–25	50–150	Amitriptyline preferred. If toxicity too great, trial of desipramine, or nortriptyline, or paroxetine.
Anticonvulsants	Lancinating neuropathic pain	Carbamazepine Phenytoin Valproate Clonazepam Baclofen	q 6–8 h qhs q 8 h q 12 h q 8 h	200 300 500 0.5 15	600–1600 300 750–2250 or higher 2–7 30–60 or higher	Baclofen is not an anticonvulsant but has potential efficacy in lancinating pain.
Oral local anesthetics	Neuropathic pain	Mexiletine Tocainide	q 8 h q 8 h	300 600	450–900 1200–1800	Mexiletine is safer than tocainide and should be tried first.
Neuroleptics	Pain complicated by delirium or nausea; refractory neuropathic pain	Fluphenazine Haloperidol Methotrimeprazine	q 8 h q 6–12 h q 6 h	2 2 20	3–6 2–10 20–60	Not first-line. Potential toxicity. Methotrimeprazine is proven analgesic and is useful for terminal pain and agitation.
Muscle relaxants	Acute musculoskeletal pain	Orphenadrine Carisoprodol Chlorzoxazone Methocarbamol Cyclobenzaprine	q 6–8 h q 6 h q 6–8 h q 6 h q 8 h	100 800 750 4000 30	100–200 800–1200 750–100 4000 30	Mechanism of action unknown.
Antihistamines	Pain complicated by anxiety or nausea	Hydroxyzine	q 6–8 h	75	200	Hydroxyzine analgesic in controlled trials of high parenteral doses. No evidence of analgesia from oral doses.
Corticosteroids	Pain from infiltration of neural structures; bone pain; pain in patients with far advanced disease	Dexamethasone	q 6–8 h	10–20, then 1–2 q 12 h, or lower or higher depending on need	2–24 2–24	Higher doses used in cord compression.
Analeptics	To reduce opioid-induced sedation	Methylphenidate Dextroamphetamine Pemoline	2/day 2/day 2/day	5 5 17.5	10–40 10–40 17.5–75	Higher doses sometimes needed.
Bisphosphonates	Bone pain	Pamidronate	60 mg IV every other week	—	—	Inhibit osteoclast activity. Need to monitor blood calcium and phosphate, magnesium, and potassium.
Radiopharmaceuticals	Bone pain	Strontium-89	Single dose	—	—	Absorbed at areas of high bone turnover. Marrow toxicity mild.
Miscellaneous	Bone pain	Calcitonin	Daily	25 I. U.	100–200 I. U.	Limited reports of efficacy in bone pain.

*Table based on clinical experience of the authors and a variety of published sources.
q = every hour; h = hour.
(Reproduced with permission from Coyle, N., Cherny, N. I., & Portenoy, R. K. [1995]. Pharmacologic management of cancer pain. In D. B. McGuire, C. H. Yarbro, & B. R. Ferrell [Eds.], *Cancer pain management* [2nd ed., pp. 118–119]. © 1995 Boston: Jones & Bartlett Publishers. Reprinted with permission.)

roleptic but early signs of extrapyramidal effects are manifesting, concurrent use of an anticholinergic drug, such as benzotropine, is suggested.

ANTIHISTAMINES

Although single-dose studies demonstrate analgesic effects of diphenhydramine, hydroxyzine, ophenadrine, phenyltoloxamine, and pyrilamine (Batterman, 1965; Beaver & Feise, 1976; Gold, 1978; Campos & Solis, 1980; Hupert, Yacoub, & Turgeon, 1980; McColl & Durkin, 1982; Sunshine et al., 1989), clinical experience does not support the use of these drugs as adjuvant analgesics for cancer pain. These drugs are of most help to patients who have anxiety, nausea, or itch associated with their pain.

PSYCHOSTIMULANTS

Controlled studies have demonstrated analgesic effects of dextroamphetamine, methylphenidate, caffeine, and intranasal cocaine (Forrest et al., 1977; Yang, Clark, Dooley, & Mignogna, 1982; Laska et al., 1983; Cantello et al., 1988; Marbach & Wallenstein, 1988). A controlled repeated dose trial of methylphenidate in patients with cancer demonstrated an improvement in analgesia and sedation (Bruera, Chadwick et al., 1987).

BENZODIAZEPINES

The use of these drugs are limited because of their marked sedative effects. The exceptions are clonazepam, which is used to relieve lancinating neuropathic pain, and diazepam, which is useful in relieving muscle spasm (Caccia, 1975; Fernandez, Adams, & Holmes, 1987; Portenoy, 1993; Swerdlow & Cundill, 1981).

ADJUVANT ANALGESICS USED PREDOMINENTLY FOR NEUROPATHIC PAIN

ANTIDEPRESSANT DRUGS

Antidepressant drugs are nonspecific analgesics that are used predominently for neuropathic pain in the cancer population (Portenoy, 1991). Analgesia associated with the antidepressants is thought to result from enhancement of neurotransmitter activity in endogenous pain-modulating pathways (Basbaum & Fields, 1984; Besson & Chaouch, 1987; Yaksh, 1979). Analgesia can occur in the absence of mood change, and the effective analgesic dose is usually much lower than that required to treat depression (Max et al., 1987; Watson et al., 1982). Some tricyclic antidepressants have also been shown to increase plasma concentration of morphine in cancer patients. Common dose-related side effects include sedation, orthostatic hypotension, constipation, dry mouth, and dizziness. Cardiotoxicity is rare (Glassman & Bigger, 1981), but in patients at risk, less cardiogenic drugs are suggested, such as desipramine. The starting dose of a tricyclic antidepressant should be low (refer to Table 57–8), with the dose increased every few days. The usual effective dosing range is 50 to 150 mg of amitriptyline, imipramine, doxepin, or desipramine daily. Analgesia is usually achieved in about a week after achieving a therapeutic

dosing level. Because of the sedative effects, most patients prefer to be treated with a single nighttime dose.

ORAL LOCAL ANESTHETICS

Oral local anesthetics are used in the management of lancinating and continuous neuropathic pain after patients have failed to respond to tricyclic antidepressants, anticonvulsant drugs, and baclofen. Their use should be avoided in patients with cardiac arrhythmias. Mexiletine is the safest of the oral local anesthetics (Portenoy, 1993).

CLONIDINE

Patients with neuropathic pain refractory to opioids and other adjuvants may benefit from a trial of oral or transdermal clonidine. Clonidine is an α-2-adrenergic agonist that has antinociceptive effects (Quan, Wandres, & Schroeder, 1993).

CAPSAICIN

Topical application of capsaicin may reduce central transmission about a noxious stimulus (Dubner, 1991). Patients with postherpetic neuralgia have benefited from this effect (Bernstein, Bickers, Dahl, & Roshal, 1987; Watson et al., 1988). An unpleasant burning sensation may follow topical application of capsaicin, making its use intolerable for some patients. Cutaneous lidocaine 5 per cent prior to treatment can be helpful.

TOPICAL ANESTHETICS

Topical local anesthetics may be effective for patients with neuropathic pain syndromes associated with a peripheral focus. EMLA, a mixture of lidocaine and prilocaine, has been used extensively to decrease venipuncture discomfort in children (Juhlin & Evers, 1990; Lycka, 1992). There has been a limited experience in its use for postherpetic neuralgia and postmastectomy pain (Watson et al., 1988, 1989).

ANTICONVULSANT DRUGS

Carbamazepine, phenytoin, clonazepam, and valproate are the anticonvulsants most frequently used in the management of lancinating dysesthetic pain. Dosing is similar to that for anticonvulsant activity (Portenoy 1993; Swerdlow, 1984; Swerdlow & Cundill, 1981).

BACLOFEN

A drug used primarily for spacticity, baclofen is potentially analgesic for lancinating or paroxysmal pains associated with neural injury of any kind. The principal side effects are sedation and confusion. Dosing is similar to that used for spacticity.

PIMOZIDE

A neuroleptic, pimozide is effective in treating patients with trigeminal neuralgia (Lechin et al., 1989). Because of the higher incidence of adverse effects, pimozide is considered a second-line drug.

Box 57–1. *Illustrative Case*

A 59-year-old man presents with arm, shoulder, and chest pain due to invasion of the chest wall and brachial plexus by an apical lung cancer. He has not responded to radiation therapy and chemotherapy. History is remarkable for a major gastrointestinal hemorrhage from a gastric ulcer 2 years earlier. Analgesic use is limited to an occasional acetaminophen for headaches. He is married and has two adult children.

Patient Encounter 1
Pain severity and descriptors: Mild, aching, (1–2/10), in arm, shoulder, amd chest.
Inferred pain pathophysiology: Somatic and neuropathic.
Analgesic selection: Acetaminophen 650 mg orally (PO), every 4 hours.
Step on Analgesic Ladder: ONE.
Rationale: Step one of the "analgesic ladder" indicated because patient had mild pain. Analgesic history indicated that he had done well with acetaminophen in the past. NSAIDs relatively contraindicated because of history of ulcer. (Note: if patient's pain was moderate to severe on the first encounter, it would have been appropriate to start the patient on Step 2 or Step 3 of the "analgesic ladder.")
Potential side effects: None.
Outcome: Good pain relief for 3 to 4 weeks.

Patient Encounter 2
Pain severity and descriptors: The patient returns to the clinic with complaints of escalating chest wall pain. The pain was described as aching and constant, moderate in severity (5–6/10).
Inferred pain pathophysiology: Somatic.
Analgesic selection: Oxycodone commenced in addition to acetaminophen and given in combination form (oxycodone 5 mg + acetaminophen 325 mg {Percocet}). To take 1 to 2 tablets PO, every 4 hours.
Step on Analgesic Ladder: TWO.
Rationale: Step 2 chosen because pain was moderate to severe.
Potential side effects: Constipation, sedation, nausea.
Outcome: Pain progressed over the next 2 to 3 days and its quality changed. Percocet intake was 12 tablets per day. No side effects were reported.

Patient Encounter 3
Pain severity and descriptors: Aching, burning, constant, radiating from chest and shoulder into arm, moderate to severe (7–8/10). Disturbed sleep and ability to concentrate.
Inferred pain pathophysiology: Neuropathic and somatic.
Analgesic selection: Percocet was changed to morphine sulphate 15 mg + acetaminophen 650 mg PO, every 4 hours, around the clock, with morphine sulfate 15 mg "rescues" every 1 to 2 hours as needed (prn). An adjuvant, amitryptyline 25 mg was added at night.
Step on Analgesic Ladder: THREE.
Rationale: Step 3 of the analgesic ladder was selected because the patient's pain was severe. An adjuvant drug was added because of the neuropathic component of the pain. The opioid dose was determined as follows: 10 mg of morphine PO is considered to be equianalgesic to 10 mg of oxycodone PO (= 2 Percocet). Because the pain was not controlled, the equianalgesic dose was increased by 50 per cent. The "rescue" dose of morphine sulphate of 15 mg PO every 1 to 2 hours prn was selected based on a 5 to 15 per cent ratio of his 24-hour baseline morphine dose. The dose, 15 mg, is in fact 17 per cent of the 24-hour dose but was chosen because of the available tablet size.
Possible side effects: Constipation, sedation, nausea, dry mouth.

ADJUVANT ANALGESICS USED FOR BONE PAIN

Bone pain is an extremely common problem for cancer patients. NSAIDs can be helpful in combination with the opioids (step 2 and 3 of the "analgesic ladder"). Corticosteroids can produce dramatic relief in difficult cases.

BISPHOSPHONATES AND RADIOPHARMACEUTICALS

Bisphosphonates inhibit osteoclast activity and thereby reduce bone resorption. They have also been shown to reduce bone pain associated with cancer (Body, 1992; Fitton & McTavish, 1991; Kanis, McCloskey, Taube, & O'Rourke, 1991). Pamidronate should be considered in patients with bone pain that has been refractory to other therapies (Fitton & McTavish, 1991). Strontium-89, a radiopharmaceutical, has also been approved for this indication (Laing et al., 1991; Fossa, Paus, Lochoff, Backe, & Aas, 1992; Robinson, Preston, Spicer, & Baxter, 1992).

CALCITONIN

A trial of calcitonin should also be considered in patients with refractory bone pain (Blomquist, Elomaa, Porkka, Karonen, & Lamberg-Allardt, 1988; Hindley, Hill, Leyland, & Wiles, 1982). Close monitoring of calcium and phosphate is needed if such an approach is to be used.

SUMMARY

Nurses have a responsibilty to understand the basic principles of pharmacolgic analgesic therapy and to constantly update their knowledge as new drugs are introduced and more effective approaches to analgesic side

---

Box 57–1. *Illustrative Case* Continued

Outcome: Thirty-six hours later the patient called to say that his pain control had markedly improved but only in the setting of frequent "rescue" doses. Overall, with "rescues," pain was 75 per cent better. He had required nine "rescue" doses in the previous 24 hours (15 mg × 9 = an additional 135 mg of morphine). Consequently his baseline morpine dose was increased by approximately the equivalent amount, to 30 mg PO every 4 hours. The dose chosen was a slightly lower dose than the total of the baseline plus "rescues" but reflected the available tablet size and was considered likely to provide adequate analgesia. Rescue medication continued to be available. His "rescue" dose was adjusted to reflect 5 to 15 per cent of the new 24-hour baseline dose of 180 mg, at 30 mg every 2 hours prn. Again, this dose, 30 mg, is in fact 17 per cent of the 24-hour dose but was chosen because of the available tablet size. Adjustment was undertaken because the 15 mg dose was not providing effective analgesia.

Good pain control was reached with "rescue" doses used only once or twice a day in relation to a specific activity. Once stable pain relief was established, he was switched to a controlled-release oral morphine preparation, allowing for 12-hour dosing. The equivalent dose he received was 90 mg Q 12 H; the "rescue" dose was left unchanged. The amitryptyline was increased every 3 to 4 days until the analgesia it provided seemed maximal and he was sleeping well; the dose reached was 100 mg qhs. Mild nausea and mental clouding resolved after a few days. Constipation was treated with a bowel regimen (refer to appropriate table for management).

He did relatively well for several months; however, his disease was progressing and intermittent upward titration of his baseline dose was undertaken based on his "rescue" requirement. Four months later he was taking controlled-release morphine 180 mg every 12 hours, and the "rescue" dose remained at 30 mg immediate release morphine every 1 to 2 hours prn (within 5 to 15 per cent of baseline and providing effective analgesia).

Patient Encounter 4

A fall at home resulted in a fractured femur. The patient elected to have surgery as a means of allowing prompt mobilization that could facilitate an improved quality of life. Preoperatively his leg pain was severe, and analgesic therapy needed to be adjusted.

Pain severity and descriptors: Sharp, 9–10/10 on movement.

Inferred pain pathophysiology: Somatic. Acute pain superimposed on chronic chest wall and arm pain.

Analgesic selection: Morphine was continued, but the route of administration was changed from an oral to an intravenous infusion. His infusion rate was started at 7.5 mg per hour with 4 mg "rescues" available every 30 minutes prn.

Step on Analgesic Ladder: THREE.

Rationale: Because of the severity of the pain, the equianalgesic dose was increased by 50 per cent when switching from the oral to the intravenous route. Using a 3:1 oral/intravenous ratio, his infusion rate was started at 7.5 mg per hour (360 mg +180 mg = 540 mg oral morphine/24 hours = 180 mg intravenous morphine/24 hours = 7.5 mg/hour), with 4 mg "rescues" available every 30 minutes prn. (The total hourly rescue was approximately 5 per cent of the total daily dose, and the first dose given provided effective analgesia. If it had not, the rescue dose would have been escalated by 30 to 50 per cent.) Although several "rescues" were required in the first few hours, the need for these subsided. Surgical recovery was uneventful. Five days after surgery, he was able to take PO medications and was using very occasional "rescue" doses. He was, however, anxious about the planned switch to oral pain medication and requested that it be done gradually. The IV infusion was initially decreased to approximately half (3.5 mg per hour) and he was given the equivalent dose, 130 mg every 12 hours, in a controlled-release oral morphine preparation. He continued to have intravenous "rescues" available to him as before. Forty-eight hours later his intravenous infusion had been discontinued, and he was taking the equivalent controlled-release morphine dosage of 260 mg every 12 hours by mouth. "Rescue" doses of oral morphine sulphate immediate release, 60 mg (5 to 15 per cent of 24-hour opioid dose) were available to him every 1 to 2 hours prn. Amitryptyline was restarted at 25 mg qhs and gradually titrated up to its previous level of 100 mg.

Outcome: The patient's pain remained well controlled at home on oral analgesics until his death 4 weeks postdischarge. Ongoing assessment and reassessment by the nurse in liaison with the paient's primary physician were critical components in managing the analgesic approach to this man's pain. The assessent included the effectiveness of relief, the duration of relief, the effectiveness of "rescue" doses, and the presence and management of side effects.

---

effect management are devised. Application of this knowledge by the bedside, in the clinic, and in the home will have a major impact on the quality of life of cancer patients and their families. Box 57–1 presents a case in which four different pharmacologic therapies were used.

REFERENCES

Adams, F., Cruz, L., Deachman, M. J., & Zamora, E. (1989). Focal subdermal toxicity with subcutaneous opioid infusion in patients with cancer pain. *Journal of Pain and Symptom Management, 4*(1), 31–33.

Agency for Health Care Policy and Research. (1994). *Management of cancer pain.* Washington, D.C.: U. S. Department of Health and Human Services.

American Pain Society. (1992). *Principles of analgesic use in the treatment of acute pain and chronic cancer pain: A concise guide to medical practice.* Skokie, IL: American Pain Society.

Arner, S., Rawal, N., & Gustafsson, L. L. (1988). Clinical experience of long-term treatment with epidural and intrathecal opioids—a nationwide survey. *Anaesthesiology Scandinavia, 32,* 253–259.

Basbaum, A. I., & Fields, H. L. (1984). Endogenous pain control systems: brainstem spinal pathways and endorphin circuitry. *Annals Review Neurosciences, 7,* 309–338.

Batterman, R. C. (1965). Methodology of analgesic evaluation: experience with orphenadrine citrate compound. *Current Therapeutic Research, 7,* 639–647.

Beaver, W. T., & Feise, G. (1976). Comparison of the analgesic effect of morphine, hydroxyzine and their combination in patients with postoperative pain. In J. J. Bonicca & D. Albe-Fessard (Eds.), *First international congress on pain* (pp. 553–557). New York: Raven Press.

Bernstein, J. E., Bickers, D. R., Dahl, M. V., & Roshal, J. V. (1987). Treatment of chronic postherpetic neuralgia with topical capsaicin. *Journal of the American Academy of Dermatology, 17,* 93–96.

Besson, J. M., & Chaouch, A. (1987). Peripheral and spinal mechanisms of nociception. *Physiology Reviews, 67,* 67–186.

Blomquist, C., Elomaa, I., Porkka, L., Karonen, S. L., & Lamberg-Allardt, C. (1988). Evaluation of salmon calcitonin treatment in bone metastases from breast cancer—a controlled trial. *Bone, 9,* 45–51.

Body, J. J. (1992). Bone metastases and tumor-induced hypercalcemia. *Current Opinion in Oncology, 4*(4), 624–631.

Breitbart, W., & Holland, J. C. (1988). Psychiatric complications of cancer. *Current Therapeutics in Hematology Oncology, 3,* 268–275.

Bruera, E., Brenneis, C., Michaud, M., MacMullen, K., Hanson, J., & MacDonald, R. N. (1988). Patient-controlled subcutaneous hydromorphone versus continuous subcutaneous infusion for the treatment of cancer pain. *Journal of the National Cancer Institute, 80*(14), 1152–1154.

Bruera, E., Brenneis, C., Paterson, A. H., & MacDonald, R. N. (1989). Use of methylphenedate as an adjuvant to narcotic analgesics in patients with advanced cancer. *Journal of Pain and Symptom Management, 4,* 3–6.

Bruera, E., Chadwick, S., Brenneis, C. Hanson, J., & MacDonald, R. N. (1987). Methylphenidate associated with narcotics for the treatment of cancer pain. *Cancer Treatment Reports, 71,* 67–70.

Bruera, E., Chadwick, S., Weinlick, A., & MacDonald, R. N. (1987). Delirium and severe sedation in patients with terminal cancer. *Current Therapeutic Research, 71,* 787–788.

Bruera, E., Fainsinger, R., Moore, M., Thibault, R., Spoldi, E., & Ventafeidda, V. (1991). Local toxicity with subcutaneous methadone. Experience of two centers. *Pain, 45,* 141–145.

Bruera, E., Macmillan, K., Hanson, J., & MacDonald, R. N. (1989). The cognitive effects of the administration of narcotic analgesics in patients with cancer pain. *Pain, 39*(1), 13–16.

Caccia, M. R. (1975). Clonazepam in facial neuralgia and cluster headache: clinical and electrophysiological study. *European Neurology, 13,* 560–563.

Calis, K. A., Kohler, D. R., & Corso, D. M. (1992). Transdermally administered fentanyl for pain management. *Clinical Pharmacology, 11*(1), 22–36.

Campora, E., Merlini, L., Pace, M., Bruzzone, M., Luzzani, M., Gottlieb, A., & Rosso, R. (1991). The incidence of narcotic induced emesis. *Journal of Pain and Symptom Management, 6*(7), 428–430.

Campos, V. M., & Solis, E. L. (1980). The analgesic and hypothermic effects of nefopam, morphine, aspirin, diphenhydramine and placebo. *Journal of Clinical Pharmacology, 20,* 42–49.

Cantello, R., Aguggia, M., Gilli, M., Delsedime, M., Riccio, A., Rainero, I., & Mutani, R. (1988). Analgesic action of methylphenidate on parkinsonian sensory symptoms. Mechanisms and pathophysiological implications. *Archives of Neurology, 45,* 973–976.

Chapman, C. R. (1989). Giving the patient control of opioid analgesic administration. In C. S. Hill & W. S. Fields (Eds.), *Drug treatment of cancer pain in a drug oriented society* (pp. 339–351). New York, Raven Press.

Cherny, N. I., & Portenoy, R. K. (1994). Practical issues in the management of cancer pain. In P. D. Wall & R. Melzack (Eds.), *Textbook of pain* (3rd ed., pp. 1437–1467). Edinburgh: Churchill Livingstone.

Citron, M. L., Kalra, J. M., Seltzer, V. L., Chen, S., Hoffman, M., & Walczak, M. B. (1992). Patient-controlled analgesia for cancer pain: a long-term study of inpatient and outpatient use. *Cancer Investigation, 10*(5), 335–341.

Cleeland, C. S. (1989). Pain control: Public and physician's attitudes. In C. S. Hill & W. S. Fields (Eds.), *Drug treatment of cancer pain in a drug-oriented society* (pp. 81–89). New York: Raven Press.

Clissold, S. P. (1986). Aspirin and related derivatives of salicylic acid. *Drugs, 32*(Suppl. 4), 70–77.

Cooper, K., & Bennett, W. (1987). Nephrotoxicity of common drugs used in clinical practice. *Archives of Internal Medicine, 147,* 1213–1218.

Cousins, M., & Plummer, J. (1991). Spinal opioids in acute and chronic pain. In M. B. Max, R. K. Portenoy, & E. Laska (Eds.), *The design of analgesic clinical trials* (pp. 457–480). New York: Raven Press.

Coyle, N., Adelhardt, J., & Foley, K. M. (1988). Disease progression and tolerance in the cancer pain patient. 2nd International Congress on Cancer Pain. *Journal of Pain and Symptom Management, 3,*S25.

Coyle, N., Adelhardt, J., Foley, K. M., & Portenoy, R. K. (1990). Character of terminal illness in the advanced cancer patient: pain and other symptoms during last four weeks of life. *Journal of Pain and Symptom Management, 5,* 83–89.

Coyle, N., Cherny, N. I., & Portenoy, R. K. (1994). Subcutaneous opioid infusions in the home. *Oncology, 8*(4), 21–27.

Coyle N., Cherny, N. I., Portenoy, R. K. (1995). Pharmacologic management of cancer pain. In D. B. McGuire, C. H. Yarbro, & B. R. Ferrell (Eds.), *Cancer pain management* (2nd ed., pp. 89–130). Boston: Jones and Bartlett.

DiPalma, J. R. (1991). Ketorolac: an injectable NSAID. *American Family Physician, 43*(1), 207–210.

Dubner, R. (1991). Topical capsaicin therapy for neuropathic pain. *Pain, 47*(3), 247–248.

Eisele, J. H., Grigsby, E. J., & Dea G. (1992). Clonazepam treatment of myoclonic contractions associated with high dose opioids: a case report. *Pain, 49*(2), 231–232.

Ettinger, A. B., & Portenoy, R. K. (1988). The use of corticosteroids in the treatment of symptoms associated with cancer. *Journal of Pain and Symptom Management, 3,* 99–103.

Fainsinger, R., Schoeller, T., Bruera, E. (1993). Methadone in the management of cancer pain: a review. *Pain, 52*(2), 137–147.

Fernandez, F., Adams, F., Holmes, V. F. (1987). Analgesic effect of alprazolam in patients with chronic, organic pain of malignant origin. *Journal of Clinical Psychopharmacology, 3,* 167–169.

Ferrell, B. R., Eberts, M. T., McCaffery, M., & Grant, M. (1991). Clinical decision making and pain. *Cancer Nursing, 14*(6), 289–297.

Fitton, A., & McTavish, D. (1991). Pamidronate: A review of its pharmacological properties and therapeutic efficacy in resorptive bone disease. *Drugs, 41*(2), 289–318.

Foley, K. M. (1985). The treatment of cancer pain. *New England Journal of Medicine, 313,* 84–95.

Foley, K. M. (1989a). Controversies in cancer pain: medical perspective. *Cancer, 63,* 2257–2265.

Foley, K. M. (1989b). The decriminalization of cancer pain. In C. S. Hill & W. S. Field (Eds.), *Drug treatment of cancer pain in a drug-oriented society* (Vol. 11, pp. 5–18). New York: Raven Press.

Foley, K. M. (1991). Clinical tolerance to opioids. In A. I. Basbaum & J. M. Bessom (Eds.), *Towards a new pharmacotherapy of pain, dahlem konfrenzen* (pp. 181–204). Chichester: John Wiley & Sons.

Foley, K. M., & Inturrisi, C. E. (1987). Analgesic drug therapy in cancer pain: Principles and practice. *The Medical Clinics of North America, 71,* 207–232.

Forrest, W. H., Brown, B. W., & Brown, C. R. (1977). Dextroamphetamine with morphine for the treatment of postoperative pain. *New England Journal of Medicine, 296,* 712–715.

Fossa, S. D., Paus, E., Lochoff, M., Backe, S. M., & Aas, M. (1992). Strontium-89 in bone metastases from hormone resistant prostate cancer: palliation effect and biochemical changes. *British Journal of Cancer, 66*(1), 177–180.

Galer, B. S., Coyle, N., Pasterak, G. W., & Portenoy, R. K. (1992). Individual variability in the response to different opioids: report of five cases. *Pain, 49*(1), 87–91.

Glassman, A. H., & Bigger, J. T. (1981). Cardiovascular effects of therapeutic doses of tricyclic antidepressants. *Archives of General Psychiatry, 38,* 815–820.

Gold, R. H. (1978). Treatment of low back pain syndrome with oral orphenadrine citrate. *Current Therapeutic Research, 23,* 271–276.

Goodwin, J. S., & Regan, M. (1982). Cognitive dysfunction association with naproxen and ibuprofen in the elderly. *Arthritis and Rheumatism, 25,* 1013–1015.

Grond, S., Zech, D., Schug, S. A., Lynch, J., & Lehman, K. A. (1991). Validation of World Health Organization guidelines for cancer pain relief during the last days and hours of life. *Journal of Pain and Symptom Management, 6*(7), 411–422.

Hanning, C. D. (1990). The rectal absorption of opioids. In C. Benadetti, C. R. Chapman, & G. Guron (Eds.), *Opioid analgesia* (pp. 259–269). New York: Raven Press.

Hardy, P. A. I., & Wells, J. C. D. (1990). Patient controlled intrathecal morphine for cancer pain. *Clincial Journal of Pain, 6,* 57–59.

Hill, C. S., & Fields, W. S. (Eds.). (1989). Advances in Pain Research and Therapy. *Drug treatment of cancer pain in a drug oriented society* (Vol. 11). New York: Raven Press.

Hindley, A. C., Hill, A. B., Leyland, M. J., & Wiles, A. E. (1982). A double-blind controlled trial of salmon calcitonin in pain due to malignancy. *Cancer Chemotherapy and Pharmacology, 9,* 71–74.

Hirsch, J. D. (1984). Sublingual morphine sulphate in chronic pain management. *Clinical Pharmacology, 3,* 585.

Hupert, C., Yacoub, M., & Turgeon, K. R. (1980). Effect of hydroxyzine on morphine analgesia for the treatment of postoperative pain. *Anesthesia and Analgesia, 59,* 690–696.

Inturrisi, C. E. (1989). Management of cancer pain. *Cancer, 63,* 2308–2320.

Inturrisi, C. E., Colburn, W. A., Kauko, R. F., Houde, R. W., Foley, K. M. (1987). Pharmacokinetics and pharmacodynamics of methadone in patients with chronic pain. *Journal of Clinical Pharmacology & Therapeutics, 41,* 392–401.

Inturrisi, C. E., Portenoy, R. K., Max, M. B., Colburn, W. A., & Foley, K. M. (1990). Pharmacokinetic-pharmacodynamic relationships of methadone infusions in patients with cancer pain. *Journal of Clinical Pharmacology & Therapeutics, 47*(5), 565–577.

Inturrisi, C. E., & Umans, J. G. (1986). Meperidine biotransformation and central nervous system toxicity in animals and humans. In K. M. Foley & C. E. Inturrisi (Eds.), *Opioid analgesics in the management of clinical pain* (Vol. 8, pp. 143–154). New York: Raven Press.

Jaffe, J. H. (1989). Misinformation: euphoria and addiction. In C. S. Hill & W. S. Fields (Eds.), *Drug treatment of cancer pain in a drug oriented society* (Vol. 11, pp. 163–174). New York: Raven Press.

Jaffe, J. H., & Martin, W. R. (1990). Opioid analgesics and antagonists. In A. G. Gelman, T. W. Rall, A. S. Nies, & P. Taylor (Eds.), *The pharmacological basis of therapeutics* (8th ed., pp. 485–521). New York: Permagon Press.

Jorgensen, L., Mortensen, M. B., Jensen, N. H., & Eriksen, J. (1990). Treatment of cancer pain patients in a multidisciplinary pain clinic. *Pain Clinic, 3,* 83–89.

Juhlin, L., & Evers, H. (1990). EMLA: a new topical anesthetic. *Advances in Dermatology, 5*(1), 75–91.

Kaiko, R. F., Cronin, C., Healy, N., Pav, J., Thomas, G., & Goldenheim, P. D. (1989). Bioavailability of rectal and oral MS-Contin. *Proceedings of the American Society of Clinical Oncology, 8,* Abstract 1307.

Kanis, J. A., McCloskey, E. V., Taube, T., & O'Rourke, N. (1991). Rationale for the use of bisphosphonates in bone metastases. *Bone, 12*(1), 8–13.

Kanner, R. M., & Foley, K. M. (1981). Patterns of narcotic drug use in a cancer pain clinic. *Annals of New York Academy of Sciences, 362,* 161–172.

Kaufman, P. N., Krevsky, B., Malmud, L. S., Maurer, A. H., Somers, M. B., Siegel, J. A., & Fisher, R. S. (1988). Role of opiate receptors in the regulation of colonic transit. *Gastroenterology, 94*(6), 1351–1356.

Kenny, G. N. (1990). Ketorolac trometamol—a new non-opioid analgesic [editorial]. *British Journal of Anesthesia, 65*(4), 445–447.

Kerr, I. G., Sone, M., Deangelis, C., Iscoe, N., Mackenzie, R., & Schuller, T. (1988). Continuous narcotic infusion with patient-controlled analgesia for chronic cancer pain in outpatients. *Annals of Internal Medicine, 108*(4), 554–557.

Laing, A. H., Ackery, D. M., Bayly, R. J., Buchanan, R. B., Lewington, V. J., McEwan, A. J., & Lacleod, P. M. (1991). Strontium-89 chloride for pain palliation in prostatic skeletal malignancy. *British Journal of Radiology, 64*(765), 816–822.

Laska, E. M., Sunshine, A., Zigkelboim, I., Rourke, C., Marrero, I., Wanderling, J., & Olson, N. (1983). Effect of caffeine on acetaminophen analgesia. *Clinical Pharmacology and Therapeutics, 33*(4), 498–509.

Lechin, F., van der Dijs, B., Lechin, M. E., Amat, J., Lechin, A. E., Cabrera, A., Gomez, F., Acosta, E., Arocha, L., & Villa, S. (1989). Pimozide therapy for trigeminal neuralgia. *Archives of Neurology, 9,* 960–962.

Ling, G. S. F. F., Spiegel, K., Lockhart, S. H., & Pasternak, G. W. (1985). Separation of opioid analgesia from respiratory depression: evidence for different receptor mechanisms. *Journal of Pharmacology and Experimental Therapeutics, 232,* 149–155.

Lycka, B. A. (1992). EMLA. A new and effective topical anesthetic. *Journal of Dermatology Oncology, 18*(10), 859–862.

Marbach, J. J., & Wallenstein, S. L. (1988). Analgesia, mood and hemodynamic effects of intranasal cocaine and lidocaine in chronic facial pain of deafferentation and myofascial origin. *Journal of Pain and Symptom Management, 3,* 73–79.

Marlowe, S., Engstrom, R., & White, P. F. (1989). Epidural patient-controlled analgesia (PCA): an alternative to continuous epidural infusions. *Pain, 37*(1), 97–101.

Max, M. B., Culnane, M., Schafer, S. C., Gracely, R. H., Walther, D. J., Smoller, B., & Dubner, R. (1987). Amitriptyline relieves diabetic neuropathy pain in patients with normal or depressed mood. *Neurology, 37,* 589–596.

McColl, J. D., & Durkin, W. (1982). The effect of pyrilamine on relief of symptoms of the premenstrual syndrome (PMS) and primary dysmenorrhea. *Federation Proceedings, 41,* 5572.

Miser, A. W., Narang, P. K., Dolthang, P. R., Young, R. C., Sindelar, W., & Miser, J. S. (1989). Transdermal fentanyl for pain control in patients with cancer. *Pain, 37,* 15–21.

Montilla, E., Frederick, W. S., & Cass, L. J. (1963). Analgesic effects of methotrimeprazine and morphine. *Archives of Internal Medicine, 111*, 725–728.

Morgan, J. P. (1989). American opiophobia: customary underutilization of opioid analgesics. In C. S. Hill & W. S. Fields (Eds.), *Drug treatment of cancer pain in a drug oriented society* (Vol. 11, pp. 181–189). New York: Raven Press.

Moulin, D. E., Inturrisi, C. E., & Foley, K. M. (1986). Epidural and intrathecal opioids: cerebrospinal fluid and plasma pharmacokinetics in cancer pain patients. In K. M. Foley & C. E. Inturrisi (Eds.), *Opioid analgesics in the management of clinical pain* (pp. 369–384). New York: Raven Press.

Moulin, D. E., Johnson, N. G., Murray, P. N., Geoghehan, M. F., Goodwin, V. A., & Chester, M. A. (1992). Subcutaneous narcotic infusions for cancer pain: treatment outcome and guidelines for use. *Cancer Medical Association Journal, 146*(6), 891–897.

Moulin, D. E., Kreeft, J. H., Murray, P. N., & Bouguillon, A. I. (1991). Comparison of continuous subcutaneous and intravenous hydromorphone infusions for management of cancer pain. *Lancet, 337*, 465–468.

Oliver, O. J. (1985). The use of methotrimeprazine in terminal care. *British Journal of Clinical Practice, 39*, 339–340.

Osborne, R. J., Joel, S. P., & Slevin, M. L. (1986). Morphine intoxication in renal failure: the role of morphine-6-glucuronide. *British Journal of Medicine, 292*, 1548–1549.

Passik, S. (1993). Post graduate course: Concepts in acute and chronic pain management. In *Pain management in patients with a history of drug abuse.* New York: NY.

Paul, D., Standifer, K. M., Inturrisi, C. E., & Pasternak, G. W. (1989). Pharmacological characterization of morphine-6 beta-glucuronide, a very potent morphine metabolite. *Journal of Pharmacology and Experimental Therapeutics, 251*(2), 477–483.

Piletta, P., Porchet, H. C., & Dayer, P. (1991). Central analgesic effect of acetaminophen but not of aspirin. *Clinical Pharmacology and Therapeutics, 49*, 350–354.

Plummer, J. L., Gourlay, G. K., Cherry, D. A., & Cousins, M. J. (1988). Estimation of methadone clearance: Application in the management of cancer pain. *Pain, 33*, 313–322.

Portenoy, R. K. (1987). Continuous intravenous infusions of opioid drugs. *Medical Clinics of North America, 71*, 233–241.

Portenoy, R. K. (1991). Issues in the management of neuropathic pain. In A. Basbaum & J. M. Besson (Eds.), *Towards a new pharmacotherapy of pain* (pp. 393–416). New York: John Wiley & Sons.

Portenoy, R. K. (1993). Adjuvant analgesics in pain management. In D. Doyle, C. W. C. Hanks, & N. MacDonald (Eds.), *Oxford textbook of palliative medicine* (pp. 187–203). Oxford: Oxford University Press.

Portenoy, R. K., Foley, K. M., Stulmow, J., Khan, E., Adelhardt, J., Layman, M., Cerlowe, D. J., & Inturrisi, C. E. (1991). Plasma morphine and morphine-6-glucuronide during chronic morphine therapy for cancer pain: Plasma profiles, steady state concentrations and the consequences of renal failure. *Pain, 47*, 13–19.

Portenoy, R. K., & Hagen, N. A. (1990). Breakthrough pain: Definition, prevalence and characteristics. *Pain, 41*(3), 273–281.

Portenoy, R. K., Thaler, H. T., Inturrisi, C. E., Friedlander-Klar, H., & Foley, K. M. (1992). The metabolite, morphine-6-glucuronide, contributes to the analgesia produced by morphine infusion in pain patients with normal renal function. *Clinical Pharmacology and Therapeutics, 51*(4), 422–431.

Porter, J., & Jick, H. (1980). Addiction rare in patients treated with narcotics (letter). *New England Journal of Medicine, 302*, 123.

Quan, D. B., Wandres, D. L., & Schroeder, D. J. (1993). Clonidine in pain management. *Annals of Pharmacotherapeutics, 27*(3), 313–315.

Robinson, R. G., Preston, D. F., Spicer, J. A., & Baxter, K. G. (1992). Radionuclide therapy of intractable bone pain: emphasis on strontium-89. *Seminars in Nuclear Medicine, 22*(1), 28–32.

Rogers, M., & Cerda, J. J. (1989). The narcotic bowel syndrome. *Journal of Gastroenterology, 11*(2), 132–135.

Roth, S. A. (1988). Nonsteroidal antiinflammatory drugs: gastropathy, deaths, and medical practice. *Annals of Internal Medicine, 109*, 353–354.

Sawe, J., Dahlstrom, B., Pazlow, L., & Rane, A. (1981). Morphine kinetics in cancer patients. *Journal of Clinical Pharmacology and Therapeutics, 30*, 629–634.

Sawe, J., Svensson, J. O., & Odar-Cedarlof, I. (1985). Kinetics of morphine in patients with renal failure (letter). *Lancet, 2*, 211.

Saxen, M. A. (1992). The clinical pharmacology of Ketorolac. *Compendium, 13*(6), 508–509.

Schug, S. A., Zech, D., & Dorr, U. (1990). Cancer pain management according to WHO analgesic guidelines. *Journal of Pain and Symptom Management, 5*, 27–32.

Schuster, C. R. (1989). Does treatment of cancer pain with narcotics produce junkies? In C. S. Hill & W. S. Fields (Eds.), *Drug treatment of cancer pain in a drug oriented society. Advances in pain research and therapy* (Vol 11, pp. 1–3). New York: Raven Press.

Seeff, L. B., Cuccherini, B. A., Zimmerman, H. I., Adler, E., & Benjamin, S. (1986). Acetaminophen hepatotoxicity in alcoholics. *Annals of Internal Medicine, 104*, 399–404.

Storey, P., Hill, H. H., St. Louis, R., & Tarker, E. E. (1990). Subcutaneous infusions for control of cancer symptoms. *Journal of Pain and Symptom Management, 5*, 33–41.

Sunshine, A., & Olson, N. Z. (1994). Non-narcotic analgesics. *Textbook of Pain* (2nd ed., pp. 923–942). New York: Churchill Livingstone.

Sunshine, A., Zighelboim, I., De Castro, A., Sorrentino, J. V., Smith, D. S., Bartigek, R. D., & Olson, N. Z. (1989). Augmentation of acetaminophen analgesia by the antihistamine phenyltoloxamine. *Journal of Clincial Pharmacology, 29*, 660–664.

Swanson, G., Smith, J., Burlich, K., New, P., & Shiffman, R. (1989). Patient-controlled analgesia for chronic cancer pain in the ambulatory setting: a report of 117 patients. *Journal of Clinical Oncology, 7*(12), 1903–1908.

Swerdlow, M. (1984). Anticonvulsant drugs and chronic pain. *Clinical Neuropharmacology, 7*, 51–82.

Swerdlow, M., & Cundill, J. G. (1981). Anticonvulsant drugs used in the treatment of lancinating pains: A comparison. *Anesthesia, 36*, 1129–1132.

Sykes, N. P. (1991). Oral naloxone in opioid associated constipation. *Lancet, 337*, 1475.

Szczeklik, A. (1986). Analgesics, allergy and asthma. Nonnarcotic analgesics today: benefits and risks. *Drugs, 32*(Suppl. 4), 148–163.

Takeda, F. (1986). Results of field-testing in Japan of WHO Draft Interim Guidelines on Relief of Cancer Pain. *The Pain Clinic, 1*, 83–89.

Turner, J. A., Deyo, R. A., Loeser, J. D., Vonkorff, M., & Fordyce, W. E. (1994). The importance of placebo effects in pain treatment and research. *Journal of the American Medical Association, 271*, 1609–1614.

Vane, J. R. (1971). Inhibition of prostaglandin synthesis as a mechanism of action for aspirin-like drugs. *Nature New Biology, 234*, 231–238.

Varvel, J. R., Shafer, S. L., Hwang, S. S., Coen, P. A., & Stanski, D. R. (1989). Absorption characteristics of transdermally administered fentanyl. *Anesthesiology, 70,* 928–934.

Ventafridda, V., Bianchi, M., Rupamontic, C., Sacerdote, P., De Conno, F., Zecca, E., & Panerai, A. E. (1990). Studies on the effects of antidepressant drugs or the antinociceptive action of morphine and on plasma morphine in rat and man. *Pain, 43,* 155–162.

Ventafridda, V., Tamburini, M., Caracenia, A., De Conno, F., & Naldi, F. (1987). A validation study of the WHO method for cancer pain relief. *Cancer, 59,* 851–856.

Walsh, T. D. (1990a). Adjuvant analgesic therapy in cancer pain. In K. M. Foley, J. J. Bonica, & V. Ventafridda (Eds.), *The second international conference on cancer pain* (pp. 155–168). New York: Raven Press.

Wall, P. D. (1994). The placebo and the placebo response. In P. D. Wall & R. Melzack (Eds.), *Textbook of pain* (3rd ed., pp. 1297–1308). Edinburgh: Churchill Livingstone.

Walsh, T. D. (1990b). Prevention of opioid side effects. *Journal of Pain and Symptom Management, 5*(6), 363–367.

Watson, C. P. N., Evans, R. J., Reed, K., Merskey, H., Goldsmith, I., & Warsh, J. (1982). Amitriptyline versus placebo in postherpetic neuralgia. *Neurology, 32,* 671–673.

Watson, C. P. N., Evans, R. J., & Watt, V. R. (1988). Postherpetic neuralgia and topical capsaicin. *Pain, 33,* 333–340.

Watson, C. P. N., Evans, R. J., & Watt, V. R. (1989). The post-mastectomy pain syndrome and the effect of topical capsaicin. *Pain, 38,* 177–186.

Weinberg, D. S., Inturrisi, C. E., Reidenberg, B., Moulin, D., Nip, T. J., Wallenstein, S. L., & Houde, R. W. (1988). Sublingual absorption of selected opioid analgesics. *Clinical Pharmacology and Therapeutics, 44,* 335–342.

Weissman, D. E., & Haddox, J. D. (1989). Opioid pseudoaddiction—an iatrogenic syndrome. *Pain, 36,* 363–366.

Willer, J., DeBroucker, T., Bussel, B., Robi-Brami, A., & Harrowyn, J. M. (1989). Central analgesic effect of ketoprofen in humans: electrophysiologic evidence for a supraspinal mechanism in a double-blind and cross-over study. *Pain, 38,* 1–8.

World Health Organization. (1986). *Cancer pain relief.* Geneva: World Health Organization.

World Health Organization. (1990). *Cancer pain relief and palliative care.* Geneva: World Health Organization.

Yaksh, T. L. (1979). Direct evidence that spinal serotonin and noradrenaline terminals mediate the spinal antinociceptive effects of morphine in the periaqueductal gray. *Brain Research, 160,* 180–185.

Yaksh, T. L. (1981). Spinal opiate analgesics: characteristics and principal action. *Pain, 11,* 293–346.

Yang, J. C., Clark, W. C., Dooley, J. C., & Mignogna, F. V. (1982). Effect of intranasal cocaine on experimental pain in man. *Anethesia and Analgesia, 61,* 358–361.

58

Nondrug Pain Interventions

Betty Rolling Ferrell • Grace E. Dean • Brandi Funk

OVERVIEW

Cancer pain, once thought of as a undimensional experience, is now viewed as a concept that involves multiple domains. A model of the impact of pain and quality of life developed by Ferrell et al. involves four dimensions of the experience of pain: physiologic well being, involving symptoms and function; psychologic well being, such as anxiety and depression; social well being, involving roles and relationships; and spiritual well being, including aspects such as suffering and the meaning of pain (Padilla, Ferrell, Grant, & Rhiner, 1990). Given the broad conceptualization of pain, limiting pain management to pharmacologic intervention alone seems inadequate.

Noninvasive or nonpharmacologic pain relief measures are one of the components of a comprehensive approach to pain relief (McCaffery, 1990). Nondrug interventions can provide cost-effective pain relief in cancer patients without the side effects associated with pharmacologic treatments (Rhiner, Ferrell, Ferrell, & Grant, 1993). Although their use may decrease the need for analgesics, they are best used as adjuvants, not substitutes, for medication (Jacox et al., 1994). It is in fact a combination of pharmacologic and nonpharmacologic methods of pain control that yields the most effective pain relief for the patient with cancer (McCaffery, 1990).

Previous research has demonstrated the importance and frequency of use of nondrug pain intervention by patients and caregivers (Rhiner et al., 1993). In a study by Ferrell, Ferrell, Rhiner, and Grant (1991), caregivers described the importance of nondrug pain relief methods they used at home to "help get his mind off the pain," to "relax," or to otherwise make the patient comfortable. This research also demonstrated that nondrug interventions are seldom initiated by health care providers but rather are generally initiated by patients themselves in a trial and error method with little guidance from professionals.

Eisenberg et al., (1993) found the frequency of use of nondrug therapy by patients with cancer to be far higher than previously reported. In fact, about one in four Americans who see their medical doctors for a serious health problem may be using unconventional therapy in addition to conventional medicine. In addition, seven out of 10 such encounters take place without patients informing their medical doctors that they are using unconventional treatments.

The use of a variety of nonanalgesic methods for pain control in people with cancer has been recommended, but there is little research to support the efficacy of such methods (Barbour, McGuire, & Kirchhoff, 1986; Mayer, 1985; McCaffery & Beebe, 1989). Nondrug pain management research is a neglected area in nursing but one that has tremendous promise (Rhiner et al., 1993). By continuing this research, nursing can make a significant contribution to overall improvement in pain relief. Due to the multidimensional nature of pain, patients with cancer need a variety of options to achieve the best and most effective pain relief specific to the etiology of their specific pain. This chapter will review both conventional and unique nondrug pain control techniques such as heat, cold, massage, counterstimulation, distraction, and relaxation as examples of critical nursing interventions. These methods have been divided into the categories of physical methods and cognitive methods of relieving pain.

METHODS OF NONDRUG INTERVENTION

PHYSICAL METHODS

SUPERFICIAL HEAT THERAPY

Superficial heat (hot tubs, hot wraps, dry heat, moist heat, hot water bottles) is a convenient, easily accessible, and inexpensive method of nondrug pain relief. Because water is an excellent conductor of heat, the effects of moist heat may be deeper than the effects of dry heat (Michlovitz, 1990). Research by Ferrell, Ferrell, Ahn, and Tran (1994) in a sample of elderly patients with cancer demonstrated that superficial heat was the most popular and was perceived as the most effective of all nondrug methods. Superficial heat is effective in providing pain relief from muscle spasm, localized infections or inflammation, pain secondary to local anesthesia, joint stiffness, reduced peristalsis and gastric acidity, and vasoconstriction and decreased blood flow.

The use of superficial heat requires great caution. Temperature must be carefully monitored to avoid burns, with a recommended range of 40° to 45° C (104° F to 113° F), especially in patients who are cognitively impaired or who have impaired sensation in the area of application (McCaffery & Wolff, 1992). Superficial heat is contraindicated in patients who have had radiation therapy, have taken various medications that alter the skin tolerance to external stimuli, and in areas of bleeding (Jacox et al., 1994).

All methods of nondrug intervention should be described to patients with an opportunity for demonstration and questions. It is also important to provide written information about nondrug methods, just as you would provide written details regarding medications. An example of written instructions for use of the heat method is provided in Table 58–1.

SUPERFICIAL COLD THERAPY

Cold is often not readily selected as the first choice for nondrug pain intervention, and most health professionals are less familiar with cold than the use of heat. However, of all the types of cutaneous stimulation, it is one of the most effective (McCaffery, 1990). The application of cold contributes to the relief of pain by numbing nerve endings and decreasing inflammation, and it may reduce muscle spasms and itching. Its use has proven to be especially effective for abdominal and lower back pain and for nerve pain (Rhiner et al., 1993). Cold therapy (cold wraps, gel packs, ice massage, cold compresses) is also recommended for reducing edema, burning type pain, and muscle spasms when superficial heat is ineffective (Jacox et al., 1994). Counterirritants such as Ben Gay, Icy Hot, and Vicks Vapor Rub are also included for use with cold. The local application of cold often relieves pain more effectively than heat, because it relieves pain faster and lasts longer after the cold is removed (McCaffery & Wolff, 1992; Ramler & Roberts, 1986).

Patients are often resistant to the use of cold. This may be due to the discomfort caused by the initial application. Patients may benefit from an explanation regarding the therapeutic efficacy of superficial cold therapy. Cold should first be applied to a small, localized area and covered adequately, assuring the first sensation the patient feels is merely cool (McCaffery, 1990).

Alternating heat and cold is even more effective than the use of heat or cold alone and may be used whenever heat and cold can be used interchangeably (McCaffery, 1990). Cold should not be applied to radiated tissue or any condition where vasoconstriction increases symptoms (Jacox et al., 1994). The use of cold is also a convenient, easily accessible, and inexpensive method of nondrug pain relief.

MASSAGE

Massage has been described as a therapy for illness since the fifth century BC. Massage is the kneading, manipulation, or application of methodic pressure and friction to the body and includes both hand massage and electric massager/vibration. Massage is convenient; one can apply it to one's self, and it is accessible with massage equipment available in local stores at a relatively inexpensive cost. The benefits of massage include relaxation, reduced swelling, decreased stress, relief of fatigue, improved sleep, and decreased pain through the stimulation of endorphins (Ferrell, Wisdom, & Wenzl, 1989; Rhiner et al., 1993).

In addition, specific massage techniques may be helpful in reducing the myofascial trigger point pain (the area within the taut band of skeletal muscle) by improving blood flow to the affected area (Travell & Simons, 1983). This increased blood flow reduces the collection of fluids, toxic metabolic waste products, and decreases ischemia. In a study of the effects of therapeutic massage on perception of pain intensity, anxiety, and relaxation, Ferrell-Torry and Glick (1993) found that the use of massage in patients with cancer reduced their perceptions of pain and anxiety and enhanced relaxation. Decreases in sympathetic nervous system activity such as heart rate, respiratory rate, and blood pressure were also noted, providing further evidence for the effectiveness of the intervention. In another study, Weinrich and Weinrich (1990) found similar results on male patients with cancer-related pain, with a significant decrease in pain levels immediately after 10 minutes of massage. However, there was no significant decrease in pain level for female patients in this study. Massage is contraindicated in cases of inflammation, fever, heart conditions, or in cases of thrombosis or phlebitis.

ACUPUNCTURE/ACUPRESSURE

Several procedures are useful for the control of pain by electrical or other forms of sensory modulation of the somatic input. The use of acupuncture and acupressure for pain relief are not new ideas. An ancient Chinese medical procedure, acupuncture, has been in continuous practice for at least 2000 years (Melzack & Wall, 1984). Acupuncture involves the insertion of fine needles through the skin adjacent to or distant from the painful area. It is believed that analgesia is produced

TABLE 58–1. *Nondrug Pain Relief*

Method: Heat/Hot Wrap

Description: Heat is the application of warmth to the skin for the relief of pain. One method of applying heat is by use of a hot wrap.

How Heat Helps: Heat can relieve pain by reducing inflammation and soreness. Heat also decreases sensitivity to pain, relieves joint stiffness, and increases blood flow to the skin. It also helps you to relax.

Special Considerations/Precautions:
- Please follow all manufacturer's directions for use. To avoid burns to your skin when heating the hot wrap, do not leave the hot wrap in the microwave or boiling water too long. To avoid burns, use only the wrap that is included with the hot pack.
- Do not use the hot wrap if the painful area is being treated with radiation therapy; it is within 24 hours of injury to that area; the painful area has decreased sensation; the painful area has open wounds or sores.

Equipment:
1. Hot wrap such as Champ Hot Wrap.
2. Microwave or boiling water.

Directions
1. The hot wrap can be heated in either a microwave or boiling water. *Microwave directions:* Unfold the hot wrap and lay it flat in the microwave. Heat with full power for 60 seconds. Note: pack will continue to heat slightly. Test it before use. If it is too warm, set it aside until it becomes cooler. If additional heating is required, use 5-second intervals to heat the hot pack. *Hot water directions:* Bring 3 quarts of water to a boil in a pot. Remove the hot pack from the wrap. Remove the pot from the heat and place the hot pack in the boiled water for no longer than 7 minutes. Remove the hot pack with kitchen tongs to prevent burns.
2. When the hot pack is ready, place the hot pack in the wrap that is provided.
3. Place the hot wrap on the area where you want relief. If the area is too painful to have the hot wrap directly on it, you can also place the hot wrap on the other side of the body that corresponds to the painful area. For example, if your right hip has pain but it is too painful to put the hot wrap on the right hip, you can put the hot wrap on the left hip.
4. If possible, secure the hot wrap on the painful area to prevent it from slipping.
5. Do not sleep on top of the hot wrap. Heat is increased with pressure, which may cause burns.
6. Once the hot wrap is cooled, if you wish to reuse it, please follow the manufacturer's directions. Do not exceed the recommended heating times, as burns may result. Do not throw the hot wrap away.
7. You may continue to use the hot wrap as long as you are comfortable, and the skin under the hot wrap is not reddened or irritated.
8. Occasionally check the skin for any signs of redness or irritation. If either are present, stop using the hot wrap, and if the redness or irritation does not disappear within an hour, call your physician or nurse.
9. You may want to alternate heat and cold (please see the instructional materials on cold) to improve comfort, or take the hot wrap off for a few minutes. By taking the hot wrap off, the skin will cool quickly, giving you the contrast between heat and cold.
10. Be certain to record the heat method and its effectiveness in the Self-Care Log.
11. Hot wraps are not intended to take the place of your pain medication; they are meant to work with your pain medication to help you achieve better pain relief.

(From Ferrell, B., & Rhiner, M. [1993]. *Managing cancer pain at home.* City of Hope National Medical Center.)

with acupuncture by activating endogenous pain-modulating pathways by direct stimulation of peripheral nerves (Melzack & Wall, 1984; Sjolund & Eriksson, 1979). Acupressure is similar to acupuncture without needles. Here, pressure is applied by exerting finger and thumb upon specific points on the surface of the skin believed to act as entrances and exits for the vital internal healing force (Sutcliffe, 1994).

TRANSCUTANEOUS ELECTRICAL NERVE STIMULATION (TENS)

Transcutaneous electrical nerve stimulation (TENS) units are frequently discussed as an adjunct for pain relief. The TENS units have shown promise in selected pain syndromes, although the duration of pain relief remains unclear (Jacox et al., 1994). TENS involves stimulating all nerves about 4 cm below the surface of the skin by placing electrodes on the skin surface. Its effects on pain are thought to be related to both excitation and inhibition of sensory nerve impulses in the central nervous system (Melzack & Wall, 1984).

Though effective in some pain syndromes, the use of TENS and acupuncture/acupressure may not be as accessible or affordable for the general public as other methods described here.

COGNITIVE METHODS

DISTRACTION

Distraction is the strategy of focusing one's attention on stimuli other than pain or the accompanying negative emotions (McCaffery & Beebe, 1989; McCaul & Malott, 1984). Distraction may be used alone to manage mild pain or as an adjunct to analgesic drugs to manage brief episodes of severe pain, such as procedure-related pain (Jacox et al., 1994). There are many effective methods of distraction discussed in the literature. In this chapter we will review two popular and effective methods, music and humor.

Music. Music has been recognized for centuries for its therapeutic property in healing the body and the mind. The use of music in the oncology setting has numerous applications in helping individuals cope with both psychologic and physiologic problems, such as pain (Cook, 1986). Recently, music therapists have found that music can alleviate the cycles of anxiety and fear that exacerbate pain. Music therapy may enhance emotional and physical tension release and induce relaxation through calming and soothing tones (Bailey, 1983; Munro & Mount, 1978). The goals of music therapy are to assist the patient in regaining a sense of control and becoming actively involved in the management of his or her pain. The aim of music therapy is to treat the varying aspects of the total pain experience (Bailey, 1986).

Though limited, studies have further demonstrated the effects of music on pain. In one study, Zimmerman, Pozehl, Duncan, and Schmitz (1989) found that 30-minute tapes of relaxing music with a positive suggestion significantly decreased pain. In another study, Beck (1991) found the effect of music on pain varied by individual, with 75 per cent having at least some response and 47 per cent of patients with cancer-related pain having a moderate or great response. When initiating music therapy it is important for the nurse to allow patients to select the type of music they prefer. If availability of equipment in the hospital setting is a problem, patients may bring their favorite tapes and their own tape players. Generally, music is a readily available, affordable, and easy intervention for pain relief.

Humor. Humor, another form of distraction, has no universal definition, but its use has been under investigation since the time of Plato and Aristotle (Bellert, 1989). Freud believed that humor developed spontaneously from the unconscious during childhood and continued its evolution on into adulthood. Various disciplines have described humor as having both a cognitive process and an emotional response that is unique to the individual (Bellert, 1989). Metcaff (1987) defines humor as a set of acquired, psychologic skills that affect the individual's ability to adapt and cope with change. He believes that humor is important for both the nurse providing care and the patient receiving that care.

Laughter is a naturally occurring, noneffortful response to a stimulus. As a nondrug intervention, laughter controls pain in three ways: by distraction, reducing tension, and increasing the production of endorphins. Laughter does not eradicate pain; rather, it makes the pain more tolerable by placing pain at the periphery of awareness. Cogan, Cogan, Waltz, and McCue (1987) found that discomfort thresholds increased for subjects in the laughter-inducing condition. Laughter, not simply distraction, reduced pressure-induced discomfort sensitivity, suggesting that laughter has the potential as an intervention strategy for the reduction of clinical discomfort.

During laughter, the facial, chest, abdominal, and skeletal muscles are stimulated, along with heart rate and blood pressure (Bellert, 1989). This increase in blood pressure and heart rate is followed by a period of relaxation that ultimately results in relaxation of muscle tension. This process results in diminished pain that may last 10 minutes or longer after laughter ceases and

a reduction in blood pressure below the prelaughter baseline. Researchers studied humor and life stress after developing their tool, the Humor Coping Scale (Bellert, 1989). They concluded that for humor to moderate the effects of stress, the individual had to place a high value on humor and needed to practice it in stressful situations encountered in daily life.

The hypothalamus is involved in the coordination of laughter. The pleasant affective experience associated with laughter is probably associated with the limbic system. Various authors have suggested that endorphins are released during laughter and are also responsible for the experience of pleasure and the relief of pain. Other health benefits of laughter include an increase in oxygenation of the blood, an increase in antibodies and immune cells, and a reduction in stress hormones (Berk, Tan, Berre, & Eby, 1991; Berk, Tan, & Fry, 1989a; Berk, Tan, Napier, & Eby, 1989b; Berk et al., 1988; Fry, 1991).

Appropriate humor may begin with a smile. Humor *is* everywhere. Nurses simply need to be alert and open to the absurdities and incongruities around them. Being able to share with patients the knowledge that humor is not only fun but therapeutic should enhance the opportunity for its implementation or continued use.

RELAXATION/IMAGERY

Relaxation strategies are thought to counteract the sympathetic nervous system activity that may accompany, and in turn exacerbate, pain (Graffam & Johnson, 1987). Extensive research has shown that muscular tension, emotional arousal, and mental confusion reduce pain tolerance and exacerbate pain and distress (Linton & Melin, 1983). Both pleasant imagery and progressive muscle relaxation have been shown to decrease self-reported pain intensity and pain distress. There are many forms of relaxation, and patients should be encouraged to decide the technique that is most appropriate for them and obtain the needed training. Some common techniques include passive relaxation, progressive muscle relaxation, guided imagery, meditation, biofeedback, and self-hypnosis. Each of these techniques will be briefly described.

Passive relaxation focuses attention systematically on the sensations of warmth and on the dissipation of tension in various parts of the body (Fishman, 1992). Progressive muscle relaxation is the active tightening and releasing of gross muscle groups while noting the differences in sensation of tension and relaxation (Graffam & Johnson, 1987). The goal is to increase the ability to identify even mild tension and to effectively reduce it. All too often patients are not in touch with their bodies enough to sense tension until it is severe enough to create or exacerbate pain.

Guided imagery or visualization is characterized as an activity in which the patient creates pleasant images through the five senses, for example, being at a beautiful beach, hearing the waves crash down, feeling the cool water on your feet, and smelling and tasting the salty ocean air. An example of a simple imagery exercise is included in Table 58–2 (Keegan, 1994). These images are used to substitute a nonpainful sensation for

TABLE 58–2. *Imagery Exercise*

1. Position yourself comfortably, loosen tight clothing, and allow your arms to be gently supported.
2. Imagine yourself in a beautiful, well-kept garden. See yourself sitting in the middle of the garden in a comfortable patio chair with your feet supported on an ottoman.
3. Look around you and see the manicured box hedges and well-designed arrangement of ornamental, flowering, dogwood trees and hanging, fucia-colored bougainvillea.
4. Feel the warm, light wind and note how the leaves of the trees sway in the breeze.
5. Heighten your gaze and note the clear, blue sky.
6. Lower your gaze and observe the beds of flowers and rosebushes in the foreground.
7. Imagine yourself now rising from your chair and walking over to the pink rosebush. Note how it is abundantly filled with roses at all stages of development. Look at the buds, the flowers in full bloom, and those that are fading. Look at the petals all over the ground at the base of the bush.
8. Focus on a mature rose in full bloom. Look carefully at the flower and lean over to smell it.
9. Inhale the scent of rose perfume that permeates the air surrounding the bush. Breathe deeply and enjoy the rich, fragrant odor.
10. Note the perfection of the flower. Feel its velvet petals and once more inhale its perfuse, lovely smell.
11. Thank the rose for offering you its gift and then return to settle in your chair in the center of the garden.
12. Feel the peace and serenity of this special place. Realize that you can return to this place whenever you desire. You need only to quiet your thoughts and relax your body-mind.
13. Say good-bye to your special place and return your attention to the present. Focus again on the here and now.

(Used with permission from Keegan, L. [1994]. *The nurse as healer.* Albany, NY: Delmar Publishers. Copyright 1994.)

pain. The patient uses imagery as a method of communicating with selected autonomic physiologic processes that occur outside of conscious awareness (Jaffe & Bresler, 1984). In support of the notion that guided imagery is a useful nondrug intervention for pain, Daake and Gueldner (1989) reported that patients who used pleasant imagery had less reported postsurgical pain and required significantly less pain medication than did the control group.

Meditation or prayer focuses the patient's attention and alters their level of awareness (Scandrett & Uecker, 1985). It may be structured or unstructured, involving mentally directed feelings and thoughts in a relaxed state through silent conversation or chants, focusing on an idea or object. Receptive meditation opens the patient up to intuition, insight, aspects of personality, guidance, inspiration, and knowledge (Scandrett & Uecker, 1985).

Biofeedback is the result of technologic advances after World War II that devised instrumentation that could detect, record, and amplify the body's internal electrical impulses and provide a corresponding signal that could be interpreted by the patient (Scandrett & Uecker, 1985). This equipment monitors information of which the patient is ordinarily unaware such as heart rate, blood pressure, temperature, electromyography (EMG [i.e., muscular tension]), and electroencephalography (EEG [i.e., brain waves]). This information is then displayed on a unit so that the patient will learn to control these physiologic responses. The ultimate goal is to train the patient to achieve the same results without the machine. Major limitations with this form of relaxation involve the availability of the equipment, cost, and accessibility of trained personnel.

Self-hypnosis involves using concentration to achieve a state of aroused, attentive focal concentration with a relative suspension of peripheral awareness. Here, subjects are aware of their environment, but their attention is turned inward. It is an advanced stage of

relaxation, as relaxation techniques are often part of the induction process (Spiegel & Bloom, 1983).

With the exception of biofeedback, in which access may be limited, these described methods of relaxation are easy to learn, are provided at minimal cost, require little or no equipment, and can be done in any setting. Most important, through teaching relaxation techniques, the nurse can play a vital role in helping patients discover effective nondrug methods for pain relief.

IMPLEMENTATION OF NONDRUG INTERVENTIONS

HOME CARE

Increasingly, cancer is managed on an outpatient basis with pain management responsibility assumed by the family at home (Buxman, 1991). Family members have often reported feeling helpless in relieving the patient's pain and are eager to learn techniques that might enhance their involvement in the patient's comfort. Nondrug pain-relieving techniques can enhance interaction and communication between patient and family while providing pain relief.

Nurses can help identify equipment available to the patient for use at home. A list of equipment used in the study of Pain Management at home by Ferrell et al. (1994) is provided in Table 58–3. A summary of the results of this study is provided in Table 58–4. This study found that simple use of distraction declined as the patients added other methods for pain relief. Imagery was viewed as the least helpful by these elderly patients.

INPATIENT CARE

Translating nondrug therapy into the inpatient setting may be best accomplished over time by implementing a few techniques at a time. For example,

TABLE 58–3. *Nondrug Equipment for Use in Intervention with Approximate Prices*

METHOD	EQUIPMENT	COST ($)
Heat		
Dry	Heating pad	14.00
Moist	Heating pad	15.00
Hot tub	Thermometer	4.00
Heat	Hot water bottle	8.00
Plastic wrap	Plastic wrap	4.00
Hot wrap	Hot wrap (Champ)	8.00
Cold		
Cold wrap	Cold wrap	7.00
Gel pack	Cold comfort packs	5.00
Ice bag	Straight ice bag	1.00
Ice massage	Paper cups	3.00
Menthol	Various ointments and salves	5.00
Massage		
Hand massage	Body massage oil	7.00
Vibration	2-speed massager	26.00
Vibration with heat	7-way massager	22.00
Relaxation		
Auditory stimulation	Variety of tapes	11.00
	with earth/nature sounds	11.00
Progressive relaxation	Deep relaxation tapes, variety of soothing classics	10.00
Guided imagery	Tapes	12.00
Distraction		
Music	A variety of choices including jazz, contemporary, classic, and country	9.00–13.00
Humor	A variety of comedians such as Will Rogers, Jack Benny, Erma Bombeck, Abbott and Costello, and W.C. Fields	4.00–17.00

humor may be introduced by bringing in humorous videos, hilarious comic strips, and inexpensive plastic wind-up toys and sharing them with patients. This is an appropriate way to "test the waters" for acceptance of humor therapy. This simple trial method may benefit both patients and staff and be an effective means of introducing the idea of nondrug interventions.

Inpatient settings with available resources may want to establish larger scale projects such as creating a humor cart or humor room. The first official humor room opened in 1980, the Living Room, at St. Joseph's Hospital in Houston, Texas (Buxman, 1991). Since then, other humor rooms have opened in many settings across the country. Resources for the room or cart include humorous books, magazines, newsletters, audiocassettes, videocassettes, games, musical instruments, costumes, toys, and creative decorations. Types of visitors to the humor room often include patients, families, and staff, as well as meetings of support groups. The humor room may also be used as a place to celebrate events, such as completion of treatment, anniversaries, or birthdays.

Once the idea for a humor cart or room is adopted, an advisory committee should be established. A budget will need to be prepared to include any needed renovations, furniture that cannot be otherwise acquired, and other more expensive items such as a television set or a video cassette recorder. Humor rooms or carts may be sponsored by outside donors, members of the hospital's Board of Directors, or hospital administrators.

SUMMARY

These nondrug methods are nursing interventions that were discussed as examples of simple, inexpensive means of pain relief. Nurses also are involved in referral of patients for more complex modalities of nondrug pain relief provided by other professionals such as psychiatrists, clinical psychologists, acupuncturists, and others. Nurses can assist patients in understanding these modalities and providing referral for these services.

One of the most basic means of nondrug intervention is simply pain education. Patient education entails giving patients and families accurate and understand-

TABLE 58–4. *Nondrug Interventions*

VARIABLE	% USING BEFORE PAIN EDUCATION	% USING AFTER PAIN EDUCATION	EFFECTIVENESS*
Heat	22	68	mean = 3.2 md = 3.0
Cold	5	19	mean = 2.9 md = 3.0
Massage	11	64	mean = 2.9 md = 3.0
Distraction	64	47	mean = 3.3 md = 4.0
Imagery/Relaxation	3	9	mean = 1.0 md = 1.0

*Effectiveness scale 0 = not helpful to 4 = very helpful.
(From Ferrell, B. R., Ferrell, B. A., Ahn, C., & Tran, K. [1994]. Pain management for elderly cancer patients at home. *Cancer, 74*[7], 2139–2146.)

TABLE 58–5. *Principles of Patient Teaching for Use of Nondrug Interventions*

1. Begin with an assessment of the patient's current use of nondrug interventions and the effectiveness of those interventions.
2. Emphasize the importance of nondrug treatments as an addition to rather than a replacement for pharmacologic treatments.
3. Offer a variety of methods for the patient's consideration including physical and cognitive methods.
4. Recommend methods of nondrug pain relief based on assessment of the pain (i.e., use of cold for nerve pain, use of distraction for pain accompanied by high anxiety).
5. Evaluate the effectiveness of nondrug methods just as you would evaluate pharmacologic treatments.
6. Emphasize the importance of "trial and error" in using nondrug treatments. If one method is ineffective, the patient should be encouraged to try other methods.
7. Provide written information to accompany verbal instruction.
8. Demonstration of nondrug methods is an integral component of patient teaching. Patients are unlikely to use methods they have not had an opportunity to try.
9. Be sensitive to issues of cost; even minimal costs such as purchase of batteries for a tape recorder may be a financial burden for patients.
10. It is generally best to introduce nondrug treatments after the patient receives adequate pharmacologic intervention.
11. Incorporate the patient's own values and beliefs in the nondrug interventions. The use of spiritual interventions such as prayer and the inclusion of culturally sensitive methods are very important.
12. Involve family caregivers in nondrug interventions. Their involvement can decrease their sense of helplessness and enhance the patient's comfort.

able information about pain, pain assessment, and the use of drugs and other methods of pain relief. Patient education empowers patients and family members to assume greater control of their pain and diminishes helplessness often associated with pain they experience. A summary of important principles in patient teaching and use of nondrug methods is provided in Table 58–5. Nondrug pain interventions are an important recognition of the role of oncology nursing in addressing the entire person.

REFERENCES

Bailey, L. M. (1983). Music therapy as an intervention in pain management. In Ashwander, P. (Ed.), *Handbook on interventions in pain management.* New York-New Jersey: Cancer Nursing Regional Committee.

Bailey, L. M. (1986). Music therapy in pain management. *Journal of Pain and Symptom Management, 1*(1), 25–28.

Barbour, L. A., McGuire, D. B., & Kirchhoff, K. T. (1986). Nonanalgesic methods of pain control used by cancer outpatients. *Oncology Nursing Forum, 13*(6), 56–60.

Beck, S. L. (1991). The therapeutic use of music for cancer-related pain. *Oncology Nursing Forum, 18*(8), 1327–1337.

Bellert, J. L. (1989). Humor: A therapeutic approach in oncology nursing. *Cancer Nursing, 12*(2), 65–70.

Berk, L. S., Tan, S. A., Berre, D. B., & Eby, W. C. (1991). Immune system changes during humor associated laughter. *Clinical Research, 39,* 124A.

Berk, L. S., Tan, S. A., & Fry, W. F. (1989a). Neuroendocrine and stress hormone changes during mirthful laughter. *American Journal of Medical Sciences, 298,* 390–396.

Berk, L. S., Tan, S. A., Napier, B. J., & Eby, W. C. (1989b). Eutress of mirthful laughter modifies natural killer cell activity. *Clinical Research, 36,* 435A.

Berk, L. S., Tan, S. A., Nehlsen-Cannarella, S. L., Napier, B. J., Lewis, J. E., Lee, J. W., & Eby, W. C. (1988). Humor associated laughter decreases cortisol and increases spontaneous lymphocyte blastogenesis. *Clinical Research, 36,* 435A.

Buxman, K. (1991). Making room for humor. *American Journal of Nursing, 91*(12), 46–51.

Cogan, R., Cogan, C., Waltz, W., & McCue, M. (1987). Effects of laughter and relaxation on discomfort thresholds. *Journal of Behavioral Medicine, 10*(2), 139–144.

Cook, J. D. (1986). Music as an intervention in the oncology setting. *Cancer Nursing, 9*(1), 23–28.

Daake, D. R., & Gueldner, S. H. (1989). Imagery instruction and the control of postsurgical pain. *Applied Nursing Research, 2*(3), 114–120.

Eisenberg, D. M., Kessler, R. C., Foster, C., Norlock, F. E., Calkins, D. R., & Delbanco, T. L. (1993). Unconventional medicine in the United States: Prevalence, costs, and patterns of use. *The New England Journal of Medicine, 328,* 246–252.

Ferrell, B. R., Ferrell, B. A., Ahn, C., & Tran, K. (1994). Pain management for elderly cancer patients at home. *Cancer, 74*(7), 2139–2146.

Ferrell, B. R., Ferrell, B. A., Rhiner, M., & Grant, M. (1991). Family factors influencing cancer pain. *Postgraduate Medicine Journal, 67*(Suppl. 2), S64–S69.

Ferrell, B. R., Wisdom, C., & Wenzl, C. (1989). Quality of life as an outcome variable in the management of cancer pain. *Cancer, 63,* 2321–2327.

Ferrell-Torry, A. T., & Glick, O. J. (1993). The use of therapeutic massage as a nursing intervention to modify anxiety and the perception of cancer pain. *Cancer Nursing, 16*(2), 93–101.

Fishman, B. (1992). The cognitive behavioral perspective on pain management. In D. C. Turk & C. S. Feldman (Eds.), *Noninvasive approaches to pain management in the terminally ill* (pp. 73–88). New York: Haworth Press.

Fry, W. F. (1991). The physiologic effects of humor, mirth and laughter. *Journal of the American Medical Association, 267*(13), 1857–1858.

Graffam, S., & Johnson, A. (1987). A comparison of two relaxation strategies for the relief of pain and its distress. *Journal of Pain and Symptom Management, 2*(4), 229–231.

Jacox, A., Carr D. B., Payne, R., et al. (1994). *Management of cancer pain: Clinical practice guideline.* No. 9. Rockville, MD: Agency for Health Care Policy and Research, U.S. Department of Health and Human Services, Public Health Services.

Jaffe, D., & Bresler, D. (1984). Guided imagery: Healing through the mind's eye. In J. Gordon, D. Jaffe, & D.

Bresler (Eds.), *Mind, body, and health* (pp. 56–69). New York: Human Sciences Press.

Keegan, L. (1994). *The nurse as healer.* New York: Delmar.

Linton, S. J., & Melin, L. (1983). Applied relaxation in the management of chronic pain. *Behavioral Psychotherapy, 11,* 337–350.

Mayer, D. K. (1985). Nonpharmacologic management of pain in the person with cancer. *Journal of Advanced Nursing, 10,* 325–330.

McCaffery, M. (1990). Nursing approaches to nonpharmacological pain control. *International Journal of Nursing Studies, 27*(1), 1–5.

McCaffery, M., & Beebe, A. (1989). *Pain: Clinical manual for nursing practice.* St. Louis: C. V. Mosby.

McCaffery, M., & Wolff, M. (1992). Pain relief using cutaneous modalities, positioning, and movement. In D. C. Turk & C. S. F. Feldman (Eds.), *Noninvasive approaches to pain management in the terminally ill* (pp. 212–153). New York: The Haworth Press.

McCaul, K. D., & Malott, J. M. (1984). Distraction and coping with pain. *Psychology Bulletin, 95*(3), 516–533.

Melzack, R., & Wall, P. D. (1984). Acupuncture and transcutaneous electrical nerve stimulation. *Postgraduate Medical Journal, 60,* 893–896.

Metcaff, C. W. (1987). Humor, life and death. *Oncology Nursing Forum, 14*(4), 19–21.

Michlovitz, S. L. (1990). Biophysical principles of heating and superficial heat agent. In S. L. Michlovitz (Ed.), *Thermal agents in rehabilitation* (pp. 88–108). Philadelphia: F.A. Davis.

Munro, S., & Mount, B. (1978). Music therapy in palliative care. *Canadian Medical Association Journal, 9,* 1029–1034.

Padilla, G., Ferrell, B. R., Grant, M., & Rhiner, M. (1990). Defining the content domain of quality of life for cancer patients with pain. *Cancer Nursing, 13*(2), 108–115.

Ramler, D., & Roberts, J. (1986). A comparison of cold and warm sitz baths for relief of postpartum perineal pain. *Journal of Obstetrics, Gynecology, and Neonatal Nursing, 15,* 471–474.

Rhiner, M., Ferrell, B. R., Ferrell, B. A., & Grant, M. (1993). A structured nondrug intervention program for cancer pain. *Cancer Practice, 1*(2), 137–143.

Scandrett, S., & Uecker, S. (1985). Relaxation training. In G. M. Bulechek & J. C. McCloskey (Eds.), *Nursing interventions: Treatments for nursing diagnoses* (pp. 22–48). Philadelphia: W.B. Saunders Co.

Sjolund, B. H., & Eriksson, M. B. E. (1979). Endorphins and analgesia produced by peripheral conditioning stimulation. In J. J. Bonica, D. G. Libeskind, & D. Albe-Fessard (Eds.), *Proceedings of the Second World Congress on Pain, Montreal, Quebec. Advances in pain research and therapy* (Vol. 3, pp. 587–592). New York: Raven Press.

Spiegel, D., & Bloom, J. R. (1983). Group therapy and hypnosis reduce metastatic breast carcinoma pain. *Psychosomatic Medicine, 45*(4), 333–339.

Sutcliffe, J. (1994). *The complete book of relaxation techniques.* Allentown, PA: People's Medical Society.

Travell, J., & Simons, D. (1983). *Myofascial pain and dysfunction: The trigger point manual.* Baltimore: Williams & Wilkins.

Weinrich, S. P., & Weinrich, M. C. (1990). The effect of massage on pain in cancer patients. *Applied Nursing Research, 3*(4), 140–145.

Zimmerman, L., Pozehl, B., Duncan, K., & Schmitz, R. (1989). Effects of music in patients who had chronic cancer pain. *Western Journal of Nursing Research, 11*(3), 298–309.

Symptom Management: Loss of Concentration[*]

Bernadine Cimprich

Loss of concentration has been identified as a distressing symptom (Holmes, 1991; McCorkle & Young, 1978) during and following cancer treatment (Mages & Mendolsohn, 1979; Oberst & James, 1985; Berglund, Bolund, Forander, Rutquist, & Sjoden, 1991). The ability to concentrate is fundamental for effective functioning, particularly in demanding life situations. In individuals with cancer, a loss of concentration can reduce ability to learn important information, adhere to complex treatment regimens, and resume valued life roles. Despite the deleterious effects of loss of concentration on functioning and quality of life, the problem has not been systematically studied. Thus, little is known about the nature and extent of this symptom in individuals with cancer. This chapter will focus on characterizing the problem of loss of the ability to concentrate in individuals with cancer including factors that place individuals at risk and nursing approaches to support and improve attentional functioning.

A THEORETIC ORIENTATION TO ATTENTIONAL PROCESSES

Concentration is a common term used synonymously with "attention" or the ability to "pay attention." Attention, however, is not a single or unitary concept, but rather involves complex neurocognitive processes (Posner & Boies, 1971; Posner & Dehaene, 1994) that are not well understood. Attentional processes operate to increase sensitivity to important information in the environment akin to a mental spotlight that focuses on one neural activity to the exclusion of others (Van Zomeren & Brouwer, 1994).

Important characteristics of attention include selectivity, intensity or concentration, limited capacity, and effort (James, 1890/1983; Posner & Boies, 1971; Van Zomeren & Brouwer, 1994). Selectivity is the ability to focus awareness on certain stimuli in the external or internal environment while ignoring other competing information. The selective operation of attention facilitates coherence of thought by protecting a person from continuous distraction caused by random environmental stimuli. Attention also involves a sustaining or intensity component that permits a person to sustain focus or "concentrate" on some mental activity while effectively ignoring any distracting stimuli. In this way a person may follow a train of thought or listen to what another is saying even in the presence of noise or when inclined to think of something else.

Limited capacity refers to the amount of information that a person can attend to at one time (Mandler, 1975). Attentional capacity is limited and thus permits active processing of only a few pieces or "chunks" of information at any one time. Miller (1956) initially proposed this was a predictable number of seven plus or minus two pieces of information. However, under optimal healthy conditions, Kaplan and Kaplan (1982) argue that in daily functioning the number is probably five plus or minus two pieces of information.

Finally, the concept of effort is particularly important in goal-directed activity (James, 1890/1983; Rothbart & Posner, 1985). Mental effort is typically at work in voluntary (James, 1890/1983), controlled, or directed attention. Directed attention here refers to the capacity to actively block or inhibit competing stimuli

---

[*]This chapter is an expanded version of an article that appeared in *Seminars in Oncology Nursing, 11*(4), 279–288, 1995.

or distractions during purposeful or goal-directed activity (Kaplan & Kaplan, 1982; Posner & Snyder, 1975). When directing attention or concentrating on some intended activity, for example, in listening to another, a person would apply mental or inhibitory effort to block out distractions such as unwanted noise or thoughts. The greater the distractions in the environment (internal or external), the more mental effort is required to concentrate on a task. Because directed attention requires effort to sustain, it is considered susceptible to fatigue (Kaplan & Kaplan, 1982; Kaplan & Kaplan, 1989).

Directed attention is essential for effective functioning in daily life. Directed attention helps a person to learn needed information, formulate goals, plan, decide, carry out tasks, and monitor and adjust behavior to meet desired goals (Cimprich, 1992a; Lezak, 1982). It has been proposed that social functioning also requires considerable directed attention, for example, in listening, exercising patience in interpersonal interactions, or delaying responses when deemed appropriate (Kaplan & Kaplan, 1989). Thus, in many life situations an individual would need to rely heavily on this critical attentional capacity to function effectively.

One term that needs to be distinguished in an attentional framework involving loss of concentration is "alertness." Alertness has been defined as: "a variable state of the central nervous system that affects general receptivity to stimulation" (Van Zomeren & Brouwer, 1994) (p. 215). Thus alertness refers to normal states of consciousness ranging from a very low level in sleep to a high level in wakefulness (Van Zomeren & Brouwer, 1994). Normal states of wakefulness are needed to support selective attentional operations; however, it is important to note that loss of concentration can occur in a normally alert and responding individual.

BRAIN MECHANISMS OF ATTENTION

Although it is not possible to relate all aspects of attention to brain structures, several anatomic systems have been associated with attentional processes (Posner & Dehaene, 1994; Van Zomeren & Brouwer, 1994). Posner and Dehaene (1994) have proposed a neurobehavioral model of attention based upon highly interconnected anatomic networks, namely the posterior and anterior attentional systems. The posterior system involves the posterior parietal cortex, specialized areas of the thalamus, and the superior colliculus, and is responsible for shifting the focus of attention from one spatial location to another or one stimulus to another. The anterior system involves the frontal lobes and basal ganglia and appears to control selection of stimuli from competing inputs and to exercise inhibitory control over other brain areas to perform complex tasks (i.e., control of attention). In this framework, "the posterior system is involved in automatic or involuntary orienting" (Van Zomeren & Brouwer, 1994, p. 53), while "the anterior system is important for focused attention" (Van Zomeren & Brouwer, 1994, p. 53). Finally, a subcortical system involving the retic-

ular formation in the brainstem is responsible for regulating alertness and waking states. The reticular formation activates the cortex and regulates the state of activity through the ascending reticular activating system, which projects via the thalamus (a major relay between the brain stem and cortex) to widespread areas of the cortex (Mesulam, 1985).

Certain central neural pathways and neurotransmitters, that is, chemical substances used for conveying signals from one cell to the next, also have been associated with attentional processes. Central cholinergic pathways that originate in the brainstem reticular core and ascend to thalamic and cortical areas are considered to be particularly important in mediating attentional tone, that is, arousal and alertness. The transmitter, acetylcholine, increases responsivity of neurons to other neural inputs (Mesulam, 1985). Thus, drugs or toxins that have anticholinergic effects, in other words, that interfere with central cholinergic transmission, are apt to reduce arousal and alertness and affect overall attentional state. The central norepinephrine system also has been linked to attentional operations (Mesulam, 1985; Sara, 1985). Central noradrenergic pathways originate in a brainstem nucleus, the locus ceruleus, innervate the thalamus, and course through the frontal areas and back toward the posterior attention system. Norepinephrine, a transmitter, enhances the signal-to-noise ratio in neural transmission, thus enhancing attentiveness. Agents that increase central noradrenergic activity such as dextroamphetamine have been shown to enhance concentration in cognitive tasks (Rapoport, Buchsbaum, Zahn, Weingartner, Ludlow, & Mikkelsen, 1978). Interruption of these pathways has been shown to interfere with the ability to ignore irrelevant stimuli, thereby heightening distractibility (Mesulam, 1985). Thus, brain tumors, metabolic imbalances, or toxic substances that interfere with these central neural pathways or with the supply, uptake, or utilization of the neurotransmitters could produce attentional disturbance.

MANIFESTATIONS OF LOSS OF CONCENTRATION

It is apparent from clinical reports that complaints of loss of concentration or distractibility in persons with cancer most often relate to loss or decline in the capacity to direct attention, that is, to exert or sustain mental effort in purposeful activity. The characteristic effect is heightened distractibility, or an impaired ability to inhibit distracting stimuli. Loss of the capacity to direct attention has widespread and often unrecognized consequences on cognitive, behavioral, and affective responses. Attention supports the successful operation of key cognitive processes such as perception and memory (Mesulam, 1985). Thus, these cognitive functions also may be impaired secondary to the loss of capacity to direct attention.

Cognitive effects related to loss of concentration would include a reduced ability to maintain a coherent train of thought in the presence of distractions. Important areas of daily functioning, such as goal-setting, planning, initiating, or persisting in effortful activity, and modifying behavior to meet desired goals (Lezak, 1982), would become more difficult with diminished directed attention, if not impossible. The ability to inhibit or delay a response also may be impaired, resulting in impatience, reduced tolerance for frustration, or impulsivity in behavioral responses. In addition, when dealing with a life-threatening situation such as cancer, lowered capacity to direct attention could lead to a declining sense of personal effectiveness and ability to master or to cope with a situation, thus having a significant impact on affective state.

Global attentional failure is manifested as an acute confusional state, often referred to as delirium (Geschwind, 1982; Lipowski, 1987; Mesulam, 1985). The salient deficits in an acute confusional state are attentional: heightened distractibility, loss of ability to maintain a coherent train of thought, and inability to carry out goal-directed activity (Mesulam, 1985). Additional cognitive and behavioral disturbances are thought to be secondary to the attentional difficulties, although some may occur independently as a result of the underlying pathologic condition (Mesulam, 1985). Although diminished alertness may eventually occur, in the early stages of an acute confusional state, impairment of selective attentional processes tends to be more pronounced than is drowsiness (Mesulam, 1985).

ETIOLOGIC FACTORS

A striking number of cancer patients appear to be at risk for attentional impairment and loss of concentration at some time during the course of treatment and illness. A diverse cancer literature exists describing acute and delayed, mild to severe alterations in cognitive functioning related to the effects of the disease and its treatment on the central nervous system. However, it is difficult to determine the true nature and extent of attentional problems, because cognitive function is defined in various ways and the aspects of cognitive functioning that are assessed vary from study to study. Furthermore, despite the apparent primacy of attention in supporting key cognitive processes, attention is sometimes not assessed. Thus, it is possible that at times reported memory or perceptual problems, or deficits in complex reasoning or analytic abilities might be secondary to an attentional impairment.

CANCER-RELATED FACTORS

When testing was conducted, cognitive dysfunction was reported in 14 to 35 per cent of hospitalized cancer patients (Folstein, Fetting, Lobo, Niaz, Capozzoli, 1984; Silberfarb, Philibert, Levine, 1980). In these reports, the cognitive problems were clinically undetected and involved attentional disturbances. Similarly, Levine, Silberfarb, and Lipowski (1978) reported that 40 per cent of 100 consecutive cancer patients referred for psychiatric evaluation were diagnosed as having a cognitive impairment rather than an affective or emotional problem.

Disease-related factors including brain tumors, particularly of the frontal lobes (Mesulam, 1985) and brain and leptomeningeal metastases (Meyers & Scheibel, 1990; Siegel, Mildworf, Stein, & Mclamed, 1985) can produce cognitive deficits of varying types (including attentional disturbances) and severity. Cognitive deficits could occur from the effects of tumor on cerebral structures and metabolism as well as from neurotoxic effects of therapy such as cranial irradiation or chemotherapy aimed at the central nervous system (Lee, Nauert, & Glass, 1986).

Acute confusional states, for example, delirium, have been related to paraneoplastic syndromes as well as metabolic and respiratory complications of advanced disease. For excellent reviews pertaining specifically to delirium and cancer, see Anderson and Holmes (1993), Zimberg and Berenson (1990), and Fleishman and Lesko (1990).

TREATMENT-RELATED FACTORS

Acute neurotoxic side effects including confusion and delirium have been related to specific chemotherapeutic agents (Goldberg, Bloomer, & Dawson, 1982; Kaplan & Wiernik, 1982; Meyers & Scheibel, 1990; Peterson & Popkin, 1980; Silberfarb, 1983), particularly intrathecal methotrexate and high-dose cytarabine (Ara-C) (Baker, Royer, & Weiss, 1991; Lazarus, Herzig, Herzig, Phillips, Roessmann, & Fishman, 1981).

Several studies have assessed the neurobehavioral effects of biologic response modifiers (BRM), in particular, α-interferon and interleukin-2. Treatment with these substances has been associated with attentional deficits and frontal lobe dysfunction including loss of concentration and impairment of goal-directed activity (Adams, Quesada, & Gutterman, 1984; Denicoff et al., 1987; Merimsky, Reider-Groswasser, Inbar, & Chaitchik, 1990; Meyers & Scheibel, 1990). Loss of concentration also was shown to persist following discontinuation of α-interferon therapy in 14 patients who received extensive neuropsychologic assessment. Meyers, Scheibel, and Forman (1991) reported that findings in 71 per cent of these patients were suggestive of frontal-subcortical dysfunction, such as impaired problem-solving and decreased flexibility in shifting attention, 18 days to 3 years after treatment was discontinued. The authors reported that since many of these patients were in demanding jobs, even mild impairments were found to be incapacitating in their usual work.

LONG-TERM EFFECTS OF CENTRAL NERVOUS SYSTEM THERAPY

A growing body of literature has documented the adverse long-term effects of cancer treatment aimed at the central nervous system on cognitive functioning, particularly in children. (See Kramer and Moore's [1989] comprehensive review of late effects of cancer therapy on the central nervous system.) Both global and specific deficits in cognitive functioning and intellectual skills have been documented. The cognitive deficits often are reflected in poor attention span, distractibility, and loss of concentration (Goff, Anderson, & Cooper, 1980; Rowland et al., 1984). Such cognitive deficits have been particularly associated with cranial irradiation (Rowland et al., 1984) and younger age at the time of treatment (less than 8 years old) (Goff et al., 1980; Eiser & Lansdown, 1977). Such deficits can have a significant impact on learning and achievement in young children.

Recent studies in adults previously treated with chemotherapy or biologic response modifiers also have revealed the presence of clinically undetected cognitive abnormalities including attentional impairment (Meyers & Abbruzzese, 1992). Meyers and Abbruzzese (1992) found that 16 (34 per cent) of 47 cancer patients with metastatic solid tumors had cognitive deficits. Of these, almost one half showed dysfunction on more complex tasks of attention, while 33 per cent had deficits on more basic tasks of attention. These patients had a good physical performance status, had no central nervous system therapy, and had not received any treatment for at least 3 weeks. Type of previous treatment, particularly biologic response modifier (BRM), was a significant risk factor. Thus, of those found to have cognitive impairment, only 18 per cent had previously received chemotherapy, while 53 per cent had been treated with a BRM (e.g., interferon, interleukin, tumor necrosis factor). Subclinical attentional problems also have been detected in untreated patients with newly diagnosed lung cancer (small cell or nonsmall cell lung cancer) who have no evidence of cerebral metastasis on a CT scan or other biochemical, respiratory, or metabolic dysfunction (Siddiqui, Deshmukh, & Karimjee, 1992). The underlying cause for these attentional problems was unclear.

ADVANCED DISEASE

Severe cognitive deficits including attentional deficits are a common complication of advanced cancer. In a study by Bruera et al. (1992), cognitive functioning was assessed three times a week in 61 consecutive patients with advanced disease admitted to a palliative care unit for symptom management. All patients were receiving opioid analgesics for pain control. Thirty-four per cent were deemed to have cognitive impairment at the time of admission. Sixty-six episodes of cognitive impairment were detected in the 47 patients who eventually died in the hospital. Cognitive impairment in these patients was detected approximately 16 days before death. Cognitive impairment was ascribed to various possible causes including multiple drugs, brain metastasis, sepsis, and metabolic abnormalities such as liver and kidney failure, hypercalcemia, and hyponatremia. The cause, however, could not be determined in 56 per cent of the observed episodes. Of interest is that severe cognitive and attentional impairment as assessed by testing was not detected by either the physician or nurse on the same day of testing in about one fifth of the instances.

PAIN AND OPIOID ANALGESICS

In a study evaluating the effects of cancer-related pain on quality of life in 84 patients hospitalized with various types of malignancies (Strang & Qvarner, 1990), 56 per cent of the patients reported that pain affected their ability to concentrate, thereby hampering normal life activities.

Bruera, Macmillan, Hanson, and MacDonald (1989) studied the cognitive effects of opioid analgesics in 40 patients with cancer pain. Patients were assessed with cognitive measures, including attentional tests, on 2 consecutive days 45 minutes before and after they received a regular morning dose of intermittent opioid. The dose ranged from 10 to 16 mg of parenteral morphine. Although there were no changes in cognitive performance in patients who were on stable doses of opioids, significant impairment occurred in persons with recent dose escalations. This effect disappeared after the narcotic dose remained stable for about a week.

IMPACT OF LIFE-THREATENING ILLNESS: ATTENTIONAL FATIGUE

Prolonged or intense use of directed attention in a demanding life situation can lead to subsequent loss of mental effort, probably from fatigue of the underlying neural inhibitory mechanism that acts to block distracting stimuli (Kaplan & Kaplan, 1982; Cimprich, 1992b, 1993). Thus, this condition is termed attentional fatigue. Individuals with cancer are considered to be at high risk for attentional fatigue because of the multiple and often intense mental demands associated with diagnosis and treatment of cancer. Various informational, affective, and behavioral factors can increase the demands for use of directed attention. Directed attention is needed for making treatment decisions and for acquiring information pertaining to treatment and self-care (Derdiarian, 1987). At the same time, affective factors such as uncertainty about future outcomes, anticipated or actual losses, and related painful thoughts and feelings serve to increase the need for directed attention to function effectively in daily life (Frank-Stromborg, Wright, Segalla, & Diekman, 1984; Northouse, 1989). Finally, constraints on usual behavior and valued life activities resulting from pain, immobility, or other effects of disease or treatment may require sustained use of directed attention to cope with necessary changes and adjustments in daily life (Heinrich, Schag, & Ganz, 1984; Mages & Mendolsohn, 1979; Northouse, 1989; Weisman & Worden, 1976-77). In addition, a loss of normal restorative activities and inadequate sleep contribute to loss of normal capacity to direct attention.

When the demands for directed attention exceed the available mental effort (directed attention capacity), the person is at risk for developing attentional fatigue. A characteristic manifestation would be loss of concentration and distractibility. Thus, a person with attentional fatigue experiences a reduced capacity to perform purposeful mental or physical activities that require mental effort, for example, planning, problem-solving, learning new information, carrying out daily life chores, and adhering to difficult or complex treatment plans.

Clinical reports reveal that patients with cancer can experience loss of concentration that cannot be explained by known effects of cancer treatment (Holmes, 1991; Kobashi-Schoot, Hanewald, Van Dam, & Bruning, 1985; Loveys & Klaich, 1991; Mages & Mendolsohn, 1979; Oberst & James, 1985; McCorkle & Young, 1978), suggesting a possible fatigue effect. Loss of concentration also has been associated with general fatigue state (Kobashi-Schoot et al., 1985; Winningham et al., 1994). Thus, patients who are already compromised due to the effects of cancer or related therapies on the central nervous system may be particularly susceptible to attentional fatigue. In such instances the development of attentional fatigue can hasten cognitive decline and increase the severity of cognitive impairment.

Cimprich (1992b, 1993) initially studied the problem of attentional fatigue in 32 women, 29 to 84 years of age, newly diagnosed with Stage I or II breast cancer who were cognitively intact. The participants, who were assessed with repeated measures, showed significant attentional deficits during the 3 months following breast cancer surgery. The attentional deficits were not related to use of narcotic analgesics, type of surgery (mastectomy vs. breast conservation), or depressed mood state, suggesting a fatigue effect. These attentional deficits were observed at a time when directed attention was most needed to learn self-care measures after surgery, to understand and deal with the demands of adjuvant therapies, and to resume important life activities and roles.

AGING AND ATTENTIONAL FUNCTIONING

Aging has been associated with declines in the capacity to direct attention in healthy, cognitively intact (no known cognitive disorder or dementia) elderly in a number of studies, particularly when the environmental demands are high. Older adults had more difficulty than younger adults in selectively attending to focal stimuli in the presence of distraction (McDowd & Filion, 1992; Rogers, 1992), were less able to ignore distracting/competing stimuli in performing various tasks (Barr & Giambra, 1990; Rabbitt, 1982; West & Crook, 1990) and were less able to sustain directed attention to an effortful task over time (Parasuraman & Giambra, 1991). Overall, the findings suggest that older people may be less efficient in directing attention, that is inhibiting competing stimuli, and thus may be more prone to attentional difficulties in demanding circumstances.

A recent study of functional status in 799 elderly patients (aged 65 years and older) newly diagnosed with cancer found that 40 per cent had some problem with cognitive functioning (Goodwin, Hunt, & Samet, 1991), suggesting an increased vulnerability for attentional disturbance in older cancer patients.

Cimprich (1992c) found that older women over 60 years of age showed significantly greater fatigue-related impairment in the capacity to direct attention during the 3 months after breast cancer surgery than did younger women. It is likely that older cancer patients may be more susceptible to attentional fatigue as a function of aging, and the detrimental impact of attentional fatigue on functioning may be even greater in older patients who already are experiencing life stresses related to comorbid illness, the loss of spouse and friends, reduced income, and/or forced dependency (Kane, 1991; Boyle, Engelking, Blesch, Dodge, Sarna, & Weinrich, 1992).

ASSESSING LOSS OF CONCENTRATION

Assessing attention and concentration in cancer patients has generally been done in the context of general cognitive assessment to detect global impairments such as delirium or psychiatric disorders (Folstein et al., 1984). Loss of concentration, however, can occur in the absence of cognitive or psychiatric disorders. Effective ways to assess this symptom in clinical practice are urgently needed. With improved assessment of attentional functioning and detection of impaired concentration, nursing interventions may be more effectively designed to meet individual needs related to patient learning, self-care, discharge planning, and adherence to treatment plan (Palmateer & McCartney, 1985). In addition, high-risk patients who will need further assistance in coping with the effects of cancer and its treatment and the added mental demands of life-threatening illness can be more readily identified.

CLINICAL ASSESSMENT

Clinical evaluation of loss of concentration may be based on observation and objective and subjective measures (Table 59–1). Van Zomeren and Brouwer (1994) propose that assessment of attention should begin with observation of the patient's behavior from the first contact. Components of the assessment include evaluating alertness, attention span, and the capacity to focus and concentrate. A normal level of alertness is necessary for effective functioning of attentional processes. Level of alertness can be estimated based on response to verbal and environmental stimuli and the patient's ability to maintain an adequate level of wakefulness over the course of a brief, few minute interaction. Folstein and colleagues (1984) have devised a valid and reliable visual analogue scale for use by the practitioner to rate the degree of drowsiness of the patient, from normally alert to very drowsy. Assessment of attention span may be made based on the patient's ability to follow simple directions or the need to repeat questions or points of information just given. The ability to sustain focus and concentrate may be observed in the presence or absence of distractibility during an interaction, for example, patient's ability to ignore irrelevant sounds or events in the environment, ability to listen, or capacity to follow a train of thought. There appear to be wide individual differences in normal attentional capacity, so noting *changes* in the ability to concentrate is particularly important.

TABLE 59–1. *General Guidelines for Clinical Assessment of Loss of Concentration*

Begin assessment at first clinical contact; assess changes or losses over time in following:
Level of alertness
    Response to verbal or environmental stimuli
    Degree of alertness/drowsiness in brief interactions
    Rating of alertness/drowsiness using a visual analogue scale (e.g., Folstein, et al., 1984)
Attention span
    Ability to follow simple directions or points of information
    Performance on standard measure (e.g., digit span forward)
Capacity to focus and concentrate on an intended activity
    Degree of distractibility (e.g., ability to ignore irrelevant sounds, listen, or follow a train of thought)
    Performance on standard measures (e.g., serial sevens, digit span backward)
Subjective perception of loss of concentration in daily life
    Self-rating of ability to concentrate using a numerical scale (e.g., McCorkle & Young, 1978)
    Perceived difficulty in planning and carrying out daily life tasks
    Perceived impatience and irritability in social interactions

Although relying on observations, interactions, and clinical judgment to determine the effectiveness of concentration in patients is in principle an acceptable clinical approach (Van Zomeren & Brouwer, 1994), milder or subtle impairments may not be detectable without more systematic assessment. Palmateer and McCartney (1985) showed that nurses did not detect cognitive impairment in 72 per cent of 65 elderly, general medical-surgical patients found to have a cognitive deficit when assessed using a screening tool.

Cognitive screening tools may be used to detect global cognitive impairments (e.g., delirium) (Lezak, 1983). Commonly used tools such as the Mini Mental Status Examination (MMSE) (11 items) (Folstein, Folstein & McHugh, 1975) or the Cognitive Capacity Screening Examination (CCSE) (30 items) (Jacobs, 1977) are valid and reliable bedside screening measures for cognitive dysfunction. Poor performance on such screening tools should be followed by more intensive diagnostic workup to determine the nature of the cognitive dysfunction including a complete physical and psychosocial assessment. Such cognitive screening tools, however, may not be able to detect more subtle impairments in attention and concentration.

Van Zomeren and Brouwer (1994) describe a group of clinical measures that may be used at the bedside to assess whether the patient is able to concentrate on a simple task demanding some mental effort. These include counting backwards from 10 (the simplest measure), the Serial Sevens task, and Digit Span. In the Serial Sevens task (part of both the MMSE and the CCSE) the patient is asked to subtract 7 from a number near 100 and stop after five answers. Foreman (1990) found that measures of concentration such as the Serial Sevens task were extremely useful in differentiating an acutely confused individual from one who was not. One important consideration, however, is that individuals having less than an eighth grade level of education have been shown to perform worse on measures involving arithmetic calculations (Anthony, LeResche, Niaz, Von Korff, & Folstein, 1982).

Digit Span is considered a valid and useful test of attention because it contains a low-demand condition requiring little mental effort (forward span) that is sensitive to impairment in attention span and a high-demand condition (backward span) that is sensitive to milder impairment in the ability to concentrate or exert mental effort (Lezak, 1983; Van Zomeren & Brouwer, 1994). It also can be done readily at the bedside. The Digit Span test is standardized and thus, general guidelines exist concerning the interpretation of Digit Span scores (Lezak, 1983). However, it is important to again note that individual differences in attentional capacity do exist and that determining changes in performance is particularly important, especially when scores are marginal or in the low normal range. For example, a person may score within a normal range on Digit Span, but still report a significant loss of concentration over time.

The patient also can be asked to provide a subjective rating of perceived ability to concentrate using a numeric scale. One such item is contained in the Symptom Distress Scale developed by McCorkle and Young (1978). Such a measure is particularly useful for repeated assessment to detect changes over time. One drawback is that subjective ratings of ability to concentrate may not be directly correlated with actual attentional performance (Cimprich, 1992b). In other words, mild losses in the capacity to concentrate and exert mental effort may not be perceived until they become more severe and the consequences are more apparent to the patient.

Another area of assessment that requires further development is evaluating the impact of loss of concentration on functioning in daily life in individuals with cancer. More systematic evaluation is needed of how a loss of the capacity to direct attention may affect specific aspects of functioning, cognitive, physical and psychosocial, including ability to return to work and to resume valued life activities and roles.

DISTINGUISHING ATTENTIONAL IMPAIRMENT FROM DEPRESSION AND MEMORY PROBLEMS

Attentional impairments need to be distinguished from other conditions such as depression and memory problems. Attentional impairment may be confused with depression and vice versa, unless a deliberate assessment is made. In a study of 100 consecutive requests for psychiatric consultation on cancer patients, cognitive impairment was diagnosed in 40 per cent of the patients (Lipowski, 1987). However, this diagnosis had been initially missed by house staff in 65 per cent of the cases, with cognitive impairment most often misdiagnosed as depression. Depressed patients also may have attentional or other cognitive problems (Cohen, Weingartner, Smallberg, Pickar, & Murphy, 1982), but changes in affect (e.g., sadness, apathy, withdrawal) usually are the dominant features. Conversely, individuals need not have depressed mood state or other affective problems to experience attentional deficits (Mesulam, 1985). Silberfarb and colleagues (1980) found little correlation between performance on various cognitive measures that tapped attention and depressed mood state in individuals with varying types of cancer. Others have found no correlation between attentional measures and depressed mood state in patients with breast cancer (Cimprich, 1992b) and in individuals with multiple sclerosis (Jansen & Cimprich, 1994).

There is a close association between attention and short-term or working memory. However, pathologic memory disorders may or may not be associated with attentional disturbance. For example, an amnesic form of Alzheimer's disease is commonly associated with attentional disturbance, but the dominant feature is the memory problem (Mesulam, 1985). In other instances, putative memory problems in daily living such as loss of a train of thought, forgetfulness (e.g., forgetting what one has started out to do, misplacing things), or difficulty finding a word may actually be attentional problems that may be ameliorated by interventions that support attentional functioning.

INTERVENTIONS FOR LOSS OF CONCENTRATION

General nursing approaches to improve cognitive functioning in persons with cancer most often have been discussed in relation to "altered mental status" such as delirium (Anderson & Holmes, 1993; Zimberg & Berenson, 1990). However, few research studies have systematically examined the effectiveness of interventions to maintain or restore the capacity to direct attention in individuals with cancer. Rehabilitation programs that address attentional deficits in other populations such as brain-damaged individuals have focused on retraining attention for specific tasks. Van Zomeren and Brouwer (1994), however, argue that it is difficult to determine the overall efficacy of such programs because they often lack a theoretic basis, incorporate multiple rather than single techniques, and focus on varying aspects of attention.

There are two promising nursing interventions for managing loss of concentration in patients with cancer. The first intervention focuses on conserving attentional capacity by reducing the environmental demands that lead to attentional fatigue. Reducing environmental demands is especially important when loss of concentration already exists due to the pathologic effects of cancer or its treatment on the central nervous system.

The second intervention focuses on controlling the overall level of attentional fatigue by promoting rest and recovery of directed attention.

CONSERVING ATTENTION: REDUCING ENVIRONMENTAL DEMANDS

Three nursing approaches may be useful for helping patients dealing with a life-threatening illness such as cancer to reduce attentional demands: (1) improving patient educational and informational interventions; (2) increasing the supportiveness of the physical environment in health care settings; and (3) instructing patients and families in attention-conserving strategies that may be applied in daily living (Table 59–2).

With shortened hospitalization for cancer treatment and the increased focus on ambulatory care, patients and families are expected to learn new information and use self-care skills within relatively short periods of time and under highly stressful conditions (Cimprich, 1992a). Such expectations place enormous demands on normal directed attentional capacity. To reduce demands for mental effort and support ease of learning and understanding, three principles should be followed (Cimprich, 1992a; Kaplan & Kaplan, 1982): (1) there should be a premium placed on economy of information in all instructional methods (verbal, written, and audiovisual) so that the main points are clear and there is little danger of getting distracted by details; (2) important information should be conveyed in a vivid and concrete manner, that is, easily imaged or visualized with liberal use of pictures, illustrations, diagrams, examples; and (3) instruction should be paced to accommodate individual levels of attentional capacity with built-in opportunities for answering questions, clarifying information, and exploring further important information. Nursing research is needed to increase understanding of how individuals learn under stressful conditions and to test strategies that might support attention and ease of learning under such conditions.

The deleterious effects of the physical environment in health care settings on attentional functioning often are unrecognized and remain poorly understood (Williams, 1988). Many health care environments contain multiple irritating distractions such as noise, traffic, multiple caregivers, and complex, technologic surroundings, to name but a few. Even under the best circumstances such conditions coerce attention and are difficult or impossible to ignore (Cimprich, 1992a). Thus, considerable vigilance and mental effort would be needed to carry out even the simplest activity, for example, finding one's way or making sense of the people, sights, and sounds in the immediate environment. Furthermore, in such environments, important activities that require directed attention such as learning, solving problems, or making decisions would be difficult, if not impossible. There is a need for nursing research to better understand ways to modify and redesign the physical environment in health care settings to reduce mental demands and support effective functioning particularly when attention is already compromised.

TABLE 59–2. *Nursing Approaches for Conserving Attention*

Reduce environmental demands in:
Patient education
    Strive for economy of information
    Provide information that is vivid (easily imaged) and concrete
    Pace instruction; use interactive techniques
Physical health care environment
    Design and modify health care environments to support functioning
    Minimize attentional demands from noise and other distractions
    Increase predictability; provide structure
Daily life activities
    Reduce or avoid time pressure
    Focus on priorities; break large tasks into smaller goals
    Create structure in daily activities, e.g., use of lists or schedules
    Prevent distractions when carrying out a task, e.g., from TV or telephone

Finally, nurses can instruct patients in certain strategies to help conserve attention in daily living. Van Zomeren and Brouwer (1994) propose strategy training for reducing unnecessary demands for directed attention. They recommend four general strategies that seem highly applicable in helping patients conserve attention and mental effort in daily life: (1) avoid time pressure when at all possible; (2) analyze priorities and direct attention to those things that are most important; (3) create or improve structure in the environment and in daily activities; and (4) prevent or minimize interruptions or distractions when carrying out a task or purposeful activity. Nurses can assist patients and families to incorporate such strategies into the home environment and activities of daily living and can assess their effectiveness in conserving attentional capacity and improving daily functioning.

ATTENTION-RESTORING INTERVENTIONS

A promising new area of nursing study involves developing interventions to counteract attentional fatigue in persons with a life-threatening illness such as cancer by restoring directed attentional capacity (Cimprich, 1993). Kaplan and Kaplan (1989) proposed that an attention-restoring experience has four important properties: (1) some source of fascination that captures involuntary or effortless attention, (2) a sense of being away from concerns that normally occupy the mind, (3) extent or sufficient scope to permit exploration, and (4) compatibility with an individual's inclinations and purposes. The natural environment appears to contain all the properties important for a restorative experience (Kaplan & Kaplan, 1989). Thus, potentially restorative activities may include walking or sitting in natural surroundings, tending plants, gardening, watching birds or other wildlife, and even a natural view from a window when a person is confined.

Preliminary research by Cimprich (1992b, 1993) and others (Hartig, Mang, & Evans, 1991) suggests that exposure to natural environment can help to counteract attentional fatigue. The effects of an intervention aimed at restoring directed attention were studied in women newly diagnosed with breast cancer who showed attentional deficits over an extended period following surgery (Cimprich, 1993). Those women who received a randomly assigned intervention that consisted of regular participation in simple nature activities showed steady improvement in attentional capacity and functioning over the 3 months following surgery, while the control group did not (Cimprich, 1993). The intervention also appeared to have a significant, positive impact on daily functioning for women in the restorative group who returned to work sooner and reported resuming jobs and valued life activities more often than those in the control group. These findings suggest that this theoretically based intervention may be beneficial for improving attentional capacity and functioning in patients with cancer. Further research, however, is needed to determine the efficacy of proposed attention-restoring activities in counteracting attentional fatigue in patients with various types of cancer and under different treatment conditions.

SUMMARY

Loss of concentration can have a significant detrimental impact on overall functioning and increase levels of distress in persons treated for cancer. Multiple factors related to cancer, its treatment, and the demands of a life-threatening illness increase the risk for loss of concentration. Attentional problems have been associated with primary and secondary brain tumors, acute and delayed effects of treatment with certain chemotherapeutic agents given intrathecally and at high doses, biologic response modifiers, cranial irradiation, and complications of advanced disease. Dose escalations in opioid analgesics also temporarily affect attentional functioning. In addition, in responding to the many demands inherent in diagnosis and treatment of cancer, a person can unknowingly overuse the capacity to direct attention resulting in attentional fatigue and loss of concentration.

Loss of concentration may be assessed clinically by observation and objective and subjective measures. Nurses can intervene to help conserve attention by reducing environmental demands. In addition, it may be possible to help counteract loss of concentration due to attentional fatigue through therapeutic application of attention-restoring activities. Finally, nursing research is needed to better understand the problem of loss of concentration and ways to support and improve attentional functioning in persons with cancer.

ACKNOWLEDGEMENT. The author thanks Barbara Therrien, Ph.D., R.N., and Stephen Kaplan, Ph.D., for their comments during the preparation of this manuscript.

REFERENCES

Adams, F., Quesada, J. R., & Gutterman, J. U. (1984). Neuropsychiatric manifestations of human leukocyte interferon therapy in patients with cancer. *Journal of the American Medical Association, 252,* 938–941.

Anderson, B., & Holmes, W. (1993). Altered mental status: An algorithm for assessment of delirium in the cancer patient. *Current Issues in Cancer Nursing Practice Updates, 2,* 1–10.

Anthony, J. C., LeResche, L., Niaz, U., Von Korff, M. R., & Folstein, M. F. (1982). Limits of the 'Mini-Mental State' as a screening test for dementia and delirium among hospital patients. *Psychological Medicine, 12,* 397–408.

Baker, W. J., Royer, G. L., & Weiss, R. B. (1991). Cytarabine and neurologic toxicity. *Journal of Clinical Oncology, 9,* 679–693.

Barr, R. A., & Giambra, L. M. (1990). Age-related decrement in auditory selective attention. *Psychology and Aging, 5,* 597–599.

Berglund, G., Bolund, C., Fornander, T., Rutquist, L. E., & Sjoden, P. O. (1991). Late effects of adjuvant chemotherapy and postoperative radiotherapy on quality of life among breast cancer patients. *European Journal of Cancer, 27,* 1075–1081.

Boyle, D. M., Engelking, C., Blesch K. S., Dodge, J., Sarna, L., & Weinrich, S. (1992). Oncology Nursing Society position paper on cancer and aging: The mandate for oncology nursing. *Oncology Nursing Forum, 19,* 913–931.

Bruera, E., Macmillan, K., Hanson, J., & MacDonald, R. N. (1989). The cognitive effects of the administration of narcotic analgesics in patients with cancer pain. *Pain, 39,* 13–16.

Bruera, E., Miller, L., McCallion, J., Macmillan, K., Krefting, L., & Hanson, J. (1992). Cognitive failure in patients with terminal cancer: A prospective study. *Journal of Pain and Symptom Management, 7,* 192–195.

Cimprich, B. (1992a). A theoretical perspective on attention and patient education. *Advances in Nursing Science, 14(3),* 39–51.

Cimprich, B. (1992b). Attentional fatigue following breast cancer surgery. *Research in Nursing and Health, 15,* 199–207.

Cimprich, B. (1992c). Restoring optimum cognitive function in the older adult with cancer. In C. D. Bailey (Ed.), *Cancer nursing: Changing frontiers* (pp. 23–26). Oxford, England: Rapid Communications of Oxford.

Cimprich, B. (1993). Development of an intervention to restore attention in cancer patients. *Cancer Nursing, 16,* 83–92.

Cohen, R. M., Weingartner, H., Smallberg S. A., Pickar, D., & Murphy, D. L. (1982). Effort and cognition in depression. *Archives of General Psychiatry, 39,* 593–597.

Denicoff, K. D., Rubinow, D. R., Papa, M. Z., Simpson, C., Seipp, C. A., Lotze, M. T., Chang, A. E., Rosenstein, D., & Rosenberg, S. A. (1987). The neuropsychiatric effects of treatment with interleukin-2 and lymphokine-activated killer cells. *Annals of Internal Medicine, 107,* 293–300.

Derdiarian, A. (1987). Informational needs of recently diagnosed cancer patients, Part II. Method and description. *Cancer Nursing, 10,* 156–163.

Eiser, C., & Lansdown, R. (1977). Retrospective study of intellectual development in children treated for acute lymphoblastic leukemia. *Archives of Disease in Childhood, 52,* 525–529.

Fleishman, S., & Lesko, L. (1990). Delirium and dementia. In J. C. Holland & J. H. Rowland (Eds.), *Handbook of psychooncology* (pp. 342–355). New York: Oxford University Press.

Folstein, M. F., Fetting, J. H., Lobo, A, Niaz, U., & Capozzoli, K. D. (1984). Cognitive assessment of cancer patients. *Cancer, 53 (Suppl. 1),* 2250–2257.

Folstein, M. F., Folstein, S. E., & McHugh, P. R. (1975). "Mini-Mental State:" A practical method for grading the cognitive state of patients for the clinician. *Journal of Psychiatric Research, 12,* 189–198.

Foreman, M. D. (1990). The cognitive and behavioral nature of acute confusional states. *Scholarly Inquiry for Nursing Practice: An International Journal, 5,* 3–16.

Frank-Stromborg, M., Wright, P., Segalla, M., & Diekman, J. (1984). Psychological impact of the "cancer" diagnosis. *Oncology Nursing Forum, 11,* 16–22.

Geschwind, N. (1982). Disorders of attention: A frontier in neuropsychology. *Philosophical Transactions of the Royal Society of London, 298,* 173–185.

Goff, J. R., Anderson, H. R., & Cooper, P. F. (1980). Distractibility and memory deficits in long-term survivors of acute lymphoblastic leukemia. *Developmental and Behavioral Pediatrics, 1,* 158–163.

Goldberg, I. D., Bloomer, W. D., & Dawson, D. M. (1982). Nervous system toxic effects of cancer therapy. *Journal of the American Medical Association, 247,* 1437–1441.

Goodwin, J. S., Hunt, W. C., & Samet, J. M. (1991). A population-based study of functional status and social support networks of elderly patients newly diagnosed with cancer. *Archives of Internal Medicine, 151,* 366–370.

Hartig, T., Mang, M., & Evans, G. W. (1991). Restorative effects of natural environment experience. *Environment and Behavior, 23,* 3–26.

Heinrich, R. L., Schag, C. C., & Ganz, P. A. (1984). Living with cancer: The cancer inventory of problem situations. *Journal of Clinical Psychology, 40,* 972–980.

Holmes, S. (1991). Preliminary investigations of symptom distress in two cancer patient populations: Evaluation of a measurement instrument. *Journal of Advanced Nursing, 16,* 439–446.

Jacobs, J. W. (1977). Screening for organic mental syndromes in the medically ill. *Annals of Internal Medicine, 86,* 40–46.

James, W. (1983). *The principles of psychology.* Cambridge, MA: Harvard University Press. (Original work published 1890.)

Jansen, D. A., & Cimprich, B. (1994). Attentional impairment in persons with Multiple Sclerosis. *Journal of Neuroscience Nursing, 26,* 95–102.

Kane, R. A. (1991). Psychosocial issues: Psychological and social issues for older people with cancer. *Cancer, 68,* 2514–2518.

Kaplan, R., & Kaplan, S. (1989). *The experience of nature: A psychological perspective.* Cambridge, England: Cambridge University Press.

Kaplan, R. S., & Wiernik, P. H. (1982). Neurotoxicity of antineoplastic drugs. *Seminars in Oncology, 9,* 103–113.

Kaplan, S., & Kaplan, R. (1982). *Environment and cognition.* New York: Praeger.

Kobashi-Schoot, J. A. M., Hanewald, G. J. F. P., Van Dam, F. S. A. M., & Bruning, P. F. (1985). Assessment of malaise in cancer patients treated with radiotherapy. *Cancer Nursing, 8,* 306–313.

Kramer, J., & Moore, I. M. (1989). Late effects of cancer therapy on the central nervous system. *Seminars in Oncology Nursing, 5,* 22–28.

Lazarus, H. M., Herzig, R. H., Herzig, G. P., Phillips, G. L., Roessmann, U., & Fishman, D. J. (1981). Central nervous system toxicity of high-dose systemic cytosine arabinoside. *Cancer, 48,* 2577–2582.

Lee, Y., Nauert, C., & Glass, J. P. (1986). Treatment-related white matter changes in cancer patients. *Cancer, 57,* 1473–1482.

Levine, P. M., Silberfarb, P. M., & Lipowski, Z. J. (1978). Mental disorders in cancer patients: A study of 100 psychiatric referrals. *Cancer, 42,* 1385–1391.

Lezak, M. (1982). The problem of assessing executive functions. *International Journal of Psychology, 17,* 281–297.

Lezak, M. (1983). *Neuropsychological assessment.* New York: Oxford University Press.

Lipowski, Z. J. (1987). Delirium (acute confusional states). *Journal of the American Medical Association, 258,* 1789–1792.

Loveys, B. J., & Klaich, K. (1991). Breast cancer: Demands of illness. *Oncology Nursing Forum, 18,* 75–80.

Mages, N. L., & Mendolsohn, G. A. (1979). Effects of cancer on patients' lives: A personological approach. In G. Stone & N. Adler (Eds.), *Health psychology-A handbook* (pp. 255–284). San Francisco: Jossey-Bass.

Mandler, G. (1975). Consciousness: Respectable, useful, and probably necessary. In R. L. Solso (Ed.), *Information processing and cognition* (pp. 229–254). Hillsdale, NJ: Erlbaum.

McCorkle, R., & Young, K. (1978). Development of a symptom distress scale. *Cancer Nursing, 1,* 373–378.

McDowd, J. M., & Filion, D. L. (1992). Aging, selective attention, and inhibitory processes: A psychophysiological approach. *Psychology and Aging, 7,* 65–71.

Merimsky, O., Reider-Groswasser, I., Inbar, M., & Chaitchik, S. (1990). Interferon-related mental deterioration and behavioral changes in patients with renal cell carcinoma. *European Journal of Cancer, 26,* 596–600.

Mesulam, M. M. (1985). *Principles of behavioral neurology.* Philadelphia: F. A. Davis Company.

Meyers, C. A., & Abbruzzese, J. L. (1992). Cognitive functioning in cancer patients: Effect of previous treatment. *Neurology, 42,* 434–436.

Meyers, C. A., & Scheibel, R. S. (1990). Early detection and diagnosis of neuro-behavioral disorders associated with cancer and its treatment. *Oncology, 4,* 115–130.

Meyers, C. A., Scheibel, R. S., & Forman, A. D. (1991). Persistent neurotoxicity of systemically administered interferon-alpha. *Neurology, 41,* 672–676.

Miller, G. A. (1956). The magical number seven, plus or minus two: Some limits on our capacity for processing information. *Psychological Review, 63,* 81–97.

Northouse, L. L. (1989). The impact of breast cancer on patients and husbands. *Cancer Nursing, 12,* 276–284.

Oberst, M., & James, R. (1985). Going home: Patient and spouse adjustment following cancer surgery. *Topics in Clinical Nursing, 7, (1)* 46–56.

Palmateer, L. M., & McCartney, J. R. (1985). Do nurses know when patients have cognitive deficits? *Journal of Gerontological Nursing, 11, (2)* 6–16.

Parasuraman, R., & Giambra, L. (1991). Skill development in vigilance: Effects of event rate and age. *Psychology and Aging, 6,* 155–169.

Peterson, L. G., & Popkin, M. K. (1980). Neuropsychiatric effects of chemotherapeutic agents for cancer. *Psychosomatics, 21,* 141–153.

Posner, M. I., & Boies, S. (1971). Components of attention. *Psychological Review, 78,* 391–408.

Posner, M. I., & Dehaene, S. (1994). Attentional networks. *Trends in Neuroscience, 17,* 75–79.

Posner, M. I., & Snyder, C. R. (1975). Attention and cognitive control. In R. L. Solso (Ed.), *Information processing and cognition* (pp. 55–85). Hillsdale, NJ: Erlbaum.

Rabbitt, P. M. A. (1982). How do old people know what to do next? In F. I. M. Craik & S. Trehub (Eds.), *Aging and cognitive processes* (Vol. 8, pp. 79–97). New York: Plenum Press.

Rapoport, J. L., Buchsbaum, M. S., Zahn, T. P., Weingartner, H., Ludlow, C., & Mikkelsen, E. J. (1978). Dextroamphetamine: Cognitive and behavioral effects in normal prepubertal boys. *Science, 199,* 560–563.

Rogers, W. A. (1992). Age differences in visual search: Target and distractor learning. *Psychology and Aging, 7,* 526–535.

Rothbart, M. K., & Posner, M. I. (1985). Temperament and the development of self-regulation. In L. C. Hartlage & C. F. Telzrow (Eds.), *The neuropsychology of individual differences-A developmental perspective* (pp. 93–123). New York: Plenum.

Rowland, J. H., Glidewell, O. J., Sibley, R. F., Holland, J. C., Tull, R., Berman, A., Brecher, M. L., Harris, M., Glicksman, A. S., Forman, E., Jones, B., Cohen, M. E., Duffner, P. K., & Freeman, A. I. (1984). Effects of different forms of central nervous system prophylaxis on neuropsychologic function in childhood leukemia. *Journal of Clinical Oncology, 2,* 1327–1335.

Sara, S. J. (1985). Noradrenergic modulation of selective attention: Its role in memory retrieval. *Annals of the New York Academy of Sciences, 444,* 178–193.

Siddiqui, T., Deshmukh, V. K., & Karimjee, N. (1992). Subclinical cognitive deficits in cancer patients: A preliminary P300 study. *Clinical Electroencephalography, 23,* 132–136.

Siegal, T., Mildworf, B., Stein, D., & Melamed, M. D. (1985). Leptomeningeal metastases: Reduction in regional cerebral blood flow and cognitive impairment. *Annals of Neurology, 17,* 100–102.

Silberfarb, P. M. (1983). Chemotherapy and cognitive defects in cancer patients. *Annual Review of Medicine, 34,* 35–46.

Silberfarb, P. M., Philibert D., & Levine, P. M. (1980). Psychosocial aspects of neoplastic disease: II. Affective and cognitive effects of chemotherapy in cancer patients. *American Journal of Psychiatry, 137,* 597–601.

Strang, P., & Qvarner, H. (1990). Cancer-related pain and its influence on quality of life. *Anticancer Research, 10,* 109–112.

Van Zomeren, A. H., & Brouwer, W. H. (1994). *Clinical neuropsychology of attention.* New York: Oxford University Press.

Weisman, A. D., & Worden, J. W. (1976–77). The existential plight in cancer: Significance of the first 100 days. *International Journal of Psychiatry in Medicine, 7,* 1–15.

West, R. L., & Crook, T. H. (1990). Age differences in everyday memory: Laboratory analogues of telephone number recall. *Psychology and Aging, 5,* 520–529.

Williams, M. (1988). The physical environment and patient care. *Annual Review of Nursing Research, 6,* 61–84.

Winningham, M. L., Nail, L. M., Burke, M. B., Brophy, L., Cimprich, B., Jones, L. S., Pickard-Holley, S., Rhodes, V., St. Pierre, B., Beck, S., Glass, E. C., Mock, V. L., Mooney, K. H., & Piper, B. (1994). Fatigue and the cancer experience: The state of the knowledge. *Oncology Nursing Forum, 21,* 23–36.

Zimberg, M., & Berenson, S. (1990). Delirium in patients with cancer: Nursing assessment and intervention. *Oncology Nursing Forum, 17,* 529–538.

Psychosocial Aspects of Cancer

Jeannie Pasacreta • Ruth McCorkle

Major changes in the understanding and treatment of cancer have led to a wider range of treatment options and increasing length of survival from time of diagnosis. While such advances are quite positive, the impact of a cancer diagnosis on the emotional lives of patients and families remains noteworthy and highlights the need to address the emotional aspects of chronic illness.

Cancer and its treatment often carry a large burden of emotional consequences due to the chronic nature of the disease. Involvement with a complicated and fragmented health care delivery system, the need for episodic and at times, aggressive treatment, remissions and exacerbations of acute and uncomfortable symptoms, family separation, financial burden, functional limitations, and role disruptions are but a few of the issues that characterize the life of many patients with cancer. Even for those considered cured or who experience lengthy disease-free intervals, the challenge of setting the cancer experience "on the back burner" can prove to be difficult.

Since most cancers are known to be fatal when untreated, the confirmation of a cancer diagnosis often leads to fear and intense psychologic concerns. Common fears and problems associated with a cancer diagnosis include threat of a premature death, discomfort from painful medical procedures, disfigurement and body image disturbances secondary to surgery and treatment effects, sexual dysfunction related to fatigue and fertility problems, and role and relationship disruptions that may occur during acute illness periods (See Chapter 18). These are just a sampling of the issues that may confront the patient with cancer and highlight the need for monitoring and increased attention to the psychosocial needs that accompany all aspects and critical phases of the illnesses.

In light of the fact that cancer poses a major public health concern in this country, health care professionals should be informed of the factors that affect psychosocial adjustment, the wide range of psychologic responses that accompany the disease during each of its phases, and the efficacy of various modes of psychosocial intervention in minimizing distress and promoting adaptation. The goal of this chapter is to provide information regarding factors that affect psychosocial adjustment among individuals with chronic illness, the wide range of psychologic responses that are possible throughout the illness trajectory, and the efficacy of various modes of psychosocial intervention in minimizing distress and promoting adaptation. Practical guidelines regarding patient management and identifying patients who may be at risk for sustaining psychosocial problems or who may require formal psychiatric consultation are offered.

CHANGES IN TREATMENT AND SOCIETAL ATTITUDES: ACCOMPANYING TRENDS IN PSYCHOSOCIAL ISSUES

The secrecy that prevailed in the 1960s and prohibited disclosure of a cancer diagnosis by most physicians (Novack, Plummer, Ochitill, Morrow, & Bennett, 1979; Oken, 1961) has given way to the practice of imparting the particulars of diagnosis, treatment options, and prognosis routinely (Krant, 1976; Oken, 1961). Despite this change, however, it has been suggested that ongoing fears and concerns among health care providers about cancer have led to a discrepancy between attitude and action, resulting in communication of emotionally laden information in a fashion ranging from overprotective and paternalistic to blunt and matter of fact (Dermatis & Lesko, 1991).

Discrepancies between attitude and practice have also been demonstrated by clinicians who have been found to avoid clear, open discussions of topics such as prognosis and death despite consistently expressed beliefs regarding the importance of openness and honesty with all mentally competent patients. Thus, although the prevailing attitude in health care supports disclosure of medical information and active involvement of patients in decisions that affect them, the actual behavior of health care providers likely reflects a more limited improvement in patient care (Holland, 1989a).

Personal views and concerns of clinicians about cancer can affect communication with patients especially at key decision-making and transition points along the continuum of care. The use of peers and other members of the health care team to assist patients with issues and concerns that are particularly upsetting for primary care clinicians are useful strategies for ensuring maximum support for patients faced with the complex decisions inherent in cancer treatment.

CLINICAL COURSE OF CANCER

The clinical course of cancer follows one of several possible courses or trajectories. Figure 60–1 outlines a scheme of clinical cancer. A number of patients respond to the curative attempt with no recurrence of disease, remain well, and are after a period of time considered cured (Course A). Some patients have a positive response to a curative attempt but then develop recurrence or metastasis (Course B). Other patients begin treatment with a hope for cure but do not respond and progressively decline (Course C). In some patients, the disease is too far advanced at the time of diagnosis, and they experience a progression of their disease (Course D).

The acute stress response has been described as a usual response to the diagnosis of cancer occurring at each transitional point of illness (beginning treatment, recurrence, treatment failure, disease progression) (Holland, 1989a). The response is characterized by shock, disbelief, anxiety, depression, sleep, appetite disturbance, and difficulty performing activities of daily living. Under favorable circumstances these psychologic symptoms should resolve within approximately 2 weeks (Holland, 1989a) to 3 months (Weissman & Worden, 1976-1977). Obviously, this time period is quite variable, but the general consensus within the literature is that once the crisis has passed and individuals know what to expect in terms of a treatment plan, psychologic symptoms diminish (Endicott, 1984; Holland, 1989a).

In one study, patient concerns and symptom distress including self-reports of affective disturbance were examined in cancer and myocardial infarction patients at 1 and 2 months postdiagnosis. Affective disturbance was greater in the cancer group on both occasions. For both groups, however, concerns and mood improved significantly at the second interview supporting the time-limited nature of the crisis associated with diagnosis (McCorkle & Benoliel, 1983). Other studies report, however, that a proportion of cancer patients continue to meet criteria for depression after 1 year (Endicott, 1984; Morris, Greer, & White, 1977). It seems reasonable to assume that despite

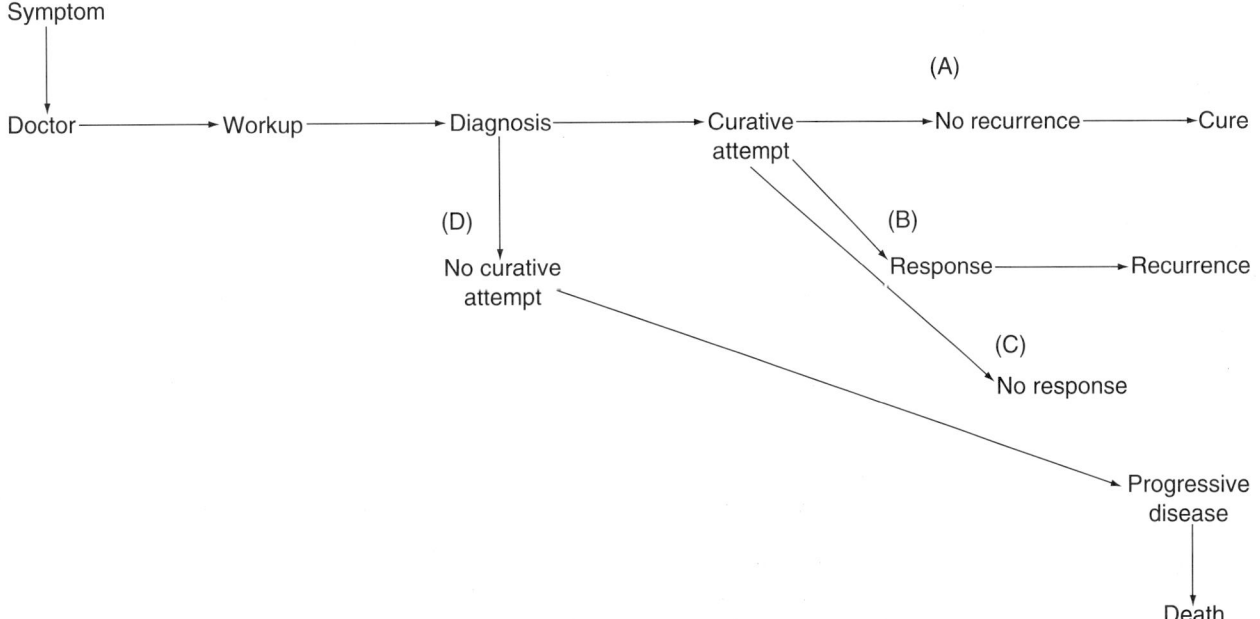

Figure 60–1. Possible clinical courses of cancer. (From Holland, J. [1982]. Psychologic aspects of cancer. In J. Holland & E. Frei, III (Eds.), *Cancer medicine*. Philadelphia: Lea & Febiger. With permission.)

adaptation by many, the potential for psychologic disturbance may be greater for cancer patients than for those with other illnesses. Additionally, it is clear from clinical and research standpoints that certain vulnerable individuals fail to adjust to the cancer experience and continue to experience ongoing psychologic symptoms after the initial crisis response associated with diagnosis. In a study by Pasacreta, Malone, and McCorkle (1991) depressive symptoms were measured using the CES-D (Center for Epidemiologic Studies of Depression) in a sample of 210 cancer patients of multiple primary diagnoses. This investigation was part of a larger, descriptive, correlational study conducted in a large northeastern city designed to examine problems and home care needs of patients and caregivers at three points in time (posthospitalization and 3 and 6 months later). At time one, 50 per cent of the sample scored above the impairment level of 16 on the CES-D, and of the patients who completed all three interviews ($n = 79$), it was quite interesting to note that mean depression scores did not change significantly over time. The fact that depression scores did not change significantly over time challenges the conceptualization of depression as a crisis response and demands attention to the ongoing nature of psychologic distress in a population with cancer, particularly for those with chronic physical symptoms.

Obviously, the stage of disease at time of diagnosis, the clinical course of illness including medical treatments, and possible recurrence will all affect the psychosocial profiles of individuals with cancer. To a large extent, these factors will determine the emotional issues that are most pressing at any given point.

The stages along the clinical course of cancer have been used to describe common events and psychosocial issues often associated with each. Such categorizations are useful, because they highlight the chronic nature of cancer and draw attention to key emotional vulnerabilities that may occur at particular times. The uniqueness of every individual, however, should always be kept in mind. The discrete stages highlighted in the literature should be acknowledged as a useful guide and conceptual framework, although limited as a result of obvious human differences.

DIAGNOSTIC PHASE

The prediagnostic phase is the time of initial symptom discovery. Initial symptoms, if subtle, are often ignored, and medical advice is usually sought when symptoms persist or worsen. The period when suspicious symptoms are associated with a definitive diagnosis is often characterized by fear, shock, and disbelief.

The period from time of diagnosis through initiation of treatment is characterized by medical evaluation, the development of new relationships with unfamiliar medical personnel, and the need to integrate a barrage of information that is at best frightening and confusing. Within the context of this anxiety-provoking situation, a decision must be made regarding treatment. As one patient aptly stated, "a decision upon which my very life or death might be based." This

statement illustrates the tremendous responsibility, concern, and isolation that many people experience during this period. Patients and their families are often particularly anxious when receiving initial information regarding diagnosis and treatment. Consequently, care should be taken by professionals to repeat information over several sessions and to inquire about the patient's and family's understanding of facts and options.

Weisman and Worden (1976-1977) describe the first 100 days after diagnosis as the period of "existential plight in cancer". During this period, patient concerns focus on existential issues of life and death more than on concerns related to health, work, finances, religion, self, or relationships with family and friends. Although it is unusual to observe extreme and sustained emotional reactions as the first response to a cancer diagnosis, it remains important to assess the nature of the patients' reactions early. Initial reactions are often predictive of later adaptation (Graydon, 1988; Northouse, 1984). Early assessment by clinicians can help to identify individuals at risk for later adjustment problems and in greatest need of ongoing psychosocial support (Weisman, Worden, & Sobel, 1980; Worden, 1983) See Table 60-1 for a listing of factors.

Initial response to diagnosis may be profoundly influenced by a person's prior association with cancer (Rowland & Holland, 1989). Those with memories of close relatives with cancer often demonstrate heightened distress, particularly if the relative died or had negative treatment experiences.

During the diagnostic and early treatment period, patients may search for explanations or causes for their cancer and may struggle to give personal meaning to their experience. Since many clinicians are guarded about disclosing information until a firm diagnosis is established, patients may develop highly personal explanations that can be inaccurate and provoke intensely negative emotions. Ongoing involvement and accurate information will minimize uncertainty and the development of maladaptive coping strategies based on erroneous beliefs.

While the literature substantiates the devastating, emotional impact of a cancer diagnosis, it is also well documented that many individuals cope effectively. Positive coping strategies such as taking action and finding favorable characteristics in the situation have been reported as effective (Gotay, 1981). Maintaining optimism (Mages et al., 1981) and having an active determination to recover (Hughes, 1982) have been

TABLE 60-1. *Factors That May Predict Poor Coping In Cancer Patients*

Psychiatric history	Inflexible, rigid coping style
Limited social support	Pessimistic outlook on life
Alcohol or drug abuse	Multiple obligations
Recent losses	

(Adapted from Rowland, J. H. [1989]. Intrapersonal resources: Coping. In J. C. Holland & J. H. Rowland [Eds.], *Handbook of psychooncology: Psychological care of the patient with cancer* [p. 53]. New York: Oxford University Press.)

associated with positive adjustment. Contrary to the beliefs of many clinicians, denial has also been found to assist patients in coping effectively with a diagnosis of cancer (Watson, Greer, Blake, & Sharpnell, 1984) unless sustained and used to an excessive degree.

With the firm establishment of the cancer diagnosis, planning for treatment begins. If patients have been given a clear explanation of their condition while encouraged to maintain hope, the initial reaction of shock, fear, and desperation can give way to a sense of optimism (Holland, 1982). Health care providers have an important role in monitoring and possibly mediating psychosocial adjustment. Keeping patients informed and actively involved in their care and being aware of the unique meaning that individuals may associate with a diagnosis of cancer are vital. Those people with pervasive and unyielding negative affect that persists long after that crisis of diagnosis may require ongoing psychosocial intervention throughout treatment and the disease course.

THE TREATMENT DECISION

Psychosocial factors are essential parameters in considering which treatment is best for a particular patient. Development of a treatment plan should include information about all aspects of the diagnostic procedures and medical/surgical treatments as well as what is known about the psychosocial sequelae.

Often, patients react to a diagnosis of cancer with feelings of fear and helplessness. The patient looks to the primary physician for a curative treatment that will also preserve quality of life. The patient may feel threatened and think nothing can be done but rely on the physician's recommendations. Combating feelings of helplessness during this period can help to alleviate painful anxiety. This is best done by a member of the health care team who has established a treatment alliance with the patient. The health care provider should make the person feel like a partner in everything that takes place. This process is especially true regarding the decision about treatment options.

RECURRENCE AND PROGRESSIVE DISEASE

The psychosocial issues experienced by the person with cancer depend in part on the clinical course of the disease process. The development of a recurrence after a disease-free interval can be especially devastating for patients and those close to them. The medical workup is often difficult and anxiety-provoking (Bope, 1987), and psychosocial problems experienced at the time of diagnosis frequently resurface, often with greater intensity (Holland, 1982; Weisman, 1984). Shock and depression often accompany relapse and require individuals and their families to reevaluate the future. This period is a difficult one during which patients may also experience pessimism, renewed preoccupation with death and dying, feelings of helplessness, and disenchantment with treatment. Patients also tend to be more guarded and cautious at this time and seem to feel as if they are in limbo (Weisman, 1984). Silverfarb,

Maurer, and Crouthamel (1980) examined emotional distress in a cross-sectional study of 146 women with breast cancer at three points in the clinical course (diagnosis, recurrence, and stage of disease progression). The point of recurrence was found to be the most distressing time with an increase in depression, anxiety, and suicidal ideation.

As the disease progresses, the person often reports an upsetting scenario that includes frequent pain, disability, increased dependence on others and diminished functional ability that often potentiate psychologic symptoms (Holland, 1982). Investigators studying quality of life in cancer patients have demonstrated a clear relationship between an individual's perception of quality of life and the presence of discomfort (McCorkle et al., 1989). As uncomfortable symptoms increase, perceived quality of life diminishes. Thus an important goal in the psychosocial treatment of patients with advanced cancer focuses on symptom control.

An issue that repeatedly surfaces among patients, family members, and professional care providers deals with the use of aggressive treatment protocols in the presence of progressive disease. Often patients and families request to participate in experimental protocols even when there is little likelihood of extending survival. Controversy continues about the efficacy of such therapies and the role health professionals can play in facilitating patients' choices about participating. These issues become even more important as changes in health care reform may limit the ability of insurance companies to reimburse patients for costly and highly technical treatments such as bone marrow transplants.

The need for health care professionals to establish structured dialogue with patients, family members, and care providers regarding treatment goals and expectations is essential. The idea that certain individuals may respond to investigational treatment with increased hope despite the existence of progressive illness should be a consideration in treatment planning. The need to separate and clarify values, thoughts, and emotional reactions of care providers, patients, and families to these delicate issues is important if individualized care with attention to psychosocial issues is to be provided. Use of resources such as psychiatric consultation-liaison nurses, psychiatrists, social workers, and chaplains can be invaluable in assisting patients, family members, and staff to grapple with these issues in a meaningful and productive manner.

It is beyond the scope of this chapter to present a comprehensive overview of the psychosocial reactions of patients to the process of dying. It should be mentioned, however, that once the terminal period has begun, it is not usually the fact of dying but the quality of dying that seems to be the overwhelming issue confronting the patient and family (Thomas, 1978). In addition, it is important that nurses recognize that working with cancer patients can be emotionally draining for them personally and professionally. See Unit XI for an overview of professional support systems.

In spite of the seemingly overwhelming nature of psychosocial responses along the cancer trajectory, most patients do indeed cope effectively, and it is important to recognize that intense emotions are not one in the same with maladaptive coping.

SURVIVORSHIP

The successful treatment of many cancers has resulted in cure for many patients and progressively longer lives for others. Longer survival, however, is not without significant emotional sequelae. Innovative and new treatments may produce long-term physiologic consequences such as infertility and organ system failure that can magnify and exacerbate the psychologic aspects initially associated with diagnosis and treatment. Many patients lack information about what to expect once they are discharged from the hospital. Clinicians need to establish ongoing mechanisms to monitor patients' symptoms, psychosocial status, and problems that they are having in terms of resuming activities and responsibilities. The clinician is then in a position to help the person to find the best solution for their situation.

Psychologic aspects of survivorship may include concern over the termination of treatment, fear of relapse, preoccupation with somatic symptoms, reentry into previous roles, lingering affinity with death, and financial, job, and insurance difficulties (Levenson & Lesko, 1990). Leventhal, Meyer, and Neremz (1980) describe the period after cessation of treatment as characterized by increased anxiety and renewed emotional concerns. These issues may manifest in a variety of ways including denial of past illness, leading to medical compliance issues, ongoing problems with anxiety, panic and depression, and inability to reenter previous roles. Health care providers should be mindful of psychologic sequelae among patients even in the context of remission and a hopeful prognosis and refer patients to a mental health specialist if indicated.

OUTCOMES ASSOCIATED WITH PSYCHOLOGIC DISTRESS IN THE MEDICALLY ILL

A number of studies equate the occurrence of psychologic distress among cancer patients with a crisis response (Holland, 1989). According to Caplan (1981), receiving catastrophic news about cancer diagnosis results in immediate problem-solving efforts; however, demands on the individual exceed the ability to respond, producing both physiologic and psychologic arousal. Problem-solving ability is consequently reduced by physiologic arousal that results in poor attention, concentration, judgment, a sense of disorganization, and erosion of self-concept. The inability to use adaptive skills results in transient dysphoria, manifested by depression and anxiety. Despite the clear documentation of significant psychologic symptoms in various cancer populations, the association of those symptoms with specific outcomes has been slow to develop. This has impeded understanding regarding the role of psychologic symptoms in the treatment, recovery, and palliative care periods and thus has impeded widespread implementation of psychosocial services in many oncology settings. The following paragraphs will review important studies that associate untoward outcomes with psychologic distress, particularly depression in various medically ill populations. Studies from a variety of medical illnesses are cited and highlight the need for more outcome-oriented research linking psychosocial distress to specific variables among patients with cancer.

In a study by Mossey, Knott, and Craik (1990), the effects of persistent depressive symptoms on hip fracture recovery were examined. Depressive symptoms were measured using the CES-D (Center for Epidemiologic Studies-Depression). After controlling for age, prefracture physical function, and cognitive status, which were found to be predictors of recovery, subjects consistently reporting few depressive symptoms were three times more likely than those with persistently elevated CES-D scores to achieve independence in walking, nine times more likely to return to prefracture levels in at least five of seven physical function measures, and nine times more likely to be in the highest quartile of overall physical function. These findings emphasize the significance of persistently elevated depressive symptoms in the recovery process and the importance of routine screening and evaluation of depressed mood states. Additionally, the need to study outcomes associated with depressive symptoms among various medical populations including patients with cancer is made clear through this study.

A recent study (Pasacreta, 1993) examined outcomes associated with depressive symptoms and syndromes in women after a diagnosis of breast cancer (Box 60–1). Women with depressive symptoms had more physical symptoms, more psychologic distress in general, and more impaired functioning than subjects with depressive disorders and without depression. A multiple regression procedure was used to examine the relative impact of clinical and demographic factors, physical symptom distress, multidimensional psychologic distress, and depressive symptoms on functional status outcomes. Two variables accounted for 35 per cent of the variance in functional status: symptom distress (28 per cent) and depressive symptoms (7 per cent) ($p < .00001$). Findings suggest that potential for depression is enhanced in physically symptomatic patients and that the combination of physical symptoms and depression are strong predictors of impaired functioning. Findings also suggest the need to broaden the definition of depression among cancer patients beyond the psychiatric depressive disorders so the spectrum of depression in the cancer patient can be recognized and treated.

Routine psychiatric evaluations of 100 adult patients undergoing allogeneic bone marrow transplantation for acute leukemia were reviewed to examine the possible relationship of psychiatric and psychosocial factors to duration of survival after the procedure (Colon, Callies, Popkin, & McGlave, 1991). Three variables were found to independently affect outcome: illness status (first remission versus other status), presence of depressed mood, and the extent of perceived social support. Patients with depressed mood ($n = 13$)

Box 60–1. *Outcomes Associated with Depressive Symptoms and Syndromes in Women Following Breast Cancer Diagnosis*

Pasacreta, J. V. (1993). *Depressive phenomena and associated functional status outcomes among women with breast cancer.* Unpublished doctoral dissertation, University of Pennsylvania School of Nursing, Philadelphia, PA.

Purpose/Objectives: Due to variable definitions and measurement, reports regarding the nature and scope of depression among cancer patients vary widely. Additionally, outcome measures associated with varying types and degrees of depression are seldom examined and are poorly understood. Based on these issues, the study purpose was to describe the nature and scope of depression and associated functional status outcomes in women with breast cancer.

Setting and Sample: Seventy-nine women were recruited from surgical offices at a large, northeastern, university-based medical center 3 to 7 months after a breast cancer diagnosis.

Method: A cross-sectional design was used. DSM-IIIR diagnostic criteria for depressive disorders and a depression rating scale, the Center for Epidemiologic Studies of Depression (CES-D), were used. To address the overlapping nature of somatic symptoms of depression with those of illness and treatment, a separate measure of physical symptom distress was obtained. Additionally, a measure of multidimensional psychologic distress characteristic of the crisis response associated with diagnosis was obtained to examine concurrent symptoms that characterize depression in this population.

Findings: Nine per cent of the sample had depressive disorder, yet 24 per cent scored above a cutoff point of 15 on the CES-D. Subjects who underwent mastectomy were more depressed than subjects who underwent lumpectomy ($p = .004$). Women with depressive symptoms had more physical symptoms ($p < .0001$), more multidimensional psychologic distress ($p < .0001$), and more impaired functioning ($p < .0001$) than subjects with depressive disorders and without depression. Subjects with current depressive disorder, depressive symptoms, or both were younger than subjects with no depression ($p = .005$). A multiple regression procedure was used to examine the relative impact of clinical and demographic factors, physical symptom distress, multidimensional psychologic distress, and depressive symptoms on functional status outcomes. Two variables accounted for 35 per cent of the variance in functional status: symptom distress (28 per cent) and depressive symptoms (7 per cent) ($p < .00001$).

Implications for Practice: Findings suggest enhanced potential for depression in physically symptomatic patients and that the combination of physical symptoms and depression are strong predictors of impaired functioning. Findings also suggest the need to broaden the definition of depression among cancer patients beyond the psychiatric depressive disorders so the spectrum of depression in the cancer patient can be recognized and treated.

Study supported by the American Cancer Society, Predoctoral Scholarship and the National Cancer Institute, F31 CA 09112.

---

as a prominent symptom at the pretransplant evaluation had significantly shorter survival after transplantation. Only one of the patients in the depressed group had a diagnosis of major depression. The authors admit that their sample is quite small and that the mechanism by which depressed mood affects outcome remains speculative. The important point is that depressive symptoms of lesser magnitude than those associated with stringent psychiatric diagnoses are being coupled with unfavorable outcomes in cancer patients. Consequently, depressive symptoms warrant attention in the clinical setting and warrant further study regarding associated outcomes and treatments.

A recent, large-scale study specifically examined and compared outcomes associated with depressive disorders, depressive symptoms, chronic medical conditions, and no chronic conditions (Wells, Stewart et al., 1989). Data from 11,242 outpatients at three health care sites were collected. The findings demonstrated significant morbidity associated with depressive symptoms and further pointed to the need to expand the study of depression among the medically ill to include depressive symptoms that do not qualify for disorder status.

Patients with either current depressive disorder or depressive symptoms in the absence of disorder tended to have worse physical, social, and role functioning, worse perceived current health status, and greater bodily pain than patients with no chronic conditions. The poor functioning uniquely associated with depressive symptoms with or without depressive disorder was comparable to or worse than that uniquely associated with eight major chronic medical conditions. For example, the unique association of days in bed with depressive symptoms was significantly greater than the comparable association with hypertension, diabetes, and arthritis. Depression and chronic medical conditions had unique and additive effects on patient functioning (Wells, Stuart et al., 1989).

The preceding information underscores the need to increase our awareness of depressive symptomatology and its consequences among oncology populations. Additionally, the need to study associations and outcomes related to depressive symptomatology among cancer patients is evident. The ultimate utility of these issues in terms of patient well being, quality of life, and health care expenditures is not within our current grasp and will not be fully appreciated until the knowledge base in this area is expanded and more thoroughly understood.

FACTORS THAT AFFECT PSYCHOSOCIAL ADJUSTMENT

Psychosocial responses to cancer vary widely and are influenced by many factors of which clinicians should be mindful when considering the responses of individual patients. A review of the literature points to key factors that may affect psychosocial adjustment. Three of the most important factors include (1) previous coping strategies and emotional stability, (2) the existence of social support, and (3) the existence of physical symptom distress.

PREVIOUS COPING STRATEGIES AND EMOTIONAL STABILITY

One of the most important predictors of psychosocial adjustment to cancer is the coping strategies and emotional stability of the person prior to diagnosis. Individuals with a history of poor psychosocial adjustment before developing cancer are at highest risk for emotional decompensation (Sinsheimer & Holland, 1987) and should be monitored closely throughout all phases of treatment. This is particularly true for people with a history of major psychiatric syndromes or psychiatric hospitalization.

Since an individual's coping style is determined relatively early in life and remains stable over time and across situations, it serves as a useful predictor of adjustment to cancer (Gorzynski et al., 1980). Several investigators have found specific personality characteristics, coping strategies, and life experiences to either enhance or inhibit positive adjustment to cancer. Coping strategies found to be most effective have included a "fighting spirit" (Penman et al., 1987) and having a feeling of control over events, resulting in active participation in treatment (Levy, Heberman, Mavlish, Schliew, & Lippman, 1985). On the other hand, poor adjustment has been associated with avoidant coping strategies (Penman et al., 1987), prior negative sexual experiences, body image problems, and inhibition in discussing personal and sexual problems (Schain, Wellisch, Pasnau, & Landsverk, 1985).

THE EXISTENCE OF SOCIAL SUPPORT

Social support has consistently been found to influence a person's psychosocial adjustment to cancer (Penman et al., 1986). The ability and availability of significant others in dealing with diagnosis and treatment can significantly affect the patient's view of himself or herself and potentially the patient's survival (Bloom, 1982).

Individuals diagnosed with all types of life-threatening, chronic disorders experience a heightened need for interpersonal support. Individuals who are able to maintain close connections with family and friends during the course of illness are more likely to cope effectively with the disease than those who are not able to maintain such relationships (Jamison, Wellisch, & Pasnau, 1978).

Living with a chronic illness often requires continuing care and management by a team of specialists, including physicians, nurses, social workers, and pharmacists. Care is usually provided through follow-up visits to ambulatory or outpatient clinics and consult-

ing rooms rather than through hospitalization. Historically, patients are often not referred to home nursing care once they are discharged from the hospital. An initial home nursing visit posthospitalization, however, may be invaluable in assisting the patient and family with the transition and help to identify areas where ongoing assistance is needed. Home care referrals can assist families who are increasingly relied upon within the present health care system to be the major provider of care outside the hospital. The phenomena of caregiver burden acknowledges that cancer affects not only the patient but members of the family as well (McCorkle, Yost, Jepson, Malone, Baird, & Lusk, 1993). The burden that caregiving places on the family highlights attention to the family's needs and the importance of targeting support and information to the family to help reduce caregiver burden. Helping to arrange respite care for the patient is also helpful in recognizing and relieving the family's caregiver burden.

THE EXISTENCE OF PHYSICAL SYMPTOM DISTRESS

The effects of treatment for cancers of all stages as well as the impact of progressive disease can inflict transient or permanent physical changes, physical symptom distress, and functional impairments in patients. It is a well-known clinical fact that excessive psychologic distress can exacerbate the side effects of cancer treatment agents. This notion has also been shown in the research literature (Andrykowski, Redd, & Hatfield, 1985). Conversely, treatment side effects can have a dramatic impact on the psychologic profiles of its recipients (Burish & Lyles, 1981).

Due to the expected and overlapping nature of somatic and affective changes secondary to cancer illness and treatment, understanding when psychologic symptoms reach clinical significance is inherently difficult. Physical symptoms imposed by illness and treatment often coexist with somatic symptoms pathognomic to depression in particular (Fig. 60–2). The coexisting and often competing nature of somatic and depressive symptoms (treatment of physical problems often assumes priority in the oncology treatment setting) has led to a lack of understanding regarding the significance of depressive symptoms among cancer patients as well as to the assumption that depression is an appropriate response to a physically and emotionally disruptive chronic illness.

Particularly during the treatment phases, patients face a range of physical symptoms based on the development of side effects and toxicities. In a study by the Psychosocial Collaborative Oncology Group, patients in over 30 chemotherapy protocols were studied at three centers (Cella et al., 1987). Patients ranked their most distressing problems to include hair loss, nausea, vomiting, fatigue, weakness, and resultant decline in stamina. Patients reported that the preceding symptoms, particularly diminished stamina, resulted in problems meeting personal and work obligations. The possible role of psychologic distress in this process

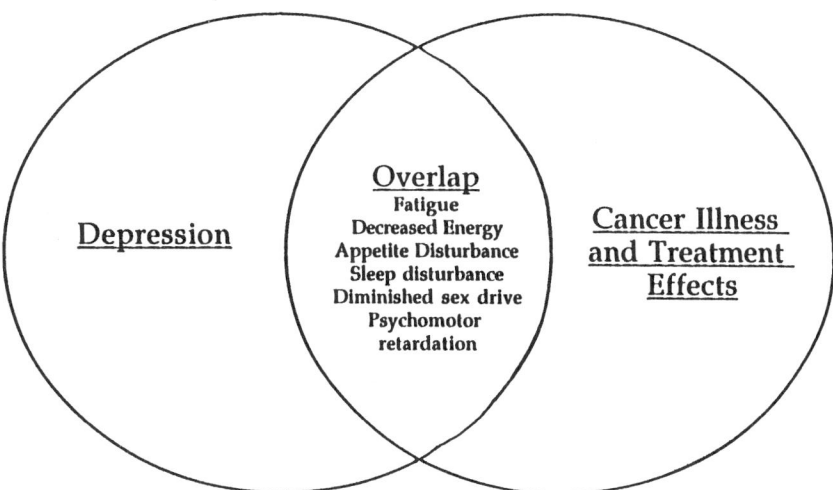

FIGURE **60–2.** Cancer, depression and somatic symptoms.

remains unclear. Some suggest that depression interferes with optimal functioning. Graydon (1988) found high rates of depression to be predictive of functioning in a sample of lung and breast cancer patients after radiation therapy. Others report, however, that diminished functioning secondary to illness and treatment enhances the potential for depression (Cella et al., 1987), and still others report that although a significant relationship between affect and functioning is evident, the direction of the relationship is unclear, and causation cannot be concluded (Northouse & Swain, 1987).

Increasingly, intensive cancer therapies given in the hospital produce severe and at times life-threatening side effects. The somatic symptoms often experienced by hospitalized cancer patients include chills, fever, stomatitis, pain, nausea, vomiting, alterations in mobility, inability to tend to self-care needs, and at times total dependence on caregivers (Sarna & McCorkle, in press).

According to information derived from prevalence studies of depression in patients with cancer, the potential for affective disturbance appears to increase in patients with advanced illness (Bukberg, Penman, & Holland, 1984; Craig & Abeloff, 1974; Derogatis et al., 1983; Plumb & Holland, 1977, 1981). Additionally, in a study that elicited information from nurses regarding psychiatric symptoms present in their patients, almost twice as many patients with metastatic disease were reported as depressed in contrast to those with localized cancers (Pasacreta & Massie, 1990). Investigators studying quality of life in cancer patients have demonstrated a clear relationship between an individual's perception of his or her quality of life and the presence of discomfort (McCorkle et al., 1989). As uncomfortable symptoms increase, perceived quality of life diminishes and depressive symptoms often increase. Symptoms frequently experienced by patients with advanced cancer include pain, confusion, dyspnea, and diminished functional ability, to name just a few. The presence of increased physical discomfort combined with a lack of control and predictability regarding the occurrence of symptoms often enhances anxiety,

depression, and organic mental symptoms in patients with advanced disease.

According to Nagi (1969), level of functioning attained after a period of disability is determined not only by physical capacity but by the individual's assessment of his or her situation as well as the assessment of the situation by significant others. An interesting hypothesis is that cancer patients who perceive somatic symptoms and associated functional alterations as being permanent are more prone to serious psychologic distress than those who view symptoms as transient.

DIFFERENTIATING PSYCHIATRIC COMPLICATIONS FROM EXPECTED PSYCHOLOGIC RESPONSES

Most patients develop transient psychologic symptoms that are responsive to support, reassurance, and information about what to expect regarding the cancer course and its treatment. Some individuals, however, require more aggressive psychotherapeutic intervention such as pharmacotherapy and ongoing psychotherapy. The following are some guidelines to assist the clinician in identifying patients who exhibit behavior suggesting the presence of a psychiatric syndrome.

Most patients do not react to a diagnosis and treatment for cancer by developing a clinically diagnosable psychiatric condition. In some cases, however, a psychiatric syndrome does occur in patients. If the patient's problems become severe, meaning that the provider feels supportive measures are insufficient and ineffective in controlling emotional distress, referral to a psychiatric clinician is indicated. Factors that may prevent adjustment to cancer illness and treatment and warrant referral to a psychiatric clinician include past psychiatric hospitalization, history of significant depression, manic-depressive illness, schizophrenia, organic mental conditions, personality disorders, lack of social support, inadequate control of physical discomfort, history of or current alcohol or drug abuse, and currently prescribed psychotropic medication.

The need for psychiatric referral among patients receiving psychotropic medication deserves specific mention here, as it is often overlooked in clinical practice. Standard cancer treatments such as surgery and chemotherapy can significantly change dosage requirements for medications used to treat major psychiatric syndromes such as schizophrenia, depression, and bipolar disorder. For example, dosage requirements for lithium carbonate, commonly used to treat the manic episodes associated with bipolar disorder and depressive episodes associated with recurrent depressive disorder, can change significantly over the course of cancer treatment. Therapeutic blood levels of lithium are closely tied to sodium and water balance. Additionally, lithium has a narrow therapeutic window, and life-threatening toxicity can develop rapidly. Side effects from cancer treatments such as diarrhea, fever, vomiting, and resulting dehydration warrant scrupulous monitoring of dosage and side effects. Careful monitoring is also indicated during preoperative and postoperative periods. Another common problem among patients treated with psychotropic medication is that medications may be discontinued at specific points in the cancer treatment process, for example, at the time of surgery, and not restarted. This may produce an avoidable recurrence of emotionally disabling psychiatric symptoms at a time when the stress of cancer and its treatment is burden enough.

Since transient symptoms of anxiety and depression are common in patients with cancer, the ability of health care providers to distinguish expected reactions from more severe psychiatric complications is crucial. As stated earlier, anxiety and depression are common symptoms particularly evident at transition points during the clinical course of cancer. Usually these symptoms subside within 2 to 4 weeks and are responsive to supportive reassurance and information regarding what to expect during the course of treatment. For a proportion of patients, psychologic distress does not subside with usual supportive interventions. Unfortunately, clinically relevant and severe psychiatric syndromes are often unrecognized by care providers who do not have psychiatric training (Wells, Hays, Burnam, & Camp, 1989). One of the reasons that it may be difficult to detect serious psychiatric reactions in patients is that several of the diagnostic criteria used to evaluate the presence of severe depression (lack of appetite, insomnia, decreased sexual interest, diminished energy) may overlap with usual disease and treatment effects. Additionally, health care providers may confuse their own fears about cancer with the emotional reactions of their patients (i.e., "I too would be extremely depressed if I were in a similar situation.").

Table 60–2 provides some general guidelines to assist in distinguishing patients who should be referred for evaluation by a trained psychiatric clinician.

ORGANIC MENTAL STATES

Organic mental impairment can have a direct causal relationship to psychologic distress in some cancer patients. Certain treatment agents including vincristine, vinblastine, L-asparaginase, amphotericin-B, interferon, steroids, as well as commonly prescribed medications (resperine, barbiturates, and valium) can produce depression, anxiety, and delirious states (Breitbart & Holland, 1988). Pancreatic and neurologic cancers, cerebral metastasis, uncontrolled pain, and certain metabolic, nutritional, and endocrine derangements are also associated with depression and organic mental states (Breitbart & Holland, 1988).

The presence of organic mental syndromes can elicit organic psychoses, personality changes, and depressive responses and are reported as significantly higher during advanced stages of cancer and during treatment than during earlier stages or nontreatment phases (Levine, Silverfarb, & Lipowski, 1978; Massie, Gorzynski, Mastrovito, Theis, & Holland, 1979; Massie, Holland, & Glass, 1983). These issues highlight the need for attention to psychologic symptoms in cancer patients particularly during active treatment periods and advanced stages of illness. The need to screen for organic impairment with a well-established, valid, and reliable instrument is also indicated.

After referral to a psychiatric specialist, one or a combination of several therapeutic modalities may be employed. Cancer and its treatment may precipitate an exacerbation of an underlying mental illness for which the patient was already predisposed and that may require extensive treatment (e.g., hospitalization for a psychosis, ongoing pharmacotherapy, or psychotherapy).

TABLE 60–2. *Guidelines Regarding Referral to a Psychiatric Clinician*

- History of psychiatric hospitalization or significant disorder.
- Persistent refusal, indecisiveness, or noncompliance with regard to needed treatment.
- Current treatment with psychotropic medication.
- Persistent symptoms of anxiety and depression that are unresponsive to usual support from health care providers, family members, or both. Symptoms may present in the form of constant fear associated with treatment and procedures or excessive crying and hopelessness that worsen rather than improve over time.
- An abrupt, unexplained change in mood or behavior.
- Insomnia, anorexia, or diminished energy out of proportion to expected treatment effects.
- Persistent suicidal ideation.
- Unusual behavior or confusion (may be indicative of an organic mental disorder).
- Excessive guilt and self-blame for illness.
- Evidence of dysfunctional family coping or complex family issues.

OUTCOMES ASSOCIATED WITH PSYCHOSOCIAL INTERVENTIONS

According to some authors, psychosocial interventions exert an important effect on the overall adjustment of patients and their families to cancer illness and treatment (Holland, Massie, & Straker, 1989). Several studies document the beneficial effect of counseling on one or more outcome measures such as anxiety, feelings of personal control (Bloom, Ross, & Burnell, 1978), and enhanced body image and satisfaction with care (Ferlic, Goldman, & Kennedy, 1979). Counseling of cancer patients has also been associated with enhanced self-image and more rapid return to premorbid levels of functioning in dimensions such as work and sexuality (Capone, Good, Westie, & Jacobsen, 1981) as well as reduced emotional distress (Linn, Linn, & Harris, 1982). Despite these favorable findings, not all studies support the positive effect of psychosocial interventions, and more studies in this area are needed. It has been difficult to draw firm conclusions regarding outcomes associated with psychotherapeutic interventions for reasons including lack of standardization and replication of the intervention, lack of control or comparison groups, and lack of specific and measurable outcomes across studies. Despite the fact that most clinicians are intuitively and experientially aware of the benefits of psychotherapeutic interventions with cancer patients, the new age of cost-containment and health care reform demand a proliferation of concrete data to justify the existence and expansion of psychosocial services.

In addition to studies that suggest a link between counseling and psychosocial outcomes, there is a small but expanding body of literature that suggests that psychosocial support may have an influence on the rate of cancer progression (Speigel, 1993) (Box 60–2). An important and widely cited study (Speigel, Bloom, Kraemer, & Gottheil, 1989) studied the effect of group counseling for women with metastatic breast cancer. Thirty women received standard care; another 50 women received standard care in addition to a weekly group therapy session. Elements of the group included the encouragement of mutual support, coping with dying, development of a life project, realigning social networks, working through physician-patient problems, and pain control. Mood was assessed at 4-month intervals over a year in both groups. The control group suffered a substantial decline in mood including anxiety, depression, fatigue, loss of vigor, and confusion. In contrast, the intervention group showed an improvement in mood. Several years after the initial intervention, survival was examined for both groups. The mean survival from time of study entry until death was 18.9 months for the control group and 36.6 months for the intervention group.

Richardson, Shelton, and Krailo (1990) similarly documented significant survival differences on the basis of psychosocial intervention in a sample of patients with leukemia and lymphoma. Patients randomized to one of several educational and home-visiting interventions survived longer than patients receiving usual care.

Despite these findings other studies have failed to show a survival advantage for patients receiving psychosocial interventions (Gellert, Maxwel, & Siegel, 1993; Morgenstern, Gellert, & Walter, 1984). More studies examining these issues are indicated before conclusions can be drawn, and it is misleading to encourage patients to participate in support programs on the basis that they will live longer.

MANAGEMENT OF PSYCHOSOCIAL PROBLEMS

Increased length of survival from time of diagnosis has highlighted the need for psychopharmacologic, psychotherapeutic, and behaviorally oriented interventions to reduce distress, promote adjustment, and improve quality of life for cancer patients. Numerous studies have documented the efficacy of a variety of modalities in managing psychosocial problems for individuals with cancer. The problems that can be managed effectively include emotional distress such as anxiety and depression, sexual dysfunction, body image disturbances, marital and family difficulties, noncompliance, pain, neurologic complications such as delirium and dementia induced by brain metastasis or treatment, anticipatory and posttreatment nausea and vomiting, anorexia, and feeding problems (Holland, 1982; Rowland & Holland, 1989).

PHARMACOLOGIC INTERVENTIONS

Pharmacotherapy, as an adjunct to one or more of the psychotherapies, can be an important aid in bringing psychologic symptoms under control. Psychopharmacologic agents for the treatment of psychiatric complications associated with cancer are reviewed only briefly here. For a thorough review as well as expanded treatment guidelines, the reader is referred to a comprehensive chapter by Massie and Lesko (1989).

For patients with excessive anxiety, factors other than a psychologic state must first be evaluated. Metabolic abnormalities, pain, hypoxia, and drug withdrawal states can all present as anxiety. Medications such as steroids and antipsychotics often used for nausea such as compazine and haldol can also cause anxiety characterized by agitation and motor restlessness. After medical or drug-induced causes for anxiety are ruled out, an anxiolytic (e.g., Valium, Ativan, Xanax) is the treatment of choice with the exception of patients who present with panic episodes, in which case tricyclic antidepressants are most efficacious. Anxiolytic agents are often fast-acting and effective. These drugs are most effective when used at adequate dosages and as standing orders. Prescribing anxiolytics on an as-needed basis places undue responsibility on patients who are already frightened and anxious. When given orally, these drugs cause minimal respiratory depression. Anxiolytic medication can help patients gain temporary control over agonizing anxiety. Use of these medications may also assist the patient in making use of psychotherapy, which can provide more permanent

---

Box 60–2. *Influence of Psychosocial Support on Survival*

Purpose/Objectives: An important and widely cited study examined the effect of group counseling for women with metastatic breast cancer.

Sample: Eighty women with metastatic breast cancer.

Design: Longitudinal.

Methods: Thirty women received standard care; another 50 women received standard care in addition to a weekly group therapy session. Elements of the group included the encouragement of mutual support, coping with dying, development of a life project, realigning social networks, working through physician-patient problems, and pain control. Mood was assessed at 4-month intervals over a year in both groups.

Findings: The control group suffered a substantial decline in mood including anxiety, depression, fatigue, loss of vigor, and confusion. In contrast, the intervention group showed an improvement in mood. Several years after the initial intervention, survival was examined for both groups. Forty-eight months after cessation of the group, all of the control patients had died, whereas one third of the intervention group was still alive. The mean survival from time of study entry until death was 18.9 months for the control group and 36.6 months for the intervention group. The mean survival times from first metastasis to death were 43.2 months for the control group and 58.4 months for the intervention group ($p<.01$). Statistical analysis controlled for factors such as baseline differences in initial staging, age, radiation, and disease-free interval.

Conclusions: The authors outline several factors that may have accounted for the survival advantage found in the intervention group such as improved diet, sleep, and appetite, better medical treatment utilization, enhancement of the neuroendocrine system, and enhanced immune function in the intervention group, all made possible by their enhanced social support.

Implications for Practice: Nurses working in oncology settings are in key positions to implement patient support groups and monitor their effectiveness including associated outcomes.

From Speigel, D., Bloom, J. R., Kraemer, H. C., & Gottheil, E. G. (1989). Effect of psychosocial treatment on survival of patients with metastatic breast cancer. *Lancet, 2,* 888–891. © The Lancet Ltd.

---

control over psychologic symptoms. When anxiety develops in the context of the terminal stages of cancer, it is often secondary to hypoxia or an untreated pain syndrome. Intravenous morphine sulfate is usually an effective treatment (Levenson & Lesko, 1990).

A number of anxiolytics are available to treat cancer patients. These drugs are all similar in their overall clinical effects. Table 60–3 reviews the anxiolytics most often recommended in clinical practice. Because of their shorter half-life, alprazolam and lorazepam have advantages for elderly patients, since toxicity from sedating medications is more common and withdrawal reactions may occur upon abrupt discontinuance unless the drug is tapered gradually (Karasu, 1989).

It is common for cancer patients to demonstrate transient depressive symptoms at various points in the illness trajectory. In patients who exhibit prolonged or severe depressive symptomatology, a major depressive illness must be considered. Depression in a cancer population can be related to a recurrence of a past depressive disorder or the stress associated with cancer treatment, or it can be a result of the illness process or treatment agents. Certain medications and cancer treatment agents can produce severe depressive states. A diagnosis of major depression in the cancer patient relies heavily on the presence of affective symptoms such as hopelessness, crying spells, guilt, preoccupation with death and/or suicide, diminished self-worth, and loss of pleasure in most activities such as being with friends and loved ones. The neurovegetative symptoms that usually characterize depression in physically healthy individuals are not good predictors of depression in the medically ill due to the fact that the cancer and its treatment can also produce these symptoms. A

combination of psychotherapy and antidepressant medication will often prove useful in treating major depression in cancer patients. Commonly used antidepressants and dosages are outlined in Table 60–4. Tricyclic antidepressants are the drugs of choice. The primary medical contraindication to their use is significant cardiac conduction delays, which should be ruled out prior to the initiation of treatment. These medications are started in low doses (25 mg to 50 mg) and are increased slowly over days to weeks until symptoms improve. Peak dosages are usually substantially lower than those tolerated by physically healthy individuals. Antidepressant medications may take 2 to 6 weeks to produce their desired effects. Patients may need ongoing support, reassurance, and monitoring prior to experiencing the antidepressant effects of medication. It is essential that patients are monitored closely during the initiation and modification of psychopharmacologic regimens by a consistent provider.

A newer class of antidepressants referred to in Table 60–4 that have achieved rapid and widespread use among the general population include specific serotonin reuptake inhibitors (SSRI's), such as fluoxitene (prozac) and sertraline (zoloft). These drugs deserve consideration only as second-line agents in the depressed cancer patient, since they have not been as well studied as the tricyclics in this population (Shuster, Stern, & Greenberg, 1992). If patients develop adverse effects from antidepressant treatment, SSRI's take longer to clear the system than tricyclics, necessitating a prolonged waiting period before beginning another, potentially effective therapy (Shuster et al., 1992). Additionally undesirable side effects for a cancer population may include agitation and anorexia.

TABLE 60–3. *Commonly Prescribed Anxiolytics In Cancer Patients*

DRUG	STARTING DOSAGES	ABSORPTION	HALF LIFE	COMMENTS
Alprazolam (Xanax)	0.25–0.5 mg PO tid	Intermediate	Intermediate	Generalized anxiety; panic attacks; mixed anxiety; depression; may be difficult to detoxify
Lorazepam (Ativan)	0.5–1.5 mg PO tid	Intermediate	Intermediate	Similar to alprazolam, can produce transient amnesia, which makes it useful with chemotherapy and before procedures. Agent of choice with hepatic impairment
Diazepam (Valium)	2.5–5 mg PO tid	Fast	Long	Because of long half-life, not ideal for patients with organic neurologic syndromes
Chlordiazepoxide (Librium)	10–25 mg PO tid	Intermediate	Long	Similar to diazepam
Triazolam (Halcion)	0.125–0.5 mg PO qhs	Intermediate	Short	Useful for severe, initial insomnia, can cause confusional state when used in elderly or medically ill

PO = orally; tid = three times a day; qhs = every night.
(Adapted from Levenson, JA, & Lesko, LM. [1990]. Psychiatric aspects of acute leukemia. *Seminars in Oncology Nursing*, 6(1), 78.)

Psychostimulants such as dextroamphetamine and methylphenidate have been useful in the treatment of depression in medically ill patients (Kaufmann & Murray, 1982; Massie & Lesko, 1989; Woods, Tesar, & Murray, 1986). Advantages include rapid onset of action and rapid clearance if side effects occur (Shuster et al., 1992). Common side effects of psychostimulants include insomnia, anorexia, tachycardia, and hypertension (Hyman & Arena, 1987), although incremental dosage increases allow adequate monitoring of therapeutic versus side effects. In patients with cardiac conduction problems, stimulants may be the treatment of choice. In cancer patients, a 1- to 2-month trial can provide remission from depression even after discontinuation of the drug (Massie & Holland, 1990).

TABLE 60–4. *Antidepressants used in Cancer Patients*

DRUG	STARTING DOSAGES	THERAPEUTIC RANGE	SEDATION	ANTICHOLINERGIC EFFECT	HYPOTENSION	CARDIAC ARRHYTHMIA
Tricyclics						
Amitryptyline (Elavil)	25 mg	75–150 mg	High	High	High	Yes
Doxepin (Sinequan)	25 mg	75–150 mg	High	Intermediate	Intermediate	Yes
Desipramine (Norpramin)	25 mg	75–150 mg	Low	Low	Intermediate	Yes
Nortriptyline (Pamelor)	10–25 mg	50–125 mg	Intermediate	Low	Low	Yes
Specific Seratonin Reuptake Inhibitors						
Fluoxetine (Prozac)	5 mg	10–20 mg	Low	Low	Low	Rare
Sertraline (Zoloft)	10 mg	30–50 mg	Low	None	Low	Rare
Trazadone (Desyrel)	25 mg	150–250 mg	High	None	Intermediate	Yes
Stimulants (Dextroamphetamine & Methylphenidate)	5 mg	5–20 mg	None	None	None	Rare

PSYCHOTHERAPEUTIC MODALITIES

According to Weisman, Worden and Sobel (1980), psychosocial interventions are defined as systematic efforts applied to influence coping behavior through educational or psychotherapeutic means. The goals of such interventions are to improve morale, self-esteem, coping ability, sense of control, and resolution of problems and to decrease emotional distress.

Two broad types of intervention strategies include educational and psychotherapeutic approaches. The educational approach is directive, utilizing problem solving and cognitive methods (Holland, Massie, & Straker, 1989). Clarifying medical information that may be missed due to fear and anxiety and clarifying misconceptions or misinformation regarding illness and treatment and normalizing emotional reactions throughout the illness trajectory are important components of the educational approach.

The psychotherapeutic approach utilizes psychodynamic and exploratory methods to help the individual understand aspects of cancer such as emotional responses and personal meaning of the disease. Psychotherapeutic interventions as opposed to educational interventions should be delivered by professionals with special training in mental health and specific interventional modalities, specifically as they are applied to patients with chronic medical illnesses.

Psychotherapy with a patient who has cancer should maintain a primary focus on the illness and its implications, utilizing a brief therapy, crisis intervention model (Massie et al., 1989). Expression of fears and concerns that may be too painful to reveal to family and friends is encouraged. Normalizing emotional distress, providing realistic reassurance and support, and bolstering existing strengths and coping skills are essential components of the therapeutic process. Gathering information about previous association with cancer through close relationships can also be instrumental in clarifying patients' fears and concerns and establishing boundaries and differences to the current situation.

Depending on the nature of the problem, the treatment modality may take the form of individual psychotherapy, support groups, family and marital therapy, behaviorally oriented therapy such as progressive muscle relaxation and guided imagery, or some combination. Table 60–5 outlines the major psychotherapeutic modalities and the advantages, goals, and indications for each.

METHODS FOR PROMOTING EFFECTIVE PATIENT COPING

A primary role for oncology nurses is to facilitate a positive adjustment in patients under their care. The

TABLE 60–5. *Psychotherapeutic Modalities in the Oncology Setting*

MODALITY	SELECTED INDICATIONS	GOALS AND ADVANTAGES	COMMENTS
Individual psychotherapy	For patients with prolonged adverse reactions to diagnosis and treatment and other aspects of chronic illness (i.e., anxiety, depression)	To support patients and enhance their ability to cope with distressing feelings Therapy usually short-term, focused, and goal-directed	In some cases pharmacotherapy and family involvement are useful adjuncts
Support groups	For patients who desire exposure to others who have been through the experience of chronic illness	To support patients and enhance coping ability Usually do not involve a fee Can be beneficial to patients to observe the coping strategies of others	Can benefit patients who have limited support systems by expanding their social network
Family and marital therapy	For patients experiencing sexual problems secondary to illness The illness is leading to increasing family tension and conflict	Can assist couples in clarifying problems and solving them together Can address role changes in family system	Problems, issues, and concerns regarding children can be addressed
Progressive muscle relaxation and guided imagery	For patients who desire assistance in enhancing personal control Useful in the management and control of pain and anxiety for some patients Has been useful in controlling anticipatory and posttreatment nausea and vomiting Can control fear associated with medical procedures	Increases sense of control and participation in treatment Individualized to meet patients' preferences and individual circumstances Time limit and goal-directed Evaluated in terms of observable changes in symptoms	Realistic goals should be stated explicitly as some patients expect relaxation and guided imagery to be curative regarding their disease process

appropriateness of periodic emotional distress and coping problems should be kept in mind and monitored routinely due to the chronic nature of cancer and the many transitions that can occur along the illness trajectory. The uniqueness of individual patients should always be kept in mind with awareness of the person's past coping style as well as the fact that emotional display is not one in the same with maladaptive coping. Understanding an individual's unique circumstances can assist nurses in supporting the constructive coping abilities that seem to work best for a particular patient. Doublsky (1985) suggests that nurses focus on specific stressors and responses to them during therapeutic interactions and also try to reinforce positive self-care behaviors.

In addition to verbal communication with cancer patients about coping strategies, written materials can be used to teach patients new coping skills. Carey and Jevne (1986) have developed an effective teaching program for postmastectomy patients to help them cope with breast cancer. The program includes specific guidelines on dealing with emotions, handling changes in family roles and relationships, encouraging family involvement in care, dealing with problems in sexuality, discussing cancer with other patients, communicating with physicians and family, and developing specific coping skills. The educational materials also advise patients to help friends and family to be comfortable with the cancer diagnosis by giving accurate information and by sharing their feelings and needs. The teaching program indicates that it helps patients to know that thoughts and emotions such as denial, anger, frustration, guilt, worry, depression, sadness, and fear are all normal reactions to cancer. Suggestions are offered to patients for dealing with these emotions by distracting themselves through activity, by talking with someone with whom they feel comfortable, by solving everyday problems as they arise and not letting them build up, and by learning specific relaxation techniques.

To enable health care providers to facilitate patients' coping, Weisman (1979, 1984) suggests the following activities for nurses: clarify problems for the patient, help patients maintain control by encouraging them to exercise whatever options they have available to them, offer a willing and noncritical ear so that patients can relieve pent-up emotions, direct patient to constructive channels to reduce anxiety, help reduce a problem to a manageable size, discourage hasty actions, and be comfortable sharing periods of silence with a patient.

In addition to providing one's own help, nurses should also encourage patients to take advantage of the many resources available for cancer patients. These may include psychologic and social work services, chaplains, patient to patient volunteers, and multiple services offered by the American Cancer Society and by local hospitals and community groups. Patients should be provided with timely and up-to-date information on all such resources. While still hospitalized, patients should be given a list of the addresses and phone numbers of important local agencies that serve their needs. Patients should also be advised of the various support groups available for cancer patients (both general and site- or procedure-specific groups). It should be kept in mind that patients may not be ready for outside support immediately and should be reminded periodically of what is available. Additionally, not all services are right for everybody; for instance, many individuals shy away from divulging personal feelings in a group setting, whereas others thrive on the support. The individual needs and preferences of each individual must always be paramount (Jalowiec & Dudas, 1991).

SUMMARY

The psychosocial issues faced by persons diagnosed with and treated for cancer are influenced by sociocultural, medical, family, and individual factors. Although involvement in decision making is clearly a positive aspect of current cancer therapies, great care should be taken to ensure the communication of timely, repeated, and relevant information that is consistent with patients' needs, tolerance, and comprehension. A multidisciplinary approach is essential to guarantee the communication of comprehensive information to all patients. Patients should be given the opportunity to speak with multiple members of the treatment team and other patients who have experienced similar management and treatment protocols. Care should be taken to provide needed information from a variety of expert perspectives while respecting the unique characteristics, psychosocial profiles, needs, and desires of each individual. In treatment settings with limited resources, every effort should be made to enlist the help and support of providers and services that can assist patients with their complex treatment decisions. Referral to community resources and support services after discharge from the hospital is often helpful, even for patients that cope well with initial treatment.

Most patients undergoing cancer treatment and their families experience expected periods of emotional turmoil that occur at transition points along the clinical course of cancer. For a small proportion of patients, more severe psychiatric complications may occur and warrant referral to a psychiatric specialist. A variety of psychotherapeutic modalities are useful in helping patients to work through the expected emotional responses to cancer as well as more severe responses. Supportive psychotherapeutic measures should be used routinely as they minimize distress and enhance feelings of control and mastery over self and environment. For these reasons alone, their utility in the care of patients with cancer is paramount. Again, in patients who are not responsive to routine support and information, referral to a psychiatric specialist may be indicated.

Throughout the clinical course of cancer, the patient's relationship with health care providers as well as the presence of a supportive social network are important factors in ensuring successful negotiation of the many physical and psychosocial demands imposed by a cancer diagnosis and treatment. Further investigation regarding the utility of systematically tested interventions aimed at promoting psychosocial adjustment to cancer are needed. Interventions aimed at enhancing understanding of the behaviors of individuals experiencing the crisis of cancer and identification of individuals in need of intensive psychosocial support are also needed.

As scientific inquiry continues to produce vast although sometimes conflicting information regarding etiology and treatment for cancer, concurrent investigation regarding the psychosocial aspects of the disease is crucial. This line of inquiry will at the very least assist in promoting emotional well being in patients faced with an extreme and unexpected life crisis. At best, expanding the knowledge base relative to the psychosocial aspects of cancer may provide some "missing links" regarding psychosocial adaptation, quality of life, and impact on survival.

REFERENCES

Andrykowski, M. A., Redd, W. H., & Hatfield, A. K. (1985). The development of anticipatory nausea: A prospective analysis. *Journal of Consulting and Clinical Psychology, 4,* 447–454.

Bloom, J. R. (1982). Social support, accommodation to stress and adjustment to breast cancer. *Social Science Medicine, 16,* 1329–1338.

Bloom, J. R., Ross, R. D., & Burnell, G. (1978). The effect of social support on patient adjustment after breast surgery. *Patient Counseling and Health Education, 1,* 50–59.

Bope, E. (1987). Follow-up of the cancer patient: Surveillance for metastasis. *Primary Care 14,* 391–401.

Breitbart, W., & Holland, J. C. (1988). Psychiatric complications of cancer. *Current Therapy in Hematology-Oncology, 3,* 268–274.

Bukberg, J., Penman, D., & Holland, J. C. (1984). Depression in hospitalized cancer patients. *Psychosomatic Medicine, 46,* 199–212.

Burish, T. G., & Lyles, J. N. (1981). Effectiveness of relaxation training in reducing adverse reactions to cancer chemotherapy. *Journal of Behavioral Medicine, 4,* 65–78.

Caplan, G. (1981). Mastery of stress: Psychosocial aspects. *American Journal of Psychiatry, 138,* 413–420.

Capone, M. A., Good, R. S., Westie, S., & Jacobsen, A. F. (1981). Psychosocial rehabilitation in gynecologic oncology patients. *Archives of Physical Medicine and Rehabilitation, 61,* 128–132.

Carey, R. L., & Jevne, R. (1986). Development of an information package for post mastectomy patients on adjuvant therapy. *Oncology Nursing Forum, 13,* 78–83.

Cella, D. F., Orofiamma, B., Holland, J. C., Silverfarb, P. M., Tross, S., Feldstein, M. A., Perry, S., Maurer, L. J., Comis, R., & Orav, E. J. (1987). The relationship of psychological distress, extent of disease and performance status in patients with lung cancer. *Cancer, 60,* 1661–1667.

Colon, E., Callies, A. L., Popkin, M., & McGlave, P. B. (1991). Depressed mood and other variables related to bone marrow transplantation survival in acute leukemia. *Psychosomatics, 32,* 420–425.

Craig, T. J., & Abeloff, M. D. (1974). Psychiatric symptomatology among hospitalized cancer patients. *American Journal of Psychiatry, 26,* 133–136.

Dermatis, H., & Lesko, L. M. (1991). Psychosocial correlates of physician patient communication at time of informed consent for bone marrow transplantation. *Cancer Investigation, 9,* 621–628.

Derogatis, L. R., Morrow, G. R., Fetting, J., Penman, D., Piasetsky, S., Schmale, A. M., Hendricks, M., & Carnicke, C. (1983). The prevalence of psychiatric disorders among cancer patients. *Journal of the American Medical Association, 249,* 751–757.

Doublsky, J. (1985). Ineffective individual coping. In J. C. McNally, J. C. Stair, & E. T. Somerville (Eds.), *Guidelines for cancer nursing practice* (pp. 62–65). Orlando, FL.: Grune & Stratton, Inc.

Endicott, J. (1984). Measurement of depression in patients with cancer. Proceedings of the working conference on methodology in behavioral and psychosocial cancer research. *Cancer, 53*(Suppl.), 2243–2248.

Ferlic, M. A., Goldman, A., & Kennedy, B. J. (1979). Group counseling in adult patients with advanced cancer. *Cancer, 44,* 760–766.

Gellert, G. A., Maxwell, R. M., & Siegel, B. S. (1993). Survival of breast cancer patients receiving adjunctive psychosocial support therapy: A 10-year follow-up study. *Journal of Clinical Oncology, 11,* 66–69.

Gorzynski, J. G., Holland, J. C., Katz, J., Weiner, H., Zumoff, B., Fukushim, D., & Levin, J. (1980). Stability of ego defenses and endocrine responses in women prior to breast biopsy and ten years later. *Psychosomatic Medicine, 42,* 323–328.

Gotay, C. C. (1981). *Causal attributions and coping behaviors in early-stage cervical cancer.* Presented at the Annual Meeting of the American Psychological Association, Los Angeles, CA.

Graydon, J. E. (1988). Factors that predict patients' functioning following treatment for cancer. *International Journal of Nursing Studies, 25,* 117–124.

Holland, J. C. (1982). Psychologic aspects of cancer. In J. F. Holland & E. Frei, III (Eds.), *Cancer medicine* (pp. 1175–1184). Philadelphia: Lea & Febiger.

Holland, J. C. (1989a). Fears and abnormal reactions to cancer in physically healthy individuals. In J. C. Holland & J. H. Rowland (Eds.), *Handbook of psychooncology: Psychological care of the patient with cancer* (pp. 13–21). New York: Oxford University Press.

Holland, J. (1989b). Clinical course of cancer. In J. C. Holland & J. H. Rowland (Eds.), *Handbook of psychooncology: Psychological care of the patient with cancer* (pp. 75–10). New York: Oxford University Press.

Holland, J., Massie, M. J., & Straker, N. (1989). Psychotherapeutic interventions. In J. C. Holland & J. H. Rowland (Eds.), *Handbook of psychooncology: Psychological care of the patient with cancer* (pp. 455–469). New York: Oxford University Press.

Hughes, J. (1982). Emotional reactions to the diagnosis and treatment of early breast cancer. *Journal of Psychosomatic Research, 26,* 277–281.

Hyman, S. E., & Arana, G. W. (1987). Other agents: Psychostimulants, beta adrenergic blockers and clonidine, In S. E. Hyman & G. W. Arana (Eds.), *Handbook of psychiatric drug therapy* (pp. 134–152). Boston: Little, Brown and Co.

Jalowiec, A., & Dudas, S. (1991). Alterations in patient coping. In S. B. Baird, R. McCorkle, & M. Grant (Eds.), *Cancer nursing: A comprehensive textbook* (pp. 806–820). Philadelphia: W. B. Saunders Co.

Jamison, K. R., Wellisch, D. K., & Pasnau, R. O. (1978). Psychosocial aspects of mastectomy: I. The woman's perspective. *American Journal of Psychiatry, 135,* 432–436.

Karasu, T. B. (Ed.). (1989). *Treatment of psychiatric disorders.* Washington, DC: American Psychiatric Press.

Kaufmann, M. W., & Murray, G. B. (1982). The use of D-amphetamine in medically ill depressed patients. *Journal of Clinical Psychiatry, 43,* 463–464.

Krant, M. J. (1976). Problems of the physician in presenting the patient with the diagnosis. In J. W. Cullen, B. H. Fox,

& R. N. Isom (Eds.), *Cancer: The behavioral dimensions* (pp. 269–274), New York: Raven Press.

Levenson, J., & Lesko, L. M. (1990). Psychiatric aspects of adult leukemia. *Seminars in Oncology Nursing, 6,* 76–83.

Leventhal, H., Meyer, D., & Nerenz, D., (1980). The common sense representation of illness danger. In S. Rachman (Ed.), *Medical psychology* (Vol. II, pp. 7–30). Terrytown, NY: Pergamon Press.

Levine, P. M., Silverfarb, P. M., & Lipowski, Z. J. (1978). Mental disorders in cancer patients. *Cancer, 42,* 1385–1391.

Levy, S., Heberman, R., Malvish, A., Schliew, B., & Lippman, M. (1985). Prognostic risk assessment in primary breast cancer by behavioral and immunologic parameters. *Health Psychology, 4,* 99–113.

Linn, M. W., Linn, B. S., & Harris, R. (1982). Effects of counseling for late stage cancer patients. *Cancer, 49,* 1048–1055.

Mages, N. L., Castro, J. R., Fobair, P., Hall, J., Harrison, I., Mendelsohn, G., & Wolfson, A. (1981). Patterns of psychosocial response to cancer: Can effective adaptation be predicted? *International Journal of Radiation Oncology Biology Physics, 7,* 385–392.

Massie, M. J., Gorzynski, R. C., Mastrovito, R. C., Theis, D., & Holland, J. C. (1979). The diagnosis of depression in patients with cancer. *Proceedings, American Association of Cancer Research of The American Society of Clinical Oncology, 20,* 432–440.

Massie, M. J., & Holland, J. C. (1990). Depression and the cancer patients. *Journal of Clinical Psychiatry, 51*(Suppl.) 12–17.

Massie, M. J., Holland, J. C., & Glass, E. (1983). Delirium in terminally ill cancer patients. *American Journal of Psychiatry, 140,* 1048–1050.

Massie, M. J., & Lesko, L. M. (1989). Psychopharmacologic management. In J. C. Holland & J. H. Rowland (Eds.), *Handbook of psychooncology: Psychological care of the patient with cancer* (pp. 470–492) New York: Oxford University Press.

McCorkle, R., & Benoliel, J. Q. (1983). Symptom distress, current concerns and mood disturbance after diagnosis of life-threatening disease. *Social Science and Medicine, 17,* 431–438.

McCorkle, R., Benoliel, J. Q., Donaldson, G., Georgiadou, F., Moinpour, C., & Goodell, B. (1989). A randomized clinical trial of home health nursing care for lung cancer patients. *Cancer, 64,* 199–206.

McCorkle, R., Yost, L. S., Jepson, C., Malone, D., Baird, S., & Lusk, E. (1993). A cancer experience: Relationship of patient psychosocial responses to caregiver burden over time. *Psycho-oncology, 2,* 21–32.

Morgenstern, H., Gellert, G. A., & Walter, S. D. (1984). The impact of a psychosocial program on survival with breast cancer: The importance of selection bias in program evaluation. *Journal of Chronic Disease, 37,* 273–282.

Morris, T., Greer, H. S., & White, P. (1977). Psychological and social adjustment to mastectomy: A two year follow-up study. *Cancer, 40,* 2381–2387.

Mossey, J. M., Knott, K., & Craik, L. (1990). The effects of persistent depressive symptoms on hip fracture recovery. *Journal of Gerontology, 45,* 163–168.

Nagi, S. Z. (1969). A conceptual framework. In S. Z. Nagi (Ed.), *Disability and rehabilitation: Legal, clinical and self concepts and measurement.* Columbus: Ohio State University Press.

Northouse, L. (1984). The impact of cancer on the family: An overview. *International Journal of Psychiatry in Medicine, 14,* 215–242.

Northouse, L. L., & Swain, M. A. (1987). Adjustment of patients and husbands to the initial impact of breast cancer. *Nursing Research, 36,* 221–225.

Novack. D. H., Plummer, R. L., Ochitill, H., Morrow, G. R., & Bennett, J. M. (1979). Changes in physicians attitudes toward telling the cancer patient. *Journal of the American Medical Association, 241,* 897–900.

Oken, D. (1961). What to tell cancer patients: A study of medical attitudes. *Journal of the American Medical Association, 241,* 897–900, 1979.

Pasacreta, J. (1993). Depressive phenomena and associated functional status outcomes among women with breast cancer. Unpublished doctoral dissertation, University of Pennsylvania School of Nursing, Philadelphia, PA.

Pasacreta, J. V., Malone, D., & McCorkle, R. (1991). *Clinical depression in a sample of cancer patients: Exploring associated risk factors and assessment strategies.* Poster presentation: American Cancer Society, 2nd Nursing Research Conference, January 31, 1991, Baltimore, MD.

Pasacreta, J. V., & Massie, M. J. (1990). Psychiatric complications in patients with cancer. *Oncology Nursing Forum, 17,* 19–24.

Penman, D. T., Bloom, J. R., Fotopoulou, S., Cook, M. R., Holland, J. C., Gates, C., Flamer, D., Murawski, B., Ross, R., Brandt, U., Muenz, L., & Pee, D. (1987). The impact of mastectomy on self concept and ego function. A combined cross sectional and longitudinal study with comparison groups. *Women's Health, 11*(3), 101–130.

Plumb, M. M., & Holland, J. C. (1977). Comparative studies of psychological function in patients with advanced cancer. I. Self-reported depressive symptoms. *Psychosomatic Medicine, 39,* 264–276.

Plumb, M. M., & Holland, J. C. (1981). Comparative studies of psychological function in patients with advanced cancer. II. Interviewer-rated current and past psychological symptoms. *Psychosomatic Medicine, 43,* 243–254.

Richardson, J. L., Shelton, D. R., & Krailo, M. (1990). The effect of compliance with treatment on survival among patients with hematologic malignancies. *Journal of Clinical Oncology, 8,* 356–364.

Rowland, J. H., & Holland, J. C. (1989). Breast cancer. In J. C. Holland & J. H. Rowland (Eds.), *Handbook of psychooncology: Psychological care of the patient with cancer* (pp. 188–207). New York: Oxford University Press.

Sarna, L., & McCorkle, R. (in press). Living with lung cancer: A prototype to describe the burden of care for patient, family and caregivers.

Schain, W. S., Wellisch, D. K., Pasnau, R. D., & Landsverk, J. (1985). The sooner the better: A study of psychosocial factors in women undergoing immediate versus delayed breast reconstruction. *American Journal of Psychiatry, 142,* 40–46.

Shuster, J. L., Stern, T. A., & Greenberg, D. B. (1992). Pros and cons of fluoxitine for the depressed cancer patient. *Oncology, 11,* 45–55.

Silberfarb, P. M., Maurer, L. H., & Crouthamel, C. S. (1980). Psychosocial aspects of neoplastic disease. I. Functional status of breast cancer patients during different treatment regimens. *American Journal of Psychiatry, 137,* 450–455.

Sinsheimer, L., & Holland, J. C. (1987). Psychosocial issues in breast cancer. *Seminars in Oncology, 14*(1), 75–82.

Speigel, D. (1993). Commentary: Psychosocial intervention in cancer. *Journal of the National Cancer Institute, 85,* 1198–1205.

Speigel, D., Bloom, J. R., Kraemer, H. C., & Gottheil, E. G. (1989). Effect of psychosocial treatment on survival of patients with metastatic breast cancer. *Lancet, 2,* 888–891.

Thomas, S. G. (1978). Breast cancer: The psychosocial issues. *Cancer Nursing, 1,* 53–60.

Watson, M., Greer, S., Blake, S., & Sharpnell, K. (1984). Reaction to a diagnosis of breast cancer: Relationship between denial, delay, and rates of psychological morbidity. *Cancer, 53,* 2008–2012.

Weisman, A. (1979). *Coping with cancer.* New York: McGraw Hill Book Co.

Weisman, A. (1984). A model for psychosocial phasing in cancer. In R. H. Moos (Ed.), *Coping with physical illness. Vol. 2. New perspectives* (pp. 107–122). New York: Plenum.

Weisman, A., & Worden, J. W. (1976-1977). The existential plight in cancer: Significance of the first 100 days. *International Journal of Psychiatry in Medicine, 7*(1), 1–15.

Weisman, A. D., Worden, J. W., & Sobel, H. J. (1980). *Psychosocial screening and intervention with cancer patients.* Final report of the Omega Project (CA 19797). Bethesda, MD: National Cancer Institute.

Wells, K. B., Hays, R. D., Burnam, A., & Camp, P. (1989). Detection of depressive disorder for patients receiving prepaid or fee-for-service care. *Journal of the American Medical Association, 262,* 3298–3302.

Wells, K. B., Stewart, A., Hays, R. D., Burnam, N. A., Rogers, W., Daniels, M., Greenfield, S., & Ware, J. (1989). The functioning and well being of depressed patients: Results from the medical outcomes study. *Journal of the American Medical Association, 262,* 914–919.

Woods, S. W., Tesar, G. E., & Murray, G. B. (1986). Psychostimulant treatment of depressive disorders secondary to medical illness. *Journal of Clinical Psychiatry, 47,* 12–15.

Worden, J. W. (1983). Psychosocial screening of cancer patients. *Journal of Psychosocial Oncology, 1*(4), 1–10.

Worden, J. W. (1984). Preventive psychosocial intervention with newly diagnosed cancer patients. *General Hospital Psychiatry, 6,* 243–249.

The theory of body image has been used commonly in nursing and other disciplines in efforts to explain the nature and behavior of the person. Body image includes all aspects of one's physical self, such as physical appearance, state of health, and sexuality (Mock, 1993). Because sexuality encompasses more than body image, a separate chapter has been devoted to sexual aspects of the person with cancer (see Chapter 62). Body image changes probably occur in most individuals with cancer, and if these changes are not effectively integrated with the self-system, they can greatly diminish the quality of life. Nursing actions based on a thorough knowledge of body image theory may be able to facilitate healthy integration of body image changes by the person with cancer, the family, and the patient's social system. This chapter explores the theoretic notions of body image, presents current knowledge from measurement and research related to body image, and explores the health consequences of alterations in body image. The nursing care of persons who are at risk of or who are experiencing difficulty in integrating body image changes within their self-structure is discussed within a nursing process framework.

THE DEVELOPMENT OF THEORETIC THOUGHT ABOUT BODY IMAGE

The recognition of body image as a mental construct first became apparent through the reported experiences of phantom body parts after amputations. The inability of persons with amputated limbs to perceive their bodies as they actually existed stimulated attempts to explain the phenomenon by scientists from a variety of disciplines. Freud (1961[1927]), in developing his psychoanalytic theory, referred to body image phenomenon, which he considered to be an element of the ego, as "body-ego." Freud explained the emergence of the body-ego primarily in terms of stages of sexual development. Head (1920), a neurologist, explained body image in terms of brain and neurologic function. According to Head, the body image develops from infancy as a result of sensory experiences and motor activities. As a portion of the body moves, the person relates both the new position of the body part and the sensation of moving it to the overall posture of the body. These experiences are accumulated, stored in the sensory cortex of the brain, and integrated with present experiences to result in the body image, which operates outside of consciousness. The body image allows the person to relate the posture of the body to objects in the environment (Jacobson, 1964). This perspective of body image includes four elements: (1) awareness of parts of the body, (2) perception of the relative size of parts of the body, (3) awareness of positions of body parts, and (4) sensation related to body parts (Arseni, Botez, & Maretsis, 1966).

Schilder (1935) built on Head's theory to include the person's personal investment in various body parts and environmental influences as factors influencing body image. He expanded Head's postural image to include sensations from the skeleton, muscles, nerves, and viscera in adding to the image of the body. Schilder proposed that people form a picture of their body appearance within their minds. This picture includes interpersonal, environmental, and temporal factors. People's views of their bodies are, in part, determined by the perceptions of their bodies by other persons in their environment, which are communicated to them.

Schilder believed that people not only perceive a body image but express a body image.

Several theorists suggest that the body and its parts are viewed by the self, or the ego, as an object (Johnson, 1976; Metcalfe & Fischman, 1985; Schilder, 1935). From this perspective, the body is viewed as a thing apart from the ego. Szasz (1957) also proposed that with maturity came an increasingly complex body-ego integration.

Fisher (1968, 1970, 1973) suggests that there are three elements of body image: (1) body boundary (or border), (2) body awareness, and (3) meanings the person places on various body parts. Fisher has developed instruments to measure each of these three elements of body image; his research indicated that they are not correlated. Fisher also found that the body image boundary may extend beyond the person to include clothing, jewelry, and even such things as the car the person drives (Crumbaugh, 1968). The space around the person and the belongings within that space may be considered part of the body image (Fisher, 1970, 1973; Horowitz, 1966). The degree of perceived vulnerability of the body or particular parts of the body is also a part of body image. Schain and Howards (1985) included two parts of the "body self": (1) the functional self (what I can do) and (2) the aesthetic self (what I look like).

The body image develops gradually as the person matures (Anthony, 1971; Erikson, 1963). Erikson (1963, 1980) has described the gradual development of the body image during childhood, using Freud's perspective of the body as primarily a sexual entity. This developmental perspective is commonly used in nursing (Blaesig & Brockhaus, 1972; Dempsey, 1972; Murray, 1972a, 1972b). Derogatis (1980) disagrees with this point of view and proposes that body image and sexuality are separate but related elements that influence a person's identity.

From experiences that begin in childhood, persons learn to place different values on various parts of their body (Fisher, 1967, 1970, 1973; Fry, 1980). Many persons learn to view parts of their body as dirty. Dirtiness carries with it a feeling of disgust (Kubie, 1937). It is often not acceptable to touch these parts of the body or look at them. Other body parts are highly valued and may be highlighted by body posture. Hair styling, cosmetics, and clothing may be selected to proudly display these body parts. The valuing of particular body parts varies to some extent from one person to another, from one culture or religion to another, and from one period of time to another (Mead, 1934; Price, 1986; Quinn, 1984; Schonfeld, 1963).

Body image is related to self-esteem, self-concept, and identity (Mathes & Kahn, 1975; Rubin, 1968). High self-esteem is a feeling of worthiness. Body image and self-esteem have been found to be highly correlated. Individuals who have poor body image also tend to have low self-esteem. Self-concept has been defined as the composite of all the feelings a person has about the self. From this point of view, body image and self-esteem are considered elements of self-concept. Others consider the four concepts as separate but constantly interacting. Schain and Howards (1985) suggest that there are four components of self-concept: (1) the body self, (2) the interpersonal self (the interaction between self and others), (3) the achieving self (goals and aspirations), and (4) the identification self (values, ethics, beliefs, spiritual behavior, and ethnic views). Self-concept and identity are sometimes viewed as interchangeable concepts. Tabachnick (1967) suggests that identity has two elements: (1) social definition, which defines the relationship with the outside world, and (2) self-realization, which reflects inner autonomy and is manifested by adherence to personal goals. Problems arise when the balance between these two elements of identity is disrupted (Weigart & Hastings, 1977).

MEASURING AND STUDYING BODY IMAGE

Numerous instruments have been developed to measure body image or specific dimensions of body image (Table 61–1). The most frequently used instrument is the Body Cathexis Scale developed by Secord and Jourard (1953). For more information about this scale, see Box 61–1. Many of the instruments designed to measure body image have interesting potential for increasing our understanding of this complex concept. An excellent critique of many of these instruments can be found in *Instruments for Clinical Nursing Research* (Frank-Stromborg, 1988).

A burst of research activity related to body image occurred in the 1960s and early 1970s. Some of these studies indicated that evaluations of body appearance and attractiveness of others were closely related to expectations of their performance and judgments of their worth (Berscheid, Walster, & Gohrnstedt, 1972, 1973; Dion, Berscheid, & Walster, 1972; Dipboye, Fromkin, & Wiback, 1975; Douty, Moore, & Hartford, 1974; Efran, 1974; Landy & Sigall, 1974). These judgments of others based on their appearance begins in childhood (Richardson, Goodman, Hastorf, & Dornbusch, 1961) and seems to be so ingrained that Fisher (1973) believes it is not possible to change them. Given this, the cancer patients' concerns about how they will be perceived by others is realistic.

In recent years, studies have moved from defining body image to examining the dynamics of body image in persons with birth defects, obesity, injuries, brain damage, hirsutism, and surgery (Adami et al., 1994; Boren, 1985; Boren & Meell, 1985; Denning, 1982; Dropkin, 1979a, 1979b, 1981, 1985; Guariglia, & Antonucci, 1992; Hoover, 1984; Kalick, Goldwyn, & Noe, 1981; Lewis, 1978; Orbach & Tallent, 1965; Piff, 1986; Polivy, 1974; Stulberg, & Caruthers, 1990; Sullivan et al., 1993).

Most methods used to treat cancer produce body image changes. The most obvious of these are the mutilating effects of surgery. Radiotherapy often leads to such consequences as skin changes, vaginal stenosis, changes in bowel habits, changes in urinary frequency, pain, fatigue, nausea and vomiting, neurotoxicity, hemorrhaging, infection, skin changes, diarrhea, sexual

TABLE 61–1. *Body Image Measurement Methods*

AUTHOR	MEASURE	STUDIES IN WHICH MEASURE IS USED
Secord (1953)	Word association procedure using homonyms	Sanger & Reznikoff (1981)
Osgood, Suci, & Tannenbaum (1957)	Body Attitude Scale	Collingwood & Willett (1971)
Secord & Jourard (1953)	Body-Cathexis Scale	Mahoney (1974), Bille (1977), Baxley, Erdman, Henry, & Roof (1984), Schwab & Harmeling (1968), Wagner & Bye (1979), Sanger & Reznikoff (1981), Ray (1977), Gerard (1982)
Fisher & Cleveland (1968)	Body Boundary Scale	Sewell & Edwards (1980)
Fisher & Cleveland (1968)	Body Awareness Scale	Sewell & Edwards (1980)
Fisher & Cleveland (1968)	Body Values Scale	Sewell & Edwards (1980)
Fisher & Cleveland (1968)	Rorschach method of measuring body boundaries	Fisher (1967), Sanger & Reznikoff (1981)
Schwab & Harmeling (1968)	Body-Image Test	
Rosen & Ross (1968)	Satisfaction with Body Appearance	Lerner, Karabenick, & Stuart (1973)
Rosen & Ross (1968)	Importance of Body Parts	Lerner, Karabenick, & Stuart (1973), Mahoney (1974)
Rosen & Ross (1968)	Importance of Body Parts in Evaluating Attractiveness of Others	Lerner, Karabenick, & Stuart (1973)
Berscheid, Walster, & Gohrnstedt (1972)	Body Image Questionnaire	Polivy (1977), Krouse & Krouse (1981), Krouse & Krouse (1982)
Tzeng (1975)	Present Body Image	Tzeng (1977), Champion, Austin, & Tzeng (1982)
Tzeng (1975)	Ideal Body Image	Tzeng (1977), Champion, Austin, & Tzeng (1982)
Allbeck, Hallberg, & Espmark (1976)	Direct measure of body image by television apparatus	
McCloskey (1976)	Body Image Assessment Tool	
Derogatis & Melisaratos (1979)	BODY (subscale of DSFI)	Andersen & Jochimsen (1985)
Schlacter (cited in Fawcett & Frye [1980])	Topographic device to measure perceived body space	Fawcett & Frye (1980), Fawcett & Chodil (1979)
Kurtz (cited in Fawcett & Frye [1980])	Body Attitude Scale	
Baird (1985)	Baird Body Image Assessment Tool	
deHaes, van Oostrom, & Welvaart (1986)	Impact of Illness on Body Image	

DSFI = Derogatis Sexual Functioning Inventory.

dysfunction, and respiratory dysfunction, all of which alter body image (Baxley, Erdman, Henry, & Roof, 1984; Beardslee & Miller, 1981; Beardslee & Neff, 1982; Griffiths, 1980). Although the manifestation of side effects of chemotherapy occur less frequently than in the past, patients receiving chemotherapy may still experience body image changes. Most of these changes are a result of normal cell/organ disruptions (e.g., bone marrow suppression, gastrointestinal disturbance, renal toxicity). Alopecia has also been associated with negative scores on body image scales (Baxley et al., 1984; Wabrek & Gunn, 1984; Wagner & Bye, 1979).

In the area of cancer, studies have focused on body image changes resulting from treatment to specific disease sites. The more obvious alterations in body structure have received the most attention in the literature. However, the serious threats to body image caused by such cancers as lung cancer, upper gastrointestinal tract cancers, hepatocarcinoma, leukemia, and lymphomas have not been adequately addressed in the literature.

BREAST CANCER

Of the numerous types of cancer that effect body image, breast cancer has been the most frequently studied (Abidin, Durham, & Dooley, 1991; Carroll, 1981; Christensen, Blichert-Toft, Giersing, Richardt, & Bechmann, 1982; de Haes, & Welvaart, 1985; de Haes, van Oostrom, & Welvaart, 1986; Ganz, Shag, Polihsky, Heinrich, & Flack, 1987; Gerard, 1982; Kennerly, 1977; Knobf, 1985; Knobf & Stahl, 1991; Krouse & Krouse, 1981; Miller & Graham, 1975; Morris, 1979; Polivy, 1977; Ray, 1977; Sanger & Reznikoff, 1981; Schain, 1985; Schain et al., 1983; Schover, 1991; Scott, 1983; Scott & Eisendrath, 1985-1986; Valanis & Rumpler, 1985). Twenty years ago, studies indicated serious, unresolved body image problems in women who had undergone a radical mastectomy. Some more recent longitudinal studies have validated these findings (de Haes et al., 1986; Goldberg et al., 1992; Kemeny, Wellisch, & Schain, 1988). Other recent studies, using

---

Box 61–1. *The Body-Cathexis Scale*

Secord, P. F., & Jourard, S. M. [1953]. The appraisal of body-cathexis and the self. *Journal of Consulting Psychology, 17,* 343–347.

Secord and Jourard define body-cathexis as "the degree of feeling of satisfaction or dissatisfaction with the various parts or processes of the body" (p. 343).

The first part of the revised scale consists of a listing of 40 parts of the body and body functions. Examples of items are hair, ears, energy level, profile, skin texture, sex activities. Each item is followed by a scale of 1 through 5. The numbers represent the following feelings:
1. Have strong positive feelings.
2. Have moderate positive feelings.
3. Have no feeling one way or the other.
4. Have moderate negative feelings.
5. Have strong negative feelings.

The second part of the scale consists of 40 items representing conceptual aspects of the self. Examples of these items are first name, life goals, general knowledge, sensitivity to opinions of others, happiness. These items are rated using the scale described above.

These scales are scored separately by summing the ratings for each item and dividing by the number of items in that part of the scale. This provides a summed score for each person on these two parts of the scale.

Secord and Jourard also report development of a homonym test, which consists of 75 homonyms, some of which have meanings pertaining to the body and some of which do not. Many of the homonyms have meanings pertaining to pain, disease, or bodily injury. Neutral homonyms are interspersed within the list "for purposes of disguise." This test is scored by totaling the number of body responses to the 75 homonyms.

In addition, an anxiety indicator score is obtained, which is scored differently for male and female subjects. Eleven items for which cathexis was most negative for men are summed for men and the 11 items that were most negative for women are summed for women.

Reliabilities for the various scales are moderately high, ranging from 0.63 to 0.92.

Some indications of validity are provided by significant intercorrelations among the various parts of the scale. Concurrent validity is demonstrated by significant correlations between each of the parts of the Body-Cathexis scale and the Maslow Test, which measures insecurity.

The Body-Cathexis scale has been used in many studies examining body image (see citations in Table 61–1).

The scale is useful for appraising the feelings of a person toward his or her body. It could be used to identify persons at high risk for difficulty in managing an alteration in body image or as a measurement tool for research.

---

repeated measure designs that follow the subjects over a 1- to 5-year period, have described a process of body image change during which body image tends to decline for about 6 months and then begins to improve. Originally, researchers assumed that the threat to body image occurred because of the sexual symbolism of the breast. However, Fallowfield and Hall (1991) found that the overriding influence on body image in women with breast cancer is a consequence of awareness of the presence of cancer in the body and experiencing the threat of death. After surgery, three fourths of women with breast cancer integrate body image changes by 1 year (Andersen & Jochimsen, 1985; Ganz, Schag, Lee, Polinsky, & Tan, 1992; Krouse & Krouse, 1981; Morris, Greer, & White, 1977; Polivy, 1974; Ray, 1977; Renneker & Cutler, 1952; Sanger & Reznikoff, 1981; West, 1977).

Four factors may be involved in the different findings of more recent studies. First, the treatment (and prognosis) have changed. Overall, breast cancer is being identified earlier, and surgery tends to be more conservative, which results in less impact on body function. Surgical treatment is often accompanied by chemotherapy, radiation, or both. Second, psychosocial care after mastectomy has improved greatly over the last 20 years, which could affect the severity of body image changes. Third, precision and objectiveness of

measurement of body image in studies have improved, allowing more accurate interpretation of findings. Fourth, examining patterns of body image across time has provided a clearer understanding of the process of body image integration.

Researchers are currently examining the differential impact of various breast cancer treatments, such as mastectomy versus breast-conserving therapy (BCT), on the severity and direction of body image changes (Bartelink, van Dam, & van Dongen, 1985; Blichert-Toft, 1992; Boman, Bjorvell, Cedermark, Theve, & Wilking, 1993; de Haes et al., 1986; Deadman, Dewey, Owens, Leinster, & Slade, 1989; Ganz et al., 1992; Ganz, Schag, Lee, & Sim, 1992; Goldberg et al., 1992; Kemeny et al., 1988; Kiebert, de Haes, & van de Velde, 1991; Lasry & Margolese, 1992; Lasry et al., 1987; Margolis, Goodman, & Rubin, 1990; Mock, 1993; Noguchi et al., 1993; Wellisch et al., 1989). When given an option, women who are most concerned about body integrity prefer BCT (Margolis, Goodman, Rubin, & Pajac, 1989; Ward, Heidrich, & Wolberg, 1989). Alterations in body image are clearly less severe in BCT. However, BCT may result in disfigurement (scar, feeling lopsided) that may cause body image problems, especially in the early postoperative period (Taylor et al., 1985). Radiation and chemotherapy, which are often components of BCT, also affect body image. Other factors also important to quality of life, such as fear of recurrence, have been found in some studies to be more severe after BCT (Fallowfield & Hall, 1991). A significant minority (25 per cent) of women who received BCT were found in one study to have psychosocial adjustment problems 2 to 11 years after treatment (Sneeuw et al., 1992).

The purpose of performing breast-conserving procedures rather than a mastectomy is to improve psychosocial outcomes, particularly body image. In terms of survival rates, studies show the two procedures to be relatively equivalent. However, Blichert-Toft (1992) cautions that since many breast cancers are multicentric, the risk of leaving cancer tissue in the breast is higher with breast-conserving therapy. Without accompanying radiation therapy and perhaps chemotherapy, the risk of recurrence in one study of 1141 patients was 43 per cent (Fisher et al., 1991). Adjuvant therapy reduced the risk to 12 per cent but also increased problems related to altered body image. Fallowfield and Hall (1991) propose that although there are increased problems with altered body image in women receiving mastectomies, this does not necessarily result in long-term psychologic distress or impairment of social functioning. The level of depression has been found to be equivalent between the two groups (Maguire, 1989; van Heeringen, Van Moffaert, & de Cuypere, 1989). Rather than altering the surgical treatment, these authors propose that more effective means be used to provide psychologic assistance, stress-reduction strategies, and antidepressant drugs that can facilitate effective coping.

GYNECOLOGIC CANCER

Women with gynecologic surgery for cancer, who are frequently used as a comparison group in studies of women with mastectomies, experience much greater difficulty integrating an altered body image than women with mastectomies (Capone, Good, Westie, & Jacobson, 1980; Krouse, 1985; Mele, Palazzanis, & Sgreccia, 1992; Sewell & Edwards, 1980). Although the appearance of the body does not usually change after gynecologic surgery (excluding pelvic exenteration and radical vulvectomy), its functioning may have changed in ways that are important to these women. Because of the emphasis put upon the uterus, many females experience a profound change in their body image as a result of a hysterectomy. One study reported that 30 per cent of the sample of women having gynecologic surgery for cancer felt they had lost a part of the self with the loss of their uterus. Of women having the same surgery but not having cancer, only 17 per cent felt a loss of self (Filiberti et al., 1991). Cervical cancer can also affect body image. Because of the postulated causal relationship between certain sexual behaviors (early age of first coitus, increased number of sexual partners) and cervical carcinoma, body image and sexual relationships can suffer after the diagnosis of cervical intraepithelial neoplasia (Palmer, Tucker, Warren, & Adams, 1993).

HEAD AND NECK CANCER

Several studies have examined altered body image in persons with head and neck cancer (Burgess, 1994; Shapiro & Kornfeld, 1987; Tierny, 1975). Eighty per cent of persons having surgery for head and neck cancer reported problems with altered body image. Responses included statements such as, "I no longer feel I'm the same person," "I look like a monster," "I hardly recognize myself." Many indicated they felt older (Gamba et al., 1992). These individuals may have problems with speech, eating and drinking, changes in taste, changes in smell, chewing, swallowing, vision, hearing, as well as appearance. Some of these individuals not only cannot verbalize, they cannot make any sound at all. The great emotions such as rage, grief, and ecstasy are not expressed in speech but in sound (Bronheim, Strain, & Biller, 1991a, 1991b; Freedlander, Espie, Campsie, Soutar, & Robertson, 1989). However, in one study, alterations of body image in this population of cancer patients was not predictive of postoperative adjustment (Krouse, Krouse, & Fabian, 1989).

CANCER IN CHILDREN

As in adults, children undergoing cancer treatment experience many bodily changes. Although some are temporary, others are permanent. Children with cancer have more knowledge of the functioning of their bodies than other children and are more concerned about their body integrity (Neff & Beardslee, 1990). Hockenberry-Eaton and Cotanch (1989) found declines over time in body image of children with cancer. Siblings of children with cancer may also experience alterations in body image (Rollins, 1990). The body image of adolescents normally undergoes rapid changes as their bodies develop and mature. Imposed changes in physical appearance as a consequence of cancer complicate their adjustment to normal body image changes. During treatment they perceive themselves as being different from other adolescents (Blotcky & Cohen, 1985). Alterations in body image are beginning to be examined in survivors of childhood cancer (Hymovich & Roehnert, 1994). Many adolescent survivors of childhood cancer have an enduring sense of fragility and vulnerability, which are expressed in a variety of ways. Some involve themselves in particularly challenging, sometimes dangerous activities. Others become exhibitionistic and flaunt a stump or scar, in part as a matter of pride but also for the shock value. Some remain highly preoccupied with their bodies and bodily functions to the point of hypochondria. About one third have negative values on measures of body image (Fritz & Williams, 1988).

HEALTH CONSEQUENCES OF ALTERATIONS IN BODY IMAGE

The powerful impact of a diagnosis of cancer can affect body image before the initiation of treatment or the obvious changes caused by progression of the disease. The person feels a higher degree of vulnerability, a decreased awareness of changes within his or her body, and a sense of decreased power to control these little-understood changes. An anticipation of overwhelming changes in the body, which no personal action can prevent, profoundly affects the patient. Following this realization, the person is confronted with major assaults to body image as the consequence of necessary treatments for the cancer and of progression of the disease. Although some body image changes are related to total body function, others differ with the cancer site and treatment choice (Christian, 1982; Clark, 1977; Murray, 1980).

The cancer process itself produces body image changes as the patient copes with pain, fatigue, weakness, susceptibility to infection, spinal cord compression, septic shock, weight gain, weight loss, and loss of body function (Hopwood & Maguire, 1988; Olson, 1967). The person may be more distressed over the body changes caused by the cancer than by the threat to survival. Because of the nurse's more immediate concern with the patient's survival and comfort, patient difficulties related to body image changes may not be noted or may be discounted. It is sometimes difficult to understand how the patient could focus on body image in the midst of a life-threatening crisis when for the patient it may be the most important concern. The focusing of the patient on body image change may be due to denial of impending death, a need for control, or simply that body image is truly the most pressing concern at that time.

An alteration in body image occurs over time, to some extent is an unconscious process, and needs to be integrated within the self-system. This process requires emotional energy, which could otherwise be invested in other pursuits. Reality for that person has changed, and uncertainty has increased. To some, it must seem as if their personal world is being torn asunder (Hart & Kenney, 1981). The process of restructuring the body image may involve changing (1) the image of the body contained within the brain, (2) body posture, (3) body movement, and (4) perceptions of body function. The person must then determine the personal meaning of the body alteration and evaluate the reaction of members of his or her social support system to the body change. All of these changes must then be integrated within the self structure, with an image of, acceptance of, and love of "this is who I am."

Studies seem to indicate that success in achieving total integration of an altered body image may be related to the person's body image, self-esteem, self-concept, and identity prior to the alteration of body image (Cantor, 1980; Champion, Austin, & Tzeng, 1982; Dropkin, 1983; Paine, Alves, & Turbino, 1985; Rosen & Ross, 1968). Because many of the studies have been retrospective and thus have not measured these concepts before the body-altering event, there is no clear understanding of how low values on these concepts before the event are associated with inability to integrate a changed body image within the self-sys-

tem. In addition, the effect of such factors as coping skills and effective social support systems before and after a body-altering event has not been studied (Brown & Bjelic, 1977).

However, it is clear that failure to integrate a changed body image is associated with long-term depression, difficulty with interpersonal interactions, withdrawal from social interaction, and overall, a lower quality of life (Beardslee & Sperhac, 1978; deHaes et al., 1986; Krouse, 1985; Krouse & Krouse, 1981, 1982; Ray, 1977; Sewell & Edwards, 1980). This outcome can be life-threatening for persons with cancer in that these persons may choose not to continue treatment. For such individuals, the body image change seems to be even more important than life itself. The depression, lack of energy, and overwhelming changes in view of self leave little strength for participating in the fight for life. From the research, it would appear that these consequences are experienced to some degree by about 25 per cent of persons who have a major body image alteration (Andersen & Jochimsen, 1985; Polivy, 1974; Schwab & Harmeling, 1968; Scott, 1983).

THE PROCESS OF CARING FOR PERSONS WITH ALTERATIONS IN BODY IMAGE

Nursing can play a pivotal role in helping the patient cope with altered body image. With knowledge and skill, the nurse can influence the outcome of altered body image at two points: (1) during the process of the initial body image–changing event, and (2) during the process of integrating the body image into the self-structure. The following section describes the nursing actions that have been found, through research or clinical practice, to assist the patient in effective integration of body image changes.

ASSESSMENT

Ideally, an initial body image assessment of the patient should occur prior to any body image changes, that is, before treatment has begun and before the devastating effects of the disease process have become evident. One purpose of the assessment is to identify patients who are at high risk of experiencing difficulty in managing body image changes. Another purpose is to gather information that can be used to provide guidance to the patient in planning strategies to facilitate effective management of the body image change when it occurs (Norris, 1978). The nurse can also make a judgment about the patient's capacity for effectively integrating the changed body image. This initial assessment should gather information related to the following:

PERSONALITY
- Self-esteem
- Self-concept
- General coping skills
- Dream content since diagnosis

BODY IMAGE FACTORS
- Significance to the patient of his or her present body image
- Importance of affected body parts
- Physical and psychologic association of the affected body part
- Body image postdiagnosis and pretreatment
- Thoughts or feelings the patient is having about possible changed body image
- Opportunities to try out new body image

CULTURAL-SOCIAL INFORMATION
- Level of social cognition
- Ability to interact with others
- Family dynamics
- Social support systems
- Perception and quantity of available help

ATTITUDES TOWARD CANCER AND ITS TREATMENT
- Patient expectations
- Attitudes toward the physician

NEED FOR INFORMATION
- Accuracy of information about the effects of cancer and its treatment (e.g., everyone loses their hair when taking chemotherapy)
- Adequacy of information provided to patient (the effect of fatigue on body image)
- Information overload (too much information is presented to the patient at a given time) (Brennan, 1994; Carroll, 1981; Price, 1986; Wilbur, 1980)

The nurse begins the assessment by asking questions that require cognition on the part of the patient. Only then does the nurse progress to questions requiring an emotional response on the part of the patient. The types of questions asked of the patient depend on the quality of the nurse-patient relationship. If a working therapeutic relationship has been established, the nurse can proceed with more probing questions (Bard & Sutherland, 1955; Knobf, 1985). Otherwise, relationship-establishing strategies must precede questioning. In assessing body image changes or risk, the nurse must be aware of both verbal and nonverbal messages the patient is communicating. Rarely will the patient clearly verbalize his or her feelings about the changes that have occurred. In fact, he or she may not be consciously aware of many of these feelings.

Open-ended questions can be used to determine the patient's perception of the impact of the cancer experience on his or her life. This can lead to questioning that can stimulate the patient to evaluate the effectiveness of current coping techniques. Questions that have been found to be useful include the following: "What does this diagnosis of cancer mean to you?" "How is it affecting your life?" "How do you feel you are coping with it?" Concurrently with questioning the patient, the nurse can judge whether the patient is avoiding

conversation about the impact of the cancer, or, conversely, is intellectualizing the impact. In some cases the patient may expend more energy in wanting to help other patients with similar concerns than in discussing personal concerns.

Comments and questions that focus directly on the body image changes can be used at this time. These should relate to the patient's particular situation and may include such comments as the following. "Frequently patients are hesitant to resume social relationships after a mastectomy or colostomy, or head and neck surgery. Although I see you as being the same person you were, how are you feeling about these changes in your life?" The nurse may share examples of questions previously asked by other patients with the patients. These may include "Will my husband still want me?" "Should I keep my scar covered during intimate times?" "Should I encourage my spouse to touch the altered part?" "What do I tell my children?" (Lamb & Woods, 1981).

Body image changes that affect internal organs, excluding the reproductive organs, or that are caused by symptoms mentioned in the previous section (fatigue, pain, and so forth) are frequently ignored because they are not directly associated with a visual change in the patient's body. In assessing the patient, these aspects must be included. The nurse should question the patient about thoughts or feelings related to the removal of internal organs, such as fears that the patient may have about the removal of the pancreas. Feelings about the self may also be influenced by experiences such as fatigue, pain, or hemorrhaging. Patients may express feelings of lowered self-esteem because of inability to perform tasks in the previous manner.

Cues that patients are experiencing difficulties include:

- Changes in patient approaches to their bodies
- Avoidance of discussion of any possible changes
- Emphatically discussing the positive aspects while denying or ignoring the negative aspects
- Displaced anger at staff members or family
- Depression
- Overcompensation, indicated by a desire to help other patients with similar problems when they have not yet resolved their own problems

It is also important to gather information about the patient from other health professionals. Interaction with nurses who cared for the patient during periods of hospitalization can provide valuable information. Information can come from a variety of sources, including housekeepers, physical therapists, respiratory therapists, and other persons in contact with the patient. Cues gathered by various members of the health care team will provide a much clearer picture of the patient's situation from which to develop effective interventions.

Of particular importance is the need to identify those persons at risk of being unsuccessful in integrating body image changes (Meyer, & Aspegren, 1989; Penman et al., 1987). Although most of the knowledge of high-risk persons was obtained by studying women with breast cancer, many of the findings may prove useful in providing care to patients with a variety of cancers. Characteristics of women who are unaccepting of their body image after breast surgery include:

- Employment in unskilled manual labor
- Few leisure time activities
- A history of broken heterosexual relationships
- Lacking confidence in spouse
- Less interest in sex after surgery than before surgery
- Avoiding being naked in front of their spouse (Meyer & Aspegren, 1989).

The number of stressful events prior to the diagnosis of cancer is related to subsequent distress. Depression and emotional lability before the surgery may be predictive of poor adjustment in the following year (Morris et al., 1977). High-risk women are described as being overwhelmed and out of control in relation to their diagnosis and treatment. However, their problems are not limited to cancer but cross all the dimensions of their life. These individuals continue to have problems with body image at 1 year (Schag et al., 1993). Those patients who experienced phantom breast syndrome also may have greater problems integrating an altered body image (Christensen et al., 1982). Persons who are dissatisfied with many body parts rather than just those affected by the illness also tend to have difficulty integrating an altered body image. This negative feeling toward the whole body can be related to high levels of emotional distress (Kolb, 1959; Leonard, 1972; Schwab & Harmeling, 1968). Individuals identified as being at high risk of not integrating body image changes may need more intensive or different nursing actions.

INTERVENTIONS THAT FACILITATE HEALTHY RESPONSE TO BODY IMAGE CHANGES

The goal of intervention is that the patient demonstrates integration of his or her altered body image. Commonly, nursing interventions that assist the patient in integrating an altered body image occur during the short period of hospitalization. A few studies indicate that such interventions do make a difference in the person's success in integrating the altered body image by increasing knowledge of the body change and how to manage it (Capone et al., 1980). However, because the process of integrating a body image change seems to occur over a 2- to 6-month period, availability of nursing care extended over this period of time, at least intermittently, would increase the effectiveness of nursing interventions.

The first and most important element for effective interventions for managing body image changes is the establishment of a trust relationship between the nurse and the patient. Maximum effectiveness can be achieved through a nurse-patient relationship that is initiated at the time of diagnosis and continues through the period of integration of the altered body image,

which, if successful, can be expected to occur between 1 and 2 years later. Effective nursing interventions focus on education, support, counseling, and referral. Within a trust relationship, the more delicate issues of body image changes can be explored (Bard & Sutherland, 1955; Donovan & Girton, 1984; Marten, 1978; Riddle, 1972; Roback, Kirshner, & Roback, 1981-1982). A landmark study supporting the use of specially trained nurses to deal with body image changes was reported by Maguire, Tait, Brooke, Thomas, and Sellwood (1980) and Hopwood and Maguire (1988). They found that specialist nurses who were trained to assess and counsel cancer patients were able to identify body image disturbances at an earlier time, thus allowing effective intervention to be initiated.

The nurse can influence the changing body image through the following actions:

- Helping the patient think through the meaning of the change
- Proposing alternative meanings not considered by the patient
- Role modeling healthy responses to the change
- Providing positive feedback as a person in the environment reacting to the change
- Helping family members and social support system members to examine the meaning of the changes
- Communicating acceptance of the changes to the patient (Hurley, Meyer-Ruppell, & Evans, 1983).

Initial interventions with a patient in the early stages of treatment for cancer should include educational preparation for the impending body image change. The nurse needs to be knowledgeable about the specific body image changes associated with the patient's situation. Frequently the alteration is so obvious that the nurse assumes that the patient is dealing with it. For example, so much information about breast disease and alteration has been published in the lay press that the nurse may assume that the patient is "educated" about the potential emotional responses to loss of a major body organ. Explanation of impending events related to the cancer process and its treatment and the expected impact on body image can be helpful. The nurse should emphasize that reactions to these changes are commonly experienced by patients with the particular diagnosis. Providing information about these changes will set the groundwork for further nurse-patient discussions at a later time (Brennan, 1994; Burgess, 1994; Erdos, 1992). Body image changes are sometimes not addressed because of the nurse's personal discomfort in dealing with the situation. In addition to knowledge about body image theory, the nurse must have worked through personal dilemmas related to body image (MacElveen-Hoehn & McCorkle, 1985).

Besides expediting assessment, open-ended questions can be used as an intervention. The questioning serves as permission granting the patient to talk about the subject. It can also be a starting point for family intervention. The inclusion of the family or significant others in assessment and intervention should be decided on in conjunction with the patient. The patient should be allowed to determine when the family is brought into the discussions about the alteration and may need assistance from the nurse in sharing fears or hopes with the family. It is important to also direct interventions towards significant members of the patient's social system. This provides a twofold benefit: (1) it helps the patient's family and friends cope with the patient's altered body image, and (2) it strengthens the support networks for the patient (Brennan, 1994).

If the patient does not respond to the nurse's introduction of the topic, the nurse needs to let the patient know that it is permissible to initiate the topic any time he or she chooses. Also, the nurse should reintroduce the topic periodically, to provide the patient with many opportunities to discuss concerns. It is important to implicitly give permission to discuss the topic but not to force discussion. The patient's not responding to the nurse's cues does not necessarily imply lack of integration of body image changes. Some patients are able to integrate the body image changes from their own mental health base and personal resources. This is confirmed by observation of healthy adaptation to the alteration (i.e., touching the altered site, open discussion about the altered part).

The nurse must also act as advocate in ensuring that the best possible care is given to the alteration site itself to minimize the severity of the body image change. This includes input regarding proper use of equipment (correct bagging techniques of ostomies, correct wound care) and observation of early breakdown of the healing process (early signs of infection, improper suture care, drainage amounts). The knowledgeable, experienced nurse cannot assume that these potential problems will be managed effectively by the physician or the other members of the health care team.

Generally the period from 2 to 6 months after diagnosis of cancer is a time of ongoing treatment or follow-up. Although sometimes the patient expresses concerns during interaction with the nurse during this period of treatment, it may be necessary for the nurse to reintroduce the topic of body image changes. Ongoing contact with other nurses who have previously cared for the patient will enable the nurse to determine what information the patient was given previously so that the information can be reinforced and expanded. This also is an ideal time to inform the patient of the availability of peer support groups. The patient needs reinforcement that his or her concerns are normal. A meta-analysis of 18 studies in which contacts between cancer patients were explored revealed that there were fewer disturbances of body image in patients who had had contact with other cancer patients (Van den Borne, Pruyn, & Van Dam-de Mey, 1986). To provide effective referral, the nurse must be aware of community resources for peer support. The American Cancer Society, local cancer treatment centers, and local hospitals usually have information about these groups. In some areas of the country, the American Cancer Society's Reach to Recovery and Dialogue programs have peer support groups as part of their services. Because of the emphasis on breast cancer nationwide, there are breast cancer support groups in many communities. These support groups spend a significant amount of time dealing with body image changes. The United Ostomy Association and the Lost Chord Club also may provide peer support groups.

Cognitive behavior therapy is an approach that is reportedly having the most success in the treatment of patients with body image problems (Glanz & Lerman, 1992; Hopwood & Maguire, 1988). This approach challenges the negative thoughts and cognitive distortions that are frequently associated with body image changes. Through this therapeutic approach, the patient learns to substitute a more positive attitude towards the new body image, which in turn progresses to an enhanced self-esteem. This type of therapy should be provided only by professionals having extensive training in therapeutic approaches.

EVALUATING THE INTEGRATION OF BODY IMAGE CHANGES

Ongoing evaluation is necessary to assess whether the goal of integration of the altered body image has been achieved (Brennan, 1994). With the exception of the study conducted by Maguire et al. (1980) and Hopwood and Maguire (1988), the outcomes of nursing care related to body image changes have not been adequately defined or examined, either clinically or through research. Because of this lack of knowledge, it is difficult to judge the effectiveness of nursing care in this area. Nurses who are actively involved in evaluating interventions for body image changes are doing so from an anecdotal, intuitive perspective. Developing a body of knowledge related to body image changes requires an understanding of desired outcomes. Because the manifestation of these outcomes typically does not occur until many months after the nursing intervention, measuring these outcomes at the present time may not be reasonable from a clinical practice perspective. The nurse may not even be in contact with the patient in any manner by the time the changes occur. In terms of nursing practice, it is important that the effectiveness of nursing interventions to facilitate the integration of altered body image be demonstrated. This can be accomplished only through research. The first step in this endeavor must be to identify measurable, desirable outcomes. These outcomes come from common sense and the nurse's observations of characteristics of patients who have successfully achieved a reintegrated body image. Although it is not certain which outcomes are actually associated with an improvement in body image, the observed outcomes will provide a starting point for research. The second step will require longitudinal studies in which the relationship between nursing interventions and desired outcomes is examined. This requires the development of clearly defined nursing interventions and multiple studies in which their effects on specific outcomes are tested. The third step will be to develop a predictive model of the impact of the nursing interventions. This step is dependent on the identification of effective nursing interventions and outcomes associated with improved body image. Many studies demonstrating a predictable outcome from a specific nursing intervention are needed. With this information, the nurse can use a specific nursing intervention with greater confidence that the desired outcome will be achieved.

From clinical practice we know that some patients are unable or unwilling to incorporate the body image change and thus could be classified as a high-risk group. Within this high-risk group will be some persons who, because of their mental health status, are unable to incorporate the body image change, and other persons who prefer the secondary gains of a poor body image to the benefits of successfully integrating the body image change. Through research, a profile of persons who are unsuccessful in reintegrating altered body image will emerge. This profile can then be used to identify high-risk patients and to determine appropriate nursing interventions.

Recognizing that this research has barely begun, we would like to propose some outcomes that from our clinical experience seem to be associated with effective integration of an altered body image:

- Resumption of former lifestyle, including relationships, employment, style of dress
- Verbalization of concerns about body image changes
- Manifestation of healthy coping ability
- Ability to touch, look at, and reveal altered body site
- Ability to incorporate necessary changes to allow activity (work, play, sex) to be satisfying
- Change in dream content to reflect reintegration of altered body image
- Incorporation of altered body part as part of the identity of the self
- Evidence of high self-esteem
- Ability to discuss and consider reconstruction
- Willingness to resume sexual relations

Alteration in body images, if not effectively integrated within the self-system, can greatly diminish the quality of life. Immediate commencement of concentrated research efforts directed toward identifying appropriate nursing intervention to facilitate the altered body image is of utmost importance. This presents an excellent opportunity for collaboration between nurse clinicians and nurse researchers. Once the knowledge derived from investigational studies is available, patients will benefit immensely from the scientifically based nursing interventions of the skilled professional nurse.

REFERENCES

Abidin, M. R., Durham, K., & Dooley, W. D. (1991). Use of immediate postoperative mastectomy prostheses. *Annals of Plastic Surgery, 27*(4), 387–388.

Adami, G. F., Gandolfo, P., Campostano, A., Bauer, B., Cocchi, F., & Scopinaro, N. (1994). Eating disorder inventory in the assessment of psychosocial status in the obese patients prior to and at long term following biliopancreatic diversion for obesity. *International Journal of Eating Disorders, 15*(3), 265–274.

Allbeck P., Hallberg, D., & Epsmark, S. (1976). Body image—an apparatus for measuring disturbances in estimation of size and shape. *Journal of Psychosomatic Research, 20,* 583–589.

Andersen, B. L., & Jochimsen, P. R. (1985). Sexual functioning among breast cancer, gynecologic cancer, and healthy women. *Journal of Counsulting and Clinical Psychology, 53*(1), 25–32.

Anthony, E. J. (1971). The child's discovery of his body. In C. B. Kopp (Ed.), *Readings in early development* (pp. 402–424). Springfield, IL: Charles C. Thomas.

Arseni, C., Botez, M. I., & Maretsis, M. (1966). Paroxysmal disorders of the body image. *Psychiatric Neurology, 151*(1), 1–14.

Baird, S. E. (1985). Development of a nursing assessment tool to diagnose altered body image in immobilized patients. *Orthopaedic Nursing, 4*(1), 47–54.

Bard, M., & Sutherland, A. M. (1955). Psychological impact of cancer and its treatment: IV. Adaptation to radical mastectomy. *Cancer: Diagnosis, Treatment, Research, 8*(4), 656–672.

Bartelink, H., van Dam, F., & van Dongen, J. (1985). Psychological effects of breast conserving therapy in comparison with radical mastectomy. *International Journal of Radiation Oncology, Biology, Physics, 11*(2), 381–385.

Baxley, K. O., Erdman, L. K., Henry, E. B., & Roof, B. J. (1984). Alopecia: Effect on cancer patients' body image. *Cancer Nursing, 7*(6), 499–503.

Beardslee, C., & Miller, S. (1981). Reactions of an adolescent girl during the initial period of treatment of a neoplastic disease. *Maternal-Child Nursing Journal, 10*(3), 175–183.

Beardslee, C., & Neff, J. A. (1982). Body related concerns of children with cancer as compared with the concerns of other children. *Maternal-Child-Nursing, 11*(3), 121–134.

Beardslee, C., & Sperhac, A. (1978). Reaction formation in a pre-adolescent girl. *Maternal-Child-Nursing, 7*(7), 31–40.

Berscheid, E., Walster, E., & Gohrnstedt, G. (1972). Body image: A *Psychology Today* questionnaire. *Psychology Today, 6*(2), 58–66.

Berscheid, E., Walster, E., & Gohrnstedt, G. (1973). The happy American body: A survey report. *Psychology Today, 7*(6), 119–131.

Bille, D. A. (1977). The role of body image in patient compliance and education. *Heart and Lung, 6,* 143–148.

Blaesig, S., & Brockhaus, J. (1972). The development of body image in the child. *Nursing Clinics of North America, 7*(4), 597–607.

Blichert-Toft, M. (1992). Breast-conserving therapy for mammary carcinoma: Psychosocial aspects, indications and limitations. *Annals of Medicine, 24*(6), 445–451.

Blotcky, A. D., & Cohen, D. G. (1985). Psychological assessment of the adolescent with cancer. *Journal of the Association of Pediatric Oncology Nurses, 2*(1), 8–14.

Boman, L., Bjorvell, H., Cedermark, B., Theve, N. O., & Wilking, N. (1993). Effects of early discharge from hospital after surgery for primary breast cancer. *European Journal of Surgery, 159*(2), 67–73.

Boren, J. A. (1985). Adolescent adjustment to amputation necessitated by bone cancers. *Orthopaedic Nursing, 4*(5), 30–32.

Boren, J. A., & Meell, H. (1985). Adolescent amputee ski rehabilitation program. *Journal of the Association of Pediatric Oncology Nurses, 2*(1), 16–23.

Brennan, J. (1994). A vital component of care: The nurse's role in recognizing altered body image. *Professional Nurse, 9*(5), 298–303.

Bronheim, H., Strain, J. J., & Biller, H. F. (1991). Psychiatric aspects of head and neck surgery. Part I. Body image and psychiatric intervention. *General Hospital Psychiatry, 13*(3), 165–176.

Bronheim, H., Strain, J. J., & Biller, H. F. (1991). Psychiatric aspects of head and neck surgery. Part II. New surgical techniques and psychiatric consequences. *General Hospital Psychiatry, 13*(4), 225–232.

Brown, A., & Bjelic, J. (1977). Coping strategies of two adolescents with malignancy. *Maternal-Child Nursing Journal, 6*(1), 77–85.

Burgess, L. (1994). Facing the reality of head and neck cancer. *Nursing Standard, 8*(32), 30–34.

Cantor, R. C. (1980). Self-esteem, sexuality and cancer-related stress. *Frontiers of Radiation Therapy Oncology, 14,* 51–54.

Capone, M. A., Good, R. S., Westie, K. S., & Jacobson, A. F. (1980). Psychosocial rehabilitation of gynecologic oncology patients. *Archives of Physical Medicine and Rehabilitation, 61*(3), 128–132.

Carroll, R. M. (1981). The impact of mastectomy on body image. *Oncology Nursing Forum, 8*(4), 29–32.

Champion, V. L., Austin, J. K., & Tzeng, O. (1982). Assessment of relationship between self-concept and body image using multivariate techniques. *Issues in Mental Health Nursing, 4*(4), 299–315.

Christensen, K., Blichert-Toft, M., Giersing, U., Richardt, C., & Bechmann, J. (1982). Phantom breast syndrome in young women after mastectomy for breast cancer. *Acta Chirurica Scandinavica, 148,* 351–354.

Christian, B. J. (1982). Immobilization: Psychological aspects. In C. Norris (Ed.), *Concept clarification in nursing* (pp. 341–356). Rockville, MD: Aspen.

Clark, C. C. (1977). *Nursing concepts and processes* (pp. 399–419). Albany, NY: Delmar.

Collingwood, T. R., & Willet, L. (1971). The effects of physical training upon self-concept and body attitude. *Journal of Clinical Psychology, 27,* 411–412.

Crumbaugh, J. (1968). The automobile as part of the body-image in America. *Mental Hygiene, July,* 349–350.

Deadman, J. M., Dewey, M. J., Owens, R. G., Leinster, S. J., & Slade, P. D. (1989). Threat and loss in breast cancer. *Psychological Medicine, 19*(3), 677–681.

deHaes, J. C. J. M., van Oostrom, M. A., & Welvaart, K. (1986). The effect of radical and conserving surgery on the quality of life of early breast cancer patients. *European Journal of Surgical Oncology, 12*(4), 337–342.

deHaes, J. C. J. M., & Welvaart, K. (1985). Quality of life after breast cancer surgery. *Journal of Surgical Oncology, 280,* 123–125.

Dempsey, M. O. (1972). The development of body image in the adolescent. *Nursing Clinics of North America, 7*(4), 609–615.

Denning, D. C. (1982). Head and neck cancer: Our reactions. *Cancer Nursing, 5*(4), 269–273.

Derogatis, L. R. (1980). Breast and gynecologic cancers: Their unique impact on body image and sexual identity in women. *Frontiers of Radiation Therapy Oncology, 14,* 1–11.

Derogatis, L. R., & Melisaratos, N. (1979). The DSFI: A multidimensional measure of sexual functioning. *Journal of Sex and Marital Therapy, 5,* 244–281.

Dion, K., Berscheid, E., & Walster, E. (1972). What is beautiful is good. *Journal of Personality and Social Psychology, 24*(3), 285–290.

Dipboye, R. L., Fromkin, H. L., & Wiback, K. (1975). Relative importance of applicant sex, attractiveness, and scholastic standing in evaluation of job applicant resumes. *Journal of Applied Psychology, 60*(1), 39–43.

Donovan, M. I., & Girton, S. E. (1984). *Cancer care nursing* (2nd ed., pp. 479–356). Norwalk, CT: Appleton-Century-Crofts.

Douty, H. I., Moore, J. B., & Hartford, D. (1974). Body characteristics in relation to life adjustment, body-image and attitudes of college females. *Perceptual and Motor Skills, 39*(Part 2), 499–521.

Dropkin, M. J. (1979a). Compliance in postoperative head and neck patients. *Cancer Nursing, 2*(5), 379–384.

Dropkin, M. J. (1979b). Compliant behavior and changed body image. *American Journal of Nursing, 79*(7), 1249.

Dropkin, M. J. (1981). Changes in body image associated with head and neck cancer. In L. B. Marino (Ed.), *Cancer nursing* (pp. 560–581). St. Louis: Mosby.

Dropkin, M. J. (1983). Body image reintegration and coping effectiveness after head and neck surgery. *The Journal, 2,* 7–16.

Dropkin, M. J. (1985). Rehabilitation after disfigurative facial surgery. *Plastic Surgical Nursing, 5*(4), 130–134.

Efran, M. G. (1974). The effect of physical appearance on the judgment of guilt, interpersonal attraction, and severity of recommended punishment in a simulated jury task. *Journal of Research in Personality, 8*(1), 45–54.

Erdos, D. (1992). Redefining identity when appearance is altered. *Dermatology Nursing, 4*(1), 41–46.

Erikson, E. J. (1963). *Childhood and society* (2nd ed.) New York: Norton.

Erikson, E. J. (1980). *Identity and the life cycle.* New York: Norton.

Fallowfield, L. J., & Hall, A. (1991). Psychosocial and sexual impact of diagnosis and treatment of breast cancer. *British Medical Bulletin, 47*(2), 388–399.

Fawcett, J., & Chodil, J. J. (1979). The topographical device: Development and research. In E. Bauwens (Ed.), *Research for clinical nursing: Its strategies and findings* (Monograph Series 1979: Three). Indianapolis: Sigman Theta Tau.

Fawcett, J., & Frye, S. (1980). An exploratory study of body image dimensionality. *Nursing Research, 29,* 324–327.

Filiberti, A., Regazzoni, M., Garavoglia, M., Perilli, C., Alpinelli, P., Santoni, G., Attili, A., & Stefanon, B. (1991). Problems after hysterectomy: A comparative content analysis of 60 interviews with cancer and non-cancer hysterectomized women. *European Journal of Gynaecological Oncology, 12*(6), 445–449.

Fisher, B., Anderson, S., Fisher, E. R., Redmond, C., Wickerham, D. L., Wolmark, N., Mamounas, E. P., Deutsch, M., & Margolese, R. (1991). Significance of ipsilateral breast tumour recurrence after lumpectomy. *Lancet, 338*(8763), 327–331.

Fisher, S. (1967). Motivation for patient delay. *Archives of General Psychiatry, 16,* 676–678.

Fisher, S. (1968). *Body image and personality.* New York: Dover.

Fisher, S. (1970). *Body experience in fantasy and behavior.* New York: Appleton-Century-Crofts.

Fisher, S. (1973). *Body consciousness: You are what you feel.* Englewood Cliffs, NJ: Prentice-Hall.

Fisher, S., & Cleveland, S. (1968). *Body image and personality.* New York: Dover.

Frank-Stromborg, M. (1988). *Instruments for clinical nursing research.* Norwalk, CT: Appleton & Lange.

Freedlander, E., Espie, C. A., Campsie, L. M., Soutar, D. S., & Robertson, A. G. (1989). Functional implications of major surgery for intraoral cancer. *British Journal of Plastic Surgery, 42*(3), 266–269.

Freud, S. (1961). *The ego and the id.* (Vol. 1). London: Hogarth. (Original work published 1927).

Fritz, G. K., & Williams, J. R. (1988). Issues of adolescent development for survivors of childhood cancer. *Journal of the American Academy of Child and Adolescent Psychiatry, 27*(6), 712–715.

Fry, W. (1980). A gift of mirrors: An essay in psychological evolution. *North American Review, December,* 53–58.

Gallagher, A. M. (1972). Body image changes in the patient with a colostomy. *Nursing Clinics of North America, 7,* 669–679.

Gamba, A., Romano, M., Grosso, I M., Tamburini, M., Cantu, G., Molinari, R., & Ventafridda, V. (1992). Psychological adjustment of patients surgically treated for head and neck cancer. *Head & Neck, 14*(3), 218–223.

Ganz, P. A., Schag, A. C., Lee, J. J., Polinsky, M. L., & Tan, S. (1992). Breast conservation versus mastectomy: is there a difference in psychological adjustment or quality of life in the year after surgery? *Cancer, 69*(7), 1729–1738.

Ganz, P. A., Schag, C. A., Lee, J. J., & Sim, M. S. (1992). The CARES: A generic measure of health-related quality of life for patients with cancer. *Quality of Life Research: An International Journal of Quality of Life Aspects of Treatment, Care & Rehabilitation, 1*(1), 19–29.

Ganz, P. A., Schag, C. C., Polinsky, M. L., Heinrich, R. L., & Flack, V. F. (1987). Rehabilitation needs and breast cancer: The first month after primary therapy. *Breast Cancer Research and Treatment, 19*(3), 243–253.

Gerard, D. (1982). Sexual functioning after mastectomy: Life vs. lab. *Journal of Sex and Marital Therapy, 8*(4), 305–315.

Glanz, K., & Lerman, C. (1992). Psychosocial impact of breast cancer: A critical review. *Annals of Behavioral Medicine, 14*(3), 204–212.

Goldberg, J. A., Scott, R. N., Davidson, P. M., Murray, G. D., Stallard, S., George, W. D., & Maguire, G. P. (1992). Psychological morbidity in the first year after breast surgery. *European Journal of Surgical Oncology, 18*(4), 327–331.

Griffiths, S. S. (1980). Changes in body image caused by antineoplastic drugs. *Issues in Comprehensive Pediatric Nursing, 4*(1), 17–27.

Guariglia, C., & Antonucci, G. (1992). Personal and extrapersonal space: A case of neglect dissociation. *Neuropsychologia, 30*(11), 1001–1009.

Hart, L. K., & Kenney, C. K. D. (1981). Loss of identity control. In L. K. Hart, J. L. Reese, & M. O. Fearing (Eds.), *Concepts common to acute illness* (pp. 9–30). St. Louis: Mosby.

Head, H. (1920). *Studies in neurology.* London: Oxford.

Hockenberry-Eaton, M. J., & Cotanch, P. H. (1989). Evaluation of a child's perceived self-competence during treatment for cancer. *Journal of Pediatric Oncology Nursing, 6*(3), 55–62.

Hoover, M. L. (1984). The self-image of overweight adolescent females: A review of the literature. *Maternal-Child Nursing Journal, 13*(2), 125–137.

Hopwood, P., & Maguire, G. P. (1988). Body image problems in cancer patients. Second Leeds Psychopathology Symposium: The psychopathology of body image. *British Journal of Psychiatry, 153*(Suppl. 2), 47–50.

Horowitz, M. J. (1966). Body image. *Archives of General Psychiatry, 14*(4), 456–460.

Hurley, M., Meyer-Ruppel, A., & Evans, E. (1983). Emma needed more than standard teaching. *Nursing, 13*(3), 62–64.

Hymovich, D. P., & Roehnert, J. E. (1994). Psychosocial consequences of childhood cancer. *Seminars in Oncology Nursing, 5*(1), 56–62.

Jacobson, E. (1964). *The self and the object world.* New York: International Universities Press.

Johnson, J. L. (1976). A research brief: The sexual concerns of the cancer patient and his or her spouse. *Counseling and Values, 20,* 186–188.

Kalick, S. M., Goldwyn, R. M., & Noe, J. M. (1981). Social issues and body image concerns of port wine stain patients undergoing laser therapy. *Lasers in Surgery and Medicine, 1,* 205–213.

Kemeny, M. M., Wellisch, D. K., & Schain, W. S. (1988). Psychosocial outcome in a randomized surgical trial for treatment of primary breast cancer. *Cancer, 62,* 1231–1237.

Kennerly, S. L. (1977). Breast cancer: Confronting one's changed image. "What I've learned about mastectomy." *American Journal of Nursing, 77*(9), 1430–1432.

Kiebert, G. M., deHaes, J. C. J. M., & van de Velde, C. J. H. (1991). The impact of breast-conserving treatment and mastectomy on the quality of life of early-stage breast cancer patients: A review. *Journal of Clinical Oncology, 9*(6), 1059–1070.

Knobf, M. K. T. (1985). Primary breast cancer: Physical consequences and rehabilitation. *Seminars in Oncology Nursing, 1*(3), 214–224.

Knobf, M. K. T., & Stahl, R. (1991). Reconstructive surgery in primary breast cancer treatment. *Seminars in Oncology Nursing, 79*(3), 200–206.

Kolb, L. C. (1959). Disturbances of the body-image. In S. Arieti (Ed.), *American handbook of psychiatry* (Vol. 1, pp. 749–769). New York: Basic Books.

Krouse, H. J. (1985). A psychological model of adjustment in gynecologic cancer patients. *Oncology Nursing Forum, 12*(6), 45–49.

Krouse, H. J., & Krouse, J. H. (1981). Psychological factors in postmastectomy adjustment. *Psychological Reports, 48*(1), 275–278.

Krouse, H. J., & Krouse, J. H. (1982). Cancer as crisis: The critical elements of adjustment. *Nursing Research, 31*(2), 96–101.

Krouse, J. H., Krouse, H. J., & Fabian, R. L. (1989). Adaptation to surgery for head and neck cancer. *The Laryngoscope, 99*(8), 789–794.

Kubie, L. S. (1937). The fantasy of dirt. *Psychoanalytic Quarterly, 6*(3), 388–425.

Lamb, M. A., & Woods, N. F. (1981). Sexuality and the cancer patient. *Cancer Nursing, 4*(2), 137–144.

Landy, D., & Sigall, H. (1974). Beauty is talent: Task evaluation as a function of performer's physical attractiveness. *Journal of Personality and Social Psychology, 29*(3), 299–304.

Lasry, J. M., & Margolese, R. G. (1992). Fear of recurrence, breast-conserving surgery, and the trade-off hypothesis. *Cancer, 69*(8), 2111–2115.

Lasry, J. M., Margolese, R. G., Poisson, R., Shibata, H., Fleischer, I. D., LaFleur, D., Legault, S., & Taillefer, S. (1987). Depression and body image following mastectomy and lumpectomy. *Journal of Chronic Disease, 40*(6), 529–534.

Leonard, B. J. (1972). Body image changes in chronic illness. *Nursing Clinics of North America, 7*(4), 687–695.

Lerner, R. M., Karabenick, S. A., & Stuart, J. L. (1973). Relations among physical attractiveness, body attitudes, and self-concept in male and female college students. *The Journal of Psychology, 85,* 119–129.

Lewis, C. W. (1978). Body image and obesity. *Journal of Psychiatric Nursing and Mental Health Services, 16*(1), 22–29.

MacElveen-Hoehn, P., & McCorkle, R. (1985). Understanding sexuality in progressive cancer. *Seminars in Oncology Nursing, 1*(1), 56–62.

Maguire, P. (1989). Breast conservation versus mastectomy: Psychological considerations. *Seminars in Surgical Oncology, 5*(2), 137–144.

Maguire, P., Tait, A., Brooke, M., Thomas, C., & Sellwood, R. (1980). The effect of counselling on physical disability and social recovery after mastectomy. *Clinical Oncology, 9,* 319–324.

Mahoney, E. R. (1974). Body-cathexis and self-esteem: The importance of subjective importance. *Journal of Psychology, 88,* 27–30.

Margolis, G., Goodman, R. L., & Rubin, A. (1990). Psychological effects of breast-conserving cancer treatment and mastectomy. *Psychosomatics, 31*(1), 33–39.

Margolis, G. J., Goodman, R. L., Rubin, A., & Pajac, T. F. (1989). Psychological factors in the choice of treatment for breast cancer. *Psychosomatics, 30*(2), 192–197.

Marten, L. (1978). Self-care nursing model for patients experiencing radical change in body image. *Journal of Obstetric, Gynecologic and Neonatal Nursing, 7*(6), 9–13.

Martin, J. P., & Ogden, S. L. (1988). Testicular cancer: From a medical model to a nursing model. *Dimensions in Oncology Nursing, 11*(2), 5–11.

Mathes, E. W., & Kahn, A. (1975). Physical attractiveness, happiness, neuroticism, and self-esteem. *Journal of Psychology, 90,* 27–30.

McCloskey, J. C. (1976). How to make the most of body image theory in nursing practice. *Nursing, 6(5),* 68–72.

Mead, G. H. (1934). *Mind, self, and society,* Chicago: University of Chicago Press.

Mele, V., Palazzani, L., & Sgreccia, E. (1992). Quality of life in gynaecological oncology: The personalist perspective of bioethics. *European Journal of Gynaecological Oncology, 13*(Supp. 1), 89–91.

Metcalfe, M. C., & Fischman, S. H. (1985). Factors affecting the sexuality of patients with head and neck cancer. *Oncology Nursing Forum, 12*(2), 21–25.

Meyer, L., & Aspergren, K. (1989). Long-term psychological sequelae of mastectomy and breast conserving treatment for breast cancer. *Acta Oncologica, 28*(1), 13–18.

Miller, S. J., & Graham, W. P., III. (1975). Breast reconstruction after radical mastectomy. *American Family Physician, 11*(5), 97–101.

Mock, V. (1993). Body image in women treated for breast cancer. *Nursing Research, 42*(3), 153–157.

Morris, T. (1979). Psychological adjustment to mastectomy. *Cancer Treatment Reviews, 6,* 41–61.

Morris, T., Greer, J. S., & White, P. (1977). Psychological and social adjustment to mastectomy: A two-year follow-up study. *Cancer, 40,* 2318–2387.

Murray, J. B. (1980). Psychosomatic aspects of cancer: An overview. *The Journal of Genetic Psychology, 136,* 185–194.

Murray, R. L. E. (1972a). Body image development in adulthood. *Nursing Clinics of North America, 7*(1), 617–630.

Murray, R. L. E. (1972b). Principles of nursing intervention for the adult patient with body image changes. *Nursing Clinics of North America, 7*(4), 697–707.

Neff, E. J., & Beardslee, C. I. (1990). Body knowledge and concerns of children with cancer as compared with the knowledge and concerns of other children. *Journal of Pediatric Nursing, 5*(3), 179–189.

Noguchi, M., Katagawa, H., Kinoshita, K., Earashi, M., Miyazaki, I., Tatsukuchi, S., Saito, Y., Mizukami, Y., Nonomura, A., Nakamura, S., & Michigishi, T. (1993). Psychologic and cosmetic self-assessments of breast conserving therapy compared with mastectomy and immediate breast reconstruction. *Journal of Surgical Oncology, 54*(4), 260–266.

Norris, C. M. (1978). Body image—its relevance to professional nursing. In C. E. Carlson & B. Blackwell (Eds.), *Behavioral concepts and nursing interventions* (2nd ed., pp. 5–36). Philadelphia: Lippincott.

Olson, E. V. (1967). The hazards of immobility. *American Journal of Nursing, 67,* 780–797.

Orbach, C. E., & Tallent, N. (1965). Modification of perceived body and of body concepts. *Archives of General Psychiatry, 12*(1), 126–135.

Osgood, L., Suci, G., & Tannenbaum, D. (1957). *The measurement of meaning.* Urbana: University of Illinois Press.

Paine, P., Alves, E., & Tubino, P. (1985). Size of human figure drawing and Goodenough-Harris scores of pediatric oncology patients: A pilot study. *Perceptual and Motor Skills, 60*(1), 911–914.

Palmer, A. G., Tucker, S., Warren, R., Adams, M. (1993). Understanding women's responses to treatment for cervical intra-epithelial neoplasia. *British Journal of Clinical Psychology. 32*(1), 101–112.

Penman, D. T., Bloom, J. R., Fotopoulos, S., Cook, M. R., Holland, J. C., Gates, C., Flamer, D., Murawski, B., Ross, R., Brandt, U., Muenz, L. R., Pee, D., & Phil, M. (1987). The impact of mastectomy on self-concept and social function: A combined cross-sectional and longitudinal study with comparison groups. *Womens Health, 11*(3-4), 101–130.

Piff, C. (1986). Facing up to disfigurement. *Nursing Times, 82*(34), 16–17.

Polivy, J. (1974). Psychological reactions to hysterectomy: A critical review. *American Journal of Obstetrics and Gynecology, 118*(3), 417–426.

Polivy, J. (1977). Psychological effects of mastectomy on a woman's feminine self-concept. *The Journal of Nervous and Mental Disease, 164,* 77–87.

Price, B. (1986). Body image: Keeping up appearances. *Nursing Times, 82*(40), 58–61.

Quinn, M. (1984). Facts, fallacies and femininity. *Nursing Mirror, 159*(1), 16–18.

Ray, C. (1977). Psychological implications of mastectomy. *British Journal of Social and Clinical Psychology, 16*(Part 4), 373–377.

Renneker, R., & Cutler, M. (1952). Psychological problems of adjustment to cancer of the breast. *Journal of the American Medical Association, 148*(10), 133–138.

Richardson, S. A., Goodman, N., Hastorf, A. H., & Dornbusch, S. M. (1961). Cultural uniformity in reaction to physical disabilities. *American Sociological Review, 26*(2), 241–247.

Riddle, I. (1972). Nursing intervention to promote body image integrity in children. *Nursing Clinics of North America, 7*(4), 654–661.

Roback, H. B., Kirshner, H., & Roback, E. (1981-1982). Physical self-concept changes in a mildly facially disfigured neurofibromatosis patient following communication skill training. *International Journal of Psychiatry in Medicine, 11*(2), 137–143.

Rollins, J. A. (1990). Childhood cancer: Siblings draw and tell. *Pediatric Nursing, 16*(1), 21–27.

Rosen, G. M., & Ross, A. O. (1968). Relationship of body image to self-concept. *Journal of Consulting and Clinical Psychology, 32*(1), 100.

Rubin, R. (1968). Body image and self-esteem. *Nursing Outlook, 16*(6), 20–23.

Sanger, C. K., & Reznikoff, M. (1981). A comparison of the psychological effects of breast-saving procedures with the modified radical mastectomy. *Cancer, 48,* 2341–2346.

Schag, C. A. C., Ganz, P. A., Polinsky, M. L., Fred, C., Hirji, K., & Petersen, L. (1993). Characteristics of women at risk for psychosocial distress in the year after breast cancer. *Journal of Clinical Oncology, 11*(4), 783–793.

Schain, W. S. (1985). Breast cancer surgeries and psychosexual sequelae: Implications for remediation. *Seminars in Oncology Nursing, 1*(3), 200–205.

Schain, W. S., Edwards, B. K., Gorrell, C. R., de Moss, E. V., Lippman, M. E., Gerber, L. H., & Lichter, A. S. (1983).

Psychosocial and physical outcomes of primary breast cancer therapy: mastectomy vs. excisional biopsy and irradiation. *Breast Cancer Research and Treatment, 3,* 377–382.

Schain, W. S., & Howards, S. S. (1985). Sexual problems of patients with cancer. In V. T. DeVita, Jr., S. Hellman, & S. A. Rosenberg, (Eds.), *Cancer: Principles and practice of oncology* (2nd ed., pp. 2066–2082). Philadelphia: W. B. Saunders Co.

Schilder, P. (1935). The image and appearance of the human body. *Studies in the constructive energies of the psyche.* London: Kegan Paul.

Schonfeld, W. A. (1963). Body-image in adolescents: A psychiatric concept for the pediatrician. *Pediatrics, 31,* 845–855.

Schover, L. R. (1991). The impact of breast cancer on sexuality, body image, and intimate relationships. *CA-A Cancer Journal for Clinicians, 41*(2), 112–120.

Schwab, J. J., & Harmeling, J. D. (1968). Body image and medical illness. *Psychosomatic Medicine, 30*(1), 51–61.

Scott, D. W. (1983). Quality of life following the diagnosis of breast cancer. *Topics in Clinical Nursing, 4*(4), 20–37.

Scott, D. W., & Eisendrath, S. J. (1985-1986). Dynamics of the recovery process following initial diagnosis of breast cancer. *Journal of Psychosocial Oncology, 3*(4), 53–67.

Secord, P. (1953). Objectification of word association procedures by the use of homonyms: A measure of body cathexis. *Journal of Personality, 21,* 479–495.

Secord, P. F., & Jourard, S. M. (1953). The appraisal of body-cathexis: body-cathexis and the self. *Journal of Consulting Psychology, 17*(5), 343–347.

Sewell, H. H., & Edwards, D. W. (1980). Pelvic genital cancer: Body image and sexuality. *Frontiers in Radiation Therapy Oncology, 14,* 35–41.

Shapiro, P. A., & Kornfeld, D. S. (1987). Psychiatric aspects of head and neck cancer surgery. *Psychiatric Clinics of North America, 10*(1), 87–100.

Sneeuw, K. C. A., Aaronson, N. K., Yarnold, J. R., Broderick, M., Regan, J., Ross, G., & Goddard, A. (1992). Cosmetic and functional outcomes of breast conserving treatment for early stage breast cancer. 2. Relationship with psychosocial functioning. *Radiotherapy and Oncology, 25*(3), 160–166.

Stulberg, D. L., & Caruthers, B. S. (1990). Hirsutism: A practical approach to improving physical and mental well-being. *Postgraduate Medicine, 87*(8), 199–205,208.

Sullivan, M., Karlsson, J., Sjstrm, L., Backman, L., Bengtsson, C., Bouchard, C., Dahlgren, S., Jonsson, E., Larsson, B., Lindstedt, S., Nslund, I., Olbe, L., & Wedel, H. (1993). Swedish obese subjects (SOS)—an intervention study of obesity. Baseline evaluation of health and psychosocial functioning in the first 1743 subjects examined. *International Journal of Obesity, 17*(9), 503–512.

Szasz, T. S. (1957). *Pain and pleasure.* New York: Basic Books.

Tabachnick, N. (1967). Self-realization and social definition: Two aspects of identity formation. *International Journal of Psychoanalysis, 48,* 68–75.

Taylor, S. E., Lichtman, R. R., Wood, J. V., Bluming, A. Z., Dosik, G. M., & Leibowitz, R. L. (1985). Illness-related and treatment-related factors in psychological adjustment to breast cancer. *Cancer, 55*(10), 2506–2513.

Tierny, E. A. (1975). Accepting disfigurement when death is the alternative. *American Journal of Nursing, 75*(12), 2149–2150.

Tzeng, O. C. S. (1975). Differentiation of affective and denotative meaning systems and their influence in personality ratings. *Journal of Personality and Social Psychology, 32,* 978–988.

Tzeng, O. C. S. (1977). Individual differences in self conception. A multivariate approach. *Journal of Perceptual and Motor Skills, 45,* 1119–1124.

Valanis, B. G., & Rumpler, C. H. (1985). Helping women to choose breast cancer treatment alternatives. *Cancer Nursing, 8*(3), 167–175.

Van den Borne, H. W., Pruyn, J. F., & Van Dam-de Mey, K. (1986). Self-help in cancer patients: A review of studies on the effects of contacts between fellow-patients. *Patient Education & Counseling, 8*(4), 367–385.

van Heeringen, C., Van Moffaert, M., & de Cuypere, G. (1989). Depression after surgery for breast cancer. *Psychotherapy and Psychosomatics, 51*(4), 175–179.

Wabrek, A. J., & Gunn, J. L. (1984). Sexual and psychological implications of gynecologic malignancy. *Journal of Obstetric, Gynecologic, and Neonatal Nursing, 13*(6), 371–376.

Wagner, L., & Bye, M. G. (1979). Body image and patients experiencing alopecia as a result of cancer chemotherapy. *Cancer Nursing, 2*(5), 365–369.

Ward, S., Heidrich, S., & Wolberg, W. (1989). Factors women take into account when deciding upon type of surgery for breast cancer. *Cancer Nursing, 12*(6), 344–351.

Weigert, A. J., & Hastings, R. (1977). Identity loss, family and social change. *American Journal of Sociology, 82,* 1171–1185.

Wellisch, D. K., DiMatteo, R., Silverstein, M., Landsverk, J., Hoffman, R., Waisman, J., Handel, N., Waisman-Smith, E., & Schain, W. (1989). Psychosocial outcomes of breast cancer therapies: Lumpectomy versus mastectomy. *Psychosomatics, 30*(4), 365–373.

West, D. W. (1977). Social adaptation patterns among cancer patients with facial disfigurement resulting from surgery. *Archives of Physical Medicine and Rehabilitation, 58,* 473–479.

Wilbur, J. (1980). Sexual development and body image in the teenager with cancer. *Frontier in Radiation Therapy Oncology, 14,* 108–114.

Cancer affects all aspects of a person's life. Most people diagnosed with cancer have concerns about the sexual ramifications of their illness as well as the proposed treatment for their disease (Auchincloss, 1991; Burbic & Polinsky, 1992; Glasgow, Halfin, & Althausen, 1987; Lamb & Woods, 1981; Smith, 1989).

In 1994 approximately 1,208,000 people were diagnosed as having cancer (American Cancer Society, 1994). More than 8 million Americans who are alive today have a history of cancer. Often health professionals focus on the disease process and its treatment. They may neglect the issue of sexuality because of a lack of information regarding the impact of the disease and its treatment on sexual functioning as well as a generalized feeling of discomfort discussing these issues with clients. This chapter outlines current knowledge regarding the impact of cancer and its treatment on sexual functioning, discusses the psychosocial factors that affect sexual functioning, enhances the practitioner's skills in the assessment and management of alterations in sexual functioning, addresses the special problems associated with alterations in sexual functioning, and presents related issues and concerns.

SEXUAL FUNCTIONING

GENERAL CONSIDERATIONS

Sexuality is a multidimensional, complex phenomenon involving biologic, psychologic, interpersonal, and behavioral dimensions. The World Health Organization's Report on Education and Treatment in Human Sexuality (1975) asserts that sexual health is the integration of the somatic, emotional, intellectual, and social aspects of sexual being in ways that are positively enriching and that enhance personality, communication, and love. A wide range of "normal" sexual functioning exists within the population. This spectrum could include the ability to maintain interpersonal relationships to the ability to sustain the closeness of an intimate, sexually active relationship.

*Supported by the Oncology Nursing Foundation and Bristol-Myers through the Bristol-Myers Oncology Division Research Grant and The Society for Gynecologic Nurse Oncologists.

PSYCHOSOCIAL ASPECTS OF SEXUALITY

Optimal sexual functioning relies on the integration of key biopsychosocial components. The psychosocial elements involved in sexual functioning vary, depending on the developmental stage of the individuals involved. A strong negative correlation ($r = -.64$) in younger women after radical gynecologic surgery was reported by Roberts, Rossetti, Cone, and Cavanagh (1992). Moderately elevated levels of psychologic distress were found to exist in most women treated for gynecologic malignancies; however, significantly higher levels were found in younger women. Developmental stage of the individuals being treated is a plausible factor in these findings.

The young adult faces an array of intimacy issues, including learning to give and receive love, choosing whether or not to marry, and choosing a marital or sexual partner or partners (Woods, 1990). In adulthood, the majority of clients will focus on the capacity to give and receive gratification in a stable relationship. This capacity is not only centered around the physiologic aspects of sexuality, to be discussed subsequently, but the individual's concept of self as a sexual being and his or her sex role. Older adults often focus on the critical task of resolving feelings of self-esteem and despair (Woods, 1990). This task includes acceptance of one's life cycle and the social factors that accompanied it. These include emancipating adolescent children, achieving a career peak, and accommodating aging parents. During the later years, from retirement to death, sexual activity and interest persist. Sexual functioning is dependent on relatively good health and an interested and interesting partner. Aging persons may find it necessary to nurture one another, to cope with bereavement and widowhood, and to find new meaning in life (Woods, 1990).

PHYSIOLOGIC ASPECTS OF SEXUALITY

The psychosocial aspects of sexual functioning are complemented by the biologic components. The human sexual response cycle comprises two principle physiologic changes: vasocongestion and myotonia. Vasocongestion is the congestion of blood vessels, usually venous, and myotonia refers to increased muscular tension (Woods, 1990). These physiologic changes are dependent on an intact neurologic system and an appropriate hormonal milieu.

An accurate assessment of sexual dysfunctions is based on a basic understanding of the normal occurrences in the sexual response cycle. Interventions are used to prevent, alleviate, or minimize the identified causes of sexual dysfunctions.

Many dysfunctions can be caused by physiologic, psychologic, or social variables or a combination of several factors. The discussion of physiologic factors is followed here by the psychosocial implications of cancer and its treatment.

The four major stages in the human sexual response cycle are excitement, plateau, orgasm, and resolution (Masters & Johnson, 1966). Excitement is characterized by the onset of erotic feelings and the attainment of erection in men and vaginal lubrication in women.

Plateau is a more advanced stage of excitement in which the sex glands become more engorged and undergo positional changes. A number of extragenital conditions also occur, including color change, respiration shifts, and generalized increase in arousal. Orgasm is experienced as the most intense and pleasurable aspect of the sexual response cycle. The male experiences expulsive contractions of the entire length of the penile urethra. Semen is rhythmically expelled from the erect penis. At the onset of ejaculation, the internal bladder sphincter closes, preventing retrograde ejaculation into the bladder. Women experience orgasm as rhythmic contractions of the circumvaginal and perineal muscles and of the swollen tissues of the orgasmic platform. The *orgasmic platform* refers to the vasocongestion of the outer third of the vagina and the labia minora. Resolution is marked by a return to normal of the genital and extragenital responses to sexual stimulation.

Sexual dysfunction occurs in the areas of desire (interest), arousal (excitement), and orgasm (tension release) (Woods, 1990). The fourth stage mentioned, resolution, is not associated with sexual dysfunction because it refers to the gradual return to the prearousal state. Physical, psychologic, social, and environmental factors may cause these dysfunctions. Neoplastic disease can cause both biologic alterations and psychosocial sequelae that can affect sexuality negatively.

The remaining sections of this chapter address (1) the biologic effects of cancer and its treatment that may interfere with sexual expression; (2) the psychosocial effects that the diagnosis of cancer may have on the client and partner; (3) the assessment and management of sexual dysfunctions related to neoplastic disease; and (4) the special problems associated with alterations in sexual functioning.

PATHOPHYSIOLOGIC FACTORS LEADING TO ALTERATIONS IN SEXUAL FUNCTIONING

CANCERS OF THE GENITOURINARY TRACT: FEMALE

Women who have been diagnosed with genitourinary cancer often harbor fears regarding the impact of the disease process and the suggested treatment on sexual functioning (Jusenius, 1981; Lamb, 1990; Smith, 1989) (see Chapters 33 and 34). Many women newly diagnosed with gynecologic cancer report a significant decrease in sexual activity and satisfaction (Box 62–1) (Andersen, 1987, Harris, Good, & Pollack, 1982; Jenkins, 1988). Gynecologic malignancies inherently affect body parts that are involved in sexual acts. The four most common types of gynecologic malignancies, in order of their occurrence, are endometrial cancer, cervical cancer, ovarian cancer, and cancer of the vulva.

ENDOMETRIAL CANCER

Abnormal vaginal bleeding is the most common symptom associated with endometrial cancer. Abnor-

---

Box 62–1. *Sexual Changes After Treatment for Gynecologic Cancer*

Jenkins, B. (1988). Patients' report of sexual changes after treatment for gynecologic cancer. *Oncology Nursing Forum,* *15*(3), 349–354.

The sexual changes experienced by 20 sexually active women following surgical and radiotherapy treatment for endometrial and cervical cancer were researched. In response to a mailed questionnaire, statistically significant negative changes were shown in four indicators of sexual function. These indicators were (1) frequency of intercourse, (2) orgasm, (3) feelings of desire, and (4) enjoyment. Fifty-nine per cent of the women reported no sexual counseling before or after treatment. Most of those who did receive sexual information reported that this information was given by the radiotherapist. No sexual counseling was given by nurses. Eighty-eight per cent of these women wanted sexual discussions initiated by the physician or the nurse.

---

mal vaginal bleeding can hinder sexual relations because either the client or the partner may feel that vaginal bleeding is aesthetically unappealing. Fear of increased bleeding, spread of the disease, or pain can also negatively affect sexual relations. Most patients diagnosed with endometrial cancer are in the early stages of the disease. The standard surgical procedure is abdominal hysterectomy with bilateral salpingo-oophorectomy. The impact of oophorectomy and hysterectomy is not limited to depression and altered body image. Removal of the uterus, compounded by the loss of estrogens and androgens, alters sensation and reactions that have long been a part of a woman's sexual response (Williamson, 1992). Pelvic irradiation for endometrial cancer may be employed in both early and late stages of the disease. Pelvic irradiation can cause vaginal thinning, dryness, and stenosis (Andersen, 1985). All of these side effects can occur and may persist as chronic problems. Sexuality will be altered as a result of these problems unless interventions to prevent or minimize them are employed.

Lamb and Sheldon (1994) explored the sexual adaptation of women treated for endometrial cancer. This study's findings indicated that the experience of sexual adaptation in women who undergo treatment for endometrial cancer is a process that evolves over time. This process begins with the onset of symptoms and continues beyond the completion of therapy. Factors that enhance this adaptational process include two discrete parts, internal factors and external factors. Internal factors include such things as viewing oneself as strong and achieving a level of contentment with life. External factors were identified as the strength derived from partner, family and friends, and religion (Lamb, 1991a; Lamb & Sheldon, 1994).

CANCER OF THE CERVIX

Cancer of the cervix is the second most common form of gynecologic cancer. By virtue of the anatomic location of this cancer, a woman diagnosed with this malignancy often perceives a threat to the core of her sense of sexuality (McMullin, 1992). Women who present with early cervical cancer are generally asymptomatic, whereas those who present with advanced disease often experience postcoital bleeding, pelvic or sciatic pain, and a thin watery discharge. All of these symptoms are likely to inhibit sexual relations (Ander-

sen, Lachenbruch, Anderson, & DeProsse, 1986). The treatment options employed for women diagnosed with cervical cancer vary, depending on the stage of the disease. Radical hysterectomy has been associated with diminished or completely disrupted sexuality in the range of 6 to 19 per cent (Andersen, 1985). Pelvic irradiation for cancer of the cervix has been associated with a 66 per cent rate of sexual dysfunction (Bertelsen, 1983). Pelvic exenteration may be employed for the treatment of locally persistent or recurrent cervical cancer. Because of the removal of the vaginal canal as well as the introduction of other profound anatomic changes, sexual activity is profoundly affected by this surgery (Andersen, 1985; Andersen & Hacker, 1983b; Jusenius, 1981; Lamb, 1985; Schrover & Fife, 1985; Wabrek & Gunn, 1984).

Pelvic exenteration may be accompanied by vaginal reconstruction to facilitate healing and continued sexual intercourse (Andersen, 1985, 1987; Andersen & Hacker, 1983b). Women who have undergone creation of a neovagina following exenteration have reported two outcomes related to sexual functioning: 57 per cent stated that the reconstruction had been a success and that they were able to continue satisfactory sexual relations; 43 per cent reported disruption in the frequency of sexual activity, dissatisfaction with the variety of the activity or with their ability to become aroused, or dissatisfaction with the neovagina itself (the length was too short; the cavity was too large; there was a chronic discharge; intercourse was painful) (Andersen & Hacker, 1983b). Continued surgical adaptations accompanied by better sexual counseling and follow-up are needed to improve the positive response rates.

CANCER OF THE OVARY

Ovarian cancer is the third most frequently diagnosed gynecologic malignancy. The symptoms most commonly associated with cancer of the ovary are anorexia, weight loss, increased abdominal girth, change in bowel function, and vague abdominal pain. These symptoms may affect sexual activity but are commonly insidious in onset and are often associated with late-stage disease. Although no studies of the sexual functioning of patients with ovarian cancer have been done to date, one can extrapolate data from studies done with women who have undergone abdominal hysterectomy and bilateral salpingo-oophorectomy. Adjuvant chemotherapy is routinely prescribed after surgery for women with ovarian cancer. This chemotherapy can have devastating effects on body image, self-image, and sexuality. Side effects include alopecia, anorexia, weight loss, lethargy, and bone marrow depression. Patients with end-stage ovarian cancer often experience a prolonged terminal stage. Many experience repeated bouts of intestinal obstruction, abdominal ascites, cachexia, pleural effusion, and sepsis. Any one of these late-stage symptoms can profoundly affect the ability to express physical love.

CANCER OF THE VULVA

Vulvar cancer is most commonly treated with radical vulvectomy and bilateral groin node dissection. This procedure has a tremendous impact on body image and sexual functioning (Andersen, 1985; Andersen & Hacker, 1983a; Andreasson, Moth, Jensen, & Bock, 1986; Jusenius, 1981; Lamb, 1985; Moth, Andreasson, Jensen, & Bock, 1983). Fifty per cent of women no longer attempted coitus after the operation, and more than two thirds of the women who did make coital attempts experienced pain and some degree of sexual dysfunction (Moth et al., 1983). Andersen and Hacker (1983a) found that, despite the fact that intercourse remained possible, sexual functioning underwent a major disruption after radical vulvectomy. These findings were confirmed by a study in Denmark (Andreasson et al., 1986) in which half of all of the participants had experienced both sexual dysfunction and psychologic problems following radical vulvectomy surgery.

CANCER OF THE BLADDER

Bladder carcinoma is the most frequent malignant tumor of the urinary tract. This disease occurs more commonly in the male population with a ratio of 2:1, males to females (Rubin, 1983). One of the more commonly prescribed treatment options for cancer of the bladder is radical cystectomy. Little information has been reported regarding female sexual functioning after radical cystectomy. Schrover, von Eschenbach, Smith, and Gonzales (1984) found that women who are sexually active before undergoing radical cystectomy can resume a satisfying sex life with appropriate counseling. Vaginal dryness, tightness, and pain were experienced by all women on initial coital attempts. Most couples were able to overcome these difficulties with the use of vaginal hormone cream, vaginal dilation, and Kegal exercises to help the women become aware of muscle tension in the pelvic floor that may contribute to coital pain. All women who made the effort to resume sexual activity experienced a complete recovery in their ability to achieve orgasm.

CANCERS OF THE GENITOURINARY TRACT: MALE

Men who have been diagnosed with genitourinary tract cancer often have sexual difficulties related to the disease itself as well as to the treatments prescribed (Shipes & Lehr, 1982; Smith & Babaian, 1992). Sexual disturbances can result in an inability to attain an erection, an ejaculation, or both. These disturbances can result from both physiologic as well as psychologic sequelae. Additionally, urinary incontinence, fertility, and sexuality are major concerns for individuals diagnosed with genitourinary malignancies. Issues of sexual body image and gender identity are frequent concerns (Ofman, 1993). The most common genitourinary cancers of the male population are cancer of the prostate, bladder, and testis (see Chapter 33).

PROSTATE CANCER

The sexual dysfunctions associated with cancer of the prostate have been studied widely (Spengler, 1983). Sexual difficulties may arise from even a diagnostic biopsy of the prostate gland. Approximately 24 per cent of open perineal biopsy patients and 32 per cent of the transurethral resection patients reported erectile failure (Andersen, 1985). The treatment for cancer of the prostate varies with the age of the patient, the extent of the disease, and the patient's preference. The current treatment options include irradiation (both external and interstitial implant), radical prostatectomy, oral estrogens, or bilateral orchiectomy. Radiation therapy to the prostate and surrounding tissues can result in erectile difficulties in 37 per cent of the population (Andersen, 1985). Fibrosis of the pelvic vasculature or damage to the pelvic nerves is believed to be the cause of these difficulties (Bachers, 1985). The impotence associated with definitive radiation for cancer of the prostate is usually insidious in onset and permanent in nature (Shipes & Lehr, 1982). The incidence of sexual dysfunction is much higher in patients who undergo a radical prostatectomy. Diminished or complete erectile failure is seen in up to 90 per cent of this population, whereas ejaculation difficulties, with or without some degree of erectile failure, are seen in 78 per cent of the population (Andersen, 1985). Postoperative impotency has been diminished recently by a nerve-sparing technique described by Shapiro (1987). Oral estrogens, bilateral orchiectomy, or both are currently used to treat metastatic or extensive disease. Of patients who reported erectile difficulties, 47 per cent were treated with orchiectomy alone, 22 per cent with estrogen alone, and 73 per cent with the combined treatment (Andersen, 1985). Gynecomastia is a common occurrence in men treated with estrogen, but this side effect has not been directly correlated with sexual dysfunctions.

CANCER OF THE BLADDER

Sexual dysfunction related to the treatment of bladder cancer is dependent on the stage and subsequent treatment of the disease. The treatment of superficial bladder cancer (transurethral resection, intravesicle chemotherapy, or fulguration) usually does not result in organic dysfunction. However, repeated cystoscopies can result in a temporarily diminished desire for sex and transient pain during erection and ejaculation (Schrover et al., 1984). More advanced bladder cancer is treated with either definitive irradiation or radical cystectomy, which usually results in sexual dysfunctions similar to those reported for the surgery and radiation used to treat cancer of the prostate (Andersen, 1985). However, an additional consideration for patients undergoing cystectomy is the necessary formation of an ostomy. Self-esteem and body image can be profoundly affected by the presence of the appliance (Shipes, 1987). Enterostomal therapists play a crucial role in the couple's adaptation to this surgery.

CANCER OF THE TESTES

Testicular cancer, although rare, is the number one cause of death from cancer in men between the ages of 20 and 40 (Wujcik, Carbonnell, Taseff, Sciarra, & Isaac, 1986). A unilateral inguinal orchiectomy, with the preservation of the disease-free testicle, maintains both organic sexual function and fertility. However, the loss of a testis can be devastating to a young man's self-image. Retroperitoneal lymphadenectomy may be used as both a diagnostic and a therapeutic tool. This surgical procedure can sever the nerves that are necessary for seminal emissions, thus decreasing the amount of ejaculate during orgasm (Bachers, 1985). Patients who require bilateral orchiectomy experience a decrease in sexual desire because of lowered levels of serum testosterone as well as an alteration in secondary sex characteristics. The effect of combined chemotherapy and surgery on the sexuality of men with testicular cancer was studied by Brenner, Vugrin, and Whitmore, (1985). Only 11 per cent of the patients sampled reported normal ejaculation following combined treatment. However, no long-term effects on sexual desire were observed. Schrover, Gonzales, and von Eschenbach (1986) studied the sexual difficulties experienced by men who had received radiotherapy for testicular cancer. Low rates of sexual activity were reported by 19 per cent of the respondents, low sexual desire by 12 per cent, erectile dysfunction by 15 per cent, difficulty reaching orgasm by 10 per cent, and premature ejaculation by 14 per cent. The two most frequently reported problems were reduced intensity of orgasm (33 per cent) and decrease in seminal volume (49 per cent).

CANCERS OF OTHER RELATED SYSTEMS

BREAST CANCER

The diagnosis of breast cancer and the subsequent surgical removal of a breast are major fears among American women (Walbroehl, 1985). Although the trend in recent years has been to offer alternative forms of treatment, any therapy involving the breasts is often viewed as disfiguring (Rutherford, 1988). The type of treatment options available are dependent on the histologic type of lesion and the extent of the disease (see Chapter 29). Treatments for breast cancer include mastectomy (either simple, modified radical, or radical), lumpectomy, radiation therapy, and chemotherapy. Breast cancer affects many psychosocial factors that have a direct impact on sexuality (Baldwin, 1990). General disruption of sexual activity, reduced frequency of intercourse, or orgasmic difficulties are estimated to occur in 21 to 39 per cent of all breast cancer patients, regardless of the treatment employed (Andersen, 1985). Body image disruption is believed to be the major factor involved in the sexual difficulties of breast cancer patients (Beckmann, Blichert-Toft, & Johansen, 1983; Golden, 1983; Holmberg, Omne-Ponten, Burns, Adami, & Bergstrom, 1989).

Reconstructive surgery following mastectomy is done on a much more frequent basis today. Little research to date has evaluated the effectiveness of reconstructive surgery in lessening the sexual disruptions previously reported. Sexual dysfunction following mastectomy has been reported in the range of 23 to 37 per cent (Schain, 1985). In addition, 36 per cent of the partners of mastectomy patients have noted a negative impact on sexuality related to the disease and subsequent treatment (Wellisch, 1985). Breast conservation through lumpectomy and adjuvant irradiation is becoming a more common practice, when feasible. The impact of this form of treatment on sexual functioning has not yet been studied extensively. Schain (1985) is currently examining the effect of this form of treatment on the partner. Clinical impressions to date have revealed some dysfunctions immediately following therapy with a gradual return to near normal function over time. Chemotherapy is often used adjuvantly and palliatively in the treatment of breast cancer. The side effects of chemotherapy can themselves cause disruptions in sexual relationships. Hormonal manipulations, as a result of either chemotherapy or oophorectomy, can cause menopausal symptoms, which can also interfere with sexual expression.

The overall psychologic impact of breast cancer on relationships is considerable. Both the patient and her sexual partner can experience temporary or permanent sexual difficulties. Wellisch (1985) described five important variables that influence the impact of breast cancer on a marital relationship: (1) the status of the relationship before the cancer developed; (2) the longevity of the marriage; (3) the stage of the breast cancer, especially as this influences the treatment required; (4) the point in the course of the illness; and (5) the interpersonal skills of the partners. Nursing care directed toward the impact of the treatment for breast cancer on sexuality should include educational information, support, and counseling. Three nursing care plans developed by Schwarz-Applebaum, Dedrick, Jusenius, and Kirchner (1984), designed specifically for couples, are shown in Tables 62–1, 62–2, and 62–3.

CANCER OF THE HEAD AND NECK

Head and neck cancer does not directly affect the sexual functioning of the client. Rather, the disease and its treatment are often severely disfiguring and thus cause a dramatic alteration in body image. Facial disfigurement can cause sexual difficulties for both the patient and the sexual partner (Metcalfe & Fischman, 1985) (see Chapter 37). Few studies have been done that directly address the impact of head and neck cancers on sexual functioning. The direct and indirect sexual implications of radiation therapy and chemotherapy for patients with head and neck cancer are addressed by Shipes and Lehr (1982). The only known

Text continued on page 1116.

TABLE 62–1. *Nursing Care Plan: Sexuality and Modified Radical Mastectomy*

ASSESSMENT	INTERVENTIONS	EXPECTED OUTCOMES
Nursing Diagnosis: Potential change in sexual self-concept due to loss of breast		
Initiate discussion of sexuality at admission; reinforce throughout hospitalization and at postsurgical follow-up visits	Initiate discussion of sexuality Explore the degree of importance of breasts in client's sexual self-concept Discuss relative importance of other areas influencing expression of sexual self-concept (health, energy, etc.)	Client discusses personal view of importance of breasts to sexual self-concept; client states ways to enlist support systems in maintaining sexual self-concept
Begin discussion at admission; expand topic throughout hospitalization Initiate discussion of appearance of incision before first dressing change; assess readiness to look at incision with each check of wound	Give adequate time for grieving for loss of breast Assess readiness to look at incision: • initiate discussion of appearance of incision • draw line picture of surgical area • help patient look at area with mirror • help patient look at actual incision when ready	Client describes appearance of incision
Discuss progress in viewing incision at postsurgical follow-up visits		Client describes plans to look at incision and chest wall and shares feelings about appearance of incision
	Explore possibility of health changes that may occur after modified radical mastectomy (temporary decrease in energy level, temporary difficulty performing routine household duties, changes in arm and hand, changes in range of motion of affected arm and shoulder, numbness or pulling in incision area with healing, decreased sensation in pectoral area and inner aspect of arm, phantom breast sensation, change in sleep patterns).	
Nursing Diagnosis: Potential diminished self-concept because of limited information about ways to enhance postoperative appearance		
Begin discussion before discharge; clarify concerns at postsurgical follow-up visits	Discuss breast prostheses: • when to purchase, relative to period of wound healing • importance of weight, consistency, size, and contour of prosthesis in promoting good posture and carriage • advantages and disadvantages of different types of prostheses • cost and possibility of insurance coverage • availability of different prostheses in geographical area (use current listings from Reach to Recovery in all of the above) Explore option of Reach to Recovery visit: • check with local unit of Reach to Recovery to determine options for referral initiation	Client lists important variables in choice of a prosthesis, taking her life style into account; client states plan for purchase of prosthesis (e.g., timing of purchase, various places to purchase prosthesis, etc.)
	Discuss attractive clothing options emphasizing remaining body strengths • need for wide shoulder straps and arm holes to prevent pressure on affected arm • wear opaque night gowns, ruffles at neckline to disguise operative area • emphasize other body parts with cut of clothing	Client describes ways to use clothing to enhance appearance
Discuss at postsurgical follow-up visit at least 4 weeks after surgery	• use of waterproof skin tone cosmetics to disguise mastectomy scar (if desired after wound has healed)	

(Modified with permission from Schwarz-Appelbaum, J., Dedrick, J., Jusenius, K., & Kirchner, C. W. [1984]. Nursing care plans: Sexuality and treatment of breast cancer. *Oncology Nursing Forum, 11* [6], 16–24.)

TABLE 62–1. *Nursing Care Plan: Sexuality and Modified Radical Mastectomy* Continued

ASSESSMENT	INTERVENTIONS	EXPECTED OUTCOMES
Initiate discussion before hospital discharge	Discuss mechanics of how to get into clothing already owned: • insert affected arm first into over-the-head clothing • use of zipper pull for items with back zippers • how to fasten bra with one hand or fasten it in front and turn bra around Discuss breast reconstruction alternatives (as appropriate to client interest): • breast mound will have normal contour underneath clothing • varying importance of construction of new nipple to self concept • no fear of shifting an external prosthesis with vigorous activity including sports	Client can dress herself by discharge and describes methods to use when dressing in clothing owned before surgery

Nursing Diagnosis: Possible reluctance to adopt positive health habits because of fear of discovery of malignancy in the other breast and limited information

	Reaffirm importance of monthly Breast Self Examination (BSE) Teach technique of BSE (as indicated) according to the normal tissue textures on unoperated breast, palpation of local incision, axilla, ribs, and intercostal area on operated side	Every month, client performs BSE on unoperated breast and examines operated side
	Teach avoidance of compressive forces on affected arm to decrease risk of lymphedema: • no blood pressure measurements on affected arm • carry heavy loads with other arm Teach avoidance of skin trauma to minimize risk of local infection: • no injections on affected arm • protect affected arm from burns and cuts	Client lists precautions to prevent injury to affected arm
	Encourage annual mammogram Encourage follow-up at scheduled postsurgical clinic visits	Client has annual mammogram Client attends scheduled appointments at postsurgical follow-up clinic appointments

Nursing Diagnosis: Potential for diminished involvement in relationships because of fear of rejection

Discuss before discharge and reinforce throughout postsurgical follow-up visits	Discuss importance to self-concept of maintaining involvement in previous activities Explore fears of mutilation and unacceptability and other concerns that might limit involvement in relationships Discuss need for others to have time to become accustomed to changes in client's body Discuss likelihood for a single woman to be reluctant to enter new sexual relationships (as appropriate to situation) Encourage recognition of client's assets List possible ways to promote resumption of former life style Role play situations likely to be encountered in establishing relationships	Client verbalizes risk for temporary disruption in former activities and states ways to promote resumption of life style

Continued on following page.

TABLE 62–1. *Nursing Care Plan: Sexuality and Modified Radical Mastectomy* Continued

ASSESSMENT	INTERVENTIONS	EXPECTED OUTCOMES
Nursing Diagnosis: Possible reluctance to participate in sexual intercourse after hospital discharge because of fear of disruption of surgical incision and pain		
Initiate discussion before discharge from hospital; reassess and continue teaching at postsurgical follow-up visits; include partner in discussion, if possible	Explore whether this is an issue for client: • whether partner is available • whether concerns exist about resuming intercourse Discuss client's usual methods of sexual expression and importance of breasts in sexual stimulation Reaffirm need for frank discussion between sexual partners and need of time for partner to become accustomed to changes in appearance of surgical area Discuss possibility that client may project own feelings onto partner Teach methods to decrease pain in surgical area or affected arm (if applicable): • use of warm soaks • warm tub baths • pain medication before intercourse • massage Explore alternate sexual positions that may be acceptable to client and partner: • male astride with small pillow over incision • female astride and supported with pillows to lessen pressure on affected arm • side lying with affected arm down and creative use of pillows to lessen pressure on affected arm • rear entry approach with woman lying on pillows to decrease pressure on affected arm	Client verbalizes methods to facilitate intercourse that are acceptable to herself and her partner Client reports satisfactory experience of intercourse or sexual expression Client discusses and role plays ways to express mutual fears and concerns about sexual intercourse with partner
Nursing Diagnosis: Possible reluctance to participate in sexual intercourse because of fear of rejection by partner		
Discuss before discharge from hospital and reinforce at postsurgical follow-up visits	Explore whether this is an issue for client Encourage honest sharing of concerns and feelings between partners Encourage rapid return to previous pattern of sexual activity and maintenance of usual patterns of modesty (as acceptable to client and partner) Assess desire for temporary options to decrease confrontation with partner during intercourse: • use of night bra • undress before partner does • sexual intercourse in the dark • use of alternate sexual positions Discuss client's and current or future partners' needs to have time to become accustomed to loss of breast and appearance of incision: • be patient with self and partner(s) • realize concerns may surface initially or resurface weeks or months after the surgery Encourage seeking professional assistance if partners cannot achieve mutually satisfying experiences	Client discusses concern about partner's reaction to changed appearance and plans ways to help partner become accustomed to changed appearance

TABLE 62–1. *Nursing Care Plan: Sexuality and Modified Radical Mastectomy* Continued

ASSESSMENT	INTERVENTIONS	EXPECTED OUTCOMES
Nursing Diagnosis: Potential reluctance for partner to participate in sexual intercourse because of misconceptions about cancer and about own reaction		
Discuss with client early in course of recovery and explore with partner or client at follow-up visits	Discuss appearance of incision with partner Reaffirm that partner's response is important to woman's self-esteem Reaffirm need for closeness and expression of caring; involve partner in touching, stroking arm, and the like Explore misconceptions about cancer etiology: • cancer is not contagious • aggressive sexual play does not cause cancer Encourage frank sharing of concerns between partners Emphasize pleasuring of partner focusing on other mutually pleasurable areas of woman's body	Client or partner describes mutually satisfactory sexual expression

TABLE 62–2. *Nursing Care Plan: Sexuality and Tyelectomy with External Beam Radiation and/or Iridium Implantation*

ASSESSMENT	INTERVENTIONS	EXPECTED OUTCOMES
Nursing Diagnosis: Potential for threatened self-concept due to changes in irradiated breast tissue and tyelectomy scar		
Initiate assessment and teaching before therapy Monitor change throughout therapy and in follow-up radiation therapy clinic visits	Explore client's self-concept and importance of breasts Assess breast tissue before therapy	Client discusses possibility of changes in breasts Client discusses importance of these changes to her self-concept
	Describe changes that can occur in appearance of irradiated breast: • change in skin color • altered consistency or texture • possible change in size of irradiated breast • possible diminished sensation or tingling in irradiated breast Review radiation treatment side effects: • skin reactions (erythema, dry or moist desquamation) • fatigue • cough secondary to pneumonitis • dry throat	
	Mention specific precautions to minimize skin reactions: • keep treatment field dry • wash treatment field only with water or mild cleansing agents (mild soaps, diluted hydrogen peroxide, saline) • avoid rubbing, friction, heat, cold, chemical irritants (perfume, laundry detergents, creams, deodorants, tape, dressings, direct sunlight exposure) Review expected skin reactions at various radiation levels Assist in managing side effects as they occur	Client lists precautions to minimize radiation skin reactions

(Modified with permission from Schwarz-Appelbaum, J., Dedrick, J., Jusenius, K., & Kirchner, C. W. [1984]. Nursing care plans: Sexuality and treatment of breast cancer. *Oncology Nursing Forum, 11* [6], 16–24.)

Continued on following page.

TABLE 62–2. *Nursing Care Plan: Sexuality and Tyelectomy with External Beam Radiation and/or Iridium Implantation* Continued

ASSESSMENT	INTERVENTIONS	EXPECTED OUTCOMES
Nursing Diagnosis: Possibility of diminished involvement in sexual relationships due to treatment logistics, fatigue, and concerns about being radioactive		
Initiate discussion prior to therapy; monitor throughout therapy	Assess effect of therapy on sexual relationships Reaffirm importance of continued involvement in relationships Clarify misconceptions about radioactivity Explore methods to promote resumption of activities and provide adequate rest: • mobilization of existing support systems (e.g., household or child care assistance, transportation resources) • temporary rearrangement of schedules • allowance for naps or rest periods as necessary	Client defines ways radiation therapy can affect involvement in current relationships and activities Client states plans to continue involvement in relationships and activities or to modify life style
Nursing Diagnosis: Possible change in satisfaction with intercourse and foreplay because of change in breast tissue and breast sensation		
Initiate discussion before therapy Continue monitoring throughout follow-up radiation therapy clinic visits	Discuss importance of breasts in foreplay and intercourse Discuss possible changes in breast tissue and breast sensation that may have an effect on satisfaction with intercourse and foreplay: • change in skin color • altered consistency or texture • possible change in size of irradiated breast • possible diminished sensation or tingling in irradiated breast Investigate ways to facilitate pleasuring using remaining body strengths (e.g., stimulation of other breast or thigh stimulation) Role play ways for client and partner to discuss effects of radiation therapy and determine mutually acceptable methods of pleasuring Determine whether alternative pleasuring activities are acceptable to client and partner	Client discusses possibility of changes in breast tissue and breast sensation Client lists ways to achieve pleasuring that are acceptable to both client and sexual partner
Nursing Diagnosis: Possible reluctance of partner to engage in intercourse, foreplay, (or both) because of concerns about radiation exposure or changes in breast tissue		
Initiate discussion before therapy Whenever possible, include partner in discussions during follow-up radiation therapy clinic visits	Reaffirm importance of closeness and intercourse in relationship Assess whether misconceptions about radiation therapy or changes in breast tissue or both have influenced partner's enthusiasm for intercourse Encourage honest sharing of concerns and feelings between partners Assure partner that there is no residual radioactivity after radiation therapy treatment Teach partner about potential change in breast tissue Discuss alternatives in pleasuring	Client and partner reestablish mutually acceptable patterns of sexual functioning Client and partner identify areas of concern with sexual functioning and discuss ways to continue to demonstrate affection and caring and to achieve mutually acceptable pleasuring

TABLE 62–3. *Nursing Care Plan: Sexuality and Adjuvant Chemotherapy Consisting of Cyclophosphamide (Cytoxan), Methotrexate, and 5-Fluorouracil (CMF)*

ASSESSMENT	INTERVENTIONS	EXPECTED OUTCOMES
Nursing Diagnosis: Potential alteration of sexual self-concept because of weight gain and alopecia		
Before initiating chemotherapy, teach likelihood of gaining weight and experiencing alopecia Reinforce teaching during therapy	Teach client potential for weight gain and alopecia Weigh at each clinic visit Encourage exercise Promote calorie reduction within the framework of a well-balanced diet Encourage reducing nausea by eating small quantities of carbohydrates to reduce excessive weight gain Encourage client to purchase wig, scarves, turbans within 2 weeks of initiating therapy: • wigs should allow for air circulation • scarves and turbans should be cotton, not polyester • a written prescription for a wig may help with insurance reimbursement	Client verbalizes signs and symptoms of chemotherapy that affect sexual self-concept immediately after teaching and 1 week after instruction Client maintains weight within 5–10 lbs. of baseline
Nursing Diagnosis: Potential for temporary or permanent amenorrhea because of ovarian suppression		
Start teaching before initiating chemotherapy	Emphasize to premenopausal clients that resumption of normal menses may take variable lengths of time after completion of chemotherapy Identify high-risk clients for permanent infertility (age 40 and over): • explore options for child rearing, if appropriate (e.g., adoption, surrogate motherhood) Teach client importance of using birth control during active therapy and for at least 12 months after therapy Discuss decision-making concepts related to pregnancy (if applicable)	Client verbalizes that CMF chemotherapy may affect fertility Premenopausal client verbalizes risks associated with becoming pregnant during adjuvant chemotherapy
Nursing Diagnosis: Occurrence of menopausal symptoms usually associated with aging (e.g., hot flashes, decreased or absent vaginal secretions) because of ovarian suppression		
Use as prescribed by physician if hot flashes become problematic	Explore use of Bellergal-5 to control hot flashes Instruct client in use of water-soluble vaginal lubricant if vaginal secretions are decreased (e.g., K-Y Jelly)	
Nursing Diagnosis: Potential disruption of sexual relationships because of depression or global anxiety regarding cancer and therapy resulting from cyclic nature of treatment		
Initiate teaching before chemotherapy; continue to reinforce throughout treatment	Assess client's understanding of disease and treatment goals; clarify misconceptions Encourage client to verbalize concerns, involve appropriate support services Reaffirm importance of client resuming pretreatment life style	Client verbalizes signs and symptoms of CMF chemotherapy that affect sexual relationship and verbalizes ways to counter these Client verbalizes that partner is supportive
Nursing Diagnosis: Possible reluctance to engage in sexual intercourse because of decreased libido, fatigue, hormonal changes, dyspareunia, and changed amount of vaginal secretions		
Initiate teaching when chemotherapy is started Continue to reinforce during subsequent cycles of chemotherapy	Teach use of intervals between chemotherapy for greatest sexual activity to optimize energy level Instruct client to monitor daily energy patterns and to use time of highest energy for sexual activity Recommend male astride position to conserve client's energy	Immediately after teaching and 1 week after initial chemotherapy treatment, client verbalizes signs and symptoms of chemotherapy that may affect sexual functioning Client verbalizes that a personally acceptable level of sexual activity is possible while proceeding with treatment regimen

(Modified with permission from Schwarz-Appelbaum, J., Dedrick, J., Jusenius, K., & Kirchner, C. W. [1984]. Nursing care plans: Sexuality and treatment of breast cancer. *Oncology Nursing Forum, 11*[6], 16–24.)

Continued on following page.

TABLE 62–3. *Nursing Care Plan: Sexuality and Adjuvant Chemotherapy Consisting of Cyclophosphamide (Cytoxan, Methotrexate, and 5-Fluorouracil (CMF)* Continued

ASSESSMENT	INTERVENTIONS	EXPECTED OUTCOMES
	Teach methods to counter vaginal dryness: • water-soluble vaginal lubricants (e.g., K-Y Jelly) • increase time or change pattern of foreplay to increase natural vaginal secretions Avoid excessive douching or perfumed douches to decrease risk of vaginal dryness or irritation or disruption of normal vaginal flora	Client does not complain of dyspareunia
Assess vaginal secretions at each treatment cycle (if oral mucositis is present, there may be other mucosal involvement)	Teach client to report increased vaginal secretions or alteration in vaginal discharge; if symptomatic, nurses should: • check temperature • culture • if yeast present, use antifungal agents as prescribed by physician (e.g., nystatin (Mycostatin), ketoconazole, yogurt) • reinforce that saliva and vaginal secretions may transmit infection	Client uses appropriate regimen as instructed for candidiasis

Nursing Diagnosis: Possibility that partner feels unable to help a loved one through crisis because of knowledge deficit concerning cancer and fear of causing infection in a potentially immunosuppressed person

Initiate discussion with partner before beginning chemotherapy or early in the course of treatment	Assess partner's understanding of disease and treatment goals; clarify misconceptions Offer partner time to express concern without presence of client Offer partner concrete suggestions on ways for him to support client: • exercise together • plan recreational activities during treatment rather than postponing until treatment stops • encourage open expression and willingness to listen • household demands should be consistent with client's energy level	Partner verbalizes potential effects of chemotherapy on sexual relationship Partner is able to state two ways he can concretely support client through treatment

direct effect of radiation therapy is a decrease in sexual desire. The indirect effects include sore, dry mouth, drooling, nausea and vomiting, loss of taste and smell, hoarseness, and malaise. Chemotherapeutic agents have also been associated with side effects that inhibit sexual functioning. These include alopecia, nausea and vomiting, diarrhea, constipation, mucositis, altered sense of taste and smell, and erectile problems. In addition, many men report fever, weakness, and fatigue associated with bone marrow suppression. Permanent or temporary sterility, a decrease in sex drive, and alterations in secondary sex characteristics such as hair distribution, voice changes, and breast development have also been noted (Shipes & Lehr, 1982). Strategies and interventions need to be identified through research that will assist couples in coping with the sexual disruptions associated with this group of diseases (Metcalfe & Fischman, 1985).

CANCERS AFFECTING THE NERVOUS SYSTEM

COLORECTAL CANCERS

Colorectal cancers and their treatment can produce major effects related to sexual dysfunction (see Chapter 32). Sexual ramifications of colorectal cancer include those related to the formation of an ostomy or those related to neurologic deficits (Dudas, 1991; Shipes, 1987). Nursing assessment and interventions related to ostomy and possible sexual dysfunction are discussed under "Special Problems Associated with Alterations in Sexual Functioning." The neural disruption is associated with anterior and posterior resection. The parasympathetic nerve damage associated with abdominal-perineal resection for cancer of the rectum results in erectile impotence in 50 to 100 percent of the patients (Grunberg, 1986). Ejaculation is lost in 50 to 75 per cent of patients who undergo abdominoperineal resection (Dobkin & Broadwell, 1986), and 25 per cent report an inability to penetrate the vagina (La Monica, Audisio, Tamburini, Filberti, & Ventafridda, 1985). Reduction in sexual desire has also been reported for both men (32 to 59 per cent) and women (28 per cent) who have undergone surgical resection for colorectal cancer (Andersen, 1985). Twenty-one per cent of this same female population reported genital numbness and dyspareunia. In addition to the pathophysiologic basis for sexual disruptions, altered body image and self-esteem on the part of the patient can affect sexuality negatively. The partner also may harbor fears and misconceptions that will result in sexual difficulties.

CENTRAL NERVOUS SYSTEM TUMORS

Both primary and metastatic lesions arising in the central nervous system can affect sexual desire and functioning (see Chapter 40). Sexual function is dependent on cortical influences, peripheral nerves, autonomic pathways, spinal cord pathways, and reflex centers (Woods, 1990). Thus pathologic lesions involving any of these structures may lead to sexual dysfunction. Scant research has been done on the impact of central nervous system tumors and sexual function. It is possible, however, to extrapolate from the immense body of knowledge on patients with spinal cord injuries and with lesions involving the brain. Much of this literature has involved male patients, probably because more males have spinal cord injuries and because women are assumed to accept more readily a passive sexual role. An intact pathway from the cortex to the sex organ is not necessary for certain components of the human sexual response cycle, for example, attainment of erection and ejaculation. Rather these functions are mediated by spinal cord reflexes. The important factor to consider is the level of the injury and the degree of interruption of nerve impulses. Sexual gratification can be experienced from feelings other than those emanating from the sex organs. A thorough assessment followed by individualized interventions can optimize sexual functioning in the client with tumors of the nervous system.

Table 62–4 contains a summary of the effects of various cancers on sexuality, including sexual function, fertility, body image, and partners.

TABLE 62–4. *Effects of Cancer on Sexuality, Including Sexual Function, Fertility, Body Image, and Partners*

SITE	DYSFUNCTION — ORGANIC	DYSFUNCTION — PSYCHOLOGICAL	EFFECT ON FERTILITY	ALTERED BODY IMAGE	IMPACT ON PARTNER	COMMENTS
Cervix	Treatment of in situ with cone biopsy will not cause dysfunction; radical hysterectomy will shorten the vagina by one third to one half; this may be appreciable but usually is not	Sometimes	No, with cone biopsy for in situ stages; yes, with hysterectomy, radiotherapy, or both	Sometimes	Sometimes (partner may feel he can "catch" cancer or be affected by its treatment, especially by radiotherapy)	Radiotherapy to the pelvis will cause thickening of the vagina and may cause stenosis, fistula formation, or both
Endometrial	Total abdominal hysterectomy with pelvic node dissection usually causes no dysfunction; radiotherapy to the pelvis will cause thickening of the vagina if it is included in the fields	Sometimes	Yes, with either radiotherapy or surgery	Sometimes	Sometimes	Because of lack of literature on female sexual response, it is very difficult to determine difference between physical and emotional dysfunction

NOTE: Chemotherapy, radiation, and analgesics are all associated with generalized feelings of malaise. This can have a profound effect on the feelings of self-esteem, self-worth, sexuality, and libido. All these factors should be taken into consideration when assessing the sexual needs and problems of cancer patients and their families.
(From Lamb, M., & Woods, N. F. [1981]. Sexuality and the cancer patient. *Cancer Nursing, 4,* 137–144. Reproduced by permission.)

Continued on following page.

| SITE | DYSFUNCTION | | EFFECT ON FERTILITY | ALTERED BODY IMAGE | IMPACT ON PARTNER | COMMENTS |
	ORGANIC	PSYCHOLOGICAL				
Ovary	In premenopausal women, bilateral oophorectomy will result in menopausal symptoms	Sometimes	Yes (except with cases with unilateral oophorectomy)	Sometimes	Sometimes	
Vulva	Simple vulvectomy can result in introital stenosis; radical vulvectomy includes removal of the clitoris	Usually	No; patient is often postmenopausal	Most often	Usually	Radical vulvectomy can cause a decrease in range of motion of lower extremities.
Breast	The absence of foreplay using nipple stimulation for arousal may cause some difficulties	Usually	None	Usually	Usually	If oophorectomy and hormonal manipulations are utilized, this can affect all aspects of sexuality
Prostate	Total prostatectomy results in impotence; simple prostatectomy usually results in retrograde ejaculation	Usually	Usually	Usually	Usually	Bilateral orchiectomy or hormonal manipulations can result in decreased libido and sexual responsiveness; if estrogen treatment is initiated, gynecomastia may result
Testicular	Nerve damage due to retroperitoneal lymph node dissection usually results in retrograde ejaculation and can cause impotence	Usually	Sometimes, if unilateral; always, if bilateral; suggest utilization of sperm bank before chemotherapy and retroperitoneal lymph node dissection	Yes	Usually	Hormonal aberration (especially decrease in androgen) will cause a decrease in libido and may cause impotence, retarded ejaculation, and a decrease in sexual responsiveness
Bladder	Local—seldom; in males, radical cystectomy involves removal of bladder, urethra, and prostate—therefore, he is impotent. In females, cystectomy usually includes urethra, uterus, and anterior vagina	Usually	Always with radiotherapy; this cancer is most common in older men	Yes (patients usually have urinary conduit with a stoma)	Usually	

TABLE 62–4. *Effects of Cancer on Sexuality, Including Sexual Function, Fertility, Body Image, and Partners* Continued

| SITE | DYSFUNCTION | | EFFECT ON FERTILITY | ALTERED BODY IMAGE | IMPACT ON PARTNER | COMMENTS |
	ORGANIC	PSYCHOLOGICAL				
Colon and Rectum	Usually; nerve damage in males negatively effects erectile ability	Usually; especially with formation of an ostomy	None; except with radiotherapy and chemotherapy	Yes (if colostomy formed)	Sometimes	Women sometimes have a hysterectomy with the operative procedure
Leukemia	The disease process and associated blood counts with chemotherapy may affect ability to have an erection	Sometimes	Chemotherapy affects sperm count and ova maturation rebound after cessation of treatment	Usually	Usually	Extensive fatigue often diminishes sex drive and function
Hodgkins	The disease process and the effects of the therapy may decrease sexual drive and ability	Sometimes	Yes, with radiotherapy to the pelvis without shielding of the gonads; chemotherapy will decrease sperm and ova maturation	Usually	Usually	Patients on chemotherapy alone should be using some form of contraception; the effect on the sperm counts and ova maturation by chemotherapy is not totally understood

CHANGES IN HORMONAL ENVIRONMENT AND VASCULATURE

An appropriate hormonal milieu and adequate vasculature to the sex organs is necessary for sexual functioning. Many cancers and treatments affect either or both of these components. A decrease in the amount of circulating estrogen, through surgical removal of the ovaries or chemical suppression by chemotherapy, can result in vaginal dryness, thinning, and other menopausal symptoms (Andersen, 1985; Feldman, 1989). Men treated with estrogen experience gynecomastia and a decrease in libido (Schrover et al., 1984). A decrease in the amount of circulating androgens, through surgical removal or chemical suppression, can also result in a decrease in sexual drive and feminization in males (Schrover et al., 1986). Hormonal replacement may be indicated or contraindicated, depending on the reason for the suppression. Patients with hormonally dependent tumors may have their systemic hormonal environment intentionally altered, or this alteration may have been an inadvertent effect of therapy. Interventions, therefore, may be either an adaptation to or a correction of the hormonal imbalance.

A decrease in the vasculature to the genitals can also interfere with sexual functioning. In the male, this decrease can result in an inability to attain or maintain an erection (Schrover et al., 1986). In the female, it will result in vaginal dryness, thinning, and dyspareunia (Andersen, 1985). The etiologic factors associated with an alteration in genital vasculature include (1) direct tumor compression of the vessels supplying the genitals, (2) surgical disruption of the genital vasculature, and (3) vascular fibrosis as a result of radiation therapy. This vascular compromise can be temporary or permanent; often the onset is insidious in nature, especially if the cause is tumor compression or radiation fibrosis. Treatments may be employed to correct the deficiency in vascularization, but correction is not always possible. Interventions aimed at adaptation to the resulting dysfunction may be the option of choice. These interventions may include use of a water-soluble lubricant if vaginal dryness is a problem or insertion of a penile implant if erectile disruption is the resulting problem.

PSYCHOSOCIAL FACTORS INFLUENCING SEXUAL FUNCTIONING

PSYCHOLOGIC FACTORS

The psychologic factors that often affect sexuality include (1) alteration in body image, (2) diminished self-esteem, (3) role change, (4) attitudes, (5) beliefs and misconceptions, and (6) anxiety or depression. Any one or combination of these factors can affect the sexual functioning of the patient with cancer (Andersen, Andersen, & de Prosse, 1989a, 1989b). Difficulties can occur at any point in the continuum of cancer care: during diagnosis, workup, treatment, or followup or during the stage of progressive or terminal disease, should this be the outcome. The client with cancer, the partner, or both can manifest sexual difficulties that are related to their psychologic responses (Quigley, 1989). The emphasis of this chapter is on the direct effect of these psychologic responses on sexual functioning.

BODY IMAGE AND SELF-ESTEEM

Body image can be viewed as a component of self-esteem (Derogatis, 1980; Drench, 1994). Self-esteem can be defined simply as the reputation we have of ourselves. The process of giving and receiving sexual pleasure is closely connected to a sense of safety, in both our person and our body (Cantor, 1980). Living with cancer produces changes in self-esteem, some transient, some permanent. These changes are based on both an immediate reality as well as an anticipation of possible further changes. Self-esteem can be affected negatively by cancer, with or without apparent changes in body image, which, in turn, may contribute to feelings of sexual inadequacy (Cooley & Cobb, 1986a, 1986b; Foltz, 1987). If in addition to altered self-esteem, the patient must adjust to changes in physical appearance, sexual functioning can be compromised further.

The identification and remediation of the patient's impoverished self-esteem, body-image disturbance, and sexual disruption are key goals of cancer care (Schain, 1980; Wood & Tombrink, 1983). An assessment of self-esteem can be achieved during an informal discussion and should be conducted at repeated intervals throughout the cancer continuum. This information will be essential in identifying and correcting sexual dysfunctions related to alterations in self-esteem. Efforts should be made directly, through counseling and behavior modification, to build self-esteem to a level compatible with a feeling of being worthwhile (Enelow, 1975).

ANXIETY AND DEPRESSION

Anxiety and depression are the two most common affective disruptions among patients with cancer (Andersen, 1985). Clinical depression can be diagnosed in 17 to 25 per cent of the hospitalized cancer population (Petty & Noyes, 1981). Anxiety about the future occurs at critical periods for patients with cancer: at diagnosis, at evidence of recurrence, and during the side effects of therapy. Both anxiety and depression have profound effects on sexual functioning (Wise, 1978).

A decrease in sexual interest, libido, and activity are all results of depressive and anxious states (Mims & Swenson, 1980). Depression and anxiety have both been associated with erectile dysfunctions; anxiety has been associated with premature ejaculation (Woods, 1990). Interventions are aimed at alleviating the anxiety and depression.

ROLE CHANGES

Social role refers to the patterns of behavior shared by individuals who occupy a certain position or fulfill a certain function in society (Enelow, 1975). Each individual may occupy a variety of social and cultural roles. Parent, wife, husband, financial provider, and homemaker are a few of the many roles that may be transiently or permanently affected by cancer and cancer treatment. During illness, some roles are relinquished and assumed by others. Role reversals are sometimes necessary (Johnson, 1986). A person's identity and sense of worth may be threatened when role changes occur. The shifting roles within families of cancer patients should be taken into account when considering the possible etiologic factors associated with sexual dysfunctions. For example, the role of the sexual partner may no longer be compatible with that of the man who is no longer the financial supporter of the family; by contrast, a women may no longer feel like a wife and sexual partner if her husband must participate in her physical care.

ATTITUDES, BELIEFS, AND MISCONCEPTIONS

The attitudes and beliefs of a person with cancer regarding cancer and its treatment often affect sexual functioning. Attitudes and beliefs are formed over time and are based on previous experience as well as on formal and informal education. In our society, many beliefs and attitudes regarding cancer are incompatible with normal sexual functioning. Cancer is often viewed as a "punishment" for past deeds, either real or fantasized (Cantor, 1980; Sewell & Edwards, 1980). Some patients may harbor misconceptions regarding the etiology of cancer and the impact that it may have on their own as well as their partner's sexual functioning. Fear of contagion is another misconception of some patients (Golden & Golden, 1980). Many people fear that they can "give" cancer to or "get" cancer from their loved ones through close physical contact, especially through sexual intercourse. A frank and open discussion between client and caregiver will often uncover the attitudes, beliefs, and misconceptions that can have a negative effect on sexual functioning. Education regarding the etiology, treatment, and long-term effects of cancer and its treatment on sexuality is an integral part of the holistic care of the cancer patient. Dispelling myths and misconceptions is a part of this educational process.

SOCIAL FACTORS

Social factors that affect the sexual functioning of the patient with cancer include (1) availability of a sexual partner; (2) evidence of anxiety or depression on the part of the partner; (3) effect of role changes on the partner; and (4) partner's attitudes, beliefs, and misconceptions. Patients who do not have a sexual partner may have difficulties establishing an intimate relationship. The stress of cancer can often cause a fragile relationship to deteriorate. People who, at the time of diagnosis, are single, widowed, or divorced often state that it is difficult to initiate an intimate relationship. Many factors may account for this phenomenon: fear of rejection due to the diagnosis or possible alteration in body image; inability to meet available people socially because of prolonged treatments and convalescence; and uncertainty about the future.

The partner, too, is vulnerable to similar psychologic factors that may impede normal sexual expression, such as anxiety, depression, guilt, and misconceptions. Anxiety and depression on the part of the partner will have detrimental effects on sexuality, similar to those experienced by the patient with these affective disorders. The partner may feel that the cancer patient is too sick for sexual activity or may feel guilty about making sexual overtures to someone who is experiencing the trauma of cancer diagnosis and treatment. Partners also may fear that the cancer is contagious or that the treatment will somehow affect them. Some spouses fear that the patient's radiation treatments will render the patient either temporarily or permanently radioactive. Other partners may have difficulty adjusting to the altered physical appearance of the patient. Role changes affect the partner in the same manner as they affect the patient. For example, the partner may not be able to switch roles easily from that of caregiver to that of sexual partner. Because of the variety of social factors to be considered, individualized interventions should be planned for the couple with sexual dysfunctions during the period of cancer care.

ENVIRONMENTAL FACTORS

Two main environmental factors that may impede sexual expression are (1) hospitalization, with its inherent lack of privacy and traditional views of the patient as an asexual being, and (2) alterations in the home environment that often lead to a decrease in the privacy necessary for intimate relations to occur. The hospital setting is notorious for the lack of quiet, uninterrupted time. Most patients are placed in semiprivate rooms and are monitored constantly by physicians, nurses, and other health care professionals. Visiting hours may or may not be structured, thereby further diminishing available time alone. Recently some hospitals have initiated policies to allow for private, uninterrupted time; however, this is an exception rather than a rule. Nurses can take an active role in policy setting to allow for intimate time in the hospital setting. This will serve to validate the humanness of their patients as well as to offer holistic care.

The home setting is sometimes altered to allow for convalescent, progressive, or terminal care. This alteration is rarely conducive to intimate relationships. A hospital bed in the family living area or first-floor den will not provide the privacy necessary for sexual activity. Couples should be encouraged to negotiate with family members, friends, and members of the health care team for private time on a regular basis. Whether or not they choose to use this time for sexual activity is not an issue. The availability of this time will allow for some degree of spontaneity and closeness otherwise lost owing to the hectic surroundings.

ASSESSMENT AND MANAGEMENT OF ALTERATIONS IN SEXUAL FUNCTIONING

SEXUAL ASSESSMENT

Assessment of sexual health begins with a sexual history and is supplemented by data regarding the person's general health, such as that obtained from a physical examination or a general health history (Lamb & Woods, 1981). The literature contains a number of articles that address sexual assessment, many of which are specific to cancer patients (Chapman & Sughrue, 1987; Greenberg, 1984; Lamb & Woods, 1981; MacElveen-Hoehn, 1985). The following is a brief sexual assessment that can be easily incorporated into a more general nursing assessment:

> Has being ill interfered with your being a (husband, father, wife, mother)?
> Has your illness changed the way you see yourself as a man/woman?
> Has your illness affected your sexual function?
> (Lamb & Woods, 1981)

The first question relates to sexual role, the second pertains to self-image, and the last addresses sexual function. Often it is necessary to ask only the first or second question, because the client will open up and freely discuss data related to the third item. If the discussion of the answers to these questions uncovers a specific sexual problem, a more in-depth assessment may be necessary. This would include the onset and course of the problem, the client or couple's ideas about what may have caused the problem and its persistence, the solutions that have been attempted to date, the solutions that are acceptable (sexual counseling, exploring alternate forms of sexual gratification), and the goals of an attempted treatment plan. A physical examination, not necessarily specific to sexual function, will also shed light onto potential sexual problems. Dyspnea on exertion, range of motion difficulties, and vaginal stenosis detected during an internal pelvic examination are all examples of physical limitations that may impede sexual functioning.

It is easy to reflect on such findings and incorporate them into a sexual assessment question. An example of this might be, "Does your difficulty breathing interfere with your sexual relations with your wife/husband/partner?" Similar information gained from the patient's records can be incorporated into the sexual history, "Often when blood counts are low, energy level is reduced. Many people find that this interferes with their sexual desire. Have you experienced this?"

To assess the sexual health of oncology patients effectively, the nurse must first be comfortable with the topic of sexuality. Comfort with self as a sexually expressive human being will convey comfort to others (Fetter, 1987). Personal beliefs and attitudes regarding sexuality are also major factors that may influence sexual assessment. Several studies have addressed the sexual attitudes held by professional nurses caring for oncology patients (Box 62-2) (Fisher, 1983, 1985;

Box 62–2. *Nurses' Attitudes Toward Sexuality*

Wilson, E., & Williams, H. A. (1988). Oncology nurses' attitudes and behaviors related to sexuality of patients with cancer. *Oncology Nursing Forum, 15*(1), 49–53.

This descriptive study explored the attitudes of 937 oncology nurses toward sexuality in cancer patients. The analysis of the responses to a mailed questionnaire revealed a positive relationship between attitudes toward sexuality in patients with cancer and number of nursing care practices related to alterations in sexuality. Nurses with more years of experience and more education reported more nursing practices related to the sexual issues of their clients. Lack of knowledge was frequently cited as a reason for not addressing sexual concerns. There was an overall lack of awareness of the presence and needs of individuals with a homosexual orientation. Nursing rounds and continuing education were two ways that were cited to increase nurses' knowledge of and comfort with discussing these issues.

Fisher & Levin, 1983; Williams, Wilson, Hongladarom, & McDonell, 1986; Wilson & Williams, 1988). Insufficient knowledge and a discrepancy between affective responses, which indicated comfort with sexuality issues, and behavioral items, which indicated actual involvement with sexual concerns, were discovered. The need for further sexual education for oncology nurses was identified. Education for oncology nurses can be gained informally via discussions with peers and consultants with expertise in the area of human sexuality. Formal training can be gained through in-service presentations, workshops, or sexual attitude reassessment programs. Individualized knowledge can be achieved by keeping abreast of the new developments within the field by attending conferences and reading journals and textbooks.

The ease of obtaining a sexual history can be enhanced by using several simple techniques: ensuring privacy and confidentiality, allowing ample, uninterrupted time, and maintaining a nonjudgmental attitude. A discussion of sexuality early in one's association with the client will legitimize sexuality as an important aspect of health care and ensure that it is an appropriate topic for concern in the nurse-client relationship. Anxiety will be reduced by moving from less sensitive to more sensitive topics. Use of language that is understandable to the client is essential. However, the use of slang or street language may be uncomfortable for the professional nurse; therefore, defining terms early in the discussion will alleviate this potential problem.

Certain communication techniques incorporated into the interview may also be helpful. Using open-ended questions, questions referring to frequency rather than occurrence, and "unloading" questions are specific examples of such techniques. An example of an open-ended question might be, "Some women are concerned that the removal of the uterus will decrease their sexual pleasure. Do you have this concern?" A question that refers to frequency rather than occurrence is, "How often do you have sexual intercourse" as opposed to "Do you have sexual intercourse?" "Unloading" the question refers to statement such as, "Some men masturbate on a regular basis, whereas others seldom or never masturbate. How often do you masturbate?" Finally, asking the client if he or she has any questions at the end of the assessment will convey a willingness to explore further those issues that were brought up during the assessment.

INTERVENTIONS

The literature contains many articles that address sexual rehabilitation and interventions. Some focus on cancer patients in general (Adams, 1980; Chapman & Sughrue, 1987; Enelow, 1975; Lamb & Woods, 1981; MacElveen-Hoehn, 1985; Smith, 1989; von Eschenbach & Schrover, 1984), and others discuss specific subgroups of oncology patients (Bachers, 1985; Capone, Westie, & Good, 1980; Cooley & Cobb, 1986a, 1986b; Donahue, 1978; Golden, 1983; Grunberg, 1986; Metcalfe & Fischman, 1985; Schain, 1985; Schrover & Fife, 1985; Schwarz-Appelbaum et al., 1984; Shipes & Lehr, 1982). The specific sexual needs or concerns of the client dictate the approach and content of the discussion. These needs and concerns can be either current or anticipated. The American Cancer Society has published two comprehensive booklets to assist cancer patients to adapt to the sexual changes that take place during cancer therapy: *Sexuality and Cancer: For the Woman Who Has Cancer, and Her Partner,* and *Sexuality and Cancer: For the Man Who Has Cancer, and His Partner.*

Intervention can be approached in many fashions. The P-LI-SS-IT model provides four levels of intervention (Annon, 1974). P-LI-SS-IT is an acronym for permission, limited information, specific suggestion, and intensive therapy. The first three levels are considered brief therapy, and the fourth is intensive therapy.

Permission. Permission to discuss sexual concerns and problems is the initial step of intervention. Open communication regarding sexuality is essential for the subsequent components of the intervention process. Often patients want to know whether their sexual practices are normal or acceptable. This includes both actual sexual behaviors as well as thoughts, desires, and dreams. Concerns may also develop about becoming sexually aroused at what is thought to be inappropriate times, for example, while the partner is hospitalized. Permission includes reassuring the patient and partner regarding all components of sexuality.

Limited Information. The second level of treatment is referred to as limited information. This level includes the first level, permission, but, in addition, gives specific information that addresses sexual concerns, myths, misconceptions, and questions that have arisen. Included in this level are basic facts on the appropriateness of sexual activity at this point and on the possibility of contagion or exacerbation of the malignancy. False assumptions about loss of sexual function and concerns about fertility are addressed. Providing anticipatory guidance regarding what to expect as a result of disease and treatment is included in this discussion.

Specific Suggestions. If the problem requires more than permission and information, the third level, specific suggestions, is initiated. This level of counseling attempts to help the couple directly to change behavior to reach a stated goal. Before embarking, the professional should have obtained a sexual problem history, as outlined previously. A clearly stated goal is also a requisite for the third level. The resultant plan will include specific activities for the couple. Usually, the couple is seen on several occasions. The subsequent sessions are used to assess progress and address related concerns. Specific suggestions usually pertain to the areas of communication, symptom management, and alternate physical expression.

Communication between partners should be fostered. This includes candid discussions regarding their emotional response to the disease and treatments, their fears and concerns, as well as their development of active listening skills. Symptom management is essential to optimize sexual expression. Cancer and its associated treatments often cause nausea and vomiting, weight loss, pain, fatigue, shortness of breath, and range of motion difficulties. The management of all of these symptoms may be necessary. Alternate physical expression is necessary if sexual disruption is due to organic changes. If intercourse is difficult or impossible, the couple will have to explore or expand alternate forms of expressing physical love. A thorough discussion of the couple's values and attitudes should be done before initiating alternative suggestions. There are many ways of stimulating and giving sexual pleasure: hugging, fondling, caressing, cuddling, kissing, and hand-holding. Genital intercourse is only one way of expressing physical love. Sexual gratification may be derived from manual, digital, and oral stimulation. Intrathigh, anal, and intramammary intercourse are also options if the female partner is unable to continue to experience vaginal penetration (Fisher, 1983).

Intensive Therapy. Intensive therapy can be instituted if adequate progress is not being made or if the couple has long-standing sexual or marital problems. At this point, the couple is referred to a professional who has received advanced training in sex therapy. This person may be a nurse, social worker, psychiatrist, psychologist, or sex therapist (Schain, 1981).

SPECIAL PROBLEMS ASSOCIATED WITH ALTERATIONS IN SEXUAL FUNCTIONING

Cancer and cancer care often have symptoms or side effects that can negatively affect sexual functioning. This section addresses specific interventions for the most commonly experienced problems associated with cancer

and its treatment. These problems include fertility concerns, range of motion difficulties, ostomy formation, nausea and vomiting, pain, fatigue, shortness of breath, and coping with progressive or terminal illness.

FERTILITY CONCERNS

Clients diagnosed with cancer during their childbearing years often have concerns regarding their future ability to parent children (Chapman, 1982; Kaempfer, 1981; Kaempfer, Hoffman, & Wiley, 1983; Kaempfer & Major, 1986; Kaempfer, Wiley, Hoffman, & Rhodes, 1985; Lamb, 1991b, 1993; Miller, 1994; Smith & Babaian, 1992; Yarbro & Perry, 1985). Surgery, radiation, and chemotherapy have all been demonstrated to cause sterility. The topic of permanent or temporary sterility should be discussed before the onset of treatment. The client or couple's attitudes and values regarding future childbearing should be explored thoroughly. Once the assessment has been completed, preventive measures and procreative alternatives should be discussed and planned. Examples of preventive measures are surgical relocation of the ovaries before pelvic irradiation or shielding of the gonads during radiation therapy. If preventive measures are not feasible, procreative alternatives can be suggested, such as contributing sperm to a sperm bank before treatment, artificial insemination, in vitro fertilization and embryo transfer, or adoption.

Storing sperm in a sperm bank is a reproductive option that should be considered when counseling male cancer patients. The banking of sperm offers the client protection from the mutagenic and antifertility effects of cancer therapy (Kaempfer, 1981). The preserved sperm can then potentially be used in subsequent artificial insemination or in vitro fertilization, as indicated. The issues related to this procedure for male cancer patients are still evolving. These issues include appropriateness of the candidate, costs, collection and storage procedures, legal considerations, and ethical issues (Kaempfer, 1981; Kaempfer et al., 1983, 1985). The American Fertility Society (1608 13th Avenue South, Birmingham, AL 35256) provides publications pertaining to infertility and lists of human semen cryobanks in the United States and facilities involved in in vitro fertilization and embryo transfer.

Artificial insemination is the next logical step after banking sperm and determining the appropriate time for conception. Artificial insemination is a procedure that usually occurs in an outpatient setting. Once the approximate date of ovulation is determined, usually via recording of basal body temperature and monitoring of cervical mucosa characteristics, the insemination is scheduled. Two inseminations are done per ovulation cycle. Six to 12 cycles of insemination are often required before pregnancy occurs (Kaempfer et al., 1983).

In vitro fertilization and embryo transfer is yet another evolving option for couples who anticipate or are actually experiencing infertility problems. An indepth discussion of this procedure is unwarranted in this text. However, to briefly summarize, the ovaries are continually monitored via periodic ultrasound to determine the appropriate time for laporascopic attainment of the ovum. Once the ripe follicles are obtained, they are mixed with the partner's semen in a culture dish, which is then incubated for 36 to 40 hours. The resultant embryo is then transferred into the uterus, and, if pregnancy occurs, it is established within 2 weeks (Kaempfer et al., 1985). A number of issues must be considered by the couple considering this procreative alternative. The overall success rate of in vitro fertilization and embryo transfer is quite low. The costs of the procedure, which is not customarily covered by insurance, are exorbitant. The cost factor alone often leaves this option available to a very few. Finally, this procedure has been found to be quite emotionally taxing. Often an exploration of the couple's coping abilities is determined before initiation into the program (Kaempfer et al., 1985). All of these factors should be taken into account by the couple considering this option.

Dramatically improved survival rates have been seen in the treatment of childhood cancer. Unfortunately, these treatments are often associated with side effects that can affect both fertility of the survivors as well as the prospective of having healthy children when fertility is preserved (Thurber, 1989). Continued research of the offspring of cancer survivors is needed to fully comprehend the impact on future generations.

RANGE OF MOTION DIFFICULTIES

The progression of the cancer as well as the surgical procedures utilized to treat it may leave the patient with limited range of motion (Chapter 63). The emphasis of this discussion is on interventions to optimize the sexual functioning of clients with range of motion difficulties. Suggestions to minimize these effects are to (1) experiment with different positions, (2) use pillows to support body weight, (3) employ relaxation techniques or massage, (4) use warm baths or hot or cold soaks to affected areas before intercourse, (5) use medications (sparingly), and (6) explore alternate ways of expressing physical love.

OSTOMY

The presence of an ostomy may affect sexual expression. Education, both before and after surgery, can prevent or minimize the detrimental effects that the presence of an ostomy may have on sexuality (Penninger, Moore, & Frager, 1985; Shipes, 1987; Stadil, 1983). Specific interventions are dependent on the patient's particular type of ostomy. Patients with continent ostomies can plan their sexual activity, remove the appliance, and cover the stoma before initiating sexual relations. If the appliance cannot be removed safely, the patient can empty the appliance before initiating intercourse, use a cover or a body stocking to conceal the appliance, or turn the appliance to the side (if the ostomate is in the dependent position). If the appliance is in the way, explore alternate positions; if a leak occurs,

continue sexual play in the shower. The United Ostomy Association (36 Executive Park, Suite 120, Irvine, CA 92714; [714]660–8624) has published several booklets that deal specifically with the sexual concerns of ostomates: *Sex, Courtships and the Single Ostomate*; *Sex, Pregnancy and the Female Ostomate*; and *Sex and the Male Ostomate*.

NAUSEA AND VOMITING

Nausea and vomiting are frequently associated with cancer treatments. These side effects can interfere directly with sexual functioning. Numerous drug and nondrug approaches have been recommended for control of nausea and vomiting (see Chapter 51). Antiemetics are often used; however, they may interfere with sexual function because of their sedative effects. Articles have been published on patient control of nausea and vomiting. If this can be done, alternate nondrug methods to control these symptoms should be explored. These include (1) recalling past strategies that were successful in controlling nausea and vomiting; (2) eating foods that are cold or at room temperature; (3) eating small, frequent meals (especially refraining from large meals before sexual play); (4) avoiding foods with strong odors; (5) avoiding sights, sounds, and smells that stimulate nausea; (6) using relaxation or distraction techniques; (7) providing for fresh air (an open window), and (8) timing sexual activities around periods of nausea (if known).

PAIN

Sexual arousal is often impaired by the presence of pain. The goal of pain therapy is to relieve pain or discomfort without hindering sexual responsiveness. The use of pain medication may decrease libido or interfere with erectile ability (Lamb & Woods, 1981). Experimenting with alternate forms of pain management, other than medication, should be explored. Relaxation techniques, such as guided imagery, may be helpful. Romantic music can be employed both for mood setting and for distraction and relaxation. Sexual activity itself is a form of distraction. Biofeedback, self-hypnosis, and application of hot and cold packs to the affected areas may substantially alleviate discomfort. The couple should be encouraged to experiment: to discover and use the most comfortable positions. The creative use of pillows should also be suggested. Massage can be both therapeutic in reducing pain as well as an arousal technique. Pain medication should be used sparingly, if at all. Finally, alternate ways of expressing physical love should be explored if the couple's traditional methods of sexual gratification are no longer feasible because of discomfort.

FATIGUE

Methods to minimize exertion are necessary if fatigue is a limiting factor in sexual activity. Providing time for rest before and after intercourse is often sufficient to minimize the detrimental effects of a decrease in available energy. Other suggestions include (1) avoid the stress of consuming heavy meals or alcohol before intercourse, (2) avoid extremes in temperature, (3) experiment with positions that require minimal exertion (male client-female astride, female client-male astride, side lying); (4) take timing into consideration (intercourse in the morning rather than at night), and (5) periodically delegate or delay household tasks such as child care and meal preparation to conserve energy for intimate relations.

SHORTNESS OF BREATH

Sexual activity can be directly impaired by dyspnea (Welch-McCaffrey, 1983). The fear of potential dyspnea itself is often a deterrent to initiating sexual play. The use of a water bed to accentuate physical movements during sexual activity can be suggested. In addition, keeping the affected partner's head and upper torso raised (via the use of pillows) will also encourage adequate oxygenation. Pulmonary hygiene before sexual activity may also be of benefit. Finally, the affected partner should be encouraged to assume a more passive role and a dependent position during sexual activity.

SUMMARY AND CONTINUING AREAS OF CONCERNS AND ISSUES

Cancer and the therapies employed to combat it often result in a compromise of quality of life. To minimize the adverse effects of these diseases and their treatments on those affected, clinicians should address the real or potential alterations in sexual functioning that occur. The more than 5 million Americans alive today who have a history of cancer should be seen as holistic beings whose needs, hopes, and concerns are the same as all others. The ramifications of withholding sexual information from clients with cancer can be profound. A little investment on the nurse's part to provide information and support can make a significant difference in the couple's ability to adjust to changes in sexual functioning (Smith, 1989).

The difficulties of a team approach in this domain are apparent. Confusion may arise as to which care provider (primary care nurse, clinical nurse specialist, physician, social worker, or others) has counseled the client or couple regarding sexual concerns. What information has been given, in what depth, to whom (client, partner, or both), regarding which actual or potential problems, and how to avoid or minimize these effects are just a few of the issues that surface. Nurses should take a leading role in the assessment and remediation of clients' concerns regarding the sexual ramifications of their disease and resultant treatments.

The sexual dysfunctions resulting from cancer are becoming less unknown and mysterious. As research in this field continues, the sexual dysfunctions experienced by oncology patients are becoming more delineated, and interventions are being explored to prevent

or minimize the adverse sexual sequelae of cancer and its treatment.

REFERENCES

Adams, A. K. (1980). The sex counseling role of the cancer clinician. *Frontiers of Radiation Therapy and Oncology, 14,* 66–78.

American Cancer Society. (1994). *Cancer facts and figures—1994.* New York: Author.

Andersen B. L. (1987). Sexual functioning complications in women with gynecologic cancer: Outcomes and directions for prevention. *Cancer, 60*(Suppl.), 2123–2128.

Andersen, B. L. (1985). Sexual functioning morbidity among cancer survivors. *Cancer, 55,* 1835–1842.

Andersen, B. L., Andersen, B., & deProsse, C. (1989a) Controlled prospective longitudinal study of women with cancer: Psychological outcomes. Part I. *Journal of Consulting and Clinical Psychology, 57*(6), 683–691.

Andersen, B. L., Andersen, B., & deProsse, C. (1989b) Controlled prospective longitudinal study of women with cancer: Psychological outcomes. Part II. *Journal of Consulting and Clinical Psychology, 57*(6), 692–697.

Andersen, B. L., & Hacker, N. F. (1983a). Psychosexual adjustment after vulvar surgery. *Obstetrics and Gynecology, 62,* 457–462.

Andersen, B. L., & Hacker, N. F. (1983b). Psychosexual adjustment following pelvic exenteration. *Obstetrics and Gynecology, 61,* 331–338.

Andersen, B. L., Lachenbruch, P. A., Anderson, B., & DeProsse, C. (1986). Sexual dysfunction and signs of gynecologic cancer. *Cancer, 57,* 1880–1886.

Andreasson, B., Moth, I., Jensen, S. B., & Bock, J. E. (1986). Sexual function and somatic psychic reactions in vulvectomy-operated women and their partners. *Acta Obstetrica et Gynecologica Scandinavica, 65,* 7–10.

Annon, J. S. (1974). *The behavioral treatment of sexual problems.* Honolulu: Mercantile Printing.

Auchincloss, S. (1991). Sexual dysfunction after cancer treatment. *Journal of Psychosocial Oncology, 9*(1), 23–42.

Bachers, E. S. (1985). Sexual dysfunction after treatment for genitourinary cancer. *Seminars in Oncology Nursing, 1,* 18–24.

Baldwin, E. (1990). Sexuality and breast cancer. *Midwife, Health, Visitor, and Community Nurse, 26*(10), 385–386.

Beckmann, J., Blichert-Toft, M., & Johansen, L. (1983). Psychological effects of mastectomy. *Danish Medical Bulletin, 30* (Suppl. 2), 7–10.

Bertelsen, K. (1983). Sexual dysfunction after treatment for cervical cancer. *Danish Medical Bulletin, 30*(Suppl. 2), 31–34.

Brenner, J., Vugrin, D., & Whitmore, W. F. (1985). Effect of treatment on fertility and sexual function in males treated with metastatic nonseminomatous germ cell tumors of the testis. *American Journal of Clinical Oncology, 8,* 178–182.

Burbie, G. E., & Polinsky, M. L. (1992) Intimacy and sexuality after cancer treatment: Restoring a sense of wholeness. *Journal of Psychosocial Oncology, 10*(1), 19–33.

Cantor, R. C. (1980). Self-esteem, sexuality and cancer-related stress. *Frontiers in Radiation Therapy and Oncology, 14,* 51–54.

Capone, M. A., Westie, K. S., & Good, R. S. (1980). Sexual rehabilitation of the gynecologic cancer patient: An effective counseling model. *Frontiers in Radiation Therapy and Oncology, 14,* 123–129.

Chapman, J., & Sughrue, J. (1987). A model for sexual assessment and intervention. *Health Care for Women International, 8,* 87–99.

Chapman, R. M. (1982). Effect of cytotoxic therapy on sexuality and gonadal function. *Seminars in Oncology, 9,* 84–94.

Cooley, M. E., & Cobb, S. C. (1986a). Sexual and reproductive issues for women with Hodgkin's disease. Overview of issues. *Cancer Nursing, 9,* 188–193.

Cooley, M. E., & Cobb, S. C. (1986b). Sexual and reproductive issues for women with Hodgkin's disease. Application of the PLISSIT model. *Cancer Nursing, 9,* 248–255.

Derogatis, L. R. (1980). Breast and gynecologic cancers. *Frontiers in Radiation Therapy and Oncology, 14,* 1–11.

Dobkin, K. A., & Broadwell, D. C. (1986). Nursing considerations for the patient undergoing colostomy surgery. *Seminars in Oncology Nursing, 2,* 249–255.

Donahue, D. C. (1978). Sexual rehabilitation of gynecologic cancer patients. *Medical Aspects of Human Sexuality, 2,* 51–52.

Drench, M. E. (1994). Changes in body image secondary to disease and injury. *Rehabilitation Nursing, 19*(1), 31–36.

Dudas, S. (1991). Rehabilitation of the patient with cancer. *Journal of Enterostomal Therapy, 18*(2), 61–67.

Enelow, A. J. (1975). Psychosocial rehabilitation for cancer patients. *Frontiers in Radiation Therapy and Oncology, 10,* 178–182.

Feldman, J. E. (1989). Ovarian failure and cancer treatment: Incidence and interventions for the perimenopausal woman. *Oncology Nursing Forum, 16*(5), 651–657.

Fetter, M. P. (1987). Reaching a level of sexual comfort. *Health Education, 18,* 6–8.

Fisher, S. G. (1983). The psychosexual effect of cancer and cancer treatment. *Oncology Nursing Forum, 10*(2), 63–67.

Fisher, S. G. (1985). The sexual knowledge and attitudes of oncology nurses: Implications for nursing education. *Seminars in Oncology Nursing, 1,* 63–68.

Fisher, S. G., & Levin, D. L. (1983). The sexual knowledge and attitudes of professional nurses caring for oncology patients. *Cancer Nursing, 6,* 55–61.

Foltz, A. T. (1987). The influence of cancer on self concept and quality of life. *Seminars in Oncology Nursing, 3,* 303–312.

Glasgow, M., Halfin, V., & Althausen, A. F. (1987). Sexual response and cancer. *CA: A Cancer Journal for Clinicians, 37,* 322–332.

Golden, J. S., & Golden, M. (1980). Cancer and sex. *Frontiers in Radiation Therapy and Oncology, 14,* 59–65.

Golden, M. (1983). Female sexuality and crisis of mastectomy. *Danish Medical Bulletin, 30*(Suppl. 2), 13–16.

Greenberg, D. B. (1984). The measurement of sexual dysfunction in cancer patients. *Cancer, 53*(Suppl.), 2281–2285.

Grunberg, K. J. (1986). Sexual rehabilitation of the cancer patient undergoing ostomy surgery. *Journal of Enterostomal Therapy, 13,* 148–152.

Harris, R., Good, R. S., & Pollack, L. (1982). Sexual behavior of gynecologic cancer patients. *Archives of Sexual Behavior, 11,* 503–510.

Holmberg, L., Omne-Poten, M., Burns, T., Adami, H. O., & Bergstrom, R. (1989). Psychosocial adjustment after mastectomy and breast-conserving treatment. *Cancer, 64*(4), 969–974.

Jenkins, B. (1988). Patients' report of sexual changes after treatment for gynecologic cancer. *Oncology Nursing Forum, 15*(3), 349–354.

Johnson, J. (1986). Sexual concerns of the cancer patient. *Nursing Republic of South Africa Verpleging, 1*(10), 24–25.

Jusenius, K. (1981). Sexuality and gynecologic cancer. *Cancer Nursing, 4,* 479–484.

Kaempfer, S. H. (1981). The effects of cancer chemotherapy on reproduction: A review of the literature. *Oncology Nursing Forum, 8*(1), 11–18.

Kaempfer, S. H., Hoffman, D. J., & Wiley, F. M. (1983). Sperm banking: A reproductive option in cancer therapy. *Cancer Nursing, 4,* 31–38.

Kaempfer, S. H., & Major, P. (1986). Fertility considerations in the gynecologic cancer patient. *Oncology Nursing Forum, 13*(1), 27.

Kaempfer, S. H., Wiley, F. M., Hoffman, D. J., & Rhodes, E. A. (1985). Fertility considerations and procreative alternatives in cancer care. *Seminars in Oncology Nursing, 1,* 25–34.

Lamb, M. (1985). Sexual dysfunction in the gynecologic oncology patient. *Seminars in Oncology Nursing, 1,* 9–17.

Lamb, M. A. (1990). Psychosexual issues: The woman with gynecologic cancer. *Seminars in Oncology Nursing, 6*(3), 237–243.

Lamb, M. A. (1991a). Sexual adaptation of women treated for endometrial cancer. In *Dissertation Abstracts International.* Boston, MA: Boston College.

Lamb, M. A. (1991b). Effects of chemotherapy on fertility in long-term survivors. *Dimensions in Oncology Nursing, 5*(4), 13–16.

Lamb, M. A. (1993a). The influence of endometrial cancer on intimate relationships: Part I. *Meniscus, 2*(1), 17–20.

Lamb, M. A. (1993b). The influence of endometrial cancer on intimate relationships: Part II. *Meniscus, 2*(2), 32–38.

Lamb, M. A. (1995). Effect of cancer on the sexuality and fertility of women. *Seminars in Oncology Nursing, 11*(2), 120–127.

Lamb, M. A., & Sheldon, T. A. (1994). The sexual adaptation of women treated for endometrial cancer. *Cancer Practice, 2*(2), 103–113.

Lamb, M., & Woods, N. F. (1981). Sexuality and the cancer patient. *Cancer Nursing, 4,* 137–144.

LaMonica, G., Audisio, R. A., Tamburini, M., Filberti, A., & Ventafridda, V. (1985). Incidence of sexual dysfunction in male patients treated surgically for rectal malignancy. *Diseases of the Colon and Rectum, 23,* 937–940.

MacElveen-Hoehn, P. (1985). Sexual assessment and counseling. *Seminars in Oncology Nursing, 1,* 69–75.

Masters W., & Johnson, V. (1966) *Human sexual response.* Boston: Little, Brown & Co.

McMullin, M. (1992). Holistic care of the patient with cervical cancer. *Nursing Clinics of North America, 27*(4), 847–858.

Metcalfe, M. C., & Fischman, S. H. (1985). Factors affecting the sexuality of patients with head and neck cancer. *Oncology Nursing Forum, 12*(2), 21–25.

Miller, K. D. (1994). Hodgkin's disease: Impact on childbearing. *Journal of Perinatal and Neonatal Nursing, 7*(4), 1–12.

Mims, F. H., & Swenson, M. (1980). *Sexuality: A nursing perspective.* New York: McGraw-Hill Book Co.

Moth, I., Andreasson, B., Jensen, S. B., & Bock, J. E. (1983). Sexual function and somatopsychic reactions after vulvectomy. *Danish Medical Bulletin, 30*(Suppl. 2), 27–30.

Ofman, U. S. (1993). Psychosocial and sexual implications of genitourinary cancers. *Seminars in Oncology Nursing, 9*(4), 286–292.

Penninger, J. I., Moore, S. B., & Frager, S. R. (1985). After the ostomy: Helping your patient reclaim his sexuality. *RN, 48*(4), 46–50.

Petty, F., & Noyes, R. (1981). Depression secondary to cancer. *Biologic Psychiatry, 16,* 1203–1220.

Quigley, K. M. (1989). The adult cancer survivor: Psychosocial consequences of cure. *Seminars in Oncology Nursing,* 5(1), 63–69.

Roberts, C. S., Rossetti, K., Cone, D., & Cavanagh, D. (1992). Psychosocial impact of gynecologic cancer: A descriptive study. *Journal of Psychosocial Oncology,* 10(1), 99–109.

Rubin, P. (Ed). (1983). *Clinical oncology: A multidisciplinary approach.* New York: American Cancer Society.

Rutherford, D. E. (1988). Assessing psychosexual needs of women experiencing lumpectomy: A challenge for research. *Cancer Nursing,* 11(4), 244–249.

Schain, W. S. (1980). Sexual functioning, self-esteem and cancer care. *Frontiers in Radiation Therapy and Oncology,* 14, 12–19.

Schain, W. S. (1981). Role of the sex therapist in the care of the cancer patient. *Frontiers in Radiation Therapy and Oncology,* 15, 168–183.

Schain, W. S. (1985). Breast cancer surgeries and psychosexual sequelae: Implications for remediation. *Seminars in Oncology Nursing,* 1, 200–205.

Schrover, L. R., & Fife, M. (1985). Sexual counseling of patients undergoing radical surgery for pelvic or genital cancer. *Journal of Psychosocial Oncology,* 3(3), 21–41.

Schrover, L. R., Gonzales, J., & von Eschenbach, A. C. (1986). Sexual and marital relationships after radiotherapy for seminoma. *Urology,* 27, 117–123.

Schrover, L. R., von Eschenbach, A. C., Smith, D. B., & Gonzales, J. (1984). Sexual rehabilitation of urologic cancer patients: A practical approach. *CA: A Cancer Journal for Clinicians,* 34(2), 66–73.

Schwarz-Appelbaum, J., Dedrick, J., Jusenius, K., & Kirchner, C. W. (1984). Nursing care plans: Sexuality and treatment of breast cancer. *Oncology Nursing Forum,* 11(6), 16–24.

Sewell, H. H., & Edwards, D. W. (1980). Pelvic genital cancer: Body image and sexuality. *Frontiers of Radiation Therapy and Oncology,* 14, 35–41.

Shapiro, E. (1987). Modified surgery curbs dysfunction. *Cope,* 1(10), 52.

Shipes, E. (1987). Sexual functioning following ostomy surgery. *Nursing Clinics of North America,* 22, 303–310.

Shipes, E., & Lehr, S. (1982). Sexuality and the male cancer patient. *Cancer Nursing,* 5, 375–381.

Smith, D. B. (1989). Sexual rehabilitation of the cancer patient. *Cancer Nursing,* 12, 10–15.

Smith, D. B., Babaian, R. J. (1992). The effects of treatment for cancer on male fertility and sexuality. *Cancer Nursing,* 15(4), 271–275.

Spengler, A. (1983). Radical prostatectomy and sexuality. *Sexuality and Disability,* 6, 155–166.

Stadil, F. (1983). Intestinal stomas. *Danish Medical Bulletin.* 30(Suppl. 2), 35–37.

Thurber, W. A. (1989). Offspring of childhood cancer survivors. *Journal of the Association of Pediatric Oncology Nurses,* 6(1), 17–19.

von Eschenbach, A. C., & Schrover, L. R. (1984). The role of sexual rehabilitation in the treatment of patients with cancer. *Cancer,* 54(Suppl.), 2662–2667.

Wabrek, A. J., & Gunn, J. L. (1984, Nov./Dec.). Sexual and psychological implications of gynecologic malignancy. *JOGN Nursing,* 371–376.

Walbroehl, G. S. (1985). Sexuality in cancer patients. *American Family Physicians,* 31, 153–158.

Welch-McCaffrey, D. (1983). Dyspnea and sexual intercourse. *Oncology Nursing Forum,* 10(1), 80.

Wellisch, D. K. (1985). The psychologic impact of breast cancer on relationships. *Seminars in Oncology Nursing,* 1, 195–199.

Williams, H. A., Wilson, M. E., Hongladarom, G., & McDonell, M. (1986). Nurses' attitudes toward sexuality in cancer patients. *Oncology Nursing Forum,* 13(2), 39–43.

Williamson, M. L. (1992). Sexual adjustment after hysterectomy. *Journal of Obstetric Gynecologic and Neonatal Nursing,* 21(1), 42–47.

Wilson, M. E., & Williams, H. A. (1988). Oncology nurses' attitudes and behaviors related to sexuality of patients with cancer. *Oncology Nursing Forum,* 15(1), 49–53.

Wise, T. N. (1978). Sexual functioning in neoplastic disease. *Medical Aspects of Human Sexuality,* 12, 16–31.

Wood, J. D., & Tombrink, J. (1983). Impact of cancer on sexuality and self image: A group program for patients and partners. *Social Work in Health Care,* 8(4), 45–54.

Woods, N. F. (1990). *Human sexuality in health and illness* (3rd ed.). St. Louis: C. V. Mosby Co.

World Health Organization. (1975). *Education and treatment in human sexuality: The training of health professionals, Report of a WHO meeting.* Technical report series no. 572. Geneva: Author.

Wujcik, D., Carbonell, M. A., Taseff, L., Sciarra, L., & Isaac, E. (1986). Managing the patient with testicular cancer. *Nursing 86,* 16(8), 42–45.

Yarbro, C., & Perry, M. C. (1985). The effect of cancer therapy on gonadal function. *Seminars in Oncology Nursing,* 1, 3–8.

Karin Dufault • Linda K. Birenbaum

Alterations in mobility present some challenging problems to the nurse caring for the person with cancer. Although they are less obvious than such problems as nutrition and pain, alterations in mobility may profoundly affect the quality of life for the person and family as they deal with the disease and its treatment (McNally, Stair, & Somerville, 1985). In this chapter the interaction between normal physiology and mobility is examined, after which some of the psychosocial factors that affect and are affected by mobility are discussed. Information related to management of specific nursing diagnoses and some of the common problems of cancer-related immobility also are presented.

THE INTERACTION OF NORMAL PHYSIOLOGY AND MOBILITY

EFFECTS OF POSITION AND WEIGHT BEARING

The maintenance of normal muscle and bone strength and structure is partially dependent on weight bearing and normal levels of activity. Both weight bearing and normal mobility help to maintain the balance between bone formation and resorption and muscle mass and strength (Potter & Perry, 1993). The effect of position on mobility is usually produced by limitation of position, which prevents weight bearing or full muscle use, thereby decreasing joint motion and muscle strength.

The direct effect of position and weight bearing is of greatest importance for mobility of the musculoskeletal system, but it is also important to keep in mind the other physical functions that are influenced by mobility: metabolic, respiratory, cardiovascular, integumentary, and eliminative (originally described by Olson in 1967 [Box 63–1 and Table 63–1]).

Metabolic functions undergo changes as the metabolic rate is decreased. Tissue atrophies and protein catabolism increases, bone demineralization begins, alteration in the exchange of nutrients occurs, and gastrointestinal disturbances develop (Olson, 1967). *Respiratory* changes then occur, partly as a direct effect of the immobility, partly as an effect of the metabolic changes. Hemoglobin decreases, lung expansion decreases, and generalized muscle weakness and stasis of secretions develop. The major changes in cardiovascular functioning are orthostatic hypotension, increased cardiac workload, and thrombus formation. Immobility has its greatest effects on the integrity of the *skin* of elderly people with altered sensory or motor function and nutritional or metabolic changes—a fair description of many persons with cancer. Any one of these factors puts the person at risk for alterations in skin integrity (Olson, 1967). In the *eliminative* processes, several changes relate to altered mobility: urine reten-

---

Box 63–1. *Classic Article: The Hazards of Immobility*

Olson, E. (1967). The hazards of immobility. *American Journal of Nursing, 67,* 780–797.

In April 1967, in the *American Journal of Nursing,* a series of articles was published that changed immeasurably the way in which nurses thought about immobility and its effect on the people for whom they were caring. With co-authors Lida F. Thompson, Joyce McCarthy, Bonnie Jean Johnson, Ruth E. Edmonds, Lois M. Schroeder, and Mildred Wade, Edith Olson presented a comprehensive look at the effects of immobility. Effects on cardiovascular, respiratory, gastrointestinal, motor, and urinary function were examined in detail. Additionally, effects on metabolic and psychosocial equilibrium were presented. The studies were thoroughly referenced, and conclusions were drawn. Nursing implications were then offered in each area.

This series of articles grew out of a symposium presented by these authors at the annual meeting of the Colorado Nurses' Association in the spring of 1966, and these authors have continued to make many contributions to nursing and nursing literature over the years.

Any nurse interested in the problems of immobility will do well to thoroughly study this series. It truly deserves the designation "classic."

---

tion, renal calculi, and urinary tract infection may result, and constipation becomes a common problem.

EFFECTS OF MUSCLE AND JOINT MOVEMENT

The general body effects of position and weight bearing on immobility have been discussed, but the

TABLE 63–1. *Potential Effects of Immobility*

Physiologic
Metabolic
    Reduced metabolic rate
    Reduced adrenal corticoids
    Stress reactions
Cardiovascular
    Orthostatic hypotension
    Increased workload
    Thrombus formation
Skin
    Decubitus ulcers
Respiratory
    Decreased respiratory movement
    Stasis of secretions
    Oxygen-carbon dioxide imbalance
Musculoskeletal
    Osteoporosis
    Contractures
Urinary
    Urinary tract stones
Gastrointestinal
    Ingestion
    Elimination
        Suppression of defecation
        Constipation

Psychosocial
Altered perceptions
Altered social roles
Altered mood states

Developmental
Delayed achievement of developmental tasks
Regression to previous developmental level

(Adapted from Olson, E. [1967]. The hazards of immobility. *American Journal of Nursing, 67,* 780–797.)

specific effects of decreased muscle and joint use also need to be considered. Normal range of motion can be maintained only with full use and normal activity. With increasing age, range of motion, particularly in the spine, tends to decrease even in persons without actual disease conditions, although these changes are extremely variable from person to person.

The mechanical effect of muscle and, indirectly, joint movement, is part of the body's mechanism for maintaining adequate venous return. Alterations result in increased venous stasis and increase the threat of thrombus formation.

Skin integrity is protected indirectly with normal mobility of the muscles and joints, as the maintenance of venous return helps prevent stasis and edema. In addition, normal movement prevents undue pressure on any particular area of the skin, again helping to guard against the dangers that pressure and ischemia present to the skin.

It is clear how important normal mobility is to the maintenance of the integrity of physical functioning. When the effects of disease, treatment, and aging are considered, they must be viewed within the context of these interactions of activity and normal systemic functioning (Gregor, McCarthy, Chwirchak, Meluch, & Mion, 1986).

PATHOPHYSIOLOGIC FACTORS THAT INTERFERE WITH MOBILITY IN THE PERSON WITH CANCER

EFFECT OF DISEASE PROCESS AND TREATMENT

Alterations in mobility stemming from the disease process may be categorized as either structural or functional. In structural effects, there is actual disease involvement of the mobilizing body parts themselves (e.g., bones, muscle, nerves, or connective tissue). These structural changes may be due to destruction of tissue, or they may be a result of pain or edema in the body part, which then leads to alterations in the mobilizing structures themselves. In functional effects, the altered mobility is an indirect effect, such as fatigue or altered mental status, that has been produced by the disease process. The alteration means that, initially, at least, there is no damage to the mobilizing structures, but because the person is unable to use those structures normally, owing to the absence of strength, coordination, and so forth, the lack of use results in structural changes, as discussed earlier.

The disease process may have a direct effect on mobility, but an equal problem may be the effect of the treatment. Again, this may be structural: surgery, radiation, and even chemotherapy may cause actual changes in the body parts that are necessary for mobility. In addition, these same treatment methods may cause various effects that indirectly produce a functional loss of mobility: pain, fatigue, and weakness all may at some time be part of the person's daily life and have a profound effect on the ability to be normally mobile.

EFFECT OF LYMPHEDEMA

Lymphedema may be produced in the person with cancer by the disease itself, with malignant involvement of lymph nodes or surrounding structures causing obstruction of lymph flow and preventing the movement of these osmotically active materials back into the systemic circulation (Kneisl & Ames, 1986). This same effect may be produced by surgery or radiation during or subsequent to the treatment process as healing and fibrosis occur. Obviously, the location of the alteration will be the most important determinant of the effect on mobility (Porth, 1994). Lymphedema, although a less common cause of lower extremity immobility in cancer survivors, is still a relatively common problem in the arms of women with radical or modified radical mastectomies. Even with less extensive breast surgery, both discomfort and decreased mobility may result in the affected arm when the patient undergoes lymph node dissection or radiation. It is important to keep in mind that in chronic edema the tissue spaces become stretched so that less filtration pressure is needed to maintain the edema. This stretching then makes permanent correction of the edema difficult (Porth, 1994). Prevention of extensive edema that may threaten mobility of any body part then becomes an important goal of posttreatment nursing care. Treatment with radiation or surgery is sometimes helpful in relieving the obstruction that is causing the edema.

EFFECT OF TUMOR INVOLVEMENT OF THE BONE

Characteristically, the person with a primary bone tumor has a painful mass. This pain often is not actually of immobilizing degree at the outset but may cause alteration in normal mobility as the person's usual activities begin to be curtailed owing to pain (Price & Wilson, 1992). Because primary lesions of the bone most commonly occur in children and young people, often in the bones of the extremities, the effect of

increasing disease and subsequent treatment on mobility is likely to be profound. As pain increases, mobility becomes much more limited. In addition, a tumor may cause pressure on a peripheral nerve, causing numbness, a limp, or limitation of movement.

Treatment is most commonly surgical and is certain to produce some modification in mobility; in addition, often some alteration will be permanent. Cryosurgery, radiotherapy, and chemotherapy may also be used at some stages of treatment and may produce either temporary or permanent alteration in mobility of the affected part. Again, treatment may cause additional pain and fatigue, which compound the total physical impact and further decrease the person's mobility. Secondary use of radiation therapy, chemotherapy, or surgery may be helpful in reducing pain and therefore increasing mobility. Both the presence of metastatic tumor and its treatment have some of the same effects on mobility as those of primary bone tumor in that bone pain will probably occur, with its immobilizing effect, and again treatment may produce side effects that compound the immobilization.

Additional threats to mobility often are present for the person with bony metastasis. The population with metastatic disease is likely to be an older group than that of patients with primary disease, so that mobility is already threatened, either from the aging process itself or from other systemic disease. Usually these people have been treated, or the disease itself may have resulted in immobilizing residual effects. Treatment options may be limited because of the previous treatment. In metastatic disease, the extremities are less likely to be affected, and the bones of the spine, rib cage, and pelvis are more commonly involved. Tumor in these locations often has a profound effect on the person's ability to be normally mobile, whether because of pain at the site or because of weakened bone structure, which may result in pathologic fractures.

EFFECT OF SPINAL CORD COMPRESSION

Some primary spinal cord tumors may cause alteration in central nervous system function. These are often relatively slowly progressive, and the neurologic deficits appear later in the course of disease because the spinal cord is able to adapt to the compression (Price & Wilson, 1992). With metastatic lesions, however, neurologic change is often rapid and progressive. Because of the anatomic structure of the spine, symptoms generally begin well below the site of the lesion, and the level of impairment ascends as the compression increases and deeper cord levels are affected. Cord compressions can also disturb the patient's sense of position, producing ataxia with its resultant disturbance of mobility. Metastatic tumors are likely to be extradural, and pain—either localized or radicular—is often the first symptom (Price & Wilson, 1992). The localized pain tends to be increased by movement and is particularly immobilizing. Actual compression of the spine may come from encroachment of the tumor, collapse of the vertebral column, or hemorrhage from the tumor. Once the compression begins it rapidly becomes total—paresthesia and sensory loss progress to irreversible paraplegia unless decompression can be accomplished (Price & Wilson, 1992). Decompression is most likely to be surgical, although radiation and chemotherapy may also be employed in this urgent situation. Fortunately, early recognition and management of the problem can prevent these serious effects. This makes the nursing responsibilities of assessment and rapid diagnosis of altered sensation and functioning critical.

EFFECT OF CENTRAL NERVOUS SYSTEM INVOLVEMENT

Because of the diversity of brain tumor types, location, and size, it is difficult to generalize about their effect on mobility. Altered mobility observed in persons with brain tumors most often is related to treatment effects occurring after the surgery, radiation therapy, or chemotherapy used to treat the primary lesion. This treatment may cause alteration in mobility because of sided weakness or seizures, just as the disease itself may. In addition, as is true for countless situations, the direct effects of either the treatment or the disease itself, such as pain and fatigue, may have considerable effect on the ability of the person to be normally mobile (Ragnarsson, 1993).

PSYCHOSOCIAL FACTORS THAT INTERFERE WITH MOBILITY IN THE PERSON WITH CANCER

Besides the pathophysiologic features that alter the ability of a person with cancer to be freely mobile, numerous psychosocial factors influence mobility. Some are described by Olson (Table 63–1). One manner of examining the psychosocial factors is to consider patterns of activities of daily living, or general lifestyle, and of coping.

PATTERNS OF ACTIVITIES OF DAILY LIVING

The degree of functional independence experienced by a person may influence both the responses to changes in mobility and the changes themselves. Functional independence encompasses the wide range of activities engaged in by persons during the course of a 24-hour day and are often described as activities of daily living and self-care. Activities of daily living capabilities often are considered in light of whether the person is independent in bed, in the home, or in the community.

Among the activities that are examined to determine functional independence are the following: (1) bathing, (2) communicating, (3) exercising, (4) grooming, (5) dressing, (6) eating, (7) bed and hygiene activities, (8) mobility, (9) transferring, (10) recreation, (11) socializing, (12) homemaking, (13) sexual activities, (14) avocational activities, and (15) vocational activities (Chiou & Burnett, 1985; Martin, Holt, & Hicks,

1980). A study by Chiou and Burnett (1985) indicated the importance of patients' values as they relate to specific activities of daily living. The value placed on the activity was an important factor to consider in identifying rehabilitation goals in this study, which involved stroke patients. The relative value of the activities that indicated functional independence for the person with cancer may also have a bearing on the response of the person to alteration in self-care and more specifically to alterations in mobility. Awareness of the degree to which alterations in mobility interfere with the functional independence activities of greatest value to the person can provide insights into understanding the real impact of the changes. The understanding can guide nursing interventions as they relate both to mobility and to enhancement of the other significantly valued activities of daily living. Among the most highly valued activities of daily living are those related to mobility.

Decreased mobility and activities of daily living ranked highest of rehabilitation problems identified in cancer patients in several studies (Cancer Rehabilitation Coordination Team, 1978; Donovan & Girton, 1984; Lehmann, DeLisa, & Warren, 1978).

GENERAL LIFESTYLE PATTERNS

Lifestyle patterns represent a complex outcome of many personal, interpersonal, environmental, and societal factors, which arise not only from the person's present situation but also from his or her life history and heredity. Carnevali and Patrick (1979) defined lifestyle as the totality of a person's approach to living. It incorporates such characteristics as preferences for independence or dependence, high or low stress levels, spontaneity and change or structure and regularity, extroversion or introversion, rapid or slow pace, and high or low physical activity. The preferences translate into observable behaviors in approaching routine as well as unusual events.

Health professionals have focused attention on the identifying elements of healthy and unhealthy lifestyle patterns. Major determinants of health include (1) nutrition, (2) physical fitness, (3) psychosocial stressors, (4) stress management or reduction, and (5) sense of purpose and will. Other important dimensions of lifestyle include the relationship network and the strength of the family structure, cultural variables, and economic and educational factors.

The Health Hazard Appraisal by Milsum (1980) is one instrument for examining lifestyle in an effort to promote health by preventing death and disability attributable to reducible risk. Three patterns are characterized: sedentary, middle-aged workers whose risk is two or more times the average risk for disease; persons who have an aggregate risk somewhat above average and whose appraised age is perhaps up to 5 years above actual age; and persons living at very low risk and for whom the emphasis is on the desirability of maintaining and improving the present good status.

It can be hypothesized that the healthier the lifestyle (before and during the cancer course), the more likely that a person will possess the physical, psychologic, social, and spiritual resources to cope with the effects resulting from the diagnosis of cancer, including alterations in mobility. Understanding the general lifestyle patterns of the person with cancer and the family can further the understanding of the impact that altered mobility has and the potential problems it imposes on the person as well as of the coping resources available to deal with the changes.

COPING PATTERNS

Coping has been described by Lazarus and Folkman (1984) as "constantly changing cognitive and behavioral efforts to manage specific external and/or internal demands that are appraised as taxing or exceeding the resources of the person" (p. 141). Weisman (1979), in speaking of coping with cancer, states that coping is "what one does about a problem in order to bring about relief, reward, quiescence, and equilibrium" (p. 27). Coping functions with a problem-solving focus when efforts are made to cope with the stress itself by dealing with obstacles and opportunities in the environment and in oneself. Coping functions with an emotion focus when efforts are made to regulate emotional stress and distress palliatively.

The Omega Project at Massachusetts General Hospital (1974-1979) provided descriptions of how cancer patients cope or fail to cope. Weisman and Worden (1977) identified the factors associated with patients who are at high risk of emotional distress (vulnerability):

- Marital problems
- Living alone
- Economic marginality
- Alcohol abuse
- Multiple problems in family of origin
- Lack of church affiliation
- Psychiatric history
- Suicidal ideation
- Low ego strength
- High anxiety level
- Pessimistic attitude
- Advanced stage of cancer
- Multiple reported symptoms
- Multiple current concerns and problems of all types with poor resolution
- Little help or support expected or received
- Health professionals seen as unhelpful or unconcerned

The greater the number of high-risk factors present, the greater the risk of suffering distress and failing to cope with the stressors of the diagnosis and treatment of cancer. Coping strategies identified by Weisman and Worden (1977) as the most likely to be *ineffective* were:

- Suppression and passivity
- Isolation and withdrawal
- Blaming others
- Blaming self

In addition to determining the least effective coping strategies, the researchers identified the three most *effective* coping strategies—that is, those that relieved distress and resolved the problem—were confrontation, redefinition, and cooperative compliance. A conclusion drawn by Weisman and Worden (1977) was that the dividing crux between good copers and bad copers is the difference between resourcefulness and rigidity and between constructive optimism versus a pessimism that expects replication of earlier defeats.

In a more recent study of 668 cancer patients, five patterns of coping with cancer were identified (Dunkel-Schetter, Feinstein, Taylor & Falke, 1992):

- Seeking or using social support
- Focusing on the positive
- Distancing
- Cognitive escape-avoidance
- Behavioral escape-avoidance

Examples of coping strategies related to these patterns are presented in Table 63–2. While attempts have been made to identify individual coping styles to predict maladaptive coping, the evidence varies. It is generally thought that cancer patients use multiple strategies to cope with cancer (Dunkel-Schetter et al., 1992).

One coping pattern, seeking social support, includes information seeking, which suggests another line of research that helps plan nursing interventions. Degner and Beaton (1987), Degner and Russell (1988), and Neufeld, Degner, and Dick (1993) identified four preferences for health care decision making:

- Provider-controlled decision making
- Patient-controlled decision making
- Family-controlled decision making
- Jointly controlled decision making.

Neufeld et al. (1993) have described how nursing intervention that fosters patient involvement in treatment decisions helps the patient to ascribe meaning and thus commit to action within the context of a cancer diagnosis.

By taking time to ascertain factors placing the patient at risk, to discover people's past patterns of coping with stress, their perception of the cancer experience (as harm, threat, or challenge), their preference for participating in health care decisions, and their available coping resources, health professionals can better help persons who are experiencing the new stress of living with alterations in mobility. Coping resources include problem-solving skills, energy, health, morale, social, spiritual, and economic support systems, and their general beliefs and specific beliefs about causes of cancer. It is possible that use of a person's least effective coping strategies can lead to the depression, apathy, hopelessness, and helplessness that result in decreased physical activity and greater immobility than his or her physical condition would suggest. By the same token, a person's psychosocial response to physiologically imposed immobility may be depression, negative behavioral changes, changes in sleep-wake cycles,

TABLE 63-2. *Examples of Coping Strategies*

Seek and Use Social Support
Talked to someone to find out more
Talked to someone about how feeling
Tried to get professional help
Looked for sympathy or understanding
Asked a friend or relative for advice
Concentrated on the next step

Distancing
Made light of it
Went on as if it were not happening
Looked for silver lining
Treated the illness as a challenge
Knew what had to be done, so increased efforts
Kept others from knowing how bad things were
Lived one day at a time

Behavioral Escape-Avoidance
Avoided being with people
Tried to make myself feel better by eating, drinking
Took it out on other people
Waited to see what would happen before acting
Criticized or lectured myself
Did something just to do something

Cognitive Escape-Avoidance
Hoped a miracle would happen
Prayed
Prepared for the worst
Wished the situation would go away or be over
Went along with fate
Depended mostly on others to handle things
Slept more than usual

Focus on the Positive
Found new faith
Rediscovered what is important
Changed or grew as a person
Changed something about myself
Was inspired to be creative
Thought of how a person I admire would act

(Adapted from Dunkel-Schetter, C., Feinstein, L. G., Taylor, S. E., & Falke, R. L. (1992). Empirical contributions: Patterns of coping with cancer. *Health Psychology, 11*(2), 79–87.)

decreased problem-solving ability, loss of interest in surroundings, increased isolation, and sensory deprivation depending on the coping resources and abilities (Table 63–1). Use of more effective coping strategies and resources results in a more positive picture, in which alterations in mobility are seen as one more challenge to be overcome or adapted to achieve yet other goals or to ensure fulfillment of treasured hopes.

PROCESS OF ASSESSMENT IN THE DIAGNOSTIC PROCESS

ASSESSMENT OF THE PROBLEM

The nurse will need to assess the level of mobility in managing the care of any client using the theoretic framework with which the nurse is most comfortable. Within that assessment, certain patterns must be discerned if an adequate nursing diagnosis is to be made. The Standards for Oncology Nursing Practice (American Nurses' Association & Oncology Nursing Society [ANA-ONS], 1987) point out the nurse's responsibility to collect data in a systematic and continuous fashion. Nursing data need to be gathered regarding both the level of mobility and the potential for sequelae related to immobility. The data collected must be both objective and subjective (ANA-ONS, 1987).

The two aspects of data gathering—history and physical assessment—must be attended to. There are many indexes for measuring the activities of daily living—probably the most useful way to examine the alteration in mobility. Because more than 43 different indexes have been developed, few of which have been documented empirically, it is difficult for the nurse to find a generally accepted means of evaluating the patient's level of activity (Feinstein, Joseph, & Wells, 1986). Probably the two most commonly used scales are the Karnofsky Scale (Table 63–3) and the Barthel Index (Table 63–4). Although few scales have been developed specifically for oncology patients, the exist-

TABLE 63-3. *Patient Performance Rating (Karnofsky)*

Able to carry on normal activity; no special care	100	Normal; no complaints; no evidence of disease
	90	Able to carry on normal activity; minor signs or symptoms of disease
	80	Normal activity with effort; some signs or symptoms of disease
Unable to work; able to live at home; cares for most personal needs; a varying amount of assistance is needed	70	Cares for self; unable to carry on normal activity or to do active work
	60	Requires occasional assistance but is able to care for most needs
	50	Requires considerable assistance and frequent medical care
Unable to care for self; requires equivalent institutional or hospital care; disease may be progressing rapidly	40	Disabled; requires special care and assistance
	30	Severely disabled; hospitalization is indicated, although death not imminent
	20	Very sick; hospitalization necessary
	10	Moribund; fatal processes progressing rapidly
	1	Unconscious
	0	Dead

(Data from Chang, S. K., & Hawes, K. A. [1983]. The adequacy of the Karnofsky rating and global adjustment to illness scale as outcome measures in cancer rehabilitation and continuing care. In P. F. Engstrom, P. N. Anderson, & L. E. Mortenson [Eds.], *Advances in cancer control: Research and development* [pp. 429–443]. New York: Alan R. Liss, Inc.)

TABLE 63–4. *Barthel Index*

INDEPENDENT		DEPENDENT		
INTACT	LIMITED	HELPER	NULL	
10	5	1	1	Drink from cup, feed from dish
5	5	3	0	Dress upper body
5	5	2	0	Dress lower body
0	0	−2	0	Don brace or prosthesis
5	5	0	0	Groom
4	4	0	0	Wash or bathe
10	10	5	0	Bladder continence
10	10	5	0	Bowel continence
4	4	2	0	Care of perineum, use of cloth at toilet
15	15	7	0	Transfer, chair
6	5	3	0	Transfer, toilet
1	1	0	0	Transfer, tub or shower
15	15	10	0	Walk on level 50 yards or more
10	10	5	0	Up and down stairs, 1 flight
15	5	0	0	Wheelchair 50 yards/if not walking
				Barthel Total Score

(Data from Jacelon, C. S. [1986]. The Barthel index and other indices of functional ability. *Rehabilitation Nursing, 11*(4), 9–11.)

ing scales often have useful approaches for the nurse's consideration in assessment of the patient with a problem of immobility (Gulick, 1986; Robinson, 1986; Williams, 1986).

The "Social Dependency Scale" was developed to allow health care providers to assess levels of social dependence in patients with progressive diseases and was tested on persons with advanced cancer (Benoliel, McCorkle, & Young, 1980). Mobility competence is one of three capacities measured and includes scores on walking, stair climbing, transferring, and traveling. Maas (1991) provides a nursing assessment guide for impaired physical mobility specifically.

Having developed the initial database that allows assessment of the person's present level of mobility and the potential for sequelae secondary to that level of mobility, the nurse is ready to move on to the identification of actual or potential health problems and formulate the nursing diagnoses on which the care plan can be built (Table 63–5).

DEFINING THE CHARACTERISTICS OF THE PROBLEM

The accepted nursing diagnosis for alterations in mobility is "impaired physical mobility"—related to pathophysiologic, treatment, situational, or maturational factors that alter lower limb or upper limb function (Carpenito, 1995, p. 492). The major characteristics that must be present are the inability to move purposefully within the environment, including bed mobility, transfers, and ambulation, or the inability to move because of imposed restrictions (e.g., bed rest, mechanical devices). Clearly these major characteristics are not uncommon in oncology patients in various stages of disease and treatment. Minor characteristics that may be present are range of motion limitations,

limited muscle strength or control, and impaired coordination. Information gathered from the assessment process should allow the nurse to identify which of these defining characteristics are present or are realistic potentials for a given client.

ETIOLOGIC AND RISK FACTORS RELATED TO THE PROBLEM

Because the diagnostic process allows the nurse to put in rational order the quantities of information accumulated in the database, it is necessary to look beyond the major and minor characteristics of the problem to examine etiologic and contributing factors, for it is toward these factors that nursing interventions are likely to be addressed. For impaired physical mobility, these factors fall into four categories: pathophysiologic, treatment-related, situational, and maturational. The *pathophysiologic* factors may relate to neuromuscular impairment or to musculoskeletal factors. The *treatment-related* factors may be associated with activity restrictions such as bed rest, physical changes such as amputation, or mechanical devices. Side effects of chemotherapy, radiation therapy, or both may be considered both pathophysiologic and treatment-related factors as seen, for example, in ataxia with the neurotoxicity from high-dose Cytosine Arabinoside (Lundquist & Holmes, 1993). *Situational* factors are personal or environmental and may consist of such things as pain or trauma. Finally, *maturational* developmental factors involve primarily the very young or the very elderly and their limitations such as lack of balance in the toddler or cautious gait in the elderly with failing eyesight (Table 63–1).

Having carefully examined the factors that contribute to defining the problem, the nurse is ready to address the planning and implementation of care for

TABLE **63–5.** *Focused Assessment Criteria*

Subjective Data	Objective Data
History of systemic disorders	Dominant hand
Neurologic	Motor function
Cardiovascular	Right arm
Musculoskeletal	Left arm
Respiratory	Right leg
Debilitating diseases	Left leg
History of symptoms that interfere with mobility	Mobility
Symptoms	Ability to turn self
Pain	Ability to sit
Muscle weakness	Ability to stand
Fatigue	Ability to transfer
Criteria	Ability to ambulate
Onset	Weight bearing (assess right and left sides)
Duration	Gait
Location	Assistive devices
Description	Restrictive devices
Frequency	Range of motion (shoulders, elbows, arms, hips, legs)
Precipitated by what?	Endurance
Relieved by what?	Assess
Aggravated by what?	Resting pulse, blood pressure, respirations
History of recent trauma or surgery	Blood pressure, respirations, and pulse after activity
Current drug therapy	After activity, assess for the presence of indicators of hypoxia
Pain	Peripheral circulation
Sedative	Capillary refill time
Laxatives	Skin color, temperature, and turgor
Chemotherapy	Peripheral pulses

the patient with altered mobility. Nursing care interventions are related to other nursing diagnoses that affect or are affected by altered mobility. The following section addresses in more detail the nursing care related to some specific problems of mobility.

MANAGING SPECIFIC PROBLEMS OF MOBILITY

ACTIVITY INTOLERANCE

Activity intolerance (the state in which the person experiences an inability, physiologically and psychologically, to endure or tolerate an increase in activity) is a commonly occurring problem for the person experiencing cancer or cancer treatment and is directly related to the impairment of physical mobility. The causative factors may relate to fatigue or problems with oxygen transport. When these factors have been adequately identified for the patient, nursing action can be taken (Table 63–5). In focusing the assessment data (both subjective and objective), it is helpful first to examine factors that increase fatigue, then to examine the effects of fatigue on the activity level, and then to examine the actual response to activity. It is here that the use of an activity index such as the Karnofsky Scale (Table 63–3) or Barthel Index (Table 63–4) can be useful.

Activity intolerance due to fatigue may be improved by (1) helping the patient to view fatigue as a normal part of treatment rather than a sign of disease progression, and (2) having patients participate in an exercise protocol that provides physical and psychologic benefit plus increased capacity to attend and function (Winningham et al., 1994). Winningham (1991) recommended that cancer patients whose performance status is at least as active as the following movements are eligible for participation in a walking program: ambulate more than 50 per cent of the time and perform instrumental activities of daily living with limited assistance and moderate fatigue. Medical conditions that contraindicate exercise such as irregular or resting heart beat >100 beats/minute were also outlined. Before starting a cancer patient on an exercise program, fitness, age, current medical and psychological status, and the type of cancer should be assessed (Winningham, MacVicar & Burke, 1986). Reading Winningham's (1991) article is also warranted.

After the assessment data are focused, it is possible to examine the results and decide which contributing factors (such as inadequate sleep or rest periods, pain, medications, daily schedule, and lack of incentive) are variably amenable to nursing action. The daily schedule and rest periods require creative problem solving with client, family, and caregivers all involved so that a satisfactory schedule can be developed. Pain management is not discussed here because it is covered extensively elsewhere in this book (see Chapters 57 and 58), but it is crucial to the achievement of optimal activity levels for the person. Further treatment, such as surgery, radiation therapy, and chemotherapy, will at times be indicated to reduce pain and allow increased mobility. Medications sometimes interfere with sleep management for the person with activity intolerance—

either because side effects of medication make adequate sleep difficult or because the scheduling of medications interferes with the sleep cycle. Usually with consideration of the goal (to increase sleep and rest, thereby increasing activity tolerance), it is possible to modify medication schedules to reduce, if not eliminate, the negative effect of the medication regimen on sleep pattern. The lack of incentive may present the greatest challenge to the nurse in motivating the client to increased levels of activity. Although it is difficult to find research documentation for many of the nursing interventions used in this challenging problem, empirically it has been found helpful to make contracts with the client about activity, identify progress, and consider concrete incentives, such as behavioral or physical rewards.

Factors other than disease or treatment also may affect activity tolerance. Age, physical strength, and cardiopulmonary status are all factors that may be of significance in altering the activity tolerance (Kozier, Erb, Blais, Johnson, & Temple, 1993). Having attempted management of the person's activity intolerance, it is essential then to evaluate, both subjectively and objectively, the response to those nursing interventions that were utilized, using both the outcomes designed with the plan and reassessment of the original measures to indicate the progress or lack of progress. The results of this kind of systematic evaluation allow for a decision to discontinue ineffective interventions or increase effective interventions on the basis of clearly identified phenomena rather than subjective impressions.

ALTERATION IN ACTIVITIES OF DAILY LIVING AND SELF-CARE

The success of persons in maintaining functional independence while coping with cancer depends in part on the effectiveness and efficiency of their mobility. When the ability to move around is compromised, so too may be initiative, self-confidence, and motivation to be involved in the activities that had significance to daily life. An essential step in caring for the cancer patient with alterations in mobility is to learn from the patient what the status of his or her mobility is in relationship to usual activities of daily living and customary lifestyle (Williams, 1986). What activities can or cannot be done independently? Which activities require assistance? Which activities are of greatest significance to the person, and which do the family consider most important? Has the patient given up some activities and at what price? Have frequency, duration, and regularity of the activities been changed because of mobility alterations? How is the family affected by the changes? What are the safety concerns related both to the alteration in mobility and the alterations in activities of daily living? One of the most obvious associations between altered mobility and activities of daily living is the fact that most activities of daily living ordinarily occur in certain places within the home, workplace, or community. If a person is unable to walk to the usual setting for whatever reason, independently or

with assistance, other modes of getting there must be used, such as wheelchair or lift. Otherwise, the activity must be performed wherever the person might be spending the majority of time, such as in bed. The extent to which this is a significant deviation from what has been normal to the person's lifestyle may indicate the difficulty of adapting to the change (Carnevali, 1985). Limitations of physical movement of the upper extremities, such as with lymphedema or pathologic fractures, also affect the ability to perform self-care activities.

Another factor to be assessed is whether the process leading to the alteration in mobility is the same process directly affecting alteration in the self-care ability. For example, if spinal cord compression damage is the cause of the alteration in mobility, it may also be the direct cause of deficits in other personal self-care abilities, such as toileting, depending on the level of spinal cord involved. Compensating for the mobility change would not necessarily correct the self-care deficit and would call for additional nursing interventions that targeted the neurologic problems. Pain may be another type of limitation on both mobility and self-care ability.

The assessment also includes objective data in the form of observing mobility factors in relationship to performance of specific activities of daily living. For purposes of this discussion, selected activities of self-care relating to feeding, bathing, toileting, and dressing are presented.

The ability to feed oneself may be affected by the partial or complete incapacity to sit up, one dimension of mobility, that could arise from central nervous system involvement; bone tumors; fractures; fatigue; or ingestion of narcotics, sedatives, or tranquilizers. Nursing interventions can be directed toward understanding the causes of the incapacity to sit up and providing the necessary assistance to place the patient in the most appropriate position for eating that is not contraindicated. Assistive and supportive devices should be used to foster maximum independence for the patient and to provide support and avoid injury for the caregiver.

In some instances a client will have a missing or disabled upper limb that will limit self-feeding. The eating environment should allow sufficient time for eating with adequate supervision and assistance necessary for relearning and adapting. Teaching the use of adaptive devices such as plate guards, utensils with large handles, and rocker knives will also foster independence.

The ability to bathe and groom, toilet, and dress oneself in the usual manner may be related to the ability to sit up, stand, transfer, position, or ambulate independently. Often the person suffering from alterations in mobility is capable of performing the activity once correctly positioned to do so. Nursing actions are directed at enhancing mobility whenever possible by physically supporting the person, using appropriate aids, minimizing environmental barriers, protecting from physical harm, providing privacy, and encouraging muscle-strengthening exercises to prevent further loss and restore function. Collaboration with other members of disciplines involved in rehabilitation, such as physical and occupation therapists, is critical.

Nurses provide assistance in a timely manner with the other self-care activities as needed until the person is able to resume self-care and teach family members how to best foster independence in the patient while at the same time helping in those areas in which the patient is dependent on others to successfully complete the task. The personal care activities of daily living are essential to maintain healthy skin, teeth, alimentary tract, and mucous membranes; to maintain continence; to prevent infection; to promote self-esteem; and to preserve self-concept.

ALTERATION IN BOWEL ELIMINATION

Probably the most significant interaction between mobility and bowel elimination is the tendency to constipation when mobility is seriously limited (Kozier et al., 1993). If the person reports hard stools fewer than three times weekly and complains of difficulty moving the bowels and also is immobile, it is likely that the two are at least partially related. The Constipation Assessment Scale (McMillan & Williams, 1989) designed to assess the presence and severity of constipation is a tool useful to nurses in a variety of settings. A therapeutic bowel regimen will need to be instituted until or unless the immobility problem can be resolved. Corrective measures should include evaluation of the diet with an attempt to increase the fiber. Bran should be used moderately at first, but fresh fruits and vegetables can be encouraged to an amount equal to 800 g per day (four to five servings). Encourage the client to identify fluids and foods that have laxative effects (see Table 63–6). Fluid intake should total at least 2 L daily, with the emphasis on water or fruit juices, not on caffeine drinks. Warm water should be drunk in the morning to stimulate the gastrocolic reflex. Lower body active or passive range of motion exercises are often helpful, especially knee to chest and other abdominal muscle strengthening exercises. Establish a regular time for elimination using the client's normal pattern as much as possible with relation to time, place, position, and equipment. Privacy is extremely important to many people. It may be necessary to use suppositories, stool softeners, or mild laxatives. Constipation should be treated early and consistently for the immobilized person so that it can be managed with the most physiologic and least irritating measures. When the patient is neutropenic or thrombocytopenic, it is particularly important to use care in managing constipation to prevent trauma to the rectal area. Diarrhea as an alteration in bowel elimination may present a problem for the client in that immobility may be increased by the fear of increasing diarrhea ("every time I move, I have another stool"). This is obviously best dealt with by managing the diarrhea effectively, to allow mobility to return to optimal levels.

ALTERATION IN PERIPHERAL TISSUE PERFUSION

One of the classic problems associated with immobility is the development of peripheral thromboses, which present the nursing problem of altered peripheral tissue perfusion. The primary nursing concern here is a preventive one to keep this a potential problem rather than an actual one. When immobility is added to the tendency toward increased clotting often present in persons with cancer (Price & Wilson, 1992), the person is at considerable risk for development of thromboses. Having established that the potential for this problem exists, the nurse will be watchful that blood pressure is maintained at optimum levels to allow adequate tissue perfusion—whether this is a problem of cardiac output or of peripheral circulation—especially as it is affected by the sympathetic nervous system. In addition, cellular perfusion, which is vulnerable to obstruction and changes in oxygen level of the circulating blood, must be maintained. Position and mobility have important effects on the optimal maintenance of tissue perfusion. Antiembolic stockings should be used by these patients. Range of motion exercises at least every shift with arm and leg exercises every 1 to 2 hours should be a part of the plan of care. If the person has a problem of immobility that decreases general activity or promotes obstruction of circulation, it is incumbent on the nurse to be alert to means of minimizing the circulatory compromise that may result, thereby minimizing the potential problem. It is also important to realize that the thrombocytopenic patient may need guidance in the kind and amount of activity that is safe.

IMPAIRMENT OF SKIN INTEGRITY

The major defining characteristics of the potential impairment of skin integrity are that the person reports fatigue and inability to move or turn and is on imposed bed rest or is immobile. Obviously the person with cancer who has altered physical mobility is at high risk for this nursing problem. Institutionalized patients with cancer have a greater risk of pressure sores than other institutionalized patients (Waltman, Bergstrom, Armstrong, Norvell, & Braden, 1991). The best predictors of pressure sores (PS) in newly admitted nursing home residents 65 years and older are the Braden scale for predicting PS risk, increasing age, hyperpyrexia, hypotension, and poor dietary intake of protein (Bergstrom & Braden, 1992). The Braden Scale for Predicting Pressure Sore Risk measures three critical determinants of pressure (mobility, activity, and sensory perception)

TABLE 63–6. *High Fiber and Bowel Stimulating Foods*

Whole grain bread and cereals
Leafy vegetables
Bananas, prunes, dates, figs, rhubarb
Fruit (raw or cooked) with skins (raw or cooked)
Processed bran products (variable amount of fiber):
   100% Bran (7%); All Bran (7.5%);
   Bran Buds (7%); Raisin Bran (3%)
Unprocessed bran (14%) or wheat germ
Nuts and seeds
Legumes: peas, beans, lentils

and three factors influencing the tolerance of the skin and supporting structures for pressure (skin moisture, nutritional status, and friction and shear) (Bergstrom, Demuth, & Braden, 1987). In cancer patients compromised tissue perfusion is an additional predictor of pressure sores (Low, 1990). For example, daunorubicin and doxorubicin can cause cardiomyopathy and congestive heart failure, resulting in decreased perfusion. Radiation therapy in lung fields causing pulmonary fibrosis also reduces oxygenation. Effects of radiation therapy are dose-dependent and can be acute, chronic, or occur as late effects because of tissue necrosis and fibrosis.

Once the person is known to either have an active problem with impaired skin integrity or be at high risk, the nurse's activity will center on trying to reduce the contributing factors involved. Obviously attempts will be made to increase mobility to the greatest extent possible, because this is one of the cardinal factors. In addition, careful management of incontinence, positioning, nutrition, and skin surveillance will be essential if the skin integrity problems are to be minimized. Protective devices will be needed, such as special mattresses and beds, as will skin care regimens. Consultation with an enterostomal skin care therapist is appropriate. Health teaching may be an important part of the management of this problem, especially if the person is being cared for at home. Evaluation of the management of impairments in skin integrity must assess both the repair and healing that occur and the success in preventing new problems.

ALTERATION IN MEANINGFULNESS—POWERLESSNESS

Alterations in mobility and the subsequent experience of dependence can lead to a perceived lack of personal control over one's life, accompanied by apathy, anger, or depression. Each change that threatens the patient's normal lifestyle, creates dependence, threatens adequacy and competence, and removes the person from the decision-making process at any level can bring varying degrees of helplessness and the sense that external forces are controlling. The powerlessness may be manifested by physical findings such as facial flushing or pallor, rapid or bounding pulse, increased blood pressure, sweating, trembling, restlessness, sleep disturbances, changes in eating habits, irritability, demanding behavior, or avoiding or leaving situations.

Powerlessness is a subjective state and therefore requires validation on the part of the person experiencing it. An assessment should include the person's usual level of control and decision making and the effects that losing control produces. By asking the patient questions related to decision-making patterns, role responsibilities, perceptions of control, and personal fears, subjective data will be obtained that will contribute to the nursing assessment of the patient's sense of potential or actual powerlessness. By observing the patient's manner of participation in activities of daily living or information seeking and responses to limits

placed on decision making and self-control, the nurse can identify the factors contributing to the sense of powerlessness and provide opportunities for patient involvement in decision making that can be followed consistently by all caregivers.

Carpenito (1993) pointed out that health care providers' routines are among the factors that can contribute to feelings of powerlessness. She advocated that patients be allowed to manipulate surrounding, such as deciding what is to be kept where; that the daily plan of activities be discussed, with the patient making as many decisions as possible about it; that patients' decisions be respected and followed once given options; and that specific choices be recorded on the care plan to ensure that all staff members will acknowledge the person's preferences. Promises must be kept and opportunities provided for the patient and family to express feelings and participate in care.

Maternalism or paternalism on the part of health professionals needs to be recognized and dealt with, and each health care professional should share actions that he or she discovered to be preferred by the patient. Realistic areas of control can be identified, paving the way for future control (hopes and goals). Enhancing problem-solving skills is also strongly indicated. Helping the person suffering from powerlessness due to altered mobility to interact with others who have also experienced a similar reaction in similar circumstances and were able to regain a sense of meaning, mastery, and power could also be extremely beneficial.

ALTERATION IN EMOTIONAL INTEGRITY—GRIEVING

The grieving process is a normal and expected response to a significant loss of something valued. Losing one's ability to be mobile is in itself a significant loss of freedom and control, which may precipitate yet other losses for the person with cancer. Becoming unable to move may result in loss of ability to perform other activities of daily living independently; loss of body image, self-esteem, and self-identity; loss of social contacts; loss of employment; loss of stable income; and loss of ability to perform usual roles, to name but a few (Baird, 1985). Altered mobility also may herald for the person with cancer the progression of disease and with it the anticipated loss of a personal future and of life itself, with all its associated grief. The family experiences the grieving process along with the patient.

Understanding the typical phases of grief described by researchers (Bowlby, 1961; Eakes, 1993; Glass, 1992; Peretz, 1970; Teel, 1991; Tucker, 1987; Worden, 1982) provides a framework for identifying behaviors that most people are likely to display or express. Common grief reactions include shock and disbelief, yearning and protest, disorganization and despair, reorganization and restitution, and resolution. Grief work involves (1) facing pain with all the sorrow and distress that that entails and recognizing the full reality of what is happening as a normal part of life, and (2) permitting emotional expression of the full range of feelings.

Nursing interventions are directed toward helping the patient and family to express the grief, to describe the meaning of the losses, to competently move through the grieving process with a sense of realistic hope, and to experience the losses as a potential for personal growth. To do so, many of the same strategies as those described in the section on coping are used.

Although most persons are successful in completing grief work, some exhibit signs that the normal grief process has been seriously delayed or disrupted (Whiting & Buckwalter, 1991). Psychiatric intervention is required when one or more of the following characteristics are present: (1) extreme depressive reactions, (2) psychotic break with reality, (3) suicidal tendencies, and (4) substance abuse. The goal of psychotherapy is to transform pathologic grief states to forms of mourning that proceed to resolution.

SENSORY-PERCEPTUAL ALTERATION— VISUAL, KINESTHETIC

Alterations in mobility can result in a decrease in the amount, pattern, and interpretation of incoming stimuli of a physiologic, sensory, motor, and environmental nature, particularly if the person is bedbound. Lack of communication and lack of touch contact may occur when the person affected by restrictions on mobility has relied on relationships outside the home as the primary source of input. Loved ones and acquaintances may be reluctant to maintain contact because of their own sense of helplessness, not knowing what to say or do to be of assistance in the situation.

Decreased mobility also may result in decreased physiologic function of the respiratory, renal, cerebral, circulatory, and sensory systems, which alter sensory-perceptual function. Immobility also may interfere with sleep-rest cycles and with fluid, electrolyte, and nutritional balances, all of which may influence the ways in which the environment is sensed and perceived. Decreased mobility, particularly in the upper extremities of older women, also significantly affects cancer detection activities such as breast self-examination (Baulch, Larson, Dodd, & Deitrich, 1992). In addition, all of these changes may be accompanied by fear of the unknown and potential and actual losses of control, income, familiar persons, objects, and surroundings. Heightened anxiety, depression, fatigue, and boredom contribute to a dulling of sensory responses.

Nursing action can be directed toward manipulating the environment to provide adequate and significant sensory stimulation and toward teaching the patient and family to do likewise. Attention needs to be paid to identifying stimulation, activity, and diversion that are meaningful to the patient. The nurse can assess the environment and make alterations so that color, lighting, sound, and windows are used to make a pleasant, interesting, and inviting environment. Availability of radio, television, videotapes, computers, and reading materials can help maintain interest in the outside world and provide both entertainment and topics for conversation with others. Active diversions with others

(both within the environment in which the person is receiving care and outside it) that do not depend on intact mobility skills can enhance sensory stimulation and decrease the sense of isolation that sensory deprivation fosters. Meaningful human interaction and the sense of value and comfort that comes from it are probably the greatest protectors against sensory-perceptual alterations. Cancer prevention activities can be maintained by teaching patients how to decrease fatigue and pain during the self-examination by taking analgesics prior to the examination, using a comfortable position, and altering actions specific to the breast self-examination (Baulch et al., 1992) or testicular examination.

This section has dealt with the interaction of a number of nursing problems resulting from altered physical mobility. It is vital for the nurse to recognize and deal with these problems concurrently if the client is to reach optimal levels of mobility and if unnecessary complications are to be prevented.

MANAGING SPECIAL PROBLEMS OF MOBILITY

LYMPHEDEMA

With improved surgical techniques and less extensive mastectomy surgery, lymphedema is not as common a problem as it was in the past, but it still does occur and may be of sufficient degree to alter mobility for the patient. The woman with axillary lymph node dissection for breast cancer and the man with prostate cancer or penectomy and groin node dissection most commonly experience this problem. Any time a lymph node dissection has occurred or tumor has interfered with lymphatic circulation, the patient has a potential problem. Physically, the problem in mobility usually occurs because of tissue edema that is secondary to obstruction, whether it is caused by scar tissue or by tumor. The edema must be minimized because it tends to become chronic once it is established in the tissue. Ironically, some of the measures used to reduce edema, such as elevation of the part or elastic bandaging, also tend to reduce mobility, so it is important to strike a balance between one treatment and another to maintain maximum range of motion.

Collateral lymphatic drainage usually develops throughout the first 3 to 4 weeks after surgery. Prevention of edema by elevation of the part, massage and exercise to encourage circulation and maintenance of function, and prevention of infection are particularly important during the first 3 months after surgery. Compliance with rehabilitation exercise is thought to reduce persistent lymphedema, which may linger in 12 per cent of women treated for breast cancer (Hladiuk, Huchcroft, Temple, & Schnurr, 1992). If necessary, postmastectomy lymphedema may be reduced as much as 25 per cent with the use of a wrist-to-shoulder elastic sleeve. A more moderate reduction of 10 to 13 per cent was found in women with postoperative weight gain (Bertelli, Venturini, Forno, Macciavello, & Dini, 1992). A pneumatic pump attached to such a support may also be useful in reducing edema and allow the client to be more comfortable and more mobile. The physical therapist may be an important resource at this point. Client teaching should include avoiding blood pressure measurement, injections, blood drawing, contact with abrasive or irritating materials, and lifting or carrying heavy objects with the affected limb.

Because the problem of lymphedema tends to increase immobility, and because immobility may increase the lymphedema for the person subject to such a problem, it is important that the nurse take early and vigorous action to assist in managing this uncommon but significant problem. A clinical trial of a new drug, (not available in the United States in 1993) 5,6-Benzp-[α]-purone, resulted in slow but safe reduction of lymphedema of the extremities (Casley-Smith, Morgan, & Piller, 1993).

MALIGNANT BONE TUMORS

Because three major symptoms of bone tumors—pain, presence of a mass, and impairment of function—may directly affect mobility, it is not surprising that these tumors present a particular challenge to nursing care with respect to mobility (Porth, 1994).

Management of pain is obviously a high priority if the person is to increase mobility successfully. This subject is covered in detail in Chapters 57 and 58, but the nurse should keep in mind that the nonsteroidal and inflammatory drugs (NSAIDs) alone or with narcotic pain medications may be most helpful for the person with bone involvement. Additionally, radiation therapy may be necessary to reduce tumor bulk and pain. Nonchemical means of pain management, such as diversion and imaging, may be of particular significance, and activity itself may be an adjunct in pain management.

Tumors may cause the bone to erode to the point it cannot withstand the stress of ordinary use or minimal trauma, precipitating a pathologic fracture. Pathologic fractures present a special problem for mobility in the person with bone tumors. In most cases the fracture treatment methods are similar to those for other fractures, but the complexity of managing pathologic fractures is greater because of the underlying disease process. The effect of the fracture and its treatment will depend largely on the location of the tumor. Prophylactic internal fixation is frequently indicated for metastatic lesions involving long bones. When metastatic disease involves the spine, compression fractures frequently occur. When more than one vertebra is involved, surgical stabilization may be difficult, leading to immobility and risk of hyperkalemia (Pritchard, & Burch, 1993).

The treatment of bone tumors, whether by surgery, radiation therapy, or chemotherapy, will usually increase mobility and decrease pain. At times these treatments negatively affect mobility by increasing pain, fatigue, and strength. Because primary bone tumors are more likely to occur in young people, often these patients have the advantage of youthful resiliency of tissue and spirit. However, this is likely to be combined with the typical impatience of youth. All of these can be assets for the nurse working with these clients if

managed wisely. Conversely, the management of metastatic bone tumor often presents real challenges because the person is likely to be older, has other disease or treatments as part of the history, and may focus on many other things besides regaining mobility. In any event, it is likely to require imaginative and careful symptom management on the part of the nurse for the client to achieve optimal mobility when bone tumors are present.

SPINAL CORD COMPRESSION

Spinal cord and nerve root compression of whatever cause (primary spinal cord tumors, metastases from lung, breast, prostate, and kidney, or lymphoma and multiple myeloma) constitutes an oncologic emergency. The characteristic initial symptom in 96 per cent of patients is pain and discomfort in the form of thoracolumbar back pain, often in a beltlike distribution and frequently extending to the groin or legs. The pain is usually worse when supine, so the patient may sleep sitting up. Lower extremity weakness is evident in approximately 74 per cent of patients usually following onset of pain by weeks to months (Henson & Posner, 1993). The weakness, reflex alterations, or paralysis results from upper or lower motor neuron damage.

Unfortunately, the condition often is not recognized until paraplegia is established. The symptoms of muscular weakness, tiredness, heaviness of the extremities, and sensory paresthesia are too often ignored by the patient, physicians, and nurses. When paraplegia or quadriplegia becomes manifest, recovery to a good level of function is unusual.

To prevent devastating complications, it is essential to provide careful nursing assessment and patient teaching emphasizing timely reporting of signs and symptoms related to potential spinal cord compression for those at risk. Other symptoms related to spinal cord compression include constipation and urinary retention with overflow incontinence, altered gait, ataxia, loss of muscle tone, and decreased sensation in the extremities.

Early diagnosis and treatment can lead to complete restoration of function. Treatment may involve an emergency decompression laminectomy, adrenocorticosteroids, radiation therapy, or chemotherapy, depending on tumor sensitivities and previous treatment. If the condition progresses without treatment or with unsuccessful treatment, irreversible paralysis occurs below the level of the spinal cord compression. The degree of compression will have a direct effect on the patient's mobility or immobility status and on the nursing measures taken to prevent loss of function, restore function, compensate for and adapt to permanent loss of elements of mobility, and prevent or minimize further complications arising from impaired mobility. In addition to other interventions, safety measures must be implemented for persons whose ambulatory ability is compromised, such as use of assistive devices, handrails, appropriately adapted chairs and furnishings, clear, wide passageways, and elimination of environmental barriers to activity.

When symptoms have had a rapid onset and treatment does not have the desired effect, patients can experience significant depression because lifestyles are abruptly disrupted and body integrity is threatened. The emotional and financial impact for the patient and family is important for health professionals to identify and acknowledge so appropriate interventions can be used to strengthen coping resources (Sullivan, 1990).

Amputation/Limb-Sparing Procedures

Improvements in histologic diagnosis, clinical staging procedures, surgical techniques, and the use of adjuvant treatments (Hockenberry & Lane, 1988) have led to increased use of limb-sparing procedures (Lawrence et al., 1985; Frieden, Ryniker, Kenan, & Lewis, 1993). The particular type of procedure depends on a variety of factors, but the nursing considerations share commonalities. Preoperative preparation is important with careful attention to type of resection, use of endoprosthesis or grafts, expected functional results, possible deficits, potential alterations in daily routine, and realistic goals of function following surgery (Hockenberry & Lane, 1988). Postoperative care is similar to that of other extensive orthopedic surgery, including pain management, with additional attention to the graft site when appropriate. Postoperative rehabilitation, once begun slowly (Hockenberry & Lane, 1988), now begins 1 day after surgery with active exercises for the unaffected extremities (Frieden et al., 1993). Exercise of the affected limb depends on the type of procedure. Frieden et al. (1993) recently reported a 10- to 14-day hospitalization for the expandable adjustable endoprosthesis. In those patients with an increased range of motion after surgery, the major contributing factor was the patient's adherence to the home exercise program (Frieden et al., 1993). The exercise adherence was facilitated by a mature attitude in the patient and a family committed to the importance of exercise. About one third of Frieden and associates' (1993) patients noted a decreased range of motion.

Lower extremity amputations have a more direct effect on general mobility than do upper extremity amputations, but the general problems are similar: adapting to a prosthesis, making necessary modifications in activities of daily living, and maintaining a positive attitude toward the rehabilitation process. Because of the belief of some health care personnel as well as lay people that rehabilitation is pointless in cancer, particularly metastatic cancer, this process may be particularly challenging for the oncology nurse. If the nursing care of the person with an amputation secondary to malignancy is to be effective, this challenge must be met. It is important to keep in mind that amputation is rarely used alone and the person is almost always treated with some combination of chemotherapy or radiation therapy. These treatments may have other implications for the client's mobility.

Additional problems of immobility are often present because of the other risk factors common to the person with cancer. These have been discussed previously but deserve highlighting—for example, the problem of trying to help the person with a lower extremity amputation to ambulate when the pain level is high, the energy level low, and the incentive to achieve mobility limited. If the oncology nurse has limited experience in working with patients who have an amputation, it is wise to consult colleagues experienced in orthopedic nursing, rehabilitation nursing, and physical therapy and to refer to related references in the literature. One of the most important areas for the nurse to keep in mind in nursing the person with an amputation is the alteration in body image and self-concept. That person has often had many other assaults on body image during the diagnostic and treatment process. Because amputation for cancer diagnoses is used almost exclusively for primary bone tumors, this group presents somewhat different nursing concerns from the person with metastatic bone tumor, who will be treated with radiation or chemotherapy. Problems with upper extremity amputations most commonly relate to retraining the person both for working with a prosthetic limb and for managing activities of daily living in a new manner. Planning for rehabilitation is essential and begins, as always, with the beginning of treatment.

Central Nervous System Tumors

The final special problem of mobility to be discussed is that of central nervous system tumors, another potential oncologic complication that can result in a neurologic emergency. Space-occupying brain malignancies can be primary tumors, but most often they result from arterial metastases from cancers of the lung, breast, prostate, and colon, malignant melanoma, lymphoma, and leukemia. Neurologic symptoms are related to the location and size of the cancer, the extent of local compression and destruction of brain tissue by the mass and edema, and the degree of increased intracranial pressure or obstruction to the normal flow of cerebrospinal fluid.

Mobility may be particularly affected with parietal lobe involvement, because sensorimotor function is under parietal control and may be manifested by weakness, atrophy, clumsiness, dysdiadochokinesia, and independent movements unrecognized by the patient. Cerebellar dysfunction can decrease mobility by reducing muscle coordination and ataxia resulting from compression of motor tracts. Frontal (precentral) lobe involvement may result in weakness, hemiparesis, disturbed gait, automatism, rigidity, tonic spasms of toes, and seizures, all of which can affect mobility. Occipital lobe damage may cause visual damage that likewise influences mobility. Unilateral cortical lesions often present strokelike symptoms.

The initial treatment of primary tumors is often surgical excision, with removal limited by the location and invasiveness of the cancer. Because most of the malignant brain tumors, both primary and metastatic, are radiosensitive, radiation therapy generally is indicated. Researchers are hopeful that radiation therapy of metastatic disease to the brain may be improved through using radiosensitizers and improved use of CT and MRI to guide therapy. Local and regional use of chemotherapy in the treatment of intracranial and spinal tumors is established for many primary tumors. However, for parenchymal CNS tumors, controversy surrounds the concept of limited antitumor efficacy for agents with restricted blood-barrier permeability. Another issue relates to toxicity when anticancer drugs are given at doses needed to circumvent the blood-brain barrier (Levin, Glutin, & Leibel, 1993).

The role of chemotherapy in the treatment of brain metastases has not been clearly defined (Wright, Delaney, & Buckner, 1993). Wright et al. (1993) identified factors that must be considered when determining appropriate treatment for patients with brain metastasis. When the general condition of the patient seems to indicate treatment of the central nervous system lesion, these investigators consider the following factors to determine the type of local treatment to be employed (namely, surgery, radiation therapy, chemotherapy, or a combination):

1. Number of lesions
2. Location of lesions
3. Primary site
4. Patient age and general functional condition
5. Pretreatment neurologic state
6. Extent of systemic disease and status of the primary tumor
7. Relative radioresponsiveness and radiocontrollability
8. Interval between treatment of the primary lesion and development of brain metastases

Nursing care of the patient with alterations in mobility related to central nervous system tumors and their treatment includes careful monitoring and reporting of existing or new symptoms, helping with mobility, and intervening to protect from injury, as previously described in other parts of this chapter. Orthotics and assistive devices may be used to substitute for lost motor function.

Assessment includes observations of any evidence of increased intracranial pressure and sensory changes as well as motor function and muscular strength of extremities. Activity tolerance and unsteady gait also need to be assessed with each contact, recording ataxia and subjective indications of weakness and fatigue (Chernecky & Ramsey, 1984).

As is true in the case of nursing care of persons with spinal cord tumors, significant nursing energies are devoted to dealing with the psychosocial and emotional impact of central nervous system tumors. Interventions are directed toward issues relating to the sense of loss of control, loss of body integrity, threats to hope, and fears associated with dying. Patient and family education concerning understanding the illness and its signs and symptoms, determining their impact on daily life, modifying expectations of work ability, lifestyle and role, and identifying ways to enhance the quality of remaining life are extremely important.

SUMMARY

Nursing care for the person with cancer who has problems of altered mobility is indeed a challenging process. Although the nursing techniques are not unique, the specialized knowledge and skills of the oncology nurse must be used to their fullest. What is unique is the importance of careful diagnosis of the problem so that nursing care is in the truest sense of the word individualized. When a problem exists, only actions carefully designed to reduce the particular contributing factors for that specific problem will be maximally effective. Probably this is the reason much of the nursing research that has been done in this area has focused on assessment and diagnosis. It is to be hoped that work will soon begin that examines the efficacy of various care techniques related to increasing mobility. Only then can selection of nursing interventions rely more on research-documented evidence of effectiveness and less on empiric experience and exchange of ideas. The latter remains a rich source of information for the oncology nurse, however, and cooperation among specialists in rehabilitation, orthopedic, and neurologic nursing is vital for the optimum care of the person with a problem of physical mobility.

REFERENCES

American Nurses' Association & Oncology Nursing Society. (1987). *Standards for oncology nursing practice.* Kansas City, MO: American Nurses' Association.

Baird, S. (1985). Development of a nursing assessment tool to diagnose altered body image in immobilized patients. *Orthopaedic Nursing, 4,* 47–54.

Baulch, Y. S., Larson, P. J., Dodd, M. J., & Deitrich, C. (1992). The relationship of visual acuity, tactile sensitivity, and mobility of the upper extremities to proficient breast self-examination in women 65 and older. *Oncology Nursing Forum, 19*(9), 1367–1372.

Benoliel, J. Q., McCorkle, R., & Young, K. (1980). Development of a Social Dependency scale. *Research in Nursing & Health, 3,* 3–10.

Bergstrom, N., & Braden, B. (1992). A prospective study of pressure sore risk among institutionalized elderly. *Journal of the American Geriatrics Society, 40,* 747–758.

Bergstrom, N., Demuth, P. J., & Braden, B. J. (1987). A clinical trial of the Braden scale for predicting pressure sore risk. *Nursing Clinics of North American, 22*(2), 417–428.

Bertelli, G., Venturini, M., Forno, G., Macchiavello, F., & Dini, D. (1992). An analysis of prognostic factors in response to conservative treatment of postmastectomy lymphedema. *Surgery Gynecology & Obstetrics, 175*(5), 455–460.

Bowlby, J. (1961). Processes of mourning. *International Journal of Psychoanalysis, 42,* 317–340.

Cancer Rehabilitation Coordination Team. (1978). *Final report to National Cancer Institute.* Unpublished document, University of Pittsburgh, School of Health-Related Professionals.

Carnevali, D. (1985). A daily functional health status perspective for nursing diagnosis and treatment in critical care nursing. *Heart and Lung, 14,* 437–443.

Carnevali, D. L., & Patrick, M. (1979). *Nursing management for the elderly.* Philadelphia: J. B. Lippincott Co.

Carpenito, L. J. (1995). *Nursing diagnosis: Application to clinical practice* (6th ed.). Philadelphia: J. B. Lippincott Co.

Casley-Smith, J. R., Morgan, R. G., & Piller, N. B. (1993). Treatment of lymphedema of the arms and legs with 5, 6-benzo-[α]-pyrone. *New England Journal of Medicine, 329*, 1158–1163.

Chang, S. K., & Hawes, K. A. (1983). The adequacy of the Karnofsky rating and global adjustment to illness scale as outcome measures in cancer rehabilitation and continuing care. In P. F. Engstrom, P. N. Anderson, & L. E. Mortenson (Eds.), *Advances in cancer control: Research and development* (pp.429–443). New York: Alan R. Liss, Inc.

Chernecky, C. C., & Ramsey, P., W. (1984). *Critical nursing care of the client with cancer.* Norwalk, CT: Appleton-Century-Crofts.

Chiou, I. L., & Burnett, C. N. (1985). Values of activities of daily living. *Physical Therapy, 65*, 902–906.

Degner, L. F., & Beaton, J. I. (1987). *Life-death decisions in health care.* New York: Hemisphere Publishing Corp.

Degner, L. F., & Russell, C. A. (1988). Preferences for treatment control among adults with cancer. *Research in Nursing & Health, 11*, 367–374.

Donovan, M. I., & Girton, S. (1984). *Cancer care nursing.* Norwalk, CT: Appleton-Century-Crofts.

Dunkel-Schetter, C., Feinstein, L. G., Taylor, S. E., & Falke, R. L. (1992). Patterns of coping with cancer. *Health Psychology, 11*(2), 79–87.

Eakes, G. G. (1993). Chronic sorrow: A response to living with cancer. *Oncology Nursing Forum, 20*(9), 1327–1334.

Feinstein, A. R., Joseph, B. R., & Wells, C. K. (1986). Scientific and clinical problems in indexes of functional disability. *Annals of Internal Medicine, 105*, 413–420.

Frieden, R. A., Ryniker, D., Kenan, S., & Lewis, M. M. (1993). Assessment of patient function after limb-sparing surgery. *Archives of Physical Medicine Rehabilitation, 74*(1), 38–43.

Glass, C. S. (1992). Applying functional analysis to psychological rehabilitation following spinal cord injury. *Journal of the American Paraplegia Society, 15*(3), 187–193.

Gregor, S., McCarthy, K., Chwirchak, D., Meluch, M., & Mion, L. C. (1986). Characteristics and functional outcomes of elderly rehabilitation patients. *Rehabilitation Nursing, 11*(3), 10–14.

Gulick, E. E. (1986). The self-assessment of health among the chronically ill. *Topics in Clinical Nursing, 8*(1), 74–82.

Henson, J. W., & Posner, J. B. (1993). Neurological complications. In J. B. Holland, E. Frei, R. C. Bast, D. W. Kufe, D. L. Morton, & R. R. Weichselbaum (Eds.), *Cancer medicine* (3rd ed.). Philadelphia: Lea & Febiger.

Hladiuk, M., Huchcroft, S., Temple, W., & Schnurr, B. E. (1992). Arm function after axillary dissection for breast cancer: A pilot study to provide parameter estimates. *Journal of Surgical Oncology, 50*, 47–52.

Hockenberry, M. J., & Lane, B. (1988). Limb salvage procedures in children with osteosarcoma. *Cancer Nursing, 11*(1), 2–8.

Jacelon, C. S. (1986). The Barthel index and other indices of functional ability. *Rehabilitation Nursing, 11*(4), 9–11.

Kneisl, C. R., & Ames, S. W. (1986). *Adult health nursing: A biopsychosocial approach.* Menlo Park, CA: Addison-Wesley Publishing Co.

Kozier, B., & Erb, G., Blais, K., Johnson, J. Y., & Temple, J. S. (1993). *Techniques in clinical nursing: A nursing process approach* (4th ed.). Redwood City, CA: Addison-Wesley Publishing Co.

Lawrence, W. Jr., (chairman) Members of the Consensus Development Panel. L. H. Baker, C. M. Balch, R. L. Scotte Doggett, E. A. Gehan, M. A. Greenly, E. D. Holyoke, A. S. Lichter, L. R. Martin, N. L. Petrakis, P. K. Teich,

R. C. Thompson, Jr., R. E. Wilson, & S. H. Winokur. (1985). Limb-sparing treatment of adult soft-tissue sarcomas and osteosarcomas. *Journal of American Medical Association, 254*(13), 1791–1794.

Lazarus, R. S., & Folkman, S. (1984). *Stress, appraisal and coping* (p. 141). New York: Springer Publishing Co.

Lehmann, J., DeLisa, J. A., & Warren, C. G. (1978). Cancer rehabilitation: Assessment of need, development and evaluation of a model of care. *Archives of Physical Medicine and Rehabilitation, 59*, 410–419.

Levin, V. A., Gutin, P. H., & Leibel, S. (1993). Neoplasms of the central nervous system. In V. T. DeVita, Jr., S. Hellman, & S. A. Rosenberg (Eds.), *Cancer: Principles and practice of oncology.* Philadelphia: J. B. Lippincott Co.

Low, A. W. (1990). Prevention of pressure sores in patients with cancer. *Oncology Nursing Forum, 17*(2), 179–184.

Lundquist, D. M., & Holmes, W. (1993). Documentation of neurotoxicity resulting from high-dose cytosine arabinoside. *Oncology Nursing Forum, 20*(9), 1409–1412.

Maas, M. L. (1991). In M. Mass, K. Buckwalter, & M. Hardy. *Nursing diagnoses and interventions for the elderly.* Redwood City, CA: Addison-Wesley Nursing.

Martin, N., Holt, N. B., & Hicks, D. (1980). *Comprehensive rehabilitation nursing.* New York: McGraw-Hill Book Co.

McMillan, S. C., & Williams, F. A. (1989). Validity and reliability of the Constipation Assessment scale. *Cancer Nursing, 12*(3), 183–188.

McNally, J. C., Stair, J. C., & Somerville, E. T. (1985). *Guidelines for cancer nursing practice.* Orlando, FL: Grune & Stratton, Inc.

Milsum, J. H. (1980). Lifestyle changes for the whole person: Stimulation through health hazard appraisal. In P. O. Davidson & S. M. Davidson (Eds.), *Behavioral medicine: Changing health lifestyles.* New York: Brunner/Mazel.

Neufeld, K. R., Degner, L. F., & Dick, J. A. M. (1993). A nursing intervention strategy to foster patient involvement in treatment decisions. *Oncology Nursing Forum, 20*(4), 631–635.

Olson, E. (1967). The hazards of immobility. *American Journal of Nursing, 67*, 780–797.

Peretz, D. (1970). Reaction to loss. In B. Schoenberg, A. C. Carr, D. Peretz, & A. H. Kutscher (Eds.), *Loss and grief: Psychological management in medical practice.* New York: Columbia University Press.

Porth, C. M. (1994). *Pathophysiology: Concepts of altered health states* (4th ed.). Philadelphia: J. B. Lippincott Co.

Potter, P. A., & Perry, A. G. (1993). *Fundamentals of nursing: Concepts, process, and practice.* St. Louis: C. V. Mosby Co.

Price, S. A., & Wilson, L. M. (1992). *Pathophysiology: Clinical concepts of disease process* (4th ed.). New York: McGraw-Hill Book Co.

Pritchard, D. J., & Burch, P. A. (1993). Orthopedic complications. In J. B. Holland, E. Frei, R. C. Bast, D. W. Kufe, D. L. Morton, & R. R. Weichselbaum, (Eds.), *Cancer medicine.* (3rd ed.). Philadelphia: Lea & Febiger.

Ragnarsson, K. T. (1993). Principles of cancer rehabilitation medicine. In J. F. Holland, E. Frei, R. C. Bast, D. W. Kufe, D. L. Morton, & R. R. Weichselbaum, (Eds.), *Cancer medicine* (3rd ed.). Philadelphia: Lea & Febiger.

Robinson, B. E. (1986). Validation of the functional assessment inventory against a multidisciplinary home care team. *Journal American Geriatric Society, 34*, 851–854.

Sullivan, J. (1990). Individual and family responses to acute spinal cord injury. *Critical Care Nursing Clinics of North America, 2*(3), 407–414.

Teel, C. S. (1991). Chronic sorrow: Analysis of the concept. *Journal of Advanced Nursing, 16*, 1311–1319.

Tucker, S. (1987). Psychological and interpersonal issues in spinal cord injury. *Topics in Acute Care Trauma Rehabilitation, 1*(3), 86–94.

Waltman, N. L., Bergstrom, N., Armstrong, N., Norvell, K., & Braden, B. (1991). Nutritional status, pressure sores, and mortality in elderly patients with cancer. *Oncology Nursing Forum, 18*(5), 867–873.

Weisman, A. D. (1979). *Coping with cancer* (p. 27). New York: McGraw-Hill Book Co.

Weisman, A. D., & Worden, J. W. (1977). *Coping and vulnerability in cancer patients: A research report.* Cambridge, MA: Shea Brothers.

Whiting, G., & Buckwalter, K. C. (1991). Dysfunctional grieving. In M. Maas, K. C. Buckwalter, & M. Hardy. *Nursing diagnoses interventions for the elderly.* Redwood City, CA: Addison-Wesley Nursing.

Williams, A. J. (1986). Self-care model: An assessment tool based on Orem's theory. *Nursing Success Today, 3*(7), 26–28.

Winningham, M. L. (1991). Walking program for people with cancer. *Cancer Nursing, 14*(5), 270–276.

Winningham, M. L., MacVicar, M. G., & Burke, C. A. (1986). Exercise for cancer patients: guidelines and precautions. *The Physician and Sports Medicine, 14*(10), 125–134.

Winningham, M. L., Nail, L. J., Burkey, M. M., Brophy, L., Cimprich, B., Jones, L. S., Pickard-Holley, S., Rhodes, V., St. Peirre, B., Beck, S., Glass, E. C., Mock, V. L., Mooney, K. H., & Piper, B. (1994). Fatigue and the cancer experience: The state of the knowledge. *Oncology Nursing Forum, 21*(1), 23–36.

Worden, J. W. (1982). *Grief counseling and grief therapy: A handbook for the mental health practitioner.* New York: Springer Publishing Co.

Wright, D. C., Delaney, T. F., & Buckner, J. C. (1993). Treatment and metastatic cancer. In V. T. Devita, Jr., S. Hellman, & S. A. Rosenberg (Eds.), *Cancer: Principles of oncology* (4th ed.). Philadelphia: J. B. Lippincott Co.

Complications of Advanced Disease

Cynthia C. Chernecky • Ruth Krech-Fritskey

ANATOMIC AND PHYSIOLOGIC FEATURES

DEFINITION OF ADVANCED DISEASE

Advanced disease is defined as at least one acute organ dysfunction caused by either metastasis or cancer treatment that results in a client's need for comprehensive management in an intensive care environment. This condition differs from metastasis alone, a single oncologic emergency, and any other circumstance that does not involve acute organ dysfunction *and* does not require comprehensive intensive care.

This chapter focuses on nursing care of the individual who experiences complications of advanced disease. The first section discusses vital organ functions. The second section includes scientific knowledge about the pathophysiologic and interfering factors that lead to advanced disease and that are caused by metastasis and sequelae of therapies. The third section of this chapter addresses associated nursing diagnoses and interventions. The final section covers special problems related to advanced disease.

NORMAL FUNCTION OF BODY ORGANS

Knowledge of the normal function of six specific organs provides the foundation for understanding the concept of advanced disease.

1. The brain is the primary center for regulating and coordinating body activities. This includes analytic thought, memory, behaviors, and communication.
2. The heart provides force so blood can be propelled through the vascular system.
3. Bones provide body support and organ protection and play an active role in the formation of blood cells.
4. The lungs exchange carbon dioxide for oxygen in the blood.
5. The liver serves many functions. In this chapter it is viewed as a return site for blood from the intestines and spleen on its way to being returned to the systemic circulation.
6. The kidneys provide for regulation of extracellular fluid, electrolyte balance, and excretion of urine.

PATHOPHYSIOLOGY AND INTERFERING FACTORS LEADING TO ADVANCED DISEASE

Dysfunctions in one vital organ generally lead to subsequent dysfunctions in other vital organs because the vital organs function interdependently. For example, a problem in the heart will decrease the amount of blood flow to the lungs. Consequently, there will be less oxygenated blood delivered to the other organs, thereby reducing their efficiency. The subsequent discussion delineates examples of specific vital organ metastasis and cancer treatment-related sequelae.

VITAL ORGAN METASTASIS

BRAIN

Two per cent of all cancers are primary brain tumors, and 15 per cent of all cancer clients develop neurologic symptoms from advanced disease (Henson & Posner, 1993). For common sites associated with brain metastasis, see Table 64–1. The most common site of metastasis in the brain occurs in the frontal lobe. Although less common, metastasis to the temporal, parietal, and occipital lobes occurs with similar frequency. The brain stem is the least likely site for metastasis (Vieth & Odom, 1965). Figure 64–1 demonstrates metastatic lesions with surrounding edema in both the frontal and parietal lobes on computed tomography (CT) scan.

Generalized signs and symptoms of brain metastasis include headache, double vision, loss of motor function, impaired mentation with lethargy, seizures, sensory loss, and increased intracranial pressure (Table 64–2). These signs and symptoms result in deficits in the following four areas: cognition, mobility, activities of daily living, and bladder and bowel control. The latter three areas are quite manageable on a general medical-surgical division. However, a deficit in cognition, known as neuropsychiatric syndrome, presents an acute situation in which the need for nursing care is greatly increased.

Neuropsychiatric syndrome can be manifested in several ways, ranging from acute anxiety disorders and personality changes to depressed consciousness, stupor, and coma (Billings, 1985). Astute nursing assessment is imperative because this syndrome can appear suddenly and can be caused by biologic response modifier therapy (Bender, 1994). Once the presence of neuropsychiatric syndrome is ascertained, general management, including orientation, hygiene, safety and suicide precautions, and constant monitoring of vital signs, can be initiated. Discussion, explanations, and support should be given to family members because the sudden onset

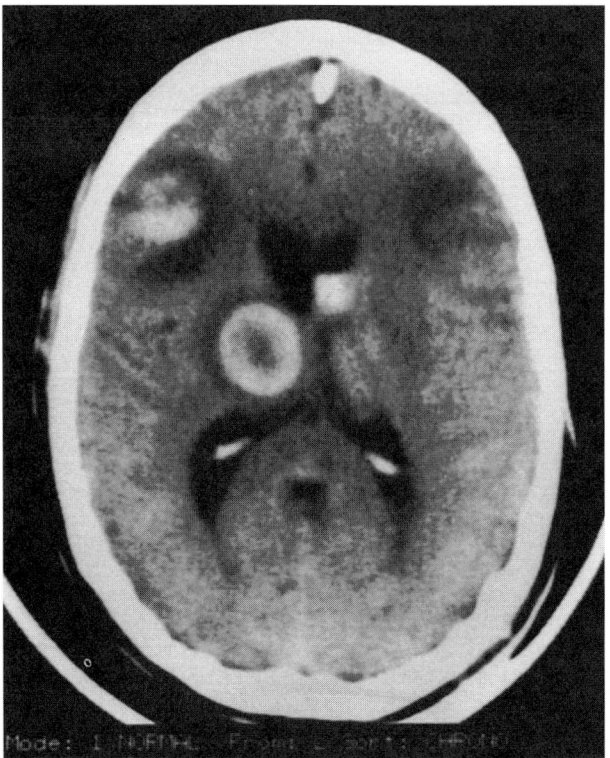

FIGURE 64–1. Brain metastasis of frontal and parietal lobes with accompanying edema surrounding frontal lobe tumor as seen on computed tomographic scan.

of this syndrome, as well as the uncertainty of the client outcome, is frightening (Newton & Mateo, 1994).

Depending on the condition of the client, the amount of systemic disease, whether the metastasis is solitary or multiple, and its location, treatment may be feasible and appropriate. Surgical removal or use of the gamma knife or photon knife (specifically targeted high-dose radiation therapy) may offer the best overall survival with the lowest morbidity in solitary and well-localized metastases. In less defined metastatic conditions, standard whole-brain irradiation may offer excellent palliation (Wright, Delaney, & Buckner, 1993; DeAngelis, 1994).

TABLE 64–1. *Types of Cancers That Metastasize to Five Specific Vital Organs*

Brain	Heart	Bone	Lung	Liver
Lung	Lung	Lung	Breast	Ovary
Breast	Breast	Breast	Lymphoma	Endometrium
Melanoma	Melanoma	Prostate	Leukemia	Breast
Renal cell	Acute leukemia	Melanoma	Mesothelioma	Colon
Sarcoma	Lymphoma	Lymphoma	Ovary	Gastric
Seminoma	Gastrointestinal	Kidney	Genitourinary	Pancreas
Uterus	Sarcoma	Thyroid	Gastrointestinal	Lymphoma
		Bladder	Melanoma	Multiple myeloma
		Cervix	Sarcoma	Melanoma
		Endometrium	Unknown primary	Unknown primary
		Pancreas	Uterus	Uterus
		Gastrinoma		
		Unknown primary		

TABLE 64–2. *Signs and Symptoms of Increased Intracranial Pressure (ICP)*

1. Decreased level of consciousness
2. Pupil dilation; occurs on the same side as the tumor
3. Increased systolic blood pressure and widening pulse pressure followed by a sharp drop in blood pressure
4. Bradycardia followed by a sharp tachycardia
5. Simultaneous bradycardia and increased systolic blood pressure*
6. Decreased respiratory rate
7. Papilledema only when increased ICP develops slowly
8. Hyperreflexia
9. Gait impairment

*Early significant finding.

HEART

Another facet of advanced disease is heart involvement. Metastases to the heart, specifically the pericardium, occur in approximately 10 per cent of all clients with cancer (Hanfling, 1960). Although cardiac metastasis can occur through any of the defined modes of metastasis (see Chapter 15), blood-borne and lymphatic metastases are most common. These two patterns of metastasis probably account for the fact that cardiac metastasis is almost always accompanied by metastasis to other organs (Bisel, Wroblewski, & LaDue, 1953). Cancers associated with heart metastasis are identified in Table 64–1.

Metastasis to the pericardium results in the accumulation of fluid in the pericardial sac. This sac is elastic and may stretch to accommodate as much as 1 L of fluid before cardiac decompensation occurs (Pursley, 1983). This results in a syndrome known as pericardial effusion, which, if ignored, can progress rapidly into cardiac tamponade (see Chapter 66). If cardiac tamponade can be avoided, the mean survival rate of clients with pericardial effusion alone is 6 to 13 months depending on the primary disease and whether the effusion can be treated to prevent reoccurrence (Vaitkus, Herrmann, & LeWinter, 1994). Because of the potential morbidity associated with the progression of pericardial effusion, a thorough knowledge of the signs and symptoms is imperative. These include dyspnea, cough, nausea, vomiting, epigastric abdominal pain, hepatomegaly, leg edema, fever, and neck vein distention.

Management of undiagnosed pericardial effusion includes treatment of the symptoms, such as providing oxygen for dyspnea, and direct bolstering of the body's hemodynamic compensatory responses with intravenous fluids and vasopressors. The most important method of management includes frequent monitoring of the client's heart rate, electrocardiogram, blood pressure, and changes in or additions to the aforementioned symptoms. Once a definitive diagnosis has been made, pericardial effusion should be treated according to the condition and treatment goals of the client. According to Vaitkus et al. (1994), the most effective treatment, if the client is well enough to endure surgery and general anesthesia, is the pericardial window. Pericardiocentesis with sclerosis or chemotherapy to the pericardium is also quite effective (Tomkowski, Szturmowicz, Fijalkowska, Filipecki, & Figura-Chojak, 1994). Radiation therapy to the pericardium may relieve the effusion but is associated with high incidences of pericarditis. The effect of systemic chemotherapy is not well known, since it is rarely employed without pericardiocentesis.

BONE

The third vital organ identified in advanced disease is the skeletal system or bones. Metastasis to the bone occurs in 70 per cent of all clients with cancer (Malawer & Delaney, 1993) (see Table 64–1). One of the most sensitive diagnostic tests in the determination of bone metastasis is the bone scan. Figure 64–2 illustrates bone metastasis to the ribs, shoulder, humerus, and lumbar spine. Bone metastasis, which deossifies and softens bones, itself is not lethal. However, the resulting pain, neurologic deficits, and immobility can significantly decrease a client's quality of life. The quality of life can be further compromised by the occurrence of a pathologic fracture.

Pathologic fractures occur in 8 per cent of all clients with cancer (Faehnrich, 1983). They occur most commonly in the spine (primarily the thoracic and lumbar regions), ribs, long bones (Fig. 64–3), and sternum. Although symptoms may vary according to the location of the fracture, there are guidelines for assessment that apply to any location. The most common symptom is pain. The assessment of other symptoms includes inspection of the bones for swelling, erythema, abnormal joint position or curvature, palpation of the joints and bones to detect pain, tenderness, change of temperature, or grating during movement, and evaluation of neurologic function distal to the affected area (Faehnrich, 1983). Signs and symptoms of spinal involvement generally include pain, progressive weakness, muscle wasting, and bladder and bowel incontinence, which should be reported immediately as they may indicate the onset of spinal cord compression (Chapter 66).

Pathologic fractures often occur without a traumatic precipitator such as a fall. Pathologic rib fractures can occur as a result of a simple cough or sneeze. The only sign of a rib fracture is pain, aggravated by breathing, which is not relieved by rest. Pathologic fractures of the long bones may be prevented by prophylactic internal fixation. Such surgery, indicated in specific situations where impending fractures are nearly certain, results in an increased survival rate when compared with that of attempts to correct these fractures after they occur (Chernecky & Ramsey, 1984; Haentjens, Casteleyn, & Opdecam, 1993). The least frequent site for metastasis is the sternum. However, when fractures occur here, they heal slowly and cause more disfigurement.

Management of pathologic fractures generally focuses on pain control, palliative chemotherapy, and localized radiation therapy. Localized radiation, in combination with good pain management techniques, is effective in the treatment of bone metastases in most clients (Malawer & Delaney, 1993). When possible,

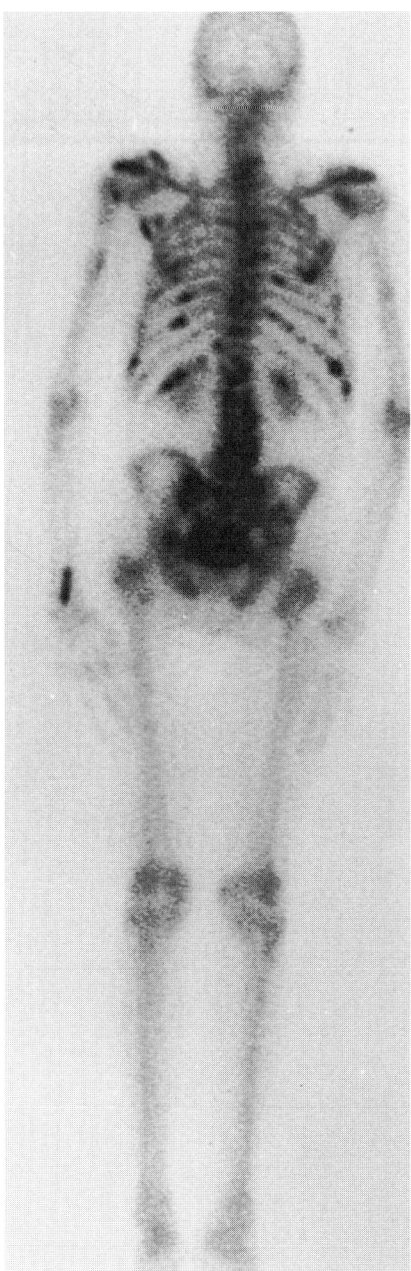

FIGURE 64–2. Bone scan shows metastatic lesions of ribs, shoulder, left humerus, and lumbar spine.

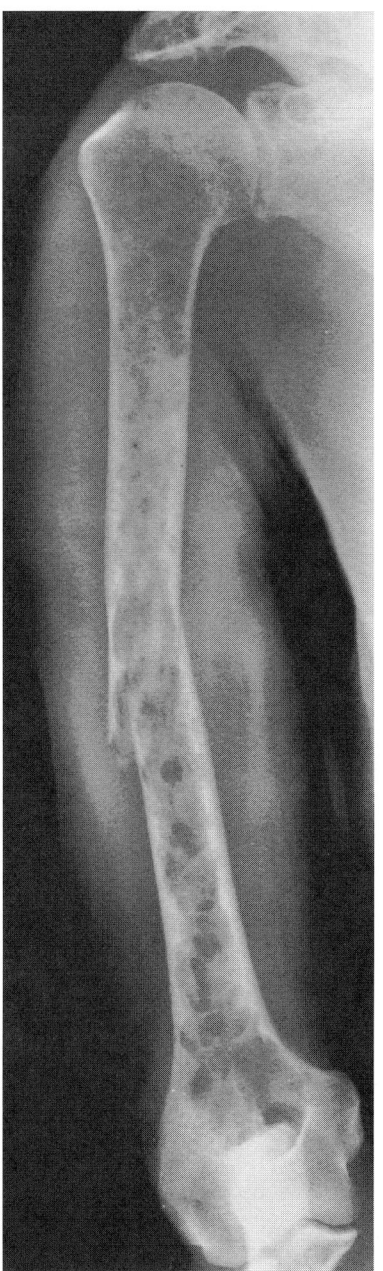

FIGURE 64–3. Plain film of humerus reveals diffuse bone metastasis and a pathologic fracture.

prevention of pathologic fractures is the ideal type of management. This can be accomplished by using principles of anatomy and physiology when caring for clients with bone metastases. Specific interventions are addressed in the nursing diagnosis portion of this chapter.

LUNG

Lung metastasis, which is the second most common site of metastasis, occurs in 30 to 40 per cent of all clients with cancer (Luce, 1994) (Fig. 64–4). The most frequent complication of advanced disease in the lungs is malignant pleural effusion (Table 64–1).

Pleural effusion is an exudative process in which irritation of the pleural membrane by cancer cells results in an increased production of fluid in the interpleural space (Chernecky & Ramsey, 1984). In Figure 64–5, the left lung is 75 per cent filled with fluid, resulting in a drastic decrease in lung expansion. Normally, the space between the visceral and parietal pleura contains 5 to 15 ml of fluid. However, when cancer cells create overproduction and underabsorption, the interpleural space can contain more than 500 ml of fluid (Broaddus & Light, 1994). Although approximately 25 per cent of clients with pleural effusion present with no symptoms, signs and symptoms for those with as much

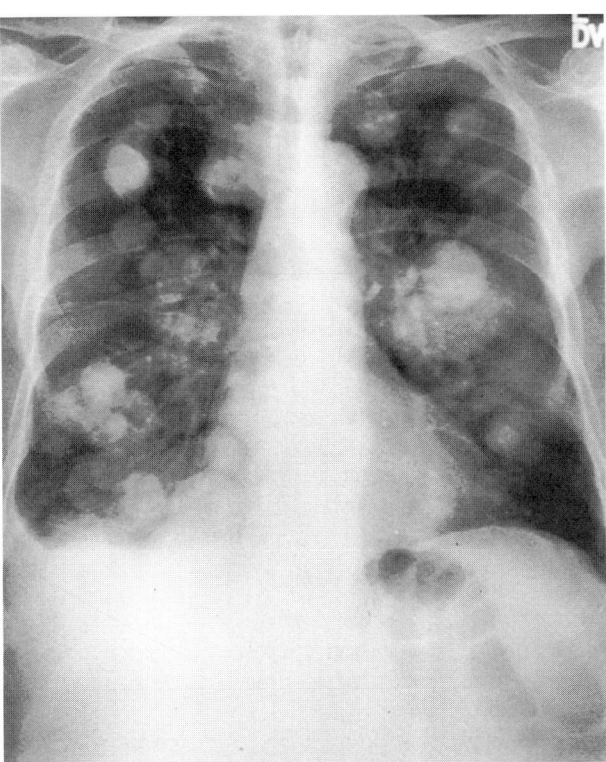

FIGURE 64-4. Anterior-posterior view of chest radiograph shows multiple bilateral metastatic lesions.

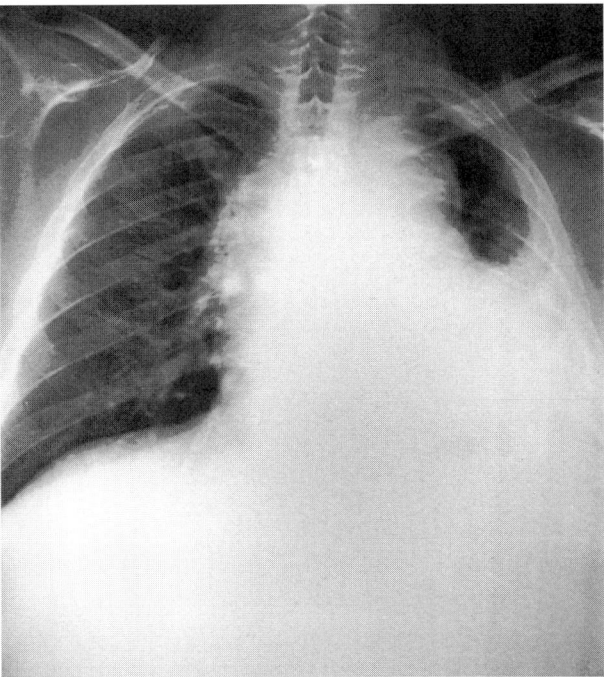

FIGURE 64-5. Anterior-posterior view of chest radiograph. Left lung space is 75 per cent replaced by fluid, as indicated by the total whitening of left lower lobes.

as 300 ml of interpleural fluid include dyspnea, pain, and hypoxia. For those with more than 300 ml of fluid in the interpleural space, signs and symptoms become more severe. These include tachycardia, tachypnea, asymmetric bulging of the intercostal spaces, diminished or absent breath sounds, and mediastinal shift.

Goals of management of malignant pleural effusion include treatment of both the symptoms and the cause (metastasis). Selection of the treatment depends on the prognosis and the present condition of the client. There are three basic treatment methods: surgical pleurectomy, needle thoracentesis, and chest tube insertion. Surgical pleurectomy is reserved for clients who have good life expectancies, are relatively healthy, and in whom less invasive methods have failed (Deslauriers, Beauchamp, & Desmeules, 1991). Needle thoracentesis and chest tube insertion relieve symptoms, but additional procedures such as sclerosis or pleurodesis are required for control of pleural effusion (Miles & Knight, 1993; Walker-Renard, Vaughan, & Sahn, 1994) (Table 64-3). Once treatment for pleural effusion has been implemented, ongoing nursing assessment of respiratory status is imperative.

LIVER

One of the most common phenomenons of advanced disease is metastatic liver involvement (see Table 64-1). This has a most profound impact on survival rates. Although prognosis is related to the primary site of disease (colorectal cancers having the best prognosis), clients will generally die within 1 year of the diagnosis of liver metastasis (Sherlock & Dooley,

1993). A CT scan can evaluate liver metastasis (Fig. 64-6).

A complication of advanced disease to the liver that may decrease the length of survival time is malignant ascites. Two types of ascites are related to liver metastasis: malignant chylous ascites and malignant clear ascites.

Malignant chylous ascites occurs because of an obstruction in the lymphatics. Consequently, the fluid is turbid milky or creamy due to the presence of lymph. This type of ascites occurs most frequently as a result of lymphoma (Baker & Weber, 1993).

Malignant clear ascites occurs as a result of a hypoalbuminemia-induced reduction in the plasma oncotic pressure. In this situation, the protein in the ascitic fluid is greater than the serum protein, and addi-

TABLE 64-3. *Agents Inserted Into the Pleural Space to Control Pleural Effusion*

RADIOACTIVE ISOTOPES	CHEMOTHERAPEUTIC AGENTS	SCLEROSING AGENTS
Gold	Bleomycin	Talc
Phosphorus	Cyclophosphamide	Tetracycline*
Yttrium	(Cytoxan)	
Yttrium gold	Doxycycline	
	5-fluorouracil	
	Nitrogen mustard	
	Thiotepa	

*No longer available in intravenous form in the United States.

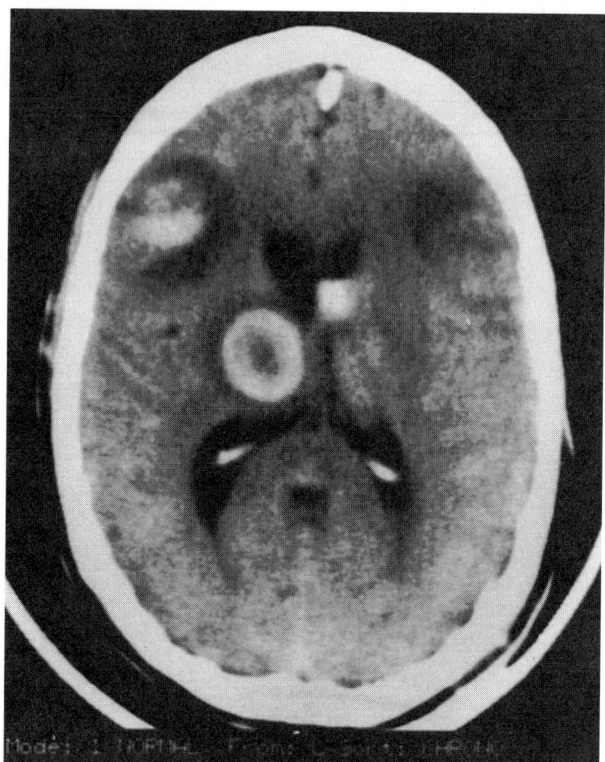

FIGURE 64-6. Computed tomographic scan shows an enlarged liver with widespread metastasis, as evidenced by the darker irregularly shaped areas of gray.

tional fluid is drawn into the abdominal cavity (Mauch, 1982).

General signs and symptoms of malignant ascites include abdominal distention, shortness of breath, and nausea. Although malignant chylous ascites may cause a rise in temperature, a diagnostic paracentesis and fluid culture should be performed to determine the type of malignant ascites.

In terms of management of malignant ascites, it should be noted that repeated paracentesis of abdominal fluid has not been effective in reducing ascites. Instead, this technique results in protein loss and risks fluid derivation. Several therapies are effective, however, in relieving ascites (Table 64-4).

SEQUELAE OF THERAPIES

As described previously, the effects of metastasis on the vital organs result in many complications of advanced disease. In addition, therapies for cancers can lead to critical complications. This section discusses complications associated with drug toxicities, radiation therapy, and bone marrow transplantation.

DRUG TOXICITIES

Drug toxicities primarily affect four major organs: heart, lung, liver, and kidney (Table 64-5). For example, chemotherapy-induced heart toxicities cause heart enlargement, which develops into congestive heart failure and pulmonary hypertension (Chernecky & Ramsey, 1984). In the lungs, antineoplastic agents damage the alveolar epithelium and the basement membrane, which decreases the amount of collagen secreted. The result is fibrosis with impaired gas exchange (Wickham, 1986). The effects of chemotherapy on the liver range from increased levels of hepatic enzymes seen with high doses of the drugs to hepatic fibrosis associated with long-term therapy due to cellular damage of the drug of one of its metabolites (Grever & Grieshaber, 1993). Each of the aforementioned types of toxicities is not uncommon in cancer therapy, but kidney toxicity is a more common cause of advanced disease and is discussed in more detail.

Drug-related kidney toxicity occurs when the chemotherapeutic agents cause direct damage to the glomerulus, tubules, or both. In addition, drugs can cause indirect damage through vascular changes. The risk of such damage increases when combination drug regimens are used (Weiss & Vogelzang, 1993).

The signs and symptoms of kidney toxicity mimic those of renal failure. They include increased blood urea nitrogen and creatinine values, decreased urinary output, fluid retention, pulmonary rales, nausea, vomiting, edema, and pruritus. In addition, the client should be monitored for metabolic acidosis and cardiac dysrhythmias.

Management of chemotherapy-induced kidney toxicity would include efforts to prevent renal toxicity such as diuretic administration and hydration before, during, and after drug administration. Of course, even though prevention efforts are employed, it is not always possible to avoid renal failure. In this instance, dialysis would be indicated.

RADIATION

Unlike systemic chemotherapy, external radiation-induced advanced disease is site-specific. That is, the areas of the body receiving the radiation will be the areas in which potential complications can occur. For

TABLE 64-4. *Therapies for Malignant Ascites*

Systemic chemotherapy	Use the chemotherapy protocol for the primary cancer
Intraperitoneal radiation	Chromic phosphate or gold
Intraperitoneal chemotherapy	Bleomycin, 5-fluorouracil, nitrogen mustard, or thiotepa; this therapy is not effective in chylous ascites
Surgery	LeVeen or Denver shunts; these shunts are used for palliation to relieve pressure; they may remain open from a few days to 3 yrs with 50% functioning for at least 1 yr (Spiro, 1983). Generally contraindicated in cytology positive ascites (Graham, 1989)
Medication	Potassium-sparing diuretic spironolactone (aldactone) as long as client is nonhyperkalemic

TABLE 64–5. *Drugs That Are Toxic to Vital Organs*

Heart	Lung	Kidney	Liver	Brain
Aclarubicin	Adenine arabinoside	Amikacin (Amikin)	Amphotericin B	Ifosfamide[†]
Amphotericin B	(Ara-A)	Aminoglycosides	Busulfan—high dose	Interleukin-2[†]
Amsacrine (AMSA)	Bleomycin	• Gentamicin*	Carmustine—high	
Busulfan	Busulfan	• Kanamycin*	dose	
Cyclophosphamide	Carmustine	• Neomycin**	Chlorambucil (Leuk-	
(Cytoxan) acts syn-	Chloramphenicol	• Streptomycin	eran)	
ergistically with	Colistin sulfate	• Vancomycin	Cyclophosphamide	
doxorubicin	(Polymixin) is asso-	Amphotericin B	Cytarabine	
Daunorubicin	ciated with respira-	Azicitidine	Cytosine arabinoside	
Doxorubicin	tory arrest	Carboplatin—high dose	(Ara-C)	
(Adriamycin)	Cyclophosphamide	Carmustine (BCNU)*	Dactinomycin—high	
5-FU	Cytosine Arabinoside	Cephaloridine	dose	
Idarubicin	Melphalan—high	Cisplatin**	Diaziquone—high	
Ifosfamide	dose (Alkeran)	Colistin sulfate	dose	
Interferon	Methotrexate	(Polymixin B)	Griseofulvin	
Mitomycin C	Mitomycin	Cyclophosphamide	Interferons—high	
Mittoxantrone—high	Procarbazine	Diaziquone—high dose	dose	
dose		Gallium nitrate	L-asparaginase	
Retinoic Acid		Hydroxyurea	Methotrexate	
Taxol		Ifosfamide	Mithramycin	
Vinblastine		Interleukin	Mitomycin—high	
		L-asparaginase	dose	
		Lomustine (CCNU)*	Pyrazinamide	
		Methotrexate—high		
		dose**		
		Mithramycin**		
		Mitomycin C**		
		Pentostatin		
		Semustine (MeCCNU)*		
		Streptozocil**		
		Vinblastine		

* High risk of nephrotoxicity with long-term use.
** High risk of immediate nephrotoxicity.
† Temporary neurotoxicity: generally stops with cessation of treatment.
(Data from Cameron, 1993; Igbal & Ironside, 1993; Lydon, 1986; Rogers, 1993; Rosetti, 1985; Sparber & Biller-Sparber, 1993.)

example, radiation to the head and neck area may cause nausea, taste changes, and stomatitis. Radiation therapy to long bones may only produce mild skin irritation. Although symptoms such as these are quite manageable, the consequences of radiation to the bowel are potentially fatal.

For clients whose cancer extends through the bowel wall, surgery alone is insufficient. Initially, radiation offers further control of the cancer with minimal danger of complications. However, even with therapeutic doses of 40 to 50 cGy, there is a 7 to 13 per cent chance of developing bowel adhesions, bowel obstruction, or fistulization that will require surgical intervention (Tepper, Cohen, Wood, Orlow, & Hedberg, 1987; Vigliotti, Rich, Romsdahl, Withers, & Oswald, 1987). In some cases, 6 to 12 months after therapy, the bowel may become increasingly friable, eliminating the possibility of further surgical intervention. The outcome is malabsorption and paralytic ileus with concomitant bowel necrosis.

Signs and symptoms of this outcome include gas, abdominal distention, abdominal pain, and absent bowel sounds. Unfortunately, this syndrome is not reversible. Instead, management focuses on symptom relief, such as nasogastric tube insertion and pain control measures.

BONE MARROW TRANSPLANTATION

The third therapeutic sequela that is related to complications of advanced disease is bone marrow transplantation (BMT). There are two types of BMT: autologous, which uses one's own bone marrow to "rescue" the immune system following high-dose chemotherapy, and allogeneic, which uses bone marrow from an HLA-matched donor to replace the damaged marrow of the recipient in a grafting process. Autologous BMTs, used to treat Hodgkins disease, lymphomas, breast cancer, and other solid tumors, carry relatively low treatment-related morbidity (Schryber, Lacasse, & Barton-Burke, 1987). The most critical complication of autologous BMTs is the reoccurrence of the primary disease. Allogeneic BMTs, used to treat leukemias and other hematologic disorders, have the potential to cause graft-vs.-host-disease (GVHD) (Chapter 27) (Armitage, 1994). Forty to 50 per cent of allogeneic BMTs develop some form of GVHD with 30 to 60 per cent of these resulting in death either from GVHD or from related infections (Wujcik, Ballard, & Camp-Sorrell, 1994; Tutschka, 1993).

Graft-versus-host-disease occurs when the donor T cells proliferate and attack various cells in the already compromised host. It can be acute, with an average onset of 25 days, or chronic, with an onset of 2 to 12 months after bone marrow engraftment. The four grades of GVHD are distinguished by the degree of organ involvement, with grade 1 involving only a skin rash and grade 4 involving multiorgan failure and extreme decrease in clinical performance.

When GVHD involves multiple organ failure it includes (1) the skin, with associated rash, sloughing, and bronze coloration; (2) gastrointestinal tract dysfunction, including nausea, pain, and malabsorption; (3) liver dysfunction, including jaundice and hemorrhage; and (4) bone marrow dysfunction, including pancytopenia and infection.

Management of GVHD is generally directed at prophylaxis. The preparative regimen for allogeneic BMT must concentrate on the best possible HLA match. Some centers use donor marrow T-cell depletion directed at elimination of the cell line responsible for the attack. Other methods of prophylaxis include antithymocite globulin and prednisone (Franko & Gould, 1994). After the transplant, GVHD prophylaxis includes cyclosporin. If GVHD cannot be controlled with cyclosporin and immunosuppression, symptom control may be the only reasonable intervention.

PROCESS OF ASSESSMENT AND MANAGEMENT OF ADVANCED DISEASE

Assessment and management of advanced disease is a complex process. Taking into account the anatomic and pathophysiologic factors and therapeutic sequelae already presented, the nurse has a basis on which to assess and care for clients with advanced disease. This portion of the chapter focuses on extending data collection, through physical assessment and diagnostics, and culminates in the presentation of selected nursing diagnoses and interventions for the client with advanced disease.

Physical Assessment, Laboratory Values, and Diagnostic Tests of Vital Organs

Physical assessment serves as a device for detecting abnormalities that may be life-threatening and for identifying signs that may suggest complications of advanced disease. Additional sources of data are necessary to complete the process of assessment. These sources include laboratory values and diagnostic tests (Chernecky, Krech, & Berger, 1993). Assessment for advanced disease, including all three aspects of data collection, is presented in Table 64–6.

Nursing Diagnoses and Interventions for Advanced Disease

The establishment of a database leads to the next phase of the nursing process: formulation of the nursing care plan. Neither the nursing diagnoses (Kelly, 1985) nor the associated interventions are intended to be all-inclusive. As each client differs, so will his or her care plan. Thus, the subsequent care plans should serve only as guidelines for care plan formulation of clients with advanced disease.

Brain: Alteration in Thought Processes

The client shows evidence of impaired thought processes related to decreased level of consciousness and impaired judgment resulting from neuropsychiatric syndrome.

Nursing interventions:

1. Assess level of consciousness every 2 to 4 hours.
2. Assess for increased intracranial pressure (see Table 64–2) every hour or with each client contact.
3. Check vital signs every 1 to 2 hours.
4. Take safety precautions: padded side rails, soft restraints, bed in lowest position, call light within easy reach.
5. Reorient the client to time, place, and reason for hospitalization with each client contact.
6. Explain the client's condition to the client and the client's family with each contact. Assist them in asking questions and expressing concerns about the present and future.

Heart: Decreased Cardiac Output

The client experiences altered cardiac output (decreased) that is related to dyspnea, tachycardia, neck vein distention, and epigastric or abdominal pain that results from pericardial effusion.

Nursing interventions:

1. Assess respiratory rate, heart rate, and blood pressure every 15 to 30 minutes and record pulse pressure.
2. Assess neck vein distention with head of bed elevated up to 60 degrees every hour.
3. Assess electrocardiogram for a decrease in QRS voltage, electrical alternans, and dysrhythmias.
4. Monitor intake and output every hour.
5. Auscultate heart and lung sounds every 2 hours.
6. Administer oxygen as prescribed.

Bone: Impaired Physical Mobility

The client has impaired physical mobility related to pain, numbness, weakness, and bladder and bowel incontinence resulting from pathologic fractures.

Nursing interventions:

1. Palpate bones for tenderness and crepitus every 4 hours.
2. Assess alignment of bones every hour.
3. Position the client using techniques of proper body alignment associated with comfort and support of wasted limbs.
4. Measure respiratory rate and quality every 4 hours.
5. Monitor intake and output every 8 hours, noting continence.
6. Splint the client within the draw sheet when transferring.
7. Medicate around the clock for pain.

TABLE 64–6. *Assessment for Advanced Disease*

ORGAN/PROBLEM	PHYSICAL ASSESSMENT	LAB VALUES	DIAGNOSTICS
Brain/neuropsychiatric syndrome	Personality changes Decision making Math computations Level of consciousness Seizure activity Increased intracranial pressure (Table 64–2)	Phenobarbital Phenytoin (Dilantin)	Computed tomography brain scan Magnetic resonance imaging of brain
Heart/pericardial effusion	Respiratory rate Liver palpation Neck vein distention Heart rate Blood pressure Heart sounds	Arterial blood gases	Electrocardiogram Echocardiogram Chest radiograph
Bone/pathologic fractures	Pain Respiratory rate Assess extremities: • motor function • tactile perception • muscle strength • bowel and bladder control	Calcium Phosphorus	Radiograph of bone Bone scan
Lung/pleural effusion	Heart rate Respiratory rate Breath sound Lung symmetry	Arterial blood gases Fluid cytology	Thoracentesis Chest radiograph Pulmonary function test
Liver/malignant ascites	Respiratory rate Abdominal girth Bowel sounds Abdominal palpation	Fluid cytology Albumin Fluid carcinoembryonic antigen	Paracentesis Computed tomography scan of liver
Kidney/renal failure	Lung sounds Palpation for edema	Blood urea nitrogen Arterial blood gases Creatinine Specific gravity of urine Electrolytes	Electrocardiogram Intravenous pyelogram

8. Schedule passive and active range of motion exercises, taking into account a client's pain and ability.
9. Encourage isometric exercises when range of motion exercises are contraindicated.

LUNG: IMPAIRED GAS EXCHANGE

The client experiences impaired gas exchange related to dyspnea, hypoxia, absent breath sounds, and altered arterial blood gases resulting from pleural effusion.

Nursing interventions:

1. Auscultate breath sounds every 2 hours. Do not expect to hear a friction rub, because fluid separates the pleura.
2. Inspect thorax for symmetry of respiratory movement, use of accessory muscles, and tracheal position every 2 hours.
3. Measure blood pressure and heart rate every 2 hours.
4. Monitor intake and output every 4 hours.
5. Elevate head of bed to 60 degrees for comfort.
6. Assess respiratory rate every 30 minutes.
7. Administer oxygen as prescribed.
8. Medicate for pain, anxiety, or both.

LIVER: ALTERED NUTRITION

The client shows effects of altered nutrition—less than body requirements—related to abdominal distention, hypoalbuminemia, shortness of breath, and nausea resulting from malignant ascites.

Nursing interventions:

1. Monitor intake and output every 4 hours.
2. Measure abdominal girth daily.
3. Record blood pressure, heart rate, and respirations every 2 hours.
4. Monitor serum albumin levels and serum and urine osmolality.
5. Restrict sodium intake.
6. Restrict fluids to less than 1500 ml per day.
7. Weigh daily.
8. Assist the client to a high Fowler's position to ease respirations.
9. Perform skin care every 4 hours.

KIDNEY: IMPAIRED SKIN INTEGRITY

The client experiences alteration in skin integrity related to fluid retention, edema, and increased blood urea nitrogen level resulting from chemotherapy-induced renal failure.

Nursing interventions:

1. Monitor intake and output every hour.
2. Weigh the client at the same time every day.
3. Record blood pressure, heart rate, and respiratory rate every 2 hours.
4. Turn and position the client every 2 hours.
5. Massage bony prominences and apply lotion to skin every 4 hours.
6. Provide hyperalimentation as prescribed.
7. Restrict dietary protein intake.

SPECIAL PROBLEMS RELATED TO ADVANCED DISEASE

Although it would seem as though the complications of advanced disease are serious in and of themselves, several problems must not be ignored. These include drainage odor, hope, and suicidal ideation.

DRAINAGE ODOR

In advanced disease in which metastases are extensive, it is not unusual to encounter direct invasion of cancer cells into the epithelium. This phenomenon occurs most commonly from primary cancers of the breast, stomach, head and neck, lung, uterus, ovary, and colon, as well as from melanoma and lymphoma. This type of metastasis causes loss of vascularity with ultimate necrosis and infection. The result is a purulent, friable, malodorous lesion (Foltz, 1980).

Because cure of these lesions is rare, the problem most significant to the client is odor. The offensive smell is noticed not only by family, hospital staff, and other visitors, but also by the client. Although others may not say anything, the client, aware of the odor, feels embarrassed, and may withdraw socially.

Management of these odors offers relief of one of the many problems a client with advanced disease must face (Anonymous, 1990). Initial management should always include wound cleansing and debridement; however, these measures alone are rarely effective. One effective method of odor control is irrigation with room-temperature yogurt or buttermilk and normal saline. Odiferous wounds, irrigated with these products at least four times a day on a regular basis, become nonproblematic within 4 days (Welch, 1981; Shulte, 1993). A second effective method is to mix a 6-g packet of Bard absorptive dressing with 10 ml of sterile water and 10 ml of puri-Clens (Sween Co.) and place this mixture in the wound, followed by a sterile dressing, twice a day. Another method of odor control is oral or topical metronidazole. This is thought to work by eradication of anaerobic infection. Oral metronidazole has unpleasant side effects such as nausea and neuropathy in long-term use. However, metronidazole, prepared in a gel, has been very effective in treating wound odor (Anonymous, 1990; Carruth, 1993). Although aerosols should not be used exclusively, commercial room deodorizers, such as Hexon odor antagonist, may be helpful.

HOPE

"Hope is a multidimensional dynamic life force characterized by a confident yet uncertain expectation of achieving a future good which, to the hoping person, is realistically possible and personally significant" (DuFault & Martocchio, 1985, p. 380). For any client with cancer, hope is an important concept. Usually the hope is for a cure or remission so that a "normal" lifestyle can be resumed. However, when a complication occurs, whether it is the first indication or a later indication of advanced disease, the hope for a cure is shattered.

It is the responsibility of nurses to help such clients and their families understand that hope is not lost. Although nurses must acknowledge the fact that cure is no longer a realistic possibility, other hopes may be kept alive. Nurses can encourage a hopeful attitude by helping clients and their families develop an awareness of life, identify reasons for living, establish support systems, incorporate religion or humor, and set realistic goals (Hickey, 1986; Poncar, 1994). Nurses must emphasize that although hopes may change in focus and direction, there is never "no hope."

SUICIDAL IDEATION

The final special problem associated with advanced disease is suicidal ideation. Suicide is 1.3 times higher in men and 1.9 times higher in women with cancer than in the general population, although this is not true of adolescents with cancer (Perrone, 1993). Cancers associated with suicide attempts include leukemia, and breast, head and neck, lung, and upper gastrointestinal tract cancers (Kline, 1984).

Suicide attempts arise in an effort to gain control over a situation in which there is no perceived control. Signs and symptoms include verbalization of the intention and the means with which to act on the intention, loss of hope, and loss of interest in any specific aspect of life.

Nursing management of the client with suicidal ideation includes constant assessment and observation because clients generally leave "clues." These clues include the client's perception of advanced illness and poor prognosis, perception of uncontrolled pain, loss of control, helplessness, feelings of failure or of being punished, and loss of interest in other people. The nurse must also take into consideration any preexisting psychopathology such as a history of self-destructive behavior, substance abuse, mental illness, as well as a history of attempted suicide (Richards, 1994). The nurse should also be available to assist in channeling aggressive feelings into constructive behaviors, fostering feelings of control, and finding hope and meaning in life. The major intervention to accomplish these goals is to encourage open communication to talk about issues. In addition to caring for the client, nurses should be attentive to the needs of the family by offering explanations and support. Family needs during the cancer illness experience have been shown to include explanations regarding comfort, pain control, family role changes, family demands such as transportation and household tasks being increased, and reaffirmation of excellence in the caregiver's skill regarding patient care (Kristjanson & Ashcroft, 1994). It is also appropriate when such a situation arises to consult a psychiatric mental health clinical nurse specialist.

SUMMARY

This chapter delineated specific complications of advanced disease according to the vital organs and the pathophysiology involved. In addition, this chapter presented guidelines for nursing management in terms of assessment, nursing diagnoses, and nursing interventions. Finally, three special problems associated with advanced disease and its management were described with subsequent guidelines for nursing management.

Advanced disease is a complex phenomenon and it often mandates decisions that will result directly in life or death. This chapter has focused on aggressive management of complications of advanced disease. However, advanced disease itself is not curable, and management of such complications has limitations. It is vital for caregivers to consider the goals of the client and family as well as the goals of aggressive management when complications are imminent. Potential risks and benefits of interventions should always be examined carefully to ensure the client maximum quality of life as he or she defines it. When there is agreement among all parties that aggressive management is no longer appropriate, invasive, disturbing interventions such as measurement of abdominal girth or frequent monitoring of vital signs should be minimized or eliminated, and supportive care approaches should be continued (see Chapter 77).

REFERENCES

Anonymous (1990). Management of smelly tumours. *The Lancet, 335*(8682), 141–142.

Armitage, J. O. (1994). Bone marrow transplantation. *The New England Journal of Medicine, 330*(12), 827–838.

Baker, A. R., & Weber, J. S. (1993). Treatment of malignant ascites. In V. T. DeVita, Jr., S. Hellman, & S. A. Rosenberg (Eds.), *Cancer: Principles and Practices of Oncology* (pp. 2255–2261). Philadelphia: J. B. Lippincott Co.

Bender, C. M. (1994). Cognitive dysfunction associated with biological response modifier therapy. *Oncology Nursing Forum, 21*(3), 515–523.

Billings, J. A. (1985). *Outpatient management of advanced cancer.* Philadelphia: J. B. Lippincott Co.

Bisel, H. F., Wroblewski, F., & LaDue, J. S. (1953). Incidence and clinical manifestations of cardiac metastases. *Journal of the American Medical Association, 153*, 712–715.

Broaddus, V. C., & Light, R. W. (1994). Disorders of the pleura: General principles and diagnostic approach. In J. F. Murray & J. A. Nadel (Eds.), *Textbook of respiratory medicine* (pp. 2145–2163). Philadelphia: W.B. Saunders Co.

Cameron, J. C. (1993). Ifosamide neurotoxicity. *Cancer Nursing, 16*(1), 40–46.

Carruth, A. K. (1993). Antifungal agent used topically to control odor. *Oncology Nursing Forum, 20*(8), 1262.

Chernecky, C. C., Krech, R. L., & Berger, B. J. (1993). *Lab-oratory tests and diagnostic procedures.* Philadelphia: W.B. Saunders Co.

Chernecky, C. C., & Ramsey, P. W. (1984). *Critical nursing care of the client with cancer.* East Norwalk, CT: Appleton-Century-Crofts.

DeAngelis, L. M. (1994). Management of brain metastasis. *Cancer Investigation, 12*(2), 156–165.

Deslauriers, J., Beauchamp, G., & Desmeules, M. (1991). Benign and malignant disorders of the pleura. In A. E. Baue, A. S. Geha, G. L. Hammond, H. Laks, & K. S. Naunheim (Eds.), *Glenn's thoracic and cardiovascular surgery* (pp. 459–485). Norwalk, CT: Appleton & Lange.

DuFault, K., & Martocchio, B. C. (1985). Hope: Its spheres and dimensions. *Nursing Clinics of North America, 20*, 379–391.

Faehnrich, J. (1983). When pathologic fractures threaten. *RN, 46*(11), 34–37.

Foltz, A. T. (1980). Nursing care of ulcerating metastatic lesions. *Oncology Nursing Forum, 7*(2), 8–13.

Franko, T., & Gould, D. A. (1994). Allogeneic bone marrow transplantation. *Seminars in Oncology Nursing, 10*(1), 3–11.

Graham, I. (1989). Edema. In T. D. Walsh (Ed.), *Symptom control* (pp. 177–194). Oxford: Blackwell Scientific.

Grever, M. R., & Grieshaber, C. K. (1993). Toxicology by organ system. In J. F. Holland, E. Frei, R. C. Bast, Jr., D. W. Jufe, D. L. Morton, & R. R. Weichselbaum (Eds.), *Cancer medicine* (pp. 683–695). Philadelphia: Lea & Febiger.

Haentjens, D., Casteleyn, P. P., & Opdecam, P. (1993). Evaluation of impending fractures and indications for prophylactic fixation of metastasis in long bones. Review of the literature. *Acta Orthopaedica Belgium, 59*(Suppl. 1), 6–11.

Hanfling, S. M. (1960). Metastatic cancer of the heart. *Circulation, 22*, 474–481.

Hickey, S. S. (1986). Enabling hope. *Cancer Nursing, 9*, 133–137.

Henson, J. W., & Posner, J. B. (1993). Neurological complications. In J. F. Holland, E. Frei, R. C. Bast, D. W. Kufe, D. L. Morton, & R. R. Weichselbaum (Eds.), *Cancer Medicine* (pp. 2268–2285). Philadelphia: Lea & Febiger.

Iqbal, J. B., & Ironside, J. W. (1993). Cerebral metastasis from a malignant mixed Mullerian tumour of the uterus. *Histopathology, 23*, 277–279.

Kelly, M. A. (1985). *Nursing diagnosis source book: Guidelines for clinical application.* E. Norwalk, CT: Appleton-Century-Crofts.

Kline, P. M. (1984). Suicidal ideation. In C. C. Chernecky & P. W. Ramsey (Eds.), *Critical nursing care of the client with cancer* (pp. 272–276). East Norwalk, CT: Appleton-Century-Crofts.

Kristjanson, L. S., & Ashcroft, T. (1994). The family's cancer journey: A literature review. *Cancer Nursing, 17*(1), 1–17.

Luce, J. A. (1994). Metastatic malignant tumors. In J. F. Murray & J. A. Nadel (Eds.), *Textbook of respiratory medicine* (pp. 1614–1621). Philadelphia: W. B. Saunders Co.

Lydon, J. (1986). Nephrotoxicity of cancer treatment. *Oncology Nursing Forum, 13*(2), 69–77.

Malawer, M. M., & Delaney, T. F. (1993). Treatment of metastatic cancer to the bone. In V. T. DeVita, Jr., S. Hellman, & S. A. Rosenberg (Eds.), *Cancer: Principles and practice of oncology* (pp. 2225–2245). Philadelphia: J. B. Lippincott Co.

Mauch, P. M. (1982). Treatment of malignant ascites. In V. T. DeVita. Jr., S. Hellman, & S. A. Rosenberg (Eds.), *Cancer: Principles and practices of oncology* (pp. 156–197). Philadelphia: J.B. Lippincott Co.

Miles, D. W., & Knight, R. K. (1993). Diagnosis and management of malignant pleural effusion. *Cancer Treatment Reviews, 19,* 151–168.

Newton, C., & Mateo, M. A. (1994). Uncertainty: Strategies for patients with brain tumor and their family. *Cancer Nursing, 17*(2), 137–140.

Perrone, J. (1993). Adolescents with cancer: Are they at risk for suicide? *Pediatric Nursing, 19*(1), 22–28.

Poncar, P. J. (1994). Inspiring hope in the oncology patient. *Journal of Psychosocial Nursing, 32*(1), 33–38.

Pursley, P. (1983). Acute cardiac tamponade. *American Journal of Nursing, 3,* 1414–1418.

Richards, S. H. (1994). Finding the means to carry on: Suicidal feelings in cancer patients. *Professional Nurse, 2,* 334–339.

Rogers, B. B. (1993). Taxol: A promising new drug of the '90s. *Oncology Nursing Forum, 20*(10), 1483–1489.

Rosetti, A. C. (1985). Nursing care of the patients treated with intrapleural tetracycline for control of malignant pleural effusion. *Cancer Nursing, 8,* 103–109.

Schryber, S., Lacasse, C. R., & Barton-Burke, M. (1987). Autologous bone marrow transplantation. *Oncology Nursing Forum, 14*(4), 74–80.

Schulte, M. J. (1993). Yogurt helps to control wound odor. *Oncology Nursing Forum, 20*(8), 1262.

Sherlock, S., & Dooley, J. (1993). *Diseases of the liver and biliary system.* Oxford: Blackwell Scientific Publications.

Sparber, A. G., & Biller-Sparber, K. (1993). Immunotherapy and neuropsychiatric toxicity. *Cancer Nursing, 16*(3), 188–192

Spiro, H. M. (1983). *Clinical gastroenterology* (3rd ed.). New York: Macmillan.

Tepper, J. E., Cohen, A. M., Wood, W. C., Orlow, E. L., & Hedberg, S. E. (1987). Postoperative radiation therapy of rectal cancer. *International Journal of Radiation Oncology Biology Physics, 12,* 5–10.

Tomkowski, W., Szturmowicz, M., Fijalkowska, A., Filipecki, S. & Figura-Chojak, E. (1994). Intrapericardial cisplatin for the management of patient with large malignant pericardial effusion. *Journal of Cancer Research and Clinical Oncology, 120,* 434–436.

Tutschka, P. J. (1993). Graft-versus-host-disease: Implications. *Recent Results in Cancer Research, 132,* 197–204.

Vaitkus, P. T., Herrmann, H. D., & LeWinter, M. M. (1994). Treatment of malignant pericardial effusion. *Journal of the American Medical Association, 272*(1), 59–64.

Vieth, R. G., & Odom, G. L. (1965). Intracranial metastases and their neurosurgical treatment. *Journal of Neurosurgery, 23,* 375–383.

Vigliotti, A., Rich, T. A., Romsdahl, M. M., Withers, H. R., & Oswald, M. J. (1987). Postoperative adjuvant radiotherapy for adenocarcinoma of the rectum and rectosigmoid. *International Journal of Radiation Oncology Biology Physics, 12,* 999–1006.

Walker-Renard, P. B., Vaughan, L. M., & Sahn, S. A. (1994). Chemical pleurodesis for malignant pleural effusions. *Annals of Internal Medicine, 120,* 56–64.

Weiss, R. B., & Vogelzang, N. J. (1993). Miscellaneous toxicities. In V. T. DeVita, Jr., S. Hellman, & S. A. Rosenberg (Eds.), *Cancer: Principles and practice of oncology* (pp. 2349–2358). Philadelphia: J.B. Lippincott Co.

Welch, L. B. (1981). Simple new remedy for the odor of open lesions. *RN, 44*(2), 42–43.

Wickham, R. (1986). Pulmonary toxicity secondary to cancer treatment. *Oncology Nursing Forum, 13*(5), 69–76.

Wright, D. C., Delaney, T. F., & Buckner, J. C. (1993). Treatment of metastatic cancer to the brain. In V. T. DeVita, Jr., S. Hellman, & S. A. Rosenberg (Eds.), *Cancer: Principles and practice of oncology* (pp. 2170–2200). Philadelphia: J.B. Lippincott Co.

Wujcik, D., Ballard, B., & Camp-Sorrell, D. (1994). Selected complications of allogeneic bone marrow transplantation. *Seminars in Oncology Nursing, 10*(1), 28–41.

Yellin, A. (1994). Doxycycline for malignant effusions [Letter]. *Annals of Thoracic Surgery, 57*(4), 1053–1054.

Symptoms of the Dying

Mary Pickett • Donna Yancey

MULTIDIMENSIONAL CARE OF THE DYING

OVERVIEW

This chapter examines the care of the dying within a framework that addresses spiritual, physical, and psychosocial concerns. Such issues as quality of life, symptoms of dying, and psycho/socio/cultural needs of patients and caregivers are examined, and specific nursing behaviors are discussed. This information will guide nurses and other health professionals as they assist dying patients and their families.

Approximately 60 per cent of cancer patients living in developed countries will die of cancer despite the advances in technology (Stjernsward & Teoh, 1991). The American Cancer Society estimates that in 1994 approximately 1.2 million Americans will be diagnosed with cancer and that more than one half million Americans will die of the disease despite the advances made in prevention, screening, and treatment (Boring, Squires, Tong & Montgomery, 1994). More than 25 years ago Dr. Cicely Saunders began her search to alleviate pain and suffering experienced by dying persons. Today hospice/palliative care philosophy and treatments designed to alleviate discomfort commonly associated with terminal illness are internationally recognized and accepted. Significant contributions to the development of new systems of personalized care for dying patients and their families and improvements in symptom management and psychosocial care have been advanced by nurses interested in improving the quality of life for terminally ill persons (e.g., Madalon Amenta, Jeanne Quint Benoliel, Inge Corless, Lesley Degner, Benita Martocchio, Ruth McCorkle, Barbara Petrosino, Mary Vachon, Florence Wald, and Joyce Zerwekh).

The concepts of loss and transition are prominent in the literature describing person-centered care designed to assist persons coping with changes associated with progressive serious illness (Benoliel, 1985; Parkes, 1988). Delivery of compassionate family-centered care is based on an appreciation of the multiple loss experiences faced by dying persons and their families. Models of nursing interventions and care delivery systems specifically designed to assist patients and their families adapt to the multiple changes resulting from advanced cancer have been reported (Benoliel, 1987; Dudgeon, 1992; McCorkle, 1988; Reimer, Davies & Martens, 1991; Saunders & McCorkle, 1985; Tornberg, McGrath, & Benoliel, 1984). Patient care that promotes quality of life during the end-of-life addresses such issues as loss of physical function and key roles that give personal meaning to life, control of distressing symptoms that interfere with ability to interact within social networks, and enforced reliance on family caregivers that results from physical changes associated with advanced cancer (Saunders & McCorkle, 1985).

McCorkle (1981) gave thoughtful consideration about how nurses can assist patients to prepare for a "good death." Despite the passage of time, McCorkle's (1981) powerful analogy between the elements of a "good birth" and a "good death" continues to be relevant as we enter the twenty-first century (see Box 65–1 for complete text of editorial).

Box 65–1. *A Good Death*

From McCorkle, R. (1981). A good death [Editorial]. *Cancer Nursing,* 4(4):267.

For some years now, I have been struggling with the question "What is a good death?" According to American psychiatrist Weisman, "A good death is one a person would choose for himself."* And yet, there is general agreement that most persons would choose not to die with cancer if they had a choice. How then can a "good death" be interpreted so it is applicable for persons dying with cancer?

In the many hours of sitting and being with persons with cancer who have died, I have felt great satisfaction in helping them remain in as much control of their dying as possible. And yet to be in control may imply not being as physically comfortable as I know I could help some of them be. In my search for an answer, I decided to take a fresh look at the question and compare the event of dying to another important transition of life, that of birth. I thought if I could identify some key characteristics of a "good birth," I could make a reasonable analogy as to what a good death is.

It was easy to recall my training in obstetrics. It was an exciting time and I quickly learned that the quality of the birth experience differed according to where it occurred, the length and type of labor, the medications used, the people present, and the mother's perception of what was happening. A good birth is influenced by at least three factors: prenatal care, help during labor and the birth, and postnatal care. Similarly, it seems for persons in whom death is expected, a good death is dependent upon care for some time prior to the actual death experience, help during the labor of dying and the death event, and care of the survivors. Nurses are assuming increased responsibility for helping persons to achieve some degree of all three factors. This is a beginning step at identifying the criteria for a good death, but more work is needed. Unlike the birth experience, the person dying may participate in the choices surrounding the death if given the opportunity.

Upon reexamining Weisman's definition, it seems to me a death one would choose for oneself would be one in which one could participate in the decisions affecting how one may live one's final days, and how one may die, and could have some degree of control over the circumstances surrounding one's dying and the death itself. For most people, opportunities for choice are limited to the presence of at least one individual knowledgeable of the alternatives available. But the presence of a knowledgeable caregiver is not enough; the caregiver must also be respectful of the dying person's right to choose and have the deepest respect for the person's choices especially when they differ from his or her own values and goals.

Many people die who do not need the help of others. For those who need help, a good death is dependent upon two criteria: (1) a relationship with a knowledgeable caregiver that is one of open continuing communication conveying the dying person's wishes; and (2) a primary caregiver who will assume responsibility for ensuring that these wishes are always taken into account when decisions are made that affect his dying.

It is a unique opportunity to help persons with cancer during the dying process. It is an enriching and growing experience to help a person achieve a good death.

---

* Weisman, A. D. (1972). *On dying and denying.* (p. 4.) New York: Behavioral Publications.

ADVANCE DIRECTIVES

The constitutional right of individuals to engage in decision making regarding medical interventions at end of life is now protected through federal legislation. The Patient Self-Determination Act (PDSA) of 1990 requires all Medicare- and Medicaid-funded health care facilities to advise patients of their legal rights to refuse or accept medical treatment. Although legislation may vary from state to state, the best sources of information to address differences across states include the individual state Attorney General's Office, Bar Association, Office on Aging, and Hospital Association (American Nurses Association, 1991). Patients are given the opportunity to prospectively determine and record their choices about end-of-life treatment in advance through such mechanisms as living wills and durable power of attorney for health care (Dimond, 1992, 1994). Cancer patients are advised to select their choices about future medical treatment before a crisis occurs. Neumark (1994) offers guidelines and patient education materials designed to increase ambulatory cancer patients' understanding about advance directives. Ideally, PSDA offers adults information about their rights and opportunities to consider documenting their choices regarding end-of-life decisions well in advance of critical decision making about initiation or continuation of life-support interventions. Advance directives offer patients the advantage of communicating their particular preferences about end-of-life care prior to the occurrence of events that might prevent them from making their wishes known (Table 65–1).

SPIRITUAL/EXISTENTIAL DIMENSIONS

QUALITY OF LIFE

A new paradigm of treatment outcome measurement that values a patient-centered approach is becoming more prevalent in cancer treatment (Schipper, Clinch, & Powell, 1990). Quality-of-life assessment attempts to represent the net effect of the disease, as well as medical and psychosocial interventions from the perspective of the patient (Schipper, 1992). In the past, treatment decisions were made without the benefit of the patient's individual assessment of dimensions of life affected by disease and treatment. Quality-of-life assessment can provide systematic evaluation of the patient's status and influence treatment decisions. Treatment decisions that are solely based on the

TABLE 65–1. *Documentation of Advance Directives*

Living Will

This document promotes the right of self-determination by preventing unwanted heroic medical interventions. The living will statute offers competent individuals a mechanism to document what medical intervention they do and do not want in case they become mentally incompetent and require medical technology to keep them alive.

When an individual signs a living will statement, within the statutory provisions, there is a hope to maintain control over medical decisions and avoid a technologic imperative that commands "that which can be done, must be done."

Specific provisions of the living will statutes allow individuals to direct withholding and withdrawal of medical treatment in the event that the patient becomes terminally ill.

Durable Power of Attorney

This document provides for an individual to control the process and content of decision making about medical interventions in case of mental incapacity by naming an authorized individual to make decisions consistent with the declarant's specific instructions documented in the statement.

---

assumption that all individuals would choose survival at any cost are flawed (Barofsky & Sugarbaker, 1990). Quality-of-life assessment in cancer patients across the illness trajectory contributes information to clinical decision making that reflects individual patient perceptions of living with serious illness.

Health-related quality of life is a multidimensional construct that typically includes physical status (symptoms), functional status, psychologic function, and social interaction (Spilker, 1990). Schipper et al.'s (1990) definitions of these terms are presented here for clarity. Physical status encompasses the level of unpleasant sensations that may detract from an individual's quality of life. Some of these somatic experiences include fatigue, pain, nausea, vomiting, and shortness of breath. Functional status indicates the level of strength, energy, and ability to carry out normal expected activities of daily living. Psychologic function refers to mood states that may include anxiety, fear, depression, as well as positive psychologic states. Social interaction refers to an individual's ability to carry out the daily person-to-person interactions with family and friends.

Cella (1992) suggests that patients who are able to adjust their expectations under duress are also likely to adapt better to their illness and experience a higher quality of life. There is evidence to suggest that patients who experience increasing levels of threat (i. e., physical decline) reduce the gap between actual and expected functional ability, which results in a better rating of quality of life (Mishel, 1990). Quality-of-life assessment in terminally ill patients requires a standardized approach that is sensitive to changes and adaptations that result during periods of physical decline. The Quality of Life Index—Cancer Version (QLI-CV) is a 35-item instrument that assesses subjective experience (Ferrans, 1990) and may be sensitive to changes that occur in the palliative care trajectory. This instrument is based on the original Quality of Life Index (Ferrans & Powers, 1985) and includes items that are pertinent to palliative care patients (i. e., health care, physical health and functioning, marriage, family, friends, stress, peace of mind, personal faith, life goals, general happiness, general satisfaction). The instrument consists of two parts: the first measures satisfaction with various aspects of life, and the second measures the importance of the same aspects to the individual. Patients select a satisfaction level and rate the importance of each aspect of life identified in each item on a six-point scale. The responses are weighted according to the "importance" value that the individual places on particular aspects of life, resulting in a summed score that reflects adaptations that may occur in advancing illness. For example, it is possible for two patients with equally low levels of physical functioning to report satisfaction scores at opposite ends of the scale, resulting in very different overall quality of life scores. Quality-of-life scores result from multiplying the satisfaction score by the importance score for each item and then summing. The QLI-CV instrument is useful in eliciting comprehensive subjective assessments from patients who are experiencing multiple changes in quality of life and provides direction for intervention. The QLI-CV holds promise for use with advanced cancer patients; however, evaluation of this instrument in a sample of advanced cancer patients is not available in the literature at this time.

Clinical situations provide support for inclusion of unique aspects of individuals that are central to personhood and meaning in life. Cohen and Mount (1992) recommend including the spiritual domain within quality-of-life assessments for palliative care patients. Quality-of-life assessment represents a shift from the medical model that places major emphasis on diagnosis and resolution of pathophysiologic processes to a model of holistic care that takes into account the patient's perception of illness and how it affects daily living.

HOPE AND MEANING OF LIFE

". . .Hope is something all people need until they take their last breath. I have seen very little evidence that most people accept death. Rather, they accept life. If they accept life well, then they die well" (Hall, 1990, p. 178). These compelling statements were written by a nurse who explored the concept of hope through an analysis of clinical, empiric, and subjective data. Hall (1990) emphasizes the importance of relating in a future-oriented way with terminally ill persons. Patients often encounter professionals in the health care setting who impose their vision of "realistic hope" for individuals living with terminal illness. Professional caregivers' perspectives on hope may not be congruent with patients' views of hope. A familiar focus in the existing literature suggests that hope should be "realistic" (Dufault & Martocchio, 1985; Herth, 1991; Hickey, 1986; Owen, 1989). Some nurses argue that the parameters of hopefulness that each individual person sets should not be limited by health care professionals' views of what constitutes "realistic hope"

(Hall, 1990; Yates, 1993). According to Dufault and Martocchio (1985) hope "is reality-based from the perspective of the hoping person" (p. 384). No universal definition of hope exists to capture the meaning of this construct for all seriously ill persons. Personal values, beliefs, experiences, and resources influence the meaning of hope for each individual.

A multidimensional model of hope, based on information obtained through interviews and observations of elderly persons with cancer, was advanced by Dufault and Martocchio (1985). Clinicians and researchers observe that maintenance of hope is instrumental in coping processes of chronically ill persons (Herth, 1989; Scanlon, 1989; Weisman, 1979). Herth's (1990) research findings about the meaning of hope and hope-fostering strategies in a convenience sample of adults (*n* = 30) enrolled in hospice programs contribute to an understanding of hope within the context of terminal care. The patients were aware that their life expectancies were projected to be 6 months or less. Hope is described as a dynamic and complex phenomenon that involves thoughts, feelings, and actions that provide a new awareness of what is possible in life, an ability to "put pieces of life into a (new) pattern," and an ability to "face the shortness of life constructively" (Herth, 1990, p. 1256). Hope-fostering strategies were identified from patient interviews and sorted into seven categories: interpersonal connectedness, attainable aims, spiritual base, personal attributes, light-heartedness, uplifting

memories, and affirmation of worth. The defining characteristics of the hope-fostering strategies provide direction for supporting persons who are terminally ill.

A critical element of hope is the presence of a caring relationship during terminal illness. Changes in interpersonal relationships may result when an awareness of advanced illness and shortened life span becomes part of an individual's life experience (Box 65–2). Nurses can influence internal and external conditions that foster caring relationships by providing the patient, family, and friends network with such approaches as physical and emotional support, information about hope and dying, encouragement to create an environment of closeness, and a sense of belonging (Herth, 1990). Active listening and being present with the terminally ill facilitate an environment in which patients define the context and meaning of their own lives (Herth, 1990; Jones, 1993). Abandonment and isolation, uncontrollable pain, and devaluation of personhood were identified by terminally ill persons as factors that interfered with their hope (Herth, 1990). The nursing strategies that Dufault and Martocchio (1985) suggest are focused on creating an environment that offers patients opportunities to express their hopes through communication of thoughts and feelings, maintenance of significant relationships, and reflection on continuity among past, present, and future hopes.

Frankl's (1963) personal narrative about meaning in life while facing desperate conditions contributes to

---

Box 65–2. *The Importance of Authentic Relationships While Living With Advanced Cancer*

The following excerpt from Martocchio (1987) provides greater insight into the experience of living with advanced cancer. Contributions from relevant theories, interviews with cancer patients, and Martocchio's own personal experience with serious chronic illness are evident in the following selection:

Dying transforms relationships. It can replace the sense of future that nourishes them with a sense of ending that impoverishes them. Many people no longer relate to the living person with a limited future, but to the dying person with no future. Such a view restricts opportunities for sharing usual human relationships and sentiments, thus isolating dying persons, even while surrounding them with people. Such persons are denied a sense of future; they are denied the opportunity to develop meaningful agendas. As a result they experience impoverishment and loss of life's meaning.

Some conditions foster development of agendas and protect the meaningfulness in situations where the future is known to be finite. First, authenticity, authentic relationships, self-representation and feelings of belonging are the fabric of meaningful living regardless of the expected length of life. Second, there is always a future whether it is minutes, days, or years. Meaning and value are preserved when dying people are respected as living with unique personalities and future goals. To develop agendas that fit reality patients must have accurate information about their well being so that they can represent themselves in decisions regarding their care *before* actions are taken. Caregivers should arrive at a consensus about information shared. Conflicting information may be more detrimental than no information. To be useful, information should be honest and on a level an individual can understand. Dying people must have freedom to choose a style or mode of dying and then be supported in that choice. The fit between the reality and agenda will be closer if family's views are considered. The dying persons may choose which decisions they *do not* want to be involved in making as well as those in which they *do wish to be involved.*

A primary agenda may be to remain autonomous human beings. . .

Another agenda may focus on being part of a social network, community, or family.

Dying persons may focus on this agenda to the exclusion of all others. They may save their energies for visits of loved ones. People derive self worth from and thus meaningfulness of living through belonging, through loving and being loved in return, touching and being touched, and sharing with others. Sharing may include telling about their philosophy of life or of death, and their memories and their family history. Sharing may be sitting together, sharing a space, thoughts, prayer, music or a sunset.

Martocchio, B. C. (1987). Authenticity, belonging, emotional closeness, and self-representation. *Oncology Nursing Forum, 14*(4), 23–27. Reprinted from the *Oncology Nursing Forum* with permission from the Oncology Nursing Press, Inc.

understanding the plight of dying persons facing grave losses and uncertainty. The experience of personal meaning as fundamental to human life is an assumption drawn from Frankl's vivid account of survival in a concentration camp. Mount (1993) suggests using Frankl's identified sources of meaning in life as a guide for discussing this topic with patients. Opportunities for patients to review key areas of their lives emerge when the following questions are asked by caring professionals and volunteers. What have you done, created, or accomplished? What do you love in life? places? people? music? ideas? What will you miss leaving behind? What do you believe in? Discussions about the particular sources of meaning for an individual can promote positive feelings of engagement in life (Mount, 1993). Life review is an approach to enhance quality of life and self-esteem of dying persons by providing an opportunity to explore the perceptions of uniqueness, value, and meaning within past life experiences. Life review approaches can also be used effectively with family members.

Lichter, Mooney, and Boyd (1993) describe a biography service that is available to hospice patients as a therapeutic intervention. This intervention is offered to patients who might benefit from the process of life review. Volunteer members of the hospice family support team receive a structured training program on interviewing techniques, practical aspects of tape recording an oral biography, and developing a written biographic sketch. No attempt has been made to objectively measure the outcomes of this process; however, patient satisfaction associated with this activity is high (Lichter et al., 1993). Patient comments indicate that the value of engaging in an oral biographic process are associated with having someone actively listening to stories about their life events and sharing favorite memories. Recounting life events may provide dying patients with an opportunity to "tie up some loose ends" and conclude some "unfinished business;" family members report that the written biographic record serves as a cherished memorial after the death of their loved one (Lichter et al., 1993).

In 1990 the Spiritual Care Work Group of the International Work Group on Death, Dying, and Bereavement developed a statement of assumptions and principles concerning spiritual care of dying persons and their families (Spiritual Care Work Group, 1990). The assumptions and principles address a range of diverse spiritual beliefs present in Western society and offer guidance to professional caregivers (see Table 65–2 for complete summary).

PHYSICAL DIMENSIONS

COMMON PHYSICAL SYMPTOMS IN TERMINAL CANCER

Patients with advanced cancer commonly experience multiple symptoms. These symptoms can result from disease progression, debility, acute organic phenomena caused by the cancer or resulting from it, and metabolic changes due to anticancer treatment

(Ventafridda, Ripamonti, DeConno, Tamburini, & Cassileth, 1990). Chart reviews and patient interviews indicate that pain, nausea, dyspnea, delirium, and drowsiness are the most common symptoms of terminal cancer patients (Coyle, Adelhardt, Foley, & Portenoy, 1990; Curtis, Krech, & Walsh, 1991; Fainsinger, Miller, Bruera, Hanson, & MacEachern, 1991; Gray, Adler, Fleming, & Brescia, 1988; Hockley, Dunlop, & Davies, 1988; Ventafridda et al., 1990). Other symptoms frequently mentioned were dysphagia, anxiety, depression, fatigue, weakness, fever, constipation, anorexia, xerostomia, and sleep problems. Analyses of 952 terminal cancer patients' symptoms revealed that pain affected most patients at some point in the terminal phase and that 56 per cent of the other symptoms involved the digestive system: nausea, vomiting, constipation, and mouth lesions (Bedard, Dionne, & Dionne, 1991). Higginson and McCarthy (1989) found pain was the most common symptom at the time of referral to the terminal support team and that it became less prominent over time. Lichter and Hunt (1990) found the common symptoms in the last 48 hours of life in 200 dying cancer patients to be pain (51 per cent), noisy and moist breathing (56 per cent), restlessness and agitation (42 per cent), urinary incontinence or retention (53 per cent), and dyspnea (22 per cent). In the last week of life, weakness and dyspnea were the most common symptoms (Higginson & McCarthy, 1989).

The foregoing studies examined symptoms of terminally ill patients by age, gender, and type of cancer. Gray et al. (1988) found that patients under 65 were more likely to have dysphagia and severe pain, while patients over 65 were more frequently found to be confused. These researchers also noted that patients with ovarian, stomach, pancreatic, and colon malignancies frequently or usually experienced nausea and that patients with cervical, prostate, and colo-rectal cancers, and bone metastases experienced severe pain. Curtis et al. (1991) showed that men and women reported major differences in frequency and severity of all symptoms except pain and xerostomia, which were equally frequent. Women in this study were more likely to have gastrointestinal (GI) symptoms such as anorexia, nausea, vomiting, early satiety, and taste change.

While some research reports note differences in symptoms, researchers in the National Hospice Study found a pattern of symptoms in end-stage cancer patients or "a terminal common pathway" (Wachtel, Allen-Masterson, Reuben, Goldberg, & Mor, 1988). The symptoms of this terminal pathway included weight loss, dyspnea, anorexia, dysphagia, xerostomia, and declining functional status. The intensity or frequency of the symptoms heightened as death neared.

DETERMINATION OF PROGNOSIS

The desire to know "how much time remains in one's life" is often an issue for the patient and family because of the need to get affairs in order and to say "good-byes." It is also important to the health care professionals who are making a determination of 6

TABLE 65–2. *Assumptions and Principles Concerning Spiritual Care of Dying Persons and their Families*

ASSUMPTIONS	PRINCIPLES
General	
Each person has a spiritual dimension.	In the total care of a person, his or her spiritual nature must be considered along with the mental, emotional, and physical dimensions.
A spiritual orientation influences mental, emotional, and physical responses to dying and bereavement.	Caregivers working with dying and bereaved persons should be sensitive to this interrelationship.
Although difficult, facing terminal illness, death, and bereavement can be a stimulus for spiritual growth.	Persons involved in these circumstances may wish to give spiritual questions time and attention.
In a multicultural society, a person's spiritual nature is expressed in religious and philosophical beliefs and practices that differ widely depending upon one's race, sex, class, religion, ethnic heritage, and experience.	No single approach to spiritual care is satisfactory for all in a multicultural society; many kinds of resources are needed.
Spirituality has many facets. It is expressed and enhanced in a variety of ways both formal and informal, religious and secular, including, but not limited to symbols, rituals, practices, patterns and gestures, art forms, prayers, and meditation.	A broad range of opportunities for expressing and enhancing one's spirituality should be available and accessible.
The environment shapes and can enhance or diminish one's spirituality.	Care should be taken to offer settings that will accommodate individual preference as well as communal experience.
Spiritual concerns often have a low priority in health care systems.	Health care systems presuming to offer total care should plan for and include spiritual care as reflected in a written statement of philosophy, and resources of time, money, and staff.
Spiritual needs can arise at any time of the day or night, any day of the week.	A caring environment shoud be in place to enhance and promote spiritual work at any time, not just at designated times.
Joy is part of the human spirit. Humor is a leaven needed even, or especially, in times of adversity or despair.	Caregivers, patients, and family members should feel free to express humor and laugh.
Individual and Family (Natural and Acquired)	
Human beings have diverse beliefs, understanding, and levels of development in spiritual matters.	Caregivers should be encouraged to understand various belief systems and their symbols, as well as to seek to understand an individual's particular interpretation of them.
Individuals and their families may have divergent spiritual insights and beliefs. They may not be aware of these differences.	Caregivers should be aware of differences in spirituality within a famiy or close relationship and be alert to any difficulties that might ensue.
The degree to which the patient and family wish to examine and share spiritual matters is highly individual.	Caregivers must be nonintrusive and sensitive to individual desires.
Health care institutions and professionals may presume they understand, or may ignore, the spiritual needs of dying persons.	Spiritual needs can only be determined through a thoughtful review of spiritual assumptions, beliefs, practices, experiences, goals, and perceived needs with the patient, or family and friends.
People are not always aware of, nor are able, nor wish to articulate spiritual issues.	Caregivers should be aware of individual desires and be sensitive to unexpressed spiritual issues.
	Individuals need access to resources and to people who are committed to deepened exploration of and communication about spiritual issues.
Much healing and spiritual growth can occur in an individual without assistance. Many people do not desire or need professional assistance in their spiritual development.	Acknowledgement and support, listening to and affirming an individual's beliefs or spiritual concerns should be offered and may be all that is needed.
Patients may have already provided for their spiritual needs in a manner satisfactory to themselves.	The patient's chosen way of meeting spiritual needs should be honored by the caregivers.
The spiritual needs of dying persons and their families may vary during the course of the illness and fluctuate with changes in physical symptoms.	Caregivers need to be alert to the varying spiritual concerns that may be expressed directly or indirectly during different phases of illness.
Patients and their families are particularly vulnerable at the time of impending death.	Caregivers should guard against proselytizing for particular types of beliefs and practices.

TABLE 65–2. *Assumptions and Principles Concerning Spiritual Care of Dying Persons and their Families* Continued

ASSUMPTIONS	PRINCIPLES
As death approaches, spiritual concerns may arise that may be new or still unresolved.	Caregivers should be prepared to work with new concerns and insights, as well as those that are long-standing. Caregivers must recognize that not all spiritual problems can be resolved.
The spiritual care of the family may affect the dying person.	Spiritual care of family and friends is an essential component of total care for the dying.
The family's need for spiritual care does not end with the death of the patient.	Spiritual care may include involvement by caregivers in the funeral and should be available throughout the bereavement period.
Caregivers Caregivers, like patients, may have or represent different beliefs as well as different spiritual or religious backgrounds and insights.	Caregivers have the right to expect respect for their belief systems.
Many health care workers may be unprepared or have limited personal development in spiritual matters.	Staff members should be offered skillfully designed opportunities for exploration of values and attitudes about life and death, their meaning and purpose. Caregivers need to recognize their limitations and make appropriate referrals when the demand for spiritual care exceeds their abilities or resources.
The clergy is usually seen as having primary responsibility for the spiritual care of the dying.	Caregivers should be aware that they each have the potential for providing spiritual care, as do all human beings, and should be encouraged to offer spiritual care to dying patients and their families as needed.
Caregivers may set goals for the patient, the family, and themselves that are inflexible and unrealistic. This may inhibit spontaneity and impede the development of a sensitive spiritual relationship.	Caregivers and health care institutions should temper spiritual goals with realism.
Ongoing involvement with dying and bereaved persons may cause a severe drain of energy and uncover old and new spiritual issues for the caregiver.	Ongoing spiritual education, growth, and renewal should be a part of a staff support program, as well as a personal priority for each caregiver.
Community Coordination Spiritual resources are available within the community and can make a valuable contribution to the care of the dying patient.	Spiritual counselors from the community should be integral members of the caregiving team.
No one caregiver can be expected to understand or address all the spiritual concerns of patients and families.	Staff members addressing the needs of patients and families should use spiritual resources and caregivers available in the community.
Education and Research Contemporary education for health care professionals often lacks reference to the spiritual dimension of care.	Health care curricula should foster an awareness of the spiritual dimension in the clinical setting.
Education in spiritual care is impeded by a lack of fundamental research.	Research about spiritual care is needed to create a foundation of knowledge that will enhance education and enrich and increase the spiritual aspect of the provision of health care.
Freedom from bias is a problem in the conduct of research into spiritual care.	Research should be carried out in the development and application of valid and reliable measures of evaluation.

months or less for entry into a certified Medicare hospice program. Some researchers tried to predict the prognosis of a terminal cancer patient by using the presence of various symptoms and the performance status of the patient (Bruera, Miller, Kuehn, MacEachern, & Hanson, 1992; Evans & McCarthy, 1985; Reuben, Mor, & Hiris, 1988; Yates, Chalmer, & McKegney, 1980). The Karnofsky Performance Scale (KPS) developed by Karnofsky, Abelmann, Craver, and Burchenal (1948) was used to measure performance. KPS applies a numeric value in tens ranging from 0 to 100 for quantifying the functional level of the patient (See Table 65–3). The use of the KPS contributed significantly to the prediction of time of death in the research reported by Evans and McCarthy (1985). They found the KPS gave a closer correlation ($r = .56$) with actual survival than estimates made by the terminal support team ($r = .44$) on 42 patients during an initial visit. Reuben et al. (1988) also found the performance status was the single best prognostic indicator of survival in the National Hospice Study. When examining the correlation of individual symptoms

TABLE 65–3. *Karnofsky Performance Status Scale (KPS)*

SCALE	CRITERIA
100	Normal; no complaints of disease.
90	Able to carry on normal activity; minor signs or symptoms of disease.
80	Normal activity with effort; some signs or symptoms of disease.
70	Cares for self. Unable to carry on normal activity or to do active work.
60	Requires occasional assistance, but is able to care for most of his or her needs.
50	Requires considerable assistance and frequent medical care.
40	Disabled; requires special care and assistance.
30	Severely disabled; hospitalization is indicated although death not imminent.
20	Very sick; hospitalization necessary; active supportive treatment necessary.
10	Moribund; fatal processes progressing rapidly.
0	Dead.

(From Karnofsky, D. A., Abelmann, W. H., Craver, L. F., & Burchenal, J. H. [1948]. The use of the nitrogen mustards in the palliative treatment of carcinoma. *Cancer, 1*[4], 634–656. Used with permission of J. B. Lippincott.)

with survival, shortness of breath correlated with the greatest reduction of survival (Reuben et al., 1988). On the other hand, Bruera, Miller, Kuehn, et al., (1992) found dysphagia, cognitive failure (score of 24 or less on the Mini-Mental State Scale), and weight loss of 10 kg or more significantly predicted survival time, while the physician's medical history and physical examination were not highly accurate in predicting short-term survival of cancer patients. Nurses and physicians assess the parameters of dysphagia, cognitive failure, weight loss, and performance status routinely, but unfortunately there is no precise way to determine length of survival.

SYMPTOM ASSESSMENT AND MANAGEMENT

Symptom management is an area of high priority in cancer patient care, especially with the terminally ill patient. It is necessary to identify and deal with the distress that the patient and family experience as a result of the symptoms. Symptom distress is not determined simply by the presence of the symptom but takes into account the patient's interpretation of the symptom. Symptom distress may be defined as the patient's self-reported interpretation of the symptom occurrence that results in physical discomfort, mental discomfort, or both (McCorkle & Young, 1978; Rhodes & Watson, 1987). Therefore, the nurse must listen and empathize with what the patient and family report and consider this step a very important process in the assessment and management of symptom distress of the terminal patient.

ALTERATION IN HYDRATION

Many symptoms experienced by the advanced cancer patient can lead to or be a result of a deficit in body fluids. Although there is great interest among lay persons and health professionals in the subject of hydration in the terminally ill patient, little is actually known about the fluid volume or distribution in dying cancer patients (Creighton, 1984; Fry, 1986; Gargaro, 1983; Jansson & Norberg, 1989; Lynn, 1984; Micetich, Steinecker, & Thomasma, 1983; Wurzbach, 1990). Terminal cancer patients frequently experience a fluid volume deficit due to the side effects of treatment or to the disease itself. The deficit may result from decreased oral intake due to nausea or anorexia or from increased fluid output due to vomiting, diarrhea, wound draining, sweating, or hyperventilation. Also, inadequate reabsorption of water and solutes in the renal tubules may result in increased fluid and solute loss.

Terminal cancer patients can also experience extracellular fluid accumulation in the interstitial spaces. This is a fluid distribution problem (Billings, 1985b; Cassileth, 1982). Fluid accumulation occurs in peripheral or dependent areas due to lack of normal muscle activity that facilitates venous and lymphatic return of fluids to the central circulation, hypoalbuminemia, venous or lymphatic obstruction, and sodium-retaining states associated with cardiac, renal, or hepatic failure. These same disease states can cause retention of fluid in the pleural, pericardial, or peritoneal cavities (Billings, 1985b). Fluid accumulation can lead to edema and taut skin in dependent or peripheral parts of the body and to associated discomfort. When the fluid accumulates in the pleural or pericardial cavities, patients often experience difficulty breathing and chest pain. Some clinicians believe lung congestion is more of a problem if the patient receives intravenous (IV) fluids (Dolan, 1983). Uncertainty exists as to whether the interstitial fluid accumulation is a result of overhydration or an inability of the body to adapt with an appropriate distribution of the body fluids due to osmotic alterations from multisystem failure (Brooker, 1992).

Waller, Adunski, and Hershkowitz (1991) attempted to examine the effects of IV fluid infusion on blood and urine parameters of dehydration in 68 terminally ill cancer patients. A state of dehydration measured by serum sodium and urine osmolality levels was present in all patients within the 24-hour period prior to death, regardless of whether they received IV fluids. There were no differences in the state of dehydration and state of consciousness between the group that received IV fluids at a keep-open rate versus those who did not receive IV fluids (Waller et al., 1991). No data were available on the actual amount of fluid intake of the two groups.

Some health care professionals caring for dying patients conclude from clinical observations that symptoms from dehydration occurring at the terminal phase of life do not contribute to pain or distress for patients (Musgrave, 1990; Printz, 1988; Schmitz & O'Brien, 1986; Zerwekh, 1983). Dehydration serves as a natural anesthesia for the central nervous system by decreasing the patient's level of consciousness (Printz, 1988; Schmitz & O'Brien, 1986; Zerwekh, 1983). Patients can remain quite alert and communicative when objectively dehydrated (Schmitz & O'Brien, 1986). Some patients consider a decrease in consciousness beneficial, while others desire mental alertness during the dying process (Wallston, Burger, Smith, & Baugher, 1988).

Clinical observations indicate that thirst and dry mouth are the only troubling and commonly encountered symptoms attributed to dehydration in terminally ill patients (Billings, 1985a). Symptom relief is gained by administering amounts of fluid too small to reverse metabolic abnormalities and by maintaining moisture in the mouth with water, ice chips, or various forms of artificial saliva (Billings, 1985b). In contrast, Yan and Bruera (1991) report the positive effects of parenteral hydration in two out of three case studies of terminal cancer patients. Administration of parenteral fluids dramatically decreased symptoms in two patients, especially in the areas of mentation, agitation, sense of well being, appetite, and anxiety. Administration of parenteral fluids did not help the remaining patient's symptoms (Yan & Bruera, 1991).

In a survey of 978 Swiss physicians chosen through a stratified random process, 42 per cent report the belief that dying patients suffer significantly from dehydration, while 33 per cent say that patients have minimal suffering (Collaud & Rapin, 1991). Essentially, there was no consensus among physicians about the assessment of suffering with dehydration. Only 28 per cent indicate that they would use artificial hydration for conscious patients, while 44 per cent would choose this treatment for comatose patients. Physicians who chose artificial hydration regardless of the patient's mental status reported a significantly higher consideration of suffering and thirst as serious than those who prefer hydration by mouth. The physicians report discomfort in dehydrated patients from dry mouth (78 per cent), thirst (43 per cent), nausea (23 per cent), and cramps (12 per cent); however, Collaud and Rapin (1991) did not look at the physicians' actual practices regarding artificial hydration. Burge, King, and Willison (1990) reviewed charts of patients ($n = 106$) who died of malignant disease and reported that 81 per cent of the patients had an IV fluid line during the last 30 days of life, and 69 per cent had an IV in place at the time of death. The most common charted reason for administering IV fluids was hydration (Burge et al., 1990).

When administering fluids by artificial methods, the nurse must consider whether the procedure itself causes distress. Artificial administration of fluids to dying patients is through the parenteral (intravenous, subcutaneous) or GI (peg tube, nasogastric tube, or jejunostomy tube) routes. Physicians generally do not view the presence of an infusion as an additional source of discomfort (Collaud & Rapin, 1991). However, a concern of patients and families is whether tubes interfere with communication and thus provoke distress.

A primary wish of the patient and the family is a comfortable death. Fluids and nutrition have many symbolic meanings for individuals, including love and sustenance. Consequently, providing fluids by artificial means and discontinuing or withholding fluids in dying cancer patients may elicit strong emotions in patients, family members, and caregivers (Brown & Chekryn, 1989; Printz, 1988).

The American Nurses' Association (ANA) position statement on artificial hydration and nutrition considers food and water as concepts closely related to caring and notes that caring is a focal point in the profession of nursing (ANA, 1992). However, it makes a distinction between providing artificial hydration and nutrition and providing food and water to a patient by mouth. The ANA (1992) supports a process of reasoned decision making by the dying patient or surrogate along with the health team. The focus of the decision-making process is the anticipated benefits and burdens of proposed interventions, such as artificial hydration and nutrition. Included in the decision-making process is an evaluation of the anticipated outcomes of the proposed intervention. The outcomes should encompass the overall well being of the patient as a person, and not be limited in scope. Lone outcomes of weight gain or increased caloric intake are examples of limited scope outcomes. Whether the patient's or surrogate's decision is to give or not to give artificial hydration and nutrition, the nurse must respect the choice and continue to provide expert care to the patient and family (ANA, 1992; Hastings Center Report, 1987).

ALTERATION IN NUTRITION

Many symptoms experienced by the advanced cancer patient can lead to or result in a nutritional deficit. Anorexia, nausea, vomiting, and cachexia are present in a significant number of cancer patients in the terminal state (Bruera & MacDonald, 1988; Reuben & Mor, 1986b; Wachtel et al., 1988). Gray et al. (1988) report that those patients with cancer of the ovaries, stomach, pancreas, and colon experienced nausea most frequently. Physiologic changes due to both the disease progression and the treatment lead to the decreased intestinal absorption and slowed gastric emptying that contribute to nausea and anorexia and ultimately cachexia (Nelson, Walsh, & Sheehan, 1994).

Artificially supplied nutrition has not resulted in a significant effect on tumor response in cancer patients receiving radiation or chemotherapy (Bruera & MacDonald, 1988). In fact, some researchers report negative aspects of shortened survival time in patients treated with total parenteral nutrition (Torosian & Daly, 1986).

The assessment of the terminal cancer patient's nutritional status includes information about the patient's disease, prognosis, pattern of metastasis, current and past therapies, effectiveness of prescribed medications, and emotional response of the patient and family dealing with the eating difficulties (Holden, 1993). This information and the desires of the patient determine the appropriateness of the intervention (Holden, 1993).

Holden (1993) recommends following the suggestions offered in *Eating Hints* (National Cancer Institute, 1986) for mild appetite loss and food aversion situations. Some medical therapies that stimulate the appetite include corticosteroids (i.e., prednisone or dexamethasone), hormones (i.e., megestrol acetate), and metoclopramide when the decreased appetite is related to delayed gastric emptying (Bruera & MacDonald, 1988; Kaye, 1990; Loprinzi et al., 1990; Nelson et al., 1994; Reitmeier & Hartenstein, 1990).

Management of the nausea and vomiting is dependent on treating the cause of these symptoms. Frequently there are multiple or untreatable causes that limit effective management. Treatment includes antiemetic therapy that will control vomiting through action on one or both areas in the brain that affect nausea and vomiting: the emetic center and the chemoreceptor trigger zone (Enck, 1994). Effective symptom relief depends on selecting the antiemetic with antagonist potencies against the various neurotransmitter receptors involved (Lichter, 1993). Lichter (1993) reports that the most frequent causes of nausea and vomiting in terminal illness are visceral (24 per cent), gastric stasis (24 per cent), biochemical (16 per cent), and constipation (13 per cent). As the disease progresses, multiple causes of nausea and vomiting may occur and require additional antiemetics to be included in the patient's regimen.

Besides the pharmacologic approach to the treatment of nausea and vomiting, Gallagher-Allred (1989) suggests avoiding fatty, greasy, and fried foods, high-bulk foods, and sweet or spicy foods. In addition, small meals of cool, odorless foods may benefit the patient who wants to eat. Because of the nausea and vomiting, medications previously administered by mouth may require an alternative route. The nurse needs to respect the decision of the patient or surrogate on providing artificial nutrition when the patient can no longer take nutrients in the normal manner.

ALTERATION IN COGNITION

Alterations in cognitive functioning at the end of life are relatively common (Massie, Holland, & Glass, 1983; Bruera, Miller, McCallion, Macmillan, Krefting, & Hanson, 1992). In a sample of hospitalized patients Massie et al. (1983) found that 85 per cent of terminally ill patients developed delirium before death. Bruera, Miller, McCallion, et al. (1992) identified cognitive failure as determined by a score of less than 24 on the Mini-Mental State Questionnaire in 83 per cent of terminally ill patients who died. Drugs, sepsis, and brain metastasis are the most frequent causes of cognitive failure. Metabolic and electrolyte imbalances, hypoxia, and fever can also alter cognition. Bruera, Miller, McCallion, et al. (1992) report that the results of treating the cause of altered cognition was variable; some patients improved, while some patients demonstrated no change. Data on the frequency of altered cognition in patients who die in the home setting are not readily available. However, it is speculated that the incidence of confused patients is higher in hospital and inpatient hospice settings because families are seeking some respite from the overwhelming burden of caring for a confused loved one at home.

In addition to assessing and, if possible, treating the cause of the cognition failure, the nurse should explain the cause of confusion to the patient and the family to help them understand the situation and to hopefully reduce their anxiety. When delirium is present, short frequent contacts with a supportive person who can reassure and reorient the patient to the environment and situation are helpful. Continuity of the caregivers is important as well (Massie et al., 1983). When severe agitation or disruptive behavior is present, sedation may be necessary (Enck, 1994).

Seizures can cause temporary loss of consciousness. While seizures are not frequently seen in the terminally ill, they can be very frightening to the patient and family (Kaye, 1990). The cause of seizures is usually a brain tumor and, less frequently, brain metastases. Anticonvulsants, such as diazepam or phenobarbital, are for controlling seizures, while phenytoin is for preventing seizures (Kaye, 1990). Carbamazepine is the prophylaxis of choice for focal seizures (Kaye, 1990).

ALTERATION IN RESPIRATION

Dyspnea is prevalent in the terminal cancer patient during the last weeks of life and is the most common severe symptom near death (Higginson & McCarthy, 1989; Reuben & Mor, 1986a). Dyspnea is a frightening problem to the patient and family. The treatment choice for dyspnea depends upon the cause, but sometimes a diagnostic workup to identify the cause is not feasible. There are some interventions that are useful. Medications such as morphine sulfate, low-dose humidified oxygen, benzodiazepines, chlorpromazine, and broncodilators can provide some relief (Bruera, Macmillan, Pither, & MacDonald, 1990; Nelson & Walsh, 1991). Nursing measures for dyspnea include (1) modifying daily activity to conserve energy, (2) using pursed lip breathing and extending exhalation, (3) clearing secretions with deep breathing and coughing, (4) cooling the face with a fan or other breeze, (5) sitting in upright and slightly leaning forward position or other position of comfort to allow maximum movement of lower chest, and (6) managing anxiety through relaxation, reassurance, and explanations (Foote, Sexton, & Pawlik, 1986; Nelson & Walsh, 1991). When the patient is unable to manage pharyngeal secretions, transdermal scopolamine can provide relief by decreasing the secretions (Blues & Zerwekh, 1984).

Anemia may contribute to the problem of dyspnea. Causes of anemia, which is often present in the terminal cancer patient, are the disease, the treatment for the disease, and/or bleeding. In the asymptomatic patient, no treatment is necessary. In the patient with symptomatic anemia, where there is a possibility of a high quality of life and death is not imminent, treatment may include blood transfusions (Gallagher-Allred, 1989). A transfusion provides red blood cells that increase the oxygen-carrying capacity of the blood, which supplements the oxygen delivery. With the improved oxygen delivery, symptoms of respiratory distress and fatigue might improve. However, in a pilot study of 24 patients in a home hospice program,

Sciortino et al., (1992) reported a significant change in hematocrit as the only clinical difference between pre-transfusion and posttransfusion variables. However, patients reported significant improvement in their quality of life.

ALTERATION IN MOBILITY

As cancer progresses, patients frequently experience overwhelming fatigue and weakness called asthenia. The incidence of asthenia is as high as 75 per cent (Bruera & MacDonald, 1988). The patient is at high risk for physical injury when performing activities of daily living due to lack of stamina and muscle control. Assistance with movement provides a safety measure for the patient who is experiencing diminished strength. Patients with severe asthenia are prone to develop pressure areas on their skin because they are immobile and require frequent positioning and protection of bony prominences. A sheepskin, an eggcrate foam mattress, or an alternating pressure mattress can be used to prevent skin breakdown. Frequently, patients avoid activity because movement may cause pain. When activity causes pain, the effectiveness of the pain management program needs to be reassessed and changes made as necessary.

ALTERATION IN ELIMINATION

Terminally ill patients frequently experience problems with bowel and bladder elimination. The causes of constipation are decreased food and fluid intake, decreased activity, muscle weakness, intestinal blockage, and use of narcotics for pain management. Patients need to be on a bowel management program of a high-fiber diet, increased fluids, increased activity, and pharmacologic therapies, such as stool softeners, laxatives, and enemas. Surfactant laxatives alone will not provide adequate evacuation in treating opioid related constipation (Canty, 1994). As death becomes apparent, it may become more difficult for patients to take food and medications by mouth. The nurse should focus on the options that are available to the individual patient and implement a bowel program designed to prevent elimination problems. Sometimes, fecal impaction can present as diarrhea when the liquid portion of the stool above the mass seeps around the hard mass. Patients should receive additional pain medication in advance if digital manipulation for fecal disimpaction becomes necessary. Diarrhea can also develop as a result of medications or the tumor itself. If laxative use causes loose stools, the dosage of the laxative needs to be decreased.

Urinary incontinence is a common problem in hospice patients (Enck, 1989). A study by Fainsinger, MacEachern, Hanson, and Bruera (1992) reports the prevalence of urinary problems and indications for use of urinary catheters in 61 consecutive terminal cancer patients on a palliative care unit. Their findings demonstrated only 16 (26 per cent) out of 61 patients died without the use of any urinary collecting device, and 14 (88 per cent) of the 16 either had a rapid deterioration

of less than 72 hours or died suddenly. The main reason for catheterization before and after admission to the palliative care unit was for patient comfort. Urinary retention was also a frequent cause (25 per cent) for catheterization (Fainsinger et al., 1992). Bacteriuria occurred in 54 per cent (28 of 52) of the patients with catheters, but the onset of the bacteriuria was undeterminable in 17 of the cases (Fainsinger et al., 1992). The bacteriuria rate is not surprising due to the debilitated state and decreased fluid intake in dying patients. While the use of catheters is helpful in maintaining the comfort of the patient and the integrity of the skin, the nurse needs to decrease the possibility of bacteriuria by taking protective measures, such as good perineal and catheter care.

ALTERATION IN COMFORT

Pain is the most feared symptom of terminal cancer patients. Pain results from the tumor, the metastasis, other pathologic processes in the body, or a combination of the three. It is important to identify the cause of the pain to initiate appropriate treatment. While Chapters 55 through 58 present comprehensive information about pain management, a few issues regarding pain in the terminal patient are included here. The primary source of pain assessment should be the patient's self-report (Jacox et al., 1994). Sometimes, as the patient becomes more lethargic, family members will request a decrease in pain medication because they want the patient more awake. Nurses should help family members to understand that the patient may still be in pain. Only patients can provide information on the amount of pain they are experiencing.

The assessment of pain at regular intervals and at suitable intervals following interventions is critical to successful pain management. An easy-to-use assessment tool to document pain intensity and pain relief is necessary to the ongoing pain management program (Jacox et al., 1994). Terminal cancer patients may benefit from administration of low-dose radiation therapy for pain relief, especially pain resulting from bone metastasis.

Use of the "prn" pain medication schedule should be avoided to eliminate a see-saw effect in the analgesic level. The desired plan for pain medication administration is "around-the-clock schedule" with "breakthrough" doses given when necessary (Jacox et al., 1994; Walsh, 1990; Walsh et al., 1992).

Side effects of opioid pain management, such as nausea, vomiting, and sedation, are usually short-lived. The patient and family should be aware of these potential side effects so that they do not assume that these symptoms are part of the disease process. Constipation and dry mouth are common side effects of opioid treatment that persist during opioid treatment. The nurse should begin immediate preventive treatment and monitor for constipation while the patient receives opioids (Jacox et al., 1994; Walsh, 1990).

The least invasive route of administration should be selected when giving pain medication (Jacox et al., 1994). Some consider morphine as the opioid of choice because of its flexibility of dosage, formulations, and routes of administration (Walsh, 1990). The availability of multiple routes of administration is especially important, since symptoms experienced by dying cancer patients may eliminate one or more routes of medication delivery.

When increased pain occurs while the patient is receiving opioids, a determination must be made as to whether the increased pain is due to tolerance to the opioid, progression of the tumor, depression, or some unrelated cause (Jacox et al., 1994). A prospective study of 29 cancer patients in a pain clinic revealed that progression of the cancer was present in most of the patients requiring increased morphine doses, while patients who did not require an increase in morphine did not have disease progression (Collins, Poulain, Gauvain-Piquard, Petit, & Pichard-Leandri, 1993). Changes in the patients' depression scores during the study did not correlate with pain intensity scores (Collins et al., 1993). Contraindications for increasing the dosage of the opioid are when the opioid-induced side effects cause or accompany the pain or when there is a need to change to another opioid or a different delivery mode (Shepard, 1994). Rapid escalation of analgesic drug therapy might be necessary to achieve a desired level of comfort in the terminal patient (Foley, 1986). Very large doses of opioids may be required to achieve optimal pain relief for the patient, even as much as several hundred milligrams of morphine every 4 hours (Foley, 1985).

Nonpharmacologic and psychosocial (cognitive and behavioral techniques) interventions are helpful adjuncts in a pain management program (see Chapter 58 for more information) (Rimer, Levy, Keintz, Fox, & Engstrom, 1987; Syrjola, Cummings, & Donaldson, 1992). As death becomes more imminent, the effectiveness of cognitive and behavioral interventions may diminish due to the decreased cognitive abilities of the patient. (Table 65–4).

PSYCHOSOCIAL DIMENSIONS

PSYCHOLOGIC CARE

In 1993 the Psychological Work Group of the International Work Group on Death, Dying, and Bereavement developed a statement of assumptions and principles concerning psychologic care of dying persons and their families (Psychological Work Group, 1993). The authors note that many of the statements apply equally to dying persons and their families but that some assumptions are not consistent with all cultures and belief systems (see Table 65–5 for complete summary).

The Life Closure Scale (LCS) was developed to measure the adaptive psychologic processes and patterns used by individuals as they accommodate to the experience of dying (Dobratz, 1990a). Two separate subscales were identified when the LCS was tested in a sample of 20 hospice patients: self-reconciling and self-restructuring. Both subscales provide information about the psychosocial well being of dying patients. Further psychometric testing of the instrument is planned in larger samples (Dobratz, 1990a). The use of this instrument may provide information to health care

professionals who attempt to enhance patients' adjustment through psychologic interventions.

Patients living in the final phase of advanced cancer may experience fears and anxiety related to uncertain future events such as unrelieved pain, loneliness, burden on family, and loss of control over life. Patient outcome studies provide evidence that psychologic interventions may reduce emotional distress, enhance coping, and improve adjustment in patients facing changes in quality of life related to cancer (Anderson, 1992). Research findings demonstrate decreased psychologic adjustment in patients with cancer diagnoses associated with decreased life span, and physical debilitation related to symptoms of advanced disease or toxic therapies when there is no intervention (McCorkle, Benoliel, Donaldson, Georgiadou, Moinpour, & Goodell, 1989; Spiegel & Bloom, 1983). The effectiveness of psychologic interventions may be related to increasing patients' sense of control, self-efficacy, and realistic appraisal while they are experiencing physical decline, social dependency, and existential distress that often accompany the last stages of living with advanced cancer. Many adjustments in feelings of control and self-efficacy may occur in patients experiencing the physical decline associated with dying. Critical factors that influence the effectiveness of psychologic intervention include empathy, warmth, genuineness, and level of comfort with difficult topics related to patients' life and death issues (Linn, Linn, & Harris, 1982; Spiegel & Yalom, 1978). The importance of social support provided by significant person(s) within the patient's existing network has been supported by research findings (Goodwin, Hunt, Key, & Samet, 1987). Social support is thought to be a contributing factor in moderating outcomes from therapeutic interventions.

Depression is not a normal reaction to life-threatening illness, nor is it caused by personal weakness. The Agency for Public Health Policy and Research (AHCPR) has provided the following list of symptoms to recognize depression (Table 65–6). Depression is suspected if these symptoms endure over a period of 2 or more weeks. Pharmacologic and psychotherapeutic modalities are available for effective treatment of depression. Treatment of depression in terminally ill patients should not be overlooked; however, assessment is more complex because some symptoms of advanced cancer overlap with symptoms of depression. Patient referral to available psychiatric consultation service for further assessment and treatment is indicated when symptoms of depression are detected in advanced cancer patients.

SOCIAL AND CULTURAL INFLUENCES

Numerous factors including personal values and beliefs, socioeconomic and cultural background, and religion or existential belief system influence patients' expectations about quality of life and palliative care. Multiple studies have demonstrated that cultural affiliation has an important influence on perception and response to pain. Bates, Edwards, and Anderson (1993) report that the best predictors of pain intensity are ethnic group affiliation and locus of control style. Some variables that contribute to effective symptom relief rely on the patient's perception of symptoms, ability to describe the symptom and accompanying level of distress, and ability to use coping methods that have been helpful in other distressing situations. A patient's stoic attitude directed toward minimizing or negating discomfort may be related to a cultural value learned and reinforced through years of family experiences.

Awareness of the patient's and family's cultural, religious, ethnic, and socioeconomic background is important to understanding their beliefs, practices, and attitudes towards illness and death. Culture may be defined as values, norms, beliefs, and practices of a particular group that are learned and shared, and that

TABLE 65–4. *Overview of Common Physical Symptoms and Interventions in Advanced Cancer*

SYMPTOM	INTERVENTION	SOURCE
Anemia	Give packed red blood cells and/or platelets as appropriate for the situation. Give multivitamin & mineral supplement. Antacids for GI bleeding. Avoid caffeine. Avoid tobacco use.	Gallagher-Allred, 1989 Sciortino et al., 1992
Anorexia/cachexia	Obtain a diet history. Encourage small frequent feedings of high nutritional foods. Eat what sounds good. Do not force-feed. Create a pleasant environment for eating. Medications to stimulate the appetite: • Corticosteroids • Megestrol acetate • Metoclopramide.	Holden, 1993 NCI, 1986 Kaye, 1990 Nelson, Walsh, & Sheehan, 1994 Bruera & MacDonald, 1988 Loprinzi et al., 1990 Reitmeir & Hartenstein, 1990
Asthenia	Assistance with movement and frequent repositioning. Plan priority activities at time of most energy. Decrease nonessential tasks. Increase dependence on others.	Winningham et al., 1994
Confusion/delirium	Correct the cause when possible such as electrolyte or metabolic imbalances, hypoxia, and fever. Explain the cause to patient & family. Short frequent contacts with supportive persons. Reassure and reorient to environment & situation. Provide continuity of caregivers. Haloperidol or chlorpromazine for relief of agitation.	Bruera, Miller, McCallion, et al., 1992 Massie et al., 1983 Enck, 1994
Constipation	Eat diet high in fiber. Increase fluid intake. Increase activity if possible. Pharmacologic therapies: • Stool softeners • Laxatives • Enemas Begin bowel regimen when initiating opioid administration.	Canty, 1994 Enck, 1994 Gallagher-Allred, 1989
Dehydration	Encourage favorite liquids as desired, such as carbonated drinks, juices, and ice chips.	Gallagher-Allred, 1989
Diarrhea	Check for and remove impaction if present. Eliminate or decrease if possible medications that may be producing the diarrhea. Eliminate foods that can be associated with diarrhea such as milk products, fruits, nuts and raw vegetables. Give antidiarrheal medication such as: Lomotil, Imodium, Paregoric, and Kaopectate as needed.	Gallagher-Allred, 1989

Continued on following page.

guide thinking, decisions, and actions in a patterned way (Leininger, 1978). Cultural assessment provides a foundation for planning care at the end of life. Role expectations, family lifestyle, child-rearing activities, patterns of authority, occupational patterns, religious requirements and beliefs, educational achievements, and dietary practices are part of cultural assessment (Tripp-Reimer & Brink, 1985). The cultural patterns of patients and their families play a significant role in determining how they will cope with terminal illness (Pickett, 1993).

Cultural factors of caregiving environments can also influence the experiences of dying patients and their families. Qualitative analysis of cultural factors in a hospital oncology unit and a free-standing inpatient hospice unit revealed differences in organizational structure, cure/care orientation, use of touch, use of rituals, and financial/political/economic barriers (Gates, 1991). The results of Gates' (1991) comparative study indicate that an inpatient hospice environment evidenced a stronger focus on interdisciplinary collaboration, care orientation, use of touch, and ritual symbolism than the conventional hospital setting.

Patient care environments are greatly influenced by health care professionals' priorities, policies, and attitudes. Most health care professionals' educational pro-

---

TABLE 65–4. *Overview of Common Physical Symptoms and Interventions in Advanced Cancer* Continued

SYMPTOM	INTERVENTION	SOURCE
Dysphagia	Dietary management to ensure diet of right consistency. Maintain good oral hygiene. Find posture best suited for patient to swallow. Dexamethasone if tumor is likely to respond or evidence of extrinsic luminal obstruction. Palliative external beam radiotherapy when appropriate.	Stykes et al., 1988
Dyspnea	Treat cause of dyspnea if possible. Medications: • Morphine sulfate • Low-dose oxygen • Benzodiazepines • Chlorpromazine • Bronchodilators Modify daily activity to conserve energy. Use pursed-lip breathing & extended exhalation to prevent airway collapse. Deep breathe & cough to clear secretions. Breeze over face to improve air circulation. Sit upright & slightly lean forward for lung expansion. Transdermal Atropine or Scopolamine for excessive secretions for "death rattle." Use Pulmocare if giving oral or tube feeding for high fat and low carbohydrate to increase calories and decrease carbon dioxide production.	Bruera et al., 1990 Nelson & Walsh, 1991 Foote et al., 1986 Blues & Zerwekh, 1984 Gallagher-Allred, 1989 Enck, 1994
Fluid accumulation	Use diuretics but avoid vigorous diuresis. Restrict sodium intake. Dietary support to increase protein and caloric intake.	Gallagher-Allred, 1989
Nausea/vomiting	Correcting the cause if possible such as metabolic or electrolyte imbalances. Use antiemetic pharmacologic therapy based on cause: • Cyclizine for CNS & visceral stimuli • Hyoscine for motion & positional sickness • Haloperidol for drugs & biochemical disorders • Domperidone & metoclopramide for gastric stasis Avoid sweet, fatty, highly salted, and spicy foods. Avoid foods with strong odors. Eat cold or room temperature foods. Use clear liquids and bland foods.	Enck, 1994 Gallagher-Allred, 1989 Lichter, 1993

TABLE 65–4. *Overview of Common Physical Symptoms and Interventions in Advanced Cancer* Continued

SYMPTOM	INTERVENTION	SOURCE
Pain	Identify the cause. Continuously assess the pain. Adjust nonopioid or opioid dosage as needed. Avoid PRN dosing and use round-the-clock dosing. Consider psychologic and social factors. Consider nonpharmacologic adjuvant measures. Use rating scale for assessment. May require very large doses of opioids to maintain severe pain. Use the least invasive modality.	Jacox et al., 1994 Enck, 1994 Foley, 1985
Seizures	Take safety precautions to protect patient in case of seizure, i.e., padded bed rails. Anticonvulsants: • Diazepam or phenobarbital for controlling • Phenytoin for prevention • Carbamazepine as prophylaxis for focal seizures.	Kaye, 1990
Skin problems	Reposition as often as appropriate. Protect bony prominences. Gently massage reddened areas with lotion to promote circulation. Keep skin clean and free of incontinent urine and feces. Keep bed clothing smooth, clean, dry and use mild detergent on bed clothes. Use sheepskin, eggcrate, air mattress, and/or special beds (Clinitron, water, Egerton) to reduce trauma. If ulcer develops—cleanse affected area with soap & water, cleanse broken skin with Betadine or other antiseptic, dry, and cover with skin prep and dress with either Op-site, Tegaderm, or semipermeable membrane (Duoderm).	Bohnet, 1986 DeConno et al., 1991
Thirst/dry mouth	Moisten lips with Vaseline, etc. Suck on hard candies and chew gum. Take sips of fluids frequently or suck on wet cloth. Use various forms of artificial saliva that contain carbonymethylcellulose and predominant electrolytes present in human saliva. Avoid use of lemon-glycerin swabs & mouthwashes that contain alcohol.	Gallagher-Allred, 1989 Billings, 1985b Poland, 1987
Urinary incontinence	Use of indwelling or external catheter. Use absorbent padding such as Attends.	Fainsinger et al., 1992 Enck, 1994

grams do not include opportunities to learn about key approaches to improving care for dying persons. It is important for professional nurses to expand their repertoire of assessment skills, communication abilities, and interventions to create environments that support terminally ill patients and their families in all settings. Professional advancement in these areas can be gained through independent study, attendance at conferences designed to increase knowledge in the care of the dying, association with local community hospice organizations, and interaction with more experienced professionals who can offer information about how they have provided care for dying patients. Observation of nurse "mentors," nurses who demonstrate knowledge

and confidence in the care of the dying, while they provide care is an effective way of increasing knowledge and personal comfort. The development and refinement of one's own skills that are based on examples of expert nursing care of the dying are attainable goals in cancer nursing practice. Patients, families, and professional colleagues benefit from efforts directed to improve care for dying patients.

TERMINAL CARE AT HOME

Delivery of terminal care in the home has been influenced by the growth of available home hospice care services and by health care delivery cost-contain-

TABLE 65–5. *Assumptions and Principles Concerning Psychologic Care of Dying Persons and their Families*

ASSUMPTIONS	PRINCIPLES
Definition of Terms	
Family: Individuals who are part of the dying person's most immediate attachment network, regardless of blood or matrimonial ties.	
Caregiver: Professionals and volunteers who provide care to dying persons and their families.	
Issues for Dying Persons	
Dying persons may choose to acknowledge or not to acknowledge their impending death.	Caregivers must recognize and respect the person's right or need to deny or not to communicate about his or her impending death. Caregivers may be helpful to family members and others in understanding or accepting the dying person's position, which may change with time.
Dying persons can communicate about their impending death in different cultural ways, encompassing verbal, nonverbal, or symbolic ways of communicating.	Caregivers must seek understanding and knowledge of the dying person's cultural and lifestyle experiences. Caregivers need to be astutely sensitive to nonverbal and symbolic ways of communicating and recognize that these modalities may be more significant to the dying person than verbal expression.
Dying persons have the right to information on their changing physical status, and the right to choose whether to be told they are dying.	Caregivers need to be sensitive and perceptive to the different ways the person may be requesting information about his or her condition.
Dying persons may be preoccupied with dying, death itself, or what happens after death.	The caregiving team needs to be aware of the dying person's concerns and fears to provide care that is responsive and supportive.
Dying persons can have a deepseated fear of abandonment. They may therefore continue treatment for the sake of the family or physician rather than in the belief that it will be of personal benefit.	Caregivers can be helpful to the dying person in identifying feelings that may affect treatment decisions. Caregivers may also be helpful in opening communication between the dying patient and family or physician that may clearly reflect the patient's goal for treatment.
Many dying persons experience multiple physical and psychologic losses before their death.	Caregivers may be helpful in facilitating the expression of grief related to the multiple losses of terminal illness. Caregivers may also be helpful in supporting the dying person's need for continued autonomy, satisfying roles and activities, and meaning despite these losses.
Dying persons exhibit a variety of coping strategies in facing death.	Caregivers need to be able to recognize the utility of adaptive coping mechanisms and be tolerant of the patient's family's need to use or abandon such mechanisms. Caregivers can help to foster an environment that encourages the use of effective ways of coping by accurately addressing the dying person's psychosocial concern.
Dying persons generally need to express feelings.	Dying persons should not be isolated but given the opportunity to communicate.
Dying persons communicate when they feel safe and secure.	Caregivers should strive to create an environment in which communication can be facilitated, paying special attention to physical comfort, symptom management, physical surroundings, privacy, confidentiality, adequate time, acceptance of feelings, and shared expectations.
Dying persons may find it helpful to communicate with others who are terminally ill.	Opportunities should be encouraged for patient interaction such as peer or professionally facilitated support groups, social functions, or designated areas within treatment settings where patients may informally gather.
A dying person's communication of concern about death may be inhibited by a number of psychosocial and culturally determined expectations.	Caregivers can be helpful in breaking through the barriers that inhibit the dying person's true expression of feelings.
Dying persons have a right to be acknowledged as living human beings until their death.	Even when they seem severely impaired, dying persons are still able to sense their own surroundings. Caregivers need to facilitate this awareness. Caregivers should encourage behavior, touch, and communication that continue to demonstrate respect for the dying person.

TABLE 65–5. *Assumptions and Principles Concerning Psychologic Care of Dying Persons and their Families*
Continued

ASSUMPTIONS	PRINCIPLES
Dying persons' psychologic suffering may be greater than their physical pain or discomfort.	Caregivers should recognize, and attend to, the psychosocial component of suffering.
Dying persons may have difficulty in dealing with the different or conflicting needs of family members.	Caregivers need to be aware of the dynamics within each family and recognize the importance of dealing with individual members as well as the family unit. Caregivers should be sensitive to the presence of conflicts between family members and may need to maintain a position of neutrality in order to be effective.
Issues for Families	
Families have fundamental needs to care and to be cared for.	Families should be encouraged to provide whatever care they can. Caregivers should not supplant the family in the caregiver role except where the family lacks physical or emotional resources, knowledge, or desire to provide care. By providing care to family members, caregivers may be better able to care for the dying person.
The need to care and the need to be cared for sometimes conflict.	Those who sacrifice their own needs for care to care for others need to be encouraged to accept help for themselves. Some need to receive care before they can give care.
People vary in their coping abilities and personal resources. Moreover, competing priorities may hamper the amount and quality of care people are able to give.	Caregivers should not impose their own expectations on a family's ability to care. Caregivers may need to explore with the family what is reasonable for each person to provide.
The approach of death may disrupt the structure and functioning of the family.	Many families need counseling and support to prepare for the dying person's death and its consequences.
Families need to have information about a dying person's condition, although in cases of conflict his or her desire for confidentiality must be respected.	The dying person and caregiving team share the responsibility for informing the family about the person's condition, depending on his or her ability to participate. Whenever possible, the dying person and appropriate caregivers need to agree on the source and extent of information to be given to families.
Families often need to be involved with the dying person in decision making.	Guided by the dying person's wishes, caregivers can be helpful in facilitating joint decision making.
Families have a right to know that their affairs will be shared only with those who have a need to know.	Confidentiality must be maintained at all times and its meaning taught to all caregivers.
Family members need to maintain self-esteem and self-respect.	Caregivers should show respect at all times. Caregivers do this by paying attention to family wishes, feelings, and concerns.
Sexual needs may continue up to the point of death.	Caregivers should acknowledge dying persons' and their partners' need to express their sexuality both verbally and physically, with easy access to privacy without embarrassment.
Families coping with terminal illness frequently have financial concerns.	Caregivers need to ensure that families have access to informed advice and assistance on financial issues. These issues represent present or anticipated problems that may or may not be realistic.
Faced with death, the family may imagine that changes will be greater than they are.	Caregivers can often allay fears with information and support.
Families have a need and a right to express grief for the multiple losses associated with illness, and for impending death.	Caregivers can help families by encouraging communication between families and the dying person about their shared losses and by encouraging the expression of grief.
Issues for Caregivers	
Caregivers need education and experience in addressing the psychosocial needs of dying persons and their families.	A combination of specialized courses in death and dying, and clinical practicums in care of the terminally ill and their families, may help to prepare caregivers to deal with the physical and psychosocial needs of dying persons.
Caregivers need to be aware of the dying person's and family's psychosocial frame of reference in acknowledging and coping with impending death.	Caregivers need to be sensitive to the dying person's and family's current willingness to acknowledge the reality of their situation. Caregivers must not impose their own expectation of how dying persons face death.

Continued on following page.

TABLE 65–5. *Assumptions and Principles Concerning Psychologic Care of Dying Persons and their Families*
Continued

ASSUMPTIONS	PRINCIPLES
Caregivers bring their own values, attitudes, feelings, and fears into the dying person's setting.	Caregivers must recognize that they cannot take away all the pain experience in the dying process. Caregivers need to be reassured that it is not a lack of professionalism to display and share emotions. Caregivers need to be aware of the way in which their coping strategies affect their communication of emotional involvement with the dying person and family.
Caregivers are exposed to repeated intense emotional experiences, loss, and confrontation with their own death in their work with dying persons.	Caregivers need to receive adequate support and opportunity to work through their accumulated emotions. Caregivers working with dying persons need sound motivation, emotional maturity, versatility, tolerance, and a special ability to deal with loss.
Caregivers dealing with family groups sometimes experience conflicting needs and requests for information and confidentiality.	Caregivers need to be prepared to deal with complex family dynamics and to assist the family in resolving their own conflicts.
Caregivers may sometimes not communicate with each other about their own needs and feelings.	Caregivers need to be tolerant, caring, and nonjudgmental with each other to promote cooperation, which will benefit the dying person's care.

(From Psychological Work Group of the International Work Group on Death, Dying and Bereavement. [1993]. A statement of assumptions and principles concerning psychological care of dying persons and their families. *Journal of Palliative Care, 9*[3], 29–32.)

ment efforts resulting in decreased length of stay and early discharge from hospitals. Successful symptom management outcomes of dying patients are enhanced if some of the following conditions exist: the patient wants to remain at home, participates in decision making, and has a supportive family network; availability of 24-hour communication with health care professionals; implementation of current symptom management medications and procedures to relieve distress; and agreement among patient, family, and professionals that the goal of care is comfort not cure (McCorkle, 1988). A comprehensive review and analysis of research examining needs reported by family caregivers of persons with cancer offers direction for planning and delivering family-oriented care (Laizner, Yost, Barg, & McCorkle, 1993). Multistudy analysis reveals that primary caregivers' gender, age, and family con-

TABLE 65–6. *Symptoms of Depression*

Depression should be suspected if a person displays several of the following symptoms for a period of 2 or more weeks. The first two symptoms listed are particularly significant.
- A depressed mood most of the day, nearly every day
- Markedly decreased interest in almost all activities
- Significant weight loss or gain
- Insomnia or hypersomnia
- Psychomotor agitation or retardation
- Excessive or inappropriate fatigue
- Feelings of worthlessness or guilt
- Indecisiveness or impaired concentration
- Recurrent thoughts of suicide or death

(From AHCPR. [1993]. *Depression in primary care: Clinical practice guideline.* No.5. AHCPR Publication No. 93–0550. Rockville, MD: U.S. Department of Health and Human Services, Public Health Service.)

stellation are important characteristics to assess when designing support most needed by family caregivers. Descriptive characteristics of the samples taken together indicate that the majority of primary caregivers are older women (mean age = 61 years) caring for spouses or parents. Female caregivers report less difficulty managing care activities for persons with advanced disease and a higher sense of purpose in life as compared with male caregivers. Examination of age differences indicates that older caregivers who perceived the caregiving experience as purposeful or time-limited cope more effectively than younger caregivers. Caregivers in households with children report additional assistance provided by extended family members, while caregivers living in caregiver-patient dyad households report no additional assistance received from extended family.

The critical time frame for reassessing caregiver's needs has been identified as the interval between 1 to 3 months posthospitalization. Caregivers report specific concerns about managing in the future, maintaining personal health, providing emotional support to the patient, and discussing concerns with the seriously ill family member (Laizner et al., 1993). Proactive approaches to these problems include development of information, support, and referral resources to assist families during a time of increased demands. Review of simple health promotion instructions designed for caregiving families is one way to open lines of communication with primary caregivers about maintenance of personal emotional and physical well being. Topics that address common emotional concerns of caregivers (e. g., uncertainty, anxiety, fear, loss), health-promoting behaviors (e. g., exercise, balanced nutrition, contact with friends and family network, avoidance of alcohol and drugs), and stress management strategies (e. g., relaxation techniques, giving self permission for "time out") may prevent health problems associated with the caregiver role.

COPING STRATEGIES OF FAMILY CAREGIVERS

Many households in America are headed by adults who work full-time or part-time outside of the home. The impact on financial income, roles, and work patterns is evident when families decide to care for a terminally ill family member at home. The Federal Family and Medical Leave Act (1993) offers working family members unpaid leave from the work place with continuation of benefits for a maximum period of 12 weeks per 12-month period. Family members who provide care to their loved ones during the final stages of life experience many stressors that challenge the limits of available family resources. Literature on caregiver burden, stress, and coping indicates that there is a need to provide family-based interventions designed to support family members providing terminal care in the home setting (Decker & Young, 1991; Dobratz, 1990b; Ekberg, Griffith, & Foxall, 1986; Gaynor, 1990; Hull, 1989; Lev, 1991; Masters & Shontz, 1989; Oberst, Thomas, & Ward, 1990; Reimer et al., 1991; Robinson, 1990; Wingate & Lackey, 1989).

Lewis (1990) identified family-focused support services needed by families facing the challenges associated with breast cancer. The following list of support services were identified by Lewis (1990) across the trajectory of the illness: information (diagnostic, treatment, and illness course), anticipatory guidance, dealing with school-age children, cognitive and emotional processing (meaning of the illness for all family members), and access to problem-focused services (physical care, psychologic care).

Anticipatory grief reactions of family members are commonly associated with the physical decline of the patient with advanced cancer (Northouse, 1984; Parkes & Weiss, 1983; Rando, 1984; Sanders, 1982-83). Family members' emotional resources are challenged by the stress associated with feelings of loss as they anticipate separation from their loved one. Although each family member has a subjective experience of loss, the family experiences dynamic shifts in expected roles and responsibilities in relation to the new demands imposed by the illness (Lewis, 1983). Care of a dying person in the home setting may strain the physical, psychosocial, and financial resources of a family. Major changes in a family's usual lifestyle patterns may be required to accommodate the demands of caring for a terminally ill loved one. Unresolved conflict and difficulties in relationships and communication patterns among family members prior to the stress of terminal illness may exacerbate. Family members need to know that the disequilibrium within the family is not unexpected and that problem-solving approaches may prevent or defuse some family tensions. Lewis (1993) emphasizes the importance of maintaining "non-illness-related aspects of family life" so that the family continues to live as a family. Additional help and respite care may be needed for families to participate in the nonillness aspects of their life.

Children require special consideration when they reside in a household with a family member living with advanced cancer. Children are especially vulnerable when the seriously ill person is a parent. In the past, many children were sheltered from the truth about the seriousness of illness by parents and professionals. However, Siegel et al. (1992) underscore that children are sensitive to changes in family dynamics and may experience distress associated with loss and separation related to hospitalizations, increasing limitations in both parents' physical and emotional availability and role functioning, changes in family routines, a shift in the family's emotional climate, and a decrease in financial resources as efforts are directed toward provision of caregiving. Depressive symptomatology and anxiety were significantly higher in children ($n = 62$) with a terminally ill parent than in a comparison sample of community children (Siegel et al., 1992). This study also identified diminished self-esteem and deficits in social competence in children with a terminally ill parent. Further complications may be expected related to decreased participation in social activities and poor school performance. Christ et al., (1993) examined the impact of parental terminal cancer on children 7 to 16 years of age. Common concerns of these children reported during interviews included the following: fears related to symptoms of the cancer and the side effects of treatment (i. e., weight loss, hair loss, vomiting, weakness), fear of parent's future death, anxiety or panic related to uncertainty and rapid changes in parent's status, guilt about the cause of the parent's illness, and concern that the well parent is also vulnerable. Clinical experience indicates that children experience greater stress during the terminal stage of cancer than following the parent's death (Christ et al., 1993). Nurses need to assess whether there are children in the dying patient's family and who has major responsibility for talking with them. Appropriate referrals may need to be made to support families during this stressful time, and age-specific needs may require special guidance from professionals skilled in family relations.

Professionals who feel comfortable talking about issues surrounding terminal illness may offer guidance to parents who are dealing with overwhelming changes within the family (Schonfeld, 1993). Bourne and Meier (1988) have developed a booklet for children (preschool to 10 years old) that addresses the topic of advanced illness in a very sensitive way. This booklet could be offered to parents to read with their children to encourage an open discussion about existing and expected changes in the family.

Coping strategies used by family caregivers providing hospice home care were reported by Hull (1992). The results of this longitudinal, qualitative study of 14 caregivers revealed that the following strategies assisted family caregivers to deal with the overall caregiving experience: "creating windows of time," social comparison, cognitive reformulation, and avoidance. The most frequently reported coping strategy by this study sample was taking time away from the caregiving responsibilities (i. e., a few hours of uninterrupted respite time at home or outside of the home to pursue life interests—hobbies, contact with friends). The strategy of downward comparison, believing that their situation was not as bad as someone else's situation, enabled some caregivers to continue their responsibilities. A cognitive reformulation process was utilized by some family caregivers to minimize the negative aspects of the situation and transform them into meaningful opportunities. Family caregivers also reported using avoidance to direct their energy away from the lack of control over their loved one's future death and actively expending their efforts toward aspects of care that were within their control. Family caregivers reported "taking 1 day at a time" to cope with the uncertainty of the situation. Family caregivers identified that when cognitive disorientation occurred in their loved one, they used attitudes of acceptance and rationalization to cope with these changes. A network of social support was identified to be a major factor in coping with the stresses associated with caring for a dying family member at home (Hull, 1992).

Warner (1992) suggests that providing information about coping strategies will enhance the effectiveness of caregivers and improve their own quality of life. Health professionals can offer anticipatory guidance about expected future events in an effort to decrease uncertainty and increase feelings of control and competence. Decision making and assertiveness skills may be reviewed with family caregivers to assist them in making the best use of available resources during this stressful time. Specific stress-management techniques (i. e., progressive relaxation, imagery), distraction techniques (i. e., music, reminiscing, reviewing photo albums), and time-management approaches are all strategies that hold potential to enhance caregivers' lives (Warner, 1992).

Caregivers of persons with AIDS (PWAs) encounter very complex situations, because many PWAs are young and face an abbreviated life span. Also, PWAs and caregivers immersed in the gay community are constantly aware of the deaths of many friends and associates. Brown and Powell-Cope (1993) identified central themes of "facing loss" and "transformed time" in a qualitative study of 53 caregivers of PWAs. The caregivers faced multiple losses including loss of interpersonal relationships, future dreams, personal freedom, and previous lifestyle. The caregivers in this study sample reported using the following strategies to cope with anticipatory grief: "taking one day at a time," "living fully in the moment," and "actualizing future dreams" (Brown & Powell-Cope, 1993).

Herth (1993) reported that family caregivers of terminally ill persons identified the following strategies as hope-fostering: sustaining supportive relationships, using cognitive reframing (i. e., positive self-talk, praying/meditating), changing perception of space, span, or focus of time (i. e., one day at a time), defining attainable goals, engaging in spiritual practices (i. e., listening to music, reading inspirational books), and balancing available internal energy with external demands (i. e., priority setting, and using available resources). Information about these approaches may be offered to increase family caregivers' range of strategies as they face the demands of terminal care of a loved one.

NURSING BEHAVIORS IN THE CARE OF DYING PERSONS

STANDARDS OF HOSPICE NURSING PRACTICE

The American Nurses' Association (1987) offers a description of the scope and standards of hospice nursing practice. Hospice nursing care is directed toward supportive management of physical, psychosocial, and spiritual issues of dying persons and their families. Dobratz (1990b) identifies four classifications of the hospice nursing role prevalent in the literature: intensive caring, collaborative sharing, continuous knowing, and continuous giving. Dobratz (1990b) emphasizes the need for a firm theoretic base to support interventions for the delivery of hospice nursing care to dying patients and their families.

Degner, Gow, and Thompson (1991) report findings from a research program designed to describe critical nursing behaviors in the care of dying persons. The study sample included 10 nurses practicing in palliative care (average of 8 years' experience in palliative care) and 10 nurse educators who taught about care of the dying. The investigators' aim is to define a model of expert nursing practice in the care of dying persons by extending this exploratory research to other samples of nurses. Seven critical nursing behaviors were identified through a qualitative analysis of responses to interview questions about care of the dying (Table 65–7).

IMMINENT DEATH

Professionals who care for dying patients require knowledge and technical skills directed to alleviate discomfort and ability to engage in empathetic interactions with patients regarding their preferences about place of death, prayers, religious rituals, and other significant issues for patients. Qvarnstrom (1988) emphasizes the importance of including the dying patient's personal wishes into the final care plan during the last stages of life and in the immediate after-death situation. The International Work Group in Death, Dying, and Bereavement has recommended that a determined effort should be made to "accede to the wishes of the patient (and family) with respect to place of death" and to provide patients with opportunities to "experience final moments in a way that is meaningful to the patient" (Qvarnstrom, 1988). Professionals and family members may initiate discussion to determine patients' preferences, or patients may clearly verbalize their choices spontaneously. It is essential for professionals to be prepared to discuss this information with patients and their families. Some family members have difficulty discussing this topic because it emphasizes the impending loss of the loved one.

As the inevitable death approaches, the most important aspect of care is comfort for the patient and family. The nurse should make the treatment regimen as simple as possible by eliminating unnecessary medications and treatments. The nurse should anticipate that the dying patient will lose the ability to swallow, and

TABLE 65–7. *Critical Nursing Behaviors in Care of the Dying*

| | OPERATIONAL DEFINITIONS | |
BEHAVIORS	POSITIVE	NEGATIVE
Responding during the death scene	Behaviors that maintain a sense of calm	Behaviors that show the nurse's horror of the death scene
	Behaviors that maintain family involvement	Controlling behavior that excludes family
Providing comfort	Behaviors that reduce physical discomfort, particularly pain	Avoidance behavior that results in neglect
		Poor symptom management due to poor knowledge base
Responding to anger	Behaviors that show respect and empathy even when anger is directed at nurse	Avoidance behavior or angry response
Enhancing personal growth	Behaviors that show the nurse has defined a personal role in care for the dying	Behaviors that show anxiety and lack of confidence in care for the dying
Responding to colleagues	Behaviors that provide emotional support and critical feedback to colleagues	Behaviors that show difficulty in providing or receiving support or criticism for colleagues
Enhancing the quality of life during dying	Behaviors that help patients do things that are important to them	Behaviors that show lack of respect for the patient or family
Responding to the family	Behaviors that respond to the family's need for information	Ignoring the family's need for information
	Behaviors that reduce the potential for future regret	Refusing to discuss dying and spiritual issues even when the family clearly wants to do so
	Behaviors that include family in care or relieve them of this responsibility according to what's best for the family	Passing judgment on family decisions and family behaviors toward the dying

(Reprinted with permission from Degner, L. F., Gow, C. M., & Thompson, L. A. [1991]. Critical nursing behaviors in care for the dying. *Cancer Nursing, 14*(5), 246–253.)

obtain suppository or injectable forms of medications (narcotic analgesics, antiseizure, etc.) in advance. This is especially important for patients who are in the home care setting. Support and companionship are important to dying patients and their families. It is also necessary to keep them informed of changing situations (Twycross, 1986). Most families want to know what to look for as death approaches, how to know when the patient is dead, and what to do after the patient has died. Written information given to the family may help to reduce stress and uncertainty (Table 65–8). Some families who are providing terminal care to their loved one in the home setting become extremely anxious as the dying process becomes evident.

TABLE 65–8. *Family Caregiver Information Sheet: Impending Death*

SYMPTOMS	ACTIONS
Decreased intake of food and drink.	Refer to nutrition sheet for information on supplements, but do not force fluids or food.
Sleeping more in daytime and more difficult to arouse.	Plan time with the patient when most alert.
Increase in confusion about time, place, and identity of familiar people.	Remind the patient of the day, time, and other people.
May become restless, pulling on linens, and having visions of people or things that do not exist.	Talk calmly and assuredly so not to startle or frighten.
Extremities become cool to touch and darker in color.	Cover with warm blankets (not electric) to prevent feeling cold.
Decrease in amount of urine.	If patient has an indwelling catheter, it may need to be irrigated to prevent blockage.
Decrease in clarity of hearing and vision.	Talk calmly and assuredly so not to startle or frighten.
Changes in breathing pattern to an irregular pace with periods of 10 to 30 seconds without breathing.	Assist patient to a position that provides good chest expansion.
Oral secretions may increase and collect in back of throat causing the "death rattle."	May use scopolamine patch to decrease secretions. Avoid suctioning patient.
Incontinence of urine and bowel movements when death is imminent.	Use pads or other items for protection of patient and environment.

(Adapted from Editor. [1992]. Preparing for the death of a loved one. *The American Journal of Hospice & Palliative Care, 9*[4], 14–16.)

Death from cancer occurs over a period of time, and generally the dying process is not rapid (Enck, 1994). As the cancer progresses, the patient will have a decreased need for food and drink. Multiple organ system failure occurs. Hypoxia, malnutrition, electrolyte imbalance, tumor burden, and toxins will overwhelm the body, and hepatic and renal failure can occur. As central nervous system failure develops, the patient will become more unresponsive. Some patients may have an increase in confusion, agitation, and restlessness that eventually leads to coma (Enck, 1994). As death approaches there is an increase in heart rate as the blood pressure drops, and peripheral coolness and cyanosis will appear. When the heart can no longer compensate, the heart rate and respirations become irregular and decrease. The irregular breathing will be more noticeable during sleep. Incontinence of urine and feces may occur when death is imminent. Pulmonary and pharyngeal secretions may increase, causing noisy breathing known as the "death rattle" (Blues & Zerwekh, 1984; Lindley-Davis, 1991); cardiopulmonary arrest follows. Death occurs when the vital organs are no longer functioning (Table 65–9).

The family caring for the dying patient at home should be aware that a call to community emergency service (911) will result in resuscitation procedures by rescue personnel who respond to the call for help. A determination of the patient's wishes about resuscitation should be known by all persons involved in the care. The hospice care team is available in most geographic locations to help the family during the dying and bereavement process. When the patient dies at home, the family member should call the hospice nurse to help confirm that the death has occurred. The nurse can initiate calls to the mortuary and the physician on behalf of the family and is available to support the family at this early point in bereavement. The actual death of a loved one has a major impact on the survivors despite the length of anticipatory grief. The reality that the loved one is no longer "dying" but dead creates another transition that family members must live through. Chapter 10 offers a comprehensive scope of loss and bereavement information and research that nursing professionals can use in the care of bereaved survivors.

Nurses who frequently encounter the care of dying patients and their families need to assess their own personal resources in the face of caregiving that requires empathy and understanding at critical transitions in persons lives. The care of dying persons presents opportunities for nurses to provide personalized care to patients and their families. It is important for nurses to take care of themselves so that they can meet the challenges that are associated with caring for terminally ill persons.

TABLE 65–9. *Family Caregiver Information Sheet: Signs of Death*

No heartbeat
No breathing
No response to shaking or shouting
Eyes fixed on a certain spot
Eyelids slightly open
Jaws relaxed and mouth slightly open
Loss of control of bowel and bladder

(Adapted from Editor. [1992]. Preparing for the death of a loved one. *The American Journal of Hospice & Palliative Care, 9*[4], 14–16.)

REFERENCES

Agency for Health Care Policy and Research. (1993). *Depression in primary care: Clinical practice guideline.* No. 5. AHCPR Publication No. 93–0550. Rockville, MD: U.S. Department of Health and Human Services, Public Health Service.

American Nurses' Association. (1992). *Compendium of position statements on the nurse's role in end-of-life decisions.* Washington, DC: American Nurses' Association.

American Nurses' Association. (1991). *Position statement on nursing and the PDSA.* Washington, DC: American Nurses' Association.

American Nurses' Association. (1987). *Standards and scope of hospice nursing practice.* Kansas City, MO: American Nurses' Association.

Anderson, B.L. (1992). Psychological interventions for cancer patients to enhance the quality of life. *Journal of Consulting and Clinical Psychology, 60*(4), 552–568.

Barofsky, I., & Sugarbaker, P. H. (1990). Cancer. In B. Spliker, (Ed.), *Quality of life assessments in clinical trials.* New York: Raven Press, Ltd.

Bates, M. S., Edwards, W. T., & Anderson, K. O. (1993). Ethnocultural influences on variation in chronic pain perception. *Pain, 52,* 101–112.

Bedard, J., Dionne, A., & Dionne, L. (1991). The experience of La Maison Michel Sarrazin (1985-1990): Profile analysis of 952 terminal-phase cancer patients. *Journal of Palliative Care, 7*(1), 42–57.

Benoliel, J. Q. (1985). Loss and terminal illness. *Nursing Clinics of North America, 20*(2), 439–448.

Benoliel, J. Q. (1987-88). Health care providers and dying patients: critical issues in terminal care. *Omega, 18*(4), 341–363.

Billings, J. A. (1985a). Comfort measures for the terminally ill: Is dehydration painful? *Journal of the American Geriatrics Society, 33*(11), 808–810.

Billings, J. A. (1985b). *Outpatient management of advanced cancer.* Philadelphia: J. B. Lippincott Co.

Blues, A. G., & Zerwekh, J. V. (1984). *Hospice and palliative nursing care.* Orlando, FL: Grune & Stratton, Inc.

Bohnet, N. L. (1986). Symptom control. In M. O. Amenta & N. L. Bohnet (Eds.), *Nursing care of the terminally ill* (pp. 67–80). Boston: Little, Brown, & Company.

Boring, C. C., Squires, T. S., Tong, T., & Montgomery, S. (1994). Cancer statistics. *CA—A Cancer Journal for Clinicians, 44*(1), 7–26.

Bourne, V., & Meier, J. (1988). What is happening? A booklet to be read to young children experiencing the terminal illness of a loved one. *Oncology Nursing Forum, 15*(4), 489–493.

Brooker, S. (1992). Dehydration before death. *Nursing Times, 88*(2), 59, 61–62.

Brown, M. A., & Powell-Cope, G. (1993). Themes of loss and dying in caring for a family member with AIDS. *Research in Nursing & Health, 16,* 179–191.

Brown, P., & Chekryn, J. (1989). The dying patient and dehydration. *Canadian Nurse, 85*(5), 14–16.

Bruera, E., & MacDonald, R. N. (1988). Nutrition in cancer patients: An update and review of our experience. *Journal of Pain and Symptom Management, 3*(3), 133–140.

Bruera, E., Macmillan, K., Pither, J., & MacDonald, R. N. (1990). Effects of morphine on dyspnea of terminal cancer patients. *Journal of Pain and Symptom Management, 5*(6), 341–344.

Bruera, E., Miller, M. J., Kuehn, N., MacEachern, T., & Hanson, J. (1992). Estimate of survival of patients admitted to a palliative care unit: A prospective study. *Journal of Pain and Symptom Management, 7*(2), 82–86.

Bruera, E., Miller, L., McCallion, J., Macmillan, K., Krefting, L., & Hanson, J. (1992). Cognitive failure in patients with terminal cancer: A prospective study. *Journal of Pain and Symptom Management, 7*(4), 192–195.

Burge, F. I., King, D. B., & Willison, D. (1990). Intravenous fluids and the hospitalized dying: A medical last rite? *Canadian Family Physician, 36*, 883–886.

Canty, S. L. (1994). Constipation as a side effect of opioids. *Oncology Nursing Forum, 21*(4), 739–745.

Cassileth, P. A. (1982). Common medical complications. In B. R. Cassileth & P. A. Cassileth (Eds.), *Clinical care of the terminal cancer patient,* (pp. 15–37). Philadelphia: Lea & Febiger.

Cella, D. (1992). Quality of life: The concept. *Journal of Palliative Care, 8*(3), 8–13.

Christ, G. H., Siegel, K., Freund, B., Langosch, D., Henderson, S., Sperber, D., & Weinstein, L. (1993). Impact of parental terminal cancer on latency-age children. *American Journal of Orthopsychiatry, 63*(3), 417–425.

Cohen, S. R., & Mount, B. M. (1992). Quality of life in terminal illness: Defining and measuring subjective well-being in the dying. *Journal of Palliative Care, 8*(3), 40–45.

Collaud, T., & Rapin, C. H. (1991). Dehydration in dying patients: Study with physicians in French-speaking Switzerland. *Journal of Pain and Symptom Management, 6*(4), 230–240.

Collins, E., Poulain, P., Gauvain-Piquard, A., Petit, G., & Pichard-Leandri, E. (1993). Is disease progression the major factor in morphine "tolerance" in cancer pain treatment? *Pain, 55,* 319–326.

Coyle, N., Adelhardt, J., Foley, K. M., & Portenoy, R. K. (1990). Character of terminal illness in the advanced cancer patient: Pain and other symptoms during the last four weeks of life. *Journal of Pain and Symptom Management, 5*(2), 83–93.

Creighton, H. (1984). Decisions on food and fluid in life-sustaining measures. *Nursing Management, 15*(6), 47–49.

Curtis, E. B., Krech, R., & Walsh, T. D. (1991). Common symptoms in patients with advanced cancer. *Journal of Palliative Care, 7*(2), 25–29.

Decker, S., & Young, E. (1991). Self-perceived needs of primary caregivers of home-hospice clients. *Journal of Community Health Nursing, 8*(3), 147–154.

DeConno, F., Ventrafidda, V., & Saita, L. (1991). Skin problems in advanced and terminal cancer patients. *Journal of Pain and Symptom Management, 6*(4), 247–256.

Degner, L. F., Gow, C. M., & Thompson, L. A. (1991). Critical nursing behaviors in care for the dying. *Cancer Nursing, 14*(5), 246–253.

Dimond, E. P. (1992). The oncology nurse's role in patient advance directives. *Oncology Nursing Forum, 19*(6), 891–896.

Dimond, E. P. (1994). Two years of the patient self-determination act. *Oncology Nursing Patient Treatment and Support, 1*(2), 1–14.

Dobratz, M. C. (1990a). The life closure scale: A measure of psychological adaptation in death and dying. *The Hospice Journal, 6*(3), 1–15.

Dobratz, M. C. (1990b). Hospice nursing: Present perspectives and future directives. *Cancer Nursing, 13*(2), 116–122.

Dolan, M. B. (1983). Another hospice nurse says. *Nursing, 13*(1), 51.

Dudgeon, D. (1992). Quality of life: A bridge between the biomedical and illness models of medicine and nursing? *Journal of Palliative Care, 8*(3), 14–17.

Dufault, K., & Martocchio, B. (1985). Hope: its spheres and dimensions. *Nursing Clinics of North America, 20*(2), 379–391.

Editor. (1992). Preparing for the death of a loved one. *The American Journal of Hospice & Palliative Care, 9*(4), 14–16.

Ekberg, J., Griffith, N., & Foxall, M. (1986). Spouse burnout syndrome. *Journal of Advanced Nursing, 11,* 161–165.

Enck, R. E. (1989). The management of urinary incontinence. *American Journal of Hospice Care, 6*(6), 9–10.

Enck, R. E. (1994). *The medical care of terminally ill patients.* Baltimore, MD: Johns Hopkins University Press.

Evans, C., & McCarthy, M. (1985). Prognostic uncertainty in terminal care: Can the Karnofsky Index help? *Lancet, 1,* 1204–1206.

Fainsinger, R., MacEachern, T., Hanson, J., & Bruera, E. (1992). The use of urinary catheters in terminally ill cancer patients. *Journal of Pain and Symptom Management, 7*(6), 333–338.

Fainsinger R., Miller, M. J., Bruera, E., Hanson, J., & MacEachern, T. (1991). Symptom control during the last week of life on a palliative care unit. *Journal of Palliative Care, 7*(1), 5–11.

Federal Family and Medical Leave Act (1993). United States.

Ferrans, C. E. (1990). Development of a quality of life index for patients with cancer. *Oncology Nursing Forum, 17,*(Suppl.), 15–21.

Ferrans, C. E., & Powers, M. J. (1985). Quality of life index: Development and psychometric properties. *Advances in Nursing Science, 8*(1), 15–24.

Foley, G. (1986). The treatment of pain in the patient with cancer. *CA-A Cancer Journal for Clinicians, 36*(4), 194–215.

Foley, K. M. (1985). The treatment of cancer pain. *New England Journal of Medicine, 313*(2), 84–95.

Foote, M., Sexton, D. L., & Pawlik, L. (1986). Dyspnea: A distressing sensation in lung cancer. *Oncology Nursing Forum, 13*(5), 25–31.

Frankl, V. (1963). *Man's search for meaning.* Boston: Beacon Press.

Fry, S. T. (1986). Ethical aspects of decision-making in the feeding of cancer patients. *Seminars in Oncology Nursing, 2*(1), 59–62.

Gallagher-Allred, C. (1989). *Nutritional care of the terminally ill.* Rockville, MD. Aspen Publishers, Inc.

Gargaro, W. J. (1983). Criminal prosecution for discontinuance of life support. Part III. *Cancer Nursing, 6*(4), pp. 311–312.

Gates, M. F. (1991). Transcultural comparison of hospital and hospice as caring environments for dying patients. *Journal of Transcultural Nursing, 2*(2), 3–15.

Gaynor, S. (1990). The long haul: The effects of home care on caregivers. *Image, 22*(4), 208–212.

Goodwin, J. S., Hunt, W. C., Key, C. R., & Samet, J. M. (1987). The effect of marital status on stage, treatment, and survival of cancer patients. *Journal of the American Medical Association, 258,* 3125–3130.

Gray, G., Adler, D., Fleming, C., & Brescia, F. (1988). A clinical data base for advanced cancer patients. *Cancer Nursing, 11*(2), 77–83.

Hall, B. A. (1990). The struggle of the diagnosed terminally ill person to maintain hope. *Nursing Science Quarterly, 3*(4), 177–184.

Hastings Center. (1987). *Guidelines on the termination of life-sustaining treatment and the care of the dying.* Briarcliff Manor, NY: The Hastings Center.

Herth, K. (1989). The relationship between level of hope and level of coping response and other variables in patients with cancer. *Oncology Nursing Forum, 16*(1), 67–72.

Herth, K. (1990). Fostering hope in terminally-ill people. *Journal of Advanced Nursing, 15,* 1250–1259.

Herth, K. (1991). Development and refinement of an instrument to measure hope. *Scholarly Inquiry for Nursing Practice: An International Journal, 5*(1), 39–51.

Herth, K. (1993). Hope in the family caregiver of terminally ill people. *Journal of Advanced Nursing, 8,* 538–548.

Hickey, S. S. (1986). Enabling hope. *Cancer Nursing, 9*(3), 133–137.

Higginson, I., & McCarthy, M. (1989). Measuring symptoms in terminal cancer: Are pain and dyspnea controlled? *Journal of the Royal Society of Medicine, 82,* 264–267.

Hockley, J. M., Dunlop, R., & Davies, R. J. (1988). Survey of distressing symptoms in dying patients and their families in hospital and the response to a symptom control team. *British Medical Journal, 296,* 1715–1717.

Holden, C. (1993). Nutrition and hydration in the terminally ill cancer patient: The nurse's role in helping patients and families cope. *The Hospice Journal, 9*(2-3), 15–35.

Hull, M. (1989). Family needs and supportive nursing behaviors during terminal cancer: A review. *Oncology Nursing Forum, 16*(6), 787–792.

Hull, M. (1992). Coping strategies of family caregivers in hospice homecare. *Oncology Nursing Forum, 19*(8), 1179–1187.

Jacox, A., Carr, D. B., Payne, R., et al. (1994). *Management of cancer pain: Clinical practice guideline.* No. 9. AHCPR Publication No. 94-0592. Rockville, MD: Agency for Health Care Policy and Research, U.S. Department of Health and Human Services, Public Health Service.

Jansson, L., & Norberg, A. (1989). Ethical reasoning concerning the feeding of terminally ill cancer patients: Interviews with registered nurses experienced in the care of cancer patients. *Cancer Nursing, 12*(6), 352–358.

Jones, S. A. (1993). Personal unity in dying: Alternative conceptions of the meaning of health. *Journal of Advanced Nursing, 18,* 98–94.

Karnofsky, D. A., Abelmann, W. H., Craver, L. F., & Burchenal, J. H. (1948). The use of the nitrogen mustards in the palliative treatment of carcinoma. *Cancer, 1*(4), 634–656.

Kaye, P. (1990). *Symptom control in hospice and palliative care.* Essex, CT: Hospice Education Institute.

Laizner, A., Yost, L. S., Barg, F., & McCorkle, R. (1993). Needs of family caregivers of persons with cancer: A review. *Seminars in Oncology Nursing, 9*(2), 114–120.

Leininger, M. (1978). *Transcultural nursing concepts, theories, and practices.* New York: John Wiley & Sons.

Lev, E. (1991). Dealing with loss: Concerns of patients and families in a hospice setting. *Clinical Nurse Specialist, 5*(2), 87–93.

Lewis, F. M. (1983). Family level services for the cancer patient: Critical distinctions, fallacies, and assessment. *Cancer Nursing, 6,* 193–200.

Lewis, F. M. (1990). Strengthening family supports: Cancer and the family. *CA-A Cancer Journal for Clinicians, 65,* 158–165.

Lewis, F. M. (1993). Psychosocial transitions and the family's work in adjusting to cancer. *Seminars in Oncology Nursing, 9*(2), 127–129.

Lichter, I. (1993). Results of antiemetic management in terminal illness. *Journal of Palliative Care, 9*(2), 14–18.

Lichter, I., & Hunt, E. (1990). The last 48 hours of life. *Journal of Palliative Care, 6*(4), 7–15.

Lichter, I., Mooney, J., & Boyd, M. (1993). Biography as therapy. *Palliative Medicine, 7,* 133–137.

Lindley-Davis, B. (1991). Process of dying: Defining characteristics. *Cancer Nursing, 14*(6), 328–333.

Linn, M. W., Linn, B. S., & Harris, R. (1982). Effects of counseling for late stage cancer patients. *Cancer, 49,* 1048–1055.

Loprinzi, C. L., Ellison, N. M., Schaid, D. J., Krook, J. E., Athmann, L. M., Dose, A. M., Mailliard, J. A., Johnson, P. S., Ebbert, L. P., & Geeraerts, L. H. (1990). Controlled trial of megestrol acetate for the treatment of cancer anorexia and cachexia. *Journal of National Cancer Institute, 82,* 1127–1132.

Lynn, J. (1984). Food and water can be withheld from dying patients: The very different situations of Claire Conroy and Karen Quinlan. *Death Education, 8,* 271–275.

Massie, M. J., Holland, J., & Glass, E. (1983). Delirium in terminally ill cancer patients. *American Journal of Psychiatry, 140*(8), 1048–1050.

Masters, M., & Shontz, F. (1989). Identification of problems and strengths of the hospice client by clients, caregivers, and nurses. *Cancer Nursing, 12*(4), 226–235.

Martocchio, B. C. (1987). Authenticity, belonging, emotional closeness, and self representation. *Oncology Nursing Forum, 14*(4), 23–27.

McCorkle, R. (1981). A good death [Editorial]. *Cancer Nursing, 4*(4), 267.

McCorkle, R. (1988). The four essentials. *Journal of Palliative Care, 4*(1), 59–61.

McCorkle, R., Benoliel, J. Q., Donaldson, G., Georgiadou, F., Moinpour, C., & Goodell, B. (1989). A randomized clinical trial of home nursing care for lung cancer patients. *Cancer, 64,* 1375–1382.

McCorkle, R. & Young, K. (1978). Development of a symptom distress scale. *Cancer Nursing, 1*(5), 373–378.

Micetich, K. C., Steinecker, P. H., & Thomasma, D. C. (1983). Are intravenous fluids morally required for a dying patient? *Archives of Internal Medicine, 143,* 975–978.

Mishel, M. H. (1990). Reconceptualization of the uncertainty in illness theory. *Image: The Journal of Nursing Scholarship, 22,* 256–264.

Mount, B. (1993). Whole person care: Beyond psychosocial and physical needs. *The American Journal of Hospice & Palliative Care, 10,* 28–37.

Musgrave, C. F. (1990). Terminal dehydration: To give or not to give intravenous fluids? *Cancer Nursing, 13*(1), 62–66.

National Cancer Institute. (1986). *Eating hints.* NCI Publication No. 86-2079. Bethesda, MD: National Cancer Institute, U.S. Department of Health & Human Services, Public Health Service.

Nelson, K., & Walsh, D. (1991). Management of dyspnea in advanced cancer. *Cancer Bulletin, 43*(5), 423–426.

Nelson, K. A., Walsh, D., & Sheehan, F. A. (1994). The cancer anorexia-cachexia syndrome. *Journal of Clinical Oncology, 12*(1), 213–225.

Neumark, D. E. (1994). Providing information about advance directives to patients in ambulatory care and their families. *Oncology Nursing Forum, 21*(4), 771–775.

Northouse, L. (1984). The impact of cancer on the family: an overview. *International Journal of Psychiatry & Medicine, 14,* 215–243.

Oberst, M., Thomas, S., & Ward, S. (1990). Caregiving demands and appraisal of stress among family caregivers. *Cancer Nursing, 12*(4), 209–215.

Owen, D. (1989). Nurses' perspectives on the meaning of

hope in patients with cancer: A qualitative study. *Oncology Nursing Forum, 16*(1), 75–79.

Parkes, C. M. (1988). Bereavement as a psychosocial transition: Processes of adaptation to change. *Journal of Social Issues, 44*(3), 53–65.

Parkes, C. M., & Weiss, R. S. (1983). *Recovery from bereavement.* New York: Basic Books.

Pickett, M. (1993). Cultural awareness in the context of terminal illness. *Cancer Nursing, 16*(2), 102–106.

Poland, J. M. (1987). Xerostomia in the oncologic patient. *American Journal of Hospice Care, 4*(3), 31–33.

Printz, L. A. (1988). Is withholding hydration a valid comfort measure in the terminally ill? *Geriatrics, 43*(11), 84–88.

Psychological Work Group. (1993). A statement of assumptions and principles concerning psychological care of dying persons and their families. *Journal of Palliative Care, 9*(3), 29–32.

Qvarnstrom, U. (1988). International standards provide guidelines for curriculum content. *Journal of Palliative Care, 4*(1), 38–40.

Rando, T. A. (1984). *Grief, dying, and death: Clinical interventions for caregivers.* Champaign, IL: Research Press Company.

Reimer, J., Davies, G., & Martens, N. (1991). Palliative care: The nurse's role in helping families through the transition of "fading away." *Cancer Nursing, 14*(6), 321–327.

Reitmeier, M., & Hartenstein, R. C. (1990). Megestrolacetate and determination of body composition by bioelectrical impedance analysis in cancer cachexia [Abstract]. *Proceedings of the American Society of Clinical Oncology, 9:*325.

Reuben, D. B., & Mor, V. (1986a). Dyspnea in terminally ill cancer patients. *Chest, 89*(2), 234–236.

Reuben, D. B., & Mor, V. (1986b). Nausea and vomiting in terminal cancer patients. *Archives of Internal Medicine, 146,* 2021–2023.

Reuben, D. B., Mor, V., & Hiris, J. (1988). Clinical symptoms and length of survival with terminal cancer. *Archives of Internal Medicine, 148,* 1586–1591.

Rhodes, V. A., & Watson, P. M. (1987). Symptom distress—the concept: past and present. *Seminars in Oncology Nursing, 3*(4), 242–247.

Rimer, B., Levy, M. H., Keintz, M. K., Fox, L., & Engstrom, P. (1987). Enhancing cancer pain control regimens through patient education. *Patient Education Counselor, 10,* 267–277.

Robinson, K. (1990). Predictors of burden among wife caregivers. *Scholarly Inquiry for Nursing Practice: An International Journal, 4*(3), 189–203.

Sanders, C. M. (1982–83). Effects of sudden vs. chronic illness death on bereavement outcome. *Omega, 13,* 227–241.

Saunders, J. M., & McCorkle, R. (1985). Models of care for persons with progressive cancer. *Nursing Clinics of North America, 20*(2), 365–377.

Scanlon, C. (1989). Creating a vision of hope: The challenge of palliative care. *Oncology Nursing Forum, 16*(4), 491–496.

Schipper, H. (1992). Quality of life: The final common pathway. *Journal of Palliative Care, 8*(3), 5–7.

Schipper, H., Clinch, J., & Powell, V. (1990). Definitions and conceptual issues. In Spilker, B. (Ed.), *Quality of life assessments in clinical trials.* New York: Raven Press, Ltd.

Schmitz, P., & O'Brien, M. (1986). Observations on nutrition and hydration in dying cancer patients. In J. Lynn, (Ed.), *By no extraordinary means: The choice to forgo life-sustaining food and water* (pp. 29–38). Bloomington, IN: Indiana University Press.

Schonfeld, D. J. (1993). Talking with children about death. *Journal of Pediatric Health Care, 7,* 269–274.

Sciortino, A. D., Carlton, D. C., Axelrod, A., Eng, M., Zhukovsky, D. S., & Vinciguerra, V. (1992). The efficacy

of administering blood transfusions at home to terminally ill cancer patients. *Journal of Palliative Care, 9*(3), 14–17.

Shepard, K. V. (1994). Increasing opioid dose in patients with malignancy. *Palliative Care Letter, 6*(1), 3.

Siegel, K., Mesagno, F. P., Karus, D., Christ, G., Banks, K., & Moynihan, R. (1992). Psychosocial adjustment of children with a terminally ill parent. *Journal of the American Academy of Child and Adolescent Psychiatry, 31*(2), 327–333.

Spiegel, D., & Bloom, J. R. (1983). Group therapy and hypnosis reduce metastatic breast carcinoma pain. *Psychosomatic Medicine, 45,* 333–339.

Spiegel, D., & Yalom, I. D. (1978). A support group for dying patients. *International Journal of Group Psychotherapy, 28,* 233–245.

Spilker, B. (1990). Introduction. In B. Spilker (Ed.), *Quality of life assessments in clinical trials.* New York: Raven Press, Ltd.

Spiritual Care Work Group. (1990). Assumptions and principles of spiritual care. *Death Studies, 14,* 75–81.

Stjernsward, J., & Teoh, N. (1991). Perspectives on quality of life and the global cancer problem. In D. Osoba (Ed.), *Effect of cancer on quality of life* (pp. 1–5). Boston: CRC Press, Inc.

Stykes, N. P., Baines, M., & Carter, R. L. (1988). Clinical and pathological study of dysphagia conservatively managed in patients with advanced malignant disease. *Lancet, 2*(8613), 726–728.

Syrjola, K. L., Cummings, D., & Donaldson, G. (1992). Hypnosis or cognitive-behavioral training for reduction of pain and nausea during cancer treatment: A controlled clinical trial. *Pain, 48,* 137–146.

Torosian, M., & Daly, J. (1986). Nutritional support in the cancer-bearing host: Effects on host and tumor. *Cancer, 58,* 1915–1929.

Tornberg, M. J., McGrath, B. B., & Benoliel, J. Q. (1984). Oncology transition services: Partnerships of nurses and families. *Cancer Nursing, 7,* 131–137.

Tripp-Reimer, T., & Brink, P. (1985). Culture brokerage. In G. Bulechek, & J. McCloskey (Eds.), *Nursing interventions treatments for nursing diagnoses.* Philadelphia: W. B. Saunders Co.

Twycross, R. G. (1986). Care of the dying: Symptom control. *British Journal of Hospital Medicine, 28,* 244–249.

Ventafridda, V., Ripamonti, C., DeConno, F., Tamburini, M., & Cassileth, B. R. (1990). Symptom prevalence and control during cancer patients' last days of life. *Journal of Palliative Care, 6*(3), 7–11.

Wachtel, T., Allen-Masterson, S., Reuben, D., Goldberg, R., & Mor, V. (1988). The end stage cancer patient: Terminal common pathway. *The Hospice Journal, 4*(4), 43–80.

Waller, A., Adunski, A., & Hershkowitz, M. (1991). Terminal dehydration and intravenous fluids. *The Lancet, 337,* 745.

Wallston, K. A., Burger, C., Smith, R. A., & Baugher, R. J. (1988). Comparing the quality of death for hospice and non-hospice cancer patients. *Medical Care, 26*(2), 177–182.

Walsh, T. D. (1990). Prevention of opioid side effects. *Journal of Pain and Symptom Management, 5*(6), 362–367.

Walsh, T. D., MacDonald, N., Bruera, E., Shepard, K. V., Michaud, M., & Zanes, R. (1992). A controlled study of sustained-release morphine sulfate tablets in chronic pain from advanced cancer. *American Journal of Clinical Oncology, 15*(3), 268–272.

Warner, J. E. (1992). Involvement of families in pain control of terminally ill patients. *The Hospice Journal, 8*(1-2), 155–170.

Weisman, A. (1979). *Coping with cancer.* New York: McGraw Hill.

Wingate, A., & Lackey, N. (1989). A description of needs of non-institutionalized cancer patients and their primary caregivers. *Cancer Nursing, 12*(4), 216–225.

Winningham, M. L., Nail, L. M., Burke, M. B., Brophy, L., Cimprich, B., Jones, L. S., Pickard-Halley, S., Rhodes, V., St. Pierre, B., Beck, S., Glass, E. C., Mock, V. L., Mooney, K., & Piper, B. (1994). Fatigue and the cancer experience: The state of the knowledge. *Oncology Nursing Forum, 21*(1), 23–36.

Wurzbach, M. E. (1990). The dilemma of withholding or withdrawing nutrition. *Image, 22*(4), 226–230.

Yan, E., & Bruera, E. (1991). Parenteral hydration of terminally ill cancer patients. *Journal of Palliative Care, 7*(3), 40–43.

Yates, J. W., Chalmer, B., & McKegney, F. P. (1980). Evaluation of patients with advanced cancer using the Karnofsky Performance Status. *Cancer, 45,* 2220–2224.

Yates, P. (1993). Towards a reconceptualization of hope for patients with a diagnosis of cancer. *Journal of Advanced Nursing, 18,* 701–706.

Zerwekh, J. V. (1983). The dehydration question. *Nursing, 13*(1), 47–51.

Oncologic Emergencies

Christine Miaskowski

Recent advances in the treatment of malignant disease have resulted in many patients being cured of their initial disease. When the disease recurs, however, it can be associated with or manifest itself as a life-threatening emergency. In other cases, the malignancy may appear initially as a medical emergency. In either case, the occurrence of oncologic emergencies is becoming more frequent in clinical practice. Careful assessment of the oncology patient is essential to diagnose emergency conditions early and initiate treatment promptly. This prompt recognition and immediate treatment can halt the progression of the oncologic emergency and often reverse potentially disabling side effects.

This chapter on oncologic emergencies is divided into three sections. The first section reviews the obstructive emergencies: superior vena cava (SVC) syndrome, intestinal obstruction, and third space syndrome. The second portion of the chapter deals with the major metabolic emergencies: the syndrome of inappropriate antidiuretic hormone (SIADH) secretion, hypercalcemia, septic shock, and disseminated intravascular coagulation (DIC). The final section concentrates on the infiltrative emergencies and covers neoplastic cardiac tamponade, spinal cord compression, and carotid artery rupture. For each oncologic emergency, the anatomy and physiology of the syndrome are reviewed briefly, the pathophysiologic mechanism is explained, the assessment and management of the oncologic emergency are discussed, and a list of actual and potential nursing diagnoses the patient may experience is presented.

OBSTRUCTIVE EMERGENCIES

Cancer can obstruct major organs, blood vessels, and lymphatic channels. When obstruction occurs, a backup occurs in the flow of blood or body fluids through the channel that is involved. The major obstructive emergencies associated with malignant disease are SVC syndrome, intestinal obstruction, and third space syndrome.

SUPERIOR VENA CAVA SYNDROME

The superior vena cava is a thin-walled, low-pressure blood vessel that lies within the confined, rigid space of the mediastinal cavity. This blood vessel collects blood from the venous vessels that drain the head and neck and the upper thoracic cavity. Because the mediastinum is a rigid anatomic structure that includes the trachea, the vertebral column, the sternum and ribs, and the lymph nodes, there is little room to expand and accommodate the growth of neoplastic tissue. The growth of a tumor within the mediastinal cavity results in compression of the superior vena cava as well as other blood vessels and organs.

Four mechanisms underlie the development of SVC syndrome. The superior vena cava can be occluded by an extrinsic mass. Occlusion of the superior vena cava can occur as a result of tumor invasion into the vessel wall. A third mechanism can involve the obstruction of the vessel lumen by a neoplastic thrombus. The final mechanism may involve the occlusion of the vessel by thrombus formation on an intravascular catheter.

Eighty to ninety per cent of the cases of SVC syndrome occur from malignant disease. The most common cancers that can cause this syndrome are bronchogenic carcinoma and lymphomas. This oncologic emergency can be observed with metastatic disease from the esophagus, colon, testes, and breast.

The primary signs and symptoms result from the obstruction of blood flow in the venous system of the head, neck, and upper trunk. The severity of symptoms depends on the rapidity, degree, and location of the obstruction and whether collateral circulation has developed. Initial symptoms occur in the early morning hours and include periorbital and conjunctival edema, facial swelling, and tightness of the shirt collar (Stoke's sign). These symptoms disappear within a few hours when the patient assumes an upright position and drainage from the face can occur.

As the obstruction worsens, the nurse should assess the patient for the following signs and symptoms: fullness of the arms, swelling of the fingers and hands, difficulty removing rings, erythema of the face, neck, and upper trunk, and epistaxis. Late symptoms of this syndrome include distention of the veins of the thorax and upper extremities, dysphagia, cough, dyspnea, tachypnea, hoarseness, cyanosis, and intracranial hypertension. In the acute, emergency situation, obstruction of the superior vena cava leads to a decrease in venous return with a marked reduction in cardiac output and a decrease in cerebral perfusion. Patients present with respiratory difficulty, hypotension, and mental status changes.

The primary form of treatment for SVC syndrome is radiation therapy. Radiation treatment is directed to the tumor plus a 2 cm margin surrounding the tumor and to the mediastinal, hilar, and supraclavicular nodes to a total dose of 30 to 50 cGy. The total dose is dependent on the patient's condition, extent of disease, response of the disease to treatment, and histology of the tumor. Relief of symptoms usually occurs within 7 to 14 days with evidence of benefit seen in 24 hours in some cases (Zaloznik, 1993).

Chemotherapy may be administered concurrently with the radiation therapy. The usual agents used are cyclophosphamide (Cytoxan), methotrexate, and nitrogen mustard (Chernecky & Ramsey, 1984). With some chemosensitive tumors (e.g., small-cell lung cancer, non-Hodgkin's lymphoma, germ-cell tumors), chemotherapy may be the primary form of treatment.

Supportive care during treatment is of primary importance. Maintenance of a patent airway or relief of airway obstruction is a major objective. Oxygen therapy may be required if the patient is hypoxic. Diuretics may be used to relieve the swelling, but they must be used with extreme caution because they can further compromise venous return to the heart. Steroids may be administered to improve the patient's condition by decreasing the amount of inflammation. In some cases, heparin may be used to minimize or prevent further thrombus formation. Recently, venographic procedures have been evaluated; during evaluation an expansile stent is placed in the lumen of the compressed vessel to maintain patency (Kishi et al., 1993).

The major potential and actual nursing diagnoses for SVC syndrome as well as the associated nursing interventions are listed in Table 66–1. Special emphasis must be placed on supporting the patient through an extremely frightening situation.

INTESTINAL OBSTRUCTION

An intestinal obstruction can involve either the large or the small intestine. The clinical picture as well as therapeutic interventions depend on the nature of the tumor and the site and degree of obstruction. An intestinal obstruction means that the bowel contents

TABLE 66–1. *Actual and Potential Nursing Diagnoses for the Obstructive Emergencies*

Superior Vena Cava Syndrome	Intestinal Obstruction
Decreased cardiac output	*Fluid volume deficit*
Monitor vital signs	Assess hydration status
Assess for pulses paradoxus	Monitor intake and output
Monitor intake and output	Administer intravenous hydration
Measure central venous pressure or other hemodynamic parameters	*Alteration in comfort*
Maintain bed rest	Maintain patency of intestinal tube
Ineffective breathing pattern	Medicate for pain as needed
Assess respiratory status	*Alteration in nutrition, less than body requirements*
Monitor arterial blood gases	Assess for protein-caloric malnutrition
Administer oxygen as necessary	Consider intravenous alimentation
Provide respiratory support (e.g., intubation, tracheostomy) as needed	**Third Space Syndrome**
Decreased cerebral perfusion	*Loss phase*
Assess mental status	Potential for fluid volume deficit
Teach patient ways to decrease intracranial pressure	Monitor intake and output to determine when the patient begins to increase urine output
Promote venous drainage from the head	Assess renal function (blood urea nitrogen, creatinine)
Severe anxiety	Monitor vital signs
Explain all procedures	Monitor for signs and symptoms of hypovolemia
Medicate for pain as necessary	Administer intravenous fluids and plasma proteins
Utilize relaxation techniques	*Reabsorption phase*
Place patient close to nurse's station	Fluid volume excess
Schedule frequent visits	Monitor intravenous hydration
Alteration in skin integrity	Monitor for signs and symptoms of hypervolemia
Perform skin assessment	Weigh patient daily
Avoid tight or abrasive clothing	
Elevate extremities to promote venous return	

cannot pass normally to the rectum. Any type of obstruction will interfere with normal peristaltic activity. Normal peristalsis is brought about by the electrical conduction of contractile stimuli from one bowel segment to the next. Within the normal bowel, there is a gradient of rhythmic, intrinsic activity that decreases from the mouth to the anus. An obstruction to the flow of gastric contents can lead to life-threatening pathophysiologic changes (Fig. 66–1).

The etiology of small-bowel obstruction is primarily nonmalignant. Ninety per cent of all small bowel obstructions result from adhesions following abdominal surgery. Only 10 to 20 per cent of all small-bowel obstructions are the result of malignant disease. Primary tumors of the small intestine account for only 1 to 3 per cent of the small bowel obstructions. Histologically, these tumors can be carcinoid, adenocarcinomas, sarcomas, lymphomas, or melanomas. The remaining small-bowel obstructions that occur as a result of malignant disease arise from metastatic tumors of the colon-rectum, ovary, or cervix. The majority of large bowel obstructions (90 per cent) occur as a result of malignant disease. The primary cancers that produce large bowel obstructions are adenocarcinomas. In addition, metastatic disease arising from ovarian or cervical tumors or from lymphomas can obstruct the large intestine.

The signs and symptoms of small- and large-bowel obstruction are listed in Table 66–2. A thorough abdominal assessment must be performed and should include a history of pain, vomiting, and frequency of bowel movements and an abdominal examination to evaluate for distention, palpable masses, and the quality and duration of bowel sounds.

The primary goals of medical therapy are to relieve the distention, correct the fluid imbalance, and, if possible, remove the obstruction. Patients will be treated initially with a nasogastric or long intestinal tube in an effort to achieve decompression. Vigorous hydration will be instituted that includes the replacement of electrolytes. If the lesion is resectable, surgery will be performed. The type of surgery performed (i.e., a resection and end-to-end anastomosis or a resection and colostomy) depends on the location and degree of the obstruction.

The major potential and actual nursing diagnoses for intestinal obstruction as well as the associated nursing interventions are listed in Table 66–1. Special emphasis must be placed on assessing the patient for signs and symptoms of strangulation or perforation, which can occur acutely. If the character of the patient's pain changes and becomes more intense and continuous and abdominal girth decreases, strangulation should be suspected. If the patient develops rebound tenderness and bowel sounds stop abruptly, bowel rupture and associated peritonitis may have occurred. The physician should be notified immediately if either of these conditions is evident.

THIRD SPACE SYNDROME

Third space syndrome is the shift in fluid from the vascular to the interstitial space owing to lowered plasma proteins, increased capillary permeability, or lymphatic blockage secondary to trauma, inflammation, or disease. Normally, body fluids are contained within three compartments: the vascular space, the intracellular space, and the interstitial space or third space. Fluid and particulate matter including plasma proteins are exchanged at the level of the capillary membrane. Fluid equilibrium is maintained at the level of the capillary membrane by a series of opposing pressures. Changes in pressures at the capillary membrane, increased capillary permeability, lowered plasma proteins, or changes in the integrity of the lymphatic system are the most common etiologic factors that produce a sequestering of fluid into the third space or interstitial space (Twombly, 1978).

Generalized third space syndrome is most commonly seen in oncology patients who have undergone major surgical procedures (e.g., abdominoperineal resection, pelvic exenteration) or who are in septic shock. Third

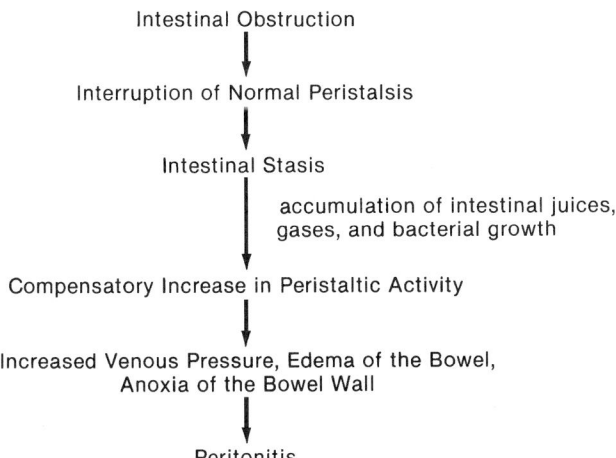

FIGURE 66–1. Consequences of an obstruction to the flow of gastric contents.

TABLE 66–2. *Assessment Parameters for Small and Large Bowel Obstruction*

SMALL BOWEL OBSTRUCTION	LARGE BOWEL OBSTRUCTION
Colicky pain, early in the obstruction	Crampy, lower abdominal pain
As obstruction progresses, pain becomes mild, non-localized, and a steady discomfort	
Obstipation	Alternating diarrhea and constipation
Distention	Marked distention
Vomiting begins early	Vomiting occurs late
Fever	
Leukocytosis	
Signs of hypovolemia	
Bowel sounds for both small and large bowel obstruction: Proximal to the obstruction they are high-pitched and hyperactive Distal to the obstruction they are diminished or absent	

space syndrome is divided into two phases: the loss phase and the reabsorption phase. The nursing assessment and management of the patient is dependent on the phase of the syndrome.

The loss phase typically occurs immediately after surgery and is usually self-limited to 48 to 72 hours. The phase is characterized by a shift in fluid from the vascular space to the interstitial space. Patients present with signs and symptoms of hypovolemia. The patient must be monitored for hypotension, tachycardia, low central venous pressure, decreased urine output, and an increased urine-specific gravity. During the loss phase, the patient's fluid intake exceeds total output by a ratio of 3:1. Active treatment during this phase of the syndrome involves the replacement of fluid and electrolytes as well as plasma proteins. The infusion of plasma proteins will increase the plasma colloid oncotic pressure and "pull" fluids from the interstitial into the vascular space. Diuretics may be prescribed to remove the excess fluid that is being reabsorbed.

As the patient begins to recover and the inflammation begins to subside, the patient enters the reabsorption phase. The injured tissue heals, the damaged capillaries begin to repair, and normal permeability returns. In addition, the degree of lymphatic blockage decreases as collateral lymphatics develop. After surgery, plasma proteins begin to return to normal levels. The end result is that capillary pressures return to normal and the fluid within the interstitial space begins to be reabsorbed. The reabsorption phase is characterized by a shift in fluid from the interstitial space into the vascular space. The hallmark sign that the patient is entering the reabsorption phase is a marked increase in urine output (i.e., greater than 200 ml/hr). The major problem that can occur is hypervolemia. The patient should be monitored for hypertension, tachycardia, elevation in central venous pressure, weight gain, rales, dyspnea, and jugular venous distention. The primary treatment is to reduce the amount of intravenous hydration and monitor the patient's fluid balance.

The major potential and actual nursing diagnoses for the two phases of third space syndrome as well as the associated nursing interventions are listed in Table 66–1. The patient must be closely monitored for signs and symptoms of hypovolemia and hypervolemic shock.

METABOLIC EMERGENCIES

Malignant disease can cause metabolic abnormalities by producing ectopic hormones that affect specific target tissues and initiate an associated list of signs and symptoms, or it can produce major derangements in all metabolic pathways. The major metabolic emergencies associated with malignant disease include the SIADH secretion, hypercalcemia, septic shock, and DIC.

SYNDROME OF INAPPROPRIATE ANTIDIURETIC HORMONE SECRETION

Normally, antidiuretic hormone (ADH) is released from the posterior pituitary gland when the plasma osmolality increases or the plasma volume decreases

(Fig. 66–2). The hormone acts on the collecting ducts of the kidney, causing a reabsorption of water and a concentrated and decreased urine volume. Antidiuretic hormone is normally released by pain, stress, trauma, hemorrhage, and certain drugs (Poe & Taylor, 1989).

The SIADH secretion is a syndrome of hypotonicity of plasma and hyponatremia that results from the aberrant production or sustained secretion of ADH (vasopressin). Inappropriate secretion is defined as secretion that continues in the face of hypotonicity of plasma. Cancer is the most frequent cause of the SIADH secretion. The type of cancer most frequently associated with the syndrome is carcinoma of the lung. Other types can include cancer of the pancreas, duodenum, brain, esophagus, colon, ovary, prostate, bronchus, and nasopharynx, and acute and chronic leukemia, mesothelioma, reticulum-cell sarcoma, Hodgkin's disease, thymoma, and lymphosarcoma. It has been shown that these cancers have the ability to synthesize, store, and release ADH. In addition, certain cancer chemotherapeutic agents can produce this syndrome. Vincristine and cyclophosphamide have been shown to stimulate the release of excess amounts of ADH (Poe & Taylor, 1989).

The signs and symptoms of the SIADH secretion are listed in Table 66–3. The signs and symptoms are reflective of water intoxication. This syndrome induces profound neurologic symptoms and should not be mistaken for a psychosis. Once the syndrome has been diagnosed, the treatment depends on the severity of the patient's symptoms. Initial treatment may simply involve water restriction. In severely symptomatic patients, 3 per cent sodium chloride solution will be administered.

The major potential and actual nursing diagnoses for the SIADH secretion as well as the associated nursing interventions are listed in Table 66–4.

HYPERCALCEMIA

Calcium is the fifth most abundant cation in the body. Ninety-nine per cent of the body's calcium is in an insoluble form in the skeleton. The remaining 1 per cent is freely exchangeable calcium. Ionized calcium is the calcium of physiologic importance and is maintained within a very precise range. The two hormones that regulate serum calcium levels are parathyroid hormone and calcitonin. The release of parathyroid hormone results in an increase in serum calcium levels. Calcitonin release produces a decrease in serum calcium levels (Fig. 66–3).

Malignancies most commonly associated with the development of hypercalcemia include squamous cell carcinomas of the lung and head and neck, breast and renal cancers, multiple myeloma, and the lymphomas. The mechanisms involved in the development of hypercalcemia of malignancy are extremely complex. Prior to 1980, hypercalcemia was thought to develop as a consequence of bone metastasis. Recent evidence suggests that while bone metastasis in some cases results in hypercalcemia, certain tumors secrete a variety of hormonal factors that stimulate osteoclast activity with

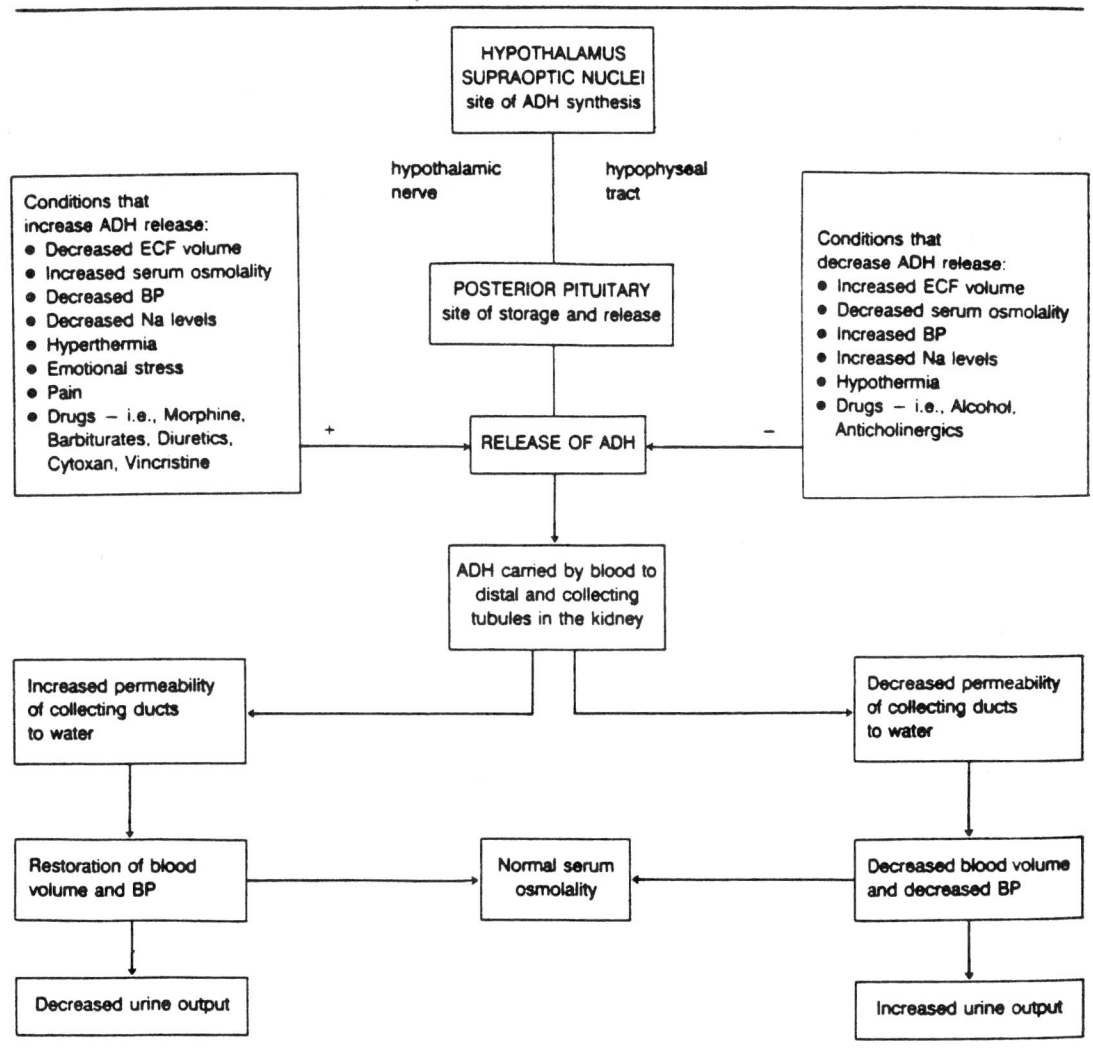

FIGURE 66–2. Mechanism of ADH release. (From Poe, C. M. & Taylor, L. M. [1989]. Syndrome of inappropriate antidiuretic hormone: Assessment and nursing implications. *Oncology Nursing Forum, 16*[3], 373–381.)

resultant release of calcium from the bone. Several humoral factors that have been identified as being associated with hypercalcemia of malignancy are parathy-

TABLE 66–3. *Assessment Parameters for SIADH Secretion*

Physical Assessment	Laboratory Assessment
Absence of edema	Hyponatremia (mild =
Mental confusion	125–134 mEq/L; moder-
Sluggish deep tendon	ate = 115–124 mEq/L;
reflexes	severe = < 110 mEq/L)
Personality changes	Serum osmolality of less
Weight gain	than 280 mOsm/kg
Weakness	Decreased blood urea nitro-
Anorexia, nausea, and vom-	gen and creatinine
iting	Increased urinary excretion
Lethargy	of sodium (> 20 mEq/L)
Seizures	Increased urine osmolality
Coma	Hypokalemia
	Hypocalcemia

roid hormone-related protein, osteoclast-activating factors, transforming growth factors, hematopoietic colony-stimulating factors, prostaglandins—E series, and 1,25-dihydroxyvitamin D.

It should be noted that two other phenomena can contribute to and worsen hypercalcemia. These are immobility and dehydration (Kaplan, 1994).

The signs and symptoms of hypercalcemia reflect the importance of calcium in the physiologic functioning of all of the body's major organ systems. The severity of symptoms often correlates with the serum calcium level. Neuromuscular symptoms can include apathy, depression, malaise, fatigue, and profound muscle weakness. Cardiovascular effects are manifested on the electrocardiogram as shortening of the Q-T interval and prolongation of the P-R interval. The kidney attempts to remove excess levels of calcium, and symptoms of polyuria and nocturia are present. The gastrointestinal system is also affected. The patient can present with anorexia, nausea and vomiting, and abdominal pain. The gastrointestinal symptoms can progress to ileus and obstipation.

TABLE 66–4. *Actual and Potential Nursing Diagnoses for Metabolic Emergencies*

SIADH Secretion
Fluid volume excess
  Monitor laboratory data
  Perform neurologic assessment
  Restrict fluids as prescribed
  Administer 3% sodium chloride as prescribed

Hypercalcemia
Fluid volume deficit
  Administer intravenous hydration
  Monitor intake and output
  Assess hydration status
  Check urine specific gravity
Potential for decreased cardiac output
  Monitor vital signs
  Assess for electrocardiogram changes associated with
    hypercalcemia
Potential for injury and decreased activity tolerance
  Institute safety measures
  Perform neurologic assessment
  Encourage mobility to prevent bone resorption of calcium

Septic Shock
Fluid volume deficit
  Administer intravenous hydration
  Monitor intake and output
  Assess hydration status
  Check urine specific gravity
Potential for decreased cardiac output
  Monitor vital signs and hemodynamic parameters
  Titrate vasopressor therapy as prescribed
Potential for alteration in renal tissue perfusion
  Monitor intake and output
  Monitor renal function (blood urea nitrogen, creatinine)
Potential for alteration in cerebral tissue perfusion
  Perform neurologic assessment
  Administer oxygen as prescribed

Disseminated Intravascular Coagulation
Alteration in tissue perfusion
  Assess patient for evidence of clotting
  Administer oxygen as prescribed
  Administer adequate hydration for renal perfusion
Potential for injury
  Assess patient for evidence of bleeding
  Initiate bleeding or thrombocytopenia precautions
  Control active bleeding
  Administer platelets and transfusions as prescribed
Alteration in comfort
  Assess patient's degree of discomfort
  Administer analgesics as needed

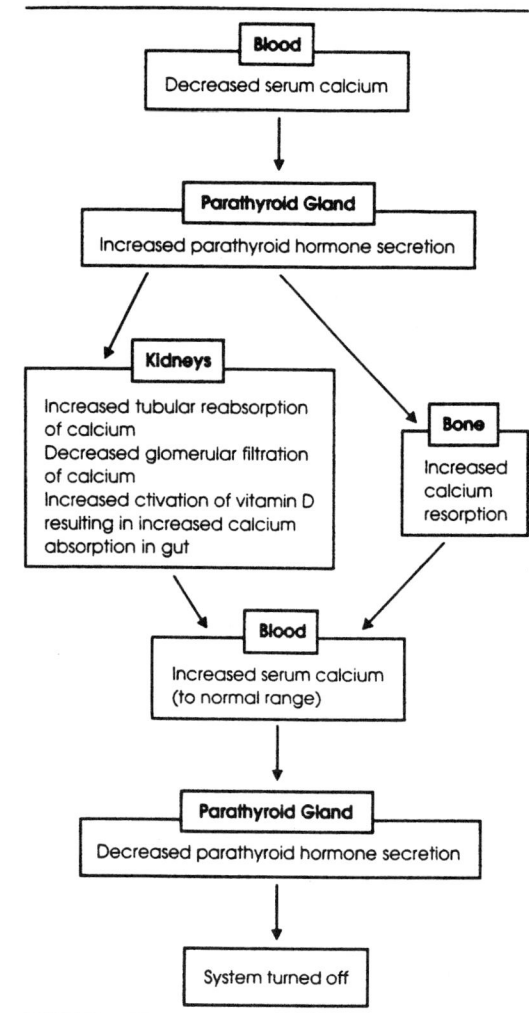

FIGURE 66–3. Negative feedback for calcium regulation. (From Kaplan, M. [1994]. Hypercalcemia of malignancy: A review of advances in pathophysiology. *Oncology Nursing Forum, 21*[6], 1039–1048.)

Treatment of hypercalcemia is focused on enhancing renal excretion of calcium and decreasing bone resorption of calcium. Increased renal excretion of calcium is accomplished through the use of intravenous hydration with normal saline and the administration of calciuretic diuretics. The rate of intravenous hydration and the dose of furosemide prescribed are based on the serum level of calcium and the severity of the symptoms exhibited by the patient. To decrease bone resorption of calcium, drug therapy is initiated.

Plicamycin, a chemotherapeutic antibiotic, is often used. Effects of the drug are seen within 24 to 48 hours, and the effects may last from 2 days to 2 weeks. The major toxicities associated with plicamycin therapy are thrombocytopenia, nausea and vomiting, hypotension, and renal and hepatic toxicity. The second drug used in the management of hypercalcemia is calcitonin. This drug also inhibits bone resorption of calcium. The major side effect associated with calcitonin is nausea and vomiting. A third drug that is used with extreme caution in managing hypercalcemia is intravenous phosphate. The primary mechanism of action of this drug is to precipitate calcium into the bone. The danger, however, is that extraskeletal calcifications can occur in the heart and kidney and produce serious and sometimes fatal consequences (Kaplan, 1994). Another drug is gallium nitrate, which blocks parathyroid hormone-induced calcium resorption of bone. This drug must be given as a continuous infusion for 5 days and has been associated with nephrotoxicity.

The major potential and actual nursing diagnoses for hypercalcemia as well as the associated nursing interventions are listed in Table 66–4.

SEPTIC SHOCK

Septic shock is the major form of distributive shock caused by a massive overwhelming infection throughout the entire body. It is the major cause of death in patients with cancer, particularly patients with leukemia and lymphoma. Shock is basically a disease of the cell. Normal cellular metabolic processes are disrupted in the shock state. This disruption results in deleterious consequences in every major organ system. The overall mechanism underlying septic shock is the death of bacteria. The death of the organism results in the release of endotoxins, which produce numerous effects.

Septic shock is divided into two phases. The first phase is referred to as *warm shock*. The release of endotoxins results in the secretion of various vasoactive substances. These vasoactive substances produce dilation of the venous and arterial systems. The release of endotoxin and the subsequent dilation of the arteries and veins result in a series of signs and symptoms including mental confusion, chills and fever, flushed and warm skin, tachycardia, tachypnea, and decreased PO_2. If the disease is not treated, the patient will progress into the second phase of the shock state, called *cold shock*. At this point, more endotoxin is released, which stimulates the release of histamine and bradykinin. These two substances are potent vasodilators that produce a series of reactions, including an increase in capillary permeability, a decrease in circulating blood volume, which results in a decrease in cardiac output, and a decrease in tissue perfusion. The patient in cold shock will exhibit the following signs and symptoms: cold skin, peripheral edema, tachycardia, hypotension, tachypnea, pulmonary congestion, hypoxemia, oliguria, and metabolic acidosis (Kahn, 1988).

The treatment of septic shock is summarized by the acronym VIP. V = ventilate. Patients in septic shock require oxygen. If the patient's respiratory status is compromised, mechanical ventilation may be required. I = infuse. The patient in septic shock is usually hypotensive. Crystalloid solutions as well as colloid solutions must be infused to maintain an adequate blood pressure.

P = perfusion. Cardiac output needs to be maintained, usually with pressor therapy. Dopamine is the vasopressor drug that is used most commonly, because it will improve cardiac output and maintain renal perfusion. The mainstay of treatment for septic shock is antibiotic therapy. Antibiotics are prescribed empirically in patients with septic shock. The usual treatment regimen includes a penicillin, an aminoglycoside, and a cephalosporin.

The major potential and actual nursing diagnoses for septic shock as well as the associated nursing interventions are listed in Table 66–4.

DISSEMINATED INTRAVASCULAR COAGULATION

Disseminated intravascular coagulation (DIC) is an alteration in the normal clotting mechanism that manifests itself as diffuse clotting occurring simultaneously with hemorrhage (Colman & Rubin, 1990). The normal clotting cascade is a tightly controlled homeostatic mechanism, which protects the body when injury has occurred. The intrinsic and extrinsic pathways of the clotting cascade are illustrated in Figure 66–4.

Disseminated intravascular coagulation is seen not as a primary disorder but as a secondary complication that requires some type of triggering event. In patients with a cancer diagnosis, DIC has been associated with intravascular hemolysis from transfusion reactions, overwhelming viral or bacterial sepsis and shock, particularly from gram-negative sepsis, and release of thrombin from malignant cells (e.g., acute myelogenous leukemia, melanoma, or cancer of the lung, stomach, colon, breast, ovary, and prostate) (Colman & Rubin, 1990).

The pathophysiologic mechanisms involved in DIC are pictured in Figure 66–5. The excessive conversion of prothrombin to thrombin and the generation of fibrin clots result in soluble clot deposition in tissue capillaries. This fibrin deposition impedes blood flow and

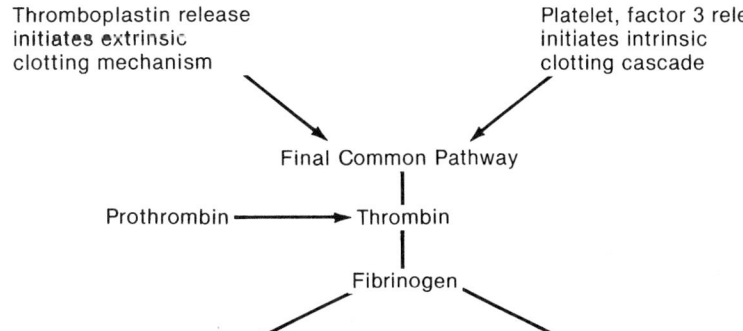

FIGURE 66–4. The intrinsic and extrinsic pathways of the clotting cascade.

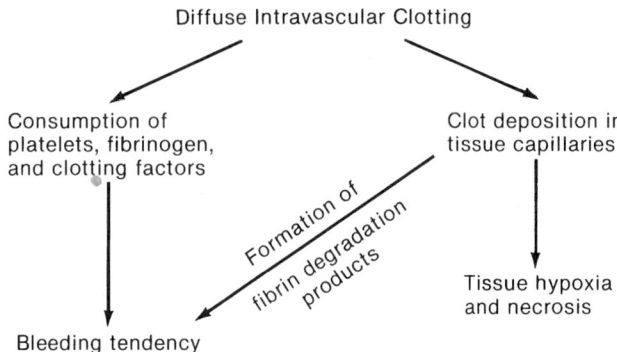

FIGURE 66–5. Pathophysiologic mechanisms in disseminated intravascular coagulation.

can result in tissue hypoxia and necrosis. As the excessive clotting proceeds, normal homeostatic controls cannot maintain an adequate supply of platelets, clotting factors, and fibrinogen. In addition, fibrin split products—natural anticoagulants that are produced as part of the normal clotting cascade—begin to accumulate, and the patient has a tendency to hemorrhage.

Patients must be observed for evidence of bleeding and clotting. The most prominent signs of bleeding are petechiae, ecchymosis, and prolonged bleeding from injection sites. The skin, gingiva, conjunctiva, and retina should be examined carefully. In addition, patients should be monitored for episodes of epistaxis, bleeding from old injection sites, bleeding from incision sites, intestinal bleeding, and signs and symptoms of a major internal hemorrhage, including hypotension, tachycardia, decreased hematocrit levels, and markedly reduced urine output. Patients have a tendency to develop clots in the microcirculation of organs with the highest blood flow (e.g., kidney, central nervous system, and skin). Assessments should be made for hematuria, changes in mental status, and acrocyanosis (i.e., generalized sweating, with cold, mottled fingers and toes). The patient's coagulation profile, including prothrombin time, activated partial thromboplastin time, fibrinogen level, platelet count, fibrin split products, and D-dimer must be monitored.

The primary treatment of DIC is to remove the precipitating factor or underlying cause, which may be difficult if the precipitating factor is the patient's cancer. The major intervention involves the administration of heparin. The rationale for this treatment is that heparin inactivates thrombin, which will inhibit the clotting process and thereby inhibit fibrinolysis. This series of reactions, in effect, stops the DIC cycle. The remaining medical interventions are supportive in nature and include platelet transfusions and interventions to prevent organ failure. The major potential and actual nursing diagnoses for DIC as well as the associated nursing interventions are listed in Table 66–4.

INFILTRATIVE EMERGENCIES

Cancers can infiltrate major organs and produce devastating, life-threatening sequelae. The major infil-

trative emergencies discussed in this section are neoplastic cardiac tamponade, spinal cord compression, and carotid artery rupture.

NEOPLASTIC CARDIAC TAMPONADE

The pericardium is a double-walled sac that surrounds the heart and the great vessels. It contains a visceral layer that directly lines the surface of the heart and an outer layer—the parietal layer—which is made of fibrous tissue and can move freely. The pericardial cavity lies between the two layers and contains approximately 25 to 35 ml of serous fluid. The pericardium provides a frictionless sac for the contractions of the heart and supports the heart in a stable position.

Neoplastic cardiac tamponade results from an accumulation of fluid in the pericardial sac, from a significant constriction of the pericardium by tumor, or from postirradiation pericarditis, which is indirectly related to the cancer (Ameli & Shah, 1991).

The signs and symptoms exhibited by the patient are extremely variable. The severity of symptoms depends on the rapidity of the development of the tamponade. The patient can exhibit any or all of the following symptoms: extreme anxiety and agitation, an oppressive feeling over the precordium, dyspnea and tachypnea, cough, dysphagia, hiccups, hoarseness, nausea and vomiting, perfuse perspiration, changes in level of consciousness, tachycardia, jugular venous distention, pulsus paradoxus, or distant or muffled heart sounds. The patient's electrocardiogram may show electrical alternans (Ameli & Shah, 1991).

Emergency management of the acutely ill patient involves rapid diagnosis and treatment with a pericardiocentesis to remove the fluid, as illustrated in Figure 66–6. The patient may require supportive therapy, including oxygen, intravenous hydration, and administration of pressor therapy. After the acute treatment, the patient may undergo surgery for a pericardial window or for placement of an indwelling pericardial catheter.

The major potential and actual nursing diagnoses for neoplastic cardiac tamponade as well as the associated nursing interventions are listed in Table 66–5.

SPINAL CORD COMPRESSION

Spinal cord compression develops in approximately 1 to 10 per cent of cancer patients. This oncologic emergency requires prompt diagnosis, evaluation, and treatment if permanent neurologic sequelae are to be prevented. Spinal cord compression can occur as a result of direct extension of the tumor from the paravertebral nodes to the spinal cord or from metastatic disease to the vertebral column. Seventy per cent of all cord compressions occur in the thoracic area. Tumors with the highest incidence of cord compression in the thoracic area are lung, breast, kidney, prostate, lymphoma, myeloma, melanoma, and gastrointestinal. Twenty per cent of all cord compressions occur in the lumbosacral area. Tumors with the highest incidence of cord compression in this area are gastrointestinal,

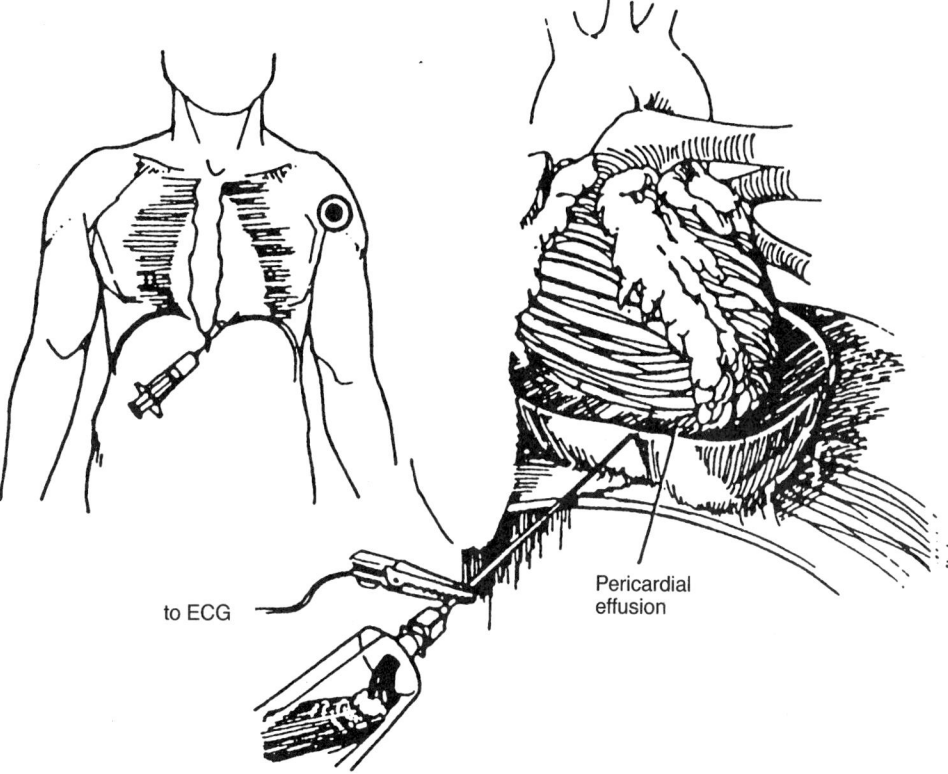

FIGURE 66–6. Emergency management of neoplastic cardiac tamponade with a pericardiocentesis to remove the fluid. (With permission from Adria Laboratories [1987]. *Understanding and managing oncologic emergencies* [p. 28]. Dublin, OH: Adria Laboratories.)

to ECG

Pericardial
effusion

TABLE 66–5. *Actual and Potential Nursing Diagnoses for Infiltrative Emergencies*

Neoplastic Cardiac Tamponade
Decreased cardiac output
  Monitor vital signs and hemodynamic parameters
  Monitor for pulsus paradoxus
  Monitor electrocardiogram for electrical alternans
Potential for alteration in cerebral tissue perfusion
  Perform neurologic assessment
  Administer oxygen as prescribed

Spinal Cord Compression
Pain
  Perform a pain assessment
  Administer analgesics as prescribed
  Utilize nonpharmacologic strategies to decrease pain
Potential for alteration in mobility
  Perform a neurologic assessment
  Institute safety measures
Potential for alteration in skin integrity
  Perform skin assessment
  Institute preventive skin care measures

Carotid Artery Rupture
Potential for decreased cardiac output
  Monitor vital signs and hemodynamic parameters
  Administer intravenous fluid and blood as prescribed
Potential for alteration in cerebral tissue perfusion
  Perform a neurologic assessment
  Institute safety measures

melanoma, lymphoma, myeloma, kidney, prostate, breast, and lung. Finally, 10 per cent of cord compressions occur in the cervical area. Tumors that produce the highest incidence of cervical cord compressions in

this area are lung, breast, melanoma, lymphoma, kidney, and myeloma (Held & Peahota, 1993).

The signs and symptoms of cord compression vary, depending on the location and degree of the infiltration. The hallmark symptom is pain, which is usually located over the site of the cord compression. The pain typically worsens when the patient moves, coughs, sneezes, or performs a Valsalva maneuver. As the cord compression progresses, the patient experiences motor weakness followed by sensory changes. Late signs and symptoms of spinal cord compression are associated with autonomic dysfunction and include bowel and bladder dysfunction.

The medical management depends on the patient's primary tumor, the level of the blockage, the rapidity of onset of symptoms, the degree and duration of the blockage, and the patient's general condition. In general, a laminectomy is performed in patients with rapidly progressing or acutely severe neurologic deficits. Following surgery, the patient receives radiation therapy. Radiation therapy, as a single agent, is used in patients with minimal or slowly progressing symptoms or in patients who have an incomplete block on myelogram. Emergency management before surgery or radiation therapy includes intravenous administration of corticosteroids. A 100 mg bolus of dexamethasone (repeated for 3 days) is given to patients with myelopathy or a complete block on myelogram. This initial dose is followed by 24 mg every 6 hours orally and is tapered through the course of radiation therapy. Patients with a partial block are treated with 5 mg of dexamethasone orally, every 6 hours (Held & Peahota, 1993).

The major potential and actual nursing diagnoses

for spinal cord compression as well as the associated nursing interventions are listed in Table 66–5.

CAROTID ARTERY RUPTURE

Rupture of the carotid artery occurs most frequently in patients with head and neck cancers. The etiologic factors include invasion of the arterial wall by tumor or erosion of the arterial vessels after surgery or radiation therapy.

In general, minor oozing is evident at the site of the invasive lesion before the true emergency situation. Attempts to control bleeding locally are rarely successful, because the site is usually at the base of infected necrotic tumor, and the bleeding is from branches of the external carotid artery. In the case of a carotid artery "blowout," treatment involves direct finger pressure over the bleeding site. The patient then receives adequate hydration and blood and blood products and is stabilized hemodynamically before surgery. The surgery involves ligation of the carotid artery above and below the site of rupture and excision of the necrotic segment (Howland & Carlon, 1985).

The major potential and actual nursing diagnoses for carotid artery rupture as well as the associated nursing interventions are listed in Table 66–5.

SUMMARY

The occurrence of an oncologic emergency in a patient with cancer can be an extremely frightening situation. The patient may associate the emergency situation with the recurrence of tumor and feel overwhelmed and unable to cope. In addition, the family may be equally alarmed at the patient's dramatic change in condition. Nursing interventions must focus on assisting the patient and family to cope with the emergency situation. Many times patients will be in an unfamiliar environment if they require attention in the intensive care unit. Oncology nurses must ease the transition for the oncology patient in the critical care environment.

The incidence of oncologic emergencies will increase as patients live longer with their disease. Oncology nurses must take an active role in assessing the patient for signs and symptoms that warn of a potential emergency situation and take steps to treat the condition before such a situation occurs to avoid serious and often deleterious consequences.

REFERENCES

Ameli, S., & Shah, P. K. (1991). Cardiac tamponade: Pathophysiology, diagnosis, and management. *Cardiology Clinics, 9*(4), 665–674.

Chernecky, C. C., & Ramsey, P. W. (1984). *Critical nursing care of the client with cancer.* Norwalk, CT: Appleton-Century-Crofts.

Colman, R. W., & Rubin, R. N. (1990). Disseminated intravascular coagulation due to malignancy. *Seminars in Oncology, 17*(2), 172–186.

Held, J. L., & Peahota, A. (1993). Nursing care of the patient with spinal cord compression. *Oncology Nursing Forum, 20*(10), 1507–1516.

Howland, W. S., & Carlon, G. C. (Eds.). (1985). *Critical care of the cancer patient.* Chicago: Year Book Medical Publishers.

Kahn, R. C. (1988). Shock as a complication of cancer. *Critical Care Clinics, 4*(1), 129–145.

Kaplan, M. (1994). Hypercalcemia of malignancy: A review of advances in pathophysiology. *Oncology Nursing Forum, 21*(6), 1039–1046.

Kishi, K., Sonomura, T., Mitsuzane, K., Nishida, N., Yang, R., Sato, M., Yamada, R., Shira, S., & Kobayashi, H. (1993). Self-expandable metallic stent therapy for superior vena cava syndrome: Clinical observations. *Radiology, 189*, 531–535.

Poe, C. M., & Taylor, L. M. (1989). Syndrome of inappropriate antidiuretic hormone: Assessment and nursing implications. *Oncology Nursing Forum, 16*(3), 373–381.

Twombly, M. (1978). The shift into the third space. *Nursing 78, 8*(6), 38–41.

Zaloznik, A. J. (1993). Superior vena cava syndrome. In G. R. Weiss. *Clinical oncology* (pp. 370–371). Norwalk, CT: Appleton & Lange.

The Phenomenon of Fatigue and the Cancer Patient

Linda A. Jacobs • Barbara F. Piper

Researchers have studied the problem of fatigue for decades, and many theories have been proposed to explain how this phenomenon occurs. Fatigue has been identified as a complex, universal experience that nearly everyone experiences on a daily basis (Piper, Lindsey, & Dodd, 1987). This commonly experienced symptom is usually attributed to physical exertion, psychologic stress, and inadequate sleep and rest (Nail & Winningham, 1993). Fatigue may also be a component of virtually any disease and can have a psychologic, physical, or mixed origin (Irvine et al., 1991).

DEFINITION OF FATIGUE

Aistars (1987) stated that it is difficult to define fatigue because it is a multifaceted problem and no general definition would apply in every situation. In addition, definitions of fatigue are derived from psychology, pathology, and physiology.

Fatigue has been described as a symptom or manifestation of many diseases. In 1988 Rhodes, Watson, and Hanson described symptoms of fatigue as subjective and apparent only to the affected individual. Symptoms or feeling states are phenomena experienced by a person and are not directly observable by another; instead, symptoms become known only through the report of the person being assessed. Irvine, Vincent, Graydon, Bubela, and Thompson (1994) defined fatigue as (1) a self-recognized phenomenon that is (2) subjective in nature and is (3) experienced as a feeling of weariness, tiredness, or lack of energy that varies in degree, frequency, and duration.

Fatigue has been accepted for clinical testing as a nursing diagnosis by the North American Nursing

Diagnosis Association (NANDA) (Table 67–1). This nursing diagnosis defines the sensation of fatigue, outlines its defining characteristics, and lists related factors. However, a major challenge that remains in defining fatigue entails differentiating among causes, indicators, and effects (Winningham et al., 1994). The definition of terms related to specific perceptual, sensory, and physiologic phenomena associated with fatigue also remains a challenge and hampers progress in research and clinical practice.

The number of fatigue studies by nurses, physicians, and members of other disciplines has increased dramatically since the 1970s when several classic studies were published addressing fatigue. In 1987 Piper et al. defined fatigue, from a nursing perspective, as a subjective feeling of tiredness that is influenced by circadian rhythm. They stated that "fatigue can vary in unpleasantness, duration, and intensity. When acute, it serves a protective function; when it becomes unusual, excessive or constant (chronic), it no longer serves this function and may lead to the aversion to activity with the desire to escape" (p. 19).

INCIDENCE AND PREVALENCE OF FATIGUE

Fatigue is one of the most prevalent and insidious symptoms reported by cancer patients (Dean et al., 1995). It is reported as a symptom experienced by cancer patients who are being treated with surgery, chemotherapy, radiation therapy, and biologic response modifiers. Fatigue is prevalent across the disease and treatment trajectory for cancer patients, yet little is

TABLE 67–1. *North American Nursing Diagnosis Association's Nursing Diagnosis for Fatigue*

Definition
An overwhelming sustained sense of exhaustion and decreased capacity for physical and mental work

Defining Characteristics
Major: verbalization of an unremitting and overwhelming lack of energy; inability to maintain usual routines
Minor: perceived need for additional energy to accomplish routine tasks; increase in physical complaints; emotionally labile or irritable; impaired ability to concentrate; decreased performance; lethargic or listless; disinterest in surroundings/introspection; decreased libido; accident prone

Related Factors
Decreased/increased metabolic energy production; overwhelming psychologic or emotional demands; increased energy requirements to perform activities of daily living; excessive social or role demands; states of discomfort; altered body chemistry (e.g., medications, drug withdrawal, chemistry)

(From NANDA. [1995]. Nursing diagnosis for fatigue. In M. E. Doenges & M. F. Moorhouse [Eds.], *Nurses' pocket guide* [4th ed., pp. 185–188]. Philadelphia: F. A. Davis Co.)

known about the pattern, intensity, duration, or predisposing factors involved in developing fatigue (Dean et al., 1995). Despite its prevalence, fatigue is poorly understood, and the relationships between fatigue and other physical, psychologic, and situational factors affecting an individual have not been conclusively determined. Research in the area of fatigue in cancer is only in its infancy (Smets, Garssen, Schuster-Vitterhoeve, & de Haes, 1993). Smets et al. (1993) proposed that further research is needed to address issues such as (1) prevalence rate of fatigue at different stages of the disease, including follow-up data after successful treatment; (2) the somatic, behavioral, and psychologic correlates of fatigue; and (3) the consequences of this particular symptom for the well-being of the patient.

CLASSIFICATIONS OF FATIGUE

There are many classification systems for fatigue found in the literature. Fatigue has been classified by many disciplines in an attempt to understand and better define this elusive problem. The symptom described as fatigue has been defined by the investigator's focus (subjective vs. neuromuscular), by its origin or cause, whether it be the central vs. the peripheral nervous system, pathologic vs. psychologic, or attentional fatigue. Chronic fatigue syndrome and all other diseases must be excluded when this phenomenon is defined, and the duration of the fatigue, acute vs. chronic, must be considered.

Muscle physiologists consider fatigue to be *central* when central nervous system mechanisms are involved and *peripheral* when peripheral nervous system mechanisms are involved (Gibson & Edwards, 1985). Central

fatigue may be caused by lack of motivation, impaired transmission down the spinal cord, and impaired recruitment of motor neurons (Gibson & Edwards, 1985) and by ". . . an exhaustion or malfunctioning of brain cells in the hypothalamic region" (Poteliakhoff, 1981, p. 94). Peripheral fatigue may be due to impaired functioning of the peripheral nerves, neuromuscular junction transmission, or fiber activation (Poteliakhoff, 1981). Figure 67–1 illustrates this classification system and the sites of impairment that may produce fatigue in healthy subjects. Little is known about how these normal physiologic mechanisms may be affected by abnormal processes such as disease states. Both central and peripheral mechanisms may be involved in chronic fatigue.

The classification system that is most useful to clinical nursing practice characterizes fatigue as acute or chronic depending on duration (Bartley & Chute, 1947; Piper, 1986, 1989). Differences between these two states have been identified in the literature, and they are summarized in Table 67–2.

The causes of acute fatigue can usually be identified and related to a specific activity or mechanism. Fatigue is perceived as a normal response to certain activities; it is rapid in onset, intermittent, of short duration, and serves as a protection from overwork or exhaustion. The symptoms produced by acute fatigue are usually localized in specific parts of the body and will usually

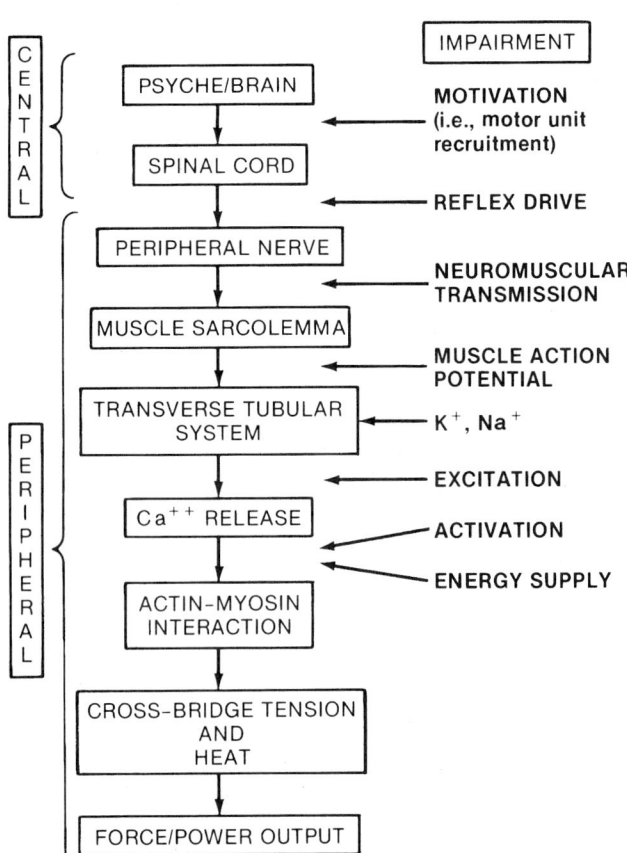

FIGURE 67–1. Central and peripheral model for fatigue.

TABLE 67–2. *Acute and Chronic Fatigue Model: Distinguishing Characteristics*

CHARACTERISTIC	ACUTE FATIGUE	CHRONIC FATIGUE
Purpose/function	Protective	Unknown, may no longer be protective May be nonfunctional
Population at risk	Primarily healthy individuals	Primarily clinical populations
Etiology	Usually identifiable	May not be identifiable
	Usually involves a single mechanism or cause	Usually multiple and additive causes
	Often experienced in relation to some form of activity or exertion	Often experienced with no relation to activity or exertion
Perception	Normal, usual	Abnormal, unusual
	Expected/anticipated with respect to specific activities or forms of exertion	Excessive or disproportionate to past experience
	Primarily localized to a specific body part or system	Generalized, whole body-mind sensation
	Pleasant or unpleasant	Unpleasant
Time dimension:		
Onset	Rapid	Insidious, gradual Cumulative Threshold model
Duration	Short; days or weeks	Long; persists over time More than 1 mo
Pattern	Intermittent/sporadic	Constant/recurrent
Relief dimension	Usually alleviated by a good night's sleep, adequate rest, proper diet, exercise program, or stress management techniques	Not completely dispelled by these methods A combination of approaches may be needed
	Resolves quickly	Does not resolve quickly
Impact on activities of daily living and quality of life.	Minor, minimal	Major

(From the American Cancer Society Monograph [1988]. *Nursing management of common problems: Fatigue in patients* [p. 26]. Reprinted with permission.)

resolve with rest (Skalla & Lacasse, 1992). In contrast, chronic fatigue has a more insidious onset and a cumulative effect, and the specific causal mechanisms are difficult to identify. Patients describe chronic fatigue as a totally overwhelming experience associated with generalized tiredness that is sometimes extreme, usually constant, and not easily resolved. The function of chronic fatigue is unknown, and a combination of approaches may be necessary to lessen the sensation (Piper, 1986; Riddle, 1982). Research is needed to determine whether these states can coexist within one individual, as may occur when cancer patients experience acute and chronic forms of pain.

Another classification system found in the literature categorizes fatigue as being normal, pathologic, situational, or psychologic in its origins (Kellum, 1985). Aistars (1987) states that fatigue includes subjective feelings such as weariness, weakness, exhaustion, and lack of energy; it results from exertion and stress; it leads to increased discomfort and decreased efficiency; and it causes deterioration of both mental and physical activities. Despite these classifications and descriptions of the phenomenon called fatigue, progress in research and clinical practice has been hindered by an inability to identify outcome measures and develop precise definitions of terms related to these specific perceptual, sensory, and physiologic phenomena associated with fatigue (Winningham et al., 1994).

NURSING RESEARCH AND FATIGUE

During the 1970s, nurses began to investigate fatigue when Hart compared fatigue patterns in multiple sclerosis (MS) patients and healthy control subjects (Hart, 1978). She later collaborated with Freel to identify indicators of fatigue in MS patients and with Haylock to identify fatigue indicators in radiation therapy patients (Freel & Hart, 1977; Haylock & Hart, 1979). In 1977 Putt published the first study examining the relationship between environmental stimulus, noise, and fatigue. During the 1980s, fatigue studies conducted by nurses and members of other disciplines increased dramatically. Fatigue became adopted as a nursing diagnosis by the NANDA, and consumers brought a new syndrome to the attention of physicians and health care professionals, chronic fatigue syndrome. During the 1990s, fatigue studies are fostering increased multidisciplinary collaboration that builds on previous work and seeks interventions for specific fatigue dimensions to better predict outcomes (Piper, in press).

In a review published in 1991, Irvine et al. stated that studies investigating fatigue in the cancer patient have been restricted primarily to those patients undergoing treatment with either chemotherapy or radiation therapy; that these studies have many design and measurement problems, i.e., cross-sectional designs with no control groups; and although several "correlates of fatigue have been postulated, research to date has failed to verify consistent relationships among fatigue, sleep deprivation, anemia, and/or psychological distress" (Irvine et al., 1991, p. 198). After the results of this study were published, Pickard-Holley (1991) used a control group to study the relationships between fatigue and various physical and psychologic factors in women undergoing treatment for cancer. Then Irvine et al. (1994), also using a control group, found a significant difference between the fatigue experienced by patients after treatment with radiation or chemotherapy and the fatigue reported by the control group of healthy persons.

Winningham (1991) conducted a study examining the effects of a walking program for people with cancer, and in 1992 St. Pierre, Kasper, and Lindsey examined the effects of tumor necrosis factor and exercise on skeletal muscle. The experience of fatigue over time in patients with cancer receiving treatment with interferon-α (Dean et al., 1995) or interleukin-2 (Piper,

Rieger et al., 1989) and the efficacy of using epoetin alpha with anemic, fatigued patients (Henry et al., 1994; Rieger & Haeuber, 1995) are currently being studied by nursing and medical researchers.

From these and other nursing studies, it is clear that nurses are interested in the acute and chronic effects of fatigue in healthy and ill populations and in identifying subjective and objective fatigue indicators. At the Oncology Nursing Society's State of the Knowledge Conference on Fatigue, participants made recommendations for future research regarding cancer-related fatigue (Table 67–3; Winningham et al., 1994).

PATHOPHYSIOLOGIC MECHANISMS OF FATIGUE

FATIGUE FRAMEWORKS

Aistars (1987) identified fatigue as a multifaceted problem and organized a theoretic framework based on energy and stress, implicating physiologic, psychologic,

---

TABLE 67–3. *Recommendations for Research Regarding Cancer-Related Fatigue*

The following areas for research regarding cancer-related fatigue are critical to the further development of theory, research, and clinical practice:

- An urgent need exists for a consistent, research-based definition of fatigue. This definition should include consideration of causes and mechanisms of fatigue that may distinguish true fatigue from expressions such as tiredness, lack of energy, and other terms.
- What is the trajectory of reported fatigue across disease, stage, and treatment? What fatigue patterns, distinct from circadian or diurnal variations, emerge in patients with cancer?
- How does chronic fatigue differ from acute fatigue?
- What are reliable and valid fatigue indicators? This research should include biophysiologic measures and self-administered questionnaires.
- Which instruments best measure fatigue and differentiate fatigue from psychologic states such as anxiety and depression?
- How does fatigue affect patient perception of other symptoms such as pain or nausea?
- What are the gender, cultural, generational, and ethnic influences on perception of fatigue?
- How does fatigue in patients with cancer differ from fatigue in other patient populations such as those with heart failure, neuromuscular diseases, or acquired immunodeficiency syndrome?
- How is perception of fatigue influenced by life events external to disease and treatment (e.g., family, financial, occupational problems)?
- What does the experience of fatigue mean to patients with cancer?
- What are reliable and valid predictors of fatigue?
- What are the adaptive functions of fatigue?
- How does education regarding fatigue as a part of disease course and treatment affect perception of fatigue?
- What are the cognitive effects of fatigue?
- What guidelines should be used for establishing the optimal activity-rest ratio for individual patients?
- What interventions are most effective in treating fatigue?
- What is the economic impact of fatigue on patients with cancer?
- What are the different mechanisms of fatigue?
- How do sleep disturbances alter perception of fatigue?
- How can fatigue and weakness be differentiated?
- How do fatigue perceptions of cancer populations differ from those of healthy individuals?
- How can the occurrence of, severity of, and response to fatigue be differentiated?
- Is fatigue a single phenomenon with different dimensions or is it multiple phenomena that are described similarly?
- Are there different types of fatigue? How are they described by individuals experiencing fatigue?
- What are the patterns of attentional fatigue exhibited by individuals receiving diverse treatments for various types of cancer?
- How does attentional fatigue affect individual, social, and occupational productivity?
- What are appropriate levels of attention-restoring activity in view of various treatment conditions and across phases of illness?
- How do limitations in physical capacity and impairment of protective mechanisms affect an individual's ability to respond to various fatigue-modifying interventions?
- How can fatigue be addressed in rehabilitation programs?

(From Winningham, M. L. et al. [1994]. Fatigue and the cancer experience: The state of the knowledge. *Oncology Nursing Forum, 21,* 32. Printed with permission from the Oncology Nursing Forum.)

and situational stressors as contributing to fatigue (Winningham et al., 1994). Aistars described fatigue as a condition characterized by subjective feelings directly or indirectly attributable to the disease process in a cancer patient. Within this framework, certain variables are identified that influence an individual's resistance and responses to stress, and the interaction of these variables ultimately determines the manifestations of the stress response (Aistars, 1987). Table 67–4 lists the physiologic, psychologic, and situational energy-depleting factors that Aistars identified as contributing to fatigue in cancer patients by the constant physical and mental stress that they produce.

Piper's Integrated Fatigue Model (IFM) is the most frequently cited theoretic framework on fatigue in cancer (Dean et al., 1995; Piper, 1991, 1993; Piper et al. 1987; Piper, Lindsey et al., 1989; Skalla & Lacasse, 1992; Winningham et al., 1994). This framework addresses many potential causes of fatigue, guides the assessment of possible etiologic factors related to fatigue, and points out the importance of considering the multiple aspects of manifestations of fatigue (Winningham et al., 1994). Factors that influence perceptions of fatigue in patients with cancer are also considered (Fig. 67–2).

Winningham's Psychobiologic-Entropy Hypothesis (PEH) builds on the central concept of energetics and

---

TABLE 67–4. *Factors Contributing to Fatigue in Cancer Patients*

Physiologic
- Accumulation of toxic waste products secondary to radiation, chemotherapy, or the tumor
- Hypermetabolic state associated with active tumor growth, infection, fever, or surgery
- Competition of the tumor with the body for nutrients
- Inadequate intake of nutrients secondary to anorexia, nausea, vomiting, or gastric obstruction
- Chronic pain
- Impairment of aerobic energy metabolism secondary to dyspnea and anemia due to various causes

Psychologic
- Anxiety
- Depression
- Anticipatory nausea and vomiting
- Grief

Situational
- Sensory deprivation due to disturbance of sleep pattern
- Immobility
- Crisis
- Problems with relationships
- Drugs—antibiotics, antidepressants, alcohol, nicotine, antianxiety agents, long-acting sleeping agents, analgesics, medications, caffeine
- Sleep deprivation
- Diagnostic tests
- Loss

(From Aistars, J. [1987]. Fatigue in the cancer patient: A conceptual approach to a clinical problem. *Oncology Nursing Forum,* *14*(6), 25–30. Printed with permission from the Oncology Nursing Forum.)

---

defines fatigue as an energy deficit, relating fatigue to concepts of disease, treatment, activity, rest, symptom perception, and functional status (Nail & Winningham, 1993). This hypothesis suggests that fatigue can be a primary symptom (a direct consequence of a pre-existing condition, disease, or treatment) or a secondary symptom (a result of the individual's physiologic or psychosocial response to other symptoms) (Fig. 67–3; Nail & Winningham, 1993).

The understanding and application of theoretic frameworks that address specific components of fatigue may enhance understanding of fatigue in patients with cancer and guide research efforts.

MANIFESTATIONS OF FATIGUE

Nurses in clinical practice continually solicit, assess, or monitor how the patient feels by gathering subjective and objective data (Rhodes et al., 1988). Sign and symptom patterns may vary according to the primary cause of the fatigue, which could include stimulation or overwork of a specific muscle group, type of occupational activity, or emotional depression (Piper, 1986; Saito, Kogi, & Kashiwagi, 1970). When fatigue becomes chronic, a combination of mechanisms may be involved; Piper (1989, p. 29) stated that "the subjective and objective indicators of fatigue may correlate with one another and further research is needed to clarify these relationships." Currently the best way to assess and measure fatigue in clinical populations is to determine the person's own perception of the fatigue experience (Piper, Reiger et al., 1989).

MECHANISMS OF CANCER AND NON–CANCER-RELATED FATIGUE

ACCUMULATION OF METABOLITES

No experimental research has identified the physiologic mechanisms that underlie the fatigue experienced by patients with cancer (St. Pierre et al., 1992). The accumulation of various metabolites has been associated with fatigue, but whether these products cause fatigue or merely parallel its occurrence remains unknown.

In cancer patients the accumulation of lactate (Burt, Aoki, Gorschboth, & Brennan, 1983; Gold, 1974; Morris, 1982), production of hydrogen ions (Karlsson, Sjodin, Jacobs, & Kaiser, 1981; Miller, Boska, Moussaui, Carson, & Weiner, 1988; Nakamura & Schwartz, 1972), and accumulation of cell destruction end products (Haylock & Hart, 1979) are likely mechanisms.

Continuous muscle work is known to produce an accumulation of lactic acid that can contribute to decreased muscle strength (Burt et al., 1983; Gold, 1974). The reason for this accelerated cycling is unknown (Gold, 1974).

Another possibility is that fatigue may be associated with changes that result from the hydrogen ions that are produced as lactate accumulates (Karlsson et al., 1981). Hydrogen ions are thought to impede muscle force by decreasing the number of calcium ions that are bound to troponin during excitation-coupling. This reduces the number of actin-myosin interactions and

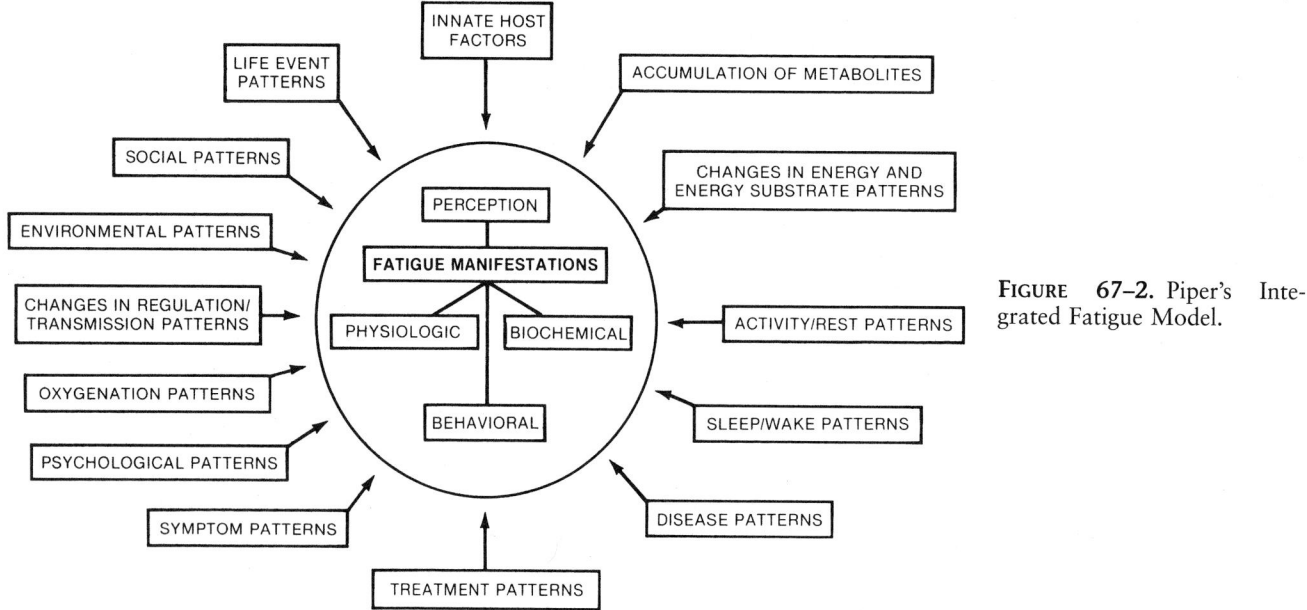

FIGURE 67–2. Piper's Integrated Fatigue Model.

results in decreased force (Nakamura & Schwartz, 1972). Skeletal muscle wasting is a part of cancer cachexia seen in advanced stages of cancer and is often accompanied by fatigue (St. Pierre et al., 1992). The specific agent that induces muscle wasting in cancer cachexia has not been definitively identified, but this

muscle wasting is believed to be mediated by tumor necrosis factor (TNF) (Beutler & Cerami 1986; Moldawer, Sherry, & Lowry, 1989). TNF is a protein that is secreted by activated macrophages, some T lymphocytes, and a few tumor cell lines (St. Pierre et al., 1992). One animal model study showed that TNF

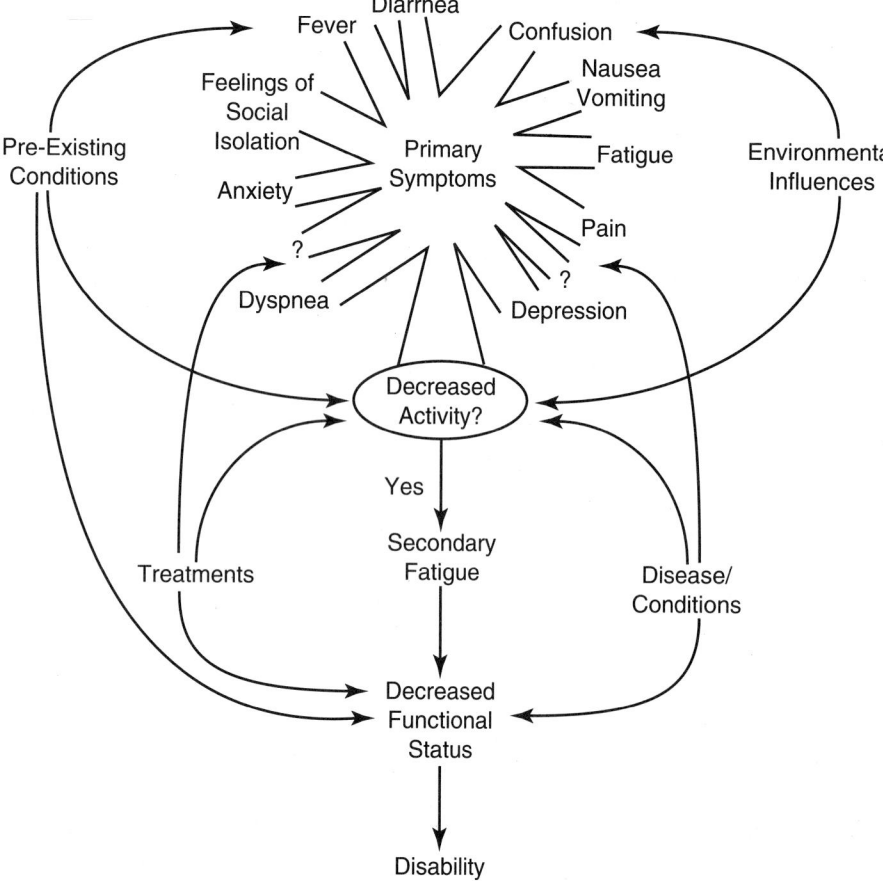

FIGURE 67–3. The Winningham Psychobiological-Entropy Model. (Copyright 1992, 1993 by Maryl L. Winningham. All rights reserved. Used with express written consent of the author.)

secreted from tumor cells can mediate skeletal muscle wasting associated with cachexia. However, the wasting could be partially the result of the local production of TNF in the muscle (Beutler & Cerami, 1986).

Fatigue may also be caused by the accumulation in the blood of cell destruction end products and toxic metabolites that inhibit normal cell functioning during lysis (Haylock & Hart, 1979). Increasing fluid intake may promote more rapid dilution and excretion of these substances and thus prevent fatigue.

ENERGY, ACTIVITY, AND REST-RELATED MECHANISMS

In 1956 Selye proposed a model for understanding the phenomenon of fatigue. According to this model, every individual is born with a finite amount of energy available for adaptation, and fatigue occurs when that energy supply is depleted. During periods of exertion, superficial energy is exhausted, and rest periods allow for that energy to be replenished from the individual's deep reserves so that adaptation can continue (Selye, 1974). Based on this hypothesis, if cancer patients rested for prolonged periods of time, they would be able to rate rest as completely effective in relieving fatigue. However, cancer patients who are receiving chemotherapy rate rest as only moderately effective in relieving fatigue (Nail, Jones, Greene, Schipper, & Jensen, 1991).

Persons with cancer describe a variety of problems that manifest themselves as changes in an individual's energy level, ability to perform and participate in certain activities, and the rest patterns necessary to maintain their functional status. "Tiredness, lack of energy, generalized lassitude, inability to sustain exertion, loss of motor power, impaired mobility, sleepiness, drowsiness, confusion, apathy, poor concentration, helplessness, a sense of inadequacy, and an inability to mobilize energy" are some of the common problems described by cancer patients (Pickard-Holley, 1991, p. 13).

Changes in energy production can profoundly influence human performance and the development of fatigue. Changes in energy patterns are common in cancer patients and may result from abnormalities in energy expenditure, cancer cachexia, anorexia, infection (Straus et al., 1985; Valdini, 1985), fever (Edwards et al., 1972), and imbalances in thyroid hormones (Axelrod et al., 1983).

Fatigue is anecdotally associated with activities that increase energy expenditure, but no studies to date have investigated this relationship in the cancer population (Piper et al., 1987). St. Pierre et al. (1992) proposed that cancer fatigue may develop or become exacerbated during exercise as a consequence of changes in the concentration of skeletal muscle metabolites as a result of endogenous TNF or from TNF administered as antineoplastic therapy. There are many variables including tumor type, tumor status, and the general condition of the patient that will determine the effects of TNF on skeletal muscle function. The involvement of muscle in the occurrence of fatigue will play a role in determining if cancer patients can participate successfully in an exercise program or can complete self-care activities (St. Pierre et al., 1992).

The development of fatigue in cachectic patients may involve changes in skeletal muscle stores that result in a tremendous increase in the effort necessary for these individuals to perform even self-care activities (St. Pierre et al., 1992). Consequently, these patients may not be able to perform any type of strenuous physical activity, and they must be taught to avoid activities that cause or exacerbate fatigue. Multiple mechanisms are probably involved in producing fatigue in cachectic cancer patients, since to date no single mechanism has been identified that alone causes cachexia. Anorexia is a common occurrence in cancer patients, and its influence on fatigue symptoms should also be investigated.

Fatigue is also associated with fever and infection. Increased energy expenditure, accumulation of toxic metabolites, and impaired neurotransmission are likely mechanisms by which fever and infection produce fatigue (Piper et al., 1987).

Activity and rest patterns can play significant roles in the prevention, cause, and alleviation of fatigue. Activity is defined broadly here and applies to work, exercise, mobility, and leisure activities. Cancer patients often report the inability to perform their usual activities of daily living, complete household chores, meet work-related demands, and continue to participate in social activities with friends and family. Whether fatigue is the underlying cause of these changes is not known, and how systematic changes in activity and rest patterns may positively affect fatigue also warrants investigation (Piper et al., 1987).

MECHANISMS ASSOCIATED WITH THE CANCER PROCESS

The actual mechanism that produces fatigue is unknown. A relationship between fatigue and the consequence of the disease has been suggested. Treatment-related factors are also important considerations when evaluating fatigue in cancer patients (Smets et al., 1993). Fatigue in the cancer patient has been studied primarily in relation to patients undergoing treatment with either chemotherapy or radiation therapy. Little is known about the correlates of fatigue or the occurrence of fatigue in cancer patients before or after treatment (Irvine et al., 1991).

Fatigue usually precedes, accompanies, or follows many adult and pediatric malignancies (Waskerwitz & Leonard, 1986). How fatigue patterns vary prospectively by disease type, site, and extent is unknown. A descriptive study on fatigue in cancer patients found no significant difference when examining fatigue and age, stage of disease and fatigue, or fatigue and the amount of treatment a patient received. This study also examined the trajectory of fatigue experienced during the 4-week period between treatments and found that fatigue levels peaked at day 7 and declined gradually back toward the baseline before the beginning of the next course of treatment. The most significant findings in this study concerned the relationship between CA 125 levels and fatigue. As the CA 125 level declined, the amount of fatigue also appeared to decline (Pickard-

Holley, 1991). In one retrospective study, patients with Hodgkin's disease indicated that energy levels took 1 to 5 years following treatment to return to normal (Fobair et al., 1986). Smets et al. (1993) proposed several somatic mechanisms for fatigue in patients with active disease or during treatment. Malnutrition resulting from anorexia, changes in metabolism, obstructions, vomiting, diarrhea, swallowing difficulties, anemia, and the accumulation of cell destruction end products and toxic metabolites that inhibit normal cell functioning have been mentioned as possible factors in fatigue (Smets et al., 1993). During the day, cancer patients may experience tiredness induced by drugs with sedative effects, including antiemetics, analgesics, or sleeping agents. Fatigue can also be a result of insomnia or pain, which can prevent the patient from getting a good night's sleep (Smets et al., 1993). Except for drug use and insomnia, none of the somatic factors proposed by Smets seem relevant for the explanation of chronic fatigue that persists after cancer treatment has ended and symptoms of disease are no longer present.

In recent years, increasing attention has been given to the role that anemia plays in fatigue for the cancer patient. This mechanism will be discussed as a related side effect of treatment.

PSYCHOSOCIAL MECHANISMS AND FATIGUE

The effects of physiologic, psychologic, and situational stressors on an individual is dependent on the perception of their presence, stress resistance, available coping mechanisms, and duration of the stress response. The patient's socioeconomic status, support network, available coping mechanisms, depression, anxiety, degree of motivation, beliefs and attitudes, and access to community resources may influence fatigue in cancer patients (Bukberg, Penman, & Holland, 1984; Petty & Noyes, 1981; Proctor, Kernahan, & Taylor, 1981; Wittenborn & Buhler, 1979). The impact of fatigue on day-to-day activities, the individual's sense of well-being, valued relationships, the meaning of fatigue to the individual, and individual cultural influences on expression of feelings of fatigue must also be considered (Winningham et al., 1994). As stated earlier, Aistars (1987) proposed that fatigue is a condition characterized by subjective feelings of generalized weakness, exhaustion, and lack of energy resulting from prolonged stress that is directly or indirectly attributable to the disease process. The outcome of this condition is an impaired functional status that ultimately has an impact on quality of life. The hypothesis that prolonged stress causes fatigue can easily be applied to people with cancer, since they frequently suffer from extreme, ongoing stress related to diagnosis and treatment (Aistars, 1987).

Many authors mention the possible influence of psychologic factors when discussing the cause of fatigue. Depression is considered to be a contributor to fatigue in cancer. However, fatigue could be a cause or a result of persistent feelings of tiredness (Smets et al., 1993). Adverse psychologic consequences can result from loss of function and loss of energy resulting directly from illness or its treatment. Fatigue is fre-

quently a presenting symptom of depression (Piper, in press). The relationship between depression or anxiety and fatigue experienced by cancer patients has not been systematically studied per se; however, most study results suggest a relation between negative affect and fatigue, and patients themselves notice a relation between psychologic patterns and their fatigue response (Smets et al., 1993). For example, tiredness, fatigue, and sleep disturbances are common symptoms of depression (Wittenborn & Buhler, 1979). Depending on the study, moderate to severe depression may range from 17 to 42 per cent in hospitalized cancer patients (Bukberg et al., 1984; Petty & Noyes, 1981). Finally, depression, lethargy, and somnolence may be related also to cranial radiation therapy, suggesting a centrally mediated mechanism for both fatigue and depression (Proctor et al., 1981).

Attitudes can influence behaviors. Chronic, unrelenting fatigue can lead to a loss of hope and a desire to escape. Chronic fatigue can prevent the person from engaging in the kinds of valued activities that give meaning to life. As a consequence, the person may lose the desire to go on living (Piper, 1986; Piper et al., 1987).

EFFECTS OF CANCER TREATMENT

Various medical treatments and forms of *diagnostic testing* can be associated with the occurrence of fatigue (Piper et al., 1987). Diagnostic testing can be quite distressing to many patients. These patients are at high risk for experiencing fatigue due to anxiety, test preparation, and duration of the testing procedures.

Fatigue is a consistent finding in patients who are recovering from *surgery* (Nail & Winningham, 1993). A number of mechanisms associated with the surgical process place the surgical patient at risk for fatigue, and it is likely that several mechanisms interact or act synergistically to produce fatigue in surgical patients. These mechanisms include tissue damage caused by the surgical procedure(s) and the effects of anesthesia, analgesia, sedation, or immobility, decreased respiratory capacity, infection, starvation, altered sleep patterns, stress, and the underlying or concurrent disease process (Piper et al., 1987). Postoperative fatigue can take up to 6 months to resolve completely. This problem is not well understood and may compound the fatigue experienced in relation to other modes of treatments for the cancer patient (Winningham et al., 1994).

In a survey of patients who received radiation therapy alone, chemotherapy alone, or radiation treatment plus chemotherapy for treatment of Hodgkin's disease, 90 per cent reported an adverse effect of treatment on energy level, and 37 per cent felt that their energy level had not returned to normal after treatment ended. The risk factors for persistent low energy included being older, presenting with more advanced disease, and receiving combined modality treatment (Fobair et al., 1986).

Irvine et al. (1991) reviewed 16 nursing studies conducted between 1978 and 1991 that examined fatigue in patients receiving *chemotherapy*. The prevalence of fatigue in cancer patients receiving chemotherapy was estimated to be 96 per cent in these studies and was supported through nonstatistical descriptive accounts and clinical observations. Despite variation among treatment regimens, disease processes, and individual variables, fatigue has been cited as one of the most frequent and distressing side effects of antineoplastic chemotherapy (Nail & Winningham, 1993; Piper et al., 1987; Winningham et al., 1994). In a 1994 study, Irvine et al. examined the prevalence and correlates of fatigue in patients receiving treatment with chemotherapy and radiation. In both treatment groups a significant increase in fatigue was observed over time compared to a nonsignificant increase in fatigue levels among the control group subjects. The strongest correlates of fatigue found in this study were distress from other symptoms and mood disturbance. Despite research findings and patient reports of feeling tired, weak, and drowsy, fatigue associated with chemotherapy is poorly understood.

There are a number of pathologic, environmental, psychologic, and nutritional factors associated with fatigue from chemotherapy (Winningham et al., 1994). Anemia, cell destruction end products, stress, mood variation, sleep pattern disturbances, chronic pain, nausea and vomiting, and cachexia have been cited by researchers as some of these factors (Haylock & Hart 1979; Nail & Winningham, 1993; Piper, 1987, 1993; Rhodes et al., 1988). Fatigue patterns often reflect chemotherapy treatment patterns. These patterns vary by disease type, site, duration, and magnitude, as well as by the specific chemotherapeutic regimen (Winningham et al., 1994). Symptom distress, emotional upset, psychosocial variables, and disruption in self-care abilities may be associated with the more long-term side effects of fatigue than from the more acute side effects such as nausea and vomiting (Rhodes et al., 1988). Boxes 67–1 and 67–2 summarize findings from two nursing studies that have investigated fatigue in patients receiving chemotherapy (Pickard-Holley, 1991; Rhodes et al., 1988). Box 67–3 summarizes findings from one nursing study that investigated fatigue in patients receiving treatment with chemotherapy and radiation (Irvine et al., 1994).

Haylock and Hart (1979), in their classic study of patients undergoing *radiation therapy,* reported that mean fatigue scores increased from baseline throughout a course of radiation treatment, declined on weekends when patients were not undergoing treatment, and increased in patients who underwent the lengthiest treatment regimens. Regardless of the specific cancer diagnosis, fatigue was the only symptom experienced by the majority of patients receiving radiation treatments, with skin problems being the other most frequently reported side effect (King, Nail, Kreamer, Strohl, & Johnson, 1985; Larson, Lindsey, Dodd, Brecht, & Packer, 1993).

Irvine et al. (1991) reviewed a number of studies that investigated fatigue among cancer patients receiving radiation therapy. Fatigue was found to be an important clinical problem in these studies, and the prospective studies identified that the prevalence of fatigue among the patients studied increased over the course of radiation treatment but gradually diminished when treatment ended. These studies also suggested that fatigue has physical, behavioral, and mental manifestations in patients receiving radiation therapy. The etiologic factors and correlates of fatigue in patients receiving radiation therapy have not been clearly identified, but some evidence suggests that fatigue is related to weight loss, negative mood, pain, and length of radiation treatment (Irvine et al., 1991). Fatigue also appears to be treatment related as reflected by the variation in prevalence rates between groups with different radiation fields and by the reduction in fatigue scores during periods without treatment (Smets et al., 1993).

More is known about the prevalence, duration, and pattern of fatigue in patients receiving radiation therapy than in patients receiving other treatments, and there is good evidence that patients become more fatigued over the course of radiation therapy. The actual mechanism or mechanisms of radiation-induced fatigue are unknown, and further research is needed to investigate the possible correlates of fatigue in this population (Irvine et al., 1991; Piper et al., 1987).

Fatigue is common, more severe, often dose limiting, and the most difficult adverse effect to manage in patients treated with *biologic response modifiers* (Dean et al., 1995; Nail, 1992; Piper, Rieger et al., 1989). Patients beginning biologic therapy will experience fever, chills, myalgias, headache, and malaise often

---

Box 67–1. *Fatigue in Chemotherapy Patients*

Rhodes, V. A., Watson, P. M., & Hanson, B. M. (1988). Patients' descriptions of the influence of tiredness and weakness on self-care abilities. *Cancer Nursing, 11,* 186–194.

Sample: Twenty cancer outpatients; status post an average of six cycles of chemotherapy at first interview; 11 patients completed second interview.

Measures: Telephone interviews conducted by research assistant.

Findings: Tiredness and weakness were the symptoms that most interfered with self-care abilities. Activities that were effective in treating these symptoms were planning and scheduling activities (spreading out activities over 1 week vs. doing them in 1 day, getting extra sleep, scheduling naps or rest periods, keeping busy); decreasing nonessential activities (housework, gardening, cooking, social activities); increasing dependence on others (obtaining assistance with cooking, cleaning, shopping, work).

Limitations: Retrospective; unclear how sample was selected from larger study sample; small sample size; no tiredness or weakness definitions provided or sample demographics (e.g., stage and type of disease or type of therapy).

Box 67–2. *Fatigue in Cancer Patients*

Pickard-Holley, S. (1991). Fatigue in cancer patients: a descriptive study. *Cancer Nursing 14*, 13–19.

Sample: Twelve ovarian cancer patients receiving chemotherapy and 12 healthy female control subjects.
Measures: Rhoten Fatigue Scale, Beck Depression Inventory, CA 125, weight change, Gynecology Oncology Group Performance Scale, Karnofsky Performance Status Scale.
Findings: Weak to moderate relationships found between level of fatigue and CA 125 levels; as CA 125 levels decrease, fatigue also appears to decrease. Fatigue trajectory found to peak at day 7 and slowly decline during the remainder of the 28-day treatment course. No significant relationship between fatigue and age, stage of disease, course of treatment, or depression.
Limitations: Rhoten Fatigue Scale did not differentiate between subjects and controls.

---

accompanied by anorexia, nausea, vomiting, diarrhea, and weight loss with some variation depending on the dose, route of administration, schedule of treatment, and individual factors such as age and performance (Dean et al., 1995).

Biotherapy exposes patients with cancer to exogenous and endogenous cytokines (Winningham et al., 1994). Cytokines have been implicated in causing fatigue in cancer patients receiving radiation and biotherapies, in patients exhibiting signs and symptoms of cognition disorders, and in patients with anemia (Piper, in press). Anorexia, weight loss, and fatigue in cancer patients are likely caused by a combination of mechanisms, particularly central neurophysiologic mechanisms (Piper, Rieger et al., 1989).

Exogenous administration of *interferon alpha* (IFN-α) has been postulated to produce fatigue, anorexia, and cognition disorders through direct toxic effects on the frontal lobe, brain structure neurons, or neurotransmitters. Peripheral neuropathies are also reported with high-dose interferon therapies (Piper, in press). When interferon is used in combination with other modalities, the exacerbation of fatigue becomes apparent, and older patients may be at higher risk (Piper, Rieger et al., 1989).

Fatigue is also a frequent side effect of treatment using *interleukin-2* (IL-2) therapy. It is dose and schedule dependent; higher doses and prolonged therapy usually intensify the fatigue. Patients treated with IL-2 may experience more severe fatigue than those receiving other biologicals and may have more adverse side effects from treatment, which may exacerbate the fatigue (Piper, Rieger et al., 1989; Winningham et al., 1994). Patients treated with IL-2 experience profound fatigue that may confine them to bed and produce a decline in cognition and orientation. Recovery for these patients may take up to 2 months after treatment (Winningham et al., 1994).

The mechanisms that cause fatigue related to IL-2 therapy remain unknown, and both peripheral and central mechanisms may be involved (Skalla & Rieger, 1995). The release of cytokines such as endogenous interferon gamma and TNF in response to IL-2 administration has been implicated in causing alterations in neuroendocrine secretion, brain electrical activity, and blood-brain barrier permeability (Piper, in press; Piper, Rieger et al., 1989; Skalla & Rieger, 1995).

The fatigue and other side effects related to treatment with *TNF* are similar to those noted with other biologicals (Piper, Rieger et al., 1989). St. Pierre et al.

Box 67–3. *Prevalence and Correlates of Fatigue in Patients Receiving Treatment with Chemotherapy and Radiotherapy*

Irvine, D., Vincent, L., Bubela, N., & Thompson, L. (1994). The prevalence and correlates of fatigue in patients receiving treatment with chemotherapy and radiotherapy. A comparison with the fatigue experienced by healthy individuals. *Cancer Nursing, 17*, 367–378.

Sample: Fifty-four radiation therapy patients (first and last weeks of treatment), 47 chemotherapy patients (before treatment and 10 to 14 days after treatment), and a control group made up of 53 healthy auxiliary staff members. The patients were being treated for breast, lung, cervical, or endometrial cancer. The control group was 100% women, and the patient group was 97% women.
Measures: Pearson-Byars Fatigue Feeling Checklist, Linear Analogue Self-Assessment Scale (LASA), a Modified Version of the Associated Symptom Subscale of the Piper Fatigue Scale, and the Sickness Impact Profile (SIP).
Findings: Cancer patients experienced a significant increase in fatigue over a 5- or 6-week course of radiotherapy and 14 days after treatment with chemotherapy, and these increases were significantly greater than the fatigue reported by healthy control subjects. Fatigue in cancer patients was found to vary with weight, symptom distress, mood disturbance, and alterations in usual functional activities.
Limitations: Patients undergoing combined modality treatment not included in this group; few men; results cannot be generalized.

(1992) stated that one physiologic mechanism in cancer-related fatigue may involve changes in skeletal muscle stores or metabolite concentration. Both TNF and IL-1 have been implicated in causing the progressive muscle wasting associated with cancer cachexia; however, the wasting could be the result of the local production of TNF in the muscle, TNF secreted from tumor cells, or the administration of TNF therapy. Fatigue in these patients may result from biochemical and morphologic changes in skeletal muscle in conjunction with other variables, including tumor type, tumor status, and general condition of the patient (Piper, in press; Piper, Rieger, et al., 1989; Skalla & Rieger, 1995; St. Pierre et al., 1992). In summary, these particular cytokines may cause fatigue secondary to their effects on the body's metabolic functions. And as a better understanding about these and other underlying fatigue mechanisms evolves, improved conceptualization, measurement, and interventions for fatigue will result (Piper, in press).

Fatigue is reported more often as a side effect of granulocyte-macrophage *colony-stimulating factor* (GM-CSF) than with other hematopoietic growth factors (Skalla & Rieger, 1995). However, it is difficult to examine the relationship between CSFs and fatigue because these agents are used most commonly to ameliorate the side effects of other forms of cancer treatment or the disease process (Winningham et al., 1994). Clinical observations of fatigue patterns in patients given CSFs are not as consistent as those reported with other biologicals, and in general, fatigue is uncommon with the administration of GM-CSF or erythropoietin. CSFs could be hypothesized to reverse fatigue when treatment is directed at reversing anemia (Piper, Rieger et al., 1989; Skalla & Rieger, 1995; Winningham et al., 1994).

RELATED SIDE EFFECTS OF TREATMENT REGIMENS AND FATIGUE

Over the course of their disease trajectory, many cancer patients undergo diagnostic testing, surgical procedures, chemotherapy, radiation therapy, or use of biologic response modifiers at different points in time. Patients receiving combined modality treatment present with a multitude of distressing symptoms mediated by a host of physiologic and psychologic factors. Many of these symptoms have been discussed throughout this chapter.

Anemia is mentioned in the literature as a possible factor in fatigue; however, it is difficult to demonstrate a significant correlation between hemoglobin, hematocrit, or serum erythropoietin levels and fatigue. Anemia may be defined functionally as a lack of sufficient red blood cells to maintain adequate tissue oxygenation (Spivak, 1994). The resulting tissue hypoxia causes symptoms of anemia, which include fatigue, weakness, lassitude, and cold intolerance (Rieger & Haeuber, 1995). Anemia develops when the demand for new red blood cells exceeds the capacity of the bone marrow to produce them. Many cancer patients develop anemia at some point during the course of their disease or treatment, and there are many other contributing factors to fatigue in these patients. For example, multiple mecha-

nisms cause anemia in patients with solid tumors. The cause of the anemia must be identified to ensure that corrective therapy is appropriate. Intrinsic or iatrogenic blood loss; nutritional deficiencies involving primarily iron or folic acid; hemolysis; bone marrow failure due to tumor encroachment, myelofibrosis, or marrow necrosis; infection and inflammation; or merely the presence of cancer elsewhere in the body are some of these mechanisms (Spivak, 1994).

Anemia associated with cancer can be characterized by a low reticulocyte count; normochromic, normocytic red blood cells without evidence of blood loss; and a normal marrow aspirate and biopsy specimens. However, anemia is most often due to an inadequate bone marrow response that can be exacerbated by myelosuppressive chemotherapy (Henry & Abels, 1994; Spivak, 1994). This type of anemia is a complication of the underlying tumor, presumably a consequence of the biochemical response initiated by the body in reaction to it. This type of anemia has been designated as the anemia of chronic illness, and it is seen in a variety of infections and inflammatory or malignant disorders (Spivak, 1994). Anemia of chronic illness is characterized by slightly shortened red blood cell survival, poor reuse of iron, and an inadequate erythropoietin response to the degree of anemia. Anecdotally, anemic cancer patients report a decrease in their functional status and feeling "tired and run-down."

Red blood cell transfusions are commonly used for symptomatic palliation, and patients generally report feeling better and having more energy (less fatigue) after receiving a transfusion. However, blood transfusions can present numerous problems for the cancer patient. Based on the success of epoetin alfa (recombinant human erythropoietin or rHuEPO) treating anemia in patients with chronic renal failure and in patients infected with human immunodeficiency virus (HIV) who receive zidovudine, the efficacy of rHuEPO for anemia in cancer patients receiving chemotherapy has been studied in the last few years (Rieger & Haeuber, 1995). A number of these studies demonstrate an increase in hematocrit values from baseline and a decrease in transfusion requirements for patients in the rHuEPO group, which led to the 1993 U.S. Food and Drug Administration approval of epoetin alfa for treatment of anemia associated with cancer chemotherapy. These studies also demonstrated that energy level, ability to engage in daily activities, and overall quality of life improved significantly for these patients. In their study of patients being treated with recombinant human erythropoietin for cancer and chemotherapy-induced anemia, Henry and Abels (1994) measured quality of life parameters to indicate energy level, ability to do daily activities, and overall quality of life. All three parameters improved significantly for patients as their hematocrit increased with the use of recombinant human erythropoietin.

Although a correlation between fatigue and degree of anemia is rarely found, the impact of anemia on quality of life issues indicates the need for further studies that examine anemia as a correlate of fatigue.

ASSESSMENT AND MEASUREMENT OF FATIGUE

ASSESSMENT OF FATIGUE

To design an effective plan of care, the nurse should perform a thorough assessment of all subjective and objective data that may influence fatigue for the patient. Frequently, family members may be more sensitive than the patient to changes in the patient's usual pattern of fatigue and its impact.

Subjective data should include an assessment of usual patterns of functioning and possible changes that have occurred as a result of illness or treatment. When assessing the patient's perception, it is important for the nurse to remember the differences that may exist between acute and chronic fatigue states and the multidimensionality of the fatigue experience. Engel and Morgan (1973) suggest that the following dimensions of a symptom must be assessed: symptom location, pattern, intensity, onset, and duration; aggravating and alleviating factors; and associated symptoms. Additional information should be collected about the person's perception of the meaning of fatigue; how distressing it is (Rhodes & Watson, 1987); and the physical, emotional, and mental symptoms experienced (Piper, Lindsey et al., 1989). Having the patient maintain a daily fatigue diary for 1 week often reveals previously unrecognized patterns of fatigue (Piper, 1986).

Physical examination, laboratory data, and the patient's past and present medical history may reveal coexisting diseases, such as hypertension or diabetes, that may be contributing to the fatigue (Kellum, 1985). Because many medications such as antiemetics, analgesics, and antihypertensives are known to produce sedation or fatigue as a side effect, it is important for the nurse to assess the patient's current medication history (Kellum, 1985). This should include information about prescription and nonprescription drugs; vitamin, caffeine, and alcohol intake (which disrupts rapid eye movement sleep); and other social or "recreational" drug use.

Behaviorally, the nurse needs to assess for any changes in the patient's physical appearance; performance status; and ways of moving, talking, or interacting that may indicate the presence of fatigue (Rhoten, 1982). Environmental factors such as heat or noise (Putt, 1977) must be assessed. Frequently, assistive devices or furniture rearrangement may prevent needless expenditure of energy.

MEASUREMENT OF FATIGUE

Several investigators stress the importance of measuring fatigue's *subjective dimension*, and one investigator has proposed that fatigue be defined based on an adaptation of Margo McCaffrey's definition of pain: "fatigue is whatever the patient says it is, whenever (the person) says it is" (Glaus, 1993, p. 306). The multidimensional nature of fatigue has made it difficult to measure or study. Thus, the dimensions of fatigue are not as well researched or conceptualized as are the dimensions for pain (Piper, in press).

Yoshitake (1969, 1971, & 1978) and other Japanese investigators were the first to develop a scale to measure symptoms of fatigue multidimensionally. These researchers conducted numerous studies on fatigue in Japanese workers that validated the symptom checklist. This instrument contains 30 fatigue symptoms arranged in a checklist format so that the presence or absence of the symptom can be indicated. Findings from these studies suggest that there are three dimensions or subscales to the instrument: general feelings of incongruity, mental fatigue, and specific feelings of incongruity. These dimensions and their representative items are shown in Table 67–5.

Although this instrument has been used in clinical studies, it is not clear how the items on this instrument were developed originally or whether this instrument is appropriate to use with different cultures or with different clinical populations (Varrichio, 1985). The items must be refactored to see if similar factors are found in the cancer population.

Subjective fatigue has been measured as a component of several instruments designed to measure other phenomena. Winningham et al. (1994) provided a review of several instruments documented in the literature.

TABLE 67–5. *Fatigue Symptom Checklist*

General Feelings of Incongruity
 1. Feel heavy in the head
 2. Feel tired in the whole body
 3. Feel tired in the legs
 4. Give a yawn
 5. Feel the brain hot or muddled
 6. Become drowsy
 7. Feel strained in the eyes
 8. Become rigid or clumsy in motion
 9. Feel unsteady while standing
10. Want to lie down

Mental Fatigue
11. Find difficulty in thinking
12. Become weary while talking
13. Become nervous
14. Unable to concentrate
15. Unable to have an interest in thinking
16. Become apt to forget things
17. Lack self-confidence
18. Anxious about things
19. Unable to straighten up in posture
20. Lack patience

Specific Feelings of Incongruity
21. Have a headache
22. Feel stiff in the shoulders
23. Feel a pain in the waist
24. Feel constrained in breathing
25. Feel thirsty
26. Have a husky voice
27. Have dizziness
28. Have a spasm of the eyelids
29. Have a tremor in the limbs
30. Feel ill

(From Yoshitake, H. [1971]. Relations between the symptoms and the feeling of fatigue. *Ergonomics, 14,*177. Reproduced by permission.)

Rhoten (1982), a nurse investigator, developed an observational checklist to measure fatigue. In this tool, patients' subjective responses are related to objective observational checklists (Table 67–6). However, the use of the observational checklist is not consistent with the definition of fatigue as a subjective phenomena. The results of data collected with the use of this tool could reflect an overlap between the reporting of fatigue sensations and responses to fatigue (Winningham et al., 1994).

Another tool used to measure fatigue is the Pearson-Byars Fatigue Feeling Tone Checklist, which is comprised of a 10-item adjective/phrase checklist (Pearson, 1957; Pearson & Byars, 1956). This tool was developed in the 1950s and has been used extensively in recent studies.

The most frequently used instrument to measure fatigue in the oncology population is the monopolar version of the Profile of Mood States (POMS). This instrument was developed for use as a mood scale, and the 65-word checklist measures the intensity of certain feelings (Burns, in review).

Piper et al. (1987) were the first to propose a multidimensional measurement model for fatigue's manifestations. In this model, subjective perception was believed to be key to understanding how fatigue might vary between healthy and ill individuals. This model was strongly influenced by what was known about pain's manifestations at the time (Melzack, 1983) and by the clinically useful "signs and symptoms" model used by medicine. The indicators of fatigue were grouped into two major dimensions, subjective and objective manifestations, each with its own subdimensions. The subjective dimension included perceptions about (1) the timing of fatigue (temporal perception); (2) the mental, physical, and emotional symptoms of fatigue (sensory dimension); (3) the emotional meaning attributed to the fatigue (affective dimension); and (4) the impact and distress fatigue had on activities of daily living (Piper, in press). This instrument is called the Piper Fatigue Scale (PFS).

Single items embedded in side effect checklists have also been used by a number of researchers to measure the severity of fatigue. The advantage of this approach is that it produces low subject burden. The selection of a research instrument for measuring fatigue has implications for both the validity of the research and the burden it places on its subjects. The ideal instrument is "reliable, valid, and short enough to be acceptable to subjects" (Winningham et al., 1994, p. 30). The timing of the measurement is also an important consideration (Winningham et al., 1994).

The *objective dimension* of fatigue includes signs of fatigue that can be validated by physiologic, biochemical, and behavioral means. As more attention has been given to the development of valid and reliable self-report scales that could be used in conjunction with physiologic or "objective" methods to measure fatigue, the need to dichotomize fatigue into subjective and objective dimensions may have lost its perceived utility. Methods designed to measure both the subjective and objective indicators (signs and symptoms) of fatigue have become more numerous, valid, and reliable. These methods must be used in combination with one another to measure fatigue's signs and symptoms in diverse populations, to specify fatigue's dimensions and their underlying mechanisms, and to target fatigue interventions to specific dimensions of fatigue that span the disease and treatment continuum. Age, educational level, language, culture, and visual, hearing, and motor coordination are factors that can influence measurement strategy, subject compliance, and findings when studying fatigue patterns and must be considered when measuring fatigue (Piper, in press).

MANAGEMENT OF FATIGUE

GOALS

The goal of nursing care is promotion of the patient's adaptation or adjustment to a condition (Aistars, 1987). A patient's perception of fatigue can be mediated by health care providers through a number of intervention strategies. Patient education on the multidimensional nature of fatigue can be helpful in both evaluating an individual's level of fatigue and setting appropriate, individualized goals. Patients should be familiar with the subjective and objective factors that cause and influence fatigue to plan these goals and manage their fatigue.

Balancing energy intake with energy output (Levine, 1973) and believing that one can mobilize energy for healing (Meleis, 1986) are essential assumptions and beliefs that underlie all nursing care. Energy conservation requires assessment of the person's current energy status, the energy-depleting factors that can and cannot be controlled, and the anticipated energy costs of various activities. All decisions about energy-conserving methods must be weighed against the negative consequences of increased patient dependence (Morris, 1982). The nurse recognizes also that what constitutes rest for one person may not constitute rest for another (Piper, 1986).

TABLE 67–6. *Categories and Subdivisions of the Rhoten Observational Checklist: Behavioral Indicators or Correlates*

General Appearance
Physical appearance
Coloring
Breathing

Communication
Eyes
Facial expression
Speech

Activity
Movements
Ambulation
Posture
Food and fluid intake

Attitude

(Data from Rhoten, D. [1982]. Fatigue and the postsurgical patient. In C. M. Morris [Ed.], *Concept clarification in nursing* [pp. 277–300]. Rockville, MD: Aspen Systems.)

Effective use of energy is needed to regenerate or maintain energy reserves. Activities should be encouraged to maintain and build on current levels of functioning (Morris, 1982). It is important for the nurse to teach patients to think about their energy stores as a bank. Deposits and withdrawals must be planned on a daily and weekly basis to ensure participation in valued activities. New goals or activities may need to be considered for those that no longer can be achieved (Morris, 1982).

Energy restoration can occur through efforts that conserve energy, promote energy expenditure (Morris, 1982), enhance nutritional status, and reduce the negative impact of physical and emotional stressors. In some patients, the goal to restore energy levels to preillness states may be unreasonable, since the restorative capacity in an individual with cancer can be diminished by the disease (Aistars, 1987). Patients, nurses, and family members must remember this to avoid setting unrealistic expectations or goals for themselves or others.

INTERVENTIONS

Providing patients with appropriate information can help them view fatigue as a normal part of cancer treatment rather than a part of disease progression. Nursing and medical research that will target appropriate interventions for the multiple mechanisms that cause fatigue is just beginning. Management of fatigue involves a wide range of nursing activities that span the treatment continuum, from preventing chronic fatigue (Kellum, 1985; Piper, 1986) and screening those who may be at high risk for it to tailoring therapies to fit the different causes of fatigue and initiating referrals on the patient's behalf.

Patient education materials provide patients with tools to manage their fatigue. Nurses have an opportunity to intervene by facilitating self-care activities that can alleviate fatigue (Skalla & Lacasse, 1992).

Exercise may be beneficial in relieving fatigue in cancer patients. In 1983 Winningham reported increased exertional and activity tolerance before onset of physiologically based fatigue in patients who participated in an exercise program. These patients reported an increase in functional capacity and feelings of internal control. For example, fatigue may be lessened in stage II breast cancer patients receiving chemotherapy by a supervised exercise program (MacVicar & Winningham, 1986). However, numerous covariables must be considered prior to prescribing an exercise program for a cancer patient.

The physical limitations resulting from anemia and its treatment can have a profound impact on a patient's quality of life by disrupting personal and professional activities (Dean et al., 1995). The therapeutic outcome from the administration of epoetin alpha in combating anemia requires further investigation.

Clearly there is a need for nurses to test fatigue interventions once existing patterns of fatigue can be documented. Until additional studies can be conducted that test specific interventions in patients with cancer, those who have the disease may be our best teachers.

Table 67–7 summarizes preliminary data on patient responses (Piper, Lindsey et al., 1989) to the question "What do you believe most directly contributes to or causes your fatigue?" The responses are listed in descending order of frequency. Average respondents identified more than one reason for their fatigue. Changes in psychologic patterns were the most common, with stress being the most frequent cause identified. This points out the importance of using the nursing strategies of therapeutic listening, counseling, and patient education to reduce anxiety and increase a patient's sense of control. One woman described how she avoided becoming unnecessarily fatigued by asking the receptionist to schedule tests only during the last 2 weeks of her treatment cycles when she was feeling better (Piper, 1987). This also gave her a sense of control, which is an important aspect of fatigue management (Kellum, 1985).

The nurse's role in controlling or preventing symptoms related to medical therapies is important also. Skin reactions (see Table 67–7) and other symptoms such as pain, shortness of breath, and headaches were frequent causes of fatigue in these patients.

Table 67–8 summarizes patient responses, again in descending order of frequency, to the question "What do you do to relieve your fatigue?" (Piper & Dodd, 1987; Piper, Lindsey et al., 1989). Clearly, there is

TABLE 67–7. *Perceived Causes of Fatigue in Cancer Patients*

Psychologic Patterns
Stress
Worry
Depression
Anxiety
Emotional strain

Treatment Patterns
Radiation
Surgery
Chemotherapy
Medical

Activity/Rest Patterns
Work
Everyday activities
Hospital/radiation therapy travel

Sleep/Wake Patterns
Insomnia

Disease Patterns
Cancer
Other

Other Patterns
Symptoms
Environment
Nutrition
Innate host factors

(From Piper, B. F. [1989]. Fatigue: Current bases for practice. In S. G. Funk, E. M. Tornquist, M. T. Champagne, L. A. Copp, & R. A. Weise [Eds.], *Key aspects of comfort: Management of pain, fatigue, and nausea* [p. 196]. New York: Springer. Reproduced by permission.)

TABLE 67–8. *Measures Used by Cancer Patients to Relieve Fatigue*

Activity/Rest Patterns
Rest
Nap
Alter activities
Sit/lie down
Read
Walk/exercise

Psychologic Patterns
Distraction
Relaxation

Sleep/Wake Patterns
Sleep

Other Patterns
Nutritional
Environmental
Social
Symptoms

(From Piper, B. F. [1989]. Fatigue: Current bases for practice. In S. G. Funk, E. M. Tornquist, M. T. Champagne, L. A. Copp, & R. A. Weise [Eds.], *Key aspects of comfort: Management of pain, fatigue, and nausea* [p. 197]. New York: Springer. Reproduced by permission.)

value in finding out what patients perceive will work for them. Distraction techniques included going to work, taking car rides, and listening to tapes or soft music.

One patient stated that chanting helped her to become distracted from her disease and other stressors that she experienced during the day. She would feel "reenergized" after these activities. Going to church sometimes had the same effect for her (Piper, 1987). Testing in patients with fatigue the efficacy of specific distraction therapies that have proven effective in patients with pain is one approach to consider.

Nursing research efforts should focus on good measurement and a better understanding of the course and correlates of fatigue that could ultimately result in recommendations for effective interventions for fatigue in cancer patients.

SPECIAL PROBLEMS RELATED TO FATIGUE

A number of fatigue-related issues have been discussed throughout this chapter that will profoundly affect many aspects of an individual's life. Fatigue can influence the *quality of a person's life* negatively by interfering in the person's ability to perform the kinds of activities and roles that give meaning and value to life. Chronically fatigued individuals may not have the same energy reserves they once had. As a consequence, fewer activities are undertaken, and those that are performed may take longer to do and may require more effort. Because many of these changes can have negative effects on a person's lifestyle and self-esteem, several quality-of-life instruments contain at least one item

on fatigue (Frank-Stromborg, 1984; Grant, Padilla, Presant, Lipsett, & Runa, 1983).

Fatigue can both result from and lead to *decreased mobility and functional status* (Davis, 1984). Prolonged inactivity and fatigue can cause decreased muscle strength, weakness, and loss of endurance. These changes can lead to a circular pattern of increased immobility, decreased activity tolerance, increased fatigue, and additional complications (Winningham, MacVicar, & Burke, 1986).

A person may become so fatigued and weak that performing the basic activities of daily living such as bathing, dressing, and eating becomes too much of an effort without additional assistance from others. Helping people decide what is most important for them to do on their own can assist in maintaining independence and self-respect for as long as possible.

As a person becomes increasingly more fatigued, the desire to engage in *social activities and interactions* declines. Increased physical dependence can lead to further declines in social activities, which can result in social isolation for both the patient and the family caregiver.

As chronic fatigue begins to alter what patients can do for themselves, family members or caregivers begin to assume many of the roles previously performed by patients. These increased physical and emotional demands on the family member can lead to *caregiver role fatigue* (Goldstein, Regnery, & Wellin, 1981). Caregivers of the chronically ill use relatively few community services that are available to them. Nurses must help direct caregivers to identify needed services and employ these resources to improve their own quality of life and well-being (McCorkle & Given, 1991).

As a result of the changes mentioned, *loss of self-esteem, depression,* and *loss of hope* can occur. A person may not have the desire to fight the disease, participate in treatment, or go on living. Maintaining hope, fighting disease, and participating in treatment protocols take energy. For chronically fatigued individuals, it simply may take too much energy to go on living.

Three studies suggest that the *presence of fatigue* as measured by one subscale on the POMS (Levy, Herberman, Maluish, Schlien, & Lippman, 1985; Temoshok, 1987) or by one item on the Symptom Distress Scale (Kukell, McCorkle, & Driever, 1986) *at diagnosis may predict a negative outcome* in breast cancer (Levy et al., 1985), lung cancer (Kukell et al., 1986), and malignant melanoma patients (Temoshok, 1987). The POMS fatigue-inertia subscale scores predicted nodal status in breast cancer patients with a 71 per cent degree of accuracy (Levy et al., 1985); higher scores were associated also with an unfavorable outcome and shorter survival time in malignant melanoma patients (Temoshok, 1987). In lung cancer patients, increased fatigue and symptom distress scores were associated with an increased risk of death and with a decreased probability of long-term survival (Kukell et al., 1986). Although future studies are needed to validate these findings with repeated measures over time, nurses clearly must recognize the importance of early recognition and treatment of acute fatigue before it becomes chronic fatigue.

SUMMARY

Fatigue is the most distressing symptom experienced by many cancer patients. Oncology nurses have a major role in recognizing and treating this pervasive, distressing, and perhaps life-threatening phenomena. Our knowledge of fatigue as experienced by the cancer patient is limited, and much work must be done to document patterns of fatigue in specific cancer populations and to test various interventions. Only through a collaborative network of oncology nurses and nurse and medical researchers can the care given to the chronically fatigued cancer patient be improved.

REFERENCES

Aistars, J. (1987). Fatigue in the cancer patient: A conceptual approach to a clinical problem. *Oncology Nursing Forum, 14,* 25–30.

Axelrod, L., Halter, J. B., Cooper, D. S., Aoki, T. T., Roussell, A. M., & Bagshaw, S. L. (1983). Hormone levels and fuel flow in patients with weight loss and lung cancer. Evidence for excessive metabolic expenditure and for an adaptive response mediated by a reduced level of 3,5,3′-triiodothyronine. *Metabolism, 32,* 924–937.

Bartley, S. H., & Chute, E. (1947). *Fatigue and impairment in man.* New York: McGraw-Hill.

Beutler, B., & Cerami, A. (1986). Cachectin and tumor necrosis factor as two sides of the same biological coin. *Nature, 17,* 146–154.

Bruera, E., Brenneis, C., Michaud, P. I., Jackson, R. N., & MacDonald, R. N. (1988). Muscle electrophysiology in patients with advanced breast cancer. *Journal of the National Cancer Institute, 80,* 282–285.

Bukberg, J., Penman, D., & Holland, J. C. (1984). Depression in hospitalized cancer patients. *Psychosomatic Medicine, 46,* 199–212.

Burns, N. (in review). *Fatigue.* University of Pennsylvania School of Nursing, Oncology Advanced Practice Nurse Program, Philadelphia.

Burt, M. E., Aoki, T. T., Gorschboth, C. M., & Brennan, M. F. (1983). Peripheral tissue metabolism in cancer-bearing man. *Annals of Surgery, 198,* 685–691.

Ciba Foundation Symposium 82. (1981). *Human muscle fatigue: Physiological mechanisms.* London: Pittman Medical.

Cimprich, B. (1990). Attentional fatigue in the cancer patient. *Oncology Nursing Forum, 17*(Suppl. 2), 218. (Abstract No. 321A)

Davis, C. A. (1984). Interferon-induced fatigue. *Oncology Nursing Forum, 11*(Suppl. 7). (Abstract No. 72).

Dean, G. E., Spears, L., Ferrell, B., Quan, W., Groshon, S., Mitchell, M. (1995). Fatigue in patients with cancer receiving interferon alpha. *Cancer Practice, 3,* 164–171.

Derdiarian, A. (1987). Informational needs of recently diagnosed cancer patients: Part II. Method and description. *Cancer Nursing, 10,* 156–163.

Edwards, R. H. T., Harris, R. C., Hultman, E., Kaijser, L., Koh, D., & Nordesjo, L. O. (1972). Effect of temperature on muscle energy metabolism and endurance during successive isometric contractions, sustained to fatigue, of the quadriceps muscle in man. *Journal of Physiology, 220,* 335–352.

Engel, G. L., & Morgan, W. L. (1973). *Interviewing the patient.* Philadelphia: W. B. Saunders Co.

Fernsler, J. (1986). A comparison of patient and nurse perceptions of patients' self-care deficits associated with cancer chemotherapy. *Cancer Nursing, 9,* 50–57.

Fobair, P., Hoppe, R. T., Bloom, J., Cox, R., Varghese, A., & Spiegel, D. (1986). Psychosocial problems among survivors of Hodgkin's disease. *Journal of Clinical Oncology, 4,* 805–814.

Frank-Stromborg, M. (1984). Selecting an instrument to measure quality of life. *Oncology Nursing Forum, 11*(5), 88–91.

Frank-Stromborg, M., & Wright, P. (1984). Ambulatory cancer patients' perception of the physical and psychosocial changes in their lives since the diagnosis of cancer. *Cancer Nursing, 7,* 117–130.

Freel, M. I., & Hart, L. K. (1977). *Study of fatigue phenomena of multiple sclerosis patients* (USDHEW Grant No. 5R02-NU-00524-02). University of Iowa, Division of Nursing, Iowa City.

Gibson, H., & Edwards, R. H. T. (1985). Muscular exercise and fatigue. *Sports Medicine, 2,* 120–132.

Glaus, A. (1993). Assessment of fatigue in cancer and non-cancer patients. *Supportive Care in Cancer, 1,* 305–315.

Gold, J. (1974). Cancer cachexia and gluconeogenesis. *Annals of the New York Academy of Sciences, 230,* 103–110.

Goldstein, V., Regnery, G., & Wellin, E. (1981). Caretaker role fatigue. *Nursing Outlook, 29,* 24–30.

Grandjean, E. P. (1970). Fatigue. *American Industrial Hygiene Association Journal, 30,* 401–411.

Grant, M. M., Padilla, G. V., Presant, C., Lipsett, J., & Runa, P. (1983). *Proceedings of the Fourth National Conference on Cancer Nursing.* New York: American Cancer Society.

Hart, L. K. (1978). Fatigue in the patient with multiple sclerosis. *Research in Nursing and Health, 1,* 147–157.

Haylock, P. J., & Hart, L. K. (1979). Fatigue in patients receiving localized radiation. *Cancer Nursing, 2,* 461–467.

Henry, D. H., & Abels, R. I. (1994). Recombinant human erythropoietin in treatment of cancer and chemotherapy-induced anemia: Results of double-blind and open-label follow-up studies. *Seminars in Oncology, 21*(Suppl. 3), 21–28.

Hubbard, S. M. (1995). Nursing research—the basis for practice. Clinical research and cancer nursing. *Oncology Nursing Forum, 22,* 505–513.

Irvine, D., Vincent, L., Graydon, J. E., Bubela, N., Thompson, L., & Graydon, J. (1991). A critical appraisal of the research literature investigating fatigue in the individual with cancer. *Cancer Nursing, 14,* 188–199.

Irvine, D., Vincent, L., Graydon, J., Bubela, N., & Thompson, L. (1994). The prevalence and correlates of fatigue in patients receiving treatment with chemotherapy and radiotherapy. *Cancer Nursing, 17,* 367–378.

Jamar, S. C. (1989). Fatigue in women receiving chemotherapy for ovarian cancer. In S. G. Funk, E. M. Tornquist, M. T. Champagne, L. A. Copp, & R. A. Weise (Eds.), *Key aspects of comfort: Management of pain, fatigue and nausea* (pp. 224–228). New York: Springer.

Karlsson, J., Sjodin, B., Jacobs, I., & Kaiser, P. (1981). Relevance of muscle fiber type to fatigue in short intense and prolonged exercise in man. In Ciba Foundation Symposium 82, *Human muscle fatigue: Physiological mechanisms* (pp. 59–74). London: Pittman Medical.

Kellum, M. D. (1985). Fatigue. In M. M. Jacobs & W. Geels (Eds.), *Signs and symptoms in nursing: Interpretation and management* (pp. 103–118). Philadelphia: J. B. Lippincott Co.

King, K. B., Nail, L. M., Kreamer, K., Strohl, R. A., & Johnson, J. E. (1985). Patients' descriptions of the experience of receiving radiation therapy. *Oncology Nursing Forum, 12*(4), 55–61.

Kogi, K., Saito, Y., & Mitsuhashi, T. (1970). Validity of three components of subjective fatigue feelings. *Journal of the Science of Labor, 46,* 251–270.

Komoike, Y., & Horiguchi, S. (1971). Fatigue assessment on key punch operators, typists, and others. *Ergonomics, 14,* 101–109.

Kukell, W. A., McCorkle, R., & Driever, M. (1986). Symptom distress, psychosocial variables, and survival from lung cancer. *Journal of Psychosocial Oncology, 4*(1/2), 91–104.

Larson, P., Lindsey, A., Dodd, M., Brecht, M., & Packer, A. (1993). Influence of age on problems experienced by patients with lung cancer undergoing radiation therapy. *Oncology Nursing Forum, 20,* 473–480.

Levine, M. E. (1973). *Introduction to clinical nursing* (2nd ed.). Philadelphia: F. A. Davis Co.

Levy, S. M., Herberman, R. B., Maluish, A. M., Schlien, B., & Lippman, M. (1985). Prognostic risk assessment in primary breast cancer by behavioral and immunological parameters. *Health Psychology, 4,* 99–113.

MacVicar, M. G., & Winningham, M. L. (1986). Promoting functional capacity of cancer patients. *The Cancer Bulletin, 38,* 235–239.

Malmquist, R., Ekholm, I., Lindstrom, L., Petersen, I., & Örtengren, R. (1981). Measurement of localized muscle fatigue in building work. *Ergonomics, 24,* 695–709.

McAdoo, B. C., Doering, C. H., Kraemer, H. C., Dessert, N., Brodie, H. K. H., & Hamburg, D. A. (1978). A study of the effects of gonadotropin-releasing hormone on human mood and behavior. *Psychosomatic Medicine, 40,* 199–209.

McCorkle, R., & Given, B. (1991). Meeting the challenge of caring for chronically ill adults. *Health Policy, Who Cares?, 4,* 59–69.

McCorkle, R., & Young, K. (1978). Development of a symptom distress scale. *Cancer Nursing, 1,* 373–377.

McFarland, R. A. (1971). Understanding fatigue in modern life. *Ergonomics, 14,* 1–10.

McGuire, D. B. (1992). Comprehensive and multidimensional assessment and management of pain. *Journal of Pain and Symptom Management, 5,* 312–319.

McNair, D. M., Lorr, M., & Droppleman, L. F. (1971). *Profile of mood states.* San Diego: Education and Industrial Testing Service.

Meleis, A. I. (1986). Theory development and domain concepts. In P. Moccia (Ed.), *New approaches to theory development* (p. 6). New York: National League for Nursing.

Melzack, R. (Ed.). (1983). *Pain measurement and assessment.* New York: Raven Press.

Miller, R. G., Boska, M. D., Moussaui, R. S., Carson, P. J., & Weiner, M. W. (1988).[31]P nuclear magnetic resonance studies of high energy phosphates and pH in human muscle fatigue: Comparison of aerobic and anaerobic exercise. *Journal of Clinical Investigation, 81,* 1190–1196.

Moldawer, L. L., Sherry, B., & Lowry, S. F. (1989). Endogenous cachectin/tumor necrosis factor-alpha production contributes to experimental cancer-associated cachexia. *Cancer Surveys, 8,* 853–859.

Morris, M. L. (1982). Tiredness and fatigue. In C. M. Norris (Ed.), *Concept clarification in nursing* (pp. 263–275). Rockville, MD: Aspen Systems Corporation.

Muncie, W. (1941). Chronic fatigue. *Psychosomatic Medicine, 3,* 277–285.

Musci, E. (1983). *Relationship between family coping strategies and self-care during cancer chemotherapy.* Unpublished doctoral dissertation, University of California, School of Nursing, San Francisco.

Muscio, B. (1921–1922). Is a fatigue test possible? *British Journal of Psychology, 12,* 31–46.

Nail, L. M. (1992). Fatigue. In S. L. Groenwald, M. H. Frogge, M. Goodman, & C. H. Yarbro. *Manifestations of cancer and cancer treatment* (pp. 485–494). Boston: Jones & Bartlett.

Nail, L. M., Jones, L. S., Greene, D., Schipper, D. L., & Jensen, R. (1991). Use and perceived efficacy of self-care activities in patients receiving chemotherapy. *Oncology Nursing Forum, 18,* 883–887.

Nail, L., & Winningham, M. (1993). Fatigue. In S. L. Groenwald, M. Frogge, M. Goodman, & C. Yarbro (Eds.), *Cancer nursing: Principles and practice.* (pp. 608–619). Boston: Jones & Bartlett.

Nakamura, Y., & Schwartz, S. (1972). The influence of hydrogen ion concentration on calcium binding and release by skeletal muscle sarcoplasmic reticulum. *Journal of General Physiology, 59,* 22–32.

Pearson, R. G. (1957). Scale analysis of a fatigue checklist. *Journal of Applied Psychology, 41,* 186–191.

Pearson, R. G., & Byars, G. E. (1956). *The development and validation of a checklist for measuring subjective fatigue* (pp. 56–115). Randolph AFB, TX: Texas School of Aviation Medicine, USAF.

Petty, F., & Noyes, R., Jr. (1981). Depression secondary to cancer. *Biological Psychiatry, 16,* 1203–1221.

Pickard-Holley, S. (1991). Fatigue in cancer patients, a descriptive study. *Cancer Nursing, 14,* 13–19.

Piper, B. F. (1986). Fatigue. In V. K. Carrieri, A. M. Lindsey, & C. W. West (Eds.), *Pathophysiological phenomena in nursing: Human responses to illness* (pp. 219–234). Philadelphia: W. B. Saunders Co.

Piper, B. F. (1987). *Perceptions of fatigue in cancer patients who are receiving radiation and chemotherapy: A qualitative study.* Unpublished S214A data, University of California, School of Nursing, San Francisco.

Piper, B. F. (1988). Fatigue in cancer patients: Current perspectives on measurement and management. In Fifth National Conference on Cancer Nursing. *Monograph on nursing management of common problems: State of the art.* New York: American Cancer Society.

Piper, B. F. (1989). Fatigue: Current basis for practice. In S. G. Funk, E. M. Tornquist, M. T. Champagne, L. A. Copp, & R. A. Wiese (Eds.), *Key aspects of comfort: Management of pain, fatigue and nausea* (pp. 187–198). New York: Springer.

Piper, B. F. (1991). Alteration in comfort: fatigue. In J. C. McNally, E. Somerville, C. Miaskowski, & M. Rostad, (Eds.), *Guidelines for oncology nursing practice* (2nd ed., pp. 155–162). Philadelphia: W. B. Saunders Co.

Piper, B. F. (1993). Fatigue. In V. Carrieri, A. Lindsey, & C. West (Eds). *Pathophysiological phenomena in nursing: Human responses to illness* (2nd ed., pp. 279–302). Philadelphia: Saunders.

Piper, B. F. (in press). Measurement of Fatigue. In M. Frank-Stromburg & K. Olsen (Eds.), *Instruments for clinical research* (2nd ed.). Boston: Jones & Bartlett.

Piper, B. F., & Dodd, M. J. (1987). *Fatigue analysis of chemotherapy and radiation therapy self-care behavior logs.* Unpublished data, University of California, School of Nursing, Department of Physiological Nursing, San Francisco.

Piper, B. F., Lindsey, A. M., & Dodd, M. J. (1987). Fatigue mechanisms in cancer patients: Developing nursing theory. *Oncology Nursing Forum, 14*(6), 17–23.

Piper, B. F., Lindsey, A. M., Dodd, M. J., Ferketich, S., Paul, S. M., & Weller, S. (1989). The development of an instrument to measure the subjective dimension of fatigue. In S. G. Funk, E. M. Tornquist, M. T. Champagne, L. A. Copp, & R. A. Weise (Eds.), *Key aspects of comfort: Man-*

agement of pain, fatigue and nausea (pp. 199–208). New York: Springer.

Piper, B. F., Rieger, P. T., Brophy, L., Haeuber, D., Hood, L. E., Lyver, A., & Sharp, E. (1989). Recent advances in the management of biotherapy-related side effects: Fatigue. *Oncology Nursing Forum, 16*(Suppl. 6), 27–34.

Poffenberger, A. T. (1928). The effects of continuous work upon output and feelings. *Journal of Applied Psychology, 5,* 450–467.

Poteliakhoff, A. (1981). Adrenocortical activity and some clinical findings in acute and chronic fatigue. *Journal of Psychosomatic Research, 25,* 91–95.

Potempa, K., Lopez, M., Reid, C., & Lawson, L. (1986). Chronic fatigue. *Image, 18,* 165–169.

Proctor, S. J., Kernahan, J., & Taylor, P. (1981). Depression as component of post-cranial irradiation somnolence syndrome [Letter to the editor]. *Lancet, 1,* 1215–1216.

Putt, A. M. (1977). Effects of noise on fatigue in healthy middle-aged adults. *Communicating Nursing Research, 8,* 24–34.

Rhodes, V. A., & Watson, P. M. (1987). Symptom distress— the concept: Past and present. *Seminars in Oncology Nursing, 3,* 242–247.

Rhodes, V. A., Watson, P. M., & Hanson, B. M. (1988). Patients' descriptions of the influence of tiredness and weakness on self-care abilities. *Cancer Nursing, 11,* 186–194.

Rhodes, V. A., Watson, P. M., & Johnson, M. H. (1984). Development of reliable and valid measures of nausea and vomiting. *Cancer Nursing, 6,* 33–41.

Rhoten, D. (1982). Fatigue and the postsurgical patient. In C. M. Norris (Ed.), *Concept clarification in nursing* (pp. 277–300). Rockville, MD: Aspen Systems.

Riddle, P. K. (1982). Chronic fatigue and women: A description and suggested treatment. *Women and Health, 7,* 37–47.

Rieger, P. T. (1987). Interferon-induced fatigue: A study of fatigue measurement. Sigma Theta Tau International 29th Biennial Convention Book of Proceedings. (Abstract A163).

Rieger, P. T., & Haeuber, D. (1995). A new approach to managing chemotherapy-related anemia: Nursing implications of epoetin alfa. *Oncology Nursing Forum, 22,* 71–81.

Saito, Y., Kogi, K., & Kashiwagi, S. (1970). Factors underlying subjective feelings of fatigue. *Journal of Science and Labour, 46,* 205–224.

Selye, H. (1956). *The stress of life.* New York: McGraw-Hill.

Selye, H. (1974). *Stress without distress.* Philadelphia: J. B. Lippincott Co.

Skalla, K. (1992). Fatigue and the patient with cancer: What is it and what can I do about it? *Oncology Nursing Forum, 19,* 1540–1541.

Skalla, K., & Lacasse, C. (1992). Patient education for fatigue. *Oncology Nursing Forum, 19,* 1537–1541.

Skalla, K., & Rieger, P. (1995). Fatigue. In P. T. Rieger (Ed.), *Biotherapy, comprehensive review* (pp. 221–242). Boston: Jones & Bartlett.

Smets, E. M. A., Garssen, B., Schuster-Uitterhoeve, A. L. J., de Haes, J. C. J. M. (1993). Fatigue in cancer patients. *British Journal of Cancer, 68,* 220–224.

Spivak, J. L. (1994). Cancer-related anemia: Its causes and characteristics. *Seminars in Oncology, 2,* 3–8.

Spross, J. A. (1987). Fatigue. In S. B. Baird (Ed.), *Decision making in oncology nursing* (pp. 76–77). Philadelphia: B. C. Decker.

St. Pierre, B., Kasper, C., Lindsey, A. (1992). Fatigue mechanisms in patients with cancer: Effects of tumor necrosis factor and exercise on skeletal muscle. *Oncology Nursing Forum, 19,* 419–425.

Straus, S. E., Tosato, G., Armstrong, G., Lawley, T., Preble, O. T., Henle, W., Davey, R., Pearson, G., Epstein, J., Brus, I., & Blaese, M. (1985). Persisting illness and fatigue in adults with evidence of Epstein-Barr virus infection. *Annals of Internal Medicine, 102,* 7–16.

Temoshok, L. (1987). In Consultation: Discussion of psychosocial factors related to outcome in cutaneous malignant melanoma: A matched samples design. *Oncology News/Update, 2*(3), 6–7.

Valdini, A. F. (1985). Fatigue of unknown etiology—a review. *Family Practice, 2,* 48–53.

Varrichio, C. G. (1985). Selecting a tool for measuring fatigue. *Oncology Nursing Forum, 12*(4), 122–123 & 126–127.

Waskerwitz, M. J., & Leonard, M. (1986). Early detection of malignancy: From birth to twenty years. *Oncology Nursing Forum, 13*(1), 50–57.

Wickham, R., Blesch, K., Paice, J., Harte, N., Barry, S., Purl, S., Mooney, M., Cahill, M., Kopp, P., & Manson, S. (1990). Fatigue and its correlates in breast and lung cancer patients. [Abstract 35A]. *Oncology Nursing Forum, 17*(Suppl. 2), 146.

Wilson, I. B., & Cleary, P. D. (1995). Linking clinical variables with health-related quality of life: A conceptual model of patient outcomes. *Journal of the American Medical Association, 1,* 59–65.

Winningham, M. L. (1983). *Effects of a bicycle ergometry program on functional capacity and feelings of control in women with breast cancer.* [Dissertation]. Ohio State University, Columbus, OH.

Winningham, M. L. (1991). Walking program for people with cancer, getting started. *Cancer Nursing, 5,* 270–276.

Winningham, M. L., MacVicar, M. G., & Burke, C. A. (1986). Exercise for cancer patients: Guidelines and precautions. *The Physician and Sportsmedicine, 14,* 125–134.

Winningham, M. L., Nail, L. M., Burke, M. B., Brophy, L., Cimprich, B., Jones, L. S., Pickard-Holley, S., Rhodes, V., St. Pierre, B., Beck, S., Glass, E. C., Mock, V., Mooney, K. H., & Piper, B. (1994). Fatigue and the cancer experience: The state of the knowledge. *Oncology Nursing Forum, 1,* 23–35.

Wittenborn, J. R., & Buhler, R. (1979). Somatic discomforts among depressed women. *Archives of General Psychiatry, 36,* 465–471.

Yoshitake, H. (1969). Rating the feelings of fatigue. *Journal of the Science of Labour, 45,* 422–432.

Yoshitake, H. (1971). Relations between the symptoms and the feeling of fatigue. *Ergonomics, 14,* 175–186.

Yoshitake, H. (1978). Three characteristic patterns of subjective fatigue symptoms. *Ergonomics, 21,* 231–233.

CHAPTER

68

Interpersonal Communication Systems

Laurel L. Northouse • Peter G. Northouse

Communication is a major concern for individuals living with cancer. These individuals have reported communication problems with health professionals (Lerman et al., 1993; McIntosh, 1974) and with significant others, such as family and friends (Hinton, 1981; Peters-Golden, 1982; Schag et al., 1993). To cope with the disease, patients must be able to communicate effectively with nurses, physicians, family, friends, and others who are important to them. Communication is an essential element in the overall treatment process and the critical factor in helping patients maintain productive relationships (Brewin, 1977; Cooper, 1982).

This chapter provides information that will help nurses understand and improve their ability to communicate with patients who have cancer. It begins with a discussion about the importance of communication in cancer nursing, and then provides a theoretic orientation to nurse-patient communication. The final section analyzes several specific communication concerns that confront patients and nurses during the cancer experience.

Given the importance of communication for nurses and patients, this chapter attempts to answer the following questions: What are the central elements of effective communication in the oncology setting? What obstacles between nurses and patients make effective communication difficult? How can oncology nurses become aware of patients' communication concerns and thereby help them adjust to their illness? What communication strategies can be used to enhance the effectiveness of nurse-patient communication?

THE IMPORTANCE OF COMMUNICATION IN CANCER NURSING

Evidence is accumulating that effective interpersonal relationships help people cope with cancer (Gotcher, 1992). Investigators have reported that supportive interpersonal relationships are associated with better survival rates (Spiegel, Bloom, Kraemer, & Gottheil, 1989), higher levels of psychosocial adjustment (Northouse, 1988; Vachon, 1986; Waxler-Morrison, Hislop, Mears, & Kan, 1991), and fewer fears of recurrence (Northouse, 1981). Within supportive relationships, communication plays a major role in helping patients cope with the effects of cancer. Through effective communication with others, patients disclose feelings, ventilate fears, and assert control in areas related to their illness.

Although interpersonal relationships are important during the cancer experience, patients have reported difficulty communicating with others about their illness. The majority of breast cancer patients in a study by Peters-Golden (1982) reported that their interactions with others became strained after the cancer diagnosis; they often felt misunderstood, received false optimism, and were avoided. Gordon and colleagues (1977) found that the lack of open family communication was a major problem cited by a sample of 136 cancer patients. Similarly, Meyerowitz, Watkins, and Sparks (1983) found that patients who were receiving adjuvant chemotherapy for breast cancer reported conflicts and negative changes in their relationships with family and friends. Cancer patients also have reported that communicating with health professionals is a problem. A sizable number of breast cancer patients (84 per cent) in one study reported difficulties communicating with members of their medical team (Lerman et al., 1993). In another study, nearly half the patients said they did not discuss their problems with a nurse (Frank-Stromborg & Wright, 1984). Among the reasons given by patients for limited nurse-patient communication were a general lack of contact with nurses and the perception that nurses were "too busy."

Although effective communication is important to patients with cancer, it is equally important to oncology nurses. Many of the nurse's daily activities require effective communication. Obtaining accurate information, providing health education, answering questions, and giving support to patients are just a few of the many nursing activities that are communication intensive. In addition, the nurse frequently serves as a patient advocate or as an intermediary with other professionals. Interacting with family members is yet another activity that requires effective interpersonal communication on the part of oncology nurses.

Although nurses recognize the importance of communication in nursing care, they often have difficulty engaging in effective therapeutic communication with patients. One major problem confronting them is that they have little time to simply interact and "be with" clients. Typically, their supportive communications must be abbreviated and fit in between many other physical tasks that occur simultaneously. In addition, they sometimes lack the communication skills necessary to deal with the complex interpersonal issues that arise during the cancer experience. Perhaps it is not surprising that oncology nurses have reported the need for further education in communication (Craytor, Brown, & Marrow, 1978).

A THEORETIC ORIENTATION TO NURSE-PATIENT COMMUNICATION

Before discussing the specific communication concerns of nurses and patients with cancer, it is important to clarify exactly what communication means and to describe the theoretic assumptions that underlie the communication process.

INTERPERSONAL COMMUNICATION DEFINED

Communication in oncology nursing settings is a complex and multifaceted process. Although the word *communication* is used often in a general way to describe a variety of events, it actually refers to an identifiable process that has specific characteristics. Because language is something people learn when they are young, they believe wrongly that effective communication is a simple, easily performed, straightforward process. In fact, effective communication is just the opposite; it is a process that demands a great deal of skill.

Interpersonal communication is the process whereby two individuals interact and share information according to a common set of rules (Northouse & Northouse, 1992). The process occurs through the use of symbolic behavior—through language. It is an ongoing process, and it involves human attitudes and feelings as well as information. Interactions between the patient with cancer and the nurse take place on many levels, including verbal and nonverbal, intentional and unintentional, content-oriented and relationship-oriented, nondirective and goal-directed, and humorous and serious. In a sense, interpersonal communication is the vehicle that connects nurse and patient. It allows them to express their thoughts and feelings with each other and to collaborate in meeting goals.

ASSUMPTIONS ABOUT INTERPERSONAL COMMUNICATION

In studying how people communicate with each other, researchers have found that several general properties form the basis for the fundamental assumptions of human communication (Berlo, 1960; Knapp & Miller, 1985; Watzlawick, Beavin, & Jackson, 1967). These assumptions govern as well as explain communication that occurs in the oncology setting.

ASSUMPTION ONE: INTERPERSONAL COMMUNICATION IS A PROCESS

To many people, the word *communication* triggers an image of one person sending a message to another person. This image is based on a linear approach to communication, which has also been referred to as the "hypodermic needle" model of communication; that is, person A instills a message into person B (Fig. 68–1). Communication is unidirectional, with one person directly influencing a second person through the use of specific messages. One problem with the linear approach is that it is too restrictive. Communication is more than a simple, one-way, or linear event; it is an

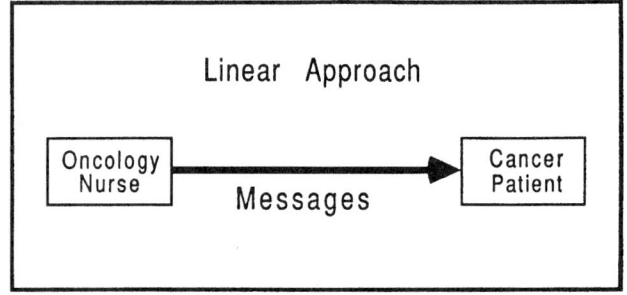

FIGURE 68–1. Linear approach to nurse-patient communication.

ongoing, continuous, dynamic, and ever-changing process.

The assumption that communication is a process is an important one, because it emphasizes the complexity of interpersonal communication in the oncology setting. The assumption directs individuals to analyze factors that affect the nurse as well as the patient and to examine how the ongoing interchange between the two will vary, depending on the nature of their relationship and the situation. During communication, the communication skills, attitudes, knowledge, social system, and culture of both the nurse and the patient influence the interaction simultaneously. Analysis of the impact of a single message created by one person and sent to another is important; however, analysis of communication as a process is even more important, because it provides a richer understanding of how messages interact with and are mediated by many other variables involved in the communication process.

ASSUMPTION TWO: INTERPERSONAL COMMUNICATION IS TRANSACTIONAL

To say communication is transactional means that both individuals in an interaction affect and are affected by each other. Communication involves reciprocal influence; each individual is both a source and a receiver at the same time. While constructing a message for a patient, the nurse is receiving cues simultaneously from the patient that influence how the message is formulated. A transactional approach emphasizes the simultaneous interplay between the sender and receiver of a message (Fig. 68–2).

From a transactional perspective, each individual perceives the other in the context of what occurs in the interaction. For example, if a nurse chooses to be dominant with a patient, it may be because the nurse desires to be dominant in general, or it may be because the nurse picks up cues from the patient indicating a preference to be submissive. In other words, the nature of the interaction can be influenced by the desires of the nurse or the patient, by each person's perceptions of the other person's desires, or by both factors working together simultaneously.

In the oncology setting, the transactional assumption helps explain the unique relationship that a nurse establishes with each patient. Each nurse brings a different set of experiences into the oncology setting, and

these experiences influence the type of relationships the nurse develops with patients. Similarly, each patient experiences cancer in a unique way, which has a significant effect on the kinds of relationships the patient wants to have with health care staff. Therefore, the communication patterns that develop are constructed mutually by nurse and patient.

ASSUMPTION THREE: INTERPERSONAL COMMUNICATION IS MULTIDIMENSIONAL

When interpersonal communication takes place, it occurs on primarily two levels; that is, it is multidimensional. One level can be characterized as the *content dimension,* the other, as the *relationship dimension* (Watzlawick et al., 1967). In interpersonal communication, these two dimensions are inextricably bound together. The content dimension of communication refers to the words, language, and information in a message; the relationship dimension refers to the aspect of a message that defines how participants in an interaction are connected to each other.

To illustrate the content and relationship dimensions, consider the following hypothetical statement made by a patient with cancer to a nurse: "Please change my nausea medication. The drug I've been taking isn't working." The *content* dimension of the message refers to the patient's desire to have the medication changed. The *relationship* dimension refers to how the patient and the nurse are affiliated. It includes the patient's attitude toward the nurse, the nurse's attitude toward the patient, and their feelings about each other. It is the relationship dimension that implicitly suggests how the content dimension should be interpreted, because the content alone can be interpreted in many ways. The exact meaning of the message emerges for the nurse and patient as a result of their interaction. If a caring relationship exists between the two, the nurse will probably interpret the content ("Please change my nausea medication. The drug I've been taking isn't working.") as a helpful suggestion from a patient who wants to be involved in his or her own care. However, if the relationship between the nurse and the patient is distant or strained, the nurse may interpret the content of the message as an inappropriate suggestion by an uninformed patient. These two interpretations illustrate how the meaning of a message is not in words alone but in how the giver and the receiver interpret the message in the context of their relationship.

In oncology settings, the implication of this assumption is that nurses need to be aware of *how* they communicate with patients in addition to *what* they communicate. In a study of helpful and unhelpful communication in cancer care, Thorne (1988) found that unhelpful communication was associated with a lack of concern toward the patient on the part of the nurse or physician. Because of the uncertain and threatening nature of cancer, it is important for health care providers to establish supportive and nurturing relationships with patients (McCorkle, 1981). Communicating both positive and negative information successfully is easier in the context of a caring relationship. For example, when telling patients about the possibility of adverse side effects of a certain chemotherapy regi-

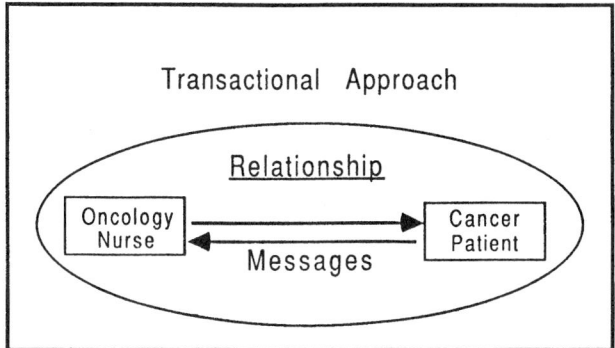

FIGURE 68–2. Transactional approach to nurse-patient communication.

men, nurses need to be sensitive to how they provide the information. The better the relationship between nurse and patient, the less threatening the information is likely to be to the patient. In other words, communication is more likely to be effective if the nurse pays equal attention to the content and the relationship dimensions of the message.

Before leaving the discussion of the multidimensionality of interpersonal communication, some attention needs to be given to the contribution of its nonverbal dimensions. Some investigators have estimated that 65 to 70 per cent of the meaning in a message is transmitted nonverbally (Birdwhistell, 1970); others have estimated that more than 90 per cent of the meaning of a message is accounted for by nonverbal aspects (Mehrabian, 1971). Nonverbal communication is relevant especially in the oncology setting, because patients and family members pay close attention to the nonverbal expressions of health care professionals to supplement the verbal communication they receive. In addition, patients commonly believe that important information is often "leaked" through nonverbal channels (Friedman, 1979); therefore, patients often scrutinize health care staff carefully to determine whether they are being completely honest. In addition to providing information, nonverbal communication such as touch can provide patients with psychosocial support and comfort (Bottorff, 1993). McCorkle and Hollenbach (1983) reported that touch had a positive effect on the self-concept, level of depression, and overall hospital stay of patients undergoing a bone marrow transplant. Hospital staff, on the other hand, rely heavily on patients' nonverbal cues to assess their needs accurately. These cues help staff members interpret and validate the verbal messages patients express.

COMMUNICATION ISSUES CONFRONTING NURSES AND PATIENTS IN CANCER CARE

In attempting to understand communication issues in nurse-patient relationships, it is important to assess these issues from the perspectives of both patient and nurse, because each brings a unique set of concerns to the relationship. An analysis of the research literature suggests that, for patients, the major communication issues are related to maintaining a sense of control, seeking information, disclosing feelings, and searching for meaning (Northouse & Northouse, 1987), whereas the primary communication issues for nurses center on imparting information, communicating hope, and dealing with emotions.

Issues Confronting Patients

Maintaining a Sense of Control

The single most important problem confronting cancer patients is loss of control (Byrne, Stockwell, & Gudelis, 1984; Ell, Mantell, Hamovitch, & Nishimoto, 1989; Fiore, 1979; Maguire, 1985; Northouse & Wortman, 1990; Speigel, 1979; Trillin, 1981)—a feeling of powerlessness resulting from the inability to predict or

have an impact on events surrounding the illness. Control issues are pronounced for cancer patients because of the clinical dimensions of the disease. Cancer carries with it a high degree of uncertainty about its cause, diagnosis, treatment, and prognosis. Patients in remission experience uncertainty about the possibility of recurrence (Harker, 1972; Mullan, 1984; Northouse, 1981; Peters-Golden, 1982; Schmale et al., 1983). In addition, the impact of the uncertainty is heightened, because cancer is often regarded as more threatening than other diseases (Brewin, 1977; Mishel, Hostetter, King, & Graham, 1984; Peters-Golden, 1982).

What are the implications of the control issue for patients' communication needs? Foremost is their need to experience an interpersonal environment that is predictable. They need contexts that allow them to regain a sense of communication competence. By promoting consistent patterns of interaction with patients, nurses can enhance patients' sense of control. Patients who are communicated with and treated in predictable ways will feel more competent about how they are handling their illness. Allowing a patient to communicate with the same nurse over the course of illness is one way of enhancing patients' sense of control. Similarly, attempts to establish routine procedures so that the same ones are followed with patients during repeated visits (e.g., taking temperatures, weighing patients, drawing blood) fosters a sense of stability. The purpose of such efforts is to give patients a sense of mastery over their environment.

In addition to providing a predictable environment, nurses can help patients gain a sense of personal control over their own internal response to the illness experience by communicating in ways that help patients to preserve a reasonable degree of emotional balance and to prepare for an uncertain future (Moos & Tsu, 1977). Although patients may not be able to control their illness, they can control, or have an impact on, their response to the illness through the messages, and therefore meanings, they give themselves about their circumstances. Nurses contribute to these meanings through their interactions with patients. For example, a newly diagnosed cancer patient expressed great relief when a nurse told him that it was normal to have irrational reactions to the diagnosis of cancer. This information confirmed for the patient that events were not out of control—that he was still in charge of what was happening.

Another aspect of control that is important for nurses to consider is that cancer patients wish to have a sense of control in their relationships with health care providers, family members, and others. Some patients want to be dominant toward providers; others want providers to be dominant. Both perspectives indicate a desire to influence the provider-patient relationship. Although many professionals are learning to share control with patients, some professionals still consider patients' desires for control a threat to their professional autonomy and power (Kelner & Bourgeault, 1993).

One major way that patients influence their relationships is to control their communication with others. By controlling what they talk about and how they talk about it, they may feel more in control of their relationships. For example, a patient may want to talk about the illness in a special way and, to that end, may force others to adapt to these expectations. Similarly, patients may want family members to play certain specific roles toward them and, as a result, communicate in ways that get family members to exhibit these roles. In other words, some patients attempt to satisfy their need for control by trying to control others.

Each patient is different, and each has an individual way of communicating. The challenge for nurses is to communicate with each patient in a way that gives the patient a sense of control. Above all, nurses must respond to patients in ways that allow patients to set the pace for the communication.

OBTAINING INFORMATION

In the last 3 decades, dramatic shifts have occurred in the amount of information providers give patients with cancer. In the early 1960s, physicians often did not inform these patients of their diagnosis (Oken, 1961); by the late 1970s, this pattern had been reversed (Novack et al., 1979). Despite this shift toward more open communication, however, acquiring sufficient medical information remains a primary concern for patients with cancer (Morrow, Hoaglund, & Carpenter, 1983; Mosconi, Meyerowitz, Liberati, & Liberati, 1991).

Obtaining information is important for patients who have cancer because it reduces their uncertainty concerning the illness. It gives them a framework for interpreting life-threatening events (Janis, 1958) and helps them feel that their responses to the uncertainties surrounding the illness are reasonable and normal (Buckalew, 1982; Dunkel-Schetter & Wortman, 1982). Waitzkin and Stoeckle (1972) go so far as to say that communicating information about illness can improve patients' physiologic and psychologic responses to therapy.

Given that information is important for patients, the following questions frequently confront oncology nurses: How much information do patients want? What kind of information is most important to them? When is it appropriate not to give information? Obviously, there are no easy or completely correct answers to these questions.

Cassileth, Zupkis, Sutton-Smith, and March (1980) studied the amount of information preferred by patients with cancer and found that most patients wanted maximum amounts of information. Those who sought detailed information tended to be younger, better educated, and more recently diagnosed than patients who avoided information. Other investigators have corroborated the finding that age is the critical factor in the amount of information desired (Derdiarian, 1986; Hopkins, 1986).

The kind of information patients want has been of interest to researchers also. Derdiarian (1986, 1987) studied the information needs of patients with cancer in four categories: disease, personal, family, and social. Of these four types of information, patients gave the

highest rank to the need for information about the disease. They were interested especially in obtaining information about treatments and prognosis. The importance of disease-related information to patients with cancer was reported also by Cassileth and colleagues (1980), who found that more than 50 per cent of the patients in their study wanted information about the side effects of treatments, treatment outcomes, the extent of disease, the potential for cure, and their day-to-day progress.

Although patients want information, they have difficulty obtaining it at times. Lerman and colleagues (1993) found that a number of communication problems existed between patients and their health care providers (Box 68–1), and these problems negatively affected patients' adjustment to their illness. In a study of a large number of individuals receiving chemotherapy, Love, Leventhal, Easterling, and Nerenz (1989) found that communication between patients and providers was often inadequate. Patients failed to receive necessary information about side effects from clinicians, and they also failed to fully inform clinicians of the complete picture of their treatment experience. Love et al., argue the need for more frequent and open provider-patient discussion of side effects and how to cope with them.

While patients usually perceive information as beneficial, some investigators have expressed the concern that information can disrupt mechanisms of denial and lead to loss of hope and depression (Bloom, Ross, & Burnell, 1978; Brewin, 1977; Kellerman, Rigler, Siegel, & Katz, 1980; McIntosh, 1974; Weisman & Worden, 1976), especially in patients who have extensive cancer. For example, Hopkins (1986) found that patients with advanced cancer sought less information than did patients with more limited disease, and she attributed

---

> ### Box 68–1. *Communication Problems Between Cancer Patients and Health Care Providers*
>
> This study examined breast cancer patients' (N=97) perceptions of their medical interactions with their health care providers. Patients completed a set of questionnaires prior to the initiation of postoperative treatment and again 3 months later. A majority of the patients (84 per cent) reported problems communicating with health professionals primarily in regard to understanding their physicians (49.5 per cent), expressing feelings (46.3 per cent), and asking physicians questions (42.6 per cent). Patients who reported more communication problems with health care professionals had higher levels of mood disturbance prior to the start of treatment and 3 months later. In addition, patients who reported a higher number of communication problems were less optimistic about their illness and felt more helpless about the disease.
>
> ---
>
> Reproduced with permission from Lerman, C. et al. (1993). Communication between patients with breast cancer and health care providers. *Cancer, 72,* 2612–2620.

this difference to the protective defense of avoidance. Similar results were reported by Gotay (1984), who compared groups of early- and late-stage cancer patients and their mates and found that information seeking was a more common coping mechanism in the early-stage group. Patients with advanced cancer used avoidance and denial relatively often. Because information can function both positively and negatively for patients, the challenge for oncology nurses is to assess each patient's unique needs for information and attempt to provide the amount and kind of information that will be most effective for that patient.

DISCLOSING FEELINGS

Another communication issue of concern to patients with cancer is self-disclosure, the process whereby one individual communicates personal information, thoughts, and feelings to others. Disclosing feelings is of critical importance for several reasons (Silver & Wortman, 1980). First, it allows catharsis, the draining of emotional tension and anxiety that often accompanies a cancer diagnosis. Second, it allows patients to receive feedback from others that their reactions to cancer are normal, which in turn lessens anxiety and tension associated with these reactions. Third, it facilitates problem solving and enables patients to view their situation from a more meaningful perspective.

Although disclosing feelings appears to help patients adjust to their illness, often they feel inhibited (Spiegel, 1979). For example, in a study of 256 patients with cancer, only 52 per cent of the patients told their friends and neighbors about the diagnosis; 32 per cent had told only their most intimate friends; and 16 per cent did not reveal the diagnosis to friends (Cassileth et al., 1980). In a study of patients undergoing radiation therapy, the majority of the patients reported that they wished they could discuss their situation more openly with someone (Mitchell & Glicksman, 1977).

Disclosure is often a problem for patients because other people may avoid them or prefer not to discuss sensitive illness-related issues with them. In a study by Byrne et al. (1984), adolescent patients reported that their friends stayed away after hearing about the diagnosis. Similarly, 52 per cent of the breast cancer patients in Peters-Golden's study (1982) said that others avoided them. The patients who did discuss the illness with others reported that the interactions were frequently uncomfortable. When others tried to cheer them up, this forced cheerfulness often made the patients feel less normal and hindered them from revealing their true feelings. Despite the problems surrounding disclosure, there is some indication that the more patients are able to discuss their illness with others, especially family members, the better their psychosocial adjustment to cancer (Gotcher, 1992) (Box 68–2).

What strategies can nurses and other health professionals use to help cancer patients disclose their feelings? First, they need to assess and adapt to each patient's unique preferences for disclosure. As Bradac, Tardy, and Hosman (1980) pointed out, different people have different styles of disclosure. Thus some patients may be able to share information, worries, and

---

BOX 68–2. *Interpersonal Communication and Psychosocial Adjustment to Cancer*

This study explored the relationship between communication, support, and psychosocial adjustment in 102 cancer patients receiving radiation therapy. Specific communication variables that were assessed included the frequency of patients' cancer-related communication, the honesty of their communication, and the degree to which they were able to discuss unpleasant topics related to their illness with their family members. Patients who reported more frequent communication, more honest communication, and who were able to discuss unpleasant topics with their family members reported fewer adjustment problems associated with the cancer. Discriminant function analysis indicated that the frequency of patients' communication with their family members and the amount of support that they perceived were the key variables that distinguished well-adjusted patients from maladjusted patients.

From Gotcher, J. M. (1992). Interpersonal communication and psychosocial adjustment. *Journal of Psychosocial Oncology, 10,* 21–39.

---

concerns about their illness without hesitation, whereas others may rely heavily on one or two family members and prefer not to disclose feelings to friends or health professionals.

A second factor to consider is the nature of the relationship between participants. Patients will feel more comfortable about disclosing their feelings within an established nurse-patient relationship. It is unrealistic to expect them to disclose personal feelings to nurses or other professionals with whom they have little contact. Therefore, nurses need to focus on increasing their relationship-oriented rather than task-oriented time with cancer patients. In addition, attention also needs to be directed toward assigning the same nurse to the same patient over an extended period.

A third important factor is the setting of the interaction. Fast-paced oncology units, which provide little privacy, are noisy, and are characterized by frequent interruptions, inhibit patients from disclosing their feelings. Thus nurses need to establish within units a private, confidential environment that allows for the expression of feelings.

SEARCHING FOR MEANING

A fourth concern confronting cancer patients is dealing with existential questions about the meaning of cancer and its impact on their lives. Cancer can disrupt virtually all aspects of the patient's life—everyday activities, short- and long-term goals, and the sense of worthiness and competence (Cantor, 1978). Everyone needs to view life as existentially meaningful, and cancer undermines this effort.

Communicating with patients about their efforts to find meaning and purpose is particularly important, because an increased sense of meaning appears to be related positively to satisfactory adjustment and coping

(Silver & Wortman, 1980; Taylor, 1993). Individuals who find personal meaning and value in their existence are better able to confront their circumstances (Frankl, 1963; Jourard, 1971; Spiegel, Bloom, & Yalom, 1981; Weisman & Worden, 1976). For example, Speigel et al. (1981) assessed the psychologic benefits of support groups for 86 patients with metastatic carcinoma and found that supportive, direct confrontation with life-and-death issues resulted in a sense of mastery rather than demoralization. In addition, they found that patients who received support felt less isolated, helpless, and worthless. Similarly, Weisman and Worden (1976) found that cancer patients who coped well accepted their diagnosis and treatment with little equivocation, talked with others to clarify their plight, and exhibited a more favorable attitude toward their illness.

The critical factor in helping patients with their struggles about meaning is effective interpersonal communication. Communication with others is the vehicle and the medium patients use to sort out, analyze, and clarify questions about meaning. In a study of two support groups composed of adolescent oncology patients, Byrne et al. (1984) found that all the group members struggled with questions such as "Why me? Why did I get cancer?" and with the development of a life-and-death philosophy. Within the context of the group, patients were able to interact with one another and sort out their existential concerns. On the basis of 4 years of experience with a therapy group for patients with metastatic carcinoma, Yalom and Greaves (1977) concluded that patients were helped by discussing existential issues. They found a greater sense of meaning and fulfillment the more they were able to move away from morbid self-absorption and into extending themselves to others. Further evidence for the significance of communication was provided by Johnson (1982), who found that patients with cancer who participated in a patient education course reported a greater sense of meaning in their lives.

ISSUES CONFRONTING NURSES

Although interpersonal communication is a transactional process, little research has been conducted on the problems confronting nurses as they communicate with patients with cancer. Most studies have focused on the patient half of the nurse-patient relationship. From the nurse's perspective, there are three issues of concern: imparting information, communicating hope, and dealing with emotions.

IMPARTING INFORMATION

Imparting information is an important aspect of the health professional's role, yet it is seldom an easy task. Many factors make imparting information a more complex process for professionals than it appears initially. First, patients have different levels of comprehension (Greenwald & Nevitt, 1982), different levels of competence (Schoene-Seifert & Childress, 1986), and, as discussed earlier, different preferences for information. Professionals should take these individual differences into consideration when imparting information.

Second, information-giving sessions typically occur within a short time period (Blanchard et al., 1983). This leaves little opportunity for questions, clarification, or even assessment of the extent to which the patient understands the information. Third, nurses' and patients' perceptions of what kind of information patients need can differ. For example, Lauer, Murphy, and Powers (1982) studied nurses' and patients' ranking of patients' educational needs and found that patients ranked information about "minimizing side effects" as their major need, whereas nurses ranked "dealing with feelings" as the patients' most important need. This example of discrepant perceptions highlights the difficulty and complexity of imparting information. Professionals need to be certain that they are addressing the patient's real informational needs, not simply projecting their own perceptions of those needs onto patients.

Nurses, in particular, face another problem in imparting information; often, they are not perceived as a legitimate source of information for patients. For years, when patients and family members asked a nurse for information about such basic facts as their blood pressure or temperature, the nurse told them to ask the physician. This practice distorted the patient's perceptions of nurses as legitimate providers of information. Although nurses' attitudes have changed and most nurses now recognize that it is within the scope of nursing practice to provide information, some evidence suggests that patients' and family members' perceptions of the nurse have not changed. For example, Dyck and Wright (1986) reported that the majority of family members of cancer patients in their study did not perceive the nurse as having a major information-giving role, and 27 per cent still believed that releasing information was contrary to the nurse's code of ethics and beyond the nurse's scope of practice. Some subjects reported that they hesitated to ask nurses for information because it would put the nurses in an awkward position. Patients perceive the physician to be the primary source of information about disease and treatment issues and less frequently cite the nurse (Dodd, 1982; Frank-Stromborg & Wright, 1984).

What strategies can the nurse use to facilitate imparting information to cancer patients and their families? First, nurses need to recognize the legitimacy of their role in providing patients with information, not only about actual and potential problems associated with cancer, but also about ways to alleviate or prevent potential problems (American Nurses Association, 1980). Next, nurses need to educate patients and family members that nurses are available to provide not only comfort and support, but also information that will enable patients to better understand and cope with their illness. Furthermore, given the hesitancy of some patients to seek information from nurses, nurses need to assume more responsibility for initiating discussions with patients and seeking out their questions about the illness. Finally, assessing patients for the amount and kind of information they want as well as for the degree to which they understand the information previously provided is an important aspect of imparting information.

COMMUNICATING HOPE

Because fear and uncertainty accompany a cancer diagnosis, communicating hope is another critical task facing nurses who work with cancer patients. Hope enables patients to move away from feeling weak and vulnerable and to function as fully as possible within the limits of their circumstances (Miller, 1985). Hope is fostered in patients through nurturing interactions with health professionals and others. It is provided by communicating in ways that enable patients to have positive expectations about their future, even though they face uncertain situations (Brewin, 1977; Holland, 1977; Nowotny, 1989). It also involves communicating in ways that help patients to feel inspired (Jourard, 1971), maintain their morale, and maximize their courage (Brewin, 1977).

In recent years there has been a growing interest in the role of hope in adjustment to cancer (Baird, 1989; Carver et al., 1993; Herth, 1989; Nowotny, 1989; Owen, 1989). Hinds and Martin (1988) studied the development of hopefulness in adolescents with cancer and found that it was a self-sustaining process that could be influenced by others, such as nurses. To achieve hopefulness in the face of health threats, adolescents went through four sequential phases: cognitive discomfort, distraction, cognitive comfort, and personal competence. Mishel and associates (1984) found a strong relationship between optimism and adjustment to illness in women with gynecologic cancer. Women who were pessimistic about their situation lacked confidence in the health care system and experienced more psychologic distress. Similar findings were reported by Carver and associates (1993), who found that breast cancer patients who were able to maintain a more optimistic outlook experienced less distress prior to surgery as well as at multiple assessment times following surgery. In a qualitative study of staff and cancer patients on a radiation therapy unit, Buehler (1975) found that patients live on a hope-doubt continuum that is strongly influenced by staff communication. Staff in this study maintained an ideology of hope exemplified by the message "we can help you," which they readily communicated to patients. The staff's hope was based on optimism about new advances in cancer research, new treatment methods, increased survival rates, and growing cooperation among cancer specialists.

What happens when health professionals fail to foster hope in cancer patients? Some reports suggest that patients may seek alternative or unorthodox methods of cancer treatment. For example, Holland (1981) contended that cancer patients who participated in a national study of Laetrile did so because they often felt that their physicians believed nothing more could be done for them. Physicians working with patients who had recurrent and disseminated cancer failed to communicate a sense of hope. Perceiving the physicians' attitude of hopelessness, patients sought alternative methods that at least offered some hope. Dunphy (1976) suggested that cancer patients' interest in Laetrile was related in part to the fact that professionals did not always inform patients that even in hopeless situations, arrests or remissions could occur.

Although hope appears to be essential for cancer patients, nurses and other health professionals hesitate to communicate hope at times for several reasons. First, some professionals believe that fostering hope in patients whose disease is extensive simply encourages denial and prevents patients from facing up to the seriousness of their illness. Although research indicates that selective denial may be a useful mechanism for protecting patients from hopelessness (Brewin, 1977; Cassileth et al., 1980; Wool & Goldberg, 1986), some professionals still view denial as maladaptive. Second, some professionals believe that they are being deceptive or providing false reassurance when they foster hope in patients who have a life-threatening disease. In an era of informed consent and malpractice suits, professionals tend to emphasize definitive disease-related information. Third, some professionals still equate hope with cure; thus they have difficulty offering hope to patients with extensive disease or to those receiving palliative treatments. Clearly, to communicate hope, professionals need to recognize that hope means the ability to maintain morale and courage (Brewin, 1977), not just the ability to eradicate disease.

To communicate hope, nurses and other health professionals need effective communication strategies. Miller and Knapp (1986) asked a sample of 60 ministers and 43 hospice workers to rate the appropriateness of seven different communication strategies used by caregivers in interactions with patients with cancer (Box 68–3). The respondents gave the highest ranking to the communication strategy called "Be Reflexive," which involved listening to the patient and "being there." This strategy was rated as the most important one during various time periods and across all emotional states. The communication strategy that received the second highest rating was "Be Demonstrative" (e.g., show affection), followed by "Be Definitive" (e.g., provide information). The communication strategy that received the lowest ranking was "Be Upbeat," which referred to focusing on happy, cheerful things and avoiding discussion of the illness. This study highlighted that communication that reflects the patient's feelings and allows the patient to control the agenda of the conversation was rated the most effective.

Other strategies help to maintain hope also. Miller (1985) suggested that nurses help patients focus on the moment, review their assets, maintain important relationships, and monitor signs of progress. Hickey (1986) encouraged nurses to foster hope by helping patients develop short-term, realistic, attainable goals. Patients with cancer, she suggested, have many interests but have difficulty planning because of the disease. Similarly, Owen (1989) encouraged nurses to help patients set temporary goals that will enable patients to cope with changing treatments or prognoses. Brewin (1977) contended that regardless of the prognosis, it is important for health care providers to give patients reassurance and encouragement, even if they have to focus on a narrow area such as symptom relief. Communicating to patients that they are not alone in their struggles facilitates hope also. No matter what their circumstances, patients need to know there is hope.

Box 68–3. *Communication Strategies with Cancer Patients*

Investigators asked 60 ministers and 43 hospice volunteers to rate the appropriateness of seven communication strategies used by caregivers in their interactions with dying cancer patients. Subjects rated the communication strategy called "Be Reflexive" (e.g., listen, be there) as the most appropriate strategy and the communication strategy called "Be Upbeat" (e.g., focus on cheerful topics) as the least appropriate strategy. Subjects also rated the appropriateness of each strategy across three stages of dying. Although "Be Reflexive" was rated as the most important strategy during each phase of dying, "Be Definitive" (e.g., provide information) and "Be Demonstrative" (e.g., show affection) were rated as important during the initial and middle phases of dying. "Be Demonstrative" was also rated important during the final phase of dying. When caregivers were asked to give advice to others on the best way to interact with dying patients, caregivers said to accept the patient, be honest and realistic, respond naturally, show emotional commitment, be with the patient as often as possible, and say little and listen.

From Miller, Y. D., & Knapp, M. L. [1986]. The post-nuntio dilemma: Approaches to communicating with the dying. In *Communication yearbook* [Vol. 8, pp. 723–738]. Beverly Hills, CA: Sage Publications. Reproduced by permission.

According to Holland (1977), another communication strategy for building hope is to offer a rational perspective of cancer. When health care providers express an attitude and a philosophy that cancer is treatable, they help patients to act rationally and to feel less anxious. Hope is provided by offering a rational course of action that reduces shock, fear, and anxiety.

DEALING WITH EMOTIONS

A third issue confronting oncology nurses is dealing with the tremendous array of emotions that surround the cancer experience. Cancer generates high levels of helplessness, fear, anger, and sadness in both patients and nurses. For the patient, these emotions emerge from the reality of having the disease. For the nurse, they arise out of the day-to-day stress of watching the patient suffering and attempting to alleviate that suffering. Nurses in one study reported that dealing with patients' feelings and managing their own feelings about cancer were formidable tasks (Craytor et al., 1978).

What difficulties do nurses encounter as they try to deal with patients' emotions? One difficulty is that they have their own fears about cancer, which can interfere with their ability to discuss and assuage patients' fears (Paulen & Kuenstler, 1978; Vachon, Lyall, & Freeman, 1978). In addition, they often feel overwhelmed when patients express strong emotions, such as anger and despair. Nurses in one study said they lacked the interpersonal and communication skills needed to handle the complex feelings expressed by cancer patients (Vachon et al., 1978). Furthermore, nurses feel frustrated and anxious when they cannot answer difficult, existential questions, such as "Why did I get cancer?" or "How long will I live?" (Paulen & Kuenstler, 1978).

Some evidence indicates that nurses use avoidance behaviors at times in attempting to deal with their feelings about cancer. Avoidance behaviors can take many forms; the most obvious one is to avoid spending time with patients. Quint (1965) found that nurses used nonverbal gestures that made it difficult for patients to initiate discussions or interrupted patients when the content of the conversations began to make them feel uncomfortable. Using linguistic analysis techniques,

Mood and Lakin (1979) found that nursing personnel engaged in avoidance by substituting pronouns such as *it* for negatively charged words such as *death*. Although such avoidance behaviors may help the nurse cope with anxiety initially, they are less useful in helping to resolve the deeper emotional issues experienced by both patients and nurses.

Although oncology nurses have difficulty at times dealing with their emotions, they are often in a position to deal with patients' feelings. Not only are they in close physical proximity to patients on a continual basis, but they are perceived by patients as the member of the health care team who is most likely to deal with emotional concerns. In a study by Karani and Wittshaw (1986), patients identified the nurse as the professional most likely to help them with concerns about sexuality, fears about their illness, and the impact of the illness on the lives of family members. Similarly, patients in a study by Frank-Stromborg and Wright (1984) reported that their interactions with the nurse provided them with emotional support.

If nurses are the professionals who are expected to deal with feelings, what communication strategies can help them to do so? First, because research suggests that the emotional profile of patients with cancer corresponds more closely to a stressed but normally functioning population than to a psychiatric population (Cassileth, Lusk, Miller, Brown, & Miller, 1985; Plumb & Holland, 1977), supportive rather than psychoanalytic techniques seem warranted. Listening appears to be among the most important supportive strategies available. Although active listening is often underrated, cancer patients and their primary caregivers identify listening consistently as one of the more important caring behaviors a nurse can demonstrate toward them (Larson, 1984; Ryan, 1992). Listening enables patients to ventilate, which in turn allows them to get a better grip on their own circumstances. Some clinicians believe that discussions about feelings should be introduced gradually (Wool & Goldberg, 1986). For example, they suggest starting with a factual question, such as "What symptom did you notice first?" then moving to questions about feelings, such as "How do you feel about your illness?" or "What effect is your illness having on your family?" Finally, the importance of the nurse's supportive presence cannot be overstated. The cancer literature is replete with personal accounts about the great value of "standing by" and "being with" patients. Patients often are helped by having another person who will tolerate their fear, uncertainty, anger, and discomfort (Wool & Goldberg, 1986).

SUMMARY

Effective interpersonal communication is essential for cancer patients and nurses. It is instrumental in helping patients cope with their fears and uncertainty about the disease, and it provides nurses with a central means for providing support as well as accomplishing health-related goals. Communication between nurse and patient is not simple; it is a complex process that involves an awareness of the many factors that affect both participants simultaneously. Effective communication depends on what is communicated (the content dimension) as well as how it is communicated (the relationship dimension).

Because communication is a transactional process, communication issues must be assessed from the perspectives of both the patient and the nurse. For patients, four concerns emerge: maintaining a sense of control; obtaining information that will reduce their uncertainty; disclosing feelings that will help them ventilate, solve problems, and receive feedback and support; and searching for meaning. Communication with supportive others enables patients to achieve a sense of mastery, obtain the information they need, disclose their feelings, and analyze and clarify the existential impact of cancer on their lives.

Nurses bring a different set of concerns and responsibilities to the nurse-patient interaction. First, they must deal with the questions of what and how much information to give patients. Second, they must determine how to communicate hope in ways that will encourage patients to function as fully as possible within the limits of their circumstances. Third, they must work through their own feelings about cancer as well as respond to patients' fears and anxieties.

Effective interpersonal communication is not a panacea for all of the problems nurses confront in the oncology setting. However, it is an important aspect of high-quality cancer care. Through an awareness of the many complex communication issues that exist in the oncology setting, nurses can help patients and family members cope with the impact of cancer.

REFERENCES

American Nurses Association. (1980). *Nursing: A social policy statement.* Kansas City, MO: Author.

Baird, S. (1989). Why hope now? *Oncology Nursing Forum, 16*(1), 9.

Berlo, D. K. (1960). *The process of communication.* New York: Holt, Rinehart & Winston.

Birdwhistell, R. L. (1970). *Kinesics and context.* Philadelphia: University of Pennsylvania Press.

Blanchard, C. G., Ruckdeschel, J. C., Blanchard, E. B., Arena, J. G., Saunders, N. L., & Malloy, E. D. (1983). Interactions between oncologists and patients during rounds. *Annals of Internal Medicine, 99,* 694–699.

Bloom, J. R., Ross, R. D., & Burnell, G. (1978). The effect of social support on patient adjustment after breast surgery. *Patient Counseling and Health Education, 2,* 50–59.

Bottorff, J. L. (1993). The use and meaning of touch in caring for patients with cancer. *Oncology Nursing Forum, 20*(10), 1531–1538.

Bradac, J. J., Tardy, C. H., & Hosman, L. A. (1980). Disclosure styles and a hint at their genesis. *Human Communication Research, 6,* 228–238.

Brewin, T. B. (1977). The cancer patient: Communication and morale. *British Medical Journal, 2,* 1623–1627.

Buckalew, P. G. (1982). On the opposite side of the bed: A nurse clinician's experiences with anxiety during chemotherapy. *Cancer Nursing, 5,* 435–439.

Buehler, J. A. (1975). What contributes to hope in the cancer patient? *American Journal of Nursing, 75,* 1353–1356.

Byrne, C. M., Stockwell, M., & Gudelis, S. (1984). Adolescent support groups in oncology. *Oncology Nursing Forum, 11*(4), 36–40.

Cantor, R. C. (1978). *And a time to live: Toward emotional well-being during the crisis of cancer.* New York: Harper & Row, Publishers.

Carver, C. S., Pozo, C., Harris, S. D., Noriega, V., Scheier, M. F., Robinson, D. S., Ketcham, A. S., Moffat, F. L., & Clark, K. (1993). How coping mediates the effect of optimism on distress: A study of women with early stage breast cancer. *Journal of Personality and Social Psychology, 65*(2), 375–390.

Cassileth, B. R., Lusk, E. J., Miller, D. S., Brown, L. L., & Miller, C. (1985). Psychosocial correlates of survival in advanced malignant disease? *New England Journal of Medicine, 312,* 1551–1555.

Cassileth, B. R., Zupkis, R. Y., Sutton-Smith, K., & March, Y. (1980). Information and participation preferences among cancer patients. *Annals of Internal Medicine, 92,* 832–836.

Cooper, A. (1982). Disabilities and how to live with them—Hodgkin's disease. *Lancet, 1,* 612–613.

Craytor, J. K., Brown, J. K., & Morrow, G. R. (1978). Assessing learning needs of nurses who care for persons with cancer. *Cancer Nursing, 1,* 211–220.

Derdiarian, A. K. (1986). Informational needs of recently diagnosed cancer patients. *Nursing Research, 35,* 276–281.

Derdiarian, A. K. (1987). Informational needs of recently diagnosed cancer patients. Part II. Method and description. *Cancer Nursing, 10,* 156–163.

Dodd, M. (1982). Assessing patient self-care for side effects of cancer chemotherapy—Part I. *Cancer Nursing, 5,* 447–451.

Dunkel-Schetter, C., & Wortman, C. B. (1982). The interpersonal dynamics of cancer: Problems in social relationships and their impact on the patient. In H. S. Friedman & M. R. DiMatteo (Eds.), *Interpersonal issues in health care* (pp. 69–100). New York: Academic Press.

Dunphy, J. E. (1976). On caring for the patient with cancer. *New England Journal of Medicine, 295,* 313–319.

Dyck, S., & Wright, K. (1986). Family perceptions: The role of the nurse throughout an adult's cancer experience. *Oncology Nursing Forum, 12*(5), 53–56.

Ell, K. O., Mantell, J. E., Hamovitch, M. B., & Nishimoto, R. H. (1989). Social support, sense of control, and coping among patients with breast, lung or colorectal cancer. *Journal of Psychosocial Oncology, 7*(4/5), 63–89.

Fiore, N. (1979). Fighting cancer—one patient's perspective. *New England Journal of Medicine, 300,* 284–289.

Frankl, Y. (1963). *Man's search for meaning: An introduction to logotherapy.* New York: Simon & Schuster.

Frank-Stromborg, M., & Wright, P. (1984). Ambulatory cancer patients' perceptions of the physical and psychosocial changes in their lives since the diagnosis of cancer. *Cancer Nursing, 7,* 117–130.

Friedman, H. S., (1979). Nonverbal communication between patients and medical practitioners. *Journal of Social Issues, 35,* 1–11.

Gordon, W., Friedenbergs, I., Diller, L., Rothman, L., Wolf, C., Ruckdeschel-Hubbard, M., Ezgchi, O., & Gerstman, L. (1977). *The psychological problems of cancer patients: A retrospective study.* Paper presented at the American Psychological Association Meeting. San Francisco, CA.

Gotay, C. C. (1984). The experience of cancer during early and advanced stages: The views of patients and their mates. *Social Science and Medicine, 18,* 605–613.

Gotcher, J. M. (1992). Interpersonal communication and psychosocial adjustment. *Journal of Psychosocial Oncology, 10*(3), 21–39.

Greenwald, H. P., & Nevitt, M. C. (1982). Physician attitudes toward communication with cancer patients. *Social Science and Medicine, 16,* 591–594.

Harker, B. L. (1972). Cancer and communication problems: A personal experience *Psychiatry in Medicine, 3,* 163–171.

Herth, K. A. (1989). Relationship between level of hope and level of coping response and other variables in patients with cancer. *Oncology Nursing Forum, 16*(1), 67–72.

Hickey, S. S. (1986). Enabling hope. *Cancer Nursing, 9,* 133–137.

Hinds, P., & Martin, J. (1988). Hopefulness and the self-sustaining process in adolescents with cancer. *Nursing Research, 37,* 336–339.

Hinton, J. (1981). Sharing or withholding awareness of dying between husband and wife. *Journal of Psychosomatic Research, 25,* 337–343.

Holland, J. C. (1977). Psychological management of cancer patients and their families. *Practical Psychology, 9,* 14–18.

Holland, J. C. (1981). Patients who seek unproven cancer remedies: A psychological perspective. *Clinical Bulletin, 11,* 102–105.

Hopkins, M. B. (1986). Information-seeking and adaptational outcomes in women receiving chemotherapy for breast cancer. *Cancer Nursing, 9,* 256–262.

Janis, I. L. (1958). *Psychological stress.* New York: John Wiley & Sons.

Johnson, J. L. (1982). The effects of a patient education course on persons with a chronic illness. *Cancer Nursing, 5,* 117–123.

Jourard, S. M. (1971). *The transparent self* (2nd ed.). New York: Van Nostrand Reinhold.

Karani, D., & Wittshaw, E. (1986). How well informed? *Cancer Nursing, 9,* 238–242.

Kellerman, J., Rigler, D., Siegel, S. E., & Katz, E. R. (1980). Disease-related communication and depression in pediatric patients. *Journal of Pediatric Psychology, 2,* 52–53.

Kelner, M. J., & Bourgeault, I. L. (1993). Patient control over dying: Responses of health care professionals. *Social Science and Medicine, 36*(6), 757–765.

Knapp, M. L., & Miller, G. R. (1985). *Handbook of interpersonal communication.* Newbury Park, CA: Sage Publications.

Larson, P. J. (1984). Cancer nurses' perceptions of caring. *Cancer Nursing, 9,* 86–91.

Lauer, P., Murphy, S., & Powers, M. (1982). Learning needs of cancer patients: A comparison of nurse and patient perceptions. *Nursing Research, 31,* 11–16.

Lerman, C., Daly, M., Walsh, W. P., Resch, N., Seay, J., Barsevick, A., Birenbaum, L., Heggan, T., & Martin, G.

(1993). Communication between patients with breast cancer and health care providers. *Cancer, 72*(9), 2612–2620.

Love, R. R., Leventhal, H., Easterling, D. V., & Nerenz, D. R. (1989). Side effects and emotional distress during cancer chemotherapy. *Cancer, 63*(3), 604–612.

Maguire, P. (1985). The psychological impact of cancer. *British Journal of Hospital Medicine, 34,* 100–103.

McCorkle, R. (1981). Communication approaches to effective cancer nursing care. In L. B. Marino (Ed.), *Cancer nursing* (pp. 405–419). St. Louis: C. V. Mosby Co.

McCorkle, R., & Hollenbach, M. (1983). Touch and the acutely ill. Paper presented at the Johnson and Johnson Pediatric Round Table #10: Touch. Key Largo, FL.

McIntosh, J. (1974). Processes of communication, information seeking and control associated with cancer: A selective review of the literature. *Social Science and Medicine, 8,* 167–182.

Mehrabian, A. (1971). *Silent messages.* Belmont, CA: Wadsworth.

Meyerowitz, B. E., Watkins, I., & Sparks, F. (1983). Quality of life for breast cancer patients receiving adjuvant chemotherapy. *American Journal of Nursing, 83,* 232–235.

Miller, J. F. (1985). Inspiring hope. *American Journal of Nursing, 85,* 22–25.

Miller, V. D., & Knapp, M. L. (1986). The *post nuntio* dilemma: Approaches to communicating with the dying. In *Communication yearbook* (Vol. 8, pp. 723–738). Beverly Hills, CA: Sage Publications.

Mishel, M., Hostetter, T., King, B., & Graham, V. (1984). Predictors of psychosocial adjustment in patients newly diagnosed with gynecological cancer. *Cancer Nursing, 7,* 291–299.

Mitchell, G. W., & Glicksman, A. S. (1977). Cancer patients: Knowledge and attitudes. *Cancer, 40,* 61–66.

Mood, D. W., & Lakin, B. A. (1979). Attitudes of nursing personnel toward death and dying: 1. Linguistic indicators of avoidance. *Research in Nursing and Health, 2,* 53–60.

Moos, R. H., & Tsu, V. D. (1977). The crisis of physical illness: An overview. In R. H. Moos (Ed.), *Coping with physical illness* (pp. 3–21). New York: Plenum Medical Book.

Morrow, G. R., Hoaglund, A. C., & Carpenter, P. J. (1983). Improving physician-patient communications in cancer treatment. *Journal of Psychosocial Oncology, 1,* 93–101.

Mosconi, P., Meyerowitz, B. E., Liberati, M. C., & Liberati, A. (1991). Disclosure of breast cancer diagnosis: Patient and physician reports. *Annuals of Oncology, 2*(4), 273–280.

Mullan, F. (1984). Re-entry: The educational needs of the cancer survivor. *Health Education Quarterly, 10,* 88–94.

Northouse, L. L. (1981). Mastectomy patients and the fear of cancer recurrence. *Cancer Nursing, 4,* 213–220.

Northouse, L. L. (1988). Social support in patients' and husbands' adjustment to breast cancer. *Nursing Research, 37,* 91–95.

Northouse, L. L., & Wortman, C. B. (1990). Models of helping and coping in cancer care. *Patient Education and Counseling, 15,* 49–64.

Northouse, P. G., & Northouse, L. L. (1987). Communication and cancer: Issues confronting patients, health professionals and family members. *Journal of Psychosocial Oncology, 5*(3), 17–46.

Northouse, P. G., & Northouse, L. L. (1992). *Health communication: Strategies for health professionals.* Norwalk, CT.: Appleton & Lange.

Novack, D. H., Plumer, R., Smith, R. L., Ochitill, H., Morrow, G. R., & Bennett, J. M. (1979). Changes in physicians' attitudes toward telling the cancer patient. *Journal of the American Medical Association, 241,* 897–900.

Nowotny, M. L. (1989). Assessment of hope in patients with cancer: Development of an Instrument. *Oncology Nursing Forum, 16*(1), 57–61.

Oken, C. (1961). What to tell cancer patients. *Journal of the American Medical Association, 86,* 86–94.

Owen, D. C. (1989). Nurses' perspectives on the meaning of hope in patients with cancer: A qualitative study. *Oncology Nursing Forum, 16*(1), 75–79.

Paulen, A., & Kuenstler, T. M. (1978). Learning to discuss the unmentionable. *Cancer Nursing, 1,* 197–199.

Peters-Golden, H. (1982). Breast cancer: Varied perceptions of social support in the illness experience. *Social Science and Medicine, 16,* 483–491.

Plumb, M. M., & Holland, J. (1977). Comparative studies of psychological function in patients with advanced cancer. I. Self-reported depressive symptoms. *Psychosomatic Medicine, 39,* 264–291.

Quint, J. C. (1965). Institutionalized practices of information control. *Psychiatry, 28,* 119–132.

Ryan, P. Y. (1992). Perceptions of the most helpful nursing behaviors in a home-care hospice setting: Caregivers and nurses. *American Journal of Hospice and Palliative Care, 9*(5), 22–31.

Schag, C. A., Ganz, P. A., Polinsky, M. L., Fred, C., Hirji, K., & Peterson, L. (1993). Characteristics of women at risk for psychosocial distress in the year after breast cancer. *Journal of Clinical Oncology, 11*(4), 783–793.

Schmale, A. H., Morrow, G. R., Schmitt, M. J., Adler, L. M., Enelow, A., Murawski, B. J., & Gates, C. (1983). Well-being of cancer survivors. *Psychosomatic Medicine, 45,* 163–169.

Schoene-Seifert, B., & Childress, J. F. (1986). How much should the cancer patient know and decide? *CA: A Cancer Journal for Clinicians, 36,* 85–94.

Silver, R. L., & Wortman, C. B. (1980). Coping with undesirable life events. In J. Garber & M. E. P. Seligman (Eds.). *Human helplessness: Theory and applications* (pp. 279–341). New York: Academic Press.

Spiegel, D. (1979). Psychological support for women with metastatic carcinoma. *Psychosomatics, 20,* 780–787.

Spiegel, D., Bloom, J. R., & Yalom, I. (1981). Group support for patients with metastatic cancer. *Archives of General Psychiatry, 38,* 527–533.

Spiegel, D., Bloom, J., Kraemer, H. D., & Gottheil, E. (1989). Effect of psychosocial treatment on survival in patients with metastatic breast cancer. *Lancet, 2* (8668), 888–891.

Taylor, E. J. (1993). Factors associated with meaning in life among people with recurrent cancer. *Oncology Nursing Forum, 20*(9), 1399–1407.

Thorne, S. (1988). Helpful and unhelpful communications in cancer care: The patient perspective. *Oncology Nursing Forum, 15*(2), 167–172.

Trillin, A. A. (1981). Of dragons and garden peas. *New England Journal of Medicine, 304,* 699–701.

Vachon, M. L. (1986). A comparison of the impact of breast cancer and bereavement: Personality, social support and adaptation. In S. Hobfoll (Ed.), *Stress, social support and women* (pp. 187–204). New York: Hemisphere.

Vachon, M. L. S., Lyall, W. A., & Freeman, S. J. J. (1978). Measurement and management of stress in health professionals working with advanced cancer patients. *Death Education, 1,* 365–375.

Waitzkin, H., & Stoeckle, J. D. (1972). The communication of information about illness: Clinical, sociological and methodological considerations. *Advances in Psychosomatic Medicine, 8,* 180–215.

Watzlawick, P., Beavin, J., & Jackson, D. D. (1967). *Pragmatics of human communication.* New York: W. W. Norton.

Waxler-Morrison, N., Hislop, G., Mears, B., & Kan, L. (1991). Effects of social relationships on survival for women with breast cancer: A prospective study. *Social Science and Medicine, 33*(2), 177–183.

Weisman, A. D., & Worden, J. W. (1976). The existential plight in cancer: Significance of the first 100 days. *International Journal of Psychiatry, 7,* 1–15.

Wool, M. S., & Goldberg, R. J. (1986). Assessment of denial in cancer patients: Implications for intervention. *Journal of Psychosocial Oncology, 4*(3), 1–14.

Yalom, I. D., & Greaves, C. (1977). Group therapy with the terminally ill. *American Journal of Psychiatry, 134,* 396–399.

CHAPTER

69

Patient and Family Education

Gloria A. Hagopian

To be active participants in health care, patients and families require knowledge. Knowledge enables patients to prevent illness, participate in early detection, adapt to illness, and manage health care problems. Providing such information to patients and their families is an important and often challenging role of the nurse.

DEFINITION OF PATIENT EDUCATION

Patient education involves providing experiences designed to help patients gain information about prevention, early detection, diagnosis, treatment, and care; cope with their diagnosis, long-term adjustments, and symptoms; and develop the skills, knowledge, and attitudes to maintain or regain health (Johnson & Blumberg, 1984; 1993). Patient education also should include the development of communication skills to enable patients to interact effectively with health care

personnel (Sharf, 1988). See definitions pertaining to patient education in Box 69–1.

THE FAMILY AND PATIENT EDUCATION

When providing cancer care, the entire family unit must be considered. The family must be involved in all phases of the teaching learning process to achieve optimum health outcomes (Billie, 1992). Although the first line of defense for the patient is the family, the entire family may be in crisis when cancer is diagnosed (Johnson & Lane, 1991). The diagnosis of cancer may create disruption and change the family forever. All aspects of family life are affected: coping patterns, communication, roles, relationships, values, and the future. The family must be assessed, and their learning needs as well as their perceptions of the patient's needs must be determined. In addition to determining needs, family strengths must be identified. It is important to assess the support and resources that

---

Box 69–1. *Definitions Pertaining to Patient Education*

Patient education. Experiences designed to help patients gain information about prevention, early detection, diagnosis, treatment, and care; cope with their diagnosis, long-term adjustments, and symptoms; and develop the skills, knowledge, and attitudes to maintain or regain health (Johnson & Blumberg, 1984, 1993).

Teaching. The passing of facts, ideas, and part of yourself to others, or the transmission of knowledge in a manner likely to stimulate interest and retention on the part of the learner.

Instruction. Any situation in which one individual intentionally influences the learning of another by structuring the environment in such a way that the latter will learn some desired behavior.

Learning. A relatively permanent change in behavior due to practice or experience.

Readiness. Being willing and able to make use of instruction.

Motivation. Emotional readiness to learn, or forces that move a person to action or inaction.

Behavioral objective. A written statement of an intended change in behavior.

Data from Hymovich, D. P., & Hagopian, G. A. (1992). *Chronic illness in children and adults: A psychosocial approach* (pp. 198–219). Philadelphia: W. B. Saunders Co.

---

the family will be able to provide (Hymovich & Hagopian, 1992).

HISTORIC PERSPECTIVE OF PATIENT EDUCATION

Historically, patient education appeared in the literature in the 1950s, when it was viewed as a factor that would enhance self-care and ultimately reduce health care costs (Johnson & Blumberg, 1984). In 1964 the American Hospital Association (AHA) decided to act as the agency to stimulate patient education programs. An outgrowth of this was "A Patient's Bill of Rights" approved by the AHA in 1973, a document that addresses patients rights (AHA, 1975). Several of these rights pertain to education and state that people have the right to know about diagnosis, treatment, prognosis, alternative treatments, and what resources are available for living with disease.

Another important document is the *Outcome Standards for Cancer Patient Education*, developed by the Education Committee of the Oncology Nursing Society to identify the knowledge needed by patients to maximize their ability to live with cancer (ONS, 1982, 1989). The standards provide guidelines for developing, implementing, and evaluating formal and informal patient/family teaching and public education programs. They are based on the premise that all people with cancer have a right to information about cancer prevention, early detection, disease process, options for treatment, consequences and prognosis of treatment, self-care activities, and community resources (ONS, 1982). The standards specify that the patient or family member should be able to:

- Describe the illness, goals, and plan of therapy, potential risks and benefits, and available alternative therapies.
- Assume an active role in decision making and identification of needs with respect to the development, implementation, and evaluation of the plan of care.

- Describe behaviors that promote a level of independence appropriate to age, developmental stage, learning ability, resources, personal preference, prognosis, and physical ability.
- Demonstrate psychomotor and coping skills required for self-care.
- Describe methods to modify behavior for health promotion and cancer prevention, detection, and control.
- Describe signs and symptoms that should be reported to the health care team.
- Discuss affective and interpersonal responses to cancer treatment and care.
- Identify community and personal resources available for health promotion and cancer care (ONS, 1989, p. 8).

BENEFITS OF PATIENT EDUCATION

There are many benefits of patient education. They include adherence to a therapeutic regimen, increased satisfaction, enhanced self-determination with increased ability to handle symptoms, enhanced outcomes after surgery, independent functioning, and self-management (Fernsler & Cannon, 1991). Studies have shown that patient education results in increased knowledge, enhanced self-care, and improved psychologic and physical status. In addition, other outcomes are more timely hospital discharges, increased productivity, more appropriate use of services, reduced need for acute care, and reduction of malpractice suits.

Several studies indicated that family involvement in the educational experience improved physiologic outcomes in children (Mahaffy, 1965); decreased hospital stay and the number of narcotics (Dziurbejko & Larkin, 1978); decreased anxiety in patients (Doerr & Jones, 1979); and decreased fears about addiction and pain medication tolerance (Rimer et al., 1987).

Lindemann (1989) reviewed the literature on patient education and summarized that:

- Education has an impact on patient learning, especially in the area of knowledge and skills.

- Most teaching strategies are effective.
- Group teaching, often preferred by patients, is as effective as individual teaching and may lead to other benefits.
- All patient groups respond to education.

SELF-CARE

More and more consumers have accepted responsibility for their own health care. This self-care approach requires education support from the health care profession, for knowledge enables people to be active participants in their care and manage their health care problems. "Self care is the practice of activities that individuals personally initiate and perform on their own behalf in maintaining life, health and well-being" (Orem, 1991, p. 13). When a patient needs assistance in learning and performing self-care activities, it is the role of the nurse to provide the necessary assistance.

Dodd (1982, 1983, 1984) studied the effects of various interventions on patients undergoing radiation and chemotherapy. She demonstrated that patients were able to initiate self-care behaviors sooner when they had an opportunity to participate in patient education (see Chapter 5, Self-Care).

SYSTEMATIC PLANNING FOR PATIENT EDUCATION

Successful patient education should be based on a systematic plan. In the first stage, assessment of patients' needs occur, and goals and objectives are identified. This crucial planning stage lays the groundwork for development of the teaching program. In the second stage, educational methods and materials are selected. Next, the materials identified are further developed and tested. The implementation stage follows. The effectiveness of the patient education is assessed in the evaluation stage. In the last stage, feedback obtained is used to revise and refine the teaching program, and the process begins again (Blumberg & Gentry, 1991).

ASSESSMENT OF NEEDS

The stress of hearing a diagnosis of cancer may inhibit a patient's ability to remember information, and often, repetition of the information is needed (Johnson & Blumberg, 1984). Family members also may be emotionally upset at the diagnosis. The family is an important source of support and care for the patient, and they also need support and information, both for themselves and to help the patient (Johnson & Blumberg, 1984). Family members must be assessed, and their learning needs as well as their perceptions of the patient's needs must be determined. The family can be a good source of information about the home environment. In addition to determining needs, family strengths must be identified. It is important to assess the potential support and resources that the family will be able to provide. Educational needs change, so

assessment must become a process throughout the diagnosis and treatment phases of illness (Morra, 1991). Assessment allows time for the nurse to establish good rapport with the patient and create a trusting, open climate that is an essential condition for learning.

KINDS OF INFORMATION PATIENTS AND FAMILIES NEED

Because people are very unique in the way they handle information, careful assessment is essential before teaching. Some people will need considerable information, whereas others may need very little. Others may need ongoing education that provides frequent contact and reinforcement.

Morra (1985) analyzed calls received by a Cancer Information Service and found that patients sought information early in the diagnostic process and that their search for information continued through treatment. Family members and friends began asking questions later and asked more questions about treatment than any other issue.

Weisman, Worden, and Sobel (1980) identified seven areas of concern that influence patients with cancer. The seven areas are:

1. health concerns including all aspects related to medical care;
2. self appraisal, self concept, and acceptance by others;
3. work and financial concerns;
4. family and significant relationships;
5. religion;
6. friends and associates; and
7. existential concerns.

The learning needs of 50 patients and family members were identified by Johnson (1979). The ten concerns identified were:

1. acquiring accurate and current information;
2. adjusting to changes in body image and self-concept;
3. learning how to express feelings about the disease;
4. readjusting major responsibilities;
5. determining the impact of disease on finances;
6. reinforcing basic life philosophy;
7. establishing a sense of hope;
8. developing meaningful interpersonal relationships with family, friends, and medical personnel;
9. identifying resources; and
10. recognizing myths about the treatment and disease.

These studies underscore the need for systematic approaches to patient and family education.

THEORIES OF PATIENT EDUCATION

Changing health behaviors is often a difficult and time-consuming challenge, for it may require changing a person's lifestyle. Several theories and models explain how, when, and why learning occurs and can provide direction when teaching patients with cancer and their families. These theories can be used in all phases of the nursing process. The Theory of Motivation, the Health Belief Model, the Protection Motivation Theory, and the Theory of Reasoned Action can be integrated into educational programs to obtain a change in behavior (Padilla & Bulcavage, 1991). Many of these value expectancy models are based on Lewin's work, founded on the assumption that people behave according to how they perceive the world, and they are most attracted to things in the world they value (Marion, 1991). That is, people look for reward and avoid things they view as negative. Action is determined by expectation. The notion of self-efficacy (believing that one can successfully perform the desired behavior), social support, and influence are important factors that can reduce stress and bolster a person's efforts to stop a harmful behavior (Marion, 1991).

The Theory of Motivation, formulated by Atkinson (1964), implies that if patients value certain outcomes, then it is expected they will be motivated to follow through on activities to achieve the outcome. The Fishbein Model or Theory of Reasoned Action states that attitudes and social norms predict behavioral intentions and, in turn, predict behavior (Ajzen & Fishbein, 1980). Using this theory, patients' values influence their intentions, and consequently their behavior. Rosenstock's Health Belief Model says that people will take health actions if they believe they are susceptible, that the disease is serious, that the benefits outweigh the barriers, and there is a cue to action (Rosenstock, Strecher, & Becker, 1988). If people believe in the benefits of taking action against a serious disease, then they will carry out the required actions, given the proper cues. The Interaction Model of Client Health Behavior addresses the relationships between the client's attributions and needs, the health professional's interventions, and the health outcomes that result (Cox, 1982). These theories can explain or predict health care behavior, and it is critical that health care professionals use these theories to guide assessment and interventions. A multitheory approach may be necessary when working with patients and their families to account for individual differences.

FACTORS THAT AFFECT LEARNING

READINESS TO LEARN

Patients must be ready to learn. The timing of teaching is important and is often determined by readiness for learning. A patient who perceives a need and is ready to learn will learn more efficiently and effectively. The nurse should assess the factors that can interfere with readiness to learn. These factors include the following.

Comfort. Discomfort and preoccupation from both physical and psychologic factors can interfere with learning. Physical factors such as nausea, pain, or other side effects of treatment may impede learning. Fear,

anxiety, depression, shock, anger, guilt, anxiety, disbelief, self-pity, grief, or bitterness are some of the emotional discomforts that can disrupt the learning process (Johnson & Blumberg, 1984).

Energy. This is often closely related to a person's physical activities and body rhythms. Patients who are fatigued, weak, or lack energy may have a decreased ability to learn.

Motivation. People have various motivations. Some motivations are internal, such as a need to return to work or to enjoy a higher level of wellness, whereas others are external, such as to be praised by others. Internal motivation is usually longer lasting than external motivation, which frequently must be reinforced by praise or rewards (Redman, 1993). In general, success is more motivating than failure, so goals should be realistic and achievable.

Capacity. A person's capacity for learning includes physical and cognitive capabilities. People with severe deficits, such as those with physical and mental handicaps, may not be able to learn as readily as those who are not handicapped (Babcock & Miller, 1994).

ESTABLISHING OBJECTIVES AND PRIORITIES

Once learning needs have been identified and readiness has been established, the next step is to identify what is to be learned and the priorities for teaching this information. Several questions should be answered (Hymovich & Hagopian, 1992). These questions include the following:

1. Who are the recipients of the teaching? Is it the patient, family, or significant other?
2. What are the content and the goals of the teaching? Specific content will be determined by the assessment of the learning needs. Goals should be mutually determined.
3. When is the appropriate time for the teaching to occur?
4. Where will the teaching take place?
5. Why is the teaching necessary? What is its purpose?
6. How will the teaching be done? What is the best method? What is available? Are there booklets, audiotapes, models, or films that can be used to supplement teaching?

DOMAINS OF LEARNING

There are three domains or categories of learning: cognitive, affective, and psychomotor (Bloom, Englehart, Furst, Hill, & Krathwohl, 1956). The cognitive domain is concerned with thinking or intellectual activity. It involves judging, recalling, making decisions, considering, and drawing inferences. The affective domain is concerned with feelings, emotions, and attitudes. Learning physical skills, tasks, and procedures composes the psychomotor domain. This type of learning is the most concrete and the easiest to teach and measure (Babcock & Miller, 1994).

BEHAVIORAL OBJECTIVES

Behavioral objectives or statements of intended change in the learner's behavior should be established. Written objectives can serve as guides in both planning and evaluating teaching. An objective should have three parts (Billie, 1992). These parts include the following: (1) A behavior or task statement that tells what the patient will be able to do. This is the most important part of establishing an objective, and it should have an action verb. An example of a task statement is "will apply a colostomy bag." (2) The criterion, or achievement statement, refers to standards, time, or amount of information to be learned. Examples of achievement statements are ". . . so it doesn't leak," or ". . . within 10 minutes," or "will list 4 of 7 side effects . . . ." (3) Conditions under which you want the patient to perform or demonstrate mastery. Not all objectives will include conditions, and sometimes the conditions will be in the form of a preface statement such as "At the end of a teaching session on chemotherapy, . . .," or "Using the daily menu, the patient will select . . . ."

ESTABLISHING PRIORITIES

Behavioral objectives should be learner-centered, realistic, individual, observable, measurable, and mutually established with the patient and family. Once they are written, the objectives should be prioritized by determining the information the patient must know, should know, and could know.

Must Know. This is core information that people must know for their own protection, safety, and well being. During an acute phase of illness, this is all of the crucial information a patient must understand and do to survive.

Should Know. This is valuable and interesting information that can be taught in the acute phase of illness if there is time. After the crisis is over, patients should have information in this category to manage their health problems.

Could Know. This consists of information that is "nice to know." These learning needs represent knowledge, skills, and attitudes that might be essential sometime in the future. If patients are interested and motivated and have learned what they must and should know, it is appropriate to teach information in this category (Hymovich & Hagopian, 1992).

LEARNING CONTRACTS

Learning contracts are mutually arrived at agreements between the patient and health provider about goals to be achieved. Contracts can be effective strategies for promoting positive health outcomes (Hymovich & Hagopian, 1992). The contract is based on the principle of positive reinforcement. Key components of a contract include focusing on the behaviors that will lead to the goal, identifying small steps that the patient believes are realistic, describing a set of steps that lead to a goal that is important to the patient, recording of patient behaviors, and providing personally meaningful rewards to the patient (Chewning, 1982). In addition, the contracts should be written, time-dated, positive, and evaluated (Herje, 1980). Although contracts can be time-consuming and require commitment, responsibility, and follow-up, patients who are actively involved in the process are more likely to internalize the new health behaviors (Chewning, 1982).

PRINCIPLES OF TEACHING AND LEARNING

There are a number of principles of teaching and learning that can guide nurses in their educational interventions (Hymovich & Hagopian, 1989). These principles include the following:

1. Individual characteristics influence learning. Heredity, environment, as well as goals, values, attitudes, beliefs, aspirations, and desires have an influence on learning. The more the nurse knows about the patient's characteristics, background, and goals, the more likely it is that teaching effectiveness can be maximized.
2. A comfortable, quiet environment enhances learning. Therefore, try to find a quiet room without distractions so the patient can concentrate. This can often be difficult to find in a busy setting.
3. Motivation influences learning. People learn those things they believe are important and interesting. They are less likely to learn those things that they believe are unimportant and are not of interest to them. A thorough assessment may make it easier to find ways to make the information more relevant to the patient.
4. Effective communication enhances teaching. Good communication skills are crucial. It is important to make no assumptions, define all terms, be succinct, and to present things as simply and clearly as possible when teaching.
5. Set aside time for teaching. Appointments should be made for teaching sessions. Teaching should not just be incidental or if time allows, but nurses should capitalize on teachable moments.
6. Teaching sessions should be short and meaningful. Attention usually starts off high, but interest drops, and fatigue and boredom set in. Make important points early, reinforce frequently, and summarize at the end of the session, for people tend to remember things said at the beginning and at the end of a teaching session. Do not try to impart too much information at one time. It is better to teach a little thoroughly than a lot superficially. Teaching basic principles is essential.
7. Involve the learner. An active person learns more effectively than a passive one. The more involved the patient is in the learning process, the more learning that will take place. Some strategies to involve the learner include frequent practice, discovery learning (letting the patient learn information on his or her own), or drawing up a written contract with the patient.

8. Transfer learning from one situation to another. Try to build on what the patient already knows by going from the simple to the complex and from the known to the unknown. Capitalize on the experiences patients bring to the situation. Use analogies to explain new concepts.

9. Provide for practice. It is important to allow the learner time to practice new skills. About 10 percent of the teaching session should be devoted to a short explanation, followed by a demonstration that takes about 25 per cent of the allotted time. The majority of time, or 65 per cent of the time should be spent allowing the patient to practice the steps of the new skill. Practice is effective because it actively involves the learner.

10. Reinforcement is important. Positive feedback will reinforce learning and increase the likelihood that the behavior will be repeated. Success enhances motivation.

11. Provide feedback. Periodic evaluation should be done to measure the attainment of the objectives. Frequent feedback about progress, mistakes, and successes will enhance learning.

MEMORY

The average adult can remember five to seven unrelated items at one time. Retention can be increased by keeping the message short and simple and using words that are familiar to the patient. Items should be arranged in a meaningful context, and concrete examples rather than abstract ones should be used. New information should be associated with information that is already known. Examples, analogies, drawings, or pictures can aid retention. Asking the patient to repeat the information in his or her own words may assist in retention (Doak, Doak, & Root, 1985).

It is easier for people to remember what they see in pictures than for them to remember what they hear. Eighty-five per cent of everything a person comprehends and remembers is learned through seeing, 11 per cent is obtained through hearing, and 4 per cent of what is remembered comes from tasting, touching, or smelling. Since hearing is one of the most passive activities we can undertake, talking alone does not encourage the optimum of learning experiences. For each sense that is added to the teaching process, the individual becomes more active and more efficient (Billie, 1981). Therefore, the nurse should supplement a discussion with visual materials to enhance the learning process.

SPECIAL CONSIDERATIONS FOR VARIOUS AGE GROUPS

While the general principles are related to all patients, there are some special considerations for various age groups.

CHILDREN

Children need information that is developmentally appropriate. Children acquire most behaviors through simple conditioning (a stimulus followed by a response), discovery learning (learning on one's own), trial and error, practice, imitation, and association. Techniques to use with children include using simple explanations that draw on the children's own experiences, supplementing verbal explanations with pictures, role playing, and having the children explain what they have been told to reveal understandings, distortions, and misinterpretations. Preschool and school-aged children who are at the preoperational and concrete operational levels of thinking have difficulty understanding abstract information, so the nurse should use concrete, familiar examples when teaching children. Cues can be taken from children by asking them what they want to know (Babcock & Miller, 1994).

THE ADULT LEARNER

Adult patients and their families also have special learning needs. Knowles (1973) makes four points about the adult learner concerning self-concept, the role of experience, readiness to learn, and orientation to learning.

Self Concept. Adults perceive themselves as self-directed people. As adults mature, their self-concept moves from one of total dependency to one of increasing self-directedness. Once people achieve this concept of self-direction, they have a deep psychologic need to be perceived by others as being self-directed. Tension develops if adults are put in a situation where they cannot be self-directing. It is, therefore, essential when working with patients and families to allow them to be as self-directing as they want to be.

Role of Experience. Adults have an accumulated reservoir of experience that is a valuable learning resource. As people mature, their accumulated experiences provide them with a broad base on which to relate new learnings. It is important to recognize family members as unique individuals with wide experience and make use of their experiences as a resource for future learnings.

Readiness to Learn. The learning motivation of adults is oriented toward the tasks of their social roles. As people mature, their readiness to learn is decreasingly the product of their biologic development and academic pressure, and increasingly the product of developmental tasks required for the performance of social roles. Adults are ready to learn the things they need to know.

Orientation to Learning. The time perspective of adult learning activities is geared to immediacy of application. While children have a subject-centered orientation to learning, adults have a problem-centered orientation. When adults experience some inadequacy in dealing with current life problems, they seek information to solve the problem, and they want to apply what they have learned immediately. The problems of patients and families are urgent and require immediate attention. See Box 69–2 for adult learning principles.

THE OLDER ADULT

Although the elderly compose 13 per cent of the population, about 55 per cent of the total incidence of cancer occurs in persons over 65 years of age (Yancik & Reis, 1991). The psychologic and physiologic effects of aging and the many attitudes and beliefs of a lifetime of acquired knowledge and experience must be considered when teaching the elderly.

PHYSIOLOGIC CHANGES IN THE ELDERLY RELATED TO TEACHING AND LEARNING

There are many physiologic changes that occur in the elderly that may interfere with the learning process. The eye lens allows less light to pass through to the retina, and structural changes impair visual acuity. Sensitivity to sound decreases with a loss of high-frequency sounds and poor discrimination of consonants. Also, the reaction time slows, short-term memory decreases, the attention span shortens, and more time is needed to process information than in younger people (Hallburg, 1976).

These age-related changes require that information be divided into short sentences, with words spoken slowly. When teaching the older patient, stand or sit directly in front of the person and speak in a low tone of voice in a quiet environment (Welch-McCaffery, 1986). During teaching sessions use simple language, a positive tone, be concrete, and give only relevant information. The information should be repeated to reinforce essential points (Theis, 1991; Weinrich & Boyd, 1992). Verbal information should be supplemented with written instructions that are in large, simple print with illustrations. Make sure the reading level is appropriate for the audience. Only one third of people 65

years and older have completed 8 years of school (United Bureau of the Census, 1989). However, by the turn of the century, 64 per cent of the elderly will be high school graduates. Like all learners, the elderly learn best when they are actively involved.

The elderly are often resistant to change, cautious in new situations, and have difficulty in unlearning well-established ways of doing things (Van Hoozer, 1994). Although the speed of learning new things decreases with age, there is little decrease in the capacity to learn (Botwinic, 1978) (see Box 69–3).

EVALUATION OF EDUCATIONAL MATERIALS

USES OF EDUCATIONAL MATERIALS

The use of educational materials is an effective method of teaching. Prepared materials may be used to teach a wide variety of subjects and are efficient in terms of saving time. Educational materials can be used to teach new information, reinforce previously taught information, or provide remedial information. Sometimes, nurses are reluctant to reteach when someone has had a health problem for a number of years. Often, it is assumed the patient is knowledgeable about the disease and its management. In these instances, educational materials can be used to provide remedial information in a nonthreatening way.

EVALUATING WRITTEN MATERIALS

Although there are many commercially prepared educational materials available for teaching patients, it is important for the nurse to evaluate existing materials and select those that are appropriate. Frank-Stromborg and Cohen (1991) list several factors to consider when

---

Box 69–2. *Adult Learning Principles*

Adults should be involved in all stages of the learning process, from planning to evaluation.
Learning should be problem-centered.
Learning should be experience-centered. Share experiences.
The learning process should be meaningful and relevant.
Objectives should be mutually set.
Inquiry should be self-directed.
The learning climate should be open. Adults should be free to explore areas of interest.
Adults like a comfortable environment.
Adults must have feedback about progress toward goals.
Treat the learner as an adult.
Adults do not like to have their time wasted.
Help adults to develop problem-solving skills.
Adults may have many things competing for their attention.
Provide a variety of learning methods.
Be a resource person to adults.
The locus of responsibility for learning lies with the learner. The teacher helps the learner learn for himself.

Data from Knowles, M. S. (1973). *The adult learner: A neglected species.* Houston: Gulf Publishing; and Hymovich, D. P., & Hagopian, G. A. (1989). The teaching role of the office nurse. *Office Nurse, 2*(5), 30–32.

Box 69–3. *Research Box*

Weinrich, S. P., Weinrich, M. C., Frank-Stromborg, M., Boyd, M. D., & Weiss, M. D. (1993). Using elderly educators to increase colorectal cancer screening. *The Gerontologist, 33*(4), 491–496.

Five older people ranging in age from 58 to 80 years were hired as educators and demonstrators for their peers in a colorectal cancer project. The study tested four educational methods on participation in fecal occult blood screening, with elderly educators used in two of the methods. One hundred seventy-one socioeconomically disadvantaged older persons participated at 11 randomly selected sites. The two groups that used elderly educators had an overall response rate of 60 per cent of participants returning the hemoccult kits, a statistically significant difference from the groups that did not use elderly educators. The authors conclude that the elderly educator method is a practical and economical intervention.

evaluating the educational materials. The following questions should be asked:

- Is the content accurate, up to date, and of sufficient breadth and depth?
- Is the content organized logically?
- Does the content achieve the objectives you want to accomplish?
- Is the material interesting?
- Is the material divided into short sections with appropriate headings?
- Are the key points emphasized?
- Is the material written at the proper level for the audience?
- Are the facts presented objectively?
- Is the print clear and readable with appropriate illustrations?
- Is there a summary?
- Is the material written by knowledgeable health professionals?
- Is there any indication of the effectiveness of the materials?
- Are the materials cost-effective?

No matter what format you use, the main purpose of the materials should be to communicate information in a manner that attracts attention, emphasizes important points, reads easily, and looks pleasing.

PRINCIPLES OF PREPARING EDUCATIONAL MATERIALS

USE OF PRINCIPLES OF PREPARING MATERIALS

In many instances appropriate patient educational materials are not available, and nurses may have to produce their own pamphlets, information sheets, posters, flip charts, self-learning modules, newsletters, or audiotapes. These materials can supplement those that are commercially available. There are several principles to keep in mind when preparing educational materials, regardless of the format. They include simplicity, unity, emphasis, balance, and legibility (Hagopian & Hymovich, 1990).

SIMPLICITY

The key to the effective presentation of educational materials is simplicity. The content, message, and design should be simple.

UNITY

Elements of the page should function together, providing unity and continuity.

EMPHASIS

Important elements can be emphasized by increasing its size and using color, space, or placement.

BALANCE

"Formal balance" is equally balanced and symmetric and is often used for titles, whereas "informal balance" is asymmetric, dynamic, and may be more attention-getting.

LEGIBILITY

Select a simple lettering style that is easy to read. Tall thin letters are difficult to read, as are square corners on letters, script writing, and gothic lettering such as calligraphy. The use of all capital letters should be avoided except for short titles (Doak et al., 1985). As a general rule, capital letters should be combined with lower case letters for phrases that are six words or more. Letters should be spaced optically to make them appear equal rather than measuring equal distances between letters. Words should be organized horizontally rather than vertically or in a stair-step fashion. Words should not be strung out across a page, but organized in columns like a newspaper.

READING LEVEL

It has been estimated that one in five Americans is illiterate and 23 million Americans read at the fifth-grade level or below (Doak et al., 1985). It is thought that people hear or read and comprehend information at a level that is two grades lower than the highest grade level completed (Hymovich & Hagopian, 1992). Several tests are available to test a person's reading ability. One quick way to measure functional reading level is the Wide Range Achievement Test (WRAT). The person is asked to pronounce words from a 100-

word graded list. When three words are mispronounced, the test is stopped and scored. The score is compared with the equivalent grade rating. Although vocabulary and comprehension are not tested, the test takes only 5 minutes to administer. It is suggested that unless the level of the audience is known, educational materials should be prepared between the sixth- and eighth-grade level (Doak et al., 1985).

READING LEVEL FORMULAS

There are several formulas to determine the reading level of written materials. They include the Frey Formula, the Ragor Readability Estimate, the Flesch Formula, and the Fog Index (Redman, 1993), although the National Cancer Institute recommends the SMOG Formula, developed by McLaughlin (1969). The quickest and easiest formula to use is the Fog Index (Redman, 1993). See Box 69–4 for the formula for the Fog Index. In addition to the above formulas, several computer programs are available that will compute a reading level analysis. For example, Berta Max produces a Reading Level Analysis Program (1985), as does Rightwriter (1990). See Box 69–5 for research that analyzes reading levels of cancer information booklets.

WRITTEN MATERIAL

Write in a conversational, active voice. Keep the concept density (ease of understanding) reduced by using short words, short sentences, and keeping the message simple. Advance organizers, such as headers or subtitles, should be used to alert the reader to what is coming. If possible, reinforcement, review, and feedback should be built into the written material. A summary should be provided (Doak, et al., 1985). Guidelines for written materials are in Box 69–6.

PREPARING EDUCATIONAL MATERIALS

PAMPHLETS AND INFORMATION SHEETS

Pamphlets and one-page information sheets are commonly used and fairly easy to produce. These handouts are good supplements to a discussion, because patients can take them home, share them with family members, and refer to them when needed.

POSTERS

Successful posters are simple, eye-catching, clear, and concise. Posters can be prepared by writing directly on a poster board, or preparing a number of items to attach to the board, such as typed information, charts, photographs, or silhouettes. The guidelines for preparing posters are in Box 69–7.

FLIPCHARTS

Almost any topic can be selected for a flipchart format, such as giving an injection, testing for blood glucose, or preparing for surgery. A flipchart can be constructed as a series of miniposters. Flipcharts can be used along with a discussion or can be read by the patient alone.

NEWSLETTERS

Newsletters can be used to share information with patients. A newsletter can be produced using a computer with a special software package or can be prepared like a pamphlet or information sheet (Hagopian, 1991).

SELF-DIRECTED LEARNING MODULES

A self-directed learning module is an instructional unit that focuses on a few well-defined behavioral objectives, contains all of the materials or directions needed to accomplish the objectives, and presents information in small segments. It provides for active involvement with the content, gives feedback about the progress and level of mastery, and is designed for independent use (Thompson, 1978).

The format for arranging the components of a learning module is as follows (deTornyay & Thompson, 1982):

1. Table of Contents. Divide the module into short sections.
2. Introduction. Include purpose, objectives, and directions for use of the module.
3. List of prerequisite knowledge and skills.

BOX 69–4. *Instructions for the Fog Index*

Select the text, then:
1. Count off 100 words (Words).
2. Count the number of sentences in these 100 words (Sentences).
3. Count the number of words with three or more syllables (Hard). Do not count proper nouns or verbs ending in "ed" or "es" that make the third syllable, or combination words.
4. Use the formula:
   Grade level = (Words/Sentences + Hard) × 0.4.

Data from Redman, B. K. (1993). *The process of patient education.* St. Louis: Mosby.

BOX 69–5. *Research Box*

Meade, C. D., Diekmann, J., & Thornhill, D. G. (1992). Readability of American Cancer Society patient education literature. *Oncology Nursing Forum, 19*(1), 51–55.

Fifty-one commonly used American Cancer Society booklets about cancer detection methods, lifestyle risks, and treatment modalities were examined for readability using the SMOG formula. The reading level ranged from grade 5.8 to 15.6 with a mean reading level of grade 11.9. Only one booklet was written at less than a sixth-grade reading level. Booklets produced since 1985 had significantly lower reading levels than earlier publications. The authors concluded that the sampled materials may be too difficult for many Americans. They suggested the nurse must be aware of patients' reading skills and develop materials that meet the needs of low-literacy groups.

---

4. Instructional objectives. Write in behavioral terms and use no more than 15 words.
5. Pretest. This should be representative of the objectives. Include answers at the end of the pretest so the learner can get immediate feedback. The pretest also can serve as the posttest.
6. Content. Present the content in an interesting way. Make sure the objectives are reflected in the content. Break the content into short segments.
7. Activities. Provide a variety of activities to keep the learner actively involved.
8. Self-evaluation of progress. Periodic self-checks or questions give the learners feedback about their progress.
9. Posttest. This will determine whether mastery of the topic has been achieved. Answers should be included at the end of the posttest so the learner can check the answers immediately.

AUDIOTAPES

Listening is a primary method of learning. As much as 70 per cent of an adult's day is spent in verbal communication. Audiotapes are relatively inexpensive, easy to use, transport, and store. The script for the audiotapes should have an introduction that explains the purpose and serves as motivation. The teaching part of the audiotape contains the content and should provide for active learner participation by including questions or practice related to the activity shown. The same principles for preparing educational materials should be applied to the preparation of an audiotape. The reading level of the audience should be kept in mind. A summary at the end of the tape should reinforce important content (Hagopian & Hymovich, 1990).

EVALUATION

Evaluation is an integral part of patient education. In addition to evaluation of the instructional materials, the effectiveness of the teacher or value of an educational program should be determined to improve effectiveness. The behavioral objectives established during the planning stage should direct the evaluation process (McMillan, 1987). When evaluating patient education programs, a systematic approach is necessary that includes the following steps:

- identify the goals of the program,
- design procedures for gathering data,
- analyze data and evaluate results, and
- report results.

DOCUMENTATION

Documentation of patient and family education is important. Patients who receive information about their disease and treatment can make contributions to

---

BOX 69–6. *Guidelines for Written Materials*

Use short words and sentences.
Use only one idea or concept in each sentence.
Use words that have few syllables.
Define all technical terms and use only meaningful words.
Break up material into short segments with frequent subtitles or headlines.
Emphasize important terms or points by underlining, bullets, or asterisks.
Make the material easy to read by using simple type with double spacing.
Enhance and augment the content with pictures and simple illustrations.
Use a ragged right margin to give a less formal appearance.
Use both upper and lower case letters to make the information easier to read. All capital letters are difficult to read.
Do not crowd information. Use plenty of white space.
Print the information in 3- to 4-inch wide columns like a newspaper rather than writing the width of a paper.

Data from Doak, C. C., Doak, L. G., & Root, J. H. (1985). *Teaching patients with low literacy skills.* Philadelphia: Lippincott; and Babcock, D. E., & Miller, M. A. (1994). *Client education: Theory and practice.* St. Louis: Mosby.

Box 69–7. *Guidelines for Posters*

Keep headlines under 10 words. Headlines should be seen from across the room.
Write headlines with brief colorful nouns and active verbs.
Do not try to say too much or crowd your material.
Use short words, short sentences, and short paragraphs.
Put the most important information at eye level.
Use upper and lower case letters. Do not use all capital letters.
Use arrows, bullets, or asterisks for emphasis.
Divide long text into shorter segments and use subheadings.
Write in columns 3 to 4 inches wide like a newspaper.
Use photographs, drawings, and color for interest and variety.

Data from Morra, M. E. (1984). How to plan and carry out your poster session. *Oncology Nursing Forum, 11*(2), 52–57.

their own self-care, prevent complications, and avoid hospitalizations. In addition, patient education and documentation are important in the context of the legal and ethical issues that sometimes arise in cancer nursing (Flynn, 1990).

SUMMARY

Cancer creates a multitude of educational needs for patients and their families. Patient education represents a major challenge and opportunity for nurses. Through education, nurses can make a significant impact on the lives of patients and their families.

REFERENCES

American Hospital Association (1975). *A patient's bill of rights* (AHA cat NO S004). Chicago: American Hospital Association.

Ajzen I., & Fishbein, M. (1980). *Understanding attitudes and predicting social behavior.* Englewood Cliffs, NJ: Prentice.

Atkinson, J. W. (1964). *An introduction to motivation.* New York: Van Nostrand.

Babcock, D. E., & Miller, M. A. (1994). *Client education: Theory & practice.* St. Louis: Mosby.

Berta Max, Inc. (1985). *Reading level analysis 3.3* (Software package). Seattle, WA: Berta Max, Inc.

Billie, D. A. (1992). Patient and family teaching in critical care. In B. M. Dossey, C. E. Guzetta, & C. V. Kenner (Eds.), *Critical care nursing: Body mind spirit* (pp. 143 154). Philadelphia: Lippincott

Billie, D. A. (1981). *Practical approaches to patient teaching.* Boston: Little Brown.

Bloom, B. S., Englehart, M. B., Furst, E. J., Hill, W. H., & Krathwohl, D. R. (1956). *The classification of educational goals. Handbook I: Cognitive domain.* New York: David McKay.

Blumberg, B. D., & Gentry, E. D. (1991). Selecting a systematic approach for educating hospitalized cancer patients. *Seminars in Oncology Nursing, 7*(2), 112–117.

Botwinic, J. (1978). *Aging and behavior.* New York: Springer.

Chewning, B. (1982). *Strategies to promote self management of chronic illness.* AHA/CDC Health Education Project. Chicago: American Hospital Association.

Cox, C. L. (1982). An interaction model of client health behavior: Theoretical prescription for nursing. *Advances in Nursing Science, 5,* 41–56.

deTornyay, R., & Thompson, M. A. (1982). *Strategies for teaching nursing.* New York: Wiley.

Doak, C. C., Doak, L. G. , & Root, J. H. (1985). *Teaching patients with low literacy skills.* Philadelphia: Lippincott.

Dodd, M. (1982). Assessing patient self-care for side effects of cancer chemotherapy. Part I. *Cancer Nursing, 5,* 263–268.

Dodd, M. (1983). Self-care for side effects in cancer chemotherapy: An assessment of nursing interventions. Part II. *Cancer Nursing, 6,* 63–67.

Dodd, M. (1984). Patterns of self-care in cancer patients receiving radiation therapy. *Oncology Nursing Forum, 10,* 23–27.

Doerr, C., & Jones, J. (1979). Effect of family preparation on the state anxiety level of the CCU patient. *Nursing Research, 28,* 315–316.

Dziurbejko, M., & Larkin, J. (1978). Including the family in preoperative teaching. *American Journal of Nursing, 78,* 1892–1884.

Fernsler, J. L., & Cannon, C. A. (1991). The whys of patient education. *Seminars in Oncology Nursing, 7*(2), 79–86.

Flynn, D. (1990). Documenting patient education: One solution. *Problem-solving in Office Oncology Nursing, 4*(2), 1–5.

Frank-Stromborg, M., & Cohen, R. (1991). Evaluating written patient education materials. *Seminars in Oncology Nursing, 7*(2), 125–134.

Hallburg, J. C. (1976). The teaching of aged adults. *Journal of Gerontological Nursing, 2*(3), 13–19.

Hagopian, G. A. (1991). The effects of a weekly radiation therapy newsletter on patients. *Oncology Nursing Forum, 18*(7), 1199–1203.

Hagopian, G. A., & Hymovich, D. P. (1990). Educational materials: Do it yourself. *Office Nurse, 3*(1), 24–27.

Herje, P. A. (1980). Hows and whys of patient contracting. *Nurse Educator, 5*(1), 30–34.

Hymovich, D. P., & Hagopian, G. A. (1989). The teaching role of the office nurse. *Office Nurse, 2*(5), 30–32.

Hymovich, D. P., & Hagopian, G. A. (1992). *Chronic illness in children and adults: A psychosocial approach* (pp. 198–219). Philadelphia: W. B. Saunders Co.

Johnson, J. (1979). *The effects of a patient-centered educational program on person's adaptability to live with a chronic disease.* Doctoral dissertation, University of Minnesota, Microfilm.

Johnson, J. L., & Lane, C. A. (1991). Helping families respond to cancer. In S. B. Baird, R. McCorkle, & M. Grant, (Eds.), *Cancer nursing: A comprehensive textbook* (pp. 921–931). Philadelphia: W. B. Saunders Co.

Johnson, J. L. B., & Blumberg, B. D. (1984). A commentary on cancer patient education. *Health Education Quarterly, 10,* 1–17.

Johnson, J. L. B., & Blumberg, B. D. (1993). Teaching strategies: Patient education. In S. L. Groenwald, M. H. Frogge, M. Goodman, & C. H. Yarbro (Eds.), *Cancer nursing: Principles and practice* (pp. 1576–1587). Boston: Jones and Bartlett.

Knowles, M. S. (1973). *The adult learner: A neglected species.* Houston: Gulf Publishing.

Lindemann, C. (1989). Patient education. J. J. Fitzpatrick, R. L. Taunton, & J. Q. Benoliel (Eds.), *Annual review of nursing research* (Vol. 6, pp. 29–60). New York: Springer.

Mahaffy, P. (1965). The effects of hospitalization on children admitted for tonsilectomy and adenoidectomy. *Nursing Research, 14,* 12–19.

Marion, L. N. (1991). Changing health behavior. Cancer prevention, early detection and screening. Proceedings of the Sixth National Conference on Cancer Nursing. 92-50M-No4503.04-PE (p. 18). Atlanta: American Cancer Society.

McLaughlin, G. H. (1969). SMOG-Grading—A new readability scale. *Journal of Reading, 12,* 639–646.

McMillan, S. C. (1987). Program evaluation. *Oncology Nursing Forum, 14*(5), 67–70.

Meade, C. D., Diekmann, J., & Thornhill, D. G. (1992). Readability of American Cancer Society patient education literature. *Oncology Nursing Forum, 19*(1), 51–55.

Morra, M. (1985). Making choices: The consumer's perspective. *Cancer Nursing, 8*(Suppl 1), 54–59.

Morra, M. E. (1984). How to plan and carry out your poster session. *Oncology Nursing Forum, 11*(2), 52–57.

Morra, M. E. (1991). Developing strategies for patient education in cancer. In S. B. Baird, R. McCorkle, & M. Grant, (Eds.), *Cancer nursing: A comprehensive textbook* (pp. 944–956). Philadelphia: W. B. Saunders Co.

Oncology Nursing Society Education Committee (1989). *Outcome standards for cancer patient education.* Pittsburgh: Oncology Nursing Society.

Oncology Nursing Society Education Committee (1982). *Outcome standards for cancer patient education.* Pittsburgh: Oncology Nursing Society.

Orem, D. E. (1991). *Nursing: Concepts of practice.* New York: McGraw-Hill.

Padilla, G. V., & Bulcavage, L. M. (1991). Theories used in patient/health education. *Seminars in Oncology Nursing, 7*(2), 87–96.

Redman, B. K. (1993). *The process of patient education.* St. Louis: Mosby.

Rightwriter. (1990). Carmel, IN: Que software, a division of Macmillan computer publishing.

Rimer, B., Levy, M. H., Keintz, M. A., Fox, L., Engstrom, P. F., & MacElwee, N. (1987). Enhancing cancer pain control regimens through patient education. *Patient Education and Counseling, 10,* 267–277.

Rosenstock, I. M., Strecher, V. J., & Becker, M. H. (1988). Social learning theory and the health belief model. *Health Education Quarterly, 15,* 175–183.

Sharf, B. F. (1988). Teaching patients to speak up: Past and future trends. *Patient Education and Counseling, 11,* 95–108.

Theis, S. L. (1991). Using previous knowledge to teach elderly clients. *Journal of Gerontological Nursing, 17*(8), 34–37.

Thompson, M. A. (1978). A systematic approach to module development. *Journal of Nursing Education, 17*(8), 20–26.

United Bureau of the Census (1989). *Statistical abstract of the United States.* 109th ed. Washington, D.C.

Van Hoozer, H. L. (1994). The teaching role of the professional nurse. In H. L. Van Hoozer, B. D. Bratton, P. M. Ostmoe, D. Weinholtz, M. J. Craft, C. L. Gjerde, & M. A. Albonese. (Eds.), *The teaching process: Theory and practice in nursing* (pp. 1–69). Kalona, IA: Kalona Graphics.

Weinrich, S. P., & Boyd, M. (1992). Education in the elderly: Adapting and evaluation of teaching tools. *Journal of Gerontological Nursing, 18*(1), 15–20.

Weinrich, S. P., Weinrich, M. C., Frank-Stromborg, M., Boyd, M. D., & Weiss, M. D. (1993). Using elderly educators to increase colorectal cancer screening. *The Gerontologist, 33*(4), 491–496.

Weisman, A., Worden, J., & Sobel, H. (1980). *Psychosocial screening and intervention with cancer patients: Research report.* Project Omega, NCI Grant # CA-19797, 1977-1980, Harvard Medical School, Department of Psychiatry, Boston.

Welch-McCaffery, D. (1986). To teach or not to teach? Overcoming barriers to patient education in geriatric oncology. *Oncology Nursing Forum, 13*(4), 25–31.

Yancik, R., & Reis, L. G. (1991). Cancer in the aged. *American Cancer Society Proceeding of the National Workshop on Cancer Control and the Older Person.* Atlanta: ACS.

Developing Strategies for Public Education in Cancer

Jayne I. Fernsler • Terri B. Ades

The impetus for public education in cancer was launched in 1913 by a small group of physicians and laypersons, who met to discuss cancer concerns and organized the American Society for the Control of Cancer, later called the American Cancer Society (ACS) (American Cancer Society [ACS], 1987). Since that time, many others have become involved in public education efforts: health care professionals; social scientists; behavioral scientists; communications specialists; federal, state, and local governmental agencies; and the general public. Now the general public expects to receive information about cancer. Those who use computer networks, read newspapers and magazines, watch television, or listen to the radio are exposed to cancer information almost daily. The openness and eagerness with which many people seek information about cancer is in itself evidence of the progress that has been made in public cancer education since 1913. Despite this progress, there is still a segment of the population that is untouched or unmotivated by the usual media. Educators must continue to try new approaches to reach both the seekers and nonseekers of information.

MAJOR INITIATIVES IN PUBLIC EDUCATION

A number of organizations, including hospitals, health maintenance organizations, and voluntary health agencies, are concerned with the provision of cancer education to the public. This section focuses on those that are the most salient to nursing: the ACS, the National Cancer Institute (NCI), and the Oncology Nursing Society (ONS). Considerable discussion is devoted to ACS and NCI because of the wide scope and availability of their programs and their evaluation efforts, and because nurses are likely to get involved in these activities.

THE AMERICAN CANCER SOCIETY

PURPOSE

The American Cancer Society was the first national organization to make a major commitment to educate the public about cancer. That commitment, dating back to the founding of the Society in 1913, was evident in its original mission statement, "to disseminate knowledge concerning the symptoms, treatment, and prevention of cancer; to investigate conditions under which cancer is found; and to compile statistics in regard thereto" (ACS, 1987).

In 1919 the President of the Society, which was then called the American Society of Cancer Control, set three axioms for its public education activities:

1. Cancer is at first a local disease.
2. With early recognition and prompt treatment, the patient's life can often be saved.
3. Through ignorance and delay, thousands of lives are needlessly sacrificed.

The Society's early printed materials, designed to educate the public, listed the first danger signals for cancer: any lump, especially in the breast; any irregular bleeding or discharge; any sore that does not heal, particularly about the tongue, mouth, or lips; and persistent indigestion with loss of weight (Ross, 1987).

Since those early days much progress has been made in educating the public about cancer. Yet, the Society believes that continued education will help accomplish its mission of eliminating cancer as a major health problem.

> The American Cancer Society is the nationwide community-based voluntary health organization dedicated to eliminating cancer as a major health problem by preventing cancer, saving lives from cancer, and diminishing suffering from cancer through research, education, advocacy, and service (ACS, 1995).

To help address the challenge of eliminating cancer as a major health problem, the American Cancer Society has adopted nationwide cancer prevention and control priorities to guide Society activities, including educational programs. These priorities focus on specific areas of cancer prevention and control that have the greatest potential for reducing cancer incidence and mortality (Table 70–1).

STRUCTURE

The American Cancer Society is composed of the National Society governed by a volunteer board of directors, 57 divisions incorporated in their respective states or metropolitan areas, and a grassroots organization of 3400 local units organized around county geographic lines. As a volunteer-driven organization, the Society depends on its 2.2 million volunteers to plan and implement its many and varied programs and to establish policies for the organization (ACS, 1995).

TABLE 70–1. *American Cancer Society Priorities for the 1990s*

Primary Cancer Prevention
Tobacco control
Comprehensive school health education
Nutrition promotion

Detection and Treatment
Breast cancer detection
Cervical cancer detection in high-risk populations
Skin cancer detection in high-risk groups
Prostate and colorectal cancer
Promotion of cancer detection tests to primary care
 providers

Patient Services
Resources, information, and guidance services
Pain control
Education and support to individuals with cancer and their
 families

Advocacy and Public Policy
Health care access related to cancer control for the uninsured and underinsured
Advocacy for the rights of cancer survivors
Legislation and regulations to control use, sale, advertising,
 and promotion of tobacco products

(Adapted from American Cancer Society. [1994]. *The strategic plan of the American Cancer Society.* Atlanta: Author.)

EDUCATION FOR ADULTS AND YOUTH

The focus of the American Cancer Society's public education programs is primary and secondary prevention of cancer; primary prevention through changing behavior in relation to known risk factors and secondary prevention through improving opportunities for early cancer diagnosis and treatment. Although the Society has information about many cancer sites, its programs focus on information and behaviors related to high-incidence cancers that can be prevented, such as lung, skin, and oral cancers, or for which early detection with effective treatment may decrease morbidity and mortality, as in colon, breast, uterus, and prostate cancers.

The programs address two major audiences—adults and youth. Adults are reached through the work sites, health sites, and community. Examples of adult education include such programs as "Taking Control," which identifies 10 steps to a healthier lifestyle; "Smart Move," a single-session stop-smoking program; and "Special Touch," which explains breast cancer and early detection techniques.

The Society's education programs for youth emphasize the importance of developing good health habits. Beginning in preschool, students learn about the dangers of tobacco use with "Starting Free: Good Air for Me." Other tobacco prevention programs include: "An Early Start to Good Health (grades K through 3), and "Health Myself" (grades 7 through 9). "Changing the Course" curricula help elementary and secondary students make good dietary choices that will reduce their risk of developing a number of diseases, including cancer. High school students can also learn in-depth about cancer through "Right Choices."

In 1993 the Society joined with the National School Health Education Coalition to promote the National Comprehensive School Health Education agenda. The Society believes that comprehensive school health education provides the structure for integrating cancer prevention information with other health topics and through a framework that widens the context of cancer prevention and control information.

REACHING UNDERSERVED POPULATIONS

While much progress has been made in cancer control, important gaps remain in the reduction of morbidity and mortality for specific populations. These gaps exist particularly for persons of low socioeconomic status who have not been reached by the Society programs in the past.

To learn more about reaching targeted populations, in 1988 the Society initiated community demonstration projects targeting African American and Hispanic groups, women of childbearing age, blue collar workers, youth, and persons with less than a high school education. The goal of the projects was to ensure the dissemination of cancer prevention and control strategies to all populations, especially the identified groups. One example of the feasibility and success of such projects was the delivery of cancer prevention, education, and early detection services by a health center to inner-city residents (Renneker et al., 1994).

Based on information gained from the demonstration projects and the use of a program development framework (Fig. 70–1), educational interventions are designed for targeted populations. One of the Society's newest programs, "Tell A Friend," offers its divisions a one-on-one breast cancer education program designed to produce a behavioral outcome. The program:

- has demonstrated, in pilot tests, a significant increase in the number of women who have mammograms
- has been proven effective with all targeted women, including lower income women
- encourages local units to target their programs, for example, to African-American and older women who have never had a mammogram
- provides units with a program that works well as a partnership with other community groups
- provides a systematic procedure to increase the likelihood that the program will reach all members of the target population.

Another new program, "Circle of Life," addresses the importance of cultural sensitivity in program development and delivery. Targeting Native American women, the program was developed with sensitivity and a realization that not only are the materials themselves important but also the method of implementation (Box 70–1).

PROGRAM DEVELOPMENT

To meet the challenge of developing and offering the very best programs for use by divisions and units, the Society has developed a standardized program development process. The title, "Partnership for Program Development," emphasizes that program development is a partnership among National, Divisions, and Units (Figs. 70–1 and 70–2). Throughout its design and processes, the program development format accommodates a number of valuable attributes for the Society:

- embodies a real partnership relationship throughout the process.
- actively espouses the values of the ACS.
- considers the ACS organization at all levels and as a whole throughout the development of a program.
- standardizes the process of developing programs.
- maintains a degree of flexibility, adaptability, and individualism for units and divisions.
- creates and maintains high-quality, effective programs that are feasible for dissemination by divisions and units.
- meets the needs of the community through ACS divisions and units.
- promotes the efficient and effective use of monies donated to the ACS (unpublished, ACS, 1994).

Through the use of the standardized format the Society ensures confidence, commitment, and involvement of staff and volunteers at all levels of the organization.

EVALUATION

Following development of its priorities, the Society developed nationwide "Measures of Success" for the

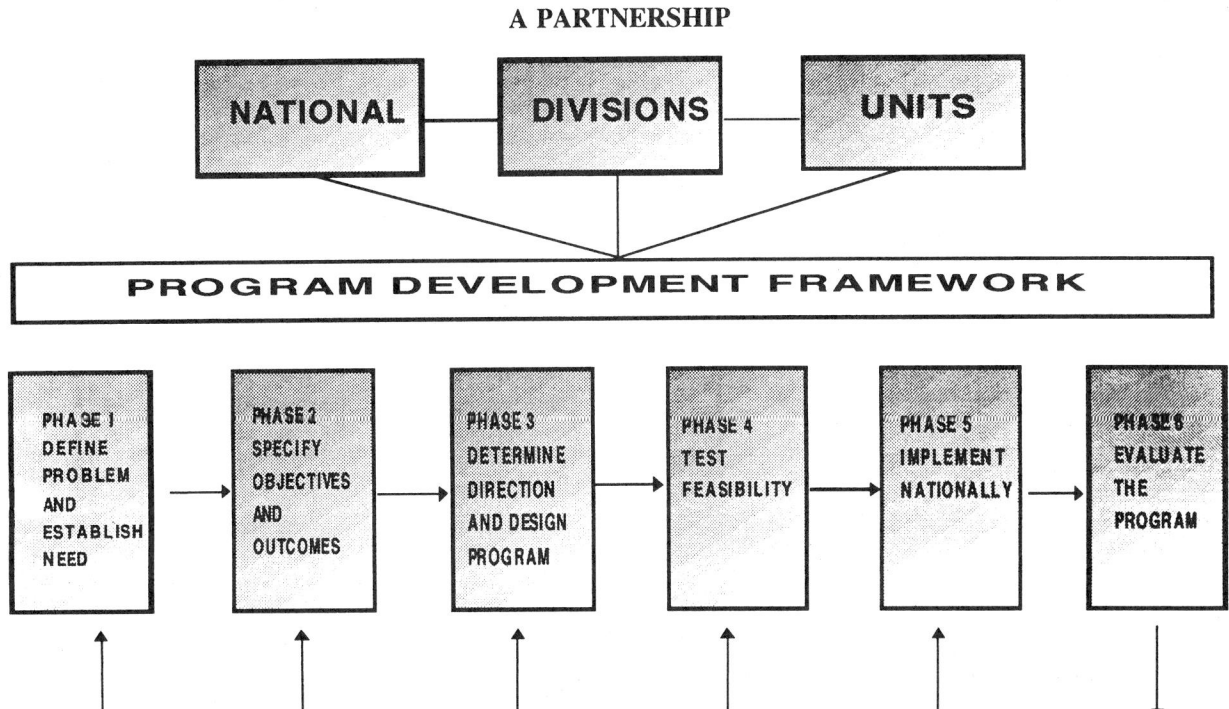

FIGURE 70–1. The American Cancer Society partnership for program development. The systematic gathering and analyzing of information about a program and its development is carried out through six sequential phases. Critical questions specific to the American Cancer Society's needs are asked at each phase to determine continuation of program development. (From American Cancer Society. [1995]. *American Cancer Society Partnership for Program Development*. Atlanta: Author.)

Many Native American women do not believe they are susceptible to breast cancer because they are not represented in the literature on breast health and screening guidelines. In part, as a result of this and the absence of an appropriate education program, their 5 year survival rate is alarmingly lower than that of white women, 46 percent compared with 76 percent, respectively.

In 1991, the Public Education Committee of the American Cancer Society's Oklahoma Division received a grant to target a cancer concern for an underserved population. Knowing the need was there, the committee chose breast cancer education for Native American women, and the *Circle of Life* program began to take shape.

Circle of Life is a culturally relevant breast cancer awareness program that stresses the importance of mammography, clinical breast exam, and breast self-exam. The program was developed by a committee of both lay and professional volunteers from several tribal and geographic areas in Oklahoma. All agreed that the education materials must be culturally sensitive and use seeing, hearing, and touching as part of the learning methods. What has resulted is a program that uses a flipchart, pamphlet, training guides, and a video and that is easily implemented through women's clinics and hospitals and the Indian Health Service.

The project has had a significant impact in Oklahoma and has also met with overwhelming acceptance in both Montana and Minnesota. According to Nancy Hane, *Circle of Life* chair, after the project was discussed at the ACS National Women's Conference to Develop Strategies in Breast Cancer Detection in New York City, June 1992, she was "getting calls from everywhere."

Circle of Life is a culturally relevant breast cancer awareness program that stresses the importance of mammography, clinical breast exam, and breast self-exam.

Native American artist Dana Tiger designed the Circle of Life logo to symbolize the courage and confidence of Native American women.

Hane believes the success results from the fact that the program was developed with sensitivity and a realization that not only are the materials themselves important but also the method of implementation; it must include a personal intervention.

This philosophy behind the program encourages recruitment of teachers who are Native American women or other personnel in the health care field, who have a good rapport with and the respect of the Native American women in their area, and who have a strong desire to help others. The training session is 3 hours long and teaches about breast growth and development, anatomy, breast cancer, mammography, clinical breast exam, breast self-exam, cultural sensitivity, and presentation preparation.

Even the artwork and title for the program were chosen with an awareness of Native American culture. The title, *Circle of Life*, stands for the idea that all women should be able to complete the full circle of their lives. Deep pink and mauve colors were used because of their significance to Indian women.

Of course, the ultimate goal of *Circle of Life*, now slated for distribution nationwide, is to increase the breast cancer survival rate of all Native American women, and the successes that have come from the very beginning arc a good sign that this will be achieved. As Hane states, "All the pieces, the stars and the moon, were all in the right place for this project. It worked from the very beginning. . . . It was blessed."

—*Karen Resha*

From Resha, K. (1994). Oklahoma's breast health program for Native American women goes nationwide. *Cancer News, 48*(2), 13.

Society's programs that would serve as benchmarks identifying specific outcomes to be achieved by the year 2000. The outcomes are consistent with the U.S. Department of Health and Human Services "Healthy People 2000" goals.

THE NATIONAL CANCER INSTITUTE

PURPOSE

The mission of the NCI with regard to public education is to provide the public with current information

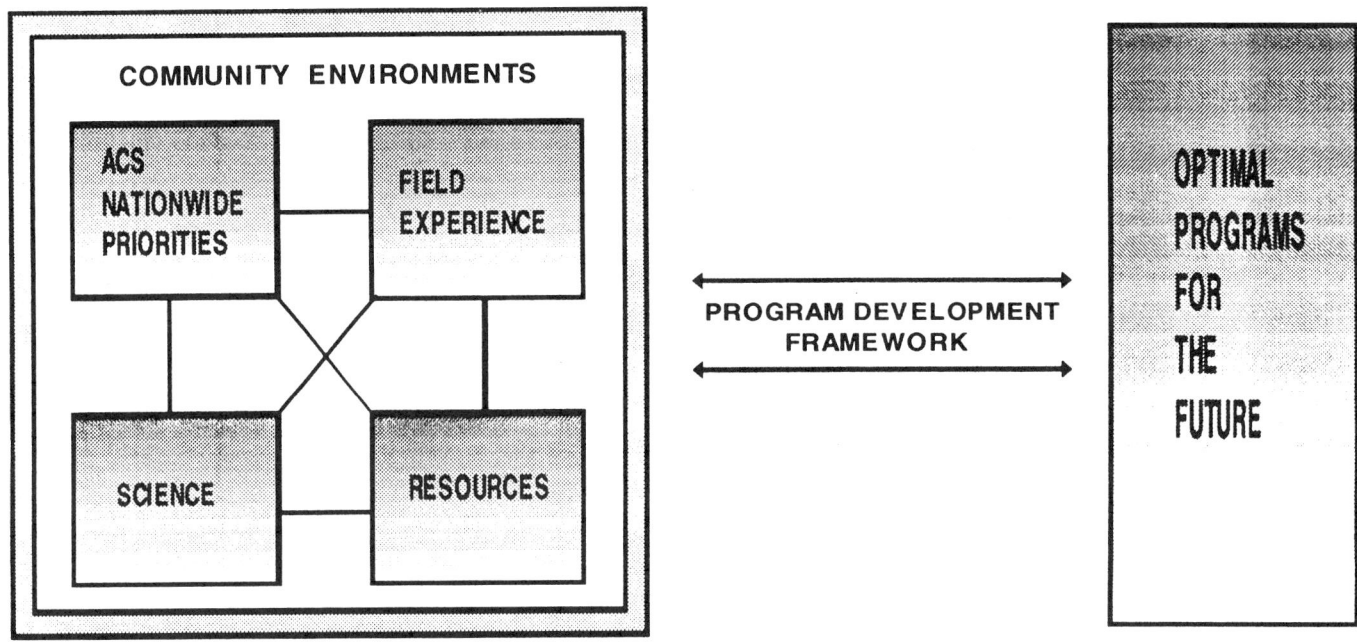

FIGURE 70–2. The American Cancer Society Partnership for Program Development. The process is designed to obtain information on a program idea from five critical sources: (1) the established direction provided by the Society's priorities; (2) current knowledge; (3) division and unit expertise in implementing effective strategies from their field experience; current activities and agendas of communities and other organizations; and available resources, including people and money. Information is systematically gathered and analyzed, and decisions are made periodically along the way as to whether to continue program development. (From American Cancer Society. [1995]. *American Cancer Society Partnership for Program Development.* Atlanta: Author.)

about prevention, detection, diagnosis, and treatment of cancer (NCI, 1994a). The Office of Cancer Communications (OCC) is the organizational component of the NCI that is responsible for public education as well as patient, family, and professional education. This section focuses on the public education component of the program.

STRUCTURE

The OCC has three major branches (Fig. 70–3). Established in 1977, the Information Projects branch is responsible for conducting audience research and developing, promoting, and evaluating education and information programs for the public (NCI, 1994b). The Reports and Inquiries branch handles all public affairs, press activities, community outreach programs, and public inquiries, including telephone inquiries received through the Cancer Information Service. Public interest in cancer care is reflected in the more than 500,000 requests for information that are processed by this branch each year (NCI, 1994a). The Information Resources branch produces NCI educational materials (books, pamphlets, audio visuals) and distributes both OCC-developed and other cancer-related publications. In fiscal year 1993, more than 18 million publications were distributed either directly by mail or indirectly through health care facilities, schools, professional meetings, supermarkets, and discount stores (NCI, 1994a).

PROGRAMS

The public education programs of the OCC focus on health promotion and information dissemination. Health promotion includes early detection, with emphasis on breast, prostate, and cervical cancer; prevention, with emphasis on smoking cessation, tobacco control, and dietary changes; and cancer risk awareness with regard to exposure to carcinogens.

A major component of the nutrition program of the OCC, 5-a-Day for Better Health, is designed to encourage the public to eat five or more daily servings of fruits and vegetables. The program is offered in partnership with the Produce for Better Health Foundation and includes educational materials and promotional strategies (NCI, 1994b).

In relation to public education about tobacco, the OCC continues to provide support for the American Stop Smoking Intervention Study (ASSIST), a combined effort of ACS, NCI, and regional as well as local coalitions working toward a smokefree environment. Additionally, smokeless tobacco campaigns are conducted in cooperation with Major League Baseball and Little League Baseball (NCI, 1994b).

A particularly exciting and timely initiative of the OCC is reflected in the development of educational programs and materials targeted to underserved and hard-to-reach populations: African-Americans, Hispanics, older Americans, and low literate people (NCI,

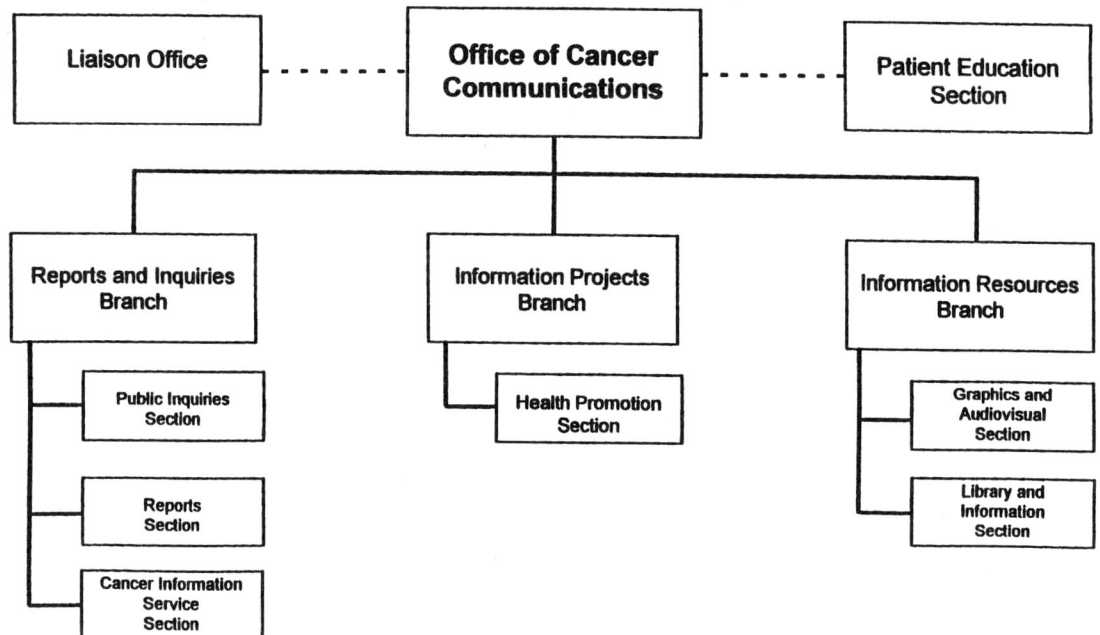

FIGURE 70–3. The Structure of the Office of Cancer Communications. (From National Cancer Institute Office of Communications, 1995.)

1994b). These programs have the potential to reduce cancer mortality among vulnerable sectors of the U.S. population.

Mass media, individual and organizational intermediaries, and community outreach programs are NCI's vehicles for communicating educational messages to the public. For example, regional summits and mini-summits, funded through grants from the NCI and the Susan G. Komen Breast Cancer Foundation, were held by medical institutions to educate business leaders and organizations about breast cancer. The NCI provided technical assistance and materials, in addition to the funding. Recipients of this education were encouraged to develop education and screening programs in their communities (NCI, 1994b).

The Cancer Information Service (CIS) of the OCC is a major source of information dissemination through a network of 19 regional offices that cover the entire U. S. population (Fig. 70–4). Since its inception in 1975, the CIS has expanded geographically and is one of the most frequently consulted telephone helplines that offers health-related information to the public (Morra, Van Nevel, Nealon, Mazan, & Thomsen, 1993). Limited research indicates that the CIS has been effective in promoting the public education initiative of the NCI (Morra, Bettinghaus et al., 1993).

EVALUATION

The NCI monitors its public education activities through formative and impact evaluation. Formative evaluation is used in planning, designing, and pretesting materials and messages. For example, in-depth interviews were conducted to evaluate a new brochure with a special educational message on prostate cancer, and a mall intercept type survey was used to pretest a

print advertisement on the 5-a-Day program. Surveys are conducted to determine baseline as well as changing levels of public awareness, knowledge, and beliefs (NCI, 1994b).

Another type of formative evaluation, Consumer-Based Health Information Profiling, is a process of combining data on cancer statistics and health practices with marketing data to identify people in a local area who are in need of cancer education. Maps are then constructed to locate specific potential audiences (NCI, 1994b).

Impact evaluation is conducted to evaluate the effectiveness of programs. Indirect measures of the influence of media campaigns include the number and type of public inquiries made to the Cancer Information Service, the number of requests for materials, the number of public service announcements made on radio and television, and the amount of exposure of the program in the print media. For example, an antismoking media campaign was evaluated as successful on the basis of a greater number of calls for smoking cessation information from the target audience in the location of the campaign (Cummings, Sciandra, Davis, & Rimer, 1993). The effectiveness of the NCI's message in changing public knowledge, attitudes, and behaviors related to cancer prevention is measured through evaluation of specific programs and through periodic national surveys by the NCI and other government and private organizations (NCI, 1994a).

THE ONCOLOGY NURSING SOCIETY

One of the goals of the ONS is to provide cancer education to the general public as well as to nurses. The Education Committee of the society developed

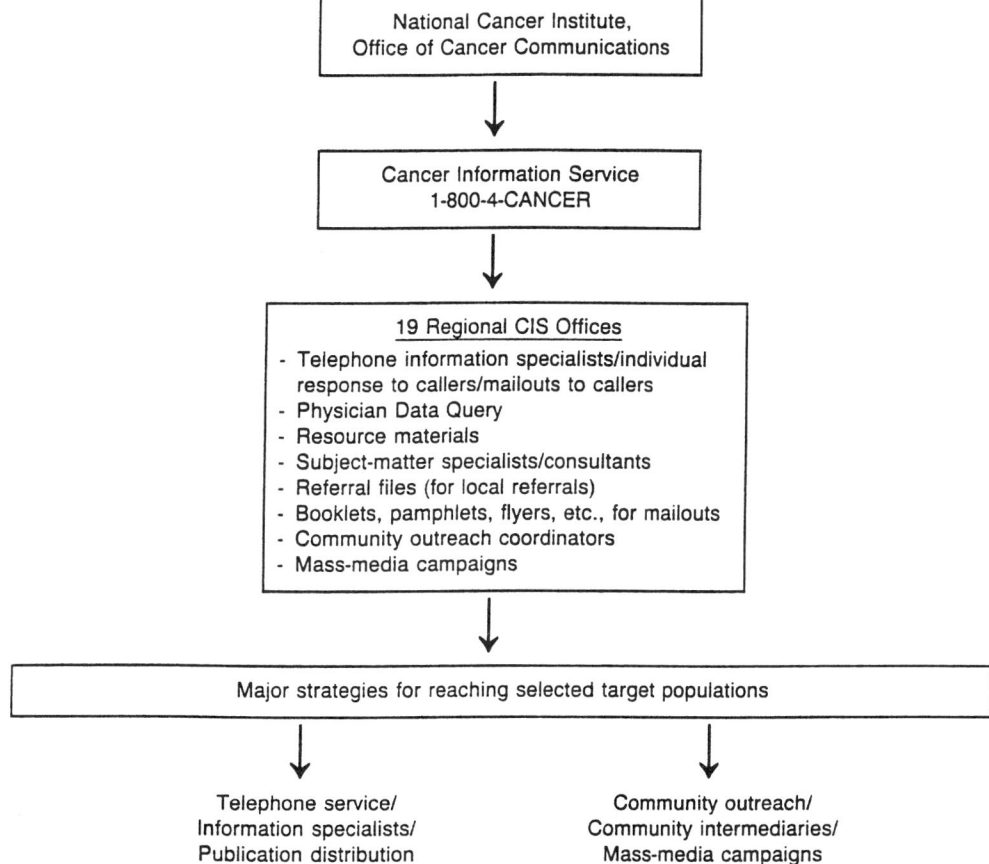

FIGURE 70–4. Overview of the CIS network. (From Marcus, A. C., Bettinghaus, E. P., Mazan, K. D., Morra, M. E., Nealon, E. O., & Van Nevel, J. P. [1993]. Introduction. *Monographs. Journal of the National Cancer Institute, 14,* 3.)

Outcome Standards for Public Cancer Education (Oncology Nursing Society Education Committee, 1983, 1989) in the belief that the public should be educated about cancer and that nurses are responsible for educating them. The target audience is all people in the community, and the major objective is to inform them about their options related to prevention, early detection, rehabilitation, and living with cancer.

The ONS suggested that the following assumptions be considered when planning a public education program (Oncology Nursing Society Education Committee, 1983):

All individuals are at risk for developing cancer at some point in their lives.

Certain individuals possess a higher risk for developing cancer by virtue of their genetic background and/or environmental exposure.

Cancer control activities are influenced by political, social, cultural, and economic factors.

Active participation by the public in the educational process enhances learning.

Public education influences the public's knowledge, skills, and attitudes about risk factors related to carcinogens.

Health care needs and cancer risk factors identified by health care providers may differ from those perceived by the public.

Individuals come to learning situations with certain knowledge and beliefs about cancer that affect their learning.

Educational strategies must reflect the culture and ethnic diversities of the public.

These assumptions are inherent in the ONS revised standards and in the society's efforts to enhance public education in cancer nursing practice. Nurses are encouraged to submit abstracts of public education projects for either oral presentations or exhibition at the ONS annual congress. Projects that reflect the assumptions are viewed favorably by the Education Committee. In addition, through funding from an NCI grant, the ONS conducted regional workshops to teach minority nurses how to develop and implement public education programs about cancer prevention and detection in their communities. As part of the evaluation of the project, minority nurses who participated in the workshops are now reporting their public education activities to the ONS.

In 1990, the ONS initiated an award to support and recognize excellence in patient or public education. The award is presented annually to a nurse member of the Society who is involved in creative programming that reflects the society's educational standards.

The Oncology Nursing Foundation, an ONS-related organization devoted to funding education and research, has a goal related to educating the general public about cancer and cancer care also. The foundation addressed this goal through a yearly request for proposals for public cancer education. The first such

RFP was awarded in 1987 for a project to educate African-American women about the early detection of breast cancer. The Oncology Nursing Foundation has reinforced its commitment to funding public education by publishing a brochure that describes the application process (Oncology Nursing Foundation, 1994).

In summary, the ONS's goal for public education is broad. The organization fosters public education indirectly by educating nurses and by providing a forum for them to share information about public education. The ONS also provides standards for nurses to use when developing or evaluating public education programs. The Oncology Nursing Foundation provides limited funding for public education projects.

INVOLVEMENT OF NURSES IN PUBLIC EDUCATION

Nurses can be pivotal in public cancer education. They constitute the largest group of health professionals involved in cancer care, and they practice in a variety of settings where they interact with the public. In addition, nurses are often approached informally by friends and neighbors who want special information about cancer. Consequently, most nurses have target audiences readily available to them.

Nursing education prepares nurses to teach both patients and the public. Many nursing curricula are organized around a framework of health maintenance and wellness. Students in such programs learn skills in these areas in the community. One recently graduated baccalaureate nurse was recognized nationally for her proposed public awareness program about testicular self-examination (Carlin, 1986). The proposal included a stepwise procedure for implementing the program at the grassroots, county, state, and national levels.

Clinical experience prepares nurses to teach also. Greene (1986) states that by virtue of their contact with patients and families, nurses know the devastating effects of cancer and the value of early detection. She states also that nurses know how to communicate with people in appropriate language. Consequently, nurses who have been in practice for many years can bring a wealth of knowledge and experience to a teaching-learning situation.

Both ACS and NCI identify nurses as important volunteers or intermediaries in their goals to educate the public about cancer prevention and detection. Nurses can influence the public as role models and as health educators. Their activities may be local, state, regional, or national in scope. Such activities have the potential to broaden nurses' skills, while empowering the public with useful information. Thus nurses' involvement in public education is mutually beneficial to nurses and society.

The nature and degree of an individual nurse's involvement in public education may depend on his or her employer, flexibility in work schedule, preparation and experience, and commitment to teaching others. A nurse's involvement may vary from leading an employee smoking cessation program at lunchtime to chairing an ACS committee that markets public education to potential audiences and develops policies and procedures for training and certifying speakers. Some institutions encourage their nurse employees' involvement in ACS public education efforts, whereas others appeal directly to the public with their own health education and prevention programs. In either situation, a nurse's participation may be limited by other demands of the job.

When the ONS board of directors asked members to report their activities with regard to cancer prevention and early detection, nursing students, practitioners, administrators, and educators responded with a variety of educational activities. The nurses reported both formal and informal teaching that was not necessarily part of their job descriptions. Specific examples of activities included informal teaching at exhibit sites in hospitals as well as in the community; making formal presentations as volunteers in cancer-related groups, such as a local ONS chapter, ACS, or NCI; answering cancer information calls; and assisting with screening and detection programs (Nevidjon, 1986).

PROGRAM DEVELOPMENT

Nurses are accustomed to using the nursing process in clinical practice. A similar systematic process is used in developing educational programs, regardless of the intended audience (professionals, patient, public). This section highlights public education program development from a nursing perspective. There is a detailed description of the stages of program development—assessment, planning, intervention, evaluation—in Chapter 69.

SETTING PRIORITIES

Nurses set priorities daily, because rarely are they able to do all that they think should be done in a clinical situation. Setting priorities in public education, as in clinical practice, is a safeguard against dissipating energy and resources by trying to do everything. Priority-setting involves asking, What are the greatest public education needs in this situation? Both ACS and NCI use national primary and secondary survey results to answer the question. At the local level, nurses can assess needs through observations made in clinical practice; data from the hospital or state tumor registry; and requests for information from family, friends, and neighbors. For example, through one or more of these methods the nurse may discover a plethora of cases of newly diagnosed, advanced breast cancer in women under the age of 30. This discovery, viewed in the appropriate context, may indicate an immediate need to educate young women about breast self-examination (BSE) and breast cancer.

Nurses in primary care settings, such as health maintenance organizations and physicians' offices, have special opportunities to assess the public's need for cancer information. They see both well and sick people and have the opportunity to assess changes in their knowledge and health behaviors over time. So-called noncompliant behaviors with regard to a health maintenance program may signal the need for education.

FORMULATING OBJECTIVES

Objectives are written in terms of what the learner is able to do at the completion of an educational program. Categories and components of objectives are discussed in Chapter 69. Objectives are useful to the teacher and the learner, because they tend to keep both focused on the topic. Limiting objectives can be difficult, because one tends to think that the learner needs to know all about the topic. In the case of the previously described need to educate young women about BSE and breast cancer, the most important objectives are that women correctly perform BSE monthly and consult a physician immediately if they discover any signs of cancer. These objectives are realistic and measurable through return demonstration and follow-up. With stepwise behavior change, however, women must first become aware of BSE and consider the practice before they try it.

The ONS public education standards (Oncology Nursing Society Education Committee, 1983, 1989) have been useful for program planning, because they provide behavioral objectives or criteria for each area of content or each standard related to public education. Nurses in one hospital used the standards as a framework for developing the purpose, content, plans, and evaluation of a multidisciplinary cancer fair (Vega, 1985).

DEVELOPING A BUDGET

Public cancer education can be done relatively inexpensively if existing resources are tapped. For example, a program to educate young women about BSE and breast cancer could be coordinated with the local ACS unit; local schools, colleges, and universities; and the county health department. With the support of experienced staff within these agencies, a nurse could coordinate the program and recruit other nurses as volunteer BSE instructors. Materials and equipment could be provided free of charge by the sponsoring organizations and by the NCI. Nevertheless, the nurse coordinator or the coordinating team should prepare a list of potential expense items, such as travel, postage, printing, educational pamphlets, audiovisual equipment, breast models, and posters. The sponsoring organizations should decide before the program who will assume the cost of items, such as postage, if follow-up information is requested from the women. Although including prepaid postage may seem expensive, it is cost-effective in terms of enhancing the response rate from participants (Elwood, Erickson, & Lieberman, 1978).

Large-scale public education programs combined with screening involve the added expense of equipment, space for screening, laboratory costs, record keeping, and follow-up. These items should be given careful consideration when considering whether to screen as well as to educate the target audience.

Depending on the nature of the program and the proposed activities, funding could be requested from the Oncology Nursing Foundation or the ACS.

SELECTING METHODOLOGIES

One method of promoting awareness and motivation among the target audience is to involve representatives of the group in program planning. Carlin (1986) reported success with soliciting artwork, from male high school students, for the cover of a pamphlet on testicular cancer and testicular self-examination. A similar approach could be used to involve high school and college females in developing materials for a BSE education program. Because the aim of the program is to encourage young women to adopt a behavior, the planners should consider a variety of strategies (Table 70–2). In this situation, a combination of lecture, audiovisual aids, discussion, demonstration, and return demonstration would be most effective.

Special considerations may need to be made when the target audience is older learners. For example, Baulch, Larson, Dodd, & Dietrich (1992) found that older women may not be able physically to perform some of the usual steps that are considered essential for proficient BSE. When these deficits are identified, the teaching strategy should be altered accordingly (Box 70–2).

STRATEGIES FOR HARD-TO-REACH POPULATIONS

Nurses are creative in reaching people who are outside the mainstream. One nurse, an ACS volunteer and patient education coordinator and outreach nurse in a small eastern community hospital, identified a need for breast cancer education among Amish women. An acquaintance of the nurse arranged her initial entry into the Amish community. She first observed the operation of an immunization clinic, which was held monthly by the public health department in the home of an Amish family. The Amish had agreed somewhat reluctantly to allow the clinic after an outbreak of whooping cough in their community. Then, with the help of a retired surgeon and a midwife who were familiar with the Amish community, a radiologic technologist, a volunteer, and a secretary, the nurse organized and implemented a BSE teaching and screening program in an Amish home.

The group planned strategies to accommodate the Amish values of privacy and simplicity. Registration and history-taking were handled individually in a private room. Women in similar age groups were taught about breast cancer and BSE in groups of four. Posters were used in lieu of slides or a film because there was no electricity in the home. Advertising of the program was limited to posters placed in Amish homes, where church services are held, and in several Amish stores. Women who required mammograms were taught about the procedure by the radiologic technologist. These women were also given slips that permitted them to have mam-

TABLE 70–2. *Strategies for Facilitating Behavior Change*

1. *Use messages tailored to the people you're trying to reach.* Attempt to see the world through their eyes and use words and examples that are familiar and meaningful to them.
2. *Give them the information they need.* There are a lot of ACS programs ready to help you.
3. *Give them specific messages about what you want them to do.* For example, set a date to stop smoking, practice BSE once a month. ACS booklets and films will help.
4. *Keep fear at a moderate level—neither too low nor too high.* Research shows that if people are too afraid, they become immobilized, but if they have no fear, they remain unconcerned. ACS public education materials have been developed carefully to strike the right balance.
5. *Involve them.* When people are involved actively in the learning process, they are more likely to recall the information and demonstrate the needed skills. Anything you can do to increase involvement will enhance learning. For example, ask the audience to list their reasons for quitting or to share ways they have to cut down on dietary fat.
6. *Show them how to do it.* Often, people are motivated to change, but they need to be shown how. For example, demonstrate the proper breast self-examination technique. Have a cooking demonstration of low-fat, high-fiber recipes. Show people how to get ready to quit smoking.
7. *Build their confidence that they can take action successfully.* If people slip up, let them know they haven't failed. This is especially true in the areas of smoking cessation and dietary change, where habits are complex and new habits must be practiced over and over.
8. *Show your target audience that you believe in them.* Let them know they have your support. That can make a difference.
9. *Reinforce the message.* Because behavior change is a long-term process, it's important to get back to people. The more you interact with a given group of people, the more likely it is that their behavior will change.
10. *Use more than one educational method to reach your target audience.* Consider using a combination of educational methods. This will give you the best chance for success.

(Adapted with permission from American Cancer Society. [1987]. *A public education planning guide for ACS unit volunteers* [pp. 18–20]. New York: Author.)

mograms done for $40.00 at a local radiology center on the days when the Amish generally go to town.

The best strategy for reaching selected populations is to consult them throughout program development. Then plan the program to accommodate their values and needs. For example, in working with Japanese-Americans, American Indians, and Hispanics, whose identity is strongly linked to the family unit, program planners should emphasize family roles and responsibilities rather than individual decision making regarding health habits. This approach fosters trust and understanding between educators and the target audience, essential ingredients for effective communication (Kagawa-Singer, 1987).

African-Americans constitute the largest minority population that could benefit significantly from education about cancer prevention and early detection. Educational efforts must avoid stereotyping individuals within this population, while acknowledging their general mistrust of professional health care, which has resulted from years of discrimination and segregation (Guillory, 1987). African-American clergy and the church are avenues for reaching a large portion of the African-American audience. In Delaware, gospelizing has been an effective medium for promoting cancer education and awareness among the African-American population in both urban and rural settings. This medium is unique; it appeals to individuals from a vari-

---

Box 70–2. *BSE Performance by Older Women*

Baulch, Y. S., Larson, P. J., Dodd, M. J., & Dietrich, C. (1992). The relationship of visual acuity, tactile sensitivity, and mobility of the upper extremities to proficient breast self-examination in women 65 and older. *Oncology Nursing Forum, 19*(9), 1367–1372.

In this descriptive correlational study, older women's ability to perform proficient BSE was examined within the framework of Orem's model of self-care. A total of 32 women (ages 66 to 69 years) from four retirement centers were interviewed and then tested for visual acuity (Snellen chart), tactile sensitivity (static two-point discrimination test), upper extremity mobility (range of motion), and ability to visually and tactilely detect abnormalities on simulated breast models (SBM). Proficiency in the latter area was scored as pass or fail according to ACS criteria for BSE. Results revealed that 94 per cent of the women had adequate or better visual acuity, which related significantly to visual detection of the lump. Although 94 per cent of the women had adequate tactile sensitivity, only 41 per cent located the 1 cm lump, and only 37 per cent located the 5 mm lump. About one third of the women failed the upper extremity mobility test, and nearly half (15) failed the corresponding component of BSE, indicating that upper extremity mobility was related to the women's ability to perform the mobility component of BSE. Mobility was limited by obesity and by pain and fatigue, which were associated with arthritis. Nurses need to address these factors when teaching BSE to older women by encouraging short sessions, rest periods, use of analgesics beforehand, and use of talc or lotion.

ety of socioeconomic and educational levels, including the illiterate. Another musical medium, rap music, has been used effectively to communicate information about breast cancer and breast self-examination to African-American adolescents (Ehmann, 1993).

EVALUATION

Several types of evaluation were discussed previously in this chapter and are discussed in Chapter 69. Evaluation is the most troublesome component of public education, even when desired outcomes are specified clearly during the planning stage. Changes in people's knowledge, attitudes, and behaviors occur over time and may not be attributable to a single educational intervention. Unplanned news events may confound evaluation efforts by prompting people to take action such as participating in a screening program (Fink et al., 1978). However, such events tend to have a short-lived effect on people's behavior. Even when well-planned educational messages, interspersed with televised news, are effective in promoting the public's awareness, public compliance with follow-up screening behaviors may be low (Winchester et al., 1980).

When dealing with hard-to-reach populations, such as the Amish community that was described previously, standards for judging program effectiveness may have to be modified. For example, about half of the Amish women who were advised to have mammograms actually had them done. By usual standards, this response indicates a low compliance rate. Nevertheless, with this population, it represents a positive outcome of the program. Another positive outcome was that the providers were invited to repeat the program in other homes in the Amish community, and several of the women have maintained contact with the nurse coordinator. The long-term impact of the program will be evaluated through clinical observation and surveillance of the tumor registry data.

FUTURE DIRECTIONS FOR PUBLIC CANCER EDUCATION

Some years ago Butler and Paisley (1977) observed that public cancer education programs were generally lacking in appropriate application of social science principles and evaluation design. They made 10 major recommendations, which have, for the most part, been considered in the public education programs of ACS and NCI. In the future, as both agencies intensify their efforts to reach nonseekers of information, particularly the socioeconomically disadvantaged and the illiterate, marketing and evaluation techniques will become even more crucial.

Continued and strengthened interagency cooperation and coordination will be needed to ensure broader coverage of the population while eliminating costly duplication of effort. One example of this cooperative effort is the recent activity by NCI and ACS to educate professionals as well as the public about available clini-

cal trials. Another example is the American Stop Smoking Intervention Study (ASSIST), which is a combined effort of ACS, NCI, and regional as well as local coalitions working toward a smokefree environment. In addition, alternative methods must be found to facilitate program implementation at the local level. ACS, NCI, and ONS all are attempting to address this need through regional committees or workshops. Educational approaches will need to be sensitive to the rapidly expanding elderly sector of the population, as well as the sector that is enticed by computers and technology.

IMPLICATIONS FOR CANCER NURSING PRACTICE

The time is right for nurses to expand their involvement in public cancer education. The public need exists, resources are available from the ACS and the NCI, and the standards for such activity are delineated by the ONS. Working collaboratively with other health care professionals, nurses have the potential to contribute significantly to the goal of reducing morbidity and mortality from cancer.

REFERENCES

American Cancer Society. (1987). *American Cancer Society fact-book for health professionals* (3076–PE). New York: Author.

American Cancer Society. (1995). *Cancer facts and figures— 1995* (No. 5008.95) Atlanta: Author.

Baulch, Y. S., Larson, P. J., Dodd, M. J., & Dietrich, C. (1992). The relationship of visual acuity, tactile sensitivity, and mobility of the upper extremities to proficient breast self-examination in women 65 and older. *Oncology Nursing Forum, 19*(9), 1367–1372.

Butler, M., & Paisley, W. (1977). Communicating cancer control to the public. *Health Education Monographs, 5,* 5–24.

Carlin, P. J. (1986). Testicular self examination: A public awareness program. *Public Health Reports, 101,* 98–102.

Cummings, K. M., Sciandra, R., Davis, S., & Rimer, B. K. (1993). Results of an antismoking media campaign utilizing the cancer information service. *Monographs. Journal of the National Cancer Institute, 14,* 113–118.

Ehmann, J. L. (1993). BSE rap: Intergenerational ties to save lives. *Oncology Nursing Forum, 20*(8), 1255–1259.

Elwood, T. W., Erickson, A., & Lieberman, S. (1978). Comparative educational approaches to screening for colorectal cancer. *American Journal of Public Health, 68,* 135–138.

Fink, R., Roeser, R., Venet, W., Strax, P., Venet, L., & Lacher, M. (1978). Effects of news events on response to a breast cancer screening program. *Public Health Reports, 93,* 318–327.

Greene, P. E. (1986). The role of the American Cancer Society in public education. *Seminars in Oncology Nursing, 2,* 206–210.

Guillory, J. (1987). Ethnic perspectives of cancer nursing: The black American. *Oncology Nursing Forum, 14*(3), 66–69.

Kagawa-Singer, M. (1987). Ethnic perspectives of cancer nursing: Hispanics and Japanese-Americans. *Oncology Nursing Forum, 14*(3), 59–65.

Morra, M. E., Bettinghaus, E. P., Marcus, A. C., Mazan, K. D., Nealon, E., & Van Nevel, J. P. (1993). The first 15 years: What has been learned about the Cancer Information

Service and the implications for the future. *Monographs. Journal of the National Cancer Institute, 14,* 177–185.

Morra, M. E., Van Nevel, J. P., Nealon, E., Mazan, K. D., & Thomsen, C. (1993). History of the Cancer Information Service. *Monographs. Journal of the National Cancer Institute, 14,* 7–33.

National Cancer Institute. (1994a). NCI Fact Book (NIH Pub. No. 94-512). Bethesda, MD: NCI Financial Management Branch.

National Cancer Institute Office of Cancer Communications. (1994b). Office of the Director Annual Report FY '93. Bethesda, MD: Author.

Nevidjon, B. (1986). Cancer prevention and early detection: Reported activities of nurses. *Oncology Nursing Forum, 13*(4), 76–80.

Oncology Nursing Foundation. (1994). *Reaching out to the communities we serve. How to apply for funding for cancer public education projects.* Pittsburgh: Author.

Oncology Nursing Society Education Committee. (1983). *Outcome standards for public cancer education.* Pittsburgh: Oncology Nursing Society.

Oncology Nursing Society Education Committee. (1989). *Standards of oncology education: Patient/family and public.* Pittsburgh: Oncology Nursing Society.

Renneker, M., Lim, N., Wheatley, B., Collins, S., Pirkle, R., Beers, L., Rambo, M., Schleper, J., Jones, T., Butler, B., Saner, H., & Hall, J. (1994). An inner city cancer prevention clinic in West Oakland, California. *Cancer Practice, 2*(6), 427–437.

Ross, W. (1987). *Crusade: The official history of the American Cancer Society.* New York: Arbor House Publishing.

Vega, T. (1985). Outcome standards for public cancer education: The foundation for community education programs. *Oncology Nursing Forum, 12*(5), 66–67.

Winchester, D. P., Shull, J. H., Scanlon, E. F., Murrell, J. V., Smeltzer, C., Vrba, P., Iden, M., Streelman, D. H., Magpayo, R., Dow, J. W., & Sylvester, J. (1980). A mass screening program for colorectal cancer using chemical testing for occult blood in the stool. *Cancer, 45,* 2955–2958.

Cancer Nursing Education Today

Ruth McCorkle • Fredrica Preston • Deborah Lowe Volker

The formalization of cancer nursing education has evolved during the second half of the twentieth century. The first college course in cancer nursing was offered at Columbia University Teachers College by Katherine Nelson in 1947. The history of cancer nursing education is included in Chapter 2. This chapter presents an overview of cancer education today at four levels: undergraduate, advanced practice, predoctoral and postdoctoral, and staff education. In addition, principles of adult learning, barriers to staff education, and Oncology Nursing Society (ONS) and Joint Commission on Accreditation of Healthcare Organizations (JCAHO) standards of professional education are discussed. The chapter includes an overview of the steps involved in developing an education program and the issues involved in providing orientation programs. The chapter concludes with a discussion of the importance of ongoing competency assurance and certification.

LEVELS OF CANCER NURSING EDUCATION

The practice of cancer nursing requires nurses to be knowledgeable about a wide range of basic content from multiple disciplines, including nursing, epidemiology, pathophysiology, sociology, pharmacology, medicine, nutrition and psychology. In 1980, the members of the Oncology Nursing Society passed a resolution declaring that nurses with baccalaureate degrees be recognized as the entry level of practice of oncology nursing. See Box 71–1 for the resolution. Staying current in cancer nursing knowledge requires a lifelong commit-

ment to learning. The building blocks of formal academic preparation are illustrated in Figure 71–1. It is important that the learner realizes that learning is a process and includes finding a balance between academic preparation and professional opportunities. There are various routes to follow as indicated by the arrows.

UNDERGRADUATE EDUCATION

Around the time when the specialty organization was assuming leadership and establishing education standards, educational institutions were making drastic changes in their curricula. In the 1980s, curricula were changed at the undergraduate level from a medical model approach (organized by body systems and diseases) to an integrative approach. During that time, nurse educators reevaluated the meaning of nursing, delineated recurring themes in nursing, and developed new strategies to transmit nursing knowledge (Pennington, 1986). Consequently, the search for common concepts diminished the specialty content included in undergraduate programs. Traditionally, cancer nursing has been taught in a limited number of hours of didactic instruction within a medical-surgical rotation, and clinical experiences with cancer patients may or may not have been planned concurrently.

The integrated approach focused on broad concepts, applicable to many patient situations, thereby making the concurrent study of specialty content and clinical assignment less critical to learning. In addition, the focus on general versus specific knowledge provided the student with a knowledge base that was not outdated quickly.

Box 71–1. *Oncology Nursing Society Entry Level of Practice Resolution*

WHEREAS,   Our stand on this issue is based upon the belief that the following recommendation must be addressed by the nursing profession; and

WHEREAS,   The development of accessible, flexible, affordable and innovative educational programs to enable nurses or potential nurses to obtain a baccalaureate degree;

WHEREAS,   The dissemination of information regarding these programs to all nurses and students seeking nursing education, especially those in rural areas and minority individuals; and

WHEREAS,   The inclusion of sufficient clinical experience and theory in the curricula of current and future educational programs to ensure that graduates are able to function at a standard level of clinical competency; and

WHEREAS,   The provision of grandfathering to ensure the Associate Degree and Diploma nurses the privileges that their current licensure provides, and the provision of state reciprocity for grandfathering; and

WHEREAS,   The active solicitation of funds from federal, state, and local sources to support baccalaureate programs in nursing; and

WHEREAS,   The provision of financial assistance for those seeking a baccalaureate in nursing; and

WHEREAS,   An accelerated effort to prepare faculty who are qualified to teach in baccalaureate degree programs; therefore, be it

RESOLVED,   That the Oncology Nursing Society believes that there should be one level of entry into professional nursing practice and that the educational preparation for the entry level shall be the baccalaureate degree in nursing.

(Adopted at ONS Congress, 1980. Report of the ONS Task Force on Entry into Practice [1980]. *Oncology Nursing Forum,* 7(3):63.)

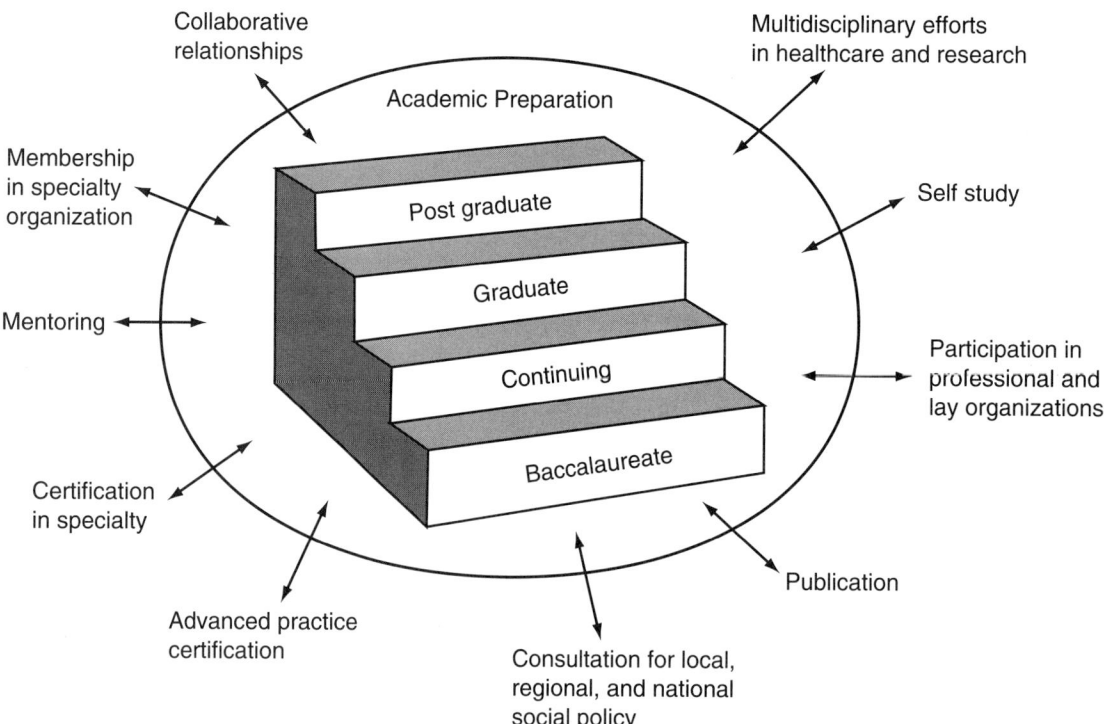

FIGURE 71–1. Life long learning: a balance between academic preparation and professional opportunities.

With all of the changes incurred with the integrated curriculum, oncology nursing content and clinical experiences in the undergraduate curriculum ranged extensively across programs (Kruse, 1986) and continues to vary today. The prevalence of cancer is such that only the rare undergraduate student finishes a program without caring for a cancer patient. If specific knowledge does, in fact, counter negative attitudes, then the integrated curriculum allows little or no time to dispel the myths and negativism associated with cancer. As a result, numerous consequences may occur, such as inadequate preparation of nurses in cancer nursing, limited understanding of theoretic content related to practice, and limited recruitment of nurses to the field of oncology nursing, to name a few.

The American Cancer Society (ACS) Professors of Oncology Nursing have recommended curriculum content that is essential for all students to learn during their basic nursing education. The first Professorship in Oncology Nursing was awarded in 1981. The purpose of a professorship is to strengthen cancer nursing content in graduate and undergraduate programs throughout the United States. In 1994, there were 10 professors. Typically, each professor is appointed for a 5-year term, which is renewable through the ACS Divisions. Their primary responsibility is to teach oncology nursing at the masters level, but most of them have responsibilities to oversee the cancer content at the undergraduate level. As a result of the professorship and related national meetings bringing them together, they identified essential content that all undergraduate students need prior to graduation. An outline of the curriculum is presented in Table 71–1. The table can be used as a guide to examine cancer content in preexisting courses and program curricula, to modify current lecture material and clinical experiences, to develop new methods of delivering cancer-specific information, to facilitate self-study by a student in a special area, and to aid in the elimination of redundant cancer content. The professors recognized that it is unlikely that all the content specific to cancer will be addressed and that some of it can be presented with other illness-related situations. For example, all students need content related to dying patients, pain management, and referrals to community resources, and this content is applicable to other patient populations. The professors also identified outcome competencies for the new baccalaureate graduate entering nursing practice. These competencies are presented in Table 71–2.

GRADUATE EDUCATION

In 1979, the American Cancer Society organized a meeting of nursing leaders in oncology and education to develop a *Masters Degree with a Specialty in Cancer Nursing Curriculum Guide and Role Definition.* This document has been updated twice. The third edition was completed in 1995 by a joint committee of the Oncology Nursing Society and the American Cancer Society. The ACS members were the 10 current American Cancer Society Professors of Oncology Nursing. Historically, the first two editions of the document focused on the role of the clinical nurse specialist in oncology. Given the changes in health care reform, the latest edition was expanded to include the skills and knowledge of the nurse practitioner. The reader is referred to Chapter 3 for a thorough discussion of the many roles that nurses assume, especially the critical distinctions between clinical nurse specialists and nurse practitioners. The curriculum guide provides nurses pursuing their masters degree with the broadest prepa-

ration to assume the potential of multiple positions in a variety of diverse cancer care settings.

Essential content for advanced practice evolves as new knowledge and innovative strategies are gained in cancer prevention, detection, treatment, and care. Graduate studies leading to a masters degree with a specialty in advanced practice oncology nursing should include a combination of didactic and supervised clinical courses. Clinical courses need to be planned in a variety of oncology settings and include supervision by experienced preceptors. Each year, the ONS Education Committee surveys the graduate programs in cancer nursing to establish a current listing. The results are published annually in the October issue of the *Oncology Nursing Forum,* the official journal of the ONS. There are over 40 nursing programs in the United States offering masters degrees with a specialty in oncology.

Programs across the country vary by cost, length, content, faculty qualifications, and focus. Potential applicants should consider a number of factors in applying for a specialty oncology nursing program. Table 71–3 lists criteria for selecting a graduate program. Ultimately, advanced practice oncology education should provide the foundation for advanced certification and for doctoral study in nursing or a related field.

PREDOCTORAL AND POSTDOCTORAL EDUCATION

Although the numbers remain small, there is an increasing number of nurses who are pursuing doctoral education in oncology nursing. The primary purpose of obtaining a doctoral degree is to gain knowledge and skills in research to develop new knowledge in cancer care. Nurse researchers are needed to develop, design, and implement research studies related to the field of cancer nursing.

A significant number of schools of nursing offering the masters degree in oncology nursing also offer doctoral and postdoctoral opportunities in oncology nursing. When selecting a school for predoctoral or postdoctoral studies, the applicant needs to consider the reputation of the school and the qualifications of the faculty he or she selects to study with. If the applicant has the ability to temporarily relocate, his or her priority should be to identify a mentor whose research is an excellent match with the applicant's interests.

Postdoctoral research training in nursing and particularly oncology nursing is relatively new (Lev, Souder, & Topp, 1990). Individual and Institutional National Research Service Awards (NRSA) are available through the National Institute of Nursing Research and the National Cancer Institute. Research opportunities are discussed in detail in Chapter 72.

STAFF EDUCATION

Despite the likelihood that nursing students will provide direct care to cancer patients during clinical experiences, most nurses are not sufficiently prepared by their undergraduate oncology nursing programs to practice oncology nursing. Thus, both academic educa-

TABLE 71–1. *Curriculum and Self-Study Guide for Core Concepts in Cancer Nursing*

I.   What is Cancer?
      Historic perspectives of cancer
      Current status of cancer as a chronic illness
      Carcinogenesis (basics of initiation and promotion)
      Alteration in cells (e.g., cell cycle)
      Immunosuppression and cancer
      Differentiation of benign from malignant tumors
      Classification of tumors
      Invasion and metastasis
II.   Cancer Prevention: Risk Reduction
      Primary prevention: Assessment of individual risk factors, assessment and exposure to carcinogens, family history
            Tobacco prevention/cessation
            Sun exposure
            Diet and weight control
            Occupational exposure
            Older age as a risk factor
III. Early Detection of Cancer (Secondary Prevention)
      Cancer epidemiology: International, national and local perspectives; differences by age, gender, socio-economic,
            racial/ethnic group; incidence, prevalence and death rates.
      Screening guidelines
      Relationship of early detection to decreased morbidity and mortality
      Early signs and symptoms of cancer
      Self-detection methods
IV.   Principles of Cancer Diagnosis and Treatment
      Importance of tissue diagnosis
      Principles of a staging workup (and TNM classification)
      Common sites of metastasis
      Purposes of treatment
            Curative, palliative and adjuvant
      Basic principles of action: risks/benefits
            Chemotherapy
            Radiation therapy
            Surgery
            Biologic response modifiers
            Bone marrow transplantation
            Ajuvant treatment
V.   Nurses' Role in Resolving Ethical Issues and Dilemmas
      Treatment decision making
      Informed consent/clinical trials
      Issues in palliative care
      Shift from cure to palliative therapy
      Questionable methods
VI.   Symptom Management
      Common side effects of treatment and tumors, especially
            Pain
            Infection/fever
            Bleeding
            Nausea/vomiting
            Cachexia/anorexia
VII. Psychosocial Aspects of Cancer Care
      The trajectory of coping with cancer as a chronic illness across the life span and in different populations
      Differences in coping and health-seeking behaviors by age, gender, culture/ethnicity, and demography
      Patient and family psychosocial responses
      Sexuality
VIII. Continuum of Care
      Economics and politics of care: access, quality of care, and outcomes
      Rehabilitation: living with cancer and lifestyle changes
      Referral to community resources
IX.   Occupational/Safety and Emotional Concerns for the Caregiver
      Radiation precautions, risk of infection/isolation precautions, occupational exposure to chemotherapy agents; coping
            with grief and loss; emotional burn-out

TABLE 71–2. *Expectations for Clinical Competencies in Cancer Care Upon Completion of Baccalaureate Program in Nursing*

Describe the principles of carcinogenesis, cancer growth, and metastasis.

Discuss concepts related to cancer prevention, assess risk factors for cancer, describe interventions to decrease cancer risk.

Specify recommendations for cancer screening, identify early signs and symptoms of cancer, describe methods for diagnosis.

Describe the purpose of staging workup for cancer, differentiate the purposes of different forms of cancer treatment.

Identify the nursing role in ethical issues and decision making in cancer care.

Describe nursing's role in symptom management of cancer, particularly pain management, describe the common side effects of cancer treatment.

Describe the major psychosocial responses of the individual and family to cancer.

Communicate effectively with people with cancer and their families.

Describe the differential impact of cancer on individuals and families in terms of culture/ethnic membership, gender, age, and socio-economic group.

Describe survivorship and quality of life issues and goals in the continuum of care.

Describe the nurse's role in palliative care and bereavement.

Practice safety to prevent risk to self in cancer settings.

---

tion and continuing staff development are important components necessary for the provision of competent cancer patient care. The process of staff development is defined by the American Nurses Association as "a process consisting of orientation, in-service education, and continuing education for the purpose of promoting the development of personnel within any employment setting, consistent with the goals and responsibilities of the employee" (ANA, 1990, p. 3). Although the degree of employer support varies greatly among agencies, most cancer nursing administrators would agree that staff development activities do enhance the provision of competent patient care, improve job satisfaction, and promote recruitment and retention of quality staff. Staff development programs for cancer patient care must be directed by advanced practice oncology nurse educators or nurse specialists who apply the ONS *Standards of Oncology Nursing Education* (1989) in the employment setting.

PRINCIPLES OF ADULT LEARNING

Teaching is an important function in the daily practice of oncology nursing. While most teaching activities are geared towards patients and caregivers, nurses at all levels may be called upon to provide education to their colleagues. The format of this education can range from brief unit-based in-services focusing on a certain procedure or treatment to a formal presentation at a national conference. Most nurses are experienced and comfortable with the content of the presentation yet have had little or no training in the principles of

adult learning. Adults differ from each other in their learning needs and styles. These differences require the educator to forgo the traditional role of transmitter of knowledge and take on the role of facilitator and resource person for the learner. The mission of the adult educator is to assist the learner in clarifying educational needs and defining means to achieve them and in so doing, develop a partnership between the learner and educator.

The following principles of adult learning will help the nurse adapt educational activities to meet the needs of the adult learner (Hagopian, 1993; Knowels, 1980; Sullivan, 1994).

- Learners must perceive a need to learn the information. The objective of the learning experience must be relevant and timely to their practice. Readiness to learn is based upon life situations that mandate a need to gain new knowledge and skills to perform more effectively.
- Commitment to the learning experience increases with learner participation in the learning process.
- Adults are problem- or task-oriented. Educational activities need to focus on the resolution of problems or completion of tasks in a timely fashion, capturing the "teachable moment." Readiness to learn corresponds to problems encountered in daily situations.
- The learning activities should recognize and build upon the experiences of the individual learners, allowing them to incorporate the new information into their experiences.
- Adult learners have multiple demands on their time. The education should be self-paced, self-directed, and provide for flexibility in scheduling.
- The learning environment should reflect mutual trust, respect, and acceptance and allow for freedom of expression. The climate should focus on the physical as well as psychologic comfort of the learners.
- Feedback is a necessary component of the learning process, and positive reenforcement can help facilitate learning.
- Adults are motivated to learn by both extrinsic (promotion, pay raise, etc.) and intrinsic (increase self-esteem, personal achievement, etc.) methods.

Incorporating these principles into the preparation, implementation, and evaluation of learning activities respects the nurse-learner as a self-directed professional and provides a foundation for meeting the educational needs of the adult learner.

BARRIERS TO STAFF EDUCATION

Participation in educational programs that serve to enhance or maintain knowledge of oncology nursing concepts and skills is a criterion of the Professional Performance Standards set forth by the American Nurses Association and the Oncology Nursing Society (1987). While this would appear to be a reasonable and attainable expectation, there are nurses who, for a variety of reasons, do not attend educational programs. For many institutions, the 1990s have seen a decrease in budgets for educational programs, which has affected both the

TABLE 71–3. *Criteria for Selecting a Graduate Program*

The School
   Is the school accredited by the NLN?
   What is the ranking of the school?
   What is the school's reputation in the community?
   Is there a doctoral or postdoctoral program?
The Faculty
   Who are the faculty?
   What are the credentials of the faculty?
   Is there more than one faculty member in the oncology program?
   Do they hold doctorates?
   Are they in leadership positions in local and national cancer organizations?
   Are they engaged in research?
   Are they engaged in clinical practice?
   What have they published?
   Where have they published?
   How many funded research grants or community education programs are ongoing?
The Program
   Are there both theory and clinical courses in oncology nursing?
   How many theory courses in oncology nursing are there?
   How many clinical courses in oncology nursing are there?
   Can the program be taken on a full- or part-time basis?
   How much time is required to complete the program?
   Does the program follow the ONS ACS curriculum guidelines?
   Are there opportunities to take elective or independent study courses?
Assignments
   Are assignments useful and meaningful?
   Are the assignments related to things that you will be doing in your future job?
   Is a masters' thesis required?
Students
   How many students are in the school?
   How many students are in the oncology program?
   Are the students happy in the program?
   What would the students like to change about the program?
   What kinds of positions do graduates of the program hold?
Clinical Experiences
   Can you specialize in the area of your interest in cancer?
   How much clinical time will be expected?
   What role does the faculty assume in the clinical area?
   Does the program use clinical preceptors?
   Are the preceptors masters' prepared in oncology?
   Do you need a car to meet your clinical obligation?
   How much flexibility is there to meet your individual needs and interests?
   What are the role options: Nurse practitioner or clinical specialist?
Resources
   What is the library like?
   Is the library open evenings and weekends?
   Does the library subscribe to journals specific to oncology nursing?
   Does the school have computers for students' use?
   Does the school have a career planning and placement office to assist you in finding a job after graduation?
   Is there a writing program to assist students with written assignments?
   Is there an international house or organization on campus?

(From Hagopian, G., & McCorkle, R. [1993]. Choosing a master's program in cancer nursing in the United States. *Cancer Nursing, 16*[6], 473–478.)

development of educational programs and attendance by graduates. These budgetary decreases have coincided with an increase in educational needs, as many oncology nurses now practice across settings. For instance, it is not unusual for the same nurse to work in both the inpatient oncology unit and outpatient chemotherapy clinic. While these new role responsibilities provide for enhanced continuity of care for oncology patients and their families, there is a required level of education and cross-training needed for nurses to function competently in multiple settings even when the patient population is similar. Prevention and detec-

tion is another area of rapid growth and development in oncology nursing, and many nurses are being called upon to incorporate sophisticated prevention and detection strategies into their practice. Again, this process requires specialized training and education to effectively prepare the nurse for this expanded role.

Many nurses and administrators do not value the worth of formal continuing education. Incidental, on-the-job training is viewed as a sufficient means of keeping current. While this is an acceptable method of learning, it tends to be task-oriented, limited to a specific area of practice, and lacking in a theoretic base transferable to other situations. Other nurses may have had a negative experience with educational programs such as irrelevant content, ineffective speakers, or lack of administrative support to attend a program.

Nurses involved in developing and implementing educational programs must remain cognizant of these and other barriers to continuing education. Strategies that the nurse educator can utilize in overcoming these barriers are: keep the content relevant to the audience; ensure accessibility of programs financially, geographically and time-wise; develop faculty who are knowledgeable, experienced, and flexible; and work with administrators in providing a means for the learners to integrate new knowledge into their practice.

ONS AND JCAHO STANDARDS OF PROFESSIONAL EDUCATION

The need for professional nursing education clearly extends beyond that of basic academic preparation. Indeed, this need is underscored by both accreditation standards and professional practice standards. JCAHO (1993) requires hospitals to ensure staff competency via orientation, in-service and continuing education efforts. Examples of JCAHO standards are listed in Table 71–4. Thus maintenance of an institution's accreditation depends, in part, on its ability to provide staff education specific to all specialty patient care services.

The importance of education specific to oncology nursing is supported further by the ANA/ONS *Standards of Oncology Nursing Practice* (1987). Oncology nurses are accountable for developing and maintaining professional skills, as evidenced by the professional performance standard: "the oncology nurse assumes responsibility for professional development and continuing education and contributes to the growth of others" (ANA/ONS, 1987, p. 17). In a broader sense, the ANA/ONS standards may facilitate professional development by identifying gaps in one's knowledge base and determining the range of practice for which one is prepared (Volker, 1992). Although the standards are useful for a wide variety of clinical, management, quality improvement, and education applications, they are particularly invaluable for curriculum planning. Both staff development and continuing education programs can be based on the standards, with specific process and outcome criteria serving as learner objectives. For example, a continuing education program on management of patient ventilation problems can be designed using the practice standards as outlined in Table 71–5. Note that the learner objectives can be modified to serve as criteria for a clinical practicum and subsequent competency validation of these knowledges and skills. For example, instead of simply describing effective measures to maintain a patent airway, the learner implements such measures successfully in the clinical setting.

TABLE 71–4. *Examples of JCAHO Standards for Leadership Development and Staff Education*

CHAPTER REFERENCE	STANDARD STATEMENT
LD*.1.9	The organization's leaders develop programs to promote the recruitment, retention, development, and continuing education of all staff members.
SE*.1	The organization provides an individual who is new to the organization or to a department/service with an orientation of sufficient scope and duration to inform the individual about his or her responsibilities and how to fulfill them within the organization or department/service.
SE.2	The organization provides for education and training designed to maintain and improve the knowledge and skills of all personnel.
SE.3	The effectiveness and appropriateness of orientation, training, and education provided for by the organization are evaluated through its quality assessment and improvement activities.
SE.4	Each individual in the organization is competent, as appropriate to his or her responsibilities.

*LD=Leadership development; SE=Staff education.

(Adapted from The Joint Commission on Accreditation of Healthcare Organizations (1993). *Accreditation manual for hospitals, Volume I: Standards* [pp. 31, 149–150]. Oakbrook Terrace, IL: Author.)

TABLE–71–5. *Application of ANA/ONS Professional Practice Standards to Staff Education*

Use of Standards IV and VI outcome criteria for teaching the nurse to care for patients with alterations in ventilation.
Goal: Upon completion of the course, the learner will be able to recognize factors that may impair ventilatory function and know how to intervene with measures that may enhance optimum ventilatory capacity (Standard VI).
Learning Objectives (Standard IV):
The learner will:
Identify reasons for altered ventilation, such as decreased hemoglobin, infection, anxiety, effusion, and an obstructed airway.
Describe plans for daily activity that demonstrate maximum conservation of a client's energy.
Describe the effects of environmental extremes on ventilatory function and oxygen utilization.
List measures to reduce or modify pulmonary irritants in the environment, such as smoke, dry air, powders, and aerosols.
Describe effective measures to maintain a patent airway.
Identify an appropriate plan of action to follow if ventilation becomes altered.
Develop a plan for managing an altered airway.

(Modified from American Nurses' Association & Oncology Nursing Society (1987). *Standards of oncology nursing practice.* [pp. 13, 15]. Kansas City, MO: American Nurses' Association.)

TABLE 71–6. *ONS Standards of Oncology Education: Generalists Level*

The faculty is prepared academically and clinically to teach oncology nursing.

Clinical and educational resources are adequate to achieve program objectives related to oncology nursing.

Basic knowledge, skills, and attitudes required for the delivery of nursing care to clients at risk for or with a diagnosis of cancer are included in the curriculum.

Teaching-learning theories are applied to the development, implementation, and evaluation of learning experiences related to oncology nursing care.

Graduates of nursing education programs assume responsibilities in oncology nursing commensurate with their educational and experiential preparation.

(Adapted from Oncology Nursing Society (1989). *Standards of oncology nursing education: Generalists and advanced practice levels.* [pp. 4–8]. Pittsburgh, PA: Author.)

A third document, the ONS *Standards of Oncology Nursing Education: Generalists and Advanced Practice Levels* (1989), also serves to enhance the quality of oncology nursing education. This document outlines standards that include structure, process, and outcomes of educational offerings for both the generalists and advanced learners. The standards provide a "comprehensive" guideline for planning and evaluating continuing education and academic programs. See Table 71–6 for the generalists practice level standards. Copies of the *Standards of Practice* can be purchased from the Oncology Nursing Society's headquarters in Pittsburgh, Pennsylvania.

PROGRAM DEVELOPMENT

Development of education programs is a systematic process that is not unlike the nursing process. The cornerstones of assessment, diagnosis, planning, intervention, and evaluation serve as a framework for the nurse educator as well as the clinician. Whether one is planning an orientation program, in-service, or continuing education offering, the process does not vary.

ASSESSMENT OF LEARNING NEEDS

Because education programs consume expensive human and material resources, it is vital to identify and validate learning needs prior to conducting any educational programs. Unfortunately, education often is viewed as the remedy for a myriad of performance problems. Mager & Pipe (1984) designed a model to analyze performance problems that is helpful in differentiating between a knowledge deficit versus poor compliance, systems barriers, or other obstacles to proper performance of a given skill. If a legitimate learning need is established, a number of strategies are available to further delineate a target group's needs and assist with program planning. It is important to identify the target group, but even in a monogeneous group of staff nurses, there will be differences in level of educational preparation and experience, to name a few. Techniques such as informal clinical observation, interview, questionnaire, patient record review, analysis of critical incidents, and so forth are well described in other references (Masten, 1992; Oncology Nursing Society, 1994; Volker, 1987). Regardless of the strategy used, the educator must always identify learner characteristics and

situational and psychosocial factors that influence learning (ONS, 1989), and delineate specific gaps in learner knowledge and skills. An analysis of the needs assessment data should differentiate findings that are amenable to an educational intervention. The result is identification (diagnosis) of cognitive, psychomotor, and/or affective learning needs (ONS, 1989).

DEVELOPMENT OF LEARNING OBJECTIVES

The program planning process then continues with the development of measurable goals and learning objectives. Depending on the learning competencies to be achieved, appropriate behaviors from the various learning domains should be selected. When possible, learner objectives should be based on established practice standards and guidelines, such as those described in the Standards section and others (e.g., ONS products such as the Cancer Chemotherapy Guidelines, Manual for Radiation Oncology Nursing Practice and Education, Access Device Guidelines, Biologic Response Modifier Guidelines, Guidelines for Cancer Nursing Practice). Programs should always include application of knowledge to the practice arena, as teaching without this tie is frustrating to the learner and conflicts with principles of adult learning.

TEACHING STRATEGY METHODS

Selection of content and learning experiences must coincide with learner characteristics, situational factors, and desired outcomes. Teaching strategies will vary but are most effective when the learner is an active participant. Teaching strategies should be matched with the objectives of the educational offering and the unique characteristics of the learner including age, developmental level, experience, and attitude. For example, behavioral objectives in the psychomotor domain such as, "the participant will demonstrate the correct procedure for accessing a vascular access device," require a method of learning that provides an opportunity to actually demonstrate the procedure in a real or simulated setting as opposed to only discussion of the procedure. Environmental factors such as room availability, lighting, noise level, and seating arrangements factor into the selection of teaching strategies. Time and economics are also important considerations, as the method chosen may require additional equipment and faculty time, all of which must be factored into the overall budget. In planning educational programs, the faculty's comfort level with different educational strategies must not be overlooked. Someone who is very comfortable and competent in presenting material to large audiences in a lecture format may be hesitant to participate in a program that requires more intimate and spontaneous involvement such as role playing. Table 71–7 summarizes the indications, advantages, and disadvantages of several teaching strategies.

The scope of the educational activity will also influence the number and type of strategies selected. For example, a 45-minute in-service on an investigational new drug for unit staff likely will include only one or two strategies. Conversely, an 8-week orientation program for novice oncology nurses should include a wide variety of learning strategies based on the specific clinical competencies to be achieved. In general, when considering which methods or strategies to use, responding to the following questions will provide guidance in selecting the method most appropriate for the program, faculty, and the learner.

- Will the method support the behavioral changes described in the objective?
- Is the method chosen the simplest approach for achieving the objectives?
- Is the method appropriate for the time allotted?
- Is the method appropriate for the level of the learner in terms of background knowledge, skills, and attitudes?
- Will both the instructional staff and the nurses be comfortable with the method chosen? (Puetz & Peters, 1981).

EVALUATION

Finally, the planning process must include an evaluation component. Two key aspects should be measured: achievement of learning objectives and resolution of the original problem or issue that gave rise to the edu-

TABLE 71–7. *Indications, Advantages, and Disadvantages of Teaching Methods*

METHOD	INDICATIONS	ADVANTAGES	DISADVANTAGES
Lecture	Presentation of standardized information.	Presents lots of material in relatively short time.	Decreases teacher-learner ratio. Not individualized for learner's needs. Can be time/cost prohibitive for some staff to attend. Learner assumes passive-observer role.
Games/simulation	Reinforce lecture material. Application of knowledge. Good for heterogenous group. Good for presentation for potentially dull, mandatory information.	Combines didactic with clinical knowledge. Fosters learner participation.	Takes time to develop. Can be perceived as "silly," not professional by some.
Internship preceptorships	New graduates. Nurses who wish to increase their knowledge in specialty (i.e., pain management).	Appreciation of knowledge in real clinical setting. Individualized. Facilitates professional role development. Recognizes expertise of staff.	Labor-intensive for host. Decreases host's productivity. Time commitment for learner.
Computer-assisted instruction	Teach basic content. Test knowledge (i.e., OCN Review). Stimulate critical thinking.	Self-paced/learner-directed. Immediately validates learning. Consistency in content. Multiple users. Commercially available.	Need special equipment (hardware, software, and maintenance). Labor/cost-intensive to develop/maintain. Decreases interaction with other learners/faculty.
Self-learning packets	Knowledge acquisition and application of specific content that does not change rapidly.	Self-paced. Decreases cost to develop. Can incorporate more than one strategy (written, AV, clinical). Commercially available. No equipment needs.	Labor-intensive to develop. Learner must be motivated. Decreases interaction with other learners/faculty.
Demonstrations	Learning psychomotor skills.	Integrates didactic with clinical skills. Involves immediate feedback on performance.	Equipment needed. May not accurately reflect performance in real clinical situation.
Case studies	Staff present specific patient and/or clinical situation.	Shares knowledge with peers in format familiar to them. Ease of relating to clinical situation.	Maintains patient confidentiality. Requires staff to have degree of comfort with public speaking.

cational offering. For example, a continuing education program on hypercalcemia may have been offered to assist novice nurses to learn the requisite patient management. Thus, one might evaluate achievement of the cognitive objectives via a posttest or presentation of a case study. But it is also imperative to examine whether these learners competently care for patients with hypercalcemia after the program is over. Do the nurses identify patients at risk for problems associated with hypercalcemia and institute appropriate interventions? Do patients with hypercalcemia receive care according to institutional standards? The answers to these questions will help the educator determine the impact of the program on patient care. The evaluation methods need to be coordinated with the documentation requirements of the institution, so when chart audits are done, the specific nurse interventions are recorded to reflect positive patient outcomes.

Selection of evaluation strategies depends on the learning objectives and scope of the program. Direct observation of changes in clinical practice is practical when both the learner and educator practice in the same agency. Evaluation of continuing education programs that draw participants from a variety of institutions presents a larger challenge. Barg et al. (1992) describe a "gaps and contract" strategy that provides the learner with a tool to transfer knowledge gained to clinical practice in a measurable format. The strategy uses a learner contract that identifies gaps in a learner's practice and a plan to close the gap via application of the newly acquired knowledge. Using this strategy, program planners (and employing agencies) can measure practice changes based on the learner's fulfillment of the contracted activity.

If the planned program is a continuing education activity, accreditation should be sought so that contact hours can be awarded to attendees. Application must be made to an American Nurses Credentialing Center (ANCC) accredited approver of continuing education; examples include ONS, state nursing associations, state boards of nursing, schools of nursing, and education departments in the larger health care organizations. Consideration of seeking accredited contact hours should be made early in program planning, as the application process can be lengthy and entails a fee. Burke et al. (1989) provide a succinct overview of the application process through ONS. If the proposed program is multidisciplinary, the planning group needs to include members from each profession involved. The continuing education application process for each discipline varies; each professional organization can provide guidance regarding application requirements.

Once the planning process is complete, the educator implements the teaching plan and adapts strategies as learner priorities or setting characteristics change. Once evaluation of learning is complete, program revisions may be required based on analysis of evaluation data.

ORIENTATION PROGRAMS

Orientation is "the means by which new staff members are introduced to the philosophy, goals, policies,

procedures, role expectations, physical facilities, and special services in a specific work setting" (ANA, 1990, p. 3). The outcome should be a competent individual who practices according to identified standards. Certainly, standards outlined by the ANA/ONS and the JCAHO support the need for a planned, systematic orientation program for nurses new to the oncology setting. Although numerous approaches to orientation exist, a competency-based strategy is most consistent with the intent of both accreditation and professional practice standards. Development of competency-based orientation programs is well described elsewhere (Alspach, 1990; ASHET, 1992; McGregor, 1990).

The program planning process for orientation should follow that described in the previous section on program development. However, one key aspect warrants emphasis: the oncology setting's nurse manager, educator, and clinical experts must begin by identifying and agreeing upon those clinical competencies that new nurses must master. The competencies must be consistent with those reflected in the job description or performance standards specific to that job category. Incongruities in these expectations can create mixed messages and chaos for the beginning nurse and the tenured staff. The end result is inconsistent patient care and expensive, early attrition of staff. Table 71–8 outlines selected competencies for orientation of the novice oncology nurse to an inpatient setting. Obviously, the novice nurse cannot achieve competency in all areas of cancer nursing practice with all types of patients. Limits must be placed on the types of patients, procedures, and standards the novice can be expected to manage.

Once learner objectives are agreed upon, development of learning activities, evaluation methodologies, and time frames for completion can be accomplished. Table 71–9 outlines a plan for orientation to chemotherapy-related competencies. Similar, specific plans can be made for knowledge, skills, and attitudes that support each learner objective.

IDENTIFICATION OF REQUISITE COMPONENTS

Given that new employees bring preexisting knowledge and abilities to the new work setting, the educator should begin the orientation process by reviewing the learner objectives with each new nurse. A learning needs assessment specific to those objectives can then be conducted via interview, pretest, and clinical observation. The product of this assessment should be an individualized orientation plan that focuses on acquiring those competencies yet to be achieved. A learning contract between educator and new employee is helpful, as specific expectations and target dates can be delineated and agreed upon by both parties.

Learning experiences should include both didactic and clinical components. Didactic materials such as self-study packages, videotapes, review of policy and procedures, and computer-assisted instruction are all appropriate, depending on the specific competency to be achieved. Teaching strategies that can be implemented with a single learner (as opposed to group or

TABLE 71–8. *Selected Clinical Competencies for Orientation to an Inpatient Medical Oncology Setting**

Provides nursing care according to standard for patients with the following problems:

Myelosuppression	Hypercalcemia
Nausea/vomiting	Renal toxicity
Alopecia	Stomatitis
Diarrhea/Constipation	Dermatitis

Implements the policies and procedures for:

Blood components	Chemotherapy administration
Infusion therapy	Handling cytotoxic agents
Medication administration	

Incorporates principles of infection control into patient care.
Documents care delivered according to policy and procedures.
Admits, transfers, and discharges patients according to standard.
Recognizes life-threatening situations and responds appropriately.

Environment	*Patient*
Internal disasters	Cardiopulmonary arrest
External disasters	Hemorrhage
	Respiratory distress
	Septic syndrome

Communicates effectively (verbal and written) with patients, families, and members of the healthcare team.

*Other non-clinical orientation information such as an agency's mission and quality improvement program should be reviewed and documented as well.

classroom activities) are the most efficient and cost-effective, because they facilitate the orientation process in a 24-hour day, 7-day-a-week framework. Consequently, orientation need not wait for groups of learners to be hired for a specific date, nor will learners be restricted to canned group presentations that may not be relevant to an individual's needs.

Given the employer's obligation to provide safe patient care, close supervision of the new nurse's clinical practice must be ensured. Although licensure provides some indication of a nurse's ability to provide minimally safe care, practice in an oncology setting requires the acquisition of additional competencies. Typically, supervision is provided either by the educa-

TABLE 71–9. *Orientation Plan for Chemotherapy Competencies*

PERFORMANCE CRITERIA	MENU OF LEARNING ACTIVITIES	COMPLETION DATES
Competency: Implement policies and procedures for the patient receiving chemotherapy.		
Administer chemotherapy to 5 patients according to policy and procedure	View chemotherapy videotapes	_____
	Complete chemotherapy computer-assisted instruction modules	_____
	Read chemotherapy programmed instruction package	_____
	Review chemotherapy administration policy and procedures	_____
	Review drug information for prescribed chemotherapy agents	_____
	Clinical practicum with preceptor	_____
	See also above items	
Provide patient and family teaching according to Chemotherapy Teaching Plan	Review chemotherapy patient teaching plan	_____
	View videotape: *Teaching the Patient About Chemotherapy*	_____
	Review care guidelines for anticipated side effects	_____
	Clinical practicum with preceptor	_____
	See also above items	
Develop nursing care plans for patients receiving chemotherapy (include management)	Review procedure for documenting care plans	_____
	Clinical practicum with preceptor	_____
	See also above items	

tor or a clinical preceptor. Preceptors are invaluable resources for orienting new nurses, provided the preceptor's practice is consistent with proscribed standards, policies, and procedures. A preceptor also must be versed in adult learning and teaching/learning principles, and the new nurse's learning contract (Hagopian, Ferszt, Jacobs, & McCorkle, 1992). As the new nurse's competencies are validated, the need for close supervision will decrease. Ultimately, the preceptor will evolve into a resource and mentor for the novice.

Evaluation of achievement of the learning objectives is conducted in the clinical setting. The new nurse must demonstrate safe, consistent practice of the required competencies according to established policy and procedure. The amount of time a learner is allowed to complete an orientation is agency-specific. A cost-benefit analysis of the orientation program will assist the administrator in deciding the amount of time and educational resources that reasonably can be committed to each new employee.

DOCUMENTATION

Documentation of the orientation process and contract completion must be forwarded to the new nurse's personnel file. The file should include the baseline needs assessment, orientation plan, competencies achieved, and plan for continued development in the new role. Documentation of orientation program specifics, such as lesson plans, instructional media, attendance rosters, and blueprints for specialty-specific activities should be maintained within the education department.

ONGOING COMPETENCY ENSURANCE: IN-SERVICE AND CONTINUING EDUCATION

Orientation is only a starting point for developing oncology nurses. Once the orientation program competencies are mastered, the nurse continues to learn and grow via in-service and continuing education programs.

FORMATS

In-service education comprises those learning activities (in the work setting) that assist the nurse in "acquiring, maintaining, and/or increasing competence in fulfilling the assigned responsibilities specific to expectations of the employer" (ANA, 1990). Thus, in-service activities for the oncology nurse may encompass annual review of the agency's fire, safety, and infection control procedures; introduction to new patient care equipment; changes in documentation forms; review of chemotherapy protocols; and so forth. The educator is challenged to communicate these updates to all staff in a time- and cost-efficient manner. Because staffing constraints hinder attendance at centralized classroom presentations, other strategies also must be used. Poster presentations, self-study packets, fliers that announce procedure changes, videotapes, and mobile teaching carts are but a few effective methods used to reach staff.

Attendance at continuing education programs is another method that promotes acquisition of new knowledge and competencies. Continuing education "builds upon varied educational and experiential bases for the enhancement of practice, education, administration, research, or theory development" (ANA, 1990, p. 1). A wide variety of programs and topics are available for oncology nurses who seek to grow beyond that which is learned in academic programs.

DOCUMENTATION

Does attendance at in-service or continuing education programs ensure competency? Decidedly not. Competency ensurance is a process that an employing agency undertakes to validate that employees practice according to established standards. The JCAHO requires that "all nursing staff members are competent to fulfill their assigned responsibilities" (1993, p. 142). The process of competency assurance begins with validation of skills and abilities in orientation and continues throughout the remainder of employment. Annual performance evaluations serve well to evaluate and verify continued competency in one's job. Artificial, periodic, clinical performance "check-offs" are unnecessary, provided the skill in question is within the scope of general nursing practice for that setting and is performed frequently enough for the nurse manager to observe implementation. A manager may opt for an annual "check-off" if the skill is high-risk yet infrequently performed (example: mock codes for resuscitation skills).

CERTIFICATION

Another method of ensuring competency is through certification. Certification is a form of credentialing that seeks to measure competence. It is a voluntary way to validate knowledge and expertise in a given clinical or functional area (Winter, Pugh, & Riley, 1992). Benefits of certification are witnessed by patients and employers as well as the certified nurse. Certification ensures patients and employers that the nurse has both the knowledge and experience consistent with the delivery of competent patient care. It demonstrates a level of commitment to the area of specialization. For the nurse, certification may enhance career development, provide opportunities for advancement, and increase self-confidence in the learner's abilities (Oncology Nursing Certification Corporation, 1995).

GENERALIST

Certification in oncology nursing was introduced by its professional organization, ONS, in 1986. Since that time, over 14,000 oncology nurses have been certified (ONCC, personal communication). The process of becoming certified involves passing a written examination designed to address general oncology nursing knowledge. The examination is based on content from seven major areas: cancer nursing practice, major cancers, treatment of cancer, issues and trends in cancer care, cancer prevention and detection, pathophysiology of cancer, and cancer epidemiology. Certification through ONS is valid for 4 years, and the nurse must retake and successfully pass the examination at that time to maintain certification. Once certified, the nurse may use the credentials OCN, Oncology Certified Nurse.

The Oncology Nursing Certification Corporation (ONCC) has added the requirement of baccalaureate degree in nursing to the eligibility requirements for taking its certification. This new requirement takes effect in the year 2000. Present criteria to sit for the examination include current RN licensure, a minimum of 1000 hours of oncology nursing experience within the past 30 months, and a minimum of 30 month's experience as an RN within the past 5 years.

This requirement is in alignment with ONS support of the baccalaureate degree in nursing as the "entry level" academic requirement for professional nursing. One of the primary reasons for establishing the new requirement is to guarantee that nurses are seen as colleagues to professionals in other disciplines. Academic preparation of nurses must conform to that mandated by other health care disciplines.

ADVANCED

The OCN certification demonstrates only entry level competence in oncology. With a large percentage of oncology nurses prepared at the masters level (15 per cent of total membership) and with the role of the advanced practice nurse being the subject of much discussion within the nursing profession, the Oncology Nursing Society has taken a lead in the development of an advanced practice certification examination. In 1993, the Job Analysis of Advanced Oncology Nursing Practice Advisory Committee was formed. The goal of this committee was to develop a conceptual framework, including roles, knowledge base, and responsibilities of advanced practice oncology nurses, to guide the development of the advanced certification examination. The results of this study served as a blueprint for the development of the advanced certification examination. The first examination was administered in 1995. This examination serves as a measurable tool for differentiating advanced from general practice. Some states have already established more rigid criteria for nurses to call themselves clinical nurse specialists or nurse practitioners. To be certified at the advanced level, an applicant must have successfully completed a masters program in nursing. In addition to education requirements, a certification component exists that mandates an applicant successfully pass the highest level practice examination in his or her area of specialization. For oncology nurses, this would be the Advanced Practice Certification Examination. The other criteria remain the same, except an applicant must have a minimum of 2000 hours of oncology nursing practice within the 5 years prior to application.

The test blueprint for the Advanced Oncology Nursing Certificate is composed of five areas of advanced practice roles: direct caregiver, administrator/coordinator, consultant, researcher, and educator. Candidates who pass the advanced test may use the certification mark "AOCN" (advanced oncology certified nurse) to verify that they have met all the eligibility and testing requirements. The certification mark can be used as long as it is valid, after which time certification must be renewed by retest (ONCC, 1995). Any potential applicants should contact ONS at their headquarters office in Pittsburgh for information about dates and locations of certification examinations.

FUTURE DIRECTION OF CANCER NURSING EDUCATION

Nurses caring for patients with cancer and their families are prepared at a variety of basic educational levels 2-, 3-, and 4-year programs). It is important to recognize that this preparation is a basic and generalist preparation and does not make a nurse expert in cancer care. Educational opportunities need to be provided at local, regional, and national levels to facilitate nurses to increase their knowledge and clinical expertise to provide the specialty care required by cancer patients or those at risk of developing cancer. For nurses who are motivated and can, they need to secure additional formal education. The American Cancer Society and Oncology Nursing Society have established a number of scholarship programs to ease the financial burden of attaining the baccalaureate and masters degrees in nursing and explore ways to facilitate additional cancer nursing education opportunities. In addition, nurses with masters degrees need to pursue doctoral studies so advances in nursing research will evolve. One goal of research is to teach nurses how to better manage persons with cancer or persons at risk for cancer.

Nurses practicing in the field of cancer nursing need to develop a commitment to lifelong learning. Nurses must be responsible for their own learning. As advances in diagnostics, treatment, and care are discovered, nurses must keep pace with the knowledge explosion. ONS has local chapters that offer a variety of educational programs and are easily accessible throughout the United States. If a nurse is not a member, one of his or her first professional responsibilities must be to join and begin to participate in the organization's activities, for example, read the specialty journal, *Oncology Nursing Forum*.

The management of all cancer patients and their families in the future will rely heavily on the development of new roles in cancer nursing. These roles will range across the full spectrum of cancer care: prevention, early diagnosis, including treatment, and recovery. Clearly a better understanding of genetic therapy, chemotherapy, and immunotherapy will have a major impact on how patients are managed. We must continue to recognize the need for "state of the art" continuing education for nurses caring for people with cancer in many settings, especially in facilities providing managed care. Often in these settings, there are limited numbers of nurses, so release time from clinical responsibilities is limited unless nurses attend on their days off. Flexible and creative educational opportunities need to be developed to reach nurses in practices where there are only one or two nurses.

In health care in general, and cancer care in particular, nurses have reached the point where it is critical to demonstrate how nursing interventions make a difference in patient outcomes. As changes in health care reform continue, cost-effectiveness and management responsibility and accountability will be extended to all cancer nurses. Nurses need to understand their individual responsibility in the financial dimension of cancer care. Innovative patient management programs need to be developed and implemented by nurses to add to the financial revenue gain of institutions. Nurses have a remarkable ability to adapt to changing scientific, social, and economic conditions. Educational programs of the future must reflect these changes and also include content about the politics, power, and organizational structures to influence and make changes in cancer care. Educational programs that are responsive to the changing trends of health care and demands of patient care will prepare nurses to demonstrate and document their unique contributions to cancer care and their impact on patient outcomes. The critical element involves every cancer nurse assuming his or her own responsibility for remaining current throughout one's career.

REFERENCES

Alspach, J. G. (1990). *A competency-based orientation program for a medical/surgical intensive care unit*. Aliso Viejo, CA: American Association of Critical Care Nurses.

American Nurses Association (1990). *Standards for nursing staff development*. Kansas City, MO: American Nurses' Association.

American Nurses Association & Oncology Nursing Society (1987). *Standards of oncology nursing practice*. Kansas City, MO: American Nurses' Association.

American Society for Healthcare Education and Training (1992). *Competency assessment: Challenges and opportunities for health care educators*. Chicago: American Hospital Association.

Barg, F. K., McCorkle, R., Robinson, K., Yasko, J., Jepson, C., & McKeehan, K. M. (1992). Gaps and contract: Evaluating the diffusion of new information. Part 1. *Cancer Nursing, 15*, 401–405.

Burke, M. B., Lillis, P. P., Wright, P. S., Paiva, D. E., Ramsey, M. M., & Bean, C. B. (1989). Applying for continuing education approval: Demystifying the process. *Oncology Nursing Forum, 16*, 733–737.

Hagopian, G. (1993). Cancer nursing education. In S. Greenwald (Ed.), *Cancer nursing principles & practice* (3rd ed., pp. 1587–1589). Boston: Jones & Bartlett.

Hagopian, G., Ferszt, G., Jacobs, L., & McCorkle, R. (1992). Preparing clinical preceptors to teach master's level students in oncology nursing. *Journal of Professional Nursing, 8*(5), 295–300.

Joint Commission on Accreditation of Healthcare Organizations. (1993). *1994 accreditation manual for hospitals*. Vol. I: Standards. Oakbrook Terrace, IL: Author.

Knowels, M. S. (1980). *The modern practice of adult education from pedagogy to andragogy*. Chicago: Follett.

Kruse, L. C. (1986). Undergraduate cancer nursing education. In R. McCorkle & G. Hongladaron (Eds.), *Issues and topics in cancer nursing*, (pp. 65–75). Norwalk, CT: Appleton-Century-Crofts.

Lev, E., Souder, E., & Topp, R. (1990). The postdoctoral fellowship experience. *Image: Journal of Nursing Scholarship, 22*(2), 116–120.

Mager, R., & Pipe, P. (1984). *Analyzing performance problems* (2nd ed.). Belmont, CA: Pitman Learning, Inc.

Masten, K. (1992). Continuing education for oncology nurses. *Oncology Nursing Forum, 19*, 1237–1241.

McGregor, R. J. (1990). A framework for developing staff competencies. *Journal of Nursing Staff Development, 6*(2): 79–83.

Oncology Nursing Certification Corporation. (1995). *Oncology nursing certification makes a difference*. Pittsburgh: Author.

Oncology Nursing Society. (1989). *Standards of oncology nursing education: Generalists and advanced practice levels*. Pittsburgh: Author.

Oncology Nursing Society. (1994). *Continuing education activities: A planning manual*. Pittsburgh: Author.

Pennington, E. A. (1986). The integrated curriculum: A 15 year perspective. In E. A. Pennington (Ed.), *Curriculum revisited: An update of curriculum design* (NLN Pub. No. 15-2165, pp. 37–38). New York: National League for Nursing.

Puetz, B. E., & Peters, F. (1981). *Continuing education for nurses*. Rockville, MD: Aspen Publications.

Sullivan, D. T. (1994). Keeping adult learning principles alive. *Staff Development Insider, 3*(3), 1–8.

Volker, D. L. (1987). Learning needs assessment. *Oncology Nursing Forum, 14*(5), 60–62.

Volker, D. L. (1992). Standards of oncology nursing practice. In J. Clark & R. McGee (Eds.), *Core curriculum for oncology nursing* (2nd ed., pp. 3–17). Philadelphia: W. B. Saunders Co.

Winter, E., Pugh, L. & Riley, O. (1992). Is certification for you? *Nursing '92, 12*(1), 88–92.

Cancer Nursing Research Today

Kathi H. Mooney • Mel R. Haberman

The advances that have been achieved in cancer care are largely the result of systematic research. Cancer investigations continue at a rapid pace today because effective approaches to the prevention, early detection, and treatment of many cancers are still elusive. Basic science studies and medical research trials endeavor to discover new knowledge about the natural history of cancer and to test the effectiveness of new screening, diagnostic, and treatment approaches, including approaches to the prevention of cancer. Similarly, cancer nursing research that focuses on the individual's and family's response to cancer risk, the experience of cancer, cancer treatment, and cancer survivorship, has as its objective the advancement of knowledge in understanding the cancer experience, and effective interventions to improve the well-being of both individuals with cancer and their families. The new knowledge that results from these investigations provides nurses in clinical practice with knowledge and skills to effectively address individual and family psychosocial and physiologic needs. Use of research findings to guide the clinical practice of nurses and physicians, also called a research-based practice, is one of the cornerstones of a professional discipline.

As with other health professions, the nursing profession has as a primary goal the improvement of clinical care by developing nursing care practices that are maximally effective. This requires the continual development and use of a scientific body of knowledge to guide nursing practice. All nurses have some responsibility to make this happen. This includes nurses in clinical practice, educators, researchers, and administrators. It also crosses all educational levels in nursing. Table 72–1 lists many types of research-related responsibilities and the way cancer nurses at all levels of education become involved in nursing research. These responsibilities are not necessarily distinct. Experience, interest, and research training of the particular nurse may increase the degree of research involvement. Rizzuto, Bostrom, Suter, and Chenitz (1994) have found that nurses' participation in research activities is influenced by prior research instruction, awareness of support for research, and positive attitudes toward research.

The purpose of this chapter is to provide an overview of cancer nursing research. Some historic highlights that have led to the development of cancer nursing research are presented. Then the complex process of research utilization is discussed, with specific suggestions for how cancer nurses in clinical practice can build a research-based practice. This is followed by an overview of the steps involved in designing research

TABLE 72–1. *Levels of Nursing Research Involvement*

AA, Diploma and BSN Level

Participate as a team member in the development of projects, focusing on issues of clinical feasibility

Act as study monitor for data collection and management

Monitor the scientific and ethical conduct of studies

Conduct pilot/feasibility studies or companion protocols with assistance of a research mentor

Read widely and critically research reports in journals, and attend conferences where research findings are presented

Conduct electronic literature searches

Participate in journal clubs

Evaluate research findings and integrate appropriate findings into clinical practice with the assistance of a mentor

Develop a clinical practice that is research-based; expect scientific evidence that nursing practices are effective

Masters Level

Identify clinical problems and gaps in existing nursing practice amenable to research

Conduct pilot/feasibility studies or companion protocols independently or with mentorship

Act as research mentor to staff nurses

Participate as a team member or leader in designing projects, focusing on clinical, educational and administrative issues

Implement studies for others as a project director or study monitor

Participate in presenting the results of studies at conferences and by publication

Facilitate journal clubs with mentorship

Coordinate research dissemination and utilization activities

Review and critique protocols for design and clinical feasibility issues

Publish integrative reviews on specific research topics

Promote a climate of critical inquiry and establish institutional expectations that value research and the establishment of research-based practice, protocols, policies and standards

Doctorate Level

Generate new nursing knowledge by implementing complex research designs for concept definition, theory and instrument development

Mentor clinical nurses, graduate students and postdoctorate fellows

Lead projects as principal investigator and obtain research funding

Ensure the scientific and ethical conduct of studies

Develop programs of research in academic and clinical settings

Review grants for scientific merit by serving on grant review study sections and site visit teams

Lead or participate in multi-institutional studies

Disseminate widely findings of research to facilitate appropriate transfer to clinical practice and into health policy

studies. An understanding of some of the basic design and methodologic issues that go into developing a research project makes cancer nurses better clinicians, reviewers of published research, and advocates for individuals with cancer and their families. Finally, the authors address the future for cancer nursing research and emphasize the importance of a commitment by all cancer nurses to participate in research development and application.

HISTORIC ROOTS AND CONTRIBUTIONS OF CANCER NURSING RESEARCH

Cancer nursing research is in its infancy. As with other specialty nursing research, cancer nursing research essentially has only a 30-year history. Visionaries in nursing's past have advocated for scientific inquiry as the base of practice as far back as Florence Nightingale, who systematically studied environmental factors and nursing interventions during the Crimean War. However, the profession of nursing and the educational preparation of nurses had to evolve for another 100 years before research on nursing practice problems became feasible. After World War II nursing education moved from hospitals to academic settings, allowing a greater emphasis on scholarship and science rather than primarily experiential training. With the recognition that a scientific base for practice was essential for the development of the profession, nursing and government leaders began to lay the foundation to support nurses in obtaining advanced degrees, including doctorates. The initial research that was conducted during this fledgling era focused more on the education, utilization, and job satisfaction of nurses rather than on clinical practice problems. However, important foundations continued to be laid that would eventually promote practice research.

It was during the 1950s that the American Nurses Foundation was formed and federal research funds were appropriated by the Division of Nursing Resources, now known as the Division of Nursing. The appearance of the first research journal for nursing came in 1952, when *Nursing Research* was published.

During the next decade important progress was made. There was increasing concern about the lack of research on nursing practice problems during the 1960s. In response, the federal Nurse Scientist Training Grants program was initiated, funding nurses to attend doctoral programs that combined nursing with biologic and behavioral disciplines. Many of the graduates of these programs are the senior leaders in nursing research today.

But it was not until the 1970s and 1980s that doctoral programs in nursing offering Ph.D.s or Doctor of Nursing Science were established. This was pivotal to the contemporary emergence of a cadre of qualified nurse researchers and was the beginning of a scientific base for the profession. Other important events of this era included congressional establishment of the National Center for Nursing Research in 1985 that more recently (1993) has been given full institute status in the National Institutes of Health and is now known as the National Institute for Nursing Research.

Cancer nurse researchers have benefited from educational and funding resources provided nursing in general. However, cancer nursing research also was fostered through nurse participation in medical cancer clinical trials (Hilkemeyer, 1982). The foundation for medical clinical trials in cancer was laid in the 1950s and 1960s with NIH establishment of the National Chemotherapy Section in 1956, which later led to the development of cooperative groups that supported medical clinical trials into the diagnosis, treatment, and prevention of cancer, utilizing a variety of modalities. An infusion of research funds into the National Cancer Institute (NCI) and urgency to find effective treatment for cancer occurred in 1971 with the federal passage of the National Cancer Act. The designation of comprehensive cancer centers occurred in 1973 by the NCI. This facilitated the development of a structure for a comprehensive clinical trials system (Jenkins & Hubbard, 1991). While the initial emphasis was on medical approaches to curing cancer, the 1980s and 1990s have brought a broader mission not only focused on cure, but also directed at decreasing morbidity and improving quality of life. Cancer nurse researchers have contributed to and received NCI research funding for this extended research agenda.

The development of nurse-initiated cancer research was a natural outgrowth of the priorities within the nursing profession for research, nurse experience with medical clinical trials, and the observation of so many unanswered nursing questions in clinical cancer care. The earliest studies by cancer nurse researchers paralleled the development of nursing research in general and did not focus on patient care problems. Farrell (1953) published a study in *Nursing Research* on the outcome of several approaches to teaching cancer nursing. Three years later Gordon (1956) developed criteria for a cancer service based upon a patient record review. It was not until 1963 that the first cancer nursing study focused on a clinical care issue appeared in the literature (Quint, 1963). This descriptive study provided the foundation for understanding the significant psychosocial adjustment to mastectomy required by women with breast cancer and the influence of information control by others on adjustment outcomes (Quint, 1963, 1965).

It is from this foundation that the contemporary era of cancer nursing research began. For excellent detailed reviews of the historic developments in cancer nursing research, consult these classic references: Benoliel, 1983; Hilkemeyer, 1982; McCorkle & Lewis, 1980; Padilla, 1990.

Since the 1970s there has been a continual expansion in the research base for cancer nursing practice. The clinical specialty of cancer nursing has simultaneously emerged during this same time frame (1970s and 1980s), increasing the demand for high-quality studies to guide specialty practice. Educational advancement and specialization in cancer has been offered through master's graduate nursing programs. These educational programs often are cancer nurses' first real experience in conducting research projects.

Cancer nurse researchers often seek federal funding for their research studies. Both the National Institute for Nursing Research and the National Cancer Institute provide research funding mechanisms and doctoral and other research training development awards. Besides this federal support, a number of other organizations have made significant contributions to the advancement of the specialty and the promotion of cancer nursing research. The International Society of Nurses in Cancer Care offers the journal *Cancer Nursing*, which publishes both clinical and research reports. The American Cancer Society (ACS) has supported cancer nursing as far back as the 1940s (Barckley, 1964). A number of ACS programs support cancer nursing research advancement. Most notable is ACS's major research grants program. Cancer nurse researchers are eligible to compete for funds, and over the years several nurses have been funded through this mechanism. Senior nurse researchers have participated in the review process by serving on the Society's research review group. The ACS provides significant educational support through its master's and doctoral scholarship program. Professorships in oncology nursing have been awarded to outstanding cancer nurse researchers in academic settings, a portion of their support going for the recipient's research activities. In addition to general nursing conferences, every few years the ACS offers a conference devoted exclusively to cancer nursing research. This conference encourages researchers and clinicians to discuss research findings and methodologic issues, and identify gaps in knowledge for practice.

The other organization that has provided essential support for the development of cancer nursing research is the Oncology Nursing Society (ONS), which was established in 1975. The official journal of ONS is the *Oncology Nursing Forum*, which publishes both clinical articles and research reports. In 1980 the Society established a research committee. Today ONS demonstrates a strong commitment to the advancement of cancer nursing knowledge through research and promotes the utilization of research findings in practice. To this end ONS and the Oncology Nursing Foundation offer research grants to support new investigations, funding, for example, 22 research studies for a total of $153,580 in 1995. ONS also provides research fellowships, doctoral scholarships, and a mentorship program for new investigators. ONS has received funding from NCI for a long-running grant that offers a 1-day "short course" in conjunction with the Society's annual congress. The course brings together doctoral students and other beginning researchers to present their research proposals and receive feedback and assistance from a panel of senior cancer nurse researchers. ONS also offers members the Advanced Research Special Interest Group that facilitates discussion and networking among cancer nurse researchers. Recently ONS developed a mechanism to promote multi-site research, instigated a special initiative to increase research on cancer fatigue, and conducted a series of state-of-the-knowledge conferences to promote knowledge synthesis and advancement.

THE FOCUS OF CANCER NURSING RESEARCH

Ideally the focus of research studies is based on clinical problems that are most urgently in need of solving. In reality, with such a short history of research, there are a vast number of problems that could be addressed. Researchers should strive to identify researchable areas with input from clinicians and an understanding of the gaps in the literature, so that programs of research are developed that provide a solid base for clinical decision making. Several published papers summarize the focus of early and more current research investigations

(Benoliel, 1983; Fernsler, Holcombe, & Pulliam, 1984; Ferrell, Rhiner, & Grant, 1992; Grant & Padilla, 1983; Hilkemeyer, 1982; McCorkle & Lewis, 1980; Padilla, 1990). Recently a meta-analysis of cancer nursing symptom management intervention research was reported by Smith, Holcombe, and Stullenbarger (1994). A meta-analysis uses statistical techniques to combine the results of similar studies to examine anew the strength of research findings in a given area.

A review of current research reports in the published nursing literature was conducted to determine major topics of interest. The search of the *Cumulative Index for Nursing and Allied Health Literature* (CINAHL) covered the years 1990 through 1994. Ninety-eight citations were found in the research report database, using the key word "neoplasms," and limiting the search to *nursing* research. The most common topics were studies of coping with cancer; prevention, risk reduction, and early detection; self-care; quality of life; symptom management, patient education and knowledge, attitudes, and practices of nurses. It should be noted that these citations do not represent all cancer nursing research studies published during this time period, since nurse researchers may publish in journals outside of those referenced by CINAHL. For example, the journal *Cancer* is not included in CINAHL's database.

Another source to determine potential areas for cancer nursing research is found in national surveys of research priorities. There have been a number of surveys of priorities for cancer nursing research reported in the literature since 1978, when Oberst (1978) published a Delphi survey. Subsequently, priority surveys have been conducted by individual researchers, the Canadian Consortium, and on a regular basis by the Research Committee of the Oncology Nursing Society (Degner et al., 1987; Dodd, 1987; Funkhouser & Grant, 1989; Grant & Stromborg, 1981; McGuire, Frank-Stromborg & Varricchio, 1985; Mooney, Ferrell, Nail, Benedict, & Haberman, 1991; Oberst, 1978; Stetz, Haberman, Holcombe, & Jones, 1995). Table 72–2 compares the top 10 research priority areas identified in the last two ONS surveys conducted during the 1990s. Commonalities between these surveys underscore the importance of cancer nursing research in the areas of quality of life, pain, prevention and early detection, and cost containment.

Cancer nursing as a specialty enjoys the contributions of a small but talented cadre of seasoned and new researchers. Mentorship of new researchers through the support and guidance of senior cancer nurse researchers adds to the quality of future research investigations. In 1992 the Oncology Nursing Society established an annual award to recognize the contributions of outstanding cancer nurse researchers. Early winners of the Distinguished Researcher Award have been Drs. Jean E. Johnson (1992), Jeanne Quint Benoliel (1993), Ruth McCorkle (1994), and Barbara A. Given (1995). All of these distinguished researchers have made significant and sustained contributions to the cancer nursing knowledge base. Table 72–3 summarizes these contributions.

USING RESEARCH FINDINGS IN PRACTICE

SOURCES OF KNOWLEDGE FOR CLINICAL PRACTICE

Historically nurses have utilized multiple sources to determine clinical practice standards and procedures. Tradition and rituals have been a common base for practice. For example, when questioned about the basis of a specific practice such as a procedure for a dressing change, the nurses may say, "We've always done it that way." This approach allows practices to be uniform and passed from nurse to nurse without the need for individual analysis. However, it discourages the critical evaluation of the effectiveness of the practice.

Authority is a second source of nursing knowledge. This is a natural extension of the historic focus on educational training where the source of learning was the expert knowledge of the teacher or from textbooks that described practices without validating the source of that knowledge. Upon graduation, nurses found that the hospital setting often provided a similar prescriptive method for nursing activities.

Nurses sometimes find that nursing care problems do not respond to traditional practices or expert advice. In these situations nurses often use their own

TABLE 72–2. *Oncology Nursing Society's 1991 and 1995 Top Ten Research Priorities*

1991 ONS RESEARCH PRIORITIES SURVEY*	1995 ONS RESEARCH PRIORITIES SURVEY[t]
1. Quality of life	1. Pain
2. Symptom management	2. Cancer Prevention
3. Outcome measures for interventions	3. Quality of Life
4. Pain control and management	4. Risk Reduction/Cancer Screening
5. Cancer survivorship	5. Ethical Issues
6. Prevention/early detection	6. Neutropenia/ Immunosuppression
7. Research utilization	7. Patient Education
8. Cost containment	8. Stress, Coping and Adaptation
9. Economic influences	9. Cancer Detection
10. AIDS	10. Cost Containment

* Mooney, Ferrell, Nail, Benedict, & Haberman, 1991.
[t] Stetz, Haberman, Holcombe, & Jones, 1995.

TABLE 72–3. *ONS Distinguished Researcher Award Recipients, 1992-1995*

RECIPIENT	CANCER RESEARCH FOCUS
J. E. Johnson (1992)	Self regulation theory
	Coping facilitation through concrete sensory information prior to treatment
J. Q. Benoliel (1993)	Psychosocial oncology
	Psychosocial impact of cancer, cancer treatment, and terminal illness on patients, families, and nurses
R. McCorkle (1994)	Psychosocial oncology
	Instrumentation for symptom distress
	Impact of home health nursing care on cancer patients and caregivers
B. A. Given (1995)	Impact, burden, and cost for family caregivers of cancer patients
	Rural cancer nursing care
	Impact of cancer in the elderly
	Compliance with cancer treatment

experience or intuition. Practices based on experience and intuition are sometimes effective and sometimes not effective. A trial and error approach can be very inefficient in solving nursing problems.

Research provides another more systematic approach to solving problems. While the development of a research investigation may draw on clinical experience, intuition, traditional practices, and expert knowledge, these assumptions are subjected to careful scrutiny and testing and may or may not hold up at the conclusion of the study. Since the primary goal of nursing is to provide nursing care that is maximally effective and safe, a scientific body of knowledge based on research is essential to meet this goal.

RESEARCH UTILIZATION AND BARRIERS TO USE

Studies of the extent to which nurses report using research findings in their clinical practices reveal a slowly increasing trend toward research utilization. In one of the earliest studies, Ketefian (1975) found that nurses were both unaware of research findings and not using findings in practice. Kirchhoff (1982) similarly found that only 21 to 35 per cent of critical care nurses had implemented research recommendations to discontinue the use of two traditional coronary precautions. By the late 1980s studies found that over half of the nurses responding reported using nine or 10 of 14 research-validated practices. However, consistent use of the practices occurred less than half of the time (Brett, 1987; Coyle & Sokop, 1990). Most recently, Walczak, McGuire, Haisfield, and Beezley (1994) found that in one comprehensive cancer center, 45 per cent of cancer nurses indicated moderate to high utilization of research in their clinical practices. Finally, the Research Committee of the Oncology Nursing Society recently completed a large national survey of research utilization patterns of cancer nurses with eight research-

based practices (Rutledge, Greene, Mooney, Nail, & Ropka, personal communication). Preliminary analysis suggests encouraging gains in the adoption of research findings in cancer nursing practice.

Even with increasing rates of research utilization in clinical practice, barriers to using research continue to hamper the development of a fully realized research-based practice in nursing (Champion, & Leach, 1989; Funk, Champagne, Wiese, & Tornquist, 1991). Historically, obtaining the research findings was the most difficult problem for nurses (Krueger, Nelson, & Wolanin, 1978; Miller & Messenger, 1978). However, with increasing numbers of research journals and improved technology for obtaining and producing personal copies of research reports, other barriers have emerged as predominate concerns, particularly job-related barriers.

The most commonly reported barrier for cancer nurses in the Walczak et al. study (1994) was a lack of time to investigate research findings for a clinical problem, cited as frequently or always a problem by 85 per cent of the respondents. Lack of rewards for applying research to practice and resistance to changing practice in the agency were also cited as common barriers by over half of the respondents.

RESEARCH UTILIZATION MODELS AND PROGRAMS

During the 1970s several research utilization projects were implemented to foster the dissemination and use of research findings in clinical practice (Nolan, Larson, McGuire, Hill, & Haller, 1994). These projects included the Western Interstate Commission for Higher Education (WICHE) Program for Nursing Research Development, the Conduct and Utilization of Research in Nursing (CURIN) Project, and a group of programs fostering use of specific neonatal and perinatal research-based practices called the Nursing Child Assessment Satellite Training Projects I and II (NCAST) and the Nursing Systems Toward Effective Parenting-Premature (NSTEP-P) Project (Barnard & Hoehn, 1978; Haller, Reynolds, & Horsley, 1979; Horsley, Crane, & Bingle, 1978; Krueger et al., 1978).

Besides these projects, Stetler and Marram proposed a process for evaluating and implementing research findings in practice (Stetler, 1994; Stetler & Marram, 1976). The model was recently revised and expanded from a three-phase process to a six-phase process (Stetler, 1994). These phases are described in Table 72–4. In a series of articles McGuire and colleagues have described their use of this model in a comprehensive cancer center (Hanson & Ashley, 1994; McGuire, Walczak, & Krumm, 1994; Reedy, Shivan, Hanson, & Haisfield, 1994; Walczak et al., 1994).

EVALUATING RESEARCH REPORTS

Tanner (1987) has proposed useful guidelines for nurses evaluating research findings for use in clinical practice. The guidelines are drawn from a combination of critique formats suggested from previous research utilization projects. Table 72–5 outlines components of

TABLE 72–4. *Phases of the Stetler/Marram Model of Research Utilization*

PHASE	DESCRIPTION
I. Preparation	Determine the need and purpose for the research review of the specific topic. Identify a time table for completion.
II. Validation	Review and critique the research literature base. Determine individual study's strengths and weaknesses, and applicability to practice.
III. Comparative evaluation	Evaluate clinical applicability on (1) four elements of feasibility, (2) fit with practice setting, (3) other support for study findings, and (4) effectiveness of current practice and need/benefit of change.
IV. Decision making	Determine whether to implement findings or reject. If use is recommended, determine level and method of use.
V. Translation/application	Specify details of application to practice.
VI. Evaluation	Specify method of evaluation. Determine if expected outcomes are achieved.

the study evaluation process. Three major components are addressed in the review, including the clinical relevance of the study findings to the clinical practice site, the rigor and scientific merit of the study, and the feasibility of implementing the study in the clinical practice site. After each evaluation component is considered, decision points require determination about whether practice should be changed or current practices should be maintained. If clinical relevance is supported by answering yes to one or more of the pertinent questions, then scientific merit is considered. If, however, the study is determined not to be clinically relevant, then further review is not necessary. It is likely that some weaknesses will be found in the rigor and scientific merit of the study. As discussed in the research process section of this chapter, there are no

perfect studies. The reviewers must make some judgment about the seriousness of study weaknesses. Consultation with experienced researchers may be beneficial in making this determination. Tanner (1987) makes the point that all criteria for generalizability (i.e., similarity to reviewers' practice setting and presence of other studies replicating the findings) may not be met. However, the study findings may still be utilized in practice if it is possible to evaluate carefully the safety and efficacy of the practice change during the trial implementation period. The risks and cost of implementation should be reasonable, and the benefits of the practice change should be anticipated. If, in contrast, the scientific merit is significantly questioned and risks or costs are of concern, then further research should be completed prior to implementing a practice change.

TABLE 72–5. *Components of the Research Review for Application to Practice*

EVALUATION COMPONENTS	QUESTIONS TO ADDRESS
Clinical relevance	Does the study assist you in solving a clinical problem in your practice setting? Does the study evaluate an intervention or have outcomes that you could use in your practice setting? Are they under nursing control? Would they be feasible to implement in your practice setting?
Scientific merit	Does the study hang together and make sense? Does the theoretic/conceptual framework make sense?
The study should make sense, have believable results, and be generalizable to your practice setting.	Do the methods make sense, including subjects, setting, sampling, instruments, procedures, and analysis? What are the strengths and weaknesses of the study? Are the research questions and study purposes accurately answered? Do the methods and conclusions lead to believable, valid findings? How similar are the study sample and setting to your practice population and setting? Are there other studies available that replicate any of the findings?
Feasibility of implementation	What is the feasibility of doing systematic evaluation of the practice change when implementing in your practice setting?
Study findings should be systematically evaluated when implemented in practice, the benefits of implementation should outweigh risks, and the cost of implementation should be reasonable.	Are there risks in implementing this practice? Are there risks in <u>not</u> implementing this practice, and continuing current practice? What are the benefits of changing practice? Are the costs of changing practice reasonable?

(Data from Tanner, C. A. [1987]. Evaluating research for use in practice: Guidelines for the clinician. *Heart and Lung, 16,* 424–430.)

STRATEGIES TO FACILITATE INCREASED RESEARCH UTILIZATION

Strategies to increase research utilization must overcome many of the barriers nurses have identified. One major barrier is the time it takes to thoughtfully evaluate research and implement a practice change. There is no getting around it: research utilization does take time. To deal with this barrier, a research-based practice must be valued. That value for research must come from all facets of nursing: staff nurses, advanced practice nurses, agency administrators, researchers, and educators. The gains achieved from a practice where clinical decision making is based on a scientific foundation, rather than tradition or authority, do outweigh the significant time cost to implement. In fact, nurses find their satisfaction with their profession, the quality of care that they offer, and the image of nursing all are heightened.

In a time when changes in the health care system are creating changes in nursing practice, nursing roles, and patient care services, research becomes even more essential to justifying staffing, cost, patient care outcomes, and satisfaction. Rather than stalling the movement towards a research-based practice, nursing needs to move forward more rapidly to embrace research as a vital tool in addressing the impact of health care change.

Numerous strategies have been suggested to increase research use in practice (Cronenwatt, 1987; Kirchhoff, 1984; McGuire, 1992; Rempusleski, 1991; Williams, 1987a, 1987b). Table 72–6 lists a number of these strategies. Clinicians, including both registered nurses and advanced practice nurses, are the cornerstone of research use, since they are the ones whose practice is changed by new clinical knowledge. Because there is a broad range in educational preparation and

TABLE 72–6. *Strategies and Responsibilities for Increasing Research Utilization*

ROLE	STRATEGIES
Clinicians	Question the basis of practice policies and standards
	Expect scientific evidence for practice decision making
	Request and join journal clubs
	Attend conferences where research results are presented
	Read widely and critically
	Advance your knowledge base about the research process
	Develop good library and computer research skills
	Recognize that the practice knowledge base is changing and that incorporation of research-based recommendations should represent positive change
	Advocate for resources, expert consultation, and procedures to facilitate research utilization
Administrators/CNS/ Staff development educators	Create a practice climate that values critical inquiry
	Incorporate research utilization into the organization
	Formalize a process
	Provide resources, literature searches, time, consultants, publications that summarize research studies, journal clubs, research-based grand rounds
	Evaluate nurse performance based on appropriate level of research adoption
	Reward role models who practice from a research base
	Expect research to provide a basis for staff development activities
	Require policies and procedures to incorporate research findings
	Negotiate and promote research utilization support among disciplines
	Involve graduate level nursing students in agency research utilization projects
	Invite researchers to your agency to promote interchange
	Use research to address your administrative practice issues
	Value the importance of research in addressing patient care problems, demonstrating nursing and patient outcomes, and evaluating cost and quality issues
Researchers	Study problems that are priority for clinical practice decision making
	Test interventions that can be transferred to clinical practice
	Add patient outcome variables and cost analysis to clinical studies
	Conduct studies that build on previous work and replication studies
	Attend to scientific merit and generalizability of studies
	Publish widely in journals read by clinicians and make findings understandable
	Present widely, including to clinician groups
	Assist clinical agencies with research utilization projects
	Develop and lead journal clubs
Educators	Provide innovative research courses at all levels of curriculum
	Provide introduction to research early in curriculum
	Socialize students to the importance and contributions of research to practice
	Promote critical inquiry and strong library skills
	Adopt textbooks that present content with a strong research base
	Promote and join journal clubs among faculty members and with clinical agencies
	Be a good role model for the use of research in teaching all courses

exposure to research, clinicians must have active support from administrators, researchers, and educators to make research utilization possible. As described earlier, currently the primary barriers to research use by clinicians are job-related. The expectations and the resources and climate nurse administrators create in the work setting will be pivotal to whether a research-based practice environment prevails. Researchers also must play a central role. Historically, researchers have not adequately assisted clinicians with the application of research findings to practice. Not only are researchers responsible for publishing their findings, but they must be more proactive in making sure relevant findings are adopted in practice. Educators, too, must renew efforts to teach from the research base, to instill an appropriate knowledge level about research, to provide skills in research utilization, and to inspire students to value a research-based clinical practice.

THE RESEARCH PROCESS

COMPONENTS OF THE RESEARCH QUESTION

Research utilizes an orderly and structured process to answer questions that contribute new knowledge. Table 72–7 lists the components of the research process, the characteristics of each component, and the sources of information for developing each component.

RESEARCH QUESTIONS

Building a scientific foundation for cancer nursing practice requires a variety of investigative skills, one of the most important being the ability to formulate a testable research question. Every stage of the research process, whether it be selecting a design, method of measurement, or statistical analysis plan, depends on the clarity of the original research question. McCorkle (1990) identified several ways for nurses to select a suitable research question. Nurses can rely on their direct observation and clinical experiences for research ideas, or they can discuss potential topics with other nurses and colleagues. Research topics can come from reading the literature and recognizing discrepancies and gaps in existing nursing knowledge or practice. Published theories can be examined and research questions formulated to test the suitability of a theory for a given specialty area. For example, three middle-range nursing theories hold exciting promise for research and practice in cancer nursing: Swanson's theory of caring (Swanson, 1991, 1993), Mishel's theory of uncertainty (Mishel, 1990), and Reed's theory of self-transcendence (Reed, 1991). As described previously in Table 72–2, research priorities also provide a useful framework for identifying potential topics for research.

A distinction must be made between generating a research question and formulating a researchable question. Research questions based on personal values, subjective opinions, and administrative policy may be valuable for clinical decision making, but they do not produce objective or generalizable topics for guiding research or practice (Wilson, 1989). To the contrary, researchable questions provide answers that describe, explain, predict, and eventually control phenomena of interest (Brink & Wood, 1988). For example, the question, "Should cancer patients enroll in experimental clinical trials?" can be reformulated into the following testable research question: "What are the potential risks and benefits of enrolling in a breast cancer prevention trial from the perspective of healthy participants?" Since the way a research question is written determines what type of research design is needed to answer the question, the next section provides a description of the three major levels of research inquiry.

LEVELS OF RESEARCH QUESTIONS

Brink and Wood (1988) classify research into one of three major levels based on the extent of knowledge, theory, or both that exists about the topic under study. Level I or basic types of research questions ask Who?, What?, When?, and Where? Basic questions are developed when a research topic is new or has not been examined before in a specific population, when little is known about the topic, or when only a scant, if any, literature base exists. Examples of basic or level I questions include: What types of ethical dilemmas occur in the treatment of persons with late-stage or terminal disease?, and, What concerns do persons undergoing chemotherapy have at different points in treatment?

The second level of research questions examines the statistical significance and direction of the relationship that exists between or among variables. The researcher must identify the variables to be examined and the theoretic rationale for proposing why an association exists between the variables (Brink & Wood, 1988). For instance, building on the findings of prior quality of life studies, Bush and colleagues examined the relationship between the side effects of therapy, physical functioning, emotional functioning, demands of recovery, and health perceptions in long-term survivors of bone marrow transplantation (Bush, Haberman, Donaldson, & Sullivan, 1995). Last, the third level of research questions examines systematically the validity of theory by the direct manipulation of a set of research variables (Brink & Wood, 1988). The investigator formulates a predictive statement or hypothesis about what will happen, identifies a theory to explain the prediction, then conducts the study to examine "why" the hypothesized relationship exists and the conditions under which the relationship holds. Level III research questions are addressed by using experimental or quasi-experimental designs and the random selection, assignment, or both of participants to either an experimental (intervention) or control group. As an example of this type of design, Shivan and colleagues (1991) examined infection rates, nursing time, and patient comfort in marrow transplant patients with an indwelling central catheter. Patients were randomized to receive either a dry sterile gauze dressing changed daily or a transparent adherent dressing changed every 4 days.

TABLE 72–7. *Components of the Research Process*

COMPONENT	CHARACTERISTICS	SOURCE
Research questions: Basic Intermediate Advanced	A researchable question must identify the topic under investigation, be testable, and provide answers that describe, explain, predict, and ultimately control the phenomenon being studied. The question guides the choice of research design, sample, selection of instruments to measure the relevant variables, and data analysis plan. Basic, descriptive level questions ask Who? What? When? and Where? Intermediate level questions examine the statistical significance and direction of the relationship that exists between key variables. Advanced questions are based on a solid theoretic foundation and written as predictive statements or hypotheses.	Direct observation, clinical experiences, reading the literature, talking with colleagues, practice guidelines, care pathways, and existing theory.
Problem statement and significance	A statement that describes the variables of interest in broad terms, the relationship or conceptual linkages among the variables, and the patient population in which the variables will be examined (McCorkle, 1990). A compelling argument about the importance of the study to improving the knowledge base for oncology nursing and, ultimately, patient care.	The statement emerges from the same sources as the research question by summarizing existing gaps in nursing knowledge and practice. Stems from an in-depth understanding of clinical practice, patient problems, and the existing state-of-the-science of the topic under study.
Review of literature	Identifies what is known and not known about the research topic and the methods of inquiry used to investigate the topic in prior research. The key concepts or variables under study become the organizing framework for the review.	Professional journals, hardbound cumulative indexes and abstracts, computerized databases, and literature retrieval software programs.
Conceptual framework	Goes beyond a simple compilation of the literature. Blends and synthesizes issues from both the existing literature and clinical practice. Elucidates the critical linkages among the key concepts.	No definitive source. Depends on the researcher's unique image of how the problem exists in the real world.
Research design and methodology: Sample size Instrumentation Controlling for sources of error Data management and analysis Protection of human rights and confidentiality Monitoring scientific and ethical conduct	Provides the blueprint for what to do and not do and what restrictions or controls are placed on experimental variables and data collection procedures (Kerlinger, 1973).	Determined by the sophistication of the research question, the amount of accumulated knowledge on the topic, and the circumstances under which the study is conducted.

PROBLEM STATEMENT AND SIGNIFICANCE OF THE PROJECT

The problem statement presents a compelling argument that explains how the proposed study will contribute to the generation of new nursing knowledge and enhance the scientific basis for practice, test the validity of an existing theory, lead to the development or refinement of a research instrument, or improve the quality of patient care (Catanzaro, 1988; McCorkle, 1990). The significance of the project addresses how the study is important to clinical practice and to further research, methodologic development, or theory development.

LITERATURE REVIEW

The published literature is examined to determine what is already known about the research topic and to critically review this literature, noting gaps and methodologic strengths and weaknesses of the published research base. The literature review can be organized around the key concepts or variables identified in the problem statement. Woods (1988a) notes that the literature review serves the following four purposes: (1) to generate the research question, (2) to identify what is already known and not known about the research topic, (3) to identify conceptual, theoretic, or empiric traditions within the discipline or literature base, and (4) to describe the methods of inquiry used to investigate the phenomenon in previous research, including both the successes and shortcomings of earlier studies.

CONCEPTUAL FRAMEWORK

The conceptual framework is designed to elucidate the critical linkages among the concepts. Batey (1977) indicates that the conceptual framework represents the researcher's unique image of how the phenomenon of interest exists in the real world. The conceptual framework is both analytical and grounded in a high-level synthesis that blends existing theory with clinical practice issues (McCorkle, 1990). The conceptual linkages identified in the framework provide the basis for selecting a research design.

RESEARCH DESIGN AND METHODOLOGY

Research design and methodology are an amalgam of interrelated components. Some aspects of research design are estimating the projected sample size, selecting methods for measuring the variables of interest, controlling for sources of measurement error, and determining procedures for data collection, management, and analysis. Other aspects of research design and methodology include the time frame for conducting the study, the protection of human rights or the welfare of animals, the informed consent process, the availability of institutional resources for successfully conducting and completing the research project, and procedures for monitoring the scientific and ethical conduct of the study. Research designs are selected once the research questions have been identified. A brief description of 10 design alternatives is presented in Table 72–8.

There is no such thing as a perfectly designed study; rather, all studies involve a series of design compromises and trade-offs. Selecting the appropriate design depends on the sophistication of the research question, the amount of research previously conducted on the topic, and the circumstances under which the study is conducted. The reader is referred to any one of a number of excellent nursing research textbooks for an in-depth discussion of research design (Brink & Wood, 1989; Grant & Padilla, 1990; Haberman, 1993, 1995; McLaughlin & Marascuilo, 1990; Polit & Hungler, 1995; Woods & Catanzaro, 1988). One specialized group of descriptive designs is qualitative designs. Because qualitative designs offer unique paradigms, design considerations, and methodologic approaches, a separate brief discussion is provided in the following section.

QUALITATIVE PARADIGMS

Qualitative approaches to descriptive research are especially suited to investigating many of the dynamic processes central to oncology nursing, including adaptation, change, decision making, transition, developmental maturation, social interaction, and holism (Haberman & Lewis, 1990). Falling under the rubric of descriptive designs, qualitative designs are shaped by a unique philosophy of science and specific methodologic perspective. Qualitative designs follow a flexible process of concept discovery and evolution (Lewis, 1990; Lincoln & Guba, 1985). Consequently, the investigator tries to avoid writing a rigid theoretic framework and relies on the study's findings to guide concept definition. Three modes of qualitative inquiry are now briefly described, including the key characteristics of phenomenology, ethnography, and grounded theory.

PHENOMENOLOGY

Phenomenology conveys both a philosophic stance and methodologic perspective. It emphasizes the subjective, holistic, and experiential nature of reality, the elucidation of the basic characteristics of phenomena, and the description of salient relationships, dynamic processes, and patterns of action that fluctuate and change over time (Haberman & Lewis, 1990). For example, The Life Cycle Research Project (Carroll-Johnson & Zichi-Cohen, 1994) sponsored by the Oncology Nursing Society used a phenomenologic methodology to interview oncology nurses about their perceptions of the meaning of oncology nursing practice.

ETHNOGRAPHY

Another type of qualitative inquiry that stems from anthropology is ethnography. Ethnographers examine the way of life of a designated cultural group and the shared knowledge and meanings that underpin the culture (Aamodt, 1982; Haberman & Lewis, 1990). Ethnographers observe and document systematically the beliefs, customs, behaviors, patterns of daily life, rituals, and objects or artifacts that constitute a given culture. In conducting ethnographic research, the investigator must abandon rigorous scientific control, adopt an improvisational and flexible style to meet unexpected situations in the field setting, and engage in prolonged periods of participant observation using himself or herself as the research instrument (Agar, 1986). Multiple triangulation is a specific research strategy used by ethnographers to collect data from a variety of empiric vantage points and perspectives (Mitchell, 1986). For example, in describing how patients adapt to protective isolation, the nurse investigator might collect data from patient interviews, medical records,

TABLE 72–8. *Ten Basic Types of Research Design*

Historical: Historical studies are designed to reconstruct the past in a systematic manner by collecting, evaluating, verifying, and synthesizing evidence. Conclusions are objective and defensible, often in regard to a specific hypothesis.

Descriptive: Descriptive designs are useful when little is known about a phenomenon. Also known as survey research, these designs are used to describe systematically the basic characteristics of a phenomenon, situation, concept or event, and to provide a conceptual foundation for subsequent intervention studies. Qualitative designs, such as ethnography, phenomenology, and grounded theory are a special case of descriptive designs.

Developmental: Developmental designs are used to examine phenomenon that fluctuate over time and are characterized by patterns of change and sequences of growth.

Correlational: Correlational designs provide a basis for investigating the noncausal relationship between or among a set of variables using correlation coefficients to establish the strength or magnitude of the relationship.

Causal Comparative or Ex Post Facto: These designs provide a basis for determining possible cause and effect relationships by examining a current phenomenon and then searching back in time to identify plausible causal factors. The designs are "ex post facto" in nature, since the data are collected retrospectively, after the event has occurred.

True Experimental or Causal: These designs are used to examine cause and effect relationships. At a minimum, they require random selection of study participants and/or random assignment to either an experimental or treatment-as-usual (control) group. They employ strategies for optimizing design control and minimizing sources of error.

Quasi-Experimental: These designs are less rigorous than true experimental designs since they often occur in clinical settings where the manipulation or control of all relevant variables is impossible. They attempt to approximate, as closely as possible, the conditions of a true experimental-control group design. Most clinical trials fall in this category.

Prescription Testing: Prescriptive designs are used to test new skills, interventions, or therapeutics for the purpose of investigating problems that are relevant to clinical practice. As a form of action research, prescriptive research provides a basis for developing nursing practice theory.

Methodological: Methodologic studies are used to develop or validate a research instrument or to test a new or existing research methodology.

Case and Field: These designs provide a framework for investigating social units such as individuals, groups, institutions or communities. The studies examine both past and current social, ethnic and cultural background and environmental issues. The studies may investigate an entire life cycle or a selected, smaller segment of time.

(Adapted from Isaac, S., & Michael, W. [1995]. *Handbook in research and evaluation* [3rd ed., pp. 46–47]. San Diego: EdITS Publishers; Haberman, M. [1995]. Nursing research. In P. C. Buchsel & M. B. Whedon [Eds.], *Bone marrow transplantation: Administrative and clinical strategies* [pp. 365–402]. © 1995 Boston: Jones and Bartlett Publishers. Reprinted with permission.)

direct observation, and interviews with staff, family members, and friends. As an example of ethnographic-type inquiry, Flaskerud and Thompson (1991) described low-income white women's beliefs about acquired immunodeficiency syndrome (AIDS), health, and illness for the purpose of discovering the impact of culture on personal beliefs about AIDS.

GROUNDED THEORY

Grounded theory development is highly popular in nursing research circles (Chenitz & Swanson, 1986; Munhall & Oiler, 1986). The term "grounded" refers to the discovery of theory from data that are anchored in empirical evidence (Glaser, 1978; Glaser & Strauss, 1967; Strauss, 1987; Strauss & Corbin, 1990). The goal of grounded theory research is to generate a parsimonious theory that describes a substantive area of human experience. Data collection and analysis usually proceed simultaneously when conducting grounded theory research. Data collection strategies include participant observation, written field notes, personal diaries, memoing, and key informant interviews. As an example of this data collection method, Haberman (1987; 1995) developed a grounded theory that describes life after the diagnosis of leukemia, factors influencing the decision to undergo a bone marrow transplantation (BMT), and the personal meaning ascribed to therapy by adults undertaking a BMT.

KEY COMPONENTS OF CLINICAL TRIALS, NURSING INTERVENTION, AND OUTCOME STUDIES

Clinical trial designs are an extension of true experimental or quasiexperimental designs. Clinical trials are the principal method for obtaining reliable evaluation of treatment effects and for examining the efficacy of new therapeutic drugs (Woods, 1988b). Stated simply, a clinical trial is a preplanned therapeutic intervention that is administered to participants who meet a firm set of eligibility criteria. Trials are conducted under controlled conditions, such as randomization and stratification, to enable well-defined questions to be answered. Clinical trials are widely used in medical research to evaluate the effectiveness of new cancer treatments; however, the use of clinical trials to evaluate the effectiveness of nursing interventions is equally important. The scientific rigor that characterizes clinical trial designs makes these designs ideal for testing the efficacy of new nursing therapeutics and for conducting nursing outcome studies.

Clinical trials evaluating cancer medical treatments are classified by phases. Phase I trials generally involve a small number of patients with advanced cancer who have exhausted other types of conventional therapy. The purposes of phase I testing are to determine the safe maximum dosage for a new drug or treatment and to identify acute toxicities. Phase II trials examine the potential efficacy of a single- or multimodal therapy regimen. The purposes of phase II studies are to conduct further testing of drug doses and schedules, evaluate antitumor activity, and further document toxicities. Grant, Padilla, and Ferrell (1993) note that in phase III trials, the emphasis shifts to large sample sizes to compare two or more therapeutic regimens. Adjuvant therapy and advanced disease regimens are included in these trials.

Researchers can choose from several solid design options when instigating a clinical trial or nursing intervention study. Optimal research designs for conducting intervention studies include randomized control-group, pretest-posttest designs; randomized Solomon four-group designs; and time-series designs. A review of these designs is beyond the scope of the current chapter, and the reader is referred to several excellent sources for a thorough discussion of these design options (Lewis, 1990; Meinert, 1986; Pocock, 1983).

HYPOTHESIS TESTING

Clinical trial and experimental designs involve the testing of hypotheses. A hypothesis is a hypothetic statement of the relationship between two or more variables (Kerlinger, 1973). Two types of hypotheses must be addressed: the research hypothesis and the statistical null hypothesis. The research hypothesis identifies the variables to be studied and the causal relationship hypothesized to exist. For instance, Hagopian (1991) hypothesized that patients receiving a weekly radiation therapy newsletter would know more about radiation therapy and its side effects, employ more self-care behaviors, and experience fewer side effects than patients not receiving the newsletter. The null hypothesis—the hypothesis of "no relationship or difference"—is the hypothesis actually tested statistically (Isaac & Michael, 1981).

The decision to accept or reject the null hypothesis is subject to type I and type II error. Type I, or α error, means the null hypothesis is rejected when it is actually true. In other words, the investigator concludes falsely that a difference exists in therapeutic efficacy when in fact it does not—a false-positive. Investigators strive to minimize the risk of committing type I error by choosing a conservative α level, such as $p = 0.05$. Type II, or β error, means the null hypothesis is accepted when it is false. In other words, the investigator concludes falsely that a difference in therapeutic effect does not exist when in fact it does—a false-negative. Large sample sizes and minimizing sources of measurement error are the easiest ways to guard against committing type II error.

RANDOMIZATION

Randomization is required for a true experimental design and quasi-experimental designs, including clinical trial designs. Randomization can occur at three levels: selection of participants, measurement occasions, and treatment conditions (Isaac & Michael, 1981). At a minimum, participants are usually allocated randomly to either a treatment group that receives the intervention or to a control group that receives treatment-as-usual. Randomization gives every member of a population an equal chance of being selected; members with distinguishing characteristics that may potentially bias the findings will, if selected, be counterbalanced by the equal selection of members with the opposite characteristic (Kerlinger, 1973).

BLINDING TECHNIQUES

Another important element of designing clinical trials is the use of blinding techniques. Potential bias exists whenever anyone involved in a trial—participant, family member, clinical staff, and researcher—is aware of which treatment the participant is receiving. In a study that uses double blinding, neither the participant nor the individuals responsible for patient care or the evaluation of the trial know which treatment the participant is receiving. In a triple-blind design, the statistician or person that is interpreting the therapeutic effect of the trial is blind to the treatment group until after all of the data are analyzed and interpreted. Regardless of the blinding procedures selected, under no circumstances should blinding produce harm or impose undue risk to the participants.

TYPES OF RESEARCH VARIABLES

INDEPENDENT AND DEPENDENT VARIABLES

Research variables can be classified into four major types: independent, dependent, control, and mediating. Independent variables are the treatment variables that the researcher manipulates in some fashion. Dependent variables are the response variables, so-called because the measured outcome presumably depends on how the independent variable is manipulated. Stated differently, variations in X (independent variable) produce variations in Y (dependent variable). For example, using a randomized experimental design, Johnson, Nail, Lauver, King, and Keys (1988) gave concrete objective information about radiation treatment to men undergoing treatment for prostate cancer. In this study, the intervention (independent variable) was the information provided about radiation therapy, and the dependent variables were mood and disruption in usual activities.

In formulating interventions, the investigator should have some conceptual basis or pilot data to suggest that the intervention is promising. The research intervention should not be so complex that it is unlikely to be transferable to practice if found effective. Complicated, multifaceted interventions, so-called "kitchen sink" interventions, make it difficult to tell whether all facets of the intervention are necessary or if effectiveness should only be attributed to specific components.

CONTROL VARIABLES

A third type of variable is known by many names, including control, extraneous, background, classificatory, or categoric variable. Control variables need to be held constant or randomized so that their effects are neutralized, canceled out, or equalized for all conditions (Isaac & Michael, 1981). Actually, the term "control variable" may be misleading, because some of these variables are under experimenter control and some are not. Typical control variables include such factors as age, gender, type of disease, disease staging, and type of conditioning regimen or therapy.

MEDIATING VARIABLES

Mediating or intervening variables are hypothetic conceptions selected to explain some mediating process that regulates the relationship between the independent and dependent variable. For example, when newly diagnosed individuals with cancer are given several options for therapy, they may experience feelings of uncertainty and some level of emotional distress. The intensity of perceived uncertainty and distress may be mediated by their individual coping skills and degree of self-mastery (Mishel, Padilla, Grant, & Sorenson, 1991).

CONCEPTUAL AND OPERATIONAL DEFINITIONS

Another key component of study development is the need to identify each variable's operational and conceptual definition (Atwood, 1990). A conceptual definition provides an abstract or nontestable definition of the variable. By contrast, an operational definition specifies exactly how a concept or variable is measured and the ways the variable is manipulated (Kerlinger, 1973). Since there are many ways to measure a given concept, the choice of a particular operational definition depends on the goodness-of-fit between the conceptual definition and available measurement instruments.

RESEARCH INSTRUMENTS

Once the variables have been identified, methods to operationally measure the variables must be chosen. Ideally, investigators select instruments that are already developed and tested in related studies with similar samples, and have been found to be reliable and valid. However, given the relatively short history of cancer nursing research, such instruments may not be available, occasionally requiring the investigator to develop a new instrument.

Potential research instruments can be found in reports of related research. In addition, Frank Strom borg and Olsen (1996) have edited a text, *Instruments for Clinical Nursing Research*, that provides an overview of existing research instruments in over 20 areas pertinent to cancer nursing research.

There are many issues in selecting and using research instruments. Consultation with an expert researcher can be very useful in refining instrumentation. Often further clarity about the phenomena of interest is needed to determine what instruments should be selected. For example, it is important to know if the phenomenon is subjective or objective. If it is subjective, such as perceptions of cancer pain or fatigue, then the researcher would select an instrument that was scored by the patient experiencing the pain or fatigue. As an alternative, an observer-scored instrument such as one scored by the nurse or family caregiver may be selected. Subjective measure can be challenging to administer in seriously ill cancer patients. Fatigue instruments are particularly problematic, since the instrument must not overwhelm the already fatigued participant.

Instruments must also be culturally relevant. Translation of instruments from one language to another involves a very detailed and complex process (Munet-Vilaro, 1988; Munet-Vilaro & Egan, 1990). Consultation should be sought in designing studies that address a broad range of cultural perspectives.

The researcher also must understand the scoring and limitations of the instrument chosen. There should be conceptual agreement with the phenomena being studied. For example, if an instrument measures the number and types of coping strategies used by newly diagnosed individuals with cancer, the investigator cannot conclude that individuals with higher scores (i.e., using more coping strategies) are more effective in coping with the diagnosis. Effectiveness was not measured by the tool, and the investigator cannot assume that the use of more coping strategies results in better coping; it may mean that nothing is effective, so the individual keeps trying other methods.

Finally, the selection of when measurement is to be taken can be extremely complicated. If a study includes multiple treatment protocols and types of cancer, it may be impossible to measure variables at specific times such as 1 month or 6 months after diagnosis. It may be more appropriate to tailor each measurement to a similar time in the various treatment cycles, such as at the expected nadir of symptoms or 1 week after the nadir. It also is important that measurement is logically planned for the time when the phenomenon is expected. If stomatitis is expected 10 to 14 days after treatment, then oral examination should continue during that time period.

INSTRUMENT RELIABILITY AND VALIDITY

Attention to issues of reliability and validity are imperative when conducting nursing research (Atwood, 1990). A comprehensive discussion of reliability and validity, and guidelines for selecting a research instrument can be found in a number of references (Frank-Stromborg & Olsen, 1996; Mateo & Kirchhoff, 1991; McLaughlin & Marascuilo, 1990; Nunnally, 1978; Strickland & Waltz, 1988; Sudman & Bradburn, 1987; Waltz & Bausell, 1981; Waltz & Strickland, 1988).

Reliability. Reliability refers to the consistency, stability, and trustworthiness of obtained data. A reliability coefficient reflects whether the obtained score is a stable indication of the person's performance on a given questionnaire. Common types of reliability include internal consistency, test-retest, and parallel/alternative forms reliability. See Atwood (1990) for a further description of reliability.

Validity. Validity determines whether an instrument actually measures what it is intended to measure. Establishing validity is a cumulative pursuit that occurs over a sequence of studies (Edwards, 1970). Several types of validity are important when considering the use of a research instrument including face, content, criterion, construct, and contrasted-groups. See Atwood (1990) for a more detailed discussion of validity.

ESTIMATING SAMPLE SIZE

Sample size determination is an essential component of designing quantitative research. In experimental designs including clinical trials, sample size estimation allows the investigator to establish beforehand the exact number of participants necessary to demonstrate the hypothesized therapeutic effect, if the effect actually exists. To maximize the likelihood of detecting a significant therapeutic effect, there are several requirements: (1) sample sizes must be large enough to demonstrate statistically significant results, (2) highly reliable outcome measures must be used, and (3) an effect size (magnitude of response) must be large enough to be detected by the appropriate analytic test. Several excellent references are available to guide investigators through the steps involved in estimating sample size (Cohen, 1988; Kramer & Thiemann, 1987; Lipsey, 1990; Munro, Visintainer, & Page, 1986).

STATISTICAL ANALYSIS PLAN

Cancer nurse researchers are relying more heavily on sophisticated analytic plans for the purpose of concept development, theoretic modeling, time-series analysis of data, and instrument development. Perhaps the best advice that can be given to all researchers is to seek consultation, whenever possible, from a statistician. Many excellent references exist that explain the actual performance of statistical tests (Brink & Wood, 1989; Hill & Metter, 1990; McLaughlin & Marascuilo, 1990; Munro et al., 1986; Woods & Catanzaro, 1988).

Descriptive analysis refers to the description of the data from a specific sample and, as such, conclusions are limited to the sample on hand. In contrast, inferential analysis focuses on drawing inferences about the larger population from which the sample is drawn. In designing a statistical analysis plan, a second distinction is needed between parametric and nonparametric statistical tests. Nonparametric tests are less powerful statistical tests than parametric tests, because they are based on fewer assumptions about the data and population.

DESCRIPTIVE ANALYSIS

All forms of descriptive analysis summarize the data in some fashion. Measures of central tendency include the mean, median, and mode. Measures of variation may include counting the number of things (categoric level variables), calculating the range of scores (nominal level variables), and standard deviation (interval/ratio level). The relationship between or among study variables can by tested by the use of chi-square (nominal level data), Spearman-rank (ordinal level data), and Pearson r (interval/ratio level data) techniques.

INFERENTIAL ANALYSIS

Brink and Wood (1988) pose a series of questions intended to guide the investigator in the choice of the most appropriate inferential statistical technique: "Are you looking for a significant difference between groups?" "Are you interested in demonstrating a correlation between variables?" "Are you seeking generalizations about the population from findings in your sample?"

When the intent of the analysis is to examine before and after changes from time 1 to time 2 in the same group, available statistical tests include the sign test, Wilcoxon test, McNemar test, chi-square, and paired t test. When trying to identify differences between groups, the investigator may use the nonpaired t test, Fisher exact test, Mann-Whitney U test, and 2×2 contingency table. When differences among more than two groups are analyzed, the following tests are available: analysis of variance or F test, Kruskal-Wallis one-way analysis of variance by ranks, chi-square, and R (row) $\times$ C (column) contingency tables. Correlational tests include the Pearson r, Spearman rank, and chi-square tests. Last, when estimating population parameters from a sample, all of the descriptive statistics described previously can be used to predict population parameters. Confidence intervals provide a range of values within which the true value of the population parameter is estimated to fall (Brink and Woods, 1988). Confidence intervals can be calculated by using a t test, Tukey's test, and the binomial test for the confidence intervals of quartiles.

INFORMED CONSENT

Potential research participants must be informed, in the context of a noncoercive environment, of the risks and benefits of participating in a study. A written consent form is developed to inform the potential participant of the specific details of the research protocol and to obtain a signature of agreement. Informed consent involves notifying potential research participants of (1) what alternative treatments, if any, are available to them if they decline participation; (2) the procedures necessary to implement the study and maintain confidentiality; (3) the risks, benefits, and financial obligations of participation; (4) the stopping-rules or conditions under which the study may be prematurely terminated; and (5) the investigator's assurance that new information, learned during the course of the study, will be provided to the participant if this information will affect care or continuing enrollment in the study. The reader is referred to several additional references for a more thorough discussion of the informed consent process (Anderson, 1990; Benoliel, 1988; Faden & Beauchamp, 1986; Meinert, 1986; Silva & Sorrell, 1984).

SCIENTIFIC AND ETHICAL CONDUCT

A final key feature in the design of all research studies is the issue of monitoring the scientific and ethical conduct of studies (Chop & Cipriano-Silva, 1991; Grady, 1991; Hawley & Jeffers, 1992; Morrison, 1993; Rennie & Gunsalus, 1993). Scientific misconduct can be defined as the "plagiarism, fabrication or deliberate falsification of data, research procedures, or data analysis; or other deliberate misrepresentation in proposing, conducting, reporting or reviewing research" (Panel on Scientific Responsibility and the Conduct of Research, Committee on Science, Engineering, and Public Policy, National Academy of Sciences, 1992, in Rennie & Gunsalus, 1993, p. 916). Examples of scientific misconduct may include a researcher who takes the findings of another and publishes them as his or her own without crediting the original investigator, an investigator who fabricates preliminary data and uses that data in a grant application for funding, an investigator who enters participants who do not meet eligibility requirements or purposely assigns participants to experimental or control conditions to increase the likelihood of favorable results, or an author who reports findings from a study that was never conducted or falsifies data by changing results or substituting fabricated data for missing data.

The potential for scientific misconduct is magnified as nurses continue to design large, complex projects that involve data collection at multiple institutions and as nurses compete for limited research dollars, for publication, and for tenure (Hawley & Jeffers, 1992). Scientific misconduct is important to all clinicians, since the practice of nursing is based on science, which means our practice is grounded in the integrity of the nursing and biomedical research community (Rennie & Gunsalus, 1993). Currently, just about every aspect of research misconduct is changing rapidly, including reaching a consensus on the definition, the procedures, the law, and professional and public attitudes (Rennie & Gunsalus, 1993).

Cancer nurses who witness a specific act of scientific misconduct or are asked to falsify data should follow their institution's policies and procedures for reporting and handling allegations of misconduct. All institutions that receive federal funding for research are required to have guidelines for handling inquiries or investigations of scientific misconduct. It is essential that nurses be aware of their institution's policies, since allegations of misconduct have direct legal implications. If your institution does not have any written policies on scientific misconduct, nursing can assume an advocacy role for developing such a policy (Chop & Cipriano-Silva, 1991). Federal policies and procedures can be obtained directly from the Public Health Service's Office of Scientific Integrity. Assistance in finding federally mandated policies can be obtained from any university with a grants office, local health science libraries, and any comprehensive cancer center's grants office or institutional review board. Moreover, the American Nurses Association recently published "Guidelines on Reporting Incompetent, Unethical, or Illegal Practices," (Scanlon, Arrindell, Carson, & Sapin, 1994). Although this document does not specifically address scientific misconduct, it provides useful guidelines for developing model institutional policies for handling allegations of clinical and research misconduct.

FUTURE DIRECTIONS

In the 25 years since Quint published her clinical study on the adjustment of women postmastectomy, cancer nursing research has made significant initial contributions to the knowledge base for practice. In the next 25 years cancer nursing, as a specialty, will achieve a strong research base. Awareness of the value of research is growing, and organizational support from professional and public organizations, notably the Oncology Nursing Society and the American Cancer Society, is providing the impetus for further growth.

Research topics, designs, and methodologies are improving in sophistication. There is a need for more programmatic research in priority areas for cancer nursing. Studies should build from previous work, and replication studies are warranted. Strategies need to be explored to increase sample size and provide greater diversity in the demographics of participants recruited for studies. Multi-site mechanisms now being implemented by the Oncology Nursing Society may begin to address this. There needs to be a stronger focus on intervention studies to provide direction for clinical decision making. The preponderance of descriptive studies in the past provides a base from which to design new intervention studies. Researchers are encouraged to conduct studies that provide direction for our practice discipline. Cancer nurses are action-oriented, and they provide care for people experiencing cancer, and therefore nurses must know that their actions are effective. With the changes that are occurring in health care, there is a critical need for studies to evaluate the impact of nursing care on patient outcomes. Work also is needed on the cost-effectiveness of care and patient satisfaction.

The importance of translating research findings into clinical practice has been strongly emphasized in this chapter. To be successful, all nurses must see the value of research and bridge the barriers to research-based cancer nursing practice. Cancer nurse leaders must also advocate for the translation of research findings into health policy at national, state, and local levels. For too long we have missed opportunities to positively affect the well-being of thousands of individuals at risk for or diagnosed with cancer because we have not taken the results of research that have implications for policy change to our legislators.

Cancer nurse researchers also need to advocate for their inclusion on policy and review panels in federal and private research funding agencies. We need to be active participants in setting forth cancer research priorities and making recommendations on funding levels and priorities. Beyond conducting the research, we must be visible in securing the resources for, and underscoring the importance of, the research knowledge that we are generating.

Every cancer nurse has a stake in the research process, from conception of the problem through the translation of findings into a practice change that improves the well-being of an individual with cancer. Clinicians, administrators, researchers, and educators must work collaboratively to produce and use the findings of the next generation of cancer nursing research studies.

Acknowledgment. The authors wish to acknowledge Dori Fortune and Kelli Wisdom for their assistance in the preparation of the manuscript. Mel Haberman is an employee of the Oncology Nursing Society. The Oncology Nursing Society assumes no responsibility for the content of this publication.

REFERENCES

Aamodt, A. (1982). Examining ethnography for nurse researchers. *Western Journal of Nursing Research, 4,* 209–221.

Agar, M. (1986). *Speaking of ethnography.* Beverly Hills, CA: Sage.

Anderson, P. (1990). Strategies for project implementation. In M. M. Grant, & G. V. Padilla (Eds.), *Cancer nursing research: A practical approach* (pp. 175–192). Norwalk, CT: Appleton & Lange.

Atwood, J. (1990). Definition of the research variables. In M. M. Grant, & G. V. Padilla (Eds.), *Cancer nursing research: A practical approach* (pp. 101–116). Norwalk, CT: Appleton & Lange.

Barckley, V. (1964). Enough time for good nursing. *Nursing Outlook, 12*(4), 44–48.

Barnard, K. E., & Hoehn, R. E. (1978). Nursing child assessment satellite training: Final Report. Hyattsville, MD: DHEW, PHS, HRA, Division of Nursing Contract No. HRA 231–77–002.

Batey, M. V. (1977). Conceptualization: Knowledge and logic guiding empirical research. *Nursing Research, 26,* 324–329.

Benoliel, J. Q. (1983). The historical development of cancer nursing research in the United States. *Cancer Nursing, 5,* 261–268.

Benoliel, J. Q. (1988). Considering human rights in research. In N. F. Woods, & M. Catanzaro (Eds.), *Nursing research: Theory and practice* (pp. 79–96). St. Louis: The C. V. Mosby Company.

Brett, J. (1987). Use of nursing practice research findings. *Nursing Research, 36,* 344–349.

Brink, P. J., & Wood, M. J. (1988). *Basic steps in planning nursing research: From question to proposal* (3rd ed.). Boston: Jones and Bartlett.

Brink, P. J., & Wood, M. J. (1989). *Advanced design in nursing research.* Newbury Park, CA: Sage Publishers.

Bush, N. E., Haberman, M. R., Donaldson, G., & Sullivan, K. M. (1995). Quality of life of 125 adults surviving 6–18 years after bone marrow transplantation. *Social Science Medicine, 40*(4), 479–490.

Carroll-Johnson, R., & Zichi-Cohen, M. (Eds). (1994). The meaning of oncology nursing: Results of the life cycle research project. *Oncology Nursing Forum, 21*(Suppl. 8), [entire issue].

Catanzaro, M. (1988). Identifying problems for nursing research. In N. F. Woods, & M. Catanzaro (Eds.), *Nursing research: Theory and practice* (pp. 35–45). St. Louis: C. V. Mosby Co.

Chenitz, W. C., & Swanson, J. M. (1986). *From practice to grounded theory.* Reading, MA: Addison-Wesley Publishing Company.

Champion, V. L., & Leach, A. (1989). Variables related to research utilization in nursing: An empirical investigation. *Journal of Advanced Nursing, 14,* 705–710.

Chop, R. M., & Cipriano-Silva, M. (1991). Scientific fraud: Definitions, policies, and implications for nursing research. *Journal of Professional Nursing, 7,* 166–171.

Cohen, J. (1988). *Statistical power analysis for the behavioral sciences* (2nd ed.). Hillsdale, NJ: Lawrence Erlbaum Associates.

Coyle, L. A., & Sokop, A. G. (1990). Innovation adoption behavior among nurses. *Nursing Research, 39,* 176–180.

Cronenwatt, L. R. (1987). Research utilization in a practice setting. *Journal of Nursing Administration, 17,* 9–10.

Degner, L., Arcand, R., Chekryn, J., Davies, E., Dyck, S., Kristjanson, L., Stewart, N., & Warren, B. (1987). Priorities for cancer nursing research. *Cancer Nursing, 10,* 319–326.

Dodd, M. (1987). Problems approaches and priorities in oncology nursing research. *AARN Newsletter, 43,* 13–14.

Edwards, A. L. (1970). *The measurement of personality traits by scales and inventories.* New York: Holt, Rinehart and Winston, Inc.

Faden, R. R., & Beauchamp, T. L. (1986). *A history and theory of informed consent.* New York: Oxford University Press.

Farrell, M. (1953). Experimentation in teaching cancer nursing. *Nursing Research, 2*(1), 41.

Fernsler, J., Holcombe, J., & Pulliam, L. (1984). A survey of cancer nursing research. *Oncology Nursing Forum, 11*(4), 46–52.

Ferrell, B. F., Rhiner, M., & Grant, M. M. (1992). Pain management: Nursing contributions through pain research. In *Proceedings of the Sixth National Conference on Cancer Nursing.* Atlanta: American Cancer Society, Inc.

Flaskerud, J. H., & Thompson, J. (1991). Beliefs about AIDS, health, and illness in low-income white women. *Nursing Research, 40,* 266–271.

Frank-Stromborg, M. & Olsen, S. (1996). *Instruments for clinical nursing research.* (2nd ed.). Boston: Jones and Bartlett.

Funk, S. G., Champagne, M. T., Wiese, R. A., & Tornquist, E. M. (1991). Barriers to using research findings in practice: The clinician's perspective. *Applied Nursing Research, 4,* 90–95.

Funkhouser, S. W., & Grant, M. M. (1989). 1988 ONS survey of research priorities. *Oncology Nursing Forum, 16,* 413–416.

Glaser, B. (1978). *Advances in the methodology of grounded theory: Theoretical sensitivity.* Mill Valley, CA: Sociological Press.

Glaser, B., & Strauss, A. (1967). *The discovery of grounded theory: Strategies for qualitative research.* Chicago: Aldine.

Gordon, D. E. (1956). Appraising a cancer service: A study to establish criteria. *Public Health Reports, 71,* 399–407.

Grady, C. (1991). Ethical issues in clinical trials. *Seminars in Oncology Nursing, 7,* 288–296.

Grant, M., Padilla, G., & Ferrell, B. (1993). Cancer nursing research. In S. L. Groenwald, M. H. Frogge, M. Goodman, & C. H. Yarbro (Eds.), *Cancer nursing: Principles and practice* (3rd ed, pp. 1599–1613). Boston: Jones & Bartlett Publishers.

Grant, M. M., & Padilla, G. V. (1983). An overview of cancer nursing research. *Oncology Nursing Forum, 10*(1), 58–67.

Grant, M. M., & Padilla, G. V. (1990). *Cancer nursing research: A practical approach.* Norwalk, CT: Appleton & Lange.

Grant, M. M., & Stromborg, M. (1981). Promoting research collaboration: ONS research committee survey. *Oncology Nursing Forum, 8*(2), 48–53.

Haberman, M. (1993). Research in ambulatory care settings: The need for and how to do research. In P. Buchsel & C. Yarbro (Eds.), *Oncology ambulatory setting: Issues and models of care* (pp. 307–340). Boston: Jones and Bartlett.

Haberman, M. (1995). The meaning of cancer therapy: Bone marrow transplantation as an exemplar of therapy. *Seminars in Oncology Nursing, 11*(1), 23–31.

Haberman, M. R. (1987). *Living with leukemia: The personal meaning attributed to illness and treatment by adults undergoing a bone marrow transplantation.* Unpublished doctoral dissertation, University of Washington, Seattle, WA.

Haberman, M. R. (1995). Nursing research. In P. C. Buchsel & M. B. Whedon (Eds.), *Bone marrow transplantation: Administrative and clinical strategies* (pp. 365–402). Boston: Jones and Bartlett.

Haberman, M. R., & Lewis, F. M. (1990). Selection of research design—Section I: Qualitative designs. In M. M. Grant, & G. V. Padilla (Eds.), *Cancer nursing research: A practical approach* (pp. 77–83). Norwalk, CT: Appleton & Lange.

Haller, K. B., Reynolds, M. A., & Horsley, J.A. (1979). Developing research-based innovation protocols: process, criteria and issues. *Research in Nursing and Health, 2*, 45–51.

Hagopian, G. A. (1991). The effects of a weekly radiation therapy newsletter on patients. *Oncology Nursing Forum, 18*, 1199–1203.

Hanson, J. L., & Ashley, B. (1994). Advanced practice nurses' application of the Stetler model for research utilization: improving bereavement care. *Oncology Nursing Forum, 21*, 720–724.

Hawley, D. J., & Jeffers, J. M. (1992). Scientific misconduct as a dilemma for nursing. *IMAGE: Journal of Nursing Scholarship, 24*, 51–55.

Hilkemeyer, R. (1982). Update on nursing issues: A historical perspective on cancer nursing. *Oncology Nursing Forum, 9*(2), 47–56.

Hill, R., & Metter, G. (1990). Analysis of data. In M. M. Grant, & G. V. Padilla (Eds.), *Cancer nursing research: A practical approach* (pp. 117–142). Norwalk, CT: Appleton & Lange.

Horsley, J., Crane, J., & Bingle, J. (1978). Research utilization as an organizational process. *Journal of Nursing Administration, 8*, 4–6.

Isaac, S., & Michael, W. B. (1981). *Handbook in research and evaluation: For education and the behavioral sciences* (2nd ed.). San Diego: EdITS Publishers.

Jenkins, J., & Hubbard, S. (1991). History of Clinical Trials. *Seminars in Oncology Nursing, 7*, 228–234.

Johnson, J. E., Nail, L. M., Lauver, D., King, K. B., & Keys, H. (1988). Reducing the negative impact of radiation on functional status. *Cancer, 61*, 46–51.

Kerlinger, F. N. (1973). *Foundations of behavioral research* (2nd ed.). New York: Holt, Rinehart and Winston, Inc.

Ketefian, S. (1975). Application of selected nursing research findings into nursing practice. *Nursing Research, 24*, 89–92.

Kirchhoff, K. T. (1982). A diffusion survey of coronary precautions. *Nursing Research, 31*, 196–201.

Kirchhoff, K. T. (1984). Using research in practice: Teaching research utilization. *Western Journal of Nursing Research, 6*, 265–267.

Kramer, H. C., & Thiemann, S. (1987). *How many subjects?* Newbury Park, CA: Sage.

Krueger, J., Nelson, A., & Wolanin, M. (1978). *Research utilization, part III in nursing research development, collaboration and utilization.* Germantown, MD: Aspen Systems.

Lewis, F. M. (1990). Selection of research design—Section II: Experimental and quasi-experimental designs. In M. M. Grant, & G. V. Padilla (Eds.), *Cancer nursing research: A practical approach* (pp. 83–100). Norwalk, CT: Appleton & Lange.

Lincoln, Y. S., & Guba, E. G. (1985). *Naturalistic inquiry.* Beverly Hills: Sage.

Lipsey, M. W. (1990). *Design sensitivity: Statistical power for experimental research.* Newbury Park: Sage.

Mateo, M. A., & Kirchhoff, K. T. (1991). *Conducting and using nursing research in the clinical setting.* Baltimore, MD: Williams and Wilkins.

McCorkle, R. (1990). Development of the research question. In M. M. Grant, & G. V. Padilla (Eds.), *Cancer nursing research: A practical approach* (pp. 27–42). Norwalk, CT: Appleton & Lange.

McCorkle, R., & Lewis, F. M. (1980). Research in cancer nursing. *Seminars in Oncology Nursing, 7*(1), 80–87.

McCorkle, R., & Young, K. (1978). Development of a symptom distress scale. *Cancer Nursing, 1*, 373–378.

McGuire, D. (1992). The process of implementing research into clinical practice. *Proceedings of the Second National Conference on Cancer Nursing Research.* Atlanta: American Cancer Society.

McGuire, D., Frank-Stromborg, M., & Varricchio, C. (1985). 1984 ONS research committee survey of membership's research interests and involvement. *Oncology Nursing Forum, 12*(2), 99–103.

McGuire, D. B., Walczak, J. R., & Krumm, (1994). Development of a nursing research utilization program in a clinical oncology setting: organization, implementation, and evaluation. *Oncology Nursing Forum, 21*, 704–710.

McLaughlin, F. E., & Marascuilo, L. A. (1990). *Advanced nursing and health care research: Quantification approaches.* Philadelphia: W.B. Saunders Co.

Meinert, C. L. (1986). *Clinical trials: Design, conduct, and analysis.* New York: Oxford University Press.

Miller, J. R., & Messenger, S. R. (1978). Obstacles to applying nursing research findings. *American Journal of Nursing, 78*, 632–634.

Mishel, M. H. (1990). Reconceptualizing of the uncertainty in illness theory. *IMAGE: Journal of Nursing Scholarship, 22*, 256–262.

Mishel, M. H., Padilla, G. V., Grant, M. M., & Sorenson, D. S. (1991). Uncertainty in illness theory: A replication of the mediating effects of mastery and coping. *Nursing Research, 40*, 236–240.

Mitchell, E. S. (1986). Multiple triangulation: A methodology for nursing science. *Advances in Nursing Science, 8*, 18–26.

Mooney, K. H., Ferrell, B. R., Nail, L. M., Benedict, S. C., & Haberman, M. R. (1991). Oncology Nursing Society research priorities survey. *Oncology Nursing Forum, 18*, 1381–1388.

Morrison, R. S. (1993). Scientific integrity in nursing research. *Journal of Neuroscience Nursing, 25*, 321–325.

Munet-Vilaro, F. (1988). The challenge of cross-cultural nursing research. *Western Journal of Nursing Research, 10*, 112–116.

Munet-Vilaro, F., & Egan, M. (1990). Reliability issues of the family environment scale for cross-cultural research. *Nursing Research, 39*, 244–247.

Munhall, P. L., & Oiler, C. J. (1986). *Nursing research: A qualitative perspective.* Norwalk, CT: Appleton-Century-Crofts.

Munro, B. H., Visintainer, M. A., & Page, E. B. (1986). *Statistical methods for health care research.* Philadelphia: J. B. Lippincott Co.

Nolan, M. T., Larson, E., McGuire, D., Hill, M. N., & Haller, K. (1994). A review of approaches to integrating research and practice. *Applied Nursing Research, 7*, 199–207.

Nunnally, J. C. (1978). *Psychometric theory* (2nd ed.). New York: McGraw-Hill Book Co.

Oberst, M. (1978). Priorities in cancer nursing research. *Cancer Nursing, 1*(8), 281–290.

Padilla, G. V. (1990). Progress in cancer nursing research. In M. M. Grant & G. V. Padilla (Eds.), *Cancer nursing research: A practical approach.* Norwalk, CT: Appleton & Lange.

Panel on Scientific Responsibility and the Conduct of Research, Committee on Science, Engineering, and Public Policy. (1992). *Responsible science: Ensuring the integrity of the research process.* Washington, DC: National Academy Press.

Pocock, S. (1983). *Clinical trials: A practical approach.* New York: Wiley.

Polit, D. F., & Hungler, B. P. (1995). *Nursing research: Principles and methods* (5th ed.). Philadelphia: J. B. Lippincott Co.

Quint, J. C. (1963). Impact of mastectomy. *American Journal of Nursing, 63*(11), 88–92.

Quint, J. C. (1965). Institutionalized practices of information control. *Psychiatry, 28,* 119–132.

Reed, P. G. (1991). Toward a nursing theory of self-transcendence: Deductive reformulation using developmental theories. *Advances in Nursing Science, 13,* 64–77.

Reedy, A. M., Shivan, J. C., Hanson, J. H., Haisfield, & Gregory, R. E. (1994). The clinical application of research utilization: amphotericin B. *Oncology Nursing Forum, 21,* 715–719.

Rempusleski, V. F. (1991). Using art and science to change practice. *Applied Nursing Research, 4,* 96–98.

Rennie, D., & Gunsalus, C. K. (1993). Scientific misconduct: New definition, procedures, and office—perhaps a new leaf. *Journal of the American Medical Association, 269,* 915–917.

Rizzuto, C., Bostrom, J., Suter, W. N., & Chenitz, W. C. (1994). Predictors of nurses' involvement in research activities. *Western Journal of Nursing Research, 16,* 193–204.

Rutledge, D. N., Greene, P., Mooney, K., Nail, L., & Ropka, M. Use of research-based practices by oncology staff nurses. (manuscript in process).

Scanlon, C., Arrindell, D. M., Carson, W. Y., & Sapin, B. J. (1994). *Guidelines: On reporting incompetent, unethical, or illegal practices.* Washington, DC: American Nurses Association.

Shivan, J. C., McGuire, D., Freedman, S., Sharkazy, E., Bosserman, G., Larson, E., & Grouleff, P. (1991). A comparison of transparent adherent and dry sterile gauze dressings for long-term central catheters in patients undergoing bone marrow transplant. *Oncology Nursing Forum, 18,* 1349–1356.

Silva, M. C., & Sorrell, J. M. (1984). Factors influencing comprehension of information for informed consent: Ethical implications for nursing research. *International Journal of Nursing Studies, 21,* 233–240.

Smith, M. C., Holcombe, J. K., & Stullenbarger, E. (1994). A meta-analysis of intervention effectiveness for symptom management in oncology nursing research. *Oncology Nursing Forum, 21,* 1201–1209.

Stetler, C. B. (1994). Refinement of the Stetler/Marram model for application of research findings to practice. *Nursing Outlook, 42,* 15–25.

Stetler, C. B., & Marram, G. (1976). Evaluating research findings for applicability to practice. *Nursing Outlook, 24,* 559–563.

Stetz, K., Haberman, M. R., Holcombe, J., & Jones, L. (1995). 1994 Oncology Nursing Society research priorities survey. *Oncology Nursing Forum, 22*(5), 785–789.

Strauss, A., & Corbin, J. (1990). *Basics of qualitative research: Grounded theory procedures and techniques.* Newbury Park: Sage.

Strauss, A. L. (1987). *Qualitative analysis for social scientists.* Cambridge: Cambridge University Press.

Strickland, O. L., & Waltz, C. F. (1988). *Measurement of nursing outcomes. (Vol. 2): Measuring nursing performance: Practice, education, and research.* New York: Springer Publishing Company.

Sudman, S., & Bradburn, N. M. (1987). *Asking questions: A practical guide to questionnaire design.* San Francisco: Jossey-Bass Publishers.

Swanson, K. (1993). Nursing as informed caring for the well-being of others. *IMAGE: Journal of Nursing Scholarship, 25,* 352–357.

Swanson, K. M. (1991). Empirical development of a middle range theory of caring. *Nursing Research, 4,* 161–166.

Tanner, C. A. (1987). Evaluating research for use in practice: Guidelines for the clinician. *Heart and Lung, 16,* 424–430.

Walczak, J. B., McGuire, D. B., Haisfield, M. E., & Beezley, A. (1994). A survey of research-related activities and perceived barriers to research utilization among professional oncology nurses. *Oncology Nursing Forum, 21,* 710–714.

Waltz, C., & Bausell, R. B. (1981). *Nursing research: Design, statistics and computer analysis.* Philadelphia: F. A. Davis Company.

Waltz, C. F., & Strickland, O. L. (1988). *Measurement of nursing outcomes. (Vol. 1): Measuring client outcomes.* New York: Springer.

Williams, C. A. (1987a). Research utilization: Preparing graduates for responsibilities in development unit policy [Editorial]. *Journal of Professional Nursing, 5,* 264.

Williams, C. A. (1987b). Research utilization: A special challenge for nursing faculty [Editorial]. *Journal of Professional Nursing, 3,* 133.

Wilson, H. S. (1989). *Research in nursing* (2nd ed.). Reading, MA: Addison-Wesley Publishing Company.

Woods, N. F. (1988a). Assessing nursing research measures: Reliability and validity. In N. F. Woods, & M. Catanzaro (Eds.), *Nursing research: Theory and practice* (pp. 246–259). St. Louis: C. V. Mosby Co.

Woods, N. F. (1988b). Designing prescription testing studies. In N. F. Woods, & M. Catanzaro (Eds.), *Nursing research: Theory and practice* (pp. 202–218). St. Louis: C. V. Mosby Co.

Woods, N. F., & Catanzaro, M. (1988). *Nursing research: Theory and practice.* St. Louis: C. V. Mosby Co.

UNIT X

THE DELIVERY OF CANCER CARE SERVICES: RESOURCES AND REFERRAL SYSTEMS

CHAPTER

73

Ambulatory Care Services

Brenda M. Nevidjon

The first half of the 1990s was an era of national debate about health care. In the fall of 1994, the media declared that health care reform was dead, but providers of health care knew that reform was continuing. Throughout the country, trends that began on the west coast were experienced. Inpatient lengths of stay shortened, more care moved to the ambulatory and home setting, and the landscape of health care blossomed with networks, alliances, partnerships, and integrated systems only hinted at in the 1980s. In cancer care, greater emphasis on ambulatory programs has resulted in more opportunities for oncology nurses.

HISTORIC PERSPECTIVE

In many respects, what is happening today returns health care to its roots. Increasingly, the diagnosis and treatment of disease is happening in outpatient and home settings. Care is being given by partnerships of professionals and family members. Emphasis on wellness and disease prevention is gaining attention. Ambulatory nursing is a full-fledged specialty with a growing national organization, American Academy of Ambulatory Care Nurses, to represent the nurses in this arena.

Ambulatory cancer nursing care has emerged as a subspecialty of oncology nursing within the past decade. Traditionally, care of people in the outpatient setting was the domain of physicians. Visits were for the purpose of symptom evaluation and treatment follow-up. When patients needed more extensive workups

or nursing care, they were admitted to the hospital. The stereotypical image of the few nurses who were in clinics or physician offices was one of overseer of patient flow from the waiting area to the examination room. Several reasons caused little incentive for care to be delivered outside the hospital: through the early 1980s the number of inpatient facilities grew steadily, inpatient beds were plentiful, and insurance covered most inpatient care, but little outpatient care.

Treatment options for cancer expanded from the dominance of surgery to radiation therapy and chemotherapy and the combination of these modalities. Advances in care necessitated frequent physician interaction and follow-up with patients. A new physician specialty, medical oncology, developed. With the increase in chemotherapy administration and expanding number of cooperative study groups, demands for oncology nurses increased. The National Cancer Act of 1971 had a major impact on cancer care, education, and research. Comprehensive cancer centers developed, and general hospitals designated units for oncology patients (McGee, 1989; Miaskowski, 1990). Advances in symptom management allowed patients the ability to spend less time in the hospital and more time at home.

During this same time, the consumer awareness movement and the breaking of taboos about discussing death and dying awakened people to quantity of time and quality of life issues. Patients and families began to question the restrictiveness of the hospital environment and forced changes in policies, such as visitation hours.

More important, they prompted health care providers to develop alternatives to lengthy hospitalizations. By 1980, ambulatory programs were increasing, and oncology nurses were routinely recruited from the inpatient setting to develop new roles. Not only had the specialty of oncology nursing been established, but the subspecialty of ambulatory oncology nursing was underway.

EMERGENCE OF AMBULATORY CARE SETTINGS

The diagnosis and treatment of cancer was often done in tertiary referral centers that had specialized services for cancer. With the National Cancer Acts, specific academic medical centers were designated with the status of comprehensive cancer center. These centers offered a full range of services from public education on cancer risk to the latest in diagnostic and treatment options. Multidisciplinary clinics and chemotherapy treatment units became cornerstones of the centers. In addition to National Cancer Institute (NCI) designated centers, other regional programs evolved. An early one was described by Isler (1977). Centers served patients from broad geographic spans and served as a center of resources for health professionals in the area. However, the drawback was that patients had to travel to these centers.

A number of factors in the 1970s and 1980s contributed to the rise in cancer providers and the emergence of ambulatory cancer care:

- Escalating cost of inpatient care—hospital costs climbed steadily causing providers to seek out alternative approaches such as medical day hospitals, outpatient treatment centers, and portable technology.
- Advances in technology/pharmacology—new drugs and technologic advances in drug delivery assisted patients to be more mobile and ultimately to be able to receive treatment totally outpatient.
- Development of the oncology nursing specialty—a body of knowledge and skills unique to cancer care was established, and increasing numbers of nurses entered the specialty.
- Restructuring of reimbursement—diagnostic related groups (DRGs) and health maintenance organizations (HMOs) were initiatives to reduce the cost of health care.
- Survivorship—treatment advances extended the disease-free intervals, and issues around long term follow-up resulted in nurse-run outpatient programs (Hobbie, 1986; Ruccione, 1985).
- Consumerism—as previously noted.

Thus far in the 1990s, more and more care that has traditionally been in the inpatient setting is becoming ambulatory. In cancer care, the reimbursement for chemotherapy, DRG 410, has produced a growth industry, outpatient infusion centers, and new business ventures for entrepreneurs. Trends in surgery clearly show the movement to ambulatory sites with prediction that more than 80 percent of surgeries will be ambulatory by the next century. For example, mastectomies are now performed as same-day surgery, and women return home with drains and dressings to manage. The care of even some of the more complex treatments, such as autologous bone marrow transplants, now occurs in the ambulatory setting (Cavanaugh, 1994; Peters et al., 1994). Office-based practices, hospital-based clinics and treatment centers, and free-standing centers that may be part of a national chain are types of ambulatory settings commonly seen today (Harvey, 1994).

Forecasters for the next century predict an intensifying effort to move care to the ambulatory and home setting. Consumers will continue to demand high-quality, cost-contained options for care. The options will, and must, extend beyond the hospital or the office setting and will tap into the interactive video and computer worlds. The structures for providing care will be further decentralized, a trend that is being seen with the proliferation of surgicenters, medical/emergency centers, and other alternate care sites. The population distribution is changing in the country, and health care must move out of being centralized in the highly populated urban areas to the small towns and rural areas, which are rapidly growing (Blendon, 1988; Boyle, Engelking, & Harvey, 1994; Callahan, 1988; Naisbitt & Elkins, 1983a, 1983b). The continued trend to ambulatory and home care opens many possibilities for the oncology nurse of today.

AMBULATORY ONCOLOGY NURSING ROLES

Distinct, defined roles for nurses who desired to work exclusively with people who had cancer evolved in academic centers. Early roles grew out of the needs associated with experimental therapies. Frequently, the route to specializing as an oncology nurse was initiated by an oncologist who sought a nurse to become a member of the cancer care team (Nevidjon, 1995). As described by Henke (1980), the first expanded oncology nursing role, associated with clinical trials, had the nurse as data collector and data administrator of experimental drugs. The growth of clinical trials resulted in a unique physician-nurse collaborative practice relationship that continues today. As oncologists established community-based practices independent of academic centers, they recruited experienced nurses to go with them. Thus began the expansion of oncology nursing and a presense in office-based practice (see also Chapter 3).

AMBULATORY ROLE DISTINCTION

Ambulatory nurses bridge the continuum of care between the hospital and home. Their practice differs from inpatient nursing and requires a set of distinct skills beyond the fundamentals of oncology nursing. Verran (1981) described the seven domains of ambulatory nursing: patient counseling, health care maintenance, preventive care, primary care, patient education, therapeutic care, and normative care. Because cancer affects the elderly, minorities, poor, and underserved in a higher proportion, ambulatory oncology nurses are challenged to develop expertise in the care of the elderly and minorities and to enhance their skills in consultation, collaboration, and team communication (Boyle, 1994; Broder, 1991; Frank-Stromborg, 1991). The development of the various roles in the ambulatory setting involves an expansion of responsibility and job descriptions that clarify the scope of the position (Harris & Bean, 1991).

As ambulatory care has expanded, a multitude of oncology nurse roles have developed. Familiar roles include staff nurses in clinics or offices and nurse managers in those settings. Clinical nurse specialists (CNS) historically have moved along the continuum of care. As the shift to ambulatory care continues, a higher percentage of their time may be spent in the outpatient arena (Welch-McCaffrey, 1986). The nurse practitioner (NP) has been used rather limitedly in cancer care and typically with the traditional focus of performing physical assessments, ordering tests, and prescribing treatments. With the public debate about health care reform, The American Nurses Association championed the NP not only in primary care, but also in specialty care. Many oncology CNSs are obtaining their NP credential to increase their marketability. A number of other roles have developed as ambulatory care has grown: product line/service line managers, research nurses, case managers/care coordinators, and subspecialty nurses, such as cancer prevention/detection program coordinators (Hogan, 1992; Nevidjon, 1986; Nielsen, 1989). Regardless of the role, there are some unique factors related to practice in the ambulatory setting: comprehensive scope of service, role in the continuity of care, and use of telephone communication.

COMPREHENSIVE SCOPE OF SERVICE

Ambulatory nursing can encompass activities related to the prevention and detection of cancer at one end of the spectrum to symptom management in terminal care at the other end. The comprehensiveness of the role is considered the most gratifying aspect of the job (Barhamand, 1991). The knowledge base of nurses in the ambulatory setting expands upon the knowledge base of inpatient nursing and includes pathophysiology and treatment of cancer, research/protocol application, safe administration of cancer treatments, management of treatment side effects/symptom control, and assessment of patients' needs for hospital and community resources (Romsaas & Juliani, 1984). Excellent observational and assessment skills are essential and must be applied in much shorter time intervals than inpatient nurses have available.

Patient and family education is an ongoing process that transcends inpatient and ambulatory boundaries. In the outpatient setting, it must be integral to every interaction and activity because of the limited time (DeMuth, 1989). Attention must be given to assisting patients to understand as much as possible about their cancer and treatment so they become partners in their plan of care. Prior to using specific written materials, ambulatory and inpatient nurses should agree about which publications to use. Also, agreement about what

to teach related to care procedures, such as how to manage pain, is helpful. Nothing confuses patients and families more than contradictory teaching by nurses in different settings.

To facilitate consistency between inpatient and ambulatory practice, effective communication is needed. A variety of mechanisms are possible. Direct communication can be achieved through patient care conferences or transfer reports. Documentation tools that consolidate information improve communication to other cancer care team members (Volker, 1991). Including the patient in this process is essential. At the Duke Comprehensive Cancer Center, a patient log has been created that combines educational resources, data from inpatient and outpatient visits, and entries by the patient (Harwood, personal communication).

Other centers have also developed similar approaches that combine education, documentation, and communication (Kiss, Dorsa, & Martin, 1993; Moore & Knopf, 1991; Skinn & Stacey, 1994).

A particular challenge to nurses in the ambulatory setting is that they deal with short episodes of care, or visits. Unlike their inpatient colleagues, they do not have days to assess, anticipate, or intervene to avoid problems. Regardless of whether a visit is scheduled, ambulatory care can be unpredictable, and the nurse must be able to respond quickly. Patient acuity is increasingly higher, and the complexity of one patient's care may limit the nurse's availability to others. Anticipating the needs of patients and flexing the nursing resources to meet them is a finely honed skill needed as much in the ambulatory setting as on inpatient units.

Although many of the nursing skills listed are also necessary in acute and community settings, it is the intense, rapid juggling of all these activities on a daily basis that makes ambulatory nursing practice unique.

LINK FOR CONTINUITY

Continuity of care provides attention to pyschosocial and rehabilitation issues as an ongoing process of comprehensive care for patients and families (Conkling, 1989). For most, cancer is a chronic illness with periodic acute events. Hospitalization is used for only the most acute episodes, such as initial treatments and complex therapies that cannot be done on an ambulatory basis, recurrence or oncologic emergencies, symptoms/treatment side effects that cannot be managed in the outpatient setting, and terminal care. The major portion of a patient's care is delivered in the ambulatory setting, allowing the nurse to build a relationship that extends for long periods of time—months or years rather than weeks. This fact gives the nurse the opportunity, and the responsibility, to be a liaison between hospital and home. Because hospitalization is used for acute care and home care is used usually for limited periods of time, the ambulatory nurse is in an ideal position to maintain the continuity with patient and family. When patients are doing well, they are still seen for follow-up visits; if they have a relapse or if problems occur, they usually reenter the system through ambulatory care or a physician's office. This liaison role demands that the ambulatory nurse be an effective communicator. One of the more important role functions is to bridge the information gap among colleagues in inpatient or home care settings when a patient's status changes (Joseph, 1990).

TELEPHONE COMMUNICATION

The third unique feature of ambulatory practice is the amount of time spent on the telephone. Little has been written about this important function, but any ambulatory nurse will tell you that the telephone is one of the most, if not the most, important pieces of equipment in ambulatory care. In support of this observation, ambulatory oncology nurses have begun to document relevant issues related to telephone use. A study by Nail, Greene, Jones, and Flannery (1989) on the delivery of nursing care by telephone reported findings on 1844 patient calls over a 6-month period (Box 73–1). Telephone triage in any ambulatory setting is vital. In a published monograph on oncology office practice, Hartigan (1987) outlined this function in detail and stated that "the skills necessary for phone triage include expert assessment, proficient communication (speaking and listening) and phone etiquette." In a university ambulatory setting, Medvec and Calzone (1989) utilized protocols developed by a primary nurse-physician team to handle a nurse-managed telephone triage system. These authors raised several issues regarding telephone care, such as the legalities of telephone advice, adequate documentation, referral support, as well as the positive outcomes relative to patient satisfaction.

No matter how carefully patient and family education is carried out, issues may arise at home that generate questions and increase anxiety. The nurse who answers questions knowledgeably and shares with the patient in decision making is able to diffuse unnecessary fears and, at the same time, anticipate problems and intervene appropriately. Frequently this process limits unnecessary emergency visits to the hospital as well. For example, the patient whose blood counts are about nadir following chemotherapy and who develops a fever will be advised to come in and be seen, whereas the patient with normal counts whose children have the flu, and who develops muscle aches and a slight fever, will probably be managed by telephone and given reassurance.

The telephone is also used for follow-up. Calling a patient the day after a treatment or a procedure gives the nurse the opportunity not only to reinforce instructions, but also to evaluate the patient's status and suggest appropriate changes. Frequently, patients are reluctant to call with questions, even if they have been encouraged to do so. By taking the initiative in this instance, the ambulatory oncology nurse is able to avert problems.

Monitoring symptom control is another area in which the telephone offers major assistance. Coyle and co-workers (1986) described their experience treating patients with chronic pain by utilizing continuous subcutaneous infusions. Treatment was initiated and the drug was titrated while the patient was hospitalized. After discharge, these patients were followed by the supportive care pain management team, which included a nurse clinician in daily telephone contact with the patient or a responsible family member.

It is well known that patients perceive calls from a consistent caretaker to be positive and supportive. The use of the telephone can offer support in its broadest sense. For the patient, it will frequently mean the difference between a night's sleep and no sleep at all. An additional benefit to using the telephone in ambulatory care is the credibility gained by the nurse. Nurses are seen as valued and knowledgeable members of the team. Another benefit described by Hartigan (1987) is that "patients gain confidence in their self-care abilities by the support they receive during these conversations."

The importance of this often neglected management tool cannot be overstated. Some researchers have begun to look at the impact that telephone use in ambulatory practice has had on both program productivity and nursing workload (Medvec & Calzone, 1989; Nail et al., 1989). Future studies in this area are critical, because findings have the potential to validate a unique role component and to support the need for additional oncology nursing staff in ambulatory settings.

Providing advice over the telephone also has its liabilities (Charmorro & Tarulli, 1990). Specific protocols for assessment and criteria for decisions about patient care need to be developed.

BOX 73–1. *Nursing Care by Telephone: Describing Practice in an Ambulatory Oncology Center*

Ambulatory oncology nursing care focuses on providing patients and families with the knowledge and resources needed to manage the symptoms of disease and the side effects of treatment. Nurses practicing in ambulatory care settings have limited face-to-face interaction with patients and families. As a result, telephone contact is used to give information, provide encouragement, and assess the patient's condition. To develop and test methods of delivering care to oncology patients by telephone, current practices must be documented. This study describes the use of the telephone in ambulatory oncology nursing in one patient care setting. Over a 6-month period, nurses reported on 1844 patient calls. Data collected on these telephone calls included duration, initiator, purpose, nurse's assessment of urgency level, impact on the nursing care plan, and changes made in the use of health care services. The *Outcome Standards for Cancer Nursing Practice* of The American Nurses' Association and the Oncology Nursing Society most frequently addressed during the calls were information, comfort, and coping. Nurses in this setting functioned independently, handling 91 per cent of the calls they received and using consultation for 52 per cent of the calls.

From Nail, L., Greene, D., Jones, L., & Flannery, M. (1989). *Oncology Nursing Forum, 16,* 387. Reproduced by permission.

MODELS OF CARE DELIVERY

In the past few years, the literature has seen an increased presence of articles and books about ambulatory care. Buchsel and Yarbro (1993) edited the first book that looked at the ambulatory setting specific to oncology nursing. Of the three sections of the book, the major one is devoted to the various types of ambulatory practice models seen today. The realm of ambulatory care encompasses office-based practice; various clinics from day programs to 24 operations; radiation therapy clinics, both free-standing and hospital-based; day surgery options; and newer practices, such as genetic screening clinics and ambulatory bone marrow transplant centers. How the various ambulatory care models fit into an integrated cancer care system is an important issue when looking at the impact health care reform will have (Spallina, 1994). Where once cancer program numbers were growing rapidly, the future may be the networking of programs and services into a comprehensive model. However current information may be, models of care delivery will continue to evolve as reimbursement and regulatory influences are felt.

In looking at models of ambulatory care, two factors must be remembered: the complexity of cancer care and the dependence on the multidisciplinary team for effective outcomes. Technology has allowed the outpatient administration of chemotherapy treatments that 5 years ago would not have been possible. Newer drugs, such as ondansetron and the colony-stimulating factors, have reduced the toxicities of treatments, thus permitting patients to remain at home.

More than ever, the ambulatory nurse has the opportunity to be the coordinator of the care among the various settings and build upon the relationship the nurse has with the patient and family.

The most effective model in the ambulatory setting is one in which the nurse, the various oncology specialty physicians, and other allied health professionals are collaborative and collegial. The nurse incorporates skills in assessment and screening, education, health promotion and disease prevention, clinical decision making for nursing care, data sharing, and care coordination (Koerner, 1987). The stereotypic picture of a task-oriented, assembly line style of ambulatory nursing care is no longer reality, nor can it be effective.

Additional considerations when designing a model of ambulatory care delivery are providing a designated, consistent person for the patients and developing the model to fit the setting versus adapting the setting to fit a model. Thus, in the ambulatory setting, primary nursing, case management, CNS-run programs, CNS/MD partnerships, or NPs with primary practices may all develop (Henne, Warner, & Frank, 1988; Hilderly, 1991; Safviet, 1992). There is no one model that is the only model for ambulatory cancer nursing.

ISSUES IN AMBULATORY ONCOLOGY NURSING

The rapidly changing health care environment is creating many challenges and opportunities for oncology nurses. Some are new, but some have existed and now are intensifying. With forecasts that 60 percent of services traditionally offered in hospitals will be offered in the ambulatory setting, attention needs to be given to how to accommodate the growth and the problems that may result (Goldsmith, 1989).

WAITING TIME

Waiting time and the effect it has on patients was written about 15 years ago as a major problem (Gardner, 1980; Welch, 1981). However, this still remains an issue today and is compounded by the increased number of patients. Overcrowded facilities, poor scheduling, and unexpected emergencies can all contribute to further delays. Automated scheduling systems may minimize the risk of poor scheduling, and various amenities in the waiting area may reduce the unpleasantness of the unit. Today, as 15 years ago, nurses still have an opportunity to help patients with the anxiety and boredom that waiting brings. One aspect to evaluate is the structure of the scheduling system. Are all patients waiting to see a physician? Are there some visits that can be handled by a staff nurse or a type of service by an advanced practice nurse?

STANDARDS OF CARE

Standards of care are well defined in the hospital, but only in the past few years has this been addressed in ambulatory nursing. The American Academy of Ambulatory Care Nursing has led the way in establishing standards of ambulatory care (*ONS News*, 1994). Standards in radiation oncology, primarily an ambulatory care setting, have also been developed (Bruner, 1990; ONS, 1992a). Hastings (1987) has described a model for quality assurance in the ambulatory setting that focuses on the appropriateness of nursing care decisions and the results of those decisions. The goals of the model were assurance of appropriate allocation of nursing resources, evaluation of the completeness of nursing care, evaluation of the effectiveness of the care, evaluation of the patient's satisfaction with care, and identification and follow-up of patients at special risk for problems.

UNIQUE RISKS

The issues of risk management in the oncology setting are described by Chamorro and Tarulli (1990). The development of nursing standards and protocols is imperative for the ambulatory care setting. Medication administration, with less control over the patient's overall medication program, is a high-risk area. Early patient release from the ambulatory setting after chemotherapy administration can be hazardous. Documentation standards are less well developed in the ambulatory setting, and the collection and recording of data is an area that needs improvement. Automation of patient data will eventually be commonplace and eliminate today's challenges. In the meantime, nurses need to adapt documentation tools to the ambulatory setting (see Chapter 80).

STAFFING

How to staff ambulatory centers is dependent on the types of services provided, patient volume, patient acuity, and time factors related to specific procedures. In a survey conducted by ONS (1992b), 54 per cent of the ambulatory centers reported using their own classification system.

An important factor to consider in staffing ambulatory centers is the indirect time that is needed for phone communication and preparation time, such as chart review. As health care dollars shrink, ambulatory centers, like hospitals, will face the question about skill mix of staff and ratio of staff to patients. Nurses have not been the dominant care provider in general ambulatory settings but have probably had a greater presence in cancer care because of the complexity of patient needs. Planning now for delivery systems that incorporate nurse assistants is an opportunity for ambulatory staff to take to clearly define the professional nurse's role and responsibilities.

The recruitment of nurses from inpatient setting to the ambulatory site is a typical approach to staffing. Success as an inpatient nurse does not predict success in the ambulatory arena. In addition to a solid foundation in oncology, ability to set priorities, flexibility, and effective communication skills are necessary. The ability to function independently is balanced by the ability to collaborate well as a member of the multidisciplinary team. With fluctuating activity levels in inpatient settings, the possibility to cross-train nurses to work in inpatient and ambulatory sites would be an asset for managing staff resources. In fact, a single manager on the inpatient and ambulatory areas in the same institution is a consideration with many benefits.

ADVANCED PRACTICE

The advanced practice nurse in the ambulatory care setting has many opportunities for role development and expansion. The two roles commonly cited are the CNS and the NP. Although coming from different traditions, they have unique and shared contributions to make in the ambulatory setting. Standards for Advanced Practice in Oncology Nursing (American Nurses Association, 1990) define professional practice standards for these groups. Currently there seems to be a trend that advocates combining the roles. *Nursing's Agenda for Health Care Reform* outlined the benefits that greater use of NPs would afford the public (Reifsnider, 1992). There are issues around combining the roles in the ambulatory setting: NP reimbursement may weaken, education programs are not designed for both content yet, core competencies could be compromised, and role confusion could result (Page & Arena, 1994).

FUTURE TRENDS

The escalating changes of the late 1980s and early 1990s will not abate as the twenty-first century approaches. Futurists predict the continued movement of care to the ambulatory setting and home (Engelking, 1994). Nurse leaders advocate that nurses must become active in creating the future, the preferred future, for patients and nurses alike (Aydelotte, 1987). Key to creating that future is dealing with issues access, cost-containment, and quality.

Access is a question that has not been answered by the health care reform debate. For the time, a two-tiered system continues in which those who can pay for services will have an easier access to care. Perhaps in the next century, the answer to this condition will be found. In the meantime, cost-containment is being felt intensely in all health care settings. With the pressure of more care being delivered in the ambulatory setting, new models of how to provide the care are needed.

How mid-level practitioners will be used needs to be defined, and the advanced practice oncology nurses will be integral to the discussion. Ambulatory oncology centers need to be prepared for the population of baby boomers who are aging and in the twenty-first century will be of the age when cancer risk and incidence increase. Quality is often combined with cost-containment as a concern of consumers. Ambulatory oncology centers will need to parallel the efforts of the inpatient setting in assessing patient satisfaction tools and using continuous quality-improvement initiatives to define the scope of their services. In particular, the academic medical centers will face unique challenges as this decade ends (Rogers, Synderman, & Rogers, 1994).

Oncology nurses will be challenged by ethical dilemmas of increasing difficulty, in particular around access to care (Rooks, 1990). Technology will continue to become commonplace in the ambulatory setting. Currently, the technology is more frequently related to the delivery of care. In the future, the education of the patient and family and the transmission of clinical data will be automated. Eventually, interactive automated education will be inexpensively and conveniently available to patients at home (Meyer, 1992; Milio, 1986).

To prepare for the future, oncology nurses need to be equal partners in the design of facilities and services. They need to articulate the roles of nurses in the ambulatory setting and be prepared to let go of traditional ways of doing things, as they discover new approaches. The foundation of oncology nursing, which has been well developed in the inpatient setting, is translating well into ambulatory care. The next decade promises to be one of exciting potential for oncology nurses and one in which ambulatory oncology nurses can be leaders for nursing.

ACKNOWLEDGMENT. The author thanks Ryan Iwamoto, RN, MN, for his contributions to the chapter, and Jennie Simpson for her assistance.

REFERENCES

American Nurses Association; Oncology Nursing Society. (1990). *Standards of advanced practice in oncology nursing.* Pittsburgh, PA: Oncology Nursing Society.

Aydelotte, M. K. (1987). Nursing's preferred future. *Nursing Outlook, 35,* 114–119.

Barhamand, B. (1991). A survey of the role, benefits, and realities of the office-based oncology nurse. *Oncology Nursing Forum, 18*(1), 31–37.

Blendon, R. (1988). The public's view of the future of health care. *Journal of the American Medical Association, 259*(24), 3587–3593.

Boyle, D. M. (1994). New identities: the changing profile of patients with cancer, their families, and their professional care givers. *Oncology Nursing Forum, 91*(1), 55–61.

Boyle, D., Engelking, C., & Harvey, C. (1994). Making a difference in the 21st century: Are oncology nurses ready? *Oncology Nursing Forum, 21*(1), 53–71.

Broder, S. (1991). The human costs of cancer and the proposal of the National Cancer Program. *Cancer, 67,* 1716–1717.

Brown, M. A., & Waybrant, K. M. (1988). Health promotion, education, counseling, and coordination in primary health care nursing. *Public Health Nursing, 5*(1), 16–23.

Bruner, D. W. (1990). *Report on the Radiation Oncology Nursing Subcommittee of the American College of Radiology Task Force on Standard Development Oncology,* 4(80), 80–81.

Buchsel, P., & Yarbro, C. (1993). *Oncology nursing in the ambulatory setting.* Boston, Jones and Bartlett Publishers.

Callahan, D. (1988). Allocating health resources. *Hastings Center Report, April/May,* 14–20.

Cavanaugh, C. (1994). Outpatient autologous bone marrow transplantation: A new frontier. *Quality of Life-A Nursing Challenge, 3*(2), 25–29.

Chamorro, T., & Tarulli, D. (1990). Strategies for risk management in cancer nursing. *Oncology Nursing Forum, 17*(6), 915–920.

Conkling, V. K. (1989). Continuity of care issues for cancer patients and families. *Cancer, 64*(1) (Suppl.), 290–294.

Coyle, N., Mauskop, A., Maggard, J., & Foley, K. (1986). Continuous subcutaneous infusions of opiates in cancer patients with pain. *Oncology Nursing Forum, 13*(4), 53–57.

DeMuth, J. S. (1989). Patient teaching in the ambulatory setting. *Nursing Clinics of North America, 24*(3), 645–654.

Engelking, C. (1994). New approaches: innovations in cancer prevention, diagnosis, treatment, and support. *Oncology Nursing Forum, 21*(1), 62–71.

Frank-Stromborg, M. (1991). Changing demographics in the United States, implications for health professionals. *Cancer, 67,* 1772–1778.

Gardner, M. E. (1980). Notes from a waiting room. *American Journal of Nursing, 80,* 86–89.

Goldsmith, J. (1989). A radical prescription for hospitals. *Harvard Business Review, May-June,* 104–111.

Harris, M. G., & Bean, C. A. (1991). Changing the role of the nurse in the hematology-oncology outpatient setting. *Oncology Nursing Forum, 18*(1), 43–46.

Hartigan, K. (1987). Administrative issues for the oncology nurse in the office setting. In S. Baird (Ed.), *The role of the oncology nurse in the office setting* (pp. 9–126). Ohio: Adria Laboratories.

Harvey, C. (1994) New systems: The restructuring of cancer care delivery and economics. *Oncology Nursing Forum, 21*(1), 72–77.

Hastings, C. E., Costa, L., & Farley, B. (1985). Developing professional practice in ambulatory care: Issues for the middle manager. *Ambulatory Nursing Administration, 7*(5), 1–3.

Henke, C. (1980). Emerging roles of the nurse in oncology. *Seminars in Oncology, 7,* 4–8.

Henne, S. J., Warner, N. E., & Frank, K. J. (1988). Ambulatory care centers: A unique opportunity for nurse practitioners. *Nursing Practice Forum, 13*(10), 43, 46, 47, 50, 51, 55.

Hilderley, L. S. (1991). Nurse-physician collaborative practice: The clinical nurse specialist in a radiation oncology private practice. *Oncology Nursing Forum, 18*(3), 585–591.

Hobbie, W. (1986). The role of the pediatric oncology nurse specialist in a follow-up clinic for long-term survivors of childhood cancer. *Journal of the Association of Pediatric Oncology Nurses, 3,* 9–12.

Hogan, C. H. (1992). An oncology clinical nurse specialist symptom management service: An advanced nursing practice [Abstract]. The First International Symposium on Symptom Management. San Francisco.

Isler, C. (1977). Emerging in cancer care: The regional ambulatory center. *Registered Nurse, 40*(2), 33–46.

Joseph, A. C. (1990). Ambulatory care: An objective assessment. *Journal of Nursing Administration, 20*(20), 27–33.

Kiss, M. E., Dorsa, B. A., & Martin, S. (1993). The development of a patient history and data base form. *Oncology Nursing Forum, 20*(5), 815–823.

Koerner, B. L. (1987). Clarifying the role of nursing in ambulatory care. *Journal of Ambulatory Care Management, 10*(3), 1–7.

McGee, R. F. (1989). Oncology nursing: Five decades of growth. *Journal of Cancer Education, 4*(3), 167–173.

Medvec, B., & Calzone, K. (1989). Effective ambulatory oncology nursing: Winning the telephone management war. *Oncology Nursing Forum, 16*(Suppl). (Abstract No: 141A).

Meyer, C. (1992). Bedside computer charting: Inching toward tomorrow. *American Journal of Nursing, April,* 38–44.

Miaskowski, C. (1990). The future of oncology nursing: A historical perspective. *Nursing Clinics of North America, 25*(2), 461–473.

Miaskowski, C., Rostad, M. (1990). *Standards of advanced practice in oncology nursing.* Pittsburgh: Oncology Nursing Society.

Milio, N. (1986). Telematics in the future of health care delivery: Implications for nursing. *Journal of Professional Nursing, January-February,* 39–50.

Moore, J. M., & Knopf, M. T. (1991). A nursing flow sheet for documentation of ambulatory oncology. *Oncology Nursing Forum, 18*(5), 933–939.

Nail, L., Greene, D., Jones, L., & Flannery, M. (1989). Nursing care by telephone: Describing practice in an ambulatory oncology center. *Oncology Nursing Forum, 16,* 387–395.

Naisbitt, J., & Elkins, J. (1983a). The hospital and megatrends: Top business forecasters examine the impact ten new directions have on health care delivery. Part 1 of 2. *Hospital Forum, 26*(3), 9, 11, 12, 17.

Naisbitt, J., & Elkins, J. (1983b). The hospital and megatrends: Top business forecasters examine the impact ten new directions have on health care delivery. Part 2 of 2. *Hospital Forum, 26*(4), 53–56.

Nevidjon, B. (1986). Cancer prevention and early detection: Reported activities of nurses. *Oncology Nursing Forum, 13,* 76–80.

Nevidjon, B. (1995). *Voices of oncology nurses . . . building a legacy.* Boston, Jones and Bartlett Publishers.

Nielsen, B. (1989). The nurse's role in mammography screening. *Cancer Nursing, 12,* 271–275.

Oncology Nursing Society. (1994). AAACN announces publication of ambulatory care standards. *ONS News, 9*(3), 3.

Oncology Nursing Society. (1992a). *The manual for radiation oncology nursing education and practice.* Pittsburgh: Oncology Nursing Press.

Oncology Nursing Society. (1992b). *The national survey of salary, staffing, and professional practice patterns in ambulatory care oncology clinics.* Pittsburgh: Oncology Nursing Press.

Page, N. E., & Arena, D. M. (1994). Rethinking the merger of the clinical nurse specialist and the nurse practitioner roles. *Image: Journal of Nursing Scholarship, 26*(4), 315–318.

Peters, W., Ross, M., Vredenburgh, J., Hussein, A., Rubin, P., Dukelow, K., Cavanaugh, C., Beauvais, R., & Kasprzak, S. (1994). The use of intensive clinic support to permit outpatient autologous bone marrow transplantation for breast cancer. *Seminars in Oncology, 21*(4) (Suppl 7), 25–31.

Reifsnider, E. (1992). Restructuring the American health care system: An analysis of nursing's agenda for health care reform. *Nurse Practitioner, 17*(5), 65–75.

Rogers, M., Synderman, R., & Rogers, E. (1994). Cultural and organizational implications of academic managed-care networks. *The New England Journal of Medicine, 331*(20), 1374–1377.

Romsaas, E. P., & Juliani, L. M. (1984). Resource utilization in an outpatient setting. *Oncology Nursing Forum, 11*(3), 45–48.

Rooks, J. (1990). Let's admit we ration health care—then set priorities. *American Journal of Nursing, June,* 39–43.

Ruccione, K. (1985). The role of nurses in late effects evaluations. *Clinical Oncology, 4,* 205–221.

Safviet, B. J. (1992). Healthcare dollars and regulatory sense: The role of advanced practice nursing. *Yale Journal on Regulation, 9*(2), 49–220.

Skinn, B., & Stacey, D. (1994). Establishing an integrated framework for documentation: Use of a self-reporting health history and outpatient oncology record. *Oncology Nursing Forum, 21*(9), 1557–1566.

Spallina, J. (1994). The cancer program leadership challenge: Preparing for system integration. Part II. *The Journal of Oncology Management, 3*(4), 28–33.

Verran, J. A. (1981). Determination of ambulatory nursing practice. *Journal of Ambulatory Care Management, 4*(1), 1–13.

Volker, D. L. (1991). Needs assessment and resource identification. *Oncology Nursing Forum, 18*(1), 119–123.

Welch, D. A. (1981). Waiting, worry and the cancer experience. *Oncology Nursing Forum, 8*(2), 14–18.

Welch-McCaffrey, D. (1986). Role performance issues for oncology clinical nurse specialists. *Cancer Nursing, 9*(6), 287–294.

CHAPTER

74

Home Care Services

Marilyn D. Harris • Carol Ann Parente

In the "good old days" the sick were cared for at home. There were no sophisticated health care facilities available. The family, neighbors, and friends provided assistance in times of need. Adequate help was available to do the housework, take care of the children, prepare meals, and care for the sick person. Many times families lived together or near one another. Wives or mothers were home to care for the sick family member and the children.

Today home care services are dramatically different. These changes are due to many factors, including changes in demographics, family structure, reimbursement for both hospital and home care services, and technologic advances that make it possible to provide safe care in the home.

In 1978 the American Nurses Association (p. 6) stated that "home care services are mobile, decentralized, and able to be dispersed to assist the patient to assume responsibility for his or her own care. Home health care services are provided to individuals and families in their places of residence for the purpose of preventing illness; promoting, maintaining, or restoring health; or minimizing the effects of illness and disability" (Box 74–1).

The National Association for Home Care (NAHC) (1993, p. 2) stated that "home care is service to recovering, disabled or clinically ill persons who need treatment and/or assistance with daily activities of living. Generally, home care is appropriate whenever a person needs assistance that cannot be easily or effectively provided solely by family or friends on an ongoing basis." This could be for a short or long period of time.

The American Nurses Association introduced its *Nursing's Agenda for Health Care Reform* in 1991. This plan states nursing's vision for a better health care system and includes universal access to a standard package of essential services such as home care, prevention services, prescription drugs, hospice, and other services, all of which are important in assisting individuals to continue to live in their homes while receiving needed nursing and related health care services.

Individuals who require health care services and choose to have these in their own homes are requiring many more nontraditional services to meet their needs. In addition to meeting the needs of patients, these services also increase the home health agency's survival prospects during this time of health care and insurance reform. Dittbrenner (1994) listed and described services that may be available to patients in the future.

The *Home Health Business Report* (Staffing Industry Analysts, Inc., 1994, p. 11) states that the "U.S. Industrial Outlook 1994, published in December 1993 by the U.S. Department of Commerce, projects home care service will be the fastest growing segment of the healthcare industry for the fifth year running, with expenditures growing 34.5% to represent only 2% of overall healthcare spending, which is forecast to top $1 trillion for the first time this year."

Although the majority of home health care services have traditionally been provided to individuals who are over 65 years of age, one of the fastest growing areas of home health care at the Visiting Nurse Association of Eastern Montgomery County, Department of Abington Memorial Hospital is the maternity "early dis-

---

BOX 74–1. *A Randomized Clinical Trial of Home Nursing Care for Lung Cancer Patients*

McCorkle, R., Benoliel, J. Q., Donaldson, G., Georgiadou, F., Moinpour, C., & Goodell, B. (1989). A randomized clinical trial of home nursing care for lung cancer patients. *Cancer, 64*(6), 1375–1382.

A randomized clinical trial was conducted to assess the effects of home nursing care for patients with progressive lung cancer. One hundred and sixty-six patients were assigned to an oncology home care group (OHC) that received care from oncology home care nurses, a standard home care group (SHC) that received care from regular home care nurses, or an office care group (OC) that received whatever care they needed except for home care. Patients were entered into the study 2 months after diagnosis and followed for 6 months. Patients were interviewed at 6-week intervals across five occasions. At the end of the study, there were no differences in pain, mood disturbance, and concerns among the three groups. There were significant differences in symptom distress, enforced social dependency, and health perceptions. The two home nursing care groups had less distress and greater independence 6 weeks longer than the office care group. In addition, the two home nursing care groups reported steadily worse health perceptions over time. Thus, it was remarkable that the office care group, which indicated more symptom distress and social dependency with time, also indicated perceptions of improved health with time. These results suggest that home nursing care assists patients with forestalling distress from symptoms and maintaining their independence longer than no home nursing care. Home care may also include assisting patients in acknowledging the reality of their situation.

---

charge" program. Many insurers are requiring that a new mother, who had a vaginal delivery, be discharged from the hospital within 24 hours of delivery. Many of the insurers contract for one or more nursing visits to these mothers and their newborns. With the increased pressure from third-party payers to decrease costs, whatever the medical diagnoses, there are increased efforts underway to decrease the length of stays on all departments within the acute care facility. This trend provides the opportunity for home care agencies to meet the increasing need for health care services in the community.

REFERRALS TO HOME CARE

Although many referrals may come from hospital staff such as discharge planning nurses, social workers, or physicians, referrals to home care can also be made by other health care professionals and the staff of the home care agency. Additional sources include patients, their families, neighbors, friends, or other community organizations. The referral process will vary with a specific agency, but in general, the process should follow the scenario in Figure 74–1.

The selection of a home health care agency is important to the patient and family and physician. When making a decision on a home care agency that will be best for everyone involved, certain questions should be asked. A list of questions as suggested by the National Association for Home Care (1993) is found in Table 74–1. A listing of additional consumer guides is found in Table 74–2.

STAFF AND SERVICES

An adequate and qualified staff of clinical, business, and administrative personnel, including contractors for specific or specialized care, is essential to the delivery of high-quality health care services in the home. The Medicare Conditions of Participation (U.S. Department of Health and Human Services, 1989, 1991a, 1991b) are used as a reference for describing home care ser-

vices recognized for reimbursement under this program. Many other insurers follow the same guidelines.

Home care services are provided by a highly professional staff consisting of representatives of many disciplines and support personnel. The Medicare program provides for reimbursement for six home health services. Providers of hospice care may also choose to seek Medicare certification for the provision of this level of care to individuals who have a terminal illness and choose to remain in their own homes.

NURSING CARE

Highly skilled registered nurses can be of immense help in speeding a patient's recovery after an operation or when illness occurs. Nurses can provide ongoing care to the aged or chronically ill of all ages. Often with the help of a visiting nurse, lengthy hospital stays and burdens on family members can be avoided. Following consultation with the physician, the nurse performs specific tasks, which include dressing surgical wounds, supervising treatment and diet, providing instructions and supervision of medication, providing intravenous therapy or chemotherapy, and offering health counseling and physical care. Staff assist patients and their families with crisis intervention such as obtaining hospice care or monitoring life-threatening illness.

PHYSICAL THERAPY

Physical therapy can help a patient regain the use of impaired muscles, increase joint motion, control pain, or perform activities of daily living. Physical therapists plan physical rehabilitation programs for patients.

OCCUPATIONAL THERAPY

Following an accident or illness, a patient often must relearn physical and general awareness skills. An occupational therapist assesses the patient's abilities and works out a comprehensive, individualized pro-

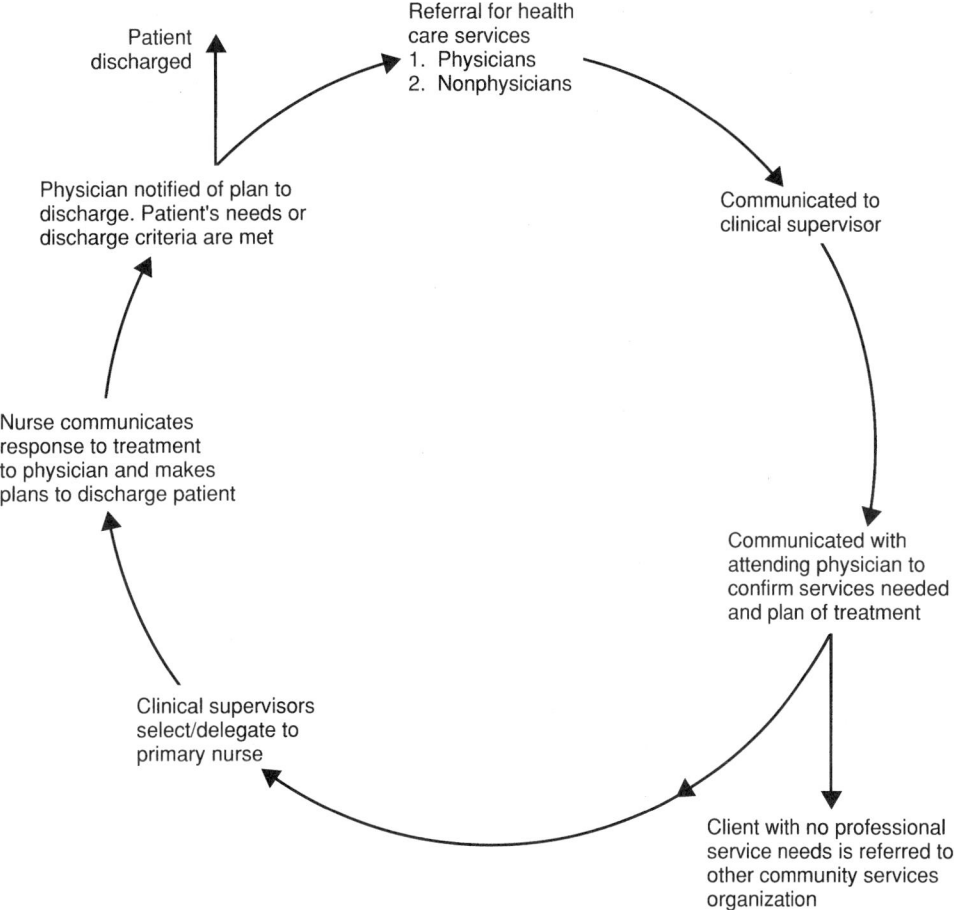

FIGURE 74–1. Home care referral flow chart.

gram that helps the patient regain many skills. With instructions, and sometimes with an adaptive device, a person can begin to do more things without help and thus become more independent.

SPEECH PATHOLOGIST

A speech pathologist helps the patient learn how to communicate after an accident or illness or in spite of a learning disability. The pathologist evaluates the patient's need and then carries out specific programs of instruction and exercise that help the patient retain speech. Speech pathologists also assist when dysphagia problems are present.

MEDICAL SOCIAL WORKER

On occasion, professional help is indicated when a patient finds it difficult to cope with the emotional and social stresses of illness or an accident. A medical social worker studies the patient's situation and works toward resolving problems. This problem-solving process entails such things as finding housing or correcting environmental problems. The social workers provide support and encouragement to both the patient and the family.

HOME HEALTH AIDES OR HOME CARE AIDES

Under the supervision of the professional staff, home health aides or home care aides help patients follow regimens prescribed by physicians, help in personal care such as bathing and exercises, and perform light housekeeping tasks and errands.

ADDITIONAL SERVICES

Additional home care services may include one or more of the following:

- Nutritional support
- Durable medical equipment
- Laboratory studies
- Radiology studies
- Portable electrocardiograms
- Medical supplies, such as catheters and dressings
- Transportation
- Emergency alert system
- Meals-on-Wheels (home-delivered meals)
- Telephone reassurance
- Electronic safety monitoring system

TABLE 74–1. *How to Choose a Home Care Agency*

Finding the best home care agency for your needs requires research, but it is time well spent. Quality of leadership and caliber of personnel will be overriding factors, of course. Fortunately, in most communities families have a variety of agencies from which to choose.

To locate home care agencies in your community, you might start by asking your doctor or consulting with a hospital discharge planner. Agencies may be licensed by the state. Contact your state licensure division within the Department of Health for a list of agencies. Home care agencies also will be listed in the yellow pages under "home care" or "home health care." If your community has any information and referral services, check with them. (Often they are affiliated with the local United Way.) Your church or synagogue may have lists of local service agencies. State Departments of Aging and Social Services also can be helpful.

State home care associations also can help you locate a good agency. Most state associations maintain directories of available home care agencies. NAHC can help you contact your state association and can provide additional information about home care.

How Do I Choose the Right Agency?

Once you have the names of a few agencies, you will want to learn more about their services as well as their reputations. Here are some questions to ask the home care agency and community leaders. Consider their answers when making a decision on which home care agency is best for you.

1. How long has the agency been servicing the community?
2. Is it certified by Medicare? Even if your care will not be paid for by Medicare, the fact that an agency is Medicare certified is one measure of quality. It means that the agency has met federal minimum requirements. You can review the agency's Medicare Survey Report at your local Social Security office. Failure to participate in Medicare does not imply that an agency provides poor care. Be careful. You must consider all factors before making a decision.
3. Is the agency licensed? In many states a home care agency must be licensed by the state, usually by the state health department.
4. Is the agency accredited? Accreditation is a voluntary process conducted by nonprofit professional organizations. Accreditation means the agency has met basic standards, especially in the area of personnel requirements, supervision, and accountability. Agencies that provide skilled nursing services may be accredited by the National League for Nursing or the Joint Commission of Accreditation of Healthcare Organizations. The National HomeCaring Council, Division of the Foundation for Hospice and Homecare accredits and approves agencies that provide home care aide services.
5. Does the agency provide written statements describing its services, eligibility requirements, fees, and funding sources? Often an annual report will offer helpful guidance on the agency. Many agencies provide patients with a detailed "Patient's Bill of Rights," outlining the rights and responsibilities of provider, patient, and caregivers alike.
6. How does an agency choose and train its employees? Does it protect its workers with written personnel policies, benefits packages, and malpractice insurance?
7. Does a nurse or therapist conduct an evaluation of your needs in the home? What is included? Consultations with family members? With the patient's physician? With other health professionals?
8. Is the plan of care written out? Does it include specific duties to be performed, by whom, at what intervals, and for how long? Can you review the plan?
9. Does the plan provide for the family to understand as much of the care as is deemed practical?
10. What are the financial arrangements? Can you get them in writing, including any minimum hour or day requirements that the agency may have and any extra charges to be involved in the home care program?
11. What plans or arrangements are made for you if your reimbursement sources are exhausted?
12. Does the agency send supervisors to visit your home and evaluate quality care regularly? Whom do you call with questions or complaints? Are your questions followed up and resolved?
13. What arrangements are made for emergencies?
14. What arrangements are made to ensure patient confidentiality?

(Copyright © 1993 by the National Association for Home Care, Washington, DC. Reproduced by permission.)

Additional personnel may also be involved in providing home care services. Homemaker-attendant care provides help with shopping and doing household chores that enables individuals to remain in their homes. Volunteers, dentists, clergy, physicians, and ophthalmologists can also provide services in the home setting.

A case study description illustrates a coordinated home health team approach for the management of a patient with an inoperable brain tumor.

CASE STUDY

Bob A. was a 56-year-old man who presented to his family physician in May with ataxia and head-aches. A neurologic workup, including a computed tomographic (CT) scan, showed no significant findings. The symptoms persisted, and a subsequent magnetic resonance image (MRI) showed a lesion on the brain.

The patient's care was assigned to a university medical center for treatment, including chemotherapy and radiation. The patient's symptoms lessened, and he was able to maintain his functional status, including a part-time job as a maintenance man.

Bob lived with his wife, Pat, in a small one-story house. Their grown son lived nearby with his family. As Bob's condition worsened, Bob and Pat asked his recently widowed mother to move from the Midwest to assist with Bob's care, because Pat worked full time to maintain their income.

TABLE 74–2. *Consumer Guides*

National Institutes of Health
   National Cancer Institute
   Bethesda, MD 20892
What You Need To Know About Bladder Cancer (1992)
What You Need To Know About Brain Tumors (1992)
What You Need To Know About Cancer of the Colon and Rectum (1989)
What You Need To Know About Hodgkin's Disease (1991)
What You Need To Know About Lung Cancer (1990)
What You Need To Know About Multiple Myeloma (1991)
What You Need To Know About Non-Hodgkin's Lymphomas (1992)
What You Need To Know About Ovarian Cancer (1990)
What You Need To Know About Cancer of the Pancreas (1992)
What You Need To Know About Prostate Cancer (1992)
What You Need To Know About Skin Cancer (1992)
What You Need To Know About Testicular Cancer (1992)
What You Need To Know About Cancer of the Uterus (1992)
When Cancer Recurs, Meeting the Challenge Again (1992)
Facing Forward, A Guide for Cancer Survivors (1992)

American Cancer Society
   1599 Clifton Road, N.E.
   Atlanta, GA 30329
Guidelines for the Cancer-Related Checkup, Recommendations and Rationale (1991)
Living with Cancer (1988)
Psychosocial Issues and Cancer (1988)

The Pennsylvania State University College of Medicine and The Central Pennsylvania Oncology Group
   Department of Behavioral Science
   Pennsylvania State University College of Medicine
   Box 850
   Hershey, PA 17033
Cancer Home Care Plan, A Guided Problem-Solving Program for Family & Friends of Persons with Cancer (1993)

U.S. Department of Health and Human Services Public Health Service
   National Institutes of Health
   National Cancer Institutes
   Bethesda, MD
Cancer Tests You Should Know About, A Guide for People 65 and Over (1992)
Chemotherapy and You, A Guide to Self-Help During Treatment (1991)
Eating Hints, Recipes & Tips for Better Nutrition During Cancer Treatment (1992)
Radiation Therapy and You, A Guide to Self-Help During Treatment (1990)

National Consumer League
   600 Maryland Avenue, S.W., Suite 202 West
   Washington, DC 20024
A Consumer's Guide to Home Health Care (1985)

Upjohn Health Care Services
   3651 Van Rick Drive
   Kalamazoo, MI 49002
A Guide to Home Health Care (1982), A. E. Nourse, M.D.

American Association of Retired Persons
   1909 K Street, N.W.
   Washington, DC 20049
A Handbook About Care in the Home (1982)

National Homecaring Council and the Better Business Bureau of Metropolitan New York, Inc.
   235 Park Avenue South
   New York, NY 10003
All About Home Care: A Consumer's Guide (1982)

National Association for Home Care
   519 C Street, N.E.
   Washington, DC 20002
Home Care (1984)
Home Health Care: A Complete Guide for Patients and Their Families (1986), JoAnn Friedman
   New York: W. W. Norton
The Home Health Care Solution (1985), Janet Zhun Nassif
   New York: Harper & Row

The referral for home care was initiated by Pat. Her call to the Visiting Nurse Association (VNA) was prompted by a sharp decline in the patient's abilities during a vacation cruise. The patient developed left-sided hemiparesis, required moderate to maximum help with his activities of daily living, and was incontinent of urine. Bob was scheduled for chemotherapy at the university hospital the following week, but it was clear to Pat that his response to treatment was lessening. She explored home care options before this hospitalization so that services and equipment would be ready at Bob's discharge.

Bob was admitted to VNA services the following day, and the initial nursing assessment showed the following problems: alteration in urinary elimination, incontinence, impaired mobility, knowledge deficit related to management of dexamethasone (Decadron)-induced diabetes, and self-care deficit.

The following week the patient was admitted as scheduled for his chemotherapy. During that hospital stay, he developed a deep vein thrombophlebitis in his left leg, with further weakness and increased difficulty in transfers. At discharge from the hospital, Bob and Pat made a decision for "no more chemotherapy." The physicians agreed that palliative care was most appropriate, and the VNA hospice team was notified.

On readmission to the VNA, the patient's mobility was of prime concern, because he was experiencing left-sided hemiplegia, and at 6 feet 2 inches in height and 200 pounds in weight he was quite a challenge to move from bed to chair. Physical therapy referral was initiated for instruction in transfers and range of motion exercises.

An occupational therapist was requested to instruct the patient and the family in adaptations of activities of daily living to promote Bob's independence. He was instructed in the use of a sling, hand splint, and adaptive eating devices.

Over the course of the next few weeks, Bob's speech deteriorated and his conversations were marked with rage and frustration with his expressive aphasia. Speech therapy assisted the patient and his family with communications, including refining a picture board Pat had devised.

Home health aides visited Bob to assist in personal care needs, including transfers to the tub for showering. Visits were initially three times each week and increased as Bob's status declined.

Nursing activities included instruction, assessment of diabetes, and insulin administration. Control of Bob's urinary incontinence became more difficult. Various external devices were tried and found to be ineffective for him, and skin deterioration necessitated a Foley catheter.

A hospice volunteer was assigned to provide companionship and respite for Bob's mother, who was far from her own circle of friends in the Midwest. Volunteers also provided transportation for Bob's mother for her own health appointments and made extended visits to Bob when she was recovering from cataract surgery and was unable to provide direct care to Bob.

The chaplain visited the family at regular intervals to offer spiritual support, sometimes praying with the patient and sometimes just listening.

As Bob's abilities declined and his care became more difficult for his mother to manage, the social worker secured added caregiving support for Bob from a county program. The social worker also focused on emotional support for Bob and his family.

In October the patient developed increased difficulty swallowing, increased aphasia, and weakness in all extremities. His wife was determined to keep Bob at home, and when he could no longer swallow, private duty nurses (also covered by his insurance plan) were provided to administer parenteral anticonvulsants.

Bob died at home 214 days after his initial VNA evaluation. The integration of multidisciplinary services offered Bob and his family the care needed to keep him at home during the terminal phase of his illness.

ROLE OF THE ADVANCED PRACTICE NURSE IN HOME CARE

The home care nurse today faces an often overwhelming onslaught of problems in the care of oncology (and other) patients in the community. Reimbursement in both acute care and home care settings dramatically influences the kind of patient seen by the home care staff nurse.

Length of stay for many hospitalized patients has been shortened. Patients are now being discharged "quicker and sicker." Recovery periods for many take place now at home rather than in acute care beds. In addition, most high-technology care equipment (e.g., intravenous lines and pumps, feeding tubes, tracheostomy tubes or "trachs," and ventilators) can accompany patients to their homes. When hospital stays are shortened, patients' families and caregivers do not always have time to receive the teaching they need to manage equipment and procedures at home. The patient's situation at home may be very confused, with many questions not yet answered, symptoms not totally controlled, and stressed family members who need help themselves.

Enter the home care nurse. Most agencies require the beginning community health nurse to have a B.S.N. degree or to be working toward a nursing degree (Yuan, 1994). Although the community nurse may be a specialist in home care, traditionally the role is one of a generalist. The typical home care nurse carries a caseload of five to seven adult patients per day with a variety of diagnoses and needs. The nurse's assessment and intervention skills must be equally well honed for a cardiac, diabetic, or oncology patient. The nursing role is independent, challenging, and frustrating when the nurse confronts the complexities of the home care patient and his or her family.

In most home care agencies, the patients with cancer represent a sizable portion of the patient population. Figures from the Pennsylvania Department of Health, Division of Primary Care and Home Health Licensing Survey (1992) of home health agencies indicate neoplasms as the second most frequently occurring diagnosis, following diseases of the circulatory system. Visit statistics from the Visiting Nurse Association of Eastern Montgomery County (1993b) closely reflect the state figures, with the top five diagnoses for patients seen in fiscal year 1994 as follows: (1) diseases of the circulatory system, (2) neoplasms, (3) respiratory diseases, (4) musculoskeletal diseases, and (5) digestive disorders.

Patient care procedures that may be commonplace in the acute care setting occur with less regularity in the home. Although the use of ventilators at home is possible, only two or three individuals of a home care agency population may have them at any one time. Intravenous therapy, home chemotherapy, feeding tubes, epidural analgesia, and associated pumps may be more commonplace in the community health setting, but they still occur with relative infrequency in any one home care nurse's caseload. The infrequency of practice of many highly technical procedures contributes to concern among supervisory and nursing staffs about the provision of safe, quality patient care.

Symptom management and patient family education play a vital part in the home care management of all patients. Oncology symptoms may present challenges to home care nurses who have a general knowledge of oncology patients from their educational and clinical background. The oncology patient population in home care may range from the newly diagnosed patient who has just had surgery, to the patient who may need chemotherapy at home, to the hospice patient. As patients with cancer at home move through different stages, their needs may vary widely, and many of their problems may be managed directly by home care nursing activities. Nutrition, activities of daily living, pain, and safety issues through oncologic emergencies may be evaluated and treated initially by the home care nurse. Other members of the home care team (e.g., home health aide; physical, occupational, and speech therapists; medical social worker; and dietitian) may be involved to further assist with symptom management. Coordination of the multidisciplinary team efforts is done by the nurse in accordance with the Medicare conditions of participation (U.S. Department of Health and Human Services, 1991a, 1991b).

Numbers of visits allotted by third-party reimbursement regulations may further compound the home care efforts for the oncology patient. Visit patterns are preset or limited to a certain schedule by some insurers. Denial of payment by Medicare for home visits that have already been made is now a fact of life for the home care agency and its staff. The home care staff must be aware of Medicare and other reimburser guidelines. For example, determination of "skilled nursing" services is often more difficult than one would first imagine. Emphasis is placed on assessment and instruction and involvement of family or other caregivers toward the goal of self-care (Della Monica, 1994) rather than on provision of maintenance level or long-term care.

NEED FOR SPECIALIZATION

As we face major health care reforms to improve access and control costs, home care and community-based care options will continue to grow in importance well into the 21st century. New coalitions of providers, patients, and insurers will also influence the delivery of health care with an emphasis on managed care (Boyle, Engelking, & Harvey, 1994).

Estimates of cancer incidence and costs show continued rises in both toward the turn of the next century (Harvey, 1994). Engelking (1994) describes a vast array of cancer prevention, diagnosis, and treatment choices for the future. From analysis of gene markers through biotechnology, stereotactic radiation, and robotics, the explosion of technology will also change the practice of oncology nursing and home care. Nurses, particularly advanced practice nurses (APN), e.g., nurse practitioners and oncology clinical nurse specialists, will play key roles in future health care delivery to cancer patients by proactively designing solutions to challenges ahead (Harvey, 1994).

Shortened acute care stays, technology advances, varied patient needs, and time constraints have an impact on the care of patients at home. To meet the needs of both patient and nursing staffs, some agencies have established high-technology teams (Weisslein, 1984). Although some agencies employ specialty teams (e.g., intravenous care teams and respiratory care teams), others may also employ APNs such as nurse practitioners, both pediatric and adult, and clinical nurse specialists (e.g., geriatric, oncologic, and psychiatric specialists). These APNs may be employed by an agency to assist visiting and supervisory staffs in the management of complex or specialized patients. The Oncology Nursing Society (ONS) Clinical Practice Committee (1990) describes four roles for the APN or oncology clinical nurse specialist (OCNS): clinician, educator, researcher, and administrator. Each role has overlapping components that may be practiced in home care, making the APN an asset to the agency and community it serves.

CLINICAL COMPETENCY

To fill the role of an APN specialist most effectively, the nurse must maintain clinical competence in the practice field. Direct caregiving may be realized for the APN in home care in a variety of ways. "Provision of direct patient care to provide expert individualized care for selected patients" (Visiting Nurse Association of Eastern Montgomery County, 1993a, p. 1) may in fact make up the bulk of the home care APN's responsibilities. The APN may choose to carry a caseload of patients with intense, multifaceted problems. In this scenario the APN manages the patient's total care needs, assessing, planning, implementing, and evaluating care for the patient and family at home. The nurse practitioner role brings added physical assessment and symptom management skills to the care of the home care cancer patient. Consultation would then be made with the patient's attending physician for changes in the patient's plan of care. McCorkle et al. (1989) describe the effectiveness of home care provided by an APN. In a randomized demonstration project, patients who received care from APNs had fewer complications and fewer hospitalizations for symptom management and remained independent at home for a longer period of time.

Another mechanism to allow the APN to provide direct care to the patient is in a consultative role to the visiting staff. In this instance the APN may visit patients on an "as-needed" basis at the request of supervisory or field staff. The APN may make home visits alone or with the primary nurse, depending on the nature of the problem. Requests for visits to patients with complex problems may be for symptom management, for specialized instruction of the patient or family or visiting staff, or for specific procedures (e.g., chemotherapy). Solo visits by the APN offer home care patients several unique opportunities. The specialist brings expanded preparation and experience into the patient's home. Because specialists usually make fewer visits per day than staff, the APN is not as constrained by time limits, and the extended home visit allows the opportunity to explore the patient's problem in some depth. Several home visits by the APN may be helpful to provide follow-up evaluation of the specialist's nursing interventions, but subsequent home visits may or may not be needed. Following a home visit, the APN may offer assistance to the primary home care nurse in problem solving and patient care management through both postvisit conferences and careful documentation of the consultation visits (McCorkle & Germino, 1984).

Joint visits with the visiting staff offer the opportunity for the APN to provide both patient and staff teaching during the same interval. This mechanism for visiting is particularly helpful if the field staff is uncertain or inexperienced in certain assessment skills or procedures.

STAFF TEACHING

Staff teaching is another focus of practice for the APN in a home care or community agency. Maintaining proficiency in myriad diagnoses is difficult for the home care nurse. Becoming well versed in a specialty such as oncology in the generalist practice base of home care is even more difficult. The presence of an APN in a home care agency setting provides a resource for staff in the formal education process, such as staff development or inservice programs, and in informal settings, such as patient care or team conferences.

STAFF CONSULTATION

Staff consultations with or without home visits provide yet another area of APN home care practice. Here the clinical specialist offers a resource in troubleshooting and problem solving to the field staff. Pain control issues challenge patients and nurses, from staff through administration, and the APN may particularly effect changes in patient pain management for a home care agency. The APN may be a model for all health team members in providing comprehensive assessment, management, and evaluation for pain control. Consultation and collaboration with other health team members (e.g., physical therapy, social service, company supply-

ing high-technology equipment) may assist the APN in providing holistic pain and symptom management, giving consideration to patients' caregiving, financial, and coping capacities. Additionally, the APN may suggest nonpharmacologic pain control measures not previously considered by patients or home care staff (Whedon, Shedd, & Summers, 1992). Frequently, the focus of the consultation is on other symptom management choices, for example, selecting an appropriate bowel regimen for an oncology patient who is receiving narcotics for pain management. Professional support offered by the APN through consultation and education is invaluable in the community setting, where nursing practice is usually a solo venture.

RESEARCH

Research in a home care setting is also an integral part of the APN role. Practice and symptom management issues that have been well explored in the acute care setting may change as the variables of home and nonprofessional (family) caregivers enter the scene. The opportunities for research in home-based nursing are many and varied. In addition to the clinical issues, the APN may contribute to administrative research efforts. As reimbursement policies continue to influence practice dramatically, research such as evaluation of costs will shape future practice and policies (Harris, Peters, Parente, & Smith, 1986). Development and evaluation of nursing strategies, for example, teaching tools and standardized care plans, specific to the agency and its population may be yet another facet of the APN role.

PROGRAM DEVELOPMENT

Opportunities for program development in the home care field are also available to the APN as agencies seek to diversify to maintain a competitive edge in the growing market. Wellness seminars for patients, nutrition hints, makeup and hair care, sexuality discussions, adult day care for patients, cancer support groups for patients and families, and hospice and bereavement programs are all within range of the home care agency (Harris, 1994a, 1994b). The APN may be instrumental in developing and participating in any of these programs.

OUTSIDE CONSULTANT

The APN may also participate in activities related to home care practice as an external consultant. Consultation may be offered to both hospital and long-term care facilities to assist with patient care management or home care planning. Staff education in other facilities or in continuing education programs enhances a home care agency's network in the community. Education programs may be related directly to home care programs (e.g., hospice) or to common patient management problems (e.g., pain or anorexia). Cooperative exchange or information between inpatient and home care may at times be facilitated by the APN, who may be called on to evaluate the patient in the inpatient facility and learn specifics about the patient's problems or highly technical procedures. This transfer of "first-hand" information may soothe the transition of patient to home for both client and staff, particularly when there are complex patient problems.

Education programs for the public in association with the American Cancer Society or local community groups also strengthen the home care agency's community ties. Topics may include cancer prevention, early detection, treatment of symptoms, and identification and use of community resources.

POTENTIAL AND CHALLENGES

For the APN, the expanding home care market represents an area of career growth. The tradition of nursing independence in the home setting lends itself to the APN role. Changes in the home care field that demand highly technical skills and reimbursement restrictions may also encourage the use of nurse specialists, thus maximizing the expertise available to patients at home. As consumers and third-party payers focus on the home care environment, the use of APNs in the field may strengthen an agency's delivery of quality patient care services.

High-technology care in the home continues to grow as a result of technologic advances and shortened hospital stays. For a home care agency seeking to develop a high-technology practice base, the clinical nurse specialist may provide one option: alone, as part of the agency's high-technology team, or in alliance with a high-technology agency. Home chemotherapy and pain and symptom management are just two areas that could require the use of high-technology equipment and advanced nursing skills.

For both APN and the home care agency, many challenges are inherent to the APN's role. In describing administrative support issues for the acute care APN, Baird (1985) raises ideas that may be applied to the home care arena as well. Where does the APN fit into the organizational structure—if not staff or supervisor, then what? In an age of cost consciousness, can a home care agency afford to support an APN position? How will the staff receive the APN's role?

The astute home care administrator and APN may use the same strategies espoused by Baird: emphasize clinical competence, document outcomes, and publish. Clinical competence for the APN in the specialty area as the home care staff nurse may be difficult to maintain, depending on the size of the agency and its oncology population. Once again, cooperative efforts between local acute care and home care settings may benefit all concerned.

A case management model (Gibson, Martin, Johnson, Blue, & Miller, 1994) by APNs providing coordination for complex patients over the continuum of their disease course could be an effective bridge between acute care and home care practice. CNS case management has been demonstrated to be a quality cost-effective tool resulting in fewer and shorter hospitalizations for patients—an outcome likely to be mandated in health care reform.

Shegda and McCorkle (1990) also discuss four models of continuity of care to patients with chronic illnesses and note the effectiveness of maintaining caregiving throughout the course of illness even when the patient is clinically stable. Extension of care to a maintenance level or stable patient is usually not a reimbursable activity for traditional payers. However, it may become an area for further research and development for an APN in a home care agency seeking to attract additional resources, e.g., grant funding or specialized third-party payer programs.

Because the APN may be "one of a kind" in an agency, peer support and continuing education for the APN through professional organizations and colleagues will be imperative. Administrative support in resources, office space, and availability will help ease the way for development of the APN role in home care. Staff, particularly the independent, experienced home care nurse, may have some difficulty accepting the APN role. Awareness of staff perceptions and sensitivity to their needs and expertise will help the APN in the home care setting and in the inpatient area. Oncology nursing practice will continue to grow in the home care field, and the role of an APN in home care can have a dynamic, positive impact on patients, staff, agency, and the community.

LEGISLATIVE AND REGULATORY ISSUES

The major change that affected the delivery of home health services was the enactment of the Medicare legislation in 1965. Between 1965 and 1994 an increasing number of legislative acts and regulations have had a major impact on the delivery of home health services. The major issues in the 1980s and 1990s, their intent, and the impact that they have had on home care services and staff are presented in Table 74–3.

Each year the NAHC prepares and publishes the *NAHC Legislative and Regulatory Blueprints for Action*. The 1994 blueprint addressed numerous issues, including health care reform, no coinsurance, managed care safeguards, consumer freedom of choice, long-term care, plus more.

In addition to national issues, some individual state issues are of concern to home care nurses. One such issue was the pronouncement of death by nurses in Pennsylvania (Harris, 1992; Independence Blue Cross, 1994). Laws in different states vary in this area. Many states still require that a physician pronounce death.

REIMBURSEMENT

Funding for home care services is a complex and dynamic process. Some of the specific stipulations that are important for nurses to understand are summarized here. Medicare legislation was signed into law by President Lyndon B. Johnson in 1965. It provides for payment for home care services for individuals who are older than 65 years or who are disabled. Specific criteria must be met; the patient must be essentially home-bound for medical reasons; he or she must require

TABLE 74–3. *Legislative or Regulatory Issues that Affect Home Care*

ISSUE	DATE	INTENT	IMPACT
Tax Equity and Fiscal Responsibility Act (TEFRA)	1982	Mandate the prospective payment system in acute care hospitals	Patients were discharged from hospitals in the acute or early recovery phase of an illness; the need for more intensive home care services increased
Peer Review Improvement Act	1982	Review care provided to Medicare patients in acute care settings	
Section 9353 (e) of Omnibus Budget Reconciliation Act (OBRA)	1986	Extended peer review organizations' (PRO) regulations to home health agencies and skilled nursing facilities	Records that are requested by PRO must be copied and returned within specified time period
		Use generic screen to review complaints or quality issues	Increased workload for office and professional staff for review and copying charts
PL97-248 Hospice Medicare Benefit	1982	Provide expanded home health services to terminally ill patients who elect this benefit in lieu of the traditional Medicare benefit	Per diem (rather than per visit) rate for services
Budget Reconciliation Act	1986		Selected care services must be provided by staff (not contract)
			Hospice must provide interdisciplinary team management and inpatient management and must assume responsibility for care of the patient until death
Social Security Amendments, Diagnosis-Related Groups (DRGs)	1983	Provide hospital payment for specific illness groups	Discharge of more acutely ill patients following a shorter length of stay in acute care facility
Omnibus Deficit Reduction Act	1984	Authorize Secretary of Health and Human Services to deem national accrediting bodies: Community Health Accreditation Program of the National League for Nursing and Joint Commission on the Accreditation of Healthcare Organizations	Decision of these accrediting bodies would determine whether a provider meets requirements for Medicare participation (implemented by 1993 for both organizations)
Omnibus Deficit Reduction Act	1984	Reduce the number of fiscal intermediaries (FI) to 10 regional FIs	All home health agencies had to transfer to a regional FI beginning in late 1988
Balanced Budget and Emergency Deficit Act (Gramm-Rudman-Hollings)	1985	Balance the federal budget by 1991 through annual reductions in the deficit	Automatic cuts to the Medicare program of 1% in the first year and 2% in subsequent years
			Home care, as a cost reimbursed program, was reimbursed at 1% and 2% below costs
Medicare Cost Limits	1993	Control Medicare spending	Health Care Financing Administration set new cost limits, lowered the adjusted wage index factor and froze the limits for 3 years
Home and Community-Based Services for the Elderly Act	1985	Establish a block grant program to provide services similar to those demonstrated under waiver programs	Make additional service available to eligible patients
Use of standardized plan of care (POC) forms: 485-6-7-8	1985 1988 (revised)	Standardize POCs throughout the United States	Initially increased costs, increased denials, poor morale for staff and administrators
Duggan vs. Bowen 691F	1987	Class action lawsuit challenging HCFA's dismantling of the Medicare benefit	Established comprehensive coverage standard allowing providers to meet patient needs
Omnibus Budget Reconciliation Act	1987	Mandate a prospective payment demonstration project to be implemented in 1990; evaluation being compiled in 1994	Payment methods for service will include per episode, per visit, and per case basis

TABLE **74–3.** *Legislative or Regulatory Issues that Affect Home Care* Continued

ISSUE	DATE	INTENT	IMPACT
Medicare Catastrophic Protection Act	1988	Expansion of Medicare program to cover catastrophic health expenses	Extended waiver of liability; catastrophic aspect was never implemented
Omnibus Budget Reconciliation Act Section 1819 (f) and 1919 (f) of the Social Security Act	1987	Direct the secretary to establish requirements for the approval of nurse aide training and competency evaluation programs plus other related matters no later than September 1, 1988	There is more demand for the home health aide level of worker in home care than there are aides available
Revised Medicare Conditions of Participation	1989		The increased cost of meeting the increased training and continuing education requirements have a financial impact on home health agencies
Clinical Laboratory Improvement Amendments of 1988 P.L. 100-578	1988	Require every facility that tests human specimens for the purpose of providing information for diagnosis, prevention, and treatment of any disease or impairment of or the assessment of the health of a human being to meet certain federal requirements	Agencies had to apply for level-specific license or waiver and pay required fee to obtain and renew license
The Patient Self-Determination Act of 1990 P.L. 101-508	1990	Requires facilities, including home health agencies to provide written information to patient/clients regarding rights under state laws, document in the medical record whether such an instrument has been executed, and educate staff and community	All staff had to have in-service regarding requirements; printing of materials for staff to distribute

skilled, intermittent services; and the services must be ordered by a physician. The Medicare program provides for covered services described earlier in this chapter. Medicaid funding provides coverage for individuals who meet specific income levels. Medicaid reimbursement varies from state to state (i.e., cost vs. a flat fee for services).

Private insurance coverage for home care services varies with the carrier. Individuals should become aware of the options included in their individual insurance policy. Private pay service is available through some agencies. Also, service agencies may adjust fees to the individual's ability to pay. Other funding sources include the Older Americans Act (Title III and Title XX), the Veteran's Administration, Worker's Compensation, health maintenance organizations, and preferred provider organizations.

Many third-party payers have now instituted managed care or case management as part of the care process. It is important that all home care nurses be aware of (and follow) these funding source requirements. It is also important that nurses serve as advocates with the insurer for patients when additional visits are needed to meet patient goals.

QUALITY ASSESSMENT/IMPROVEMENT (QAI)

The assessment and improvement of the quality of patient care is an on-going challenge. The elusive nature of quality and the difficulty in reaching a consensus on the definitions used by various sources including the insurer, patient, physician, nurses, regulatory agencies, professional review organization, and home health agencies make it challenging to describe and evaluate quality in a consistent manner.

Although structure and process criteria are used to measure the quality of home care delivered to the patient, the emphasis on outcome measures is increasing. Accrediting bodies such as the Joint Commission on Accreditation of Healthcare Organizations, the Community Health Accreditation Program (CHAP), and the National HomeCaring Council (NHCC) stress the importance of evaluating patient outcomes and monitoring the outcomes of care provided to high-volume and high-risk cases. The Medicare Conditions of Participation (U.S. Department of Health and Human Services, 1989, 1991a, 1991b) are also patient outcome focused.

Agency, professionals, and individual standards are important to a QAI program. These include agency certification and accreditation standards (U.S. Department of Health and Human Services, 1989, 1991a, 1991b; Joint Commission on Accreditation of Healthcare Organizations, 1992; National League for Nursing, 1993) and professional standards from national organizations such as the American Nurses Association (American Nurses Association, 1986a, 1986b), national and state trade organizations (National Association for Home Care, 1986; Pennsylvania Association of Home Health Agencies, 1986), and individual licensure and certification (Fickerssen, 1985) (Tables 74–4

TABLE 74–4. Organizational Standards

STANDARD	CREDENTIAL
Community Health Accreditation Program (CHAP) of the National League for Nursing	Accreditation
Joint Commission on the Accreditation of Healthcare Organizations (JCAHO)	Accreditation
National HomeCaring Council (NHCC) Foundation for Hospice & Home Care (home care aide agencies)	Accreditation
Medicare Conditions of Participation (COP) for home health agencies	Certification
Medicare COP for hospice	Certification
State licensure laws	Licensure

TABLE 74–5. Professional Standards

ORGANIZATION	CREDENTIAL
American Nurses' Credentialing Center	Certification
Individual states	Certification Licensure
Professional associations (Fickerssen, 1985)	Certification

and 74–5). Administration and staff must be committed to the QAI program, which includes a commitment of time, money, and personnel to monitor progress toward established goals on an ongoing basis.

A report published by Arthur Anderson and Company and the American College of Health Care Executives (1987, p. 21) included some findings that must be considered when discussing quality. Seventy-three per cent of the respondents agree that providers in 1995 will sacrifice quality of care for financial viability. Seventy-two per cent believe that future capitation systems will sacrifice quality of care for financial viability.

In light of these projections, the quality issue and the agency's QAI program must receive high priority in the 1990s. The evaluation of quality must include both clinical and financial data related to patient care and patient outcomes. This is especially important because the Omnibus Budget Reconciliation Act (OBRA) of 1987 mandated that a prospective payment demonstration project be implemented for home care services in mid-1988. As of 1994 the demonstration project is being evaluated (Remington, 1994).

Tongues (1985) stated that in a cost-containment atmosphere, providers must either lower their standards or find ways to provide quality care more economically. The challenge in the 1990s continues to be to provide quality care in a more economical manner, not to lower our standards of care.

REFERENCES

American Nurses Association. (1978). *Health care at home: An essential component of a national health policy* (p. 6). Kansas City, MO; Author.

American Nurses Association. (1986a). *Standards—community health nursing practice*. Kansas City, MO: Author.

American Nurses Association. (1986b). *Standards—home health nursing practice*. Kansas City, MO: Author.

American Nurses Association. (1991). *Nursing's agenda for health care reform* (pp. 1–24). Kansas City, MO: Author.

Arthur Anderson & Company & The American College of Health Care Executives. (1987). *The future of healthcare, changes and choices*. American College of Health Care Executives.

Baird, S. B. (1985). Administration support issues and the oncology clinical nurse specialist. *Oncology Nursing Forum, 12*(2), 51–54.

Boyle, A. M., Engelking, C., & Harvey, C. (1994). Taking command of the future: Getting ready NOW for the 21st century. *Oncology Nursing Forum, 21*(1), 77–79.

Della Monica, E. (1994). Home health care documentation and record keeping. In M. Harris (Ed.), *Handbook of home health care administration* (pp. 117–142). Gaithersburg, MD: Aspen Publishers.

Dittbrenner H. (1994, June). Ensuring survival: Expansion into nontraditional services. *Caring, 13*(6), 54–58.

Engelking, C. (1994). New approaches: Innovations in cancer prevention, diagnosis, treatment, and support. *Oncology Nursing Forum, 21*(1), 62–71.

Fickerssen, J. L. (1985). Getting certified. *American Journal of Nursing, 85*, 265–269.

Gibson, S. J., Martin, S. M., Johnson, M. B., Blue, R., & Miller, D.S. (1994) CNS-directed case management: Cost and quality in harmony. *Journal of Nursing Administration, 24*(6), 45–51.

Harris, M. (1992). Death pronouncement by registered nurses. *Home Healthcare Nurse, 10*(2), 57–59.

Harris, M. (Ed.). (1994a). *Handbook of home health care administration*. Gaithersburg, MD: Aspen Publishers.

Harris, M. (1994b). Medicare update. Medicare and the nurse. *Home Healthcare Nurse, 12*(2), 47–50.

Harris, M., Peters, D., Parente, C., & Smith, J. (1986). *Cost of home care by nursing diagnoses*. Paper presented at the Second National Nursing Symposium on Home Health Care. University of Michigan School of Nursing, Ann Arbor.

Harvey, C. (1994). New systems: the restructuring of cancer care delivery and economics. *Oncology Nursing Forum, 21*(1), 72–77.

Independence Blue Cross. (1994, March 31). Medicare provider bulletin. *Home Health Agency Bulletin, 94*–14.

Joint Commission of Accreditation of Healthcare Organizations. (1992). *1993 accreditation manual for home care* (Vols. 1 & 2). Oakbrook Terrace, IL: Author.

McCorkle, R., Benoliel, J.Q., Donaldson, G., Georgiadou, F., Moinpour, C., & Goodell, B. (1989). A randomized clinical trial of home nursing care for lung cancer patients. *Cancer, 64*(6), 1375–1382.

McCorkle, R., & Germino, B. (1984). What nurses need to know about home care. *Oncology Nursing Forum, 11*, 63–69.

National Association for Home Care. (1986, August). *Code of ethics*. Washington, DC: Author.

National Association for Home Care. (1993). *How to choose a home care agency*. Washington, DC: Author

National League for Nursing. (1993). *Standards of excellence for home care organizations*. New York: Author.

Oncology Nursing Society Clinical Practice Committee. (1990). *Standards of advanced practice*. Pittsburgh, PA: Author.

Pennsylvania Association of Home Health Agencies. (1986). *Home health service provider standards*. Harrisburg, PA: Author.

Pennsylvania Department of Health. (1992). *Division of primary care and home health licensing survey*. Harrisburg, PA: Author.

Remington, L. (1994). Feature interview—Henry Goldberg. *The Remington Report, 10,* 35–40.

Shegda, L. M., & McCorkle, R. (1990). Continuing care in the community. *Journal of Pain and Symptom Management, 5*(5), 279–286.

Staffing Industry Analysts, Inc. (1994). *Home Health Business Report, 1*(1), 11.

Tongues, M. (1985). Quality with economy. Doing the right thing for less. *Nursing Economics, 3,* 205–211.

U.S. Department of Health and Human Services. Health care financing administration, Part II. 42 CFR Part 484. Medicare program: Home health agencies: Conditions of participation and reduction in recordkeeping requirements: Interim final rule. *Federal Register,* 54:155; Monday August 14, 1989.

42 CFR Part 494. Medicare program: Home health agencies: Conditions of participation. *Federal Register,* 56:138; Thursday July 18, 1991a.

42 CFR Parts 409, 418, 484. Medicare program: Medicare coverage of home health services, Medicare conditions of participation and home health aide supervision. *Federal Register,* 56:188, Friday September 27, 1991b.

Visiting Nurse Association of Eastern Montgomery County. (1993a). *Position description: Nurse practitioner.* Abington, PA: Author.

Visiting Nurse Association of Eastern Montgomery County. (1993b). *Visit statistics by diagnosis.* Abington, PA: Author.

Weisslein, S. (1984). Home care today. *American Journal of Nursing, 94,* 341–345.

Whedon, M., Shedd, P., and Summers, B. (1992). The role of the advanced practice oncology nurse in pain relief. *Oncology Nursing Forum, 19*(7) (Suppl.) 12–19.

Yuan, J. (1994). Staff development in a home health agency. In M. Harris (Ed.), *Handbook of home health care administration* (pp. 401–410). Gaithersburg, MD: Aspen Publishers.

Rehabilitation Services

Pamela G. Watson

Comprehensive cancer care should include a rehabilitation component that *begins with diagnosis, accompanies definitive cancer treatment, extends through the posttreatment recuperative phase, and prepares the individual for survivorship.* Recognition of the need to link rehabilitation with cancer care can be traced to the work of selected oncology physicians who observed the presence of significant cancer-related disabilities in many individuals who were treated for cancer (Dietz, 1981; Rusk, 1984). These physicians joined with specialists in rehabilitation medicine, known as physiatrists, to establish model cancer rehabilitation systems (Kudsk & Hoffmann, 1987; McLaughlin 1984). At the same time, survey studies revealed a widespread gap between disabilities that developed in individuals with cancer and rehabilitation services provided. As shown in Table 75–1, more than 50 per cent of the cancer patients in one study were found to have a range of moderate to severe physical disabilities. However, many of the patients did not receive appropriate rehabilitation services because of a lack of referrals (Lehmann et al., 1978). The problem of referrals was also pointed out in a study by Harvey, Jellinek, and Habeck (1982) that revealed cancer patients' access to rehabilitation services is dependent on the awareness of need for services by health care providers (Table 75–1). Thereafter, a few model cancer rehabilitation programs began to appear, but such programs have never been available to the extent needed (Hickey, 1986; McLaughlin, 1984). Even the state and federal vocational rehabilitation system has yet to adequately reach out to the potential pool of clients with cancer-related disabilities who would benefit from services (Conti, 1990; Taylor, 1984). In contrast to the lack of action with regard to cancer rehabilitation, research findings have continued to reveal that cancer patients

have marked rehabilitation needs and that those who are exposed to rehabilitation interventions benefit from them. Several studies, summarized in Table 75–1, have shown cancer patients often require episodic or long-term assistance with selected aspects of physical functioning, self-care, and activities of daily living (Mor, Guadagnoli, & Wool, 1987; Mor et al., 1992; Guadagnoli & Mor, 1991). Similarly, the presence of cancer-related symptoms, treatment side effects, and concomitant conditions has been found to magnify the rehabilitation needs of cancer patients (Kurtz, Kurtz, Given, & Given, 1993; Vinokur, Threatt, Caplan, & Zimmerman, 1989). Rehabilitation interventions shown to be helpful for cancer patients (Table 75–1) have included aerobic exercises, moderate walking programs, health-promoting lifestyles programs, and psychosocial support (Johnson & Kelly, 1990; Mock et al., 1994; Winningham, MacVicar, Bondoc, Anderson, & Minton, 1989; Young-McCaughan, & Sexton, 1991).

Although barriers to cancer rehabilitation have been identified (Mayer, 1992), lack of more widespread enthusiasm for the concept can be attributed to a dearth of understanding about what rehabilitation actually means. Rehabilitation is as much a way of thinking as it is a set of services or interventions. This chapter *identifies fundamental principles of rehabilitation as a basis for understanding cancer rehabilitation, provides a core definition for cancer rehabilitation, and presents a framework for combining rehabilitation and cancer care.* The core components of the rehabilitation process are discussed, namely the measurement of functional abilities, the development of a rehabilitation program plan, and delivery of rehabilitation services by an interdisciplinary team, measurement of outcomes, and establishment of follow-up activities. Since this chapter is intended to furnish a rehabilitation perspective for *all*

TABLE 75–1. *Studies on Rehabilitation and Cancer Care*

REFERENCE	PURPOSE	SAMPLE	PERTINENT FINDINGS
Lehmann et al., 1978	To determine the type and frequency of physical disabilities and psychosocial problems that occur in cancer patients	805 randomly selected cancer patients from four general hospitals	More than 50% of the patients in the study sample had cancer-related disabilities including paralysis, paresis, intellectual or perceptual deficits, communication impairments, contractures, pressure sores, ambulation or transfer difficulties, self-care deficits, fractures, and lymph edema. More than half the patients with physical disabilities also had psychologic problems. Many of the patients did not receive appropriate rehabilitation interventions for the cancer-related disabilities they developed. Gaps in rehabilitation services were found to be due to a lack of referral for services.
Harvey, Jellinek, & Habeck, 1982	To identify rehabilitation services provided to cancer patients	Convenience sample of 36 institutions with known cancer rehabilitation facilities	In addition to physical therapy, most rehabilitation programs identified patient education as the key feature of their programs; family involvement was encouraged by the majority of the programs; rehabilitation protocols were established for particular cancer sites; pain control methods were used by about 50% of the programs. The most common methods of initiating patient contact for rehabilitation services were consultations and referrals.
Mor, Guadagnoli, & Wool, 1987	To determine specific rehabilitation service needs of patients diagnosed with cancer	A random sample of 217 patients drawn from lists of patients currently receiving either psychosocial support or financial services since 1984	The majority of cancer patients surveyed needed assistance in at least one activity of daily living and one area of physical functioning; about half needed help with walking and with various aspects of self-care; all needed some assistance with housekeeping tasks; more than 90% indicated a need for one or more community resource.
Winningham et al., 1989	To determine the effect of aerobic exercise on the body weight and composition of women undergoing chemotherapy for breast cancer	A convenience sample of 24 stage II women with breast cancer receiving adjuvant chemotherapy	Aerobic exercise may have potential as an intervention for stabilizing body weight and decreasing body fat deposits in individuals with cancer.
Vinokur et al., 1989	To examine the long-term effects of breast cancer on physical functioning and social psychologic well-being.	Sample of 10,056 women from the state of Michigan who entered a breast cancer screening program who were screened annually between 1974–1981.	Younger patients with more *recent* disease are at greater risk of poor mental health, whereas older patients with more *advanced* disease are at greater risk of physical health problems than either of their age counterparts with less recent and less advanced disease.
Johnson & Kelly, 1990	The purpose of this study is to promote rehabilitation following treatment for cancer by encouraging women to adopt a long-term lifestyle emphasizing wellness and a sense of control over changes	A convenience sample of 12 women with breast cancer who completed a wilderness program designed to enhance the wellness process through invigorating physical activity	Women who completed the rehabilitation program expressed a sense of competence, invigoration, determination, courage, and willingness to take risks.

Continued on following page.

TABLE **75–1.** *Studies on Rehabilitation and Cancer Care* Continued

REFERENCE	PURPOSE	SAMPLE	PERTINENT FINDINGS
Young-McCaughan & Sexton, 1991	To determine whether women with breast cancer who experience a higher quality of life as compared with similar women who do not exercise	A convenience sample of 71 women from two institutions irrespective of disease stage, type of treatment, or phase of treatment	Women who exercised had a significantly higher quality of life than those who did not exercise.
Mor et al., 1992	To investigate the daily living needs of 629 patients with advanced cancer and to calculate the point prevalence of need and unmet need for assistance with personal care, instrumental activities, transportation, and home health tasks	629 patients with cancer in three northeast locations (central Pennsylvania, Rhode Island, and New York)	The need for assistance with personal care activities was minimal at the beginning of chemotherapy and radiation therapy but increased substantially at follow-up; the prevalence of new needs for personal care grew as cancer advanced. A high proportion of the patients with needs for assistance with self-care or activities of daily living did not receive enough assistance to meet their needs.
Kurtz et al., 1993	To further investigate symptoms and loss of physical functioning over time in cancer patients	A convenience sample of 279 patients with cancer from six community-based cancer treatment centers located in lower Michigan	The most frequently occurring symptoms were fatigue, pain, insomnia, nausea, and poor appetite. Coexisting medical conditions most frequently identified were arthritis, hypertension, heart disease, gastrointestinal problems, and emphysema. Over time, age was significantly correlated with loss of physical functioning but not with the presence of symptoms. However, symptoms present and loss of physical functioning were significantly correlated.
Mock et al., 1994	To examine the effects of a comprehensive rehabilitation program to facilitate physical and psychosocial adaptation of women with breast cancer	A convenience sample of 14 women being evaluated for postsurgical adjuvant chemotherapy protocols from medical centers in the northeast	Breast cancer patients receiving adjuvant cytotoxic chemotherapy can acquire physical and psychosocial benefits from a modest walking exercise program and support group participation. Benefits derived included favorable levels of physical functioning, psychosocial adjustment, and lowered levels of distressful symptoms.

individuals with cancer, it does not contain information regarding specific cancer site rehabilitation issues. For such information, the reader is referred to the chapters in Unit VI.

CANCER REHABILITATION PHILOSOPHY AND PRINCIPLES

To explain cancer rehabilitation, it is necessary to consider the concepts of *impairment, disability,* and *handicap* as defined by the World Health Organization (1980). *Impairment* pertains to the organ level, anatomic, and physiologic deficits caused by disease or injury. *Disability* derives from the impairment and embodies restrictions in the ability to function optimally. *Handicap* is a societal concept that represents the extent to which a disability interferes with the ability to be a fully functioning member of society. Accordingly, reha-

bilitation aims to prevent the extent to which a *disability,* produced by an impairment, becomes a *handicap.*

A disability is a state of being or a condition that can be objectively measured by physical examination or functional assessment. A disability may be physical or psychologic, temporary or permanent, minor to severe, relatively static, or characterized by declining functional abilities. From a rehabilitation standpoint, disabilities produced by cancer, or its treatment, are often complex. The nature of the disease is such that the individual with cancer may be frail and may require management of symptoms not usually part of the rehabilitation process with other disabilities. Often cancer prognoses are guarded, and for the individual with cancer the threat of recurrence is always present (Gamble, Brown, Kinney, & Mahoney, 1990).

Rehabilitation is appropriately linked with cancer care as a parallel process. Although cancer treatment

TABLE 75-2. *Principles of Rehabilitation*

1. Every individual needs hope, encouragement, and the opportunity to learn to function at the highest level possible. The presence of disease and disability, no matter how severe, does not alter these fundamental rights.
2. The process of rehabilitation begins with the diagnosis of illness or the onset of disability; it is an ongoing process that does not end until the individual dies.
3. The severity of a disability can be increased or diminished by conditions that exist in the person's environment.
4. The healthy physical and mental attributes of an individual should be the basis of each rehabilitation effort.
5. Consumers of rehabilitation should participate as fully as possible in all aspects of the rehabilitation process from planning through the provision of services and evaluation of outcomes.
6. Because each individual with a disability has unique characteristics, variability and flexibility are required for all rehabilitation programs.
7. Predictions of rehabilitation gains based on group outcome data should be applied with caution to individual cases.
8. Interdisciplinary and interagency collaboration and coordination of services are essential elements of the rehabilitation process.
9. Self-help organizations and coalitions are important allies in the rehabilitation effort.
10. Consumers of rehabilitation should have the opportunity to evaluate the rehabilitation services they receive.

(Data from Wright, B. (1983). Principles of rehabilitation. In *Physical disability—A psychosocial approach,* [2nd. ed.]. New York: Harper & Row.)

targets the arrest or elimination of the disease, rehabilitation focuses on physical and psychosocial well-being. Rehabilitation has been characterized as an education and training process aimed at enabling patients to become as independent as possible in self-care and the resumption of customary life activities (Anderson, 1975). The practice of rehabilitation is guided by a set of well-established principles, examples of which appear in Table 75-2 (Wright, 1983). These principles are intended to make explicit certain fundamental beliefs about disability situations and the needs and rights of individuals with disabilities. When applied to the person with cancer, rehabilitation principles have the potential to facilitate the achievement of improved quality of life, maximum productivity, and minimum dependency regardless of life expectancy (Dietz, 1981).

A GENERIC DEFINITION FOR CANCER REHABILITATION

Varying definitions for the term *cancer rehabilitation* have been suggested (Gunn, 1984; Kurtzman, Gardner, & Kellner, 1988; Rusk, 1984). Common to most definitions is the notion that cancer diagnosis and prognosis are not focal points in rehabilitation. Instead, cancer rehabilitation is based on the fundamental rehabilitation principle that every person who is treated for

cancer has the potential to function at a level that is individually optimal.

The Oncology Nursing Society (ONS) has offered a succinct cancer rehabilitation definition that includes the fundamental concepts noted above and has broad applicability in cancer care: "Cancer rehabilitation is a process by which individuals within their environments are assisted to achieve *optimal functioning* within the limits imposed by cancer" (Mayer & O'Connor, 1989, p. 433; Mayer & O'Connor-Kelleher, 1993).

The ONS definition captures the essence of the rehabilitation process and is broad enough to be relevant for individuals of all ages with all types of cancer (Watson, 1990). The definition connotes *optimal functioning* as the central target of cancer rehabilitation efforts. Optimal functioning is a concept rooted in each individual's unique situation; it can be characterized as one's highest level of physical, cognitive, and psychosocial well-being. For the individual with cancer, the core elements that comprise *optimal functioning* may be summarized as follows:

- Achievement of personal goals
- Increased or sustained functional abilities
- Improved physical conditioning
- Adequate nutrition
- Satisfactory psychosocial adjustment
- Appropriate health promotion and health protection
- Effective management of symptoms

Preillness level of functioning, existing functional abilities, cancer status, productivity aspirations, and social support are factors that determine what is actually *optimal functioning* for an individual with cancer.

FRAMEWORK FOR COMBINING REHABILITATION AND CANCER CARE

As depicted in Figure 75-1, rehabilitation and cancer care can be joined together by an organizing framework that consists of rehabilitative cancer care with two additive rehabilitation pathways to optimal functioning.

REHABILITATIVE CANCER CARE

As noted earlier, cancer care becomes *rehabilitative* when a rehabilitation component is added at the time of diagnosis. This incremental part of cancer care begins with functional assessment.

Functional assessment constitutes the first step in the rehabilitation process. The term refers to the measurement of functional status or functional abilities. Stewart, Ware, and Brook (1981) have pointed out that functional status is an individual's ability to perform a spectrum of activities considered normal for healthy people. These activities fall in the categories of *self-care activities* (eating, bathing, dressing, using a bathroom); *mobility* (getting around indoors, outdoors, and in the community); *physical activities* (walking, using stairs, lifting, bending, running); *societal role activities* (em-

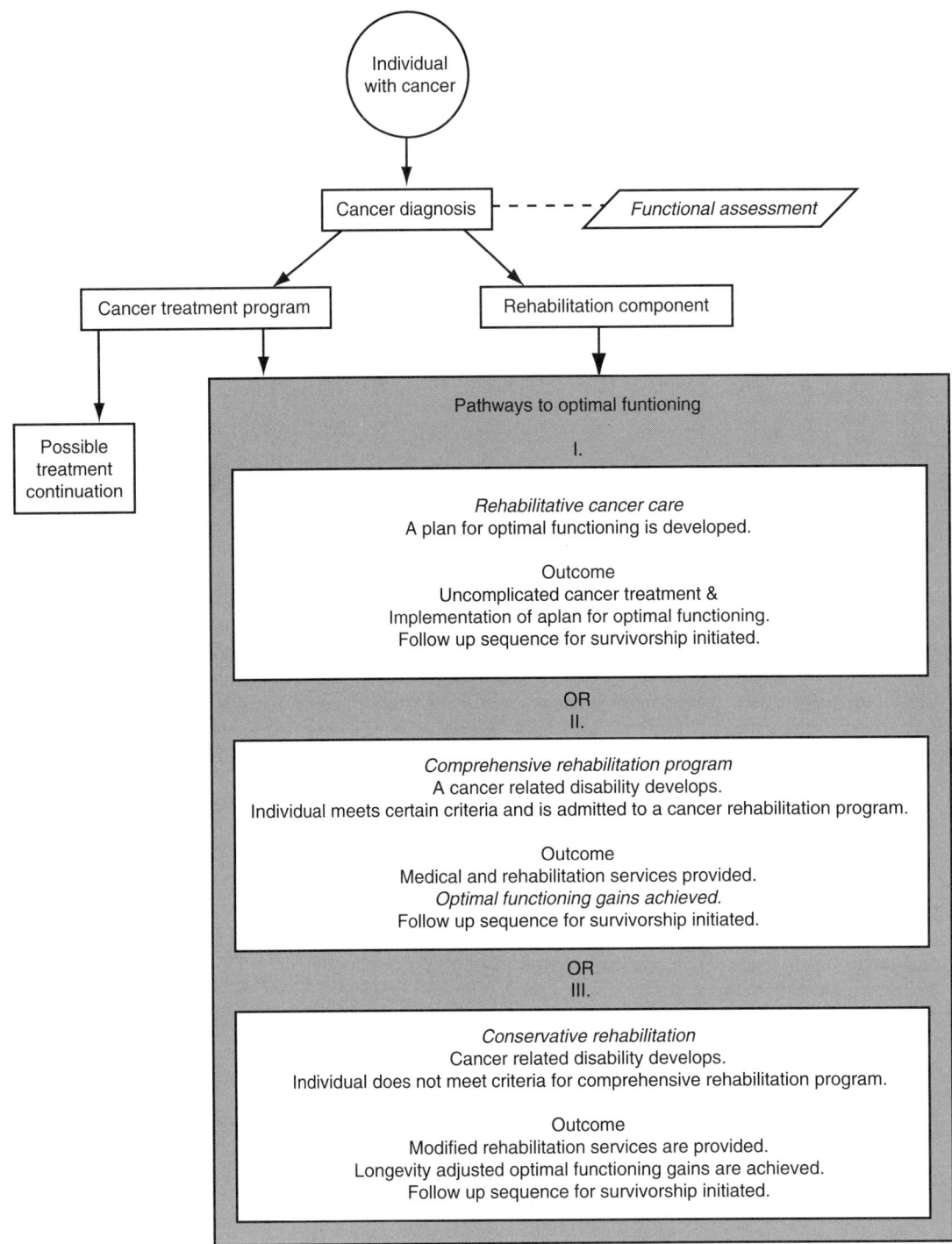

FIGURE 75–1. Combining rehabilitation and cancer care.

ployment, school or household activities); *leisure activities* (hobbies, sports, social activities) (Stewart et al., 1981). Functional assessment instruments are available for all age groups and for varying disability populations (Applegate, Blass, & Williams, 1990; Brown, Gordon, & Diller, 1983; Katz, 1983; Spitzer, 1987). Reviews of many such instruments are found in the rehabilitation and primary care literature (Fleming, 1991).

Over the last decade, the importance of functional assessment in relation to cancer care has increased.

There has been a growing recognition that functional status should be measured at the outset of the cancer experience. For rehabilitative cancer care, functional status provides an objective assessment of the individual's physical and psychosocial strengths, apart from the cancer diagnosis. Because most generic functional assessment instruments do not adequately measure functional status in cancer patients, instruments designed specifically for cancer patients have now been developed (Moinpour, McCorkle, & Saunders, 1988).

The reader is urged to refer to Chapter 6 for a thorough discussion of functional status measurement in cancer patients.

PLAN FOR OPTIMAL FUNCTIONING

Functional assessment data should provide the basis for creating a plan for optimal functioning (POF). In the context of rehabilitative cancer care, a POF is actually a formula for meeting the initial rehabilitation needs of the individual undergoing cancer treatment. To be congruent with rehabilitation principles, shown in Table 75-2, the POF should reflect the viewpoint and personal goals of the individual for whom it is developed. The POF is based on a set of generic goals that are aimed at optimal functioning and the ability of the individual to reach and maintain the best possible health and functional status before, during, and after cancer treatment (Watson, 1992a). To be complete, a POF should address the following optimal functioning goals.

Best Degree of Physical Fitness Possible. The therapeutic value of exercise for individuals with cancer has been documented in several studies (MacVicar & Winningham, 1986; MacVicar, Winningham, & Nickel, 1989). Guidelines for appropriate exercises are now available (American College of Sports Medicine, 1991; Skinner, 1987; Winningham, 1990, 1991). A program of exercise is an integral component of rehabilitative cancer care. When feasible, individuals with cancer should also be encouraged to participate in muscle strengthening and joint flexibility programs. Depending on the cancer situation, some individuals may also require physical therapy and occupational therapy services to achieve optimal levels of mobility (McGarvey, 1990).

Promoting the best degree of physical fitness also means that the individual with cancer must be ready for the transition from patient to cancer survivor. This requires attention to possible long-term residual effects of the disease and its treatment. The reader is referred to Chapter 76 for information on survivorship issues.

Highest Level of Nutrition Attainable. The need for attention to the nutritional challenges that confront many cancer patients is well recognized. The subject is discussed in Chapter 51. Here it is important to note that *food and eating* should be incorporated in the POF in a positive manner. A nutritional enhancement program should be presented to the patient as armament for the course of cancer treatment and for healthy life afterward as a cancer survivor (Watson, 1992b).

Optimistic Outlook. Chapter 60 describes the psychologic responses to cancer that bring about a need for psychosocial support in all individuals with cancer. This dimension of cancer care must be made explicit in the POF and continue throughout all phases of the cancer experience (Watson, 1992b). The goals of psychosocial intervention include acceptance of the cancer diagnosis, participation in decision making, and maintenance of a personal sense of control (Gamble, Brown, & Mahoney, 1990). In addition, psychosocial support that promotes an optimistic outlook should include preparation for survivorship as discussed in Chapter 76. Psychosocial support may encompass episodic therapeutic communication with an oncology nurse, visits from a cancer survivor, support group participation, short-term one-to-one counseling, or psychotherapy. Pharmacologic measures and behavioral approaches such as relaxation, biofeedback, and hypnosis may also be used (DeVita, Hellman, & Rosenberg, 1989).

Independence in Self-Care and Activities of Daily Living. From a rehabilitation standpoint, self-care and activities of daily living are two distinct concepts of critical importance in the life of an individual with a disability. Basically self-care refers to the ability to bathe, dress, and take care of oneself on a daily basis. The term generally also refers to active involvement in the promotion of one's health and the prevention of disease (Dodd, 1988). Self-care is discussed in Chapter 5. Activities of daily living (ADL) are a more global concept that connotes the spectrum of activities that constitute an individual's customary way of life. The POF should include strategies for ensuring that the individual will be independent in self-care and prepared to carry out ADL that are part of personal goals for survivorship. For many individuals, ADL include employment. Increasing numbers of cancer patients are returning to the work force or continuing to perform job responsibilities while being treated for cancer (Brown & Tai-Seale, 1992). Therefore, the POF should include attention to vocational issues, particularly protected employment rights, of individuals with cancer under the Americans With Disabilities Act (P.L. 101-336).

Effective Side Effect and Symptom Management. For the individual with cancer, optimal functioning cannot occur in the absence of effective symptom and side effect management. Therefore, symptom side effect management should be incorporated in the POF, and conveyed to the patient, as another component of the rehabilitation dimension of cancer care. Frequently, pain is the most troublesome symptom with which the cancer patient must contend. Because pain interferes with almost every aspect of one's life, it is particularly problematic from a rehabilitation standpoint (Williams & Maly, 1994). The assessment and management of pain is thoroughly discussed in Chapters 55 through 58. Many of the other chapters in Unit VIII also contain important information regarding other aspects of appropriate symptom and side effect management. Preparation for survivorship management of late onset symptoms and residual side effects should also be part of the POF.

LIMITS OF REHABILITATIVE CANCER CARE

For many individuals with cancer, *rehabilitative cancer care*, with a POF is sufficient to produce the desired outcome of a return to preillness levels of functioning (Watson, 1990). In Figure 75-1, it can be seen that such individuals are able to move directly to a follow-up sequence. However, as noted at the outset of this chapter, a sizable number of individuals who undergo cancer treatment develop cancer-related disabilities (Harvey et al., 1982; Lehmann et al., 1978).

For these cancer patients, rehabilitative cancer care is not enough to produce optimal functioning. These individuals are candidates for comprehensive or conservative rehabilitation programs.

COMPREHENSIVE CANCER REHABILITATION

Comprehensive cancer rehabilitation programs consist of coordinated and integrated medical and rehabilitation services provided by an interdisciplinary team. Designated as medical rehabilitation programs (Commission on the Accreditation of Rehabilitation Facilities [CARF], 1994), these programs are designed to produce optimal functioning in individuals who have significant functional limitations caused by cancer. Examples of disabilities in cancer patients that may be indicative of the need for a comprehensive inpatient cancer rehabilitation program include the following:

- Generalized musculoskeletal deconditioning
- Self-care limitations
- ADL deficits
- Paralysis or loss of sensation and balance
- Mechanical eating problems
- Bowel or bladder dysfunction
- Communication disorders
- Uncontrolled pain

Comprehensive cancer rehabilitation programs are becoming available on selected rehabilitation units in tertiary care settings and in freestanding rehabilitation hospitals. These programs are usually accredited by the Commission on the Accreditation of Rehabilitation Facilities (CARF). Cancer patients enter rehabilitation programs through a referral process that requires an initial assessment of eligibility. To be admitted to a comprehensive program, the individual with a cancer-related disability must meet the criteria listed below. These criteria are fairly standard and are largely dictated by accreditation standards and third-party payers who cover the costs of the rehabilitation services provided.

- Capable of achieving rehabilitation gains
- Expected to live more than 6 months
- Medically stable (patients undergoing radiation, chemotherapy, or total parenteral nutrition are usually considered on an individual basis)
- Not severely debilitated
- Evidence of declining abilities is readily apparent
- Significant functional improvement can be expected in a timely manner; usually 2 to 3 weeks
- Able to participate in 3 hours of therapy 5 days per week
- Active and sustained caregiver support is present
- Post discharge plans are in place

Once an individual becomes part of a comprehensive program, an extensive assessment and individualized rehabilitation process begins. A coordinated interdisciplinary team, of which the patient is a member, is the major decision-making body for the entire rehabilitation program.

INTERDISCIPLINARY TEAM

An interdisciplinary team has been the hallmark of the rehabilitation effort. Use of the team approach is based on the belief that individuals with disabilities have multiple needs that require the coordinated input of a variety of disciplines. The team is considered the key to successful rehabilitation. Still, to be effective, the team must share a common philosophic approach to cancer rehabilitation, meet on a regular basis, document the results of its meetings, and be receptive to the ongoing evaluation of its programs. In the absence of a coordinated team, rehabilitation services are apt to be provided by individual therapists in an uncoordinated manner and without a guiding set of rehabilitation goals.

The person with cancer, and his or her designees, are members of the rehabilitation team. Interdisciplinary membership on the team is based on the professional expertise needed to develop and carry out each individual's cancer rehabilitation plan. Most teams include the following core members who provide services to every patient: patient care coordinator or case manager, oncology advanced practice nurse specialist, oncology physician, physiatrist, rehabilitation clinical nurse specialist, staff nurse, psychologist, nutritionist, social worker, and pastoral counselor. The other team members provide services in accordance with individual needs identified in the diagnostic assessment: physical therapist, occupational therapist, respiratory therapist, speech or language pathologist, audiologist, and vocational rehabilitation counselor.

DIAGNOSTIC ASSESSMENT

The comprehensive rehabilitation process begins with an extensive intake assessment that builds on the preadmission assessment. Customarily, the diagnostic assessment is coordinated by the patient care coordinator or case manager, who conducts the overall assessment and then requests assessments by other members of the team in accordance with the needs of the person being served.

Functional Assessment. Functional status measurement is the core component of the diagnostic assessment (Granger & Gresham, 1984). Functional assessment findings are used to develop the individualized rehabilitation plan, select rehabilitation services, monitor response to therapies, modify rehabilitation plans, and evaluate the achievement of rehabilitation goals (Halpern & Fuhrer, 1984). For this reason, the functional assessment instrument used should yield comprehensive baseline data that will be useful in predicting rehabilitation outcome. The instrument should be sensitive to changes in status and appropriate for use over time.

Functional Independence Measure. For individuals in comprehensive cancer rehabilitation programs, it is worthwhile to consider using the functional independence measure (FIM) for functional assessment (O'Toole & Golden, 1991). The FIM measures self-care, mobility, ambulation, bowel and bladder dysfunction, cognition, social interaction, and emotions. The FIM yields an estimate of burden of care and measures progress in rehabilitation. The score produced ranges from 18 (total assistance required) to 126 (maximally independent). Currently, the FIM is used by a number of facilities that offer definitive cancer rehabilitation programs.[1] Fucile (1992) has observed that the FIM is an appropriate functional assessment instrument for individuals with cancer-related disabilities. However, she also pointed out that the FIM does not measure pain, which means that a separate pain assessment is necessary.

The FIM was developed for the Uniform Data System (UDS) (Granger & Hamilton, 1994). Sponsored by the American Congress of Rehabilitation Medicine and the American Academy of Physical Medicine and Rehabilitation, the UDS was created to meet a long-term need to document severity of disability and rehabilitation outcome (Hamilton, Granger, & Sherwin, 1987). In turn, the FIM was developed to be a valid, clinically relevant instrument applicable to various populations of individuals with disabilities (Linacre, Heinemann, Wright, Granger, & Hamilton, 1994). Use of the FIM with individuals with cancer is recommended because to date there is a paucity of aggregate data on disability severity and rehabilitation outcomes for cancer patients. The FIM allows cancer rehabilitation data to become part of the UDS, thus bringing individuals with cancer-related disabilities into the mainstream of rehabilitation.

Other Assessment Areas. An integral part of the diagnostic assessment is the identification of the individual's personal goals and aspirations, including expectations and desired outcomes for the rehabilitation process. Initial estimates of overall strengths, limitations, and preferences are made by the patient care coordinator or case manager. To provide for continuity of care, oncology, medical, and nursing referral data are analyzed and incorporated into the assessment. All data are then used for the development of the individualized rehabilitation plan.

INDIVIDUALIZED REHABILITATION PLAN

The individualized rehabilitation plan (IRP) is the blueprint for the effective delivery of rehabilitation services. Careful planning and coordination is required for the development and implementation of the IRP. According to standards established by CARF, an IRP should include two components: (1) an overall plan that addresses the personal goals and outcome expectations of the patient, as well as the outcomes expected by the interdisciplinary team, and (2) a plan for each rehabilitation service that specifies the need for the service, identifies goals and objectives, provides an anticipated time frame for goal accomplishment, and notes

outcomes measured (CARF, 1994). As noted earlier, the interdisciplinary team, of which the patient is a member, is the decision-making body for the development, implementation, and ongoing modification of the IRP. To achieve optimal functioning, patients with cancer-related disabilities usually require a spectrum of rehabilitation services beyond those provided by core team members. For example, Table 75–3 shows typical indications for physical therapy and occupational therapy services. The functional limitations shown in Table 75–3 are common rehabilitation problems for many cancer patients. These limitations may indicate the need for a number of cancer rehabilitation services.

To illustrate, using optimal functioning as the outcome, a sampling of possible rehabilitation services, appears in Table 75–4.

Once developed, the IRP is communicated to all members of the team and the patient in an understandable manner. Overall responsibility for implementation of the IRP is assumed by the patient care coordinator or case manager. On successful implementation of the IRP, optimal functioning gains can be expected, and the individual progresses to the follow-up sequence.

CONSERVATIVE REHABILITATION

The second additional pathway to optimal functioning, shown in Figure 75–1, pertains to individuals with cancer-related disabilities who cannot meet eligibility criteria for *comprehensive cancer rehabilitation*. Efforts are now being directed toward measures that enable patients with advanced or metastatic disease to continue to function as optimally as possible (Mellette & Parker, 1992). These are the frail cancer patients with guarded prognoses, who none the less, are candidates for modest rehabilitation efforts.

Conservative rehabilitation programs derive from the same concepts that are fundamental to rehabilitative cancer care and comprehensive cancer rehabilitation programs. Today, conservative rehabilitation programs are becoming available under the heading of *subacute rehabilitation* (Salcido & Jenkins, 1994). Subacute rehabilitation programs offer less intense specialized rehabilitation services that can help to strengthen or stabilize cancer patients to the point where *longevity adjusted optimal functioning gains can be achieved.* CARF mandates the use of an interdisciplinary team and IRPs for all patients in subacute programs. A minimum of 1 to 3 hours of rehabilitation services 5 days per week are provided to patients. Even for the most difficult, guarded cancer situations, conservative ongoing rehabilitation is warranted to maintain optimal functioning as rehabilitation services give way to supportive care services (Chapter 77) or hospice care services (Chapter 78).

MEASUREMENT OF OUTCOMES

Typically, rehabilitation outcomes for disabilities caused by disease are measured in terms of medical morbidity, mortality, length of hospitalization, cost, functional ability, and placement after discharge (Cifu

---

[1]Good Samaritan Hospital and Medical Center Comprehensive Cancer Program, Portland, OR 97210.
Harmerville Rehabilitation Center, Pittsburgh, PA 15240.
New England Rehabilitation Hospital, Woburn, MA 01801.
The FIM, a Guide for Its Use and an IBM-compatible disk for inputting data can be obtained from the UDS Data Management Service, 82 Farber Hall, State University of New York, Main Street, Buffalo, NY 14214. (716) 829-2076.

TABLE 75–3. *Examples of Functional Problems in Cancer Patients that Indicate a Need for Physical Therapy or Occupational Therapy Services*

Physical Therapy
Head and Neck Problems:
  Musculoskeletal deficits, and loss of function related to surgical severance of nerves; decreased head and cervical range of motion due to pain; poor posture and ligamentous strain; chronic shoulder girdle pain.
Respiratory Problems:
  Ineffective cough; decreased chest expansion; poor breathing ration; decreased upper trunk mobility.
Upper Body Problems:
  Decreased mobility of one or both upper extremities; fibrotic skin changes on the chest wall; lymphedema; neuropathic changes; superficial sensory loss and radiating pain; asymmetric posture.
Lower Body Problems:
  Decreased mobility of one or both lower extremities; amputation; edema; neuropathic changes; joint dysfunction; contractures; chronic pain.
Generalized Deconditioning:
  Loss of strength and endurance; weakness and loss of motor control; disequilibrium.

Occupational Therapy
Self-Care Deficits:
  Inability to perform daily hygiene routine and to get dressed; need for clothing adaptation or special garment construction.
Activities of Daily Living Limitations:
  Problems with obtaining groceries or preparing meals; difficulties performing household tasks; barriers to entering and leaving the home; need for therapeutic leisure activity; need for work simplification strategies.
Need for Adaptive Equipment or Assistive Devices:
  Upper extremity splints, specialized eating and drinking apparatus.

(Data from McGarvey, C. L. [1990]. *Physical therapy for the cancer patient.* New York: Churchill Livingstone; and Strong, J. [1987]. *Occupational therapy and cancer rehabilitation. British Journal of Occupational Therapy, 50*[1], 4–6.)

& Lorish, 1994; Whiteneck, 1994). Recently, increased attention has been directed at adding quality of life to the spectrum of variables used to judge the effectiveness of rehabilitation efforts (Mellette, 1993; Spitzer, 1987). However, with cancer rehabilitation all outcome variables must be measured in the context of cancer status. The need for valid measures that quantify outcomes cannot be overemphasized. Returning to the definition for cancer rehabilitation, it is clear that optimal functioning is governed by the limits of the cancer situation. Yet, as emphasized elsewhere in this chapter, it is critical to establish aggregate databases on individuals with cancer and their related disabilities. For as Stineman & Granger (1994) have noted, accountability requires outcome analysis. Cost-effective care requires an examination of variations in the process and results of rehabilitation through analyses of large databases.

FOLLOW-UP SEQUENCE

Those who provide services to individuals with disabilities have traditionally placed great importance on the value of follow-up activities. For the individual who has been treated for cancer, a well-designed follow-up sequence is essential. The follow-up process allows for evaluation of rehabilitation outcomes and monitoring of the individual's progress as a cancer survivor. Follow-up provides an opportunity for the following:

1. Monitor the individual's overall health and cancer status.
2. Oversee the individual's progress as a cancer survivor and explore survivorship issues.

3. Assess the individual's functional status and ability to sustain rehabilitation gains.
4. Evaluate the adequacy of community resources.
5. Assess the need for additional services.
6. Provide ongoing informal psychosocial support.
7. Evaluate the individual's satisfaction with rehabilitation services provided.

FUTURE OF CANCER REHABILITATION

For cancer rehabilitation, the emerging health care reform environment can be a positive force. It is becoming common for managed care organizations and their subsidiaries to judge health care services in terms of the ability to favorably *shift patient survival curve.* Cancer rehabilitation can be seen as complementing this objective by aiming to favorably *shift the independence and quality of life curve.* Similarly, the performance of health care providers will be increasingly measured in relation to patient access to interventions, institutional capabilities to provide services, appropriateness of services provided, outcomes, patient satisfaction, and cost (Zatz, 1994). For cancer rehabilitation, this trend will mean that rehabilitation services will be subjected to the same scrutiny as acute care services. We will need to be ever more mindful of the need to provide cost-effective care and to quantify outcomes. However, based on all that has been stated in this chapter, cancer rehabilitation has the potential to be an indispensable element of the cancer care product line for the future. Throughout this chapter, emphasis has been placed on the fact that all individuals treated for cancer have rehabilitation needs. In the best of situa-

TABLE 75–4. *Sampling of Possible Rehabilitation Services*

Achievement of Personal Goals
Personal adjustment counseling
Vocational counseling
Self-image counseling
Couples counseling
Cosmetic devices
Stress management
Legal and financial counseling
Adaptive driver education
Home modifications

Increased or Sustained Functional Abilities
Joint mobility exercise
Postural education
Movement therapy
Retrograde massage
Lymphedema management
Activities of daily living retraining
Transfer skills training
Ambulation training
Orthotic intervention
Dynamic or static splinting
Skin care procedures
Electric stimulation
Bowel and bladder retaining
Colostomy or urostomy training
Self-care skills restoration
Adaptive equipment

Improved Physical Conditioning
Therapeutic strengthening exercises
Stretching programs
Upper body strengthening exercises
Endurance self-monitoring
Chest physiotherapy
Aerobic exercise
Aquatic therapy
Cryotherapy

Adequate Nutrition
Diet consultation
Dietary prescriptions
Nutrition workshops
Dysphagia intervention
Swallowing retraining
Taste change management
Enteral nutrition
Total parenteral nutrition

Satisfactory Psychosocial Adjustment
Patient and family support groups
Stress management
Meditation and imagery techniques training
Psychologic consultation
One-to-one counseling
Structured leisure activity
Cognitive behavioral therapy
Pastoral counseling

Appropriate Health Promotion and Health Protection
Ongoing medical management of oncology and general health issues
Administration of chemotherapy
Patient and family oncology education

Effective Management of Symptoms
Pain management
Relaxation techniques
Energy conservation
Pharmacologic intervention

tions, a *rehabilitative approach* during cancer treatment suffices to return the individual to preillness levels of functioning. However, when cancer-related disabilities develop, *comprehensive cancer rehabilitation* is indicated. When advanced or metastatic disease is present, a need for *conservative cancer rehabilitation* exists. Finally, this chapter has also pointed out that rehabilitation is as much a way of thinking as a set of services and intervention. Thus, it is appropriate to end on the reflective note put forth by Wells (1990, p. 505): ". . .we must help others realize that rehabilitation is not a functional phenomenon; rather it is a philosophy of care that must be relevant to all healthcare providers. . . ."

REFERENCES

Anderson, T. P. (1975). An alternative frame of reference for rehabilitation: The helping process vs. the medical model. *Archives of Physical Medicine and Rehabilitation, 56*(1), 101–104.

American College of Sports Medicine. (1991). Exercise prescriptions for special populations. In *Guidelines for exercise testing and prescription* (4th ed.). Philadelphia: Lea & Febiger.

Applegate, W. B., Blass J. P., & Williams, T. F. (1990). Instruments for the functional assessment of older patients. *New England Journal of Medicine, 322*(17), 1213.

Brown, M., Gordon, W. A., & Diller, L. (1983). Functional assessment and outcome measurement: An integrative review. In E. L. Pan, T. E. Backer, & C. L. Vash (Eds.), *Annual Review of Rehabilitation* (Vol. 3). New York: Springer.

Brown, H. G., & Tai-Seale, M. (1992). Vocational rehabilitation of cancer patients. *Seminars in Oncology Nursing, 8*(3), 202–211.

Citu, D. X., & Lorish, T. R., (1994). Stroke rehabilitation. 5. Stroke outcome. *Archives of Physical Medicine and Rehabilitation, 75*(5S), S56–59.

Commission of the Accreditation of Rehabilitation Facilities. (1994). *Standards manual and interpretive guidelines for organizations serving people with disabilities.* Tucson: Author.

Conti, J. V. (1990). Cancer rehabilitation: Why can't we get out of first gear. *Journal of Rehabilitation, 56*(4), 19–22.

DeVita, V. T., Hellman, S., & Rosenberg, S. A. (Eds.). (1989). *Cancer: Principles and practice of oncology.* Philadelphia: J. B. Lippincott Co.

Dietz, J. H. (1981). *Rehabilitation oncology.* New York: Wiley.

Dodd, M. J. (1988). Measuring self care activities. In M. Frank-Stromborg (Ed.), *Instruments for clinical nursing research.* Norwalk, CT: Appleton & Lange.

Fleming, J. (1991). Overview of functional health status measures in nursing. In H. Hibbard, P. Nutting, & M. L. Grady (Eds.), *Conference proceedings: Primary care research: Theory and methods.* Washington DC: U.S. Department of Health and Human Services, P.H.S., Agency for Health Care Policy and Research.

Fucile, J. (1992). Functional rehabilitation in cancer care. *Seminars in Oncology Nursing, 8*(3), 186–189.

Gamble, G. L., Brown, P. S., Kinney, C. L., & Mahoney F. P. (1990). Cancer rehabilitation: Principles and psychosocial aspects. *Archives of Physical Medicine and Rehabilitation, 71,* S245–247.

Granger, C. V., & Gresham, G. E. (1984). *Functional assessment in rehabilitation medicine.* Baltimore: Williams & Wilkins.

Granger, C. V., & Hamilton, B. B. (1994). The Uniform Data System for medical rehabilitation report of first admissions for 1992. *American Journal of Physical Medicine and Rehabilitation, 73*(1), 51–55.

Guadagnoli, E., & Mor, V. (1991). Daily living needs of cancer patients. *Journal of Community Health, 16*(1), 37–47.

Gunn, A. E. (1984). *Cancer rehabilitation.* New York: Raven Press.

Halpern, A. S., & Fuhrer, M. J. (1984). *Functional assessment in rehabilitation.* Baltimore: P.H. Brookes.

Hamilton, B. B., Granger, C. V., & Sherwin, F. S. (1987). A uniform national data system for medical rehabilitation. In M. J. Fuhrer (Ed.), *Rehabilitation outcomes: Analysis and measurement* (pp. 137–147). Baltimore: Brookes Publishing Co.

Harvey, R. F., Jellinek, H. M., & Habeck, R. V. (1982). Cancer rehabilitation: an analysis of 36 program approaches. *Journal of the American Medical Association, 247*(15), 2127–2131.

Hickey, R. C. (1986). Historical basis for cancer rehabilitation at the University of Texas M. D. Anderson Hospital and Tumor Institute. *Cancer Bulletin, 38*(5), 239–240.

Johnson, J. G., & Kelly, A. W. (1990). A multifaceted rehabilitation program for women with cancer. *Oncology Nursing Forum, 17*(5), 691–695.

Katz, S. (1983). Assessing self maintenance: Activities of daily living, mobility, and instrumental activities of daily living. *Journal of the American Geriatrics Society, 31*(12), 721–727.

Kudsk, E. G., & Hoffmann, G. S. (1987). Rehabilitation of the cancer patient. *Primary Care, 14*(2), 381–390.

Kurtz, M. E., Kurtz, J. C., Given, C. W., & Given, B. (1993). Loss of physical functioning among patients with cancer. *Cancer Practice, 1*(4), 275–281.

Kurtzman, S. H., Gardner, B., & Kellner, W. S. (1988). Rehabilitation of the cancer patient. *American Journal of Surgery, 155*(6), 791–803.

Lehmann, J. F., DeLisa, J. A., Warren, C. G., deLateur, B. J., Bryant, P. L., & Nicholson, C. G. (1978). Cancer rehabilitation: Assessment of need, development and evaluation of a model of care. *Archives of Physical Medicine and Rehabilitation, 59*(9), 410–419.

Linacre, J. M., Heinemann, A. W., Wright, B. D., Granger, C. V., & Hamilton, B. B. (1994). The structure and stability of the functional independence measure. *Archives of Physical Medicine and Rehabilitation, 75*(2), 127–132.

MacVicar, M. G., & Winningham, M. L. (1986). Promoting the functional capacity of cancer patients. *Cancer Bulletin, 38*(5), 235–239.

MacVicar, M. G., Winningham, M. L., & Nickel, J. L. (1989). Effects of aerobic interval training in cancer patients functional capacity. *Nursing Research, 38*(6), 348–351.

Mayer, D. K. (1992). The healthcare implications of cancer rehabilitation in the twenty-first century. *Oncology Nursing Forum, 19*(1), 23–27.

Mayer, D., & O'Connor, L. (1989). Rehabilitation of persons with cancer: Oncology Nursing Society position statement. *Oncology Nursing Forum, 16*(4), 33.

Mayer, D. K. & O'Connor-Kelleher, L. (1993). *Rehabilitation of people with cancer: An Oncology Nursing Society position statement.* Pittsburgh, PA: Oncology Nursing Society.

McGarvey, C. L. (1990). *Physical therapy for the cancer patient.* New York: Churchill Livingstone.

McLaughlin, W. J. (1984). Cancer rehabilitation: People investing in people. *Journal of Rehabilitation, 50*(4), 57–59.

Mellette, S. J., (1993). Cancer rehabilitation. *Journal of the National Cancer Institute, 85*(10), 781–784.

Mellette, S. J., & Parker, G. G. (1992). Future directions in cancer rehabilitation. *Seminars in Oncology Nursing, 8*(3), 219–233.

Mock, V., Burke, M. B., Sheehan, P., Creaton, E. M., Winningham, M. L., McKenney-Tedder, S., Schwager, L. P., & Liebman, M. (1994). A nursing rehabilitation program for women with breast cancer receiving adjuvant chemotherapy. *Oncology Nursing Forum, 21*(5), 899–907.

Moinpour, M. C., McCorkle, R., & Saunders, J. (1988). Measuring functional status. In M. Frank-Stromborg (Ed.), *Instruments for clinical nursing research* (pp. 23–45). Norwalk, CT: Appleton & Lange.

Mor, V., Guadagnoli, E., & Wool, M. (1987). An examination of the concrete service needs of advanced cancer patients. *Journal of Psychosocial Oncology, 5*(1), 1–17.

Mor, V., Laliberte, L., Morris, J. N., & Wiemann, M. (1984). The Karnofsky Performance Status Scale—An examination of its reliability and validity in a research setting. *Cancer, 53,* 2002–2007.

Mor, V., Masterson-Allen, S., Houts, P., & Siegel, K. (1992). The changing needs of patients with cancer at home: A longitudinal study. *Cancer, 69*(3), 829–838.

O'Toole, D. M., & Golden, A. M. (1991). Evaluating cancer patients for rehabilitation potential. *Western Journal of Medicine, 155*(4), 348–387.

Rusk, H. A. (1984). *Rehabilitation medicine* (5th ed., pp. 621–642). St. Louis: The C. V. Mosby Co.

Salcido, R., & Jenkins, S. C. (1994). The subacute rehabilitation boom. *Journal of Subacute Care, 1*(1), 3–6.

Skinner, J. S. (Ed.). (1987). Exercise testing and exercise prescription for special cases. In *Theoretical basis and clinical application.* Philadelphia: Lea & Febiger

Spitzer, W. O. (1987). State of science 1986: Quality of life and functional status as target variables for research. *Journal of Chronic Diseases, 40*(6), 465–471.

Stewart, A. L., Ware, J. E., & Brook, R. H. (1981). Advances in the measurement of functional status: Construction of aggregate indexes. *Medical Care, 19*(5), 473–478

Stineman, M. G., & Granger, C. V. (1994). Outcome studies and analysis: Principles of rehabilitation that influence outcome analysis. In G. Felsenthal, S. J. Garrison, & F. U. Steinberg (Eds.), *Rehabilitation of the aging and elderly patient.* Baltimore: Williams & Wilkins.

Strong, J. (1987). Occupational therapy and cancer rehabilitation. *British Journal of Occupational Therapy, 50*(1), 4–6.

Taylor, C. M. (1984). The rehabilitation of persons with cancer: Is this the best we can do? *Journal of Rehabilitation, 50*(4), 60–71.

Vinokur, A. D, Threatt, B. A., Caplan, R. D., & Zimmerman, B. L. (1989). Physical functioning and adjustment to breast cancer. *Cancer, 63*(2), 394–405.

Watson, P. G. (1990). Cancer rehabilitation: The evolution of a concept. *Cancer Nursing, 13*(1), 2–12.

Watson, P. G. (1992a). Cancer rehabilitation, an overview. *Seminars in Oncology Nursing, 8*(3), 167–173.

Watson, P. G. (1992b). The optimal functioning plan: A key element in cancer rehabilitation. *Cancer Nursing, 15*(4), 254–263.

Wells, R. (1990). Rehabilitation: Making the most of time. *Oncology Nursing Forum, 17*(4), 503–507.

Whiteneck, G. G. (1994). Measuring what matters: Key rehabilitation outcomes. *Archives of Physical Medicine and Rehabilitation, 75,* 1073–1076.

Williams, F. H., & Maly, B. J. (1994). Pain rehabilitation: 3. Cancer pain, pelvic pain, and age related considerations. *Archives of Physical Medicine and Rehabilitation, 75*(5S), S20.

Winningham, M. L. (1990). Cancer and exercise. In L. Goldberg & D. L. Elliot (Eds.), *Exercise and medical therapy: Physiologic principles and clinical considerations.* Philadelphia: F. A. Davis.

Winningham, M. L. (1991). Walking program for people with cancer. *Cancer Nursing, 14,* 270–276.

Winningham, M. L., MacVicar, M. G., Bondoc, M., Anderson, J. I., & Minton, J. P. (1989). Effect of aerobic exercise on body weight and composition in patients with breast cancer on adjuvant chemotherapy. *Oncology Nursing Forum, 16*(5), 683–689.

World Health Organization. (1980). *International classification of impairments, disabilities and handicaps (ICIDH).* Geneva: Author.

Wright, B. A. (1983). *Physical disability—A psychosocial approach* (2nd ed.). New York: Harper & Row.

Young-McCaughan, S., & Sexton, D. (1991). A retrospective investigation of the relationship between aerobic exercise and quality of life in women with breast cancer. *Oncology Nursing Forum, 18*(4), 751–757.

Zatz, S. L. (1994). Performance-based hospital contracting for quality improvement. *USQA Quality Monitor, 1*(1), 4–7.

Survivorship and Quality of Life Issues

Marcia Grant • Geraldine V. Padilla • Eva R. Greimel

This chapter focuses on cancer survivorship as it relates to the stages or seasons of survival (Bushkin, 1993; Dow, 1990; Mullan, 1985). Survivorship is described within a framework of quality of life research (Padilla, Grant, Ferrell, & Presant, 1995). Interest by health professionals in cancer survivorship has emerged as the number of survivors has increased, the consumer movement in the United States has begun focusing on cancer, as physiologic and psychosocial effects of cancer survival have been described by cancer researchers, and quality of life measurement for cancer patients has evolved. Each of these aspects is described.

SURVIVAL: DEFINITIONS AND DESCRIPTIONS

About 1,252,000 Americans will be diagnosed with new cases of cancer this year (American Cancer Society, 1995; Wingo, Tong, & Bolden, 1995). Of these, approximately 54 per cent will survive. In 1995 approximately 8 million Americans now living have a history of cancer, with 5 million diagnosed 5 or more years ago. Most of this group of 5 million survivors are considered "cured," while some still have evidence of disease. "Cured" is defined as someone who has no evidence of disease and has the same life expectancy as a person who never had cancer (American Cancer Society, 1995). Survivors, then, include patients "cured" of cancer and patients who still have disease.

Cure rates differ across cancer diagnoses, age groups, ethnic background, and socioeconomic status. Survivors thus represent these differences. Table 76–1 identifies the percentage of estimated survivors for all cancers and some commonly occurring cancers based on estimated new cases for 1995. One can expect from these estimates, for example, that survivors in general will include a higher proportion of breast and prostate cancer patients than lung cancer patients.

Cancer rates increase as age increases. One can expect therefore that survivors will include a large number of older patients. Survival statistics also vary according to ethnic status. Table 76–2 identifies relative 5-year survival percentages comparing whites and African-Americans from 1960 to 1990. While both groups illustrate increases in survival percentages, survival percentages in the white group are considerably higher. This difference has been attributed primarily to late diagnosis in the black population (American Cancer Society, 1995). Differences in incidence and survival also occur in other ethnic populations, such as Hispanics. These differences may reflect cultural variations, various lifestyles, or genetic characteristics and provide important clues in research on the development of cancer across populations.

Socioeconomic status also appears to have an impact on survival. Figure 76–1 illustrates the relationships between poverty, race, and cancer, and how decreased survival may be attributed to a number of factors. A study of patterns of cancer care among the poor revealed that the poor reported more tobacco-related cancers, more advanced disease, less desirable treatment, and poorer survival rates (American Cancer Society, 1994).

These descriptions on the impact of cancer site, age, ethnic status, and socioeconomic status on survival percentages provide information useful in understanding the nature of the population of survivors and point to some of the concerns and needs of various subgroups. Problems faced by survivors are just beginning to be described. The impact both the cancer and the resultant problems have on the cancer survivors' quality of life is an area of increased research activity.

TABLE 76–1. *Selected New Cancer Cases and Percent Survival, United States, 1995*

CANCER SITE	ESTIMATED NEW CASES	ESTIMATED SURVIVORS
All sites	1,252,000	705,000 (56.0%)
Prostate	244,000	203,600 (83.0%)
Breast	183,400	137,160 (74.8%)
Lung	169,900	12,500 (7.4%)
Colo-Rectal	138,200	82,900 (60.0%)
Bladder	50,500	39,300 (77.8%)
Uterus	48,600	37,900 (77.9%)
Melanoma	34,100	26,900 (78.9%)
Oral	28,150	19,780 (70.0%)
Thyroid	13,900	12,780 (91.9%)
Hodgkins disease	7,800	6,350 (81.4%)
Testis	7,100	6,730 (94.8%)
Eye	1,870	1,630 (87.0%)

(From American Cancer Society. [1995]. *Cancer facts and figures, 1995.* Atlanta: Author.)

SURVIVORSHIP: STAGES AND PHASES

Mullan (1985) defines a cancer survivor as anyone diagnosed with cancer, regardless of the stage or course of illness. Confrontation with one's own mortality begins when the cancer is diagnosed, and one becomes a cancer survivor. Separating survivors into different phases is useful in defining the different concerns survivors have (Dow, 1990; Mullan, 1985).

Surviving the diagnosis and the initial treatment is the first phase of survival. During this phase, the survivor concentrates on the initial diagnosis and the initial treatment. Surviving surgery, radiation, and chemotherapy are patient goals, with the outcome for cure being the driving force. During this phase, the survivor works closely with health care professionals involved in implementing medical treatment and helping the patient to withstand the toxic side effects. The patient is busy learning self-care skills to survive surgery, daily radiation therapy, and chemotherapy side effects such as infections and hair loss. Survival also includes the beginning adjustments of placing cancer in the context of other aspects of life: work, family relationships, role adjustments. During this phase, the survivor has more in common with other survivors than those who have not experienced cancer (Mullan, 1985). This first phase involves facing the possibility of a shortened life.

The second phase involves extended survival and occurs when the patient has completed initial therapy and has gone into remission or completed initial treatment (Dow, 1990; Mullan, 1985). This phase is dominated by the fear of recurrence. Every symptom is evaluated in terms of a recurrence. The focus is less on health professionals and more directed toward adapting to the physical limitations associated with the tumor and treatment, such as hair loss, amputation, and chronic fatigue. Support services such as the American Cancer Society "I Can Cope" program and the support groups held at the Wellness Community are valuable during this phase.

The final phase, permanent survival, is roughly equated with "cure" and occurs when the disease is considered to be permanently arrested. This is a gradually occurring perspective and involves the likelihood that cancer is permanently arrested. Some patients are able to put their cancer experience into perspective and are able to thrive despite their history of cancer (Dow, 1990). Other problems, however, present formidable challenges. Employment problems and insurance problems are common, and discrimination of various sorts occurs (Mullan, 1985). The long-term secondary effects of cancer become more of a focus during this phase. Long-term effects of radiation, sterility, possibility of second cancers, and cardiopulmonary complications are among the secondary effects that can compromise quality of life.

Each of these phases presents a different set of challenges for health care professionals involved in assisting patients in the progression through these phases. Resources and support issues differ across phases. Phases may not always occur linearly, and progress may be gradual (Hassey-Dow, 1991). An understanding of the different issues and concerns of each phase can assist health professionals in evaluating survivors' needs and planning appropriate interventions.

CONSUMER MOVEMENT IN CANCER SURVIVORSHIP

The National Coalition of Cancer Survivorship (NCCS) is an organization founded in 1986 by Mullan, a physician and a cancer survivor. The current president is Susan Leigh, a nurse and a cancer survivor consultant. This organization represents a grass roots movement aimed at providing health care professionals with accurate information about what it is like to experience cancer and live with it as a chronic disease. Leigh identifies the recurrent theme of cancer survivors to be that of quality of life issues (Leigh & Logan, 1991). The NCCS is located in Washington D.C., where involvement with such issues as work, third-party cov-

TABLE 76–2. *Trends in Relative 5-year Cancer Survival, by Race: All Sites Diagnosed*

	1960–1963	1970–1973	1974–1976	1977–1979	1983–1990
White	39%	43%	50%	51%	56%
African-American	27%	31%	39%	39%	40%

(From American Cancer Society. [1995]. *Cancer facts and figures, 1995.* Atlanta: Author.)

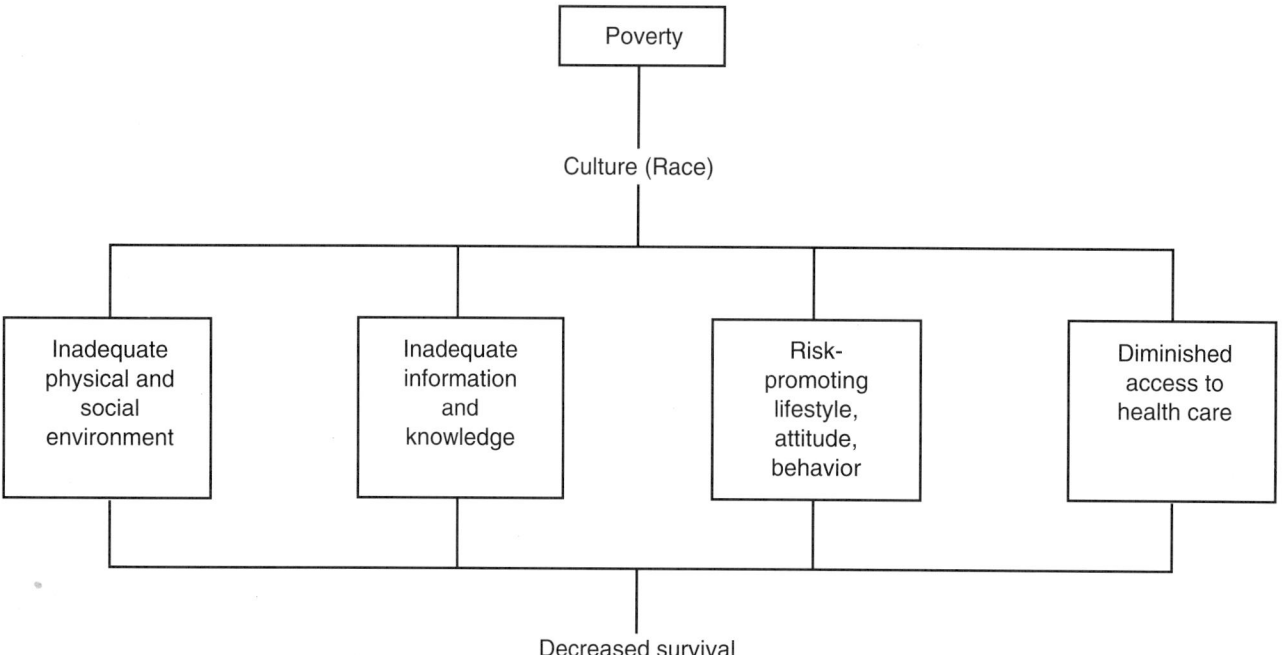

FIGURE 76–1. The interrelationship among poverty, race, and cancer. Poverty acts through the prism of culture/race. (From Steele, G. D., Osteen, R. T., Winchester, D. P., Mench, H. R., & Murphy, G. P. [1994]. *National cancer data base: Annual review of patient care, 1994.* Atlanta: American Cancer Society.)

erage of off-label drugs, and coverage of patient costs during clinical trials can be addressed at the national level.

PHYSIOLOGIC AND PSYCHOSOCIAL ASPECTS OF CANCER SURVIVORSHIP

One of the more extensive reviews of effects of cancer survivorship was conducted by Loescher and colleagues and reported in separate articles on physiologic effects (Loescher, Welch-McCaffrey, Leigh, Hoffman, & Meyskens, 1989) and psychosocial effects (Welch-McCaffrey, Hoffman, Leigh, Loescher, & Meyskens, 1989). A review of 285 articles was done to determine long-term and late effects of cancer. These problems were classified into eight groups: sex and reproductive, neurologic, vascular, cardiac, pulmonary, urologic, gastrointestinal including hepatic, and other. The occurrence, frequency, and severity of each effect varied across cancer diagnoses and disease stages, intensity and type of therapy, age, and overall health of the individual. Multiple effects were identified. They varied from mild effects that had little impact on daily life to potentially lethal complications. The need to conduct prospective studies to predict physiologic complications in specific cancer populations and to explore treatment choices that decrease long-term side effects was a recommendation (Loescher et al., 1989).

A review of 58 articles was done to identify the psychosocial implications of surviving adult cancers (Welch-McCaffery et al., 1989). Data were sparse compared with the physiologic studies examined above.

Problems identified were classified as follows: fear of recurrence and death, relationships with the health care team, adjustment to physical compromise, alterations in customary social support, isolationism, psychosocial reorientation, and employment and insurance problems. Most studies were descriptive. Additional studies were recommended on interventions to improve the psychosocial responses of cancer survivors.

Since this early descriptive work, some information on survivors of specific cancers and cancer treatments has become available. Breast cancer patients have been the focus of several studies (Dow, Ferrell, Leigh, Ly, & Gulasekaram, 1995; Ferrans, 1994; Wyatt, Kurtz, & Liken, 1993). The study by Wyatt et al. (1993) of 11 long-term breast cancer survivors used a focus group discussion to uncover quality of life issues, concerns, and needs of women who had survived breast cancer for over 5 years. Themes included integration of the disease process into current life, change in relationship with others, restructuring of life perspective, and unresolved issues such as relationships with health care providers and fears of susceptibility to cancer. Ferran's study reports findings of breast cancer survivors resulting from content analysis of two questions: "All things considered, do you think that all you have gone through to treat the cancer was worth it?" Responses revealed that 95 per cent of the 38 respondents answered yes. The second question, "Is there anything else you would like to tell us about your life or your health care?" resulted in validating the conceptual model of four dimensions of quality of life: health and functioning domain, psychological/spiritual domain, family domain, and social and economic domain. Both positive and negative aspects of each of these domains were identified during content analysis. Ferrans concluded that the majority of the women interviewed were getting on with life, and even thriving. Dow et al. reported findings of a study of 294 breast cancer survivors. This quantitative design used a 41-item 10-point scale representing the conceptual model of four dimensions: physical well being, psychologic well being, social well being, and spiritual well being. Physical well being had the highest quality of life scores, followed by social, spiritual, and then psychologic well being. The resolution of physical symptoms common during therapy illustrated that this population had moved away from the acute survival symptoms of disease, treatment, or both and were in the more permanent phase of survival.

Studies have also focused on various quality of life aspects in patients with cancer in other sites. Schag, Ganz, Wing, Sim, and Lee (1994) used a cross-sectional approach to examine quality of life and rehabilitation in patients with lung, colon, and prostate cancer. Differences across diagnoses were revealed, with lung cancer patients reporting stable quality of life scores across a short survival period, colorectal cancer patients experiencing improved quality of life as they lived longer, and a declining quality of life for patients with prostatic cancer. Other researchers have provided evidence of patterns of quality of life in relation to treatment and specific kinds of cancer (Danoff, Kramer, Irwin, & Gottlieb, 1983; Grant, et al, 1992; Haberman, Bush, Young, & Sullivan, 1993; Johanssen, et al., 1992; Kornblith et al., 1992; Padilla, Grant et al., 1992). These studies provide beginning information on quality of life status among many patient groups and illustrate the individual responses and the need to plan interventions for specific patient problems.

SURVIVORSHIP AND QUALITY OF LIFE

Quality of life has become a frequent and important measurement of survival. Research has provided a beginning foundation for definitions, conceptual approaches, and changes that occur among various cancer populations. This scientific foundation has provided the basis for shaping nursing approaches and evaluating nursing interventions aimed at improving quality of life for cancer survivors.

CONCEPTUAL DEFINITIONS OF HEALTH-RELATED QUALITY OF LIFE

Quality of life is a broad concept that reflects a subjective evaluation of well being. In the context of cancer survival, health-related quality of life (HRQL) is more narrowly defined as, "a personal, evaluative statement summarizing the positivity or negativity of attributes that characterize one's psychological, physical, social, and spiritual well-being at a point in time when health, illness and treatment conditions are relevant" (Padilla et al., 1995, p. 301). The HRQL domains were identified in previous work (Grant et al.,

1992; Ferrell, Rhiner, Cohen, & Grant, 1991; Ferrell, Cohen, Rhiner, & Rozak, 1991; Ferrell, Grant, Schmidt, Rhiner et al., 1992; Ferrell, Grant, Schmidt, Whitehead et al., 1992; Padilla, Ferrell, Grant, & Rhiner, 1990; Padilla et al., 1995).

Other investigators support this view of HRQL as a subjective, multidimensional experience. For example, Gill and Feinstein (1994) described quality of life as ". . . . a uniquely personal perception, denoting the way that individual patients feel about their health status and/or nonmedical aspects of their lives" (p. 619). The Division of Mental Health of the World Health Organization (1993), defined quality of life as, "an individual's perception of their position in life in the context of the culture and value systems in which they live and in relation to their goals, expectations, standards and concerns" (p. 1).

OPERATIONAL DEFINITIONS OF HEALTH-RELATED QUALITY OF LIFE

Numerous measures of quality of life have been developed over the last 40 years. Rather than discuss all of them here, the reader is referred to a number of helpful summaries and reviews of measures of quality of life. Padilla and Frank-Stromborg (in press) reviewed single measures of quality of life, whereas Dean (in press) discussed multiple measures. Grant, Padilla, Ferrell, and Rhiner (1990) and Cella and Tulsky (1990) summarized the definitions and dimensions, reliability, validity, and format of quality of life instruments commonly used in cancer research. Gotay and Moore (1992) reviewed instruments that assess quality of life in head and neck cancer. Hays and Shapiro (1992) provide an overview of generic health-related quality of life measures for HIV research. Revicki, Turner, Brown, and Martindale (1992) tested the reliability, validity, and responsiveness of a battery of depression-specific health-related quality of life scales. In 1990, Spilker, Molinek, and Johnston published a quality of life bibliography that indexes references under quality of life instruments and subject headings.

The variety of instruments available to measure quality of life provide a valuable resource that makes it possible to match research or clinical questions with an appropriate quality of life measurement. Selection of which instrument to use depends on the specific project. The research question posed or the clinical use proposed need to be defined carefully, following which the instrument or instruments selected that match the questions are selected.

THEORETIC BASIS OF HRQL CHANGE

The authors view HRQL as essentially a dynamic construct affected by one's ability to cope with the "gap" between expected and experienced levels of well-being (Michalos, 1986) brought about by disease severity, comorbid conditions, or treatment-related symptoms. Whether good or poor, one's level of HRQL is a function of the extent of the perceived gap between expectations and experiences (Padilla, Mishel, & Grant,

1992) surrounding the four dimensions of well-being (psychologic, physical, social, and spiritual well being). Improvements in HRQL can be brought about by narrowing the gap.

Closing the gap between actual and expected outcomes means that the expected outcome or the actual experience change(s) in a direction that serves to close the gap. Cella (1991) suggests that there are four ways to improve quality of life: treat the disease, treat the symptoms and side effects, enhance communication, and reframe attitudes. In the context of gap theory, treating the disease and the symptoms moves the experience closer to expectation, whereas enhancing communication and reframing attitudes moves the expectation closer to experience. Cella (1991) suggests that when the disease no longer responds to treatment and symptom control efforts fail, communication can clarify, provide reassurance, demonstrate care, and support the patient. In addition, communication contributes to the reframing of attitudes. Patients can place their suffering in a different context so that they modify their expectations to be more in line with their experience. The quality of survival depends on finding ways to narrow the gap between actual experience and expected outcomes of survival.

The gap between actual experience and expected outcomes of survival can be operationally defined as subjectively perceived needs. Needs can also be identified by others, such as family caregivers and health care providers. But the most meaningful needs, in the context of HRQL, are those identified by the person with cancer.

The HRQL of survivors and their caregivers is linked to the satisfaction of survivor needs. The model of quality of survivorship proposed here is based on the model proposed by Greimel and Padilla (1995) linking HRQL outcomes to home care needs, resources, and interventions. Gap theory would predict that meeting survivor needs would result in improved quality of life (Michalos, 1986). Cella's (1991) strategies for improving quality of life are included as a way of categorizing interventions. Home care needs follow the Wingate and Lackey (1989) classification scheme modified by Hileman, Lackey, and Hassanein (1990, 1992). In this model, Figure 76–2, survivor needs influence HRQL outcomes directly as well as indirectly through resources and interventions. Survivor needs are met through the use of survival resources and HRQL interventions. As needs are met, HRQL outcomes improve because the gap between actual and desired outcomes narrows.

SIGNIFICANCE OF QUALITY OF LIFE FOR SURVIVORS

From a personal viewpoint, quality of life is the most important outcome by which to measure the success of survival. Stewart (1992), emphasized that, "The ultimate goal [of health care] is to help patients function in their daily activities and feel as good as possible within the constraints of their illness. This means that quality of life outcomes are the most relevant given the goals of health care" (p. 3).

Patient satisfaction with health care depends largely on whether, as a result of treatment, one feels better and functions better. To properly evaluate the effectiveness of treatment on survival, one must consider the effect of treatment on the disease as well as the person with the disease (Wenger, Lawton, Kaplan & Mulley, 1993). The significance of quality of life in the context of survival is reflected in Strickland's comments that, "Nursing focuses on changing or modifying human behaviors and responses to positively affect the quality of life" (Strickland, 1992, p. 145).

Four quality of life themes expressed by 11 survivors of breast cancer support the view of HRQL as a dynamic construct affected by the survivor's ability to cope with the "gap" between expected and experienced levels of well being following the diagnosis and treatment of the cancer (Wyatt, Kurtz, & Liken, 1993). The first theme, integration of the disease process into current life, focused on physical aspects of the disease to which the women had to adjust. The women felt they had coped with the physical loss and change required by the disease and did not continue to struggle. In this case the women had changed their expectations to fit the experience. The second theme dealt with changes in relationships with others. This second theme addressed the social and psychologic dimensions of HRQL. In some cases the women changed their perception of health/illness, whereas in other cases actual relationships changed, growing closer or farther apart to fit the individual's changed ideas about the importance of relationships. The third theme, restructuring of life perspective, involved the psychologic, social, and spiritual domains of HRQL. In this case, the women changed both actual experiences and expectations, bringing each side of the equation closer. Everyday experiences were infused with special meaning befitting a new philosophic view of life that cherished simple experiences. In addition, the women expressed a desire to be of service to others, a change in their perception of health/illness, and a need for spiritual guidance for health decisions. The fourth theme focused on unresolved issues related to the psychologic and social domains. The women talked of their relationship with health care providers and their fears of susceptibility to cancer. In these cases their quality of life was affected negatively by the discrepancy between their expectations regarding health care and health information and the actual care and information received. Quality of life was also negatively affected by their fear of recurrence.

CLINICAL IMPLICATIONS

These beginning descriptions of survivorship provide the scientific foundation for planning clinical interventions that improve quality of life for cancer survivors. In a recent survey in Minnesota, 1400 cancer survivors participated. Respondents reported experiencing the following: fear of recurrence 69 per cent, priority changes 56 per cent, lifestyle changes 53 per cent, self-image issues 42 per cent, treatment-related health problems 35 per cent, insurance problems 31 per cent, sexuality issues 30 per cent, financial issues 25

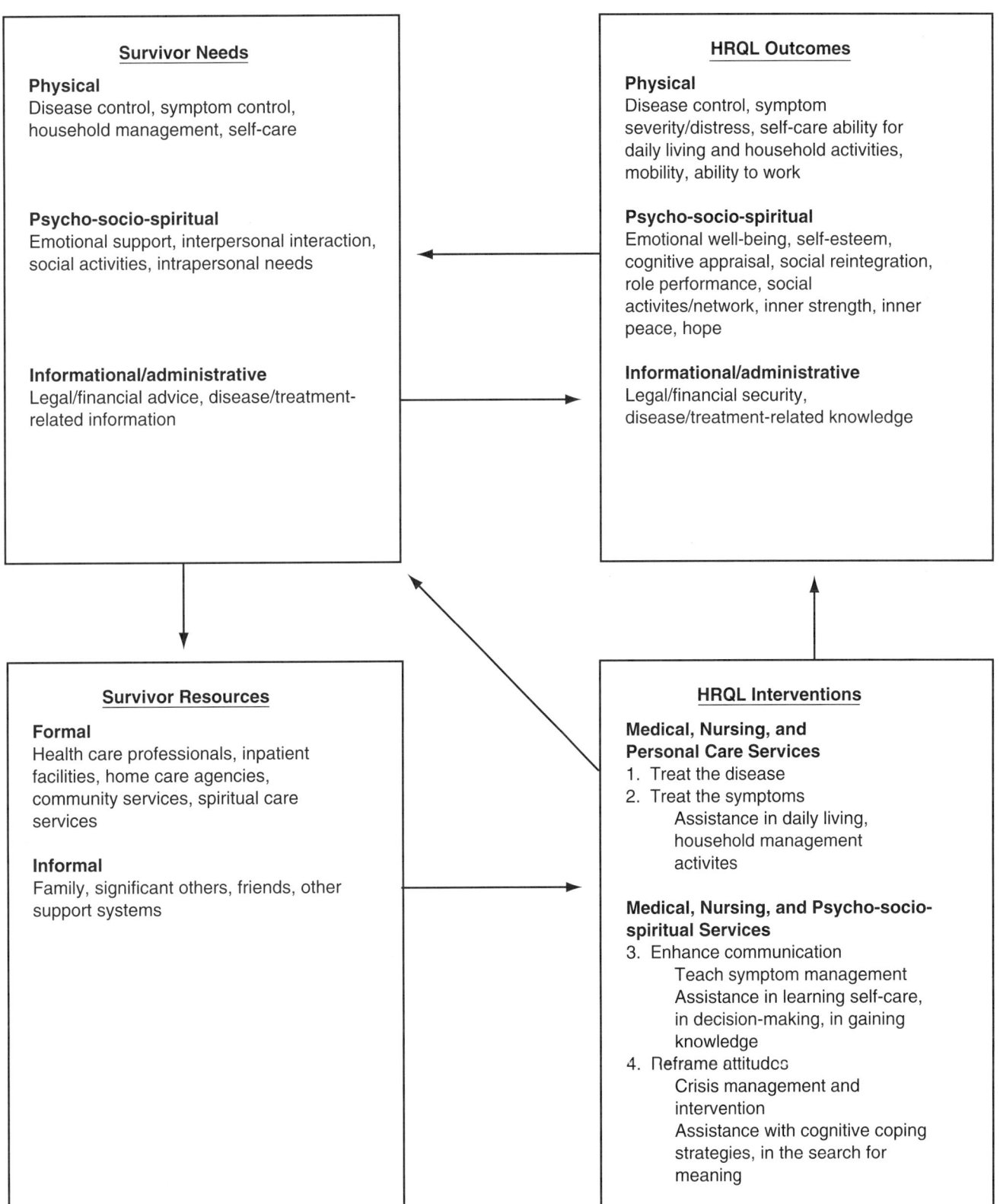

Survivor Needs

Physical
Disease control, symptom control, household management, self-care

Psycho-socio-spiritual
Emotional support, interpersonal interaction, social activities, intrapersonal needs

Informational/administrative
Legal/financial advice, disease/treatment-related information

HRQL Outcomes

Physical
Disease control, symptom severity/distress, self-care ability for daily living and household activities, mobility, ability to work

Psycho-socio-spiritual
Emotional well-being, self-esteem, cognitive appraisal, social reintegration, role performance, social activites/network, inner strength, inner peace, hope

Informational/administrative
Legal/financial security, disease/treatment-related knowledge

Survivor Resources

Formal
Health care professionals, inpatient facilities, home care agencies, community services, spiritual care services

Informal
Family, significant others, friends, other support systems

HRQL Interventions

Medical, Nursing, and Personal Care Services
1. Treat the disease
2. Treat the symptoms
    Assistance in daily living, household management activites

Medical, Nursing, and Psycho-socio-spiritual Services
3. Enhance communication
    Teach symptom management
    Assistance in learning self-care, in decision-making, in gaining knowledge
4. Reframe attitudes
    Crisis management and intervention
    Assistance with cognitive coping strategies, in the search for meaning

FIGURE 76–2. Quality of survivorship model. HRQL-health-related quality of life. (Data from Cella, 1991; Greimel & Padilla, 1995; Hileman, Lackey, & Hassanein, 1992; Hileman, & Lackey, 1990; Michalos, 1986; Wingate & Lackey, 1989.)

per cent, difficulty being diagnosed 24 per cent, loss of friends 22 per cent, employment issues 20 per cent, and fertility issues 16 per cent (American Cancer Society, 1994). Interventions should target the major issues that confront survivors: emotional consequences, social consequences, and physical consequences. Lifelong monitoring of physical and psychosocial status is a part of the cancer survivor's appropriate medical care.

Teaching the survivor about the importance of these regular checkups, providing timely and sensitive feedback following tests and examinations, and providing reminders and support during checkups are important nursing interventions. During the early survival period, physical symptoms are usually interpreted by the survivor as a return of the cancer. This may decrease as survivorship extends, but the fear of recurrence persists (Northouse, 1981; Rose, 1989; Quigley, 1989). Some strategies have been described for providing psychosocial support for cancer survivors (Table 76–3). These strategies need to be implemented during discharge planning, clinic follow-up visits, and home visits.

Reproductive issues differ according to the disease and treatment. Appropriate sexual assessment and interventions are essential (see Chapter 62 for specific assessments and interventions). These issues may be identified during long-term follow-up evaluations and illustrate the need for availability of referral and consultation services.

Another major issue for survivors is related to work and insurance issues. Employment discrimination includes dismissal, denial of new jobs, demotions, loss of benefits such as insurance, undesirable transfers, isolation, hostility in the workplace, and mandatory medical examinations unrelated to job performance (Hoffman, 1991). Discrimination by employers has resulted in federal laws prohibiting these employment practices in some situations. The Federal Rehabilitation Act of 1973 prohibits discrimination by employers who receive federal funding or are implementing federal contracts (Hoffman, 1991). To address other employers who do not receive federal monies, the American Disabilities Act of 1990 prohibits discrimination because of disability or history of disability for all private employers regardless of whether they receive federal monies (Hoffman, 1991). The nurse can assist the survivor in working through the benefits and risks of discussing the diagnosis of cancer at work (Box 76–1). In

some instances, coworkers' support can be life-saving, whereas in others, the diagnosis can bring about fear and hostility from coworkers. Disclosing a cancer diagnosis is a very personal decision. Many factors are important in selecting appropriate nursing interventions (Table 76–4). Helping the survivor evaluate the

TABLE 76–3. *Strategies for Prevention and Intervention of Psychosocial Morbidity*

Educate health care providers regarding survivorship issues
Adopt rehabilitation model of patient care
Facilitate early identification of those at risk
Educate survivors about disease, treatment, and signs and symptoms of recurrence
Encourage family involvement in illness/treatment discussions
Facilitate open communication of sexual issues
Identify community programs and resources
Provide for/identify forums for ongoing support and education
Facilitate discussions concerning reproduction and fertility issues prior to treatment
Provide ongoing multidisciplinary plan of care
Advocate in community on issues related to employment and insurance
Facilitate discussion relative to reductions of potential physical sequelae
Minimize lifestyle disruptions through flexible scheduling of treatment appointments
Assist survivors through identification and anticipation of potential sequelae
Encourage adaptive coping strategies and effective problem-solving
Participate in and conduct research to clarify issues and design interventions
Participate actively in advocating changes in public policies

(From Quigley, K. M. 1989. The adult cancer survivor: Psychosocial consequences of cure. *Seminars in Oncology Nursing, 5*(1), 63–69.)

Box 76–1. *Returning to Work After a Cancer Diagnosis*

Berry, D. L. (1991). Return-to-work experiences of people with cancer. *Oncology Nursing Forum, 30*(6), 905–911.

Purpose: The purpose of this exploratory, longitudinal study was to explore and further the understanding of the dimensions and process of the experience of returning to work after a cancer diagnosis.

Sample: Twelve individuals diagnosed with a genitourinary cancer were recruited from two urban areas in the Pacific Northwest. All 12 were employed on a full-time basis. Initially, purposive sampling was used with variations in age, gender, and length of time since diagnosis. Theoretic sampling guided the later accrual of participants.

Procedures: The naturalistic paradigm and qualitative research methods were used, employing a grounded theory approach. Data were collected via open ended interview questions and a demographic/medical history form. Initial face-to-face interviews were audiotaped. Follow up interviews were conducted from 6–16 weeks later, with some of these being telephone interviews. Analysis was done using the Ethnograph, a computer software program for qualitative analysis. The constant comparative analysis approach was used.

Major Findings: The core social process suggested by the data is one of *mobilizing social support* in the workplace. This process was described in various ways by participants. The dimensions identified in relation to telling others in the workplace about their diagnosis included comments about (1) why tell, (2) why not tell, (3) who was told, (4) who had to know, (5) when to tell, and (6) how to tell. This process in the workplace facilitated the individual's reintegration into normal activities after a cancer diagnosis. Results can guide nurses to focus not only on related dimensions of the return-to-work experience, such as time off for treatment, but on central concerns, such as the social benefits of returning to work.

TABLE 76–4. *Nursing Interventions for Factors Relevant to the Return to the Workplace for a Person with a Cancer Diagnosis*

FACTORS	NURSING INTERVENTIONS
Personal	Collaborate with medical and other discipline modalities to modify disease extent and meet other therapeutic goals.
	Address knowledge deficits, particularly regarding accomodations for side effects and for discrimination issues, providing resources to patients regarding legal rights and support (e.g., *Charting the Journey*).
	Discuss the meaning of work for the person with cancer to understand the unique characteristics of their experience relevant to the workplace.
Environmental	Facilitate reintegration of therapy with life activities, e.g., streamline treatment schedules.
	Encourage the worker with cancer to establish regular communication with occupational health professionals at the workplace.
	Communicate with occupational health professionals regarding abilities and necessary accommodations such as bathroom access.
	Communicate with patient's supervisor, if desired by the patient.
Human Responses	Discuss options regarding work absences, termination, and/or reentry with the worker who has a cancer diagnosis.
	Management of early and late treatment toxicities with attention to the workplace environment.
	Plan to monitor return-to-work efforts at regular follow-up visits in the therapeutic or workplace setting.

(From Berry, D. L., & Catanzaro, M. (1992). Persons with cancer and their return to the workplace. *Cancer Nursing, 15*(1), 40–46.)

situation, supporting choices available, and assisting the survivor in making an informed decision are appropriate nursing interventions.

RESOURCES AVAILABLE

Several resources are available for oncology nurses in providing care for cancer survivors. The Oncology Nursing Society has a Special Interest Group (SIG) on Survivorship. This SIG publishes a newsletter three times a year that provides stories on survivors, discusses issues and solutions, identifies books, videos, and other information available for health professionals as well as survivors and their families, publishes poems and other literary works related to survivorship, and gives information on Survivor Programs located across the United States. Both patients and health professionals can derive valuable information from this newsletter. In addition, the SIG meets at the Annual Oncology Nursing Society Clinical Congress, where issues are discussed, action plans voted on and put into place, and general networking about survival issues takes place.

The National Coalition for Cancer Survivorship is a nonprofit organization that allows patients, families, and health professionals to join forces in dealing with the issues of cancer survivorship. Annual meetings provide the structure for identifying key issues, conducting workshops on such topics as pain management and ethical challenges, and planning special projects related to survivorship.

SUMMARY

Survivorship represents success for medical treatment and challenges for survivors. Inclusion of quality of life as one measure of the impact of cancer and cancer treatment has provided a sound scientific basis for identifying physical, psychologic, and social issues surrounding cancer survivorship. The nurse plays a major role from the detection of cancer through long-term follow-up care in assisting cancer survivors in adapting to the emotional, physical, and social consequences of cancer and cancer treatment. Testing related to nursing interventions is an important next step.

REFERENCES

American Cancer Society. (1994). Minnesota Division, Inc., Survivorship Survey, Concept, Initial Results

American Cancer Society. (1995). *Cancer facts and figures, 1995.* Atlanta: author.

Berry, D. L., & Catanzaro, M. (1992). Persons with cancer and their return to the workplace. *Cancer Nursing, 15*(1), 40–46.

Bushkin, E. (1993). Signposts of survivorship. *Oncology Nursing Forum, 20*(6), 869–873.

Cella, D. F. (1991). Functional status and quality of life: Current views on measurement and intervention. In *(Proceedings) Functional Status and Quality of Life in Persons with Cancer,* Atlanta, 1985, American Cancer Society, 1–12.

Cella, D. F., & Tulsky, D. S. (1990). Measuring quality of life today: Methodological aspects. *Oncology, 4*(5), 29–38.

Danoff, B., Kramer, S., Irwin, P., & Gottlieb, A. (1983). Assessment of the quality of life in long-term survivors after definitive radiotherapy. *American Journal of Clinical Oncology (CCT), 6,* 339–345.

Dean, H. (In press). Multiple instruments for measuring quality of life. In M. Frank-Stromborg & S. Olsen (Eds.), *Instruments for clinical research in health care* (2nd ed.), Boston: Jones & Bartlett.

Dow, K. H. (1990). The enduring seasons in survival. *Oncology Nursing Forum, 17*(4), 511–516.

Dow, K. H., Ferrell, B. R., Leigh, S., Ly, J., Gulasekaram, P. (in press) An evaluation of the quality of life in long-term breast cancer survivors. Submitted for review.

Ferrans, C. E. (1994). Quality of life through the eyes of survivors of breast cancer. *Oncology Nursing Forum, 21*(10), 1645–1651.

Ferrell, B., Grant, M., Schmidt, G. M., Rhiner, M., Whitehead, C., Fonbuena, P., & Forman, S. J. (1992). The meaning of quality of life for bone marrow transplant survivors. Part 2. Improving quality of life for bone marrow transplant survivors. *Cancer Nursing, 15*(4), 247–253.

Ferrell, B., Grant, M., Schmidt, G. M., Whitehead, C., Fonbuena, P., & Forman, S. J. (1992). The meaning of quality of life for bone marrow transplant survivors. Part 1. The impact of bone marrow transplant on quality of life. *Cancer Nursing, 15*(3), 153–160.

Ferrell, B. R., Cohen, M., Rhiner, M., & Rozak, A. (1991). Pain as a metaphor for illness. Part II: Family caregivers' management of pain. *Oncology Nursing Forum, 18*(8), 1315–1321.

Ferrell, B. R., Rhiner, M., Cohen, M., & Grant, M. (1991). Pain as a metaphor for illness. Part I: Impact of cancer pain on family caregivers. *Oncology Nursing Forum, 18*(8), 1303–1309.

Gill, T. M., & Feinstein, A. R. (1994). A critical appraisal of the quality of quality-of-life measurements. *Journal of the American Medical Association, 272*, 619–626.

Gotay, C. C., & Moore, T. D. (1992). Assessing quality of life in head and neck cancer. *Quality of Life Research, 1*, 5–17.

Grant, M., Ferrell, B., Schmidt, G. M., Fonbuena, P., Niland, J. C., & Forman, S. J. (1992). Measurement of quality of life in bone marrow transplant survivors. *Quality of Life Research, 1*(6):375–384.

Grant, M., Padilla, G. V., Ferrell, B. R., & Rhiner, M. (1990). Assessment of quality of life with a single instrument. *Seminars in Oncology Nursing, 6*, 260–270.

Greimel, E. R., & Padilla, G. V. (1995). Quality of life and home care needs of cancer patients after discharge from hospital. Unpublished report, University of California Los Angeles, Los Angeles, CA.

Haberman, M., Bush, N., Young, K., & Sullivan, K. M. (1993). Quality of life of adult long-term survivors of bone marrow transplantation: A qualitative analysis of narrative data. *Oncology Nursing Forum, 20*(10), 1545–1553.

Hassey-Dow, D. (1991) The growing phenomenon of cancer survivorship. *Journal of Professional Nursing, 7*, 54–61.

Hays, R. D., & Shapiro, M. F. (1992). An overview of generic health-related quality of life measures for HIV research. *Quality of Life Research, 1*, 91–97.

Hileman, J. W., & Lackey, N. R. (1990). Self-identified needs of patients with cancer at home and their home caregivers: A descriptive study. *Oncology Nursing Forum, 17*, 907–913.

Hileman, J. W., Lackey, N. R., & Hassanein, R. S. (1992). Identifying the needs of home caregivers of patients with cancer. *Oncology Nursing Forum, 19*, 771–777.

Hoffman, J. D. (1991). Employment discrimination: another hurdle for cancer survivors. *Cancer Investigation, 9*(5), 589–595.

Johansson, S., Steineck, G., Hursti, T., Fredrikson, M., Furst, C. J., & Peterson, C. (1992). Aspects of patient care: Interviews with relapse-free testicular cancer patients in Stockholm. *Cancer Nursing, 15*(1), 54–60.

Kornblith, A. B., Anderson, J., Cella, D. F., Tross, S., Zuckerman, E., Cherin E., Henderson, E., Weiss, R. B., Cooper, M. R., Silver, R. T., Leone, L., Canellos, G. P., Gottlieb, A., & Holland, J. C. (1992). Survivorship: Hodgkin disease survivors at increased risk for problems in psychosocial adaption. *Cancer, 70*, 2214–2224.

Leigh, S., & Logan, C. (1991). The cancer survivorship movement. *Cancer Investigation, 9*(5), 571–579.

Loescher, L. J., Welch-McCaffrey, D., Leigh, S. A., Hoffman, B., & Meyskens, J. L. (1989). Surviving adult cancers. Part 1: Physiologic effects. *Annals of Internal Medicine, 111*(5), 411–432.

Michalos, A. C. (1986). Job satisfaction, marital satisfaction, and the quality of life: A review and a preview. In FM, Andrews (Ed.), *Research on the quality of life.* Ann Arbor, MI: Institute for Social Research, University of Michigan, 57–83.

Mullan, F. (1985). Seasons of survival: Reflections of a physician with cancer. *New England Journal of Medicine, 313*(4), 270–273.

Northouse, L. L. (1981). Mastectomy patients and the fear of cancer recurrence. *Cancer Nursing, 4*(3), 213–220.

Padilla, G. V. (1992). Validity of health-related quality of life subscales. *Progress in Cardiovascular Nursing, 7*, 13–20.

Padilla, G. V., Ferrell, B., Grant, M. M., & Rhiner, M. (1990). Defining the content domain of quality of life for cancer patients with pain. *Cancer Nursing, 13*(2), 108–115.

Padilla, G. V., & Frank-Stromborg, M. (In press). Single instruments for measuring quality of life. In M. Frank-Stromborg, & S. Olsen, (Eds.), *Instruments for clinical research in health care.* Boston: Jones & Bartlett.

Padilla, G. V., Grant, M. M., Ferrell, B. R., & Presant, C. A. (1995). Quality of Life—Cancer. In B. Spilker, (Ed.), *Quality of life and pharmacoeconomics in clinical trials,* (2nd ed. pp. 301–308), New York: Raven Press.

Padilla, G. V., Grant, M. M., Lipsett, J., Anderson, P. R., Rhiner, M., & Bogen, C. (1992). Health quality of life and colorectal cancer. *Cancer, 70*(5), 1450–1456.

Padilla, G. V., Mishel, M. H., & Grant, M. M. (1992) Uncertainty, appraisal and quality of life. *Quality of Life Research, 1*(3), 155–165.

Quigley, K. M. (1989), The adult cancer survivor: Psychosocial consequences of cure. *Seminars in Oncology Nursing, 5*(1), 63–69.

Revicki, D. A., Turner, R., Brown, R., & Martindale, J. J. (1992). Reliability and validity of a health-related quality of life battery for evaluating outpatient antidepressant treatment. *Quality of Life Research, 1*, 257–266.

Rose, M. A. (1989). Health promotion and risk prevention: Applications for cancer survivors. *Oncology Nursing Forum, 16*(3) 335–340.

Schag, C. A. C., Ganz, P. A., Wing, D. S., Sim, M. S., & Lee, J. J. (1994) Quality of life in adult survivors of lung, colon and prostate cancer. *Quality of Life Research, 3*,127–141.

Spilker, B., Molinek, F. R. Jr., & Johnston, K. A. (1990). Quality of life bibliography and indexes. *Medical Care, 28* (Suppl. 12), DS1–DS77.

Steele, G. D., Osteen, R. T., Winchester, D. P., Mench, H. R., & Murphy, G. P. (1994). *National cancer data base: Annual review of patient care, 1994.* Atlanta: American Cancer Society.

Stewart, A. L. (1992). Conceptual and methodologic issues in defining quality of life: State of the art. *Progress in Cardiovascular Nursing, 7*(1), 3–11.

Strickland, O. L. (1992). Measures and instruments. In *Patient outcomes research: Examining the effectiveness of nursing practice, Proceedings of the State of the Science Conference,* sponsored by the National Center for Nursing Research, September, 1991, NIH Publication No. 93-3411.

Welch-McCaffery, D., Hoffman, B., Leigh, S. A., Loescher, L. J., & Meyskens, F. I. (1989). Surviving adult cancers. Part 2: Psychosocial implications. *Annals of Internal Medicine, 111*(6), 517–524.

Wenger, N. K., Lawton, M. P., Kaplan, R. M., & Mulley, A. G., (1993). Quality of life assessment: Interpretation and implications. In Furberg, C. D. & Schuttinga, J. A. (Cochairmen),

Quality of life assessment: Practice, problems, and promise. Proceedings of a workshop, October 15–17, 1990, Sponsored by the Office of the Director, National Institutes of Health, NIH Publication 93–3503, pp 65–80.

Wingate, A. L., & Lackey, N. R. (1989). A description of the needs of noninstitutionalized cancer patients and their primary care givers. *Cancer Nursing, 12*, 216–225.

Wingo, P. A., Tong, T., & Bolden, S. (1995). Cancer Statistics, 1995. *CA: A Cancer Journal for Clinicians, 45*(1), 8–30.

World Health Organization. (1993). *WHOQOL study protocol: The development of the World Health Organization Quality of Life assessment instrument.* Division of Mental Health, World Health Organization, MNH/PSF/93.9. Geneva, Switzerland.

Wyatt, G., Kurtz, M. E., & Liken, M. (1993). Breast cancer survivors: An exploration of quality of life issues. *Cancer Nursing, 16*(6), 440–448.

Supportive Care Services

Paul H. Coluzzi • Michelle Rhiner

Oncology care in the United States for decades has focused on the reversal, stabilization, or cure of the malignant disease process. Equally important during these aggressive, anticancer approaches is the relief of symptoms experienced by the patient. The palliation of symptoms associated with these regimens historically has often been overlooked or deemphasized.

Heightened awareness of our limited success in curing cancer coupled with our improved delivery of oncology services has refocused our attention on the relief of symptoms associated with both the active treatment and long-term care of patients with cancer (National Cancer Institute [NCI], 1990). The World Health Organization definition of palliative medicine "the active total care of patients whose disease is not responsive to curative treatment" (World Health Organization [WHO], 1990, p. 11) inherently creates conflict between the curative and the palliative universe. The future of American oncology care demands an integration of these two approaches.

Key to the conflict is the disease focus of American medicine. Physicians are trained to value the reversal of the malignant process as the overriding principle. Nursing models have balanced the focus between the disease process and the patient's personal experience, emphasizing the role of the nurse as a care provider for the patient's medical, psychosocial, and nursing needs. During this evolution of oncologic services, the nurse plays an important role in furthering the integration of palliative and curative strategies.

At present, the scope of palliative care services is poorly defined, with the actual services themselves ranging from pain and symptom management programs to wound care, psychosocial support systems, cancer rehabilitation, and terminal care services. For successful integration, not only must the scope of services be defined, but the proper language in which to describe these services must be established. This chapter attempts to define not only the evolution of these services but the current definition, integration, and scope of services impacting cancer nursing care, interdisciplinary assessment, and development of a plan of care.

EVOLUTION OF SUPPORTIVE CARE SERVICES

The evolution from the curative to the palliative care universe has been debated for many years. Most recently the World Health Organization focused attention on this potential conflict when in 1982 an expert panel on cancer pain relief in palliative care was convened (Schug, Zech, & Dorr, 1990; Takeda, 1986; Ventafridda, Tambunni, Caraleni, DeComno, & Naldi, 1987; Walker, Hoskin, Hanks, & White, 1988). The World Health Organization in describing the allocation of oncologic resources in the developed countries noted that 80 per cent of all resources allocated were to anticancer or curative treatments (Fig. 77–1). Cancer pain relief and palliative care, therefore, received only 20

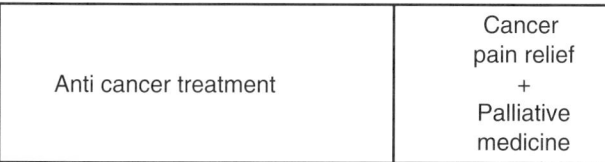

FIGURE 77–1. Oncology services: present allocation of resources. (Data from World Health Organization Expert Committee. [1990]. *Cancer pain relief and palliative care.* Geneva: WHO.)

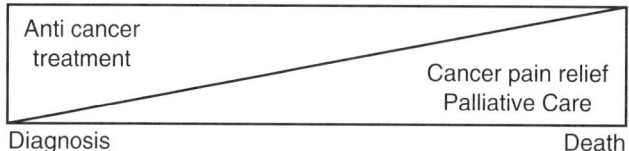

FIGURE 77–3. Oncology services: proposed allocation of resources. (Data from World Health Organization Expert Committee. [1990]. *Cancer pain relief and palliative care.* Geneva: WHO.)

per cent of those resources (WHO, 1990). Realizing that the age-adjusted mortality from cancer is 50 per cent in the United States, this allocation seems inappropriate. Considering that anticancer or curative treatments are more expensive and labor intensive than palliative care, this relative focus on curative therapies reflects our philosophic approach to oncologic care and the treatment of persons with life-threatening or life-limiting illnesses.

One model from Europe suggests that one third of our focus should be curative therapies, one third active palliation, and one third palliative care (MacDonald, 1993) (Fig. 77–2). In this model, palliative care becomes essentially those terminal care services known as hospice, and active palliation includes all those therapies for whom cure is not possible. Active symptomatic programs may include anticancer or therapeutic interventions. These interventions include chemotherapy, surgery, or radiotherapy for hematologic or solid malignancies.

The World Health Organization in its final recommendations very clearly stated that at diagnosis, anticancer treatment should be the focus of most of our care. At the same time, however, the relief of pain and other symptoms is essential. If the patient is expected to follow the continuum from diagnosis to death from their cancer, the focus on palliative care will increase as the focus on anticancer or curative therapies diminishes (Fig. 77–3). At present, the current practice of oncology in the United States suggests that anticancer treatments are offered when very little hope of response is expected. This approach often eliminates the possibility of emphasizing symptom relief. The integration of cancer pain relief and palliative care in the general oncologic model, therefore, is left unoffered to patients and families.

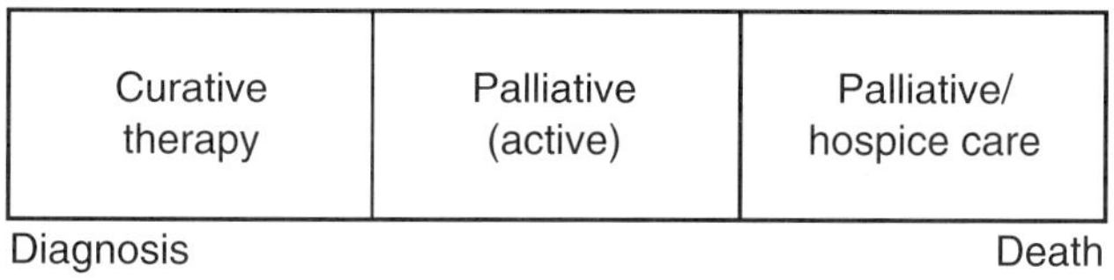

GOAL-ORIENTED ONCOLOGIC CARE

The paradigm shift that is required philosophically from the curative to palliative care universe is challenging today's health care professionals. This reform is problematic since over the decades technologic advances have allowed the cure of diseases that were never considered curable. For example, the introduction of antibiotics cured numerous infections previously considered fatal in the immunocompromised patient. The introduction of chemotherapies have now led to the induction of remission in Hodgkin's disease, non-Hodgkin's lymphoma, testicular carcinoma, and leukemia. Despite these advances the majority of illnesses that cause death of Americans, including diabetes, heart disease, neurologic illness, and cancer, essentially involve active palliation of the disease.

Palliation in the words of the World Health Organization is "the active total care of patients for whom cure is not possible" (WHO, 1990, p. 11). Philosophically, this definition is often inappropriately equated to "giving up" or not attempting to actively reverse or stabilize disease. What modern medical knowledge suggests, however, is that curative therapies and palliative therapies must coexist. Advancements in technology have focused on the disease process, not on patient's symptoms. The process of integration of these concepts is further clouded by the promise of a cure overriding the clinician's need to simply care for the patient. The professional must determine what the presenting symptoms mean, how they define a possible disease process through diagnostic studies, and ultimately develop a plan that focuses on the palliation of symptoms and possible reversal or cure of the disease process.

QUALITIES AND REDEFINITION OF PALLIATIVE CARE

The qualities embodying palliative care focus on maternalism or patient choice, collaboration, interdisciplinary approaches, holism, and a patient/family/system orientation. These factors contrast with the traditional scope of oncologic services, which include paternalism, or authoritarianism, single practitioner focus, traditional consultative services, and patient focus (Table 77–1). Other attributes often linked with palliative care include fringe, limitation, death, and hospice. Understanding the negative connotations of these synonyms for palliative care reiterates the importance for medical and nursing professionals to redefine this area of practice.

Curative therapy	Palliative (active)	Palliative/ hospice care

Diagnosis   Death

FIGURE 77–2. Oncology services: proposed allocation of resources. (Adapted from MacDonald, N. [1993]. Palliative care: The case for coordination. *Cancer Treatment Review, 19*[Suppl. A], 35.)

TABLE 77–1. *Unique Qualities: Supportive Care vs. Traditional Oncology Service*

SUPPORTIVE CARE	TRADITIONAL ONCOLOGY SERVICE
Patient's choice	Authoritarian
Interdisciplinary	Single practitioner
Collaborative	Traditional consultation
Holistic	Traditional Western medicine
Patient/family/system focused	Patient focused

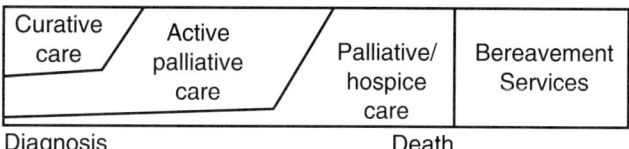

FIGURE 77–4. Goal oriented medical therapies—oncology. (From Coluzzi, P. H., Grant, M. M., Doroshow, J., Rhiner, M., Ferrell, B. F., & Rivera, L. [1995]. Survey of the provision of supportive care services at national cancer institute-designated cancer centers. *Journal of Clinical Oncology,* 13[3]. 756–764.)

Since nurturing, support, and patient/family focus cross both curative and noncurative boundaries, the term *supportive care* has in fact been suggested as an appropriate describer of these services. Supportive care is not linked with death or "giving up" but rather embodies those positive attributes listed above.

American oncologic practices must therefore provide direct care based on realistic goals set by the patient, family, and health care professionals once a comprehensive medical and psychosocial assessment and diagnosis have been established. The clinician should be clear as to the reversibility of disease and subsequently offer either curative, active palliation, or palliative/hospice care. The primary goals of curative therapy are reversal of the disease process and prolongation of life with the secondary goals of symptom control. Active palliation and hospice strategies focus goals not on the reversal of the disease process and the prolongation of life but rather to the control of symptoms. At the core of palliative/hospice strategies is the patient and family choice (Table 77–2 and Fig. 77–4).

TABLE 77–2. *Goals of Curative, Active Palliative, and Palliative/Hospice Care*

Curative
Primary
  Reversal of disease process
  Prolongation of life
Secondary
  Symptom control
  Clear delineation of goals/outcome of therapy

Active Palliative
Primary
  Clear delineation of goals/outcome of therapy
  Reversal of disease process
  Symptom control
Secondary
  Prolongation of life (possible)

Palliative/Hospice
Primary
  Clear delineation of goals/outcome of therapy
  Symptom control
  Psychosocial/medical/spiritual support
Secondary
  Prolongation of life (unlikely)

(From P. H. Coluzzi, personal communication, January, 1995.)

DEFINITION OF SUPPORTIVE CARE

The term *supportive care services* best describes a variety of services that are available to patients whether applied to curative or palliative modes of therapy. Supportive care services are those medical and psychosocial services that through education, research, and clinical service promote and enhance the quality of life for patients with cancer.

Supportive care has been applied in pediatric oncology to describe a variety of services, including the support of the patient with blood products, antibiotics for fever, and traditional palliative or symptom control programs. Supportive care also focuses on the whole person within their family system allowing for the inclusion of psychosocial programs.

Within the National Cancer Institute (NCI) designation, supportive care coexists with cancer rehabilitation and survivorship as defined by the Extramural Committee to Assess Measures of Progress Against Cancer. This committee developed a model by which to evaluate outcomes in oncology care related to research projects (Fig. 77–5). The schematic applies also to the clinical practice of American oncology. Pertinent to supportive care is a major emphasis on prevention, detection, diagnosis, and treatment management that includes rehabilitation, continuing care, and outcomes (including cancer death and noncancer death). Supportive care focuses on the concept of cancer control, which encompasses both prevention, detection, and management of symptoms. Supportive care programs, therefore, include a wide variety of clinical and research programs. The model suggests that compatible terminology to describe a similar scope of services is *cancer rehabilitation*. The purpose of cancer rehabilitation is to maximize the patient's quality of life by restoring physical and emotional well-being while understanding possible functional limitations (see Chapter 75).

PROVISIONS OF SUPPORTIVE CARE SERVICES IN THE UNITED STATES

Despite the NCI's direction, the exact scope of services has yet to be definitively established in the United States. In England, Addington-Hall and colleagues reported in a survey of 170 health districts the most

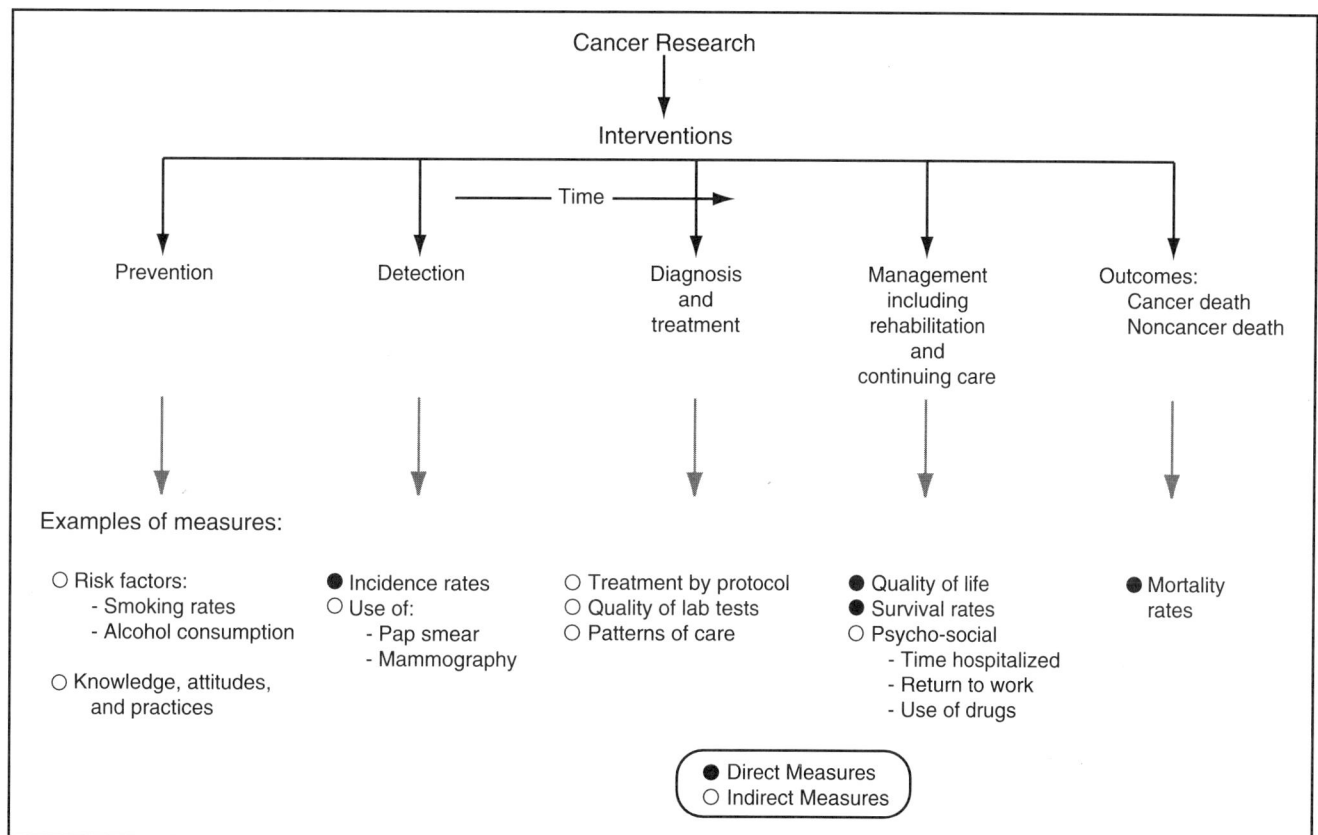

FIGURE 77–5. NCI conceptual model of cancer interventions and measures. (From Extramural Committee to Assess Measures of Progress Against Cancer. [1990]. Special report: Measurement of progress against cancer. *Journal of the National Cancer Institute, 82*(10), 825–835.)

commonly provided supportive care services were post-mastectomy and ostomy care for cancer patients. The authors concluded that psychosocial support and complementary therapies were offered sporadically and were often times, in the words of the authors, inadequate (Addington-Hall, Weir, Zollman, & McIllmurray, 1993; Smith, 1990).

In the United States, at NCI-designated cancer centers, supportive care services are provided in an uncoordinated, nonsystematic manner. A recent survey of NCI-designated cancer centers examined the provision of supportive care services at these institutions (Coluzzi et al., 1995). A 60-question survey was developed based on the survey conducted of British health districts and NCI-based criteria. The questionnaire contained 13 areas of interest including center characteristics, specific supportive care services, terminal illness management, personal image services, reconstructive surgery, emotional support/counseling, community programs, other supportive care services, spiritual care, educational services, research, survivor services, and funding sources.

Thirty-nine questionnaires were received for a total response rate of 75 per cent. Of the respondents, 17 (45 per cent) of 26 were from comprehensive cancer centers, 9 (24 per cent) of 11 were from clinical cancer centers, and 11 (29 per cent) of 15 were from P20 planning centers. One center did not identify their NCI des-

ignation. The number of beds dedicated to cancer care varied from 0 to 530. Hospital-based ambulatory care services were offered by 72 per cent of those responding. Sixty-eight per cent of centers offered day hospital services. The average number of visits per month in the outpatient setting varied from 120 to 3923 visits. Forty-seven per cent of the respondents offered a home care program. Radiation oncology was offered by 92 per cent of the respondents.

GENERAL SUPPORTIVE CARE SERVICES

The most frequently offered personal support services were dietary (95 per cent), ostomy care (84 per cent), rehabilitation including postmastectomy care (84 per cent), sexual counseling (74 per cent), and specialized pain management team (77 per cent). Sixteen per cent of the centers did not offer postmastectomy care or ostomy care. Twenty-three per cent did not offer sexual counseling, and 24 per cent did not have specialized cancer pain management services (Fig. 77–6).

CANCER PAIN MANAGEMENT

Of the 30 (77 per cent) centers offering specialized cancer pain management services, the number of team members varied from 2 to 22. One center identified their services as being part of a palliative care/supportive care program. The team most frequently consisted

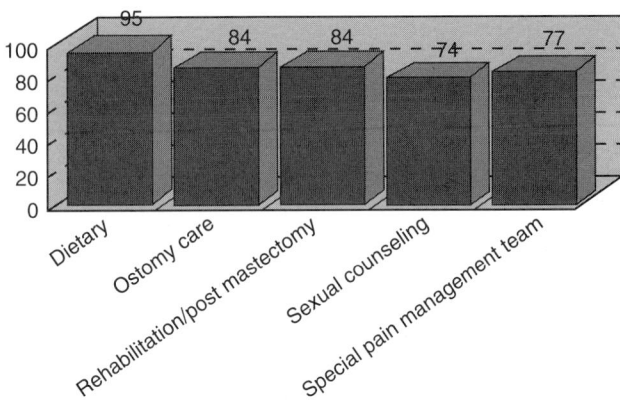

FIGURE 77–6. Supportive care services: most frequently offered services.

of anesthesiologists, nurses, and pharmacists (67 per cent, 67 per cent, and 49 per cent, respectively). Social workers, medical oncologists, and neurologists were the next most frequently found members of the team at 41 per cent, 39 per cent, and 26 per cent frequency. Chaplains were found only 10 per cent of the time and psychologists only 18 per cent of the time. Clinical nurse specialists were found on the teams only 49 per cent of the time. Unique pain clinics were offered 79 per cent of the time, with inpatient consultative services being offered 90 per cent of the time. Of those with specialized pain teams that specified a director, the most frequently identified chiefs of the program were anesthesiologists (8), followed by medical oncologists (2), neurologist (1), psychologist (1), and nurse (1) (Fig. 77–7).

Only 13 per cent of the pain management services had special funding. Sixty-two per cent of the institutions had written policies and procedures related to pain, and 82 per cent had written patient education materials related to pain management. Fifty per cent of the facilities performed quality assurance pain audits

with the frequency occurring from monthly to yearly. The symptoms of nausea and vomiting were identified as the most frequently formulated symptom management programs in these institutions (72 per cent and 74 per cent, respectively). Constipation, diarrhea, and depression had specialized treatment and management programs 53 per cent of the time (Fig. 77–8).

TERMINAL ILLNESS MANAGEMENT

The respondents identified Medicare-certified hospice as being available in 44 per cent of the institutions, with non–Medicare-certified hospice being available 11 per cent of the time. Hospice services were, therefore, not offered specifically by these institutions in 46 per cent of the instances.

SPECIAL IMAGES SERVICES AND RECONSTRUCTIVE SURGERIES

Development of prostheses was offered in 39 per cent of the institutions. Reconstructive surgery was offered in the areas of breast cancer 87 per cent of the time, head and neck cancer 77 per cent of the time, and general reconstructive surgery 80 per cent of the time.

EMOTIONAL SUPPORT COUNSELING

Emotional support counseling was provided through both in-house services and community services. Counseling was offered at the institutions primarily by masters-prepared social workers (84 per cent); in addition, nurses, psychologists, and psychiatrists provided the remainder of the counseling (85 per cent, 72 per cent, and 67 per cent). Collaborative efforts with other facilities, as evidenced by referrals to other centers, occurred 77 per cent of the time.

On-site support groups were offered by 90 per cent of the respondents. Additionally, 76 per cent of the facilities referred to outside programs for additional support. A range of topics was evident in the support groups, namely survivor programs, smoking cessation and prevention, bone marrow transplantation, newly diagnosed support groups for patients and families, breast and prostate cancer, and bereavement groups.

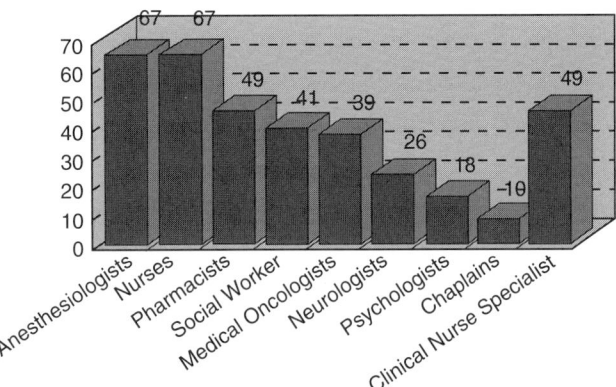

FIGURE 77–7. Cancer pain management team members. (Adapted from Coluzzi, P. H., Grant, M., Doroshow, J., Rhiner, M., Ferrell, B., & Rivera, L. [1995]. Survey of the provision of supportive care services at national cancer institute designated cancer centers. *Journal of Clinical Oncology, 13*[3], 756–764.)

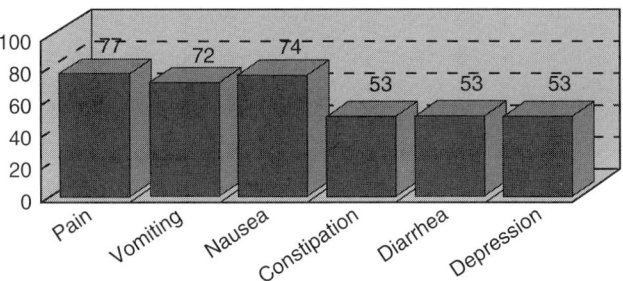

FIGURE 77–8. Symptom management programs offered. (Adapted from Coluzzi, P. H., Grant, M., Doroshow, J., Rhiner, M., Ferrell, B., & Rivera, L. [1995]. Survey of the provision of supportive care services at national cancer institute designated cancer centers. *Journal of Clinical Oncology, 13*[3], 756–764.)

The most frequently supported community programs included the American Cancer Society's "I Can Cope"(74 per cent) and "Reach to Recovery"(80 per cent) programs. Counseling to cancer survivors was offered by 68 per cent of the institutions, support groups by 63 per cent.

COMPLEMENTARY SERVICES

Other supportive care services were defined as those services felt to be complementary and adjunctive to the overall enhancement of quality of life. These nondrug strategies usually have direct application in symptom control. The most frequently offered services included relaxation/meditation (82 per cent), transcutaneous electrical nerve stimulation (76 per cent), and guided imagery (56 per cent). Hypnotherapy, music therapy, and art therapy were represented at lesser frequencies (46 per cent, 36 per cent, and 39 per cent). Heat/cold and massage were offered by less than one third of the centers (31 per cent and 26 per cent). The centers also identified special programs including child life specialists, therapeutic touch, humor carts, movie nights, and play therapy.

SPIRITUAL CARE

An actual department of spiritual care was established in 90 per cent of the facilities. The number of professional staff ranged from 1 to 25. The spiritual care departments were active in counseling, both on-site as well as on-call (85 per cent).

EDUCATIONAL SERVICES

Educational programs for the health care professional should include those programs that promote the specialized skills needed to practice in clinical oncology and include topics such as rehabilitation, pain management, psychosocial services, and quality of life considerations (NCI-Designated Comprehensive Cancer Center, 1992). Public information services should cooperate with existing cancer information services (CIS) to provide accurate information on cancer prevention, diagnosis, treatment, and rehabilitation (NCI, 1992). Educational services targeting professionals were offered by 97 per cent of the institutions; patient programs represented 89 per cent of the efforts, and community programs, 66 per cent.

RESEARCH

"A comprehensive cancer center fosters a strong clinical research program(s) which utilizes patient resources of the community . . . and which derives significant research support from external sources that were peer reviewed by the NIH standard" (NCI-Designated Comprehensive Cancer Center, 1992, p. 5). General research programs in supportive care were offered by 62 per cent of the institutions. The number of professional staff in these areas varied from 1 to 10. Outside funding was noted by 51 per cent of the respondents: 39 per cent of which was peer reviewed, and 28 per cent of which was from private industry. Fifty-one per cent did not respond to funding queries.

Although a wide range of services were provided, the frequency with which these services were provided varied. Pain is the most frequent symptom associated with palliative care, but surprisingly only 79 per cent of the time were pain management services offered by a dedicated interdisciplinary, collaborative team. Interestingly, on this team, medical oncologists were represented only 39 per cent of the time; however, nurses and advanced practitioners were represented the most frequently. A variety of other medical clinicians were represented, with psychosocial and spiritual support being minimal. This one study suggests that in the United States, the provision of these services needs further definition.

CORE OF SUPPORTIVE CARE SERVICES

INTERDISCIPLINARY ASSESSMENT

The core of supportive care is patient choice, collaboration, and interdisciplinary models. The term *interdisciplinary* reflects a multidisciplinary approach yet requires active interaction among the disciplines with consensus building. Operationally, both in nursing and medical models, this translates into the team concept. Team work has developed over the years, with hospice as the primary model in palliative care (Fig. 77–9). In these models the patient and family in their system are the focus, and an interdisciplinary collaborative group of health care professionals offers advice and direction. This team concept has been applied successfully to oncologic models as evidenced at traditional tumor board and multidisciplinary conferences. This team approach has been applied to the treatment of cancer patients experiencing pain and other symptomatology. The team approach allows for comprehensive assessment by multiple professionals, with recommendations being made to meet and complement the needs of the patient and family.

PATIENT/FAMILY EXPERIENCES: PAIN AS THE CLINICAL MODEL

Pain and other symptoms may be present to some degree throughout all phases of cancer treatment. Pain may be evident in upward of 50 per cent of patients in the early stages of cancer, and the incidence of moderate to severe pain increases to 80 per cent of patients with advanced cancer (Portenoy, 1989). The effect of pain on individuals has been studied extensively, demonstrating that patients do not suffer alone with their pain. Pain affects the patient's family and all other related systems (Ferrell, Rhiner, Cohen, & Grant, 1991). This phenomenon is apparent when the initial pain assessment and interview is conducted with the patient and family. Although the caregiver does not experience the physical pain of the patient, he or she expresses suffering based on several factors such as prior pain experiences, culture, relationship of the caregiver to the patient, meaning of pain, and understand-

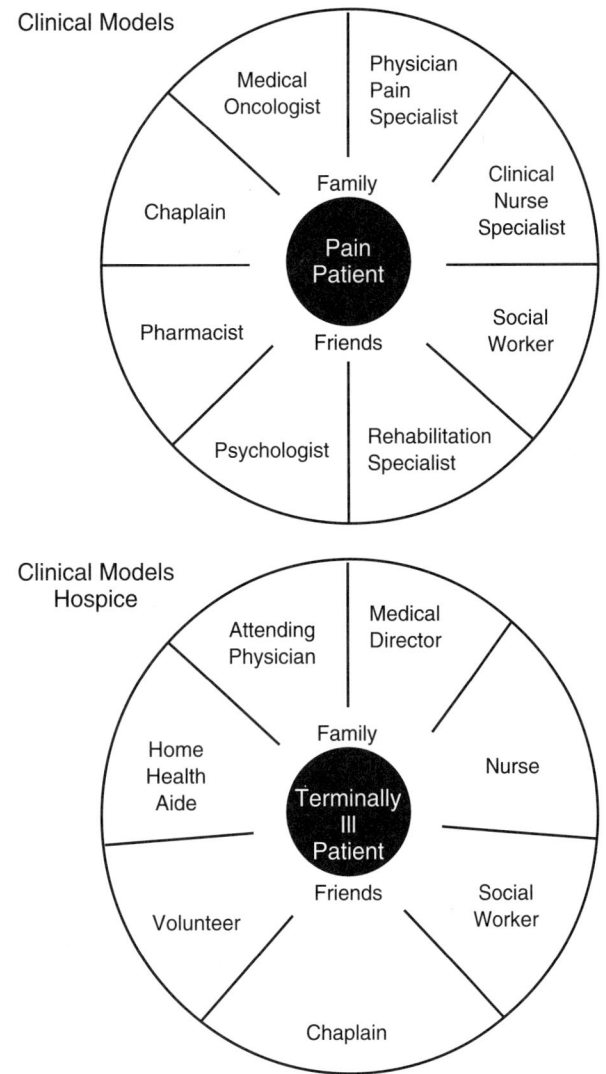

Clinical Models

Clinical Models
Hospice

FIGURE 77–9. Models of interdisciplinary approaches to care.

ing of the pain. These factors influence the expression of pain, which can be manifested as suffering, anxiety, depression, and caregiver burden (Ferrell, Cohen et al., 1991; Ferrell, Ferrell, Rhiner, & Grant, 1991; Ferrell, Rhiner et al., 1991). Despite the progress in diagnosis and treatment over the past six decades resulting in cures for more than 50 per cent of patients overall affected, individuals and their families still associate cancer with death. Since pain is associated with poor outcomes in most medical situations, especially cancer care, the association of pain with death is not surprising. The persistence of pain only serves to strengthen this metaphor. Patients and families often deny the presence of pain because pain is seen to mean the cancer is progressing and death is becoming more imminent (Ferrell, Rhiner et al., 1991).

The impact of cancer on the family has many dimensions including inherent physical and psychosocial burdens. Additionally, survival may come at the price of suffering chronic pain or side effects from curative therapy or surgeries. These experiences are a con-

stant reminder to the patient of the risk of recurrence, reinforcing the "sick role."

SUPPORTIVE CARE SERVICES THROUGHOUT THE PHASES OF CANCER

The trajectory of the cancer patient can be chronicled in five stages: (1) initial diagnosis, (2) treatment phase, (3) posttreatment reactions, (4) relapse, and (5) terminal phase (Biegel, Sales, & Schulz, 1991). Often patients experience distressing or painful symptoms that prompt them to seek professional advice. Experienced clinicians and practitioners will acknowledge that patients come to them with symptoms and rarely ever with a complaint such as "my cancer hurts." This phase of *initial diagnosis* is extremely stressful and emotionally charged with feelings of shock, fear, anger, and denial (Northouse, 1984). The patient may be required to endure painful diagnostic procedures such as biopsies, numerous venipunctures, and radical diagnostic surgeries. This phase is perceived by many as receiving the "death sentence," a time when meaning is being established, and potential causes (e.g., smoking) of the cancer are formulated, often adding to the person's self-blame. Patients will often avoid people, believing that the cancer may be contagious (Abrams, 1974; Kerson, 1985; Schnaper, Legg-McNamara, Dutcher, & Kellner, 1983). The opposite has also been found to exist in clinical practice, where social acquaintances or friends abandon the patient with cancer because of the feared contagion of cancer. The diagnosis of cancer is a threat to the family system due to the constant disruption of the family's normal routine and may contribute to the disintegration of the family at a time when integration is most vital for the patient's adjustment to the diagnosis and treatment (Bruhn, 1977; Johnson & Lane, 1991; Lewis, 1990). A psychosocial assessment at this phase will help to identify any underlying factors that could be barriers to the patient receiving the support needed at this time. Barriers such as coping strategies and economic difficulties can be identified and a supportive relationship can be established (Barg, Cooley, Pasacreta, Senay, & McCorkle, 1994).

The *treatment phase* is based on trust and hope. The patient places trust in the physician to know how to use the appropriate modalities to increase survival or to obtain a cure. These modalities may include chemotherapy and radiotherapy with their various local and systemic side effects such as fatigue, skin excoriation, wound dehiscence, and secondary pain from intractable nausea, vomiting, and diarrhea. The patient may struggle to maintain normalcy despite physical losses or deficits occurring from treatment. The patient also deals with physical disabilities or psychologic manifestations such as depression and anxiety that occur throughout this phase. Finally, there is often a decline in functional status, increasing the patient's fears of becoming a burden to their families. Nye (1976) identified eight different roles within the family system. Each member of the family is responsible for a certain number of these roles. When a family member is unable to perform his/her role, other members of the family must assume those roles. The degree to which a family adjusts to the change in roles depends on the availability and ability of other family members to perform the roles, external support, and resources for those assuming the new roles (Lewis, 1983; Nye, 1976). Nursing plays a vital role during this phase of the patient's treatment continuum to supply the information in minimizing and preventing the negative sequelae that often occurs (see Unit VIII regarding management of major nursing problems).

In the *posttreatment phase* the patient's adjustment to cancer and ability to cope are often directly proportional to prognosis and functional level. A person who has not suffered any permanent disability from the cancer treatment and is able to return to a normal lifestyle may still have a fear of cancer and its recurrence. For other patients, subsequent phases may involve pain and functional impairment from conditions such as chronic postthoracotomy syndrome, wound and dermal fibrosis, chronic abdominal adhesions, and phantom pain syndromes. Patients' priorities may change and life in general may be more precious when faced with a life-threatening situation (Ferell et al., 1992). Individuals challenged with permanent disabilities may have difficulty dealing with an altered self-image, changes in their family or work roles, and sexuality. If the family is resilient, there is an adaptation to the various role changes. As physical alterations and demands of the patient are made in the treatment phase, a transition is made from the precancer state to the new family identity (Germino, 1991). Rehabilitation aimed at minimizing disabilities and strengthening after long and arduous treatment regimens should be implemented. Mild stretching, strengthening exercises, the use of nondrug interventions such as heat, cold, massage, ultrasound, compression devices, and transcutaneous electrical nerve stimulation (TENS) for pain relief are measures used to support the patient during this phase.

If a *relapse* occurs, further disruption and feelings of helplessness may result. Communication between health care providers and patients may become guarded as patients realize that their cancer may not be controlled by medical intervention (Gotay, 1984). Depression, denial, and a withdrawal from family may result as patients face their own imminent mortality. Pain may be the most significant problem in this phase, and interventions should be aimed at its relief. If a rapport has been established with a clinician during the initial phase, issues related to an uncertain future, anticipatory grief, fear, anger, unpredictability of the disease, and limited availability of treatment options the family experiences can be moderated (Germino, 1991; Gotay, 1984; Woods, Lewis, & Ellison, 1989).

The *terminal phase* is marked by an increasing loss of independence and increase in dependence on family members. Pain syndromes such as tumor compression, extensive bony metastases, and hepatic distension are among the most painful experiences (Portenoy, 1990). Treatment may focus primarily on pain, and supportive care to the family is imperative. The patient's withdrawal from the family that began in the relapse phase may continue, causing the family to feel rejected and unable to comfort the patient (Germino, 1987). The family's concerns are focused on management of side effects, the patient's decreased mobility, death, and the emotional demands of the other family members (Germino, 1991; Gotay, 1984; Lewis, 1990). This is the phase most closely identified with supportive care. It is at this time an interdisciplinary approach is recognized as being vital in providing the symptom management and psychosocial support required at this stage.

The psychosocial reactions of the family (e.g., anxiety, fear, depression, stress) to the different stages of disease are similar to the patient's reactions, except in the terminal phase when the caregiver's stress, anxiety, and psychosocial reactions may exceed the patient's levels (Biegel et al., 1991).

DEVELOPMENT OF A PLAN OF CARE

To provide the patient and family with supportive care services, a plan of care must be initiated based on six steps.

STEP 1—OBTAIN A COMPREHENSIVE INTERDISCIPLINARY ASSESSMENT

An interdisciplinary assessment from all members of the supportive care team is crucial to understanding the patient experience with disease and the subsequent treatment of symptoms. Experts in the area of pain have written extensively on the multiple approaches used to elicit an accurate description of cancer pain (Cleeland, 1984; Foley, 1989; McCaffery, 1979; McGuire, 1992; Melzack & Wall, 1982; Payne, 1989). Similar rating scales have been developed to help assess and communicate other symptoms (Bruera, 1991). Quantification of pain using an objective pain rating scale is now a necessity; however, the personal, unique experience of pain cannot always be measured using rating scales. Experienced health care professionals learn from cancer patients that pain affects all dimensions of their physical, psychologic, social, and spiritual lives, or in essence their overall quality of life.

PAIN AND SYMPTOM INTERVIEWS

In the conventional interview with the patient, spouse, or surrogate, the physician or nurse learns the true impact of pain and other symptoms. To gain the most information, the clinician should listen after asking simple questions regarding pain. For example, open-ended questions such as "Describe the meaning of the pain you're experiencing now," or "Describe your mood" will reveal valuable information to the listener. Patients invariably describe fear, interruption in daily routine, anxiety, or depression. The fear of cancer and the treatment seems secondary to these expressions of suffering. To be effective, the clinician must be willing to be available often by simply being present and supportive to deal with tears, silence, anger, or hostility. If the patient and family can feel safe in the relationship, the more likely an appropriate intervention can be identified and family adaptation enhanced.

In addition to a pain assessment, a psychosocial assessment by the clinicians or a social worker is recommended. It should include (1) the patient's overall appearance and behavior, (2) financial considerations, (3) social support, (4) activities of daily living, (5) emotional concerns, and (6) coping strategies, including spiritual beliefs or concerns. The authors use a comprehensive psychosocial assessment form developed at City of Hope to address these concerns; the form is administered by the clinical social worker on the interdisciplinary pain team. (Readers can obtain the form by writing the May Day Pain Resource Center, City of Hope National Medical Center, 1500 East Duarte Road, Duarte, CA 91010.)

This focused interview will often illuminate conflicting goals and concerns between patient and family. The family caregiver is also interviewed to obtain a better picture of the impact the cancer is having on the family system. The information elicited from the comprehensive nursing and psychosocial assessment is discussed at the interdisciplinary pain team meeting. The members from the various disciplines provide input on how to respond to and resolve the issues identified. Through clinical practice and research, the authors have identified the following steps that should be taken by the health care team before, during, and after formulating a treatment plan.

STEP 2—DETERMINE PATIENT/FAMILY GOALS

An understanding of the patient's disease and its course is crucial in establishing a treatment plan. Once this understanding is established, the patient is then able to develop goals. The family's objectives should be explored, as they may differ from the patient's desires. The collaboration of the entire team of physicians, nurses, social workers, and chaplains is tantamount at the initial steps of contemporary supportive care. The establishment of goals is vital to an enduring relationship among the team, the patient, and the family.

STEP 3—ADDRESS DIFFICULT ISSUES EARLY

Experienced cancer care and pain specialists know that avoiding troublesome topics can be dangerous to the establishment of a lasting therapeutic relationship. The one dimension that should always be discussed with the patient and family is the issue of depression and suicidal ideation. Many patients with chronic cancer pain are currently or may become depressed. This depression may be in response to the pain or other symptoms or the psychologic association of pain with serious illness. Introduction of the topic in a caring and supportive manner will allow crucial clinical data to be obtained. Open-ended questions such as "How is the pain affecting you and your family" or "Please describe your mood" can lead to a rich discussion of the

patient's mood and reveal therapeutic avenues. Occasionally, patients may feel suicidal obligation because of the perception that they have become a costly, unnecessary burden to the family.

To determine the impact of pain and other symptoms on the patient within the family system, the health care professional should ask the same question of the patient's family. Divergent answers are common. Inherent in the same line of questioning should be a direct assessment of suicidal potential. Strong suicidal ideation is usually a result of severe depression and a sense of hopelessness, isolation, and frustration. Candid discussions with patient and family will allow the health care professional to adequately assess the suicidal or depressive origins and motivation and intervene appropriately. As with any severely depressed or suicidal patient, involvement of a psychiatrist or appropriate mental health professional is imperative when establishing a contract to prevent personal harm. It is important to remember, however, that this referral to the psychiatrist or mental health professional is made as an adjunct to treatment and that pain control remains a priority in the patient's plan of care. Although possibly difficult and uncomfortable for those involved, the establishment of this caring and supportive relationship is critical.

STEP 4—ASSESS FAMILY DYNAMICS AND POTENTIAL BARRIERS TO PROPER PAIN CONTROL

When assessing a patient's cancer symptoms, clinicians are often forced to determine the essence of the patient's needs in an artificial setting, e.g., the hospital or physician's office. A variety of dynamics are established in this environment that are false and often hinder correct treatment planning. For example, when considering family interactions, this problem is particularly evident. Although home visits may not always be possible, the clinician must strive to include the patient's family in the initial interview to establish ground rules and emphasize that the patient will be treated in a comprehensive manner, which includes the patient's family. This approach gives the clinician a clearer picture of the potential challenges that lie ahead.

STEP 5—ASSESS THE HOME ENVIRONMENT

In the hospital environment, virtually all therapies discussed can be provided safely. This is not the case, however, in the home setting. Unless an assessment of the patient's home is made and the resources identified for continued care, the health care provider can unwittingly compromise a patient's safety. A basic understanding of home conditions will allow the clinician to determine whether certain therapies can be used. For example, a person who lives in a suboptimal, unsafe home or who has no primary caregiver will be a poor candidate for intravenous, subcutaneous, or epidural infusions of analgesics. Unreliable caregivers or family members may lead to the isolation of a patient and compromised care.

Another concern is that of divergent spiritual beliefs within the same family. In these instances, the potential for nonsupport of the medical plan is great. Such conflicts add to the many existing barriers to pain and symptom management (e.g., physician and patient lack of knowledge regarding pain control) and underscore the need to assess special attributes and dynamics of each family. Failing to assess the meaning of the cancer experience to the patient and family and the family dynamics before a therapeutic plan is developed would be negligent. The best collaborative efforts must therefore always be comprehensive in nature.

STEP 6—IMPLEMENT A PATIENT/FAMILY PAIN EDUCATION PROGRAM

An educational plan based on patient and family needs is important. Educational interventions can be classified into three categories: (1) cognitive information only, (2) cognitive information or behavioral management skill or both, and (3) self-enhancement or behavioral management skills or both (Biegel et al., 1991). Clinical experience indicates that families require information specific to their loved one's care that will answer questions concerning specific symptom management (rationale as to why the symptom is occurring and how to manage the symptom), instructions necessary to provide the physical care of the patient, and information regarding community resources and respite assistance. Educational interventions that address the specific needs of the patients and caregivers are useful in increasing knowledge and skills and are generally helpful in relieving caregiver stress and burden (Lovett & Gallagher, 1988; Pohl, 1980).

SUMMARY

Patients require support throughout the continuum of a cancer treatment. Supportive care services clarify the curative and palliative universe, offering goal-oriented, patient/family-focused care. These services address the symptoms patients and their families experience throughout the trajectory of the cancer illness, whether the symptoms are manifested either physiologically or psychosocially. The introduction of an inter disciplinary team approach provides a comprehensive framework for assessment and planning. The provision of these services varies from one health care setting to another. Understanding of the importance of multidimensional symptom control will guide efforts to standardize programs both regionally and nationally.

REFERENCES

Abrams, R. (1974). *Not alone with cancer*. Springfield, IL: Charles C. Thomas.

Addington-Hall, J. M., Weir, M. W., Zollman, C. & McIllmurray, M. B. (1993). A national survey of the provision of support services for people with cancer. *British Medical Journal, 304,* 1649–50.

Barg, F. K., Cooley, M., Pasacreta, J., Senay, B., & McCorkle, R. (1994). Development of a self-administered psychosocial cancer screening tool. *Cancer Practice, 2*(4), 288–296.

Biegel, D. E., Sales, E., Schulz, R. (1991). Caregiving in cancer. *Family Caregiving in Chronic Illness, 1,* 62–104.

Bruera, E. (1991). The Edmonton symptom assessment system: A simple method of assessment of palliative care patients. *Journal of Palliative Care, 7*(2), 6–9.

Bruhn, J. G. (1977). Effects of chronic illness on the family. *Journal of Family Practice, 4,* 1057–1060.

Cleeland, C. S. (1984). The impact of pain on the patient with cancer. *Cancer, 54,* 2635–2641.

Coluzzi, P. H., Grant, M. M., Doroshow, J., Rhiner, M., Ferrell, B. F., & Rivera, L. (1995). Survey of the provision of supportive care services at National Cancer Institute-designated cancer centers. *Journal of Clinical Oncology, 13*(3), 756–764.

Ferrell, B. R, Cohen, M. Z., Rhiner, M. et al. (1991). Pain as a metaphor for illness. Part II: Family caregivers' management of pain. *Oncology Nursing Forum, 18,* 1315–1321.

Ferrell, B. R., Ferrell, B., Rhiner, M., & Grant, M. (1991). Family factors influencing cancer pain. *Postgraduate Medical Journal, 67*(Suppl. 2), S64–S69.

Ferrell, B., Grant, M., Schmidt, G., Rhiner, M., Whitehead, C., Fonbuena, P., & Forman, S. (1992). The meaning of quality of life for bone marrow transplant survivors. Part I: The impact of bone marrow transplant on quality of life. *Cancer Nursing, 15,* 153–160.

Ferrell, B. R., Rhiner, M., Cohen, M. Z., & Grant, M. M. (1991). Pain as a metaphor for illness. Part I: Impact of cancer pain on family caregivers. *Oncology Nursing Forum, 18,* 1303–1309.

Foley, K. M. (1989). The treatment of cancer pain. *New England Journal of Medicine, 313,* 84–95.

Germino, B. (1991). Cancer and the family. In S. Baird, R. McCorkle, & M. Grant (Eds.), *Cancer nursing* (pp. 38–44). Philadelphia: W. B. Saunders Co.

Gotay, C.C. (1984). The experience of cancer during early and advanced stages: The view of patient and their mates. *Social Science and Medicine, 18,* 605–613.

Johnson, J. L., & Lane, C. A. (1991). Helping families respond to cancer. In S. Baird, R. McCorkle, & M. Grant (Eds.), *Cancer nursing.* (pp. 921–931). Philadelphia: W. B. Saunders Co.

Kerson, T. S. (1985). Cancer. In D. Turk & R. Kerns (Eds.), *Health, illness and families: A life space perspective* (pp. 338–353). New York: John Wiley.

Lewis, F. M. (1983). Family level services for the cancer patient: Critical distinctions, fallacies and assessment. *Cancer Nursing, 6,* 193–199.

Lewis, F. M. (1990). Strengthening family supports: Cancer and the family. *Cancer, 65,* 752–759.

Lovett, S., & Gallagher, D. (1988). Psychoeducational interventions for family caregivers: Preliminary efficacy data. *Behavior Therapy, 19,* 321–330.

MacDonald, N. (1993). Oncology and palliative care: The case for coordination. *Cancer Treatment Review, 19* (Suppl.A), 29–41.

McCaffery, M. (1979). *Nursing management of the patient in pain*. New York: J. B. Lippincott Co.

McGuire, D. B. (1987). The multidimensional phenomenon of cancer pain. In D. B. McGuire & C. H. Yarbro (Eds.), *Cancer pain management* (pp. 1–20). Orlando, FL: Grune & Stratton.

McQuire, D. B. (1992). Comprehensive and multidimensional assessment and measurement of pain. *Journal of Symptom Management, 7,* 312–319.

Melzack, R., & Wall, P. D. (1982). *The challenge of pain.* (pp. 9, 71, & 235). New York: Basic Books.

National Cancer Institute Extramural Committee To Assess Measures of Progress Against Pain. (1990). Special report: Measurement of progress against cancer. *Journal of the National Cancer Institute, 82*(10), 825–835.

National Cancer Institute-Designated Comprehensive Cancer Center. (1992). Guidelines. Baltimore: National Cancer Institute, National Institutes of Health, & Department of Health and Human Services.

Northouse, L. (1984). The impact of cancer on the family: An overview. *International Journal of Psychiatry in Medicine, 14,* 215–242.

Nye, P. Z. (1976). *Role structure and analysis of the family.* Beverly Hills, CA: Sage Publications.

Payne, R. (1989). Cancer pain: Anatomy, physiology and pharmacology. *Cancer, 63,* 2266–2274.

Pohl, C. R. (1980). The "WTL" model of cancer care. *Journal of Religion and Health, 19,* 3304–312.

Portenoy, R. K. (1989). Cancer pain: Epidemiology and syndromes. *Cancer, 63,* 2298–2307.

Portenoy, R. K. (1990) The management of cancer pain. *Comprehensive Therapy, 16,* 53–65.

Schnaper, N., Legg-McNamara, C., Dutcher, J., & Kellner, T. (1983). Emotional support of the patient and his survivors. In P. H. Wiernik (Ed.), *Supportive care of the cancer patient* (pp. 1–15). Mt. Kisco, NY: Futura Publishing.

Schug, S. A., Zech, D., & Dorr, U. (1990). Cancer pain management according to WHO analgesia guidelines. *Journal of Pain and Symptom Mangement, 5*(1), 27–32.

Smith, T. (1990). Cancer services. *British Medical Journal, 301,* 1406–1407.

Takeda, F. (1986). Results of field testing in Japan of the WHO draft interim guidelines on relief of cancer pain. *The Pain Clinic, 1,* 83–89.

Ventafridda, V., Tambunni, M., Caraleni, A., DeComno, F., & Naldi, F. (1987). A validation study of the WHO method for cancer pain relief. *Cancer, 59,* 851–856.

Walker, V. A., Hoskin, P. J., Hanks, G. W., & White, I. D. (1988). Evaluation of WHO analgesic guidelines for cancer pain in a hospital-based palliative care unit. *Journal of Pain and Symptom Management, 3,* 145–149.

Woods, N. F., Lewis, F. M., & Ellison, E. S. (1989). Living with cancer: Family experiences. *Cancer Nursing, 12,* 28–33.

World Health Organization Expert Committee. (1990). *Cancer pain relief and palliative care.* Geneva: World Health Organization.

Hospice Services: The Place of Hospice Care in Cancer Treatment

Madalon Amenta

HISTORY OF THE HOSPICE MOVEMENT IN THE UNITED STATES

EXPANSION OF TECHNOLOGY AND DENIAL OF DEATH

During the period that began shortly after the end of World War II until the late 1960s, there was a pervasive taboo against open acknowledgment of death in health care settings in the United States and Great Britain. Caregiving staff at all levels set the tone of denial, and patients and families went along by never mentioning what research was beginning to document: the point at which everyone knew that there was no realistic hope that the patient would recover or live much longer (Fiefel, 1959; Foster, Wald, & Wald, 1978; Glaser & Strauss, 1965; Hinton, 1965; Kalish & Reynolds, 1976; Kubler-Ross, 1971; Wald, 1981).

While conducting a nationwide study of health care institutions and of education of nursing and medical students, Brown (1978) was stunned to find that the word *death* was almost never used. She found patients who had received mechanical life support for many days characterized as "doing poorly." When patients finally died, it was said they had "expired" or "passed on." She noted also that the word *cancer* was never used in direct interaction with patients and families.

During this period, the overriding objective of care was the application of high-technology "heroic" invasive measures to maintain physical function. This maintenance of biologic life was regarded by physicians not only as their professional obligation but also evidence of their skill. The organizing principle of nursing care was the monitoring of machines, tubes, lines, and wires and the meticulous documentation of laboratory, pharmacologic, and radiologic data. "The patient as a person" was a concept taught in schools of nursing, but one that was rarely observed in the real world of practice. Furthermore, dying patients who were not receiving mechanical life support tended to be neglected outright (Kastenbaum & Aisenberg, 1972; Quint, 1967) (Box 78–1).

The emotional, social, and financial implications of this "treat always and at any cost" philosophy were never questioned or examined. Patients and families were not regarded as people with significant needs other than medical, nor were their personally held values or the quality of their lives ever considered. Visiting hours were brief and rigidly maintained. When professionals knew patients' families at all, they knew them by sight and treated them formally and at best politely as guests, not as integral parts of the patient's life and recovery process.

Because the apparatus was more important than anything else in the caregiving mix, visiting family and friends were shooed out of the room to wait in the hall when a crisis did occur. Behind the closed door, the staff, unencumbered by the presence of laypersons, worked on both the apparatus and the patient. "When the miracle-working technology failed, the families were on their own. They signed the necessary forms, took the deceased's belongings, and left as quickly as possible. The modern hospital got right on with its proper function—curing" (Amenta & Bohnet, 1986, p. 2).

THE 1960s AND SOCIAL CHANGE

By the mid-1960s, however, the social climate of the United States began to change. Antiauthoritarianism in the form of social protest found expression in the civil rights movement, women's liberation activity, and protest against the Vietnam War. The major themes and subliminal messages of these causes, thanks largely to television, spread throughout all socioeconomic levels of society.

The new antiauthoritarianism expressed itself in the health care sector as antiscience. People began to question the value of the application of an all-out life-saving technology in every instance, and they came to challenge the validity of physician-dominated policies in the organization of health care. Natural foods and natural remedies gained new interest and popularity. The option for natural or anesthesia-free childbirth became widely available also. The American Hospital Association began to take a formal interest in patients' rights, and new organizations such as the Society of Health and Human Values (Amenta & Bohnet, 1986) and the Hastings Institute, which studies emerging biomedical ethical issues, were founded.

The ancient common law precept of a person's primacy in the right to make decisions about his or her body was prominently revived with the women's movement's insistence that women be allowed to control their own bodies, especially in the area of reproductive health. New self-help groups like Make Today Count and Widow to Widow came into being. Awareness of the right to and the presumed healthiness of free and authentic communication was gaining ground at the same time that social science research was validating the need and desire of dying patients and families to be able to talk frankly about death and, later, bereavement (Fiefel, 1959; Raphael, 1977) (Box 78–2).

EVOLUTION OF A SCIENCE OF PALLIATIVE CARE

In the United States where much of the research on attitudes about death, dying, bereavement, pain control, and effective communication techniques was being

---

BOX 78–1. *Nursing Research Note*

Quint, J. (1967). *The nurse and the dying patient.* New York: Macmillan.

As an outgrowth of her work with B. Glaser and A. Strauss on a larger study of how hospital personnel gave care to dying patients (funded by a Public Health Service Grant from the Division of Nursing), the author concentrated on nursing education to discover what formal preparation students received in the care of the dying. She was concerned particularly with communication skills in relation to the dying process.

Some of the research questions included the following:

- What are nursing students taught about death?
- In the course of the curricular progression, when is the material taught?
- What situations with dying patients give the students satisfaction?
- What situations with dying patients cause them difficulty?

Starting in 1961, data were collected from five schools of nursing in the San Francisco Bay area. One was a university school with both graduate and undergraduate programs. The other four were hospital schools selected for diversity of locale, organizational pattern, and type of facility.

Results indicated that nursing students (and by extension, graduates) found it difficult under most circumstances to communicate meaningfully with dying patients and their families. Only when the patient had already come to terms with death or was very old or when the student could assure the patient that she or he would die easily, did the students find it professionally satisfying or less difficult.

The author recommended increased work in the specifics of psychosocial support and communication skills in all elements of the curriculum. She particularly urged planned and organized faculty attention to and amplified and deepened student experiences in the care of the terminally ill.

Box 78–2. *Research Note*

Raphael, B. (1977). Preventive intervention with the recently bereaved. *Archives of General Psychiatry, 34*, 1450–1454.

Nonselected widows in a large urban area were contacted in the early weeks following their husbands' deaths and assessed for risk of poor bereavement outcome. In addition to a description of the course of the bereavement thus far, the semistructured, nondirective interview sought information about level of risk in terms of the preexisting relationship with the husband, the circumstances of the death, the presence of concurrent crises, and the griever's perception of availability of social support. Those who either ranked high on perception of nonsupportiveness of the social network or ranked somewhat lower but high on the other characteristics were considered to be at high risk. They were randomly assigned to intervention and nonintervention control groups.

The intervention consisted of supportive counseling that averaged four sessions of about 2 hours in each widow's home. The goals of the counseling were encouragement of the expression of grief, promotion of mourning, and direct discussion of the specific areas of risk for the particular widow. Interviews were recorded and rated by an independent evaluator for level of goal achievement. All subjects were contacted 13 months later and reevaluated on general health and adjustment dimensions.

At follow-up the high-risk subjects in the treatment group were significantly more likely to have had a good outcome than those who were not visited. Those at risk in the nontreatment group were worse off in terms of the health and adjustment scores than the non–high-risk control subjects, whereas the health of the intervention group approximated that of the non–high-risk subjects. Among the treatment subjects, those who had the highest scores for perception of lack of a supportive network were especially likely to have benefited from the intervention.

---

conducted, a body of knowledge was developing slowly about palliative—comforting, not curing—care. A persistent and growing concern with human and social values accompanied the increasing awareness that the organization of health care had a direct influence on patient outcomes. In addition, it was becoming apparent that to make organizational changes, caregivers themselves had to change their attitudes.

QUESTIONS OF COST OF CARE VS. QUALITY OF LIFE

In the meantime, the costs of care due to continuing advances in technology were escalating rapidly. A trend toward high costs of care in conventional settings, notably in the last year of life, first identified in studies published in the early 1970s, was solidly confirmed by later research (Mor & Masterson-Allen, 1987). Health care economists began to question the value of this highly intensive care in relation to quality of life, especially for very elderly people.

INFLUENCE OF SAUNDERS AND KUBLER-ROSS

In London during these years, Saunders was developing an organizational model of humane care for the dying (DuBoulay, 1984). Her synthesis of modern pharmacology to ease the pain of terminal illness with the historical religious-hospice functions of fastidious personal care, companionship, and spiritual support is generally accepted as the theoretic basis of modern hospice care. St. Christopher's, founded in 1967, is an inpatient facility with a homelike atmosphere where visiting schedules are flexible and families and patients are treated holistically and compassionately.

During the 1960s in the United States, Dr. Elisabeth Kubler-Ross's work with dying patients resulted in her assertion that coping with death and dying can take place only in a climate that encourages and supports open communication. Her book, *On Death and Dying*, published in 1969, fostered a disseminated general interest in the subject.

In the 1960s both Kubler-Ross and Saunders spoke at seminars at Yale University, where a small group of clergy, nurses, physicians, students, and concerned laypeople were discussing the issues of mechanically and bureaucratically controlled death and dying. As a result of these sessions, the dean of the Yale School of Nursing, along with others, visited St. Christopher's to get a grounding in its organization and clinical practice.

At St. Christopher's, Saunders was applying her theory that treating the whole person, rather than just the disease or the physical pain, brings beneficial results (DuBoulay, 1984). She and her staff had learned that pain is not just physical but emotional, spiritual, and economic as well. By paying attention to the treatment of these other domains in a patient's and family's life, they found that the intensity of the patient's physical pain was often decreased. Over and over again, they were able to demonstrate that if patients perceived themselves to be heard and understood, physical pain was diminished.

SAUNDERS AND THE REGULAR GIVING OF PAIN MEDICATION

The sensitively balanced and highly sophisticated pharmacologic pain control techniques developed by Saunders in her earlier research were also being systematically applied. Part of Saunders' innovative contribution to modern medicine was the regular giving of pain medication that she had observed during her student days in a nursing home. This system strives for prescribed medications, in whatever dosage or combination, to be given whenever possible by mouth on a regular schedule that anticipates the reemergence of pain. If the patient requires 60 or 90 mg morphine every 2 hours because the pain has been documented to "bleed through" the analgesia barrier every 2 hours and 15 minutes, the patient gets it. Because this eliminates the anticipatory anxiety that enhances physical pain, the patient remains pain free.

FIRST AMERICAN HOSPICE

Soon after visiting St. Christopher's, some of the New Haven study group, with the help of a small grant from the National Cancer Institute, mounted a demonstration of what the new system of care could accomplish (Brown, 1978). Although home care was not the emphasis of the St. Christopher's model, it became the most reasonable setting for the Connecticut project because no available physical structure would meet state building code standards as an inpatient facility and also because there was no category in the licensure and reimbursement structures for hospice care. So in November 1971, Hospice, Inc. was incorporated as an independent, nonprofit organization to provide hospice services as a supplement to the services provided by home health agencies and hospitals. Still later, in 1974, when a building was being planned, the organization changed its name to Connecticut Hospice, Inc., and in the fall of 1979 it opened its new 44-bed facility (Amenta & Bohnet, 1986).

In 1975 the second hospice program in the United States, the Hospice at St. Luke's, St. Luke's-Roosevelt Hospital in New York City, began offering services. This program, too, although housed in an acute care hospital, devised another uniquely American hospice care organizational variation, the scatter bed consultation model. Soon hospice planning groups sprang up all over the country, and the growth in the number of new operational hospices has been steady (Fig. 78–1).

In fact, hospice care remains one of the most rapidly growing segments of the health care system ("NHO Reports," 1988).

CHARACTERISTICS OF THE MODERN AMERICAN HOSPICE

PHILOSOPHY

The contemporary American hospice—with several elements of care that distinguish it from traditional care—is an array of services rooted in a holistic health care philosophy of living, dying, and living while dying (Amenta & Bohnet, 1986). It is a concept that unites treatment of terminally ill patients and their families, taken together as the unit of care, with modern science, belief, and caring. Its goal is the prolongation of meaningful life as the patient and family define it, not physiologic dying. As a general rule—and there are always exceptions in hospice care—no "active curative" measures or invasive diagnostic procedures are employed except for palliative or comfort-inducing reasons. For example, both radiation and chemotherapy may be used, not only for reduction of tumor size, but also for control of pain.

PROGRAM ELEMENTS

PAIN AND SYMPTOM CONTROL

The overall objective of pain and symptom control in hospice care is the balance of the potential side effects of palliative therapeutic treatments with the maintenance of an alert state in the patient. Ideally, patients should be as much like themselves as feasible so that they can be in control of as much of the remaining time and as many of the remaining choices as possible.

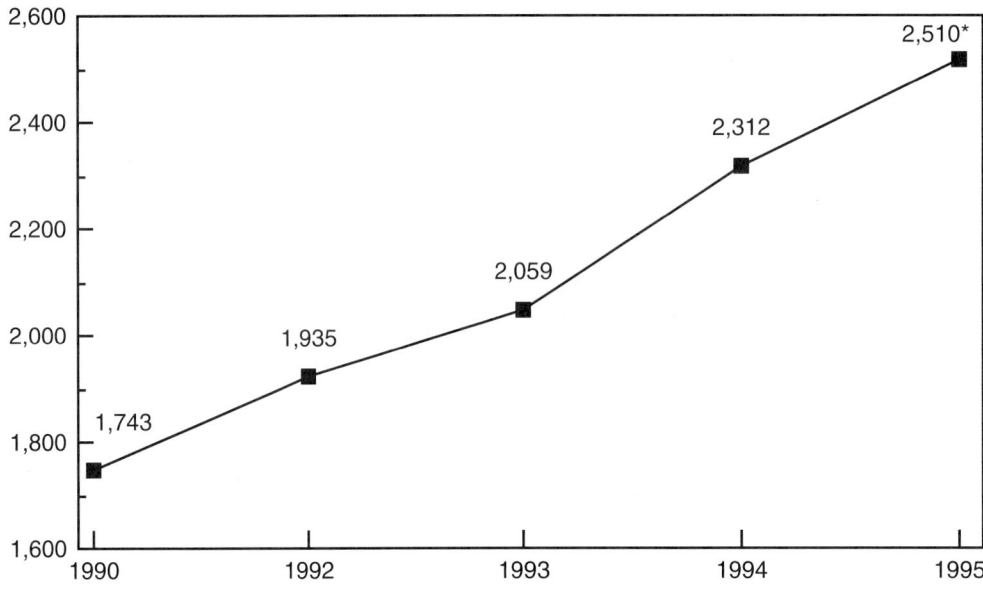

FIGURE 78–1. Hospice growth in the United States, 1990–1995. (Copyright 1995, National Hospice Organization. All rights reserved.)

SPIRITUAL SUPPORT

A strong emphasis on spiritual support, individualized to meet patient and family need, is another prominent characteristic of hospice care (Amenta & Bohnet, 1986). As patients and their families approach death in an open and forthright way in a freely communicating atmosphere, they should have the opportunity to examine the dimensions of meaning, relatedness, forgiveness, and transcendence if they wish, whether or not they are conventionally religious (Box 78–3).

HOME CARE, INPATIENT CARE, AND BEREAVEMENT SUPPORT

Hospice services are available in the home or inpatient facility when needed either for stabilization of symptoms, development of pain control regimens, or for brief periods of respite for the primary caregiver. In addition to home and inpatient care, all bona fide hospice organizations must offer bereavement support on a regular basis not only to selected, usually high-risk individual survivors, but also to the entire family. In 1992, 69 per cent of hospice families accepted bereavement services ("NHO Newsline," 1993).

In the 1992 National Hospice Organization (NHO) census, 81 per cent of responding hospices claimed to be providing bereavement support services not only to their hospice patient families, but to the wider community, as well. Eighty per cent of that group conducted bereavement groups, 63 per cent presented educational programs, 60 per cent offered individual and family counseling, 43 per cent offered crisis counseling, 35 per cent presented programs for children, and 15 per cent offered emergency room support ("NHO Newsline," 1993).

INTERDISCIPLINARY TEAM

All the above-mentioned services are provided by an interdisciplinary team of nurses, physicians, social workers, counselors and other therapists, clergy, and volunteers.

VOLUNTEERS

Volunteers play a major role in this country in the administration and delivery of all aspects of hospice care. Often bereavement components are completely managed by volunteers. Data compiled by the NHO 1992 census showed the average number of volunteers per hospice program in the United States was 50 ("NHO Newsline," 1993), with these volunteers contributing approximately 5.25 million service hours during the year.

STAFF STRESS AND STAFF SUPPORT

Another hallmark of hospice care is support for staff to help them deal with the work-related stress many of them experience. Although some of the stress may be due to the wearing effect of losing one patient after another to death, more often it is team-related. A 1987 survey conducted by Dr. Dale Larson supports the findings of Vachon (Beresford, 1988; Vachon, 1987) (Box 78–4). The greatest impediments to effective hospice team functioning are the members' difficulty in openly and comfortably dealing with conflict and their lack of trust in the team.

COORDINATION OF CARE

The interdisciplinary team coordinates and supervises all hospice services 7 days a week, 24 hours a day. Careful monitoring of clinical care from one level to another is essential. There should be effective informal and formal two-way communication between the hospice organization and inpatient facilities, traditional home care agencies, physicians, and other community professionals such as pharmacists, clergy, and funeral directors.

Box 78–3. *Nursing Research Note*

Johnston T. E., & Amenta, M. (1994). Midwifery to the soul while the body dies: Spiritual care among hospice nurses. *American Journal of Hospice and Palliative Care, 11*(6), 28–36.

In a 1992 study of 181 (26 per cent) Oncology Nursing Society staff nurse members to determine attitudes and beliefs about the relationship of the spiritual domain to the application of spiritual care behaviors in their clinical practice, the authors observed several statistically significant differences between the total sample and a small subset (16 respondents, 9 per cent) who worked in hospice home care settings. In 1993, using the same questionnaire, they surveyed the 1160 members of the Hospice Nurses Association, receiving 641 responses (55 per cent).

Results of the latter study demonstrated that the hospice nurses believed strongly that all patients, including those who were not religious, had spiritual needs and that it is appropriate and important for nurses to provide spiritual care. They regarded themselves as more spiritual than religious, although 68.4 per cent held formal membership in a religious organization, 60.1 per cent attended religious services frequently or more often, and 64.4 per cent prayed frequently.

Higher educational level, low religious service attendance, disbelief in an after life, and infrequent praying were strongly related to the attitude that agnostics and atheists are spiritually healthy and that one need not believe in a higher power to be spiritually healthy.

These nurses (59.2 per cent) reported that support for spiritual care was adequate at work. Their most frequent sources of spiritual support were fellow nurses (77.3 per cent), patients (57.7 per cent), and chaplains (57.5 per cent).

Overall these findings indicate that hospice nurses have high positive regard for spiritual care. Spirituality and religiosity were directly correlated with positive attitudes and beliefs about spiritual care in the clinical setting. We do not know whether this is due to the high value the hospice philosophy places on the spiritual domain or whether the more spiritually evolved are strongly attracted to hospice care.

Box 78–4. *Nursing Research Note*

Vachon, M. L. S. (1987). *Occupational stress in the care of the critically ill, the dying, and the bereaved.* Washington, DC: Hemisphere Publishing.

On the basis of what she had perceived in several years of providing staff support and consultation of team issues for workers in high-stress health care treatment centers—palliative care facilities, intensive care units, and chronic care hospitals—Vachon tried to validate her impressions systematically. She explored four questions about workplace-related stress:

- What were workers' perceptions of what caused them stress?
- How were these stresses affected by factors in their personal lives?
- How did these stresses manifest themselves?
- How did the workers cope with the stresses?

The author conducted unstructured interviews based on these questions with workers in oncology (25 per cent), palliative care (18 per cent), critical care (17 per cent), and other specialties in many parts of the world—Canada, the United States, Western Europe, Australia, India, South Africa, and the West Indies. Forty-nine per cent of the subjects were nurses, 24 per cent were physicians, and 71 per cent were women. Fifty-four percent were clinicians, and another 21 per cent combined clinical work with teaching, research, or administrative activities. Fifty per cent were 30 to 45 years old, and 35 per cent were older than 45 years, thus increasing the likelihood that the group would have had experience in identifying and managing to cope with workplace-induced stresses.

There were 327 interviews with 600 caregivers, many in groups, that yielded a total of 8912 anecdotes, which were coded and analyzed. The anecdotes fell into four major categories: coping strategies (38 per cent), work environment stress (37 per cent), manifestations of stress (18 per cent), and personal mediating variables (7 per cent).

Of the anecdotes relating to stress in the work environment, 36 per cent dealt with the work setting itself, 26 per cent with occupational roles, and 23 per cent with issues connected with patients and families. Only 15 per cent were associated with patients' illnesses. The highest ranking item in this category was "problems with team communication," which had as the most frequently cited underlying source "control issues." Other work-setting stresses cited were nature of the unit, role ambiguity, role conflict, inadequate resources (staffing), and communication problems with others in the institution.

AVAILABILITY AND ORGANIZATION OF HOSPICE SERVICES IN THE UNITED STATES

PROFILE OF HOSPICE PATIENTS

AGE, ETHNICITY

More than 275,000 terminally ill patients were treated in American hospices in 1993 (Lubieniecki, 1994). Seventy per cent of them were 61 years and older, and 18 per cent were between 45 and 60 years ("Hospice Forum," 1994). There were slightly more women (51.6 per cent) than men (48.7 per cent); 84.5 per cent were Caucasian, 10.4 per cent African-American, and 3.5 per cent Hispanic—reflecting the proportions of these groups in the 1990 United States Census; 1.1 per cent of all hospice patients served in 1993 were children under the age of 18 ("Hospice Forum," 1994).

DIAGNOSTIC CATEGORIES AND PROGNOSIS

Although few hospice programs explicitly reject applicants by disease category, 78 per cent of all hospice patients have cancer ("NHO Newsline," 1993). In fact, in 1992, 37 per cent of all Americans who died of cancer received hospice care. This is because admission requirements in the majority of hospice programs include a 6 month or less prognosis. This also reflects either the willingness or the ability of physicians to predict approximate time of death more accurately for advanced cancer than for other life-threatening diseases such as hypertension, diabetes, end-stage renal disease, and amyotrophic lateral sclerosis.

PERSONS WITH AIDS

The NHO has called on hospices nationwide to serve the needs of persons with acquired immunodeficiency syndrome (AIDS), their families, and significant others through existing hospice program structures; in 1992, 98 per cent of hospices in the United States had policies that encouraged the admission of AIDS patients. Of the estimated 29,763 AIDS patients who died in 1992, hospices cared for 9340 (31 per cent) ("NHO Newsline," 1993). AIDS patients accounted for 4.5 per cent of hospice patient caseloads nationally ("Hospice Forum," 1994). This relatively small number may reflect certain problems inherent in the average American hospice's capacity to treat persons with AIDS (Martin, 1991).

A prominent deterrent lies with these patients themselves. Many do not want to forfeit the possible benefits of intensive technical care, nor are they prepared to abandon the goal of cure. They avidly and persistently seek out scientific and nontraditional therapies. A lucky few get the interferon injections or zidovudine provided by the scientific medical care establishment, but they too may drink herbal teas, take acupuncture treatments, go to faith healers, and consume large quantities of vitamin C, as do the majority who do not get the experimental treatments.

A second significant difficulty facing hospices in the care of persons with AIDS is that they require much more care and many more labor-intensive services for longer periods of time than the types of dying patients that have been traditionally served. The symptoms of AIDS are so severe, diverse, and unremitting and the downhill course is so rapidly progressive that treatment is extremely, arguably prohibitively, costly. There is a real fear among hospice administrators that just one too many of these patients might "break the bank."

The work-related group insurance of persons with AIDS is canceled when they become too ill to continue at their jobs. Once out of a group plan, they cannot find individual coverage. Many of them do not live the 2 years from diagnosis required to claim disability under Medicare, and for the most part they are too young to claim the traditional Medicare benefits for those older than 65. One hope for relief of this situation is the growing number of states that are developing a new Medicaid hospice option benefit made possible by the 1986 Consolidated Omnibus Budget Reconciliation Act legislation (Beresford, 1988) (explained further in this chapter in the section "Reimbursement for Hospice Services").

ECONOMIC CONSIDERATIONS

The issue of cost savings for the total health care system through hospice care is not insignificant. Part of the reason for the great growth in the availability of the hospice option in the last 20 years has been the presumed cost effectiveness of hospice care through the substitution of home care days for inpatient days in acute care facilities during the last weeks of life (Mor & Masterson-Allen, 1987). In 1984 Lubitz and Prihoda found in an in-depth analysis of Medicare reimbursement statistics that 5.9 per cent of Medicare beneficiaries who had died within the year incurred 28 per cent of all Medicare expenditures. Those who died with cancer had the highest acute care hospital use and also the highest total Medicare reimbursements.

Recent analyses fault the cost studies of the 1980s for their omission of data related to private-pay personal attendants and time lost from work for caregivers (Emanual & Emanuel, 1994). The very latest research (Manard & Perone, 1995) has found that terminally ill patients in hospice programs cost Medicare less than those in conventional medical treatment. On a daily basis the Medicare hospice benefit saved $1.65 for every dollar spent for Part A benefits in the last months of life. For hospice-enrolled cancer patients dying from July through December, 1992, Medicare saved $1.41 per dollar spent on Part A services. The conclusion was that even with increasingly more patients being cared for in Medicare benefit hospices every year, longer lengths of stay, and unlimited days of coverage, cancer patients being cared for in hospices continued to save Medicare expenditures.

ORGANIZATION

The various shapes and sizes that hospice programs have assumed historically have depended more on the caregiving assets and the leadership structure of the communities in which they have developed than on rational planning and scientifically based needs assessments.

GENERIC PROGRAM CHARACTERISTICS

Because organizational structure is related to both clinical and cost of care outcomes, it is important to have a knowledge of hospice programs in general and knowledge of the major administrative types in particular. Hospices have typically been small, labor-intensive organizations. The majority (60 per cent) of hospice programs in 1992 reported annual operating budgets of less than $500,000; 19 per cent had budgets between $500,000 and $1 million; 14 per cent, between $1 and $3 million; and 7 per cent, between $3 and $7 million ("NHO Newsline," 1993). The average length of stay was 59 days in 1990 and 64 days in 1992.

PROGRAM AVAILABILITY

In 1995 the NHO identified 2510 programs in various stages of development, planning through fully operational, in all 50 states. In 1990 there were 1743; in 1991, 1874; and in 1992, 1935 (NHO, 1995).

OWNERSHIP AND MAJOR MODELS

Despite 20 years of hospice experience in the United States, there is still considerable variability in the extent of services offered by individual hospice agencies. Eligibility requirements, nature and organization of inpatient services, reimbursement arrangements, and service to children, patients with AIDS, and patients living alone differ (Beresford, 1993). The following basic categories, however, influence the range of services.

Of the 1700 NHO member hospices that supplied data in 1994, 39 per cent were independently owned, 30 per cent were divisions of hospitals, 24 per cent were divisions of home health agencies, 2 per cent were divisions of a hospice corporation, and 1 per cent were nursing home based. Four per cent did not supply these data. (G. Gillen [personal communication, Communications Coordinator, NHO, February 25, 1995]).

HOSPITAL-BASED HOSPICES

Hospice programs based administratively in acute care hospitals enjoy the built-in advantage of having easy access to shared support services and various treatment specialties. There are three major types. The first is the discrete unit. In this type, from one to ten beds located together are designated for hospice care exclusively. The staff is specially trained and is assigned to the unit permanently. Characteristically, these units have nurse-to-patient ratios that are similar to those for acute and critical care levels.

In the second type of acute care hospital-based hospice, there is neither a designated contiguous group of beds nor a designated hospice team. In these programs, patients appropriate for hospice care are identified in all units of the institution and are treated palliatively through the existing caregiving structures.

The third type of acute care hospital-based hospice is what is known as the scatter bed model. In these programs a specially trained, designated hospice care team—at a minimum, a nurse, a physician, a social worker, and associated volunteers—sees appropriate patients anywhere in the hospital. Rather than give direct care, they consult about palliative measures with the regular staff. In general, they do assessments, teach patients and families and unit staff, coordinate care, and act as patient advocates. A growing number of hospitals also provide the continuum of hospice services to patients in their homes through their home care divisions.

HOSPICES BASED IN LONG-TERM CARE FACILITIES

Hospice programs in the few long-term care facilities have from one to four dedicated beds and may or may not have a specially trained, designated staff. For home care follow-up, they make arrangements with home health agencies or independent community-based hospices.

As a result of the 1986 Omnibus Budget Reconciliation Act (OBRA) legislation extending Medicare benefits to the terminally ill, a growing number of community-based hospices care for patients in nursing homes. They assume professional responsibility for the management of the patient's entire continuum of hospice services, the only difference being that the nursing facility is regarded as the patient's home and nursing home staff become the functional equivalent of the patient's family caregivers. The nursing home must provide 24 hour a day supervision to the patient, and the hospice is accountable for all Medicare- and Medicaid-mandated hospice benefit core services. The hospice must supply all needed drugs and biologics, and it must arrange for inpatient acute care when it is indicated (Beresford, 1993).

COMMUNITY-BASED COMPREHENSIVE HOME HEALTH AGENCY HOSPICES

There are two types of program organizations in the community-based, home health agency–owned hospices. In the first type, there is a designated hospice care team, selected and trained for work with hospice patients and families exclusively. Because of the time involved in the care of hospice patients, these nurses on average see fewer patients and families per day than do regular home care nurses. Often three to five visits are all that can be managed realistically.

In other community-based comprehensive home health agencies that offer hospice services, the entire nursing staff, after appropriate orientation, carries one or two families in their districts as part of their generalized caseload. Usually there is ongoing education and consultation and staff support to help these nurses remain current in the hospice-specific aspects of care.

INDEPENDENT COMMUNITY-BASED HOSPICES

Community-based independent hospice programs treat hospice patients and their families exclusively. Because many of these programs are also licensed and certified by Medicare as home health agencies, they may provide the full range of traditional home care services, as well as the hospice-specific services arrayed above. Some supply only part of the home care and arrange with other comprehensive home health agencies to provide the rest.

FREESTANDING HOSPICES

In addition to the Connecticut Hospice, approximately 200 other programs have reported themselves to the NHO as "freestanding" models (G. Gillen [personal communication, Communications Coordinator, NHO, February 25, 1995]). These independently managed hospices have their own inpatient care buildings and integrated home care services. A prominent factor in the growth of this model is the hospice's desire to treat the estimated 10 per cent of patients who would benefit from hospice care but who do not have primary caregivers.

HOSPICE IN THE CHANGING HEALTH CARE ENVIRONMENT

With so many people in the United States moving from the traditional fee-for-service insured systems of care to managed care, many questions present themselves to the hospice community. Mergers are taking place, with several small hospices in a community joining into one larger agency (Lubieniecki, 1994). In other cases, individual hospices form cooperative purchasing and information sharing systems. Still others are incorporating themselves into vertical alliances in which they become a part of a larger health care system. One thing is clear, all hospice programs are seriously revisiting their mission statements, program structures, standards of care, and costs.

REIMBURSEMENT FOR HOSPICE SERVICES

HISTORIC ASPECTS

Early in the history of the hospice movement in the United States, hospice services were reimbursed from many sources. Existing third-party payers covered the traditional medical, social, and nursing care charges generated by physicians, inpatient facilities, and home health agencies, but they did not pay for the hospice-specific elements of care (Amenta, 1985). The costs of managing extensive pain and symptom control consultation, volunteer components, family care, interdisciplinary team support, bereavement follow-up, and round-the-clock availability were met largely through donations and memorials, grants from foundations and philanthropic organizations, religious groups, and the United Way. In many instances, patients and families themselves paid out of pocket for these services. A small number of hospices had either state or federal funding for limited periods as pilot programs or research projects. Several local Blue Cross–Blue Shield organizations supported pilot projects, and although many did not acknowledge hospice programs officially, often they turned benign blind eyes and were frequently lenient in honoring claims.

Slowly and sporadically other insurance companies, industry, and unions began adopting hospice benefits not only as humane options for their beneficiaries but also as cost savers for their group plans. A deterrent to more rapid proliferation of reimbursement for hospice care as an alternative in the private sector was the lack of a legal definition of the nature and scope of hospice services and a lack of generally accepted standards (Blum & Robbins, 1985).

MEDICARE HOSPICE BENEFIT

In 1982, however, with the passage of the Medicare Hospice Benefit, an official definition of hospice as a discrete set of services was established, federal regulations were promulgated, and a steady stream of funding for hospice care became available (Cummings, 1985).

SCOPE OF SERVICES AND FLOW OF PAYMENT

Under the terms of this legislation, the qualified hospice program provides eligible beneficiaries with the following benefits: physician services; nursing care; medical social services; counseling; spiritual support; physical, occupational, and speech therapies; homemakers and home health aides; pharmaceutics and biologics required for the control of pain and other symptoms; medical equipment and supplies; and short-term inpatient care either for the management of acute or chronic symptoms or pain control or for respite for the patient's caregivers. The hospice program must provide continuous care in the home during periods of crisis, as well as bereavement counseling, volunteer services, and continuity of inpatient and home care. For every day the patient is enrolled, the hospice is reimbursed at a fixed rate for one of four levels of care. In turn, the hospice program pays for services of all other agencies, professionals, and vendors.

ELIGIBILITY, ELECTION, AND DURATION OF SERVICE

Eligibility is conferred on those entitled to Medicare Part A who are certified by an attending physician as terminally ill with a 6 month or less prognosis. The patient must sign an "election" statement indicating that she or he understands the palliative nature of the hospice program and that certain other traditional Medicare benefits, with the exception of the attending physician, who will continue to be reimbursed for services under Medicare Part B, will be waived.

There are four discrete benefit periods, three of which are 90, 90, and 30 days. The final period, an indeterminate one, is for patients who outlive the first 210 days of hospice treatment. At the beginning of each new benefit period, the patient's terminal prognosis and projected longevity of 6 months or less must be reconfirmed by the physician. During these benefit periods, the patient may revoke the hospice option and resume traditional Medicare coverage. The patient may also reelect hospice care at any time.

CORE SERVICES AND HOSPICE PROGRAM HEGEMONY

Those professionals providing the core services— medicine, nursing, medical social services, and counseling—must be employees of the hospice. The hospice is responsible for coordinating and controlling the quality of all other services. This makes the hospice organization responsible legally, clinically, and financially for all care.

AVAILABILITY OF THE MEDICARE HOSPICE BENEFIT

According to the statistics in the 1992 NHO database, 72 per cent of the 1935 operational hospices in the nation were either currently billing under the Medicare benefit or in the application process ("NHO Newsline," 1993).

OTHER PUBLIC SOURCES OF REIMBURSEMENT FOR HOSPICE CARE

TRADITIONAL MEDICARE AND COMPREHENSIVE CANCER CENTERS

In addition to the Hospice Medicare Benefit, other sources of reimbursement for hospice or hospice-like care exists in the wholly and partially publicly insured sector. Regular Medicare provides both inpatient and home care for indefinite periods, and many terminally ill patients and their families are satisfied with this traditional benefit. Patients and families are satisfied especially with the comprehensive cancer centers, where the strong commitment to patient and family psychosocial support from the day of diagnosis, the interdisciplinary team approach, and the integrated home care services are incorporated into total care (Beresford, 1988).

VETERANS ADMINISTRATION

For many years a few Veterans Administration Hospitals had discrete hospice programs, and others had "closet" hospices that provided palliative care (Knowles, 1985). A 1991 internal mandate requires all Veterans Administration facilities to establish hospice care. This means that all Veterans Administration patients who are appropriate for hospice care should receive it under those auspices (C. Cody [personal communication, Technical Assistance Manager, NHO, February 28, 1995]).

MEDICAID

As a result of the 1986 Consolidated Omnibus Budget Reconciliation Act (COBRA) legislation, 38 states are already paying for hospice care under Medicaid, and several others are developing a Medicaid hospice benefit to reimburse hospice care for low-income persons of any age (G. Gillen [personal communication, Communications Coordinator, NHO, February 25, 1995]). Many of these Medicaid schemes duplicate the structure of the Medicare benefit, but some have modifications imposed by the states.

PRIVATE SOURCES OF REIMBURSEMENT FOR HOSPICE CARE

The role of private insurers in funding hospice services has also grown with the establishment of hospice care as a discrete cluster of services. A 1978 survey found only 17 per cent of insurance companies offering coverage specifically designated for the terminally ill, and coverage was limited to traditional medical and nursing care, not hospice-specific services (Cummings, 1985). In 1985

Box 78–5. *Questions Consumers Can Ask Regarding a Hospice Program*

There are a number of questions people might want to ask regarding a hospice program before they let this team of strangers into their homes and their lives. The hospice's certification of accreditation can provide some assurance that it is a credible and reliable provider. But one should also ask about the hospice's admission policies and see how well they fit the individual's situation. How flexible is this hospice in applying its policies to each patient or negotiating over differences? If the hospice imposes up front a lot of conditions that do not feel comfortable, that may be a sign that it is not going to be a good fit.

How does the hospice respond to the very first call? Do telephone staff convey an attitude of caring, patience, and competence from the first contact, even if they need to ask the intake coordinator to return the patient's call? Do they speak in simple language, or do they use a lot of jargon about the requirements that patients must meet? How a hospice responds to that first call for help may be a good indicator of the kind of care to expect. If you are not certain whether your loved one qualifies for hospice—or whether you even want it—is the agency willing to make an assessment visit to help clarify these issues?

How quickly can the hospice initiate services? What are its geographic service boundaries? Can the hospice respond to unusual needs, such as putting in a telephone line for families who do not have one already but need one to manage the patient's care at home? Does the hospice offer specialized extras such as rehabilitation therapists, pharmacists, dietitians, family counselors, or art therapists when these could improve the patient's comfort? Are any of these extras likely to be needed in your case? Does the hospice offer to lend used medical equipment, audiovisuals, or other items that might also enhance the patient's quality of life?

Ask what the program's policies are regarding inpatient care, where such care is provided, what the requirements are for an inpatient admission, and how long patients ordinarily can stay—especially if you think the patient's situation is likely to require a lengthy inpatient stay. Find out the average length of stay in the inpatient unit and what happens to patients who no longer need inpatient care but cannot return home. If the hospice has its own inpatient unit or residential facility, you may want to request a tour, although there is little value in touring a home care hospice's administrative offices. If the patient needs to go back to the hospital, which hospitals contract with the hospice for inpatient care? Families also need to know what kind of follow-up the hospice provides when its patients are in the hospital if it does not operate an inpatient unit itself. Does the hospice have a residential facility or contractual agreements with nursing homes to provide a safe setting of care for patients who cannot be at home? Find out which nursing homes contract with the hospice and how much of a difference the hospice actually makes in the lives of their terminally ill residents. Does the hospice provide as much nursing, social work, and aide care for each patient in the nursing home as it does in the home setting?

You will want to know whether the hospice requires a family primary caregiver as a condition of admission, and if so, how much responsibility is expected from that family caregiver. What help can the hospice offer in coordinating and supplementing the family's efforts or filling in around job schedules, travel plans, or other responsibilities? If a patient lives alone, what alternatives can the hospice suggest?

You may also want to look into the hospice's relationship with the patient's physician and the physician's past relationship with the hospice. Has your physician referred other patients to hospice recently and was the experience a positive one?

---

the Washington Business Group on Health reported that 59 per cent of the Fortune 500 companies offered a hospice benefit to their employees (Freudenhaim, 1986). In 1994 Manard and Perone reported that coverage for hospice care was provided to 80 per cent of employees in medium-to-large-sized businesses and to 82 per cent of enrollees in managed care plans.

Health maintenance organizations (HMOs) tend to include hospice care in their benefits packages even more than traditional insurers. A 1990 survey by the Group Health Association of America indicated that 83 per cent of HMOs covered hospice (Beresford, 1993). Some HMOs, such as Kaiser Permanente in California and Group Health Cooperative of Puget Sound, Washington, have maintained hospice care divisions in their programs for several years. All HMOs that participate in Medicare, although not required to provide "hands-on" hospice care to their Medicare enrollees, must inform them of the availability of local Medicare-certified hospices.

HOW TO FIND HOSPICE CARE

A 1994 Medicare Technical Amendment requires that starting in November of 1995 hospitals evaluate a patient's appropriateness for hospice care and notify the patient and family of the availability of hospice services during the discharge planning process.

If hospice care is desired but not suggested at the time the patient is diagnosed with a terminal condition, the nurse or the family should know that there are several ways to find help. The NHO publishes and sells an annual *Guide to the Nation's Hospices* that lists all known hospice organizations by state and town, contact person, phone number, type of hospice, operational status, scope of service, and counties served. The 1994–1995 NHO guide also lists the names, addresses, and phone numbers of the officers of the 50 state (plus District of Columbia) hospice organizations, most of which also maintain directories of hospices by location, contact person, and scope of services.

Other national organizations that assist families and professionals in the search for satisfactory hospice care through national telephone referral services are the Hospice Association of America (a subsidiary of the National Association for Homecare) and the National Institute for Jewish Hospice.

When choosing a hospice, the family should be alerted to standards of care expressed in national accreditation, certification, and state licensing creden-

Box 78–5. *Questions Consumers Can Ask Regarding a Hospice Program*   Continued

Can they work together comfortably, or should you expect conflicts? You should ask whether the hospice medical director will visit patients when this is appropriate.

It may also be worth asking who provides nursing on-call coverage for the hospice and what their qualifications are. How accessible are they? How does the hospice respond to after-hours emergencies? A hospice that only uses an answering machine for handling medical emergency calls after hours will probably have a hard time responding to emergencies. Although operator-staffed answering services can get very busy at times, if there is always a long wait to get emergency calls answered, or if there is a busy signal or disconnection, that, too, is a problem. Remember that when you call the hospice after hours and reach its answering service, the operator must then contact the on-call nurse at home or by pager, perhaps even getting the nurse out of bed. Such a process can take 10 to 20 minutes or more; but there should always be a nurse accessible this way, and that nurse should be willing to come to the home quickly if the medical situation warrants.

How frequently do the nurse and social worker come to the patient's home for routine visits? What is the average length of nursing visits? Will it be the same nurse for every visit? What is the average caseload carried by each nurse? The fewer patients a nurse manages, the more time and energy there will be for each case. Hospice nurses who have to manage more than 12 to 14 cases may find themselves having to cut corners just to keep up. How often will the home health aide or personal care aide visit if the patient's physical care needs are heavy? The hospice's willingness to provide extra aide shifts to help the family through rough spots is one of the best indicators of its commitment to truly meet the patient's needs. Does the hospice guarantee to provide scheduled aide services, even if the person originally scheduled for that visit calls in sick or fails to show up?

It may also be important to know whether the hospice has policies excluding treatments such as enteral or parenteral nutrition, blood transfusions, radiation therapy, chemotherapy, antibiotics, dialysis, ventilators, resuscitation—or anything else that might figure prominently in your care needs. This may or may not pose a problem, since some patients seek out hospices to help them wean from dialysis, ventilators, or other invasive treatments. However, each hospice defines covered palliative services in its own way, and some are more or less restrictive in the kinds of treatments that are excluded from hospice coverage.

Ask about the actual out-of-pocket costs for hospice care, if any. If you have Medicare or private insurance, what additional charges might there be? Does the hospice accept Medicaid? Will the hospice accept insurance "assignment," meaning that it will settle for whatever the insurance company offers as payment in full, without asking the family to make up the difference? Will the hospice handle all the billing and paperwork or negotiate on the patient's behalf with the insurer? If there is no insurance, how do they handle that? Are fees charged per visit, per day, or some other way? Do they have a sliding fee scale or a payment plan? Will they care for patients who have no ability to pay for the care as cheerfully and as thoroughly as they do for paying clients?

Adapted from Beresford, L. (1993). *The hospice handbook* (pp. 96–100). Boston: Little, Brown & Co.

---

tials. In a state that licenses hospices, the state health department will have up-to-date lists of all caregiving organizations that meet this basic standard. The state health department will also have lists of all Medicare-certified hospices, and the Joint Commission on the Accreditation of Healthcare Organizations (JCAHO) lists all those that are accredited as subsets of accredited home care agencies.* As a rule, a hospice will provide this information when contacted.

Some communities may have hospices at various levels of operation; some may be providing only referral, volunteer, and bereavement services, whereas others offer comprehensive programs that are fully certified, accredited, and licensed if applicable. Still others may be offering services through nursing homes. The family should be assisted in making the decision, if there is a choice, based on their needs and their resources, human as well as financial.

For a comprehensive list of questions consumers should ask about hospice care see Box 78–5.

REFERENCES

Amenta, M. (1985). Hospice in the United States: Multiple models and varied programs. *Nursing Clinics of North America, 20,* 269–279.

Amenta, M. & Bohnet, N. (1986). *Nursing care of the terminally ill.* Boston: Little, Brown & Co.

Beresford, L. (Ed.). (1988, January). *Hospice Letter, 9,* 10.

Beresford, L. (1993). *The hospice handbook: A complete guide.* Boston: Little, Brown & Co.

Blum, J., & Robbins, D. (1985). Considerations in licensure. In P. Torrens (Ed.), *Hospice programs and public policy* (pp. 73–79). Chicago: American Hospital Publishing.

Brown, E. (1978, May). Hospice in the United States—its origin and promise. In *Hospice as a social health care institution. Report of the pre-forum institute of the 105th annual forum of the National Conference of Social Welfare* (pp. 80–90). Los Angeles: Hillhaven Foundation.

Cummings, M. (1985). Current status of hospice financing. In P. Torrens (Ed.), *Hospice programs and public policy* (pp. 137–175). Chicago: American Hospital Publishing.

---

*Useful Addresses: National Hospice Organization, Membership Department, 1901 North Fort Myer Drive, Arlington, VA 22209, (703)243-5900; Hospice Association of America, 210 7th Street, SE, Washington, DC 20003, (202) 547-5263; National Institute for Jewish Hospice, 8723 Alden Drive, Suite 562, Los Angeles, CA 90048, (800)446-4448; Hospice Nurses Association, 5512 Northumberland Street, Pittsburgh, PA, 15217, (412)687-3231.

DuBoulay, S. (1984). *Cicely Saunders—founder of the modern hospice movement.* New York: The Amaryllis Press.

Emanuel, E. J., & Emanuel, L. L. (1994). The economics of dying. The illusion of cost savings at the end of life. *New England Journal of Medicine, 330,* 540–544.

Fiefel, H. (1959). *The meaning of death.* New York: McGraw-Hill.

Foster, A., Wald, F., & Wald, H. (1978). The hospice movement—a backward glance at its first two decades. *New Physician,* pp. 176–21.

Freudenhaim, M. (1986, February 12). Hospice care as an option. *New York Times,* p. 30.

Glaser, B., & Strauss, A. (1965). *Awareness of dying.* Chicago: Aldine.

Hinton, J. (1965). *Dying.* Baltimore: Penguin.

Hospice Forum, June 30, 1994.

Kalish, R., & Reynolds, D. (1976). *Death and ethnicity.* Los Angeles: University of Southern California Press.

Kastenbaum, R., & Aisenberg, R. (1972). *The psychology of death.* New York: Springer.

Knowles, C. (1985). Reimbursements and the Medicare certified hospice. *American Journal of Hospice Care, 2*(5), 15–21.

Kubler-Ross, E. (1969). *On death and dying.* New York: Macmillan.

Kubler-Ross, E. (1971). What is it like to be dying? *American Journal of Nursing, 71,* 54–59.

Lubieniecki, K. (1994). Hospice at twenty: Looking back at the birth and development of hospice in the United States. *Hospice Magazine, 5*(4), 31–32.

Lubitz, J., & Prihoda, R. (1984). The use and costs of Medicare services in the last 2 years of life. *Health Care Finance Review, 5,* 117–131.

Manard, C., & Perone, P. (1994). *Hospice care: An introduction and review of the evidence.* Arlington, VA: National Hospice Organization.

Manard, C., & Perone, R. (1995). *An analysis of the cost savings of the Medicare hospice benefit.* Arlington, VA: National Hospice Organization.

Martin, J. P. (1991). Issues in the current treatment of hospice patients with HIV disease. In M. Amenta & C. Tehan (Eds.), *AIDS and the hospice community* (pp. 31–41). Binghamton, NY: Harrington Park Press.

Mor, V., & Masterson-Allen, S. (1987). *Hospice care systems.* New York: Springer.

NHO Newsline, 3(16), October 1993.

NHO reports 7 per cent growth in hospice programs. (1988, February.) *Hospice News,* pp. 1–3.

NHO. (1995). *1994–1995 hospice statistics.* Arlington, VA: author.

Quint, J. (1967). *The nurse and the dying patient.* New York: Macmillan.

Raphael, R. (1977). Preventive intervention with the recently bereaved. *Archives of General Psychiatry, 34,* 1450–1454.

U.S. General Accounting Office. (1989). *Report to the Subcommittee on Health, Committee of Ways and Means, House of Representatives. Medicare: Program Provisions and Payments Discourages Hospice Participation* (GAOHRD-89-111). Washington, DC: Author.

Vachon, M. (1987). *Occupational stress in the care of the critically ill, the dying, and the bereaved.* Washington, DC: Hemisphere Publishing.

Wald, F. (1981). Hospice care concepts. In *Hospice education program for nurses.* Hyattsville, MD: U.S. Department of Health and Human Services.

CHAPTER

79

Understanding Cancer Reimbursement

Lee E. Mortenson

Without question, reimbursement affects one's career in the health care professions. It determines whether facilities for work and research are open. It determines a hospital's ability to provide adequate care. It affects patient management and is likely to determine the settings in which a patient is treated. It affects research and availability of new therapies. In more and more cases, it may be a deciding factor in life and death resource judgments. Reimbursement, more than any other factor, influences the ability to provide quality care to patients with cancer.

UNCONTROLLED GROWTH: HEALTH CARE EXPENDITURES

As we enter the mid-1990s, approximately 14 per cent of the annual United States gross domestic product is spent on health care. Few other industries can claim such a huge share of the economy. There are major economic concerns about the health care industry. Significant cutbacks are underway, and political figures intend to find ways to trim health care expenditures. Hospitals are closing. Major layoffs of nursing personnel are taking place, physicians are working for less money and are working longer hours. More patients are being treated under managed care plans—health maintenance organi-

zations (HMOs), preferred provider organizations (PPOs), and independent practitioner associations (IPAs)—all of the time. Concern over access of patients to health care and the creation of levels of care is mounting.

The costs of medical care have expanded radically since 1965 when the federal government first began to underwrite the costs of the financially indigent (Medicaid) and of individuals older than 65 years of age (Medicare). During the following 2.5 decades, health care costs continued to increase as benefits have been extended to more people and as new, more expensive technology has been introduced.

Over the next 3 decades, a greater percentage of the United States population will be older than 65 years of age, whereas the percentage of individuals younger than age 65 who will pay for their care will drop. In the mid 1980s, 13 per cent of the United States population was older than 65 years; by 2030, more than 25 per cent will be in the Medicare-eligible age group. Moreover, the largest portion of this population will be older than 75 years, a group that typically includes a significant percentage of chronically impaired individuals and the frail elderly. This is also the group with the highest incidence of cancer. With more people requiring care, fewer people contributing to the payment pool, and more technology, it is not surprising that cost issues are a national concern.

THE CHANGING FORMS OF REIMBURSEMENT: FROM RETROSPECTIVE TO PROSPECTIVE

Reimbursement is bewildering because it is done a variety of different ways through an ever-changing series of mechanisms. Moreover, reimbursement is in the midst of a major series of changes that began in the 1980s and will continue for at least the next decade.

The basic concept of health insurance was to provide financial coverage if an individual became ill. An insurance company pools together the premiums of a group of people, and actuaries compute the price of insurance based on the kinds of illnesses the group is statistically likely to have.

As individuals use physician and hospital services, they submit bills to their insurance companies, which, in turn, pay them. When insurance was first introduced, the patient selected the physician, and the physician selected the tests, the hospital, the consultants, the therapies, and the rest. Payment to all of these health care providers was retrospective (after the fact) and based on the treatments given. Of course, layer on layer of bureaucracy and rules have complicated this simple concept.

PHYSICIAN REIMBURSEMENT: A CONTINUING SERIES OF CHANGES

To make certain that physicians do not charge whatever they please, insurance companies have developed profiles of charges by specialty, region of the country, and procedure. Now they issue checks based upon "usual and customary" fees and, in some cases, "prevailing" fees. *Usual and customary* fees relate to what the physician has charged in the past for the same procedure, so that he or she cannot suddenly increase the rates. *Prevailing* fees are used when a new physician tries to establish a payment schedule and the insurance companies want to make certain the charges remain close to the average profile.

Physicians have been restricted in a variety of ways over the past decade. Perhaps the most significant cost-containment step has been taken by the federal government, which pressured physicians to "take assignment." Fundamentally, this means that when a physician treats a Medicare patient, reimbursement will be made only for the amount allowed by Medicare.

Until the end of the 1980s, physician payment remained primarily retrospective, with few direct controls imposed on services provided on an outpatient basis except by insurance companies that indicated an unwillingness to pay for some procedures or drugs.

The federal government implemented a relative value scale (RBRUS) in the early 1990s. This system installed regional and then national reimbursement profiles for each physician procedure and activity. The plan puts pressure on physician incomes, especially those of specialists in internal medicine. In conjunction with these changes, Medicare is now beginning to pay less of the overhead medical oncologists charge for giving drugs in their office. These financial pressures are lowering the income potential of private practice at the same time managed care proliferation is cutting fees, limiting access to patients, and removing follow-up care from the purview of specialists.

HOSPITAL PAYMENT: TRYING TO INSPIRE COST CONSCIOUSNESS BY DIRECT INCENTIVES

Initially, the federal government tried to pay hospitals on the basis of their charges (i.e., what they billed the patient). Looking at approximate hospital-wide costs, the federal government reimbursed hospitals at 70 to 80 per cent of charges, roughly what the federal government assumed were the actual, rough costs for delivering the care.

Under retrospective reimbursement, hospitals received a percentage of whatever they charged. If the patient's bill was $10,000 and the hospital was reimbursed for 70 per cent of the charges (a rate that takes into account Medicare, overhead, charitable care, etc., by negotiated agreement with the federal government) the hospital received a check for $7000. If it charged $100,000, it received $70,000. No one asked if these charges had any basis in reality or any relation to the costs of providing the actual care. Both the federal government and hospitals were certain that no one had any idea what the actual costs of care were.

Indeed, hospitals are still having difficulty ascertaining their real costs, because most have been "cost shifting" from one department or procedure to another since the beginning of their operations. For example, the cost of a simple laboratory procedure may be only 13 cents but billed to the patient at $50; the actual cost of a room (overhead, facility, direct labor, etc.) may be $450 per day but billed at $250. When there is plenty of money, there is plenty of room for error. Hospitals had little incentive to cost account because the more they billed, the more they received.

The outcome of this system was the creation of a series of incentives for hospitals to charge as much as possible, because this method would allow them to receive the maximum reimbursement and profit. There were no incentives to reduce charges to the end users, so the spiral of inflationary costs and inflationary insurance premiums continued.

FROM REGULATION TO COMPETITION

The first attempts to limit the costs of care were initiated in the early 1970s. The basic philosophy was to regulate the health care industry, especially the establishment of new, high-cost facilities (Feldstein, 1980). The federal government established a network of professional standards review organizations (PSROs) to issue certificates of need to hospitals that wished to build new buildings, buy major new equipment, or expand existing facilities. Local decisions were made by local appointees, and decisions could be appealed to statewide review organizations. As might be predicted, this approach was highly political. In the long run, almost all requests were approved.

One analysis by Salkever and Bice (1978) indicated that hospital investment was, at best, deflected to other facilities and services by the certificate of need process. Other analyses indicated that more than 90 per cent of the projects that were initially proposed were eventually allowed to go ahead. Indeed, delays caused by the lengthy political review process caused the costs of the facilities and equipment to increase substantially, thereby producing the opposite of the cost-savings effect intended. The PSROs were widely criticized as restraints on the free market economy of health care. The bulk of opinion about ways to contain health care costs began to shift away from regulation and toward competition as the Reagan era of government began.

The total amount of federal and state commitment to health care rose precipitously from $5.7 billion in 1967 to $37 billion in 1977. Given this kind of environment, few hospitals could not make a profit. The rich got rich, and, with only a few exceptions, the poor got rich as well. At the same time, federal legislators began to realize the health care expenditures were growing at an incredible rate, one that could contribute to major national budgetary problems.

PROSPECTIVE REIMBURSEMENT SYSTEM VARIATIONS

In the early 1980s, Congress decided to take an entirely different approach to health care and switched strategies from regulation to competition as the major method of cost control. Before the Tax Equity and Fiscal Responsibility Act of 1982, it did not matter whether a hospital was efficient or inefficient. Almost all hospitals survived. Moreover, efficiency was not necessarily rewarded. The more a hospital charged, the more it was reimbursed. Congress figured that competition would drive out inefficient caregivers in favor of efficient ones and voted to establish a prospective payment system (PPS).

During the late 1970s and early 1980s, the federal government initiated a number of investigations into methods of cost containment that were not based on regulation. Several states were given the option to reimburse all of their Medicare patients with a single formula or to use some other mechanism. Waivers were granted to New York, New Jersey, and Maryland (Mortenson & Winn, 1983, 1984). New York and Maryland developed state rate review mechanisms. These rate reviews entailed the establishment of all-inclusive single-payment rates for each hospital that reflected all of their ongoing, approved activities.

The PPS was mandated by Congress in 1982. By 1983, the administration had selected diagnosis-related groups (DRGs) as the mechanism for prospective payment. The Health Care Financing Administration

(HCFA) felt that it was a compromise between a retrospective system that had thousands of categories of payment and a form of prospective payment that had a single hospital rate system applied to each patient that allowed for very little case variation.

Work at Yale University in 1975 to develop a method for predicting the average length of stay for patients offered an interesting alternative, which was utilized by the state of New Jersey. Working with a large computer budget and medical faculty, the Yale research team developed a series of clinically cohesive groupings of length of stay. These DRGs pulled thousands of clinical diagnoses into 365 groups. These clusters were later refined into 470 DRGs by the federal government.

Length of stay is an important predictor of cost. Moreover, researchers determined that the groupings defined by the DRG system could be used to analyze current practice patterns and to assign average costs. Under a waiver from the federal HCFA, the state of New Jersey began to use these DRG categories as a method of reimbursing hospitals. Essentially the state took all reimbursement for patients in New Jersey for a year, determined which procedures (and billing) fell into which categories, and told hospitals that the state would reimburse the average of each category.

The theory was that hospitals regularly see cases that cost more than the average and others that cost less than the average, but in the long run, these differences even out. At the same time, once the average reimbursement is established, hospitals have incentives to perform more and more efficiently in the delivery of care. Whenever a case falls below the average reimbursement, the hospital makes money. Whenever a case costs more than the average, the hospital loses money. Obviously there are significant incentives for the hospital to minimize costs for cases that are costing them more than the average. There are also incentives to avoid patients who are too costly and to seek "high-profit" patients.

The debate over which form of prospective payment as well as the entire concept of PPS raged during the later 1970s and the early 1980s. Pollard (1980) suggested that "the challenge for the future is to learn how to use competition to achieve a more efficient health care system without abandoning commitments to equity and access." As we shall see, this goal appears to be a significant challenge in the cancer care area.

HEALTH MAINTENANCE ORGANIZATIONS AND MANAGED CARE PLANS

At the same time the federal government was changing from retrospective to prospective payment, it was promoting competition by loosening up some of the rules for alternative delivery systems. When HMOs were first promoted in the 1970s, the federal government imposed a series of restrictions that forced them to take a balanced group of patients, not just those who were likely to want the fewest services.

To open competition, many of these restrictions were lifted. In the 1980s, HMOs and similar organizations began an enormous expansion, one that has accelerated in the 1990s. The two other HMO-type organizations are PPOs and IPAs. Although the classic HMO model has all of the health care resources necessary for care under central control, the other models piggyback on current provider resources and employ utilization review and discounts to lower their prices. All three types are collectively known as *managed care*. Managed care plans may restrict physician choice, hospital choice, tests, treatment, and other forms of care. All three types of organizations (HMOs, PPOs, and IPAs) guarantee lower costs through utilization review, preadmission review, and careful control of hospital and physician resources. Some also require that hospitals and physicians discount their usual fees 5 to 10 per cent or more. Health maintenance organizations receive a fixed cost per person, so there are very specific reasons to prevent disease and to minimize use of resources. Physicians usually work exclusively for the classic HMO at a very limited number of locations. Although PPOs and IPAs also work from a fixed cost per person, their physicians are usually independent contractors who work in their own office settings.

By the late 1980s, many hospitals found that 70 per cent of their reimbursement was coming from DRGs or managed care sources (some of which were also using the DRG format for reimbursement). The remaining 30 per cent came from retrospective reimbursement by companies and individuals who were willing to pay higher premiums to give their employees or themselves a choice of physicians and hospitals. Whatever costs were not paid through DRGs and managed care revenues were shifted to standard third-party insurance, making these plans less cost-competitive.

COMPETITIVE DYNAMICS AND INCENTIVES

All of these competitive dynamics have caused great upheavals in care, some with special significance for cancer care providers. The economic incentives of various groups in the health care system include the following:

- The *federal government* has every incentive to keep increases in DRG payments as low as possible while shifting the burden of responsibility for selecting the right form of care to health care providers (e.g., the hospital, the physician, the nurse).
- *Hospitals* have significant incentives to shorten the length of stay, to minimize resource utilization, to attempt to attract patients who are economic "winners," and to avoid attracting "losers."
- *Businesses* have significant incentives to switch their employees to managed care plans and to continually shop around for the best-priced alternatives.
- *Third-party insurers* have major incentives to cut costs to compete with low-cost managed care plans and to gain more of a market share.
- *HMOs, PPOs, IPAs, and other managed care plans* have major incentives to contain costs, limit resource utilization, and select low-risk subscribers.

Some of these incentives are predictable and "good"; others are unintended consequences of the system and can be a cause for major problems or dysfunctions in it. For example, when it became apparent that managed care was likely to dominate the marketplace, many large hospitals launched managed care plans in an attempt to manage their own future. Unfortunately many of these met with rapid and significant losses.

Third-party insurers and managed care plans have both attempted to find new ways of cost-cutting. Some of these have made the health care system more efficient, whereas others are threatening the quality of health care and the future of research.

REIMBURSING CANCER CARE AND CANCER RESEARCH—THE CHALLENGES OF THE 1990S

A number of key factors about cancer care make it difficult to understand from a reimbursement perspective.

1. Cancer care involves hundreds of site and stage variations, uses many treatment methods, and includes a full spectrum of activities from prevention through terminal care. As a consequence, cancer patients are discharged under a wide spectrum of DRGs (Mortenson, 1985, 1986a; Mortenson & Baum, 1985; Mortenson, Yarbro, Clarke, & Cahill, 1985; Mortenson, Young, & Ney, 1988; Young, Mortenson, & Ney, 1988), making it difficult for hospital administrators to know whether they are making or losing money on cancer patients.
2. Cancer care has a significant outpatient component but is also likely to remain an important portion of hospital inpatient revenues.
3. Patients with cancer are chronically ill and require many admissions (Katterhagen, Clarke, & Mortenson, 1989) and long-term follow-up.
4. Typically patients with cancer are managed in many facilities (on average, 1.5 to 1.8 hospitals).
5. To advance cancer care, a large number of patients are annually enrolled in clinical research trials.
6. Some types of cancer management are well established, whereas others are highly variable.
7. Treatment patterns, reimbursement, and cooperative research group experience vary widely by region (Mortenson, Anderson, & Novak, 1986; Mortenson et al., 1988).

These factors cause confusion to health care policymakers, providers, insurers, and hospital executives. Some of the problems that face each of these decision-making groups will be considered.

HOSPITAL CANCER PROGRAMS: DEFINING THE CANCER PROGRAM PRODUCT LINE

Hospital administrators are often confused about the importance of patients with cancer to their hospital's survival. Much of this confusion stems from the diverse nature of cancer care. Over the past decade, hospitals have moved toward identifying three or four important diseases or services that they wish to emphasize. Cardiology, women's services, oncology, and trauma are examples of this concept (Mortenson & Yarbro, 1983; O'Leary, 1987). Unlike cardiology, however, cancer patients are discharged under a wide variety of DRGs.

Our research indicated that 40 DRGs include strictly cancer discharges, whereas 26 more have a significant proportion of cancer discharges but also include patients with other diagnoses (Mortenson et al., 1985). Yet, when patients with cancer are tracked over numerous admissions, records indicate that they are admitted under a wide variety of complications, making it exceedingly difficult to track their actual costs and reimbursement.

Non-small-cell lung cancer patients admitted to one midwestern medical facility were discharged under DRG 82 (Lung Cancer) and 28 other categories (Fig. 79–1) (Katterhagen et al., 1989). If a hospital administrator attempted to determine whether lung cancer was an economic "winner" by examining only the data from DRG 82, the administrator would see an incomplete picture of the revenues and costs generated.

Indeed, hospitals chronically underestimate the financial importance of their cancer programs, many by as much as 50 per cent. In tertiary care hospitals, it is not uncommon for cancer to account for 15 to 20 per cent of total gross revenues; however, in many cases, hospital administrators are unable to follow patients with cancer through their accounting systems across multiple admissions, and they lose track of a significant portion of their associated revenues.

Hospital administrators are beginning to recognize that oncology will be one of the top two product lines, perhaps number one, by the year 2000, consuming 20 per cent of all health care costs. In part, this is a product of changing demographics, with the baby boomer population reaching the cancer years.

Figure 79–2 illustrates one facility's top DRG billings by cancer site. Although these sites have generated the highest volume of charges, they are not necessarily the most profitable. Figure 79–3 illustrates the most profitable cancer sites for this same facility, and Figure 79–4 illustrates the "losers."

It is important to note that even losers can be important to a facility's survival. When hospitals attempt to determine their costs of care, they develop a formula that is roughly half their fixed costs and half variable costs. A fixed cost is something that cannot be changed easily, such as the annual cost of maintaining the building itself and the amortized cost of construction. Therefore, half of the costs cannot be altered no matter what administrators do. The other half of hospital costs might be categorized into variable and semivariable costs. An example of a variable cost is the level of staffing of an oncology unit. An administrator can readily alter one or two positions up or down without too much difficulty. A semivariable cost might be the unit itself. Opening or closing a unit is a much bigger decision and has greater implications.

NATIONAL POLICY SETTERS: A CONFUSION OF GOALS AND VALUES

The shift from retrospective to prospective and managed care reimbursement has had major implications for cancer care and research. Although the National Institutes of Health (NIH) is mandated to encourage research, technology transfer, and preventive care, the HCFA refuses to pay for patients on NIH experimental therapy (Wagner & Power, 1986), develops regulations that slow down the dissemination and use of new technologies, and pays for routine detection and prevention tests only when Congress mandates payment. All of these issues affect current and future cancer care.

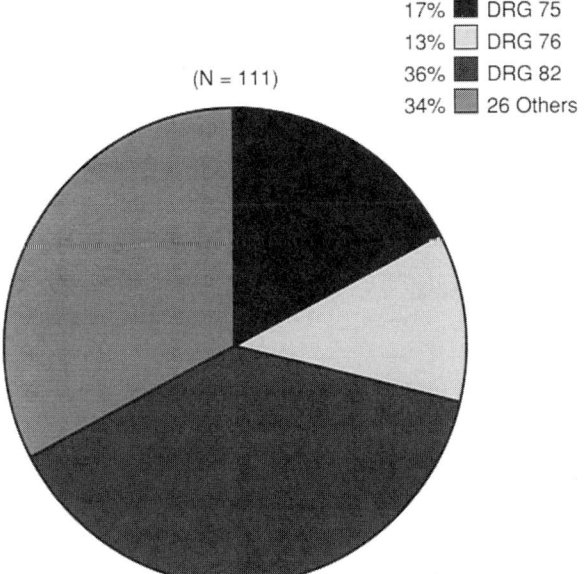

FIGURE 79–1. Frequency of non-small-cell lung cancer diagnosis-related groups (DRG).

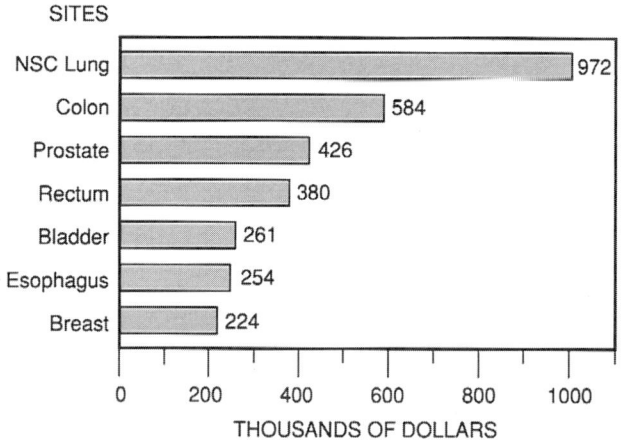

FIGURE 79–2. Top diagnosis-related group billings by cancer site. *NSC* = non-small-cell.

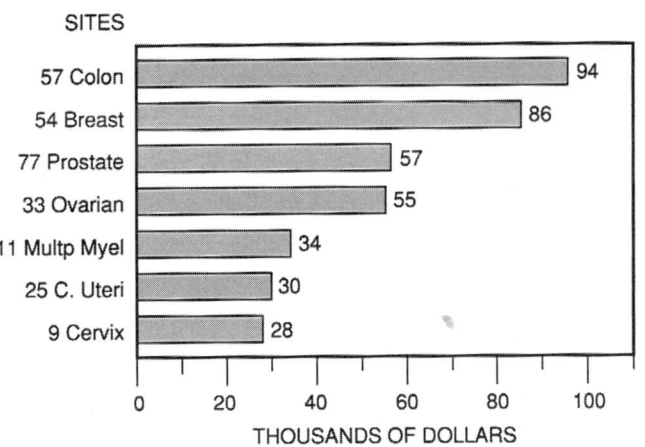

FIGURE 79-3. Diagnosis-related group major profit sites. *Multp. Myel* = multiple myeloma; *C. Uteri* = *corpus uteri.*

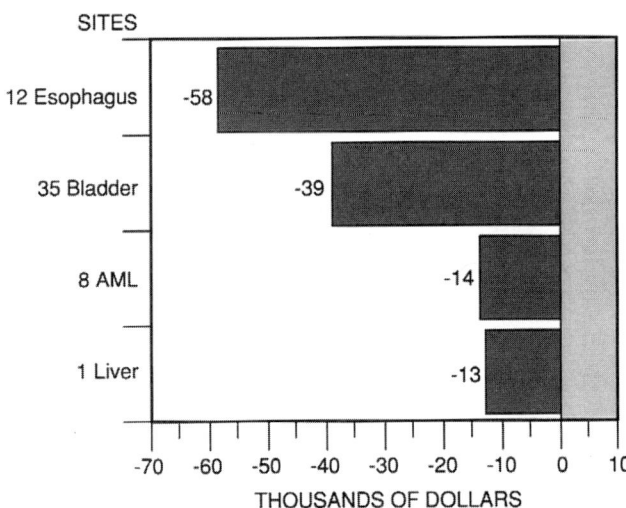

FIGURE 79-4. Diagnosis-related group major loss sites. *AML* = acute myelogenous leukemia.

Between 1982 and 1988, the NIH did not acknowledge a problem with reimbursement for patients who participate in formal clinical trials. Medicare will not pay for the extra costs of patients in trials, and many insurance plans specifically exclude payment for such patients. Until the mid 1980s, this was not a big problem because the policy was not generally enforced. As finances tightened, however, insurers began to identify patients in formal clinical research trials and to deny payment for tests, hospitalizations, and even physician fees (Antman, Schnipper, & Frei, 1988; Katterhagen & Mortenson, 1984; Lee & Mortenson, 1984; Mortenson, 1988c, 1989a; Wagner & Power, 1986; Yarbro & Mortenson, 1985). A recent survey indicates that managed care providers are most likely to prohibit patients from entering trials (Mortenson, 1994).

Concern over the potential impact of fixed-price (DRG or capitated) reimbursement on cancer patient management and clinical research led to a series of investigations by the Association of Community Cancer Centers (ACCC). Two specific concerns emerge from the concept of a fixed-price system of reimbursement.

Progress in management of patients with cancer depends on a significant number of research innovations. If innovative methods of care are more expensive than the prevailing methods of care, there is little likelihood that the new methods will be adopted unless the fixed price shifts. In many cases, it seems likely that the more expensive forms of care will be foregone unless the therapeutic advantage is significant. Yet who determines significant therapeutic advantage? Recently, one pharmaceutical company reported that reimbursement for a new form of therapy that extended the lives of patients with prostate cancer by 7 months was being refused by insurers despite the fact that it was lower in cost on a monthly basis than the prevailing forms of therapy (Mortenson, 1989a). The problem was that patients on the new therapy lived longer, so the total cost of therapy was higher.

If clinical research (vital to the development of new innovations) is more costly than conventional patient management, it is likely to be discouraged by hospital administrators or managed care executives who are trying to contain costs wherever possible (Yarbro & Mortenson, 1985). An overt federal policy that denies payment for patients in clinical trials and sets an example to other insurers is likely to lead to obstacles that impede clinical research.

PROBLEMS WITH REIMBURSEMENT FOR CANCER RESEARCH

Before the introduction of PPS, there were already prohibitions on research for new drugs. In an article entitled, "Federal Regulation and Pharmaceutical Innovation," the president of Pfizer noted that regulation was shortening the effective patent life of a product from 13.8 years in 1966 to about 8.9 years in 1977, seriously affecting the viability of the American pharmaceutical industry and reducing the incentives for new drug development in the United States (Laubach, 1980). Recognizing these problems with the new PPS in 1982, the ACCC asked the Department of Health and Human Services (DHHS) to make some exceptions in the PPS law for cancer research.

Starting in 1982, the association and others began a series of studies aimed at determining the impact of DRG (fixed price) reimbursement on both treatment and clinical research (Katterhagen & Mortenson, 1984; Mortenson & Winn, 1984; Yarbro & Mortenson, 1985). Using this data, a case was then made to the Congress, the DHHS, the HCFA, the NIH, and the National Cancer Institute (NCI) regarding the difficulties uncovered.

Congress took several measures to ensure that innovation in health care would continue and that research in general, and cancer research in particular, would not be curtailed. One of the measures instructed the secretary of DHHS to exempt hospitals doing a considerable amount of cancer research and treatment from the new PPS. Another established the Prospective Payment

Assessment Commission as an arm of the congressional Office of Technology Assessment and mandated that this new agency target required changes in the DRG to ensure that quality of care is appropriately compensated and that innovation continues.

The Secretary of DHHS (then Margaret Heckler) and HCFA administrator Carolyn Davis recommended that nothing be done about providing extra compensation to hospitals engaged in research (Davis, 1985; Yarbro & Mortenson, 1985). Regulations formulated by DHHS required extremely high levels of cancer research for an institution to receive an exemption from PPS. Only five NCI-designated comprehensive cancer centers were declared exempt from PPS by the initial regulations.

After some pressure from Senator Robert Dole (then Chairman of the Health Appropriations Subcommittee), the secretary established a panel to review the potential problems; it met once and decided to take a "wait and see" attitude. Members of the panel from the ACCC, the American Medical Association, and other specialty societies argued that there were already concrete examples of innovations and research being halted when DRGs were in force. Yet other representatives of hospitals and medical schools remained publicly silent.

Members from the NIH, the NCI, the Assistant Secretary for Planning and Evaluation, the HCFA, and the DHHS secretary's office generally exhibited a "party line" approach to the problem during the commission meeting. However, at one point, the director of the NIH turned to the assistant secretary of DHHS and said, "I hope you are right about this policy because there is no way my budget can stand the stress of all the additional patient care costs of patients on research protocols." In the final analysis, however, the director of NIH said he perceived no problem. The DHHS secretary's office maintained that the "teaching supplement" provided to university medical schools for training was a proxy compensation for research activities and was sufficient to cover the extra costs of new research approaches.

Subsequent to the DHHS commission, only one adjustment was made to the regulations developed to compensate hospitals and centers that performed a great deal of cancer research. This was to drop the formula required to qualify for an exemption from the PPS from 75 per cent of all discharges to 50 per cent so that the M. D. Anderson Tumor Institute would qualify for an exemption and Congressman Jake Pickle would be satisfied. No other political accommodations were made, and only six university-based cancer institutes throughout the nation were declared exempt. Although the National Cancer Advisory Board issued a statement of concern that some hospitals and research institutions were in jeopardy, NCI officials publicly stated that they did not perceive a problem.

Studies initiated by the ACCC were followed by large-scale studies of cancer DRG reimbursement undertaken by the NCI to determine whether any past change in reimbursement had affected research. Although critics suggested that the NCI studies were developed to serve as an apologist for the administration's position on DRGs, the Prospective Payment Assessment Commission (ProPAC) urged Congress to make several moves to compensate for new innovations and inadequacies in reimbursement for new innovations. The results of the NCI studies were never published.

Data developed by the ACCC were utilized by ProPAC as the basis for recommending that the reimbursement of leukemia patients be altered. The NCI and other research officials began to appraise the cost-effectiveness of proposed new protocols to determine whether new institutions would be likely to undertake them.

Researchers at Johns Hopkins University issued research findings that pointed out that patients at organized cancer programs were more expensive to treat and that DRGs did not compensate for differences in severity (Horn & Sharkey, 1986; Mortenson, 1986b). Their data noted the significant disparities in funding for research patients that could be prohibitive.

Throughout the early 1980s, no public statement was made that departed from the policy expressed by HCFA Administrator Davis's article in the *Journal of the American Medical Association* (1985). In a response to an article in that journal by Yarbro and Mortenson (1985), Davis said that there was no cause for concern. Patient care costs of research patients were included in the national pool when the initial calculations of DRGs were made and thus they were covered by the PPS system.

In 1986, two researchers from the Office of Technology Assessment reported ". . . cost-based payment permitted subsidy of some clinical research costs by Medicare, but the same data limitations that allowed such subsidies to occur also preclude accurate estimation of the magnitude of the subsidy. Yet, the impact of PPS on clinical research depends to a great extent on how large the subsidy was to begin with" (Wagner & Power, 1986, p. 66). Noting that "it is not altogether clear at this time whether such 'fixes' are necessary or even desirable," the authors added the following:

> The Association of Community Cancer Centers has suggested the establishment of a separate DRG for patients participating in research, and the National Cancer Advisory Board has suggested that research-related expenses for cancer patients be reimbursed as a cost pass through. Of course, either of these alternatives requires official recognition of Medicare reimbursement for research-related costs. Since DHHS has interpreted the Medicare law as prohibiting payment for most kinds of research, these options are infeasible without regulatory or legislative changes (p. 66).

Subsequently, federal and pharmaceutical research leaders have watched as clinical researchers report increasing difficulties in conducting their research trials. Medicare intermediaries are now denying all payments for research drugs even if they are commonly used for this indication. In many cases, individual physician fees and entire hospital stays are being denied on the basis that Medicare does not pay for research patients. Third parties are now denying payments for all of their clinical research patients. Clearly, the policy is having a major negative impact on NIH's mission. Yet it was not until 1988 that some leading NCI researchers broke ranks and began to discuss the problem in a series of federally sponsored forums.

In 1988, the NCI and other NIH officials began a series of national meetings in an attempt to draw attention to the growing problems faced by the NIH. If the policy remains in effect, a great many innovations will be scrapped because they are too costly to test or appear initially to be more costly than the prevailing therapy. Of course, experience teaches that some higher-cost therapies are greatly reduced in price once in widespread use.

The HCFA is now suggesting that cost-effectiveness be proved before a drug can be reimbursed. Because research methodologies for cost-effectiveness are widely variable, significant problems in new drug approvals and reimbursements will occur.

As health care reform bills move through Congress in 1994, ACCC, ASCO, and other cancer care organizations have stressed the need to protect research and off-label use of chemotherapeutic agents. In the early 1990s, ACCC was successful in passing federal and widespread state legislation to protect patient access to proven agents for off-label indications. Congress continues to debate various mechanisms for research protection, but regardless of their legislated solution, the reality of rapid reform suggests that research and use of new technologies may continue to be threatened.

The problems with health care policymaking are likely to continue. The HCFA's job is to contain costs. The NIH's job is to develop and promote the use of new technologies. National priorities in the 1990s will continue to focus on balancing the United States budget and reducing the budget deficit. These goals will require major economies in health care, and they are likely to take precedent over other priorities such as research. The best guess is that when clinical research is significantly crippled, some action will likely be taken to alleviate the problem.

PROBLEMS WITH REIMBURSEMENT FOR NEW TECHNOLOGIES

In addition to the problems with reimbursement for patients on clinical trials, reimbursement for the use of new technologies that have proved to be more effective has faced increasing obstacles as third-party intermediaries and other insurers attempt to find some uniform criteria for payment. These groups wish to establish Food and Drug Administration (FDA) labeling as the criteria for payment, which would cause a major problem for cancer care. The FDA has traditionally reviewed and approved new drugs, judging their safety and efficacy for a particular use or indication. This is a lengthy process, involving data analysis from highly controlled studies.

Once a drug is approved, pharmaceutical companies can market it for approved indications, and physicians can use it as they see fit. Although pharmaceutical manufacturers cannot market their drugs outside of the approved FDA labeling, physicians and scientists have often used drugs for indications that were not listed on the label. In cancer, cooperative group research provides a strong basis for the use of chemotherapeutic and biologic agents, well beyond the indications approved by the labeling. In fact, our research indicates that approximately 47 per cent of all chemotherapy use is outside of the approved labeling (Mortenson, 1988a, 1988b).

The U.S. Pharmacopeia's *Drug Information for the Health Care Professional*, the *AMA Drug Evaluations*, and the *American Hospital Formulary Service Drug Information* all involve scientists and clinicians in evaluations of the literature. All three compendia were cited in the ill-fated federal Catastrophic Insurance Act as standard references. Data from the USPDI suggest that 25 per cent of the accepted indications are not on the FDA label. These other accepted indications could readily account for 40 to 50 per cent of all drug use. These three compendia are cited as sources in recently passed ACCC legislation affecting Medicare, Medicaid, and 16 states' insurance plans. Recently the National Association of Insurance Commissions (NAIC) adopted ACCC's uniform language as their model bill, making universal acceptance of the three compendia a likelihood.

If insurance companies force pharmaceutical and biotechnology manufacturers to seek FDA approval before they pay for every new use, proven technologies will take a great deal of time to gain widespread use. Indeed, physicians are reporting major difficulties in obtaining reimbursement for new cancer technologies and major increases in the administrative time required to cajole insurance companies into paying for new technology and care.

One three-member oncology group's experience may be indicative. Over the past 3 years, this group's members have seen a steady increase in the volume of patients they are managing; their total consultations and practice have increased by 30 per cent. Yet their revenues have remained the same, and they report an additional 20 per cent of their time is now being spent attempting to secure payment for drugs and agents for their patients. From a national policy standpoint, reimbursement for all current cancer therapy, all patients on clinical trials, and all new therapies would account for less than one tenth of 1 per cent of the national health care bill (Mortenson, 1989b), surely a good investment.

NEW LOCATIONS FOR CANCER CARE

As patients with cancer have been removed from hospital settings, alternative delivery systems have sprung up. Freestanding cancer centers represent a move away from hospitals to outpatient centers. Although the primary method of care in many of these centers is radiation therapy, medical oncology and, in a few rare instances, outpatient surgical facilities are also included.

Home care is emerging as a major mechanism for delivery of chemotherapy because of the inability of hospitals to receive adequate reimbursement. Thus radiation therapy and chemotherapy have both moved away from the hospital setting to lower-cost outpatient settings.

THE IMPACT ON PROVIDERS

As noted earlier, physicians are finding that setting up practice is more difficult, revenues are going down, patient load is going up, and more time is being spent on administration. Physicians are also faced with the reality of delivering very different levels of care to groups of patients. In some cases, HMOs and other managed care plans have indicated that they will not pay for the care of patients with cancers that have poor prognoses. Thus physicians may be restricted from providing the types of care that might ensure a small percentage of these patients longer survivals or remissions. Without a doubt, this consideration also adds to the stress of the job.

THE FUTURE OF HEALTH CARE REIMBURSEMENT

What do we face in the 1990s? All of the change in reimbursement schemes has a real impact on nurses, their patients, and the kind of care they can provide. It will also have an impact on the types of care that will be available in the future.

First, it should be noted that both Medicare and Medicaid are in significant financial trouble. Throughout the last decade, a number of individuals have suggested that Medicare benefits would have to be cut. This problem has been exacerbated by the debate and repeal of the Catastrophic Insurance Act, which attempted to provide additional benefits to patients but which also increased the premiums required by individuals who are eligible for Medicare. Health care reform bills are explicit in cutting Medicare and Medicaid reimbursement to pay for more patient access.

Medicaid is a major financial drain on the states, and talk of reform is just beginning. Given that AIDS patient management is approximately 40 per cent covered by Medicaid, many states are seeing their financial problems compounding rapidly. It is possible that several states will not be able to handle the burden of cost under the current system.

Second, as patients have been forced out or kept out of hospitals, outpatient costs have exploded. As the federal government attempts to deal with this growing problem, it is exploring systems such as ambulatory visit groups, which are similar to DRGs. Without question, the federal government will concentrate on categorizing outpatient care into some system with a limited number of options that will allow payment to be fixed to diagnoses and paid for on a fixed-price basis. The other alternative is to attempt to move a major portion of all health care into managed care plans. This is the intent of health care reform.

Third, insurers are looking for ways to standardize approaches to care to minimize variations in costs and uncertainty. They are aware that 50 per cent of the average cost of care covers the last 6 months of life, and they often suggest that physicians and hospitals take too many measures that do not affect the ultimate outcome but do affect the cost. More and more insurers are attempting to cut costs by limiting the availability of care, restricting the use of new therapies, and insisting on a standardization of therapy. Using a variety of review mechanisms, patients are being kept out of high-cost settings (such as hospitals), discharged earlier, and provided with limited care whenever possible. Given the proliferation of managed care, ACCC, ASCO, ONS, and other national associations are now beginning to work collaboratively on patient management guidelines. These guidelines will serve as pathways for evaluating which patients can receive standard care and which need careful, specialized attention. They will also serve as a means of standardizing pricing of care and are likely to be tools used by nurses in lieu of physician intervention.

Fourth, as the costs of health care continue to rise inexorably as our population grows steadily older, as AIDS becomes more prevalent, and as new technology emerges, insurance plans of all types will be put under greater pressure. Of course, although federal and state governments pick up a major portion of the costs of care through Medicare and Medicaid, third-party insurance plans pick up a substantial portion of the total for industry. And industry has seen the costs of health care insurance skyrocketing. General Motors loudly complains that health care insurance absorbs more of the cost of its cars than steel. Industry leaders are eager to promote competition among health care providers and find alternative forms of care that are more cost-effective. Insurance plans that provide consumers with options are likely to become less and less viable as cost shifting from fixed price and capitated systems to these patients continues.

Everyone involved in the competition to provide lower insurance premiums has been in a race since 1982. Each of the insurance companies and managed care plans has been trying to obtain the greatest possible market share (i.e., the percentage of consumers or businesses subscribing to their plan), pushing as many competitors out of the market as possible. At the same time that everyone was cutting prices to get more customers, new technology and other market forces continued to force up the costs of care. The result is that many hospital and private insurance plans have lost significant amounts of money. In 1988, the National Blue Cross and Blue Shield plans announced that they had lost $1 billion in the previous year (Mortenson, 1988d).

Fifth, hospitals have also had their reimbursement from the federal government radically cut as the DRG system starts to crank down the lid on variations. Initially hospital and regional variations in length of stay and practice were allowed, but the DRG system is now national, and many hospitals that are used to operating with a profit margin will begin to operate below the break-even point. Many hospitals are experiencing losses now, and increasing numbers of them will fold (Mortenson, 1984). With tighter margins, hospitals will have to focus more attention on "winners" and on lowering the costs of care. They will have less funding for programs and new ventures and less funding for extras. This is likely to affect oncology units and their staffing, for example.

Not all of the news is bad. Many hospitals are still interested in supporting clinical research because they perceive it to be useful in positioning their cancer programs as superior. A whole new range of jobs has opened up in home care. Some of the deinstitutionalization of patients has allowed them greater freedom, and new and innovative ways to deliver lower cost and ambulatory or outpatient therapies are constantly emerging.

What Will Happen to the Insurance Industry?

In the 1990s, health insurance plans will continue to encounter major difficulties with survival. Self-insured companies will put increasing pressure on the current mechanisms of care, as will managed care organizations, both of which are steadily increasing their share of the marketplace.

As their reserves and margins go down, insurance plans will continue to cut services and restrict access to care while they attempt to force providers to maintain publicly acceptable quality standards (Futurist predicts, 1988). In the early 1990s, a number of states initiated their own health care reform plans, beginning a wide variety of experiments. Oregon's plan rations care. Washington state is a miniature of President Clinton's initial proposal. Under several reform bills in Congress, states will have the option of being "sole providers," putting further pressure on insurers. Sole providers will have only one single universal insurer in that state.

Unfortunately for patients with cancer, as with so many other aspects of the reimbursement system over the past decade, yesterday's good news is today's bad news. Because cancer was a life-threatening illness with no sure cure, insurance companies in the past allowed almost any cancer claim to be paid. Today, recognizing that many cancers are incurable and that the public perceives that cancer is most likely to be fatal, insurance companies are taking advantage and denying therapies and reimbursement. Only consumer or business pressure can force insurance companies to alter this trend, and the complexity of the issue militates against consumers understanding how their care is being manipulated and driven by inadequate reimbursement.

Concerns about Quality of Care

In the mid 1990s, increasing numbers of elderly, sick patients with significant health care problems are being seen on an inpatient basis. More patients will be seen as outpatients or at home. Care will be restricted. Different levels of care will be available to various patient groups.

Although a number of measures have been taken to cut costs, the federal government and insurers want to ensure that quality is not sacrificed. The Joint Commission on Accreditation of Healthcare Organizations is leading this charge, developing clinical indicators based on appropriate outcomes (Mortenson, Kerner, & Novak, 1987; O'Leary, 1987). Oncology clinical indicators were completed in 1989 and went into initial testing in 1989 and 1990. These clinical indicators are worthy of more discussion than can be managed here. However, it should be noted that clinical indicators and guidelines are likely to be used by insurers to determine what they will pay for and where.

Although health care providers have classically disdained discussions of reimbursement, marketing, and advertising, they can no longer afford this luxury. Incentives drive the system. Quality care and research are directly affected by payment. Keeping up with these reimbursement and practice issues will help nurses understand the dynamics of cancer care and give them an opportunity to affect it by working within their professional organizations and the oncology community.

REFERENCES

Antman, K., Schnipper, L., & Frei, E. (1988). The crisis in clinical cancer research: Third-party insurance and investigational therapy. *New England Journal of Medicine, 319*, 46.

Davis, C. (1985). The impact of prospective payment on clinical research progress. *Journal of the American Medical Association, 253*, 686–687.

Feldstein, P. J. (1980). The political environment of regulation. In A. Levin (Ed.), *Regulating health care: The struggle for control* (Proceedings of The Academy of Political Science), *33*(4).

Futurist predicts significant changes in health care. (1988). *Oncology Issues, 3*, 26.

Horn, S. D., & Sharkey, P. D. (1986). A study of patients in cancer-related DRGs. *Journal of Cancer Program Management, 1*(2), 8–14.

Katterhagen, J. G., Clarke, R. T., & Mortenson, L. E. (1989). Understanding the economics of inpatient cancer care. *Oncology Issues, 4*, 11–14.

Katterhagen, J. G., & Mortenson, L. E. (1984). Clinical research patients generate significant losses under diagnosis related groups (DRGs). *Seminars in Oncology, 11*, 330–331.

Laubach, G. D. (1980). Federal regulation and pharmaceutical innovation. In A. Levin (Ed.), *Regulating health care: The struggle for control* (Proceedings of The Academy of Political Science), *33*(4).

Lee, C., & Mortenson, L. E. (1984). Clinical research patients exceed costs of cancer patients within the same DRG category. *Cancer Program Bulletin, 10*(3), 6–7.

Mortenson, L. E. (1984). Can oncology nursing survive DRGs? *Journal of Oncology Nursing, 11*, 14–15.

Mortenson, L. E. (1985). *Cancer diagnosis related groups*. Washington, DC: Association of Community Cancer Centers.

Mortenson, L. E. (1986a). Cancer diagnosis related groups. In L. E. Mortenson, P. N. Anderson, & P. F. Engstrom (Eds.), *Advances in cancer control health care financing and research* (pp. 149–155). New York: Alan R. Liss, Inc.

Mortenson, L. E. (1986b). Without severity-adjusted DRGs, prospective payment may severely impair state-of-the art cancer care. *Journal of Cancer Program Management, 1*(2), 1.

Mortenson, L. E. (1988a). Audit indicates half of current chemotherapy users lack FDA approval. *Journal of Cancer Program Management, 3*(1), 21–26.

Mortenson, L. E. (1988b). Audit indicates many users of combination therapy are unlabeled. *Journal of Cancer Program Management, 3*(2), 33.

Mortenson, L. E. (1988c). The grocery store syndrome. *Oncology Nursing Forum, 15,* 545–546.

Mortenson, L. E. (1988d). The impact of reimbursement on quality cancer care. *Business and Health,* 38–40.

Mortenson, L. E. (1989a). Starve them or shoot them. *Oncology Issues, 4*(1), 2.

Mortenson, L. E. (1989b). Tight-money casualties in the war on cancer: Insurers target chemotherapy payments. *Wall Street Journal,* A14.

Mortenson, L. E. (1994). Health care policies affecting the treatment of patients with cancer and cancer research. *Cancer, (Suppl.), 74*(7).

Mortenson, L. E., Anderson, P. N., & Novak, C. (1986). What the research bases have to say about CCOPs. *Cancer Program Bulletin, 12*(1), 4–5.

Mortenson, L. E., & Baum, H. M. (1985). Cancer DRG's: 1985 analysis. *Cancer Program Bulletin,* 7–11.

Mortenson, L. E., Kerner, J. F., & Novak, C. M. (1987). Striving for excellence: Evaluating quality of care in oncology. *Journal of Cancer Program Management, 2*(1), 21–29.

Mortenson, L. E., & Winn, R. (1983). The potential negative impact of prospective reimbursement on cancer treatment and clinical research progress. *Cancer Program Bulletin, 9*(3), 1–4.

Mortenson, L. E., & Winn, R. (1984). DRGs: How will they affect your practice—and cancer care. *Your Patient and Cancer, 4*(2), 28–38.

Mortenson, L. E., & Yarbro, J. W. (1983). Oncology DRG research produces key findings for cancer program managers and policy makers. *Journal of Cancer Program Management, 1*(2), 6–7.

Mortenson, L. E., Yarbro, J. W., Clarke, R. T., & Cahill, E. (1985). Conventional cancer patient management and DRG's: A first report of ACCC's DRG research program. *Cancer Program Bulletin, 11,* 3–5.

Mortenson, L. E., Young, J. L., Jr., & Ney, M. S. (1988). Variations in cancer DRG profit and loss by hospital size and region of the nation. *Journal of Cancer Program Management, 3*(4), 16–19.

O'Leary, D. S. (1987). Quality control challenges in the new competitive marketplace. *Journal of Cancer Program Management, 2*(1), 6–10.

Pollard, M. R. (1980). Fostering competition in health care. In A. Levin (Ed.), *Regulating health care: The struggle for control* (Proceedings of The Academy of Political Science), *33*(4).

Salkever, D., & Bice, T. (1978). Certificate-of-need legislation and hospital costs. In M. Zubkoff, I. Raskin, & R. Hanft (Eds.), *Hospital cost containment.* New York: PRODIST.

Wagner, J. L., & Power, E. (1986). Diagnosis-related groups (DRG) payment and clinical research: In search of the problem. *Cancer Investigation, 4*(1), 61–67.

Yarbro, J. W., & Mortenson, L. E. (1985). The need for DRG 471—protection for clinical research. *Journal of the American Medical Association, 253,* 684–685.

Documentation Issues in Cancer Nursing

Barbara A. Barhamand

Documentation is commonly defined as a systematic gathering, classifying, and storing of information. To document is to support with written references or to serve as evidence or proof. In the realm of current professional nursing practice, documentation is each of these definitions and more. Early in one's nursing education, documentation is expanded from the methodic recording of what was actually done in terms of measurements (i.e., vital signs, input and output [I & O]) and tasks (i.e., IV tubing changed, ambulated × 1), to more complex assessments based on observations and information processing. Documentation in this framework is the essence of communication amongst health professionals to facilitate quality patient care (Edelstein, 1990).

This chapter explores a variety of methods used in nursing documentation, the advantages of each, and considerations for different practice arenas based on standards of care. Basic principles of effective and protective documentation are reviewed, as are the resulting legal issues.

METHODOLOGIES OF DOCUMENTATION

The Standards for Nursing Services developed by the Joint Commission for Accreditation of Health Care Organizations (JCAHO) provide the overall goals for documentation of each step of the nursing process (1990). These are generic in nature and are meant to be used as a guideline for the development of standards specific to the setting in which care is provided (Miaskowski & Nielsen, 1991). The American Nurses' Association and the Oncology Nursing Society (ANA-ONS) *Standards of Oncology Nursing Practice* (1987) were developed specifically for oncology nursing. They provide the guidelines for oncology nurses to develop

oncology patient assessment tools, oncology nursing care plans, and criteria for outcome evaluation. The patient's records should document the written care plan, indicating that nurses respond to the specific patient's needs (Edelstein, 1990).

The act of documentation is commonly referred to as "charting." In the clinical inpatient setting, this traditionally included the recording and plotting of vital signs and input and output measurements on a graph-like sheet. Medications given were accounted for on a medication record. A long narrative account of the nurse's tasks and patient's activities throughout the shift were recorded in "Nurse's Notes," which were often summarized and written at the end of the shift. These continue to be important elements of documentation, but there are numerous variations and rationales for accomplishing it.

The chronologic narrative method of charting requires that the patient's care is documented in the order that it occurred, taking into account the nurse's assessments and interventions, and the patient's response (Burke & Murphy, 1988). Although information is presented in an orderly fashion, notes tend to be lengthy, with pertinent data lost amongst the impertinent. Bailey-Allen (1990) discourages this type of documentation, which frequently results in vague descriptions and assessments. The practical nature of nursing results in a "do-it-now, write-it-down-later" mentality. Specific data are often incorrectly timed when using this method.

PROBLEM-ORIENTED RECORDS

Problem-oriented records (POR) were introduced to help physicians decrease redundancy in their documentation (Burke & Murphy, 1988). This type of documentation was adapted for many other medical disciplines, including nursing, as it concisely organized the information into a nursing process format: each assessment, intervention, and evaluation was problem-centered. The commonly-used SOAP (subjective, objective, assessment, and planning) format is an example of problem-oriented charting that has been revised by some to add an evaluation component (SOAPE) and revised again to include interventions, evaluation, and revisions (SOAPIER). Although more complete, this type of documentation remains repetitive and wordy (Coles & Fullenwider, 1988). Nurses often find it difficult to use when they have incidental information to record that does not necessarily fit a designated problem.

A variation of POR is known as focus charting (Lampe, 1985). Replacing the SOAP format with DAE (data, action, and evaluation), is particularly useful when documenting patient behaviors, types of therapy and response to therapy, and patient education. Nurses, according to Montemuro (1988), found it reflected their thinking in relation to clinical problem solving more effectively than the SOAP format. It also integrates well with the use of flow sheets.

FLOW SHEETS

Abbreviated charting methods using graphlike sheets for vital signs adds a visual perspective for quick reference and analysis (i.e., febrile patterns) and is well known to nurses. The expanded use of flow sheets has more recently encompassed any part of nursing care that is routine for that setting. Deane, McElroy, and Alden (1987) estimate that 15 per cent of a nurse's hours worked are used for documentation activities. Flow sheets can reduce documentation time significantly by eliminating the narrative format for routine patient care. By reserving Nurses' Notes for identified problems and observed responses, the narrative portion of charting is also less repetitive (Edelstein, 1990).

The limited space available on a flow sheet is a disadvantage of their use. Nonroutine observations may be incompletely charted due to the mandated brevity. Notations also tend to be duplicative and lack individuality. The flow sheet format, however, provides an organized presentation of data that not only improves accuracy, saves time, and enhances patient care (Miller & Pastorino, 1990; Ozuna & Adkins, 1993). Assessment cues or "triggers" minimize omissions in charting and eliminate unnecessary information. The utilization of flow sheets for alternative uses in oncology nursing has burgeoned. The creative development and use of flow sheets in a variety of clinical settings has streamlined documentation significantly.

Patient Education. Documentation of patient and family teaching is commonly inadequate or overlooked (Edelstein, 1990; Pevny, 1993). In an effort to conform with JCAHO standards, nurses have attempted to include this aspect of patient care in their documentation, but found it to be a time-consuming task in a narrative format. It is conceivable to conform this aspect of documentation to a flow sheet format, but an accepted standard of care must be in place.

Moore and Knobf (1991) and Lynch and Yanes (1991) allocated space for patient education on their flow sheets, but space is extremely limited for a lengthy initial contact. A separate flow sheet limited to the patient education component is a reasonable alternative (Fig. 80–1) but is most appropriate for initial contacts, with follow-up teaching documentation integrated with nursing assessments as they occur. A flow sheet specifically for documenting the patient education component of outpatient cisplatin therapy, including instructions for self hydration (Frogge, 1989), is an example of designing a tool that meets the needs of a specific patient population and the nurse. It is imperative that any forms used must accommodate the specific setting in which care is provided, and follow the accepted standards of that setting.

Nursing Assessment. The initial assessment made of the patient in an acute care setting is typically done using an "Admission sheet" and interviewing the patient for background information. Miaskowski and Nielsen (1991) present a complex format for collection of this initial data. This tool is structured around 11 high-incidence problem areas in an oncology population and presents an organized and comprehensive format for the interview process. The physical assessment/medical history provides a systematic database to use to develop nursing diagnoses. A final portion of the tool provides information about psychosocial needs, which evolves into a discharge plan.

A second format, described by Holton-Smith (1992), provides a component of information for the nurse that might otherwise be overlooked. Questions are psychosocial in nature (i.e., "Who is your main support?"; "Has anyone close to you ever had cancer, and how did they do?"; "What upcoming events do you have planned that may interfere with treatment scheduling?") and can be self-completed or serve as directives for a nurse's interview and assessment.

A self-reporting health history is encouraged by Skinn and Stacey (1994) and Kiss, Dorsa, and Martin (1993). Nurses commonly skip over questions that are sensitive in nature, and patients are more likely to respond accurately when they can be self-recorded. Questions geared toward sexuality, safety, and pain status are frequently omitted or only briefly addressed. By allowing patients to privately report their own assessments, nurses are more apt to follow up when a need is already identified.

A self-reporting Toxicity Assessment Tool was developed by Brinkman, Hay, and Laubinger (1994) to enhance the documentation of chemotherapy side effects. For those patients who are enrolled in clinical trials, it is vital that information about toxicities be graded and all-inclusive. By offering the tool to the patient, the investigator or data manager is assisted in grading the toxicities accurately.

CHARTING BY EXCEPTION

Standards of Nursing Practice provide a minimum level of routine care for patients when using a Charting By Exception (CBE) method of documentation (Burke & Murphy, 1988). Generalized protocols list standardized nursing interventions used for a specific patient

NAME:		Also present:						
(√ signifies topic covered with apparent understanding from patient and/or significant other)		Initial instruction			Followup instruction			
		√	Initials	Needs Reinf.	Date each			
Rationale for prescribed chemotherapy protocol								
Effect of chemotherapy on cancer/normal cells								
Variability/manageability of side effects								
Potential/rational for occurrence of								
Fatigue								
Infection								
Bleeding/bruising								
Alopecia								
Kidney function								
Mouth sores								
Weight loss/gain								
Nausea/vomiting								
Diarrhea								
Neuropathy/constipation								
Extravasation								
Reproductive changes								
Instructed regarding the use of:								
Tylenol								
Birth control								
Alcohol								

Rx given (with instruction) for: Written materials provided:

   Antiemetics _____   ____ Chemotherapy & You

   Sedative _____   ____ Drug info sheets

   Antidiarrheal _____   ____ _____

   Chemotherapy _____   ____ _____

   Hormonal _____   ____ _____

   Hair prosthesis _____   ____ _____

Additional notes:

_____

_____

_____

_____

_____

Initials	Nurse's Signature

Figure 80–1. Chemotherapy teaching documentation. (Used with permission of Hematology-Oncology Consultants, Ltd., Naperville, IL)

population during a typical clinical course. Initial information is collected using a format similar to that of Miaskowski and Nielsen (1991), with an area reserved for "within normal limits." Exceptions to the normals are developed into nursing diagnoses and become the identifiable areas in need of documentation. The underlying philosophy of CBE is to chart only significant findings, but requires a variety of flow sheets specific to each patient population to establish the norms (Burke & Murphy, 1988). This type of system is quite adapt-

able to an outpatient oncology setting where standards of care are well delineated and the patient population is relatively homogeneous.

COMPUTERIZATION

While the overwhelming majority of a nurse's documentation is done with traditional pen and paper, computers are more frequently being used than ever before. In the current cost-conscious health care environment, nurses are held accountable for their time. According to Volden, Esslinger, Johnson, Busch, and Doepke, (1988), the completion of charting was the single primary reason given for nursing overtime. Institutions and practice settings are looking at electronic alternatives to reduce the time spent on the documentation process.

Computers are used in hospital settings most commonly for patient admitting, billing, medical records and coding, and laboratory (Kahl, Ivancin, & Fuhrmann, 1991). More recently, bedside computer charting has been introduced. "Point of care" (POC) systems, as they are referred to, have several obvious advantages, although primary is the time saved for the nurse (Meyer, 1992). Patient data (i.e., vital signs, I & O) are also immediately recorded and are instantly available to other health care providers. Information is not jotted on worksheets or note paper for later transfer to the chart. Some bedside systems actually record vital signs using their own thermometers and blood pressure cuffs and transfer data directly from monitors and infusion pumps.

Another advantage to the POC system is the accuracy and completeness that it ensures. Computerized records allow for standardized terminology, system prompts reduce charting omissions, entries outside normal limits are "flagged" and questioned to reduce charting errors, and duplicative entries are eliminated (Meyer, 1992). Ancillary benefits (and disadvantages) to a computerized system are detailed in Table 80–1. Specifically, hospitals value the ability to retrieve information for quality assurance or research purposes, the availability of patient information from unit to unit, monitor drug usage, evaluate staff productivity and efficiency, and abstract information into report format (Latz, 1992; Willey & Winstead, 1990).

Computerized nursing care plans with diagnosis-related interventions and expectations have reduced documentation time significantly. Nurses in alternative practice sites, such as home care, utilize laptop computers to access a patient's permanent record and enter data from the home. Patient records can also be accessed via modem from a physician's home, if computerization has been accomplished in the office setting (Willey & Winstead, 1990).

Voice-activated systems, originally developed for use by the physically challenged and orthopedically impaired, are now being increasingly used in the medical field. Equipped with a microphone or headset, the user utilizes voice commands to prompt specific portions of the medical record, then dictates the information to fill each field. Information can be immediately printed to include in the patient record. Certain commands can be formatted to include a cluster of descriptives. For example, the spoken command "Port Flushed" could actually chart "Port-a-cath flushed with 10 cc normal saline, followed by 5 cc Heplock solution, 100u/ml." Programmed "forms," such as a chemotherapy flow sheet, prompt the user if a field is bypassed or content omitted. A physician's or nurse's progress notes can be dictated and are immediately available, unlike traditional dictation that requires a time delay for transcription. Obvious advantages of this type of system include legibility and completeness, both of which are ideals in the documentation process from a professional and legal standpoint.

The use of computers in health care is ever-changing. Systems are now interfaced, unit to unit, hospital to clinic, office to hospital, office to lab, etc. Although a costly investment, its impact on information management as well as nursing documentation, will likely prove to be worth its price. Nurses should involve themselves, providing a nurse's perspective, from the planning phase if computerization becomes a possibility in the workplace.

TABLE 80–1. *Considerations Before Computerization*

Conveniences
Minimizes paperwork
Immediate availability of patient information
Multiple users have access to "chart"
Standardized care plans are diagnosis-specific
Standardized terminology
System prompts minimize charting omissions
System prompts query abnormal entries
Remote access to patient records via modem or laptop
Legibility
Minimizes errors due to transcription error
Availability of system-generated reports for QA
Automated data source for retrospective research
Monitoring of supplies or drug usage

Concerns
Initial cost
Ongoing maintenance expense
Unexpected system failure ("the computer is down")
System becomes obsolete
Confidentiality/unauthorized access to medical records
Staff training and orientation

PRINCIPLES OF EFFECTIVE DOCUMENTATION

Regardless of the method of documentation used and the setting in which one practices, the general principles of documentation remain unchanged. The basics demand that the charting done be accurate and comprehensive, but brief. Accuracy is imperative regarding timing, amounts, and descriptions (Eggland, 1988). Vague terminology such as "apparently" or "appears to" can be misinterpreted to mean that the nurse was not sure of what was observed, and should be avoided. Use definitive wording in describing observations and assessments, such as "port-a-cath site edematous; swelling noted in circular area, 5 cm in diameter; site is not hot to touch." This allows for concise comparisons and precisely defines what is seen.

All observations should be followed with a nursing action and evaluation of that action (Eggland, 1988). The above notation should also include "Patient reports slight discomfort; infusion of normal saline stopped; needle repositioned, back of access device confirmed; blood return is observed and infusion restarted. Patient reports resolution of discomfort." Being brief keeps charting direct and succinct, but details should never be omitted for the sake of lengthiness. Incomplete statements are acceptable, and actually prevent verbose, run-on sentences that can be misunderstood and cause confusion.

Timeliness is another factor in effective documentation. Narrative, shift-end notes are written in summary of what has happened, but may not give precise details of what was done when. Frequent charting will help keep details in a correct perspective, but flow sheets and computers may provide the best format for documenting what time a dressing was changed, medication was given, etc. If charting is done promptly, errors in recall and documentation are reduced (Iyer, 1991).

LEGAL ISSUES

Documentation and compliance with an institution's policies and procedures are the two single-most important strategies in avoiding professional malpractice (Schulmeister, 1987). Although the process of documentation is time-consuming and time spent away from patient care, it must be viewed as a component of patient care, rather than a separate act in itself. Each nursing entry relates a portion of the patient's medical history. Each entry, if done correctly, provides communication for other health care workers, to update the plan for care. Each entry is a vital link to subsequent entries.

Incorrect entries and omissions will promote inconsistencies in care, miscommunications, and possibly, negligence and harm to the patient. If an error is made while charting, corrections should be made by crossing out the incorrect information with the notation, "error" and your initials. If a complete entry is made into the wrong chart, do not discard the page. Cross out the entire entry with a single line, make the notation "error—wrong chart," add your initials, and keep it with the original record. Correction fluid to "white out" an error is a "red flag" to an attorney reviewing records and should not be used under any circumstances. Late entries are not ideal, but outweigh the option of the omission of relevant information. Such entries should be designated as such by the notation "Late entry" or "addendum." Omissions and errors will happen in day-to-day practice but can be minimized by thoughtful and careful charting done as events progress, rather than hours after-the-fact. By documenting the care provided in a correct manner, the patient ultimately benefits and the nurse is protected.

The most common legal complaints brought against nurses include medication errors, breach of a patient's safety, failure to recognize or report a change in the patient's condition, or failure to comply with the standard of care or an institutional policy (Burke & Murphy, 1988). Nurses commonly chart what has been done in a defensive manner to protect themselves from malpractice. Care should be taken, though, to avoid any critical language and to document concisely what has been done and what has been said. Attorneys will peruse medical records for any slanted presentation of facts if the chart is being examined for possible legal action.

It is important in an outpatient or home care setting to carefully document what the patient was told about self-care issues, and that the caregiver understood the directions given. Home care and ambulatory care nurses routinely provide face-to-face evaluations and instructions, as well as by phone, that should be well documented. Telephone triage is an important aspect of the nurse's role that carries a high potential for liability. To minimize this risk, established protocols for complaint-specific calls should be used for offering advise and the subsequent documentation (Chamorro & Tarulli, 1990). In the physician's office, pharmacy calls for prescription refills are common interruptions for the nurse. Clerical staff should present the patient's chart with such requests so that immediate documentation can be done (Barhamand, 1992).

Physicians have been advised to carry a memo-type form when on call to document what interventions have been recommended when the chart is not immediately available (Daugrid, 1988). These should then be entered into the patient's outpatient record, which can provide vital information (i.e., new medications prescribed) to the nurse taking future calls or making further assessments. Nurses have developed similar forms for telephone triage, as shown in Figure 80–2, which facilitates the documentation process (Pfeifer, 1992).

IMPACT OF EFFECTIVE DOCUMENTATION

The obvious result of quality documentation is enhanced patient care. The process of planning for a patient's care, implementing it, and evaluating it are consolidated into the patient's record. This allows for each health care provider to work effectively as a team member, providing his or her unique input and observations. The patient ultimately benefits. There are ramifications of optimal documentation, however, that affect health care from other perspectives.

REIMBURSEMENT STRATEGIES

The current health care climate has produced an acute awareness of cost containment in every health care setting. Now, more than ever, it is mandatory that documentation accurately denotes what was done for the patient. Under the current system payment made for patient care is based on medical diagnoses. Documentation must consistently support the diagnoses and the services provided. Reimbursement for nursing services will be based on the documentation that supports the need for care, based on the diagnoses (Campbell & Dowd, 1993).

Medicare regulations state that hospitals cannot hold a patient liable for the cost of hospitalization; however, the hospital is ultimately responsible to ensure that the admission of the patient was truly justified (Hoke, 1985). Accurate nursing assessment and

TRINITY LUTHERAN HOSPITAL

Allergies
Time of Call
Time Call Returned
Length of Call
PURPOSE OF CALL
☐ PT Problem

Call initiated by:
☐ PT
☐ Family
☐ MD
Phone #
☐ Pharmacy #
☐ Visiting RN #

Urgency
☐ Emergency
☐ ASAP
☐ Today

Name

ADDITIONAL NOTES:

☐ Drug Refill
Test Results

DISPOSITION OF CALL
☐ See Orders   ☐ Medication Change
☐ Drug Refill   ☐ Test Results Given:
  ☐ TLH   ☐ By RN Per MD OK
  ☐ Called   ☐ To Be Given By MD
  ☐ Script   Notified_____
  Mailed

☐ Question About Appt/Tests
☐ Update on PT Status
☐ Special
Instructions_____
_____
☐ F/U Required_____

☐ Other

NURSE SIGNATURE: DATE:

PHONE CALL DOCUMENTATION

FIGURE 80–2. Documentation of telephone interventions. (Used with permission of P. Eldredge and Trinity Lutheran Hospital, Kansas City, MO)

documentation are needed to support the diagnosis-related groups (DRGs) for each patient. If more than one diagnosis is listed, each one should be addressed in the ongoing nursing evaluation and documentation. Optimal documentation will increase revenues, just as lost revenues will result when data are not accurately or completely recorded or communicated to physicians.

In the outpatient setting, reimbursement is somewhat similar, although much more procedure-oriented. For instance, reimbursement is made based on Current Procedural Terminology (CPT) codes, which designate the level (complexity) of care provided by the physician and separate procedures done (i.e., chemotherapy administration, venipuncture for specimen collection). A predetermined rate is allowed for each code, although each code's approval is dependent on specific diagnoses. Utilizing a CPT code does not guarantee reimbursement, and payment will be denied if not listed with a correlated diagnosis code. Subsequently, adequate documentation must again support the diagnosis, and monetary penalties will result if documentation is lacking at the time of a chart audit by a third-party payor.

In a hospital-based ambulatory care center, documentation must support the actual procedures done and durable medical goods and equipment used, as those are billed and reimbursed separately. In a physician's practice setting, reimbursement is based on procedures done and a level of care provided, with durable medical goods included in the actual procedural charge. There is little reimbursement made for the actual nursing component of care, although documentation of the care provided may influence the level of care, which in turn will increase reimbursement made.

QUALITY ASSURANCE

Quality assurance (QA) is the systematic evaluation of clinical practice (Pevny, 1993). This process of self-assessment is used to measure the extent to which poli-

cies and procedures are followed, and high-quality patient care is achieved. Hospitals have an ongoing QA program that monitors patient care and resolves problems when they occur. This ongoing evaluation is necessary for accreditation by the JCAHO. Accurate and comprehensive documentation of the patient care delivered will result in a high level of approval and will enhance the accreditation process (Eggland, 1988). A lack of consistent documentation reflects poorly on even the best patient care.

While a Quality Assurance program is mandatory at most institutions, they are usually lacking at free-standing centers and private practices, unless they are subject to accreditation of some type. The overall goal of QA is quality patient care; however, alternative practice settings should consider initiating QA to directly measure the care they are providing. A substandard level in any specific area would indicate that (a) the policy or procedure is not being followed, or (b) that staff members are not charting what is being done.

Pevny (1993), through a quality assurance review, found that documentation of chemotherapy administration was deficient in the areas of verification of informed consent, IV site placement, and patient/family teaching. This prompted the development of a tool that included "prompts" addressing these subjects, encouraging the nurse to be more inclusive.

INDIVIDUALIZING DOCUMENTATION SYSTEMS

The ideal documentation system is comprehensive yet streamlined. In an attempt to achieve consistently high-quality documentation, nurses have developed numerous variations of each aspect of the documentation system. These systems must be continually updated to meet the changing requirements of accreditation organizations (DiBlasi & Savage, 1992). Although one system cannot work efficiently for all practice settings, a tool that works effectively in one setting (i.e., radiation therapy) would ultimately work universally in similar settings. Some alternative settings (beyond inpatient/outpatient hospital-based practice) have a distinct advantage of not dealing with a hierarchy when instituting change. Although the developmental stage may be somewhat arduous, the efforts toward improving a documentation system that does not work efficiently is usually time well spent. Each setting, however, has unique needs that should be considered when developing a documentation system.

RADIATION THERAPY

The nursing care provided in a radiation therapy setting includes initial patient assessments, patient and family teaching, and ongoing evaluation. The patient-to-nurse ratio is high, and side effects experienced are often chronic and predictable in nature (Dudjak, 1988). The documentation of patient care and teaching can be lengthy and repetitious but can be accomplished with a variety of flow sheets.

Because side effects are often treatment site-specific (i.e., pelvis), an effective documentation tool would address the needs of the patient receiving radiation to that site. A national work group organized by the Radiation Oncology Nursing Special Interest Group (SIG) of the Oncology Nursing Society (ONS) has developed a series of standardized documentation tools for nurses to use in their workplace. The forms are available for purchase through the ONS office. Computer software has also been developed by IMPAC utilizing the same standardized documentation system, with a QA component.

Collegial sharing in a project such as this has many benefits. Cooperative development allows the input of experts in the field working collaboratively to fine-tune and perfect a system utilizing years of work experience and individual perspectives. According to a study by Grant, Dodd, Hilderly, and Patterson (1984), radiation oncology nurses commonly work "solo" (one nurse per center), lacking the day-to-day professional support of other nurses. By standardizing forms, nurses need not "reinvent the wheel" to have a quality documentation system specific to their needs.

AMBULATORY/OFFICE ONCOLOGY PRACTICE

Physicians have used a flow sheet format for documentation of chemotherapy administration and corresponding hematology data for many years. This has extended to use in ambulatory oncology clinics and offices where treatments are repetitive, and information can be concisely recorded. Hematologic response to therapy and subsequent dosage modifications are clearly portrayed in a space-conservative manner. Typically, multiple treatment dates are displayed, which facilitates cross-comparison of dosages and lab data.

Cooperative oncology research groups utilize flow sheets to also record the incidence of side effects, con-comitant therapies, and tumor response. Lynch and Yanes (1991) adapted the ECOG (Eastern Cooperative Oncology Group) flow sheet to include patient teaching and symptom management, which better reflected the nursing process.

An alternative format for chemotherapy administration documentation is a one-treatment-per-sheet layout, as described by Cushman (1991) and Pickett (1992). Assessment cues (i.e., lab parameters, side effects) may be listed, providing the inexperienced nurse with the necessary prompts for complete documentation. Detailed areas for IV sites, vascular access devices, and patient teaching, subjects that are commonly omitted from documentation in hectic ambulatory care settings, can also be included. While this format encourages comprehensive and complete charting, it does not enhance treatment-to-treatment comparison of lab values and dosage modification.

Advantages of a single treatment flow sheet for the patient on a complex regimen and requiring continuing patient education are offset by the disadvantages for the patient on adjuvant or repetitive treatments with few or no side effects and little need for patient education after the initial weeks of therapy. Specifically, a patient on adjuvant therapy for colorectal cancer would accumulate over 50 pages of chemotherapy administration flow sheets over the 1-year course, creating a significant paper burden with possibly minimal variance in side effects and hematologic values.

Chemotherapy treatments that require documentation of frequent monitoring (i.e., vital signs for paclitaxel infusions) or fluid balance records (i.e., I & O for cisplatin therapy) can be difficult to conform to an abbreviated flow sheet format. An expanded format using standing orders, as shown in Figure 80–3, minimizes documentation time, yet concisely records the information required.

The ONS Special Interest Group for Ambulatory/Office nurses has a work group assigned to develop a standardized tool for documentation in their work setting. Similar to the efforts made by the Radiation Oncology SIG, this attempt to provide a common documentation system would be helpful to oncology nurses in like settings. A collaborative effort reduces time spent unnecessarily developing tools from "scratch." Although not yet available at the time of this printing, another foreseeable advantage will be a common patient record, recognizable to professionals elsewhere, as patients frequently consult second opinions, move, or travel in today's mobile society.

HOME AND HOSPICE CARE

In the current health care environment, where the patient at home is more acutely ill than ever before, nurses must verify and document the patient's and family's ability to provide the necessary care that has been prescribed (Chamorro & Tarulli, 1990). Family members-turned-caregivers often seem to understand what is being taught as it is presented, yet forget or panic when left alone to actually implement the plan. Written instructions should be left with the caregiver to refer to

HEMATOLOGY ONCOLOGY CONSULTANTS, LTD.
TAXOL FLOW SHEET

NAME: DATE: CYCLE:

SITE: PORT   IV _____   MD: FB   DA

STANDING ORDERS: RN INITIALS

     Decadron 20 mg po X 2 doses at 9pm-12am last noc and between 6-9am today   _____

     Epinephrine 1: 1000/sub-q; Benadryl 50 mg for IV/IM inj.:
     Hydrocortisone 100 mg IV/IM injection at bedside   _____

(TIME)

_____   Access IV: draw CBC, if necessary   _____

_____   100 cc 0.9 NS with Benadryl 50 mg + Cimetadine 300 mg over 30 min.   _____

     Preinfusion vitals, then at 5 min, 15 min, 30 min, 60 min and hourly
     up to 2 hrs. post infusion until discharged home.   _____

_____   Taxol_____ mg (135 mg/m2; 150 mg/m2; 175 mg/m2) in 500 cc 0.9 NS
     using filter, non-PVC tubing, and infusion pump, over 3 hours.   _____

TIME	BP	P	R	Notes:	INITIAL

NURSES' SIGNATURES   PORT CARE:

_____ _____   Cleanse site with Betadine X 3   _____
                                               1% Lidocaine 0.5 cc sub-q over site   _____
_____ _____   Blood return ascertained   _____
                                               Flush: 10cc NS/5cc Heplock   _____
_____ _____

                                               RN INITIALS   _____

FIGURE 80–3. Documentation of paclitaxel administration. (Used with permission of Hematology-Oncology Consultants, Ltd., Naperville, IL)

later. The nurse should document concisely what was said, what written materials were left, and that return demonstrations were successfully achieved.

Coker and Lampert (1990) developed a checklist for documentation of patient teaching done in the home care setting for infusion therapy, which could be adapted to most topics in similar settings. It features an area for documenting return demonstrations. Future instructions at subsequent sessions can be added by other nurses, as its intention is to be cumulative, rather than for isolated incidences. Patients must also receive information that enables them to make decisions regarding their care, and information about the safe use of medical supplies, which is JCAHO-mandated.

The checklist format eliminates the lengthy narrative note that would be otherwise necessary to accomplish all that is required.

SUMMARY

Documentation issues for cancer nurses are as varied as the settings in which nurses practice. A common thread is the desire to document in a manner that enhances communication between the health care team and ensures quality patient care. Oncology nurses must acquaint themselves with institutional policies and procedures, if they exist. Critical evaluation of the documentation system in place should answer such questions as, "What takes the most time to document?"; "What is most commonly omitted or insufficiently charted?"; and "What already exists that could be adapted for use in this setting?" Options, such as standardized formats and computerization of patient records, deserve consideration.

Nurses must no longer view documentation as a separate, time-consuming entity. Documentation is a vital component of the care that is provided to the patient and a key to communication amongst health care providers.

REFERENCES

American Nurses' Association and Oncology Nursing Society. (1987). *Standards of oncology nursing practice.* Kansas City, MO: American Nurses' Association.

Bailey-Allen, A. M. (1990). Changing liability of the nurse over the past decade. *Orthopaedic Nursing, 9*(2), 13–15.

Barhamand, B. (1992). Optimizing the use of the telephone for oncology nurses in an office setting. In R. M. Carroll-Johnson, (Ed.), *Meeting the expanding needs of the office-based oncology nurse* (pp. 8–14). Pittsburgh: Oncology Nursing Press.

Brinkman, P., Hay, D., & Laubinger, P. (1994).Chemotherapy toxicity assessment using a self-report tool. *Oncology Nursing Forum, 21*(10), 1731–1733.

Burke, L. J., & Murphy, J. (1988). *Charting by exception: a cost-effective, quality approach.* Milwaukee, WI: Aurora Health Care.

Campbell, J. M., & Dowd, T. T. (1993). Capturing scarce resources: Documentation and communication. *Nursing Economics, 11*(2), 103–106.

Chamorro, T., & Tarulli, D. (1990). Strategies for risk management in cancer nursing. *Oncology Nursing Forum, 17*(6), 915–920.

Coker, M., & Lampert, A. (1990). Teaching checklist for home infusion therapy. *Oncology Nursing Forum, 17*(6), 923–926.

Coles, M., & Fullenwider, S. (1988). Documentation: Managing the dilemma. *Nursing Management, 19*(12), 65–72.

Cushman, K. E (1991). A tool for documenting chemotherapy administration quickly and completely. *Oncology Nursing Forum, 18*(3), 599–600.

Daugrid, A. (1988). Patient telephone call documentation. *Journal of Family Practice, 27*, 420–421.

Deane, D., McElroy, M. J., & Alden, S. (1987). Documentation: Meeting requirements while maximizing productivity. *Nursing Economics, 4*(4), 175.

DiBlasi, M., & Savage, J. (1992). Revitalizing a documentation system. *Rehabilitation Nursing, 17*(1), 27–29.

Dudjak, L. (1988). Radiation therapy nursing care record: A tool for documentation. *Oncology Nursing Forum, 15*(6), 763–777.

Edelstein, J. (1990). A study of nursing documentation. *Nursing Management, 21*(11), 40–46.

Eggland, E. T. (1988). Charting: How and why to document your care daily—and fully. *Nursing88, 88*(11), 76–84.

Frogge, M. H. (1989). Streamlining outpatient cisplatin therapy to meet the challenges of today. *Seminars in Oncology Nursing, 5*(2 Suppl.), 21–28.

Grant, M., Dodd, M., Hilderly, L., & Patterson, P. (1984). Radiation oncology nurses' role: A national survey. *Oncology Nursing Forum Supplement: Proceedings of the Tenth Annual Congress, 11*(2), 107.

Hoke, J. L. (1985). Charting for dollars. . . documentation can bring in money—or lose it. *American Journal of Nursing, 885*(6), 658–660.

Holton-Smith, D. (1992) Enhancing nursing assessments in the oncology office practice. In R. M. Carroll-Johnson, (Ed.), *Meeting the expanding needs of the office-based oncology nurse* (pp. 1–7). Pittsburgh: Oncology Nursing Press.

Iyer, P. W. (1991). Thirteen charting rules to keep you legally safe. *Nursing91, 91*(6), 40–44.

Joint Commission for Accreditation of Hospitals. (1990). *Nursing care scoring guidelines.* Oakbrook Terrace, IL: Author.

Kahl, K., Ivancin, L., & Fuhrmann, M. (1991). Automated nursing documentation system provides a favorable return on investment. *Journal of Nursing Administration, 21*(11), 44–51.

Kiss, M. E., Dorsa, B. A., & Martin, S. (1993). The development of a patient history and data base form. *Oncology Nursing Forum, 20*(5), 815–823.

Lampe, S. (1985). Focus charting: Streamlining documentation. *Nursing Management, 16*(7), 43–46.

Latz, P. (1992). Computerized nursing documentation systems. *Association of Operating Room Nurses, 56*(2), 300–311.

Lynch, M., & Yanes, L. (1991). Flowsheet documentation of chemotherapy administration and patient teaching. *Oncology Nursing Forum, 18*(4), 777–783.

Meyer, C. (1992). Bedside computer charting: Inching toward tomorrow. *American Journal of Nursing, 92*(4), 38–44.

Miaskowski, C., & Nielsen, B. (1991). Documentation of the nursing process in cancer nursing. In S. B. Baird, R. McCorkle, & M. Grant (Eds.), *Cancer nursing: A comprehensive textbook* (pp. 1126–1138). Philadelphia: W.B. Saunders Co.

Miller, P., & Pastorino, C. (1990). Daily nursing documentation can be quick and thorough. *Nursing Management, 21*(11), 47–49.

Montemuro, M. (1988). CORE documentation: A complete system for charting nursing care. *Nursing Management, 19*(8), 28–32.

Moore, J. M., & Knobf, M. T. (1991). A nursing flow sheet for documentation of ambulatory oncology. *Oncology Nursing Forum, 18*(5), 933–939.

Ozuna, L. A., & Adkins, A. T. (1993). Development of a vital-sign/fluid balance flow sheet. *Oncology Nursing Forum, 20*(1), 113–115.

Pevny, V. (1993). Outcome of a quality assurance review: Development of a documentation tool for chemotherapy administration. *Oncology Nursing Forum, 20*(3), 535–541.

Pfeifer, P. (1992). Documentation of care in an oncology outpatient setting. *Oncology Nursing Forum, 19*(5), 809–818.

Pickett, R. R. (1992). Outpatient oncology chemotherapy documentation tool. *Oncology Nursing Forum, 19*(3), 515–517.

Schulmeister, L. (1987). Litigation involving oncology nurses. *Oncology Nursing Forum, 14*(2), 25–28.

Skinn, B., & Stacey, D. (1994). Establishing an integrated framework for documentation: Use of a self-reporting health history and outpatient oncology record. *Oncology Nursing Forum, 21*(9), 1557–1566.

Volden, C. M., Esslinger, V. M., Johnson, M. E., Busch, D. E., & Doepke, L. A. (1988). Decentralization of patient charts: What does it accomplish? *Applied Nursing Research, 1*(3), 132–139.

Willey, B., & Winstead, W. W. (1990). Computer-based clinical charting and patient case management. *CARING, June,* 44–47.

The Generation of Stress in the Provision of Care

Patricia J. Larson • *Bonnie Mowinski Jennings*

Perhaps more than any chronic disease other than acquired immunodeficiency syndrome (AIDS), the diagnosis of cancer evokes a tremendous amount of fear. This fear may be based, in part, on the long history of negative connotations that surround cancer. These include visions of pain, disfigurement, helplessness, altered consciousness, financial distress, isolation, and death. As Schoenberg and Senescu (1970) asserted more than 2 decades ago, the word *cancer* stimulates thoughts of an eroding, devouring, and mutilating disease. Given this rather gruesome image of cancer as an illness, it is not surprising that individuals caring for patients with cancer are faced with a multitude of challenges and questions.

Caring—both the attitude and the activity—has been identified not only as the dominant theme of clinical nursing but also as a salient feature of cancer nursing (Larson, 1984; Styles, 1982). The demands facing nurses who care for patients with cancer are a complex composite of the patient's physical and psychosocial needs. Amid the flurry of checking doctors' orders, striving to control pain, writing myriad nursing notes, comforting families, making beds, formulating nursing diagnoses, and giving prescribed treatments, nurses must also confront personal issues concerning the care versus cure dichotomy and recognize their own mortality. These diverse and demanding responsibilities have generated a belief that nurses caring for patients with cancer experience a great deal of stress.

The purpose of this chapter is to examine the stress experienced by nurses in providing care to patients with cancer. This will be accomplished by reviewing stress research that pertains to nurses in general, evaluating empiric evidence of the stress of cancer nursing in particular, and examining how the patient's cancer tra-

jectory may influence the nurse's stress. To focus the discussion, a definition of stress and a brief mention of pertinent conceptual issues are offered.

THE MEANING OF STRESS

Defining stress is considerably more difficult than it may seem, because there is no agreed on definition. In fact, the concept is thickly veiled in conceptual confusion. Stress has been viewed as an antecedent or stimulus, a consequence or response, and an interactive process between the person and the environment (Lazarus & Launier, 1978; Mason, 1975). The last-mentioned perspective is particularly useful when considering stress in occupations as well as a more holistic view of individuals. Stress, then, occurs when there is a perceived imbalance between demands and abilities (Harrison, 1978).

In addition, there are two sides to stress; one is the positive, stimulating aspect, and the other is the negative, threatening component. The negative consequences of stress tend to receive more attention because they are more likely to lead to dysfunctional problems. Perhaps the most dangerous consequence is the potentially deleterious effect of stress on health (Holt, 1982; Pelletier, 1984). No one is immune from stress. It can affect both persons whose health is unimpaired as well as those whose health is compromised by disease.

The issue of perception and the subjective nature of stress must be emphasized. As Sutterley (1979, p. 8) articulates, "Stress lies in the perception of events, not in events themselves." Therefore, situations are not inherently stressful; rather, a dynamic process is involved. How one evaluates an occurrence—the event itself, the context in which it occurs, the circumstances preceding it, the incidents that are taking place concurrently—influences whether stress is evoked. Potential sources of stress range from demanding physical activities to draining emotional experiences, such as the death of a patient, to disturbing professional exchanges among persons with whom one works.

The opinions or assertions in this chapter are the private views of the authors and are not to be construed as official or as reflecting the views of the Department of the Army or the Department of Defense.

Stress, therefore, is a complex, ubiquitous phenomenon that is experienced by patients and nurses alike. The stresses experienced by the patient with cancer are many and varied and require study and interventions from a variety of health care professionals. The focus of this chapter, however, is on the stress generated by the nurse in the process of providing care.

STRESS IN NURSING

Despite its complexity, or perhaps because of it, stress in nursing has captured the interest of innumerable researchers dating back to 1960. It is useful to review the themes of these investigations as they have evolved over 3 decades to provide a background for more specifically evaluating stress generated by providing care to patients with cancer.

THE 1960S

Menzies (1960) was the first investigator to examine stress in nursing. Using a participant observation approach, data were collected from an unknown number of nurses in one British hospital over a 4-year period. The findings suggested that the nurses experienced anxiety from (1) caring for patients, (2) making decisions, (3) taking responsibility, and (4) dealing with change. The stress generated by patient care was a finding common to all 1960 accounts of stress in nursing (Cleland, 1965; Holsclaw, 1965; Jones, 1962; Kornfeld, Maxwell, & Momrow, 1968; Koumans, 1965; Strauss, 1968; Vreeland & Ellis, 1968).

With the exception of Cleland's (1965) experimental investigation of the effects of stress on medical-surgical nurses' job performance and ability to think, the understanding of stress in nursing in the 1960s was based on studies using participant observations, case reports, and anecdotal accounts of nurses in intensive care units (ICUs). These studies, generated during the initial surge of nursing research, must be primarily appreciated for their heuristic value rather than for their scientific merit.

Nevertheless, the studies were the first to identify stresses experienced by nurses. The stressors, which were subsequently corroborated in ensuing decades, could be categorized by four themes: physical and emotional aspects of patient care, complexity of equipment used in providing patient care, inadequate staff support, and interpersonal relationships. Cleland's (1965) work departed from the trend of enumerating what factors evoked stress in nurses and instead considered the effects of stress. More precisely, Cleland demonstrated that nurses' ability to think deteriorated as the quantity of environmental stress increased. Table 81–1 depicts the major findings from the research on stress in nursing.

THE 1970S

During the 1970s, the nursing unit of interest in studies of stress was almost exclusively some form of an ICU (Bilodeau, 1973; Cassem & Hackett, 1972;

Huckabay & Jagla, 1979; Jacobson, 1978; Michaels, 1971; Olsen, 1977; Oskins, 1979). Most of these studies were descriptive accounts, using either interviews and questionnaires with some semblance of validity and reliability. Furthermore, although the number of participants remained low (n = 16 to 46) except in the case of Robinson's (1972) nationwide survey of 1111 directors of nursing, sample sizes were routinely reported.

The increased scientific merit of studies from this era corroborated the themes concerning nurses' stress that had emerged in the preceding decade (Table 81–1). Patient care remained a potent source of stress. In addition, interpersonal relationships and the care environment were also stress-producing. These stresses were also identified as being problematic for nurses working with critically ill neonates (Jacobson, 1978). A study of operating room nurses found that in addition to interpersonal relationships, missing and malfunctioning equipment was also a source of stress (Olsen, 1977).

Three new ideas concerning stress among nurses emerged during the 1970s. First, positive aspects of nursing—particularly ICU nursing—were addressed by Michaels (1971). These included expanding one's knowledge, being closer to patients, and experiencing the exciting features of the work. In searching for sources of frustration and satisfaction in ICU nursing, Bilodeau (1973) identified a fascinating dichotomy: those things that frustrated the nurses—patients, families, co-workers—were also the sources of satisfaction. For example, patient care was frustrating insofar as it involved repetitive routines, whereas it was satisfying when the pace quickened and crises occurred.

The second unique contribution of the 1970s was that coping strategies within the nurse's repertoire were

TABLE 81–1. *Stress in Nursing*

1960s: First Studies of Stress among Nurses
Identified sources of stress:
    Physical and emotional aspects of patient care
    Complex equipment
    Inadequate support for staff
    Interstaff relationships
1970s: New Dimensions of Stress in Nursing
    Inadequate knowledge and skills
    Sources of satisfaction
    Coping strategies
    Initial ICU/non-ICU comparison
1980s: Changing Trends in Nursing Stress Studies
    Renaissance of ICU/non-ICU comparisons
    Effects of personality
    Burnout
    Initial studies of stress in oncology nursing
1990s: New Issues and Challenges
    ICU, oncology, AIDS setting demonstrated little effect on
      increasing stress for nurses
    Naming the domains of stress
    Health care changes such as managed care systems, capitated budgets, emphasis on efficiency and cost-effectiveness present major challenges

ICU, intensive care unit.

also identified. Oskins (1979), in a study of 79 critical care nurses from five hospitals, discerned that nurses coped by talking with others, taking definite action, drawing on past experiences, and acknowledging their anxiety. This was an important beginning to the development of an understanding of what mechanisms protect nurses from succumbing to the deleterious effects of stress.

Finally, it was in the 1970s that the first comparison between ICU and non-ICU nurses was made. Gentry, Foster, and Froehling (1972) explored the emotional responses of 34 nurses working in three ICUs ($n = 26$) and one non-ICU ($n = 8$). This study came to be regarded as the hallmark report that established that ICU nurses were more stressed than their non-ICU colleagues. The caution with which these results should have been regarded, particularly with respect to the disproportionately small size of the non-ICU group, was not adequately communicated, thus giving rise to the myth that the ICU was the most stressful nursing environment.

THE 1980s

Interest in studying stress in nurses burgeoned during the 1980s. Descriptive studies from this decade continued the emphasis on ICU nursing and supported existing beliefs: the main stress experienced by nurses was related to patient care; inadequate knowledge and skills; interpersonal relations; and the environment, which included unit management (Anderson & Basteyns, 1981; Bailey, Steffen, & Grout, 1980; Kelly & Cross, 1985). Other themes that continued to prevail included appraising both stress and coping (Albrecht, 1982; Stockton, 1986), and corroborating that satisfaction was derived from the same features that provoked stress (Bargagliotti & Trygstad, 1987; Norbeck, 1985) (Table 81–1).

The new ideas that emerged in the 1980s included considering how personality affected one's perception of stress (Ivancevich & Matteson, 1980; Keane, DuCette, & Adler, 1985; Maloney & Bartz, 1983; Numerof & Abrams, 1984; Rich & Rich, 1987) and examining an increasingly popular concept called *burnout* (Albrecht, 1982; Bartz & Maloney, 1986; Cronin-Stubbs & Rooks, 1985; Stone, Jebson, Walk, & Belsham, 1984). Investigators began to consider the need to view the pervasive stress phenomenon in relation to outcomes; what were the effects of that stress? For example, stress was considered in regard to the way it affected job satisfaction (Norbeck, 1985) and produced psychologic symptoms (Esteban, Ballesteros, & Caballero, 1983; Norbeck, 1985).

Perhaps the most significant contribution from the 1980s, however, was a renewal of curiosity regarding stress in ICU and non-ICU nursing environments. Repeated studies conducted in a variety of institutions consistently reported the same finding; there was no detectable difference in the stress experienced by ICU and non-ICU nurses (Albrecht, 1982; Fawsey, Wellisch, Pasnau, & Licbowitz, 1983; Maloney, 1982; Mohl, Denny, Mote, & Coldwater, 1982; Vincent & Cole-

man, 1986). Comparisons of ICU and non-ICU nurses in regard to job satisfaction (Nichols, Springford, & Searle, 1981) as well as personality (Jones, 1962; Maloney & Bartz, 1983) also indicated that nurses in general were more similar than they were different.

It was during this period of renewed interest in stress experienced by nurses outside the ICU setting that studies began to consider oncology units. Concomitantly, interest in oncology as a nursing specialty was escalating. Momentum had been building over several years, but in the 1980s oncology nursing gained a heightened prestige because of the unique talents and knowledge required to meet the challenge of caring for patients with cancer. The needs of these patients are complex and numerous; they cover all aspects of the psychologic and physiologic spectra. As it became more evident that stress was indeed a common phenomenon among nurses and as the interest in oncology nursing grew, studies began to focus on the world of caring that is unique to cancer nurses.

THE 1990s

Stress associated with nursing continued to be of interest in the 1990s. The issues of stress and burnout as universal nursing concerns were presented in a variety of international journals (Fletcher, Jones, & McGregor-Cheers, 1991; Larsson, Starring, & Wilde, 1991; Tsai & Crockett, 1993). New nursing stress situations evolved such as the Gulf War and care associated with natural disasters (Wassel, 1993). Care setting effect on nursing stress was broadened to include nurses in psychiatric, operating room, and home health settings (Fletcher et al., 1991; Sullivan, 1993; Walcott-McQuigg & Ervin, 1992). The ICU setting stress effect compared with other settings, was revisited, and outcomes were similar to the earlier studies of this population. ICU was no more stressful than comparative medical-surgical, oncology, and hospice settings (Boumans & Landeweerd, 1994; Boyle, Grap, Younger, & Thornby, 1991; Fornes, Gallego, Barcelo, Crespie, Guttierrez, 1994; Glass, McKnight, & Valdimarsdottir, 1993; Snape & Cavanagh, 1993; van Servellen & Leake, 1993).

The 1990s also began to demonstrate a more sophisticated approach to stress-related research. Conceptualization of the domains of stress in nursing were identified and tested; sample sizes increased; and analysis included correlations, analysis of variance, and factor analysis. Two studies in particular demonstrate this refinement. A study of 104 nurses from three practice settings (a university hospital, a cancer center, and a home health agency) focused on identifying major domains of nursing stress associated with clinical care (Benoliel, McCorkle, Georgiadou, Denton, & Spitzer, 1990). Using factor analysis, the responses on the major instrument of the study (Nursing Stress Checklist [NSC]), indicated there are five domains of nurse stress: personal reactions, personal concerns, work concerns, role competence work completion concerns, and schedule of recent events. However, only 41.8 per cent of the variance was accounted for by these five factors.

Burnout was revisited in a study of 237 nurses from 18 units (AIDS, special care, oncology, medical ICU, and general medical) in seven hospitals, using the Maslach Burnout Inventory (Van Servellen & Leake, 1993). Nurses, regardless of unit setting, reported similar levels of distress and burnout, with one exception: medical ICU nurses scored significantly lower on the Personal Accomplishment subscale. These studies continue to raise ongoing concerns relative to the stress associated with caregiving. Are there additional, as yet unidentified, domains of stress for nurses?

Concern about stress in oncology nursing continued to be of interest. Studies of oncology nurses providing care to pediatric patients found that personalized relationships with a patient, while often desired by nurses, may in turn create stress for the nurse. For instance, in a national study of randomly selected members of the Association of Pediatric Oncology Nurses (N = 92) intensity of work stressors was determined. Results indicated that seeing patients suffer and not being able to do anything about it; having a favorite patient die; and making mistakes were the most stressful issues for these pediatric nurses (Bond, 1994; Hinds et al., 1990).

Rapidly evolving health care events in the 1990s began to create new potential stressors for oncology nurses. For example, in many instances oncology nurses were the first nurses to care for patients with AIDS because many of their needs are very similar to oncology patient needs. The stress issues associated with the care of patients with AIDS became the focus of several studies (Haddock & McGee, 1992; van Servellen & Leake, 1993). Similarly, the narrative literature on stress associated with AIDS caregiving, like the earlier literature on cancer care, was often focused on approaches to managing the stress, based on the apparent assumption that the care of this population would be stressful to nurses providing their care. The care of this population raises many complex issues, and the dimensions of stress associated with AIDS caregiving is still being explored.

In the mid 1990s another major source of potential stress for nurses began to be discussed, written about, and experienced: the impact of the evolving health care reform on nurses, nursing roles, and nursing jobs. The reform under the rubric of managed care, mandated that patient care become less costly. As a result increasing numbers of patients began to receive their care outside of the acute care setting. The center of care quickly moved to ambulatory care and the patient's home. Stays in acute care settings, when needed, were often short. In addition to the mandate to decrease costs, high-technology diagnostic and surgical procedures began to emerge to additionally shorten the amount of hospitalization needed for procedures that previously required lengthy hospital stays.

Nurses, particularly those practicing in acute care settings, often found themselves, their nursing unit, and not infrequently their entire hospital affected by this health care reform. Nurses quickly begin to hear and be affected by the corporate language and actions of down-sizing (wherein nursing positions and/or nursing units are eliminated); out-placement (assistance provided by an institution to aid employees to find a new position in a different setting); and, cross-training (becoming proficient in two or more types of patient care). There seemed to be no time, and no money, to study the effect of all of this on nurses. What was known was: nurses were experiencing a great deal of stress!

What effect these rapidly and continuing changes and challenges have on nurses—individual and/or nursing units—may truly never be known from a scientific perspective. For with the increased emphasis on mandating decreased costs there is little money available for conducting research on nurses—even as it relates to the potential stress the changes have on nurses providing the care.

However, as this is written, many oncology nurses are demonstrating a resiliency to these challenges. They are finding that their skills of the past—ability to establish good interpersonal relationships, competent hands-on skill (e.g., IV and central line care), promoting the hallmark of oncology care: interdisciplinary teamwork—work well in the "new" system. While the patient, and often the nurse, is more often found in an outpatient oncology or home setting than an acute care setting, the application of these established skills, enhanced by creative approaches to patient care such as coaching, advice nurse service, desktop publishing, or increased use of existing information service networks, work well. The caregiving experience continues to provide many oncology nurses with a sense of pride, satisfaction, and a commitment to continue providing quality care to patients. Additionally, many of the oncology nurses who survived the extreme challenges presented in the early stages of the health care revolution have become more politically astute, proactive, and creative. Perhaps in the new health care milieu stress will continue to be of concern for nurses. However, based on the premises demonstrated in the research of the past decades, the stress associated with providing care to patients with cancer will continue to be balanced by the satisfaction gained from caring for these very same patients.

STRESS IN CANCER NURSING

The premise underlying most studies of oncology nurses is that the prolonged exposure to very ill people and death puts them at particular risk for experiencing the negative effects of stress. In fact, Stockton's (1986) anecdotal account of burnout among oncology nurses refers to this syndrome as bereavement overload. However, others have found that belief about stress associated with oncology nursing appears to be more myth than fact when the empiric evidence is considered (Vachon, 1986; van Servellen & Leake, 1993).

Although the essays by McElroy (1982) and Newlin and Wellisch (1978) are representative of the anecdotal accounts of the stress that is purported to exist in oncology nursing, a different impression is conveyed by the data-based studies that have evaluated the world of cancer nursing (Table 81–2). Overall, three approaches have prevailed in the study of stress experienced by oncology nurses. These are identification of the sources

TABLE 81–2. *Stress Issues Among Cancer Nurses*

Personal reactions
Personal concerns
Work environment
Role competency
Questioning the reality of burnout

of stress, comparison of oncology nurses with nurses in other specialties, and evaluation of the extent of burnout experienced by oncology nurses.

The sources of stress for oncology nurses have been studied less extensively than those for ICU nurses, which may account for the difficulty in discerning a pattern among the stressors. Donovan's (1981) study was designed to identify sources of stress among 22 oncology nurses—11 from an inpatient setting and 11 involved with home care. The stressors could be encompassed in three broad categories—work-related issues such as scheduling and paperwork, interpersonal encounters at work, and personal problems such as car trouble. Data from a study of three hospices evaluated the stressful events reported by 93 care providers, 70 of whom were nursing personnel (Yancik, 1984). The three major sources of stress among these individuals concerned lack of staff support, emotional issues arising from patient and family interactions, and frustrations with the disease process. Barstow (1980) examined stress in 26 hospice nursing personnel. The sources of stress were many and varied in intensity depending on the stage of the patient's illness.

Vachon (1986) found that the work environment and occupational role, not patients and families, were the dominant sources of stress among 100 hospice care providers. Furthermore, in the same study, it was reported that oncology nurses experienced more stress than nurses providing care in the hospice setting. Therefore, it may be that a complex combination of many factors contributes to stress rather than simply the fact of caring for persons with cancer.

Just as studies of ICU nurses have not, overall, demonstrated greater stress among critical care staff compared with other nurses, so too it is difficult to demonstrate that oncology nurses experience greater stress than those in other nursing specialties (Benoliel et al., 1990; Fawsey et al., 1983; Stewart, Meyerowitz, Jackson, Yarkin, & Harvey, 1982; Vachon, 1986; van Servellen & Leake, 1993). These studies demonstrate that oncology may be no more stressful than other nursing specialties.

A particularly eloquent portrayal of the positive side of cancer care was reported by Trygstad (1986), who interviewed 17 oncology nurses. Koocher (1979) also elucidated a number of the rewards that may balance the demands of caring for persons with cancer. The positive aspects of working on a cancer unit were reflected in a classic study of 190 clinical staff members at a comprehensive cancer center (Box 81–1). The nurses in the study, like their physician and social work colleagues, uniformly rated their job satisfaction as high. Neither death itself nor staff conflict were problems (Peteet et al., 1989).

Evaluating the extent of burnout is a strategy that is common in studies of stress in oncology nurses. Ogle (1983) studied 22 nurses from two hospitals with patient oncology units. Data were collected using the Maslach Burnout Inventory (Maslach & Jackson, 1986). Findings indicated some evidence of emotional exhaustion, the first stage of burnout, but even then scores were low compared with normative data. In studies of Oncology Nursing Society members—oncology clinical nurse specialists and oncology staff nurses—there was minimal evidence of burnout, demonstrating that oncology nurses are probably not at great risk for burnout (Jenkins & Ostchega, 1986; van Servellen & Leake, 1993; Yasko, 1983).

It is important to consider the degree to which support from staff members has been cited as a means of ameliorating burnout and other manifestations of stress (Barstow, 1980; Jenkins & Ostchega, 1986; Ogle, 1983; Yancik, 1984; Yasko, 1983). Although it may be that burnout is less prevalent than has previously been surmised, it is also possible that this conclusion reflects

---

Box 81–1. *Job Stress and Satisfaction*

Peteet, J. R., Murray-Ross, D., Medeiros, C., Walsh-Burke, K., Rieker, P., & Finkelstein, D. (1989). Job stress and satisfaction among the staff members at a cancer center. *Cancer, 64,* 975–982.

The rewards and discomforts of working with cancer patients in a comprehensive cancer center were explored in a study of clinical staff that was composed of 94 registered nurses (RNs), 33 medical doctors (MDs), 11 social workers, and 45 allied health care workers. The dimensions of staff characteristics, patient care experience, and work environment on goal attainment and job satisfaction were examined. The study's conclusions were as follows:

- Helping patients was the most rewarding aspect of working in oncology for all subjects.
- RNs ranked emotional care as being their most valued goal; MDs selected treatment as their prime goal.
- Having high-technology procedures take precedence over patient comfort and experiencing ethical concerns over do-not-resuscitate status were the most discomforting for the RNs; inability to help patients was the most discomforting for the MDs.
- An interdisciplinary team approach was identified by both RNs and MDs as being most helpful in achieving goals.
- Job satisfaction was uniformly high (8.2 [SD = 1.9] on a scale of 1 to 10).

the way rewards, satisfaction, coping, and staff support attenuate the effects of stress and thwart the evolution of burnout. Also, because these nurses were all attracted to oncology, an alternate explanation is that they may be more resilient to the negative aspects of cancer care that could be deleterious to those not inclined to pursue this nursing specialty.

This assertion is defensible based on findings from two studies. Although burnout was low overall among nurses studied by Jenkins and Ostchega (1986), they found that as stressors, such as the number of deaths, escalated, levels of burnout increased. Concurrently, burnout was mitigated by satisfaction and support. Yasko (1983) also found that burnout was more intense among nurses who were dissatisfied with their role, under more stress, and not perceiving adequate psychologic support.

Throughout the studies of oncology nurses, it is unclear to what extent patient care is a source of stress. As noted, patient care has both positive and negative aspects for nurses; patients are both a source of pride and reason for being a nurse as well as a key source of demands—the hard, physical care and the constant emotional bombardment that accompany involvement with persons who face illnesses that are often the precursors to death. The studies of nurses who care for pediatric patients indicate that personalizing the relationship with a patient who eventually dies increases the stress potential for nurses (Bond, 1994; Hinds et al., 1990). The reality of oncology is that nurses care for patients with a number of disease entities, each with its own trajectory of events, ranging from precancerous conditions to cure or to death. Larson (1987) contends that the cancer trajectory may help to explain why stress does indeed exist among oncology nurses and yet has not been found in previous inquiries.

THE CANCER TRAJECTORY

Larson asserts that each cancer disease and each patient's resulting illness experience has a unique trajectory that ranges from prevention through a number of possible outcomes that include cure or death. Each disease's trajectory, although unique, has common critical points, consisting of prevention, detection, diagnosis, treatment, remission, cure, relapse and treatment, or death (Fig. 81–1). Each of these trajectory points places different demands on the persons involved. The treatment and terminal care dimensions of the trajectory have the potential to be especially stressful for nurses. During these two points, nurses often have intense and involved interactions with patients and their families, who are also experiencing a period of high stress.

Research concerning the critical points of the trajectory has generally focused on patient needs. Examples of this are Stillman's (1977) work on health beliefs and breast self-examination, Dodd's and Larson's work on self-care and caring needs during treatment (Dodd, 1982, 1984a, 1984b; Larson, 1984, 1995; Larson, Viele, Cebulski, & Coleman, 1993), and Burns and Carney's (1986) focus on hospice costs. These studies,

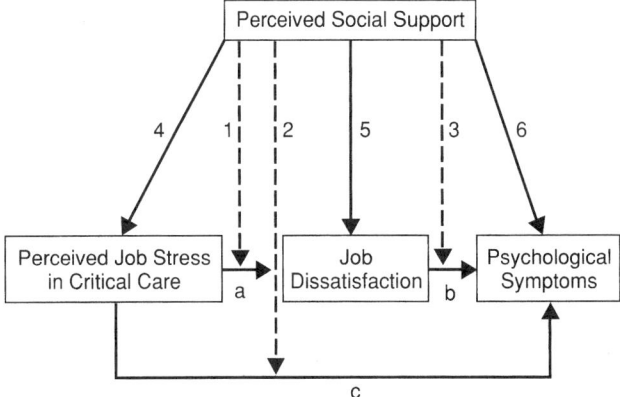

FIGURE 81–1. The cancer trajectory and nurse-patient interaction. (From Patricia J. Larson, R.N., D.N.Sc., University of California, San Francisco. Reproduced by permission.)

although not addressing the cancer trajectory perspective per se, do demonstrate that the various disease entities have a unique impact on the patient. It would therefore seem reasonable to expect that each trajectory point for each disease entity would also place unique demands on those providing the care. This expectation is especially true for nurses, because they are the most consistent care providers throughout patients' illness experiences.

There are approximately 1,050,000 new cases of cancer diagnosed each year; all of these individuals will need nurses to help with their care (American Cancer Society, 1994). At the opposite end of the trajectory, more than 500,000 cancer-related deaths occur annually (American Cancer Society, 1994). Again, almost all of these individuals will have nurses provide care throughout the course of their dying. Many of the nurses providing care for the dying will be involved with more than one patient death; some nurses may experience more than 20 deaths per year. The magnitude of this death experience must surely have some effect on the nurses as they experience the process of attachment, loss, and mourning. In fact, Jenkins and Ostechega (1986) found that as patient deaths increased, nurses did indeed experience more stress.

In the middle of these extremes, the patients will encounter various modes of therapy. Surgical intervention, medical modalities, and radiation therapy can generate intense illness experiences for the patient. Again, nurses are the primary care providers during these times that require ingenious approaches to symptom control as well as emotional support for patients and their families. Furthermore, interactions between patients and families may become so difficult that anger and rage provoked by the illness and all that it implies are turned on the nurse, who is a convenient source on whom feelings can be released. Is it reasonable to believe that such emotional outpourings have no effect on the nurse?

Because the cancer trajectory is variable for each disease, nursing care may be provided intermittently or continuously. For example, the person with lung cancer or acute leukemia may have a shortened but almost continuous trajectory that is very intense, whereas someone with breast cancer or Hodgkin's disease may have a lengthy intermittent trajectory that ultimately is marked only by sporadic follow-up care. These patients have very different nursing needs, but the needs are there nevertheless. Is it possible that nurses who have the difficult task of helping people deal with both dying and living are not affected by the intensity of the experience?

As noted in the 1990s discussion of stress associated with providing care to patients with cancer, many influences beyond the nurse-patient relationship may be major determinants of whether the oncology nurse experiences stress. In the 1980s there was a belief that the oncology nurse would be faced with increasing numbers of patients on inpatient units and that many of these patients would become well known to the nurses providing their care throughout their cancer trajectory experience. Now the opposite may be the case: oncology nurses may become stressed because they will not have multiple opportunities to interact with patients. As care moves to the home and the interactions with the patient are more sporadic and of a shorter length, oncology nurses may feel they never have the opportunity to get to "really know" the patient—which in the past has been demonstrated to create a sense of satisfaction for the nurse. The cancer trajectory will, however, remain a reality for the patient. If continuity of care and knowing the patient are important stress detractors for the nurse, oncology nurses will have to develop new strategies to interact and support the patient through this experience.

In sum, the cancer trajectory, with its demanding critical points for patients, has the potential to place stresses on the nurses responsible for the varying treatment and management aspects required at each point. Empirically, little is known about how the cancer trajectory affects nurses. Clinically, it is evident that nurses approach each point with different and varying skills and attitudes. It is therefore reasonable to expect that nurses would experience stress from a variety of sources, depending on where the care is delivered and at what point the patient is in his or her cancer trajectory.

SUMMARY

Stress engendered in the course of providing care to cancer patients is a topic that has intuitive appeal, especially for those nurses who have experienced the joys and the sorrows, the successes and the losses that are commonplace in working with oncology patients. It is startling to realize that empiric investigations only modestly support the notion that oncology nurses encounter stress. That is not to say that stress is absent but merely that it is an elusive phenomenon.

In oncology, it would appear that perhaps the approaches used in studying stress among nurses should be reconsidered. First, the sources of stress need to be better identified, with the understanding that the same issues—patients, for example—may represent both sources of satisfaction and frustration. Future research

must also address the not yet identified sources of stress. Jennings' (1987, 1990) investigation of mental health in head nurses is a case in point. The study was conceptualized to include nonwork sources of stress as well as work-engendered stress in predicting mental health for a group of 300 head nurses. This premise is supported by the recent work of Benoliel and her colleagues (1990) and van Servellen and Leake (1993).

Second, looking at the relationship between stress and outcome measures is important. As Norbeck (1985) noted, from a list of 16 stressors reported by critical care nurses, only seven were related to either job satisfaction or psychologic symptoms. Previous research in oncology has taken outcomes into account; however, the focus has been almost exclusively on burnout. Would other outcome measures better demonstrate the effects of stress?

A third need is to move away from single point in time studies to better capture the dynamic process of stress. Clearly the cancer trajectory makes this need all the more compelling. Either longitudinal studies in the quantitative tradition or grounded theory or phenomenologic studies in the qualitative tradition would help to better address this process. Bargagliotti and Trygstad (1987) both studied work stress, but the former investigator used a quantitative approach, and the latter researcher used a qualitative method. The findings, although not in conflict, were very different because the methodologies exposed varying facets of stress.

A fourth issue concerns coping. Although coping strategies have been identified, they have not been studied with regard to effectiveness. In the early 1980s Albrecht (1982) noted that common suggestions for reducing burnout, such as taking time off or talking with individuals other than unit staff, did not in fact attenuate it. The need remains to explicate ways to moderate stress and to evaluate the actual effectiveness of these methods.

Finally, the radical changes occurring in health care during the 1990s impact all of nursing. Although the speed of change has not allowed careful research-based examination of stress, the effects of downsizing, centering care in the ambulatory setting, and assessing the cost of care cannot be ignored.

For nurses committed to the care of patients with cancer, several realities will continue. Cancer remains a leading cause of death, one that elicits many emotional and physical responses in the patient. Some cancers will race through the patient's body, causing a rapid downward course that quickly concludes in a fatal outcome. However, many cancers are being viewed as chronic diseases that, it is hoped, will allow the patient to have a longer but an ever-vigilant life. Curative-intent therapies will continue to be aggressive, demanding much from patients, families, and caregivers. Perhaps by taking a cue from the realities of oncology nursing, that the care of patients with cancer requires a fine balance between what is caring to patients—the competent know-how demonstrated in knowledgeable nursing actions—and what is caring to nurses—the personalized affective dimensions of talking, listening, and comforting (Larson, 1984, 1986; Mayer, 1987)—it may be possible to identify what is unique about oncology nurses and stress. Researchers will need to utilize old, new, and evolving methodologies to glean the aspects of oncology nursing that should remain unchanged and to delineate carefully those aspects that generate stress too burdensome for the nurse to remain a productive, caring, and vital person.

REFERENCES

Albrecht, T. L. (1982). What job stress means for the staff nurse. *Nursing Administration Quarterly, 7*(1), 1–11.

American Cancer Society. (1994). *Cancer facts and figures—1994.* Atlanta: Author.

Anderson, C. A., & Basteyns, M. (1981). Stress and the critical care nurse reaffirmed. *Journal of Nursing Administration, 11*(1), 31–34.

Bailey, J. T., Steffen, S. M., & Grout, J. W. (1980). The stress audit: Identifying the stressors of ICU nursing. *Journal of Nursing Education, 19*(6), 15–25.

Bargagliotti, L. A., & Trygstad, L. N. (1987). Differences in stress and coping findings: A reflection of social realities or methodologies? *Nursing Research, 36,* 170–173.

Barstow, J. (1980). Stress variance in hospice nursing. *Nursing Outlook, 28,* 751–754.

Bartz, C., & Maloney, J. P. (1986). Burnout among intensive care nurses. *Research in Nursing and Health, 9,* 147–153.

Benice, S. W., Longo, C. B., & Barnsteiner, J. H. (1992). Perceptions and significance of patient deaths for pediatric critical care nurses. *Critical Care Nurse, 12*(3), 72–75.

Benoliel, J. Q., McCorkle, R., Georgiadau, F., Denton, T., & Spitzer, A. (1990). Measurement of stress in clinical nursing. *Cancer Nursing, 13*(4), 221–228.

Bilodeau, C. B. (1973). The nurse and her reactions to critical-care nursing. *Heart and Lung, 2,* 358–363.

Bond, D. C. (1994). The measured intensity of work-related stressors in pediatric oncology nursing. *Journal of Pediatric Oncology Nursing, 11*(2), 44–52.

Boumans, N. P., & Landeweerd, J. A. (1994). Working in an intensive or non-intensive care unit: Does it make any difference? *Heart and Lung, 23*(7), 71–79.

Boyle, A., Grap, M. J., Younger, J., & Thornby, D. (1991) Personality hardiness, ways of coping, social support and burnout in critical care nurses. *Journal of Advanced Nursing, 16*(7), 850–857.

Burns, N., & Carney, K. (1986). Patterns of hospice care—The RN role. *The Hospice Journal, 2*(1), 37–61.

Cassem, N. H., & Hackett, T. P. (1972). Sources of tension for the CCU nurse. *American Journal of Nursing, 72,* 1426–1430.

Clcland, V. S. (1965). The effect of stress on performance. *Nursing Research, 14,* 292–298.

Cronin-Stubbs, D., & Rooks, C. A. (1985). The stress, social support, and burnout of critical care nurses: The results of research. *Heart and Lung, 14,* 31–39.

Dodd, M. J. (1982). Cancer patients' knowledge of chemotherapy: Assessment and informational interventions. *Oncology Nursing Forum, 9*(3), 39–44.

Dodd, M. J. (1984a). Patterns of self care in cancer patients receiving radiation therapy. *Oncology Nursing Forum, 11*(3), 23–27.

Dodd, M. J. (1984b). Self-care for patients with breast cancer to prevent side effects of chemotherapy: A concern for public health nursing. *Public Health Nursing, 1,* 202–209.

Donovan, M. I. (1981). Stress at work: Cancer nurses report. *Oncology Nursing Forum, 8*(2), 22–25.

Esteban, A., Ballesteros, P., & Caballero, J. (1983). Psychological evaluation of intensive care nurses. *Critical Care Medicine, 11,* 616–620.

Fawsey, F. I., Wellisch, D. K., Pasnau, R. O., & Leibowitz, B. (1983). Preventing nursing burnout: A challenge for liaison psychiatry. *General Hospital Psychiatry, 5,* 141–149.

Fletcher, B. C., Jones, F., & McGregor-Cheers, J. (1991) The stressors and strains of health visiting: Demands, supports, constraints and psychological health. *Journal of Advanced Nursing, 16*(9), 1078–1089.

Fornes, V. J., Gallego, C. G., Barcelo, O. M., Crespie, C. M. & Guttierrez, C. A. (1994) Causal and emotional factors related to work stress in ICU nursing staff: The importance of accurate measurements. *Intensive and Critical Care Nursing, 10*(1), 41–50.

Gentry, W. D., Foster, S. B., & Froehling, S. (1972). Psychologic response to situational stress in intensive and nonintensive nursing. *Heart and Lung, 1,* 793–796.

Glass, D. C., McKnight, J. D., & Valdimarsdottir, H. (1993) Depression, burnout, and perceptions of control in hospitals nurses. *Journal of Consulting and Clinical Psychology, 61*(1), 147–155.

Haddock, C. C., & McGee, G. W. (1992). HIV-related knowledge, attitudes, and stress among health care providers: A literature review and research agenda. *Journal of Health Administration Education, 10*(1), 59–76.

Harrison, R. V. (1978). Person-environment fit and job stress. In C. L. Cooper & R. Payne (Eds.), *Stress at work* (pp. 175–205). New York: John Wiley & Sons.

Hinds, P. S., Fairclough, D. C., Dobos, C. L., Greer, R. H., Herring, P. L., Mayhall, J., Arheart, K. K., Day, L. A., & McAulay, L. S. (1990). Development and testing of the stressor scale for pediatric oncology nurses. *Cancer Nursing, 13*(6), 354–360.

Holsclaw, P. A. (1965). Nursing in high emotional risk areas. *Nursing Forum, 4*(4), 36–35.

Holt, R. R. (1982). Occupational stress. In L. Goldberger & S. Breznitz (Eds.), *Handbook of stress. Theoretical and clinical aspects* (pp. 419–444). New York: The Free Press.

Huckabay, L. M. D., & Jagla, B. (1979). Nurses' stress factors in the intensive care unit. *Journal of Nursing Administration, 9*(2), 21–26.

Ivancevich, J. M., & Matteson, M. T. (1980). Nurses and stress: Time to examine the potential problem. *Supervisor Nurse, 11*(6), 17–22.

Jacobson, S. P. (1978). Stressful situations for neonatal intensive care nurses. *Maternal Child Nursing Journal, 3,* 144–150.

Jenkins, J. F., & Ostchega, Y. (1986). Evaluation of burnout in oncology nurses. *Cancer Nursing, 9,* 108–116.

Jennings, B. M. (1987). *Stress, social support, and locus of control: Effects on head nurses' mental health.* Unpublished doctoral dissertation, University of California, San Francisco.

Jennings, B. M. (1990). Stress, locus of control, social support, and psychological symptoms among head nurses. *Research in Nursing and Health, 13,* 393–401.

Jones, E. M. (1962). Who supports the nurse? *Nursing Outlook, 10,* 476–478.

Keane, A., DuCette, J., & Adler, D. C. (1985). Stress in ICU and non-ICU nurses. *Nursing Research, 34,* 231–236.

Kelly, J. G., & Cross, D. G. (1985). Stress, coping behaviors, and recommendations for intensive care and medical surgical ward registered nurses. *Research in Nursing and Health, 8,* 321–328.

Koocher, G. P. (1979). Adjustment and coping strategies among the caretakers of cancer patients. *Social Work in Health, 5*(2), 145–150.

Kornfeld, D. S., Maxwell, T., & Momrow, D. (1968). Psychological hazards of the intensive care unit. *Nursing Clinics of North America, 3,* 41–51.

Koumans, A. J. R. (1965). Psychiatric consultation in an intensive care unit. *Journal of the American Medical Association, 194,* 633–637.

Lansdown, R., Kike, S., & Smith, M. (1990). Reducing stress in the cancer ward. *Nursing Times, 86*(38), 34–38.

Larson, P., Viele, C., Cebulski, C., & Coleman, S. (1993). Comparison of bone marrow transplant patients' perceptions of symptoms. *Oncology Nursing Forum, 20*(1), 81–87.

Larson, P. (1995). Perceptions of need of hospitalized patients undergoing bone marrow transplant. *Cancer Practice, 3*(3), 173–179.

Larson, P. J. (1984). Important nurse caring behaviors perceived by patients with cancer. *Oncology Nursing Forum, 11*(6), 46–50.

Larson, P. J. (1986). Cancer nurses' perceptions of caring. *Cancer Nursing, 9,* 86–91.

Larson, P. J. (1987, May). *Patients and nursing stress: The paradox of cancer nursing.* Paper presented at the Twelfth Annual Congress, Oncology Nursing Society, Denver, CO.

Larsson, G., Starrin, B., & Wilde, B. (1991) Contributions of stress theory to the understanding of helping. *Scandinavian Journal of Caring Sciences, 5*(2), 79–85.

Lazarus, R. S., & Launier, R. (1978). Stress-related transactions between person and environment. In L. A. Pervin & M. Lewis (Eds.), *Perspectives in interactional psychology* (pp. 287–327). New York: Plenum.

Mallett, K., Price, J. H., Jurs, S. G., & Slenker, S. (1991). Relationships among burnout, death anxiety, and social support in hospice and critical care nurses. *Psychological Reports, 68*(3), 1347–1359.

Maloney, J. P. (1982). Job stress and its consequences on a group of intensive care and nonintensive care nurses. *Advances in Nursing Science, 4*(2), 31–42.

Maloney, J. P., & Bartz, C. (1983). Stress-tolerant people: Intensive care nurses compared with non-intensive care nurses. *Heart and Lung, 12,* 389–394.

Maslach, C., & Jackson, S. E. (1986). *The Maslach Burnout Inventory* (2nd ed). Palo Alto, CA: Consulting Psychologists Press.

Mason, J. W. (1975). A historical view of the stress filled. Part I. *Journal of Human Stress, 1*(1), 6–12.

Mayer, D. K. (1987). Oncology nurses' versus cancer patients' perceptions of nurse caring behavior: A replication study. *Oncology Nursing Forum, 14*(3), 48–52.

McElroy, A. M. (1982). Burnout—A review of the literature with application to cancer nursing. *Cancer Nursing, 5,* 211–217.

Menzies, I. E. P. (1960). Nurses under stress. *International Nursing Review, 7,* 9–16.

Michaels, D. R. (1971). Too much in need of support to give any? *American Journal of Nursing, 71,* 1932–1935.

Mohl, P. C., Denny, N. R., Mote, T. A., & Coldwater, C. (1982). Hospital unit stressors that affect nurses: Primary task vs. social factors. *Psychosomatics, 23,* 366–374.

Newlin, N. J., & Wellisch, D. K. (1978). The oncology nurse: Life on an emotional roller coaster. *Cancer Nursing, 1,* 447–449.

Nichols, K. A., Springford, V., & Searle, J. (1981). An investigation of distress and discontent in various types of nursing. *Journal of Advanced Nursing, 6,* 311–318.

Norbeck, J. S. (1985). Perceived job stress, job satisfaction, and psychological symptoms in critical care nursing. *Research in Nursing and Health, 8,* 253–259.

Numerof, R. E., & Abrams, M. N. (1984). Sources of stress among nurses: An empirical investigation. *Journal of Human Stress, 10*(2), 88–100.

Ogle, M. E. (1983). Stages of burnout among oncology nurses in the hospital setting. *Oncology Nursing Forum, 10*(1), 31–34.

Olsen, M. (1977). OR nurses perception of stress. *AORN Journal, 25,* 43–48.

Oskins, S. L. (1979). Identification of situational stressors and coping methods by intensive care nurses. *Heart and Lung, 8,* 953–960.

Pelletier, K. (1984). *Healthy people in unhealthy places.* New York: Delacorte.

Peteet, J. R., Murray-Ross, D., Medeiros, C., Walsh-Burke, K., Riekeo, P., & Finkelstein, D. (1989). Job stress and satisfaction among the staff members at a cancer center. *Cancer, 64,* 975–982.

Rich, V. L., & Rich, A. R. (1987). Personality hardiness and burnout in female staff nurses. *Image, 19,* 63–66.

Robinson, A. M. (1972). Intensive care today—and tomorrow: A summing-up. *RN, 35*(9), 56–60.

Saunders, J. M., & Valente, S. M. (1994). Nurses' grief. *Cancer Nursing, 17*(4), 318–324.

Schoenberg, B., & Senescu, R. A. (1970). The patient's reaction to fatal illness. In B. Schoenberg, A. C. Carr, D. Peretz, & A. H. Kutscher (Eds.), *Loss and grief: Psychological management in medical practice.* New York: Columbia University Press.

Snape, J., & Cavanagh, S. J. (1993) Occupational stress in neurosurgical nursing. *Intensive and Critical Care Nursing, 9*(3), 162–170.

Stewart, B. E., Meyerowitz, B. E., Jackson, L. E., Yarkin, K. L., & Harvey, J. H. (1982). Psychological stress associated with outpatient oncology nursing. *Cancer Nursing, 5,* 383–387.

Stillman, M. J. (1977). Women's health beliefs about breast cancer and breast self-examination. *Nursing Research, 26,* 121–127.

Stockton, M. V. (1986). Who's taking care of you? *Caring, 5*(10), 60–63.

Stone, G. L., Jebsen, P., Walk, P., & Belsham, R. (1984). Identification of stress and coping skills within a critical care setting. *Western Journal of Nursing, 6,* 201–211.

Strauss, A. (1968). The intensive care unit: Its characteristics and social relationships. *Nursing Clinics of North America, 3,* 7–15.

Styles, M. M. (1982). *On nursing. Toward a new endowment.* St. Louis: C. V. Mosby Co.

Sullivan, P. (1993). Stress and burnout in psychiatric nursing. *Nursing Standard, 8*(2), 36–39.

Sutterly, D. (1979). Stress and health: A survey of self-regulation modalities. *Topics in Clinical Nursing, 1*(1), 1–21.

Tsai, S. L., & Crockett, M. S. (1993) Effects of relaxation training, combining imagery, and meditation on the Taiwan. *Issues in Mental Health Nursing, 14*(1), 51–56.

Trygstad, L. (1986). Professional friends. The inclusion of the personal into the professional. *Cancer Nursing, 9,* 326–332.

Vachon, M. L. S. (1986). Myths and realities in palliative/hospice care. *The Hospice Journal 2*(1), 63–79.

van Servellen, G., & Leake, B. (1993). Burn-out in hospital nurses: A comparison of acquired immunodeficiency syndrome, oncology, general medical, and intensive care unit nurse samples. *Journal of Professional Nursing, 9*(3), 169–177.

Vincent, P., & Coleman, W. F. (1986). Comparison of major stressors perceived by ICU and non-ICU nurses. *Critical Care Nurse, 6*(1), 64–69.

Vreeland, R., & Ellis, G. L. (1968). Stresses on the nurse in the intensive-care unit. *Journal of the American Medical Association, 208,* 332–334.

Walcott-McQuigg, J. A., & Ervin, N. E. (1992) Stressors in the workplace: Community health nurses. *Public Health Nursing, 9*(1), 65–71.

Wassel, M. L. (1993) A stress management incentive program for nursing staff during Operation Desert Storm. *Aaohn Journal, 41*(8), 393–395.

Wolf, Z. R. (1986). Nurses' work: The sacred and the profane. *Holistic Nursing Practice, 1*(1), 29–35.

Yancik, R. (1984). Sources of work stress for hospice staff. *Journal of Psychosocial Oncology, 2*(1), 21–31.

Yasko, J. M. (1983). Variables which predict burnout experienced by oncology clinical nurse specialists. *Cancer Nursing, 6,* 109–116.

Role Clarification: Rights and Responsibilities of Oncology Nurses

Jean K. Brown

Role clarification is a supportive strategy for managing stressors associated with the work environment. One facet of this process is to be cognizant of one's rights and responsibilities as a professional nurse and to apply them in practice. Knowledge of rights and responsibilities gives nurse clinicians at all levels of practice self-confidence regarding the scope of nursing practice, guidelines for dealing with role conflicts, and power to advocate for patients and negotiate changes in the work environment. Nurse managers use this knowledge to support their staff, evaluate performance, resolve conflicts, develop policies and procedures, negotiate with hospital administrators and representatives from other health care disciplines, meet regulatory standards, and ensure occupational safety. The purpose of this chapter is to provide an overview of responsibilities and rights of registered professional nurses that are particularly relevant to cancer nursing practice.

In many ways, the responsibilities and rights of professional nurses specializing in cancer care are similar to those of other nurses; however, there are significant differences in application. Many nursing specialties practice in areas in which procedures and treatment regimens are well-established and nursing responsibilities and rights are well understood and incorporated into practice. Cancer nurses, however, often practice at the forefront of scientific knowledge and technology, where policies and procedures may not have been developed, and subsequently nursing responsibilities and rights may not have been fully incorporated into

practice. Cancer nurse clinicians and managers must be highly vigilant regarding their practices to be sure that their actions are within their legal and professional responsibilities and that their rights are protected.

RIGHTS VERSUS RESPONSIBILITIES

Inherent in professionalism is the integral relationship between rights and responsibilities. Characteristics of professionalism include maximal competence in the service provided, provision of a service of significant value to society, and performing the service with a high degree of autonomy (Jameton, 1984). All of these imply that the professional is legally and ethically responsible for a level of performance that meets specified standards and societal expectations. In the United States, these responsibilities are defined by state law and by ethical codes and standards developed by professional societies.

Increased concern with human rights has contributed to society's changing view of the rights of persons in the helping professions such as nursing (Fagin, 1975). The nurse is an individual who has both individual and professional rights. Some of these rights are given by the law, for example, the right to express oneself freely or refuse to carry out a physician's order that is contrary to acceptable nursing practice (Annas, Glantz, & Katz, 1981).

Other rights must be asserted or acted on by the individual nurse. "People seem to obtain rights by having an image of themselves as worthy of rights, through sharing positive information and publicity about themselves, through pressure, and through doing something for society which society values" (Fagin, 1975). For example, job satisfaction and professional growth are rights that cannot be given but require effort on the part of the individual. Job satisfaction requires a positive attitude about work, and professional growth requires learning. Neither can be given but must be acted on by the individual.

When functioning as a professional, the individual's rights and responsibilities must be considered together. The right to refuse a physician's order also has the responsibility to communicate with the physician about the order, take the matter to a higher authority if necessary, and document personal observations and responses of others in the manner in which institutional policy dictates (Annas et al., 1981). Job satisfaction is a right that must be weighed against obligations for patient care. The dissatisfied nurse cannot walk away from responsibilities, leaving the patient without the care required (Creighton, 1986). The professional's individual rights must be considered within the framework of legal and ethical responsibilities.

RESPONSIBILITIES OF PROFESSIONAL NURSES

LEGAL GOVERNANCE

Legislation regarding the practice of nursing occurs at the state level and consists of statutes enacted by the legislature as well as decisions and rulings of administrative agencies and common law. The statutes deal primarily with licensure and definitions of the scope of nursing practice. These vary from state to state. Individual nurses must be knowledgeable about the licensure and nurse practice laws in the state in which they practice.

Licensure statutes describe the criteria that must be met to be given and maintain the privilege of practicing nursing. Licensure can be mandatory or permissive (Creighton, 1986; Rhodes & Miller, 1984). Mandatory licensure requires that anyone practicing nursing must be licensed. Permissive licensure protects the title of registered nurse (RN) by allowing only licensed individuals to represent themselves as RNs; however, the practice of nursing by unlicensed individuals is not prohibited. Mandatory licensure exists in 48 states; permissive licensure exists in Oklahoma, Texas, and the District of Columbia (Creighton, 1986).

Nurse practice acts define nursing practice using three approaches (Rhodes & Miller, 1984). The traditional approach uses the 1955 American Nurses' Association (ANA) definition.

> The term "practice of professional nursing" means the performance, for compensation, of any acts in the observation, care, and counsel of the ill, injured, or infirm, or in the maintenance of health or prevention of illness in others or in the supervision and teaching of other personnel, or the administration of medications and treatments prescribed by a licensed physi-

cian or dentist, requiring substantial specialized judgment and skill and based on knowledge and application of the principles of biological, physical, and social science ("ANA Board," 1955).

The second approach identifies specific acts that nurses may perform beyond the traditional definition and allows for nursing practice governed by standing physician orders (Rhodes & Miller, 1984). More modern, administrative approaches broaden the traditional definition to allow for expanded nursing roles and empower appropriate state regulatory agencies to authorize additions to nurse practice acts. An example of such a broad definition is the New York State Nurse Practice Act passed in 1972 and later adopted by the ANA. "Nursing is the diagnosis and treatment of human responses to actual or potential health problems" (American Nurses' Association, 1980).

STATE BOARDS OF NURSING

The nurse practice acts create regulatory agencies—the state boards of nursing—to control licensure, develop rules and regulations, and deal with violations of rules or professional standards (Rhodes & Miller, 1984). Professional nurses need to be knowledgeable about the rules and regulations in their state as well as the statutes, or they may jeopardize their licenses unknowingly. For example, in the state of New York a nurse is reported to the State Board of Nursing if convicted of driving while intoxicated, which is a felony. Action taken by the State Board of Nursing ranges from censure and reprimand to revocation of license and permanent listing of the offense on the individual's professional record ("Nurses warned," 1987). The advice of an attorney should be obtained in such situations.

STATE HEALTH DEPARTMENTS

The role of state health departments varies from state to state, but all are concerned with the health of the public. These agencies set standards that must be met by health care agencies, institutions, and professionals. In New York one of the duties of the state health department is the enforcement of the Patient Abuse Law. To accomplish the increasingly stricter enforcement of this law, the health department reviews all institutional and agency incident reports. Nurses responsible for an incident are advised of a health department hearing. No matter how minor the incident, the nurse should attend and may wish to seek legal counsel. Any nurse found guilty at such a hearing is guilty of malpractice and may be in danger of a reprimand or loss of license from the New York State Board of Nursing ("Nurses warned," 1987).

OTHER REGULATORY BODIES

Two other regulatory bodies that have a great influence on the practice of nursing are the Joint Commission on Accreditation of Healthcare Organizations (JCAHO) and the Health Care Financing Administration (HCFA). The JCAHO accreditation is extremely important to hospitals because loss of accreditation may jeopardize reimbursement for services from health care insurance. Many standards set by JCAHO have a direct impact on nursing practice and also promote ANA standards of practice. For example, evidence of the nursing process must be documented in the medical record, and policies and procedures must include information on current scientific knowledge and findings from quality assessment and improvement activities (Joint Commission on Accreditation of Healthcare Organizations, 1993). Because JCAHO standards are usually incorporated into the policies and procedures of the hospital, nurses practicing in settings accredited by JCAHO are responsible for meeting these standards in their practice.

The HCFA is a federal agency responsible for overseeing the Medicare law and related prospective payment based on diagnosis-related groups (DRGs). Because cancer is a disease with a high incidence among elderly individuals, changes in the Medicare law have an influence on cancer nursing practice (Donley, 1984). Prospective payment based on DRGs has raised many economic issues and concerns among hospital administrators that have led to efforts for more cost-effective health care delivery. This has created both a threat to and a potential enhancement for nursing practice to which nurses have a responsibility to respond. Threats might include elimination of nursing positions to reduce costs. In this case, nurses, especially those in management, have a professional responsibility to ensure that the work environment is conducive to high-quality nursing care (ANA, 1985a). Potential enhancement of nursing practice includes an increased need and recognition of the positive results of high-quality nursing care in shortening hospital length of stay and providing high-quality ambulatory and home care. Nurses have a responsibility to clients and to the profession to develop and implement efficient, cost-effective approaches to high-quality nursing care; evaluate client outcomes for the use of these approaches; and publicize the outcomes for educate hospital administrators, other health care providers, and the public about the effectiveness of nursing care (Yasko & Fleck, 1984).

PROFESSIONAL STANDARDS AND GUIDELINES

The ANA and the Oncology Nursing Society (ONS) have established professional standards and guidelines that are applicable to cancer nursing. These are developed for a variety of purposes. The most common is to define what the profession believes to be high-quality nursing practice and to provide a model for nurses in their practice. Legally, RNs must comply with the standard of care practiced by a reasonably prudent and competent RN, or they will be considered professionally negligent (Annas et al., 1981). Professional standards provide a basis for legislation, court decisions, and rules adopted by state boards of nursing. An example of the latter is the adoption of the ANA's entry into practice resolution by the North Dakota State Board of Nursing in 1986 that requires registered professional nurses to have a baccalaureate degree. There are four

documents describing professional standards and guidelines of particular relevance to the cancer nurse.

CODE OF ETHICAL CONDUCT

The ANA *Code for Nurses* (1985a) is a code of ethical conduct that delineates the primary goals and values of the profession of nursing (Table 82–1). There are four themes in this document: respect for human dignity and worth, safeguarding the client, responsibility for nursing practice, and responsibilities to nursing and society. Assistance in applying this code to specific situations can be obtained from the ANA.

Respect for human dignity and worth and safeguarding the client are two fundamental principles of nursing practice that have special significance in oncology. Nurses are obligated to protect and preserve human life as long as there is hope for recovery or benefit from treatment (ANA, 1985a). Self-determination is inherent in respect for human dignity and requires full involvement of clients in their health care. Thus the nurse is obligated to involve clients fully in their plan of care and its implementation and ensure informed consent. If a nurse is ethically opposed to specific procedures used in a client's care, refusal to participate is justified only if advance notice is given and other satisfactory arrangements are made for nursing care.

TABLE 82–1. *American Nurses' Association Code for Nurses*

The nurse provides services with respect for human dignity and the uniqueness of the client, unrestricted by considerations of social or economic status, personal attributes, or the nature of health problems.

The nurse safeguards the client's right to privacy by judiciously protecting information of a confidential nature.

The nurse acts to safeguard the client and the public when health care and safety are affected by the incompetent, unethical, or illegal practice of any person.

The nurse assumes responsibility and accountability for individual nursing judgments and actions.

The nurse maintains competence in nursing.

The nurse exercises informed judgment and uses individual competence and qualifications as criteria in seeking consultation, accepting responsibilities, and delegating nursing activities to others.

The nurse participates in activities that contribute to the ongoing development of the profession's body of knowledge.

The nurse participates in the profession's efforts to implement and improve standards of nursing.

The nurse participates in the profession's efforts to establish and maintain conditions of employment conducive to high quality nursing care.

The nurse participates in the profession's effort to protect the public from misinformation and misrepresentation and to maintain the integrity of nursing.

The nurse collaborates with members of the health professions and other citizens in promoting community and national efforts to meet the health needs of the public.

(Reprinted with permission from *Code for nurses with interpretive statements*, © 1985 [p. 1]. Kansas City, MO: American Nurses' Association.)

The *Code for Nurses* clearly indicates that nurses are responsible for their practice. They are answerable for their judgments and behaviors and are not relieved of this accountability by physician's orders or institutional policies. If unprepared to provide the nursing care needed because of lack of knowledge or experience, the nurse has the responsibility to seek consultation. Individual competency and experience must also be assessed in delegating responsibilities to others. Nurses are responsible for maintaining their own competence and should be open to peer review of their practice.

Nurses also have a responsibility to the profession of nursing and society to promote high-quality nursing care and health care of the public. All nurses have a role in the development of knowledge, whether as researchers, data collectors, subjects, or users of knowledge. The use of research findings in practice, or research utilization, is extremely important to validate new scientific knowledge and to use new knowledge to improve patient care. Increasing attention to this essential component of knowledge building is evident in cancer nursing practice. Nursing research utilization committees have been implemented in practice settings to educate nursing staff about research utilization, identify clinical research findings that could be applied to cancer nursing practice, identify clinical research findings that could not be applied to practice, and develop recommendations for practice changes (Hanson & Ashley, 1994; McGuire, Walczak, & Krumm, 1994; Reedy, Shivnan, Hanson, Haisfield, & Gregory, 1994; Walczak, McGuire, Haisfield, & Beezley, 1994).

Nurses are responsible to the public and the profession for the delivery of high-quality patient care. Knowledge, skills, and commitment essential to nursing practice must be demonstrated by those wishing to enter the profession. Nurse educators, in particular, have an obligation to ensure that their students demonstrate these qualities. Practicing nurses have the duty to implement and maintain standards of nursing care and to promote a practice and community environment in which these standards can be achieved.

Some institutions have developed a code of ethics for their health care providers. The University of Texas System Cancer Center became the first comprehensive cancer center to develop and adopt an ethical code. The purpose was "to help guide staff members in making professional decisions" ("University of Texas," 1984). Such action is highly relevant in a cancer treatment setting, where complex dilemmas and decision making are common.

SOCIAL POLICY STATEMENT

In 1980, the ANA published *Nursing: A Social Policy Statement*, which sought to clarify the evolving role of nursing. It was endorsed by the ONS in 1983 (Oncology Nursing Society, 1983a). This statement deals with the social context of nursing, the nature and scope of nursing practice, and the issue of specialization. It is important to the clarification of nursing responsibilities because it is the most modern discussion of overall nursing practice obligations.

The core of nursing practice is the "diagnosis and treatment of human responses to actual or potential health problems" (ANA, 1980). This was reaffirmed and applied to the practice of the individual nurse in a report to the ANA House of Delegates in 1987. "The depth and breadth to which the individual nurse engages in the total scope of the clinical practice of nursing are defined by the knowledge base of the nurse, the role of the nurse and the nature of the client population within the practice environment" ("Report to house," 1987). Nursing functions include physical care, health teaching, anticipatory guidance, counseling, and other related activities. The method by which nursing is practiced is the nursing process.

The difference between generalists and specialists in nursing is also important in role clarification, especially since the public, other health professionals, and even some nurses are often confused about this. These roles were defined in *Nursing: A Social Policy Statement* and affirmed by the general membership of the ONS (ONS, 1983b). Generalists provide "a comprehensive approach to health care and can meet diversified health concerns of individuals, families, and communities" (ANA, 1980). The ONS gave cancer nurse generalists the title of "oncology nurse clinician" (ONS, 1983b).

Specialists "are experts in providing care focused on specific clusters of phenomena drawn from the range of general practice" (ANA, 1980). Specialists become expert in a specific clinical area through graduate study and supervised practice. The ONS (1983b) entitled the cancer nurse specialist role "oncology clinical nurse specialist" (OCNS). Because the role of the graduate prepared nurse specialist is relatively modern, having been conceptualized in the 1940s (Reiter, 1967) and debated through the 1970s, the ANA went on to define the functions of this role as follows:

- Identification of populations at risk
- Direct care of selected patients or clients in any setting, including private practice
- Intraprofessional consultation with nurse specialists in different clinical areas and with nurses in general practice
- Interprofessional consultation and collaboration in planning total patient care for individual and groups of patients, and in planning and evaluating health programs for population groups at risk related to the specialty or the public in general
- Contribution to the advancement of the profession as a whole and to the specialty field (ANA, 1980)

A national invitational conference held in 1984 analyzed the role of the OCNS and made recommendations for the future (Donoghue & Spross, 1985). This conference endorsed the aforementioned ANA-defined functions and described how the OCNS could accomplish these functions in regard to cost-containment, consumerism, client populations, role development, type of practice, nontraditional settings, practice standards, and professional issues. A second invitational conference was held in 1990 to update recommendations.

In recent years, the nurse practitioner role has received more attention in cancer nursing specialist practice. In fact, in many areas of the United States OCNS practice has been evolving to include nurse practitioner skills. New titles for these hybrids are also being used such as advanced practice nurse and acute care nurse practitioner. In response to this need identified primarily by clinical nurse specialists, many schools of nursing have added an acute care nurse practitioner/advanced practice track to their graduate programs and are offering postgraduate certificate programs for clinical nurse specialists to learn nurse practitioner skills to add to their expertise. OCNSs appear to see many advantages in this role evolution, such as increased independence in their practice, increased prescriptive privileges, and potential for third-party reimbursement for their services. However, there is much controversy in nursing about this role merger (Page & Arena, 1994). Potential disadvantages have been identified such as weakening of reimbursement policies, increasing role confusion, and supporting hospital medical practice at the expense of nursing practice. Continued discussion among nurses and the forces of health care reform and the market place will continue to clarify this evolution.

STANDARDS OF ONCOLOGY NURSING PRACTICE

The ONS, in collaboration with the ANA Council on Medical-Surgical Nursing Practice, developed practice standards intended for the oncology nurse clinician. These standards are focused on both professional practice and performance, with emphasis on 11 high-incidence problems common among individuals with cancer (Table 82–2). According to the ANA ethical code of conduct, it is the responsibility of oncology nurses to use these standards to guide practice.

Standards for the advanced practice of oncology nursing have also been developed by the ONS (Table 82–3). Advanced oncology practitioners include master's or doctorally prepared nurses with any or all of the following roles: clinical nurse specialist, nurse practitioner, educator, administrator, and researcher.

In addition to the standards and their rationale, these documents include structure, process, and outcome criteria to assist in implementation and evaluation of practice through quality assurance, peer review, or self-evaluation. The ONS has also published nursing practice guidelines that provide care plans for a large number of nursing diagnoses common to oncology nursing (McNally, Somerville, Miaskowski, & Rostad, 1991). For example, the guidelines provide the information needed by the nurse to assess and teach the individual who has a knowledge deficit related to the prevention and early detection of many forms of cancers.

RESEARCH GUIDELINES

Cancer nurses are frequently involved in caring for individuals participating in medical, pharmacologic, or nursing research or conducting research themselves. They are obligated to have a special concern and vigi-

---

TABLE 82–2. *Standards of Oncology Nursing Practice*

Professional Practice Standards

The oncology nurse applies theoretical concepts as a basis for decisions in practice.

The oncology nurse systematically and continually collects data regarding the health status of the client. The data are recorded, accessible, and communicated to the appropriate members of the multidisciplinary team.

The oncology nurse analyzes assessment data to formulate nursing diagnoses.

The oncology nurse develops an outcome-oriented care plan that is individualized and holistic. This plan is based on nursing diagnoses and incorporates preventive, therapeutic, rehabilitative, palliative, and comforting nursing actions.

The oncology nurse implements the nursing care plan to achieve the identified outcomes for the client.

The oncology nurse regularly and systematically evaluates the client's responses to intervention in order to determine progress toward achievement of outcomes and to revise the database, nursing diagnoses, and the plan of care.

Professional Performance Standards

The oncology nurse assumes responsibility for professional development and continuing education and contributes to the professional growth of others.

The oncology nurse collaborates with the multidisciplinary team in assessing, planning, implementing, and evaluating care.

The oncology nurse participates in peer review and interdisciplinary program evaluation to assure that high-quality nursing care is provided to clients.

The oncology nurse uses the code for nurses and "A Patient's Bill of Rights" as guides for ethical decision making in practice.

The oncology nurse contributes to the scientific base of nursing practice and the field of oncology through the review and application of research.

(Reprinted with permission from *Standards of oncology nursing practice,* © 1987 [pp. 6–20]. Kansas City, MO: American Nurses' Association.)

---

lance for human rights related to research as well as support the development of knowledge through research. The ANA's *Human Rights Guidelines for Nurses in Clinical and Other Research* (1985b) addresses ethical guidelines, mechanisms for protecting rights, and responsibilities of nurses. Human rights refer to both research subjects and workers who are expected to participate in the research process. The protection of these rights includes the right to freedom from injury, right to privacy and dignity, and right to anonymity. Potential subjects must be informed about the degree of risk and benefits related to the study; be given full information about the study proposal, procedures, and instruments; and be assured of the confidentiality of their responses.

When nurses are involved in activities that are part of the research process, such as administering experimental cancer chemotherapeutic agents, their rights must be protected as well as those of the subjects. Informed consent applies to the nurse as well as the client. Nurses need to be informed in writing of the

TABLE 82–3. *Standards of Advanced Practice in Oncology Nursing*

Professional Practice Standards

The advanced practice oncology nurse who functions as:

A *direct caregiver* provides, guides, directs, and evaluates the nursing practice delivered to clients with actual or potential diagnoses of cancer.

A *coordinator* uses systems theory and the change process with the interdisciplinary oncology team to determine and achieve realistic healthcare goals for the client, the community, or the healthcare system.

A *consultant* provides expert knowledge about oncology to colleagues, health professionals, allied health personnel, healthcare consumers, and professional and public organizations.

An *educator* assesses the learning needs of the client, health professionals, or the community and then designs, implements, and evaluates educational activities.

A *researcher* identifies current researchable problems in oncology nursing, tests relevant theories related to oncology nursing, collaborates in research, and evaluates and implements research findings that have an impact on cancer care and cancer nursing.

An *administrator* uses management theory to create an environment that provides quality care to the client and the community and that promotes professional nursing practice.

Professional Performance Standards

The advanced practice oncology nurse:

Assumes responsibility for individual professional development and continuing education and serves as a role model and mentor to other health professionals.

Applies the *Code for Nurses* and the *Patient's Bill of Rights* to ethical decision making in cancer nursing practice.

Demonstrates knowledge of legal issues in cancer nursing practice.

Monitors and evaluates oncology nursing practice to ensure that high quality care is provided to clients and the community.

Demonstrates knowledge of the political process as a mechanism to address healthcare policy and issues to improve health care.

(Reprinted with permission from *Standards of advanced practice in oncology nursing.* ©1990 [pp. 7, 23]. Pittsburgh: Oncology Nursing Press.)

conditions of employment, expectations related to research studies, risks, and risk management.

There are three mechanisms for ensuring the protection of human rights: informed consent, institutional review boards (IRBs), and vigilant practicing professionals. Free and voluntary informed consent must be obtained from all potential research subjects before they participate in a research study. This requires:

> . . . an explanation of the study and the procedures to be followed and their purposes; a description of physical risk or discomfort, any invasion of privacy, and any threat to dignity; and an explanation of the methods used to protect anonymity and ensure confidentiality. The subject should also receive a description of expected benefits to himself or to the development of new knowledge. In instances in which control groups are used and therapeutic measures such as

drugs are withheld, appropriate alternative procedures that might be advantageous to the subject should be discussed. Also, subjects need to know they are free to discontinue participation in the study at any time without jeopardy (ANA, 1985b).

Institutions and agencies are responsible for establishing procedures to protect human rights and create IRBs to be responsible for this function. The IRBs should have representatives from all occupational groups, including nursing, that may conduct research or participate in the research process. The IRB must review all research proposals before data collection is initiated, and any problems occurring in the implementation of a study should be reported to the IRB.

In addition to the IRB review, many institutions have instituted a review by specialty groups for the purpose of preventing the overstudy of specific populations as well as ascertaining the scientific merit of the study. These groups should also consist of members from all occupations involved in conducting or participating in the research. In agencies with specialty review committees, research proposals must be approved by both review groups.

Practicing professional nurses must be vigilant regarding the protection of human rights. They often have much more contact with clients than investigators and may observe known or unknown violations of human rights. For example, an individual who is confused and unable to give true informed consent may be enrolled in a study. The nurse is responsible for notifying the investigator and being sure the situation is corrected. For situations in which notification or correction is not possible, a mechanism should be established in which nurses can report the violation of human rights and action be taken to deal with them.

RIGHTS OF PROFESSIONAL NURSES

RIGHT TO PRACTICE NURSING

DEFINED DUTIES AND EXPECTATIONS

Nurses have a right to written job descriptions, policies, and procedures that describe their practices. This clarifies the nurse's role, gives direction for specific situations, and protects the nurse. This right is not always given and must be asserted by the nurses involved. For example, there are times in cancer nursing practice when a new procedure is implemented for which no written institutional procedures are developed. This problem frequently occurs when new technologies such as vascular access devices or implanted pumps become available and physicians are eager to use them in patient care. In these situations, nurses must insist on adequate training and preparation for all nurses involved so that safe nursing care can be given. Nurses should take the initiative in reviewing the literature, contacting other institutions that use the technology, and obtaining information from the company that makes the device to determine what constitutes optimal nursing practice. If nurses take these steps and incorporate their findings into practice, they will be practicing as reasonable and competent nurses; however, written policies and procedures should be developed as quickly as possible.

Cancer nurses practicing in ambulatory-care centers have special needs regarding the job description, policies, and procedures that guide their practice. Often these nurses have a great deal of autonomy, and their patient care functions occur in physician- and nurse-client visits as well as by telephone (Brown, 1985; Nail, Greene, Jones, & Flannery, 1989). Nurses functioning in this role have a right to a job description and policies that recognize the autonomy with which they are expected to function. It is also useful for them to have nursing protocols with physician standing orders, if needed, that can be used in the management of common patient problems and emergencies such as allergic reactions (Medvec, 1987). Often these rights are achieved by nursing management and clinicians working together to identify needs and develop the written, institutionally approved guidelines necessary.

Oncology clinical nurse specialists and nurse practitioners also have special problems in clarifying their roles with specific job descriptions. Of necessity, their job descriptions may be very broad. They may be establishing a new, incompletely defined role. A strategy that has been successful in this situation is to develop goals, objectives, and a plan of action that is mutually agreed on by the OCNS and employer that guides the OCNS's or nurse practitioner's work ("Recommendations for administrative," 1985). This requires documentation of steps taken toward goal achievement and evaluation of outcomes. Over time this can contribute to the development of a clear, comprehensive job description.

REASONABLE TIME FOR DUTIES

Nurses have a right to a work environment that minimizes physical and emotional stress (Fagin, 1975) and should participate in efforts to create and maintain a work environment that is conducive to high-quality nursing care (ANA, 1985a). Legally, employers are responsible for providing sufficient nursing coverage to meet patients' needs (Creighton, 1986). Although nurses' rights and employer responsibilities are clear, nurse clinicians often believe that they do not have enough time to provide high-quality nursing care. As nursing shortages increase, these beliefs will become more prevalent.

A reasonable amount of time to perform one's duties is a right that may need to be asserted by sharing information with administrators and the public, using pressure, and having an image of oneself as being worthy of this right. Nurses may need to provide information and exert pressure on management by analyzing client needs with respect to nursing time required. They may also need to publicize their findings in their community. However, nurse clinicians and managers also need to examine their practice areas in terms of nursing care priorities and efficiency. Nursing care goals need to be reasonable with respect to the clients' length of stay and capabilities, and more efficient methods for routine aspects of nursing responsibilities may

need to be developed and implemented. Job descriptions may need to be redefined to include fewer responsibilities. For example, in a new physician practice, a nurse may be hired to provide nursing care, administer chemotherapy, and collect and manage data for collaborative group studies. As the number of clients grows, the nurse may need to negotiate to have the job redefined to exclude data collection and management. Finally, if nurses believe they have exhausted their endurance and change strategies without establishing an environment in which they have a reasonable amount of time to perform their duties, their self-image of being worthy of this right could lead them to leave the position.

AUTONOMOUS PROFESSIONAL ROLE

Refusing Physician Orders. Nurses have the legal right to refuse physician orders that are believed to be contrary to good nursing practice (Annas et al., 1981). Such an order might be the prescription of high-dose methotrexate without the essential order for leucovorin rescue. If this very dangerous order were followed, the nurse would be professionally negligent. When a nurse refuses an order, there is also the obligation for follow-up. The nurse should contact the physician and discuss concerns about the order. If unsatisfied with the outcome of the discussion with the physician, the nurse must report the matter to a higher authority, such as the nurse manager. For the nurse's and client's protection, complete documentation of the details observed and responses given by the physician and others should be done in the manner directed by the institution's policies.

Reporting Incompetent Conduct. Nurses have the right and obligation to report incompetent, illegal, and unethical conduct on the part of health-care providers, such as physicians, nurses, agencies, and institutions (ANA, 1985a; Annas et al., 1981). When nurses become aware of such conduct, concern should be expressed to the individual or agency whose practice is being questioned, pointing out negative effects on the client. If the situation is not resolved in a satisfactory manner, it should be reported to a higher authority. The nurse must complete written documentation of the problem. There should be a mechanism for reporting incompetent, illegal, or unethical conduct in the institution or agency that protects the reporting individual from reprisals (ANA, 1985a).

In spite of the right and obligation to report professional wrongdoing, whistle-blowers take substantial risks in their actions and need to be aware of them (Bandman, 1985). Whistle blowing is often seen as evidence of disloyalty to the team or institution, and whistle-blowers often rightly fear retaliation. Nurses, however, need to take a broader moral and ethical point of view. Their primary responsibility as professionals is to respect human dignity and worth and to safeguard their clients. This clearly places their responsibility to clients at a higher level than their loyalty to professional colleagues and health care institutions.

There is no risk-free method for whistle blowing, but Bandman (1985) has identified some considerations that could improve effectiveness and safety based on the work of consumer rights activist Ralph Nader. First, one should identify the misconduct, the related threats to clients, and the amount of harm that could result from lack of disclosure. If the amount of harm is great, the likelihood of support for disclosure is greater. Second, one should be sure knowledge of the misconduct is accurate, have documentation of the misconduct, and obtain support from others. This action will allow the case to stand on its own merit even if the motives of the whistle-blower are questioned. Third, one should use nursing standards for practice, statutes, rules, and regulations to support the decision to disclose misconduct. Fourth, one should consider the responses of others and the risk to self in developing a plan of action. It is useful to exhaust all options within an agency or institution to remedy a situation, starting at the lowest levels and working up, before going to outside authorities. Anonymity in disclosure may also be a useful strategy for self-protection, but if used, it is imperative that the information disclosed can stand alone in evaluating the case. Finally, it would be helpful to locate a source of external support such as professional societies, legal counsel, state agencies, or special-interest groups.

OCCUPATIONAL SAFETY

As advances in cancer treatment have been made, occupational hazards to health care professionals providing cancer care have increased. Cancer nurses may be exposed to hazards such as radiation, antineoplastic drugs, and hepatitis B, and they have the right to protect themselves. Institutional policies and procedures for protection against hazards in the work environment should be consistent with those recommended by regulatory agencies such as the Occupational Safety and Health Administration (OSHA) or the National Council of Radiation Protection (NCRP).

Maximum permissible dose limits of radiation for occupational and general exposure have been established for many years by the NCRP (1976, 1977). Nurses may be in either the occupational or the general category depending on the nature of their position and the institution in which they are employed. Nurses working in a radiation treatment center or caring for patients receiving brachytherapy have the right to a radiation monitoring device, such as a film badge, provided by their employer. A written report of monthly exposure and a permanent cumulative record of exposure should be available to personnel. When filing any new application for radiation monitoring, the nurse should be sure to note previous radiation monitoring and the location of exposure records, so a cumulative lifetime exposure record can be maintained. Radiation safety procedures for nurses are described in Chapter 20.

The OSHA has developed guidelines for the safe mixing and administration of antineoplastic drugs, which are discussed in depth in Chapter 22 (U.S. Department of Labor, OSHA, 1986). Compliance with these guidelines has varied according to the setting, with nurses working in physicians' offices handling more drugs and using fewer precautions than nurses in other settings (Valanis & Shortridge, 1987). Although it has

been reported that the OSHA guidelines are not mandatory standards and that there are no penalties for noncompliance (Gullo, 1988), OSHA has cited and fined an oncology physician for failure to protect employees who were exposed to hazardous materials in his office ("Oregon physician," 1988). In this case, a ventilated hood for mixing antineoplastic drugs, separate refrigeration, and separate trash receptacles for needle disposal had not been provided. Although nurses are often sympathetic to the expense their employer must incur for employee protection (Barhamand, 1986), they have a right to this protection.

In 1983, OSHA identified nurses as high-risk employees in a hazard alert on hepatitis B (Richardson, 1987). Oncology nurses who administer chemotherapy are at high risk for this hazard. OSHA has mandated that nurses and other high-risk health care providers must be vaccinated with hepatitis B vaccine and receive education and training in protective practices. The ANA, American Public Health Association, and several unions have urged OSHA to make this recommendation a standard and to mandate employers to provide the vaccine free of charge to high-risk employees (Richardson, 1987).

JOB SATISFACTION

There are both great satisfactions and emotional hazards for nurses practicing in the field of oncology. According to studies of oncology nurse clinicians and oncology clinical nurse specialists, the stressors encountered in cancer care are similar in quantity and character to those experienced in other specialties (Donovan, 1981; Jenkins & Ostchega, 1986; Yasko, 1983a). The major stressors for oncology nurse clinicians were identified as lack of psychologic support, lack of work satisfaction, and high work stress (Donovan, 1981; Jenkins & Ostchega, 1986). Sources of stress for oncology clinical nurse specialists included lack of psychologic support, complex bureaucratic organizational structures, and role development and expectations (Yasko, 1983a).

To minimize these stressors and enhance job satisfaction, nurses need to use strategies to cope with work stress effectively (Yasko, 1983b). "A good stress management plan has three objectives: eliminate those stressors you can eliminate, learn to master those situations which routinely produce stress, and develop a mechanism for relieving the residual stress response" (Donovan, 1981, p. 24). At a personal level, training in time management, conflict resolution, and relaxation strategies are useful. At the management level, a commitment to providing adequate staffing for the workload, developing innovative strategies for recruitment and retention, and providing counseling for high-risk employees are needed to reduce employee work stress.

The development and maintenance of a professional support system is also helpful in decreasing stress and enhancing job satisfaction. Some institutions provide psychologic support in formal support groups led by a trained group leader such as a psychologist. More often oncology nurses must develop their own support network. Professional colleagues are often able to be more supportive than family and friends because of their depth of understanding of the day-to-day experiences and stressors in cancer care. In some settings, oncology nurses may not have colleagues who are readily available to provide support. Oncology nurses may need to reach out to their local or regional community of nurses or other health care providers to identify a support system. In this case, nurses need to negotiate with their employer for time or make a personal time commitment to use their support system on a regular basis.

PROFESSIONAL GROWTH

Professional growth is both a right and a responsibility identified by the *Standards of Oncology Nursing Practice* (ANA & ONS, 1987). Many opportunities for professional growth are available in oncology nursing. There are many continuing education opportunities provided by the ONS and American Cancer Society as well as a large number of journals in various disciplines that can be used for independent study and to keep current about research findings and new technology, treatment, and procedures. Another means for professional development is participation in professional and community organizations. This demonstrates professional responsibility, serves as a method for exchange of new knowledge among professional colleagues and the public, and provides a forum for heightening awareness of political, cultural, social, and ethical issues related to oncology.

Other mechanisms for professional growth are peer review and program evaluation. Although the primary goal of these activities is to ensure high-quality care of clients, a secondary outcome is self-evaluation. Critical evaluation of one's practice leads to the identification of factors critical to high-quality care and areas of needed growth that can contribute to improved practice.

RIGHTS IN THE NURSE-CLIENT RELATIONSHIP

COMMUNICATING WITH CLIENTS AND FAMILIES

Answering Client Questions. The nurse has the right and obligation to answer clients' questions about their condition, treatment, and nursing care honestly, but there are limitations based on what would be expected of the reasonable and prudent nurse (Annas et al., 1981; Payton, 1985). For example, the reasonable nurse would not advocate alternative treatments that were dangerous or ineffective. In fact, nurses are obligated by their professional code of ethics to advise clients against the use of such treatments.

The dilemma nurses often face is who should tell what (Payton, 1985). The best solution to this dilemma is multidisciplinary collaboration, especially between oncology nurses and physicians. The American Hospital Association's *Patient's Bill of Rights* (1975) affirms the right of patients to obtain current information regarding their diagnosis, treatment, and prognosis

from their physician. If the physician appears reluctant to answer a client's question or the client does not understand the information provided by the physician, the nurse should discuss the situation with the physician, encourage an honest and clear discussion between physician and patient, and be sure that it takes place. Often it is helpful to the client for the nurse to be present when such a discussion occurs. When it is clear that clients have not received information they need and want, nurses have the right and obligation to ensure that the client receives that information (Payton, 1985).

In the case of Tuma v. Idaho Board of Nursing a significant legal decision about answering client questions was made that is relevant to cancer nursing (Annas et al., 1981; Jameton, 1984). Ms. Tuma, a clinical nursing instructor, was assigned to a woman dying of myelogenous leukemia whose physician had told her that chemotherapy was her last hope. When Ms. Tuma approached the woman for the purpose of administering the chemotherapy and discussed the side effects, the woman was emotionally distraught and apprehensive about the treatment. She told the nurse that the leukemia had been controlled for 12 years by natural foods and that she believed God would cure her. Ms. Tuma then discussed several alternative cancer therapies with the woman and said they were not sanctioned by the medical profession. The family reported Ms. Tuma's actions to the physician, who reported them to the hospital. Action was taken against Ms. Tuma by the State Board of Nursing, and she was suspended from practice for 6 months for unprofessional conduct. The state nurses' association supported this action. Ms. Tuma appealed to the Idaho Supreme Court, and the decision was reversed. The basis for the reversal was that neither the licensing statute nor the state board regulations defined unprofessional conduct in such a way that forbade Ms. Tuma's actions. Because the court did not seek expert testimony, it is believed that there was concern about a nurse being disciplined for talking to a patient (Annas et al., 1981). Although Ms. Tuma acted within her moral and ethical rights, it is reasonable to believe that the resulting disciplinary action could have been avoided if communication between the physician and Ms. Tuma had taken place (Jameton, 1984).

Disclosure to Families. The maintenance of confidentiality of client information is both a legal and an ethical obligation specifically identified in the ANA *Code for Nurses* (1985a). Disclosure to spouses is an area of legal controversy, with the American Medical Association contending that such disclosure is not a breach of confidentiality. Annas and colleagues (1981) advised that the best rule from the perspective of the rights of health care providers is that disclosures of confidential information to spouses and families should be made only with the client's express permission. Nurses should always determine and follow the client's wishes. When clients do not give permission for sharing of information with their spouse or family, the nurse has the right to discuss the family's need for information with the client and to promote open communication among family members.

CARE OF THE DYING

Clients' Right to Know Their Condition. Clients have the right to know their prognosis, and they also have the right to refuse this knowledge. Because nurses' primary obligation is to their clients, physicians have no authority to order nurses to withhold information that the patient wishes to have (Annas et al., 1981). Thus nurses have the right and obligation to answer client questions about prognosis honestly and openly. This information is important to the individual's ability to make informed decisions about consent or refusal of further treatment (Otte & Allen, 1987).

Honoring Client Directives for Treatment. Competent adult patients have the right to accept or refuse treatment, and health care providers have the right to honor a patient's directive for treatment (Annas, 1991). The right to refuse treatment has been consistently upheld in court and is perceived as an absolute constitutional right (Annas et al., 1981).

Dying individuals do not lose this right when they become incompetent. If they have made their wishes to refuse treatment known before they became incompetent, health care providers have the right to honor these wishes. Federal enactment of the Patient Self-Determination Act in 1991 encourages individuals to complete advance directives (living will) and durable power of attorney (health care proxy) (Annas, 1991). It also requires health care providers and institutions to increase their efforts to honor advance directives (LaPuma, Orentlicher, & Moss, 1991). If individuals' wishes are not known, their right to accept or refuse treatment must be exercised for them by the next of kin, guardian, family members, physician, ethics committee, or court of law (Annas et al., 1981). The decision is made on the basis of what most competent people would do and what decision the individual would make if able.

Nurses have an excellent opportunity for opening the topic of advance directives during admission and routine health assessments of individuals with cancer. Quality of life issues and advance directive goals can be integrated into discussions of goals for nursing care. At that time, patient teaching about advanced directives can be initiated (Haisfield et al., 1994).

Ethics Committees. Institutional ethics committees have been initiated to deal with the dilemmas and resolve conflicts that often arise in caring for the dying. These committees usually have the following functions: policy development, education, and case consultation (Vaux & Savage, 1989). Committee members should be from a number of disciplines and should include nurse representatives. Nurses should have the right to bring cases to the committee for consultation.

Many ethics committees have been instrumental in developing do-not-resuscitate (DNR) policies. The JCAHO has mandated that hospitals have policies stating that DNR orders are permissible and describing exactly what these orders mean ("New policy," 1987). Advance discussion with the patient, family, and health care providers is needed to make DNR decisions. Nurses often initiate DNR discussions because they are frequently the health care providers that must begin resuscitation measures. Do-not-resuscitate orders should be written by the primary physician and communicated to all health care providers involved (Otte & Allen, 1987). If the patient improves or has a better prognosis, the DNR order should be reviewed. Also, DNR orders should not be automatically carried over from one hospitalization to another.

RIGHTS REGARDING PROFESSIONAL LIABILITY AND COMPENSATION

LIABILITY

A review of litigation involving oncology nurses indicated that the incidents involved medication discrepancies, incorrect follow-up or referral, and failure to provide reasonable care after chemotherapy extravasation (Schulmeister, 1987). Most nursing negligence falls under the rule of respondeat superior. This rule in essence states that employers are responsible for wrongful acts of their employees that occur in the course of performance of work duties. However, nurses are liable for patient injuries resulting from medication errors or not following the written policies and procedures of their hospital or agency (Hogue, 1986).

Nurses have a right to written policies and procedures that determine the standard of care in their workplace. They can reduce their liability by being sure that policies and procedures are comprehensive and cover all their responsibilities. If these are not complete, they can initiate and contribute to the development of those policies and procedures needed.

Many institutions have very specific guidelines for risk management. Familiarity with these guidelines can also be helpful in reducing liability. Guidelines for reporting and documenting patient injuries should be followed carefully.

Nurses also have a right to adequate liability insurance coverage. They should carefully investigate coverage provided by their employer and may need to engage their own attorney to understand these complex policies. Although many employers discourage nurses from carrying their own liability insurance, it is in the nurses' best interest to do so because they may be sued individually. Also, the employer's insurance company may seek restitution from the nurse if damages are paid (Schulmeister, 1987).

ADEQUATE COMPENSATION

Nurses have a right to adequate compensation, and the ANA has worked toward this goal through the legislative and legal systems since the 1950s and continues to do so. Although compensation has improved over this time period, many nurses believe they are undervalued. The ANA recommends four ways in which nurses can work to achieve pay equity: educate other nurses and the general public, pursue legal changes through the courts and government agencies, lobby for legislation, and use collective bargaining (Flanagan & Barnett, 1987).

As a result of a 1974 amendment to the National Labor Relations Act, employees of both profit and nonprofit hospitals and health care institutions have the right to be represented by unions (Annas et al., 1981). They also have the right to strike and picket. However, they must give a 10-day advance notice so provisions can be made for continuity of health care. In some cases, unions bargain away the right to strike and substitute grievance and arbitration procedures. When returning to work after a strike, employees are entitled to return to their previous positions.

SUMMARY

The rights and responsibilities of professional nurses are very closely related. Having a clear understanding of these rights and responsibilities can assist nurses in clarifying their roles, enhancing their self-confidence in their practice, and providing the fortitude to assert their professional rights. Because oncology nurses often practice at the forefront of scientific knowledge and technology, these actions enhance high-quality care for individuals with cancer and high standards for oncology nursing practice.

REFERENCES

American Hospital Association. (1975). *A patient's bill of rights* (AHS Cat. No. 2415). Chicago: American Hospital Association.

American Nurses' Association. (1980). *Nursing: A social policy statement.* Kansas City, MO: Author.

American Nurses' Association. (1985a). *Code for nurses with interpretive statements.* Kansas City, MO: Author.

American Nurses' Association. (1985b). *Human rights guidelines for nurses in clinical and other research.* Kansas City, MO: Author.

American Nurses' Association & Oncology Nursing Society. (1987). *Standards of oncology nursing practice.* Kansas City, MO: American Nurses' Association.

ANA board approves a definition of nursing practice. (1955). *American Journal of Nursing, 55,* 1474.

Annas, G. J., Glantz, L. H., & Katz, B. F. (1981). *The rights of doctors, nurses and allied health professionals: A health law primer.* New York: Avon.

Annas, G. J. (1991). The health care proxy and living will. *New England Journal of Medicine, 324,* 1210–1213.

Bandman, E. (1985). Whistle-blowers take risk to halt wrongdoing. In American Nurses' Association Committee on Ethics, *Ethical dilemmas confronting nurses* (pp. 18–22). Kansas City, MO: American Nurses' Association.

Barhamand, B. A. (1986). Difficulties encountered in implementing guidelines for handling antineoplastics in the physician's office. *Cancer Nursing, 9,* 138–143.

Brown, J. K. (1985). Ambulatory services: The mainstay of cancer nursing care. *Oncology Nursing Forum, 12*(1), 57–59.

Creighton, H. (1986). *Law every nurse should know* (5th ed.). Philadelphia: W. B. Saunders Co.

Donley, S. R. (1984). The effects of changing health care policy on cancer nursing. *Oncology Nursing Forum, 11*(4), 64–66.

Donoghue, M., & Spross, J. A. (1985). A report from the first national invitational conference: The oncology clinical nurse specialist role analysis and future projections. *Oncology Nursing Forum, 12*(2), 35–73.

Donovan, M. (1981). Stress at work: Cancer nurses report. *Oncology Nursing Forum, 8*(2), 22–25.

Fagin, C. (1975). Nurses' rights. *American Journal of Nursing, 75,* 82–85.

Flanagan, L., & Barnett, E. (1987). *Pay equity: What it means and how it affects nurses.* Kansas City, MO: American Nurses' Association.

Gullo, S. M. (1988). Safe handling of antineoplastic drugs: Transplanting recommendations into practice. *Oncology Nursing Forum, 15,* 595–601.

Haisfield, M. E., McGuire, D. B., Krumm, S., Shore, A. D., Zabora, J., & Rubin, H. R. (1994). Patients' and health care providers' opinions regarding advanced directives. *Oncology Nursing Forum, 21,* 1179–1187.

Hanson, J. L., & Ashley, B. (1994). Advanced practice nurses' application of the Stetler model for research utilization: Improving bereavement care. *Oncology Nursing Forum, 21,* 720–724.

Hogue, E. (1986). Lessons you can learn from court decisions. *Nursing 86, 16*(4), 45–47.

Jameton, A. (1984). *Nursing practice: The ethical issues.* Englewood Cliffs, NJ: Prentice-Hall, Inc.

Jenkins, J. F., & Ostchega, Y. (1986). Evaluation of burnout in oncology nurses. *Cancer Nursing, 9,* 108–116.

Joint Commission on Accreditation of Healthcare Organizations. (1993). *The Joint Commission 1994 accreditation manual for hospitals* (Vol. 1). Oakbrook Terrace, IL: Author.

LaPuma, J., Orentlicher, D., & Moss, R. J. (1991). Advance directives on admission: Clinical implications and analysis of the Patient Self-Determination Act of 1990. *Journal of the American Medical Association, 266,* 402–405.

McGuire, D. B., Walczak, J. R., & Krumm, S. L. (1994). Development of a nursing research utilization program in a clinical oncology setting: Organization, implementation, and evaluation. *Oncology Nursing Forum, 21,* 704–710.

McNally, J. C., Somerville, E. T., Miaskowski, C., & Rostad, M. (1991). *Guidelines for oncology nursing practice* (2nd ed.). Philadelphia: W. B. Saunders Co.

Medvec, B. R. (1987). Nursing protocols. *Outpatient Chemotherapy, 1*(4), 7.

Nail, L. M., Greene, D., Jones, L. S., & Flannery, M. (1989). Nursing care by telephone: Describing practice in an ambulatory oncology center. *Oncology Nursing Forum, 16,* 387–395.

National Council of Radiation Protection. (1976). *Radiation protection for medical and allied personnel* (NCRP Report No. 48). Washington, DC: U.S. Government Printing Office.

National Council of Radiation Protection. (1977). *Review of NCRP radiation dose limit for embryo and fetus in occupationally exposed women* (NCRP Publ. No. 53). Washington, DC: U.S. Government Printing Office.

New policy set on DNR orders. (1987). *Cope Magazine, 2*(1), 19.

Nurses warned that ignorance of law can jeopardize license to practice. (1987). *NYSNA Reports, 18*(1), 3.

Oncology Nursing Society. (1983a). Resolution to endorse. *Nursing: A Social Policy Statement. Oncology Nursing Forum, 10*(3), 89–90.

Oncology Nursing Society. (1983b). Titles in oncology nursing practice. *Oncology Nursing Forum, 10*(3), 90.

Oregon physician cited for violations. (1988). *Cope Magazine, 2*(10), 38.

Otte, D. M., & Allen, K. S. (1987). Ethical principles in the nursing care of the terminally ill adult. *Oncology Nursing Forum, 14*(5), 87–91.

Page, N. E., & Arena, D. M. (1994). Rethinking the merger of the clinical specialist and nurse practitioner roles. *Image, 26,* 315–318.

Payton, R. (1985). Truth essential for trust between nurse, patient. In American Nurses' Association Committee on Ethics, *Ethical dilemmas confronting nurses* (pp. 23–26). Kansas City, MO: American Nurses' Association.

Recommendations for administrative support of the oncology clinical nurse specialist. (1985). *Oncology Nursing Forum, 12*(2), 71–73.

Reedy, A. M., Shivnan, J. C., Hanson, J. L., Haisfield, M. E., & Gregory, R. E. (1994). The clinical application of research utilization: Amphotericin B. *Oncology Nursing Forum, 21*, 715–719.

Reiter, F. (1967). The nurse clinician. *American Journal of Nursing, 67*, 274–280.

Report to house outlines scope of nursing practice. (1987). *The American Nurse, 19*(6), 13–14.

Rhodes, A. M., & Miller, R. D. (1984). *Nursing & the law* (4th ed.). Rockville, MD: Aspen Publishers, Inc.

Richardson, D. (1987). Technology produces occupational hazards for nurses. *American Nurse, 19*(4), 7–8.

Schulmeister, L. (1987). Litigation involving oncology nurses. *Oncology Nursing Forum, 14*(2), 25–28.

University of Texas adopts formal code of ethics to help people. (1984). *Oncology Times, 6*(11), 12.

U.S. Department of Labor, Office of Occupational Medicine, Occupational Safety and Health Administration. (1986). *Work practice guidelines for personnel dealing with cytotoxic (antineoplastic) drugs* (Publication No. 8-1.1). Washington, DC: Occupational Safety and Health Administration.

Valanis, B., & Shortridge, L. (1987). Self protective practices of nurses handling antineoplastic drugs. *Oncology Nursing Forum, 14*, 23–27.

Vaux, K. L., & Savage, T. A. (1989). Initiating and maintaining an ethics committee. *Seminars in Oncology Nursing, 5*, 82–88.

Walczak, J. R., McGuire, D. B., Haisfield, M. E., & Beezley, A. (1994). A survey of research related activities and perceived barriers to research utilization among professional oncology nurses. *Oncology Nursing Forum, 21*, 710–715.

Yasko, J. M. (1983a). A survey of oncology clinical nurse specialists. *Oncology Nursing Forum, 10*(1), 25–30.

Yasko, J. M. (1983b). Burnout and oncology nursing. *Cancer Nursing, 6*, 109–116.

Yasko, J. M., & Fleck, A. (1984). Prospective payment (DRGs): What will be the impact on cancer care? *Oncology Nursing Forum, 11*(3), 63–72.

CHAPTER
83

Legal Responsibilities of the Nurse

Marilyn Frank-Stromborg • Terry Chamorro

Changes within the nursing profession itself have forced nurses to consider the legal ramifications of their professional and business actions. Health care reform, managed care, and the national emphasis on cost-containment in health care have spurred the growth of nurse-run clinics, nurses in advanced practice roles, and nurses in collaborative practice with physicians (Kindig, Cultice, & Mullan, 1993). Nurses in advanced practice roles are increasingly entering into partnership arrangements with physicians or setting up independent practices, and thus further subjecting themselves to legal action. There are also a multitude of legal issues surrounding the advanced practice role such as scope of practice and the state's Nurse Practice Act, prescriptive authority, and reimbursement for services (Heffernan, 1995). Advanced practice nurses (APNs) are as vulnerable to lawsuits for malpractice as physicians have been.

PRACTICE DIMENSIONS IN CANCER NURSING

COMPETENCE IN NURSING

Advancements in cancer treatment have dictated a reformulation of responsibilities among the various clinicians attending to this spectrum of diseases. The shift in responsibilities has expanded the scope of cancer nursing across all practice settings. Treatment advances demand change and extension of nurse competencies and skills. The oncology nurse undertakes more functions than before in administering treatment previously delivered solely by the physician (Sheidler, McGuire, Grossman, & Gilbert, 1992). This statement is especially true of oncology nurses in advanced practice roles. In general, autonomy in the practice arena is becoming commonplace to many oncology nurses whether or not they are in the advanced practice role, especially in ambulatory and home care settings. In addition to the physical care, the nurse now provides emotional support and teaching programs for patients undergoing complex cancer treatment that carries significant morbidity (Sharp, DePriest, Potts, & Willeford, 1994; Walker, Roethke, Sandman, Clark, & Martin, 1994). The dimensions of cancer nursing have changed in conjunction with the whole of nursing, perhaps more so, in response to the rapid technologic changes in oncology treatment and movement of oncology treatment out of the acute care setting into the community. Changes of this nature bring greater exposure in the legal arena, where the public will demand a remedy in event of an adverse outcome in health care.

SOCIETAL EXPECTATIONS

Society expects of its professionals a standard of competence as persons possessing special skills and knowledge. This conduct, the duty of care, forms the basis for the professional's legal responsibilities (Northrop & Kelly, 1987). Legal obligations demanded of the oncology nurse in the various practice settings are not dictated solely by legal regulation. The complex of professional regulation, less direct in authority and obscure in nature, has powerful legal implications as well. Risk management in cancer nursing is based on understanding legal and professional regulations of practice plus recognition of potentially sensitive issues that may lead to liability exposure. In concert, legal and professional regulations determine the dimensions of nursing practice. This chapter addresses the essentials in defining legal responsibilities from the perspective of cancer nursing. It is meant to guide the nurse in instituting personal risk evaluation that can enhance professional security in the face of ever-changing conditions in cancer care.

NURSE PRACTICE ACTS

Competence in nursing is a reflection of decisions the nurse makes in practice. Many of those decisions are bound by public law, which is society's way of imposing its goals, compelling individuals and organizations to follow specified courses of actions. Statutory law, a variety of regulations enacted by legislative bodies, is the first legal boundary nurses should evaluate. A state's nurse practice act is statutory law that defines nursing performance in its most fundamental terms and exerts primary control over practice. Statutes vary in the language used to define the scope of professional nursing. Hall (1993) recommends that when analyzing state statutes to determine the practice environment of the state, that the nursing, medical, and pharmacy practice statutes for that state be examined. When nurse practice acts are examined:

1. The established rules of statutory interpretation require statutes first to be given their plain meaning (Morse & Kane, 1995).

2. Look at the general purposes or intent of the legislation. This requires looking at the legislative history behind the statute.
3. Identify the problem the legislature most likely sought to remedy as well as the conditions existing at the time of the enactment of the statue.
4. Interpret amendment(s) to the statutes on the theory that the legislature intended to substantially change the law by adding the amendment(s).
5. Try and harmonize the various statutes that govern nursing practice (Hall, 1993, p. 34).

Many practice acts stem from the model definition of nursing formulated by the American Nurses Association (ANA) in 1955. It contained a broadly constructed phrase stating that nursing practice is "acts based on knowledge and application of scientific principles." This phrase may not provide sufficient legal weight for the new tasks and functions nursing continually assumes as a result of scientific and technologic advances (Trandel-Korenchuk & Trandel-Korenchuk, 1980) or justify all facets of the expanding role of oncology nursing.

There are two types of statutes governing nursing practice: licensure statutes and registration or certification statutes. Licensure statutes limit practice to people with specific qualifications, whereas registration or certification statutes merely provide a definition and limit who can use a title, without limiting practice (Hall, 1993).

Because of the increasing emphasis on advanced practice in nursing, state nurse practice acts have been closely scrutinized in terms of their regulation of nurse practitioners, certified nurse-midwives, and certified registered nurse anesthetists and the barriers to practice that these statutes create for advanced practice nurses. As the practice of nursing evolved over the past decades, the needs of patients changed and the role of the nurse expanded to meet those demands. However, the restricted scope of practice in many Nurse Practice Acts does not recognize the new roles nurses are assuming. This has created a continuing legal tension between what is allowed and what is actually occurring (Heffernan, 1995).

Sekscenski, Sansom, Bazell, Salmon, and Mullan (1994) analyzed variations in the regulation of nurse practitioners, physician assistants, and certified nurse-midwives in all 50 states and the District of Columbia. When analyzing state practice acts they looked at the legal status, reimbursement, and authority to prescribe in the statute:

1. *Legal status.* 20 points were allocated if practitioners had legal status as professionals.
2. *Reimbursement.* 40 points were allocated if reimbursement for their services was required.
3. *Authority to prescribe.* 40 points were allocated if practitioners had the authority to write prescriptions.

A score of 100 points represented the most favorable environment and a score of 0 the least favorable practice environment.

As expected, there was wide variation among the states. For physician assistants, the practice-environment scores ranged from a high of 100 in the state of Washington to 0 in Mississippi. Practice-environment scores for nurse practitioners ranged from 100 in Oregon to 14 in Ohio and Illinois, while practice-environment scores for certified nurse-midwives ranged from 100 in Minnesota to 25 in Indiana. In general, the researchers found that favorable state practice environments for physician assistants, nurse practitioners, and certified nurse-midwives were strongly associated with a greater supply of these practitioners (Sekscenski et al., 1993).

PROTOCOLS FOR COMPLEX CARE

The statutes of many states recognize that greater interdependence in the position and role of nursing is important in modern health care. States prepare for this interdependence by specifying the extent of physician involvement and supervision required as the role of the registered nurse expands. Specialization in any area of nursing denotes minimally acceptable conduct in the performance of professional services. Oncology nurses in independent situations must clearly interpret the limit of practice dimensions defined by regulatory statutes of their state. If they determine that the outer bounds of their practice extend beyond that of traditional nursing, it may be wise to consider placing on file written protocols and specific documentation attesting to their specialized skills and mode of acquisition.

Procedures that questionably exceed the scope of traditional nursing or overlap with medicine should be secured by a written protocol. Some states, such as California, term these "standardized procedures." Standardized procedures, written protocols, or practice guidelines are used by health care professionals to decrease variation in practice, to improve the quality of care by standardizing practice, and in the hopes that the expense of malpractice litigation will be decreased because the protocols delineate the standard of care (West, 1994).

Written protocols may protect against claims of illegal practice of medicine in that they convey some authority for a nurse with appropriate skills and knowledge to undertake certain functions (Kelly & Garrick, 1984). The protocol should define the exact procedure and delineate circumstances that require a report or referral to the physician. Nurse practitioners have worked under such protocols for some time. Investigational cancer treatment may especially require protocols that define nurse-performed procedures. In other instances, oncology nurses may be delegated independent authority in cancer screening, physical assessment, or treatment.

A protocol is merely a guide that recommends an explicit set of actions. Instruction for some far-reaching function performed independently by the oncology nurse such as paracentesis may have been given by a collaborating physician. Documentation on file of a skills check by the supervising physician argues strongly as to nurse competency in these tasks if a challenge should occur on legal grounds. The relationship

of protocols to law may be along the lines of "standing orders" (Greenfield, 1980). Because protocol guides performance along a sequential decision-making process, it becomes a standard, outlining nursing practice and demanding a measure of competence. Nurses may overlook the value of a written protocol in planning a sound basis for legal protection or, in the busy workplace, may postpone the formality of writing one.

There are several problems with standards/written protocols and these include (1) standards set by national organizations may not take into account regional differences, (2) standards tend to be based on typical textbook patients, (3) standards that were developed for urban research centers may not be appropriate for community hospitals, (4) standards may be idealistic and not oriented to the real world of health care and the diminishing financial resources, and (5) departures from standards do not imply wrong or inappropriate care, nor does adherence always indicate excellent care or favorable outcomes (Moniz, 1992; Rosoff, 1995).

In a malpractice suit, the patient suing a health care provider (the plaintiff) must prove four elements. First, the health care professional must owe a duty to the patient. This element is almost always present in a health care setting. Second, the health care professional must have breached the duty owed the patient. Third, the patient must have sustained damage. Fourth, the patient must prove that the damage was "more likely than not" caused by the health care professional's breach of that duty (Moniz, 1992). Written protocols or standards can be used in court to measure the nurse's care. The written protocols are used to establish the standard of care and argue that the nurse breached that standard, thus satisfying the second element of a malpractice suit.

Because the written protocols can be used against the health care professional in court, Moniz (1992) recommends that:

1. minimal protocols be developed,
2. protocols should be the minimum requirements for safe care and not the maximum for ideal care,
3. protocols should be updated as scientific knowledge develops,
4. realistic protocols be developed that mirror the clinical practice setting, and
5. once the protocols are adopted in the clinical setting they *must* be followed, since any deviation from the protocols is a deviation from the legal standard of care (Moniz, 1992, p. 60).

CERTIFICATION

Many registered nurses have strengthened their professional positions by attaining certification. Certification requires testing for evidence of knowledge that other professionals consider essential and reflects a certain level of acumen and experience in the specialty. The process is standardized, and bias is diminished by use of a professional testing service. Fulfilling the criteria and passing the test for certification as an Oncology Certified Nurse is significant to a cancer nursing career.

The Oncology Nursing Society now offers both certification in basic oncology and advanced oncology practice. Legal connotations may be applied to the certification, however, if it is interpreted to attest to a specific level of competence in practice. Society will then hold the oncology nurse to the professional accountability denoted by the certification. Court opinion or rule has yet to test this premise, but the notion is suggestive that the information on which the nurse is tested may in fact imply the job description and responsibilities within that specialty. A lawyer in litigation involving a professionally certified nurse would be wise to use the implications of certification in attempting to prove or disprove the level of nurse competence and expectation of job-related functions.

STANDARDS OF CARE

DEFINING NURSING STANDARDS

The dimensions of nursing practice are defined by the accepted standards of care. Standards are in constant change as a result of influences such as the institution of new federal health care programs for groups of patients, consumer directives, new medical discoveries, or nurses' demands for greater involvement in health care decisions (Cantor, 1978). The decision on a malpractice suit is shaped by the arguments about standards of care. The outcome of litigation may, in turn, reshape nursing standards of practice. This becomes case law. It is also generally established that a nurse's conduct will not be measured by the standard of care required of a physician or surgeon, but by that of other nurses in the same or similar locality and under similar circumstances (*Alef v. Alta Bates Hospital*, 1992).

The leading case that recognizes the separate standard of care for professional nurses is *Fein v. Permanente Medical Group* (1985). In *Fein*, a family nurse practitioner examined a man who complained of chest pain and diagnosed the pain as due to muscle spasms. The next day when the patient was seen by the physician, the physician also diagnosed the chest pain as due to muscle spasms. On the third day, the patient was diagnosed as having a myocardial infarction. The *Fein* court held that the trial court was in error in telling the jury that "the standard of care required of a nurse practitioner was that of a physician and surgeon . . . when the nurse practitioner is examining a patient or making a diagnosis" (*Fein* at 673). In *Fein*, the court held that a nurse practitioner was to be judged by the standard of care applied to a reasonably prudent nurse practitioner in conducting the examination and prescribing the treatment "in conjunction with her supervising physician" (*Fein* at 674). The case was sent back to the trial court for rehearing.

Standards of care and *standards of practice* are interchangeable terms broadly interpreted as implying a level of performance. The standard of care determines the *minimum* level of care to which the patient is entitled (*Alef v. Alta Bates Hospital,* 1992). Although disturbing for patients, patients are not entitled to the best possible care, or even to average care. Such an approach would create malpractice cases in at least half

of all patient contact. A patient is only entitled to the care that a minimally qualified health care professional would render under the same or similar circumstances (West, 1994).

A health care facility may adopt written standards for governance of nursing practice, or there may be standards not specifically delineated but clearly operant in the setting. Sometimes both exist, and practice is found to deviate from the written standards or policies.

In a suit involving negligence all the elements listed above must be met. Once the relationship between the patient and the health care professional exists, the health care professional has a duty to exercise the same degree of care and skill in managing the patient as would be exercised by a competent health care professional in similar circumstances (Osuch & Bonham, 1994). Courts refer to the degree of care and skill that should be exercised as the "standard of care." *Cooper v. The National Motor Bearing Co.* (1955) is an example of a suit involving the standard of care.

Cooper was a suit against an employer and the employer's trained nurse by the employee who incurred a basal-cell carcinoma at the site of a puncture wound treated by the nurse.

> The standard of good nursing care in the community required the nurse to examine the wound for foreign bodies. If a wound persisted and did not heal, proper nursing care would require that the workman be sent to the doctor, . . . Appellant nurse admitted that she was familiar with the seven danger signals of cancer, one of which is "any sore that does not heal." Nevertheless, she continued to treat the wound for 10 months before sending respondent to the doctor (*Cooper* at 583).

The *Cooper* court opined that a nursing diagnosis of any condition must meet the standard of learning, skill, and care to which nurses practicing that profession in the community are held. The jury verdict against the nurse was held.

The health professional who breaches the standard of care with an extremely harmful state of mind may be liable for punitive damages. Punitive damages are awarded when the breach can be characterized as being done deliberately or willfully or with malice or gross negligence (*Manning v. Twin Falls Clinic & Hospital*, 1992). Punitive damages are monetary awards given in addition to the monetary awards for negligence. In *Manning*, a nurse disconnected the oxygen when she moved a terminally ill patient to a private room. The family had pleaded with the nurse not to remove his oxygen while moving him. The patient went into respiratory failure and died. The court found that the nurse's conduct was grossly negligent and that she acted with disregard for the consequences that were likely to follow. Punitive damages were awarded in this case.

> Evidence was . . . presented that nurse Anderson disconnected Manning's oxygen despite the pleadings of family members present who claimed he could not survive without his oxygen, and who requested that he be provided a portable oxygen unit preparatory to

the move . . . we agree a jury could have found nurse Anderson's conduct was grossly negligent and that she acted with disregard for the consequences that were likely to follow (*Manning* at 1191).

THE EXPERT WITNESS

The standard of care is the measure on which malpractice law bases its decisions. Standards are established from evidence of usual and customary practice. In litigation, an attempt is made to define what the "reasonably prudent" professional would do under certain circumstances—what is common practice. Experts in the field express opinions as to generally accepted practice and actions appropriate to a situation. Both prosecution and defense will use the testimony of expert witnesses to help the court make an informed decision about particular issues of the litigation. Experts base their opinions on knowledge drawn from a variety of sources, experience being the most weighty. Experts cite facts of the case derived from medical documents and records placed in evidence. Testimony also introduces specialized literature, research, and scientific inquiry, and general consensus on standards (Gosnell, 1987).

In an effort to limit frivolous suits and claims, states have responded by enacting legislation restricting those who may offer expert testimony in medical suits. Today almost all claims of medical negligence must be supported by expert testimony that documents the case has merit (Beyer & Popp, 1990). The plaintiff may be required to review his or her case with an expert who testifies the case has merit and to attach evidence of that review with the complaint.

If the conduct in question is within the common knowledge of laymen, an expert witness may not be required at trial. Courts have routinely held that no expert testimony is necessary in circumstances that fall within the common sense of the jury (Beyer & Popp, 1990). Examples of this are "fall out of bed" cases or the use of nursing judgment as to restraining a patient, assisting a patient in and out of bed, or how closely to monitor a medicated patient.

Czubinsky v. Doctors Hospital (1983), is an example of a negligence case involving a nurse who failed to monitor a postsurgical patient. A 28-year-old patient was admitted to the hospital for surgery to remove an ovarian cyst. The routine procedure was done by the surgical team of a surgeon, anesthesiologist, an OR technician, and a circulating nurse. Following the surgery, the surgeon left the room, yelled for the nurse to come and assist him in the other operating room, and the nurse left. When the patient developed a postoperative cardiac arrest, the OR technician left the anesthesiologist alone to perform CPR while he went to get help. The patient suffered severe loss of oxygen and total and permanent paralysis. The appellate court opined that expert testimony was not needed in this case because the nurse's failure to follow the proper procedure with ordinary care and diligence was evident without an expert testifying.

On such facts as a conceded abandonment-neglect in the purest sense—of a patient by nursing personnel at

a life-endangered time, no expert testimony is required either on the issue of neglect or causation. Want of care is so obvious as to render expert testimony unnecessary (Cox, 1989).

The likelihood the court will require expert testimony increases with the technical complexity of the case. Another situation where expert testimony will be required is where the nurse is performing functions that are also being performed by physicians. The emerging issue in litigation involving nurses is the ability to use a nurse expert witness to establish the applicable standard of care based on the argument that nursing is a separate profession from medicine.

There are states (e.g., Ohio, Michigan, West Virginia) that have statutes that specifically require a physician to provide expert testimony in any case involving professional liability as to the standard of care (Beyer & Popp, 1990). In these select states, the statutes have prevented nurses from assisting juries in determining whether nurses have met the standard of care. However, many states have statutes that require that the expert be familiar with the standard of care to testify. One argument used to support the separate profession argument is the existence of separate professional nursing insurance coverage.

The nurse needs to be aware that there are presently obstacles to the use of nurse experts in both state statutes and judicial interpretations in the rules of evidence. Any arguments made to the use of nurse experts must bolster the concept of nursing as a separate profession.

A persuasive argument for the use of nursing experts may include:

- Citation to the state professional nursing statute or advanced nursing practice statute to establish the concept of nursing as a separate profession;
- Use of particular facts of the case, such as certification in a nursing subspecialty or existence of individual professional liability coverage, to further enhance separate professional concept (Beyer & Popp, 1990, p. 366).

COMMUNITY STANDARDS

Standards of care, both written and implied, are the most important factor in molding the legal responsibilities of the nurse. Aside from explicit written standards, many people believe that professional nurses will be held to certain implicit standards that prevail in their community or locale. This is no longer true in matters under litigation. National and community standards are the same. The community cannot expect more or less than nationally accepted criteria in nursing practice (Fiesta, 1983). Nursing education and licensure are now standardized among all states through schools accredited through the National League of Nurses and licensing examinations given concomitantly across the nation. Nursing journals and other media have eliminated the basis for variance in professional practice. In cancer nursing, information about practice is disseminated through several scholarly journals pertaining to the specialty. The most important tactic nurses can employ to avoid a legal encounter is to be aware of and to adhere to the standard of care generally applicable to the clinical situation (Northrup, 1986). The standard of care dictates the extent of the nurse's duty of care.

A case that illustrates the expectation that nurses will adhere to a standard of care that transcends community standards is *Daniel v. St. Francis Cabrini Hospital of Alexandria, Inc.* (1982). In *Daniel*, the nurse left a patient who was taking a number of drugs at the same time—including pills that caused him to feel dizzy and weak—alone in the bathroom. The patient had metastatic prostate cancer, a missing left arm, and chronic organic dementia. The nurse administered an enema to the patient and then left the patient alone in the bathroom while he evacuated the enema and the contents of his bowel. The patient became dizzy in the bathroom, fell, and lacerated his penis. The nurse (Morgan) appealed the trial court's decision in favor of the patient (Mr. Daniel) on the grounds that the trial court had failed to prove the duty owed by the nurse to the patient was that owed by registered nurses licensed to practice in the State of Louisiana and actively practicing in a similar community or locale and under similar conditions (*Daniel* at 590). The *Daniel* court rejected the "locality rule."

> [W]e have serious doubts as to whether any "locality rule" is applicable to registered nurses. Morgan's duty, owed to decedent, was identical to that owed by the defendant-hospital to any patient, i.e., to exercise the requisite amount of care toward a patient that the particular patient's condition may require and to protect the patient from dangers that may result from the patient's physical and mental incapacities as well as from external circumstances peculiarly within its control (*Daniel* at 590).

PROFESSIONAL PRACTICE STANDARDS

Written professional practice standards provide the foundation of nursing performance today. Beginning with the 1974 ANA *Standards: Medical-Surgical Nursing Practice*, professional organizations, especially specialty societies, have defined standards that represent current principles in nursing practice. The standard bearer in cancer nursing is the *Outcome Standards for Cancer Nursing Practice* developed by the Oncology Nursing Society (ONS) (1979). These differ in format from ANA standards, which are arranged in the sequencing of steps in nursing "process." The ONS standards are product-oriented rather than process-oriented and delineate desired outcomes that patients may achieve with professional nursing planning and intervention. In 1990, the Oncology Nursing Society developed *Standards of Advanced Practice in Oncology Nursing*.

The ONS outcome standards and the ANA process standards are stated in broad terms. Both imply a sophisticated level of nursing. Some believe that the existence of practice standards in nursing specialties introduces potential legal exposure because they emphasize professionalism and set the groundwork for quality assurance evaluation (Marks, 1987). Knowledge of ONS professional practice standards is, there-

fore, of the greatest importance to the individual nurse in formulating the goals and purposes of patient care in cancer. Although not always explicitly stated, the standards imply the various activities and functions desired in meeting those goals. Familiarity with ANA medical-surgical standards and ONS outcome standards provides a strong armamentarium for nurses who wish to establish a sound practice that minimizes the risk of litigation. Furthermore, nurses should have a clear concept of the ways they operationalize the standards in the course of daily practice.

The courts have held that professionals who specialize will be held to the standards established by other health professionals in the same specialty area. It is to be expected that the standards of care for specialized areas of nursing would be based on nationally accepted practice standards generated by specialty's national organization. *Gibson v. Bossier City General Hospital* (1991) illustrates the general expectation that nurses who specialize will be held to the standard of care possessed by members of his or her profession actively practicing in such a specialty service under similar circumstances. In *Gibson* the parents of an infant who died sued the pediatrician, hospital, and nursery nurse for failure to timely diagnose and treat the infant's hypoglycemia. The *Gibson* court specifically stated that nurses who specialize in an area will be held to the standard of care of nurses in the same specialty service who use reasonable care and diligence, along with his or her best judgment, in the application of his or her skill to the case (*Gibson* at 1342).

INSTITUTIONAL STANDARDS

Standards of nursing practice are shaped by agency policy, nursing procedure manuals, and job descriptions. These will be the first sources an attorney will refer to when challenging nursing performance in litigation. Probably the most important policies and procedures that influence cancer nursing practice are those pertaining to administration of chemotherapy and control of extravasation. Most facilities are sensitive to the potential for liability and have developed written guidelines for these treatments. Deviation from the prescribed guidelines invites challenge by attorneys if a situation of concern arises. Nurses must be cognizant of this governance, because the court considers these documents as partial evidence of the standard of care. With continual advances and more efficacious ways of administering these treatments, the sophisticated nurse would be well advised to ensure that institutional policies are kept updated in conformity with state-of-the-art tactics outlined in professional texts and journals. Methodology outlined in the nurse's institutional policy, even though outdated in large measure, will likely prevail over techniques outlined in a recent journal. Job descriptions also delineate nursing practice. Nurses often briefly review the facility's written job description when accepting employment but seldom refer to it thereafter. Nurses should periodically reread the job description to ensure that it matches the current performance of functions on the unit or area. As with other policies, these documents are infrequently upgraded in conformity to changing technologies and practice requisites. When confronted with litigation, the nurse using newer techniques that differ from the written policy or job description could be open to accusation of exceeding practice limits. Another institutional standard affecting oncology nursing practice is that of certification. Nurses may be designated by the employment facility as "chemotherapy certified" on completion of certain didactic content and accompanying skills demonstration. This type of certification carries no distinction outside the facility. It is, however, among the battery of standards that will be used as evidence of the assumed level of nurse competence in a negligence charge. Ensuring that proper documents attesting to institutional certification standards are on file adds a measure of legal security to one's practice.

In *Guzeldere v. Wallin* (1992) the father of an infant who died in the hospital after contracting bronchopneumonia brought a malpractice suit against the doctor, nurses, and hospital. The jury verdict was in favor of the pediatrician, primarily because the nurse did not call the pediatrician concerning the infant's condition even though she should have called and thus given the pediatrician an opportunity to be at the hospital when the infant's condition deteriorated. One of the issues in the trial was whether the nurse should have called the physician and the hospital's policies and procedures were used as evidence at the trial.

> Dr. Wallin had worked with both Nurse Draudt and Nurse Ramirez for many years at La Grange Community Hospital. He trusted them and believed they were experienced and well trained. Dr. Wallin stated that the hospital's policies and procedures did not require that he write orders to nurses asking them to call if patient's condition significantly deteriorated (*Guzeldere* at 635).

THE NURSE IN THE EXPANDED ROLE

EXTENDING NURSING ROLES

Advanced Practice Nurse. A nursing role is profiled through its functions, and expanded nursing practice is an outgrowth of job responsibilities (Chamorro, 1979). Critical care nursing, now sanctioned by certification, is an example of an extension of job responsibilities dictated by need and advancing technology. Generally, the oncology nurse in an expanded role independently assumes some level of patient management in accordance with the medical regimen initiated by a physician, and certain aspects of diagnosis and prescription become a daily part of the nursing practice, particularly in the ambulatory setting where chemotherapy is administered (Chamorro, 1979). M.D. Anderson developed a nurse-run, follow-up clinic for breast cancer patients (Long Term Breast Evaluation Clinic) that exemplifies this trend. The advanced practice nurse in this clinic is responsible for monitoring the x-rays, laboratory tests, and physical body changes, as well as for helping the patients to develop an awareness of her physical and psychosocial patterns (Judkins, 1995). If a problem is detected by the nurse, the nurse orders a series of tests to evaluate and diagnose the abnormality.

In this nurse-managed clinic, the physician has relinquished primary responsibility for the patient's care to the nurse.

In 1993, the ANA Board of Directors defined advanced practice registered nurses as "professional nurses who have successfully completed a graduate program of study in a nursing specialty or related health care field that provides specialized knowledge and skills forming the foundation for expanded practice roles in health care" (American Nurses Association, 1993). The designation APRN is an umbrella term used to refer to a registered nurse who has met advanced educational preparation, usually a masters or doctoral degree, and clinical experience requirements beyond the basic education required of all registered nurses (Heffernan, 1995). In addition to graduate education, NPs often choose to obtain national certification, because 31 states require current certification to practice. Advanced practice registered nurse (APRN) is an umbrella term for nurse practitioners, clinical nurse specialists, certified nurse midwives, and certified registered nurse anesthetists (O'Connor, 1994). In 1995 the Oncology Nursing Society issued a position statement on advanced practice in oncology nursing. ONS endorsed the title "Advanced Practice Nurse to designate clinical nurse specialist (CNS) and nurse practitioner (NP) roles in oncology nursing (Spencer-Cisek, 1995).

Many oncology nurses carry out the activities of assessment, diagnosis, and treatment autonomously without the supervision or support of even a junior physician on the premises. This may be true especially of nurses in research settings undertaking clinical trials (Johnson, 1986). Diagnosis of adverse effects from treatment may be made and medications prescribed by telephone under the general guidelines of the investigational study. In the event of a patient injury and a resulting legal challenge, the question of nursing practice beyond the limits of the state practice act is in the hands of court opinion. Professional support for soundness of the procedure or skill of the individual nurse performing the procedure may be insufficient to influence the court's judgment to the contrary.

Nurse practitioners (NPs) and often other advanced-practice nurses have formal status authorized under special laws by some states and under existing nurse practice acts in other states (Northrop & Kelly, 1987). By 1995, NPs had specific statutory practice authority in 47 states including the District of Columbia and some degree of prescriptive authority in 43 states including the District of Columbia (excluding Alabama, Illinois, and Oklahoma) (Pearson, 1995). Also in 1995, 12 states either added independent prescriptive authority for Advanced Practice Nurses (APN) (where none had existed previously) or passed less restrictive legislative statutes (in APN scope of practice, reimbursement, or prescriptive authority). Additionally, 10 more states have specific plans for 1996 to seek independent APN prescriptive authority (Fig. 83–1) (Pearson, 1995).

Reimbursement for the services of a nurse practitioner using Medicare or Medicaid are addressed by federal legislation. Medicare reimburses for NPs who

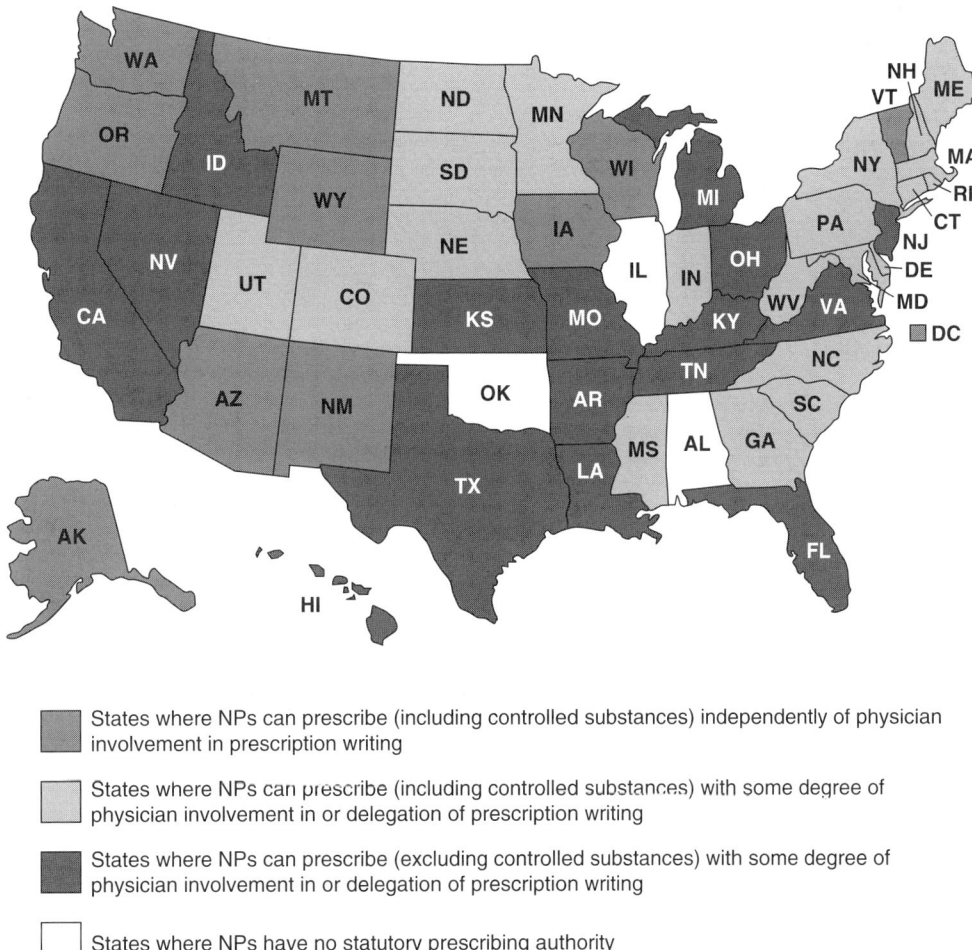

States where NPs can prescribe (including controlled substances) independently of physician involvement in prescription writing

States where NPs can prescribe (including controlled substances) with some degree of physician involvement in or delegation of prescription writing

States where NPs can prescribe (excluding controlled substances) with some degree of physician involvement in or delegation of prescription writing

States where NPs have no statutory prescribing authority

FIGURE 83–1. Nurse practitioner prescriptive privileges. (From Pearson, L. [1995]. Annual update of how each state stands on legislative issues affecting advanced nursing practice. *Nurse Practitioner, 20*[1], 51.)

provide services within their scope of practice, incident to physician services; services under a contract with a health maintenance organization; services in a nursing home; and services in rural areas (Heffernan, 1995). Medicare regulations require that all the services delivered by the NP must be in collaboration with a physician. Medicaid reimbursement differs from that required for Medicare reimbursement. Medicaid directs reimbursement to certified PNPs and NPs, which the advanced practice nurse is legally authorized to perform under state law regardless of whether it is under the supervision of a physician. Advanced practice nurses presently receive Medicaid reimbursement in 49 states. Thirty-nine of these states reimburse at 80 to 100 per cent of a physician's rate, but reimbursement is very limited in 10 of these 39 states (Heffernan, 1995).

Illinois and Washington illustrate the significant differences between states in terms of the legislative legal, prescriptive authority, and reimbursement of the advanced nurse practitioner. In Illinois, there is no specific prescriptive authority within the Illinois Nursing Act of 1987 and the Department of Professional Regulation (Board of Medical Examiners) does not recognize prescriptive authority for nurses. Neither Medicaid

nor Medicare reimbursement has been implemented according to the federal guidelines. The Health Care Financing Administration cited Illinois out of compliance for failing to reimburse NPs providing services to Medicaid clients. Presently in the state of Illinois a debate rages on whether the nursing practice statute, as amended in 1984, allows specialty nurses to diagnosis and prescribe (Heitland, Villarreal, & Rzonca, 1993; Morse & Kane, 1995).

In contrast in the state of Washington, nurses have prescriptive authority and Medicaid reimbursement is available to Advanced Practice Registered Nurses at 100 per cent and Medicare reimbursement following federal guidelines (Pearson, 1995). Furthermore in this state, NPs can prescribe, including controlled substances, independently of physician involvement in prescription writing. In fact if there is a difference in payment between a doctor and a nurse who provide the same services, it must result from the "disparity of fees actually charged by medical doctors and registered nurses rather than from an arbitrary formula based on assumptions concerning the relative worth of doctor-provided services versus nurse-provided services" (WAC 284-44-05) (Pearson, 1995, p. 49).

Safriet (1992) has recommended state statutory changes that are necessary for full advanced practice nursing to exist in a state. These recommendations are:

1. Eliminate references to mixed-regulator entities, and vest regulatory authority solely with the Board of Nursing (BON).
2. Amend the Nurse Practice Act to specifically acknowledge Advanced Practice Nursing (APN) and include a basic definition of APN.
3. Amend the Nurse Practice Act definition of nursing to include APN regulated by the BON with empowerment to the BON to promulgate all regulations for APNs.
4. Eliminate statutory requirements for any APN/MD collaboration, practice agreements, supervision, or direction (Safriet, 1992, p. 478).

Advanced practice nurses in states with statutory language that does not permit independent practice will need to challenge the statute's language to reflect the language recommended by Safriet (Table 83–1). In the past few decades, nursing education has broadened to include practices historically limited to the realm of medicine. It follows that nursing should maintain its own legal jurisdiction over what nurses now educate and practice (Birkholz & Walker, 1994).

Sermchief v. Gonzales (1983) is a case where nurses practicing in an agency that provided family planning and obstetric and gynecologic services were charged with violating the nursing law of the state of Missouri and engaged in the unauthorized practice of medicine. The nurses had received postgraduate special training in the field of obstetrics and gynecology. Everything the nurses did in the clinic (histories, physicals, prescribing medications, etc.) were done pursuant to written standing orders and protocols signed by the physicians. The Supreme Court of Missouri examined the Missouri Nursing Practice Act, the legislative history of the act, and the amendments to the act. They con-

TABLE 83–1. *Statutory Characteristics Necessary for Full APN Independent Prescriptive Authority*

1. The NPA grants the APN plenary prescriptive authority (to administer, prescribe and distribute) including controlled substances on Schedules II through V.
2. The NPA regulates prescriptive practice by the Board Of Nursing (BON) and no other board.
3. There is no language requiring mutual agreement, collaboration, or direction of physicians.
4. If a drug formulary is legislatively necessary, the BON selects the drugs with no joint Board permission required.
5. In BON regulations the NP is the sole name required on the prescription script.
6. The BON has the authority to verify practitioners eligible for Drug Enforcement Agency (DEA) registration.

Federal language for controlled substances can be found in the DEA Mid-level Practitioners Manual.
(From Birkholz, G., & Walker, D. [1994]. Strategies for state statutory language changes granting fully independent nurse practitioner practice. *Nurse Practitioner, 19*[1], 55. Reproduced with permission from the January, 1994 issue of *The Nurse Practitioner,* © Springhouse Corporation.)

cluded that most significant feature of the act was the redefinition of the term "professional nursing." The Sermchief court interpreted the expanded definition of nursing to mean that "a nurse may be permitted to assume responsibilities heretofore not considered to be within the field of professional nursing so long as those responsibilities are consistent with her or his "specialized education, judgment and skill" (*Sermchief* at 689). The Court believes that it is significant that while at least forty states have modernized and expanded their nursing practice laws during the past fifteen years neither counsel nor the Court have discovered any case challenging nurses' authority to act as the nurses herein acted (*Sermchief* at 690).

The court found that the nurses' acts were authorized by the Missouri Nursing Practice Act and did not constitute the unlawful practice of medicine.

Malpractice claims related to nurses in advanced practice are presently extremely low. But with the current climate of health care and litigation, malpractice insurance premiums for nurses in advanced practice are climbing steadily (Smrcina, 1993). There is a national computer data bank that tracks health care providers' malpractice payments by insurers and adverse actions by licensing boards, hospitals, or professional societies since September 1, 1990 (Birkholz, 1995). The National Practitioner Data Bank (NPDB) must be checked by any hospital initially granting clinical privileges and every 2 years thereafter.

The NPDB shows that nurses had less than 3 per cent of the reported malpractice payments, whereas physicians had more than 97 per cent from September 1990 to February 1992 and March 1992 to July 1993. In fact, registered nurses had more reports than advanced practice nurses in both time periods (Birkholz, 1995). However, Birkholz makes the point that malpractice reports of RNs and APNs may be underreported due to "targeting deep pockets, lack of a duty for insurers to report payment on identifiable but unnamed health care providers, and possible confusion on including nurses in reports when nursing licensing boards are not required to report" (1995, p. 34).

A 1994 survey of the malpractice experiences of the readership of *The Nurse Practitioner* had 25 NPs report that there were 29 claims against them; 21 of the claims were brought since 1986 (Pearson & Birkholz, 1995). Twenty-three of the 26 claims (three claims were second claims against the same NP) divide into two main alleged claims: failure to properly diagnose and negligent treatment. The majority of claims were failure to properly diagnose, and most were not reported to the NPDB because either the NP was dropped from the suit or the case was settled before the data bank required reporting. Table 83–2 shows the advice that these 25 NPs gave to other advanced practice nurses to prevent being sued. One important point brought up by these NPs was to be certain that the physicians with whom you consult or to whom you refer patients are excellent clinicians (Pearson & Birkholz, 1995). This is especially important today since the "captain of the ship" doctrine is no longer a legal reality.

TABLE 83–2. *Physician and Nurse Responsibilities in Informed Consent*

PHYSICIAN RESPONSIBILITIES	NURSE RESPONSIBILITIES
Determining whether the patient (or appropriate decision maker) is competent and able to understand the explanation fully enough to make an informed choice	Clarifying the physician's explanations
	Providing additional information, especially on the management of side effects
Explaining the protocol to the patient and significant others without using force, deceit, fraud, or constraint, while emphasizing voluntary participation	Answering the patient's and significant others' questions and notifying the doctor of questions that the nurse cannot answer
Describing conventional treatment options that might be beneficial	Helping the patient and significant others explore their feelings with respect to the impact that the various risks and benefits may have on their lives
Explaining the risks and benefits of the various treatment options	Signing the consent form as a witness (if requested)
Answering the patient's and significant others' questions and obtaining the patient's (or surrogate decision maker's) signature on the consent form	Reassessing the patient's willingness to participate in the research protocol (immediately before administering the treatment) and notifying the doctor if the patient expresses uncertainty
Countersigning the consent form	
Monitoring the patient's willingness to continue participating in the protocol as the patient proceeds through the program	Providing ongoing support to the patient and significant others, and reassuring them that the patient can withdraw from the study at any time without compromising his or her care

(From Winters, G., Glass, E., & Sakurai, C. [1993]. Ethical issues in oncology nursing practice: An overview of topics and strategies. *Oncology Nursing Forum, 20* [Suppl. 10], p. 28.)

The "captain of the ship" phrase was first used by the Pennsylvania Supreme Court in a medical malpractice and refers to admirality law, under which the master of a vessel is in total command of the crew and the ship and is liable for the acts of the crew (Heitland et al., 1993). The physician in the operating room or in control of hospital personnel was liable for the negligence of the other personnel. This concept has been universally rejected (Heitland et al., 1993). The clinical implications of the loss of this legal concept is that the nurse in the expanded role cannot shift all the responsibility for alleged malpractice onto the physician if the patient sustains an injury connected to the nurse's care provider encounter.

Nurses as Case Managers. With the changes in the delivery of health care in the United States, many nurses are being reassigned to case management positions within the hospital. Case management is relatively new as a cost-containment/utilization review tool. St. Paul, the nation's largest medical liability insurance company, has developed a Case Management Liability Coverage policy. To receive coverage, the individual must have a valid nursing or professional license or national certification in a health or human services profession and at least 1 year of case manager experience and/or 4 years of clinical experience in the medical profession (Hinden, 1994).

The liability issues that are emerging with this new expanded role include (1) negligent referral (Hyatt, 1994), (2) liability surrounding experimental treatment and technology, (3) liability surrounding sensitive information and confidentiality, (4) fraud and abuse involving the use of improper financial incentives to direct referrals for needed services to a particular provider or the furnishing of services of poor quality or other conduct that is fraudulent, unethical, wasteful, or improper (Sollins, 1994).

A case that exemplifies a negligent referral is *Siklas v. Ecker* (1993). In this case it was alleged that the plaintiff patient's case manager had negligently placed him with a dangerously psychotic roommate, who was also a patient of the institution. The appellate court held that the mental health center that employed the case manager had a duty to exercise reasonable care in performing services which made up its undertaking on behalf of the patient and sent the case back to the trial court.

Of particular importance to oncology nurses who assume case management positions is the recent California case of *Fox v. Health Net* (Wynstra, 1994). In this case, the patient was denied coverage of a bone marrow transplant for breast cancer. A multimillion dollar ($89.1 million) jury award was given to the patient's survivors. The lawyer for the patient argued that Health Net refused to pay for the treatment to save money and that company executives received financial incentives and bonuses when they refused to authorize expensive treatments.

Saue (1994) cites the following legal risks that commonly arise in connection with reviewing this kind of treatment or technology:

1. Failure to apply the contractual definition of "experimental" treatment found in the patient's insurance policy.
2. Failure to review the sources of information referenced in the applicable insurance policy.
3. Failure to review the patient's complete medical records.
4. Failure to make a timely determination of coverage.
5. Failure to accurately convey the coverage determination to the insured or participant.
6. Improper economic consideration influencing the coverage determination (p. 106).

There are several risk-reduction behaviors that are recommended for requests from oncology patients that can be considered experimental. Case managers are urged to check the contractual definition of "experimental" before reviewing the patient's request. They are also urged to solicit and review all relevant information including medical records, expert opinions cited by the patient, opinions of independent medical experts, and information referenced in the patient's insurance policy. Case managers should adjudicate the request in a *timely manner, document everything* that has constituted the adjudication, and *promptly inform the patient* of the coverage determination.

COLLABORATIVE PRACTICE

Opportunity for the highest level of professional independence is offered to the nurse in collaborative practice with an oncologist in an office or clinic. The practice departs significantly from that of the staff nurse in that the nurse assumes considerable autonomy in decision making (Chamorro, 1979). Many nurses in this role may be prepared at the master's degree level as clinical specialists or nurse practitioners and possess considerable nursing skills in diagnosing or determining the importance of certain patient symptoms.

It is wise to base any collaborative practice on a collection of standing orders, standardized procedures, or protocols. The specific job description and responsibilities should be drafted, along with educational and specialty certification. The documents should demonstrate that any state statutory requirements have been met but need not be limited to the minimal requirements. Such a documentary packet proves that the nurse is serious in asserting professional status and the full accountability that goes with it.

LIABILITY ISSUES IN CANCER NURSING

LIABILITY IN GENERAL

The nurse needs to be aware that there are multiple theories of liability that can be applied in a malpractice case against the nurse when the nurse is employed by the hospital, institution, or some other entity. First the hospital may be liable based on the *principal-agency* relationship between the hospital (Weaver, 1992). This is called contract liability. The courts will look at whether there is actual authority granted by the hospital to the nurse; is there a formal contract, formal arrangement, or was the relationship terminated prior to the injury?

If there is not actual authority, is there apparent authority arising from the hospital's holding out of the nurse as the hospital's agent to patients. In this situation, the court will ask if the hospital "held out" the nurse in such a manner that it induced the patient to believe that the nurse was an agent of the hospital. Some of the questions the courts will ask are the following. (1) Was the reliance by the patient reasonable?

(2) Did something happen that terminated the nurse's employment with the hospital, and were patients given notice? (3) Did the hospital place the nurse in a position that has customary responsibilities that would lead the public to believe the nurse had authority from the hospital? Apparent authority differs from actual authority in that apparent authority arises out of the reasonable belief of third parties (the patient), whereas actual authority arises out of reasonable beliefs of the agent (the nurse).

If there is not actual or apparent authority, was there ratification by the hospital after the unauthorized act of the nurse, thus making the hospital liable for the act of the nurse? The courts will look to see whether the hospital knew all the material facts at the point of ratification and whether the hospital ratified the entire transaction (Agency, 1995).

If there is not contract liability, the courts will look to see whether there is tort liability under the doctrine of respondeat superior. For there to be liability under the doctrine of respondeat superior, there must be an employer-employee relationship, and the wrongful conduct must be within the nurse's scope of employment. The hospital is not generally liable for the wrongful acts of independent contractors. The courts will first investigate whether the nurse was an employee or an independent agent. Some questions the courts will ask are the following. (1) Was the wrongful act intentional? (2) Was it criminal? (3) Was there fraud?

Vicarious liability accrues when the legal relationship between two individuals is governed by the rules of respondeat superior.

> The generally accepted rule is that, where an employment relationship exists between the physician [or nurse] and the hospital, the hospital will be liable, under the traditional rule of respondeat superior, for any negligence or malpractice which results in injury to a hospital patient. Conversely, no liability attaches to the hospital when the physician [or nurse] is an independent contractor (*Jackson v. Power*, 743 P.2d 1376 Supreme Court of Alaska, 1987).

Courts have shown a strong trend toward liability against hospitals that permit or encourage patients to believe that independent contractor/physicians are, in fact, authorized agents of the hospitals. The courts have held such hospitals vicariously liable under a doctrine labeled either "ostensible" or "apparent" agency or "agency by estoppel."

Pace v. Hazel Towers, Inc. (1992) is a case that illustrates the concept of vicarious liability. In *Pace* the patient brought suit for the alleged injury received from the nurse's negligent injection of medicine into the patient's right arm. The *Pace* court opined that the hospital was vicariously liable for the nurse's alleged negligence and thus could be sued even when the claim against the nurse was withdrawn. Not all states follow the vicarious liability theory. For instance, Illinois courts require actual negligence on the part of the surgeon/specialist and allow the surgeon/specialist to be found vicariously liable only under the traditional respondeat superior theory, that is, where the negligence alleged is attributable to one in the actual employ of the physician (Plaintiff's Medical Malpractice Litigation, 1986).

In contrast, *McDaniel v. Sage* (1981) is a case illustrating an attempt to base liability on the agency theory. In *McDaniel*, a company employee brought action against a nurse and a doctor who were also company employees, alleging the nurse negligently administered an injection prescribed by the doctor, who the employee claimed was also liable on an agency theory. The court held that as a licensed registered nurse, Watters, the nurse in the case, was engaged in an "independent profession" (*McDaniel* at 1325). The court acknowledged that while the nurse was a salaried employee of the company, the company did not control her placement of the injection. Rather Watters relied on her training, experience, and skill of a professional, licensed registered nurse to determine the placement of the injection. Thus the court reasoned Watters acted as an independent contractor and was not an agent of the doctor when she administered the injection to the employee. An agency relationship can exist only if the agent is subject to the principal's control with respect to work details. This ruling by the *McDaniel* court enabled the injured patient to sue the nurse directly.

In *Williams v. St. Claire Medical Center* (1983) the nurse anesthetist was an independent contractor, but the court opined that since the hospital gave the patient the impression the nurse anesthetist was an employee of the hospital, the doctrine of apparent authority applies and the hospital is vicariously liable. The patient suffered permanent brain damage when he was anesthetized by a nurse who was not a certified registered nurse anesthetist at the time of the incident causing the injury. The nurse was not an employee of the hospital but rather was employed by a professional service corporation that supplied nurse anesthetists to the hospital. However, since the "patient justifiably believed nurse to be hospital employee, and hospital took no action to give patient notice otherwise, thus creating apparent agency" (*Williams* at 591).

As *Pace* (1992), *McDaniel* (1981), and *Williams* (1983) illustrate, practicing nurses need to be aware of the liability doctrine(s) recognized in the state in which they practice.

FAILURES IN COMMUNICATION

DETECTION OF DISEASE

Beyond the legal establishment of dimensions of practice, competence, and standards of care in cancer nursing, there are other relevant issues that impose a legal burden on the nurse. These are potential liability issues suggested by the needs and rights of patients with cancer in the continuum from diagnosis to the terminal phase. At the center of much health care litigation are failures in communication. If test results indicating a cancer diagnosis or recurrence are not communicated to appropriate persons and cause a delay in treatment, charges of negligence may be brought. Professional nurses in office settings are frequently the first line of contact with patients and their presenting symptoms. They are responsible for gathering test data or receiving calls from patients, which may require triage or referral. Staff nurses also bear a similar responsibility. Sound professional judgment is called for in determining abnormal laboratory and diagnostic results or interpreting symptoms reported by the patient.

Overlooking important data or misjudging the severity of patient complaints that require immediate physician attention may carry serious legal consequences for nurses, particularly nurses in advanced practice roles. The value of delayed or missed opportunity for treatment has been contested in several cancer cases (delayed diagnosis is also referred to as "lost chance for cure or of a longer period of disease-free survival") (*Savelle v. Heilbrunn*, 1989). The physician Insurers Association of America's 1990 breast cancer study of 273 paid claims by 21 companies found that women younger than age 50 represented 69 per cent of the patients who sued physicians for delay in diagnosis of breast cancer (Osuch & Bonham, 1994). Other studies report the same trends. Although women younger than 40 years of age make up only about 7 per cent of those with breast cancer, they comprise 39 to 52 per cent of published series of patients suing for delayed diagnosis. Advanced practice nurses need to remember that in terms of actual numbers, in 1993, there were 12,810 women younger than 40 and 45,750 women younger than 50 diagnosed with breast cancer (Osuch & Bonham, 1994). It is important for advanced practice nurses in family settings to know that many of these women presented with symptoms during periods of pregnancy and lactation, when diagnosis of breast cancer is difficult. Another factor that may account for the large percentage of younger women who are suing for delayed diagnosis is that diagnosis of breast cancer can be difficult, particularly in young women with dense breasts.

Risk management strategies for nurses in primary care settings or in advanced practice include (1) a tracking system of outstanding test results and recommended follow-up visits so that patients are not "lost," (2) communication between providers when a referral is initiated, (3) a meticulous medical record keeping system and documentation, (4) follow-up of all breast complaints to resolution and familiarity with the absolute and relative indications for referral of breast complaints, and (5) the communication of abnormal findings to the patient in a timely manner that is both oral and written (Gargaro, 1981, 1982).

The question of evaluating prospects for cure had earlier diagnosis allowed timely initiation of treatment is a difficult issue for the courts. One approach that is used is to have an oncology expert present the nature and the progression of the disease cancer. In *Chudson v. Ratra* (1988) the physician was sued for negligently failing to timely diagnose breast cancer in a 36-year-old woman. To bolster the argument that earlier detection would have made a difference, the plaintiff had an expert describe each of the four stages of breast cancer and the biology of the cancer cell. In *Chudson*, while the court found that the physician had failed to timely diagnose and treat breast cancer, the patient's delay in seeking further medical treatment at a time when there was a better-than-even chance that the cancer could have been cured was contributory negligence on the patient's part.

DISCLOSURE AND INFORMED DECISIONS

Cancer carries such negative connotations that family members frequently enjoin the medical or nursing staff to conceal the diagnosis from the patient. A conspiracy of silence may ensue, even though disclosure is desired by patients as well as mandated by law. Oncology nurses report being placed in this position especially when the patient is non-English-speaking and cultural overtones prevail. A conspiracy of silence is an ethical issue but becomes a legal issue under the doctrine of informed consent. This guarantees competent patients the right to receive sufficient information to make intelligent decisions about their care (Northrop & Kelly, 1987). The law requires that patients be told about risks of proposed treatment and additional options or alternative forms of treatment. There are situations when consent is not necessary because it is "implied" or is compulsory (Wallace, 1991). In medical emergencies, consent is implied by law using the legal fiction that patients would consent to life-saving or limb-saving treatment if they were able to consent. "A patient who has made an informed, competent refusal cannot later be treated pursuant to the emergency privilege simply because the patient later lapses into incompetence" (Gregory, 1992, p. 590).

How much disclosure is required and whether the nurse as well as the treating physician has a duty to disclose are two important considerations. Extreme positions have been taken by courts across the United States regarding the scope of disclosure. The majority approach taken by courts of this country requires a physician to disclose information to patients to the same extent that other physicians, practicing the same specialty if applicable, in the same or similar community, in the same or similar circumstances, would disclose. This "professional" standard is consistent with the negligence standard generally applicable to medical and other professional malpractice (Merz, 1993). The overwhelming majority of the states have held that failure to secure informed consent properly is negligence. There are two states that characterize the lack of an informed consent as battery. The minority approach, "prudent patient" approach, allows the judge or jury in a case to determine whether particular information would be "material" to the reasonable person in the patient's position, therefore requiring disclosure (Merz, 1993).

The point has been made that consent is a process that is ongoing between the patient and health care providers. Both parties in the process must actively participate. The emphasis of informed consent should be communication, not the form used to obtain the written consent.

The "informed consent" precept has now been extended to include what the court calls "informed refusal," in which the client is to be informed of risks or consequences inherent in refusing treatment or diagnostic tests. When cancer is in question, it is important for the oncology nurse to be knowledgeable of potentially adverse outcomes for the patient who refuses a diagnostic test or treatment.

The World Medical Assembly in 1978 proposed five points as of central importance in obtaining consent from a patient to medical intervention.

1. There should be explanation of the proposed treatment.
2. The risks and benefits of treatment should be clearly detailed.
3. Any alternatives to treatment should be included in the presentation.
4. There should be adequate time for patient questions.
5. Patients should be aware of the option to withdraw (McGrath, 1995, p. 97–98).

McGrath (1995) writes that because the prevailing philosophy of medicine centers around the concept of the "technological imperative," support for the patient who refuses treatment runs counter to the prevailing medical milieu.

To date, the clinician in charge of the treatment has been held responsible for obtaining informed consent. The legal duty to obtain full consent rests on the treating physician, not the hospital. When nurses, because of their knowledge and expertise, possess information that can improve a patient's ability to make rational decisions regarding treatment, the obligations of the nurse-patient relationship generally demand that the information be transmitted either directly by the nurse or by the physician through the nurse (Gargaro, 1978). A documented notation in the patient record regarding the nurse's assessment and advisement in informed consent or refusal is an important safeguard of the nurse. See Table 83–2 for the physician and nurse responsibilities in informed consent.

Clearly, the oncology nurse must not support any misrepresentation of a procedure or treatment. In controversies, the nurse should first discuss the problem with the physician. If it is not resolved, the nursing supervisor should be notified or, finally, the matter brought to the attention of the patient, who may further pursue it.

One issue that is brought up in any discussion of informed consent and consent forms is the readability of the forms (Grossman, Piantadosi, & Covahey, 1994; Meade & Howser, 1992). Currently, approximately 20 per cent of Americans have an estimated reading ability below fifth-grade level. Another way to look at this issue is that about one of five adult Americans is functionally illiterate and lacks the reading and writing skills necessary to deal with routine daily activities (Meade & Howser, 1992). Two recent studies of consent forms found that the majority were at grade levels that would have prevented a substantial number of patients from understanding what they were signing. Meade and Howser (1992) looked at 44 consent forms from the Medicine Branch and Clinical

Pharmacology Branch at the National Cancer Institute and report that mean estimate of consent form reading level was grade 14.3, which is considered to be a professional reading level. Grossman et al. (1994) assessed the readability of 137 consent forms from eight clinical oncology protocols. They report that readability was at or below an eighth-grade level in 6 per cent of the consent forms. Nurses involved in helping to obtain informed consent need to be aware of the difficulty patients may have reading the material if it is at a reading level beyond their educational ability. Consent forms need to be evaluated using readability formulas and forms that are beyond the fifth-grade reading level changed.

Encouraging informed decision making about treatment or care is part of the rationale for providing patient education. Oncology nurses have a special obligation to teach patients at the time of discharge to minimize any potential for injury when the patient assumes self-care. The merits of patient education as a quality assurance issue are well understood, and the legal foundation for patient teaching has been established as well by court opinion as early as 1944 (Creighton, 1985). Some believe that negligence in discharge instruction and health teaching will increase liability as nurses become legally accountable in more situations (Ficsta, 1983). Patient education, especially discharge teaching, should be documented in the medical record. In disputed testimony, reference to the written note overrides mere verbal confirmation.

CONSENT FOR INVESTIGATIONAL STUDIES

Liability may be imposed when the nurse dispenses investigational or experimental drugs without ensuring that the hospital's procedure regarding protection of human subjects has been followed (Fiesta, 1983). The facility's institutional review board will approve an informed consent document relating to the specific clinical trial. A copy of this document bearing the patient's signature along with that of a witness should be in the medical record for verification by clinicians administering the treatment.

CONFIDENTIALITY

MEDICAL RECORD DISCLOSURE

Confidentiality about the facts of a patient's case is a mandate well understood by most nurses in practice. Sensitivity issues associated with a diagnosis of cancer or acquired immune deficiency syndrome (AIDS) render a violation of confidence particularly grave. One frequently finds that patients prefer to keep a cancer diagnosis secret even from significant persons in their lives. This request should be documented in the record and other members of the health team informed of the wishes. Such wishes must be honored to the limits feasible. Charges may be brought by patients and family against the indiscreet oncology nurse who shares this information inappropriately with a third party or to satisfy public curiosity. The law interprets this invasion as public disclosure of private facts (Fiesta, 1983).

Nurses who are functioning as case managers should refrain from giving assurances to the patient that the information would be kept confidential. "Any such assurance . . . could be construed as a contract with the patient that the information would be kept confidential" (Scheutzow, 1994, p. 109). The nurse could be subject to a breach of contract action if the information is released to other health care providers.

DIRECTIVES IN HEALTH CARE

Congress passed the "Patient Self-Determination Act of 1990" as an amendment to OBRA 1990 (Wallace, 1991). This act placed the burden upon institutions at the time of admission to a facility, to ensure that patients are aware of their rights to consent to or to refuse treatment, primarily in the terminal care setting, and to assure them that, when they wish to specify their choices, those choices will be implemented (Gregory, 1992). This information must be provided at the time of admission to a hospital or nursing home, at the time of enrollment in an HMO, prior to the initiation of care by a home care or personal care provider, or at the onset of hospice care. The act sets forth new requirements for health care providers regarding advance directives, such as living wills and health care powers of attorney. An advanced directive is a statement made by a competent person that directs his or her medical care in the event that he or she becomes incompetent (Dimond, 1992).

The American Nurses Association's Code of Ethics urges nurses in their role as patient advocates to support patients in their self-determination and decision making. The ANA views nurses as critical to the implementation of the Patient Self-Determination Act. It is recommended that nurses include questions regarding advanced directives as part of their initial assessment of the patient. In cases where advance directives are already part of a patient's medical record, the responsible staff nurse, nurse practitioner, or other health care professional periodically should review these documents and verify their validity (Gobis, 1992).

With the recent national emphasis on patient autonomy, health care professionals who oppose or contradict valid advanced directives may be sued for negligence or battery.

WILLS

At times, nurses involved with patients experiencing progressive disease may likely encounter a request to draw up or witness a will. The nurse-patient relationship places a nurse in a good position to act as witness because of knowledge about the patient's physical and mental capacity at the time of the signing. If not a beneficiary, the nurse may witness a will but also has the equal right to refuse such a position without penalty. It is inappropriate, however, for the nurse to take part in drawing up a will, because this may constitute the practice of law. The nurse may work through the facility's legal department to obtain legal assistance for the patient in constructing such a document (Northrop & Kelley, 1987).

Living Wills

The passage of so-called "right to die" laws allows competent persons in terminal illness to refuse the use of extreme life-sustaining procedures to remain alive. The purpose of a living will is to provide direction to caregivers and to promote dialogue among patients, family members, and the health care team (Dimond, 1992). Several landmark cases have debated this issue. As a consequence, many states recognize a document known as a "living will," requesting the withholding or discontinuance of artificial measures when the patient's lack of physical or mental competence prevents the specific expression of these wishes. A living will may have been executed at an earlier date, or some patients may request assistance in preparing one when disease progression is noted. It is the nurse's legal responsibility to bring a prepared living will to the attention of the attending physician and other health care personnel. Any nurse assisting a patient in preparing or witnessing a will needs some knowledge of statutory requirements of the particular jurisdiction involved (Bernzweig, 1987). Generally, the living will cannot take force until the patient has been examined and certified in writing by two physicians (one of whom is to be the attending physician) as to the terminal condition. Documentation of the patient's desires in these matters and any prepared living will should be prominent in the medical record.

Orders Not to Resuscitate

"Do not resuscitate" (DNR) orders should not be confused with measures designed to sustain life. The use of artificial means of nutrition and hydration or measures to improve ventilation or cardiac function in the absence of a respiratory or cardiac arrest qualify as life-sustaining measure, not resuscitative measures (Meehan, 1991).

DNR orders may be instituted based on a patient's expressed wishes even if they are not backed by a signed document. The physician must write the order and record a brief note regarding the circumstances. Under common law, a physician has the duty to preserve his or her patient's life by appropriate means. Under certain circumstances a negligence suit could be filed if the physician fails to provide life-saving means to the patient. Since 1988 all facilities that are accredited by the Joint Commission on the Accreditation of Healthcare Organizations (JCAHO) must have a policy concerning the withholding of resuscitative services.

Problems frequently develop when the patient is incompetent and not able to indicate his or her wishes. In these cases the health care professionals should look to either an advance directive or to a legally appointed guardian to obtain a court order for proper consent (Meehan, 1991). In circumstances where the patient is incompetent, the courts have stipulated that another person, usually a close family member, can substitute his or her judgment for that of the patient who is unable to consent.

Most health care facilities recognize consent by next of kin when a patient is determined to be incompetent. The determination of incompetence should be determined and well documented. *Payne v. Marion General Hospital* (1990) is an example of what happens when the incompetence of the patient is not formally determined and documented. In *Payne*, the sister of the patient requested a DNR order, and the physician went along with this but did not determine the competence of the patient. At that time, the patient was competent. When the patient had a cardiac arrest, no CPR was performed. The patient's estate sued the physician and the hospital for malpractice. The Appellate Court held that the hospital was not liable, but the case against the physician could go back to the trial court to determine whether the patient was incompetent at the time the DNR order was entered.

A frequent omission in caring for the patient is the failure to obtain the written order when circumstances dictate. An exception exists in facilities whose written policy allows the physician's telephone order to be enforced for a brief period until arrival on the premises to make written notation in the medical record. Under these specially defined conditions, the nurse accepting the verbal orders must execute care that the order is given directly by the physician, not his agent or other inappropriate individual. Failure to initiate resuscitation on the terminal patient without the written order may put the nurse in the legal position of practicing medicine without a license (Fiesta, 1983). Evaluating the patient and his or her desires regarding life-sustaining measures and preparing for the moment of death with appropriately written orders should be part of care planning by the professional nurse.

Durable Power of Attorney

The living will honors the patient's wishes in a serious illness but is limited in meeting all medical contingencies that may occur if the patient becomes incapacitated or incompetent. Forty-six states and the District of Columbia have enacted Durable Power of Attorney legislation for health care (Dimond, 1992). A competent person may give a specified individual the durable power to act as his or her agent in medical decision making in the event he or she becomes incompetent to act in his or her own behalf. It is recommended that the appointed agent should not have a conflict of interest with the patient; thus, nurses and physicians are not appropriate choices for this role. These decisions extend beyond life-sustaining procedures to include the power to select treatments, seek other therapeutic opinions and options, and remove physicians from the case (Bernzweig, 1987). The nurse is unlikely to become involved in the actual directives of the power of attorney but must understand that it is an acceptable legal mechanism in some jurisdictions. Health care workers are protected from liability when relying on this authority.

NEGLIGENCE IN CARE

ADVERSE OUTCOMES OF TREATMENT

Some oncology nurses have questioned whether liability exists if there is an adverse outcome of treatment that is otherwise expected to bring about a positive result. Battery can be claimed when medical treatment is performed without lawful authority or patient consent. The charge has no merit unless, as in the circumstances of "conspiracy of silence," the patient's implied consent does not even exist. A patient's severity of treatment side effects will not have legal consequence for any nurse, per severity, unless negligence is charged because a nurse breaches the duty of care. In negligence, the plaintiff has several conditions to prove. If injury occurs because a nurse failed to enact the usual and customary set of actions consistent with the circumstance at hand, it could be proved that duty was breached. It must be clearly established, however, that the injury was a direct result of the deviation from duty.

MEDICATION ERRORS

Medication injuries are frequently the cause of litigation. It is estimated that one out of every seven medication orders in hospitals is erroneously carried out (Bernzweig, 1987). One review of litigious actions against oncology nurses showed that administration of chemotherapy or narcotics to the wrong patient, in incorrect doses, or through the wrong route, or extravasation that caused tissue damage constituted 75 per cent of the cases (Schulmeister, 1987). Administering medications is considered the most potentially hazardous therapeutic activity nurses perform (Fiesta, 1983). Particular care must be taken in administering chemotherapeutic agents because of their toxic effect. Double- and triple-checking of patient identification physician orders, drug name, dose, and route cannot be overemphasized. Legal charges may be initiated, especially when a patient experiences life-threatening toxicities from administration of the wrong drug. In extravasation injuries, negligence may be proved if it is shown that the nurse failed to take due care in administering the drug or proper measures when infiltration of the vesicant was discovered. Aside from the pain and suffering associated with the injury, there may be a delay in reinstituting chemotherapy, leaving the nurse open to charges that the patient ostensibly is deprived of therapeutic benefit during postponement. Extravasation of drug is sometimes an unfortunate occurrence even with the nurse's impeccable technique (Lind & Bush, 1987).

In the event of an extravasation or an error in chemotherapy administration, immediate reporting and documentation of the event and the condition of the patient, following the facility's policy, become the immediate legal responsibilities of the nurse. Demonstration of a caring attitude to the patient is simply quality nursing care, but additionally it is often a successful strategy in the management of potentially litigious situations. Full disclosure of the event to appropriate supervisory persons and filing of an incident report in conformity with prescribed policy are also important tactics. Failure to do so may substantiate the court's opinion of negligence.

Several recent incidents have focused national attention on nurses negligently administering incorrect amounts of chemotherapy to patients, which resulted in the patient's death (Altman, 1995). As mentioned in Chapter 1, a young women at Dana-Farber Cancer Institute in Boston was given four times the intended dose of Cytoxan for several days. At least a dozen physicians, nurses, and pharmacists counter-signed the order for the Cytoxan including some of the institution's senior staff. The physicians continued to pursue the Cytoxan treatment despite "her warnings that something was drastically wrong" and in the face of tests that indicated heart damage. Incidents such as this point out the importance of the nurse knowing exactly what they are administering, the usual dosages, and any other pertinent information. Certification in the administration of chemotherapy may offer some protection for the nurse in terms of arguing that the institution and nurse followed the national standard of care in terms of having only certified nurses administer chemotherapy.

Several cases that resulted in costly settlements are illustrative of how the courts view the incorrect administration of chemotherapy drugs. In a Virginia case, *Lynwood V. Shaw v. Richmond Memorial Hospital* (1991), the patient was awarded $200,000 when intravenous chemotherapy infiltrated his hand (Medical Malpractice Verdicts, Settlements & Experts, 1991). The infiltration resulted in multiple surgeries and treatments and, ultimately, an above-the-elbow amputation. In Michigan, a settlement of $475,000 was awarded to a 63-year-old female patient who had received chemotherapy that infiltrated. The patient's chemotherapy infiltrated and caused chemical burns to tendons and necrosis of tissue, which resulted in multiple plastic surgeries, severe abdominal scarring, and disfigurement on the left forearm and both legs. The case, *Mary and Willie Latham v. Southwest Detroit Hospital and Jane Doe* (1991), points out the importance of continually checking the IV site, telephone follow-up of all patients who have experienced an extravasation, and documentation of follow-up.

> The plaintiff alleged that the . . . nurse was negligent in allowing the needle to go subcutaneous and that the hospital was negligent in failing to properly treat her hand after the incident. The defendants contended that the nurse checked for good blood flow before administering the chemicals and the plaintiff reached for a telephone during the administration of the drugs, causing the needle to go subcutaneous. . . The nurse had instructed the plaintiff to treat the hand by soaking it in hot water. The plaintiff attempted that treatment for six days and failed to seek medical care as the condition worsened (Medical Malpractice Verdicts, Settlements & Experts, 1991).

Nurses can also be held accountable for failure to medicate and control pain. The case that illustrates this point is *Administration of the Estate of Henry James v. Millhaven Corporation et al* (Cushing, 1992). This case involves a nurse making the assessment that Mr. James was addicted to morphine and then instituting her own "pain management" plan that included withholding opioid analgesics, substituting a placebo for pain medications, and substituting a mild tranquilizer for the prescribed opioid medication.

> When Mr. James was admitted, an employee nurse assessed him as being "addicted to morphine," and on that basis alone instituted a "pain management" plan without the advice, consent, or orders of a physician. Her plan was to minimize the use of pain medication, substitute a mild tranquilizer, and delay or withhold the administration of an analgesic. The patient's personal physician had prescribed Roxanol (Roxame Laboratories, Columbus, Ohio) in the dosage of 7.5 cc Roxanol every 3 hr as needed for pain. During the trial, the jury heard that this nurse withheld opioid analgesics and also substituted a placebo for pain medications (Angarola, 1991, p. 407).

Mr. James had cancer of the prostate with metastasis to the left femur as well as to the lumbosacral spine. At trial, Mr. James's family proved that the failure of the nurse and her employer to meet their responsibility caused the patient to experience increased pain and suffering, as well as "emotional and mental anguish." The North Carolina jury awarded $15 million in damages to the family of Mr. James. Later the $15 million jury verdict was resolved by an undisclosed settlement between the parties. The award documents the serious consequences of not providing appropriate pain control or following the "standard and accepted practice in the treatment of intractable pain" (Cushing, 1992, p. 22).

REPORTING PATIENT'S CONDITION

Failure to communicate the patient's condition to the physician is another breach of duty resulting in nurse liability. Management of specified patient complaints, a major component in oncology nursing, is especially common in office or clinic nursing. Advice about a symptom is given to the patient via telephone and then frequently dismissed from the nurse's mind in the busy office setting. Telephone instructions given to patients should be noted in the medical chart, no matter how minor the complaint. Astute nursing judgment is required to determine the significance of any complaint. For instance, a complaint of persistent nausea 1 week following chemotherapy may not be drug-induced but may imply impending bowel obstruction. Failure to communicate essential data to the physician may result in delay in treatment and patient harm, leaving both physician and nurse liable.

ENACTING PROFESSIONAL JUDGMENT

Professional judgment is an obscure concept difficult to define out of specific context. Clinical judgment by a nurse is the outcome derived from the process of collecting and analyzing data about the patient for the purpose of determining nursing needs. Careful examination of most potentially litigious situations reveals frequent omissions or lack of competent judgment rather than commissions or errors in judgment. Professional judgment is demanded at every juncture of practice. Sound problem identification and reaffirmation of the desired outcomes for the patient are fundamental to professional nursing practice. The evidence of planned care for the patient is the stalwart providing the best defense against potential error and liability exposure.

SUPERVISION

There is confusion among nurses about liability exposure when the professional nurse supervises nurse aides, vocational or practical nurses, or other registered nurses involved in direct patient care. The rule is that if the supervising nurse assigns duties to an otherwise competent nurse in conformity to his or her training and experience, the supervisor cannot be held liable for the subordinate's negligence. However, liability for negligence in supervision can be charged if the supervising nurse fails to determine the patient's needs adequately or fails to give closer personal attention to a subordinate who demonstrates need for such supervision (Bernzweig, 1987). The complexity of care required by patients with cancer may necessitate closer surveillance by supervising nurses than in other patient situations. There is special concern about liability exposure should harm come to a patient when the oncology nurse is supervising students. The instructing nurse must take care to assign only tasks clearly within the student's capabilities or provide the extra measure of supervision and direction required of the situation. Orientation of new staff to the care of cancer patients is another area of concern in supervision. Orientation should be well planned and backed by documentation of completion of each new experience. Orienting to chemotherapy administration is an area requiring particularly close attention so that exposure is diminished for both preceptor and orientee. Consequently, there have been a number of institutional programs in chemotherapy certification established.

DEFENSIVE STRATEGIES FOR ONCOLOGY NURSES

CLINICAL COMPETENCE SETTING THE STANDARDS

Superior expertise in oncology nursing will diminish the likelihood of a malpractice claim against a nurse; however, real risk prevention is achieved by careful thought and a well-planned program. Many of the legal responsibilities a nurse may incur in the oncology setting have been previously defined and discussed. It is possible for the nurse to construct strategies that will improve the potential of remaining free from litigation during a professional career. In-depth knowledge of the standards of care is, perhaps, the prime defensive measure of all. The oncology nurse today has the advantages of journals and texts detailing guidelines for virtually every aspect in nursing care of patients with cancer, no matter what the site of malignancy or clinical problem. Through association or active participation in local and national professional societies, the nurse has further access to advanced techniques and perspectives within the specialty. This is a primary tactic for amassing knowledge of nursing standards in oncology. Professional goals and purposes are defined by such a society, which helps the practicing nurse realize the standards of practice to which the professional will be held in a court of law. The ONS Outcome Standards for Cancer Nursing Practice (1979) delineates the specific goals in caring for the patient with cancer.

The oncology nurse is advised to take inventory of the myriad functions and activities encountered in the individual clinical setting. On the basis of this inventory, the nurse must determine whether most activities are carried out in conformity to applicable policies and procedures or standards referenced in the literature of the specialty profession. In addition, the nurse might organize and collect references, maintaining a library of guidelines or care plans to upgrade and authenticate his or her practice. In the expanded role, the nurse engaging in more far-reaching procedures must ensure written standing orders and protocols for some diagnostic or treatment functions. These applications in essence define or set the standards commensurate with the characteristic practice of the nurse.

JOB DESCRIPTION

Another strategy to establish competence is through the job description. The job outline may be either broad or specific in defining nurse activities. It is important that what the nurse actually does is contained and easily interpreted within the description. Scope of practice problems may continue to arise for nurses working in expanded or advanced roles, in which functions are traditionally viewed as within the domain of physicians or not generally recognized as legitimate nursing functions by an accredited professional organization (Bernzweig, 1987). Anticipating this, delineating the current scope of the job may diminish some legal exposure. Job descriptions should be updated as health care delivery continues to reorganize in cancer care.

PERSONAL RISK ASSESSMENT

The judicious oncology nurse should make a personal risk assessment listing the parameters and all influencing factors on the individual nursing practice. Guidelines for making this personal assessment are outlined in Table 83–3.

DEFENSIVE DOCUMENTATION

COMPREHENSIVE DOCUMENTATION

The duty to keep accurate records of a patient's physical and mental status is one of the most fundamental of a nurse's legal responsibilities. It reflects the professional nurse's accountability for interpreting and evaluating the patient's symptoms. Nurses often believe that charting is simply a function they perform as part of procedural rules. Many nurses have been taught to doc-

TABLE 83–3. *Personal Risk Assessment*

Do you know the state Nurse Practice Act and its legal interpretation?
Do you have an expanded role in cancer nursing?
Do you have on file documents attesting to any of your specialized training?
Are standardized procedures required for your unique practice?
Are you certified in your area of expertise?
Have you identified the facility's policies most influential to your practice?
Is your job description up to date and accurate?
Are you familiar with written professional standards of care?
Have you operationalized the written standards in your practice?
Do the written standards dominate your practice framework?
Do you have guidelines for the significant activities of your practice?
Do you give proper attention to those you supervise?
Do you know your patients; are your assessments sharp?
Do you plan patient care and follow-up on the plan?
Is your documentation evaluative and interpretive?
Do you keep an open line of communication to patient, family, and team members?
Do you foster excellent public relations?

ument only what was actually seen, not to interpret or diagnose. Frequently, the notion prevails that charting is done to "cover" oneself, to indicate that an activity was executed, no matter how well or poorly done or how successful the outcome. These are erroneous concepts. In litigation, testimony concerning the standards of care carries great weight, but the medical record notes of the nurse accused of negligence are the major chronicle of the situation. The nursing chart is the hard evidence that follows the jury into the deliberation room.

The best defense will lie not in flimsy documentation solely of what the nurse sees when delivering patient care but the interpretation and evaluation of that which is seen. This documentation provides the rationale or substantiation for activities the nurse subsequently carries out. As discussed previously, planned patient care by its very nature is activated by professional judgment. When clinical judgment is put into play, logic implies that this reflective approach will lead to a higher level of care, and liability exposure potentially will be held in greater check.

Patient assessment is particularly important. In charting, common errors concern omissions of the observations of significance and what is selective and relevant in patient signs and symptoms in relationship to the medical problem or treatment. In assessment, positive or negative indicators associated with a particular problem should be emphasized. Nursing documentation must be continually reflective of the medical diagnosis, because this will provide the experienced nurse with associated signs and symptoms for ongoing assessment. Nurses' notes devoid of comments about these anticipated symptoms will lead the court to form an unfavorable opinion about nursing competence.

MEDICAL AND NURSING DIAGNOSES

The use of nursing diagnoses has been avoided by some nurses or facilities for fear that "diagnosing" oversteps the bounds of nursing. However, there is the contrary opinion that the use of nursing diagnoses notably demonstrates a high level of professional functioning by meeting the nursing responsibility to interpret and evaluate assessment findings. Nursing diagnostic labels are a direct way to report not only patient symptoms but response and reactions to the nursing or medical regimen. The use of nursing diagnoses, furthermore, clearly indicates the planning activities the nurse applies to patient care. Nursing diagnoses are a defensible, even desirable, method of conveying information about the patient in the medical record. Their use leads to high-quality nursing by encouraging care on the basis of patient reactions and response. There is always greater legal protection in distinctive charting; a lawsuit may be avoided or won on the merits of nurses' notes. Unfortunately, there has not been wide acceptance of the use of nursing diagnoses by nurses in general and oncology nurses in particular; therefore, their application to cancer problems has been limited (Daeffler & Petrosino, 1989).

PUBLIC RELATIONS

HARM VERSUS MISTREATMENT

The most important defensive strategy the nurse may undertake is the formation of a superior public relations stance. Anger breeds thoughts of legal recourse in patients and families who feel an affront by their health care provider. Often without justification, hurt feelings will occur through a lack of communication between nurse or physician and patient. The issue of mistreatment often surfaces, and the patient or family will threaten suit. This frightens the nurse, and further damage is potentially done to the relationship as the nurse reacts to the hostility. The nurse must clearly evaluate whether mistreatment has occurred or the more serious offense of harm. Basic to every nursing malpractice suit is a failure to meet the standard of care such that real harm or injury to the patient has occurred as a result of that failure.

The nurse must not compound the sensitive situation by retreating or covering up when confronted by a patient who has undergone actual or perceived mistreatment. Many malpractice suits involving nurses are traceable to the patient's psychologic dissatisfaction with the nursing care. Nurturing patient relations is key in such instances. There is the belief that patients with cancer seldom initiate legal proceedings. This may be true because patients generally receive definitive psychologic support from oncology nurses and physicians during the course of their health care. According to one authority, the success in preventing malpractice claims may lie in a patient-centered approach that encourages a more wholesome, therapeutic interaction between patient and nurse (Bernzweig, 1987).

SENSITIVITY TO THE ISSUES

The oncology nurse shoulders multiple legal responsibilities while providing complex care and maintaining sensitive patient interactions. It is difficult to anticipate every influencing factor in potentially litigious situations. The professional nurse meets this challenge by assembling an armamentarium consisting of discerning attention to the standards of care underlying a situation coupled with meticulous documentation of assessment, nursing care, and patient response. There must be judicious knowledge of the bounds of the traditional nursing role so that appropriate education and supporting policies or procedures are developed as nursing practice expands from advancing technology. Equally important is the nurse's regard for the powerful expectations the patient brings to the cancer treatment program. The greatest strategy for limiting liability exposure lies in sensitive communication and the establishment of sound nurse-patient relations.

REFERENCES

Agency. (1995). *Barbri bar review.* Harcourt Brace Legal and Professional Publications, Inc.

Alef v. Alta Bates Hospital, 6 Cal. Rptr. 2d 900 (Cal. App. 1 Dist. 1992).

Altman, L. (1995, March 24). Big doses of experimental drug killed patient, hurt second. *New York Times National,* A18.

American Nurses' Association. (1993). *National nursing summit on the nurse of the future: Summary of proceedings.* Washington, DC: The Association. (Unpublished).

American Nurses' Association. (1974). *Standards: Medical-surgical nursing practice.* Kansas City, MO: Author.

Angarola, R. (1991). Inappropriate pain management results in high jury award [Letter]. *Journal of Pain and Symptom Management, 6*(7), 407.

Bernzweig, E. P. (1987). *The nurse's liability for malpractice.* New York: McGraw-Hill.

Beyer, E. W., & Popp, P. W. (1990). Nursing standard of care in medical malpractice litigation: The role of the nurse expert witness. *Journal of Health and Hospital Law, 23*(12), 363–367.

Birkholz, G. (1995). Malpractice data from the National Practitioner Data Bank. *The Nurse Practitioner, 20*(3), 32–35.

Birkholz, G., & Walker, D. (1994). Strategies for state statutory language changes granting fully independent nurse practitioner practice. *The Nurse Practitioner, 19*(1), 54–58.

Cantor, M. M. (1978). *Achieving nursing standards: Internal and external* (pp. 3–15). Wakefield, MA: Nursing Resources, Inc.

Chamorro, T. (1979). The role of a nurse-clinician in joint practice with gynecologic oncologists. *Cancer, 48,* 622–631.

Chudson v. Ratra, 548 A.2d 172 (Md. App. 1988).

Cooper v. National Motor Bearing Co., 238 P. 2d 581 (1955).

Cox, M. D. (1989). Did nursing follow the standard of care, or was the patient abandoned? *The Nurse, The Patient, & the Law, 14*(7), 4–6.

Creighton, H. (1985). Law for the nurse manager: Patient teaching. *Nursing Management, 16,* 12–18.

Cushing, M. (1992). Pain management on trial. *American Journal of Nursing, February,* 21–22.

Czubinsky v. Doctors Hospital, 130 Cal. App. 3d 362 (Jan. [1983]).

Daeffler, R., & Petrosino, B. (1989). *Manual of oncology nursing practice: Nursing diagnoses and care.* Rockville, MD: Aspen Publishers.

Daniel v. St. Francis Cabrini Hosp., 415 So.2d 586 (1982).

Dimond, E. P. (1992). The oncology nurse's role in patient advance directives. *Oncology Nursing Forum, 19*(6), 891–896.

Fein v. Permanente Medical Group, 695 P.2d 665 (1985).

Fiesta, J. (1983). *The law and liability: A guide for nurses.* New York: John Wiley & Sons.

Gargaro, W. J. (1978). Informed consent: Parts I, II, III. *Cancer Nursing, I*(1), 81–82; *I*(2), 167–172; *I*(3), 249–250; *I*(6), 467.

Gargaro, W. J. (1981, 1982). Valuing the missed opportunity for treatment. *Cancer Nursing, 2*(6), 491–492; *5*(1), 65–66.

Gibson v. Bossier City General Hosp., 594 So.2d 1332 (La.App.2 Cir. 1991).

Gobis, L. J. (1992). Recent developments in health law relevant to health care providers. *Nurse Practitioner, 17*(3), 77–80.

Gosnell, D. J. (1987). Acting as an expert witness: A professional responsibility. *Nursing Outlook, 35,* 102.

Greenfield, S. (1980). Protocols as analogs to standing orders. In B. Bullough (Ed.), *The law and the expanding nursing role* (pp. 186–202). Norwalk, CT.: Appleton-Century-Crofts.

Gregory, D. R. (1992). Patient care decision-making: A legal guide for providers, C. C. Obade author. *Journal of Legal Medicine, 13,* 589–597.

Grossman, S., Piantadosi, S., & Covahey, C. (1994). Are informed consent forms that describe clinical oncology research protocols readable by most patients and their families? *Journal of Clinical Oncology, 12*(10), 2211–2215.

Guzeldere v. Wallin, 593 N.E.2d 629 (Ill. App. 1 Dist. 1992).

Hall, J. K. (1993). How to analyze nurse practitioner licensure laws. *Nurse Practitioner, 18*(8), 31–34.

Heffernan, L. (1995). Regulation of advanced practice nursing in health care reform. *Journal of Health and Hospital Law, 28*(2), 73–84.

Heitland, A. R., Villarreal, J. A., & Rzonca, L. E. (1993). The legal limits of advanced nursing specialty practice in Illinois. *Illinois Bar Journal, 81,* 22–29.

Hinden, R. A. (1994). Liability for managed care. *Topics in Case Management, July/Aug/Sept,* 99–100.

Hyatt, T. K. (1994). Negligent referral. *Topics in Case Management, July/Aug/Sept,* 102–105.

Jackson v. Power, 743 P.2d 1376 (Supreme Court of Alaska, 1987)

Johnson v. Power, 743 P.2d 1376 (Supreme Court of Alaska 1987).

Johnson, J. M. (1986). Clinical trials: New responsibilities and roles for nurses. *Nursing Outlook, 34,* 149–152.

Judkins, A. F. (1995). Advance practice nurses for follow-up care of breast cancer patients. *Nursing Interventions in Oncology, 8,* 17–20.

Kelly, M. E. & Garrick, T. R. (1984). Nursing negligence in collaborative practice: Legal liability in California. *Law, Medicine & Health Care, 12,* 260–267.

Kindig, D., Cultice, J., & Mullan, F. (1993). The elusive generalist physician: Can we reach a 50% goal? *Journal of the American Medical Association, 270,* 1069–1073.

Lind, J., & Bush, N. J. (1987). Nursing's role in chemotherapy administration. *Seminars in Oncology Nursing, 3,* 83–86.

Lynwood V. Shaw v. Richmond Memorial Hospital. (1991). *Medical malpractice verdicts, settlements & experts, 7*(4), 45.

Lynwood V. Shaw v. Richmond Memorial Hospital, City of Richmond (VA) Circuit Court, Case No. LS-11-12-2.

Manning v. Twin Falls Clinic and Hospital, 830 P. 2d 118 5 (Idaho 1992).

Marks, D. T. (1987). Legal implications of increased autonomy. *Journal of Gerontological Nursing, 3,* 83–86.

Mary and Willie Latham v. Southwest Detroit Hospital and Jane Doe. (1991). *Medical malpractice verdicts, settlements & experts, 7*(1), 45.

McDaniel v. Sage, 419 N.E.2d 1322 (Ind. App. 1981).

McGrath, P. (1995). It's ok to say no! A discussion of ethical issues arising from informed consent to chemotherapy. *Cancer Nursing, 18*(2), 97–103.

Meade, C. D., & Howser, D. M. (1992). Consent forms: How to determine and improve their readability. *Oncology Nursing Forum, 19*(10), 1523–1528.

Meehan, F. (1991). Comment: DNR orders-judicial authorization or statutory mandate? *Journal of Health and Health Law, 24*(5), 144–146, 167.

Merz, J. (1993). On a decision-making paradigm of medical informed consent. *The Journal of Legal Medicine, 14,* 231–264.

Moniz, D. M. (1992). The legal danger of written protocols and standards of practice. *The Nurse Practitioner, 17*(9), 58–60.

Morse, S. J., & Kane, J. K. (1995). Nurses lack medical diagnosis and prescriptive authority under Illinois law. *Illinois Bar Journal, 83,* 130–134.

Northrop, C. (1986). Legal outlook: Malpractice and standards of care. *Nursing Outlook, 34,* 160.

Northrop, C., & Kelly, M. E. (1987). *Legal issues in nursing.* St. Louis: CV Mosby Co.

O'Connor, K. S. (1994). Advanced practice nurses in an environment of health care reform. *Maternal Child Nursing, 19,* 65–68.

Oncology Nursing Society & American Nurses' Association (1979). *Outcome standards for cancer nursing practice.* Kansas City, MO: American Nurses' Association.

Oncology Nursing Society (1990). *Standards of advanced practice in oncology nursing.* Pittsburgh: Author.

Osuch, J. R., & Bonham, V. L. (1994). The timely diagnosis of breast cancer. Principles of risk management for primary care providers and surgeons. *Cancer Supplement, 74*(1), 271–278.

Pace v. Hazel Towers, Inc., 584 N.Y.S.2d 23 (A.D. 1 Dept. 1992).

Payne v. Marion General Hospital, 549 N.E. 2d 590 (Ind. 1990).

Pearson, L. J. (1995). Annual update of how each state stands on legislative issues affecting advanced nursing practice. *The Nurse Practitioner, 20*(1), 13–51.

Pearson, L. J., & Birkholz, G. (1995). Report on the 1994 readership survey on NP experiences with malpractice issues. *Nurse Practitioner, 20*(3), 18–30.

Plaintiff's Medical Malpractice Litigation (1981 with 1986 Supplement). Springfield, IL: Illinois Institute for Continuing Legal Education.

Rosoff, A. J. (1995). Review of standards of care in emergency medicine. In H. Wigder & J. Moffat (Eds.). *Journal of Legal Medicine, 16,* 167–173.

Safriet, B. J. (1992). Health care dollars and regulatory sense: The role of advanced practice nursing. *Yale Journal of Regulation, 9,* 417–487.

Saue, J. (1994). Experimental treatment and technology. *Topics in Case Management, Jul/Aug/Sept,* 105–106.

Savelle v. Heilbrunn, 552 So.2d 52 (La.App. 3 Cir. 1989).

Scheutzow, S. O. (1994). Confidentiality. *Topics in Case Management, July/Aug/Sept*, 108–109.

Schulmeister, L. (1987). Litigation involving oncology nurses. *Oncology Nursing Forum, 14*(2), 25–28.

Sekscenski, E. S., Sansom, S., Bazell, C., Salmon, M. E., & Mullan, F. (1994). State practice environments and the supply of physician assistants, nurse practitioners, and certified nurse-midwives. *New England Journal of Medicine, 331*, 1266–1271.

Sermchief v. Gonzales, 660 S.W. 2d 683 (Mo. banc 1983).

Sharp, E., DePriest, C., Potts, L., & Willeford, R. (1994). A teaching tool for patients receiving continuous IV infusion recombinant interleukin-2 therapy. *Oncology Nursing Forum, 21*(5), 911–914.

Sheidler, V., McGuire, D., Grossman, S., & Gilbert, M. (1992). Analgesic decision-making skills of nurses. *Oncology Nursing Forum, 19*(10), 1531–1534.

Siklas v. Ecker, 617 N. E. 2d 507 (Ill. 1993).

Smrcina, C. (1993). Licensure of advanced practice nursing: What's our position. *Orthopaedic Nursing, 12*(1), 9–13.

Sollins, H. L. (1994). Fraud and abuse. *Topics in Case Management, July/Aug/Sept*, 109–110.

Spencer-Cisek, P. (1995). Conference urges unity among advanced practice nurses: ONS position statement: Advanced practice in oncology nursing. *ONS News, 10*(4), 14.

Trandel-Korenchuk, D., & Trandel-Korenchuk, K. (1980). State nursing laws. *Nurse Practitioner, 5*, 39–41.

Walker, F., Roethke, S., Sandman, V., Clark, K., & Martin, G. (1994). Guiding patients and their families through peripheral stem cell transplantation with the help of a teaching booklet. *Oncology Nursing Forum, 21*(3), 585–591.

Wallace, T. E. (1991). Consent to treatment: A practical guide (2nd ed.). In F. Rozovsky (Ed.). *Journal of Legal Medicine, 12*, 249–255.

Weaver, T. A. (General Ed.) (1989 with 1992 Supplement). *Medical malpractice.* Springfield, IL: Illinois Institute for Continuing Legal Education.

West, J. C. (1994). The legal implications of medical practice guidelines. *Journal of Health and Hospital Law, 27*(4), 97–128.

Williams v. St. Claire Medical Center, 657 S. W. 2d 590 (Ken. App. 1983).

Wynstra, N. A. (1994). Breast cancer. Selected legal issues. *Cancer Supplement, 74*(1), 491–511.

CHAPTER
84

Cancer Legislation

Mary S. McCabe • Joan A. Piemme

Nurses constitute the largest number of health care professionals in the country, numbering approximately 2,239,816 registered nurses (American Nurses' Association, Personal Communication, March 1995). Additionally, one in every 44 registered women voters is a registered nurse. To activate this political force, nurses must learn how to use and influence the legislative process effectively.

In April of 1993, the American Nurses Association (ANA) initiated the Nurses Strategic Action Team (N-STAT), a grassroots effort to influence legislation. In addition, many nursing subspecialty organizations have legislative committees and are members of the National Federation of Nursing Subspecialty Organizations. In oncology nursing what is now the Government Relations Committee of the Oncology Nursing Society (ONS) began its legislative focus in 1980 and is now represented by full-time legislative staff.

The nursing literature has devoted most of its attention to nursing's potential leverage at the federal or national level. While this arena is important and powerful, nurses can "learn the ropes" gaining skill and confidence at the local level and progress with this political savvy to the state and national levels. A voter exerts far more influence than a nonvoter. At the very basis of influence is the nurse's responsibility as a citizen to exercise the right to vote and to determine how tax dollars will be spent. As a group, nurses have become more sophisticated in the political process and are capable of exerting even more influence over the shaping and monitoring of policy affecting the public and the profession. Simply stated, "Those who produce the votes, contribute money and communicate with their legislators, develop political clout" (Vance, 1985, p. 170).

HISTORIC PERSPECTIVE

The role of the government in the organization, financing, and delivery of health services in the United States was initially very constricted and involved a limited provision of services and oversight of the public health. It now has assumed a major financial role in the payment of health care services. The traditional basis for such involvement has been a remedial one focused on areas where private institutions either cannot or choose not to undertake responsibility (Litman, 1991). Many milestones have occurred that have shaped the role and responsibility of the government today. The marriage of politics and health care in America has evolved as a major public policy issue, and Table 84–1 clearly outlines some of the important legislative landmarks that established the government's role in health care.

In the early 1900s, the Sheppard-Towner Act, which established the government's role in providing funds to the states, was enacted and served as the model system for the funding of all programs through the Public Health Service. Within a few years after enactment of this law, the National Institutes of Health (NIH) was authorized under the Randall Act and established the role of government funding for research as a cornerstone to the improved health of the nation. It is within the NIH that the National Cancer Institute

TABLE 84–1. *Major Legislative Milestones in Health Care*

1872	Establishment of the American Public Health Association
1898	Establishment of the U.S. Public Health Services and several PHS hospitals in East Coast seaports
1906	Legislation was passed regulating the Food and Drug Industry
1912	Establishment of the Childrens Bureau within the Department of Labor (forerunner of the Department of Health and Human Services)
1921	Enactment of the Sheppard-Towner Act (first legislation to provide federal financial aid to the states)
1930	Randall Act changed the Hygienic Laboratory on Staten Island, New York into the first National Institute of Health
1934	Blue Cross begun under the direction of the American Hospital Association
1935	Social Security Act (American Medical Association opposed Federal government's involvement in health care)
1938	Kaiser-Permanente Medical Care Program begun as first prepaid comprehensive health plan
1939	Blue Shield established by state medical societies
1946	Hill-Burton Hospital Construction Act
1956	Congress authorized student aid to public health schools
1963	Health Professions Educational Assistance Act
1964	The Nurse Training Act
1965	Title XVIII and XIX of the Social Security Act
1971	National Cancer Act
1971	Comprehensive Health Manpower Training Act
1973	Health Maintenance Organization Act
1974	Health Planning and Resources Development Act
1982	Tax Equity and Fiscal Responsibility Act
1986	Nurse Training Act
1988	Catastrophic Health Care Reform (Repealed in 1989)
1990	The Americans with Disabilities Act passed
1990	Establishment of the Office of Research on Women's Health
1990	Comprehensive AIDS Relief Emergency Act (Ryan White CARE Act)
1994	Proposed Health Security Act defeated by Congress

(NCI) and the National Institute for Nursing Research (NINR) are located. These two NIH institutes are the source of Federal funding for our National Cancer Program and provide much of the resources available to support nursing research.

Over time, many federal efforts have been made to address the nation's health care needs in a comprehensive manner. Although the Social Security Act was passed in 1935, there was ongoing opposition to presidential proposals of health care reform. For instance, Franklin D. Roosevelt excluded health insurance out of his new deal to extensive opposition (Jennings, 1991).

President Truman also unsuccessfully made health insurance an issue, and it was not until the Kennedy-Johnson era that successful legislation was passed. These presidents were able to develop a major focus for the health problems of the elderly, and the result was the enactment of Medicare and Medicaid in 1965 (Title XVIII and XIX of the Social Security Act). President Nixon contributed to a growing interest in Health Maintenance Organizations (HMOs), but his major health care accomplishment clearly was passage of the National Cancer Act.

President Carter supported national health insurance in his presidential campaign in 1976 but was unable to develop a consensus around this issue while in office and as health care costs continued to increase (Lammers, 1991). During the Reagan and Bush administrations, the efforts to control costs in health care became acute and included the repeal of the Catastrophic Health Care Act in 1988, which had been intended to expand the catastrophic health benefit under Medicare. In 1994, the Clinton administration was defeated in its extensive

attempt to reform health care with the very public defeat of the Health Security Act.

So with a continuing lack of consensus of how to address health care coverage and services nationally, the population needing care has increased, the costs of technologies has skyrocketed, and the government's share of health care has grown to be in excess of 14 per cent of the Gross National Product (GNP). As a result, efficiency of services, reimbursement, and cost containment continue to be the focus of the health care debate as they have been for over the past 15 years.

Due to a lack of a national consensus and no national health policy, cost containment continues to be the most significant single factor driving the health care system in the twenty-first century. It will be incumbent upon the nursing profession to play a key role in the development of this system as the many facets of the system attempt to redefine themselves (Greenhouse, 1993).

THE LEGISLATIVE PROCESS

To maximize the effectiveness of political action, one must know the process of making laws. For when one knows the process, the commitment to become actively involved is more likely and therefore is a greater opportunity to be effective. According to Carolyne K. Davis, who was the first woman and first nurse to be administrator of the Health Care Financing Administration (HCFA), "By learning the art of politics, nurses can exert political influence and have a major effect on such health policy areas as nurses training, research, Medicaid and Medicare, and other legislation and regulations that affect both acute and long-term care agencies" (Davis, Oakley, & Sochalski, 1982, p. 15). First, one must know the legislative process.

WHO ARE THE PLAYERS?

At the national level, this process takes place in Washington, D.C. The task and responsibility of writing laws and regulating government operations lies in the Congress of the United States, "the peoples branch" of the government. These 535 congressional lawmakers are the only federal officials elected directly by the people; even votes for the President are passed through the Electoral College. The authority to levy federal taxes and to decide how those revenues will be spent lies with Congress. Its members hold the "power of the purse."

WHAT ARE THE ISSUES?

Where do the issues come from? Bills originate in many diverse quarters, and the sources of ideas are limitless. In the Burson-Marsteller Report, *Communicating with Congress*, Congressmen identified and rated their sources of information.

• The number one source of ideas is *constituents*. Congressional offices pay more attention to personal communication from constituents than any other source.
• Rated number two are *government employees* including congressional aides, members of the Administration, or other members of Congress.
• Numbers three and four are the *print media* and the *broadcast media*.
• The number five rated source is *special interest groups*. Special interests in this country are very important and should not be underestimated (Burson-Marsteller, 1992). These special interest groups are organized in a variety of ways. They include *coalitions* and *lobbying groups*, which exert a continuing influence on Congress.

HOW DO YOU COMMUNICATE?

Once the issue has been identified and developed, it is important to know how to communicate about it. Spontaneous, individually composed letters from constituents are the most effective way of communicating with congressional decision makers (Goldwater & Zusy, 1990). These letters receive more attention than any other form of written communication, although orchestrated mail also receives high ratings.

Coalitions have become a powerful communication medium. Coalitions comprise a variety of groups and organizations that may be very broad in purpose but "sign on" to provide unanimity to a specific policy issue or legislative initiative. For example, the Coalition on Smoking OR Health comprises three organizations, the American Cancer Society, the American Lung Association, and the American Heart Association, with 12 additional health-related organizations on its legislative advisory council. As the coalition name implies, these organizations are concerned with issues related to smoking and tobacco products. The ONS supports an official liaison with this coalition who serves as a representative at coalition meetings and is a communication link with ONS. Recently, in response to a request for action, ONS signed on to a coalition-driven letter writing effort to encourage legislators to support H.R. 2147, the Fairness in Tobacco and Nicotine Regulation Act, which could classify tobacco products as drugs that would therefore be subject to regulation under the Food, Drug, and Cosmetic Act.

In the past 10 years, advocacy groups have developed, evolving largely as a result of the acquired immunodeficiency syndrome (AIDS) epidemic. Advocacy groups are similar to coalitions in that organizations are formed with the expressed intent to influence Congress, the president, and the regulatory agencies to take specific actions related to a particular disease or health problem. ACT-UP (AIDS Coalition to Unleash Power), for example, has had a very powerful political influence despite widespread criticisms about their militant activism and radical tactics. Their efforts have resulted in the "fast tracking" by the FDA of some AIDS-related experimental drugs, the expansion of federally funded AIDS clinical trials, and the overall increased recognition of human immunodeficiency virus (HIV) infection and AIDS as a political and social issue as well as a disease condition. Advocacy has come more recently to oncology, and two cancer-related advocacy groups are the National Coalition for Cancer Survivorship and the National Breast Cancer Coalition.

Once an issue is identified and a communication route is established, it then becomes crucial to make contact with the appropriate individuals through visits. Visits can be made to promote familiarity with an organization's purpose, or they can be scheduled to coincide with an individual grassroots organization or coalition effort to support a particular piece of legislation under consideration. It would seem most logical and beneficial to address the legislator directly, especially during visits. But that is not necessarily so, because accompanying the rise of congressional power in the last decade has been the rise in the power and influence of the congressional staff, commonly known as the legislative aide.

It is both important and practical to realize that most congressional offices are organized so that the staff control the communication lines to and from the legislator. Some of the most experienced lobbyists value a 10-minute visit with a key staff person as much as equal time with a member of Congress. By profile, this staff person is young and well educated. Unfortunately, only a small minority of these legislative aides are trained in any health profession. In addition, they handle at least four other issue areas in addition to health. These individuals are key to nurses in conveying ideas and registering support for the wide spectrum of health care issues.

In summary, there are four general principles for communicating with Congress either as an individual or as part of a group. These are:

- *Keep it local.* Local issues brought by local constituents are most important to members of Congress.
- *Keep it personal.* Because personal communication involves a commitment of time and energy, it is taken seriously.
- *Keep it concise.* Communication that is direct and to the point is most likely to receive attention.
- *Put it in writing.* A personal, hard copy of the request provides a reading available record for the legislator.

WHAT IS THE PROCESS OF LAWMAKING?

The work of Congress as defined by the "development of a bill" can be summarized in one important word—*compromise*. This point becomes obvious as a bill passes through the many groups and committees that have the opportunity to shape it (summarized in Fig. 84–1).

Bills can be proposed in either house of Congress, but the large majority of laws originate in the House of

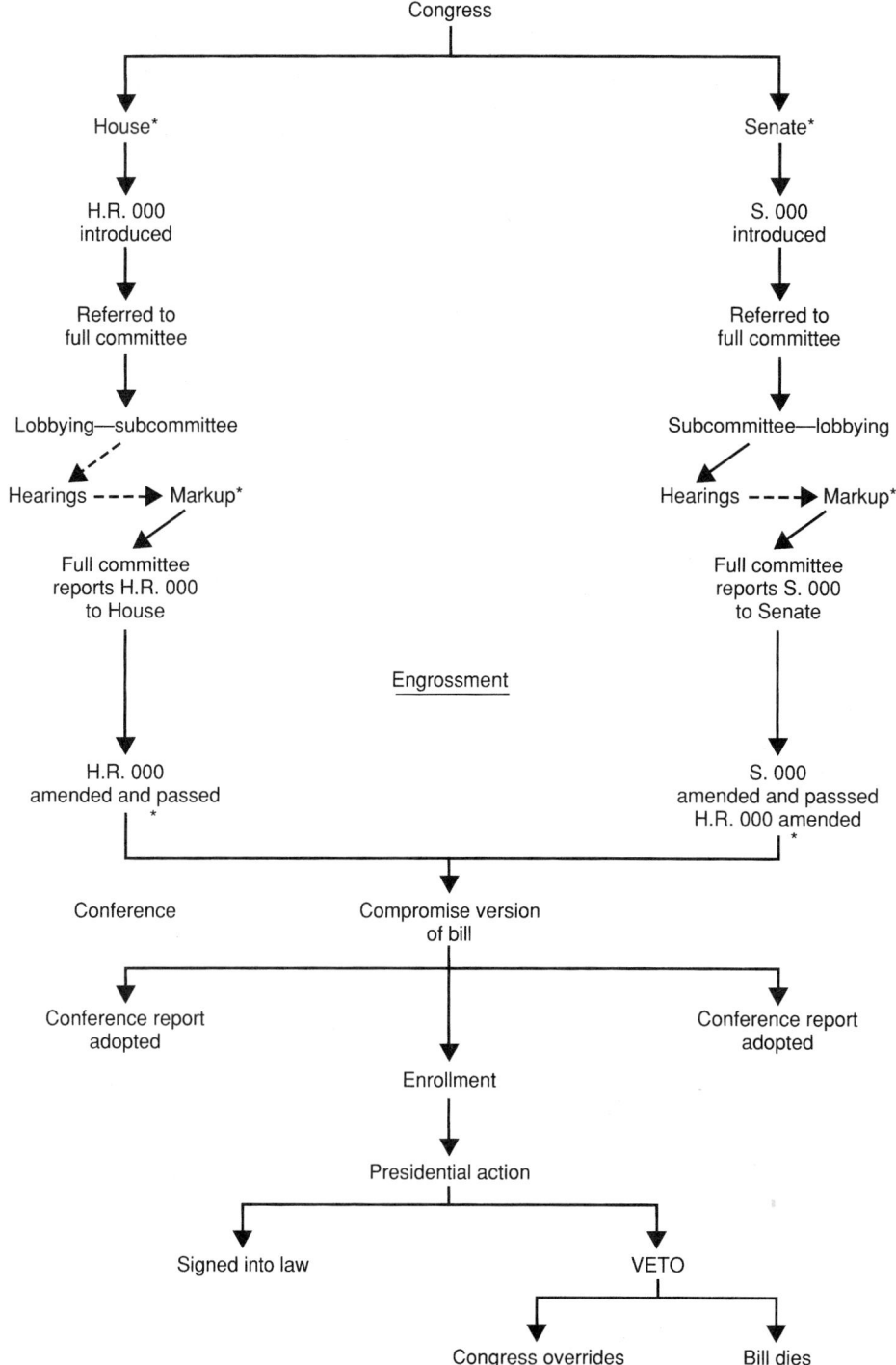

FIGURE 84–1. The making of a law. *Lobbying efforts appropriate at these stages.

Representatives. In the House, a bill may be introduced at any time while the House is actually in session by simply placing it at the side of the clerk's desk in the House Chamber. Permission is not required to introduce the measure or to make a statement at the time of introduction. The bill is then assigned its legislative number by the clerk and referred to the appropriate committees by the Speaker. In the Senate, a Senator usually introduces a bill or a resolution by presenting it to the clerk at the presiding officer's desk or by introducing it more formally on the floor of the Senate. It is then referred to the appropriate committee.

Most crucial and important to the legislative process is the action by the committees. It is here that the most intensive consideration is given to the proposed measures and at this point that citizens are given their opportunity to be heard. Each committee is responsible for certain subject matters of legislation and has jurisdiction over a particular area of the law. Most of the committees have two or more subcommittees that specialize in a particular class of bills. Each standing committee of the House, except the Committee on the Budget, must establish at least four subcommittees. In regard to health care issues, there are specific committees that initiate and review health legislation. It is these committees and their members that nurses want to access (Table 84–2). If the bill is important or controversial, the committee reviewing it will usually set a date for public hearings. Each hearing is required to be open to the public except when the testimony may endanger national security or defame or incriminate an individual (U.S. Printing Office, 1986). After hearings are completed, the bill will then go to a "mark-up" session. Here the legislators review both sides of the issue in detail and make amendments to the bill as introduced based upon their discussion. At the conclusion of this deliberation, a vote is taken to determine the action of the subcommittee. The subcommittee may decide to report the bill favorably to the full committee, with or without amend-

TABLE 84–2. *Congressional Health Committees*

Senate
Committee on Appropriations
   Subcommittee on Labor, Health and Human Services,
   Education and Related Agencies
Committee on the Budget
Committee on Finance
   Subcommittee on Medicaid and Health Care for Low-
   Income Families
   Subcommittee on Medicare, Long-Term Care and Health
   Insurance
Committee on Labor and Human Resources
House
Committee on Appropriations
   Subcommittee on Labor, Health and Human Services, and
   Education
Committee on the Budget
Committee on Commerce
   Subcommittee on Health and the Environment
Committee on Ways and Means
   Subcommittee on Health

ment, or unfavorably, or suggest that the committee table it, that is, postpone action indefinitely. Each member of the subcommittee has *one* vote, and if he or she is unable to attend the mark-up, the committee chairperson can have their "proxies," or vote on their behalf. Mark-up of legislation must also be open to the public. The bill, with or without amendments, goes back to full committee, which reports it to the entire membership with adequate opportunity for debate and proposing amendments.

The Senate then receives a copy of the bill precisely as it passed the House. Then the Senate committees give the bill the same kind of detailed consideration it received in the House. After the Senate passes its version of the bill, a conference is called to resolve the differences between the two Houses. When the conferees, by majority vote, have reached complete agreement, they prepare a report that must be signed by a majority of the conferees appointed by each body.

When the bill has been agreed to in identical form by both bodies and in conference and has been passed on the floor of each chamber, a copy of the bill is enrolled for presentation (enrollment) to the President for his signature or veto.

This general information of the legislative process can be directly related to health care and the action of nurses. The important points to remember as one gains expertise are:

- develop the issue that is important;
- know the political process;
- network and build coalitions;
- cover the political territory where impact is most likely;
- respond and act when legislation is moving;
- gain support on the Hill for your issues.

The success nursing has in achieving a legislative knowledge base will relate directly to its ability to participate.

USING THE LEGISLATIVE PROCESS

For nurses interested in becoming involved in the legislative process, it is wise to think of starting out at the local level, where the issues can be clearly identified and where it is more feasible to gather a ground swell to rally around an issue of importance in the community.

LOCAL GOVERNMENT

Local government, the unit of government closest to the people, is profoundly influenced directly by its constituency. Local governments are very involved in health care. Together with professional organizations (e.g., local American Cancer Society chapters), oncology nurses can raise the consciousness of local officials as to the prevalence of specific malignancies. In Washington, D.C., a multiorganizational effort was initiated to highlight the prevalence of colorectal cancer in the African-American population. In this endeavor, public and private health care agencies joined together to provide low-cost screening to residents for a designated period of time.

The nurse concerned about professional issues, the quality of care, and the public well-being of consumers needs to know the structure and function of local government. Few generalizations concerning formulas for local success can be made due to the variation in specific localities. Therefore, nurses need to learn the particular structure and political climate in their community. A city charter provides for one of four forms of city government: major-council (most common), commission, council-manager, or major-manager (Majewski, 1993). The next level of local government is the county (with most states being divided in this manner), which is the oldest form of local government in the country.

An elected member of the District of Columbia city council had some very helpful advice for a group of local nurses. This councilwoman pointed out that the local medical society was "visible" to the members of city council (i.e., present at hearings, at open sessions of council) on a weekly basis, yet nurses were never seen. The point was also made that the physicians' presence was felt whether or not they were seeking support on a particular issue or piece of legislation. As a result of this observation, the nurses developed an action plan delegating responsibility for monitoring sessions of interest to nurses and ensuring a nursing presence as often as possible. After a period of increased visibility, nurses were requested to attend sessions to provide input and feedback to council members. Additionally, nurses realized the importance of being a visible presence and the long-term benefits that accrue from offering assistance to promote issues where nursing is *not* asking for something in return!

Reading the newspaper on a daily basis keeps the individual abreast of what is happening in the community. If the reader has unanswered questions about an issue, an effort needs to be made to become fully informed as quickly as possible. After getting the necessary data, an individual nurse or a nursing group can write a letter to the newspaper editor or submit an entry to the opinion page or whatever avenue the newspaper may have. Often one letter will prompt another, or, if the letter was signed by an organized group, the organization may be contacted directly by interested parties.

The board of education is elected in many counties or appointed by the governor. An ongoing interest of many pediatric and adult oncology nurses is the adoption by the Board of Education of policies regulating school attendance and emergency care of children with AIDS. Because some children with HIV infection have been refused admission to schools, nurses interested in policy development can assume an active role in guaranteeing that the policy of the board of education reflects the most current information about the transmissibility of HIV as well as the emergency care and precautions in the event of illness or injury at school.

STATE GOVERNMENT

Every nurse has a professional relationship with state government. The right to practice and the parameters of professional practice are determined by the state Board of Nurse Examiners and embodied in the state's Nurse Practice Act.

Nurses need to expand their understanding of state governments and increase their political power at the state level to influence health policy development and resource allocation as well as to ensure the proper state regulation of nursing practice (Long & Hinds, 1993). The structures of state governments vary; therefore, as with local governmental structure, the first step is to learn the organization.

All states have equal powers through the U.S. Constitution and have similar government power and structure, that is, each state has an executive, legislative, and judicial branch of government with the organization and power of each defined by the state constitution (Long & Hinds, 1993).

The legislative branch of the state government is similar to the structure on the federal level with two houses composed of the Senate and the Assembly (or designated as House of Delegates or Representatives). Each elected legislator represents people in a predetermined geographic location or district. The regular sessions of the legislature vary in length. Knowing the schedule is particularly important when planning nursing lobbying efforts.

Reapportionment or the redrawing of district lines occurs every 10 years using the U.S. Bureau of Census figures. Nursing can be potentially aided or hindered as a result of reapportionment. In one state, recently this process was felt to be partly responsible for the defeat of a multiterm state senator known for her efforts in education and health and human services. She has long been a "friend" of nursing and could be counted on to champion nursing positions in the state capitol.

It is instructive to realize that hundreds or perhaps more than 1000 bills will be introduced to a State Assembly or House and Senate during a session. Many of these bills will not be enacted into law but may be reintroduced at a subsequent session. To decrease one's frustration, it is helpful to look upon the energy spent on efforts that may not have materialized into law as effective training and experience upon which to build. Even though a bill may not be passed the first time it is introduced, it is also helpful to reflect on the "education" of the legislators that has occurred as a result of nursing's lobbying efforts. Some newspapers report the major bills in the state legislature, the action taken, and the current status of the bill. The vote of the legislator on a bill may be publicized or will be available through the legislator's office. Most elected officials send newsletters to voters indicating current issues and the stand or vote taken on bills. Additionally, legislators hold periodic open forums to hear directly from constituents. It may be politically astute to write the legislator a letter of appreciation acknowledging their stand on a specific issue.

The committee structure and function is of major importance, since much of the legislative process occurs in committees. Each state capitol or League of Women Voters can provide the name and domains of the state committees. In addition to committees dealing with health and welfare, the education committee concerns itself with professional practice, and the insurance committee often deals with reimbursement legislation.

The executive branch, with the governor as the chief executive officer, relates to the two branches of state government. In many states, governors select health professionals as political appointees as well as for membership on commissions and task forces. This process provides a unique opportunity for nurses to become involved. Most often nurses gain attention through professional achievements, political or professional activities, or are recommended by professional organizations. When nurses have been appointed, it has provided the opportunity for nursing input into recommended policy as well as having a highly visible forum for nursing expertise and influence. It is becoming increasingly common for nurses to hold political office at the local and state levels.

The regulatory process of state government under the secretary of state is as essential to monitor as the legislative process. The state board of nursing is accountable to the secretary of state. The education department frequently governs the credentialing of nursing education programs in the state (Long & Hinds, 1993). Nurses need to become known to these department staff as knowledgeable and reliable sources of information. It is a good rule of thumb to build these relationships over time in an organized fashion, rather than becoming visible only at periods that are deemed critical for nursing.

More than one objective can often be achieved at the state level because of the opportunity for direct contact. The following example illustrates how nurses can simultaneously network and have the opportunity to have an information-sharing session with a state-elected legislator. A nurse from an acute care center convened a group of nurses from a variety of community health care agencies to discuss state health issues with this official during his recess from the state House of Delegates. Prior to his arrival, the nurses agreed upon the health care issues that were a priority in the legislator's district and presented these during the subsequent discussion. Not only was this informative to the legislator, but the nurses broadened their scope of understanding and developed a greater appreciation for nursing activities in the community.

FEDERAL GOVERNMENT

At the Federal level, the government is structured into three branches: the executive, the legislative, and the judicial. As on the state level, the legislative branch is the lawmaking body, the Congress. The individual nurse can make the greatest contribution by maintaining frequent contact with the appropriate elected representatives and senators regarding issues as well as pending legislation that merit legislative action (Tables 84–3 and 84–4).

Much of the organized impact on the Federal level will come about from the efforts that national nursing groups make through their legislative liaisons or lobbyists. Therefore, it is important not only to belong to the professional organizations but also to take an active role in helping to shape the priorities of those organizations (Table 84–5).

Nurses have a variety of ways to keep informed about what is upcoming or the progress of key issues on the national level. The generic nursing journals (e.g., *The American Journal of Nursing* and *Nursing Outlook*) report on national legislative issues. *The American Nurse*, the monthly newsletter of the ANA sent to all ANA members, carries a "Capitol Commentary" column written by members of the ANA Washington office, the professional organization's lobbying group. Many national nursing organizations have newsletters, journals, or both that may carry legislative updates as a regular feature of issues of interest to the particular specialty. The *ONS News* carries a legislative update in its monthly publication, and a legislative summary is compiled by the Director of Government Relations.

TABLE 84–3. *Activities for Individual Political Involvement*

Vote at each election
Join organizations that will provide development, e.g., PAC, League of Women Voters
Secure accurate information on each issue
Become knowledgeable and conversant on issues
Demonstrate that an issue is important to the community—get a petition signed
Monitor meetings—city council, school boards, commissions
Monitor officials' performance on health issues—voting record, public statements, news accounts
Testify—city council, public hearings on social, educational or health-related topic
Know structure and function of health related committees
Communicate with elected officials—telephone, fax, letter, visit
Identify yourself as a nurse in verbal and written communications
Maintain contact with specific legislators, legislative aides, and staff
Invite legislators and staff to visit health care agency (include media if approved)
Have professional calling cards printed
Work on election campaign
Provide financial support to candidate of choice
Attend a fund-raising party for candidates running for office
Attend open forums sponsored by elected officials
Become a consultant on health care issues
Run for elected office

TABLE 84-4. *Group Political Activities*

Monitor meetings to learn issues
Develop position statements on health issues
Monitor performance of official on health issues
Participate in election process—publicly endorse candidates, organize work banks for candidates, make financial contributions in key races
Propose member for seat on commission, task force, or board
Establish and join coalitions—nursing, woman's political caucus, NOW, local political clubs
Mobilize group to lobby
Arrange for a social event for legislator and other key figures
Organize a telephone tree for member information or for political legislative action
Develop fact sheet about your professional organization—send to nurses and have available for legislative visits
Organize voter registration drives
Organize letter writing campaign

TABLE 84-5. *Helpful Hints for Writing Your Legislator*

Type letter—include home address on letter
Identify yourself as a nurse—in body of letter or with signature
Use own words—avoid form letters or modify model being circulated
Clearly and concisely state pro or con stand on issue or bill
Limit letter to one issue
If a bill has been introduced, know bill number.
  HR _____ : S _____
Be proactive and positive; avoid harsh, negative statements
Enclosed pertinent documentation for position
Offer assistance for providing additional information
Send copy of letter to nursing organization
Send thank-you letter for support given to specific health legislation

TABLE 84-6. *Access to Capitol Hill*

Federal Publications and Reports
Government Printing Office
  Superintendent of Documents
  U.S. Government Printing Office
  Washington, D.C. 20402
  (202) 275-3030
General Accounting Office (GAO) Reports
  U.S. General Accounting Office
  P.O. Box 6015
  Gaithersburg, M.D. 20877
  (202) 275-6241

Bills, Reports and Public Laws
Senate Document Room
  Hart Senate Office Building, B-04
  Washington, D.C. 20510
  (202) 224-7860
House Document Room
  H-226 Capitol
  Washington, D.C. 20515
  (202) 225-3456
Status of Bills "Legis"
  (202) 225-1772

Elected Officials
Office of the President
  (202) 456-1414
Capitol Switchboard
  Senate (202) 224-3121
  House (202) 225-3121
Supreme Court—Office of the Clerk
  (202) 479-3011

Examples of publications exclusively addressing legislative, nursing, and health policy issues of interest to nurses are the *Capitol Update,* published biweekly by the AMA Washington Office, and the *Legislative Network for Nurses,* published by LNN, Inc. A sampling of additional contacts that nurses will find useful are found in Table 84-6.

The executive branch is responsible for administering the laws passed by Congress and may also appoint commissions to investigate areas of concern or interest. Health care policies related to financing, disease prevention, education of health professionals, medical research, and children are coordinated under the Department of Health and Human Services (DHHS) (Richardson, 1993). For legislation supporting nursing education, DHHS is responsible for implementing the legislation. This responsibility is further delegated to the NINR at the NIH and the Division of Nursing of the Bureau of Health Professions of the Health Resources and Services Administration. The Division of Nursing is the operating program unit with knowledge and expertise in this area. In 1989, the Agency for Health Care Policy and Research (AHCPR), formerly the National Center for Health Service Research and Health Care Technology Assessment, was established under DHHS to establish medical practice guidelines and to conduct research on effectiveness of care and patient outcomes. Nursing is included in its Medical Treatment Effectiveness Program (MEDTEP), which to some extent has influenced the appointment of nurses to various advisory and guideline panels (Richardson, 1993). The agency has recently established a Senior Nursing Scholar Program with the American Academy of Nursing, which will begin in the 1995 academic year (Legislative Network for Nurses, 1994).

What is very clear in dealing with legislators at the federal level is that they and their staff have little first-hand knowledge of the health care delivery system and the complex issues with which health professionals deal on a daily basis. Yet, this is the group of policy makers that are responsible for shaping what the health care system of the next decade and the next century will look like.

One of the most vital roles that a nurse can assume from initial involvement in the legislative process is that of an educator. Through the professional nurse's expertise, legislators and their staff can gain pertinent insight and make informed policy decisions as they shape the government's continued role in the health and welfare of the United States.

When dealing with legislators, educate about the basics and build upon them. For instance, if a nurse is seeking the support of a legislator to expand federal funding of cancer prevention efforts, the following information would be useful.

- What is cancer prevention?
- What types of cancer are prevalent in the legislator's district as evidenced by the nurses experience in the workplace? How prevention and education programs could impact this incidence of cancer?
- How cancer prevention programs would be made available? (Through the ACS, school programs, community outreach, hospital public information programs).
- What role the legislator might play in the implementation of cancer prevention programs in his or her district. This could range from press coverage at the time that federal funding is increased to actually encouraging constituents to participate in the program as a proactive health platform.

Although the benefit of this time-consuming investment may not be immediate, it may lay the groundwork for very important decisions in the future. For example, senators, representatives, and their staff who are interested in health legislation are very responsive when invited to a health care facility. It can be useful and productive to select a unique health care facility that reflects the specific health topic of concern such as a cancer research unit, a palliative care unit, a bone marrow transplant program, an AIDS clinic, a day hospital, etc. In conjunction with the public relations department of the facility, schedule activities that will (1) provide the greatest exposure for the elected official (a tour, meetings with patients, nurses, and physicians), and (2) enhance the important messages to be conveyed to the delegation in a limited period of time. This type of activity is important as a long-term investment, because it creates lasting impressions and continuing relationships between health care providers and legislators.

LEGISLATIVE INITIATIVES THAT HAVE SHAPED THE FACE OF ONCOLOGY NURSING

EDUCATION

Nursing's first government affairs office was established by the ANA in 1951 with a major purpose to maintain funding of nursing education programs

(Richardson, 1993). The Nurse Training Act of 1964 (Public Law 88-581) is the most significant federal legislation in support of nursing ever enacted in peacetime. This legislation postdated another significant peacetime law, the Health Amendment Act of 1956, which included a professional nurse traineeship program that provided funds for nurses pursuing leadership careers in teaching, administration, clinical practice, and public health (Miller, 1985).

Federal funds for nursing are often in jeopardy. Over the years, the percentage of allocation of the health care dollar for nursing has decreased. For many years the president's proposed budget did not include monies for the Nurse Training Act; however, as a result of nurses' lobbying efforts, Congress appropriated money to continue funding nursing education. In the 1988 reauthorization, the legislation became known as the Nursing Education Act (NEA, Title VIII of the Public Health Service Act). It is likely that subsequent Nurse Education Act reauthorization will consolidate specific sections of the current NEA; however, projects to be funded would be similar to those currently funded (TriCouncil, 1995). It is anticipated that what has been known as the NEA will be incorporated into a Health Professions Consolidation Act. These nursing funds are for research and education primarily, with the greatest allocation for education. Emphasis is currently placed on primary and preventive care, education for advanced practice, and programs that support the preparation of minority and disadvantaged nurses.

If nursing is going to continue to establish itself as a scientific discipline, then nursing research is essential. Research studies are costly to conduct, and individual nursing researchers cannot afford the expense out of their department budgets alone or from their personal income. The institutions in which nursing research is conducted generally pick up some expense, if only some of the indirect costs. Financial support for nursing research is supported substantially through grant funds from multiple foundations and from federal funds (e.g., NINR).

It would be proactive for nursing to put forth a view of increased self-sufficiency rather than having it done for us through diminishing funding overall. A decrease in overall funding could limit initiatives in both education and research; affirmative action toward research efforts would help us to establish our professional priorities for federal support while providing concrete evidence that nursing understands the need to tighten the belt.

RESEARCH

For over 100 years, since the National Institutes of Health was established, biomedical research has received federal funding and therefore been an ever-present policy issue for presidents and elected officials to oversee and direct. In 1980, federal funding for research and development for defense and domestic programs was par, but by 1989, the federal government was spending more in 24 months for defense research and development than had been spent for medical and nursing research in the 100-year history of the National Institutes of Health. There has been a continuing decline in the commitment of federal funds to support medical research, which has a direct effect on cancer research specifically. This is occurring at a time when cancer research opportunities are enormous, and yet the viability of laboratories and clinical investigative groups are threatened (Ultman, Donoghue, & Lierman, 1993). This trend is likely to continue, and for persons with cancer and the professionals who care for them, this limiting of research opportunities will continue to mean that important components of the National Cancer Institute and the NINR will continue to go unfunded. It is frequently said that how a nation allocates its budget reveals its true priorities.

NATIONAL CANCER PROGRAM

The legacy of our National Cancer Program began over 50 years ago, when President Franklin D. Roosevelt signed into law the National Cancer Institute Act. This began a rich history of involvement by presidents and the Congress in the growth and development of our current Cancer Program to "conduct research, investigations, experiments and studies relating to the cause diagnosis and treatment of cancer."

In 1971, this effort was reenergized by the passage of the National Cancer Act, which was enacted as a result of the joint advocacy efforts of the Congress, the scientific community, and, more importantly, "the people" (Table 84–7). The key supporters of this legislation, Mary Lasker, Senators Warren Magnuson, Claude Pepper, and Randolph Jennings, believed that the government had no direction or effective policy to manage this disease at the federal level.

The National Cancer Act codified their belief that special presidential authorities were necessary to manage this epidemic and that additional resources were necessary in the area of cancer control, basic and applied research, and outreach. Perhaps the single most important authority of this act is the bypass bud-

TABLE 84–7. *Authorities of the National Cancer Act*

Presidential Authorities
Bypass budget
Presidential appointment of Director, NCI
Presidential appointment of National Cancer Advisory Board
President's Cancer Panel

Special Authorities
Special peer review authority for grants and contracts
Ability to establish cancer research centers and prevention and control programs
Ability to fund construction programs
Authority to train clinicians and researchers
Authorization to conduct research in foreign countries
Develop, support, and disseminate cancer education programs
Authority to convene experts, consultants, and special advisory groups

get, a needs budget that is sent annually by the National Cancer Advisory Board directly to the president and is not under the control or "editorial" licensure of any part of the administration. This legislation has also enabled the establishment of a nationwide network that consists of cancer centers, community oncology programs, training for researchers, physicians, and nurses, clinical cooperative groups, cancer prevention and control programs, and cancer information systems.

NATIONAL INSTITUTE FOR NURSING RESEARCH

As the United States achieved worldwide preeminence in health, science, and technology, it became apparent to nurses within the government and in academia that nursing research needed to be expanded and that it merited federal support. In 1955, the Division of Nursing, an arm of the Public Health Service, was given the lead responsibility for developing a national program of nursing research and until 1987 was the sole source of federal funding for nursing research and education (Brown, 1985).

In 1983, an Institute of Medicine study recommended that a National Center for Nursing Research (NCNR) was needed at a high level in the federal government to be a focal point for promoting the growth of quality research (Institute Of Medicine, 1983). Based upon recommendations of this report, Congressman Madigan (R-IL) introduced an amendment to the National Institutes of Health Reauthorization Bill, H.R. 2350, to create an Institute for Nursing. (Brown, 1985).

In the words of Congressman Madigan in his statement on the floor of the House of Representatives, "the purpose of the Institute is to conduct basic and clinical nursing research and training related to prevention of disease, health promotion and care of individuals and families with acute and chronic illness. This is a straightforward amendment that seeks to put nursing research into the mainstream of scientific investigations. . . It is in our national interest for the Federal government to assume a major responsibility for developing the nursing leadership in the nation" (Madigan, 1983).

Although adoption of this amendment failed, the NCNR, later to become the National Institute of Nursing Research, was established by law after a 3-year struggle and two presidential vetoes. It was a triumph of strong coalition building lead by the Tri-council on Nursing, which includes the ANA, American Association of the Colleges of Nursing (AACN), and the National League for Nursing (NLN). The NCNR was authorized in 1985 under the Health Research Extension Act. Secretary Bowen, Department of Health and Human Services, announced its establishment as part of the National Institutes of Health (NIH) on April 18, 1986. Its broad purpose is to support a program of grants and awards promoting nursing research. The Division of Extramural Programs is the administrative branch responsible for program management of research and research training activities. The program comprises four major branches:

- Health Promotion and Disease Prevention
- Acute and Chronic Illness
- Nursing Systems and Special Programs
- Research Development and Review (Merritt, 1986).

The ultimate realization of the National Institute of Nursing Research in 1993 provides the visibility and support that nursing research requires to meet the demands of the next century.

CLINICAL PRACTICE

It is nearly impossible within the scope of this chapter, to discuss all the state and federal legislation that has imported upon the practice of oncology nursing. The reason for this is that any legislation that relates to patients and nurses, even in the general sense, may ultimately affect how oncology nurses care for their patients. Therefore, it is often important to have a broad interest in legislative issues related to health and not just those issues that are specifically related to cancer.

The general legislative headings that are of ongoing importance to oncology nursing are the nursing role, patient care services, and health care costs.

These topics are discussed in detail elsewhere in this book as content areas of oncology nursing practice and are discussed here as issues in which elected officials share an interest with the nursing profession. It therefore becomes necessary that nurses join legislators in shaping the future health care delivery system and the role of the professionals who will deliver that care.

NURSING ROLE

The establishment of state nurse practice acts (see Chapter 83) set the historical standard that demonstrates how legislation can affect the professional practice of nursing. As the arena for health care delivery continues to change, it is essential that nursing put forth a clear, articulate description of nursing practice at all levels or run the risk of being swept aside as the current of change gains momentum. Nursing's role must be clearly understood and deemed vital by patients, families, other health care providers, health care institutions and organizations, and legislative bodies.

Legislation continues to address the advanced professional skills and the increasingly independent roles of nurses. An advanced practice nurse is a registered nurse who has advanced education and clinical practice skills beyond basic nursing education (American Nurses Association Nursing Facts, 1993). At present, this advanced practice role applies to the certified registered nurse anesthetists (CRNA), the certified nurse midwives (CNM), clinical nurse specialists (CNS), and nurse practitioners (NP); the latter two are of particular interest to oncology nursing practice. "A clinical nurse specialist is a masters prepared nurse who has expert knowledge, experience and skills for a specific patient population. A nurse practitioner is a registered nurse with advanced educational preparation who performs physical examinations, diagnosis and treats acute and minor illness and stable chronic illness and provides counseling and education to clients" (Galassi & Wheeler, 1994, p. 2). The

development of both roles originated in the 1960s, and indeed, there are many similarities in the roles of the CNS and the NP. In fact, the boundaries that did exist between the practice of the roles are blurring further today (Galassi & Wheeler, 1994).

A key to distinguishing these advanced practice roles from others labeled as "physician extenders" is certification. The ANA's American Nurses Credentialing Center (ANCC) offers certification examinations for clinical nurse specialists, and three organizations offer certification as nurse practitioners in midwifery, anethesia, and pediatrics. Certification of advanced practice nurses should not be confused with specialty certification (e.g., OCN). Advanced education (masters degree or higher in nursing) is a prerequisite for CNS and NP certification; however, advanced education is not required for specialty certification (Galassi & Wheeler, 1994).

The current and predictably the future focus of legislative proposals revising practice acts is the broadening of the nurses role and the further development of certification in nursing specialties. Both these issues are of importance to oncology nurses and necessitate cancer nursing involvement to direct the future definition and direction of nursing into the twenty-first century.

Timely as well is the issue of reimbursement for nursing services. It is a topic to be addressed as bills are proposed for altering patterns of health care delivery. But it must be addressed with the somber awareness that the health dollar is contracting and the number of groups seeking continued as well as expanded compensation for services is growing.

PATIENT CARE SERVICES

Beginning with the implementation of Prospective Payment as the system for Medicare reimbursement for inpatient hospitalization, there have been continuing legislative and regulatory initiative contributing to a massive movement of patient services to the outpatient, home care, and hospice settings. Hospitals, in fact, are rapidly becoming acute care settings for oncology with most of the care provided outside of this traditional structure. Even autologous bone marrow transplants for solid tumors are being done as outpatient procedures at some institutions. Points of service are expanding and evolving, with the leading incentive being an economic one. The issue of health care costs has moved from the form of a debate to an action of enormous dimension. There is a serious rethinking of what services should be provided, in what setting, and under what circumstances. None of this is occurring in a national coordinated manner, but rather it is occurring largely at the regional (state) level. Therefore, it is essential that oncology nurses be intimately involved in the legislative initiatives affecting the standards of care oncology nurses are committed to deliver.

HEALTH CARE COSTS

Any discussion of patient care in this country is overshadowed by the potential costs of such care. The problem of escalating health care costs cannot be ignored, and it has set into motion a continuing series of legislative and business initiatives focused on cost containment and not always focused on the resulting impact on quality of care or the potential rationing of services.

At the federal level, diagnostic related groups (DRGs) have become the accepted method of payment, and many states have cost-containment mechanisms in place for Medicaid as well.

Insurance companies now scrupulously review claims using technology assessment programs to determine whether payment will be made for patient care services. Managed care is rapidly becoming the chief structure for health care delivery, with HMO membership growing from 6 million to 40 million in recent years (Iglehart, 1992).

Managed care is defined as a system that focuses on the cost-effective delivery of care "through organizations that closely monitor how physicians treat specific illnesses, by limiting referrals to costly specialists, and requiring preauthorization for hospital care" (Colburn, 1993). It means cost containment and careful scrutiny of treatment options for cancer patients and therefore has enormous implications for oncology nursing practice. Because of the intensity of services, HMOs often consider cancer patients to be "high cost enrolles" (Vendelaan, 1992). As summarized by McDermott, "Oncology nurses who practice in managed care settings will face many challenges including an increased emphasis on outcome based research to determine effective and appropriate care, the development of information technology to support the delivery of patient care and enhance nursing knowledge and research, and increased clinical and financial accountability" (McDermott, 1994, p. 830). To ensure an integrated system that includes quality as well as cost-effective care, oncology nurses must participate and contribute to the political debates that will directly impact both services and clinical practice.

ISSUES AND ACTIONS

THE PARTICIPATION OF ONCOLOGY NURSING IN POLITICAL ACTIVITY

There have always been individual oncology nurses who have participated in political activities at the local, state, and even national level. Now there is the strength and leadership of the Oncology Nursing Society to support and encourage oncology nurses as they actively seek to impact the health issues that affect them and their patients (Table 84–8).

Members are encouraged to recommend and submit issues to be considered as priorities by the ONS. The issues may have clinical, educational, or research relevance to oncology and nursing. Once approved by the board as a priority, activities may involve one or multiple approaches to action. These include mobilizing the corresponding members of the Government Relations Committee to take a specific stand (usually through a letter writing campaign). It may involve joining an active coalition to bring together the voice of cancer nurses with multiple organizations such as the National Coalition for Cancer Research. Alternatively, it may involve direct lobbying efforts orchestrated with the professional staff of ONS. One example of such an orchestrated activity is the long-term, concerted efforts on ONS in support of antitobacco and antismoking legislation. It may also involve testifying in support of an ONS priority issue to a legislative Committee, Commission, or Agency (Table 84–9).

TOBACCO

Tobacco use is the single most preventable cause of illness and premature death in the United States. Tobacco products are the single most dangerous and least regulated consumer products in this country. Despite extensive scientific studies on the effects of using tobacco products, the Surgeon General's goal to achieve a smokefree society by the year 2000 remains highly unlikely.

The issue of smoking has had a long winding course through consumer awareness, concern by health care providers, and ultimately to legislative actions. In 1964, Surgeon General Luther Terry warned the country about the hazard of smoking with the result that warning labels were placed on all packages of cigarettes. In the mid-1980s, the NCI adopted the elimination of smoking as one of its Year 2000 objectives to increase survival by 50 per cent, since it has been estimated that cigarette smoking is responsible for 87 per cent of lung cancer cases (American Cancer Society, 1994).

The next significant step was to ban the advertising of all tobacco products on the electronic media. Over the past few years, there have been successful legislative and voluntary restrictions developed to prohibit smoking in public facilities. In April 1995, Maryland became the first state to ban smoking in all public buildings except for permitting separate smoking sections in restaurants and bars. For a number of years, smoking has been prohibited in federal health care facilities. Many private health care facilities have followed suit, often at the behest of nurses.

The 101st Congress marked a significant milestone in extending the smoking ban on commercial flights in the United States from flights lasting less than 2 hours to flights lasting 6 hours or less. This affects virtually all domestic flights. The 103rd Congress passes legislation banning smoking on all international flights originating in this country. We have come a long way from the time when mini-packs of cigarettes were distributed on airlines.

At the state level, Minnesota is working toward being a banner state with their official policy of being smokefree by the year 2000. This could well be a model for other states and a project in which nurses are a natural for involvement.

Nurses, individually and collectively, have played a significant role in the drive toward a smokefree society. First of all, they have frequently set the example by changing their own smoking habits. Additionally, nurses across the country have supported such activi-

TABLE 84–8. *Development of Legislative Activity of the Oncology Nursing Society (ONS)*

1980	Resolutions and legislation committee formed—the purpose was to "receive, determine appropriateness, clarify and respond to resolutions submitted by members"
1981	Meeting held to develop "legislative" focus
1982–1983	Political—educational activities and priority setting of legislative issues began
1984	Series of instructional sessions at Congress began. Participation in NFSNO-Nurse in Washington Internship
1985	Legislative training begun. Corresponding committee structure established. Board approval to track legislation and represent ONS in Washington. First lobbying efforts for Nurse Training Act and National Cancer Act. Letter writing campaign to support appointment of a nurse to NCAB
1986	ONS joined Coalition on Smoking or Health and Nurses Coalition for Legislative Action. Legislative column in ONS publications
1987	Separate Government Relations Committee established
1988	Political action workshop, Washington, D.C. Professional "Director of Government Relations" hired—formal legislative priorities identified. "Legislative Summary" begins publication
1989	Political activities expanded—include mammography, antismoking, reauthorization of National Cancer Act, reimbursement for clinical trials
1990	Fact Sheets developed for priority issues and revised annually. Participation in bill signing ceremony at White house for H.R. 5444—Breast and Cervical Cancer Mortality Prevention Act
1991	First Nurse appointed to the National Cancer Advisory Board of the National Cancer Institute. ONS joins the Breast Cancer Coalition
1992	Corresponding members for Special Interest Groups and Chapters formalized
1993	Government Relation Task Force report presented to the Board of Directors
1994	Capitol Coordinator appointed
1995	Legislative Educational Program begun. Network Nurse Pilot begun

TABLE 84–9. *Key Points in Presenting Effective Testimony*

Know what objectives you want to achieve
Have accurate information and have the facts well organized
Know the text well enough to not have to read it
Be brief and to the point
Be prepared to expand on the issue during the question period
Speak in precise but understandable terms (do not use jargon)
Have support material available for the committee
Have written text ready to submit for the record

ties as the American Cancer Society's Great American Smokeout. The national meetings of ONS have been smokefree since 1985, and ONS has initiated a variety of collaborative efforts through its affiliation with the Coalition on Smoking OR Health in addition to passing several tobacco/smoking resolutions at ONS Congress over the years, the most recent having been adopted in April 1995.

In recent years, the issue of environmental (secondhand or passive) smoke has achieved increased attention. In January 1993, the Environmental Protection Agency (EPA) declared that environmental tobacco smoke is a known human carcinogen. Other substances with this designation have been subject to strict regulation. An estimated 3000 lung cancer deaths annually among nonsmoking is attributed to second-hand smoke. The nonsmoking public is becoming increasingly vocal about this exposure. Oncology nurses can actively support these concerns through education and visible advocacy for this nonsmoking population.

While laudable efforts have resulted in increased numbers of adults breaking the nicotine habit, greater attention must be directed toward the use of tobacco products by our youth. Smoking among school-aged children, especially girls, is increasing. Enforcement of the regulations restricting the sale of tobacco products to minors needs to be accomplished. This enforcement along with passage of legislation to significantly increase the tax on tobacco products will go a long way toward discouraging the use of tobacco products among our youth.

The tobacco issue serves as an effective model to demonstrate how the individual nurse and nursing organizations can work to bring significant and lasting changes. This issue will continue to require energistic leadership until there is truly a smokefree society.

AIDS

Perhaps the most striking issue to affect political tides over the past decade and a half has been the onset of the AIDS epidemic. The political momentum that has been mobilized in response to the epidemic has enabled a massive research, treatment, and civil rights program to chart the future of HIV infection in this country. In fact, many believe that the AIDS epidemic will chart the course for how chronic and catastrophic diseases are managed in this nation.

It is remarkable to realize that in the 15 years since the first case of HIV infection was recognized that our legislative process has:

- established and funded programs that provide for AIDS research, education, and prevention, training of health professionals and access to treatment that are *equal to* those for cancer research;
- convened and received the Report of the Presidential Commissions on the Human Immunodeficiency Virus;

- mandated a Congressional AIDS Commission to work with the Congress and the Administration to carry out the recommendations of the Presidential AIDS Commission, which concluded its 4-year history with a series of reports detailing specific aspects of the epidemic;
- enacted Law 100-607, a broad comprehensive bill that dictates several of the key policy issues confronted by this epidemic;
- created a position of AIDS Policy Coordinator to oversee and unify government-wide AIDS efforts;
- created a National Task Force on AIDS Drug Development whose mission is to identify and remove any barriers to developing effective treatment;
- enacted the NIH Revitalization Act of 1993 (PL103-43), which established the Office of AIDS Research (OAR) at the NIH. OAR identifies scientific priorities, conducts evaluation, and ensures the effective allocation of AIDS research funds among the NIH Institutes and Centers.

Many believe that the HIV epidemic has realized so many successes in such a short period of time because of one factor—grassroots support. Clearly the gay community, the community with the most significant rate of HIV infection, has put into operation a tremendously sophisticated network that has wielded substantial clout with policy makers. In essence, they have made the system work, in a way unequaled by any other constituency group in recent memory.

BREAST CANCER

Breast cancer in the United States has reached epidemic proportions. By the year 2000, nearly 2 million American women will be diagnosed with the disease, and 460,000 women will have died. Advances in breast cancer detection and treatment have been modest in recent years with mortality rates remaining stable for the last 2 decades (Langer & Dow, 1994). These facts have led to an increased national awareness and concern about this disease, especially among women. In the 1980s, as breast cancer statistics became more widely disseminated to the general public, women began to organize and mobilize national breast cancer groups to expand their efforts from patient support to include public advocacy. Groups such as Y-ME and the National Alliance of Breast Cancer Organizations (NABCO) began to have more frequent requests for women for information about funding for breast cancer research (McCabe, Varricchio, Peedberg, & Simpson, 1995).

Then in 1991, the National Breast Cancer Coalition (NBCC) was cofounded by eight organizations and defined its mission to "join women and concerned others in a grass roots movement that would increase funding for breast cancer research; improve access to diagnosis and treatment for all women, especially those uninsured and undeserved; and increase the involvement and influence of breast cancer survivors in medical and regulatory decisions" (Langer & Dow, 1994). This organization immediately had broad-based support, not only from breast cancer and oncology-related groups, but also women's organizations in general. Momentum built rapidly, and initiatives were developed to bring attention of women's health and to target federal legislators to increase funding for breast cancer research. Very quickly women with breast cancer became knowledgeable advocates and lobbyists.

As a result of the lobbying efforts of the Coalition and its dedicated membership, federal breast cancer research funding increased by more than $300 million in 1992, including a unique appropriation of $210 million for breast cancer research awarded to the Department of Defense (Marshall, 1992). In 1994, reflecting the increasing awareness of breast cancer research as a national priority, the NCI requested $449 million for women's health in the bypass budget, a 228 per cent increase from the previous year, and $498 million for fiscal year 1995.

In 1992, the President's Cancer Panel established a Special Commission on Breast Cancer. Its specific charter was to provide a comprehensive report on the status of breast cancer research, detection, and treatment, and to recommend government actions to reduce breast cancer morbidity and mortality. The final report of this panel was released in October 1993 and contained recommendations related to etiology, prevention, detection and diagnosis, treatment, psychosocial effects, access, public policy, information dissemination and empowerment, and development of a partnership of breast cancer advocates and breast cancer scientists.

In response to this report, the Department of Health and Human Services (HHS) convened the "Secretary's Conference to establish a National Action Plan on Breast Cancer." This conference was a unique undertaking that brought together advocates, consumers, clinicians, scientists, government officials, educators, members of Congress, the media, and others to develop an HHS-wide comprehensive plan for fighting breast cancer. This conference developed a National Action Plan on Breast Cancer with a framework for activities in three major areas: the delivery of health care, the conduct of research, and the enactment of policy.

The enormous national success of this breast cancer initiative is impressive in its results. The lesson is that multiple diverse groups can join together and make a national impact. The breast cancer advocates have learned from the AIDS advocates. There are lessons here for other oncology groups, oncology professionals, and the cancer patient community as a whole. Nurses have been active as professionals and leaders in this national breast cancer effort. There will continue to be important and necessary contributions for nurses to make in this arena.

THE FUTURE

What issues are on the horizon? Where should nursing and particularly oncology nurses focus their attention in an effort to influence health care policy and thus patient care delivery and the image of oncology nursing?

In 1989, Dr. Louis Sullivan, former Secretary of HHS, outlined five health care priorities of national concern: HIV infection, illicit drug use, health care for the poor and minorities, health care costs, and care for the elderly (Sullivan, 1989). These are still concerns today and doubtless will be priorities into the year 2000. These issues are not separate entities but rather are inextricably interrelated and, in varying degrees, affect oncology nurses individually and collectively as a specialty.

The HIV epidemic within the decade of the 1990s will involve an ever-increasing number of nurses. While not a malignant disease in the classic sense, ONS has put forth the position for involvement and responsibility by oncology nurses. The ever-expanding problem of substance abuse is increasingly recognized as a health problem that affects nurses in every practice setting as an entity in and of itself or as a correlate to other health problems (e.g., HIV infection).

There is an increasing focus in oncology on the issues of special populations such as the economically disadvantaged, rural communities, and cultural groups. However, there is not a systematic approach to either addressing them or resolving their unique health care issues (Baldwin, 1994). Health problems of the poor and minority groups seem never-ending, as does the continuing spiraling cost of health care (McCabe, 1991). At the close of the 1980s more people were uninsured or underinsured then in any other time in the history of our nation. Without any national policy of health care coverage, the question of health care as a right or privilege almost becomes moot, except for philosophic discourse. The reorganizing of health care systems into managed care entities raises serious questions about maintenance of quality while at the same time controlling costs and ensuring access.

Cancer in the elderly has achieved more of a focus in oncology nursing recently and will command greater attention as the numbers of elderly increase. By the year 2030, there will be 30 million more Americans over the age of 65.

Women's health has become a special focus in health care in the last decade and will continue to merit attention in the future. Nursing, primarily a woman's health profession, should be a powerful lobbying force in advocating for legislation that affects women and their health, for example, efforts toward a smokefree society in light of lung cancer being the number one cause of cancer deaths in women and greater allocation of the health care dollar to cancer screening measures such as mammography for earlier detection of the number one form of cancer in women. Although underrepresented in nursing, African-American and Hispanic women make up a significant population of the underserved, uninsured, and largely ignored health care consumer group All of these factors impact upon the practice of oncology nursing and provide a mandate for oncology nurses.

The challenges are many, and so are the opportunities. We have the chance to learn from the past and shape tomorrow. It is only through thoughtful and deliberate consideration of policy issues as well as understanding how the system works and where we can and should have an impact that nurses will realize their full potential, which could be substantial.

As Charles Francis Kettering stated, "We should all be concerned about the future because we will have to spend the rest of our lives there."

SUMMARY

In this rapidly changing health care environment it is imperative for nurses to become involved in the creation and implementation of health care policy at the local, state, and national level. Clearly, nurses are becoming more visionary and proactive in articulating the issues that impact on health care. As the largest group of health care professionals with a strong history of advocacy, nurses have a mandate to become increasingly expert in organized political activity. This involvement will shape public policy, promote the professionalization of nursing, and benefit the health consumer.

ACKNOWLEDGMENT. The authors thank Marguerite Donoghue for her valuable contributions to the original chapter on which this revision is based.

REFERENCES

American Cancer Society. (1994) *Cancer facts and figures, 1994.* Atlanta: Author.

American Nurses Association Nursing Facts. (1993). *Advanced practice nursing: A new age in health care.* Kansas City, MO: American Nurses Association.

Baldwin, P. D. (1994). Caring for the indigent patient: Resources to improve care. *Seminars in Oncology Nursing, 10*(2), 130–139.

Brown, B. J. (1985). Past and current status of nursing's role in influencing governmental policy for research and training in nursing. In J. C. McCloskey & H. K. Grace (Eds.), *Current issues in nursing* (2nd ed., pp. 697–712). Boston: Blackwell Scientific Publications.

Burson-Marsteller Report. (1992). *Communicating with Congress: A survey of Congressional offices.*

Colburn, P. (1993, Dec 14). Is my doctor on the list? *Washington Post,* 10–13.

Davis, C. K., Oakley, D., & Sochalski, J. A. (1982). Leadership for expanding nursing influence on health policy. *Journal of Nursing Administration, 12,* 15–21.

Galassi, A., & Wheeler, V. (1994). Advanced practice nursing: history and future trends. *Oncology Nursing, 1*(5), 1–10.

Goldwater, M., & Zusy, M. J. L. (1990). *Prescription for nurses—effective political action.* St. Louis: C. V. Mosby Co.

Greenhouse, S. (1993, May 3) Mandated insurance faces fight: Small concerns fear costs of healthcare. *The New York Times,* 1, 3.

Iglehart, J. K. (1992) Managed care. *New England Journal of Medicine, 327,* 742–747.

Institute of Medicine. (1983). *Nursing and nursing education: Public policies and private actions.* Washington D. C.: National Academy of Science Press.

Jenning, S. P. (1991) My job, my health and an answer from government. *The Health Quarterly,* Spring, 1–15.

Lammers, W. (1991) Presidential leadership in health policy. In T. Litman & L. S. Robins (Eds.), *Politics and policy* (2nd ed., pp. 95–115). Albany, NY: Delmar Publishers.

Langer, A. S., & Dow, K. H. (1994). The breast cancer advocacy movement and nursing. *Oncology Nursing, 1*(3), 1–13.

Legislative Network for Nurses. (1994). Silver Spring, MD: Business Publishers, Inc.

Litman, T. (1991) Government and health: The political aspects of health care—a sociopolitical overview. In T. Litman & L. S. Robins (Eds.), *Health politics and policy* (2nd ed., pp. 3–37). Albany, NY: Delmar Publishers.

Long, M. N., & Hinds, M. (1993). State government. In D. J. Mason., S. W. Talbott, & J. K. Leavitt (Eds.), *Policy and politics for nurses* (pp. 433–450). Philadelphia: W. B. Saunders Co.

Madigan, E. R. (1983, November 17) House of Representatives. Congress of the United States.

Majewski, J. (1993). Local government. In D. J. Mason, S. W. Talbott, & J. K. Leavitt (Eds.), *Policy and politics for nurses* (2nd ed., pp. 421–432). Philadelphia: W. B. Saunders Co.

Marshall, E. (1992). Breast cancer's forced march? *Science, 258*, 732–734.

McCabe, M. S. (1991). The economics of cancer care. *Current Issues in Cancer Nursing Practice, February*, 1–9.

McCabe, M. S., Varricchio, C. G., Peedberg, R., & Simpson, N. (1995). Women's health advocacy: Its growth and development in oncology. *Seminars in Oncology Nursing, 11*(2), 137–143.

McDermott, K. C. (1994). Healthcare reform: Past and future. *Oncology Nursing Forum, 21*(5), 827–832.

Merritt, D. H. (1986). National Center for Nursing Research. *Image, 18*(3), 84–85.

Miller, P. G. (1985). The nurse training act: A historical perspective. *Advances in Nursing Science, 7*(2), 47–65.

Richardson, D. R. (1993). Federal government. In D. J. Mason, S. W. Talbott, & J. K. Leavitt (Eds.), *Policy and politics for nurses* (2nd ed., pp. 451–466). Philadelphia: W. B. Saunders Co.

Sullivan, L. W. (1989). Shattuck lecture—The health care priorities of the Bush administration. *New England Journal of Medicine, 321*, 125–128.

Tri-Council for Nursing. (1995). Funding recommendations for nursing education. *Nursing Practice and Nursing Research*. Fiscal Year 1966.

Ultman, J. E., Donoghue, M., & Lierman, T. L. (1993). Government and cancer medicine. In J. F. Holland, E. Frie, R. C. Bast, D. W. Kufe, D. L. Morton, & R. R. Weichselbaum (Eds.), *Cancer medicine* (3rd ed., pp. 2481–2491). Philadelphia: Lea and Febiger.

U.S. Government Printing Office. (1986). *How our laws are made* (Rev. ed.) Washington, DC: Willett.

Vance, C. N. (1985). Political influence: Building effective interpersonal skills. In D. J. Mason & S. W. Talbott (Eds.), *Political action handbook for nurses* (p. 170). Menlo Park, CA: Addison-Wesley Publishing Co.

Vandelaan, B. F. (1992). *Oncology practice and managed care*. Illinois: Blue Cross Blue Shield, HMO.

PROFESSIONAL ORGANIZATIONS
NOT-FOR-PROFIT ORGANIZATIONS AND FOUNDATIONS
GOVERNMENT AGENCIES

Over the last two and a half decades, since the identification of cancer by Congress as a national health problem, several organizations have been formed, ranging from professional societies to international agencies, all with a focus on some aspect of cancer care.

Cancer organizations provide important functions for the health professional involved with caring for the patient with cancer. Although a number of organizations exist today with diverse purposes, each addresses two common objectives: (1) to generate new knowledge by providing education to both members and nonmembers, and (2) to enhance the level of cancer care for a specific group of patients.

Two categories of cancer organizations exist: professional associations, which include both nursing and multidisciplinary groups, and voluntary health organizations. Professional associations have a common interest, are private, are nonprofit, and have a professional membership requirement. Unlike the professional association, a voluntary health agency is composed of both lay and professional persons and supported by voluntary contributions from the public. Voluntary organizations expend resources for education, research, and service programs relevant to a specified disease. Both types of organizations are dedicated to the prevention, alleviation, and cure of a particular disease or disability.

Several cancer organizations predate the National Cancer Act of 1971, including the American Cancer Society, which celebrated 80 years of service in 1993; the Leukemia Society of America, which dates back to 1949; and the International Union Against Cancer, founded in 1933. The long history of these organizations, with the current expansion of new organizations, points to the increased interest and growth occurring in the field of oncology. Nurses are challenged to assess the impact of these organizations on cancer care.

The organizations are a primary source of reference for the nurse. A listing of organizations, their addresses, and overall objectives follow.

PROFESSIONAL ORGANIZATIONS

1. American Association for Cancer Education, Inc. (AACE)
   Robert M. Chamberlain, Ph.D., Secretary
   University of Texas
   M.D. Anderson Cancer Center-189
   1515 Holcombe Boulevard
   Houston, TX 77030-4095
   Telephone: 713/792-3020

   The association provides a forum for health-related professionals concerned with the study and improvement of cancer education at the undergraduate, graduate, continuing professional, and paraprofessional levels. Cancer education efforts are related to prevention, early detection, treatment, and rehabilitation. The association conducts annual meetings and publishes the *Journal of Cancer Education.*

2. American Association for Cancer Research (AACR)
   Public Ledger Building, Suite 816
   150 South Independence Mall West
   Philadelphia, PA 19106-3483
   Telephone: 215/440-9300

   The American Association for Cancer Research is the largest professional society of scientists specializing in both basic and clinical research. The purposes of the association are to facilitate communication and dissemination of knowledge among scientists and others dedicated to the cancer problem; to foster research in cancer and related biomedical sciences; to encourage the presentation and discussion of new and important observations in the field; to foster public education, science education, and training; and to advance the understanding of cancer etiology, prevention, diagnosis, and treatment throughout the world. The association publishes three journals, *Cancer Research, Cell Growth & Differentiation,* and *Cancer Epidemiology, Biomarkers, & Prevention.*

3. American Pain Society
5700 Old Orchard Road, First Floor
Skokie, IL 60077-1057
Telephone: 708/966-5595

A multidisciplinary not-for-profit educational and scientific organization comprising clinicians and researchers whose mission is to serve people in pain by advancing research, education, treatment, and professional practice.

4. American Society of Clinical Oncology (ASCO)
Robert E. Becker, Executive Director
435 North Michigan Avenue, Suite 1717
Chicago, IL 60611
Telephone: 312/644-0828

The American Society of Clinical Oncology is a group of more than 9000 professionals who are dedicated to leading and advancing the study of human neoplastic diseases. The society promotes and fosters the exchange of information related to neoplastic diseases with particular emphasis on human biology, diagnosis, and treatment. The society publishes the *Journal of Clinical Oncology.*

5. American Society of Hematology (ASH)
1200 19th Street, NW, Suite 300
Washington, DC 20036-2401
Telephone: 202/857-1118

A society that engages exclusively in charitable, scientific, and education activities and endeavors including promoting and fostering, among the many scientific and clinical disciplines, the exchange and diffusion of information and ideas relating to blood and blood-forming tissues and encouraging investigations of hematologic matters.

6. Association of Community Cancer Centers (ACCC)
11600 Nebel Street, Suite 201
Rockville, MD 20852
Telephone: 301/984-9496

A national organization that provides a mechanism for the exchange of information among health care professionals who believe that high-quality cancer care should be available in the community. The ACCC's mission is to promote quality, comprehensive, multidisciplinary care for patients with cancer and the community. ACCC publications include *Cancer DRGs, Community Cancer Programs in the United States, Oncology Issues, The Compendia Based Drug Bulletin,* and *Cancer Treatment Your Insurance Should Cover: Information for Patients and Their Families.*

7. Association of Oncology Social Work (AOSW)
1910 East Jefferson Street
Baltimore, MD 21205
Telephone: 410/614-3990

The Association of Oncology Social Work (formerly the National Association of Oncology Social Workers) is an organization that seeks to enable professional social workers in oncology to better serve the needs of clients, practitioners, managers, educators, and researchers; advocate sound public policy and professional programs; promote high professional standards and ethics; foster communication and support among members and between members and other oncology and social work organizations; encourage continuing education and research on psychosocial issues in oncology. Membership includes a subscription to the *Journal of Psychosocial Oncology* and *AOSW News,* a national membership directory.

8. Association of Pediatric Oncology Nurses (APON)
5700 Old Orchard Road, 1st Floor
Skokie, IL 60077-1057
Telephone: 708/966-3723

The Association of Pediatric Oncology Nurses is dedicated to promoting optimal nursing care for children and adolescents with cancer and their families. Membership in the organization is open to all registered nurses interested in or active in pediatrics or pediatric oncology. The association holds an annual conference; publishes a newsletter and journal, *The Journal of Pediatric Oncology Nursing;* and conducts local chapter activities.

9. Association of Pediatric Oncology Social Workers (APOSW)
c/o Lynda Walker, President
All Children's Hospital
St. Petersburg, FL 33701
Telephone: 813/892-4147

The purpose of the Association of Pediatric Oncology Social Workers is to advance the practice, enhance knowledge, and develop policy and programs of pediatric oncology social work; foster quality and effectiveness of the social work practice of pediatric oncology; promote solidarity among social workers; provide community and professional education; formulate and record local and federal legislation related to pediatric oncology. The association publishes a quarterly newsletter and convenes an annual conference.

10. International Association for the Study of Pain (IASP)
IASP Secretariat
909 NE 43rd Street, Suite 306
Seattle, WA 98105 USA
Telephone: 206/547-6409

A nonprofit, international organization dedicated to fostering and encouraging research of pain mechanisms and pain syndromes and helping improve the management of patients with pain and promoting and facilitating the dissemination of new information. Membership is open to health care professionals who have a special interest in pain syndromes.

11. International Society of Nurses in Cancer Care
    (ISNCC)
    The Secretariat
    Mulberry House
    The Royal Marsden Hospital
    Fulham Road
    London SW3 6JJ
    Telephone: 071-352-8171 X 2123

    A society of cancer nurses worldwide established to
    advance the knowledge and understanding of can-
    cer nursing and to foster the dissemination of this
    knowledge. Membership is open to cancer nursing
    societies, universities, and institutions involved in
    cancer care and other groups whose work affects or
    involves the care of people with cancer. The society
    publishes the journal *Cancer Nursing*.

12. International Union Against Cancer (UICC)
    3, rue du Conseil-General
    1205 Geneva, Switzerland
    Telephone: (41-22) 320 18 11

    A unique organization of voluntary cancer leagues
    and societies, cancer research, and/or treatment cen-
    ters and ministries of health devoted to advancing
    scientific and medical knowledge in research, diag-
    nosis, and treatment in all aspects of the worldwide
    fight against cancer.

13. National Hospice Organization
    1901 North Moore Street, Suite 901
    Arlington, VA 22209
    Telephone: 703/243-5900
    1/800/658-8898 (Hospice Helpline)

    A nonprofit public benefit membership organization
    made up of hospice providers and professionals
    who promote and maintain humane and compas-
    sionate care for terminally ill individuals and their
    families. The National Hospice Organization pro-
    vides literature and information about hospice care
    to patients and their families as well as referral to
    other local, regional, and national resources.

14. Oncology Nursing Society (ONS)
    501 Holiday Drive
    Pittsburgh, PA 15220-2749
    Telephone: 412/921-7373

    A national organization dedicated to excellence in pa-
    tient care, teaching, research, administration, and
    education in the field of oncology. The purpose of the
    organization is to promote the highest professional
    standards of oncology nursing. In addition to guide-
    lines and standards for oncology nursing practice and
    education, the society publishes a journal, the *Oncol-
    ogy Nursing Forum*, and a newsletter, the *ONS
    News*. ONS holds an annual national congress and
    fall institute. ONS also has a computerized national
    speakers bureau and is an ANA-accredited approver
    and provider of continuing education credits.

15. Wound Ostomy and Continence Nurses Society
    (WOCN)

2755 Bristol Street, Suite 110
Costa Mesa, CA 92626
Telephone: 714/476-0268

A national organization for nurses who specialize in
the prevention of pressure ulcers and the management and rehabilitation of persons with ostomies,
wounds, and incontinence. WOCN supports its
members by promoting educational, clinical, and
research opportunities to guide the delivery of
expert health care to individuals with wounds,
ostomies, and incontinence.

NOT-FOR-PROFIT ORGANIZATIONS AND FOUNDATIONS

1. American Brain Tumor Association (ABTA)
   2720 River Road, Suite 146
   Des Plaines, IL 60018
   Telephone: 708/827-9910 and 1/800/886-2282

   The American Brain Tumor Association is a
   national organization that provides written information about brain tumors and their treatments.
   Services include patient education publications, listing of brain tumor support groups, a Pen-Pal program, and information about treatment facilities.
   ABTA also funds brain tumor research.

2. American Cancer Society (ACS)
   1599 Clifton Road, NE
   Atlanta, GA 30329-4251
   Telephone: 404/320-3333 and 1/800/ACS-2345

   The American Cancer Society is a nationwide community-based voluntary health organization dedicated to eliminating cancer as a major health problem by preventing cancer, saving lives from cancer,
   and diminishing suffering from cancer through
   research, education, advocacy, and service. The
   American Cancer Society offers programs to educate the public and health professionals and provides programs and services to individuals with cancer and their families. Among its publications are a
   Cancer Source Book for Nurses, *Textbook of Clinical Oncology*, and a newsletter, *Cancer Nursing
   News*.

3. American Foundation for Urologic Disease, Inc.
   300 West Pratt Street, Suite 401
   Baltimore, MD 21201-2463
   Telephone: 410/727-2908

   The American Foundation for Urologic Disease provides printed information to both the public and
   health professionals related to urologic problems,
   including cancer. The organization also provides
   information concerning the availability of scholarships for research that focuses on urologic problems.

4. International Myeloma Foundation
   2120 Stanley Hills Drive

Los Angeles, CA 90046
Telephone: 1/800/452-CURE

The International Myeloma Foundation promotes education for both health professionals and patients regarding myeloma, its treatment, and management. The foundation funds research, holds clinical and scientific conferences, and publishes a quarterly newsletter.

5. Leukemia Society of America
600 Third Avenue, Fourth Floor
New York, NY 10016
Telephone: 212/573-8484 or 1/800-955-4LSA

A national volunteer health organization dedicated to curing leukemia and its related cancers, lymphomas, multiple myeloma, and Hodgkin's disease, and to improving the quality of life of patients and their families through research, patient aid, public and professional education, and community service.

6. National Alliance of Breast Cancer Organizations
Amy S. Langer, Executive Director
Nine East 37th Street, 10th Floor
New York, NY 10016
Telephone: 212/719-0154

A nonprofit central resource for information about breast cancer and a network of more than 300 organizations that provide cancer detection, treatment, and care to many of the nation's individuals with breast cancer and survivors. The alliance works on the local, state, and national level as an advocate for regulatory change and legislation that benefits breast cancer survivors. Membership is available to individuals and organizations.

7. National Brain Tumor Foundation (NBTF)
323 Geary Street, Suite 510
San Francisco, CA 94102
Telephone: 415/296-0404
1/800/934-CURE

The National Brain Tumor Foundation supports research related to causes of and treatments for brain tumors. The foundation offers information and resources to patients with brain tumors and their families. A network of nurses, patients with brain tumors, and family members provides individual support by phone. NBTF also sponsors a biennial conference for patients with brain tumors, their families, and health professionals.

8. The National Coalition for Cancer Research (NCCR)
Capitol Associates, Inc.
426 C Street, NE
Washington, DC 20002
Telephone: 202/544-1880

The National Coalition for Cancer Research is a coalition of cancer research, cancer care, and lay groups representing cancer survivors, children with cancer and their families, cancer researchers, nurses

and physicians, cancer hospitals, centers and clinics, and specialized research institutions. The NCCR directs its efforts at making widely known the value of cancer research and the major contributions made by the National Cancer Program to the basic biomedical sciences and related fields, patient care, and to the reduction of cancer incidence, morbidity, and death.

9. National Coalition for Cancer Survivorship (NCCS)
1010 Wayne Avenue, Fifth Floor
Silver Springs, MD 20910
Telephone: 301/650-8868

The National Coalition for Cancer Survivorship is a network of individuals, organizations, and treatment centers working in the area of cancer survivorship and support. The primary goal of NCCS is to generate a nationwide awareness of survivorship, showing that there can be vibrant productive life after a cancer diagnosis. NCCS facilitates communication among people involved with cancer survivorship, promotes peer support, serves as an information clearinghouse, advocates the interests of survivors, and encourages the study of survivorship.

10. National Lymphedema Network (NLN)
2211 Post Street, Suite 404
San Francisco, CA 94115
Telephone: 1/800/541-3259

NLN is a nonprofit organization that disseminates information on the prevention and management of primary and secondary lymphedema to the general public as well as to health care professionals. NLN provides a quarterly newsletter and a toll-free hotline (1/800/541-3259) that provides individuals with emotional support, educational information, and referrals to healthcare professionals, treatment centers, local support groups, and exercise programs.

11. The Skin Cancer Foundation
245 Fifth Avenue, Suite 2402
New York, NY 10016
Telephone: 212/725-5176

The Skin Cancer Foundation, a nonprofit foundation, is the only national organization concerned solely with the world's most prevalent malignancy—cancer of the skin. The Foundation develops public and medical education programs and provides support for research to help reduce the incidence, morbidity, and mortality of skin cancer. The Foundation offers patient education materials including newsletters, books, brochures, pamphlets, slide presentations, and a video presentation.

12. The Susan G. Komen Breast Cancer Foundation
5005 LBJ Freeway, Suite 370
Dallas, TX 75244
Telephone: 214/450-1777
Helpline: 1/800/I'M AWARE (1/800/462-9763)

A national volunteer-based nonprofit organization raising funds to provide educational programs, mammography screening, and treatment for medically underserved women. The Foundation awards grants and fellowships annually in basic and clinical research and works in the legislative arena to increase federal funds for breast cancer research and screening. National Toll-Free Breast Care Helpline offers information and resources to individuals with breast health or breast cancer concerns.

13. United Ostomy Association (UOA)
    36 Executive Park, Suite 120
    Irvine, CA 92714
    Telephone: 714/660-8624
    1/800/826-0826

The United Ostomy Association is a nonprofit organization that provides speakers, literature, and monthly information meetings for people with ostomies. Volunteers, most of whom are ostomates, may visit patients with ostomies in the hospital or at home with the consent of the patient's physician.

GOVERNMENT AGENCIES

1. Agency for Health Care Policy and Research (AHCPR)
   P. O. Box 8547
   Silver Spring, MD 20907
   Telephone: 1/800/358-9295

A government organization of the U.S. Public Health Service established to enhance the quality, appropriateness, and effectiveness of health care services and access to these services. AHCPR conducts and supports general health services research, including medical effectiveness research, facilitating development of clinical practice guidelines, and disseminating research findings and guidelines to health care providers, policymakers, and the public.

The Office of the Forum for Quality and Effectiveness in Health Care, within AHCPR, has primary responsibility for facilitating the development, periodic review, and updating of clinical practice guidelines. The guidelines will assist practitioners in the prevention, diagnosis, treatment, and management of clinical conditions.

2. Centers for Disease Control and Prevention (CDC)
   Division of Cancer Prevention and Control
   National Center for Chronic Disease Prevention and Health Promotion
   3rd Floor Davidson Building
   4770 Buford Highway, NE, MS-K52
   Atlanta, GA 30341-3724
   Telephone: 404/488-4226

The Division of Cancer Prevention and Control (DCPC) at the Centers for Disease Control and Prevention plans, directs, and supports cancer control efforts through collaborations with prevention partners in state health agencies, federal agencies, academic institutions, and national, voluntary, and private sector organizations. DCPC is responsible for directing, monitoring, and reporting on activities associated with the implementation of The Breast and Cervical Cancer Mortality Prevention Act of 1990 (PL 101-354) and The Cancer Registries Amendment Act (PL 102-515).

The Division plans and conducts epidemiologic studies and evaluations to identify the feasibility and effectiveness of cancer prevention and control strategies. DCPC provides technical consultation, assistance, and training to state and local public health agencies and other health care provider organizations related to improved education, training, and skills in the prevention, detection, and control of selected cancers, including colorectal, prostate, and skin cancers.

3. Combined Health Information Database (CHID)
   Attn: Richard Pike
   National Institutes of Health
   Box CHID
   9000 Rockville Pike
   Rockville, MD 20892
   Telephone: 301/468-6555
   301/770-5164 (fax)

CHID is a computerized bibliographic database containing references to health information and health education resources, many of which are not referenced in any other computer system or print resource. CHID is intended to serve health professionals, patients, and the general public.

4. Food and Drug Administration (FDA)
   Office of Consumer Affairs
   HFE-88
   5600 Fishers Lane
   Rockville, MD 20857
   Telephone: 301/443-3170

FDA is a consumer source on publications dealing with food-related subjects, FDA regulations, cosmetics, general medical drug information, medical devices, radiologic health, and health fraud.

5. National Cancer Institute (NCI)
   Cancer Information Service (CIS)
   Building 31, Room 10A07
   Bethesda, MD 20892
   1/800/4-CANCER
   1/800/422-6237
   Attn: Chris Thomsen
   301/496-8664

The Cancer Information Service is a nationwide telephone service for cancer patients and their families, the public, and health care professionals. CIS information specialists have extensive training in providing up-to-date and understandable information about cancer. The toll-free number of the CIS is 1/800/4-CANCER (1/800/422-6237). Callers are automatically routed to the office that serves their region.

CancerFax[R]
NCI International Cancer Information Center
Attn: Jean Baum
Building 82, Room 123
Bethesda, MD 20892
Telephone: 301/402-5874 (on fax machine handset)
301/496-8880 (for technical assistance)

This service enables individuals to retrieve current cancer treatment information directly from NCI's source of cancer information—Physician Data Query database. Summaries are available for health care professionals and one that is written in language geared toward the general public. Information is available on screening, supportive care, patient publications, and other information services provided by NCI. Selected fact sheets for patients on various cancer-related topics are also available.

CancerNet™
NCI International Cancer Information Center
Building 82, Room 123
Bethesda, MD 20892
Telephone: 301/496-4907
E-Mail address: cancernet@icicb.nci.nih.gov

CancerNet is a service that enables health professionals to access cancer information from the National Cancer Institute via Internet. CancerNet contains cancer information from the PDQ (Physician Data Query) database. Users can access state-of-the-art treatment summaries geared to the health professional as well as summaries written in basic language appropriate for the general public. Information is available concerning cancer screening, supportive care, patient publications, investigational drugs, and other NCI information services.

NCI Information Associates Program
Building 82, Room 123
Bethesda, MD 20892
Telephone: 1/800/NCI-7890 (U.S.)
301/816-2083 (international)

The NCI Information Associates Program provides easy access to all of NCI's scientific information services for health professionals through one point of contact and for one low yearly fee. Information associates can receive the *Journal of the National Cancer Institute,* all forthcoming *Journal of the National Cancer Institute* monographs, and access to the PDQ database through a toll-free dial-up bulletin board system. Toll-free access to both Cancer-Fax and a customer service desk staffed by specially trained representatives is also available.

National Black Leadership Initiative on Cancer (NBLIC)
National Outreach Initiatives Branch
NCI, DCPC 9000 Rockville Pike
Bethesda, MD 20892
Telephone: 301/496-8680

The National Black Leadership Initiative on Cancer is the work of the National Institutes of Health's National Cancer Institute. It is one of the institute's community outreach initiatives, responsible for increasing cancer awareness among African-Americans. Its purpose is to enlist community-based leadership to become active in organizing cancer education and services within their local town.

PDQ (Physician Data Query): NCI's Computerized Database for Health Professionals
Attn: Jean Baum
Building 81, Room 123
Bethesda, MD 20892
Telephone: 301/496-4907

PDQ is NCI's comprehensive cancer information database that provides access to state-of-the-art cancer treatment information. The database includes summaries of the most current treatment approaches for over 80 types of cancer, ongoing clinical trials that are open to patient entry, and a directory of physicians involved in oncology and health care organizations that have cancer care programs. Also included in the database are screening and prevention information for a variety of cancers, as well as extensive information about a number of investigational drugs. PDQ is updated monthly.

6. National Marrow Donor Program
Suite 400
3433 Broadway Street NE
Minneapolis, MN 55413
Telephone: 1/800/526-7809 or 612/627-5800

Partially funded by the federal government, the National Marrow Donor Program was created to improve the effectiveness of the search for bone marrow donors so that a greater number of bone marrow transplants can be performed. The program maintains a registry of more than 1 million potential bone marrow donors and provides free information on bone marrow transplantation.

7. U.S. Department of Labor Occupational Safety and Health Administration (OSHA)
Directorate of Technical Support
200 Constitution Avenue, NW
Washington, DC 20210
Telephone: 202/219-7047

OSHA is involved in the development and enforcement of occupational safety and health standards and strives to ensure safe and healthful working conditions for every worker in the United States, The directorate of technical support can provide information regarding work-related hazards and occupational injuries and illnesses.

Index

Note: Page numbers in *italics* refer to illustrations; page numbers followed by t refer to tables.

A

Aβ fiber, in pain impulse transmission, 1010, 1010t, 1012
Aδ fiber, in pain impulse transmission, 1010, 1010t
Abdominoperineal resection, in rectal cancer, 664, *664*
abl oncogene, 163
ABO blood group system, 488–491, 489t, *490*, 490t, *491*
Absorbable gelating sponge (Gelfoam), 1000t
5-AC (azacitidine), 367t, 384t, 385
Acculturation, 41
Acetaminophen, 1036, 1037t
Acetylcholine, in attentional processes, 1065
Acinar cells, T-antigen genes of, 164
Acquired immunodeficiency syndrome (AIDS), 870–883
  antiretroviral therapy in, 882–883, 882t
  CD4+ lymphocyte count in, 871, 871t, 872–873
  cervical cancer in, 877t
  clinical definition of, 870–871, 871t
  clinical spectrum of, 874–882
  coccidioidomycosis in, 878t
  cryptococcosis in, 879t
  cryptosporidiosis in, 879t
  cytomegalovirus in, 880t
  definition of, 870–871, 871t
  dementia in, 877t
  esophageal candidiasis in, 879t
  etiology of, 872
  frequency of, 871
  herpes simplex in, 881t
  histoplasmosis in, 879t
  immune profile in, 874, 874t
  immunopathogenesis of, 872–873, *872*
  Kaposi's sarcoma in, 877t
    interferon-α for, 442
  lymphadenopathy in, 875
  microsporidiosis in, 880t
  Mycobacterium avium complex in, 878t
  Mycobacterium tuberculosis in, 878t
  non-Hodgkin's lymphoma in, 747, 877t, 878t
  nursing management of, 883
  nursing stress and, 1368
  opportunistic infections in, 875, 876, 878t, 879t, 880t, 881t
  Pneumocystis carinii pneumonia in, 880t
  political activity on, 1421–1422
  progressive multifocal leukoencephalopathy in, 881t
  retinitis in, 880t
  surveillance definition of, 870, 871t
  thrombocytopenia in, 875
  toxoplasmosis in, 880t
  treatment of, *876*, 882–883, 882t
  varicella zoster in, 881t
  wasting syndrome in, 877t
Acromegaly, 806

Actinic keratosis, 222
  5-fluorouracil treatment of, 866
  in squamous cell carcinoma, 863
Actinomycin-D (dactinomycin), 369t, 382–383, 382t, 422t
  extravasation of, 425–426
  myelosuppression with, 388t
Actions, in Health Belief Model, 215, *215*
Activities of daily living. See also *Functioning*.
  immobility effects on, 1131, 1136–1137
  in rehabilitation, 1305
Activity intolerance, immobility and, 1135–1136, 1135t
Acupressure, for pain, 1057–1058
Acupuncture, for pain, 1057–1058
Acute lymphoblastic leukemia, 753–760. See also *Leukemia, lymphoblastic, acute*.
Acute myelogenous leukemia, 759–763. See also *Leukemia, myelogenous, acute*.
Adaptation, definition of, 40
Addiction, iatrogenic, 1022–1023, 1023t
Adenocarcinoma, 154, 154t
  clear-cell, of vagina, 720, *721*
  in unknown primary malignancies, 853–855
  of lung, 617
  of small bowel, 640, 641
Adenoma, parathyroid, 807–808, 808t
  pituitary, 805–807
Adenosis, vaginal, 720
Adenoviruses, in gene therapy, 166
Adhesion, cellular, in metastasis, 195–196
Adjuvant analgesics, 1047–1050, 1048t
Adjuvant therapy. See *Chemotherapy; Radiation therapy*.
Administration of the Estate of Henry James v. Millhaven Corporation et al., 1403–1404
Administration role component, 30
Admission sheet, 1357
Adrenocortical carcinoma, 801–804
  biology of, 801
  classification of, 802, 803t
  clinical presentation of, 802–803, 803t
  diagnosis of, 803
  incidence of, 801
  staging of, 802, 803t
  treatment of, 803–804, 804t
Adrenocorticosteroids, 387, 387t
Adrenocorticotropic hormone (ACTH), hypersecretion of, 802, 803t, 806
  in immune response, 185, *186*
Adriamycin (doxorubicin), 370t, 382–383, 382t, 388t, 422t
  extravasation of, 425–426
  in breast cancer, 589–590
Adrucil (5-fluorouracil), 370t—371t, 384–385, 384t, 388t

Advance directives, 1158, 1159t
  before bone marrow transplantation, 512
Advanced beginner, 26
Advanced directives, 1385, 1401
Advanced disease, 1145–1155
  ascites in, 1153t
  assessment of, 1152–1154, 1153t
  bone marrow transplantation in, 1151–1152
  bone metastases in, 1146t, 1147–1148, *1148*
  brain metastases in, 1146, *1146*, 1146t, 1147t
  cardiac metastases in, 1146t, 1147
  cardiac output in, 1152, 1153t
  definition of, 1145
  drainage odor in, 1154
  drug toxicity in, 1150, 1151t
  fractures in, 1153t
  gas exchange impairment in, 1153
  graft-versus-host disease in, 1151–1152
  hepatic metastases in, 1146t, 1149–1150, *1150*
  hope in, 1154
  immobility in, 1152–1153
  intracranial pressure in, 1146, 1147t
  malignant ascites in, 1149–1150, 1150t
  neuropsychiatric syndrome in, 1146, 1152, 1153t
  nutrition in, 1153
  pathophysiology of, 1145–1152
  pericardial effusion in, 1153t
  pleural effusion in, 1148–1149, *1149*, 1153t
  prognosis for, 1161, 1163–1164, 1164t
  pulmonary metastases in, 1146t, 1148–1149, *1149*
  radiation toxicity in, 1150–1151
  renal failure in, 1153t
  skin integrity in, 1153–1154
  suicidal ideation in, 1154–1154
  supportive care services for, 1326, 1329
  symptoms of, 1161
Advanced Oncology Nursing Certificate, 1259
Advanced practice certification, 1259
Advanced practice oncology nurse, 25, 31–35, 32t
  for ambulatory care services, 1284
  for home care services, 1292–1298
  legal issues and, 34–35, 1394–1398
  legislation on, 1419
  prescriptive authority of, 35, 1395–1396, *1395*, 1396t
  regulation of, 35
  reimbursement for, 1394–1395
  reimbursement of, 35
  role definition of, 35
Affinity, in antigen-antibody binding, 176
Aflatoxin, in carcinogenesis, 142

Mortality rates, 35
  by age, 123, 123t, 127t, 221, 221t
  by gender, 123, *127*
  by geographic region, *129*
  calculation of, 122–123
  in breast cancer, 134
  in lung cancer, 130, *131*
  leading causes in, 122, 122t
  screening reduction of, 273
Motivation, in learning, 1226, 1227
Mouth. See *Oral cavity*.
Mouth blindness, 950
Mouth cancer. See *Oral cavity cancer*.
MTX (methotrexate), 374t—375t, 383–384,
      384t, 388t, 399t
  in graft-versus-host disease, 523
  tumor cell resistance to, 362
Mucosal erythroplasia, in oral cavity cancer,
      777
Mucositis. See *Stomatitis*.
Multifocal myoclonus, opioid-associated,
      1047
Multiple endocrine neoplasia, 467, 467t,
      800t, 808–809
Multiple myeloma, 840–848
  activity intolerance in, 848
  bone involvement in, 843, *844*
  bone marrow involvement in, 844
  bone marrow transplantation in, 846
  chemotherapy in, 845–846
  clinical manifestations of, 843–845, *844*
  constipation in, 848
  differential diagnosis of, 842–843, 842t,
      843
  electrolytes in, 847–848
  epidemiology of, 840
  etiology of, 840–841
  fluids in, 847–848
  hypercalcemia in, 843–844, 847
  hyperviscosity in, 845, 847
  immunotherapy in, 846–847
  infection in, 845
  injury potential in, 847
  mobility problems in, 847
  nursing care in, 847–848
  occupation and, 841
  pain management in, 847
  pathophysiology of, 841–842
  postirradiation, 841
  radiation therapy in, 846
  radiography in, 843
  renal failure in, 844
  risk factors for, 840–841
  signs and symptoms of, 842
  staging of, 843, 843t
  treatment of, 845–847
Multiple sclerosis, fatigue in, 1195
Multipotential stem cell, 964–965
Muscle relaxants, for pain, 1048t, 1049
Muscle relaxation, 1086, 1086t
Music, for pain, 1058–1059
Mustargen (mechlorethamine), 365,
      373t—374t, 388t, 422t
  extravasation of, 426
Mutagen, 139t
Mutamycin (mitomycin-C), 375t, 382–383,
      382t, 388t, 422t
  extravasation of, 426
Mutation, 160
  in oncogene formation, 162
  tumor cell, 362
Mutuality, in caregiving, 96
myb oncogene, 163
myc oncogene, 163
Mycobacterium avium complex, in AIDS,
      878t

Mycobacterium tuberculosis, in AIDS, 878t
Mycosis fungoides, 749
Myelitis, after radiation therapy, 625
Myeloma cells, lymphokine secretion by,
      840–841
Myeloperoxidase stain, in acute leukemia,
      753t
Myelosuppression, 486. See also *Thrombocy-
      topenia*.
  blood transfusion in, 486–487
  chemotherapy-associated, 967–969, 968t,
      969t, 983
  infection-associated, 983–984
  radiotherapy-associated, 969–970, 970t,
      983
  surgery-induced, 970–971
Myleran (busulfan), 365, 367t, 397t
  in breast cancer, 587–588, 587t
  side effects of, 388t, 521
Mylosar (azacitidine), 367t, 384t, 385
Myoclonus, multifocal, opioid-associated,
      1047

N

Nabumetone, 1037t
*NAHC Legislative and Regulatory Blueprints
      for Action*, 1295
Nalbuphine, doses for, 1041t
Naphthol AS-D chloracetate esterase stain, in
      acute leukemia, 753t
Naproxen, 1037t
Nasal cavity, *775*
Nasal cavity cancer, 782–783
Nasoenteric tube feeding, 932, 932t
Nasopharyngeal cancer, detection of, 789t
  incidence of, 238t
  signs and symptoms of, 777, 779
  staging of, 778t
  treatment of, 780
Nasopharynx, *775*
National Alliance of Breast Cancer Organiza-
      tions, 1428
National Black Leadership Initiative on Can-
      cer, 1430
National Brain Tumor Foundation, 1428
National Breast Cancer Coalition, 1422
National Cancer Institute, 474–475,
      1238–1240, 1429–1430
  alternative therapy research of, 534
  as educational resource, 28
  cancer intervention model of, 1324–1325,
      1325
  educational programs of, 1239–1240, *1241*
  evaluation of, 1240
  Nursing Section of, 16
  screening guidelines of, 267, 269t,
      270t—271t
  structure of, 1239, *1240*
National Cancer Institute Information Asso-
      ciates Program, 1430
National Cancer Nursing Conference, 20
National Cancer Program, 1418, 1418t
National Center for Nursing Research, 1262
National Coalition for Cancer Research,
      1428
National Coalition for Cancer Survivorship,
      1313–1314, 1319, 1428
National Death Index, 120
National Hospice Organization, 1427
National Institute for Nursing Research,
      1418–1419
National Lymphedema Network, 1428
National Marrow Donor Program, 1430
Natural environment, in attentional restora-
      tion, 1071

Natural killer cells, 181
  breast cancer recurrence and, 187
  in immune response, 186
Naturopathy, 533t
Nausea, 934
  assessment of, 934, 935t
  chemotherapeutic agents and, 934t
  in bone marrow transplantation, 516
  in dying patient, 1165–1166, 1170t
  management of, 934, 936t—937t, 938t
  nonpharmacologic interventions for, 938t
  nursing care plan for, 935t
  opioid-associated, 1047
  pathophysiologic mechanisms of, 934
  pharmacologic interventions for,
      936t—937t
  radiation-induced, 342–343
  sexual functioning and, 1124
Navelbine (vinorelbine), 378t, 381, 381t
Neck, dissection of, 323t
Neck cancer, 773–792. See also *Head and
      neck cancer*.
Negligence, 1403–1404
  elements of, 1391
Neoplasm. See also specific cancers.
  definition of, 150–151, 157
  differentiation of, 153
  transformation of, 154–157, *155*
Neopterin, in AIDS, 874, 874t
Neosar (cyclophosphamide), 365, 368t, 397t
  administration error with, 1403
  in breast cancer, 587–588. 587t
  side effects of, 388t, 949
Neurogenic pain, 1015
Neuroleptics, for pain, 1047, 1048t, 1049
Neurons, crossexcitation of, 1014
Neuropathic aftersensation, 1014
Neuropathic pain, 1014–1015
Neuropathy, chemotherapy-induced, 949
  in AIDS, 875
Neuropsychiatric syndrome, in advanced dis-
      ease, 1146, 1152, 1153t
Neutropenia, 968, 968t
  infection and, 972–973, 973t
  management of, 973, 976–977, *976*
Neutrophils, 173t, 174, 486t, *981*
  absolute count of, 968, 968t
  granulocyte colony stimulating factor en-
      hancement of, 968–969
  normal range of, 966t
Never fibers, in pain impulse transmission,
      1010, 1010t
Nevus (nevi), dysplastic, 862, 862t, 863–864
Newsletters, for patient education, 1231
Nicotine patch, 229
Nipent (pentostatin), 376t, 384t, 385
Nitrogen balance, 929–930
Nitrogen mustard (mechlorethamine), 15–16,
      365, 373t—374t, 388t, 422t
  extravasation of, 426
Nitrosourea, 380
NM-23 tumor suppressor gene, 203
  in metastasis, 198t
Nociception, 1010, 1010t
  vs. pain, 1009
Nolvadex. See *Tamoxifen*.
Nonbacterial thrombotic endocarditis, 987
Nonspecific esterase stain, in acute leukemia,
      753t
Nonsteroidal antiinflammatory drugs
      (NSAIDs), 1036–1038, 1037t
  administration of, 1036–1038
  central nervous system effects of, 1036
  doses for, 1038
  gastrointestinal effects of, 1036
  gastroprotective therapy with, 1038

ISBN 0-7216-5668-4

90038

9 780721 656687